# Online Supplements

evolve http://evolve.elsevier.com/Rothrock/Alexander

- *Surgical Instrumentation Photos*
- *Surgical Technology Resources*
- *Printable Surgical Pharmacology Tables*
- *Printable Patient and Family Education Tables*
- *Content Updates*
- *WebLinks*

## *Animations*

Abdominal aortic aneurysm
Acute coronary syndrome (ACS), acute myocardial infarction (AMI), coronary ischemia, coronary artery disease
Anatomy of the throat
Angioplasty without stent
Appendicitis, symptoms
AVM, arteriovenous malformation; subarachnoid hemorrhage
Cesarean delivery, cesarean section
Closed reduction/pinning of hip fracture
Coronary oxygenation
CPR, cardiopulmonary resuscitation
Diverticulitis
Epidural hematoma
Epigastric auscultation
Hypoxia and brain damage
Insertion of Foley catheter (male and female)
Intravenous antibiotic therapy
Intubation, normal; endotracheal intubation
Laparoscopic cholecystectomy; gallbladder removal
Nephrostomy
ORIF (Open reduction internal fixation) of ankle fracture
Ovarian cyst
Perforated duodenal ulcer with bleeding
Phagocytosis
Posterior cruciate ligament tear, PCL tear
Pulmonary embolus
Quadrants of body; organs in each quadrant
Renal anatomy and function
Resection of pancreatic tumor
Retinal detachment
Spine
Stereotactic brain biopsy
Subaortic stenosis
Subdural hematoma
Surgery to repair liver laceration
Ventriculoperitoneal shunt; relief of hydrocephalus
Visual pathway
Volvulus, pediatric

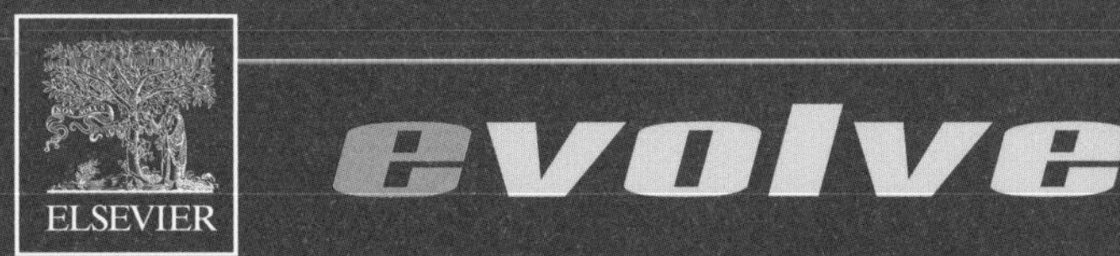


*To access your Student Resources, visit:*

**http://evolve.elsevier.com/Rothrock/Alexander**

Evolve Student Learning Resources for Rothrock: *Alexander's Care of the Patient in Surgery,* Thirteenth Edition, offers the following features:

## Student Resources

- **Surgical Instrumentation Photos**
  View a variety of surgical instruments not pictured in the book.
- **Content Updates**
  The latest content updates from the author to keep you current with recent developments in perioperative nursing.
- **Surgical Technology Resources**
  Additional activities for the surgical technology student.
- **Printable Surgical Pharmacology and Patient and Family Education Tables**
  Print useful information that you can easily take with you for use in clinical settings.
- **State-of-the-Art Animations**
  Refer to the reverse side of this page for a complete listing of animations.
- **WebLinks**
  An exciting resource that lets you link to hundreds of websites carefully chosen to supplement the content of the textbook. The WebLinks are regularly updated, with new ones added as they develop.

# ALEXANDER'S
# CARE *of the* PATIENT *in* SURGERY

# ALEXANDER'S
# CARE *of the* PATIENT *in* SURGERY

THIRTEENTH EDITION

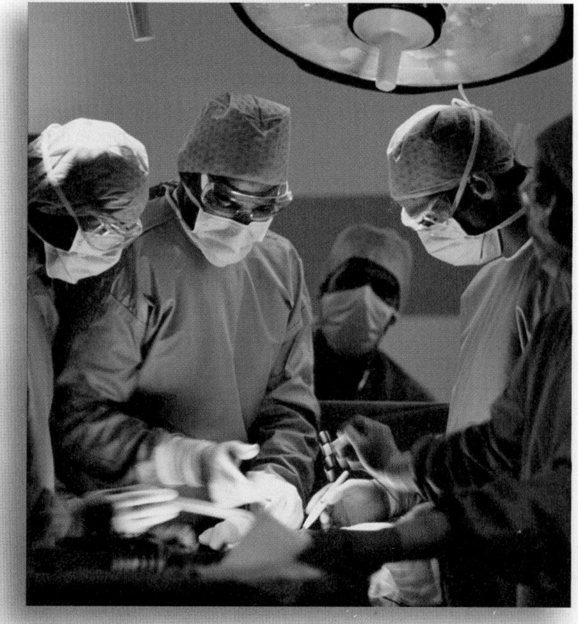

**JANE C. ROTHROCK,** DNSc, RN, CNOR, FAAN
Professor and Director, Perioperative Programs
Delaware County Community College
Media, Pennsylvania

***Associate Editor:***
**DONNA R. McEWEN,** RN, BSN, CNOR
Educational Instructional Designer, Specialized Care Services
United Health Care
San Antonio, Texas

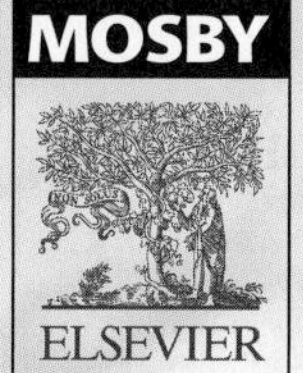

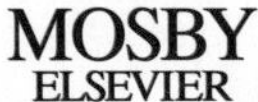


11830 Westline Industrial Drive
St. Louis, Missouri 63146

ALEXANDER'S CARE OF THE PATIENT IN SURGERY

ISBN-13: 978-0-323-03927-7
ISBN-10: 0-323-03927-8



**Notice**

Knowledge and best practice in this field are constantly changing. As new research and experience broaden our knowledge, changes in practice, treatment and drug therapy may become necessary or appropriate. Readers are advised to check the most current information provided (i) on procedures featured or (ii) by the manufacturer of each product to be administered, to verify the recommended dose or formula, the method and duration of administration, and contraindications. It is the responsibility of the practitioner, relying on their own experience and knowledge of the patient, to make diagnoses, to determine dosages and the best treatment for each individual patient, and to take all appropriate safety precautions. To the fullest extent of the law, neither the Publisher nor the Editors/Authors assume any liability for any injury and/or damage to persons or property arising out or related to any use of the material contained in this book.

The Publisher

ISBN-13: 978-0-323-03927-7
ISBN-10: 0-323-03927-8

*Acquisitions Editor:* Kristin Geen
*Developmental Editor:* Jamie Horn
*Editorial Assistant:* Jennifer Stoces
*Publishing Services Manager:* Jeff Patterson
*Senior Project Manager:* Anne Konopka
*Design Direction:* Teresa McBryan

Printed in China

Last digit is the print number: 9 8 7 6 5 4 3 2 1

# Contributors

**SHEILA L. ALLEN, RN, BSN, CNOR, CRNFA**
Self-employed Consultant, Speaker
The Memorial Hospital
Craig, Colorado
Colorado Northwestern Community College
Meeker, Colorado
*Ch 30 Geriatric Surgery*

**KAY A. BALL, RN, BSN, MSA, CNOR, FAAN**
Perioperative Consultant/Educator
K&D Medical Inc.
Lewis Center, Ohio
*Ch 7 Surgical Modalities*

**BARBARA BOWEN, CRNP, CRNFA**
President
Perioperative Consulting & Surgical Services, LLC
Collegeville, Pennsylvania
Staff Development Instructor
Jefferson University Hospital
Philadelphia, Pennsylvania
*Ch 22 Orthopedic Surgery*

**SUSAN K. CHANDLER, RN, BSN, CRNFA, CPSN**
Nurse Clinician
Virginia Commonwealth University Medical Center
Richmond, Virginia
*Ch 24 Plastic and Reconstructive Surgery*

**SUSAN M. CRAIG, RN, BSN, CNOR, RCT**
Staff Nurse
The Everett Clinic Surgery Centers
Everett, Washington
*Ch 32 Integrated Health Practices: Complementary and Alternative Therapies*

**BRENDA S. GREGORY CRUM, RN, MSN, CNOR**
Vice President, Patient and Nursing Safety
Sandel Medical Industries, LLC
Chatsworth, California
*Ch 25 Thoracic Surgery*

**LINDA M. DeLAMAR, CRNA, MSN, MS**
Certified Registered Nurse Anesthetist
Mount Laurel, New Jersey
*Ch 4 Anesthesia*

**ALTHEA R. DUNSCOMBE, PhD, RN, CRNFA, LNC**
RN First Assistant, Professor Clinical Education, Legal Nurse Consultant, Professional Assistants PRN
Southwest Florida College
Gainesville, Florida
*Ch 6 Sutures, Needles, and Instruments*

**DIANE L. FERRARA, RN, MSN, BA, CRNP, RNFA, APRN,BC**
Nurse Practitioner, RN First Assistant for Neurosurgery
Thomas Jefferson University Hospital
Philadelphia, Pennsylvania
*Ch 23 Neurosurgery*

**VICKI J. FOX, MSN, RN, ACNP-BC**
Acute Care Nurse Practitioner
Tyler, Texas
*Ch 10 Patient Education and Discharge Planning*

**CHARLOTTE L. GUGLIELMI, RN, BSN, CNOR**
Perioperative Nurse Specialist/Educator
Beth Israel Deaconess Medical Center
Boston, Massachusetts
*Ch 20 Rhinologic and Sinus Surgery*

**PAULINE ANNE HEIZENROTH, RN, MSN, CNOR**
Perioperative Nurse
Paoli Surgery Center
Paoli, Pennsylvania
*Ch 5 Positioning the Patient for Surgery*

**THERESA M. JASSET, MSN, RN, CNOR**
Nursing Informatics Coordinator
New England Baptist Hospital
Boston, Massachusetts
*Ch 20 Rhinologic and Sinus Surgery*

**DONNA R. McEWEN, RN, BSN, CNOR**
Educational Instructional Designer, Specialized Care Services
United Health Care
San Antonio, Texas
*Ch 8 Wound Healing, Dressings, and Drains*
*Ch 14 Gynecologic and Obstetric Surgery*
*Ch 19 Otologic Surgery*
*Ch 21 Laryngologic and Head and Neck Surgery*
*Ch 28 Ambulatory Surgery*

**GRATIA M. NAGLE, CRNFA, CURN, BA**
CURN, James R. Bollinger, MD, FACS, PC
Paoli, Pennsylvania
*Ch 15 Genitourinary Surgery*

**JANICE A. NEIL, RN, PhD**
Associate Professor
East Carolina University
Greenville, North Carolina
*Ch 12 Surgery of the Liver, Biliary Tract, Pancreas, and Spleen*

**LILLIAN H. NICOLETTE, RN, MSN, CNOR**
Cardiovascular Specialist—Cardiovations, a division of Ethicon, a Johnson & Johnson Company
Faculty, Perioperative Nursing
Delaware County Community College
Newton, Pennsylvania
*Ch 3 Infection Prevention and Control in the Perioperative Setting*

**JAN ODOM-FORREN, MS, RN, CPAN, FAAN**
Perianesthesia Nursing Consultant
Louisville, Kentucky
*Ch 9 Postoperative Patient Care and Pain Management*

**DIANE CATHERINE SAULLO, RN, BSN, MSN (CNOR, CPD)**
Clinical Education Specialist
New Hanover Health Network
Wilmington, North Carolina
*Ch 31 Trauma Surgery*

**PATRICIA C. SEIFERT, RN, MSN, CNOR, CRNFA, FAAN**
Education Coordinator
Inova Heart and Vascular Institute
Falls Church, Virginia
*Ch 27 Cardiac Surgery*

**MICHELLE SLOAN, RNFA, BSN, CNOR**
Nurse Manager
Specialty Orthopaedics Surgery Center
Gainesville, Georgia
*Ch 13 Repair of Hernias*

**CHRISTINE E. SMITH, RN, MSN, CNOR**
Perioperative Clinical Nurse Specialist
Fox Chase Cancer Center
Philadelphia, Pennsylvania
*Ch 11 Gastrointestinal Surgery*

**SARAH C. SMITH, RN, MA, CRNO, COA**
Nurse Manager, Department of Ophthalmology and Visual Sciences
University of Iowa
Iowa City, Iowa
*Ch 18 Ophthalmic Surgery*

**KATHERINE STEGNER, RN, BSN**
Nurse Clinician IIe
The Johns Hopkins Hospital
Baltimore, Maryland
*Ch 26 Vascular Surgery*

**JOANNE STOW, BSN, RN, CNOR**
Clinical Nurse III
The Children's Hospital of Philadelphia
Philadelphia, Pennsylvania
*Ch 29 Pediatric Surgery*

**WENDELYN A. VALENTINE, RN, MS, CNOR, CWCN**
QI/QA Nurse Manager
The Everett Clinic Surgery Centers
Everett, Washington
*Ch 32 Integrated Health Practices: Complementary and Alternative Therapies*

**PATRICIA WIECZOREK, RN, BSN, CNOR**
Nurse Manager
The Johns Hopkins Hospital
Baltimore, Maryland
*Ch 26 Vascular Surgery*

# Clinical Consultants

**MARIA ALVAREZ, RN, BSN, CNOR, CRNFA**
Chief, RN First Assistant
Robert Wood Johnson University Hospital
New Brunswick, New Jersey

**DAVID W. ANDREWS, MD**
Assistant Professor of Neurosurgery, Vice Chairman for Clinical Services, Department of Neurosurgery
Thomas Jefferson University
Philadelphia, Pennsylvania

**SUE BALLATO, RN, MBA, PhDc**
Director, Trauma Services
New Hanover Health Network
Wilmington, North Carolina

**RICHARD A. BERGER, MD**
Midwest Orthopaedics at Rush
Chicago, Illinois

**J. ALLEN BUTTS, MD**
General Surgery
Northeast Georgia Medical Center
Gainesville, Georgia

**DAVID S. CARADONNA, MD, DMD, FACS**
Attending Otolaryngologist
Beth Israel Deaconess Medical Center
Harvard Medical School
Boston, Massachusetts

**JANE COLLINS, RN**
Staff Nurse
Pennsylvania Hospital
Philadelphia, Pennsylvania

**DEBRA COSTON, RN, CCRN**
Educator STICU
New Hanover Health Network
Wilmington, North Carolina

**JEFF DUPERON**
Healthcare Policy and Economics Manager
Ethicon (Endo-Surgery), Inc., a Johnson & Johnson Company
Somerville, New Jersey

**JAMES J. EVANS, MD**
Assistant Professor of Neurosurgery, Department of Neurosurgery
Thomas Jefferson University
Philadelphia, Pennsylvania

**BETH FITZGERALD, RN, BSN, CNOR**
Perioperative Nurse Internship Manager
Christiana Care Health System
Newark, Delaware

**PATRICIA S. FRITZ, RN, BS, CNOR**
Clinical Education Consultant
Advanced Sterilization Products
Johnson & Johnson
Lansdowne, Pennsylvania

**EILEEN GHENN**
Urology Specialist
Ethicon (Endo-Surgery), Inc., a Johnson & Johnson Company
Somerville, New Jersey

**CHRISTINE GRAKOFF, RN, BSN**
Adjunct Faculty, Surgical Technology Program
Delaware County Community College
Media, Pennsylvania

**PETER B. GRAVES, RN, BSN, CNOR**
Clinical Nurse Consultant
Corinth, Texas

**BILL GRAY**
Interstin Specialist
Medtronic, Inc.
Minneapolis, Minnesota

**VESNA MILICA HESS, RN, BSN, CNOR, RNFA**
Thomas Jefferson University Hospital
Philadelphia, Pennsylvania

**NORMA HOLMES, RN, BSN, CNOR, HNC**
OR Specialty Team Coordinator: Urology, Plastics, General and Gynecology
Paoli Hospital
Paoli, Pennsylvania

**EDWARD A. LEFRAK, MD**
Professor of Surgery
Virginia Commonwealth University School of Medicine—Inova Campus
Medical Director of Cardiac Surgery
Inova Heart and Vascular Institute
Falls Church, Virginia

**ANTONIO LUCIANO, BSNA, CRNA, CNOR, LNC**
President
Independent Anesthesia Services
Manalapan, New Jersey

**HELENE KOREY MARLEY, RN, CNOR, CRNFA**
Clinical Service Coordinator, Orthopaedics
Pennsylvania Hospital
Philadelphia, Pennsylvania

**PAUL S. MASSIMIANO, MD**
Chief of Vascular Surgery Section, Cardiovascular Surgery
Inova Heart and Vascular Institute
Falls Church, Virginia

**RAYMOND MOORE, CST**
CST, ORTHO
Pennsylvania Hospital
Philadelphia, Pennsylvania

**JANICE A. NEIL, PhD, RN**
Associate Professor
East Carolina University
Greenville, North Carolina

**MARY PATRICIA O'CONNELL-SIMON, CRNA**
Paoli Hospital
Paoli, Pennsylvania

**BRUCE PERLER, MD**
Chief, Division of Vascular Surgery
The Johns Hopkins Hospital
Baltimore, Maryland

**ANDREW L. POZEZ, MD**
Professor, Plastic and Reconstructive Surgery
Virginia Commonwealth University Health System
Richmond, Virginia

**CHRIS RAISER**
Urology Consultant
C.R. Bard, Inc.
Covington, Georgia

**RYLAN REYNOLDS, RN, BSN, CNOR**
Inova Heart and Vascular Institute
Falls Church, Virginia

**JEFFREY L. ROSENBLUM, MD, FACS**
Board Certified Urologic Surgeon
Paoli Hospital, Chester County Hospital, Brandywine Hospital, Bryn Mawr Hospital, Lankenau Hospital
Exton, Pennsylvania

**SHEILA SANDERS, RN, BSN, ONC**
Midwest Orthopaedics at Rush
Chicago, Illinois

**GINNY SCHUSTER**
Clinical Consultant
American Medical Systems
Minnetonka, Minnesota

**SARAH SMITH, RN, BSN, CRNA, LNP**
President, S. Smith Anesthesia Services, LLC
Virginia Commonwealth University Health System
Richmond, Virginia

**CHRISTY SPIVEY, RN, BSN, CEN, EMT**
SERAC Manager
New Hanover Health Network
Wilmington, North Carolina

**MARGOT SWEED, CRNP, MSN**
Adult Nurse Practitioner—GI
Fox Chase Cancer Center
Philadelphia, Pennsylvania

**BARBARA TRATTLER, RN, MS, CNOR**
Vice President, Surgical Services
Monmouth Medical Center
Monmouth, New Jersey

**KAARE J. WEBER, MD**
Assistant Professor of Surgery, General and Endocrine Surgery
Mount Sinai Medical Center
New York, New York

# Reviewers

**DIANA BECK, RN, BSN, CNOR**
Clinical Educator, Surgical Services
St. Mary's Good Samaritan, Inc.
Centralia, Illinois

**CAROL BOWLING, RN**
Thoracic Clinic
Vanderbilt University Medical Center
Nashville, Tennessee

**MICHELLE BYRNE, RN, PhD, CNOR**
Associate Professor of Nursing
North Georgia College and State University
Dahlonega, Georgia

**DEBORAH CASWELL, MSN**
Assistant Director, Vascular Surgery, UCLA Gonda Vascular Center
UCLA Center for Health Sciences
Los Angeles, California

**CAROLYN CLARY-MACY, RN, OCN**
Special Projects Coordinator, Thoracic Surgery
University of California San Francisco
San Francisco, California

**MARY B. CONDRON, BSN, CNOR, RNFA**
Specialty Team Supervisor, Orthopedics, Perioperative Services
Thomas Jefferson University Hospital
Philadelphia, Pennsylvania

**NANCY COUCH, RN, AAS-ORT, BSN, CNOR**
Perioperative Educator, Surgical Technology Director, Instructor
Health Science Center
Trinity Valley Community College
Kaufman, Texas

**HEATHER C. EVERS, RN, BSN, CNOR**
Staff Nurse, Surgery
Rockford Memorial Hospital
Rockford, Illinois

**MICHELLE HAUN-HOOD, RN, MA, CCRN**
Director Life Flight Network, Director Trauma and Transport
Legacy Emanuel
Portland, Oregon

**R. MARK HOVIS, CRNA**
Department of Anesthesiology
Washington University School of Medicine
St. Louis, Missouri

**SHERRY M. LAWRENCE**
Clinical Specialist, Surgical Services
University of South Alabama Knollwood Hospital
Mobile, Alabama

**LEIGH W. MOORE, RN, MSN, CNOR**
Assistant Professor of Nursing
Southside Virginia Community College
Alberta, Virginia

**SHIRLEY A. MORGAN, RN, MSN, CS, CNOR**
Staff Nurse Operating Room, Perioperative Nursing
Thomas Jefferson University Hospital
Philadelphia, Pennsylvania

**JANICE NEIL, RN, PhD**
Associate Professor
East Carolina University
Greenville, North Carolina

**KELLY RODRIGUES, RN, CNOR**
Coordinator, Surgical Technology
Galveston College
Galveston, Texas

**DIANNE SHARP, RN, CNOR, BS**
Staff Nurse, Surgical Services
Boone County Hospital
Boone, Iowa

**SARAH SMITH, RN, MA, CRNO, COA**
Nurse Manager, Department of Ophthalmology and Visual Sciences
University of Iowa
Iowa City, Iowa

**BETH ANN SWAN, PhD, CRNP**
Associate Professor, Department of Nursing, Jefferson College of Health Professions
Thomas Jefferson University
Philadelphia, Pennsylvania

**SARAH R. TVEDT-POOL, MS, RN**
Nursing Education Specialist, Cardiac Surgery, Department of Surgical Services
Mayo Medical Center
Rochester, Minnesota

**NANCY WALLACE, RN, BSN, CORLN**
Nurse Coordinator, Head and Neck Oncology/Laryngology, Otolaryngology/Head and Neck Surgery
University of Michigan Health System
Ann Arbor, Michigan

**DENISE WITT, RN, CNOR, CST**
Associate Professor, Allied Health Sciences
Nassau Community College
Garden City, New York

**JOANNA JIEHONG YANG, RN, MS, NP**
APN Department, Neurosurgery and Neurology
Loma Linda University Medical Center
Loma Linda, California

*To* **Jan,**
*my sister and best friend,*
*for whom I have enormous love and esteem.*
*She embodies what one thinks of when they describe a bright, successful woman,*
*an incredible mother and wife, a woman of spirit and soul,*
*who moves through life touching those she encounters*
*and leaves them different for knowing her.*

# About the Author

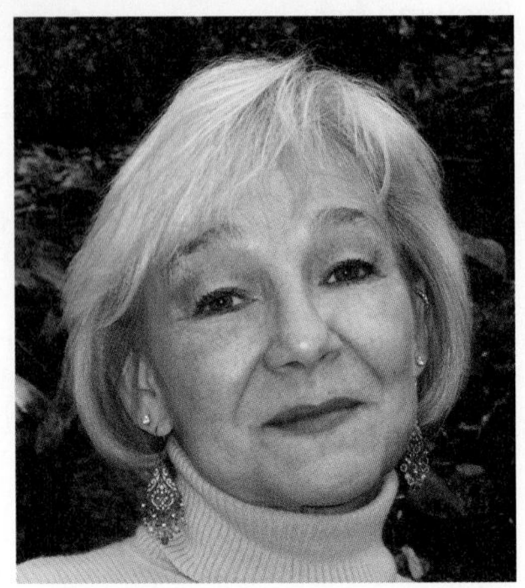

## JANE C. ROTHROCK, DNSc, RN, CNOR, FAAN

Dr. Jane Rothrock has been in perioperative nursing since 1969. In 1978, she joined the faculty at Delaware County Community College, where she is currently Professor and Director of Perioperative Programs. Her responsibilities include entry-level, postbasic RN education for perioperative nursing and advanced skill preparation for RN first assistants. These courses are offered both in Pennsylvania and at various sites around the United States in host institutions. During her tenure at the college, Jane has been involved with the education of more than 3500 registered nurses for professional practice in perioperative patient care.

Jane has years of experience as a faculty member, author, and speaker. She has taught at the University of Pennsylvania, been an OR Director, and served as the preceptor for a number of graduate students. She has authored four perioperative nursing textbooks, published more than 50 articles, and presented a wide range of topics to nursing audiences across the United States and at international meetings. Jane is an AORN past president, served in 1996-1997 as the Chair of the AORN Project Team on Professional Practice Issues, chaired the AORN Project Team on a Professional Practice Model for Perioperative Nursing in 1998-1999, and chaired the Perioperative Academic Curriculum Task Force in 2006. She has multiple Who's Who listings, has received a number of distinguished awards, and is very active in both nursing and community organizations. She is a past vice chair of NOLF, a past member of the ANCC Magnet Commission, and a past president of the ASPAN Foundation. Jane served on ASPAN's National Clinical Guideline Panel to develop a Guideline on Prevention of Unplanned Hypothermia in Adult Surgical Patients. She is a member of the Editorial Board for *Advance for Nurses, the American Nurses' Publishing Group,* as well as the *AORN Journal.* In 2000, she became a Fellow of the American Academy of Nursing (FAAN). She currently serves as the president of the AORN Foundation, serves as an "Ask the Expert" for Medscape Nursing, and is an editor of *Tea & Toast for the Perioperative Nurse's Spirit,* a book of inspirational stories published in 2006.

Jane began her nursing education with a diploma from Bryn Mawr School of Nursing. She received her BSN and MSN from the University of Pennsylvania and was the first recipient of a doctoral degree from Widener University, earning her Doctor of Nursing Science in 1987.

# Preface

The thirteenth edition of *Alexander's Care of the Patient in Surgery* has been extensively updated to reflect new concepts in perioperative nursing practice and increased sophistication and complexity of surgical procedures. An exciting new addition to the thirteenth edition is a multimedia resource, enhancing the elemental goal of this textbook: to provide a comprehensive basic reference that will assist perioperative practitioners with safely, cost-effectively, and efficiently meeting the needs of the patients they care for during surgical interventions.

The standard in perioperative nursing for more than 50 years, *Alexander's Care of the Patient in Surgery* is written primarily for professional perioperative nurses but is also useful for nursing students, surgical technologists, health care industry representatives, medical students, interns, residents, and government officials concerned with health care issues. Perioperative nurses, RN first assistants, clinical nurse specialists, nurse practitioners, surgeons, surgical technologists, and educators from many geographic areas of the United States have served as contributors and reviewers for this text, providing a vast range of perioperative nursing knowledge and procedural information.

This thoroughly revised edition highlights current techniques and innovations in surgery. Hundreds of illustrations, including many new photographs and drawings, help familiarize the reader with new procedures, methods, and equipment. Classic illustrations, particularly of surgical anatomy, have been preserved to enhance the text. New to this edition, each clinical chapter now has a Surgical Pharmacology and a Patient Safety feature. Continuing from previous editions, there are also Best Practices, Research Highlights, Sample Plans of Care, Patient and Family Education features, and History Boxes in each clinical chapter, so our readers can look back, as well as forward, as they explore perioperative patient care.

New in the thirteenth edition is the *Evolve Website.* With its learner resources, readers will be able to access content updates, surgical instrumentation photos, printable surgical pharmacology tables, printable patient and family education material, resources for surgical technology students, and WebLinks.

Also new in the thirteenth edition are resources for instructors and clinical educators. In addition to the learner resources listed above, there is an instructor's manual containing the following elements: chapter focus, key terms, learning objectives, chapter outline/teaching strategies, critical thinking activities, learning activities, case studies or quizzes, PowerPoint lecture slides, an image collection (more than 950 images), and animations to use in teaching. Instructors and clinical educators will also find a test bank with more than 500 questions, including rationales.

Overall, this textbook imparts state-of-the-art information and resources that reflect contemporary practice and promotes the delivery of comprehensive perioperative patient care.

Unit I, *Foundations for Practice,* provides information on basic principles and patient-care requisites essential to the care of all recipients of perioperative patient care. The nursing process, a model for developing therapeutic nursing interventional knowledge, reflects a six-step process that includes the identification of desired patient outcomes. Interest in patient outcomes and their improvement continues to be an essential element of nursing as reformation of the health care delivery system escalates. Realizing that the collection of health data in an expansive information age requires clear identification of contributions to patient outcomes and quantification of these in data-driven improvement of quality patient care, perioperative nurses must continue to link their interventions to clearly identified outcomes. This relationship is presented in Chapter 1 and explicated in each Sample Plan of Care throughout the text. Research Highlights continue to be included in every chapter, reflecting the steady increase in the amount and quality of research relevant to perioperative patient care. Because the findings of research are important to use in clinical practice, the editors and authors of *Alexander's Care of the Patient in Surgery* are committed to supporting this research-practice relationship. The Research Highlights will help perioperative nurses read about and implement research findings in their practice and patient care activities. Chapter 1 also sets the stage for an emphasis on patient and family education and discharge planning throughout the text, with a subsequent entire chapter dedicated to this important topic. All chapters in Units II and III address specific patient and family education and discharge planning relevant for patients undergoing one or more of the respective specialty surgical procedures. As the responsibilities of perioperative nurses become greater with regard to those important care components, it is imperative that we effectively educate patients and families. With the length of stay in health care facilities continuing to decrease, patients and families must be informed and prepared to appropriately deal with postoperative needs after discharge. Pain management, addressed in Chapter 9, is also reflected in many of the chapters on surgical specialties, as all perioperative nurses recognize the importance of this in planning patient discharge.

Coverage of emergency preparedness and bioterrorism is incorporated in Chapters 2 and 3 of Unit I and in Chapter 31, *Trauma Surgery.*

The chapters within Unit II, *Surgical Interventions,* include more than 400 contemporary and traditional specialty surgical interventions and numerous minimally invasive surgical procedures. Each chapter provides a helpful review of pertinent anatomy and details the steps of each procedure. Perioperative nursing considerations are once again presented within the nursing process framework. Current NANDA-approved nursing diagnoses and Sample Plans of Care for each surgical specialty are intended to help perioperative nurses plan, implement, and evaluate individualized perioperative patient care. Each of these chapters also provides an example of a Best Practice related to the surgical specialty. In 2007 and beyond, perioperative nurses can expect to find a continuing emphasis on evidence-based nursing as a means to provide care that is effective and yields improved outcomes. Much of the "evidence" in the Best Practice boxes is medical in nature, since nursing has just begun its intense focus on this effort. However, the integration of evidence-based practice with the perioperative nurse's individual clinical expertise will lead to optimal care provision, which is the foundation of perioperative patient care. Improving the quality of patient care and effecting safe outcomes are at the heart of all of our efforts to achieve excellence in whatever setting we encounter the patient undergoing an operative or other invasive procedure.

The incorporation of Surgical Pharmacology in the thirteenth edition reflects the ongoing emphasis on medication safety in the United States. *Alexander's Care of the Patient in Surgery* joins the nationwide health professional education campaign aimed at reducing the number of common but preventable sources of medication errors. Providing information about select medications used in surgical specialties, the Surgical Pharmacology features are intended to promote safe medication practices among perioperative practitioners to help avoid serious and even potentially fatal consequences of medication errors. Medication errors can occur anywhere in the medication-use system, from prescribing to administering a drug. Readers will find the Joint Commission's "Do not use" list, assisting perioperative practitioners in eliminating the use of potentially confusing abbreviations. Other areas covered in the new Surgical Pharmacology feature address the use of written medication orders, read-back, repeat-back recommendations, suggestions for proper labeling of medications on and off the sterile field, and uses of, dosages for, and other information regarding perioperative medications.

To further facilitate the perioperative nurse's focus on safe patient care, the Patient Safety feature in each chapter succinctly reviews a practice to assist perioperative practitioners in developing a core body of knowledge regarding safe patient care. We hope this new feature not only raises awareness about patient safety applications, but also simultaneously fosters communication and ongoing dialogue in perioperative practice settings regarding application of recommended patient safety strategies.

The unique needs of ambulatory, pediatric, geriatric, and trauma surgery patients are presented in Unit III, *Special Considerations*. The chapter on *Integrated Health Practices: Complementary and Alternative Therapy* was introduced in the twelfth edition. Perioperative nurses frequently encounter patients who use such therapies, some of which are nonpharmacologic and some of which are consumed as medications. This chapter explores alternative medical systems, mind-body interventions, biologically based therapies, manipulative and body-based methods, and energy therapies. Numerous treatments and systems within each category are discussed.

Many expert perioperative practitioners, RN first assistants, clinical nurse specialists, and educators have contributed to this thirteenth edition, and I owe a debt of gratitude to all of them for sharing their expertise in the development of this text. Special thanks to Alan Zulick for his help during page proofs! I also acknowledge the valuable assistance of editors, reviewers, photographers, and illustrators who have contributed their time and expertise to the revision of this text. The team I had the privilege of working with at Elsevier is talented and eager to support perioperative practitioners in their commitment to excellence in patient care.

*Alexander's Care of the Patient in Surgery* is written by and for perioperative nurses. Its premise is underscored by the clear understanding that perioperative nursing is a caring and intellectual endeavor, requiring critical thinking, technical acumen, and clinical decision making to improving patient outcomes. With the multimedia package accompanying this thirteenth edition, *Alexander's Care of the Patient in Surgery* invites you to walk with us as we meet the challenges and opportunities of perioperative nursing in this first decade of the twenty-first century.

**Jane C. Rothrock**

# Contents

## 16 *Thyroid and Parathyroid Surgery,* 553



## 17 *Breast Surgery,* 566

## 18 *Ophthalmic Surgery*, 585



## 19 *Otologic Surgery*, 630



## 20 *Rhinologic and Sinus Surgery*, 657

## 24 *Plastic and Reconstructive Surgery,* 863



## 25 *Thoracic Surgery,* 906

CHAPTER 1

# Concepts Basic to Perioperative Nursing

JANE C. ROTHROCK

The term *perioperative nursing* now is used in nursing and medical circles. Perioperative nursing is recognized and practiced in surgical suites, ambulatory surgery centers, endoscopy suites, laser centers, interventional radiology departments, mobile surgical units, and physicians' offices across the United States. Remote surgery, virtual endoscopy, robotics, computerized navigation systems during knee replacement surgery, electronic medical records,[20] biologic materials that are absorbed to replace worn-out body parts, radiofrequency identification (RFID) technology to mark the surgical site,[9] and face transplants for severely burned victims are just some of the innovations developed as part of a vast array of futuristic technology.[11] In this new millennium, perioperative patient care is very different from what it was in the past.

In the past, the term *operating room (OR) nursing* was used to describe the care of patients in the immediate preoperative, intraoperative, and postoperative phases of the surgical experience (Figure 1-1). Such a term intimated, however, that nursing care activities were circumscribed to the geographic limits of the surgical suite. The term may have contributed to stereotypic images of an OR nurse who took care of the operating room and had little interface or nursing responsibility for medicated and anesthetized patients in the surgical suite (Research Highlight). With such a perspective, nursing practitioners outside the OR had difficulty ascribing important elements of the nursing process and patient care accountability to the nurse who practiced behind the doors of the surgical suite. The current view of perioperative nursing connotes the delivery of patient care in the preoperative, intraoperative, and postoperative periods of the patient's experience during operative and other invasive procedures using the framework of the nursing process. In such a framework, the perioperative nurse assesses the patient—collecting, organizing, and prioritizing patient data; establishes nursing diagnoses; identifies desired patient outcomes; develops and implements a plan of nursing care; and evaluates that care in terms of outcomes achieved by the patient (Figure 1-2). In these activities, the perioperative nurse functions independently and interdependently. The perioperative nurse collaborates with other health care professionals, makes appropriate nursing referrals, and delegates and supervises nursing care.

When perioperative nursing is practiced in its broadest scope, nursing care may begin in the patient's home, a clinic, a physician's office, the patient care unit, the presurgical care unit, or the holding area. After the surgical intervention, nursing care may continue in the perianesthesia care unit (PACU) or in patient evaluation on the patient care unit, in the physician's office, in the patient's home, in a clinic, or through written or telephone patient surveys.

When perioperative nursing is practiced in the narrower sense, patient care activities may be confined to the common areas of the surgical suite. Assessment and data collection may take place in the holding area; evaluation may take place on discharge from the OR. Despite the way perioperative nursing is practiced in a health care setting, it is underscored by the nursing process and all the care activities inherent in that process.

## OVERVIEW OF PERIOPERATIVE NURSING PRACTICE

The various perioperative nursing roles all subsume elements of the behaviors and technical practices that characterize professional nursing. Probably no other area of nursing requires the broad knowledge base, the instant recall of nursing science, the need to be intuitively guided by nursing experience, the diversity of thought and action, the stamina, and the flexibility needed in perioperative nursing endeavors. Whether a generalist or a specialist, the perioperative nurse depends on knowledge of surgical anatomy, physiologic alterations and their consequences for the patient, intraoperative risk factors, potentials for patient injury and the means of preventing them, and psychosocial implications of surgery for the patient and significant others. This knowledge enables the perioperative nurse to anticipate needs of the patient and surgical team and initiate safe and appropriate nursing interventions rapidly. This is part of patient advocacy—of doing for the patient what needs to be done to provide a safe and caring environment. The Association of periOperative Registered Nurses (AORN) has asserted the significance of such safety by affirming that staffing skill mixes must ensure that patients undergoing surgical and invasive procedures have a perioperative nurse as the circulator, and that the core activities of perioperative nursing care (assessment, diagnosis, outcome identification, planning, and evaluation; discussed subsequently) are completed by the perioperative nurse.[2]

Perioperative nursing is a purposeful and dynamic process. By planning patient care and identifying required nursing interventions and actions, perioperative nurses ensure that surgical patients receive scientific, evidence-based professional nursing care. Perioperative nurses historically have assumed responsibility for providing a safe, efficient, and caring environment for

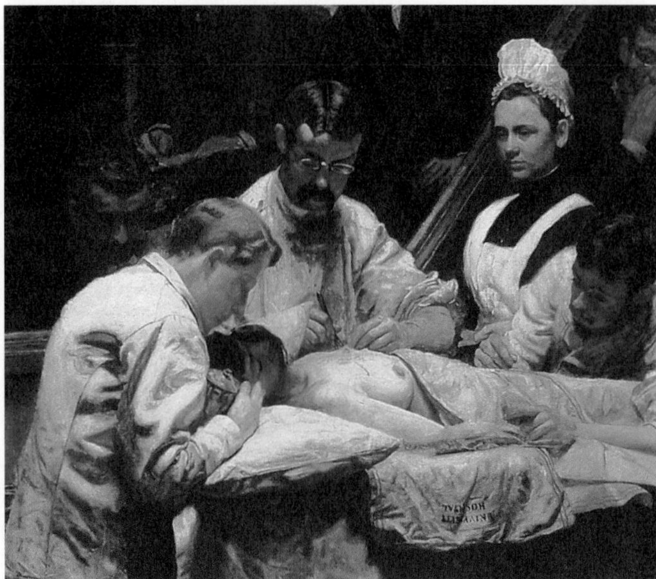

FIGURE 1-1 Thomas Eakins, *The Agnew Clinic*, 1889. In this painting, reforms and advancements in surgical techniques and procedures are apparent. Surgeons wear gowns, instruments are sterilized, ether is used, and the patient is covered. An OR nurse is a prominent member of the team.

surgical patients, one in which the surgical team functioned effectively and efficiently to achieve positive patient outcomes. Such mutuality between nursing and other health care disciplines and the role of patient advocacy continue to be part of the essence of perioperative nursing and will remain so.

A significant part of perioperative nursing is the delivery of scientifically based care: understanding the necessity for certain techniques of care; knowing how and when to initiate them; being creative in maintaining a technique when the situation calls for flexibility; and evaluating the safety, cost, and outcomes of the care delivered. Knowledge of surgical interventions, instruments, and equipment is essential during the implementation phase of nursing care. Without such knowledge, the perioperative nurse cannot prepare for or anticipate the steps in the surgical procedure, with their concomitant implications for the patient and for the surgical team. Scientific nursing interventions and caring, comforting behaviors are at the heart of perioperative nursing.[8] The chapters in Unit II focus on surgical interventions common to patients in inpatient and ambulatory settings. Each of the chapters on surgical interventions contains a *Sample Plan of Care* with suggested nursing interventions. A fundamental assumption is that perioperative nursing is a blend of the technical and behavioral; it is critical thinking as well as doing and caring for patients. Clinical judgment derives from critical thinking,[10] which requires purposeful, outcomes-directed thought; is driven by patient need; is based on the nursing process and nursing science; requires knowledge, skills, and experience; is guided by professional standards and ethics; and is underscored by constant reevaluation, self-correcting, and striving to improve.

## Perioperative Patient Focused Model

The Perioperative Patient Focused Model (Figure 1-3) consists of domains (areas) of nursing concern: nursing diagnoses, nursing interventions, and patient outcomes. These domains are in continuous interaction with the health system encircling the focus of perioperative nursing practice: the patient.

Three of these domains—behavioral responses, patient safety, and physiologic responses—reflect phenomena of concern to perioperative nurses and comprise the nursing diagnoses, interventions, and outcomes that surgical patients or their families experience. The fourth domain, the health system, comprises the structural data elements and focuses on clinical processes and outcomes. Looking at the model, note the heavy line that indicates a differentiation between the health system and the patient.

The model as a whole illustrates the dynamic nature of the perioperative patient experience and the nursing presence throughout that process. Working in a collaborative manner with other members of the health care team and the patient, the nurse establishes outcomes, identifies nursing diagnoses, and provides nursing care. The nurse intervenes within the

## RESEARCH HIGHLIGHT

### Historical Analysis of Preoperative Patient Preparation

Over the past 150 years, nurses have worked to extend and develop the professional practice base of nursing. As clinical specialization developed, roles and responsibilities evolved and adapted. It is important for nurses to understand historical and contemporaneous depictions of their professional roles. In this historical analysis, four periods were reviewed to identify the changing focus of preoperative patient preparation. From 1900 to 1919, preparation of the patient for surgery took place primarily in the patient's home, where much of surgery also was done. The patient took light, nourishing food; baths; and frequent rest periods to build up the body. The nurse arrived at the home a few hours before surgery, choosing and preparing a room, emptying it of furniture, boiling sheets and instruments, and preventing excitement on the patient's part. The nurse also obtained a personal and family history from the patient, although little patient teaching took place. Between 1920 and 1939, physicians became affiliated with hospitals, and minimum standards of preoperative patient preparation began to evolve. Physical and mental preparation of the patient were stressed, the concept of patient consent for surgery was initiated, and preparation of the OR and instruments was addressed. Nursing manuals on care of the surgical patient included normal anatomy and physiology, pathophysiology, medical and surgical treatments, and nursing interventions. The years between 1940 and 1959 witnessed enormous scientific medical discoveries; nursing care of surgical patients became more complex to accommodate rapid changes in surgical care. Patient teaching became part of preoperative patient preparation, individual patient needs were emphasized, and the psychologic preparation of the patient was increasingly recognized as important. From 1960 to 1979, nursing research was being conducted and emphasized; early research demonstrated a link between preoperative preparation and improved postoperative recovery. Patients' emotional needs were recognized as they related to individual patients, and concepts of structured preoperative instruction were introduced and validated by nursing research.

Modified from Oetker-Black SL: Preoperative preparation: historical development, *AORN Journal* 57(6):1402-1410, 1993; Nelson S, Gordon S: The rhetoric of rupture: nursing as practice without a history, *Nursing Outlook* 52(5):255-261, 2004.

| | |
|---|---|
| **Assessment...** | Review medical record, validate important findings, corroborate with patient.<br>Analyze, interpret, and prioritize information. |
| **Nursing Diagnosis...** | Synthesize data collected; then label clinical judgment about the patient as a nursing diagnosis.<br>Can be actual or risk for.<br>Based on patient assessment and perioperative nurse's clinical judgment. |
| **Outcome Identification...** | Because perioperative nursing is largely preventive, generic outcomes have been identified that apply to all patients undergoing an operative or other invasive procedure.<br>Additional outcomes are identified based on individual patient assessment and nursing diagnosis.<br>Some outcomes are mutually formulated by the nurse and patient.<br>Guide implementation of nursing interventions.<br>Should be specific, realistic, and measurable. |
| **Planning...** | Incorporate information into a plan for the patient's care.<br>Identify nursing interventions to achieve identified outcomes. |
| **Implementation...** | Carry out nursing plan of care.<br>Gather equipment and supplies; participate in/guide/supervise patient preparation, transfer to OR bed, anesthesia induction, antimicrobial skin preparation, draping, patient positioning, monitoring of physiologic alterations during surgery, and patient discharge (transfer from OR bed, discharge to postanesthesia or postoperative unit). |
| **Evaluation...** | Determine whether outcomes were met; use outcome statements.<br>Incorporate outcomes that have been met and those that are pending in report to nurse in postanesthesia care unit/ discharge area. |

**FIGURE 1-2** The steps of the nursing process are interrelated, forming a continuous cycle of thought and action.

context of the health care system to help the patient achieve the highest attainable health outcomes (physiologic, behavioral, and safety) throughout the perioperative experience.

The model is outcome-focused, emphasizing the outcomes-driven nature of perioperative patient care. Perioperative nurses possess a unique knowledge base of desired outcomes that apply to all patients. In contrast to traditional nursing practice, in which nursing diagnoses are evidenced by signs and symptoms, perioperative nurses "know" that many surgical interventions and other invasive procedures carry inherent risks. They identify these risks and potential problems in advance and direct nursing interventions at prevention. From these or in addition to these, relevant nursing diagnoses are selected by the perioperative nurse, based on individual patient assessment. This information guides the nursing interventions for each particular patient for whom the nurse provides care. The practice of perioperative nursing encompasses traditional and expanded nursing activities during intraoperative care, preoperative and postoperative patient education, counseling, assessment, planning, and evaluation functions. The perioperative nurse's activities address the psychologic, social, and physiologic problems that may result. Perioperative nurses scrub, circulate, assist during surgery (registered nurse first assistant [RNFA]), manage, teach, and conduct research. From admission through discharge and home follow-up, the perioperative nurse plays a significant role in managing the patient's care. Research based on the Patient Focused Model will test and validate the contributions of perioperative nurses to patient care outcomes in all settings where patient care is practiced.

## STANDARDS OF CLINICAL NURSING PRACTICE

Perioperative nursing is a systematic, planned process—a series of integrated steps. For professional nursing, standards set forth the expectations of the full professional role within which the nurse practices. In the 1960s, the American Nurses Association (ANA) engaged in standards development. First published in 1973, these standards have helped to shape nursing practice. Specialty nursing organizations such as the AORN have worked with the ANA to develop their own standards and guidelines using the ANA framework. This collaboration has resulted in the use of common language and a consistent format for the profession. The AORN *Standards of Clinical Nursing Practice*[1] comprise the standards of care and professional performance. The standards of care are based on the nursing process.

### Nursing Process

The nursing process is a way of looking at nursing and bringing it into perspective as methodic critical thinking that guides actions. The focus of the nursing process is on the patient, and the nursing interventions prescribed are those that meet patient needs. Because of the setting and the nature of the work, perioperative nursing is particularly vulnerable to being considered only a conglomeration of mechanical techniques and an execution of surgeons' orders. By using the nursing process, perioperative nurses focus on the patient and, at the same time, use skills and knowledge in caring for patients and making clinical decisions. Use of the nursing process, nursing plans of care, clinical pathways, and best practices (discussed later in this chapter) has become an integral part of patient care.

In its simplest form, the nursing process defined by the ANA consists of six steps: assessment, nursing diagnosis, outcome identification, planning, implementation, and evaluation (see Figure 1-2). The process is circular and continuous. In all areas of nursing practice, responsibilities inherent in the nursing process include (1) providing culturally and ethnically sensitive care[12] that is also age appropriate, (2) maintaining a safe environment, (3) educating patients and their families or significant others, (4) ensuring continuity and coordination of care through discharge planning and referrals, and (5) communicating information.

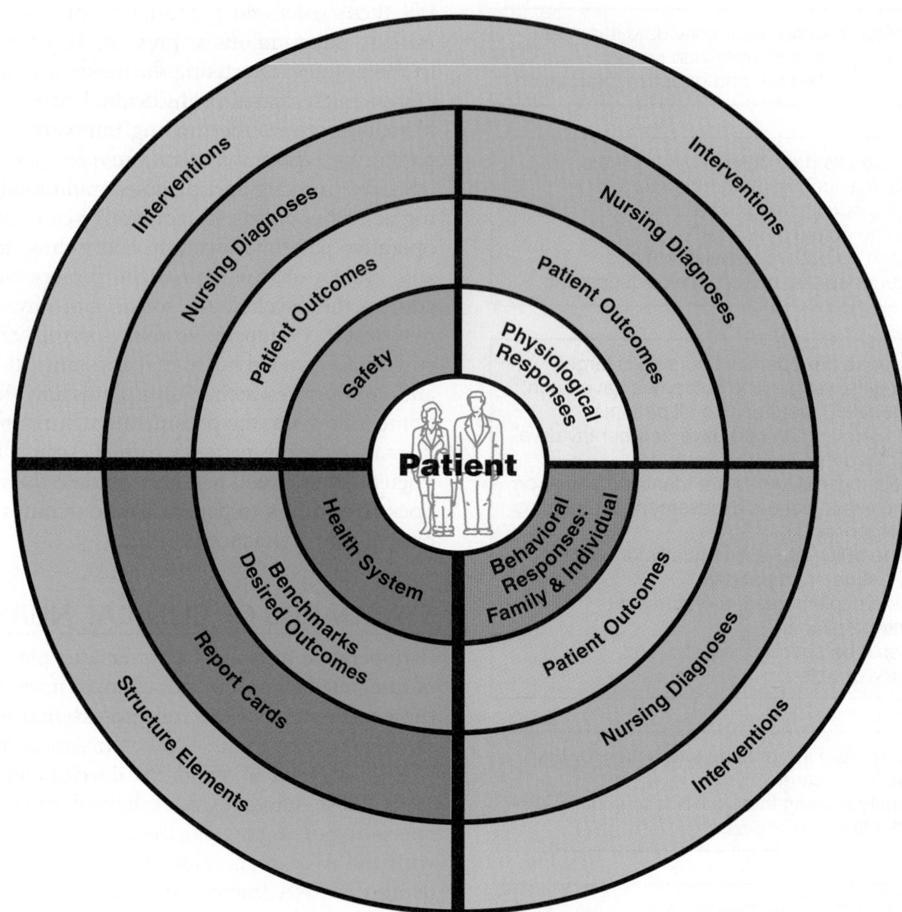


**FIGURE 1-3** The AORN Perioperative Patient Focused Model.©

***Assessment.*** *Assessment* is the collection of relevant health data about the patient. Sources of data may be a preoperative interview with the patient and the patient's family by a perioperative or unit nurse; review of the nursing plans of care and patient's medical record; examination of the results of presurgical diagnostic studies; and consultation with the surgeon and anesthesia provider, unit nurses, or other personnel. The focuses of data collection are (1) the patient's current diagnosis, physical status, and psychosocial status (including literacy level; language skills; and spiritual, ethnic, cultural, and life-style information relevant to the delivery of patient-specific care) and (2) previous hospitalizations or surgical interventions. Of primary importance is the patient's and family's understanding of the scheduled intervention and their ability to participate in activities such as marking the surgical site (the Universal Protocol for correct site surgery is discussed in Chapter 2). Implementing the concept of patient-centered care mandates that perioperative nurses encourage the patient's active involvement in his or her own care as part of patient safety.[15] The perioperative nurse also reviews laboratory data and reports deviations to the surgeon. The nurse should document all data that are collected and should note any referrals that he or she makes.

The format this assessment takes may vary from institution to institution but always includes the physiologic and the psychosocial aspects of the patient. For a perioperative nurse caring for a healthy patient, assessment may mean a thoughtful, quick scan of the patient and medical record; a review of the surgical procedure; and a mental rehearsal of the resources and knowledge necessary to direct the patient through an operative course. At other times, the perioperative nurse must thoroughly assess all aspects of the patient and the patient's condition, along with preoperative and postoperative reviews. Assessment may be performed by a perioperative nurse in the presurgical care unit or by telephone before the day of surgical admission.

When developing guidelines for preoperative assessment, patient and family education, and discharge planning, the perioperative nurse should consider the following:

- Is relevant, concise patient information already available to the perioperative nursing staff?
- Is enough information available to allow perioperative nurses to consider patient care needs when setting up the room (e.g., special equipment, accessory items, instruments, sutures)?
- Is sufficient time available to initiate a meaningful perioperative nurse–patient interaction?
- Are surgical patients satisfied with their perioperative nursing care (do they express feelings of comfort and satisfaction regarding their care in the surgical setting), and do they have knowledge of the perioperative nurse's role?
- Is there continuity of care between the perioperative unit and other nursing care units?

Being able to exchange information about their patients in face-to-face meetings, by telephone, or by written messages is helpful for unit and perioperative nurses. A thorough assessment, made and recorded by the unit nurses, can accompany inpatients to the OR and serve as a guide to perioperative nursing personnel. The perioperative nurse completes a more focused preoperative patient assessment. With the burgeoning number of ambulatory surgery procedures, preoperative assessment is often integrated in preadmission testing (PAT). In some institutions, group preoperative sessions are held. These not only help nurses get to know the patients but also permit nurses to impart information on common routines, reactions, sensations, and nursing procedures that will take place preoperatively, intraoperatively, and postoperatively. The perioperative setting determines the type of interaction that may occur. The use of preoperative phone calls and questionnaires has gained wide acceptance. Soliciting information before the patient's arrival in the perioperative setting and this one-on-one contact with the perioperative nurse can affect patient outcomes. The important point is that some form of assessment, patient and family education, and discharge planning should be done. How it is accomplished is determined by the particular facility and nursing staff.

Assessment is knowing and understanding the patient as a feeling, thinking, and responsible individual and as a candidate for a surgical procedure. Data identified through assessment help the perioperative nurse meet unique patient needs throughout the surgical intervention. Based on the data collected, recorded, and interpreted during patient assessment, nursing diagnoses are formulated.

***Nursing Diagnosis.*** *Nursing diagnosis* is the process of identifying and classifying data collected in the assessment in a way that yields a focus for the planning of nursing care. Nursing diagnoses have been evolving since they were first introduced in the 1950s. They have now reached the stage of development of being identified, named, and classified according to human response patterns and functional health patterns. The organization responsible for delineating the accepted list of nursing diagnoses is the North American Nursing Diagnosis Association (NANDA) (Box 1-1). Each NANDA-approved nursing diagnosis has a set of components, as follows: definition (meaning of the diagnostic term), defining characteristics (pattern of signs and symptoms or cues that make the meaning of the diagnosis clear), and related or risk factors (causative or contributing factors that can be useful in determining whether the diagnosis is applicable to a particular patient). For perioperative patients, many nursing diagnoses are "risk" diagnoses; that is, they are not evidenced by signs or symptoms because the problem has not occurred, and nursing interventions are directed at prevention.

Not all patient problems encountered in the perioperative setting can be described by the list of accepted nursing diagnoses. Perioperative nurses must participate in describing and naming new nursing diagnoses that characterize unique perioperative patient problems. NANDA has established a "to be developed" category to designate nursing diagnoses that are partially developed and deemed useful to the nursing profession; perioperative nurses may develop unique diagnostic labels and definitions and work to develop and validate them further through this process. This process becomes even more important as health care moves toward the use of information systems to document nursing practice.

***Outcome Identification.*** *Outcome identification* is a statement that describes the desired or favorable patient condition that can be achieved through nursing interventions. The study of patient outcomes is not new (History box). To be useful for assessing the effectiveness of nursing care, patient outcomes should be "nursing-sensitive"; that is, they should be influenced by nursing and describe a patient state that can be measured and quantified. Nursing-sensitive patient outcomes are derived from nursing diagnoses and direct the interventions to resolve the nursing diagnoses. They are the standards or criteria by which the effectiveness of the interventions is measured. Outcomes should be stated in terms of expected or desired patient behavior and be specific and measurable in time. The appropriate time to measure perioperative nursing-sensitive outcomes varies. Some outcomes from intraoperative nursing interventions can be evaluated immediately. Others occur over a longer period. In this textbook, the use of "the patient will . . . " indicates an outcome that is expected to occur over time. Identification of expected and desired outcomes unique to the surgical patient provides the opportunity to prioritize care, becomes a basis for continuity of care, and directs evaluation (outcomes research). In this type of research, the relationship between patient characteristics, the processes of care (what the perioperative nurse does, described in the implementation section), and the outcomes of that care are studied, enhancing the perioperative nurse's ability to improve care (Figure 1-4). In many instances, outcomes research efforts result in the identification of "best practice" for improving patient care.[23]

**EVIDENCE-BASED PRACTICE.** In 1996 the ANA and other nursing organizations held a nursing summit to address the delivery of safe, high-quality, accessible, and cost-effective health care. An outcome of this meeting was the creation of a *best practices network,* where institutions could share better or new ways of providing a particular health care service or program. At that time, a "best practice" represented an innovative health care practice, process, or service that had been implemented successfully and viewed as a creative solution. In the twenty-first century evidence-based practice (EBP) is in the forefront of contemporary discussions of nursing research and practice.[21,23]

The underpinnings of the movement toward EBP, in nursing and other disciplines, is an intent to know which interventions are most effective clinically and economically. Ingersoll[13] defined evidence-based nursing practice as "the conscientious, explicit and judicious use of theory-derived, research-based information in making decisions about care delivery to individuals or groups of patients in consideration of individuals' needs and preferences." Figure 1-5 shows a model that builds on such a definition. Perioperative nurses can view EBP as a problem-solving method that involves identifying a clinical problem, searching the literature, evaluating the evidence from multiple studies, and deciding on the most appropriate intervention. The subsequent "best practice" is one that enables the perioperative nurse to make decisions that have the "best" possible impact on patient care. The goal is improving the care of the patient and the outcome of that care.[7]

In a general framework for EBP, clinical decision making and patient care delivery interact with the processes of *measuring* patient outcomes and quality clinical indicators; *establishing best practices,* which involves clinical problem analysis via review of nursing theory, research, literature, and expert opinion; *implementing* via educating health care providers and patients about the EBP and providing feedback on it; and *perfor-*

BOX 1-1

## NANDA Nursing Diagnoses Taxonomy II

**A**ctivity intolerance
Risk for **A**ctivity intolerance
Impaired **A**djustment
Ineffective **A**irway clearance
Latex **A**llergy response
Risk for latex **A**llergy response
**A**nxiety
Death **A**nxiety
Risk for **A**spiration
Risk for impaired parent/infant/child **A**ttachment
**A**utonomic dysreflexia
Risk for **A**utonomic dysreflexia
Disturbed **B**ody image
Risk for imbalanced **B**ody temperature
**B**owel incontinence
Effective **B**reastfeeding
Ineffective **B**reastfeeding
Interrupted **B**reastfeeding
Ineffective **B**reathing pattern
Decreased **C**ardiac output
**C**aregiver role strain
Risk for **C**aregiver role strain
Impaired **C**omfort
Impaired verbal **C**ommunication
Decisional **C**onflict
Parental role **C**onflict
Acute **C**onfusion
Chronic **C**onfusion
**C**onstipation
Perceived **C**onstipation
Risk for **C**onstipation
Ineffective **C**oping
Ineffective community **C**oping
Readiness for enhanced community **C**oping
Defensive **C**oping
Compromised family **C**oping
Disabled family **C**oping
Readiness for enhanced family **C**oping
Ineffective **D**enial
Impaired **D**entition
Risk for delayed **D**evelopment
**D**iarrhea
Risk for **D**isuse syndrome
Deficient **D**iversional activity
Disturbed **E**nergy field
Impaired **E**nvironmental interpretation syndrome
Adult **F**ailure to thrive
Risk for **F**alls
Dysfunctional **F**amily processes: alcoholism
Interrupted **F**amily processes
**F**atigue
**F**ear
Deficient **F**luid volume
Excess **F**luid volume
Risk for deficient **F**luid volume
Risk for imbalanced **F**luid volume
Impaired **G**as exchange
**G**rieving
Anticipatory **G**rieving
Dysfunctional **G**rieving
Risk for dysfunctional **G**rieving
Delayed **G**rowth and development
Risk for disproportionate **G**rowth
Ineffective **H**ealth maintenance
**H**ealth-seeking behaviors
Impaired **H**ome maintenance
**H**opelessness
**H**yperthermia
**H**ypothermia
Disturbed personality **I**dentity
Functional urinary **I**ncontinence
Reflex urinary **I**ncontinence
Stress urinary **I**ncontinence
Total urinary **I**ncontinence
Urge urinary **I**ncontinence
Risk for urge urinary **I**ncontinence
Disorganized **I**nfant behavior
Risk for disorganized **I**nfant behavior
Readiness for enhanced organized **I**nfant behavior
Ineffective **I**nfant feeding pattern
Risk for **I**nfection
Risk for **I**njury
Risk for perioperative-positioning **I**njury
Decreased **I**ntracranial adaptive capacity
Deficient **K**nowledge
Readiness for enhanced **K**nowledge of (specify)
Sedentary **L**ifestyle
Risk for **L**oneliness
Impaired **M**emory
Impaired bed **M**obility
Impaired physical **M**obility
Impaired wheelchair **M**obility
**N**ausea
Unilateral **N**eglect
**N**oncompliance
Imbalanced **N**utrition: less than body requirements
Imbalanced **N**utrition: more than body requirements
Risk for imbalanced **N**utrition: more than body requirements
Impaired **O**ral mucous membrane
Acute **P**ain
Chronic **P**ain
Impaired **P**arenting
Risk for impaired **P**arenting
Risk for **P**eripheral neurovascular dysfunction
Risk for **P**oisoning
**P**ost-trauma syndrome
Risk for **P**ost-trauma syndrome
**P**owerlessness
Risk for **P**owerlessness
Ineffective **P**rotection
**R**ape-trauma syndrome
**R**ape-trauma syndrome: compound reaction
**R**ape-trauma syndrome: silent reaction
Impaired **R**eligiosity
Readiness for enhanced **R**eligiosity
Risk for impaired **R**eligiosity
**R**elocation stress syndrome
Risk for **R**elocation stress syndrome
Ineffective **R**ole performance
Bathing/hygiene **S**elf-care deficit
Dressing/grooming **S**elf-care deficit
Feeding **S**elf-care deficit

BOX 1-1

### NANDA Nursing Diagnoses Taxonomy II

Toileting **S**elf-care deficit
Chronic low **S**elf-esteem
Situational low **S**elf-esteem
Risk for situational low **S**elf-esteem
**S**elf-mutilation
Risk for **S**elf-mutilation
Disturbed **S**ensory perception
**S**exual dysfunction
Ineffective **S**exuality patterns
Impaired **S**kin integrity
Risk for impaired **S**kin integrity
**S**leep deprivation
Disturbed **S**leep pattern
Impaired **S**ocial interaction
**S**ocial isolation
Chronic **S**orrow
**S**piritual distress
Risk for **S**piritual distress
Readiness for enhanced **S**piritual well-being
Risk for **S**uffocation
Risk for **S**uicide
Delayed **S**urgical recovery
Impaired **S**wallowing
Effective **T**herapeutic regimen management
Ineffective **T**herapeutic regimen management
Ineffective community **T**herapeutic regimen management
Ineffective family **T**herapeutic regimen management
Ineffective **T**hermoregulation
Disturbed **T**hought processes
Impaired **T**issue integrity
Ineffective **T**issue perfusion
Impaired **T**ransfer ability
Risk for **T**rauma
Impaired **U**rinary elimination
**U**rinary retention
Impaired spontaneous **V**entilation
Dysfunctional **V**entilatory weaning response
Risk for other-directed **V**iolence
Risk for self-directed **V**iolence
Impaired **W**alking
**W**andering

NANDA International: *NANDA nursing diagnoses: definition and classification 2005-2006,* Philadelphia, 2005, NANDA.

*mance reporting.* Thurston and Long[22] described a six-step process that may be used to implement evidence-based nursing practice:

- Assess need for change—identify practice problem; collect and analyze data.
- Link problem to nursing interventions and outcomes—use a standardized classification system or language (e.g., the Perioperative Nursing Data Set, which is discussed later).
- Synthesize best evidence—critique and rate research (determine if research is relevant to your practice problem, if research can be applied to a broad population, what outcomes were studied, and if results used tests of statistical significance),[17] then assess feasibility of change for your practice setting.
- Design practice changes—plan a pilot change or demonstration.
- Implement the proposed practice change—evaluate it and decide whether to adopt or not.
- Integrate the change—policy or procedure changes may be required; change needs to be widely communicated with staff education; measure and monitor outcomes.

***Planning.*** After collecting and interpreting patient data, arriving at appropriate nursing diagnoses, and establishing desired outcomes, the perioperative nurse is prepared to *plan* the nursing care for the patient. Planning requires use of nursing knowledge and information about the patient and planned surgical intervention to prepare the surgical environment. Perioperative nurses check equipment, have requisite supplies and positioning devices ready, and use their knowledge of anatomy to have proper instruments and sutures on hand for the procedure to be performed. They know the sequence of steps in the operative or other invasive procedure and use surgeons' preference cards, nursing care guides, and other resources such as computerized data sheets to ready the room and equipment for the patient.

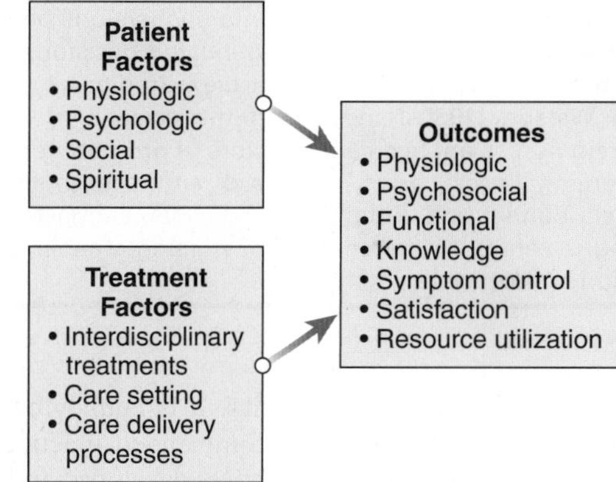


**FIGURE 1-4** A conceptual model to illustrate visually elements in outcomes research.

Planning is preparing in advance for what will happen and determining the priorities for care. Planning, based on patient assessment, results in knowing the patient and the patient's unique needs so that alterations in events such as positioning requirements or the surgical process are anticipated and readily accommodated. Planning also requires knowledge of the patient's psychosocial state and feelings about the proposed operation so that an extra needed explanation, comforting, or emotional support can be provided when patient care is being implemented.

***Implementation.*** *Implementation* is performing the nursing care interventions that were planned and responding with critical thinking and orderly activities to changes in surgical routine,

## HISTORY

### Nurses' Responsibilities to Their Patients

Although theoretic perspectives regarding patient outcomes have been described by nursing scholars, a recognition and appreciation of the contributions and legacy of the past should not be disregarded. Early in our nursing history, the foundation was clearly laid for nurses' responsibility and accountability to their patients.

- The Order of St. John (1000s) had as its mission the relief of sickness, suffering, distress, and danger.
- Florence Nightingale (1800s) analyzed health care conditions and patient outcomes related to morbidity and mortality in the Crimean War.
- Clara Weeks-Shaw (1900s) described in some detail the measures perioperative nurses should take when surgery was being done in the patient's home, noting actions to alleviate anxiety and provide for patient comfort.
- Dorothy Johnson (1950s) introduced the concepts of internal and interpersonal equilibrium to relieve discomfort and tension in patients.
- Virginia Henderson (1970s) described nursing as a substitute for self-care, assisting in the outcome of bringing the patient toward independence.
- Dorothy Orem (1970s) identified self-care needs of patients and nursing measures to support them: partially compensatory, wholly compensatory, and supportive-educative. Perioperative nurses act therapeutically in all three ways with their surgical patients.
- Imogene King (1980s) noted the interconnections between nurse and patient, identifying goal-related decisions to attain, maintain, or restore health or die with dignity.
- Jean Watson (1980s) introduced the science of caring, wherein nurses applied caring factors in promoting health, preventing illness, caring for the sick, and restoring health.
- Patricia Benner and Judith Wrubel (1980s) suggested that caring is central to the essence of nursing, enabling connection and concern.

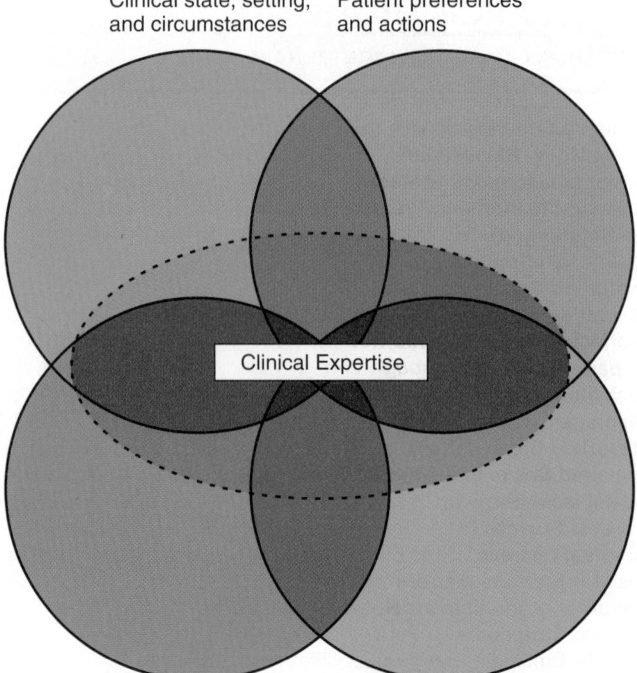


**FIGURE 1-5** Evidence-based clinical decision making should incorporate consideration of the patient's preferences, clinical status, and circumstances; evidence from research; and health care resources. The perioperative nurse's clinical expertise integrates the other four components, as the nurse uses clinical skills and past experience to design nursing care.

the patient's condition, or emergencies. It is employing established standards of nursing care, recommended practices, and other clinical guidelines and best practices developed and maintained by the nursing profession. During this phase of the nursing process, the perioperative nurse continues to assess the patient to determine the appropriateness of selected interventions and to alter the intervention as necessary to achieve the desired outcomes of care. Nursing interventions are the "work of nursing." The study of nursing interventions can link nursing diagnoses with interventions and outcomes and lead to the validation of selected interventions or the development of new ones. Clinical practice, decision making, and research-based practice are enhanced. The study of nursing interventions also assists in the delivery of cost-effective care by quantifying resource allocation. Implementation also means being the patient's advocate by recognizing and acknowledging the patient's concern or unmet need. Advocacy is part of nurse-caring, and it encompasses nursing interventions that promote emotional and physical comfort. Caring behaviors include establishing a "connection" with the patient, responding to the individuality of the patient, and meeting the expectations of the patient and family (Research Highlight). The role of patient advocate is especially important in surgical settings when patients are sedated or unconscious and unable to speak for themselves. Perioperative nurses, as patient advocates, act in ways that advance the best interests of their patients.[3]

**DELEGATION.** During the implementation of patient care, the perioperative nurse may delegate certain nursing interventions. Perioperative patient care is delivered by a team; numerous categories of personnel assist in various direct and indirect patient care activities. Often referred to as *unlicensed assistive personnel (UAP)*, these health care workers emerged during the nursing shortages of World War I and World War II and were part of the team model of delivering patient care. In the 1980s, delivery models shifted the skill mix away from assistive personnel; RNs were the principal caregivers in primary nursing models. During the fiscally constrained 1990s, health care facilities began to reintroduce assistive personnel, who have less training and who receive a lower salary. Instead of using UAP in narrowly defined job categories (e.g., clerical, housekeeping, orderly, patient transport), the trend in the late 1990s was to create a set of multiskilled assistive personnel who could assist the nurse in various activities rather than just a single activity.

As the use of UAP quickly burgeoned in the 1990s, questions and concerns arose regarding delegation of activities that were formerly performed by the registered nurse. In each state, the board of nursing defines the scope of practice for registered nurses based on the nursing process. The legal definition of nursing is contained in the state's nurse practice act—a state law that protects the health and safety of the public by establishing legal qualifications for who can practice nursing. Because imple-

## RESEARCH HIGHLIGHT

### Clinical Decision Making: Caring and Advocacy

Clinical judgment and decision making are hallmarks of professional nursing. In one qualitative study, Parker, Minick, and Kee asked the question, "What are the processes used by expert perioperative nurses in clinical decision making?" A structured interview guide was used with six perioperative nurses who had a minimum of 5 years of experience and considered themselves expert circulating nurses. After in-depth interviews, four levels of data analysis were used to sort through and interpret findings. The single, overriding pattern for these expert nurses was captured as *Seeing the big picture: engendered through caring.* Three themes emerged as essential to the expert decision making of the study participants: (1) connecting with patients (subthemes were the use of touch, conducting a perioperative interview, and humanizing the patient's care), (2) advocating for patients, and (3) embodied knowing (knowing through personal experience and through the experience of similar situations).

Another study by Boyle explored perioperative nurses' definition of, role in, and personal experiences with advocacy. A sample of 33 perioperative nurses participated in tape-recorded interviews. Four overarching themes of advocating for surgical patients emerged: protection, communication/giving voice, doing, and comfort and caring.

Seeing the big picture through connecting to and advocating for the patient and depending on one's own experience embody essential elements of critical thinking. Expert perioperative nurses actively and skillfully conceptualize, analyze, synthesize, and evaluate information gathered from and generated by observation, experience, reflection, and intellectual reasoning as a guide to their belief about their practice and the actions they take with patients. Advocacy, as reflected in both of these studies, underscores the perioperative nurse's acts in informing and supporting patients they care for and taking action to achieve goals on behalf of those patients. The pattern, themes, and subthemes identified in these studies support the cognitive, psychomotor, and affective skills used by perioperative nurses as they make decisions about patient care.

Modified from Parker CB and others: Clinical decision-making processes in perioperative nursing, *AORN Journal* 70(1):45-62, 1999; Boyle HJ: Patient advocacy in the perioperative setting, *AORN Journal* 82(2):250-262, 2005.

mentation of the plan of care and the interventions to accomplish it are part of the nursing process, guidelines for delegating some of these interventions were required. Delegation is transferring, to a competent person, the authority to perform a selected nursing task in a selected situation according to the five "rights" of delegation (Box 1-2). When the perioperative nurse delegates a task, he or she retains the accountability for delegation. Nursing functions of assessment, determining nursing diagnoses, establishing nursing care goals and patient outcomes, developing the plan of care, and evaluation and nursing interventions that require independent nursing knowledge, skills, or judgment cannot be delegated.[6] It is important for perioperative nurses to understand that institutional policy cannot contradict the nurse practice act of their state. Although tasks and procedures may be delegated to unlicensed members of the surgical team, the perioperative nurse is responsible for supervising care; supervision cannot be delegated. The perioperative nurse must assess the patient and the competency level of personnel to determine which team member has the skill to provide the necessary care. Using unlicensed personnel appropriately assists the

### BOX 1-2

### The Five Rights of Delegation

1. **The Right task.** The perioperative nurse determines that this task is one that is delegable for a specific patient, taking into consideration such factors as potential for harm, the complexity of the task, necessary problem solving, and the predictability of the outcome. Routine tasks that are performed according to a standardized procedure and that have predictable outcomes are the safest to delegate.
2. **The Right circumstances.** The perioperative nurse considers the patient care setting, the resources available, and other relevant factors. Tasks delegated must be ones that do not require independent nursing judgment.
3. **The Right person.** The perioperative nurse is the right person to delegate the right task to the right person to be performed on the right patient. The perioperative nurse must be familiar with the job description of the UAP along with the person's capabilities, knowledge and skill level, and learning needs to ensure that safe, quality patient care is provided. In this way, the nurse matches tasks to the UAP's skills, qualifications, and competence.
4. **The Right communication and direction.** The perioperative nurse provides a clear, specific, and concise description of the task, with key information relating to its objectives, rationale, limits, and expectations. There should be an opportunity for questions and clarifying instructions. Information the perioperative nurse needs to know from the person performing the task must be identified. Communication should be direct and not provided through others.
5. **The Right supervision and evaluation.** The perioperative nurse appropriately monitors the task or person performing it, evaluates the results or patient's outcome or both, intervenes if necessary, and provides feedback. Providing immediate feedback or identifying a problem with performance as it occurs is essential to upholding standards of care and performance expectations.

Perioperative nurses must be actively involved in providing the assessment, evaluation, and judgment needed to coordinate and supervise perioperative patient care. When delegating care activities, the perioperative nurse retains accountability for analyzing and evaluating the outcome of the delegated task. Activities that rely on the nursing process, such as assessment, nursing diagnosis, establishing plans of care, extensive patient and family education, and discharge planning, cannot be delegated.

Modified from the *National Council of State Boards of Nursing Response to the PEW Taskforce Principles and Vision for Health Care Workforce Regulation,* Chicago, 1996, The Council, pp. 4-5; Cherry B, Jacob SR: *Contemporary nursing: issues, trends and management,* St Louis, 2005, Mosby.

profession of perioperative nursing to be better prepared for the challenge of maintaining high quality in patient care services even when nurse shortages occur.

**DOCUMENTING INTERVENTIONS.** Accurate documentation of nursing care is an integral part of all phases of the nursing process, especially implementation of the plan of care. A description of the patient, the nursing diagnoses and desired patient outcomes, the nursing care given, and the patient's response to care (outcomes) should be included in the patient's record (Chapter 2 has a fuller review of documentation). Documentation of the nursing care given should include more than the technical aspects of care, such as the sponge count or the application of the electrosurgical dispersive pad. Nursing care documentation should be related to assessment and nursing diagnoses, with preestablished outcomes against which the appropriateness and effectiveness of care may be judged. The form for this documentation may include standardized protocols and interventions as noted on clinical pathways; space should be provided to write in interventions that are unique to individual patients or to describe variances in care. Documentation should require little time to complete, be specific to the perioperative setting, and provide continuity across the various areas in surgery, from presurgery holding areas to perianesthesia care units.

**PERIOPERATIVE NURSING DATA SET.** In 1993 the AORN recognized the need to describe and define the unique contributions of perioperative nurses to patient outcomes. After 6 years of research and validation, the perioperative nursing data set (PNDS) was recognized as a specialty nursing language in 1999, providing a uniform and systematic method of collecting basic elements of perioperative nursing care.[4,16] Similar to the Perioperative Patient Focused Model, the PNDS begins with patient outcomes (Figure 1-6). Each outcome is defined and interpreted and presents criteria by which to measure outcome achievement. Subsequently, nursing interven-

**Explanation of PNDS Layout**

| | |
|---|---|
| Patient outcome. → | **OUTCOME O7** The patient is free from signs and symptoms of radiation injury. |
| Definition provides further explanation of the outcome. → | **OUTCOME DEFINITION**<br>The patient is free from signs or symptoms of injury related to use of radiation. Radiation exposure is limited to the target site. |
| Interpretive statement describes the scope of the current problem or need. → | **INTERPRETIVE STATEMENT**<br>Prevention of radiation injury requires the application of principles of physics and radiologic safety standards. Policies addressing education, credentialing, and radiologic safety and maintenance must be in accordance with national regulatory standards and manufacturers' documented instructions. Preexisting patient conditions (e.g., length of and/or previous exposure) can influence the patient's susceptibility to radiologic injury. |
| Outcome indicators are derived from assessment data and provide a framework for evaluating the patient's progress or a clinical standard. → | **OUTCOME INDICATORS**<br>• Skin condition (general): smooth, intact, and free from unexplained edema, redness, blistering, or tenderness in nontargeted areas.<br>• Cognition: responds appropriately to questioning; memory intact. |
| Examples of interim outcome statements provide outcomes that reflect a patient's family member's* status at a specific point and time across the surgical continuum. → | **EXAMPLES OF INTERIM OUTCOME STATEMENTS**<br>• The patient's skin remains smooth, intact, free from unexplained redness, blistering, or tenderness in targeted areas between admission and discharge from the OR. |
| Nursing diagnoses are linked to each outcome and provide possible human responses linked with surgical experiences. → | **POTENTIALLY APPLICABLE NURSING DIAGNOSES**<br>• Risk of impaired skin integrity (X51)<br>• Impaired skin integrity (X50)<br>• Acute confusion (X11) |
| Nursing intervention statements are in bold print. Each intervention statement has a definition. An intervention statement is generally the data element that is documented. → | **NURSING INTERVENTIONS AND ACTIVITIES**<br>**Implements protective measures to prevent injury due to radiation sources.**<br>Provides safety equipment such as gonadal protection for diagnostic and therapeutic uses of radiation.<br>• Assembles proper protective equipment. |
| Activity statements are the bulleted points under interventions. Activities support interventions, but do not necessarily need to be documented. → | • Limits exposure to radiation to therapeutic levels (e.g., fluoroscope is off when not in use, radioactive elements remain in lead-lined containers until ready for implantation).<br>• Provides shields to protect body areas from scatter radiation or focused beam whenever possible (fetus/gonadal shields, thyroid/sternal shields, lead aprons, lead gloves).<br>• Implements appropriate procedures for handling of radiated tissue specimens.<br>• Implements measures to protect the patient from direct and scatter radiation.<br>• Manages body fluids and tissue removed from patients who have undergone recent diagnostic studies using radioactive materials according to recommendations of the radiation safety department.<br>• Documents protective measures on clinical record. |

*Family member—AORN defines *family* as the person or people that the patient identifies as their family. *Family member(s)* replaces the term *support person* or *significant other* and indicates the same meaning.

**FIGURE 1-6** An explanation of the layout of the Perioperative Nursing Data Set (PNDS).

tions to achieve the desired patient outcomes are noted, along with suggested nursing activities to support the intervention. Of special import is the opportunity for perioperative nurses to use the PNDS to support standardized documentation. When this is accomplished, databases allow comparison of clinical outcomes from large patient populations within an institution or across institutions.[5] The databases can be used to guide research, develop best practices and practice guidelines, and support the work of EBP.

***Evaluation.*** *Evaluation* is checking, observing, and appraising the results of what was done. Although evaluation is traditionally listed as the last phase of the nursing process, it is an integral, systematic, and ongoing component of providing perioperative patient care. Evaluation is directed toward the patient's progress in attaining identified outcomes. When feasible and appropriate, the patient and family or significant others should be involved in the evaluation process. The attainment of outcomes or the need to revise nursing diagnoses or modify outcomes and the plan of care must be documented. Because perioperative patient care processes and interventions often are multidisciplinary, additional evaluation methods may be used in health care facilities.

Performance improvement activities, notably monitoring important aspects of care, problem identification, problem solving, and peer review, may be part of the overall system evaluation. Often referred to as *quality improvement (QI) programs,* multidisciplinary teams address areas for improvement in patient care, identify problems, propose solutions, and monitor and evaluate the effectiveness of the improvements. This topic is discussed in more detail later.

## Perioperative Nursing Practice Standards

Perioperative nurses are responsible for identifying, interpreting, and implementing contemporary professional standards. The AORN[1] has established standards for perioperative nursing practice that can serve as guidelines for measuring the quality of patient care. These sound principles are broad in scope, attainable, definitive, and relevant for perioperative nurses. The standards represent a comprehensive approach to meeting the health care needs of surgical patients. Nursing care standards consist of three elements: structure, process, and outcome. The AORN[1] *Standards of Perioperative Administrative Practice* are *structure* standards, describing organizational characteristics, administrative and fiscal accountabilities, personnel qualifications, and facilities and environmental requirements. These standards provide guidance for evaluating operational systems.

*Process* standards relate to nursing activities, interventions, and interactions and are used to explicate clinical, professional, and quality objectives in perioperative nursing. Examples of process standards are the AORN[1] *Standards of Perioperative Clinical Practice, Standards of Perioperative Professional Performance,* and *Quality Improvement Standards for Perioperative Nursing.*

*Outcome* standards identify desirable and measurable physiologic and psychologic responses of patients to nursing interventions. Patient outcomes are an essential indicator of the quality of care. The AORN[1] *Patient Outcomes: Standards of Perioperative Care* provide outcome statements, interpretations, and criteria guidelines for measuring patient responses. The common goal of standards is quality care for the surgical patient.

## Standards of Professional Performance

The pace and complexity of advances in surgical procedures, minimally invasive surgery, newly developed technology with surgical applications, professional nursing issues, ongoing health care reform measures, changes in recommended practices, and the burgeoning body of nursing research and best practice guidelines demand constant attention to professional education and development. Perioperative professionals must continue to (1) research patient outcomes tenaciously, (2) link nursing interventions to outcomes, and (3) determine methods that conserve resources when implementing interventions. The AORN[1] *Standards of Professional Performance* expect, in part, that the perioperative nurse evaluates the effectiveness of nursing practice and the quality of that practice. Professional performance standards also require perioperative nurses to evaluate their own practice in relation to AORN's professional practice standards. Achieving certification (Certified Nurse, Operating Room [CNOR]), lifelong learning, and maintaining competency and current knowledge in perioperative nursing are the hallmarks of a professional. Other standards of professional performance address ethics, collaboration, and collegiality.

***Patient and Family Education and Discharge Planning.*** As part of the AORN[1] *Standards for Professional Performance,* the nurse is expected to collaborate with the patient and family in formulating goals, the plan of care, decisions regarding care, and delivery of health care services. In a patient-centered care philosophy, it is strongly recognized that emphasizing patient education and prevention is a key to improving outcomes; longitudinal care, prevention of problems, and providing emotional and physical support for the patient and family are integral components. As the number of short-stay, same-day admission, and ambulatory surgeries continues to grow, patient and family education and discharge planning become crucial perioperative nursing activities. Many procedures that were previously done in an acute-care, inpatient setting are now performed on an ambulatory basis. Patient education and discharge planning also must consider the environment to which the patient will be returning (usually the home), resources available, and self-care requisites.

In developing a plan for patient and family education and discharge planning, the perioperative nurse must consider an educational assessment (what the patient needs to know and wants to know and the factors that influence the patient's readiness and ability to learn), an environmental assessment, the level of information provided to the patient and family (materials should be between sixth-grade and eighth-grade reading levels), supportive patient education materials (print, video, computer, and Web-based), and the participation of the family or significant others. Goals of patient education include providing information and support, correcting misconceptions, and assisting the patient in understanding self-care roles and responsibilities. To be an effective educator, the perioperative nurse should be caring and empathetic and should have knowledge of the subject, unconditional positive regard, good verbal and nonverbal communication skills, and counseling skills. Technology has made it possible for patients and nurses to obtain clinical information from the Internet. In the twenty-first century, perioperative nurses need to be familiar with Web-based health care information, facilitating patient and family access to and support for information translation and validation.

Chapter 10 provides a comprehensive discussion of patient and family education and discharge planning. In each of the chapters in Unit II, a section summarizes important features of patient and family education and discharge planning for selected surgical interventions.

***Clinical Pathways.*** Another expectation in the AORN[1] *Standards of Professional Performance* is that the nurse uses the best available evidence, preferably research data, in planning patient care and participates in research activities. Clinical pathways (also referred to as *care maps* or *care protocols*) lead to improvement in patient care because they are based on research and outcomes. In general, clinical pathways are multidisciplinary practice guidelines that allow one to recommend key resources and activities with targeted time frames during various phases of a patient's care. Their intent is to improve quality of care, improve patient and family satisfaction, and reduce or control costs.

### Institutional Standards of Care

Perioperative departments have delegated responsibility, through the governing board of the institution, for the development of policies and procedures. Often referred to as *surgical services standards of care,* these serve as the institution's standards for delivering quality care. Policies are written statements that outline responsibilities and appropriate actions for specific circumstances. To be effective, a policy should be consistent with national and state practice standards, be realistic and achievable, be consistently followed except where prior approval has been obtained, be based on evidence and reasoned and rational thinking, and be related to the long-term intent of the surgical services department.

Procedures are the guides to implementing a policy; they set forth the detailed chronologic sequence of activities as they relate to a particular policy. Policies and procedures are usually combined into a manual that is kept readily available as a perioperative care resource in departments where operative or other invasive procedures are performed. Participation of staff members in policy and procedure development increases their knowledge of the subject matter and generates a sense of ownership. This results in meaningful interpretation of the approved policy or procedure to peers and its successful implementation.

## PERFORMANCE MEASUREMENT

Trends in health care have mandated increased control of costs, efficient use of resources and supplies, decreased length of stay for surgical patients, and shifting of many surgical procedures from inpatient to ambulatory care settings. Along with this shift has come an increasing awareness of the need for continued improvement in the provision of perioperative patient care. The Joint Commission on Accreditation of Healthcare Organizations (JCAHO) has taken a strong position on the need for continuously monitoring and evaluating the quality and appropriateness of care delivery to resolve any identified problems, while striving constantly to improve delivery systems and processes. In 1994 the JCAHO instituted performance assessment, measurement, and improvement as the core of its standards. This represented an evolution from quality assurance, to continuous quality improvement, to performance improvement (PI). Such a transition was underscored by the belief that measuring outcomes and improving care are the essential purposes of health care delivery. Performance improvement efforts encompassed improvements in quality and effectiveness, based on ethical and economic perspectives.

The surgical services performance improvement program should be based on established standards of care. The intent of each standard should be reflected in realistic and measurable outcomes. A plan to measure and improve care, which includes the scope of care and the important aspects of care, should be in place. Specific quality indicators should be identified that reflect these important aspects of care. Thresholds that identify the level of acceptability of variance for each indicator are then established. Measurement methods include retrospective review, review of incident reports, utilization review, patient surveys and interviews, and peer review. Emphasis has evolved from process auditing to the current emphasis on structure, process, and outcome indicators. These efforts underscore nursing's commitment to improving processes and outcomes of care.

A performance measurement and improvement approach facilitates the delivery of safe, high-quality perioperative patient care. When processes are understood, they can be improved through a systematic plan of action. Involvement on teams that work on the surgical services performance assessment and improvement plans can strengthen the staff's commitment to meeting standards and enhance program effectiveness. The JCAHO supports the evolution to an information technology infrastructure (i.e., an electronic health record) in which performance measurement becomes a natural part of the care delivery process. As current uses of data are expanded and enhanced, objectives still will include the use of data for research activities directed toward improving the quality of care and identifying and disseminating evidence-based practices. Perioperative nurses can anticipate that measurement requirements and performance expectations will be modified over time to reflect evolving technologies and care practices as they affect the quality and safety of care. The JCAHO also is expected to add measurement of patient perception of care to the required set of core measures over the next several years. The objectives of future activities will be focused on the following:

- Continuing expansion and coordination of nationally standardized core measurement capabilities.
- Increasing the use of measurement data for quality improvement, benchmarking, accountability, decision making, accreditation, and research.

## EVOLVING PERIOPERATIVE NURSING ROLES

The nursing profession and the health care culture in the United States continue to undergo rapid transformation, changing in response to many elements. An aging population, with the over-65 population already topping 40 million, will continue to create a significant increase in the demand for health services. As baby boomers turn 65, the over-85 segment of the population is projected to triple by 2050. Referred to as the "longevity revolution," in 2030 it is anticipated that one in five residents in United States will be over 85. New ambulatory settings for delivery of health services, including operative and other invasive procedures, will continue to develop, as will community-based clinics, school-linked clinics, mobile clinics, and drive-in health centers. Health care organizations that are agile and flexible and able to respond quickly to change will have an edge in the health care industry of the future. Perioperative nurses who understand the need for clinical and service quality, cost-effectiveness, information management, coordinating care, efficiency, special needs of an aging surgical population, and the importance of patient satisfaction will be able to anticipate and position themselves for this future. Roles in nursing research, industry, consulting, informatics,[5] case management,[14] and advanced practice are all possibilities for perioperative nurses. Perioperative nurses need personal strategic plans for enhancing their education, skill sets, and professional goals as they expand their practice horizons and move into some of these roles that directly or indirectly support perioperative patient care.

### Registered Nurse First Assistant

The role of the perioperative nurse as assistant at surgery is a good example of an evolving role. In 1984 the AORN approved an official statement on the RNFA; the statement has been revised on an ongoing basis to reflect changes in role evolution. The RNFA, who must have formal education for role preparation in an academic setting, works collaboratively with the surgeon (and the patient and surgical team) by handling and cutting tissue, using instruments and medical devices, providing exposure and hemostasis, and suturing as components of assisting-at-surgery behaviors.[1] Many experienced perioperative nurses have obtained education to prepare themselves for this role. Performing as an RNFA allows an experienced perioperative nurse to advance in clinical knowledge and skill, while still remaining directly involved with the provision of perioperative nursing care and undertaking responsibility for preoperative and postoperative patient management. The role of the RNFA has gained wide acceptance and is just one of the ways perioperative nurses are developing themselves to meet the changing needs of health care delivery.

### Nursing Informatics Specialist

Pressures for more efficient management of fiscal, material, and human resources have stimulated the development of automated information systems for diverse functions in perioperative patient care settings. Prompt access to accurate data is essential to maintain and improve the management and functioning of a surgical suite. A well-designed management information system can efficiently synthesize large volumes of data into meaningful reports. Ad hoc delivery reporting capabilities are a vital component that can enhance decision making. Administrative systems were probably the first area of nursing informatics. Newer nursing applications include point-of-care clinical systems, electronic health records, Internet-based patient education, research, and telemedicine and telenursing. Fueling the need for information systems is managed care, in which decisions to "purchase" health care from an institution rely heavily on information that shows cost-effectiveness and efficiency of care provided. The growing field of nursing informatics is an interaction of cognitive science, computer science, and informatics, all of which is based on a foundation of nursing science. Perioperative nurse informatics specialists have the opportunity to develop clinical nursing systems that incorporate nursing care protocols, critical paths, best practices, the PNDS and patient education materials that track patients over time. Such systems allow sharing information across wide networks as patients access health care at different points and times over a continuum of care. Perioperative practice settings require structural data (e.g., specimens collected, equipment used) and patient care data (care processes, interventions, outcomes). Future technology systems may include interactive computer/television, by which perioperative nurses can communicate with their patients over phone or cable lines, allowing the perioperative nurse to "view" the patient's wound or "discuss" overall recovery and rehabilitation from surgery. Many surgical patients themselves are information-literate in the age of the Internet, using this technology to search out health care providers, best institutions, and knowledge about their disease process and up-to-date information on treatment options. Perioperative nurse informatics specialists can assist in developing information infrastructures that support a broad range of information technology.

### Advanced Practice

Advanced nurse practitioners, either nurse practitioners (NP) or clinical nurse specialists (CNS), have become valuable members of health care teams in multiple settings. Traditionally, NPs practiced in primary care or outpatient settings, whereas CNSs were employed in acute-care settings. As residency programs have been downsized and part of the revenue stream for specialty preparation (surgical residents) diverted to primary care medicine, acute-care NPs have begun to fill the gap in providing care for patients who are more acutely ill and whose medical-surgical problems are more complex. NPs and CNSs have graduate nursing education and, as a result of the Balanced Budget Act of 1997, receive Medicare reimbursement in a variety of settings. This legislation also provides for Medicare reimbursement of RNFAs when they are an NP or CNS. The AORN has developed competency statements for the perioperative advanced practice nurse. These include managing health or illness status, competency in helping and healing, competency in teaching and coaching disease prevention and health promotion, competency in organization and work role, and competency in monitoring and promoting the quality of perioperative practice.[1]

## CONCLUSION

The perioperative nurse works in collaboration with surgeons, anesthesia providers, and other health care providers to plan the best course of action for each patient. To ensure the highest quality of care, input from each of the health care disciplines represented in the perioperative practice setting is crucial. The perioperative nurse serves in a leadership role in fostering collegiality, creativity, and collaboration among a variety of disciplines. With energy, enthusiasm, and fortitude, perioperative nurses contribute to building a surgical team and caring environment that achieves safe patient outcomes.

Perioperative nurses are accountable to their patients and demonstrate it by using standards, recommended practices, guidance statements, performance measurement and improvement activities, best practices, and clinical guidelines. They constantly strengthen their professional skills through education. As the transformation of health care continues, new perioperative nursing roles will emerge, but perioperative nurses in any role will continue to demonstrate humanized care for surgical patients and their families. Perioperative nursing care honors the patient as a whole person; it combines caring, healing, theory, ethics, and practice in a nursing role that values the sacred relationship that exists between the nurse and his or her patient.[18,19] *Scrubbing* and *circulating* (discussed in Chapter 3) may become obsolete terms; already we know that they define circumscribed functions that are only a part of the perioperative nurse's sphere of responsibility. The future may bring new titles and functions but will never erase the critical function in surgical patient care that every perioperative nurse fulfills: coordinating interventions, ensuring patient safety and comfort, prioritizing and planning care, and managing multiple aspects of the patient's and team's needs in each surgical intervention. The future of perioperative nursing is directly related to the sophistication of its practitioners. Sophistication means that perioperative nurses must be superior thinkers (knowledge) and doers (clinical skills). Outcomes of surgical interventions are related to the quality of perioperative nursing care provided, which reflects the aptitudes and motivations of perioperative practitioners. With this perspective, the reader should consider the remainder of this book as one part of a perioperative nurse's knowledge bank. The remaining chapters in this textbook contain vital information related to nursing practices and care processes that are needed to function in perioperative practice settings.

## REFERENCES

1. *AORN standards, recommended practices and guidelines,* Denver, 2006, The Association.
2. AORN statement on operating room staffing skill mix for direct caregivers, *AORN Journal* 81(6):1204-1205, 2005.
3. Beyea SC: Patient advocacy—nurses keeping patients safe, *AORN Journal* 81(5):1046-1047, 2005.
4. Beyea SC: *Perioperative nursing data set: the perioperative nursing vocabulary,* Denver, 2002, AORN.
5. Bowen ME, Elkind E: Opportunities in nursing informatics, *Nursing Spectrum* 13(20):13, 2004.
6. Cherry B, Jacob SR: *Contemporary nursing: issues, trends and management,* St Louis, 2005, Elsevier Mosby.
7. Duffy ME: Resources for building a research utilization program, *Clinical Nurse Specialist* 18(6):279-281, 2004.
8. Duffy WJ: The importance of keeping our hand in the scrub role, *AORN Journal* 80(5):817-819, 2004.
9. FDA clears new surgical marker; uses RFID to protect patients, *FDA Talk Paper.* Accessed 2004, Nov. 19, on-line: www.fda.gov.
10. Fesler-Birch D: Critical thinking and patient outcomes: a review, *Nursing Outlook* 53(2):59-65, 2005.
11. Gorner P: Surgery's next step: face transplants. *Chicago Tribune,* Accessed June 12, 2005, on-line: www.chicagotribune.com.
12. Hascup VA: Transcultural nursing, *Advance for Nurses* 6(24):31-32, 2004.
13. Ingersoll GL: Evidence-based nursing: what it is and what it isn't, *Nursing Outlook* 48(4):151-152, 2000 (Op-Ed).
14. James E: Coordinating care, *Advance for Nurses* 6(23):30-31, 2004.
15. JCAHO proposal for patient-centered care brings concept to mainstream healthcare settings, *The Risk Management Reporter* 24(3):1-7, 2005.
16. Kleinbeck SVM, Dopp A: The perioperative nursing data set—a new language for documenting care, *AORN Journal* 82(1):51-60, 2005.
17. Krugman M: Follow the evidence to up-to-date practice, *Nursing Spectrum* 14(5):21-23, 2005.
18. Mariano C: Jean Watson discusses her model of caring-healing, *Nursing Spectrum* 14(10):41, 2005.
19. McGarvey HE and others: The influence of context on role behaviors of perioperative nurses, *AORN Journal* 80(4):1103-1120, 2004.
20. McLane S: Designing an EMR planning process based on staff attitudes toward and about computers in healthcare, *Computer Informatics in Nursing* 23(2):85-92, 2005.
21. Olade RA: Evidence-based practice and research utilization activities among rural nurses, *Journal of Nursing Scholarship* 36(3):220-225, 2004.
22. Thurston NE, Long KM: Implementing evidence-based practice: walking the talk, *Applied Nursing Research* 17(4):239-247, 2004.
23. Whittemore R: Combining evidence in nursing research, *Nursing Research* 54(1):56-62, 2005.

CHAPTER 2

# Patient and Environmental Safety

JANE C. ROTHROCK

The safety and welfare of patients during surgical interventions are primary concerns of members of the surgical team. The health care imperative, "first, do no harm," depends in part on the perioperative nurse's clinical competence. In surgical settings, individual clinical competence is not enough, however, to ensure patient safety. All members of the surgical team must understand and contribute to the improvement of the systems in which they practice and work, contribute to effective teamwork, and enhance individual and collective ability to recognize and respond to patient safety issues.[33] Risk management and risk reduction, systematic ways of identifying, analyzing, and controlling potential problems to ensure safe patient care, have become increasingly important in health care environments.[27] Such efforts are likely to accelerate with implementation of electronic health records, integration of best practices with surgical team training, and the movement to full disclosure to patients after an injury (Research Highlight).[22]

Patient injuries during operative or other invasive procedures have serious consequences, necessitating a clear understanding of prevention strategies by perioperative personnel. Patients entering perioperative settings are presented with numerous risks, including risk for infection; impaired skin integrity; ineffective thermoregulation; deficient (or excess) fluid volume; latex allergy response; and injury related to perioperative positioning and chemical, electrical, and physical hazards. Patients also are vulnerable to medical errors, such as medication errors, wrong-site surgery, diagnostic and treatment errors, and equipment malfunctions.[8] In this context, the importance of competence on the part of the perioperative nursing staff and the surgical team becomes clear because patient protection and advocacy depend on the nurse's and team's ability to integrate knowledge and skills and apply standards of care and appropriate policies and procedures in patient care activities.[7]

Policies and procedures are designed to ensure the safety of patients and personnel and to provide a setting in which all activities of the surgical team and ancillary personnel fit together, resulting in an efficient course of action for the benefit of each patient. Such policies and procedures are the institutional standard of care (SOC) and are part of a systematized approach to reducing errors and improving patient safety. Organizational factors and complex systems can contribute to medical errors and adverse events in surgical settings. The Association of periOperative Registered Nurses (AORN) Perioperative Patient Focused Model (see Chapter 1) includes a structural component that represents the organization's role in supporting staff with clinical processes that assist in achieving patient safety goals. The Joint Commission on Accreditation of Healthcare Organizations (JCAHO) also has recognized the importance of staffing effectiveness in relationship to clinical/service screening indicators.[1] Data from monitoring indicators such as adverse drug events (ADE), injuries to patients, and patient complaints may be used to identify potential staffing effectiveness issues when the institution conducts an analysis of sentinel events.

Regulations are mandated activities with which the institution must comply to meet certain standards set by outside agencies. Several agencies regulate the health care environment and affect practice in perioperative settings, including the following:

- The Environmental Protection Agency (EPA) regulates the use of chemicals for disinfection and sterilization and the disposal of medical wastes.
- The JCAHO sets standards related to the structure, process, and outcomes of services provided by health care facilities. Accreditation is voluntary but recommended for Medicare and Medicaid reimbursement for services.
- The Occupational Safety and Health Administration (OSHA) regulates safety and health issues in the workplace. OSHA's regulations regarding preventing exposure to bloodborne pathogens and permissible levels of exposure to toxic substances in the environment most directly affect operating room (OR) practices.
- The U.S. Food and Drug Administration (FDA) regulates implantable medical devices and requires surgical facilities to track them.
- Many state health agencies have strict regulations affecting health care facilities and practices in surgical suites, including staffing and sterilization practices. In addition, local fire departments often have regulations that control corridor clearance and the storage of combustible supplies. It is important to become familiar with local and state regulations affecting perioperative practice.

## SAFE ENVIRONMENT

Patient-centered processes create the product and service of health care—the delivery of safe and effective care, the attainment of desired outcomes, and the achievement of patient satisfaction. To ensure that these processes fulfill their function, they need to be designed, implemented, and executed consistently. As part of a system-wide approach to patient and staff safety, the environment in which care is delivered needs to be carefully controlled.[5]

### Safety Design Features

Designing a safe environment incorporates features that prevent or control the risk of infection, fire, explosion, and chemical and electrical hazards. Well-devised traffic patterns; material-handling systems; disposal systems; positive-pressure, filtered ventilation; and high-flow, unidirectional ventilation

## RESEARCH HIGHLIGHT

### Apologizing After Adverse Events

The objective of this study was to explore patient perceptions of patient-provider communication after an actual adverse medical event. The researchers recruited study participants using a statewide postinjury program database in Colorado. Three geographic sites were identified, and every other patient from each site was contacted to participate in the research (for a total of 50 contacts). Twenty-two patients initially agreed to participate; for the final analysis, 16 adults participated, representing 13 cases of adverse medical events. The researchers conducted four patient focus groups using a semistructured guide. Transcripts were analyzed using an editing approach to identify themes.

The study results uncovered complex issues and processes that were involved in resolution attempts resulting from an adverse event. Effective communication was an important factor in whether professional relationships between the patient and the health care provider continued after an adverse event. The nature and quality of the communication influenced whether patients defined the adverse event as "an honest mistake" or "an error." Two types of trauma (physical and emotional) were expected in the population of patients experiencing an adverse event and confirmed in the study. Besides the physical implications of an unanticipated outcome, emotional trauma included feelings of anger, betrayal of trust, frustration at not receiving information after the event, and a relational "disconnect." A third type of trauma, labeled *financial trauma,* was identified and proved in some cases the most salient factor influencing patients' subsequent actions. Caring, honest, quick, personal, and repeated provider responses during disclosure of an adverse event were linked to patient satisfaction.

In this study, the timeliness and quality of provider communication were important influences on patients' responses to adverse events. Confronting an adverse medical event collaboratively helped patients and providers with patients' emotional, physical, and financial trauma and minimized the anger and frustration commonly experienced. The researchers recommended that health care organizations, providers, investigators, and policymakers should consider the patient experience when developing provider training or evaluating processes in disclosure policies and patient resolution. In her review of legislating apologies, Sparkman notes that other studies have confirmed that apologies encourage settlement of perceived grievances by patients and their families, sometimes avoiding litigation.

The Joint Commission on Accreditation of Healthcare Organizations (JCAHO) recommends encouraging open communication between practitioners and patients when an adverse event occurs. In the JCAHO's vision for tort resolution and injury prevention, four areas are identified:

- Patient safety becomes the priority in all health care organizations.
- When a medical injury occurs, the injured patient is informed promptly and receives an apology. Error analysis guides the prevention of such error in the future.
- An early offer of compensation for losses is provided to the patient.
- If a claim of injury remains in dispute, an alternative dispute mechanism is used to bring the claim to a swift and fair resolution.

The JCAHO also recommended pursuing legislation that protects disclosure and apology from being used as evidence against the practitioner in litigation. The Patient Safety and Quality Improvement Act of 2005 amended the Public Health Service Act to encourage a culture of safety in health care organizations. The bill included provision of legal protection of information voluntarily reported to designated patient safety organizations (PSOs). The U.S. government will develop and maintain the voluntary reporting system.

Modified from Duclos CW and others: Patient perspectives of patient-provider communication after adverse events, *International Journal of Quality Health Care,* 2005. Accessed July 21, 2005, on-line: AHRQ Patient Safety Network; JCAHO: *Health care at the crossroads—strategies for improving the medical liability system and preventing patient injury,* Chicago, 2005, The Commission; Patient Safety and Quality Improvement Act of 2005. Accessed August 3, 2005, on-line: AHRQ Patient Safety Network www.psnet.ahrq.org; Sparkman CAG: Legislating apology in the context of medical mistakes, *AORN Journal* 82(2):263-272, 2005.

systems for special applications all contribute to a safe surgical environment. In addition, a reliable and adequate emergency power source must be available for use during electrical interruptions and must be tested regularly to ensure working order. Emergency shutoffs for piped medical gases, such as oxygen and nitrous oxide, must be clearly labeled and readily accessible. Education designed to familiarize staff with all safety and hazard-prevention programs is required by the JCAHO. Although flame and explosion hazards have decreased significantly in recent years as a result of the use of nonflammable anesthetics and skin-preparation solutions, fire safety protocols are essential in the oxygen-enriched atmosphere of the OR. Electrical hazards also are of concern and are discussed later.

## Physical Plant Design Elements

Individuals who design surgical suites should consider the need for adequate space to accommodate the technology to be employed, such as video monitors, microscopes, lasers, robotic devices, and cardiopulmonary bypass machines. ORs that are too small compromise the safety of staff and patients. It is difficult to maneuver around equipment and to monitor and maintain the sterile field in a crowded room. Generally, the standard modern OR is recommended to be 400 to 600 square feet.[6] Specialty ORs, such as those used for minimally invasive, orthopedic, neurologic, or cardiac surgery procedures, require 600 to 750 square feet of floor space, with at least a 20-foot clear floor space. Specialty rooms designed for endoscopy and cystoscopy may be 350 square feet. ORs designated for ambulatory surgery previously were designed at the lower range of square footage; however, as increasing numbers of minimally invasive procedures are done on an ambulatory basis, larger surgery rooms have become necessary to accommodate this technology.

Surface materials used in ORs must be nonporous, smooth, easy to clean, waterproof, and fire resistant. High-impact vinyl materials and flexible wall coverings, together with new adhesives, permit completely sealed wall, ceiling, and floor joints so that the surfaces may be washed effectively with disinfectant solutions. The surfaces should be as free as possible of seams, joints, and crevices to prevent the harboring of microorganisms. Bumper guards should be placed on the corridor walls and corners to avoid damage from movement of surgical equipment and stretchers. Damaged walls cannot be cleaned properly and can harbor microorganisms.

Floor coverings also should be nonporous, seamless, and easy to clean. They should be made of slip-proof materials to prevent injuries to personnel. The color of the floor covering should be such that surgical needles are readily visible against its surface should they fall to the floor. The juncture between the floor and the wall should be curved to prevent material from gathering in the floor-to-wall juncture and to facilitate cleaning. Floors should be kept dry, clean, and unobstructed.

Sliding doors are recommended to eliminate the air turbulence caused by swinging doors. A pronounced increase in microbial counts has been noted when swinging doors are opened or closed. Doors should be made of the surface-sliding type, if possible, to facilitate cleaning of all surfaces.

Supply cabinets inside ORs should be enclosed, with wire shelving to facilitate cleaning and minimize dust collection. Stainless steel cabinets with sliding glass doors are preferred, to provide for ease of cleaning and ready visibility of contents to the circulating nurse.

When the supplies for a specific procedure are chosen in the central sterile department and sent to the OR on an enclosed cart (case cart), the amount of supplies that is stocked in each OR can be minimized. Fewer supplies in each OR centralizes and reduces excess inventory for the facility, allows for greater control, and makes it easier to keep the environment clean and dust-free. Ideally, clean carts with clean and sterile supplies are brought to the OR via a clean lift system (elevator, dumbwaiter, or cart lift). At the end of the procedure, contaminated instruments and supplies are placed into the cart and returned via a contaminated lift, where they are reprocessed, and the cart is washed. Case carts work well when preference cards, or computerized data sheets that are specific to a given procedure and surgeon, are accurate and routinely updated. Communication and collaboration between perioperative staff and central processing staff are crucial to the success of a case cart system.

Operating suite design with a sterile core is the most common design of modern ORs. This design eliminates cross traffic of staff and supplies from the contaminated or soiled areas to the clean or sterile areas. Because decontamination and clean assembly processes occur outside the OR (in a central processing department), design of the suite needs to allow for the flow of items from clean to dirty areas without compromising principles of infection control, standard precautions, or aseptic technique (see Chapter 3).

The surgical services department must be designed with consideration for adequate space for storage of supplies and equipment. Storage space usually is underestimated when a new facility is being planned, resulting in clutter and inefficient movement of staff to gather equipment from distant storage spaces. One method to determine the amount of storage space needed in an OR is to add 50% of the total square footage of the surgical suite into the design for storage. Storage space should be adjacent to the ORs. Several medium-size storage rooms are preferable to one large room, to avoid the difficulty of retrieving items from the back of a large room.

### Emergency Signals

Every surgical suite should have an emergency signal system that can be activated inside each OR. A light should appear outside the door of the room involved, and a buzzer or bell should sound in a central nursing or anesthesia area. The signals should remain on until the alarm is turned off at the source. All personnel should be familiar with the system and should know how to send a signal and how to respond to it. Such a system, restricted to use in life-threatening emergencies, saves invaluable time in bringing additional personnel and resources for assistance.

## STAFF SAFETY

All perioperative personnel should be educated in the use of good body mechanics to avert common falls and strains when standing in one position for long periods, reaching, stretching, lifting, or moving or positioning heavy patients or other articles.[25] Where possible, mechanical devices should be used for lifting patients and other heavy objects. Good body mechanics and application of ergonomic principles conserve energy, protect the worker, and promote good performance. Personnel also should be educated and supervised in proper use of equipment to prevent injuries, such as burns from autoclaves and electrical equipment, abrasions from contact with metal accessory levers, injuries from swinging doors, cuts from knife blades, needle sticks,[29] and splash exposures.

Personnel must be cognizant of and use appropriate protective apparel in the surgical suite in accordance with OSHA's rule on exposure to bloodborne pathogens and the Centers for Disease Control and Prevention (CDC) Standard and Transmission-Based Precautions. Eye protection, facemasks, head and shoe covers, gowns, gloves, and any other protective wear must be used whenever the potential for blood and body fluid contact exists. These precautions are applied to all patients receiving care regardless of their diagnosis or presumed infection states. A blood and body fluid exposure control plan for the institution should be developed, identifying areas of high risk in the perioperative environment (see Chapter 3 for a thorough discussion of these elements). Such actions not only protect personnel but also keep patients safe from hospital-acquired infections.

The maintenance and cleaning program should be clearly defined and understood by the perioperative staff. Promptly attending to spills, immediately drying wet floors, using warning signs in danger areas, and keeping corridors and traffic areas clear of obstacles are important parts of maintaining a safe environment.

Effective disposal procedures for disposable items contaminated with blood, tissue, or other potentially infectious materials and hazardous waste are essential to render the area safe for patients and personnel. Biohazardous medical waste must be placed in leak-proof containers or bags that are color-coded, labeled, or tagged for easy identification. State and federal regulations for transport and disposal of regulated medical waste serve as the institution's guideline; state regulations, if they are more stringent than federal regulations, must be followed.[4] Any disposable sharps must be placed in a puncture-resistant container that has a biohazard label.

The professional nursing staff has a responsibility to work with the designated facility committees in establishing appropriate policies and reporting occurrences. Cleaning, disinfection, and sterilization of equipment; control of contaminants; hand hygiene; and application of Standard and Transmission-

Based Precautions and aseptic practices are basic to an effective infection control program that helps protect patients and staff from the transmission risk of bloodborne and other pathogens (see Chapter 3).[23]

## EMERGENCY AND DISASTER PREPAREDNESS

All surgical services departments need a plan for emergency and disaster preparedness. The essential first step is identifying who needs to know how to do what. The department plan should address surgery cancellations, standby capacity for incoming patients, and the chain of command. The entire surgical services staff should be familiar with the department's emergency response plan and should be able to describe their individual roles and functions in an emergency and demonstrate these in regularly scheduled drills. Such drills and testing of the emergency management plan enable the department to assess the appropriateness of the plan, the adequacy of the plan, the effectiveness of logistics, human resources, training, policies, procedures, and protocols. Simulated situations should use plausible and realistic scenarios. Such planned exercises allow the surgical services department to identify deficiencies and take corrective action to improve the plan's effectiveness continuously.

Competence in the use of equipment should be part of these drills. Emergency and disaster preparedness plans also should include a response to terrorist activity and contamination with biologic or chemical agents. In this venue, perioperative staff should be educated to recognize symptoms of nuclear, biologic, or chemical terrorism; triage procedures should be developed; and a decontamination area should be identified. Disposable or easily cleaned equipment should be used for victims, and perioperative staff should wear personal protective equipment appropriate to the source of contamination. As part of emergency and disaster preparedness, the institution should ensure a 48- to 72-hour stand-alone capability through stockpiling of necessary medications and supplies.[18] If the source is not immediately known, patients should be isolated until a determination of the source and transmissibility are identified. The JCAHO standards focus on cooperative emergency management planning among health care organizations in a community (community-based emergency preparedness). As such, local government officials, emergency management officials, health care organizations, police, fire, and emergency medical services work together to create command structures and control centers and resources and assets that can be shared or pooled.

### Electrical and Fire Hazards

The types of electrical hazards encountered in the OR environment include electric shock, fire, explosions, and burns. Electric shock results from current flowing through the body and can result from touching a damaged plug or an ungrounded piece of metal equipment. Fires can result from faulty wires, inappropriate use of extension cords, and careless use of electrical equipment such as lasers and electrosurgical units (ESUs), particularly in the presence of an oxygen-enriched atmosphere (OEA) or flammable liquids (Box 2-1). Referred to as the "fire triangle," these conditions represent a heat or ignition source (e.g., a laser), an oxygen source, and a fuel source (e.g., drapes, preparation solutions, dressings).

The electrical and fire safety plan for the OR includes the following practices:

1. Prohibit smoking and the use of any apparatus or device producing an open flame.
2. Evaluate and test all new equipment to ensure optimal safety and performance.
3. Inspect all electrical equipment, regardless of the source, for safety and proper functioning before use, and label with an inspection sticker according to institutional procedure.
4. The biomedical technician or electrical safety officer should determine whether electrical equipment, cameras, lights, and electrosurgical units are safe for use in a given situation.
5. Establish inventory control, regular inspection, preventive maintenance, and safety approval systems.
6. Instruct personnel in the safe use of all equipment, and require a return demonstration of their proficiency.
7. All personnel must be familiar with the procedure for prompt removal from use and expeditious repair of defective equipment.
8. A qualified electrician should inspect electrical outlets and equipment at designated intervals or as requested and should file written reports with the director of surgical services.
9. A standard procedure for care and use of electrical equipment should include the following:
   The plug, cord, and connections of electrical equipment must be checked before each use for insulation integrity and secure connections.
   All electrical cords should be of adequate length and flexibility to reach an outlet without stress and without the use of extension cords. Kinks and curls should be removed from electrical cords before the plugs are inserted into wall outlets.
   The plug, not the cord, should be handled when electrical cords are plugged into or removed from an outlet. Pulling on the cord may cause it to break at the point where the wire is attached to the plug.
   Cords should not be wrapped tightly around equipment, which causes the protective covering to wear and breaks the wires inside the covering.
   Cords always should be removed from traffic pathways before equipment such as a bed or a machine is moved. If the position of electrical equipment necessitates cords lying on the floor where people will be walking during surgery, the cords should be taped down to prevent tripping.

***Isolated Power System.*** An isolated power system, although no longer required by the National Fire Protection Agency in nonflammable anesthetizing locations, may be found in older ORs. These systems may reduce the hazard of shock or burn from electrical current flowing through the body to ground by allowing identification of a piece of equipment in the system that is not appropriately grounded. Each isolated power system must have a continually operating line-isolation monitor that indicates possible leakage or fault currents to ground. Most monitors have a green signal lamp that indicates when the system is isolated from ground. A red signal lamp and an audible warning signal indicate when a ground fault is detected. All perioperative personnel must know the procedure to follow when this occurs.

BOX 2-1

### Reducing the Risk of Surgical Fires

The fire triangle identifies the three elements required for a fire—fuel, oxygen, and an ignition source. The surgical suite contains a wide range of combustibles and flammables. Ignition sources include devices and equipment such as electrosurgery, lasers, and light sources. All disciplines involved in perioperative patient care need to be educated on controlling ignition sources, including fuels, oxygen, and surgical devices. Policies and procedures should be current and reviewed annually in an education session. Attendance at the session should be documented. The following actions assist in reducing the risk of surgical fires:

- Use prepackaged unit-dose skin preparation (prep) applicators to control the amount of flammable skin preparation solution used.
- Ensure that skin prep solutions, which might contain alcohol, are dry before applying the surgical drapes. Inspect the prepped area before draping. Some prep solutions change appearance when dry (e.g., change from shiny to matte). Follow any instructions or warnings provided by the manufacturer. As part of the "time out," ensure that any flammable prep solution used in the presence of a heat source has dried.
- If towels placed at the bed line are soaked with prep solution, consider removing them from the OR/procedure room.
- Coat head and facial hair (e.g., eyebrows, beard, moustache) with water-soluble surgical lubricating jelly. Use an incise drape to isolate head and neck incisions from oxygen and alcohol vapors from prep solutions.
- Be aware of potential oxygen-rich environments, such as under the drapes near the surgical site and in the drape fenestration, especially in head and neck surgery. Oxygen under the drapes can seep to the area of the fenestration in the surgical drape and reach the surgical site. Arrange drapes to minimize oxygen buildup; keep fenestration/towel edges as far from incision site as possible.
- Question the need for 100% oxygen during surgery, especially during head and neck surgery and monitored anesthesia care (MAC). An oxygen-rich environment can vastly increase the flammability of drapes, plastics, and hair. The surgeon and anesthesia provider should communicate with one another about oxygen concentrations under the drapes.
- Complete all connections to fiberoptic light sources before activating the source. Place the device in standby mode when disconnecting cables.
- Moisten sponges to make them ignition resistant in oropharyngeal surgery and pulmonary/upper chest surgery. If an uncuffed endotracheal tube is used, soak sponges or gauze to minimize gas leakage into the oropharynx, and keep them wet.
- Control heat sources by holstering surgical equipment (e.g., the electrosurgical active electrode) or placing it in standby mode (e.g., the laser).
- When using electrosurgery, lasers, or cautery:
  - If supplemental oxygen is at a concentration greater than 30%, stop it, if possible, at least 1 minute before and during activation of the unit.
  - Activate a unit only when the tip is in view (especially during microscopic or endoscopic procedures).
  - Deactivate the unit before the tip leaves the surgical site.
- Create a fire response plan to ensure staff is trained in preventing and extinguishing fires. Include the following in education programs:
  - Location and use of fire extinguishers. Carbon dioxide fire extinguishers are recommended. These fire extinguishers can extinguish small OR fires on cloth, plastic, or paper; burning liquids; and electrically energized fires. They leave no residue and do not harm the patient, staff, or equipment.
  - Rescuer methods
  - Location and operation of medical gas panels
  - Locations and operation of ventilation and electrical systems and personnel authorized to shut them off
  - Initiation of the fire alarm or "code red"
  - Procedures for contacting the local fire department
- Conduct mock scenarios, such as a surgical drape fire.

Modified from Association of periOperative Registered Nurses (AORN): *Position Statement on Fire Prevention,* Denver, 2006, The Association; Emergency Care Research Institute [ECRI]: A clinician's guide to surgical fires [guidance article], *Health Devices* 32(1):5-24, 2003; ECRI: Only you can prevent surgical fires. Accessed on-line August 8, 2005: ecri.org, 2004; Joint Commission Perspectives on Patient Safety 5(8), 2005; NFPA adopts new language on alcohol-based surgical preps, *OR Manager E-bulletin,* August 2005. Accessed August 12, 2005, on-line: www.ormanager.com.

***Volatile Liquids.*** Flammable liquids, including alcohol, must be properly stored. Volatile liquids, such as acetone and aerosol sprays, are prohibited for cleaning and incidental use in hazardous locations. Skin preparation solutions should be applied with care to prevent pooling, which can lead to a chemical burn.[31] Towels should be tucked under the patient along the area to be prepared to catch any dripping solution and removed as soon as the preparation is completed. In addition to being a chemical irritant, the preparation solution may be ignited by a spark from an active electrode of the electrosurgical unit or from a charge of static electricity. Ignition of vapors can occur as the solution evaporates. Solutions used for skin preparation always should be permitted to dry before application of the surgical drapes.[3]

The *Right to Know* directive published by OSHA sets the standard for providing information to employees about hazardous substances encountered in the workplace. Material Safety Data Sheets (MSDSs) are information sheets that are the basis for the standard. Each manufacturer of a chemical or solution is required to provide safety information about its products, and employers are required to have this information available to employees to review at any time. Personnel should be familiar with the MSDSs for chemicals and solutions used in the OR because they provide valuable patient and personnel safety information.

## RADIATION SAFETY

Radiation presents environmental safety concerns for patients and staff. Many surgical procedures use radiologic studies that are performed immediately before, during, or after surgery, increasing the potential for radiation exposure. X-rays of all frequencies can damage tissues and may produce long-term effects. The effects of radiation are dose dependent and cumulative; the larger the dose or the more frequent the exposure, the greater the risk of the effects of radiation. Exposure should be kept as low as reasonably achievable (ALARA).

Sources of radiation exposure in the OR include (1) ionizing sources—portable radiography (x-ray) machines and portable fluoroscopy units (C-arm)—and (2) nonionizing sources—lasers (see Chapter 7 for a thorough discussion of laser safety). Members of the surgical team should avoid unnecessary exposure to radiation sources and comply with practices that reduce potential for exposure—time, distance, and shielding. Personnel present in the OR must maintain the greatest practical distance (at least 6 feet) from the radiation source or remain behind leaded shielding when ionizing radiation is used during surgery. Nonessential personnel should leave the room, and members of the scrubbed team should wear protective devices and move as far from the radiation source as is possible, while still adhering to aseptic technique.

Protective equipment is used to reduce the intensity of radiation exposure. Radiation safety devices include but are not limited to special eyewear, radioprotective gloves, leaded aprons, and thyroid shields. Careful handling and regular examination of leaded garments are important to ensure the integrity of shielding; they should not be folded during storage, and they should undergo regularly scheduled radiologic testing. Staff-development programs on radiation safety should be conducted periodically to reinforce radiation safety practices and to correct misconceptions or unrealistic practices relating to radiation exposure and monitoring.

Personnel who may be exposed to radiation use radiation-monitoring devices (film badges) in accordance with radiation safety standards. The radiation-monitoring device should be worn consistently in the same area of the body. When a leaded apron is worn, two monitoring devices may be used. One is worn on the neckline outside the apron, and the other is worn inside the leaded apron. Film badges are collected monthly and sent to a monitoring company. A written monthly report provides a permanent record of an individual's occupational exposure.

Patient protection during procedures in which radiation is used is accomplished by shielding and by using machines that limit the size of the beam, reducing the amount of tissue being exposed to direct radiation. Shields should be placed (1) over reproductive organs (fetus or gonadal shields) during radiographic studies of the abdomen, hips, and upper legs where possible and (2) over the thyroid/sternum during radiographic studies of the head, neck, and upper extremities. A careful preoperative history is an important part of radiation safety, especially related to a woman's reproductive status. If a woman might be pregnant, especially during the first trimester, it is crucial to avoid radiation exposure if possible. Measures taken to protect patients from radiation exposure should be documented on the perioperative nursing record.

## LATEX ALLERGY

Latex allergy is a subject crucial to the health and safety of the patient and the health care worker (Box 2-2). Latex has been the material of choice for surgical gloves because it is flexible, maintaining the wearer's tactile sensitivity. Although natural rubber latex has been a common component in thousands of medical and consumer products for many years, latex sensitivity is a relatively new problem for patients and health care personnel. Although some individuals experience an irritant contact dermatitis, this is often the result of a chemical irritation and does not involve the immune system. In a *type IV* allergic reaction, the response is a delayed cell-mediated reaction, which includes symptoms of contact dermatitis (e.g., pruritus, edema, erythema, vesicles, drying papules, crusting and thickening of the skin) that spread beyond the areas of contact. A true latex reaction is *type I*: immediate, IgE-mediated, and anaphylactic. The onset of an anaphylactic reaction usually occurs within minutes, with symptoms of generalized urticaria, wheezing, dyspnea, laryngeal edema, bronchospasm, tachycardia, angioedema, hypotension, and cardiac arrest. Many serious anaphylactic reactions have occurred when a latex product (e.g., surgical gloves) is in direct contact with mucous membranes during surgical procedures. This situation permits a rapid introduction of latex antigen directly into the vascular circulation.

Individuals at high risk for latex allergy include health care workers; patients who have undergone multiple surgical procedures, including procedures to treat spina bifida and other congenital neural or genitourinary tract anomalies; and rubber factory workers. Until more recently, it was assumed that the sensitization to latex resulted only from cutaneous absorption in health care workers or from direct mucosal contact during clinical treatments. Recent studies confirm that latex protein allergens effectively bind to glove powder and when airborne can remain suspended for prolonged periods. Inhalant exposure is an additional risk factor for sensitization to latex allergens. The prevalence of type I latex allergy among health care workers has been estimated to be 10% to 30%, which is much higher than that found in the general population.[37]

Institutions need to develop strategies for limiting health care workers' occupational exposure to latex. If a latex-free environment cannot be created, the goal is to create a latex-safe environment, where all reasonable efforts have been made to remove high-allergen and airborne latex sources.[4] This includes switching to low-allergen, powder-free gloves. The cornstarch powder on powdered latex gloves is an efficient allergen carrier and contributes to airborne contamination, especially in ORs and invasive procedure rooms where glove use is high. The use of low-allergen, powder-free gloves reduces the airborne latex allergen content (to below detectable levels), reducing occupational exposure.

Health care facilities also need to develop policies and procedures for caring for latex-sensitive patients, and all staff members must adhere to these policies. One of the first steps to protect latex-sensitive patients is to replace latex-containing devices and products with alternate synthetic materials for surgical procedures. Latex-safe carts that contain alternate products should be set up, maintained, and used with known allergic or high-risk patients (Box 2-3). If the surgical facility is not latex-safe, it is preferable for patients who are latex-sensitive to have their procedures performed as the first procedure of the day. Prominent signs identifying a "latex-precautions environment" should be posted at all entrances to an OR where the latex-allergic patient is having surgery. The patient should wear a latex allergy identification band, and the transport vehicle and chart should be clearly labeled. The perioperative nursing plan of care is developed and implemented using the nursing diagnosis "Risk for latex allergy response."

BOX 2-2

## Latex Allergy

Latex allergy is an immunoglobulin E (IgE)-mediated reaction to proteins retained in finished natural rubber latex products.

**ETIOLOGY AND INCIDENCE**

Latex is the milky sap of the rubber tree *Hevea brasiliensis.* This natural rubber product contains proteins. Latex allergy is the reaction to certain proteins in the latex rubber. These allergies emerged in the 1990s as one of the most pervasive problems in health care. It is a serious and growing problem, and health care workers are at increasing risk of acquiring latex allergies. It is currently estimated that an allergy caused by repeated exposure to latex protein allergens develops in at least 1 in 10 health care professionals, and 53% of health care workers reported some type of reaction to latex gloves when surveyed. Children with spina bifida and individuals with chronic illnesses who require frequent operations are especially susceptible to sensitization toward latex.

**PATHOPHYSIOLOGY**

The amount of latex exposure necessary to produce sensitization or an allergic reaction is unknown. Increasing exposure to latex proteins increases the risk of developing allergic symptoms. Although latex-containing products have only 2% to 3% protein, it is this protein that is thought to be the allergen in type I hypersensitive individuals. The precise protein responsible for causing allergic contact dermatitis latex type I hypersensitivity has not yet been identified and may be different for individual patients.

**RISK FACTORS**

- Health care professionals; surgical workers, emergency care workers, and obstetrics workers are at highest risk
- Children with spina bifida or others with conditions requiring frequent operations
- Persons with congenital urogenital abnormalities requiring indwelling catheters
- Employees in the rubber industry
- Persons with history of other IgE-dependent allergies (e.g., rhinitis, asthma, or food allergies) with a positive skin test

**CLINICAL MANIFESTATIONS**

Clinical signs include local skin redness, dryness, and itching after contact with latex. Inhalation of particles results in respiratory symptoms, such as rhinitis, sneezing, itchy eyes, scratchy throat, or asthma. More severe manifestations include anaphylaxis with bronchospasm, laryngeal edema, respiratory distress, or respiratory failure.

**COMPLICATIONS**

Complications include anaphylactic shock and respiratory and cardiac arrest leading to death.

**DIAGNOSTIC TESTS**

**History**

Items of diagnostic significance in the history include atopic history, hives under rubber or latex gloves, hand dermatitis related to gloves, allergic conjunctivitis after rubbing eye with hand that has been in contact with latex, swelling around mouth after dental procedures or blowing up a balloon, and vaginal burning after pelvic examination or contact with condom.

**Immunologic Evaluation**

Immunologic evaluation comprises skin prick, intradermal, and patch contact skin tests and serologic testing (e.g., radioallergosorbent test [RAST] or enzyme-linked immunosorbent assay [ELISA]). The Food and Drug Administration (FDA) has approved a standardized latex reagent for skin testing to be used for research only. This is not yet available for public use.

**THERAPEUTIC MANAGEMENT**

**Medications**

Medications include epinephrine for reaction (may be autoinjector and carried by individual), β-agonist inhaler, prednisone, and other anaphylactic life-supporting medications.

**General**

Immediate assessment and interventions for acute reaction include cardiac monitoring and, if needed, respiratory support.

**PREVENTION AND PROMOTION**

For latex-sensitive individuals:

- Avoid latex products.
- Avoid environments with high levels of circulating aeroallergens (e.g., ORs, emergency departments, blood banks).
- Wear Medic-Alert bracelet or tag.
- Carry autoinjector for use at first signs of anaphylaxis.

Modified from Langford RW, Thompson JD: *Mosby's handbook of diseases,* ed 3, St Louis, 2005, Elsevier Mosby, pp. 372-374.

## PATIENT SAFETY

The Institute of Medicine (IOM) report, "To Err Is Human: Building a Safer Health System," described patient *safety* as freedom from accidental injury and *error* as a failure of planned actions to be completed as intended or the use of the wrong plan to obtain the desired outcome. A safe environment for perioperative patient care depends on a safety program with well-defined policies and procedures and a well-trained staff.[35] All staff members, regardless of their position, need to recognize potential hazards in the surgical environment and prevent accidental injury and contribute to making the environment safe for themselves, their co-workers, and the patients.

### Patient Safety Standards

In 2001 the JCAHO revised its standards in support of patient safety and medical and health care errors, requiring an integrated and coordinated approach to an organization-wide safety program. Such programs consist of at least the following:

- Designation of one or more individuals or an interdisciplinary group to manage the safety program
- Identification of the types of occurrences to be addressed
- Description of the mechanisms used to ensure that all components/departments of the organization are integrated into and participate in the safety program
- Procedure for immediately responding to medical/health care errors
- Clear systems for internal and external reporting
- Defined mechanisms for analysis of the various types of occurrences and for conducting risk-reduction activities
- Mechanisms for supporting staff who have been involved in an adverse event
- At least an annual report to the governing body on occurrences and actions taken to improve patient safety

BOX 2-3

### Latex-Safe Cart

Use of a dedicated *latex-safe cart* facilitates the care of perioperative patients with a latex allergy. The FDA requires manufacturers to label latex-containing supplies and devices. It is advisable to establish a latex consultant in the institution. The following departments should be notified so that they can use appropriate procedures when preparing supplies for the patient: pharmacy, radiology, central processing, housekeeping, and PACU. In general, *latex-allergic* and *latex-risk* patients are scheduled as the first surgical procedures in the morning. All latex products should be removed from the room. The room should be labeled *latex precautions* to avoid personnel bringing rubber products (e.g., wrist bands, chart labels, bed, room signs) into the room. The dedicated *latex-safe cart* should then be brought into the room. The cart contents should include, at a minimum, the following basic items:

**Gloves**—Neoprene, nitrile, or nonlatex gloves of various sizes (sterile and nonsterile)

**Syringes**—Glass syringes or other nonlatex syringes (most regular syringes have latex-tipped plungers)

**Drugs**—Most common medications come in vials with Neoprene stoppers. If a medication has a rubber stopper, glass ampules should be used, or the rubber stopper should be removed.

**IV tubing**—Regular IV tubing has latex ports. Tubing without ports should be used. If this is unavailable, tape over and do not use the ports; use stop cocks for injection. Tourniquets used for inserting IV tubes should be latex-free.

**IV bags**—IV bags that have rubber injection ports should be taped and labeled "Do not inject or withdraw fluid from the latex port."

**Breathing systems**—Latex-free reservoir bag, nonlatex breathing circuit, with plastic mask and bag. Anesthesia circuits are usually latex-free, but the reservoir bag may be latex. Some valves in self-inflating resuscitation bags (Ambu, Laerdal) may contain latex. The anesthesia provider needs to determine whether the anesthesia ventilator has latex bellows.

**Airway supplies/equipment**—Most endotracheal tubes are disposable and made of polyvinyl chloride (PVC). The laryngeal mask airway (LMA) is made of silicone. Red rubber nasopharyngeal tubes contain latex.

**Stethoscope**—Latex-free stethoscopes must be used.

**Webril**—Webril or other protective material, such as stockinette, should be on the cart to place under a latex blood pressure (BP) cuff or tourniquet and other monitoring devices to prevent direct skin contact (e.g., cords/tubes, pulse oximeter, wire from ECG leads).

**Nonlatex surgical items**—Nonlatex substitutes should be available for the following commonly used items, which may contain latex:

- OR caps, masks, other personal protective equipment
- Indwelling urinary catheters and drainage systems
- Penrose drains
- Instrument mats (to keep instruments from slipping off the sterile field)
- Rubber-shod clamps
- Vascular loops/tags
- Bulb syringes
- Underpads or Chux placed at the bed line during surgical skin preparation
- Surgical tape

Modified from AORN latex guideline, in *AORN standards, recommended practices and guidelines,* Denver, 2006, The Association; AANA Latex protocol, American Association of Nurse Anesthetists. Accessed August 15, 2005, on-line: www.aana.com.

In this context, patient safety is a leadership priority. Processes such as reporting, investigating, analyzing, and reducing hazards reflect an organizational commitment to patient safety. To ensure that appropriate problems and areas are targeted by preventive measures, routine identification of errors must be part of practice by all health care professionals. Confidential, no-fault reporting is one of the best ways to adopt an institutional culture that encourages incident/occurrence/event reporting (Box 2-4).[21]

***National Patient Safety Goals.*** In 2003 the JCAHO first introduced National Patient Safety Goals (NPSGs) as part of its ongoing effort to improve patient safety in accredited organizations. An expert panel, the Sentinel Event Advisory Panel, advises the JCAHO in developing the goals and their requirements. This panel includes national patient safety experts, nurses, physicians, risk managers, pharmacists, and other health care professionals who have hands-on experience in addressing patient safety. Each year, the National Patient Safety Goals are reviewed, and specific recommendations are made for goals for the ensuing year. Recommendations are based on data obtained from the JCAHO's Sentinel Event Database and other established sources of information on patient safety. For each goal, a limited set of evidence-based, practical, cost-effective recommendations is identified.

***Protecting Patients' Rights.*** Protection of patients' personal, moral, and legal rights begins at the time of admission. The course of action involves correctly identifying patients, safeguarding their right to privacy and their right to make choices regarding their care, and keeping confidential all records and reports.

The Health Insurance Portability and Accountability Act (HIPAA) granted patients significant rights over how their health information is used.[17] Involving rules regarding transaction, security, and privacy of health care data, patients must grant consent for their protected health information to be used for treatment, payment, or health care operations. To limit the use or disclosure of protected health information and to ensure patients' rights with respect to this information, health care facilities must have in place administrative procedures to protect the privacy and confidentiality of such information, including protocols for the presence of health care industry representatives in the OR.

Advance directives and consent forms for treatment or surgical procedures are other important measures that protect the patient and the caregiving personnel. OR personnel who witness consent forms should be aware of the conditions that ensure validity of the consent. A signed consent also must be an informed consent, which implies adequate communication with the patient regarding the procedure for which the consent is being signed. Consent is not only a legal mandate but also one that prepares patients psychologically for the planned surgical intervention by ensuring that they have a thorough understanding of that planned intervention. Surgical procedures should not be performed without a signed and witnessed informed consent (Figure 2-1). The surgeon or practitioner performing the procedure is responsible for informing the patient about the proposed operation or other invasive procedure and its inherent risks, benefits, alternatives, and complications and for obtaining consent. The patient must receive this infor-

BOX 2-4

### Incident/Occurrence/Event Reports

A commitment to patient safety requires prevention and mitigation of harm to patients. Harm is any physical or psychologic injury or damage to the health of an individual, including temporary and permanent injury. A threat to patient safety is any risk, event, hazardous condition, or set of circumstances that could lead to patient harm. The objective of incident/occurrence/event reports is primarily to determine the cause of a problem and prevent its recurrence. An incident or occurrence is an unusual event, condition, or set of circumstances that has the potential for patient injury. Incident/occurrence/event reports should be completed as soon as possible. The person who witnessed, first discovered, or is most familiar with the incident should complete the form. After completion, the report should be submitted to the individuals in the institution responsible for reviewing and following up on incidents; this is often the risk management department. These reports are not part of the medical record; they are administrative documents. An objective description of the incident/occurrence/event should be in the medical record, however, along with any follow-up diagnostic studies or related treatments. The report form submitted to risk management should include the following:

- The date and time of the event and of the report
- A brief, factual narrative of the details of the incident/occurrence/event, consisting of an objective description of the facts:
  - *What* (type of incident/occurrence/event)
  - *Where* (location where discovered or occurred)
  - *When* (date, time, other relevant information)
  - *Who* (identification of person affected [patient, visitor, staff], functions of staff persons involved)
- Quotes where applicable with unwitnessed incidents ("The patient states . . .")
- The names of any witnesses of the incident (who discovered the incident/occurrence/event, their role[s])
- Any findings as a result of patient assessment/examination
- Actions taken at the time of the incident to provide care (identify physician to whom incident/occurrence/event reported, if applicable, and response, such as orders given, treatments)
- Ancillary information (e.g., product information, if relevant, including devices, blood [include batch number], medications; if a medical device is involved, the manufacturer, model, and lot number should be noted)
- Condition of the person affected, including any complaints of injury, observed injury, and a brief comment on follow-up care

Modified from Emergency Care Research Institute, Incident reporting and management, May 2003. Accessed July 24, 2006 on-line: www.ecri.org/Patient_Information/Patient_Safety/IncRep1.pdf; Institute of Medicine: *Patient safety: achieving a new standard of care,* Washington, DC, 2004, National Academy Press.

mation in terms that he or she can understand.[32] The patient also must be informed as to who will perform the procedure and when practitioners other than the primary surgeon will perform important parts of the procedure, even when under the primary surgeon's supervision.[13] Consent forms must be signed before the administration of preoperative medications. On the patient's arrival in the OR, the circulating nurse and anesthesia provider are responsible for verifying that the consent is on the chart and is correct, properly signed, and witnessed before the administration of anesthesia. If properly done, the consent form should include the following:[16]

- The patient's name (and legal guardian, if applicable)
- Name of the facility where the procedure is being performed
- Specific name of the surgical procedure (or, where multiple procedures are being done, the names of those procedures)
- Site/side of the planned procedure
- Name of the practitioner or practitioners performing the procedure or important aspects of it
- Risks of the procedure
- Alternative procedures, treatments, or therapies
- Signature of the patient (or legal guardian, if applicable)
- Date and time consent is obtained
- Statement that procedure was explained to the patient (or legal guardian or both, if applicable)
- Name and signature of person who explained the procedure
- Signature of professional witnessing the consent

If telephone consent is necessary, two persons who will sign as witnesses should hear the consenting person verbalize the consent. Speaker phones may be used, or the consenting person may repeat the information to each person who is serving as a witness. The name and relationship of the consenting person should be obtained and documented, and both witnesses sign the "witness" portion of the consent form.[10] Special permits for anesthesia administration, specific operations such as sterilization and therapeutic abortion, disposal of severed body parts, organ donation, administration of blood products, videotapes or photographs, and autopsy provide additional safeguards for the patient, staff, and institution.

***General Patient Safety Measures.*** Minimizing human error helps eliminate hazardous conditions for the patient undergoing operative or other invasive procedures. In all perioperative settings, where the patient is unable to protect himself or herself, nursing personnel must protect the patient.

Communication of vital medical information to surgical team members is essential to safe patient care. An allergy identification band is used to communicate a patient's allergy to a given medication or substance. This is a safety measure that prevents the administration of drugs or the use of materials that would evoke an allergic reaction in the patient. Even in the absence of an allergy band, patients must be queried regarding allergies to medications or food products.

All medications must be checked three times before administration: (1) when removed from the drug cabinet or case cart, (2) before being drawn up in the syringe or otherwise dispensed to the sterile field, and (3) before being given to the patient. Medications that are on the sterile field should be labeled or identified such that the correct solution is used for the intended purpose (see Medication Safety, later).

Patients' hearing tends to become more acute after the administration of the preoperative medication and in the induction stage of anesthesia. A quiet environment is essential for all patients awaiting surgery. Studies indicate that some patients' hearing is acute throughout the surgical procedure. Even with the use of amnesia-invoking drugs, a small percentage of the population report auditory recall and sensations (e.g., not being able to breathe, pain) that occurred during their surgery.[24] (See Chapter 4 for a discussion of awareness during anesthe-

**GENERAL REQUEST AND CONSENT**

**FOR OFFICE USE ONLY:**
**Patient Name:** ______
**Date of Birth:** ______
**Date of Procedure:** ______

I ______ (Type or print patient name) request and give consent to ______ (Type or print Doctor or Practitioner Name(s))

to perform the following procedure(s) ______ (Please list site and side if appropriate)

The benefits, risks, complications, and alternatives to the above procedure(s) have been explained to me.

I understand that the procedure(s) will be performed at Christiana Care by and under supervision of my doctor or practitioner. My doctor or practitioner may use the services of other doctors or practitioners, or members of the resident staff as he or she deems necessary or advisable.

I authorize my doctor or practitioner and his or her associates and assistants to perform such additional procedures, which in their judgment are necessary and appropriate to carry out my diagnosis or treatment.

I authorize the hospital to retain, preserve and use for scientific, teaching or transplant purposes, or to make other dispositions of, at their convenience, any specimens, tissues, or parts taken from my body during the course of this operation.

I consent to observers in the operating room in accordance with hospital policy. I consent to photography or video taping of my surgical procedure for educational purposes, provided my identity remains anonymous and confidential.

I agree to being given blood or blood products as deemed advisable during the course of my procedure. The risks, benefits, and alternatives to receiving blood or blood products have been explained to me.

I consent to the administration of sedation or analgesia during my procedure. The risks, benefits, and alternatives to receiving sedation or analgesia have been explained to me.

If anesthesia is required, I consent to the administration of anesthesia by members of the Department of Anesthesiology. I also consent to the use of non-invasive and invasive monitoring techniques as deemed necessary. I understand that anesthesia involves risks that are in addition to those resulting from the operation itself including, but not limited to, dental injury, hoarseness, vocal cord injury, infection, nerve injury, corneal abrasion, seizures, heart attack, stroke and even death.

Please initial one of the following statements (females only):

______ To the best of my knowledge I am not pregnant. ______ I believe I am pregnant.

I certify that I have read and understand the above consent statements. In addition, I have been offered the opportunity to ask my doctor or practitioner any questions I have regarding the procedure(s) to be performed and they have been answered to my satisfaction. I acknowledge that I have been given no guarantee or assurance as to the results that may be obtained from the procedure(s).

Signature of Patient or Decision Maker — Date and Time

Doctor or Practitioner Signature — Date and Time

Relationship to Patient if Decision Maker

Doctor ID # or Print Name

Witness Signature — Date and Time

Practitioner Print Name/Title

Witness Print Name

**Telephone Consent:** ______
Name of person obtained from/Relationship to Patient

Witness(s') Signature(s) — Date and Time

Witness(s') Signature(s) — Date and Time

Witness(s') Print Name(s)

Witness(s') Print Name(s)

FIGURE 2-1 Surgical consent form.

sia). In addition, high noise levels interfere with accurate communication with the patient and among members of the surgical team and may increase the likelihood of error. For both of these reasons, noise in the OR should be controlled and conversations kept to a minimum.

Transport vehicles (stretchers) and OR/procedure beds must be stabilized with the wheels locked when a patient is moved from one to another. One person must stabilize the transport vehicle while another stands on the opposite side of the OR/procedure bed to receive the patient. Patient transfer devices, such as rollers, hoists, or slides, are useful for patients who are unable to assist with their own transfer. All safety devices on transport vehicles and OR/procedure beds must be in proper working order. Locking mechanisms, side rails, safety straps, hydraulic controls, armboards, and other protective devices should be used whenever necessary. It is essential to have an adequate number of personnel present to ensure patient safety during transfer activities.

**ADMISSION OF THE PATIENT TO THE OPERATING/INVASIVE PROCEDURE ROOM.** Admission of patients to the operating/invasive procedure room is a crucial time for the perioperative nurse to gather and verify data to help plan for the patient's care and safety. Information collected during preadmission testing and preoperative patient care may be reviewed using a perioperative information system.[14] The patient's arrival in the preoperative holding area allows an opportunity to collaborate with the patient by identifying and verifying his or her needs and planning care to meet those needs. Empathic communication, good listening skills, being alert to nonverbal communication, offering gentle reassurance, providing explanations, and using comforting behaviors are essential responsibilities of perioperative nurses.

Institutional policy and procedure for patient admission should include a preoperative verification process, which may encompass the following steps:

1. The perioperative nurse verifies the patient's identification orally with the patient (if feasible) and compares the name on the surgical schedule with the name on the patient's armband and medical record. Two unique identifiers must be used. Information on the surgical schedule pertaining to the patient's name, hospital number, date of birth, and physician's name must match the information on the patient's identification band and medical record.
2. The procedure to be performed (including the operative site, side, and surgical approach) is verified by the patient and matched with the surgical schedule, medical record, and consent form. Similar validation is undertaken by the anesthesia provider and the surgeon. The surgical site should be marked, and the patient should be involved in the marking process. The institutional procedure for marking the skin at or near the incision site should be followed. Special equipment, positioning needs, or implants also are verified at this time.
3. The consent form, history and physical (H&P) examination record, laboratory results, and other examination or diagnostic results should be complete before surgery and reviewed by the perioperative nurse as part of patient assessment. The H&P must be performed within 30 days before admission or within 24 hours of the inpatient admission. If the history and physical examination was done within 30 days before admission, it must be updated at the time of admission, before surgery.[20] In addition, the medical record and laboratory and diagnostic tests, especially x-ray films and other imaging studies, should be verified and matched to the patient's name and identification (ID) number. Facility policy determines which examinations are mandatory as part of the patient's preoperative preparation. These may include recent blood and urine testing, chest x-ray, and electrocardiogram (ECG).
4. Allergies; previous unfavorable reactions to anesthesia or blood transfusions; previous reactions to latex; religious, cultural, spiritual, or ethnic preferences; and any relevant advance directive must be carefully noted.
5. The patient should be queried about personal effects, including clothing; money; jewelry; wigs; religious symbols; and prostheses such as dentures, lenses, glass eyes, and hearing aids. The nurse is responsible for ensuring the safe handling and proper disposition of patient property and valuables.
6. The perioperative nurse should review the orders and results concerning preoperative skin preparation, medication administration, and elimination, such as enema results and the amount of urine voided or collected through a catheter.
7. It is important to determine whether preoperative dietary and fluid restrictions have been maintained; this is crucial in preventing the aspiration of gastric contents during anesthesia induction.
8. The nurse should meticulously document any medications, fluids, blood, or blood products administered as ordered during the immediate preoperative period.
9. The nursing staff should apply side rails, locking devices, and safety straps on stretchers to prevent falls and injury to the patient during transport.

The intent of the preoperative verification process is to ensure that all relevant parts of the medical record are available before starting the surgical procedure, and that they have been reviewed and are consistent with each other. A preoperative checklist (Figure 2-2) (a list of the important patient care measures to be checked and verified preoperatively) is frequently used to prevent oversights, omissions, and sentinel events (Box 2-5). This form is usually completed on the patient care unit if the patient is an inpatient or in the preadmission area for ambulatory or admit-on-day-of-surgery patients.

**MEDICATION ADMINISTRATION.** Medication administration in the OR/invasive procedure room is unique in that it often requires that the circulating nurse and scrub person prepare a medication that is being administered by the surgeon. Vigilance in following established safe medication practices is an important part of perioperative patient care (Box 2-6). Policies and procedures should be followed for checking the medication or solution before it is dispensed to the sterile field. Medications on and off the sterile field must be labeled and processes established for verifying the labels. Scrub persons should identify medications when they are passed to the surgeon. A repeat-back confirmation from the surgeon can ensure that the correct dose of medication or solution is being used. The JCAHO's "Do Not Use" list must be applied to all medication orders and medication-related documentation that are handwritten or on preprinted forms (Table 2-1).

**CORRECT SITE SURGERY.** All institutions that perform operative or other invasive procedures must have policies and procedures to prevent wrong-site surgery. Surgery on the wrong

## PRESURGICAL CHECKLIST

Date: ______________

Side 1

| | INITIALS: UNIT | INITIALS: Prep & Holding | COMMENTS |
|---|---|---|---|
| 1. Allergies: ☐ Latex ☐ Environmental ☐ Medications<br>______________ | | | Green allergy band intact if allergies are present |
| 2. Isolation/Precautions: ☐ MRSA ☐ VRE ☐ C-diff<br>Other: ______________ | | | ☐ Operating Room notified (OR)<br>☐ Post-Anesthesia Care Unit notified (PACU) |
| 3. Side/Site identification form completed | | | |
| 4. Pre-Surgical Testing (RESULTS ON CHART)<br>☐ CBC ☐ SMA6 ☐ Glucose ______ ☐ Chest X-ray ☐ UA<br>☐ ECG ☐ Hemoglobin & Hematocrit ☐ Other: ________ | | | Pending Results:<br>______________<br>______________ |
| 5. Vital Signs: Time performed: ________<br>Temperature: ________ Blood Pressure: ________<br>Pulse: ____ $SpO_2$: _____% Respiratory Rate: ________ | | | |
| 6. NPO since: ________ Solids: ______ Liquids: ______ | | | |
| 7. Weight (last 24 hours): ________kg Height: ________ cm | | | |
| 8. Last Menstrual Period: ________ | | | |
| 9. Patient's belongings including valuables secured/removed:<br>☐ wedding band taped ☐ dentures<br>☐ contact lenses ☐ glasses<br>Drawer number (Surgicenter only): ________ | | | Secure all valuables. |
| 10. ☐ Type & Cross-Match ☐ Blood consent on chart<br># of autologous units available: ________ | | | |
| 11. Voiding or catheter: ________ (Time) | | | |
| 12. Preoperative surgical antimicrobial prophylaxis guideline checklist instituted and faxed to pharmacy. | | | Call placed to physician if not ordered<br>________ (time) ________ initials |
| 13. Intravenous antimicrobials should be administered within 0-60 minutes prior to surgical incision. | | | |
| 14. Surgical site prep:<br>☐ Prep ordered by physician<br>☐ If no prep ordered, call placed to physician for Surgical Site prep order | | | ☐ Clip Only ☐ Scrub Only<br>Location: ________<br>☐ Site prep location: ________<br>☐ Clip & Scrub-Betadine<br>☐ Clip & Scrub-Hibiclens<br>Signature: ________ Time: ______ |
| 15. Equipment to go to OR with patient<br>☐ X-ray films ☐ Old records ☐ Chart volumes | | | |

| Signature/Initials | Signature/Initials |
|---|---|
| Print Name | Print Name |

FIGURE 2-2 Presurgical checklist.

**BOX 2-5**

## Sentinel Events

Perioperative nursing practice has a fundamental goal of protecting patients from injury related to numerous events, equipment, and activities, such as physical hazards, extraneous objects, chemicals, electrical equipment, positioning, radiation (ionizing and nonionizing), inadvertent hypothermia, wrong-site/wrong-person surgery, incorrect administration of medications, fluid therapy, and medical devices. The Joint Commission on Accreditation of Healthcare Organizations (JCAHO) defines a *sentinel event* as an "unexpected occurrence involving death or serious physical or psychological injury, or risk thereof." Organizations accredited by the JCAHO are expected to undertake a thorough root cause analysis (Research Highlight), implement improvements to reduce risk in the future, and monitor the effects of the improvements. Under the JCAHO policy, the following subset of events is subject to review by the JCAHO:

- Suicide in a setting where the patient receives around-the-clock care
- Infant abduction
- Infant discharge to the wrong family
- Rape (as defined by the health care organization)
- Hemolytic transfusion reaction
- Surgery on the wrong patient or wrong body part

*Risk thereof* includes any process variation for which a recurrence would carry a significant chance of a serious adverse outcome. The JCAHO sentinel event program supports the institution in its efforts to examine errors that occur, consider contributing factors, and make recommendations to prevent subsequent errors. When a sentinel event has occurred, the facility must perform a root cause analysis and submit an action plan to the JCAHO. The analysis must focus on systems and processes, with identification of process improvements that could reduce the likelihood of a similar event occurring in the future. The JCAHO issues *Sentinel Event Alert* recommendations, which reflect a root cause analysis and offer strategies to reduce similar errors in other facilities. Institutions are often assessed on their knowledge of these recommendations and plans for implementing them. The JCAHO also develops annual National Patient Safety Goals (NPSGs); accredited health care organizations are required to implement (if applicable) one or two recommendations drawn from *Sentinel Event Alerts* or to implement an acceptable alternative. In determining the annual NPSGs, the evidence to support the goal, the availability of adequate solutions to achieve the goal, and the feasibility of implementing the solutions are considered. After introduction as an NPSG, the goal may become part of the JCAHO Standards.

Modified from Beyea SC: Learning from sentinel event statistics, *AORN Journal* 80(2):315-318, 2004; JCAHO: *What every health care organization should know about sentinel events,* Chicago, 2005, The Association; Wengert W: Inside JCAHO, *Advance for Nurses* 6(22):40-41, 2004.

site includes any operative or other invasive procedure performed on the wrong patient, wrong body part, wrong side of the body, or at the wrong level of the correctly identified anatomic structure, such as in spinal surgery.[2] All institutions accredited by the JCAHO must follow the Universal Protocol for Preventing Wrong Site, Wrong Procedure, Wrong Person Surgery.[36] The Universal Protocol requires the following activities:

- *Preoperative verification process* to ensure that all relevant documents (e.g., the history and physical examination, surgical consent) and imaging studies (properly labeled and displayed) are available before the start of the procedure. These must be reviewed and be consistent with the patient's stated expectations (when the patient is awake and aware, the patient should actively participate in the verification process). The surgical team must agree that this is the correct patient, the planned procedure, on the specified side and site. Any additional special equipment, supplies, or implants also must be confirmed as being correct and available.
- *Marking the surgical site* must be done such that the intended site of incision or insertion is unambiguous. Procedures that involve left/right distinction, multiple structures, or multiple levels must be marked. The mark also must be unambiguous; initials, a "yes," or a line at or near the incision site may be used. The person doing the procedure should do the site marking. The method of marking should be consistent throughout the institution. The mark must be visible after the patient has been prepared and draped. Institutions should have procedures in place for patients who refuse site marking.

The JCAHO has identified numerous risk factors that contribute to an increased risk of wrong-site surgery, including the following:[21]

- More than one surgeon involved in the procedure (multiple procedures or care of patient transferred to another surgeon)
- Multiple procedures conducted on the same patient
- Unusual time pressures
- Unusual patient characteristics, such as physical deformity or massive obesity

Figure 2-3 shows a sample form used to identify the patient, procedure, and surgical site/side that is used from preadmission through the intraoperative time out conducted by the surgical team. This form also includes a surgical site fire risk assessment (discussed earlier). Some institutions have implemented a "hard stop" rule to the verification process. If any discrepancies are discovered, or if all the steps in the protocol are not followed, everything is stopped until the discrepancy is rectified.[26]

**TIME OUT.** When the patient is positioned, prepared, and draped, the entire surgical team participates in a time out just before starting the procedure. The patient's identity is rechecked. The procedure to be done, operative side and site, and correct patient position are verified by the entire surgical team. The patient must be positioned such that the marking of the operative site (e.g., with the word "yes" or the surgeon's initials) is visible on the patient's skin. The availability of implants, special equipment, or other requirements (e.g., blood, if it has been ordered) is verified. It is determined and verified that any flammable prep solution used in the presence of a heat source has dried. When all of these tasks have been completed, the procedure can begin. The time out should be documented according to institutional protocol (see Figure 2-3).

**CLINICAL DOCUMENTATION.** Institutions where operative and other invasive procedures are performed maintain records of each operation, including the preoperative diagnosis, the surgery performed, a description of findings, the specimens removed, the postoperative diagnosis, and the names of all individuals participating in intraoperative care. This operative record is a permanent part of the patient's chart. The AORN Recommended Practices for Documentation of Periop-

## RESEARCH HIGHLIGHT

### Root Cause Analysis

Since 1995, the Joint Commission on Accreditation of Healthcare Organizations (JCAHO) has reviewed 3044 sentinel events. An analysis of the events reported in 2003 indicated that approximately 15% of events occurred perioperatively. These are voluntary reports and do not include near-misses, in which the possible event is averted but could have happened. For this reason, well-designed systems that are thoughtfully developed and based on research, evidence, and best practices are essential in prevention of the occurrences themselves and the near-misses.

In one analysis of such a system-wide development process, management shifted to a proactive methodology. Brainstorming by involved staff members and reports of their experiences with possible contributing factors were combined with an intensive literature review. This led to the identification of sentinel events that were targeted for action:

- Wrong-site surgery
- Operative complications
- Medication errors

For each of the targeted areas, proactive measures were identified. Root cause analysis indicated 12 possible causes of sentinel events. For wrong-site surgery, the top three causes, in order of frequency, were attributable to communication problems, orientation/training/education inadequacies, or compliance with procedures. For operative complications, the top three causes, in order of frequency, were attributable to orientation/training/education inadequacies, communication problems, or compliance with procedures. For medication errors, the top three causes, in order of frequency, were attributable to communication problems, orientation/training/education inadequacies, or compliance with procedures.

A *root cause* is the most fundamental reason for the failure or inefficiency of a process. A *root cause analysis* is a process for identifying the basic or causal factors that underlie variation in performance, including the occurrence or possible occurrence of a sentinel event. The analysis begins with a brief description of the event, then focuses on the steps in the process. These are often illustrated on a flowchart, diagramming the key steps involved in the specific process related to the event. It is recommended that the flowchart be done as the process is designed, then as it is actually done, then as it was done if there was or is a risk for a sentinel event. Participants next identify risk points in the process, and re-chart it with suggested improvements. Because communication problems are listed as causes in the aforementioned three events, participants might look at the quality and quantity of verbal or written communications. Questions to ask include whether key communication was completed in a timely manner and whether there were misunderstandings resulting from the use of abbreviations or terminology that was confusing. Policies and procedures also are methods of communication, and they should be reviewed for adequacy of information and currency of the recommendations they contain. When potential risk factors are identified, participants explore whether there are barriers to communication, such as fear of reprisal. Each participant in the process also must evaluate the degree to which prevention of adverse outcomes is communicated throughout the institution as a high priority. The root cause analysis is transferred into an action plan, noting the root cause/opportunity for improvement, the risk reduction strategies that have been identified, who is responsible for implementation, when the implementation will occur, and what the measurement strategies will be to determine if the plan has been successful.

In 2004 the Association of periOperative Registered Nurses (AORN) sponsored the first National Time Out Day, which focused on implementation of the JCAHO's Universal Protocol. In 2005 the AORN developed a Safe Medication Administration Toolkit, intended to assist perioperative nurses by highlighting medication administration competencies, common medication conversion calculations, herbal interactions, and common perioperative medications. These are excellent resources to consider in assessing risk reduction strategies in a plan for improvement.

Perioperative nurses are in a unique position to improve patient safety because of their inherent proximity to patients. This position gives them the needed insight to identify problems in perioperative processes and to be part of patient safety solutions. Reviewing sentinel event alerts and root cause data, taking a proactive stance, involving staff, reviewing the literature, reaching consensus on proactive measures to be instituted for targeted areas, and researching the effectiveness of these measures enhance the OR staff's ability to "first, do no harm."

Modified from Beyea SC: Best practices for safe medication administration, *AORN Journal* 81(4):895-898, 2005; JCAHO: *What every health care organization should know about sentinel events,* Chicago, 2005, The Association; Karanfil L and others: Creating a patient-safe environment in a perioperative setting, *AORN Journal* 81(1):168-180, 2005; Meltzer B: Wrong site surgery: are your patients at risk? *Outpatient Surgery Magazine* 3(2):26-35, 2002.

erative Nursing[4] suggest that the intraoperative patient care record should include the following information:

1. Evidence of a patient assessment on arrival in the OR, which includes an assessment of the patient's skin condition immediately before and after the procedure
2. Confirmation by members of the surgical team before starting surgery ("time out") that they have the correct patient, surgical site, procedure, equipment, specials needs such as implants, and proper surgical position. The surgical site mark should be clearly visible.
3. Evidence of a plan of care individualized for the patient and considering the patient's baseline psychosocial, physical, emotional, and religious or cultural status/preferences. The plan of care, along with identified outcomes, might include data elements and nursing interventions based on the Perioperative Nursing Data Set (PNDS) (see Chapter 1).
4. Any sensory aids or prosthetic devices worn by the patient on admission to the OR and their subsequent disposition
5. Patient position, including supports or restraints/immobilizing devices used
6. Location of dispersive electrode pad placement and identification of electrosurgical unit and settings used
7. Use of temperature-regulating device placement, with identification of unit used and recording of time and temperature, on admission and discharge from the OR
8. Placement of monitoring electrodes (noninvasive and invasive)

BOX 2-6

## Medication Safety

- Follow the five "Rs" of medication delivery: right patient, medication, dose, route, and time.
- Use at least two patient identifiers when administering medications. Identifiers include the patient's name, assigned identification number, or bar coding in a patient ID bracelet that includes two or more specific patient identifiers.
- Identify/verify any patient allergies and sensitivities (e.g., medications, latex, foods, adhesives, chemicals).
- Review patient's medication history (including herbal remedies, over-the-counter drugs); identify any possible medication interactions or contraindications.
- When receiving a verbal or telephone order for a medication, write the complete order or enter it into the computer, then "read back" the medication order, receiving confirmation from the person who gave the order that it is correct.
- When writing the complete order or entering it into the computer, comply with the institution's "Do not use" list and the list of look-alike/sound-alike drugs. Look-alike and sound-alike drugs should be stored separately.
- The circulating nurse and scrub person should audibly review and confirm the medication ordered before transfer to the sterile field. Medication verification should include drug/solution/agent name, strength, dosage, and expiration date.
- Label all medications and containers with solutions (e.g., syringes, medicine cups, basins) on and off the sterile field, even if there is only one medication being used.
- Verify any medication listed on the physician's preference card/pick list with the physician before delivery to the field, labeling, or administration.
- Label any medication or solution when it is transferred from its original package to another container.
- Label each medication or solution one at a time. Verify name and concentration, complete preparation for administration, deliver to the sterile field, and label on the field before another product is prepared.
- Use medication vial transfer devices to dispense medications onto the sterile field without contaminating the medication during dispensing.
- Keep original packages from medications or solutions available for reference in the perioperative area until the conclusion of the procedure.
- Labels should contain the drug name, strength, amount (if not apparent from the container), expiration date when not used within 24 hours, and expiration time when expiration occurs in less than 24 hours.
- Differentiate look-alike and sound-alike products by using tall man lettering on products or highlighting/circling the distinguishing information to prevent errors when drug or solution names are similar.
- All labels are verified verbally and visually by two qualified individuals.
- Discard any unlabeled medication or solution immediately.
- The scrub person should actively communicate the medication name, amount, and dose when transferring the medication or solution to the surgeon.
- At shift change or when personnel are relieved ("hand-offs"), all medications and solutions on and off the sterile field and their labels should be reviewed by entering and exiting staff.
- Document all medications on the perioperative nursing record.
- Monitor patients for adverse medication reactions, and document interventions to treat adverse reactions.
- Discard all labeled containers used during the surgical procedure at the procedure's conclusion.
- Follow procedures for reporting and responding to medication errors (adverse drug events [ADE]), including near misses.

Modified from AORN guidance statement: safe medication practices in perioperative practice settings, in *AORN Standards, Recommended Practices, and Guidelines*, Denver, 2005, The Association; *AORN Safe Medication Administration Toolkit,* Denver, 2005, The Association; Beyea SC: *Perioperative nursing data set*, ed 2, Denver, 2004, The Association; Giarrizzo-Wilson S: Clinical issues—medication practices, *AORN Journal* 81(6):1326-1329, 2005; ISMP Medication Safety Alert: NurseAdvise-ERR: positive identification—not just for patients, but for drugs and solutions, 3(8), 2005; JCAHO: *What every health care organization should know about sentinel events,* Chicago, 2005, The Association.

TABLE 2-1

## JCAHO Five "Do Not Use" Abbreviations

| Do Not Use | Potential Problem | Use Instead |
|---|---|---|
| U (unit) | Mistaken for "0" (zero), the number "4" (four) or "cc" | Write "unit" |
| IU (International Unit) | Mistaken for IV (intravenous) or the number 10 (ten) | Write "International Unit" |
| Q.D., QD, q.d., qd (daily) | Mistaken for each other | Write "daily" |
| Q.O.D., QOD, q.o.d, qod (every other day) | Period after the Q mistaken for "I" and the "O" mistaken for "I" | Write "every other day" |
| Trailing zero (X.0 mg)† | Decimal point is missed | Write X mg |
| Lack of leading zero (.X mg) | Decimal point is missed | Write 0.X mg |
| MS | Can mean morphine sulfate or magnesium sulfate | Write "morphine sulfate" |
| MSO4 and MgSO4 | Confused for one another | Write "magnesium sulfate" |

*Applies to all orders and all medication-related documentation that is handwritten (including free-text computer entry) or on preprinted forms.
†*Exception:* A "trailing zero" may be used only where required to show the level of precision of the value being reported, such as for laboratory results, imaging studies that report size of lesions, or catheter or tube sizes. It may not be used in medication orders or other medication-related documentation.

**Identification of Patient, Procedure and Surgical Side/Sites, and Fire Risk Assessment**

Procedure: ______________________ ______________ Date of Procedure

Preoperative verification process to be completed by assigned personnel in designated areas. Mark appropriate blocks. Side 1

| PEP | Sending Unit | Prep & Holding/Admission Area |
|---|---|---|
| ☐ Posting Card | ☐ Patient verbalizes | ☐ Patient verbalizes |
| ☐ Patient verbalizes | ☐ ID Bracelet (eg Name & DOB) | ☐ ID Bracelet (eg Name & DOB) |
| ☐ Other | ☐ OR Schedule | ☐ OR Schedule |
| | ☐ Surgical Consent | ☐ Surgical Consent |
| | ☐ Site marked with "Yes" ☐ N/A | ☐ Site marked with "Yes" ☐ N/A |
| | ☐ H & P | ☐ H & P |
| | ☐ X-ray Report / X-ray | ☐ X-ray Report / X-ray |
| | ☐ Other studies | ☐ Other studies |
| Signature: | Signature: | Signature: |
| Print Name: | Print Name: | Print Name: |
| Date/Time: | Date/Time: | Date/Time: |

**Surgical Site Marking Verification**

* Not applicable (N/A) meets exemption criteria (see instructions on side 2).
* After 2 methods of verification (patient verbalized, consent, H & P, other), the patient (in presence of RN) will write "Yes" with a permanent marker on or as near to surgical site:

☐ N/A ☐ RIGHT ☐ LEFT

Signature ______ Print Name ______ Date / Time

Side/Sites Marked by: ______________

**COMMENTS**

Signature ______ Date/Time

**ANESTHESIA (Time-out)** — **CONFIRMATION OF PATIENT IDENTIFICATION, PROCEDURE & SURGICAL SITE PRIOR TO THE START OF ANESTHESIA BLOCK**

The anesthesiologist ______________ (Provider Name(s)) and the identification assistant (perianesthesia nurse, operating room RN, another anesthesia provider, another physician or physician assistant) have verbally agreed that ______________ (Patient Name) will have the following block performed: ______________ Identification Assistant ______________

Re-verification completed ________ Re-verification completed ________ Re-verification completed ________

**SURGICAL TEAM (Time-out)** — **CONFIRMATION OF PATIENT IDENTIFICATION, PROCEDURE SURGICAL SITE AND AS APPLICABLE, IMPLANT WITH START OF PROCEDURE**

The surgical team (Surgeon/Resident, Anesthesia Provider, and Circulating RN) has verbally agreed that ______________ (Patient Name) will have the above procedure performed.
**Document procedure/site only if the procedure/site is different or left blank at top of form.** ______________

Circulating RN: ______________ Signature / Print Name ______ Date / Time

**SURGICAL TEAM** — **SURGICAL SITE FIRE RISK ASSESSMENT SCORE**

Alcohol based prep solution had sufficient time for fumes to dissipate. ☐ YES ☐ NO ☐ N/A

| (Circle appropriate option) | Y | N | Verified by: |
|---|---|---|---|
| • Surgical site or incision above the xiphoid | 1 | 0 | (Circulating RN Signature) |
| • Open oxygen source (Patient receiving supplemental oxygen via any variety of face mask or nasal cannula) | 1 | 0 | Print Name: |
| • Available ignition source (i.e., electrosurgery unit, laser, fiberoptic light source) | 1 | 0 | |
| **Scoring** 3 = High risk; 2 = Low risk w/potential to convert to high risk; 1 = Low risk — Total Score | | | ☐ High Risk Fire Protocol initiated |

**(Complete this section if Risk Score increases to "3" during procedure)**
☐ High Risk Fire Protocol Initiated Signature/Title: ______________ Print Name: ______________ Time: ________

FIGURE 2-3 Identification of patient, procedure, and surgical side/site and fire risk assessment.

9. Medications administered or dispensed by the perioperative nurse, complying with the JCAHO "Do Not Use" list for abbreviations (see Table 2-1)
10. Presence of catheters, drains, packing, and dressings
11. Location of tourniquet cuff placement, identification of unit, pressure setting, and inflation and deflation times
12. Blood products administered and fluid output, including blood loss estimates, as appropriate. Unused blood that is returned to the blood bank or taken with the patient to the perianesthesia care unit (PACU) should be noted.
13. Implant type, size, expiration date (if applicable), name of manufacturer or distributor, and identification information used by the manufacturer (e.g., lot, batch, model, serial number). A separate implant logbook entry also should be completed with FDA-required information, noting the name and address of the facility where the surgery took place; identification information used by the manufacturer; the patient's name, address, and social security number (unless the patient refuses permission to use this information); and the name, address, and telephone number of the implanting surgeon.[9]
14. Skin-preparation solutions used, areas prepared, and any reactions to prep solution
15. Known allergies to medications, prep solutions, tape, latex, dyes, and other substances
16. Sponge, sharp, and instrument counts taken and results obtained
17. Wound classification (see Chapter 8) and anesthesia classification (see Chapter 4)
18. Time of discharge and disposition of patient from OR, including mode of transfer and patient status

Perioperative nursing documentation needs to describe the assessment, planning, and implementation of perioperative care that reflects individualization of care and the evaluation of patient outcomes. Any unusual or significant incidents/events/occurrences pertinent to patient outcomes should be documented. Careful thought should be given to the design of perioperative nursing documentation tools that include the identified elements in a format that minimizes time needed for the documentation process (e.g., checklists). Ideally, collaboration with the preoperative, perianesthesia, and postoperative nursing units would produce one documentation tool that is used across the areas, avoiding duplication of patient data by different nursing staff. Figure 2-4 is a sample intraoperative/perioperative nursing record. Increasingly, settings where operative and other invasive procedures are performed are using computerized charting, with terminals in each individual room to enter and track patient data. Such point-of-care technology helps streamline workflow and reduces errors.

## Maintaining Fluid and Electrolyte Balance

Fluid and electrolyte balances within the body are important to the health and safety of the patient in surgery. The body's fluids and electrolytes play a key role in maintaining homeostasis, transporting necessary oxygen and nourishment to the cells, removing waste products of cellular metabolism, and helping to maintain the temperature of the body. Electrolytes are essential to the processes of transmitting nerve impulses, regulating water distribution, contracting muscles, generating adenosine triphosphate (needed for cellular energy), regulating acid-base balance, and clotting blood. The intake, distribution, and output of water and electrolytes, regulated by the renal and pulmonary systems, normally maintain fluid and electrolyte balance.

Fluid and electrolyte imbalances may occur rapidly in the surgical patient, caused by numerous factors, including preoperative fluid and food restrictions, intraoperative fluid loss, or the stress of surgery. The surgical patient is unable to regulate the body's fluid and electrolyte requirements by normal activities of drinking, eating, excreting, and breathing unaided. It is imperative that the perioperative nurse monitor and collaborate in controlling the fluid and electrolyte status of the patient intraoperatively.

***Body Fluids.*** The adult human body is approximately 60% water, although water content varies by age, gender, and body mass. In the elderly, body water content averages 45% to 55% of body weight, whereas it is 70% to 80% in infants. Older adults are at risk because they have less fluid reserve, and the very young are at risk for fluid problems because a greater percentage of their body weight is water. Both age groups have a decreased ability to compensate for fluid loss. Muscular tissue contains more water than the same amount of adipose tissue; men generally have higher water content because they usually have more lean body mass (more muscular tissue) than women.

Body fluids are distributed in two main functional compartments: intracellular and extracellular. *Intracellular fluids* (ICF) are liquids within cell membranes that contain dissolved substances essential to fluid and electrolyte balance and metabolism. Intracellular fluids constitute approximately 70% of the body's fluid. Consequently, anything that affects water loss at the intracellular level has significant implications for the entire body. *Extracellular fluids* (ECF) (30% of the body's fluid) are fluids in compartments outside the cells of the body, including plasma, intravascular fluids, fluids in the gastrointestinal (GI) tract, and cerebrospinal fluid (CSF). *Fluid spacing* is a term used to classify the distribution of body water. *First spacing* is the normal distribution of fluid in the extracellular and intracellular compartments. *Second spacing* refers to an excess accumulation of interstitial fluid (edema), and *third spacing* occurs when fluid accumulates in areas that normally have no fluid or only a minimal amount of fluid. This fluid accumulation occurs with burns, ascites, peritonitis, or small bowel obstructions. Third spacing traps fluid away from the normal fluid compartments and results in a deficit in extracellular fluid volume.

***Electrolytes.*** Electrolytes (Table 2-2) are substances found in intracellular fluids and extracellular fluids that, when dissolved in water, dissociate into ions and are able to carry an electric current. Positively charged ions are cations, and negatively charged ions are anions. The electrolytes found in the ECF and ICF are essentially the same, but the concentration of each electrolyte differs in extracellular and intracellular fluids. The primary intracellular cation is potassium, and the primary extracellular cation is sodium. The primary intracellular anion is phosphate, and the primary extracellular anion is chloride. Fluids and electrolytes move between the intracellular and extracellular spaces to facilitate body processes, such as acid-base balance, tissue oxygenation, response to drug therapies, and response to illness. Diffusion, active transport, and osmosis control this movement.

Operating Room
**OPERATION REPORT (Long Form)** Page 1 of 2

Date: ___/___/___ OR Room #:______ Patient Type: ☐ Inpatient ☐ Outpatient To OR via: ☐ Stretcher ☐ Bed ☐ Wheelchair ☐ AMB (with escort)

Procedure Type: ☐ Elective ☐ Emergency ☐ Return to OR Class ☐1 ☐2____ ☐3 | A.S.A. (Physical status) ☐1 ☐2 ☐3 ☐4 ☐5 | Wound Classification ☐1 ☐2 ☐3 ☐4

Patient Time in:______ Anesthesia Induct Time:______ Procedure Start Time:______ Procedure Stop Time:______ Patient Time Out:______ Delay Code:______ Delay Time:______

☐ Allergies verified; Comments: ______
☐ Interdisciplinary Admission Data Base/Outpatient Preoperative Record (local anesthesia) reviewed.
☐ Implemented standard plan of care for the operative patient.

Exception(s) noted: ______ Intervention(s) ______

RN Initials:

**ANESTHESIA TYPE:** ☐ GEN ☐ SPINAL ☐ EPIDURAL ☐ M.A.C. ☐ LOCAL ☐ BLOCK (type): ______
☐ OTHER ______

| | |
|---|---|
| **Preoperative Diagnosis:** | Attending Surgeon: |
| | Attending Surgeon: |
| | Attending Surgeon: |
| | Resident: |
| **Procedure:** | Resident: |
| | Assistant: ☐ M.S. ☐ P-A ☐ S-A ☐ RNFA |
| | Assistant: ☐ M.S. ☐ P-A ☐ S-A ☐ RNFA |
| | Assistant: ☐ M.S. ☐ P-A ☐ S-A ☐ RNFA |
| | |
| | Anesthesiologist: |
| | Anesthetist: |
| | Perfusionist: |
| **Postoperative Diagnosis:** | Autotransfusionist: |
| | **Cell Saver** ☐ Yes ☐ No |
| | |
| **Circulating Nurse:** | **Scrubperson** |
| Relief by: Time in: out: | Relief by: Time in: out: |
| Relief by: Time in: out: | Relief by: Time in: out: |
| Relief by: Time in: out: | Relief by: Time in: out: |
| Relief by: Time in: out: | Relief by: Time in: out: |

Others/Observers: ______

Comments: ______

**X - RAYS:** ☐ Portable ☐ Fluoro ☐ Self Image ☐ Yes ☐ No
By: ______

**LASERS:** Type: ______ Total Time: ______ ☐ Yes ☐ No

**FIGURE 2-4** Intraoperative record.

Operating Room

**OPERATION REPORT (Long Form)**

Page 2 of 2

**POSITION:** ☐ Supine ☐ Prone ☐ Lithotomy ☐ Sitting ☐ Lateral ☐ R↑ ☐ L↑

| **ARMS** | Side | Board | Arm Holder | Chest |
|---|---|---|---|---|
| Right | ☐ | ☐ | ☐ | ☐ |
| Left | ☐ | ☐ | ☐ | ☐ |

☐ Other ______
Positioned by: ______
Comments: ______

Pre-op Skin condition: ☐ Intact ______
Post-op Skin condition: ☐ Intact ______

**POSITIONING AIDS/DEVICES:** Location

☐ Safety Strap ______
☐ Tape ______
☐ Blankets ______
☐ Pillow(s) ______
☐ Sandbag(s) ______

☐ Vac Pac
☐ Stirrups
☐ Lami Rolls
☐ Foam Headrest
☐ Eggcrate

☐ Donut ☐ Fracture Table ☐ Mayfield Headrest
☐ Axillary Roll ☐ Andrews Bed ☐ Hall Relton Frame
☐ Gel Pad ☐ Stryker Frame ☐ McGuire Positioner
☐ Other ______

Comments: ______
RN Initials

**PREP:** ☐ Betadine ☐ Iodine____% ☐ Alcohol ☐ Duraprep ☐ Other:______ ☐ None

**EQUIPMENT**

**ESU** ☐ Bipolar Setting: ______ Serial/I.D.#______ ☐ Yes ☐ No

☐ Monopolar Coag ______ Cut______ Serial/I.D.#______

☐ Argon Beam Setting:______ Serial/I.D.#______

Dispersive Pad
Location: ______ Applied by:______

**TOURNIQUET:** Cuff Location______ ☐ Yes ☐ No

Pressure:______ Time up: ______ Time down: ______
Pressure:______ Time up: ______ Time down: ______

Applied by: Serial/I.D. #

**COMPRESSION BOOTS:** ☐ Yes ☐ No Pressure: ______

Applied by: Serial/I.D. #

**URINARY CATHETER**

To O.R. with catheter ☐ Yes ☐ No Inserted in O.R. by:______

Type/Size: ______ Amount: ______ mL Color:______

Removed in O.R. by:______ Time: ______

**PACKING/TUBES/DRAINS**

Type: ______ Size: ______ ☐ None

Location: ______ Amount of Packing:______

Comments: ______

**SPECIMENS**

Examined and Disposed Per Dr.______
# & Type of spec to Lab: ☐ None

______ Tissue ______ Culture______ FB ______ Fluid ______ Frozen Section

☐ Skin/Bone Freezer, describe: ______

☐ Explant, describe:______

Comments: ______

**MEDICATIONS**

OTHER THAN THOSE GIVEN BY ANESTHESIA ☐ None

| | Dosage | Route | Time | Given by |
|---|---|---|---|---|
| | | | | |
| | | | | |
| | | | | |
| | | | | |

IRRIGATION:______

Amount in: ______ Estimated amount out: ______

IRRIGATION:______

Amount in: ______ Estimated amount out: ______

RN Initials: ☐ None

**IMPLANTS/EXPLANTS**

☐ Yes See Implant/Explant Record ☐ None

**SPECIAL COMMENTS:** ______

**FAMILY COMMUNICATION DURING PROCEDURE (If applicable)**

Status discussed with ______
Name/Relation

RN Signature Time

Comments: ______ ☐ N/A

**DISCHARGE VIA:**

☐ Stretcher ☐ Patient Bed ☐ Crib ☐ Wheelchair ☐ Other ______

Verbal orders for intraoperative interventions given by: ______
Physician Signature Print Name/ID# Time Date

RN Initials & Signature Print Name Time Date

RN Initials & Signature Print Name Time Date

**FIGURE 2-4, cont'd** Intraoperative record.

***Diffusion, Active Transport, and Osmosis.*** *Diffusion* is the movement of molecules from an area of high concentration to one of low concentration across a permeable membrane. Movement continues until there is an equal concentration of molecules on both sides of the membrane.

*Active transport* is a process by which molecules are moved across a cell membrane, against a concentration gradient, with the use of external energy. The sodium-potassium pump moves sodium out of the cell and potassium into the cell to maintain the intracellular and extracellular concentration differences of sodium and potassium. Adenosine triphosphate is the energy source for the sodium-potassium pump.

*Osmosis* is the movement of a fluid through a semipermeable membrane from a solution that has a lower solute concentration to one that has a higher solute concentration (Figure 2-5). The semipermeable membrane prevents movement of

**TABLE 2-2**

**Electrolyte Functions and Regulators**

| Electrolyte | Reference Range | Functions | Regulation |
|---|---|---|---|
| Sodium ($Na^+$) | 135-145 mEq/L | Maintains blood volume<br>Controls water shifting between compartments<br>Major cation involved in sodium-potassium pump necessary for nerve impulses<br>Interacts with calcium to maintain muscle contraction<br>Major cation in bicarbonate and phosphate acid-base buffer system | Renin-angiotensin-aldosterone system |
| Potassium ($K^+$) | 3.5-5 mEq/L | Affects osmolality<br>Major cation involved in sodium-potassium pump necessary for transmission of nerve impulses<br>Promotes nerve impulses, especially in heart and skeletal muscles<br>Assists in conversion of carbohydrates to energy and amino acids into protein<br>Promotes glycogen storage in liver<br>Assists maintenance of acid-base balance through cellular exchange with hydrogen | Renin-angiotensin-aldosterone system |
| Calcium ($Ca^{2+}$) | 9-10.5 mg/dL<br>4.5-5.5 mEq/L | Nonionized form promotes strong teeth and bones<br>Promotes blood coagulation<br>Promotes nerve impulse conduction; decreases neuromuscular irritability<br>Strengthens and thickens cell membrane<br>Assists in absorption and use of vitamin $B_{12}$<br>Activates enzymes for many chemical reactions<br>Inhibits cell membrane permeability to sodium<br>Activates actin-myosin muscle contraction | Parathormone<br>Increases calcium reabsorption from bone<br>Increases calcium reabsorption by inhibiting phosphate reabsorption from kidney tubules<br>Increases calcium absorption from gastrointestinal tract |
| Chloride ($Cl^-$) | 98-106 mEq/L | Inhibits smooth muscle contraction<br>Regulates extracellular fluid volume<br>Promotes acid-base balance through exchange with bicarbonate in red blood cells (chloride shift)<br>Promotes protein digestion through hydrochloric acid; acid pH required for activation of protease | Renin-angiotensin-aldosterone system |
| Magnesium ($Mg^{2+}$) | 1.5-2.5 mEq/L | Promotes metabolism of carbohydrates, fats, and proteins<br>Activates many enzymes (vitamin $B_{12}$ metabolism)<br>Promotes regulation of Ca, $PO_4$, K<br>Promotes transmission of nerve impulses and heart function<br>Powers sodium-potassium pump<br>Promotes conversion of adenosine triphosphate to adenosine diphosphate for energy release | Parathormone<br>Increases or decreases magnesium reabsorption in kidney tubules relative to body need |
| Phosphate ($HPO_4^-$) | 1.2-3 mEq/L<br>3-4.5 mg/dL | Nonionized form promotes bone and teeth rigidity<br>Promotes acid-base balance through phosphate buffer system<br>Necessary for adenosine triphosphate production | Parathormone<br>Increases phosphate resorption from bone<br>Inhibits phosphate reabsorption in kidney tubules<br>Increase phosphate absorption in gastrointestinal tract as needed |

From Harkreader H, Hogan MA: *Fundamentals of nursing: caring and clinical judgment,* ed 2, St Louis, 2004, Saunders.

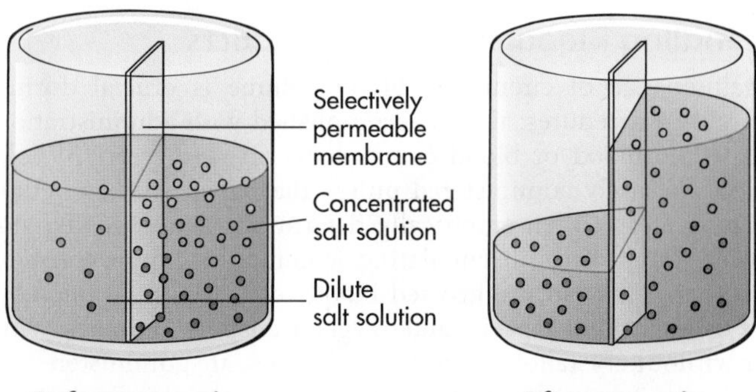


FIGURE 2-5 Osmosis is the movement of solvent molecules across a membrane to an area of higher solute concentration. The solvent moves because the solute cannot pass through the membrane. The result of osmosis is two solutions, separated by a selectively permeable membrane, which are equal in concentration.

solute particles. The number of particles is measured in a unit called the *osmol*. *Osmolality* is the term used to express the concentration of a solution in milliosmoles per kilogram (mOsm/kg) of water. A solution with the same osmolality as blood plasma is called *isotonic*. Isotonic solutions, such as 0.9% normal saline or lactated Ringer's solution administered intravenously (IV), prevent the shift of fluid and electrolytes from intracellular compartments. A hypotonic IV solution (0.45% saline or 2.5% dextrose) has a lower concentration of solutes than plasma does and moves water into the cells. Administration of a hypertonic IV solution (5% dextrose in normal saline or 5% dextrose in lactated Ringer's solution) with a greater concentration of solutes than that of plasma moves water out of the cells.

***Preoperative Considerations.*** A crucial part of assisting the surgical patient to maintain fluid and electrolyte balances is preoperative assessment and identification of risk factors for fluid and electrolyte imbalances. Preoperative laboratory analysis of electrolyte levels should be checked and abnormalities corrected to within normal limits before any surgical procedure, unless the surgery is needed to correct a life-threatening problem. Preexisting conditions, such as diabetes mellitus, liver disease, or renal insufficiency, may be aggravated by surgical stress, increasing a patient's risk of fluid and electrolyte imbalances. Diagnostic procedures that require the administration of IV dyes may produce osmotic diuresis, with a resulting urinary excretion of water and electrolytes. Preoperative steroids or diuretics affect the excretion of water and electrolytes; diuretics, used in the management of hypertension, cause the loss of potassium. Preoperative surgical regimens, such as administration of enemas or laxatives, may act to increase fluid loss from the gastrointestinal tract. Medical management of preexisting conditions, such as gastric suction, can affect fluid and electrolyte balance in the surgical patient, just as preoperative fluid restriction can.

Preoperative fluid restrictions are used to reduce nausea, vomiting, and aspiration risk in the surgical patient. This practice is being modified in many health care settings because newer anesthetic agents cause less nausea and vomiting than in the past. Prolonged fluid restrictions may not be necessary in healthy patients before surgery; black coffee or pulp-free juice may be ingested 2 to 3 hours before surgery safely, without an increase in gastric volume (see Chapter 4).

***Deficient Fluid Volume.*** The most common patient problems associated with fluid and electrolyte balance during surgery include deficient fluid volume (DFV), water imbalances, and potassium imbalances. DFV is an imbalance in isotonic body fluids related to decreased intravascular, interstitial, or intracellular fluid. Very young and very old surgical patients are affected most rapidly by fluid losses from bleeding; inadequate intake because of previous nothing-per-mouth (NPO) status; inadequate IV fluid replacement; excessive cutaneous losses from fever and sweating; third-space losses attributable to bowel obstructions, ascites, or peritonitis; excessive GI losses resulting from diarrhea, vomiting, GI suctioning, or fistulas; evaporation of fluid from the exposed peritoneum during abdominal surgery; shifting of intravascular fluid into the surgical site (third-space edema); and inhalation of dry gases. Third-space fluid shift cannot be measured directly, but it can be considerable after extensive dissection of tissue. Intraoperative use of an electrolyte solution, such as lactated Ringer's solution, for fluid replacement can help correct intraoperative third-space fluid losses.

The effect of fluid loss on the surgical patient depends on the amount of fluid lost and the speed at which the fluid is lost. A patient who loses a large amount of fluid (>500 ml) or loses fluid rapidly exhibits symptoms of shock; fluid replacement therapy is required. A slow loss of fluid may be compensated for through albumin synthesis and erythropoiesis.

***Sodium and Water Imbalances.*** Sodium is a cation in extracellular fluid, which plays a major role in maintaining the osmolality and water balance of the extracellular fluid. Because cell membranes are permeable to water, it also affects the intracellular fluid volume. Sodium also helps maintain acid-base balance in the body. The sodium-potassium pump plays a vital role in neuromuscular activity.

Hyponatremia (serum sodium level <135 mEq/L) can be caused by increased excretion of sodium with diuretic therapy and the abnormal loss of sodium through nasogastric suctioning and third spacing. Patients undergoing transurethral resection of the prostate (TURP) and uterine endoscopic laser surgery are at risk for dilutional hyponatremia and volume overload, caused by absorption of the irrigation solution used in those procedures. Because saline is a good conductor of electrical current, fluids that contain no electrolytes, such as glycine, sorbitol, and mannitol, must be used to irrigate in the presence of the electrical current used in the dissection during these procedures.

***Potassium Imbalances.*** Potassium is the major intracellular cation and is necessary for the contraction of skeletal muscle and smooth muscle. It is necessary for cardiac contractions and for movements of the GI tract. It plays a role in the transmission of nerve impulses by regulating neuromuscular excitability and in the formation of muscle protein by transporting glucose into the cells with insulin. It also is involved in the maintenance of acid-base balance and intracellular osmotic pressures.

Hypokalemia (serum potassium <3.5 mEq/L) can occur intraoperatively because of suctioning large amounts of body fluids or using diuretic therapy and other drugs (e.g., mannitol) that increase renal flow. Signs and symptoms of hypokalemia include cardiac effects, such as ectopy, dysrhythmias, conduction abnormalities, and altered sensitivity to digitalis. The neuromuscular effects of hypokalemia include muscle weakness; smooth muscle effects include gastric distention, paralytic ileus, and urinary retention.

Treatment of hypokalemia includes IV replacement when the deficit is severe, as in the development of cardiovascular or other serious symptoms. Potassium is irritating to veins on infusion; the infusion site should be monitored for redness, heat, swelling, or site pain—all signs of chemical phlebitis. Overcorrection and subsequent hyperkalemia must be avoided by monitoring serum potassium levels at frequent intervals (often every 2 to 4 hours).

Hyperkalemia, a serum potassium of more than 5 mEq/L, can be caused during surgery by massive transfusions of stored blood; decreased excretion of potassium caused by hypovolemia or renal failure; and shifting of potassium from the cells into the extracellular fluid caused by acidosis, tissue breakdown from surgery, crush injuries, or burns. Drugs infused during surgery can induce hyperkalemia, including anti-inflammatory agents, β-adrenergic receptor blockers, digitalis, succinylcholine, heparin, and the penicillins.

The signs and symptoms of hyperkalemia include neuromuscular symptoms, such as weakness and paresthesias in the arms and legs. Smooth muscle symptoms include diarrhea and abdominal distention. Excess potassium can cause serious cardiac symptoms, including ventricular dysrhythmias, heart block, and asystole. Cardiac side effects of hyperkalemia are treated by calcium gluconate. Sodium bicarbonate or insulin-glucose infusions can be given to shift the extracellular potassium into the cells, reducing the level of potassium in the plasma.

## Estimating Blood Loss

Measuring blood loss is a vital procedure in the surgical management of critically ill or elderly patients, patients undergoing complex extensive surgery, trauma and organ transplant patients, patients with abnormal bleeding or clotting time or extensive renal/liver disease, and infants. Weighing sponges provides a reliable means of judging the amount of blood lost and of gauging the need for replacement of fluids and blood products. The weight of the unit of dry sponges and the plastic bag for soiled sponges must be determined and excluded from the weight tally. Grams (g) measured are converted to milliliters (ml) on a 1:1 basis, and blood loss estimates are reported to the anesthesia provider. If necessary, the setup for weighing sponges requires a gram scale and plastic bags and twist ties to hold soiled sponges.

### *Procedure*

1. Weigh the unit of dry sponges and the plastic bag, and adjust the scale to register zero.
2. Place bagged sponges on the scale.
3. Record the scale reading: 1 g equals 1 ml of blood loss.
4. Note the blood loss on the record.
5. Add subsequent weight to the preceding weight each time sponges are weighed so that a running total blood loss, calculated from sponges, is available.
6. Measure blood in the suction bottles at regular intervals, subtracting the amount of irrigating solution used.
7. Add the amount of blood loss calculated from suction bottles to the total recorded from sponges to obtain accurate blood loss estimates.

## Handling Blood and Blood Products

Maintenance of circulating blood volume is crucial during surgical procedures; this is accomplished with administration of whole blood or blood components (History box). Whole blood is rarely administered unless the patient has an acute, massive loss (often empirically determined as a loss that exceeds one third of circulating volume, or approximately 1500 ml). Instead, packed red blood cells (RBCs) to improve oxygen-carrying capacity and oxygen transport to tissues, with or without crystalloid or colloid solutions, are administered to maintain intravascular blood volume. Crystalloid solutions include normal saline and lactated Ringer's solution; colloid solutions include albumin, purified protein factors, dextran, and hydroxyethyl starch (hetastarch). When blood must be given, appropriate precautions are necessary to reduce the hazards of its administration.

Safe administration of blood or blood products begins with the pretransfusion blood sample that is sent for typing and crossmatching (compatibility testing). Elective surgery patients have this sample taken 3 to 5 days before surgery to ensure compatibility and to avoid antibodies that may emerge in response to exposure through blood transfusions, pregnancy, or environmental factors or resulting from the patient's

**HISTORY**

### Blood Transfusion

The safe transfusion of blood and blood products is commonplace in surgery. It is a relatively recent advance, however, compared with other surgical milestones. Bloodletting and phlebotomy, described in many historical references, were recommended for many ailments, including insanity. Transfusions were attempted several hundred years ago to change the nature of an individual; for example, they were used for individuals accused of being witches, to infuse them with the proper sprits. In 1825 Dr. Philip Syng Physick of Philadelphia administered what might have been the first successful transfusion of human blood. In the 1900s, the A, B, AB, and O blood types were discovered, and by the 1940s techniques for crossmatching, anticoagulation, storage of blood, and blood banks made routine blood transfusion possible. A 1942 nursing textbook noted, "blood transfusion is a procedure employed in the treatment of severe shock, especially when accompanied by haemorrhage, whether due to injury or some such emergency. . . ." The textbook showed a procedure for "taking blood," wherein a cuff was applied to the arm to distend the veins, a venesection needle with rubber tubing attached was inserted, and the blood was drained by gravity into a glass bottle that was rotated by an assistant to ensure that it mixed properly with the citrate solution already in it. A second assistant was shown who "may suck the air out of the bottle and so hasten the flow of blood" during the taking procedure. After the blood was taken, the glass bottle had beads added to it to prevent clots from passing out, glass tubing was placed in the rubber tubing so that the flow of blood could be observed, and a flattened end was placed at the administration part of the tubing so that blood but not the beads could pass into the patient. It was noted that a syringe could be used to blow air into the bottle if blood was running too slowly.

Modified from Fakhry SM and others: Hematologic principles in surgery. In Townsend CM, editor: *Sabiston textbook of surgery,* ed 16, Philadelphia, 2001, Saunders; Houghton M: *Aids to tray and trolley setting,* ed 2, London, 1942, Bailliere, Tindall & Cox.

disease process. *Typing* refers to the test to determine the ABO and Rh blood type compatibility. *Crossmatching* refers to testing the compatibility of the recipient's serum with the donor's red blood cells. It is crucial to identify the patient correctly before the pretransfusion blood sample is drawn and to ensure that the sample is properly labeled. Improperly identified pretransfusion blood samples can result in acute hemolytic transfusion reactions at the time of transfusion.

A patient having an elective surgical procedure for which blood has been requested should not be anesthetized without verification that the requested blood products are typed, crossmatched, and available. The appropriate institutional blood requisition form, with complete and accurate patient identification information, should be sent to the blood bank when blood or blood components are being requested. Included on or with this requisition should be the number of units desired. Many institutions have computerized ordering; the same information is required when blood is requested by computer.

If the patient is sent to the OR directly from the emergency department or trauma admitting area without a chart, all patient identification information must be printed plainly on a piece of paper. The perioperative nurse should contact the blood bank to explain the emergency situation and facilitate release of the needed blood products.

The storage of blood products is important to ensure the safety of the patient and to avoid wasteful discarding of improperly stored blood units. Whole blood, packed red blood cells, and thawed fresh frozen plasma (FFP) must be stored under continuously monitored conditions, according to the American Association of Blood Banks (AABB) and the FDA regulations. Temperatures should be documented and all storage equipment for blood products properly maintained and tested, including function checks on the alarms. When blood components have been out of monitored refrigeration for more than 30 minutes, they cannot be returned to the blood bank for reissue.

Before the administration of any blood product, the circulating nurse and the anesthesia provider (or a second licensed individual) must confirm the following:

- The number on the unit of blood corresponds with the number on the blood requisition.
- The name, birth date, and number on the patient's identification band agree with the name, birth date, and number on the unit of blood.
- The patient's name on the unit of blood corresponds with the name on the requisition.
- The blood group indicated on the unit of blood corresponds with that of the patient.
- The date of expiration has not been reached.
- The blood bag is free of leaks, damage, or signs of possible bacterial contamination (e.g., presence of fine gas bubbles, discoloration, clots, or excessive air in the bag).

Both individuals reviewing the above-listed identification information must sign the slip that comes with the blood, verifying that the information is correct.[11] If a discrepancy is identified with any of these checks, the blood product must not be infused until the discrepancy is resolved.

When it becomes apparent that more blood will be needed than originally anticipated, the perioperative nurse should request the blood bank to prepare a specified number of units in advance of the actual need to transfuse. This procedure allows the blood bank time to crossmatch the units carefully without rushing and jeopardizing patient safety. Crossmatch requisitions should be sent for any additional units requested. A new, properly labeled sample with a blood grouping requisition also may need to be sent to have adequate serum for crossmatching or to ensure antibody compatibility after a significant amount of transfusion has been required.

The need for rapid blood transfusion necessitates the warming of blood to prevent hypothermia, which may induce cardiac arrest. Blood should be warmed during its passage through the transfusion set. The warming device should incorporate a temperature monitor and, ideally, an audible warning system. The probability of a transfusion reaction increases in direct proportion to the number of units transfused. The circulating nurse should be alert to any signs of reaction, including the following:

- Increased intraoperative bleeding
- Weak pulse
- Hypotension
- Visible hemoglobinuria
- Vasomotor instability
- Greatly decreased or absent urinary output

If any suspicious reactions occur, the circulating nurse should assist the anesthesia provider to do the following:

1. Stop the transfusion. The tubing is disconnected and a new infusion of fluid, such as 0.9% sodium chloride, is begun to maintain venous access.
2. Report the reaction to the surgeon and the blood bank.
3. Return the unused portion of the blood, the IV tubing used during transfusion, and a sample of the patient's blood to the blood bank.
4. Send a urine sample to the laboratory as soon as possible.
5. Complete an incident/occurrence/event report covering the details of the reaction. These might include time and date of reaction, type and amount of blood/blood product infused, and time transfusion started and time stopped. Signs and symptoms, in the order of occurrence, along with the patient's vital signs, any urine or blood samples sent to the laboratory for analysis, any treatment given, and the patient's response also should be noted. Some facilities also require the completion of a transfusion reaction report to be sent to the blood bank.[12]
6. Monitor the patient's reaction carefully.

Any unused blood should be returned to the blood bank as soon as the patient leaves the operating suite. Returned blood can be reissued if it has not been allowed to warm to a temperature greater than 10°C. New external blood bag thermometers (e.g., HemoTemp II), similar to a skin contact tape thermometer, are being used on blood bags by many blood banks to identify quickly blood that has exceeded safe storage temperatures.

Autotransfusion—the reinfusion of a patient's own blood—is being used with increasing frequency. In autologous blood donations, the blood is predonated up to 1 month before surgery for use in the patient's own planned surgery. Using normovolemic hemodilution, the patient's blood is "thinned" before the surgery by collecting blood through a closed system and replacing it with fluid. During surgery, the blood that is lost is "thin" (i.e., fewer cells are lost). At the same time, the anesthesia provider reinfuses the precollected blood of the patient.[30] During intraoperative autotransfusion (cell salvage), blood is collected as it is lost during the surgical procedure and reinfused to the patient after it is filtered or washed. This technique can be lifesaving in emergency situations, such as major trauma, or in procedures with major blood loss, as in liver transplantation. It also is used for patients who refuse blood based on religious beliefs.

## Maintaining Normothermia in a Surgical Patient

An important component of patient safety is the avoidance of hypothermia. Studies have shown that perioperative hypothermia contributes to increased postoperative discomfort, increased surgical bleeding, incidents of postoperative cardiac events (ischemia and tachycardia), and impaired wound healing with susceptibility to surgical site infection and longer lengths of stay in the PACU (Research Highlight) (see Chapter 9).

The temperature and humidity in the OR, the number of room air exchanges occurring per hour, open body cavities, the use of anesthetics (all of which impair thermoregulation), and cool air currents contribute to the loss of body heat. Patients at greatest risk include patients undergoing complex surgeries lasting long periods because body cavities are exposed to cold temperatures for extended times. Other patients at risk include thin patients (fat acts as insulation to conserve heat), elderly patients (shivering occurs less in the elderly because the vasoconstrictive response to cold is blunted), and patients whose positioning causes them to have a greater body surface exposed to cool room temperatures.

Nursing interventions to reduce inadvertent hypothermia include the following:

1. Identify risk factors for hypothermia.
2. Keep the patient warm preoperatively.
3. Assess the patient's body temperature frequently.
4. Increase the ambient room temperature of the OR.
5. Use forced-air warming blankets over the upper or lower body or a temperature-regulating blanket under the patient.
6. Apply warm blankets immediately postoperatively.
7. Use warm irrigation fluids.
8. Assist the anesthesia provider to infuse warm intravenous fluids and use heated humidified gases.

Patient temperature should be included in the hand-off report[19] (Best Practice) to the nurse in the PACU or ambulatory surgery recovery area.

## Care and Handling of Specimens

The proper care and handling of specimens is important to the safe outcome of a patient's surgical experience. It is the responsibility of the circulating nurse to identify, document, and care for properly specimens collected in the OR. Commonly handled specimens include blood, soft tissue, bone, body fluids, and foreign bodies. Complete and accurate identification and labeling of specimens and timely delivery to the proper laboratory for analysis are the responsibilities of the perioperative nurse. A mislabeled specimen could result in misdiagnosis and subsequent inappropriate treatment of the patient. The circulating nurse must ensure that each specimen is labeled with the correct patient name and specific origin of the specimen (e.g., Jane Doe, 100001, right breast biopsy). The surgeon should provide descriptive information about the specimen (e.g., suture tag at 6 o'clock). The nurse should "repeat-back" information (patient, type of specimen, source/location, re-

## RESEARCH HIGHLIGHT

### Significance of Inadvertent Hypothermia

Inadvertent hypothermia is a common patient complication experienced by surgical patients. Hypothermia is defined as a core temperature of 36°C (98.6°F). Complications associated with inadvertent hypothermia include postoperative surgical site infection, cardiac events related to myocardial ischemia, and increased intraoperative blood loss. This study examined the adverse patient outcome of a prolonged stay in the PACU. When patients are required to stay in the PACU longer than the average time for length of stay (LOS), there are increased economic implications and inherent staffing issues. If the LOS is prolonged, the PACU nurse-to-patient ratio is overloaded, which has implications for patient safety.

When PACU LOS was examined in other studies, the most important factors influencing prolonged stay included duration and type of anesthesia and amount of intraoperative fluid replacement. This study sought to explore two research questions:

- Does the actual and appropriate LOS in the PACU differ between patients who are hypothermic and patients who are normothermic?
- What are the differences between subgroups of patients according to age, gender, and type of anesthesia received?

The study sample included 150 elective orthopedic surgery patients who were 18 years old or older, had a normal preoperative core temperature, and were extubated before leaving the OR. Temperatures were measured with infrared thermometers at the tympanic membrane just before patients entered the OR and on admission to the PACU. Other monitoring included routine parameters for PACU patients (heart rate, blood pressure, oxygen saturation). Criteria for PACU discharge included an 8 or greater Aldrete score (see Chapter 9), oxygen saturation of 90% or better on room air, control of postoperative pain (reports of none or mild discomfort), no vomiting, and complete recovery of sensation and mobility of the lower limbs for patients having regional anesthesia.

The researchers found that 74% of patients in this study arrived in the PACU with unplanned hypothermia. A commonality among these patients was duration of surgery, age (≤60 years old), and type of anesthesia (general anesthesia). Length of stay for hypothermic patients was increased from what a normal amount of time for recovery would be, which is similar to findings in other research.

Perioperative nurses should find this research affirmative for initiating early strategies to prevent hypothermia. Measures should begin in the preoperative phase and continue intraoperatively. As noted in the AORN Position Statement on Patient Safety, perioperative nurses form a bond with patients, who place their physical and emotional needs in the hands of the nurse and other members of the surgical team.[4] The Perioperative Nursing Data Set discusses the physiologic outcome related to achieving normothermia as a patient whose core body temperature is within expected range, recommending thermoregulation measures to warm the patient as indicated and reporting the patient's temperature to the PACU nurse for determination of appropriate postoperative treatment methods.

Modified from Beyea SC: *Perioperative nursing data set: the perioperative nursing vocabulary,* Denver, 2002, AORN; Panagiotis K and others: Is post-anesthesia care unit length of stay increased in hypothermic patients? *AORN Journal* 81(2):379-392, 2005.

quired tests, special handling needs). All specimens and their disposition are documented on the OR record.

Each specimen is cared for according to the specific protocol established by the receiving laboratory. Generally, all tissue should be handled with caution to preserve its integrity, kept moist, and transported to the laboratory as soon as possible. Standard transmission-based precautions should be used to protect individuals handling the specimen. Labels should identify the need for precautions and the presence of biohazardous material.

Formalin, a combination of methanol, water, and formaldehyde, is frequently used to preserve specimens if they are not taken to the laboratory immediately. Formaldehyde is considered a hazardous substance that can cause watery eyes and respiratory irritation. Care must be taken in handling to avoid exposure to skin and the respiratory tract. Gloves must be worn and adequate ventilation provided in areas where formaldehyde is handled. Exposure to formaldehyde fumes should be monitored at least quarterly, and an MSDS should be available. Institutional policy should describe procedures to follow in case of formaldehyde spills.

When immediate tissue identification or the identification of malignancy is needed, specimens are quick-frozen, sliced, stained, and examined in the laboratory under a microscope—a method of tissue examination known as *frozen section*. Specimens for frozen section usually are placed on Telfa or into a dry specimen container. They are *never* placed in saline solution or formalin. The results of frozen-section reports are communicated to the surgeon intraoperatively. If the perioperative nurse receives the telephone report of a frozen section, it is considered a critical test result. The nurse should "read-back" the test result to the pathologist to verify the result.

## Sponge, Sharp, and Instrument Counts

Sponge, sharp, and instrument counts are performed to prevent patient injury from a retained foreign object. The Perioperative Nursing Data Set (PNDS) (see Chapter 1) domain of "safety" applies to counts; the desired patient outcome is "freedom from signs and symptoms of injury caused by extraneous objects," and the outcome is defined as "the patient is free from signs or symptoms of injury due to instrumentation, sponges, or sharps." The National Quality Forum has identified leaving a retained item in a patient a serious reportable event, and one that should *never happen* to patients in health care facilities.[28] Every OR should have established written policies and procedures for sponge, sharp, and instrument counts that define materials to be counted, the times when counts must be done, and the documentation required. The Council on Surgical and Perioperative Safety has developed guidelines to assist perioperative personnel in preventing unintentional retention of foreign bodies in the surgical wound, noting that "No thing is left behind" without the full knowledge and agreement of the team.[34] The American College of Surgeons has issued a statement on prevention of retained foreign bodies, urging health care organizations to take steps to prevent retained foreign bodies in the surgical wound. Preventive strategies include good communication among the surgical team, application of standardized processes, counting, wound exploration before the closure of the operative site and use of technology such as x-rays as indicated.[15] Prevention of retained foreign bodies is a crucial part of patient safety, advocacy, and teamwork in perioperative settings.

### BEST PRACTICE

#### Hand-Off Communication and Reports

In 1999 the Institute of Medicine (IOM) issued its landmark report, "To Err Is Human: Building a Safer Health System." The report was a clarion call to renew efforts in pinpointing medical errors and adverse events. Following that report, the IOM issued *Crossing the Quality Chasm,* suggesting that patient hand-offs provide opportunity for error. In the health care setting, hand-offs include nursing shift changes, temporary relief or coverage, nursing and physician hand-offs from one department to another, various transfers of information at the inpatient settings, and transfers to different hospitals. The purpose of hand-off communication and reports is to provide appropriate, up-to-date, and specific information.

To improve care, ORs should standardize hand-off communications and include an opportunity to ask and respond to questions. Following are strategies to assist in effective and efficient hand-off communication and reports:

1. Use clear language. Avoid unclear or potentially confusing terms ("she's a little unstable," "he's doing fine," or "she's lethargic"). Define the terms you are using. Do not use abbreviations or jargon that could be misinterpreted.
2. Incorporate effective communication techniques. Limit interruptions, focus on the information being exchanged, and allocate sufficient time to this important task. Keep the report patient-centered, and avoid irrelevant details. Use read-back, report-back, or check-back techniques to ensure there is a common understanding about information exchanged.
3. Standardize shift-to-shift reporting. A consistent format increases the amount of information staff members accurately record and recall and improves their ability to plan patient care. Keep the report concise and accurate.
4. Standardize perioperative nursing reports to the PACU or ambulatory surgery units. Consider essential information such as reporting the procedure done, the duration (and whether it was longer or shorter than expected), the complexity of the procedure (was it greater than, less than, or as expected), whether there were events or deviations from the expected course, implants, medications administered, current status of vital signs (including temperature and warming methods used), pulses, incision/dressings/drains, blood/fluids administered, and urinary output. During any hand-off, there must be an opportunity for each nurse to ask and respond to questions.
5. Use technology to your advantage. Communication systems that transmit information across settings and care providers bring consistency and coordination to care practices. Automated electronic perioperative records can facilitate transitions by providing consistent, accessible information about surgical patients and their care in the OR. Staff members should be able to access readily essential components of care, such as whether a newly ordered medication was administered, whether laboratory studies were done, or if a do-not-resuscitate order is in place.

Modified from Committee on the Quality of Health Care in America, Institute of Medicine: *Crossing the Quality Chasm.* Washington, DC, 2001, National Academy Press; JCAHO comments on hand-off requirement, *OR Manager* 21(8):8, 2005; Moore DT: Clinical issues—national patient safety goals, *AORN Journal* 82(2):275-277, 2005; Strategies to improve hand-off communications: implementing a process to resolve questions, Joint Commission International Center for Patient Safety, Accessed August 9, 2005, on-line: www.jcipatientsafety.org.

Certain general guidelines are pertinent to counting all three categories of items. The scrub person and the circulating nurse should count all items in unison and aloud, quietly, as the scrub person touches each item. Counting should not be interrupted. If any uncertainty exists about a count, it should be repeated. The circulating nurse should record the count for each type of item immediately on the count record or worksheet (Figure 2-6). If additional sponges, instruments, sharps, or other items are dispensed during the procedure, they are similarly counted, and the circulating nurse records the number added. The names of the circulating nurse and the scrub person are recorded as soon as each count is completed. Additional counts should be performed whenever there is a change in personnel.

When items are counted, linen or trash bags should not be removed from the OR until the procedure is completed, and the patient has been taken out of the room. Emergency or trauma surgery sometimes may necessitate omission of counts. If this occurs, it should be documented on the operative record, and an x-ray film should be obtained after the procedure to ensure that items are not left in the patient. Institutional policy often requires completion of an incident/occurrence/event report for omission of counts during emergency and trauma surgery.

***Sponge Counts.*** Sponges should be counted in all procedures in which there is a possibility that a sponge may be inadvertently retained. The scrub person and the circulating nurse should count sponges simultaneously and audibly as each sponge is separated from others in the pack before the beginning of the operation, before any closure begins, and when skin closure is begun. Additional counts may be indicated according to individual institutional policy and circumstance. Additional counts always should be done before a cavity within a cavity is closed, as when the uterus is closed after a cesarean birth. Types and sizes of sponges used should be kept to a minimum. All soft goods that are used within a wound and are not intended to be left in the wound after closure must contain a radiopaque marker. Radiopacity allows a retained item to be identified or the surgeon to rule out a retained item with an x-ray film taken after

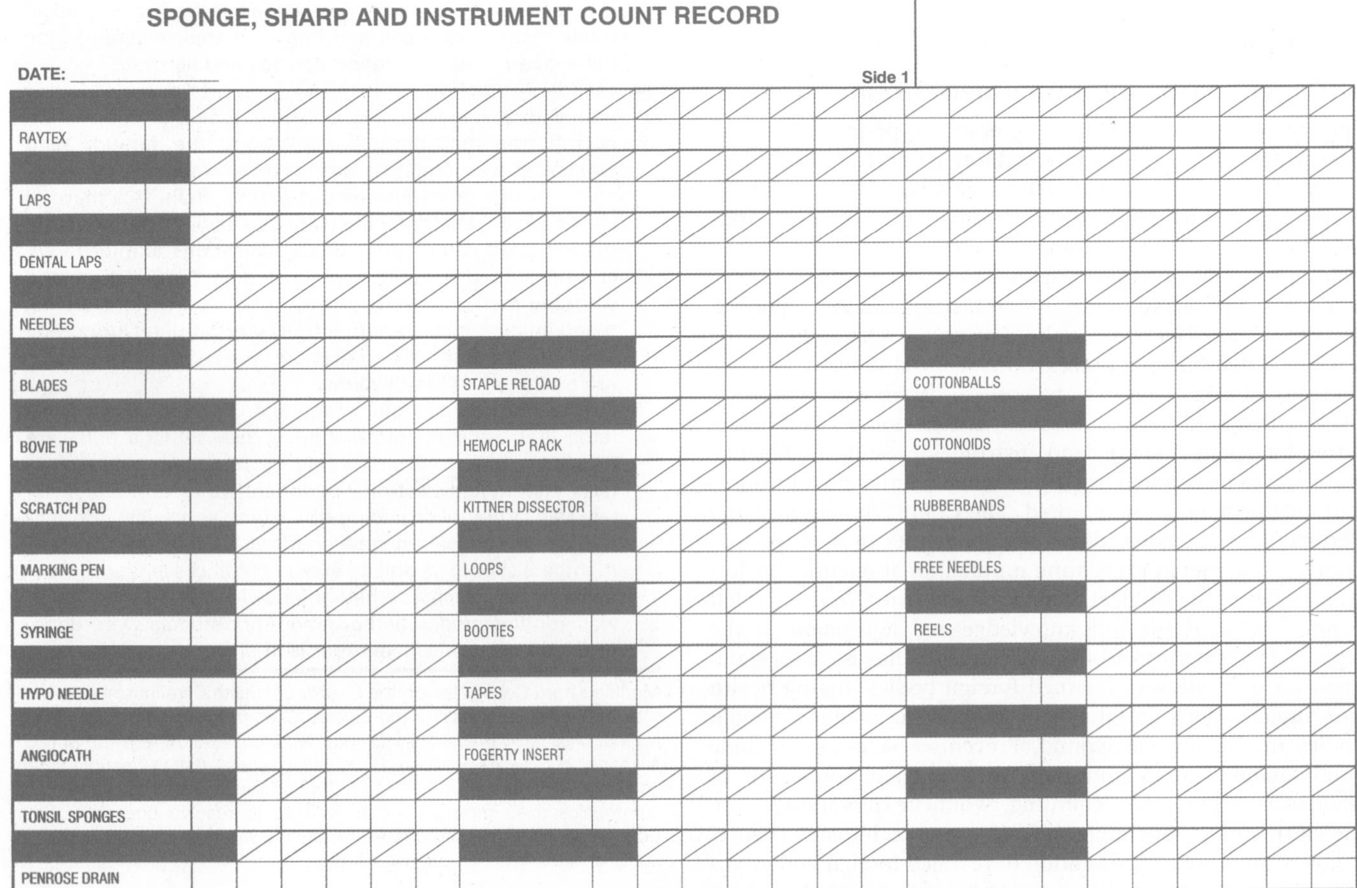

SPONGE, SHARP AND INSTRUMENT COUNT RECORD

DATE: ______________ Side 1

- RAYTEX
- LAPS
- DENTAL LAPS
- NEEDLES
- BLADES
- BOVIE TIP
- SCRATCH PAD
- MARKING PEN
- SYRINGE
- HYPO NEEDLE
- ANGIOCATH
- TONSIL SPONGES
- PENROSE DRAIN
- STAPLE RELOAD
- HEMOCLIP RACK
- KITTNER DISSECTOR
- LOOPS
- BOOTIES
- TAPES
- FOGERTY INSERT
- COTTONBALLS
- COTTONOIDS
- RUBBERBANDS
- FREE NEEDLES
- REELS

**FIGURE 2-6** Sponge, sharp, and instrument count record.

an incorrect count. X-ray–detectable sponges should never be used for dressings to avoid the appearance of a retained item on postoperative x-ray studies.

Each type and size of sponge should be kept separate from the other types. Sponges must be kept away from other supplies, such as towels and drapes, to prevent a sponge from being misplaced or carried inadvertently into the wound. To minimize the possibility of an incorrect count, counted sponges should never be taken from the OR for any reason during surgery.

If an incorrectly numbered package of sponges is dispensed to the field, it should be handed off the field in its entirety, not included in the count, bagged, labeled, isolated, and reported to the nurse manager (or other designated person) for follow-up with the manufacturer (quality control). This practice reduces the potential for error by using only standard multiples of sponges.

During surgery, the scrub person should discard soiled sponges into a plastic-lined bucket or receptacle. Throughout the procedure, the circulating nurse transfers the discarded sponges from the bucket into impermeable plastic bags or other appropriate containers, according to type and prescribed number, counting them with the scrub person. The bag is closed, secured, and labeled with the type and number of sponges. The bag can be set aside, and unless a discrepancy occurs, the sponges need not be taken out and counted again at the time of the closure sponge counts. Bagging of sponges reduces the possibility of airborne contamination arising from the sponges as they become dry, facilitates weighing of sponges for estimating blood loss, and enables the anesthesia provider to assess the patient's blood loss visually.

The circulating nurse should tally the number of each type of sponge dispensed, as recorded on the count worksheet before the closure counts are taken. As the first layer of closure is begun, the scrub person and the circulating nurse should count all sponges consecutively, proceeding from the sterile field to the Mayo stand to the back table and then to the bagged sponges off the field. The circulating nurse should inform the surgeon of the results of the count. The procedure should be repeated as skin closure is begun. The scrub person is responsible for knowing where sponges are on the sterile field during the procedure. Regardless of whether a formal count is done, all sponges must be accounted for at the end of each surgical procedure. This avoids the possibility that a sponge that fell on the floor and ended up under the OR bed would be mistakenly considered "discovered" in the event of an incorrect count for another patient procedure.

***Sharp Counts.*** The scrub person and the circulating nurse should count sharps in all procedures at the same time as sponges are counted. In addition to suture needles, sharps include scalpel and electrosurgical blades, hypodermic needles, and safety pins. When needles are counted before surgery begins, opening every package of suture dispensed onto the field is unnecessary. The needles may be counted according to the number indicated on the package. If a package indicates that five needled sutures are contained within, five needles should be documented on the worksheet. The scrub person is responsible for verifying the number of needles at the time the package is opened. The scrub person should count needles continually during the procedure and hand them to the surgeon on an exchange basis. Hands-free transfer of sharps by using an emesis basin or magnetic pad is recommended to prevent staff and surgeon needle-stick injuries.

Collecting used needles on a needle pad or container facilitates counting and helps to ensure their containment on the table. In procedures that may require use of a high volume of needles, the scrub person can count any filled needle pad with the circulating nurse and hand it off the field. The circulating nurse should bag it and label it with the number of needles contained and the initials of the individuals who counted them.

Needles broken during the procedure must be accounted for in their entirety. Similar to sponges, needles should never be taken from the room for any reason during a procedure. Closure counts are conducted in the same format as that for sponges.

SHARPS SAFETY. In addition to hands-free transfer of sharps, through the creation of a neutral zone, many ORs have adopted the use of blunt needles, skin staples, or adhesives for skin closure to reduce the amount of suturing; safety types of IV access systems; and syringes with protective features. Scalpels with blade-shielding features and disposable scalpels that do not require manual blade removal also are available. Many surgeons, scrub persons, and RNFAs routinely double-glove to decrease the risk of inadvertent glove puncture and contact with a bloodborne pathogen. These measures are discussed more fully in Chapter 6.

***Instrument Counts.*** The policy of some institutions specifies that instrument counts be taken only when a major body cavity is entered or when the depth and location of the wound are such that an instrument could inadvertently be left in the patient. Individual facility policy must be followed without deviation. Instrument sets should be standardized for ease in counting, with the minimum number and type of instruments in each set. Instruments should be counted in the instrument room as sets are being assembled, in the OR by the scrub person and circulating nurse before the beginning of the operation, and before closure begins. Additional counts may be indicated according to facility policy or individual circumstance. Instruments that are broken or disassembled during the procedure must be accounted for in their entirety. No instruments should be taken from the OR during a procedure. Printed instrument count sheets with the names of all items to be counted help expedite the count procedure. Instrument counts follow the same sequence as just described for sponge counts.

***Incorrect Counts.*** An incorrect count occurs when the number of items on the count record or worksheet does not match the number of items actually counted. Any incorrect closure count should be repeated immediately, and attempts must be made to resolve the discrepancy. If it remains incorrect, the circulating nurse should notify the surgeon of the incorrect count, and a search should be made for the missing item, including the surgical wound, field, floor, linen, and trash (if they can be searched safely). All personnel should direct their immediate attention to locating the missing item. If it is not found, an x-ray film may be taken and read by the radiologist or surgeon as specified in institutional policy. If the x-ray is negative, the count is recorded as incorrect, and the x-ray results are noted on the OR record. An incident/occurrence/event report (see Box 2-4) should be initiated according to institution policy. Accurate counting and recording of sponges, sharps, and instruments are essential for the protection of the patient, personnel, and the institution.

## Cardiopulmonary Resuscitation

An important part of a patient safety plan is training staff in cardiopulmonary resuscitation (CPR). CPR is the immediate restoration of circulatory and respiratory functions by means of manual and mechanical methods and the administration of drugs to provide for ventilation and conversion of the heartbeat to normal sinus rhythm. Cardiac arrest, standstill, or fibrillation may occur in patients undergoing surgery because of the hazards of surgery, including blood loss and shock, or because of unfavorable reactions to anesthesia, such as hypoxia and poor ventilation. CPR is vital to the survival of these patients.

All body organs and tissues must receive sufficient oxygen through the circulatory system for life to be sustained. The circulating blood must carry the oxygen supplied by pulmonary ventilation. Ventilation may be reestablished by mouth-to-mouth breathing or by other means of mechanical ventilation, such as oxygen apparatus, facemask, and intubation (artificial airway and endotracheal tube), with the use of an Ambu bag or mechanical ventilator. Cardiac compression is directed toward the reestablishment of circulation.

The resuscitation protocol should be understood by all personnel. Periodic practice sessions (mock codes) for delegated duties should be scheduled as part of the safety program. A movable emergency cardiopulmonary arrest cart (crash cart) containing all items that may be needed for CPR should be immediately available. The surgical committee, the perioperative nursing staff, and the anesthesia department collaboratively determine the equipment needed and supplies needed. Institutions use advanced cardiac life support (ACLS) protocols as a guideline, updating drugs and drug doses as ACLS protocols change. Others also include the pharmacy in determining the cart's contents. The cart should be in a central location and be routinely checked per the protocol established in the facility for completeness, medication expiration dates, and properly functioning equipment. It is important to stress the team approach for successful CPR of the patient in surgery. Items on or with the emergency cart usually include ventilation equipment (to establish an airway if the patient is not already intubated), syringes and needles, emergency drugs (often with prefilled syringes), IV infusion supplies, and cardiac support equipment. The primary priorities in a cardiac arrest situation are airway management, chest compression, defibrillation when needed, and treatment of any dysrhythmia.

### *Procedure*

1. Activate the emergency alarm to alert appropriate surgical and anesthesia personnel. Record the exact time of arrest, and obtain additional assistance as required.
2. Nursing personnel responding to the alarm should bring the cardiopulmonary arrest cart to the room. The circulating nurse should stay with the patient. The scrubbed person remains sterile and moves sterile items (Mayo stand, back table) out of the way.
3. If not already established, an airway should be established and ventilation of the patient begun by means of artificial ventilation to restore and maintain oxygenation. Mouth-to-mouth resuscitation is begun if resuscitative equipment is not immediately available.
4. Perform closed-chest massage to maintain circulation and provision of oxygen to vital tissues.
5. Designate one person to direct the resuscitation efforts, that is, "run the code" (usually the anesthesia provider) and another to record (usually the circulating nurse). The recorder should document the sequence of events and interventions as they occur, including medications given and procedures performed.
6. Prepare and administer medications as ordered.
7. Procure and prepare infusions or transfusions as ordered.
8. Assist the surgeon and anesthesia provider as needed.
9. Document the event, care given, and patient outcomes.
10. Notify appropriate personnel as the situation requires. This may include a request to the pastoral care service and notification to the proper personnel of the change in the patient's condition and the need to inform the patient's family.

Successful CPR of the patient in surgery depends on a coordinated team effort, starting with early recognition of impending danger and rapid response by all team members.

## Malignant Hyperthermia

A separate cart or box for malignant hyperthermia (MH) (see Chapter 4 for a full discussion) also is recommended to facilitate prompt initiation of treatment protocols for a patient diagnosed with MH. Emergency drugs and equipment include dantrolene sodium, sterile water (bacteriostatic-free) for injection, sodium bicarbonate, furosemide, insulin, 50% dextrose or glucose, mannitol, calcium carbonate, and antidysrhythmic agents. Equipment and supplies to cool the patient are typically stocked with the MH cart, as are tubes for laboratory tests, temperature probe, several sizes of nasogastric (NG) tubes, three-way Foley catheters, and other items required for patient treatment.

# CONCLUSION

The OR is a complex environment with many hazardous substances and equipment. The perioperative nurse, through the activities described in this chapter, plays a crucial role in helping maintain a safe environment for the patient in surgery and for other members of the surgical team.

# REFERENCES

1. Aiken LH: The unfinished patient safety agenda, *AHRQ Morbidity and Mortality Rounds on the Web,* Accessed July 22, 2005, on-line: www.webmm.ahrq.gov/printviewperspective.aspx?perspectiveID=7.
2. Association of periOperative Registered Nurses (AORN): Correct site surgery position statement, *AORN Journal* 81(6):1188-1190, 2005.
3. Association of periOperative Registered Nurses (AORN): *Position Statement on Fire Prevention,* Denver, 2005, The Association.
4. Association of periOperative Registered Nurses (AORN): *Standards, Recommended Practices and Guidelines,* Denver, 2006, The Association.
5. Barron WM and others: Critical success factors for performance improvement programs, *Joint Commission Journal on Quality and Patient Safety* 31(4):220-226, 2005.
6. Berger J: Tips for planning new surgical facilities, *OR Manager* 21(5):20-21, 2005.

7. Beyea SC: Patient advocacy—nurses keeping patients safe, *AORN Journal* 81(5):1046-1047, 2005.
8. Buerhaus PI: Lucian Leape on patient safety in U.S. hospitals, *Journal of Nursing Scholarship* 36(4):366-370, 2004.
9. Burlingame BL: Clinical issues—implant documentation, *AORN Journal* 82(1):109-110, 2005.
10. Burlingame BL: Clinical issues—who is allowed to witness the patient's signature on the consent form? *AORN Journal* 81(1):215-216, 2005.
11. Chart smart: documenting a blood transfusion, *American Journal of Nursing* 35(1):27, 2005.
12. Chart smart: documenting a transfusion reaction, *American Journal of Nursing* 35(3):25, 2005.
13. CMS consent guidelines riles hospitals, *OR Manager* 21(3):7, 2005.
14. Cobb D: Improving patient safety—how can information technology help? *AORN Journal* 80(2):295-302, 2004.
15. College of Surgeons issues statement on retained foreign bodies, *OR Manager E-Bulletin,* Accessed August 8, 2005, on-line: www.ormanager.com.
16. Dunbar C: CMS expands scope of informed consent; hospitals must comply, *OR Management Connections* 1(4):1, 5, 2005.
17. Harman LB: HIPAA—a few years later, *Online Journal of Issues in Nursing* 10(2), 2005.
18. *Health care at the crossroads: strategies for creating and sustaining community-wide emergency preparedness systems,* Chicago, 2003, JCAHO.
19. Helpful solutions for meeting the 2006 National Patient Safety Goals, *Joint Commission Perspectives on Patient Safety* 5(8):2-8, 2005.
20. JCAHO posts new H&P FAQ, *OR Manager* 21(6):32, 2005.
21. JCAHO: *What every health care organization should know about sentinel events,* Chicago, 2005, JCAHO.
22. Leape LL, Berwick DM: Five years after *To Err is Human*—what have we learned, *JAMA* 293:2384-2390, 2005.
23. Lyons EN and others: Front-line safety, *Advance for Nurses* 16(22):38-40, 2004.
24. Mathias JM: Take steps to prevent anesthesia awareness, JCAHO says in alert, *OR Manager* 20(12):1, 8-9, 2004.
25. Mathias JM, Patterson P: New research looks at ergonomic stresses on operating room staff, *OR Manager* 21(7):1, 6-8, 2005.
26. Minnesota takes extra steps on wrong surgery, retained items. *OR Manager* 21(4):1, 18-20, 2003.
27. Miranda F and others: Risk management, *Advance for Nurses* 16(24):19-20, 2004.
28. National Quality Forum: *Serious Reportable Events in Healthcare: A Consensus Report*. Washington, DC, 2002, National Quality Forum.
29. Nelson R: Needlestick injuries: going but not gone? *American Journal of Nursing* 104(11):25-26, 2004.
30. Ringler RD: Bloodless survival, *Nursing Spectrum* 14(7):30-31, 2005.
31. Risk of fire from alcohol-based solutions, *Patient Safety Authority* 2(2):13-14, 2005.
32. Sallady SA: Informed consent, *Nursing 2005* 35(3):22-23, 2005.
33. Schyve PM: Teamwork—the changing nature of professional competence, *Joint Commission Journal on Quality and Patient Safety* 31(4):183-184, 2005.
34. Statement on the prevention of foreign body retention in surgical wounds from the Council on Surgical Patient and Perioperative Safety, *The Surgical Technologist* 37(4):16-19, 2005.
35. Stone PW: IOM data standards for patient safety and nursing, *Applied Nursing Research* 17(3):217-220, 2004.
36. Universal protocol for preventing wrong site, wrong procedure, wrong person surgery, JCAHO, Accessed July 1, 2004, on-line: www.jcaho.org.
37. Yip E: Choices, choices—how to select the right gloves to minimize latex allergy, *Advance for Nurses* 7(10):41-42, 2005.

CHAPTER 3

# Infection Prevention and Control in the Perioperative Setting

LILLIAN H. NICOLETTE

Information and knowledge associated with the fact that bacteria could cause disease that was transmissible were not acquired until the nineteenth century. The concept that there were tiny creatures that could cause disease had existed for thousands of years, however (History box). The work of leaders such as Lister, Semmelweiss, and Nightingale provided the structure for modern infection control practices.[26,57]

Although various forms of surgery were practiced throughout the centuries, the first period of surgical prominence occurred during the 1500s, when a French military surgeon used ligatures to control bleeding when amputations were done. In that same era, Fracastorius, the world's first epidemiologist, proclaimed that diseases were spread in three ways: by direct contact, by handling articles that infected individuals had handled previously, and by transmission from a distance. The seventeenth century brought advances in anatomy, physiology, and medical instrumentation. The most momentous advance was the discovery and fundamental understanding of the anatomy and physiology of human circulation. The invention of the microscope by van Leeuwenhoek also contributed to the evolution of surgery.[55] During the seventeenth century, specialized anatomic research was conducted, and a movement from unsubstantiated theory to more scientific thinking occurred. During the eighteenth century, the close relationship between surgeons and anatomic research continued. The profession of medicine became more organized and more scientific. The first tentative movement toward public health, surgical cleanliness, and surgical statistics occurred during this period. Surgery came to be associated more closely with the field of military medicine.[57]

In the mid-nineteenth century, a new era began, greatly expanding the horizons of surgery. Anesthesia became a beneficial tool of the surgeon, permitting pain-free operations and decreasing the need for speed during surgery. Interest in surgical techniques and the development of new operations flourished. The preservation of life was still not being fulfilled, however. Wound infections were so common that they were considered normal. When pus appeared in the incision, it was believed to be a healthy sign, signaling the beginning of clinical improvement. *Hospitalism* was a term coined by Simpson to describe the array of infections that developed among hospitalized patients. Today these infections are referred to as *health care–associated* (formerly known as *nosocomial*) infections.[57]

## CAUSES OF INFECTION

### Asepsis

The term *asepsis* means the absence of infectious organisms. Asepsis is directed at cleanliness and the elimination of all infectious agents. With the knowledge that bacteria could be destroyed by heat, it was only a short intellectual jump from the antiseptic practice of Lister to current aseptic practice. In 1889 Halstead at the Johns Hopkins Hospital asked the Goodyear Rubber Company to make rubber gloves for his operating room (OR) scrub nurse because she was allergic to the corrosive hand rinse being used. Gradually the idea of wearing gloves to protect the patient emerged. White aprons and gowns replaced the usual morning coat worn by surgeons. Later the color was changed to green for eye comfort. Masks were added in 1897 as microbiologists measured the microbial soil that occurred during conversation. Before the use of masks, many procedures were performed in total silence to decrease the probability of surgical wound infection. Sterilizers completed the transition to a truly aseptic approach to surgery, with all items coming into contact with the patient being sterile. By 1910 use of sterile instruments, gowns, masks, and gloves was standard practice in large university hospitals.[55]

Surgical asepsis is designed to exclude all microbes, whereas medical asepsis is designed to exclude microbes associated with communicable diseases. Practices that restrict microorganisms in the environment and on equipment and supplies and that prevent normal body flora from contaminating the surgical wound are termed *aseptic techniques*. The goal of each aseptic practice is to optimize primary wound healing, prevent surgical infection, and minimize the length of recovery from surgery. For perioperative practitioners, surgical aseptic principles and practices are the foundation for infection control efforts in the perioperative arena.

The human body has three lines of defense to combat infection. The first line of defense consists of *external barriers,* such as the skin and mucous membranes, which are usually impervious to most pathogenic organisms. The second line of defense is the *inflammatory response,* which prevents an invading pathogen from reproducing and possibly involving other tissue. The third line of defense, the *immune response,* is triggered after the inflammatory response. When there is a break in this defense mechanism, the possibility for infection increases. (See Box 3-1 for definitions of terms.)

## HISTORY

**FIRST CENTURY BC**
It was believed that swampy land contained minute animals not visible to the naked eye. These invisible animals were thought to become airborne, enter humans through the mouth, and cause disease.

**450 BC**
Hippocrates, the father of surgery, used wine or boiled water to irrigate wounds, laying the foundation for the rudiments of aseptic technique and infection control.

**SECOND CENTURY**
Galen, a Roman, is reported to have boiled his instruments before use.

**MIDDLE AGES**
The practices of segregating lepers, avoiding areas of pestilence, and isolating the severely ill indicated an awareness that diseases were transmissible.

**SIXTEENTH CENTURY**
Thomas Moffett identified and described lice, fleas, and mites.

**SEVENTEENTH CENTURY**
Antony van Leeuwenhoek, inventor of the microscope, discovered previously unseen creatures in his microscopic observations.

**EIGHTEENTH CENTURY**
Angostino Bassi linked a disease of the silkworm with a fungal parasite; he went on to suggest that many contagious diseases, such as smallpox, typhus, and cholera, were the result of live organisms.

**1850s**
Louis Pasteur, founder of the science of microbiology, theorized that fermentation was caused by particles of living matter so small that they could not be seen but could be carried freely in the air. He referred to these microorganisms as germs and found that heat killed them. The relationship between the fermentation process and the putrefaction of tissue was not understood at that time.

**1860s**
Joseph Lister learned about Pasteur's work, recognized the analogous relationship between the two processes, and set out to investigate the relationship of the germ theory to the process of infection. By 1867 Lister was advocating carbolic acid soaks and sprays for hands, wounds, dressings, sutures, and the OR itself. Although Lister's antiseptic methods and principles were crude and undeveloped, their use resulted in a decrease in surgical mortality from 45% to 15%.

Ignaz Semmelweis made a simple but momentous contribution to infection control by advocating that hands be washed between examinations of patients and that a clean gown be worn for each patient.

Florence Nightingale instigated radical changes in sanitation, resulting in reductions in mortality from contagious diseases.

**MID-NINETEENTH CENTURY**
The pathogenic nature of bacteria was first studied when Casimir Davaine and Pierre Rayer studied the anthrax bacillus.[60]

## Microorganisms That Cause Infection

Microorganisms are living organisms that are too small to be seen with the naked eye. These organisms include bacteria, fungi, protozoa, algae, and viruses. Microorganisms are classified to determine appropriate treatment for an infection. Each organism is assigned two names; the genus is the first name, and the specific epithet (species) is the second. Scientific names can be assigned to organisms in various ways. *Staphylococcus aureus* is a microorganism commonly found on the skin. *Staphylo* describes the clustered arrangement of the cells; *coccus* (Greek *kokkos*, "berry") indicates that they are shaped like spheres. The species *aureus* is Latin for "golden," the color of the colonies of the bacterium. Bacteria cause most surgical site infections (SSIs). Gram-positive cocci, as a group, are the most common cause of SSIs. The organisms most commonly found in postoperative SSIs include staphylococcal, enterococcal, pseudomonal, and streptococcal species. *S. aureus* is the most frequently identified organism.

***Staphylococci.*** Staphylococci are gram-positive cocci. They are facultative anaerobes but grow best under aerobic conditions. Staphylococci can be found in the indigenous flora of the skin and mucous membranes of the nasopharynx, urethra, and vagina. They are resistant to drying, heat, and high salt concentrations.

The two recognized species of staphylococci are *S. aureus* and *S. epidermidis*. Staphylococci are called *coagulase positive* when they are capable of clotting plasma and *coagulase negative* when the plasma clumps them. Coagulase-positive staphylococci are more virulent or pathogenic than coagulase-negative staphylococci. *S. aureus* is hemolytic, parasitic, pathogenic, and coagulase positive. *S. epidermidis* is parasitic, less pathogenic, and coagulase negative. *S. aureus* is a long-recognized cause of surgical site infections. More recently, *S. epidermidis* has been implicated in infections of prosthetic devices.[42]

The skin surface is the most common site of *S. epidermidis*. Thirty percent to 70% of individuals carry staphylococci on their skin. This can lead to contamination of clothing and dispersal of the microorganisms. For no known reason, individuals who are skin carriers of staphylococci differ in the rate at which they shed the microorganisms. There is no obvious difference in hygiene and skin condition between light and heavy shedders, and no other contributing factor is apparent. Heavy shedders seem to be in normal good health.

*S. aureus* infections in hospitals can lead to prolonged hospital stays and may result in death. *S. aureus* has been found in the nasal passages of 30% to 50% of the adult population.[30] Human nasal and throat cavities are the most important reservoirs that continually replenish the external environment. Among OR personnel, *S. aureus* has been found most commonly in the respiratory passages. The potential for patient infection increases greatly as the personnel carrier rate increases. Nasal carriers also may be skin carriers. Carriers usually harbor either coagulase-positive (pathogenic) or coagulase-negative (nonpathogenic) staphylococci; seldom are there both types and rarely more than one strain is identified. Because an individual may be a carrier of staphylococci one day and a noncarrier the next, frequent swab testing of the nose as an infection control measure is impractical. Staphylococci sur-

BOX 3-1

**Definition of Terms**

**Aeration:** Method by which absorbed ethylene oxide (EO) is removed from EO-sterilized items.

**Aerobes:** Microorganisms unable to live and reproduce without access to free atmospheric oxygen, such as *Mycobacterium tuberculosis.*

**Anaerobes:** Bacteria able to survive only in the absence of molecular oxygen, such as *Clostridium perfringens.*

**Biologic indicator:** A sterilization process–monitoring device commercially prepared with a known population of highly resistant spores to test the effectiveness of the sterilization process being used.

**Carrier:** Person who harbors one or more specific pathogens in the absence of discernible clinical disease.

**Contamination:** Presence of pathogenic microorganisms on or in animate or inanimate objects. This term generally is used in reference to a specific object, substance, or tissue that contains microorganisms, especially disease-producing microorganisms.

**Deep incisional SSI:** Infection involving deep soft tissue, fascia, and muscle.

**Facultative bacteria:** Bacteria with enzyme systems that permit them to live and reproduce with or without free oxygen.

**Flash sterilization:** An abbreviated cycle; a sterilization process that is designed for immediate patient use employing the steam sterilization method.

**Infection:** Invasion and multiplication of microorganisms in body tissues causing cellular injury attributable to competitive metabolism, toxins, intracellular replication, or antigen-antibody response.

**Infectious agent:** Parasite (bacterium, spirochete, fungus, virus, or any other type of organism) that is capable of producing infection.

**Health care–associated infections:** Infections acquired by patients during hospitalization, with confirmation of diagnosis by clinical or laboratory evidence. The infective agents may originate from endogenous sources, as from one tissue to another within the patient (self-infection), or from exogenous sources, as acquired from objects or other patients within the hospital (cross-infection). Health care–associated infections, which are often referred to as *hospital-acquired* or *nosocomial infections,* may not become apparent until after the patient has left the hospital.

**Opportunists:** Microorganisms of low virulence and requiring large numbers to produce infection.

**Organ or space SSI:** Infection involving any part of the anatomy other than the incision.

**Parasites:** Microorganisms that reside on or within the bodies of living organisms called *hosts* to find the environment and food they require for life and reproduction. Some microorganisms are *obligatory* parasites, meaning that they depend on their hosts for survival and reproduction. Other microorganisms are *facultative* parasites, meaning that they normally reside on dead matter, but may receive nourishment from living matter. All disease-producing microorganisms are parasites; however, not all parasites are disease producing.

**Pathogen:** Any disease-producing agent or microorganism.

**Primary pathogens:** Highly virulent organisms that are capable of producing disease in low numbers.

**Resident microorganisms:** Organisms that habitually live in the epidermis, deep in the crevices and folds of the skin.

**Source:** Object, substance, or individual from which an infectious agent passes to a host. In some cases, transfer is direct from the reservoir, or source, to the host.

**Superficial SSI:** Infection involving skin and subcutaneous tissue as opposed to deep tissue.

**Surgical-site (incisional) infection (SSI):** Infection involving body-wall layers that have been incised.

**Transient microorganisms:** Organisms with a very short life span, such as the normal flora present on the skin surface of humans. Gram-negative bacteria are transient on the hands of hospital personnel and account for 60% of infections.

vive for long periods in the air, dust, debris, bedding, and clothing. Pathogenic staphylococci grow in the sweat, urine, and tissue and on the skin of humans. They are more difficult to destroy than many other non–spore-forming organisms. Cleanliness of the environment; proper handling and, when appropriate, sterilization of linens and equipment; and adherence to adequate hand hygiene are important controls to prevent transmission of infection.

***Enterococci.*** Enterococci are gram-positive organisms that are found in the normal flora of the gastrointestinal and female genital tracts. These organisms are responsible for many serious health care–associated infections, including surgical site infections, bacterial endocarditis, septicemia, and urinary tract infections (UTIs).[42] In older men who have undergone urinary tract instrumentation, 40% of UTIs are the result of enterococci. This organism also has been implicated in polymicrobial wound infections.[42] Enterococcal infections are most often health care-associated. They are usually seen in patients with co-morbid conditions.

***Pseudomonads.*** The most common aerobic species of pseudomonads pathogenic to humans is *Pseudomonas aeruginosa.* It thrives in moist environments and is found frequently in soil, water, sewage, debris, and air. It also can be found in the normal flora of the skin and intestines. *P. aeruginosa* was considered a microorganism of slight pathogenic power. More recently, it has been found growing in intravenous fluids and soap solutions. Aqueous solutions, such as benzalkonium chloride, support the growth of pseudomonads. *P. aeruginosa* is now known to be associated with many infections in humans, including surgical site infections. *P. aeruginosa* seems to be pathogenic only when it is introduced into areas where normal defenses are absent, when it is superimposed on staphylococcal infection, or when it is present in a mixed infection. It may attack a debilitated patient who has extensive burns or major trauma. The organism is often seen in critical care and burn units. *P. aeruginosa* is resistant to most antimicrobial agents. Other species of pseudomonads have been associated with intravascular cannula infections, as with the use of pressure transducers, or infections in lumens of equipment, such as endoscopes used in gastrointestinal (GI) suites. An important preventive measure is proper environmental sanitation and strict adherence to aseptic technique.

**Streptococci.** Most streptococci are gram-positive, non–spore-forming, facultative microorganisms. They are normally found in the indigenous flora of the upper respiratory, genitourinary, and gastrointestinal tracts. Streptococci are classified as *alpha, beta,* or *gamma* according to chemical factors, biochemical tests, and their action on red blood cells.

Group A streptococci account for most streptococcal infections in humans. Known as the *flesh-eating bacteria* because of their ability to cause necrotizing fasciitis, group A streptococci are of concern because of the sporadic and deadly outbreaks of community-acquired and health care–associated infection.[42] An example is *Streptococcus pyogenes,* which is responsible for most soft tissue infections, otitis media, pharyngitis, impetigo, septicemia, and surgical site infections. Virulent streptococci are more serious invaders than staphylococci. Streptococci tend to involve wide areas of tissue and cause necrosis without localization. Streptococci are usually sensitive to penicillin, whereas staphylococci may not be. Streptococci also occur in mixed infections with other pathogens.

In surgical wounds, streptococci can be introduced into the incision and spread via the lymph vessels and nodes. This spread can result in inflammation, cellulitis, and sometimes suppuration. Streptococcal transmission occurs by droplet transmission and by contamination of the environment. Inhalation of infectious droplets expelled from the nose and mouth of an infected individual is considered direct contact. Indirect contact occurs when infected air and dust from the environment enter a susceptible host. Group A streptococcus can be carried in the nasal passages, anus, or vagina. The upper respiratory tract is not a significant reservoir for microorganisms that cause surgical site infections except in the presence of an acute upper respiratory infection. In several randomized, controlled studies, it was found that surgical wound infection rates are unaffected by the use or nonuse of surgical masks by noninfected individuals during the operative procedure. It is not always possible to know who might be infected, and the use of masks during operative procedures continues to be strongly recommended in the prevention of SSIs. Most bacteria in the OR environment are shed from the skin of perioperative personnel.[19,20]

**Clostridia.** The clostridia bacteria are spore-forming, anaerobic gram-positive bacilli that are quite virulent as a result of the toxins they produce. *Clostridium difficile* is a bacterium in the *Clostridium* genus, which also includes *C. perfringens* (gas gangrene), *C. tetani* (tetanus), and *C. botulinum* (botulism). *C. difficile* refers to an overgrowth of *C. difficile* in the colon that can manifest symptoms of diarrhea, colitis, toxic megacolon, dehydration, colonic perforation, and death. The overgrowth of *C. difficile* in the colon usually results from alterations in the normal flora of the colon, which is associated with the use of antibiotics. For this organism to cause disease, *C. difficile* must already be in the gastrointestinal system. Subsequently, there must be a change in the normal flora of the colon to allow the organism to grow and produce toxins. The two toxins produced are toxin A, which is an enterotoxin causing excretion of large amounts of fluid from the bowel, and toxin B, which is cytotoxic. Toxin B attacks and disintegrates cells of the intestines. Additionally, *C. difficile* produces tissue-degrading enzymes, which produce an inflammatory response within the colon that can result in a spectrum of disease entities.[48,52]

In its spore form, *C. difficile* can withstand drying and heat and may be resistant to many disinfectants. The spores can survive 5 months in the environment. *C. difficile* can be transmitted between individuals and by touching objects contaminated with the organism. In the health care environment, *C. difficile* has been cultured in rooms of infected individuals 40 days postdischarge. *C. difficile* also has been cultured from health care workers' shoes, fingernails, fingertips, and the underside of rings.[48,52]

Several interventions can assist in the prevention of *C. difficile* transmission in the health care environment, including contact precautions, handwashing with antimicrobial soap and water, use of personal protective equipment (PPE), cleaning and disinfection of all surfaces and equipment, and cleaning and disinfection of reusable devices in the perioperative suite. The use of disposable equipment only is recommended for infected patients.[52,67]

**Mycobacterium Tuberculosis.** *Mycobacterium tuberculosis* is a non–spore-forming, nonmotile, aerobic bacillus. Establishment and proliferation of virulent microorganisms within the host produce disease. Tubercle bacilli spread in the host through the lymphatic channels and bloodstream and by way of the alveoli and gastrointestinal tract. These bacilli can infect almost any tissue, including skin, bones, kidney, lymph nodes, intestinal tract, and fallopian tubes.

Tubercle bacilli are transmitted directly by means of discharge from the respiratory tract, by inhalation of droplets expelled during coughing, by kissing, and, less frequently, through the digestive tract. They are transmitted indirectly by means of contaminated articles and particles (e.g., lint, dust, glove powder) floating through the air. *M. tuberculosis* is carried via airborne droplet nuclei when infected persons sneeze, cough, or speak. These nuclei particles are less than 5 microns in size and contain up to three bacteria, allowing them to be kept airborne for a prolonged period.[30] Infection occurs when individuals inhale these infected droplet nuclei. The droplet nuclei travel through the nasal passages, upper respiratory tract, and bronchi to reach the lung alveoli, where they are taken up by macrophages and spread throughout the body.

Generally 2 to 10 weeks after initial infection, an immune response limits additional multiplication and spread of the bacilli. Some of the bacilli can remain dormant for many years, however, a condition referred to as *latent tuberculosis infection.* Individuals with latent tuberculosis usually have positive purified protein derivative (PPD) results, but they exhibit none of the symptoms of active tuberculosis (TB) and are considered noninfectious. The probability that a person who is exposed to *M. tuberculosis* will become *infected* depends on the concentration of infectious droplet nuclei and the duration of exposure.[1] When infected, an individual has approximately a 10% risk of developing active TB in his or her lifetime. The risk is greatest during the first 2 years after initial exposure. In individuals with compromised immune systems, there is a higher risk that latent tuberculosis will progress into active tuberculosis.

**Viruses.** Viruses are classified as small particles, rather than living cells, because viruses have no metabolic activity and must receive all sustenance for survival from a host cell. Viral pathogens are transmitted via the oral and respiratory tracts (e.g., poxvirus, rhinovirus), the intestinal and urinary tracts (e.g., poliovirus, hepatitis A virus [HAV], hepatitis E virus [HEV]), and the genital tract (e.g., herpes simplex 2, human immunodeficiency virus [HIV]) and through blood and some blood products (e.g., HIV, hepatitis B virus [HBV], hepatitis C virus [HCV], hepatitis D virus [HDV], and others). Some viruses have multiple routes of transmission.

When a virus invades a host cell, it combines with the host cell's nucleic acid (deoxyribonucleic acid [DNA] or ribonucleic acid [RNA]) and reprograms the host cell metabolism to accommodate virus replication. Virus replication stimulates antibody defense in the host. The presence of viruses may be detected by identification of the virus-specific antibodies that are produced by the infected individual's immune system, by detection of the antigens elaborated by the virus and present in the blood, or by growing of a culture of the virus itself. Detection of virus-specific antibodies or antigens is termed *seropositivity,* or *seroconversion.* Viruses are susceptible to destruction by high-level disinfection—a process that destroys most disease-producing microorganisms.

**HEPATITIS.** Hepatitis is a frequently reported infectious disease in the United States, with six identified strains (A through E and G). HAV is the causative agent of what is referred to as *infectious hepatitis*. HAV is spread through the fecal-oral route and can be prevented by proper hand hygiene. HAV constitutes slightly less than half of all hepatitis cases reported in the United States. Vaccination is available for HAV.

HBV is the causative agent for what is sometimes referred to as *serum hepatitis*. This worldwide virus has reached near-epidemic levels but is preventable via vaccination and the strict use of Universal Precautions. HBV can be transmitted by blood or body fluids, such as serum, saliva, semen, and vaginal fluids. It has an incubation period of 6 weeks to 4 months, depending on the amount of inoculum received. Almost 30% of infected individuals are asymptomatic; individuals with symptoms experience fatigue, abdominal pain, nausea, vomiting, and jaundice. Chronic hepatitis infection leads to progressive liver disease and possible death and is a leading cause of liver transplants. HBV vaccine is recommended, by government regulation, for health care workers who may be exposed to blood and body fluids. Postexposure prophylaxis for percutaneous or permucosal exposure to HBV depends on the vaccination status of the health care worker. The Occupational Safety and Health Administration (OSHA) mandates that all health care workers report blood and body fluid exposures, and perioperative personnel should follow the institutional protocol for exposure reporting.

HCV transmission is most often associated with direct exposure to blood or other infectious materials. Currently there is no vaccine for the prevention of HCV. Individuals who contract HCV infection are prone to develop chronic infection. A high proportion of this population is asymptomatic and develops chronic liver disease, such as cirrhosis, hepatocellular carcinoma, and portal hypertension. As with HBV, a small proportion of individuals infected with HCV die. Prevention of HCV requires strict use of Universal Precautions, implementation of and adherence to sharps safety programs, compliance with exposure reporting protocols, and completion of a post-exposure treatment plan. It is crucial that education of all perioperative personnel occur about the risk for and prevention of all bloodborne infections, including HCV. These education sessions should be conducted routinely and updated for accuracy of information.

HDV requires the co-infection of HBV. HDV is transmitted by blood and body fluids. Individuals immunized against HBV have protection against contracting HDV. HDV is suspected when individuals present with HBV superinfection. Treatment is supportive for acute infections. With chronic HDV infections, antiviral therapies and liver transplants may be required.

HEV is spread by the fecal-oral route. HEV is similar to HAV in the transmission and disease process. Most outbreaks have occurred in developing countries, where fecally contaminated water was found to be the source for these outbreaks. No vaccine is available for the prevention of HEV. Prevention is similar to that for HAV, with the use of hand hygiene. Treatment is supportive. Frequency of HEV in the United States is low.

Hepatitis G virus is a bloodborne pathogen, with a comparable rate of infection as that of HCV in units of banked blood. It is spread in a manner similar to HBV and HCV by percutaneous or permucosal exposure. There is no vaccine to prevent hepatitis G virus infection. Similar to HBV and HCV, prudent and consistent use of barrier protection (e.g., standard precautions) is recommended. There are no data yet on the chronic nature of this viral disease.

HIV is a latent virus that attacks the immune system by destroying T helper lymphocytes. The period from HIV exposure to actual disease has been reported to be 12 years or longer. During this time, the individual is a carrier of the virus.[29] HIV has been isolated from all body fluids (e.g., blood, semen, vaginal secretions, saliva, tears, breast milk, cerebrospinal fluid, amniotic fluid, and urine) of infected individuals. Transmission of HIV can occur by percutaneous injury (e.g., a needle stick or cut with a sharp instrument) or mucous membrane or nonintact skin exposure (e.g., exposed skin that is abraded) to blood, tissue, or other body fluids that are potentially infectious. The Centers for Disease Control and Prevention (CDC) estimates that at least 5000 needle-stick exposures to HIV occur annually in the United States.[42] If an exposure incident occurs, appropriate postexposure management should take place as a part of workplace safety. The source patient should be informed of the incident. Serology testing should be done according to institutional policy and governmental requirements. Policies should be established for instances in which source patient consent cannot be obtained. The health care worker should be counseled about the risk of infection, and he or she should be evaluated clinically and serologically for evidence of HIV infection as soon as possible after exposure. Postexposure prophylaxis (PEP) regimens should be supervised by an expert in the management of exposures; follow-up should be provided for adherence to PEP; and adverse events, including seroconversion, should be monitored. Timely postexposure management and administration is important, and an exposure incident should be treated as an urgent medical condition.

## Drug-Resistant Bacteria: Emerging and Resurging Organisms

***Historical Perspective.*** In 1935 sulfonamides were introduced, resulting in a cure for staphylococcal and streptococcal infections. In the 1940s during World War II, the introduction of penicillin was even more significant.[55] Streptomycin was discovered in the mid- to late 1940s.[42] When the concept of using antibiotics before surgery to prevent infection after surgery was introduced, the practice of surgery flourished with "miracle" drugs to prevent septicemia and cure infections, many of which had proved fatal up until this time.[42,55]

In the mid-1940s, strains of previously susceptible microorganisms began showing resistance to penicillin. In the 1950s, severe epidemics of staphylococcal infections in pediatric and surgical units occurred in Europe and the United States.[57] Strains of *S. aureus* that were resistant to penicillin, tetracycline, streptomycin, and erythromycin were isolated. At the same time, resistant strains of gram-negative bacteria, such as *Klebsiella, Proteus,* and *Pseudomonas,* emerged as leading causes of health care–associated infections.[42,55]

During the 1960s, cephalosporin and semisynthetic penicillins were developed, and it was believed that the problem of health care–associated infections was solved. Many gram-negative bacteria were found to be susceptible to these new drugs. By the late 1970s, however, strains of *S. aureus* resistant to penicillin, methicillin, cephalosporins, aminoglycosides, clindamycin, erythromycin, and other antibiotics were isolated in hospital outbreaks of infection. This situation led to the development of new antibiotics, including carbapenems, cephamycins, and fluoroquinolones. These broad-spectrum antimicrobials were bactericidal at low concentrations and led to a false sense of euphoria during the 1980s, when it was believed that, at last, resistance to these antimicrobials would be impossible.[42]

In the 1990s, it became evident that the potential for resistance to any and all antimicrobials existed as health care–associated outbreaks of multidrug-resistant tuberculosis (MDR-TB) began to occur. Significant outbreaks of methicillin-resistant *S. aureus* (MRSA) (Surgical Pharmacology) and vancomycin-resistant *Enterococcus faecalis* (VRE) also occurred in the 1990s. In some cases, organisms seem to acquire resistance almost immediately on exposure to the particular antibiotic. As fewer new antimicrobial drugs are being developed by the pharmaceutical industry, many consider the 1990s to be the beginning of the postantibiotic era.[42]

***Mechanisms of Resistance.*** Similar to their unwilling human hosts, pathogenic bacteria have an instinct to survive. When faced with an antimicrobial attack, they assemble their defensive resources. These microorganisms have the remarkable capability to incapacitate the threatening antibiotic and to mutate and outwit the most lethal clinical weapons. Although carrying only a single chromosome, bacteria by nature have extra minichromosomes called *plasmids.* These plasmids are hearty, and some may survive even the most aggressive antibiotic attack. Surviving plasmids are resistant and reproduce in kind, creating dominant organisms within the host. In addition, incompletely or ineffectively treated infections create the potential for reinfection with resistant organisms.[1,26,42]

Microbial resistance can be divided into three categories: (1) presence of a naturally resistant strain of an organism before any drugs are administered, (2) acquisition of a drug-resistant strain from an external source, and (3) drug resistance from treatment-related causes. Occurrence of naturally resistant strains of organisms without any exposure to drugs can occur by intrinsic resistance, genetic mutation, or transfer of genetic material. Some microorganisms possess genes that make them resistant to an antibiotic. These genes may always be present in the microorganism but remain in an inactive stage until challenged by an antibiotic. Genetic mutation can occur spontaneously in the course of rapid multiplication of the microbe. These antibiotic-resistant mutants reproduce

## SURGICAL PHARMACOLOGY

### Treating Methicillin-Resistant *Staphylococcus aureus*

In the past, vancomycin was the only alternative for treating methicillin-resistant *Staphylococcus aureus* (MRSA). With the increased use of vancomycin, however, strains of *S. aureus* with reduced susceptibility to vancomycin began to appear. Newer antibiotics include daptomycin, linezolid, teicoplanin, and quinupristin-dalfopristin. Of these, linezolid has excellent activity against vancomycin-intermediate and vancomycin-resistant *Staphylococcus* and is approved for skin and soft tissue infection and for pneumonia caused by MRSA.

**LINEZOLID (ZYVOX): NURSING CONSIDERATIONS**

**Assessment**

Assess central nervous system symptoms: headache, dizziness
Monitor liver function studies: aspartate aminotransferase (AST), alanine aminotransferase (ALT)
Monitor allergic reactions: fever, flushing, rash, urticaria, pruritus
Assess for pseudomembranous colitis: severe diarrhea, cramping
Monitor complete blood count (CBC) weekly, assess for myelosuppression (anemia, leukopenia, pancytopenia, thrombocytopenia)

**Nursing Diagnoses**

Infection, risk for (uses)
Knowledge, deficient (teaching)

**Implementation**

*PO route:* Store reconstituted oral suspension at room temperature, use within 3 weeks
*IV route:* Give over 30-120 minutes; do not use intravenous infusion bag in series connections, do not use with additives in solution; do not use with another drug, administer separately

**Patient Family Education**

Advise patient if dizziness occurs to ambulate and perform activities with assistance
Advise patient to complete full course of drug therapy
Advise patient to contact prescriber if adverse reaction occurs
Advise patient to avoid large amounts of tyramine-containing foods (give list)

Data from Skidmore-Roth L: *Mosby's drug guide for nurses,* ed 6, St Louis, 2005, Elsevier Mosby; Stevens DL: Infections due to gram-positive cocci, *What's New in ACP Medicine* 27(9), September 2004 (on-line journal www.acpmedicine.com).

within the host. New genetic material also can be transferred into bacteria by means of free DNA that contains resistant genes.[1,42]

Introduction of drug-resistant microorganisms can occur through a person or an inanimate object. Bacteria become mobile and accessible to humans on the hands or clothing of care providers, through instruments and procedures, or through food. Resistant microorganisms may travel from distant lands by means of infected travelers. Surgical instruments that have been ineffectively cleaned and processed can contribute to the spread of resistant organisms. Use of antibiotics in agriculture and in animal feed products also has contributed to the development of resistant organisms. When the food is ingested, resistant genes may be spread to humans.[1,26,42]

Drug resistance from treatment-related causes is often the result of misuse (e.g., incorrect use, overuse, or underuse) of antibiotics. It is believed that 50% of all antibiotic use in the United States is characterized by misuse in one form or another, and efforts to reduce surgical site infections include appropriate prophylactic antibiotic use in surgical patients (Best Practice). It is estimated that half of all prescriptions written are not needed.[42] During antibiotic therapy, the patient may have had a few resistant organisms. By natural selection, that is, as the susceptible organisms are killed, the resistant organisms multiply and become predominant. Inadequate drug therapy may contribute to the phenomenon and may be the fault of the patient, the provider, or both. Failure to perform sensitivity testing and prescription of an inappropriate drug can be a contributing factor. Inappropriate dosing also can contribute to resistance. If the patient is noncompliant with the prescribed regimen or discontinues the drug prematurely, he or she may be contributing to drug resistance.[42]

### *Perioperative Considerations*

**METHICILLIN-RESISTANT *STAPHYLOCOCCUS AUREUS*.** MRSA infections, a serious public health problem in the United States since the mid-1970s, occur in surgical patients with increasing frequency. Common sites in which MRSA can be found include wounds (e.g., burns, surgical incisions, abrasions), chest tubes, intravenous catheter tips, intraabdominal

## BEST PRACTICE

### Prevention of Surgical Site Infections: Surgical Care Improvement Project

Surgical site infections (SSIs) occur in 2% to 5% of clean, nonabdominal surgical procedures and in 20% of intraabdominal procedures. Some studies show even higher infection rates, suggesting that SSIs account for 14% to 16% of all hospital-acquired infections and are among the most common complications of surgical patient care. SSIs increase morbidity and consume additional resources. Infectious complications result in an increased median hospital stay of 2.8 days and an increased cost of $1398. Medicare spent an estimated $326.7 billion on hospital-acquired infections in 2005.

SSIs include superficial incisions, deep incisional, and organ/space infections. These have been defined in the Centers for Disease Control Prevention (CDC) National Nosocomial Infections Surveillance (NNIS) System and are recognized worldwide. Surgical patients often receive some form of antibiotic prophylaxis. Studies indicate that in 25% to 50% of cases antibiotic selection, timing of administration, or duration of use is inappropriate. The Surgical Care Improvement Project (SCIP) is a partnership of organizations committed to improving surgical patient care. In 2005 the SCIP launched a multiyear campaign to reduce surgical complications by 25% in 2010. One of the targeted areas is SSI.

**BEST PRACTICES IDENTIFIED BY SURGICAL CARE IMPROVEMENT PROJECT TO REDUCE SURGICAL SITE INFECTIONS**

Although some surgical complications are unavoidable, surgical care can be improved through better adherence to evidence-based practice recommendations. Research shows that delivering antibiotics to a patient within 1 hour of beginning surgery can dramatically decrease SSI rates, yet this practice is not universal.

Numerous more recent, successful projects have shown that institutional implementation of evidence-based practices can have a significant impact on surgical complications.

- Application of the National Surgical Quality Improvement Program (NSQIP) within the Veterans Health Administration resulted in a 27% reduction in mortality related to surgery.
- Hospitals participating in the CDC and NNIS have shown reductions of 44% in device-associated infection rates and SSI rates.
- The national network of Medicare quality improvement organizations (QIOs), working under contract to Centers for Medicare and Medicaid Services (CMS), conducted a surgical infection prevention collaborative that effectively reduced SSI by 27% at 56 centers across the United States.

The purpose of antibiotic prophylaxis is to reduce intraoperative microbial contamination sufficiently to preclude microbial presence from overwhelming host defenses and causing infection. The antimicrobial used should be safe, inexpensive, and bactericidal against a broad spectrum of the most probable contaminants for the procedure. Key measures identified in the SCIP to reduce surgical site infections are the following:

- Administer a prophylactic antibiotic within 1 hour before the incision.
- Ensure that the bactericidal concentration of antibiotic in the serum and tissues is maintained until a few hours after the incision is closed.
- Stop prophylactic antibiotics within 24 hours after surgery (48 hours for cardiac surgery).
- Cardiac surgical patients should have their 6 AM postoperative glucose level controlled.
- Remove hair at the surgical site by an appropriate method.
- Ensure that patients undergoing colorectal surgery achieve immediate postoperative normothermia.

Modified from Dimick JB and others: National Surgical Quality Improvement Project, *Journal of the American College of Surgeons* 199:531-537, 2004; Goldstein J: Cost of infections staggering, *The Philadelphia Inquirer,* November 19, 2005; Centers for Disease Control and Prevention National Nosocomial Infections Surveillance System. Accessed December 1, 2005, on-line: www.cdc.gov/ncidod/hip/SURVEILL/NNIS.HTM; Surgical Care Improvement Project—A National Quality Partnership. Accessed December 1, 2005, on-line: www.medqic.org/scip. Other resources with links to other tools, including success stories on improving the antibiotic process and resources from the CMS Surgical Infection Prevention Collaborative are available at: www.ihi.org/IHI/programs/campaing/campaign.htm.

abscesses, nasal passages, and the groin. *S. aureus* is one of the most frequently isolated organisms in postoperative surgical site infections. Surgical patients at risk for the development of MRSA infection include high-risk patients with underlying disease, patients who have a prolonged hospitalization, patients who have had previous antimicrobial therapy, patients who receive care in an intensive care unit, and patients who have been in proximity to another patient colonized with MRSA.[24] Patients may present with unrecognized colonization or become infected by caregivers who carry MRSA in their nose or on their skin. The ambient environment is rarely a source of MRSA except for some burn units.[42]

The primary mode of transmission for MRSA is most likely direct contact transmission from the hands of health care personnel. The organism has been recovered from the hands of personnel after they touched contaminated material and before they washed their hands. It also has been shown that MRSA can be carried in the nares of personnel and transferred to patients by hand contact.[42] The importance of handwashing cannot be overemphasized.

Because MRSA is transmitted by contact, perioperative protocols to be used when caring for these patients should include the following:

- Segregate the patient, using Contact Precaution guidelines.
- Wear a gown and gloves whenever there is potential for contact with contaminated fluids or materials.
- Implement strict hand hygiene practices.
- Limit patient transportation to essential movement only.
- Clean and disinfect patient-care equipment as close as possible to the time of use.[26]

In health care facilities, MRSA causes serious and sometimes fatal infections, including necrotizing fasciitis. MRSA resists almost every antibiotic except intravenous vancomycin. In 2005 the U.S. Food and Drug Administration (FDA) approved a new treatment for hospital patients with serious bacterial infections, including infections caused by MRSA. The drug tigecycline (Tygacil) is an antibiotic related to the tetracycline family. This drug is formulated to retain activity against some bacteria that are resistant to tetracyclines.[54]

VANCOMYCIN-RESISTANT ENTEROCOCCI. Enterococci are intrinsically resistant to cephalosporins, semisynthetic penicillins, and clindamycin. Some strains also have acquired resistance to erythromycin, chloramphenicol, tetracycline, fluoroquinolones, and vancomycin.[42] The incidence of vancomycin-resistant enterococci (VRE) infections in the United States has increased rapidly in recent years. Patients at greatest risk of VRE infection are patients with a critical care unit stay, intraabdominal or cardiothoracic surgical procedures, presence of indwelling central venous catheters, presence of urinary catheters, extended hospital stays, multiple antimicrobial therapies, and proximity to infected individuals. Because the enterococcal plasmid carrying the resistant gene can be transferred to organisms such as *S. aureus,* VRE infections are of serious concern.[4,42]

The CDC has issued recommendations regarding the use of vancomycin, including identifying situations in which vancomycin should and should not be used; establishing education programs for practitioners, susceptibility testing, isolation procedures, and dedication of equipment and devices; verifying procedures for cleaning and disinfecting the environment; and minimizing movement of personnel between patients with and without VRE.[28]

VRE can be transmitted directly from patient to patient or through the hands of health care providers or through contact with contaminated environmental surfaces and equipment used for patient care.[83] As with MRSA, Contact Precautions should be followed when caring for patients infected with VRE. Perioperative protocols are similar to protocols for MRSA patients and should include the following:

- Segregate patients, using Contact Precaution guidelines.
- Wear gown and gloves when in contact with contaminated materials.
- Implement strict hand hygiene practices.
- Limit patient transportation to essential movement only.
- Clean and disinfect patient-care equipment as close as possible to the time of use.[12,26]

Germicides commonly used for cleaning and disinfecting in hospitals are effective against VRE. Isopropyl alcohol and sodium hypochlorite (bleach) are highly effective. With a 10-minute exposure time, some phenolic and some quaternary ammonium compounds also are effective. These are less effective at shorter exposure times. Hydrogen peroxide has been found to be ineffective.[26] No relationship seems to exist between microbial resistance to antibiotics and increased resistance to germicides.[54] Perioperative personnel should routinely consult the manufacturer's written instructions and follow Environmental Protection Agency (EPA) recommendations when selecting germicides for surface cleaning.

VANCOMYCIN–INTERMEDIATE RESISTANT *STAPHYLOCOCCUS AUREUS.* In 1996 the first known incidence of vancomycin–intermediate resistant *S. aureus* (VISA) occurred in Japan when the organism was isolated from a surgical site infection and undrained abscess. Treatment with vancomycin for 29 days left the condition unchanged. Further treatment with other antibiotic agents and abscess drainage led to patient recovery.[70] In 1997 the first occurrence of the organism was seen in the United States. A patient having been treated with vancomycin for multiple episodes of peritoneal MRSA developed bacterial strains moderately resistant to vancomycin, the treatment of choice for MRSA. Although the organism showed only intermediate levels of resistance, the CDC viewed this occurrence as an early warning that strains of *S. aureus* with full resistance to vancomycin may emerge.[30]

MULTIDRUG-RESISTANT *MYCOBACTERIUM TUBERCULOSIS.* Outbreaks of TB have heightened concern about health care–associated transmission of this disease. The incidence of MDR-TB is increasing in the United States. Transmission is most likely to occur from patients with unrecognized pulmonary or laryngeal tuberculosis. Populations at greatest risk of developing TB or MDR-TB are the elderly, indigent, minorities, immigrants from countries where TB and MDR-TB are prevalent, and HIV-infected individuals.[26,27] Transmission also occurs as a result of procedures such as bronchoscopy, endotracheal intubation, endotracheal suctioning, and open abscess irrigation or from inadequate equipment disinfection.

The CDC *Guidelines for Preventing the Transmission of* Mycobacterium tuberculosis *in Health Care Facilities*[27] emphasize the following:

- Importance of control measures, including engineering controls and personal respiratory protection, including fit-tested, personal respirators when indicated
- Use of risk assessment to develop a tuberculosis-control plan

- Early detection and treatment of patients with tuberculosis
- Screening programs for health care workers
- Training and education for health care workers
- Evaluation of the tuberculosis-control program

**CREUTZFELDT-JAKOB DISEASE.** Creutzfeldt-Jakob disease (CJD) is an infectious, neurodegenerative, and fatal disease of the central nervous system.[35] CJD is one of a group of encephalopathies known as *transmissible spongiform encephalopathies (TSEs)*. Other human forms of TSE are Gerstmann-Sträussler-Scheinker syndrome and *new variant CJD (nvCJD)* or *variant CJD (vCJD)*.[72]

CJD is considered a "slow viral infection" caused by a self-replicating protein known as a *prion*.[46] Prions are a unique class of organisms that have no detectable DNA or RNA.[79] These small, proteinaceous agents are abnormal isoforms of normal cellular proteins. The incubation period for CJD varies from months to years to decades. Symptoms include rapidly progressing dementia, memory loss, rapid physical and mental deterioration, and a distinctive electroencephalogram reading. Positive diagnosis can be made only by direct examination of affected brain tissue. Most cases occur randomly and for unknown reasons when the patient is between 50 and 75 years old. The average duration of illness after the patient becomes symptomatic is 6 months, always ending in death. In contrast, vCJD has an earlier onset (between 18 and 41 years of age). Patients exhibit initial psychiatric symptoms and then neurologic symptoms differing from those of CJD, and the course of illness averages 14 months. The disease is always fatal.[72] According to the CDC, there is strong epidemiologic and laboratory evidence for a causal association between vCJD and bovine spongiform encephalopathy (also known as *mad cow disease*).

CJD can be familial (i.e., inherited in the form of a mutant gene) or sporadic (no family history and no known source of transmission). Approximately 90% of cases are sporadic. Only about 1% of cases result from person-to-person transmission, and those are primarily the result of iatrogenic (medically related) exposure. Exposures have occurred via transplantation of contaminated central nervous system tissue, such as dura mater or corneas; from injections of pituitary hormone extracts; and by use of contaminated surgical instruments or stereotactic depth electrodes.[35]

CJD and other TSEs are unusually resistant to conventional chemical and physical decontamination methods. The causative prions are resistant to steam autoclaving, dry heat, ethylene oxide gas, and chemical disinfection with formaldehyde or glutaraldehyde as normally used in the health care environment.[85] Glutaraldehyde and formaldehyde act as fixatives, causing the prions to become more stable and less susceptible to normal sterilization/disinfection protocols. Special protocols for instrument care after exposure to prions should be followed.[46] Some institutions use disposable instrument sets for diagnostic brain biopsies to rule out CJD or TSE. A process using radiofrequency (RF) gas plasma to eliminate prions that cause CJD from surgical instruments has been developed. The technique removed contamination to levels 1000 times lower than that achieved by existing decontamination methods.[22,56] Other processes being investigated include the use of an alkaline cleaning agent before sterilization and vaporized hydrogen peroxide (VHP) sterilization. Protocols for dealing with CJD are evolving as researchers learn more about prions and their destruction. Table 3-1 lists options from which an acceptable protocol for care of instruments and equipment exposed to the CJD prion can be developed.

## CONTROLLING INFECTION

Infection control practices should focus on prevention. Transmission of infection involves a chain of events, including presence of a pathogenic agent, reservoir, portal of exit, transmission, portal of entry, and host susceptibility. Prevention occurs when there is a break in the chain of transmission. Infection control practices involve personal and administrative measures. Personal measures should include fitness for work and application of aseptic principles. Administrative measures should include provision of adequate physical facilities, appropriate surgical supplies, and operational controls in the perioperative area.

### Universal, Standard, and Transmission-Based Precautions

***Universal Precautions.*** In 1985, in response to the growing number of individuals testing positive for HIV, the CDC published recommendations for the use of Universal Precautions.[29] Reports of hospital personnel becoming infected with HIV after a needle stick or skin exposure to a patient's blood created an urgent need for new and better measures to protect personnel from patient transmission of infection. With knowledge that many patients with bloodborne infections are undiagnosed, Universal Precautions, for the first time, placed emphasis on applying Blood and Body Fluid Precautions (one of the categories in the 1993 *Guidelines for Isolation Precautions in Hospitals*) universally to all individuals regardless of their presumed infection status.[26] Universal precautions expanded the Blood and Body Fluid Precautions by recommending masks and eye protection to prevent mucous membrane exposures in addition to the routine use of barrier protection, such as gowns and gloves. Universal Precautions also emphasized the prevention of needle-stick injuries and the use of ventilation devices when resuscitation was done. The CDC continued to recommend the use of Universal Precautions until 1987, when a new system of isolation called *Body Substance Isolation* (BSI) was proposed. BSI directed isolation of *all* moist and potentially infectious body substances (e.g., blood, feces, urine, sputum, saliva, wound drainage, other body fluids) for all individuals regardless of their infection status. This was accomplished primarily with the use of gowns and gloves. Because of the similarities yet differences between Universal Precautions and BSI, confusion reigned.

OSHA issued a rule for Occupational Exposure to Bloodborne Pathogens.[63] This document was based on the concept of Universal Precautions. OSHA subsequently revised its final rule to include a special focus on needle stick and other percutaneous exposures to bloodborne pathogens.[63] The revised rule addressed "sharps with engineered sharps injury protections" (nonneedle sharps or needle devices with built-in safety features to reduce the potential for injury) and "needleless systems" (alternative delivery devices using blunt cannulae, catheter ports or connectors, or other nonneedle devices). Other revisions focus on revision and updating of exposure control plans, solicitation of employee input, and improved record keeping. The following is a summary of the require-

**TABLE 3-1**

## Care of Items Exposed to the Creutzfeldt-Jakob Disease Prion

| Tissue Infectivity | Item/Device (Using Spaulding Classification System)[75] | Cleanable | Heat/ Moisture Stable | Disposition |
|---|---|---|---|---|
| High infectivity | Critical/semicritical instruments/devices | If easily cleaned | If yes | 1. Thoroughly clean with detergent germicide<br>2. Autoclave at 134°C (272°F) immersed in water in prevacuum sterilizer for 18 minutes (extended cycle) *or*<br>3. Autoclave instruments immersed in water at 121°C (250°F) in gravity sterilizer for 20 minutes; 60 minutes if not immersed in water *or*<br>4. Immerse in 1N NaOH (1 normal sodium hydroxide) for 60 minutes at room temperature. After 60 minutes, remove items from NaOH, rinse, and steam sterilize at 121°C (250°F) in gravity sterilizer for 30 minutes<br>5. After the process as selected from the above, prepare instruments in the usual fashion and sterilize for future use |
| | | | If no | Discard |
| | Critical/semicritical instruments/devices | If difficult to clean | If yes | 1. Discard *or*<br>2. Decontaminate initially by:<br>a. Autoclaving at 134°C (272°F) in prevacuum sterilizer for 18 minutes *or*<br>b. Autoclaving at 121°C (250°F) in gravity sterilizer for 60 minutes *or*<br>c. Immersing in 1N NaOH for 60 minutes at room temperature. After 60 minutes, remove items from NaOH, rinse, and steam sterilize at 121°C (250°F) in gravity sterilizer for 30 minutes<br>3. After initial decontamination as above, thoroughly clean, wrap, and sterilize by conventional methods for future use |
| | | | If no | Discard |
| | Critical/semicritical instruments/devices | If impossible to clean | NA | Discard |
| | Noncritical instruments/devices | If cleanable | NA | 1. Clean according to routine procedures<br>2. Disinfect with a 1:10 dilution of sodium hypochlorite or 1N NaOH, according to which solution would be least damaging to the items<br>3. Continue processing according to routine procedures |
| | | Noncleanable | NA | Discard |
| | Environmental surfaces | NA | NA | 1. Cover surface with disposable, impermeable material<br>2. Incinerate material after use<br>3. Disinfect surface with 1:10 dilution of sodium hypochlorite (bleach)<br>4. Wipe entire surface using routine facility decontamination procedures for surface decontamination |
| Medium/low/no infectivity | Critical/semicritical/noncritical instruments/devices | Cleanable | NA | 1. Clean, disinfect, or sterilize according to routine procedures |
| | | Noncleanable | NA | Discard |
| | Environmental surfaces | NA | NA | 1. Cover surface with disposable, impermeable material<br>2. Dispose of material according to facility policy<br>3. Disinfect surface with OSHA-recommended agent for decontamination of blood-contaminated surfaces (e.g., 1:10 or 1:100 dilution of sodium hypochlorite) |

*NA,* not applicable; *OSHA,* Occupational Safety and Health Administration.

Data from Favaro MS, Bond WW: Chemical disinfection of medical and surgical materials. In Block SS, editor: *Disinfection, sterilization, and preservation,* ed 5, Philadelphia, 2001, Lippincott Williams & Wilkins, pp. 910-913; New clues on how to inactivate prions, *OR Manager* 20(11):23, 2004; Rutala WA, Weber DJ: Creutzfeldt-Jakob disease: recommendations for disinfection and sterilization, *Clinical Infectious Diseases* 32(9):1348-1349, 2001; World Health Organization Department of Communicable Disease Surveillance and Response, *WHO Infection Control Guidelines for Transmissible Spongiform Encephalopathies.* Access on-line: www.who.int/site-search/data-who-hq-live/search.shtml.

ments of the Final Rule: Occupational Exposure to Bloodborne Pathogens:

1. Each facility must develop and implement an exposure control plan that defines exposure and implements the requirements of the final rule. This plan is to be reviewed and revised annually with information provided to all employees. The plan must reflect changes in available technology to reduce exposure to bloodborne pathogens and implementation of appropriate technology to that end. Nonmanagerial employee input must be solicited in selecting technology to be implemented in the practice setting.
2. Engineering and work practice controls must be used to eliminate or minimize employee exposure. Examples follow:
   a. The employer must provide everything necessary for proper hand hygiene.
   b. Contaminated needles must not be recapped or removed unless such action is required by a specific medical procedure. Such recapping or removal must be accomplished by the use of a mechanical device or one-handed technique.
   c. A clamp or other mechanical device should be used to disassemble a knife blade and handle.
   d. Sharps are to be placed in labeled or color-coded, puncture-resistant, leak-proof containers for disposal.
   e. Specimens of blood or body fluids must be placed in containers that prevent leakage and are labeled or color-coded. Warning labels must be affixed to containers of regulated waste, refrigerators and freezers containing blood or potentially infectious material, and other containers used to transport blood or potentially infectious material (Figure 3-1). The labels must be fluorescent orange or orange-red.
   f. Food and drink are not to be kept in the same storage area where blood or other potentially infectious materials are present.
   g. PPE must be provided by the employer at no cost to the employee. Appropriate PPE shall include but is not limited to gloves, gowns, face shields or masks, and eye protection. Protective eyewear must have solid side shields. Gloves are to be worn when contact with blood or body fluids is anticipated. Disposable gloves are to be replaced as soon as possible after contamination occurs. Disposable gloves are not to be washed or decontaminated for reuse. Some facilities may have educational signs posted to assist employees in recognition of appropriate PPE (Figure 3-2).
   h. Signs must be posted at the entrance to work areas of potential contamination. These signs are to bear the biohazard legend with the following information: name of infectious agent, special requirements for entering the area, and name and telephone number of the responsible individual.
   i. Housekeeping provisions are to ensure that the workplace is maintained in a clean and sanitary condition. A written schedule for cleaning and a method of decontamination must be established. All equipment and working surfaces must be cleaned and decontaminated after contact with blood or other potentially infectious materials.
   j. Contaminated laundry must be placed in a labeled or color-coded container that is recognized by all employees.
   k. All employees are to receive education and training about safe handling of hazardous substances and materials. Information must be provided to all occupationally exposed employees at no cost to them. Individuals must receive training at the time of employment and annually thereafter. Individual employee training records are to be maintained by the employer for the duration of employment plus 30 years. The health care worker is highly encouraged to receive the HBV vaccine after receiving the required information about the risk of exposure and about the vaccine. If the employee chooses not to accept the vaccination, the employer must have the employee sign a letter of declination.
   l. Employees should report all exposures to blood and body fluids for postexposure evaluation.[63]
   m. Employers who are required to maintain a log of occupational injuries and illnesses must maintain a sharps injury log that acts as a tool for identifying high-risk practice areas and for evaluating various devices in use. This log must protect the confidentiality of the injured employee. Log information should include the type and brand of the device, the practice area in which the injury occurred, and an explanation of how the incident occurred.

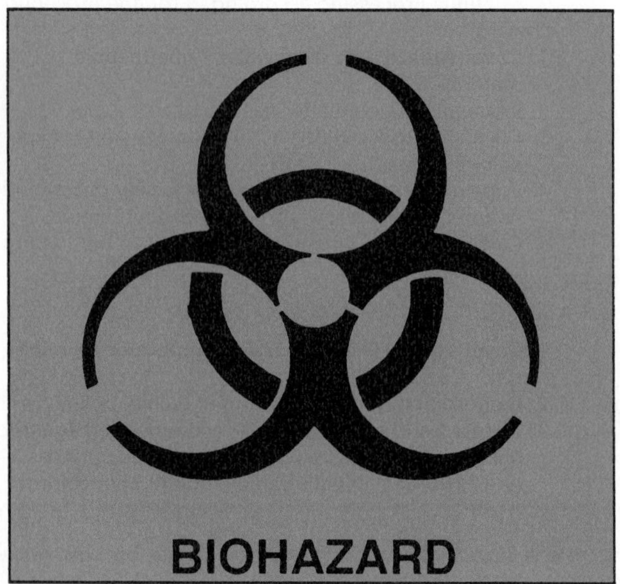


**FIGURE 3-1** Biohazard label.

The bloodborne pathogen regulation is enforceable by OSHA at the federal and state levels. This regulation is based on the concept of Universal Precautions to serve and protect health care providers and to minimize the transfer of pathogens from one patient to another. Surveyors for OSHA may engage in on-site visits to health care facilities. Unannounced visits may occur at any site where an employee exposure occurs. The visit may be a result of a verbal or written employee concern, referral from another regulatory agency, or random inspections of facilities.

***Standard Precautions.*** By the early 1990s, the controversy regarding Universal Precautions and BSI had escalated. There was considerable confusion about which body fluids required

**BODY SUBSTANCE ISOLATION IS FOR ALL PATIENT CARE** | **BODY SUBSTANCES INCLUDE ORAL SECRETIONS, BLOOD, URINE AND FECES, WOUND OR OTHER DRAINAGE.**

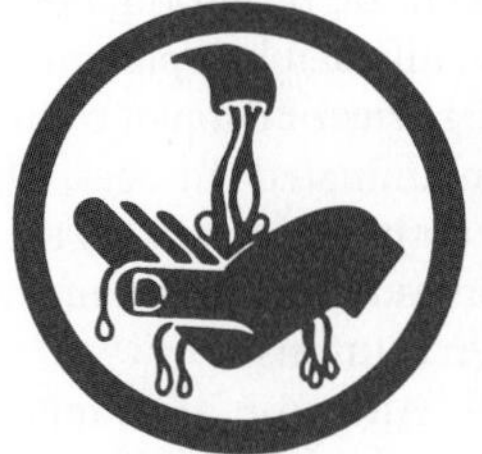

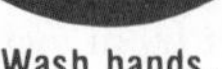

**Wash hands.**

Wear gloves when likely to touch body substances, mucous membranes or nonintact skin.

Wear plastic apron when clothing is likely to be soiled.

Wear mask/eye protection when likely to be splashed.

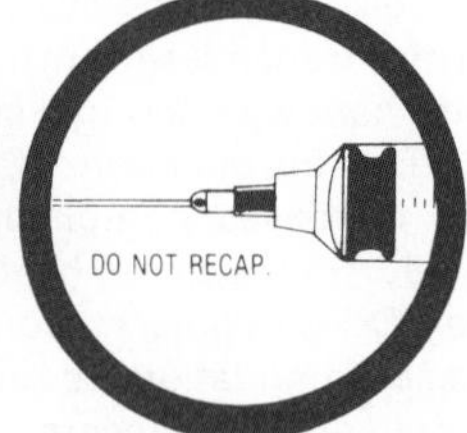


Place intact needle/syringe units and sharps in designated disposal container. **Do not** break or bend needles.



**FIGURE 3-2** Example of universal symbols for blood and body fluid protection.

special care under either Universal Precautions or Body Substance Isolation. There were also concerns about the need for additional precautions to prevent airborne, droplet, and contact transmission of other infectious agents. With this need in mind, the CDC developed a single set of precautions incorporating the major features of Universal Precautions and BSI.[26] These precautions are called *Standard Precautions,* and they are designed to reduce the transmission risk of bloodborne and other pathogens. Additional precautions based on routes of transmission for patients known or suspected to be infected or colonized with highly transmissible or epidemiologically significant pathogens are included in the document.

Standard Precautions are intended to reduce the transmission of microorganisms from recognized and unrecognized sources of infection. Standard Precautions should be applied to all patients receiving care regardless of their diagnosis or presumed infection status. They are considered the first, and most important, tier of precautions and as such are a primary strategy for successful infection prevention and control. Standard Precautions apply to (1) blood, (2) all body fluids and secretions and excretions (except sweat) regardless of whether they contain visible blood, (3) mucous membranes, and (4) nonintact skin. Standard Precautions include the following:

1. *Hand hygiene.* Hand hygiene is the most important factor in preventing the spread of infection. Hands are to be washed whenever they are in contact with blood, body fluids, secretions, excretions, and contaminated items, whether or not gloves are worn. Hands are washed immediately after gloves are removed, between patient contacts, and when otherwise indicated to avoid transfer of microorganisms to other patients or environments. Sometimes it is necessary to wash hands between tasks and procedures on the same patient to prevent cross-contamination of different body sites. A plain (nonantimicrobial) soap should be used for routine handwashing. When special circumstances such as hyperendemic conditions occur, an antimicrobial soap or an antiseptic hand rub (waterless antiseptic agent) should be used. The hand rub antiseptic agent is most effective if the hands are clean before the antimicrobial agent is applied. For effectiveness, a sufficient amount of the agent must be used for the hand rub. Manufacturers' written instructions should be followed. An additional amount of hand rub agent may be necessary (Research Highlight).
2. *Gloves.* Clean, nonsterile gloves should be worn when touching blood, body fluids, secretions, excretions, and contaminated items. Freshly donned gloves should be worn when touching mucous membranes and nonintact skin. Gloves should be changed between tasks and patient procedures and after contact with material that may contain high concentrations of organisms. Gloves should be removed immediately after use and hands washed before engaging in another task or giving care to another patient.
3. *Masks, eye protection, face shields.* A mask and eye protection or a face shield is to be worn at any time patient care activities are likely to generate sprays or splashes of blood or body fluids, secretions, and excretions. These protective devices help protect the mucous membranes of the nose, mouth, and eyes.
4. *Gowns.* Clean, nonsterile gowns are to be worn at any time patient care activities are likely to generate sprays or splashes of blood or body fluids, secretions, and excretions. Gowns help protect the skin and prevent soiling of clothing. The activity to be performed and the amount and type of fluid likely to be encountered dictate the degree of protective barrier necessary in the gown. Gowns should be removed immediately after use and hands washed before engaging in other activities or giving care to another patient.
5. *Sharps.* Needles, scalpels, and other sharps should be handled in a manner to avoid injury. Needles should never be recapped using any technique that directs the point of the needle toward any body part. If recapping is necessary, it should be done using a mechanical device or a one-handed scoop technique. Used needles should not be removed from disposable syringes, and they should not be bent, broken, or otherwise manipulated by hand. Used disposable sharps should be placed in puncture-resistant containers located as close as possible to the point-of-sharps use. Reusable sharps should be contained in a puncture-resistant container for transport to the point of decontamination.

## RESEARCH HIGHLIGHT

### Handwashing Compared with Alcohol-Based Hand Rubs

It has been reiterated often that handwashing is the most important measure that health care providers can implement to prevent the transmission of infections. Nonetheless, compliance with handwashing has been less than 50% in numerous studies. The introduction of waterless alcohol-based hand products increased compliance with hand hygiene, and in 2005 the JCAHO required health care organizations to comply with the CDC Category I recommendations for hand hygiene. These recommendations require monitoring health care workers' compliance with recommended hand hygiene practices, making improved hand hygiene practices an institutional priority, and providing easier methods for hand hygiene, such as alcohol-based hand rubs.

One of the objectives of this study was to evaluate the comparative microbial efficacy of handwashing with an unmedicated soap and hand rubbing. Before and after handwashing or hand rubs, imprints of the participants' palms and fingertips were taken and sent for colony counts and identification of transient flora. Handwashing was considered to be satisfactory if both hands were washed together for 30 seconds (±5 seconds), rinsed under running water, and dried with a paper towel. Hand rubs were considered satisfactory if 2 to 3 ml of the alcohol-based agent was applied to both hands, and all surfaces of the hands were rubbed together until the alcohol was dry. Observation was used for this part of the study.

Before hand hygiene procedures, the mean colony counts were 87 for the palms and 85 for the fingertips. During the study, it was observed that hand rubbing was performed more vigorously than handwashing. Transient flora levels were 4% after handwashing and 0% after hand rubbing. The results of this study support the CDC Category I recommendations, indicating that hand rubbing with a waterless, alcohol-based hand hygiene product is more effective than handwashing with an unmedicated soap.

Modified from Kac G and others: Microbial evaluation of two hand hygiene procedures achieved by health care workers during routine patient care: a randomized study, *The Journal of Hospital Infection* 60:32-39, 2005.

6. *Patient-care equipment.* Single-use items should be discarded after use. Reusable equipment must be cleaned and reprocessed to ensure safe use for another patient. Equipment soiled with blood, body fluids, secretions, and excretions should be handled carefully to prevent exposure of skin and mucous membranes, clothing contamination, and transfer of organisms to patients, personnel, and the environment.
7. *Linens.* Linens soiled with blood, body fluids, secretions, or excretions should be handled in a manner to avoid skin and mucous membrane exposure, clothing contamination, and transfer of microorganisms to other patients, personnel, and the environment.
8. *Environmental control.* Adequate procedures for routine care and cleaning of environmental surfaces, beds, and associated equipment are to be developed, and the use of these procedures is monitored on a regular basis.
9. *Patient placement.* Patients who contaminate the environment or who are unable to maintain appropriate hygiene or environmental control are to be housed in a private room with appropriate air handling and ventilation. If a private room is unavailable, the infection-control professional may determine a method for cohorting patients with similar infectious organisms.[26,30]

***Transmission-Based Precautions.*** Transmission-based precautions are the second tier of infection prevention, designed for patients known or suspected to be infected by epidemiologically important pathogens spread by airborne or droplet transmission or by contact with dry skin or contaminated surfaces. They may be used singly or in combination with one another if the patient has a disease that has multiple routes of transmission and are to be used in addition to Standard Precautions.

AIRBORNE PRECAUTIONS. Airborne transmission occurs by dissemination of droplet nuclei from evaporated droplets that can remain suspended in the air for long periods or by dissemination of dust particles that contain the infectious agent. Droplet nuclei are particles 5 μ or smaller in size. Airborne microorganisms can be dispersed widely depending on air currents and can be inhaled by or deposited on a susceptible host. In addition to Standard Precautions, Airborne Precautions include the following:

1. Patients are to be placed in private, negative-pressure rooms. The air exchange should be at a rate of 6 to 12 exchanges per hour with air discharged to the outdoors or circulated through high-efficiency particulate-arresting (HEPA) filters before being circulated to other areas of the facility.
2. Caregivers must wear OSHA-specified respiratory protection when caring for patients with known or suspected tuberculosis. If susceptible personnel care for patients with rubeola (measles) or varicella (chickenpox), respiratory protection should be worn. If the caregiver is immune to rubeola and varicella, respiratory protection is unnecessary.
3. All precautions for preventing transmission of tuberculosis should be implemented if the patient is known or suspected to have tuberculosis.[26,27]
4. A surgical mask should be placed over the patient's nose and mouth for Airborne Infection Isolation Precautions when the patient must be transported from one location to another. Patient transport should be limited to essential purposes only.

DROPLET PRECAUTIONS. Droplet Precautions are used for patients known or suspected to be infected with microorganisms that are transmitted by large droplets (>5 μ). These droplets can be generated when the patient sneezes, coughs, or talks. Droplet Precautions are used in addition to Standard Precautions. Droplet Precautions[26] include the following:

1. Patients are to be placed in private rooms when available. If this is not possible, the patient should be placed in a room with another patient who is infected with the same organism and with no other infection. If this is not possible, a 3-foot spatial separation should be maintained between the infected patient and other patients in the same room. For Droplet Precautions, no special air handling is required.
2. Caregivers should wear a mask when working within 3 feet of the patient.
3. Patients should be transported only for essential purposes. When transport is necessary, a mask should be placed over the patient's nose and mouth to minimize dispersal of droplets.

CONTACT PRECAUTIONS. In addition to Standard Precautions, Contact Precautions should be used for patients known or suspected to be infected or colonized with epidemiologically important organisms that can be transmitted by (1) direct contact as occurs when the caregiver touches the patient's skin or (2) indirect contact as occurs when the caregiver touches patient care equipment or environmental surfaces in the patient's room. Contact Precautions include the following:

1. Patients should be placed in a private room. If this is not possible, the patient should be placed in a room with another patient who is infected with the same organism and with no other infection. If this is not possible, patient placement must be determined on an individual basis, depending on the organism involved.
2. Gloves should be worn on entering the patient's room. Gloves should be changed after handling infective material that might contain a high concentration of microorganisms. When patient care activities have been completed, gloves should be removed before leaving the patient's room. Hands should be washed after glove removal. To avoid transferring microorganisms to others, no environmental surfaces in the patient's environment should be touched after the hands have been washed.
3. Gowns should be worn on entering the patient's room if there is a probability that the caregiver's clothing will be in contact with the patient or the environmental surfaces or if the patient is incontinent, has diarrhea, or has an ileostomy or colostomy. The gown should be removed before leaving the patient's room, and care should be exercised to avoid contact with environmental surfaces.
4. Patient transportation should be limited to essential transport only and Contact Precautions maintained to avoid contamination of personnel, visitors, or the environment.
5. Patient-care equipment should be dedicated to a single patient and not be shared between patients. If this is impossible, equipment must be cleaned and disinfected thoroughly before being used for another patient.

**PROTECTIVE ENVIRONMENT.** The purpose of creating a protective environment for allogeneic HSCT (hematopoietic stem cell transplantation) patients is to minimize fungal spore counts in the environment. These immunocompromised patients are highly susceptible to environmental fungi, and such an infection can cause morbidity. Implementation of the following helps create a protective environment:

- Place patients in specifically designated private rooms.
- Filter incoming air using HEPA filters.
- Maintain positive air-pressure gradient in relation to surrounding areas. Rooms should be well sealed to prevent air leakage into rooms.
- Maintain unidirectional airflow with air entry on one side of the room, across patient, and exit on the opposite side of the room.
- Maintain more than 12 air exchanges per hour.
- Lower dust levels by using smooth, washable surfaces as opposed to textured surfaces.
- Prohibit dried and fresh flowers and potted plants.
- Place N95 respirators on patients during transport.

Perioperative staff members historically have relied on numerous types of precautions to protect themselves and others from bloodborne pathogens and other infectious diseases. Implementing these precautions within the surgical environment requires critical thinking skills and nursing judgment. Consistent application of these precautions by all members of the perioperative team serves to protect the health care provider and to minimize cross-infection of pathogens among patients.[14]

## Engineering Practices to Control Infection

***Environment of Care.*** The surgical suite should be designed in such a way as to minimize and control the spread of infectious organisms. Either a central-core or a single-corridor design may be used. With the central-core design, sterile equipment and supplies should be contained within the central-core area, which is surrounded by ORs and a peripheral corridor. The single-corridor design places the ORs on either side of a single corridor, with separate storage rooms, usually along the corridor, to house sterile equipment and supplies. If a single-corridor design is used, sterile and contaminated items must be separated by either space or time. That is, sterile, wrapped, or containerized items can pass contaminated items in the corridor when the contaminated items are covered or otherwise contained.

Floors in the ORs should be hard, seamless, easily cleaned, and contiguous with the walls. This design eliminates the sharp angle where the floor and walls meet, where bacteria can become lodged and proliferate. If floors must be seamed, all seams should be heat-sealed. Walls may be constructed of any hard surface that is easily cleaned and hard enough to withstand the impact of surgical equipment that may accidentally be pushed into the wall during transport. If ceramic tile is used, smooth-surface grouting mortar should be used. This grout provides a surface nearly as smooth as the tile itself, eliminating concerns that surface roughness may attract and retain bacteria. Painted walls are less desirable because the paint flakes and peels, particularly in areas of higher humidity. If a hard-finish, epoxy paint is used, it is only as good as the surface beneath it. Equipment banged into a wall may cause damage and expose construction material to the environment. A soft-colored, matte-finished wall may be preferred to reduce reflectance and glare.[2]

Doors in the ORs may swing or slide. If sliding doors are used, they should not recess into the wall but should slide over the adjoining wall to facilitate housekeeping.[2] Cabinets should be recessed into the wall if possible. This configuration allows for maximum use of open floor space in ORs. Size and configuration of ORs are discussed in detail by the American Institute of Architects Academy of Architecture for Health.[2] Stainless steel cabinets are preferred because the surfaces remain smooth and are easily cleaned. Wooden cabinets quickly become damaged with cracks and crevices where bacteria can collect and proliferate. Wooden cabinets are difficult to clean and disinfect and should be avoided in ORs. Cabinet doors may be of either the swinging or the sliding type. A cleaning protocol should be established for the tracts if sliding doors are used. For noncabinet shelving, open wire shelves are preferred because dust and bacteria do not accumulate, and air can circulate freely around shelf contents.[2]

Scrub sinks should be located adjacent to each OR with a single area serving two ORs if possible. Ideally, scrub sinks are located in a room or alcove adjacent to the peripheral or single corridor of the OR. Scrub sinks should not be within the central-core area because aerosolization and splashing may occur where sterile items are stored, contaminating the environment.

Each surgical suite must contain an enclosed soiled workroom exclusive for its own use. The workroom should contain a flushing hopper, receptacles for waste and soiled linen, a handwashing sink, and a work counter. If the area is used as a holding area as part of a larger system for collection and disposal of soiled materials, the flushing hopper is not required.[2]

***Heating, Ventilation, Air Conditioning.*** To control bioparticulate matter in the OR environment, ventilating air should be delivered to the room at the ceiling and exhausted near the floor and on walls opposite to those containing inlet vents. Airflow should be in a downward directional flow, moving down and through the location with a minimum of draft, to the floor and exhaust portals.[2]

Air pressure in the OR should be greater than that in the surrounding corridor; this is called "positive pressure" in relation to corridors and adjacent areas. This positive pressure helps maintain the unidirectional airflow in the room and minimizes the amount of corridor air (less clean area) entering the OR (more clean area). Each OR should have a minimum of 15 total air exchanges per hour, with the equivalent of at least three replacements being of outside air to satisfy exhaust needs of the system. No recirculating devices, such as cooling fans or room humidifiers or dehumidifiers, are to be used. These units create a turbulent airflow and may recirculate settled bacteria. Doors to ORs should be kept closed to maintain correct ventilation, airflow, and air pressure. To minimize static electricity and to reduce the potential for bacterial growth, relative humidity in the OR should be maintained between 30% and 60%. A lower relative humidity may support accumulation of static electricity, whereas presence of a higher humidity may cause condensation of ambient moisture, which may result in damp materials and supplies. This dampness supports bacterial growth. Temperatures in ORs should be maintained at 68°F (20°C) to 73°F (23°C).[2]

## Practices to Prevent Infection

***Sterilization.*** Sterilization is defined as the complete elimination or destruction of all forms of microbial life. The concept of what constitutes "sterile" is measured as the *probability* of sterility for each item to be sterilized. This probability is known as the *sterility assurance level* (SAL). For terminal steam sterilization processes, $10^{-6}$ is the recommended probability of survival for microorganisms on a sterilized device.[84] A probability of microorganism survival of $10^{-6}$ means that there is less than or equal to 1 chance in 1 million that an item is contaminated or unsterile. The SAL of $10^{-6}$ is considered appropriate for items to be used on compromised body tissue. For items not intended to come into contact with compromised tissue, a SAL of $10^{-3}$ is sometimes accepted. A SAL; of $10^{-3}$ represents a 1 in 1000 chance of a surviving microorganism.[6,10]

STEAM STERILIZATION. Steam sterilization is the oldest, safest, most economical, and best understood method of sterilization available in health care. It is the preferred method of sterilization for items that are heat and moisture sensitive. The efficacy of steam sterilization depends on lowering and limiting the bioburden on the item to be sterilized, using effective sterilization cycles, and preventing recontamination of sterile items before delivery to the point of use.[6]

**Theory of Microbial Destruction.** Microorganisms are believed to be destroyed by moist heat through a process of denaturation and coagulation of the enzyme-protein system within the bacterial cell. Microorganisms are killed at a lower temperature when moist heat is used as opposed to when dry heat is used. This fact is based on the theory that all chemical reactions, including coagulation of proteins, are catalyzed by the presence of water.

**Principles and Mechanisms.** At standard atmospheric pressure (sea level) when water is heated, the water temperature increases as heat energy is added. After the boiling point of 100°C (212°F) is reached, additional heat energy evaporates the water to form steam. At this point, the steam and the water are at the same temperature, but the steam has more energy than the water. This difference in energy is known as the *latent heat of vaporization.* When a cold item is introduced into the steam, some of the steam gives up its latent energy to the object and changes back to liquid water. This phenomenon allows items to be heated much more rapidly in steam than in dry heat. The phenomenon of steam changing to liquid water is called *condensation,* and the steam and the liquid water are at a temperature of 100°C (212°F) when this occurs. At this point, the steam is said to be saturated. This 100°C (212°F) temperature is insufficient to kill microorganisms, however. To achieve a saturation temperature sufficient to kill microorganisms (250°F [121°C]), it is necessary to have a sealed container. When water is boiled in a vessel from which the steam cannot escape, a higher temperature is reached. As more steam is generated with no escape route, pressure in the vessel increases. The higher the steam pressure, the higher the temperature. The steam is the sterilizing agent. Any compressed air remaining in the vessel mixes with the steam and lowers the steam temperature. This reduced-temperature steam is incapable of sterilization. Air acts as a barrier to steam sterilization.[74,84]

Steam entering the sterilizer chamber should contain little or no entrapped liquid water. The term *steam quality* describes the amount of steam vapor and liquid water in the mixture. A steam quality of 100% indicates that no liquid water is present in the steam. A steam quality of 97% or greater (i.e., <3% of the mixture is liquid water) is recommended to achieve an efficient sterilization process. Causes of low steam quality include improper boiler operation and inadequate or poorly maintained steam distribution lines to the sterilizer.[74,84]

**Presterilization Preparation.** Efficacy of the sterilization process depends in part on lowering or limiting the amount of bioburden present on the item to be sterilized. Items to be sterilized should be precleaned to lower the bioburden to the lowest possible level.

To prevent infection, all items that come into contact with the patient or sterile field should be systematically decontaminated after a surgical procedure. Handling, transport, and cleaning methods must be selected to prevent cross-contamination to other patients, exposure of personnel to bloodborne pathogens, and damage to instruments.[9] The cleaning and decontamination methods chosen should be economic and of demonstrated effectiveness. Items may be cleaned by hand, by mechanical means, or by a combination of the two.[6] Increased productivity, greater cleaning effectiveness, and increased employee safety may result from use of mechanical cleaning methods. Some mechanical cleaning equipment is designed to remove microorganisms through a cleaning and rinsing action, whereas others destroy specific types of microorganisms by thermal or chemical means. Types of mechanical cleaning equipment include washer-sterilizers, washer-disinfectors/

washer-decontaminators, or washer-sanitizers; ultrasonic cleaners; utensil washers; and cart washers.

All workers handling soiled surgical instruments, whether in the OR, the substerile room, or a central decontamination area, must wear PPE sufficient to prevent contact with any blood or other body fluid. This generally means scrub attire covered with a liquid-proof gown, coverall, or sleeved apron; hair covering; surgical face mask; eye protection; and rubber or latex gloves suitable to the task. In the event that fluids may pool on the floor, liquid-proof boots or shoe covers are recommended.

Instruments should be kept as free as possible from gross soil and other debris during the surgical procedure. Throughout the surgical procedure, used instruments should be wiped with sponges moistened with sterile water. When blood is allowed to dry on the instrument, it may cause pitting, rusting, or corrosion. Sterile water is preferred to saline solution, which can cause pitting and damage to instrument surfaces. Initial decontamination should begin immediately on completion of the surgical procedure.[9,12] All instruments that can be immersed are disassembled, and box locks are opened to allow solution to contact all soiled surfaces. These instruments should be placed in a basin, solid-bottom container system, or bin with a lid. Scissors and lightweight instruments should be placed on top. Heavy retractors should be placed in a separate tray. An enzyme solution, foam, or spray can be added to the instruments to begin the process of breaking down any proteinaceous materials that may remain on the instruments.

Some instruments have sharp or pointed edges, such as scissors, forceps with teeth, perforating towel clamps, curettes, and rongeurs. These items can penetrate the gloves and skin, creating a portal of entry for infectious organisms. A different process is used for these instruments. They must not be placed in a basin or tray in such a way that a worker would have to reach into the container to retrieve the instrument, risking injury. Instead, they are placed with points down in a basin small enough that the handles are outside the basin, allowing individual instruments to be grasped. An alternative is to place all instruments together and not handle them until after they have been through a mechanical cleaning process.

All soiled instruments should be transported from the OR for cleaning and decontamination. They should be contained in leak-proof containers or trays inside plastic bags. If sharps are being transported, the container should be puncture-resistant. Means of containing instruments include plastic, rubber, or metal bins with lids; solid-bottom sterilization container systems with the lids in place and filters in place; or simply placement of the instrument tray in a plastic bag. All soiled containment packages should be labeled with the biohazard symbol to warn handlers as to the nature of the contents. Transporting instruments while they are soaking in water is discouraged because of the possibility of a liquid spill, its associated clean-up problems, and the difficulty of safely disposing of the contaminated liquid unless a flushing hopper is available.

In the decontamination area, an initial cold water rinse with tap water or a soak in cool water with a protein-dissolving and blood-dissolving enzyme helps remove blood, tissue, and gross debris from device lumens, joints, and serrations.[6] After this pretreatment, the instruments may be processed mechanically, which is preferred, or washed by hand.

Mechanical processing is completed with the use of washer-sanitizers or washer-decontaminators. In most facilities, these units have replaced manual washing of instruments and the use of washer-sterilizers. They may have a single chamber where several phases of a rinsing, cleaning, rinsing, and drying process occur. Alternatively, they may have multiple chambers, each specialized for a specific function in the cleaning process, including initial cool water rinse to remove protein debris, enzymatic-solution soak, washing with detergent, ultrasonic cleaning, sustained hot water (80°C to 95°C) rinse, perhaps a liquid chemical germicide rinse (e.g., sodium hypochlorite solution), a lubrication cycle, and drying. Soiled utensils such as basins and trays similarly should pass through a utensil washer, washer-disinfector-sanitizer, or a washer-sterilizer.[6,9] When laparoscopic items or other items with a lumen are cleaned, a cleaning apparatus for these items can be attached to the newer washer-sanitizers/decontaminators.

If manual cleaning is done, instruments should be submerged in warm water with an appropriate detergent and cleaned and rinsed while submerged. Cleaning in this manner helps protect personnel from aerosolization or splashing of infectious material and from injury by sharp objects. Harsh abrasives should not be used for manual cleaning because they damage the protective surfaces of instruments, contribute to corrosion, and impede sterilization.[12]

If a washer-sterilizer is to be used, gross debris should be removed with a cold water rinse before the instruments are placed in the washer-sterilizer, with care used to minimize splashing during rinsing. Instruments are placed in perforated or meshed-bottom trays or baskets and positioned so that the cleaning portion of the washer-sterilizer cycle can reach all parts of the instrument. The two types of washer-sterilizers are (1) those configured like a tunnel, with doors at each end and rotating spray arms on the sides, top, and bottom of the chamber, and (2) those that cover the instruments with water and blow steam and air through the water to cause agitation that produces the cleaning effect (Figure 3-3). The former machines are generally found in central decontamination areas and may be connected to an automatic or manual conveyer. The second type of machine is generally small (about 16 to 20 inches in diameter) and located in the instrument-processing room of the surgery suite.

After cleaning the instruments with detergent and water and rinsing them, the washer-sterilizer begins a steam sterilization cycle. The exposure time for this cycle depends on the temperature at which the cycle is run. Some washer-sterilizers of the tunnel type operate at 285°F (140°C) for less than 1 minute. Others, including all of the second type of washer-sterilizers, operate at 270°F (132°C) for 10 minutes. All rely on gravity displacement to remove air from the chamber. Debris remaining on the instruments because of possible inefficiencies of the cleaning process is baked on by the sterilization portion of the process and may be difficult to remove. Instruments processed through a single cycle of a washer-sterilizer are safe to handle and may be sterile, depending on presterilization bioburden. They are not suitable, however, for immediate use in another surgical procedure. They must be inspected, arranged in a manner convenient for the surgical team to use, and steam-sterilized again.

Not all instruments tolerate this process, and not all hospitals have access to mechanical washers that incorporate hot

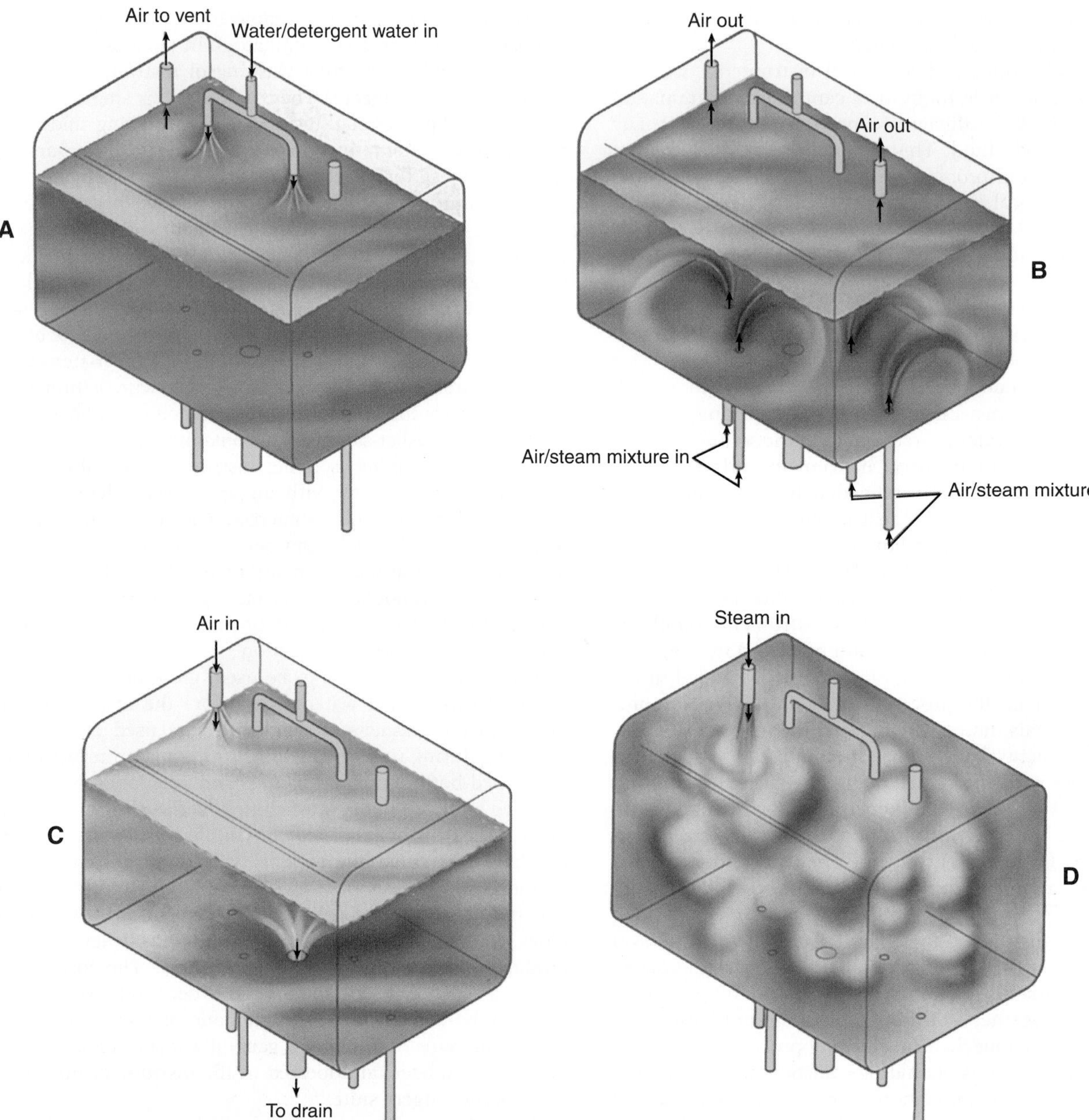


**FIGURE 3-3** Automatic washer-sterilizer. **A**, The cycle in this machine begins with a cold water rinse entering through the top of the chamber to loosen and remove gross soil, such as blood and tissue, without coagulating proteinaceous material, which would cause it to adhere to instruments. Then warm water and detergent enter the chamber to a level to cover the instruments. **B**, Next, jets of steam and air are injected into the filled chamber through ports in the floor of the chamber. Violent turbulence in the detergent-water solution removes any debris remaining on the instruments after the initial rinse. **C**, At the conclusion of the wash time, the water drains out of the chamber. Newer models of washer-sterilizers may have microprocessor controls that allow the user to set the duration of wash time based on the nature of soil on the instruments. A final rinse coming in through the top of the chamber carries any detergent residues and soil away from the instruments and out the drain. **D**, Finally, saturated steam begins to fill the chamber. Air in the chamber and load is heavier than the steam and, because of gravity, is displaced downward and out the drain. As pressure builds in the chamber from the incoming steam, the temperature rises to 132°C (270°F), the chamber drain closes, and the temperature is held for the duration of the sterilization exposure time selected by the user. Then steam is exhausted through the automatic condenser exhaust. Some machines have the capability of selecting drying times for the instruments. At the conclusion of the cycle, an audible signal indicates that the unit is ready for unloading. Instruments and the inside of the sterilizer are very hot, and if no dry time was used, the instruments and trays are also wet. Use extreme caution in handling.

water or chemical decontamination as part of the cleaning cycle. Some instruments do not tolerate immersion in water or cannot take the heat or pressures involved in mechanical processes. These items must be handwashed using an appropriate detergent for the type of material and the type of soil on the item. If protein or other organic soil is present, the detergent should have an alkaline pH (>7). If inorganic soil is present, the detergent should have an acid pH (<7). The degree of alkalinity or acidity should be selected so that the instrument or item itself is not damaged in the cleaning process. Stainless steel instruments with organic soil are best cleaned by alkaline detergents with a pH range of 7 to 10, according to most U.S. surgical instrument manufacturers. Using acidic or harshly alkaline solutions can remove the protective passivation layer from the instrument, resulting in irreparable pitting and other corrosive activity. This advice regarding detergent selection applies to mechanical washing also. Although a neutral pH detergent is often selected for the foregoing reasons, written instructions from the instrument manufacturer should be consulted to determine appropriate cleaning products and procedures.

Items that were soiled with blood or body fluids and that have been cleaned only may not have been sufficiently decontaminated to allow handling by workers not wearing protective attire. If such an item tolerates steam sterilization, it can be decontaminated further by processing through an unwrapped steam-sterilization cycle (flash sterilized). It is then safe to handle. The item also can be soaked in a liquid chemical germicide, such as 2% alkaline glutaraldehyde or ortho-phthalaldehyde (OPA) to disinfect it; the manufacturer's written recommendations for immersion time must be followed. If none of these methods is suitable for the item, because of damage to the item, cost, or unavailability, workers in the preparation area should wear protective gloves when handling, inspecting, assembling, and packaging these items for sterilization.

The ultrasonic cleaning process is designed to remove fine soil from crevices and box-lock areas of instrumentation. It should be used only after instruments have had gross debris removed. Ultrasonic energy occurs in waveforms and is generated by transducers on the sides or bottom of a specially constructed chamber that is filled with water or a water and detergent solution. The ultrasonic waves pass through the water, creating tiny bubbles that collapse or implode. This creates a negative pressure, which pulls debris away from surfaces. This process is known as *cavitation*. Ultrasonic cleaning is not biocidal, and after the cleaning process is done, the instruments should be rinsed to remove the loose debris. Some ultrasonic consoles have chambers for rinsing and drying instruments.

Not all items tolerate the energy waves of the ultrasonic process. Chromium-plated instruments should not be cleaned ultrasonically because the energy waves can loosen the chromium from the base metal underneath. Dissimilar metals, such as stainless steel, titanium, copper, and lead, should not be ultrasonically processed at the same time. The energy waves, combined with the heat and detergent solution, can cause electrolysis to occur, plating one metal onto others, potentially ruining the instruments. Some manufacturers recommend that microsurgery instruments not be placed in the ultrasonic cleaner because of their delicate design and the fact that they may contain several types of metal. The detergent or enzyme cleaner used in the ultrasonic machine should be selected carefully. The corrosiveness and overall effectiveness of some solutions can be dramatically affected by the combination of heat and ultrasonic energy in such a machine.

The final step before sterilization for reuse includes instrument preparation and packaging. These activities occur in a clean area, separate from the area where decontamination occurred. Instruments are inspected carefully for cleanliness and functionality. Soiled instruments are returned for further cleaning. Instruments with movable parts are treated with a water-soluble lubricant solution that contains an antimicrobial agent to retard growth in the lubricant solution. Broken or worn instruments are set aside for repair. Instruments are assembled into sets according to set content lists prepared by perioperative nursing staff.

**Packaging and Sterilizer Loading.** Packaging of surgical supplies and their arrangement in loads in the sterilizer are factors that govern the effectiveness of steam sterilization. The prime function of a package containing a surgical item is to permit sterilization of the contents and to ensure the sterility of the contents up to the time the package is opened.[8,9] Provision must be made for the contents to be removed without contamination. To be effective, packaging material should have the following characteristics:[15]

- Allows for adequate air removal and steam penetration
- Provides an adequate microbial barrier
- Resists tearing or punctures
- Has proven seal integrity (does not delaminate when opened and does not allow a reseal after opening)
- Allows for aseptic delivery of package contents
- Is free of toxic ingredients and nonfast dyes
- Is low-linting
- Is cost-effective by cost and value analysis

Sterilization container systems are one method of packaging instrumentation. Rigid packaging systems can be sterilized, stacked, and stored and offer a simple, effective packaging method. Because of the rigid material of the container, they cannot be punctured, abraded, or easily contaminated by environmental microbes. Studies have indicated that, properly initiated, container systems are a cost-effective packaging method. Recommendations and written instructions for sterilizing should be obtained from the container manufacturer. Performance testing should be carried out in the sterile processing department of the health care facility to ensure that all conditions essential for sterilization and drying are effectively achieved. Before opening a container, the perioperative nurse should check for evidence of integrity and sterility. The lid should be removed with care. The scrub person should examine the contents to verify that the indicator or integrator has changed to connote that steam or ethylene oxide has reached the interior, then maintain a margin of safety between himself or herself and the unsterile outer container when removing the inner basket.

If textile wrappers are used, they must be laundered between sterilization exposures to ensure sufficient moisture content of the fibers. This prevents superheating and absorption of the sterilizing agent. Rehydrated materials also deteriorate at a slower rate. All wrappers must be checked for holes or tears before use. Many in-hospital packaging materials—woven and nonwoven, reusable and disposable—are marketed today. Materials should be evaluated carefully before a product is chosen.

The size and density of woven textile packs must be restricted to ensure uniform steam penetration. The pack should not exceed 12 × 12 × 20 inches (30 × 30 × 50 cm) and should not weigh more than 12 lb (5.4 kg). When the items in the pack are being assembled, the lighter materials should be placed near the center of the pack. Each succeeding layer of dry goods should be placed crosswise on the layer below to promote free circulation of steam and removal of air. Pack density should not exceed 7.2 lb per cubic foot. A chemical indicator or integrator that accurately reflects one or more of the physical parameters of sterilization should be inserted into the center of each pack. These parameters are time, temperature, and steam saturation.

The pack should be wrapped sequentially in two barrier-type wrappers, which may be disposable or reusable. A single-textile reusable wrapper is defined as one layer of 270- to 280-thread count woven fabric. Cross-stitching and raw edges are unacceptable. Sequential double-wrapping creates a package within a package, providing for ease in presenting the wrapped item to the sterile field. Wrappers are made in suitable dimensions for the various items that must be packaged. The familiar envelope wrap is made by placement of the article diagonally in the center of the wrapper. The near corner, which should point toward the worker, is brought over the item, and the triangular tip is folded back to form a cuff. The two side flaps are folded to the center in like manner. The far corner of the wrapper is then folded on top of the other three. The process is repeated with the second wrapper, and the package is secured with autoclave indicator tape.

When the pack is opened for use, the flaps at the corners are used to form a protective cuff over the person's hands during dispensing of the sterile contents. When the items are wrapped, the wrappers should be folded securely about the contents. The package should be firm and sealed securely to prevent contamination in handling and storage. Single, disposable, nonwoven wrappers composed of fused material layers are available and widely used to wrap surgical supplies. These single wrappers provide a bacterial barrier at least equivalent to the sequential double wrap and allow for safe and easy presentation of the package contents to the sterile field, providing an alternative to the sequential double-wrapping procedure. Careful wrapping to prevent tenting and gapping of the package is essential. Nonwoven, single-use wrappers should not be reused.

Sterilization process (chemical) indicator tape should be used to hold wrappers in place on packages and to indicate that the packages have been exposed to the physical conditions of a sterilization cycle. When packages are opened, these tapes should be first torn so that the package cannot be retaped and then removed from reusable wrappers because they create laundry problems, such as occluding screens and filters. In some cases, the tapes leave a dye on the wrappers that may cause deterioration of the material. Tapes also may leave an adhesive residue that can interfere with future sterilizations of the fabric. Every package intended for sterile use should be imprinted or labeled with a load-control number that identifies the date of sterilization, the sterilizer used, and the cycle or load number. Load-control numbers facilitate identification and retrieval of supplies, inventory control, and appropriate rotation to ensure that older packages are used first.

Some instruments or packaging systems may present challenges to the sterilization process. Special preparation or loading procedures may be necessary to meet these challenges. Hinged instruments must be arranged so that the steam can contact all surfaces of the instrument, including the tips, hinged surfaces, and ratchets. To accomplish this, these instruments must be sterilized in the open position. If the instruments have ringed handles for the fingers, the instruments may be placed on a "stringer," which is a U-shaped metal rod made especially for this purpose. When using closed container systems for sterilization, basket attachments may be used to immobilize instruments in the proper position for sterilization. Tubular instruments with lumens can trap air, which interferes with the sterilization process. To avoid this problem, lumens should be moistened with water immediately before sterilization. As the instrument is heated, the water turns to steam and forces the air out of the lumen. Instruments with concave or other surfaces that can hold water must be carefully placed on edge to facilitate removal of air, which may become trapped in the concave surface. Placing the instrument on edge also facilitates drainage of condensate. Items such as basins, which may be stacked for sterilization, should be stacked with sufficient space between all surfaces so that steam can contact all surfaces.[60]

When packaging is complete and the sterilizer chamber is loaded, the bundles and packages should be arranged to minimize resistance to steam, which must pass through the load from the top of the chamber toward the bottom of the sterilizer. All packages should be placed on a vertical edge in the sterilizer in a loose-contact position. This allows free circulation and penetration of steam, enhances air elimination, prevents entrapment of air or water, and precludes excessive condensation. A second or upper layer may be placed crosswise on the first or lower layer. All jars, tubes, canisters, and other nonporous objects should be arranged on their sides with their covers or lids removed to provide a horizontal path for the escape of air and the free flow of steam and heat. To guard against superheating, surgical packs and supplies should not be subjected to preheating in the sterilizer with steam in the jacket before sterilization.

Rigid container systems should be placed flat on the sterilizer shelf. These containers should not be stacked during sterilization unless the manufacturer specifically recommends this practice. Containers should be stacked only in the manner recommended by the manufacturer's written instructions. Stacking may interfere with air removal and steam penetration. In addition, condensation from upper containers may drip down and contaminate lower containers when the sterilizer door is opened and the cooler room air contacts the containers.[74]

**Sterilizing.** When steam enters the autoclave, it is at the same pressure as the atmosphere. As the valves and doors to the outside close, steam pressure rises inside the chamber, increasing the temperature of the steam. Evacuation of air from the sterilizer is necessary to permit proper permeation of steam. If a sterilizer is improperly loaded, mixing of air with steam acts as a barrier to steam penetration and prevents attainment of the sterilization temperature.

The three factors necessary to achieve steam sterilization are *time, temperature,* and *moisture.* The microbial destruction period is based on the known time and temperature necessary to accomplish sterilization in saturated steam. Authorities have shown that definite laws determine the order of death in a given bacterial population subjected to a sterilizing process. If the temperature is increased, the time may be decreased.

To provide a safety margin, the minimum estimated exposure is extended to cover the lag between the attainment of the selected temperature in the chamber and the temperature of the load. The length of exposure varies with the type of sterilizer, cycle design, altitude, bioburden, packaging, and size and composition of items to be sterilized. Written instructions for sterilization parameters should be obtained from the sterilizer manufacturer. If a closed container system is used as packaging for items to be sterilized, the container manufacturer's written instructions for exposure times should be consulted and reconciled with those of the sterilizer manufacturer.[6]

Sterilizers vary in design and performance characteristics. Use of rigid container systems may alter the come-up and exposure times in steam sterilizers. The configuration of some instruments or medical devices may hinder air removal and steam penetration, making sterilization more difficult. In such circumstances, the device manufacturer must be able to specify the necessary parameters to achieve steam sterilization. The most common time and temperature parameters are provided in Table 3-2. Certain instruments and implants require extended time cycles, however. The manufacturer's written instructions for extended time cycles must be followed.

The recording thermometer, not the pressure gauge, is the important guide to the sterilizing phase. The recording clock on the sterilizer gives information about the run of the load and to what temperature the goods were exposed and the exposure time. The temperature inside the chamber must be maintained throughout the determined time of exposure.[6] The sterilization printout documents the come-up time, exposure time, and exhaust time.

**Drying, Cooling, and Storing.** On completion of the sterilization cycle, the steam inside the chamber is removed immediately so that it does not condense and produce wet packs. To assist in the drying process, the jacket pressure should be maintained to keep the walls of the chamber hot as the steam from the chamber is exhausted. When the chamber pressure has been exhausted, the door may be opened slightly to permit vapor to escape. Another method is to introduce clean, filtered air by means of a vacuum dryer (ejector) device in conjunction with the operating valve on the sterilizer. The minimum drying time for all methods is approximately 15 to 20 minutes.

After removal from the sterilizer, freshly sterilized packs should be left untouched on the loading carriage until they have cooled to room temperature. This is usually accomplished in 30 to 60 minutes, depending on the load contents. If freshly sterilized packages are placed on cool surfaces such as metal tabletops, vapor still inside the essentially dry package may condense to water. This water may dampen the package from the inside to the outside. When the outside is wet, bacteria may follow the moist tract into the contents of the package. Because bacteria are capable of passing through layers of wet material, any packages that are wet must be considered unsterile.

A written record of existing conditions during each sterilization cycle should be maintained. It should include the sterilizer number, the cycle or load number, the time and temperature of the cycle, the date of sterilization, the contents of the load, and the initials of the operator. These records should be retained for the length of time designated by the statute of limitations in each state.

Sterile packages must be handled with care and only as necessary. They should be stored in clean, dry, limited-access areas that are well ventilated and have controlled temperature and humidity. Closed cabinets are preferred to open shelves for sterile storage. If open shelves must be used, the lowest shelf should be 8 to 10 inches from the floor to avoid floor contamination. The highest shelf should be at least 18 inches from the ceiling to allow for circulation around the stored items. All shelves should be at least 2 inches from outside walls to facilitate air circulation and avoid any condensation that might accumulate on the walls during periods of severe temperature change. Shelving should be smooth and well spaced, with no projections or sharp corners that might damage the wrappers. Sterilized packs should never be stacked in close contact with each other. Their arrangement on the shelves should provide for air circulation on all sides of each package. Excessive handling, crowding, dropping, and stacking of sterile packs tend to force particles through the mesh or matrix of the wrapping material, which might contaminate the contents. Sterile items should not be stored near or under sinks or in any area where they can become wet. Storage on nondesignated shelving, counters, carts, or areas of possible contamination should be avoided.

*Shelf life* refers to the length of time a pack may be considered sterile. Loss of package sterility is event-related as opposed to time-related; that is, what happens to the package after sterilization determines its continued sterility—not the length of time the package remains on the shelf ready for use. Variables that must be considered in determining shelf life are the type and number of layers of packaging material used, the presence or absence of impervious protective covers, the number of times a package is handled before use, and the conditions of storage. Impervious protective covers known as *dust covers* may extend shelf life by protecting the sterile package from a contaminating event. When used to protect sterilized items, impervious covers should be designated as such to prevent their being mistaken for a sterile wrap. They should be

**TABLE 3-2**

**Common Time-Temperature Parameters for Steam Sterilization**

| Type of Sterilizer | Load Configuration | Temperature, in °C (°F) | Time, in Minutes |
|---|---|---|---|
| Gravity displacement | Porous or nonporous | 121-123 (250-254) | 15-30 |
| | | 132-135 (270-275) | 10-25 |
| Prevacuum | Porous or nonporous | 132-135 (270-275) | 3-4 or manufacturer's instructions |
| Steam flush/pressure pulse | Porous or nonporous | 121-123 (250-254) | 20 |
| | | 132-135 (270-275) | 3-4 |

applied only to thoroughly cooled, dry packs at the time of removal from the sterilizer cart, after the required cooling period.

Supply standards should be planned to maintain adequate stock with prompt turnover. Appropriate volume and proper rotation of supplies reduce the need for concern about shelf life. The longer an item is stored, the greater the chances of contamination. For proper rotation, the most recently dated sterile packages should be placed behind those already on the shelves.

**Quality Control Practices: Physical Monitoring.** Physical monitoring includes checking items such as time, temperature, and pressure recorders, digital printouts, and gauges. All mechanical parts of sterilizers, including gauges, steam lines, and drains, should be checked periodically by the engineering department within the facility. The individual responsible for the sterilizers should keep reports of these inspections. Temperature, humidity, and vacuum should be measured with control equipment, independently of the fixed gauges. There are several methods of keeping a constant check on the proper functioning of a sterilizer and ensuring the efficiency of the sterilizing process. *Mechanical, chemical,* and *biologic* controls assist in identifying and preventing sterilizer malfunction and operational errors made by personnel.

Automatic controls are a type of mechanical control that, by a predetermined program, control all phases of the sterilizing process. The controls allow the steam to enter, monitor the time of the sterilizing cycle, exhaust the steam, and initiate drying. Some lock the door so that it cannot be opened until the cycle is complete.

On older sterilizers, recording thermometers were the mechanical control that indicated and recorded the temperature throughout the sterilizing cycle on a dial on the front of the sterilizer. Sterilizers today provide a digital readout as opposed to a graphic depictor of the sterilizing cycle. The digital readout records a decrease in temperature when and if it occurs; this can warn of sterilizer failure. The digital readout records the time the sterilizer reaches the desired temperature and the duration of each exposure. It can be determined if a decrease in temperature occurred, warning of sterilizer failure. These recordings are proof that the exposure time of loads has been correct and proper temperature limits have been maintained. The daily record should show the number of the sterilizer, the number of cycles run, the time, and the date. Mechanical monitoring devices provide real-time assessment of sterilizer-cycle conditions and permanent records by means of either the chart recording or computer printouts.[6] This evidence can be used for detection of malfunctions as soon as possible so that alternative procedures can be implemented while the cause of the malfunction is identified and corrective action is taken. Recordings cannot detect air pockets within the load or pack, however. Air is a poor conductor of heat; it is one of the most common causes, other than human error, of sterilization failure.

Chemical controls, also commonly known as *chemical indicators* or *integrators,* include devices such as pellet-containing, sealed glass tubes; sterilizer indicator tapes; color-change cards or strips, which may or may not provide a line of demarcation to indicate use or nonuse of the sterilizer load; and indicators containing color-changing enzymes, which mimic or provide a representation of bacterial kill. Some enzyme indicators contain a biologic component; others do not. Chemical indicators are used to detect failures in packaging, loading, or sterilizer function, such as presence of cool air pockets inside the sterilizing chamber. Chemical indicator cards or strips that are impregnated with a material that changes color or moves up a gauge when steam initiates a chemical reaction are placed in instrument trays or other packages. No chemical monitor verifies that an item is actually sterile.[6] Integrators are so named for their ability to integrate time, temperature, and the presence of steam. They reduce the risk of using an unsterile pack and may be used with numerous types of sterilization processes. Because they vary in color changes for each type of sterilizer or words used on the integrator to denote that an instrument set or other item is acceptable for use, perioperative nurses and scrub persons should always refer to the manufacturer's written instructions when relying on indicators and integrators.

AORN's Recommended Practices for Sterilization in the Perioperative Practice Setting do not recommend flash sterilizing implantable devices. In the event that there is no other reasonable alternative but to flash sterilize an implant, a biologic indicator should be run with the cycle. The Association for the Advancement for Medical Instrumentation (AAMI) recommends that the sterilized implant be quarantined until the biologic test results are obtained. In an emergency situation or event in which the patient is on the OR bed and under anesthesia, it may pose a patient safety issue to wait for the results of the biologic test. One option may be to use a biologic indicator with enzyme-based early readout capabilities that can provide early indications of the adequacy of the sterilization process in approximately 1 to 3 hours. Rapid-read biologic indicators incorporate a dual system: spore associated enzymes that indicate sterilization effectiveness and conventional *Geobacillus stearothermophilus* spores. The biologic indicator should continue to be incubated for the full time. Documentation should reflect patient follow-up if the final biologic test indicates a failure. Appropriate perioperative planning along with communicating and working with implant vendor representatives may help decrease unplanned flash sterilization of implantable devices.[6,7,18]

An external chemical indicator (class 3, 4, or 5) should be used on all packages to be sterilized except for those that allow direct visualization into the package, where an internal indicator is used (e.g., paper or plastic pouches). The primary purpose of the external indicator is to differentiate between processed and nonprocessed packages. This indicator should be checked after the sterilization process and before a package is opened for use to determine that the package has been exposed to a sterilization process.

An internal chemical indicator or integrator (class 3, 4, or 5) should be placed within each package to be sterilized in the area of the package believed to be the least accessible to steam penetration. The indicator or integrator should be located and interpreted by the user at the time the package is opened and before use of the contents.[6,18]

A biological indicator is the most accurate method of checking sterilization effectiveness. Commercially prepared biologic indicators (manufactured in accordance with minimum performance criteria of the *United States Pharmacopoeia*) should be stored and used according to the manufacturer's written instructions. They contain a known population of *G. stearothermophilus,* a highly heat-resistant, spore-forming microorganism that does not produce toxins and is nonpathogenic. Rapid-action indicators are available commercially for certain types of sterilizers. These indicators provide a preliminary enzymatic reaction that is highly correlated to biologic kill. Reaction times range from 20 seconds to 3 hours. The length of time necessary for an initial reading depends on the type of indicator used, the type of sterilizer, and the cycle used.[6] For a true indication of biologic kill, only indicators having a biologic component should be used, and the indicator should be incubated after the initial reading according to the manufacturer's instructions to ensure biologic results.

Biologic testing should be done after initial installation of steam sterilizers, after any major repair of the sterilizer, and with all loads of implantable devices. Whenever possible, implantable devices should be quarantined until the results of the biologic testing are available.

Biologic testing for steam sterilizer loads should be conducted at least weekly and preferably daily on the first run of the day. The biologic indicator should be placed in a test pack that is positioned on edge in the front, bottom section of a routinely loaded steam sterilizer. This area of the sterilizer most challenges all sterilization parameters. The AAMI has defined the challenge test pack composition, configuration, and use.[6] Commercially prepared test packs are available on the market.

After the sterilization cycle, the biologic indicators are removed from the pack and incubated according to the manufacturer's instructions. Negative reports (failure to recover any spores from the indicators in the test pack) indicate that the sterilizer is functioning properly. Results of these tests should be filed as a permanent record. A positive report does not indicate sterilizer failure because false-positive results sometimes occur. The sterilizer should be retested immediately, however, and taken out of service until it is operationally inspected and the results of retesting are negative. If a sterilizer malfunction is found, all items prepared in the suspect load should be considered unsterile. They should be retrieved if possible and washed, repackaged, and resterilized in another sterilizer. All items in any load processed since the last negative result also should be considered suspect and should similarly be retrieved if possible.

When a prevacuum sterilizer is used (see the discussion of the prevacuum sterilizer next), a test designed to detect residual air in the chamber should be run daily. The test, generally known as a *Bowie-Dick* test, is run with an otherwise empty chamber so that residual air is not forced into other packs or materials, degrading the test results. The Bowie-Dick test pack and procedure have been described by AAMI.[10] The Bowie-Dick test determines the efficacy of the vacuum system of the prevacuum sterilizer. The Bowie-Dick test is *not* a sterility-assurance test.

**Types of Steam Sterilizers.** For sterilization to occur, steam must contact all surfaces of the item to be sterilized. To accomplish this, the air in the sterilizer chamber must be evacuated. The terms *gravity displacement* and *dynamic air removal* describe the methods by which air leaves the sterilizer chamber. Dynamic air removal sterilizers use preconditioning techniques to remove air from the sterilizing chamber. This may be through a vacuum pump (prevacuum) or above atmospheric pressure process, such as the steam-flush pressure-pulse process.

At the beginning of the cycle in a gravity sterilizer, steam begins to enter the chamber after the door is closed and locked (Figures 3-4 and 3-5). An initial burst of steam enters the chamber and forces out much of the free air in the chamber. Air is heavier than steam, and the two do not mix well. As more steam enters the chamber, the air that is held by gravity at the bottom of the chamber exits down the drain, which is at the bottom of the sterilizer—hence the name *gravity displacement sterilizer.*[74]

In a prevacuum cycle, rather than passive air removal as is the case with the gravity sterilizer, air is actively removed from the sterilizer (Figure 3-6). When the cycle is initiated, steam is injected with force into the chamber. At the same time, the drain at the bottom of the chamber is automatically closed. As more steam enters the chamber, pressure increases, and the steam and air form a turbulent mixture. When a specific pressure is reached, the drain opens, and the pressurized steam and air rush from the chamber, aided by a water ejector or a vacuum pump. This sudden rush of gas from the chamber creates a vacuum within the chamber. This is the basis for the name *prevacuum sterilizer.* The sterilizer repeats this injection and vacuum process four times in succession in an effort to evacuate all air from the chamber.[74]

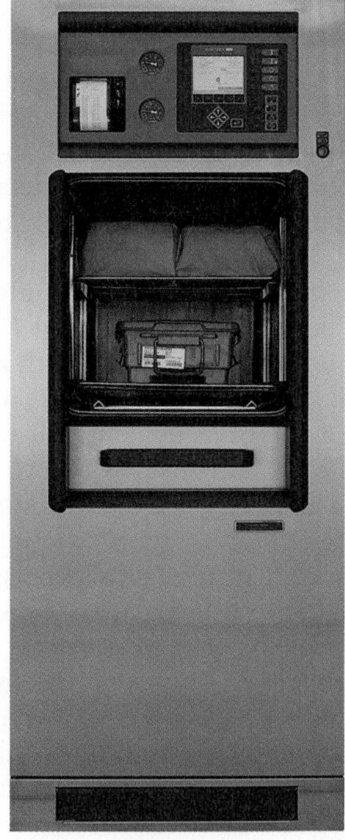

**FIGURE 3-4** General-purpose gravity air displacement steam sterilizer. This type of sterilizer can be used to sterilize wrapped or unwrapped instruments and utensils, linen packs, and solutions in specially designed vented flasks. These units come in several sizes, from the small unit similar in size to the washer-sterilizer described in Figure 3-3 to large, floor-loading units. A medium-size unit is pictured here. Some units have sophisticated microprocessor controls that allow maximum flexibility in selecting sterilization and drying times and help in troubleshooting if a problem occurs during a cycle. Digital readouts and heat-sensitive paper printouts have replaced the round chart and pen found on older models. These changes have helped the operator more easily determine and document that the conditions needed for proper sterilization were met.

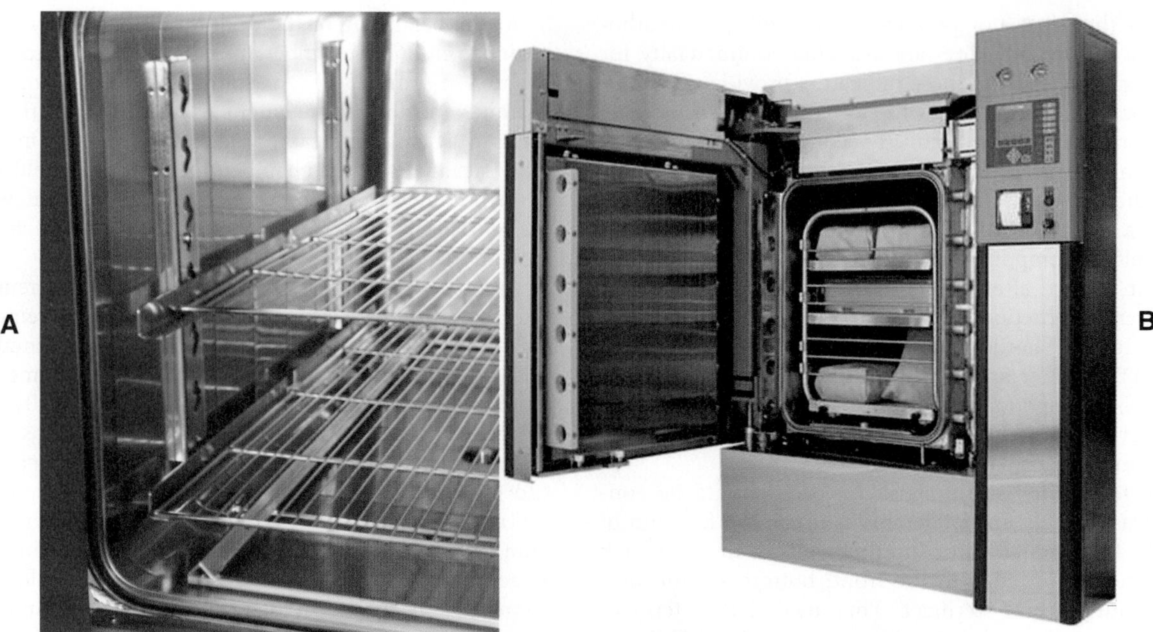


FIGURE 3-5 A, Adjustable racks are designed to permit maximum loading efficiency. B, Instrument baskets or trays should have either wire-meshed bottoms or a sufficient number of perforations in the sheet metal to allow for air removal and drainage of condensate during the sterilization cycle.

Some prevacuum sterilizers have the capability of providing an *abbreviated prevacuum cycle.* In this cycle, there are two rather than four pulses of the steam injection-vacuum process. This cycle may be used only for simple metal or glass instruments. No instruments with a lumen should be sterilized using this cycle.[6,74]

The *high-speed steam sterilizer,* commonly referred to as a *flash sterilizer,* can be adjusted to operate at 132°C (270°F) and 27 psi of pressure for shortened cycles with no accompanying drying cycle. Flash sterilization can be accomplished in either a gravity displacement or a dynamic air-removal sterilizer. Flash sterilization is most frequently used in the OR for sterilizing urgently needed unwrapped instruments. This method of sterilization is intended for use with unwrapped items or sterilizing pans or container systems developed specifically for the flash cycle. Flash sterilized items are to be used immediately after sterilization; they may not be stored for future use. Flash sterilization should be used only in situations when time does not permit processing by the preferred wrapped presterilization.[7,18] Implantable devices should not be flash sterilized. If, in an emergent situation, an implantable device must be flash-sterilized, a biologic indicator should be included in the tray and the item quarantined until, at a minimum, a preliminary result from a rapid-indicator system is available. Although flash sterilizing is considered a rapid method of sterilization for unwrapped items, some pulsing gravity and the abbreviated prevacuum cycles have been designed with a brief drying cycle intended to dry the single wrapper, which may be used to cover the tray holding instruments being sterilized. Even with the brief drying cycle, however, the tray itself and its contents still may be wet. The tray should be transported to its point of use only by individuals wearing sterile gloves. The tray should be placed on a sterile impervious drape that will not melt with the heat of the tray. The wrapper should be removed by the individual handling the tray so that the scrub person can remove the tray contents in an aseptic manner.[74] Routine cycle parameters for flash sterilization are shown in Table 3-3.[7,74]

**CHEMICAL STERILIZATION.** Materials that cannot be heat-sterilized are continually being introduced for use in health care. These materials require the use of other methods of sterilization. Chemical agents provide an effective alternative to steam sterilization. Chemical sterilization is frequently referred to as *low-temperature sterilization.* This term refers to the maximum temperature of 54°C to 60°C (130°F to 140°F) of gaseous sterilization compared with temperatures of 121°C to 132°C (250°F to 270°F) for steam sterilization.

Sterilization can be achieved by many agents when only vegetative cells are present. If the microbial population is unknown, however, a sporicidal agent must be employed to ensure sterilization. An antimicrobial agent must exhibit a wide microbiologic spectrum and sporicidal activity to qualify as a chemosterilant.

**Ethylene Oxide.** Gaseous chemical sterilization has had considerable application for heat-labile and moisture-sensitive items, such as intricate, delicate surgical instruments; large pieces of equipment used in the hospital; plastic and porous materials; and electrical instruments—all of which are difficult to steam-sterilize without deterioration and damage. Ethylene oxide (EO) is a gas frequently used for this purpose. It is colorless at ordinary temperatures, has an odor similar to that of ether, and has inhalation toxicity similar to that of ammonia gas. EO gas is an effective sterilant but must be used with care because of its toxicity. It is easily stored as a liquid, which boils at 10.73°C (51.3°F) and freezes at −111.3°C (−168.3°F). It is highly explosive and very flammable in the presence of air. These hazards are greatly reduced by dilution of EO with inert gases such as carbon dioxide and hydrochlorofluorocarbons (HCFCs). Neither of these two inert gases seems to affect the

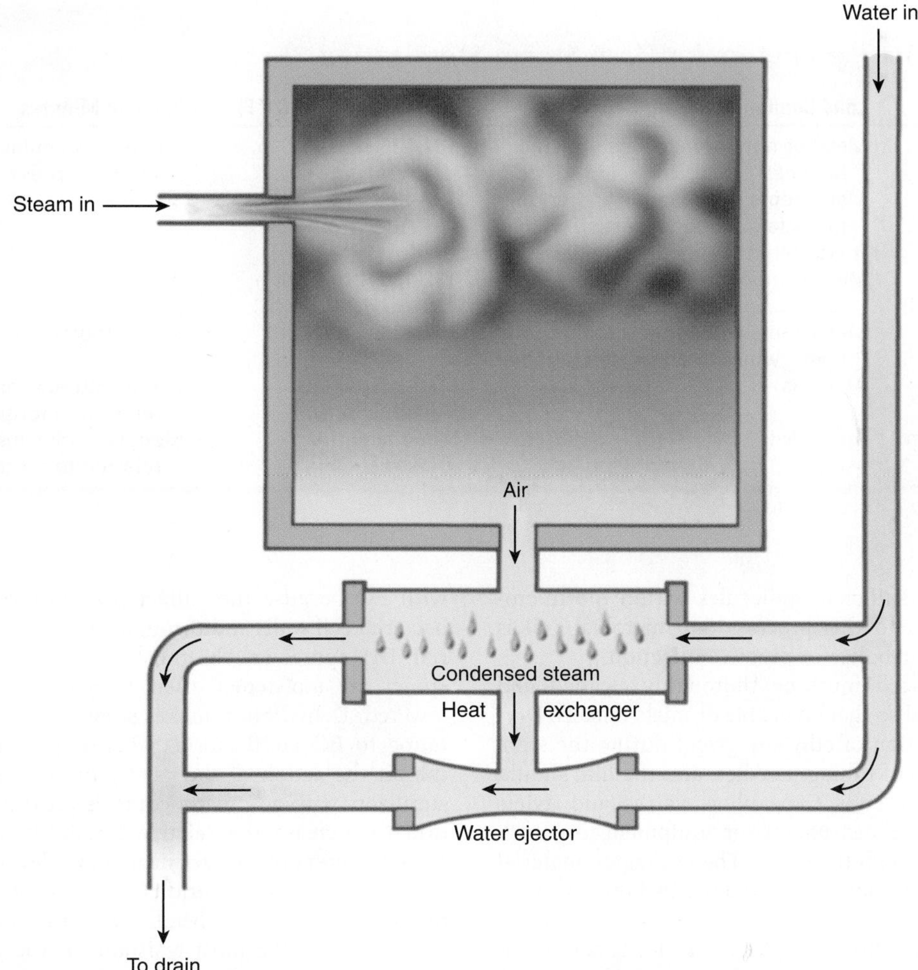


**FIGURE 3-6** Prevacuum steam sterilizer. This type of sterilizer features active, aggressive removal of air rather than relying on the passive action of gravity. When the cycle is initiated, steam is injected with force into the chamber. At the same time, the drain at the bottom of the chamber is automatically closed. As more steam enters the chamber, pressure increases and the steam and air form a turbulent mixture. When a specific pressure is reached, the drain opens, and the pressurized steam and air rush from the chamber, aided by a water ejector or a vacuum pump. This sudden rush of gas from the chamber creates a vacuum within the chamber. This process is repeated several times and deepens the level of vacuum drawn with each pulse. The effect of this pulsing cycle is to displace any air in the load and rapidly increase the chamber and load temperatures. At the conclusion of this conditioning phase, steam flows into the chamber and raises the temperature to sterilization levels, usually 132°C (270°F). The temperature is maintained for at least 3 minutes for unwrapped, nonporous materials and 4 minutes for wrapped or porous items. Steam is removed from the chamber to draw a partial vacuum again. Heated, filtered air is introduced into the chamber to dry the load. Drying times are selected and set by the user, depending on the nature of the load. Some units have a special cycle designed for rapid sterilization of an instrument tray in a single wrapper. This express cycle has fewer conditioning pulses, a 4-minute exposure time, and 1 or 2 minutes of dry time, for a total cycle time of approximately 12 minutes. Although the wrapper feels warm and dry to the touch, the contents may not be totally dry. This package should be handled by individuals wearing sterile gloves and using sterile towels for protection from burns. The instruments sterilized in this express cycle must be used immediately. Because the contents are not dry, the package is not suitable for storage.

bactericidal activity of EO, serving only as inert diluents that reduce the flammability hazard.

Several theories on how EO kills bacteria have been proposed. The killing rate of bacteria is generally believed to be relative to the rate of diffusion of the gas through their cell walls and the availability or accessibility of one of the chemical groups in the bacterial cell walls to react with the EO. The killing rate also depends on whether the bacterial cell is in a vegetative or spore state. Destruction takes place by alkylation through chemical interference and probably inactivation of the reproductive process of the cell. In the process of alkylation, a hydrogen atom within the microbial cell is replaced with a portion of the EO molecule (e.g., an alkyl group). This process alters the structure of the microbial molecule and renders it

**TABLE 3-3**

**Time-Temperature Parameters for Flash Steam Sterilization**

| Type of Sterilizer | Load Configuration | Temperature, in °C (°F) | Time, in Minutes |
|---|---|---|---|
| High-speed gravity displacement | Metal or nonporous items only (no lumens) | 132-135 (270-272) | 3 (follow manufacturer's instructions for the express cycle) |
| | Metal items with lumens and porous items (e.g., rubber, plastic), which are sterilized together | 132-135 (270-272) | 10 |
| Prevacuum (Dynamic air removal) | Metal or nonporous items only (no lumens) | 132-135 (270-272) | 3 |
| | Metal items with lumens and porous items, which are sterilized together | 132-135 (270-272) | 4 or manufacturer's instructions |
| Pulsing gravity | All loads | Manufacturer's instructions | Manufacturer's instructions should be referred to for time and temperature |
| Abbreviated prevacuum | All loads | Manufacturer's instructions | Manufacturer's instructions should be referred to for time and temperature |

nonfunctional. When sufficient molecules within the microbial cell are subjected to this process, the microbial cell is rendered unable to metabolize or produce infection.

Items to be sterilized must be thoroughly cleaned and towel-dried or air-dried so that no visible droplets remain. Drying inhibits the formation of ethylene glycol during the sterilization cycle. Lumens of tubing, needles, and the like should be dry and open at both ends. Caps, plugs, valves, and stylets should be removed from instruments or equipment to permit the gas to circulate through the items. The packaging material used should possess the characteristics described previously in this chapter.

Items to be sterilized should be placed in a loose configuration within the confines of metal baskets or sterilizer carts. Packages should not touch the chamber walls when loaded into the sterilizer. An excessively large load or a load that is tightly packed interferes with proper air removal, load humidification, sterilant penetration, and sterilant evacuation at the conclusion of the cycle. Penetration of gas throughout the load is essential. Compression of packages prevents penetration of the gas. If packages are wrapped in plastic, compression hinders evacuation of air and causes packages to open during the decrease in chamber pressure when a vacuum is drawn. Proper loading is essential so that sterilized items do not fall from the container or cart after sterilization, requiring personnel to handle them before aeration. Because metal baskets or carts do not absorb ethylene oxide, they can be handled before aeration. An EO-sensitive chemical indicator should be used with each package to indicate that the package was exposed to the gas. The chemical indicator does not indicate achievement of sterility.[5,85]

Factors affecting sterilization with EO are time of exposure, gas concentration, temperature, humidity, and penetration. The exposure time required depends on temperature, humidity, gas concentration, the ease of penetrating articles to be sterilized, and the type of microorganisms to be destroyed. Gas concentration is affected by the temperature and humidity inside the sterilizing chamber. If the concentration of gas is doubled, the exposure time may be shortened. Temperature and humidity have a pronounced influence on the destruction of microorganisms. They are important in gaseous sterilization with EO because they affect penetration of the gas through bacterial cell walls and through wrapping and packaging material. Dry spores are the most difficult to kill, but when such spores are moistened, their resistance to gas penetration is lowered. Dehydration makes some microorganisms nearly immune to EO sterilization, whereas droplets of moisture can inhibit the action of the gas by protecting the organism. EO sterilizers with automatic controls provide for moisture injection to increase the relative humidity within the chamber. Manufacturers of gas sterilizers have developed recommended exposure periods for various EO concentrations in relation to the material to be sterilized. Exposure time is set for absolute destruction of the most resistant microorganisms, which is a very slow process.

The adequacy of every EO cycle should be verified by the use of biologic monitors that contain *Bacillus atrophaeus*. Where feasible, implantable or intravascular items should not be used until the results of the test are known. The AAMI has defined two standard test packs for use in monitoring the EO sterilization cycle.[6] The sterilizer manufacturer's instructions regarding cycle parameters should be followed. The most common parameter ranges are shown in Table 3-4.[5]

EO-sterilized items must be aerated to make them safe for personnel handling and patient use. At the conclusion of the sterilization cycle, items may be removed safely from the chamber to a separate aerator. Certain models of sterilizers may have an internal aeration cycle. The sterilizer manufacturer's recommendations relating to opening the sterilizer door after completion of the sterilization cycle and subsequent transferring of items to the aerator must be followed closely. Excessive exposure to EO represents a health hazard to personnel. It is a known carcinogen and has been linked to reproductive problems and other disorders in animals. Inhalation of EO should be avoided or minimized, and direct contact with items sterilized by EO should be avoided during transfer to the aerator. Various safety features, such as a purge system, an audible alarm at the end of the sterilization cycle, and automatic door-locking and door-sealing mechanisms, are used on EO sterilizers to protect personnel. Opening the sterilizer door within the capture zone of the scavenging hood for a period of 5 to 10 minutes can reduce operator exposure to the sterilizing

TABLE 3-4

## Common Parameters for Ethylene Oxide Sterilization

| Time, in Minutes | Temperature, in °C (°F) | Humidity, in % | Gas Concentration, in mg/L |
|---|---|---|---|
| 105-300 | 37-63 (99-145) | 45-75 | 450-1200 |

gas. If the sterilizer contents are not removed at that time, they begin to "outgas," resulting in increased EO concentration within the chamber.

Aeration may be accomplished in a mechanical aerator or in the ambient environment. Length of aeration for each item should be based on the manufacturer's instructions. Typical aeration times when a mechanical aerator is used are 8 to 12 hours at 50°C to 55°C (122°F to 131°F) or 12 to 16 hours at 38°C (100.4°C). Aeration in the ambient environment should be for 7 days. Ambient aeration should be carried out in a limited-access, well-ventilated room with a controlled temperature of 18°C to 22°C (65°F to 72°F) and vented to the outside. When moving items from the sterilizer to the aerator, items should be handled minimally. Personnel should not breathe the air that passes over baskets or carts containing EO-sterilized items. To avoid breathing this air, carts should always be pulled as opposed to pushed. Depending on the sterilization-cycle temperature used, items may be warm to the touch at the end of the cycle. Butyl rubber gloves are recommended to protect personnel from contact with liquid EO and from thermal injury.[18]

Because of the highly explosive and flammable nature of EO, the sterilizer and aerator should be installed in a well-ventilated room and should be vented to the outside atmosphere as recommended by the manufacturer and requirements of the National Institute for Occupational Safety and Health (NIOSH). Only authorized personnel are allowed access, and hazard signs should be posted. Compliance with other administrative controls to ensure safety is essential.

Because of EO's carcinogenicity and its potential as a reproductive hazard, OSHA has issued standards regulating personnel exposure to EO. These standards set the permissible exposure level (PEL) (the amount of EO in the air) at 1 part per million (ppm) and the action level (AL) (monitored value at which corrective action should occur) at 0.5 ppm. These are calculated as time-weighted averages (TWA) over an 8-hour period. OSHA requires that monitoring and surveillance be performed to ensure that exposure levels do not exceed 1 ppm over an 8-hour period.[65] In addition, occupational exposure level to EO may not exceed 15 ppm in any 15-minute period. This is known as the *excursion level* (EL).[66] EO-monitoring badges are available. Adherence to these guidelines helps protect patients and personnel from problems associated with EO sterilization.

In general, EO sterilization should be used only if the materials are heat-sensitive and unable to withstand sterilization by saturated steam under pressure. Any item that can be steam-sterilized should never be gas-sterilized. EO's advantages are that it is easily available; it is effective against all types of microorganisms; it easily penetrates through masses of dry material; it does not require high temperatures, humidity, or pressure; and it is noncorrosive and nondamaging to items. Sterilization with EO also has numerous disadvantages. The long exposure and aeration periods make it a lengthy process. Compared with other methods of sterilization, EO sterilization is expensive. Liquid EO may produce serious burns on exposed skin if not immediately removed; insufficiently aerated materials can cause skin irritation, burns of body tissue, and hemolysis of blood; and diluents used with EO cause damage to some plastics. Human error and mechanical breakdown can enhance these disadvantages.

**Aqueous Glutaraldehyde.** When used properly, liquid chemosterilants can destroy all forms of microbial life, including bacterial and fungal spores, tubercle bacilli, and viruses. Although formaldehyde is one of the oldest chemosterilants known to destroy spores, it is rarely used because it takes 8 to 24 hours to be effective, its pungent odor is objectionable, and it may cause irritant or allergic reactions. Glutaraldehyde works more rapidly and is less irritating than formaldehyde solutions.

Activated aqueous glutaraldehyde 2% is recognized as an effective liquid chemosterilant. It is most useful in the disinfection of lensed instruments, such as cystoscopes and bronchoscopes, because it has minimal deleterious effects on the lens cement and is noncorrosive. Its low surface tension permits easy penetration and rinsing.

Instruments must be free from bioburden and completely immersed in activated aqueous glutaraldehyde solution for 10 hours to achieve sterilization. Any period of immersion less than 10 hours does not kill spores that may be present and must be considered as only a disinfection procedure. During immersion, all surfaces of the instrument must be contacted by the liquid chemosterilant. After immersion, instruments must be rinsed thoroughly with sterile distilled water before being used.

**Peracetic Acid.** Liquid peroxyacetic (peracetic) acid is a biocidal oxidizer that maintains its efficacy in the presence of high levels of organic soil. The mechanism of action of peracetic acid is not well understood. Because peracetic acid is highly corrosive to instruments, it must be used in combination with anticorrosive additives.[12,80] Commercially available sterilization systems using peracetic acid have found increasing use in recent years because of their relatively short cycles and subsequent ability to ready items for use quickly. These systems should be maintained and used according to the manufacturer's instructions. Although peracetic acid does not leave toxic residues on items that have been adequately rinsed, the agent may cause serious injury if not handled, neutralized, and rinsed properly. Items processed in peracetic acid systems should be used immediately after processing because the item containers are wet and are not sealed from the environment.[18] Some controversy regarding internal-process monitors has existed with peracetic acid sterilization systems. *B. atrophaeus* indicators should be used on installation of a peracetic acid sterilization unit and after any major repairs. Manufacturer recommendations should be sought and carefully followed for routine sterilizer monitoring.

**Gas Plasma Sterilization.** Plasma is the fourth state of matter, the sequence being solid, liquid, gas, and plasma. Gas plasmas are highly ionized gases composed of ions, electrons, and neutral particles. In this process, microbial life is disrupted when free radicals created from hydrogen peroxide gas plasma interact with microbial cell membranes, enzymes, or nucleic acids.[18,50,51] To create gas plasma for sterilization, a precursor solution, such as hydrogen peroxide, is introduced into a closed area in the sterilizer under low vacuum conditions. This precursor is injected into the chamber via an injection/flow mechanism, becomes vaporized, and remains within the sterilization chamber. RF energy is used to create an electromagnetic field to excite the precursor. In hydrogen peroxide gas plasma sterilization, hydrogen peroxide vapor kills microorganisms. Hydrogen peroxide vapor is charged with radiofrequency, and a plasma is created that removes hydrogen peroxide residuals from the sterilized items. The by-products of this process are oxygen and water (in the form of humidity). Packages are dry at the end of the cycle.[56,59,61]

Plasma sterilization has the potential of displacing ethylene oxide sterilization for most but not all applications. It is designed to provide nontoxic, dry, low-temperature sterilization in a shorter turnaround time than that of ethylene oxide. The hydrogen peroxide gas plasma process rapidly destroys a broad spectrum of microorganisms, including gram-negative and gram-positive vegetative bacteria, mycobacteria, yeasts, fungi, lipophilic and hydrophilic viruses, and highly resistant aerobic and anaerobic bacterial spores.[50,51] Cycle times for gas plasma sterilization range from 28 minutes to more than 1 hour depending on the model. At the completion of the sterilization process, no toxic residues remain on the sterilized items. No aeration is necessary, making it a safe process for patients and health care workers. Preparation of instrumentation for sterilization includes cleaning and decontaminating procedures, drying, reassembly, and wrapping with nonwoven polypropylene wraps or Tyvek/Mylar pouches (Figure 3-7). Cellulosic-based products, such as paper and linen, are not recommended for use with plasma systems because they tend to absorb the vapor and cause the sterilization cycle to abort. Manufacturer's written instructions for use should always be followed.[50,51,56]

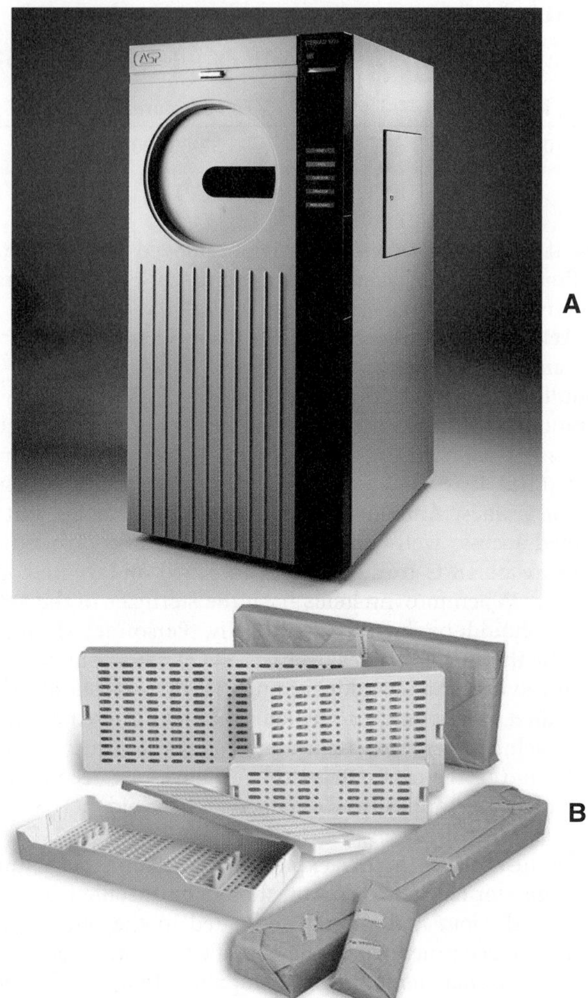


**FIGURE 3-7** A, Gas plasma sterilizer. B, Supplies for use in low-temperature, gas plasma sterilization systems.

Biologic and chemical indicators for process verification are used in the same manner as indicators for steam and ethylene oxide sterilization procedures. Plasma sterilization processes should be tested with biologic indicators at intervals similar to the intervals used for steam and ethylene oxide sterilization. Manufacturer recommendations should be followed in determining the specific monitor to be used. For hydrogen peroxide plasma sterilization systems, *G. stearothermophilus* spores show the greatest resistance to kill. The importance of consulting the system manufacturer for specific instructions cannot be overemphasized.[56,59,61]

**DRY HEAT STERILIZATION.** Dry heat sterilization should be used only for materials that cannot be sterilized by other methods, when the moisture of other processes would damage the materials, or the materials would be impermeable to the process.[53] These materials include grease, anhydrous oils, powders, and some glassware. Dry heat is not a suitable sterilization method for fabrics and rubber goods because the high temperatures necessary for sterilization cause deterioration of these materials. There are two kinds of dry heat (also known as *hot air*) sterilizers—the gravity convection type and the mechanical convection type. Both heat by electricity to achieve accurate and dependable temperature control.

In the *gravity convection sterilizer,* convection is created by the temperature differences within the sterilizing chamber. The heating apparatus present in the bottom of the chamber warms the air within the chamber. The warmed air rises, contacting the items in the chamber to be sterilized. At contact, heat is transferred from the air to the items. With this loss of heat, the cooled air descends toward the bottom of the chamber where it is warmed again by the heating coils.

In the *mechanical convection sterilizer,* the heating apparatus is outside the chamber, in a compartment separated from the chamber by a diffusing wall placed in front of a motor-driven turbine blower. Through an internal process, air is heated and forced into a chamber on the opposite wall. From this chamber, the air is discharged into the chamber uniformly over the vertical plane of the chamber. This system provides for uniform delivery of heated air and equal transfer of heat to all regions of the chamber.[10,69] This system offers the maximum in functional efficiency at a minimum cost and is the system most often used in hospitals.

Because of the variation in items to be sterilized and packaging methods and materials, parameters for dry heat sterilization vary. Temperature parameters refer to the temperature of the load, not sterilizer chamber temperature. When sterilizing by the dry heat method, the parameters provided in Table 3-5 are believed to be adequate.[10,53]

Spore tests may be used with dry heat sterilization. *B. atrophaeus* is the most commonly used challenge microorganism. The sterilizer manufacturer's instructions should be carefully followed for sterilizer monitoring.[10,53]

***Disinfection.*** High-level disinfectants play a key role in the processing of semicritical medical devices. They must be practical, fast, safe, and easy to use. Appropriate cleaning, disinfecting, and sterilizing of reusable devices are crucial to ensure their safe use and to maintain equipment integrity. Advances in instrument processing, specifically in the area of high-level disinfectants, continue to support better patient care in the clinical setting.

Disinfection is defined as the process of eliminating many or all pathogenic organisms except bacterial spores from inanimate objects.[73] In health care facilities, equipment is usually soaked in liquid chemicals for a specified period to achieve disinfection of the equipment or item. The disinfection process may destroy tubercle bacilli and inactivate hepatitis viruses and enteroviruses but usually does not kill resistant bacterial spores. The term *disinfection* also may refer to treatment of body surfaces that have been contaminated with infectious material. Chemicals used to disinfect inanimate objects are referred to as *disinfectants*. Chemicals used for body surfaces are known as *antiseptics*. The term *germicide* refers to any solution that destroys microorganisms. Some germicides are disinfectants and antiseptics.

Disinfectants are categorized as high-level, intermediate-level, or low-level, depending on their disinfecting capability.[73] High-level disinfectants kill all microorganisms except high numbers of bacterial spores. Intermediate-level disinfectants may kill tubercle bacilli, vegetative bacteria, and most viruses and fungi but not bacterial spores. Low-level disinfectants kill most vegetative bacteria and some viruses and fungi.

Just as with sterilization, an item must be cleaned first before it can be disinfected. Proper cleaning removes all foreign substances, such as soil or organic material, from an object. This is usually accomplished by the use of soap and water or an enzymatic detergent. The term *decontamination* refers to the removal of pathogenic organisms from an object, making the object safe to handle.

**TABLE 3-5**

**Time-Temperature Parameters for Dry Heat (Hot Air) Sterilization**

| Temperature, in °C (°F) | Time |
|---|---|
| 180 (356) | 30 minutes |
| 170 (340) | 1 hour |
| 160 (320) | 2 hours |
| 150 (300) | 2½ hours |
| 140 (285) | 3 hours |
| 121 (250) | 6 hours (preferably overnight) |

Items to be sterilized or disinfected have been classified as critical, semicritical, and noncritical, based on the risk of infection for the patient. This classification system, known as the *Spaulding classification system* and named for its developer, Earle Spaulding,[73,77] has withstood the passage of time and continues to be used today to determine the correct processing method for preparing instruments and other items for patient use. According to the Spaulding system, the level of disinfection required is based on the nature of the item and the manner in which it is to be used.

*Critical items* are items that enter sterile tissue or the vascular system. These items should be subjected to a sterilization process and be sterile at the time of use. Many critical items are purchased from the manufacturer as sterile. Unsterile critical items should be steam-autoclaved if they are heat-stable and moisture-stable. If the items cannot withstand heat or moisture, they may be sterilized by one of the other methods discussed earlier. Examples of critical items include surgical instruments, needles, implants, and certain types of catheters.

*Semicritical* items are items that contact nonintact skin and mucous membranes but do not ordinarily penetrate the blood barrier. Examples of semicritical items include anesthesia breathing circuits, fiberoptic endoscopes, and laryngoscopes. Semicritical instruments require high-level disinfection; that is, these items must be free of microorganisms other than bacterial spores. Examples of high-level disinfecting agents include glutaraldehyde, ortho-phthalaldehyde, stabilized hydrogen peroxide, peracetic acid, and chlorine or chlorine compounds.[73,77]

*Noncritical* items are items that come into contact only with intact skin. Because skin is an effective barrier to most microorganisms, most noncritical, reusable items can be cleaned at the point of use. Intermediate-level or low-level disinfectants may be used to process noncritical items. Examples of noncritical items include blood pressure cuffs, bedpans, linens, utensils, furniture, and floors. Although it is unlikely that infection will be transmitted to patients with intact skin by means of noncritical items, noncritical items can contaminate the hands of health care workers or medical equipment that will be used on other patients who may be at greater risk for infection. Examples of low-level disinfectants include alcohols, sodium hypochlorite, phenolic solutions, iodophor solutions, and quaternary ammonium solutions.[73,77]

TYPES OF DISINFECTANTS

**Alcohols.** For disinfection in health care, the term *alcohol* refers to either 70% or 90% isopropyl alcohol. Both of these compounds are water-soluble and have a high degree of antimicrobial activity. They are bactericidal as opposed to bacteriostatic against vegetative forms of bacteria. They are also tuberculocidal, fungicidal, and virucidal. Isopropyl alcohol (isopropanol) and ethyl alcohol (ethanol) are effective against HBV and HIV. The alcohols do not destroy spores or kill certain hydrophilic viruses, such as echovirus and coxsackievirus. Alcohols are flammable and must be stored in a well-ventilated area. Because they evaporate rapidly, extended contact time is difficult to achieve unless items are immersed. Alcohols lack residual effect and are easily inactivated by protein material. Alcohols tend to damage the coating on lensed instruments and may cause hardening of certain rubber and plastic tubing after repeated exposure to the compound. Alcohols are considered intermediate-level disinfectants. They are often used to disinfect thermometers and rubber stoppers on medication vials. Alcohol also is used in processing flexible endoscopes. After high-level disinfection and a tap water rinse, alcohol is effective in inactivating water contaminants. Its speed of evaporation also assists in rapid drying of the endoscope channels.[13,71,75] Guidelines from the Association of Practitioners in Infection Control (APIC) should be followed.

**Chlorine Compounds.** In health care facilities, hypochlorites are the most widely used of the chlorine compounds. Hypochlorites are available in a liquid form (sodium hypochlorite [liquid household bleach]) and in a solid form (calcium hypochlorite). Hypochlorites have a broad-spectrum antimicrobial activity. They are inexpensive and fast-acting. Low concentrations of free chlorine (50 ppm) are effective against vegetative bacteria and *M. tuberculosis*. Free chlorine at 50 ppm inactivates HIV, whereas a 500-ppm concentration is needed to inactivate HBV. Concentrations of 1000 ppm are recommended for inactivation of bacterial spores. Household bleach contains 5.25% sodium hypochlorite. A dilution of 1:1000 provides 50 ppm of available chlorine. A dilution of 1:50 provides 1000 ppm of available chlorine, which is considered adequate to achieve high-level disinfection. The CDC recommends a 1:10 solution, which provides 5000 ppm of available chlorine. Hypochlorite solutions are stable for 30 days in opaque containers. Beyond that time, a new solution should be prepared. Hypochlorites are inactivated in the presence of organic matter. All organic material should be removed before application of the disinfecting solution. Hypochlorites are used sparingly on instruments because of the corrosive action of the compound. Hypochlorites are most often used for countertops, floors, and other surfaces to be disinfected. Other chlorine compounds that may be used include chlorine dioxide and chloramine-T. Chlorine compounds are the preferred disinfectant in water treatment.[71,75]

**Glutaraldehyde.** Glutaraldehyde is a saturated dialdehyde that has gained prominence as an overall effective disinfecting agent for high-level disinfection. Aqueous solutions of glutaraldehyde are acidic and as such are not sporicidal. The solution is said to be "activated" when alkalizing agents are added to make the solution alkaline. Glutaraldehyde has a broad antimicrobial range, being effective against vegetative bacteria, *M. tuberculosis*, fungi, and viruses. Although glutaraldehyde is effective against most bacteria in 10 minutes, some species of mycobacteria require a longer exposure time. To achieve high-level disinfection, a minimum exposure time of 20 to 45 minutes is recommended, based on the manufacturer's written instructions.[75] Glutaraldehyde is noncorrosive to endoscopic equipment, thermometers, rubber, and plastic. Glutaraldehyde phenate is a related compound that has been shown to lose efficacy against certain organisms in the recommended dilution. Another compound, glutaraldehyde with *ortho*-phenylphenol and *para-tertiary* amylphenol, provides a wide range of antimicrobial activity similar to 2% glutaraldehyde. The compound is odorless and minimizes irritation and allergic reactions in users.[71,75]

**Ortho-phthalaldehyde.** Ortho-phthalaldehyde is a 0.55% ortho-phthalaldehyde solution in an aqueous buffer with a pH of 7.5. The solution is bactericidal, virucidal, and fungicidal. It is tuberculocidal in 12 minutes, at room temperature. Minimum exposure time is 12 minutes at room temperature. As with any high-level disinfectant, PPE should be employed when using ortho-phthalaldehyde. Ortho-phthalaldehyde can be used for most applications for which glutaraldehyde is used and has broad materials compatibility. The manufacturer's written instructions should be read before use. The compound is odorless and minimizes the irritating qualities that glutaraldehyde possesses.[13]

**Hydrogen Peroxide.** Unstable and low concentrations of hydrogen peroxide (<3% solution) may be used as low-level disinfectants for work-surface cleaning and disinfection. More concentrated (6%) and stable solutions of hydrogen peroxide show an antimicrobial effect against some bacteria, fungi, and viruses. Stabilized 6% hydrogen peroxide is sporicidal and can be used as a liquid sterilant with sufficient exposure time. The solution is corrosive, however, to copper, zinc, and brass. It also can damage rubber and plastic. Hydrogen peroxide is not used widely as a disinfectant in today's health care environment.

**Iodine and Iodophors.** An iodophor is a water-soluble combination of iodine and a solubilizing agent or carrier that allows for a slow but continuous release of free iodine over time. Iodophors may be used as disinfectants or antiseptics, depending on the concentration of free iodine. As disinfectants, iodophors have the advantage of having the germicidal efficacy of iodine without the disadvantages of toxicity and surface irritation. Iodophors are usually nonstaining and effective against vegetative bacteria, *M. tuberculosis*, and most viruses and fungi. Iodophors are not considered suitable for high-level disinfection because they have no sporicidal capability.[71,75]

**Phenolics.** Phenol (carbolic acid) was first used by Lister in the mid-1800s. Since that time, many phenol derivatives (phenolics) have been developed. Phenolics are assimilated by porous material, making their removal difficult. Residual disinfectant can cause tissue irritation. Most phenolic formulations are tuberculocidal, bactericidal, viricidal, and fungicidal. Certain viruses, including echovirus and coxsackievirus, are resistant to phenolics. Phenolics are not sporicidal, and they are not considered effective as high-level disinfectants. They are used primarily as intermediate-level and low-level disinfectants for environmental disinfection. They are known to have toxic effects, however, and their use has been associated with depigmentation and hyperbilirubinemia in newborns. Because of this, phenolics are not recommended for cleaning incubators or infant bassinets.

**Quaternary Ammonium Compounds.** Quaternary ammonium compounds ("Quats") have been used for many years as a result of a reputation for microbicidal activity, good detergent action, and low-level toxicity. In more recent times, it has been noted that environmental factors, such as hard water, soap residues, and protein soils, reduce or nullify the efficacy of these compounds. Quaternary ammonium compounds are ineffective against *M. tuberculosis* and the lipophilic viruses. They are not sporicidal. Quaternary ammonium compounds are not recommended for high-level, intermediate-level, or low-level disinfection. They are good cleaning agents and are used most often for noncritical surfaces such as floors, walls, and furniture.[71,75]

**DISINFECTION OF ENDOSCOPES.** In today's technologically advanced environment, flexible fiberoptic endoscopes and their associated instrumentation allow for myriad minimally invasive surgical procedures. The list of these procedures grows almost daily. Current technology allows not only for direct visualization of internal sites but also for diagnostic biopsies and therapeutic procedures to be performed with reduced pain and shorter recovery time for patients. Along with advances in technology, complications also have occurred. Some complications, such as bleeding or tissue perforation, are immediately obvious. Infectious complications may be more difficult to identify.

Endogenous and exogenous microorganisms can cause infections related to endoscopic procedures. When an infection occurs from endogenous sources, organisms normally present in the procedure area gain access to the bloodstream. Examples of endogenous infections resulting from endoscopy include cholangitis, pneumonia, endocarditis, brain abscess, and subdural empyema. Infections also can be caused by organisms introduced into the patient via the endoscope (exogenous organisms). Organisms commonly associated with exogenous infection include *Pseudomonas, Klebsiella, Enterobacter, Salmonella,* and *M. tuberculosis*. Because HAV, HBV, HCV, and HIV are inactivated by commonly used chemical germicides, documented endoscopic transmission of these viruses is uncommon. HBV transmission via the endoscope has been reported,[60] as has the transmission of tuberculosis via a contaminated bronchoscope.[1]

For an endoscope to be thoroughly disinfected, the disinfecting agent must contact all internal and external surfaces of the endoscope for the prescribed length of time. Organic soil, such as blood, feces, or respiratory secretions, harbors embedded microorganisms and prevents penetration of the disinfecting agent. Some disinfectants are inactivated by organic material. Rigorous mechanical cleaning is essential to remove soil and debris from the outside of the scope and from the lumens of all accessible channels.[23,73]

Endoscopes and their accessories should be cleaned immediately after use to prevent drying of secretions or other organic soil. They should be cleaned with a nonabrasive enzymatic detergent as recommended by the endoscope manufacturer.[13,73] If a powdered detergent is used, all granules must be dissolved completely before washing begins. Undissolved granules can block the internal channels of the instrument. To soften, moisten, and dilute organic debris, endoscope channels should be flushed with copious amounts of water and detergent. The external surfaces of the endoscope should be washed with a detergent solution and rinsed. Internal channels should be brushed to loosen and remove organic matter. The detergent solution should be suctioned or pumped through all channels to remove loosened debris. Special attention should be given to convoluted areas and crevices where contaminated organic material may lodge. The tip of the endoscope should be gently wiped or brushed to remove any debris or tissue that may be lodged around the air and water outlets. Brushes used for cleaning should be disposable or be thoroughly cleaned and sterilized daily. Detachable parts of the endoscope, such as hoods and suction valves, should be removed and soaked in a detergent solution. They should be thoroughly cleaned with a detergent, using a brush to remove any organic material.[13,60,73]

Before immersion in any liquid, endoscopes should be pressure tested (leak tested) to determine integrity of seals and minimize the potential for damage to the head of the scope. If damage is detected, the scope should not be immersed or reused. The endoscope should be removed from service and returned to the manufacturer for repair. An endoscope sent for repair is considered a contaminated item and must be labeled as such for shipping.

Immediately after decontamination and cleaning, endoscopes should be rinsed of residual debris and cleaning agent. After a tap-water rinse, endoscopes should be rinsed with 70% or 90% alcohol and forced air dried. Alcohol inactivates organisms normally found in tap water and helps dry the internal channels of the scope. After being cleaned, endoscopes and accessories should be sterilized or high-level disinfected before being stored. Care must be taken to dry internal channels of the scopes after being processed and before being stored. Endoscopes should be stored in a vertical position in an area in which recontamination is unlikely. Endoscopes should be processed immediately before patient use, including first use of the day, to preclude the possibility that the scope may have been recontaminated during storage or handling or both. Endoscopes should be sterilized or high-level disinfected depending on their intended use (see discussion of the Spaulding classification system earlier). Because of pressure and heat sensitivity, for many years the sterilization method of choice for endoscopes was EO. More recently, liquid peracetic acid with anticorrosive buffers also has been used to process endoscopes. As endoscopic surgery grows, and the need for sterile endoscopes increases, additional processing methodologies are expected to become available.

Activated glutaraldehyde was long considered the agent of choice for high-level disinfection of endoscopes. A manual or an automated system may be used. Regardless of whether a manual or automated system is used, meticulous manual cleaning must precede the disinfection process. The solution manufacturer's written instructions should always be followed.[60,73]

The facility should maintain a log for each procedure with the patient's name, medical record number (if available), type of procedure being performed, endoscopy physician's name, and serial number or other identifier of the scope. If an automatic endoscope reprocessor is used, identification of this device should be included in the record. This documentation assists in the investigation in the event of an outbreak or safety concern.[18]

**PASTEURIZATION.** Pasteurization is a process that uses hot water at temperatures between 65.5°C (150°F) and 76.6°C (170°F) for 30 minutes to achieve high-level disinfection. The actual time/temperature relationship depends on the items to be disinfected. Contact time is inversely related to temperature. For equivalent microbial destruction, longer exposure times are required when the temperature is decreased. Controversy exists as to whether pasteurization results in high-level or intermediate-level disinfection. The CDC definition of high-level disinfection requires destruction of all microbial life except for large populations of bacterial spores. Because pasteurization, by definition, does not kill bacterial spores, some would consider the process to result in only intermediate-level disinfection. Some semicritical items, such as respiratory therapy and anesthesia devices, are ready for patient use after cleaning and pasteurization. High numbers of bacterial spores are not found often on these devices after use. Cleaning before pasteurization reduces the bioburden, and the low number of spores that might be present on a properly pasteurized device of this type would not represent an infective dose when contacting intact mucous membranes. Advantages of pasteurization include absence of toxic residues and the associated need for postprocess rinsing. Disadvantages of pasteurization include the lack of sporicidal activity and the potential for splash burns to personnel involved with the process.[8,75]

***Reprocessing/Reuse of Items Labeled for Single-Use Only.*** Health care trends reflect cost-driven market forces and consumer-driven demands for quality, safety, and effectiveness. Facilities in today's marketplace are reprocessing and reusing devices labeled for single use. The practice of reprocessing and reusing single-use items is controversial. Each facility must decide whether to reprocess and to what extent the practice should be instituted. Three basic tenets must underlie any reprocessing/reuse program, as follows:[11]

- If a device cannot be cleaned, it cannot be reprocessed and reused.
- If sterility of a postprocessed device cannot be shown, the device cannot be reprocessed and reused.
- If the integrity and functionality of a reprocessed single-use device cannot be shown and documented, the device cannot be reprocessed and reused.

Although some savings may be realized by reusing certain single-use devices, any cost-benefit analysis necessarily would include consideration of the labor costs associated with reprocessing; program costs, including quality systems requirements such as sterility and postprocessing testing, documentation, and record-keeping costs; and the cost of device failure. The results of this cost analysis are helpful when making a decision about reprocessing/reusing single-use devices (Research Highlight).

The FDA views any reprocessor as a manufacturer and subject to federal regulations governing manufacturers. Hospitals and third-party reprocessors are subject to the same regulation as the original equipment manufacturer. These requirements include the following:

- Registration and listing
- Medical device tracking
- Medical device reporting
- Corrections and removals
- Device labeling
- Quality system regulation
- Premarket notification requirements

Each requirement has associated resource needs. An in-depth discussion of these requirements is beyond the scope of this book. Details of the FDA requirements for reprocessors can be found in the Code of Federal Regulations.

## RESEARCH HIGHLIGHT

### Reprocessing Single-Use Items

The practice of reprocessing single-use, disposable devices has been controversial for more than 25 years. Authors favoring the practice cite substantial cost savings and the absence of adverse patient outcomes. Authors who oppose the practice cite concerns about cleaning and sterilizing the devices and concerns about product integrity. Other authors cite the ethical issues of multiple charging for the same device. The purpose of this study was to determine whether reprocessed single-use devices could be sterilized and whether the devices would meet the same standards as a new device.

Single-use and reusable biopsy forceps and papillotomes and a reusable stone-retrieval basket were selected for the study. Eleven instruments, including a sterile control device, were used for the cleaning test. Devices were first contaminated with a radionuclide product and then cleaned under running tap water at 30°C to 35°C (86°F to 95°F) for 3 minutes. The inner lumens were flushed using a 10-mL syringe filled with enzymatic cleaner. The instrument was submerged in the same enzymatic cleaner for 10 minutes. After the enzymatic soak, the devices were placed in an ultrasonic bath of tap water at 30°C to 35°C (86°F to 95°F) for 5 minutes. After this ultrasonic treatment, lumens were flushed again with a syringe, and external surfaces were cleaned under running water at 30°C to 35°C (86°F to 95°F) for 3 minutes. Lumens were blown dry with a syringe, and the outer surfaces of the devices were dried. After processing, cleaning results were measured using a gamma camera to determine the distribution and intensity of radioactivity of the radionuclide-contaminating product used before cleaning.

To evaluate disinfection of the devices, channels were filled with 2% glutaraldehyde solution, and the devices were submerged in the glutaraldehyde solution for 20 minutes at a temperature of 20°C to 25°C (68°F to 77°F). After this treatment, lumens were flushed, using a syringe with tap water; the outside was cleaned under running tap water. Water was blown from the lumens with a dry syringe, and the outer surface of the devices was dried. Disinfection was measured in terms of log reduction factors calculated from the difference in colony-forming units before and after processing.

To evaluate sterilization, devices were placed in appropriate packaging materials and exposed to half-cycle in either a steam or an ethylene oxide sterilizer. After sterilization, devices were placed in appropriate culture media and incubated for the designated length of time. Sterilized devices were evaluated for growth or no growth. Finally, scanning electron microscopy and x-ray photoelectron spectroscopy were used to evaluate device surfaces and the microstructure of materials after processing.

Results of this study showed that all devices remained contaminated after being cleaned, although the level of contamination differed according to type of device. Testing after disinfection and sterilization indicated that reusable devices were adequately disinfected using the described protocol, but single use devices were not. Sterilization reduced the number of spores on devices, but spores could not be totally eliminated. Finally, single-use and reusable devices were physically damaged during sterilization. Compared with unused devices, surfaces of soiled and reprocessed devices showed increased concentrations of carbon and nitrogen, which were explained as traces of residual peptides from blood or other body materials.

The authors of this study conclude that when using the described standards for cleaning, disinfection, and sterilization, none of the reprocessed single-use devices in this study are suitable for use with subsequent patients. Disinfection and sterilization of disposable devices could not be accomplished to required levels, and reprocessing procedures resulted in material changes adding to degradation and reduced functional integrity of the devices.

Modified from Heeg P and others: Decontaminated single-use devices: an oxymoron that may be placing patients at risk for cross-contamination, *Infection Control and Hospital Epidemiology* 22:539-542, 2001.

If a user facility chooses to engage a third-party reprocessor as opposed to conducting the program at the facility, it is the user facility's responsibility to assess the quality of the services provided under the contractual arrangement with the third-party reprocessor. The user facility must review the processes used by the contracted agency and determine whether correct procedures are being followed.[16,30]

## ASEPTIC PRACTICES TO CONTROL INFECTION

### Surgical Aseptic Principles

Asepsis has been defined as the absence of infectious organisms. Surgical aseptic practices are based on the premise that most infections are caused by organisms exogenous to the surgical patient's body. To avoid infection, surgical procedures must be done in a manner that minimizes or eliminates the patient's exposure to exogenous organisms. Opening sterile supplies as close to the time of their use as possible, using sterile drapes to create a sterile field around the incision site, using sterile instruments for the surgical procedure, and placing the operative team in sterile attire after their hands and arms have been cleansed of surface bacteria aid in avoiding infection.

Aseptic technique stems from the principles of asepsis derived over time from microbiologic and epidemiologic concepts. Although some investigators may believe that current aseptic practices and techniques have become too ritualistic or lack scientific research to support their use, present-day infection-control statistics support the application of aseptic principles for safe perioperative nursing practice. Until empiric research shows that a technique is unnecessary or ineffective, the basic aseptic principles should be followed. These principles follow:

1. Only sterile items are used within the sterile field. Individuals dispensing sterile items to the sterile field must look at the sterilization indicator on or visible in the package, check for package integrity, and check for package expiration date (or appropriate marking for event-related shelf life) before dispensing the item to the field.
2. Items of doubtful sterility must be considered unsterile. Examples include sterile items found in unsterile work areas, sterilized packages wrapped in pervious materials that have become wet, sterilized items without an integrator or other internal indicator, and sterilized packages wrapped in pervious materials that are dropped. If a package wrapped in an impervious material is dropped, and the area of contact is dry, the package may be opened and the contents used. The package should not be returned to sterile storage for future use.
3. Whenever a sterile barrier is permeated, it must be considered contaminated. This principle applies to packaging materials and to draping and gowning materials. Obvious contamination occurs from direct contact between sterile and unsterile objects. Other less apparent modes of contamination are the filtration of airborne microorganisms through materials, passage of liquids through materials, and undetected perforations in materials. Moisture soaking through a drape, gown, or package is considered a strike-through, and the item must be considered contaminated.
4. Sterile gowns are considered sterile in front from shoulder to level of the sterile field and at the sleeves from 2 inches above the elbow to the cuff. The cuff should be considered unsterile because it tends to collect moisture and is not an effective bacterial barrier. The sleeve cuffs should always be covered by sterile gloves. Other areas of the gown that must be considered unsterile are the neckline, shoulders, areas under the arms, and back. These areas may become contaminated by perspiration or by collar and shoulder surfaces rubbing together during head and neck movements. Wrap-around gowns that completely cover the back may be sterile when first put on. The back of the gown must not be considered sterile, however, because it cannot be observed by the scrub person and protected from contamination. The sterile area of the front of the gown extends to the level of the sterile field because most scrub personnel work adjacent to a sterile table. For this reason, the scrub person should avoid changing levels, as would occur while moving from footstool to floor. To maintain sterility, scrub persons should not allow their hands or any sterile item to fall below the level of the sterile field. Scrub persons should neither sit nor lean against unsterile surfaces because the threat of contamination is great. The only time scrub persons may be seated is when the entire surgical procedure is performed at that level. Self-gowning and gloving should be done from a sterile surface separate from the sterile field. This method eliminates reaching over the sterile field to retrieve the sterile towel and then the sterile gown. It also eliminates the potential for water to be dripped on sterile items or on any part of the sterile field, preventing inadvertent contamination. When prepared, the scrub person's hands should be kept in sight at or above waist level. Elbows should be kept close to the body, and the hands should be kept away from the face. Hands should not be folded under the arms because axillary perspiration may permeate the bacterial barrier of the gown.
5. Tables are sterile only at table level. Sterile drapes are used to create a sterile field. Only the top surface of a draped table is considered sterile. Although the drape extends over the sides of a table, the sides cannot be considered sterile. Any portion of the drape that falls below the top edge of the table cannot be brought back up to the table level. When placed, a drape should not be shifted or moved. Items should be dispensed to a sterile field by methods that preserve the sterility of the items and the integrity of the sterile field. Good judgment must be used when dispensing items by presenting them to the scrub person or by placing them securely on the sterile field. A sterile field should be created as close as possible to the time of use. If a sterile field must be covered because of unavoidable case delay, the cover should be placed in such a manner that it can be removed without contamination. Using a wide cuff on the cover and draping only the top of the table allow for aseptic removal of the cover. In some instances, two covers may be needed to cover all sterile items on the tabletop. Sterile drapes also are used to create a sterile field when placed over the patient and operative bed. Any item that extends beyond the sterile boundary is considered contaminated and cannot be brought back onto the sterile field. A contaminated item must be lifted clear of the operative field without contacting the sterile surface and must be dropped with minimal handling to an nonscrubbed surgical team member, an unsterile area, or a designated receptacle. Interpretation of sterile areas

versus unsterile areas on a draped patient requires astute observation and use of good judgment.

6. The edges of a sterile enclosure are considered unsterile. Items should be dispensed to the field in a manner that preserves the sterility of the item and the integrity of the sterile field. After a sterile package or container is opened, the edges are considered unsterile. Sterile and unsterile boundaries are often intangible. A 1-inch safety margin is usually considered standard on package wrappers, whereas the sterile boundary on a wrapper used to drape a table is at the table edge. When opening a sterile wrapper, the top flap is first opened away from the operator. The side flaps follow. The inside or proximal flap is opened last. All flaps are secured in the hand by the operator, so as not to dangle and contaminate other items. When removing items from a sterile package, the scrub person should lift it straight up from the package. On peel-pack pouches, the inner edge of the heat seal is the line of demarcation. Peel-pack edges should be pulled back as opposed to being torn. The contents of the package should be flipped by the nonscrubbed person or lifted directly upward by the scrub person. Its contents should not be allowed to slide over the side of the package. Interpreting sterile boundaries requires good judgment based on an understanding of aseptic principles.

7. Sterile individuals touch only sterile items or areas; unsterile individuals touch only unsterile items or areas. All members of the surgical team must understand which areas are considered sterile and which are considered unsterile. All must maintain a continual awareness of these areas. Scrub individuals must guard the sterile field to prevent any unsterile item from contaminating the field or the individuals themselves. Unsterile individuals must not touch or reach over a sterile field or allow any unsterile item to contaminate the field. When a circulating nurse opens a package, hand and arm motions are always from unsterile to sterile objects. The circulating nurse avoids contact with the sterile area by placing the hands under the cuff to provide a protected wide margin of safety between the inside of the pack (sterile) and the hands (unsterile) (Figure 3-8). As the unsterile circulating nurse opens a sterile article that is wrapped sequentially in two wrappers with the corners folded toward the center of the article, the corner farthest from the body is opened first and the corner nearest the body opened last. When a scrub person opens a sterile wrapper, the side nearest the body is opened first. This portion of the wrapper then protects the gown and enables the individual to move closer to the table to open the opposite side (Figure 3-9). If a solution must be poured into a sterile receptacle on a sterile table, the scrub person holds the receptacle away from the table or sets it near the edge of a waterproof-draped table (Figure 3-10). This procedure eliminates the need for the unsterile circulating nurse to reach over the sterile field. Maintaining a safe margin of space can reduce accidental contamination when items are passed between sterile and unsterile fields. An instrument may be used as an extension of a team member's hands to ensure a safe margin between fields. The use of transfer forceps is unacceptable, however. Maintaining the sterility of these forceps is questionable because of many variables, such as sterilization method, type of container, and type and amount of soaking solution

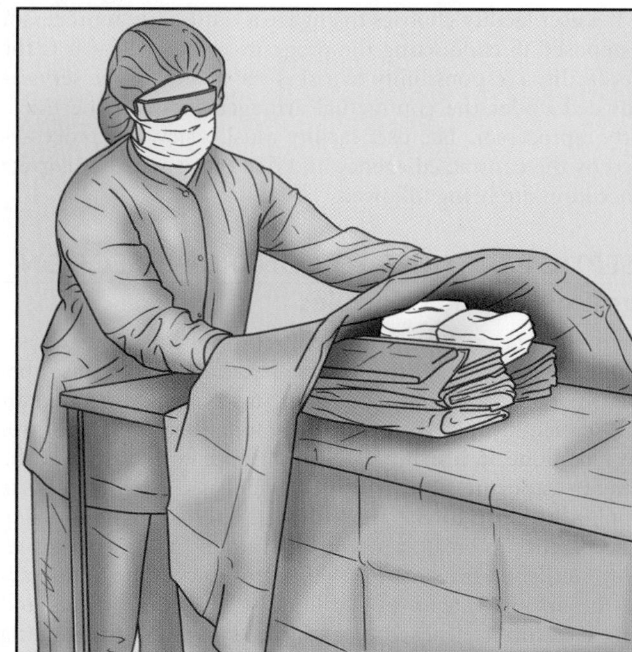

**FIGURE 3-8** Circulating nurse is shown opening the cover of a pack containing sterile drapes for surgery. The cover is cuffed to provide protection for sterile contents. The circulating nurse avoids contact with the sterile area by keeping all fingers under the cuff as the cover is drawn back over the table to expose the pack contents.

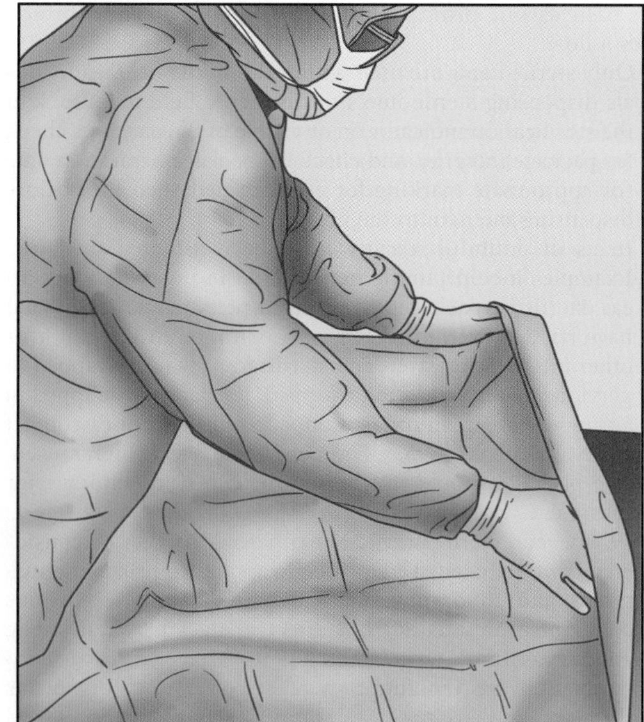

**FIGURE 3-9** Scrub person opens near side of the wrapper first, providing protection for the sterile gown. The scrub person protects gloves with the cuff of the drape as the drape is opened to provide sterile table cover.

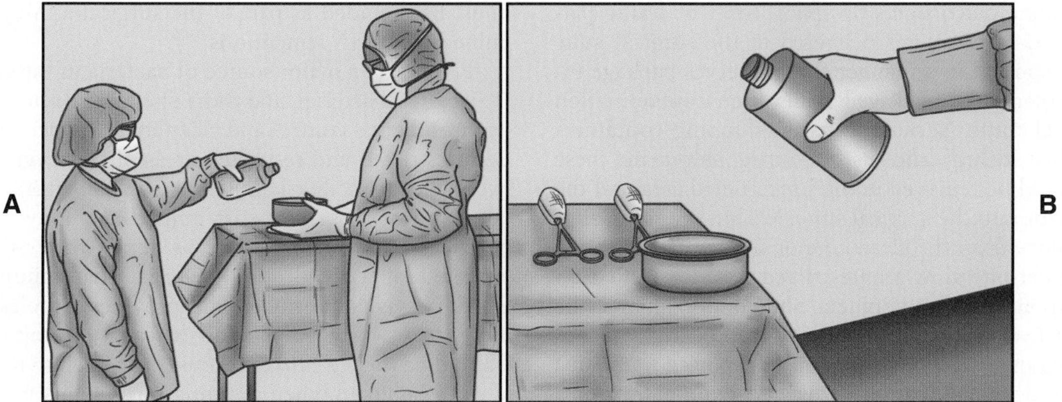


FIGURE 3-10 A, When pouring solution into the receptacle held by the scrub person, the circulating nurse maintains a safe margin of space to avoid contamination of sterile surfaces. B, Care must be used when pouring solution into a receptacle on a sterile field to avoid splashing fluids onto the sterile field. Placement of the receptacle near the edge of the table permits the circulating nurse to pour solution without reaching over any portion of the sterile field.

used. Incorrect handling of soaked forceps results in contamination. The preferred procedure is for single use of a packaged, sterile ring forceps, which is discarded into a container for reprocessing.

8. Movement within or around a sterile field must not contaminate the field. The patient is the center of the sterile field during an operative procedure; additional sterile areas are grouped around the patient. If contamination is to be prevented, patterns of movement within or around this sterile grouping must be established and rigidly practiced. Scrub persons stay close to the sterile field. If they change positions, they turn face to face or back to back with another individual while maintaining a safe distance between themselves and other objects. Accidental contamination is a threat to any scrub person who wanders into a traffic pathway or out of the clean area of the OR. Circulating nurses approach sterile areas facing them and never walk between two sterile fields. Keeping sterile areas in view during movement around the area and maintaining a safe distance from sterile fields help prevent accidental contamination. Bacterial fallout from the body or clothing is a source of contamination when an unsterile individual leans over a sterile field. All perioperative personnel must maintain vigilance over sterile areas and point out any contamination immediately. Movement within and around a sterile area should be kept to a minimum to avoid contamination of the field or the sterile members of the surgical team.

Close adherence to principles of asepsis and consistent observance of the boundaries established in the principles provide protection against infection. Application of the basic principles of aseptic technique depends primarily on the individual's understanding and conscience. Every person on the surgical team must share the responsibility for monitoring aseptic practice and initiating corrective action when a sterile field is compromised.

## Traffic Control

The surgical suite should be designed to minimize the spread of infectious organisms and to facilitate movement of patients and personnel within that framework.[21] Ideally, the suite is divided into three areas, each defined by the activities occurring within the area. The *unrestricted* area includes areas outside of the surgical suite and a control point to monitor the entrance of patients, personnel, and materials. Street clothes are appropriate attire in this area, and traffic is not limited. The *semirestricted* area comprises the peripheral support areas within the surgical suite. These may include storage areas, work areas, and corridors leading to restricted areas of the surgical suite. Traffic in the semirestricted area is limited to appropriately attired personnel and patients. Personnel must wear surgical attire and cover all head and facial hair when in this area. Patients should have their hair covered, wear clean hospital attire, and be covered with clean hospital linens. The *restricted* area includes the ORs, procedure rooms (if any), the central core, and the scrub sink area. Personnel must wear surgical attire including hair coverings when in the restricted area. Masks are worn where open sterile supplies or scrub persons may be present. Patients should wear hospital attire as just described. Masks are not required for patients because a mask could hinder access to the patient's face and airway and cause additional patient anxiety.

Personnel entering semirestricted or restricted areas of the surgical suite should do so through prescribed routes. These routes contain vestibular areas, which serve as transition zones between the outside and inside of the suite. Offices, holding rooms, and locker rooms act as transition zones. Personnel entering the OR should access the locker room via the unrestricted area. After donning clean, hospital-laundered surgical attire, personnel should exit directly into the OR suite without retracing steps through the unrestricted area.

Air is a potential source of microorganisms that can result in a surgical site infection. Airborne contamination increases with movement of the surgical team. This movement should be kept to a minimum during operative procedures. Each OR door should remain closed except during movement of patients, personnel, supplies, and equipment. The positive-pressure gradient of air in the OR is disrupted if the door remains open. The turbulent flow occurring as the pressure equalizes can increase airborne contamination.

Surgical equipment and supplies also are potential sources of contamination. Clean and sterile supplies should be separated from contaminated items by space, time, or traffic patterns. Clean and sterile items delivered to the surgical suite should be transported in a manner that preserves package integrity and protects the packaged items from contamination along the travel route. Because external shipping containers may collect dust, debris, and insects during shipment, these containers should be removed in the unrestricted area and the contents brought into the surgical suite. Within the suite, supplies should move from the clean core or storage area through the OR to the peripheral or semirestricted corridor. Soiled instruments, supplies, and equipment should not reenter the clean core. Instead, soiled items should be covered or contained in closed carts or containers and transported to an area designated for decontamination. This decontamination area should be separate from personnel and patient traffic areas, as should be the soiled linen and trash collection areas.

## Surgical Attire

Every surgical department should have a written policy and procedure regarding proper attire in the surgical suite. According to OSHA regulations and institutional policy and to prevent transmission of organisms from the patient to personnel, it is required that personnel wear personal protective equipment (PPE) when it can be reasonably anticipated that the individual may come in contact with blood or other potentially infectious materials. PPE, which includes protective eyewear; gloves; and fluid-resistant gowns, aprons, and shoe covers, must be included as part of the surgical attire policy as determined by OSHA regulations.[19,63]

People are a major source of bacteria in the surgical setting. To reduce bacterial and skin shedding (scurf) and promote environmental control and cleanliness, all persons entering the semirestricted and restricted areas of the surgical suite should wear clean, facility-laundered, surgical attire (Figure 3-11) made of multiuse fabric or limited-use nonwoven material.[19] Surgical attire, also known as *scrub attire,* should be constructed of a low-linting material that minimizes bacterial shedding, is comfortable, and provides a professional appearance. If a two-piece pantsuit is worn, the top of the pantsuit should be tucked into the trousers or fit close to the body. Care should be taken when donning scrub pants to avoid dragging the pant legs on the floor. If nonscrubbed perioperative personnel wear long-sleeved shirts, the sleeves of the warm-up jackets should cover the shirtsleeves. Long sleeves are not appropriate for scrub personnel because the surgical scrub extends beyond the edge of the long sleeves.[19] A head cover, mask, and, if required, shoe covers complete the surgical attire ensemble. Shoe covers are required if there is a risk of blood or body fluid contamination as set forth in OSHA regulations. To protect the patient and the health care worker, surgical attire must be changed whenever it becomes soiled or wet with blood, any body fluid including perspiration, or food. Nonscrubbed personnel should wear long-sleeved jackets that are buttoned or snapped closed during wear. These jackets help

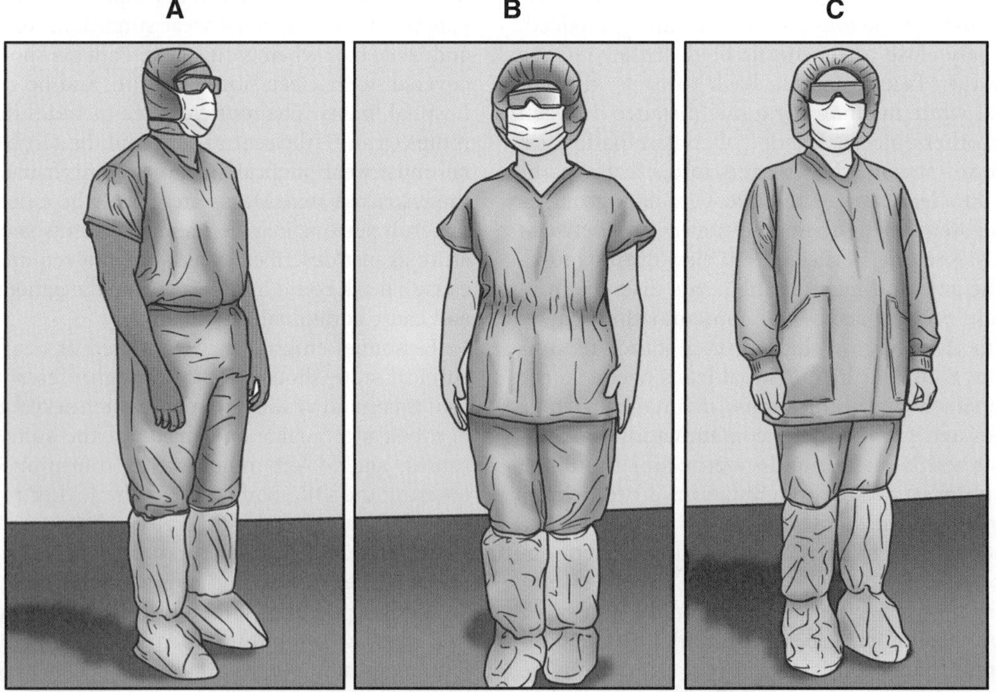


**FIGURE 3-11** Proper surgical attire consists of a two-piece pantsuit, a scrub dress, or a one-piece coverall suit. Shoe covers should be worn when it is reasonably anticipated that spills or splashes will occur. If worn, they should be changed whenever they become wet, torn, or soiled. All head and facial hair should be covered in semirestricted and restricted areas. In restricted areas, all personnel should wear masks. Jewelry should be removed or totally confined. Artificial nails should not be worn. **A,** When a two-piece scrub suit is worn, loose-fitting scrub tops should be tucked into pants. **B,** Tunic tops that fit close to the body may be worn outside of pants. **C,** Nonscrubbed personnel should wear long-sleeved jackets that are buttoned or snapped closed.

decrease bacterial and skin shedding from bare arms. Closing the jackets helps prevent inadvertent contamination, which can occur if the loose fabric brushes against a sterile area. All jewelry should be confined within scrub attire or removed when personnel enter the semirestricted or restricted areas of the surgical suite. This includes any visible jewelry associated with body piercing. Confinement reduces the possibility of jewelry falling or shedding bacteria into a sterile field or wound. Before handwashing, rings, watches, and bracelets should be removed because organisms can be harbored beneath these pieces of jewelry.[19]

Before scrub attire is donned, a clean, lint-free surgical hat or hood that completely covers all head and facial hair should be donned. Hair acts as a filter when left uncovered and collects bacteria, which are released into the air during activity. Hair attracts, harbors, and sheds bacteria in proportion to its length, curliness, and oiliness. A head cover eliminates the possibility of hair or dandruff being shed on the scrub suit. The design and composition of the hat or hood should minimize dispersal of bacteria, be comfortable to wear, and confine and contain all hair. Head covers should always be worn in areas where equipment and supplies are processed and stored. Disposable bouffant and hood types of head covers are preferred. They are discarded in a designated receptacle immediately after use. Skullcaps that fail to cover the side hair above the ears and hair at the nape of the neck should not be worn in the OR. If reusable hats or hoods are worn, they should be laundered daily. If they become contaminated with blood or body fluids, they must be laundered according to OSHA regulations.

For personnel safety, shoes that provide protection should be worn. Cloth shoes provide little protection against spilled liquids or sharp items that may be accidentally dropped to the floor. Shoes with enclosed toes and heels help minimize injury. Shoe covers may be worn to help keep shoes clean and may decrease the amount of soil and bacterial tracking throughout the suite. It is easier to change a shoe cover than to stop to clean or change a shoe that has become soiled. If it is reasonably expected that the feet may become contaminated with blood or body fluids, shoe covers are required as part of personal protective attire. Shoe covers should be kept in an area adjacent to the semirestricted area entrance. They should be removed and discarded in the appropriate receptacle on leaving the restricted area.

A surgical mask is worn to reduce the dispersal of microbial droplets expelled from the mouth and nasopharynx of personnel and to protect health care workers from aerosolized pathogenic organisms and particles from the surgical environment. Single, high-filtration surgical masks are worn in ORs and other designated areas where open sterile supplies or scrub persons may be located. A single mask provides a filter; double-masking creates a barrier, causing the exhaled air to be expelled through tents and gaps around the mask. Although some studies indicated that oral bacteria expelled by personnel in the OR are of no threat to the surgical patient and that surgical masks for nonscrubbed personnel in the OR may not be necessary,[62] OSHA regulations mandate the use of surgical masks as part of personal protection.

When a mask is being chosen, one with a microbial filtration efficiency of 95% or greater should be selected. Aerosol particles generated by the surgical team, sometimes visible to the naked eye, are most likely 10 μm or larger. The plume of lasers or the electrosurgical unit has been found to contain particles with a mass of 0.31 μm, smaller than that expelled by the surgical staff. The filtration efficiency of masks should ensure protection against aerosol particles 0.1 μm.[41] The most effective filter mask is relatively useless if worn incorrectly, however, and can be dangerous if handled improperly. Figure 3-12 illustrates the proper application and removal of a surgical mask.

The mask must cover the mouth and nose entirely and have facial compliance, fitting comfortably around the contours of the nose and cheeks. The mask is tied securely without crossing the strings. Crossing strings allows the sides of the mask to gap (tenting) and consequently permits nonfiltered air to escape through venting. Air should pass only through the filtering system (the faceplate) of the mask. A pliable metal or adhesive strip in the top hem of some masks provides a firm, contoured fit over the bridge of the nose. This strip may help prevent fogging of protective eyewear. Masks should be either on (properly) or off. They should not be saved from one operation to the next by being left hanging around the neck or being tucked into a pocket. Bacteria that have been filtered by the mask become dry and airborne if the mask is worn necklace-fashion. Touching only the strings during removal of the mask reduces contamination of the hands. Masks should be changed between procedures and sometimes during a procedure, depending on the length of the operation and the amount of talking done by the team. The facepiece, which is contaminated with droplet nuclei, should not come into contact with the hands of personnel. Immediately after removal, masks should be discarded directly into a designated covered waste receptacle. After discarding the mask, the wearer must wash and dry the hands thoroughly.

Gloves should be selected according to the task to be done: sterile gloves for sterile procedures, unsterile gloves for other tasks. Gloves should be changed between patient contacts and after contact with any infectious material. Hands should be washed thoroughly after gloves are removed. To reduce the risk of mouth, nose, and eye mucous membrane exposure, protective eyewear, masks, or face shields are worn whenever there is opportunity for contamination by splash or aerosols. When the protective devices become contaminated, they should be discarded or decontaminated as soon as possible to prevent contamination to the wearer. Other protective equipment such as liquid-resistant attire, including gowns and shoe covers, should be worn whenever there is a reasonable expectation of exposure to infectious materials.

## Surgical Hand Antisepsis

Skin is a major source of microbial contamination in the surgical environment. Although members of the surgical team at the sterile field wear sterile gowns and gloves, the skin of their hands and forearms should be cleaned preoperatively to reduce the number of microorganisms in the event of glove failure. The purposes of surgical hand antisepsis are to remove dirt, skin oil, and transient microorganisms from the nails, hands, and forearms; to reduce the resident microbial count to as near zero as possible; and to leave an antimicrobial residue on the skin to prevent regrowth of microbes for several hours.[20] The skin can never be rendered sterile, but it can be made surgically clean by reducing the number of microorganisms present.

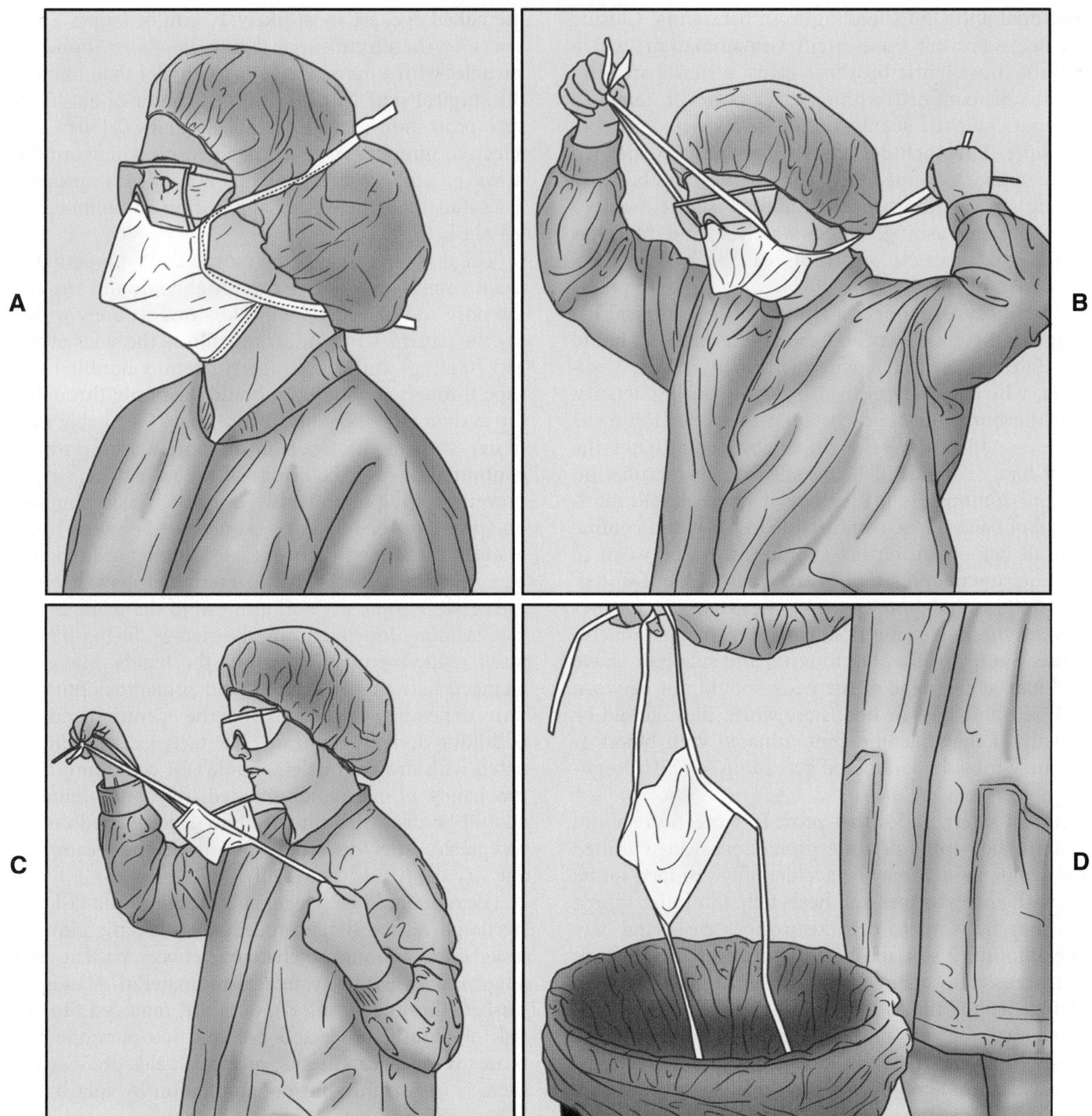


**FIGURE 3-12** Proper handling of a mask. **A**, Edges of a properly worn mask conform to facial contours when the mask is applied and tied correctly. **B** and **C**, Personnel should avoid touching the filter portion of the mask when removing it. **D**, Masks should be discarded on removal.

Scrub persons should be in good health and possess healthy, intact skin. Cuts, abrasions, and hangnails tend to ooze serum, a potential risk for infection. Because microorganisms may be protected and harbored by rings, watches, body-piercing jewelry and bracelets, these items should be removed before scrubbing.[20] Fingernails of scrub persons should be short, clean, and healthy. The subungual region of the nails harbors most microorganisms found on the hands. Soap, running water, and a nail-cleaning device are necessary to clean under the fingernails. Nails that extend beyond the tips of the fingers are more difficult to clean and increase the risk of glove tears. Longer nails also may scratch patients during the positioning or transfer process. Artificial nails or synthetic nails should not be worn. Higher numbers of gram-negative organisms have been cultured from the nails of individuals wearing artificial nails or nail additives than from individuals with natural nails before and after handwashing.[20,45] Fungal growth also occurs under artificial nails as a result of trapped moisture between the natural and artificial nail. The length of artificial nails may interfere with effective hand scrubs and handwashing.

Facility infection control procedures govern the selection of materials and the methods used for surgical hand antisepsis. This may be accomplished by a surgical scrub or with the use of an approved hand rub agent.

***Surgical Hand Rub.*** All hand rub products that are alcohol-based are not indicated for use in lieu of the traditional hand scrub. Rubs come in many forms, combinations, and concentration of alcohols, which may influence the antimicrobial strength and kill factor. Many of these products contain isopropanol, ethanol, n-propanol, or combinations at various concentrations. Subsequently, the effectiveness of each product should be evaluated. A review of each product by the infection control committee should include an analysis of its effectiveness, ease of use, concentration, and cost-benefit ratio.[81,82] When hand rubs are used for surgical hand antisepsis, only a FDA-compliant, alcohol-based surgical hand rub product should be used. Alcohols in 60% to 90% concentrations are highly effective in lowering skin bacterial counts immediately after application. Alcohols do not have a persistent activity, but bacteria continue to die or reproduce slowly after exposure to alcohol. Prescrub bacterial levels can occur, however, after gloves are worn for 1 to 3 hours. In addition, alcohol is irritating to the skin. By combining alcohol with appropriate concentrations of other antimicrobials having a persistent activity (e.g., chlorhexidine gluconate) and adding compatible emollient agents, manufacturers have produced effective, nonirritating, hand-hygiene agents with persistent activity. The manufacturer's written instructions for contact time and amount of product to be used should be followed. The basic steps of a surgical hand antisepsis/hand rub are as follows:

1. Turn on the faucet, bringing water to a comfortable temperature. Most scrub sinks have automatic or knee controls for the faucets.
2. Moisten hands and forearms and wash with soap and running water to create lather.
3. Clean nail beds with a disposable nail cleaner under running water. Discard nail cleaner after use.
4. Rinse hands and forearms under running water.
5. Dry hands and forearms thoroughly.
6. Apply the hand rub product to the hands and forearms. Manufacturer's written instructions should be followed regarding the amount of time the product should be applied and whether water should be used as part of the hand rub process. Rub thoroughly until dry.

***Surgical Hand Scrub.*** For the traditional surgical scrub, individually packaged disposable brushes and sponges or synthetic sponges without a brush may be used. The use of synthetic sponges in place of brushes has gained wide acceptance, especially where long and repeated scrubbing may be traumatic to the skin. Disposable brushes or sponges are available with a variety of antimicrobial soap or antiseptic solutions impregnated into the sponge. A thorough hand wash with an antimicrobial agent may be as effective as the traditional surgical scrub using a brush or sponge.[58]

Surgical hand-scrub agent selection should be based on the effectiveness of the product, recommended contact time, and user-friendliness of the product. The antimicrobial soap or detergent used for the surgical hand scrub should:

- Reduce microorganisms on the skin
- Be fast acting
- Have a broad range of activity
- Not depend on cumulative action
- Have a minimally harsh effect on skin
- Inhibit regrowth of microorganisms

Antimicrobial agents used for surgical hand scrubs include povidone-iodine complex and chlorhexidine gluconate (CHG). These agents are broad-spectrum, rapid-acting antimicrobials that are effective against many gram-positive and gram-negative microorganisms. For individuals who have skin sensitivity to these agents, another broad-spectrum antimicrobial agent, parachloro-metaxylenol (chloroxylenol, PCMX), may be used as an effective alternative agent for surgical scrubbing. Many individuals who previously were unable to use any surgical hand scrub other than hexachlorophene (which is ineffective against gram-negative microorganisms) are now safely using PCMX. It significantly reduces skin flora with an antibacterial effect that persists after prolonged surgery. Moisturizing agents are now being incorporated into various surgical scrub agents to reduce the potential of skin irritation resulting from multiple scrubs.

An anatomic scrub, using a prescribed amount of time or number of strokes plus friction, is employed for effective cleansing of the skin. The fingers, hands, and arms should be visualized as having four sides; each side must be scrubbed effectively. Individual attention to detail is essential. The prescribed number of strokes with a brush is usually 30 strokes to the nails and 20 strokes to each area of the skin. When using the timed approach, the institution's protocol should be followed. Surgical hand-scrub procedures should be documented and available within the perioperative setting.

***Scrub Procedure.*** Before beginning the surgical hand scrub, members of the surgical team should inspect their hands to ensure that their nails are short, their cuticles are in good condition, and no cuts or skin problems exist. All jewelry is removed from the hands and forearms. The cap or hood is adjusted to cover and contain all hair. A fresh mask is placed carefully over the nose and mouth and tied securely to prevent venting. Protective eyewear, such as goggles with side shields or a full-face shield, is adjusted to ensure clear vision and to avoid lens fogging. Personnel confirm that the scrub shirt is tucked into the trousers to prevent potential contamination of the scrubbed hands and arms from brushing against loose garments. The basic steps of the scrub procedure follow:

1. Turn on faucet, and bring water to a comfortable temperature. Most scrub sinks have automatic or knee controls for the faucets.
2. Moisten hands and forearms.
3. Using a foot control, dispense the manufacturer's recommended amount of the antimicrobial agent into the palms. Add small amounts of water to create lather.
4. Wash hands and forearms using the antimicrobial soap or detergent. Rinse before beginning the surgical hand scrub. The amount of time needed varies with the amount of soil and the effectiveness of the cleansing agent.
5. If a packaged scrub brush or sponge is used, open the package, remove the brush and nail cleaner, and discard the package. Hold the brush in one hand while cleaning the nails on the other hand (Figure 3-13). Clean all nails and subungual spaces. If a disposable nail cleaner is unavailable, a metal nail file can be used.
6. Rinse the hands and arms thoroughly, exercising care to hold the hands higher than the elbows. Avoid splashing water onto the scrub suit because this moisture may cause subsequent contamination of the sterile gown.
7. If the brush or sponge is impregnated with antimicrobial soap, moisten the brush or sponge and begin scrubbing. If the brush or sponge is not impregnated with soap, apply antimicrobial soap or detergent solution to hands. Starting

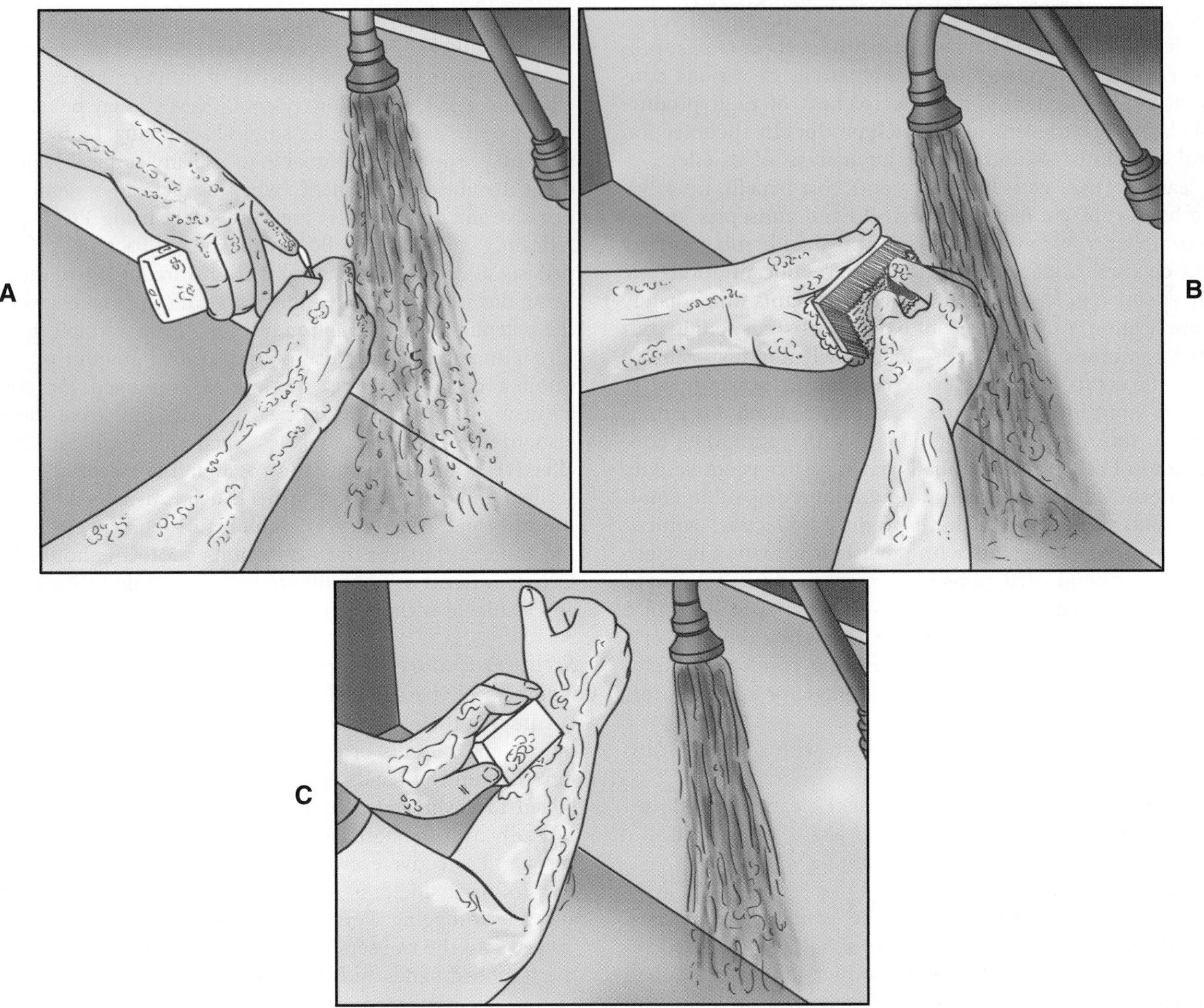


FIGURE 3-13 Traditional surgical scrub technique. A, Cleaning nails with plastic nail cleaner. B, Holding brush/sponge perpendicular to nails facilitates thorough scrubbing of underside of nails. C, Holding brush/sponge lengthwise along arm covers maximum area with each stroke.

at the fingertips, scrub the nails vigorously, holding the brush perpendicular to the nails. Scrub all sides of each digit, including the connecting webbed spaces. Next scrub the palm and back of the hand.

8. Scrub each side of the forearm with a circular motion (see Figure 3-13) up to the elbows.
9. Hold the hands and arms away from the body, with the hands above the level of the elbows while scrubbing, allowing the water and detritus to flow away from the first-scrubbed and cleanest area. Add small amounts of water during the scrub to develop suds and remove detritus.
10. Rinse the hands and arms thoroughly.
11. If the sink is not automatically timed, turn off the faucet by using the knee control or by using the edge of the brush on a hand control. Discard the brush or sponge.
12. Hold the hands and arms up in front of the body with elbows slightly flexed and enter the OR.

***Drying the Scrubbed Area.*** Moisture remaining on the cleansed skin after the scrub procedure should be dried with a sterile towel before donning sterile gown and gloves. The gown and gloves should be opened on a flat surface before the surgical scrub is completed. A small sterile field is created by the gown wrapper, which is opened over the flat surface. The gown and gloves should not be opened on the sterile back table because of the increased chance of contamination to the field. The towel must be used with care to avoid contaminating the clean skin. The folded towel is grasped firmly near the open corner and lifted straight up and away from the sterile field without dripping contaminated water from the skin onto the sterile field. The person steps away from the sterile field and bends forward slightly from the waist, holding the hands and elbows above the waist and away from the body. The towel is allowed to unfold downward to its full length and width (Figure 3-14).

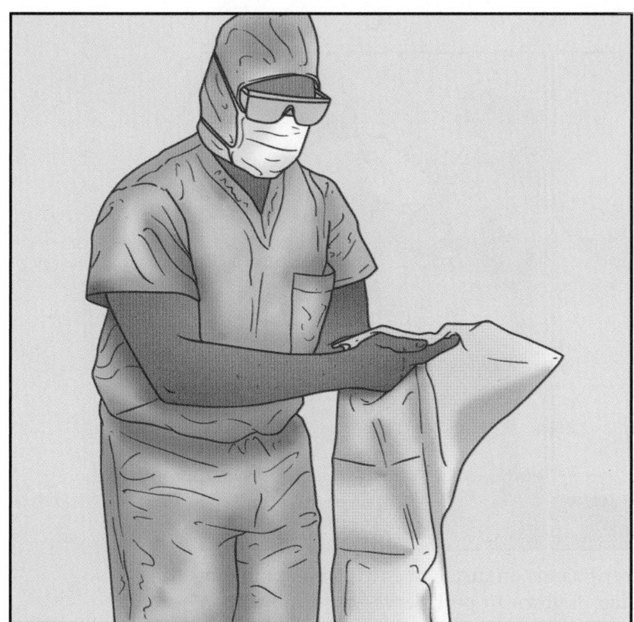

**FIGURE 3-14** Drying hands and forearms. Fingers and hand are dried thoroughly before forearm is dried. Extending arms reduces possibility of contaminating towel or hands.

The top half of the towel is held securely with one hand, and the opposite fingers and hand are blotted dry; ensure that they are thoroughly dry before moving to the forearm. To avoid contamination, use a rotating motion while moving up the arm and do not retrace an area. The lower end of the towel is grasped with the dried hand, and the same procedure is used for drying the second hand and forearm. Care must be taken to prevent contamination of towel and hands. On completion, discard the towel without dropping the hands below waist level.

## Gowning

Before scrub personnel can touch sterile equipment or the sterile field, they must put on sterile gowns and sterile surgical gloves to prevent microorganisms on their hands and clothing from being transferred to the patient's wound during surgery. The sterile gowns and gloves also protect the hands and clothing of personnel from microorganisms present in the patient or in the atmosphere.

The surgical gown should be made of a combustion-resistant material that establishes an effective barrier to minimize the passage of microorganisms, particulate matter, and fluids between unsterile and sterile areas. Reusable fabrics must allow complete penetration of steam during the sterilization process and should withstand multiple launderings and other processing. Tests indicate that 280-thread count, water repellent–treated materials lose their barrier quality when subjected to multiple laundering, and sterilizations, usually at about 75 to 100 cycles. Original barrier quality of the material must be maintained until the manufacturer's recommended number of processings has been reached. A mechanism should be established to monitor the number of times the fabric is processed. The manufacturer must provide the facility with instructions for testing the material at periodic intervals during the life of the product to ensure continued barrier quality. The particular item should be removed from circulation when the maximum number of processings as noted by the manufacturer has been reached. If possible, the item may be used in circumstances where surgical-barrier quality is not needed. With each processing, reusable materials also must be examined for holes or fraying. If these occur, the material should be removed from service. To reduce particle dissemination into the wound and the environment, materials used for surgical gowns should be tear-resistant and puncture-resistant and as lint-free as possible.[16,19] Regardless of the gown's material, the shape and size should fit the wearer and allow freedom of movement. To provide extra protection, the gown's front from the waist upward and the forearms of the sleeves can be reinforced with additional or different water-repellent material. Each sleeve should be finished with a tight-fitting cuff that prevents the inner side of the sleeve from slipping down onto the outer side of the sterile glove. Cotton tapes, snaps, or Velcro fasteners are attached to the back of the gown to hold it closed. A wraparound gown may be used to achieve better coverage of the back. Once donned, however, the back of the gown is never considered sterile.

Because the outer side of the front and sleeves of the gown come into contact with the sterile field during surgery, the gown must be folded so that the scrub person can put it on without touching the outer side with bare hands. For in-house wrapping and sterilization, the gown is folded with the inner side out and the back edges together. The sleeves are not turned inside out; consequently, they remain within the folded gown. The side folds of the gown are folded lengthwise toward the center back opening, overlapping slightly at the center. With the open edges of the gown remaining on the inside, the bottom third of the gown is folded upward and the top third of the gown is folded over the bottom portion. The gown is then folded in half widthwise so that the inside front neckline of the gown is visible on top. Gowns with wraparound backs are prepared in the same manner, with care taken to tie the tape securely on the wraparound back flap to the external side tie of the gown before initial folding. A folded hand towel with its free corners facing up is usually placed on top of the folded gown before the gown is wrapped and sterilized.

***Self-Gowning Procedure.*** The procedure for donning a wraparound sterile surgical gown follows (Figures 3-15 and 3-16). The scrub person should do the following:

1. Grasp the sterile gown at the neckline with both hands and lift from the wrapper. Step into an area where the gown may be opened without risk of contamination.
2. Hold the gown away from the body, and allow it to unfold with the inside toward the wearer.
3. Keep hands on the inside of the gown while it completely unfolds.
4. Slip both hands into the open armholes, keeping the hands at shoulder level and away from the body.
5. Push the hands and forearms into the sleeves of the gown, advancing the hands only to the proximal edge of the cuff.

The circulating nurse should do the following:

6. Pull the gown over the scrub person's shoulders, touching only the inner shoulder and side seams.
7. Tie or clasp the neckline and tie the inner waist ties of the gown, touching only the inner aspect of the gown. The

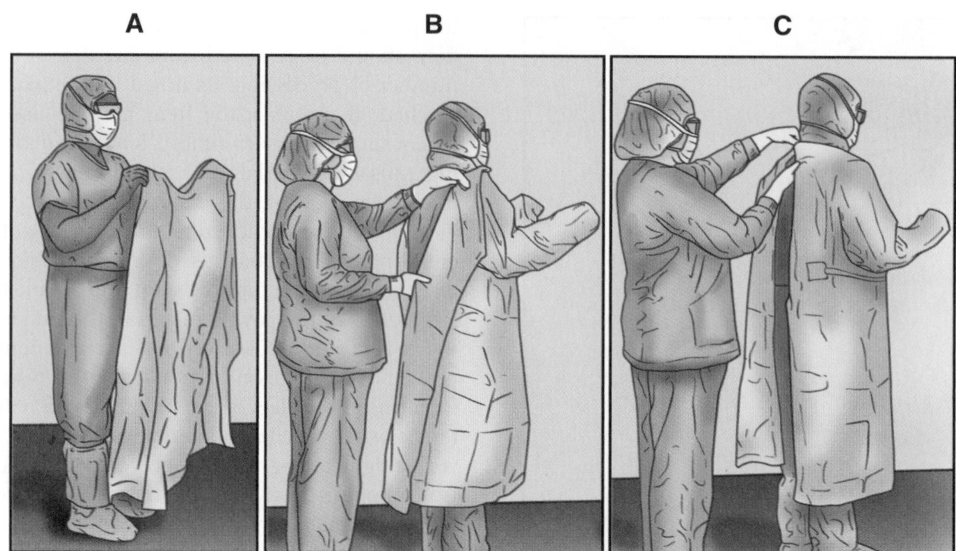


**FIGURE 3-15** Gowning procedure. A, Scrub person keeps hands on inside of gown while unfolding it at arm's length. B, Circulating nurse reaches under flap of gown to pull sleeves on scrub person. C, Circulating nurse snaps neckline of gown, touching only snap section of neckline.

gown should be completely fastened by the circulator before the scrub person dons gloves, to prevent contamination from the gown flapping.

To secure the gown, the scrub person and the circulating nurse should do the following:

8. After gloving, the scrub person hands the tab attached to the back tie of the gown to the circulating nurse. The scrub person then makes a three-fourths turn to the left while the circulating nurse extends the back tie to its full length. This action effectively wraps the back panel of the gown around the scrub person and covers the previously tied inner waist ties. The scrub person retrieves the back tie by carefully pulling it out of the tab held by the circulating nurse and ties it with the other tie, which had been secured to the front top of the gown.

When a reusable gown is used, absence of a tab on the back tie necessitates use of an alternative procedure for securing the gown (see Figure 3-16 *C, D,* and *E*). If the closed gloving technique and commercially prepared, double-wrapped gloves are employed, the inner wrap can be used as a protective extension for the gown tie when the circulating nurse assists with tying a wraparound gown. After gloving, the scrub person unties the exterior gown ties (which were tied at the front of the gown before it was folded, wrapped, and sterilized) and holds both in the hands. The end of the back tie is placed in the center crease of the empty glove wrapper, approximately two-thirds of the way up to the edge of the opened wrapper. The glove wrapper is then closed so that the tie is concealed. The closed wrapper is handed to the circulating nurse, who firmly grasps the folded edge of the wrapper without touching the tie. The scrub person pivots in the opposite direction from the circulating nurse, who extends the back tie to its full length. The scrub person grasps the exposed portion of the back tie, pulls it out of the glove wrapper while taking care to avoid touching the glove wrapper or the circulating nurse, and ties both ties. If a sterile glove wrapper is unavailable, a sterile hemostat or ringed forceps may be clamped to the back tie and used in the same manner as a glove wrapper. After the gowning procedure has been completed, the circulating nurse retains the instrument in the room to avoid problems with the subsequent instrument count.

If another scrub person is gowned and gloved, that individual, instead of the circulating nurse, may assist with the wraparound procedure. The assisting individual must extend the back tie to its fullest length before the scrub person turns, to avoid any potential contamination.

***Assisted-Gowning Procedure.*** A gowned and gloved individual may assist another individual in donning a sterile gown (Figure 3-17). The gown is opened in the manner previously described. The inner side with the open armholes is turned toward the individual who is to be gowned. A cuff is made of the neck and shoulder area of the gown to protect the gloved hands. The gown is held until the person's hands and forearms are in the sleeves of the gown. The circulating nurse assists in pulling the gown onto the shoulders, adjusting the back, and tying the tapes. The wraparound back on the gown is fixed into position by the scrub person after gloving is completed.

## Gloving

Sterile surgical gloves are worn to provide a barrier between the patient and the health care worker, decreasing the probability of exposing the patient to exogenous organisms with a resulting surgical site infection or the health care worker to exposure to blood or other potentially infectious material. Nonetheless, many surgeons, first assistants, and scrub personnel have encountered blood on their hands at the conclusion of a surgical procedure without being aware of any breech in the glove barrier (glove puncture, tear, or rip). Increasing evidence supports and recommends the practice of double-gloving to offer a degree of protection from this common event. Although a breech may occur in the outer glove, the inner glove remains intact and continues to serve as a barrier. Some surgeons who work in areas where perforation risk is high,

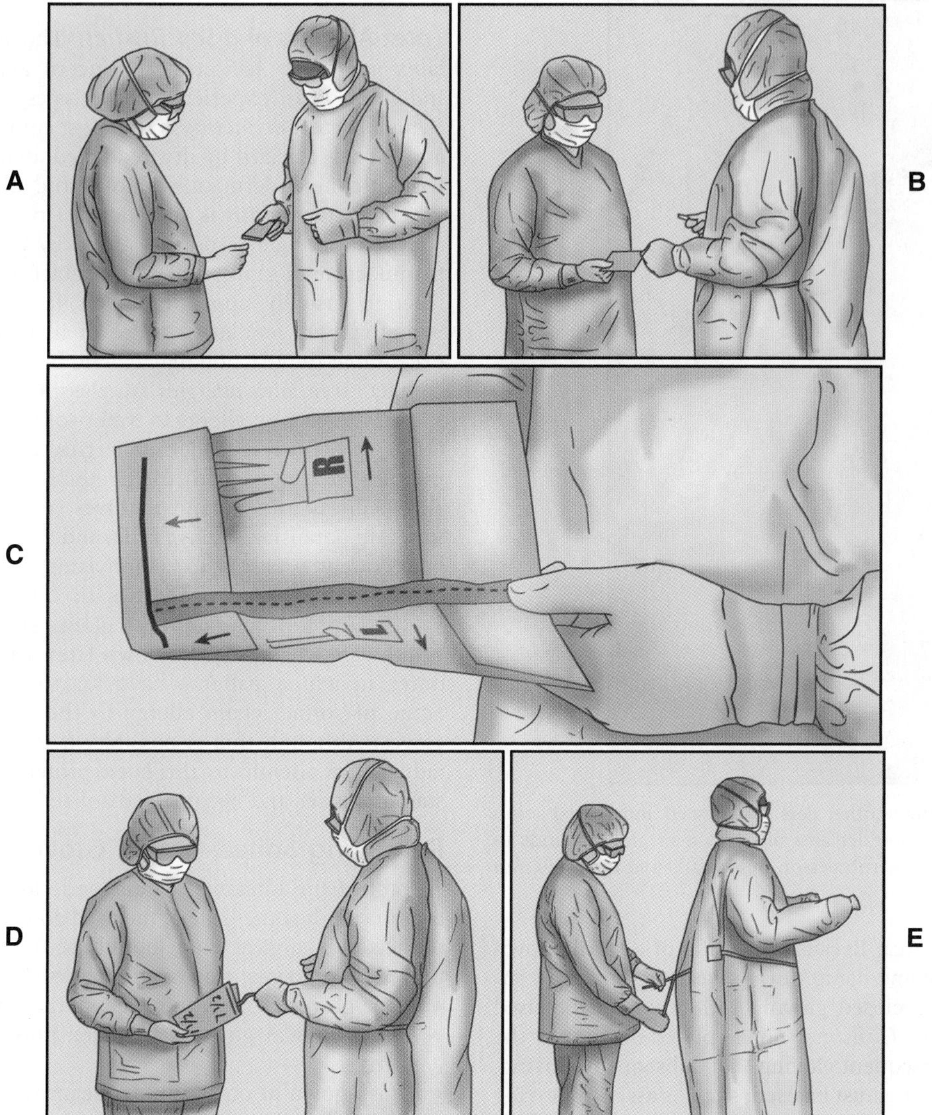


**FIGURE 3-16** Methods of tying a wraparound gown. **A,** After handing tab on back tie of gown to circulating nurse, scrub person makes a three-fourths turn toward the left. **B,** Sterile back panel now covers previously tied unsterile ties; scrub person retrieves back tie by carefully pulling it out of the tab held by circulating nurse and ties it securely with other tie. **C,** For gowns having no tab on back tie: using sterile inner glove wrapper, scrub person places the end of the back tie in the crease of the wrapper. **D,** After closing the wrapper, scrub person hands tie to circulating nurse, who grasps it carefully, touching neither the tie nor the gloved hand of the scrub person. **E,** After making a three-fourths turn to the left, scrub person carefully pulls back tie from wrapper and ties it with other tie as in step **B.**

such as orthopedics or thoracic surgery, opt to wear double-layer gloves, with the inside glove being a colored glove, which allows the wearer to recognize perforations to the outer glove. In orthopedic surgery, surgeons may wear a glove liner between two layers of gloves to reduce perforations to the inner glove. On completion of the case, both pairs of gloves should be discarded, and hand antisepsis should be performed.

The use of powder as a glove lubricant is not recommended because of three primary hazards: the potential for postoperative complication of powder granulomas; powder fallout from hands and gloves, which provides a convenient vehicle for dissemination of microorganisms throughout the OR; and the ability of powder to carry and disperse latex proteins, contributing to an increased latex sensitivity among health care workers and others. Powder-free gloves are widely available. If powdered gloves are chosen, any glove film or powder must be removed. The gloves must be wiped thoroughly after they are put on and before approaching the sterile field.

***Closed-Gloving Technique.*** The closed method of gloving (Figure 3-18) is the technique of choice when initially donning sterile gown and gloves. Using this technique, the gloves are handled through the fabric of the gown sleeves. The hands are not extended from the sleeves and cuffs when the gown is put on. Instead, the hands are pushed through the cuff openings as the gloves are pulled into place. The woven cuff should remain

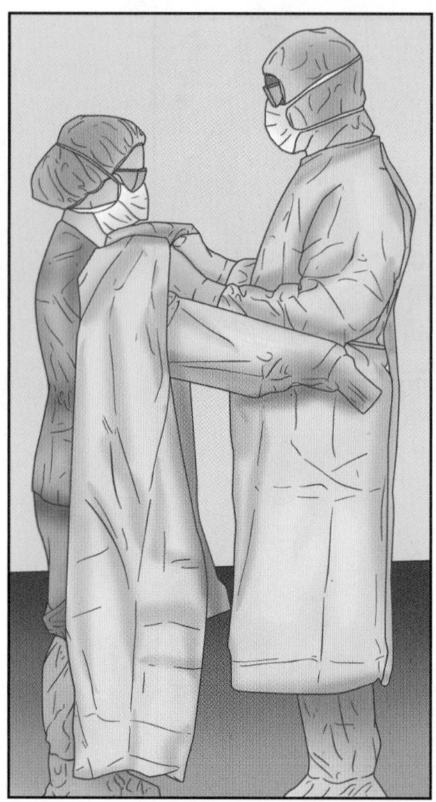

FIGURE 3-17 Gowning another person. Gowned and gloved scrub person cuffs neck and shoulder area of gown over gloved hands to prevent contamination as scrub person puts hands and forearms into sleeves.

in the natural wrist area. Because the cuffs of a sterile gown collect moisture, become damp during wearing, and are considered unsterile, the closed gloving technique can be used only for initial gloving. Cuffs may not be pulled down over the wearer's hand for subsequent gloving. For subsequent gloving, an alternative technique must be used, such as assisted gloving or open gloving.

***Open-Gloving Technique.*** With the open-gloving technique, the everted cuff of each glove permits a gowned individual to touch the glove's inner side with ungloved fingers and to touch the glove's outer side with gloved fingers (Figure 3-19). Keeping the hands in direct view, no lower than waist level, the gowned individual flexes the elbows. Exerting a light, even pull on the glove brings it over the hand, and using a rotating movement brings the cuff over the wristlet. Extreme caution is necessary when using the open method to prevent contamination by the exposed hands. This gloving technique can be used by individuals not wearing a gown.

***Assisted-Gloving Technique.*** A gowned and gloved individual may assist another gowned individual with gloving. To assist another individual, grasp the glove under the everted cuff. Ensure the palm of the glove is turned toward the ungloved individual's hand with the thumb of the glove directly opposed to the thumb of the individual's hand. Using fingers, stretch the cuff to open the glove. The ungloved individual can insert his or her hand into the glove. The procedure is repeated for the other hand (Figure 3-20).

***Latex Allergies and Sensitivities.*** The increased reporting of latex sensitivity has created concern among OR personnel. Individuals can experience three types of reactions to latex. *Irritant contact dermatitis* is the most common type of reaction and is characterized by dry, reddened, itchy, or cracked hands. Irritant contact dermatitis is not a true allergic reaction. *Allergic contact dermatitis* is considered a type IV allergic reaction and is an allergic response caused by chemicals used in the manufacture of gloves. Allergic contact dermatitis is a delayed reaction, usually appearing 6 to 48 hours after exposure. Symptoms are similar to those of irritant contact dermatitis except that the reaction may extend beyond the actual point of contact. *True latex allergies* are classified as type I allergic responses. This is an allergy to water-soluble natural rubber latex (NRL) proteins. True latex allergies are usually seen within minutes of contact with the proteins. Symptoms range from skin redness and itching to hives, dyspnea, gastrointestinal upset, hypotension, tachycardia, and anaphylaxis. Reactions to latex rarely progress to anaphylaxis because the wearer is treated with appropriate drugs to interrupt the allergic response. Appropriate latex-free gloves should be provided for health care workers with known latex sensitivity or for procedures in which patients have known sensitivity or allergy. Some personnel claim allergy to the starch powder in latex gloves. Although this is possible, it is more likely that individuals are allergic to the latex proteins that bind with the starch powder and become aerosolized.[76]

## Removing Soiled Gown, Gloves, and Mask

To protect the forearms, hands, and clothing from contacting bacteria on the outer side of the used gown and gloves, members of the scrub surgical team should use the following steps to remove soiled gowns, gloves, and masks (Figure 3-21):

- Wipe gloves clean with a wet, sterile towel.
- Untie surgical gown. Circulator must unfasten back closures.
- Grasp gown at one shoulder seam without touching scrub clothing.
- Bring neck and sleeve of the gown forward, over, and off the gloved hand, turning the gown inside out and everting the cuff of the glove.
- Repeat above two steps for the other side.
- Keep arms and gown away from body while turning the gown inside out and discarding carefully in the designated receptacle.
- Using the gloved fingers of one hand to secure the everted cuff, remove the glove turning it inside out. Discard appropriately.
- Using the ungloved hand, grasp the fold of the everted cuff of the other glove and remove the glove, inverting the glove as it is removed. Discard appropriately.
- After leaving the restricted area, remove the mask by touching the ties or elastic only.
- Discard in the designated receptacle.
- Wash hands and forearms.

## Patient Skin Disinfection and Preparation

To prevent bacteria on the skin surfaces from entering the surgical wound, the skin area at and around the proposed incision site must be cleaned and disinfected. Skin preparation methods

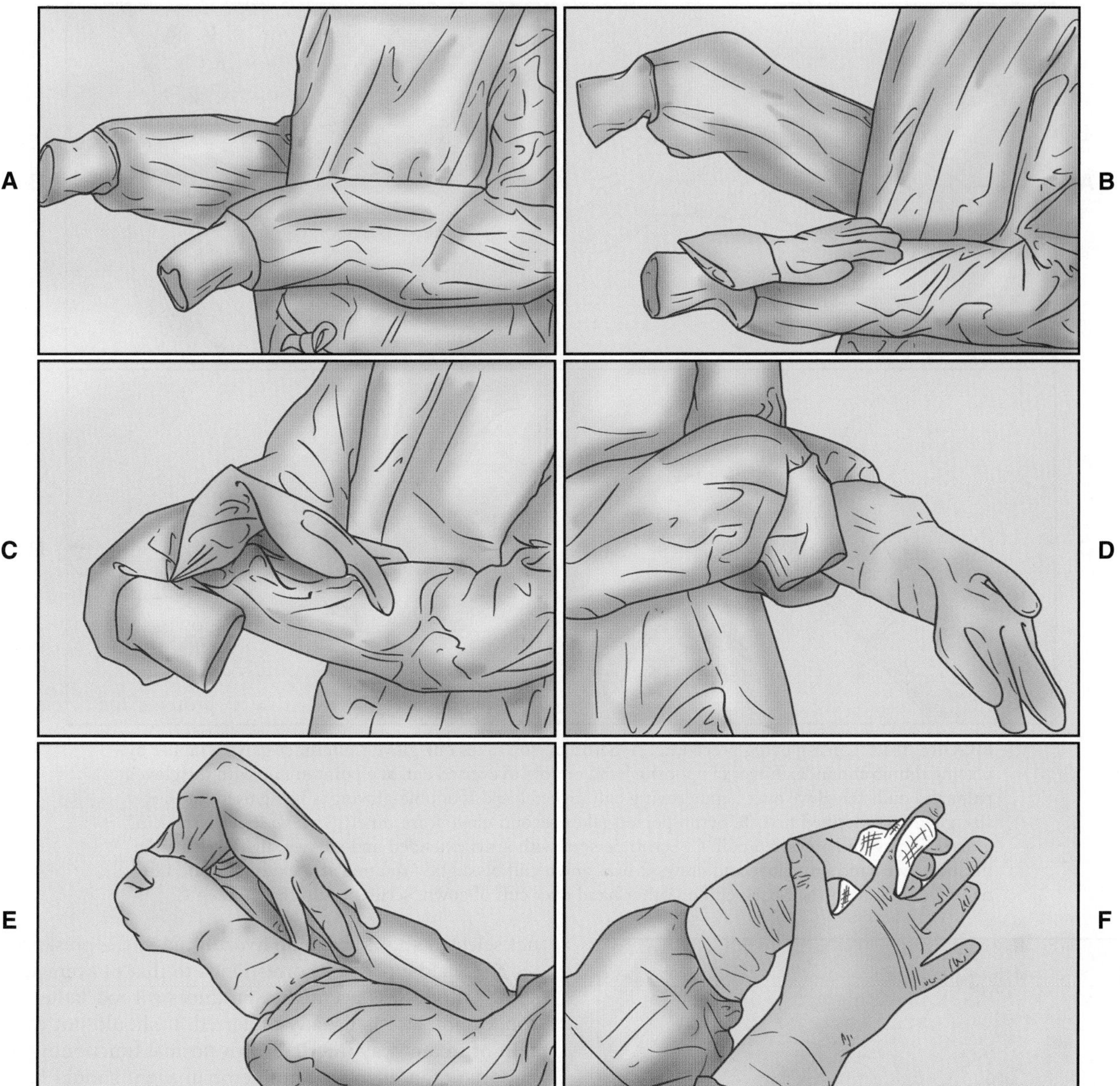


FIGURE 3-18 Closed-gloving procedure. **A,** When donning gown, scrub person does not slip hands through gown cuffs. Hands are not extended from sleeves. **B,** First the glove is lifted by grasping it through the fabric of the sleeve. Cuff on glove facilitates easier handling of glove. The glove is placed palm down along forearm of matching hand, with thumb and fingers pointing toward elbow. Glove cuff lies over gown cuff. If double-gloving is being used, the larger size gloves are donned first. **C,** Glove cuff is held securely by hand on which it is placed, and with the other hand, the cuff is stretched over the opening of the sleeve to cover gown cuff entirely. **D,** As cuff is drawn back onto wrist, fingers are directed into their cots in the glove, and the glove is adjusted to the hand. **E,** Gloved hand is used to position remaining glove on opposite sleeve in the same fashion. Glove cuff is placed around gown cuff. The second glove is drawn onto the hand, and cuff is pulled into place. **F,** Fingers of gloves are adjusted, and gloves are wiped with wet gauze sponge or commercially prepared sterile, disposable, glove wipe to remove any powder that may be on them.

vary, but all are based on the same principles and share the same objectives: to remove dirt and transient microbes from the skin, to reduce the resident microbial count as much as possible in the shortest time and with the least amount of tissue irritation, and to prevent rapid rebound growth of microbes. Factors to be considered in skin disinfection are as follows:

1. Condition of the involved area
2. Number and kinds of contaminants
3. Characteristics of the skin to be disinfected
4. General physical condition of the patient

Many soaps and detergents are available for skin cleansing. Although most of them produce similar results for the immedi-

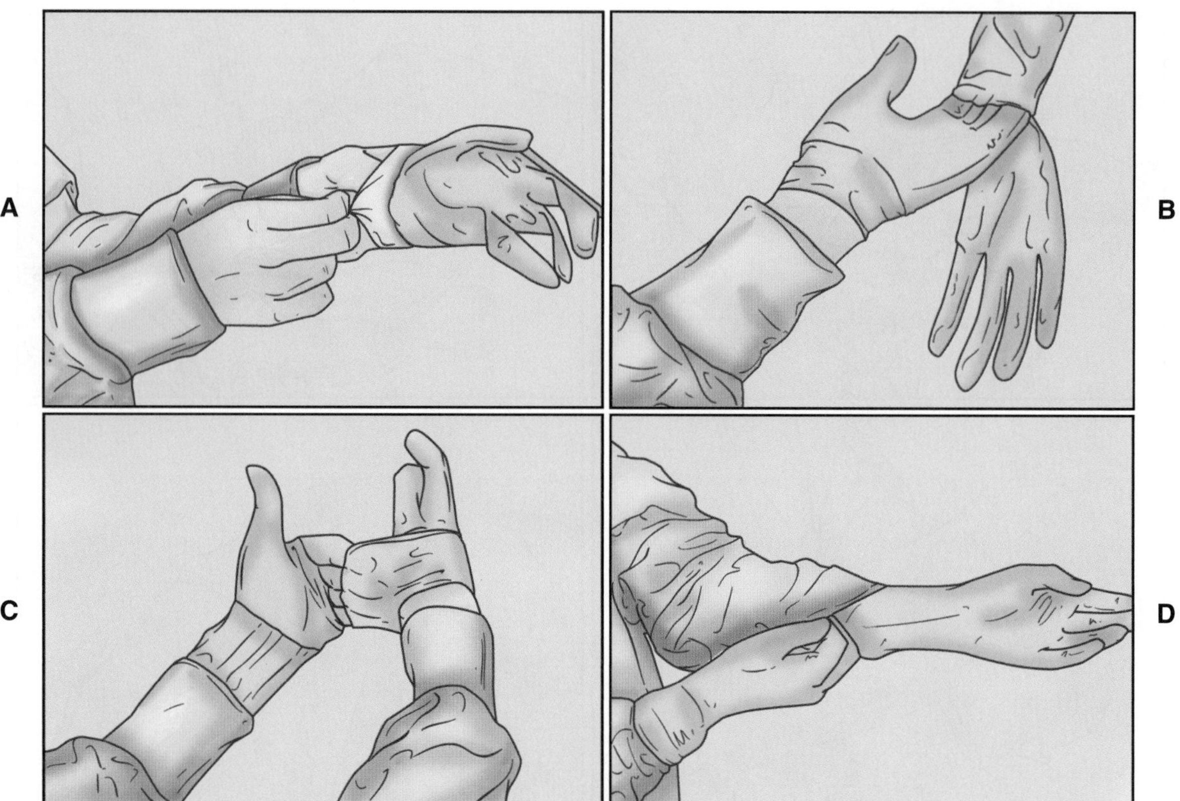


FIGURE 3-19 Open-gloving procedure. **A**, Scrub person takes one glove from inner glove wrapper by placing thumb and index finger of opposite hand on fold of everted cuff at a point in line with the glove's palm and pulls the glove over hand, leaving cuff turned back. If double-gloving is being used, the larger size gloves are donned first. **B**, Scrub person takes second glove from inner glove wrapper by placing gloved fingers under everted cuff. **C**, Scrub person, with arms extended and elbows slightly flexed, introduces free hand into glove and draws it over gown cuff by slightly rotating arm externally and internally. **D**, To bring turned-back cuff on other hand over cuff of gown, scrub person repeats step **C**.

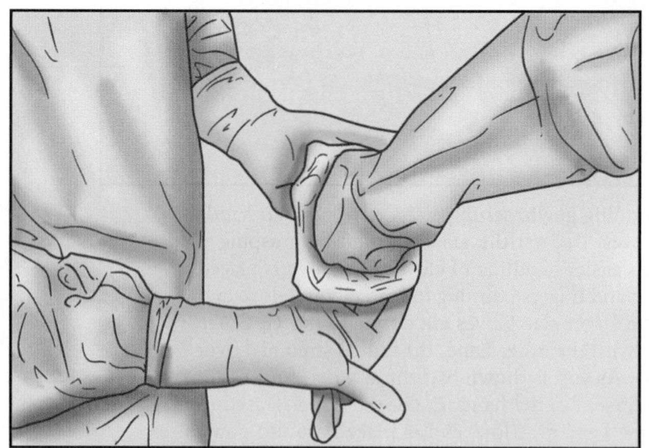

FIGURE 3-20 Gloving another person. Gowned and gloved scrub person places fingers of each hand beneath everted cuff, keeping thumbs turned outward and stretching cuff as gowned person slips hand into sterile glove, using firm downward thrust. If double-gloving is being used, the larger size gloves are donned first.

ate removal of soil and microorganisms, certain factors require further consideration in selecting a product for surgical use. Most soaps and detergents emulsify and peptize waste products and oils that are absorbed in surface soil and permit the detritus to be rinsed off the skin with running water. The product selected should become hydrolyzed in the presence of water and yield a pH that corresponds to that of average, normal skin. An odorless agent that produces a good lather for easy, comfortable use is usually preferred. It should not irritate the skin or in any way interfere with normal functioning. Equally important, an effective antimicrobial agent should be used to achieve appropriate disinfection of skin. The antimicrobial agent employed for disinfection of the skin should be selected according to its ability to decrease the microbial count of the skin rapidly, be applied quickly, and remain effective throughout the operation. The agent should not cause irritation or sensitization or be incompatible with or inactivated by alcohol, organic matter, soap, or detergent.[78,81]

Hair should not be removed from the surgical site unless required. The necessity for hair removal depends on the amount of hair, the location of the incision, and the type of surgical procedure to be performed.[17] If hair is to be removed, an electric or battery-operated clipper with a disposable or detachable reusable head that can be disinfected is the recommended method, not shaving. Clipping, immediately before surgery, is the simplest and least irritating method of hair removal. Wound infection rates are considerably higher for patients who are shaved preoperatively than for patients who have no preoperative shave preparation or a small amount of hair clipped or for patients on whom a depilatory is used. Use of a depilatory requires a pretest to ascertain that the patient is

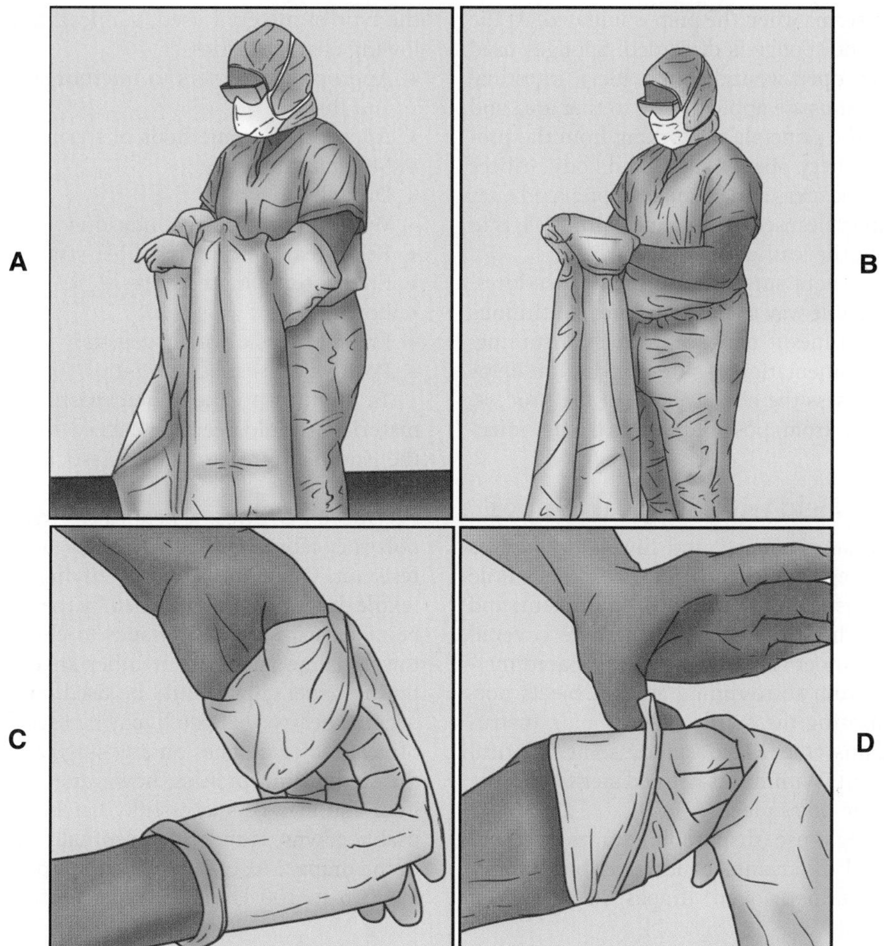


**FIGURE 3-21** Removing soiled gown and gloves. **A,** To protect scrub suit and arms from bacteria that are present on outer side of soiled gown, the gown is grasped without touching the scrub clothes. **B,** Scrub person turns outer side of soiled gown away from body, keeping elbows flexed and arms away from body so that soiled gown will not touch arms or scrub suit. **C,** To prevent outer side of soiled gloves from touching skin surfaces of hands, the scrub person places gloved fingers of one hand under everted cuff of other glove and pulls it off hand and fingers. **D,** To prevent ungloved hand from touching outer side of soiled glove, the scrub person hooks bare thumb on inner side of glove and pulls glove off.

not sensitive to the depilatory product. The specific manufacturer's written instructions should be carefully followed. If a shave is desired by the surgeon, some institutions require a written order. The patient should be shaved as close to the time of surgery as is possible. The shave should be performed in an area within the surgical suite that affords privacy and is equipped with good lighting. The amount of time between the preoperative shave and the operation has a direct effect on the surgical site infection rate. Hair removal should be performed by skillful personnel, with great care taken to avoid scratching, nicking, or cutting the skin because cutaneous bacteria proliferate in these areas and increase the chances of infection. The method of hair removal and the condition of the skin before and after removal should be documented.

The surgical principle followed when preparing the patient's skin for surgery ("prepping") is to prepare ("prep") the cleanest area first and then move to the less clean areas (clean to dirty). The skin at the surgical site should be exposed and inspected before beginning the skin prep. Patients should have been instructed to remove any body jewelry. Surgical departments often stock snap-ring pliers to remove jewelry from piercings for emergency situations or when a patient has neglected to remove body jewelry. The skin prep usually begins at the point of the incision and continues to the periphery of the area. When the patient's skin is being prepped, the antimicrobial agent is applied using commercially prepared devices or applicators that have handles to distance the operator's hand from the area being prepared. Gloves should be worn. A soiled applicator is never brought back over a previously prepped surface. On completion of the skin prep, any lather is blotted with dry, sterile sponges or a sterile towel. Depending on the surgeon's preference, a topical antimicrobial solution or "paint" may be carefully applied to the prepped area, using care to avoid any pooling of solution beneath the patient. All wet drapes should be removed from the patient area after the skin preparation is complete.

When a stoma or other contaminated area is involved in the prep procedure, a sponge soaked in the antimicrobial agent of choice is placed over the stoma when the prep is initiated. At the completion of the prep, the sponge is discarded. Sponges used to cleanse or disinfect an open wound, sinus, ulcer, intestinal stoma, the vagina, or the anus are applied once to that area and discarded. In contrast to the principle of working from the proposed incision to the periphery, open wounds and body orifices are potentially contaminated areas and as such are prepared after the peripheral intact skin is cleansed. The surgical principle is to work from the cleanest to the least clean area.[43,78,81]

It is important to document surgical skin prep procedures. Documentation is an effective way to promote safe, continuous patient care. Although at times it may seem time-consuming, periodic audits of the documentation of skin preparation helps the perioperative nurse assess the effectiveness of the process, while protecting patients from possible surgical site infections.[78]

## Creating the Sterile Field with Surgical Drapes

To create a sterile field, sterile sheets and towels, known as surgical drapes, are strategically placed to provide a sterile surface on which sterile instruments, supplies, equipment, and gloved hands may rest. The patient and OR bed are covered with sterile drapes in a manner that exposes the prepared incision site and isolates it from surrounding areas. Objects normally draped and composing the sterile field include instrument tables, trays, basins, the Mayo stand, some surgical equipment, and the patient. Within this defined sterile area the actual operative procedure takes place.

Today, reusable and single-use (disposable) drapes are used. There are advantages and disadvantages for reusable (fabric) and single-use (disposable, nonwoven) drapes. Regardless of the type of material used, surgical drapes should have the following characteristics:[11]

- Appropriate barriers to microorganisms, particulate matter, and fluids
- Appropriate to methods of sterilization
- Maintain integrity
- Durable
- Withstand physical conditions
- Resist tears, punctures, fiber strains, and abrasions
- Free of toxic ingredients
- Low linting
- Free of holes or other defects
- Positive cost-to-benefit ratio[16]

In addition to the characteristics just mentioned, draping materials should meet or exceed the current requirements of the National Fire Protection Association (Patient Safety).

***Reusable Drapes.*** Chemically treated cotton or cotton-polyester fabrics provide a barrier to liquids and are abrasion-resistant. Quantitative data verifying the barrier quality of any textile drape must be provided by the manufacturer. Care should be taken with reusable drapes to eliminate pinholes caused by towel clamps, needles, or other sharp objects. Only nonpenetrating towel clips should be used. Should breaks in the fabric occur, a heat-sealed patch may be used for repair. An abundance of heat-sealed patches on any surgical drape may interfere with the sterilization process, however. The exact percentage of any item that may be successfully patched is unknown. As with reusable gowns, laundering eventually impairs the barrier quality of the drape. Most manufacturers report a loss of barrier quality after 75 to 100 laundry or sterilization cycles. The process of

### PATIENT SAFETY

#### Preventing Surgical Fires

The fire triangle—fuels, ignition sources, and oxidizers—is present in almost all ORs. The use of oxygen, via nasal cannulas or in nitrous oxide, medical air, or anesthetizing gases must always be considered as part of the oxygen-enriched environment in the OR. Ignition sources in the form of the electrosurgical unit, lasers, fiberoptic lights, drills, or other electrical equipment are also common. The third element—a fuel—can be provided in the form of preparation agents[68] and surgical drapes. Approximately 100 surgical fires occur annually. In June 2003, the JCAHO issued a sentinel event alert to prevent surgical fires, and in 2005 it incorporated surgical fire prevention as a National Patient Safety Goal (NPSG). Surgical fires can be prevented if one of the elements of the fire triangle is eliminated or reduced.

To reduce the risk of a surgical fire from an agent used to prepare the surgical site antiseptically, steps should be taken as follows:

- Use only necessary amounts of preparation solution. Flammable preparation solutions should be packaged for controlled delivery, such as in unit-dose applicators or swabs.
- Avoid any pooling of preparation solution. If linens on the OR bed or patient become soaked with solution, remove them from the OR.
- Allow preparation solution to dry completely (3 to 5 minutes) before surgical drapes are applied. This may be incorporated as a time out or "all-clear" announcement before proceeding with draping.
- Activate an ignition source, such as an electrosurgical unit (ESU), cautery device, or laser, only when vapors from preparation solution have dissipated.
- Perform periodic hazard assessments of safe processes and the OR environment.

If a surgical fire occurs, the *RACE* (*R*escue, *A*lert/*A*larm, *C*ontain, and *E*xtinguish) method can be used. Fire policies and fire drills should be reviewed continually. Each member of the surgical team is responsible for communicating with one another about surgical fire risk and for knowing the steps for extinguishing a surgical fire on a patient and in the airway. Key concepts in establishing a culture of safety include evaluation, education, standard processes, and tools to foster interdisciplinary communication. A culture of safety requires rapid identification of errors and root causes, successful implementation of improvement strategies, strong leadership, critical thinking, and commitment to excellence.

Modified from Ball MJ: Culture of safety, *Advance for Nurses* 7(23):31-32, 2005; Giarrizzo-Wilson S: Clinical issues—fire protection standards, *AORN Journal* 82(4):673-674, 2005; Lypson ML and others: Preventing surgical fires: who needs to be educated? *Joint Commission Journal on Quality and Patient Safety* 31(9):522-527, 2005; Kostka J: Take advantage of surgical-fire safety and prevention resources, *AORN Connections,* April 2005, p. 6.

laundering and steam-sterilization swells the fabric fibers, whereas drying and ironing shrink the fibers. Over time, these processes loosen fabric fibers, altering the fabric structure and decreasing the barrier properties and fluid impermeability of the fabric. As with surgical gowns, a system to monitor the number of times an item has been processed is essential for quality control of the barrier and fluid impermeability.

***Single-Use (Disposable) Drapes.*** Many synthetic single-use (disposable) drapes prevent bacterial penetration and fluid breakthrough, also known as *strikethrough.* These versatile materials can be manufactured to meet different specifications in absorbent and nonabsorbent forms. Disposable products are packaged and sterilized by commercial sources. Disposable drapes reduce the hazards of contamination in the presence of known infectious microorganisms in body fluids and excretions and in situations where laundering of grossly contaminated textiles is problematic. The danger inherent in the use of synthetic drapes is that solvents, volatile liquids, and sharp instruments tend to penetrate the barrier. Loss of effectiveness may be caused by cracking at the folds or by pinholes from the use of regular, perforating towel clamps. Manufacturers are continually improving disposable drapes to permit easy handling and adaptability to the body. When considering the purchase of single-use drapes, the buyer must determine whether they will meet the needs of the surgical procedure, be acceptable to users, and be cost-effective versus laundering and processing reusable drapes. A cost-benefit ratio analysis may warrant their use in the health care facility. Availability of items, storage facilities, and disposal methods must be analyzed.[16]

Compactors provide a relatively inexpensive method of discarding disposable drapes. They accept any material and reduce its volume substantially. Storage, collection, and transportation of compacted waste materials can be a problem. Hospital engineers must establish methods of controlling odor and maintaining sanitation in the compactor area. Because a portion of the compacted material may be grossly contaminated, city or county codes may prohibit transporting this potentially infectious material through city streets or dumping it at landfills. Incineration is an alternative method for destroying waste disposables. If incinerators are used, they must be managed properly to prevent environmental contamination. Facilities choosing to incinerate must follow specific guidelines established for medical waste incinerators. Many hospital incinerators do not meet federal pollution standards, and their use is prohibited.

The environmental effect of disposable items can be only roughly estimated. Each facility must carefully evaluate its capabilities and restrictions for handling single-use and reusable supplies and equipment to make an informed decision about the products it will use.

Preassembled, sterile, disposable custom packs are used in many health care facilities. Advantages of these packs include reduced setup and room-turnover times, less risk of contaminated waste resulting from fewer individually wrapped items, improved inventory control, and fewer lost charges. Although custom packs may be more expensive than multiple separate items, indirect savings related to increased efficiency can offset those costs. Health care facilities choosing to use custom packs should determine and document ownership of liability for the function and integrity of individual items within the packs.

***Drape Configurations.*** Careful planning by perioperative personnel helps determine the desired types and sizes of surgical drapes required for surgical procedures. Standardized draping methods provide management control that ensures patient safety, simplifies staff education, and conserves human and material resources.

A whole, or plain, sheet is used to cover instrument tables, operating tables, and body regions. The sheet should be large enough to provide an adequate margin of safety between the surrounding physical environment and the prepared operative field. Surgical towels should be available in several sizes to drape the operative site. Four surgical towels of woven or nonwoven material are usually sufficient (Figure 3-22).

Fenestrated, or slit, sheets are used for draping patients. They leave the operative site exposed. A typical fenestrated (laparotomy) sheet is large enough to cover the patient and operating bed in any position, extend over the anesthesia screen at the head of the bed, and extend over the foot of the bed (Figures 3-23 to 3-25). The typical fenestrated laparotomy

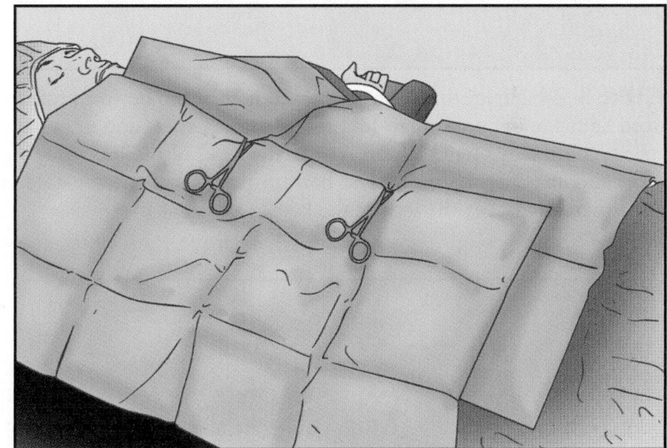

**FIGURE 3-22** Abdomen may be draped with four sterile towels, which are secured with nonperforating towel clamps. Standard method of placement of disposable towels is used.

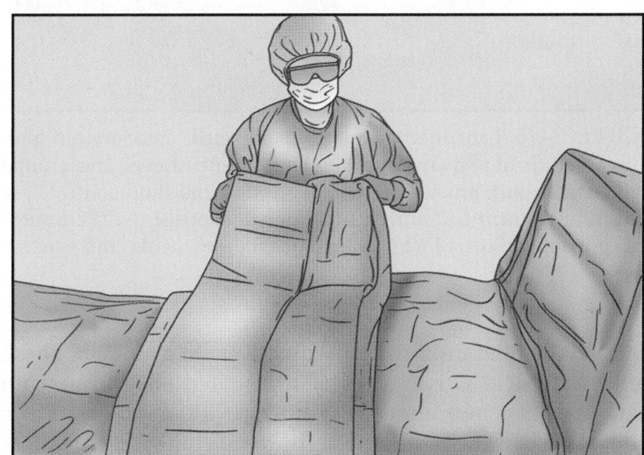

**FIGURE 3-23** Placement of laparotomy sheet. Identification of top portion of laparotomy sheet helps the scrub person readily determine correct placement of the drape. After placing the folded laparotomy sheet on the patient, with fenestration of sheet directly over site of incision outlined by sterile towels, the scrub person unfolds drape over sides of patient and bed.

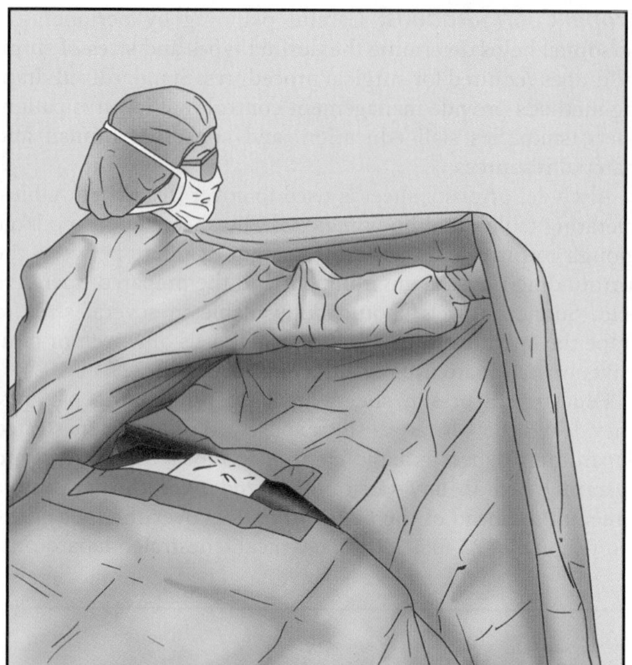

FIGURE 3-24 Laparotomy draping continued. Scrub person protects gloved hands under cuff of fan-folded laparotomy sheet and draws the upper section above fenestration toward the head of the bed, draping it over the anesthesia screen. The bottom portion of the fan-folded sheet is extended over the foot of the bed in a similar manner.

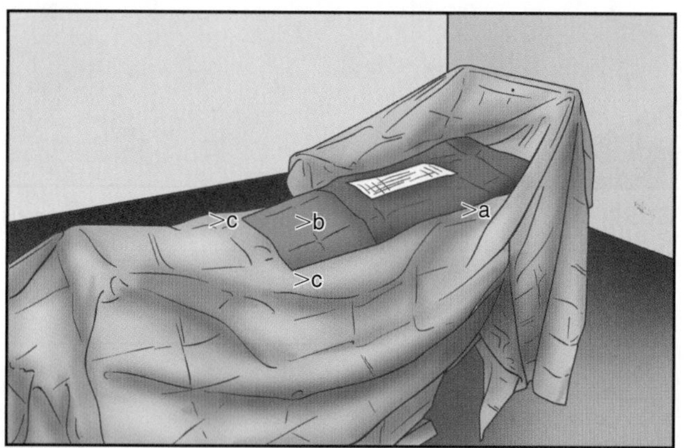


FIGURE 3-25 Laparotomy draping completed. Fenestration provides exposure of prepared operative site. >*a*, Reinforced area around drape fenestration provides greater protection and fluid control. >*b*, Built-in instrument pad prevents instrument slippage. >*c*, Perforated tabs provide means of controlling position of cords and suction tubes.

sheet can be used for most procedures on the abdomen, chest, flank, and back. Other types of fenestrated sheets but with small or split fenestrations may be used for the limbs, head, and neck when the patient is in the supine or prone position. The size of the fenestration is determined by the use for which the sheet is intended. The fenestrated sheet is fan-folded and handled as a typical laparotomy sheet. A perineal drape is needed for procedures on the perineum and genitalia when the patient is in the lithotomy position. A lithotomy drape consists of a fenestrated sheet and two triangular leggings. Although a three-piece drape is less costly and is easier to handle and launder, a single drape with attached leggings may be used.

Several types of impermeable polyvinyl chloride (PVC) sheeting are available in the form of sterile, prepackaged surgical drapes. Plastic incisional drapes are available as a plain impermeable drape or impregnated with iodophor. These plastic drapes are useful adjuncts to the conventional draping procedure. They can be applied after the fabric drape, alleviating the need for towel clamps. They obviate the need for skin towels and sponges to separate the surgeon's gloves from contact with the patient's skin. Skin color and anatomic landmarks are readily visible, and the incision is made directly through the adherent plastic drape. These materials facilitate draping of irregular body surfaces, such as neck and ear regions, extremities, and joints (Figure 3-26).

***Draping Procedure.*** Drapes should be folded so that the gowned and gloved members of the team can handle them with ease and safety. The larger, regular sheet is usually fan-folded from bottom to top. The bottom folds may be wider than the upper ones. The small sheet is folded in half and quartered, with the top corners of the sheet turned back or marked for easy identification and handling. To provide for safe, easy handling and a wide margin of safety between the unsterile item and the scrub person's gloved hands, the open end of the Mayo stand cover should be cuffed or folded back on itself (Figure 3-27). Most fenestrated sheets are fan-folded to the opening from the top and the bottom, and the folds are rolled or fanned toward the center of the opening. The edges of the top and bottom folds of the sheet are fanned to provide a cuff under which the scrub person may place gloved hands. The top and lower sections should be identified by a marking to facilitate easy handling.

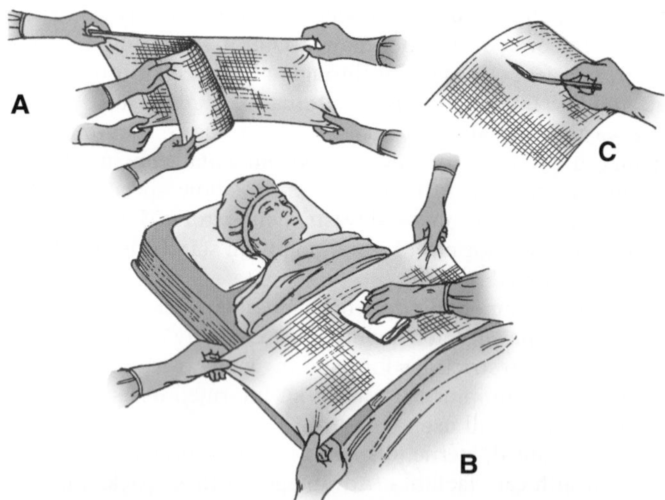


FIGURE 3-26 Sterile, impermeable adhesive drape. For maximum sealing to prevent wound contamination, prepared skin must be dry, and the drape must be applied carefully, preventing wrinkles and air bubbles. **A**, Surgeon and assistant hold plastic drape taut while another assistant peels off back paper. **B**, Surgeon and assistant apply plastic drape to operative site and, using folded towel, apply slight pressure to eliminate air bubbles and wrinkles. **C**, Surgeon makes incision through plastic drape.

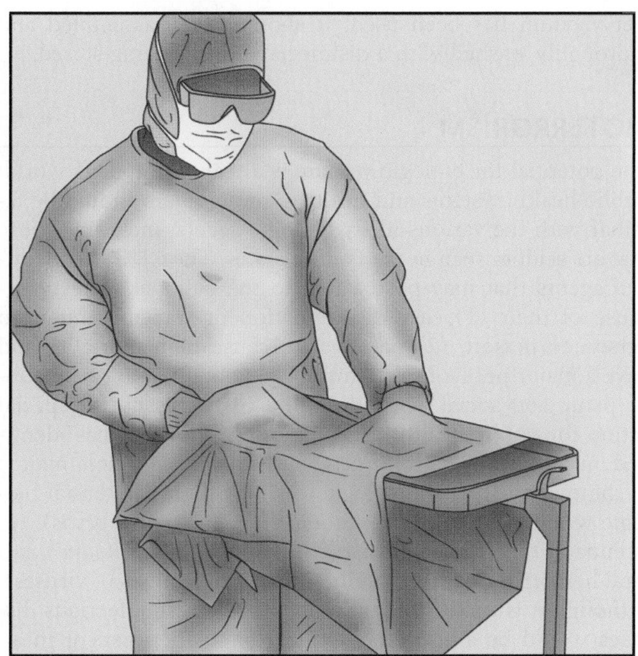

**FIGURE 3-27** Draping Mayo stand. Folded cover is slipped over frame. Scrub person's gloved hands are protected by cuff of drape. Cover is unfolded to extend over upright support of stand.

When applying drapes to create the sterile field, these principles should be followed:

- Allow sufficient time and space to permit careful draping and proper aseptic technique.
- Handle sterile drapes as little as possible.
- Carry the folded drape to the operative site. Carefully unfold the drape, and place it in the proper position. Do not move the drape after it has been placed. Shifting or moving the drape may bring bacteria from an unprepared area of the patient's skin into the surgical field.
- Hold sterile drapes above waist level until properly placed on the patient or object being draped. If the end of a drape falls below waist level, it should not be retrieved because the area below the waist is considered unsterile.
- Without contaminating the gloves or other sterile items, immediately discard a drape that becomes contaminated during the draping procedure.
- Protect the gown by distance and the gloved hands by cuffing drapes over them. Control all parts of the drape at all times during placement, using precise and direct motions.
- Do not flip, fan, or shake drapes. Rapid movement of drapes creates air currents on which dust, lint, and droplet nuclei may migrate. Shaking a drape causes uncontrolled motion of the drape, which may cause it to come into contact with an unsterile surface or object. A drape should be carefully unfolded and allowed to fall gently into position by gravity.
- Drape the incisional area first and then the periphery. Always drape from a sterile area to an unsterile area by draping the near side first. Never reach across an unsterile area to drape. When draping the opposite side of the OR bed, go around the bed to drape.
- Use nonperforating towel clamps or devices to secure tubing and other items on the sterile field. The low portion of a sheet that falls below the safe working level should never be raised or lifted back into the sterile area.
- When sterility of a drape is questionable, consider it contaminated.

After the patient is positioned, prepared and draped, a time out is conducted to verify patient identification, correct position, and correct surgical site (and side if applicable) and that required equipment is available (see Chapter 2).

## Environmental Cleaning

Contamination in the OR can occur from various sources. The patient, health care workers, and inanimate objects all are capable of introducing potentially infectious material onto the surgical field. Techniques have been established to prevent some of the transmission of microorganisms into the surgical area, such as proper surgical attire and controlled traffic patterns in the surgical suite. During the surgical procedure, traffic within and through the room should be kept to a minimum to reduce air turbulence and to minimize human shedding. All doors in and out of the OR should be kept closed to decrease air turbulence and the potential for contamination. HEPA filters placed between outside air processing and the OR vents are used in many facilities and are recommended for newly constructed systems/facilities.[2] HEPA filters are capable of screening out particles larger than 0.3 μm.

All surgical patients are potentially infected with bloodborne or other infectious material. For patient and personnel safety, cleaning procedures should be uniform throughout the OR and for all patients. Using a uniform procedure designed to protect persons from visible or invisible contamination eliminates the need for special cleaning procedures for so-called dirty cases. Cleaning procedures should be carried out in a manner that protects patients and personnel from exposure to potentially infectious microorganisms. Cleaning measures are needed before, during, and after surgical procedures and at the end of each day. Overall housekeeping procedures, such as wall and ceiling washing, should be done on a defined, regular basis.[14]

Transmission-based precautions are designed for patients who have a documented infection or who are suspected to be infected with a highly transmissible pathogen for which additional precautions are necessary. There are three types of transmission-based precautions: airborne, droplet, and contact. The CDC guidelines should be followed when all policies and guidelines are developed.[47]

Before beginning the first procedure of the day, horizontal surfaces in the ORs should be dusted with a cloth dampened with a facility-approved disinfecting agent. Dust and lint deposited on horizontal surfaces during the night can become airborne vectors for organisms if not removed. During surgery, efforts should be made to confine contamination to as small an area as possible around the patient. Sponges should be discarded in plastic-lined containers. As they are counted, they should be contained in an impervious receptacle. The circulating nurse must use protective eyewear and gloves, instruments, or both when collecting and counting sponges or handling contaminated items. Spills should be cleaned up immediately, and the cleaned area should be disinfected with a broad-spectrum disinfectant or germicide. Specimens of blood or other potentially infectious tissue should be placed in a container that prevents leakage. The container must be color-coded or labeled using the biohazard symbol (see Figure 3-1). If the outside of the container becomes contaminated, the primary container must be placed within a second container that prevents leakage and is labeled or color-coded. Some facilities use biohazard-labeled impervious bags to transport blood or other potentially infectious material.

On completion of the surgical procedure, soiled linens should be discarded in fluid-impervious bags to eliminate potential contamination from wet linen soaking through to the outside of the bag. Contaminated items should be placed in leak-proof, color-coded, or labeled containers. Sharps (e.g., needles, scalpels, electrosurgical tips) are considered infectious and should be placed in special puncture-resistant containers.[64] Bulk blood or suctioned fluid may be poured carefully down a drain connected to a sanitary sewer unless prohibited by environmental regulations. Local and state environmental regulations may exist and should be consulted before establishing guidelines for waste disposal. Wall suction units should be disconnected to eliminate contamination of the wall outlet. Suction contents should be disposed of during the flushing of a hopper. Depending on local and state regulations, powder treatments of a chlorine compound are available to solidify liquid material before transport. This chemical also may be tuberculocidal, virucidal, and bactericidal. Suction tubing should be discarded; reusable suction tubing should be avoided because of difficulties in cleaning the lumen properly. Personnel should remove their gowns and gloves and place them in the proper receptacles before leaving the OR, then go wash their hands. Instruments and supplies should be contained and taken to the decontamination area, where appropriately educated personnel wearing personal protective attire begin the instrument decontamination process. Care should be taken to arrange sharp instruments in such a manner that personnel need not reach into basins where sharp instruments are unexposed and could cause injury. Equipment and furniture in the OR should be cleaned with an EPA-approved hospital disinfectant, and the floor should be cleaned in a 3-foot to 4-foot perimeter around the operating bed and where visibly soiled. A standard practice of cleaning helps prevent surgical site infections and maintains a clean and safe environment.

At the end of each day's operative schedule, all rooms where procedures may be performed should be cleaned by appropriately trained and supervised personnel. Areas to be cleaned include the following:

- Surgical lights and external tracks
- Fixed and ceiling-mounted equipment
- All furniture and equipment including wheels and casters
- Equipment
- Handles of cabinets and push plates
- Ventilation faceplates
- Horizontal surfaces (e.g., countertops, fixed shelving, autoclaves)
- Floor
- Kick buckets
- Scrub sinks

If refillable liquid soap dispensers are used, they should be disassembled and cleaned before being refilled because they can serve as reservoirs for microorganisms. At the conclusion of the housekeeping protocol, cleaning equipment and supplies should be properly cleaned, disinfected, and stored. If a wet vacuum has been used, it should be disassembled and thoroughly washed with a disinfectant before being stored.

## BIOTERRORISM

The potential for biologic warfare is a reality in today's world. Public health systems and health care providers should be familiar with the various likely biologic agents, including those that are seldom seen in the United States. The CDC has identified agents that may pose a risk to the national security because of their (1) easy dissemination or transmission from person to person, (2) potential to cause high mortality and have a major public health impact, (3) potential to cause public panic and social disruption, and (4) necessity for special action for public health preparedness.[40] The CDC has identified anthrax (*Bacillus anthracis*) and smallpox (variola major) as the two most likely biologic weapons. Other potential biologic weapons include pneumonic plague (*Yersinia pestis*), tularemia (*Francisella tularensis*), botulism (*C. botulinum*), and viral hemorrhagic fevers (multiple distinct families of viruses). Although it is unlikely that patients with these infectious diseases would be among the surgical population except in an extreme circumstance, it is likely that, given a national crisis or epidemic, perioperative personnel could and would be mobilized to serve in a variety of locations and roles as part of the emergency preparedness plan. Perioperative personnel should have a basic knowledge and understanding of the agents most likely to be encountered and the levels of precautions required for patient and personnel safety.

### Anthrax

Anthrax is caused by *B. anthracis*, a gram-positive, spore-forming, bacterial rod. Anthrax spores can survive for many decades in the soil. Anthrax presents in three clinical forms: cutaneous, inhalation, and gastrointestinal. Spores can enter the system through nonintact skin, resulting in progressive cutaneous lesions. Spores can become easily aerosolized and inhaled, resulting in the inhaled form of disease. Gastrointestinal disease can occur as a result of ingesting infected animals. If untreated, all forms can result in bloodstream infection and death. Anthrax is not transmitted from an infected person to a noninfected person via body fluids. A powdered preparation of anthrax may disseminate from a common source, however, including a person contaminated with that powder. Small particles may become aerosolized, leading to any form of the disease, depending on the portal of entry. When encountering a credible threat of exposure or a person having been exposed, N95 masks or positive air pressure respirators and protective clothing should be used until the threat is obviated.[34]

Inhalation anthrax is the most likely form of the disease to be employed in a bioterrorism event. The usual incubation period for inhalation anthrax is 1 to 6 days, but disease has appeared 43 days after exposure. Early symptoms are influenza-like, but progress to high fever, dyspnea, stridor, cyanosis, and shock. Chest wall edema and hemorrhagic meningitis may be present. Chest x-ray examination shows pleural effusions and a widened mediastinum. Death is universal in untreated cases and may occur in 95% of cases not treated in the first 48 hours. Early treatment with antibiotics is essential for survival.

Because person-to-person transmission of confirmed inhalation anthrax does not occur, these patients are cared for using Standard Precautions. Patient isolation is unnecessary, and routine cleaning procedures are sufficient.[31,34] Special attention should be given to protection and containment of any draining wounds, including cutaneous lesions. Transmission has occurred after contact with cutaneous lesions.

## Smallpox

Smallpox is caused by variola major and is a viral disease unique to humans. The virus is transmitted from person to person by inhalation of droplets, droplet nuclei, aerosols, and direct or indirect contact. The incubation period for the disease is typically 12 to 14 days. The disease begins with high fever, malaise, abdominal pains, and, in some cases, delirium. A rash develops over the face and spreads to the extremities. The rash soon becomes vesicular and then pustular. All lesions progress at the same rate. The fever continues throughout the course of the disease, and the growing and expanding pustules are very painful. In 5% to 10% of patients, a rapidly progressive disease develops, which is almost always fatal within 5 to 7 days. Smallpox is contagious from onset of the rash until all scabs have fallen off.

The only treatment for smallpox is vaccination, isolation, and quarantine. Vaccination within 7 days after exposure is recommended. Vaccine against smallpox contains another live virus called *vaccinia.* The vaccine does not contain the smallpox virus. Other than vaccination, there is no treatment for smallpox. Research into new antiviral agents continues. Because it is impossible to vaccinate the entire population, vaccinations should be given according to the "ring of vaccination" concept. According to this concept, individuals having close contact with infected individuals should be vaccinated first. Individuals with face-to-face contact or in the household with the infected individual are at greatest risk of developing the disease. Individuals coming into contact with contacts or household members (contacts of the contacts) of the infected individual also should be vaccinated. Household members of contacts of the contacts having contraindications for vaccination should be removed from the home until after the incubation period.

Because of the highly infectious nature of smallpox, Standard, Droplet, Airborne, and Contact Precautions should be followed. Patients should be placed in negative-pressure, private rooms with the door closed. If a private room is unavailable, patients may be cohorted with "like" patients. Patient transport should be limited to essential movement only, and the patient should wear a surgical mask to minimize dispersal of droplets and droplet nuclei. Patient equipment should be dedicated to the specific patient and disinfected before being removed from the room. Linens should be bagged and labeled "smallpox."[40] Routine environmental cleaning with an EPA-registered hospital disinfectant is adequate. If the patient dies, Standard and Contact Precautions should be maintained throughout the postmortem period. Autopsy is not recommended and, if done, should be done using Standard, Airborne Infection Isolation, and Contact Precautions in a HEPA-filtered room. Cremation is recommended whenever possible.

Smallpox is considered an exceedingly dangerous, potential biologic weapon, with far-reaching ramifications.[38] If a patient with smallpox must have an emergent surgical procedure, the following precautions are recommended:

- Perioperative personnel involved in the patient's care, including patient transport and personnel cleaning the OR, should wear an N95 mask, gowns, gloves, and shoe covers.
- All nonessential equipment should be removed from the room. Each OR door should be labeled with Airborne and Contact precaution signs. Only one door should be used in that OR; if there is more than one door, the other doors should be taped shut.
- A HEPA filter may be placed in front of the designated door access. Only essential personnel may enter this door.
- An outside circulator may be assigned to bring equipment and supplies to the designated access door. This nurse does not enter the room.
- All waste material, including tape from the doors, unopened supplies, packaging material, regardless of contamination, is red-bagged.
- At the conclusion of the procedure, PPE is red-bagged. Personnel who were involved in the patient's care and who were not previously vaccinated against smallpox should be vaccinated.
- Instrument containers should be labeled "smallpox" before being transported to central processing.

## Plague

Plague is an infectious disease of humans and animals. It is caused by the *Y. pestis*, which is found in rodents and their fleas. Plague occurs in various forms, separately or in combination.

*Pneumonic plague* occurs when the bacteria infect the lungs. It is transmissible from person to person through aerosolized bacteria carried on respiratory droplets from the infected person. Symptoms include fever, headache, and weakness, with rapid progression to pneumonia with dyspnea, chest pain, cough, and bloody or watery sputum. Respiratory failure and shock may follow within 2 to 4 days. Early treatment is essential for survival, with administration of antibiotics recommended within the first 24 hours. Individuals in direct contact with the infected person also should receive antibiotics. Standard and Droplet Precautions should be followed when caring for these patients. Patients should be placed in private rooms or cohorted with "like" patients. Transport should be limited to essential movement only, and the patient should wear a mask during transport. No special precautions for environmental cleaning and linen management are necessary.[37]

*Bubonic plague* is the most common type of plague and occurs when an infected flea bites a person or when the bacteria enter through already broken skin. Symptoms include swollen, tender lymph nodes (buboes), fever, headache, chills, and weakness. Bubonic plague is not transmitted from person to person, and use of Standard Precautions is sufficient in caring for these patients.

*Septicemic plague* occurs when the bacteria multiply in the blood. It can occur in conjunction with pneumonic plague or bubonic plague. When it occurs alone, it is caused in the same manner as bubonic plague. Symptoms include fever, chills, prostration, abdominal pain, shock, and bleeding into the skin and other organs. Septicemic plague is not transmitted from person to person, and patients are cared for using Standard Precautions.[33,37]

## Tularemia

Tularemia was first described in 1911 and soon thereafter recognized to be a potentially severe and fatal disease in humans.[3] Tularemia is caused by *F. tularensis,* found in mice, water rats, squirrels, rabbits, and hares. These animals acquire the infection by being bitten by flies, mosquitos, and ticks and by contact with contaminated environments. The bacteria can be recovered from contaminated water, soil, and vegetation. Humans become infected through the bites of ticks, deerflies, and other arthropods that have eaten infected animal tissue; by handling infected animal carcasses; by eating or drinking contaminated food or water; or by inhaling infected aerosols.

Tularemia is highly infectious. It can infect humans through the skin, mucous membranes, gastrointestinal tract, and lungs. The incubation period for tularemia is 1 to 14 days (average 3 to 5 days). Depending on the route of exposure, symptoms of tularemia include skin ulcers, inflamed eyes, sore throat, oral ulcers, swollen and painful lymph nodes, and pneumonia. When the bacteria are inhaled, symptoms include sudden fever, chills, headache, muscle aches, joint pain, cough, and progressive weakness. Symptoms may progress to chest pain, dyspnea, bloody sputum, and respiratory failure. Without antibiotic treatment, 40% or more of individuals with lung or systemic forms of the disease are likely to die. If used as a biological weapon, the bacteria would likely be used in an aerosol form for exposure by inhalation.

Human-to-human transmission of tularemia is unknown, and use of Standard Precautions when caring for these patients is appropriate. Patient transport is not restricted, and environmental cleaning with a hospital disinfectant is sufficient.[3,39]

## Botulism

Botulism is a neuroparalytic disease characterized by symmetric, descending, flaccid paralysis of motor and autonomic nerves, usually beginning with the cranial nerves. It is caused by a neurotoxin produced by *C. botulinum,* an anaerobic, spore-forming bacterium. Early symptoms of botulism include gastrointestinal distress, nausea, and vomiting. Symptoms progress to diplopia, blurred vision, drooping eyelids, slurred speech, difficulty swallowing, dry mouth, and muscle weakness. If not treated, the disease progresses to respiratory paralysis and paralysis of the arms and legs. Botulinum toxin is the most poisonous substance known.[25] There are three types of botulism:

- Foodborne botulism occurs as a result of ingesting the preformed toxin. Disease occurs within a few hours of ingesting the food but can occur 8 days after ingesting the food, depending on the amount of bacteria or toxin or both present.
- Infant botulism occurs in susceptible infants who harbor *C. botulinum* in their intestinal tract.
- Wound botulism occurs when wounds are infected with *C. botulinum* that secretes the toxin. Injection drug users are at risk for wound botulism.[25,36]

Because botulism is not transmitted from person to person, use of Standard Precautions is sufficient when caring for these patients.

## Viral Hemorrhagic Fevers

Viral hemorrhagic fevers (VHFs) are a group of illnesses caused by four distinct families of viruses: (1) arenaviruses, (2) filoviruses, (3) bunyaviruses, and (4) flaviviruses. Viruses causing VHFs naturally live in animal hosts and depend on their hosts for survival and replication. The viruses are transmitted to humans via arthropods, such as mosquitos or ticks. Arthropods also may infect livestock, and humans may contract disease during the slaughtering process. These viruses also can be transmitted via urine, feces, saliva, or other body excretions from infected rodents. The animal hosts of some VHFs are unknown (e.g., Ebola hemorrhagic fever [HF], Marburg HF).

Symptoms of viral hemorrhagic fevers vary by the type of viral hemorrhagic fever, but initial symptoms often include high fever, fatigue, dizziness, muscle aches, weakness, and exhaustion. More progressive symptoms include bleeding under the skin, into internal organs, and from body orifices (e.g., mouth, nose, eyes); shock; nervous system malfunction, such as coma, delirium, and seizures; and renal failure.

Human-to-human transmission of some VHFs occurs (e.g., Ebola HF, Marburg HF, Lassa HF, Crimean-Congo HF). Transmission is through direct or indirect contact with infected individuals or infected body fluids. Contaminated syringes and needles have been linked to spread of Ebola HF and Lassa HF. Standard, Droplet, Contact, and Airborne Precautions should be followed when caring for patients with VHFs. Patients should be placed in negative-pressure rooms with the door closed. Patient transport should be limited to essential transport only, and the patient should wear a mask to prevent dispersal of droplets or droplet nuclei or both. Environmental surfaces should be cleaned with a 10% bleach solution or a phenolic disinfectant. Dedicated equipment should be used for each patient, and the equipment should be disinfected before being brought from the room. If the patient dies, autopsy is not recommended and, if done, should be done using Standard, Airborne Infection Isolation, and Contact Precautions in a HEPA-filtered room. These precautions should be maintained throughout the postmortem period. The body should be sealed in leak-proof material and handled as little as possible.[32,49]

## Emergency Preparedness

Communication, collaboration, and coordination are required in the face of any bioterrorist activity or natural disaster. Communities need emergency plans for such matters as guarding patient data and protecting information systems, linking quickly and easily with state and federal resources, ensuring culturally competent communication and care, accessing mental health resources, and identifying agencies that can partner with one another to provide services. Each institution must be compliant with the JCAHO's requirements for periodic testing of emergency management plans. Plausible scenarios that are realistic and relevant to the institution are recommended to evaluate the effectiveness of the plan should an actual emergency situation occur.[44]

## Progressive Knowledge

The information about bioterrorism and the identified biologic weapons presented in this chapter represents current knowledge at the time of publication. Practitioners are encouraged to update their knowledge continually by consulting the CDC website (www.cdc.gov) and other experts in the field. The Health Alert Network (HAN) is the CDC's surveillance system. It connects local, state, and national public agencies with high-speed and satellite Internet access. The extent of precautions necessary can be quickly determined by using this system.

## SUMMARY

Advancements in surgical interventions and the science of infection prevention and control continue to evolve over time. This chapter provides an overview of the causes of infection, including emerging drug-resistant bacteria, and identifies a variety of methods to control infection in the perioperative environment. Use of Standard Precautions along with engineering and work-practice controls assist perioperative practitioners in reducing the transmission of pathogenic organisms. Perioperative patient care is based on surgical aseptic principles. Careful adherence to these principles supports infection prevention and control, ultimately improving surgical patient safety and outcomes. Each member of the surgical team must demonstrate the utmost integrity in application of this knowledge. Finally, in today's world, the potential for bioterrorism has forced the United States and the rest of the world to strengthen security and emergency readiness. If a bioterrorism attack resulted in massive exposure or illness, perioperative personnel could and would be mobilized to serve in a variety of locations as in the New York World Trade Center attacks of 2001 and the London tube attacks in July 2005. These attacks redefined the meaning of disaster preparedness for all nurses. Perioperative personnel need to be familiar with the most likely biologic weapons and the levels of precautions required for patient and personnel safety.

## REFERENCES


1. Agerton T and others: Transmission of a highly resistant strain (strain WI) of *Mycobacterium tuberculosis, JAMA: The Journal of the American Medical Association* 278:1073-1077, 1997. Accessed October 1, 2005, on-line: www.jama.com.
2. American Institute of Architects Academy of Architecture for Health; U.S. Department of Health and Human Services: *Guidelines for design and construction of hospital and health care facilities,* Washington, DC, 2001, American Institute of Architects. Accessed October 1, 2005, on-line: www.aia.org/release.
3. American Medical Association: Tularemia as a biological weapon: medical and public health management, *JAMA: The Journal of the American Medical Association* 285(21):2763-2773, 2001. Accessed October 1, 2005, on-line: www.jama.com.
4. Anglim AM and others: A hospital epidemic of vancomycin-resistant enterococcus: risk factors and control. *Infection Control and Hospital Epidemiology* 22 (3) 140-147, 2001. Accessed October 10, 2005, on-line: www.chejournal.com.
5. Association for the Advancement of Medical Instrumentation (AAMI): *Good hospital practice: ethylene oxide sterilization in healthcare facilities: safety and effectiveness,* Arlington, Va, 2002, The Association. Accessed October 1, 2005, on-line: www.aami.org.
6. Association for the Advancement of Medical Instrumentation (AAMI): *Good hospital practice: steam sterilization and sterility assurance in healthcare facilities,* Arlington, Va, 2002, The Association. Accessed October 1, 2005, on-line: www.aami.org.
7. Association for the Advancement of Medical Instrumentation (AAMI): *Flash sterilization in steam sterilization and sterility assurance in health care facilities,* Arlington, VA, 2005, The Association. Accessed October 1, 2005, on-line:www.aami.org.
8. Association for the Advancement of Medical Instrumentation (AAMI): *Packaging for terminally sterilized medical devices,* Arlington, Va, 2000, The Association.
9. Association for the Advancement of Medical Instrumentation (AAMI): *Safe handling and biological decontamination of medical devices in health care facilities and in nonclinical settings,* Arlington,Va, 2003, The Association.
10. Association for the Advancement of Medical Instrumentation (AAMI): *Table top dry heat (heated air) sterilization and sterility assurance in health care facilities,* Arlington, Va, 2004, The Association. Accessed October 1, 2005, on-line: www.aami.org.
11. Association of periOperative Registered Nurses (AORN): AORN guidance statement: reuse of single-use devices. In: *Standards, recommended practices and guidelines,* Denver, Colo, 2006, The Association.
12. Association of periOperative Registered Nurses (AORN): Recommended practices for the care and cleaning of instruments and powered equipment. In: *Standards, recommended practices and guidelines,* Denver, Colo, 2006, The Association.
13. Association of periOperative Registered Nurses (AORN): Recommended practices for cleaning and processing endoscopes. In: *Standards, recommended practices and guidelines,* Denver, Colo, 2006, The Association.
14. Association of periOperative Registered Nurses (AORN): Recommended practices for environmental cleaning in the surgical practice setting. In: *Standards, recommended practices and guidelines,* Denver, Colo, 2006, The Association.
15. Association of periOperative Registered Nurses (AORN): Recommended practices for selection and use of packaging systems. In: *Standards, recommended practices and guidelines,* Denver, Colo, 2006, The Association.
16. Association of periOperative Registered Nurses (AORN): Recommended practices for selection and use of surgical gowns and drapes. In: *Standards, recommended practices and guidelines,* Denver, Colo, 2006, The Association.
17. Association of periOperative Registered Nurses (AORN): Recommended practices for skin preparation of patients. In: *Standards, recommended practices and guidelines,* Denver, Colo, 2006, The Association.
18. Association of periOperative Registered Nurses (AORN): Recommended practices for sterilization in the perioperative practice setting. In: *Standards, recommended practices and guidelines,* Denver, Colo, 2006, The Association.
19. Association of periOperative Registered Nurses (AORN): Recommended practices for surgical attire. In *Standards, recommended practices and guidelines,* Denver, Colo, 2006, The Association.
20. Association of periOperative Registered Nurses (AORN): Recommended practices for surgical hand antisepsis. In: *Standards, recommended practices and guidelines,* Denver, Colo, 2006, The Association.
21. Association of periOperative Registered Nurses (AORN): Recommended practices for traffic patterns in the perioperative practice setting. In: *Standards, recommended practices and guidelines,* Denver, Colo, 2006, The Association.
22. Baxter HC and others: Elimination of transmissible spongiform encephalopathy infectivity and decontamination of surgical instruments using radio-frequency gas plasma treatment, *Journal of General Virology* 86:2393-2399, 2005.
23. Bond WW and others: Effective use of liquid chemical germicides on medical devices: instrument design problems. In Block SS, editor: *Chemical disinfection of medical and surgical materials,* ed 5, Philadelphia, 2001, Lippincott, Williams & Wilkins. Accessed October 1, 2005, on-line: www.simaaldrich.com/catalog/search.
24. Boyce JM: Are the epidemiology and microbiology of methicillin-resistant *Staphylococcus aureus* changing? *JAMA: The Journal of the American Medical Association* 279:623-624, 1998. Accessed October 1, 2005, on-line: www.jama.com.
25. Center for Civilian Biodefense Strategies: Botulinum toxin, 2000. Accessed October 1, 2005, on-line: www.upmc.-biosecurity.org/.
26. Centers for Disease Control and Prevention: Guideline for isolation precautions in hospitals, *Infection Control and Hospital Epidemiology* 17(1):53-80, 1996. Accessed October 10, 2005, on-line: www.cdc.gov/ncidod.
27. Centers for Disease Control and Prevention: *Guidelines for preventing the transmission of* Mycobacterium tuberculosis *in health care facilities,* Atlanta, 1994, CDC. Accessed October 10, 2005, on-line: www.cdc.gov/search.

28. Centers for Disease Control and Prevention: Recommendations for preventing the spread of vancomycin resistance: recommendations of the Hospital Infection Control Practices Advisory Committee (HICPAC), *Morbidity and Mortality Weekly Report* 44(RR-12):1-13, 1995. Accessed October 10, 2005, on-line: www.cdc.gov/ncidod.
29. Centers for Disease Control and Prevention: Recommendations for preventing transmission of infection with human T-lymphotropic virus type III/lymphadenopathy-associated virus during invasive procedures, *Morbidity and Mortality Weekly Report* 34:681-695, 1985. Accessed October 1, 2005, on-line: www.cdc.gov/search.
30. Centers for Disease Control and Prevention: *Staphylococcus aureus* with reduced susceptibility to vancomycin—United States, 1997, *Morbidity and Mortality Weekly Report* 46(33):765-766, 1997. Accessed October 10, 2005, on-line: www.cdc.gov/search.
31. Centers for Disease Control and Prevention, Disease Information: Anthrax, 2002. Accessed October 10, 2005, on-line: www.cdc.gov/ncidod/ dbmd/diseaseinfo/anthrax_t.htm.
32. Centers for Disease Control and Prevention, Disease Information: Viral hemorrhagic fever, 2002. Accessed October 10, 2005, on-line: www.cdc.gov/ncidod/dvrd/spb/mnpages/dispages/vhf.htm.
33. Centers for Disease Control and Prevention, Division of Vector-borne Infectious Diseases: Plague, 2002. Accessed October 1, 2005, on-line: www.cdc.gov/ncidod/dvbid/plague/index.htm.
34. Centers for Disease Control and Prevention, Emerging Infectious Diseases: *Clinical and epidemiological principles of anthrax.* Accessed October 10, 2005, on-line: www.cdc.gov/ncidod/EID/vol5no4/cieslak.htm.
35. Centers for Disease Control and Prevention, Hospital Infections Program, National Center for Infectious Diseases: *Creutzfeldt-Jakob disease: epidemiology, risk factors, and decontamination,* Atlanta, 1997, CDC. Accessed October 10, 2005, on-line: www.cdc.gov/ncidod/dbm/diseaseinfo/cjd/.
36. Centers for Disease Control and Prevention, Public Health Emergency Preparedness and Response: Facts about botulism, 2002. Accessed October 10, 2005, on-line: www.bt.cdc.gov/DocumentsApp/FactSheet/Botulism/About.asp.
37. Centers for Disease Control and Prevention, Public Health Emergency Preparedness and Response: Facts about plague, 2002. Accessed October 10, 2005, on-line: www.bt.cdc.gov/DocumentsApp/FactSheet/Plague/About.asp.
38. Centers for Disease Control and Prevention, Public Health Emergency Preparedness and Response: Facts about smallpox, 2002. Accessed October 10, 2005, on-line: www.bt.cdc.gov/DocumentsApp/FactSheet/Smallpox/About.asp.
39. Centers for Disease Control and Prevention, Public Health Emergency Preparedness and Response: Facts about tularemia, 2002. Accessed October 10, 2005, on-line: www.bt.cdc.gov/DocumentsApp/FAQTularemia.asp.
40. Centers for Disease Control and Prevention, Public Health Emergency Preparedness and Response: Biological diseases/agents listing, 2002. Accessed October 10, 2005, on-line: www.bt.cdc.gov.Agent/Agentlist.asp.
41. Chen CC, Willeke K: Aerosol penetration through surgical masks, *American Journal of Infection Control* 20(4):177-184, 1992. Accessed October 15, 2005, on-line: www.journals.elsevierhealth.com/periodical.
42. Cohen ML and others: Antimicrobial resistance: are the pathogens winning? In: *Infection control sourcebook.* Atlanta, 1997, American Health Consultants. Accessed October 15, 2005, on-line: www.journals.elsevierhealth.com/periodicals.
43. Conner R: How to select a patient skin prep solution for your OR, *Outpatient Surgery Magazine,* June 2003. Accessed April 1, 2006, on-line: www.outpatientsurgery.net..
44. Dennis DT and others: Working group on biodefense, *JAMA: The Journal of the American Medical Association* 285(6):2763-2773, 2001.
45. Edel E and others: Impact of a 5-minute scrub on the microbial flora found on artificial, polished, or natural fingernails of operating room personnel, *Nursing Research* 47:54-58, 1998.
46. Favaro MS, Bond WW: Chemical disinfection of medical and surgical materials. In Block SS, editor: *Disinfection, sterilization, and preservation,* ed 5, Philadelphia, 2001, Lippincott, Williams & Wilkins.
47. Horan TC and others: CDC definitions of healthcare-associated surgical site infections, 1992: a modification of CDC definitions of healthcare-associated surgical site infections, *American Journal of Infection Control* 20(5):271-274, 1992. Accessed October 15, 2005, on-line: www.ajic.com.
48. Hurley BW, Nguyen CC: The spectrum of pseudomembranous enterocolitis and antibiotic-associated diarrhea, *Archives of Internal Medicine* 162(19):2177-2184, 2002.
49. Institute for Biosecurity: Isolation guidelines, November 2001. Accessed October 5, 2005, on-line: www.bioterrorism.slu.edu/anthrax/key-ref/isolation.PDF.
50. Jacobs PT: Plasma sterilization, *Journal of Healthcare Materials Management* 7(5):49, 1989.
51. Jacobs PT: STERRAD sterilization system—a new technology for instrument sterilization, Arlington, Tex, 1993, Johnson & Johnson Medical, Inc.
52. Jenkins L: The prevention of *Clostridium difficile* associated diarrhea in hospitals, *Nursing Times* 100(26):56-57, 59, 2004.
53. Joslyn LJ: Sterilization by heat. In Block SS, editor: *Disinfection, sterilization, and preservation,* ed 5, Philadelphia, 2001, Lippincott, Williams & Wilkins.
54. Kaufman M: FDA approves new antibiotic for resistant bacteria. *Washington Post,* June 17, 2005; A14.
55. LaForce FM: The control of infections in hospitals: 1750-1950. In Wenzel RP, editor: *Prevention and control of nosocomial infections,* ed 4, Philadelphia, 2003, Lippincott, Williams & Wilkins.
56. Lagergren E: Gas plasma sterilization, *Surgical Services Management* 1(2):18-20, 1995. Accessed October 10, 2005, on-line: www.ssmonline.org.
57. Larson E: Innovations in healthcare: antisepsis as a case study, *American Journal of Public Health* 79(1):92-99, 1989. Accessed October 10, 2005, on-line: www.ajph.org/cgi/content/abstract.
58. Loeb M and others: A randomized clinical trial of surgical scrubbing with a brush compared to antiseptic soap alone, *American Journal of Infection Control* 20:11-15, 1997. Accessed October 10, 2005, on-line: www.journals.elsevierhealth.com/periodicals.
59. Lynch MM: Gas plasma sterilization, *Surgical Services Management* 1(2):16-17, 1995.
60. Martin MA, Reichelderfer M: APIC guideline for infection prevention and control in flexible endoscopy, *American Journal of Infection Control* 22(1):19-38, 1994. Accessed October 15, 2005, on-line: www.ajic.com.
61. McCormick PJ, Wilder JA: Gas plasma sterilization, *Surgical Services Management* 1(2):13-15, 1985. Accessed October 15, 2005, on-line: www.ssmonline.org.
62. Mitchell NJ, Hunt S: Surgical face masks in modern operating rooms—a costly and unnecessary ritual? *Journal of Hospital Infection* 18:239-242, 1991.
63. Occupational Safety and Health Administration (OSHA): Occupational exposure to bloodborne pathogens: final rule, *Federal Register* 56(235):64175-64182, 1991. Accessed October 10, 2005, on-line: www.osha.gov.
64. Occupational Safety and Health Administration (OSHA): Occupational exposure to bloodborne pathogens: needlestick and other sharps injuries: final rule, *Federal Register* 66:5317-5325, 2001. Accessed October 10, 2005, on-line: www.osha.gov.
65. Occupational Safety and Health Administration (OSHA): Occupational exposure to ethylene oxide, final standard, *Federal Register* 49(122):25737-25768, 1984. Accessed October 10, 2005, on-line: www.osha.gov.
66. Occupational Safety and Health Administration (OSHA): Occupational exposure to ethylene oxide, final standard, *Federal Register* 53(66):11414-11438, 1988. Accessed October 10, 2005, on-line: www.osha.gov.

67. *Patient Safety Authority (PSRS),* produced by ECRI and ISMP under contract to the Patient Safety Authority, Vol. 2, June 2005, pp. 1-8.
68. *Patient Safety Authority (PSRS),* produced by ECRI and ISMP under contract to the Patient Safety Authority, Vol. 2, June 2005, pp. 13-14.
69. Perkins JJ: *Principles and methods of sterilization in health sciences,* ed 2, Springfield, Ill, 1969, Charles C. Thomas.
70. Pugliese G, Favaro MS: First isolate of vancomycin-resistant *Staphylococcus aureus*—Japan, *Infection Control and Hospital Epidemiology* 18(7):527, 1997. Accessed October 10, 2005, on-line: www.iche.org.
71. Rutala WA: APIC guideline for selection and use of disinfectants, *American Journal of Infection Control* 24(4):313-342, 1996. Accessed September 30, 2005, on-line: www.apic.org.
72. Rutala WA, Weber DJ: Creutzfeldt-Jakob disease: recommendations for disinfection and sterilization, *Clinical Infectious Diseases* 32(9):1348-1349, 2001.
73. Rutala WA, Weber DJ: Disinfection of endoscopes: review of new chemical sterilants used for high-level disinfection, *Infection Control and Hospital Epidemiology* 20(1):69-76, 1999.
74. Schultz JK: Steam sterilization: recommended practices. In Reichert M, Young JH, editors: *Sterilization technology for the health care facility,* ed 2, Gaithersburg, Md, 1997, Aspen Publications.
75. Sharbaugh RJ: Decontamination: principles of disinfection. In Reichert M, Young JH, editors: *Sterilization technology for the health care facility,* ed 2, Gaithersburg, Md, 1997, Aspen Publications.
76. Shoup AJ: Guidelines for the management of latex allergies and safe use of latex in the perioperative practice setting, *AORN Journal* 66(4):726-731, 1997. Accessed October 1, 2005, on-line: www.aorn.org.
77. Spaulding EH: Chemical disinfection of medical and surgical materials. In Lawrence CA, Block SS, editors: *Disinfection, sterilization, and preservation,* Philadelphia, 2001, Lippincott, Williams & Wilkins.
78. Spry C: Brush up your skin prep protocol: manager's guide to infection prevention, *Outpatient Surgery Magazine,* 2005. Accessed April 1, 2006, on-line: www.outpatientsurgery.net.
79. Steelman VM: Creutzfeldt-Jakob disease: recommendations for infection control, *American Journal of Infection Control* 22(5):312-318, 1994. Accessed October 3, 2005, on-line: www.ajic.org.
80. Steris Corporation: Peracetic acid sterilization, *Surgical Services Management* 1(2):21-23, 1995.
81. Taylor D: Evaluating surgical skin preps, *Outpatient Surgery Magazine,* February 2005. Accessed April 1, 2006 on-line: www.outpatientsurgery.net.
82. Taylor D: Three steps to success with surgical rubs, *Outpatient Surgery Magazine,* February 2005. Accessed April 1, 2006, on-line: www.outpatientsurgery.net.
83. Weber DJ, Rutala WA: Role of environmental contamination in the transmission of vancomycin-resistant enterococci, *Infection Control and Hospital Epidemiology* 18(5):306-309, 1997. Accessed October 3, 2005, on-line: www.ishe.org.
84. Young JH: Steam sterilization: scientific principles. In Reichert M, Young JH, editors: *Sterilization technology for the health care facility,* ed 2, Gaithersburg, Md, 1997, Aspen Publications.
85. Young ML: Ethylene oxide sterilization: recommended practices. In Reichert M, Young JH, editors: *Sterilization technology for the health care facility,* ed 2, Gaithersburg, Md, 1997, Aspen Publications.

CHAPTER 4

# Anesthesia

LINDA M. DeLAMAR

Without anesthesia, most modern surgical procedures would not be feasible. As an integral part of the patient care team in operative and other invasive procedure settings, perioperative nurses need to be familiar with the principles and practices of anesthesia and the perioperative functions of the anesthesia provider. This chapter presents an overview of the modern practice of anesthesia, the factors involved, and the interrelationship with the perioperative nurse. This chapter includes discussions of the major types of anesthesia, an introduction to the more commonly used drugs, a review of the standards of anesthesia care, and an overview of some of the problems that can occur during the perioperative period. Descriptions of the anesthesia machine and monitoring equipment also are included so that the perioperative nurse can become familiar with their basic functions for potential use during local anesthesia or conscious sedation procedures.

The sections of this chapter are organized so that they can be referred to independently without reading the entire chapter. Experienced perioperative nurses are familiar with the commonly used abbreviations employed in this chapter. To provide a single reference source for the student or novice perioperative nurse, most abbreviations are defined in Box 4-1.

## HISTORY OF ANESTHESIA

The early history of modern anesthesia was fraught with controversy. Surgeons in the early nineteenth century frequently used alcohol or opium to intoxicate the patient for procedures involving intense pain or when muscle relaxation was needed. In some cases, hypnotism also was employed. Successful surgery was related directly to the speed of the surgeon (see the History box for a brief overview of anesthesia history).

In March 1842, Crawford W. Long, a physician in Danielsville, Georgia, using ether as an anesthetic, removed a cystic tumor from the neck of a patient named James Venable. As confirmed by other physicians in the area, Dr. Long subsequently used ether for other procedures, but did not publish reports of his experiences.[6,14]

In 1844 Horace Wells, a dentist in Hartford, Connecticut, began to use nitrous oxide ($N_2O$) for anesthesia and communicated his results to his former partner, William T.G. Morton. After a death with $N_2O$, however, Wells quit the practice of dentistry and later committed suicide. Morton subsequently studied medicine and learned of the anesthetic effects of chloric ether from his preceptor, Charles T. Jackson, a chemist. In 1846, while employing this new drug, Morton was able to fill a tooth without the patient experiencing pain. He later learned from Jackson that sulfuric ether had similar properties and used it while extracting a deeply rooted bicuspid tooth from another patient.[6,14]

Morton contacted John C. Warren, a surgeon at the Massachusetts General Hospital, and persuaded him to give the new anesthetic a trial during a surgical procedure. With Morton as the anesthetist, this historic operation took place in the amphitheater (subsequently renamed "The Ether Dome") of Massachusetts General Hospital on October 16, 1846. In 5 minutes, Warren operated on an unconscious, quiet patient and dissected "a congenital but superficial vascular tumor just below the jaw on the left side of the neck." As the patient regained consciousness, Warren exclaimed, "Gentlemen, this is no humbug." The next day, Haywood, with Morton as the anesthetist, removed a large fatty tumor from the shoulder of another patient.[14]

Based on these events, the first medical report of anesthesia was announced to the world on November 18, 1846, by Henry J. Bigelow in the *Boston Medical and Surgical Journal.* An era had ended in which successful surgery was largely predicated on the lightning speed of the surgeon while working on a struggling, distressed patient. Anesthetic techniques gave the surgeon more time to operate and permitted new procedures to be undertaken that would have been impossible before. Many modern surgical techniques have become feasible because of the advances in the art and science of anesthesia.

The word *anesthesia* is derived from the Greek word *anaisthesia*, which literally means "no sensation." Anesthesia was listed in *Bailey's English Dictionary* in 1721. When the effects of ether were discovered, Oliver Wendell Holmes suggested *anesthesia* be used as a name for the new phenomenon. Some believed that he coined this term; others believed that he knew of the Greek word that Plato had employed. In any case, anesthesia was, in the memorable phrase of Werr Mitchell, the "death of pain." From these early beginnings, anesthesia has developed into a sophisticated science and "clinical art" that interfaces with many other medical specialties.

## ANESTHESIA PROVIDERS

In the United States, anesthesia care usually is provided by an anesthesiologist, a certified registered nurse anesthetist (CRNA) working under the direction of an anesthesiologist or a physician, or an anesthesiologist's assistant (AA) working under the direction of an anesthesiologist. An anesthesiologist is a physician with 4 or more years of specialty training in anesthesiology after medical school.

Nurse anesthesia programs are now a minimum of 2 years in length. They require a bachelor of science (BS) degree in nursing or other appropriate field and a minimum of 1 year of critical care experience before acceptance. All nurse anesthesia programs are at the master's degree level, usually within a school of nursing or allied health. Some programs are based in

BOX 4-1

## Abbreviations Used in This Chapter

AANA—American Association of Nurse Anesthetists
ABG—arterial blood gas. Usually includes pH, $PaO_2$, $PaCO_2$, $HCO_3^-$, $K^+$, and ionized $Ca^{++}$
ACLS—advanced cardiac life support; a protocol for resuscitation from the American Heart Association
APL—adjustable pressure-limiting valve; a valve on anesthesia machines that limits the maximum pressure in the patient breathing circuit; frequently referred to as the "pop-off valve"
ASA—American Society of Anesthesiologists
cm—centimeter; $1 \times 10^{-2}$ m; 2.54 cm = 1 inch
CRNA—certified registered nurse anesthetist
CSF—cerebrospinal fluid; the fluid surrounding the brain and spinal cord; for spinal anesthesia, local anesthetics are injected into the CSF
EGTA—esophageal (gastric tube) airway; a cuffed tube that is inserted blindly into the esophagus and connected to a mask; this permits ventilation through the mask and gastric suctioning through the cuffed tube
$ETCO_2$—end-tidal carbon dioxide reported as a partial pressure; see "Capnography" section
ETT—endotracheal tube
$FIO_2$—fraction of inspired oxygen; this is a fraction (0.00 to 1.00) that corresponds to the percent (0% to 100%) of inspired oxygen
FO—fiberoptic
μg—microgram; the nonstandard abbreviation is mcg
kg—kilogram; 1 kg = 2.2 lb
LED—light-emitting diode; an electronic device that emits light at a predetermined frequency
LMA—laryngeal mask airway or laryngeal airway
MAC—monitored anesthesia care; see "Monitored Anesthesia Care" section
mg—milligram; $1 \times 10^{-3}$ g
MH—malignant hyperthermia; see "Malignant Hyperthermia" section
MHAUS—Malignant Hyperthermia Association of the United States
MMS—master of medical science degree
MRI—magnetic resonance imaging
NIOSH—National Institute for Occupational Safety and Health
nm—nanometer; $1 \times 10^{-9}$ m
NMS—neuroleptic malignant syndrome; see "Malignant Hyperthermia" section
$N_2O$—nitrous oxide
NSAID—nonsteroidal antiinflammatory drug
PA—pulmonary artery
$PaCO_2$—partial pressure of arterial carbon dioxide; lower case "a" denotes "arterial"; an uppercase "A" denotes "alveolar"
$PaO_2$—partial pressure of arterial oxygen; lower case "a" denotes "arterial"; an uppercase "A" denotes "alveolar"
PCA—patient-controlled analgesia; see "Pain Management" section
ppm—parts per million; 1 ppm = $1 \times 10^{-6}$
psi—pounds per square inch; a measurement of pressure
QA—quality assurance; this function also may be identified as quality improvement (QI), continuous quality improvement (CQI), or similar names
$SpO_2$—saturation (pulse) of oxygen or in a pulsating vessel, expressed as a percentage; see "Pulse Oximetry" section
$SvO_2$—saturation of mixed venous oxygen in percentage; this measurement is made from a special pulmonary artery catheter
torr—1 mm Hg

## HISTORY

### A Brief Look at Anesthesia History

In *Nursing, The Finest Art,* Donahue notes that "The first nursing specialists have existed since the late nineteenth and early twentieth centuries: the nurse midwife and the nurse anesthetist. . . . The role of the nurse anesthetist developed as part of the increasing sophistication of surgery in the early 1900s, when it was recognized that trained assistants were needed to administer anesthetics. No longer was it safe or satisfactory to have untrained medical students or attendants providing anesthesia. These early specialists were recruited from the available pool of trained nurses to meet very specific societal demands and needs."

**1861-1865**
Catherine S. Lawrence and other nurses provided anesthesia for surgeons during the Civil War.

**1887**
Sister Mary Bernard was the first nurse known to specialize in anesthesia.

**1893**
Alice Magaw began as a nurse anesthetist for Dr. Mayo, who would later give her the title "The Mother of Anesthesia" for her mastery of open drop ether.

**1899**
Magaw published the first paper by a nurse anesthetist in the Northwestern *Lancet.*

**1909**
St. Vincent's Hospital in Springfield, Illinois, began a nurse anesthetist program.

**1911**
Frances Hoeffer McMelhan began to push for physician anesthetists.

**1914-1917**
Agatha Hodgins and many other nurse anesthetists in volunteer American medical units provided anesthesia to casualties during World War I.

**1931**
Agatha Hodgins and 47 nurse anesthetists founded the National Association of Nurse Anesthetists (NANA).

**1936**
The American Society of Anesthesiologists (ASA) was founded.

**1939**
The NANA became the American Association of Nurse Anesthetists (AANA).

**1941-1945**
Second Lieutenant Mildred Clark became the first nurse anesthetist to serve as the Chief of the Army Nurse Corps. Nurse anesthetists provided anesthesia to World War II casualties.

**1945**
AANA administered its first certification examination (CRNA).

Modified from American Association of Nurse Anesthetists: A brief look at nurse anesthesia history (*AANA Archives-Library,* June 15, 2005). Accessed on-line: www.aana.com/archives/timeline.asp; Bankert M: *Watchful care: a history of America's nurse anesthetists,* New York, 2000, Continuum Publishing Company; Gunn IP: Nurse anesthesia: a history of challenge. In Nagelhout JJ and others, editors: *Nurse anesthesia,* ed 3, Philadelphia, 2005, Saunders.

community hospitals and are affiliated with a university. On completion of the program, graduates must successfully complete the American Association of Nurse Anesthetists Council on Certification National Certification Examination. Nurse anesthetists must maintain their certification by obtaining 40 continuing education credits every 2 years.

In recent years, AAs also have been trained. These are assistants to anesthesiologists. Acceptance into an AA program requires a BS degree including a college-level "premed" education. AAs are graduate students within a medical school and typically receive a master of medical science (MMS) degree from the medical school. They also take a national certification examination administered by the National Commission on Certification of Anesthesia Providers' Assistants under the supervision of the National Board of Medical Examiners.

In this chapter, the term *anesthesia provider* denotes the individual *providing* the continuous anesthesia care for the patient. Depending on the practice in a given hospital, this may be an anesthesiologist, a CRNA, or an AA. In many hospitals, an *anesthesia care team* includes CRNAs with or without AAs supervised by anesthesiologists. In small rural hospitals in some states, an anesthesiologist may not be present, and a CRNA may be the sole anesthesia provider.

The anesthesia provider is the patient's advocate in the perioperative period; as such, he or she must be concerned with many divergent factors when the patient's own sensory and cerebral functions are obtunded by anesthesia. The field of anesthesia has become so complex that in many large hospitals an anesthesia provider may specialize further in obstetric, neurosurgical, pediatric, cardiovascular, regional, or ambulatory anesthesia. Anesthesiologists also may subspecialize in acute and chronic pain management or in critical care medicine.

## PATIENT SAFETY

Patient safety is always a concern during surgery and anesthesia. Approximately 26 million anesthetics are administered each year in the United States. Of these, data from several sources indicate a death rate ranging from 1 per 35,000 to about 1 per 40,000. These rates represent a significant decline during the past 30 years, despite surgical procedures being performed on increasingly higher risk patients than in the past.

The general public still considers anesthesia to be a major risk of surgery. This attitude may be attributable to sensationalized reports in the news media and in magazine articles. In addition, people may have a heightened awareness of anesthesia-related deaths because these often occur acutely in the perioperative period, whereas surgical or medical problems may not result in death until days after the procedure.

## AWARENESS DURING ANESTHESIA

The possibility of being awake during anesthesia is a concern of patients and anesthesia providers (Research Highlight). Some patients are so anxious about being aware of anything during surgery that it affects their reasoning when discussing the options for anesthesia. Many procedures, such as biopsies, inguinal hernias, or procedures on the lower extremities, can be done under regional anesthesia or monitored anesthesia care (MAC). These patients may want general anesthesia, however, because they do not want to be aware of anything during the procedure. In rare cases during general anesthesia, the patient may be paralyzed but be aware of what is going on and be unable to indicate this to anyone. Intraoperative awareness (IOA) has been reported with many anesthetic techniques. Several

### RESEARCH HIGHLIGHT

#### Anesthesia Awareness

Awareness during anesthesia is a constant concern for anesthesia providers. Intraoperative awareness (IOA) was recognized in 1846, when Morton demonstrated ether anesthesia and the patient later reported that he had been half-awake during the procedure. Although rare with modern anesthetic agents and techniques, IOA does occur. Multiple studies have found IOA to occur in 0.1% to 0.2% of patients undergoing general anesthesia. Of 21 million patients who receive general anesthesia, 20,000 to 40,000 experience awareness each year. Of patients who experienced awareness, 48% reported auditory recollections, 48% reported the sensation of not being able to breathe, and 28% reported feeling pain. Greater than 50% of these patients were reported to experience mental distress, including an indeterminate number with posttraumatic stress syndrome. More recent dramatized accounts in the lay press have caused an increasing number of patients to voice their concern during preoperative interviews. To evaluate this issue, investigators have used a variety of approaches, including the following:

- The effects of intraoperative therapeutic suggestions on the length of postoperative hospitalization or the level of pain
- Positive suggestions during anesthesia for changes in lifestyle (e.g., smoking cessation, weight loss)
- Assessment of inadequate amnesia or recall of intraoperative conversation or events or both
- Intraoperative memory analyzed by recall of specific words or phrases spoken during anesthesia
- Intraoperative physiologic changes or postoperative recall evaluated under hypnosis when a mock crisis was staged during anesthesia
- Learning of new information during anesthesia

Many of these studies employed changes in the latency and amplitude of middle-latency, auditory-evoked potentials. They found that even under seemingly adequate general anesthesia, implicit memory may be retained along with the ability to process auditory stimuli subconsciously. Based on these studies, it would seem prudent to avoid anesthetic techniques that rely solely on receptor-based drugs (i.e., benzodiazepines, opioids, nitrous oxide [$N_2O$]) and to include volatile anesthetics.

In an effort to reduce the risk of anesthesia awareness, the American Society of Anesthesiologists (ASA) and the American Association of Nurse Anesthetists (AANA) have provided guidelines for administering and monitoring anesthesia.

Studies in the area of patient memory are ongoing. While a patient is anesthetized, it is important that all persons in the OR and procedure room always conduct themselves in a professional manner. There is a possibility that the patient may remember conversations conducted during the anesthesia experience.

Modified from Lennmarken C, Sandin R: Neuromonitoring for awareness during surgery, *Lancet* 363:1747-1748, 2004; Sebel PS and others: The incidence of awareness during anesthesia: a multicenter United States study, *Anesthesia and Analgesia* 99:833-839, 2004; Stanski DR, Shafer SL: Measuring depth of anesthesia. In Miller RD, editor: *Anesthesia*, ed 6, Philadelphia, 2005, Churchill Livingstone.

factors may contribute to its occurrence. Overall, 0.2% of all patients may experience awareness during general anesthesia.[26] The incidence of awareness may increase to 1% to 1.5% in higher risk patient populations, such as patients requiring anesthesia for obstetrics, major trauma, and cardiac surgery.[17,26]

For many years, the electroencephalogram (EEG) has been the standard for assessing a person's hypnotic and sleep state. To employ an EEG routinely for all surgical procedures is unrealistic, however. For years investigators have attempted to analyze and process the EEG mathematically to develop a usable monitor. In the late 1990s the bispectral index system (BIS) was developed, which analyzes the relationship and frequency of the signals using a sophisticated algorithm to generate a composite, numeric value that seems to correlate with the cerebral state. Five electrodes are positioned across the forehead, and the monitor gives an index (0 to 100) of the hypnotic state or sedation level; an index of 40 to 60 is considered optimal anesthesia. The BIS seems to monitor the effects of anesthetics and sedatives on the hypnotic status of the brain but is less informative about the level of analgesia. This monitor is used mostly for general anesthesia. Motion artifacts and mental changes cause erratic changes under the lighter level of sedation commonly used with MAC. Use of the BIS monitor has increased over the past next few years. Often patients wake up more quickly and experience less nausea and vomiting because drugs can be titrated using BIS.[17, 27] It is hoped that ongoing studies will show a reduced incidence of perioperative awareness during anesthesia.

## PREOPERATIVE PREPARATION

### Patient Evaluation

It is common to perform the preoperative evaluation in advance of the scheduled surgical procedure. One or more days before the procedure, the patient visits a preadmission clinic. (This also may be called *preadmission testing, preanesthesia clinic,* or *anesthesia-assessment unit.*) All the admission data and appropriate consent forms are completed, a preoperative history is obtained, a physical examination is done, a preanesthesia evaluation and examination are completed, and appropriate diagnostic or laboratory tests are processed. "Routine" preoperative testing is less extensive than previously because numerous studies have shown limited benefits of extensive routine testing. More extensive testing is indicated for patients who have higher than average risk based on their history. The patient's physical status is assessed, and the most appropriate anesthetic technique is selected. The patient's questions and concerns are resolved, and instructions are given to expedite admission on the day of surgery. This preadmission processing has become popular because third-party payers have agreed to reimbursement for outpatient laboratory testing. In addition, the patient usually is more relaxed and rested after sleeping at home rather than adapting to a strange hospital environment before surgery.

Before elective surgery, the patient should be in optimal medical condition. Anesthesia, even in healthy patients, presents risks. Inhaled general anesthetics are myocardial depressants; these may lead to dose-dependent decreases in myocardial contractility and blood pressure. This response may be accentuated in patients who are volume depleted, who are overdiuresed, who have poor ventricular function, or who have autonomic neuropathy, such as found in diabetics. If it is determined that the patient's physical status should be improved to reduce the risks involved, this is discussed with the patient's primary physician or the surgeon, and if necessary, elective surgery is deferred until the patient's condition is optimized. If the intended surgery is emergent, however, any benefits gained from a delay must be weighed carefully with the hazards of waiting.[11]

The assignment of a physical status classification is based on the patient's physiologic condition independent of the proposed surgical procedure. The physical status classification was developed by the American Society of Anesthesiologists (ASA) to provide uniform guidelines. It is an evaluation of the severity of systemic diseases, physiologic dysfunction, and anatomic abnormalities. The ASA classification system is widely used by many clinicians to estimate perioperative risk (Table 4-1). In recent years the validity of this practice has been questioned because many other variables affect perioperative risks and outcomes as well.

Preadmission clinics are commonly used by many hospitals and ambulatory surgery centers. In some metropolitan areas where travel and congestion are problems and for patients in reasonably good health, nurses may conduct preoperative telephone interviews with patients. Questions are asked relating to pulmonary and cardiac disease; medication (prescription, over-the-counter, herbal, and homeopathic remedies) and alcohol use; medication, latex, or anesthetic allergies; pregnancy; and personal or family history of anesthetic reactions. On the day of surgery, patients arrive 1 to 2 hours before the scheduled surgery time to complete other preoperative processes. In some facilities, certain ambulatory patients are evaluated just before surgery. These are usually healthy patients having minor procedures or patients with stable, chronic conditions having a procedure (e.g., cataract removal, skin lesion excision) under MAC. These preadmission processes have reduced the cost of health care, decreased the risk of nosocomial infections associated with longer hospital admissions, increased the use and efficiency of health care resources, improved patient relations, and enhanced the chances of having a well-informed patient in optimal health status.[11]

In larger hospitals and ambulatory surgery centers, the individual who evaluates the patient in the preanesthesia clinic is often not the anesthesia provider for the patient's surgical procedure. Immediately before surgery, the anesthesia provider (1) reviews the patient's chart, laboratory data, and diagnostic studies, such as electrocardiogram (ECG) and chest x-ray; (2) confirms that the appropriate consent forms (surgery, anesthesia, use of blood products) have been signed; (3) identifies the patient; (4) verifies the surgical procedure; (5) reviews the choice of anesthesia; (6) examines the patient; and (7) administers preoperative medications if appropriate.[11,30]

### Choice of Anesthesia

The choice of anesthesia for a given surgical procedure is made by the patient, the anesthesia provider, and the surgeon. A variety of factors influence this choice, including the following:

1. Patient's wishes and understanding of the types of anesthesia that could be used
2. Patient's physiologic status
3. Presence and severity of coexisting diseases
4. Patient's mental and psychologic status

**TABLE 4-1**

**Physical (P) Status Classification of the American Society of Anesthesia (ASA) Providers**

| Status*† | Definition | Description and Examples |
|---|---|---|
| P1 | Normal healthy patient | No physiologic, psychologic, biochemical, or organic disturbance |
| P2 | Patient with mild systemic disease | Cardiovascular disease with minimal restriction of activity. Hypertension, asthma, chronic bronchitis, obesity, diabetes mellitus, or tobacco abuse |
| P3 | Patient with a severe systemic disease that limits activity, but is not incapacitating | Cardiovascular or pulmonary disease that limits activity. Severe diabetes with systemic complications. History of myocardial infarction, angina pectoris, poorly controlled hypertension, or morbid obesity |
| P4 | Patient with a severe systemic disease that is a constant threat to life | Severe cardiac, pulmonary, renal, hepatic, or endocrine dysfunction |
| P5 | Moribund patient who is not expected to survive 24 hr with or without the operation | Surgery is done as last recourse or resuscitative effort. Major multisystem or cerebral trauma, ruptured aneurysm, or large pulmonary embolus |
| P6 | Patient declared brain dead whose organs are being removed for donor purposes | |

*In statuses 2, 3, and 4, the systemic disease may or may not be related to the reason for surgery.

†For any patient (P1 through P5) requiring emergency surgery, an E is added to the physical status, such as P1E, P2E. ASA 1 through ASA 6 or I-VI is often used for physical status.

Modified from American Society of Anesthesia (ASA) Providers: *Manual for anesthesia departments,* Park Ridge, Ill, 1997, The Association. Accessed June 15, 2005, on-line: www.asahq.org/profinfo/physicalstatus.html.

5. Postoperative recovery from various kinds of anesthesia
6. Options for management of postoperative pain
7. Type and duration of surgical procedure
8. Patient's position during surgery
9. Particular requirements of the surgeon

## Premedications

The primary purpose of premedication before anesthesia is to sedate the patient and reduce anxiety. Medications that may be given preoperatively include sedatives and hypnotics, anxiolytics, amnestics, tranquilizers, narcotics or other analgesics, antiemetics, and anticholinergics. A single drug may possess the properties of several classes. Midazolam (Versed) is administered frequently to relieve apprehension and to provide amnesia. An analgesic or narcotic may be ordered if preoperative discomfort is anticipated during invasive procedures or during the administration of a regional anesthetic. An anticholinergic, such as atropine or glycopyrrolate, may be used to prevent bradycardia in pediatric patients, to control secretions in patients undergoing oropharyngeal procedures, or to control cardiac reflex that may cause bradycardia (e.g., during ophthalmic procedures).[30,31]

To decrease the risk of aspiration, metoclopramide (Reglan) may be given to empty the stomach and to reduce nausea and vomiting. In addition, an antacid or an $H_2$-receptor–blocking drug, such as cimetidine (Tagamet), ranitidine (Zantac), or famotidine (Pepcid), may be included to decrease gastric acid production or the acidity of the gastric contents or both. Should aspiration occur, a gastric pH greater than 2.5 decreases the resultant pulmonary damage.[31]

Before a premedication is given, any last-minute questions from the patient concerning surgery and anesthesia should be answered, and the preoperative verification process should be completed to ensure that all relevant documents (e.g., the history and physical examination, surgical consent) and imaging studies (properly labeled and displayed) are available before the start of the procedure. These must be reviewed and be consistent with the patient's stated expectations (when the patient is awake and aware, the patient should actively participate in the verification process). The surgical team must agree that this is the correct patient, the planned procedure, on the specified side and site. Any additional special equipment, supplies, or implants also must be confirmed as being correct and available. Marking the surgical site also must be done before administering premedication (see Chapter 2 for a full discussion of the Joint Commission on Accreditation of Healthcare Organizations [JCAHO] Universal Protocol for preventing wrong site, wrong procedure, wrong person surgery).

Premedication may be administered intramuscularly (IM), intravenously (IV), intranasally, or orally (PO) with 15 to 30 mL of water. The patient usually prefers oral premedication, and the small amount of water is readily absorbed directly across the gastric mucosa. Premedication usually is given 30 to 90 minutes before surgery but may be given IV in the preoperative holding area or after the patient arrives in the surgical suite. Except for the small amount of water needed to swallow any medications, adult patients traditionally have been required to maintain nothing by mouth (NPO) status for a minimum 4 to 6 hours before elective surgery. More recent data indicate, however, that clear liquids may be acceptable 2 hours before surgery. Breast milk may be acceptable 4 hours before surgery. Infant formula, nonhuman milk, or a light meal (toast and clear liquids) should not be consumed within 6 hours of surgery.[11]

Although premedications commonly are used, studies have shown that visits before surgery by the anesthesia provider and the perioperative nurse are far more important in relieving patient anxiety and concern. Major patient concerns include fear of the unknown, relinquishing control of one's life to someone else, being awake during surgery, not awakening from anesthesia, and concerns related to the surgery (e.g., diagnosis, prognosis). Premedication may be unnecessary for older patients because their anxiety levels are lower, their responses to medications are unpredictable, and sedation can be given IV in the operating room (OR) if required.

## TYPES OF ANESTHESIA CARE

The JCAHO *Comprehensive Accreditation Manual for Hospitals* has Anesthesia Care Standards that apply when patients receive, in any setting, moderate or deep sedation or general, spinal, or other major regional anesthesia. Descriptions of the frequently used classifications of anesthesia care follow.

### General Anesthesia

General anesthesia is a reversible, unconscious state characterized by amnesia (sleep, hypnosis, or basal narcosis), analgesia (freedom from pain), depression of reflexes, muscle relaxation, and homeostasis or specific manipulation of physiologic systems and functions. Most patients think of general anesthesia when they are scheduled to have a surgical procedure; that is, they expect to be "put to sleep." As such, they experience a drug-induced loss of consciousness during which they are not arousable. Their ability to maintain ventilatory function is often impaired, requiring assistance maintaining a patent airway. Positive-pressure ventilation may be required because of decreased spontaneous ventilation or drug-induced depression of neuromuscular function.

### Regional Anesthesia

Regional anesthesia is defined broadly as a reversible loss of sensation in a specific area or region of the body when a local anesthetic is injected purposefully to block or anesthetize nerve fibers in and around the operative site. Common regional anesthesia techniques include spinals (subarachnoid block [SAB]), epidurals, caudals, and major peripheral nerve blocks.

### Monitored Anesthesia Care

MAC is provided when infiltration of the surgical site with a local anesthetic is performed by the surgeon, and the anesthesia provider supplements the local anesthesia with IV drugs that provide sedation and systemic analgesia. (*Local standby* and *anesthesia standby* are older, less accurate terms frequently used interchangeably with MAC.) The anesthesia provider also monitors the patient's vital functions and may use additional medication to optimize the patient's physiologic status. MAC is often used for healthy patients undergoing relatively minor surgical procedures. This technique also may be used for some procedures for critically ill patients who may tolerate a general anesthetic poorly without extensive invasive monitoring and pharmacologic support.

### Conscious Sedation/Analgesia

Conscious sedation/analgesia is being administered increasingly for specific short-term surgical, diagnostic, and therapeutic procedures within a hospital or ambulatory center. The ASA has developed *Practice Guidelines for Sedation and Analgesia by Non-Anesthesiologists*. These guidelines were approved by the ASA House of Delegates and last amended in October 2001. In these guidelines, the ASA defines moderate sedation/analgesia (*Conscious Sedation*) as "a drug-induced depression of consciousness during which patients respond purposefully to verbal commands, either alone or accompanied by light tactile stimulation." No interventions are required to maintain a patent airway, and spontaneous ventilation is adequate. Cardiovascular function is usually maintained." Patients whose only response is reflex withdrawal from a painful stimulus are sedated to a greater degree than encompassed by sedation/analgesia.[30] The demand for appropriate providers to administer and monitor the patient receiving conscious sedation/analgesia has grown over the past few years, exceeding the supply of anesthesia providers. This demand has resulted in the increased use of nonanesthesia providers (usually professional registered nurses with additional training in administering conscious sedation/analgesia medications and monitoring these patients) for these functions. Various medications and techniques may be used to achieve conscious sedation, each with advantages and disadvantages. Competency-based education programs and assessment should be established for nurse-monitored conscious sedation. The Association of periOperative Registered Nurses (AORN) has established Recommended Practices for managing patients undergoing conscious sedation/analgesia, which should be used by health care facilities in developing such programs.[5]

### Local Anesthesia

*Local anesthesia* refers to the administration of an anesthetic agent to one part of the body by local infiltration or topical application. The surgeon usually administers it. Local anesthesia is used (1) for minor procedures, (2) if the patient's cooperation is necessary for the procedure, or (3) if the patient's physical condition warrants its use. An anesthesia provider is not involved in the patient's care. A perioperative nurse monitors the patient's vital signs and provides supportive care during the procedure. AORN has established Recommended Practices for managing patients undergoing local anesthesia and documenting care, which should be used by health care facilities in establishing policies and procedures for patient care in operative and other invasive settings.[4]

## PERIOPERATIVE MONITORING

Significant advances in perioperative monitoring have been made in recent years. (See also "Awareness During Anesthesia" earlier in this chapter.) Among the medical specialties, anesthesiology has been a pioneer in the review and analysis of perioperative mishaps and the implementation of improved monitoring techniques and guidelines. These advances have resulted in significant decreases in mortality and morbidity. In several states, malpractice insurance carriers have recognized the significance of these improvements and have decreased premiums if certain monitors are used routinely. These monitors include pulse oximetry, which measures oxygen saturation in a pulsating vessel ($Spo_2$), and capnography, which measures end-tidal carbon dioxide ($ETco_2$).[16]

The ASA has adopted the Standards for Basic Anesthetic Monitoring (Patient Safety) as guidelines for patient care. Perioperative nurses should be familiar with these standards and understand their significance in patient safety. If routine or

## PATIENT SAFETY

### Standards for Basic Anesthetic Monitoring

These standards for basic anesthetic monitoring apply to all anesthesia care, although in emergency circumstances, appropriate life support measures take precedence. These standards may be exceeded at any time based on the judgment of the responsible anesthesia provider. They are intended to encourage quality patient care, but observing them cannot guarantee any specific patient outcome. They are subject to revision from time to time, as warranted by the evolution of technology and practice. They apply to all general anesthetics, regional anesthetics, and monitored anesthesia care. This set of standards addresses only the issue of basic anesthetic monitoring, which is one component of anesthesia care. In certain rare or unusual circumstances, (1) some of these methods of monitoring may be clinically impractical, and (2) appropriate use of the described monitoring methods may fail to detect untoward clinical developments. Brief interruptions of continual[a] monitoring may be unavoidable. *Under extenuating circumstances, the responsible anesthesia provider may waive the requirements marked with an asterisk (*); it is recommended that when this is done, it should be so stated (including the reasons) in a note in the patient's medical record.* These standards are not intended for application to the care of an obstetric patient in labor or in the conduct of pain management.

**Standard I**

Qualified anesthesia personnel shall be present in the room throughout the conduct of all general anesthetics, regional anesthetics, and monitored anesthesia care.

***Objective***

Because of the rapid changes in patient status during anesthesia, qualified anesthesia personnel shall be continuously present to monitor the patient and provide anesthesia care. In the event there is a direct known hazard (e.g., radiation) to the anesthesia personnel that might require intermittent remote observation of the patient, some provision for monitoring the patient must be made. In the event that an emergency requires the temporary absence of the person primarily responsible for the anesthetic, the best judgment of the anesthesia provider will be exercised in comparing the emergency with the anesthetized patient's condition and in the selection of the person left responsible for the anesthetic during the temporary absence.

**Standard II**

During all anesthetics, the patient's oxygenation, ventilation, circulation, and temperature shall be continually evaluated.

***Oxygenation***

*Objective*

To ensure adequate oxygen concentration in the inspired gas and the blood during all anesthetics

*METHODS*

1. *Inspired gas:* During every administration of general anesthesia using an anesthesia machine, the concentration of oxygen in the patient breathing system shall be measured by an oxygen analyzer with a low oxygen concentration limit alarm in use.*
2. *Blood oxygenation:* During all anesthetics, a quantitative method of assessing oxygenation, such as pulse oximetry, shall be employed.* Adequate illumination and exposure of the patient are necessary to assess color.*

***Ventilation***

*Objective*

To ensure adequate ventilation of the patient during all anesthetics

*METHODS*

1. Every patient receiving general anesthesia shall have the adequacy of ventilation continually evaluated. Although qualitative clinical signs, such as chest excursion, observation of the reservoir breathing bag, and auscultation of breath sounds, may be useful, quantitative monitoring of the carbon dioxide content or volume of expired gas or both is strongly encouraged.
2. When an endotracheal tube or laryngeal mask is inserted, its correct positioning must be verified by clinical assessment and by identification of carbon dioxide in the expired gas. Continual end-tidal carbon dioxide analysis, in use from the time of endotracheal tube/laryngeal mask placement, until extubation/removal or initiating transfer to a postoperative care location shall be performed using a quantitative method, such as capnography, capnometry, or mass spectroscopy.*
3. When ventilation is controlled by a mechanical ventilator, a device that is capable of detecting disconnection of components of the breathing system shall be in continuous use. The device must give an audible signal when its alarm threshold is exceeded.
4. During regional anesthesia and monitored anesthesia care, the adequacy of ventilation shall be evaluated by continual observation of qualitative clinical signs or monitoring for the presence of exhaled carbon dioxide or both.

***Circulation***

*Objective*

To ensure the adequacy of the patient's circulatory function during all anesthetics

*METHODS*

1. Every patient receiving anesthesia shall have an electrocardiogram continuously displayed from the beginning of anesthesia until preparing to leave the anesthetizing location.*
2. Every patient receiving anesthesia shall have arterial blood pressure and heart rate determined and evaluated at least every 5 minutes.*
3. Every patient receiving general anesthesia shall have, in addition to the aforementioned, circulatory function continually evaluated by at least one of the following: palpation of a pulse, auscultation of heart sounds, monitoring of a tracing of intraarterial pressure, ultrasound peripheral pulse monitoring, or pulse plethysmography or oximetry.

***Body Temperature***

*Objective*

To aid in the maintenance of appropriate body temperature during all anesthetics

*METHODS*

Every patient receiving anesthesia shall have temperature monitored when clinically significant changes in body temperature are intended, anticipated, or suspected.

[a] *Continual* is defined as "repeated regularly and frequently in steady rapid succession," whereas *continuous* means "prolonged without any interruption at any time."

From the American Society of Anesthesia Providers (ASA), Park Ridge, Illinois. Approved by ASA House of Delegates on October 21, 1986, and last amended on October 27, 2004.

frequent deviations from such standards occur, a performance assessment and improvement (also known as *quality assurance* [*QA*]) review should be considered.

Monitors and basic anesthetic monitoring considered appropriate include the following:

- Inspired oxygen analyzer ($FIO_2$), which is calibrated to room air on a daily basis
- Low-pressure disconnect alarm, which senses pressure in the expiratory limb of the patient circuit
- Inspiratory airway pressure
- Respirometer (these first four devices are an integral part of most modern anesthesia machines)
- Electrocardioscope
- Blood pressure (usually measured with a noninvasive automated unit)
- Heart rate
- Precordial or esophageal stethoscope
- Temperature
- Peripheral nerve stimulator if muscle relaxants are used
- $SpO_2$
- $ETCO_2$

More recent models of anesthesia machines have most of the basic monitors integrated into a computerized system. This system generally includes $FIO_2$; inspired and expired $CO_2$; inspired and expired volatile agents; airway pressure and disconnect alarms; tidal volume, respiratory rate, and minute ventilation; noninvasive blood pressure (systolic, diastolic, and mean); $SpO_2$ and pulse rate; temperature; and an event marker. A sophisticated, prioritized system displays caution or alarm conditions in one location, making it unnecessary to scan numerous individual monitors with a variety of displays when an alarm sounds.

Based on the cardiovascular and pulmonary status of the patient, the surgical procedure, and the chance of significant physiologic changes, additional invasive monitors may be used. These include direct arterial and venous pressure measurements, a pulmonary arterial (PA) catheter, and continuous mixed venous $O_2$ saturation ($SvO_2$) measured with a special PA catheter. A recently developed PA catheter can provide a continuous measurement of cardiac output. This new technology employs pulsed thermodilution to provide intermittent heat along a distal segment of the catheter. The small changes in the temperature of the blood are proportional to the blood flow (cardiac output). These changes are sensed by a thermistor on the tip of the catheter.[16]

For certain conditions, other equipment, such as transcutaneous $O_2$ and $CO_2$, transesophageal echocardiography, evoked potentials, EEG, and cerebral or neurologic function monitors, may be used. For procedures posing a risk of venous air embolism, special monitors (e.g., a Doppler probe over the right atrium) may be used. An indwelling urinary catheter also provides a useful indication of renal function and hemodynamic status.[16]

Despite some controversy, most anesthesia providers believe that the monitoring employed depends on the physiologic status and stability of the patient, the surgical procedure planned and its potential for sudden changes in cardiopulmonary functions, the anticipated blood loss and major fluid shifts, and the anticipated monitoring needs for postoperative management. Although not yet a standard of care, many facilities use the BIS monitor (see the Anesthesia Awareness Research Highlight earlier). This monitoring modality is a processed EEG obtained noninvasively from scalp electrodes. It provides a measure of the sedative and hypnotic effects of anesthetic drugs on the central nervous system. Monitoring of some parameters may be negated by the anesthetic technique selected.[12,16]

## Pulse Oximetry

Pulse oximetry is based on the principles of spectrometric oximetry, plethysmography, and the Lambert-Beer law, which relates the concentration of solute in suspension to the intensity of light transmitted through the solution. It gives a continuous noninvasive indication of the arterial $O_2$ saturation of functional hemoglobin and the pulse rate and provides an early warning of hypoxemia.

The $O_2$-dissociation curve relates the percentage of totally saturated hemoglobin with $O_2$. The following values are approximations with the $O_2$ saturation ($SpO_2$) in percentage and the $PaO_2$ in torr: 98% to 100% ($\geq$95 torr), 90% (60 torr), 75% (39 torr), 50% (26 torr), and 25% (16 torr). Most pulse oximeters are accurate within $\pm$2% greater than 70% and $\pm$3% from 50% to 70% but correlate poorly at less than 50%. On room air, the $SpO_2$ for a young, healthy individual should be 98% to 100%; a value for an elderly patient may be in the low 90s, whereas a value for a heavy smoker or a patient with severe lung disease may be in the 80s. It is wise to note the baseline $SpO_2$ of a patient before any $O_2$, medications, or stimulation is introduced. Maintenance of a $SpO_2$ greater than 90% corresponds to a $PaO_2$ of 60 torr or greater.[16,23]

The sensor combines two low-intensity, light-emitting diodes (LEDs) as light sources and a photodiode as a receiver or light detector. One LED emits red light (approximately 660 nm), and the other LED emits infrared light (approximately 940 nm). These light sources alternate about 480 times a second. When the two frequencies of light are transmitted through blood and tissue, they are absorbed differently by the tissue components and by the reduced hemoglobin and the oxyhemoglobin. Because absorption by the other tissue components is essentially constant, the major variable is the saturation of the hemoglobin with $O_2$. The internal microprocessor analyzes the variations in the absorption of light emitted from both LEDs and provides a readout of the percent saturation of hemoglobin with $O_2$. The pulse rate also is indicated. Many units also display a waveform that correlates with the arterial pulsations.[16,23]

The pulse oximeter reading can be adversely affected by any event that significantly reduces vascular pulsations, such as hypoperfusion, hypotension, hypovolemia, vasoconstriction, or hypothermia. Electrosurgery, motion, or ambient light also may artifactually decrease the readout. Carboxyhemoglobin (carbon monoxide bound to hemoglobin) falsely elevates the indicated $SpO_2$ saturation, and methemoglobin (hemoglobin that has an oxidized iron molecule and cannot reversibly combine with $O_2$) falsely lowers the $SpO_2$. Intravenous dyes affect the pulse oximeter. Methylene blue may cause a drop to 65% for 1 to 2 minutes; indigo carmine, a very slight decrease; and indocyanine green, a slightly greater decrease. Nail polish also can decrease the $SpO_2$. Blue, black, or green polish significantly decreases the $SpO_2$, whereas red polish has only a slight effect. Opaque, acrylic nail coverings may block the light beam. If nail polish or coverings seem to cause problems, the sensor can be turned sideways so that the fingernail is parallel to the light path.[16,23]

The sensor usually is placed on a finger or a toe. Some manufacturers have sensors for the ear lobe and the bridge of the nose and smaller ones for soles and palms of infants and children. The pulse oximeter does not require user calibration. Care must be taken to prevent localized neurovascular or ischemic damage. A hard-cased sensor placed on a finger may cause ischemia when the arms are tightly secured at the patient's side during a long procedure.

If trouble with the pulse oximeter is encountered during a local anesthetic, the perioperative nurse should evaluate the patient's ventilatory status, verify proper placement of the sensor, and rule out the items just listed that adversely affect operation of the unit. Pulsatile blood flow in the extremity may be inadequate because of hypovolemia, decreased cardiac output, malpositioning, constriction by the blood pressure cuff, or hypothermia. As a final step, the pulse oximetry unit, cable, and sensor can be checked by the nurse placing the sensor on his or her own finger to verify satisfactory function.[16,23]

## Capnography

A capnometer measures $CO_2$, and a capnograph displays the $CO_2$ waveform. For patients with normal circulation and pulmonary function, capnography is an excellent method to evaluate alveolar ventilation because the gradient between the arterial and the alveolar $CO_2$ is small. With forced expiration, the $ETco_2$ provides a close approximation of the arterial $CO_2$ ($Paco_2$). During general anesthesia, expiration is passive, and the point of measurement is near the connection between the patient's circuit and the endotracheal tube (ETT), laryngeal mask airway (LMA), or mask. The $ETco_2$ is 5 to 10 torr lower than the $Paco_2$ measured in arterial blood.[23] During other types of anesthesia, in which oxygen may be administered via a nasal cannula, there is a small-bore tube connected to the cannula, which can be attached to the anesthesia machine so that $ETco_2$ can be measured.

The $ETco_2$ can be measured by a mass spectrometer, a Raman spectrometer, or an infrared analyzer. Advances in the technology of infrared analyzers and microprocessors have resulted in compact units that provide a continuous indication of the $ETco_2$ and have made these the most widely used units for perioperative monitoring. These units measure the amount of infrared light absorbed by the $CO_2$ in the sample of gas. Two types of monitors are in use. In the *mainstream* unit, all respired gas passes through the detector, whereas with the *sidestream* unit, a portion of the gas is aspirated at a constant rate (50 to 250 mL/min) through small-bore tubing into the unit. Each design has advantages. Most units display a waveform of the expiratory $CO_2$ partial pressure relative to time after a short sampling and processing delay. The waveform is important for correctly interpreting the output data. Digital readouts usually give the $ETco_2$ and respiratory rate. Daily user calibration is rarely required with the newer units. Clinically the units confirm proper endotracheal intubation and are useful to detect anesthesia circuit disconnection, alveolar ventilation, early return of respiratory function after muscle relaxants are used, and acute alterations in metabolic functions, such as malignant hyperthermia (MH) or thyrotoxicosis.[12,23]

## ANESTHESIA MACHINES AND ANESTHETIC GASES

The first apparatus resembling an anesthesia machine was used in 1905. Since then, innumerable changes and improvements have been made. The anesthesia machines used for general anesthesia look complicated, but the basic functions are similar and simple to understand. Perioperative nurses should be familiar with the basic function of anesthesia machines because they may need to administer $O_2$ during procedures with local anesthesia or conscious sedation/analgesia. A modern anesthesia machine is shown in Figure 4-1 to help perioperative nurses become familiar with the basic components of it.

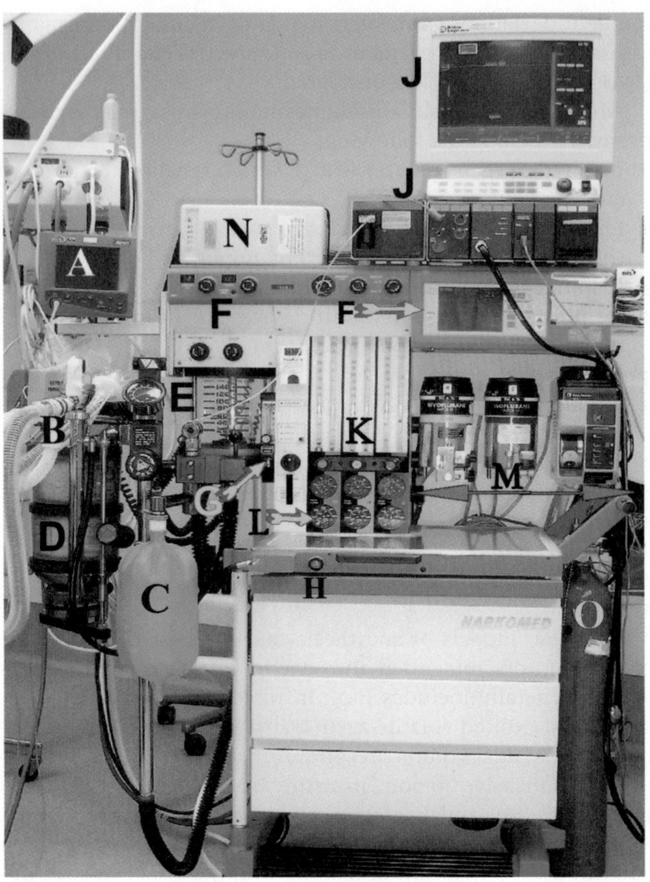


**FIGURE 4-1** Modern anesthesia machine. **A,** BIS monitor display. **B,** Patient breathing circuit. **C,** Reservoir ("breathing") bag. **D,** $CO_2$ absorber. **E,** Ventilator. **F,** Integrated ventilator controls, monitor, and displays. **G,** $O_2$ flowmeter for nasal cannula. **H,** $O_2$ flush valve. **I,** On/off switch. **J,** Monitor display and controls for ECG, temperature, blood pressure, pulse oximetry, and end tidal $CO_2$. Other modules can be inserted for additional pressures, cardiac output, and BIS. **K,** Flowmeters for air, $N_2O$, and $O_2$. **L,** Gauges for pipeline and E-tank pressures (air, $N_2O$, and $O_2$). **M,** Flow-through vaporizers (desflurane, isoflurane, and sevoflurane). **N,** Power surge protector for anesthesia machine. **O,** E-cylinder with $O_2$.

Oxygen, $N_2O$, and air usually are supplied from the facility's pipelines to the anesthesia machine at pressures of 50 to 55 pounds per square inch (psi). The gas hoses going to the machine are color-coded: green ($O_2$); blue ($N_2O$); and yellow (air). The connectors are specific for each gas so that they cannot be inadvertently cross-connected. If a central gas supply is not available or the hospital piping system fails, the machines are equipped with E-size cylinders of $O_2$ and $N_2O$. One or two cylinders of each gas are connected to yokes on the machine. These yokes are pin-indexed so that only the correct gas can be connected in that position. In the pin-indexing safety system, two steel pins are in a unique location on the yoke assembly. The mating gas cylinder (e.g., the $O_2$ tank) has two matching holes in the same locations so that the cylinders cannot be mounted in the wrong place.[12]

In cylinders, $O_2$ is stored as a compressed gas. A full E-size cylinder contains about 660 L of $O_2$ at approximately 2000 psi. As the $O_2$ is used, the pressure decreases in direct proportion to the remaining volume. Because the E-size cylinder is used to provide $O_2$ while patients are being transported, one should know how much $O_2$ is left in a partially used tank; 1000 psi would indicate 330 L remaining, and 500 psi would indicate 165 L remaining, or sufficient $O_2$ at 5 L/min flow for approximately 30 minutes. When the pressure has decreased to about 250 psi, the cylinder should not be used because it no longer has an adequate reserve.[12]

$N_2O$ is stored as a liquid in cylinders, and the pressure above the liquid is 745 psi. A full, E-size cylinder contains about 1600 L of $N_2O$. As the $N_2O$ is used, the pressure above the liquid remains constant. Only when the liquid has been completely vaporized does the pressure begin to decrease. The $N_2O$ can be almost gone but still show the same pressure. In contrast to $O_2$, the amount remaining in the tank cannot be readily determined.[12]

The gases in the cylinders flow through regulators that reduce the pressure to about 45 psi as the gas enters the machine. The hoses from the hospital gas sources are connected to the machine at the outlet of these regulators. In machines sold after January 1, 1984, a safety interlock device shuts off the $N_2O$ flow if $O_2$ pressure is not present or proportionately lowers the $O_2$ and $N_2O$ flow rates to maintain 30% $O_2$. The gases flow through individual flowmeters (or rotameters) on the front of the machine so that the gas flows and the ratio of $O_2$ to $N_2O$ or air can be selected by the anesthesia provider. From the top of the flowmeters, the gases are mixed and then flow through a vaporizer in which the inhalational anesthetic of choice is vaporized and added to the gas mixture. The total gas flow is delivered from the machine to the patient. With a flow-through vaporizer, by definition, all the fresh gas going from the anesthesia machine to the patient flows through the vaporizer. The control dials usually are located on top of these vaporizers and are calibrated in percentages. The filling ports on the vaporizers are usually key-indexed so that only the appropriate volatile agent can be used. More recently manufactured vaporizers are flow and temperature compensated, meaning that they are reasonably accurate at all flows and temperatures used clinically.[12]

Desflurane (Suprane) is a unique inhalational anesthetic because it boils at 22.8°C, near room temperature, and its vapor pressure (669 mm Hg) approximates atmospheric pressure (760 mm Hg). The vaporizer for desflurane is pressurized and contains an electric heater. Desflurane also has several other unique characteristics: (1) The solubility in blood (blood-gas partition coefficient) is lower (0.42) than that of $N_2O$ (0.47), sevoflurane (0.63 to 0.69), isoflurane (1.41), and halothane (2.30), which means that it has a faster "wash-in" (induction) and "wash-out" (emergence) than the other agents do; (2) metabolism is far less (0.02%) as a percentage of the anesthetic taken up than that of isoflurane (0.2%), sevoflurane (5%), and halothane (15 to 20%); (3) emergence and recovery from general anesthesia and discharge from postanesthesia care unit (PACU) is significantly faster than when thiopental is used; (4) the cardiovascular effects are similar to those of isoflurane; and (5) the muscle relaxation seems similar to that which occurs with other inhalational agents. The pungency of desflurane precludes its use as an inhalational induction agent.[29]

Sevoflurane (Ultane) is the newest volatile agent available in the United States. Its pleasant odor and low solubility in blood make it a popular volatile agent for inhalational induction in pediatric patients. In contrast to any of the other volatile agents, it also can provide a rapid, pleasant mask induction in adults.

Another important feature of the anesthesia machine is the $O_2$ flush valve. With all new machines and on most earlier models, pushing the $O_2$ flush valve allows 100% $O_2$ from the 50 psi line to flow directly to the *fresh gas outlet* on the machine and to the patient. This $O_2$ flow completely bypasses the flowmeters and vaporizers. ***Caution must be exercised because the pressure is 35 to 50 psi, and the flow rate is 35 to 75 L/min.***

In most hospitals and ambulatory surgery centers in the United States, a semiclosed-circle system is used to deliver the fresh gas flow (including anesthetic gases) to patients. The circle system is composed of a container filled with a $CO_2$-absorbing material (e.g., soda lime or Baralyme), two one-way (unidirectional) valves, an adjustable pressure-limiting (APL) valve, a reservoir bag, an inlet connection for fresh gas flow, and two connections to the patient through corrugated breathing (or anesthesia circuit) tubing. As the patient inspires, gases are drawn through the $CO_2$ absorber and from the fresh gas supply through the inspiratory limb of the corrugated tubing. As the patient exhales, the one-way valve on the inspiratory limb prevents backflow, and the exhaled gases flow into the expiratory limb and through the expiratory one-way valve. The expiratory limb and valve are easily identified by the condensation of water vapor along this portion of the circuit. The reservoir bag absorbs the peak flow of expired gases and allows the anesthesia provider to force gas through the $CO_2$ absorber, along the inspiratory limb of the circuit, and to ventilate the patient. The expired gases flow through the $CO_2$ absorber where $CO_2$ is removed. Substances used in the $CO_2$ absorbent include an indicator that changes color as the soda lime or Baralyme is exhausted. The soda lime may turn from white to blue, indicating that the absorbent material must be changed to prevent a buildup of $CO_2$ in the patient. Any excess gas is vented through the APL valve into the gas-scavenging system. The APL valve usually is mounted just ahead of the $CO_2$ absorber.[12]

The $FIO_2$ sensor usually is mounted in the inspiratory limb just after the one-way valve. It measures the fraction of inspired $O_2$ ($FIO_2$) and can be set to alarm if a low concentration is detected. A low-pressure sensor usually is mounted in the expiratory limb near the one-way valve to detect a ventilator malfunction or a circuit disconnection.

On some new machines, volumeters are mounted in the inspired and expired limbs where the patient breathing circuit is connected. When the ventilator is used, the electronic circuitry measures the inspiratory and expiratory volumes to ensure that they correspond with the tidal volume and respiratory rate selected. With a cuffed ETT, the ventilator compensates for changes in fresh gas flow or small leaks in the breathing circuit and alarms if a disconnect or inadequate flow occurs.[12]

The advantage of the circle system is that much lower flows of $O_2$, $N_2O$, and anesthetic gases can be used, which conserves the patient's body heat and respiratory moisture and reduces the cost of expensive, volatile agents. A *semiclosed circuit* (or circle system) typically is used when the fresh gas flows into the system range from 0.5 to 6 L/min. During exhalation, some of the expired gases are recycled through the $CO_2$ absorber, and the excess gas is scavenged or eliminated (hence *semiclosed*). With a *closed-circle system,* all of the $CO_2$ is absorbed.

No gas is vented from the system, and only enough $O_2$ is added to the system to meet the basal requirements of the patient (approximately 3.5 mL/kg/min). In a *semiopen circuit* (e.g., Ayres T-piece, Magill, Bain circuits), a relatively high flow of fresh gas is used and most of the exhaled gas is vented from the circuit. The fresh gas flow rate per minute varies from approximately two thirds of the patient's minute volume with the Magill circuit to at least 100 mL/kg with the Bain T-piece circuit. The semiopen circuit system is commonly used for neonates, infants, and small children.[12] With all these circuits, the final connection to the patient is by a mask, ETT, or LMA.

## GENERAL ANESTHESIA

### Mechanism of Action

Numerous theories have been proposed to explain the action of general anesthetics. Many more recent investigations have involved inhalation anesthetics. (The terms *volatile anesthetic, potent agent,* and *inhaled* or *inhalational anesthetic* are synonymous with *inhalation anesthetic.*) Evidence indicates that the synaptic transmission of nerve impulses is reversibly inhibited in several areas of the central nervous system. The extent of inhibition and consequently the progressive depression of function are correlated with the partial pressure of the inhaled anesthetic at various sites. The inhibition is believed to occur at a lipophilic site on the biologic membrane of synapses and possibly on small, unmyelinated nerve fibers. Suppression of spinal reflex activity is believed to produce some relaxation of skeletal muscles. Although no single concept explains all of the phenomena, a few theories explain many of the actions that have been observed.[29] The following are some of the more widely accepted theories.

***Protein Receptor Theory.*** The protein receptor theory proposes that hydrophobic areas of specific proteins in the central nervous system act as receptor sites. The steep, dose-response curve of inhaled anesthetics seems to support this theory by indicating that a critical number of receptor sites must be occupied before patient movement in response to noxious stimuli is obtunded.[29]

***Meyer-Overton Theory.*** The Meyer-Overton theory is also called the *critical volume hypothesis*. It explains the correlation between the lipid solubility (oil-to-gas partition coefficient) and the anesthetic potency. This theory proposes that when enough anesthetic molecules dissolve (i.e., a critical volume is reached) at a crucial hydrophobic site, such as the lipid cellular membrane, anesthesia is achieved. As the cell membrane expands in response to the dissolved anesthetic molecules, changes in the ionic channels occur and alter the sodium flux involved in cellular depolarization. Because some lipid-soluble compounds are not anesthetics, this theory does not completely explain anesthetic action.[29]

***Endogenous Endorphins.*** Endogenous endorphins, or opiate-like substances, suppress various pain pathways. Several classes of endorphins have been identified. The action of beta-endorphins is antagonized by naloxone or nalmefene, specific narcotic antagonists, but the relative potency of inhaled anesthetics is not altered. Although some degree of analgesia may be explained by this mechanism, it does not correlate well with the level of anesthesia achieved by inhaled anesthetics.

Intravenous anesthetics also may function by some of the mechanisms proposed for the inhaled anesthetics. Factors involved in the pharmacokinetics of IV drugs include the volume of distribution, biotransformation, and clearance of the drug by metabolism, excretion, or elimination of the drug and its metabolites.[29]

No single theory for the mechanism of action can explain all of the effects observed with anesthetic agents. The range of anesthetic activity varies with the different anesthetics; the effects on the central nervous system and skeletal muscles are similar but not identical; structural and spatial differences exist among agents; changes at the membrane and cellular levels occur; and optical isomers produce different responses. Although similar in many respects, anesthetic agents are individually unique and probably work through numerous mechanisms and at multiple sites to produce their effects.

### Levels of General Anesthesia

Guedel integrated the signs and stages of ether anesthesia into a system that was used clinically for more than 60 years. This system applied only to unpremedicated patients breathing spontaneously during ether anesthesia, a technique that is rarely used in modern practice except in developing countries. By evaluating the physiologic changes and reflex responses, one can estimate the depth of anesthesia. Stage 1 is from the initial administration of anesthetic agents to loss of consciousness. Stage 2 is from the loss of consciousness to the onset of regular breathing and loss of the eyelid reflex. Stage 2 also is called the *delirium* or *excitement* stage, and thrashing movements may occur. No auditory or physical stimulation should occur during this stage, especially in children. Stage 3, which begins with the onset of a regular breathing pattern and lasts until cessation of respiration, is divided into four planes and is the stage of surgical anesthesia. Stage 4 is from cessation of respiration to circulatory failure that leads to death.[23a]

Although Guedel's system gives us an appreciation for the interrelationships of numerous signs during anesthesia, the variety of drugs and anesthetic techniques used today do not provide such uniform responses suitable for estimating the exact depth of anesthesia. Narcotics and anticholinergic drugs given as premedicants alter the pupillary responses. Evaluation of respiratory responses and muscle tone is not valid when controlled ventilation and muscle relaxants are used. Today, general anesthesia usually is induced with the IV injection of a rapid-acting drug, such as thiopental or propofol (Diprivan), which takes the patient rapidly to stage 3 and eliminates the untoward responses often seen during stage 2.

For optimal anesthesia and good surgical conditions, several different but interrelated factors are involved. These include hypnosis (sleep), analgesia (freedom from pain), amnesia (lack of recall or awareness), appropriate surgical conditions including muscle relaxation and positioning of the patient, and continued homeostasis of the patient's vital functions. Different drugs and anesthetic agents possess various properties that facilitate the just-mentioned conditions. Combinations of drugs are used to obtain the desired effects. Hypotensive or hypertensive drugs and cardioactive agents also may be included to achieve the optimal depth of anesthesia, while affecting physiologic homeostasis as little as possible. Drugs commonly used in anesthesia are briefly described in Table 4-2.

**TABLE 4-2**

## Commonly Used Anesthetic Gases and Drugs

| | Common Usage | Advantages | Disadvantages | Comments |
|---|---|---|---|---|
| **INHALATION GASES** | | | | |
| Air | Maintenance with $O_2$; laser surgery near airway | Less support of combustion than $N_2O$ | No anesthetic qualities | Possibly less nausea than $N_2O$[13,15] |
| Oxygen ($O_2$) | Essential for life | Can slightly ↑ $O_2$ available to tissues in low cardiac output states | Can cause retinopathy in premature infants | High concentrations hazardous with lasers in surgery of head, neck, and pulmonary areas[13,15] |
| Nitrous oxide ($N_2O$) | Maintenance; frequently for induction | Rapid induction and recovery; additive effects to other anesthetics | No relaxation; can depress myocardium | Hypoxia if overdose given; ↑ uptake of other volatile agents[13,15] |
| Enflurane (Ethrane) | Maintenance; occasionally for induction | Good relaxation; allows more epinephrine to be used than does halothane; 2.4% metabolized | Can cause ↑ HR and ↓ BP; lowers seizure threshold; slightly irritating odor | Abnormal EEG at high concentrations; used less often today[15] |
| Desflurane (Suprane) | Maintenance in short cases | Rapid emergence; good relaxation; 0.02% metabolized | May cause transient ↑ HR and ↓ BP; airway irritation; requires heated vaporizer | Rapid recovery phase; can use for emergence after maintenance with another volatile agent[15] |
| Halothane (Fluothane) | Maintenance; frequently for induction in pediatric patients | Rapid induction and recovery; pleasant, nonirritating odor; fair relaxation | May cause ↓ HR and ↓ BP; PVC and ventricular fibrillation may occur with epinephrine[15] | Narrow margin of safety; sensitizes myocardium to epinephrine; rare cause of liver damage; 15%-20% metabolized |
| Isoflurane (Forane) | Maintenance | Good relaxation; allows more epinephrine to be used than does halothane; maintains cardiac output; 0.2% metabolized | ↑ HR; slightly irritating odor | Isomer of enflurane; commonly used agent |
| Sevoflurane (Ultane) | Induction and maintenance | Rapid induction and emergence; good relaxation; ~5% metabolized | Metabolite (compound A) is nephrotoxic in rats; effect in humans unknown | Rapid and smooth mask induction in children and adults[15] |
| **OPIOID ANALGESICS** | | | | |
| Morphine sulfate | Perioperative pain; premedication | Inexpensive; duration of action 4-5 hr; euphoria; good cardiovascular stability | Nausea and vomiting; histamine release; postural ↓ BP (↓ SVR); high first-pass effect with PO administration | Used intrathecally and epidurally for postoperative pain; elimination half-life 3 hr[4,15] |
| Alfentanil (Alfenta) | Surgical analgesia in ambulatory patients | Duration of action 0.5 hr; used as bolus or infusion | — | Potency: 750 mcg = 10 mg morphine sulfate; elimination half-life 1.6 hr[4,15] |
| Fentanyl (Sublimaze) | Surgical analgesia; epidural infusion for postoperative analgesia; add to SAB | Good cardiovascular stability; duration of action 0.5 hr | — | Most commonly used opioid; potency: 100 mcg = 10 mg morphine sulfate; elimination half-life 3.6 hr[4,15] |
| Remifentanil (Ultiva) | 0.25-1 mcg/kg/min infusion for surgical analgesia; small boluses for brief, intense pain | Easily titratable; metabolized by blood and tissue esterases; short duration; good cardiovascular stability | Expensive; requires mixing | Potency: 25 mcg = 10 mg morphine sulfate; 20–30 × potency of alfentanil; elimination half-life 3–10 min[4,15] |
| Sufentanil (Sufenta) | Surgical analgesia | Good cardiovascular stability; duration of action 0.5 hr; prolonged analgesia | Prolonged respiratory depression | Potency: 15 mcg = 10 mg morphine sulfate; elimination half-life 2.7 hr[4,15] |

*BP,* blood pressure; *CSF,* cerebrospinal fluid; *CNS,* central nervous system; *EEG,* electroencephalogram; *HR,* heart rate; *IM,* intramuscular; *IV,* intravenous; *MAC,* monitored anesthesia care; *PO,* oral; *PVC,* premature ventricular contractions; *SAB,* subarachnoid block; *SVR,* systemic vascular resistance.

*Continued*

**TABLE 4-2**

## Commonly Used Anesthetic Gases and Drugs—cont'd

| | Common Usage | Advantages | Disadvantages | Comments |
|---|---|---|---|---|
| **DEPOLARIZING MUSCLE RELAXANTS** | | | | |
| Succinylcholine (Anectine, Quelicin) | Intubation; short cases | Rapid onset; short duration | Requires refrigeration; may cause fasciculations, postoperative myalgias, and dysrhythmias; ↑ serum $K^+$ with burns, tissue trauma, paralysis, and muscle diseases; slight histamine release | Prolonged muscle relaxation with serum cholinesterase deficiency and certain antibiotics; trigger agent for malignant hyperthermia[15] |
| **NONDEPOLARIZING MUSCLE RELAXANTS—INTERMEDIATE ONSET AND DURATION** | | | | |
| Atracurium (Tracrium) | Intubation; maintenance of relaxation | No significant cardiovascular or cumulative effects; good with renal failure | Requires refrigeration; slight histamine release | Breakdown by Hofmann elimination and ester hydrolysis[15] |
| Cisatracurium (Nimbex) | Intubation; maintenance of relaxation | Similar to atracurium | No histamine release | Similar to atracurium[15] |
| Mivacurium (Mivacron) | Intubation; maintenance of relaxation | Short-acting; rapid metabolism by plasma cholinesterase; used as bolus or infusion | Expensive in long cases | Rarely need to reverse; prolonged effect with plasma cholinesterase deficiency[15] |
| Rocuronium (Zemuron) | Intubation; maintenance of relaxation | Rapid onset (dose-dependent); elimination via kidney and liver | Vagolytic; may ↑ HR | Duration similar to atracurium and vecuronium[15] |
| Vecuronium (Norcuron) | Intubation; maintenance of relaxation | No significant cardiovascular or cumulative effects; no histamine release | Requires mixing | Mostly eliminated in bile, some in urine[15] |
| **NONDEPOLARIZING MUSCLE RELAXANTS—LONGER ONSET AND DURATION** | | | | |
| Tubocurarine | Maintenance of relaxation | — | May cause histamine release and transient ganglionic blockade | Mostly used for pretreatment with succinylcholine[15] |
| Metocurine iodide (Metubine Iodide) | Maintenance of relaxation | Good cardiovascular stability | Slight histamine release | Large bolus may cause ↓ BP[15] |
| Pancuronium (Pavulon) | Maintenance of relaxation | — | May cause ↑ HR and ↑ BP | Mostly renal elimination[15] |
| **INTRAVENOUS ANESTHETICS** | | | | |
| Etomidate (Amidate) | Induction | Good cardiovascular stability; fast, smooth induction and recovery | May cause pain with injection and myotonic movements[13,15] | — |
| Diazepam (Valium, Dizac) | Amnesia; hypnotic; preoperative medication | Good sedation | Prolonged duration | Residual effects for 20-90 hr; ↑ effect with alcohol[13,15] |
| Ketamine (Ketalar) | Induction, occasional maintenance (IV or IM) | Short-acting; patient maintains airway; good in small children and burn patients | Large doses may cause hallucinations and respiratory depression | Need darkened, quiet room for recovery; often used in trauma cases[13,15] |
| Midazolam (Versed) | Hypnotic; anxiolytic; sedation; often used as adjunct to induction | Excellent amnesia; water-soluble (no pain with IV injection); short-acting | Slower induction than thiopental | Often used for amnesia with insertion of invasive monitors or regional anesthesia[13,15] |
| Propofol (Diprivan) | Induction and maintenance; sedation with regional anesthesia or MAC | Rapid onset; awakening in 4-8 min | May cause pain when injected | Short elimination half-life (34-64 min)[13,15] |

*BP*, blood pressure; *IM*, intramuscular; *IV*, intravenous; *MAC*, monitored anesthesia care; *PO*, oral; *PVC*, premature ventricular contractions; *SAB*, subarachnoid block; *SVR*, systemic vascular resistance.

**TABLE 4-2**

## Commonly Used Anesthetic Gases and Drugs—cont'd

| | Common Usage | Advantages | Disadvantages | Comments |
|---|---|---|---|---|
| Sodium methohexital (Brevital Sodium) | Induction | Ultrashort-acting barbiturate | May cause hiccups | Can be given rectally[15] |
| Thiopental sodium (Pentothal) | Induction | Induction | May cause laryngospasm; can be given rectally[15] | Large doses may cause apnea and cardiovascular depression |
| **LOCAL ANESTHETICS** | | | | |
| Bupivacaine (Marcaine, Sensorcaine) | Epidural, spinal, or local infiltration | Good relaxation; long-acting | Overdose can cause cardiac collapse | Maximum dose 200 mg and 150 mg/70 kg with and without epinephrine; duration 240-480 min[14] |
| Chloroprocaine (Nesacaine) | Epidural anesthesia | Ultrashort-acting; good relaxation | May cause neurotoxicity if injected into CSF | Maximum dose 600 mg; duration 30-45 min[14] |
| Lidocaine (Xylocaine) | Epidural, spinal, peripheral, IV anesthesia, and local infiltration | Short-acting; good relaxation; low toxicity | Overdose can cause convulsions; possible transient neurologic changes with spinal anesthesia | Also used for ventricular dysrhythmias; maximum dose 7 mg/kg and 5 mg/kg with and without epinephrine; duration 60-120 min[14] |
| Tetracaine (Pontocaine) | Spinal anesthesia | Long-acting; good relaxation | — | Maximum dose 1-1.5 mg/kg (epinephrine rarely used); duration 60-180 min[14] |
| **ANTICHOLINERGICS** | | | | |
| Atropine | Block effects of acetylcholine; ↓ vagal tone; reverse muscle relaxants; treat sinus bradycardia | ↑ HR; suppresses salivation, bronchial and gastric secretions | Depresses sweating; may cause dry mouth, flushing, dizziness, CNS symptoms | Quite selective at muscarinic receptor in smooth and cardiac muscle and exocrine glands[15] |
| Glycopyrrolate (Robinul) | Similar to atropine | Slightly ↑ HR; does not cross blood-brain barrier; can ↑ gastric pH > atropine | Prolonged duration of effects | Lower incidence of dysrhythmias than atropine[15] |
| **CHOLINERGIC AGENT** | | | | |
| Neostigmine (Prostigmine) | Reverses effects of nondepolarizing neuromuscular blocking agents | Prevents breakdown of acetylcholine by inhibiting acetylcholinesterase | — | Given with either atropine or glycopyrrolate[15] |

*BP,* blood pressure; *IM,* intramuscular; *IV,* intravenous; *MAC,* monitored anesthesia care; *PO,* oral; *PVC,* premature ventricular contractions; *SAB,* subarachnoid block; *SVR,* systemic vascular resistance.

## Phases of General Anesthesia

General anesthesia may be divided into three phases: *induction, maintenance,* and *emergence. Induction* begins with administration of anesthetic agents and continues until the patient is ready for positioning or prep, surgical manipulation, or incision. The surgical prep is often started after the induction drugs are given. This end point of induction may vary with the surgical procedure. The *maintenance* phase continues from this point until near completion of the procedure and may be accomplished with inhalation agents or with IV drugs given in titrated doses or by continuous infusions. *Emergence* varies in length and depends on the patient's state and the depth and duration of anesthesia. Emergence starts as the patient begins to "emerge" from anesthesia and usually ends when the patient is ready to leave the OR. Intubation occurs during the induction phase, and extubation usually is performed during emergence. Recovery from anesthesia can be considered a fourth phase of general anesthesia.

## Types of General Anesthesia

The type of general anesthesia employed often is described as IV technique, inhalation technique (with a volatile anesthetic agent), or a combination of IV and inhalation techniques. An IV technique traditionally includes (1) an induction agent such as thiopental, combined with 30% to 40% $O_2$ and $N_2O$, (2) an amnestic drug such as diazepam, (3) an analgesic such as fentanyl or morphine sulfate, and (4) a muscle relaxant.

In contrast, an inhalation technique may use thiopental or propofol to facilitate a rapid induction, or patients may "breathe themselves down" with a potent agent, such as sevoflurane or halothane, plus $N_2O$ and $O_2$. An inhalation induction is often used with children to avoid inserting an IV catheter when they are awake. Depending on the kind of surgical procedure, maintenance of anesthesia may be accomplished with only inhalation agents and spontaneous, assisted, or controlled ventilation. Effects of the volatile agents are dose related and provide differing levels of anesthesia, amnesia, analgesia, muscle relaxation, and hemodynamic responses. If supplemental muscle relaxation is needed, the relaxant dose required is significantly less than the dose necessary during IV anesthesia.

In the past, the term *balanced anesthesia* was used when various combinations of IV drugs were "balanced" to provide complete anesthesia. Today, the term is often used to describe a combination of IV drugs and inhalation agents employed to obtain specific effects for each patient and procedure.

Today, many anesthesia providers may use *total IV anesthesia (TIVA)*. This technique may be used in the OR but is commonly employed for pediatric, uncooperative, or trauma patients in remote locations, such as the magnetic resonance imaging (MRI), radiology, or surgical laser suite where a waste-gas evacuation system is not available. TIVA also is used in the expanding area of office-based surgical procedures. With TIVA, short-acting drugs such as propofol with remifentanil or alfentanil are used for induction. These drugs may be administered by continuous infusion. Anesthesia is maintained by an infusion plus $O_2$ alone or with $N_2O$. An intermediate-acting muscle relaxant (mivacurium, cisatracurium, atracurium, rocuronium, or vecuronium) also may be given. As surgery nears completion, the maintenance drugs are titrated off, and emergence from anesthesia occurs.

## Muscle Relaxants

Muscle relaxants are used by anesthesia providers primarily to facilitate intubation and to provide good operating conditions at lighter planes of general anesthesia. These drugs may be used elsewhere for emergency intubation or less frequently when a patient is being mechanically ventilated. Muscle relaxants affect primarily skeletal muscle and have little effect on cardiac or smooth muscle. Although not always dose dependent, many of these drugs have adverse side effects. The route of metabolism and elimination varies, and this may be important for patients with hepatic or renal disease. Muscle relaxants are classified as *depolarizing* or *nondepolarizing*.

Succinylcholine is the only *depolarizing* muscle relaxant in clinical use. Its action is similar to acetylcholine, and at the neuromuscular junction it causes depolarization of the postjunctional membrane.[29] Generalized skeletal muscle contractions known as *fasciculations* result from the simultaneous depolarization of all the muscle fibers. These fasciculations and associated postoperative myalgias may be attenuated when a pretreatment dose of a nondepolarizing relaxant (such as tubocurarine 0.04 mg/kg) is given 3 to 5 minutes before administration of the intubating dose of succinylcholine. Onset of paralysis (30 to 90 seconds) is faster and the duration of action (5 to 10 minutes) is shorter than with other relaxants. The speed of onset makes it a preferred drug for rapid-sequence inductions. Adverse side effects associated with the use of succinylcholine include cardiac dysrhythmias; hyperkalemia; myalgias (particularly in young and muscular ambulatory patients); and increases in intraocular, intracranial, and intragastric pressures. It also can trigger MH in susceptible patients. It can be infused for longer procedures, but an excessive dose may cause prolonged relaxation (known as *phase II blockade*). Succinylcholine is hydrolyzed by plasma cholinesterase, and the rare patient with an abnormal or absent enzyme (plasma cholinesterase) has prolonged muscle paralysis.[29]

*Nondepolarizing* muscle relaxants competitively block the depolarizing action of acetylcholine at the neuromuscular junction, which results in skeletal muscle paralysis. Fasciculations do not occur. These drugs can be subdivided by the duration of action into intermediate (mivacurium, atracurium, cisatracurium, rocuronium, and vecuronium) and long-acting (tubocurarine, metocurine, pancuronium, pipecuronium, and doxacurium).[19,29] The potency, duration (metabolism and elimination), and side effects of these drugs vary and may be individually altered in patients with hepatic or renal dysfunction, electrolyte imbalance, or hypothermia or by other drugs administered perioperatively (inhalation and local anesthetics, aminoglycoside antibiotics, calcium-entry blockers, magnesium, and cardiac antidysrhythmics). Generally, nondepolarizing relaxants can be used for patients with MH or plasma cholinesterase deficiencies (except for mivacurium). Side effects vary with the individual drugs. They usually are dose dependent and include alterations in blood pressure and heart rate. The effect of the muscle relaxants (neuromuscular blockade) can be monitored with a peripheral nerve stimulator. Paralysis caused by the nondepolarizing relaxants may be antagonized by IV anticholinesterases, such as edrophonium, neostigmine, or pyridostigmine. These antagonists allow acetylcholine to accumulate and compete for receptor sites at the neuromuscular junction and may be associated with bradycardia, for which atropine or glycopyrrolate is routinely given.[29]

## Typical Sequence of General Anesthesia

After arriving in the preoperative area or the OR suite, the patient is again identified, the chart is checked to ensure that the preoperative verification process is complete (e.g., a re-check is done to verify signed consents or an operative permit or both), and the latest results of laboratory tests and diagnostic studies are reviewed. Although the patient may have been evaluated several days earlier in a preanesthesia clinic, the perioperative nurse must verify certain information immediately before surgery. The anesthesia provider also reviews the pertinent medical history and data and confirms that there have been no interval changes in the patient's status. Depending on the practice of the anesthesia department and institutional policy, an IV infusion may be started in a preoperative area or after the patient is transferred to the OR. After the patient arrives in the OR, the appropriate intraoperative monitors are connected to the patient before induction of anesthesia. In the perioperative period, nearly all anesthesia-related drugs are given IV except the inhalation agents.

Before induction, the patient usually is preoxygenated (actually denitrogenated) using a mask with 100% $O_2$ for 3 to 5 minutes. This practice permits washout of most of the gaseous nitrogen from the body and provides a large reserve supply of $O_2$ in the lungs. Opioids and benzodiazepines usually are administered at this time. A test dose of the induction agent (e.g., 50 mg of thiopental) often is given to check for any unusual or exaggerated response. If succinylcholine is to be used for intubation, a small pretreatment dose of a nondepolarizing muscle relaxant (e.g., 3 mg of tubocurarine, 0.5 to 1 mg of pancuronium or vecuronium or 5 mg of rocuronium) usually is given. If the patient can be safely ventilated with a mask, many anesthesia providers avoid the adverse effects of succinylcholine and use one of the nondepolarizing muscle relaxants for intubation.[24,29]

To induce anesthesia, a short-acting barbiturate, such as thiopental (2 to 6 mg/kg) or propofol (1.5 to 2.5 mg/kg), is given. When the patient becomes apneic and the eyelash reflex is gone, the airway is checked for patency by ventilating the patient with a mask. Depending on several factors, such as the airway and the type and duration of surgery, $O_2$ and anesthetic gases may be delivered to a spontaneously breathing patient through a mask that is held in place with a head strap. Positioning of the head or insertion of an oral or nasal airway may be used to maintain a patent airway. If spontaneous or assisted ventilation is planned, an LMA may be inserted without a muscle relaxant. A mask or LMA may be used for a patient with a good airway who is at minimal risk of aspiration and is undergoing a relatively short procedure, and when the surgical site is not located in the head or neck area.

If mask anesthesia or an LMA is not suitable or appropriate, an ETT may be used to facilitate ventilation and to prevent aspiration. (Typical equipment used for intubation and airway control and monitoring is shown in Figure 4-2.) An intubating dose of a muscle relaxant is administered, which results in temporary paralysis. When the patient is paralyzed, ventilation is controlled during the procedure.

To facilitate intubation, the patient's head is placed in a "sniffing" position. The laryngoscope is held in the left hand. The laryngoscope blade is inserted into the right side of the mouth and moved to the midline, "sweeping" the tongue to the left. The ETT is introduced on the right side of the mouth and gently inserted into the trachea so that the cuff is approximately 1 cm below the vocal cords. The cuff is inflated just enough to occlude any air passage with the peak pressures used for ventilation. Location of the ETT in the trachea is verified by an appropriate level and waveform of $ETco_2$, bilaterally equal breath sounds and absence of sounds over the stomach (using a stethoscope), symmetric movement of the thorax with positive-pressure ventilation, and condensation of moisture from expired air in the ETT and breathing circuit. Proper placement of the ETT is shown in Figure 4-3. The vocal cords are the narrowest portion of an adult trachea; however, the smallest portion of a child's airway is below the vocal cords at the cricoid cartilage. Uncuffed ETTs usually are selected for children. After the initial paralysis from the muscle relaxant has worn off, the patient may be allowed to breathe spontaneously with intermittent assistance, or additional muscle relaxant may be given and ventilation controlled mechanically.

If the procedure is an emergency or the patient is at risk for aspiration (as in cases of a full stomach, intestinal obstruction, hiatal hernia, or significant esophageal reflux) (Research Highlight), a rapid sequence induction or an "awake" fiberoptic intubation may be planned. In these instances and in routine intubation, the perioperative nurse must be ready to assist by applying cricoid pressure (Figure 4-4). The nurse exerts downward pressure on the cricoid cartilage with the thumb and index finger of one hand (Sellick maneuver). The cricoid cartilage is the only complete ring in the trachea, and downward pressure occludes the esophagus, which lies immediately posterior (or dorsal) to the trachea. The pressure should not be released until proper placement of the ETT has been con-

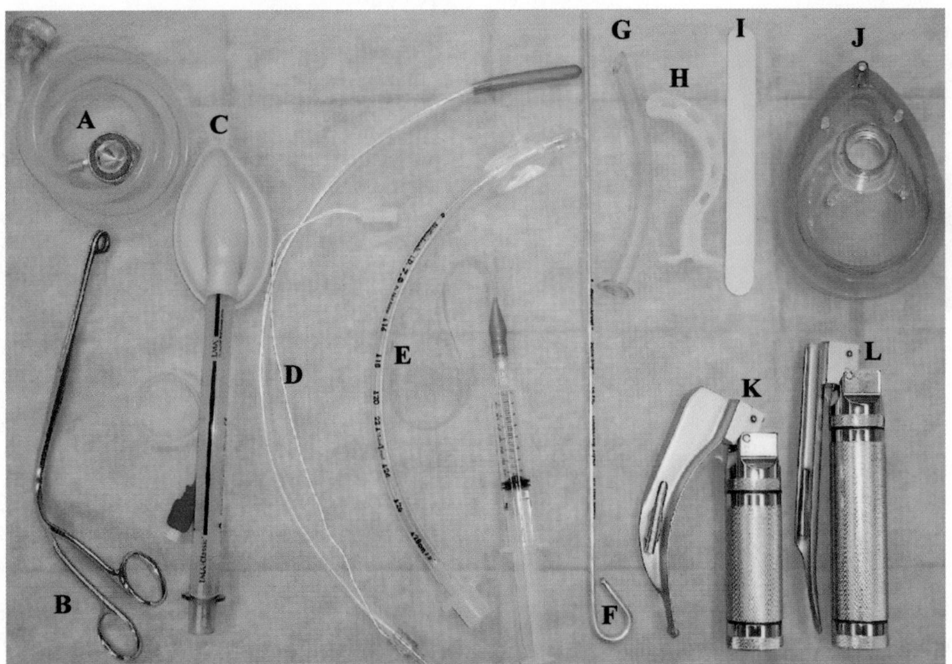


**FIGURE 4-2** Commonly used anesthesia equipment. **A,** Precordial stethoscope. **B,** McGill forceps. **C,** Laryngeal mask airway (LMA). **D,** Esophageal stethoscope with esophageal temperature monitor. **E,** Endotracheal tube (ETT). **F,** Intubating stylet for endotracheal tube. **G,** Nasal airway. **H,** Oral airway. **I,** Tongue blade. **J,** Mask. **K,** "Stubby" laryngoscope handle with MacIntosh (curved) fiberoptic laryngoscope blade. **L,** Miller (straight) fiberoptic laryngoscope blade and handle.

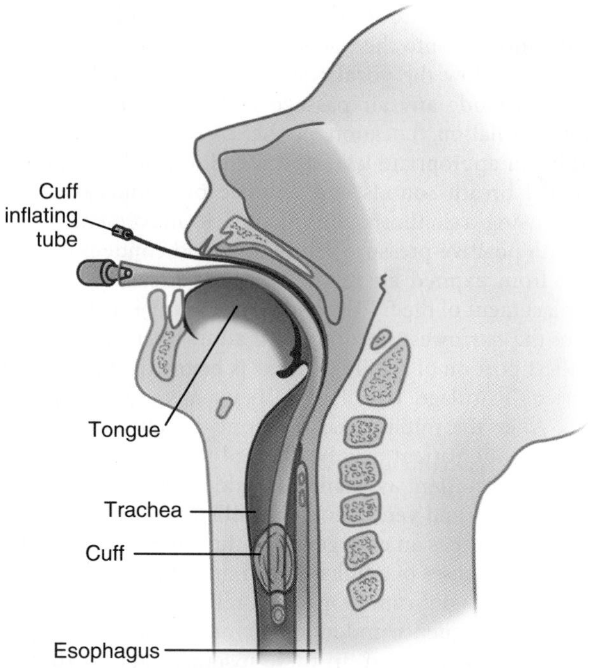


**FIGURE 4-3** ETT in position.

firmed, and the cuff has been inflated. This procedure has been widely accepted among anesthesia providers. More recently, some research studies have shown that this maneuver is difficult to do correctly and effectively.[25,34]

The perioperative nurse may provide additional assistance if an unexpected difficult intubation occurs or the patient cannot be ventilated adequately with a mask. Emergency airway equipment should be brought into the room immediately. The perioperative nurse should be familiar with the location of the various pieces of equipment and how to assemble them for use and should assist the anesthesia provider in securing the patient's airway. Securing the airway in an emergency situation requires an intense team effort. Contents of a typical difficult-airway cart are listed in Box 4-2. If invasive monitors (e.g., an arterial line) are to be placed after induction, the perioperative nurse may assist by properly positioning the patient or extremity; prepping the area or areas; and assisting with placement, connection, and calibration of the monitors. If the procedure is emergent, the perioperative nurse also may assist by obtain-

## RESEARCH HIGHLIGHT

### Perioperative Pulmonary Aspiration

Pulmonary aspiration is an infrequent perioperative event, occurring at a rate of approximately 1 per 3000 patients undergoing general anesthesia. Patients who are sicker and undergoing emergency procedures are at the greatest risk and have the highest incidence. Complications of aspiration have been reported to cause 10% to 30% of anesthesia-related deaths. Approximately 25% of patients who aspirate gastric contents develop significant complications. About 10% of patients who aspirate require mechanical ventilation support for more than 24 hours.

Unconsciousness interferes with multiple biologic mechanisms that normally guard the airway against aspiration. Aspiration may occur at any time, but it is most common during tracheal intubation and extubation. A common factor during intubation is when muscle relaxation is inadequate, which may cause the patient to gag and vomit. During extubation, aspiration may occur because the patient is weak or unresponsive. Consequences of aspiration include aspiration pneumonia, acute respiratory distress syndrome, pulmonary edema, and long-term complications such as laryngotracheal damage and decreased lung compliance.

The perioperative nurse assists the anesthesia provider if the procedure is an emergency or the patient is at risk for aspiration (as in cases of a full stomach, intestinal obstruction, hiatal hernia, or significant esophageal reflux). For these patients, a rapid sequence induction or an "awake" fiberoptic intubation may be planned. In these instances and in routine intubation, the perioperative nurse must be ready to assist by applying cricoid pressure, exerting downward pressure on the cricoid cartilage with the thumb and index finger of one hand (Sellick maneuver). When cricoid pressure is used to prevent aspiration, it should not be released until the intubation is accomplished (or the anesthesia provider directs release, as a patient vomits), the cuff on the endotracheal tube is inflated, and proper placement of the endotracheal tube has been verified by the anesthesia provider.

Modified from Pisegna JR, Martindale RG: Acid suppression in the perioperative period, *Journal of Clinical Gastroenterology* 39(1):10-16, 2005; Warner MA: Is pulmonary aspiration still an important problem in anesthesia? *Current Opinions in Anesthesiology* 13:215-218, 2000.

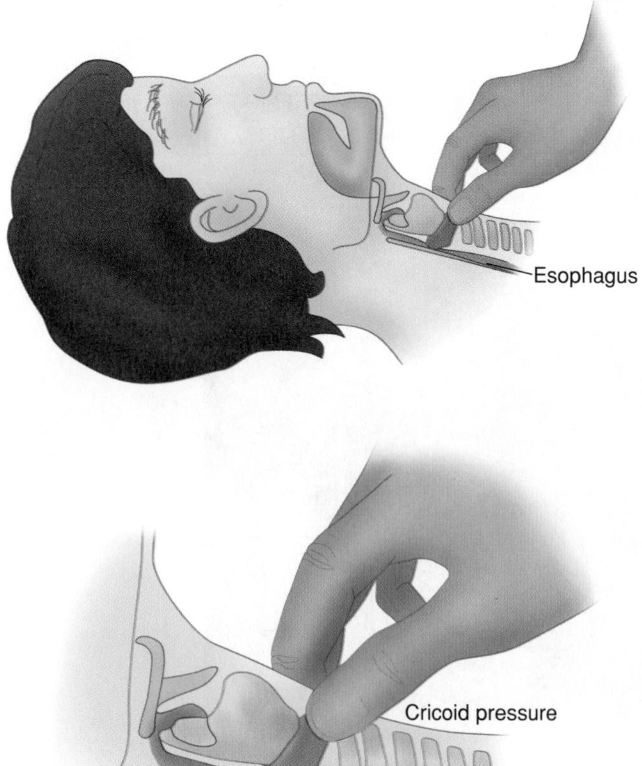


**FIGURE 4-4** Applying cricoid pressure.

ing additional IV access, connecting fluid-warming or patient-warming units, double-checking blood products, and "pumping" IV fluids as needed. In situations in which the anesthesia provider is involved with a critical procedure, such as a difficult airway/airway emergency, the perioperative nurse can perform a valuable service by ensuring 100% $O_2$, having suction available, observing the monitors, recording data ($SpO_2$ and $ETCO_2$), and communicating significant changes to the anesthesia provider (Best Practice).

## BEST PRACTICE

### Difficult-Airway Management

Best practices, clinical guidelines, and evidence-based patient care are all forms of systematically developed recommendations that assist practitioners in making decisions about treatments and interventions. Although they are not standards or absolute requirements, they are utilitarian for the clinical situation they represent. In 1992 the ASA developed Practice Guidelines for management of the difficult airway. Airway emergencies can occur at any time during the perioperative period. Serious airway problems can result in adverse outcomes, including death, brain injury, myocardial injury, and airway trauma. The ASA difficult-airway algorithm has recommended sequences of activity for recognized and unrecognized difficult airways and primary and alternative strategies for awake intubation and intubation attempts after induction of general anesthesia. Although patient management is the responsibility of a member of the anesthesia department, all perioperative nurses should know about necessary equipment, including location, setup, and function. Most institutions have a difficult-airway cart (see Box 4-2), centralizing items and supplies necessary to manage airway emergencies. The ASA Practice Guideline suggests contents for this cart, but anesthesia providers may add or modify preference items.

The anesthesia provider assesses the likelihood and clinical impact of potential airway problems by evaluating the patient's airway. Questions related to congenital, acquired, and traumatic disease states are posed to detect factors that might indicate the presence of a difficult airway. The patient is examined to detect physical characteristics that may make intubation or mask ventilation difficult. The pharyngeal structures may be assessed, the distance from the mandible to the hyoid noted, and the ability to extend the neck determined. An obese patient is more likely to require a shoulder roll to align the three axes of the airway (oral, pharyngeal, and laryngeal). With a shoulder roll, the scapulae, shoulders, and nape of the neck are supported, resulting in an improved sniff position. Anticipatory action on the part of the perioperative nurse in assisting with shoulder roll placement is an example of the hallmark teamwork and collaboration that characterize good patient care. The perioperative nurse also should anticipate equipment and assistance required should an awake intubation be necessary or if the emergency pathway must be followed. Finally, patients who experience a difficult airway may be recommended to wear a Medic-Alert bracelet. The National Medic Alert Registry for Difficult Airway/Intubation can be contacted. Information regarding why it was difficult to secure an airway and what technique finally worked is recorded in the Foundation's data bank and can be accessed by future anesthesia providers.

Modified from American Society of Anesthesiologists: Practice guidelines for management of the difficult airway, *Anesthesiology* 98:1269-1277, 2003.

BOX 4-2

### Typical Contents of a Difficult-Airway Cart

**FIBEROPTIC (FO) EQUIPMENT**
- Flexible FO bronchoscopes (adult and pediatric)
- FO light source
- Bullard scope (FO)
- Siliconized spray

**LARYNGOSCOPE EQUIPMENT**
- Assorted pediatric and adult laryngoscope handles and blades
- Extra alkaline batteries

**ENDOTRACHEAL TUBES (ETT)**
- Regular ETT: uncuffed, 2.5-6 mm
- Regular ETT: cuffed, 5-9 mm
- Oral RAE ETT: uncuffed, 3-7 mm
- Oral RAE ETT: cuffed, 6-8 mm
- Nasal RAE ETT: uncuffed, 3-7 mm
- Nasal RAE ETT: cuffed, 6-8 mm
- Reinforced ETT: cuffed, 7-8 mm
- Controllable-tip ETT (Endotrol)
- Combitube

**AIRWAYS**
- Regular oral: assorted pediatric and adult
- Regular nasal: assorted adult
- Intubating airways: assorted (e.g., Ovassapian, Williams)
- Nasopharyngeal airway with inflatable introducer
- Laryngeal mask airways (LMAs): assorted sizes
- Tongue blades
- Water-soluble lubricant (K-Y)

**INTUBATING EQUIPMENT**
- Intubating stylets
- McGill forceps: pediatric and adult
- Esophageal (gastric tube) airway (EGTA)
- Hollow ETT changers with removable Luer-Lok connectors for $O_2$ insufflation

**SUCTION EQUIPMENT**
- Assorted flexible suction catheters to fit ETT and LMA
- Stiff suction catheters (Yankauer)

**TOPICAL ANESTHESIA EQUIPMENT**
- Atomizers and pressurized topical anesthetic spray
- Long Q-tips
- Lidocaine 4%
- Lidocaine 4% with phenylephrine
- Lidocaine 2%—viscous
- Lidocaine 5%—ointment
- Lidocaine 10%
- Tetracaine 1%

**TRANSTRACHEAL AIRWAY EQUIPMENT**
- Transtracheal $O_2$ jet ventilator with pressure regulator, manual control valve, and Luer-Lok male connector
- Assorted large IV catheters
- Assorted long guidewires, epidural needles, and epidural catheters (for retrograde intubation)

**MISCELLANEOUS**
- Safety glasses
- Heat-moisture exchanger (Humidivent)
- Assorted facemasks with port for FO scope
- Right-angled connector (for facemasks) with port for FO scope
- $ETCO_2$ chemical indicators (Easy Cap)
- Twill tape (to secure ETT)
- Skin adhesive (Mastisol)

The LMA is a major advancement in airway management. Placement is relatively simple and does not require laryngoscopy or muscle relaxation. When comparing ease of use, invasiveness, and airway protection, the LMA ranks between the facemask and an ETT. It is ideal for a supine patient under general anesthesia with spontaneous ventilation. The LMA also may be useful in a difficult-airway situation in which tracheal intubation cannot be achieved. It is available in six sizes, it can be autoclaved, and it is reusable. A disposable LMA also is available.

Before insertion, the LMA must be deflated carefully so that there are no wrinkles in the cuff. The recommended technique for insertion of the LMA is shown in Figure 4-5, and correct placement is shown in Figure 4-6. For adults, it is recommended that a 2.5-cm to 3-cm diameter roll of gauze sponges be used as a "bite block" and inserted beside the LMA tube.[6,20] The LMA and gauze roll can be secured with tape.

Maintenance of anesthesia can be accomplished with IV or inhalational anesthetic techniques or a combination of both, with or without additional muscle relaxation. The anesthesia provider considers a variety of factors when selecting the anesthesia technique for each situation.

Whichever technique is selected for general anesthesia (or any of the other anesthesia types discussed subsequently), the entire surgical team participates in a time out just after the patient is positioned, prepped, and draped and before starting

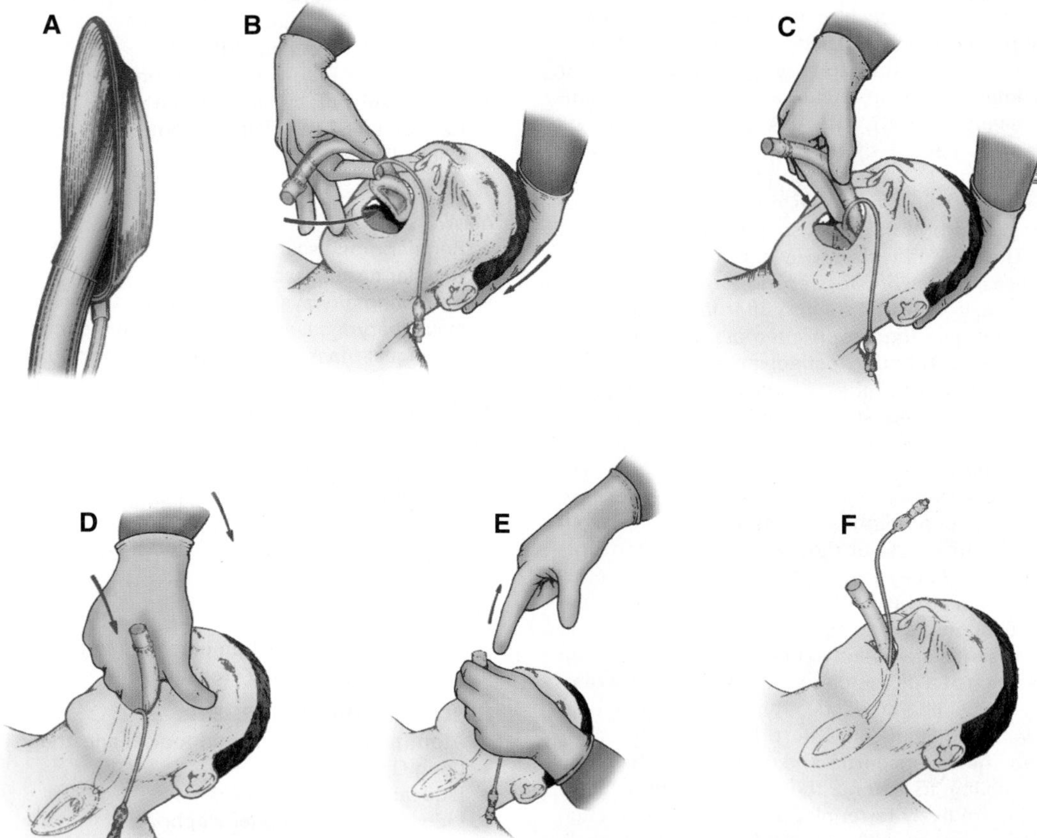


FIGURE 4-5 Insertion of the laryngeal mask airway (LMA). Select the appropriate-size LMA (*1*, neonates ≤5 kg; *1.5*, infants 5 to 10 kg; *2*, infants and children 10 to 20 kg; *2½*, children 20 to 30 kg; *3*, children and small adults >30 kg; *4*, normal-size to large adults; *5*, large adults). **A,** Carefully deflate the LMA as flat as possible so that the rim faces away from the mask aperture as shown. There should be no folds near the tip. **B,** Under direct vision, press the tip of the LMA cephalad against the hard palate to flatten it out. Using the index finger, continue pressing the LMA against the palate as the LMA is advanced into the pharynx to ensure that the tip remains flattened and avoids the tongue. **C,** Keeping the neck flexed and the head extended, use the index finger to press the LMA into the posterior wall. **D,** Continue pushing with the ball of the index finger guiding the LMA posteriorly into position. By withdrawing the other fingers and slightly pronating the forearm, it is usually possible to push the LMA fully into position in one fluid movement. **E,** Firmly grasp the tube with the other hand, then withdraw the index finger from the pharynx. Gently press the LMA posteriorly to ensure that it is fully inserted. **F,** Carefully inflate the LMA with the recommended volume of air for size (*1*, 2 to 4 mL; *2*, ≤10 mL; *2½*, ≤14 mL; *3*, ≤20 mL; *4*, ≤30 mL; *5*, ≤40 mL). Do not overinflate. Do not touch the LMA tube while inflating, unless it is obviously unstable (as with elderly edentulous patients with loose oropharyngeal tissues). Usually the LMA moves slightly forward out of the hypopharynx as it is inflated. Insert a bite-block (roll of gauze) alongside the LMA tube to minimize occlusion of the tube as the patient is awakening.

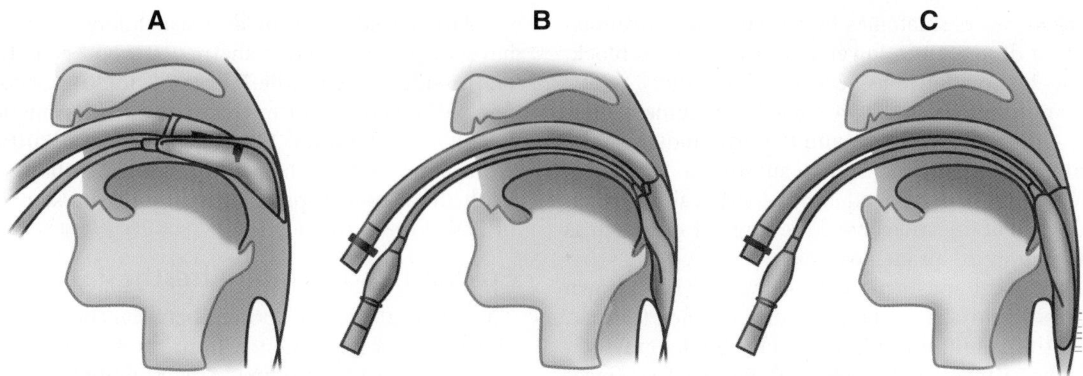


FIGURE 4-6 Sagittal views of insertion and proper placement of the laryngeal mask airway (LMA). **A,** Insertion of LMA. **B,** Proper location of LMA (deflated). **C,** Properly placed and inflated LMA.

the procedure. The patient's identify is re-checked. The procedure to be done, operative side and site, and correct patient position are verified by the entire surgical team. The patient must be positioned such that the marking of the operative site (e.g., with the word "yes" or the surgeon's initials) is visible on the patient's skin. The availability of implants, special equipment, or other requirements (e.g., blood, if it has been ordered) is verified. When this has all been completed, the procedure can begin. The time out should be documented according to institutional protocol.

Many factors influence emergence. The objective is to be able to move the patient from the OR bed to the post anesthetic unit (PACU) bed as soon as the dressing is applied. During emergence, the anesthesia provider suctions the oropharynx before extubation to decrease the risk of aspiration and laryngospasm after extubation, reverses any residual neuromuscular blockade, and allows the washout of $N_2O$ and volatile agents by giving 100% $O_2$ for several minutes before extubation. After extubation, the patient is transported to the PACU to awaken from the anesthetic experience. In some situations, the patient may be transferred to the PACU before extubation and the ETT removed when the patient is fully awake.

Untoward events that can occur with general anesthesia include hypoxia; respiratory, cardiovascular, or renal dysfunction; hypotension; hypertension; fluid or electrolyte imbalance; residual muscle paralysis; dental damage; neurologic problems; hypothermia; and MH. The anesthesia provider usually directs the treatment and management of such events.

## REGIONAL ANESTHESIA

Regional anesthesia (also called *conduction anesthesia*) can be accomplished by injecting a local anesthetic anywhere along the pathway of a nerve from the spinal cord (spinal anesthesia), epidurally, peripherally. It can also be administered topically on the mucous membranes or skin.[28] This injection provides anesthesia to a region of the body. Preoperative preparation for regional anesthesia is essentially the same as that for general anesthesia. Preoperative medication frequently is ordered before regional anesthesia to ease any discomfort that may be experienced during placement of the block. The criteria for monitoring during regional anesthesia are similar to those during general anesthesia. Whenever regional anesthesia is performed, resuscitative equipment and drugs must be immediately available. During preparation and placement of the regional anesthetic, the perioperative nurse can provide valuable assistance. This assistance may include placing the appropriate monitors, such as pulse oximetry, ECG, and blood pressure; providing supplemental $O_2$ if indicated; reassuring the patient; administering sedation, such as midazolam, as directed; and properly positioning the patient, which is crucial for a successful block.

Peripheral blocks on the lower or upper extremities or on the head frequently are done in a preoperative holding area to allow adequate time for the local anesthetic to penetrate the peripheral nerve before the patient is transferred to the OR. For peripheral blocks, the perioperative nurse may need to perform aspiration during needle placement (to detect vascular puncture) and inject the local anesthetic while the anesthesia provider is stabilizing the needle in the precise location. After an initial period of evaluation by the anesthesia provider, the nurse monitors the patient for any substantial change in vital signs or untoward reactions until the patient is transferred to the OR. For regional anesthesia and general anesthesia, an anesthesia provider continuously monitors the patient during the surgical procedure.

### Spinal Anesthesia

A local anesthetic (usually lidocaine, tetracaine, or bupivacaine) injected into the cerebrospinal fluid (CSF) in the subarachnoid space is termed a *spinal anesthetic* or a *subarachnoid block (SAB)*. To provide additional analgesia, fentanyl or preservative-free morphine often is added to the local anesthetic. A spinal needle is inserted into a lower lumbar interspace with the patient either lying on one side or in a sitting position. The local anesthetic generally is mixed with a dextrose solution for a total of 1 to 4 mL to make a *hyperbaric* (heavier than the CSF) solution. These hyperbaric mixtures settle in a gravity-dependent manner after injection into the CSF. By changing the patient's position, the block can be directed up, down, or to one side of the spinal cord. With prostate surgery, the patient may remain in the sitting position for a minute or so after the local anesthetic is injected. A bilateral block of the S1-S5 dermatomes results.

For surgery in the upper abdomen, the patient may be placed in a slightly (5 to 10 degrees) head-down position to allow the anesthetic to move cephalad while the anesthesia provider carefully checks the level of sensory block. When an adequate level is obtained, the bed is leveled to minimize further spread. After 10 to 15 minutes, the block is usually "set" and does not extend farther. The sympathetic nervous system usually is blocked two dermatomes higher and the neuromuscular system two dermatomes lower than the sensory block. The patient may be positioned as necessary for surgery.

If the local anesthetic is mixed with a larger volume of sterile water, the solution is *hypobaric,* and the drug moves to the nondependent area. Hypobaric spinal anesthesia usually is done after the patient is positioned and the surgical site is exposed (with the site of injection above the surgical site, such as in perianal surgery in the prone position).

By mixing the local anesthetic with some CSF withdrawn from the subarachnoid space, the solution becomes *isobaric.* Distribution of this solution is minimally affected by gravity.

Spinal anesthesia may evoke several physiologic responses that can result in major problems if not properly managed. A description of these follows.

***Hypotension.*** Hypotension may occur rapidly after an SAB. It is caused by vasodilation because the sympathetic nerves that control vasomotor tone are blocked. Peripheral pooling of blood occurs, resulting in a reduced venous return to the heart and a decrease in cardiac output. The hypotensive response usually can be avoided by infusing 750 to 1500 mL of balanced salt solution immediately before the block and placing the patient in a 5-degree head-down position to improve venous return to the heart. A vasopressor, such as ephedrine, also may be administered.

***Total Spinal Anesthesia.*** Total spinal anesthesia (or an inadvertently high block) may cause paralysis of the respiratory muscles and necessitate immediate intubation and ventilation. Any sign or symptom of respiratory distress occurring shortly after instituting spinal anesthesia should alert the anesthesia provider to the possibility of a high spinal block.

***Positioning Problems.*** Positioning problems can occur because pain and sensory inputs to a portion of the patient's body are blocked. Care must be taken in positioning the patient intraoperatively to avoid neurologic damage, burns, loss of skin integrity, or other trauma. Positioning the surgical patient is a collaborative effort among the anesthesia provider, the surgeon, the assistant, and the perioperative nurse (see Chapter 5 for a comprehensive discussion of positioning the surgical patient).

***Postdural Puncture Headache.*** Postdural puncture headache (PDPH) (also called *postspinal cephalgia* or *spinal headache*) is a frequent postoperative complaint after spinal anesthesia. It occurs more commonly in young parturients or other patients younger than 40 years. The incidence is about 1% when a 25- or 27-gauge blunt-bevel needle is used. It is unrelated to how soon the patient is ambulated. The headache is believed to result from leakage of CSF through the hole in the dura and typically occurs when the patient assumes an upright position. The incidence, severity, and duration of the headache seem to correlate with the size of the hole left in the dura. The headache is usually in the occipital area and generally resolves over 1 to 3 days but may last 2 weeks. A variety of treatment modalities have been used to relieve the headache, including strict bed rest for 24 to 48 hours, vigorous hydration, abdominal binders, epidural infusion of saline, PO or IV caffeine, and injection of 5 to 20 mL of autologous blood into the epidural space at the puncture site ("blood patch").[9]

Many anesthesia providers use different spinal needles that have a tip shaped like a sharpened wood pencil with the hole on the side of the needle. These 24- to 26-gauge spinal needles (e.g., Whitacre, Sprotte, Gertie Marx) presumably separate or go between the dural fibers as opposed to cutting the fibers, which may occur when a blunt-bevel spinal needle is used. With these "pencil-point" needles, the incidence and severity of PDPH are extremely low.[9]

## Epidural and Caudal Anesthesia

The epidural space is located between the ligamentum flavum and the dura and extends from the foramen magnum to the sacrococcygeal membrane. This potential space is filled with epidural veins, fat, and loose areolar tissue. For *epidural* anesthesia, the local anesthetic usually is injected through the intervertebral spaces in the lumbar region, although it also can be injected into the cervical or thoracic regions. The anesthetic spreads cephalad and caudad from the site of injection. A comparative location of the needle points and injected anesthetic is shown in Figure 4-7.

For *caudal* anesthesia, the local anesthetic also is injected into the epidural space, but the approach is through the caudal canal in the sacrum. Compared with a lumbar epidural, this approach requires a greater volume of anesthetic to fill the epidural space. Caudal anesthesia has a 5% to 10% technical failure rate. Because of the ease of administration, however, it is often employed for pediatric surgical procedures on the lower extremities or the perineal area.[33]

Several techniques may be used for epidural or caudal anesthesia. A "single-shot epidural" involves administration of the local anesthesia through the needle before its removal. For

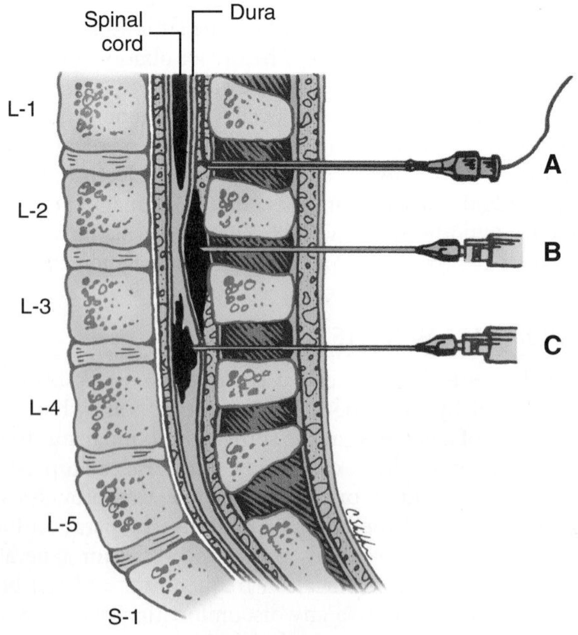


FIGURE 4-7 Location of needle point and injected anesthetic relative to dura. **A,** Epidural catheter. **B,** Single injection epidural. **C,** Spinal anesthesia. (Interspaces most commonly used are L4-L5, L3-L4, and L2-L3.)

intermittent injections or continuous infusions, a small catheter is inserted into the epidural space for administration of the local anesthetic.

For a combined spinal and epidural anesthesia, the epidural needle is inserted into the epidural space, and a special, long 26-gauge spinal needle is inserted through the epidural needle into the CSF. A small amount of fentanyl or preservative-free morphine may be injected and provides good analgesia for several hours. The spinal needle is removed, and an epidural catheter is inserted. This technique is especially useful for obstetric anesthesia.[8,9]

Techniques used to identify the epidural space include the "hanging drop" and the "loss of resistance" to injection of either air or liquid (saline or local anesthetic) as the needle is advanced slowly through the ligamentum flavum. With the hanging-drop technique, the needle is filled with liquid to form a meniscus at the needle hub. As the needle is slowly advanced into the epidural space, the negative (less than atmospheric) pressure draws the liquid inward toward the epidural space. Location of the needle tip within the epidural space is verified by injection of an additional 1 to 2 mL of air or saline.[8,9]

When local anesthetics are injected into the epidural space, the major sites of action are probably the nerve roots as they leave the spinal cord and proceed out the intervertebral foramina beyond the meningeal sheath. Some of the anesthetic diffuses into the subarachnoid space, however, to the spinal cord. Because local anesthetics diffuse away from the site of injection, segmental anesthesia may be possible in specific areas. In contrast to spinal anesthesia, much larger volumes of local anesthetic are needed with epidural anesthesia; the head-up, head-down, or lateral position of the patient does not affect the level of the epidural anesthetic as much, and the onset of anesthesia is much slower with epidural anesthesia. As with spinal anesthesia, hypotension can occur with epidural anesthesia, but the onset is much slower and usually can be managed with the rapid IV infusion of a balanced salt solution or repositioning of the patient.[9,28]

The local anesthetics most frequently used for epidural anesthesia are lidocaine, bupivacaine, and chloroprocaine. Ropivacaine and levobupivacaine are newer local anesthetics that may prove to be less cardiotoxic than bupivacaine and possess a larger therapeutic ratio. Although much of their pharmacologic profile is similar to bupivacaine, levobupivacaine and ropivacaine seem to possess more selective action in terms of neural blockade (Research Highlight).[9,19,28] Depending on the concentration of the anesthetic agent, the effect can range from loss of sensory input to complete motor blockade. To help verify that the anesthetic is not being injected into the subarachnoid space or into an epidural vein, a test dose of 3 to 5 ml of lidocaine with a 1:200,000 concentration of epinephrine is frequently used. Injected intravascularly, this test dose causes a transient tachycardia. If injected into the subarachnoid space, it produces a low level of spinal anesthesia. Complications associated with the use of local anesthetics in the epidural and subarachnoid spaces are unique to the agent used. Permanent neurologic sequelae have been reported when chloroprocaine with a preservative was injected into the subarachnoid space. Bupivacaine is associated with pronounced cardiac toxicity if injected intravascularly.[8,9,28] With epidural anesthesia, several complications can occur, including inadvertent dural puncture, subarachnoid injection, and vascular injection.

## RESEARCH HIGHLIGHT

### Epidural Anesthesia with Ropivacaine During Labor

Epidural analgesia is a popular and effective method of pain relief during labor. Epidural analgesia is often desired so that the parturient may remain awake and interact immediately with her newborn. Bupivacaine has been used and provides effective analgesia; however, adverse effects of potential cardiovascular toxicity and motor nerve blockade limit its usefulness. Unintentional intravenous injection of bupivacaine has been reported as resulting in cardiac arrest and death. The motor blockade that results, reducing maternal mobility, has been shown to increase instrument and surgical deliveries.

Ropivacaine is structurally related to bupivacaine, but it is a stereoisomer, whereas bupivacaine is a racemic mixture. Ropivacaine has a similar potency and duration, but less cardiac toxicity. Ropivacaine has greater selectivity for sensory fibers than motor fibers, producing less motor blockade. These properties make it a desirable drug for obstetric analgesia.

In this study, 500 records for each group, comparing ropivacaine and bupivacaine, were reviewed. The instrument delivery rate for the bupivacaine group was 14.2% (71 of 500) and 9.8% for the ropivacaine group (49 of 500). The cesarean section rate was 14% (70 of 500) for the bupivacaine group and 10.2% (51 of 500) for the ropivacaine group. The use of ropivacaine decreased surgical and instrument delivery rates compared with bupivacaine. The ability to use lower infusion rates and the decrease in re-dose boluses compared with bupivacaine reduced the risk of systemic and intravascular exposure of the patient to local anesthetic.

Modified from Litwin AA: Mode of delivery following labor epidural analgesia: influence of ropivacaine and bupivacaine, *AANA Journal* 69(4):259-261, 2001.

***Inadvertent Dural Puncture.*** Inadvertent dural puncture with the epidural needle (a wet tap) can cause a PDPH. This headache is significant in about 50% of patients, and the intensity can be incapacitating. Treatment is essentially the same as discussed in the "Spinal Anesthesia" section earlier.[9]

***Subarachnoid Injection.*** Subarachnoid injection occurs if the needle or catheter is unintentionally inserted into the subarachnoid space. If a large volume of local anesthetic is injected as a bolus, it causes "total spinal" anesthesia. This condition is associated with a rapid onset of hypotension caused by vasodilation, profound bradycardia as the sympathetic nerves to the heart are blocked, and a totally paralyzed patient. Treatment includes intubation, control of ventilation, support of blood pressure and the cardiovascular system, and administration of amnestic drugs until the block has resolved. If properly managed, this problem is not life-threatening, but use of the test dose described previously and injection of only 3 to 5 mL at a time usually avert this problem. With patient movement over time, the epidural catheter may migrate through the dura. A small test dose should be given each time additional local anesthetic is injected through the catheter. In addition, each subsequent dose should be injected in increments of 3 to 5 mL each.

***Vascular Injection.*** Vascular injection of the local anesthetic into an epidural vein may occur inadvertently with the initial dose or with subsequent injections. Intravenously injected bupivacaine is associated with cardiac arrest. Toxicity from other local anesthetics can cause sudden and profound hypotension, convulsions from the effects on the central nervous system, and tachycardia if the solution contains epinephrine. The convulsions usually dissipate rapidly as the local anesthetic is redistributed throughout the body. Intravenous thiopental or a benzodiazepine may be given to reduce these effects. A vasopressor (e.g., ephedrine or phenylephrine) can be used to restore blood pressure. If the patient becomes paralyzed, intubation and ventilation may be required until the toxic effects are gone. Use of the test dose with each injection usually prevents these problems.

### Peripheral Nerve Blocks

A wide variety of peripheral nerves can be blocked effectively by injecting local anesthetic around them to provide adequate surgical anesthesia. Onset and duration of the block are related to the drug used, its concentration and volume, the addition of epinephrine, and the site of injection. Complications usually are caused by an inadvertent intravascular injection or an overdose of the local anesthetic. Rarely, nerve damage may occur from trauma caused by the needle or compression from the volume of local anesthetic injected.

### Intravenous Regional Anesthesia

Intravenous regional anesthesia was first described by Bier in 1908 and is frequently referred to as a *Bier block*.[8] Although it can be used on a lower extremity, it is used more often on the upper extremities. It is highly reliable and easy to accomplish.

A small IV catheter is inserted as distal as feasible, and a single-cuffed or double-cuffed pneumatic tourniquet is placed around the limb proximal to the surgical site. The limb is raised upward and is exsanguinated by wrapping it with an Esmarch bandage. The tourniquet is inflated to approximately 100 mm Hg above the patient's systolic blood pressure, and the Esmarch bandage is removed. Approximately 50 mL of 0.5% lidocaine is injected through the catheter. Onset of anesthesia is rapid and lasts until the tourniquet is deflated.[8,28]

When a double-cuffed pneumatic tourniquet is used, the proximal cuff is initially inflated. When the patient experiences discomfort from the cuff pressure (usually about 35 to 40 minutes after inflation of the cuff), the distal cuff, which is located over an anesthetized area, is inflated. Then the proximal cuff is deflated. The proximal cuff must remain inflated until the distal cuff has been inflated to prevent loss of the IV anesthetic from the limb. Two single-cuffed tourniquets can be used instead of a double-cuffed tourniquet. If the patient experiences pain from the tourniquet, an IV analgesic or sedative can be used to supplement the block.[8,28]

Although problems can occur from an overdose or toxic reaction to the lidocaine, these are rare if the tourniquet has been inflated more than 20 minutes. The risk also is minimized by intermittently deflating the cuff for a few seconds at a time for several cycles when the surgical procedure is over. This method reduces the transient peak blood level of the local anesthetic in the central nervous system and the heart. Loss of pneumatic pressure in the tourniquet can cause a toxic reaction and a loss of anesthesia.

## MONITORED ANESTHESIA CARE

A gentle and patient surgeon can safely accomplish minor and even some major procedures with a peripheral nerve block or when the surgical site is infiltrated with a local anesthetic. This technique can be employed for normal, healthy individuals and sicker, unstable patients who may require extensive invasive monitoring and pharmacologic management if general anesthesia is employed. For these patients, the issue is the relative risks and benefits of monitored anesthesia care (MAC) versus general anesthesia.

During MAC, the anesthesia provider may supplement the local anesthetic with an IV analgesic (e.g., fentanyl) and with sedative and amnestic drugs (e.g., midazolam or propofol). In addition, the anesthesia provider carefully monitors the patient's vital signs, respiratory and cardiovascular status, and positioning and may give supplemental low-flow $O_2$. Depending on the clinical situation, the anesthesia provider may have to induce general anesthesia or use one of the regional techniques described previously if a greater degree of anesthesia is necessary during the procedure.

## CONSCIOUS SEDATION/ANALGESIA

*Conscious sedation/analgesia* refers to the IV administration of certain sedatives and analgesics that produces a condition in which the patient exhibits a depressed level of consciousness but retains the ability to maintain a patent airway independently and respond appropriately to verbal commands or physical stimulation. An anesthesia provider is not involved in the patient's care. These functions may be performed under the direction of a physician by perioperative nurses who have additional training and demonstrated competencies in (1) administering medications to achieve conscious sedation/analgesia and (2) monitoring these patients.[5] Objectives for a patient receiving conscious sedation/analgesia include alteration of mood, maintenance of consciousness, enhanced cooperation, elevation of pain threshold, minimal variation of vital signs, some degree of amnesia, and a rapid and safe return to activities of daily living.

Selection of patients for conscious sedation/analgesia should be based on established criteria developed by an interdisciplinary team of health care professionals. These patients must be thoroughly assessed physiologically and psychologically before the procedure. The assessment should include a review of physical examination findings; current medications taken; existing allergies; current medical problems; history of smoking or substance abuse; current chief complaint; baseline vital signs, height, and weight; age; emotional state; any communication deficits; and the patient's perceptions of the procedure and conscious sedation/analgesia. The monitoring methods used for patients receiving conscious sedation, the medications administered, and the interventions initiated must be within the scope of nursing practice as defined by the respective state board of nursing. If the nurse does not feel comfortable managing the care and monitoring of a particular patient, the attending physician and an anesthesia provider should be consulted.

When monitoring a patient who is receiving conscious sedation/analgesia, the nurse should have no other responsibilities that would leave the patient unattended or compromise continuous patient monitoring during the procedure. The nurse must be clinically competent in the use of monitoring equipment and oxygen-delivery devices, medications used for conscious sedation/analgesia and resuscitation, and airway management. Advanced cardiac life support (ACLS) certification of nurses responsible for monitoring patients receiving conscious sedation/analgesia may be required by some health care institutions. If not, health care professionals with ACLS skills should be readily available to render support if needed in an emergency situation.[5]

The nurse who administers conscious sedation/analgesia medications should understand the usual dosages, contraindications, interactions with other medications, onset and duration of action and desired effects, and adverse reactions and emergency management techniques. Benzodiazepines (e.g., diazepam, midazolam) and opioids (e.g., fentanyl, meperidine hydrochloride) are used for conscious sedation/analgesia.[5] Equipment that should be present and ready for use in the room where conscious sedation/analgesia will be administered includes a noninvasive blood pressure device, an ECG, a pulse oximeter, oxygen-delivery devices, and suction.

Before conscious sedation/analgesia is administered, an IV access line should be established to facilitate administration of conscious sedation/analgesia medications and emergency medications and fluids if needed. Parameters that should be monitored during conscious sedation/analgesia are respiratory rate, cardiac rate and rhythm, blood pressure, oxygen saturation, level of consciousness, and condition of skin. An emergency cart with appropriate resuscitative medications and equipment (e.g., a defibrillator) should be immediately available to every location where conscious sedation/analgesia is administered.

Nursing documentation of care provided should include the preprocedure assessment; dosage, route, time, and effects of all medications administered; type and amount of fluids administered; physiologic data from continuous monitoring at 5- to 15-minute intervals and on significant events; level of consciousness; nursing interventions initiated and the patient's responses; and any untoward significant patient reactions and their resolution.[4]

Postprocedure monitoring should be provided until the patient has returned to preprocedure baseline parameters as identified by individual institutional policy. Patients and family members or significant others should receive appropriate oral and written discharge instructions and be able to verbalize understanding of the instructions. It is helpful if the instructions can be given before and after the procedure because conscious sedation/analgesia medications may cause amnesia, which affects recall ability.

Discharge criteria should be established by an interdisciplinary team and should include adequate respiratory function, stable vital signs, return to preprocedure level of consciousness, intact motor reflexes, return of motor and sensory control, absence of protracted nausea, acceptable skin color and condition, absence of significant pain, and satisfactory surgical site and dressing condition (when present). A responsible adult must be available at discharge to accompany the patient home.

## LOCAL ANESTHESIA

The terms *local anesthesia, local,* and *straight local* are used interchangeably to describe the administration of an anesthetic agent to a specific area of the body by topical application, local infiltration, regional nerve block, or "field" block. Local anesthesia is administered by the surgeon. In addition, other physicians, such as cardiologists, pulmonologists, proctologists, and gastroenterologists, may perform local procedures in the OR suite. No anesthesia provider is involved in the care of these patients.

Hospitals and ambulatory centers should have established interdisciplinary guidelines for the selection of patients who are appropriate for local anesthesia procedures and should have monitoring criteria for these procedures. The decision to monitor the patient receiving local anesthesia, the parameters that need to be monitored, and the frequency of observation and monitoring should be tailored to the patient, the surgical procedure, and the medications used. Patients receiving local anesthesia during a surgical procedure should be assessed preoperatively and monitored continually by the perioperative nurse during the procedure.

Local anesthesia usually is employed for minor, short-term surgical, diagnostic, or therapeutic procedures. Because the patient does not lose consciousness with local anesthesia, it is frequently preferred when the patient's cooperation is necessary for the procedure. Local anesthesia is economical and eliminates the undesirable effects of general anesthesia. Adverse reactions may occur from large amounts of local agents, however. If the agent enters the bloodstream directly, convulsions, circulatory and respiratory distress, cardiovascular collapse, or even death can result.

The surgeon chooses local anesthetics based on the desired duration of action, surgery site, potency potential, and the patient's physical status. Topical agents, such as cocaine hydrochloride, tetracaine, or lidocaine, may be applied to mucous membranes of the nose, throat, trachea, and urethra. Lidocaine 0.5% to 2%, with or without epinephrine, is the drug most commonly used for local infiltration anesthesia, although bupivacaine (Marcaine) has seen increased use in recent years. Epinephrine may be added to the local anesthesia agent for vasoconstricting properties in the area injected, slower rate of absorption of the local anesthetic agent, and lower incidence of toxicity; this allows for a longer duration of action for the agent by reducing blood flow to the area injected. Epinephrine should be used with caution in patients with hypertension, diabetes, or heart disease. A general recommendation is that no more than 50 mL of a 1% solution, or 100 mL of a 0.5% solution, of an anesthetic drug such as lidocaine be injected per hour for local anesthesia. For maximum adult dosages, see Table 4-2. All local anesthetic containers or syringes should be clearly labeled when on the sterile table.

Preoperatively, the perioperative nurse should review the patient's history and physical examination findings and the results of laboratory or other diagnostic tests if indicated. Patients should be assessed carefully to determine their physiologic baseline, presence of any allergies (to medications, latex, or other substances), and emotional status. They should have an IV infusion started before the procedure because adequate venous access can be crucial in life-threatening situations when resuscitative drugs must be given immediately.

The perioperative nurse should be clinically competent in the function and use of the monitoring equipment to be used, the placement of equipment connections, and the interpretation of data. When indicated, intraoperative monitoring should include heart rate and regularity, respiratory rate, and mental status. Additional monitoring parameters should be based on the patient's condition and may include blood pressure, skin condition, and oxygen saturation.[5] Any changes in the patient's condition should be communicated immediately to the surgeon.

The perioperative nurse should be familiar with the drugs to be administered during the procedure. This knowledge should include the usual dosages, limits on the rate of injection and maximum dosage (usually stated on a per-kilogram basis), duration of action, physiologic and psychologic changes to be expected, normal and abnormal reactions to the drugs used, and appropriate action to take should an untoward reaction occur. The nurse should monitor the dosage, route, and time of administration of all local anesthetic medications given to the patient. In addition, the patient should be observed for the presence of side effects, such as central nervous system disturbances, cardiovascular problems, hypersensitivity to medication, and toxic reaction resulting from high levels of the local anesthetic agent. Emergency drugs, suction apparatus, and resuscitation equipment should be readily available. Symptoms of adverse drug reactions include restlessness, unexplained anxiety or fearfulness, diaphoresis, nausea, palpitations, disturbed respiration, pallor or flushing, syncope, and convulsive movements. The nurse also should be aware of signs and symptoms of allergic reaction, such as urticaria, tachycardia, laryngeal edema resulting in breathing difficulties, nausea, vomiting, and elevated temperature. In some instances, anaphylactoid symptoms, including severe hypotension, can occur. If any significant change occurs in the patient's physiologic or psychologic status, the nurse should notify the physician immediately. Good communication is essential for optimal patient care. Because the patient is awake during the procedure, extraneous or irrelevant conversation and noise should be kept to a minimum.

Documentation of care provided to a patient receiving a local anesthetic should be consistent with the AORN Recommended Practices for Documentation of Perioperative Nursing Care.[4] In addition, the drug dosage, route, and time of administration and patient monitoring used and its results should be properly documented.

After completion of the procedure, the patient's postoperative status must be assessed carefully. This evaluation and any special needs of the patient should be documented properly on the chart, and a report should be called to the receiving unit before the patient's transfer. The hand-off report should include the type and amount of drugs given and any adverse reaction noted, the site and condition of the IV infusion (if applicable), the type and amount of solution infused in the OR, the range of intraoperative vital signs, the surgical procedure performed, and the condition of the dressing. Any special postoperative orders, allergies, and a general statement of the patient's tolerance of the procedure also should be included. The patient may be transferred to the day-surgery and discharge area or returned directly to the hospital room. Local anesthesia patients are rarely transferred to the PACU for recovery or observation.

## PAIN MANAGEMENT

Many anesthesia providers have applied their expertise in analgesia and regional anesthesia to the management of acute and chronic pain. Chronic pain is often a multifactorial entity that may occur after a discrete injury (or trauma), amputation, laminectomy, or other surgical procedure. It also may result from prolonged repetitive stress, such as "low back pain." Chronic pain frequently has complex psychologic components that are unrecognized by patients or individuals closely associated with them. Diagnosis and treatment of such chronic pain problems usually involve multiple medical disciplines and prolonged management.

Acute perioperative pain is a different problem. Traditionally, postoperative pain has been treated with IM narcotics every 3 to 6 hours as needed. This treatment is often associated with undesirable side effects, including oversedation, respiratory depression, deep venous thrombosis secondary to decreased mobility, and variable degrees of pain relief. Other pain-management modalities are being used successfully. Patient-controlled analgesia (PCA) uses a programmable electronic pump that can continuously infuse a small amount of IV narcotic (at a basal rate); in addition, the patient can administer a predetermined bolus "on demand." Safety interlocks limit the frequency of the boluses and the total dose per hour.[13]

When spinal or epidural anesthesia is employed for a surgical procedure, a small amount of preservative-free narcotic, such as fentanyl, sufentanil, or morphine, may be added to the local anesthetic mixture. The narcotic acts via central opiate receptors and provides analgesia for 24 to 36 hours.

Continuous epidural analgesia also may be used for prolonged postoperative pain management. This technique is employed for extensive procedures, including total hip or knee replacements; knee reconstruction; and major abdominal, thoracic, or gynecologic operations. In addition, it can be used for acute trauma, such as multiple rib fractures.

Typically, a lumbar or thoracic epidural catheter is inserted before surgery, covered with a transparent occlusive dressing, and injected with local anesthetic. Because of the duration, manipulation, or positioning required for the operative procedure, general anesthesia is often induced for patient comfort. The epidural greatly reduces the analgesic requirements of general anesthesia. For postoperative pain control, the epidural infusion of local anesthetic is usually one eighth to one sixteenth the concentration used for surgical anesthesia.[13] A small dose of preservative-free narcotic, such as fentanyl, sufentanil, or morphine, is usually added to enhance analgesia. After the surgical procedure, the infusion rate is adjusted to provide analgesia during the early recovery phase. As the level of pain decreases over time, the infusion rate is reduced. The catheter is removed after 2 to 5 days to minimize the risk of infection. Benefits of epidural analgesia for acute postoperative pain include good analgesia with minimal sedation, early ambulation and physical therapy, and excellent patient satisfaction. Possible side effects include nausea, pruritus, and areas of slight numbness. These are controlled with drugs such as diphenhydramine (Benadryl) or naloxone (Narcan) and by adjusting the infusion rate. A nonsteroidal antiinflammatory drug (NSAID), such as ketorolac (Toradol), frequently is given for any "breakthrough pain" instead of increasing the epidural infusion.

A single caudal injection is often used in pediatric patients having surgery of the lower abdomen, pelvis, or lower extremities. It usually is administered after the induction of general anesthesia, and a long-acting local anesthetic, such as bupivacaine with epinephrine, typically is used. This injection provides good analgesia for 8 to 24 hours postoperatively and greatly decreases the intraoperative requirements for general anesthesia. If the procedure requires prolonged recovery, a lumbar epidural catheter can be placed intraoperatively. Postoperatively, management is similar to that for adult patients, although for younger patients the level of analgesia and the presence of side effects must be assessed by someone other than the patient.[13,33]

Epidural infusions also have been used for patients experiencing the intense pain of terminal malignancies. These patients may experience pain that is often so severe that parenteral analgesics provide inadequate pain relief and produce deep respiratory depression. Epidural infusions for prolonged periods have been used in these patients. Transdermal fentanyl patches also may be used for these patients and for patients experiencing chronic pain.

## TEMPERATURE CONTROL

Monitoring temperature is an important part of anesthesia monitoring. The monitoring of temperature was not routinely practiced until malignant hyperthermia (MH) was described in the 1960s. This complication eventually led to the routine monitoring of body temperature in the OR.[16] Increased attention has been directed toward maintaining a normal temperature range perioperatively for pediatric and adult patients. Hypothermia is the most common disorder of temperature homeostasis. It may be intentional or unintentional. Unintentional hypothermia can cause patient discomfort, untoward cardiac events, adrenergic stimulation, impaired platelet function, altered drug metabolism, and impaired wound healing. A multidisciplinary task force has developed a clinical guideline for preventing unplanned hypothermia in the adult surgical patient (see Chapter 9).

Contributing risk factors for the development of inadvertent hypothermia include age extremes (elderly and pediatric patients), co-morbidity, length of the surgical procedure, cachexia, fluid shifts, cold irrigating fluids, and general and regional anesthesia. Agents such as skeletal muscle relaxants interfere with shivering mechanisms. Agents that depress the central nervous system decrease autonomic reflexes that ordinarily autoregulate body temperature. Vasodilation, which accompanies various anesthetic agents, including the inhalation agents, enhances heat transfer from the core to the periphery, where it is lost to the atmosphere. Cold, unhumidified inhalation gases further promote hypothermia through convection and evaporation.

The room temperature can be increased and infrared warming lamps used for pediatric patients. Fresh-gas flow rates of cool, dry anesthetic gases can be lowered. A heat and moisture exchanger (e.g., Humidivent) helps to maintain the heat and moisture of inspired gases. A variety of IV fluid warmers are available to warm crystalloid solutions or refrigerated blood products. Some of these units, originally designed for major trauma procedures, warm fluids at flow rates of 500 mL/min. Units that blow heated air onto the upper or lower body surface also are available. These units are effective in maintaining body temperature even during a long abdominal procedure and can be used subsequently in the PACU (see Chapter 9). Forced-air warming units must be used according to manufacturers' instructions. They must be used with the appropriate disposable patient warming blankets and should *not* have the hose inserted under the surgical drapes to warm the patient (this directs the heat on the patient, with the risk of a burn, rather than filtering it through the blanket). The blanket air temperature is typically a couple of degrees lower than that coming directly from the hose because heat is dissipated as it moves through the blanket.

## MALIGNANT HYPERTHERMIA

First identified in the late 1960s, malignant hyperthermia (MH) is a rare, life-threatening complication that may be triggered by drugs commonly used in anesthesia. Inhalational anesthetics and succinylcholine are the most frequently implicated triggering agents. Trauma, strenuous exercise, or emotional stress also may induce MH. It is a multifactorial disease and is genetically transmitted as an autosomal dominant trait with variable expression in affected individuals. Incidence of MH is increased in patients with central core disease (a congenital myopathy) and some muscular dystrophies.[15,22,32]

The syndrome begins with a hypermetabolic condition in skeletal muscle cells that involves altered mechanisms of calcium function at the cellular level. Characteristics of the syndrome include cellular hypermetabolism resulting in hypercarbia, tachypnea, tachycardia, hypoxia, metabolic and respiratory acidosis, cardiac dysrhythmias, and elevation of body temperature at a rate of 1°C to 2°C every 5 minutes. The increase in body temperature is a late manifestation of MH. These signs may occur during induction or maintenance of anesthesia, although the syndrome can occur postoperatively or even after repeated exposures to anesthesia. It is seen most frequently in children and adolescents.[15,22,32] The signs and symptoms associated with MH are listed in Box 4-3.

It is important to remember that (1) MH is a rare, multifaceted syndrome and can have variable clinical presentations; (2) many of the signs and symptoms associated with MH can have other causes; and (3) other disorders, such as neuroleptic malignant syndrome (NMS), may have similar presentations. (NMS occurs after use of neuroleptic drugs, such as haloperidol, and is characterized by muscular rigidity, akinesia, hyperthermia, and autonomic dysfunction.) Because MH is such a life-threatening disorder, many anesthesia providers initiate a

**BOX 4-3**

**Signs and Symptoms Often Seen with Malignant Hyperthermia**

- Hypercarbia
- Tachycardia
- Tachypnea (may not be seen in a paralyzed patient)
- Muscle stiffness or rigidity
- Hypoxia and dark (desaturated) blood in operative field
- Unstable or elevated blood pressure
- Cardiac dysrhythmias
- Changes in $CO_2$ absorbent (temperature, color)
- Metabolic and respiratory acidosis
- Peripheral mottling, cyanosis, or sweating
- Rising body temperature (1°C to 2°C every 5 minutes)
- Myoglobinuria
- Hyperkalemia, hypercalcemia, lactic acidemia
- Pronounced elevation in creatine kinase

BOX 4-4

### Emergency Management of Malignant Hyperthermia

1. Immediately discontinue all triggering agents (inhalational anesthetics and succinylcholine).
2. Terminate surgery if possible, or continue with safe anesthetic drugs.
3. Hyperventilate with 100% $O_2$ at highest flow rate. It is not necessary to change any anesthesia equipment.
4. Immediately give dantrolene sodium (Dantrium) 2 to 3 mg/kg IV. Give additional incremental doses up to 10 mg/kg total or until the signs of malignant hyperthermia (MH) are controlled.
5. Give sodium bicarbonate IV to correct the metabolic acidosis. Refer to arterial blood gas (ABG) values to determine dosage. If ABG are not available, consider administering 1 to 2 mEq/kg IV.
6. If the patient is hyperthermic, begin active cooling.
   a. Inject iced saline (not lactated Ringer's solution) IV 15 mL/kg every 15 minutes × 3.
   b. Use iced saline to lavage the stomach, bladder, rectum, and open body cavities as feasible.
   c. Cool the body surface with a hypothermia blanket. Rub with cold, wet towels or ice.
   d. Monitor the temperature to avoid hypothermia.
7. Cardiac dysrhythmias usually resolve with correction of acidosis and hyperkalemia. If not, antidysrhythmic agents, such as procainamide 3 mg/kg (maximum 15 mg/kg), may be used. Avoid calcium-entry blockers because they may cause hyperkalemia and cardiovascular collapse.
8. Closely monitor temperature, $ETco_2$, arterial or central venous blood gases, urine output, $K^+$, $Ca^{++}$, and coagulation studies. Insert a urinary catheter. Consider arterial line and a central venous or pulmonary arterial (PA) catheter.
9. Hyperkalemia is common. Treat with hyperventilation, sodium bicarbonate, or 10 units of regular insulin in 50 mL of 50% dextrose ($D_{50}$) IV titrated to $K^+$ level or regular insulin 0.15 units/kg in $D_{50}$ 1 mL/kg. Life-threatening hyperkalemia also may be treated with calcium (e.g., 2.5 mg/kg of $CaCl_2$).
10. Maintain urine output >2 mg/kg/hr. Consider volume of urine output to determine need for mannitol or furosemide.
11. Children <10 to 12 years old who have a sudden cardiac arrest without hypoxia after succinylcholine may have subclinical muscular dystrophy. Treat for acute hyperkalemia first. Give $CaCl_2$ with other treatments in Step 9.
12. Transfer patient to intensive care unit (ICU) when stable. Monitor at least 24 hours for recurrence of MH and for late complications.
13. Administer dantrolene 1 mg/kg IV every 6 hours for 24 to 48 hours. Then dantrolene 1 mg/kg every 6 hours for 24 hours may be given orally as necessary.
14. Monitor core body temperature (continuously), ABG, $K^+$, $Ca^{++}$, creatine kinase (CK), serum and urine myoglobin, and coagulation studies until values return to normal.
15. Counsel the patient and family about MH and further precautions. Refer the patient to MHAUS, and submit an Adverse Metabolic Reaction to Anesthesia (AMRA) report to the North American Malignant Hyperthermia Registry at 1-888-274-7899.

Modified from Malignant Hyperthermia Association of the United States: Emergency therapy for malignant hyperthermia. 2005. Accessed June 10, 2005, on-line: www.mhaus.org. MHAUS 24-hour hotline: 1-800-MH-HYPER (1-800-644-9737); Redmond MC: Malignant hyperthermia: perianesthesia recognition, treatment, and care, *Journal of PeriAnesthesia Nursing* 16(4):259-270, 2001.

treatment protocol when some of these early signs and symptoms occur that cannot otherwise be readily explained.

Time is crucial when MH is diagnosed. All OR and anesthesia personnel should be familiar with the protocol for its management. In the past, mortality ranged up to 80%, but the immediate infusion of dantrolene (Dantrium) and proper treatment have reduced the mortality rate to about 7%. Dantrolene is a hydantoin skeletal muscle relaxant that also has effects on vascular and heart muscle. In addition to dantrolene, the major modalities of treatment include cooling the patient with ice packs and cold IV solutions, administering diuretics, treating cardiac dysrhythmias, correcting acid-base and electrolyte imbalances, and monitoring fluid intake and output and the body temperature. Many hospitals maintain an emergency MH kit or cart that contains the drugs, laboratory tubes, other supplies, and instructions to treat MH in the OR area. Location of the iced or cold saline and other equipment also should be listed with the emergency kit. Chilled saline is often kept in the refrigeration unit for blood products.[15,22] An outline for emergency treatment of MH is provided in Box 4-4. The Malignant Hyperthermia Association of the United States (MHAUS) has names of on-call physicians available for consultation in MH emergencies at 1-800-MH-HYPER (1-800-644-9737). For patient-referral or nonemergency calls, 1-607-674-7910 should be used.

Patients known or suspected to have MH can be anesthetized with minimal risk if appropriate precautions are taken. If the syndrome is suspected, a muscle biopsy specimen should be obtained to make a diagnosis before the patient is electively anesthetized. For their own safety, relatives of persons with MH should be evaluated for presence of the syndrome.[22] MHAUS announced that a molecular genetic diagnostic test is now available. This new test would allow patients and their families who are uncertain about whether or not they are at risk for MH to determine their risk by means of a DNA analysis obtained from a blood sample.[18] According to Rosenberg, president of MHAUS, "the genetics test does not take the place of the current muscle biopsy, but it could identify the 50% of those at risk in an MH susceptible family. It is not a screening test. However, it is a first step...."[18,21,22]

## SAFETY OF HEALTH CARE WORKERS

The transmission of diseases including hepatitis B virus, hepatitis C virus (HCV), and human immunodeficiency virus (HIV) from body fluids is a major concern for health care workers. An estimated 3.9 million Americans have been infected with HCV.[10] HCV infection is the most common chronic bloodborne infection in the United States.[10] All health care workers should observe Standard and Transmission-Based Precautions for body fluids. It has been shown that blood, serum, and CSF have higher concentrations of HIV than saliva, tears, urine, breast milk, amniotic fluid, and vaginal secretions. Precautions include use of protective eyewear, facemasks, and gloves and use of a needleless system, stopcocks, or one-way injection devices for all IV medications given to infected patients.

With the implementation of Standard and Transmission-Based Precautions among health care workers, a new problem has arisen. The increased need to use latex gloves and products has created a rapidly growing segment of health care workers who are allergic to latex products. This is seen most frequently in dental or medical (e.g., anesthesia, perioperative) personnel who repeatedly change inexpensive, disposable latex gloves. Alternatives, such as vinyl gloves, are not satisfactory. Polyvinyl gloves are probably the least expensive and most widely used non-latex glove alternative. Their main disadvantages are inflexibility and permeability to fluids and infectious agents. Vinyl gloves may also contain colorants and formaldehyde, which may produce delayed-type allergy.[35] Patients with certain congenital deformities or who require multiple surgical procedures have an increased risk of developing a latex allergy. Management of an anaphylactic reaction to latex during anesthesia is described in Box 4-5. (See Chapter 2 for more information on latex allergies.)

## OPERATING ROOM POLLUTION

Contamination and pollution of the OR environment can come from many sources. Every chemical should be considered harmful until proved otherwise. Reaction to chemicals and irritants may vary with age, gender, race, season of the year, and concurrent exposure to other substances. Disinfectants, antiseptics, soaps, aerosol or pressurized sprays, and other compounds contribute to the pollution potential. Attention also is being paid to noise pollution. Of particular interest in the present context is the pollution of the OR with anesthetic gases, such as $N_2O$ and the inhalation anesthetics. Various surveys taken among personnel exposed to these anesthetic gases (anesthesia providers, other anesthesia personnel, perioperative nurses, dentists, dental assistants who work with anesthetic gases) and their spouses have implicated such pollution as a possible contributing factor to an increased abortion rate and incidence of lymphoma and other conditions. The interpretation of these surveys is controversial, however.

To minimize the hazards of bacteria, other airborne pollutants, and waste anesthetic gases, most OR suites condition and filter their own air and provide more than 15 air exchanges each hour. To minimize contamination, the air pressure inside each OR is usually greater than that in adjacent hallways. To reduce pollution from trace anesthetic gases and to contain costs, many anesthesia providers use "low-flow" anesthetic techniques that greatly reduce the volume of waste gases. Air

**BOX 4-5**

### Latex Allergy

The incidence of allergic reactions to latex products has escalated rapidly. Occupational asthma caused by natural rubber latex (NRL) has been reported in health care workers. It is the most frequent cause of anaphylaxis in children. There are two high-risk groups: (1) health care workers (especially workers who repeatedly change latex gloves or products to implement Standard Precautions) and (2) compromised patients who are exposed to latex products through multiple surgical or invasive procedures. Seventy percent of children with myelomeningocele are reportedly allergic to latex, compared to 1% to 5% of healthy children. The risk of latex allergy in health care providers is 13.7% for dental personnel, 7.5% for physicians, 5.6% for nurses, and 1.3% for hospital workers compared with 10% for workers in the rubber industry and 0.08% for the general public. Latex allergy occurs in 18% to 40% of patients with spina bifida and in 35% to 83% of patients with a history of atopy (e.g., allergic response to balloons, rubber gloves, or certain foods or fruits).

Latex-induced anaphylaxis comprises about 10% of the life-threatening anaphylactic reactions that occur during anesthesia. The intensity of the reactions varies and may include contact dermatitis, conjunctivitis, asthma, angioedema, anaphylaxis, perioperative hemodynamic collapse, or death. Allergy is an undesirable physiologic response to a foreign substance, which may be nonimmunologic (initial exposure) or immunologic (reexposure). Reactions mediated by IgE antibodies are called *anaphylactic reactions* and can be confirmed by IgE antibody titers or allergy skin tests. Reactions that may be similar but not proved to result from IgE antibodies are called *anaphylactoid reactions.*

A careful preoperative evaluation should be done of all "high-risk" patients (e.g., patients with spina bifida, urogenital abnormalities; patients who have had multiple surgeries; health care workers; individuals with atopy, extensive exposure to rubber products, or a history of latex allergy). If indicated by the evaluation, a latex allergy can be confirmed by tests such as radioallergosorbent test (RAST) for latex-specific immunoassays, AlaSTAT test for latex-specific IgE allergens, skin-prick testing (SPT) for IgE-mediated latex hypersensitivity, or a patch test for delayed hypersensitivity reactions.

Preoperative prophylaxis with steroids or histamine ($H_1$ and $H_2$) blockers does not prevent IgE-mediated anaphylactic reactions to latex. Such reactions usually occur 10 to 40 minutes after induction of anesthesia, but may occur up to 290 minutes later. The severity and intensity of the reactions vary.

Management of an anaphylactic reaction to latex should include stopping all anesthetics, giving 100% $O_2$ with controlled ventilation, changing to latex-free gloves and products, and infusing intravenous fluids to sustain blood pressure. Most anesthesia machines that have been serviced recently by factory-authorized personnel should be "latex-free," and changing anesthesia machines should not be required. If necessary, the following intravenous drugs may be given: epinephrine 3 to 5 mcg/kg, plus an infusion of 1 to 4 mcg/kg/min; diphenhydramine 0.5 to 1 mg/kg; aminophylline 1 to 6 mg/kg over 20 minutes, followed by an infusion of 0.5 to 0.9 mcg/kg/hr if bronchospasm continues; steroids such as methylprednisolone 1 to 2 g, hydrocortisone 1 g, or dexamethasone 4 to 20 mg; and sodium bicarbonate 0.5 to 1 mEq/kg if acidosis or hypotension persists.

Arterial blood gases should be obtained. Blood analyses for tryptase and specific IgE antibodies should be obtained. Urinary methylhistamine should be measured within 3 hours. Because laryngeal edema can occur, the airway should be evaluated carefully. The patient should be monitored in the ICU for 24 to 48 hours after an anaphylactic reaction.

The National Institute for Occupational Safety and Health (NIOSH) released a medical alert titled "Preventing Allergic Reactions to Natural Rubber Latex in the Workplace" on June 23, 1997. A copy may be obtained from the NIOSH homepage at www.cdc.gov/niosh/homepage.

Modified from Amr S, Bollinger ME: Latex allergy and occupational asthma in healthcare workers: adverse outcomes, *Environmental Health Perspective* 112(3):378-381, 2004; AORN Latex Guideline. In: *AORN standards, recommended practice and guidelines*, Denver, Colo, 2005, The Association; Warshaw EM: Latex allergy, *SkinMed Dermatology for the Clinician* 2(6):359-366, 2003.

pollution with waste anesthetic gases is still a major concern, however, and all anesthesia machines should have a waste-gas-scavenging system. In modern OR suites, a dedicated vacuum line is used to scavenge such gases. Evacuation hoses are connected to the ventilator and the adjustable pressure-limiting (APL) valve. When the patient is not intubated, however, air pollution may occur from a loose mask fit on the patient's face. According to the National Institute for Occupational Safety and Health (NIOSH), pollution levels should be less than 25 parts per million (ppm) (time-weighted average) for $N_2O$ and 2 ppm for halogenated agents. These levels are difficult to achieve during induction and emergence.[13]

Chronic occupational exposure to trace concentrations of anesthetic gases is of particular concern to pregnant women. A safe exposure level below which one can be assured that no adverse effects would occur has not been established. Individuals with questions about exposure levels should consult a knowledgeable member of the anesthesia department for the latest information.

## PERIOPERATIVE NURSING CONSIDERATIONS

Care of the surgical patient is a cooperative effort, and personnel involved in the perioperative period should function as a smooth, well-coordinated team. As part of conducting the preoperative patient assessment and developing the nursing plan of care, the perioperative nurse participates with the anesthesia provider in the preoperative verification process. As part of this process, the nurse checks the chart to verify the patient's identity, the surgeon, and the scheduled procedure; confirms that the operative and anesthesia permits are properly signed; identifies and communicates any patient allergies; ensures that the surgical site is marked; and ensures that current reports of laboratory tests and diagnostic studies are complete and on the chart.

In many OR suites, a preoperative preparation or *holding area* is used for procedures such as the insertion of arterial, central venous, or pulmonary arterial catheters and placement of epidural catheters or peripheral nerve blocks. Nursing personnel from the OR, PACU, or anesthesiology department may staff this area. The purpose of this area is to improve patient care delivery, optimize the perioperative flow of patients, and provide support services for the just-mentioned procedures. The minimum requirement for monitoring should be an ECG, noninvasive blood pressure, and pulse oximetry. Equipment for emergency airway management should be readily available. It is important that the nursing staff be familiar with such equipment and be readily available to assist in its use.

A patient should never be left alone in the OR suite. When an anesthetized patient is in the OR, a perioperative nurse always should be immediately available to provide assistance if needed. During the insertion of IV, arterial, central venous, or pulmonary arterial catheters, the nurse should assist as required.

During induction of anesthesia, particularly with a traumatized patient or for an emergency procedure, the perioperative nurse should be ready to apply cricoid pressure to prevent regurgitation of stomach contents and assist the anesthesia provider in visualizing the vocal cords. When cricoid pressure is used to prevent aspiration, it should not be released until the intubation is accomplished, the cuff on the ETT is inflated, and proper placement of the ETT has been verified. When two anesthesia providers are present, one of them usually provides this support.

OR personnel should never move an unconscious patient without first coordinating the positioning or move with the anesthesia provider. When the patient is positioned for surgery, the perioperative nurse always should collaborate with the anesthesia provider in checking the arms and legs to ensure that no pressure points exist and that the extremities are appropriately positioned and padded (see Chapter 5). After positioning, prepping, and draping, the time out is conducted and documented.

Before transporting the patient from the OR to the PACU, the circulating nurse, in some institutions, may call the PACU and give a preliminary status report of the patient's condition. This report includes the surgical procedure performed, type of anesthesia care provided, information specific to the patient's preoperative diagnosis and subsequent outcome related to intraoperative intervention, and any special equipment required (e.g., ventilator, T-piece, arterial pressure monitor). Postanesthesia recovery care and functions are described in Chapter 9.

## REFERENCES


1. American Association of Nurse Anesthetists: AANA archives-library: a brief look at nurse anesthesia history. Accessed June 4, 2005, on-line: www.aana.com/archives/timeline.asp.
2. American Society of Anesthesiologists: Practice guidelines for management of the difficult airway, *Anesthesiology* 98:1269-1277, 2003.
3. Amr S, Bollinger ME: Latex allergy and occupational asthma in health-care workers: adverse outcomes, *Environmental Health Perspective* 112(3):378-381, 2004.
4. Association of periOperative Registered Nurses: Recommended practices for documentation of perioperative nursing care. In: *Standards, recommended practices and guidelines,* Denver, Colo, 2005, AORN.
5. Association of periOperative Registered Nurses: Recommended practices for managing the patient receiving conscious sedation/analgesia. In: *Standards, recommended practices and guidelines,* Denver, Colo, 2005, AORN.
6. Bankert M: *Watchful care: a history of America's nurse anesthetists,* New York, 2000, Continuum Publishing Company.
7. Brain A and others: *LMA instruction manual,* San Diego, 1996, Gensia, Inc.
8. Brown DL: *Atlas of regional anesthesia,* ed 2, Philadelphia, 1999, Saunders.
9. Burkard J and others: Regional anesthesia. In Nagelhout JJ and others, editors: *Nurse anesthesia,* ed 3, St Louis, 2005, Mosby.
10. Centers for Disease Control and Prevention: Hepatitis C: what clinicians and other health professionals need to know. 2005. Accessed May 25, 2006, on-line: www.cdc.gov/ncidod/diseases/hepatitisc_training/edu/default.htm.
11. DeLamar LM: Preparing your patient for surgery, *Topics in Advanced Practice Nursing eJournal, Medscape* 5(1), 2005.
12. Dosch M: Anesthesia equipment. In Nagelhout JJ and others, editors: *Nurse anesthesia,* ed 3, St Louis, 2005, Mosby.
13. Faut-Callahan M, Hand WR: Pain management. In Nagelhout JJ and others, editors: *Nurse anesthesia,* ed 3, St Louis, 2005, Mosby.
14. Gunn IP: Nurse anesthesia: a history of challenge. In Nagelhout JJ and others, editors: *Nurse anesthesia,* ed 3, St Louis, 2005, Mosby.
15. Karlet MC: Musculoskeletal system, anatomy, physiology and pathophysiology. In Nagelhout JJ and others, editors: *Nurse anesthesia,* ed 3, St Louis, 2005, Mosby.
16. Kossick MA, Wright EL: Clinical monitoring in anesthesia. In Nagelhout JJ and others, editors: *Nurse anesthesia,* ed 3, St Louis, 2005, Mosby.

17. Lennmarken C, Sandin R: Neuromonitoring for awareness during surgery, *Lancet* 363:1747-1748, 2004.
18. Litman RS, Rosenberg H: Malignant hyperthermia: update on susceptibility testing, *JAMA* 293:2918-2924, 2005.
19. Litwin AA: Mode of delivery following labor epidural analgesia: influence of ropivicaine and bupivicaine, *AANA Journal* 69(4):259-261, 2001.
20. *LMA airway instruction manual*. 2004. Accessed May 26, 2006, on-line: www.lmana.com.
21. Malignant hyperthermia susceptibility testing via RYRI (MHS1) gene screening. 2005. Accessed on-line: www.preventiongenetics.com/.
22. Malignant Hyperthermia Association of the United States. 2005. Accessed July 22, 2006 on-line: www.mhaus.org.
23. Moon RE, Camporesi EM: Respiratory monitoring. In Miller RD, editor: *Anesthesia,* ed 6, Philadelphia, 2005, Churchill Livingstone, pp. 1437-1474.

23a. Nagelhout JJ and others, editors: *Nurse Anesthesia,* ed 2, Philadelphia, 2001, Saunders.

24. Naguib M, Lien CA: Pharmacology of muscle relaxants and their antagonists. In Miller RD, editor: *Anesthesia,* ed 6, Philadelphia, 2005, Churchill Livingstone.
25. Pisegna JR, Martindale RG: Acid suppression in the perioperative period, *Journal of Clinical Gastroenterology* 39(1):10-16, 2005.
26. Sebel PS and others: The incidence of awareness during anesthesia: a multicenter United States study, *Anesthesia and Analgesia* 99:833-839, 2004.
27. Stanski DR, Shafer SL: Measuring depth of anesthesia. In Miller RD, editor: *Anesthesia,* ed 6, Philadelphia, 2005, Churchill Livingstone.
28. Stoelting RK: Local anesthetics. In: *Pharmacology and physiology in anesthetic practice,* ed 3, Philadelphia, 1999, Lippincott-Raven.
29. Stoelting RK: Pharmacokinetics and pharmacodynamics of injected and inhaled drugs. In: *Pharmacology and physiology in anesthetic practice,* ed 3, Philadelphia, 1999, Lippincott-Raven, pp. 1-30.
30. Stoelting RK, Miller RD: Preoperative preparation and intraoperative management. In: *Basics of anesthesia,* ed 4, New York, 2000, Churchill Livingstone.
31. Stoelting RK, Miller RD: Preoperative medication. In: *Basics of anesthesia,* ed 4, New York, 2000, Churchill Livingstone, pp. 121-134.
32. Theroux MC: Malignant hyperthermia. In Litman RS, editor: *Pediatric anesthesia, the requisites in anesthesiology*, ed 1, Philadelphia, 2004, Saunders..
33. Tobias JD, Litman RS: Pediatric regional anesthesia. In Litman RS, editor: *Pediatric anesthesia, the requisites in anesthesiology*, ed 1, Philadelphia, 2004, Saunders.
34. Warner MA: Is pulmonary aspiration still an important problem in anesthesia? *Current Opinions in Anesthesiology* 13:215-218, 2000.
35. Warshaw EM: Latex allergy, *SkinMed Dermatology for the Clinician* 2(6):359-366, 2003.

CHAPTER 5

# Positioning the Patient for Surgery

PAULINE ANNE HEIZENROTH

## OVERVIEW

Proper patient positioning is essential for safe, successful surgical procedures. The surgical team plays a significant role in ensuring uncompromised and physiologically safe patient positioning by understanding the systems affected by positioning and their associated risks. Because surgery may be performed on all anatomic areas, the body may be positioned in multiple and sometimes unnatural configurations to expose a surgical site. Positioning, combined with anesthesia and its physiologic effects, can yield undesirable changes if safety factors are not considered. This chapter discusses some of the risks and prevention strategies associated with standard surgical positions.

The goals of surgical positioning include providing optimal exposure and access to the surgical site, maintaining body alignment, supporting circulatory and respiratory function, protecting neuromuscular and skin integrity, and allowing access to intravenous sites and anesthesia support devices. Meeting these goals while maintaining the patient's comfort and safety is the responsibility of every member of the surgical team.

## ANATOMIC AND PHYSIOLOGIC CONSIDERATIONS

The perioperative nurse must thoroughly understand the anatomic and physiologic changes associated with positioning the patient. These changes are affected by numerous factors, such as the type of surgical position; the length of time the patient is in that position; the operating room (OR) bed, padding, and positioning devices used; the type of anesthesia given; and the operative procedure. These changes most frequently involve (1) the skin and underlying tissue; (2) the musculoskeletal system; (3) the nervous system; (4) the cardiovascular system; (5) the respiratory system; and (6) other vulnerable areas, such as the eyes, breasts, perineum, and fingers.

### Skin and Underlying Tissue

The physical forces used to establish and maintain a surgical position can injure the skin and underlying tissue. These forces include *pressure, shear,* and *friction.* Additionally, OR conditions such as moisture, heat, and negativity further increase the vulnerability of the skin and underlying tissues to injury.

- *Pressure* is the force placed on underlying tissue. Pressure can come from the weight of the body as gravity presses it downward toward the surface of the bed. Pressure also can come from the weight of equipment resting on or against the patient, such as drills, Mayo stands, surgical instruments, rigid edges of the OR bed or its attachments, or vertical posts for self-retaining retractors. Positioning devices, such as stirrup bars, leg or arm holders, and edges of laminectomy frames, can rest against the patient under tension. Surgical team members can lean on the patient and cause various degrees of pressure.
- *Shear* is the folding of underlying tissue when the skeletal structure moves while the skin remains stationary. A parallel force creates shear compared with a perpendicular force created by pressure. This can happen when the head of the bed is raised or lowered and when the patient is placed in Trendelenburg (head down, supine) or reverse Trendelenburg (head up, supine) position. As gravity pulls the skeleton down, the stretching, folding, and tearing of the underlying tissues as they slide with the skeleton occlude vascular perfusion, which leads to tissue ischemia.
- *Friction* is the force of two surfaces rubbing against one another. Friction on the patient's skin can occur when the body is dragged across bed linen instead of being lifted.[18] Friction can denude the epidermis and make the skin more susceptible to higher stages of pressure ulcer formation and pain and infection.
- *Moisture,* in excess, can exacerbate the effects of pressure, shear, and friction. Maceration occurs when prolonged moisture on the skin saturates the epidermis to the point that the connective tissue fibers dissolve[15] and can be easily torn apart. The skin becomes weakened and more vulnerable to the detrimental effects of external forces. In surgery, maceration can occur by the patient perspiring or lying in a pool of prep solution, blood, irrigation solution, urine, or feces. If this moisture also is located in an area of high pressure, the risk of pressure ulcer expansion into higher stages increases. If friction occurs on macerated skin, it becomes more vulnerable to denuding into the dermal layer. Every effort should be made to avoid pooling of prep solution. Prolonged exposure to the chemicals in the skin prep under the pressure area also can increase the likelihood of chemically induced contact dermatitis.[18]
- *Heat* on the body surface can increase the metabolism of the tissue and increase the oxygen and nutritional demands. If the tissue is also under pressure, constriction of vessels may impede blood flow enough that those demands are not met. Preexisting vascular impairment and the hypotensive effects of anesthesia may exacerbate the tissue further and lead to cellular tissue damage. This is especially true when the heated surface is under the weight of the body. Excessive heat can cause thermal damage as well, resulting in burns.
- *Cold* environmental conditions, such as those found in the OR, can lead to hypothermia. Major surgery can cool the

patient further by exposing the core of the body to the cold air. A cold core temperature can reduce peripheral circulation, reducing oxygen delivery to the skin and underlying tissue.[29]

- *Negativity* occurs when layers of materials, such as extra sheets or blankets, are placed over the OR mattress or padding. Extra linen can add rigidity and diminish the pressure-reducing properties of the mattress or padding. It is absorbent and abrasive and can produce high and inconsistent pressure. Eliminating extra layers of material between the patient and the OR bed can reduce sacral pressure readings.[15,18]

***Pressure Ulcers.*** A pressure ulcer (pressure sore) is an injury to the skin and underlying tissue as a result of unrelieved pressure (see History box). Between 1990 and 2000, the prevalence rate of pressure ulcers in acute care settings was 15%. Prevalence in the OR was 8.5%. The most frequently reported location was the sacrum or coccyx; the second most frequent location was the heels.[12]

Pressure ulcers have a tremendous cost and impact on patients and health care institutions. Patients may endure often needless pain, suffering, and lost productivity. Health care institutions expend countless billions of dollars annually in treatment and increased hospital stays. Because it costs more to treat than to prevent pressure ulcers, research has focused on trying to determine causes of pressure ulcer development and effective preventive strategies.[28]

Pressure ulcer development depends on extrinsic and intrinsic contributing factors. *Extrinsic* factors include the physical forces and conditions the patient is subjected to during surgery as described earlier. *Intrinsic* factors include the internal health conditions and the physical body structure of the patient. The interaction of these factors contributes to the overall risk of developing pressure ulcers.

**EXTRINSIC FACTORS.** Pressure is the physical force most responsible for pressure ulcer formation. Its intensity and duration are the primary factors involved.[29] An inverse relationship exists between pressure and time. The greater the pressure, the shorter the amount of time it takes to cause ischemic changes. Pressures greater than 32 mm Hg (capillary interface pressure) can occlude the flow of the arterioles, which nourish and oxygenate the tissue at the capillary level. An individual can endure relatively large amounts of pressure for a short time or low amounts of pressure for a longer time without sustaining tissue damage.[3] A point in time can be reached, however, when the tissue no longer can withstand the pressure (especially if it is >32 mm Hg), and cells die from the lack of oxygen and nutrients. Such prolonged pressure can result in tissue ischemia manifested as a pressure ulcer.[1]

The intensity of pressure is contingent on the size of the surface area being compressed. The smaller the surface area in which pressure is applied, the greater the force (pressure per surface area). Compression of tissue between an external surface and a bony prominence of the body tends to create high forces of pressure in the local tissue surrounding that bone. Pressure ulcers are most likely to develop around protruding bony prominences such as the heels, elbows, and sacrum in the supine position. The tissue injury is highest in the deep areas immediately adjacent to the bone. Because the deeper ischemia progresses outward toward the skin, the damage may not be visible for several days. If pressure could be distributed more evenly over other surfaces of the body, the force of the pressure in those vulnerable areas could be reduced. This theory fuels manufacturers to create OR mattresses, overlays, and padding materials that are designed to distribute the forces of pressure more evenly (see "Operating Room Beds" later in this chapter for a more detailed discussion).

The amount of time that is required for OR-acquired pressure ulcer development has been a topic of much research.

## HISTORY

One of the most emphasized aspects of surgical positioning has been that of maintaining tissue integrity by preventing pressure ulcers. In the past, terms for this condition included *decubitus ulcers* and *bedsores.* The early term, *decubitus,* is a Latin derivative of the word *cumbere,* which means "to lie down." In 1749 the Frenchman Quesnay coined the term *bedsores* to distinguish between sores caused by lying down and sores caused by other diseases. *Decubitus ulcer* and *bedsore* both implied that recumbency was the primary reason for this condition. The true source of the injury, *pressure,* can be achieved through other means, however (e.g., sitting in a wheelchair; unrelieved pressure from a rigid surface, such as an appliance or cast). *Pressure sore* and *pressure ulcer* became the more accurate terms used to describe this condition.

Pressure ulcers are known to have been a problem as far back as the time of the pharaohs. Pressure ulcers were discovered on the mummy of an Egyptian princess. In the 1800s, Brown-Séquard identified pressure and moisture as causing ulceration of the skin, and Paget described these ulcers as the sloughing and death of a part resulting from pressure. In 1930 Lanis determined that 32 mm Hg is the average capillary pressure at arterial inflow. This value is still accepted as the threshold beyond which tissue trauma occurs. In 1946 Guttman appreciated the importance of relieving pressure in the bedridden patient by initiating a lifting and turning team on a spinal cord injury unit in England. In 1953 Husian showed that there was an inverse relationship between pressure and time for the development of pressure ulcers. In studies using rats, he found that low pressures maintained for long periods produced more tissue damage than high pressures for short periods. He also found that the smaller the surface area over which the compressive force was applied, the greater the damage to the tissue. In 1959 Kosiak experimented with dogs and found that their tissue, when subjected to 60 to 70 mm Hg pressure for an average of 2 hours, began to show microscopic damage. Two-hour turning schedules were used to reduce pressure ulcer development in bedridden patients.

The findings of these early studies laid the foundation for many of the pressure ulcer prevention strategies practiced today. Continued research and technologic advances in support materials have focused on reducing the incidence of pressure ulcers originating in all settings, including the OR.

Modified from Allman RM: Pressure sores among the elderly, *New England Journal of Medicine* 320:850-853, 1989; Copeland-Fields LD, Hoshiko BR: Clinical validation of Braden and Bergstrom's conceptual schema of pressure sore risk factors, *Rehabilitation Nursing* 14(5):257-260, 1989; Goodman T and others: Skin ulcers: overview and nursing implications, *AORN Journal* 50(1):24-37, 1990; Makleburst J: Pressure ulcers: etiology and prevention, *Nursing Clinics of North America* 22(2):359-375, 1987; Narcete TA and others: Pressure sores, *American Family Physician* 28(3):135-139, 1983; Souther SG and others: Pressure, tissue ischemia, and operating room pads, *Archives of Surgery* 107(10):544-547, 1973; Torrance C: *Pressure sores: aetiology, treatment, and prevention,* London, 1983, Croom Helm.

Generally, surgeries lasting 2 hours or longer have been linked with pressure ulcer formation. As the time on the OR bed increases, so does the prevalence of pressure ulcers.[30] Duration is considered more of a causative factor than is the intensity of the pressure. Healthy individuals may tolerate high external pressures (e.g., 100 mm Hg) over bony prominences for short periods. Constant, unrelieved pressure is most responsible for microscopic necrosis. Lowered pressures over extended periods also may cause tissue damage, particularly if tissue tolerance is diminished.[1] Frequent repositioning of an immobilized patient can protect against the adverse effects of pressure. Surgical procedures that extend beyond 2 hours often do not afford the opportunity for repositioning the patient, however. The perioperative nurse should plan ahead to ensure that preventive measures are taken to reduce pressure ulcer risks. Pressure-relieving OR mattresses or overlays may reduce pressure in dependent areas. Padding applied under or around vulnerable areas, such as the heels, elbows, and sacrum and areas in contact with hard surfaces, can reduce localized pressure.

The type of positioning devices used can increase pressure ulcer development risk. Rigid, unpadded objects that press against a body surface, such as stirrup bars, compressed beanbags, or rolled sheets, can cause tissue injury if the pressure is not relieved periodically. Negativity, as explained earlier, can override the pressure-relieving capabilities of mattresses and padding. Placing a warm blanket under a patient may be soothing initially, but if a surgical procedure is long, pressure to the bony prominences resting on the blanket will be higher than if only a sheet and draw sheet are used. Additionally, wrinkles and folds can cause further pressure points.

When a patient is placed in a shear-producing position (e.g., semi-Fowler) before being prepped and draped, measures can be taken to reduce the shear forces. One technique is to lift the patient slightly momentarily to allow the skin to realign with its surrounding skeletal structures. When the patient is placed in these positions *during* a surgical procedure, however, interventions to reduce shearing are limited. Reducing the time that shearing forces are in place is the best countermeasure to reduce tissue injury.

The type of surgery being performed can have an impact on pressure ulcer development. The longer the procedure, the more at risk the patient becomes. Also, procedures that involve significant blood loss, extracorporeal circulation, and clamping of major vessels can contribute to the lack of blood flow to tissue under pressure. Patients who have cardiac surgery face a high risk for pressure ulcers, which occur in 9.2% to 38% of patients. This high risk is attributed to the diagnostic procedures these patients undergo, the long surgical time, and the extended period of restricted movement postoperatively.[25]

Anesthesia alters mobility by removing patients' protective mechanisms to shift their weight in response to pressure. Patients often are placed in situations that they would not be able to tolerate comfortably if they were awake or even asleep without the presence of anesthetics. Anesthesia also alters blood pressure, tissue perfusion, and oxygen and carbon dioxide exchange. All of these anesthetic effects can exacerbate the impact of pressure forces, particularly if other co-morbid conditions are present.

The vascular effects of anesthesia combined with the cool environment of the OR, exposure of external and internal body surfaces, and irrigation with unwarmed solutions can cause hypothermia, which increases the patient's heat metabolism. This increased metabolism leads to increased tissue needs for oxygen, nutrients, and metabolic waste-product removal.[29] When tissue is under pressure, these needs are not easily met. If a warming blanket is used under the patient in the area where the pressures are the greatest, the tissue requirements become even more intense, and the impact of tissue ischemia may be more profound. Research has shown that the use of a warming blanket under the patient can be the greatest predictor of pressure ulcer development. Warming the patient with forced-air warming therapy in nonpressure areas can decrease the risk of pressure ulcer development by offsetting many of the detrimental effects of hypothermia (Research Highlight).[29]

**INTRINSIC FACTORS.** Intrinsic factors can lower a patient's tissue tolerance to pressure and decrease the time and pressure required for tissue breakdown. Studies that associate particular comorbid medical conditions with pressure ulcer development in the OR show conflicting results. This may be because, as was just described, so many other intraoperative factors come into play, such as the length of the surgical procedure, positioning devices used, and physiologic changes encountered during the surgical procedure. Still, certain preexist-

## RESEARCH HIGHLIGHT

### Effects of Warming Therapy on Pressure Ulcer Prevention

Scott and colleagues conducted a randomized experimental study to test whether intraoperative control of hypothermia would reduce the incidence of postoperative pressure ulcers. Data were obtained on 324 patients, all undergoing major surgery that required a usual hospital stay of at least 5 days. The control group consisted of 163 patients who received standard care that consisted of automatic regulation of ambient air, minimal exposure during preparation time, and the use of blankets stored in warming units for immediate postoperative care. The warming of some intravenous infusions, particularly blood products, was determined by clinical need. The treatment group consisted of 161 patients who received standard care as described with the addition of forced-air warming blanket therapy and warmed intravenous fluids. Patient characteristics in both groups were similar.

The study results showed that 17 patients in the control group (10.4%) developed pressure ulcers compared with 9 patients in the treatment group (5.6%). Although not achieving statistical significance, the incidence of pressure ulcers was reduced by almost half by the use of intraoperative warming therapy, which was clinically significant. Neither duration of surgery nor individual health status seemed to be significantly related to pressure ulcer development. The percentage of affected patients increased, however, with higher American Society of Anesthesiologists (ASA) status (see Chapter 4). There was a significant correlation between patients with low body mass index (BMI) and the lowest temperatures recorded during surgery. This correlation suggests that patients with low body fat content are less likely to maintain body temperatures. The researchers concluded that all patients undergoing major surgery would benefit from intraoperative warming therapy, particularly patients with low BMI and high ASA grades, regardless of the expected duration of surgery.

Modified from Scott EM and others: Effects of warming therapy on pressure ulcers: a randomized study, *AORN Journal* 73(9):921-938, 2001.

ing conditions continue to be regarded as intrinsic risk factors for OR-induced pressure ulcer development. These conditions include respiratory and circulatory disorders, diabetes mellitus, anemia, malnutrition (serum albumin levels <3.5 g/dL), advanced age, body size (obesity and thin, frail build), body temperature (hypothermia), and impaired mobility.[3,25,28]

Various scales exist for determining pressure ulcer potential. One that is widely used is the Braden scale.[1,8] This scale scores a patient's potential for pressure sore development based on various intrinsic factors. A scale such as the Braden scale (Table 5-1) can be used during the preoperative assessment to guide perioperative nursing interventions. The Best Practice box explains how to interpret the Braden scale score and use the score to plan perioperative interventions. Assessment using this scale must be done before the induction of general anesthesia. Otherwise, all perioperative patients would receive the lowest possible scores on all but the moisture and nutrition subscales.[9]

Assessment for pressure ulcer risk factors and development should occur during three periods: *preoperative, intraoperative,* and *postoperative.* Preoperative assessment for intrinsic risk factors using a scale such as the Braden scale can determine if the patient may be at higher risk for tissue breakdown. This assessment can guide the nurse in the degree of padding and thermoregulation required. Consideration of expected OR events must be included in such assessments. Research indicates that *all* surgical patients should be considered at risk because of the variables inherent to the OR experience that often cannot be controlled. These variables include the need for vasoactive medications, the patient's hemodynamic state, and the length of the procedure.[3] The intraoperative assessment can include variables that occurred during surgery that could have an impact on tissue perfusion, such as the length of surgery, rigidity of positioning devices and length of time they were used, amount of blood loss, hypothermia, and anesthetic events such as ongoing diminished blood pressure. This information should be communicated with the hand-off report to the nurse in the postanesthesia care unit (PACU) receiving the patient (see Chapter 2 for a discussion of hand-off communication). Included in the postoperative assessment would be inspections for altered tissue integrity. These inspections would continue beyond the PACU to discharge.

**STAGING.** The Agency for Healthcare Research and Quality (AHRQ), formerly known as the Agency for Health Care Policy and Research (AHCPR), gives the following guidelines for the identification and staging of pressure ulcers:[1]

- *Stage 1:* Nonblanchable erythema (redness) of intact skin, is the heralding lesion of skin ulceration. In individuals with darker skin, discoloration of skin, warmth, edema, induration, and hardness also may be indicators. The definition according to the National Pressure Ulcer Advisory Panel (NPUAP)[23] is as follows: "A stage I pressure ulcer is an observable pressure-related alteration of intact skin whose indicators as compared to the adjacent or opposite area on the body may include changes in one or more of the following: skin temperature (warmth or coolness), tissue consistency (firm or boggy feel) and/or sensation (pain, itching). The ulcer appears as a defined area of persistent redness in lightly pigmented skin, whereas in darker skin tones, the ulcer may appear with persistent red, blue or purple hues."
    - Assessment of stage 1 pressure ulcers is difficult in patients with darkly pigmented skin. In lighter skinned individuals, a stage 1 pressure ulcer may change skin color to a dark purple or red area that does not become pale under fingertip pressure. In dark-skinned individuals, this area may become darker than normal. The affected area may feel warmer than surrounding tissue. When an eschar is present, accurate staging is impossible.
- *Stage 2:* Partial-thickness skin loss involving epidermis, dermis, or both (e.g., abrasion, blister, or shallow crater).
- *Stage 3:* Full-thickness skin loss involving damage to or necrosis of subcutaneous tissue that may extend down to but not through underlying fascia (deep crater with or without undermining). The ulcer presents clinically as a deep crater with or without undermining of adjacent tissue.
- *Stage 4:* Full-thickness skin loss with extensive destruction, tissue necrosis, or damage to muscle, bone, or supporting structures (e.g., tendon or joint capsule).

## BEST PRACTICE

### Braden Scale Assessment: Perioperative Implications

When using the Braden Scale (see Table 5-1) to assess pressure ulcer risk, the tool should not be altered. Because the tool has been tested for reliability and validity in its complete form, minor changes to shorten or otherwise alter it could affect the accuracy of the results. (This would violate copyright restrictions as well.) The lower the score, the greater the risk of developing pressure ulcers. The levels of risk according to scores are as follows:[8]

19-23, not at risk
15-18, mild risk
13-14, moderate risk
10-12, high risk
≤9, very high risk

All surgical patients should be considered at risk for pressure ulcer development. If, during the preoperative assessment, a patient's score is 18 or lower, the patient is at an increased risk for skin breakdown. The perioperative nurse should do the following with *all* surgical patients:

1. Before positioning, assess skin for evidence of diminished tissue integrity, particularly in areas over bony prominences.
2. Pad and protect any fragile skin areas, and limit the amount of time these areas are under pressure to the extent possible.
3. Pad under or around all areas in contact with a firm surface.
4. For immobile patients, do passive range of motion every 1½ to 2 hours to any accessible limbs and slight repositioning of the head if this does not interfere with the surgical procedure or the sterile integrity of the drapes.
5. Reassess skin postoperatively, document findings, and communicate any changes to appropriate personnel.

During the preoperative assessment, if the patient has a score of 18 or lower and an existing pressure ulcer (any stage) or areas of skin breakdown over bony prominences or has had muscle flap surgery, the perioperative nurse *additionally* should do the following:

1. Support and protect all existing wound dressings.
2. Arrange for the patient to be placed on a specialty bed designed for extreme pressure reduction postoperatively (e.g., alternating air mattress, flotation support bed).

**TABLE 5-1**

## Braden Scale for Predicting Pressure Sore Risk

| Category | 1 Point Per Square | 2 Points Per Square | 3 Points Per Square | 4 Points Per Square | Scores* |
|---|---|---|---|---|---|
| **SENSORY PERCEPTION** Ability to respond meaningfully to pressure-related discomfort | **COMPLETELY LIMITED** Unresponsive (does not moan, flinch, or grasp) to painful stimuli, owing to diminished level of consciousness or sedation, *or* limited ability to feel pain over most of body surface | **VERY LIMITED** Responds only to painful stimuli. Cannot communicate discomfort except by moaning or restlessness, *or* has a sensory impairment that limits the ability to feel pain or discomfort over half of body | **SLIGHTLY LIMITED** Responds to verbal commands but cannot always communicate discomfort or need to be turned, *or* has some sensory impairment that limits ability to feel pain or discomfort in one or two extremities | **NO IMPAIRMENT** Responds to verbal commands. Has no sensory deficit, which would limit ability to feel or voice pain or discomfort | **SCORE** ____ |
| **MOISTURE** Degree to which skin is exposed to moisture | **CONSTANTLY MOIST** Skin is kept moist almost constantly by perspiration or urine. Dampness is detected every time patient is moved or turned | **MOIST** Skin is often but not always moist. Linen must be changed at least once a shift | **OCCASIONALLY MOIST** Skin is occasionally moist, requiring an extra linen change approximately once a day | **RARELY MOIST** Skin is usually dry. Linen requires changing only at routine intervals | **SCORE** ____ |
| **ACTIVITY** Degree of physical activity | **BEDFAST** Confined to bed | **CHAIRFAST** Ability to walk severely limited or nonexistent. Cannot bear own weight or must be assisted into chair or wheelchair | **WALKS OCCASIONALLY** Walks occasionally during day but for very short distances, with or without assistance. Spends most of each shift in bed or chair | **WALKS FREQUENTLY** Walks outside the room at least twice a day and inside room at least once every 2 hr during waking hours | **SCORE** ____ |
| **MOBILITY** Ability to change and control body position | **COMPLETELY IMMOBILE** Does not make even slight changes in body or extremity position without assistance | **VERY LIMITED** Makes occasional slight changes in body or extremity position but unable to make frequent or significant changes independently | **SLIGHTLY LIMITED** Makes frequent although slight changes in body or extremity position independently | **NO LIMITATIONS** Makes major and frequent changes in position without assistance | **SCORE** ____ |
| **NUTRITION** Usual food intake pattern | **VERY POOR** Never eats a complete meal. Rarely eats more than a third of any food offered. Eats ≤2 servings of protein (meat or dairy products) per day. Takes fluids poorly. Does not take a liquid dietary supplement, *or* is NPO or maintained on clear liquids or IV for >5 days | **PROBABLY INADEQUATE** Rarely eats a complete meal and generally eats only about half of any food offered. Protein intake includes only 3 servings of meat or dairy products per day. Occasionally takes a dietary supplement, *or* receives less than optimum amount of liquid diet or tube feeding | **ADEQUATE** Eats more than half of most meals. Eats a total of 4 servings of protein (meat, dairy products) each day. Occasionally refuses a meal, but usually takes a supplement if offered, *or* is on a tube feeding or total parenteral nutrition (TPN) regimen, which probably meets most nutritional needs | **EXCELLENT** Eats most of every meal. Never refuses a meal. Usually eats a total of ≥4 servings of meat and dairy products. Occasionally eats between meals. Does not require supplementation | **SCORE** ____ |
| **FRICTION AND SHEAR** | **PROBLEM** Requires moderate to maximum assistance in moving. Complete lifting without sliding against sheets is impossible. Frequently slides down in bed or chair, requiring frequent repositioning with maximum assistance. Spasticity, contractures, or agitation leads to almost constant friction | **POTENTIAL PROBLEM** Moves feebly or requires minimum assistance. During a move skin probably slides to some extent against sheets, chair, restraints, or other devices. Maintains relatively good position in chair or bed most of the time but occasionally slides down | **NO APPARENT PROBLEM** Moves in bed and in chair independently and has sufficient muscle strength to lift up completely during move. Maintains good position in bed or chair at all times | | **SCORE** ____ |
| | | | | **Total Score** | ____ |

*See Best Practice box on page 133 for scoring implications.

Source: Barbara Braden and Nancy Bergstrom, Copyright 1988. Reprinted with permission.

Stage 1 or stage 2 pressure ulcers may be evident immediately after surgery. These areas must be kept free from additional pressure for healing to occur and to keep them from advancing to higher stages. They are sometimes misidentified and treated inappropriately. Stage 1 pressure ulcers can look like normal reactive hyperemia (excessive redness), which generally fades on its own in one half to three fourths the time that the area was under pressure, with little or no permanent tissue damage.[18] Reactive hyperemia needs to be distinguished from a stage 1 pressure ulcer. In reactive hyperemia, the healthy tissue blanches when compressed. As the compression is released, the blood rushes back to the area, causing it to become erythematous again. Stage 1 pressure ulcers do not blanch when compressed. This is a serious sign, indicating that the compromised tissue is not receiving adequate oxygen and nutrients.[10] The blistering that sometimes occurs in stage 2 pressure ulcers is often misidentified as a chemical or thermal burn. The lack of contact with a chemical or thermal agent in that area and its location under a bony prominence or near where a hard surface had been during surgery can help distinguish it as a pressure ulcer.[17]

Full manifestation of pressure ulcers may be delayed hours to days after the triggering injurious event. Because deep tissue damage extends from the bony prominence to the skin, when the deeper necrosis finally erupts to the skin level, what first appeared to be a stage 1 pressure ulcer, normal reactive hyperemia, or even uninjured skin may be a stage 3 or stage 4 pressure ulcer. Lack of postoperative pressure relief can contribute to this advance. Because of the delayed manifestation, the connection that the surgical experience was the triggering event may be overlooked.[17]

When a pressure ulcer has reached its highest stage, that stage does not reverse as it heals. In other words, as a stage 3 pressure ulcer reepithelializes, it does not sequentially revert from stage 3 to stage 2, stage 1, and stage 0. When it is a stage 3, it could worsen to a stage 4, but it can never reverse to a lower stage. The process of healing can be documented only by the improved characteristics of the healing wound (i.e., depth, width, and presence of granulation tissue).[22]

Pressure alopecia (pressure-induced hair loss of the scalp) can result from prolonged local pressure to the scalp during and after surgery. Symptoms can occur between postoperative days 3 and 28.[31] Occipital scalp pain, swelling, exudate, crusting, or focal ulceration may precede the actual loss of hair. Pressure alopecia is most commonly reported in cases that require prolonged intubation and head immobilization. In cardiac surgery, the anesthesia induction-to-extubation time may extend more than 24 hours. The longer the time, the greater the risks are that the alopecia will be permanent. Repositioning the patient's head every 30 minutes and the use of soft, contoured head padding can reduce the potential for pressure-induced local alopecia.

Circular shaped head rests (ring cushions or donuts) are often used for head immobilization during surgery to the head and neck or for protecting the ear when the head is placed in a lateral position. When a ring cushion is used as a head rest, the weight of the portion of the head that sits inside the hole is supported by the portion of the head that rests on the edge of the inner circle, potentially causing higher pressures to that area. Caution should be taken when using ring cushions for long procedures. The weight of the head is distributed more evenly on a cushion with an indentation rather than a hole in the center.

***Compartment Syndrome.*** Compartment syndrome can develop if the perfusion to an extremity is inadequate. This syndrome is characterized by ischemia, hypoxic edema, and elevated tissue pressure within the fascial compartments of the extremity, which can cause extensive damage to the muscles and the nerves. Toxic byproducts from myoglobin destruction can cause renal damage. Because this process occurs at a cellular level in the tissues, distal pulses and capillary refill may appear normal as the process begins to develop in the extremity. The most effective means of terminating this syndrome is a decompressive fasciotomy.

Certain positioning factors can contribute to causing compartment syndrome, as follows:

- A tight strap on an armboard
- Elevation of an extremity coupled with systemic hypotension
- Compression on an elevated extremity by straps or leg wrappings that are too tight
- Pressure from the weight of an extremity against an edge of a leg holder
- Pressure from the arm of a surgical assistant holding an extremity too tightly
- Excessive popliteal pressure from a knee crutch stirrup
- Excessive flexion of the knees or hips
- Prolonged lithotomy position (especially >5 hours)[11,31]

Preventive interventions include paying careful attention to the tightness of straps on extremities. Limit the time the patient is in the lithotomy position, especially high lithotomy. Ensure that legs placed in stirrups are well padded and adequately supported without undue pressure on the calf or popliteal fossa.[31]

## Musculoskeletal System

The musculoskeletal system of the patient may be subjected to unusual stress during operative positioning. Normal range of motion is maintained in an alert patient by pain and pressure receptors that warn against overstretching and twisting of ligaments, tendons, and muscles. The tone of opposing muscle groups also acts to prevent strain and stress to the muscle fibers. When pharmacologic agents such as anesthetics and muscle relaxants depress the pain and pressure receptors and muscle tone, the normal defense mechanisms cannot guard against joint damage and muscle stretch and strain. A patient safety goal is to keep the body in as much natural alignment as possible, while providing adequate access to the surgical site. The perioperative team needs to be aware of resistance to range of motion and not extend a joint beyond what is absolutely necessary.

Every time a patient is transferred to or from the OR bed, the alignment of the body needs to be maintained. This is especially true when the transfer involves moving the patient from a supine position to lateral or prone. Quick, jerky movement of unsupported limbs can cause strain to the muscles and ligaments. If the transfer vehicle and the OR bed are not adequately locked and supported, the patient could fall, potentially causing fractures and other severe bodily injuries.[6]

## Nervous System

Nervous system depression accompanies the administration of anesthetic agents and other drugs. The degree of depression depends on the type of regional anesthesia or the level of general anesthesia. Pain and pressure receptors may be affected regionally or systemically. The most important factor for the perioperative nurse to remember is that when nervous system depression occurs, the body's communication and command system becomes totally or partially ineffective. Compensatory reactions to changes in the physical status no longer respond normally. Lifesaving, physiologic adaptive mechanisms are altered. The stresses of operative positioning are not automatically compensated.

***Peripheral Neuropathies.*** Peripheral nerves can be injured during positioning, resulting in impaired sensory function or motor function or both. The basic types of injuries to peripheral nerves in clinical practice are stretch-related injuries, compression, and lacerations.[5] Stretching and compression tend to be the main culprits in position-induced nerve injuries. Prolonged stretching from hyperabduction of an extremity or compression from pressure results in ischemia, which can progress to necrosis. In addition, collateral damage to the surrounding tissue and capillaries can affect the circulation and nourishment to the nerves. These pathologic forces combine to result in structural or functional damage to the nerves. Depending on the degree of damage, subsequent injuries may be temporary or permanent.[16]

During surgery, all patients are at risk for nerve injury if sustained compression is placed on nerves. Numerous patient characteristics have been identified, however, as potentially increasing the risk for intraoperatively acquired neuropathies. These include diabetes mellitus, cancer, alcoholism, smoking, vitamin deficiencies, previous nerve injuries, preexisting limitations in flexion or extension of joints, personal/occupational habits that require repeated bending of an extremity, obesity, thin habitus, and male gender (for ulnar nerve injuries).[31,32] Possible risk factors associated with the patient's hospital experience include lengthy surgical procedures, the use of abdominal pelvic self-retaining retractors, long duration in the lithotomy position, sternal retraction from a median sternotomy, surgical procedures in which shoulder braces are used for support while the patient is in steep Trendelenburg, prolonged hospitalization, and prolonged bed rest postoperatively.[32] Damage usually is not discovered until the patient reaches the PACU. Sometimes there is a delayed onset of symptoms in which the injury does not manifest until days or weeks after the suspected insult. This delay can lead to some confusion as to whether the injury occurred during surgery or convalescence.[31] The most commonly reported OR-related nerve injuries involve the upper extremities (primarily the ulnar nerve and the brachial plexus) and the lower extremities (primarily the common peroneal, sciatic, and femoral nerves).

UPPER EXTREMITY NEUROPATHIES. Upper extremity neuropathies generate from lesions to the brachial plexus and the nerves that emerge from it. The brachial plexus consists of a bundle of nerve cords that run through the shoulder and innervate the lower shoulder, arm, and hand (Figure 5-1). This bundle originates from cervical spinal nerves C5-C8. The nerve cords emerge to form peripheral nerves. The axillary nerve innervates the deltoid muscle. The musculoskeletal nerve innervates the biceps muscle. Three main peripheral nerves run down the arm to the fingers: median, radial, and ulnar (Figure 5-2).

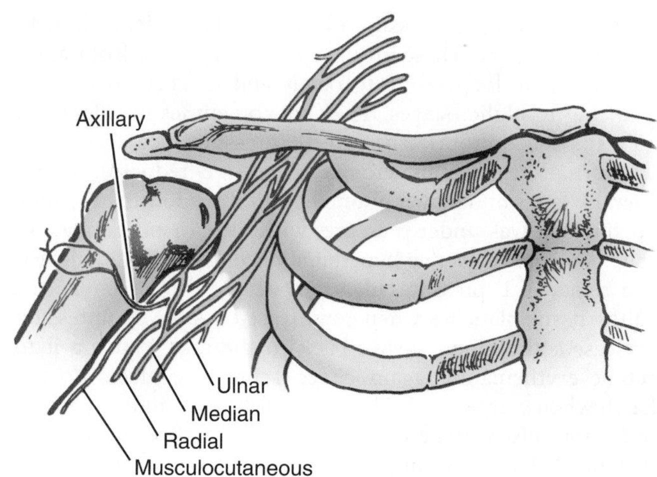


**FIGURE 5-1** Brachial plexus on the right with associated bone structures and nerve branches that extend down the right arm.

The *median nerve* runs through the antecubital space to the fingers and provides sensory and motor ability to the distal and palmar surfaces of the thumb and adjacent two fingers. A normally perceived pinprick to the palmar surface of the distal index finger generally would show that the median nerve was intact (Figure 5-3).

The *radial nerve* loops around the posterior humerus before it runs through the antecubital space to the fingers. It provides motor and sensory function to the triceps and the muscles of the posterior forearm and hand. Injury to this area can cause difficulty extending the wrist and thumb. If the distal thumb can be actively extended, this generally indicates an intact radial nerve (see Figure 5-3).

The *ulnar nerve* runs behind the elbow and innervates the third, fourth, and fifth fingers and the muscles of the medial forearm. It is responsible for wrist flexion and, along with the radial nerve, enables the thumb to oppose the other four fingers. A normally perceived pinprick over the plantar surface of the distal fifth finger generally indicates an intact ulnar nerve (see Figure 5-3).

Injury to any of these nerves along their course can result in sensory or motor defects in the areas that they innervate. In surgical positioning, the most common areas of injury are the brachial plexus and the ulnar nerve.[11] The major reason is that the brachial plexus resides in the shoulder, which is subject to abduction, manipulation, and sometimes pressure, depending on the position. As the ulnar nerve circles behind the elbow, it lies superficially in the shallow cubital tunnel of the humerus, where it is subject to pressure and to stretching from flexion of the elbow.

Improper positioning techniques, such as the following, can place the brachial plexus at risk for injury:

- Placing the arms on armboards that extend beyond a 90-degree angle to the body
- Surgical team members leaning against the shoulder or the arm while it is tucked against the body
- Shoulder braces used for supporting the patient in steep Trendelenburg position, which can put pressure on the brachial plexus if the braces are medial or lateral to the acromioclavicular joint
- If, in lateral position, the dependent shoulder and arm are directly under the rib cage

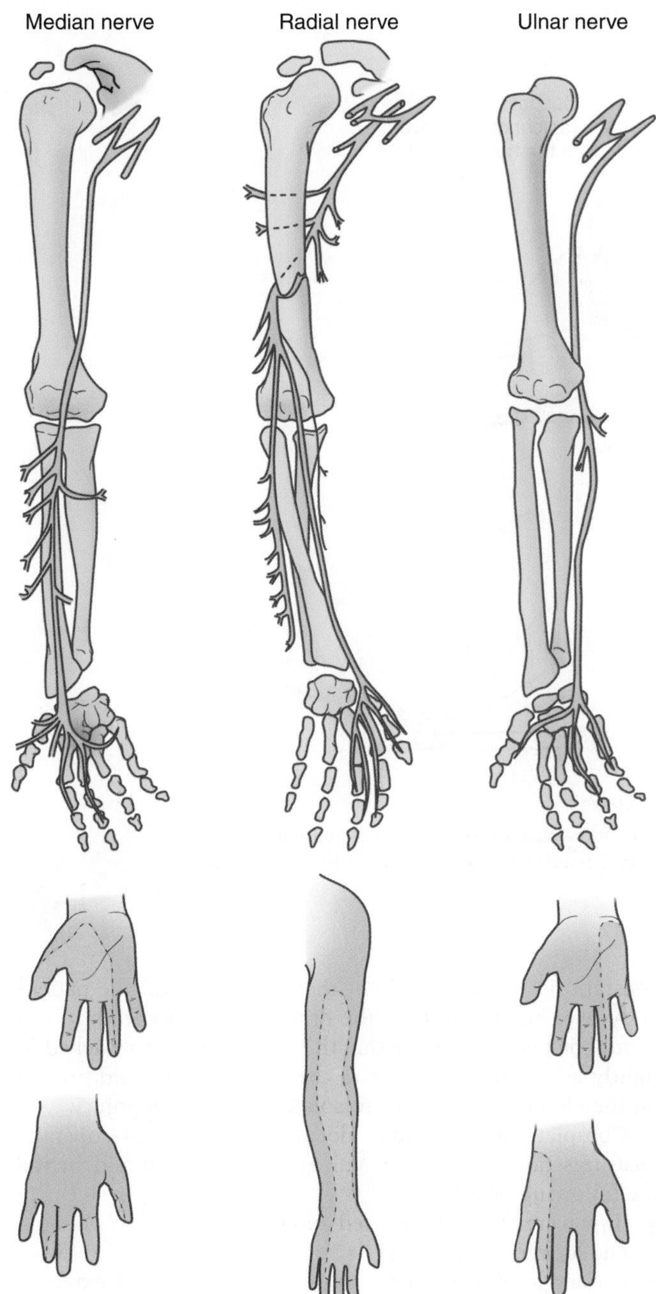


FIGURE 5-2 Median, radial, and ulnar nerves and nerves of the right arm with areas of sensory distribution shaded.

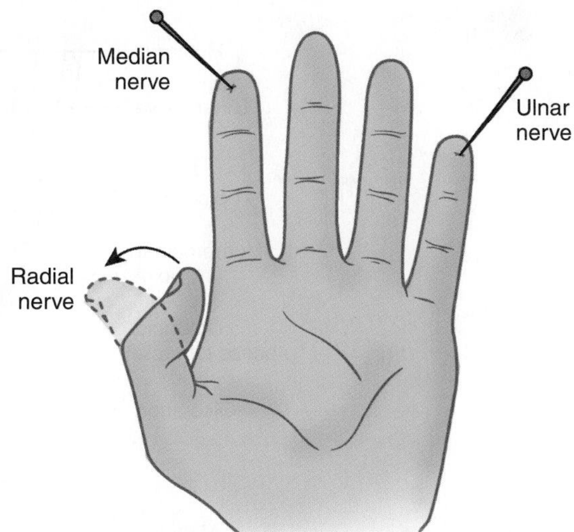


FIGURE 5-3 A quick way to check for injuries to the major peripheral nerves of the upper extremity. The ability to actively extend the thumb indicates an intact radial nerve. A normally perceived pinprick to the distal palmar surface of the index finger indicates an intact median nerve. A normally perceived pinprick to the distal palmar surface of the fifth finger indicates an intact ulnar nerve.

- Rotation and lateral flexion of the patient's head, which can pull and compress the brachial plexus at its cervical origin

The brachial plexus also can be injured by the separation of the sternum during open cardiac procedures that require a median sternotomy. When the sternum is split, a retractor is used to separate it, allowing access to the heart. This separation forces the ribs to move laterally. If internal mammary artery dissection is done as part of the procedure, there is additional asymmetric retraction of the rib cage. The first rib compresses the brachial plexus nerve bundles and, in particular, the nerve cord that emerges into the ulnar nerve. When brachial plexus and ulnar neuropathies develop as a result, they generally are not preventable by proper positioning of the patient's arm.[14,31] Improper arm positioning could add to the insult of the injury.

Isolated ulnar nerve injuries occur primarily from pressure on the vulnerable location of that nerve (Figure 5-4). The ulnar nerve becomes quite superficial as it runs behind the elbow, nesting in the epicondyle groove of the humerus. Predisposition specific to ulnar nerve injuries exists in patients whose occupational or personal habits require repeated bending of the elbow. In addition, there is a 2:1 predominance of ulnar nerve injuries in male versus female patients. This is probably attributable to three anatomic differences between the elbows of men and women:

1. The tubercle of the coronoid process is larger in men than in women, creating a smaller cubital tunnel around the ulnar nerve (see Figure 5-4).
2. Men have less adipose tissue over the medial aspect of the elbow compared with women with similar body fat composition; this provides less natural padding to that area.
3. Men have a thicker, more developed cubital tunnel reticulum, which can reduce further the space for the ulnar nerve in the cubital tunnel. This becomes a greater risk when the elbow is flexed.[31]

The main goal in protecting the ulnar nerve is to eliminate pressure on it. As Figure 5-4, *C* illustrates, pressure on the medial aspect of the elbow can compress the ulnar nerve. Figure 5-5 illustrates ways to prevent this pressure. Supination (palms up) of the forearms on an armboard (Figure 5-5, *A*) places the olecranon of the elbow on the flat surface instead of the cubital tunnel, which contains the ulnar nerve. When the arm of a supine patient rests on the trunk, direct trauma can occur to the ulnar nerve as the weight of the arm presses the flexed elbow against the surface of the bed. Placing padding under the upper arm, proximal to the elbow (Figure 5-5, *B*), leaves a free space under the elbow, eliminating pressure on the nerve. When a patient is prone with arms pronated on arm-

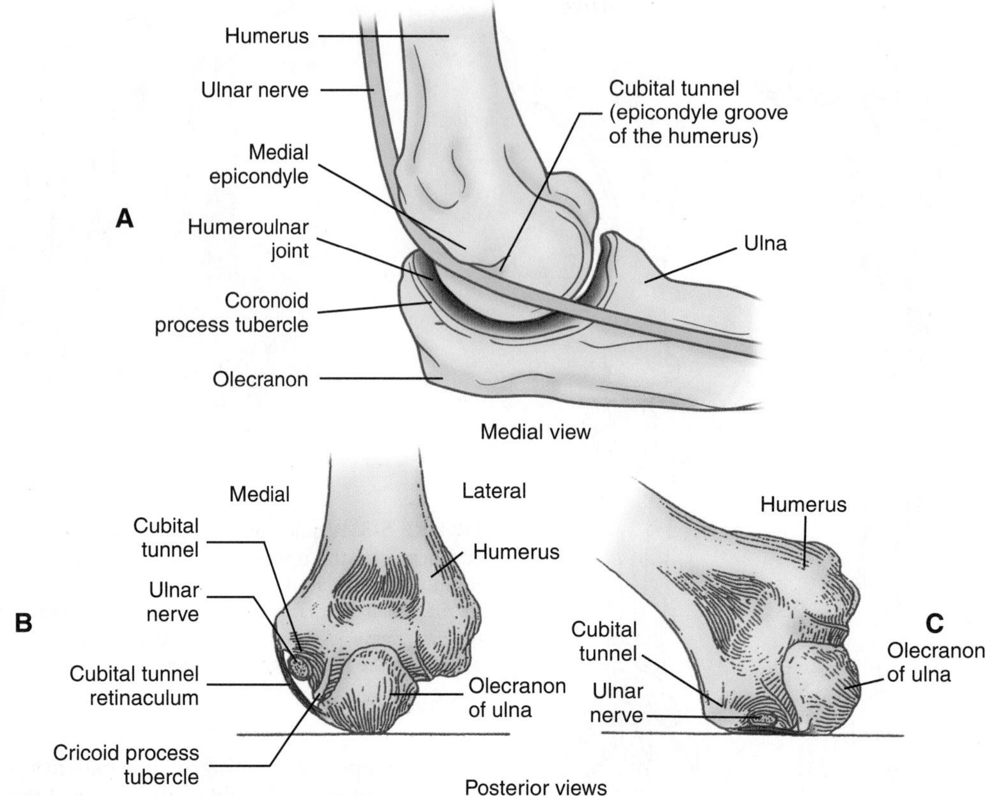


**FIGURE 5-4** The ulnar nerve at cubital tunnel. **A,** Medial view. **B,** Posterior view. Note cubital tunnel retinaculam over the ulnar nerve in the cubital tunnel. **C,** Posterior view with elbow tilted on medial side. Note the ulnar nerve compressed.

boards, the ulnar nerve is vulnerable to pressure from the elbow. Placing padding proximal and distal to the elbow (Figure 5-5, *C*) frees the nerve from pressure. If the patient has a history of thoracic outlet syndrome or pain when lifting the arms overhead, the arms should not be pronated, but rather restrained and tucked alongside the trunk.[31]

Ulnar neuropathies may manifest symptoms in the immediate postoperative period. Sometimes symptoms are delayed until 2 to 7 days after surgery, however, which makes it difficult to isolate the exact event that triggered the complication. The postoperative course cannot be completely ruled out as a possible causative or contributing factor. Some patients are forced to lie on their backs for prolonged periods postoperatively because of devices such as endotracheal tubes and abdominal drains. Often they rest with their elbows flexed and their hands on their chest. This places pressure on that superficial section of the ulnar nerve under the elbow, which may cause or contribute to injury to the nerve during the postoperative period.

Many OR-induced peripheral upper extremity nerve injuries can be avoided by properly securing the arms when they are tucked at the patient's side. The arms should be tucked in a way that prevents them from sliding down the side of the OR bed and contacting the bed edge or rigid table attachments. An effective technique to prevent arm slippage during surgery is to wrap the draw sheet smoothly around the arm and then tuck the draw sheet under the patient's body instead of under the mattress (Figure 5-6). This technique can be used with the supine and prone positions. It is best accomplished with an assistant on the other side of the OR bed to roll the patient's body over enough to tuck the draw sheet underneath it. Care should be taken to ensure that the draw sheet is not tucked too tightly as to cause pressure to the arms. A tight fold pressing on the elbow could cause an isolated ulnar nerve injury.

Complete and thorough documentation of intraoperative measures taken to protect vulnerable nerves should include the following details:

- How were the arms secured and by whom
- The location of padding
- The angle of armboards (approximate degree of extension from body), the position of the palms, and the location of arm straps
- Times and type of repositioning or passive range of motion done
- Presence of distal pulses, color, and temperature of arms and hands when procedure is long or extremity is compressed or both

The upper extremities should be evaluated postoperatively. Any changes from the preoperative condition should be verbally reported and documented.

**LOWER EXTREMITY NEUROPATHIES.** Lower extremity neuropathies result most frequently from prolonged lithotomy positioning and tend to manifest symptoms within hours after surgery. The common peroneal, sciatic, and femoral nerves are most frequently implicated.

*Intrinsic* risk factors include thin body build, smoking, diabetes, rheumatoid arthritis, previous hip surgery, presence of

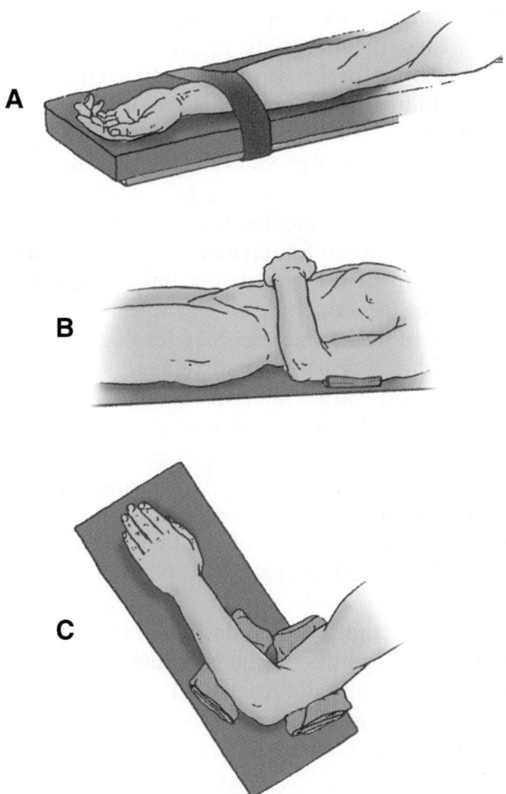


**FIGURE 5-5** Three ways to protect the ulnar nerve. **A,** Arm of supine patient on armboard with palms up. **B,** Elbow lifted free from bed surface by padding upper arm when arm is resting on trunk. **C,** Arm of prone patient pronated on armboard. Padding above and below elbow frees the ulnar nerve from the pressure of the armboard surface.

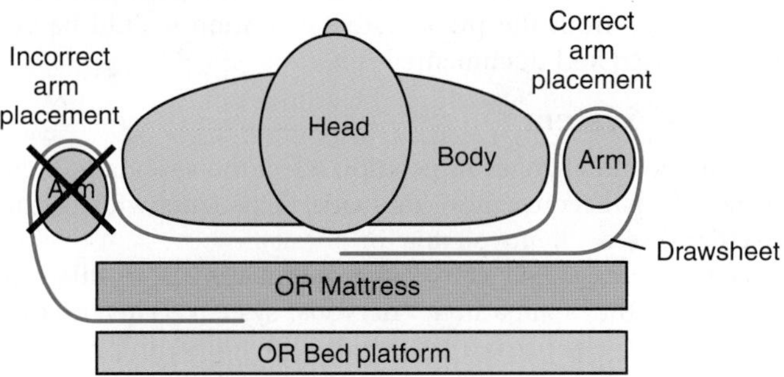


**FIGURE 5-6** Correct method for tucking arms in at the patient's side.

familiar or subclinical neuropathies, and presence of anatomic anomalies. *Extrinsic* intraoperative risk factors include the length of time in lithotomy, high or exaggerated lithotomy, and positioning the extremities beyond their comfortable range of motion when awake.[4,19,21,31,32] Different types of stirrups vary in the degree to which they control hip flexion (see "Lithotomy" section later for further discussion). Hip extension should be limited to only the amount required for adequate access to the operative area.

The *common peroneal nerve* branches from the sciatic nerve behind the knee and becomes superficial as it wraps around the lateral head of the fibula (Figures 5-7, 5-8, and 5-9). At this level, it is quite vulnerable to direct compression by stirrup bars. This risk may be increased in extremely thin patients who have minimal overlying tissue in this area. It is important to ensure that the lateral head of the fibula does not rest against stirrup bars or any other rigid surface. Compressive leg wraps (i.e., pneumatic compressive devices, elastic wrappings, or stockings) also can put pressure on this nerve if the wrapping is too tight in this area. In addition, pressure behind the knee can compress the common peroneal and tibial nerves where they run through the popliteal fossa, so only *soft* padding or pillows should be used for knee support. The ability to dorsiflex the great toe (point it upward) generally indicates that the common perineal nerve is intact.

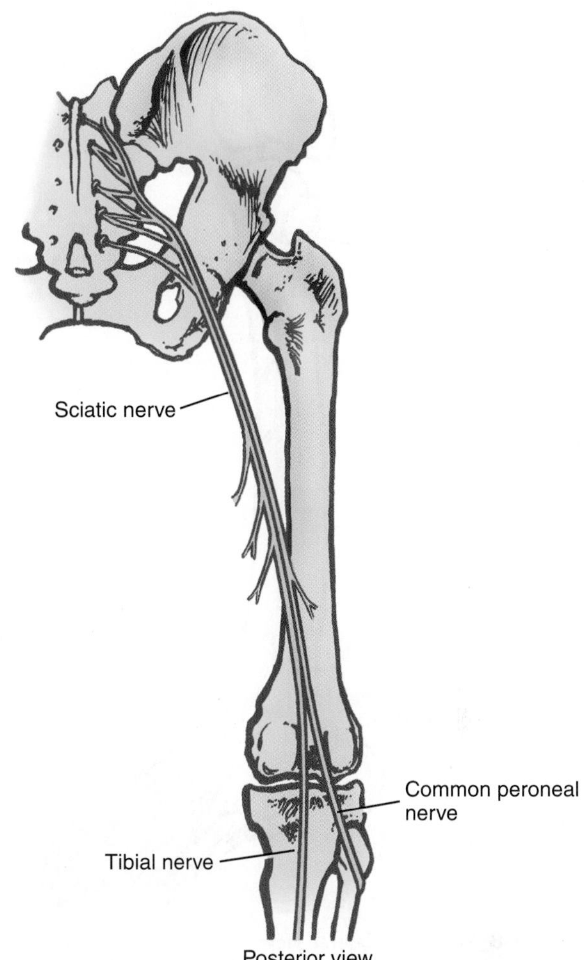


**FIGURE 5-7** Right sciatic nerve and right thigh and upper leg, posterior view. Note the division of the sciatic nerve into the tibial and common peroneal nerves.

The *sciatic nerve* originates from the L4-S3 spinal nerve roots and travels down the buttock and posterior thigh before it divides into the common peroneal and tibial nerves (see Figure 5-7). It may be injured by the stretching that occurs during hyperflexion of the hip. A patient who has had a total hip replacement may have some preexisting sciatic nerve damage as a result of the excessive rotation of the femur that is part of that operative procedure. Additionally, patients with a history of hip trauma who have required surgery such as open reduction and internal fixation may be at increased risk for sciatic neuropathy because of the potential presence of scar

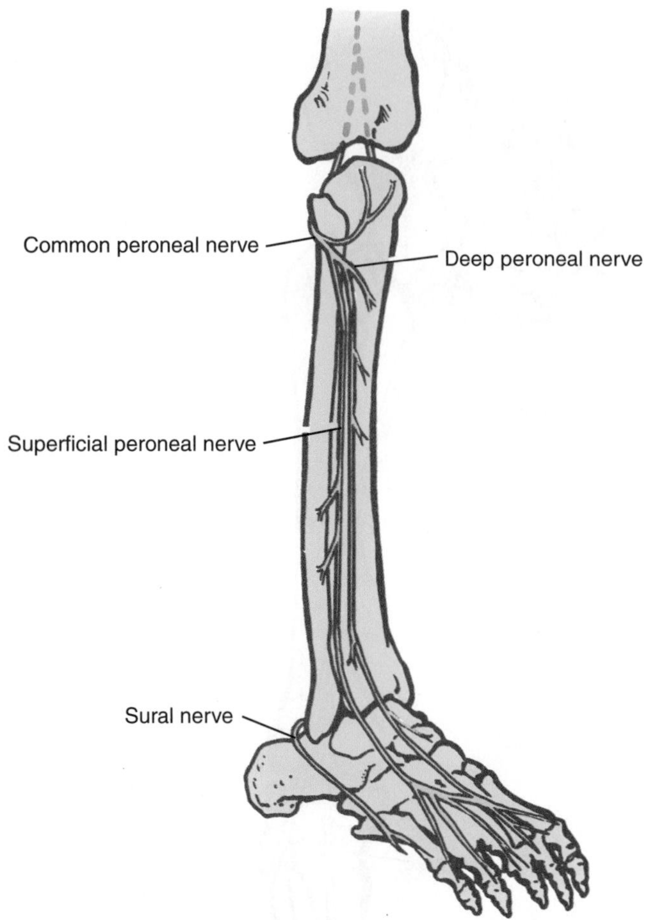


**FIGURE 5-8** Right leg, lateral view. Note the common peroneal nerve pathway around the lateral fibular head. The nerve is very susceptible to injury when the patient is in lateral position. Also note the sural nerve in the heel area. This nerve is susceptible to injury from stirrup straps.

tissue around the nerve area.[4] Because the branches of the sciatic nerve run from the thigh to the hamstring, the ability to flex the thigh generally would indicate an intact sciatic nerve.

The *femoral nerve* arises from the L2-L4 spinal nerve roots and runs through the medial thigh. Injury to the deep femoral nerve may occur more as a result of inappropriate placement of abdominal pelvic retractors and vaginal retractors in the pelvic cavity than inappropriate positioning.[19] The femoral nerve and the obturator nerve can be subjected to excessive stretching and injury, however, as a result of inappropriate lithotomy positioning (see Figure 5-9). The ability to flex the thigh to the trunk generally would indicate an intact femoral nerve.

The *obturator nerve* originates from L2-L4 nerve roots. It runs through the obturator foramen of the ischium to innervate the adductor group of muscles in the inner thigh. It can be subjected to excessive stretching when the patient is in lithotomy position. Scrubbed personnel may lean against the inner thigh while holding vaginal or anal retractors, causing additional stretching and compression of the nerve. The ability to adduct the leg generally means the obturator muscle is intact.

The *tibial nerve* branches from the sciatic nerve behind the knee and runs along the posterior tibia to the foot. There it branches into the medial and lateral plantar nerves. Normal sensation to the plantar surface of the foot and the ability to curl the toes downward generally would indicate an intact tibial nerve.

The perioperative nurse should document measures taken to protect the lower extremities from injury, such as the following:

- Location and type of padding used (i.e., pillow to support knees or calves, padding under heels)
- Type of stirrups used, names of persons placing legs in stirrups
- Type of lithotomy position (low, standard, high, or exaggerated)
- Presence of distal pulses, color, and temperature of legs and feet
- Use of sequential compressive devices or antiembolic compression stockings

The lower extremities should be evaluated postoperatively. Any changes from the preoperative condition should be verbally reported and documented.

## Vascular System

Anesthesia and changes in position affect the vascular system. These effects become more dramatic in patients with cardiovascular disease, hypovolemia, or obesity.

General anesthesia causes peripheral vessels to dilate by depressing the sympathetic nervous system. This dilation

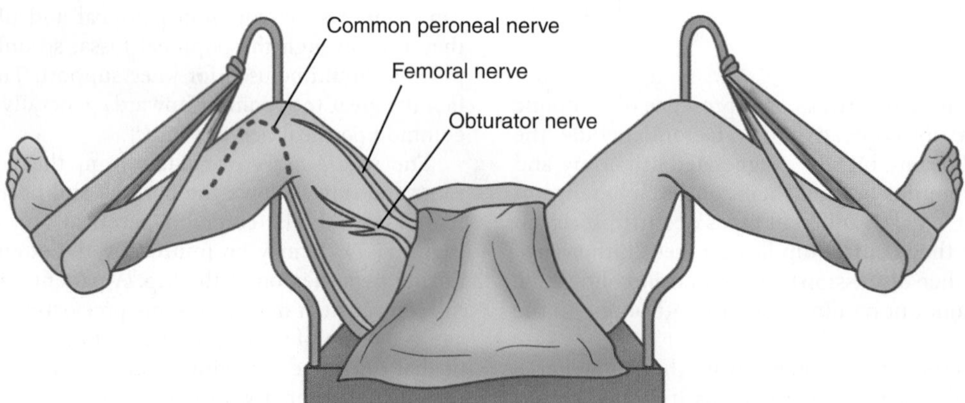


**FIGURE 5-9** Nerves of the inner thigh. The femoral and obturator nerves can be overstretched by hyperextending the hips or by staff leaning against the thighs. If the lateral knee rests against a stirrup bar, the common peroneal nerve can be compressed.

causes an overall decrease in blood pressure by the pooling of blood in dependent areas of the body. In general anesthesia, these effects are systemic, whereas in regional anesthesia, such as spinal and epidural, these effects are more limited to the areas anesthetized.

Position changes affect where the pooling of blood occurs. Muscle tone and peripheral vascular resistance are no longer effective in counteracting the forces of gravity on blood pooling. Blood pooling shifts to whatever part of the body is lowest. If the head of the OR bed is raised, the lower torso has increased blood volume, and the upper torso becomes more compensated. Hypovolemia and cardiovascular disease can compromise the patient's status further.

The anesthesia provider can treat some of the hypotensive effects of positioning through pharmacologic agents and increased intravenous infusion. Vital signs, intravenous intake, and urinary output need to be monitored closely. Position changes may need to be delayed until the blood pressure is stabilized.

Venous thrombosis is a serious complication of surgical positioning. Compression to deep and peripheral vessels (i.e., tight safety strap or wrist restraints) can predispose the patient to venous thrombosis. When the legs are in a dependent position (i.e., legs lowered during knee arthroscopy, sitting position), venous return is slowed, and thrombosis can occur. Compressive antiembolic stockings or sequential compressive devices can reduce this risk. Thrombosis also can occur as a result of hyperabduction of the arms beyond 90 degrees. Subclavian and axillary vessels pass through the brachial plexus; vessel constriction can occur by compression between the clavicle and the first rib. Radial pulses need to be checked whenever arms are extended to ensure that the radial pulse is not obliterated.

The vascular status of upper and lower extremities should be assessed preoperatively. Measures taken to reduce assessed risks should be documented. Vascular status should be evaluated intraoperatively and postoperatively. Any changes from the preoperative condition should be verbally reported and documented.

## Respiratory System

The respiratory system can be compromised during positioning. In almost all types of positions, except semi-Fowler, sitting, and reverse Trendelenburg, the abdominal viscera are shifted upward toward the diaphragm. Subsequently, the diaphragm shifts upward and outward such that it contributes only about two thirds of the ventilatory force and significantly reduces tidal volume (the volume of air inhaled or exhaled).[11] Patients who are obese or pregnant or have pulmonary disease have additional respiratory compromise in these positions. Any patient who experiences dyspnea should have the head of the bed elevated during transport and during local, regional, or spinal anesthesia if this does not interfere with surgical access. During general anesthesia, the anesthesia provider generally ventilates these patients mechanically.

External chest movement during surgery needs to be as unrestricted as possible to avoid even further reduction in tidal volume. The placement of arms across the chest should be avoided or very time-limited. Arms resting on the chest not only restrict chest expansion but also place pressure on the ulnar nerve at the elbow area. Some positions (i.e., lateral, fracture table) require the placement of straps or tape around the chest area to secure the patient to the OR bed without obstructing the surgical site. Efforts are needed to ensure that the straps or tape is not excessively tight, and that these positions are not maintained any longer than necessary. Anesthesia personnel closely monitor the respiratory status of these patients.

The portions of the lung that are perfused with blood also are affected by position. As blood is pumped into the lungs, the areas of the lung that are most dependent have a greater pulmonary arterial pressure. The greater the pressure, the greater the perfusion. The alveoli in the bases of the lungs are more compliant; ventilation is generally highest in those areas. An even distribution of ventilation and perfusion (ventilation-perfusion ratio) is needed for efficient gas exchange. If the position causes a pathologically compromised area of the lung to be dominant and most perfused, the balance between perfusion and ventilation may be disrupted, and respiratory status may be diminished. The rest of the lung fields may or may not have the capacity to compensate. Oxygen therapy or mechanical ventilation can help compensate, but the amount of time a patient can tolerate a certain position and maintain adequate gas exchange may be limited.

Monitoring of respiratory status should always include pulse oximetry. In some cases, intraoperative arterial blood gas monitoring may be necessary.

## Other Vulnerable Areas

Certain other body structures, including the eyes, breasts, genitalia, and fingers, are placed at risk during surgical positioning and warrant special discussion.

***Eyes.*** Eye injuries during positioning can range from corneal abrasions to blindness. The eyes do not always close during anesthesia, so they may be vulnerable to abrasions from the movement of the face on the sheets, pillows, or drapes in certain positions and from being brushed by intravenous lines, masks, fingers, or the clothes of personnel. When the patient is unconscious, the eyelids should be taped shut to reduce this risk. Eye patches or shields can provide additional protection.

Eyes should be checked to ensure that they are not under pressure when the prone or lateral position requires the face to be in a dependent position. Direct pressure on the globe of the eye could displace the intraocular lens in a patient who has had cataract surgery. Direct pressure on the eye, especially coupled with systemic hypotension, could cause retinal ischemia or thrombosis of the central retinal artery, which could result in temporary or permanent blindness.[21,24] In the prone position, the head should be turned, as long as cervical injuries are not an impacting factor. If turning the head is not an option, and the head must be pronated in a device such as a horseshoe-shaped headrest, it should be adjusted in such a way as to free the eyes from pressure. Periodically, the head should be checked for slippage into a position that puts pressure on the eyes.[11,21,31]

***Breasts.*** In the prone position, the female breasts are compressed between the weight of the body and the bed or ventral chest supports. If the breasts are displaced laterally, the medial borders can be stretched and injured. If the patient has a mammary prosthesis, direct pressure can rupture the implant. Soft ventral supports on the lateral sides of the breasts, diverting the breasts toward the midline, are generally better tolerated.[31]

***Genitalia.*** Crush injuries can occur to the genitalia in certain positions. In prone position on a laminectomy frame, male genitalia can be compressed between the pelvis and the frame. Patients positioned supine on the fracture table have the pelvis stabilized by a vertical post placed close to the perineum. This post should be placed between the genitalia and the uninjured leg so that the pressure is not directly on the genitalia. If the post is not well padded, the intense pressure placed on the pelvis during traction of the injured leg can crush and severely injure the genitalia and pudendal nerve. Loss of penile sensation has been reported after positioning in the fracture table.[31]

***Fingers.*** Fingers are vulnerable to injury during surgical positioning. When the arms are tucked at the patient's side, the fingers should be straightened with palms toward the patient's body. Curled fingers can put pressure on the finger joints and allow fingernails to press into other fingers or the body.

Another risk for finger injury can occur during lithotomy positioning. If the fingers hang over the edge after the leg section of the OR bed is lowered, there is a potential for the fingers to be caught in the joint of the bed as the leg section is raised at the end of the procedure. This situation could result in a crushing injury or amputation of the fingers. A general precaution should be employed that the leg section is never raised without the fingers being visualized and secured away from the OR bed leg section hinge.

# *Perioperative Nursing Considerations*

## ASSESSMENT

Assessment for positioning needs should be made before the patient is transferred to the OR bed.[2] The perioperative nursing assessment includes a patient interview, physical examination, and review of medical records. Key points of assessment that are related to surgical positioning include age, height and weight, skin condition, nutritional status, preexisting conditions (e.g., conditions of the vascular, respiratory, circulatory, neurologic, or immune system), and physical/mobility limits (e.g., prostheses, implants, range of motion). It also should be determined if there are any particular areas of discomfort that may be affected by a particular position and what interventions might alleviate or reduce that discomfort.

The assessment also should alert the perioperative nurse to patients and situations that could contribute to problems caused by positioning. Vulnerable patients include the following:

1. Geriatric patients, whose thin skin layer and increased arteriosclerosis make them more prone to skin breakdown because of pressure
2. Pediatric patients, whose size and weight must be considered when selecting positioning aids
3. Patients who have respiratory and circulatory disorders, diabetes mellitus, malnutrition, advanced age, and anemia because they are more prone to skin breakdown caused by pressure
4. Patients with limitations to mobility because of congenital anomalies, preexisting injuries, arthritis, or prosthetic implants, who need special considerations during positioning
5. Patients with edema, infection, cancer, or conditions of lowered cardiac or respiratory reserves who have poor general health, making them vulnerable to tissue injury
6. Patients with demineralizing bone conditions, such as malignant metastasis or osteoporosis, which puts them at higher risk for skeletal fractures
7. Patients who will be subjected to anticipated high-risk surgical situations, such as the following:
   - Lengthy surgical procedures (≥2 hours) because of the increased risk of pressure-related injuries
   - Lengthy time in the lithotomy position because of the increased risk of lower extremity nerve injury
   - Vascular surgery because optimal blood perfusion already may be compromised as a result of the patient's disease process
   - Excessive sustained pressure to certain body areas because of the surgical procedure or retraction
   - Cool environment or exposure of large body surfaces or both because of the risk of hypothermia and its related complications

## NURSING DIAGNOSIS

The encompassing nursing diagnosis related to the care of the patient during surgical positioning is the risk for perioperative-positioning injury. Other potentially applicable nursing diagnoses include the following:

1. Impaired comfort
2. Impaired transfer ability
3. Risk for falls
4. Risk of wrong-site surgery
5. Disturbed sensory perception
6. Risk for impaired skin integrity
7. Risk for impaired tissue integrity
8. Hypothermia
9. Impaired gas exchange
10. Impaired physical mobility
11. Risk for peripheral neurovascular dysfunction

## OUTCOME IDENTIFICATION

The outcome identified for safe surgical positioning may be stated as "the patient is free from signs and symptoms of perioperative positioning injury." Primary outcome indicators mandate a review of the skin condition and cardiovascular and neuromuscular status, along with other considerations. The perioperative nurse may define freedom from injury, noting that the patient will

1. Be comfortable.
2. Experience a safe transfer to and from the OR bed.
3. Be protected from falls.
4. Have surgery on the correct site.
5. Resume preprocedural patterns of mobility.
6. Not experience tingling, numbness, or pain unrelated to the surgical procedure.
7. Maintain normal skin and tissue integrity.
8. Maintain normothermia.
9. Maintain adequate gas exchange.
10. Regain normal physical mobility postoperatively.
11. Maintain normal peripheral neurovascular function.

## PLANNING

The perioperative nurse needs to plan activities that will protect the patient from injury and provide physiologic support and comfort, while allowing for optimal exposure and access to the surgical site. Although carrying out safe surgical positioning involves all members of the surgical team, the circulating nurse plans and coordinates this teamwork. Knowledge of any preexisting risk factors that may affect positioning strategies (e.g., obesity, diabetes, paralysis, advanced age) should be considered when planning for (1) additional staff assistance that would be required during positioning and (2) support devices or padding that would be needed.

It is imperative that the exact location of the operative site be identified so that access to that site is not obstructed. If a secondary surgical procedure is involved, such as a graft donor site, that area needs to be exposed and accessible as well. There are times when all the anticipated sites of incision cannot be exposed during initial positioning. Plans need to be made for repositioning an anesthetized patient (i.e., assisting personnel, additional padding devices, additional sterile drapes) so that repositioning occurs quickly and smoothly without unnecessarily prolonged anesthesia time.

Planning for physiologic support involves collaborating with the anesthesia provider. Sometimes chest rolls are needed for adequate lung expansion while the patient is in the prone position. Supports and padding for the head, arms, hands, and axilla should be anticipated and easily accessible.

Planning for the patient's comfort can involve communicating with the patient as to potential areas for discomfort and possible remedies. An awake patient receiving local anesthesia can give feedback on the comfort of the position before, during, and immediately after the procedure. In some cases, all or part of the positioning for a patient who is to be anesthetized can be done before induction if it does not interfere with the anesthesia process. A patient could be placed in the lithotomy position before induction if he or she has a history of discomfort with leg abduction or lower back pain. If this is done, privacy must be ensured by covering the patient with a sheet or blanket and covering or pulling the blinds on room windows. A Sample Plan of Care for the patient undergoing surgical positioning follows.

## SAMPLE PLAN OF CARE

**NURSING DIAGNOSIS**

Risk for perioperative-positioning injury

**OUTCOME**

The patient will be free from injury related to perioperative positioning.

**INTERVENTIONS**

1. Identify surgical site, and determine appropriate position.
2. Identify and document specific risk factors that may predispose the patient to position-related injuries.
3. Identify areas of potential discomfort/limitations in mobility and possible remedies. Note condition of patient's skin and presence of peripheral pulses, as applicable.
4. Check OR bed for proper functioning and availability of all needed attachments.
5. Obtain any needed positioning aids and padding materials; verify that these are clean and in working order.
6. Ensure a safe transfer between the transport vehicle to OR bed, and document mode of transfer.
7. Safely secure the patient to the OR bed without compromising circulation underneath restraining straps.
8. Provide the patient with warmth, privacy, and reassurance.
9. If the patient is repositioned after being anesthetized, support all body parts, and maintain body alignment throughout the move.
10. Use slow, smooth movements in making all position changes, using a team approach.
11. Avoid pulling or dragging the patient; use lifting techniques instead.
12. Pad bony prominences and all areas in contact with a solid surface.
13. Protect anatomic areas containing superficial vessels and nerves.
14. Protect the eyes.
15. Monitor physiologic effects of position changes, and be prepared to intervene when necessary.
16. Ensure access to airway, intravenous catheters, and monitoring devices.
17. Prevent pooling of fluids under dependent areas or any area under pressure by doing the following:
    Place absorbent towels or pads under the area to be prepped to catch excess prep solution that drips from the prep site. Remove these towels or pads after the prep and before the application of sterile drapes.
    When intraoperative fluid runoff is expected (e.g., arthroscopic surgery, intraabdominal irrigation), secure the edges of the sterile drape to the skin so that the fluid will run *over* instead of *under* the drapes. Sterile, impervious fluid collection pockets incorporated into the drapes aid in reducing the spillage of this fluid onto the floor.
18. Document in detail patient position, including the following:
    Position of extremities
    Type and location of restraints, positioning aids, and padding materials
    Frequency of passive range of motion and other injury prevention interventions
    Site of electrosurgical dispersive pad
    Use and location of warming or cooling blankets or devices
    Positional changes made during procedure (e.g., supine to lithotomy to supine)
    Adverse physiologic responses to positions and interventions taken
19. If the patient needs to be repositioned back into supine position at the completion of the procedure, do so slowly and smoothly, supporting body alignment and monitoring physiologic responses.
20. Visually inspect skin for any changes, particularly around areas under pressure; document and communicate any changes.
21. Document method of transfer at time of discharge from OR.

## IMPLEMENTATION

The nursing actions involved in positioning should reflect the individualized plan of care, which is designed to ensure injury prevention, while maintaining optimal surgical access, patient comfort, and physiologic support. Patient comfort measures need to include physical and emotional aspects. Direct communication with the patient regarding his or her positioning concerns can help to reassure the patient and provide the nurse with insight into possible comfort strategies. Providing the patient warmth and privacy can help the patient feel more comfortable and relaxed and feel respected and cared for.

Assemble all necessary positioning aids, such as padding, pillows, bed accessories, and stirrups, before the patient's induction because the patient is generally positioned immediately after anesthesia is administered. Ensure that all positioning devices are clean and in proper working order.[2] Ensure extra staff members are available if needed for lifting or turning the patient.

When the patient enters the OR suite, the circulating nurse identifies the patient, using two identifiers, and verifies the correct person, procedure, and operative site. Institutional procedures for preventing wrong-site, wrong-procedure, and wrong-person surgery must be followed. The patient is prepared for transfer onto the OR bed, which should be positioned in the room in such a way that relocation after the patient is anesthetized is kept to a minimum. During transfer, the OR bed and transport vehicle should be next to each other and locked. At least one individual should stand on either side to assist the patient in the transfer. If the patient is unable to assist in the transfer, a four-person lift should be done using a draw sheet and supporting the head and feet.

Falls are an important consideration during all stages of patient transfer and positioning. Prevention of falls is listed as one of the Joint Commission on Accreditation of Healthcare Organizations (JCAHO) National Patient Safety Goals.[6] Falls can occur during transfers if the two beds are not locked. Falls also can occur while the patient is on the OR bed, whether awake or anesthetized. An awake patient may not fully appreciate the narrowness of the OR bed and can continue to move beyond the bed edges. Someone needs to stand on either side of the patient until a safety strap is applied. Falls also are a risk during induction and emergence from anesthesia. Lighter stages of anesthesia can result in patient movement. Often the movement is strong enough that safety straps alone do not offer adequate security. Infants and toddlers are particularly at risk because standard safety straps frequently are not used on them because of their small stature. Other means of securing a pediatric patient could be employed depending on the area needed for surgical access. Constant personnel presence immediately at the patient's side and the use of safety straps or portable cushioned side rails can minimize the risk of patient falls during vulnerable times.

When the patient is on the OR bed, the safety strap is placed 2 inches above the knees. The strap should be snug but not so tight as to place pressure on nerves or restrict venous return. One should be able to slide two fingers comfortably beneath the strap. The patient's ankles must not be crossed because vessel and nerve constriction and skin pressure could result. The patient should be reminded of this because many patients automatically cross their ankles while lying down.

Movement of the patient should be slow and smooth, ensuring that the whole body is supported during movements. Quick, jerky movements can cause musculoskeletal injury and put the patient at risk for bruises, pinches, abrasions, fractures, or falls. Any lateral, anterior, or posterior movement of the patient on the OR bed should be done by lifting the patient with the draw sheet rather than by pulling or dragging the patient. Vulnerable areas, such as the eyes, breasts, perineum, and fingers, should be protected during all movement.

When the desired position is obtained, the patient should be secured so that movement off the OR bed cannot occur from any direction. Safety straps and other support accessories should be checked for pressure against the patient, particularly in areas adjacent to bony prominences. Padding or adjustment needs to be done at this point because it is the last opportunity to do so before prepping and draping are done. In addition, consider how the position may cause certain body parts to sustain more gravitational weight. If a pillow elevates the knees, the heels bear additional weight from the calves. Heel padding may be needed to help dissipate this additional pressure. Placing the pillow under the calves elevates the knees and lifts the heels off the surface of the OR bed at the same time.

When the patient is positioned, prepped, and draped, the entire surgical team participates in a time out just before starting the procedure (see Chapter 2 for a full discussion of guidelines for preventing wrong-site, wrong-procedure, and wrong-person surgery). The patient's identity is re-checked. The procedure to be done, operative site and side, and correct patient position are verified by the entire surgical team. The patient must be positioned such that the marking of the operative site mark (e.g., with the surgeon's initials or the word "yes") is visible on the patient's skin. Confirm the availability of implants, special equipment, or other special requirements (e.g., blood, if ordered). When all of this has been completed, the procedure can begin.[7,20] The time out should be documented according to institutional protocol.

During the procedure, the circulating nurse monitors and assists with any modification to the position that is required. Periodically, the nurse checks pressure points that are accessible and adjusts the patient or padding as needed. Passive range of motion can be done to accessible extremities. This is particularly important during long procedures ($\geq$2 hours). The position, all padding, positioning devices, and methods used to secure the patient to the OR bed are documented. If the patient needs to be repositioned during the procedure, the circulating nurse coordinates the move by calling additional personnel to the OR to assist, ensuring additional positioning devices and padding are available, and protecting the patient from injury as the move commences. All interventions for the repositioning are documented.

After the surgical procedure is completed, all pressure sites, especially those under bony prominences, should be checked before transfer to the PACU. Any changes in the skin integrity should be documented and verbally communicated during the hand-off report so appropriate interventions can occur immediately to reduce further injury. The mode of transfer, time of discharge, and patient status on discharge also need to be documented.

## EVALUATION

Actions, observations, and patient responses to treatment should be clearly documented to enable nurses to evaluate and measure the outcomes of the care processes. The evaluation of the plan of care should be ongoing during the procedure and conclude with a written and verbal report to the PACU nurse. The outcome of successful implementation of the plan of care may be documented as follows:

The patient is free from injury related to perioperative positioning, as evidenced by the following:

1. The skin and tissue integrity are consistent with the preoperative status, particularly at bony prominences and pressure areas.
2. There are no complaints of strained muscles or ligaments, altered range of motion, or peripheral sensory/motor deficits that were not present preoperatively.
3. The circulation in extremities is consistent with preoperative status.
4. The patient's respiratory status is consistent with preoperative status.
5. There are no adverse changes in hemodynamics; the heart rate and blood pressure are within expected ranges.

Any abnormalities should be documented on the postoperative assessment and reported to the surgeon and the PACU nurse.

## OPERATING ROOM BEDS

Modern OR beds are designed to support and accommodate the various anatomic configurations required in surgical positioning. Their height can be raised or lowered, they can tilt laterally, and they can be placed in the Trendelenburg or reverse-Trendelenburg position. Generally, OR beds are electrically or battery operated with a manual mechanical backup. They have roller wheels, which allow them to be moved easily, and brakes that can lock them in place.

### Operating Room Bed Parts and Accessories

General OR beds are composed of a flat platform divided into three major sections: the head, torso, and leg sections (Figure 5-10). Each section has a corresponding removable mattress pad, which usually attaches to the main platform by Velcro or straps. The area between each section is called a "break." Raising or lowering sections is called "breaking the table."

Along the edges of the bed are flat metal side rails that separate at each break and run horizontally along both sides of the entire OR bed. Armboards lock directly onto the side rails at any level of the OR bed. The side rails also accommodate sockets, triclamps, and locks that can secure a multitude of attachments, including stirrups, anesthesia screens, armboards, and various retractors. Underneath the OR bed platform is a tunnel that runs under the entire body and leg sections to support x-ray cassettes. In addition, in newer models, the entire OR bed platform is radiopaque to accommodate the use of intraoperative radiologic fluoroscopy.

The OR bed width is narrow to allow ease of access to the operative site. For some patients, this width may not be enough to support their whole body adequately (see Chapter 11 for a discussion of special considerations for OR beds and positioning of bariatric surgery patients). Armboards or table width extenders can be secured parallel to the OR bed at the waist and hip levels to give additional lateral support to such patients if a bariatric surgical bed is not available. Some OR beds have weight limitations and cannot accommodate patients of certain weights.

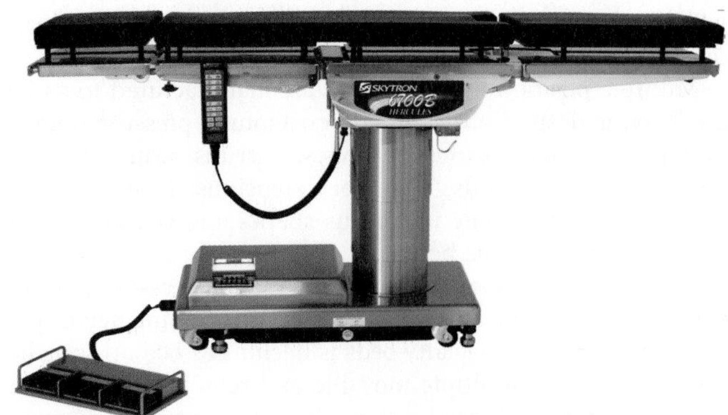


**FIGURE 5-10** OR bed adaptable to a wide range of surgical procedures.

The torso section is attached to the base of the OR bed because this section supports the heaviest parts of the body: the chest, abdomen, and pelvis. This section also has a break in the center at the hip level that can be flexed or lowered to allow the head and chest areas to be elevated or lowered. At this central break in the torso section, there is a crossbar, called a *kidney bridge* (body elevator), which can be raised or lowered for kidney or gallbladder exposure. The kidney bridge is concave and can accommodate lateral braces that slide vertically onto the bridge to maintain the patient in a lateral position. The distal portions of the torso section's platform and mattress have concave perineal cutouts to accommodate access to the perineum when the patient is in the lithotomy position. Drainage trays may be fitted into this section for gynecologic, urologic, and proctologic procedures.

The head section of the OR bed can be flexed, lowered, or removed. It is connected to the bed by two horizontal posts that fit into corresponding grooves in the front of the torso section. Special headrests, such as a craniotomy or ophthalmic headrest, can slide into these grooves to be used for special procedures.

The leg section of the OR bed can be flexed or lowered to the extent that it folds deeply beneath the torso section to allow leg room for a sitting surgeon to gain access to the perineal area when the patient is in the lithotomy position. The leg section also has grooves in the distal-most platform to accommodate a foot extension for tall patients. The foot extension attachment can be flexed upward to give plantar support if needed. The distal grooves also accommodate the head section in case the patient is to be positioned with the head where the feet usually are. Such positioning allows for movement of C-arm radiologic fluoroscopy around the patient's chest and abdomen because the leg section protrudes farther away from the base than the head section does. Another use for placing the head section at the foot of the OR bed is to enable the patient to be positioned with the buttocks in the perineal cutout immediately on transfer to the OR bed; this extends the leg section so that the patient's legs do not hang over the end of the bed and eliminates the need for the patient to be moved down on the bed after induction. The shearing and friction risks of such a move are reduced.

Multiple positioning accessories are manufactured to assist in achieving desired positions and cushioning pressure points. Examples include various headrests, stirrups, arm supports, hand tables, footboards, and foot extensions. Foam and gel pads and overlays come in various shapes and sizes designed for specific areas of the body.

Because new state-of-the-art OR beds and accessory devices can accommodate most types of surgical positioning needs, the need for additional specialty beds is declining. The orthopedic fracture table has multiple movable and removable parts and suspended frames. Special orthopedic extensions and accessories that duplicate the functions of the features on traditional orthopedic fracture tables are available for some OR beds. Although urologic procedures can be done on a general OR bed set up in the lithotomy position, specialty urology beds are still beneficial to the OR because they have built-in drainage trays and radiologic equipment.

## Mattress Materials and Their Pressure-Reducing Properties

OR mattresses should meet certain basic characteristic requirements. They should be durable, versatile to many intended uses, nonflammable, resistant to bacterial growth, radiolucent with low x-ray attenuation, compatible with warming and cooling devices, and covered with nonallergic antistatic fabric. OR mattresses should have pressure-reduction capabilities.

Durability can lead to increased longevity and cost-efficiency. The cover should be made of durable but pliable material that is easily washed and resistant to deterioration from various prep solutions and chemical cleaning agents. The covering material should be resistant to the effects of heat and reduce friction and shear. Covers also should be waterproof and completely intact. Seams should be heat sealed or bonded instead of stitched to inhibit entry of solutions into the core of the mattress. The mattress core also should be resistant to fungal and bacterial growth.

Mattress pad versatility can be evaluated by its ability to flex easily and extend with its accompanying OR bed platform. The more lightweight it is, the easier it is to remove and reposition the pads. Some pads must be stored horizontally because of gel components.

Pressure reduction is a prime consideration in OR mattress pads. Neither the position of the patient nor time spent on the OR bed can be altered easily during surgery. Varying the type of pressure-reducing mattress may be the most appropriate method to prevent pressure ulcers during the perioperative period.[13] With more attention being directed toward optimal pressure relief, manufacturers are improving OR mattresses to be more protective of tissue integrity. As mentioned earlier, distributing pressure over a larger surface of the body decreases the force of that pressure. Overall interface pressure can be reduced by providing even pressure distribution without "bottoming out" (i.e., flattening or collapsing such that parts of the body rest on the underlying surface, defeating the purpose of the mattress).[13,18] Generally, the thinner the foam, the easier it is to "bottom out." Mattress materials vary in their pressure-reducing characteristics. Following are some examples of materials currently on the market.

***Standard Foam Operating Room Mattress Pads.*** Standard foam OR mattress pads have greatly improved in quality over the years. They are usually purchased with OR beds, or replacement pads can be purchased. Years ago these mattresses used to be about 2 inches thick, made of standard foam, and covered with a relatively rigid vinyl covering. Today's mattresses are 3 or more inches thick and have greater protection against the effects of pressure. They have a soft, pliable waterproof cover. The more pliable the cover, the greater the patient benefit from the pressure-reducing properties of the foam or other material inside the mattress. Many pads are made with new advanced foam technology. The foams have contouring properties, which allow the bony prominences to sink into the surface of the foam so that they no longer are the sole "landing gear." Because other body surfaces also are in contact with the resting surface, the overall interface pressures are reduced. These foam pads have pliable covers, which allow the body surfaces more contact with the foam and help reduce shear.[18] The benefits of these pads are causing many manufacturers to use them as their new "standard" OR pads.

***Gel Products.*** Gel products, which comprise dry polymer elastomer gels, generally are used as overlays to mattress segments and positioning devices. Some OR bed mattress pads are being made with a layer of gel over the foam and a pliable cover. Gel products seem to reduce the effects of shearing forces because they are pliable and similar to the qualities of body fat. Results are inconclusive regarding their effectiveness in reducing pressure compared with other pressure-reducing surfaces. Compared with a standard OR mattress, however, research has shown that gel pads do reduce pressure ulcers.[3,18] Because gel pads are expensive, heavy, and slow to adapt to temperature, they are more practical for spot protection and overlays for smaller positioning devices.[15]

***Air Support Surfaces.*** Air support surfaces comprise pads with thousands of air cells that are either static (providing consistent dry flotation) or dynamic (providing constantly changing pressure points through a pump or motor).[13] Studies have shown these surfaces to be effective in reducing pressure ulcer development compared with other available products.[3,27] They have a durability advantage as well. The plastic air cells do not degrade as rapidly as foam. Their life span is about 5 years compared with that of foam, which is about 2 years.[18]

## Pressure-Reduction Considerations

Because OR mattress compositions vary widely, it is difficult to know which products provide the best results, especially in reducing pressure. It is helpful to refer to studies (preferably by independent researchers) that compare the pressure-reducing features of various products. Broader studies, comparing a wider variety of products, tend to be more useful because products change and improve continuously (Research Highlight).

Mattress companies and independent researchers use various interface pressure-monitoring instruments to measure and compare products. The interface pressure can be measured under selected sites by electropneumatic sensors that can convert pressures to mm Hg. Because capillary interface pressure is about 32 mm Hg, the lower the interface pressure sustained by the mattress, the better. Another type of instrument used to show relative interface pressure is a table in which a computerized image of the table shows as a color-coded scan. The entire surface of the body in contact with the mattress on this table displays various colors ranging from light to dark. The darker the color, the higher the pressure. It can locate areas of highest pressure for selected positions and provide a comparative pressure analysis between different products.

Whatever pressure-reducing properties exist in a mattress, a stiff outer covering can reduce these properties. Thin, pliable yet durable outer coverings maximize the benefits of the mattress. In addition, the overuse of bedding materials can contribute to increased interface pressures. The more layers of sheets, absorbent pads, and/or blankets placed between the patient and the mattress, the more resistance there is to the pliability and effectiveness of the mattress material. Bedding should be kept to a minimum. With some products, such as certain dry polymer overlays, bedding should not be used at all. Manufacturer's recommendations should be reviewed and implemented.

## STANDARD SURGICAL POSITIONS

This section discusses standard positions and their variations in terms of their requirements for certain surgical procedures, the unique risks that they present to various body systems, and nursing interventions that diminish risks to the patient. Table 5-2 provides an abbreviated summary of standard surgical positions.

## RESEARCH HIGHLIGHT

### Effectiveness of Operating Room Pressure-Reduction Surfaces

Through a systematic and critical synthesis and evaluation of literature on pressure relief in surgical patients, three types of intraoperative risk factors for surgical patients were identified. These were quantified as *intrinsic* (e.g., age, comorbidity, nutritional status, body size, mobility and activity levels, body temperature), *extrinsic* (e.g., heat, shearing, friction, moisture), and *OR-specific* factors (e.g., type and length of surgical procedure, surgical position, type of OR mattress, positioning, and warming devices). As a result of this integrative analysis, findings related to pressure-reduction surfaces used in ORs suggested that the use of a static air overlay during surgery best reduces tissue interface pressure. Foam overlays and standard OR mattresses were found to have the lowest pressure reduction capabilities. Dry viscoelastic polymer pads or gel pads reduce pressure better than foam overlays or standard OR mattresses but not as efficiently as air overlays.

Modified from Armstrong D, Bortz P: An integrative review of pressure relief in surgical patients, *AORN Journal* 73(3):645-670, 2001.

**TABLE 5-2**

**Risks and Interventions of Surgical Positions**

| Position | Risks | Interventions |
|---|---|---|
| Supine | 1. Pressure to head, shoulders, elbows, back, sacrum, coccyx, and heels | 1. Pressure-reducing OR mattress. Additional padding as needed |
| | 2. Pressure to peripheral vessels and nerves, primarily brachial plexus and ulnar nerves | 2. Armboards level with OR mattress, <90 degrees extension and palms up. Ankles uncrossed |
| Supine variations | *Risks in addition to above* | |
| Trendelenburg | 1. Diminished lung capacity | 1. Close respiratory monitoring |
| | 2. Venous pooling shifts toward head | 2. Slow, smooth postural transitions to diminish cardiovascular effects |
| | 3. Sliding and shearing | 3. Flex knees slightly. Limit time in position |
| Reverse Trendelenburg | 1. Deep vein thrombosis (DVT) in lower extremities | 1. Antiembolic or sequential compression stockings |
| | 2. Sliding and shearing | 2. Padded footboard |
| Fracture table | 1. Pressure to foot and ankle in traction | 1. Adequate padding. Appropriate foot cuff inflation |
| | 2. Pressure to genitalia | 2. Properly padded and positioned perineal post |
| Lithotomy | 1. Hip dislocations, fractures, and muscle and nerve injuries | 1. Securely fasten stirrups to OR bed. Avoid hyperabduction of hips and leaning against inner thighs. Avoid candy cane stirrups when possible. Avoid leg contact with stirrup bars. Limit time in position |
| | 2. Pressure injuries to foot, ankles, and knees | 2. Use stirrups that disperse support and pressure over wide areas. Check distal pulses before and after positioning |
| | 3. Back strain | 3. Buttocks should not hang off the edge of the torso section of the bed |
| | 4. Diminished lung capacity | 4. Close respiratory monitoring |
| | 5. Venous pooling shifts toward head | 5. Slow, smooth postural transitions to diminish cardiovascular effects |
| | 6. DVT in lower extremities | 6. Antiembolic or sequential compression stockings if in position >2 hr |
| | 7. Crushed fingers | 7. Ensure fingers are away from break of bed when leg section is elevated |

*Continued*

**TABLE 5-2**

## Risks and Interventions of Surgical Positions—cont'd

| Position | Risks | Interventions |
|---|---|---|
| Fowler (sitting) | 1. Pressure to scapulae, sacrum, coccyx, ischium, back of knees, and heels | 1. Pressure-reducing OR mattress. Additional padding as needed |
| | 2. Air embolism if venous sinus is opened | 2. Doppler probe over chest wall, insert central venous catheter, saline-soaked sponges available |
| | 3. Shearing | 3. Momentarily tilt torso slightly away from OR bed to allow skin to realign with skeletal structures |
| | 4. DVT in lower extremities | 4. Sequential compression stockings |
| | 5. Venous pooling shifts toward lower body | 5. Slow, smooth postural transitions to diminish cardiovascular effects |
| Semi-Fowler (beach chair) | Risks similar to Fowler position, but generally not as severe | Same interventions |
| Prone | 1. Pressure to cheeks, eyes, ears, breasts, genitalia, patellae, and toes | 1. Pressure-reducing OR mattress. Additional padding as needed. Check ears, cheeks, eyes, and genitalia for pressure. Tape eyes closed |
| | 2. Falls and dislodgment of airway and monitoring cords and intravenous lines | 2. Lock both beds. Use a minimum of 4 people for turning patient. Secure airway and all cords and lines |
| | 3. Diminished lung capacity | 3. Chest rolls and close respiratory monitoring |
| | 4. Injury to shoulders, arms, and upper extremity nerves | 4. Arms never hang off the side of the OR bed. Arms on armboard are flexed and pronated with upper arm <90 degrees to the OR bed. Pads placed above and below elbow to free ulnar nerve |
| Prone variations | *Risks in addition to above* | |
| Jackknife | 1. DVT in lower extremities | 1. Check distal pulses before, during, and after positioning. If position maintained for extended time, antiembolic or sequential compression stockings |
| Knee-chest | 1. Extreme pressure on knees and ankles | 1. Additional padding to these areas |
| | 2. DVT in lower extremities | 2. Check distal pulses before, during, and after positioning. Antiembolic or sequential compression stockings |
| Lateral, lateral chest, and lateral kidney | 1. Pressure to structures on dependent side: ears, shoulder, ribs, hips, greater femoral head, knees, and ankles | 1. Pressure-reducing OR mattress. Additional padding as needed. Check that earlobes are not folded over. Place pillow between knees and under ankles. Be sure neck is in alignment |
| | 2. Risk of tilting and falling during procedure | 2. Flex dependent leg for support. Support abdomen and back to prevent lateral movement. May require additional straps or wide tape to secure patient further in addition to hip area |
| | 3. Brachial plexus injury | 3. Place padded roll under lower axilla. Bring lower shoulder slightly forward. Support lower arm on armboard with palm up. Support upper arm on elevated armboard or pillow |
| | 4. Venous pooling shifts toward dependent side | 4. Slow, smooth postural transitions to diminish cardiovascular effects |
| | 5. Diminished lung capacity of dependent lung | 5. Ventilator support provider includes positive-end expiratory pressure (PEEP). Anesthesia inserts double-lumen endotracheal tube to ventilate dependent lung if thoracotomy performed |
| | 6. DVT in lower extremities | 6. Check distal pulses before, during, and after positioning. Antiembolic or sequential compression stockings |

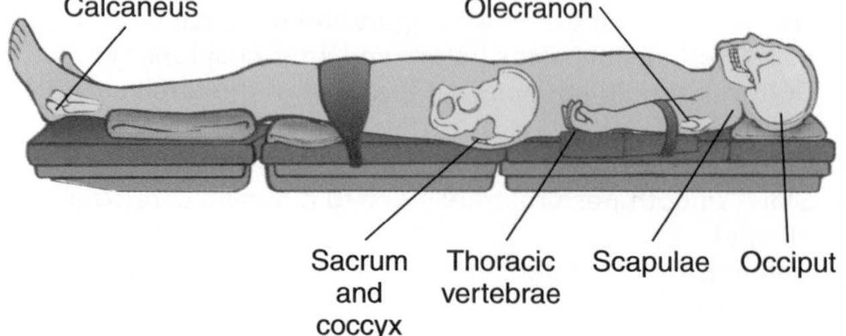


**FIGURE 5-11** Potential pressure areas: supine position. A pillow under the calves frees popliteal areas and heels from pressure.

## Supine

The supine (dorsal recumbent) position is the most common. The patient lies with the back flat on the OR bed. The arms may be tucked at the side or placed on armboards. This is the most natural position of the body at rest and is the position in which the patient is usually anesthetized.

The supine position allows access to the major body cavities (peritoneal, thoracic, pericardial). It also allows access to the head, neck, and extremities. Vulnerable pressure areas in the supine position are the occiput, scapulae, olecranon, thoracic vertebrae, sacrum, coccyx, and calcaneus (Figure 5-11).

A safety strap should be placed 2 inches above the knees. A sheet or blanket should always be placed between the safety strap and the patient's skin. The strap should be applied with enough tension to secure the patient to the OR bed but without compromising circulation underneath the strap. If the knees are to be flexed, caution should be taken in placing a pillow directly under the patient's knees. The popliteal artery, common peroneal nerve, and tibial nerve all run superficially through the popliteal space. Compression of these structures between a pillow and the safety strap theoretically could cause nerve damage, impaired circulation, and possibly venous thrombosis. Although there is no evidence that such injury has been reported, using a soft pillow under the knees and ensuring that the safety strap is not too tight or placing the pillow proximal to the popliteal space reduce the likelihood of such an occurrence.

The head generally rests on a small pillow or head cushion to support cervical alignment, reduce occipital pressure, and reduce strain on neck muscles. The eyes must be protected from textiles, solutions, and other foreign objects by applying eye patches or eye shields or by taping the eyelids closed.

If the arms are placed on armboards, the armboards should be padded with the pad level equal to that of the OR bed. Extension should be less than a 90-degree angle to prevent stretching and compression of the brachial plexus. Wrist restraints should be soft and nonocclusive. It is preferable that the rotational position of the hand on an armboard be in supination (palms up). If the arms rest with the forearms across the trunk, padding should be placed proximal to the elbow (see Figure 5-5 and "Upper Extremity Neuropathies" for more details). If the arms are tucked at the side, the fingers should be straight, and the palms should lie neutral against the body. The drawsheet should be brought next to the body, over and around the arm, and tucked under the body (see Figure 5-6).

Sometimes the patient's legs need to be flexed in a frog-leg fashion to provide access to the groin, perineum, and medial aspects of the lower extremities. The thighs are externally rotated, and the knees are flexed and supported with a pillow under each leg. This position is used when access to the genitals is required during abdominal gynecologic and urologic procedures. During coronary artery bypass graft procedures, this position allows access for harvesting the saphenous vein. Sometimes a special contoured positioning pad is used instead of pillows.

In the supine position, blood volume to the heart and lungs is increased compared with the erect position because the venous blood from the lower body flows back to the heart without the counterforce of gravity. This increased blood volume is what increases the cardiac output and the cardiac workload. The weight of the chest in obese patients can cause increased intrathoracic pressure and increase the cardiac workload further. If a patient has cardiovascular deficiencies, this position can increase the risk for cardiac failure further.

Increased pressure on the inferior vena cava from abdominal viscera, abdominal masses, or a fetus in a pregnant woman may decrease blood return to the heart; blood pressure would then be lowered. The inferior vena cava lies slightly to the right of the vertebral column. Tilting the patient slightly to the left by placing a small roll or wedge under the right flank can divert the weight away from the vena cava. An example is tilting a supine cesarean section patient slightly to the left until the fetus is delivered.

Respiratory function is compromised in the supine position because the tidal volume is less than that in the erect posture. The supine position allows a more even distribution of ventilation from the apex to the base of the lungs. Anterior and upward excursion of the chest during inspiration is not greatly impeded except in obese patients, whose chest wall weight significantly compresses the rib cage. The abdominal viscera lessen diaphragmatic excursion, particularly when an abdominal retractor is used and packs are placed toward the diaphragm.

## Trendelenburg

Trendelenburg position is a variation of the supine position in which the upper torso is lowered and the feet are raised. This position facilitates visualization of the pelvic organs during open or laparoscopic surgeries in the lower abdomen or pelvis. Trendelenburg position can be used to improve circulation to the cerebral cortex and basal ganglia when the blood pressure is suddenly lowered. In this position, the knees are often bent by flexing the leg section of the bed (Figure 5-12). The patient must have the knees over the break in the bed to maintain safe anatomic positioning. As the lower section of the bed is elevated, the Mayo stand should be raised to prevent pressure on the feet.

Shearing is a significant risk in this position. The skeletal structure slides up toward the head of the bed. If the patient is draped, lifting the patient to realign the tissue cannot be done. If necessary, shoulder braces may be used to limit upward sliding; however, they pose their own risk to the brachial plexus (as described in "Upper Extremity Neuropathies" section earlier) and should be used with caution. To protect the brachial plexus from compression injury if shoulder braces must be used, it is important to ensure that they are well padded and placed above the supraclavicular joint, not the soft tissue of the neck. They should *not* be used if the arms are extended on armboards.

Any variation of Trendelenburg position should be maintained only as long as necessary. In this position, blood pools in the upper torso, increasing blood pressure and intracranial pressure. Although the head-down position facilitates drainage of secretions from the bases of the lungs and the oropharyngeal passages, the weight of the abdominal viscera further impedes diaphragmatic movement; as the abdominal viscera push the diaphragm up and compress the lung bases, pulmonary compliance and tidal volume are diminished. Fluid shifts into the alveoli, causing edema, congestion, and atelectasis. Slow, smooth postural transitions allow sufficient time for the body to adjust to physiologic changes. If this is not done when the patient is being placed in Trendelenburg position, blood rapidly shifts from the lower extremities, causing a reflexive de-

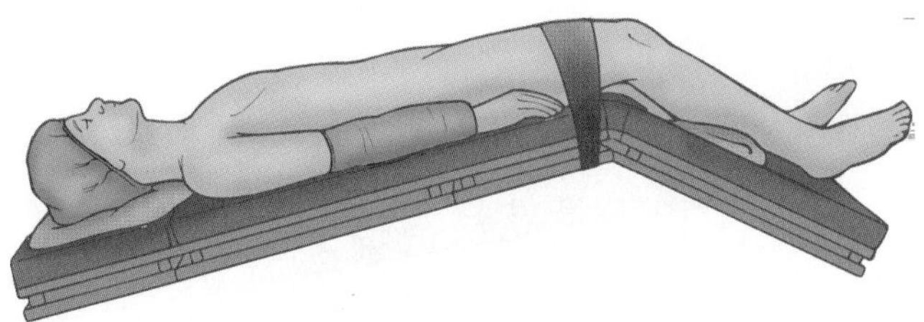

**FIGURE 5-12** Trendelenburg position.

creased cardiac output. Conversely, hypotension may result if the patient is not returned slowly to the supine position.

## Reverse Trendelenburg

Reverse Trendelenburg position is described as the head-up, feet down, supine position (Figure 5-13). It is frequently used to provide access to the head and neck and to facilitate gravitational pull on the viscera away from the diaphragm and toward the feet. When the foot of the bed is tilted toward the floor, a padded footboard supports the patient's body.

For patients having thyroid, neck, or shoulder surgery, a pillow or soft roll is placed horizontally under the shoulders to hyperextend the neck. The knees can be slightly flexed to counteract sliding forward and minimize shearing. The arms generally are tucked at the side to allow for closer access to the surgical site.

In the reverse Trendelenburg position, respiratory function is similar to that in the erect position. Venous circulation may be compromised by extended time in the legs-downward position. When this situation is anticipated, the superficial venous return can be aided by the preoperative application of antiembolic stockings, elastic bandages, or sequentially inflatable stockings. If the legs are wrapped, compression of the common peroneal nerve at the head of the fibula must be avoided.

For minimally invasive approaches to the esophagus, such as laparoscopic Nissen fundoplication, steep reverse Trendelenburg position is required. The OR bed is modified by the addition of leg holders, and the surgeon stands between the legs. To prevent the patient from sliding as a result of the steep position, a Vac-Pac (beanbag) is inflated under the patient, and the knees are slightly flexed to a range of 20 to 30 degrees (this surgical positioning system is described later). In this position, the combination of increased abdominal pressure from pneumoperitoneum and steep reverse Trendelenburg position decreases venous return. Sequential compression stockings are applied as prophylaxis against deep vein thrombosis. Return to the supine position from reverse Trendelenburg position should be accomplished slowly and smoothly to avoid overload to the cardiovascular system.

## Fracture Table Position

The orthopedic fracture table allows the patient to be positioned for hip fracture surgery or closed femoral nailing (Figure 5-14). The patient may be brought into the OR in the hospital bed with traction applied. Before transfer, the patient can be anesthetized. During transfer to the fracture table, manual traction to the injured leg can be applied. Distal lower extremity pulses should be evaluated before, during, and after this position.

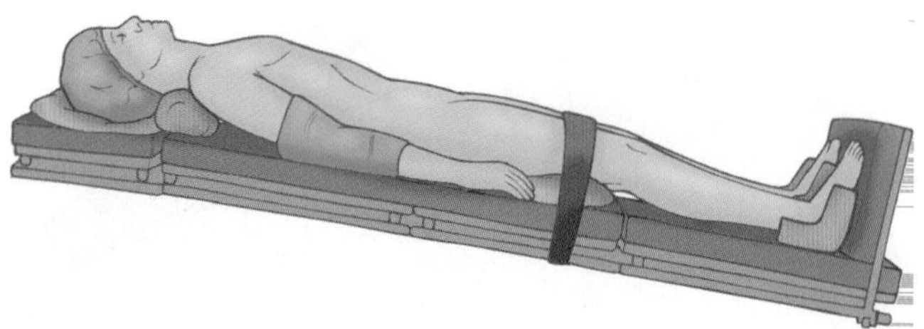

FIGURE 5-13 Reverse Trendelenburg position with soft roll under shoulder for thyroid, neck, and shoulder procedures.

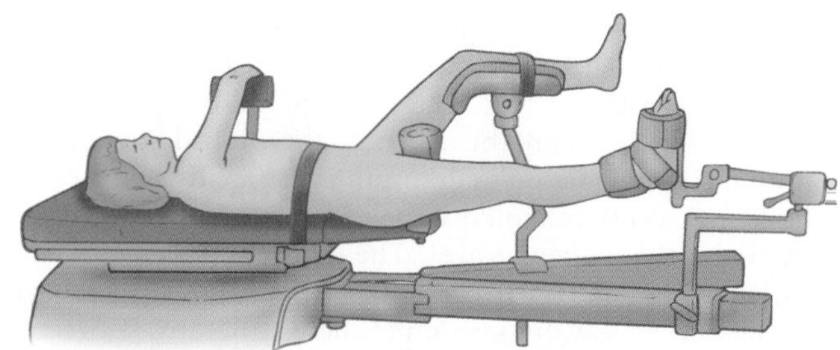

FIGURE 5-14 Fracture table position. The unaffected leg is raised, abducted, and supported in a padded leg rest.

The patient is positioned supine with the pelvis stabilized against a well-padded vertical perineal post. Pressure on the genitalia from the perineal post can injure the genital structures. Pressure on the perineal and pudendal nerves can cause fecal incontinence and loss of perineal sensation (see "Genitalia" section on page 142 for more details).

Traction is achieved by restraining the foot of the injured leg in a well-padded, bootlike device that is connected to the traction bar so that the leg may be rotated, pulled into traction, or released, as the surgery requires. One method of securing the foot in this device is the use of a boot-shaped cuff that wraps around the entire foot and connects to the traction device. It is inflated with air to secure the foot. Another method is to cushion the foot and secure it to the device with restraining straps, Ace bandages, or a self-adhering wrap. Whatever method is used, excessive pressure can be placed on the foot and ankle, especially while traction is being applied. Adequate padding must be used. If the boot-shaped cuff is used, care should be taken that it is not inflated beyond the manufacturer's recommendations. Distal lower extremity pulses should be evaluated before, during, and after this position.

The unaffected leg rests on a well-padded, elevated leg holder or is secured in a well-padded, bootlike device. C-arm fluoroscopy examinations can be done during surgery because the unaffected leg is abducted well out of the field of the x-ray machine.

The arm on the operative side is generally secured over the patient's body in a padded sling or a post-supported arm holder to reduce obstruction of the operative area. Care should be taken to avoid pressure on the ulnar nerve. The edges of the sling should not be right on the bend of the elbow. If a post is supporting the arm holder, the post and arm holder should be distal to the elbow, freeing the cubital tunnel from pressure.

## Lithotomy

The lithotomy position is used for gynecologic, rectal, and urologic procedures. With the patient supine, the legs are raised and abducted to expose the perineal region. The legs are placed in stirrups to maintain this position. There are four levels of lithotomy: low, standard, high, and exaggerated (Figure 5-15). *Low lithotomy* is used for most urologic procedures and for procedures that require access to the perineum and abdomen simultaneously. The thighs are elevated approximately 30 to 45 degrees. *Standard lithotomy* is the most commonly used position for gynecologic procedures. The thighs are flexed approximately 90 degrees from the trunk, and the calves remain horizontal. For improved perineal access, some surgeons prefer a *high lithotomy* position. The thighs are often

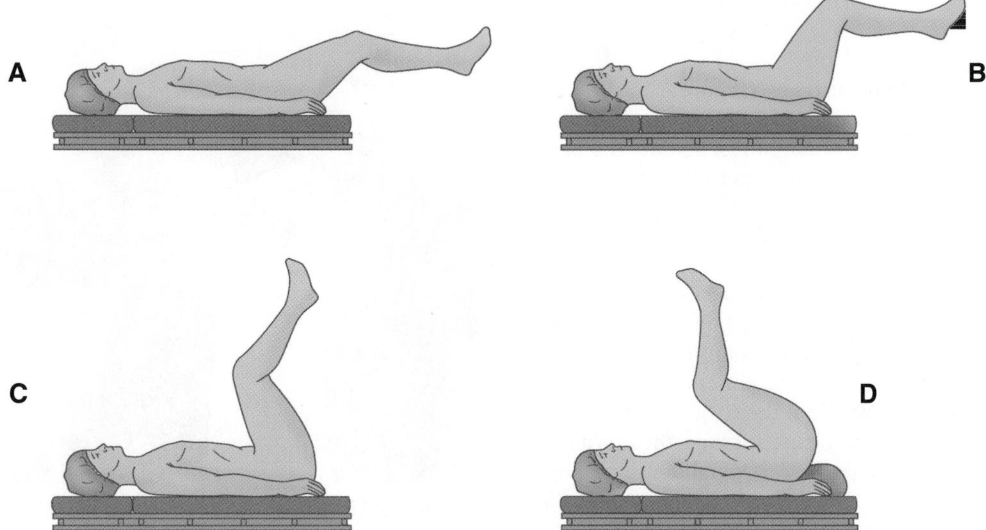


**FIGURE 5-15** The four basic types of lithotomy position with progressively increasing leg elevation. **A,** Low. **B,** Standard. **C,** High. **D,** Exaggerated.

flexed beyond 90 degrees, and the legs are suspended high toward the ceiling. The *exaggerated lithotomy* position is sometimes used for transperineal access to the retropubic area. This extreme position moves the legs completely out of the way of the surgical field. The thighs are flexed toward the abdomen; the calves are suspended vertically; and the pelvis is flexed vertically at the spine, propped upward on a pillow or pad.[31]

The stirrups should be checked before use so that they are securely fastened to the side rails of the OR bed. Slippage of the stirrups or dropping of the legs during stirrup adjustments could cause hip dislocation, muscle or nerve injury, or bone fractures. Both stirrups should be at equal height and attached to the OR bed at the same level (Figure 5-16). The legs should be raised simultaneously to prevent strain on the patient's lower back; this requires two people so that both legs are totally supported throughout the move. Each person should grasp the sole of the foot with one hand and support the calf near the knee with the other. The legs should be raised and the knees flexed in slow, smooth movements.

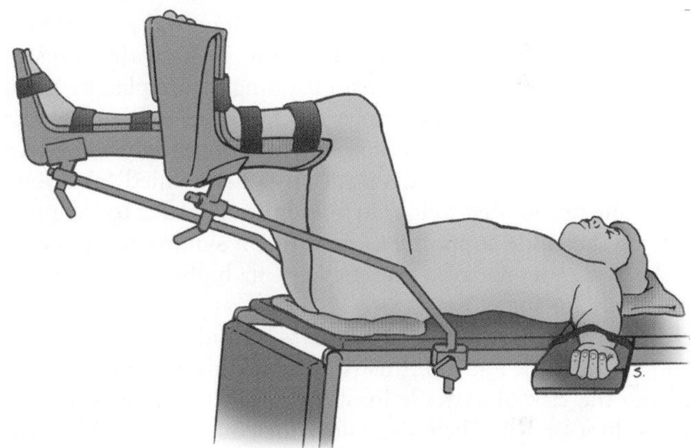

**FIGURE 5-16** Lithotomy position using boot-type stirrups.

When the legs are secured in the stirrups, the mattress of the leg section of the OR bed is removed, and the leg section platform is lowered. The buttocks should be even with the edge of the OR bed to reduce the risk of lumbosacral strain.

The arms are supported on armboards (see Figure 5-16), placed across the trunk, or tucked at the patient's side. When the arms are tucked, extreme caution should be taken when the leg section of the bed is elevated back to a horizontal position at the conclusion of the procedure. The hands and fingers can be caught in the break of the bed and pinched or crushed (see "Fingers" section on page 142).

Various types of stirrups are used for lithotomy positioning (Figure 5-17). The most common include posts with knee crutches, candy cane-shaped bars with straps that wrap around the ankles and plantar surface of the foot, and boot-type stirrups that cradle the lower foot and heel and extend to the midcalf area. The type of stirrup used can create unique hazards.

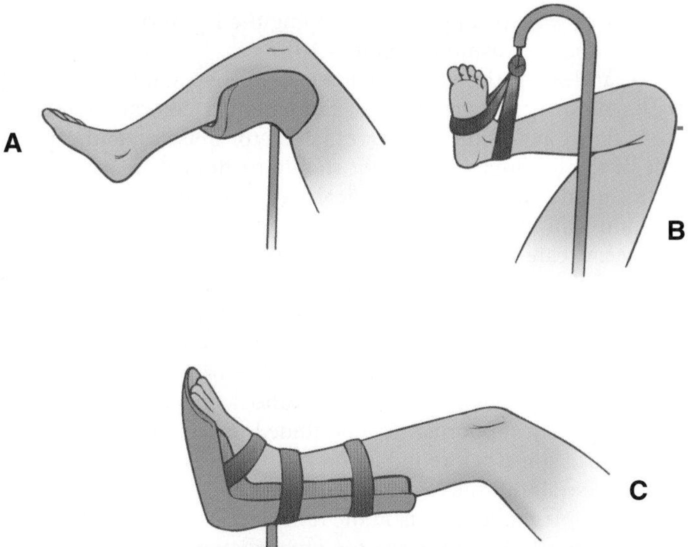


**FIGURE 5-17** Types of stirrups used. **A,** Knee crutch. **B,** Candy cane. **C,** Boot.

Knee crutch stirrups (Figure 5-17, *A*), in which the weight of the leg rests solely on the knee supports, can put pressure on the posterior tibial and common peroneal nerves and the popliteal artery in the popliteal fossa. This pressure predisposes the patient to complications, such as neuropathies and compartment syndrome.

When using the candy cane stirrups (Figure 5-17, *B*), the knees can drop close enough to the vertical stirrup bars that the lateral side of each knee or calf might rest against the bars. This can put pressure on the common peroneal nerve as it curves laterally over the fibula, resulting in footdrop and a lack of sensation below the knee. If the medial aspect of the knee or calf rests against a stirrup bar, the saphenous branch of the femoral nerve can be compressed against the tibia. Stirrup bar pads can soften the rigidity of the bars, but do not totally eliminate the pressure if the legs rest against the stirrup bars.

The relaxed hips of an anesthetized patient may separate further than they comfortably would if the patient were awake. When the legs hang freely in candy cane stirrups, there is a risk of external rotation of the hips and hyperabduction. Hips should not be flexed more than 90 degrees. Exaggerated rotation and flexion can stretch the sciatic and obturator nerves and strain the hip joint and muscles.

When relatively thin ankle straps support the weight of the entire leg, this can put pressure on the ankles and distal sural and plantar nerves. Neuropathies of the foot and pressure ulcers of the ankle support sites can result. Using wide straps or cradling the feet with gel or foam padding before placing them in the stirrup straps can reduce the localized pressure to the nerves in the foot. This is especially important when the legs are highly elevated and this position is maintained for a long time. The heavier leg weight in obese patients adds to the pressure on the ankle supports. Compartment syndrome can be an undesired outcome of a patient kept in high or exaggerated lithotomy for many hours.[26]

Boot-type stirrups (see Figures 5-16 and 5-17, *C*), which support the foot and calf, distribute pressure more evenly, reducing the risk of extreme localized pressure on any one area of the foot or leg. They also allow for controlled and limited abduction. Newer designs of boot stirrups allow the user to adjust the degree of hip flexion and abduction without the need to release the side rail socket. This safety feature reduces the risk of stirrup slippage or dropping the leg during adjustment of the leg position (Figure 5-18).

Regardless of the type of stirrup used, hyperabduction of the legs can cause stretching of the femoral, femoral cutaneous, sciatic, and obturator nerves; abductor muscles; and capsule of the hip joint. Abduction should be limited to only the degree needed for adequate surgical access, and the time in this position should be minimized.

Special care is needed for the patient who has a limited range of motion attributable to a hip prosthesis, cast, amputation, or obesity. Severe hip flexion and abduction of the joint must be avoided. The stirrup should be as low as possible and tilted slightly outward. Preexisting lumbar backache also can be worsened in this position if the buttocks or lower back is not adequately supported. Several folded towels placed under the lumbar spine before induction can retain lordosis and reduce the strain on the lower back. An exception is the patient with palpable tender points in the lumbar region. The pressure of a pad in this area may cause too much distress. Elevating the legs may aggravate the pain of a herniated nucleus pulposus. In each of these situations, the patient could be placed in the lithotomy position before induction to assess areas of discomfort and implement appropriate therapeutic measures before the procedure begins. If the patient will be in this position for longer than 2 hours, Ace bandages or antiembolic stockings/devices should be applied to the patient's legs. The flexing of the knee may impede venous return.

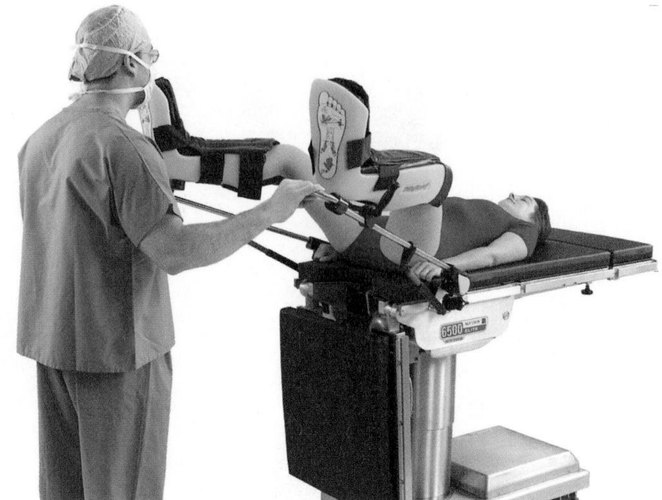

**FIGURE 5-18** Yellofin boot-type positioner allows one to raise and lower boot and abduct and adduct intraoperatively without needing to release the side rail socket.

The lithotomy position poses significant risk for respiratory and circulatory compromise. The risks increase as the position is exaggerated for radical surgery of the groin, vulva, or prostate. Extreme flexion of the thighs impairs respiratory function by increasing intraabdominal pressure against the diaphragm, decreasing the tidal volume. Interference with gravity flow of blood from the elevated legs causes pooling in the trunk of the body during the operative procedure. This effect is greater when hip and knee flexion is extreme, as in high or exaggerated lithotomy positions. Blood loss during surgery may not be immediately manifest because of this increased trunk volume. When the legs are lowered, and 500 mL or more of blood is diverted to more total leg circulation, however, the circulating volume is depleted, and the blood pressure may decrease. The effects of anesthesia on the nervous system depress normal compensatory mechanisms, and hemodynamic adjustment may not be achieved easily.

The arms must not impede chest movement and respiration. The weight of the limbs on the chest, especially in infants and children, may fatigue the muscles used in respiration and induce respiratory problems. In addition, the elevation of the legs pushes abdominal viscera toward the diaphragm. Lowering the head of the bed can exaggerate this shift further as diaphragmatic excursion is reduced.

Releasing the patient from the position must be done slowly and with adequate assistance. The legs must be taken out of stirrups and lowered simultaneously, with support given to the joints to prevent strain on the lumbosacral musculature, which can stretch and tilt, placing the pelvis and limbs in imbalance. The legs should be lowered slowly to allow for gradual hemodynamic adjustment as more blood shifts into the lower extremities. Distal lower extremity pulses should be evaluated before, during, and after this position.

## Semi-Fowler

Semi-Fowler (lawn chair or beach chair) position may be used for some cranial, shoulder, nasal, abdominoplasty, or breast reconstruction procedures. This position is accomplished first with the patient supine. The upper body section of the bed is flexed 45 degrees, and the leg section is lowered slightly, flexing the knees. The arms may rest on a pillow in the lap or be secured on armboards parallel to the OR bed. A footboard may be flexed at the bottom of the OR bed to act as a footrest and prevent footdrop. The entire OR bed is tilted so that the head of the bed is not so erect. This can reduce sliding and shearing effects and diminish the hemodynamic effects of anesthesia.

When this position is used for shoulder surgery, the arm of the affected shoulder is prepped and draped to allow for intraoperative shoulder manipulation. The head and cervical spine need to be aligned properly and supported to prevent neuromuscular strain. Rotation of the head in an opposite direction of a shoulder that the surgeon is manipulating can cause injury to the brachial plexus. A shoulder chair attachment allows for vertical torso support and drop-away shoulder panels, which can be removed on the affected side during shoulder procedures to allow full access to the shoulder. This attachment also includes a padded head restraint, which secures the head from forward and lateral movement while the patient is in sitting position, and arm supports (Figure 5-19).

Diaphragmatic excursion is improved in this position compared with the supine position. Although pressure points remain similar to the pressure points of the supine position, additional pressure is placed on the ischial tuberosities, calcanei, and coccyx.

## Fowler

Fowler (sitting) position is used for some ear and nose procedures and craniotomies involving a posterior or occipital approach (Figure 5-20). This position is accomplished initially with the patient supine. Slowly, the upper body section of the OR bed is raised 90 degrees, while the knees are slightly flexed and the legs lowered. A footrest is used to prevent footdrop. The arms either rest in the lap on a pillow with the elbows flexed 90 degrees or less or are supported on the side with padded armboards. The cervical, thoracic, and lumbar sections of the spine should be in alignment when the position is established. When this position is used for posterior fossa craniotomy or cranial ventricular procedures, a special craniotomy headrest is used to secure and immobilize the head.

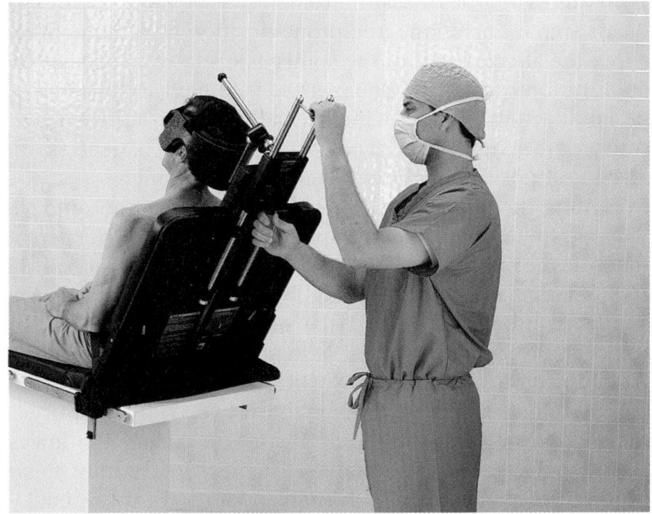

FIGURE 5-19 Shoulder Chair with drop-away shoulder support panels to allow surgical access to shoulder while maintaining torso support. Padded U-shaped head restraint with adjustable Velcro straps holds head secure and reduces undue stress on the neck when the back section is positioned.

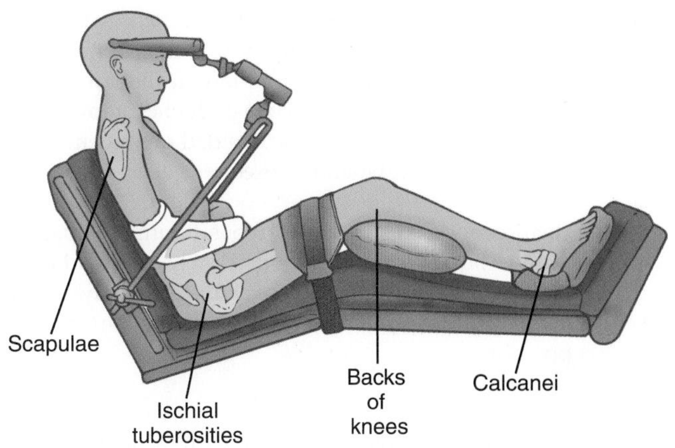


FIGURE 5-20 Potential pressure areas: Fowler (sitting) position.

The main pressure points include the scapulae, ischial tuberosities, calcanei, and coccyx. Also, pressure is increased on the sciatic nerve. Padding should be adequate at the lumbar area and under the elbows, knees, buttocks, and heels. The popliteal space needs to be checked to ensure that no pressure is sustained from the edge of the mattress at the bottom of the torso section.

This position poses some significant circulatory compromises and risks. Blood pooling occurs in the lower torso and legs, which causes significant orthostatic hypotension and diminished perfusion to the brain. Venous return from the lower extremities is impeded, and such hindrance causes an increased threat of venous thrombosis. Antiembolic stockings or Ace bandages along with a sequential venous compression device assist in supporting venous return.

Because the operative site is elevated compared with the heart, gravity causes a negative venous gradient between the operative site and the right atrium; this creates a potential for an air embolism if a venous sinus is opened. During a craniotomy, this potential increases when tissue is dissected free from the cranium, bone is removed, the dura is tacked up, or a highly vascular tumor bed is entered. Additional monitoring for venous air embolism includes the insertion of a central venous catheter into the pulmonary artery or right atrium and the placement of a Doppler probe over the chest wall. If air embolism is diagnosed, the scrub nurse should irrigate the area quickly with normal saline to prevent further venous aspiration of air. The exposed area should be packed with saline-soaked sponges or cottonoids. If the air embolism occurred during bone entry, bone wax should be placed immediately over the exposed bone to seal it. The anesthesia provider may aspirate air from the right atrium through the central venous line. The circulator should assist and support the endeavors of the anesthesia provider and scrub team.

Respirations are probably least impeded in the Fowler position than in any other surgical position. It is important to ensure that if the arms are resting on a pillow in the lap and secured with tape, this position does not restrict chest movement. Flexion of the head and neck must be avoided to prevent kinking of the endotracheal tube and subsequent airway obstruction.

When the procedure is concluded, repositioning the patient back to a supine position must be done slowly so that the patient can make hemodynamic adjustments gradually. Distal lower extremity pulses should be evaluated before, during, and after this position.

## Prone

In the prone position, the patient is lying with the abdomen on the surface of the OR bed mattress (Figure 5-21). Modifications of the position allow approaches to the cervical spine, back, rectal area, and dorsal areas of the extremities.

Anesthesia is induced with the patient in the supine position, usually on the transport vehicle. Before the patient is turned, the anesthesia provider secures the endotracheal tube with tape, applies eye ointment in each eye, and tapes the eyelids closed to prevent corneal abrasions. The transport vehicle is locked adjacent to the locked OR bed. Four people using the "log-roll" technique can accomplish turning the supine patient to prone position safely, smoothly, and gently. The anesthesia provider supports the head and neck during the turn. A second person stands at the side of the stretcher with hands at the patient's shoulders and buttocks to initiate the roll of the patient. A third person stands at the opposite side of the OR bed, with arms extended to support the chest and lower abdomen as the patient is rolled forward and over. The fourth person stands at the foot of the stretcher to support and turn the legs. At the completion of the turn, the stretcher is removed.

The perioperative nurse should not allow the patient's arms to hang over the edge of the bed because the radial nerve can be compressed quickly by the weight of the humerus against the OR bed side rails. The arms are secured at the sides or placed on armboards. If the arms are to remain at the patient's side, they should be close to the body and secured with the draw sheet pulled smoothly around the arms and tucked under the patient's body. The elbows are facing upward in this position, so there is less risk of pressure on the ulnar nerve from the mattress; however, compression still can occur from a tight draw sheet or from scrubbed personnel leaning on the elbow. Padding the elbow can minimize this risk. If the arms are to be placed on armboards, the arms are brought down and forward slowly and with minimal abduction to prevent shoulder dislocation and brachial plexus injury. The armboards should be at the same height as the OR bed, and the arms rest with elbows flexed and hands pronated. Elbows should not be flexed beyond 90 degrees to avoid stretching the ulnar nerve. Pads should be placed distal and proximal to the elbow so that the ulnar nerve is not in contact with the armboard (see Figure 5-5, *C*). The head is turned and positioned on a pillow or concave headrest with the neck kept in alignment with the spinal column. The eyes are carefully protected because they are most vulnerable to pressure injuries in this position (see "Eyes" section on page 141). Other areas that require special attention and padding are the cheek, ear, patellae, and toes.

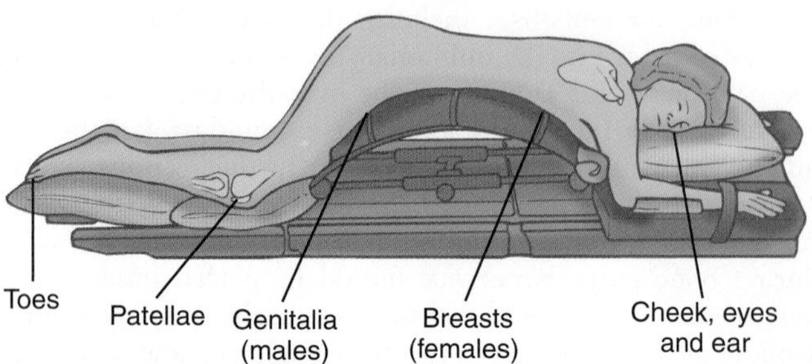


**FIGURE 5-21** Potential pressure areas: prone position using laminectomy frame for spinal procedures.

Generally, when the patient is placed in prone position, the patient is placed on a laminectomy frame or chest rolls that extend lengthwise from the acromioclavicular joint to the iliac crest. These positioning devices raise the chest and permit the diaphragm to move more freely and the lungs to expand. Supports must not press against male genitalia. Female breasts should be angled toward the sternum to reduce compression. These areas should be checked after final positioning to ensure that they are free from pressure. A bolster or pillow under the pelvis can decrease abdominal pressure on the inferior vena cava, especially in obese patients with large abdominal girths. A cushion or pillow is placed under the ankles to prevent pressure on the toes. The safety strap is placed across the dorsal aspects of the thighs so that the patient is secured but superficial venous return is not impaired.

The prone posture is initially hazardous as the anesthetized patient is turned from the supine position to the prone position. Endotracheal tubes, intravenous lines, and monitoring devices can be dislodged easily. Normal compensatory mechanisms are depressed, and the patient cannot readily adjust to imposed hemodynamic changes and the resulting hypotension.

The respiratory system is most vulnerable in the prone position because normal anterior lateral respiratory movement is restricted, and the compressed abdominal wall and rib cage inhibit normal diaphragmatic movement. This position generally requires ventilator assistance.

For spinal operations, the prone position may be modified to flex the affected part of the spine. The surgeon specifies the modifications preferred. One method is to increase the arch on the laminectomy frame, which usually can be adjusted by a hand crank. Another method is to place the patient in the knee-chest position without a laminectomy frame.

Turning the patient back into the supine position onto the PACU stretcher requires a four-person team effort. One person stands at the side of the OR bed and another at the side of the stretcher that is adjacent to the OR bed and is locked. The anesthesia provider supports the head, and a fourth person supports the feet. The patient is log-rolled onto the stretcher. If a laminectomy frame was used, it can be tilted in the direction of the stretcher to initiate the move. Skin integrity is checked over all pressure-point areas, particularly the knees, chest, breasts, and male genitalia. Distal lower extremity pulses should be evaluated before, during, and after this position.

## Jackknife

The jackknife (Kraske) position is a modification of the prone position that is often used for hemorrhoidectomy and pilonidal sinus procedures (Figure 5-22). The patient's hips are placed

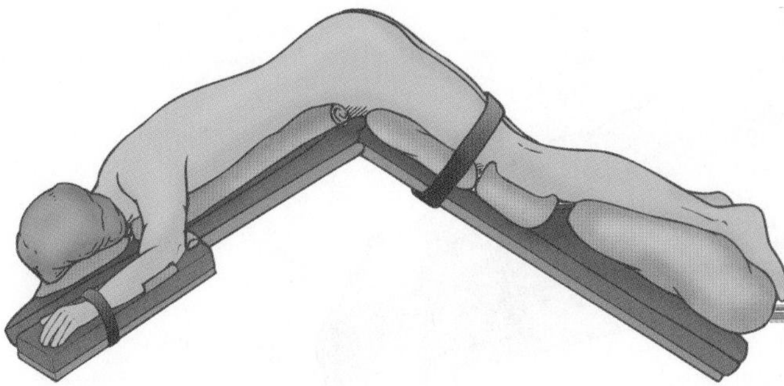
FIGURE 5-22 Jackknife (Kraske) position.

on a bolster or pillow over the break in the lumbar section of the OR bed, and the bed is flexed at a 90-degree angle, raising the hips and lowering the head and trunk. The patient's head, chest, and feet need the usual supports in this position. Chest rolls or a small roll placed under each shoulder relieve pressure on the brachial plexus from the clavicle. A pillow should be placed under the lower legs to prevent pressure on the toes. The restraint strap is placed across the posterior thighs.

For anal procedures, the buttocks may be separated with strips of 3-inch tape secured firmly at the level of the anus a few inches from the midline on either side. These strips are pulled tight simultaneously and are fastened to the underside of the bed surface. The strips are released at the end of the procedure to facilitate approximation of the wound edges.

This position causes circulatory changes because the head and the feet are in dependent positions, causing cephalad and caudad venous pooling. Antiembolism stockings assist in venous return and decrease the risk of venous thrombosis.

Respirations are severely compromised because anterior lateral chest movement is restricted. In addition, pressure is exerted on the diaphragm from the abdominal viscera, and that stress is exacerbated further by the pressure from the flexed OR bed.

When the procedure is completed, the patient is placed on the recovery stretcher in the supine position. The OR bed is first straightened very slowly so that the body can adjust hemodynamically. Four people using the log-roll technique turn the patient. Distal lower extremity pulses should be evaluated before, during, and after this position.

## Knee-Chest

The knee-chest position, a further exaggeration of the jackknife position, is used primarily for sigmoidoscopies and occasionally for lumbar laminectomy procedures (Figure 5-23). An extension platform is placed on the end of the foot section. The patient is positioned prone with the hips at the break of the body section. The leg section is lowered, and the extension platform is flexed at a right angle so that the patient kneels on the lower platform. The entire bed is tilted cephalad to expose the posterior pelvis. The safety strap is placed around the posterior area of the thighs.

The arms are placed on armboards and flexed at the elbows to lie adjacent to the head. The chest rests directly on the OR bed. Pressure points are a vital consideration for this position. They include the anterior rib cage, anterior iliac crests, anterior tibial aspects of the calves, anterior tali, toes, and especially the knees. All of these areas need to be well padded and supported.

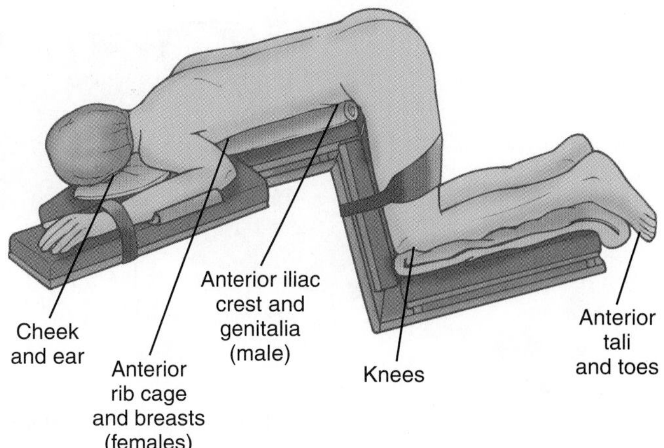

FIGURE 5-23 Potential pressure areas: knee-chest position.

Respiratory and circulatory compromise is similar to that of prone position. Lower extremity venous return is more restricted, however, because of bending of the knees. Antiembolic stockings/devices can reduce the risk of venous thrombosis. Distal lower extremity pulses should be evaluated before, during, and after this position.

## Lateral

In the lateral (lateral recumbent, lateral decubitus, or Sims) position, the patient is lying on the nonoperative side, providing access to the upper chest, the kidney (Figure 5-24), or the upper section of the ureter. Reference to right or left lateral position depends on the side on which the patient lies. In the right lateral position, the patient lies with the right side down. In left lateral, the patient lies with the left side down.

After induction of anesthesia with the patient in the supine position on the OR bed, the patient is turned to the side. A four-person team uses a liftsheet that is under the patient to facilitate a safe, smooth, gentle turn.

A pillow is placed under the patient's head to maintain good alignment with the cervical spine and the thoracic vertebrae; this alignment also helps to minimize stretching on the dependent brachial plexus. The bottom leg is flexed at the knee and hip to stabilize the patient on the bed. The top leg is straight or slightly flexed. A pillow is placed lengthwise between the patient's legs. The lateral aspect of the bottom knee must be padded to prevent pressure on the peroneal nerve, located superficially at the head of the fibula. A person should remain at the patient's back to steady and support the torso during positioning of the lower extremities.

Pillows, rolled blankets, padded kidney braces, or a surgical positioning system, sometimes referred to as a Vac-Pac, or beanbag, support the torso. A beanbag is a soft pad filled with tiny beads. When suction is attached to a port on the pad, it conforms to the shape of whatever it is wrapped around. A valve is closed to maintain the vacuum. It acts as an immobilizer until air is reintroduced, and then it softens back into its original shape. During the time that it is rigid, it increases the interface pressures of all the tissue it contacts, and the risk of pressure ulcer development increases. Large gel pads placed between the beanbag and the skin can reduce this risk.

The shoulders, hips, and legs may be secured with wide tape fastened to the platform of the OR bed. The upper arm is

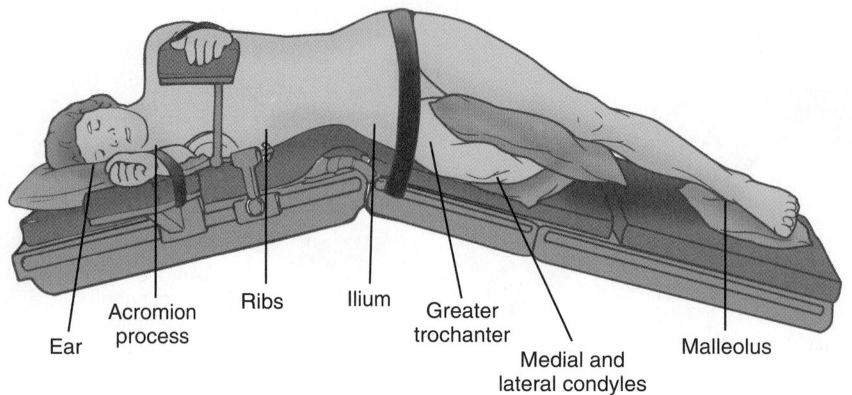


**FIGURE 5-24** Potential pressure areas: lateral kidney position.

placed on an elevated armboard or rests on a pillow in front of the patient. The lower arm is flexed and rests on an armboard. The lower shoulder should be brought slightly forward, and a small bolster should be placed slightly posterior to the axilla to relieve pressure on the nerves and vessels along the brachial plexus and to facilitate chest expansion. Radial pulses should be monitored to confirm adequate circulation in the arms. A pulse oximeter may be used to check perfusion in the dependent hand.

Systolic and diastolic pressures decrease when the lateral position is assumed because pharmacologic agents and pathophysiologic processes depress normal compensatory mechanisms. The patient may not readily compensate for abrupt postural changes. Respiratory function is compromised by the weight of the body on the lower chest. Chest movements are limited, and the chest size may be decreased. Distal lower extremity pulses should be evaluated before, during, and after this position and all modifications of this position.

***Lateral Chest.*** The lateral chest position is a modification that allows an operative approach to the uppermost part of the thoracic cavity. A variation in the upper arm placement is that it is flexed slightly at the elbow and raised above the head to elevate the scapula, provide access to the underlying ribs, and widen the intercostal spaces. The uppermost arm may be supported on a raised armboard or pillow. Slanting the upper section of the bed downward places the trachea and mouth at a lower level than the lungs—a position that enables bronchial secretions and fluids from the lung bases to drain into the mouth and not pass into the unaffected side of the chest.

A respiratory effect of this position is that the dependent lung is more perfused because of the gravitational pooling of blood. The nondependent lung is more easily ventilated, however, because it is less compressed. This results in a ventilation-perfusion mismatch. The anesthesia provider applying positive end-expiratory pressure (PEEP) to both lungs helps to compensate for this decrease in functional lung capacity. When the nondependent lung is the site of the operation and decompressed, however, functional lung capacity is aggravated further.

***Lateral Kidney.*** The lateral kidney position (see Figure 5-24) allows approach to the retroperitoneal area of the flank. While being turned from the supine to the lateral position, the anesthetized patient is positioned so that the lower iliac crest is just below the lumbar break where the kidney bridge is located. To render the kidney region readily accessible, the kidney bridge is raised, and the bed is flexed so that the area between the twelfth rib and the iliac crest is elevated. Raising the kidney bridge depends on the cardiovascular response of the body to the increased pressure transmitted from this area. It should be raised slowly and the blood pressure monitored frequently by the anesthesia provider. The bed is flexed to lower the patient's head and legs. The patient's affected side presents a straight horizontal line from shoulder to hip. In this position, the gravitational force on the head and torso opposes that on the extended limb to facilitate operative exposure.

For torso stabilization, well-padded kidney braces may be used. A longer one is placed anteriorly, against the iliac crest. A shorter one is placed against the back. Wide adhesive tape is placed across the hips and secured to the undersides of the OR bed. Before wound closure, the adhesive strap is released, the kidney elevator is lowered, and the bed is straightened to facilitate approximation of the wound edges.

Diaphragmatic movement is limited by the increased intraabdominal pressure evoked by the kidney bridge and by the flexion of the lower limbs toward the abdomen. The acute angulation of the body in the lateral kidney posture and the effect of gravity also may decrease blood return to the right side of the heart.

## SUMMARY

Carefully planned positioning results in maximum patient safety and surgical-site exposure and access to the head and neck to administer anesthesia care. All members of the surgical team share the responsibility to protect the patient from injury during positioning. All team members should be familiar with possible risks to maintain patient safety. The perioperative nurse should actively participate in monitoring the patient body alignment and tissue integrity during and after positioning.[2] Following is a summary of important nursing interventions when positioning patients:

1. Determine the patient's risk factors for tissue and nerve damage before the procedure, and adjust nursing plans accordingly.
2. Assess and document the patient's tissue, mobility, and pain status before induction and positioning.
3. Ensure the OR bed in the room is appropriate for the procedure, and that it is in good working order.
4. Gather all positioning accessories before the patient is brought into the OR.

5. Remain at the patient's side during induction, and check with the anesthesia provider before moving the patient.
6. Provide the number of personnel needed to position the patient safely and effectively.
7. Maintain patient privacy and dignity by avoiding unnecessary exposure.
8. Ensure the transfer vehicle and the OR bed are aligned and locked.
9. Use slow, smooth movements, using a team approach; lift (do not drag) the patient.
10. Use good body mechanics.
11. Secure the patient to the OR bed to prevent falls or slippage of extremities over the OR bed's edge.
12. Ensure that the body is in good alignment.
13. Pad all bony prominences and areas under pressure to prevent disruption to tissue integrity.
14. Protect all superficial nerves from strain or pressure.
15. Ensure that legs are not crossed to prevent pressure on nerves and blood vessels.
16. Maintain normothermia without placing a warming blanket underneath the patient's body.
17. Ensure that no equipment, Mayo stand, or personnel are creating pressure on the patient throughout the procedure.
18. Monitor changes in respiratory and hemodynamic status, and assist in needed interventions.
19. Periodically re-check position, extremities, straps, and padding to ensure that the patient remains protected, and that nothing has slipped or moved.
20. During long procedures, periodically do passive range of motion on accessible extremities if it does not interfere with the surgical procedure or sterile integrity of the drapes.
21. Document all pressure and injury prevention interventions and intraoperative assessments.
22. At the end of the procedure, any repositioning should be done slowly for the patient to accommodate hemodynamically to the change.
23. The patient should remain secured and personnel should remain at the patient's side because patient movement is likely when emerging from anesthesia.
24. Transfers should be done using a team approach.
25. Secure the patient in the transfer vehicle.
26. Reassess for changes in tissue integrity; document and verbally communicate any changes to the surgeon and postanesthesia care providers.
27. Document postoperative outcome evaluation.

## REFERENCES


1. Agency for Health Care Research and Quality: *Clinical practice guidelines: treatment of pressure ulcers.* Accessed July 13, 2005, on-line: www.guideline.gov/summary/summary.aspx?view_id=1&doc_id=3457&nbr=2683.
2. AORN (Association of periOperative Nurses): Recommended practices for positioning the patient in the perioperative practice setting. In: *AORN Standards, recommended practices and guidelines,* Denver, Colo, 2005, The Association.
3. Armstrong D, Bortz P: An integrative review of pressure relief in surgical patients, *AORN Journal* 73(3):645-670, 2001.
4. Barrack RL, Butler RA: Avoidance and management of neurovascular injuries in total hip arthroplasty, *AAOS Instructional Course Lectures* 52:267-274, 2003.
5. Burnett MG, Zager EL: Pathophysiology of peripheral nerve injury: a brief review, *Neurosurgery Focus* 16(5):1-7, 2004.
6. Beyea SC: Preventing falls in perioperative settings, *AORN Journal* 81(2):393-395, 2005.
7. Beyea SC: Ensuring correct site surgery, *AORN Journal* 76(11): 880-882, 2002.
8. Braden BJ, Maklebust J: Preventing pressure ulcers with the Braden Scale, *American Journal of Nursing* 105(6):70-72, 2005.
9. Byers PH and others: Pressure ulcer research issues in surgical patients, *Advances in Skin and Wound Care* 13:115-121, 2000.
10. Calianno C: Assessing and preventing pressure ulcers, *Advances in Skin and Wound Care* 13:244-246, 2000.
11. Cucchiara RF, Faust RJ: Chapter 26: Patient positioning. In Miller RD, editor: *Anesthesia,* ed 5, vol 1, Philadelphia, 2000, Churchill Livingstone.
12. Cuddigan J, Berlowitz DR: Pressure ulcers in America: prevalence, incidence and implications for the future, *Advances in Skin and Wound Care* 14(4):208-215, 2001.
13. Defloor T, De Schuijmer JDS: Preventing pressure ulcers: an evaluation of four operating-table mattresses, *Applied Nursing Research* 13(3): 134-141, 2000.
14. Episcopio JV: Nerve damage from coronary artery bypass surgery can affect arm functioning, *Geriatric Times* 4(4), 2003. Accessed May 2, 2005, on-line: www.geriatrictimes.com/g030824.html.
15. Goodman T: Pressure damage in surgery. *Advance for Nurses: Pennsylvania, New Jersey, Delaware* 39-40, July 11, 2005.
16. Heizenroth PA: Surgery: it's got some nerve! *Nursing 2001* 31(10):1-4, 2001.
17. Heizenroth PA: Rising above the pressures of surgery, *Nursing 2000* 30(5):1-4, 2000.
18. Hill Rom Surgical Surfaces: *OR pressure management study guide,* Denver, CO, 2001, Educational Design.
19. Irvin W and others: Minimizing the risk of neurologic injury in gynecologic surgery, *Obstetrics and Gynecology* 103(2):374-382, 2004.
20. Joint Commission on Accreditation of Healthcare Organizations: *Universal protocol for preventing wrong site, wrong procedure, wrong person surgery.* 2003. Accessed July 13, 2005, on-line: www.jcaho.org/accredited+organizations/patient+safety/universal+protocol/faq_up.htm.
21. Morgan GE and others, editors: *Clinical anesthesia,* ed 3, 2002, New York, Lange Medical Books/McGraw Hill.
22. National Pressure Ulcer Advisory Panel: *NPUAP: the facts about reverse staging in 2000.* Accessed July 14, 2005, on-line: www.npuap.org/positn5.html.
23. National Pressure Ulcer Advisory Panel: *NPUAP statement on pressure ulcer prevention.* Accessed July 14, 2005, on-line: www.npaup.org/positn5.html.
24. Plambeck A: VI. Potential injuries related to anesthesia or anesthetic procedures. In: *Risks of anesthesia.* Accessed July 14, 2005, on-line: www.corexcel.com/courses3/html/body_anesthesia_title.htm.
25. Pokorny ME and others: Skin care intervention for patients having cardiac surgery, *American Journal of Critical Care* 12(6):535-544, 2003.
26. Roeder RA and others: Heel and calf capillary-support pressure in lithotomy positions, *AORN Journal* 81(4):821-830, 2005.
27. Russell JA, Lichtenstein SL: Randomized controlled trial to determine the safety and efficacy of a multi-cell pulsating dynamic mattress system in the prevention of pressure ulcers in patients undergoing cardiovascular surgery, *Ostomy/Wound Management* 46(2):46-55, 2000.
28. Schultz A: Predicting and preventing pressure ulcers in surgical patients, *AORN Journal* 81(5):985-1012, 2005.
29. Scott EM and others: Effects of warming therapy on pressure ulcers—a randomized study, *AORN Journal* 73(9):921-938, 2001.
30. Stevens J and others: Risk factors for skin breakdown after renal and adrenal surgery, *Urology* 64(2):246-249, 2004.
31. Warner MA, Martin JT: Chapter 24: Patient positioning. In Barash PG and others, editors: *Clinical anesthesia,* ed 4, Philadelphia, 2001, Lippincott Williams & Wilkins.
32. Warner MA and others: Lower extremity neuropathies associated with lithotomy positions, *Anesthesiology* 93(4):938-942, 2000.

CHAPTER 6

# Sutures, Needles, and Instruments

ALTHEA R. DUNSCOMBE

## SUTURE MATERIALS

The development of surgical sutures has been closely allied with the development of the art of surgery. Medical writings of ancient Egyptian and Assyrian cultures dating back to 2000 BC mention the various materials used, to a limited extent, for suturing and ligating. The concept of suturing and ligating also is recorded in the writings of the father of medicine, Hippocrates (born 460 BC). Gut of sheep intestines was first mentioned as suture material in the writings of the ancient Greek physician Galen. The Persian physician and philosopher Rhazes is credited with employing surgical gut, or catgut, in AD 900 for suturing abdominal wounds. The word *catgut* is a misnomer, and its use is inappropriate. According to the *Oxford English Dictionary,* it matches the Dutch *kattedarm,* "cat-intestine." *Catgut* entered English around 1560 to 1600 under obscure conditions, possibly connected humorously with caterwauling (History box).

*Suture* is a generic term for all materials used to sew severed body tissue together and to hold these tissues in their normal position until healing takes place; to *suture* is to stitch together cut or torn edges of tissue.[14] A *ligature* is a strand of suture material used to tie off (seal) blood vessels to prevent hemorrhage and simple bleeding or to isolate a mass of tissue to be excised (cut out). A variety of suture materials are available for ligating, suturing, and closing the wound. The appropriate suture is selected according to numerous characteristics: whether it is absorbable or nonabsorbable, its breaking (tensile) strength, whether it is monofilament or multifilament, its knot-tying facility, and its tissue reactivity. An understanding of these characteristics of suture materials and knowledge of the risk factors of wound healing and the interaction between the tissues and suture materials is essential for the perioperative nurse and proper wound healing.

### Characteristics of Suture Material

The three main features to evaluate the general properties of suture material are (1) physical characteristics, (2) handling characteristics, and (3) tissue-reaction characteristics (Box 6-1). The ideal suture material is one that causes minimal inflammation and tissue reaction, while providing maximum strength during the lag phase of wound healing (see Chapter 8). Although the ideal suture has not yet been found, perioperative nurses should evaluate the characteristics of suture as they relate to what would be ideal in surgical patient care and incorporate research findings into clinical practice.

**Physical Characteristics.** Physical characteristics of sutures, defined and described by the *United States Pharmacopeia* (USP), which is the official compendium for suture manufacture, can be measured or visually determined and include the following properties:

- *Physical configuration.* Single-stranded (monofilament) or multistranded (multifilament), containing numerous fibers rendered into a single thread by twisting or braiding (Figure 6-1).
- *Capillarity.* Ability to transmit fluid along the strand.
- *Diameter (size).* Determined in millimeters, and expressed in USP sizes with zeroes; the smaller the cross-sectional diameter, the more zeroes; sizes range from #7, the largest, to 11-0, the smallest; sizes 0 to 4-0 are the most commonly used sutures in general surgery. (The surgeon usually selects the finest suture possible for the tissue being closed. The finer diameter [smaller size] provides better handling qualities and small knots. Improved suturing techniques are possible with sutures of finer diameter.)
- *Tensile strength.* The amount of weight (breaking load) necessary to break a suture (breaking strength); varies with type of suture material (Table 6-1).
- *Knot strength.* The force necessary to cause a given type of knot to slip, either partially or completely.
- *Elasticity.* Inherent ability to regain original form and length after having been stretched.
- *Memory.* Capacity of a suture to return to its former shape after being re-formed, as when tied; high memory yields less knot security.

**Handling Characteristics.** Handling characteristics of suture material are related to pliability (how easily the material bends) and the coefficient of friction (how easily the suture slips through tissue and can be tied). A suture with a high friction coefficient tends to drag through tissue. It is more difficult to tie because its knots do not set easily. Some suture materials are coated to reduce their coefficient of friction. This coating not only improves the way they pull through tissue on insertion but also lessens the force needed to remove the suture after the wound is healed. The coefficient of friction should not be too low, however, because knots come undone more easily.

**Tissue Reaction Characteristics.** Because it is a foreign substance, all suture material causes some tissue reaction. Tissue reaction begins when the suture inflicts injury to the tissue during insertion. In addition, tissue reacts to the suture material itself (Table 6-2). This reaction begins with an infiltration of white blood cells into the area; macrophages and fibroblasts then appear; and by about the seventh day, fibrous tissue with chronic inflammation is present. The reaction persists until the suture is encapsulated (nonabsorbable material) or absorbed (absorbable material) by the body.

## HISTORY

During the sixteenth century, Ambrose Paré reintroduced the use of ligatures to stop hemorrhage and abandoned the use of cauterizing hooks. Subsequently the nurse in the OR became responsible for the time-consuming task of preparing suture material. The following are references to suture and its preparation (or removal from the operative wound) as chronicled in select nursing and medical textbooks.

**1879**
Sutures are composed of various materials and are applied in many different ways, according to circumstance. Some surgeons prefer hempen thread or silk; others prefer an animal membrane, such as catgut; and others prefer a fine wire. The advantages claimed for the last-mentioned are that it does not irritate the tissues, and that it does not absorb the secretions.

**1890**
The method most commonly used by surgeons for the arrest of hemorrhage from an artery of any size is ligation. The artery is picked up by a pair of forceps, and a ligature is tied firmly about it. Ligatures should be about 18 inches long. A ligature is most often made of strong, soft silk, although catgut or wire is sometimes used. Its strength should be tested well, so as to leave no chance of its breaking when strained.

**1918**
Catgut is wound evenly on glass spools, 1 yard of catgut on each spool, and each spool is placed in a glycerin-jelly jar. Each jar is filled with absolute alcohol; the cap is lightly screwed on; and the jars are placed, cap down, in a 2-quart glass jar and covered with absolute alcohol. The glass jar is placed in a water bath on a gas stove . . . at a distance from the flame . . . The catgut is boiled in alcohol three successive times for 1 hour at intervals of 24 hours.

**1961**
Skin sutures (black silk thread, fine wire, or metal skin clips) are removed from abdominal wounds on about postoperative day 7, from head and neck wounds on about postoperative day 3 to 5, and from wounds of the extremities on postoperative day 8 to 10. Retention sutures composed of heavy wire and passed deep into muscle tissue usually are not removed until postoperative day 14 to 21. Most patients are apprehensive when they know the sutures are to be removed.

**1961**
The ligatures used in a surgical operation are of two main kinds: absorbable and nonabsorbable. Absorbable sutures are made of catgut, which is prepared from the muscle coat in the wall of the sheep's intestine. Catgut is now provided already sterilized in ampoules that are stored in antiseptic solution and have to be broken open at the time they are required. When the ampoule is opened, the catgut must be rinsed in warm sterile saline or water to remove the fluid in which it is preserved. This fluid has a penetrating odor because of the cresol in it.

**1971**
Skin stitches, Mersilene or nylon, are removed when the wound has healed, usually on postoperative day 8 to 10. It is advisable to remove alternate stitches on one day and the remainder the next day if the wound is sound.

**1972**
The word *catgut* is a misnomer. The Arabic word *kit* means a "dancing master's fiddle," but the word *catgut* has no relation to a cat.

Modified from Ballinger WF and others: *Alexander's care of the patient in surgery,* ed 5, St Louis, 1972, Mosby; Clarke WF: *A manual of the practice of surgery,* New York, 1879, William Wood & Co; Fowler RS: *The operating room and the patient,* ed 3, Philadelphia, 1918, Saunders; Moroney J: *Surgery for nurses,* ed 12, Baltimore, 1971, Williams & Wilkins; Shafer KN and others: *Medical-surgical nursing,* ed 2, St Louis, 1961, Mosby; Taylor S, Worrall O: *Principles of surgery and surgical nursing,* London, 1961, The English Universities Press Ltd; Weeks CS: *Textbook of nursing,* New York, 1890, Appleton.

BOX 6-1

### Characteristics of Suture Material

**PHYSICAL CHARACTERISTICS**
Physical configuration
Capillarity
Fluid absorption ability
Diameter (caliber; also referred to as size)
Tensile strength
Knot strength
Elasticity
Plasticity
Memory

**HANDLING CHARACTERISTICS**
Pliability
Tissue drag (related to the coefficient of friction)
Knot tying (related to the coefficient of friction)
Knot slippage (related to the coefficient of friction)

**TISSUE-REACTION CHARACTERISTICS**
Inflammatory and fibrous cell reaction
Absorption
Potentiation of infection
Allergic reaction

Modified from *Ethicon wound closure manual,* Sommerville, NJ, 2004, Ethicon.

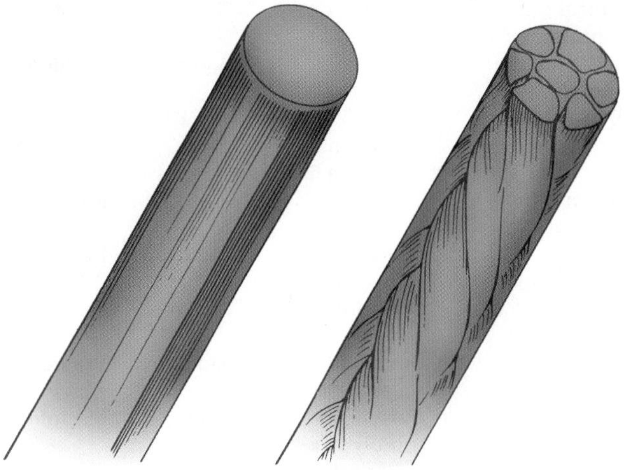

FIGURE 6-1 *Left,* Monofilament suture; *right,* multifilament (braided) suture.

## Types of Suture Material

Suture materials are classified into two broad groups: *absorbable* and *nonabsorbable.*

***Absorbable Sutures.*** The USP defines an absorbable surgical suture as follows: sterile, flexible strand prepared from collagen derived from healthy mammals, or from a synthetic polymer. . . . It is capable of being absorbed by living mammalian tissue but may be treated to modify its resistance to absorption. . . . It may be modified with respect to body or texture. It may be impregnated with a suitable coating, softening, or antimicrobial agent. It may be colored by a color

**TABLE 6-1**

### Relative Straight-Pull Tensile Strength of Suture Materials

| | Greatest → Least | | | | | | |
|---|---|---|---|---|---|---|---|
| **Nonabsorbable** | Steel | Polyester (Mersilene) | Nylon (monofilamentous) | Nylon (braided) | Polypropylene (Prolene) | Silk | |
| **Absorbable** | | Polyglycolic | Polyglactin 910 (Vicryl) | | Polydioxanone (PDS) | Poliglecaprone (Monocryl) | Catgut |

Modified from *Ethicon wound closure manual,* Sommerville, NJ, 2004, Ethicon. Accessed May 28, 2006, online: www.jnjgateway.com.

**TABLE 6-2**

### Relative Tissue Reactivity to Sutures

| | Greatest → Least | | | | | |
|---|---|---|---|---|---|---|
| **Nonabsorbable** | | Silk, cotton | Polyester coated | Polyester uncoated | Nylon | Polypropylene (Prolene) |
| **Absorbable** | Catgut | | Polyglactin 910 (Vicryl) | Polyglycolic acid | Poliglecaprone (Monocryl) | |

Modified from *Ethicon wound closure manual,* Sommerville, NJ, 2004, Ethicon. Accessed May 28, 2006, online: www.jnjgateway.com.

**TABLE 6-3**

### Comparison of Absorbable Sutures

| Ethicon | Syneture (U.S. Surgical) | Package Color | Configuration | Tensile Strength | Absorption Rate | Degradation |
|---|---|---|---|---|---|---|
| Surgical gut (plain) | Plain gut | Yellow | Twisted | 0% at 2-3 wk | Unpredictable (12 wk) | Proteolytic |
| Surgical gut (chromic) | Chromic gut | Tan | Twisted | 0% at 2-3 wk | Unpredictable (12 wk) | Proteolytic |
| Vicryl* *Rapide* (polyglactin 910) | | Violet | Braided | 0% at 14 days | Complete at 42 days | Hydrolytic |
| | Caprosyn (polyglytone 6211) | Pink | Monofilament | 0% at 21 days | Complete at 56 days | Hydrolytic |
| Monocryl (poliglecaprone) | | Rose | Monofilament | 20-30% at 2 wk | Complete in 91-119 days | Hydrolytic |
| | Dexon-S (polyglycolic acid) | Gold | Braided or monofilament | 20% at 3 wk | Complete in 60-90 days | Hydrolytic |
| | Polysorb (polyester) | Violet | Braided | 30% at 3 wk | Complete in 56-70 days | Hydrolytic |
| | Dexon-II (polycaprolate) | Gold | Braided | 35% at 3 wk | Complete in 60-90 days | Hydrolytic |
| | Biosyn (Polydioxanone) | Red | Monofilament | 40% at 3 wk | Complete in 90-110 days | Hydrolytic |
| Vicryl (polyglactin 910) | | Violet | Braided or monofilament | 50% at 3 wk | Complete in 56-70 days | Hydrolytic |
| PDS (polydioxanone) | | Black | Monofilament | 60% at 3 wk | Complete within 6 mo | Hydrolytic |
| | Maxon (polyglyconate) | Black | Monofilament | Excellent until 6 wk | Complete within 6 mo | Hydrolytic |

Modified from: Ethicon wound closure manuel, Sommerville, NJ, 2004, Ethicon, Inc. Accessed on-line www.jnjgateway.com; Absorbable suture, accessed May 28, 2006, on-line: www.syneture.com.

additive approved by the federal Food and Drug Administration.

Absorbable sutures can be digested (by enzyme activity) or hydrolyzed (by reaction with water in tissue fluids to breakdown) and assimilated by the tissues during the healing process. Absorbable sutures vary in treatment, color, size, packaging, and resistance to absorption, according to their purpose. Types of absorbable suture include plain or chromic surgical gut, collagen, and glycolic acid polymers (Table 6-3).

**SURGICAL GUT.** Surgical gut is obtained from the collagen of the submucosal layer of the small intestine of sheep or the intestinal serosa of cattle or hogs. The processed strands or ribbons of collagen are either untreated (plain, type A) or treated with chromium salts (chromic, type C).

Chromatization delays absorption of the suture in living mammalian tissue. The strength of the chromium salt content and the duration of the chromatizing process are accurately controlled and tested. Proper chromatizing of gut ensures the integrity of the suture and maintenance of its strength during the early stages of wound healing. It enables a wound with slow healing power to heal sufficiently before the suture is entirely absorbed.

The elaborate processes of mechanical and chemical cleaning of the raw gut are followed by sterilization, usually with ionizing radiation, and storage in hermetically sealed packages. Modern manufacturing processes also ensure tensile strength, more controlled absorption, and more predictable results.

Absorption occurs by digestion of the gut by tissue enzymes. The absorption rate of surgical gut is influenced by the type of body tissue it contacts and, to some extent, by the patient's general physical condition. Studies also show that surgical gut is absorbed faster in serous or mucous membranes than in muscular tissues. When fine chromic gut is properly buried in successive layers of the gastrointestinal tract, it retains its strength long enough for primary union to take place.

Surgical gut suture is wet-packaged in an alcohol solution to provide maximum pliability and should be used immediately after removal from the packet. When a gut suture is removed from its packet and is not used at once, the alcohol evaporates, which causes the strand to lose its pliability. If required, the strand's pliability may be restored just before use by immersing it in sterile water or normal saline solution, preferably at body temperature, for only a few seconds. This immersion is recommended only for eye sutures; in other areas, tissue fluids moisten the gut sufficiently as it passes through the tissue when the surgeon sews. Excessive moisture reduces tensile strength.

**COLLAGEN SUTURES.** Collagen sutures are derived from the tendons of cattle. They are chemically treated to remove noncollagenous material, purified, and processed into strands that have physical properties superior to surgical gut. Collagen suture is used most often as a fine suture material for the eye.

**SYNTHETIC ABSORBABLE SUTURES.** To produce synthetic absorbable sutures, specific polymers are extruded into suture strands. The base material for synthetic absorbable suture is a combination of lactic and glycolic acid polymers (Vicryl, Dexon, Polysorb). The molecular structure of these products has a tensile strength sufficient for approximation of tissues for 2 to 3 weeks, followed by rapid absorption.

The newer synthetic polymers (PDS, Maxon, Monocryl) provide wound support for longer periods (3 months). They

| Tissue Reactivity | Handling | Knot Security | Contraindications |
|---|---|---|---|
| Moderate | Fair | Poor | Not used where extended approximation of tissue under stress is required. Not used in patients with known allergies or sensitivities to collagen or chromium |
| Moderate | Fair | Fair | Not used where extended approximation of tissue under stress is required. Not used in patients with known allergies or sensitivities to collagen or chromium |
| Minimal | Excellent | Good | Not used where extended approximation of tissue under stress is required or where wound support beyond 7 days is required |
| Minimal | Excellent | Excellent | Not used where extended approximation of tissue is required. Not for use in cardiovascular surgery, neurologic surgery, microsurgery, or ophthalmic surgery |
| Minimal | Excellent | Good | Not used where extended approximation of tissue is required. Undyed not indicated for use in fascia |
| Minimal | Good | Good | Not used where extended approximation of tissue is required. Not for use in cardiovascular or neural tissues |
| Minimal | Excellent | Excellent | Not used where extended approximation of tissue is required. Not for use in cardiovascular or neural tissues |
| Minimal | Good | Good | Not used where extended approximation of tissue is required. Not for use in cardiovascular or neural tissues |
| Minimal | Excellent | Excellent | Not used where extended approximation of tissue is required. Not for use in cardiovascular or neural tissues |
| Minimal | Good | Good | Not used where extended approximation of tissue is required. Undyed not indicated for use in fascia |
| Slight | Good | Good | Not used where extended approximation of tissue is required. Not used with prosthetic devices, such as heart valves or synthetic grafts |
| Minimal | Good | Good | Not used where extended approximation of tissue is required. Not for use in cardiovascular surgery, neurologic surgery, microsurgery, or ophthalmic surgery |

## RESEARCH HIGHLIGHT

### Evaluating Suture Material for Perineal Repair

Best practices are part of the growing movement in evidence-based medicine (EBM) and evidence-based nursing (EBN). This initiative tracks down, critically appraises, and incorporates a rapidly growing body of scientific evidence into clinical practice. The *Cochrane Review* is one source for such a review. Approximately 70% of women experience some degree of perineal trauma after vaginal delivery and require stitches, which may result in perineal pain and superficial dyspareunia. The object of this review was to assess the effect of absorbable synthetic suture material compared with catgut on the amount of short-term and long-term pain experienced by mothers after perineal repair. Eight randomized trials comparing absorbable synthetic (polyglycolic acid and polyglactin) with plain or chromic catgut suture for perineal repair were included in this review of the Cochrane Pregnancy and Childbirth Group trials register. Compared with catgut, the polyglycolic acid and polyglactin groups were associated with less pain in the first 3 days. Fewer analgesics were required, and less suture dehiscence was noted, although removal of suture material was significantly more common. There was no significant difference in long-term pain or the amount of dyspareunia experienced by the women.

The review concluded that absorbable synthetic suture material in the form of polyglycolic acid and polyglactin for perineal repair after childbirth seemed to decrease women's experience of short-term pain. The length of time taken for the synthetic material to absorb remains of concern, however.

Modified from Kettle C, Johanson RB: Absorbable synthetic versus catgut suture material for perineal repair. *Cochrane Rev Abstract* 2004. Accessed July 22, 2006 on-line: www.medscape.com/viewarticle/484957.

are used when prolonged support for wound healing is desired, as with fascial closure, or for elderly or oncology patients. They combine the desirable qualities of extended wound support and eventual absorbability.

Synthetic absorbable sutures are absorbed by slow hydrolysis in the presence of tissue fluids. Hydrolysis is the chemical process whereby the polymer reacts with water to cause an alteration of breakdown of the molecular structure. These sutures are degraded in tissue by this process at a more predictable rate than surgical gut (or collagen) and with less tissue reaction (Research Highlight). These sutures are dry-packaged in sizes 10-0 to #3. They should not be dipped in solutions because moisture reduces their tensile strength. Some polymers have additional coatings to reduce drag in tissue.

**TABLE 6-4**

### Comparison of Nonabsorbable Sutures

| Ethicon | Syneture (U.S. Surgical) | Package Color | Configuration | Tensile Strength | Absorption Rate |
|---|---|---|---|---|---|
| Perma-Hand (silk) | Sofsilk | Light blue | Braided; Sofsilk is available with wax coating | Progressive degradation with gradual loss over time | Hydrolysis leads to gradual encapsulation by fibrous connective tissue |
| Ethilon (nylon) | | Light green | Monofilament | Progressive degradation with gradual loss over time | Hydrolysis leads to gradual encapsulation by fibrous connective tissue |
| Nurolon (nylon) | Dermalon, Surgilon, Monosof (nylon) | Light green | Braided; Dermalon, Surgilon, Monosof silicone coated | Progressive degradation with gradual loss over time | Hydrolysis leads to gradual encapsulation by fibrous connective tissue |
| Mersilene (polyester) | Surgidac (polyester) | Turquoise, orange (Surgidac) | Braided or monofilament | No significant loss in vivo | Gradual encapsulation by fibrous connective tissue |
| Ethibond (polyester) | Ti-Cron (polyester) | Orange, orange stripe (Ti-Cron) | Braided; uncoated or coated with silicone | No significant loss in vivo | Gradual encapsulation by fibrous connective tissue |
| Prolene, Pronova (polypropylene) | Surgipro, Surgipro II (polypropylene) | Deep blue | Monofilament | Not subject to degradation or weakness by hydrolysis | Nonabsorbable |
| | Novafil (polybutester) | Blue green | Monofilament | Not subject to degradation or weakness by hydrolysis | Nonabsorbable |
| Stainless steel | Stainless steel | Mustard | Monofilament, twisted, or braided | Indefinite | Nonabsorbable |

Modified from Ethicon Wound Closure Manual, Sommerville, NJ, 2004, Ethicon, Inc, accessed on-line: www.jnjgateway.com; nonabsorbable suture. Accessed May 28,2006, on-line: www.syneture.com.

***Nonabsorbable Sutures.*** Nonabsorbable sutures are strands of material that effectively resist enzymatic digestion in living animal tissue. The USP classifies nonabsorbable surgical suture as follows:

- Class I suture is composed of silk or synthetic fibers of monofilament, twisted, or braided construction.
- Class II suture is composed of cotton or linen fibers or coated natural or synthetic fibers, in which the coating significantly affects thickness but does not contribute significantly to strength.
- Class III suture is composed of monofilament or multifilament metal wire.

The strand of suture material may be uncoated or coated with a substance to reduce capillarity and friction when passing through the tissue. Several products are used for coating, including silicone, polytef (Teflon), and various polymers. Fibers may be uncolored, naturally colored, or impregnated with a suitable dye.

Nonabsorbable suture material is encapsulated or walled off by the tissues around it during the process of wound healing. Skin sutures, for which nonabsorbable materials are often the choice, are removed before healing is complete. The most common nonabsorbable suture materials are silk, nylon, polyester fiber, polypropylene, and stainless steel wire (Table 6-4).

**SILK.** Silk is prepared from thread spun by the silkworm larva in making its cocoon. Top-grade raw silk is (1) processed to remove natural waxes and gum, (2) manufactured into threads, and (3) colored with a vegetable dye. The strands of silk are twisted or braided to form the suture, which gives it high tensile strength and better handling qualities. Silk handles well, is soft, and forms secure knots.

Because of the capillarity of untreated silk, body fluid may transmit infection along the length of the suture strand. For this reason, surgical silk is treated to eliminate its capillarity properties (able to resist the absorption of body fluids and moisture). It is available in sizes 9-0 to #5, in sterile packets or precut lengths, and with or without attached needles. The scrub person should keep the silk dry. Wet silk loses 20% in strength.

Silk is not a true nonabsorbable material. When buried in tissue, it loses its tensile strength after about 1 year and may disappear after several years. Silk sutures, more commonly than less reactive suture materials, occasionally form tracts as the suture migrates gradually to a wound's exterior surface. This spontaneous migration is called *spitting* and may occur weeks, months, or years after the suture was placed.[12] Spitting is annoying and sometimes frightening to the patient but has no deleterious effect on wound healing.

**COTTON.** Surgical cotton sutures are made from individual cotton fibers that are combed, aligned, and twisted to form a finished strand. Because new types of fibers have been introduced, cotton suture is rarely used. Some companies no longer manufacture it.

Umbilical tape, although not used for suturing, is produced by suture manufacturers and packaged in the same way as su-

| Degradation | Tissue Reactivity | Handling | Knot Security | Contraindications |
|---|---|---|---|---|
| Progressive | Acute inflammatory reaction | Good | Good | Not used in patients with known sensitivities or allergies to silk. Not used in contaminated or potentially contaminated wounds. Not used where permanent retention of tensile strength required |
| Progressive | Minimal | Poor | Poor | Not used where permanent retention of tensile strength required |
| Progressive | Minimal | Fair; Syeneture products coated for better handling | Fair; Syneture products coated for increased knot security | Not used where permanent retention of tensile strength required |
| None | Minimal | Good | Good | None known |
| None | Minimal | Good | Good | None known |
| None | Minimal | Poor | Poor | None known |
| None | Minimal | Fair | Poor | Not used in patients with known sensitivities or allergies to its components. Not used in microsurgery or neurologic surgery |
| None | Minimal | Poor | Good | Not used in patients with known sensitivities or allergies to steel or its principal metallic components, chromium and nickel |

ture. It consists of long woven ribbons of cotton, 1/16 to 1/8 inch wide, and is used for retraction or suspension of small structures and vessels. (Other soft, pliant products, such as vessel loops, are available and more common for this purpose.)

NYLON. Surgical nylon (Dermalon, Ethilon, Surgilon, Nurolon, Bralon, Monosof) is a synthetic polyamide material. It is available in two forms: multifilament (braided) and monofilament strands. Multifilament nylon is relatively inert in tissues and has a high tensile strength. It is used in conditions similar to those in which silk and cotton are used. Monofilament nylon is a smooth material that is particularly well suited for closing skin edges and for tension sutures. Because of its poor knot security, the surgeon usually ties three knots in small sutures and a double square knot in large sutures. It is used frequently in ophthalmology and microsurgery because it can be manufactured in fine sizes. Size 11-0 nylon is one of the smallest suture materials available.

POLYESTER FIBER. Surgical polyester fiber (Ti-Cron, Dacron, Mersilene, Tevdek, Polydek, Ethibond, Surgidac) is available in two forms: a nontreated polyester fiber suture and a polyester fiber suture that has been specifically coated or impregnated with a lubricant to allow smooth passage through the tissue. Polyester fiber is available in fine filaments that can be braided into various suture sizes to provide good handling properties.

Polybutester (Novafil) is a special type of polyester suture that possesses many of the advantages of polyester and polypropylene. Because it is a monofilament, it induces little tissue reaction.

Polyester material has many advantages over other braided, nonabsorbable sutures. It has greater tensile strength, minimal tissue reaction, and maximum visibility and does not absorb tissue fluids. It is used frequently as a general-closure fascia suture and in cardiovascular surgery for valve replacements, graft-to-tissue anastomoses, and revascularization procedures.

POLYPROPYLENE. Polypropylene is a clear or pigmented polymer. This monofilament suture material (Prolene, Surgilene, Surgipro, Dermalene) is used for cardiovascular, general, and plastic surgery. Because polypropylene is a monofilament and is extremely inert in tissue, it may be used in the presence of infection. It has high tensile strength and causes minimal tissue reaction. Sizes range from 10-0 to #2.

STAINLESS STEEL. Surgical stainless steel is formulated to be compatible with stainless steel implants and prostheses. This formula, 316L (L for "low carbon"), ensures absence of toxic elements, optimal strength, flexibility, and uniform size. Monofilament and multifilament surgical stainless steel are known for their strength, inert properties, and low tissue reaction. Stainless steel–suturing technique is very exacting, however. Steel can pull or tear out of tissue, and necrosis can result from a suture that is too tight. Barbs on the end of steel can traumatize surrounding tissue or tear gloves. Torn or cut gloves fail to provide an adequate and effective barrier for the patient or the surgeon and assistant and can remain undetected. Kinks in the wire can render it practically useless. For this reason, packaging has played an important part in the development of surgical stainless steel sutures. Surgical stainless steel is available in packets on spools or in packages of straight, precut, sterile lengths, with or without swaged needles. This packaging affords protection to the strands and delivery in straight, unkinked lengths.

Before surgical stainless steel was available from suture manufacturers, it was purchased by weight with the Brown and Sharp (B&S) scale for diameter variations. Today the B&S gauge, along with USP size classifications, is used to distinguish diameter ranges. Table 6-5 compares steel suture sizes.

**TABLE 6-5**

**Steel Suture Comparison**

| Size (USP) | B&S Gauge | Size (USP) | B&S Gauge |
|---|---|---|---|
| 6-0 | 40 | 0 | 26 |
| 6-0 | 38 | 1 | 25 |
| 5-0 | 35 | 2 | 24 |
| 4-0 | 34 | 3 | 23 |
| 4-0 | 32 | 4 | 22 |
| 000 | 30 | 5 | 20 |
| 00 | 28 | 7 | 18 |

*B&S,* Brown and Sharp; *USP,* United States Pharmacopeia.

## PACKAGING, STORAGE, AND SELECTION OF SUTURES

Manufacturers now supply suture materials in some form of sterile package ready for immediate use. The USP specifies, "Preserve . . . dry or in fluid, in containers so designed that sterility is maintained until the container is opened."

### Types of Packaging

For packaging, the suture material is sealed in a primary inner packet, which may or may not contain fluid; placed inside a dry, outer, peel-back packet; and sterilized. This method permits easy dispensing onto the sterile field. Various forms of foil, plastic, and special paper are used for the inner and outer packets.

Each primary suture packet is self-contained, and its sterility for each patient is ensured as long as the integrity of the packet is maintained. Some suture packets have expiration dates that relate to stability and sterility. Packages should be stored in moisture-proof and dust-proof containers in units of one size and type.

Suture packets may contain single or multiple strands, with or without a needle attached to the strand. The needle may be permanently attached (swaged) to the suture and may need to be cut off for removal, or it may be designed to separate easily from the suture with a quick tug of the needle holder (Controlled Release, D-Tach, Pop-off). Some sutures may be double-armed, with a needle at each end of the strand.

**TABLE 6-6**

**Suture Packaging Color Codes**

| Fiber | Color Code |
|---|---|
| Plain gut | Yellow |
| Chromic gut | Tan |
| Polyglactin 910 (Vicryl) | Violet* |
| Silk | Medium blue |
| Cotton | Pink |
| Polypropylene (Prolene) | Royal blue |
| Polyester (Mersilene) | Medium green* |
| Polydioxanone (PDS) | Black |
| Poliglecaprone (Monocryl) | Rose |
| Nylon | Light green |
| Stainless steel | Mustard* |

*These color codes may change from one manufacturer to another.

***Color Codes.*** Color-coded packaging based on suture fiber is used by most companies to make identification quicker and easier (Table 6-6). Each individual packet is color-coded, as the dispenser box is. Although most color codes are universal across companies, there are some exceptions. Ethibond, a coated polyester, is coded orange, whereas most polyesters are coded in shades of green. Dexon, a glycolic acid polymer, is gold, whereas Vicryl, a comparable polymer, is violet.

### Selection of Suture

The choice of suture material, size, and type depends on the procedure, the tissue being sutured and type of reapproximation required, the general condition of the patient, and the surgeon's preferences. A surgical services committee or project team may be responsible for establishing standard suture uses for various operations. Current guides published by suture manufacturers should be consulted. These guides list the specific suture materials recommended for various wounds and are based on current clinical practice and research. Although the perioperative nurse is not responsible for choosing the suture material used, he or she must be knowledgeable of the suture properties to ensure the best possible outcome for the surgical patient. For more efficient delivery of sutures to the field for specific procedures and surgeons, one can request that suture companies prepare custom packets of mixed sutures in advance.

## HEMOSTASIS

Hemostasis is an ongoing process during surgery. In addition to the damaging physiologic effects of blood loss for the patient, bleeding from cut vessels obscures visualization of the operative site for the surgeon and must be controlled. Hemostasis may be accomplished with suture materials, electrosurgical devices, lasers, and chemical agents. Before wound closure, the surgeon carefully checks the operative site to ensure that all active bleeding has been stopped.

### Methods of Ligating Vessels

A ligature is a strand of suture material used to encircle and close off the lumen of a vessel to effect hemostasis, close off a structure, or prevent leakage of materials. Ties may be on a reel—a spool or disk containing a long length of suture that the surgeon may use to ligate several superficial vessels, or they may be free ties—precut lengths of suture handed to the surgeon one at a time, usually for bleeders in deeper tissues.

Following are several techniques used to secure a ligature in deep tissues:

- A hemostat is placed on the end of the structure; the ligature is then placed around the vessel. The knot is tied and tightened with the surgeon's fingers or with the aid of forceps.
- A slipknot is made, and its loop is placed over the involved structure by means of a forceps or clamp.
- In deeper cavities, ties are often placed on clamps with the long end extending from the tip. These are sometimes called *ties on a pass* or *bow ties*. The extending long end is held tightly against the rings by the surgeon (creating the bow), who then passes the tip of the clamp under the vessel or duct to be ligated. The first assistant grasps the extending tie with a forceps, the surgeon releases it, and the tie is pulled under and up to the wound surface and tied.
- A forceps or a clamp is applied to the structure, and transfixion sutures are applied and tied. A *suture ligature, stick tie,* or *transfixion ligature* is a strand of suture material threaded or swaged on a needle. This is usually placed through the vessel and around it to prevent the ligature from slipping off the end.

When two ligatures are used to ligate a large vessel, usually a free ligature is placed on the vessel, and a suture ligature is placed distal to the first ligature. To ligate a blood vessel situated in deep tissues, the strand must be of sufficient strength and length to allow the surgeon to tighten the first knot. See the discussion of preparation of ligatures and suture ligatures in "Perioperative Nursing Considerations" later in this chapter.

### Ligating Clips

Ligating clips are small, V-shaped, staple-like devices that are placed around the lumen of a vessel or structure to close it off. They may be made of one of several metals, such as stainless steel, tantalum, or titanium. Stainless steel clips are the most economical to use. Although more expensive, titanium clips are used frequently in specific surgical procedures because the starburst reflection on postoperative radiographs is less with titanium than with other metals. Absorbable clips made of synthetic absorbable suture material also are available.

Ligating clips are available in several sizes; each size requires its own applier, which must be loaded by the scrub person. These clips are available in disposable, prepackaged units. Preloaded, disposable clip appliers that can be used in open wounds or through endoscope trocar cannulae are available. Ligating clips afford a rapid and secure method of achieving hemostasis when arteries, veins, nerves, and other small structures are ligated.

Metal Cushing or Frazier clips are made of small-diameter pieces of stainless steel or silver wire and are heat sterilized. They must be hand-loaded onto special rack dispensers. Frazier

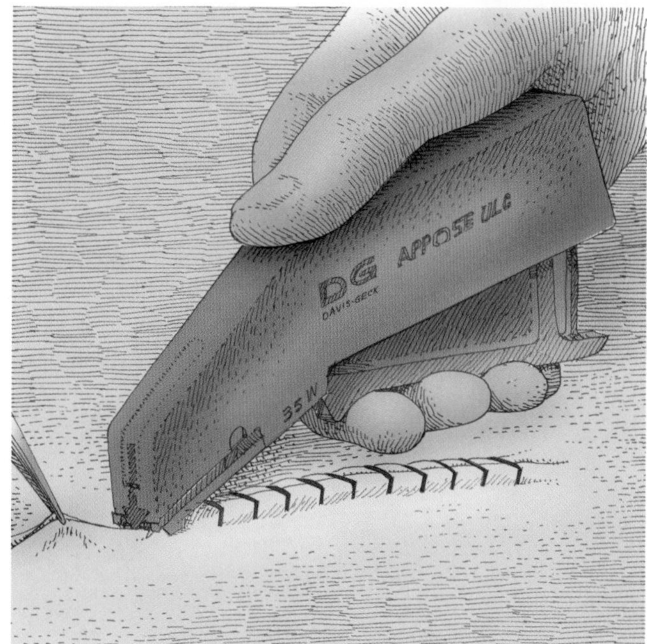


**FIGURE 6-2** Application of skin staples. The stapler is lightly positioned over everted skin edges. It is not necessary to press the staple, or stapler anvil, into the skin to get a proper "bite" (just "kiss" the skin). Center the staples over the incision line, using the locating arrow or guideline, and place approximately ¼ inch apart.

clips are applied to the ends of severed nerves and blood vessels by means of a forceps designed for the purpose. They are used in neurosurgery and orthopedic procedures. Since the introduction of prepackaged ligating clips, their use is declining.

## SKIN STAPLES

Skin staples are one of the most frequently chosen methods of skin closure. They can be used on many types of surgical incisions. The staple appliers are easy to use. They reduce operating time and tissue trauma, allowing uniform tension along the suture line and less distortion from the stress of individual suture points. When properly applied (Figure 6-2), they provide excellent cosmetic results. Some staplers use bioabsorbable staples that are placed under the skin and absorb similar to suture. Others use stainless steel staples. With these, the length of time the staples stay in place depends on the part of the body affected; they are usually removed within 5 to 7 days. An extractor is required for their removal.

Most staplers employ a similar anvil-type mechanism for forming the staple, but the application device varies from company to company. Device choice usually is determined by the weight, handling characteristics, ease of application, and unobstructed view of the site during application. Staplers are packaged in various assortments of numbers and types of staples, depending on the length of the incision and the type of tissue encountered.

## SKIN TAPES

Wounds that are subjected to minimal static and dynamic tension are easily approximated with skin tape. The selection of surgical tape for skin closure is based on the tape's adhesive ability, tensile strength, and porosity. The tape must provide a firm tape-to-skin bond to keep the wound edges closely adhered. The tensile strength must be sufficient to maintain wound approximation. A tape that is too occlusive limits moisture or vapor transmission; fluid may accumulate under the tape and lead to maceration and bacterial growth. Microporous tapes prevent this problem. The tape must be applied to dry skin; an adhesive adjunct (e.g., tincture of benzoin or Mastisol liquid adhesive) may be applied in a thin film to the skin at the wound edges before tape application. Edema at the surgical site may cause taped wound edges to invert; supplemental skin sutures may be used to enhance closure. Tapes may be cut to accommodate smaller incisions. Tapes are applied perpendicularly to the wound edge, first on one side and then the other, so that the edges can be pulled together (Figure 6-3).

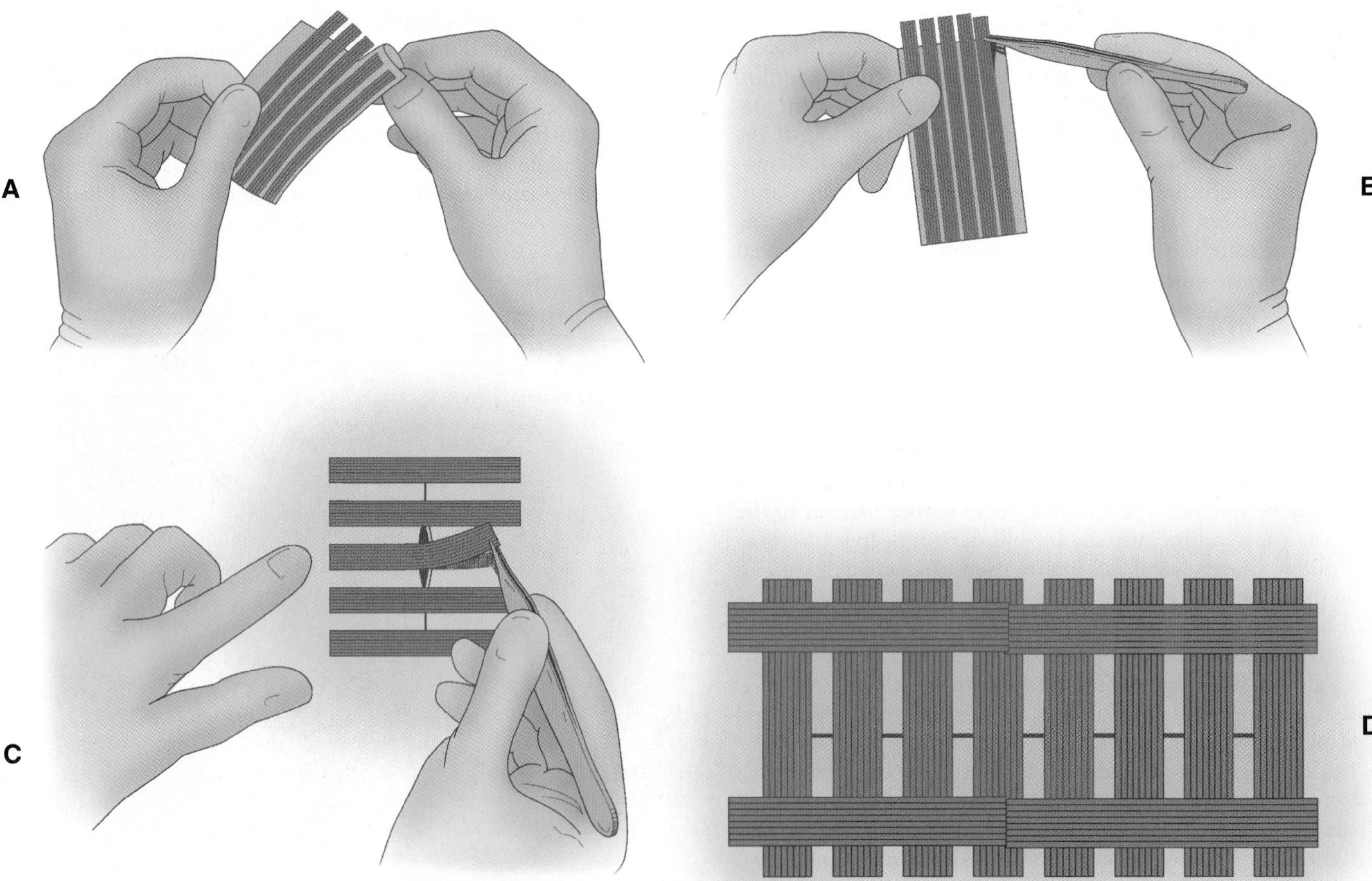


FIGURE 6-3 Application of skin tapes. **A,** Perforated tab is bent and removed. **B,** Tape is peeled from the card. **C,** Tape is applied to wound. **D,** Additional tape is placed parallel to wound to limit shear stress on the skin.

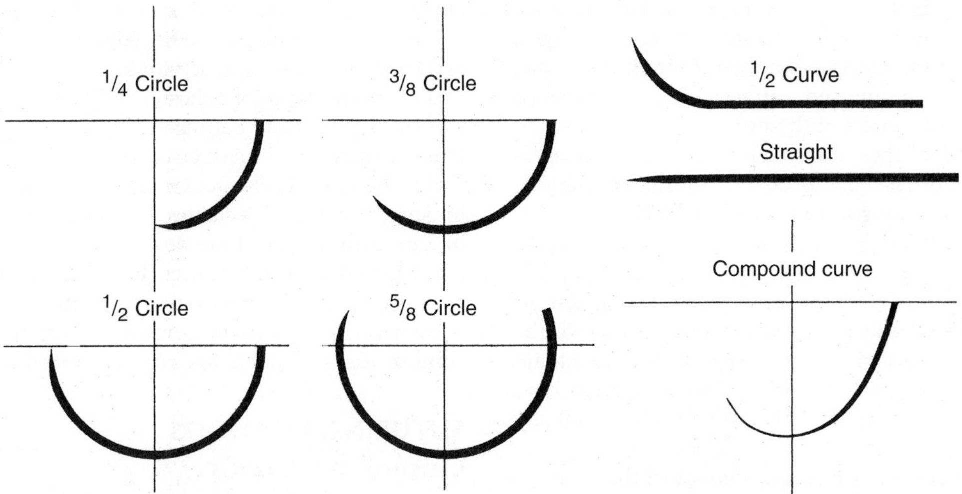


**FIGURE 6-4** Surgical needles vary in shape, size, type of point and body, and how the suture is attached.

## SURGICAL ADHESIVES

Tissue adhesives may be applied topically to intact skin at the wound edges to hold surfaces together. Care must be taken to avoid any contact with the open wound; adhesive in the wound creates a barrier to wound healing. When used in areas that are not subject to stress (e.g., areas that penetrate the fascia) or movement (e.g., on the hands or joints, where there is repetitive movement), tissue adhesives provide for fast closure and less pain for the patient.[13,19]

## SURGICAL NEEDLES

Surgical needles vary in shape, size, point design, and wire diameter (Figure 6-4). The appropriate needle is selected depending on the type and location of tissue being sutured. Surgical needles are made from stainless steel or carbon steel. Various metal alloys used in manufacturing surgical needles determine their basic characteristics. They must be strong, ductile, and able to withstand the stress imposed by tough tissue. Stainless steel is the most popular, not only because it provides these physical characteristics but also because it is noncorrosive. The three basic parts of a surgical needle are the *eye,* the *body,* and the *point* or *tip.*

### Eye

The eye of the surgical needle falls into three general categories:

- Eyed needles, in which the needle must be threaded with the suture strand, and two strands of suture must be pulled through the tissue (Figure 6-5, *A*)
- Spring, or French, eyed needles, in which the suture is placed or snapped through the spring (Figure 6-5, *B*)
- Eyeless needles, a needle-suture combination in which a needle is swaged (permanently attached) onto one or both ends of the suture material (Figure 6-5, *C*)

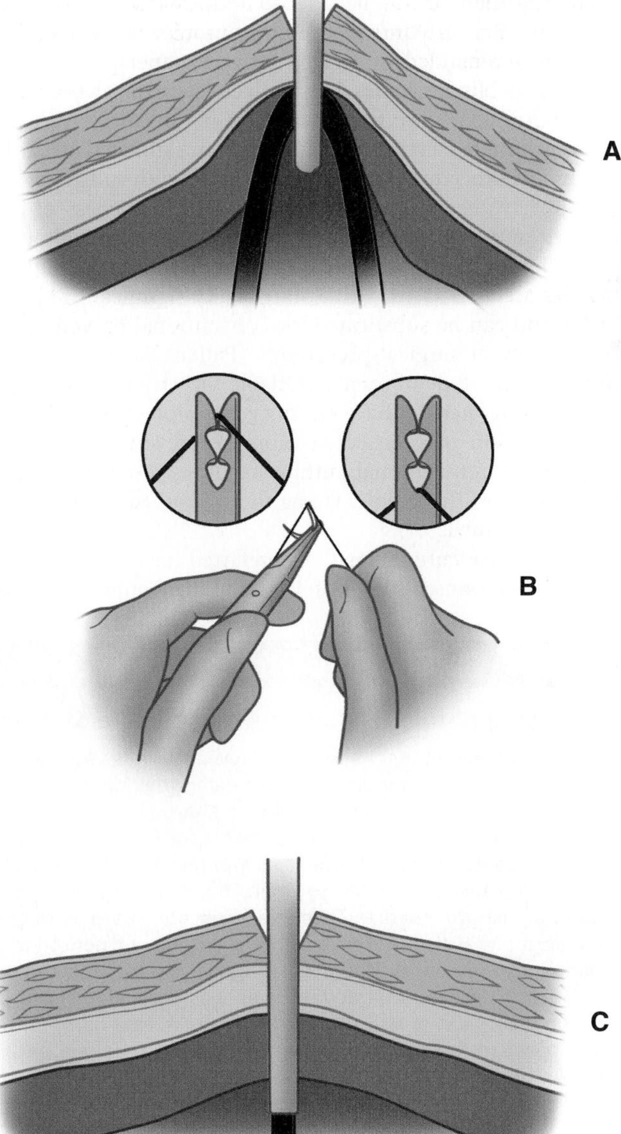


**FIGURE 6-5** Types of needles. **A,** Eyed needle. Greater tissue trauma is caused by the double suture strand threaded through eyed needles. **B,** Spring eye. Holding suture strand taut with left hand, bring strand down over top and spring into eye. **C,** Atraumatic (eyeless) needle causes minimal tissue trauma by eliminating the double suture strand.

The swaged needle is the most universally used needle type, eliminating threading eyed needles before and during surgery. A single strand of suture material is drawn through the tissue, and tissue damage is minimized (atraumatic). The swaged needle may need to be cut off with suture scissors or swaged for controlled release of the suture (semiswaged). With semiswaged suture, the needle remains attached until the surgeon releases it with a straight tug of the needle holder.

## Body

The body, or shaft, of the needle may be round, triangular, or flattened. Surgical needles also may be straight or curved; the curve is described as part of an imaginary circle (see Figure 6-4). As the radius of the imaginary circle increases, the size of the needle also increases. The body of a round needle gradually tapers to a point.

Choice of needle point relates to the density of the tissue to be penetrated. Delicate tissue, such as bowel or kidney, requires a taper or blunted point, whereas skin, which is dense in structure, requires a cutting edge. Taper points tend to tear tissue less than cutting needles do and leave a smaller hole in the tissue. Recently introduced blunt protect-point needles are being recommended as an alternative to taper point needles. Interest in blunt needles has evolved because of the risk of bloodborne exposure from percutaneous injuries (PIs). Such injuries have been reported to occur in an estimated 1% to 15% of surgical procedures—mostly associated with suturing. Some studies have been done to evaluate the effectiveness of blunt needles in preventing PIs and to assess their clinical acceptability by surgeons. Results of these studies indicate that blunt needles are associated with a statistically significant reduction in PIs and can be substituted for conventional curved needles in a variety of surgical procedures (Patient Safety). Table 6-7 illustrates the type of points available for various tissues.

Triangular needles have cutting edges along three sides. The cutting action may be conventional or reverse. The cutting edge of the conventional cutting needle is directed along the inner curve of the needle, facing the wound edge when suturing is performed.

The reverse cutting needle is preferred for cutaneous suturing. When it transects the skin lateral to the wound, the outside cutting edge is pointed away from the wound edge, and the inside flat edge is parallel to the edge of the wound. This cutting action reduces the tendency for suture to tear through tissue.

For certain types of delicate surgery, needles with exceptionally sharp points and cutting edges are used. Microsurgery, ophthalmic surgery, and plastic surgery require needles of this type; special honing wheels provide needles of precision-point quality for surgery in these specialties. In some instances, the application of a microthin layer of plastic to the needle surface provides for easier penetration and reduces drag of the needle through tissue.

Most surgical services departments have instituted standardization programs to control the variety of needle-suture combinations available for surgical procedures.

# SUTURING METHODS

## Closure of Wounds

The *primary suture line* refers to sutures that obliterate dead space, prevent serum from accumulating in the wound, and hold the wound edges in approximation until healing takes place (Figure 6-6). Surgical wounds that have skin edges immediately closed with sutures or staples have minimal scarring; this method of wound closure is used in clean or clean-contaminated wounds that are expected to heal by primary intention (see Chapter 8).[10] The *secondary suture line* refers to sutures that supplement the primary suture line. They are placed on each side of the primary suture line, passing through several layers of tissue at once. A secondary suture line helps eliminate tension on the primary sutures and reduces the risk of evisceration or dehiscence. Retention sutures are a type of secondary suture line.

An *interrupted suture* is inserted into tissues or vessels in such a way that each stitch is placed and tied individually. This type of suture is widely used and generally considered the strongest and most secure (Figure 6-7, *A*). Various techniques used for the insertion of interrupted sutures in the tissue are designed to alter the angle of pull and the relationship of the wound's edges to each other. Such maneuvers cause the edges of the wound to invert or to evert and aid in wound healing because fewer sutures are used. This type of stitch generally is used on skin and may be used on any underlying tissue layer.

## PATIENT SAFETY

### Using Blunt Needles to Avoid Needle-Stick Injuries

Analysis of percutaneous injuries shows that rates for the most part have decreased in many device categories. Suture needles have failed to show a major decline in sharps injury rates, however. Of the top six devices responsible for 80% of all injuries, suture needles ranked second, accounting for 19% of needle sticks. A safer alternative to sharp-tip suture needles is the blunt-tip suture needle. These needles are sharp enough to pierce internal tissue, but not sharp enough to penetrate the skin. They are now available in a range of bluntness. In the past, a challenge for perioperative nurses was their inability to persuade a surgeon to use a safer device, such as a blunt-tip needle, because the surgeon chose which devices to use. In 2005 the American College of Surgeons (ACS) issued a *Statement on Blunt Suture Needles,* addressing the need for methods of reducing the rate of cuts and needle-stick injuries that occur during operations. This statement noted that cuts and needle-stick injuries occur in approximately 1% to 15% of all operations, with the most common cause of suture needle injury being the suturing of fascia, during which 59% of all suture needle injuries occur. The ACS believes that blunt suture needles should be available in various sizes and with a range of suture adequate for different surgical applications, and that the use of blunt suture needles is an important factor in reducing or eliminating a prevalent occupational hazard for surgeons and perioperative nurses.

Modified from Cowles L: The point of the matter, *Advance for Nurses* 6(17):43-44, 2004; Perry J, Jagger J: Sharps safety update—are we there yet? *Nursing 2005* 35(6):17, 2005; News from the American College of Surgeons: ACS issues patient safety statement on preventing needlestick injuries. Accessed August 4, 2005, on-line: www.facs.org/news/patientsafetystatements.html.

**TABLE 6-7**

## Atraumatic Needles

| Needle Type | Description of Body | Use |
|---|---|---|
| Taper point | Round shaft, straight or curved, taper point, no cutting edge | Soft tissue closure, such as gastrointestinal, fascial, vascular, and most soft tissues below the skin surface |
| Penetrating point | Taper body with finely sharpened point; optimum penetration with less tissue wound | Ligaments, tendons, calcified, fibrous, and cuticular tissue; mostly used for vascular, thoracic, plastic, obstretrics/gynecology, and orthopedic surgery; excellent penetration through synthetic grafts and scar tissue during repeat surgeries |
| Blunt point | Taper body with a rounded point, no cutting edge | Friable tissue, fascia, liver, intestine, kidney, muscle, uterine cervix. Note recommendations regarding use of blunt needles, p. 168. |
| Protect-point | Taper body with a blunted point, no cutting edge | Primarily in fascia and mass closure to minimize the potential of needle sticks |
| Reverse cutting | Triangular point with cutting edge on the outer curvature | Skin closure, retention sutures, subcutaneous, ligamentous, or fibrous tissues |
| Cutting taper | Reverse cutting tip with taper shaft | In microsurgery for excellent penetration through tough tissue, such as vasovasostomy, tuboplasty |
| Hand-honed reverse cutting | Same as reverse cutting but hand-honed for added sharpness | Primarily in plastic surgery for delicate work and where a good cosmetic result is a concern |
| Spatula side cutting | Two cutting edges in a horizontal plane | Ophthalmic surgery for muscle and retinal repair; also for delicate eyelid or plastic surgery; cutting edges "ride" along scleral layers |
| Regular cutting | Triangular point with cutting edge on the inner curvature | General skin closure, subcutaneous tissue, sometimes for ophthalmic surgery, plastic or reconstructive surgery |
| Lancet, inverted lancet | Spatula needle with the cutting edge (lancet) or outer (inverted lancet) curvature | Ophthalmic surgery and microsurgery |

Modified from *Ethicon wound closure manual,* Sommerville, NJ, 2004, Ethicon.

A *continuous suture* consists of a series of stitches, of which only the first and last are tied (Figure 6-7, *B*). With this type of suture, a break at any point may mean a disruption of the entire suture line. It is used to close tissue layers where there is little tension but tight closure is required, such as the peritoneum, to prevent the intestinal loops from protruding, or on blood vessels to prevent leakage.

*Retention* (or *stay*) sutures are placed at a distance from the primary suture line to provide a secondary suture line (Figure 6-7, *C*), relieve undue strain, and help obliterate dead space. Wound dehiscence, the partial or total disruption of any or all layers of the surgical wound, is the result of a combination of factors, including technical problems with closure, local wound factors (infection or hematoma), poor wound healing, and undue stress caused by increased intraabdominal pressure on the wound (abdominal distention, dilated bowel, vomiting, coughing, chronic obstructive pulmonary disease [COPD]). Predisposing factors to wound dehiscence include age (>60 years old), obesity, poor nutrition, diabetes, chemotherapy or radiation therapy, renal or hepatic insufficiency, infection, and corticosteroid use.[9] With patients in whom these factors exist, retention sutures are likely to be used. They are placed in such a way that they include most if not all layers of the wound. A simple interrupted or figure-of-eight stitch is used. Usually heavy, nonabsorbable suture materials, such as silk, nylon, polyester fiber, or wire, are used to close long, vertical abdominal wounds and lacerated or infected wounds. To prevent the suture from cutting into the skin surface, a small piece of rubber tubing (bumper, bolster, bootie) or other type of device (bridge, button) is passed over or through the exposed portion of the suture. The bridge device allows the surgeon to adjust tension over the wound postoperatively.

*Subcuticular sutures,* sometimes referred to as *buried,* are sutures placed completely under the epidermal layer of the skin (Figure 6-7, *D*).

A *purse-string suture* is a continuous circular suture placed to surround an opening in a structure and cause it to close (Figure 6-7, *E*). This type of suture may be placed around the appendix before its removal. Or it may be used in an organ such as the cecum, gallbladder, or urinary bladder before it is opened so that a drainage tube can be inserted; then the purse-string suture is tightened around the tube.

The Nursing Interventions Classification (NIC) lists suturing as a nursing intervention, defined as "approximating edges of a wound using sterile suture material and a needle."[5] The NIC was developed to classify nursing interventions so that the work of nursing could be documented and nursing knowledge improved through the evaluation of patient outcomes. In perioperative nursing practice, the act of suturing is considered part of the education and subsequent role of the registered nurse first assistant.[16]

## Endoscopic Suturing

Suturing through an endoscope is a learned skill, not an innate talent. The ports must be placed and used to maximize the precision and efficiency of the suturing motions. An array of

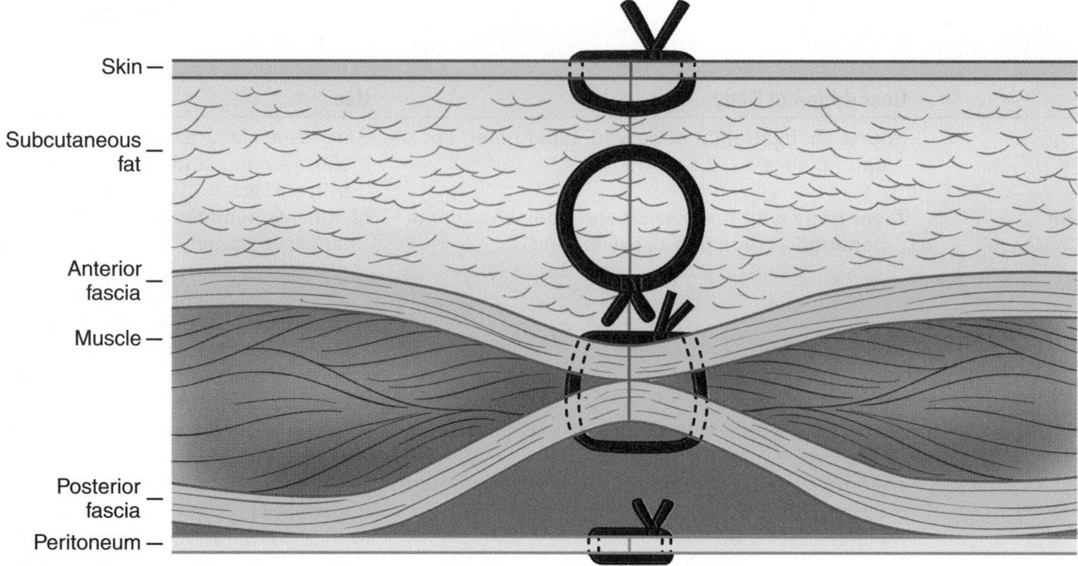


FIGURE 6-6 Primary suture line on the abdominal wall, midline incision.

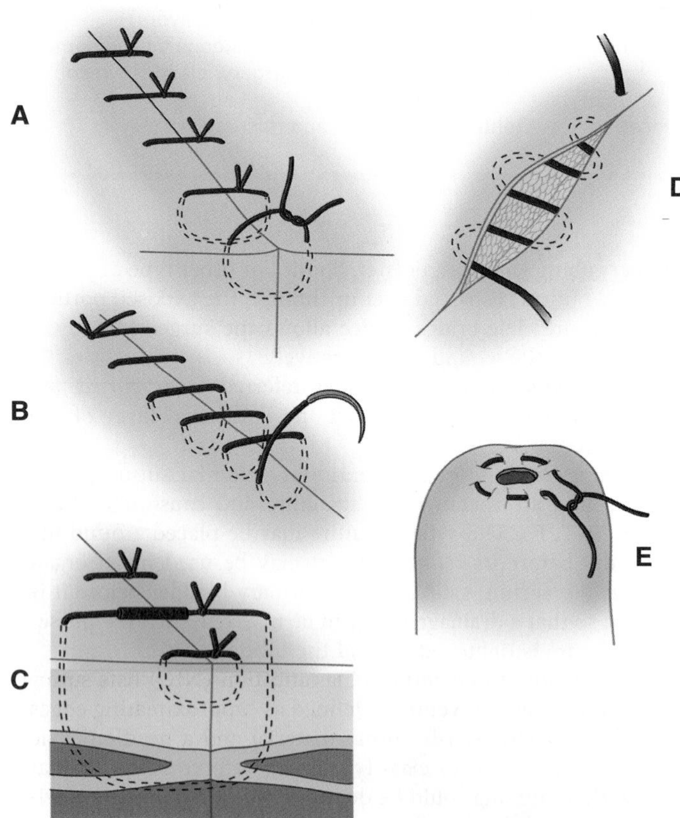


FIGURE 6-7 Types of stitches. **A,** Interrupted. Each stitch is made with a separate piece of suture material, which is tied separately. **B,** Continuous or "running." A stitch is made with one uninterrupted length of suture material. **C,** Retention. Stitches are used to reinforce the primary suture line; heavy, strong suture material is used. **D,** Subcuticular. Stitch is placed completely under the epidermal layer of the skin. **E,** Purse-string. A stitch runs parallel to the edge and encircles a circular wound.

needles and suture materials is available for endoscopic suturing so that the surgeon is not disadvantaged by a lack of choice. Research and development of technique, instrumentation, needles, and suture materials are ongoing as the types of procedures done endoscopically increase and methods are perfected.

## Holding a Drain in Place

If a drainage tube is inserted into a wound, the tube may be anchored to the skin with a nonabsorbable suture so that it will not slip in or out. A tube left in a hollow viscus, such as the gallbladder or common duct, may be secured to the wall of that organ with an absorbable suture.

## Knot-Tying Technique

The successful use of the many varieties of suture materials depends, in final analysis, on the skill with which the surgeon or first assistant ties the knot. The completed knot should be firm to prevent slipping and should be small, with ends cut short, to minimize the bulk of suture material in the wound. The suture may be weakened by inappropriate handling. One should avoid excessive tension, sawing, friction between the strands, and inadvertent crushing with clamps or hemostats.

## Endoscopic Knot Tying

Knot tying is one of the most challenging aspects of endoscopic surgery. Preformed ligature loops are used in ligating the appendix or blood vessels. Extracorporeal knots are tied outside the abdomen and slid into the abdomen using a knot pusher. They can be tied rapidly and securely; the square knot is normally used as the locking loop knot. Intracorporeal knotting is done completely within the abdominal cavity whenever fine sutures are being placed in tissues for reconstruction purposes. All suturing and knot-tying techniques performed through the endoscope require excellent hand-eye coordination, practice, and the ability to perform these techniques while the operative site is being viewed on a television monitor.

## PERIOPERATIVE NURSING CONSIDERATIONS

### General Considerations

In the preparation and use of sutures in surgery, every precaution must be taken to keep the sutures sterile, to prevent prolonged exposure and unnecessary handling, and to avoid waste. Before perioperative personnel prepare any suture materials, they should review the sutures listed in the card file or computerized data sheet for a particular procedure and surgeon. The scrub person should prepare only one or two sutures during the preliminary preparation, but the circulator should have an adequate supply of sutures available for immediate dispensing to the sterile instrument table.

Customized suture kits that contain a designated number and variety of sutures for particular procedures, surgeons, or both are available for use when suture preferences are consistently the same. These kits may be more economical than individually packaged sutures because of reduced packaging costs, decreased gathering and dispensing times, and less capital outlay for inventory.

### Opening Primary Packets

The scrub person tears the foil packet across the notch near the hermetically sealed edge and removes the suture. Some sutures are now packaged for delivery to the field in their inner folders, ready to load, with no foil wrapper.

### Handling Suture Materials

To remove suture strands to be used for ties when they are not on a reel or disk, the loose end is pulled out with one hand while the folder is grasped with the other hand. To straighten a long suture, the free end is grasped (using the thumb and forefinger of the free hand), the kinks, caused by package memory, are removed by gentle pulling with the free ends secured, one in each hand, and then the arms are slowly abducted to straighten the strands.

Kinks should never be removed by running gloved fingers over the strand because this action causes fraying.[18] The tensile strength of a gut suture should not be tested before it is handed to the surgeon. Sudden pulls or jerks may damage the suture so that it will break when in use.

To prepare individual lengths of ligature or suture, the strand is folded in equal parts and held between the fingers and then divided. Standard 54-inch lengths of suture may be cut into quarters, thirds, or halves by the scrub person to meet most procedure needs. For general surgery, a continuous suture threaded on a needle is usually about 24 inches long, and its short end is 3 to 4 inches long (half-lengths). An interrupted suture is 12 to 14 inches long, with 2 or 3 inches threaded through the needle (quarter-lengths). To ligate a vessel in the epidermal and subcutaneous layers, the ligature may be quarter-lengths. Vessels or structures deep in the wound are ligated with a suture or ligature that is 24 to 30 inches long (third-lengths to half-lengths). Sutures also are provided in 12- to 60-inch precut lengths by the manufacturer. Also supplied are the more commonly used 54-inch lengths on reels or disks (discussed earlier) and labyrinth packs, where precut strands may be removed one at a time from the package rather than all at once.

To remove a suture-needle combination from the package, the scrub person grasps the needle with a needle holder and gently pulls (Figure 6-8). To straighten the suture in a suture-needle combination, the scrub person grasps the suture 1 to 2 inches distal to the needle and pulls gently on the other end of the strand with the other hand to remove kinks. The jaws of the needle holder grasp the flattened surface of the needle to prevent breakage and bending. To facilitate suturing, the needle is secured about ⅛ inch down from the tip of the needle holder (Figure 6-9). The holder is placed on the needle about a third of the distance in from the eye or swaged end.

A suture or free ligature should not be too long or too short. A long suture is difficult to handle and increases the possibility of contamination because it may be dragged across the sterile field or fall below it. A short suture makes tying difficult; if threaded on a needle, it may slip out of the eye. The depth and distance to the site of tying or suturing guide the scrub person in preparing ties or sutures of the correct length.

### Threading Surgical Needles

Free needles, which come packaged separately from the suture, must be threaded by the scrub person for the surgeon. A curved needle is threaded from within its curvature so that the short end falls away from the outside curvature (Figure 6-10). This practice helps to prevent accidental pullout. The scrub

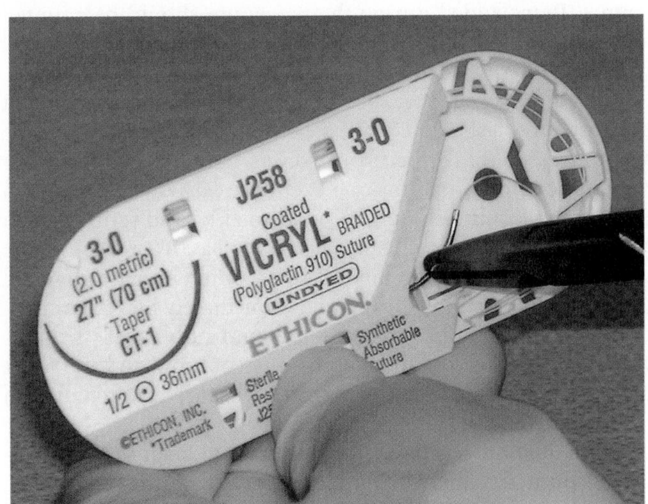


**FIGURE 6-8** Loading a suture directly from packet.

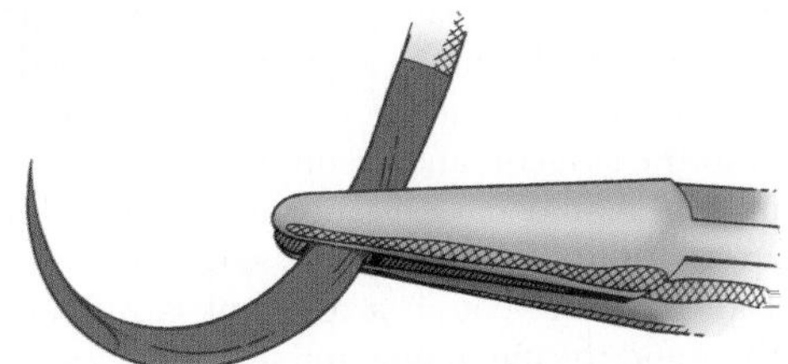

**FIGURE 6-9** Loading a needle holder. Clamp needle holder approximately one-third the distance from the swage or eye to point of needle.

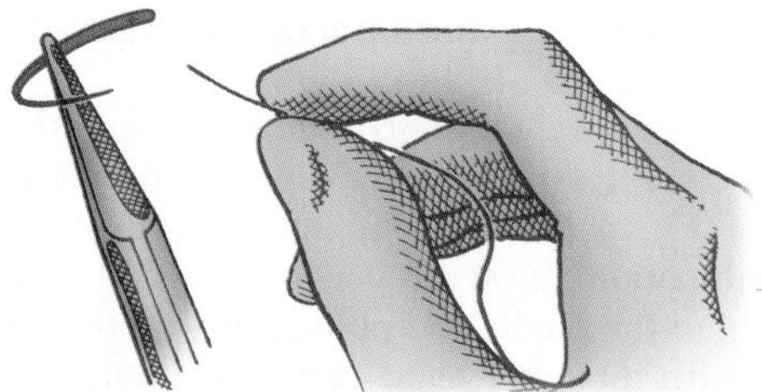

FIGURE 6-10 Eyed needle is threaded from inside curvature. Take care to avoid pricking glove on sharp needle point.

person pulls the suture about 4 inches through the eye of the needle to prevent the suture from being pulled out of the eye during suturing.

## Counting Needles

A patient outcome identified in the Perioperative Nursing Data Set (PNDS) is that "the patient is free from signs and symptoms of injury due to extraneous objects."[3] Among the many perioperative nursing activities undertaken to achieve this patient outcome is the performance of counts to ensure that the patient is free from injury related to retained sponges, sharps, or instruments. Institutions vary in their policies regarding needle and sharps counts during operative procedures, but most follow established procedures based on the Association of periOperative Registered Nurses (AORN) Recommended Practices for Sponge, Sharp, and Instrument Counts.[2] Initial counts before the start of the procedure provide the basis for subsequent counts. Items added during the procedure should be counted and documented. The count should be performed audibly and with each sharp visualized by the scrub person and circulator.

During the procedure, the scrub person should be aware of the location of sharps on the sterile field. Needles should be accounted for by the scrub person as they are placed in the neutral zone on a one-for-one exchange basis when possible. Subsequent counts should be performed by the scrub person and circulator before closure of a body cavity or deep, large incision, after closure of a body cavity, when either individual is relieved by other personnel, and immediately before completion of the surgical intervention. It is imperative that two individuals be involved in the count—one counting and the other witnessing that the count is correct. All sharps are retained in the OR during the surgical procedure.

Many institutions have printed forms to keep track of routinely counted items. Others use erasable count boards visible to all personnel. Recording the count is the responsibility of the circulator. The count sheet may become part of the patient's record. To facilitate counting, needles are counted according to the number indicated on the package; the scrub person verifies this number with the circulating nurse when the package is opened. Used needles should be kept on a needle pad or counter on the scrub person's table. Broken or missing needles must be reported to the surgeon and accounted for in their entirety. Each institution should have established policies for dealing with incorrect counts. In general, the surgeon is immediately notified of an incorrect count; a re-count is initiated. Sterile team members and the circulating nurse initiate a search of the sterile and unsterile field. If the missing item is not revealed after a re-count and search, the surgeon is asked to explore the wound. If the missing item is not found, agency policy may dictate that an x-ray film be taken. Documentation of these activities should be completed according to institutional policy and procedure.

## Sharps No-Touch Technique

Scalpel blades and suture-needle injuries account for most hospital-based sharps injuries reported in the OR.[4,15] Because sharp instruments used in surgery are a frequent cause of injury, recommendations for eliminating hand-to-hand passing have been developed (Best Practice).

### BEST PRACTICE

#### Preventing Sharps Injuries

The Exposure Prevention Information Network (EPINet) is a voluntary surveillance system used to track needle-stick injuries. During the period from 1993 to 2001, 29% of OR injuries occurred between steps in the procedure, such as when passing sharp devices. Another 29% of injuries occurred after the device was used, but before it was disposed—that is, while disassembling the device. Suture needles caused 34% of injuries to perioperative nurses, whereas scalpels were responsible for 19% of injuries.

Although 2002 data revealed that injuries from reusable scalpels had declined, the proportion of injuries to perioperative nurses from suture needles increased. Perioperative nurses should use the following best practices for handling sharps:

- Double glove; inspect gloves for punctures frequently.
- Use standardized sterile field setups.
- Keep all sharps on instrument tables or trays with the points away from staff members.
- Use a neutral zone or hands-free method for passing sharps. Establish the neutral zone before the incision (a magnetic pad or basin may be used to create the neutral zone; if a basin is used, it should be placed on the field and not held by the scrub person).
- Dedicate the neutral zone for sharps only (these include suture and hypodermic needles, scalpels, and other sharp instruments). Include identification of the neutral zone during hand-off communications to relief scrub persons.
- Only one sharp at a time should be in the neutral zone.
- Avoid handling suture needles manually whenever possible. Instead, use a needle holder, forceps, or suturing assist device.
- Do not hold a sharp and any other instrument simultaneously.
- Announce the transfer of a sharp before placing it in the neutral zone. After the announcement, orient the sharp in the correct position in the neutral zone. The scrub person and surgeon or assistants should communicate about the best placement of sharps in the neutral zone.
- Do not use fingers to touch tissue being cut or sutured.
- Know where all sharps are throughout the procedure.
- Confine and contain all sharps in a disposable, puncture-resistant needle container.
- Pass sharp, long laparoscopic instruments handle first, keeping the tip down.
- At the conclusion of the procedure, verify that the container holding sharps is securely closed.

Modified from AORN guidance statement: Sharps injury prevention in the perioperative setting. In: *AORN standards, recommended practices and guidelines*, Denver, CO, 2005, The Association; Perry J, Jagger J: Exposure safety—pass with care in the OR, *Nursing 2005* 35(2):70, 2005.

Based on Occupational Safety and Health Administration (OSHA) regulations and the Standard Precautions of the Centers for Disease Control and Prevention (CDC), institutions should have written policies regarding the handling of sharp instruments and needles at the surgical field. In a no-touch technique, sharps are placed in a predesignated basin, tray collection device, or safe "neutral" zone on the field, from which the surgeon can retrieve the sharps. After use, the item is placed back in the neutral zone, and the scrub person retrieves it. This technique eliminates hand-to-hand passing of sharps between the surgeon and the scrub person, such that no two individuals touch the same sharp at the same time, reducing the chance of accidental needle punctures and cuts. All sharps should be accounted for and properly disposed of before the room is prepared for the next patient.

The Needlestick Safety and Prevention Act was signed into law November 6, 2000, and changes to OSHA's Bloodborne Pathogens Standards mandated by this Act took effect in April 2001.[7,8] Considerations for the perioperative health care team include the following:

- Blunt needles, stapling devices, adhesive strips (skin tapes), and tissue adhesives are used whenever clinically feasible to reduce the use of sharp suture needles.
- Scalpel blades with safety features are used.
- Alternative cutting methods are used when appropriate.
- Manual tissue retraction is avoided by using mechanical (self-retaining) retraction devices.
- All equipment that is unnecessarily sharp is eliminated.
- Double-gloving is employed.
- Eye protection and face shields are used by all health care team members.
- Appropriate use and disposal of all sharps is mandated (Box 6-2).

The risk of transmission after a needle-stick or sharps injury is estimated to be 6 to 30 out of every 100 people for hepatitis B virus (HBV); 3 to 10 out of every 1000 people for hepatitis C virus (HCV), and 1 out of every 300 people for human immunodeficiency virus (HIV). If an occupational exposure or injury occurs that could result in a bloodborne pathogen exposure, the injured person should do the following:[11]

- Immediately flood the exposed area with water.
- Clean the wound with an antimicrobial skin disinfectant or soap and water.
- Alert the nurse manager or other appropriate person.
- Identify the source patient.
- Immediately report to employee health (or the appropriate institutional department).

An immediate evaluation and risk assessment is done. A postexposure treatment plan is initiated with counseling, education, and follow-up testing 1 year after exposure.

All OR personnel should work collaboratively to select the least dangerous device that would accomplish the intended function (i.e., cutting, providing hemostasis, retracting, suturing) efficiently and effectively. By doing so, perioperative personnel may significantly reduce the rates of injuries in the OR and exposures to blood and bloodborne pathogens.

**BOX 6-2**

**Sharps Disposal Containers**

- Durable, closable, leakproof, and puncture resistant
- Appropriate size for user and type of sharps
- Lids allow sharps to enter by gravity without need for additional manipulation
- Within horizontal reach of health care team members (close to the point of use) who dispose of sharps
- Container, level of fullness (full line), proper warning labels (biohazard labels), and color coding (orange, orange-red) must remain visible to health care team members
- Self-closing lids to prevent overfill if container is not "see-through" to observe fill line
- Ease of assembly and operation, including one-handed disposal

Modified from AORN guidance statement: sharps injury prevention in the perioperative setting. In: *AORN standards, recommended practices and guidelines,* Denver, Colo, 2005, The Association; Davis MS: *Advanced precautions for today's O.R.,* ed 2, Atlanta, 2001, Sweinbinder.

## INSTRUMENTS

### Historical Perspective

The history of surgical instruments dates back to 2500 BC. The first instruments were sharpened flints and fine animal teeth. Ancient Greek, Egyptian, and Hindu instruments are amazing in their resemblance to contemporary instruments.

In the late 1700s, to be equipped for the practice of surgery, the surgeon had to employ various skilled artisans, such as coppersmiths; steelworkers; needle grinders; turners of wood, bone, and ivory; and silk and hemp spinners. The surgeon had to explain the mechanisms of the instruments and supervise their manufacture. The resulting instruments were crude, expensive, and time-consuming to make. Each artisan used hand labor exclusively, devoted time to making only one type of instrument, and gained proficiency. A cutter would keep a small supply of surgical knives. Thus began physicians' supply houses and surgical instrument making.

In the mid-1800s, physicians' principal tools were their eyes and ears. Official records show that amputation, the trademark of the Civil War, was the result in three of four operations. Surgeons were scarce, and medical instruments were almost nonexistent. Kitchen knives and penknives, carpenter saws, and table forks did the job. After the Civil War, the advent of the administration of ether and chloroform brought a demand for new ideas and methods in surgery and instruments. The division of general surgery into specialties occurred in the late 1800s and early 1900s. Delicate instruments were seen as more useful than the force of crude and heavy instruments. So that instruments could withstand repeated sterilization, handles of wood, ivory, and rubber were discontinued.

The development of stainless steel in Germany ensured a better material for surgical instruments and other equipment. Today, surgeons and perioperative nurses assist manufacturers in research, design, and development of new and better instrumentation. Most instrument companies design an instrument to a physician's specifications. Advancement in endoscopic surgery continually requires the development of instrumentation specifically designed for this type of surgery.

Throughout the history of surgery, the tools of the surgeon and the manual aspects of the surgical technique have influenced the evolution of practice. Along with innovative wound closure materials and tools in recent decades, there have been unprecedented developments of new and improved instrumentation. The benefits of minimally invasive surgery are well documented, especially in surgical procedures that typically required lengthy hospital stays, required long and sometimes difficult postoperative recovery or rehabilitation, and exposed the patient to increased risk of surgical infection. One example is the advancements that have taken place in spinal fusion surgeries. Originally performed through a large incision, under direct vision, removing a portion of the lamina and taking bone graft material from the pelvis through a second incision, spinal fusion has progressed to a minimally invasive procedure. Foley, in collaboration with instrumentation companies, developed the Sextant Instrumentation used in the most minimally invasive lumbar fusion surgeries performed today. The incision is the size of a trocar site; two on each side, lateral to the spine. Key instrumentation for this procedure is shown in Figure 6-11. With fluoroscopic guidance, screws are placed on the end of the screw extender rods (center of Figure 6-11) and placed in the lamina. The screw extender rods are locked together, and the rod templates (Figure 6-12) are used to determine the length of the rod. The sextant (left component in Figure 6-12) replaces the rod template, and a sharp trocar is placed in the tip. With proper alignment assured by the fixation of the instrumentation, the trocar is moved through the tissues to the point of rod insertion and back. The rod is placed in the sextant, and this procedure is repeated, all with fluoroscopic guidance. Proper alignment is confirmed, and the fixation screws are tightened. The trocar sites are closed. Advantages of having the procedure performed in this manner include a 1- to 2-day hospitalization with almost no postoperative pain. The disadvantages are that a maximum of two levels can be done at one time, there is no crosslink bar that would provide additional stabilization, and there is a sharp learning curve for this procedure.[17]

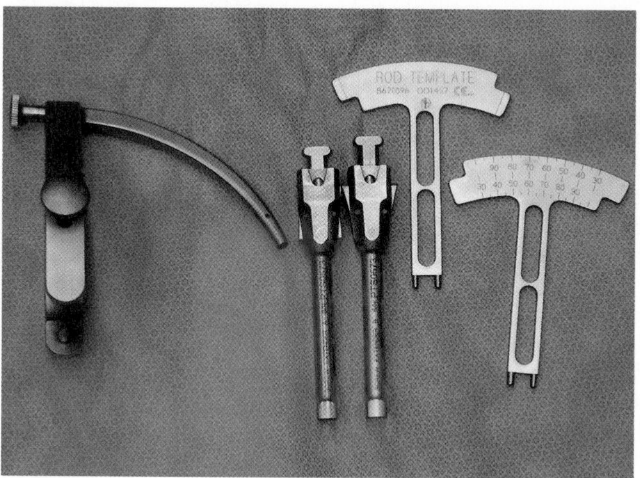


**FIGURE 6-11** Selected components of the Sextant Instrumentation. *Left to right,* Sextant, screw extender rods, rod templates.

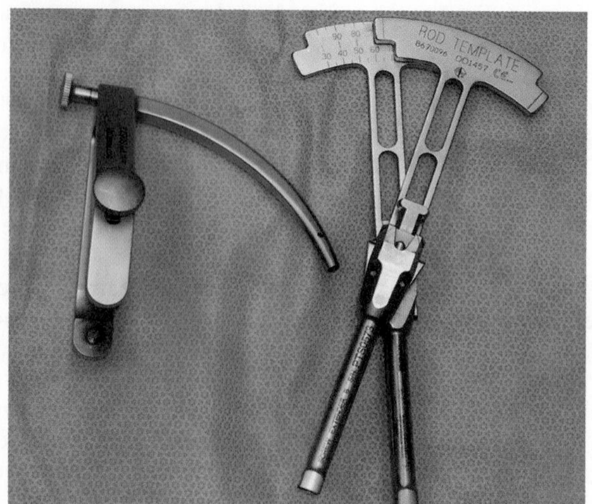


**FIGURE 6-12** Selected components of the Sextant Instrumentation. *Left to right,* Sextant, screw extender rods with rod templates in place.

## Composition of Surgical Instruments

Perioperative nurses are responsible for the use, handling, and care of hundreds of surgical instruments a day. A basic knowledge of how these instruments are manufactured can help in their selection and maintenance. Surgical instruments are expensive and represent a major investment for every institution.

Instruments used today are made in the United States, Germany, France, and Pakistan. The United States does not have an agency that reviews or sets standards for surgical instruments. The quality is set by the individual manufacturer. A reputable company stands behind its product. A properly cared for instrument should last 10 years or more.

Most instruments are manufactured from stainless steel. Stainless steel is a compound of iron, carbon, and chromium, which means that stainless steel can have varying qualities. These qualities are designated by grading the steel into series by the American Iron and Steel Institute (AISI). The 400 series stainless steel has some noncorrosive characteristics and good tensile strength. It resists rust, produces a fine point, and retains a keen edge. Handheld ringed instruments, such as scissors and clamps, should be 400 series stainless steel.

For ringed instruments, the raw steel is converted into instrument blanks by a machinist making an impression of the piece in a stainless steel blank. These blanks are die-forged into specific pieces—male and female halves. The excess metal is trimmed away, and the instrument parts are ready for the final steps.

The two halves are milled to prepare the box lock fittings, jaw serrations, and ratchets, and the jaws and shanks are properly aligned. After this is done, the halves are assembled by hand. A hole is drilled through the box lock, and a pin or rivet is inserted through the hole. Final grinding and hardening, accomplished by heat-treating, bring the object to proper size, weight, spring temper, and balance.

The last part of the process is called *passivation*. The instruments are put into nitric acid to remove any residue of carbon steel. The nitric acid also produces a surface coating of chromium oxide. Chromium oxide is important because it produces a resistance to corrosion in the stainless steel instrument. The instrument is then polished.

There are three types of instrument finishes. The first is the bright, highly polished mirror finish, which tends to reflect light and may interfere with the vision of the surgeon. The second is the satin or dull finish, which tends to eliminate glare and lessen eyestrain for the surgeon. The third finish is ebonized, which produces a black finish. Ebonized instruments are

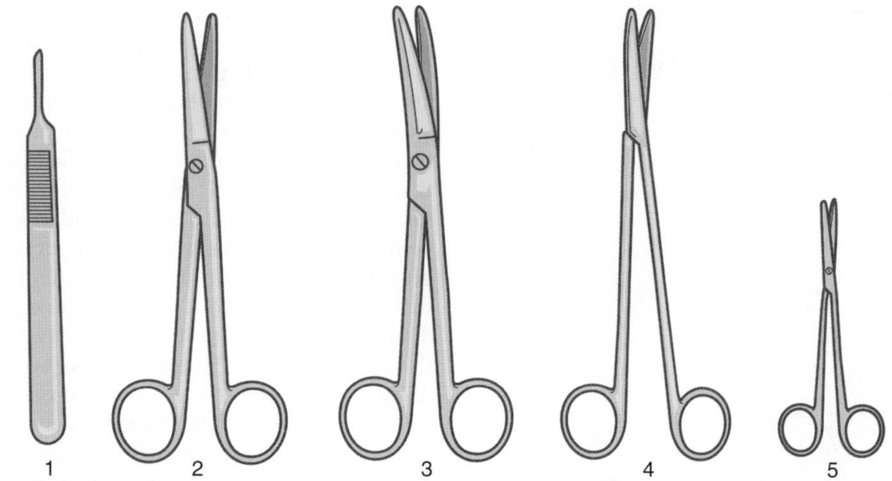


**FIGURE 6-13** Basic cutting instruments. *1,* Knife handle; *2,* Mayo scissors, straight; *3,* Mayo scissors, curved; *4,* Metzenbaum scissors, curved; *5,* Suture scissors, straight.

used during laser surgery to prevent deflection of the laser beam.

The final inspection and testing are for hardness, proper jaw closure, and smooth lock-and-ratchet action. The instrument is then ready for sale.

## Instrument Categories

Although there is no standard nomenclature for specific instruments, there are four main categories: *cutting instruments* (also called *dissectors*), *clamps, retractors,* and *accessory* or *ancillary* instruments.

***Cutting Instruments (Dissectors).*** Dissectors, which may be sharp or blunt, are instruments used to cut or separate tissue. The largest categories of sharp dissecting instruments are scalpels and scissors. Scalpels are probably the oldest of all surgical instruments (Figure 6-13). Most scalpels are handles (knife handle) with one end suited to the attachment of disposable blades (Figure 6-14). During an operation, the blades may be conveniently changed by the scrub person as often as necessary. The blades come prepackaged and sterile and are passed onto the sterile field as needed by the circulator. Careful handling of blades during the procedure and disposal of blades at the end of a procedure are important in the implementation of Standard Precautions.

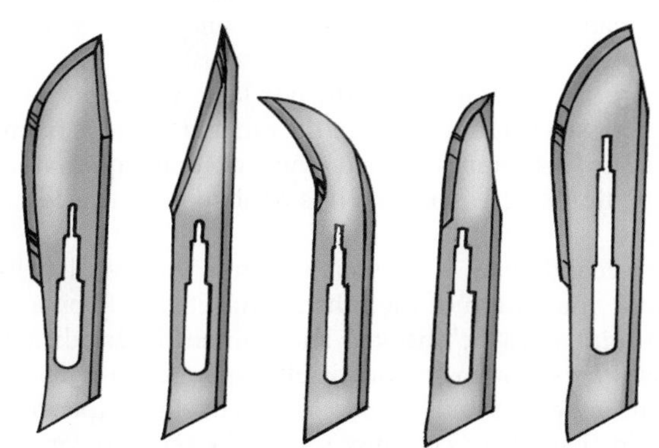

**FIGURE 6-14** Scalpel/knife blades: size numbers 10, 11, 12, 15, 20 (actual size).

Scissors are designed in various shapes and sizes for different purposes in cutting body tissues and surgical materials (see Figure 6-13). The basic design consists of two blades, each having a chisel-shaped edge with the bevel consistent with the structure or material it has to cut. Scissor tips may be blunt or sharp, and the blades may be straight or curved. Conventional scissors require two movements in use: one to open and another to close the jaws. Other scissors may have a spring action in the body design that holds the jaws in an open position. A single movement pressing the spring together closes the jaws to cut. Scissors designed for delicate plastic and eye surgery are often of the latter type. A basic instrument set usually includes a curved Mayo scissors for dissection of heavy tissues, a Metzenbaum scissors for dissection of delicate tissues, and a straight scissors for cutting suture. For surgery in deep areas of the body, scissors with long handles and short blades are used for better control and easier use.

Other sharp dissectors include drills, saws, osteotomes, rongeurs, and other instruments such as adenotomes and dermatomes. Some instruments in the dissecting category are produced in sharp or blunt form, such as curettes and periosteal elevators. Instruments or devices used for blunt dissection include gauze dissectors (peanuts, pushers, kitners), a sponge on a stick, the back of a knife handle, and the surgeon's finger or hand.

***Clamps.*** Clamps are instruments specifically designed for holding tissue or other materials, and most have an easily recognizable design. They have finger rings, for ease of holding; shanks, whose length is appropriate to the wound depth; ratchets on the shanks near the rings, which allow for the distal tip to be locked on the tissue or object grasped; a joint, usually a box lock (described later), which joins the two halves of the instrument and allows opening and closing of the instrument; and a jaw, which is the working portion of the instrument and defines its use (Figure 6-15). Clamps are divided into the following categories.

*Hemostats* are used to close the severed ends of a vessel with a minimum of tissue damage (Figure 6-16). They prevent the excessive loss of blood in the course of dissection. The jaws have deep transverse cuts so that the bleeding vessels may be

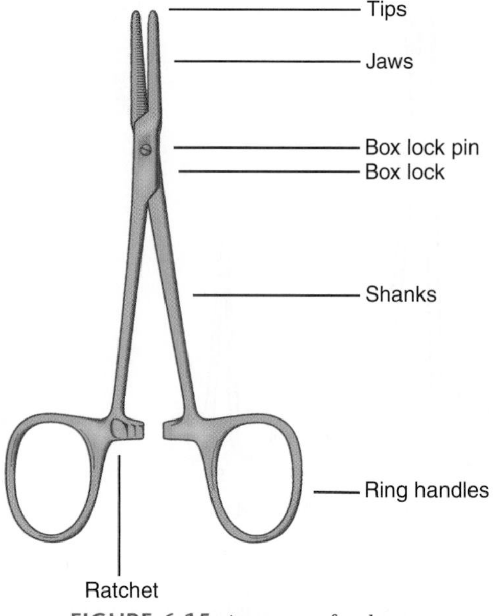


**FIGURE 6-15** Anatomy of a clamp.

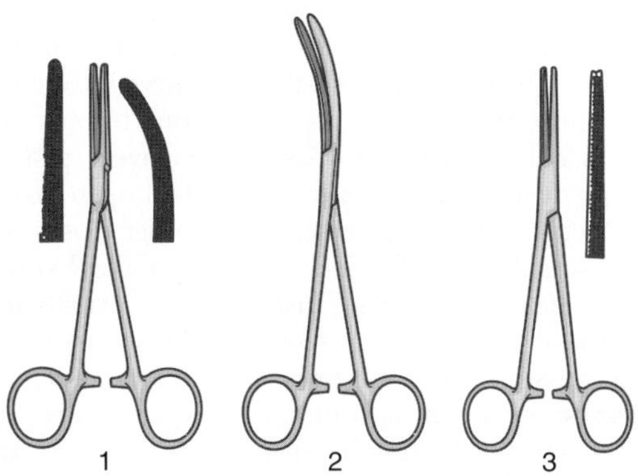


**FIGURE 6-16** Basic clamping instruments. *1,* Crile hemostatic forceps; *2,* Rochester-Pean forceps; *3,* Ochsner or Kocher hemostatic forceps.

compressed with sufficient force to stop bleeding. The serrations must be cleanly cut and perfectly meshed to prevent the tissue from slipping free from the jaws of the clamp.

*Occluding clamps* usually have vertical serrations or special jaws that have finely meshed, multiple rows of longitudinally arranged teeth to prevent leakage and to minimize trauma when clamping bowel, vessels, or ducts that are to be re-anastomosed.

*Graspers* and *holders* are used for tissue retraction and generally have jaws of specific design based on their use (Figure 6-17). The Kocher (also referred to as an Ochsner) clamp has transverse serrations and large teeth (1 × 2) at its tip to grasp tightly on tough, slippery tissue such as fascia. The Allis clamp has multiple, interdigitating short teeth on the tip, minimizing crushing or damaging tissue. The Babcock clamp has broad, flared ends with smooth tips, and it atraumatically grips or encloses delicate structures, such as bowel, ureters, or fallopian tubes. Other holding forceps have handles like clamps with specialized tips or jaws, which may be triangular, straight, angular, or T-shaped.

Nonclamp graspers and holders are known as *forceps* or *pickups* because they are used to lift and hold tissue (see Figure 6-17). Often, while the surgeon is cutting with scissors or sewing with a needle, forceps are used in the other hand. Forceps are held like a pencil. The most common kinds are the various two-arm spring forceps. Tweezer-like, they vary in length and thickness and are available with and without teeth. Nontoothed forceps create minimal damage and hold delicate, thin tissues. Toothed forceps hold thick or slippery tissues that need extra grip. The toothed forceps ("rat tooth") has interdigitating teeth that hold tissue without slipping; these are used to hold skin or dense tissue. Adson tissue forceps have small serrated teeth on the edge of the tips; these are designed for light, careful handling of tissue and are commonly used during skin closure.

Grasper and holder clamps may hold objects as well. Sponge-holding forceps with ring-shaped jaws (see Figure 6-17) are available in 7- and 9-inch lengths. They can be used to grasp or handle tissue but are commonly used as sponge holders. A gauze sponge is folded and placed in the jaws and is used to retract tissue, to absorb blood in the field, and occasionally to perform blunt dissection.

*Needle holders* (Figure 6-18), because they must grasp metal rather than soft tissues, are subject to greater damage. As a result, needle holders must be repaired and replaced regularly. For maximum usage, needle holders must retain a firm grip on the needle. Many types of jaws have been designed to meet this need. The so-called *diamond jaw* needle holder has a tungsten carbide insert designed to prevent rotation of the needle. In needle holders of standard design, a longitudinal groove or pit in the jaw releases tension, prevents flattening of the needle, and holds the needle firmly. Needle holders may have a ratchet similar to that of a hemostat, or they may have a spring action that may or may not lock.

Towel clamps also are considered holding instruments. Of the two basic types, one is a nonpenetrating towel clamp used for holding draping materials in place. The other has sharp tips (see Figure 6-17) used to penetrate drapes and tissues, but it is damaging to both. The use of sharp towel clamps to penetrate drapes is highly discouraged because they penetrate the sterile field.

**INSPECTION AND CARE.** The apposition of a clamp's tips is necessary for its functioning and must be periodically checked. When a hemostat is held up to the light and the handles are fully closed, no light should be visible between the jaws. These instruments, if used for purposes other than that for which they are intended, can be damaged and need to be repaired. The instrument's joint also must be checked. Instruments made up of two halves have one of three types of joints.

- The most common joint is the box lock, where one arm has been passed through a slot in the other arm and is riveted or pinned. This joint is needed where accurate approximation of the tips is necessary, and it is basic to most ringed instruments.
- The second type is the screw joint. The two halves are placed one on top of the other, connected only by a screw. The joint must be checked and tightened periodically because the screw may work itself loose. Screw-joint instruments are easy to make and comparatively inexpensive.
- The final and least common type is the semibox, or aseptic, joint. It has the advantage that the two halves can be separated for easy cleaning.

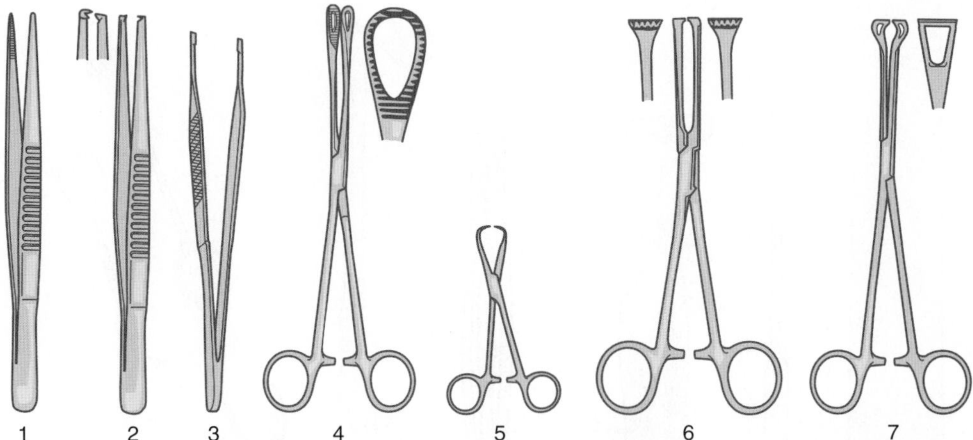


FIGURE 6-17 Basic holding instruments. *1,* Tissue forceps, smooth; *2,* tissue forceps with teeth; *3,* Adson tissue forceps; *4,* Sponge-holding forceps; *5,* Towel clamp; *6,* Allis forceps; *7,* Babcock intestinal forceps.

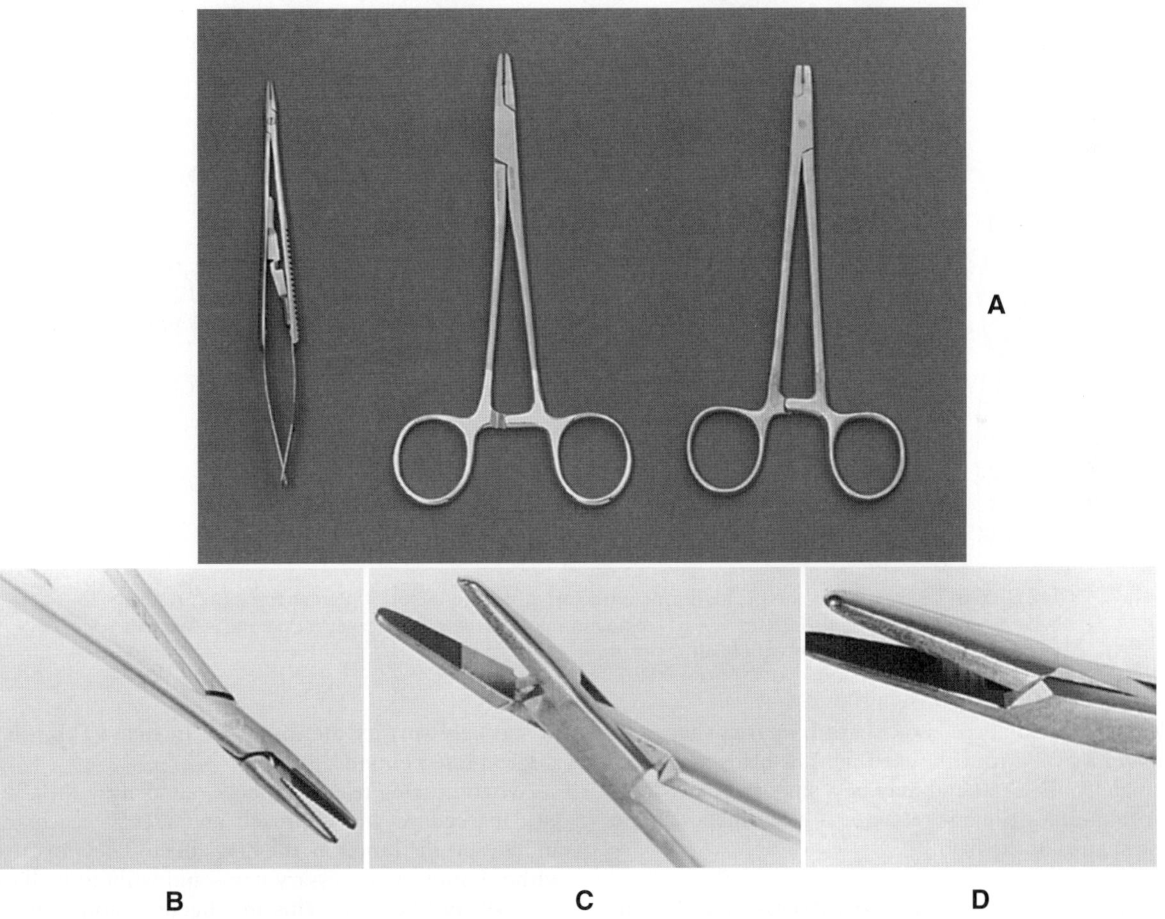


FIGURE 6-18 **A,** Needle holders. **B,** Fine. **C,** Regular. **D,** Heavy.

All types of joints must be cleaned regularly. Protein deposits or rust collecting at the site must be removed to ensure proper functioning.

***Retractors.*** Retractors are used to hold back the wound edges, structures, or tissues to provide exposure of the operative site. A surgeon needs the best exposure possible that inflicts a minimum of trauma to the surrounding tissue. Retractors are self-retaining (Figure 6-19) or manually held in place by a member of the surgical team. The two types of self-retaining retractors are (1) retractors with frames to which various blades may be attached, and (2) retractors with two blades held apart with a ratchet. An example of the latter is a Weitlaner retractor. Today there are very large self-retaining retractors, such as the Omni or Bookwalter, with multiple blades of varying lengths and sizes. With handheld retractors,

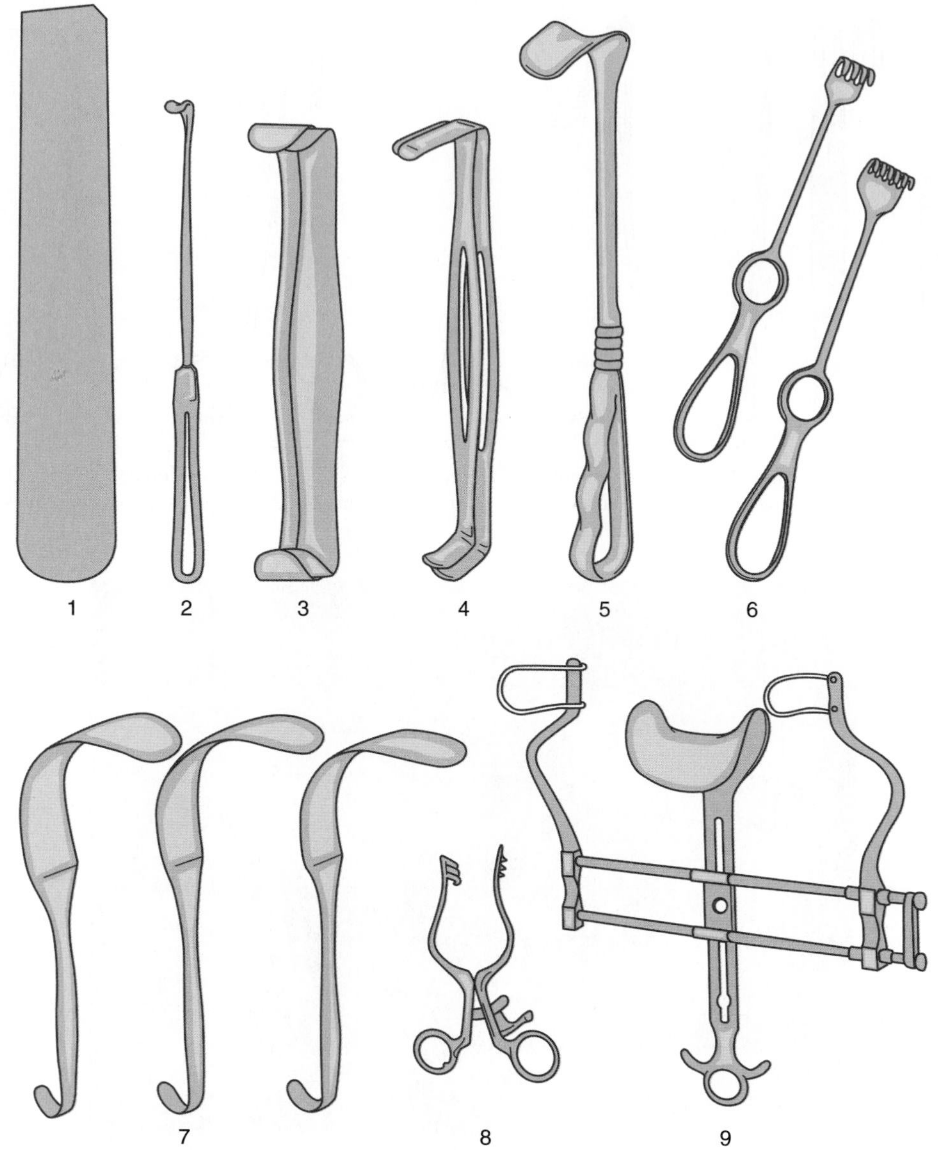


**FIGURE 6-19** Basic retractors. *1,* Malleable retractor; *2,* vein retractor; *3,* Parker retractor; *4,* Army-Navy retractor; *5,* Richardson retractor; *6,* Volkmann rake retractors; *7,* Deaver retractors; *8,* Weitlaner retractor; *9,* Balfour retractor with blades.

the handles may be notched, hook-shaped, or ring-shaped to give the holder a firm grip without tiring. The blade is usually at a right angle to the shaft and may be a smooth blade, rake, or hook. A malleable (ribbon) retractor is a flat metal ribbon that may be shaped at the field.

***Accessory and Ancillary Instruments.*** Accessory and ancillary instruments are designed to enhance the use of basic instrumentation or to facilitate the procedure (Figure 6-20). These include suction tips and tubing; irrigators-aspirators; electrosurgical devices; and special-use devices, such as probes, dilators, mallets, and screwdrivers.

Many miscellaneous instruments or specialty items are particular to a certain specialty but generally fall into one of the categories just mentioned. Microsurgical instruments are delicate and expensive. They are extremely fine and should be handled separately from other instruments. Instruments used in specialty surgery are discussed in each of the chapters on surgical interventions.

When nursing team members can analyze the planned surgical procedure and approach and identify each instrument and its specific function, they are able to select instrument sets without omitting necessary items and without including items that will not be used. This intelligent, planned approach ensures economy of time and motion, protects instruments from misuse, and prevents unnecessary handling. During the operation, the informed scrub person who anticipates instrument needs becomes a more valuable member of the surgical team.

## Endoscopic Instrumentation

Laparoscopy has introduced new equipment and instrumentation to the surgical suite (see Chapter 7 for a full discussion of laparoscopic equipment). In addition to insufflation equipment, an optical system, and a documentation system, perioperative

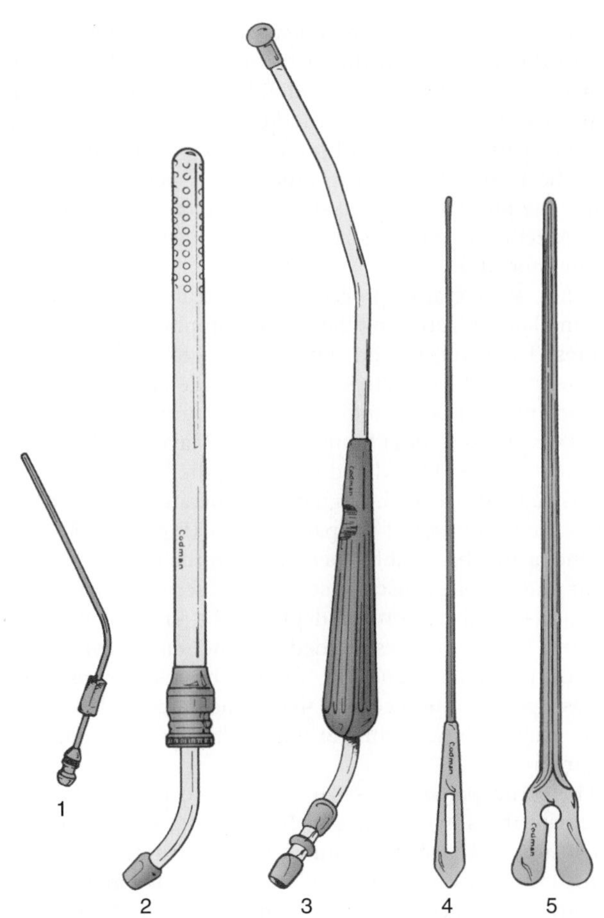


**FIGURE 6-20** Accessory items. *1,* Frazier suction; *2,* Poole suction; *3,* Yankauer suction; *4,* Silver probe; *5,* Grooved director.

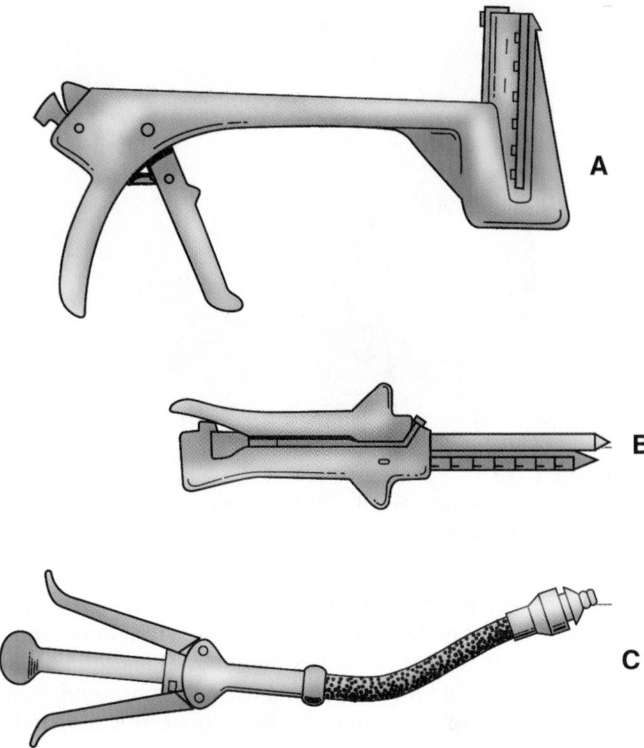


**FIGURE 6-21** Internal staplers. **A,** Terminal end stapler, designed for closing the end of a hollow organ, such as the stomach, with a double staggered line of staples. **B,** Internal anastomosis stapler, designed to connect hollow organ segments to fashion a larger pouch or reservoir. **C,** End-to-end stapler, designed to staple two hollow, tubelike organs, such as bowel, to create a continuous circuit.

personnel must be familiar with the instrumentation used by the surgeon to perform surgery through the scope. Basic instrumentation, which may be disposable or reusable, includes trocars, forceps or graspers, clip appliers, stapling devices, scissors, needle holders, and aspiration-irrigation systems.

Verres needles and trocars provide access to the peritoneal cavity. A retractable safety shield protects abdominal structures from being inadvertently punctured during insertion. Forceps or graspers are available in 3-mm, 5-mm, and 10-mm sizes. Atraumatic graspers provide appropriate retraction and little risk to tissues. Bipolar coagulation forceps are used to control bleeding. The forceps are available with different tips, including ring, paddle, dolphin nose, claw, spoon, DeBakey, Allis, Pollack, Pennington, Glassman, Maryland, Reddic-Saye, Duval, and Babcock. Some dissectors are available with coagulation capability. Scissors also come with different tips: hook, straight and microtipped, serrated, and curved. Also, several disposable instruments coagulate and cut the tissue. One such instrument is the Harmonic Scalpel (discussed in Chapter 7).

Needle holders come with a hinged-jaw tip to allow easy positioning of the needle before intracorporeal suturing and the sliding sheath. The sliding sheath holds the needle in a distal notch and inner spring-loading mechanism. To aid with extracorporeal knot tying, the surgeon may use a knot pusher (e.g., a Clarke-Reich) to deliver tied knots into the abdomen. A slide and cinch pusher (Gazayerli) also is used to deliver and secure the preformed knot. Intraabdominal stapling devices have been modified to fit and perform through the endoscope.

## Stapling Instruments

Instrumentation for internal stapling, first introduced in 1908, has been refined and is now widely used (Figure 6-21). Various instruments to suture tissue mechanically are used for ligation and division, resection, anastomoses, and skin and fascia closure. In general, these instruments may be classified as follows:[19]

- Ligating and dividing staplers (LDSs)
- Gastrointestinal anastomosis (GIA) staplers (Figure 6-22)
- Thoracoabdominal (TA) staplers
- End-to-end anastomosis (EEA) staplers
- Laparoscopic hernia mesh staplers
- Open hernia mesh staplers
- Endo-GIA devices

Employed in many surgical specialties, the mechanical application of these instruments reduces tissue manipulation and handling. The edema and inflammation that usually accompany anastomoses are minimized because the noncrushing B shape of the staples allows nutrients to pass through the staple line to the cut edge of the tissue.

Mechanical staplers (nondisposable and disposable) use cartridges of tiny stainless steel or absorbable, nonmetallic staples that are commercially preloaded, prepackaged, and presterilized. The staples are essentially nonreactive; metal

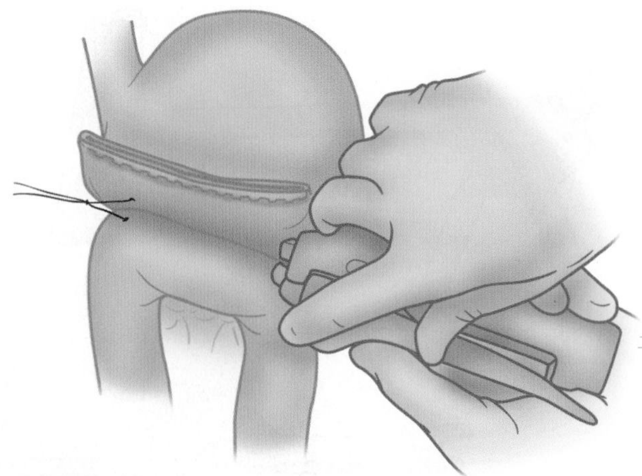

FIGURE 6-22 Using the GIA stapler to staple and join stomach and jejunum. At the same time, the blade in the GIA cuts between double staple lines, creating a stoma for a gastrojejunostomy.

staples remain permanently in the tissue. The staplers may fire individually or lay down multiple rows in a straight or circular pattern. Devices to cut or anastomose bowel and other structures are available for open-wound use or through endoscopic cannulae. The use of staplers significantly decreases operating time and may shorten postoperative stays.

## Selecting and Preparing Instruments for Patient Use

Designated OR or central supply personnel arrange the various instruments into trays or sets. The trays are named according to their functions. Three basic OR instrument sets are the minor/plastic, the basic laparotomy, and the dilation and curettage (D&C). A minor (or plastic surgery) set includes instruments needed for simple superficial incision, excision, and suturing. A basic laparotomy set includes instruments to open and close the abdominal cavity and repair any gross defects in the major body musculature. A D&C set, in addition to its use for dilation and curettage, is often used as the basic instrumentation for vaginal surgery.

According to each procedure's needs, more individualized instruments or specialty sets, such as an intestinal set or a vascular set, may be added. In the same way, basic instrument sets may be selected for opening other body cavities, such as the skull, chest, and pelvis.

Instruments are selected according to the size of the patient's body structures and the nature of the organs involved. Proper selection requires a general understanding of surgical procedures and approaches and knowledge of anatomy, possible pathologic conditions, and the design and purpose of instruments.

## Basic Table Setups

In most ORs, the instruments are set up on Mayo stands and back tables in a planned, standardized, organized, functional manner to maintain continuity when the original scrub person is replaced by another. The teaching manual should have illustrations or diagrams to which all personnel may refer. Each item used by the scrub person should have its own placement on the table to prevent the mass clutter that would occur if instruments and supplies were randomly placed.

A proficient scrub person must know the instrument inventory of the department, the instruments routinely needed for each type of operation, the individual surgeon's preferences, correct use and handling, method of preparation, and aftercare of the instruments. A file of preference cards or computerized data sheets usually list the procedures each physician performs, the physician's glove size, the preferred skin prep solution, specific draping instructions, and instruments required for the procedure.

Before an operative procedure, the scrub person may assist the circulator in gathering the needed supplies, equipment, and sutures. The scrub person scrubs; dons gown and gloves (see Chapter 3); and begins to set up the sterile tables with drapes, instruments, supplies, and sutures. Instruments are arranged with those most frequently used on the Mayo stand. When the patient is on the OR bed and is draped, the Mayo stand, set up for instrument use at the immediate operative site, is brought across the lower part of the patient's legs (Figure 6-23).

One or two back tables, according to the number of instruments and supplies, also are set up. The scrub person prepares the sutures and ligatures and places the knife blades on the handles. Other supplies needed are suction tubing and tips, electrosurgical cord and tip, drains, basins, gowns, gloves, drapes, sponges, and needles, all of which are sterile and set up on the back table according to standardized institutional policy (Figure 6-24).

The scrub person must be attentive to the sterile field to anticipate the surgeon's needs. Instruments should be passed in a positive and decisive manner. Each instrument is placed or slapped firmly into the surgeon's palm in such a manner that it is ready for immediate use with no wasted motion. When a curved instrument is passed to the surgeon, the curve should be pointing in the direction of intended use; there should be no need for readjustment. It is necessary to know if a surgeon or assistant is left-handed or right-handed to pass instruments efficiently and in the correct position.

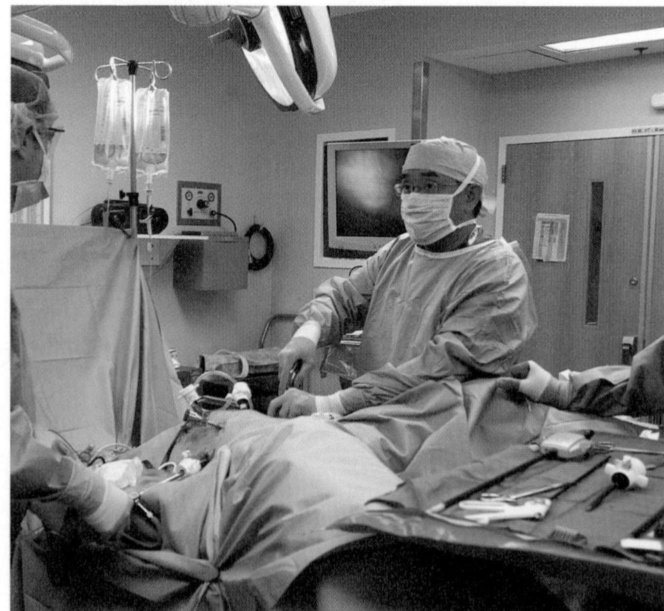

FIGURE 6-23 Mayo stand, with instruments required for start of surgical procedure, is moved into place across the lower part of the draped patient.

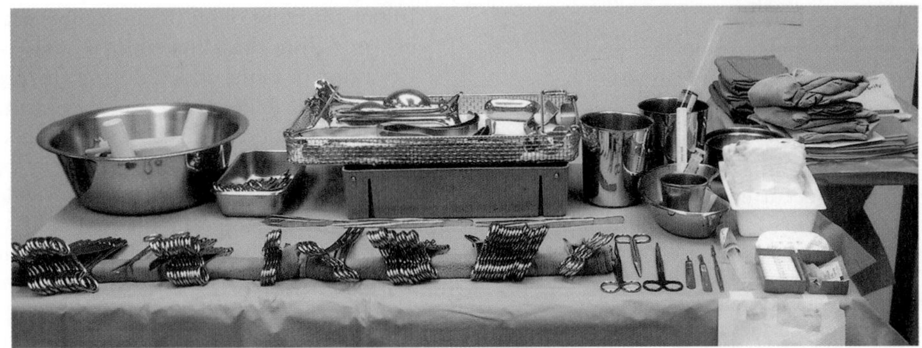

**FIGURE 6-24** Back table setup.

Often the surgeon or assistant uses hand signals for the type of instrument desired, to eliminate unnecessary talking. Scrub persons should become familiar with the basic signals for knife, scissors, suture, forceps, and clamp.

## Care and Handling of Instruments

An instrument should be used only for the purpose for which it is designed. Proper use and reasonable care prolong its life and protect its quality. Scissors and clamps, which are most frequently misused, can be forced out of alignment, cracked, or broken when used improperly. Tissue scissors should not be used to cut suture or gauze dressings. Hemostatic clamps should not be used as towel clamps or to clamp suction tubing.

Instruments must be handled gently. Bouncing, dropping, and setting heavy equipment on top of them must be avoided. During the procedure, used instruments should be wiped with a damp sponge or placed in a basin of sterile distilled water to prevent blood from drying on them. Saline solution should never be used on instruments because the salt content is corrosive and increases rusting or deterioration of the metal. As time allows during the procedure, the scrub person should rinse and dry the used instruments and replace them on the back table to facilitate closing counts.

At the end of a procedure, the instruments should not be thrown together in a tangled heap. They should be handled individually or in small groups. Sharp and delicate instruments should be set aside for individual handling and cleaning to avoid damage and accidental injury. Standard Precautions should be applied as dictated by institutional policy. All instruments set up for the procedure should be terminally sterilized or disinfected before reassembly. Instruments must be completely clean to ensure effective sterilization.

Each instrument should be inspected before and after each use to detect imperfections. An instrument should function perfectly to prevent needlessly endangering a patient's safety and increasing operative time because of instrument failure.

Forceps, clamps, and other hinged instruments must be inspected for alignment of jaws and teeth. Instrument jaws and teeth should meet perfectly so that blood flow is occluded without damaging the vein or artery. Ratchets should hold firmly yet release easily. Instrument joints should work smoothly.

The edges of scissors should be tested for sharpness by cutting smoothly through four layers of gauze. All instruments should be checked for worn spots, chips, dents, cracks, or sharp edges.

Damaged instruments should be set aside and sent for repair or replacement. An instrument repair service should be selected carefully and used for regular maintenance, such as sharpening and realignment.

With today's focus on cost containment, perioperative nurses must assess the care and handling of instrumentation carefully. Instrument sets can be monitored for use, and instruments that are used infrequently can be removed and packaged separately to prevent continued wear from unnecessary resterilization.

## Instrument Counts

Most institutions perform instrument counts as standard practice. Establishing standardized instrument sets with the minimum numbers and types of instruments in them facilitates instrument counts and reduces the amount of time and space required for a setup. Initial counts should be carried out concurrently by the circulator and scrub person before the procedure, with each person simultaneously viewing the instrument and audibly counting it. This is the baseline count. To facilitate the baseline count, the scrub person needs to be in the OR or other invasive procedure room in a timely manner to complete the instrument setup. Items added during the procedure are counted and immediately recorded. Subsequent counts should be taken before closure of a cavity or large, deep incision; when the scrub person or circulator is relieved by other personnel; and at the completion of the procedure. The method of counting should be consistent for every procedure, beginning at the surgical site and immediate surrounding area and moving to the Mayo tray, back table, and to items discarded from the field. Rushing at the end of a surgical procedure can result in incorrect or incomplete counts. When the scrub person and circulating nurse are rushed, it may be necessary to call for a "pause for the count," enabling counts to be carried out in an orderly manner.

Instruments that are disassembled during surgery, such as certain retractors, must be accounted for in their entirety. All counts are documented on the appropriate record by the circulator.

## Patient Safety

In 2002, AORN initiated its *Patient Safety First Program* and has continued to assist perioperative nurses in maintaining a safe environment for surgical patients. Retained foreign bodies after surgery are a complication with serious potential consequences for the people involved (Research Highlight). Several steps are taken to ensure that needles, sponges, and instruments are not retained in the patient, as follows:

- Identification and counting of instrumentation in instrument sets before sterilization

## RESEARCH HIGHLIGHT

### Retained Surgical Instruments and Sponges

In 2001, Suzanne Beyea, PhD, RN, then Director of Research at AORN, noted, "If nurses had to record certain types of information each time a near miss or an actual incidence of a retained instrument or sponge occurred, processes could be improved to reduce risks. Perhaps they would discover that extremely obese patients or those undergoing abdominal surgery are at the greatest risk for retaining an instrument or a sponge. Reliable and valid data might direct clinicians to be more attentive to counts during certain types of surgical procedures. Furthermore, specific clinicians or clinical services might be at greater risk for being involved in procedures in which instruments or sponges are retained. This type of information could assist clinicians in developing practices and procedures to ensure patient safety related to counts."

There were known risk factors associated with retained foreign bodies. Among those were changes in nursing personnel during a surgical procedure, excessive loss of blood, lack of a complete count of sponges and instruments, surgical team member fatigue, and urgency of the surgery. Anecdotal data collected from surgeon interviews suggested other risk factors, such as patient obesity, unexpected intraoperative developments, procedures that involve multiple teams, and performance of more than one major procedure at a time.

In 2003, a research study was published that examined risks using a retrospective, case-control methodology. Malpractice claims and incident reports involving retained instruments and sponges were reviewed to identify cases. Cases from 10 hospitals (54 patients who had incurred a retained foreign body) were matched with controls (i.e., patients who had undergone the same type of procedure during the same 6-month period but who had not experienced the complication of a retained foreign body). Every case was matched with approximately four randomly selected controls so that there were 235 patients in the control group. Univariate and multivariate conditional regression modeling procedures were used to analyze the data.

The study findings confirmed that the risk of leaving a foreign object behind significantly increased in procedures that were considered emergencies (risk of a retained foreign object was nine times as high), when unplanned changes in the procedure occurred (risk of a retained foreign object was four times as high), and in patients with obesity as determined by body mass index. Sixty-one retained foreign bodies were identified. Of foreign bodies, 69% were sponges, and 31% were instruments. Of patients in whom a foreign body was left, 69% required reoperation, and 22% had small bowel fistulas, obstructions, or visceral perforations. The findings further suggested that emergency procedures and procedures involving unexpected changes were significantly more likely to involve a failure to perform counts.

Perioperative nurses can use this information proactively to take steps when surgical procedures involve one of the identified risk situations. In addition to following count protocols carefully and engaging in detailed communication during hand-off reports when personnel are changed, consideration should be given to routine radiographic screening in these situations as part of the process to prevent retention of foreign bodies.

Modified from Gawande AA and others: Risk factors for retained instruments and sponges after surgery, *The New England Journal of Medicine* 348:229-235, 2003.

- Initial counting of all items at table setup, before the surgical procedure (baseline count)
- Counting of items added during the procedure
- Counting of items as the wound closure is initiated
- Final counting of items as wound closure is completed

Despite these efforts, items still may be retained in the patient after surgery. The Agency for Healthcare Research and Quality (AHRQ) has established quality indicators based on literature review, expert input, and empiric evaluation. Patient Safety Indicators (PSI) constitute a set of measures that can be used to screen for problems that patients experience. One of these is "Foreign body left during procedure."[6] In 2005, the American College of Surgeons issued a patient safety statement regarding the prevention of retained foreign bodies after surgery. Paramount to preventing retained foreign bodies are good communication, consistent practices, and wound exploration before closure of the surgical site.[1]

## Storing Instruments

Instruments should be stored safely. Cabinet shelving should be adjustable and properly spaced for storage of various sizes and types of instruments. Most institutions store instruments in presterilized trays or containers. Attached labels and diagrams in cabinets assist personnel. An inventory of all instruments should be taken at periodic intervals.

## REFERENCES

1. American College of Surgeons: Patient safety statement on preventing retained foreign bodies after surgery. Accessed August 4, 2005, online: www.facs.org/news/patientsafetystatements.html.
2. Association of Perioperative Registered Nurses (AORN): Recommended practices for sponge, sharp and instrument counts. In: *AORN standards, recommended practices and guidelines,* Denver, CO, 2005, The Association.
3. Beyea SC: *Perioperative nursing data set,* Denver, CO, 2002, Association of periOperative Registered Nurses.
4. Davis MS: *Advanced precautions for today's OR,* ed 2, Atlanta, 2001, Sweinbinder.
5. Dochterman JM, Bulechek GM: *Nursing interventions classification (NIC),* ed 4, St Louis, 2004, Mosby.
6. Elixhauser A and others: Using the AHRQ quality indicators to improve health care quality, *Joint Commission Journal on Quality and Patient Safety* 31(9):533-538, 2005.
7. Farley K: Evaluating the risks of bloodborne pathogens, *Point of View* 40(3):16-22, 2001.
8. Goulett C: Safety first, *Advance for Nurses* 6(22):28-30, 2005.
9. Harken AH, Moore EE: *Abernathy's surgical secrets,* ed 4, Philadelphia, 2000, Hanley & Belfus.
10. Hwang KO: *Surgery cue cards,* Philadelphia, 2001, FA Davis.
11. Kenny P: Safe needles save lives, *The Pennsylvania Nurse* 60(3):12, 2005.
12. Lawrence PF: *Essentials of general surgery,* ed 3, Philadelphia, 2000, Lippincott Williams & Wilkins.
13. Lawrence WT and others: Acute wound care. In Souba WW and others: *ACS surgery principles and practices,* New York, 2005, WebMD.
14. *Mosby's medical dictionary,* ed 7, St Louis, 2006, Mosby.
15. Nelson R: Needlestick injuries—going but not gone, *American Journal of Nursing* 104(11):25-26, 2004.
16. Official Statement on RN first assistants. In: *AORN standards, recommended practices and guidelines,* Denver, CO, 2005, The Association.
17. Salerni A, Rock T: Personal communication. August 16, 2005.
18. Semer NB: *Practical plastic surgery for nonsurgeons,* Philadelphia, 2001, Hanley & Belfus.
19. Weintraub SL and others: Principles of preoperative and operative surgery. In Townsend CM, editor. *Sabiston textbook of surgery,* ed 17, Philadelphia, 2004, Saunders.

CHAPTER 7

# Surgical Modalities

KAY A. BALL

Surgery continues to evolve as less invasive procedures and instrumentation are introduced and accepted. A variety of modalities have been developed that have enhanced and advanced surgical procedures. This chapter provides detailed information about the evolution of some popular surgical modalities, including endoscopy, video technology, and energies used during surgical intervention.

## ENDOSCOPIC MINIMALLY INVASIVE SURGERY

In the late 1980s, the "laparoscopy revolution" began in the United States (Box 7-1). General surgeons developed techniques to perform procedures using the laparoscope, eliminating the need for a large incision.

As surgeons and perioperative nurses were accessing knowledge and information, the surgical industry concomitantly was working to accommodate the rapid change from open surgical procedures to the newer techniques of minimally invasive surgery (MIS). Perioperative nurses and surgical technologists experienced a marked opportunity for competence acquisition during this period. Since the 1990s, equipment, instrumentation, surgical skills, and perioperative nursing knowledge have markedly expanded as MIS has become a safe approach for a multitiude of surgical interventions.[4] Ongoing changes in surgery to incorporate endoscopic procedures continue to present multiple and complex challenges for the surgical team, while offering patients potentially shorter hospital stays, reduced postoperative pain, and faster recuperation (Table 7-1). A thorough understanding of the goals of endoscopic MIS, clinical competence, and preoperative patient assessment establish the basis for the perioperative plan of care.

### Endoscopes

An endoscope is a tube that is inserted into a natural body orifice or through a tiny incision to access internal organs or structures. Endoscopes can be flexible, rigid, or semirigid. Flexible endoscopes include but are not limited to angioscopes, bronchoscopes, choledochoscopes, colonoscopes (Figure 7-1), cystonephroscopes, hysteroscopes, mediastinoscopes, ureteroscopes, and ureteropyeloscopes. Rigid endoscopes include but are not limited to cystoscopes, laparoscopes, sinuscopes, arthroscopes, bronchoscopes, laryngoscopes, and hysteroscopes (Figure 7-2). Some endoscopes may be manufactured in flexible and rigid forms. A semirigid endoscope, such as the ureteroscope, provides some movement, although it remains fairly rigid (Figure 7-3).

Endoscopes can be diagnostic or operative. *Diagnostic* scopes are for observation only and have no operating channels. The system is sealed at both ends. A diagnostic scope can be used, however, when multiple access sites are planned for the introduction of other instrumentation to perform a surgical procedure. *Operative* endoscopes are channeled for irrigating, suctioning, inserting, and connecting accessory instrumentation (Figure 7-4). For example, when a neodymium:yttrium-aluminum-garnet (Nd:YAG) laser is used, the laser fiber is inserted into the operating port of the laparoscope.

Endoscopes come in a variety of diameters and lengths depending on access to the area being visualized and the requirements of the procedure. Optical capability through a rigid scope is controlled by the lens system and can be direct (0-degree angle) or angled (e.g., 30, 70, 120 degrees) (Figure 7-5). Flexible scopes by their nature of being able to be angulated allow for a more panoramic view.

There are two types of flexible endoscopes: fiberoptic endoscopes and videoscopes. A fiberoptic endoscope has an eyepiece with a lens for visualization; the image is carried through the endoscope via a bundle of tiny glass fibers. A videoscope has, at the scope's distal end, a video chip that provides an image that is directly viewed on a monitor; a videoscope does not have an eyepiece for direct viewing.

Flexible endoscopes have four distinct components:

1. Control body (e.g., angulation knobs, air-water channels, biopsy port, eyepiece for fiberoptic endoscopes)
2. Insertion tube (e.g., flexible tube containing channels for suction, biopsy, irrigation, air and water, image bundles for the fiberscope, light bundles)
3. Bending section at distal tip (e.g., bending rubber, lenses, air-water nozzle, C-cover, charged coupled device [CCD] chip for videoscopes)
4. Light-guide connector unit (e.g., suction, air-water channel)

Flexible endoscopes also have three different systems that include some of the various components within the endoscope:

1. Mechanical system (provides ports to introduce accessories to perform treatments and procedures)
2. Angulation system (allows the endoscope's distal tip to be moved in different directions)
3. Illumination system (provides light for viewing internal structures)

Rigid endoscopes also have four distinct components:

1. Eyepiece (e.g., ocular lenses; rigid videoscopes are being developed today without an eyepiece)
2. Body (e.g., light-guide connector, valves)
3. Shaft (e.g., rod lenses, spacers)
4. Distal end (e.g., objective lens, negative lens)

Understanding the anatomy of an endoscope can help assess technical problems that can occur during an endoscopic procedure. The internal components are complex, sophisti-

BOX 7-1

### History of the Evolution of Endoscopic Minimally Invasive Surgery

Endoscopy, the examination of body organs or cavities by means of an endoscope, has been practiced for several centuries. Although primitive, the first use of reflected light for inspection of the vagina and uterine cervix is credited to Abul Kasim (936-1013), an Arabian physician. From this new conquest came instrumentation to examine the nasal sinuses and urinary bladder. Of primary concern during this initial era of endoscopy was the thermal tissue injury caused by the intense heat emitted by the light sources that were used. Incandescent lighting was eventually incorporated into the tips of certain endoscopes (e.g., cystoscopes, ureteroscopes) that could be cooled by continuous irrigation. Modifications allowed for examination of the nasal sinuses, larynx, bronchus, and sigmoid colon. Procedures were restricted, however, to those performed through endoscopic placement in external body orifices.

In 1910 Jacobaeus, a Swedish physician, first reported using a cystoscope to examine the peritoneal cavity. He was able only to diagnose conditions because the ability to create a pneumoperitoneum (the introduction of a gas into the peritoneum to increase visualization and operative exposure) was yet to be developed. Numerous complications were associated with these brave attempts to perform this rudimentary form of laparoscopy. Some common injuries during these pioneering activities were to the bowel and vascular structures—complications that today, although not unknown, are rare.

In an attempt to reduce morbidity, gynecologists introduced the cul-de-sac approach to pelvic endoscopy (culdoscopy). Instead of inserting the scope through the abdomen, they did so through the cul-de-sac. During this era, the importance of introducing air into the abdomen was recognized. Air was introduced through the use of a syringe and needle. Knee-chest and Trendelenburg positions were used to facilitate this procedure.

In 1964 an automatic insufflation device was developed by the German surgeon Semm. Laparoscopy was still considered to be "blind" surgery and because of this did not gain rapid popularity in North America or Europe. During the 1960s, two other developments enhanced the endoscopic revolution. In 1966 the rod-lens system designed by the British optical physicist Hopkins improved brightness and clarity. Fiberoptic (cold) light sources also were introduced that reduced further the risk of visceral and bowel burns.

In the late 1970s to early 1980s, endoscopic surgery moved from the category of diagnostic to that of operative. Semm termed his pioneering work *pelviscopy.* His work led to many technologic advances in instrumentation, equipment, and practice. Diagnostic and operative laparoscopies were becoming the techniques of choice for gynecologists throughout the world. Flexible and rigid endoscopic procedures also were increasing for urologists, internists, and otorhinolaryngologists. In the 1970s, orthopedic surgeons began to appreciate the art of arthroscopy.

In the 1980s, the laparoscope was introduced in general surgery. General surgeons were familiar with laparoscopy because many were consulted to assist gynecologists when evaluating right lower quadrant pain in young women. That experience enabled surgeons to perform their own laparoscopic procedures to diagnose acute appendicitis.

Modified from Ball KA: *Endoscopic surgery,* St Louis, 1997, Mosby; White RA, Klein SR: *Endoscopic surgery,* St Louis, 1991, Mosby; Semm K: Advances in pelviscopic surgery, *Progress in Clinical and Biological Research* 112(Pt B):127-129, 1982; Zucker KA: *Surgical laparoscopy,* St Louis, 1991, Quality Medical Publishing.

TABLE 7-1

### Advantages of Minimally Invasive Surgery Over Open Surgery

| Minimally Invasive | Open |
|---|---|
| Ambulatory or short hospital stay | Hospital admission |
| Short postoperative recuperation | 4- to 6-wk recuperation |
| Reduced postoperative pain; reduced need for pain medications | Postoperative pain related to surgical site; more analgesics required |
| Earlier return to normal life-style | Return to normal life-style varies with recuperation period |

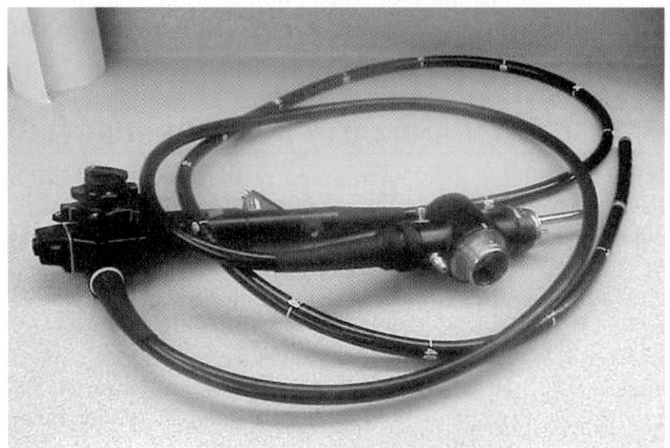

FIGURE 7-1 Flexible colonoscope.

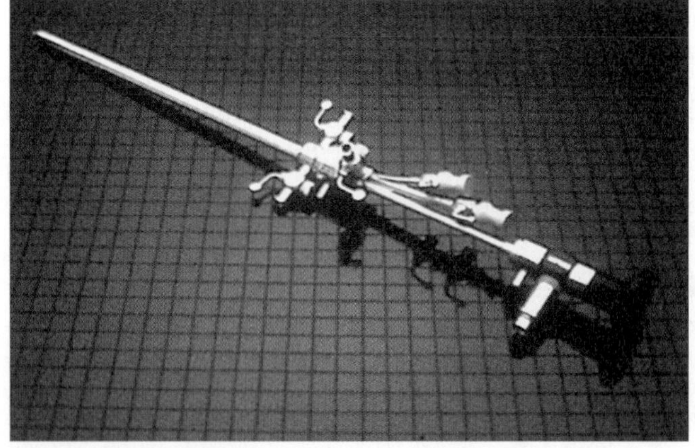

FIGURE 7-2 Rigid endoscope.

cated, and sometimes delicate (Figure 7-6); the endoscope must be treated with care.

## Light Sources and Fiberoptic Cables

Endoscopic light is often referred to as *cold light,* meaning that the heat from the light source is not transmitted through the length of the scope; therefore, tissue damage from heat at the distal tip of the endoscope is minimized. When the ends of

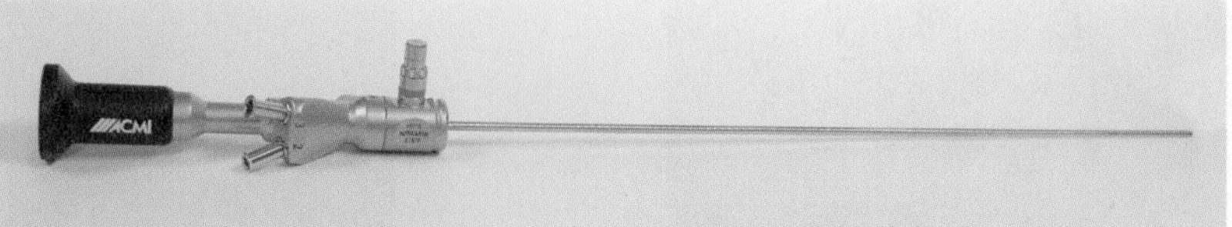


FIGURE 7-3 Semirigid ureteroscope.

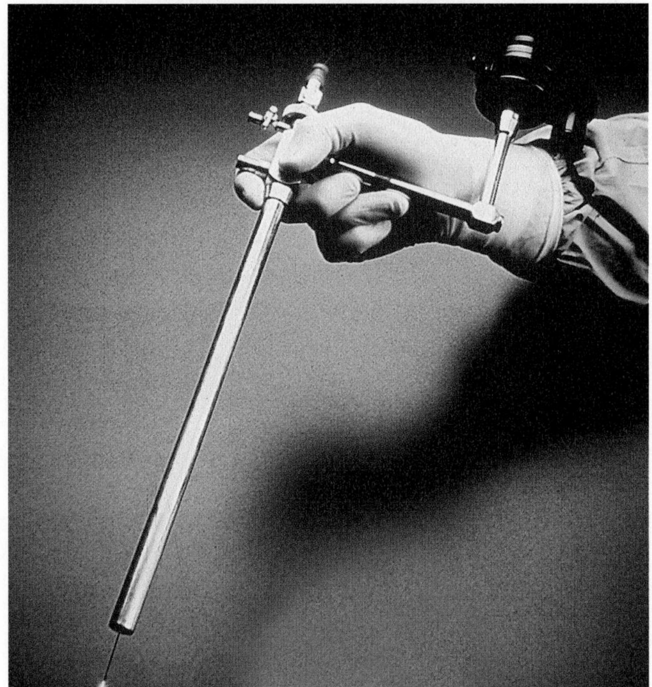

FIGURE 7-4 Operative laparoscope.

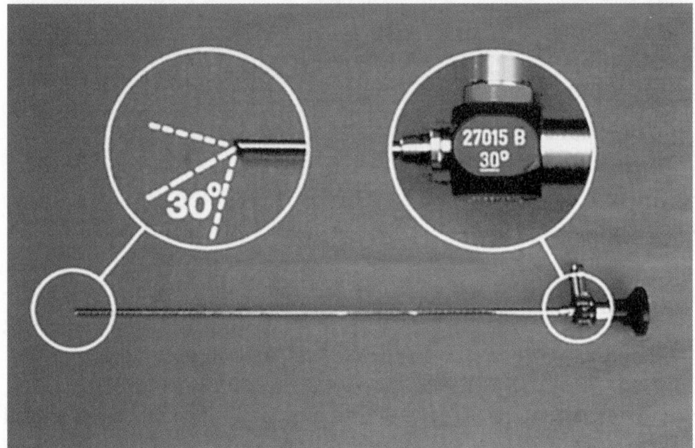


FIGURE 7-5 The lenses inside the endoscope determine the angle of view.

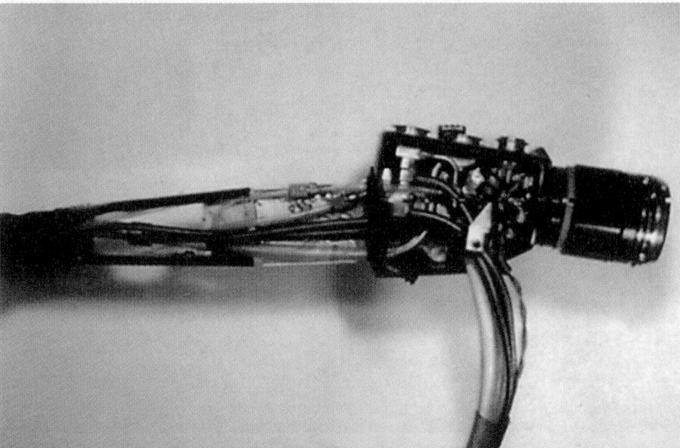

FIGURE 7-6 Dissected flexible endoscope, showing the complexity of the internal structure and design.

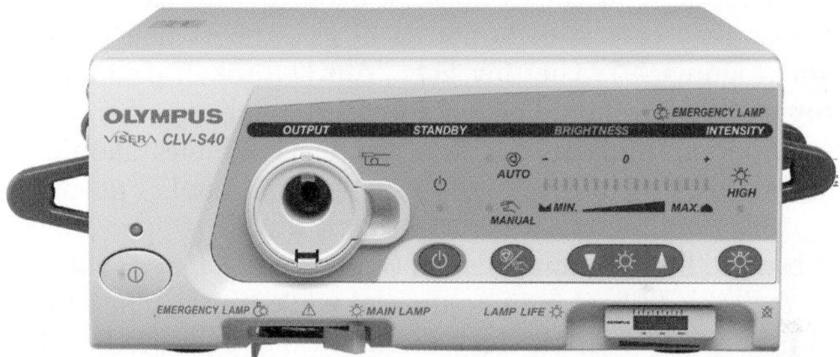


FIGURE 7-7 Light source with universal light cable adapter.

the fiberoptic cables are disconnected from the scope, however, they are very hot. The surgical team must use extreme caution to keep the ends of the cables out of contact with the patient's skin and any flammable materials or liquids. If the fiberoptic cable is disconnected from the endoscope during surgery, the scrub person must ensure that the cable end is held away from drapes or placed on a moist towel to prevent burns and fires. Ideally the light should be turned off whenever disconnected from the endoscope. The ECRI (formerly the Emergency Care Research Institute) recommends labeling all fiberoptic light sources to prevent fires from the hot light source energy. According to the ECRI, high-intensity fiberoptic light sources and cables can ignite drapes and other materials. All cable connections must be completed before activating the light source to prevent a fire. The light source must be placed in standby when the cables are disconnected.

Light sources should have adjustable manual and automatic brightness modes. The automatic mode adjusts brightness according to the video image. If the light source is set in this mode, the circulating nurse does not need to make adjustments constantly.

When selecting a light source, certain options should be considered. A light source that can adapt to several rigid endoscopic systems is desirable, such as one with a universal light cable adapter, which enhances flexibility and usage (Figure 7-7). If a previously purchased unit does not provide this feature, universal light cables with connectors to an interchangeable light source and endoscope adapters are available (Figure 7-8). A generic cord can be used with most scopes and light sources. Light sources also must have connection capability with different camera units.

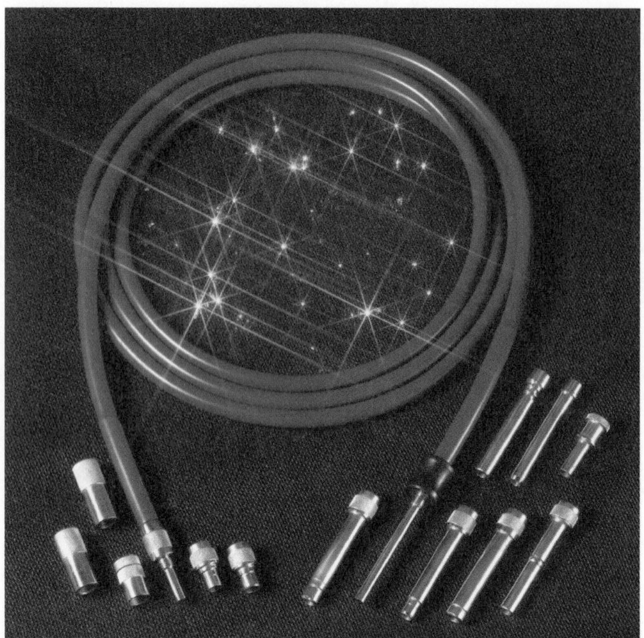
**FIGURE 7-8** Universal light cable with interchangeable light source connectors and endoscope adapters.

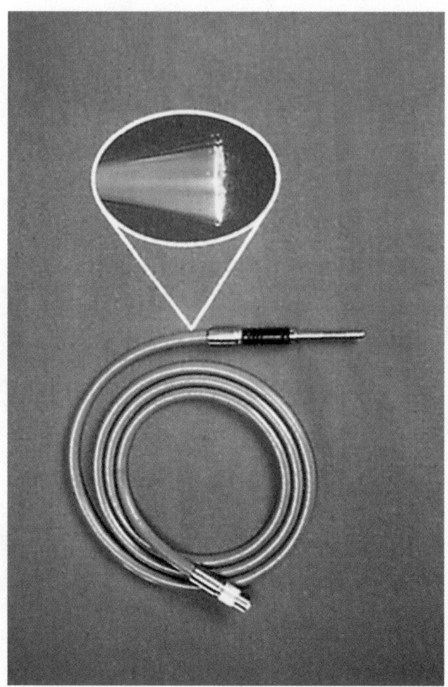
**FIGURE 7-9** Inside the light cable are hundreds of glass fibers that transmit light.

Fiberoptic light cables must be handled with extreme care because they consist of hundreds of glass fibers that transmit light (Figure 7-9). The tiny fibers can be broken if kinked or dropped. Cables should be loosely coiled, not bent, when not in use. After multiple uses, fibers can break. Cables should be checked after each use. To do this, one should hold one end of the cable pointing toward a bright light while the opposite end is observed for light transmission (Figure 7-10). One should not test the cable by looking into the end while it is attached to the light source. The visible light and ultraviolet light produced by the light source could be harmful to the eye if directly viewed for extended periods. "Peppering" on the light cable end indicates broken fibers. When approximately 20% of the fibers are broken, the cable should be replaced because adequate light for visualization would not be transmitted through fractured fibers.

Bulbs within the light source usually are easy to replace. Most bulbs are located in lamp-assembly drawers, which are readily accessible. The bulb itself should not be touched because (1) it may be very hot, and (2) the oils on an individual's hands and fingers can adhere to the bulb, causing the bulb to burn out more quickly. Nonmetal handles usually are built into the light source for bulb removal and replacement.

Three popular types of light sources are available today: xenon, metal halide, and halogen. Advantages and disadvantages are associated with each. Xenon bulbs are more expensive but can last longer. A xenon light is better for smaller diameter endoscopes (≤2 mm) because the light can focus down to a smaller spot size. Xenon light also is a preferred light for video or picture taking. Metal halide bulbs have a shorter life span (about 250 hours) and are less expensive. These bulbs are easier than the others to handle and replace and do not require large fans for cooling. Halogen light sources are used for office and some hospital applications. They do not offer the light intensity required for many endoscopic and video applications, however. Personal preference and conditions for use are the parameters to consider when choosing an appropriate light source for endoscopy. A light source that incorporates a lamp-life status–testing mode is desirable so that bulb replacement can be anticipated.

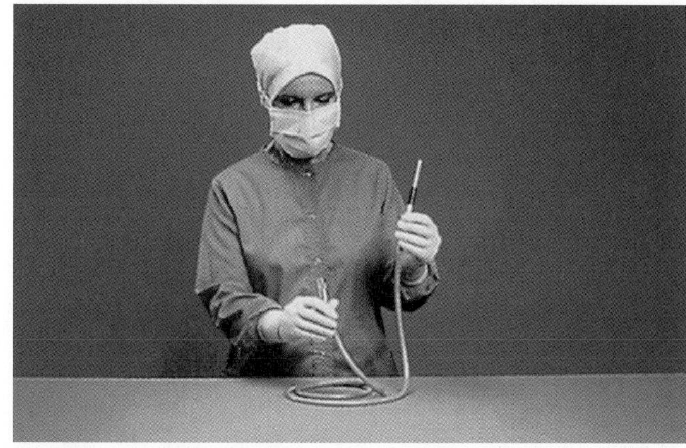
**FIGURE 7-10** The light cable can be checked for broken fibers by holding one end toward a bright light while looking at the other end.

Because light sources produce different colors of light, whenever a camera is used, *white balancing* must be performed during each procedure. White balancing is merely adjusting the camera to all other optical components (endocoupler, light cable, laparoscope). This is a method for the camera to reference white so that it can identify all primary colors properly. White balancing should be performed only when the scope and light cable are connected, the light source is turned on, and the lens is held close to a white gauze or drape (for white color referencing).

## Endoscopic Instrumentation

Endoscopic instrumentation has been designed to correspond with the surgical site and technique. The length and working end of the instrument must be adequate to perform surgery at the target site. The hand control is designed for the comfort of the operator. Graspers and other instrumentation used by the assistant in surgery often are built for a shorter hand span because many women function in this role.

Because endoscopic surgical approaches differ from the traditional open surgical equivalents, modifications of existing instruments have been made as endoscopic procedures have evolved. Some basic patterns have been used for years and continue to be popular, whereas others have been designed to accommodate the new endoscopic approaches. The full effect of this new era in surgery was realized in the 1990s and instrument designs are in their fifth and sixth generations. As surgery becomes more sophisticated, so do the instruments required for successful, less invasive techniques (Figure 7-11).

***Trocars and Cannulas.*** When a natural orifice does not exist for diagnostic or operative procedures, one or several orifices can be created. To do so, a trocar and cannula are necessary. They provide a mechanism for inserting and removing instrumentation while endoscopic surgery is performed. The cannula, or sheath, is inserted to access the operative site by use of a trocar as an obturator. When the port of entry has been made, the trocar is removed, and the cannula is left in place.

If reusable trocars and cannulas are used, the trocar tip must be sharpened routinely. The stopcock and trumpet valves must be inspected before and after each use to ensure proper functioning. Internal gaskets may need occasional replacement. The trocar and cannula must fit properly and may not always be interchangeable. Component parts must be kept together, but they must be disassembled completely for cleaning and sterilization.

Disposable trocar and cannula units offer several advantages (Figure 7-12). A popular feature is that the trocar is always sharp. When multiple ports of the same size are used, the same trocar can be reused on the same patient. Some manufacturers package one trocar and two or more sheaths of the same size. The same trocar is used to establish multiple access ports. Disposable units also may provide siliconized trocar tips and safety features when entry has been made. Systems are available that (1) engage a safety shield to advance automatically over the trocar tip when entry is made (Figure 7-13) or (2) provide retractility of the trocar tip when entry is made.

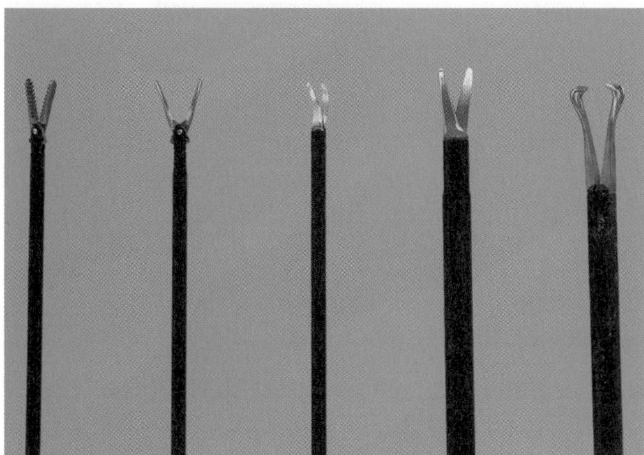

**FIGURE 7-11** Disposable endoscopic instruments are designed to meet procedural needs during endoscopic surgery.

Many disposable cannulas have gripping devices that can reduce the risk of accidental cannula removal during repeated advancement and withdrawal of the endoscopic instrumentation. Grippers are incorporated into the cannula or as separate entities. Grippers can be used with reusable cannulas as long as the fit is appropriate.

Disposable cannulas have a stopcock assembly for the insufflation gas, similar to the reusable system. One-way flapper valves in disposables provide leak-proof protection and operate automatically for instrument insertion, specimen removal, or rapid desufflation. Because the diameters of instrumentation vary with design and use, various sizes of trocar and cannula units may be required for one procedure. Reusable and disposable systems come in a variety of diameters and lengths. To increase flexibility, converters and reducers are used to adapt the size of the instrument. Converters can be separate or built into the cannula as a diaphragm seal. Both systems are designed to reduce the chance of $CO_2$ leaks so that the pneumoperitoneum can be maintained.

Radiolucent disposable cannulas offer the ability to visualize tissue and lesions without obstruction. This feature may be crucial during an endoscopic cholangiogram to avoid obstructing the view during fluoroscopy. During other procedures, this design may not be necessary.

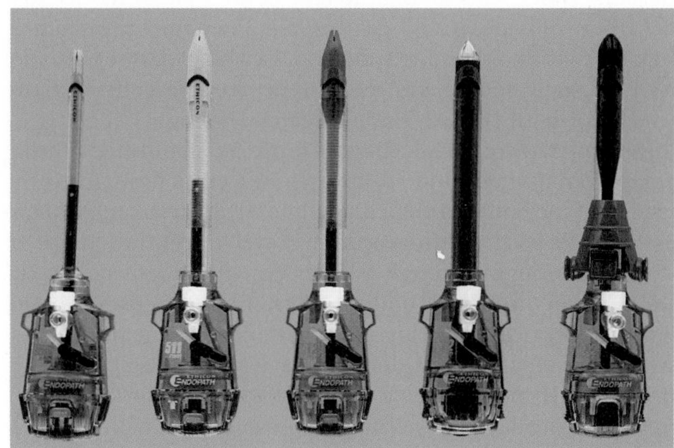

**FIGURE 7-12** Disposable trocars and cannulas.

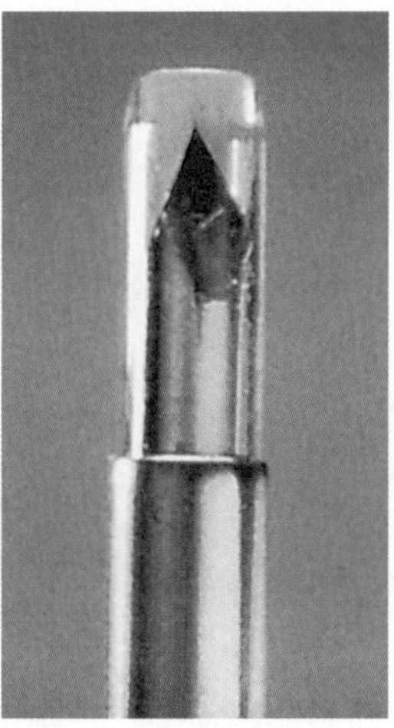

**FIGURE 7-13** A close-up view of the trocar safety shield in place.

Radially expanding dilator systems, consisting of a cannula with a blunt obturator and an insufflation/access needle with a radially expandable sleeve, have been shown to cause less traumatic abdominal wall entry. Intraabdominal entry is accomplished using an access needle with a radially expandable sleeve. When insufflation is achieved, the needle is withdrawn, leaving the expandable sleeve in place. While the sleeve and tissue are expanded, a tapered, blunt-tipped dilator is inserted, providing a large working channel for an access port. Because a sharp-tipped trocar is not used, the muscles are spread and not cut, and the risk of abdominal wall or vascular damage is minimized. Bladeless trocars, which separate tissue in a sequential fashion rather than cut or stretch tissue, also are available in an optical version that allows the surgeon to visualize all tissue layers being separated.

Occasionally a procedure is scheduled as an open laparoscopy. Patients who have had multiple surgeries, patients who have developed adhesions, and pediatric patients can present an added risk. When a surgeon is unsure of underlying structures, the laparoscopy may be done in an open fashion. A small paraumbilical incision is made, and tissues are dissected. The peritoneum is opened, and a large, blunt-tipped trocar-sheath assembly is inserted (Figure 7-14). The sheath is designed to fit snugly against the peritoneum from underneath and against the skin from above. Stay sutures are used to close any excess incision. Wafer seals (similar to colostomy wafers) reduce loss of carbon dioxide ($CO_2$) gas further. Pneumoperitoneum is then created. If a reusable system is used, stay sutures also are used to stabilize the system. S-type retractors usually are needed for both (Figure 7-15; Research Highlight).

When extracorporeal surgery must be performed during laparoscopy (when tissue to be operated on is brought to the outside of the body through a small hole), an even larger diameter port is used. During certain bowel resections, loops of bowel are brought through a larger port to be resected or sutured. When the chest is entered, shorter blunt trocars are used with grippers that provide stabilization while in the pleural cavity. This type of trocar does not have insufflation ports (Figure 7-16). If insufflation is required to assist the anesthesia provider in collapsing the lung, regular trocars with insufflation ports are used.

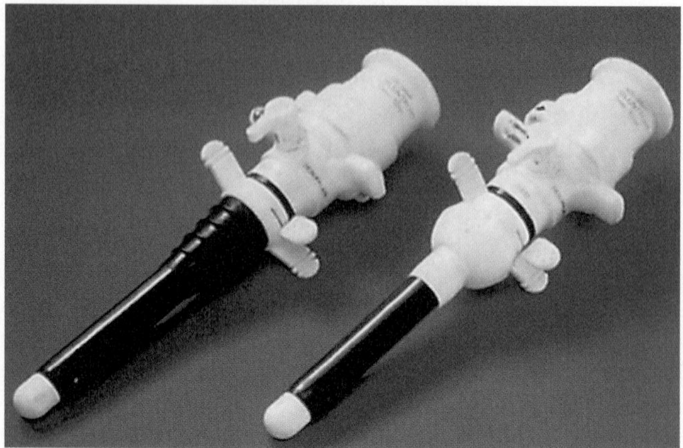

FIGURE 7-14 Blunt-tipped trocars can be used to minimize injuries during insertion.

***Dissecting Instruments.*** Dissecting instruments for endoscopy are used to cut, divide, or separate tissue. Scissors and dissectors that are similar to their open-procedure counterparts have been designed for endoscopic use.

Endoscopic scissors are available for blunt or sharp dissection. They can be straight or curved (including hook scissors),

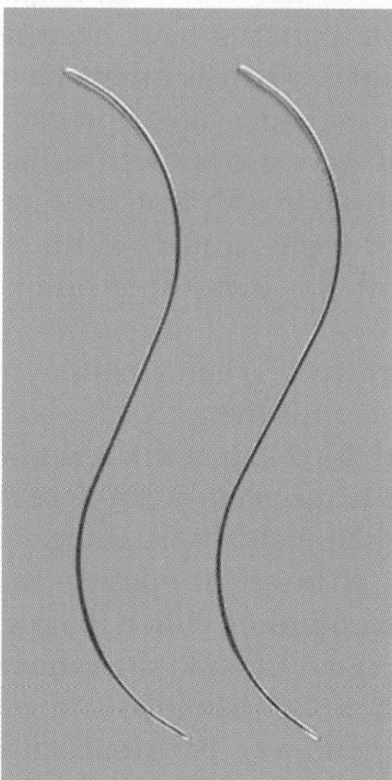

FIGURE 7-15 S-type retractors.

## RESEARCH HIGHLIGHT

### Laparoscopic Access in Children

This study was performed to describe a variation of the Hasson technique for laparoscopic access in children. A small semicircumferential incision was made in the inferior part of the umbilicus of the pediatric patients. The peritoneum was opened under direct visualization without an incision using a blunt trocar that was easily introduced into the peritoneal cavity without any forceful manipulation. This retrospective study noted that this technique offers easy and safe access to the peritoneal cavity with good cosmetic results, even in obese pediatric patients.

Modified from Franc-Guimond J and others: Experience with the Bailez technique for laparoscopic access in children, *Journal of Urology* 171 (2 Pt 1):806, 2004.

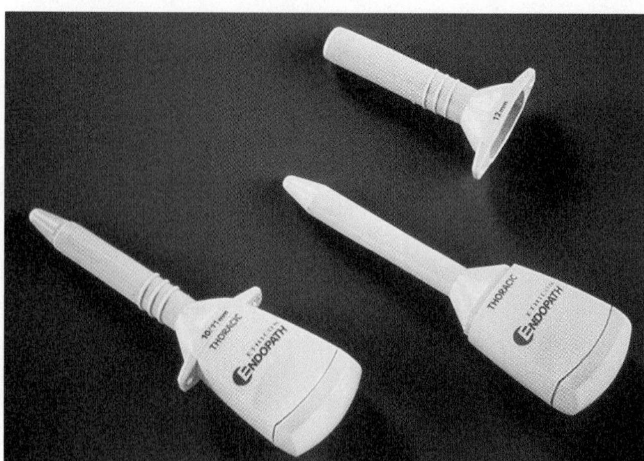


FIGURE 7-16 Thoracic blunt trocar and gripper assembly. Notice absence of stopcock insufflation capability.

depending on the location of the target tissue and technique used (Figure 7-17). Scissors usually have a rounded tip when closed so that they also can be used to manipulate tissue without trauma. When open, both jaws of the scissors should be visualized to prevent inadvertent injury. Some scissors are designed to be connected to an electrosurgical energy source so that coagulation can be provided during cutting.

Dissectors are used to separate or divide tissue. Many different tip shapes are available for dissecting, spreading, dividing, grasping, retracting, and coagulating structures (Figure 7-18). Other dissecting instruments, such as balloon dissectors, have been developed for blunt dissection or creation of a space so that surgery can be performed. A balloon dissector may be used to create a preperitoneal space during laparoscopic herniorrhaphy (Figure 7-19).

***Clamping Instruments.*** Endoscopic clamping instruments are used to grasp and hold tissue or other materials. Ratchets are used in the instrument design to allow the distal tip to be locked onto the tissue or whatever is being grasped. Graspers, forceps, and biopsy forceps are classified as clamping instruments.

Graspers and forceps can be (1) traumatic, with sharp teeth, or (2) atraumatic, with a smooth, serrated jaw surface (Figure 7-20). Traumatic graspers and forceps customarily are used to hold tissue that will be excised, whereas the atraumatic versions are used to hold structures such as the bowel or liver gently. Some clamping instruments are insulated so that electrosurgical energy can be transmitted to provide coagulation.

***Suturing and Stapling Instruments.*** Suturing or stapling instruments are used to deliver sutures, staples, or clips to join, hold, and secure tissue. Needle holders, clip appliers, and staplers all are in this category.

Needle holders have been designed to deliver and place sutures within body cavities during endoscopic procedures. Tungsten carbide jaw inserts on the needle holders are often used to prevent rotation of the suture needle. These inserts often can be replaced when they become worn. Some needle holders have been designed to transfer the needle from one jaw to the other during suturing (Figure 7-21). Suture passers and curved needle holders also are available.

A clip applier is used to provide hemostasis and tissue security. Using a clip applier represents the safest, easiest, and quickest way to occlude small vessels and structures. Reusable appliers exist, but many must be removed from the cannula each time to be reloaded. This process adds time, contributes to loss of pneumoperitoneum (if used), and causes frustration when the clip is dislodged on reinsertion. For this reason, the automatic-feed, reloadable, disposable version is the most popular today (Figure 7-22).

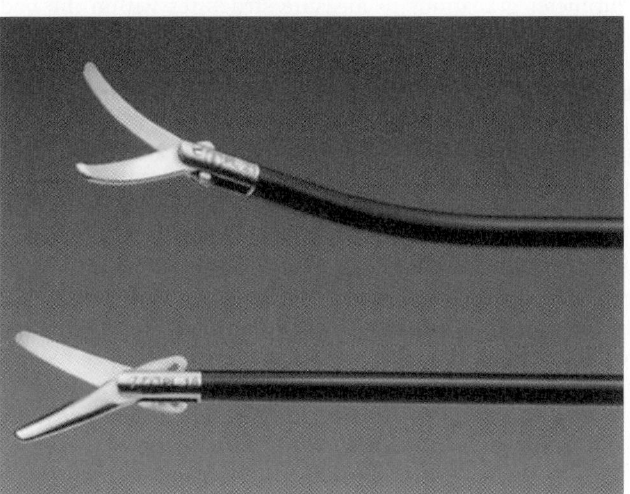

**FIGURE 7-17** Straight and curved endoscopic scissors.

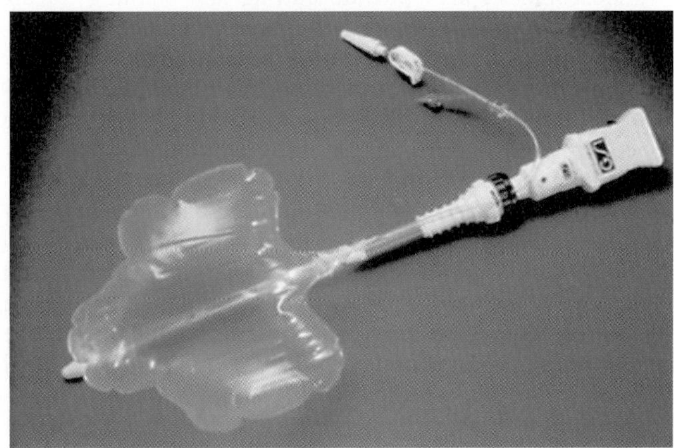

**FIGURE 7-19** Balloon dissecting instrument.

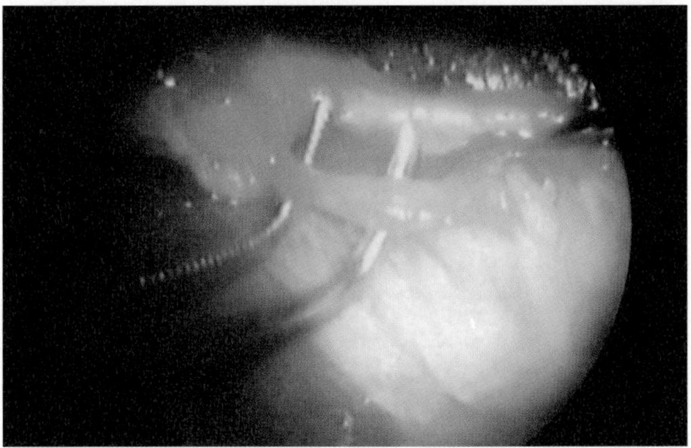

**FIGURE 7-18** Dissector with jaws open to divide and separate tissue.

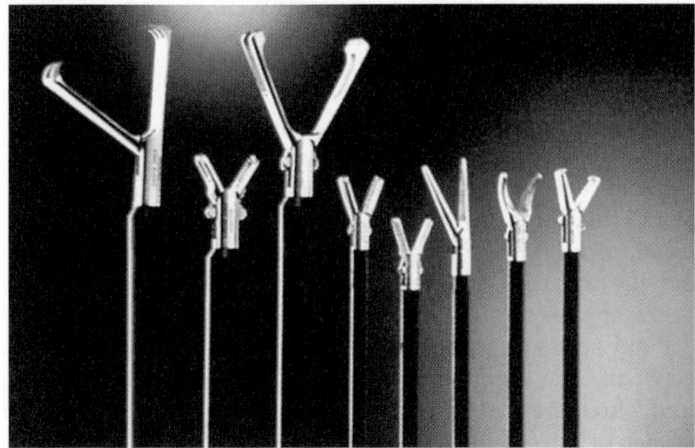

**FIGURE 7-20** Endoscopic grasping instruments.

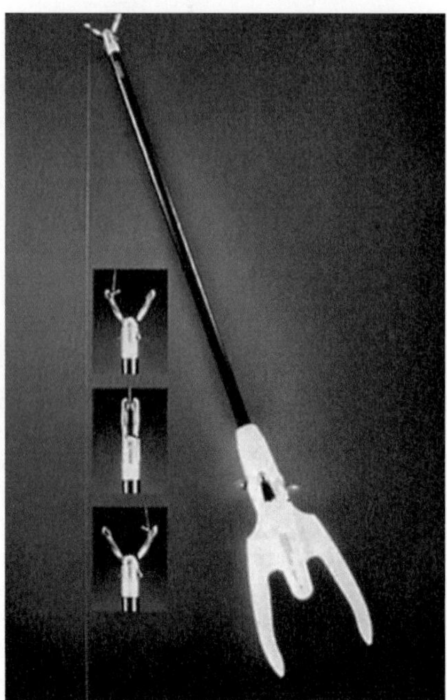

**FIGURE 7-21** Endoscopic needle holder that transfers the needle from one prong of the jaw to the other.

Endoscopic staplers provide cutting and stapling during endoscopic resections (Figures 7-23 and 7-24). Certain structures can be easily resected intracorporeally (e.g., the ovary and appendix). Others may necessitate extracorporeal resection or reanastomosis; if this is necessary, traditional stapling devices are used.

The evolution of more complex endoscopic surgical techniques has challenged traditional suturing and ligation methods; therefore several devices and techniques have been developed for laparoscopic tissue suturing. When surgical clips and staples cannot be used, a laparoscopic suture may have to be substituted. Conditions that preclude the use of clips include large arteries and edematous or inflamed ducts. Most general surgeons prefer to use nonabsorbable sutures and ligation materials to prevent rapid absorption. The three basic types of laparoscopic suturing materials are *loop ligatures, extracorporeal sutures,* and *intracorporeal sutures.*

LOOP LIGATURES. Preknotted suture loops (loop ligatures) are used to ligate pedicle tissues. The suture loop is packaged with an introducer sleeve, which can be inserted through one of the trocars. The loop is passed over the targeted tissue or pedicle by means of a grasping forceps to assist. When the loop is in position, the existing suture knot is pushed down the introducer sleeve until it is cinched tightly around the tissue. The suture is cut with endoscopic scissors (Figure 7-25).

EXTRACORPOREAL SUTURES. Tissue can be approximated intraabdominally when the knot is tied extracorporeally (outside the body). To accomplish this, endoscopic swaged sutures are used. The suture is grasped proximally to the needle, and both are inserted through one of the trocars into the abdomen. The needle is held with the grasper or laparoscopic needle holder and driven through the desired tissue. A second grasper or needle holder inserted through a second trocar is used to assist. The needled end of the suture is pulled through the tissue and out through the trocar. The needle is removed, and a knot is tied extracorporeally. The knot is advanced down the trocar and onto the tissue. The suture is cut by use of laparoscopic scissors (Figure 7-26). The three types of knots tied extracorporeally are the *slip knot,* the *fisherman's knot,* and the *surgeon's knot.* The surgeon determines which knot is used.

INTRACORPOREAL SUTURES. Suture ligature also can be passed through the trocar to be tied while it is inside the body. The tissue is approximated in the same fashion but tied intracorporeally (inside the abdomen) using grasping forceps or laparoscopic needle holders. Some surgeons prefer this simplified technique.

***Retractors and Accessory Instruments.*** Retractors are used to hold tissue and expose the operative target site (Figure 7-27). Retractors can be traumatic to some structures, such as the bowel and liver, so they must be used with caution. Miniretractors and balloon retractors have been designed for use on delicate structures. A miniature version of a surgical clamp with blades that splay the incision open beneath the tissue has been approved by the U.S. Food and Drug Administration (FDA).[14] Other accessory instruments have been designed to enhance the use of basic endoscopic instruments and to facilitate the surgical procedure. Probes that are used to manipulate tissue should be blunt to minimize tissue trauma. Some probes have centimeter gradations to measure structures within the body. Irrigation-aspirator probes are used to enhance visualization of the internal structures, and electrosurgical probes provide hemostasis. Endoscopic specimen bags are available to contain specimens to minimize cross-contamination. Special accessory instruments are being designed continually to enhance endoscopic procedures.

***Care and Handling of Endoscopes and Instrumentation.*** Endoscopes and instruments must be clean and free from all bioburden (contaminating organisms) before sterilization or high-level disinfection. During routine use, bioburden accumulates in channels, ports, crevices, and other movable parts of scopes and instruments. Periodically throughout the procedure, gross blood and bioburden should be removed by flushing the channels and wiping the surfaces with sterile water. Saline should never be used routinely to remove gross debris during the procedure because this salt solution can leave mineral deposits on or in the device. Keeping instruments and endoscopes relatively clean during the procedure helps to prevent debris from drying, thus facilitating the cleaning process.

After each procedure, all instrumentation and devices must be decontaminated thoroughly. Immersible equipment should be cleaned or flushed with an enzymatic or other appropriate detergent solution; this loosens organic material and makes it easier to remove. Instruments that can withstand cavitation

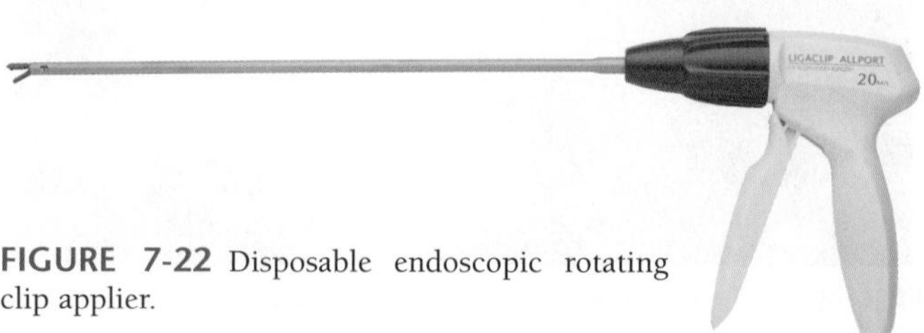

**FIGURE 7-22** Disposable endoscopic rotating clip applier.

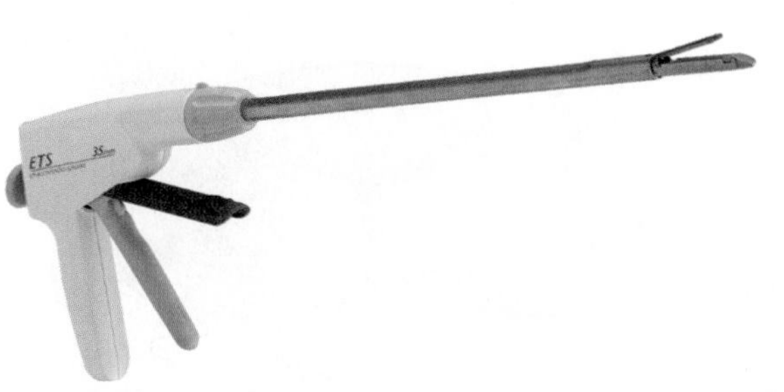


FIGURE 7-23 Disposable linear cutter with reloading unit.

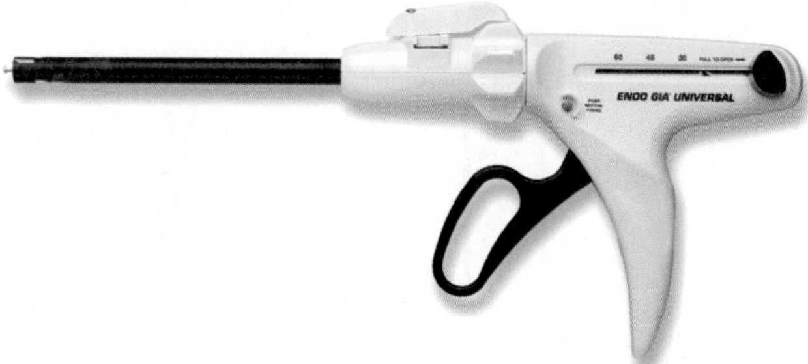


FIGURE 7-24 Disposable endoscopic stapling device.

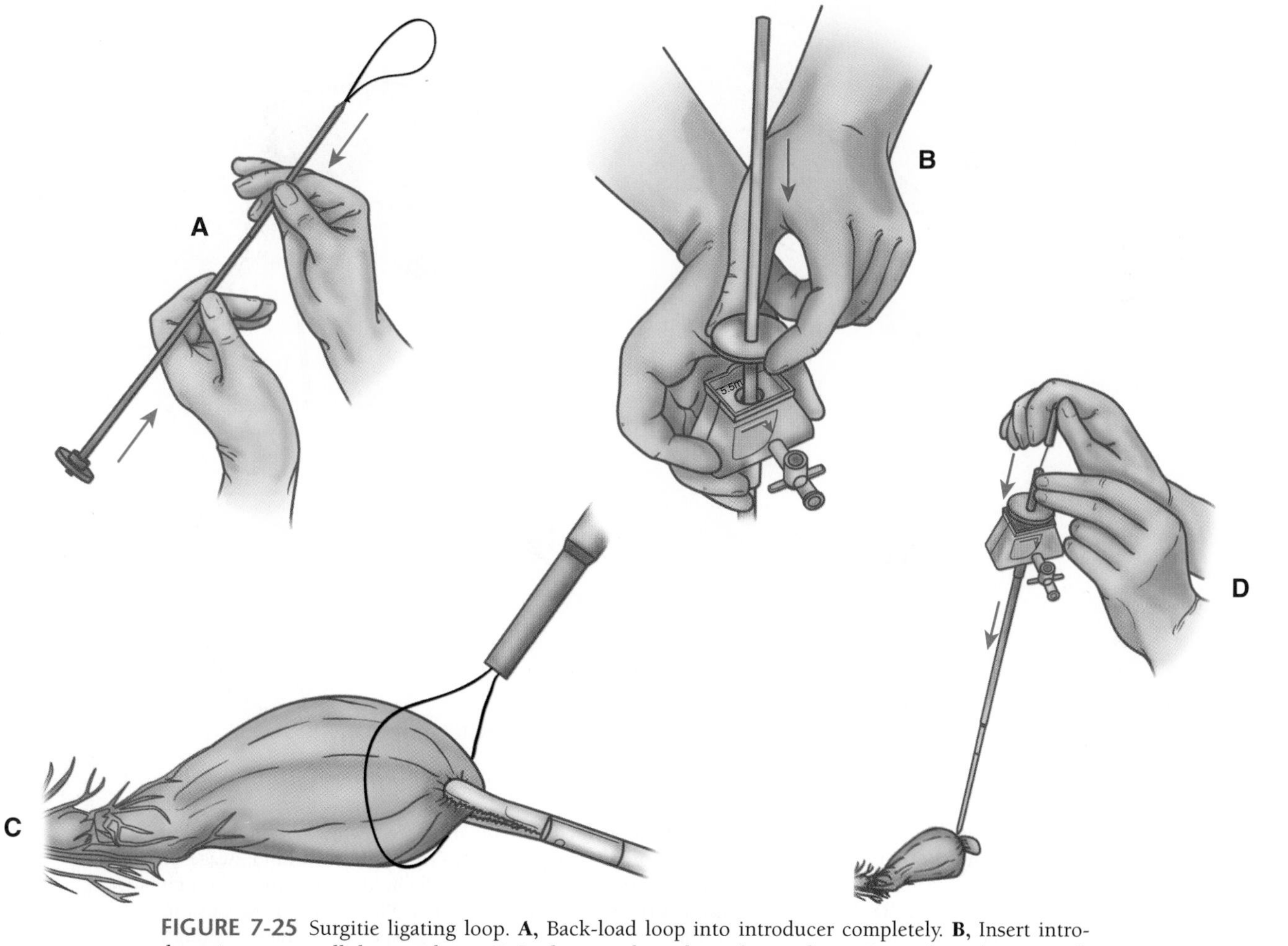

FIGURE 7-25 Surgitie ligating loop. **A,** Back-load loop into introducer completely. **B,** Insert introducer into trocar, all the way down. **C,** Push suture loop through introducer. Grasp desired tissue with grasping forceps (passed through another trocar), and maneuver loop over tissue. **D,** Push down knot by advancing nylon carrier all the way until knot is cinched. Cut suture.

(process whereby high-frequency energy causes microscopic bubbles) or ultrasonic cleaning can be placed in an ultrasonic device. Fiberoptics and endoscopes usually cannot be placed in an ultrasonic machine because the ultrasonic vibration can damage the tiny fiberoptic bundles.

Careful rinsing and flushing with copious amounts of water must follow the cleaning process. Often deionized or demineralized water is recommended for the final rinse to minimize any mineral buildup from tap water. The manufacturer's written recommendations for cleaning and processing always should be followed. Instruments must be dried before disinfection or sterilization.

Automatic cleaning devices that flush the ports of instruments provide an economic, practical, and effective way initially to clean reusable channeled instruments (Figure 7-28). Although instruments have flush ports, debris can become lodged distally. Some automatic systems provide a means to flush in a retrograde fashion, forcing debris out the larger

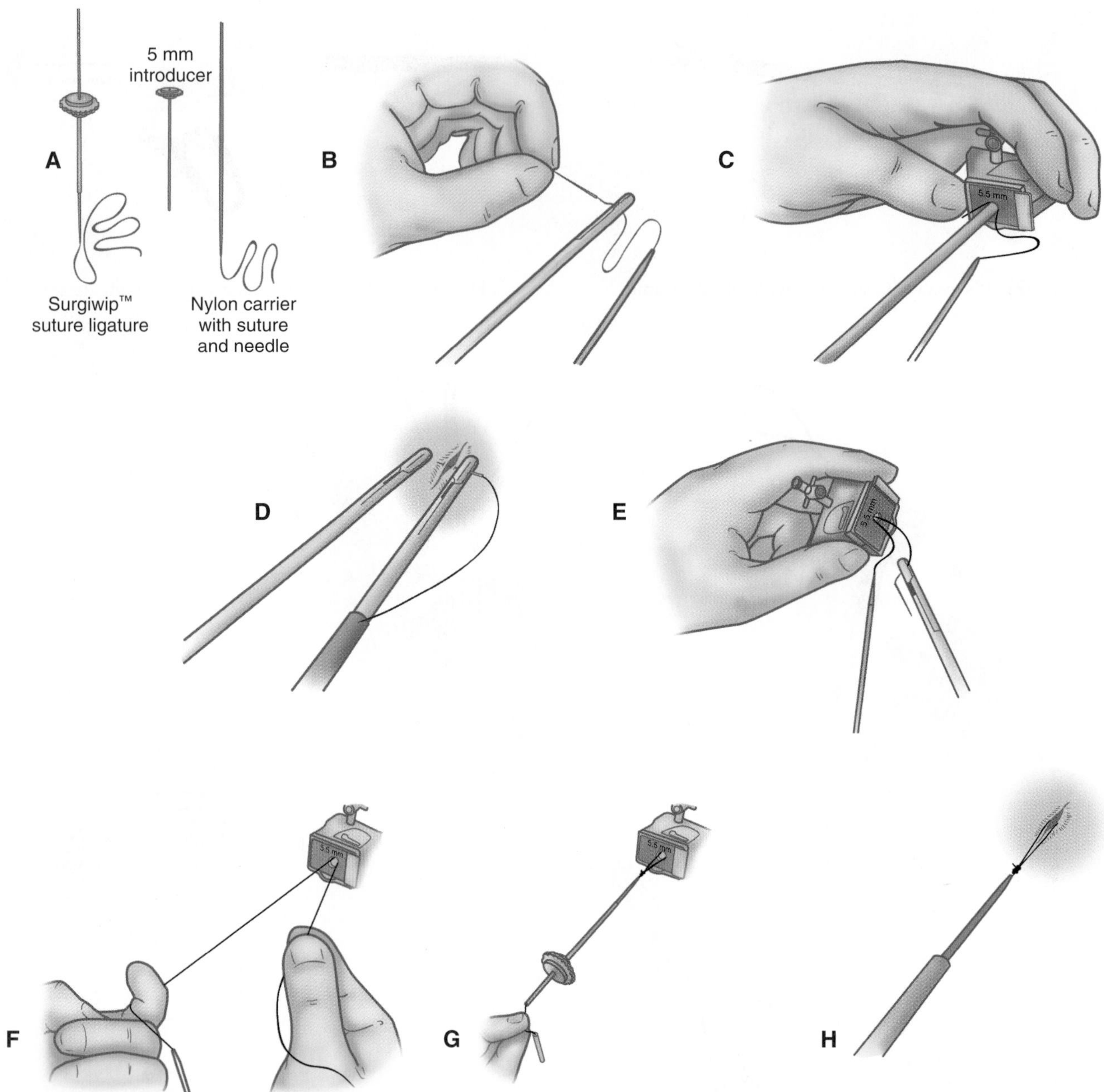


**FIGURE 7-26** Surgiwip suture ligature application for approximating tissue intraabdominally by extracorporeal knot-tying (outside body). **A,** Component pieces. **B,** Grasp suture behind swage of needle with tissue grasper or needle holder. **C,** Introduce grasper or needle holder and suture through trocar into abdomen. **D,** Drive needle through tissue to be approximated. Place instrument close to center of needle for control. Pull needle through tissue using second grasper (introduced through another trocar). **E,** Regrasp needle behind swage intracorporeally, and pull it through and out the same trocar. (Allow for slack of suture to avoid tissue tears.) **F,** Remove needle. Tie knot. **G,** After knot is tied, break end of nylon carrier. **H,** Push knot down with nylon carrier and out onto tissue. Cut suture. For additional suturing, repeat **B** through **H** until tissue is satisfactorily approximated.

proximal port. Sealed instruments also can be tested for seal integrity using this type of system.

After the device has been thoroughly cleaned, the integrity and functionality of the instrument must be assessed. Personnel involved with reprocessing endoscopic devices must be aware of the instrument composition, design, and use. Any laparoscopic device with electrosurgery capabilities must be checked to ensure the length of insulation has not been compromised. Equipment is now available to scan these instruments to note electrical leakage through any breaks in the insulation.

Often new endoscopic accessories are purchased and put into use without educating the staff responsible for their reprocessing. A staff member cannot understand the design and use of a device without proper instructions. The FDA requires that any device purchased as reusable must have written instruc-

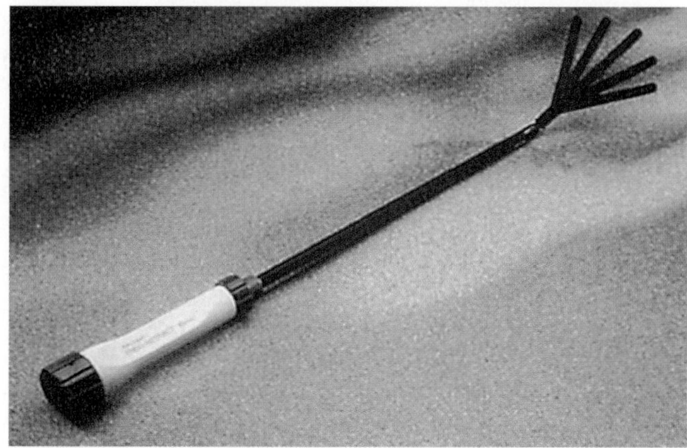

FIGURE 7-27 Endoscopic fan retractor with five fingers.

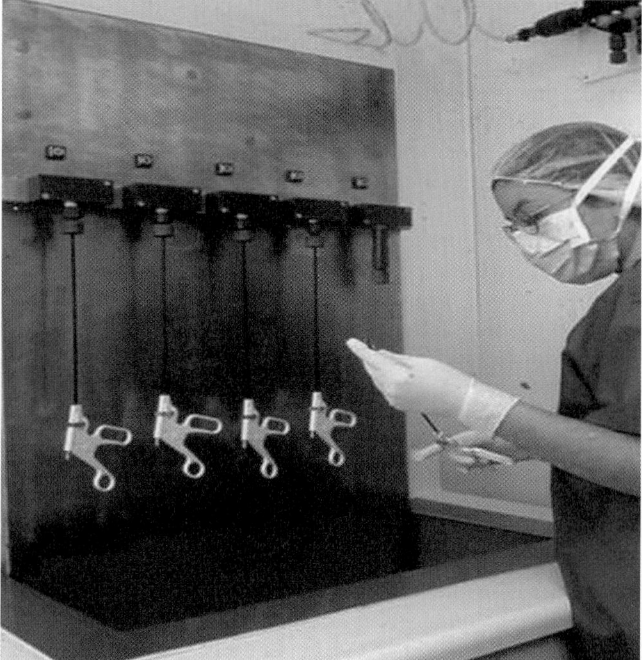

FIGURE 7-28 Commercial endoscopic instrument cleaner used by a reprocessing company.

tions for reprocessing. The staff must understand how the instrument works to ensure that the functionality of the device has not changed during reprocessing. Compliance with federal, professional, and regional standards cannot be ignored for reprocessing.

Instruments and devices coming into contact with sterile tissues and the vascular system should be sterile. Instruments coming into contact with intact mucous membranes can be processed using high-level disinfection. This means that sterility is required for all laparoscopy, angioscopy, thoracoscopy, and arthroscopy procedures. High-level (cold-soak) disinfection may be acceptable for colonoscopy, laryngoscopy, bronchoscopy, cystoscopy, and other diagnostic procedures. Because more invasive procedures that access the vascular system (biopsies) are performed during many endoscopy procedures, however, the adequacy of high-level disinfection must be evaluated. Viruses and microorganisms, such as human immunodeficiency virus (HIV), hepatitis B and C viruses, Mycobacterium (tuberculosis bacteria), and antibiotic-resistant organisms, are not easily destroyed during high-level disinfection. Even though high-level disinfection has been the accepted primary standard for some endoscopic instrumentation, the concern over viruses and microorganisms has caused debate about the adequacy of merely disinfecting devices.

Thermal pasteurization, using a washer/pasteurizer, may be selected for thermal high-level disinfection. An FDA-approved chemical germicide should be selected for chemical high-level disinfection. Glutaraldehyde, used for many years, has hazards that must be considered when it is the agent selected for high-level disinfection. The maximum recommended exposure level of glutaraldehyde determined by the Occupational Safety and Health Administration (OSHA) is 0.2 ppm. When solution is being poured after mixing or when devices are being submerged, the level rises to approximately 0.4 ppm, which is double the exposure level. The odor of glutaraldehyde becomes an irritant at 0.3 ppm, causing tearing, nausea, and other effects. Hooded systems to house the glutaraldehyde solutions have been designed to absorb the odor and fumes that are emitted. When using this or any other chemical germicide, the item must be totally immersed and soaked for the specified time (contact time), following the manufacturer's recommendations for cleaning protocols, preparing the solution, maintaining contact time, and calculating expiration dates.

Institutional policy sets the guidelines from which practitioners work. Insight and coordination are required to provide comparable levels of care when there are too few instruments for the number of scheduled procedures. If sterile instruments are required for a particular endoscopic procedure, sterile instruments should be used for all patients undergoing that procedure. Enough instrumentation and equipment must be purchased to accommodate the endoscopic patient volume, or other reprocessing measures must be implemented.

When sterile devices and instrumentation are needed, multiple options provide sterilization today, including steam, ethylene oxide, peracetic acid, gas-plasma, and ozone sterilization methods.[2] Often steam cannot be used on delicate endoscopes, but the endoscopic accessory instrumentation may be able to withstand the heat produced during this type of sterilization. Some arthroscopes and laparoscopes have been designed that can withstand the high temperatures of steam sterilization. For items that cannot withstand high temperatures, options include the following:

- *Ethylene oxide sterilization*—used for many years to sterilize endoscopes and instruments. Past rulings to eliminate the agents that have been combined with the ethylene oxide, such as chlorofluorocarbon (CFC) and halogenated CFC (HCFC) to decrease flammability, have led to the use of 100% ethylene oxide to provide safe and effective ethylene oxide sterilization. One limitation of ethylene oxide sterilization is the prolonged time needed for aeration of the ethylene oxide.
- *Peracetic acid sterilization*—for instruments and endoscopes that are immersible but are sensitive to heat. This method provides sterility within approximately 30 minutes. Instruments are placed into removable trays where the solution is purged over all surfaces and within all lumens and ports. A four-rinse cycle with sterile water removes all the sterilizing diluent. Devices sterilized in this manner should be used

soon after sterilization because this process does not ensure a sterile shelf life for later use (Figure 7-29).

- *Plasma sterilization system*—creates hydrogen peroxide gas plasma, which sterilizes within 50 to 75 minutes and breaks down into nontoxic by-products. Understanding the advantages and limitations (e.g., lumen restrictions) of this type of system is important when determining if it would meet the needs of endoscope or endoscopic instrument sterilization. Generally, flexible endoscopes cannot be sterilized in the plasma sterilization system.
- *Ozone sterilizer*—involves oxygen that is used in a natural process to produce ozone. When oxygen is exposed to an intense electrical field, the oxygen molecule separates into atomic oxygen (O). This atomic oxygen combines with other oxygen molecules ($O_2$) to create a triatomic oxygen ($O_3$), which is ozone. Ozone reverts quickly back to its oxygen state while producing no toxic residuals. Ozone is a powerful sterilizing agent because it creates an oxidative action on organic matter (fungi, bacterial spores, viruses). Key features of this new type of ozone sterilizer include: easy to use, low temperature sterilization, cost-effective, and compatible with anodized aluminum containers. The manufacturer's instructions must be followed regarding the operation of the ozone sterilizer, instrument and device preparation, and device limitations.

***Single-Use Versus Reusable Instrumentation.*** Many facilities use a combination of reusable and single-use laparoscopic instruments. Advantages of single-use items include sharpness, reliability related to function, guaranteed sterility, and safety. Indirect advantages include no reprocessing time and effort, no associated repair costs, and the provision of comparable levels of patient care. Upgraded designs also are more easily accepted if the device is labeled for single use. Disadvantages may include the need for increased storage space, budgetary implications, and environmental concerns related to disposal and biohazardous waste.

Advantages of reusable instruments include less storage space required, a reduced budgetary effect (except for initial purchase and repair), and minimal waste. With reusable instruments, the decontamination and reprocessing system must be reliable, must be compatible with the devices being processed, and must be monitored for effectiveness. Above all, safe and effective patient outcomes should be the criteria with which all else is compared.

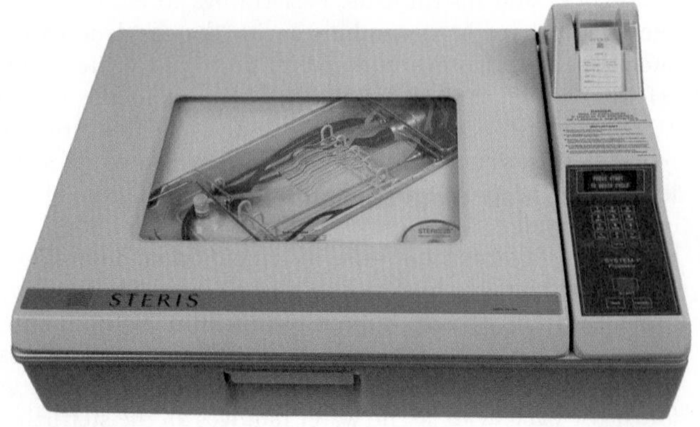


**FIGURE 7-29** STERIS System 1 sterile processing system.

The advantages and disadvantages of reusable versus single-use devices must be explored, using a risk-to-benefit analysis, before purchasing decisions can be made. Institutional policy may dictate whether reusable or single-use items are chosen. The choice between single-use and reusable instrumentation and equipment must be evaluated thoroughly in each individual practice setting and justified accordingly.

***Reprocessing Single-Use Devices.*** Reprocessing single-use devices is a practice that has grown steadily in acceptance during the past decade. The General Accounting Office, in a Congressional Report, stated, "The evidence suggests that some SUDs (single-use devices) can be safely reprocessed if appropriate cleaning, testing, and sterilization procedures are carefully followed."[10]

In the United States, the practice is highly regulated by the FDA, which published a Guidance Document entitled, "Enforcement Priorities for Single-Use Devices Reprocessed by Third Parties and Hospitals." This document outlines the regulatory requirements, which are enforceable by the FDA, for reprocessing previously used single-use medical devices. (The FDA also has related publicly that open/unused devices eventually will fall under similar regulations.)

The FDA defines a reprocessor as a third-party reprocessing company or hospital that reprocesses single-use devices.[13] Hospitals rarely pursue the challenges of becoming listed as a reprocessor owing to the expense involved with this activity. Reprocessing organizations are considered manufacturers and are subject to the same regulatory requirements as the original device manufacturer and must comply with the following[9]:

1. Registration and listing with the FDA—any organization reprocessing single-use devices must be registered with the FDA and provide a comprehensive list of all single-use medical devices that they reprocess.
2. Medical device reporting (MDR)—all organizations reprocessing single-use devices must comply with FDA's manufacturer reporting requirements and report not only all patient injuries from device malfunctions or failures but also any event that potentially could have led to a patient injury or death.
3. Device tracking—the FDA can issue a tracking order for any specific device, if applicable. These devices are typically high-risk, class III medical devices, such as implants. Reprocessing companies usually refrain from reprocessing class III devices.
4. Corrections and removals—all reprocessors must have a formal procedure in place for recalling or correcting affected devices.
5. Quality system regulation (QSR)—all reprocessors must develop and maintain comprehensive quality system controls that comply with the FDA's requirements for all aspects of their reprocessing operation.
6. Labeling requirements—all reprocessors must provide instructions-for-use documents (IFUs) with the reprocessed medical devices and must comply with the specific requirements for what should appear on the device label. Any reprocessed single-use device must be labeled "prominently and conspicuously" with the following statement: "Reprocessed device for single use. Reprocessed by (name of manufacturer that reprocessed the device)."
7. FDA premarket submission of a premarket notification (510[k]) or premarket approval (PMA)—the FDA has de-

veloped a device classification system (class I, II, or III) to determine what level of review is required before the device can be marketed. Class I devices are considered no risk or very low risk and in most cases require no premarket submission. Examples of class I devices are needle counters, most noninvasive devices, and some drill bits and chisels. Class II devices require all reprocessors to submit a 510(k) and include devices such as arthroscopic shavers and burrs, sequential compression sleeves, and laparoscopic dissectors. Class III devices require all reprocessors to submit a PMA. This classification includes devices that could pose the greatest risk to the patient, such as electrophysiology ablation catheters, and requires valid scientific data to include the completion of prospective clinical study data. Submitting the required paperwork for a PMA may cost an organization or company many millions of dollars and take years to complete.

Reprocessors also repackage and resterilize items with an expired shelf life date or when sterility of the outer packaging has been compromised, segregating their single-use devices into two categories for reprocessing: *open/not used* and *open/used* devices. The devices that have been used should be grossly decontaminated before they are sent for reprocessing. If devices are not grossly decontaminated, they must be collected in approved containers and transported by a licensed biohazardous material hauler using appropriate packaging materials and labeling.

Liability is an important concern for reprocessing single-use items. A hospital or surgery center is liable for this practice if reprocessing is performed within the confines of the facility. If a third-party company provides this service, it is likewise liable and should present documentation verifying insurance coverage for this service. Although the original manufacturer of a device warrants a disposable product for one use, a reprocessing company also warrants the reprocessed device for one use.

Questions to ask when determining whether to reprocess single-use items include the following:

- Can the disposable device be adequately cleaned?
- Can the device withstand disinfection or sterilization? Can the item be adequately aerated if ethylene oxide sterilization is used?
- Can the device be tested and checked for proper form and function after cleaning has been completed?
- Has the device integrity been destroyed during reprocessing, or is equipment available to test the integrity of the device? How is the integrity of the insulation checked on an electrosurgical probe?
- Can the device be returned to its original intended use (Figure 7-30)?
- Will cost savings be passed on to the patient, if appropriate?
- Have the maximum number of safe reuses been determined through comprehensive testing?
- Should the patient be informed that a reprocessed device may be used? The FDA does not require informed consent for the use of reprocessed single-use devices. Many providers contend that because reprocessing is so regulated and the risk of using a reprocessed device is the same as using the device for the first time, there is no need to seek an informed consent from the patient.

No matter where reprocessing is performed, appropriate equipment must be available to ensure that the form and function of the device has not been compromised. Customers should inquire about the reprocessing and quality assurance practices if dealing with a third-party reprocessor. Usually these companies have the appropriate equipment to perform comprehensive device and validation testing. They must be registered with the FDA and must comply with the Quality System Regulations (QSR).[9] Reprocessors should provide documentation of FDA registration, any reports of FDA inspection such as an Establishment Inspection Report (EIR), FDA warning letters, or the all-important 510(k) or PMA documentation.

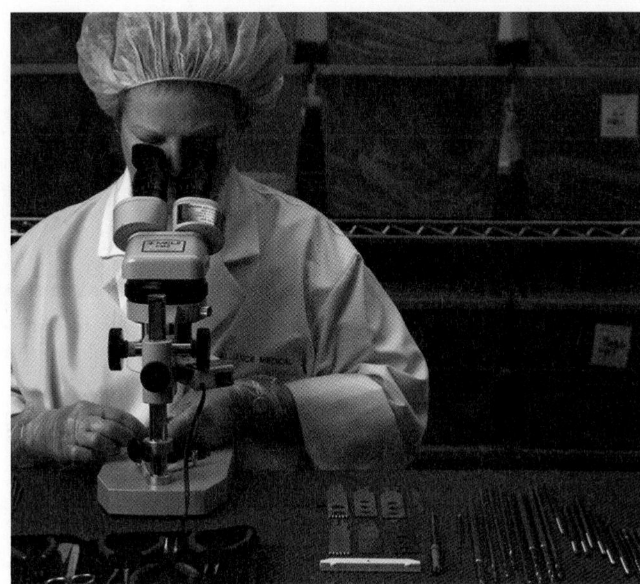

**FIGURE 7-30** Single-use device is carefully sharpened during reprocessing at a third-party company.

The practice of reprocessing single-use devices will continue to grow in popularity as significant cost savings are realized by all sizes of health care facilities. Surgical team members must work closely with their purchasing agent, infection control officer, financial administrator, and others to decide if reprocessing single-use devices is an appropriate option for their facility.

## VIDEO TECHNOLOGY

### Evolution of Video Technology

A basic medical video system includes the scope, light cable, light source, camera head, camera cord, camera-scope coupler, camera control unit, and video monitor. Additional peripheral equipment is necessary for specific surgical procedures and is discussed later. Because video technology can be so complex, a glossary of terms is provided in Box 7-2.

A video system takes light energy from a beginning source and converts it into electrical energy and then back into light energy to provide a picture. The camera head contains a sensor, which is light sensitive. The sensor is a solid-state unit, or chip, called a *charged coupled device (CCD);* it produces the unprocessed video signal. The CCD is composed of small picture elements called *pixels,* which in the presence of light become conductive and in the absence of light remain nonconductive. Each pixel is capable of sensing red, blue, or green light. The picture is transformed into a matrix made up of the conductive and nonconductive pixels. This matrix may scan at a rate of 525 lines per frame, 30 frames per second, generating a signal frequency. The scanning rate is standardized by the National Television Standards Committee (NTSC). The picture is reproduced at its terminal destination.

BOX 7-2

## Video Glossary

**Autoexposure**—An electronic circuit built into cameras to eliminate electronically (within the camera) excess light from the picture; sometimes referred to as *electronic shutter.*
**Automatic gain control**—Ability to increase or decrease the video output level depending on the average light level of the viewed object.
**Blooming**—A glaring effect on the monitor caused by excessive light.
**Boost**—The ability to increase the signal strength of the camera. When used under low light conditions, boost provides increased sensitivity.
**Chroma**—Saturation of a color.
**Chromiance**—Defines the video camera's ability to handle the color red, the most difficult color to reproduce. The more accurate the color reproduction, the higher is the chromiance.
**C-mount**—Standard thread size and diameter for a standard video camera lens.
**Color bars**—A test pattern used to adjust controls on the monitor for color, brightness, and contrast.
**Color reproduction**—Ability of an imaging device to reproduce colors exactly as the human eye perceives them.
**Composite video output**—The most commonly used video signal; the typical television video signal.
**Electronic shutter**—Ability of a camera to freeze image information within fractions of a second ($^1/_{60}$, $^1/_{125}$, $^1/_{1000}$, $^1/_{10,000}$).
**Foot-candle**—Standard measure of luminance; the amount of light emitted by a standard candle at a distance of 1 foot from the flame; 10 luxes equals 1 foot-candle.
**Light gain**—Another circuit within the camera to amplify the picture electronically to show a brighter image; sometimes referred to as *automatic gain control (AGC),* or *boost circuit.*
**Luminance**—Intensity or effectiveness of a given light on the eye.
**NTSC**—National Television Standards Committee; type of television signal used in the United States.
**Orientation**—A mark or ridge on the camera head to orient the top portion of the video monitor.
**Pixel**—A signal-sensor element on a solid-state video chip; most solid-state chips used in medical videography have about 400,000 pixels on their surface. Each pixel is light-sensitive and sees its own small part of the total picture.
**Resolution**—An optical device's ability to separate fine detail; usually expressed in TV lines. Resolution traditionally is measured by aiming the camera at a target chart with squares of fine lines. The maximum resolution of the optical device is determined at the point where it begins to blur the lines together. If a box showing 400 lines per inch is still clear with spaces between the lines, the optical device has at least 400 lines-per-inch resolution.
**Sensitivity**—The response to low light levels by a video system.
**S-VHS output**—A signal from the camera that splits the chroma and luminance, allowing for a richer resolution recording; Super Video Home System (Japan Victor Co.)
**White balance**—Different light sources produce different temperatures of light and different colors of light. White balancing is an adjustment of the camera for various sources of light.

The NTSC is the standard video format in the United States, Canada, Japan, and most of South America and Asia. It was established to be used for broadcast purposes. A format is the way electronic camera signals carry brightness and color information. The three most commonly used formats are the composite, the Y/C, and the RGB. The standard format is termed *composite* because it carries color and brightness on the same signal (Figure 7-31). The advantage is that it is standard. The disadvantage is that when color and brightness information are combined on one signal, cross-talk, or interference between the two, can result in increased video noise (disturbance).

Another commonly available signal transmission method is *Y/C. Y* stands for the brightness signal, and *C* stands for the color signal. Video information is carried on two different signals and is commonly referred to as *Super Video Home System* (S-VHS) (Figure 7-32). This transmission method does not have cross-talk problems and produces sharper pictures with higher resolution on video recorders and hard copy producers. These systems require more expensive monitors and recorders. Another disadvantage is that color and brightness travel at different speeds and, over longer cord distances, may be out of synchronization, requiring extra electronic circuitry.

The third commonly used video format, *RGB,* also a component system, separates video information into red, green, and blue signals and carries each separately (Figure 7-33). Brightness is generated as a percentage of the three colors (30% red, 59% green, 11% blue). An advantage of this format is less noise interference, resulting in sharper pictures with distinct color separation. It is the format of choice for computer interfacing, which has become more popular and accepted. Some RGB components are more expensive compared with the other formats because the three signals must be synchronized.

Several cameras are available with all three formats, which allows for flexibility. Accompanying equipment must be compatible with the camera's format. For the Y/C or RGB camera format to be advantageous, the monitor used also must be capable of handling these formats and the composite signals. System compatibility is crucial. For this reason, the basic composite format is still very desirable.



FIGURE 7-31 Standard composite signal format.



FIGURE 7-32 Component Y/C (S-VHS) signal format.



FIGURE 7-33 Component RGB signal format. Brightness is generated as percentage of three primary colors.

## Visualization Systems

Endoscopes previously offered visualization only to the operating physician. The introduction of the teaching arm provided direct visualization not only for the physician but also for the assistant, perioperative nurse, or other surgical team members. Often images seen through the teaching arm were not identical, however, to the images seen through the primary optics. The inability to interact effectively with the physician and anticipate surgical needs was frustrating and time consuming.

In the late 1960s and early 1970s, medical video and still cameras were being introduced to the marketplace; this allowed for still photography and video documentation of select surgical procedures. The tube style of cameras was large, bulky, and heavy—not adequately meeting the video needs of the surgery. Video technology rapidly changed with the introduction of the chip TV camera. Its lightweight, low-profile design triggered the era of video-guided surgery. Cameras that previously weighed several pounds now weigh only a few ounces (Figure 7-34).

The rapid developments in video imaging also have resulted in higher resolution monitors. Together this integrated system provides increased assurance of maintenance of sterility during direct visualization, enhanced participation by assistants, and promotion of accurate assessment and planning by the perioperative nursing staff. Today video technology has evolved to the point of being almost mandatory during endoscopic procedures. All surgical disciplines have been enhanced by the availability and capability of video systems.

***Camera, Cable, and Control Unit.*** The video camera represents the optical-electronic interface of the video system. A camera cable transfers the signal frequency to a camera control unit (processor), which modifies the signal and then transmits the image to a video monitor, recorder, or hard copy picture, or all three. The camera is the most important component of the video system. Camera options vary according to available technology, specialty, and personal preference.

Cameras have either one or three CCD chips. Three-chip cameras provide enhanced color and image quality but are larger, can cost three times that of a single-chip camera, and are not as light sensitive as the single-chip type. Color and the resulting image are enhanced because each chip is dedicated to one of the primary colors—red, green, or blue. For this reason, three-chip cameras are often used with microscopes when higher magnification requires increased resolution.

Newer single-chip cameras are available with digital processing in their control units, which boosts resolution. In essence, this technology incorporates three-chip quality in a single chip. Although the signal processing in the control unit may be digital, the video output from most cameras is an analog signal.

Digital processing refers to the way information is delivered through the various components of the control unit. This processing format allows for image enhancement and manipulation of the video image. It also allows multiple video signals to be shown on one monitor and has electronic zoom capability. Digital processing also provides the user with freeze-frame capability when using video printers and when using picture-in-picture systems. The disadvantage of complete digital processing of images is the inability to refresh the picture on the monitor in real time. This processing method produces a jumpy, jittery picture. Most cameras convert the digital image back to an analog signal before sending it to the video monitor.

Most cameras also feature the ability to adjust to changes in light intensity while in use. This adjustment is done by an automatic shutter (iris), which measures the availability of light and adjusts accordingly. Automatic shutter activation also helps reduce glare from reflected light off instrumentation and moist viscera. The ability for continuous variable shutter speeds rather than discrete shutter speeds allows for instruments to be brought into the field without glare, while still maintaining adequate illumination of background objects. The shutter's response should be rapid and without perceptible stepping of image intensity.

Camera heads have buttons to control certain functions. Some of these are white balancing, light-sensitivity boosting (ability to provide a brighter picture when the image requires more light, especially when a scope <3 mm is used during sinuscopy), starting and stopping the VCR, and taking hard copy prints. The surgeon controls these functions instead of requesting the circulating nurse to do so each time. The surgeon also has the ability to capture events exactly when they occur (Figure 7-35).

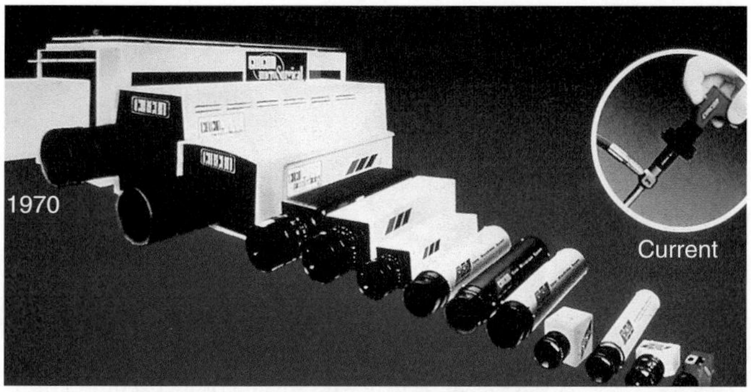

**FIGURE 7-34** Evolution of medical video cameras.

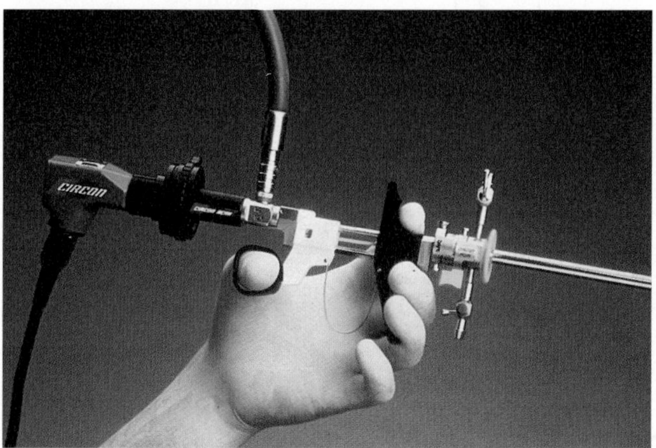

**FIGURE 7-35** Microdigital I RGB color video camera with fingertip control.

Remote-control handheld devices also are available for additional functions. These mimic the familiar household VCR remote control. These devices take time to master. If used routinely, they can become the perioperative nurse's best friend.

All cameras have focusing capability at the camera-coupler interface. Some also have zoom capability, allowing for closer visualization of specific structures or pathologic conditions. A camera cable connects the camera head to the camera control unit (Figure 7-36). Most camera malfunctions are cable-related, not camera-related. For this reason, a system that provides field-replaceable cables is most appealing (Figure 7-37). If wires in the cable break, a new cable can be quickly exchanged, reducing downtime from having to ship the camera and cable for repair. Because wires in the flexible cable can break, the cable must be handled with care. Cables should never be twisted, crimped, or kinked. They also should be long enough to allow sufficient space between the sterile field and the visualization system.

***Couplers (Adapters).*** Endocouplers are optical coupling devices used to connect cameras to various endoscopes. They are usually available in 28-mm and 35-mm focal lengths and with different optical magnifications.

The specific type of coupler required depends on the type of surgery or diagnostic procedure performed and endoscope to be used. When the surgeon is viewing only on a monitor, a direct-link coupler between the telescope and camera head is required (Figure 7-38). For the surgeon to look directly through the endoscope and have monitor-viewing capability, a beam-splitter coupler is necessary (Figure 7-39). Beam splitters often are used with flexible endoscopes. There are rotating beam splitters designed for the surgeon who operates in a sitting position. Zoom couplers provide variable focal lengths, usually from 22.5 to 50 mm.

A videoscope is a design of camera-to-scope connection without the use of a coupler (Figure 7-40). Because a coupler

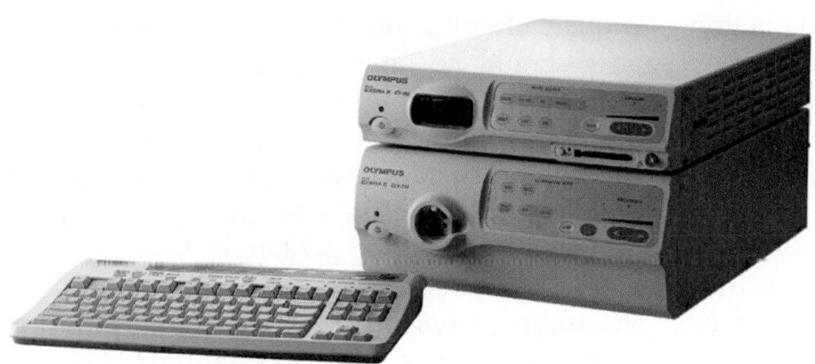


FIGURE 7-36 Camera control unit.

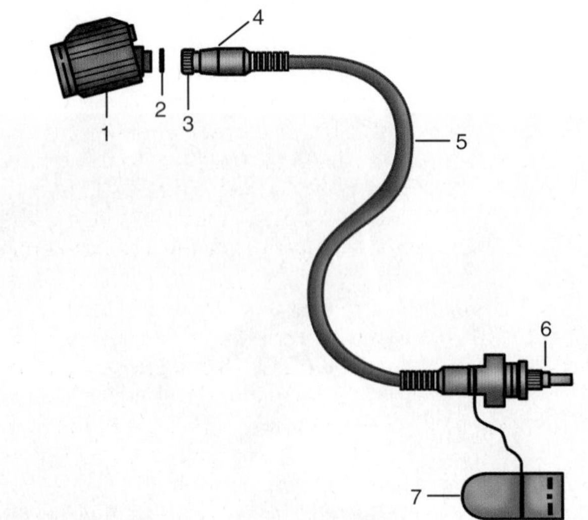


FIGURE 7-37 Camera and field-replaceable cable. *1*, Camera head; *2*, O-ring; *3*, Knurled ring; *4*, Cable connector; *5*, Replaceable cable; *6*, Camera connector; *7*, Soak cap.

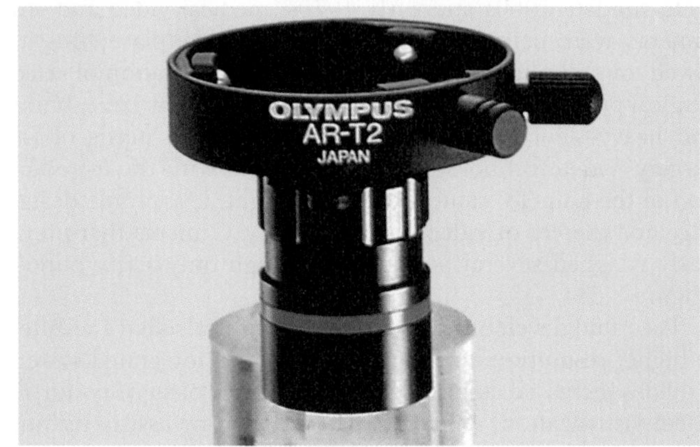


FIGURE 7-38 This camera adapter provides a direct link from the camera to the monitor when eyepiece viewing is not desired.

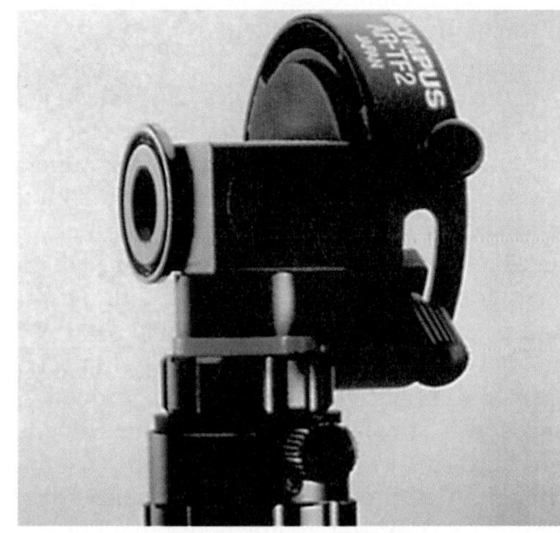


FIGURE 7-39 The camera adapter with a beam splitter allows the physician to look through the eyepiece, while others view the procedure on the monitor.

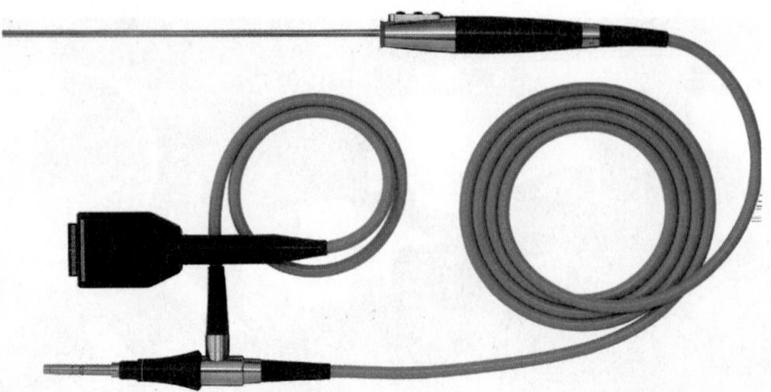

FIGURE 7-40 A one-piece design with a camera incorporated into the endoscope provides consistent, superior image quality.

adds one more link to the chain, this connection can cause loss of light and lens fogging. Connecting the camera and scope with a screw-in design instead of the coupler clamp achieves a tighter fit. This design requires, however, that the camera and scope be bought as a unit; there is no interchangeability between systems. It also does not allow for sterile bagging of the camera because the camera is part of the endoscope.

Lens fogging can be frustrating. It occurs because a cool metal scope is introduced into a warm body. Several ways to handle this phenomenon have been developed. The elimination of a coupler already has been discussed. Sterile defogging solutions are available for application to the telescope and coupler lenses (Figure 7-41). These provide a coating and reduce the incidence of fogging. Other options on the market include O-ring seals at connections, sapphire lenses, and various water seals. Warming of the telescope before insertion also may help reduce fogging. The telescope can be warmed by wrapping it with lap sponges that have been soaked in warm, sterile water. Also available are scope warmers, such as thermos jugs that warm the scope while maintaining the scope sterility. Another method is to use a $CO_2$ insufflator, which warms the gas (if used) before it enters the body. It may be sufficient to change the insufflation site to a secondary port, after the initial pneumoperitoneum has been achieved. The surgeon also may opt to warm the lens of the telescope by gently touching an intraabdominal structure that requires visualization, obviating the need to withdraw the scope to wipe or defog the outer lens.[16]

***Video Monitor.*** High-resolution video monitors represent the end of the chain in video endoscopy. They have become the "windows of observation" during minimally invasive surgery (MIS). Monitors should match closely the resolution quality of the camera being used. A high-resolution monitor that meets or exceeds the horizontal resolution specification of the camera used should be purchased. The camera-monitor system always has the resolution of the least-detailed element. Determining the picture quality of monitors is difficult unless the monitors are side by side. The picture-tube design is the component that alters the monitor's picture quality. Monitors must be able to handle the camera/recorder format (composite, Y/C, or RGB).

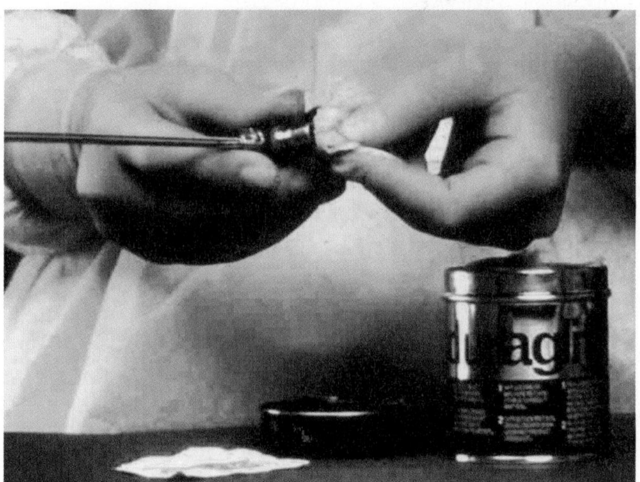

**FIGURE 7-41** Sterile defogging solutions are available for endoscopic procedures.

Operating room (OR) monitors are designed for sharper imagery, increased edge enhancement, increased contrast, and true color reproduction. Video monitors used for endoscopy differ from televisions in that they are capable of receiving input only through direct cables. They usually cannot receive broadcast signals.

Many operative procedures require two video monitors. One is placed on each side of the patient so that the primary surgeon and assistant can view the screen comfortably and simultaneously. The second monitor is called the *slave monitor.* Abdominal and thoracic procedures are performed in this manner. Certain procedures can be performed with only one monitor. Whenever the monitor can be placed comfortably in a position of visibility to the surgeon and assistant, only one is necessary. This is usually the method of choice for urologists, endoscopists, gynecologists, and otorhinolaryngologists. Most general surgeons require only one monitor whenever they perform surgery with the endoscope directed toward the patient's feet (as in endoscopic herniorrhaphy).

Monitors should be at least 13 inches (diagonal measurement of screen) for adequate visualization. When the endoscopic revolution began, most institutions purchased 19-inch or 20-inch main monitors and 13-inch slave monitors. Today many institutions purchase only 19-inch or 20-inch monitors. This size increases flexibility in usage and provides excellent visibility from most observational angles and distances.

When only one monitor and a composite signal is being used, the 75-ohm termination on-off switch must be in the *on* position. When multiple monitors are being used, the switch on the last monitor in line to receive the video signal should be in the *on* position, and all others should be in the *off* position to enhance picture quality. Some monitors are self-terminating and do not have termination switches (Figure 7-42).

***Recording Systems.*** Some recording devices allow for archiving the surgical procedure or selected portions of it. The most commonly used is the video printer, or Mavigraph (Figure 7-43). The video printer is similar to a Polaroid camera in that it takes still photography instantly. The printer stores the selected image and reprints it onto special paper. Many units can be programmed to print 1, 4, 9, or 25 pictures on one piece of $5\frac{1}{2} \times 8$ inch paper in split-screen fashion. Comparisons can be made as the pathologic condition changes. Information such as patient name, date, time, and operating surgeon usually also can be superimposed on top of the print. These prints can be used for teaching purposes or remain as a permanent record on the patient's chart. Some patients are interested in seeing prints of the "before and after" images of their condition.

Video disk recorders are available when one is considering storage and easy access to information. The disk recorder may become the documentation format of the future. To use this format, one also must use a video printer because the images are limited to video.

The VCR is used when moving-image documentation is needed. The VCR format usually is required for teaching purposes and is not used as often as the printer. Image quality is not as clear when one is using a commercial VCR. Professional-grade VCRs differ in that they do not have tuners and radiofrequency (RF) converters. Although rarely used, the best

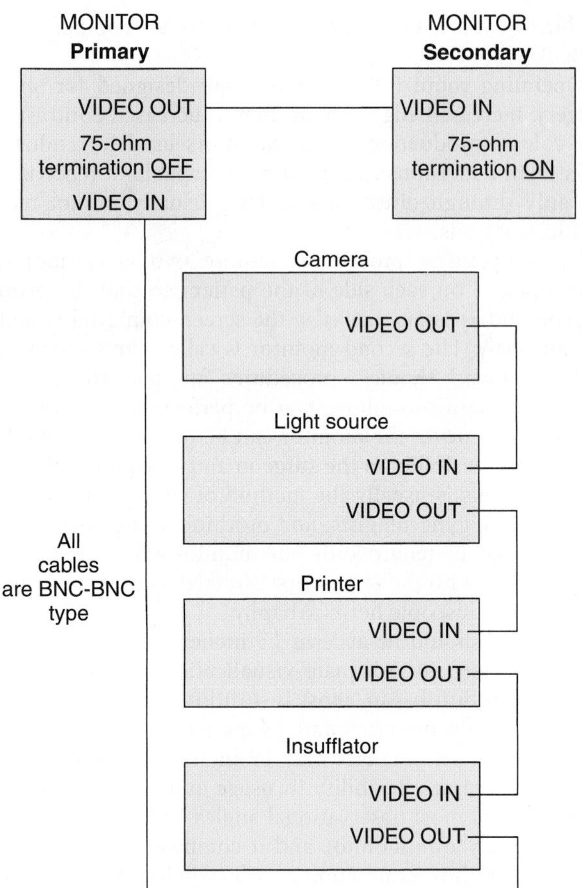


**FIGURE 7-42** Basic wiring configuration.

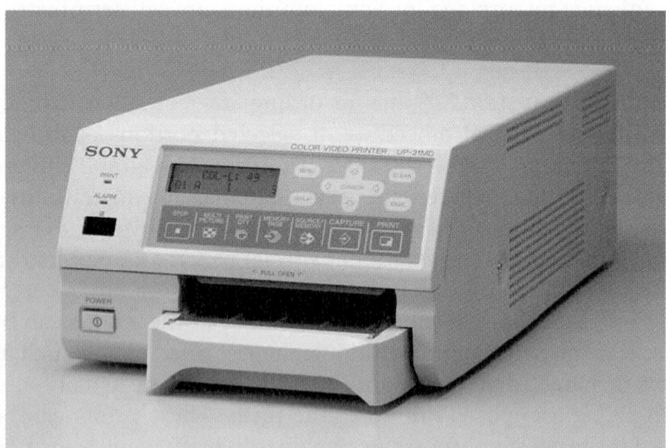


**FIGURE 7-43** Video printer producing a picture of the endoscopic image.

quality recorder available is the ¼-inch U-matic cassette recorder. It provides the best resolution available but also has advantages and disadvantages. It is an expensive piece of equipment, but it has low theft incentive because it cannot be used with standard ½-inch VCR tapes. This feature becomes a deterrent because videos recorded in surgery are ¾-inch and usually cannot be reviewed in surgeons' offices or at home. If security and quality resolution are issues, the best VCR is the professional grade ½-inch S-VHS. It costs more, but is not subject to theft because it cannot be connected to household televisions. S-VHS recorders have the ability to record in the standard VHS format and the S-VHS format. When recorded in the S format, tapes can be played back only on an S-compatible VCR.

***Storage Systems.*** Space, storage capability, security, and required components determine the type and size of video storage carts needed. Purchasing a cart that can house multiple components of the video system is beneficial (Figure 7-44). This eliminates clutter from multiple smaller carts and tables. It also eliminates the number of cord connections to wall outlets because most carts have power strips incorporated in the electrical setup. If the cart has a power strip, an on-off main switch usually is located near the base. The power switch must be in the *on* position for the equipment that is plugged into the strip to work. Because of the location of the switch, it can be turned off easily during transport and cleaning. Time and embarrassment can be avoided if this switch position is checked before each use.

Articulating arms can be used as monitor mounts. Surgeon preference and room space determine if this option is necessary. If a surgical or treatment room has been set aside for endoscopy, the monitor can be suspended from the ceiling on a swivel mount. The mount should be placed in a location where the monitor can be easily and comfortably viewed and cleaned. Care must be taken to ensure the swivel mount would be able to withstand the weight of the monitor and other equipment.

Carts have either a locked (Figure 7-45) or an open (Figure 7-46) shelf design. Institutional security determines this need.

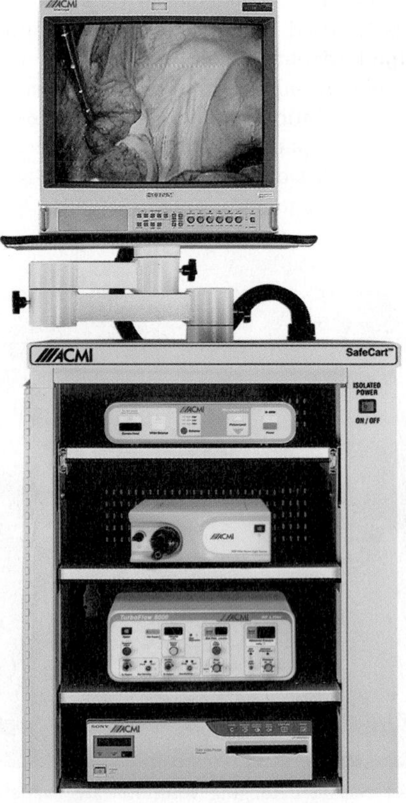


**FIGURE 7-44** Video laparoscopy cart.

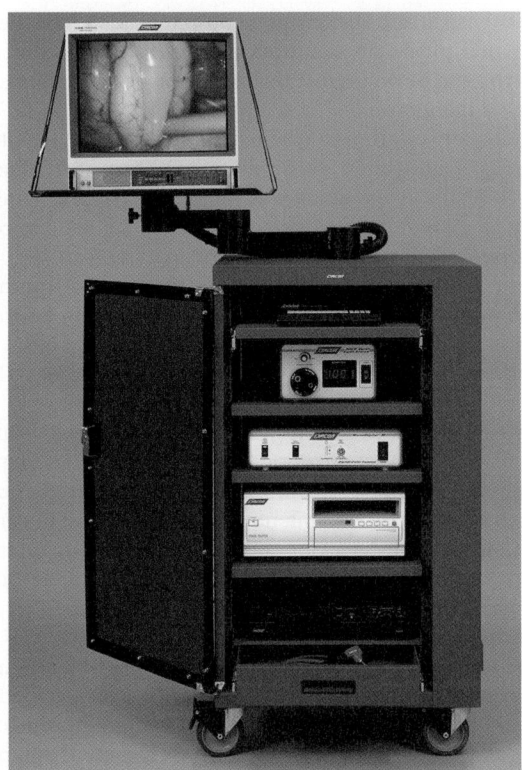

FIGURE 7-45 Video storage cart with swivel monitor arm and lockable door.

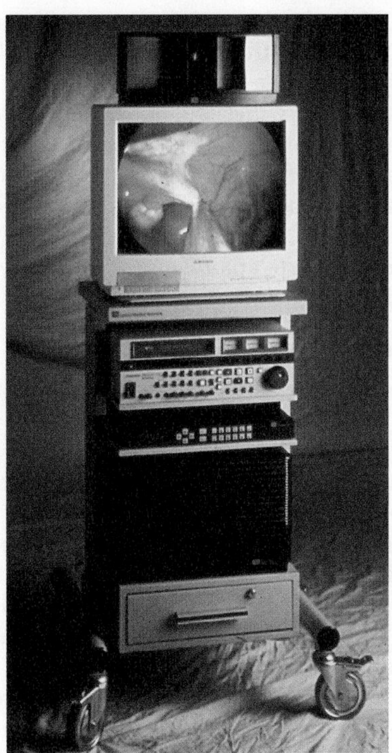

FIGURE 7-46 Open shelf design video cart.

Considerations of storage capability, tampering with equipment, and key availability are important. A locked drawer may be an ideal area to store VCR tapes, printing paper, and the computer disk if these options are available. Carts also should be selected for ease in movement, component accessibility, and cleaning. They should include an optional storage bracket for E-cylinders when insufflation is required. Secondary (slave) monitor carts usually do not contain multiple shelving and cabinet components.

## Robotics

Robotic devices to assist with holding and maneuvering a laparoscope have been introduced to free up team members to perform other roles and attend to other responsibilities. The robotic arm minimizes problems with shaky video images and reduces miscommunication and misunderstanding between the surgeon and the assistant. The robot's movement is controlled directly by foot pedals, handheld control panels, and voice activation (Figure 7-47). This advancement in laparoscope stabilization and movement facilitates the procedure, promotes safety, and minimizes the time needed to perform the procedure.[11]

The robotic arm chassis houses the power system and the computerized control unit. An electromechanical positioner bar attaches to the surgical bed and connects to the laparoscope with a magnetic coupling device. A sterile drape covers this arm to maintain a sterile field. The robotic arm maintains the laparoscope in proper orientation—a problem experienced with manual scope maneuvering.

Advantages of using a robotic device for laparoscope positioning are as follows:

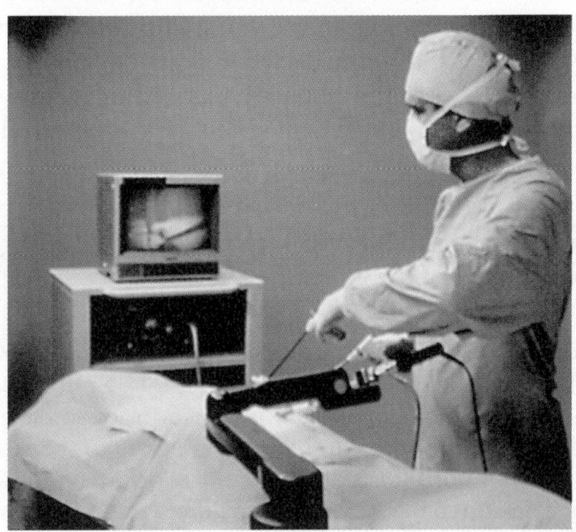

FIGURE 7-47 By being able to command the movement of the robotic arm, the surgeon has complete control over laparoscopic positioning.

- Minimizes fatigue associated with endoscope holding and moving
- Returns scope control to the physician
- Can accommodate quick scope movements through a computerized memory
- May shorten the procedure time by minimizing scope-positioning time
- Provides a steady image that enhances the video quality
- Ensures the same level of care for every patient (consistent scope positioning and movement), which is not always possible with different assistants
- Frees the surgeon's hands to perform other tasks

In September 2001, an Internet news source reported that surgeons at Mount Sinai Hospital in New York City used a remote-controlled robot to operate successfully on a patient in France. The New York surgeons removed the gallbladder of a 68-year-old woman at the European Institute for Tele-Surgery in Strasbourg, France, which was more than 4000 miles away from the operating surgeons. Physicians were amazed at this defining moment in medical history that advanced remote telepresence surgery to a new level.[15] Research and experimentation continue to be conducted to determine if robotics can assist with more delicate and precise procedures, such as during endoscopic surgeries (Research Highlight).

## Videoconferencing

Videoconferencing is a relatively new method to reach distant sites through two-way interactive communications using live audio and video signals. Communications between two or more sites may be live, or one site may play a videotape for the other sites connecting to the videoconference. This relatively new technology requires basic videoconferencing equipment and a network mode to transmit the communication signal to different sites. The higher the network bandwidth used by the participating sites, the better the audio and video motion-handling capabilities, and the resolution of the video signal that can be transmitted to each. A videoconference may be held between two sites or dozens of sites simultaneously. Videoconferencing applications in health care include education, remote assessments and consultation, administrative meetings, and product development.

Because formal education and continuing education are the foundations of quality health care, providing education to and from distant sites has gained tremendous popularity. Health care workers practicing in remote areas do not feel so isolated because educational videoconferencing is now available to many of these areas. Distant preceptorships also have been offered as one physician monitors and oversees another physician learning a new surgical technique or using advanced surgical instrumentation.

Remote consultation to evaluate patients at remote sites has been used as assessment technology has been introduced and accepted. A physician can assess heart sounds of a patient located at a distant place through the use of a telemedicine stethoscope. The retina of a diabetic patient can be viewed from afar by use of a special remote-assessment ophthalmoscope. A perioperative nurse practitioner located in a rural area can consult with a specialty physician located in a large urban teaching institution regarding treatment of a patient (Figure 7-48).

Another videoconferencing application is conducting administrative and other meetings to minimize travel expenses and time away from work. Product development also can be enhanced through videoconferencing. A company that manufactures surgical devices can communicate on a regular basis with key customers who are conducting trials of the devices. Device malfunctions and limitations can be assessed easily through real-time audio and video communication.

Some issues need to be addressed as videoconferencing becomes accepted universally. Standardization must be adhered to so that videoconferencing equipment can communicate and be compatible with each other. Some governmental and professional organization recommendations and mandates have guided manufacturers to meet the agreed-on criteria so that global interactivity can be accomplished. Confidentiality is another concern as the popularity of this technology increases. Patient information, assessment data, and treatment results are being shared among providers by means of videoconferencing today. Patient confidentiality and privacy must be maintained. HIPAA (Health Insurance Portability and Accountability Act of 1996) compliance is vital when transmitting patient records. Private networks, advanced coding systems, and other technology can help address this issue. Practicing across state lines also has become a concern as videoconferencing in health care evolves.[12] State boards of nursing, medicine, pharmacy, and other professions are addressing this situation and are proposing methods to facilitate licensing so that providers can practice across state boundaries. Finally, reimbursement for remote consultation and assessment is being analyzed by many third-

### RESEARCH HIGHLIGHT

**Feasibility of Robotically Assisted Laparoscopy**

Laparoscopic surgery was accepted in 1987, whereas robotic technology in surgery was introduced in 1991. Robotic devices are used primarily in minimally invasive procedures to hold and manipulate the scope under the guidance of the surgeon. They are often voice activated or controlled by handheld devices or a foot pedal. This study was conducted to determine the feasibility of performing simple laparoscopic maneuvers during laparoscopic cholecystectomies using the robotic surgical system. Three robotic arms were fixed at the OR table and controlled remotely by the surgeon using 3-mm laparoscopic instruments to remove the gallbladders from seven female pigs. The mean operating time was 46 minutes, and no complications were experienced. All maneuvers with the robotics were performed without difficulty, and the movements were stable and with good control. The researchers noted that robotic activities during laparoscopy, such as tying, dissection, suturing, clipping, and electrosurgery, could be performed as quickly and accurately as laparoscopic techniques done without robotics. This study confirmed the feasibility that laparoscopic cholecystectomy can be performed with robotic assistance.

Modified from Lomanto D and others: Robotically assisted laparoscopic cholecystectomy, *Archives of Surgery* 136:1106-1108, 2001.

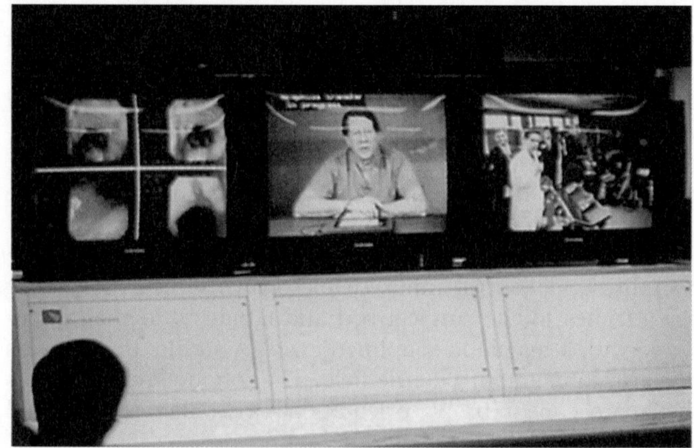

**FIGURE 7-48** A nurse practitioner can consult with a physician at a remote location about a patient's treatment.

party carriers and reimbursers. Pilot project sites have been established by the Centers for Medicare and Medicaid Services (formerly the Health Care Financing Administration) to study this predicament. When reimbursement can be provided, more health care providers and facilities will get involved with videoconferencing for health care applications.

## ENDOSCOPIC PRACTICES AND POTENTIAL RISKS

### Insufflation

To help visualize abdominal structures and for safe operative functions during laparoscopic procedures, a pneumoperitoneum is created. To do so, the surgeon makes a paraumbilical incision and inserts an insufflation (Verres) needle into the abdomen (Figure 7-49). Trendelenburg position is selected to reduce the risk of visceral perforation. Appropriate positioning devices should be used (see Chapter 5). While the surgeon inserts the needle, he or she lifts up the patient's abdomen by grasping a fold of tissue on either side of the umbilicus. Preoperative patient education should include the possibility of finger-pinched bruising at the site where the abdominal tissue is grasped.

The needle safely enters the peritoneum if positioned at a 45-degree angle. Placement usually is confirmed by a negative bowel and blood return on aspiration and by a saline instillation that meets no resistance. This is a relatively blind procedure because no scope can be introduced until pneumoperitoneum has been established.

When needle confirmation is established, the insufflation tubing is connected, and the process is begun. $CO_2$ gas is used for insufflation because it does not support combustion, can be absorbed at large volumes per minute without serious side effects, and is fairly inexpensive. The peritoneal cavity is filled by starting at a low flow rate which is then increased to a high flow rate of at least 9 L/min ideally. Flow rate refers only to how quickly a predetermined intraabdominal pressure can be reached. Intraabdominal pressure is the actual parameter that must be closely monitored and should be maintained between 14 and 16 mm Hg. High flow rates are important because during the procedure, the insufflation $CO_2$ gas can escape. The more quickly the gas can be replaced, the less time will be spent waiting for the abdomen to be redistended. Perioperative nurses must demonstrate competence in insufflation and understand and manage the potential risks.

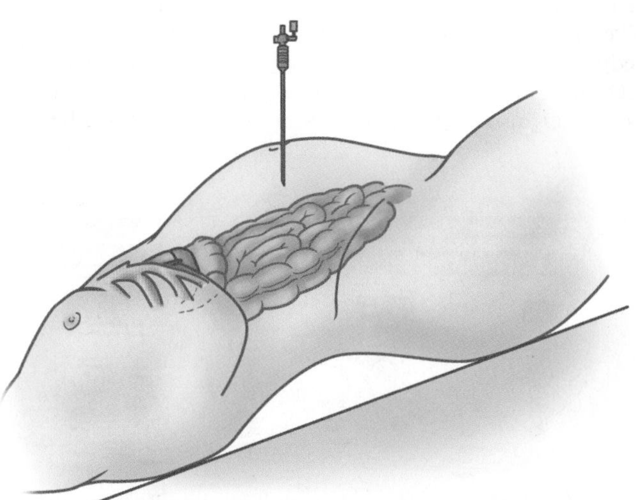
**FIGURE 7-49** Verres needle insertion into abdomen.

Insufflator control panels should monitor and display the following variables:

1. Rate of flow
2. Volume delivered
3. Intraabdominal pressure

Selection of an insufflator that can accommodate a high flow rate is important. In the initial phases of the endoscopic revolution, flow rates of 6 L/min were adequate. Today, because of the increased complexity of endoscopic procedures, increased numbers of secondary ports, and longer procedures (attributable to surgical complexity), pneumoperitoneum must be maintained over longer time frames. This requires flow rates of at least 9 L/min. Insufflators delivering 15 to 20 L/min are much more supportive and effective than those delivering gas at the slower rate.

Of even greater concern during the insufflator selection process should be the guarantee that an insufflator can and will monitor insufflation pressure continuously, stop the insufflation process when the predetermined set pressure has been reached, and release pressure if there is an inadvertent increase (called "taking a breath"). Intraabdominal pressure can be increased for reasons other than $CO_2$ insufflation; leaning on the abdomen and additional gas introduction from other sources, such as an argon-beam coagulator or a $CO_2$ laser with a purge gas system, can inadvertently increase intraabdominal pressure.

Overpressurization can be extremely hazardous to the patient and must be avoided. Excess pressure can force $CO_2$ to diffuse into the blood, resulting in hypercarbia. End-tidal $CO_2$ monitoring becomes a crucial assessment parameter to detect increased $CO_2$ absorption. Excess pressure also increases diaphragmatic pressure, which could result in gastric regurgitation and aspiration of stomach contents. It also could reduce intrathoracic space, resulting in decreased respiratory effort and cardiac output. The phrenic nerve innervates the diaphragm and is responsible for some motor activity associated with respiration. $CO_2$ gas irritates this nerve, causing postoperative pain in the shoulder and neck. Although a common complaint, excessive pressure could cause tremendous postoperative discomfort and more severe nerve damage. The surgeon or assistant should press on the patient's abdomen to release as much residual $CO_2$ gas as possible before removal of the last trocar when the procedure is completed. Insufflators that automatically vent excessive $CO_2$ gas into the air provide assurance that many potential complications can be avoided. Special smoke evacuators can provide a safe and quick method to remove the insufflated gas using a closed system so that no gas escapes into the environment.

A two-way, single-use disposable filter should be incorporated into the insufflation tubing (Figure 7-50). This hydrophobic filter provides patient protection from harmful gas-tank contamination, such as chromium particles. It also provides protection from the colonization of organisms in the insufflator itself. Without a filter, when the insufflator is turned on, organisms such as *Klebsiella, Pseudomonas,* and *Staphylococcus aureus* can be blown into the patient. This contamination could jeopardize the patient's welfare and surgical outcome. It could be deadly for a very ill, elderly, or immunocompromised patient. The manufacturer's written instructions must be followed when implementing $CO_2$ insufflation. Steps perioperative nurses should consider to reduce cross-contamination of the patient and insufflator during $CO_2$ insufflation include the following:

- *Before* the procedure, verify that the cylinder is medical grade $CO_2$; note the level of gas in the cylinder.
- Flush insufflator and tubing with $CO_2$ gas *before* attaching to patient.
- Use a disposable hydrophobic filter on insufflation tubing. Discard after procedure.
- *During* the procedure, monitor level of $CO_2$ remaining in cylinder; have second cylinder readily available.
- Disconnect tubing from insufflator *before* turning off, at end of procedure.
- Keep insufflator *elevated* above the patient to prevent fluid backflow.

An insufflator capable of warning the operative team of insufflation parameter problems throughout the procedure is highly desirable. If these parameters are periodically visualized on the monitor, information can be processed immediately and action taken. Alarms that sound when there is a deviation from predetermined parameters also call attention to the need for immediate intervention, such as an alarm ringing and a monitor blinking "Gas supply low." An alarm sounding when overpressurization occurs from a secondary source (e.g., by leaning on the abdomen) also alerts the team to the need for corrective action.

Insufflators also are available with $CO_2$ warming devices (Figure 7-51). Cylinder $CO_2$ is in liquid form, and as it is released, it expands into a gas. During this conversion from liquid to gas, energy is lost, and the gas becomes colder. The higher the flow, the colder the gas. Some warming does occur as the gas travels through the insufflation tubing. Use of cold $CO_2$ gas can easily cause a decrease in patient temperature, especially with prolonged laparoscopy. Although many factors contribute to the reduction of body temperature during endoscopic procedures (e.g., cold irrigation, room temperature, surface exposure, length of the procedure, patient's age and medical history, anesthetic choice), cold $CO_2$ represents an additional one. The best way to reduce patient heat loss and the risk for hypothermia is to address all the variables and intervene wherever possible.

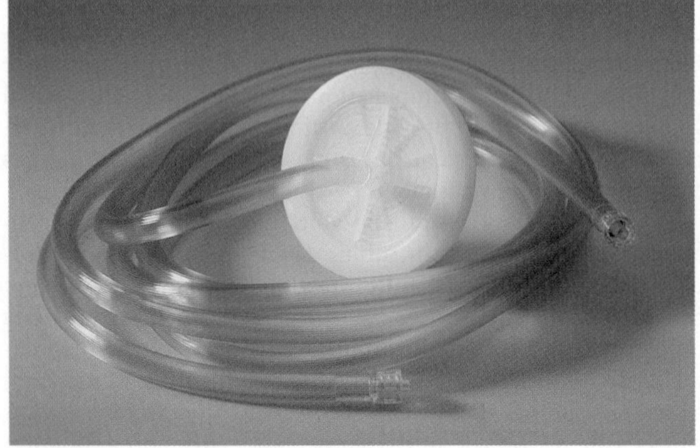

FIGURE 7-50 Disposable insufflation tubing with two-way filter.

Cold $CO_2$ gas also contributes to the fogging of telescope lenses. Fogging occurs whenever a cold instrument enters the warm, moist environment of the body. Methods to reduce this condensation process were discussed previously. Moving the insufflation site to a secondary port away from the scope often is sufficient.

## Complications and Anesthetic Considerations During Endoscopic Minimally Invasive Surgery

Although anesthetic technique and delivery are the responsibility of the anesthesia provider, the perioperative nurse must anticipate and respond appropriately to associated risks during endoscopic intervention. Many open surgical procedures, which require lengthy hospitalization and result in substantial postoperative pain, are now performed endoscopically as ambulatory or short-stay surgeries. Postoperative pain has been minimized for most patients. Because of these changes, anesthetic technique also has changed. Today there is an emphasis on minimal anesthesia during surgery. Short-acting drugs are used so that the patient awakens quickly and experiences as few side effects as possible (see Chapter 4).

The three major goals of the anesthesia provider during endoscopic procedures remain the same: *respiratory stability, appropriate muscle relaxation,* and *hemodynamic stability.* In addition, during many laparoscopic and pelviscopic procedures, it is necessary to control diaphragmatic excursion. Patient monitoring includes an electrocardiogram (ECG) and assessment of end-tidal $CO_2$, blood pressure, oxygen saturation, and temperature.

When Trendelenburg position is used, intraabdominal pressure is increased, which can result in respiratory complications, including hypoxia. $CO_2$ absorption from the peritoneal cavity can aggravate this situation further. Reverse Trendelenburg position could result in decreased venous return, cardiac output, and blood pressure. $CO_2$ insufflation in this position could lead to an increase in total peripheral resistance, especially if intraabdominal pressure is high, and the aorta is compressed. The perioperative nurse must be prepared to change the position of the OR bed when necessary and decrease the $CO_2$ flow rate of the insufflator. The anesthesia provider may require assistance with medications and extra supplies.

$CO_2$, highly soluble in blood, generally does not become a hazard when used during laparoscopic insufflation because it is rapidly absorbed in the splanchnic vascular region. Excessive intraabdominal pressure or any anesthetic technique that reduces splanchnic blood flow could increase the potential for $CO_2$ gas emboli, however. This could lead to circulatory collapse. $CO_2$ also could advance from the heart to the pulmonary

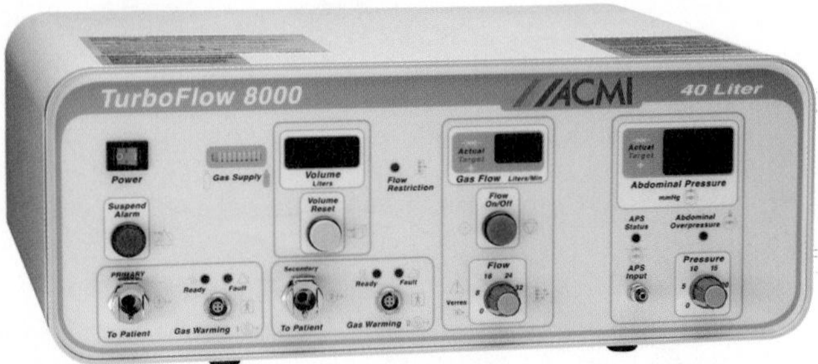


FIGURE 7-51 Computerized high-flow insufflator with $CO_2$ warmer.

circulation, causing acute pulmonary hypertension with right-sided heart failure. If these effects are undetected and $CO_2$ insufflation continues, cardiac arrest and death could occur.

Signs of $CO_2$ embolus (pulmonary embolism) include sudden decrease in blood pressure, dysrhythmia, heart murmurs, cyanosis, pulmonary edema, and an abrupt increase in end-tidal $CO_2$. If an embolus is suspected, continuous monitoring of heart sounds, blood pressure, and end-tidal $CO_2$ can help the anesthesia provider make a rapid diagnosis. Immediate deflation of pneumoperitoneum is necessary. Treatment may include immediate placement of the patient in a left lateral position and aspiration of the $CO_2$ gas through a central venous catheter. The perioperative nurse should assist in patient repositioning while maintaining sterility of equipment and the surgical field wherever possible. Assistance may be required during central venous catheter placement. Debilitated patients may require preoperative invasive monitoring.

Hypotension can result from excessive bleeding, excessive intraabdominal pressure, and hypoxia. $CO_2$ insufflation rates may have to be reduced. Extra intravenous fluids may be needed. Hypertension resulting from increased intraabdominal pressure and increased $CO_2$ gas absorption also may be evident. Increased bleeding may result. The perioperative nurse can help by decreasing $CO_2$ insufflation flow rates; additional hemostatic agents and endoscopic clips may be required.

Gastric reflux is a concern if the patient is obese, a hiatal hernia is present, or excessive pneumoperitoneum occurs. Hiatal hernia could be discovered during the preoperative assessment. A nasogastric or orogastric tube may be inserted after general anesthesia is administered. Postoperative discomfort is less if an orogastric tube is used. During epidural and regional anesthesia, patients are usually awake, and insertion of a gastric tube may be poorly tolerated. For this reason, the tube is not inserted unless gastric distention occurs. The perioperative nurse must be quick to respond if assistance is required during gastric tube insertion. Intercostal nerve blocks offer surgical pain relief and abdominal muscle relaxation when the patient is awake during surgery. This anesthetic technique requires extreme patient cooperation because several injections are necessary. The perioperative nurse's role during intercostal nerve block induction is to remain at the patient's side and help to reduce anxiety. Other potential risks include hypercarbia, subcutaneous emphysema, and pneumoscrotum. The perioperative nurse's understanding of the potential risks along with appropriate nursing interventions can have a significant effect on the patient's outcome.

## ENERGIES USED DURING SURGERY

### Laser

A health care revolution that has occurred in the past 5 decades is the birth and evolution of an amazing tool called the *laser* (History box). The perioperative nurse must be keenly aware of the expanded responsibilities associated with laser applications. The laser has had an impact on surgery by making possible less invasive procedures, decreasing inpatient hospitalization, diminishing postoperative complications, and saving health care dollars.

#### *Laser Biophysics*

PRINCIPLES OF LIGHT. *LASER* is an acronym that describes a process in which light energy is produced—*l*ight *a*mplification by *s*timulated *e*mission of *r*adiation. This term also refers to the device that generates the laser energy.

Light is a form of electromagnetic energy that can be graphically illustrated on a continuum known as the *electromagnetic spectrum* (Figure 7-52). The unit of measurement that delineates the continuum is called a *wavelength,* which is the distance between two successive peaks of a wave. The wavelength determines color and usually is measured in nanometers ($10^{-9}$ m) or micrometers (1000 nm). The various wavelengths of laser energy extend from the shorter waves in the ultraviolet area to the longer waves in the infrared region along this perpetual line (Box 7-3). The visible laser wavelengths occupy only a small

**BOX 7-3**

**Electromagnetic Spectrum Wavelengths**

| Type of Light | Wavelength (nm) |
|---|---|
| Ultraviolet (UV) | 100-400 |
| Visible | 400-750 |
| Near-infrared (NIR) | 750-3000 |
| Mid-infrared (MIR) | 3000-30,000 |
| Far-infrared (FIR) | 30,000 nm-1 mm |

**HISTORY**

**Laser Technology**

During the early 1900s, Einstein first described a theory that involved the stimulation of matter to cause the release of energy. In 1957, Gould developed the principle of *LASER,* which was derived from the acronym for *l*ight *a*mplification by the *s*timulated *e*mission of *r*adiation. In 1958 Schawlow and Townes investigated this concept of stimulated atoms and the creation of photons. They suggested that mirrors be used to amplify the stimulated emission of radiation to multiply the photons at an accelerated rate.

In 1960 Maiman developed the first laser for medicine and surgery using a ruby crystal. The ruby laser was used for dermatologic applications and for retinal photocoagulation in patients with diabetic retinopathy. It was not very efficient, however. Other lasers, such as the argon, $CO_2$, Nd:YAG, KTP, holmium, erbium, excimer, and diode lasers, have been developed and now are being used in many surgical disciplines. Continued advancements in laser technology have provided the physician with a precision tool for cutting, coagulating, vaporizing, and welding tissue during surgical intervention.

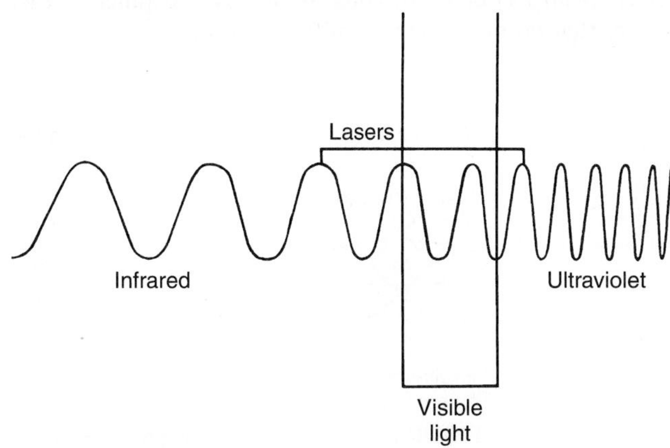


FIGURE 7-52 Electromagnetic spectrum.

portion of this continuum. The radiation used in laser technology in health care is nonionizing in that it does not present the hazard of cellular DNA disruption through continual tissue exposure. Pregnant women can work with lasers because laser energy does not produce harmful ionizing radiation.

Briefly, the laser functions in the following way. A negatively charged electron orbits a positively charged nucleus while the atom is in its ground or resting state, which is at its lowest possible level of energy. An outside source of energy (e.g., electricity, flash lamps, other lasers) can excite the atom and cause an electron to jump to a higher, less stable orbit. The electron almost immediately returns to its stable orbit, and the atom resumes its normal resting state. As the unstable electron returns to its ground state, it spontaneously releases a tiny packet of light energy known as a *photon,* which travels away from the source in the form of waves. If the photon is close to another similar atom while it is still in the excited state, it interacts with this atom. The photon triggers the excited second atom to return to its resting state, and in this process another photon of laser light is emitted. These two photons of identical energy travel together. The process of stimulated emission has occurred, and laser energy has been initially formed (Figure 7-53). This process continues to repeat itself over and over again creating more photons of laser energy.

This activity occurs in the resonating chamber of the laser, where the lasing medium is contained. The name of the laser usually is derived from the actual medium that causes the lasing action. The photons that are generated during the stimulated emission process are reflected back and forth between mirrors at each end of the resonating chamber as the process is amplified, until the number of excited atoms surpasses the number of resting atoms. This is known as *population inversion.* One of the mirrors in the chamber is partially reflective and, when activated, allows a stream of laser photons to escape the unit. These photons are introduced to the target area by means of a specific delivery system.

**CHARACTERISTICS OF LASER LIGHT.** Three distinct characteristics distinguish laser light from ordinary light. Laser light is monochromatic, collimated, and coherent.

- *Monochromatic light* is composed of photons of the same wavelength or color. In contrast, ordinary light consists of many different colors or wavelengths. When white light is passed through a prism, an array of different colors is displayed. White light is the presence of all colors, whereas laser light consists of one color or wavelength.
- A *collimated* laser beam consists of waves parallel to each other that do not diverge significantly, minimizing any loss of power. When a collimated beam is passed through a lens, the light pattern is changed, allowing the light to be focused into a tiny spot that tremendously concentrates the energy. In comparison, the light waves from a flashlight are not parallel and lose intensity as they travel away from the source. A lens cannot easily focus these noncollimated waves to concentrate the light into a small area.
- Laser light is *coherent*—all the waves are orderly and in phase with each other as they travel in the same direction. All peaks and troughs of the waves are opposite each other in time and space. This property provides an additive effect that gives the laser beam power. Ordinary light is incoherent because the waves radiate away from the source without being in phase or in an orderly pattern.

**LASER POWER.** The power, or energy, of a laser beam is measured in watts. An important factor in laser application is the concept of power density, or irradiance of the beam. *Power density* is the amount of power that is concentrated within an area and is described by the following formula:

$$\text{Power density} = \text{watts/spot size (cm}^2)$$

The spot size of the laser beam can be controlled when the beam is passed through a special lens that causes the beam to converge. The focal configuration of the lens determines at what distance from the lens the beam would be most intense; this is called the *focal point.* If the beam is defocused into a larger spot size, the laser energy is spread over a greater area, decreasing the intensity or power density of the beam. In contrast, a small spot size of the beam concentrates the laser energy into a smaller area, increasing the intensity or power density of the beam. When the power density is increased, the beam has a greater depth of penetration into the tissue.

A *joule* is the unit of measurement used to describe the total energy used. A joule is expressed by the power multiplied by the time duration of the beam exposure (see equation). Often the laser energy used during ophthalmic procedures is expressed in millijoules.

$$\text{Joule} = \text{watts} \times \text{time}$$

*Fluence* is a term that involves the power and duration of exposure of the beam and measures the specific amount of energy that is delivered to the tissue. The following equation calculates the fluence:

$$\text{Fluence} = \text{watts} \times \text{duration time/spot size (cm}^2)$$

**TISSUE INTERACTION.** When laser energy is delivered to the target site, four different interactions can occur: reflec-

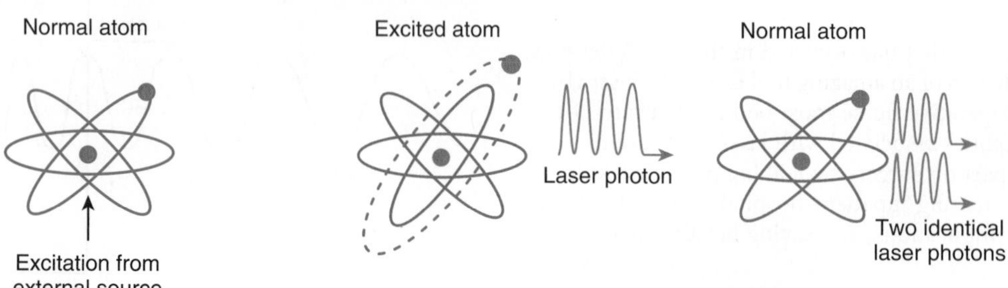


**FIGURE 7-53** Laser energy is produced when an external source excites the atom to emit a photon spontaneously. This photon can "stimulate" the emission of two identical photons.

tion, scattering, transmission, or absorption (Figure 7-54). The extent of the reaction of the beam on the target depends on the laser wavelength, power settings, spot size, length of time the beam is in contact with the tissue, and the characteristics of the tissue.

*Reflection* of the laser beam occurs when the direction of the beam is changed after it contacts an area. Specular reflection occurs when the angle of the incoming light is equal to the angle of the reflected light. Laser light can be intentionally reflected in this manner off a reflective mirror to contact hard-to-reach areas. This type of reflection also can pose safety problems by inadvertently striking untargeted areas if it is not controlled at all times. The $CO_2$ laser beam can be reflected off of the surface of a shiny instrument and impact a surgery team member's mask, causing it to ignite. Eye and fire safety measures are mandatory when the potential for laser beam reflection is high.

*Scattering* of the laser light occurs when the beam spreads over a large area as the tissue causes the beam to disperse. The intensity of the beam is decreased as the waves travel in different directions. The Nd:YAG laser beam can backscatter up an endoscope and possibly cause damage to the end of the scope, the optics, or the operator's eye. The noncontact Nd:YAG beam also can scatter through tissue causing a great depth of penetration of 3 to 5 mm.

*Transmission* of the laser beam occurs when the beam passes through fluids or tissue without thermally affecting the area. The argon beam can be transmitted through the clear fluids and structures of the front part of the eye and the vitreous to cause thermal photocoagulation on the retina, while the cornea, lens, and vitreous are unaffected by the transmission of this beam.

*Absorption* of the laser light results when the tissue is altered from the absorption of the beam. As the amount of energy delivered to the tissue (fluence) increases, different tissue effects can be produced.[18] The lowest level of energy produces a photochemical reaction, then as the fluence increases, a photothermal reaction occurs. With the highest level of fluence, a photoacoustic effect is produced. The reactions from the lowest level of energy to the highest include the following:

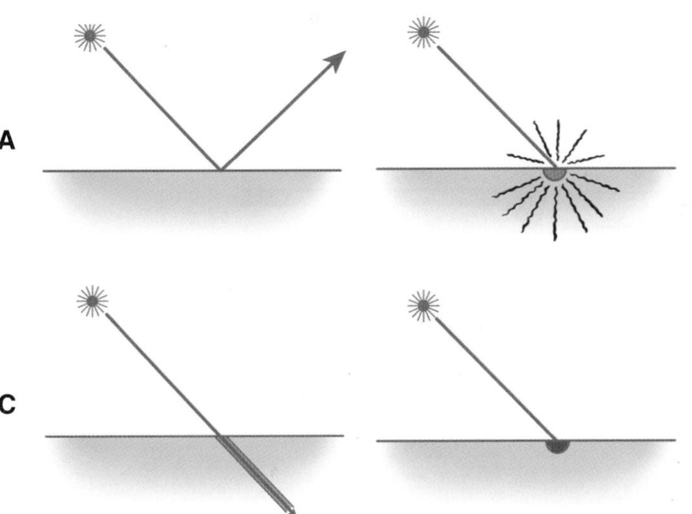


FIGURE 7-54 Laser tissue interaction. **A**, Reflection. **B**, Scattering. **C**, Transmission. **D**, Absorption.

1. *Photochemical effect*—the laser energy is selectively absorbed by tissue containing a light-sensitive dye, leading to a chemical change that produces singlet oxygen, which ultimately causes tissue destruction.
2. *Photothermal effect*—the laser energy is absorbed by the tissue, heating the tissue.
3. *Photoacoustic effect*—the laser energy is absorbed and produces a snapping sound, disrupting the tissue without a significant thermal effect.

The consistency, color, and water content of the target tissue often determine the rate of absorption of the laser energy. The laser wavelength also affects the absorption of the beam. Certain laser light, such as that from the argon laser, is highly absorbed by pigmented tissues. The $CO_2$ laser is independent of color-selective absorption, however. The $CO_2$ laser light is absorbed superficially by tissue to a shallow depth of approximately 0.1 to 0.2 mm, whereas the holmium laser beam is absorbed to about 0.4 to 0.6 mm. Argon laser light is readily absorbed by pigmented tissue to a depth of approximately 1 to 2 mm, whereas that of the noncontact Nd:YAG laser beam is more readily absorbed by darkened tissue to a depth of 3 to 5 mm.

Photothermal tissue reaction becomes more pronounced as the temperature of the target area increases during absorption of the laser beam (Table 7-2). As the laser energy is absorbed, the water within the cell is heated. As the temperature increases, the intracellular protein is destroyed, and the water inside the cell turns to steam. Eventually the cellular membrane ruptures from increased pressure, spewing cellular debris and plume (smoke) from the tissue. The surrounding tissue also is heated through conduction because it borders the impingement site. The degree of adjacent tissue damage depends on the duration of the laser-beam exposure that causes the thermal injury.

***Laser Systems.*** New laser systems are being introduced into health care regularly. Constant efforts by researchers and physicians to explore the use of different wavelengths are changing surgical approaches in a variety of specialties. Table 7-3 describes popular lasers used in medicine and surgery today.

PARTS OF A LASER SYSTEM. The five major components of a laser system are the laser head, excitation source, ancillary components, control panel, and delivery system.[3] When a laser malfunctions, an organized investigation of each of these parts (Figure 7-55) usually can determine the source of the problem.

The *laser head,* or resonating chamber, is the part where the laser energy is generated and amplified. The laser head con-

**TABLE 7-2**

**Tissue Changes with Temperature Increases**

| Temperature (°C) | Visual Change | Biologic Change |
|---|---|---|
| 37-60 | No visual change | Warming, welding |
| 60-65 | Blanching | Coagulation |
| 65-90 | White/gray | Protein denaturization |
| 90-100 | Puckering | Drying |
| >100 | Smoke plume | Vaporization, carbonization |

From Ball KA: *Lasers: the perioperative challenge,* ed 3, Denver, Colo, 2004, AORN.

TABLE 7-3

## Description of Laser Color and Wavelength

| Laser | Color | Wavelength (nm) |
|---|---|---|
| Excimer | Ultraviolet | |
| ArF | | 193 |
| KrCl | | 222 |
| KrF | | 248 |
| XeCl | | 308 |
| XeF | | 351 |
| Helium-cadmium | | 325 |
| Argon | Blue | 488 or 457 |
| | Green | 514.5 or 528 |
| Frequency-doubled YAG (KTP) | Green | 532 |
| Krypton | Green | 531 |
| | Yellow | 568 |
| | Red | 647 |
| Dye laser | Variable with dyes | 400-1000 |
| Gold vapor | Red | 628 |
| Helium neon | Red | 632 |
| Ruby | Deep red | 694 |
| Diode | Visible to near-infrared | 532-908 |
| Alexandrite | Near-infrared | 760 |
| Nd:YAG | Infrared | 1064 or 1318 |
| Holmium:YAG | Infrared | 2140 |
| Erbium:YAG | Infrared | 2940 |
| Carbon dioxide | Infrared | 10,600 |

From Ball KA: *Lasers: the perioperative challenge,* ed 3, Denver, Colo, 2004, AORN.

tains the active medium or substance that actually produces the photons that generate the laser light. The active medium can be a gas ($CO_2$ or argon), a solid crystal (Nd:YAG), a liquid (tunable dye), or a semiconductor crystal (diode).

Many lasers used in health care today work in the following manner. The *excitation source* supplies the energy to excite the active medium in the laser head. Different sources include flash lamps, electricity, radio waves, batteries, chemicals, and other laser systems. The $CO_2$ laser gas mixture is excited by electrical current or radio waves, and the Nd:YAG laser crystal is excited by flash lamps. Diode lasers, such as the gallium arsenide laser, are solid-state lasers that are excited by electrical energy.

The *ancillary components* are the other laser parts that are needed to help produce the laser energy. A cooling system maintains the appropriate temperature of the laser head to keep the unit from overheating. Usually lasers are air cooled or water cooled. A vacuum pump may be required in a $CO_2$ free-flowing laser to pull the gas mixture from an external cylinder into the laser head for laser light production. The current sealed-tube $CO_2$ lasers do not require a vacuum pump because the laser gas mixture is catalyzed to regenerate the mixture necessary for the lasing action to continue, using the same gas mixture over and over again.

The *control panel* consists of the board that regulates the delivery of laser energy. Various power settings, modes, durations, and other parameters can be selected as desired. Most laser panels are computerized, allowing the laser to be controlled quickly and accurately. Wireless control modules that can be placed into a sterile plastic bag have been developed so that the surgical team can control the laser from the sterile

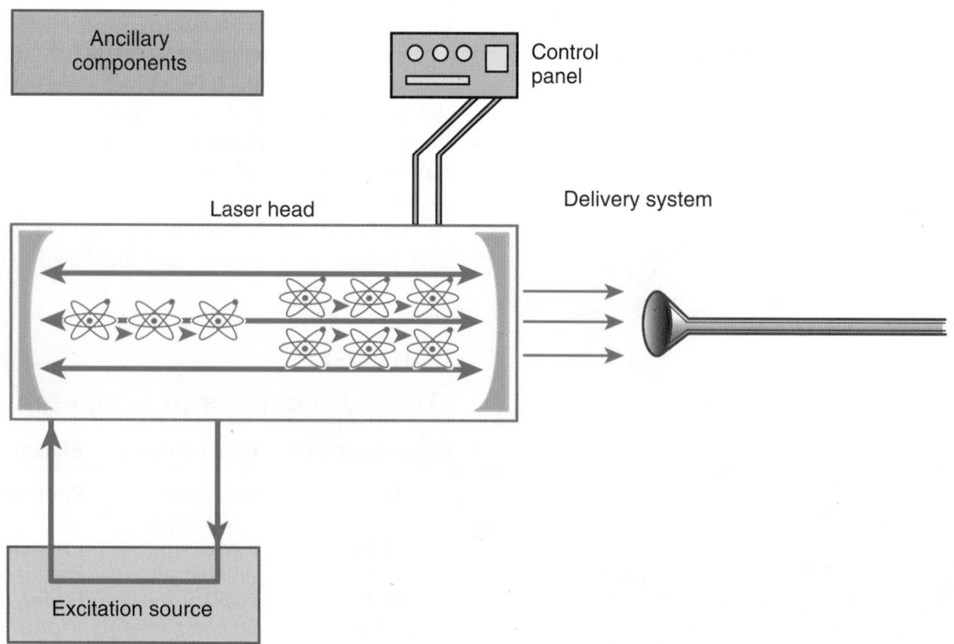


FIGURE 7-55 Parts of a laser system.

operating field. The laser team should be exceedingly familiar with the operation of the laser control panel or module.

The *delivery system* of the laser is the device or accessory that conducts the laser energy from the laser head to the target area. $CO_2$ laser energy usually is delivered to the tissue through an articulated arm with a series of special mirrors at each joint. The commonly used argon, KTP, Nd:YAG, and holmium lasers deliver energy through a fiber system. Advancements in laser technology are refining delivery systems to make them more adaptable, convenient, and user friendly. Various lasers are described in the next section, beginning with lasers in the infrared region with long wavelengths, through the visible wavelengths, and finally to the short ultraviolet wavelengths.

**$CO_2$ LASER.** The $CO_2$ laser is versatile and widely used. Its wavelength of 10,600 nm is located in the infrared region of the electromagnetic spectrum. Because this light is invisible, a visible helium-neon laser beam is transmitted co-axially with the $CO_2$ laser energy to serve as an aiming beam.

The $CO_2$ laser is characterized by its superficial tissue interaction (0.1 to 0.2 mm) because the beam is highly absorbed by water. The degree of tissue response is related to the photothermal effect (the amount of heat buildup) from absorption of the $CO_2$ laser beam. The longer the $CO_2$ beam is in contact with tissue, as with other laser wavelengths, the more destruction is noted, and a greater depth of penetration can be achieved. The tissue reaction is visible and has been described as "what you see is what you get." The $CO_2$ beam is independent of color selectivity, meaning that lighter tissue absorbs the beam as readily as darker tissue.

The two types of $CO_2$ lasers that use electricity or radio waves as the excitation source are described next:

1. *Free-flowing $CO_2$ laser system*—an older model that requires an external cylinder of a special laser gas mixture of $CO_2$, helium, and nitrogen. The concentrations of these gases must be specific to the particular laser unit so that the laser operates properly. The gas is pulled into the laser head by a vacuum pump, laser energy is generated, and harmless disassociated by-products are discharged from the unit. The laser gas cylinder is replaced when empty.
2. *Sealed-tube $CO_2$ system*—contains a special mixture of $CO_2$, helium, and nitrogen within a tube that is sealed. A catalyst is added to the tube to cause regeneration of the mixture so that lasing action can be produced again. The shelf life (functional period) of this type of tube is usually 1 to 5 years or more. At the end of this time, the tube can be serviced by the manufacturer to replace the special gas and catalyst mixture.

The $CO_2$ laser beam is delivered to the target site through a hollow tube called an *articulated arm*. Mirrors are positioned within the arm to reflect the laser energy forward. Because the helium-neon aiming beam runs co-axially with the $CO_2$ beam, care must be taken when moving the laser so that the mirrors are not jarred out of alignment.

The articulated arm can be attached to a microscope or a special handpiece. A lens system within these attachments causes the beam to converge at the focal point. A special coating on the lens maintains the beam's integrity and intensity and must be cared for carefully so that the coating is not disrupted. The manufacturer's instructions that provide information on lens care must be followed closely. The articulated arm is connected to a microscope through the use of a microslad (or micromanipulator). The laser energy is conducted through the articulated arm to a mirror within the microslad that directly reflects the beam to the tissue. The position of the beam is controlled by moving a joystick. The articulated arm also may be attached to a scanner for more precise delivery of the laser energy.

The focal length of the lens is the distance from the lens to the focal point where the beam converges and is most concentrated and intense within a small spot. The size of the spot can be changed by focusing or defocusing the lens to allow the spot to become larger or smaller. When the $CO_2$ handpiece is moved toward and then away from the tissue, the spot size changes.

Sometimes tubing is connected to the handpiece or microscope adapter to conduct a purge gas or compressed air that blows the laser smoke away, keeping the lens cool and free from debris. If this tubing is unavailable, a smoke evacuator can be used to prevent the plume from coating the focusing lens.

The $CO_2$ laser beam also can be conducted through a narrow wave guide, which consists of a hollow, semiflexible tube that allows the energy to "wiggle" down its path by being reflected off the surface of the inner lumen. Because of this reflection, some of the power of the beam is lost as it exits this delivery device. Solid fibers that conduct the $CO_2$ wavelength to the target site still are being developed.

The $CO_2$ laser energy can be delivered to tissue in a variety of modes. The continuous mode allows the laser energy to be delivered continuously as long as the foot pedal is depressed. The timed pulsed mode delivers the energy one pulse at a time or in a repeat manner that specifically controls the duration of exposure. The superpulse or ultrapulse mode delivers the energy in an extremely quick sequence of interrupted pulses that may appear to be a continuous mode. The energy may peak 5 to 10 times higher than the desired wattage, but the duration of exposure is extremely limited, providing great precision. This type of interaction allows the adjacent tissue to cool so that tissue destruction is minimized.

**ERBIUM:YAG LASER.** One of the newer YAG lasers in health care is the erbium:YAG solid crystal laser that generates a wavelength of approximately 2940 nm. The laser energy is usually delivered in a pulsed mode. The erbium laser beam is highly absorbed by water, allowing a shallow penetration of the energy into tissue. The erbium was first introduced after research was published on the response of dental tissue (teeth) to erbium laser energy. The erbium laser has gained acceptance in dermatology for skin resurfacing and ablation.

**HOLMIUM:YAG LASER.** A solid crystal YAG laser that has been widely accepted into the surgical arena is the holmium: YAG laser. The YAG crystal is doped with holmium, which is a rare earth element. This laser produces a wavelength of 2140 nm and is delivered to the tissue in a quick, pulsed mode. The holmium wavelength is absorbed intensely by water, so the depth of penetration is limited to approximately 0.4 to 0.6 mm. It has many of the same benefits of $CO_2$ laser technology in that it can ablate tissue precisely. The difference is that it can be conducted to the target through a flexible fiber. This wavelength can be delivered to tissues in a fluid environment because it produces a vapor bubble that transmits the laser energy within a short distance. If the fiber is held almost in contact or directly in contact with the tissue, cutting occurs. If sculpting or ablating is needed, the fiber is held at a distance of approximately 2 mm from the target. Adjacent tissue is left significantly unharmed, enhancing the precision of this wavelength. If the fiber is held 5 mm from the target, no tissue response is noted. The holmium:YAG laser also is being used to produce a photoacoustical effect to fragment urinary stones and gallstones.

**ND:YAG LASER.** The Nd:YAG laser wavelength is in the near infrared region of the electromagnetic spectrum at approximately 1064 nm. This invisible wavelength usually is accompanied by a visible helium-neon beam or other colored light, such as white light, to provide an aiming source. The Nd: YAG laser consists of a solid crystal of YAG that is doped with neodymium, which produces the lasing energy when exposed to bright flash lamps.

The noncontact Nd:YAG wavelength is transmitted through clear fluids and structures and is more highly absorbed by darker tissue. This laser light tends to scatter within the tissue and cause thermal damage from approximately 3 to 5 mm. Tissue absorption produces a homogeneous coagulative effect as tissue is heated to the point of coagulation without vaporization occurring. The noncontact Nd:YAG beam can backscatter, posing an eye safety concern when used through an endoscope.

The Nd:YAG energy is delivered to the tissue through a fiber system. The core fiber, usually made of quartz, is surrounded by a polytetrafluoroethylene (Teflon) silicone coating or cladding that keeps the light in. This is known as a *bare fiber.* If the bare fiber is encased by a catheter sheath, a purge gas, air, or fluid can be conducted down the length of the fiber. This purge is used to cool the fiber tip and keep debris from accumulating.

The Nd:YAG laser wavelength can be delivered to the tissue in a noncontact mode, meaning that the fiber does not touch the tissue. If the noncontact fiber comes in contact with the tissue, any debris on the end of the fiber can cause the fiber to heat to the point of destroying the tip.

Nd:YAG laser energy also can be delivered to the tissue using the contact method. A synthetic sapphire contact probe or scalpel can be attached to the end of a fiber with a special connector to deliver the Nd:YAG laser energy directly to the tissue in a more concentrated manner. The depth of penetration from the laser energy is limited to less than 1 mm. These contact tips are available in a variety of configurations. Depending on the desired tissue effects, the appropriate contact tip is chosen. A scalpel is used to cut, and a rounded probe is used to vaporize. A flat probe may be used to coagulate tissue.

The end of the quartz fiber also may be sculpted into a configuration that can be used in direct contact with the tissue. Contact technology provides precision because the power output of the beam is confined to a small area and less wattage is needed. It causes less thermal buildup, so adjacent tissue is relatively unaffected. The beam does not scatter as readily as the noncontact Nd:YAG laser fiber energy, and less plume is generated.

Besides the continuous-mode Nd:YAG laser, a special pulsed-mode Nd:YAG laser for ophthalmic applications (class 3B laser) delivers the energy to the tissue in extremely short pulsations of nanoseconds. This laser works with an acoustic effect instead of a thermal effect. A clouded membrane behind an artificial lens implant can be ruptured quickly and painlessly with this ophthalmic Nd:YAG laser beam through the production of an acoustic effect at the target site.

**KTP LASER.** The frequency-doubled YAG laser also is popular in health care. An Nd:YAG beam of 1064 nm is passed through a potassium titanyl phosphate (KTP) crystal to produce an intense green laser light of 532 nm. This process of delivering the Nd:YAG incident beam of 1064 nm through the KTP crystal shortens the wavelength in half, to 532 nm, while doubling the beam's frequency. The emergent beam then is visible. If the original Nd:YAG beam is again desired, the crystal is rotated out of the way when a button is pressed on the control panel (if this feature is available). The aiming system of the KTP laser can be a low-power KTP laser beam or a helium-neon beam.

The 532-nm wavelength responds to tissue in the same manner as the argon beam. It is color selective and is highly absorbed by hemoglobin, melanin, and other similar pigmentation. The beam is conducted to tissue through a fiber, and this wavelength can be transmitted through clear solutions and structures. The depth of penetration is approximately 1 to 2 mm.

**ARGON LASER.** The argon laser is a popular visible laser beam system for ophthalmology, dermatology, and general applications. This laser produces an intense, visible, blue-green light of approximately 488 nm and 514.5 nm (or 457 nm and 528 nm). In clinical applications, this combination of light wavelengths allows for more complete tissue absorption. The depth of penetration is usually 1 to 2 mm. The aiming system can be a low-power argon laser beam or a helium-neon beam.

The argon energy is highly absorbed by hemoglobin, melanin, and other similar pigmentation and is less absorbed by lighter tissue. The absorbed laser energy is converted to heat to cause coagulation or vaporization. Because of the high color selectivity of the beam, adjacent tissue injury is reduced significantly when the laser is being used on a localized pigmented area.

The argon wavelength, similar to the Nd:YAG laser, is transmitted through clear fluids and structures while being delivered to the target site through a fiber system. The fiber can be attached to a slit lamp, microscope, or handpiece, depending on the surgical approach. As with other fiber-directed lasers, the argon light diverges 10 to 14 degrees when leaving the fiber. The size of the spot can be altered by changing the distance of the fiber tip from the tissue. Special handpieces that contain an internal lens can be adjusted to change the spot size of the beam for dermatology and other procedures.

**TUNABLE DYE LASER.** The tunable dye laser allows the operator to dial in the desired wavelength within a limited range of visible light (e.g., 400 to 1000 nm). By changing dyes or other certain parameters, the wavelength can be changed. Tunable dye lasers produce a range of colors by exposing a liquid dye to an intense light source, such as an argon laser beam. The dye then absorbs the laser light and fluoresces over a broad spectrum of colors. By using special crystal prisms, diffraction gratings, or birefringent filters within the laser, a specific wavelength can be produced.

Flash lamp pulsed dye lasers have become popular in treating pigmented dermatologic conditions. A yellow laser beam can be generated at 585 nm, which is readily absorbed by hemoglobin and less absorbed by the epidermal melanin, resulting in less scarring. These tunable dye lasers have been refined to provide quick pulsations in milliseconds that allow increased power to be used. Automatic scanners attached to the delivery system have been perfected for this quick pulsation while moving the beam over the target area. Less adjacent tissue damage is achieved with shorter durations of exposure, and greater tissue response occurs through the increased wattage used. Advancements to produce an array of different wavelengths with a variety of pulsation modes are continually being developed to treat dermatologic conditions successfully and fracture urinary stones or gallstones.

DIODE LASER. Because they are extremely compact and reliable, diode lasers are being used in consumer products, such as video disc players and computers. This technology also is being used for surgical lasers, with approximately 30 W of output in the 532 to 908 nm range. With the efficiency, small size, and reliability of these systems, increasing medical applications have been introduced. With the advent of the high-power semiconductor diode lasers in the gallium arsenide family (840 to 910 nm), smaller laser photocoagulators for ophthalmic, urologic, and other applications have been developed. This laser energy can be delivered directly to the tissue through a fiber or can be attached to an existing slit lamp microscope for ophthalmic applications. Other clinical applications that allow this type of laser to be used in place of other wavelengths, such as the Nd:YAG or argon lasers, are available.

EXCIMER LASER. The excimer laser wavelengths are located in the ultraviolet area (short wavelengths) of the electromagnetic spectrum. The excimer laser derives its name through the use of an active medium that is an excited dimer. This laser also is known as a rare gas-*n*-halide laser in that it combines a rare gas with a halide, usually a halide-oxide or a halide-halide dimer. The dimeric media are excited to emit the laser energy. Depending on the chemical composition of the active medium, a variety of short ultraviolet wavelengths can be produced. Four of the most popular wavelengths are argon fluoride (ArF) at 193 nm, krypton fluoride (KrF) at 248 nm, xenon chloride (XeCl) at 308 nm, and xenon fluoride (XeF) at 351 nm. One of the hazards of the excimer laser is that these gases are extremely toxic; appropriate protective laser housings have been manufactured.

Excimer lasers are popular for their significant ablative capabilities. The beam penetrates less than 1 mm into the tissue and disassociates the molecular bonds of the cells. The adjacent tissue is not significantly damaged because the beam provides a sharp, clean-cutting action at the target site without any significant thermal damage. This laser has been used successfully to sculpt corneas for refractive purposes and to ablate plaque in arteries. Excimer lasers producing wavelengths from 308 to 311 nm are being used to treat psoriasis and vitiligo. Other applications continue to be developed and researched for FDA approval.

FUTURE LASERS. As technology continues to advance, laser wavelengths are being combined into one unit so that a selection of wavelengths, such as the Nd:YAG, erbium:YAG, or holmium:YAG, can be offered easily during a procedure. The delivery systems must be compatible for this type of setup. A variety of wavelengths are being developed as other active media are being explored. New delivery systems are being perfected as different material combinations that more efficiently conduct the laser energy to the tissue are being perfected.

***Benefits of Laser Technology.*** Laser technology continues to evolve as more surgical applications are explored and introduced. Previously controversial, the laser has now become a respected and valued medical device that is advancing and refining surgical techniques. As physicians become more adept in laser applications, use continues to grow. The laser has fostered the development of new minimally invasive procedures and endoscopic techniques along with ophthalmic and dermatologic applications. The true potential of the laser has yet to be realized as health care practitioners explore different procedures that can use laser technology. Following are some advantages that have been associated with laser technology, depending on the procedure performed:

- Seals small blood vessels (less intraoperative and postoperative blood loss)
- Seals lymphatics (decreases postoperative edema and the chance of spread of malignant cells in the lymphatic system)
- Seals nerve endings (on selective procedures, decreases postoperative pain)
- Sterilizes tissue (from the heat generated at the laser tissue impact site)
- Decreases postoperative stenosis (by decreasing the amount of scarring that could lead to stenosis)
- Produces minimal tissue damage (from precision of the laser beam)
- Reduces operative and anesthesia time
- Allows a shift to more ambulatory surgery procedures
- Allows more use of local anesthesia instead of general anesthesia
- Provides quicker recovery and return to daily activities

As new laser technology is introduced and refined, perioperative nurses have the responsibility of expanding their knowledge base by keeping current with the safety requirements and operation of these systems. Laser technology is a challenge to the perioperative nurse's professional growth. As the full potential of the laser in health care is being realized, the perioperative nurse continues to play an instrumental role in the safe application of this technology.

***Laser Safety.*** Because laser systems are capable of concentrating high amounts of energy within very small areas, they present hazards. Safe and appropriate use of the laser during surgical intervention is the responsibility of the entire health care team. Each member must be acutely aware of the many controls needed to prevent accidental injury. Often the laser team member is given the responsibility and authority to shut down the laser system if safety policies are not being followed.

The laser is a class III medical device that is subdivided into four subclasses. The lasers designated as subclasses 3 and 4 have the potential to cause injury. Some ophthalmic Nd:YAG lasers that cause a photoacoustic instead of a photothermal reaction are classified in the subclass 3B category and can cause injury with sustained interaction. Most of the lasers used in surgical applications are subclass 4 lasers and can cause photothermal reactions that can lead to fire, skin burns, and optical damage by either direct or scattered radiation. Specific safety precautions must be followed to prevent injury from these laser systems.

Many agencies address the regulation of laser safety. Health care facilities must develop safety protocols in anticipation of mandates by these regulatory agencies as the technology advances and grows.

The American National Standards Institute (ANSI), a nongovernmental organization of experts, first published standards (Z136.1) in 1973 as safety guidelines for laser use in warfare, industry, and health care. Standards were expanded to provide specific recommendations for laser use in health care environments (ANSI Z136.3).[1] The appendix of ANSI Z136.3 (revised and published in 2005) discusses a consensus on laser safety in each of the special areas of medicine and surgery. These standards are reviewed periodically and revised as surgical trends change. It is recommended that the most current versions of both ANSI standards be acquired for reference because the Z136.3 document often refers to the Z136.1 publication.

Other guidelines have been suggested by the Center for Devices and Radiological Health (CDRH), Association of periOperative Registered Nurses (AORN), American Society for Laser Medicine and Surgery (ASLMS), Laser Institute of America (LIA), FDA, OSHA, and individual state and local regulatory bodies.

Hospitals and other health care delivery facilities need to create laser safety policies and procedures using these groups of experts as resources. In the development of safety guidelines for a facility, protocols should address situations individually without being too general or too specific. A policy or procedure must be general enough to address the need, but not so detailed that the surgical team cannot follow it. The staff of health care facilities must realize that they can be held liable for following their own safety policies and procedures. Basic education on the written laser policies and procedures for all personnel in the surgical environment (including orderlies, aides, and housekeeping personnel) should be mandatory within the health care facility. Policy and procedure topics can include the following:

- Eye protection
- Controlled access
- Fire safety
- Smoke (plume) evacuation
- Documentation
- Laser team responsibilities
- Skin/tissue protection
- Electrical safety
- Education/training
- Credentialing

**EYE PROTECTION.** Because the eye is extremely sensitive to laser radiation, great care must be taken to protect the eyes during laser intervention. Even low levels of laser radiation can lead to permanent optical damage. The area of possible ophthalmologic injury depends on the type of wavelength. The $CO_2$ laser can damage the cornea because this beam is absorbed readily by water within the surface cells, causing a burn. Immediate pain is associated with this corneal injury. The argon and Nd:YAG laser beams, in contrast, are transmitted through the clear optical structures and fluids and can be refocused by the lens of the eye. The intensity of the beam after refocusing can permanently damage the retina. Sometimes pain is not felt during this destruction (Figure 7-56).

Adequate eye protection requires understanding the two concepts of maximum permissible exposure (MPE) and nominal hazard zone (NHZ). According to the ANSI Z136.3 standards, the MPE is the level of laser radiation to which a person may be exposed without hazardous effects to the eye or skin. The MPE levels are determined through consideration of the laser wavelength, power, exposure time, and pulse repetition.

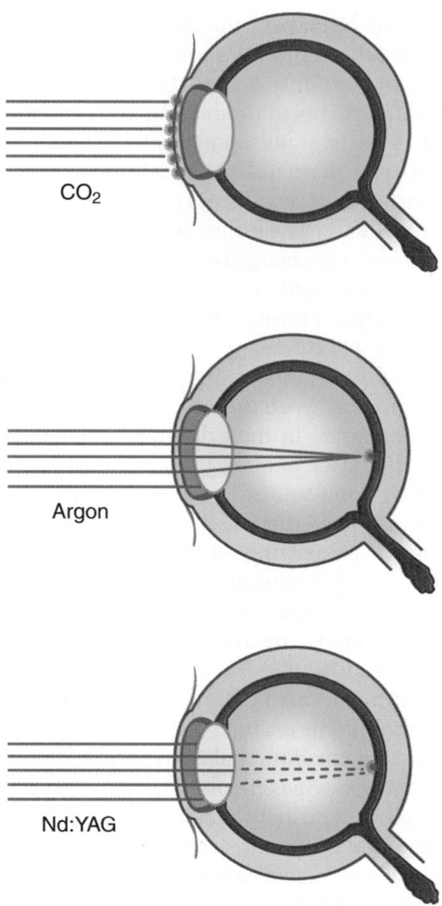


**FIGURE 7-56** The $CO_2$ laser beam can damage the cornea; the argon and Nd:YAG beams can injure the retina.

The NHZ is the space where the level of the direct, reflected, or scattered radiation during normal laser operation exceeds the MPE; eye, skin, and fire safety precautions must be followed while one is working within this hazard zone. The NHZ can be calculated mathematically to determine the distance from the laser beam emission in which the beam can cause skin and eye damage. Because the power, operating modes, and other parameters are changed frequently during a procedure, this calculation also would change. The area inside the surgical room usually is considered to be within the NHZ so that consistency and simplicity can be maintained when lasers are used in health care.

Recommendations suggest that protective goggles and glasses should be inscribed with the appropriate filtering capabilities and adequate optical densities for the specific wavelength being used. A pair of Nd:YAG goggles may be inscribed "1064 nm, optical density 4." The optical density of the lens is the capability of the lens material to absorb a specific wavelength. The darker lens shades do not have higher optical density or give more protection than the lighter ones do. Technology has introduced lighter lens shades with high optical densities that provide adequate safety. The laser team members must ensure that eyewear is properly labeled, handled, and stored so that hazards are minimized, and scratching and damage of the eyewear are avoided.

During surgical procedures using multiple wavelengths, protective eyewear must be changed as the wavelengths are changed. Some types of eyewear protect against a limited range of wavelengths. If the range is expanded to block a greater variety of wavelengths, the eyewear is more difficult to see through.

Controversy exists as to the appropriateness of using one's own prescription glasses to serve as $CO_2$ laser eye protection when the wearer is not in the immediate vicinity of the laser beam emission (e.g., the circulating nurse). Prescription eyeglasses do not have the wavelength protection inscribed on them and have not been tested to determine the protective ability of the lens; adequate protection cannot be guaranteed. Opponents state that the NHZ is so limited when the $CO_2$ beam is passed through the focusing lens that individuals who are not close to the laser emission port are not at a high risk for eye damage. Facilities must address this controversial issue and develop a policy for the surgical team to follow. Contact lenses and half glasses do not offer adequate protection against $CO_2$ laser energy.

During a microscopic procedure, the optics of the microscope provides eye protection against $CO_2$ laser energy. When other wavelengths are used, such as argon or Nd:YAG, an automatic lens shutter can be connected to the microscope head. During the laser activation, the shutter allows a lens filter to drop into place to provide a shield from any laser backscatter, protecting the eyes of the laser operator. When this device is attached to the microscope head, any observer tube being used also must be placed above the filter so that all portal optics have protection provided. Any others involved with the procedure must wear the appropriate eyewear.

A lens filter can be placed over the eyepiece of a rigid or flexible endoscope. The lens must offer the appropriate protection for the specific laser being used. Guidelines suggest that the other surgical team members also wear eye protection, even though the laser energy seems to be confined within an enclosed cavity. Optical injury is always possible if a fiber or articulated arm becomes separated from the endoscope while the laser is being activated, or if a fiber is fractured, and the beam escapes at the fracture site.

Sometimes a baseline eye examination is recommended, including visual acuity and retinal health, for health care professionals who routinely work with laser systems. Another eye examination can be performed after any ophthalmic accident or on termination of employment. The baseline examination provides a foundation for comparison with abnormal findings from subsequent examinations. Performing baseline eye examinations merely documents the ocular health of the laser team member so that it can be used during a potential Workers' Compensation claim for retinal damage from accidental beam reflection. Some facilities have opted not to follow this expensive and difficult-to-monitor guideline of performing baseline eye examinations. Instead they strictly enforce their eye safety policy, minimizing the chance of any ophthalmic accidents. These facilities usually state in an eye safety policy that an eye examination will be performed if an ocular accident occurs.

The patient's eyes also must be protected during laser intervention. When general anesthesia is used, patients should have the eyes covered with wet gauze, eye pads, or a towel; the eyelids should be taped closed. If awake or under local anesthesia, the patient should wear appropriate eye protection. Explanations regarding this safety action should be provided to the patient. If the laser is to be used in the immediate vicinity of the eye, such as to lighten a port-wine stain on the eyelid, a special laser eye shield can be placed on the surface of the eye after instillation of a drop of an ophthalmic local anesthetic. If the laser eye shields are sterilized with steam sterilization, these devices must be cooled completely before being placed on the cornea to prevent accidental burns. Box 7-4 summarizes actions to promote eye safety during laser surgery.

**CONTROLLED ACCESS.** Inadvertent access to rooms where laser treatments are being performed should be prevented. Laser warning signs must be placed at all entrances to the treatment area so that access is granted only to individuals who have been appropriately educated in laser safety. The word "Danger" and the universally accepted laser symbol should be present on any laser warning sign to indicate the possibility of hazards (Figure 7-57). Laser signs should be removed when the procedure has been completed.

Windows and ports into rooms where lasers are used must be covered with appropriate protection for the specific laser being used. The $CO_2$ laser beam that is passed through a lens and the holmium laser beam delivered through a fiber provide a limited NHZ, so window coverage is not required. Argon, Nd:YAG, and certain other laser wavelengths can be transmitted through the window glass. Windows and ports must be covered with a blocking barrier that stops the transmission of specific wavelengths with extensive NHZs.

**BOX 7-4**

### Guide to Eye Safety During Laser Surgery

- Ensure that everyone in the laser room is wearing the appropriate eye protection with side shields before activating the laser. The eyewear should have the laser wavelength protection and optical density of the lens material inscribed on it.
- Place a special lens cover over the eyepiece of an endoscope to protect the physician's eye from laser backscatter. Remember the physician's other eye is unprotected.
- Everyone in the laser room should wear eye protection during laser endoscopic procedures.
- An automatic lens shutter can be connected to a microscope head to provide eye protection for individuals viewing the procedure through the microscope.
- When general anesthesia is used, cover the patient's closed eyes with moistened gauze pads. When the patient is awake, place the appropriate glasses or goggles on the patient. Explain the need for eye protection to the patient.
- During laser surgery near the eye, place a special laser eye shield directly on the anesthetized eye surface.
- The laser team members ensure that the appropriate protective eyewear is available at all entrances to the laser room for anyone entering this area.
- Cover windows in the laser treatment area appropriately, depending on the wavelength of the laser used.
- To prevent reflection of the laser beam, special precautions must be followed (i.e., using anodized or ebonized instruments near the laser-tissue impact site, covering large reflective retractors with wet towels or sponges).
- When storing protective eyewear, guard against scratches and mishandling. Scratches on the lenses may decrease their effectiveness. The laser team members should inspect the eyewear regularly to ensure the integrity of the eyewear lenses has not been compromised.

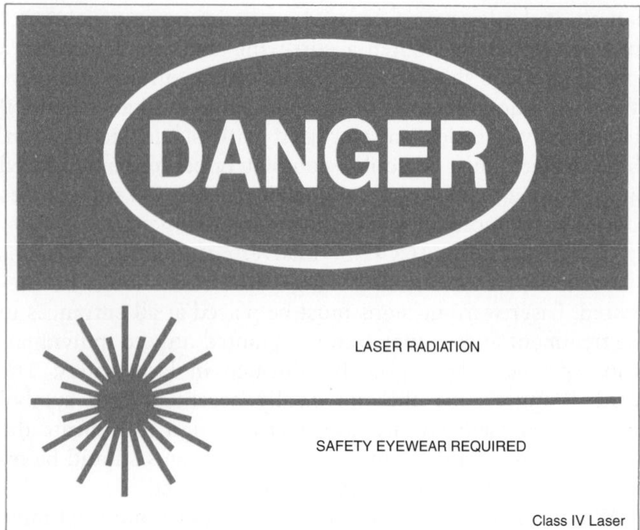


FIGURE 7-57 Warning signs should be placed at all entrances to the surgical room to notify personnel that a laser is being used, and that appropriate eye protection is needed before entering the room.

The laser key must not be left in the laser during storage. The key should be available only to authorized personnel who have the appropriate education and training to operate the laser. Laser keys can be stored in the narcotics cabinet or in a special key lockbox to control access. Box 7-5 summarizes actions that should be initiated to control access to laser rooms.

**FIRE SAFETY.** An awareness of laser biophysics and tissue interaction is necessary to understand the actions needed to prevent laser fires. A fire can be started by a reflected beam as easily as from a direct impact. The laser team must be able to respond quickly if a fire occurs. Immediate action is the key to minimize injury to the patient and the surgical team. Box 7-6 summarizes important measures to support fire safety during laser surgery.

Sterile water or saline solution should be readily available to douse a small fire on the patient. A laser-appropriate fire extinguisher, such as a halon fire extinguisher, should be available to control a fire within the laser system. During the surgical intervention, combustibles, such as sponges or towels, near the laser tissue impact site should be kept wet to prevent ignition. The surgical team should monitor constantly the moisture level of the sponges and other materials to prevent drying, which eventually could support a fire.

A laser beam can ignite flammable draping material easily. Some water-repellent drapes and other laser-safe materials are able to withstand laser impact, and the flammability of the material is decreased. If the restrictions of draping material or any other supplies are questionable, such as plastic tooth protectors, the item can be tested for flammability in the manufacturer's or researcher's laboratory.

Instrumentation used in the immediate vicinity of the laser tissue impact site should be nonreflective to decrease the chance of the laser beam bouncing off the surface and accidentally impacting another area. The laser beam can easily be reflected off shiny instrument surfaces and can cause skin or eye injury or ignite flammable materials. An instrument may be ebonized by coating the instrument with a special substance (usually black) to decrease reflectivity during laser use. Many

BOX 7-5

### Guide to Controlled Access During Laser Surgery

- Laser warning signs are posted at all entrances to the laser room to prevent unauthorized individuals from entering.
- Ideally the warning sign should include the word *Danger* along with the universal laser symbol.
- Windows or ports must be covered with the appropriate protection for the specific laser wavelength being used.
- The laser key is not stored in the laser ignition port. The laser key must be available only to authorized individuals.

BOX 7-6

### Guide to Fire Safety During Laser Surgery

- Have sterile water or saline immediately available to douse a small fire near or on the patient.
- Have a laser-appropriate fire extinguisher available in the department in case the laser catches fire. Surgical team members must understand the operation of the fire extinguisher.
- Do not place fluids or solutions on the laser unit. The laser system should be protected from spillage or splatter, which could cause short-circuiting and fire.
- Do not place dry combustibles in the vicinity of the laser impact site. Use wet towels, nonflammable drapes, or special laser-retardant materials near the laser target area. Moisten dry drapes and sponges with sterile saline or water to prevent ignition. Monitor the moisture level constantly throughout the procedure. Remoisten as needed.
- Do not use flammable materials near the laser tissue impact site.
- Use nonreflective instrumentation in or near the laser tissue impact site to decrease accidental direct reflection of the laser beam. Cover larger instruments, such as retractors, with wet sponges or towels to protect against reflection.
- Do not use flammable skin preparations, such as alcohol, as prepping solutions.
- A wet pack may be inserted into the rectum as a tamponade to prevent methane gas from escaping into the surgical area. A cleansing bowel prep before surgery also decreases this risk.
- Use appropriate laser-resistant endotracheal tubes during upper airway surgery. Follow the directions in the product literature and on the labels, which typically include information regarding the tube's laser resistance, use of dyes in the cuff to indicate a puncture, use of a saline fill to prevent cuff ignition, and immediate replacement of the tube if the cuff becomes punctured.
- Protect the endotracheal tube cuff with wet gauze sponges.
- Use nonexplosive anesthesia gases during laser procedures.
- Keep oxygen concentrations between 21% and 30% to minimize the possibility of an airway fire during laser procedures of the airway.
- Nitrous oxide supports combustion and should not be used.
- Place the laser in the standby mode when it is not in active use.
- The laser foot pedal is identified to the operating physician to avoid accidental activation. Allow only the individual using the laser to activate it. The laser should be activated only when the tip is under this individual's direct vision.

companies offer this service at a low cost. The instrument should be inspected regularly to ensure the integrity of the coating. Any scratched surface or area where the ebonization has worn off should be recoated as needed.

An instrument also may be anodized or surfaced with a matte finish to decrease reflectivity. Other coatings and surfaces that cause the laser light to scatter and diffuse on impact are being introduced. Larger retractors can be covered with wet sponges or towels so that the laser beam cannot be accidentally reflected off the shiny surface.

Special instruments have been designed to provide backstops for laser energy to decrease adjacent tissue damage and the chance of fire. Titanium rods are effective backstops and can be reprocessed easily. Quartz rods often are used as backstops for the $CO_2$ laser beam, but argon and Nd:YAG beams may be transmitted through them. Glass rods must never be used with a $CO_2$ laser because the glass material heats and shatters after continuous impact by the laser beam. Teflon backstops should not be used because they can melt when heated and produce toxic fumes. Wet sponges also can be used as backstop material.

Special laser mirrors that directly reflect the beam onto a hard-to-reach area have been introduced. Mirrors may be made of rhodium or stainless steel. Glass-surface mirrors do not withstand laser impact and heat and shatter instead. Using a laser mirror requires skill because the beam must be focused on the target area and not on the mirror to deliver the full impact of the laser energy. A laser beam that is misdirected off a mirror can easily cause a fire.

Flammable skin preparations should not be used for laser procedures. During skin cleansing, the prep solution can pool underneath a patient, and ethanol vapors from alcohol-based preparations can become trapped beneath the drapes. The volatility of these vapors increases the risk of a surgical drape fire. Iodophor or any other tinted prep solution should be rinsed before argon or Nd:YAG lasers are used because the tint unexpectedly may increase laser absorption by the skin.

When a laser is used in the rectal area, a wet pack may be used to tampon the methane gas, which could enter the surgical area from the colon and cause an explosion. The wet sponges used for the pack must be counted so that the packing is not inadvertently left in place after the surgery is completed. Some practitioners disagree with this practice, stating that the wet sponges cause stretching of the colonic tissue, increasing peristalsis and the movement of methane gas into the surgical area. Whatever method is chosen, a cleansing bowel preparation before surgery also helps to decrease this potential hazard.

Airway explosion caused by the laser beam igniting the endotracheal tube can cause a potentially lethal accident for the patient. A polyvinyl chloride (PVC) endotracheal tube is highly flammable, especially when a high concentration of oxygen flows through it during anesthesia administration (Figure 7-58). Specific laser-retardant endotracheal tubes should be used during oral, tracheal, or esophageal laser procedures that require general anesthesia. The laser power limitations of a commercially prepared endotracheal tube must be followed closely to ensure proper performance of the protective material. The cuff of the endotracheal tube should be inflated with sterile saline to provide a heat sink and retard a fire if perforated by the laser beam. Saline may be tinted with methylene blue to note a cuff rupture more quickly by the presence of the blue dye escaping. A protocol should be developed to describe the emergency procedure steps needed to control an endotracheal fire. Immediate considerations include the following:

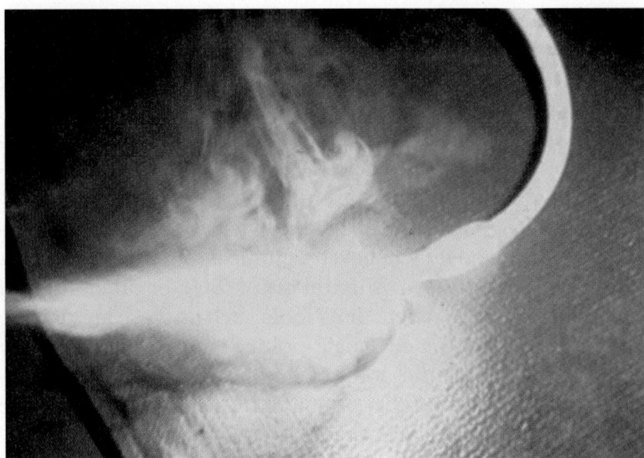

**FIGURE 7-58** A polyvinyl chloride endotracheal tube can become a blowtorch if ignited by a laser beam.

- Stop ventilation (disconnect the gas flow).
- Extinguish all flames with saline if needed.
- Remove the endotracheal tube, ensuring the entire tube is removed.
- Ventilate the patient by mask or reintubate immediately to prevent laryngospasm.
- Examine the airway (mouth, oral cavity, bronchial tree) for burns or foreign bodies or both.
- Decide on the next course of action (by the anesthesia provider and surgeon):
  - Cancel the procedure.
  - Continue with the procedure.

A nonintubation technique involving jet ventilation also may be used during a laser microlaryngoscopy. A jet ventilator is a mechanical ventilation unit that delivers the anesthetic gases through a small metal needle used with a rigid laryngoscope. Under pressurization, the jet ventilator is set to deliver a determined amount of anesthesia gas while setting the rate, pressure (in pounds per square inch [psi]), and percentage of inspiratory time. The needle is positioned between the vocal cords on the side opposite the lesion. The needle extends into the trachea so that the proper amount of anesthesia gas can be delivered easily. After the surgery, the patient may be intubated to maintain an open airway if postoperative edema or tracheal spasm is anticipated.

Other nonintubation techniques, such as apneic methods, can be used to avoid intubation. The patient's oxygen saturation must be monitored closely when these techniques are used.

**ENDOSCOPE SAFETY.** Special precautions should be followed when using the laser during an endoscopic procedure. When a laser fiber is introduced through the biopsy port of a flexible or rigid endoscope, the operator must view at least 1 cm of the tip of the fiber before activating the laser (Figure 7-59).[7] If the end of the fiber is still within the sheath of the endoscope and the laser is fired, the heat from the laser energy quickly damages the optics and channel of the endoscope.

When a "bare" fiber is placed down the biopsy channel of a flexible endoscope, the sharp tip possibly can tear the inside lumen of the channel. A length of medical-grade tubing can be placed over the fiber with the tip recessed within the sheath. The entire unit is passed through the endoscope. When the end of the tubing is observed, the medical-grade tubing is withdrawn sufficiently to expose the end of the fiber. This procedure effectively protects the inside lumen of the endoscope channel during fiber insertion.

**SMOKE EVACUATION.** Smoke evacuation and odor control must be adequate whenever a plume is generated, whether it is from the laser, electrosurgical unit (ESU), or other surgical devices being used. When "hot" tools such as these are used to cut, excise, ablate, or coagulate tissue, the cells of the target tissue are heated to the point of boiling. This causes the cellular membranes to rupture, spewing the cell contents into the air and producing surgical smoke (Box 7-7).

One of the most crucial elements in providing adequate smoke evacuation is determining the method of smoke evacuation needed. A variety of choices are available depending on the amount of plume produced.

An *in-line smoke evacuation filter* is appropriate only when small amounts of plume are generated, similar to what is produced during a microlaryngoscopy vaporization of vocal cord polyps. The in-line filter is connected to the existing suction line by positioning it between the wall connection and the suction canister (Figure 7-60). If the filter gets wet from placing it between the patient and the suction canister, it loses its effectiveness.

If an in-line plume filter is not used, the particulate matter from the surgical smoke can occlude and corrode the suction pipes and contaminate the building. Also the suction flow may not be forceful enough to capture the plume adequately. Wall suction usually generates 2 cubic feet per minute (cfm) of air movement, whereas an individual smoke evacuator may move air at 35 to 50 cfm. Usually an in-line filter is changed after each procedure or according to the manufacturer's instructions.

When greater amounts of surgical smoke are generated, an *individual smoke evacuator* is used. Individual smoke evacuators today have a filtration system that includes a charcoal filter and an ultra-low penetration air (ULPA) filter (Figure 7-61). The charcoal filter removes the toxic gases and odor, whereas the ULPA filter removes the small particulate with filtration of 0.01 μ-size matter at 99.9999% efficiency.[4]

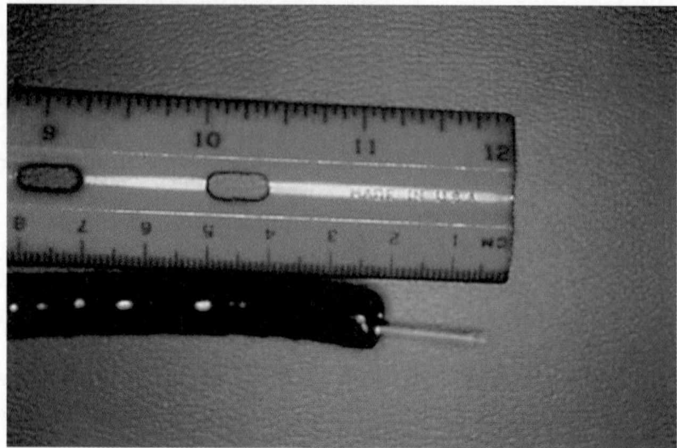

FIGURE 7-59 The laser fiber should extend past the end of the endoscope before the laser is activated.

Maintenance of a smoke evacuator involves changing the filter per the manufacturer's written instructions. Protective gloves and clean technique should be used when discarding a contaminated filter because this is an occupational hazard. Usually the used filter can be placed in a plastic disposal bag and discarded in the general waste receptacle. Some practitioners believe that a contaminated filter need not be treated as infectious or as regulated medical waste (biohazardous) because it is not listed as an environmental hazard. Some manufacturers have provided contaminated filter disposal guidelines, however, that suggest the filter be treated as biohazardous. A contaminated filter is an occupational hazard; gloves should be worn when handling it, but it is not designated as an environmental hazard, so it really does not need to be treated as biohazardous medical waste.[4]

Centralized smoke evacuation systems have been designed to provide smoke evacuation for several surgical rooms at the same time. The smoke evacuation line needs to be routinely flushed and cleaned to prevent debris buildup and pathogen growth within the system. This type of system is convenient because it is always available, but if the central system malfunctions or breaks down, smoke evacuation is not available to multiple surgical areas.

Contamination by the surgical plume and tissue splatter is decreased when the surgical team wears gloves, gowns, and masks. The surgical team must ensure that the smoke evacuation wand or suction device is close to the target site so that all plume is evacuated. Devices are available that attach or are

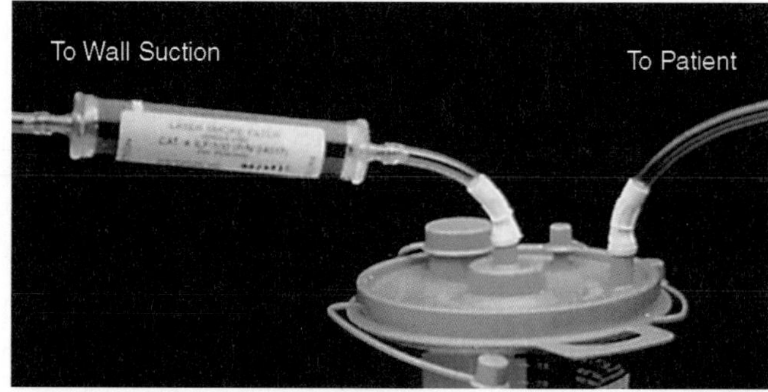


FIGURE 7-60 An in-line filter is placed between the suction canister and the wall outlet and is used to evacuate small amounts of surgical smoke.

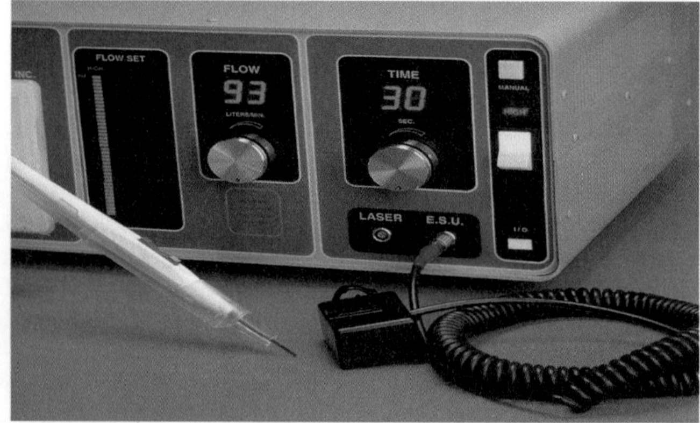


FIGURE 7-61 Individual smoke evacuator.

BOX 7-7

## Concerns About Surgical Smoke and Its Chemical By-Products: A Review

**1975**
Mihashi and associates vaporized tissue with a $CO_2$ laser in a laboratory setting to note the size of the particles within the smoke. Their results determined that approximately 77% of the particulate matter in the plume was less than 1.1 μ in size. *Note:* A regular surgical mask may filter particulate matter that is 5 μ in size; surgical smoke can pass easily through these masks and be deposited in the alveoli of lungs when inhaled. This potentially can cause chronic irritation, bronchitis, or emphysema-like or allergic-like conditions.

**1985**
The National Institute for Occupational Safety and Health (NIOSH) published and distributed a Health Hazard Evaluation Report, which stated there is "potential hazard from exposure to smoke generated by electrosurgery knives."

**1988**
The NIOSH issued a Health Hazard Evaluation Report, which stated "smoke generated during laser surgery presents a potential health hazard."

**1988**
Baggish and associates conducted research to compare the effects of unfiltered laser smoke on rat lungs with plume that had been filtered. The rats breathing in unfiltered plume developed hypoxia and pulmonary congestion with bronchial hyperplasia and hypertrophy. The rats subjected to plume that was filtered down to 0.1 μ in size (similar to smoke evacuators) developed no lesions and remained identical to the control rats.

**1988**
Garden's research team used the $CO_2$ laser to vaporize bovine fibropapillomavirus. Intact viral DNA was extracted from the plume that was emitted. The viral DNA material was injected back into the cow at another site, and the same papilloma viral lesion grew again. This significant study showed that viral DNA can cause viral growth in the host if the transmission mode is through injection.

**1989**
Tomita and associates compared the hazards of cigarette smoke with the hazards associated with laser and electrosurgery smoke. Results noted that the $CO_2$ laser vaporization generated a plume that had the same hazard potential as smoking three unfiltered cigarettes. The ESU created a plume that was equivalent to smoking six unfiltered cigarettes.

**1991**
A report described a 44-year-old surgeon in Norway who developed laryngeal papillomatosis, probably at the workplace where he used the laser to vaporize condylomas. The surgeon's own laryngeal biopsy report revealed human papillomavirus DNA types consistent with the anogenital condylomas that were being lased on his patients.

**1993**
Ott and his team showed that when surgical smoke is not evacuated during a laparoscopic procedure, the patient's methemoglobin and carboxyhemoglobin increase, while oxygenation of the tissues decreases. The patient usually responds to this problem with nausea, vomiting, or headaches.

**1995**
Hoglan's analysis indicates that perhaps more than 600 more compounds within surgical smoke have yet to be identified.

There are four issues of concern associated with the hazards of surgical smoke:

- Odor
- Size of the particulate matter
- Viability of the particulate matter
- Endoscopy concerns

When surgical smoke is generated, a noxious odor is emitted with the smoke. This odor results from tissue destruction that produces chemical by-products and toxins. Some of these chemical by-products already have been identified as toxic carcinogens, such as polycyclic aromatic hydrocarbons, benzene, toluene, formaldehyde, and acrolein. The question of whether the particulate within surgical smoke is viable has yet to be conclusively proven. Further studies are needed to note if inhalation of surgical smoke containing viral DNA can be transmitted and lead to regrowth. Nonetheless, surgical smoke continues to be recognized as being hazardous as the results of more research studies are published. The following professional organizations, agencies, and research groups have consistently recommended guidelines and statements regarding these hazards and how to minimize them:

- ANSI Z136.3 "Safe Use of Lasers in Healthcare Facilities," 2005
- NIOSH, *Control of Smoke From Laser/Electric Surgical Procedures,* March 1998.
- AORN "Recommended Practices for Laser Safety in Practice Settings," 2005
- ASLMS
- OSHA

Modified from Baggish M and others: Protection of the rat lung from the harmful effects of laser smoke, *Lasers in Surgery and Medicine* 8:248-253, 1988; Garden J and others: Papillomavirus in the vapor of carbon dioxide laser-treated verrucae, *Journal of the American Medical Association* 259:1199-1202, 1988; Hallmo P, Naess O: Laryngeal papillomatosis with human papillomavirus DNA contracted by a laser surgeon, *European Archives of Otorhinolaryngology* 248(7):425-427, 1991; Hoglan M: Potential hazards from electrosurgical plume, *Canadian Operating Room Nursing Journal* 13:10-16, 1995; NIOSH: *Health Hazard Evaluation Report,* Washington, DC, 1985, The Institute; Mihashi S and others: *Some problems about condensates induced by $CO_2$ laser irradiation,* Karume, Japan, 1975, Department of Otolaryngology and Public Health, Karume University; NIOSH: *Health Hazard Evaluation Report,* Washington, DC, 1988, The Institute; Ott D: Smoke production and smoke reduction in endoscopic surgery: preliminary report, *Endoscopic Surgery and Allied Technologies* 1:230-232, 1993; Tomita Y and others: Mutagenicity of smoke condensates induced by $CO_2$ laser irradiation and electrocauterization, *Mutation Research* 89:145-149, 1981.

built into the electrosurgery or laser delivery system that effectively evacuate the surgical smoke as it is being generated (Figure 7-62). Using an appropriate smoke evacuation method to ensure that all plume is eliminated is the only practice that protects the surgical team members from continual exposure to the hazards of surgical smoke. Box 7-8 highlights practices for effective smoke evacuation.

The presence of surgical smoke during flexible endoscopic procedures or laparoscopic applications causes visibility problems. Hand control suction devices and valve filters have been

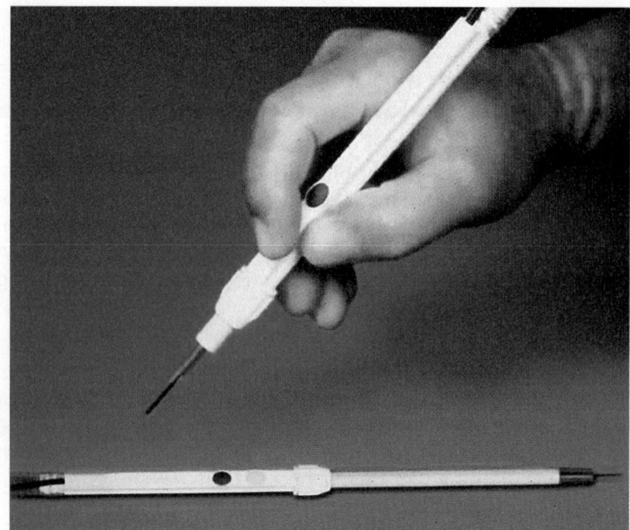

FIGURE 7-62 Electrosurgery pencil with the smoke evacuation system built into the device.

designed to provide a gentle movement of the plume during a laparoscopic procedure without destroying the pneumoperitoneum. A high-flow insufflator also is recommended for a continual replacement of the $CO_2$ gas. A special smoke evacuator also may be used that automatically provides a slow evacuation of the smoke when plume is generated.

**OTHER SAFETY MEASURES.** Foot pedals also can present safety problems if mistakenly activated. The number of foot pedals placed on the floor for the physician often can be confusing and can easily lead to accidents. The laser pedal should be identified clearly for the physician and should be used by only the physician who is delivering the laser energy to the target area.

Laser team members should appreciate the potential for electrical hazards because the laser, similar to the ESU, is a high-voltage piece of equipment. Water and other solutions should not be placed on the laser unit, and the components of the laser should be protected against spillage or splatter, which could cause short-circuiting. The outside housing of the laser should never be removed by unauthorized personnel because the potential for electrical shock or electrocution is high.

Transportation hazards are always a threat because some systems are quite heavy. When these units need to be moved from one area to another, proper body mechanics must be employed to prevent injury to the transporter. The laser unit should be pushed instead of pulled to provide less stress on the transporter's back muscles. The laser should never be bumped against a wall because the internal components can be damaged or thrown out of alignment.

**DOCUMENTATION.** Closely following written laser safety procedures is crucial for safety and medicolegal reasons, as with any potentially hazardous piece of equipment. Specific notes about laser safety can be written on a laser log form or as part of the existing intraoperative nursing notes. Either record should be placed on the patient's chart so that safety activities that were performed can be recorded. Often safety measures are not specifically documented if listed in the facility's policies and procedures.

BOX 7-8

### Guide to Smoke Evacuation During Laser Surgery

- Use the appropriate smoke evacuation system depending on the amount of plume generated. If small amounts of plume are generated and room suction is to be used, an in-line suction filter is positioned between the suction canister and the wall outlet to capture the surgical smoke particulate. An individual smoke evacuation system is used if larger amounts of plume are generated.
- Change the smoke evacuation filter or filters according to the manufacturer's written instructions.
- Hold the smoke evacuation suction tube close (<1 inch away) to the tissue interaction site to remove as much plume (odor and particulate matter) as possible.
- Smoke evacuation tubing should have a smooth inner lumen to eliminate any whistling noise.
- Use a reducer fitting to adapt a large smoke evacuation tube to a smaller suction or evacuation tube.
- The scrub person or first assistant can operate the smoke evacuation foot pedal (if available) to minimize the wear and tear on the smoke evacuator motor and to decrease noise. Some smoke evacuators have sensing mechanisms that automatically activate the smoke evacuator when plume is generated.
- Evacuate surgical smoke generated during endoscopic or laparoscopic procedures. Endoscopic smoke evacuation instruments, such as suction tubes, help decrease the presence and retention of plume inside a body cavity or organ. A low-pressure suction valve can be used to remove plume gently during a laparoscopic procedure without destroying the pneumoperitoneum. A high-flow insufflator is recommended to replace any lost insufflation gas quickly. A special smoke evacuator that provides automatic plume removal also can be used to evacuate the intraabdominal smoke.
- Wear a surgical mask that provides adequate filtration (0.1 μ filtration) to protect against any residual smoke particulate matter that has not been evacuated. The high-filtration mask must fit snugly around the face. Wearing a high-filtration mask does not replace the need to use a smoke evacuation system to remove the surgical smoke from the environment.
- Continuing education helps health care personnel understand the hazards of surgical smoke and encourages the use of appropriate methods for evacuation.

Modified from AORN: *AORN standards, recommended practices and guidelines,* Denver, Colo, 2005, The Association; Ball KA: *Lasers: the perioperative challenge,* ed 3, Denver, Colo, 2004, AORN.

A special laser log can be designed to be a permanent part of the patient's record and could include information such as the laser used, power, pulse duration, and other laser parameters. The use of smoke evacuation, fibers, and contact tips also may be documented, especially if specific charges for these items are made. A sample laser log is shown in Box 7-9.

**ROLE OF THE LASER TEAM MEMBER.** As the popularity of laser technology continues to grow, the role of the laser team member becomes increasingly important. The backbone of a progressive and successful laser program is the enthusiastic and dedicated laser team. Expanded responsibilities are being assumed by the laser team member to provide consistency and promote a safe environment for the patient and the surgical team. Some of the roles of the laser team member may

BOX 7-9

### Sample Laser Log

Date ____________________ OR Room No. __________

**PATIENT INFORMATION:**
Name ____________________ Patient ID No. __________
Zip Code ____________________ Sex: M F Age __________
Status: IP OP

**SURGERY INFORMATION:**
Physician __________ Anesthesia: General MAC Local
Procedure ____________________

**LASER INFORMATION:**
Laser and wavelength____________________
Power __________ Duration __________
Total spots __________ Total energy __________
Laser time on __________ Laser time off __________

**DELIVERY SYSTEM:**
Laser fiber ____________________
Contact tip ____________________
Microscope handpiece ____________________

**LASER SAFETY:**
Eye protection____________________
Smoke evacuation ____________________
Fire safety____________________
Other safety measures ____________________
____________________

**COMMENTS:**
____________________
____________________
Laser team member ____________________

include becoming the laser safety officer, serving on the laser committee, becoming actively involved with laser procurement, and promoting the laser program through marketing.

Perioperative nurses who are part of the laser team often are involved with patient education. The perioperative nurse reinforces what the physician has described to the patient before the laser procedure. When told that surgery is needed, the patient is often anxious because of the unknown. When it is mentioned that laser surgery is needed, the anxiety may be compounded because the patient is confronted with two alarming unknowns. Many patients develop an uneasiness about laser procedures based on information from science-fiction movies, talk shows, and other such sources. The patient always should have the opportunity to discuss the laser procedure to allay any worries. The perioperative nurse may provide additional information if the patient has any further questions about laser technology. After the physician has explained the procedure, the surgical consent is signed by the patient. Sometimes the consent form reflects that a laser will be used during the surgical experience. Some physicians have noted that a laser is merely a tool used during the surgical intervention and do not believe it is necessary to list the laser use on the consent form.

An adequate amount of time should be allotted for patient questions before the procedure. If local anesthesia is used, the patient should understand what to anticipate during the surgery, what sounds or odors will be present, why eye protection is needed, and what the patient's role is during the procedure. If the patient understands the application, the role of the laser, and his or her responsibility during and after the procedure, the perioperative nurse can expect better compliance and diminished anxiety in the patient.

Discharge instructions are required for any ambulatory procedure; laser discharge instructions may be preprinted for each surgical application. These written instructions should be reviewed and given to the patient on discharge. A follow-up phone call helps the perioperative nurse evaluate the care delivered during the laser intervention and the patient's compliance with the postoperative instructions.

Sometimes the perioperative nurse is placed in a compromising position by being expected to circulate during the surgical procedure and operate the laser. This nurse has the tremendous responsibility of being accountable for two crucial roles in the OR; the risk of a laser incident may be increased. In the traditional setting, one nurse circulates while another nurse or a technologist, who is part of the laser team, operates the laser. The health care facility must determine what procedures require more staffing to handle each perioperative nursing role.

## Electrosurgery

Electrosurgical devices have been popular for many years to cut and coagulate tissue (Box 7-10), but this energy also has been associated with numerous patient injuries and accidents. The same procedures used to prevent fires and to evacuate surgical smoke for laser surgery are needed when electrosurgery is performed. (See the laser safety section in this chapter for detailed information.) Education is vital to ensure the safe use of electrosurgery by understanding the principles and actions of this surgical energy.

***Physics of Electrosurgery.*** The basic principles of electricity must be understood to comprehend how an ESU works. Electricity involves the motion of subatomic particles that behave

BOX 7-10

### History of Electrosurgery

Around 1926 Dr. Harvey Cushing, a neurosurgeon, and Dr. William T. Bovie, a biophysical engineer, combined their talents and knowledge to develop electrosurgical technology for use during neurosurgical procedures. In 1928, they published a series of 500 neurosurgical procedures performed using an electrical device developed by Bovie. This primitive electrosurgical tool provided hemostasis for surgery in highly vascular areas. The first commercial ESU was produced in the early 1930s. The unit stood chest high, weighed about 300 lb, and was set in a beautifully crafted wooden cabinet. In the third edition (1958) of *Alexander's Care of the Patient in Surgery,* it was noted, "Electrocoagulation has become an essential part of the neurosurgical setup. The nursing personnel must understand the construction of the machine before attempting to regulate it and they must carry out proper safety measures." Electrosurgery began to gain acceptance as the benefits of tissue coagulation producing a drier surgical field became recognized by many surgical disciplines and remains one of the most important and basic surgical modalities used in operative and other invasive procedures.

in a consistent and predictable manner. Electrons are negatively charged and orbit the nucleus of an atom. As electrons jump from one atom to the orbit of another, an electrical current is generated.

Three terms help to describe the properties of electricity—current, voltage, and impedance. *Current* is the flow of electrons measured in amperes. *Voltage* is the force or push that moves the electrons from one atom to another and is measured in volts. *Impedance* is the opposition to the flow of current (electrons) and is measured in ohms.[17] As electrons encounter impedance, heat is produced, and a tissue effect results. These terms can be compared with terms related to the cardiovascular system, with current being compared with the cardiac output, voltage being compared with the movement of blood through the circulatory system, and resistance being compared with the internal lumen size of the vessels in the cardiovascular system.

One characteristic of electricity is that it must have a complete circuit or pathway so that the electrons can flow. That is, if an electrical current originates from earth, the electricity must be returned to ground to complete the circuit. Two forms of electrical current are used today—direct current (DC) and alternating current (AC). With DC, the electrons flow in only one direction, whereas with AC, the electrons flow back and forth as the polarity changes. During electrosurgery, the AC enters the patient's body, causing the patient to become part of the circuit as the energy is returned to the source of the energy.

Electrocautery often is misused as a reference for electrosurgery. Electrocautery devices use DC because electrons flow in one direction through a wire. The wire provides resistance, heating up. As the hot wire is held in contact with tissue, coagulation results. Electrocautery units are usually battery-operated, such as the small disposable units used during ophthalmic procedures to coagulate small blood vessels.

Frequency is the number of waves passing through a given point over a specified time. This is measured in hertz (Hz) or cycles per second. Electrosurgical systems operate at frequencies greater than 100,000 Hz, which also is the frequency at which nerve and muscle stimulation ceases. In comparison, the electrical current in a normal household wall outlet in the United States alternates at 60 cycles per second, or 60 Hz. An ESU generator takes the 60-cycle current and increases the frequency to greater than 200,000 Hz so that it can be passed through the patient's body without muscle or nerve stimulation and without the risk of electrocution (Figure 7-63).

***Electrosurgical Modes.*** The two modes used for electrosurgery are *monopolar* and *bipolar.* Electrosurgical instruments provide cutting and coagulating abilities by using monopolar or bipolar modes.

In a monopolar electrosurgery system, the electrical energy flows from the generator through an active electrode to the patient (Figure 7-64). If the energy is concentrated in a small area, and the tissue provides increased impedance, controlled heat is generated, and cutting or coagulation is achieved. The electrical energy passes through the patient to a dispersive electrode (pad) or patient return electrode (PRE) placed on the patient's body. The dispersive electrode surface area is larger so that the energy is not concentrated enough to generate significant heat. The energy is then returned to the generator as the circuit is completed. If the dispersive electrode is tented, or only a small part of the pad is in contact with the patient's body, the electrical energy becomes concentrated, and a burn can result. Monopolar electrosurgery includes the patient to complete the electrical circuit and is the most common mode of electrosurgery used today.

In a bipolar system, a dispersive electrode is not needed because the electrical energy flows from one tine (or prong or blade) of the bipolar instrument to the other tine as it passes through the tissue located between these tines (Figure 7-65). The energy is returned directly through the instrument to the generator to complete the circuit, eliminating the flow of current through the patient's body. During bipolar electrosurgery, the flow of electricity is stopped if a certain impedance level is reached. This is frequently 100 ohms but may be different for the various types of bipolar generators available today. Although the ESU seems to be activated because an audible sound is heard while the pedal is depressed, the flow of current is significantly decreased when the specified impedance is met. Impedance meters (or ammeters) are often used today to alert the physician when tissue desiccation is occurring or when complete desiccation has been achieved.

***Tissue Effects.*** As electrosurgery variables change, different tissue effects can be achieved. The electrosurgery variables include the following:

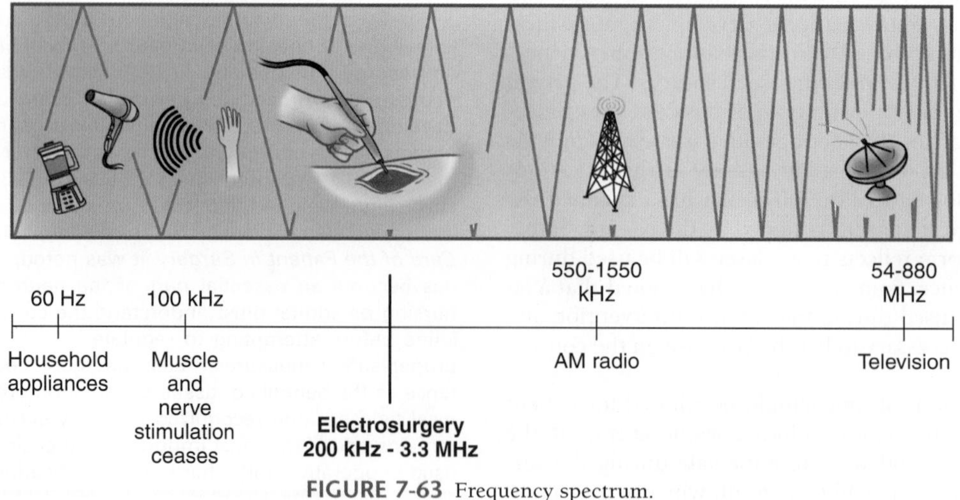


**FIGURE 7-63** Frequency spectrum.

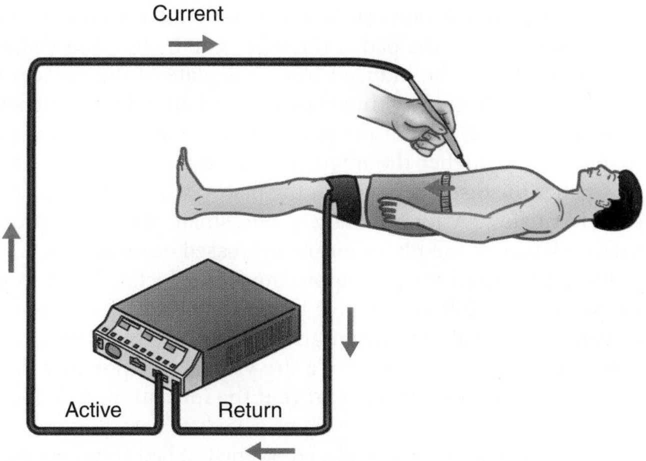

FIGURE 7-64 Monopolar electrosurgical circuit.

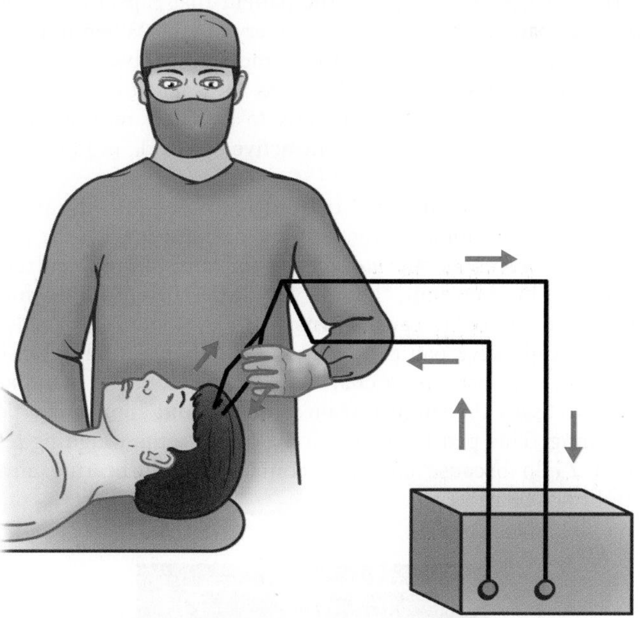
FIGURE 7-65 Bipolar electrosurgical circuit.

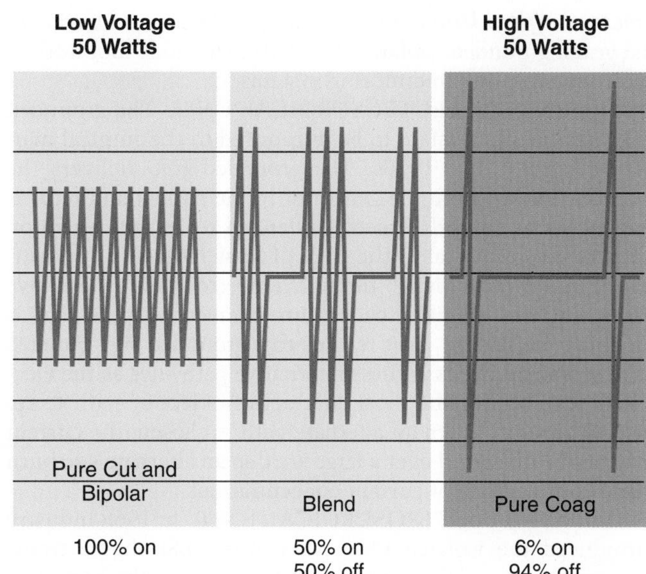

FIGURE 7-66 Electrosurgery waveforms: typical examples.

- Waveform
- Power setting
- Length of exposure
- Active electrode size
- Type of tissue
- Eschar presence

As the waveform changes, so does the tissue effect. Waveforms can range from pure cut to pure coagulation. To produce a pure-cut mode, the generator must be on a 100% duty cycle, meaning that the electrical flow is continually being applied, and heat is quickly being generated for cutting and tissue vaporization (Figure 7-66). The frequency is high, but the voltage is low. Because less force is being used to push the current, the cut mode may be considered safer than the other modes. As the cut mode produces a constant bombardment of electrons on the tissue, heat is produced, cells are ruptured, and the tissue is cut. For maximum activity, the active electrode used to deliver the current should be held slightly above the tissue so that the electrons have to jump through the impedance of the air to reach the target site. This generates even more heat. Most of the heat dissipates as steam as tissue cells are vaporized.

In a pure coagulation mode, the frequency is decreased, but the voltage is increased. The duty cycle is on only about 6% of the time, leaving 94% of the time with no flow of electrons to the surgical site (see Figure 7-66). To compensate for this "off" duty cycle, the voltage, or force of the push, must be increased to produce the desired wattage setting. During coagulation, this intermittent delivery of electrons causes the cells to heat up and then cool, producing a coagulative effect. Higher voltage allows the active electrode to be held over the area while a fulguration or spraying effect delivers the electrical energy to coagulate a larger area. The tissue effect is superficial, collapsing the cells and producing a coagulum.

Most ESUs have a blend mode that allows the operator to achieve differing levels of simultaneous coagulation in the cut mode. Increasing the voltage and decreasing the duty cycle provide increased coagulation effects (see Figure 7-66).

The power setting also influences the tissue effect. Higher power settings produce more extensive tissue effects. Long activation of electrical current increases the thermal effects in the tissue. Thermal energy can spread from the target site, causing damage to adjacent tissue. Smaller active electrodes concentrate the electrical energy and require lower power settings; larger electrodes disperse the electrical energy and require higher power settings.

Tissue type also influences the tissue effect. Tissue, such as adipose tissue, that is not well vascularized offers more impedance. As a result, electrical energy is not conducted well, and higher power settings may be required. Muscle tissue is well vascularized and requires less power to achieve a tissue effect. Eschar is less conductive and impedes the flow of electrons, requiring more power to be used to achieve the desired tissue effect. Electrosurgical tips on the active electrode must be kept clean and free from debris to function properly. Electrode tips with nonstick coating make removal of eschar easier.

***Electrosurgical Units.*** Four types of ESUs have evolved over the years: grounded, isolated, dispersive electrode monitoring, and tissue response monitoring systems.

**GROUNDED ELECTROSURGICAL UNIT.** The grounded ESU was the first system to be introduced to the surgical market during the late 1920s. The grounded ESU delivers the electrical energy from the generator to the patient and returns the energy to ground, which is intended to be the generator. Because electricity takes the path of least resistance, the current can flow or divide through any grounded alternative paths, such as an ECG pad or an intravenous pole that is touching the patient, as it returns to a grounded site. Patients have sustained burns at these alternative path sites as the electricity searches for the most conductive object or path to return to ground. When an alternate path is chosen, the current may not be dispersed over a large area, so an alternate site burn may result because of current concentration.

**ISOLATED ELECTROSURGICAL UNIT.** In 1968 industry introduced the isolated ESU. An isolated ESU has a transformer that causes the current to return only to the generator and not use alternate pathways to return to its source. The current flows through the patient's body and must return to the generator to complete the circuit. If this is not possible, the generator shuts down, adding to the safety of this type of unit. An isolated ESU prevents alternative site burns but not PRE (patient return electrode) burns. The function of the dispersive electrode is to remove the electrical current from the patient safely. This may not always happen, however. If the pad is tented, the electrical current arcs from the patient's skin to the pad to complete the circuit. The current is concentrated in the reduced pad-patient interface surface area and may cause a burn at this site. The surgical team became more focused on proper dispersive electrode placement by choosing a well-vascularized site with a secure pad-patient interface. Monitoring the pad placement became a crucial responsibility of the perioperative nurse.

**DISPERSIVE ELECTRODE MONITORING.** In the 1980s, different dispersive electrode monitoring systems were introduced using a variety of names, including dispersive pad monitoring, REM (return electrode monitoring), RECQMS (return electrode contact quality monitoring system), contact quality monitoring system, and patient safety system. This type of ESU protects the patient from dispersive electrode site burns caused by inadequate contact of the dispersive electrode. The system continually monitors the impedance under the split pad as it sends out an interrogation circuit to measure the impedance level. The system deactivates the current flow when the impedance level under the pad increases to an unsafe level, thus preventing a burn.

The placement of a dispersive electrode (pad) is crucial to prevent patient injuries. The pad should be placed over an area that is well vascularized, such as a muscle mass. Sites with excessive hair, bony prominences, excessively dry skin, or adipose tissue should be avoided. When a patient is being repositioned after the pad has been placed, the pad site must be inspected to ensure proper adherence.

A new capacitance pad working on the principle of "bulk resistivity" and "capacitive coupling" has been introduced to the surgical arena. Capacitive coupling is the technology on which this new technology is based. A capacitor is defined as two conductors separated by an insulator. In an electrosurgical circuit, the patient is one conductor (plate), and the conductive mesh (plate) inside the pad is the other conductor. The ability for current flow to be induced from one plate of the capacitor to the other is affected by three primary variables: (1) frequency of the current, (2) size of the plates, and (3) distance between the plates. The higher the frequency, the larger the plates, and the smaller the distance between the plates, which leads to better current flow. A low frequency, one small plate, or a great distance between the plates means decreased current flow.

The large capacitive pad, approximately 2 feet × 3 to 4 feet, consists of a flexible conductive fabric surrounded by a nonlatex, urethane insulating material. The pressure reduction version of this pad is composed of a dry viscoelastic polymer that is one of the best materials to prevent the formation of decubitus ulcers.

This large reusable pad is placed on the OR bed (Figure 7-67) with a linen sheet and drawsheet placed on top of the pad. When the patient is lying on the OR bed, the electrode pad forms a large capacitor with the patient that capacitively couples the patient into the electrosurgery circuit. When in place, this type of dispersive electrode induces a flow of current (>30,000 cycles per second) across the capacitor (patient to electrode), allowing the electricity to be safely returned from the patient to the ESU while the active electrode produces the surgical effect desired.

The amount of induced current that goes into the pad is directly proportional to the amount of contact with the pad. The pad serves as the gatekeeper for this induced current. With too little current, there is very little current flow, which would be too low to cause burns.

The capacitive pad can be used for patients in all types of positions. A positioning chart is available from the manufacturer to assist the surgical team with safe and appropriate positioning. This pad is inappropriate for patients weighing less than 25 lb because adequate contact (weight-bearing area) could not be achieved.

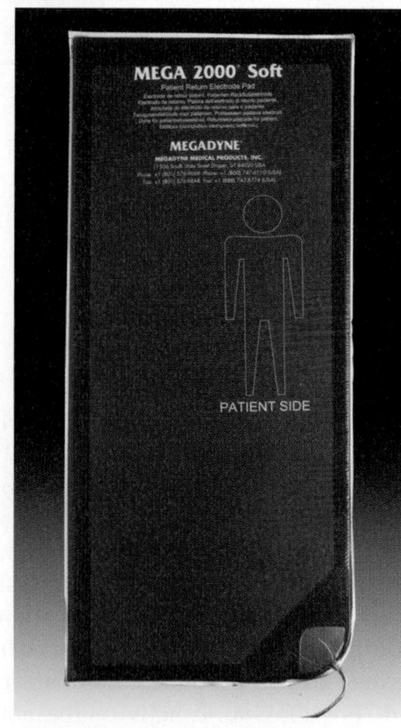


**FIGURE 7-67** New capacitance pad.

This large capacitive pad eliminates the need for an individual adhesive dispersive electrode pad that may become a safety problem if it becomes tented during a procedure. The bulk resistivity of this unique capacitive pad ensures that current densities are kept to a clinically safe level such that no pad site burns can occur. Adhesive pads also can irritate sensitive skin, may require a shaved area for placement, or may become a hazard if not placed on the patient appropriately. As surgical teams are learning more about the use and the safety features of the capacitance pad, its acceptance continues to grow.

TISSUE RESPONSE MONITORING SYSTEM. An advancement in electrosurgery generator technology is the tissue response monitoring system. The generator uses a computer-controlled tissue feedback system that senses the impedance of the tissue and automatically adjusts the current and output voltage to maintain a constant surgical effect. The need to adjust power settings for different tissue types is reduced through this advanced feedback system. Because of the improved performance at lower power settings and voltages, the risk of patient injury is reduced (Figure 7-68).

Another advanced feedback-controlled generator has been combined with a bipolar instrument to seal vessels and tissue bundles reliably for surgical ligation during open and laparoscopic procedures (Figure 7-69). The feedback system is used to achieve a reliable tissue seal using a minimal amount of time, reducing thermal spread compared with traditional bipolar systems. With a single activation, this system has provided stable seals on tissue bundles or on vessels up to and including 7 mm in diameter. The seal site is often translucent, allowing the operating physician to evaluate hemostasis before cutting (Figure 7-70). The strength of the seal is comparable to mechanical ligation methods, such as suture or clips, and is significantly stronger than standard bipolar coagulation.

***Special Electrosurgery Considerations During Endoscopic Minimally Invasive Surgery.*** Three unique problems can occur during endoscopic procedures involving electrosurgery: direct coupling, insulation failure, and capacitive coupling.

DIRECT COUPLING. Direct coupling occurs when the active electrode accidentally touches a noninsulated metal instrument, allowing the electrical energy to flow from one to the other (metal-to-metal sparking) (Figure 7-71). Direct coupling also can occur if an active electrode is activated while in contact with a clip. When the metal instrument or clip receives the electrical energy, a burn can easily result. This type of coupling is often referred to as "pilot error" because it is within the surgeon's control to avoid this problem. The surgeon should not activate the active electrode until the target site is within the field of vision, and the active electrode is in direct contact with the targeted tissue and not a metal object.

INSULATION FAILURE. Insulation failure can occur when the insulation coating of an endoscopic instrument has been compromised. If a crack or break is present in the insulation along the shaft of the instrument, the electrical energy can

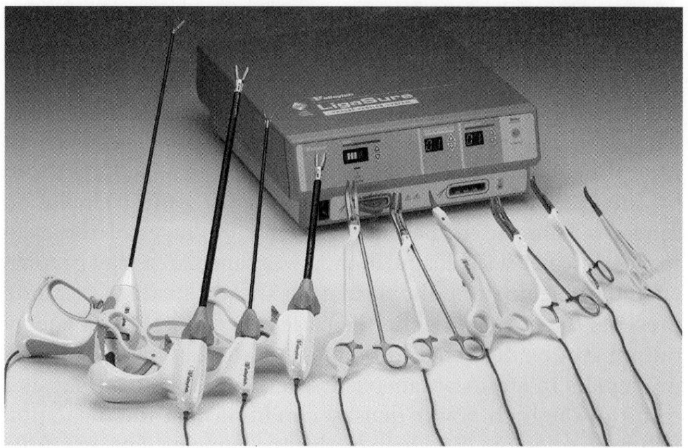

**FIGURE 7-69** Vessel sealing generator with instruments—Valleylab LigaSure.

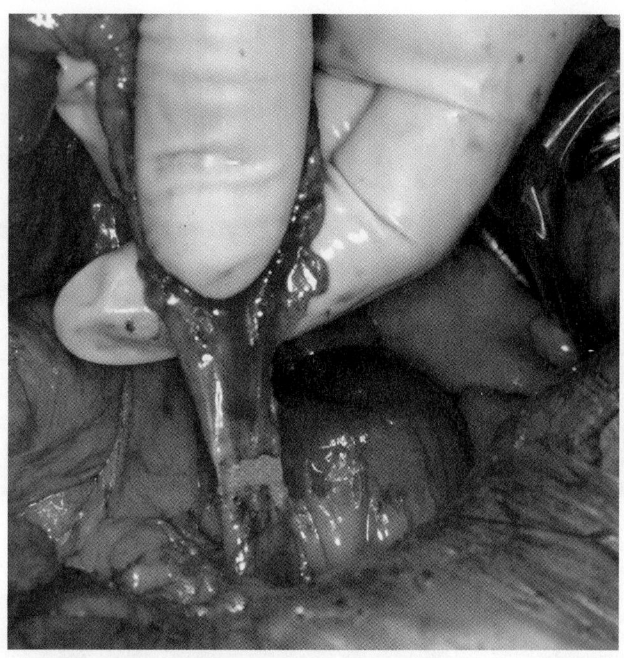

**FIGURE 7-70** Bowel seal using vessel-sealing system.

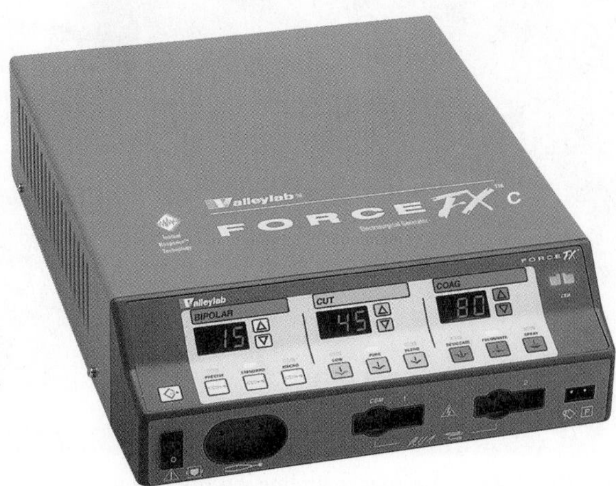


**FIGURE 7-68** Tissue response monitoring system—Valleylab Force FX-C Electrosurgical Generator with Instant Response technology.

escape at the point of the defect and burn untargeted tissue (Figure 7-72). The insulation must be inspected before, during, and after each use of the endoscopic electrosurgical tool. A scanning device can be used to ensure the integrity of the insulation is not compromised during reprocessing. Even an area of insulation that is merely weakened may be penetrated by the electrical flow if a high voltage, or pure coagulation mode, is being used. Because the force (voltage) of the electrons is greater with coagulation, a weakened area may become an actual break along the insulation sheath. Insulation failure presents the greatest risk to the patient because the full energy output can be delivered to nontargeted tissue. Insulation failure results in an instantaneous irreversible death to tissue as a result of the high power density condition that the insulation failure creates on the shaft of the instrument. The resulting tissue burn may not be observed or realized by the operating physician because it may not be within the field of vision.

One manufacturer has introduced a dual layer of insulation on laparoscopic instruments. The outer black insulation layer lies on top of a bright yellow insulation layer. When the top black layer is penetrated, the bright yellow layer can be seen easily and alerts the user that insulation failure may be imminent.

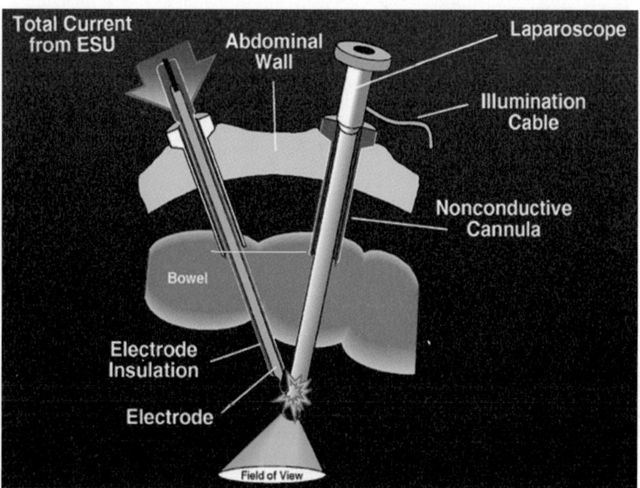


FIGURE 7-71 Direct coupling during laparoscopy.

**CAPACITIVE COUPLING.** Capacitive coupling is a natural RF (electrosurgical energy) phenomenon that can occur when energy is transferred through intact insulation on the shaft of a laparoscopic instrument to nearby conductive materials (Figure 7-73).[8] A capacitor consists of the following: *two conductors* separated by an *insulator.* The metal active electrode is one conductor, and an adhesion, an adjacent organ, or a conductive trocar/suction irrigation cannula can represent the second conductor. The primary insulation on the instrument represents the insulator. When an electrode is activated within a narrow suction irrigator, the RF energy can flow from the active electrode through the intact insulation and transfer 20% to 80% of the power displayed on the ESU to the metal suction irrigator. The induced current on the suction irrigator can cause a burn even though the outer insulation on the first instrument has been inspected and determined to be intact.

The use of monopolar electrosurgical instrumentation through metal suction irrigators or shafts increases the risk of visceral burns through capacitive thermal energy. The laparoscope also can cause alternate-site burns if the electrosurgical electrode is used through a narrow-lumen scope. Instruments that are long and narrow with thin insulation combined with high voltage increase the incidence of capacitive coupling.

The electrical charge stays in the second metal instrument until a path to the dispersive electrode is found to complete the circuit. Usually this energy can be dispersed safely through the large surface of the abdominal wall from the conductive cannula. If a nonconductive device, such as a plastic stability collar, is in this path, the energy cannot be safely discharged and burns any tissue touched by the metal instrument within the body. These burns often go undetected by the operating physician, and the problem is not diagnosed until the patient presents with complications after the surgery. The use of hybrid instruments (combination of plastics and metals) during laparoscopy is avoided to minimize the problem of capacitive coupling.

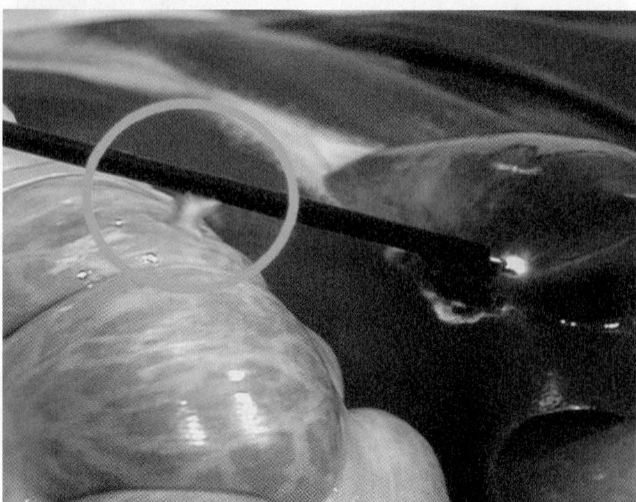

FIGURE 7-72 Insulation failure during laparoscopy.

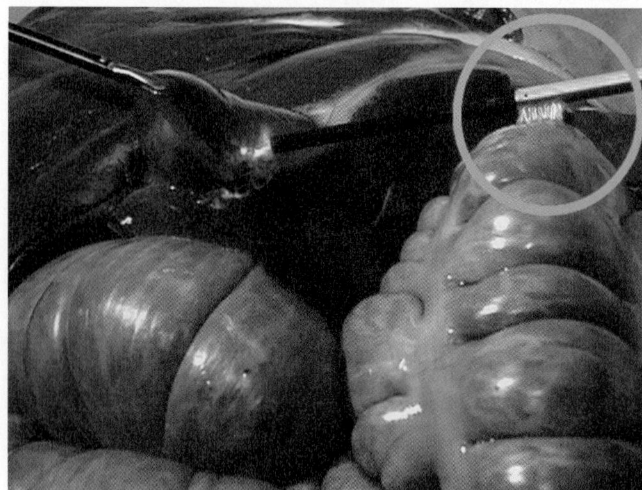

FIGURE 7-73 Capacitive coupling occurs when electrical energy flowing from an instrument charges a nearby metal trocar sheath or laparoscope.

To eliminate the hazard of capacitive coupling, special instruments that provide active electrode monitoring (AEM) are available to capture stray energy that is transferred from one conductive device to another.[5,6] AEM laparoscopic instruments are shielded and monitored to detect stray RF current and prevent electrosurgical burns. The protective shield that is built within an AEM instrument provides the neutral path for capacitive-coupled energy and returns it to the ESU (Figure 7-74). These safety devices also detect insulation failure and provide a path for this stray current back to the generator. Active electrode monitoring is the only fail-safe technology currently designed to address the concerns of insulation failure and capacitive coupling. AEM ensures that 100% of the electrosurgical energy is delivered at the surgeon's intended site.

***Argon-Enhanced Electrosurgery.*** An argon-enhanced electrosurgical device combines argon gas with electrosurgical energy to improve the effectiveness of the electrosurgical current. Because argon gas is heavier than air, inert, and noncombustible, it creates an efficient pathway for the electrosurgical energy from the electrode to the target tissue. The flow of argon gas clears the surgical site of blood and fluids, allowing for greater visibility of the bleeding site or target area. It also blows away the oxygen, decreasing the chance of combustion and the formation of surgical smoke.

The most popular benefits of argon-enhanced electrosurgery include the following:

- Rapid coagulation of diffuse bleeding site with reduced blood loss
- Reduced risk of rebleeding
- Noncontact tissue coagulation
- Reduced surgical plume
- Reduced depth of penetration by the electrical energy and less adjacent tissue damage

When the argon-enhanced electrosurgical device is used during laparoscopic procedures, care must be taken not to overinsufflate or overpressurize the abdomen because there is a constant flow of argon gas that could cause the formation of a gas embolism. Often another port is left open during activation of the argon-enhanced electrosurgical device to allow any excess gas to escape. An insufflator with an audible alarm indicating overpressurization should be used. The patient also should be monitored closely so that any early symptoms of an embolism can be detected and treated.

## Ultrasonic Device Surgery

Vibrating energy devices have been developed to provide a safe option for cutting and coagulation. High-frequency sound waves are propagated to a blade tip to produce ultrasonic energy. These ultrasonic waves have a frequency of greater than 20,000 Hz and cannot be sensed by the human ear.

The production of ultrasonic energy begins with an electrical current that generates an electrical signal sent through a co-axial cable to a transducer in a handpiece. The transducer converts the electrical energy to mechanical motion through the contraction and expansion of ceramic elements. A longitudinal vibratory response that moves the tip at the end of the handpiece from 23,000 Hz to greater than 55,000 Hz is produced (Figure 7-75). As the power is increased, the frequency remains the same, but the longitudinal excursion of the tip becomes longer.

Because the tip is in contact with tissue, the mechanical motion causes the tissue protein to become denatured as the hydrogen bonds are broken. This action causes the protein molecules to become disorganized, and a sticky coagulum forms, which welds and coagulates the smaller bleeding vessels. No tissue plume is generated during the cellular destruction, but a small amount of water vapor is produced and dissipates quickly. Because such a small amount of thermal energy is produced, the adjacent tissue damage is minimal.

Different tip configurations are available, including a blade, ball, and hook. To obtain optimal tissue response, countertraction must be applied to the structure being treated. A shear-grasper to hold the tissue between a blade and tissue pad can be used to eliminate the need for countertraction.

The advantages of using an ultrasonic device for cutting and coagulation are as follows:

1. No surgical plume or odor is generated.
2. Less adjacent tissue is damaged compared with that which occurs with use of laser and electrosurgical devices.
3. Tactile feedback is provided.
4. No nerve or muscle stimulation is present because no electrical current is delivered to the target area.
5. No stray electrical or laser energy is produced.
6. Precise cutting and control are offered.

***Plasma Coagulation.*** In 2004, the FDA approved a plasma coagulator called PLASMAJET, made by Plasma Surgical Limited. PLASMAJET consists of a range of disposable handpieces that are used for coagulation by neutral argon or thermal plasma. In the PLASMAJET system, anode (where current flows in) and cathode (where current flows out) electrodes used to generate the argon plasma are contained within the handpiece,

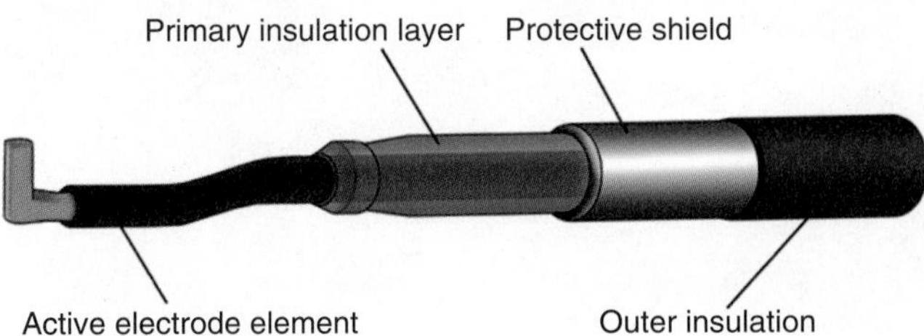


**FIGURE 7-74** Cross section of active electrode monitoring instrument.

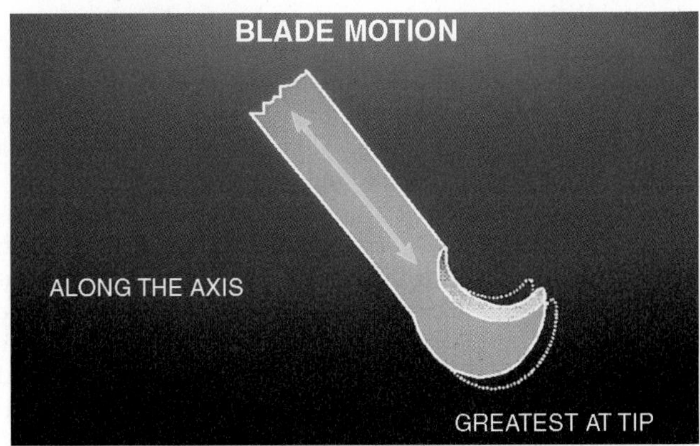


**FIGURE 7-75** An ultrasonic blade may move longitudinally more than 55,000 times per second.

no ground plate is used, and the level of risk for the patient is greatly reduced because no electrical current passes through the patient. When the PLASMAJET reaches the bleeding tissue, it gives up its kinetic energy as heat and causes coagulation of the bleeding surface, reducing blood loss in the patient.

## Hydrodissection and Irrigation

Irrigation is essential during most open and endoscopic procedures. Irrigation is accomplished through irrigation probes for open procedures; through irrigating channels built into endoscopes; or by irrigating systems inserted through an operating port, cannula sheath, or operative endoscope.

Irrigating fluid can be introduced manually through an endoscope by a syringe and stopcock attached to irrigation tubing on one end and an irrigation bag and tubing assembly on the other (original intravenous pole, Y-tubing, and irrigation system). Fluid flows by gravity and is manually forced through the distal tubing.

A pressure bag can be used to increase flow, if desired. Irrigation through a flexible endoscope also can be delivered directly by a syringe attached to the irrigation port. Fluid travels through a specific channel built into the scope. Rigid scopes, such as ureteroscopes, cystoscopes, and hysteroscopes, also have this capability, just as operative laparoscopes do.

Pumps are available when large quantities of fluid are used and manual operation is cumbersome and time-consuming. Pumps are beneficial when irrigation is used for hydrodissection because more fluid can be introduced to the surgical site under pressurization. More force can be exerted over longer periods, and the pressure is adjustable.

A common pump irrigation system includes the irrigation pump ($CO_2$ or electric), irrigation bottle caps, irrigation probe with dual trumpet valves, and Y-tubing irrigation set. When a $CO_2$-controlled system is in use, an E-cylinder of $CO_2$ gas must be attached by means of a tank yoke and input hose. A wrench always should be available to turn off the tank when not in use. It is important to check tank pressure before and after each use. The pump usually has an adjustable pressure on-off capability and dual irrigation bottle selection. As one bottle is emptied, a flip of the switch redirects $CO_2$ flow to the second bottle. Bottles can be replaced as needed. The system operates by the displacement of water or saline with $CO_2$ gas.

When an electric setup is used, a carrier bag with an inflatable bladder surrounds the solution bag (Figure 7-76). When the bladder is inflated, an adequate pressure can be achieved and controlled to provide irrigation and hydrodissection.

The distal tubing attaches directly to an irrigation probe. The time and amount of irrigation are controlled by a trumpet valve (Figure 7-77). Probes are available as reusable, disposable, or a combination of both. All three types incorporate a second trumpet valve for suctioning purposes.

If reusable probes are used, they must be completely disassembled for cleaning and sterilization or disinfection. Each trumpet valve has a spring mechanism (almost like a ballpoint pen). The springs are under pressure when the trumpet valve is inserted. During disassembly, it is important to hold one's hand over the valve so that the spring does not become ejected and lost or cause eye injury. Protective eyewear should be worn during this process. Extra springs should be available.

Completely disposable units also are available. Some systems incorporate disposable with reusable. Tubing and pistol-grip handles containing the trumpet valves are disposable, and the suction and irrigation probes are reusable. The disposable and disposable-reusable units also may incorporate electrosurgical capability into the system (Figure 7-78). This allows the device to be used for three separate functions.

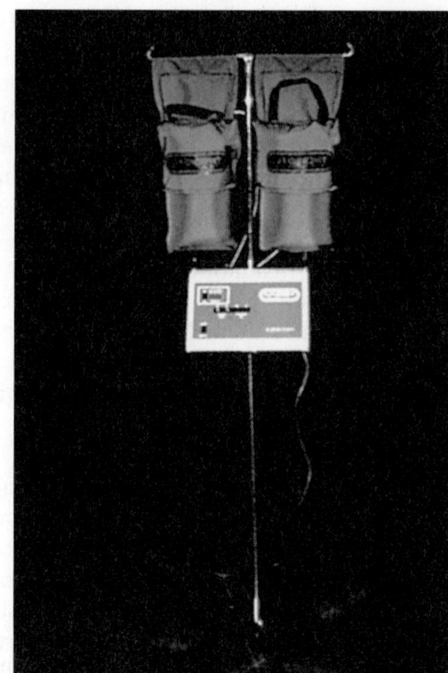

FIGURE 7-76 Hydrodissection system.

The type of irrigation fluid depends on surgeon preference. Traditionally, normal saline has been used. Because saline is a conductive fluid, there is concern when monopolar electrosurgery is used. The disadvantage rests with the risk from the transfer of heat and current to adjacent tissues. Because of this, sterile water or other nonconductive solutions should be considered to prevent electrosurgical energy from being transferred to alternative sites whenever excessive monopolar electrosurgery is anticipated. Sorbitol, which also is used as an irrigation medium during hysteroscopy, can be absorbed rapidly into the vascular system, especially during excessive venous bleeding. The patient must be monitored carefully because of the potential for congestive heart failure from fluid overload.

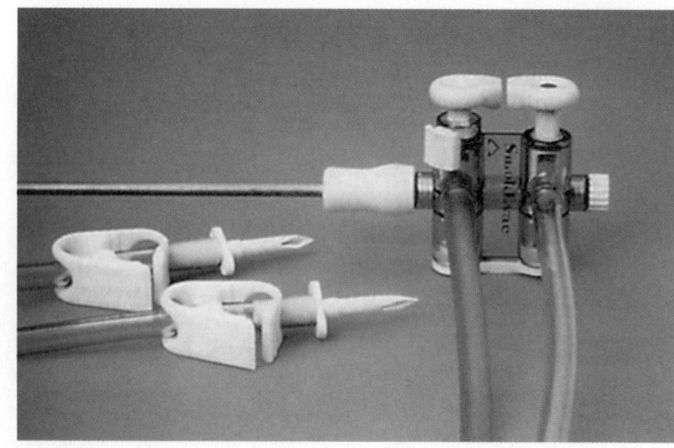

FIGURE 7-77 A trumpet valve controls the flow of irrigant and suction.

## Cryosurgery

Cryosurgery has been used in health care for many years, even though it may appear to be a space-age surgical technique. Archeological evidence indicates that in 2500 BC, freezing tissue was probably employed as an anesthetic. In the early 1800s, cancer was treated using different freezing techniques. Today cryosurgery systems are being used successfully to destroy small quantities of unwanted tissue, such as unwanted skin tumors, and are being perfected to ablate larger tissue targets, such as liver tumors, prostatic cancer, and cervical dysplasia.

To freeze tissue properly, a cooling device or cryosurgical probe must produce an iceball capable of destroying tissue at approximately −50°C and colder. Some systems produce freezing effects down to −240°C (−400°F). The cooling source of the system is usually gaseous nitrogen or supercooled liquid nitrogen systems.

For external tumors, the liquid nitrogen is applied directly to the dysplastic tissue with a cotton swab or through a spraying device. For internal tumors, liquid nitrogen is circulated through the length of a cryoprobe with an insulated shaft to confine the freezing to the distal tip. Ultrasound imaging often is used to guide the cryoprobe and to monitor the freezing of the cells. By localization of the freezing effects, nearby healthy tissue is spared. Smaller cryoprobes that can be inserted through small trocar sites are being perfected.

The effects produced by cryosurgery cause tumor death by freezing it. When internal tumors (e.g., liver cancer) are treated, the dead tumor cells eventually are absorbed into the surrounding tissue. Cryosurgery often involves cycles or steps during the treatment as a tumor is frozen, allowed to thaw, and then frozen again. Research continues to validate the effectiveness of this technology.

Cryosurgery has been used successfully to treat early-stage skin cancers (basal cell and squamous cell carcinomas) and retinoblastoma (a childhood cancer that attacks the retina of the eye). Precancerous lesions, such as actinic keratosis and cervical intraepithelial neoplasia, also have been treated effectively with this technologic method. Cryosurgery has been explored to treat a variety of cancers, including prostate, liver, bone, brain, spinal, lung, and tracheal. It also is being used in combination with other cancer treatments, such as radiation, hormone therapy, chemotherapy, and surgery.

The primary advantage of cryosurgery for cancer treatment over other therapies is that it is less invasive because only a small incision is needed to introduce the cryoprobe through the skin; less bleeding, pain, and other complications are experienced. Cryosurgery is less expensive compared with other treatments and often requires shorter hospital stays and recovery time. The main disadvantage of cryosurgery is the uncertainty of its long-term effectiveness because microscopic cancer cells can spread easily if these cells are missed during the freezing application. Cryosurgery is an evolving technique that will continue to be explored for treatment cures and palliative therapy.

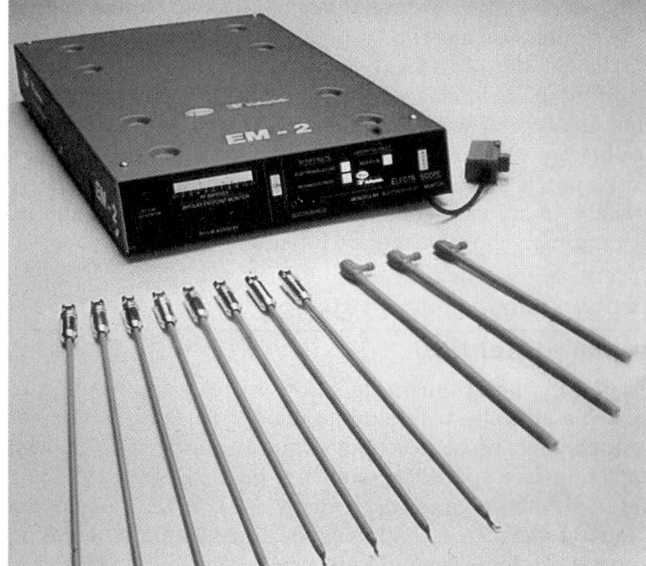


**FIGURE 7-78** Disposable laparoscopic system with irrigation, suction, and monopolar electrosurgical capability. Electrosurgical probes are available in a variety of tips.

## REFERENCES


1. American National Standards Institute, Inc: *American national standard for the safe use of lasers in health care facilities,* ANSI Z136.3, New York, 2005, ANSI.
2. AORN: *AORN standards, guidelines and recommended practices,* Denver, Colo, 2005, The Association.
3. Ball KA: *Lasers: the perioperative challenge,* ed 3, Denver, Colo, 2004, AORN.
4. Chang C, Rege RV: Minimally invasive surgery. In Townsend CM and others, editors: *Sabiston textbook of surgery,* ed 17, Philadelphia, 2004, Saunders.
5. Dennis V: Electrosurgery safety and your staff, *Outpatient Surgery Magazine* 5(9):75-81, 2004.
6. Dennis V: Implementing active electrode monitoring: a perioperative call, *Surgical Services Management* 7(2):32-38, 2001.
7. ECRI: A clinician's guide to surgical fires: how they occur, how to prevent them, how to put them out, *Health Devices* 32(1):5-24, 2003.
8. ECRI: Electrosurgery using capacitively coupled return electrodes, *Health Devices* 29(12):448, 2000.
9. FDA: *Enforcement priorities for single-use devices reprocessed by third parties and hospitals,* Rockville, Md, 2000, US Department of Health and Human Services.
10. General Accounting Office (GAO): *Single-use medical devices: little available evidence of harm from reuse, but oversight warranted,* Washington, DC, June 2000, GAO.
11. Gomez G: Emerging technology in surgery: informatics, electronics, robotics. In Townsend CM and others, editors: *Sabiston textbook of surgery,* ed 17, Philadelphia, 2004, Saunders.
12. Jenkins RL, White P: Telehealth advanced nursing practice, *Nursing Outlook* 49:100-105, 2001.
13. Mayworm D: SUD reprocessing update, *Outpatient Surgery Magazine* 5(8):86-87, 2004.
14. Riordan T: Improving laparoscopic surgery, *New York Times,* March 29, 2004. Accessed March 29, 2004, on-line: www.nytimes.com/2004/03/29/technology/29patent.html.
15. Scheeres J: Surgeons here, patient there, *Wired News,* Sept 19, 2001. Accessed on-line: www.wired.com/news/print/0,1294,46946,00.html.
16. Taylor D: Troubleshooting your laparoscope's hitches and glitches, *Outpatient Surgery Magazine* 5(9):66-71, 2004.
17. Ulmer BC: *The Valleylab Institute of Clinical Education Electrosurgery Continuing Education Module,* Boulder, CO, 2004, Valleylab. Accessed on-line: www.valleylabeducation.org.
18. Weintraub SL and others: Principles of preoperative and operative surgery. In Townsend CM and others, editors: *Sabiston textbook of surgery,* ed 17, Philadelphia, 2004, Saunders.

CHAPTER 8

# Wound Healing, Dressings, and Drains

DONNA R. McEWEN

The ability to heal wounds is one of the most powerful defensive properties humans possess. Wound healing is a complex, highly organized response by an organism to tissue disruption caused by injury. This process is highly reliable in the absence of endogenous and exogenous infections, mechanical interferences, or certain disease processes. Apposition and maintenance of the edges of a cleanly incised wound almost always result in prompt healing. A primary goal of perioperative patient care is the prevention of surgical wound infections. Surgical wound infections are an important cause of illness, death, and excessive health care costs. Surgical wound infections have been complicated further by the potential for infection from new strains of antibiotic-resistant bacteria, such as methicillin-resistant *Staphylococcus aureus* (MRSA) and vancomycin-resistant enterococci (VRE).

Postoperative surgical site infections (SSIs) are a major source of complications for the millions of individuals undergoing surgery annually in the United States and frequently are related to health care–associated infection. Health care–associated infections are increasing, affecting approximately 2 million patients every year, causing an estimated 90,000 deaths, and adding an estimated $4.5 billion to $5.7 billion per year to the costs of patient care and treatment. Although many surgeries are performed on an outpatient basis, and the average number of admissions to hospitals and length of stay have decreased since the 1980s, the incidence of health care–associated infections has increased. Currently, 5% to 10% of all patients admitted to U.S. facilities acquire at least one infection.[3] Actions taken by perioperative personnel sometimes can mean the difference between developing an SSI and the normal healing process. A clear understanding of these actions and a solid knowledge of wound healing and factors adversely affecting healing is important for the appropriate management of patients undergoing surgery.

## ANATOMY

The skin is the largest organ of the body and acts as the first line of defense against infection. It provides protection and sensation, regulates fluid balance and temperature, and produces vitamins (i.e., vitamin D) and immune system components.[7] The skin of the average adult covers approximately 3000 square in., weighs about 6 lb, and receives one third of the body's circulating blood volume. It varies in thickness from 0.5 mm in the tympanic membrane to 6 mm on the soles of the feet and the palms of the hands. Key structures of the skin are the primary layers of the epidermis, the dermis, and the subcutaneous. The *epidermis* is the outermost layer of the skin, lines the ear canals, and is contiguous with the mucous membranes. The epidermis is composed of several layers consisting of keratin and lipids. Keratin is the primary substance that hardens nails and hairs and protects the body from fluid loss and against invasion by pathogens. The epidermis is supported by the *dermis,* which is thicker than the epidermis and composed of collagen. The dermis is the largest portion of the skin, providing strength and structure. Contained within the dermis are blood vessels, lymph ducts, hair roots, nerves, and sebaceous and sweat glands. The dermis is vascularized and innervated (Figure 8-1). The innermost layer is the *subcutaneous,* which is composed of adipose tissue that merges with the deepest layer of the dermis to provide insulation, shape, and support.[2,7] Any wound or disruption of the skin can provide a portal for bacteria and possible infection.

## ETIOLOGY OF WOUNDS

The causes of wounds can be described as follows:

- *Surgical*—caused by an incision or excision
- *Traumatic*—caused by mechanical, thermal, or chemical destruction
- *Chronic*—caused by underlying pathophysiologic condition (e.g., pressure ulcers or venous leg ulcers) over time

The amount of tissue loss, the existence of contamination or infection, and damage to tissue are some factors that determine the type of wound closure selected by the surgeon. The healing process is inherently related to whether the wound is closed or left open. This process occurs in one of three ways: primary intention, secondary intention (granulation), and delayed primary closure (tertiary intention).

## TYPES OF WOUND CLOSURE

### Primary Intention

Healing through primary intention occurs when wounds are created aseptically, with a minimum of tissue destruction and postoperative tissue reaction. Wounds closed with sutures, staples, or tape applied as soon after the time of injury as possible fall into this category (Figure 8-2). When wounds are created under sterile conditions, healing is optimized and begins almost immediately. This type of healing is known as primary intention and occurs under the following conditions:

- Edges of an incised wound in a healthy individual are promptly and accurately approximated

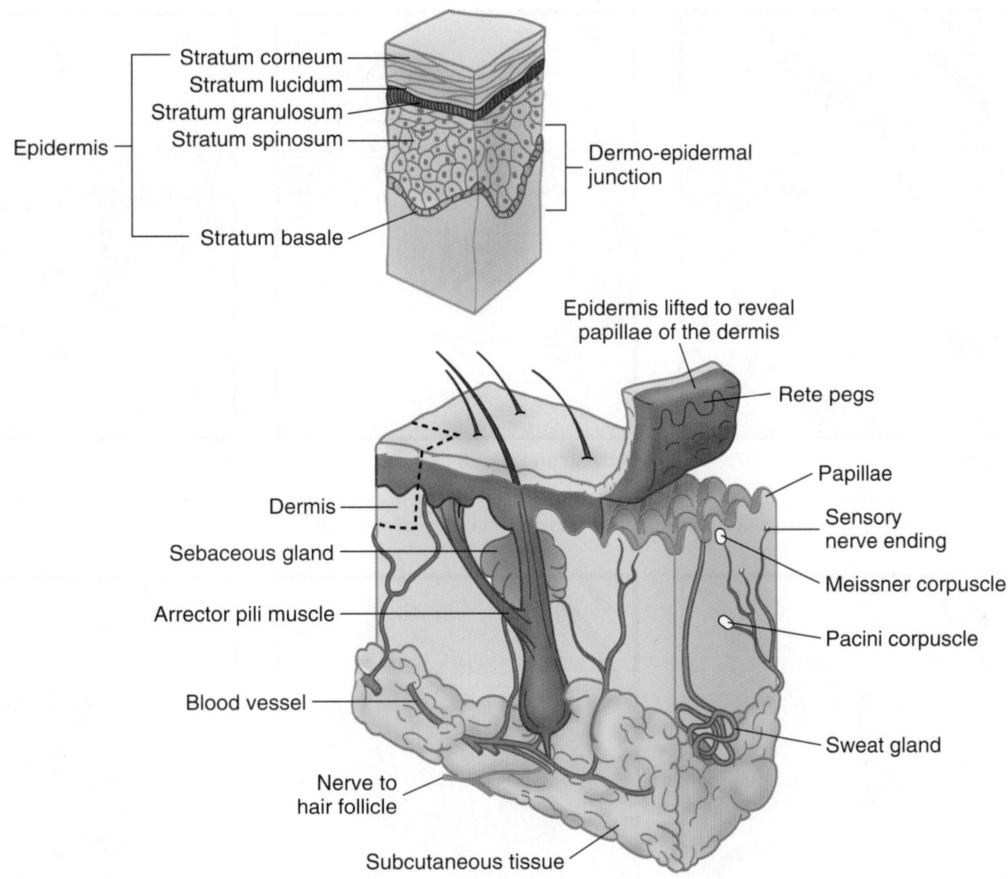


**FIGURE 8-1** Schema of skin and subcutaneous tissue.

- Contamination is held to a minimum by rigid adherence to aseptic technique
- Trauma is minimal
- No tissue loss
- On completion of closure, no dead space is left to become a potential site of infection
- Drainage is minimal

### Secondary Intention (Granulation)

When surgical wounds are characterized by tissue loss with an inability to approximate wound edges, healing occurs through secondary intention (see Figure 8-2). This type of wound is usually left open and allowed to heal from the inside toward the outer surface. In infected wounds, this process allows the proper cleansing and dressing of the wound as healthy collagen tissue builds up from the inside. The area of tissue loss gradually fills with granulation tissue, comprising fibroblasts and capillaries. Scar tissue is extensive because of the size of the tissue gap that must be closed. The scar is referred to as a *cicatrix*. Contraction of surrounding tissue also occurs. Consequently, this healing process takes longer than primary intention healing. Healing by secondary intention is often seen in chronic wounds, dirty wounds, and traumatic wounds where large areas of tissue are lost.

### Delayed Primary Closure or Tertiary Intention

As the name *delayed primary closure* implies, this healing process occurs when approximation of wound edges is intentionally delayed by 3 or more days after injury or surgery (see Figure 8-2). These wounds may require debridement and usually require a primary and secondary suture line, such as when retention sutures are used. The conditions leading to a decision for a delayed closure are as follows:

- Removal of an inflamed organ
- Heavy contamination of the wound
- The critical nature of the patient's intraoperative condition, such as with hemodynamically unstable trauma patients

## PHASES OF HEALING

Clean, full-thickness wound healing is an intricate biologic process that occurs in three overlapping phases: (1) inflammatory (also known as the reactive stage), (2) proliferative (also known as the regenerative or reparative stage), and (3) remodeling (also known as the maturation stage) (Figure 8-3).[11]

### Inflammatory Phase

In the inflammatory phase, an exudate containing blood, lymph, and fibrin begins clotting and loosely binds the cut edges together. Blood supply to the area is increased, and the basic process of inflammation is set in motion. Inflammation is a prerequisite to wound healing and is a vascular and cellular response to dispose of bacteria, foreign material, and dead tissue. Leukocytes increase in number to fight bacteria in the wound area and by phagocytosis help to remove damaged tissues. The severed tissue is quickly glued together by strands of fibrin and a thin layer of clotted blood, forming a scab. Plasma seeps to the surface to form a dry, protective crust. This seal

Healing by First Intention

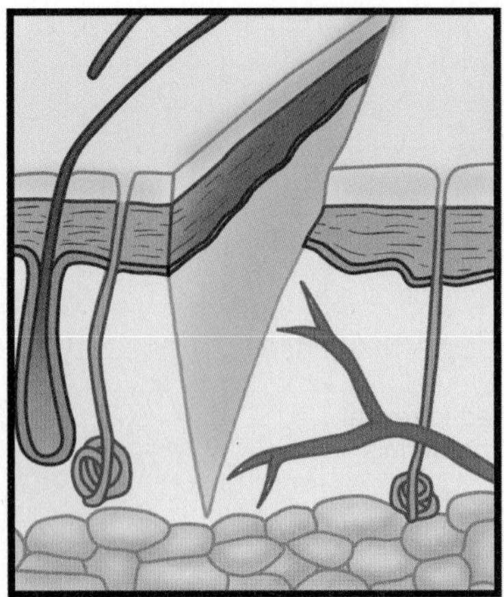

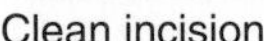

Clean incision

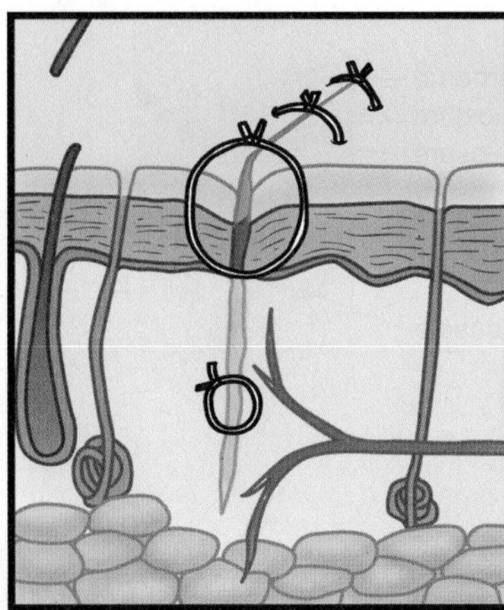

Early suture

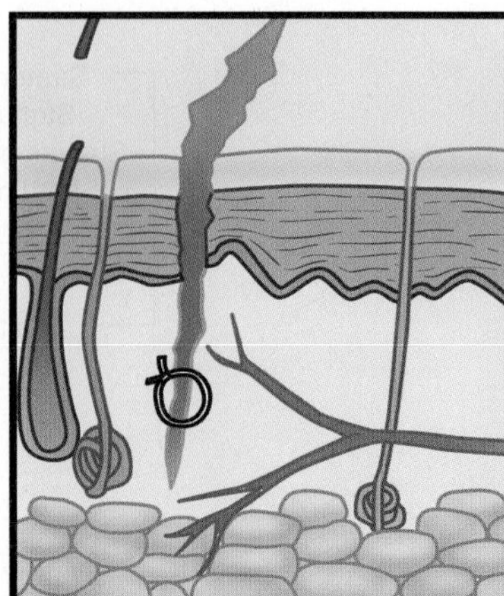

"Hairline" scar

An aseptically made wound with minimal tissue destruction and minimal tissue reaction begins to heal as the edges are approximated by close sutures or staples. No open areas or dead spaces are left to serve as potential sites of infection.

Healing by Second Intention (Granulation) and Contraction

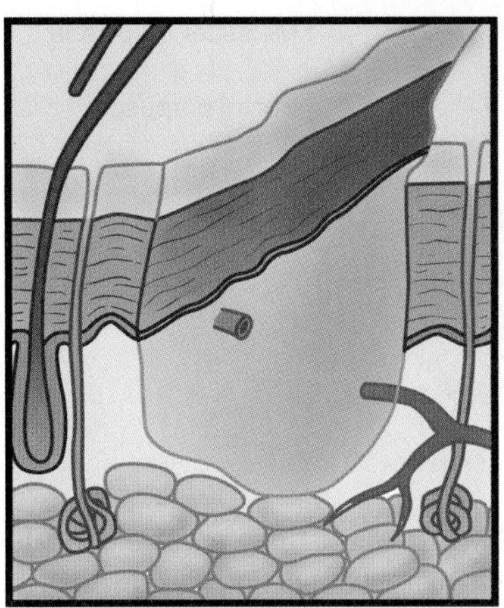

Gaping, irregular wound

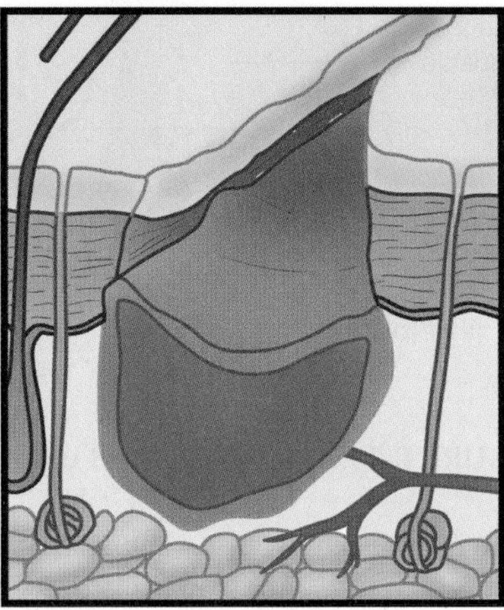

Granulation and contraction

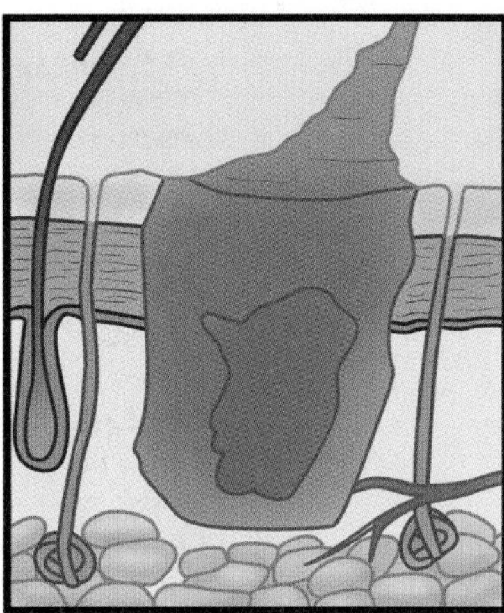

Growth of epithelium over scar

An infected or chronic wound or one with tissue damage so extensive that the edges cannot be smoothly approximated is usually left open and allowed to heal from the inside out. The nurse periodically cleans and assesses the wound for healthy tissue production. Scar tissue is extensive, and healing is prolonged.

Healing by Third Intention (Delayed Closure)

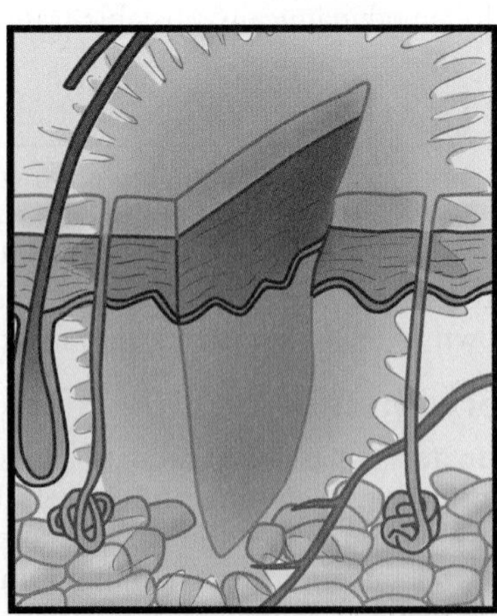

Infected wound

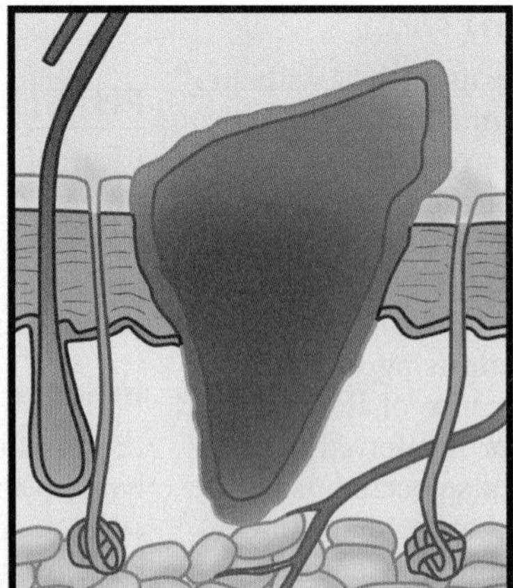

Granulation

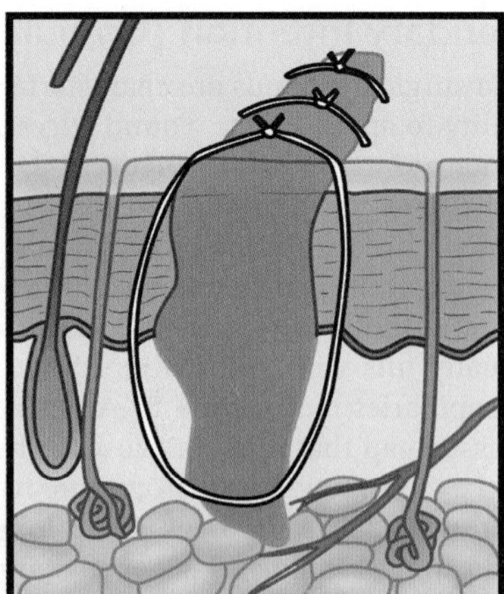

Closure with wide scar

A potentially infected surgical wound may be left open for several days. If no clinical signs of infection occur, the wound is then closed surgically.

**FIGURE 8-2** The process of wound healing.

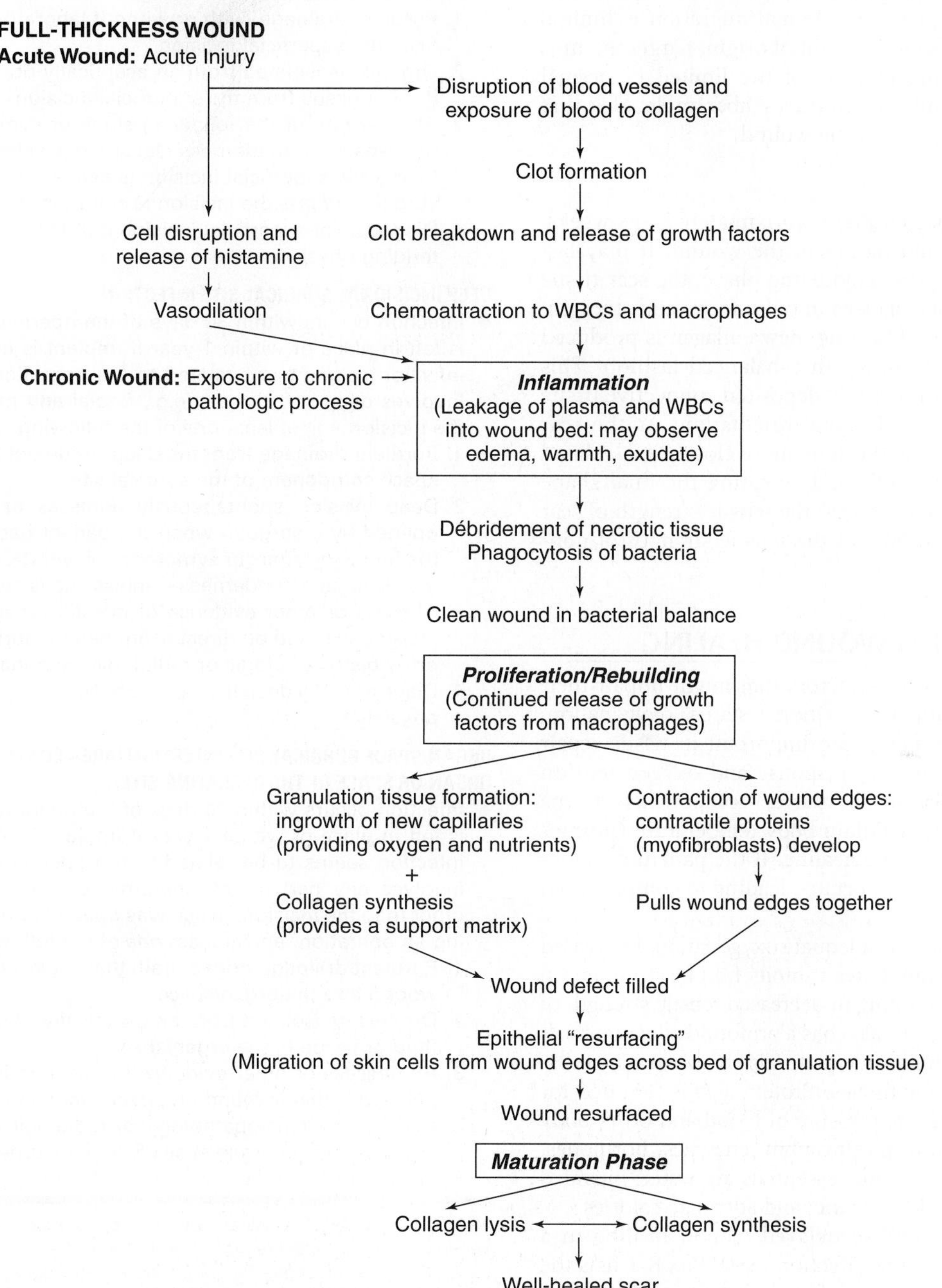


**FIGURE 8-3** Flow diagram of normal wound healing. *WBCs,* White blood cells.

helps to prevent fluid loss and bacterial invasion. During the first few days of wound healing, however, the seal has little tensile strength. The inflammatory phase normally lasts 1 to 4 days. The skin edges may appear mildly swollen and slightly red in this phase as a result of the inflammatory processes at work. Many chronic wounds "stall" at this phase.

## Proliferative Phase

The proliferative phase allows for new epithelium to cover the wound, beginning the process within hours of the occurrence of injury. Epithelial cells migrate and proliferate to the wound area covering the surface of the wound to close the epithelial defect. Epithelialization also provides a protective barrier to prevent fluid and electrolyte loss and to reduce the incidence of infection. While the reepithelialization takes place, collagen synthesis and wound contraction are occurring. Contraction begins approximately 5 days after the wound onset and peaks at 2 weeks, gradually pulling the entire wound into a smaller area. Granulation tissue forms under the edges of the incision and can be palpated as a hard ridge, which eventually resolves during the remodeling phase. Epidermal migration is limited to approximately 3 cm from the point of origin. Larger wounds may require skin grafting because of the limited epidermal migration. Collagen synthesis produces fiber molecules that crosslink to provide strength to the wound.

### Remodeling Phase

The remodeling phase begins after approximately 2 to 4 weeks, depending on the size and nature of the wound. It may last 1 year or longer. During the remodeling phase, the scar tissue formed during fibroplasia changes in bulk, form, and strength. Throughout normal wound healing, new collagen is produced while old collagen breaks down in a balanced fashion. This collagen turnover allows randomly deposited connective tissue to be arranged in linear and lateral orientation. As the scar ages, fibers and fiber bundles become more closely packed and form a crisscross pattern, ultimately creating the final shape and function of the wound. At best, the tensile strength of scar tissue is never more than 80% of the tensile strength of non-wounded tissue.

## FACTORS AFFECTING WOUND HEALING

Patients should be assessed for factors that might impair their wound healing. The patient's nutritional status, oxygenation, and overall recuperative power are important in tissue repair and healing. The inflammatory response and oxygen tension depend on microcirculation to deliver components to the wound. It is important to maintain body temperature (normothermia) in the OR to promote healing. If the patient becomes hypothermic, vasoconstriction occurs, leading to compromised wound healing.[16]

Wound healing depends on adequate oxygenation. Decreased oxygen tension to the wound area inhibits fibroblast migration and collagen synthesis, resulting in decreased tensile strength of the wound. Nutritional status also has a profound effect on healing because of the need for an adequate supply of protein necessary for the growth of new tissues. Protein also is required for the regulation of the osmotic pressure of blood and other body fluids and the formation of prothrombin, enzymes, hormones, and antibodies. Other nutritional essentials are water; vitamins A, C, $B_6$, and $B_{12}$; iron; calcium; zinc; and adequate calories.

The most common cause of delayed wound healing in a surgical patient is surgical site infection (SSI). Box 8-1 lists the types of SSIs and defines criteria for classification. There are many possible causes of SSIs, including patient susceptibility and severity of illness, microbial contamination by the patient's microflora, and exogenous wound contamination from the OR environment and personnel. Adherence to strict aseptic principles, careful observation of sterile technique, and thorough antimicrobial preparation of the patient and operative site are essential to minimize the risk of postoperative SSI. Perioperative personnel who are not scrubbed at the sterile field must maintain meticulous handwashing techniques when possible during the procedure to decrease the transmission of bacteria to the surgical field or the patient (Patient Safety).

Wound healing also can be impaired by poor surgical technique. Rough handling of tissue causes trauma that can lead to

**BOX 8-1**

### Criteria for Defining a Surgical Site Infection

**SUPERFICIAL INCISIONAL SURGICAL SITE INFECTION**

- Occurs within 30 days after the operation
- Involves only the skin and subcutaneous tissue of the incision *and* at least one of the following:
  1. Purulent drainage, with or without laboratory confirmation, from the superficial incision
  2. Organisms isolated from an aseptically obtained culture of fluid or tissue from the superficial incision
  3. At least one of the following signs or symptoms of infection—pain or tenderness, localized swelling, redness, or heat—*and* superficial incision is deliberately opened by the surgeon, *unless* the incision is culture negative
  4. Diagnosis of superficial incisional SSI by the surgeon or attending physician

**DEEP INCISIONAL SURGICAL SITE INFECTION**

- Infection occurs within 30 days of the operation if no implant is left in place or within 1 year if implant is in place, and the infection seems to be related to the operation, *and* infection involves deep soft tissues (e.g., fascial and muscle layers) of the incision *and* at least *one* of the following:
  1. Purulent drainage from the deep tissue not from the organ/space component of the surgical site
  2. Deep incision spontaneously dehisces or is deliberately opened by a surgeon when the patient has at least one of the following signs or symptoms—fever (>38°C [>100.4°F]), localized pain, tenderness—unless site is culture-negative
  3. Abscess or other evidence of infection involving the deep incision is found on direct examination, during reoperation, or by histopathologic or radiologic examination
  4. Diagnosis of a deep incisional SSI by a surgeon or attending physician

**ORGAN/SPACE SURGICAL SITE INFECTION (AREA CONTIGUOUS WITH ORGAN OR SPACE OF THE OPERATING SITE)**

- Infection occurs within 30 days of the operation if no implant is left in place or within 1 year if implant is in place, and the infection seems to be related to the operation, *and* infection involves any part of the anatomy (e.g., organs or spaces), other than the incision, which was opened or manipulated during an operation, *and* at least *one* of the following:
  1. Purulent drainage from a drain that is placed through a stab wound into the organ/space
  2. Organisms isolated from an aseptically obtained culture of fluid or tissue in the organ/space
  3. An abscess or other evidence of infection involving the organ/space that is found on direct examination, during reoperation, or by histopathologic or radiologic examination
  4. Diagnosis of an organ/space SSI by a surgeon or attending physician

Modified from Mangram AJ and others: *Special report: guidelines for prevention of surgical site infection, 1999,* National Centers for Infectious Diseases, Hospital Infections Programs. Accessed August 21, 2005, on-line: www.cdc.gov.nciod/hip/ssi/ssi.pdf; National Nosocomial Infections Surveillance System, Centers for Disease Control and Prevention. Accessed October 6, 2005, on-line: www.cdc.gov/ncidod/hip/SURVEILL/NNIS.HTM.

## PATIENT SAFETY

### Perioperative Handwashing

The Joint Commission on Accreditation of Healthcare Organizations has made patient safety a priority through annual National Patient Safety Goals (NPSGs). One NPSG is the goal of reducing the risk of health care–associated infections. One of the criteria for meeting this goal is for organizations to comply with the current Centers for Disease Control and Prevention (CDC) hand hygiene recommendations. The OR typically is considered a "sterile" environment, but perioperative nurses must be cautious and vigilant about complying with hand hygiene guidelines. Patients are vulnerable anytime the intact skin barrier is breached. Activities that are not conducted in a sterile situation, such as application of surgical dressings to a fresh incision, provide an opportunity for the establishment of pathogens. Health care workers (HCWs) often have a false sense of security about the protection that gloves offer and may think that frequent hand hygiene is unnecessary. The use of gloves cannot replace the act of effective hand hygiene. Other reasons cited for noncompliance with hand hygiene include the following:

- Too busy
- Dry skin caused by hand hygiene agents
- Forgetfulness
- Denial about risks
- Inadequate time/staff
- Lack of supplies for hand hygiene
- Patient is a higher priority than infections

Effective hand hygiene is the easiest, least expensive, and most effective tool that perioperative nurses have at their disposal when acting in the role as a patient advocate. The goal of hand hygiene is a sufficient reduction of microbial counts on the skin to prevent cross-contamination of pathogens. Good hand hygiene practices also provide safety and protection to the HCW.

After extensive research, the CDC published guidelines for hand hygiene. The guidelines are ranked by category ratings, which provide direction to facilities for implementation.

Category I rankings (IA and IB) are applicable to all settings and should be adopted. Subcategories A and B differ only in the strength of supporting research and evidence. Category II rankings are supported by less research and evidence. They may be appropriate for addressing specific situations or patient populations. The Unresolved category offers no recommendation for some practices, either because little research is available to support the effectiveness, or because there is no consensus regarding their efficacy. Perioperative nurses must exercise judgment in determining policies and practice interventions based on the Unresolved category.

**Rankings**

***Indications for Handwashing and Hand Antisepsis***

*CATEGORY IA*

- When hands are visibly dirty or contaminated with proteinaceous material or are visibly soiled with blood or other body fluids, wash hands with a nonantimicrobial soap and water or an antimicrobial soap and water.
- If hands are not visibly soiled, use an alcohol-based hand rub for routinely decontaminating hands in all other clinical situations. Alternately, wash hands with an antimicrobial soap and water.
- Decontaminate hands after contact with body fluids or excretions, mucous membranes, nonintact skin, and wound dressings if hands are not visibly soiled.

*CATEGORY IB*

- Decontaminate hands before having direct contact with patients.
- Decontaminate hands before donning sterile gloves when inserting a central intravascular catheter.
- Decontaminate hands before inserting indwelling urinary catheters, peripheral vascular catheters, or other invasive devices that do not require a surgical procedure.
- Decontaminate hands after contact with a patient's intact skin (e.g., when taking a pulse, measuring blood pressure, and lifting a patient).
- Decontaminate hands after removing gloves.
- Before eating and after using a restroom, wash hands with a nonantimicrobial soap and water or with an antimicrobial soap and water.
- Antimicrobial-impregnated wipes (i.e., towelettes) may be considered as an alternative to washing hands with nonantimicrobial soap and water. Because they are not as effective as alcohol-based hand rubs or washing hands with an antimicrobial soap and water for reducing bacterial counts on the hands of HCWs, wipes are not a substitute for using an alcohol-based hand rub or antimicrobial soap.

*CATEGORY II*

- Decontaminate hands if moving from a contaminated body site to a clean body site during patient care.
- Decontaminate hands after contact with inanimate objects (including medical equipment) in the immediate vicinity of the patient.
- Wash hands with nonantimicrobial soap and water or with antimicrobial soap and water if exposure to *Bacillus anthracis* is suspected or proven. The physical action of washing

| Category | Supporting Research and Evidence |
|---|---|
| IA | Strongly recommended for implementation and supported by well-designed experimental, clinical, or epidemiologic studies |
| IB | Strongly recommended for implementation and supported by some experimental, clinical, or epidemiologic studies and strong theoretic rationale |
| IC | Required for implementation, as mandated by federal or state regulation or standard |
| II | Suggested for implementation and supported by suggestive clinical or epidemiologic studies or theoretic rationale |
| No recommendation; unresolved issue | Practices for which insufficient evidence or no consensus regarding efficacy exists |

Modified from Boyce JM, Pittet D: *Centers for Disease Control and Prevention guideline for hand hygiene in health-care settings: recommendations of the Healthcare Infection Control Practices Advisory Committee and the HICPAC/SHEA/APIC/JDSA Hand Hygiene Task Force.* Accessed August 21, 2005, on-line: www.cdc.gov.mmwr/preview/mmwrhtml/n5116a1.htm; Clark AP, Houston S: Nosocomial infections: an issue of patient safety, part 2, *Clinical Nurse Specialist* 18(2):62-64, 2003;Trampuz A, Widmer AF: Hand hygiene: a frequently missed lifesaving opportunity during patient care, *Mayo Clinic Procedures* 79:109-116, 2004.

*Continued*

## PATIENT SAFETY

### Perioperative Handwashing—cont'd

and rinsing hands under such circumstances is recommended because alcohols, chlorhexidine, iodophors, and other antiseptic agents have poor activity against spores.

*UNRESOLVED ISSUE*

- No recommendations can be made regarding the routine use of nonalcohol-based hand rubs for hand hygiene in health care settings.

***Hand Hygiene Techniques***

*CATEGORY IB*

- When decontaminating hands with an alcohol-based hand rub, apply product to palm of one hand, and rub hands together, covering all surfaces of hands and fingers until hands are dry. Follow the manufacturer's recommendations regarding the volume of products to use.
- When washing hands with soap and water, wet hands first with water, apply an amount of product recommended by the manufacturer to hands, and rub hands together vigorously for at least 15 seconds, covering all surfaces of the hands and fingers. Rinse hands with water, and dry thoroughly with a disposable towel. Use towel to turn off faucet. Avoid using hot water because repeated exposure to hot water may increase the risk of dermatitis.

*CATEGORY II*

- Liquid, bar, leaflet, or powdered forms of plain soap are acceptable when washing hands with a nonantimicrobial soap and water. When bar soap is used, soap racks that facilitate drainage and small bars of soap should be used.
- Multiple-use cloth towels of the hanging or roll type are not recommended for use in the health care setting.

***Surgical Hand Antisepsis***

*CATEGORY IB*

- Surgical hand antisepsis using an antimicrobial soap or an alcohol-based hand rub with persistent activity is recommended before donning sterile gloves when performing surgical procedures.
- When performing surgical hand antisepsis using an antimicrobial soap, scrub hands and forearms for the length of time recommended by the manufacturer, usually 2 to 6 minutes. Long scrub times (e.g., 10 minutes) are unnecessary.
- When using an alcohol-based surgical hand-scrub product with persistent activity, follow the manufacturer's instructions. Before applying the alcohol solution, prewash hands and forearms with a nonantimicrobial soap, and dry hands and forearms completely. After application of the alcohol-based product as recommended, allow hands and forearms to dry thoroughly before donning sterile gloves.

*CATEGORY II*

- Remove rings, watches, and bracelets before beginning the surgical hand scrub.
- Remove debris from underneath fingernails using a nail cleaner under running water.

***Selection of Hand Hygiene Agents***

*CATEGORY IA*

- Do not add soap to a partially empty soap dispenser. This practice of "topping off" dispensers can lead to bacterial contamination of soap.

*CATEGORY IB*

- Provide personnel with efficacious hand hygiene products that have low irritancy potential, particularly when these products are used multiple times per shift. This recommendation applies to products used for hand antisepsis before and after patient care in clinical areas and to products used for surgical hand antisepsis by surgical personnel.
- To maximize acceptance of hand hygiene products by HCWs, solicit input from these employees regarding the feel, fragrance, and skin tolerance of any products under consideration. The cost of hand hygiene products should not be the primary factor influencing product selection.

*CATEGORY II*

- When selecting nonantimicrobial soaps, antimicrobial soaps, or alcohol-based hand rubs, solicit information from manufacturers regarding any known interactions between products used to clean hands, skin care products, and the types of gloves used in the institution.
- Before making purchasing decisions, evaluate the dispenser systems of various product manufacturers or distributors to ensure that dispensers function adequately and deliver appropriate volume of product.

***Skin Care***

*CATEGORY IA*

- Provide HCWs with hand lotions or creams to minimize the occurrence of irritant contact dermatitis associated with hand antisepsis or handwashing.

*CATEGORY IB*

- Solicit information from manufacturers regarding any effects that hand lotions, creams, or alcohol-based hand antiseptics may have on the persistent effects of antimicrobial soaps being used in the institution.

***Other Aspects of Hand Hygiene***

*CATEGORY IA*

- Do not wear artificial fingernails or extenders when having direct contact with patients at high risk (e.g., patients in intensive care units or ORs).

*CATEGORY IB*

- Remove gloves after caring for a patient. Do not wear the same pair of gloves for the care of more than one patient, and do not wash gloves between uses with different patients.

*CATEGORY IC*

- Wear gloves when contact with blood or other potentially infectious materials, mucous membranes, and nonintact skin could occur.

*CATEGORY II*

- Change gloves during patient care if moving from a contaminated body site to a clean body site.

*UNRESOLVED ISSUE*

- No recommendation can be made regarding wearing rings in health care settings.

PATIENT SAFETY

### Perioperative Handwashing—cont'd

***Health Care Worker Educational and Motivational Programs***

*CATEGORY IA*

- Monitor HCWs adherence to recommended hand hygiene practices, and provide personnel with information regarding their performance.

*CATEGORY II*

- As part of an overall program to improve hand hygiene practices of HCWs, educate personnel regarding the types of patient care activities that can result in hand contamination and the advantages and disadvantages of various methods used to clean their hands.
- Encourage patients and their families to remind HCWs to decontaminate their hands.

***Administrative Measures***

*CATEGORY IA*

- As part of a multidisciplinary program to improve hand hygiene adherence, provide HCWs with a readily accessible, alcohol-based hand rub product.
- To improve hand hygiene adherence among personnel who work in areas in which high workloads and high intensity of patient care are anticipated, make an alcohol-based hand rub available at the entrance to the patient's room or at the bedside, in other convenient locations, and in individual pocket-sized containers to be carried by HCWs.

*CATEGORY IB*

- Make improved hand hygiene adherence an institutional priority, and provide appropriate administrative support and financial resources.

*CATEGORY IC*

- Store supplies of alcohol-based hand rubs in cabinets or areas approved for flammable materials.

bleeding and other conditions conducive to infection. Examples of surgical technique promoting wound healing include adequate hemostasis, precise cutting and suturing techniques, efficient use of time to minimize wound exposure to air, elimination of dead spaces, and minimal pressure from retractors and other instruments. Additional factors affecting wound healing are the patient's age, stress level, immunologic status, and smoking history. Preexisting conditions, such as diabetes, anemia, malnutrition, cancer, obesity, certain drug therapies (e.g., steroid therapy), and cardiovascular or respiratory impairments also contribute to poor wound healing. Additional terms used in connection with wound healing are shown in Box 8-2.

BOX 8-2

### Additional Terms Used in Connection with Wound Healing

The following are additional terms used in connection with wound healing:

**Adhesions**—Adherence of serous membranes to one another, causing fibrous tissue to form; sometimes occurring in healing and inflammatory processes; commonly occurring in or about gastrointestinal tract, where adhesions may form bands and cause obstructions and subsequent surgical emergencies

**Dead space**—Air or empty space between layers of tissue or beneath wound edges that have been approximated

**Dehiscence**—Separation of layers of surgical wound (Figure 8-4)

**Evisceration**—Extrusion of internal organs, or viscera, through gaping wound (see Figure 8-4)

**Gangrene**—Anaerobic infection process that may occur instead of healing; implies necrosis (death of tissue) and putrefaction (decomposition); usually caused by failure of nutriment or blood to reach a part

**Keloid**—Dense, unsightly connective tissue or excessive scar formation that is often removed surgically

**"Proud flesh"**—A mass of excessive granulation formed when a wound shows no other sign of healing or excessive cicatrization

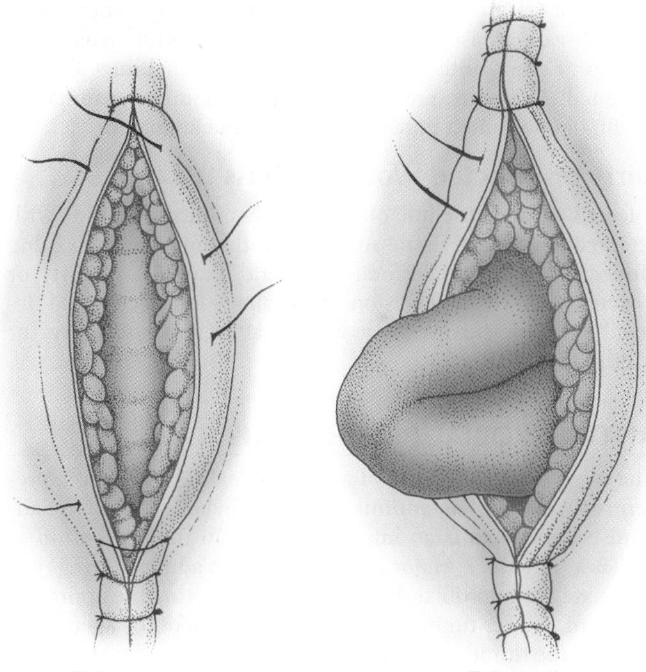


FIGURE 8-4 Complications of wound healing.

## WOUND CLASSIFICATION

The Centers for Disease Control and Prevention (CDC) recommends four surgical wound classifications: clean wounds, clean contaminated wounds, contaminated wounds, and dirty or infected wounds.[12] This classification scheme reflects the probability of infection and enables appropriate preventive measures to be taken. The *AORN Recommended Practices for Documentation of Perioperative Nursing Care* note the importance of documenting the wound classification in the patient record.[1] Following are descriptions of each classification.

### Clean Wounds (Class I)

Clean wounds are uninfected operative wounds in which no inflammation is encountered, and the respiratory, alimentary, and genitourinary tracts are not entered. They are primarily closed and can be drained with a closed wound drainage system. Clean wounds show no sign of infection. Examples are breast biopsy, total hip replacement, and open-heart surgery.

### Clean Contaminated Wounds (Class II)

Clean contaminated wounds are operative wounds in which the respiratory, alimentary, or genitourinary tract is entered under controlled conditions. There is no sign of infection and no break in surgical aseptic technique. Examples of clean contaminated wounds are nonperforated appendectomy, hysterectomy, and thoracotomy.

### Contaminated Wounds (Class III)

Contaminated wounds are open, fresh, accidental wounds, such as penetrating trauma, open fractures, or operations with major breaks in aseptic technique. Incisions with signs of infection or gross spillage from the gastrointestinal tract also are included. Examples are a penetrating abdominal trauma involving bowel and a gunshot wound to the abdomen.

### Dirty or Infected Wounds (Class IV)

Infected wounds include old physically induced wounds with retained devitalized tissue and wounds that involve an existing clinical infection or perforated viscera. Examples of dirty or infected wounds are excision and drainage of abscess and delayed primary closure of a wound after appendectomy for ruptured appendix.

## ANTIMICROBIAL PROPHYLAXIS

The most effective course of action in dealing with SSI is prevention. Appropriate antimicrobial prophylaxis (antibiotic administration) also is an important factor in the prevention of SSI (Best Practice). Major considerations in administering prophylactic antimicrobial therapy include selecting the appropriate agent, proper timing of the administration of the agent, and limiting the duration of the therapy.

Antimicrobial prophylaxis agent selection is based on clinical efficacy, safety, cost, and whether the agent is broad spectrum. The surgeon commonly takes into consideration the nature of the surgical procedure, noting the most common pathogens associated with that procedure (e.g., common pathogens of the small bowel in undertaking a small bowel resection). Cephalosporins often are used for elective clean or clean contaminated surgical procedures. For these procedures, a single dose usually is administered during the immediate preoperative period.

To enhance the effectiveness of prophylactic antimicrobial therapy, it is necessary for the optimal level of the antibiotic to be present in the tissue at the time of the incision. Equally important is the need to maintain circulating blood levels throughout some procedures. The antibiotic of choice should be administered within 1 hour before the skin incision. The anesthesia provider administers the antibiotic intravenously. If the surgical procedure is longer than the half-life of the antibiotic, another dose usually is administered intravenously during the procedure.

Antibiotic therapy usually is discontinued within 24 hours. There is little evidence that ongoing administration contributes to a decrease in SSI rates in clean or clean contaminated procedures. Equally as important is the need to evaluate carefully the need for antibiotics with the emergence of antibiotic-resistant microorganisms (see Chapter 3).

## BEST PRACTICE

### Antimicrobial Prophylaxis

A best practice based on evidence is important for improving patient outcomes. The long established practice of administering antimicrobials (i.e., antibiotics) prophylactically (antimicrobial prophylaxis [AMP]) in surgical patients is used to enhance the host defense by reducing any microbial burden that may result from surgical intervention. AMP should be viewed as an adjunct to other measures that nurses use to promote successful outcomes for their patients and can never substitute for strict adherence to aseptic technique. Optimizing AMP is a form of patient advocacy and can be maximized by understanding and implementing recommendations from the Centers for Disease Control and Prevention.

**CENTERS FOR DISEASE CONTROL AND PREVENTION RECOMMENDATIONS FOR ANTIMICROBIAL PROPHYLAXIS**

Use an AMP agent for all operations or classes of operations in which its use has been shown to reduce surgical site infection (SSI) rates based on evidence from clinical trials (i.e., trauma, thoracic, general surgery, head and neck procedures with incisions through the oropharyngeal mucosa, obstetrics and gynecology) or for operations after which incisional or organ/space SSI would represent a catastrophe (i.e., when intravascular prosthetic materials or a prosthetic joint will be inserted, all cardiac operations including pacemaker insertion, limb revascularization.)

Use an AMP agent that is safe, inexpensive, and bactericidal with an in vitro spectrum that covers the most possible intraoperative contaminants for the operation.

Time the infusion of the initial dose of antimicrobial agent within 1 hour before the surgery so that a bactericidal concentration of the drug is established in serum and tissues by the time the skin is incised.

Maintain therapeutic levels of the antimicrobial agent in serum and tissues throughout the operation and until, at most, a few hours after the incision is closed in the OR. Because clotted blood is present in all surgical wounds, therapeutic serum levels of antimicrobial agents are logically important in addition to therapeutic tissue levels. Fibrin-enmeshed bacteria may be resistant to phagocytosis or to contact with antimicrobial agents that diffuse from the wound space.

Do not use AMP for operations classified as contaminated or dirty. In such operations, patients frequently are receiving therapeutic antimicrobial agents perioperatively for established infections.

Modified from A consensus on improving antibiotic use, *OR Manager* 20(11):7, 2004; Mangram AJ and others: *Special report: guidelines for prevention of surgical site infection, 1999,* National Centers for Infectious Diseases, Hospital Infections Programs. Accessed August 21, 2005, online: www.cdc.gov.nciod/hip/ssi/ssi.pdf; National surgical QI project rolls out, *OR Manager* 21(9):5, 7-8, 2005.

## NURSING DIAGNOSES

The nursing diagnoses—risk for infection, risk for impaired skin integrity, imbalanced nutrition, ineffective tissue perfusion, and hypothermia—point the perioperative nurse toward strategies that can be used to prevent wound infections and promote healing.

The Centers for Medicare and Medicaid Services (CMS) and the CDC provide SSI prevention guidelines for consideration in planning and implementing nursing interventions to optimize successful patient outcomes (Box 8-3). Attention also should be given to controlling perioperative serum glucose in major cardiac procedures, maintaining skin integrity through proper positioning, the use of pressure-reducing mattresses as needed (see Chapter 5), and the safe use of electrosurgery (see Chapter 7). The perioperative nurse plays a vital role in the prevention of adverse events and patient injury by using intellectual and technical knowledge.

## PATIENT AND FAMILY EDUCATION AND DISCHARGE PLANNING

Because more patients are discharged from the acute care setting to the home care setting much earlier in their recovery, more surgical wound care is delivered by patients, their families, and home care providers instead of by the hospital nurse.

**BOX 8-3**

### Guidelines for Surgical Site Infections

SSIs account for 14% to 16% of all hospital-acquired infections. An understanding of the Centers for Disease Control and Prevention guideline ranking system enables nurses to weigh factors that are viewed as effective in preventing SSIs. Category I rankings (including IA and IB) are applicable to all settings and should be adopted. Subcategories A and B differ only in the strength of supporting research and evidence. Category II rankings are supported by less research and evidence. They may be appropriate for addressing specific situations or patient populations. The Unresolved category offers no recommendation for some practices, either because little research is available to support the effectiveness, or because there is no consensus regarding their efficacy; that category is not addressed here.

**RANKINGS**

| Category | Supporting Research and Evidence |
|---|---|
| IA | Strongly recommended for implementation and supported by well-designed experimental, clinical, or epidemiologic studies |
| IB | Strongly recommended for implementation and supported by some experimental, clinical, or epidemiologic studies and strong theoretic rationale |
| II | Suggested for implementation and supported by suggestive clinical or epidemiologic studies or theoretic rationale |

**RECOMMENDATIONS**

Preoperative—partial and modified

**PREPARATION OF THE PATIENT**

**Category IA**

- When possible, identify and treat infections remote to the surgical site before elective operation; postpone surgery until resolved. Do not remove hair from operative site unless necessary to facilitate surgery. If hair is removed, do immediately before surgery, preferably with electric clippers.

**Category IB**

- Adequately control serum blood glucose in diabetics and particularly avoid hyperglycemia perioperatively.
- Encourage cessation of tobacco use (cigarettes, cigars, pipes, chewing/dipping) 30 days before surgery.
- Do not withhold necessary blood products from surgical patients to prevent SSIs.
- Require patients to shower or bathe the night before operative procedure.
- Wash incision site to remove gross contamination before performing antiseptic skin preparation.

**Category II**

- Prepare skin in concentric circles from incision site.
- Keep preoperative stay in hospital as short as possible.

**SURGICAL TEAM MEMBERS**

**Category 1B**

- Keep nails short and do not wear artificial nails.
- Perform a preoperative surgical scrub/surgical hand antisepsis (hands and forearms up to the elbows) for at least 2 to 5 minutes using an appropriate antiseptic. After performing the surgical scrub/surgical hand antisepsis, keep the hands up and away from the body. Dry hands with a sterile towel, and don a sterile gown and gloves.
- Educate and encourage surgical personnel who have signs and symptoms of transmissible infections to report conditions promptly to supervisory personnel.
- Develop well-defined policies concerning patient care responsibilities when personnel have potentially transmissible infectious conditions.
- Do not routinely exclude surgical personnel who are colonized with organisms such as *S. aureus* or group A streptococcus, unless such personnel have been linked epidemiologically to dissemination of the organism in the health care setting.

**Category II**

- Clean underneath each fingernail before performing the first surgical scrub of the day.
- Do not wear hand or arm jewelry.

**POSTOPERATIVE INCISION CARE**

**Category IB**

- Protect with a sterile dressing for 24 to 48 hours postoperatively incisions that have been closed primarily.
- Wash hands before and after dressing changes and any contact with the surgical site.

**Category II**

- When an incision dressing must be changed, use sterile technique.
- Educate the family regarding proper incision care, symptoms of SSI, and the need to report such symptoms.

Modified from Mangram AJ and others: *Special report: guidelines for prevention of surgical site infection, 1999,* National Centers for Infectious Diseases, Hospital Infections Programs. Accessed August 21, 2005, on-line: www.cdc.gov.nciod/hip/ssi/ssi.pdf.

Early planning and teaching regarding wound care, standard precautions, and medical waste disposal have become a vital component of preparing the patient for continuity of care after discharge (Patient and Family Education).

## WOUND MANAGEMENT

A variety of treatment modalities exist for acute and chronic wound management. Perioperative nurses often care for patients with infected wounds and are familiar with surgical wound debridement and sterile dressing changes performed under anesthesia. Patients also may come to the OR with chronic wounds being managed with a combination of surgical interventions and other treatment modalities. An understanding of adjunct wound therapies is essential to planning perioperative nursing care. These therapies include hyperbaric oxygenation (HBO), negative pressure therapy, hydrotherapy, engineered living skin substitute, and the topical application of growth factors.

### Debridement

Debridement is the act of removing dead and devitalized tissue from a wound and is necessary because the dead tissue in the wound provides a nidus for wound infection. Perioperative nurses often care for patients scheduled for surgical wound debridement (i.e., the sharp excision of dead or devitalized tissue). Debridement also can be accomplished through mechanical means (forceful irrigation, wet-to-dry dressings), enzymatic action (application of debriding agents containing papain and collagenase), and biologic methods (sterile maggot debridement therapy).[17,18] There are advantages and disadvantages to each method. Surgical debridement may not always be precise, and healthy tissue may be sacrificed. Additionally, the act of surgical debridement may shower organisms into the

#### PATIENT AND FAMILY EDUCATION

#### Patient Education for Wound Care and Dressing Changes

Although the surgeon may perform the initial dressing change after surgery, patients or their caregivers are often responsible for subsequent dressing changes and wound care. Patient compliance with wound care and dressing change techniques is important to prevent infection.

**HOME CARE**

Provide *written* and *verbal* instructions to the patient and the caregiver. Patients may be anxious about wound care. Provide reassurance and encouragement to the patient to bolster confidence in implementing this procedure at home. Assess the availability of dressing materials in the home care setting, and assist the patient with the appropriate referral if necessary to obtain the needed materials.

**Warning Signs**

Review the signs and symptoms that should be reported to a physician or a nurse:

- Redness, marked swelling (beyond ½ inch from the incision site), tenderness, increased warmth around the wound, or red streaks near the wound
- Temperature greater than 37.7°C (>100°F) or chills
- Purulent drainage or foul odor

**Special Instructions**

- Advise patients to ask the physician if bathing or showering is allowed.
- Review dressing change and wound care products with the patient and caregiver; explain the procedure and frequency to be performed.
- Emphasize the need to keep the wound dry and clean.
- Instruct patients not to remove casts and splints unless instructed to do so by the physician.
- Advise patients to assemble all supplies needed for the dressing change before starting. Explain how to maintain sterility of dressing supplies, and provide instruction on disposal of soiled dressings.
- Teach proper handwashing techniques, and instruct the patient to wash hands before changing the dressing.
- Instruct the patient to remove tape gently to avoid traumatizing the skin. Remove the old dressing and discard. Wash hands.
- Advise the patient to inspect the wound, and review the warning signs that should be reported to the physician.
- Describe how to clean the wound as ordered by the physician (i.e., with saline, povidone-iodine [Betadine], or alcohol, using cotton swabs, gauze, or other materials). Discuss how to clean around drain sites if applicable.
- Provide instruction on how to reapply the dressing, with emphasis on the order of materials used (i.e., nonadherent pad, gauze, any packing, top layer of dressing, and tape).
- Instruct the patient to wash hands after completing the dressing change.

**Interventions to Reduce Swelling After Extremity Surgery**

To avoid venous congestion and to enhance wound healing, advise patients recovering from extremity surgery to elevate the affected limb:

- Hand or arm
  - Sleep—elevate the arm on pillow at side
  - Sitting—place arm on pillow on adjacent table
  - Standing—rest affected hand on opposite shoulder, support elbow with unaffected hand
- Leg or Foot
  - Sitting—place a pillow on the facing chair; provide support underneath the knee
  - Lying—place a pillow under affected leg

**Wound Care After Suture/Staple Removal**

- Remind patient that although the wound appears healed, it still may be tender and will continue to heal and strengthen for several weeks.
- Instruct the patient to keep the suture line clean; do not rub vigorously; pat dry after bathing or showering. Provide education about the appearance of the wound at this stage. Remind the patient that the wound edges still may be red and slightly raised.
- If allowed by the physician, advise the patient to massage around the wound gently using bland baby oil, petroleum, or moisturizing cream twice a day.
- Recommend that the patient report any swelling, redness, tenderness, or excessive scar thickening that persists beyond 8 weeks to the physician.

Modified from Canobbio MM: *Handbook of patient teaching,* ed 3, St Louis, 2006, Mosby.

bloodstream resulting in bacteremia. Mechanical debridement is painful and nonselective in the tissue it removes. Enzymatic debridement may be uncomfortable for the patient and may macerate surrounding tissue. Biologic debridement is not well accepted by most patients.[19] Patients with chronic, nonhealing wounds may become well known to the perioperative staff as they are scheduled for procedures such as debridement, grafting, flaps, and other wound coverage. Perioperative nurses play a key role in wound care and must be familiar with the various wound care treatment modalities to support patients throughout the course of their recovery.

## Hyperbaric Oxygenation (HBO)

HBO has been used to enhance healing in problem wounds for many years. Although some form of HBO treatment for wounds has been used since 1662, the era of HBO use in wound healing began in 1961 when it was used to treat gas gangrene.[8] HBO increases the capacity of blood to carry oxygen to the tissues. The increased oxygenation assists in cellular restoration, is directly bactericidal to anaerobes, and improves leukocyte migration and phagocytocis to the wound bed.[6] HBO therapy is administered in a pressurized chamber with the patient breathing 100% oxygen. Chambers may be monoplace to accommodate a single patient or multiplace to allow simultaneous treatment of multiple patients. Patients who undergo HBO therapy may require the insertion of myringotomy tubes to manage pressure changes while in the chamber. Perioperative nurses may be involved in the placement of the tubes and may be involved in wound debridement procedures for these patients.

## Negative Pressure Wound Therapy

Also known as vacuum-assisted closure (VAC), negative pressure wound therapy is used for difficult-to-manage wounds that do not respond to traditional wound care methods. Negative pressure wound therapy works by using a device to apply constant controlled negative pressure to a wound that is filled with a drainage sponge and sealed with an occlusive dressing. The VAC system has three main mechanisms of action that promote wound healing. First, the act of negative pressure results in mechanical tension on the tissues causing the development of new blood vessels, mitosis, and dilation of the arterioles. The pressure also produces a centripetal force that helps to pull the wound edges together. Second, VAC therapy promotes evacuation of excess wound fluid, such as the interstitial fluid that accumulates in a wound and prevents the circulatory and lymph systems from delivering nutrients and oxygen. A third beneficial mechanism is the reduction of bacterial colonization in the wound bed. The stagnant exudates are eliminated, stunting bacterial growth and proliferation.[10] The therapy may be used for acute and traumatic wounds, subacute wounds, pressure ulcers, chronic open wounds, meshed skin grafts, and skin flaps. The therapy is contraindicated in the presence of necrotic tissue, cancer in the wound edges, untreated osteomyelitis, or fistulas to organs or body cavities.

The negative pressure unit may be applied in the OR after wound debridement. All nonviable tissue must be removed to reduce bacterial load in the wound bed. The skin area around the wound is dried, and specialized reticulated foam is cut to fit the wound bed, including all tunnels and tracks. The surgeon must be careful not to overfill the wound with the sponge because this could cause further mechanical trauma. When the sponge is in place, the surgeon covers the entire sponge, wound bed, and surrounding skin with a transparent occlusive drape, taking care to seal the edges completely. A 2-cm or greater edge of intact periwound skin must be available to ensure an airtight seal of the dressing. A 2-cm cut is made through the occlusive dressing into the sponge for insertion of the drainage tube, which has side and end ports. The tubing is connected to a VAC pump (Figure 8-5). A portable, battery-operated unit also is available for more ambulatory patients. A canister collects the fluid and exudate. The cycle may be used on a continuous or intermittent setting. For best results, the patient must use the unit at least 22 hours a day.[13]

## Hydrotherapy

Traditionally hydrotherapy is undertaken via immersion in a whirlpool tank or tub. The mechanism of the agitated water and injected air is thought to dilute bacterial loads and remove debris, while increasing circulation to the area. Because immersion in a tank is not practical from an intraoperative perspective, the hydrotherapy method most frequently used in the OR is pulsatile lavage. A variety of manufacturers provide systems to deliver pulsatile lavage. Most systems consist of a motor that creates pressure within a tubing set to allow the delivery of fluid at 10 to 15 psi through a handpiece to the wound bed. The handpiece is equipped with a splash shield to help concentrate the spray and minimize droplet aerosolization of the irrigant. While the system is delivering the fluid, it simultaneously suctions it away to remove debris and bacteria. Standard precautions must be observed by all health care team members while using pulsatile lavage, and the patient should be protected from areosolization (Research Highlight).[5,8]

## Skin Substitutes

A more recent technology for the treatment of wounds is the use of an engineered skin substitute. The skin substitute stimulates wound epithelialization and is capable of producing growth factors.[9] The skin substitute may be used in lieu of a split-thickness skin graft for wound coverage. Skin substitutes

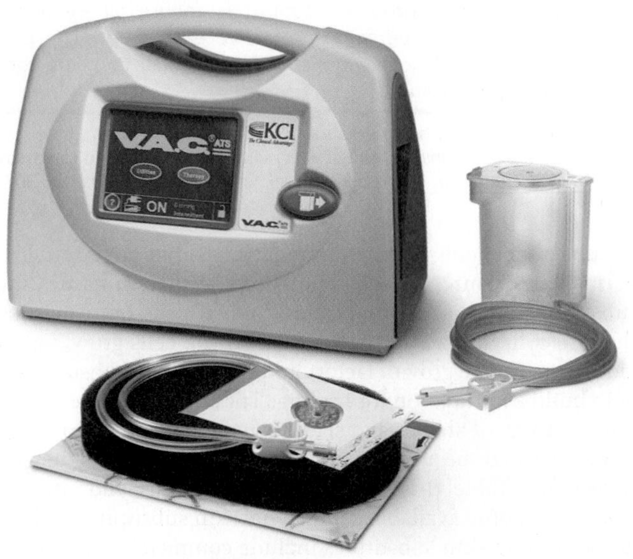


**FIGURE 8-5** The VAC pump.

## RESEARCH HIGHLIGHT

### Pulsatile Lavage and Bacterial Aerosolization

Perioperative nurses frequently are involved in the use of pulsatile lavage as a mechanism for cleansing and débriding wounds. These devices deliver irrigation solution via a handpiece under pressure and are equipped with a splash shield to minimize scatter and aerosolization. The possibility of transmission of irrigant contaminated with organisms from the patient exists, however. In many cases, the organisms that are aerosolized can be life threatening.

This clinical investigation used approved case-control outbreak methodology to determine the mode of transmission in a hospital cluster of multidrug-resistant *Acinetobacter baumannii* bacteria (MDR-Ab). *A. baumannii* is an emerging pathogen implicated in ventilator-associated pneumonia, bloodstream infections, and wound infections. It survives on environmental surfaces for months, making transmission difficult to prevent and control.

The investigation was conducted in a 1000-bed tertiary care hospital and included 11 patients who had positive MDR-Ab cultures. Eight patients had received pulsatile lavage treatment in the physical therapy department wound care room. The same strain of MDR-Ab was cultured from all wounds and from multiple surfaces in the wound care area. The primary diagnoses for the patients involved included solid organ transplant, coronary artery bypass graft, stroke, diabetes, end-stage renal disease, and paraplegia. Investigation revealed a change in the pulsatile lavage procedure approximately 2 months before the outbreak. As a cost savings measure, the designated single-use disposable suction canisters were changed only when they became full or once a day, whichever came first.

Although only a few patients were affected by this outbreak, the nature of the organism and severity of the outcomes were significant. Three of the patients became septic and required admission to the intensive care unit. The outbreak was thought to contribute to the death of two other patients.

The correlation of pulsatile lavage and MDR-Ab dissemination shows the possibility of the spread of other aquaphilic organisms, such as *Pseudomonas,* via the same mechanism and spotlights the need for stringent infection control measures, including terminal cleaning of solid surfaces of associated equipment. Perioperative nurses involved in pulsatile lavage must take appropriate action to ensure all involved parties are wearing personal protective equipment. The patient and his or her intravenous lines also must be protected from any aerosolization.

Modified from Maragakis LL and others: An outbreak of multidrug-resistant *Acinetobacter baumannii* associated with pulsatile lavage wound treatment, *JAMA:* The *Journal of American Medical Association* 292(24):3006-3011, 2004.

are not permanent solutions in most cases, but are a bridge to permanent closure with skin grafts or granulation tissue. Skin substitutes are formed by placing human cells onto matrices that are collagen or synthetic based. As the cells grow and divide, they secrete growth factors and other useful substances to help build a foundation for healing. The substitutes are formed into a variety of shapes and sizes to facilitate wound coverage. They also may be used to cover donor sites from skin graft harvesting. Table 8-1 summarizes the actions and uses for some commonly available commercial skin substitutes. Advantages to using skin substitutes include commercial availability, effectiveness in wound contracture management, decreased risk of donor area morbidity, provision of long-term coverage of the wound, and compatibility with autologous tissues.[15]

### Growth Factors

Growth factors are naturally occurring proteins (cytokines and peptides) that are signaling molecules that stimulate cycles of mitosis of fibroblasts and epidermal cells, smooth muscle cells, and vascular endothelial cells. Human or recombinant growth factors may be applied to wounds in the OR, but are more typically administered in the clinic setting. Growth factors initiate wound healing by accelerating the formation of granulation tissue and work most effectively in the proliferative phase of wound healing. The factors improve the cellular or molecular environment of the wound and signal target cells to begin tissue repair. Growth factors generally are categorized by their source (i.e., if obtained from platelets, they are designated as platelet-derived growth factors [PDGF]; from the epidermis, epidermal growth factor [EGF]). To obtain PDGF, typically 50 to 200 mL of venous blood is withdrawn. The platelets are separated and activated with thrombin to make a gel that is applied to a clean wound bed. The wound is covered with a nonadherent gauze dressing and left on for 12 hours.[7] The average wound healing time in acute skin wounds can be shortened by 1 to 4 days when locally treated with growth factors.[4] Healing time for chronic wounds also is substantially shortened when growth factors are applied (Research Highlight).

## DRESSINGS

Application of surgical dressings is often the responsibility of the perioperative nurse (History box). The dressing may serve one or more of the following purposes:

1. Cushioning and protection of the wound from trauma and gross contamination
2. Absorption of drainage
3. Debridement of the wound
4. Support, splinting, or immobilization of the body part and incisional area
5. Aid in hemostasis and minimize edema and dead space, as in a pressure dressing
6. Enhance the patient's physical comfort and aesthetic appearance
7. Maintenance of a moist environment and prevention of cell dehydration
8. Application of medications

Dressings are selected based on the characteristics of the surgical site, depth, and area and the patient's overall condition (Table 8-2). Questions to ask when choosing a dressing are as follows:[14]

1. What does the wound need?
2. What does the product do?
3. How well does it do it?
4. What does the patient need?
5. What is available?
6. What is practical?

Dressings can be grouped into two main categories: primary and secondary dressings. *Primary* dressings are placed directly over or in the wound. A variety of dressing materials are available on the market today. The function of these dressings is to absorb drainage and allow it to wick away from the wound edge. Cotton gauze or synthetic dressings may be used for this

**TABLE 8-1**

**Skin Substitutes**

| Name | Description | Use/Application |
|---|---|---|
| Dermagraft | Single layer, contains cultured fibroblasts on cultured synthetic matrix. Provides cells and growth factors to the wound | Approved only for use in diabetic foot ulcers |
| Transcyte | Two-layer product. Outside layer is semipermeable and synthetic allowing fluid and gas exchange and promoting a moist healing environment. Inner layer is a bioengineered cell matrix that adheres quickly to wound surfaces | Superficial to mid–partial thickness burns, temporary coverage of excised burns |
| Apligraft | Living, two-layer product. Inside layer combines bovine type I collagen with human fibroblasts to produce matrix proteins. Outside layer stimulates epidermal cells to replicate | Widely used for wounds of the ankle and foot. Also used to treat donor sites and surgical excisional wounds |
| Alloderm | Cadaver donated product that is processed to remove all epidermal and dermal cells while leaving the cellular matrix intact | Can be used on large areas, comes in large sheets |
| Oasis | Made from pig small intestinal submucosa. Consists of naturally occurring growth factors and collagen | Superficial burns, donor sites |
| Integra | Two-layer dressing consisting of dermal layer and epidermal layer. Inner, dermal layer is composed of bovine tendon collagen and synthetic chondroitin 6-sulfate. As healing progresses, inner layer degrades. Outer layer is a synthetic (silicone) that serves to control moisture loss from the wound | Useful in burn coverage |

Information from www.burnsurgery.org accessed August 28, 2005; Jimenez PA, Jimenez SE: Tissue and cellular approaches to wound care, *American Journal of Surgery* 187(5 Suppl 1), 2004; accessed August 28, 2005, online www.woundhealer.com/sknsub.

## RESEARCH HIGHLIGHT

### Topical Treatment of Pressure Ulcers with Nerve Growth Factor

Pressure ulcers often are related to increased morbidity and mortality in susceptible populations, and management of the condition is a challenge, even in light of many technologic and scientific advances in wound care. This randomized, double-blinded study evaluated the daily topical use of nerve growth factor compared with conventional topical treatment of severe, noninfected pressure ulcers of the foot.

Patients were considered for the study if they had a pressure ulcer of the foot that ranged from 1 to 30 cm in total area. After screening for ulcer size and other factors (i.e., demographic characteristics, functional and cognitive status, and nursing needs relevant to care planning), a treatment group of 18 patients and a control group of 18 patients were established. Most patients had a pressure ulcer on the heel (14 in the treatment group and 15 in the control group) or lateral malleolus (4 in the treatment group and 3 in the control group). Ulcer size and stage were recorded at baseline and every subsequent week for 6 weeks. Digital photographs also were taken weekly for progress comparisons. Two wound cultures, performed at different parts of the ulcer, showed no bacterial growth. The ulcers showed a range of stages from stage 1 to stage 5.

Dressings were changed daily in both groups until the wound healed or for a maximum of 6 weeks. All patients received irrigation with normal saline, use of débriding enzymes, and application of hydrocolloid occlusive barriers. The patients in the treatment group underwent application of the growth factor dissolved in a balanced salt solution, dropped on the wound, and allowed to dry. The control group had a plain balanced salt solution that was dropped on the wound and allowed to dry.

After 6 weeks of treatment, the mean area of the ulcers in the treatment group was 274 ± 329 $mm^2$ compared with 526 ± 393 $mm^2$ in the control group. All the ulcers treated with topical application of nerve growth factor showed a statistically significant acceleration of the healing process. Within 4 weeks of initiation of treatment with growth factor, the total area of ulceration was reduced by nearly 50%. The results of this study indicate a use for growth factors in the treatment of chronic severe pressure ulcers.

Modified from Landi F and others: Topical treatment of pressure ulcers with nerve growth factor, *Annals of Internal Medicine* 139(8):635-641, 2003.

purpose. The layer of dressing directly contacting the wound should be nonadherent, unless debridement is desired.

*Secondary* dressings are placed directly over the primary dressing. These function to absorb excessive drainage, provide hemostasis by compression, and protect the wound from further trauma. These functions usually are accomplished with a bulky dressing, such as an abdominal pad. These pads have a cotton filling that provides extra absorbency.

Dressings may be secured with a variety of products, including tape, Elastoplast, Ace bandages, or soft roll products. Tape is available with a variety of backing materials (cloth, paper, taffeta, plastic) and with regular or nonallergenic adhesive. The amount of strength and elasticity required, patient allergies, the condition of the patient's skin, and anticipated frequency of dressing change influence which type is selected. When applying tape to the dressing, the nurse should apply pressure evenly from both sides of the tape and away from the direction of the incision. Applying tape with excessive pressure may result in stretching and trauma to the skin. The tape should cover the edges of the dressing and be placed at right angles to the direction of motion when applied over a joint. When frequent dressing changes are anticipated, Montgomery straps can be selected to secure the dressing (Figure 8-6). When compression of the wound for hemostasis or reduction of edema is desired, a polyurethane dressing, elastic tape, or elastic bandage may be used to secure the secondary dressing.

## HISTORY

One of the duties of the perioperative nurse in the 1900s was the manufacture, sterilization, and maintenance of bandages and drains. Typical classifications of bandages were roller bandages, compound bandages (e.g., many-tailed bandages and slings), immobilizing bandages (e.g., gauze rolls impregnated with plaster, paraffin, or starch), and pressure bandages.

Roller bandages were made from muslin, crinoline, flannel fabric, or gauze. Pressure and occlusive bandages were made from India-rubber cloth. To make roller bandages from muslin, crinoline, or flannel, the nurse obtained 4 to 6 yards of uncut fabric and washed it first in a hot saline solution. When the fabric dried, it was cut to the desired width and was rolled by hand or on a bandage-rolling machine operated by a foot treadle. An expedited method of making multiple roller bandages was to roll the entire length of fabric without cutting it into individual strips and placing it into a carpenter's miter box and cutting the desired width with a bread knife. Roller bandages were steam sterilized and wrapped in paraffin-coated paper. The paper was made by spreading the paper over a flat surface, pouring wax on it and ironing it evenly with a flat iron. Compound dressings (e.g., the Scultetus binder) were cut and sewn by hand. The nurse made immobilizing bandages by manually applying plaster of Paris to crinoline strips and placing the rolled bandage in an airtight metal container. India-rubber cloth and other rubber goods were maintained in drawers dusted with powdered sulfur. To prepare drains, the nurse obtained the desired length and diameter of tubing from the rubber goods drawer, scrubbed the drain in soap and water, rinsed, and boiled the drainage tube in a solution of 1% carbonate of soda for 1 hour. The drain was removed and sealed in a jar containing a solution of normal saline and carbolic acid. The solution in the jars was changed once a week. Any fenestrae or other modifications were made at the time of use. Cigarette drains were made by impregnating four 9-inch lengths of lamp wicking with antiseptics, such as iodoform powder, zinc oxide powder, carbolic crystals, resin, or castor oil, and enclosing the bundle in green silk or rubber tissue stitched in place.

To apply muslin bandages, the nurse saturated the bandage in warm water to enhance the patient's comfort and wound the bandage in a circular, figure-of-eight, or spiral fashion to cover the affected area. Muslin roller gauze was used to bandage all parts of the body. When the bandage was complete, the nurse secured it by sewing it closed, fastening it with safety pins, or knotting the tails. Removal of the bandage was accomplished by unrolling the muslin instead of cutting it, to facilitate disinfection and reuse.

Modified from Fowler FS: *The operating room and the patient,* ed 3, Philadelphia, 1913; Saunders, Witkowski JA, Parish LC: Occlusive therapy in historical perspective, *International Journal of Dermatology* 37:555-558, 1998.

**TABLE 8-2**

## Comparing Wound Dressings

| Products | Advantages | Disadvantages | Nursing Considerations |
|---|---|---|---|
| **COTTON MESH GAUZE** | Low cost, readily available | Woven forms may leave lint in wound | Can be used as wet-to-dry dressing for wound débridement and granulation |
| Woven and nonwoven | Wicks away moisture | May dry out | Frequent dressing changes may be needed if gauze dries out |
| | Can be used for mechanical debridement | Nonwoven not as effective as woven for debridement | May be used with saline and amorphous gels to keep moist |
| **NONADHERENT DRESSING** | Less traumatic for the patient | Poor absorption of fluids | Nonimpregnated can be used as primary or secondary dressing |
| *Nonimpregnated:* Telfa | | Impregnated form cannot be used as primary dressing | Useful for donor sites, skin grafts |
| *Impregnated:* Adaptic, Scarlet Red, Vaseline Gauze, Xeroform | | Impregnated form may cause maceration if left on wound for prolonged period | |
| **TRANSPARENT FILMS** | Resistant to shearing and friction | Cannot absorb exudate, which may lead to maceration | May wrinkle on application |
| Bioclusive, Op Site, Tegaderm | Conforms well to irregular surfaces<br>Wound is easily monitored through film<br>May be more cost-effective because of decreased frequency of dressing change | Exudate may leak through seal | Use with caution on fragile skin |
| **HYDROCOLLOID** | Insulates and cushions | May melt and leave residue in wound | Should not be used in the presence of infection because of occlusive properties |

*Note:* The products included here are representatives of what is available; the lists under each category are not meant to be inclusive.
Modified from Lionelli GT, Lawrence WT: Wound dressings, *Surgical Clinics of North America* 83:617-638, 2003; Worley CA: So what do I put on this wound? Making sense of the wound dressing puzzle: part I, *Dermatology Nursing* 17(2):143-144, 2005; Worley CA: So what do I put on this wound? Making sense of the wound dressing puzzle: part II, *Dermatology Nursing* 17(3):204-205, 2005; Worley CA: So what do I put on this wound? Making sense of the wound dressing puzzle: part III, *Dermatology Nursing* 17(4):299-300, 2005.

**TABLE 8-2**

## Comparing Wound Dressings—cont'd

| Products | Advantages | Disadvantages | Nursing Considerations |
|---|---|---|---|
| Comfeel, Sorbex, DuoDerm, Tegasorb | Available in a variety of sizes and forms | May bunch or wrinkle at edges | Need 1- to 2-in. border of intact skin beyond wound to seal edge of dressing |
| | Useful on all stages of wounds | May not adhere well to irregular shapes or contours | Can be used as a primary or secondary dressing |
| | Adheres in the presence of moisture | May be bulky | May react with wound proteins and develop an odor that can be mistaken for infection |
| **HYDROGEL** | Can be used to fill shallow wounds and cavities | Excessive application can lead to maceration | Should be applied to wound surface only |
| Carrasyn, Solosite Gel, Tegagel, Vigilon, Nu-gel, Curagel | Cooling, soothing action may decrease pain | May be difficult to keep in shallow wounds | Viscosity varies among products |
| | May be used to rehydrate wounds | | Compatible with a variety of medications, so can be used as a carrier for antibiotics |
| **ALGINATES** | Highly absorbent | May cause burning sensation for patient | Available in pastes, pads, ropes, powders, starches |
| Algiderm, Algosteril, Curasorb, SeaSorb, Kaltostat, Sorbsan | Useful for increased levels of exudate | Requires secondary dressing | Product swells, so apply lightly in cavities and undermined areas |
| | Moisture retentive | Easily dislodged by mechanical force | Saturate with saline for removal if dried |
| **FOAM** | Highly absorbent | Contraindicated for desiccated wounds | Dressing should be 2-3 cm larger than wound |
| Lyofoam, Curafoam Allevyn, Flexan, Biopatch, Vigifoam | Helps contain exudate | Leakage may occur if not covered with waterproof protection | Use with packing in undermining, tunneling wounds |
| | Can be left in place for 7 days | | Available as pads, sheets, or rolls |
| | Comfort for patient | | |
| **SILICONE** | Easy to apply, reusable | May adhere to itself | May be used to reduce pain when wound vacuum system is used |
| Cica-Care Adhesive Silicone Gel Sheet, Mepiform, Oleeva | Variety of sizes, promotes scar reduction | Can be difficult to apply | Marketed to consumers as a way to reduce scar formation |
| **COLLAGEN** | May accelerate wound repair | May have unpleasant odor | Requires a secondary dressing |
| Fibracol, Promogran Cellerate | Effective in recalcitrant wounds | | Available in gels, pastes, pads, powder |
| | | | Source is bovine, porcine, or avian collagen |
| **COMPOSITES** | Thin, nonadherent attached adhesive | Not recommended for heavily draining wounds | May be used as primary or secondary dressing |
| Alldress, Primapore Op-Site Post Op | | | One-hand application in some cases |
| | | | Use with caution with fragile skin |

Immobilization is accomplished with the addition of soft padding, elastic bandages, splints, and casting materials (splints and casts are discussed in greater detail in Chapter 22).

In some situations, the wound is not dressed at all. The air-exposed wound heals, and having no dressing (1) allows for optimal observation of the incisional area, (2) aids bathing, (3) prevents possible adhesive-tape reactions, (4) increases comfort and maneuverability for many patients, and (5) seems to minimize adverse responses by the patient to the operation.

## DRAINS

Drains control ecchymosis and provide exits through which air and fluids, such as serum, blood, lymph, intestinal secretions, bile, and pus, can be evacuated from the operative site. Drains also may be used to prevent the development of deep wound infections. They usually are inserted at the time of surgery, primarily through a separate small incision known as a *stab wound,* close to the operative site. Drains may or may not be sutured to the skin.

In some instances (chest, common bile duct, bladder), drainage is directly through the lumen of the tube (as with a Foley retention catheter) or via perforations or fenestrations in the tubing into a closed drainage system. In other instances (peritoneal cavity or skin wound), drainage of pus or blood is primarily along the outside surface of the drain by capillary action and gravity (as with the simple Penrose drain) into a dressing. The selection of a simple versus a closed drainage system depends on the needs of the site to be drained, patient activity, and overall healing capability. Many types of drains are

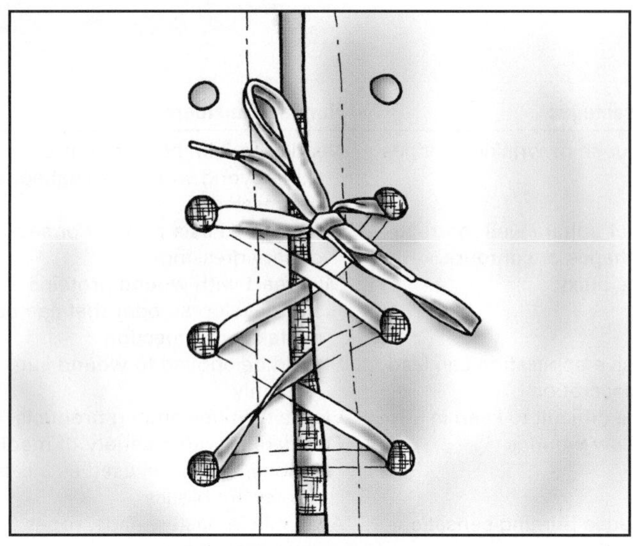

FIGURE 8-6 Montgomery straps.

available. The most common are made of latex, polyvinyl chloride (PVC), or silicone (Figure 8-7). Particular care should be taken to ensure that the patient is not allergic to latex when selecting any latex drain. For many wounds, a portable, self-contained, closed wound suction unit is selected. These units create a negative pressure in a reservoir attached to the drain. Fluid is gently drawn out of the wound and collected in the reservoir.

The perioperative nurse must document clearly on the operative record the location and type of drain and ensure the drain is working properly before the patient leaves the OR. This information is important to nurses caring for the patient in the postanesthesia and postoperative nursing units. Some wounds yield significant amounts of drainage and must be monitored closely during the postoperative course. A disadvantage of wound drains is that they create a portal for entry and exit of infectious microorganisms. Extreme care must be taken in emptying drain reservoirs to avoid contamination.[7] Closed autologous drains allow for collection of blood from a surgical wound and the return of that blood to the patient; this minimizes the need for transfusion of blood from outside donors, reducing the risk of bloodborne pathogen transmission.

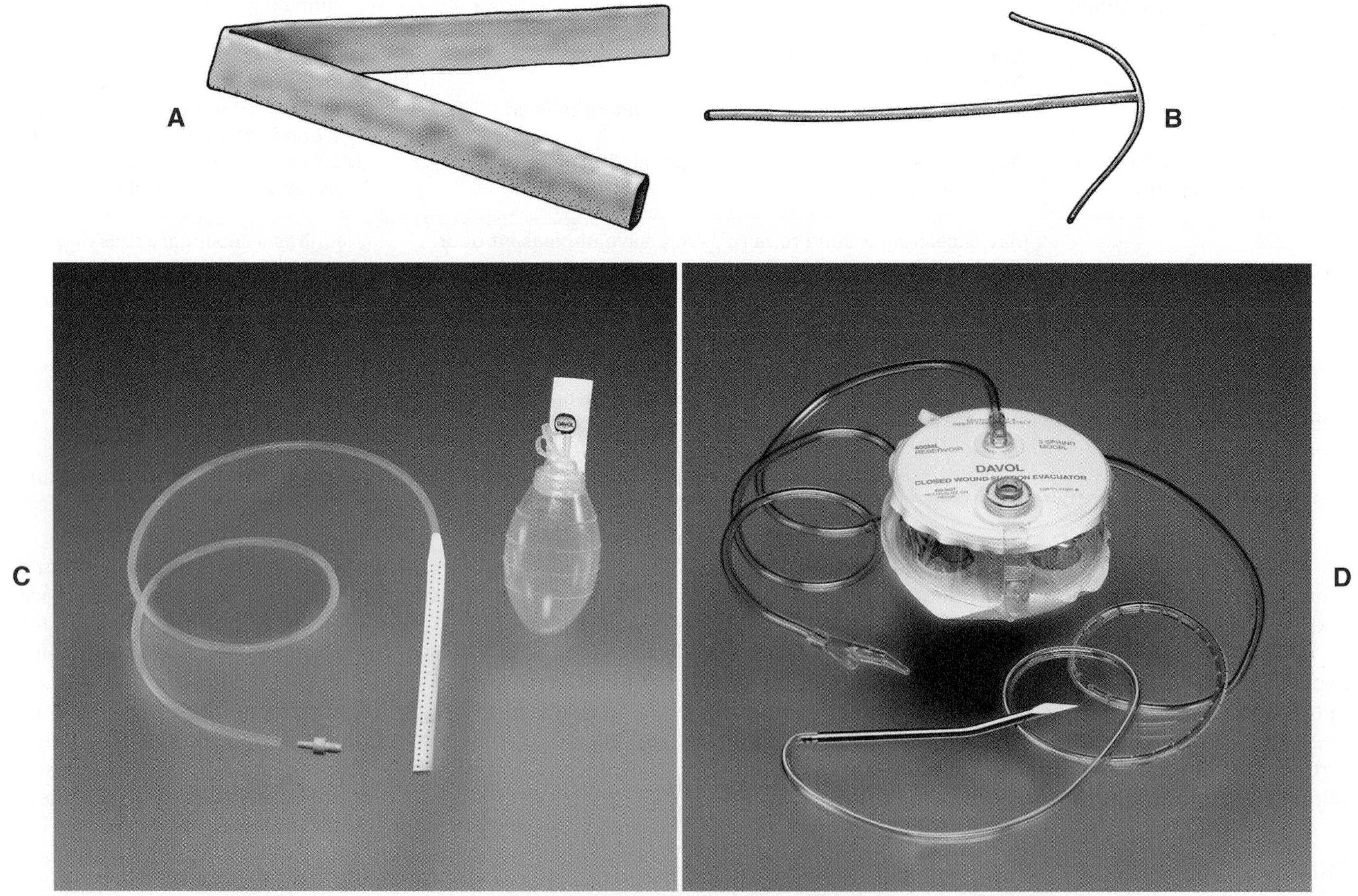

A

B

C

D

FIGURE 8-7 Drains are available in a variety of styles. Pictured are Penrose **(A)** and T-tube **(B)**, which drain by gravity, and Jackson Pratt **(C)** and Hemovac **(D)**, which represent closed drainage systems.

## SUMMARY

Wound healing is an essential part of the surgical experience. The perioperative nurse should vigilantly guard and enhance the patient's ability to heal with an eye toward prevention of problems before they occur. There is no more important time to prevent surgical wound infections than in the perioperative period.

## REFERENCES

1. AORN: *AORN standards, recommended practices, and guidelines,* Denver, Colo, 2005, The Association.
2. Cameron J, Newton H: Dermatological aspects of wound healing. In Morison MJ and others, editors: *Chronic wound care: a problem based learning approach,* St Louis, 2004, Mosby.
3. Clark AP: Nosocomial infections: an issue of patient safety, part 1, *Clinical Nurse Specialist* 17(6):284-285, 2003.
4. Fu X and others: Engineered growth factors and cutaneous wound healing: success and possible questions in the past 10 years, *Wound Repair and Regeneration* 13(2):122-130, 2005.
5. Fuller J: Cover up and clean up to prevent deadly infections, *Nursing* 35(1):31, 2005.
6. Gottrup F: Oxygen in wound healing and infection, *World Journal of Surgery* 28(3):312-315, 2004.
7. Harvey C: Wound healing, *Orthopaedic Nursing* 24(2):143-157, 2005.
8. Hess CL and others: A review of mechanical adjuncts in wound healing: hydrotherapy, ultrasound, negative pressure therapy, hyperbaric oxygen therapy, electrostimulation, *Annals of Plastic Surgery* 51(2), 2003.
9. Jimenez PA, Jimenez SE: Tissue and cellular approaches to wound care, *American Journal of Surgery* 187(5 Suppl 1), 2004.
10. Kaufman MW, Pahl DW: Vacuum-assisted closure therapy: wound care and nursing implications, *Dermatology Nursing* 15(4):317-325, 2003.
11. Leong M, Phillips LG: Wound healing. In Townsend CM and others, editors: *Sabiston textbook of surgery,* ed 17, Philadelphia, 2004, Saunders.
12. Mangram AJ and others: *Special report: guidelines for prevention of surgical site infection, 1999,* National Centers for Infectious Diseases, Hospital Infections Programs. Accessed August 21, 2005, on-line: www.cdc.gov.nciod/hip/ssi/ssi.pdf.
13. Mendez-Eastman S: Using negative pressure wound therapy for positive results, *Nursing* 35(5):48-50, 2005.
14. Ovington LG and Eisenbud D: Dressings and cleaning agents. In Morison MJ and others, editors: *Chronic wound care: a problem based learning approach,* St Louis, 2004, Mosby.
15. Ozerderm OM and others: Use of skin substitutes in pediatric patients, *Journal of Craniofacial Surgery* 14(4):517-520, 2003.
16. Sessler DI: Temperature monitoring. In Miller RD, editor: *Miller's anesthesia,* ed 6, Philadelphia, 2005, Churchill-Livingstone.
17. Sosin J: Ancient remedy heals today's wounds, *Nursing Spectrum* 15(6):32-33, 2005.
18. Steed DL: Debridement, *American Journal of Surgery* 187(Suppl to May):71S-74S, 2004.
19. Stotts NA: Wound infection: diagnosis and management. In Morison MJ and others, editors: *Chronic wound care: a problem based learning approach,* St Louis, 2004, Mosby.

CHAPTER 9

# Postoperative Patient Care and Pain Management

JAN ODOM-FORREN

The postoperative phase of care begins as soon as the surgical procedure is concluded and the patient is transferred to the postanesthesia care unit (PACU). The PACU has been known in the past as the *recovery room* or *postanesthesia room*. A postanesthesia area was first described by Florence Nightingale:[23] "It is not uncommon, in small country hospitals, to have a recess or small room leading from the operating theater in which the patients remain until they have recovered, or at least recovered from the immediate effects of the operation" (History box).

An assigned area for the care of the postoperative patient is a relatively recent addition to surgical patient care. Although surgical procedures have been performed for thousands of years, and general anesthesia has been available for almost 150 years, PACUs became common only in the past 30 to 40 years. A few recovery rooms were opened in the 1920s and 1930s. In the 1940s, numerous PACUs opened because of the shortage of nurses during the war years and the need to centralize patients, equipment, and personnel for postoperative care. It was soon realized that use of the PACU decreased patient morbidity and mortality and shortened the length of hospitalization of some patients.[28] Many hospitals opened PACUs after this discovery was reported.

PACUs have flourished since that time. Technologic innovation has had a profound effect on PACUs, as in other critical care areas. The complexity of anesthesia management demands specially trained nurses who have expertise in the prompt recognition and management of postoperative complications. Most patients who receive general anesthesia, major regional anesthesia, or monitored anesthesia care are transferred to a PACU.

The PACU should be adjacent to the surgical suite with easy access for patient transport. The patient's status should be assessed for needs during transfer (e.g., oxygen, manual positive-pressure ventilation device, a bed instead of a stretcher).

The perioperative nurse accompanies the patient to the PACU with an anesthesia provider and gives a hand-off report on the status of the patient to a perianesthesia nurse. The nurse in the PACU assumes the care of the patient after an initial assessment of the patient and a report from the transferring team.

## PERIANESTHESIA CONSIDERATIONS

### Assessment

***Admission to Postanesthesia Care Unit.*** The initial assessment of the postoperative patient begins with an immediate determination of airway and circulatory adequacy. The airway is assessed for patency, humidified oxygen is applied, and respirations are counted. Pulse oximetry is initiated on all patients, and the quality of breath sounds is determined. The patient is connected to the cardiac monitor, and cardiac rate and rhythm are evaluated. Blood pressure is measured by means of a manual cuff or an automatic cuff (e.g., a Dinamap). If the patient has an arterial line, it can be connected to the monitor at this time.

After the PACU nurse has assessed the *ABCs* (*a*irway, *b*reathing, *c*irculation), the perioperative nurse and anesthesia provider give a comprehensive hand-off report on the patient. The perioperative nurse should collaborate and add and verify important information about the patient. The American Society of PeriAnesthesia Nurses (ASPAN)[7] recommends that the report contain the following:

- Relevant preoperative information, such as vital signs and temperature, radiology findings, laboratory values, oxygen saturation, allergies (including latex), effect of preoperative medication, disabilities, substance abuse, mobility limitations, prostheses, and communication disabilities and, in the pediatric patient: birth history, development stages, and parent/child interactions
- Anesthesia technique and agents administered
- Length of time anesthesia was administered and time reversal agents were given
- Type of operative or other invasive procedure performed
- Estimated fluid or blood loss and replacement therapy
- Complications occurring during anesthesia, treatment initiated, and patient response
- Emotional status on arrival to operating room (OR) or procedure room
- Numeric score, if used

The patient's American Society of Anesthesiologists (ASA) physical classification status (see Chapter 4) also should be provided during the patient report. Other useful information that the perioperative nurse can provide includes the status of the airway; presence of tubes, drains, and catheters; and intravascular lines. Any postoperative orders to be initiated in the PACU can be discussed at this time.

The anesthesia provider should not leave the patient until the PACU nurse accepts responsibility for the patient's care. Standard III-3 of the ASA *Standards for Postanesthesia Care*[4] states, "the member of the anesthesia care team shall remain in the PACU until the PACU nurse accepts responsibility for the nursing care of the patient."

## HISTORY

Separate care for postsurgical patients can be dated back to 1751, when it is noted that New Castle Infirmary, in New Castle, England, had rooms reserved for dangerously ill or major surgery patients. Florence Nightingale in 1863 suggested separate rooms for patients to recover from the immediate effects of anesthesia. During the twentieth century, the complexity of surgeries increased in direct relation to technical discoveries. The number of recovery units gradually grew, especially after their value was established in the 1940s. The Anesthesia Study Commission of the Philadelphia County Medical Society reported in 1947 that one third of preventable postsurgical deaths during an 11-year period could have been prevented by improved postoperative nursing care. The Operating Room Committee for New York Hospital in 1949 stated that adequate recovery room service was necessary for any hospital that provided surgical services. By the 1970s, recovery rooms were managing routine postanesthesia patients and critically ill postanesthesia patients receiving respiratory and circulatory support. Currently, recovery rooms are known as *postanesthesia care units (PACUs)* and sometimes, because of space constraints and cost containment, also manage the care of overflow intensive care unit/telemetry patients.

Modified from Odom-Forren J: The evolution of perianesthesia nursing. In Quinn DMD, Schick L, editors: *Perianesthesia nursing core curriculum: preoperative, phase I and phase II PACU nursing,* St Louis, 2004, Saunders.

***Initial Assessment.*** After the immediate assessment of ABCs and completion of the report, the PACU nurse begins a more thorough postanesthesia assessment. The assessment is performed quickly and is specific, in part, to the type of operative procedure. Recommended elements of an initial assessment in the PACU are presented in Box 9-1.

Some PACUs use a head-to-toe assessment to organize the data obtained (Figure 9-1). Other PACUs have adopted a major body systems approach to assessment (Figure 9-2). In any case, the PACU nurse assesses the admitting vital signs and the ABCs, beginning with the respiratory system. Respiratory assessment comprises rate, rhythm, auscultation of breath sounds for ventilatory adequacy, and oxygen saturation level. Presence of an artificial airway and type of oxygen delivery system are noted.

The cardiovascular system is assessed by monitoring heart rate and rhythm. The patient's initial blood pressure is compared with one or more preoperative readings. Body temperature is obtained, skin condition is examined, and peripheral pulses are checked, if indicated. The patient is assessed for neurologic function: Has the patient reacted (awakened from anesthesia)? Can the patient follow commands? Is the patient oriented, at least to name and hospital? Can the patient move all extremities and lift the head? Are there deviations from preoperative neurologic functioning? Some operative procedures require a more detailed assessment.

To assess renal function, intake and output are measured. The total intraoperative fluid intake and estimated blood loss are assessed. The intravenous lines, infusions, and irrigation solutions are reviewed and recorded. Presence of all lines, drains, and catheters is noted; output is noted for color, amount, and consistency.

The surgical site is assessed. Any drainage on the bandage is noted, including amount and color. The area around the incision is assessed so that any future changes may be compared. A patient undergoing a vaginal hysterectomy requires that the abdomen be assessed for firmness. In the event of hemorrhage, one indication of the type of problem may be a rigid abdomen. Comparisons of the firmness of the abdomen on admission and later findings of a rigid abdomen lead to accurate and important comparisons. The patient also is assessed for signs or symptoms of pain or discomfort, such as nausea, and is medicated as appropriate.

All the information obtained from the admission assessment is documented in the PACU record. An example of a PACU record is shown in Figure 9-3.

**BOX 9-1**

### Initial Assessment in the Postanesthesia Care Unit

The initial assessment in the PACU is to include documentation of the following:

1. Integration of data received at transfer of care
2. Vital signs
   a. Respiratory status—airway patent, breath sounds, type of artificial airway, mechanical ventilator settings, and oxygen saturation
   b. Blood pressure—cuff or arterial line
   c. Pulse—apical, peripheral
   d. Cardiac monitor, rhythm documented
   e. Temperature/route
   f. Pain/comfort assessment
3. Level of consciousness
4. Pressure readings—central venous, arterial blood, pulmonary artery wedge, and intracranial pressure if indicated
5. Position of patient
6. Condition and color of skin
7. Patient safety needs
8. Neurovascular—peripheral pulses and sensation of extremity or extremities as applicable
9. Condition of dressings
10. Condition of suture line, if dressing absent
11. Type, patency, and security of drainage tubes, catheters, and receptacle
12. Amount and type of drainage
13. Muscular response and strength
14. Pupillary response as indicated
15. Fluid therapy—location of lines, condition of intravenous site, and security and amount of solution infusing (including blood)
16. Level of physical and emotional comfort
17. Postanesthesia scoring system if used
18. Procedure-specific assessment

Modified from American Society of PeriAnesthesia Nurses: *Standards of perianesthesia nursing practice,* Cherry Hill, NJ, 2004, The Society.

## Nursing Diagnosis

Common nursing diagnoses related to the care of postanesthesia patients include the following:

- Ineffective Breathing Pattern
- Decreased Cardiac Output
- Ineffective Thermoregulation
- Disturbed Thought Processes
- Acute Pain

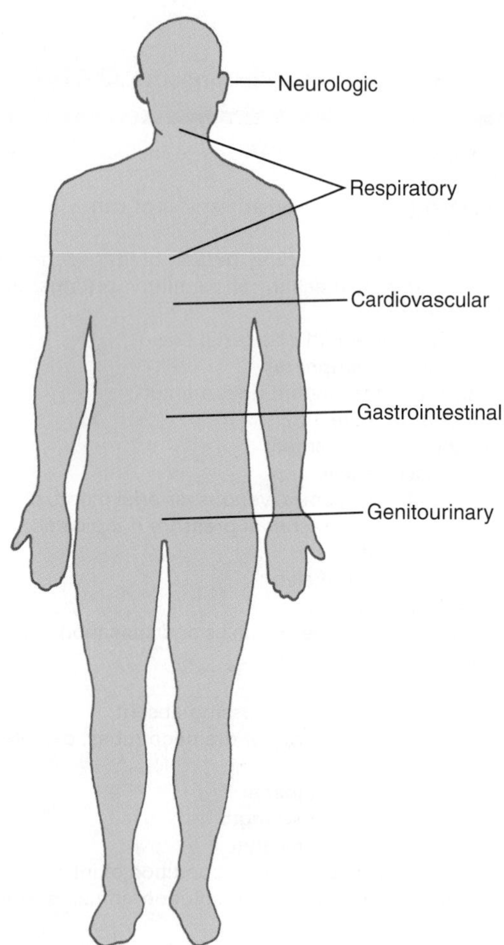


FIGURE 9-1 Head-to-toe assessment.

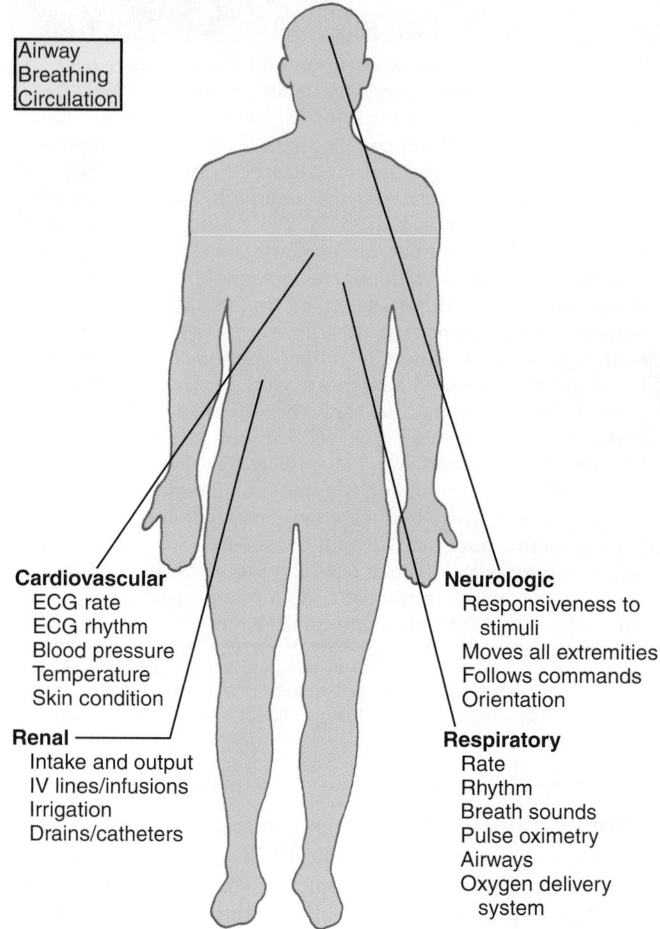


FIGURE 9-2 PACU major body systems assessment. *ECG*, electrocardiogram; *IV*, intravenous.

## Outcome Identification

Outcomes identified for the selected nursing diagnoses can be stated as follows:

- The patient will demonstrate adequate ventilation, perfusion, and expansion of the lungs on discharge from the PACU.
- The patient will achieve and maintain adequate cardiac output on discharge from the PACU.
- The patient will attain a normal body temperature (96.8°F to 100.4°F) (36°C to 38°C) on discharge from the PACU.
- The patient will demonstrate appropriate cognitive function on discharge from the PACU.
- The patient will exhibit 4 or less on a numeric pain rating scale of 0 to 10 (or a comfort level established by the patient as "acceptable") on discharge from the PACU.

## Planning

When the nursing diagnoses and desired outcomes are identified for the postoperative patient, a plan of care is designed for the specific patient. Some nursing diagnoses are appropriate for all postanesthesia patients. A Sample Plan of Care for the postanesthesia patient follows on p. 252.

## Implementation

Dramatic and life-threatening changes can occur rapidly in the postanesthesia setting. The following complications are pertinent to the care of all patients during the postoperative period. Prompt recognition and immediate intervention are imperative for the well-being of the patient.

### *Postoperative Complications*

#### RESPIRATORY

**Airway Obstruction.** The first priority in the care of the postanesthesia patient is to establish a patent airway. A common cause of airway obstruction is the tongue, which is relaxed because of anesthetic agents and muscle relaxants used during surgery (Figure 9-4 on p. 253). The patient may present with snoring, little or no air movement on auscultation of the lungs, retraction of intercostal muscles, asynchronous movements of the chest and abdomen, and a decreased oxygen saturation level. The nursing action taken may be simple, such as stimulating the patient to take deep breaths, positioning the patient on the side, or providing supplemental oxygen. If the patient is still unresponsive, the nurse may need to open the airway with a chin tilt or jaw thrust. A chin tilt is accomplished by lifting the chin with one hand while tilting the forehead back with the other. A jaw thrust is accomplished by displacing the temporomandibular joint forward bilaterally. The patient also can be repositioned on the right side. This position is called the recovery position. Placing the patient in this position allows the tongue to move forward and the airway to remain open.

## FORREST GENERAL HOSPITAL
## POST ANESTHESIA CARE UNIT RECORD

| POST ANESTHESIA RECOVERY SCORE | | MINUTES in | 30 | 60 | 90 | out |
|---|---|---|---|---|---|---|
| **Activity** | | | | | | |
| Able to move 4 extremities voluntarily or on command | = 2 | | | | | |
| Able to move 2 extremities voluntarily or on command | = 1 | | | | | |
| Able to move 0 extremities voluntarily or on command | = 0 | | | | | |
| **Respiration** | | | | | | |
| Able to deep breathe and cough freely | = 2 | | | | | |
| Dyspnea or limited breathing | = 1 | | | | | |
| Apneic | = 0 | | | | | |
| **Circulation** | | | | | | |
| BP ± 20 of Preanesthetic level | = 2 | | | | | |
| BP ± 20-50 of Preanesthetic level | = 1 | | | | | |
| BP ± 50 of Preanesthetic level | = 0 | | | | | |
| **Consciousness** | | | | | | |
| Fully Awake | = 2 | | | | | |
| Arousable on calling | = 1 | | | | | |
| Not Responding | = 0 | | | | | |
| **$O_2$ Saturation** | | | | | | |
| Able to maintain $O_2$ Sat > 92% on room air | = 2 | | | | | |
| Needs $O_2$ to maintain $O_2$ Sat > 90% | = 1 | | | | | |
| $O_2$ Sat < 90% even with $O_2$ | = 0 | | | | | |
| TOTAL | | | | | | |

Pre-op B.P. ______
Allergy

Airway: On Adm.
Jawthrust ______
Chin Hold ______
Endotracheal ______
Oral Airway ______
Mask Oxygen ______
Nasal Oxygen ______
Trach ______
T-Tube ______
Nasal Airway ______
Ventilator Settings ______

Addressograph

Time In ______ Time Out ______

Accompanied by ______

Type of anesthesia ______

Surgical Procedure:

PULSE - RESPIRATION - BLOOD PRESSURE

| | 15 | 30 | 45 | | 15 | 30 | 45 | | 15 | 30 | 45 | | 15 | 30 | 45 |
|---|---|---|---|---|---|---|---|---|---|---|---|---|---|---|---|
| 240 | | | | | | | | | | | | | | | |
| 220 | | | | | | | | | | | | | | | |
| 200 | | | | | | | | | | | | | | | |
| 180 | | | | | | | | | | | | | | | |
| 160 | | | | | | | | | | | | | | | |
| 140 | | | | | | | | | | | | | | | |
| 120 | | | | | | | | | | | | | | | |
| 100 | | | | | | | | | | | | | | | |
| 80 | | | | | | | | | | | | | | | |
| 60 | | | | | | | | | | | | | | | |
| 40 | | | | | | | | | | | | | | | |
| 20 | | | | | | | | | | | | | | | |
| $O_2$ Sat. | | | | | | | | | | | | | | | |
| Pain score | | | | | | | | | | | | | | | |
| PAP | | | | | | | | | | | | | | | |

CODES: ⊥ A-line, T B.P. | V Manual or Λ NBP | Pulse • Resp. ○ | Siderails: Yes No | Restraints:: Yes No

IV Type ______

Total IV in OR ______ cc
Blood in OR ______ units
Urinary Output in OR ______ cc
Est. Blood Loss ______ cc

Foley Cath. ______
Suprapubic ______
Ureteral ______
Levine ______

**DRAINS**

______ RN Signature

______ RN Signature

### MEDICATIONS AND TREATMENTS

| | AMT. | ROUTE | TIME |
|---|---|---|---|
| Demerol | | | |
| Morphine | | | |
| Phenergan | | | |
| Droperidol | | | |
| Zofran | | | |
| Toradol | | | |

**FIGURE 9-3** PACU record. *Continued*

If these actions do not open the airway, an artificial airway may need to be inserted. An oral or a nasal airway may be used. An oral airway is indicated for use with an unresponsive patient (Figure 9-5 on p. 253). A nasal airway, better tolerated by an awake patient, is indicated for patients who are arousable.

Hemorrhage after neck surgery or carotid endarterectomy also can cause acute obstruction of the airway. The perianesthesia nurse should assess these patients carefully for bleeding. In certain situations, such as apnea, intubation with ventilation may be required. If intubation is impossible, the patient may require a tracheostomy, although this rarely is needed.

**Laryngospasm.** A serious complication that can occur in the PACU is laryngospasm, usually the result of an irritable airway. The muscles of the larynx contract and partially or

FORREST GENERAL HOSPITAL

| DATE | TIME | DESCRIPTIVE NOTES (SIGN EACH ENTRY) |
|---|---|---|
| | | |

| Report to Family:<br>Time: | GU IRRIGANT | FOLEY OUTPUT |
|---|---|---|
| | TOTAL INFUSED: | TOTAL OUTPUT: |

FIGURE 9-3, cont'd. PACU record.

# PACU DISCHARGE SUMMARY

| VITAL SIGNS ON DISCHARGE | PACU OUTCOME | COMFORT LEVEL |
|---|---|---|
| B/P: P: R: T: | UNEVENTFUL ☐ | PAIN FREE ☐ PAIN CONTROLLED ☐ |
| OXIMETER: PAR SCORE: | COMPLICATIONS ☐ | SLEEPING BUT C/O PAIN WHEN AWAKEN ☐ PAIN SCORE ________ |

| REPORT TO: TIME: | SKIN CONDITION: WARM COOL DRY MOIST | COLOR: PINK PALE JAUNDICED DUSKY |
|---|---|---|

DRESSINGS / SURGICAL SITE / PUNCTURE SITE

| X-RAYS TAKEN IN PACU | LABS DRAWN IN PACU | $O_2$ ORDERED YES NO ________ L/MIN PER ______ <br> $O_2$ TRANSPORT YES NO |
|---|---|---|

| TOTAL IV IN PACU | TOTAL OUTPUT IN PACU | | |
|---|---|---|---|
| | URINARY | LEVINE | DRAINS |
| TOTAL BLOOD IN PACU | | | |
| TOTAL PO INTAKE IN PACU | IV SITE: <br> ________ cc LTC | | |

| ORDERS FAXED TO PHARMACY YES NO | EQUIPMENT ORDERED | TRANSPORT BY: AMBASSADOR <br> RN LPN TECHNICIAN |
|---|---|---|

| DIAGNOSIS (Circle number of any diagnosis made) | GOAL | Goal Achieved YES | Goal Achieved NO |
|---|---|---|---|
| 1 Alteration in neurological status | | | |
| 2 Alteration in comfort level | | | |
| 3 Alteration in emotional status | | | |
| 4 Alteration in circulation | | | |
| 5 Alteration in fluid volume | | | |
| 6 Alteration in mobility | | | |
| 7 Alteration in respiratory function | | | |
| 8 Alteration in skin integrity | | | |
| 9 Alteration in temperature | | | |
| 10 Alteration in elimination | | | |
| 11 Alteration in gastrointestinal function | | | |
| 12 Alteration in injury | | | |
| 13 Alteration in bleeding | | | |
| 14 Other | | | |

RHYTHM STRIPS

**FIGURE 9-3, cont'd.** PACU record.

## SAMPLE PLAN OF CARE

### IMMEDIATE POSTOPERATIVE PATIENT CARE

#### Nursing Diagnosis

**Ineffective Breathing Pattern** related to medications associated with anesthesia, type of surgical procedure, pain, tracheobronchial obstruction

#### Outcome

The patient will maintain ventilation, perfusion, and adequate expansion of lungs on discharge from the PACU as evidenced by regular respiratory rate and pattern, bilateral breath sounds clear and equal, blood pressure and pulse within preoperative range, oxygen saturation at least 92% or equal to preoperative status, patent airway, and pain controlled.

#### Interventions

- Assess respiratory status on admission to the PACU and at intervals until discharge.
- Determine level of consciousness (to assess for need to reverse opioid, benzodiazepine, or muscle relaxant).
- Administer humidified oxygen; assess need for continued oxygen after discharge.
- Elevate head of bed (if not contraindicated).
- Encourage patient to take deep breaths or sustained maximal inspiration.
- Determine need for chin tilt or jaw thrust if patient is nonreactive without patent airway. Insert artificial airway if needed. Call physician for further assistance.
- Assess patient for level of comfort. Administer pain medication as needed, per order or protocol.

#### Nursing Diagnosis

**Decreased Cardiac Output** related to anesthetic agents and other medications, fluid or blood loss or replacement, peripheral pooling of blood, alteration in preload or afterload, alterations in rate or rhythm

#### Outcome

The patient will maintain adequate cardiac output on discharge from the PACU as evidenced by blood pressure within preoperative range, skin warm and dry, oriented to person and place, and pulse strong and regular.

#### Interventions

- Monitor vital signs, electrocardiogram, and central venous pressure, with or without pulmonary artery catheter.
- Assess level of consciousness to determine effect of medication still in circulation.
- Monitor and record drainage from surgical site.
- Monitor and record intake and output.
- Administer fluid or blood products if indicated.
- If hypotensive, elevate legs unless contraindicated; increase rate of fluid administration.
- Maintain patency of intravenous lines.
- Administer medication if needed to improve depressed myocardial contractility, increase cardiac output, and promote diuresis.
- Administer vasodilators, vasocontrictors, or antidysrhythmics as ordered.
- Warm patient to temperature 36°C (96.8°F).
- Administer humidified oxygen.

#### Nursing Diagnosis

**Ineffective Thermoregulation** related to surgical procedure: anesthetic agents, length of surgery, age of patient, environment, irrigation, type of surgery, or genetic predisposition to malignant hyperthermia

#### Outcome

The patient will maintain normothermia, a core temperature of 36°C to 38°C (96.8°F to 100.4°F) on discharge from the PACU.

#### Interventions

- Measure body temperature on admission; document temperature and route of measurement.
- Assess peripheral circulation.
- Monitor vital signs and oxygen saturation.
- Observe for shivering.
- Initiate measures to warm patient if hypothermic: place warmed blankets on patient's body and head; use forced-air warming device to rewarm patient.
- Initiate appropriate measures for malignant hyperthermia, if indicated (see Chapter 4).
- Maintain ongoing temperature monitoring until discharge.

#### Nursing Diagnosis

**Disturbed Thought Processes** related to the surgical procedure: anesthetic agents, hypoxia, pain, anxiety, bladder distention

#### Outcome

The patient will demonstrate appropriate cognitive functioning on discharge from the PACU and will be oriented to person and place and responsive to commands and requests.

#### Interventions

- Assess level of consciousness.
- Determine type of anesthetic agents used.
- Monitor oxygen saturation level.
- Evaluate level of anxiety and pain.
- If there is a policy regarding family visitation in the PACU, a family member may be brought into the PACU at an appropriate time for visitation.
- Offer reassurance; allow anxious patient or family member (if visitation policy in place) to vent feelings, concerns, or questions.
- Determine if bladder is distended; catheterize if appropriate.
- Reorient patient to person and place.
- Administer humidified oxygen.
- Administer sedation for anxiety or appropriate pain medication.

#### Nursing Diagnosis

**Acute Pain** related to operative or other invasive procedures

#### Outcome

The patient will exhibit a decreased level of pain or pain at a tolerable level on discharge from the PACU.

#### Interventions

- Assess for subjective signs of pain: patient reports to the nurse that he or she is in pain; patient is given a visual analogue or numeric scale to determine perception of level of pain.
- Assess for objective signs of pain: protective guarding behavior, moaning, crying, whimpering, restlessness, irritability, diaphoresis, dilated pupils, facial expression of pain, change in vital signs (blood pressure, respiratory rate, or pulse).
- Refer to agency protocol for assessing and treating pain based on patient's pain rating.
- Monitor for pain relief and adverse reactions (respiratory depression, oversedation), and document.
- Administer pain medication as prescribed: titrate intravenous doses; initiate patient-controlled analgesia or continuous epidural analgesia (this may be patient-controlled epidural analgesia).
- If epidural analgesia is used, assess for numbness, leg weakness, pruritus, and respiratory depression. Document findings, and notify physician if findings are positive.
- If patient is intubated but conscious, collaborate in pain rating scale by pointing to a number or face and having patient indicate *yes* or *no*. If patient is unconscious, be especially attentive to signs such as grimacing.
- Initiate alternate methods of pain relief: transcutaneous electrical nerve stimulation (TENS), music, massage, relaxation, guided imagery.
- Reposition patient for comfort if not contraindicated.
- Assess causes of pain (e.g., surgical site versus chest pain).
- Document medications administered, dose, route, time, and effectiveness of pain relief.

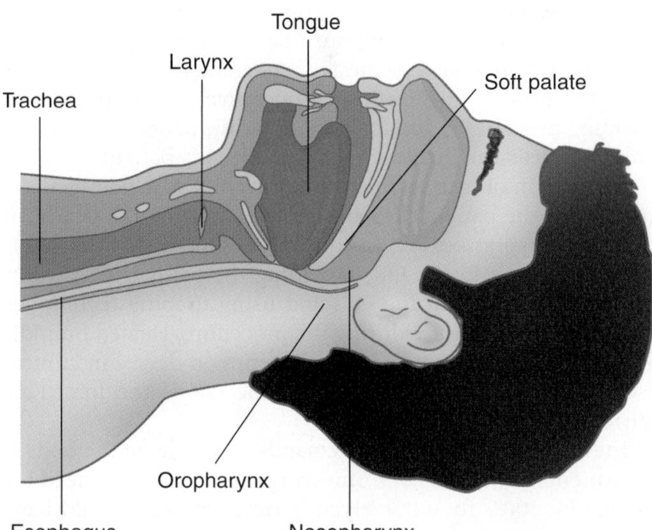

FIGURE 9-4 Obstruction of airway by tongue.

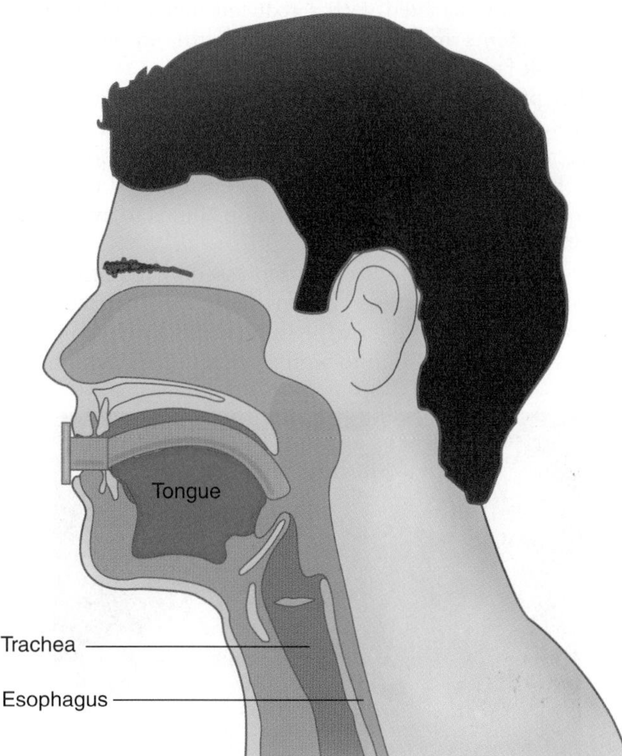

FIGURE 9-5 Oropharyngeal airway in place.

completely obstruct the airway; the patient becomes hypoxemic quickly. Nursing actions include removing the irritating stimulus, suctioning secretions that may be triggering a glottic response, hyperextending the patient's neck, oxygenating the patient, and possibly administering an aerosol with racemic (optically inactive) epinephrine. An awake patient experiencing a laryngospasm is terrified and needs reassurance and a calm demeanor from nurses and physicians.[21] Other treatment suggested for the patient includes pressure in the depression just posterior to the condyle of the mandible and doxapram intravenously.[2] In many cases, positive-pressure ventilation must be delivered per mask and bag. If the symptoms last longer than 1 minute and are unrelieved by positive pressure, administration of a muscle relaxant, such as succinylcholine, is required to relax the muscles of the larynx. Reintubation is undesirable and is used only as a last resort.[21]

**Bronchospasm.** Bronchospasm is a lower airway obstruction caused by spasms of the bronchial tubes. These spasms can cause complete closure because of the lack of cartilaginous support in the bronchioles. The patient presents with wheezing, dyspnea, use of accessory muscles, and tachypnea.[19] Bronchospasm can result from aspiration, pharyngeal suctioning, or histamine release secondary to allergic response or related to medication use. Inhaled bronchodilators are the first choice of therapy for these patients, followed by intravenous aminophylline. In some cases, epinephrine and methylprednisolone also may be administered.

**CARDIOVASCULAR.** Cardiovascular system instability is a frequent finding after surgery because many anesthetic agents exert a depressive effect on the heart and vascular system.[13] Common problems include hypotension, hypertension, and dysrhythmias.

**Hypotension.** Hypotension has been defined as a blood pressure 20% less than baseline or preoperative blood pressure and indicates either relative or absolute hypovolemia.[19] Clinical signs of hypotension include a rapid, thready pulse; disorientation; restlessness; oliguria; and cold, pale skin. Because hypovolemia is the most common cause of postoperative hypotension, the first initial intervention is to open the intravenous fluids to maximum rate while a specific diagnosis is being determined.

Cardiac output and vascular resistance determine blood pressure. Hypotension may be caused by cardiac dysfunction, such as myocardial infarction, tamponade, embolism, ischemia, dysrhythmias, congestive heart failure, valvular dysfunction, or medications, including anesthetic agents. In this case, the heart is no longer pumping effectively. Hemodynamic monitoring, supplemental oxygen, and cardiac stimulants are used as needed.

**Hypovolemia.** Hypovolemia reduces cardiac output and may be caused by hemorrhage, dehydration (inadequate fluid replacement), or increased positive end-expiratory pressure (PEEP). Fluid or blood replacement is used to treat hypovolemia. If the patient is hemorrhaging at the surgical site, a return to the OR is indicated.

Decreased vascular resistance, which causes relative hypovolemia (interference with venous return to the heart), can be related to medications, general and regional anesthesia, or anaphylaxis.[19] Vasodilation can be treated with fluids, vasopressors, or elevation of the patient's legs. Anaphylactic reactions are treated with epinephrine, antihistamines, and additional fluids.

**Hypertension.** The normal ranges for systolic blood pressure and diastolic pressure are generally 100 to 140 mm Hg and 60 to 95 mm Hg, although these may vary with individual patients.[13] Hypertension has been defined as a 20% to 30% increase above baseline blood pressure.[19] Hypertension is among the most common postoperative complications and often occurs early in the recovery phase. Blood pressure must be verified, and the rapidity of the change must be noted. Clinical signs and symptoms are the most important indicators of the severity of the hypertension. Headache, mental status changes, and substernal pain all are indicators of end-organ damage.

Asymptomatic hypertension is a common occurrence in the PACU and usually is considered to be harmless. The solution usually is determined by the cause. Elevated blood pressure causes increased ventricular wall tension, afterload, and myocardial work. The patient with a history of cardiac disease is more at risk for adverse results.

Hypertension may be caused by volume overload or pulmonary edema, which causes an increase in the cardiac output. In this case, the patient is given diuretics, put on fluid restriction, and is hemodynamically monitored.

Pain is one of the most common causes of hypertension. Other causes of hypertension are anxiety, reflex vasoconstriction from hypothermia, hypoxemia, hypercapnia, and viscus distention, all of which cause increased vascular resistance. Patients in pain are medicated, and patients with hypothermia are warmed. Patients are oxygenated well and ventilated if necessary to improve hypoxemia or hypercapnia. Patients are encouraged to void or are catheterized to empty a full bladder.

Antihypertensive drugs are used as necessary to control blood pressure. Patients should resume taking prescribed preoperative antihypertensives as soon as possible after surgery. Ambulatory surgery patients and inpatients usually are directed to take their prescribed antihypertensives the day of surgery.

**Dysrhythmias.** Most dysrhythmias seen in the PACU have an underlying cause that is not related to myocardial injury.[19] A common dysrhythmia after surgery is sinus tachycardia (rate >100 beats/min in an adult). Frequent causes include pain, hypoxemia, hypovolemia, increased temperature, and anxiety. The underlying cause is treated. Propranolol, metoprolol, or esmolol may be given. Sinus bradycardia (heart rate <60 beats/min in an adult) also is a common dysrhythmia in the PACU. Causes include hypoxemia, hypothermia, high spinal anesthesia, vagal stimulation, and some medications that are commonly given during or after surgery. The underlying cause is treated. Atropine is the drug of choice to increase the heart rate, and usually no other treatment is required. Temporary or permanent pacemakers sometimes may be required.

Premature ventricular contractions (PVCs) are represented by wide, bizarre-looking QRS complexes. The most common causes in the postoperative period are hypoxemia and hypokalemia. These underlying conditions should be treated. Often, if cardiac disease or hypotension is not present, PVCs do not require medication. If intervention is required, amiodarone is the drug of choice.[3]

Treatment of dysrhythmias begins with determining and removing any source of the problem. Antidysrhythmic drugs, resuscitation equipment, and monitoring equipment should be immediately available.[21]

### THERMOREGULATION AND TEMPERATURE ABNORMALITIES

**Hypothermia.** Postoperative hypothermia, defined as a temperature less than 36°C (96.8°F),[5] continues to be a widespread problem in the PACU. Often hypothermia is not life threatening; however, it does cause physiologic stress. Hypothermia can prolong recovery time and contributes to postoperative morbidity. Especially vulnerable to the effects of hypothermia are the elderly and children 2 years old or younger. It is believed that the four most important risk factors for hypothermia are neonate less than 1 month of age, low ambient temperature of the OR, burn patient, and a general anesthesia with neuraxial anesthesia.[20] Assessment of the patient's need for prewarming begins preoperatively with preventive warming measures begun for normothermic patients and active warming measures instituted for hypothermic patients.[5]

Prevention of heat loss continues in the OR. Under general anesthesia, the patient does not produce heat and depends on ambient temperature. Prevention includes increasing the ambient temperature in the OR, providing the patient with warm blankets on arrival in the OR, and using draping techniques that minimize exposure during the procedure. Heated humidifiers and fluid warmers add heat. A common device in clinical use for preventing hypothermia in the OR is the forced-air warming device (Figure 9-6).

In the PACU, tremendous demands are made on the body if the patient begins to shiver. Shivering can increase the need for oxygen by 300% to 400%. Hypothermic patients should have oxygen therapy initiated immediately on admission. For a patient with a healthy heart, there may be no untoward effects. For a patient with coronary artery disease or cardiomyopathy, however, decompensation can occur. Perioperative normothermia has been associated with a reduced incidence of morbid cardiac incidents and ventricular tachycardia in patients with cardiac risk factors.[18,29]

Other problems are associated with hypothermia. Intravascular volume loss, attributable to a fluid shift from the extracellular space, is probably related to vasoconstriction. As the patient begins to rewarm, vasodilation ensues, and the patient can require large amounts of intravenous fluids to avoid hypovolemia.

The central nervous system is depressed by hypothermia. A cold postanesthesia patient remains more anesthetized than a warm patient while recovering. Nitrogen loss and hypokalemia can cause a predisposition to wound infection.[12] Hypothermia

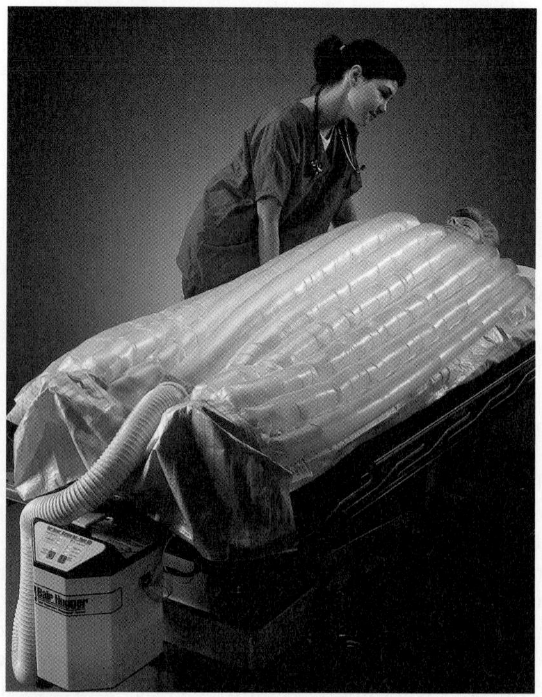


**FIGURE 9-6** Bair Hugger; focused thermal environment.

delays metabolism and alters effects of some anesthetic drugs. Of special interest is the prolonged elimination of muscle relaxants in hypothermic patients. Clotting abnormalities can occur. Platelet activity declines, and fibrinolysis increases with hypothermia. Both of these conditions enhance the tendency to bleed.[30]

Rewarming is a priority in the immediate care of the postoperative patient because hypothermia may augment the risk of adverse outcomes.[30] Wet and cold gowns and blankets should be removed, and warm, dry gowns and blankets should be applied to the head and body. Several external rewarming techniques are available. Application of warm cotton blankets has been the tradition in the PACU. The warm blankets are applied every 5 to 10 minutes until the patient is normothermic. Cotton blankets gradually increase the patient's temperature. They do not actively heat patients, however, and warming can be a slow process. Forced-air warming devices have been effective in rewarming patients,[29] producing a thermal-focused environment that transfers heat to a patient by blowing warm air through a plastic and tissue paper blanket that covers the patient. Forced-air warming devices are a standard hypothermia treatment in the PACU setting (Best Practice).

Continuous fluid-circulating blankets or warm-water mattresses have been shown to have little value in rewarming patients because of the size of surface area in contact with the heat source. Radiant heat lamps depend on exposure of large areas of body surface, which is of limited use to adult patients. Fluid and blood warmers are useful for large volumes of cool fluids but not to reverse hypothermia.

**Hyperthermia.** Hyperthermia may be an indication of an infectious process or sepsis, or it may indicate a hypermetabolic process—malignant hyperthermia (MH). MH is a serious emergency that is genetic in origin and is triggered by volatile anesthetic agents and the depolarizing muscle relaxant *succinylcholine.* Death ensues unless MH is immediately recognized and treated (see Chapter 4).

**DISTURBED THOUGHT PROCESSES.** The PACU patient may be disoriented, drowsy, confused, or delirious. Causes range from residual effects of anesthesia to pain and anxiety. Hypoxemia always should be ruled out first; it remains the most common cause of postoperative agitation. Patients who are chemically dependent or substance abusers often awaken in an agitated state. Viscus distention also can contribute to agitation in a drowsy, confused patient. The PACU nurse should identify and eliminate the cause of the agitation or confusion, if possible. The patient can be engaged in short conversations and reoriented to place and person. Baseline preoperative data are important to determine cause. Persistent changes from preoperative status require thorough assessment and possible intervention from the physician.

**NAUSEA AND VOMITING.** Postoperative nausea and vomiting (PONV) is a problem that affects approximately 30% of patients in the PACU.[24] For patients with four risk factors, the incidence can be 70% to 80%.[8] The management of nausea and vomiting begins preoperatively and continues into the intraoperative period. Preventive therapy for patients at high risk of PONV has been effective in reducing the incidence. There is no single method of prevention or treatment of PONV. Many causative factors are related to anesthesia and surgery.

It is important not to oversedate the patient when medicating for nausea and vomiting. Antiemetic drugs have chemically diverse modes of action and may be chosen by their mechanism of action. If the patient is hypotensive with nausea and vomiting, the patient may be given ephedrine with additional fluid administration. Metoclopramide (Reglan) blocks stimulation of the chemotrigger receptor zone by antagonizing central and peripheral dopamine receptors. The phenothiazines prochlorperazine (Compazine) and promethazine (Phenergan) can be used but must be titrated to avoid sedation. Ondansetron (Zofran) and dolasetron (Anzemet), 5-hydroxytryptamine (5-HT3) serotonin antagonists, have become popular because of the lack of side effects such as sedation, hypotension, and tremors.[13] Dexamethasone (Decadron) also has proved to be a useful addition to the drug arsenal because of inhibition of prostaglandin synthesis in the higher central nervous system.[33] Other useful medications include dimenhydrinate (Dramamine), hydroxyzine (Vistaril, Atarax), and scopolamine (Transderm Scop). A new neurokinin-1 antagonist, aprepitant, is now available for use with chemotherapy patients and is undergoing testing with positive results for PONV. Palonosetron, a second-generation 5-hydroxytryptamine receptor antagonist, also has been approved in the United States.

**ASPIRATION.** Aspiration, or passage of regurgitated material into the lungs, can occur during the perioperative period, with most aspirations occurring during tracheal intubation or extubation.[15] The PACU nurse must protect the airway of an unconscious or semiconscious patient to prevent the possibility of aspiration of gastric contents. Prevention of aspiration postoperatively includes responding quickly to reports of nausea and vomiting, avoiding conversations that could elicit nausea and vomiting, and preventing rapid movement and head elevation of the patient. Nonreactive patients can be placed on their sides in the recovery position.

The volume and acidity of the aspirate determine the extent of damage to the lungs. The most severe damage seems to be in cases in which the pH was less than 2.5 or the volume was greater than 25 ml.[15] Preoperatively, patients may receive clear, nonparticulate antacids, such as Bicitra, to raise the gastric fluid pH. Histamine ($H_2$)-receptor antagonists, such as cimetidine, ranitidine, or famotidine, decrease gastric acid production. Metoclopramide increases gastric-emptying time.[21] Aspiration does not occur in patients with normal protective reflexes. Risk factors can be divided into general and specific (Table 9-1).

Signs and symptoms of aspiration include tachypnea and hypoxemia attributable to a decrease in lung compliance. Wheezing, coughing, dyspnea, hypotension, apnea, and bradycardia may occur. Treatment centers around promoting tissue oxygenation. Supplemental oxygen is given. Positive pressure applied by use of a mask or an endotracheal tube may be needed to maintain arterial oxygenation, and a chest x-ray may be done. If intubated, the trachea can be suctioned. Bronchoscopy is performed if the particles aspirated are large and causing an airway obstruction. Neither steroids nor antibiotics are warranted.[15] Tracheal secretions can be cultured, and if the results are positive, an appropriate antibiotic can be started. Bronchodilators are used as required. Recovery of the patient depends on recognition of the problem, quantity of aspirate, pH of the aspirate, physical condition of the patient before the event, and rapidity with which medical care is initiated.[15]

**ACUTE PAIN.** Pain is a subjective experience and may or may not be verbalized. Often health care providers require

## BEST PRACTICE

### Clinical Guideline for Prevention of Unplanned Perioperative Hypothermia

**Background**

In February 1998, the American Society of PeriAnesthesia Nurses (ASPAN) and ASPAN Foundation held the first Consensus Conference on Perioperative Thermoregulation. At the conference, a panel of experts shared research data with participants. The conference ended with an interdisciplinary development panel appointed to create the clinical guideline. The development panel consisted of representatives from interested nursing and medical organizations. After development, the guideline was peer reviewed by colleagues and clinicians with expertise in thermoregulation. The guideline was pilot tested at six different institutions. This guideline is a "bedside tool for clinicians to use in the prevention and management of the adult surgical patient at risk for the development of unplanned hypothermia." The guideline was published in October 2001 in the *Journal of PeriAnesthesia Nursing.*

**Endorsements**

The guideline has been endorsed by ASPAN, Association of periOperative Registered Nurses (AORN), and American Association of Nurse Anesthetists (AANA). Endorsements are pending from American Society of Anesthesiologists (ASA), American Nurses Association (ANA), American College of Surgeons (ACS), and American Association of Critical-Care Nurses (AACN). The guideline has been endorsed by the National Guideline Clearinghouse and can be accessed at www.guideline.gov/summary/summary.aspx?doc_id=5527&nbr=3 or www.aspan.org.

**Definitions**

Normothermia—core temperature range from 36°C to 38°C (96.8°F to 100.4°F)

Hypothermia—core temperature less than 36°C (<96.8°F)

**Thermal Management Flow Chart**

The thermal management flow chart identifies appropriate preoperative, intraoperative, and postoperative patient management, including assessments, interventions, and expected outcomes.

**THERMAL MANAGEMENT FLOW CHART**

**Preoperative Patient Management**

Identify patient's risk factors for hypothermia
Measure patient's temperature on admission
Determine patient's thermal comfort level (ask patient if he/she is cold)
Observe for signs/symptoms of hypothermia (shivering, piloerection, and/or cold extremities)

↓

**Patient Normothermic**

Institute preventive warming measures:
- Passive insulation (apply warm cotton blankets, socks, and head covering, and limit skin exposure)
- Increase ambient room temperature (minimum 68°F-75°F)

**Patient Hypothermic**

Institute active warming measures:
- Apply forced-air warming system
- Apply passive insulation
- Increase ambient room temperature (minimum 68°F-75°F)

**Intraoperative Patient Management**

**Assessment**

Identify patient's risk factors for hypothermia
Monitor patient's temperature (see guideline)
Determine patient's thermal comfort level (ask the patient if he/she is cold)
Observe for signs/symptoms of hypothermia (shivering, piloerection, and/or cold extremities)

↓

**Interventions**

Passive insulation (apply warm cotton blankets, socks, and head covering, and limit skin exposure)
Increase ambient room temperature (minimum 68°F-75°F)
Institute active warming measures: apply forced-air warming system
Warm fluids: intravenous and irrigants
Humidify and warm gases: anesthetic

↓

**Expected Outcomes**

The patient's core temperature should be maintained at 36°C (96.8°F) or above during the intraoperative phase unless hypothermia is indicated

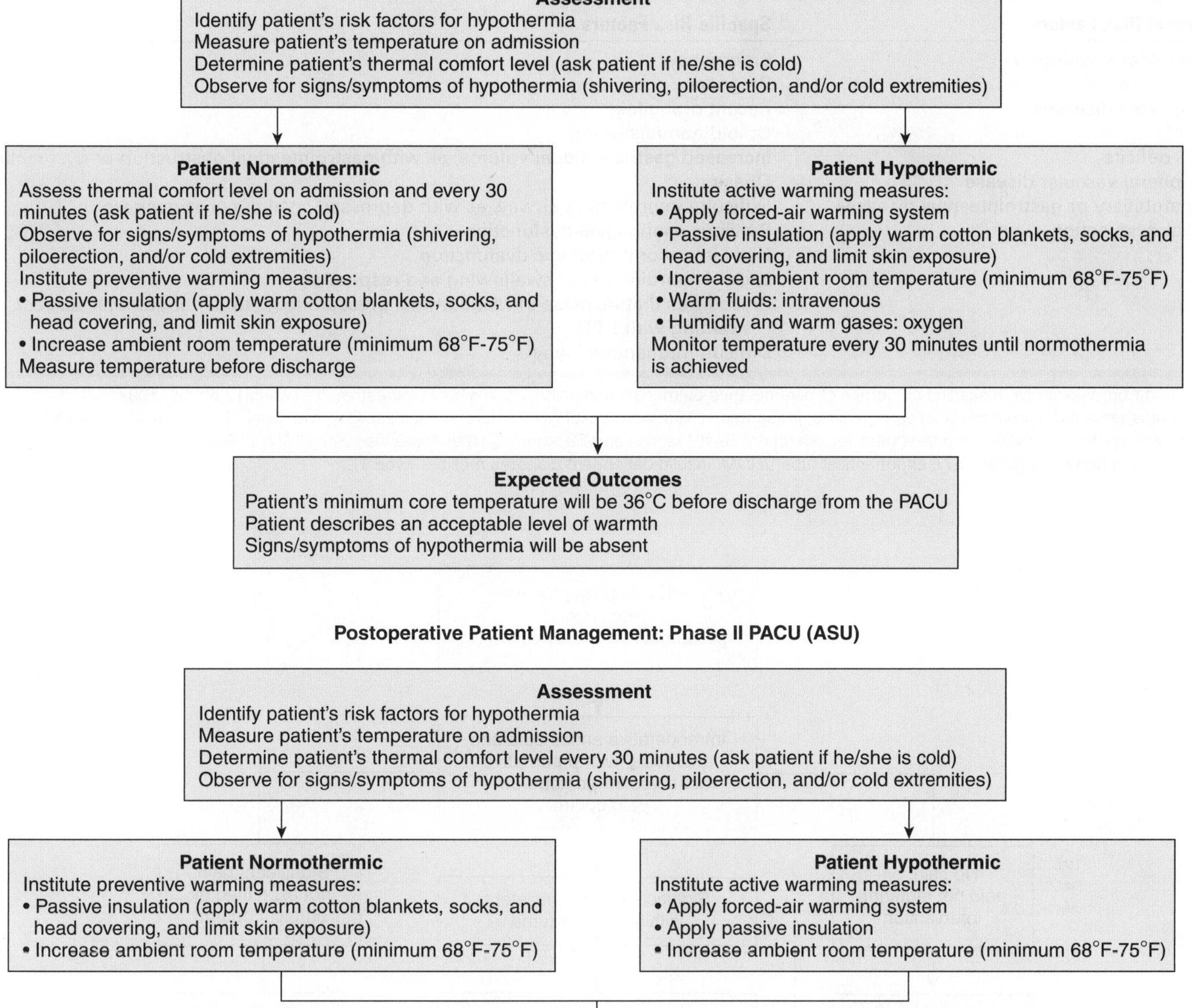
Postoperative Patient Management: Phase I PACU
Assessment
Identify patient's risk factors for hypothermia
Measure patient's temperature on admission
Determine patient's thermal comfort level (ask patient if he/she is cold)
Observe for signs/symptoms of hypothermia (shivering, piloerection, and/or cold extremities)
Patient Normothermic
Assess thermal comfort level on admission and every 30 minutes (ask patient if he/she is cold)
Observe for signs/symptoms of hypothermia (shivering, piloerection, and/or cold extremities)
Institute preventive warming measures:
• Passive insulation (apply warm cotton blankets, socks, and head covering, and limit skin exposure)
• Increase ambient room temperature (minimum 68°F-75°F)
Measure temperature before discharge
Patient Hypothermic
Institute active warming measures:
• Apply forced-air warming system
• Passive insulation (apply warm cotton blankets, socks, and head covering, and limit skin exposure)
• Increase ambient room temperature (minimum 68°F-75°F)
• Warm fluids: intravenous
• Humidify and warm gases: oxygen
Monitor temperature every 30 minutes until normothermia is achieved
Expected Outcomes
Patient's minimum core temperature will be 36°C before discharge from the PACU
Patient describes an acceptable level of warmth
Signs/symptoms of hypothermia will be absent
Postoperative Patient Management: Phase II PACU (ASU)
Assessment
Identify patient's risk factors for hypothermia
Measure patient's temperature on admission
Determine patient's thermal comfort level every 30 minutes (ask patient if he/she is cold)
Observe for signs/symptoms of hypothermia (shivering, piloerection, and/or cold extremities)
Patient Normothermic
Institute preventive warming measures:
• Passive insulation (apply warm cotton blankets, socks, and head covering, and limit skin exposure)
• Increase ambient room temperature (minimum 68°F-75°F)
Patient Hypothermic
Institute active warming measures:
• Apply forced-air warming system
• Apply passive insulation
• Increase ambient room temperature (minimum 68°F-75°F)
Expected Outcomes
Patient's minimum core temperature will be 36°C before discharge from Phase II PACU (ASU)
Patient describes an acceptable level of warmth
Signs/symptoms of hypothermia will be absent
Patient should describe methods of maintaining normothermia at home

objective signs of discomfort in addition to subjective reports of pain from the patient, which can lead to undertreatment of pain. The guiding principle in pain care is that pain is whatever the patient says it is.[1,25] The Agency for Health Care Policy and Research (now known as the Agency for Healthcare Research and Quality)[1] reports that the most reliable indicator of the existence and intensity of pain is the patient's self-report. The Agency for Health Care Policy and Research developed clinical practice guidelines on acute pain management and contends that all patients should be assessed for severity of pain using a verbal rating scale or a visual analogue scale (Figures 9-7 and 9-8). Approximately 80% of patients in one study experienced acute postoperative pain with most patients experiencing moderate, severe, or extreme pain.[9]

Pain management is one of the highest priorities of postanesthesia care.[11] Patients should be assessed for pain on admission to the PACU and at frequent intervals (Box 9-2). It is important to remember that not all patients respond to pain in the same manner, despite comparable surgical procedures. Basic measures of pain intensity should be prioritized with the patient's self-report as the most important measure. Other measures of pain intensity include exposure to a painful procedure;

**TABLE 9-1**

## Risk Factors for Pulmonary Aspiration

| General Risk Factors | Specific Risk Factors |
|---|---|
| Age (older > younger) | Emergency |
| Gender (female > male) | Pregnancy |
| Co-morbid diseases | Recent oral intake |
| IDDM | Opioid administration |
| CNS deficits | Increased gastric residual volume, as with gastrointestinal obstruction or dysfunction |
| Peripheral vascular disease | Obesity |
| Hepatobiliary or gastrointestinal diseases | Difficulty in protecting airway, as with depressed level of consciousness |
| Renal dysfunction | Previous esophageal dysfunction |
| | Head injury or neurologic dysfunction |
| | Lack of coordination of swallowing and respiration |
| | Procedures that increase intraabdominal pressure (e.g., upper abdominal surgery, straining with ETT) |
| | Difficult intubation/airway |

Modified from Warner M: Risks and outcomes of perioperative pulmonary aspiration, *Journal of Perianesthesia Nursing* 12(5):355, 1997; Schick L: *Calling 911: management of common PACU emergencies,* presented at 19th Annual ASPAN Conference, Kansas City, Mo, April 19, 2000; Kalinowski CPH, Kirsch JR: Strategies for prophylaxis and treatment for aspiration, *Best Practice and Research Clinical Anaesthesiology* 18(4):719-737, 2004.
*CNS,* Central nervous system; *ETT,* endotracheal tube; *IDDM,* insulin-dependent diabetes mellitus (type 1).

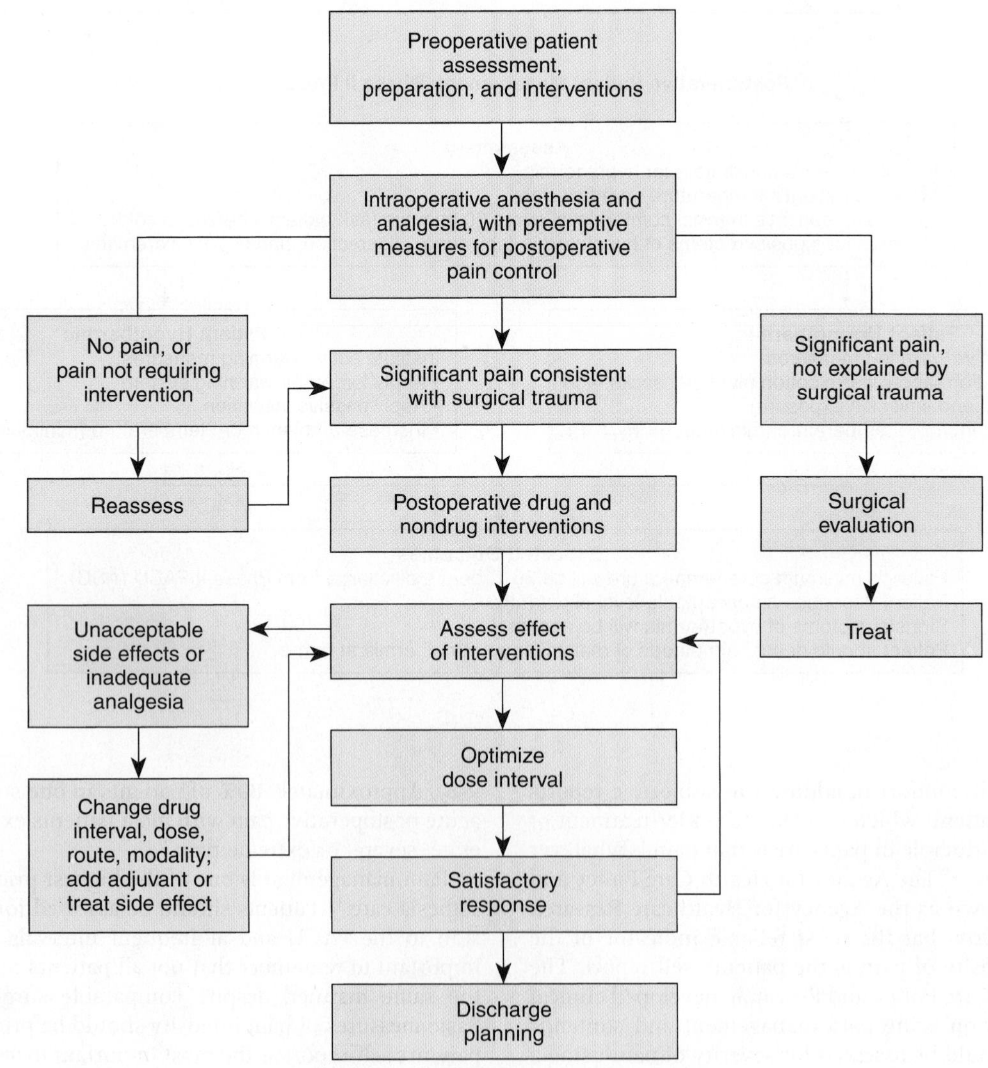


**FIGURE 9-7** Acute pain management in adults.

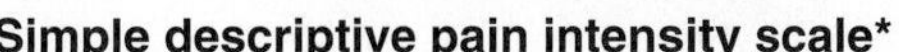


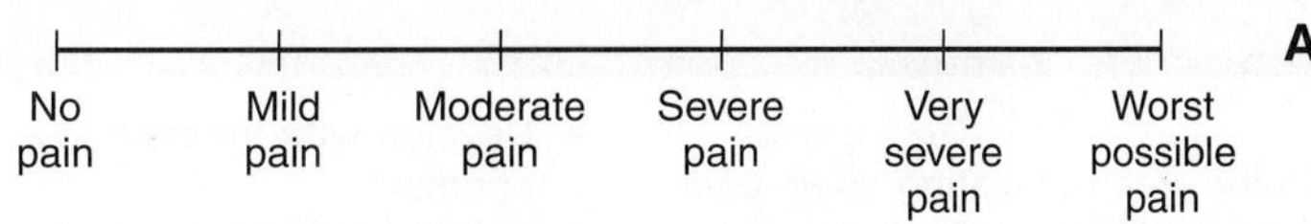




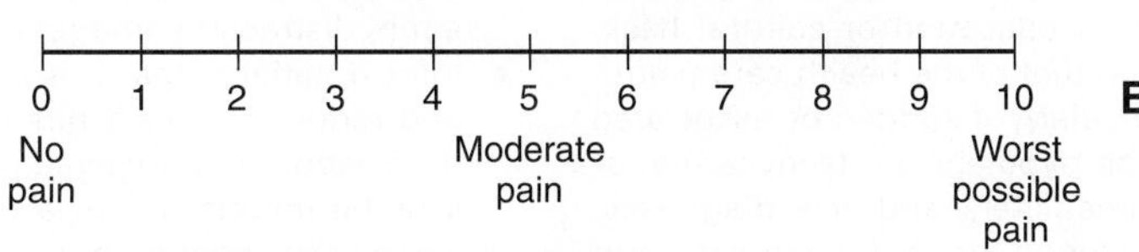




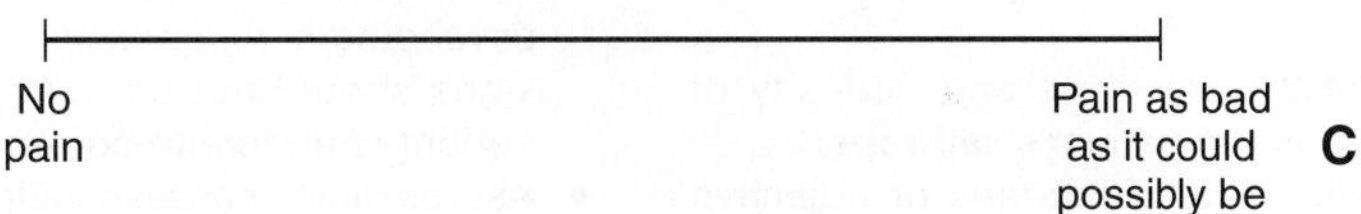

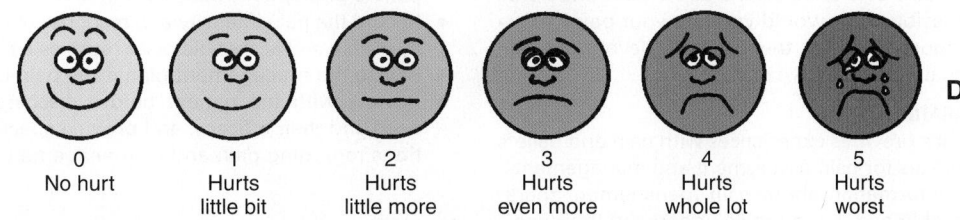


**FIGURE 9-8** **A-C,** Examples of pain intensity and pain distress scales. **D,** FACES Pain Rating Scale.

behavioral signs, such as crying or restlessness; a proxy pain rating by someone who knows the patient well; and physiologic indicators, such as elevated vital signs.[25]

Evidence indicates that early analgesia reduces postoperative problems. Nonsteroidal antiinflammatory drugs (NSAIDs), or cyclooxygenase type 2 (COX-2) inhibitors for patients who have experienced adverse effects from conventional NSAID use, and opiates are the analgesics of choice and generally are used in combination (multimodal therapy) in the PACU (Tables 9-2 and 9-3). Using NSAIDs in combination with opiates can reduce opioid requirements by 20% to 40%.[14] The COX-2 inhibitors were developed with selective inhibition of the COX enzyme, with resulting analgesia and decreased inflammation without gastrointestinal and bleeding risks.[10] Until more recently, there were three COX-2 inhibitors available: celecoxib, rofecoxib, and valdecoxib. Rofecoxib and valdecoxib have been withdrawn from the U.S. market because of excess cardiovascular risk, and celecoxib is the only COX-2 inhibitor currently available in the United States. It is believed that the risk with celecoxib is small and comparable to traditional NSAIDs.[10] Parecoxib is another COX-2 inhibitor currently approved for use in Europe and undergoing trials in the United States. If approved, parecoxib would be the first COX-2 inhibitor to be given intravenously.[14]

Traditionally, pain has been treated with intramuscular (IM) injections of opioids at intervals from 3 to 6 hours as needed. It is now recognized that the inadequate pain relief experienced by postoperative patients using IM injections is attributable to varying blood levels. Other methods of pain relief have become more widespread. The most common form of an opioid-delivery system is by way of patient-controlled analgesia (PCA). PCA allows a patient to control the analgesic administration. Dosage, time between doses, and the maximum dosage that can be administered are programmed into the machine. This form of analgesia also allows for a basal rate of opioids to infuse continuously, if ordered. The PCA pump also can be set to deliver continuous infusion and patient boluses. This setting allows the patient to use the bolus function to premedicate before an activity or for breakthrough pain. When PCA devices are started in the PACU, delays in preventing pain are avoided, effectiveness of the PCA device can be evaluated, and the patient's understanding and ability to use PCA can be assessed.

Other forms of postoperative pain relief may involve use of spinal analgesia, usually in the form of epidural opioid or local anesthetic administration. Patients who have had extensive procedures, including total hip or knee replacements, knee reconstruction, and major abdominal or thoracic operations, have been shown to profit from this method of pain control.

BOX 9-2

## Pain Assessment and Reassessment

**PRINCIPLES**

- Patients who may have difficulty communicating their pain require particular attention. This includes patients who are cognitively impaired, psychotic, or severely emotionally disturbed; children; the elderly; patients who do not speak English; and patients whose level of education or cultural background differs significantly from that of the health care team.
- Unexpected intense pain, particularly if sudden or associated with altered vital signs, such as hypotension, tachycardia, or fever, should be evaluated immediately, and new diagnoses, such as wound dehiscence, infection, or deep venous thrombosis, should be considered.
- Family members should be involved when appropriate.

**PAIN ASSESSMENT TOOLS**

- The most reliable indicator of the existence and intensity of pain and any resultant distress is the patient's self-report.
- Self-report measurement scales include numeric or adjective ratings and visual analogue scales.
- Tools should be reliable, valid, and easy for the patient and the nurse or physician to use. One may use these tools by showing a diagram to the patient to indicate the appropriate rating. One also may use the tools by simply asking the patient for a verbal response: "On a scale of 0 to 10 with 0 as no pain and 10 as the worst pain possible, how would you rate your pain?"
- Tools must be appropriate for the patient's developmental, physical, emotional, and cognitive status.

**PREOPERATIVE PREPARATION**

- Discuss the patient's previous experiences with pain and beliefs about and preferences for pain assessment and management.
- Give the patient information about pain management therapies that are available and the rationale underlying their use.
- Develop with the patient a plan for pain assessment and management.
- Select a pain assessment tool, and teach the patient to use it.
- Provide the patient with education and information about pain control, including nonpharmacologic options, such as relaxation, distraction, imagery, and massage.
- Inform patients that it is easier to prevent pain than to chase and reduce it after it has become established, and that communication of unrelieved pain is essential to its relief. Emphasize the importance of a factual report of pain, avoiding stoicism or exaggeration.

**POSTOPERATIVE ASSESSMENT**

- Assess the patient's perceptions, along with behavioral and psychologic responses. Observations of behavior and vital signs should not be used instead of a self-report, unless the patient is unable to communicate.
- Assess and reassess pain frequently during the immediate postoperative period. Determine the frequency of assessment based on the operation performed and the severity of the pain. Pain should be assessed every 2 hours during the first postoperative day after major surgery.
- Increase the frequency of assessment and reassessment if the pain is poorly controlled or if interventions are changing.
- Record the pain intensity and response to intervention in an easily visible and accessible place, such as a bedside flow sheet.
- Revise the management plan if the pain is poorly controlled.
- Review with the patient before discharge the interventions used and their efficacy, and provide specific discharge instructions regarding pain and its management.

Modified from Acute Pain Management Guideline Panel: *Acute pain management in adults: operative procedures. Quick reference guide for clinicians*, AHCPR Pub. no. 92-0019, Rockville, Md, 1992, Agency for Health Care Policy and Research, Public Health Service, U.S. Department of Health and Human Services. Accessed November 18, 2005, on-line: www.ahrq.gov/clinic/medtep/acute.html.

Benefits of epidural analgesia for acute postoperative pain include good analgesia with minimal sedation, early ambulation and physical therapy, and excellent patient satisfaction. The U.S. Food and Drug Administration approved a new extended-release epidural morphine (EREM) that provides pain relief for 48 hours after a single bolus injection.[27] Side effects of intrathecal administration of opioids include nausea, pruritus, urinary retention, areas of slight numbness, and respiratory depression. These side effects can be controlled by adjusting the infusion rate or with drugs such as diphenhydramine, ondansetron, or naloxone. Naloxone is the opioid antagonist used most frequently to reduce opioid-induced respiratory depression. It is administered slowly, never as a bolus, while the nurse observes the patient response. The patient should be able to open his or her eyes and talk to the nurse within 1 to 2 minutes; the naloxone is discontinued when the patient can take deep breaths on instruction and respond to physical stimulation.

Other techniques that have been shown to reduce the level of pain for the surgical patient include infiltration of the site of incision with a local anesthetic even before the initial incision and use of a long-acting local anesthetic at the site at the conclusion of the surgical procedure. Local anesthetics as part of a multimodal approach to pain management can contribute to a considerable decrease in opioid dosage with minimal side effects.[26] One option is perineural local anesthetic infusion, in which a catheter is threaded along or into the wound. A diluted concentration of a long-acting local anesthetic is delivered to the surrounding nerves by a mechanical infusion pump for inpatients or a disposable infusion pump for ambulatory surgery patients.[26] Thorough patient education is imperative, including removal of the catheter for patients who will be discharged home with the pump. It also is important to know the type of anesthesia the patient received during surgery and the type of local anesthetic in the pump to prevent overdose of local anesthetic. Multimodal analgesia allows a smaller dose of each component, which helps to minimize adverse effects.[32]

Nonpharmacologic interventions that may be used to relieve pain include positioning for comfort, verbal reassurance, touch, applications of heat or cold, massage, and transcutane-

**TABLE 9-2**

## Surgical Pharmacology: Dosing Data for Nonopioid Analgesics

| Drug | Usual Adult Dose | Usual Pediatric Dose* | Comments |
|---|---|---|---|
| **ORAL** | | | |
| Acetaminophen | 650-975 mg q4hr | 10-15 mg/kg q4hr | Acetaminophen lacks the peripheral antiinflammatory activity of NSAIDs |
| Aspirin | 650-975 mg q4hr | 10-15 mg/kg q4hr† | The standard against which other NSAIDs are compared. Inhibits platelet aggregation; may cause postoperative bleeding |
| Choline magnesium trisalicylate (Trilisate) | 1000-1500 mg bid | 25 mg/kg q12hr | May have minimal antiplatelet activity; also available as oral liquid |
| Diflunisal (Dolobid) | 1000 mg initial dose followed by 500 mg q12hr | — | — |
| Etodolac (Lodine) | 200-400 mg q6hr | — | — |
| Fenoprofen calcium (Nalfon) | 200 mg q4-6hr | — | — |
| Flurbiprofen | 100 mg bid, tid, qid | — | — |
| Ibuprofen (Motrin, others) | 400 mg q4-6hr | 10 mg/kg q6-8hr | Available as several brand names and generic forms; also available as oral suspension |
| Ketoprofen (Orudis) | 25-75 mg q6-8hr | — | — |
| Magnesium salicylate | 650 mg q4hr | — | Many brands and generic forms available |
| Meclofenamate sodium (Meclomen) | 50 mg q4-6hr | — | — |
| Mefenamic acid (Ponstel) | 250 mg q6hr | — | — |
| Naproxen (Naprosyn) | 500 mg initial dose followed by 250 mg q6-8hr | 5 mg/kg q12hr | Also available as oral liquid |
| Naproxen sodium (Anaprox) | 550 mg initial dose followed by 275 mg q6-8hr | — | — |
| Oxaprozin | 600 mg q24hr | — | Long half-life, so can be given once daily |
| Salsalate (Disalcid, others) | 500 mg q4hr | — | May have minimal antiplatelet activity |
| Sodium salicylate | 325-650 mg q3-4hr | — | Available in generic form from several distributors |
| **SELECTIVE COX-2 INHIBITOR** | | | |
| Celecoxib | 100-200 mg twice daily | — | Reduces risk of gastrointestinal side effects and renal toxicity. No effects on platelet aggregation. May have a higher risk of having heart attack or stroke |
| **PARENTERAL NSAID** | | | |
| Ketorolac | 30 or 60 mg IM initial dose followed by 15 or 30 mg q6hr<br>Oral dose after IM dose: 10 mg q6-8hr<br>IV dose 30 mg IV for healthy adults and 15 mg for adults >65 years | — | IM dose not to exceed 5 days. IV administration comparable to 10 mg IM morphine |

Modified from Acute Pain Management Guideline Panel: *Acute pain management in adults: operative procedures. Quick reference guide for clinicians,* AHCPR Pub. no. 92-0019, Rockville, Md, 1992, Agency for Health Care Policy and Research, Public Health Service, U.S. Department of Health and Human Services. Accessed February 20, 2006, on line: www.ahrq.gov/clinic/medtep/acute.htm. National Pharmaceutical Council, Inc, Joint Commission on Accreditation of Healthcare Organizations: *Pain: Current understanding of assessment, management, and treatments.* December 2001. Accessed July 30, 2006, on-line: www.npcnow.org/resources/PDFs/PainExecSummary.pdf.

*Note:* Only the above NSAIDs have Food and Drug Administration approval for use as simple analgesics, but clinical experience has been gained with other drugs as well.

*Drug recommendations are limited to NSAIDs for which pediatric dosing experience is available.

†Contraindicated in presence of fever or other evidence of viral illness.

*COX-2,* Cyclooxygenase type 2; *NSAID,* nonsteroidal antiinflammatory drug

**TABLE 9-3**

## Surgical Pharmacology: Dosing Data for Opioid Analgesics

| Drug | Approximate Equianalgesic Oral Dose | Approximate Equianalgesic Parenteral Dose | Recommended Starting Dose (Adults >50 kg Body Weight) | | Recommended Starting Dose (Children and Adults <50 kg Body Weight)* | |
|---|---|---|---|---|---|---|
| | | | *Oral* | *Parenteral* | *Oral* | *Parenteral* |
| **OPIOID AGONIST** | | | | | | |
| Morphine† | 30 mg q3-4hr (around-the-clock dosing)<br>60 mg q3-4hr (single dose or intermittent dosing) | 10 mg q3-4hr | 30 mg q3-4hr | 10 mg q3-4hr | 0.3 mg/kg q3-4hr | 0.1 mg/kg q3-4hr |
| Codeine‡ | 130 mg q3-4hr | 75 mg q3-4hr | 60 mg q3-4hr | 60 mg q2hr (IM/Sub-Q) | 1 mg/kg q3-4hr§ | NR |
| Hydromorphone† (Dilaudid) | 7.5 mg q3-4hr | 1.5 mg q3-4hr | 6 mg q3-4hr | 1.5 mg q3-4hr | 0.06 mg/kg q3-4hr | 0.015 mg/kg q3-4hr |
| Hydrocodone (in Lorcet, available Lortab, Vicodin, others) | 30 mg q3-4hr | NA | 10 mg q3-4hr | NA | 0.2 mg/kg q3-4hr§ | NA |
| Levorphanol (Levo-Dromoran) | 4 mg q6-8hr | 2 mg q6-8hr | 4 mg q6-8hr | 2 mg q6-8hr | 0.04 mg/kg q6-8hr | 0.02 mg/kg q6-8hr |
| Meperidine (Demerol) | 300 mg q2-3hr | 100 mg q3hr | NR | 100 mg q3hr | NR | 0.75 mg/kg q2-3hr |
| Methadone (Dolophine, others) | 20 mg q6-8hr | 10 mg q6-8hr | 20 mg q6-8hr | 10 mg q6-8hr | 0.2 mg/kg q6-8hr | 0.1 mg/kg q6-8hr |
| Oxycodone (Roxicodone, also in Percocet, Percodan, Tylox, others) | 30 mg q3-4hr | NA | 10 mg q3-4hr | NA | 0.2 mg/kg q3-4hr§ | NA |
| Oxymorphone† (Numorphan) | NA | 1 mg q3-4hr | NA | 1 mg q3-4hr | NR | NR |
| **OPIOID AGONIST—ANTAGONIST AND PARTIAL AGONIST** | | | | | | |
| Buprenorphine (Buprenex) | NA | 0.3-0.4 mg q6-8hr | NA | 0.4 mg q6-8hr | NA | 0.004 mg/kg q6-8hr |
| Butorphanol (Stadol) | NA | 2 mg q3-4hr | NA | 2 mg q3-4hr | NA | NR |
| Nalbuphine (Nubain) | NA | 10 mg q3-4hr | NA | 10 mg q3-4hr | NA | 0.1 mg/kg q3-4hr |
| Pentazocine (Talwin, others) | 150 mg q3-4hr | 60 mg q3-4hr | 50 mg q4-6hr | NR | NR | NR |

Modified from Acute Pain Management Guideline Panel: *Acute pain management in adults: operative procedures. Quick reference guide for clinicians,* AHCPR Pub. no. 92-0019, Rockville, Md, 1992, Agency for Health Care Policy and Research, Public Health Service, U.S. Department of Health and Human Services. Accessed February 20, 2006, on line: www.ahrq.gov/clinic/medtep/acute.htm.

*Note:* Published tables vary in the suggested doses that are equianalgesic to morphine. Clinical response is the criterion that must be applied for each patient; titration to clinical response is necessary. Because there is not complete cross-tolerance among these drugs, it is usually necessary to use a lower equianalgesic dose when changing drugs and to retitrate to response.

*Caution:* Recommended doses do not apply to patients with renal or hepatic insufficiency or other conditions affecting drug metabolism and kinetics.

**Caution:* Doses listed for patients with body weight <50 kg cannot be used as initial starting doses in infants <6 months of age. Consult the AHCPR *Clinical practice guideline for acute pain management: operative or medical procedures and trauma* section on management of pain in neonates for recommendations.

†For morphine, hydromorphone, and oxymorphone, rectal administration is an alternate route for patients unable to take oral medications, but equianalgesic doses may differ from oral and parenteral doses because of pharmacokinetic differences.

‡*Caution:* Codeine doses >65 mg often are inappropriate because of diminishing incremental analgesia with increasing doses but continually increasing constipation and other side effects.

§*Caution:* Doses of aspirin and acetaminophen in combination opioid/NSAID preparations also must be adjusted to the patient's body weight.

*NA,* Not available; *NR,* not recommended.

ous electrical nerve stimulation (TENS). If the patient was taught preoperatively, other techniques that can be used are relaxation, imagery, music distraction, and biofeedback. Interventions that can be useful for the postanesthesia patient in the PACU are preoperative education, which reduces the fear of the unknown; relaxation with deep breathing; distraction; and therapeutic massage.[22] Nonpharmacologic interventions are designed to supplement, not substitute, pharmacologic intervention (Research Highlight).[1]

Physiologic effects of pain can be harmful for the postoperative patient and include the following: decreased thoracic movement, increased splinting, reduced lung compliance and volume leading to atelectasis, decreased mobility, increased risk of thromboembolism, exaggerated catecholamine response (which increases cardiac work and myocardial oxygen demand), increased risk for myocardial ischemia, impaired immune system, and delayed return of bowel and gastric function. Physiologic responses with acute pain include increased blood pressure and heart rate, dilated pupils, perspiration, increased respiratory rate, and decreased respiratory excursion.[16,22] Psychologically, the patient still in pain may display fear, helplessness, anxiety, anger, or frustration.[16]

## RESEARCH HIGHLIGHT

### Nonpharmacologic Methods for Pain Management

Laurion and Fetzer conducted an experimental pilot study to determine the effects of guided imagery and music therapy on postoperative pain, postoperative nausea and vomiting (PONV), and length of stay for patients undergoing gynecologic laparoscopy. Patients were randomly assigned to one of three interventions: guided imagery audiotapes, music audiotapes, or standard care. Outcome measures were evaluated. Results indicated that patients in the guided imagery and music groups had significantly less pain on PACU discharge to home than patients in the control group. Although no significant difference was found with respect to PONV or length of stay, these findings suggest that guided imagery and music are effective strategies in improving pain management.

Modified from Laurion S, Fetzer SJ: The effect of two nursing interventions on the postoperative outcomes of gynecologic laparoscopic patients, *Journal of PeriAnesthesia Nursing* 18(4):254-261, 2003.

With the advent of the Joint Commission on Accreditation of Healthcare Organizations (JCAHO) standards for pain management, health care providers are required to become more knowledgeable about pain assessment and management. An excellent resource is the monograph developed by the National Pharmaceutical Council as part of a collaborative project with JCAHO.[22] Patients of differing cultures respond to pain and express pain differently.[17] A patient may believe that nonverbal communication is expressing the pain to the nurse, but the nurse may not recognize the clues. Common misconceptions about pain also abound. These misconceptions must be recognized and corrected. A summary of misconceptions is listed in Table 9-4.

Buss and Melderis[11] developed a tool to allow perianesthesia nurses to assess cognitively impaired postanesthesia patients to determine the presence of pain. This tool is limited to use in the phase I PACU but adds to the PACU nurse's ability to deal with acute postoperative pain. The tool, an algorithm, was developed to "assist perianesthesia nurses with the assessment and management of pain during the patient's emergence from anesthesia"[11] (Figure 9-9). The American Society of PeriAnesthesia Nurses established the first comprehensive pain and comfort guideline. The guideline addresses the assessment, expected outcomes, and appropriate interventions for pain in the preoperative phase, postanesthesia phase I, and postanesthesia phases II and III.[6]

**TABLE 9-4**

### Misconceptions About Pain

| Misconception | Correction |
|---|---|
| The best judge of the existence and severity of a patient's pain is the physician or nurse caring for the patient | The patient is the authority about his or her pain. The patient's self-report is the most reliable indicator of the existence and intensity of pain |
| The clinician must believe what the patient says about pain | The clinician must accept and respect the patient's report of pain and proceed with an appropriate assessment and treatment. The clinician is entitled to a personal opinion but should not allow it to guide practice |
| Patients should not receive analgesics until the cause of pain is diagnosed | Symptomatic relief of pain should be provided while the investigation of cause proceeds |
| Visible signs, either physiologic or behavioral, accompany pain and can be used to verify its existence and severity | Even with severe pain, periods of physiologic and behavioral adaptation occur, leading to periods of minimal or no signs of pain |
| Pain never killed anyone | Unrelieved pain may be dangerous and is unacceptable. Postoperative pain can delay healing and contribute to complications that can be life threatening. Acute pain warns of actual or potential tissue damage and resolves when healing has occurred. Unrelieved postoperative pain is a complication or risk, not an acceptable consequence of surgery |
| If the patient requires higher doses of opioids than other patients, "he's hitting the PCA button too much" | There is no set dose of opioid that is effective for all patients. Even an opioid-naïve patient may require 6× more opioid than another patient. A patient who is opioid-tolerant may require 100× the opioid of an opioid-naïve patient |

Modified from Canobbio MM: *Mosby's handbook of patient teaching,* ed 3, St Louis, 2006, Mosby; McCaffery M, Pasero C: *Pain clinical manual,* ed 2, St Louis, 1999, Mosby.

Effective management of postoperative pain occurs if the following are addressed and accomplished:[1,22]

1. Regular assessment and reassessment of pain intensity and relief
2. Respect for patient preferences for method of pain management
3. Development of an organized program to evaluate effectiveness of pain assessment and management

### Evaluation

The patient is evaluated based on the outcomes identified as significant after the initial assessment. For the desired outcomes presented previously in this chapter, these might be stated as follows:

- The patient maintained an adequate oxygen saturation while receiving room air.
- The blood pressure and heart rate are within normal range for the patient.
- The patient is normothermic.
- The patient is oriented to time and person.
- The patient's pain is 4 or less (on a scale of 0-10) or at a comfort level established by patient. The patient is relaxed and sleeping at intervals. The patient verbalizes pain relief.

## DISCHARGE FROM THE POSTANESTHESIA CARE UNIT

The PACU nurse completes a thorough assessment immediately before the patient's discharge and transfer to the surgical unit. The nurse assesses the patient's vital signs, level of consciousness, condition of the operative site, pain and comfort level, intake and output, respiratory function and oxygen saturation, and mobility. If the patient requires ongoing oxygen therapy, a transport oxygen canister is provided, and oxygen supply is prepared in the hospital room.

The patient usually is discharged from the PACU by an anesthesiologist, who may be present and write a discharge order. Alternatively, a numeric scoring system approved by the department of anesthesia may be used to determine if the patient is ready for discharge. The most common scoring system in use is the Aldrete score. Activity, respiration, circulation, consciousness, and oxygen-saturation level are scored from 0 to 2 (see Figure 9-3). A total score of 8 to 10 is generally acceptable for PACU discharge, with exceptions made by the physician's order.

A hand-off report on the patient's condition is given to the nurse who will assume care for the patient on the surgical or short procedure unit. This report may be given by telephone before the patient leaves the PACU or person-to-person after the patient reaches the unit. The report should include a preoperative history, pertinent information regarding the patient's surgery and recovery, medications the patient was given, physician's orders, and any other appropriate information.

## ADMISSION TO THE SURGICAL OR SHORT PROCEDURE UNIT

The patient's room is prepared for admission, and any necessary equipment is obtained. The patient is assisted into the bed. The bed rails should remain raised until the patient is fully awake, to prevent patient falls. The patient is informed to notify the nurse for assistance to ambulate. Family members also are instructed and enlisted to maintain safety for the patient. The equipment and condition of the patient should be explained to the family members who are present. A special concern is the use of PCA. Family members should be instructed that the PCA is for the patient's use only; that pushing the PCA button for the patient can have a detrimental effect on the patient's well-being.

## POSTOPERATIVE NURSING CONSIDERATIONS

### Assessment

The nurse makes an immediate assessment as soon as the patient is transferred to the bed. The nurse may choose a head-to-toe or systems assessment. Parameters include respiratory, cardiovascular, and neurologic status. The condition of the dressing and surgical site and patient comfort and safety also are assessed (Box 9-3).

### Nursing Diagnosis

Nursing diagnoses related to the care of the postoperative patient include the following:

- Risk for Infection
- Ineffective Breathing Pattern
- Acute Pain
- Imbalanced Nutrition: Less Than Body Requirements
- Impaired Physical Mobility

### Outcome Identification

Outcomes identified for the selected nursing diagnoses could be stated as follows:

- The patient will be free from infection as indicated by normal vital signs; temperature within normal range; normal white blood cell count; clear breath sounds; clear, yellow urine; and warm, dry skin.
- The patient's respirations will be easy, unlabored, and adequate.
- The patient will state subjective assertions of comfort: "I am in no pain." "My pain is a 2 on the scale of 0-10." The patient will have no objective signs of discomfort (e.g., grimaces, tachycardia).
- The patient will eat well from prescribed diet; weight loss will be minimal.
- The patient will ambulate at an appropriate level and carry out activities of daily living appropriate for condition.

### Planning

Planning for the postoperative patient requires not only knowledge of surgical techniques but also knowledge regarding underlying medical conditions. Throughout the patient's stay, planning must always involve the family or significant others, with measurable goals determined by discharge. A Sample Plan of Care for the postoperative patient follows.

### Implementation

***Wound Healing.*** Nursing care of the postoperative patient includes a focus on wound healing. Nursing interventions focus on prevention and monitoring for wound complications. The nurse should use strict aseptic technique when placing a new dressing and monitor signs and symptoms of infection (e.g., elevated body temperature; red, swollen, warm area sur-

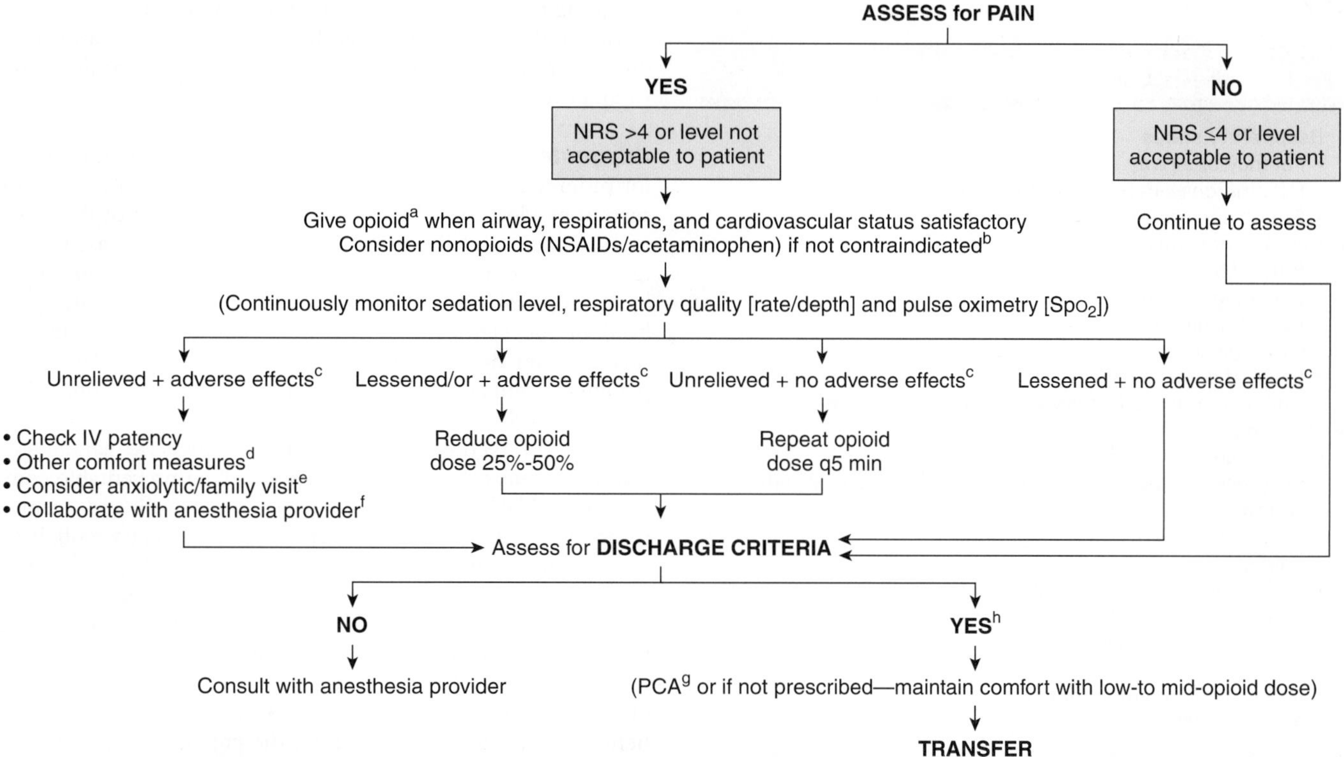
ASSESS for PAIN
YES
NO
NRS >4 or level not acceptable to patient
NRS ≤4 or level acceptable to patient
Give opioid[a] when airway, respirations, and cardiovascular status satisfactory
Consider nonopioids (NSAIDs/acetaminophen) if not contraindicated[b]
Continue to assess
(Continuously monitor sedation level, respiratory quality [rate/depth] and pulse oximetry [$Spo_2$])
Unrelieved + adverse effects[c]
Lessened/or + adverse effects[c]
Unrelieved + no adverse effects[c]
Lessened + no adverse effects[c]
• Check IV patency
• Other comfort measures[d]
• Consider anxiolytic/family visit[e]
• Collaborate with anesthesia provider[f]
Reduce opioid dose 25%-50%
Repeat opioid dose q5 min
Assess for DISCHARGE CRITERIA
NO
YES[h]
Consult with anesthesia provider
(PCA[g] or if not prescribed—maintain comfort with low-to mid-opioid dose)
TRANSFER

**Perianesthesia Pain Management Considerations (for Use in Conjunction with PACU Pain Algorithm)**

- Using the Sedation Scale, level of sedation (LOS) 3 requires proceeding with opioid cautiously (reduce opioid dose 25%-50%/increase interval between doses). LOS 4 requires holding opioids, and other sedatives, regardless of numeric rating scale (NRS); administer naloxone if physical stimulation fails to reverse respiratory depression and sedation.
- Respiratory function in an emergent tachypneic patient can improve through use of opioids by reducing respiratory rate, the depth increases, and the $Spo_2$ rises.
- During preadmission testing/preparation, staff should identify candidates for PCA and teach its use. Include in teaching the benefits of effective pain control, use of the pain scale, and the importance of reporting pain early. This information should be reinforced before surgery/procedure and again in the PACU.
- Encourage patients preoperatively to consider and discuss with anesthesia provider the use of local, regional, or epidural anesthesia/analgesia for preemptive analgesia, because the most effective pain control is achieved through multimodal approach (combined use of local anesthesia, opioids, and nonopioids).
- Give nonopioids (acetaminophen, salicylates, NSAIDs) on admission to the PACU when not contraindicated or previously administered. Encourage anesthesia providers to administer intraprocedure for preemptive analgesia.
- Preferred opioids are morphine, fentanyl, and hydromorphone. Avoid meperidine except for treatment of shivering or allergy to other opioids; meperidine metabolite, normeperidine, is toxic to the central nervous system and can cause seizures and death.
- Determine patient's preoperative use of opioids, nonopioids, and substance/alcohol use for possible higher opioid requirements.
- Give feedback to anesthesia provider when a patient has prolonged pain with an NRS higher than 4 for collaborative solutions.
- Avoid sedatives and use of antiemetics that produce sedation. Avoid IM injections.
- Pain goal: Level of comfort should allow patient to deep breathe, cough, turn, and move into/out of bed. Opioid side effects should be minimal.
- Appearing to sleep may not equal comfort. Always ask patients to rate their pain.
- Initiate PCA early when possible for evaluating effectiveness of programmed dose. Opioid loading is indicated first for severe escalating pain with minimal opioids on board.
- This algorithm is a suggested guide. Interventions should be individualized to each patient.

[a]For a numeric rating scale (NRS) of 5 or higher, use the higher opioid dose range; for an NRS lower than 5, use the mid-to-low dose range.
[b]Acetaminophen, salicylates, or NSAIDs (which include ketorolac, ibuprofen, salsalate, nabumetone, choline magnesium trisalicylate, and so on), or the cyclooxygenase type 2 (COX-2) inhibitor rofecoxib. Contraindications to NSAIDs are aspirin-sensitive asthma, bleeding, coagulopathy disorders, history of gastrointestinal bleeding, renal compromise, and hypovolemia.
[c]Adverse effects include but are not limited to increasing sedation (LOS 3), respiratory depression, local histamine reaction, and uncontrolled nausea and vomiting.
[d]Comfort measures include the following: reassurance, reposition, warm/cold applications, relaxation measures, and music therapy.
[e]Use anxiolytics for anxiety and muscle spasms only.
[f]Collaborate for other adjuvants or regional block. Consult also with surgeon.
[g]Start PCA early or after opioid loading (PCA pump or syringe) per anesthesia provider orders for rapidly escalating pain higher than an NRS of 4.
[h]Discharge criteria include the following: NRS of pain of 4 or less, LOS of 3 or less, respiratory rate of 10 or higher, $Spo_2$ of 93% or higher, and minimal other opioid side effects.

FIGURE 9-9 PACU pain algorithm.

**BOX 9-3**

**Patient Assessment on Return from the Postanesthesia Care Unit**

- Respiratory status
  - Patency of airway
  - Respirations—depth, rate, character
  - Breath sounds—presence, character
- Circulatory status
  - Pulse, blood pressure
  - Skin color, temperature
  - Capillary filling
- Neurologic status
  - Level of consciousness
  - Ability to move extremities, peripheral pulses (as applicable)
- Dressing
  - Presence of drainage
  - Presence of tubes to be connected to drainage systems
- Comfort
  - Presence of pain, nausea, vomiting
  - Pain score
  - Patient positioned for comfort and to facilitate ventilation
  - Other comfort measures as determined by patient preference (e.g., warm blanket, music, massage)
- Safety
  - Use of two patient identifiers
  - Necessity for side rails
  - Call cord within reach and instructions on operation reviewed
- Equipment
  - Monitors connected and functioning
  - Intravenous fluids—location of insertion site, type and size of intravenous device, type of infusion, rate, amount in bag, patency of tubing, assessment of site
  - Drainage systems (e.g., nasogastric, chest, urinary)—type, patency of tubing, connection of appropriate container, character and amount of drainage

rounding the incision; elevated white blood cell count; tachycardia; and purulent drainage from wound).[31] For a detailed discussion of the pathophysiology of wound healing, see Chapter 8.

***Adequate Respirations.*** The postoperative patient is at risk for pulmonary complications because of increased respiratory secretions, decreased lung expansion, depression of the respiratory center, and the possibility of aspiration of gastric contents. The occurrence of these complications can be minimized by appropriate nursing management, including elevating the head of the bed whenever possible; encouraging coughing, turning, and deep breathing every 2 hours; ambulating the patient as soon as possible; and encouraging hydration.[31]

***Circulation.*** Venous stasis in the postoperative patient can lead to thrombophlebitis, which is usually a preventable complication. Platelets adhere to the venous wall and form a thrombus, with a resultant potential for pulmonary embolus.

Prevention may include administration of prophylactic heparin, aspirin, dextran, or warfarin. Application of an intermittent external pneumatic sequential compression device may be ordered, or application of antiembolic (AE) hosiery may be required. Nursing measures that can prevent formation of a thrombus include using the AE hosiery whether the patient is in or out of bed, teaching the patient not to cross the legs, having the patient do isometric leg exercises, and encouraging early ambulation.

If thrombophlebitis is suspected (pain or tenderness, presence of Homan's sign, erythema, localized area of warmth, swelling), the patient should return to bed, and the physician should be notified. Treatment consists of rest, heat, AE hosiery, and anticoagulant therapy.

## SAMPLE PLAN OF CARE

### ADMISSION TO THE POSTOPERATIVE PATIENT CARE UNIT

**Nursing Diagnosis**

**Risk for Infection** related to altered skin integrity, compromised aseptic technique, or malnutrition

**Outcome**

The patient will be free from infection, as indicated by normal vital signs; temperature within normal range; normal white blood cell count; clear breath sounds; clear, yellow urine; and warm, dry skin.

**Interventions**

- Monitor vital signs every 4 hours or as prescribed.
- Monitor temperature every 4 hours as needed; document and report increased temperature.
- Monitor laboratory values for evidence of infection; report variance from normal.
- Encourage patient to take deep breaths or sustained maximal inspiration or use respiratory aids.
- Preserve closed urinary system, and provide catheter care. Remove catheter as soon as possible.
- Encourage patient to eat foods high in protein and vitamin C.
- Avoid antiinflammatory drugs such as steroids to facilitate healing.
- Use aseptic technique when changing dressings, and change soiled dressings immediately.
- Monitor suction of wound catheters to provide drainage from wound.
- Teach patient and family members how to care for surgical site, what to expect, and who to call if drainage at incision or drain sites increases or if other symptoms develop, such as fever, increased pain at site, redness, and swelling of incision.

**Nursing Diagnosis**

**Ineffective Breathing Pattern** related to postoperative pain, decreased energy or fatigue, decreased lung expansion, surgery

**Outcome**

The patient's respirations will be easy, unlabored, and adequate.

**Interventions**

- Monitor respirations and chest expansion frequently for 24 to 48 hours after the surgical intervention.
- Place the bed in high Fowler position if possible.
- Auscultate lungs, and evaluate the productiveness of the cough; document any adventitious breath sounds and nature and amount of sputum associated with cough (as appropriate).

*Continued*

## SAMPLE PLAN OF CARE—cont'd

- Have patient cough and deep breathe at regular intervals; collaborate with patient to identify cues to remember to undertake these activities or recommend 10 deep breaths each hour.
- Encourage use of respiratory aids (e.g., incentive spirometry, if appropriate).
- Treat underlying conditions, such as pain.
- Demonstrate splinting incisional area with pillow before cough.
- Encourage patient to turn and change positions at least every 2 to 3 hours.
- Encourage early ambulation, and explain rationale to patient.

**Nursing Diagnosis**

**Acute Pain**

**Outcome**

The patient will state subjective assertions of comfort: "I am in no pain." "My pain is a 2 on a scale of 0-10." The patient will have no objective signs of discomfort (e.g., grimaces, tachycardia).

**Interventions**

- Discuss the concept of pain and what it means for patient (e.g., throbbing, aching, stabbing, burning, tight).
- Educate patient and family members on the use of pain rating scale:
  - Show pain rating scale, and explain its purpose.
  - Explain the components of scale (if numeric scale used, explain what the numbers mean).
  - Set realistic comfort goals (pain rating score should be ≤4).
- Encourage patient to report pain, emphasizing that this is an important part of his or her care.
- Consider personal, cultural, spiritual, and ethnic beliefs in developing a pain management plan with patient.
- Document assessment of pain (intensity, duration, location, frequency) and response to pain management therapies.
- If patient has continuous local anesthetic infusion therapy (also known as *site-specific infusion therapy*) (common with select orthopedic procedures, abdominal hysterectomy, mastectomy, or hernia repair):
  - Assess site to ensure dressing intact and catheter site clean and dry.
  - Query patient to determine if symptoms of local anesthetic toxicity are present (dizziness, ringing in the ears, metallic taste, tingling or numbness of lips, slowed speech); contact physician to initiate immediate treatment if assessment positive.
- If patient is to be discharged with infusion therapy, provide verbal and written instructions.
- Support patient in the use of personally effective nonpharmacologic pain management strategies (e.g., relaxation techniques, distraction, massage, biofeedback, music, guided imagery, meditation).

**Nursing Diagnosis**

**Altered Nutrition: Less Than Body Requirements** related to surgery

**Outcome**

The patient will eat well from prescribed diet; weight loss will be minimal.

**Interventions**

- Encourage patient to eat foods high in protein and vitamin C.
- Offer frequent, small amounts of food or high-protein liquids to patient with little or no appetite.
- Encourage ambulation (improves appetite).
- Schedule procedures not to conflict with mealtime.
- Administer medication for pain as needed.
- Determine patient's previous history of nausea and vomiting after surgery; consult with physician regarding preventive measures for discharge if history positive.
- Refer to nutritional support team if appropriate; dietary consultation may be important for patient with cultural or ethnic food preferences.

**Nursing Diagnosis**

**Impaired Physical Mobility** related to surgical procedure or pain

**Outcome**

The patient will ambulate at appropriate levels and carry out activities of daily living appropriate for condition.

**Interventions**

- Encourage muscle-strengthening exercises before ambulation. Encourage ambulation or position changes and extremity exercises at least every 8 hours.
- Encourage leg exercises in bed.
- Have patient dangle legs over side of bed until pulse has stabilized and patient is not dizzy before attempting to ambulate.
- Have two people to help ambulate if patient is weak or obese.
- Encourage patient to walk further with each ambulation.
- Teach proper use of appropriate devices (e.g., crutches, slings, Ace bandages), and observe return demonstration.

***Urinary Function.*** One of the priorities during surgery and immediately afterward is to keep the patient well hydrated so that voiding takes place 6 to 8 hours after surgery. Usually intake is greater than output for 48 hours, when the fluid and electrolyte balance returns to normal. Every effort is made to refrain from use of a catheter because of the risk of urinary tract infection. Measures to help the patient void include warming the bedpan, letting water run, applying warm water to the perineum, and allowing the patient up to the bathroom whenever possible. If discomfort is present, and the bladder is palpable, catheterization becomes necessary. In the event several catheterizations are required, an indwelling catheter is inserted. Hydration of the patient becomes a priority. Intake and output are recorded accurately. A urine output of less than 30 ml/hr is reported to the physician.

***Bowel Elimination.*** The postoperative patient who has had abdominal or pelvic surgery may have decreased peristalsis for at least 24 hours; this may persist for several days for the patient who has had gastrointestinal surgery.[31] Increased fluid intake and early ambulation can promote the return of peristalsis. Bowel sounds should be auscultated with a stethoscope to ensure that peristalsis has returned, and the abdomen should be assessed for distention.

Constipation occurs frequently after surgery because of the effects of the anesthetic agents, narcotics, immobility, and decreased gastrointestinal motility. Fluids, roughage, and bulk laxatives can be given to relieve constipation. Occasionally a suppository or an enema may be needed to empty the lower bowel.

***Early Ambulation.*** Early ambulation can expedite recovery and prevent complications. Early ambulation increases muscle tone, improves gastrointestinal and urinary tract function, stimulates circulation, and increases vital capacity.[31] Benefits are shown in Figure 9-10. Ambulation usually is postponed in the event of severe infection or thrombophlebitis.

### Evaluation

Evaluation of the postoperative patient on the surgical unit involves evaluating the outcomes identified as the patient was assessed:

- The patient's vital signs and laboratory values were within normal limits; the surgical site showed no signs or symptoms of infection.
- The patient's breath sounds were clear bilaterally.
- The patient verbalized freedom from pain and was free from facial grimaces, moaning, and other evidence of pain or discomfort.
- The patient was eating well; there were no complaints of nausea or vomiting.
- The patient ambulated as appropriate and was assessed as being capable of performing the appropriate activities of daily living.

## PATIENT AND FAMILY EDUCATION AND DISCHARGE PLANNING

Ideally, patient and family education and discharge planning should begin before the patient's admission for surgery. The patient and family should be prepared to assume any care that may be needed after discharge. If needed, community resources should be used. Home health care is a valuable resource for patients with treatment needs after discharge. The nurse responsible for the patient's care in the acute care setting collaborates and communicates with the home health team as soon as the need is identified so that the patient's care will be consistent and continue as needed.

The patient and family members should be instructed in the proper care of the wound or incision and signs and symptoms of a wound infection. They should know how to take a temperature and when the physician should be notified for elevated temperature. They should be knowledgeable about medication that the patient will be using at home, including analgesics (Patient Safety). Appropriate nonpharmacologic methods of pain control, such as imagery, distraction, massage, and relaxation, also can be taught. An appointment for the return visit should be scheduled as ordered, and the patient should be taught the importance of the return visit. Normal activities are resumed gradually according to the physician's protocols. Chapter 10 describes patient education and discharge planning in further detail. The chapters on surgical interventions have incorporated important elements for patient and family education and discharge planning. These elements assist the perioperative nurse in identifying and teaching what patients need to know and facilitate safe self-care during recovery from operative and other invasive procedures (Research Highlight).

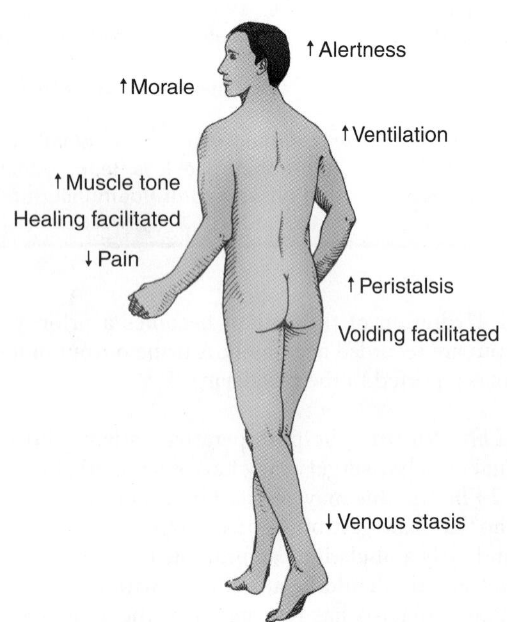


**FIGURE 9-10** Benefits from early postoperative ambulation.

## RESEARCH HIGHLIGHT

### Patient Retention of Discharge Instructions

Lee and Bokovoy conducted a study to describe patient responses to predischarge instructions and teaching. The study sample included patients who had undergone either femoropopliteal bypass or abdominal aortic aneurysm repair. All patients in the study received standardized prewritten discharge instructions and verbal education from a staff nurse on the day of discharge. Items discussed on the discharge instructions included pain control, diet, bowel elimination, medications, activity limitations and progression, driving, sexual activity, bathing, incision care, clothing, foot care, and reasons to contact the surgeon. Three days after discharge, patients were contacted and surveyed to determine their understanding of the education provided.

The overall mean of comprehension was 67% with no significant difference between surgery groups. Further research on patient knowledge retention of preprinted patient education materials needs to be conducted. The authors also call for more research to test the association of patient knowledge with objective outcomes, such as wound infection rates. Nurses need to be aware of patients' knowledge of discharge instructions because understanding is vital to the patient's outcome. Strategies such as "teach-back" are part of patient safety. In this type of strategy, the patient and family members, as applicable, or the individuals responsible for providing continuing care should be asked to recount in their own words what they have been told or reviewed as part of discharge education and planning.

Modified from Lee TL, Bokovoy J: Understanding discharge instructions after vascular surgery: an observational study, *Journal of Vascular Nursing* 23(1):25-29, 2005.

## PATIENT SAFETY

### Educating Patients About Medications for Pain Management

- Explain the purpose, dosage, schedule, and route of administration of any prescribed drugs and side effects to report to a physician or nurse.
- Give the patient general guidelines for the use of pain medications.
  - Provide information from the Agency for Healthcare Research and Quality guidelines for patients.
  - Explain that a variety of pain relief measures may be necessary for some types of pain.
  - Instruct the patient to use pain relief measures before pain becomes severe. Determine the patient's ability or willingness to participate actively in the use of pain relief measures, and suggest pain relief measures the patient believes would be helpful.
  - Rely on patient behavior that indicates pain severity rather than on known physical stimuli.
  - Encourage the patient to try a pain relief measure at least twice before abandoning it as ineffective. Instruct the patient to keep an open mind as to what may relieve pain.
  - Urge the patient to keep trying to relieve the pain and not to become discouraged.
- Discuss the use of nonopioid analgesics.
  - Inform the patient that nonopioid analgesics include acetaminophen, aspirin, and nonsteroidal antiinflammatory drugs, such as ibuprofen, indomethacin, and naproxen.
  - Explain that these medications are generally well tolerated, but have the potential to cause gastrointestinal ulceration, renal and hepatic toxic effects, and inhibition of platelet aggregation.
  - Tell the patient that if the nonopioid drug does not have a therapeutic effect initially, the dosage should be increased before another type of drug is tried.
- Discuss the use of opioids, which are indicated for severe postoperative pain or intractable pain such as that associated with cancer.
  - Inform the patient that opioids include morphine, hydromorphone, and methadone, and that these may be administered by oral route, intravenous drip, intrathecally, or epidurally to enhance the analgesic effect.
  - Explain that fixed dosage schedules with adequate doses for pain relief provide more constant blood levels and predictable pain relief. Suggest that additional doses may be needed for breakthrough pain.
  - Discuss the side effects of narcotic analgesics, including constipation, vomiting, and respiratory and central nervous system depression.
  - Review the use of opioid agonists and antagonists, including nalbuphine (Nubain), butorphanol (Stadol), pentazocine (Talwin), and buprenorphine (Buprenex).
- Explain the use of analgesic potentiators.
  - Inform the patient that these drugs include hydroxyzine (Vistaril), diazepam (Valium), lorazepam (Ativan), diphenhydramine (Benadryl), and phenothiazine derivatives, such as promethazine (Phenergan), prochlorperazine (Compazine), and chlorpromazine (Thorazine).
  - Discuss the use of stimulants.
  - Inform the patient that these drugs include cocaine, methylphenidate (Ritalin), dextroamphetamine, and caffeine.
- Discuss other types of drugs used in pain control, including tricyclic antidepressants, such as amitriptyline (Elavil), imipramine (Tofranil), and doxepin (Sinequan), and butyrophenones, such as droperidol (Inapsine) and haloperidol (Haldol).
- Discuss and demonstrate the use of equipment for administering pain relief medications.
  - External and implantable pumps for intravenous, epidural, and intrathecal administration of opioid analgesics
  - Patient-controlled analgesia, particularly for the management of acute pain, such as postoperative pain
  - Continuous subcutaneous infusion with an ambulatory infusion pump
  - Transcutaneous electrical nerve stimulation (TENS)
  - Discuss the side effects of narcotics. For example, constipation requires the use of laxatives and stool softeners (e.g., senna [Senokot]).

From Canobbio MM: *Mosby's handbook of patient teaching,* ed 3, St Louis, 2006, Mosby.

## REFERENCES


1. Acute Pain Management Guideline Panel: *Acute pain management: operative or medical procedures and trauma. Clinical practice guideline,* AHCPR Pub. No. 92-0032, Rockville, Md, 1992, Agency for Health Care Policy and Research, Public Health Service, U.S. Department of Health and Human Services. Accessed November 18, 2005, on-line: www.ahrq.gov/clinic/medtep/acute.html.
2. Ahmed I: Prevention and management of laryngospasm, *Anaesthesia* 59:920, 2004.
3. American Heart Association: *ACLS provider manual,* Dallas, Tex, 2001, The Association.
4. American Society of Anesthesiologists: *Standards for postanesthesia care* (amended by House of Delegates, 2004), Park Ridge, Ill, The Society. Accessed July 28, 2006 on-line: www.asahq.org/publicationsAndServices/standards/36.pdf.
5. American Society of PeriAnesthesia Nurses: *Clinical guideline for the prevention of unplanned perioperative hypothermia.* Accessed November 21, 2005, on-line: www.aspan.org/HypoThermia.htm.
6. American Society of PeriAnesthesia Nurses: *ASPAN pain and comfort clinical guideline.* Accessed November 21, 2005, on-line: www.aspan.org/PDFfiles/pain&comfort.pdf.
7. American Society of PeriAnesthesia Nurses: *Standards of perianesthesia nursing practice,* Cherry Hill, NJ, 2004, The Society.
8. Apfel CC and others: Comparison of predictive models for postoperative nausea and vomiting. *British Journal of Anaesthesia* 88:234-240, 2002.
9. Apfelbaum JL and others: Postoperative pain experience: results from a national survey suggest postoperative pain continues to be undermanaged, *Anesthesia and Analgesia* 97:534-540, 2003.
10. Brophy JM: Celecoxib and cardiovascular risks, *Expert Opinion on Drug Safety* 4(6):1005-1015, 2005.
11. Buss HE, Melderis K: PACU pain management algorithm, *Journal of PeriAnesthesia Nursing* 17(1):11-20, 2002.
12. Doufas AG: Consequences of inadvertent perioperative hypothermia. *Best Practices in Research and Clinical Anaesthesiology* 17(4):535-549, 2003.
13. Ferrara-Love R: Immediate postanesthesia care. In Burden N and others, editors: *Ambulatory surgical nursing,* ed 2, Philadelphia, 2000, Saunders.
14. Joshi GP: Multimodal analgesia techniques and postoperative rehabilitation, *Anesthesiology Clinics of North America* 23:185-202, 2005.
15. Kalinowski CPH, Kirsch JR: Strategies for prophylaxis and treatment for aspiration, *Best Practice and Research Clinical Anaesthesiology* 18(4):719-737, 2004.

16. Krenszichek DA: Pain and comfort management. In Quinn DMD, Schick L, editors: *Perianesthesia nursing core curriculum,* St Louis, 2004, Mosby.
17. Laschke KE: *Pain clinical updates: culture and pain,* Vol X(5), 2002. Accessed June 14, 2006, on-line: www.iasp-pain.org/PCU02-5.html.
18. Leslie K, Sessler D: Perioperative hypothermia in the high-risk surgical patient, *Best Practices in Research and Clinical Anaesthesiology* 17(4):485-498, 2003.
19. Litwack K: Postanesthesia recovery. In Nagelhout JJ, Zaglaniczny KL, editors: *Nurse anesthesia*, ed 2, Philadelphia, 2001, Saunders.
20. Macario A, Dexter F: What are the most important risk factors for a patient's developing intraoperative hypothermia? *Anesthesia* and *Analgesia* 94:215-220, 2002.
21. Mamaril ME: Clinical emergencies and preparedness. In Burden N and others, editors: *Ambulatory surgical nursing,* ed 2, Philadelphia, 2000, Saunders.
22. National Pharmaceutical Council, Inc, Joint Commission on Accreditation of Healthcare Organizations: *Pain: current understanding of assessment, management, and treatments,* December 2001. Accessed online: July 30, 2006 www.npcnow.org/resources/PDFs/PainExecSummary.pdf www.jcaho.org/news+room/health+care+issues/pain_mono_npc.pdf.
23. Nightingale F: *Notes on hospitals,* ed 3, London, 1863, Longman, Green, Longman, Roberts, & Green.
24. Odom-Forren J, Moser DK: Postdischarge nausea and vomiting: a review of current literature, *Journal of Ambulatory Surgery* 12:99-105, 2005.
25. Pasero C: The challenge of pain assessment in the PACU, *Journal of PeriAnesthesia Nursing* 17:348-350, 2002.
26. Pasero C: Perineural local anesthetic infusion: when close is almost perfect, *American Journal of Nursing* 104(7):89-92, 2002.
27. Pasero C, McCaffery J: Extended-release epidural morphine, *Journal of Perianesthesia Nursing* 20:245-250, 2005.
28. Ruth HS and others: Anesthesia study commission, *JAMA: The Journal of the American Medical Association* 35:881-884, 1947.
29. Siew-Fong N and others: A comparative study of three warming interventions to determine the most effective in maintaining perioperative normothermia. *Anesthesia* and *Analgesia* 96:171-176, 2003.
30. Sessler DI: Complications and treatment of mild hypothermia, *Anesthesiology* 95:531-543, 2001.
31. Smith DJ: Nursing management postoperative care. In Lewis SM and others, editors: *Medical-surgical nursing: assessment and management of clinical problems,* ed 6, St Louis, 2004, Mosby.
32. Viscusi ER: Emerging techniques in the treatment of postoperative pain, *American Journal of Health-System Pharmacy* 61(Suppl 1):S11-S14, 2004.
33. Wang J and others: The effect of timing of dexamethasone administration on its efficacy as a prophylactic antiemetic for postoperative nausea and vomiting, *Anesthesia and Analgesia* 91:136-139, 2000.

CHAPTER 10

# Patient Education and Discharge Planning

VICKI J. FOX

## IMPORTANCE OF PATIENT EDUCATION

Patient education and discharge planning are vital components of perioperative nursing care. In the 1980s, the growing emphasis on shortened hospital stays, the increasing number of ambulatory surgery procedures, and managed care made it clear that the process of patient education needed to accommodate to changing health care delivery systems. Today, patient education is a standard of nursing practice. A growing body of research describes what is effective in this nursing undertaking, as studies concentrate on why and which nursing interventions are selected and how they improve patient outcomes. To assess their usefulness, nursing-sensitive patient outcomes (outcomes that are responsive to nursing care) should be identified as part of patient education efforts.[16] The perioperative nurse has the unique opportunity and knowledge base to coordinate efforts to meet the education needs of surgical patients and their families or significant others. This chapter examines four questions about patient education:

1. Why teach?
2. When should patient education occur?
3. What is the appropriate content for patient teaching?
4. How should perioperative nurses teach?

### Historical Development

One answer to the question, "Why teach?" is that patient education is a long-standing nursing tradition. Nursing has used patient education as a tool for providing safe, cost-effective, and quality health care since the middle of the nineteenth century (History box). Nurses themselves value patient education highly and consider it an important part of their professional responsibility.[14] Patient education began in an era when the sick were cared for in the home. Operative procedures were often done at home. Nurses taught families about sanitation and cleanliness when caring for the sick and how to care for patients convalescing from home surgery. The National League of Nursing Education, in its 1918 *Standard Curriculum for Schools of Nursing*, considered "preventive and educational factors" an essential element of routine nurse training,[17] especially in new specialties, such as public health, school nursing, infant welfare, and industrial welfare. In 1937 the *Curriculum Guide* described the nurse as a teacher and an agent for health.[18] By 1950 the *Guide* identified teaching and contributing subject matter, such as psychology, knowledge of principles of teaching and learning, and teaching skills, as areas common to all nursing curricula.[19]

***Legal and Ethical Mandates.*** In answering the question, "Why teach?" one could argue that, as health care providers, nurses are ethically and legally bound to teach. Illness prevention and patient education have long been nursing priorities. Traditionally, however, the physician's first priority was protecting the patient from harm. Complete disclosure about the disease and treatment was a secondary concern. More recently, the emphasis in medical care has changed from simply treating the disease to health maintenance and wellness. The American Hospital Association's *The Patient Care Partnership* (formerly known as *The Patient's Bill of Rights*) affirms the patient's right to information about his or her medical condition and to information about the surgical treatment plan and consenting to it.[2] If a health care facility adopts that partnership as policy, it becomes an ethical duty to uphold it. Several nurse practice acts have made patient education an explicit legal responsibility for the individual nurse.[21] Failure to teach or to document that teaching was done may be considered below reasonable and prudent nursing practice and become the basis of malpractice litigation involving nurses. Courts repeatedly have maintained that the right of self-determination in a democratic society is fundamental. To limit it in health care decision making is an injustice. Nowhere is this better shown than in the perioperative setting when obtaining informed consent. All patients have the right to receive accurate, easily understood information that enables participation in treatment decisions (Patient Safety). By 2000, the Joint Commission on Accreditation of Healthcare Organizations (JCAHO) *Accreditation Manual for Hospitals* (AMH) consolidated functions of patient and family education from eight chapters in the previous AMH into one new chapter, "Patient and Family Education."[12] This chapter set a distinct set of standards for patient and family education and an even higher degree of accountability for institutions.

***Definitions and Goals.*** A third answer to the question, "Why teach?" comes from the ultimate goal of patient education, which is to enable patients to be responsible for their own health care. Patient education is a planned experience, based on the best information (evidence-based practice) designed to change or improve health behaviors and health status.[24] Patient education may use a combination of methods to accomplish this, including behavior modification, counseling, and teaching. Patient teaching is an activity that aims to increase the patient's knowledge. The goals of patient teaching are to provide information and to improve knowledge. Changes in

## HISTORY

This brief overview affirms nursing's early emphasis on protecting the patient's privacy and dignity; preventing injury; providing information; performing patient assessment; and addressing issues of consent, early ambulation, and discharge planning.

**1879**
Clarke, in his discussion of the practice of surgery, notes, "The most trivial operations have occasionally been followed by death, and the possibility of such a contingency ought always to be present to the surgeon's mind. He should, therefore, try to convey to the patient, or his friends, a fair idea of the risk to be incurred, whether it be great or small."

**1890**
Jones notes, "The patient is prepared by the nurse, who gives a full bath, braids the hair, puts on clean and suitable clothing, and arranges her on a table, where she is always covered by a sheet or single blanket if necessary."

**1897**
Weeks, in describing preparation for surgery in the patient's home, notes, "The instruments, and as far as possible everything that is disagreeably suggestive, should be covered."

**1898**
In a paper considering the management of patients before and after laparotomy, Wiggin notes, "In the early days of the decade now drawing to a close, it was generally believed that abdominal operations could not safely be performed outside of hospitals . . . but it is now known . . . it is perfectly safe to do such operations in ordinary houses."

**1899**
Fullerton notes the nurse should never cut sponges because this would make the count incorrect.

**1903**
In an account of practical suggestions for preparing for an operation in a private house, McCallum (a nurse) suggests many creative ideas, one being, "The windows can be frosted by rubbing Sapolio on the inner surface, thus preventing any possible observation from the outside."

**1918**
In discussing postoperative recovery, Fowler recommends, "The stay in bed should be as short as is compatible with wound rest. If wound rest can be maintained with the patient in a chair or walking about this is preferable. As soon as possible, the patient should get into the open air and sunshine."

**1943**
In her book, *Operating Room Technique,* Alexander discusses attributes of an operating room nurse, stressing conscientiousness in patient care activities, noting that, "One cannot take a single chance regardless of how great the pressure of orders or time."

**1961**
Taylor and Worrall remind the nurse, "It is important that an even temperature be maintained in the operating theatre because the patient is often exposed for a long time and it would add to the likelihood of shock occurring if there was much cooling of the skin."

**1961**
In discussing the nurse's contribution to prevention and release of anxiety, Shafer notes, "The nurse cannot possibly know all the factors contributing to anxiety or their particular application for each patient. However, by recognizing anxiety and understanding that all behavior has some meaning, the nurse may be guided by some rules. She must remember that it is the patient, his family, and his friends who are primarily concerned with his welfare, and she must try to keep them informed."

**1970**
LeMaitre and Finnegan stress the role of the operating room nurse in conducting the patient interview, noting that, "A purposeful interview will go far toward determining any nursing problems that may follow the surgical procedure. More importantly, the manner in which this interview is carried out will, in large part, determine the degree of anxiety which the surgical procedure will engender in the patient. In no area of surgical care are the nurse's services more valuable than in this subtle creation of confidence and security in the patient."

**1971**
In discussing discharge planning, Moroney cautions, "It is surprising at times to see what at 'home' means, and the advice given to a patient on leaving hospital must be considered against this background."

Modified from Alexander EL: *Operating room technique,* St Louis, 1943, Mosby; Clarke WF: *A manual of the practice of surgery,* New York, 1879, William Wood; Fowler RS: *The operating room and the patient,* Philadelphia, 1918, Saunders; Fullerton A: *Surgical nursing,* Philadelphia, 1899, Blakiston's Son; Jones MC: The training of a nurse, *Scribner's Magazine* 8:613-624, 1890; LeMaitre G, Finnegan J: *The patient in surgery: a guide for nurses,* Philadelphia, 1970, Saunders; McCallum J: An improvised outfit for operation in a private house, *AJN* 3:619-621, 1903; Moroney J: *Surgery for nurses,* London, 1971, Churchill Livingstone; Shafer KN and others: *Medical-surgical nursing,* St Louis, 1961, Mosby; Taylor S, Worrall O: *Principles of surgery and surgical nursing,* London, 1961, The English Universities Press Ltd; Weeks CS: *A textbook of nursing,* ed 2, New York, 1897, Appleton; Wiggin FH: The management of patients before and after laparotomy, *Journal of the American Medical Association* 30:378-379, 1898.

## PATIENT SAFETY

### Informed Consent: National Quality Forum Safe Practice 10

Informed consent is a central element of safe, high quality care of surgical patients. In 2003, the National Quality Forum published a report identifying 30 evidence-based practices that would reduce the risk of health care errors. Among these was Safe Practice 10—specifying the need for improved communication during the informed consent process. Patients who are well informed are more likely to receive care that reflects their own values, are better prepared for requisite self-care, are more satisfied with the care they receive, and are more likely to have increased trust in their caregivers.

**Safe Practice 10**
Ask each patient or his or her legal surrogate to recount what he or she has been told during the informed consent discussion.

- Use informed consent forms written in simple sentences and in the primary language of the patient or legal surrogate.
- Engage the patient in a discussion about the nature and scope of the procedure covered by the consent form.
- Provide an interpreter or reader to assist non–English-speaking patients or legal surrogates, vision-impaired or hearing-impaired patients, and low-literacy patients.

Modified from Wu HW and others: *Improving patient safety through informed consent for patients with limited health literacy,* Washington, DC, 2005, National Quality Forum.

knowledge may be needed before the patient is motivated to change behaviors. Teaching is a systematic way of introducing new information, events, skills, or objects into the patient's environment. When viewed as an interpersonal interaction between the patient and nurse, teaching is a distinctive form of communication that is uniquely structured and sequenced to produce learning. Theoretically, teaching should meet the patient's need for new information and skills. Neither the definition of patient education nor patient teaching contains assurance that the patient will actually learn or that behavior will change.[21]

Learning, on the patient's part, is shown in changed behavior. Nurses can assess educational needs; provide information, instruction, and resources; and communicate with family and colleagues to enable learning, all as part of patient-centered care.[1] Nurses cannot force patients to learn, however. Ultimately, patients are responsible for changing their own behaviors.

***Benefits of Preoperative Patient Education.*** A fourth answer to the question, "Why teach?" relates to the benefits for the patient; for the patient's family, support system, and significant others; for nurses; and for institutions. Early nursing research confirmed the value of preoperative patient teaching when based on scientific content and structured either for a group or for an individual. The benefits of patient education for the patient undergoing a surgical intervention include the following: education (1) speeds recovery, (2) relieves anxiety,[25] (3) increases self-esteem by increasing self-efficacy, (4) reduces cost of hospitalization, (5) prevents complaints about care, and (6) decreases the amount of perceived immediate and residual pain.

The benefits of education for the patient's family and support system are as follows: education (1) alleviates anxiety and fear, (2) reduces cost, (3) hastens the family's return to normal functioning, (4) increases self-esteem, and (5) develops support for the caregiver's efforts. A primary benefit of patient education for nurses is increased job satisfaction. Patient education makes the nurse's job easier in the long run by saving time. It reduces the nurse's stress level and increases self-esteem. The institution benefits from patient education by increased patient and family satisfaction, decreased length of hospital stay, fewer re-hospitalizations (Patient Safety), and compliance with JCAHO requirements.

## Trends in Patient Education

The focus of health care moved from the home to institutions between 1925 and 1975; in the 1990s, the focus returned to the home setting. Ambulatory surgery and shortened hospital stays required creative strategies for preadmission teaching and preparation for convalescence at home. Homes also became the site of preventive care, such as reducing the risk of highly communicable diseases (e.g., human immunodeficiency virus [HIV] infection), appropriate nutrition for specific health states (e.g., diabetes), and early screening for diseases (e.g., breast self-examination). The home is the site of follow-up care (e.g., long-term intravenous antibiotic therapy; long-term care of the frail elderly). Home care is based on a self-care philosophy aimed at moving the patient from the dependent role limited to compliance with instruction into a more contractual arrangement with the health care provider.[21] Self-care philosophy is based on self-reliance, personal responsibility, and individual initiative. Educational support is an integral part of the self-care philosophy. The perioperative nurse has a unique opportunity to manage the educational partnership among health care professionals, patients, and their families. Patient perceptions of care and information received also are included in patient satisfaction surveys. The National Quality Forum, in its standardized survey of patients' perceptions of their hospital experience and discharge information, suggested three survey items for patients transitioning from a health care facility to home:[20]

- The hospital staff took my preferences and those of my family into account in deciding what my health care needs would be when I left the hospital.
- When I left the hospital, I had a good understanding of the things I was responsible for in managing my health.
- When I left the hospital, I clearly understood the purpose for taking each of my medications.

## PATIENT SAFETY

### Patient Education and Patient Safety

Perioperative nurses collectively value patient safety. One way to facilitate this goal is to improve patient self-care through information and education.[23] In one study, findings suggested that many patients leave the hospital not knowing their diagnosis, the names of their medications, the purpose of the prescribed drugs, or the side effects of the drugs.[9] The Joint Commission on Accreditation of Healthcare Organizations (JCAHO) Speak-Up campaigns are safety initiatives that encourage patients to take an active role in their health care. The JCAHO launched "Planning Your Recovery" in 2005, noting that patients who understand and follow directions about follow-up care are likely to heal faster and require fewer re-admissions.[13] The JCAHO advised patients to:

- *Know your condition*—which includes when the patient should expect to feel better, when to resume normal activity levels (e.g., walking, climbing stairs, driving, returning to work), and activity progression. All patients should know warning signs and symptoms, and what to do if they have them. A phone number should be provided for any problems after leaving the hospital. A family member or friend should be with the patient when he or she first gets home; discharge planning should determine whether the home is set up to accommodate any physical restrictions or limitations the patient may have.
- *Find out about new medicines*—and how to take them. All medications (not just new ones) should be listed. Written directions should be provided, and verification of understanding should be confirmed. Precautions (e.g., foods, sunlight, alcohol) should be reviewed, as should side effects and what to do if they occur.
- *Find out about follow-up care*—such as wound care, special equipment, further tests, and postoperative visits and checkups. Transportation issues should be discussed. If required, insurance coverage and home care or other services should be planned.

## ASSESSMENT

This section examines what content is appropriate for patient teaching and when a patient is ready to learn, introducing the interrelatedness of the nursing process and the process of teaching. The first step in the teaching process is assessment.

### Assessment of Individual Patient Education Needs

The most important activity the perioperative nurse can carry out is *assessment* because it is the foundation for the entire patient education process. Collecting accurate assessment data about what a patient needs to know and the level of readiness to learn assists the perioperative nurse in setting realistic priorities. Not all patient needs are the same, and not all patients need or desire to know everything. The key question the nurse must ask when assessing the patient's educational needs is, "What does this patient *need* to know?" Most patients need to know enough to (1) grant informed consent to an invasive procedure, (2) facilitate intraoperative cooperation, (3) provide self-care at home (Research Highlight), and (4) survive until more teaching can be provided. A patient's admission for a surgical procedure may involve enough discomfort and anxiety to prevent retention of any information on complicated subjects, such as pathophysiology. Highly technical content may confuse the patient. Patients learn information about events directly related to their admission for surgery. The need-to-know assessment should be based on crucial activities the patient would be expected to accomplish in the immediate postoperative period (Best Practice). Naturally the plan is different if the patient actively seeks highly technical information or if the patient is a child (Research Highlight). Assessment also should include determining what the patient already knows.

## RESEARCH HIGHLIGHT

### Information Patients Want to Know

The purpose of this study was to find out what specific questions patients about to undergo a total hip arthroplasty (THA) or total knee arthroplasty (TKA) wanted answered about their care. The researchers planned to use this information in developing a Web-based educational program. The researchers assembled a set of questions, then asked patients to rate the importance of the questions. Patients used a Likert scale, with 1 being least important and 5 being most important. The sample comprised 29 THA patients and 19 TKA patients. Four questions ranked most important by both groups follow:

1. Will the surgery affect my abilities to care for myself?
2. Am I going to need physical therapy?
3. How mobile will I be after my surgery?
4. When will I be able to walk normally again?

Most of the remaining questions were judged to be of high importance by at least one person in each group. Some patients wrote additional questions they wanted answered.

The researchers concluded there was enough agreement to define a core set of questions that should be addressed. Perioperative nurses should keep in mind, however, that the core set of information may not be enough to satisfy any one patient's essential information needs adequately. As with all planning of patient care, individual patient need for information must be integrated into patient-centered education.

Modified from Macario A and others: What questions do patients undergoing lower extremity joint replacement surgery have? *BMC Health Services Research*, June 24, 2003. Accessed July 28, 2006 on-line: www.biomedcentral.com/1472-6963/3/11.

### Assessment of Individual Readiness to Learn

The timing of preoperative teaching is crucial. When to teach has more to do with the patient's readiness to learn than the number of weeks, days, or hours before a surgical procedure. The literature is replete with articles on the importance of assessing the learner's readiness to learn. Assessment of readiness to learn requires expertise in observation, communication skills (especially listening), collaboration with nurse and physician colleagues, and assimilation of chart data. Much of the literature on readiness to learn refers to healthy students in the classroom setting. Although some similarities exist between readiness to learn in an academic setting and readiness to learn in the context of health care, there are notable differences—*time* and *health*. Health affects readiness to learn because the patient and family may be profoundly concerned, rationally or irrationally, about basic issues such as pain, disability, self-esteem, and dying. Time constraints are different. In the academic setting, the teacher and learner have agreed on a time period—6 weeks, a semester, or a year. In the health care setting, the nurse most often is concerned with the patient's readiness to learn at this moment in time. The moment may be the brief span of time the perioperative nurse sees the patient preoperatively and postoperatively. The nurse's assessment must be brief, basic, concrete, specific, and useful.

***Factors That Influence Readiness to Learn.*** Assessing the patient's readiness to learn should occur before each teaching interaction as a distinct activity. Assessment often occurs as the perioperative nurse is assessing other needs or providing other kinds of nursing care. The assessment may be done quickly. The quality, nature, method, and scope of instruction may affect the patient's future levels of readiness to learn. Readiness to learn is being willing and able to make use of instruction. Readiness establishes evidence of motivation. The degree of readiness to learn depends on the degree of willingness and ability.

Several factors influence readiness to learn. The first is *comfort*—physical and psychologic. The six most common sources for physical discomfort are the following:

- Pain
- Nausea or dizziness
- Itching
- Fatigue or weakness
- Hunger or thirst
- Need to urinate or defecate

Because these conditions are not always directly observable, the perioperative nurse may be able to obtain information regarding physical discomfort from the medical record or by asking the patient directly. One cannot assume that absence of complaints indicates comfort.

Psychologic comfort implies that the patient is not currently having uncomfortable emotions to a degree that would impair abilities. The six most common uncomfortable emotions are the following:

- Fear
- Anxiety

## BEST PRACTICE

### Patients Identify Areas Unmet in Postoperative Teaching

In one prospective, descriptive study, published in 2000, patient reports of educational information received after surgery were examined. A convenience sample included 45 patients who underwent common surgical procedures requiring short hospital stays. Patients were surveyed for the type of information received and their satisfaction with the level of information provided.

Patients indicated that predischarge teaching did occur, but that some of the greatest areas of concern to them were not sufficiently addressed before they were discharged. Overall, discharge instructions stressed medication regimens. Patients indicated that more information regarding self-monitoring of specific postoperative parameters, such as activity restrictions, wound care, potential complications, pain management, and elimination, was needed for them to feel confident in their abilities to manage an early discharge after their surgery.

In a larger study by Clark assessing patient satisfaction with ratings of "instructions given about how to care for yourself at home," patient satisfaction decreased over a 5-year period (1997-2001, $n$ = 4,901,178). Patients gave lower scores to the quality of discharge instructions than to their overall satisfaction with their hospital stay. Patient age, sex, self-described health status, and length of stay did not predict evaluation of discharge instructions.

Another study examined the relationship between patient-centered care and satisfaction with information among women with a history of breast cancer. A questionnaire was administered to 182 women who had completed treatment for breast cancer. Findings suggested that, although breast cancer survivors were highly satisfied with information related to treatment, they were less satisfied with information related to the long-term physical, psychologic, and social sequelae of the disease and its treatments. In multivariate analysis, patients' perception of patient-centered behaviors was strongly associated with satisfaction with information. These results provide additional support for the theory that patient satisfaction is improved when perioperative nurses incorporate patient-centered behaviors into their care.

**IMPLICATIONS FOR PERIOPERATIVE NURSES**

With the reality of shorter postoperative stays, patient teaching has become more challenging for perioperative nurses. When patients are discharged more quickly, they still must be adequately prepared to take responsibility for their postdischarge care. Monitoring for postoperative complications and problems previously had been part of the postoperative hospital stay. Information and instruction regarding medications are important because there is a significant potential for confusion regarding medication regimens. Other issues of patient education are equally as important for safe and effective recovery at home. As noted in this chapter, perioperative nurses need to focus on what patients and their families *need* to know. The results of these studies and others provide evidence that perioperative nurses need to construct patient education materials and content that address these patient information needs. Satisfaction with information is an important patient outcome and may be related to the perioperative nurse's ability to elicit the patients' concerns, to consider the patients' psychosocial needs, and to involve patients in treatment decision making; these communication techniques are crucial to "patient-centered" care.

Modified from Clark PA and others: Patient perceptions of quality discharge instruction, *Patient Education and Counseling* 59(1):56-58, 2005; Mallinger JB and others: Patient-centered care and breast cancer survivors' satisfaction with information, *Patient Education and Counseling* 57(3):342-349, 2005; Patton RM: Interventions for postoperative clients. In Ignatavicius DD, Workman LM: *Medical-surgical nursing: critical thinking for collaborative care,* Philadelphia, 2006, Saunders; Rodehaver C: Medication reconciliation in acute care—ensuring an accurate drug regimen on admission and discharge, *Joint Commission Journal on Quality and Patient Safety* 31(7):406-413, 2005.

## RESEARCH HIGHLIGHT

### Preparing Children for Surgery

O'Conner-Von reviewed 63 research studies pertaining to the preparation of children for surgery published between 1974 and 1995. Her meta-analysis included a review of the methodology and characteristics of these studies comparing them with a landmark 1965 review by Vernon. This review concluded that there are three key elements of preparation: (1) providing information to children about the experience, (2) encouraging emotional expression of concerns, and (3) establishing a trusting relationship with the health care provider. The earlier review delineated seven primary weaknesses with the research. The more recent research studies were better designed, used advanced statistical procedures, were more concerned with reliability and validity, controlled observer bias better, and measured the direct effects of experimental conditions and psychologic benefits better. O'Conner-Von's review confirms that children and their parents need preparation before the surgical experience. Recommendations from the meta-analysis include using proven preparation strategies that effectively reduce anxiety for children, flexible preparation strategies for cultural diversity, methods that can be adapted for children undergoing emergency or repeat surgery, and developing methods to solicit patients' and parents' satisfaction with the preparation strategy. The population sample in the integrative review comprised mostly healthy, white, middle-class children between ages 3 and 12 years. Future research should include children with chronic or acute illness; children from a variety of ethnic, cultural, and socioeconomic groups; children whose second language is English; and children younger than 3 years and older than 12 years.

Preparing children for surgery, particularly when they have a chronic condition, can be challenging because of demanding regimens, their progressing developmental stages, and varying family perspectives and relationships. Perioperative nurses should focus on building trust in the nurse-patient-family relationship. It also is important to understand beliefs and attitudes in shaping acceptance of educational strategies, social and cultural norms, barriers and pressures faced by patients and their families, the role of social networks and social support, and the effects of family cohesiveness and family conflict.

Modified from DiMatteo MR: The role of effective communication with children and their families in fostering adherence to pediatric regimens, *Patient Education and Counseling* 55(3):339-344, 2004; O'Conner-Von S: Preparing children for surgery: an integrative research review, *AORN Journal* 22:334-343, 2000.

- Worry
- Grief
- Anger
- Guilt

The perioperative nurse may be able to observe behaviors or body language that indicates the presence of psychologic discomfort. Any intense emotion, including pleasant ones, precludes the possibility of effective involvement in learning. A skillful perioperative nurse modifies a planned intervention to accommodate the patient's comfort. If the patient is physically or psychologically uncomfortable, the appropriate intervention is to relieve the discomfort before proceeding. Consider the patient in the surgeon's office who has just learned he should have a thoracotomy for a suspected malignant lesion. He may be so overwhelmed with the fear of cancer that listening to procedural information may be impossible. The wise intervention is to be supportive and schedule another clinic visit to discuss treatment options. The patient should be allowed to process the fear and advance to a higher level of readiness to learn.

The amount of *energy* currently available to the learner is a second crucial factor. If large amounts of physical or psychologic energy are being expended, none may be available for learning. The amount of energy patients have is closely related to their physical condition, their reaction to the stage of illness, the current number of stressors in their lives, and the degree of the situational or maturational crisis. A patient who is fighting for every breath has no energy for anything else; a person actively denying the illness has little energy to learn about it.

A third factor influencing readiness to learn is *motivation.* The following behaviors may indicate a person is motivated to learn:

- Leaning forward
- Asking questions or for a more complete explanation
- Taking notes
- Seeking out the perioperative nurse for help or information
- Requesting books or pamphlets.

Remember the patient's cultural values, beliefs, and customs when observing behavior to assess readiness to learn.[8] Culture-based health behavior and communication patterns are closely intertwined and include culture-specific verbal and nonverbal behaviors. The perioperative nurse's goal is to provide culturally competent teaching that helps the patient and family members learn whatever they need or wish to learn. The goal is to assess the level of, not the reason for, motivation.

The patient's *capability* to learn is a fourth crucial factor affecting the readiness to learn. Obstacles to learning include vision or hearing problems, limited manual dexterity, vocal or language limitations, and neurologic deficit. The first three factors that influence readiness to learn can be assessed primarily by the use of subjective data. The patient's capabilities can be assessed on more or less objective data. Prerequisite capabilities include physical ability, intellectual ability, knowledge, attitudes, and skill. Capability is influenced or determined by age, maturation, stage of development, past learning, physical and mental health, and environment. When assessing physical capability, the perioperative nurse should ask the following questions:

1. Are the patient's height and weight adequate to accomplish the task involved? (Can this child reach the light switch?)
2. Is the patient strong enough? (Can this frail, elderly woman lift a long leg cast?)
3. Does the patient have the coordination and dexterity to accomplish the task? (Can this patient whose hands are crippled with arthritis manage to change a colostomy bag?)
4. Can the patient see, hear, smell, taste, and feel well enough to accomplish the task?
5. Can the patient see well enough to compare adequately the color chart on a reagent strip for urinalysis?

Assessment of intellectual capability includes the following:

1. *Basic math skills.* (Can this patient read a thermometer?)
2. *Reading skills.* (Can this patient read the directions on a prescription bottle?)
3. *Verbal skills.* (Can this patient communicate with others who are involved in care and express himself?)
4. *Problem-solving skills.* (Can this patient recognize situations in which she should seek help, and would she know how to seek help? For example, would this patient know what to do if she became febrile at home?)
5. *Comprehension and ability to follow instructions.* (Is there some factor, such as recently administered pain medication, that may impair this patient's ability to receive the information the perioperative nurse has to offer?)

Knowledge influences readiness to learn. Does the patient have the basic concepts and facts to understand the new material? Does the patient know where the organ to be operated on is located? A related factor influencing the patient's readiness to learn is the patient's acquired skills. Has this patient already acquired skills from past experiences? Would past experiences attract or detract the patient from the goal? Discrepancies between expectations and capabilities should be discovered early as a result of careful assessment, rather than later as a result of the patient's failure to reach the goals. The patient's attitude and value system are powerful influences on readiness to learn. These are influenced by factors such as ethnicity; spiritual, cultural, and religious beliefs; values about health care; and socioeconomic status.[5] What is important to the patient? In teaching a new mother about immunizations for her infant, does the mother share the belief that immunizations are safe? The discussion on the *health belief model* in this chapter helps illustrate this concept.

***Motivation.*** Motivation is the force that "initiates, directs, and maintains behavior."[21] No single motivation theory, but rather a combination of two or more of these theories, is likely to account for a patient's behavior. The six theories are reinforcement, needs, cognitive dissonance, attribution, personality, and expectancy.[21] Behaviors that have been positively reinforced, rather than punished or ignored, are far more likely to be repeated. The positive social reinforcement a cardiac rehabilitation patient gets from exercising in groups, rather than alone, provides motivation to continue the behavior. Another powerful way to reinforce behavior is verbal encouragement from other patients and the cardiac rehabilitation nurse.

According to Maslow, a hierarchy of needs motivates individuals; higher level needs emerge as lower level needs are met. In other words, unmet needs create motivation. A satisfied need has no power to motivate, but it permits a higher level need to emerge, which motivates the individual. If the patient perceives that a surgical procedure is life threatening, safety needs motivate him or her to learn more about it, rather than to interact in meaningful ways with friends, which serves to meet a higher level social need.

Cognitive dissonance theory maintains that individuals become uncomfortable when a deeply held value or belief is challenged. To resolve the discomfort, an individual may rationalize to justify the belief or behavior: "Well, everybody has to die of something. I'll really enjoy smoking while I'm alive and just die a little sooner." An individual also may be motivated to change the behavior or belief: "Smoking is less socially acceptable than it used to be. It does contribute to heart disease and lung cancer. I will quit smoking."

Attribution is identifying a cause for what is happening. Patients frequently do this after the diagnosis of a condition, an accident, or cure of a disease. Attribution answers the question, "Why did this happen to me?" A concept essential to understanding attribution is locus of control. Individuals with an internal locus of control believe that their own efforts contribute to the success or failure of a situation. A postoperative patient with an internal locus of control may be highly motivated to cough, deep breathe, and ambulate. This patient believes these activities are in her control and will positively affect her health. Individuals with an external locus of control attribute success or failure to causes external to themselves, such as luck, the difficulty of the task, or other people's behavior. A postoperative patient with an external locus of control may be poorly motivated to cough, deep breathe, and ambulate. This patient may see these activities as something the nurse requires of him, rather than being in control of his own recovery. He may not connect participation in those activities to quicker recovery and a shorter hospital stay.

In personality theory, motivation is a relatively stable characteristic that exhibits a tendency toward a desire for one of the following: (1) affiliation—having positive relationships with others, (2) achievement—being productive and reaching goals, or (3) power—influencing and controlling others. Patients with strong affiliation desires may be motivated to learn if they believe it would improve their relationships with their family or health care provider. A patient with strong achievement desires may be motivated to learn because of a sense of accomplishment. This is especially true of learning specific tasks. Coping styles can be a stable personality characteristic. Table 10-1 summarizes various coping styles individuals use in the face of illness. Dysfunctional coping occurs when coping styles do not change as one matures or adapts in new situations, such as illness.

**TABLE 10-1**

**Coping Styles When Faced with Illness**

| Coping Style | Description | Strategy |
|---|---|---|
| Confronting | Making an observation about one's behavior | Not useful in dealing with the illness itself; useful in dealing with another's positive or negative response to illness |
| Distancing | Separating oneself from the problem | Patients convince themselves that their problem is unique, and they believe that they cannot learn from someone else's experience |
| Self-control | Taking an active interest in something by taking control | Practicing self-care and participating in decision making; patient must learn the difference between what can be controlled and what cannot |
| Seeking social support | Through supportive interaction with friends, family, church groups | Perception of having support is more important than the actual support received |
| Accepting responsibility | Buying into the treatment plan | Useful when encouraging life-style changes; harmful when used for blaming |
| Escape or avoidance | Failing to deal with or address the problem | May be useful as short-term strategy but harmful in the long run |
| Problem solving | Critical thinking skills | One of the more useful strategies; most educational programs teach solutions—not the problem-solving process |
| Positive reappraisal | Reinterpreting or reframing a negative to a positive | Instead of dwelling on what one cannot do, emphasize what one is successful at doing; looking at the illness as a challenge |
| Activity or distraction | Physical activity, such as walking, jogging, swimming, or other activity, such as painting or reading; humor, laughter, and relaxation are other forms | The idea that doing something is better than doing nothing; especially helpful in dealing with pain, depression, and changing habits such as eating or smoking; keeps the mind occupied |
| Self-talk | Variation of positive thinking | Can be either positive or negative; goal is to change negative self-talk to positive self-talk |
| Prayer | Private conversations with a higher power; meditation | Useful for segments of the population who find it a source of inner strength |
| Reframing | Changing the meaning of an experience | Useful for focusing on a strength rather than a weakness |
| Cognitive optimizing | Comparing oneself favorably with others | Useful in helping to see that one is better off than others with the same condition |

Modified from Lorig K: *Patient education: a practical approach,* ed 2, Thousand Oaks, Calif, 1992, Sage; Perry CK, Rosenfeld AG: Learning through connections with others—women's cardiac symptoms, *Patient Education and Counseling* 57(1):143-146, 2005; Shea K: Reframing: a fresh outlook helps patients envision positive outcomes, *Nursing Spectrum* 13(22):21-23, 2004.

Expectancy theory maintains that a person's motivation is based on an expectation of success or failure. A patient who expects to go home the morning after a laparoscopic cholecystectomy is more likely to do so than a patient who expects to stay in the hospital 2 or 3 days. Learners try to live up to the expectations set by themselves and by others. Learned helplessness is the idea that one is doomed to failure, no matter what. Depression is a common result. Learned helplessness may be attributed to three causes. The first separates helplessness caused by the patient and helplessness caused by other factors. A smoker may believe he has a personality flaw—lack of willpower—that will defeat his efforts to quit smoking. He believes his inability to quit smoking is caused by his own personal failure. He may blame his inability to quit smoking, however, on peer pressure. His inability to quit is caused by factors out of his control or external to himself. Notice how similar these concepts are to locus of control discussed earlier. The second cause of learned helplessness differentiates between global and specific causes. Global helplessness means that a patient lacks confidence in his or her ability to do a wide range of things—from losing weight, to graduating from school, to quitting smoking. Specific helplessness focuses on one activity. A patient may be certain he can quit smoking but does not believe he can graduate from school. The third cause of learned helplessness distinguishes between what occurs occasionally and what occurs consistently, or a trait-state distinction. A trait is a stable personality characteristic. A state is temporary or transitory. Occasional or transient helplessness accounts for a patient's inability to lose weight during holidays, even though he or she may be able to at other times during the year.

Self-efficacy is a concept closely related to learned helplessness and locus of control. Perceived self-efficacy is a person's judgment of his or her capabilities to organize and follow through a course of action required to achieve a designated level of performance. Perceived self-efficacy has to do with the person's belief that he or she is capable of accomplishing the goal rather than with his or her actual skill (efficacy expectancy), and that the goal will result in beneficial changes (outcome expectancy).[4] Self-efficacy has been positively related to activities such as coughing, deep breathing, and ambulating to prevent postoperative complications and dietary modification and is a useful framework to view the effects of preoperative teaching on behavior change.

***Stages of Psychosocial Adaptation to Illness.*** Stages in emotional adjustment occur in all patients; however, the duration of each stage varies depending on the patient, the support system, and coping patterns. Transitions between stages are usually gradual and not clearly defined. The perioperative nurse can assess the correct stage by listening to the patient. Lee describes these four stages as (1) impact, (2) regression, (3) acknowledgment, and (4) reconstruction. Figure 10-1 compares Lee's four stages with Maslow's hierarchy of needs.

*Impact* corresponds with the foundation of Maslow's pyramid—physiologic and safety needs. Patients experience fear, anxiety, and loss of control. They may feel threatened. This may be a patient's first encounter with mortality. Patients may be very discouraged and become present-oriented, seeing only the here and now. They focus all their energy inward because they perceive survival as their primary goal.

*Regression* corresponds to Maslow's third level—social needs. Regression occurs when patients are forced to deal with their present reality and attempt to return to a time when they felt more emotionally comfortable. After regressing for a short time, they usually are able to handle the reality of their disease process and mourn the loss of body image or self-esteem. In this stage, the sense of belonging is threatened. Patients may lash out in anger at the family or staff. If they succeed in driving individuals away, their fears of not being able to give or receive love will be reinforced. Accept the patient, but do not support the behavior. To help the patient through this stage, use realistic terms and specific time frames: "It will be 3 or 4 days before your intestines start to work again." They may joke about their illness or reveal unrealistic plans on discharge: "I plan to play golf with my buddies on Wednesday." Respond in realistic terms, but try not to overwhelm them. Having been provided with a measure of psychologic safety, patients move on to the next stage.

Many perioperative nurses do not recognize teaching as such during the impact and regression stages. Although little response is produced, therapeutic instruction helps the patient when moving into subsequent stages. At this point, families may benefit from teaching more than the patient does because families may be ahead of patients in terms of adjusting to the crisis. They will be able to reinforce information when the patient is ready.

*Acknowledgment* parallels Maslow's fourth level—esteem needs. Patients have little self-confidence and self-respect and may express loss and fear of abandonment: "I'm such a burden to my family like this." As unlikely as it seems, this is the time when effective teaching, in the traditional sense, may begin. Patients realize that they have survived their crisis and are reviewing the events in an attempt to prevent them from recurring. Patients give subtle signs that they have accepted changes in body image: "I thought the colostomy would be bigger." This indicates the patient has actually looked at it. They also begin to make provisions for the future: "Can I get this incision wet? I'd like to take a shower." Soon they will perceive their own need for information, leading them to the last stage.

*Reconstruction* parallels Maslow's fifth level—self-actualization. This is the most creative and positive stage because patients perceive hope for the future. Even though many patients cannot resume their lives exactly where they left off, they experience a renewed sense of self-worth. Patients start to plan new approaches for old behaviors. They are concerned about the future; instruction should be positive.

## Discharge Planning

Although discharge planning is often considered a postoperative activity, assessment of the patient's needs on discharge should begin in the preoperative phase. A preliminary assessment of the patient's and family's understanding of the knowledge and skills required for convalescence often make educational needs apparent. Discharge planning must be more than just preparing the patient to leave the health care setting. Discharge planning is preparing for moving the patient from one level of care to another within or outside the current health care agency. Perioperative nurses are becoming more responsible for discharge planning because of the tremendous increase in same-day surgical procedures. The most significant contribution the perioperative nurse can make is to begin dis-

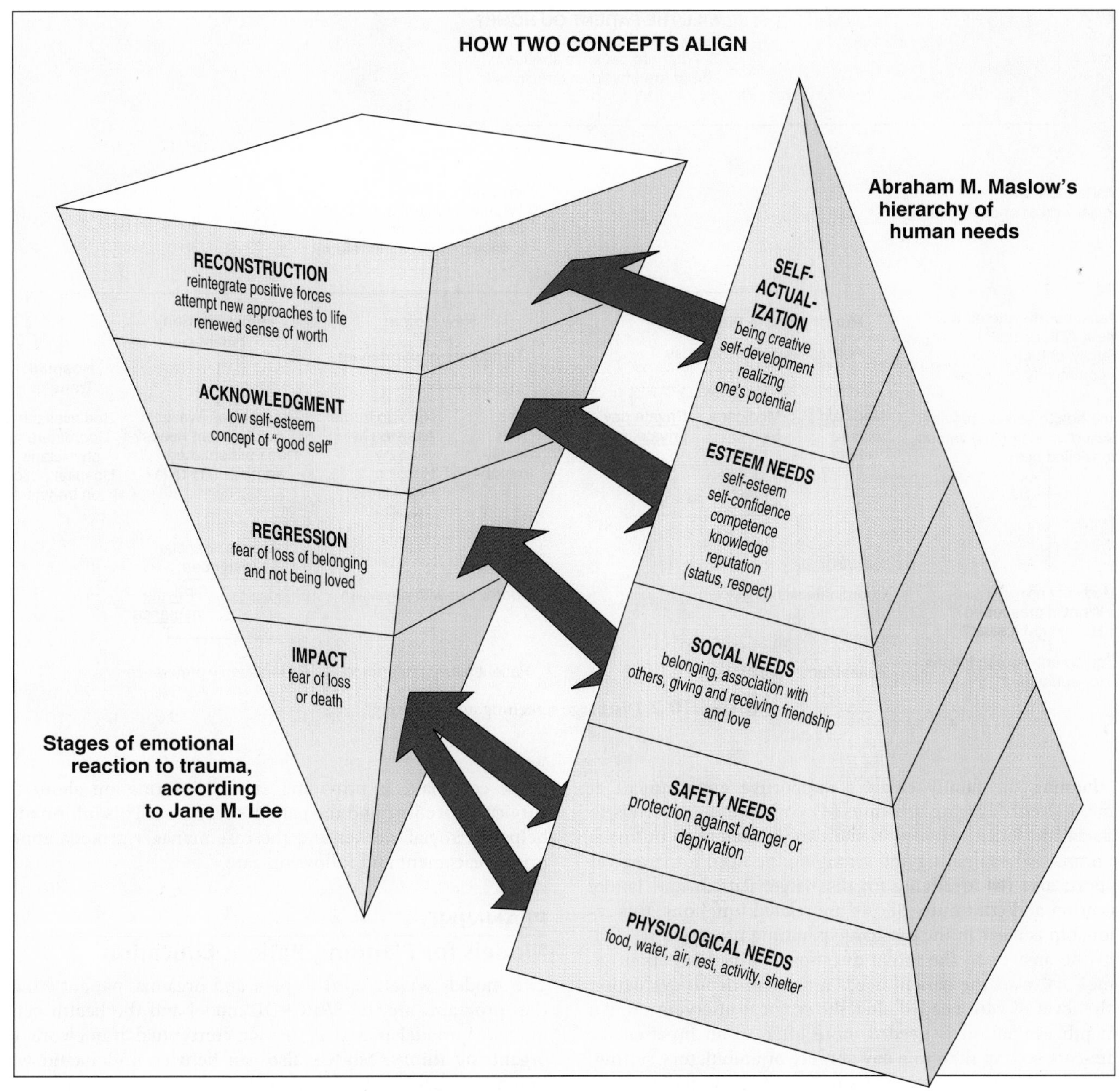


**FIGURE 10-1** How two concepts align.

charge planning early in the treatment process, preferably before or on admission. The perioperative nurse may be the individual who determines if the patient meets the criteria for discharge and communicates and documents discharge plans. The development of nursing knowledge also requires that the perioperative nurse evaluate the effectiveness of various interventions in achieving particular outcomes.[11]

The perioperative nurse is in a unique position to begin the discharge planning process by asking a single question: "Will this patient go home?" Considering the patient's physical and mental abilities previously discussed, the patient's preferences and rights, and the physician's recommendations, can the patient function well enough after surgery to accomplish activities of daily living in the environment from which he or she came? If the answer is "yes," a brief appraisal can determine if existing support systems are adequate (Figure 10-2). Does the family have enough resources to assist the patient at whatever level of care he or she would need on discharge? Required resources may range from providing taxi services to and from the physician's office for follow-up visits to changing dressings, cooking meals, and shopping for groceries. Does the family need unskilled assistance, such as transportation or housekeeping? What community resources, such as church ministries, are available to the patient and family? Does the patient need skilled care, such as complicated wound management provided by a registered nurse? Can the patient get the prescribed medications? Does the patient need home health equipment, such as a bedside commode or wheelchair? Discharge activities include (1) arranging for maintenance or follow-up care with the physician or nurse practitioner;

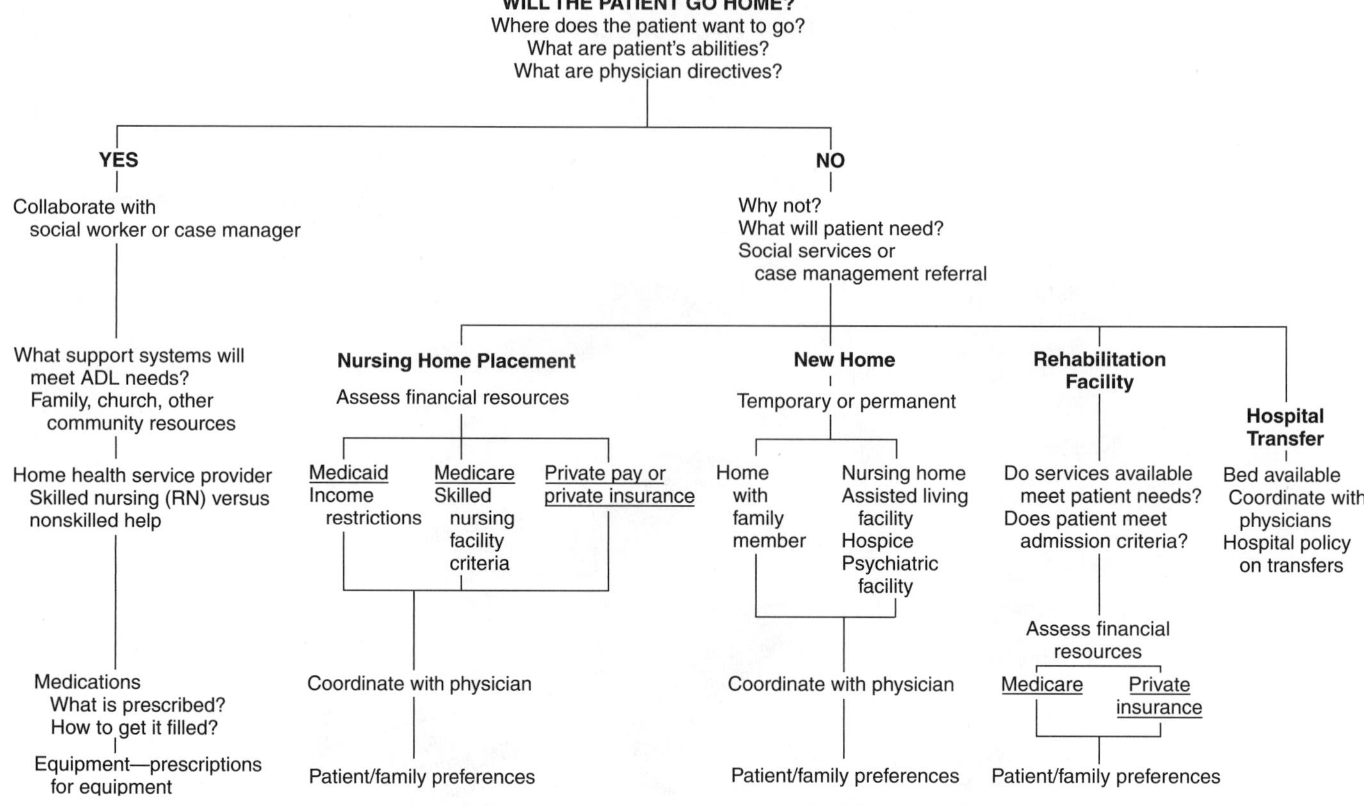


**FIGURE 10-2** Discharge screening and planning.

(2) helping the family create a supportive environment at home; (3) encouraging self-care; (4) coordinating referrals to financial or social services, home care agencies, or outreach programs; (5) evaluating and arranging the need for caregiver support; and (6) arranging for discharge. Patient and family education and continuity of care are related functions; this relationship is clear in the discharge planning process.

If the answer to the initial question, "Will this patient go home?" is "no," the patient needs a more in-depth evaluation of the level of care needed after the surgical intervention. An in-depth evaluation is needed more often in an inpatient or acute-care setting than in a day-surgery or ambulatory setting. When the perioperative nurse suspects that the patient may not be able to return to his or her presurgical environment, early referral is essential. The perioperative nurse's partners in discharge planning are the case manager and social worker; early referral can shorten the length of stay and prevent readmissions. Perioperative nurses often have little information about community resources, Medicare and Medicaid regulations, extended-care facilities, and subacute-care units. They may find themselves overwhelmed by the maze of rules and regulations faced when discharge planning. Social workers are familiar with community resources and regulations but know little about the patient's educational needs, physical capabilities, nursing requirements, or home care needs. The case manager coordinates the activities of all hospital services, including social services, and provides clinical expertise about patient physical and psychologic needs during an acute-care episode. The second most important contribution the perioperative nurse can make is providing clinical information about the surgical procedure and the patient's response. This information helps the social worker and the case manager arrange appropriate placement and follow-up care.

## PLANNING

### Models for Planning Patient Education

Two models widely used to plan and organize patient education programs are the PRECEDE model and the health belief model. A model is a structure or conceptual framework for organizing things. Models also can help us understand why individuals behave the way they do and what works when they are changing behaviors. The *PRECEDE model* (Figure 10-3) is a means of looking at predisposing, enabling, and reinforcing factors when planning an educational program.

*Predisposing factors* can be beliefs or benefits. The perioperative nurse's goal is to determine what the predisposing factors are and in which category they fall. Individuals generally have rational reasons for doing what they do. If a patient believes spinal anesthesia always causes headaches, it is not surprising when the patient chooses general anesthesia instead. To change beliefs, the nurse must first find out what they are. An excellent way to do this is simply to ask, "What do you think will happen if . . ." (then adding the desired behavior)?" When you know the belief, the plan can include information to change it: "Headaches after a spinal happen only rarely." Be prepared for times when you cannot change a belief, particularly if it is a dearly held spiritual, cultural, or religious belief.

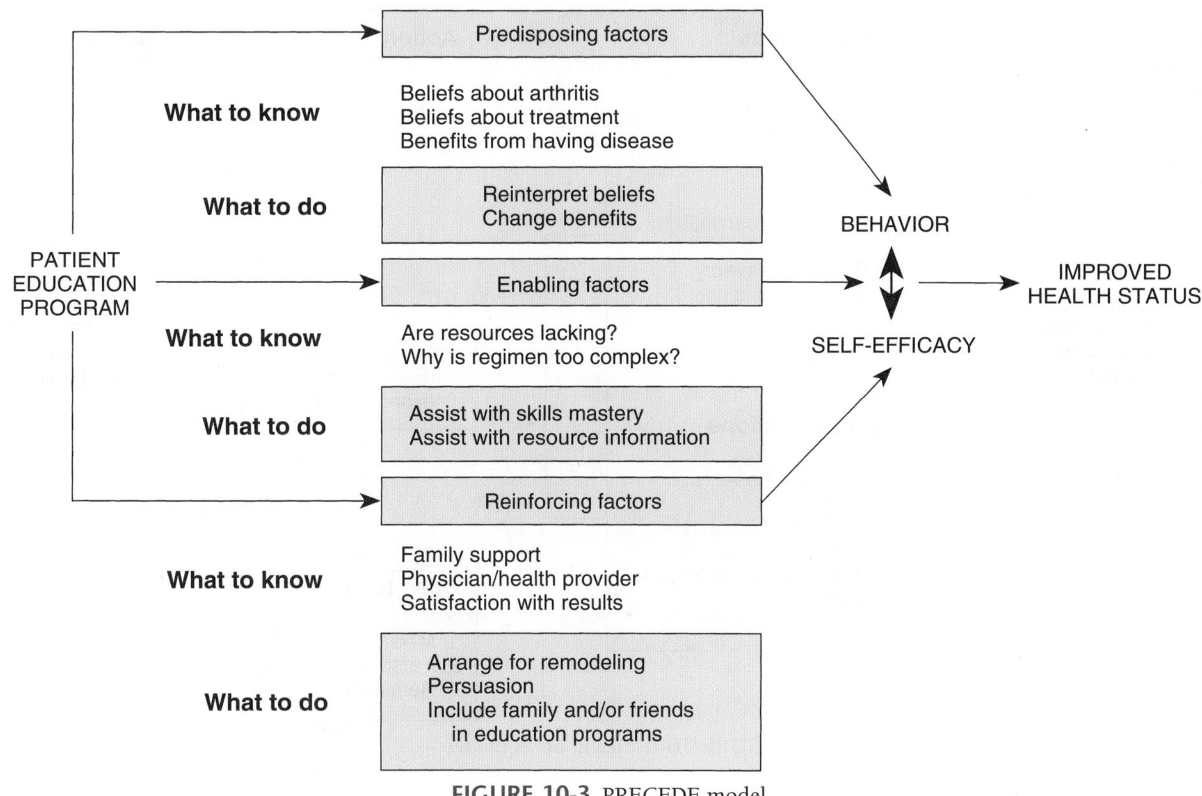


**FIGURE 10-3** PRECEDE model.

A good example is refusal of blood products. In these cases, helping an individual broaden an interpretation of the belief may accomplish behavior change and improve self-efficacy. Some religious beliefs allow for use of autologus blood transfusions but not donor transfusions. The second category of predisposing factors is benefits—the secondary gain from having this illness: Is this illness being used to get out of work or get attention from family and friends? Behavior change is unlikely to occur until the benefits for maintaining the behavior cease. For example, the number of smokers has decreased as smoking has become less socially acceptable.

*Enabling factors* help individuals do what they should do and want to do but are unable to do. Two ways to enable individuals are by finding resources and by mastering skills. Putting resources where the person is can enable learning; skills mastery enables problem solving rather than simply fixing the situation at hand. Being too helpful can encourage dependence.

*Reinforcing factors* support the individual's decision to change. Perioperative nurses can reinforce change by modeling, persuasion, and including families and friends and other health care providers in educational efforts. (More examples of reinforcement are discussed in "Facilitating Learning" later in this chapter.) One final reinforcing factor is that, if behavior changes, individuals feel better. If a person consents to a cholecystectomy, the acute attacks of cholecystitis should stop.

The *health belief model* is one of the oldest and best-known educational models (Figure 10-4). It is based on the concept that individuals act according to perceived threats or expectations. Perceived threat has two components: perceived susceptibility and perceived severity. Although most health care providers believe that bloodborne pathogens may transmit a severe disease (high perceived severity), many demonstrate low perceived susceptibility by failing to wear gloves when they should. To change behaviors, individuals must have expectations that the new behavior would reduce their susceptibility or the severity of the condition, that the benefits to changing are greater than the barriers, and that the behavior change can be accomplished. Individuals engage in a subconscious or conscious cost-to-benefit analysis, such as: "If I have my uterus removed, it will hurt for several days and I will miss several weeks of work. On the other hand, if I have my uterus removed, I will stop bleeding so much. I will feel better and do a better job at work." Difficulty arises when the barriers to behavior change are obvious and the benefits are unpredictable. A good example is exercising and eating properly now to avoid vascular disease later in life.

## Nursing Diagnosis

The nursing plan of care provides a structured framework through which the nurse delivers nursing care. The perioperative nurse diagnoses the patient's educational needs, identifies desired outcomes, and plans nursing interventions. Only one of the nursing diagnoses that follows deals directly with an educational need. The other nursing diagnoses indirectly reflect the need for patient teaching. Many nursing diagnoses

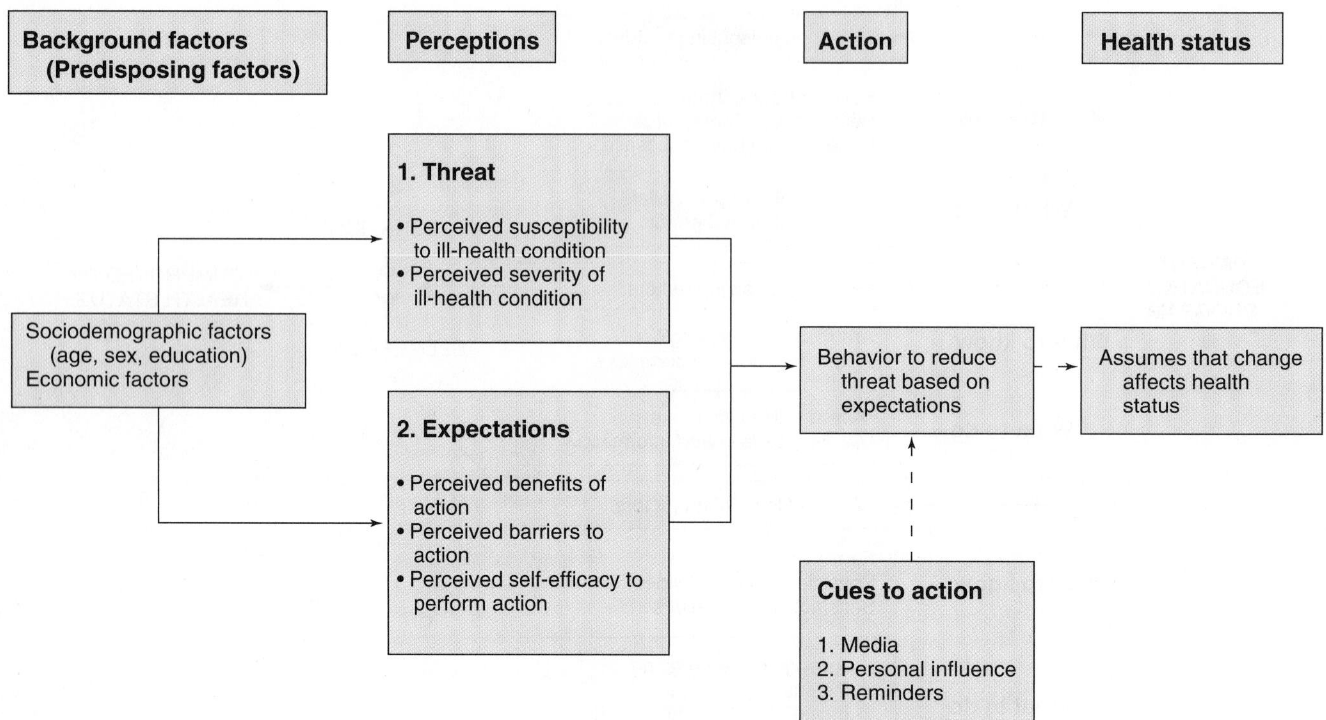


**FIGURE 10-4** Health belief model.

used by perioperative nurses have an inherent educational component. The perioperative nurse cannot isolate planning interventions to meet educational needs from the continuous reassessment and planning that occurs when providing other patient care.

Nursing diagnoses related to the educational needs of the perioperative patient may include the following:

- Decisional Conflict Regarding the treatment options
- Anxiety
- Deficient Knowledge regarding planned surgical intervention

*Decisional conflicts* arise when the decision maker must consider one or more options. A classic example is the surgical treatment options for breast cancer with a tumor mass less than 2 cm in size and no skin involvement. Different options afford the patient an excellent 10-year survival rate. The options have advantages and disadvantages. The decision maker may take or avoid opportunities to seek further information. Decisional conflict and the accompanying emotional distress occur when one of three conditions is present. First, a conflict can arise when the patient has a treatment preference, such as nutritional or faith healing, but was not offered this option or was discouraged from using it. Second, a conflict can arise when neither treatment option seems to have any advantages from the patient's perspective, and yet, the patient must choose one. Third, conflict can occur when the patient prefers one of the offered treatment options, but a significant person, such as the surgeon, recommends an alternative. Families also can contribute to the conflict by adding their views regarding what the patient should do. A patient's decision-making ability may be so impaired by anxiety, fear, and interpersonal conflict that the patient is unable to make the choice, and definitive treatment is significantly delayed.

*Anxiety* is present in most surgical patients to a certain degree. Anxiety is the uneasiness and apprehension a patient feels without being able to identify the precise cause. Anxiety interferes with the patient's ability to concentrate, recall information, and process new information. In the preoperative patient, anxiety may be attributed to threats to the patient's self-concept, socioeconomic status, role functioning, patterns of interacting, or fear of the diagnosis or of dying. The surgical patient may be anxious about the way the surgical intervention would alter essential values and life goals. Clues that the patient is experiencing high levels of anxiety are increased heart and respiratory rates, elevated blood pressure, voice and hand tremors, insomnia, and poor eye contact. The patient may be able to say that he or she is "uptight" or "nervous" or may express concern about changes in his or her life.

*Deficient knowledge* occurs when the patient lacks specific information. Signs of deficient knowledge include inappropriate or exaggerated behaviors, such as hysteria, overt hostility, agitation, apathy, inaccurate follow-through of instruction, inadequate return demonstration, a request for more information, or verbalization of the problem. When the knowledge deficiency relates directly to the surgical procedure, the surgeon is responsible for informing patients of the nature, risks, and benefits of the procedure. The perioperative nurse's role is to enhance and reinforce this information. To assist patients in obtaining and demonstrating essential knowledge, the perioperative nurse undertakes many of the activities already described in this chapter, such as assessing the patient's current status, identifying any barriers to communication, noting readiness to learn, determining personally effective coping mechanisms and reinforcing those, and eliciting and clarifying misperceptions. Education focuses on patient/family-specific requirements and includes a description of the sequence of perioperative events, wound and pain management, nutritional requirements to promote convalescence, activity restrictions, appropriate and effective methods for managing postoperative nausea and vomiting,[7] and follow-up appointments. The perioperative nurse also may be responsible for ensuring that an informed consent has been obtained and documented in the health record according to institutional policy.

## Outcome Identification

The Association of periOperative Registered Nurses (AORN) in *Perioperative Patient Outcomes* addresses outcome identification. The Perioperative Patient Focused Model (see Chapter 1) provides the framework for the outcome statements. The domain of patient and family behavioral responses specifies the needs of the patient and family for information related to expected responses to the operative or invasive procedure, pain management (Box 10-1 presents various pain scales; the patient should be involved in selecting the preferential scale and introduced to it before surgery), the rehabilitation process, and wound care, all with respect for value systems, lifestyle, ethnicity, and culture. Outcome identification based on these patient/family needs should state explicitly the desired behavior; however, as with nursing diagnoses, outcomes may not indicate explicitly that an educational need was met. The desired outcome for the standard, "The patient demonstrates knowledge of wound healing,"[3] may be stated explicitly as, "The patient communicates anticipated events during wound healing of his or her midline abdominal incision and abdominal drain site." The AORN outcome statements are each accompanied by outcome indicators that assist in developing more explicit outcome statements. Often, a behavior in the outcome may indicate that the educational need was met ("verbalizes expected sequence"; "describes plan for wound care"). Many outcomes imply that learning occurred, and the patient was motivated to change a behavior. Outcomes identified for the selected nursing diagnoses could be stated as follows:

- The patient will consent to a specific treatment option.
- The patient will verbalize feeling a lower level of anxiety.
- The patient will communicate the sequence of events in the perioperative period.

BOX 10-1

### Examples of Pain Assessment Scales

The Joint Commission on Accreditation of Healthcare Organizations began surveying compliance with its pain management standards in 2001. The pain scales presented here are for use with patients who can give a report of pain. For patients who cannot report pain, the nurse should devise an alternative, standardized pain assessment method that evaluates underlying pathology, identifies potentially painful procedures, and observes behaviors that may indicate pain.

**SIMPLE DESCRIPTIVE PAIN-INTENSITY SCALE***

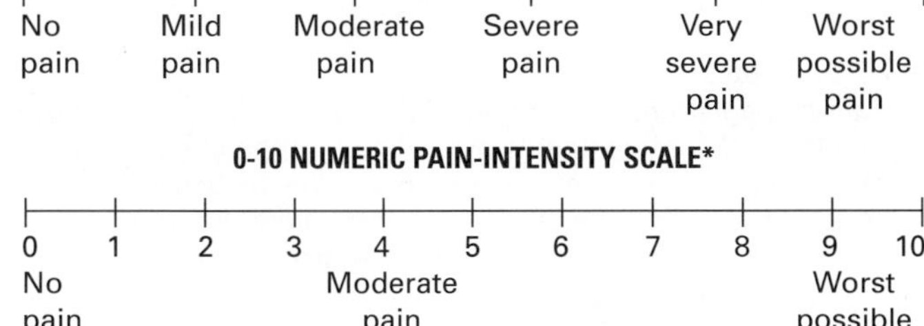


**VISUAL ANALOGUE SCALE (VAS)†**

No pain — Pain as bad as it could possibly be

Modified from Acute Pain Management Guideline Panel: *Acute pain management in adults: operative procedures: quick reference guide for clinicians,* AHCPR Publication no. 92-0019,Rockville, Md, 1992, Agency for Health Care Policy and Research; Pasero C, McCafferey M: No self-report means no pain-intensity rating, *American Journal of Nursing* 105(10):50-53, 2005.

*If used as a graphic rating scale, a 10-cm baseline value is recommended.

†A 10-cm baseline value is recommended for VAS scales.

## Plans of Care Specific to Each Diagnosis

After diagnosing the educational needs and specifying outcomes, the perioperative nurse must plan interventions to help the patient achieve those outcomes. The University of Iowa's Nursing Interventions Classification (NIC) research project defines nursing interventions, nursing activities, nurse-initiated treatments, and physician-initiated treatments as follows.[6]

***Nursing Interventions.*** Nursing interventions are any direct care treatment that a nurse performs on behalf of the client. Nursing interventions include nurse-initiated treatments and physician-initiated treatments. Nursing intervention labels are at the conceptual level and require a series of actions or activities to carry them out.

***Nursing Activities.*** Nursing activities are behaviors or actions that nurses do to assist clients to move toward a desired outcome. Nursing activities are at the concrete level of action.

***Nurse-Initiated Treatment.*** Nurse-initiated treatment refers to interventions initiated by the nurse in response to a nursing diagnosis: "an autonomous action based on scientific rationale that is executed to benefit the client in a predicted way related to the nursing diagnosis and stated goals."

***Physician-Initiated Treatment.*** Physician-initiated treatment refers to interventions that are initiated by the physician in response to a medical diagnosis and carried out by the nurse in response to a "doctor's order."

A Sample Plan of Care for a perioperative patient that incorporates the selected diagnoses and outcomes follows. Suggested interventions indicate how the nurse may directly or indirectly meet the patient's educational needs for each diagnosis. Planning to meet the educational needs of the patient is impossible to separate from planning other interventions. Each intervention is defined according to the NIC.

## SAMPLE PLAN OF CARE

### NURSING DIAGNOSIS
**Decisional Conflict** regarding the treatment options

### OUTCOME
The patient verifies consent for the planned procedure.

### INTERVENTIONS
- *Active listening.* Attending closely to and attaching significance to a patient's verbal and nonverbal messages: Note any sensory impairment (visual, auditory, speech); determine any barriers to communication that may affect ability to comprehend/understand; assess readiness to learn; determine coping mechanisms; implement measures to provide emotional/psychologic support.
- *Cognitive restructuring.* Challenging a patient to alter distorted thought patterns and view self and the world more realistically: Elicit perceptions of surgery; determine knowledge level; clarify misperceptions; provide frequent explanations of the sequence of care.
- *Decision-making support.* Providing information and support for a patient who is making a decision regarding health care: Provide and explain the Patient Self-Determination Act; provide information based on age and identified needs; maintain patient confidentiality.
- *Family involvement.* Facilitating family participation in the emotional and physical care of the patient: Include family members in preoperative teaching and discharge planning; provide status report to family during surgery or other invasive procedure; identify capacity for home care.
- *Referral.* Arrangement for services by another care provider or agency: Obtain consultations from other health care providers; ensure continuity of care.
- *Self-esteem enhancement.* Assisting a patient to increase his or her judgment of self-worth: Encourage patient to identify own values and wishes regarding care.
- *Teaching: sequence of events to expect before, during (awake patient), and after surgery.* Assisting the patient to understand information related to a specific process: Explain expected sequence of events, routines, and protocols related to perioperative patient care.

### NURSING DIAGNOSIS
**Anxiety**

### OUTCOME
The patient will verbalize feeling a lower level of anxiety.

### INTERVENTIONS
- *Admission care.* Facilitating entry of a patient into a health care facility: Determine knowledge of patient/family regarding surgical or invasive procedure.
- *Anxiety reduction.* Minimizing apprehension, dread, foreboding, or uneasiness related to the unidentified source of anticipated danger: Use a calm, reassuring approach; seek to understand the patient's perception of a stressful situation; listen attentively.
- *Learning-readiness enhancement.* Improving the ability and willingness to receive information: Determine the patient's decision-making ability; control external stimuli that interfere with enhancement of a learning environment; assist patient to articulate realistic description of information needed/desired.
- *Surgical preparation.* Providing care to a patient immediately before surgery and verifying required procedures, tests, and documentation in the clinical record: Explain all procedures, including sensations likely to be experienced; provide factual information; stay with the patient to reduce anxiety and fear.
- *Teaching: preoperative.* Assisting the patient to understand and mentally prepare for surgery and the postoperative recovery period: Provide information regarding time of surgery; verify food and fluid restrictions; clearly state expectations for patient/family involvement; encourage verbalization of feelings, perceptions, and fears; clarify misperceptions; elicit understanding of expectations.
- *Touch.* Providing comfort and communication through purposeful tactile contact: Administer a back rub/neck rub (as appropriate); support the patient in using personally effective relaxation techniques; hold the patient's hand; offer a warm blanket or pillow.

### NURSING DIAGNOSIS
**Deficient Knowledge** with regard to planned surgical intervention

### OUTCOME
The patient will communicate the sequence of events in the perioperative period.

### INTERVENTIONS
- *Learning facilitation.* Promoting the ability to process and comprehend information.
- *Teaching: preoperative.* Assisting a patient to understand and mentally prepare for surgery and postoperative recovery period: Determine knowledge level of patient/family; explain anticipated sequence of events; provide information on preoperative verification process and marking of the surgical site.
- *Teaching: disease process.* Assisting the patient to understand information related to a specific process: Allow the patient to express any concerns, questions; communicate these to appropriate members of the health care team.

### NURSING DIAGNOSIS
**Acute Pain**

### OUTCOME
The patient will communicate/demonstrate knowledge of pain management and identify an acceptable level of pain on a pain-intensity scale.

### INTERVENTIONS
- *Pain management.* Alleviation of pain or a reduction in pain to a level of comfort that is acceptable to the patient: Determine cultural components of pain; describe the use of a pain scale; provide pain management information; describe institution's pain management guideline; assist patient into position of comfort.
- *Patient-controlled analgesia (PCA).* Facilitating patient control of analgesic administration and regulation: Determine whether intravenous (this method of PCA is the most common for postoperative pain management), epidural, and oral PCA[15] is planned; provide instructions to the patient regarding method for PCA.
- *Touch.* Providing comfort and communication through purposeful tactile contact: Determine previously used methods to cope with pain and facilitate these (as appropriate); administer a back rub/neck rub (as appropriate).
- *Simple relaxation therapy.* Use of techniques to encourage and elicit relaxation for the purpose of decreasing undesirable signs and symptoms, such as pain, muscle tension, or anxiety: Determine methods the patient prefers (music, guided imagery, relaxation exercises); facilitate individually preferred method.

## IMPLEMENTATION

### Nursing Activities: Case Studies

Nursing interventions are conceptual labels that require activities to carry them out. Nursing activities are how nurses help patients reach a specified outcome. They are concrete behaviors. Nursing activities can be nurse-initiated or physician-initiated. This section is an analysis of the implementation of nursing activities for selected nursing interventions in the planning section. In the case studies that follow, there may not be a separate nursing intervention that deals with meeting education needs. There are nursing activities within every intervention, however, that deal directly or indirectly with meeting educational needs. These nursing activities involve more than merely instructing or informing the patient. Teaching is an interpersonal interaction that includes assessing readiness and current knowledge; facilitating learning; establishing rapport, trust, and mutual respect; reducing anxiety; and evaluating learning and the activities of instruction. The perioperative nurse adjusts nursing activities to meet the educational needs of the individual patient in the following case studies. Many nursing activities specific to one diagnosis overlap nursing activities specific to another diagnosis.

***Decisional Conflict.*** Mrs. Adams, a 44-year-old bookkeeper, had a left breast biopsy 1 week ago. The pathologic diagnosis is invasive intraductal carcinoma. The surgeon discussed treatment options with Mr. and Mrs. Adams. Mrs. Adams has been scheduled for a quadrantectomy and left axillary lymphadenectomy at a freestanding ambulatory surgery center. The perioperative nurse visits Mr. and Mrs. Adams in the preoperative admitting area. As soon as Mr. Adams leaves the room, Mrs. Adams confides to the nurse that she is not all that sure about having this procedure. She then berates herself for being "wishy-washy" about making a decision. She confesses that she and her mother have had considerable conflict over her original decision to have lumpectomy and radiation rather than mastectomy. Mrs. Adams asks the nurse if she has heard anything about radiation causing cancer rather than curing it.

NURSING DIAGNOSIS. Decisional conflict regarding the treatment options.

OUTCOME. The patient will consent to a specific treatment option.

INTERVENTION. ***Decision-making support:*** Providing information and support for a patient who is making a decision regarding health care.

NURSING ACTIVITIES

*Patient:* "I'm really not sure I want this radiation stuff."

*Nurse:* "Having radiation scares you?"

*Patient:* "Yes, my mother says radiation can cause cancer rather than cure it."

*Nurse:* "Are you fearful of getting cancer somewhere else if you choose radiation over mastectomy?"

*Patient:* "Yes. I meant to ask my doctor about that, but I was too upset at the time. Have you ever heard of that?"

*Nurse:* "The research done on this treatment option looks very good when the cancer is found as early as yours. This type of radiation has not been shown to cause cancer in other places. How about my asking your surgeon to step in here for a few minutes to help you get comfortable with your decision?"

*Patient:* "That would be great. Would you get my husband in here, too?

Begin decision-making support by establishing a therapeutic communication with Mrs. Adams on first contact. Identify discrepancies in the patient's view of her options and the physician's. Provide the patient with the information she requests. To obtain consent for the procedure and facilitate collaborative decision-making, the nurse serves as a liaison between the patient, her husband, and her physician.

INTERVENTION. ***Cognitive restructuring:*** Challenging a patient to alter distorted thought patterns and view self and the world more realistically.

NURSING ACTIVITIES

*Patient:* "I hate being so wish-washy. I'll never be able to make such an awful decision."

*Nurse:* "Hey, go easy on yourself. Some uncertainty is normal when dealing with a difficult illness. Seems to me that you've done a great job of deciding what's in your best interest despite some hefty opposition from family members."

Help the patient accept that self-statements elicit emotional arousal, and that comments about the inability to make this decision may be irrational self-statements. Help the patient recognize that some of her beliefs are inaccurate. Overgeneralization, polarized thinking, and magnification of the problem can lead to dysfunctional thinking.

*Nurse:* "What evidence supports your mother's belief that radiation to the breast will cause you to have cancer somewhere else?"

*Patient:* "Well, now that you mention it, none that I know of. I guess I'm just scared and angry about the whole thing. I wish I had my mother's support right now. "

Replace faulty interpretations with accurate information and reality-based interpretations of the situation. Help the patient label the uncomfortable emotions and identify perceived stressors (e.g., interactions with family, the diagnosis).

*Nurse:* "You have your husband's full support. That must feel good."

INTERVENTION. ***Family involvement:*** Facilitating family participation in the emotional and physical care of the patient.

NURSING ACTIVITIES. Identify which family members would be capable and willing to participate in Mrs. Adams' care. Mrs. Adams has expressed a preference for her husband's involvement. The patient's preferences give the nurse a good starting point for assessing the family's learning needs regarding Mrs. Adams' care, the strengths and weaknesses in the family's coping skills, and situational stressors on the family that would affect Mrs. Adams' care.

***Anxiety.*** Mr. Caldwell is a 66-year-old retired football coach scheduled for a left inguinal herniorrhaphy through the ambulatory surgery department of a small community hospital. Ambulatory surgery patients are admitted directly to the holding area for admission procedures. Mr. Caldwell is to have local anesthesia and intravenous sedation monitored by a certified registered nurse anesthetist (CRNA). His wife and adult son accompany him. When the perioperative nurse enters the holding area, Mr. Caldwell is pacing beside the stretcher and has refused to change into a hospital gown.

NURSING DIAGNOSIS. Anxiety related to the surgical intervention.

OUTCOME. The patient will verbalize feeling a lower level of anxiety.

INTERVENTION. *Admission care:* Facilitating entry of a patient into a health care facility.

NURSING ACTIVITIES. Begin by introducing yourself and briefly describing the role you will play in Mr. Caldwell's procedure. Briefly orient the patient and family to the immediate environment and the expectation of care.

*Nurse:* "Hello, Mr. Caldwell. I'm Claire O'Connell. I'm an RN. I'll be in charge of your nursing care while you are in surgery today. This is the preoperative holding area where we help you get ready for surgery. You're here to get that hernia on the left fixed—is that correct? Here is the nurse call button. Just press it if you need us for any reason. The family waiting room is just outside those double doors and on your right."

Pull the drapes around the bed to provide privacy for the patient and family. In the initial interview, document the admission history, nursing assessment (physical examination, psychosocial history, educational needs), and informed consent as required by institutional policy. Ensure that the patient is properly identified. At this point, the nurse has enough information to create a formal plan of care, including nursing diagnosis, outcomes, and interventions. Carry out the admitting physician's orders. Begin planning for Mr. Caldwell's needs on discharge.

INTERVENTION. *Anxiety reduction:* Minimizing apprehension, dread, foreboding, or uneasiness related to the unidentified source of anticipated danger.

NURSING ACTIVITIES. Establish the patient and nurse relationship through active listening while providing admission care. Create an atmosphere of trust by displaying respect. Allow Mr. Caldwell to remain in his street clothes as long as possible. He may feel safer, less vulnerable, and more in control in his own clothes. Stay with the patient as long as possible. Allow time for addressing his concerns. Begin by making an observation about his behavior and stating your expectations for his behavior. Seek to understand Mr. Caldwell's perspective of this stressful situation.

*Nurse:* "You seem awfully jittery. I'd like to help you feel calmer. Is there anything I can do to help?"

*Patient:* "Yeah. They brought me in here and told me to undress and put this flimsy little gown on. What am I supposed to do? Flash the whole room? I just don't see any need in undressing until it's time to go back to the room."

Explain all procedures, including the sensations likely to be experienced during the procedure.

*Nurse:* "You will feel a burning sensation while the numbing medicine is being injected. After that, you may feel pressure and pulling. You should not feel anything sharp. If you do, just tell us, and the surgeon will put in more numbing medicine."

Reinforce his behavior when his anxiety level decreases.

*Nurse:* "You seem calmer. You are sitting down instead of pacing."

Judicious use of humor also can lower anxiety levels.

*Nurse:* "I'm here to take you to the room. That means it's about 5 minutes to kickoff."

INTERVENTION. *Simple relaxation therapy:* Use of techniques to encourage and elicit relaxation for the purpose of decreasing undesirable signs and symptoms, such as pain, muscle tension, or anxiety.

NURSING ACTIVITIES. Describe the reason for and benefits of relaxation therapy. Determine if Mr. Caldwell has any previous experiences with relaxation therapy. Consider his willingness and ability to participate. Create a quiet, soothing atmosphere by dimming lights and closing the door. Use a slow, rhythmic tone of voice. Use one of the relaxation exercises in Box 10-2, or consider using a guided imagery tape to assist Mr. Caldwell in coping and relaxing.[22]

INTERVENTION. *Surgical preparation:* Providing care to a patient immediately before surgery and verification of required procedures and tests and documentation in the clinical record.

NURSING ACTIVITIES. Verify Mr. Caldwell's identity orally and by checking his armband. Reinforce preoperative teaching information. Complete preoperative documentation as required by the institution, such as checklists, consent forms, and nursing assessment. Administer, explain, and document the use of preoperative medications as appropriate. Ensure that the results of required preoperative laboratory work and electrocardiogram and history and physical examination are on the chart. Start intravenous therapy, explaining the procedure, tubing, and equipment as needed. List allergies on the front of the chart. Note special care needs, such as sight or hearing impairments. Support the family's needs with reassurance and information. Use supportive touch as appropriate. Solicit family assistance in keeping Mr. Caldwell's personal valuables. Explain any preoperative medications given. Apply antiembolism stockings as needed. Assist the patient to the transport vehicle.

INTERVENTION. *Teaching: preoperative:* Assisting the patient to understand and mentally prepare for surgery and the postoperative recovery period.

NURSING ACTIVITIES. Involve Mr. Caldwell and his family in this intervention. Inform them of the scheduled time of surgery, keeping them updated if delays occur. Ensure that they know the approximate length of the procedure and stay in the postanesthesia care unit (PACU). Familiarize the family with the locations of the waiting room and cafeteria. Discuss postoperative routines (medication, surgical dressings, ambulation, diet, activity). Discuss how Mr. Caldwell can assist in his own recovery (early ambulation, techniques for incision splinting and getting out of bed, coughing and deep breathing, limits on activity). Determine Mr. Caldwell's expectations of surgery, and correct unrealistic expectations. Discuss possible pain control measures. Provide information on what Mr. Caldwell will hear, see, taste, and feel during the procedure and immediately after.

***Deficient Knowledge.*** Mrs. Rhines is a 77-year-old retired English literature professor. She is a widow and has no children. Mrs. Campbell, a friend who lives across the street, accompanies her. Mrs. Rhines still enjoys an occasional round of golf. She experienced a transient ischemic attack (TIA) that caused her to faint in her kitchen last week. She was admitted through the ambulatory surgery department for carotid arteriograms this morning. She is scheduled for a right carotid

BOX 10-2

**Relaxation Exercises**

Exercises such as the ones listed here are part of nonbiologic therapies that treat patients in a holistic fashion. Such therapies are often referred to as *mind-body therapies.*

**EXAMPLE 1: DEEP BREATHE/TENSE, EXHALE/RELAX, YAWN FOR QUICK RELAXATION**

1. Clench your fists; breathe in deeply and hold it a moment.
2. Breathe out slowly and go limp as a rag doll.
3. Start yawning.

*Additional points:* Yawning becomes spontaneous. It is also contagious, and so others may begin yawning and relaxing too.

**EXAMPLE 2: SLOW RHYTHMIC BREATHING FOR RELAXATION**

1. Breathe in slowly and deeply.
2. As you breathe out slowly, feel yourself beginning to relax; feel the tension leaving your body.
3. Now breathe in and out slowly and regularly, at whatever rate is comfortable for you. You may wish to try abdominal breathing. If you do not know how to do abdominal breathing, ask your nurse for help.
4. To help you focus on your breathing and breathing slowly and rhythmically: Breathe in as you say silently to yourself, "in, two, three." Breathe out as you say silently to yourself, "out, two, three," or each time you breathe out, say silently to yourself a word such as "peace" or "relax."
5. You may imagine that you are doing this in a place you have found very calming and relaxing for you, such as lying in the sun at the beach.
6. Do steps 1 through 4 only once or repeat steps 3 and 4 for up to 20 minutes.
7. End with a slow, deep breath. As you breathe out, say to yourself, "I feel alert and relaxed."

*Additional points:* If you intend to do this for more than a few seconds, try to get in a comfortable position in a quiet environment; you may close your eyes or focus on an object. This technique has the advantage of being very adaptable in that it may be used for only a few seconds or for up to 20 minutes.

**EXAMPLE 3: PEACEFUL PAST**

Something may have happened to you a while ago that brought you peace and comfort. You may be able to draw on that past experience to bring you peace and comfort now. Think about these questions:

1. Can you remember any situation or place, even when you were a child, when you felt calm, peaceful, secure, hopeful, comfortable?
2. Have you ever daydreamed about something peaceful? What were you thinking of?
3. Do you get a dreamy feeling when you listen to music? Do you have any favorite music?
4. Do you have any favorite poetry that you find uplifting or reassuring?
5. Have you ever been religiously active? Do you have favorite readings, hymns, or prayers? Even if you have not heard or thought of them for many years, childhood religious experiences still may be very soothing.

*Additional points:* Very likely some of the things you think of in answer to these questions can be recorded for you, such as favorite music, poetry, or a prayer. Then you can listen to the tape whenever you wish. You should listen for 15 to 20 minutes. You also simply may close your eyes and recall the place, events, or words.

Modified from Lindquist R, Synder M: Introduction to complementary and alternative therapies in nursing. In Ignatavicius DD, Workman ML: *Medical surgical nursing,* ed 5, St. Louis, 2006, Saunders; McCaffery M, Beebe A: *Pain: clinical manual for nursing practice,* St Louis, 1989, Mosby.

endarterectomy this afternoon. During the preoperative assessment, Mrs. Rhines says, "I wish I understood more about this block in the vein in my neck. My surgeon explained some of it, but I didn't understand it all."

NURSING DIAGNOSIS. Deficient knowledge regarding planned surgical intervention.

OUTCOME. The patient will demonstrate knowledge of the physiologic and psychologic responses to surgery.

INTERVENTION. *Teaching: disease process:* Assisting the patient to understand information related to a specific process.

NURSING ACTIVITIES. Begin by determining what Mrs. Rhines knows about carotid artery disease. Reinforce and elaborate on information provided by other health care team members.

*Nurse:* "Tell me what you'd like to know."

*Patient:* "I know it's in my neck, but where exactly?"

*Nurse:* "Good. You already know where the problem is. Let me show you some pictures."

Acknowledge the patient's existing knowledge of the condition. Show her a drawing of the vessel. Point out on her neck where it is located. Draw in the distribution of plaque around the bifurcation. Use the arteriogram to show her the exact location of the lesion.

*Patient:* "That's odd. Why did my left hand feel numb when the problem is on the right side? Shouldn't my right hand have been numb?"

Explain the disease process and the cause of the TIAs. Discuss the anatomy and physiology, and how the right side of the brain controls the left side of the body. Determine what she understands about the surgical procedure. Preoperative teaching may be necessary and can be included in this intervention.

*Patient:* "Well, now it makes sense that the surgeon would need to operate on that vessel. Thanks so much for your help. I'm ready to sign the consent form."

## Selecting Content in Preoperative and Postoperative Teaching

Nursing research has recommended that selection of content for preoperative teaching be based on what the patient wants and needs to know. The perioperative nurse can select content for an individual patient based on input from not only the patient and family and the nurse's own observations but also from other health care team members. Other variables influencing teaching content include what is appropriate by institutional standards, the amount of time allotted, and resources available.

Preoperative information falls into four broad categories: (1) procedural, (2) sensory and temporal, (3) coping, and (4) reassurance. Procedural information is a concrete description of which procedures are to be carried out and why. The Patient and Family Education box "Procedural Information in Preoperative Teaching" below lists possible procedural information that could be included in preoperative and postoperative content. Sensory and temporal information includes how the procedures will feel and how long they will take (Patient and Family Education box "Sensory and Temporal Information in Preoperative Teaching" below). The Patient and Family teaching table "Selecting Content for Teaching" on pp. 289-293 has procedural, sensory, and temporal content for specific surgical procedures. Coping suggestions inform the patient of ways to control emotional responses. Perioperative nurses frequently provide reassurance rather than specific information they believe the patient will find alarming or when time is extremely limited, as in emergency situations such as trauma. "Your surgical team is highly skilled at this procedure. This hospital has the latest equipment." A combination of the salient points of all categories is the appropriate content. Patients welcome booklets that provide simple procedural information, sensory and temporal experiences, suggestions on how to cope, and practical information about hospital admission procedures.

## Facilitating Learning

Facilitating learning can take a variety of forms. Because readiness to learn is an essential factor, nurses can enhance readiness to learn by addressing the patient's specific concerns first, minimizing sensory overload in the environment, providing time for the patient to ask questions, assisting the patient to realize what ability he or she has to control the illness, and helping the patient to have confidence in his or her judgment. Creating a positive learning environment, limiting teaching objectives to the patient's concerns and what must be taught, communicating clearly and simply, using multiple methods, and verifying patient understanding all assist the perioperative nurse in facilitating learning.

The perioperative nurse can use basic principles of motivation to enhance teaching and learning interactions. Use the environment to focus the patient's attention on what he or she needs to know. A warm yet businesslike atmosphere is a suc-

*Text continued on p. 294*

### PATIENT AND FAMILY EDUCATION

### Procedural Information in Preoperative Teaching

- Location of surgery suite
- Location of holding area
- Location of surgery waiting area
- Location of postanesthesia care unit (PACU)
- Location of surgical family waiting area and postsurgical unit
- Incision site
- Planned alterations to anatomy and physiology by surgical intervention
- Use of patient-controlled analgesia (PCA) pump
- Splinting of the incision
- Technique for getting out of bed postoperatively
- Coughing and deep breathing
- Use of incentive spirometer
- Leg exercises and early ambulation
- Description of preoperative routines
  - Bowel preparation
  - Diet and NPO
  - Preoperative laboratory tests and diagnostic procedures
  - Preoperative verification process and marking of the surgical site
  - Voiding
  - Skin preparation
  - ECG
  - Invasive procedures (e.g., intravenous lines, indwelling urinary catheters)
  - Preoperative sedation
- Anesthesia
- Description of postoperative routines
- PACU nursing care
- Support hose/pneumatic compression devices
- Surgical dressings, tubes (e.g., urinary catheter), and drains (as applicable)
- Diet
- Medications
- Pain management
- Respiratory treatments
- Activity progression
- Nature of postoperative nursing assessments

### PATIENT AND FAMILY EDUCATION

### Sensory and Temporal Information in Preoperative Teaching

- Date and time of surgery
- Time patient will leave room or ambulatory surgical unit (ASU)
- Amount of time spent in the preoperative holding area
- Length of surgical procedure
- Length of stay in postanesthesia care unit (PACU)
- Length of hospital or ambulatory surgery center (ASC) stay
- Estimated time to full recovery
- When diet can resume
- When such items as drains, cast, or dressings will be removed
- Hours of family visitation
- Sights, sounds, and smells of preoperative holding area, operating room, and PACU
- Sensations during administration of local anesthesia
- Sensations produced by preoperative medications
- Taste of certain drugs used in anesthesia induction
- Postoperative pain sensations
- Sensations of the stretcher transport to and from surgery
- Postoperative sensations specific to certain procedures (e.g., sore throat from endotracheal intubation)

PATIENT AND FAMILY EDUCATION

## Selecting Content for Teaching

| | Inguinal Herniorrhaphy | Sigmoid Colectomy | Thoracotomy | Cholecystectomy (Open or Laparoscopic) | Carotid Endarterectomy |
|---|---|---|---|---|---|
| **PREOPERATIVE POINTERS** | | | | | |
| **Medical Diagnosis** | Inguinal hernia | CA of sigmoid colon; diverticulitis | CA, primary or metastatic; for diagnosis; drain abscesses | Cholecystitis; cholelithiasis | Carotid stenosis |
| **Diagnostic Tests** | History and physical examination | Barium enema, colonoscopy<br>CT abdomen and pelvis | CT of chest, bronchoscopy, needle biopsy, CME, thoracoscopy | Sonogram, HIDA scan, oral cholecystogram, blood amylase and bilirubin | Doppler scan, arteriogram, CT of head |
| **Routine Preoperative Tests** | CBC, ECG if >50 yr | SMA 6/20, T&C if H&H low, bowel prep, ECG | Pulmonary functions, SMA 20, T&C, ECG | SMA 20, ECG | SMA 6/20, ECG |
| **Incision Site** | Right or left lower quadrant | Lower midline or transverse | Lateral chest, fourth or fifth interspace | Open: right subcostal; laparoscopic: umbilicus, right subcostal, RLQ, upper midline | Neck |
| **Resume Eating** | ASAP | 4-5 days or when ileus resolves | 1-3 days | Open: 2-3 days; laparoscopic: 2-6 hr | ASAP |
| **Pain Control** | PO or IM | IM, PCA, or epidural catheter | PCA or epidural | IM, PCA, or PO | IM or PO |
| **Estimated Length of Procedure** | 1-1½ hr | 2½-3 hr | 3-4 hr | 1-1½ hr | 1-1½ hr |
| **Estimated Length of Hospital Stay** | Day surgery or 23 hr | 6-8 days | 5-8 days | Open: 3-5 days; laparoscopic: 12-23 hr | 2-4 days |
| **Long-term Effects of Surgery** | Return to normal activities | Potential for temporary colostomy | Potential for reduced pulmonary functions | Rare bile salt imbalance | Potential for permanent or temporary neurologic deficit |
| **Drains or Tubes** | None | Potential for colostomy bag; Foley catheter | Two chest tubes and suction; needed 2-4 days | Open: potential for T-tube/ surgical drain; laparoscopic: drainage tube rare | Potential for drain; needed 1-2 days |
| **POSTOPERATIVE POINTERS—HOME INSTRUCTIONS** | | | | | |
| **Food** | ASAP | Regular or low-residue diet | Regular diet | Regular diet | Regular or cardiac diet |
| **Wound Care** | Change dressing PRN × 1-2 days, then none required except for comfort; ice pack is okay | Shower daily | Shower daily | Bathe or shower daily | Bathe or shower daily |
| **Bathing** | 24-48 hr | Shower | Shower | Daily | Daily |
| **Driving** | 2-4 wk and within limits of pain | 10-14 days when soreness less | 6-8 wks when soreness less | Open: 1-2 wk when soreness less; laparoscopic: 2-4 days | 5-7 days when soreness less |
| **Sex** | Restricted 2-3 wk and within limits of pain | Restricted 4-6 wk and within limits of pain | 4-6 wk when soreness less | Restricted 2-3 wk and within limits of pain for open | Restricted within limits of pain |

*ASAP,* As soon as possible; *CA,* cancer; *CBC,* complete blood cell count; *CEA,* carcinoembryonic antigen; *CME,* cervical mediastinal exploration; *CT,* computed tomography; *ECG,* electrocardiogram; *ERCP,* endoscopic retrograde cholangiopancreatography; *H&H,* hematocrit and hemoglobin; *HIDA,* hepatobiliary imaging (HIDA is the acronym for the radioisotope hepato-iminodiacetic acid used in a hepatobiliary scan); *IM,* intramuscular; *IOL,* intraocular lens; *IVP,* intravenous pyelogram; *MRI,* magnetic resonance imaging; *PCA,* patient-controlled analgesia; *PO,* by mouth; PRN, as needed; *PSA,* prostate-specific antigen; *PT,* prothrombin time; *PTCA,* percutaneous transluminal coronary angioplasty; *PTT,* partial thromboplastin time; *RLQ,* right lower quadrant; *T&C,* type and crossmatch.

*Continued*

PATIENT AND FAMILY EDUCATION

**Selecting Content for Teaching—cont'd**

| | Inguinal Herniorrhaphy | Sigmoid Colectomy | Thoracotomy | Cholecystectomy (Open or Laparoscopic) | Carotid Endarterectomy |
|---|---|---|---|---|---|
| **Return to Work** | 2-6 wk, depending on nature of work | 6-8 wk | Restricted 6-8 wk and within limits of pain | Laparoscopic: restricted within limits of pain | 2-4 wk |
| **Medications** | Oral analgesics | Oral analgesics | 6 wks | Oral analgesics | Oral analgesics: aspirin |
| **Follow-up** | 7-10 days | 7-10 days | Oral analgesics | 7-10 days | 7-10 days |
| **Special Restrictions** | Heavy lifting 4-6 wk | Within limits of pain and energy; heavy lifting 4-6 wk | 10-14 days | Walking within limits of pain and energy | Within limits of pain and energy |
| **Worrisome but Normal** | Swelling and bruising of penis and scrotum | Temporary colostomy closure 6-8 wk | Walking within limits of pain and energy; heavy lifting 4-6 wk<br>Noticeable incision pain 3-6 mos | | Temporary or permanent numbness of earlobe |

| | Mastectomy | Ventral Herniorrhaphy | Small bowel resection | Abdominal Perineal Resection | Open Common Duct Exploration |
|---|---|---|---|---|---|
| **PREOPERATIVE POINTERS** | | | | | |
| **Medical Diagnosis** | CA of breast | Incisional hernia | Small bowel obstruction; small bowel strangulation | CA of rectum | Common duct stone; common duct stricture |
| **Diagnostic Tests** | History and physical examination, mammogram, breast biopsy | History and physical examination | History and physical examination, abdominal x-ray | Digital rectal examination, colonoscopy, rigid sigmoidoscopy | History and physical examination, ERCP |
| **Routine Preoperative Tests** | CBC, ECG if >50 yr | CBC, ECG if >50 yr | CBC, ECG if >50 yr | CEA, SMA 6/20, CBC, ECG, T&C, bowel prep | SMA 6/20, ECG, CBC, amylase, bilirubin |
| **Incision Site** | Right or left upper chest | Previous abdominal incision site | Midline or transverse | Midline or transverse; perianal | Right subcostal |
| **Resume Eating** | ASAP | ASAP | 4-5 days or when ileus resolves | 4-5 days or when ileus resolves | 1-3 days |
| **Pain Control** | PO or IM | PO, IM, or PCA | IM or PCA | IM, PCA, or epidural | IM or PCA |
| **Estimated Length of Procedure** | 1-1½ hr | 1½-2 hr | 1-2 hr | 3-4 hr | 1-1½ hr |
| **Estimated Length of Hospital Stay** | 24-48 hr | 24-48 hr | 5-7 days | 6-8 days | 1-3 days |
| **Long-term Effects of Surgery** | Potential for restricted movement in arm, lymphedema | Possibility of recurrence | Possibility of recurrence | Permanent colostomy | Potential for common duct stricture |
| **Drains or Tubes** | 1-2 Jackson-Pratt drains to stay 2-5 days | Jackson-Pratt drain to stay 2-5 days | Unlikely | Colostomy bag; Jackson-Pratt drain to stay 2-4 days; possible posterior wound drain | T-tube to stay 10 days; potential for other surgical drain to stay 2-3 days |
| **POSTOPERATIVE POINTERS—HOME INSTRUCTIONS** | | | | | |
| **Food** | Regular diet | Regular diet | Regular diet | Regular diet | Regular diet |
| **Wound Care** | Empty drain and re-dress daily for comfort; ice pack is okay | Shower daily and re-dress | Bathe or shower daily | Shower daily; change perineal pad to posterior wound PRN | Shower daily; re-dress T-tube daily |
| **Bathing** | Daily—lower body | Shower | Shower | Shower | Shower |

| | | | | | |
|---|---|---|---|---|---|
| **Driving** | 2-4 wks when soreness less | 7-10 days when soreness less | 10-14 days when soreness less | 2-3 wk when soreness less | [illegible] less |
| **Sex** | Restricted within limits of pain | Restricted 4-6 wk and within limits of pain | Restricted 2-3 wk and within limits of pain | Restricted 2-3 wk and within limits of pain | Restricted 2-3 wk and within limits of pain |
| **Return to Work** | 4-6 wk | 6-10 wk | 4-6 wk | 6-10 wk | 2-4 wk |
| **Medications** | Oral analgesics | Oral analgesics | Oral analgesics | Oral analgesics | Oral analgesics |
| **Follow-up** | 7-10 days; 2-4 days if discharged with drain | 7-10 days; 2-4 days if discharged with drain | 10-14 days | 10-14 days | 10-14 days |
| **Special Restrictions** | Begin arm and shoulder exercises within prescribed limits | Walking within limits of pain and energy; heavy lifting 6-10 wk | Walking within limits of pain and energy; heavy lifting 2-3 wk | Walking within limits of pain and energy; heavy lifting 2-3 wk | Walking within limits of pain and energy |
| **Worrisome but Normal** | Numbness and tingling from elbow to axilla | Unlikely | Unlikely | Drainage from posterior wound, particularly if left open | Leaking of bile around T-tube |

| | **Cesarean Delivery** | **Vaginal Hysterectomy** | **Total Hip Replacement** | **Cataract Extraction** | **Craniotomy** |
|---|---|---|---|---|---|
| **PREOPERATIVE POINTERS** | | | | | |
| **Medical Diagnosis** | Cephalopelvic disproportion; cord prolapse; fetal distress; abruptio placentae; placenta previa; breech presentation; previous cesarean section; failure to progress | Uterine prolapse; dysfunctional uterine bleeding; benign or malignant lesions | Degenerative joint disease | Cataracts | Subdural hematoma; malignant or benign lesions; closed head injury |
| **Diagnostic Tests** | History and vaginal examination, fetal monitor | History and pelvic examination, biopsy of lesions, transvaginal sonogram | History and physical examination, x-ray | History and slit-lamp eye examination, keratometer, A-scan | CT of head, neurologic assessment, MRI |
| **Routine Preoperative Tests** | CBC, T&C | SMA 6/20, T&C if H&H low | SMA 20, T&C, ECG, blood for autotransfusion | SMA 6, ECG if warranted | SMA 20, ECG |
| **Incision Site** | Vertical, Pfannenstiel or transverse | Through the vaginal opening; abdominal punctures if laparoscopic-assisted | In line with vertical axis of joint | Conjunctival flap | Head, depending on location of lesion |
| **Resume Eating** | ASAP | 1 day postoperative | ASAP | ASAP | ASAP |
| **Pain Control** | PO or IM | IM, PO, or intrathecal morphine (ITM) | PCA, epidural, IM, PO | PO, nonnarcotic | IM, PO, PCA |
| **Estimated Length of Procedure** | 1 hr | 1-1½ hr | 2-3 hr | ½-1 hr | 1-1½ hr |
| **Estimated Length of Hospital Stay** | 3-4 days | 2-4 days | 4-7 days | 4-6 hr | Variable depending on diagnosis and neurologic status |
| **Long-term Effects of Surgery** | May require subsequent cesarean delivery | Permanent sterilization | Reduced pain; potential for dislocation of prosthesis | Improved or restored vision; rarely change IOL | Potential for permanent or temporary neurologic deficit |
| **Drains or Tubes** | Foley catheter | Foley catheter | Hemovac for 2 days | Unlikely | Possible intracranial pressure monitor |
| **POSTOPERATIVE POINTERS—HOME INSTRUCTIONS** | | | | | |
| **Food** | Regular diet | Regular diet | Regular diet | Regular diet | Regular diet |
| **Wound Care** | Change dressing PRN × 1-2 days; then none required | Bathe or shower daily | Shower may be easier than bathing | Eye patch and shield for 24 hr; then shield at night; sunglasses | Bathe or shower daily |

*Continued*

PATIENT AND FAMILY EDUCATION

## Selecting Content for Teaching—cont'd

| | Cesarean Delivery | Vaginal Hysterectomy | Total Hip Replacement | Cataract Extraction | Craniotomy |
|---|---|---|---|---|---|
| **POSTOPERATIVE POINTERS—HOME INSTRUCTIONS—cont'd** | | | | | |
| **Bathing** | 12-24 hr | Daily | Shower | Bathe or shower after 24 hr | Daily |
| **Driving** | 1-4 wk | 7-14 days when soreness less | Varies with MD preference; may be 2-6 wk | 2-7 days because of impaired depth perception | Depends on existence and extent of neurologic deficit |
| **Sex** | Restricted within limits of pain | Restricted 3-6 wk and within limits of pain | MD preference; limited by restrictions on internal and external rotation of joint | Restrictions by limitations on rigorous activity | Restricted within limits of pain |
| **Return to Work** | 6 wk, depending on nature of work | 2-4 wk | 6-12 wk | 3-7 days if work does not require rigorous activity | 6-12 wk |
| **Medications** | Oral analgesics | Oral analgesics | Oral analgesics; anticoagulant | Antibiotic and antiinflammatory drops; artificial tears | Oral analgesics |
| **Follow-up** | 7-10 days | 7-10 days | 7-10 days | First day postoperative; then 7 days; then in 3-4 wk | 7-10 days |
| **Special Restrictions** | Within limits of pain and energy; heavy lifting 4-6 wk | Within limits of pain and energy; heavy lifting 2-4 wk | Must keep knees lower than hips; may recline but may not sit in low chair or commode seat if lower than knees | Heavy lifting, bending, or rigorous activities 7 days | Within limits of pain and energy |
| **Worrisome but Normal** | Vaginal drainage | Vaginal drainage | Prolonged discomfort | Foreign-body sensation; dry eye; may see floaters | Lingering neurologic deficit |
| | **Retropubic Prostatectomy** | **Nephrectomy** | **Radical Neck Dissection** | **Arthroscopy of Knee** | **Coronary Artery Bypass Graft** |
| **PREOPERATIVE POINTERS** | | | | | |
| **Medical Diagnosis** | Malignant lesions | Malignant lesions; infectious or inflammatory processes that destroy kidney function | Malignant lesions of the mouth and neck | Torn meniscus; diagnostic purposes | Coronary artery occlusive disease |
| **Diagnostic Tests** | Rectal sonogram control for needle biopsy | Arteriogram, sonogram, CT, IVP with retrograde pyelogram, radionucleotide renogram | Physical examination, CT, nasopharyngoscopy | Physical examination, MRI | ECG, stress test, chest radiograph, thallium scan, cardiac catheterization, interventions: PTCA, atherectomy, laser |
| **Routine Preoperative Tests** | CBC, ECG, T&C, PSA, acid phosphatase | Renal functions (creatinine, electrolytes) | SMA 20, ECG | SMA 6, ECG if indicated | SMA 20, ECG, T&C, pulmonary function studies, PT, PTT |
| **Incision Site** | Pfannenstiel or midline | Lateral for inflammatory disease; anterior for malignant lesions | T shape; horizontal extends along underside of mandible; verticle from jaw to sternal notch | 3-4 stab incisions around patella | Midsternal, multiple leg incisions for vein harvest |
| **Resume Eating** | ASAP | Lateral: ASAP; anterior: 2-3 days | ASAP | ASAP | 2-3 days after removal of endotracheal and na- |

| | | | | | |
|---|---|---|---|---|---|
| **Pain Control** | PO or IM | IM or PCA | IM or PO | PO | IM, PO, or PCA |
| **Estimated Length of Procedure** | 2-2½ hr | 2 hr | 2-2½ hr | 1-2 hr | 4-6 hr |
| **Estimated Length of Hospital Stay** | 4-6 days | 5-7 days | 3-5 days | 4-6 hr | 5-7 days |
| **Long-term Effects of Surgery** | Probably impotence; possibly incontinence | Remaining kidney hypertrophies up to one third in size | Poor cosmetic effect; possible loss of trapezius muscle | Possibility of arthritic changes | Loss of saphenous vein, possible intermittent lower leg edema |
| **Drains or Tubes** | Jackson-Pratt for 2-4 days; Foley catheter | Jackson-Pratt or other surgical drain for 2-4 days | Jackson-Pratt for 2-4 days | None | 2 days: mediastinal chest tube; 2-3 days: pleural chest tube; 2-3 days: Hemovac in leg wounds |
| **POSTOPERATIVE POINTERS—HOME INSTRUCTIONS** | | | | | |
| **Food** | Regular diet | Regular diet | Regular diet | Regular diet | Cardiac diet |
| **Wound Care** | Shower daily | Bathe or shower daily | Bathe or shower daily | Bathe or shower daily | Wounds covered if draining; re-dress after shower or bath |
| **Bathing** | Shower | Shower | Daily | Daily | Daily |
| **Driving** | 2-3 wk when soreness less | 2-3 wk when soreness less | 5-10 days when soreness less | 2-4 days when soreness less | 4-6 wk (automatic shift only) |
| **Sex** | Restricted 2-3 wk and within limits of pain and ability | Restricted 2-3 wk and within limits of pain | Restricted within limits of pain | Restricted within limits of pain | Restricted within limits of ability to bear weight on upper arms and chest |
| **Return to Work** | 6-8 wk | 4-6 wk | 3-4 wk | 2-4 days, depending on nature of work | 8-12 wk |
| **Medications** | Oral analgesics | Oral analgesics | Oral analgesics | Oral analgesics | Aspirin anticoagulant; cardiac drugs |
| **Follow-up** | 7-10 days | 7-10 days | 7-10 days | 7-10 days | 7-14 days |
| **Special Restrictions** | Within limits of pain and energy | Within limits of pain and energy; should always avoid dangerous contact sports | Within limits of pain and energy | Limited weight bearing as tolerated; crutch or walker training | Upper body movement restricted for 6 wk for sternal healing |
| **Worrisome but Normal** | Impotence; incontinence | — | Inability to raise shoulder | — | Fatigue, swelling in leg, leg discomfort 4-6 wk |

cessful strategy. Visual and tactile aids, such as a drawing of the biliary system or a sample of a vascular prosthesis, capture and hold the learner's interest. Incentives stimulate the motivation to learn. For some individuals, the payoff for learning is approval and praise from family members or health care providers. For others the enjoyment of reaching a goal is motivation enough. Internal, self-directed motivation to learn lasts longer than external motivation. External motivation requires frequent positive reinforcement.

An individual learns most effectively when he or she is ready to learn. Factors affecting readiness to learn and ways to enhance readiness have been discussed. If the need for change is urgent, the perioperative nurse is in a good position to encourage the development of readiness and to supervise the patient's progress. Structured educational materials enhance motivation. Better organized material is more meaningful and effective. Success motivates better than failure. Design a learning experience that allows the learner to succeed. Learning takes place in small increments. The patient can be overwhelmed by too much, too soon. Practice and return demonstrations done in sequence allow the patient to succeed one step at a time. Learning is likely to create anxiety when changes in beliefs and behavior are required. During high-anxiety or stress periods, keep teaching and learning interactions to a minimum.

The perioperative nurse must help the learner set personal goals and provide feedback about progress toward those goals. Goals are more likely to be met if the patient's behavior is reinforced and praised, if the content is tailored to the individual, if the perioperative nurse helps the patient take action, if the content is relevant, and if the teaching methods are meaningful and appealing to the patient.

As discussed earlier, there are three ways to enhance self-efficacy that, when used properly, can enhance learning. Skills mastery, based on the principle that success motivates better than failure, is accomplished by breaking the task into small, manageable subtasks and ensuring that each subtask is completed successfully. Modeling is another way to enhance self-efficacy. Ideally the model should be an ordinary person who has the same problem as the patient and has to cope with it daily. An excellent example of learning enhancement through modeling is the American Cancer Society's *Reach for Recovery* program. Women who have had mastectomies teach new mastectomy patients how to do arm and shoulder exercises. A third way of facilitating learning by enhancing self-efficacy is through persuasion. This is probably the most used and least effective. It can be used to urge patients to do more than they are currently doing.

Teaching materials are divided into two major categories: printed and nonprint materials. Printed materials include booklets, brochures, and pamphlets. Although printed material can limit feedback, it is always available to the learner and can be referred to as often as needed. The following should be considered when selecting printed material.

Is the content written at the appropriate skill level of the target audience? The mean literacy level in the United States is the eighth-grade level or below; 20% of adult learners are functionally illiterate; and 34% have marginal reading skills. Materials should be written for a sixth-grade level or lower. Simplify printed material by eliminating medical terminology and using familiar words, short sentences, the second person pronoun ("you"), and active tense ("take" rather than "should be taken").[10] In addition, illness or stress can lower one's ability to comprehend even more. For patients with higher levels of literacy and the desire to know, additional information can be provided. Avoid too much information; material presented should be the least needed to convey the message. Use a font size that is easy to read and illustrations or pictures that are simple. Focusing on required behaviors, such as "Do not eat or drink anything after midnight the day of your surgery," increases the chances the patient will follow through. Is the material logically organized? The most important points should be presented first and highlighted. Headings and graphics can draw attention to important content and clarify instructions. Visuals should relate to the topic and not detract from the message. Is the content accurate? Does the material foster interaction between the perioperative nurse and patient? This helps develop the nurse-patient relationship and assists the patient to individualize and personalize the instructions.

Nonprint materials include Web-based resources (see *www.evolve.elsevier.com/rothrock* for numerous patient education sites) and audio and visual programs, such as videotapes, television, flip charts, pictures and slides, cassette tapes, and models. Videotapes combined with print materials are effective tools (Research Highlight). These may be rented or purchased. Some hospitals are part of a nationwide satellite network that televises patient-education programs, and some produce their own videotapes and live broadcasts. Audiotapes and telephone teaching are available in some hospitals by means of a toll-free dial-access system. Another technique is to tape an educational session and give it to the patient when the session is completed. Cassette

## RESEARCH HIGHLIGHT

### Effectiveness and Satisfaction with Education Methods

This study compared three methods of conducting a preanesthesia visit by the anesthesia provider. The sample consisted of 284 patients undergoing elective surgery with general anesthesia, with endotracheal intubation and mechanical ventilation. Patients with cognitive or speech barriers, disoriented patients, and patients who were expected to have a postoperative critical care stay were excluded from the study. Patients were randomly assigned to one of three groups: (1) routine face-to-face visit, (2) an informational brochure read before the face-to-face visit, and (3) a documentary video seen before a face-to-face visit. After the visit, patients rated the degree of satisfaction and information gain they obtained by completing a questionnaire. The questionnaires were administered before preoperative medication and anesthesia were given. The patients in the interview-only group scored the satisfaction with the visit 91% and information gain 72%. Patients in the brochure plus interview group scored satisfaction at 93% and information gain at 80%. The patients in the video plus interview group scored satisfaction at 98% and information gain at 93%. This study suggests that teaching aids, such as videos, used in conjunction with a face-to-face interview enhance patient learning.

Modified from Snyder-Ramos SA and others: Patient satisfaction and information gain after the preanesthetic visit: a comparison of face-to-face interview, brochure and video, *International Anesthesia Research Society* 100:1753-1758, 2005.

tapes or videotapes of the teaching session can be replayed at the patient's convenience. Select audio or video programs that are appropriate to the subject matter, accurate in content, simple, and appealing to the target audience. When referring patients to websites, readability and reliability need to be considered. Much information found on patient-education websites is written at the tenth-grade level or higher.

## Documentation

Patient education is often not thoroughly documented. Perioperative nurses, while recognizing the value of teaching and learning, may fail to consider their patient interactions as "patient education" because they did not conduct a formal process with written objectives. As the JCAHO focuses on quality of care and outcomes, standardized documentation of all kinds of patient education is becoming very important. A simple narrative in the nursing notes is adequate for informal teaching and learning interactions. Include the outcomes of the interaction and assessment data and content. Effective forms for documentation combine teaching protocols, objectives, and outcomes on a single page. Equally as important to document are times when the patient was not ready to learn. It should include the assessment data that indicated lack of readiness and what the perioperative nurse did to enhance readiness. Document when portions of the content are referred to another provider. Referral is an important nursing intervention for perioperative nurses, given the limited amount of time available to spend with patients. (Figure 10-5 shows an example of

**GENERIC CARE PLAN** **The patient demonstrates knowledge of the physiologic and psychologic responses to surgery**

**KEY ASSESSMENT POINTS**

Physiologic condition
Presence of anxiety/fear/concern
Level of formal education
Cultural/ethnic/language barriers
Current knowledge and understanding
Psychologic response to current condition
Interest in learning
Motivation/readiness to learn
Experience with surgery

**NURSING DIAGNOSIS**

Deficient knowledge regarding planned surgical intervention

**PATIENT OUTCOMES**

The patient will demonstrate knowledge of the physiologic and psychologic responses to the planned surgical intervention as evidenced by:

1. Remaining oriented to person, place, and time
2. Confirming, in writing or verbally, consent for the operative procedure
3. Describing the sequence of events during the perioperative period
4. Stating outcomes in realistic terms
5. Expressing feelings about the surgical experience

| NURSING ACTIONS | Yes | No | N/A |
|---|---|---|---|
| 1. Patient identified? | ☐ | ☐ | ☐ |
| 2. Sensory aids/prosthetic devices removed? | ☐ | ☐ | ☐ |
| 3. Sensory impairments? | ☐ | ☐ | ☐ |
| 4. LOC: Alert? | ☐ | ☐ | ☐ |
| 5. Verification of operative site? | ☐ | ☐ | ☐ |
| 6. Consent signed? Advance directive? | ☐ | ☐ | ☐ |
| 7. Language barrier? | ☐ | ☐ | ☐ |
| 8. Special religious/spiritual needs? | ☐ | ☐ | ☐ |
| 9. Special cultural/ethnic needs? | ☐ | ☐ | ☐ |
| 10. Perioperative routine explained? | ☐ | ☐ | ☐ |
| 11. Patient expressed understanding? | ☐ | ☐ | ☐ |
| 12. Patient has additional questions? | ☐ | ☐ | ☐ |

Document additional nursing actions/care plan revisions here:

______________________________

______________________________

______________________________

| EVALUATION OF PATIENT OUTCOMES | Outcome met | Outcome met with additional outcome criteria | Outcome met with revised nursing care plan | Outcome not met | Outcome not applicable to this patient |
|---|---|---|---|---|---|
| 1. The patient remained oriented to person, place, and time. | ☐ | ☐ | ☐ | ☐ | ☐ |
| 2. Physical and emotional factors which impacted on the patient's response to the planned surgical intervention were alleviated. | ☐ | ☐ | ☐ | ☐ | ☐ |
| 3. The patient was physically and emotionally prepared for the planned surgical intervention. | ☐ | ☐ | ☐ | ☐ | ☐ |
| 4. The patient correctly reviewed anticipated perioperative events. | ☐ | ☐ | ☐ | ☐ | ☐ |
| 5. The patient signed the operative permit. | ☐ | ☐ | ☐ | ☐ | ☐ |

Signature: ____________________ Date: ________

FIGURE 10-5 Example of checklist documentation.

how to document the nursing diagnosis, activities, and outcomes in an easily used checklist format.) To meet the JCAHO requirements, some institutions have created interdisciplinary documentation forms.

## EVALUATION

Evaluation of patient education activities should be considered early in the teaching process. Evaluation measures if and how well a patient learned the desired behavior. Evaluation can serve many purposes. It can motivate continued learning or behavior change because it provides concrete evidence that the patient accomplished or failed to accomplish the goal. It reinforces desired behavior on the part of the patient and helps the perioperative nurse determine the adequacy of the instruction and teaching materials. Evaluation also may serve to identify an especially beneficial or particularly worthless educational process. In evaluation, the evidence of learning is compared with the outcome criteria. Although a variety of methods measure learning, the method most frequently used by the perioperative nurse is some form of observation. Direct observation is more effective in evaluating learning in health care than in other areas. Although it may be difficult to evaluate cognitive skills and thinking processes by direct observation, we know that motor skills rely on and reflect cognitive processes. For the outcome criterion, "The patient will consent to a specific treatment option," the nurse can observe directly whether the patient signed the operative permit.

Recording observations or documenting outcomes is essential when using observation as the evaluation method. Narrative form is the best method to document critical incidents or anecdotal events that do not lend themselves to a simpler, quicker method of documentation. Checklists and rating scales save time and produce uniform documentation. The perioperative nurse rarely would be able to evaluate using more extensive self-reports and self-monitoring methods. Although these are excellent methods of evaluation, they are time-consuming. Time is a resource in critically short supply. These methods are best used for group educational programs. Although evaluation is the final step in the teaching and nursing process, it rarely means the end of the process. Evaluation frequently points the perioperative nurse back to other steps in the process.

## SUMMARY

This chapter examines four basic questions about patient education for the perioperative nurse: *Why teach?* Teach because it is the right thing to do for the patient, family, nurse, and institution. *When should patient education occur?* Teach when the patient is ready to learn. *What is the appropriate content for patient teaching?* Teach what patients and families want and need to know to accomplish the tasks of daily living and return to their "usual self." *How should nurses teach?* Teach so that patients and families can actively participate in what they are learning.

## REFERENCES


1. American Hospital Association: *Patient and family-centered care,* Chicago, 2004, The Association.
2. American Hospital Association: *The patient care partnership,* Chicago, 2003, The Association.
3. Association of periOperative Registered Nurses: Patient outcomes: standards of perioperative care. In: *Standards, recommended practices and guidelines,* Denver, Colo, 2006, The Association.
4. Burke LE and others, I think I can, I think I can—using self-efficacy theory to lower lipid levels, *Patient Education and Counseling* 57(1): 134-142, 2005.
5. Clark PA and others: Addressing patients' emotional and spiritual needs, *Joint Commission Journal on Quality and Safety* 29(12):659-667, 2003.
6. Dochterman JM, Bulechek GM, editors: *Nursing interventions classification (NIC),* ed 4, St Louis, 2004, Mosby.
7. Fetzer SJ and others: Self-care activities for postdischarge nausea and vomiting, *Journal of PeriAnesthesia Nursing* 20(4):249-254, 2005.
8. Flowers L: Giving culturally competent care another element in patient safety, *OR Manager* 21(2):1, 17-24, 2005.
9. Friedman EI and others: Discharged patients often unaware of diagnosis and prescribed medication, *Mayo Clinic Proceedings* 80:991-995, 2005. Accessed August 23, 2005, on-line: www.medscape.com.
10. Hochadel M: Educating patients, *Advance for Nurses* 6(18):46-47, 2004.
11. Johnson M and others: *Nursing diagnoses, outcomes, and interventions—NANDA, NOC, and NIC linkages,* ed 2, St Louis, 2006, Mosby.
12. Joint Commission on Accreditation of Healthcare Organizations: *2001 Accreditation Manual for Hospitals,* Chicago, 2000, The Commission.
13. Joint Commission on Accreditation of Healthcare Organizations: *Speak up: planning your recovery,* Chicago, 2005, The Commission.
14. Lewis SM and others: *Medical-surgical nursing—assessment and management of clinical problems,* ed 6, St Louis, 2004, Mosby.
15. Miakowski C: Patient-controlled modalities for acute postoperative pain management, *Journal of PeriAnesthesia Nursing* 20(4):255-267, 2005.
16. Moorhead S and others: *Nursing outcomes classification (NOC),* St Louis, 2004, Mosby.
17. National League for Nursing Education: *Standard curriculum for schools of nursing,* Baltimore, 1918, Waverly.
18. National League for Nursing Education: *A curriculum guide for schools of nursing,* New York, 1937, The League.
19. National League for Nursing Education: *Nursing organization curriculum conference,* Glen Gardener, NJ, 1950, Libertarian Press.
20. National Quality Forum: *Hospital CAHPS,* Washington, DC, 2005, National Quality Forum.
21. Redman BK: *The practice of patient education,* ed 9, St Louis, 2001, Mosby.
22. Rothrock JC: Generic care planning: AORN patient outcome standards. In Rothrock JC, editor: *Perioperative nursing care planning,* ed 2, St Louis, 1996, Mosby.
23. Schmid RE: Steps to reduce medical errors urged. Accessed January 11, 2005 on-line at *Yahoo News.*
24. Steefel L: The case for expanding evidence-based practice, *Nursing Spectrum* 14(18):3, 2005.
25. Winslow EH: Patient education materials, *American Journal of Nursing* 101(10):33-38, 2001.

CHAPTER 11

# Gastrointestinal Surgery

CHRISTINE E. SMITH

Surgery of the gastrointestinal (GI) system may be indicated to establish a diagnosis, cure disease, relieve symptoms, restore function, or afford palliative measures to provide nutrition and promote quality of life. Advances in scientific knowledge, research, pharmacology, technologic developments in the interventional disciplines, and successful outcomes based on clinical evidence continue to broaden the spectrum of modalities and approaches to managing patients with GI disorders.

GI surgery is a subspecialty within the domain of general surgery, traditionally concerned with surgical management of the esophagus, stomach, small intestine, large intestine, and rectum. Gastroenterology is a medical specialty that diagnoses and manages GI disorders and conditions through endoscopic and pharmacologic approaches. Many surgical procedures that formerly required laparotomy and extensive postoperative recovery have been replaced or duplicated by endoscopic access and intervention. Endoscopic examination enhanced with fluoroscopy, ultrasound, and video magnification in conjunction with interventional radiology is a critical component of surgical diagnosis and postoperative evaluation. Laparoscopy, a minimally invasive approach to the intraabdominal compartment, has revolutionized the practice of GI surgery. Medical and surgical specialties have evolved to embrace and facilitate these advancements. Although clinicians may specialize in the discipline of laparoscopy, gastroenterology, general surgery, bariatrics, GI surgical oncology, or colorectal surgery, it is important for the perioperative nurse to be knowledgeable of the basis of GI surgery and the interventional options available to patients, as well as the care requirements common to all GI patients.

## Surgical Anatomy

The GI tract, or alimentary canal, is a continuous tubelike structure that extends the entire length of the trunk (Figure 11-1). The alimentary tract includes the mouth; pharynx; esophagus; stomach; small intestine, consisting of the duodenum, jejunum, and ileum; and large intestine, which comprises the cecum, ascending colon, transverse colon, descending colon, sigmoid colon, rectum, and anus. The length of the GI tract in a cadaver is about 9 meters, or 30 feet. In a living person it is shorter because of sustained muscle contraction and tone. The six basic functions of the GI tract are ingestion, secretion, mixing and propulsion, digestion, absorption, and defecation.[45]

The esophagus extends from the pharynx, at the level of the sixth cervical vertebra, and passes through the neck, posterior to the trachea and heart, and anterior to the vertebral column. The lower portion of the esophagus passes in front of the aorta and through the diaphragm, slightly to the left of the midline, to join the cardia of the stomach.

Blood is supplied to the esophagus from branches of the inferior thyroid arteries, bronchial arteries, thoracic aorta, and branches of the left gastric and inferior phrenic arteries. The nerve supply comes from branches of the vagus and sympathetic nervous system. The length of the esophagus in an adult is about 25 cm, or 10 inches. The esophagus is a collapsible musculomembranous tube, and its primary function is to transport ingested material, by way of peristalsis, from the pharynx to the stomach.

The stomach is an expanded J-shaped organ situated between the esophagus and the duodenum and lies in the upper left abdominal cavity, slightly to the left of the midline and beneath the diaphragm. The stomach is divided into three parts: the fundus, the body, and the antrum (Figure 11-2). The fundus lies beneath the left dome of the diaphragm, behind the apex of the heart. The body and antrum lie in an oblique direction within the abdominal cavity. The stomach is stabilized indirectly by the lower portion of the esophagus and directly by its attachment to the duodenum, which is anchored to the posterior parietal peritoneum. The omentum, the peritoneal ligaments, and branches of the celiac vessel provide additional support to the stomach.

The convex, or lower, margin of the stomach is known as the *greater curvature;* the concave, or upper, margin is the *lesser curvature.* Attached to the greater curvature is the greater omentum, which is a double fold of peritoneum containing fat. It covers the intestines loosely and is not to be confused with the mesentery, which connects the intestines with the posterior abdominal wall. The left gastroepiploic branch of the splenic artery and the right gastroepiploic branch of the hepatic artery run through the greater omentum. The lesser omentum, which is attached to the lesser curvature of the stomach, contains the left gastric artery, a branch of the celiac axis, and the right gastric branch of the hepatic artery. During a gastrectomy, these vessels are clamped and ligated.

The stomach functions include acceptance and storage of ingested material; chemical and mechanical digestion through the production of gastric lipase, pepsinogen, hydrochloric acid, gastrin, and intrinsic factor, responsible for the absorption of vitamin $B_{12}$; plus peristaltic waves, which both mix and propel stomach contents, or chyme, into the duodenum.

The small intestine, the longest part of the digestive tract, begins at the pylorus and ends at the ileocecal valve (Figure 11-3). The small intestine varies in size with the degree of contraction but is usually about 3 meters in length and 2.5 cm in diameter. It is divided into three parts: the duodenum, which is

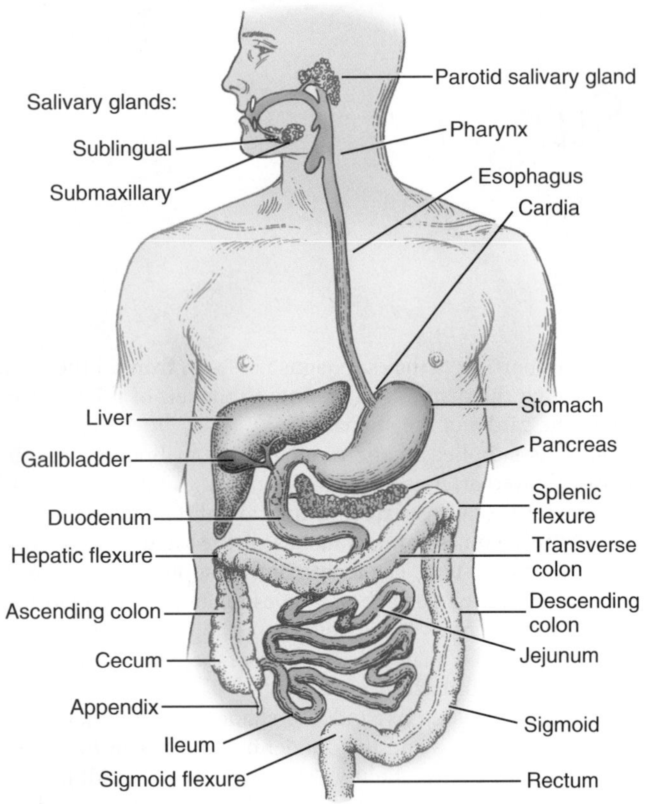


FIGURE 11-1 Alimentary canal and its appendages.

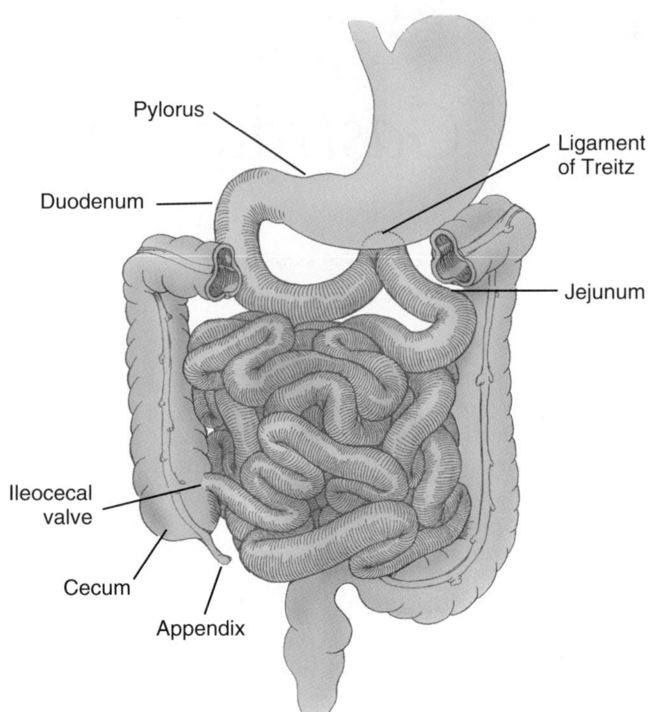


FIGURE 11-3 Illustration of the small bowel; the duodenum originates at the pylorus and flexes at the ligament of Treitz where the jejunum begins. The jejunum extends into the ileum, which terminates at the ileocecal valve at the cecum.

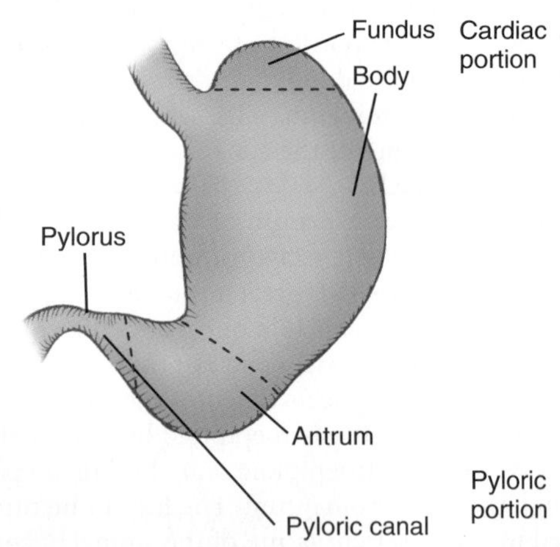


FIGURE 11-2 Regional anatomy of stomach.

about 25 cm long; the jejunum, which is about two fifths of the length of the entire small intestine; and the ileum, which makes up the remaining length in an adult. The duodenum, the proximal portion of the small intestine, begins at the pylorus, is contiguous with the jejunum, and is stabilized by a fusion between the pancreas and the posterior parietal peritoneum. The duodenum is divided into four portions: superior (I), descending (II), transverse (III), and ascending (IV) (Figure 11-4). Nearly all of the superior portion mucosa is characterized by the lack of folds; it appears slightly dilated and is referred to as the *duodenal bulb*. The characteristic circular folds of the small intestinal mucosa begin just proximal to the end of the superior portion of the duodenum and extend through the jejunum. They become less prominent in the ileum. The purpose of the circular mucosal folds, called *plicae circulares of Kerckring*, or *valvulae conniventes*, is to provide greater mucosal surface area.

The common bile duct and the main pancreatic duct enter the medial wall of the middle of the second portion of the duodenum at the ampulla of Vater. The first, second, and third portions of the duodenum curve in a C-loop concavity in which the head of the pancreas lies. The fourth portion of the duodenum ascends to the duodenojejunal flexure. The duodenojejunal flexure is stabilized by the ligament of Treitz, which suspends the duodenum from the posterior body wall. The ligament of Treitz serves as an important landmark during any abdominal exploration because it provides the surgeon with a reliable orientation of the patient's anatomy.

The blood supply of the duodenum comes from the arterial branches of the celiac axis (Figure 11-5). The gastroduodenal artery branches off the hepatic artery and is located behind the duodenal bulb. At the inferior margin of the bulb the gastroduodenal artery divides into the right gastroepiploic artery and a superior pancreaticoduodenal branch. The superior pancreaticoduodenal artery supplies blood to the proximal duodenum and head of the pancreas. The inferior pancreaticoduodenal artery branch of the superior mesenteric artery supplies blood to the third and fourth portions of the duodenum as well as to the head and body of the pancreas.

The jejunum, which is situated in the upper portion of the abdomen, joins the ileum, which is situated in the lower portion of the cavity. The ileum empties into the large intestine through the ileocecal valve. The jejunum and ileum are sus-

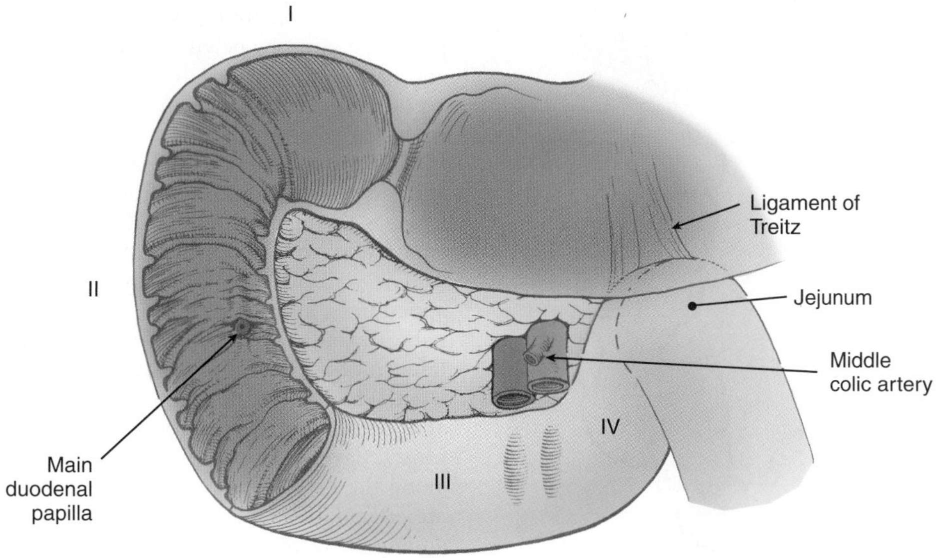


FIGURE 11-4 The duodenum consists of four portions, as illustrated.

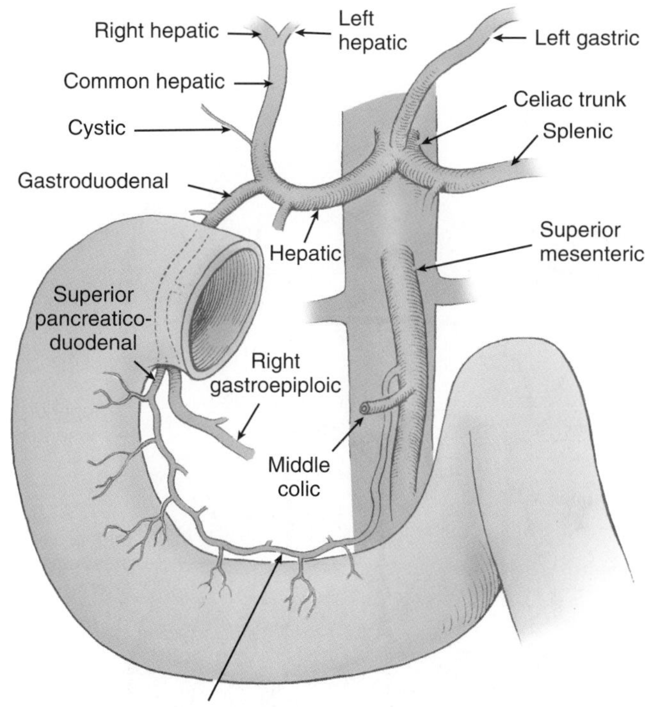


FIGURE 11-5 Blood supply of the duodenum.

pended by the mesentery, which is attached to the posterior abdominal wall. The free border of the mesentery, which is about 5.5 meters (18 feet) long, contains branches of the superior mesenteric artery, many veins, lymph nodes, and nerve fibers. The blood supply to the jejunum and ileum comes entirely from the superior mesenteric artery. The small bowel contains major deposits of lymphatic tissue, known as *Peyer's patches,* in the ileum. The rich lymphatic drainage of the small bowel plays a major role in fat absorption. Lymphatic drainage from the mucosa proceeds through the wall of the small intestine to lymph nodes adjacent to the mesentery. Lymphatic drainage then proceeds to larger lymphatics that communicate with the retroperitoneal cisterna chyli and from there to the thoracic duct. The lymphatics of the intestine play a major role in the body's immune defense as well as in the spread of cells arising from intestinal neoplasms.

The jejunum has a larger circumference and is thicker than the ileum. The mesenteric vessels usually form only one or two arcades, a series of anastomosing arterial arches, compared with the multiple vascular arcades of the ileum. The jejunal mucosa is thick and has prominent plicae circulares. The ileum mucosa is thinner with few plicae.

The small intestine serves two important but opposite functions simultaneously. It absorbs essential nutrients at 95% efficiency while providing an effective barrier from harmful ingested environmental elements. The remarkably large surface area of the combined small and large intestinal mucosa is estimated to be 200 square meters, or the size of a doubles' tennis court.[21]

The large intestine begins at the ileocecal valve and terminates at the anus. It is divided into the cecum, colon, and rectum. The cecum is attached to the ileum and extends about 7 cm below it. The cecum in an adult is usually adherent to the posterior wall of the peritoneal cavity and has a serosal covering on its anterior wall only. The cecum forms a blind pouch from which the appendix projects.

The colon, approximately 1.5 meters long, is divided into four parts: the ascending colon, the transverse colon, the descending colon, and the sigmoid colon (Figure 11-6).

The ascending colon extends upward from the ileocecal valve to the hepatic flexure. The upper portion of the ascending colon lies behind the right lobe of the liver and in front of the anterior surface of the right kidney.

The transverse colon begins at the hepatic flexure and ends at the splenic flexure. It lies below the stomach and is attached to the transverse mesocolon.

The descending colon extends downward from the splenic flexure to the area just below the iliac crest. The iliac portion of the sigmoid colon lies on the inner surface of the left iliac

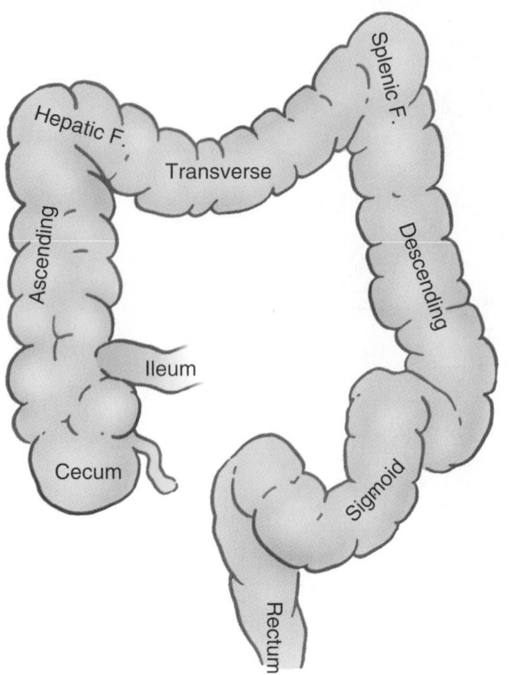


**FIGURE 11-6** Anatomic division of large intestine, showing placement of hepatic flexure and splenic flexure. *F*, Flexure.

muscle. The remaining portion of the colon passes over the pelvic rim into the pelvic cavity and lies partly in the abdomen and partly in the pelvis. It then forms an S curve in the pelvis and terminates in the rectum at the level of the third segment of the sacral vertebrae.

The blood supply to the ascending colon, hepatic flexure, and transverse colon comes from the superior mesenteric artery, whereas the blood supply to the descending colon and rectum comes from the inferior mesenteric artery (Figure 11-7).

The wall of the colon is made up of taeniae coli, epiploic appendices, and haustra. The taeniae coli are three longitudinal, or axial, strips of muscles distributed around the circumference of the colon. They represent the longitudinal muscle layer, which is not complete in the colon. The small intestine and rectum have both circular and complete longitudinal muscle layers. The epiploic appendices are fatty appendages along the bowel that have no particular function; the haustra are sacculations that are the outpouchings of bowel wall among the taeniae coli. The diameter of the colon varies in size from about 9 cm (3½ inches) in the cecum to an average of about 1.25 cm (½ inch) in the sigmoid colon.

The rectum originates at the sigmoid colon and terminates in the anus. This slightly curved passage is surrounded by the pelvic fascia as it lies on the anterior surface of the sacrum and

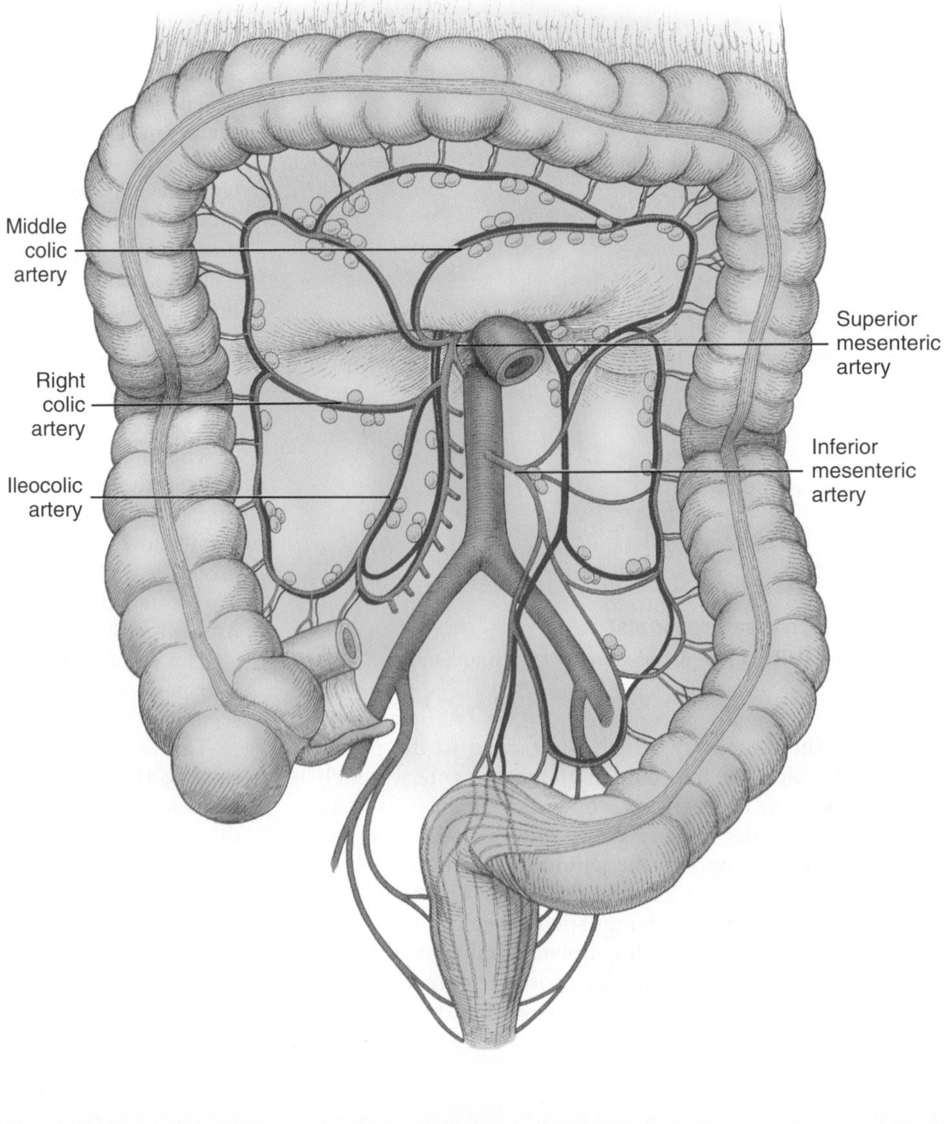

**FIGURE 11-7** Blood supply of the colon.

coccyx. In the male the rectum lies behind the prostate gland, seminal vesicles, and bladder. In the female the rectum lies behind the uterus and the vagina. A septum rectovesicale, also called *Denonvilliers fascia,* separates the rectum from the urogenital structures. The rectum is suspended in the pelvis by fascia extending from the right and left pelvic sidewalls. Rectosacral fascia extending from the sacrum to the anorectal junction suspends the rectum posteriorly. The rectum dilates just before it becomes the anal canal, and this dilation, or ampulla, presents folds called *Houston valves.* The wall of the rectum consists of four layers, similar to those of the small intestine.

The anal canal is a narrow passage that passes downward and slightly posteriorly. It is surrounded and controlled by two circular muscle groups, which form the external and internal anal sphincters. The internal sphincter is a continuation of the longitudinal muscle layer.

The primary function of the large intestine is to reabsorb water and electrolytes, form solid waste into feces, synthesize K and B-complex vitamins, and propel and eliminate solid food residue and waste through defecation.[13]

The GI tract harbors a complex microbiologic ecosystem that supports and maintains the essential digestive and protective functions necessary for life yet presents significant risk and challenge during diagnostic and surgical intervention. Substantial populations of microorganisms, both obligate anaerobes and facultative bacterial spores, exist in the intestinal lumen. The organisms of the upper tract differ from those of the lower tract, with the highest concentration in the distal bowel. These organisms can contribute to contamination and disease processes within the intestinal tract and throughout the body.[33] Gastric and intestinal pH, while indicated for digestive benefit and protection from selected organisms, can compromise peritoneal tissues and structures when unplanned spillage or leakage occurs. The pH of the stomach ranges from 1.5 to 3, whereas the pH of the intestines can range from 7 to 8.5.

# Perioperative Nursing Considerations

GI surgery and endoscopic procedures present special considerations related to the planned procedure, instrumentation, approach, anatomic structures involved, primary and secondary diagnoses or health status of the patient, surgeon and patient preferences, and availability of special institutional resources. Special institutional resources might include a bariatric program, an oncology program with research protocols, a transplant program, or a technologically advanced integrated operating room (OR) with robotics. Optimum care of the patient undergoing GI surgery and other invasive GI procedures relies on sound knowledge and experience, thorough assessment of the patient with identification of care needs, preplanning and preparation, and follow-through with competent care and evaluation of the completed process and its results. The risks for injury or failure to achieve the intended outcome are equally present in GI surgery as in any surgical or invasive procedure. Perioperative nurses have long recognized that no procedure is routine and that unexpected outcomes can occur even when planning and preventive measures have been employed under the most optimal circumstances. Although it is prudent to address and review the vulnerabilities faced by all surgical patients, additional selective considerations may be a concern for patients undergoing GI surgery and other invasive GI procedures.

## Assessment

Nursing care for patients undergoing GI surgery begins with assessment. Individualized care, integrating physiologic with psychologic preparation, is given to each patient. Patients undergoing GI surgery should understand why they need preoperative preparation, what the intended surgical intervention will be, and how it will affect them and their family postoperatively. A preoperative nursing assessment of the patient is essential for appropriate planning and implementation of intraoperative nursing care and evaluation of patient outcomes. The nurse will ensure that the patient understands the nature of the surgery, the intended approach with the expected site of the incision(s), the expected outcome(s), and follow-up recovery and care. Turning, coughing, and deep breathing are taught preoperatively and reinforced after surgery. If an ostomy is anticipated, a wound ostomy continence nurse (WOCN, formerly called an *enterostomal therapist*) will be consulted to site-mark the abdomen for optimal stoma placement (Box 11-1)

### BOX 11-1

### Criteria for Ostomy Site-Mark Selection

- Determine planned surgical procedure and ostomy (refer to surgeon's notes and preferences).
- Explain procedure to patient, and establish privacy.
- Provide ostomy appliance and literature for patient and family to read and examine.
- Verify patient's knowledge and understanding of surgery and planned ostomy.
- Examine abdominal skin integrity and surface for scars, lesions, bulges, implants, and stomas.
- Locate waistline and patient's preferred beltline. Patient may have to put on pants to illustrate.
- Locate abdominal skinfolds, creases, and bulges as patient lies flat, stands, bends forward, and sits upright.
- Identify the lateral margins of the rectus abdominis muscle. Palpate while patient coughs.
- Select a site within the rectus margin on the crest of the infraumbilical or infraabdominal bulge.
- Place finger tip on proposed site, and verify patient can see site when standing or sitting.
- Avoid belt or waistline, bony prominences, scars, excoriated lesions, creases, folds, below pendulous breasts, umbilicus, hernia, or horizontal plane with existing stoma or fistula.
- Position ostomy pouch faceplate on proposed site as template to ensure avoidance of umbilicus, beltline, and waistline. At least 2 inches of smooth skin should surround stoma for good seal. (Patients who wear their pants low below the waistline can wear suspenders or sweat pants postoperatively to pull pants loosely above stoma to prevent irritation when lower quadrant sites are appropriate.)
- Mark site boldly with indelible or permanent skin marking pen. Cover with clear adhesive dressing to protect from shower or wear.
- Verify site by having patient stand, sit, and twist, noting avoidance of creases and interference. Patient must be able to see site for later self-care.
- Document skin assessment, teaching, patient's understanding and level of acceptance, site selected, and rationale for choice.

and prepare the patient for the postoperative management and care. The WOCN can also assist in allaying fears and anxieties for the patient and the family.[11]

The nursing assessment of the patient before GI surgery or invasive procedures includes the following information:

- Demographic data
- Present problems, chief complaint, or symptoms that led the patient to seek medical attention (Box 11-2)
- Medical history, including nutrition and allergies to foods, drugs, latex, or other substances

BOX 11-2

**Assessment Data**

**GENERAL DATA**

Usual height and weight

Nutrition

- Types of food usually eaten at each meal or snack
- Food likes and dislikes
- Alcohol consumption
- Tobacco use
- Religious, cultural, ethnic, or medically prescribed food restrictions
- Food intolerances or allergies
- Patient's perception and concerns pertaining to diet and weight
- Effects of life-style on diet and weight gain or loss
- Vitamins and other nutritional or herbal supplements used

Oral hygiene

Bowel elimination patterns

Use of medications or laxatives

- Stool softeners
- Antiemetics
- Antidiarrheals
- Antacids
- Histamine blockers or proton pump inhibitors
- Frequent or high doses of aspirin, acetaminophen, or ibuprofen

**SPECIFIC DATA**

Oral lesions

Appetite

Digestion or indigestion

Dysphagia

Nausea

Vomiting

Hematemesis

Change in stool

- Color (clay color, black)
- Contents (undigested food, blood, mucus)

Constipation

Diarrhea

Flatulence

Hemorrhoids

Abdominal pain

Hepatitis

Jaundice

Ulcers

Gallstones

Polyps

Tumors

Anal discomfort

Fecal incontinence

Exposure to infectious disease

- History of chronic disease or other medical conditions
- Surgical history, including prior surgeries, invasive procedures, and anesthesia experiences
- Medications, including use of nonsteroidal antiinflammatory drugs (NSAIDs), antacids, histamine blockers, proton pump inhibitors, steroids, or anticoagulants
- Family history
- Personal and social history, including use of alcohol, nicotine, herbal nutraceuticals, and illicit substances
- Focused GI assessment, including bowel sounds, pain, abdomen appearance, and GI risk factors

Examination of the patient's abdomen should include inspection, palpation, and auscultation of bowel sounds. Systematic investigation, with open-ended questions, should cover descriptions of pain with or without palpation; digestion; presence of nausea, vomiting, diarrhea, or constipation; bleeding; recent trauma; and nutrition.[7]

Pertinent serum studies related to the patient with GI disease might include a complete blood count (CBC) with differential, serum electrolytes, platelet count, cholesterol level, vitamin and mineral levels, liver function, serum proteins, coagulation studies, pancreatic function, and indices of nutritional status (Table 11-1).

Diagnostic endoscopic examinations, radiologic studies with or without contrast markers, abdominal ultrasound, endoscopic ultrasound (EUS), magnetic resonance imaging (MRI), positron emission tomography (PET), computed tomography (CT) imaging scans, plus GI secretion laboratory studies will add further information about the patient's health or disease process to help formulate the surgical plan. Advances in endoscopic technology provide enhanced details of GI anatomy and pathology. EUS combines endoscopy and ultrasound, using sound waves to generate an image of the histologic layers of the esophageal, gastric, and intestinal walls. The frequencies used are higher than those used in traditional ultrasound, providing high-level accuracy of depth of mucosal invasion.[8] EUS is of critical importance in staging of GI malignancies, determining surgical options and potential for therapeutic resection. Endoscopic image-enhancement techniques include high-resolution endoscopes and magnification to identify mucosal surface details; narrow band filters to see capillary patterns, pits, and villi; and chromoendoscopy or staining techniques and fluorescence to differentiate between normal and dysplastic tissue.[25]

An emerging technology and noninvasive diagnostic test use a small camera in the shape of a capsule, the size of a large vitamin pill. It is swallowed with a few sips of water and propelled along the GI tract by normal peristalsis. The Pill Cam ESO glides down the esophagus taking 14 color digital pictures per second, which are transmitted to a recording device worn by the patient. This device is suitable for imaging the mucosal surface of the esophagus and takes 20 to 30 minutes.[23] The capsule is eventually passed naturally within 24 to 72 hours.[39]

The M2A Given Imaging, also called wireless capsule endoscopy, has dramatically altered the ability to visualize the mucosal surface of the small intestine. M2A refers to mouth-to-anus. The small bowel makes up 90% of the mucosal surface of the entire GI tract and had formerly been constrained by the limits of traditional diagnostic modalities.[38] The only preprocedure preparation is an 8-hour fast. The M2A capsule is swallowed with a full glass of water, a data recorder is worn around the patient's waist, and the patient is permitted to leave the facility if an outpatient.

**TABLE 11-1**

## Common Serum Studies with Gastrointestinal Function Relevance

| Test | Normal Adult Values | Significance of Abnormal Values |
|---|---|---|
| **COMPLETE BLOOD COUNT WITH DIFFERENTIAL (CBC WITH DIFF)** | | |
| **Red Blood Cell Count (RBC)** | *Men:* 4.7-6.1 million/mm$^3$<br>*Women:* 4.2-5.4 million/mm$^3$ | Low indicates anemia from blood loss, hemolysis, dietary deficiency, drug ingestion, bone marrow failure, or chronic illness.<br>High indicates compensation for high altitudes, chronic anoxia, or polycythemia vera. |
| **Hemoglobin (Hb) Concentration** | *Men:* 14-18 g/dl<br>*Women:* 12-16 g/dl | Low and high values tend to be caused by the same processes that cause low or high values for RBCs. Artificially high in dehydration. |
| **Hematocrit (Hct)** | *Men:* 42%-52%<br>*Women:* 37%-47% | Low and high values same as above. |
| **Mean Corpuscular Volume (MCV)** | *Adults:* 80-95/mm$^3$ | High in megaloblastic anemias (vitamin $B_{12}$ deficiency).<br>Low in iron-deficiency anemia or thalassemia. |
| **Mean Corpuscular Hemoglobin (MCH)** | *Adults:* 27-31 pg | Low and high values tend to be caused by the same processes that cause low or high values for MCV. |
| **Mean Corpuscular Hemoglobin Concentration (MCHC)** | *Adults:* 32-36 g/dl | Low indicates hemoglobin deficiency seen in iron-deficiency anemia or thalassemia. |
| **White Blood Cell Count (WBC) Differential** | *Adults:* 5000-10,000/mm$^3$ | Elevated WBC level indicates infection or leukemia. Decreased WBC may indicate bone marrow failure, overwhelming infection, dietary deficiency, or autoimmune disease. |
| Neutrophils<br>Lymphocytes<br>Monocytes<br>Eosinophils<br>Basophils | 20%-40%<br>2%-8%<br>1%-4%<br>0.5%-1%<br>55%-70% | Elevated neutrophil count may indicate acute suppurative infection.<br>Decreased neutrophil count may indicate overwhelming bacterial infection (especially in the elderly) or dietary deficiency.<br>Elevated lymphocyte count may indicate chronic bacterial or viral infection.<br>Decreased lymphocytes may indicate sepsis.<br>Elevated eosinophils may indicate parasitic infestation, allergic reactions, or autoimmune diseases. A "shift to the left" means the percentage of neutrophils and immature leukocytes is increased, which occurs with infection. |
| **Platelet Count** | 150,000-400,000/mm$^3$ | Reduced levels of platelets may result from decreased platelet production, increased sequestration (as seen in hypersplenism), increased platelet destruction or consumption (e.g., disseminated intravascular coagulation [DIC]), or loss of platelets through hemorrhage.<br>Elevated levels may indicate severe hemorrhage, polycythemia vera, postsplenectomy syndromes, and some malignant disorders. |
| **SERUM ELECTROLYTES** | | |
| **Sodium (Na)** | 136-145 mEq/L | Elevated levels may be seen with excessive sweating, extensive burns, osmotic diuresis, and excessive sodium intake or reduced sodium excretion.<br>Reduced levels may be seen with inadequate sodium intake, increased sodium losses (e.g., vomiting, nasogastric suction, diarrhea, renal disease, third-space losses of sodium). |
| **Phosphate ($PO_4$)** | 3-4 mg/dl | Decreased levels in long-term antacid ingestion. |
| **Potassium (K)** | 3.5-5 mEq/L | Elevated levels may indicate excessive intake or reduced excretion of potassium (e.g., renal failure). Crush injuries cause release of intracellular potassium, or metabolic acidosis.<br>Reduced levels may indicate inadequate intake or excessive losses (e.g., diarrhea, vomiting, use of diuretics, hyperaldosteronism) or result of metabolic alkalosis or administration of glucose, insulin, or calcium (which causes a shift of potassium from the bloodstream into cells). |
| **Chloride (Cl)** | 98-106 mEq/L | Changes in chloride concentration usually parallel changes in sodium concentration. Decreased in long-term gastric suctioning. |
| **Carbon Dioxide ($CO_2$)** | 23-30 mEq/L | Elevated levels are seen with acidosis.<br>Reduced levels are seen with alkalosis. |

Data from Pagana KD, Pagana TJ: *Mosby's diagnostic and laboratory test reference,* ed 7, St Louis, 2005, Mosby.

*Continued*

**TABLE 11-1**

## Common Serum Studies with Gastrointestinal Function Relevance—cont'd

| Test | Normal Adult Values | Significance of Abnormal Values |
|---|---|---|
| **ARTERIAL BLOOD GASES** | | |
| **Ph** | 7.35-7.45 | High levels indicate alkalosis.<br>Low levels reflect acidosis. |
| **Partial Pressure of Carbon Dioxide ($Pco_2$)** | 35-45 mm Hg | High levels indicate carbon dioxide retention caused by respiratory depression or pulmonary disease (respiratory acidosis).<br>Low levels reflect excessive loss of carbon dioxide through hyperventilation (respiratory alkalosis from overventilation or emotional trauma; may also be seen as compensatory response in metabolic acidosis). |
| **Bicarbonate ($HCO_3$)** | 22-26 mEq/L | Low levels indicate metabolic acidosis caused by excessive acid production, resulting in depletion of $HCO_3$ (e.g., diabetic acidosis); failure to eliminate $H^+$ ions, resulting in depletion of $HCO_3$ (e.g., renal failure); or excessive loss of $HCO_3$ (e.g., intestinal losses through diarrhea, fistula drainage). Low levels may also be seen with insulin overdose, insulinoma, hypothyroidism, hypopituitarism, Addison's disease, and extensive liver disease.<br>High levels indicate metabolic alkalosis resulting from bicarbonate overdose or excessive gastric losses; may also be seen as a compensatory response in a patient with prolonged respiratory acidosis; pancreatic disorders (e.g., adenoma, pancreatitis), corticosteroid therapy, diuretics, Cushing disease, and hyperthyroidism. |
| **COAGULATION STUDIES** | | |
| **Prothrombin Time (PT)** | 85%-100% or 11-12.5 sec | Elevated times with anticoagulant, acetylsalicylic acid (ASA), and nonsteroidal antiinflammatory drug (NSAID) use. Decreased times may be seen in malignant disease caused by unidentified hypercoagulability factors. |
| **Partial Prothrombin Time (PTT)** | 60-70 sec | Increased in acquired or congenital clotting factor deficiencies, cirrhosis, vitamin K deficiency, leukemia, DIC, heparin administration, hypofibrinogenemia, von Willebrand's disease, hemophilia. Decreased in early stages of DIC, extensive cancer. |
| **Activated Partial Prothrombin Time (APTT)** | 30-40 sec | Same as for PTT. |
| **OTHER SERUM STUDIES** | | |
| **Albumin** | 3.5-5.5 mg/day | Decreased levels seen in protein malnutrition and hepatocellular injury. |
| **Alkaline Phosphatase (ALP)** | 30-120 units/L | Slightly elevated in elderly. Elevated in intestinal ischemia. Decreased with excess vitamin B ingestion. |
| **Amylase** | 60-120 Somogyi units/dl | Increased in penetrating or perforated peptic ulcer, perforated or necrotic bowel, or duodenal obstruction. |
| **Ammonia** | 10-80 mcg/dl | Increased in gastrointestinal (GI) bleeding, GI obstruction, or liver disease. |
| **Carcinoembryonic Antigen (CEA)** | $<$5 ng/ml | Elevated in GI cancer, colitis, diverticulitis, cirrhosis, peptic ulcer, hepatobiliary and pancreatic cancer. |
| **Complement Assay (C3 and C4)** | C3: 55-120 mg/dl<br>C4: 20-50 mg/dl<br>Total complement: 75-160 mg/dl | Elevated in ulcerative colitis and cancer. |
| **Cortisol (Hydrocortisone)** | 8 AM: 5-23 mcg/dl<br>4 PM: 3-13 mcg/dl | Elevated in obesity. |
| **C-Reactive Protein** | $<$1 mg/dl | Elevated in Crohn's disease, postoperative wound infection, malignant disease. |
| **Transferrin (Serum)** | 250-300 mg/dl | Decreased levels may indicate protein malnutrition; transferrin levels may be used to monitor a patient's response to nutritional support therapy since the half-life of transferrin is 8-10 days, whereas the half-life of albumin is 19-20 days (this means that transferrin levels reflect changes in the patient's visceral protein status much faster than albumin levels do). |

Data from Pagana KD, Pagana TJ: *Mosby's diagnostic and laboratory test reference*, ed 7, St Louis, 2005, Mosby.

**TABLE 11-1**

**Common Serum Studies with Gastrointestinal Function Relevance—cont'd**

| Test | Normal Adult Values | Significance of Abnormal Values |
|---|---|---|
| **OTHER SERUM STUDIES—CONT'D** | | |
| **Prealbumin (Serum)** | 15-32 mg/dl | Decreased levels seen in protein malnutrition. Because the half-life of prealbumin is 2-3 days, these values reflect changes in the patient's visceral protein status even faster than transferrin levels do. |
| **Total Lymphocyte Count (Serum)** | >150,000/mm$^3$ | Decreased levels may be seen in protein malnutrition; however, many other conditions affect the total lymphocyte count (e.g., infections, conditions affecting WBC production). |

The 8-hour video collects 50,000 images, significantly improving diagnostic yield of information.[49]

Contraindications to capsule endoscopy include small bowel strictures, narrowing, fistulas, swallowing disorders, suspected intestinal obstruction, or pacemakers.

Reports and images of study results should be available at the time of surgery.

## Nursing Diagnosis

Perioperative nurses often are challenged to assess, diagnose, and plan care in a short preoperative time frame, usually sharing the patient and their attention with other members of the surgical team and the patient's family. They must be aware of the care considerations general to all surgical patients plus those implications relevant to patients anticipating GI surgery. A focused preoperative assessment provides the data to formulate the nursing diagnoses, identify desired outcomes, and organize and prioritize the plan for intraoperative care.

Nursing diagnoses related to the care of patients undergoing GI surgery might include the following:

- Anxiety related to perioperative events
- Deficient Knowledge related to impending surgery
- Pain
- Disturbed Body Image related to intestinal diversion (when diversion possible or planned)
- Risk for Imbalanced Body Temperature
- Risk for Surgical Site Infection
- Risk for Perioperative Positioning Injury
- Risk for Impaired Tissue Integrity related to lasers, thermal devices, electrosurgery, radiation, or chemical solutions
- Risk for Injury from retained surgical items, wrong procedure, wrong site, or administration of wrong or incorrect medications
- Risk for Imbalanced Fluid Volume

## Outcome Identification

Outcomes identified for the selected nursing diagnoses could be stated as follows:

- The patient will demonstrate or verbalize decreased anxiety immediately before and after surgery.
- The patient will demonstrate or verbalize knowledge of physiologic and psychologic responses to surgery.
- The patient will demonstrate or report pain control throughout the perioperative period.
- The patient will demonstrate coping patterns and acceptance of appearance.
- The patient will be at or returning to normothermia at the conclusion of the immediate postoperative period.
- The patient will be free from signs and symptoms of surgical site infection.
- The patient will be free from perioperative positioning injury.
- The patient will be free of evidence of impaired tissue integrity.
- The patient will be free from injury related to retained surgical items, wrong procedure, wrong site, and medication errors.
- The patient's fluid volume, electrolyte, and acid-base balance will be consistent with or improved from preoperative baseline levels.[6,12]

Rationales guide the interventions aimed at achieving the nursing outcomes for the surgical patient. Rationales identified for the selected nursing outcomes are presented in Box 11-3.

## Planning

The nursing plan of care is an organized framework of nursing activities designed to guide the nurse in selecting materials and supplies and providing interventions based on evidence of credible scientific research and successful outcomes. Planning and preparation extend beyond the list of items and informational notes on the surgeon's preference card/pick list.

Preoperative assessment enables the perioperative nurse to plan for the specific physiologic, psychologic, and technical needs of the individual patient. For example, the size of the patient influences positioning during surgery and may necessitate additional instruments, such as deeper retractors and longer forceps and scissors. Provisions for a safe, clean, and equipped surgical environment require meticulous planning, integrating information specific to the individual patient, structural materials typically used on this procedure by this surgical team, and those standards and recommended practices indicated for the care of all surgical patients. The perioperative nurse is proactive in organizing, prioritizing, ensuring safety, and expediting all aspects of the surgical experience for the patient.

BOX 11-3

**Rationales for Perioperative Nursing Interventions**

- Providing emotional support and promoting sharing may help clarify fears. Fears may be based on inaccurate information.
- Anxiety and sensory deficits may impair the patient's readiness to learn or retain new knowledge.
- Patients who are prepared for painful procedures by an explanation of the actual sensory experience have less stress than those with vague information.
- The use of noninvasive pain management measures can enhance comfort and therapeutic effect of pain medications.
- Pain management should be aggressive and individualized at regular intervals of administration rather than as needed (PRN).
- Frequent contact with the patient conveys trust, and encouraging sharing can provide an outlet for fears and misinformation.
- Divert focus from the change to positive characteristics that reinforce the self-concept and control.
- The surgical and anesthesia experience, with exposure of body surfaces, introduction of fluids and instruments, and an open wound, will decrease core body temperature.
- The physiologic stress of surgery may impair normal thermal regulating mechanisms.
- The surgical and anesthesia experience challenges the immune system and poses many opportunities to introduce endogenous and exogenous microorganisms.
- Hyperextension of limbs, mechanical pressure, and prolonged positioning can cause skin, nerve, vascular, and musculoskeletal compromise.
- Repositioning and transfer can cause shearing force and skin injuries.
- Directed energy modalities such as electrosurgery, lasers, radiation, and fiberoptic light cords can cause tissue burns and fire.
- Antimicrobial prep solutions, chemical sterilants, and alcohol can cause tissue irritation and burns.
- Surgical patients are at risk for wrong procedure and wrong-site surgery when patient identification practices are flawed and not repeated at each level of perioperative care.
- Multiple surgical items, such as instruments, sharps, and sponges, present the potential to be retained when counting practices are flawed.
- Anesthetized patients are vulnerable and unable to advocate for themselves.
- The physiologic stressors of surgery and anesthesia can result in fluid shifts from excess to depletion along the continuum throughout the entire time frame of the procedure.[6,12]

A typical plan of care for a patient undergoing GI surgery follows on pp. 307-308.

## Implementation

Nursing activities involved with the preparation of the surgical environment; procurement of the supplies, equipment, materials, and devices; and communication with the team are based on structural materials and processes typical for this procedure and team, plus individualized data gathered from the patient, family, and medical record.

Open laparotomy and laparoscopic surgical approaches are usually accomplished with general endotracheal or spinal anesthesia. The choice of anesthesia will be determined by the patient's health status, planned incision site, length of surgery, the patient's choice, and the collaborative judgment of the anesthesia provider and surgeon. Procedures done by the endoscopic approach, such as EGD (esophagogastroduodenoscopy [upper endoscopy]) or colonoscopy, are typically accomplished with intravenous (IV) moderate sedation. Monitoring devices and parameters typical to those anesthesia plans will be used. Patients at risk for fluid and electrolyte shifts and significant loss of blood will require arterial monitoring and frequent intraoperative sampling of hemoglobin and hematocrit, arterial blood gases, coagulation studies, and electrolytes. Preoperative fasting and bowel cleansing preparation, combined with alterations in nutritional status of this patient population, may severely deplete the patient of fluids and electrolytes. These elements will have to be measured, replaced, and balanced throughout and after the procedure. A nasogastric tube may be inserted to decompress the stomach and suction collected gastric secretions. A urinary catheter may be inserted to decompress the bladder and provide accurate measurement of urinary output and renal function.

Preoperatively, the physician may order that blood be available for those patients anticipating open laparotomy or laparoscopic GI surgery where blood replacement is predicted. Selected elective surgery patients may be requested to donate 1 or 2 units of autologous blood. Patients' friends and family may donate donor-directed blood. Autotransfusion, or cell salvage, of the patient's own blood during surgery may not be appropriate because of potential for contamination from bowel contents with their organisms or malignant cells from a GI neoplasm. Blood replacement will be augmented, managed, and balanced as needed with IV colloids and crystalloids, albumin, platelets, fresh frozen plasma, and appropriate electrolytes.

IV antibiotics will be given before the incision is made and throughout the procedure (Surgical Pharmacology). Antibiotic irrigation solutions may be used intraabdominally during the procedure and before closure. Additional intraoperative medications may be indicated as per institutional standard or the surgeon's preference. Hemostatic agents, anticoagulant solutions, steroid preparations, and local anesthetics may be prepared for administration. The best guide will be a comprehensive and frequently updated plan of care, pick list, or surgeon/procedure preference sheet. (See Chapter 2 for a review of medication safety practices.)

For laparotomy and laparoscopic approaches, the patient typically is placed in the supine position with the arms abducted less than 90 degrees to the sides. Modifications may include flexion of the knees to a modified lithotomy position with the legs in self-balancing, or Allen, stirrups or Yellow Fins for procedures where access to the rectum is necessary. Check for presence of bilateral posterior popliteal, posterior tibial, and dorsalis pedis pulses, and document. Monitor and document circulation throughout the procedure. Intraoperative access and exposure may require frequent alterations of patient position with side-to-side tilt, elevation of the kidney rest, and shifts to Trendelenburg or reverse Trendelenburg position to permit gravity displacement of abdominal organs for surgical exposure. Entry into the thoracic and abdominal space is often approached through a thoracoabdominal access. The patient will be placed and immobilized in lateral or side-lying position. Gastroscopy (EGD) is

## SAMPLE PLAN OF CARE

### NURSING DIAGNOSIS
**Anxiety** related to perioperative events

### OUTCOME
The patient will demonstrate or verbalize decreased anxiety.

### INTERVENTIONS
- Explain preoperative activities and expectations (e.g., intravenous [IV] lines, skin preparation, positioning), sequence of sensory experiences and activities in the operating room (OR), and postoperative expectations (e.g., postanesthesia care unit [PACU], drains, catheters, dressings).
- Determine effective coping strategies used by patient in the past; support these as appropriate.
- Minimize stimuli in the OR that can contribute to anxiety (e.g., high noise levels, excessive talking, music that is not of the patient's preference).
- Remain with the patient during induction; convey caring behaviors (e.g., touch; a soft, reassuring voice; warm blankets).
- Maintain the patient's dignity, privacy, and modesty.
- Encourage expression of feelings and concerns.

### NURSING DIAGNOSIS
**Deficient Knowledge** related to impending surgery

### OUTCOME
The patient will demonstrate or verbalize knowledge of physiologic and psychologic responses to surgery.

### INTERVENTIONS
- Verify information the patient and family need and want to know. Determine current knowledge level and perceptions of surgery.
- Initiate preoperative education and discharge planning early in the perioperative process.
- Assess readiness to learn and patient's preferred learning style.
- Include family or patient's accompanying responsible adult in teaching. Use simple language. Present information in the patient's dominant language (use an interpreter if necessary). Note any sensory impairments, and accommodate same. When possible, provide written information that replicates verbal education.
- Verify patient's understanding of material presented by having the patient repeat back, in his or her own words, information that has been presented. Correct misunderstandings.
- Communicate patient or family's concerns to appropriate surgical team members, or make appropriate referral.

### NURSING DIAGNOSIS
**Pain**

### OUTCOME
The patient will demonstrate or report adequate pain management throughout the perioperative period.

### INTERVENTIONS
- Identify cultural components related to pain.
- Provide pain management information (purpose, methods of administration, desired effects). Review pain assessment scales that will be used postoperatively. Have patient verbalize, in his or her own words, understanding of pain management. Encourage questions; clarify information.
- Use, as appropriate to individual patient, nonpharmacologic methods of pain management (relaxation, massage, imagery, music, other preferred comfort measures). These may also promote comfort and enhance pain medication effect.
- Evaluate response to pain management interventions.

### NURSING DIAGNOSIS
**Disturbed Body Image** related to intestinal diversion (when diversion possible or planned)

### OUTCOME
Patient will demonstrate coping patterns and acceptance of appearance and self-care.

### INTERVENTIONS
- Encourage verbalization of feelings about anticipated alterations in body function if diversion procedure planned.
- Elicit patient and family's (if appropriate) perceptions of planned surgical intervention.
- Identify effective sources of support.
- Encourage patient to implement cultural, religious, ethnic, or social customs associated with perceived loss.
- Provide accurate information relevant to patient's postoperative expectations (general principles of ostomy care and solutions to concerns that may be worrying patient).
- Refer patient to wound, ostomy, and continence nurse (WOCN) if this has not already been done.

### NURSING DIAGNOSIS
**Risk for Imbalanced Body Temperature**

### OUTCOME
Patient will be at or returning to normothermia at the conclusion of the immediate postoperative period.

### INTERVENTIONS
- Regulate ambient room temperature in range between 20°C and 25.6°C (68°F and 78°F) as appropriate.
- Monitor patient temperature during surgery.
- Minimize patient exposure to room air. Keep patient covered with warm blankets before induction. Ask patient if he or she is comfortable.
- Use forced-air warming blanket over patient's upper body and head or legs as appropriate.
- Use warmed irrigating solutions and fluid replacements as appropriate.
- Cover patient with a warm blanket before transport to the PACU.

### NURSING DIAGNOSIS
**Risk for Surgical Site Infection** related to operative or other invasive procedure

### OUTCOME
Patient will be free from signs and symptoms of surgical site infection.

### INTERVENTIONS
- Identify patient-specific risk factors for infection (e.g., altered nutritional status, chronic diseases, preoperative radiation therapy, total parenteral nutrition [TPN]).
- Initiate practices required for creating and maintaining a sterile field.
- Protect the patient from cross-contamination—employ bowel/GI technique as appropriate.

*Continued*

## SAMPLE PLAN OF CARE—cont'd

**INTERVENTIONS—CONT'D**

- Designate appropriate wound classification (clean, clean-contaminated, contaminated, dirty/infected) at end of procedure.
- Practice Standard Precautions with attention to handling of contaminated instruments, specimens, and cultures.
- Administer medication as prescribed (e.g., antibiotic prophylaxis), and document.

**NURSING DIAGNOSIS**

**Risk for Injury** related to perioperative positioning

**OUTCOME**

Patient will be free from signs of perioperative positioning injury.

**INTERVENTIONS**

- Position patient in body alignment with attention to possible modifications of surgical position, patient limitations, and safety.
- Use adequate body supports, restraints, and padding of pressure sites specific to planned position. Reassess position status throughout procedure.
- Lift and transport patient carefully with sufficient assistance and lifting aids as needed.
- Reassess patient for signs and symptoms of injury at conclusion of procedure.

**NURSING DIAGNOSIS**

**Risk for Impaired Tissue Integrity** related to lasers, thermal devices, electrosurgery, radiation, and chemical solutions

**OUTCOME**

The patient will be free from evidence of tissue injury.

**INTERVENTIONS**

- Inspect skin condition, and determine patient's risk factors related to skin injury.
- If hair must be removed from surgical site, select removal method most likely to preserve skin integrity.
- Protect patient from thermal, electrical, laser, and chemical injury by following institutional practice guidelines. Implement fire precautions with skin prep solution.
- Before applying dressings, clean and dry skin at incision site or sites.
- Prevent stretching of the skin when securing dressings with tape.
- Reassess patient for signs of skin injury at conclusion of procedure.

**NURSING DIAGNOSIS**

**Risk for Injury** from retained surgical items, wrong procedure, wrong site, or medication administration

**OUTCOME**

The patient will be free from injury.

**INTERVENTIONS**

- Confirm patient identity.
- Initiate preoperative verification process. Verify surgical procedure, and involve patient in marking surgical site.
- Identify any allergies to medications.
- Perform and document required counts. If necessary, take a "pause for the count" to avoid distractions.
- Administer medications and solutions as prescribed. Label all medications and solutions on and off the sterile field.
- Verify and record implants.
- Perform accurate specimen care, handling, and transfer.

**NURSING DIAGNOSIS**

**Risk for Imbalanced Fluid Volume**

**OUTCOME**

The patient's fluid and electrolyte and acid-base balance will be consistent with or improved from preoperative baseline levels.

**INTERVENTIONS**

- Review baseline laboratory data from the chart; confer with surgeon or anesthesia provider regarding deviations from normal.
- Assess nutritional status, skin turgor, renal status, and other conditions or medications affecting fluid and electrolyte balance.
- Collaborate with surgeon and anesthesia provider in accurately estimating fluid and blood loss and maintaining or correcting losses (administration of fluid replacement therapies, electrolytes, or medications).
- Record all solutions administered from the surgical field.

## SURGICAL PHARMACOLOGY

### Gastrointestinal-Specific Antibiotics

- Ampicillin—prophylaxis against *Salmonella and* shigellosis
- Cephalosporin—prophylaxis against aerobes and anaerobes
- Clindamycin—prophylaxis against aerobes and anaerobes
- Fluoroquinolone—prophylaxis in combination with metronidazole or clindamycin
- Gentamycin—prophylaxis against gram-negative rods and enterococci
- Metronidazole—prophylaxis in Crohn's disease, pseudomembranous colitis
- Tetracycline—prophylaxis against shigellosis, cholera
- Tobramycin—prophylaxis against aerobic gram-negative bacilli
- Vancomycin—prophylaxis in penicillin allergy, pseudomembranous colitis

typically done with the patient in slight semi-Fowler position, whereas colonoscopy is accomplished with the patient in left lateral position with the knees flexed.

Patients who are morbidly obese pose a positioning challenge for their safety, exposure, and access and the safety of the staff who must transfer and position the patient. These patients require a surgical bed that can accommodate their weight and size, protect them from falls, and support their frame while preventing skin and musculoskeletal injury. More than four staff persons may be needed to safely transfer and position the patient. Transfer aids, such as rollers, sliders, liftsheets, and hydraulic lifts, should be used when available. Encourage patients to assist in their transfer. Determine the patient's level of comfort, and make appropriate adjustments before anesthesia induction.

The patient will arrive with or have compression stockings and a sequential compression device (SCD) ordered for use during surgery. Apply and institute this preventive treatment as soon as possible to prevent deep vein thrombosis (DVT). Smooth the stockings and sleeves over the legs, and prevent folds when the legs are positioned in stirrups. Place the unit to hang on the OR bed or place on the floor under the OR bed in an area away from team members' feet and areas that may be wet. The vibration noise can be buffered with a bath blanket under the unit.

Positioning is accomplished with attention to body alignment; access and exposure to the intended incision site; positioning of the surgical light and instrument accessories and equipment, which may be attached to the OR bed; and padding and protection of potential pressure sites.

The vast amount of skin exposure required for either a laparotomy or laparoscopic approach presents a risk for hypothermia in the compromised surgical patient. A forced-air warming unit, such as the Bair Hugger patient warming system, may be positioned over the patient's legs or across the chest and arms under the sterile drapes. Temperature settings range from low at 32°C (89.6°F) to high at 43°C (109.4°F). Keep the ambient room temperature warm (between 20°C [68°F] and 26°C [78°F]) until after the patient is prepped and draped. Keep the patient covered with warm bath blankets until the skin prep is begun. Expose only the areas to be prepped. Warm all irrigation fluids to a temperature not greater than 40.5°C (105°F). Consult with the anesthesia provider for an assessment of the patient's body temperature before adjusting the room temperature during the procedure. Raise the room temperature before the conclusion of the procedure. IV fluids and blood products will be administered by way of a fluid warming system with blood warmed to 37°C (98.6°F) and IV fluids between 37°C (98.6°F) and 40°C (104°F).

If prescribed, hair removal from the proposed operative site will be accomplished as close as possible to the time of incision. Hair should be removed according to institutional protocol and surgeon's preference; many institutions require a physician's order for this procedure. Direct special attention to existing or intended ostomy sites, avoiding further skin injury. Existing ostomy stomas may be covered and protected with an occlusive sterile plastic dressing or a collection bag or isolated with a plastic drape with adhesive strip. Antimicrobial skin preparation follows general protocol for laparotomy, with generous borders in the event that the incision must be extended. Precautions for the protection of skin at and under the bed line are taken to prevent accumulated fluid, skin injury, and surgical fires. Sites within the prep area that provide concentrated microorganisms, such as an existing ostomy, draining fistula, or the rectum, will be prepped last.

Intraoperative draping will typically follow the usual standard for draping the patient undergoing laparotomy or laparoscopy. Extra drapes will be indicated when the patient is placed in a modified lithotomy position and where bowel isolation precautions are taken. The patient may be redraped or the existing drapes reinforced before incision closure.

All surgical team members pause for a "time out" before the incision is made. Full participation is required by all members, and a comprehensive review and consensus include the following: patient identification, intended surgical procedure or procedures, marked site (and laterality if appropriate), patient position, pertinent medical conditions or concerns, availability of implants or any special equipment or devices, and verification that prep solutions have dried.

GI surgery instrumentation, for both the laparotomy and laparoscopic approach, requires a basic laparotomy instrument set. Sharp cutting instruments include #3 and #4 knife handles, curved tissue dissection scissors, and curved and straight utility scissors. Clamps include curved and straight hemostats: Kelly clamps; Kocher, right angle, and Crile (tonsil) hemostats; Babcock and Allis clamps; towel clamps; ring or sponge forceps; and assorted needle holders. Tissue-grasping forceps include short-, medium-, and long-toothed, plain, DeBakey, Adson, and Russian forceps. Handheld retractors include Army-Navy, Richardson, Deaver, malleable, rake, and selected self-retaining retractors. Additional accessory instruments may include but are not limited to various grooved and nontraumatic curved, straight, and angled bowel clamps (Figure 11-8).

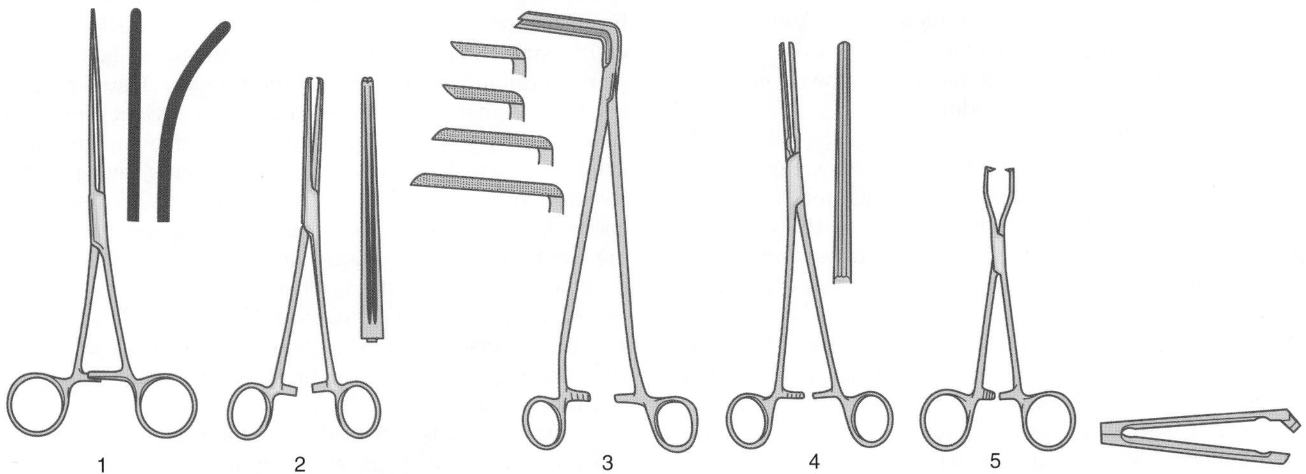


**FIGURE 11-8** Instruments for stomach and intestinal operations. *1,* Doyen intestinal forceps, straight and curved; *2,* Allen intestinal anastomosis clamp; *3,* Best colon clamps; *4,* Dennis intestinal clamp; *5,* Pace-Potts clamp.

Suction tips may include a Yankauer tonsil suction, Frazier tip, cardiac suction tip, or a Poole, intestinal sump suction. Protective nontraumatic covers or shods may be slipped over the jaws of selected clamps to protect and stabilize organ tissue during dissection or suturing. Longer versions of many of the basic instruments will be required for low abdominal procedures, obese patients, and thoracoabdominal approaches.

Laparoscopic surgery of the GI tract requires laparoscopic instruments intended for abdominal surgery. These instruments may be disposable, reusable, hybrid "resposables" (reusable instruments with disposable cutting or coagulation tips), or a combination. Laparoscopic instruments are designed to offer operating tips that function similarly to the basic laparotomy instruments but are designed to fit through a narrow trocar and extend into all quadrants of the abdominal cavity from the skin surface. Several laparoscopic dissectors and scissors have electrosurgical capability. Bipolar or monopolar electrosurgery may be used, with bipolar considered the safer alternative. Accessories to the laparoscopic instruments, telescopes, and trocars are the light cord, insufflation tubing, camera and cord, suction-irrigation tubing, and harmonic ultrasound scalpel handpiece with cord. When laparoscopic procedures necessitate extracorporeal (outside the abdomen) assistance for inspection, dissection, anastomosis, or specimen manipulation, a hand-assisted port may be used to offer the surgeon a sterile, protected entry into the abdomen for his or her nondominant hand, while maintaining pneumoperitoneum.[30] Referred to as hand-assisted laparoscopic surgery (HALS), the hand-assisted port is suitable for laparoscopic surgeries that require a mini-laparotomy to remove an organ or specimen or for extracorporeal anastomoses. A primary advantage is the tactile sensation afforded the surgeon (and assistant). These devices have an adhesive base to attach the sleeve and a protractor to expose the wound and to protect against contamination. Additional small incisions, or port sites, are made to introduce standard laparoscopic instruments.

Robotic or telerobotic surgical systems can provide technologic advancements to laparoscopic surgery, enhancing the surgeon's performance and precision by promoting an ergonomically comfortable hand position, three-dimensional virtual field, replacing the camera holder with a stable platform, and unlimited motion of instrumentation.[5,15] Magnification and full-field lighting enhance the surgeon's orientation.[47] Since 1997, robotic systems have been successfully employed in a broad range of GI procedures of the esophagus, stomach, and bowel, including fundoplication and bariatric procedures.[19]

A tall, multishelf video cart, or primary tower, will contain the primary video monitor, light source, video camera, video cassette recorder (VCR), printer, and insufflator. The tower may also contain a bipolar electrosurgical unit (ESU), pulsed irrigation system, or harmonic ultrasound dissection unit. A second tower or cart will display a second monitor, often called the *slave monitor,* to stand on the opposite side of the OR table to allow the surgical team on the other side to view the procedure. These monitors, if not attached and wired to a ceiling boom system, are joined with a co-axial cable that will connect the two systems. The surgeon may prefer to use one monitor, placed between the patient's legs, when lithotomy position is used.

Meticulous planning is needed to ensure that all equipment is in working order. Equipment may have to be positioned after the patient is transferred to the OR bed; it should be done quickly and quietly to expedite the procedure, without provoking anxiety in the patient. Place the insufflator unit on a tower shelf above the level of the patient's abdomen. This precaution will prevent backflow of gas, fluid, and organic debris if the unit is turned off before the tubing is disconnected from the patient. Run electrical cords and tubing from all equipment to the nearest outlet, with consideration for staff and patient safety. Avoid areas that may be wet. Secure cords to the floor to prevent falls. Do not overload an outlet with plugs from several units that each draws considerable current, such as units that produce heat. Be prepared to connect all equipment cords and tubing after the patient is draped, and white-balance the camera. Provide a source of light for anesthesia and the scrub person when the overhead room lights are turned off.

It is prudent to have an open laparotomy set with instruments and accessories available, should conversion to an open laparotomy or laparoscopic-assisted procedure be necessary. The laparotomy instruments may be opened and counted on the laparoscopy back table or a separate sterile table as per institutional protocol.

The surgeon may request ureteral catheters to be placed by a urologist before a GI procedure is begun. The catheters enable the surgeon to see and palpate the ureters during the procedure. A basic cystoscopy setup with sterile ureteral catheters, two of each size, will be needed.

Intraluminal examination of the bowel may be necessary during the procedure. The surgeon may request a sterile colonoscope or sigmoidoscope to insert into an opening made through the bowel wall, after the abdomen is open. Set up the scopes and accessories on a separate sterile table. This table will be considered contaminated after the scope is removed. Team members who have directly participated in the endoscopic procedure must change gown and gloves before proceeding with the remainder of the surgical intervention.

Additional accessory instruments or devices may include a sterile plastic drawstring intestinal bag to confine loops of normal bowel from the operative segment, combination suction/irrigator, or irrigator/bipolar coagulation. Ultrasound-guided probes and ultrasonic dissection instruments are commonly used in GI surgery. Automatic stapling devices have streamlined the process of tissue ligation, cross-clamping, and creating anastomoses and reservoir pouches. These instruments can deliver single staples and single or double rows of closely staggered linear and circular rows of inert staples. The staple appliers may be single-fire or accept multiple cartridges for successive use. They may be designed for open laparotomy or endoscopic use. Surgical stapling instruments have greatly influenced the technical aspects of GI surgery. For some surgeons the use of these devices has replaced conventional suturing techniques. The B-shaped design of the implanted staple does not compromise the vascularity of the approximated tissue edges. These devices are available in reusable and disposable units. Personnel must be familiar with the types of available stapling equipment, applications, assembly if indicated, and proper loading.

Electrosurgery is a critical component in the achievement and maintenance of hemostasis. Optimal dispersive pad sites include the thigh, flank, shoulder, upper arm, and buttocks. The pad should be placed over a fleshy muscular site as close as possible to the incision yet out of the prep area. Avoid dependent areas that may have a bony prominence or affinity for pooled solution. Choose power settings that achieve the best tissue response at the lowest setting. Smoke evacuation apparatus should be available. Provide long and angled ESU tips. Other hemostatic and dissection equipment and devices may include the argon beam coagulator, ultrasonic tissue dissector, radiofrequency ablation, and laser (see Chapter 7).

Suture materials used on GI tissue have traditionally been chromic gut and silk. With the increased number of synthetic absorbable and nonabsorbable suture materials available, surgeons have a variety of materials from which to choose. Polyester fiber sutures and polyglycolic acid sutures are frequently employed on GI tissue. Generally, 3-0 and 4-0 sutures on a semicircular taper needle are used on intestinal tissues. Ligatures for small vessels usually require a 3-0 or 4-0 braided material, whereas 0 or 2-0 braided ligatures are used for larger vessel occlusion. For closure or anastomosis of GI layers, 3-0 or 4-0 synthetic absorbable suture with a curved intestinal needle is commonly used on the mucosa. A 3-0 or 2-0 continuous synthetic absorbable suture and 4-0 or 3-0 nonabsorbable suture with curved or straight intestinal needles may be used for the seromuscular layer. Some surgeons may prefer interrupted silk sutures on intestinal (semicircular taper) needles for anastomosis procedures. For abdominal closure #1 or 0 braided or monofilament suture is commonly used. Retention sutures may be indicated when there is potential for compromised tissue or wound healing. Checking the surgeon's preference/procedure card or pick list for appropriate suture materials not only ensures the availability of necessary supplies but also is a cost-effective measure.

Sponges used in open laparotomy procedures may include large packs (18″ × 18″), large laps (12″ × 12″), or small elongated tape sponges (4″ × 18″). These items may vary in size according to the product available. Blunt fine tissue dissection may be accomplished with Kittner gauze dissectors (peanuts) on a Kelly clamp or right angle. Meticulous care and vigilance must prevent the incidental misplacement of these items. Gauze sponges (Raytex) are not recommended for use in the abdominal cavity. In the case of significant bleeding or isolation of bowel during anastomosis, lint-free radiopaque cloth towels can be used. Towels must be counted.

Bowel technique, also referred to as a *contamination* or *isolation* technique, is employed to prevent cross-contamination of the wound or abdomen with bowel organisms. This technique is also employed during cancer procedures to prevent mechanical metastasis, or "seeding" of malignant cells throughout the abdomen. Bowel technique begins as soon as the GI tract is clamped and transected and proceeds through wound irrigation, before wound closure. The wound edges and surrounding drapes are protected with extra drapes, and the instruments used for the GI tract resection and anastomosis are sequestered and used only for this part of the procedure. The rest of the sterile back table remains untouched and is maintained as sterile throughout the anastomosis. Separate instruments and drapes are saved for the closure. Gowns, gloves, and drapes will be changed before closure. The contaminated GI tract instruments may be handed off or left on a separate Mayo stand. Preplanning during preoperative setup will provide extra and separate instruments ready for anastomosis and also for closure. These must all be included in the instrument count with provisions for accomplishing the closing count of the contaminated set. Provide for the containment and display of the needles used for the anastomosis. Surgeon's preference and institutional protocol will determine details of the technique.

Specimens are handled carefully and prepared for examination by the pathologist. Consider that the specimen may be contaminated with microorganisms or malignant cells. Prevent contamination of the sterile field and instruments. The surgeon usually determines how the specimen will be handled before examination. It may be sent to the pathology department fresh, in saline, or in a preservative solution. Tissue also may be sent for frozen-section examination to verify the pathologic condition and determine whether tissue margins are free from malignant cells. Specimens may also be entered into research protocols, which will require special handling, storage, and transport.

Verify specimen accuracy with the surgeon by reading back the label and pathology form before removing the specimen from the room or before the surgeon leaves the room, and document according to institutional protocol.

Drains may be indicated for evacuation of gastric secretions or serosanguineous fluid. A closed suction wound drain may be used. A Malecot, Pezzer, or Foley catheter in desired size may be inserted as a gastrostomy tube for drainage until normal bowel peristalsis returns. A jejunostomy tube may be placed in the jejunum after gastric resection to provide access for enteral nutrition.

## Evaluation

Evaluation of nursing care is ongoing throughout the procedure and before the patient is transported to the postanesthesia care unit (PACU) or a surgical intensive care unit (SICU). The dressing and drains are securely placed to avoid damage during transfer to the PACU stretcher or SICU bed. Skin is assessed for reddened or bruised areas; if such areas are present, treatment is initiated immediately. The electrosurgical dispersive pad is removed, the site is inspected, and the condition of the skin is documented. The circulating nurse ensures that the patient is covered with a clean, warm blanket before being transported to the PACU or SICU. Any variances are reported to the surgeon, documented in the nursing record, and included in the hand-off report given to the nurse in the PACU, SICU, or nursing unit. Patient outcomes, based on the perioperative nursing diagnoses, will be reviewed. Postoperative documentation will reflect and measure how each outcome was met and note significant variations to the desired expectation.

## Patient and Family Education and Discharge Planning

Patients undergoing surgical intervention for GI disorders vary greatly in the length of time and complexity of their recovery. Recovery and convalescence vary according to the type of procedure, site of surgery, type of anesthesia, pain management, and individual health status.

GI structures may have varying degrees of edema, decreased peristalsis, and alterations in tissue oxygenation and lymphatic drainage, depending on the amount of manipulation, resection, and trauma to the normal anatomic structures of the GI tract. General anesthesia is commonly administered to the patient undergoing surgical interventions of the GI tract. Smooth muscle relaxation is imperative for most major GI procedures. The patient will usually experience decreased GI peristalsis for

2 to 5 days after laparotomy and intestinal resection. A nasogastric tube or gastrostomy tube is inserted to evacuate the gastric secretions. Diet is introduced only after bowel sounds return. The patient may experience nausea and vomiting if food or drink is introduced too early for the GI system to function with normal absorption and motility. Small bowel function typically returns 1 to 2 days after surgery. Postoperative outcomes can be improved when nutritional status is maximized. When bowel sounds are present, the patient will receive nutritional support as tolerated by way of oral feeding, total enteral nutrition (TEN), or total parenteral nutrition (TPN).[37]

Coughing and deep breathing are important for the patient recovering from general anesthesia. Splinting of the abdominal muscles and the use of incentive spirometry will assist the patient in postoperative coughing and deep breathing initiatives and moving pooled secretions. Early ambulation will assist the patient in regaining overall muscle tone and strength, support cardiac and pulmonary function, prevent DVT in the lower extremities, and boost a general sense of well-being.

Pain management is a critical factor in the patient's recovery. An epidural catheter may be placed immediately before surgery for postoperative pain control. For most major GI procedures, patient-controlled analgesia (PCA) or patient-controlled epidural analgesia (PCEA) is used for consistent control of pain and discomfort in the first 1 to 3 postoperative days of hospital recovery. Narcotics may add to the length of time after which normal bowel peristalsis returns and are monitored closely after the third postoperative day.

The patient with a newly created ostomy will need consultation with the WOCN to assist both the patient and family or significant others in the care and management of the ostomy and surrounding skin. Many life-style changes are associated with an ostomy. The WOCN consultation is essential in the successful recovery and rehabilitation of the patient with a new ostomy. The WOCN first teaches the patient and family to accept the ostomy. Skin care, appliance application, ostomy irrigation, diet, and bowel training are but a few of the topics that must be taught for care and management of an ostomy. Clothing, self-esteem, body image, sex and intimacy, travel, public toileting, and odor control are some of the social issues for which the WOCN will provide the patient and family or significant others with strategies and resources to ensure quality and fulfillment in their lives.[11]

Patients with resected small bowel may require TPN because their ability to absorb nutrients from ingested food is compromised. Referral to homecare agencies that are expert in administering TPN is essential for this patient population.

General discharge instructions for the patient undergoing GI surgery may include the following:

- Swelling inside the GI tract may produce a feeling of tightness; this should dissipate in 6 to 8 weeks.
- Solid foods should be added to the diet gradually. Chew solid foods well, and avoid gulping or eating fast or swallowing large bulk portions.
- Avoid carbonated beverages for 3 to 4 weeks to help prevent gas bloating.
- Plan small, frequent meals, because the feeling of fullness will come quickly.
- Keep the incisional area clean and dry.
- Increase exercise gradually to return to activities of daily living. Exercise regularly.
- Make an appointment for follow-up care with the surgeon.
- Follow written instructions with phone numbers as to whom to call and when. The patient should call the physician if any of the following develop:
  - Persistent fever (38.4°C [101°F] or higher)
  - Bleeding
  - Increased abdominal swelling or pain
  - Persistent nausea or vomiting
  - Chills
  - Persistent cough or shortness of breath

Procedure-specific instructions are usually necessary to fully assist the patient and caregivers with recovery and rehabilitation at home.

# Surgical Interventions

## ABDOMINAL INCISIONS

The abdominal cavity is surgically entered more than any other anatomic region. The site of the incision (Figure 11-9) is chosen to gain quick, easy access and exposure to underlying pathologic conditions; to minimize trauma, bleeding, and postoperative discomfort; to maximize wound strength; and to afford ample room to accomplish the intended surgery. Each incision has advantages and disadvantages regarding adequacy of exposure, length of time required for closure, disruption of surrounding blood and nerve supply, underlying muscles that must be cut or split, incidence of postoperative wound hernia, effect on pulmonary function, and cosmesis. Abdominal incisions permanently change the blood supply of the anterior abdominal wall and impact future surgeries and reconstructive options available to the patient. Any compromise of the skin, muscle, or blood supply by a prior incision may preclude the use of an otherwise optimal tissue flap for reconstruction after radical thoracic, breast, or GI surgery.[24] Developments in technology and surgical technique have advanced the use of minimally invasive approaches, which decreases the use and extent of abdominal incisions and preserves the integrity of the abdominal wall.

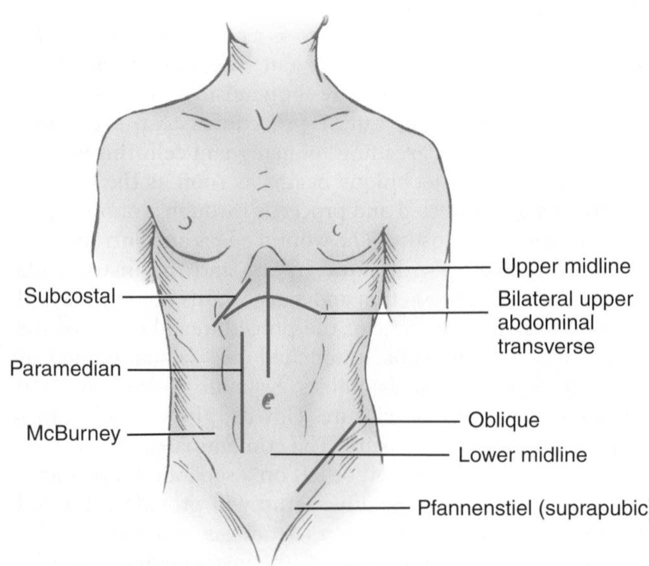


**FIGURE 11-9** Incisions made through the abdominal wall.

The abdominal wall consists of various tissue layers through which dissection is necessary to enter the abdominal cavity (Figure 11-10). Beneath the skin and subcutaneous fat, the layers include the fascia, muscles (internal and external oblique, rectus abdominis, transverse abdominis), preperitoneal fat, and peritoneum. The fascia layer, consisting of bands of tough fibrous connective tissue, surrounds the muscle anteriorly and posteriorly (Figure 11-11). The peritoneum is a serous membrane lining the abdominal cavity (parietal peritoneum) and the surface of the abdominal organs (visceral peritoneum).

## Vertical Midline Incisions

The vertical midline incision is the simplest abdominal incision to perform. It is an excellent primary incision and offers good exposure to any part of the abdominal cavity. Hemostasis

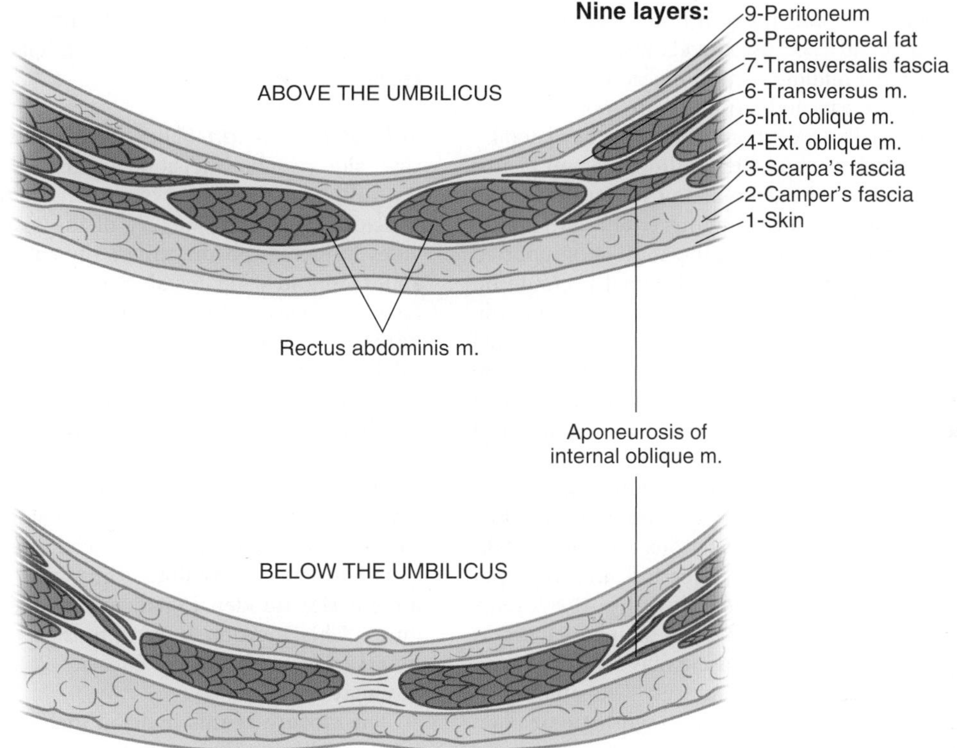


**FIGURE 11-10** Horizontal section of abdominal wall. Aponeurosis of internal oblique muscle splits into two sections, one lying anterior and the other posterior to rectus abdominis muscle, thereby forming an encasing sheath around muscle above umbilicus. Below umbilicus, aponeuroses of all muscles pass anterior to rectus. *m.*, Muscle. *Int.*, Internal; *Ext.*, external.

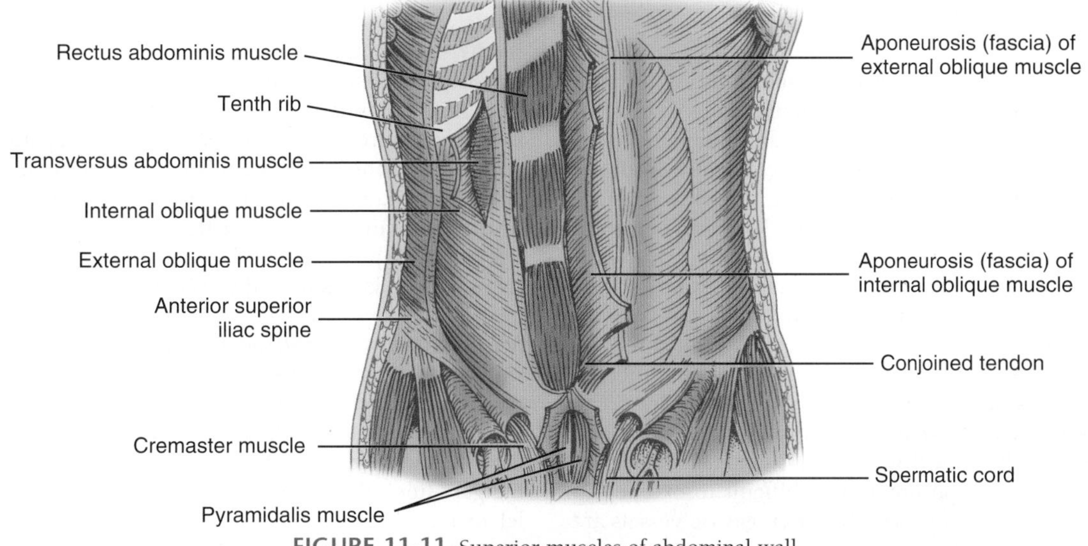


**FIGURE 11-11** Superior muscles of abdominal wall.

is easily achieved, and fewer layers are traversed. The incision can be extended from just below the sternal notch, distally around the umbilicus (which is avascular, tough connective tissue), back to the midline, and down to the symphysis pubis. The peritoneum is incised, and the round ligament of the liver may be divided. Postoperative hernias are more common above the umbilicus than below it. The midline crossover vasculature is permanently altered with this incision.

The paramedian incision, also called a *rectus* incision, is a vertical incision placed approximately 4 cm (2 inches) lateral to the midline on either side of the upper or lower abdomen. This incision is used infrequently because it adds little to the exposure obtained by way of a midline vertical incision. Paramedian incisions take longer to create and close and are more prone to herniation; this is especially true when they are farther lateral.

Closure of the paramedian and the midline incision begins with the peritoneum. The peritoneum and posterior fascia may be sutured as a single layer in a continuous stitch with an absorbable suture material. The suture line may be supported with retention sutures when outward abdominal pressure on the suture line is anticipated, bringing the risk for herniation, dehiscence, or evisceration. Retention sutures are placed through all layers of the wound, using a heavy #2-gauge nylon, polypropylene, or wire suture material. Wound dehiscence, a potential complication of abdominal surgery, is separation of the unhealed incision. When dehiscence is severe, bowel or other abdominal structures may protrude (evisceration). Dehiscence and evisceration are most common with midline vertical incisions. Risk factors include serious nutritional deficiencies, diabetes, steroid use, obesity, infection, and improper surgical closure.

Anterior fascia, subcutaneous tissue, and skin are closed as separate layers. Anterior fascia and muscle may be closed with interrupted nonabsorbable synthetic sutures. The subcutaneous layer may be closed with an absorbable synthetic or plain gut interrupted suture. Skin edges will be approximated and secured with interrupted nonabsorbable sutures, skin staples, subcuticular continuous closure with an absorbable suture material, skin-bonding adhesive, or sterile skin tape strips. There are many alternatives and variations to abdominal incision closure, based on the individual patient's need and the surgeon's preference.

### Oblique Incisions

***McBurney Incision.*** The McBurney muscle-splitting incision is used most commonly for open appendectomy. It is an 8-cm oblique incision that begins well below the umbilicus, goes through McBurney point (two thirds of the distance from the umbilicus to the anterior iliac spine in the right lower quadrant), and extends upward toward the right flank. The external oblique muscle and fascia are divided bluntly (split in the direction of their fibers) and are retracted. The internal oblique muscle, transverse muscle, and fascia are also split and retracted. When muscles are divided in line with their direction of pull, as is the case with muscle-splitting incisions, there is less chance of postoperative herniation or disruption. The peritoneum is incised transversely. This incision is quick and easy to close and allows a firm wound closure. However, it does not permit good exposure and is difficult to extend. To extend the incision medially, the inferior epigastric vessels are ligated and the rectus sheath incised transversely.

***Lower Oblique Inguinal Incision.*** An oblique right or left inguinal incision extends from the pubic tubercle to the anterior iliac crest, slightly above and parallel to the inguinal crease. This is the standard incision for open inguinal herniorrhaphy. Incision through the external oblique muscle gives access to the cremaster muscle, inguinal canal, and cord structures. This incision does not typically interrupt major abdominal arteries.

Long, lower abdominal oblique incisions may be used for transplant, urologic, and vascular procedures. These incisions require transection of the abdominal wall and flank musculature. These incisions may result in ligation of the deep inferior epigastric artery.

***Subcostal Incision.*** The subcostal incision is made on the right side (Kocher incision) when used for open procedures of the gallbladder, biliary system, and pancreas. A left subcostal incision is used for surgery of the spleen. This incision provides limited exposure unless the patient is short with a wide abdomen and wide costal margins. It provides good cosmetic results because it follows the skin lines and nerve damage is minimal. Tension on the skin edges is less than that of a vertical incision, permitting wider retraction and exposure with less respiratory impairment during the procedure.

This oblique incision begins in the epigastrium, extending laterally and obliquely downward to just below the costal margin (Figure 11-12). It continues through the rectus muscle, which is retracted or transversely divided. The superior epigastric artery is occasionally sacrificed. A chevron incision (joined right and left subcostal incisions) provides excellent exposure for gastric, duodenal, pancreatic, and portal system procedures. This incision interrupts the lateral blood supply and innervation to the rectus muscle. Postoperative muscle atrophy may occur.

The closure of this incision includes approximation of the falciform ligament, peritoneum, posterior rectus sheath, and anterior rectus sheath. Postoperatively, this is a strong yet painful incision.

### Transverse Incisions

***Pfannenstiel Incision.*** The Pfannenstiel incision is used for pelvic surgery. It is a curved transverse incision across the lower abdomen through the skin, subcutaneous layer, and rectus sheath, approximately 1 cm (½ inch) above the symphysis pubis, usually within the pubic hairline (Figure 11-13). This is the standard incision for open obstetric and gynecologic procedures. The rectus muscles are separated along the midline, and the peritoneum is entered through a midline vertical incision. This incision does not alter the vascular supply to the abdominal wall if the deep inferior epigastric artery is left intact. It provides good exposure and a strong postoperative scar that is cosmetically acceptable.

***Midabdominal Transverse Incision.*** The midabdominal transverse incision is used on the right or left for a retroperitoneal approach. The incision begins slightly above or below the umbilicus on either side, is carried laterally to the lumbar region at an angle between the ribs and the iliac crest, follows Langer's lines of tension of the abdominal wall, and runs parallel to vessels and nerves, rarely causing permanent damage. This is a standard incision for transverse colectomy or colos-

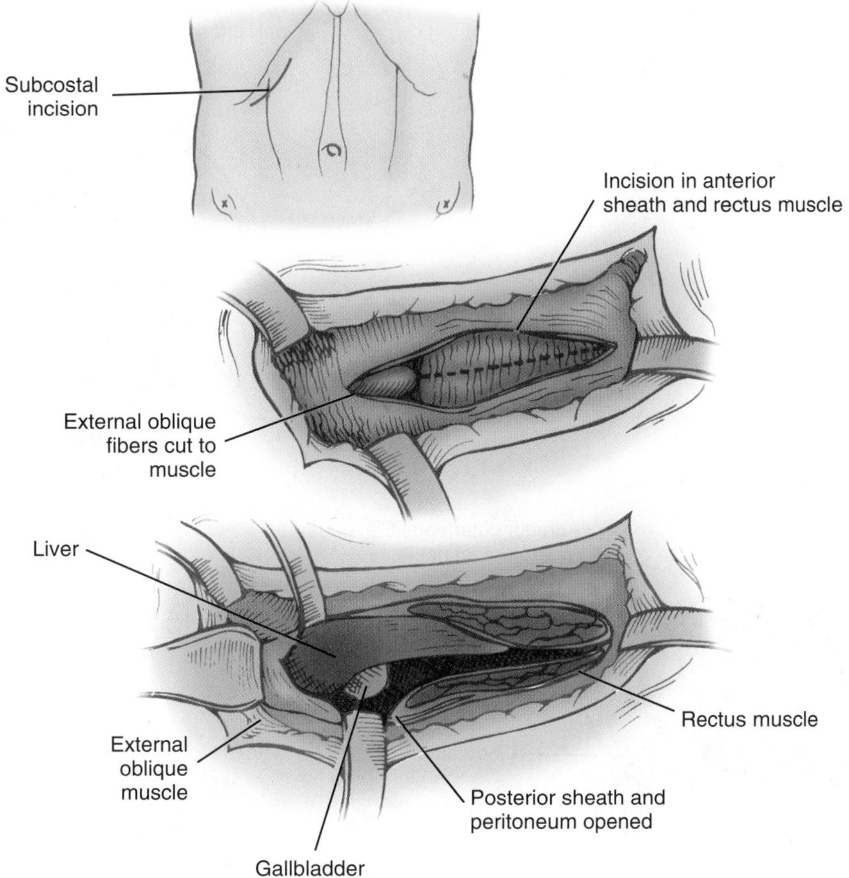


**FIGURE 11-12** Subcostal incision in upper right quadrant. Anterior sheath has been divided transversely, and muscle is exposed. Posterior sheath and peritoneum have been opened transversely.

tomy and choledochojejunostomy. The skin and subcutaneous tissue are incised, the anterior sheath is split, the rectus muscle is divided, and the vessels within the rectus are clamped and ligated. The posterior rectus sheath and peritoneum are cut in the direction of the fibers, preserving the intercostal nerves. The peritoneum is incised along the midline, and the incision is extended laterally to the oblique muscle.

***Thoracoabdominal Incision.*** The thoracoabdominal incision is the standard incision for surgery of the proximal stomach, distal esophagus, and anterior spine. The patient is placed in a lateral position. The incision begins at a midpoint between the xiphoid and umbilicus and extends posteriorly, across the seventh or eighth interspace and the midscapular line into the chest. The rectus, oblique, serratus, and intercostal muscles are divided down to peritoneum and pleura. The costal cartilage and diaphragm are then divided (Figure 11-14). This incision sacrifices the superior epigastric artery.

The wound is closed in layers with an interrupted suture technique. The peritoneum and pleura may be closed with an absorbable suture material, whereas the muscle and fascia layer may be closed with either an absorbable or nonabsorbable synthetic suture material. Skin edges are approximated and secured with suture, staples, skin bonding adhesive, or skin tape strips.

## LAPAROTOMY

An opening made through the abdominal wall into the peritoneal cavity is called a *laparotomy*. Surgical intervention may be necessary to repair or remove traumatized tissue, to cure disease processes by organ removal, or to examine by biopsy or otherwise visualize internal organs for diagnosis. Surgery may be indicated for diagnostic, therapeutic, palliative, or prophylactic reasons. Most procedures requiring a laparotomy involve the organs of the alimentary canal.

### Procedural Considerations

A basic laparotomy instrument set is used. An electrosurgical unit and suction are basic to performing laparotomy. The patient is positioned supine with arms extended on locked armboards at less than a 90-degree angle. General anesthesia with endotracheal intubation is the usual choice, although spinal or epidural anesthesia may be used. An indwelling urinary catheter may be inserted before the abdominal prep, which extends from above the nipple line to above the symphysis pubis. A forced-air warming blanket may be applied over the patient's upper body, arms, and head for thermoregulation. Synchronous compression leggings may be ordered and applied before induction to prevent deep venous blood pooling in the lower extremities.

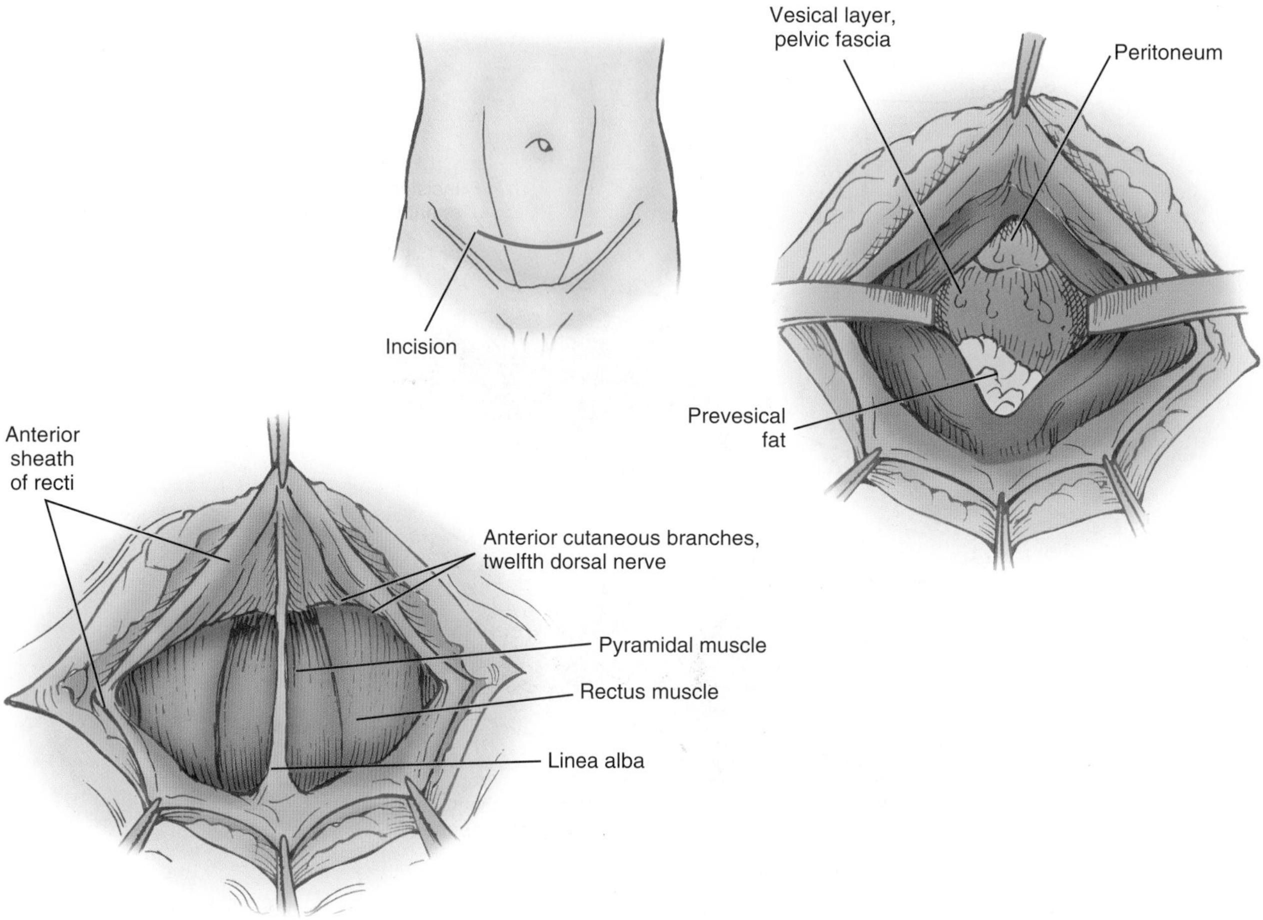

**FIGURE 11-13** Pfannenstiel incision (suprapubic).

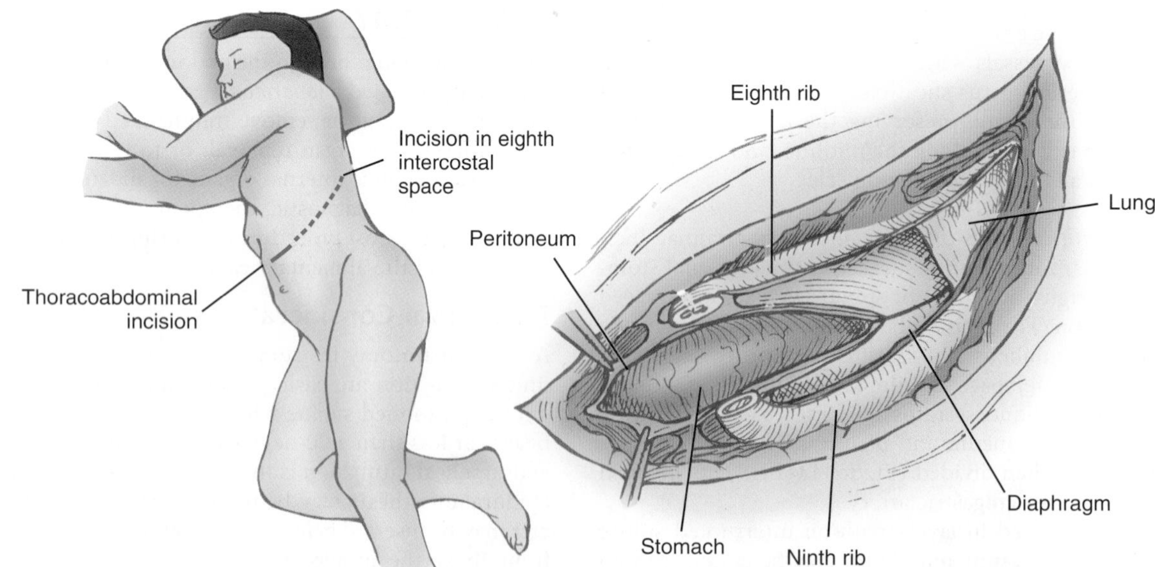


**FIGURE 11-14** Thoracoabdominal incision. Patient is placed on unaffected side. Incision is usually made from point midway between xiphoid process and umbilicus to costal margin at site of eighth costal cartilage. Dissection is carried down to peritoneum and pleura. Costal cartilage and diaphragm are divided, and stomach is exposed.

For a select population of patients, laparotomy leads to the formation of adhesions and the consequent potentials of chronic pain, infertility, or small bowel obstruction. Adhesions are fibrous bands of filamentous protein tissue that form a network of fibers, causing separate tissues and organs to adhere to one another in the abdominal cavity. Surgical separation of individual adhesions, called *adhesiolysis,* is not always effective, with adhesions re-forming, causing a cycle of symptoms and recurrent adhesive disease. Adhesion formation is caused by a defect in the process of normal tissue healing, prompted by tissue injury, inflammation, infection, or ischemia. The peritoneum is most associated with abdominal and pelvic adhesions. Introduction of microscopic particles, such as glove starch, gauze fibers, and suture materials, seems to promote their development.

Preventive measures include the following:

- Minimizing tissue trauma and inflammation with meticulous surgical technique
- Reducing the time that the abdomen is open
- Irrigating the abdomen with copious amounts of warmed solution before closure
- Administering antiinflammatory drugs such as corticosteroids and NSAIDs
- Mechanically separating the organs before closure with physical barriers such as omentum, polytetrafluoroethylene (PTFE), cellulose, or sodium hyaluronate membrane

## Operative Procedure

### *Laparotomy Opening*

1. The skin incision is made and carried to the fascia (Figure 11-15, *A*).
2. Hemostats may be used to control bleeding vessels. Clamped vessels are ligated with fine nonabsorbable ligatures (ties), or they are electrocoagulated.
3. The wound edges are retracted with small retractors.
4. With tissue forceps and scalpel, the external fascia is incised (Figure 11-15, *B*).
5. With Metzenbaum or curved Mayo scissors, electrosurgery, or a knife, the external oblique muscle is split the length of the incision. Bleeding vessels are controlled with hemostats, ligating clips, medium or fine ligatures, or electrocoagulating current.
6. The external oblique muscle is retracted.
7. The internal oblique and transverse muscles are split, parallel to the fibers, up to the rectus sheath with a scalpel or scissors. These muscles are then retracted.
8. The peritoneum is exposed, grasped with smooth tissue forceps, and nicked with a #10 blade (Figure 11-15, *C*).
9. Sponges, laparotomy pads, and suction are used as needed. Culture samples may be taken at this time.
10. The peritoneal incision is extended the length of the wound with Metzenbaum or Mayo scissors.

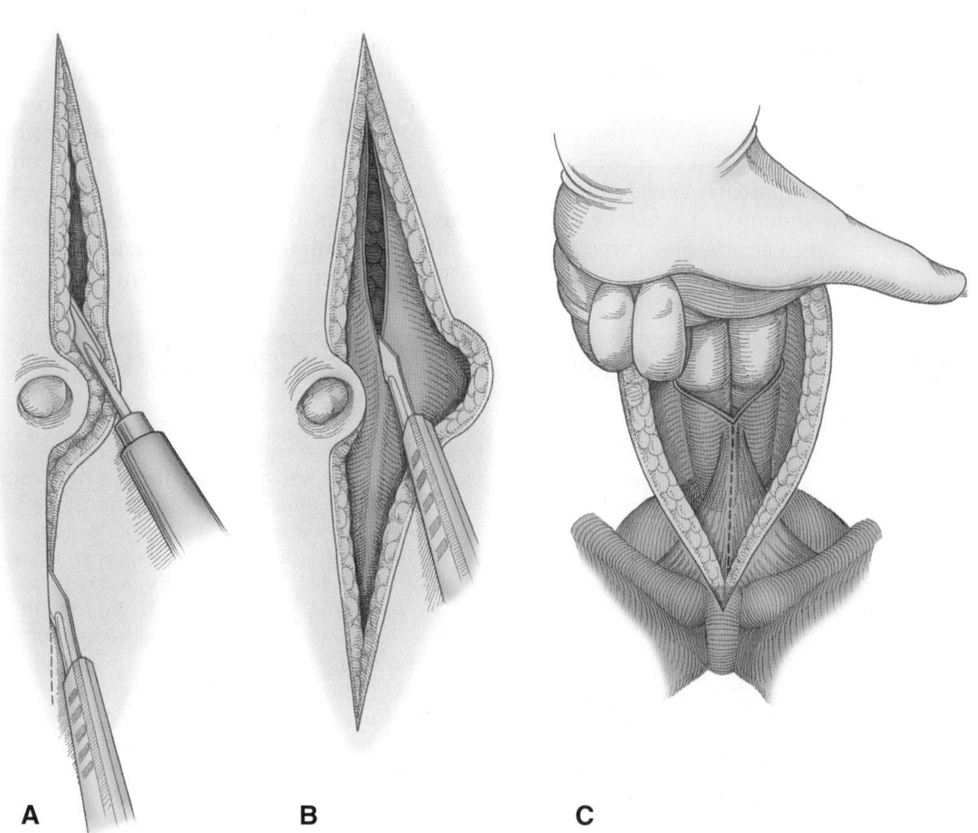


**FIGURE 11-15** **A,** Midline laparotomy incision around the umbilicus. **B,** External fascia is incised. **C,** Entry into the peritoneal cavity.

11. The peritoneum is retracted with large Richardson retractors for initial exploration.
12. Once the affected organs are identified, a self-retaining retractor, such as a Balfour or the Bookwalter retractor system, may be used to establish adequate and hands-free exposure.

### *Laparotomy Closure*

1. Two tissue forceps or clamps are used to approximate the peritoneal edges, and the peritoneum is closed with a continuous synthetic absorbable suture or interrupted nonabsorbable sutures. The internal oblique fascia is usually closed with the peritoneum. Muscle tissue is approximated and may or may not be sutured.
2. The external oblique fascia is closed with interrupted sutures, staples, or both. Retraction is necessary as the various layers are closed. Richardson retractors are commonly used.
3. Fine (3-0 or 4-0) absorbable sutures are usually employed to close the subcutaneous or subcuticular tissue. Retraction is provided with laparotomy pads or small retractors.
4. Skin edges are held with Adson, Russian, or medium-toothed forceps and approximated with interrupted 3-0 or 4-0 silk, nylon, or other nonabsorbable sutures on a cutting needle. A cosmetically pleasing wound closure may be achieved in patients with limited tension on the incision by using a subcuticular closure with a 3-0 or 4-0 nonabsorbable suture. Skin staples or clips, sterile adhesive strips, or skin-bonding adhesive is often used to approximate skin edges. Retention sutures of #1 or #2 nonabsorbable suture material may be used. Prepackaged retention bridges or rubber-tubing bolsters are used to protect the incision site.

## LAPAROSCOPY

Laparoscopy is a technique-based approach to abdominal surgery for minimal access into the abdomen to achieve the same surgical result as open laparotomy. Laparoscopic surgery is often referred to as minimally invasive surgery (MIS), wherein the surgery is performed with instruments (rather than the surgeon's hands) inside the body, yet manipulated from outside the body. Procedures described as "laparoscopically assisted" combine laparoscopic surgical manipulation of tissue with enlargement of one of the port incisions, permitting the surgeon direct access, or hand contact, to the operative tissue. The surgeon may bring a portion of the surgical tissue out onto the abdominal surface to achieve the repair outside the body (*extracorporeal* repair). *Intracorporeal* refers to inside the abdomen. Laparoscopically assisted surgery may also refer to laparoscopic dissection and resection with an open approach to remove the surgical specimen.

Laparoscopy is typically contraindicated in patients with extensive adhesions from prior surgeries. Patients with bleeding disorders or pregnancy also pose a risk.[14] Advanced cardiac or pulmonary disease may preclude the option of a minimal access approach. Potential complications include trocar site bleeding (Patient Safety), vascular injury, hemorrhage, perforation or laceration of organs, infection, anastomotic leaks, ileus, strictures, and pulmonary problems. The surgeon may have to convert to an open procedure in the presence of adhesions, hemorrhage, fixed small bowel, unusual anatomy, unexpected findings, or instrument failure. The potential for conversion to an open approach is discussed with the patient before surgery and documented on the consent form by the surgeon.

Laparoscopy offers advantages over the conventional open approach in many GI procedures in a variety of selected areas. Surgical repair of the involved GI system, postoperative recurrence of disease, and overall survival are similar between open and laparoscopic approaches for the same surgery. Operative times may vary, dependent on many variables, including unusual occurrences, the surgeon's skill and technique, and instrumentation. Parenteral analgesia needs are the same or may be less than in the open laparotomy approach. These patients typically report less postoperative discomfort because of the absence of a large abdominal incision yet may report muscle discomfort in the area of a working-port incision where significant manipulation of instruments occurs. Postoperative flatus and first bowel movement may occur 1 day sooner than

### PATIENT SAFETY

#### Perioperative Considerations in Trocar Safety

Trocars may be bladed, bladeless, or blunt-tipped. To gain access to the abdominal cavity, the selected trocar must pass through the abdominal wall layers without injuring blood vessels or internal organs. Although the surgeon has primary responsibility for preventing these and other trocar injuries, the perioperative nurse should understand the risks related to such instrumentation, as well as have a basic understanding of the techniques for trocar insertion. The perioperative nurse's review of the patient's history should focus on previous surgeries that might have contributed to the formation of adhesions, patient weight (in thin patients, the distance between vascular structures and the abdominal wall is considerably short; in obese patients, more force may be required), and patients with enlarged livers or spleen. Of special concern is any trocar with a shield. With this device, the scrub person and surgeon must ensure that the shield is retracted before insertion and kept retracted. If it is not, too much force is required. Further, the shield itself may lock into place prematurely when pressure is reduced before full penetration into the abdomen.

Other important safety issues with trocars are how far they reach into the abdomen. Registered Nurse First Assistants (RNFAs) assisting in access procedures during minimally invasive surgery (MIS) should develop skills to detect the passage of the tip through the peritoneum, avoiding possible injury to internal organs. When working in the upper abdomen, the RNFA should use maximum countertraction when inserting a trocar toward the diaphragm. This assists in avoiding major blood vessels. Often, aiming the trocar parallel to the spine and off midline helps avoid vascular injury.

Modified from Chang C, Rege RV: Minimally invasive surgery. In Townsend CM: *Sabiston textbook of surgery,* ed 17, Philadelphia, 2004, Saunders; Laparoscopic access, *Point of View* 44(1):20-26, 2005; Rad BN, Beart RW: Minimally invasive surgery—laparoscopic colectomy. In Souba WW and others: *ACS surgery—principles and practice*, New York, 2005, WebMD.

for conventional surgery patients. Resumption of oral intake may also be sooner in this group.[22,31] The minimal access approach offers a faster recovery of pulmonary function, fewer postoperative complications, less potential for surgical site infections, improved cosmesis, shorter recovery period, and quicker return to former activities of daily living.

### Procedural Considerations

Minimal access surgery requires the use of specially designed instruments, telescopes, trocars with cannulas, suction and irrigation devices, retractors, electrosurgery, $CO_2$ introduction devices, stapling instruments and appliers, and video image equipment. Surgeons must train to become proficient and develop a two-dimensional working knowledge of surgical anatomy. The video camera, light source, and monitors provide indirect visualization of the surgical site, enhanced with magnification and bright illumination.

### Operative Procedure

1. Initial entry is made in the periumbilical region with percutaneous puncture with an insufflation (Verres) needle (closed technique) or a sharp trocar in a sheath (direct technique). A cut-down technique (Hasson technique) may be used with a small incision through to the fascia with a #15 blade. The trocar is then introduced through and into the peritoneal cavity. In the direct optical technique, an optical trocar is inserted to visualize trocar placement before insufflation.
2. Pneumoperitoneum is established with insufflation of 3 to 4 liters of $CO_2$ into the peritoneal cavity to achieve an intraabdominal pressure of 12 to 15 mm Hg.
3. The needle is removed and replaced with a 10-mm or 11-mm trocar. The rigid laparoscope, with a video camera and cord coupled to the telescope eyepiece end, is inserted into the port for visualization. Two to six more ports may be established to facilitate the entry and use of an endoscopic fan retractor; various grasping, dissection, cutting, and electrosurgery instruments; ultrasonic scalpel dissector; suction-irrigation devices; laser fibers; endoscopic clip and staple appliers; and specimen retrieval graspers. The port sites are selected to permit all the instrument tips to converge at the primary surgical working spot, maximizing the surgeon's ergonomics and enhancing performance.[16]
4. The surgical exploration, dissection, resection, anastomosis, inspection, and irrigation are accomplished.
5. $CO_2$ is exhausted, and the ports are removed. The umbilical incision is closed with a 3-0 or 4-0 nonabsorbable synthetic suture. The remaining port incisions are closed with the same suture, adhesive strips, or skin-bonding adhesive. A small dressing or bandage is applied.

## ENDOSCOPIC PROCEDURES

GI endoscopy has transformed all aspects of diagnosis and treatment of patients with diseases of the GI system. Endoscopic procedures that permit direct or video visual inspection of the contents and walls of the esophagus, stomach, duodenum, and colon are significant tools in (1) routine screening for individuals at risk for GI disease[34] (Research Highlight), (2) establishing a diagnosis, (3) determining preferred treatment of a disease process, or (4) follow-up on completion of a treatment regimen or surgery. GI endoscopy, enhanced by technologic advances in imaging, instrumentation, and accessory devices, has evolved into an interventional discipline, offering nonsurgical approaches to cure and palliation of symptoms of selected GI diseases and conditions. Common GI endoscopy procedures include esophagogastroduodenoscopy (EGD) (also referred to as gastroscopy or upper endoscopy), small bowel endoscopy (also referred to as push enteroscopy or double-balloon enteroscopy), colonoscopy (also referred to as lower endoscopy), and sigmoidoscopy (also referred to as a "flex sig").

Endoscopic procedures may be performed with the patient under local anesthesia, with IV moderate sedation/analgesia, or with general anesthesia in selected patients. This permits a safe

### RESEARCH HIGHLIGHT

#### Colonoscopic Screening of Average-Risk Women for Colorectal Neoplasia

This study compared the diagnostic results of flexible sigmoidoscopy alone with colonoscopy in a large sample of women and compared those results with an equally matched population of men in a similar study (the Veterans Affairs Cooperative Study 380) for age-matched men and women with negative fecal occult blood tests (FOBTs) and no family history of colon cancer.

The primary aim was to compare the presence of advanced neoplasia in the proximal colon in patients without distal presence with those with distal presence of neoplasia. The secondary aim was to determine if a patient with advanced neoplasia would have had this lesion found if she only had a flexible sigmoidoscopy. Flexible sigmoidoscopy examines the distal rectosigmoid colon distal to but not always as far as the splenic flexure. This segment of bowel represents one third of the entire colon.

A total of 1483 women received complete colonoscopy with no significant complications. The mean age was 58.9 years, and 15.7% had a family history of colorectal cancer (CRC); 20.4% had a total of 446 advanced neoplastic findings, and 15.5% had small adenomas.

If all the 1483 women had only had a flexible sigmoidoscopy, advanced neoplastic lesions would have been missed in 47 patients, or 33%, and only 25 would have been identified. This means that of 72 women who were identified with advanced disease only 25 would be detected with flexible sigmoidoscopy.

After matching men and women who had no family history of CRC and negative FOBTs, men were found to have more advanced lesions than women. Also, the diagnostic yield was higher in men. Men 50 to 69 years old had a higher prevalence of advanced lesions than women, but prevalence was similar for both men and women after 70 years of age. This trend suggests that women's biologic or behavioral factors may delay advanced disease.

The findings of this comparative study suggest that the majority of cases of advanced neoplasia would be missed if women only underwent flexible sigmoidoscopy; however, flexible sigmoidoscopy seems to be a more effective screening tool in men than women. This study recommends colonoscopy for CRC in asymptomatic average-risk women (see Best Practice).

Modified from Schoenfoeld P and others: Colonoscopic screening of average risk women for colorectal neoplasia, *New England Journal of Medicine* 352:2061-2068, 2005. Accessed May 26, 2005, on-line: www.healthorbit.ca/NewsDetail.asp?opt=1&nltid=013230505.

and complete examination. IV moderate sedation provides a depressed level of consciousness and tolerance of a potentially uncomfortable procedure, yet patients retain their ability to maintain their airway and respond appropriately to physical and verbal stimuli. The goal of IV moderate sedation is to use the least amount of sedation while providing comfort to the patient. Sedation is administered by the attending physician/interventionalist, anesthesia provider, or a registered nurse competent in monitoring the patient under IV moderate sedation. The patient is monitored for heart rate and rhythm, oxygen saturation, blood pressure, respirations, level of consciousness, and comfort during and immediately after the procedure until the patient is stable and ready for discharge or transfer.

Preprocedure preparation for elective procedures includes limiting ingestion of solid foods and liquids for a prescribed period. Bowel preparation with diet limitation, bowel cleansing preparations, and sometimes enemas will be prescribed before lower endoscopy procedures.

Flexible endoscopes are semicritical patient care devices that must undergo high-level disinfection before each patient use. They are easily damaged by misuse and should be handled according to the manufacturer's recommendations. They must be leak-tested, decontaminated, reprocessed, and dried after each patient use. They must be stored in an appropriate secure and ventilated endoscope closet. Endoscopic accessories, such as biopsy forceps, snares, cytology brushes, and fine needle aspiration (FNA) catheters, must be sterile because they are considered critical devices that invade the mucosal barrier.

## Esophagogastroduodenoscopy (Upper Endoscopy)

EGD is visualization of the esophagus, stomach, and proximal duodenum. It is used for diagnosis, treatment, and documentation of abnormalities with biopsy, brush cytology, polypectomy, electrosurgery, thermal coagulation, laser therapy, dilation, banding or sclerosing of esophageal varices, removal of foreign bodies, insertion of an esophageal prosthesis, and various interventional procedures for gastroesophageal reflux disease (GERD), Barrett's esophagus, and percutaneous endoscopic gastrostomy (PEG) tubes. When an EGD is performed with local anesthesia or sedation, the patient is usually given no solid food for 6 to 8 hours before the procedure but may drink liquids up to 2 hours before.

***Procedural Considerations.*** The patient's position for EGD may depend on the areas to be visualized, but a left lateral supine or low Fowler position is commonly used. For inspection of lesions in the gastric fundus and cardia, an upright sitting position may be used. A protective bite-block is placed in the patient's mouth to protect the scope and the patient's teeth from injury. Instrumentation will include a gastroscope and video system (optional), biopsy forceps, suction, water-soluble lubricant, saline and water for irrigation, and electrosurgery capability.

A topical local anesthetic (applied to the posterior pharynx) along with IV moderate sedation is the most common technique. Monitoring of airway, vital signs, and oxygenation is done by a perioperative or endoscopy nurse skilled and credentialed in moderate sedation and advanced cardiac life support or an anesthesia provider.

A light source with air and water infusion capability and a water bottle for irrigation are required. Suction, aspiration tubes, and a cup of saline for the biopsy specimen should be available. Lubricating jelly is placed over the sheath of the gastroscope for ease in placement. An electrosurgical unit and cord should be available for fulguration of a lesion or coagulation of a bleeding site.

#### *Operative Procedure*

1. The gastroscope is completely covered with a thin coat of water-soluble lubricating jelly.
2. During introduction of the gastroscope, the patient's head and neck must remain in the sagittal plane of the spine so that the axis of the mouth is in line with the esophagus.
3. The gastroscope is slowly passed down through the nasopharynx into the esophagus, stomach, and duodenum.
4. The mucosal surface is inspected, and contents may be aspirated for cytologic analysis. A biopsy may be performed.
5. After the procedure the patient will be monitored and the gag reflex checked for return before fluids are offered.

## Small Bowel Enteroscopy

The small bowel has traditionally been a difficult segment of the GI tract to reach for endoscopic visualization. Enteroscopy can be approached orally or through the anus using an adult or pediatric colonoscope, or a push enteroscope that measures 200 to 250 cm in length. Push enteroscopy advances the scope deep into the small bowel. A balloon on the tip of the scope permits it to be held in place. The patient receives IV metoclopramide (Reglan), promoting peristaltic advancement of the scope. The small bowel is examined as the scope is slowly withdrawn. This procedure may take 6 to 8 hours.[43] Push enteroscopy is useful for examining areas of bleeding and strictures.

Double-balloon enteroscopy employs an enteroscope with a balloon on the end of the scope and on the end of the overtube, which creates a traction system permitting the small bowel to pleat itself onto the overtube, preventing overstretching of the small intestines. This technique permits visualization and therapeutic maneuvers such as biopsies, coagulation of small bleeders, and lysis of strictures.[27,44]

## Colonoscopy and Sigmoidoscopy (Lower Endoscopy)

Colonoscopy is an endoscopic examination of the colon from the rectum to the ileocecal valve. The bowel wall is inspected for abnormalities such as bleeding, polyps, inflammation, ulceration, or tumors during both the insertion and withdrawal of the colonoscope (Best Practice). Colonoscopy facilitates biopsy, removal of polyps, electrocoagulation or laser treatment of tumors or bleeders, dilation, decompression, and provision for a video and photographic record of the procedure and findings. Sigmoidoscopy, both flexible and rigid, provides access and visualization of the sigmoid or descending colon to the level of the splenic flexure. Colonoscopy or sigmoidoscopy may be performed before colon or sigmoid resection for surgical localization of tumor site with India ink tattooing or clip placement. This permits the surgeon to identify the tumor site, viewing the marked site from the serosal side of the colon by laparotomy or laparoscopy access.

Endoscopy can be performed through an ostomy stoma to inspect an anastomosis site or identify recurrence of disease or bleeding. Reservoir pouches can also be inspected after surgi-

BEST PRACTICE

### Colonoscopy as Best Test for Colorectal Cancer

Colorectal cancer is the third most commonly diagnosed cancer and the second leading cause of cancer death in the United States. Approximately 104,950 colon cancers and 40,340 rectal cancers were predicted to occur in 2005.[1] The incidence of colorectal cancer is increasing, while the mortality rate is decreasing, probably in part because of the increase in screening. Incidence is higher in men than in women. Colorectal cancer survival is closely related to early clinical diagnosis. Survival rate is 90% for early localized cancers, yet only 39% of colorectal cancers are diagnosed at this stage.[1] There are many risk factors, yet about 75% of colorectal cancer cases occur in people with no risk factors.

Screening studies, including fecal occult blood test (FOBT), sigmoidoscopy, and colonoscopy, have been recommended for those at risk as well as for all adults past the age of 50 years.[34] Several experts have recommended combined screening with FOBT and sigmoidoscopy.

The American Cancer Society[1] recommends that starting at age 50 years men and women should begin screening with one of the studies below:

- FOBT or fecal immunochemical test (FIT) every year
- Flexible sigmoidoscopy every 5 years
- Annual FOBT or FIT and flexible sigmoidoscopy every 5 years
- Double-contrast barium enema every 5 years
- Colonoscopy every 10 years

A study of 2885 veterans, ages 50 to 75 years, who volunteered for colonoscopy found that sigmoidoscopy and FOBT missed 25% of tumors and precancerous growths detected by colonoscopy. Colonoscopy offers the potential to view the entire colon and both identify and remove premalignant lesions throughout the colon and rectum. Colonoscopy proved far superior to the other common tests for detection of colon cancer.

With the development of unique new technologies and sciences, such as fecal DNA testing and virtual CT colonoscopy, many options are available to yield diagnostic data. Polypectomy surveillance will have future implications for routine screening. At this time, evidence, guidelines, and practice promote colonoscopy as the preferred screening for colorectal cancer.

Modified from Agency for Health Care Policy and Research: *AHCPR Publication no. 97-0302: colorectal cancer screening, summary, evidence report: number 1,* Rockville, Md, 1996.The Agency. Accessed February 15, 2006, on-line: www.ahrq.gov/clinic/colorsum.htm; American Cancer Society: *Cancer facts and figures 2005,* Atlanta, 2005, American Cancer Society; Crim R, Hurley J: *Does everyone need a colonoscopy? A surgeon's view.* Accessed May 6, 2005, on-line: surgery.medscape.com/ACCC/OncIssues/2001/v16.n02/oi1602.02.crim/pnt-oi1602.02.c; Lieberman DA, Weiss DG: One-time screening for colorectal cancer with combined fecal occult-blood testing and examination of the distal colon, *The New England Journal of Medicine* 345(8):555-560, 2001.

cal healing for anastomosis integrity, inflammation, bleeding, and other abnormalities.

The patient must receive a clear liquid diet the day before the colonoscopy and sigmoidoscopy and may receive bowel-cleansing agents such as citrate of magnesia or a commercial bowel prep solution. Enemas may be necessary before the procedure.

***Procedural Considerations.*** The instruments and equipment that must be available for performing colonoscopy and sigmoidoscopy include a colonoscope or flexible sigmoidoscope, video camera and monitors (optional), a light source, an air-insufflation device with water bottle for irrigation, a biopsy forceps, snares, cytology brush, electrosurgical-fulguration-desiccation unit and appropriate accessories, lubricating jelly, and suction.

#### *Operative Procedure*

1. The patient is positioned on the left side with knees bent.
2. The well-lubricated colonoscope is passed slowly into the anal canal and advanced continuously until it reaches the cecum for colonoscopy. The endoscopist or surgeon may ask the nurse or technician to apply gentle abdominal pressure to assist advancement of the scope around the splenic or hepatic flexures. With sigmoidoscopy, only the left colon is examined. Flexible sigmoidoscopy may be accomplished in a cooperative patient without the benefit of sedation.
3. After the endoscopic examination, the patient will be observed for postprocedural bleeding, pain, signs of perforation, or reaction to medications.

## Procedures for Gastroesophageal Reflux Disease

Gastroesophageal reflux disease (GERD) is described as a condition of backflow of gastric or duodenal contents into the distal esophagus, causing pain, heartburn, coughing, and respiratory distress. GERD may also present with an incompetence of the distal esophageal valve to the stomach or lower esophageal sphincter (LES). Chronic GERD can lead to erosive esophagitis, asthma, dysphagia, aspiration pneumonia,[42] and Barrett's esophagus. Several innovative, nonsurgical interventional endoscopic techniques have been developed to minimize or prevent the reflux of stomach acid into the esophagus, controlling GERD symptoms by enhancing the competency of the LES. These procedures, accomplished through an EGD, or upper endoscope, reinforce the LES by plicating and sewing the inner lumen of the esophageal junction to re-fashion the valve, tightening the tissue above the LES to create a stricture, or implanting devices to narrow the LES lumen.

The Stretta (Curon Medical) procedure is a radiofrequency therapy–delivering heat energy through an endoscopically introduced balloon catheter to the distal esophagus creating thermal lesions to tighten the tissue.[29]

The EndoCinch (Bard Medical) technique involves dilating the lumen of the esophagus before passing the EndoCinch device through an EGD scope. The device is a sewing capsule that pinches or pleats mucosal folds and anchors them in place with a suture. Several plications are placed in a circumferential or staggered vertical pattern.[18,40]

The Wilson-Cook Sewing System (Wilson-Cook Medical) is another submucosal plication device that suctions a small fold of tissue into the lumen of the scope accessory, plicates, sutures, and knots the tissue pleat.[40]

## Procedures for Barrett's Esophagus

Cellular changes, or dysplasia, of the mucosa of the distal esophagus is called Barrett's esophagus, a precursor for cancer of the esophagus. Twenty percent of patients with GERD may develop Barrett's.[42] Patients who experience progression of dysplasia in spite of medical therapies such as histamine blockers and proton pump inhibitors, may be treated with one of several endoscopic techniques targeted to eliminate the dysplastic tissue, prevent or eliminate strictures, and promote the regrowth of normal esophageal mucosa.

Endoscopic mucosal resection (EMR) is an interventional technique to remove submucosal flat or depressed lesions.[35] EUS is used to determine depth of invasion into the esophageal wall, and the lesion or dysplastic tissue is then injected with isotonic saline, hypertonic saline, or saline with epinephrine to lift the lesion away from the muscle layer, creating a polyplike lesion. This tissue bulge is then suctioned into a cap secured to the end of the scope and resected with a rigid wire snare and removed. The saline creates a cushion to protect the muscle wall from perforation and facilitates snare resection. This technique also provides a tissue specimen for histologic examination. Areas of bleeding can be endoscopically electrocoagulated.[34]

Photodynamic therapy (PDT) is a technique using laser light ablation of dysplastic tissue that uptakes a photosensitizer drug, Photofrin II (sodium porfimer), which is activated by the laser. The drug is administered 48 hours before the procedure to allow for tissue uptake. Normal tissue will excrete the drug sooner than abnormal or dysplastic tissues. The drug is retained in the mucosal layer, which limits the depth of the laser effect. After 48 hours the patient returns for the endoscopic procedure. The laser fiber is introduced through the scope channel, and laser light is directed toward the mucosa, causing tissue destruction and cell death of those areas identified by the uptake of the photosensitizer. The patient may continue to be sensitive to light for 60 to 90 days following the injection and must take precautions to prevent cutaneous burns.[20,42,46] Unlike EMR, PDT does not provide a tissue specimen. PDT is often combined with endoscopic mucosal resection. PDT and EMR can also be used to treat the gastric and colonic mucosa.

### Self-Expanding Metal Stents

Self-expanding medical stents (SEMSs) are medical devices that expand within a lumen to maintain patency in an area constrained by stricture or tumor. They are used in the esophagus or colon, advanced across the obstruction, and released to remain in place. They are preloaded in a constrained, or closed, position on a delivery catheter, introduced through an endoscope with fluoroscopy guidance, and deployed, applying radial force that holds them in place. Stents may also be made of silicone. Although initial complications are low, stents may migrate, perforate, become impacted with food, cause bleeding or fistula development, or become obstructed with tumor overgrowth. Stent placement is frequently a palliative procedure.[42]

## SURGERY OF THE ESOPHAGUS

### Esophagectomy

Esophageal cancer is the sixth most common cancer worldwide and is notorious for its aggressive progression of intramural invasion of the esophageal wall and lymphatic metastasis.[50] Esophageal cancer may be of adenocarcinoma or squamous cell type, each with an equally poor prognosis when treated in late stages. As many as 50% of patients with esophageal cancer may be ineligible for surgery because of late stage of disease at diagnosis, debilitating multisystem conditions, infection, and malnutrition.[50]

Esophagectomy can be accomplished by several different approaches and procedures: transthoracic, transhiatal, and video-assisted thoracotomy surgery (VATS) or laparoscopic-assisted approach. A segment of the colon or jejunum may be used as a reconstructive conduit in the patient with prior partial or total gastrectomy.

***Procedural Considerations.*** Instrumentation includes a basic thoracotomy set, basic laparotomy set, vascular instruments, and a GI instrument set. Long versions of the basic instruments, deep retractors, linear stapling devices, and vascular ligating clips should also be available. Laparoscopic and thoracoscopic instrumentation and video equipment should be available for the VATS approach. The patient will be positioned and secured in the preferred position for the intended surgical approach after induction of general anesthesia. A double-lumen endotracheal tube will be placed with the patient under anesthesia in order to deflate the lung for a thoracotomy approach. Critical monitoring devices, such as arterial lines and pulmonary artery catheters, will be inserted. An indwelling urinary catheter is inserted. Measures are taken to ensure that the patient's body temperature is maintained. Any of these procedures may be modified with laparoscopic, thoracoscopic, or mini-laparotomy or mini-thoracotomy access. Postoperative pain management may be augmented with interscalene perineural blockade for shoulder pain. Patients undergoing esophagectomy usually go to the intensive care unit (ICU).

### Transhiatal Esophagectomy

1. Transhiatal esophagectomy removes two thirds to the entire thoracic esophagus through an upper midline abdominal incision and an incision in the neck above the left clavicle. The abdominal component may be approached laparoscopically. Thoracotomy is avoided.
2. Accessible lymph nodes are removed for staging purposes. Not all lymph nodes can be reached.
3. The stomach is mobilized and fashioned into a tubular shape at the greater curvature with surgical staples.
4. The tubular stomach segment is tunneled up through the posterior mediastinum to the left cervical incision. This procedure is often called a gastric pull-up.
5. The stomach is reconstructed with the fundus of the stomach attached to the remaining cervical portion of the proximal esophagus with an end-to-side anastomosis. The fundus is also sutured to the cervical prevertebral fascia.
6. A pyloromyotomy or pyloroplasty is then done to increase stomach emptying. This often results in postoperative "dumping syndrome" and reflux.
7. A jejunostomy tube is placed for postoperative enteral nutrition.
8. Postoperative hoarseness and dysphagia are common because of ipsilateral nerve damage.

### Transthoracic Esophagectomy

Transthoracic esophagectomy is indicated for disease of the middle third of the esophagus and high-grade dysplasia in Barrett's esophagus. This approach permits complete lymph node dissection under direct vision and combines a left-sided thoracoabdominal incision or separate right posterior lateral thoracotomy and a midline abdominal incision. The latter describes the traditional Ivor Lewis approach. Another variation, sometimes called the "three-hole esophagectomy," combines a cervical, right thoracotomy, and midline laparotomy approach for proximal tumors. The single incision thoracoabdominal incision provides the best exposure for low gastroesophageal junction tumors and is indicated for patients with cardiac and pulmonary disease.

### *Operative Procedure*

1. The skin incision is carried downward midway between the vertebral border of the scapula and the spinous processes to the eighth rib and then forward along this rib to the costochondral junction. The extent of the vertical portion of the incision depends on the location of the tumor.
2. The wound is retracted, and bleeding vessels are ligated or coagulated.
3. The chest cavity is opened, and the rib spreader is placed. Moist packs are placed, and the lung is retracted with a Deaver or Harrington retractor.
4. The mediastinal pleura is incised with long Metzenbaum scissors and long plain forceps in line with the esophagus and the lesion.
5. The esophagus is dissected free from the aorta with dry gauze dissectors.
6. Suture ligatures of 2-0 and 3-0 nonabsorbable material are used for controlling bleeding vessels.
7. The diaphragm is opened, and a series of traction sutures are attached.
8. The stomach is mobilized by dissection of its ligamental attachment with long scissors and curved thoracic clamps.
9. The left gastric artery is clamped, cut, and doubly ligated with 2-0 nonabsorbable suture and a suture ligature of 3-0 nonabsorbable material. The sterile field is prepared for the open method of anastomosis.
10. The stomach is transected well below the lesion with the selected resection instruments.
11. Closure of the stomach is completed with two rows of intestinal sutures of 2-0 synthetic absorbable suture and sometimes with an additional row of 3-0 nonabsorbable sutures for reinforcement. A linear stapling device may be used as well.
12. A separate circular opening is usually made in the upper portion of the stomach for anastomosis to the esophagus.
13. Two Allen clamps or a stapler type of clamp is applied above the stricture, and the freed esophagus is divided.
14. The circular opening in the stomach and the transected end of the esophagus are anastomosed. The mucosal layers are approximated. The muscular layers of the esophagus and stomach are closed by two rows of interrupted sutures. A mechanical end-to-end anastomosing (EEA) surgical stapling device may also be used to accomplish the gastroesophageal anastomosis.
15. The stomach is anchored to the pleura, and the edges of the diaphragm are sutured to the wall of the stomach with interrupted sutures of 3-0 or 2-0 nonabsorbable material.
16. The pleura is cleansed with warm normal saline irrigation that is suctioned off.
17. A thoracic catheter is inserted for closed drainage. The chest wall is closed as described for thoracotomy.

## Video-Assisted Thoracotomy Surgery (VATS)

1. VATS is accomplished in three stages beginning with thoracoscopic dissection and mobilization of the esophagus.
2. The second stage is the laparoscopic dissection, mobilization, and tubular construction of the stomach. Pyloroplasty will also be performed laparoscopically.
3. The third stage is the open cervical incision anastomosis.[50]

## Excision of Esophageal Diverticulum

Excision of an esophageal diverticulum, sometimes referred to as *Zenker diverticulum,* is removal of a weakening in the wall of the esophagus that collects small amounts of food and causes a sensation of fullness in the neck. Because diverticula usually occur in the cervical portion of the esophagus, excision completely relieves symptoms.

***Procedural Considerations.*** Instrumentation includes a thyroid set (see Chapter 16) with the addition of two Pennington clamps, six Halstead curved mosquito hemostats, two 5-inch Adson forceps, and two lateral retractors. The patient is positioned supine with a shoulder roll placed to assist with hyperextension of the neck. The head may be turned to the side and supported with a padded headrest. This procedure may be done endoscopically.

### *Operative Procedure*

1. An incision is made over the inner border of the sternocleidomastoid muscle and is extended from the level of the hyoid bone to a point 2 cm above the clavicle.
2. The sac of the diverticulum is freed and ligated.
3. The pharyngeal muscle and surrounding tissues are closed.
4. In conjunction with this procedure, an esophageal myotomy is often performed distal to the diverticulum to minimize the likelihood of recurrence.

## Esophageal Hiatal Hernia Repair and Antireflux Procedure

Hiatal herniorrhaphy is performed to restore the cardioesophageal junction, or LES, in its correct anatomic position in the abdomen, to secure it firmly in place, and to correct GERD. A hiatal hernia (also called a *diaphragmatic hernia*) is a defect, either congenital or acquired, in the diaphragm where a portion of the stomach protrudes up into the thoracic cavity.

Hiatal hernias are usually of two distinct types—paraesophageal and sliding. Symptoms vary from none to severe heartburn, reflux (backward flow), regurgitation, and dysphagia. When symptoms are severe, a repair of the hernia is done, usually through a transabdominal approach. A transthoracic approach is used for patients with prior left upper quadrant surgery and for those who are extremely obese.

An antireflux procedure, which prevents reflux of gastric juices into the esophagus, is also done when the hernia is repaired. The three most frequently performed antireflux procedures are the Nissen, Hill, and Belsey Mark IV procedures.

***Procedural Considerations.*** The patient is positioned supine but may need to be repositioned to lateral if the gastroesophageal sphincter cannot be accessed through a high midline position. An indwelling urinary catheter is inserted after induction of general anesthesia.

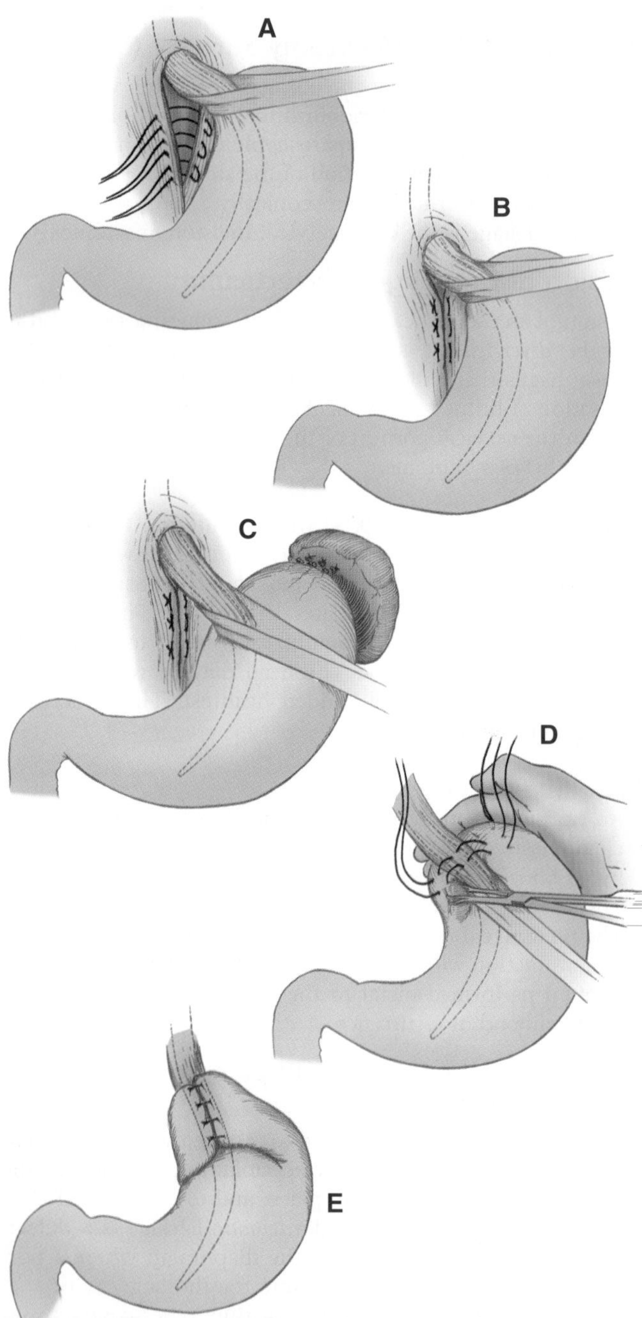


**FIGURE 11-16** The Nissen fundoplication procedure begins with oral passage of a Maloney dilator (40 Fr to 48 Fr) into the lumen of the stomach. **A,** The esophagus is then mobilized. A Penrose drain is placed around the gastroesophageal junction to pull the esophagus down and out of the hernia. **B,** Shown are three heavy sutures (#0 braided absorbable) placed to narrow the hiatal aperture but not so tight as to constrict the esophagus, thus the purpose of stenting the esophagus with the Maloney dilator. **C,** Further traction is applied to the distal esophagus while the proximal stomach and fundus are freed from all peritoneal attachments. **D,** The posterior wall of the stomach is brought up around the distal esophagus. **E,** The stomach walls are wrapped and sutured around the intraabdominal esophagus, with the Maloney stent in place.

Instrumentation includes a basic laparotomy set, Maloney or Hurst dilators in 32 Fr to 42 Fr, a self-retaining retractor system, and a 1-inch Penrose drain. If a transthoracic approach is planned, a basic thoracic set is required.

#### *Operative Procedure*

1. Through a transabdominal incision, the hernia is located and a crural repair is done.
2. The fundus of the stomach is wrapped around the lower 4 to 6 cm of the esophagus and is sutured in place (Nissen fundoplication); the upper part of the lesser curvature of the stomach and the cardioesophageal junction are sutured to the median arcuate ligament (Hill procedure); or the stomach is plicated around approximately 270 degrees of esophageal circumference (Belsey Mark IV procedure). The Nissen fundoplication procedure is illustrated in Figure 11-16.
3. Vagotomy, pyloroplasty, or both may be performed at the same time.
4. The wound is closed.

### Laparoscopic Nissen Fundoplication

Recent advances in minimal-access surgery, using laparoscopic visualization, have prompted adaptations for laparotomy procedures. The Nissen fundoplication previously described was developed in the early 1990s. The Nissen-Rosetti fundoplication and several other laparoscopic procedures were developed for the management of GERD. The Nissen fundoplication procedure is also used for repair of paraesophageal hernias, to reduce the hernia, to eliminate the hernia sac, and to repair the large defect in the diaphragm hiatus. Gastroesophageal reflux can also be treated with a silicone prosthetic implant placed around the distal esophagus under the diaphragm and above the stomach. This prosthesis, a small donut-shaped device with an open end that is sutured to be continuous, allows the passage of food but prevents the stomach from sliding into the chest cavity. This procedure may be done as an open laparotomy.

The patient having laparoscopic Nissen fundoplication is usually admitted the day of surgery. The surgery is performed through five trocar sites in the abdomen, which greatly reduces the postoperative recovery period. The healthy patient is typically discharged by the second postoperative day if there are no complications. A postoperative upper GI series is performed to verify the functioning of the newly constructed antireflux valve.

***Procedural Considerations.*** The surgery is performed with the patient under general anesthesia. A nasogastric tube and urinary drainage catheter are placed after induction and intubation. The patient is positioned supine or in the modified lithotomy position.

Instrumentation and supplies required for a laparoscopic Nissen fundoplication include a basic laparotomy set, laparoscope, laparoscopic camera, five trocars (trocar size or sizes depend on the surgeon's preference), a light cord, filtered insufflation tubing, and an electrosurgery cord. Laparoscopic instruments commonly used for the procedure include grasping forceps, endoscissors, endo-Babcock forceps, endodissecting forceps, endoclip appliers, an endosuturing device, and endoretractors, such as the fan retractor. Suction and a suction irrigator are commonly used. A Penrose drain or a 12-Fr red

Robinson catheter is used to assist in isolating and retracting the distal esophagus. Bougie dilators (large sizes, such as 40 Fr to 60 Fr) may be used to act as an esophageal stent in which to secure the fundoplication. A water-based lubricating jelly is used to assist the anesthesia provider in placing the bougie. Equipment needed for the procedure includes an electrosurgical unit, an insufflation unit with $CO_2$ gas, and two video monitors (one placed on each side of the patient).

### *Operative Procedure*

1. A stab wound is made with a #11 blade for insertion of the first trocar.
2. The trocar is placed, and insufflation is achieved. This may be performed before placing the trocar by inserting a Verres needle for the purpose of insufflation.
3. The laparoscope is placed through the port, and the camera is attached to the laparoscope.
4. Two trocars are placed below the xiphoid process, in the right upper quadrant of the abdomen, high in the costal margin, about 5 to 6 mm to the right and left of the midline. Another trocar is placed on the lateral plane to the midline in the left abdomen (left midclavicular), and the last trocar is placed in the lateral abdominal wall for use by the assistant.
5. A fan-shaped endoretractor is inserted through the right midclavicular port site and used to retract the left lobe of the liver for exposure of the gastroesophageal junction.
6. An endo-Babcock forceps is inserted through the left midclavicular port and is used to grasp the upper aspect of the fundus of the stomach. The stomach is retracted laterally and downward. This port site is also used for insertion of a grasper to hold the Penrose drain, the clip applier, and the ultrasonic coagulating shears.
7. The surgeon mobilizes the distal esophagus by opening the hiatus and employs an endodissector forceps to bluntly dissect the tissue along the right and left crura.
8. Endoclips are used to ligate the most distal portion of the pericardiophrenic vessel before it is divided.
9. The posterior vagus is identified but left intact.
10. The dissection is continued to expose the posterior esophagus.
11. The upper aspect of the greater curvature of the stomach is mobilized, and dissection is continued to the posterior esophagus.
12. The Penrose or Robinson catheter is inserted through a sheath and is passed behind the gastroesophageal junction. The ends are brought together and secured with an endoclamp that is then locked and used as a traction retractor during the procedure.
13. Another grasping forceps is used to grasp the apex of the gastric fundus and retract it downward to expose the short gastric vessels. The vessels are ligated with endoclips and divided with endoscissors.
14. The upper portion of the mobilized greater curvature is grasped and passed through the opening that has been created at the hiatus.
15. Tension and adequate mobilization of the greater curvature of the stomach are assessed. The portion of the greater curvature of the stomach that has been brought around the posterior esophagus at the proximal part of the gastroesophageal junction is then manipulated over the anterior distal esophagus.
16. A nonabsorbable endosuture is passed through a 5-mm port and used to place a row of interrupted sutures to join the aspects of the greater curvature of the stomach in a 2-cm to 3-cm "wrap" around the esophagus.
17. The anesthesia provider passes a large bougie down the lumen of the esophagus. The sutures are secured with the bougie in place.
18. The catheter (or drain) and bougie are removed. The abdomen is deflated.
19. Final inspection is completed, hemostasis obtained, and the instruments and ports removed under direct vision so that any bleeding from the abdominal wall can be readily detected. The trocar sites are then closed and dressings applied.

## Esophagomyotomy (Heller Procedure)

Esophagomyotomy (Heller cardiomyotomy) is myotomy of the esophagogastric junction to correct esophageal obstruction resulting from achalasia, a motility disorder of aperistalsis of the esophagus and elevated LES pressure. These patients have dysphagia, esophageal fullness, regurgitation, and weight loss.[42]

***Procedural Considerations.*** Selection of a transthoracic or transabdominal incision depends on the patient's general condition and other existing pathologic factors. The surgeon may elect to perform a pyloroplasty to prevent reflux by promoting stomach emptying. Instrumentation includes a basic laparotomy set and instruments to enter and retract the thorax if necessary. Laparoscopic and thoracoscopic approaches are a safe and effective alternative to the open procedure. The laparoscopic approach offers the advantage of adding fundoplication.[26] Potential postoperative complications include esophageal perforation and reflux.

### *Operative Procedure*

1. A midline abdominal incision is made from the xiphoid process to the umbilicus.
2. After exposure of the esophagogastric junction, a Maloney dilator is inserted through the patient's oral cavity to distend the esophagus.
3. A scalpel with a #15 blade is used to make a longitudinal incision through the muscular wall of the distal esophagus and proximal stomach, leaving the mucosa intact.
4. A small portion of the fundus of the stomach may be plicated to the lateral wall of the esophagus.
5. The wound is closed.
6. VATS is approached with the patient positioned and secured in a right lateral position.
7. A 30-degree thoracoscope is inserted in the left eighth intercostal space along the left posterior axillary line.
8. The lung is retracted through a working port placed in the left anterior axillary line of the fifth space.
9. Dissection is done through a mini-thoracotomy in the left ninth intercostal space to sweep the muscular layer from the mucosa from 6 cm above and 1 cm below the gastroesophageal junction. This dissection is made halfway around the circumference of the esophagus.
10. A chest tube is placed and the incision and port sites closed.

## Esophageal Dilation

Esophageal dilation may be indicated in patients who have an esophageal stricture related to past surgery, chemical or thermal injury, or anatomic anomalies. An upper GI series is required before the procedure to determine the location of the stricture.

*Procedural Considerations.* Esophageal dilation is a clean procedure performed in the operating room or endoscopy unit. General anesthesia or moderate sedation is usually indicated. An esophageal perforation is a complication that could require an open repair.

The patient is positioned supine.

A flexible gastroscope and light source with video camera and monitor, bougie dilators (Hurst or Maloney dilators are commonly used) in graduated sizes, water-soluble lubricant, gauze sponges, and gloves are required to perform the procedure. An esophageal stent that can be inserted through a large-channel gastroscope or along a guidewire may be requested. The surgeon may use fluoroscopy to demonstrate that the dilation site is accurate by combining esophagoscopy with fluoroscopy and marking the site of stricture distally and proximally with radiopaque markers taped to the patient's skin.

### *Operative Procedure*

1. The perioperative nurse arranges the bougies in graduated order beginning with the smallest size (24 Fr) and progressing to the largest size (60 Fr).
2. The surgeon may first perform gastroscopy and pass a guidewire through the esophageal stricture.
3. The bougies are then passed one at a time gently but firmly through the stricture in an attempt to dilate the esophageal lumen.
4. Continuation of the dilation to the largest bougie depends on ease of passage and the patient's tolerance.
5. Laser therapy may be indicated for palliation if a tumor mass is causing the stricture. The neodymium:yttrium-aluminum-garnet (Nd:YAG) laser energy may be delivered to the mass or stricture by way of a flexible quartz fiber passed through the operative channel of the gastroscope.

An esophageal stent may be placed at the stricture site to decrease the chance of recurrence.

# SURGERY OF THE STOMACH

## Vagotomy

Truncal vagotomy is the identification of the two vagal trunks on the distal esophagus and resection of a segment of each, including any additional nerve fibers running separately from the trunks. By interrupting the parasympathetic innervation, this procedure reduces gastric acid secretion in patients with duodenal ulcers. When truncal vagotomy was initially performed alone, a high incidence of gastric stasis resulted from the loss of cholinergic innervation to the smooth muscle of the stomach; thus pyloroplasty or another gastric drainage procedure almost always accompanies truncal vagotomy. Truncal vagotomy deprives not only the stomach but also the liver, gallbladder, bile duct, pancreas, small intestine, and half of the large intestine of the parasympathetic nerve supply (Figure 11-17). Truncal vagotomy with antrectomy or a drainage procedure is the most common operation for duodenal ulcers.

Selective vagotomy is the transection of each abdominal vagus at a point just beyond its bifurcation into the gastric and extragastric divisions. Thus the hepatic branch of the anterior vagus and the celiac branch of the posterior vagus are preserved. Selective vagotomy possesses theoretic advantages over truncal vagotomy because vagal innervation of the viscera other than the stomach is preserved. However, selective vagotomy also denervates the entire stomach, so the addition of a drainage procedure is still necessary. Selective vagotomy may cause less postvagotomy diarrhea than truncal vagotomy does, but the incidence of dumping syndrome is probably the same or even higher. Both procedures are about equally effective in controlling duodenal ulcers.

Parietal cell vagotomy is the vagal denervation of only the parietal cell area of the stomach. The technique spares the main nerves of Latarjet but divides all vagal branches that terminate on the proximal two thirds of the stomach. The operation has also been called *proximal gastric vagotomy* (Figure 11-18) and *highly selective vagotomy.* Because antral innervation is preserved, gastric emptying is unimpaired and a drainage procedure is unnecessary. The incidence of dumping and diarrhea after parietal cell vagotomy is much lower than after truncal or selective vagotomy.

*Procedural Considerations.* Instrumentation for vagotomy includes a basic thoracotomy set (if a thoracoabdominal incision is to be used), a laparotomy set, a GI instrument set, two blunt nerve hooks (Smith-Wick), two 10-inch vessel clip appliers with clips, and 10-inch Metzenbaum dissecting scissors. A 1-inch Penrose drain is used to retract the esophagus. The patient is positioned supine under general anesthesia. A laparoscopic approach is an alternative.

### *Operative Procedure*

1. A midline incision is made, and the esophagus is identified and retracted with a 1-inch wide Penrose drain.
2. The vagus nerves or their branches, depending on which type of vagotomy is being done, are identified, clamped with either a ligature or a hemostatic clip, and resected.
3. The wound is closed in layers.

## Pyloroplasty (Pyloromyotomy)

Pyloroplasty is the formation of a larger passageway between the prepyloric region of the stomach and the first or second portion of the duodenum. A pyloroplasty may be performed for the treatment of a peptic ulcer under selected conditions but is more frequently employed to remove cicatricial bands in the pyloric ring, thus relieving spasm and permitting rapid emptying of the stomach. In adults a vagotomy is usually performed with a pyloroplasty.

*Procedural Considerations.* A laparotomy set and a GI instrument set are required. The patient is positioned supine, and general anesthesia is administered. A nasogastric tube is placed by the anesthesia provider. An indwelling urinary catheter is inserted.

### *Operative Procedure*

1. The abdominal cavity is opened through a midline incision.
2. The pylorus of the stomach is isolated.
3. An incision is made through the stomach and the duodenum.

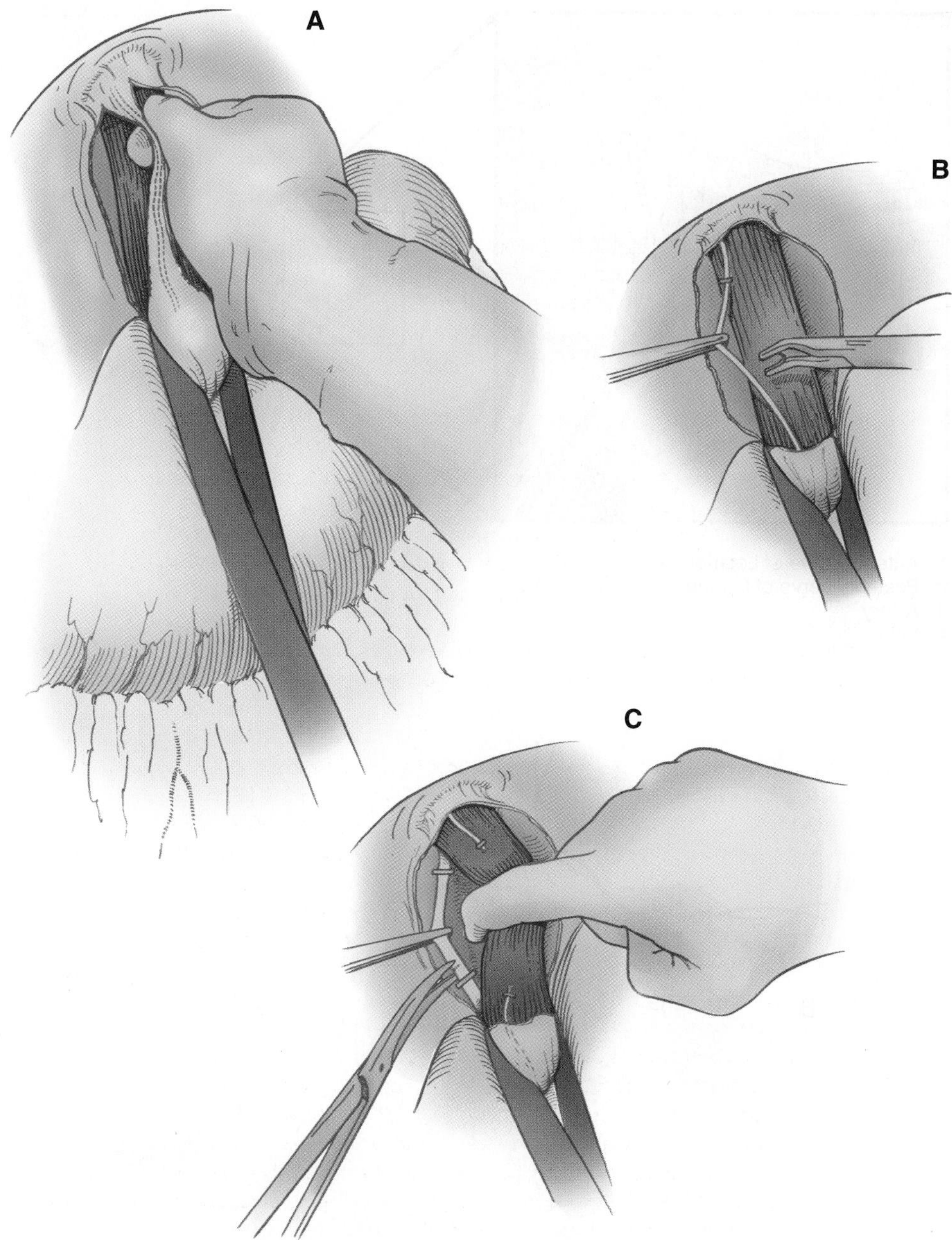


FIGURE 11-17 Truncal vagotomy. **A,** The phrenoesophageal ligament is lifted from the surface of the esophagus, and the vagal trunks are identified. **B,** Ligating clips are applied to the vagus nerve. **C,** Ligating clips have been applied to the larger posterior nerve in preparation for resecting a 2-cm segment between the clips.

4. The pyloroplasty is closed with nonabsorbable or synthetic absorbable intestinal sutures.
5. The abdominal wound is closed in layers, and a dressing is applied.

## Gastrostomy

Through a high left rectus abdominal or midline incision, a temporary or permanent channel is established from the gastric lumen to the skin. This lumen permits liquid feeding or retrograde dilation of an esophageal stricture. Gastrostomy is a palliative procedure performed to prevent malnutrition and starvation, which may be caused by a lesion or stricture situated in the esophagus or in the cardia of the stomach. A temporary procedure is done when the obstruction can be corrected.

For an extensive lesion of the esophagus, some surgeons advise a permanent gastrostomy in which a stomach flap is formed around the catheter. The catheter is brought out of the abdomen through a separate stab wound. When the incisional area is avoided, tissue healing is improved and the incidence of postoperative wound healing problems decreases.

***Procedural Considerations.*** The patient is positioned supine under general anesthesia or IV moderate sedation/analgesia with local anesthesia. A basic laparotomy instrument set and a catheter and drainage reservoir are required.

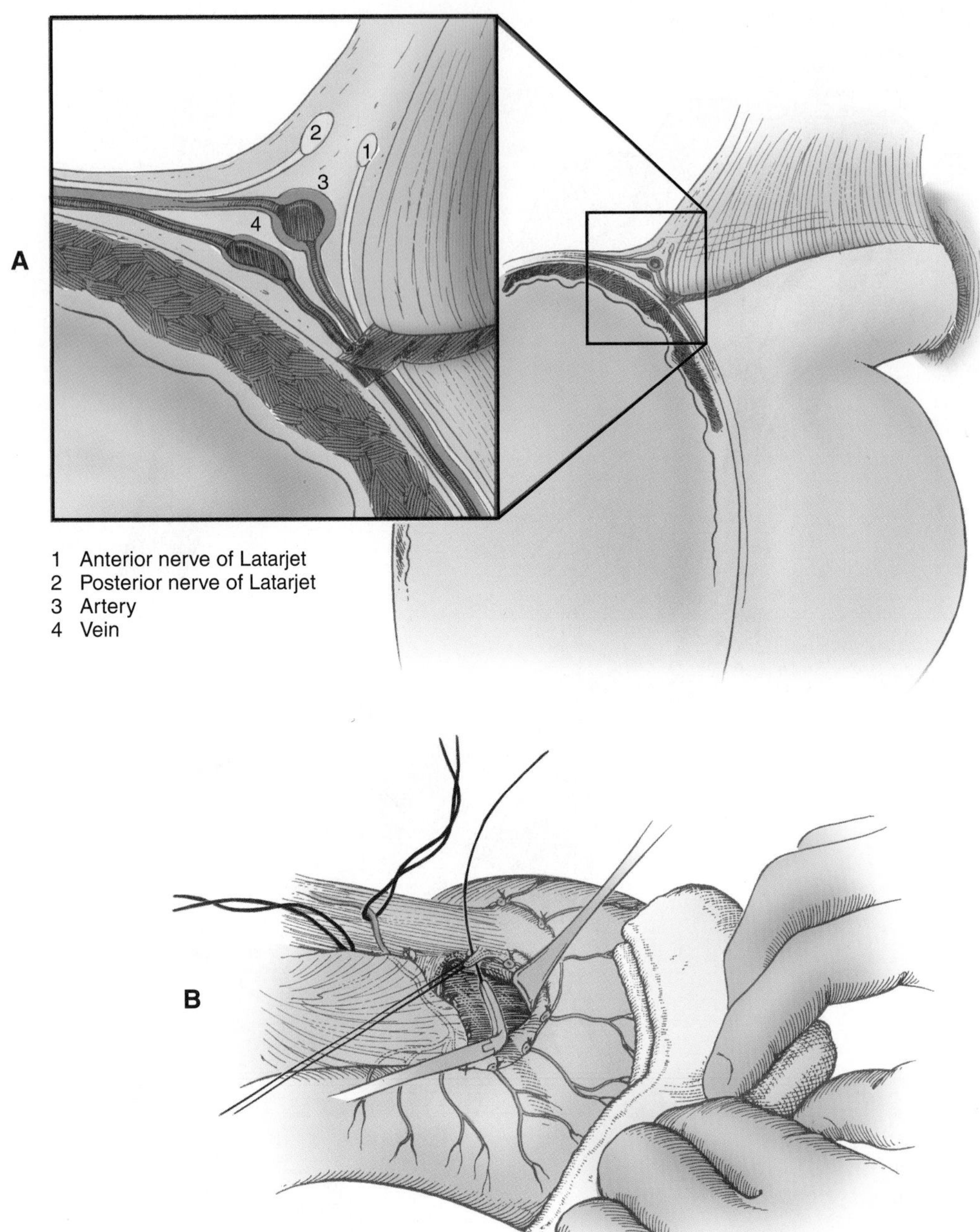


FIGURE 11-18 Selective proximal vagotomy. **A,** Illustrates the junction of the gastrohepatic ligament with the lesser curve of the stomach and demonstrates the anterior *(1)* and posterior *(2)* nerves of Latarjet, along with the artery *(3)* and vein *(4)*. **B,** The lesser curve is lifted with a vein retractor to facilitate serial ligation of the intermediate and posterior neurovascular attachments.

### *Operative Procedure*

1. The abdominal cavity is opened through an upper midline or transverse incision.
2. The stomach is held with an Allis or Babcock forceps, and a purse-string suture is placed at the proposed site for the catheter.
3. A scalpel with a #15 blade is used to make an incision within the purse-string suture, and the contents of the stomach are suctioned.
4. Bleeding points are controlled using electrocoagulation.
5. The catheter is inserted, and the purse-string suture is tied around it.
6. The catheter is brought through a stab wound in the area of the left rectus muscle.
7. The stomach may be sutured to the peritoneal layer, and the abdominal wound is closed in layers.

## Percutaneous Endoscopic Gastrostomy (PEG)

The PEG method has become the most popular gastrostomy tube placement approach. This tube is placed endoscopically with the patient under local anesthesia or moderate sedation/analgesia. It can be used for gastric decompression and enteral feedings.[10] PEG uses a flexible gastroscope and a uniquely designed gastrostomy tube for placement through the abdominal wall and requires a push-pull technique to insert. This procedure may be done in the endoscopy suite, in the OR, or at the bedside in a critical care unit if necessary.

***Procedural Considerations.*** A PEG tube kit containing the following is required: a percutaneous needle, a long silk suture with end strengthened for feeding it down the lumen of the needle, a percutaneous gastrostomy tube, and a bolster. A flexible gastroscopy system is required as well as snare forceps.

The patient is positioned supine under IV moderate sedation. A bite-block is inserted into the patient's mouth.

#### Operative Procedure

1. The gastroscope is passed.
2. The end of the scope is angled anteriorly to the left anterolateral wall of the stomach's fundus so that the light from the gastroscope can be seen through the abdominal wall.
3. The stomach is insufflated with air through the gastroscope.
4. Local anesthesia is injected at the site of the intended gastrostomy if the patient is awake.
5. A small stab wound is made with a #11 blade.
6. The percutaneous needle is inserted into the abdominal wall and into the stomach lumen under direct visualization of the gastroscope.
7. The long silk suture is threaded into the lumen of the needle and passed into the stomach, where it is snared with the forceps.
8. A clamp is applied to the exterior distal end of the suture after the needle is removed.
9. The gastroscope is removed, and the suture extends out of the patient's oral cavity.
10. The suture is then attached to the tapered end of the gastrostomy tube.
11. The gastrostomy tube is gently guided into the patient's oral cavity, down the esophagus, and into the lumen of the stomach and pulled through the abdominal wall (push-pull technique).
12. The tube is secured with an internal bolster by reinserting the gastroscope and snugging it up to the gastric wall under direct visualization.
13. An external bolster is applied over the tube and snugged to the abdominal wall. Care is taken to ensure the bolsters are not compressing the tissues because such compression could compromise tissue integrity and perfusion.
14. The distal end of the tube is cut, and a connector is applied.
15. The patient's stomach is deflated, and the procedure is complete.

### Gastrotomy

Gastrotomy is the opening of the anterior stomach wall through a left paramedian abdominal incision and exploration of the interior. This procedure is usually done to explore for upper GI tract bleeding, perform a tissue biopsy, or remove a gastric lesion or foreign body.

***Procedural Considerations.*** A laparotomy set and a GI instrument set are required.

#### Operative Procedure

1. The abdominal wall is incised and the stomach exposed. A longitudinal incision is then made through the anterior wall of the stomach, halfway between the curvatures.
2. The stomach wall is grasped and elevated by an Allis or Babcock forceps.
3. An incision is made, and a suction tube is inserted into the stomach to remove gastric contents.
4. The lesion or foreign body is removed.
5. The stomach wall and abdominal wall are closed.

### Closure of Perforated Gastric or Duodenal Ulcer

Closure of a perforation in the stomach or duodenum is performed through a high right rectus or midline abdominal incision.

***Procedural Considerations.*** A perforated gastric or duodenal ulcer is treated as a surgical emergency, and the operation is performed as soon as the diagnosis is made. The patient will be typed and cross matched so that an adequate supply of blood will be available for emergency replacement. A gastric lavage is not performed, but continuous suction is used. A laparotomy set and a GI instrument set are required. Linear stapling instruments should be available.

#### Operative Procedure

1. Through a right rectus or midline abdominal incision, the perforation is located.
2. Suction is used to remove exudate in the peritoneal cavity.
3. The perforation is closed with a purse-string suture by inverting the raw edges and suturing a piece of omentum over the closure.
4. The ulcerated area may be resected using linear stapling devices.
5. The abdomen is copiously irrigated with warm saline, which may contain a broad-spectrum antibiotic.
6. The abdominal wound is closed in layers, and a dressing is applied.

### Gastrojejunostomy

Gastrojejunostomy is the establishment of a permanent communication, either between the proximal jejunum and the anterior wall of the stomach or between the proximal jejunum and the posterior wall of the stomach, without removing a segment of the GI tract (Figure 11-19). It is accomplished through a midline or paramedian abdominal incision.

Gastrojejunostomy may be performed to treat a benign obstruction at the pyloric end of the stomach or an inoperable lesion of the pylorus when a partial gastrectomy would not be feasible. It also provides a large opening without sphincter obstruction.

***Procedural Considerations.*** A laparotomy and a GI instrument set are required. Linear stapling instruments should be available. The patient is positioned supine under general anesthesia. The anesthesia provider inserts a nasogastric tube after intubation. An indwelling catheter is placed into the urinary bladder before abdominal skin prep.

#### Operative Procedure

1. Through an upper midline or paramedian abdominal incision, exploration of the peritoneal cavity is completed, as described for routine laparotomy.

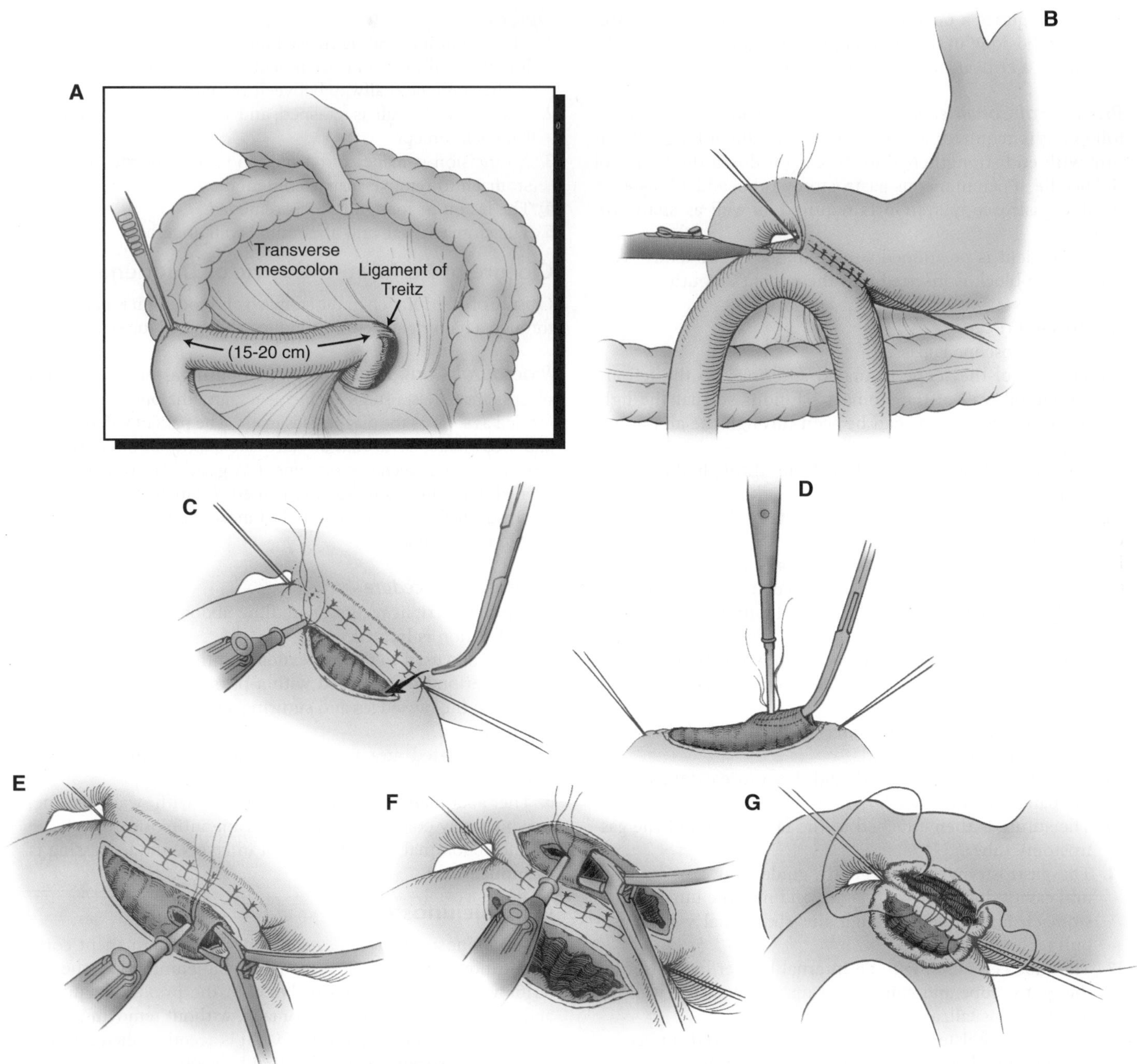


**FIGURE 11-19** Gastrojejunostomy. **A,** Illustrates the selection of a segment of jejunum that will be anastomosed to the stomach; the distance between the ligament of Treitz and the anastomosis should not be excessively long or under any tension. **B,** A posterior row of interrupted sutures is placed between the gastric and jejunal serosae, and the sites of the gastric and jejunal stomas are scored with the electrosurgical pencil. **C,** The jejunal stoma is created by dissecting through the serosa and muscularis with the electrosurgical pencil. An opening is made in the mucosa, and a right-angled clamp is inserted into the lumen. **D,** The clamp is opened and elevated. **E,** Electrosurgery is applied between the two jaws of the clamp. **F,** The procedure is repeated for creating the gastric stoma. **G,** Full-thickness anastomosis is begun posteriorly.

2. The pathologic condition is confirmed.
3. Warm, moist packs are placed, and a self-retaining retractor is positioned.
4. A loop of proximal jejunum is grasped with a Babcock forceps and freed from the mesentery.
5. The loop of jejunum is approximated to either the anterior or posterior stomach wall several centimeters from the greater curvature of the stomach.
6. Nonabsorbable 2-0 traction sutures are placed through the serosal layers at each end of the selected portion of the jejunum and stomach.
7. Gastroenterostomy clamps may be placed before insertion of the posterior interrupted 3-0 or 2-0 nonabsorbable serosal sutures.
8. The field is draped for open anastomosis (GI technique).
9. The jejunum and stomach are opened.

10. Bleeding points are clamped with mosquito or Crile hemostats and ligated with 3-0 synthetic absorbable sutures.
11. The inner posterior row of sutures is placed, using continuous 2-0 or 3-0 synthetic absorbable suture with atraumatic intestinal needles, and continued for the first anterior row.
12. The anastomosis is completed with anterior serosal sutures of 3-0 or 2-0 nonabsorbable material.
13. Traction sutures are removed.
14. Interrupted 4-0 nonabsorbable sutures may be used for reinforcement.
15. The contaminated instruments are discarded into a basin.
16. The abdominal wound is closed in layers, and a dressing is applied.

## Partial Gastrectomy—Billroth I and Billroth II

A Billroth I gastrectomy is the resection of a diseased portion of the stomach through a right paramedian or midline abdominal incision and the establishment of an anastomosis between the stomach and duodenum. It is performed to remove a benign or malignant lesion located in the pylorus, or upper half of the stomach. One of several techniques may be followed to establish GI continuity, including the Schoemaker, the von Haberer–Finney, and other modifications of the Billroth I procedure (Figure 11-20).

***Procedural Considerations.*** A laparotomy set and a GI instrument set are required. Linear stapling instruments should be available. The patient is positioned supine under general anesthesia. The anesthesia provider inserts a nasogastric tube after intubation. An indwelling urinary catheter is inserted before the abdominal skin prep.

### *Operative Procedure*

1. The abdominal wall is incised, and the peritoneal cavity is opened and explored.
2. Bleeding vessels are clamped and ligated or coagulated.
3. The abdominal wound is retracted, and the surrounding organs are protected with warm, moist packs.
4. The gastrocolic omentum is freed from the colon mesentery to prevent injury to the middle colic artery.
5. With hemostats and Metzenbaum scissors, the right and left gastroepiploic arteries and veins are clamped, divided, and ligated with 2-0 nonabsorbable sutures and 2-0 and 3-0 suture ligatures, thereby freeing the greater curvature of the stomach.
6. The gastric vessels are clamped, divided, and ligated to free the diseased portion of the stomach.
7. The operative field is prepared for open anastomosis (GI technique).
8. After sectioning of the stomach from the greater to lesser curvature, two Allen intestinal anastomosis clamps or other suitable clamps are placed on the upper portion of the duodenum just distal to the pylorus.
9. The duodenum is divided by scalpel, electrosurgery, or a linear cutting and stapling device (e.g., gastrointestinal anastomosis [GIA]).
10. Additional moist packs are placed for protection, and two sets of anastomosis clamps are placed across the stomach.
11. Division of the stomach is completed.
12. At the lower margin the opened stomach is approximated to the duodenum by a series of interrupted sutures placed in the serosal layers. An atraumatic intestinal needle with 3-0 nonabsorbable suture is used. Suture ends are held with hemostats, and the intestinal clamps are removed.
13. Stumps of the stomach and duodenum are cleansed with moist sponges, and bleeding vessels are ligated with fine suture or coagulated.
14. During the anastomosis of the stomach and remaining duodenum, the involved segments may be held with rubber-shod clamps. The excess of the lesser curvature of the stomach is closed on completion of the anastomosis.
15. Instruments used in the open portion of the GI tract are discarded into a separate basin.
16. Routine laparotomy closure is completed.

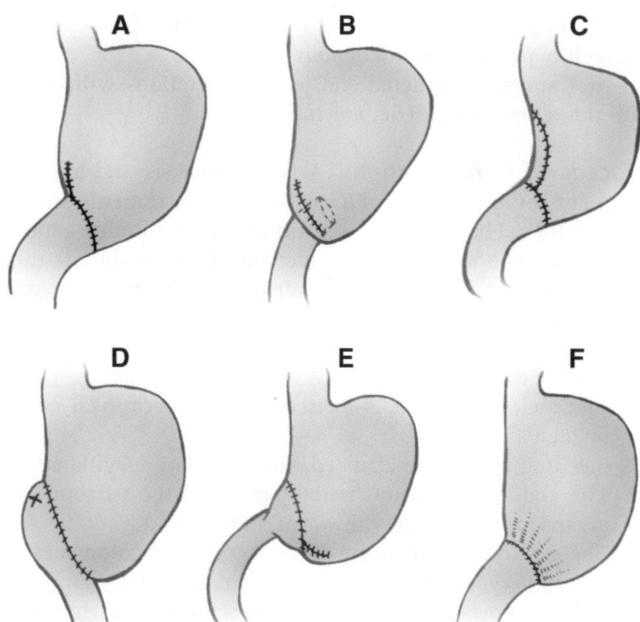


**FIGURE 11-20** Diagrams illustrating resections of stomach with anastomosis of stomach and duodenum (gastroduodenal anastomosis). All are modifications of Billroth I technique, in which stomach is brought to duodenum. **A,** Billroth I: after pylorus is removed, lesser curvature is partially closed and duodenum is sutured to open end of stomach at its lower margin. **B,** Kocher: distal end of stomach is closed, and duodenum is brought up to posterior margin of closed stomach. **C,** Schoemaker: lesser curvature of stomach is sutured and brought down to same size as duodenum, and end-to-end anastomosis is done. **D,** von Haberer–Finney: side of duodenum is brought up to end of stomach so that entire end of stomach is open for direct anastomosis. **E,** Horsley: lesser curvature end of stomach is used to suture to duodenum and closes greater curvature end. **F,** von Haberer: modification of operation shown in **D**. Stomach is, so to speak, narrowed or puckered so that it fits end of duodenum. Modification of this is done by some as follows: duodenum is split longitudinally, and its ends are flared open so that opening is large enough to fit open end of stomach.

A Billroth II gastrectomy is a resection of the distal portion of the stomach through an abdominal incision and the establishment of an anastomosis between the stomach and jejunum. It is performed to remove a benign or malignant lesion in the stomach or duodenum. This technique and modifications may be selected because the volume of acidic gastric juice will be reduced and the anastomosis can be made along the greater curvature or at any point along the stump of the stomach. Modifications of the Billroth II procedure include the Polya and Hofmeister operations, which also establish GI continuity through bypassing the duodenum.

After surgery, duodenal and jejunal secretions will empty into the remaining gastric pouch.

***Procedural Considerations.*** A laparotomy set and a GI instrument set are required. Linear stapling instruments should be available. The patient is positioned supine under general anesthesia. The anesthesia provider inserts a nasogastric tube after intubation. An indwelling urinary catheter is inserted before the abdominal skin prep.

### *Operative Procedure*

1. The abdominal wall is incised and the peritoneal cavity opened and explored.
2. Bleeding vessels are clamped and ligated or coagulated.
3. The abdominal wound is retracted, and the surrounding organs are protected with warm, moist packs.
4. The gastrocolic omentum is freed from the colon mesentery to prevent injury to the middle colic artery.
5. With hemostats and Metzenbaum scissors, the right and left gastroepiploic arteries and veins are clamped, divided, and ligated with 2-0 nonabsorbable suture and 2-0 and 3-0 suture ligatures, thereby freeing the greater curvature of the stomach.
6. The distal portion of the stomach is isolated.
7. Moist packs are placed for protection of the viscera, and two sets of anastomosis clamps are placed across the distal stomach.
8. The stomach is resected just distal to the pylorus using a scalpel, electrosurgery, or a linear stapling and cutting device (GIA) (Figure 11-21, *A*).
9. A proximal loop of jejunum is positioned for anastomosis to the posterior wall of the remaining stomach.
10. An anastomosis is established between the stomach and jejunum using mechanical linear stapling devices (GIA and thoracic abdominal [TA] instruments) (Figure 11-21, *C*).
11. The abdomen is closed.

## Total Gastrectomy

Total gastrectomy is the complete removal of the stomach and establishment of an anastomosis between the jejunum and the esophagus (esophagojejunostomy) (Figure 11-22). It may include an enteroenterostomy if indicated. Total gastrectomy is done with curative intent or as a palliative procedure to remove a malignant lesion of the stomach and metastases in the adjacent lymph nodes (Research Highlight).

***Procedural Considerations.*** The incision may be bilateral subcostal, long transrectus, long midline, or thoracoabdominal. A basic thoracotomy set, a GI instrument set, and a laparotomy set are necessary. Mechanical linear stapling devices should be available. In addition, two long, blunt nerve hooks and two 10-inch needle holders are required. The patient is positioned supine under general anesthesia. The anesthesia provider inserts a nasogastric tube after intubation. An indwelling urinary catheter is inserted before the abdominal skin prep.

### *Operative Procedure*

1. The abdomen is opened through an incision of choice.
2. The wound edges are protected and retracted.
3. Careful and complete exploration for metastasis is performed.
4. The omentum is freed from the colon, using sharp dissection; vessels are ligated with 2-0 nonabsorbable suture.
5. The splenic vessels are ligated and transfixed with 2-0 and 3-0 nonabsorbable suture at the tail of the pancreas; the spleen is left attached to the omentum.

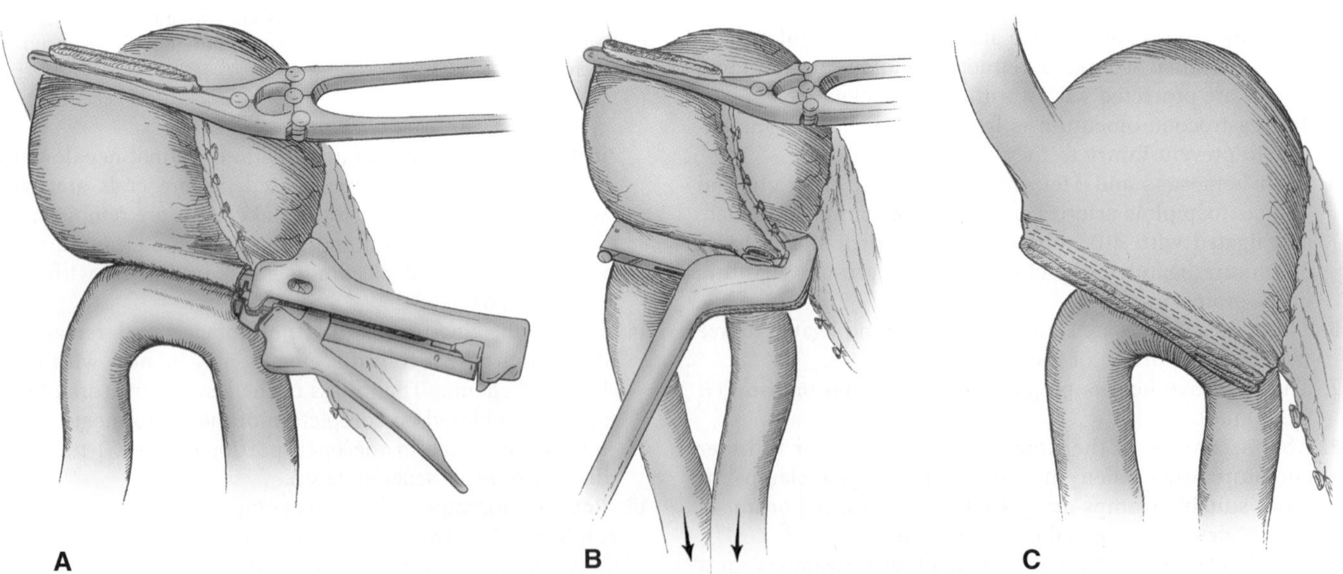


**FIGURE 11-21** Subtotal gastrectomy with stapled Billroth II anastomosis. **A,** The distal stomach has been dissected free and resected just distal to the pylorus. A proximal limb of jejunum is brought up to anastomose to the posterior wall of the stomach with a linear stapling instrument that transects between two parallel staple lines. **B,** The stomach is elevated, and a 90-staple mechanical stapling device is placed across the distal stomach. **C,** Illustration of the completed subtotal gastrectomy with stapled antecolic gastrojejunostomy.

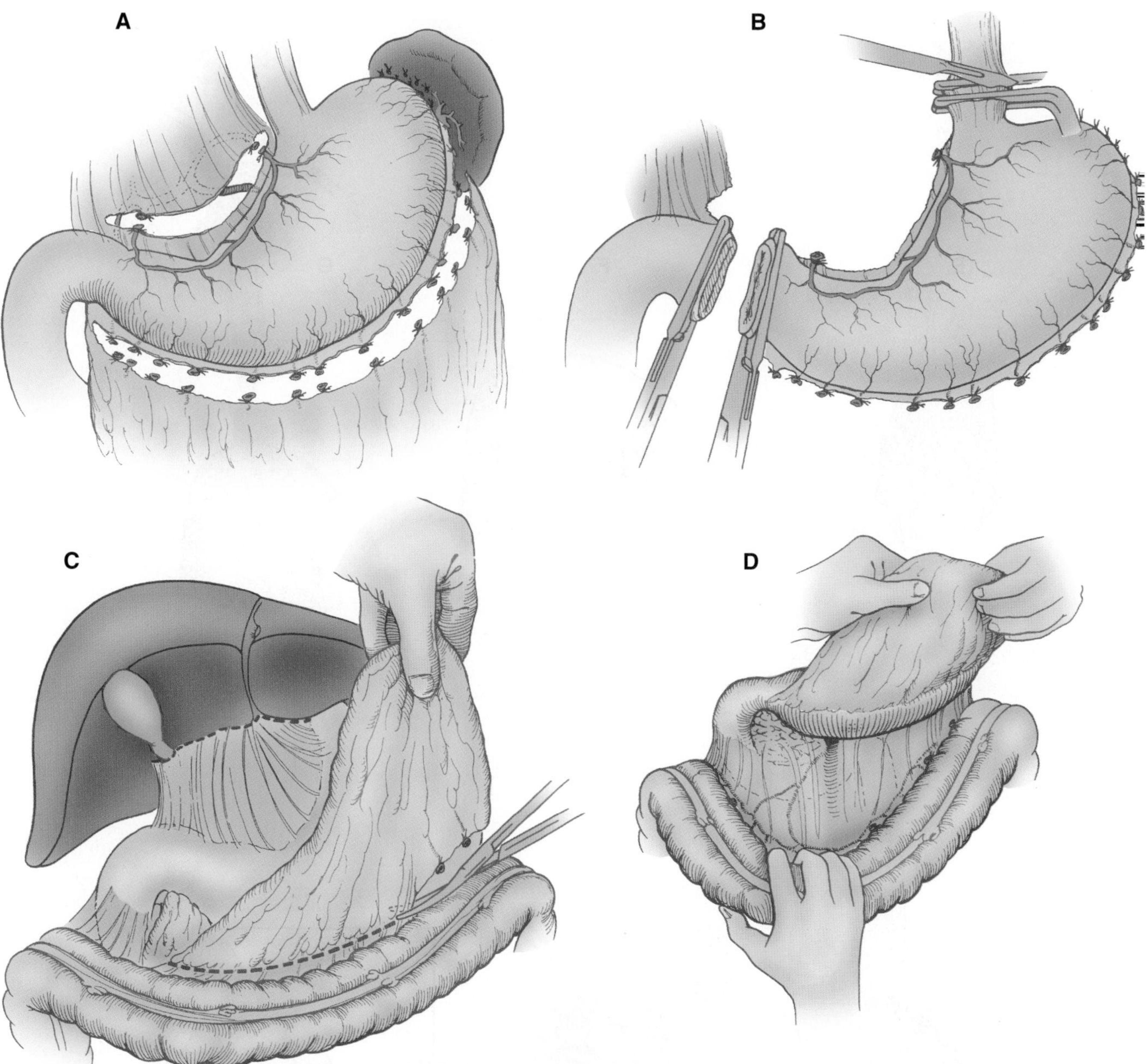


FIGURE 11-22 Total gastrectomy may be performed for benign or malignant disease. **A,** Demonstrates the mobilization of the stomach for benign disease. Serial division of the vessels in the gastrocolic ligament and gastrohepatic ligament is performed to free the greater and lesser omentum. The short gastric vessels connecting the stomach to the spleen are divided, and the spleen is preserved. **B,** The duodenum is divided distally to the pylorus, and the proximal line of division is at the distal intraabdominal esophagus. **C,** For malignancies, the line of resection includes both the lesser and greater omentum. **D,** The retrogastric area is inspected for tumor involvement. The spleen and tail of the pancreas may be included in the resection.

*Continued*

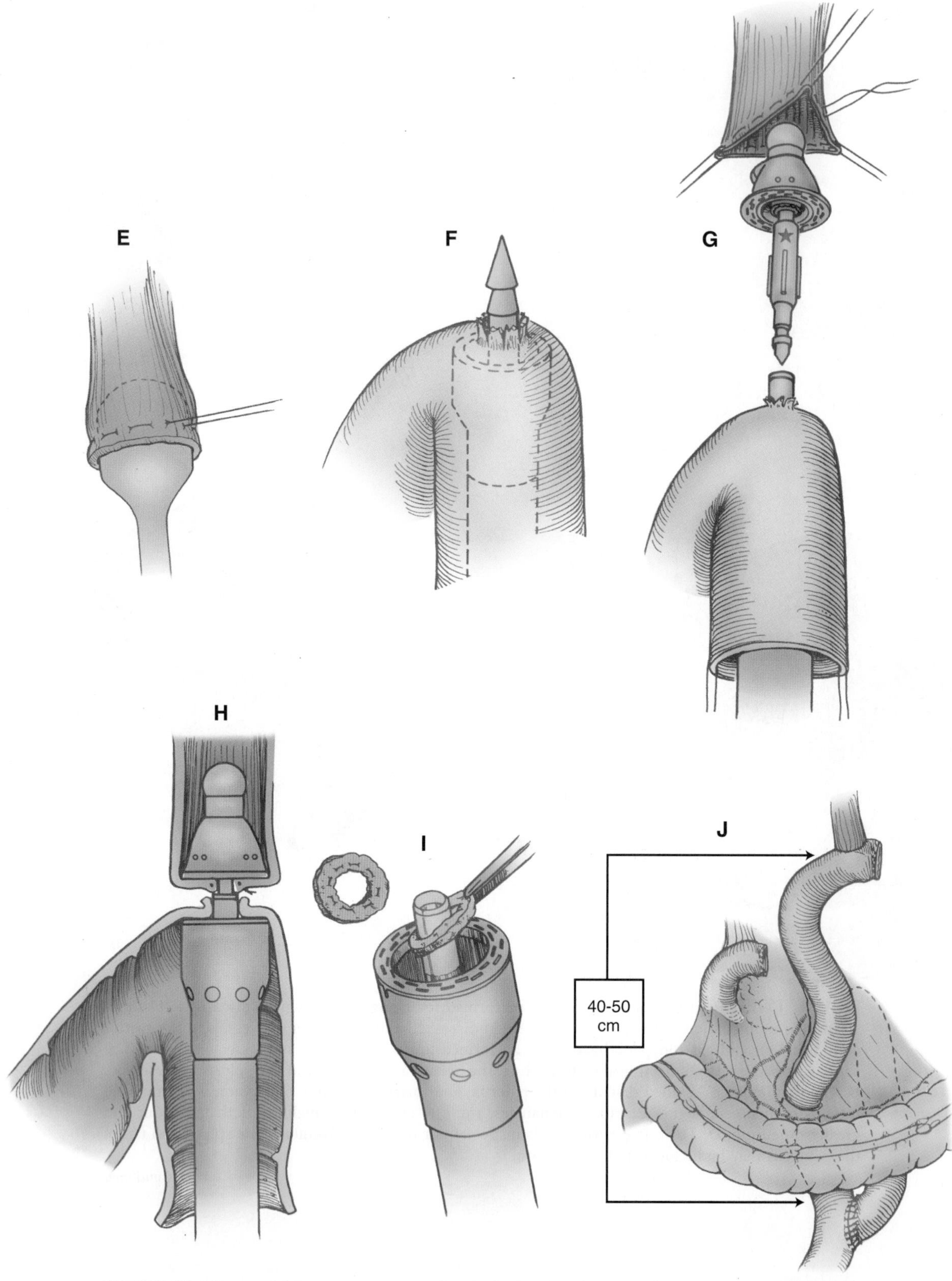


FIGURE 11-22, cont'd **E,** A sizer is inserted into the lumen of the distal esophagus. **F,** The EEA or intraluminal anastomosis (ILA) is inserted into the lumen of the jejunum to facilitate esophagojejunostomy. **G,** The anvil is inserted into the distal esophagus where purse-string sutures will be snugged around the protruding arm of the anvil. **H,** The distal esophagus and the jejunum are brought together by the mechanism of the stapling device, and the interluminal anastomosis will be performed. **I,** The "donuts," distal esophagus and jejunal tissues, are examined for integrity and completeness. **J,** Illustration of the esophagojejunostomy completed.

## RESEARCH HIGHLIGHT

### Quality of Life and Symptoms After Gastroesophageal Cancer Surgery

This pilot study was designed to provide preliminary descriptions of quality of life (QOL) and symptoms of patients with gastroesophageal surgery, comparing individual QOL and symptom experiences between total gastrectomy versus esophagogastrectomy. It also sought to describe the frequency of symptoms and health-related QOL questions to evaluate QOL after gastroesophageal surgery and determine what symptoms were frequently experienced by patients.

This exploratory descriptive study used retrospective chart review and mailed surveys. Ninety-four patients were identified during a 10-year period. Surveys were sent to 32 surviving patients with 27 returns. Of the 27 surviving patients 25 were men. The majority were white, and the mean age was 69.7 years. Eleven had had a total gastrectomy, and 16 had an esophagogastrectomy.

The gastroenterology QOL index measures health-related QOL as it relates to general gastrointestinal (GI) function, symptoms, emotions, and physiologic and social function in a 36-item Likert-type scale. The authors developed a Life After Gastroesophageal Surgery (LAGS) tool designed to measure symptoms and psychosocial impact resulting from gastroesophageal surgery. The scale, a 24-item Likert-type scale, also contains two questions investigating global life satisfaction after surgery.

Generally, as a combined group, the 27 patients had a high QOL level, with the total gastrectomy group presenting higher than the esophagogastrectomy group. The gastrectomy group reported significantly less abdominal pain and fullness, choking, coughing, and depression and were able to eat more meals per day. The most common bothersome symptoms for both groups included weakness, cramping, loose stools, weight loss, vomiting, belching, and sensitive thoracic scar. There were significant differences in symptom experience and QOL between the two surgery groups. This study also revealed that patients with increased symptom frequency had a considerably lower QOL.

This study supported literature findings claiming weight loss, dysphagia, and altered eating patterns in this surgery population. The evidence also suggests that esophagogastrectomy patients will have considerably more negative postoperative symptoms than patients with total gastrectomy, and the former group will go on to have poorer life satisfaction.

Comments from the LAGS tool requested more patient education and suggested that a support group might be beneficial.

Modified from Spector NM and others: Quality of life and symptoms after surgery for gastroesophageal cancer, *Gastroenterology Nurse* 2(3):120-125, 2002.

6. The duodenum is mobilized, intestinal clamps are applied, and the operative field is protected for transection and closure of the distal duodenum (GI technique).
7. The right gastric artery is ligated and transfixed with 2-0 and 3-0 nonabsorbable suture, and the gastrohepatic omentum is separated from the liver.
8. After ligation of the left gastric artery, the mobilized stomach, spleen, omentum, and lesser and greater curvature ligamentous attachments are delivered into the wound.
9. Division of the coronary ligament of the left lobe of the liver permits exposure of the diaphragmatic peritoneum over the esophagogastric junction.
10. The liver is protected by moist packs, and gentle retraction is maintained with a Harrington, Deaver, or malleable retractor.
11. A flap of peritoneum is freed from the diaphragm, and branches of the vagus nerves are divided.
12. A loop of jejunum is selected and delivered antecolic to the esophagogastric junction for anastomosis.
13. Traction is placed on the specimen, and the posterior layer of interrupted 3-0 nonabsorbable sutures is inserted, or stapling devices are used.
14. As the jejunum and the esophagus are incised, mosquito or Crile hemostats and ligatures of 3-0 synthetic absorbable suture control bleeding.
15. The posterior layer is reinforced with 3-0 intestinal synthetic absorbable sutures or a linear staple line.
16. Division of the esophagus is completed, and the entire specimen is removed.
17. The mucosal anterior wall of the anastomosis is also approximated with 4-0 interrupted synthetic absorbable sutures. An end-to-end anastomosis circular stapling device may be used to complete the anastomosis between the esophagus and jejunum.
18. A second layer of sutures, 3-0 nonabsorbable or synthetic absorbable, is placed anteriorly in the seromuscular and muscular coat of the intestine.
19. A flap of the peritoneum is attached to the jejunum with interrupted 3-0 nonabsorbable sutures to relieve traction on the anastomosis.
20. A lateral jejunojejunal anastomosis is completed to permit irritating bile and pancreatic fluids to bypass the anastomosis line, thereby preventing esophageal regurgitation.
21. The alternative to using suture materials is the use of mechanical stapling devices. Another method of establishing continuity is a combination of a Roux-en-Y jejunojejunostomy and a jejunoesophagostomy.
22. The abdominal wound is closed in layers. If retention sutures are used, they must be placed extraperitoneally because of the absence of omentum to protect the small bowel.

A Roux-en-Y, also written RNY, is any Y-shaped anastomosis in which small bowel is included.

## BARIATRIC SURGERY

Bariatric surgery is the surgical treatment of obesity, also termed *weight loss* or *weight reduction surgery* (History box). Morbid obesity is a disease affecting more than 20 million people in the United States in 2004; in that same year, more than 200,000 weight loss surgeries were performed.[9,41] Morbid obesity is defined as 45 kg (100 lb) over ideal body weight or a body mass index (BMI) of 40 kg/m$^2$. Obese patients typically present with serious co-existing health conditions, such as diabetes, cardiopulmonary disease, obstructive sleep apnea (OSA), gallstone disease, hypertension, lipidemia, respiratory problems, or joint disease.

Eligibility criteria for patients seeking bariatric surgery include morbid obesity complicated by medical conditions secondary to obesity, history of failed dietary therapy, psychologic stability and motivation, acceptable operative risks, and a patient who is well-informed about the procedure, recovery, and postsurgery life-style modifications.

HISTORY

**The History of Bariatric Surgery**

**1950s** J. Kremen, MD, performs jejunoileal bypass.
It is recognized that patients with short-bowel syndrome lose weight because of impaired absorption.
Similar procedure is performed in Sweden, excising redundant portion of intestine.

**1960s** Ten jejunocolic shunt procedures are reported.
Shunts are eventually converted to jejunoileostomies to control diarrhea, electrolyte imbalance, and dehydration.
Patients continue to experience postoperative anemia, cholelithiasis, vitamin depletion, and renal and liver disease.
E. Mason, MD, performs partial gastrectomy with staples, creating a pouch anastomosed to small intestine.
Early complications promote refinement of gastroplasty.

**1970s** E. Mason, MD, develops vertical-banded gastroplasty (VBG).
L. Wilkinson, MD, uses mesh strip for the band to reduce size of gastric reservoir.
Biliopancreatic diversion is developed in Italy.

**1980s** Gastric banding is refined to limit food intake.
L. Kuzmak, MD, develops first adjustable gastric band and later a hollow band with inflatable ring.
American Society for Bariatric Surgery (ASBS) is formed in 1983.

**1990s** Laparoscopic access becomes approach of choice.
Some procedures move to ambulatory surgery units.

**2000s** *Bariatric* becomes common medical terminology.
Many institutions develop interdisciplinary programs specifically for weight loss surgery.
Bariatric boutique surgery centers enter surgical market.
Long-term studies begin to evaluate persistence of surgery results over time.
Insurance reimbursement continues to evolve as studies evaluate risks, complications, and rehospitalization rates and costs.

Modified from Association of periOperative Registered Nurses: AORN bariatric surgery guideline. In *AORN standards, guidelines and recommended practices*, Denver, 2005, The Association; Barclay L: Bariatric surgery may be a viable treatment option for severe obesity, December 2004, Accessed December 30, 2004, on-line: www.medscape.com/viewarticle/496590?src=mp; Rundle RL, Spencer J: Concerns grow over weight-loss surgery, *Wall Street Journal*, pp. D1, D6, October 19, 2005.

Contraindications are not clearly generalized because morbidly obese patients are typically at greater risk for surgery. Patients at greatest risk are those with end-stage heart and lung function, inability to ambulate, weight more than 272 kg (600 lb), age younger than late teens or older than 65 years, and presence of Prader-Willi syndrome.[41]

The three categories of bariatric procedures are restrictive, malabsorptive, or a combination of both. Restrictive procedures reduce the size of the stomach. When the patient eats, food is digested and absorbed normally, but the small capacity of the stomach gives the feeling of fullness; therefore the patient eats less. In malabsorptive procedures, absorption capacity of the small intestine is reduced with a bypass of a segment or segments of the proximal small bowel.

Adjustable gastric banding is a restrictive procedure. The adjustable band surgery uses a silicone strip and elastic ring called the *LAP-BAND* (INAMED Health). It is placed laparoscopically around the top of the stomach. A fold of stomach is sutured around the band to secure it in place (Figure 11-23). The band has a connected implanted port that is inflated with saline 4 weeks postoperatively. The constriction created by the inflated band restricts the amount of ingested food permitted to enter the stomach, preventing overeating. This procedure is adjustable and reversible.

## Laparoscopic Roux-en-Y Gastric Bypass

The Roux-en-Y gastric bypass (RYGB) is a largely restrictive and mildly malabsorptive procedure that reroutes the passage of ingested food and fluid from a small pouch created with surgical staples or sutures in the proximal stomach to a segment of the proximal small bowel. Jejunum or ileum may be used as described under "Gastrojejunosotomy." Laparoscopic RYGB has become a commonly performed bariatric procedure in the United States.[41]

***Procedural Considerations.*** All patients undergoing bariatric surgery need special consideration, since they usually have associated serious co-morbidities that place them at risk during the operative procedure. A special OR bed is required that can accommodate patients who weigh more than 350 lb (159 kg). Other special equipment required, in addition to the laparoscopic instrumentation and accessory supplies, includes extra-large blood pressure cuffs and extra-long trocars. Posi-

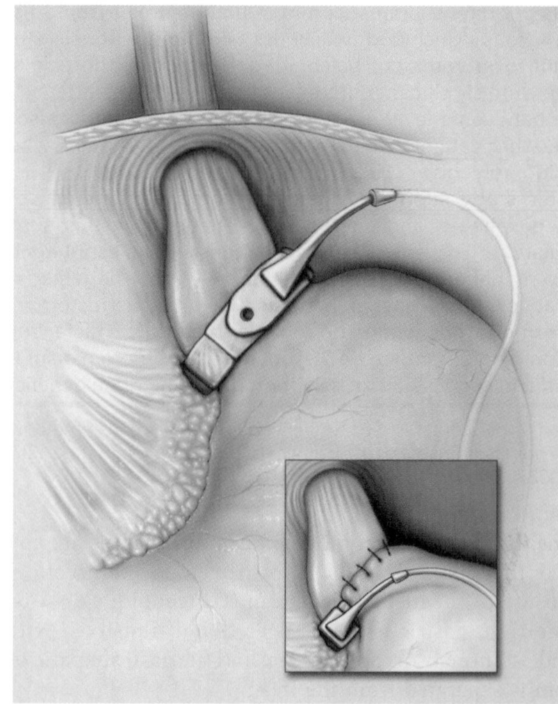

**FIGURE 11-23** Proper position of the LAP-BAND. The silicone band around the stomach of the fundus creates a small gastric pouch. The inner lining of the band contains an inflatable balloon that is connected to a subcutaneous port on the patient's abdomen (not shown). The band can be inflated or deflated, adjusting the stomach size as needed.

tioning requires additional padded safety restraints, pressure reduction devices to reduce the risk of pressure injury, and proper fitting SCDs. The perioperative nurse should anticipate the potential for anesthesia assistance during intubation and airway management.

### *Operative Procedure*

1. Five trocars are placed above the umbilicus: two on the midline, two in the left upper quadrant, and one in the right upper quadrant; and an incision is made for the liver retractor (Figure 11-24).
2. The omentum is mobilized and the ligament of Treitz identified.
3. The jejunum is divided 40 cm distal to the ligament with a vascular stapler (Figure 11-25). The proximal jejunum is left to lie in the patient's right side and the Roux limb lifted superiorly and passed through the transverse colon mesentery (Figure 11-26).
4. A gastric pouch is created with several loads of a linear stapler.
5. The Roux limb is anastomosed to the proximal gastric pouch. The stapler defect is closed, and methylene blue is used to check for leaks. The gastrojejunostomy may alternatively be accomplished with traditional suturing technique or a circular EEA stapler.
6. Mesenteric defects are closed, the abdomen is inspected, and the port sites are closed.

With the RYGB, a critical segment of the calorie- and nutrition-absorbing mucosal surface is avoided. The gastric pouch is generally less than 30 cc in volume. This procedure results in considerable weight loss for the patient. Serious complications include hemorrhage, anastomotic leaks, pulmonary embolism, pneumonia, infection, small bowel obstructions or stenosis, and incisional hernia.[41] Nutritional deficits, nausea, flatus, diarrhea, and dumping syndrome are other common complications following this procedure.

The biliopancreatic diversion (Figure 11-27) and the duodenal switch (Figure 11-28) procedures are largely malabsorptive and mildly restrictive. In these procedures, both the Roux limb and the biliopancreatic limb are long in length, leaving a shortened common channel where digestion and absorption of proteins, fats and carbohydrates can occur. These procedures present more risk of complications, nutritional deficiencies, liver abnormalities, anemia, and lactose intolerance.[4]

## SURGERY OF THE SMALL BOWEL

### Meckel's Diverticulectomy

Meckel's diverticulum is removed to prevent inflammation and obstruction from intussusception of the diverticulum, which consists of an unobliterated congenital duct at the umbilicus that is attached to the distal ileum (Figure 11-29). The diverticulum may contain gastric mucosa, which may ulcerate, perforate, or bleed.

***Procedural Considerations.*** A laparotomy set and a GI instrument set are required. Linear stapling devices should be available. The patient is positioned supine under general anesthesia. The anesthesia provider inserts a nasogastric tube after intubation. An indwelling urinary catheter is inserted before the abdominal skin prep.

#### *Operative Procedure*

1. The abdomen is opened through a midline incision or laparoscopically accessed, and the diverticulum is identified.
2. If the diverticulum is long and narrow with a narrow base, the procedure is similar to that of an appendectomy (see the following discussion). If the base is broad, the loop of bowel

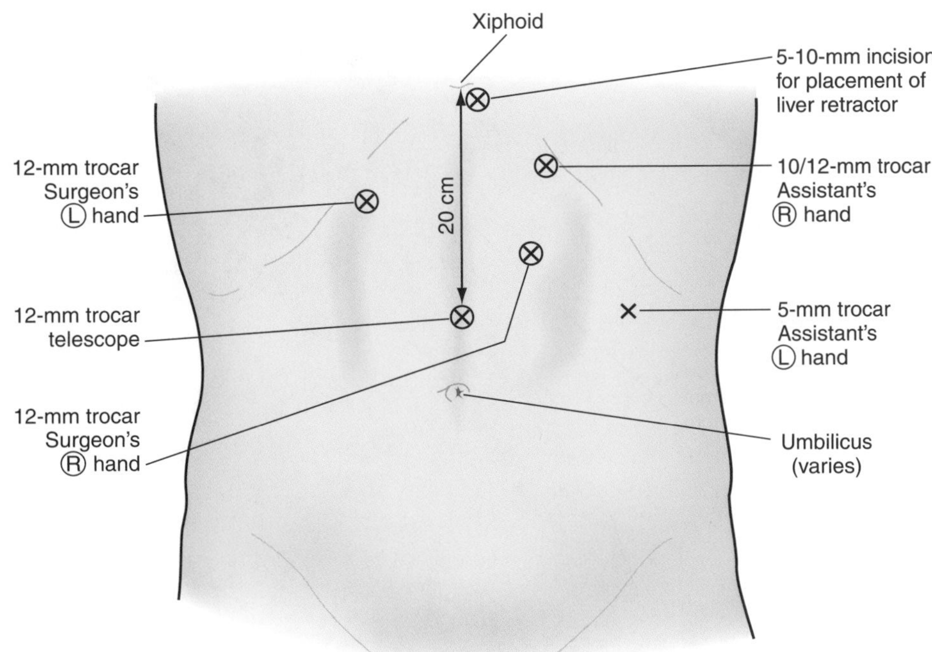


**FIGURE 11-24** Trocar configuration for laparoscopic Roux-en-Y gastric bypass.

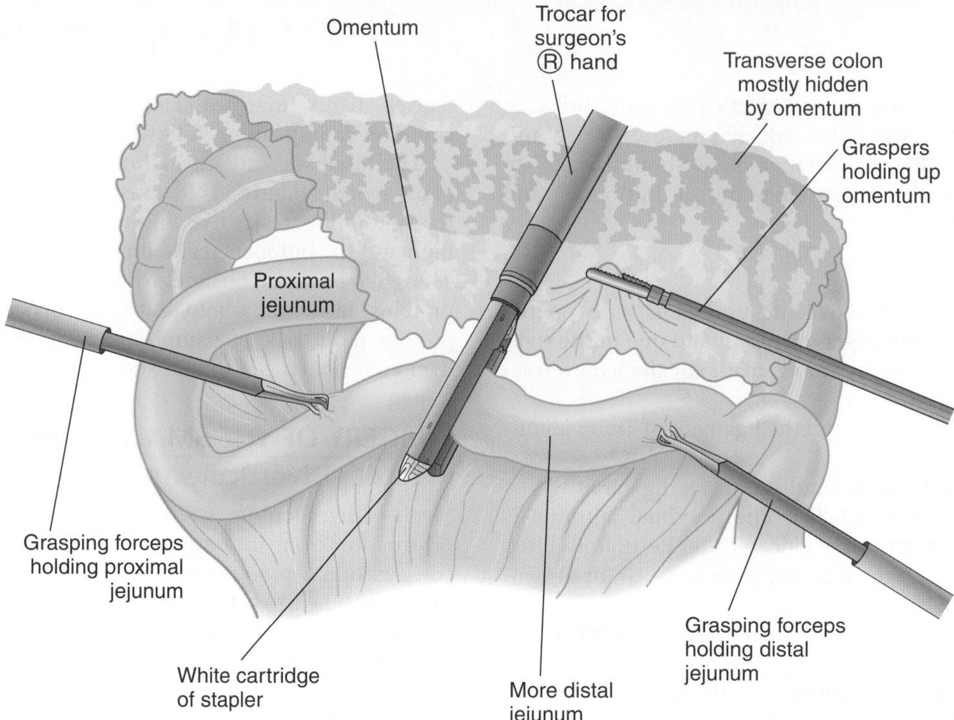


**FIGURE 11-25** Placing stapler to divide jejunum to create Roux limb.

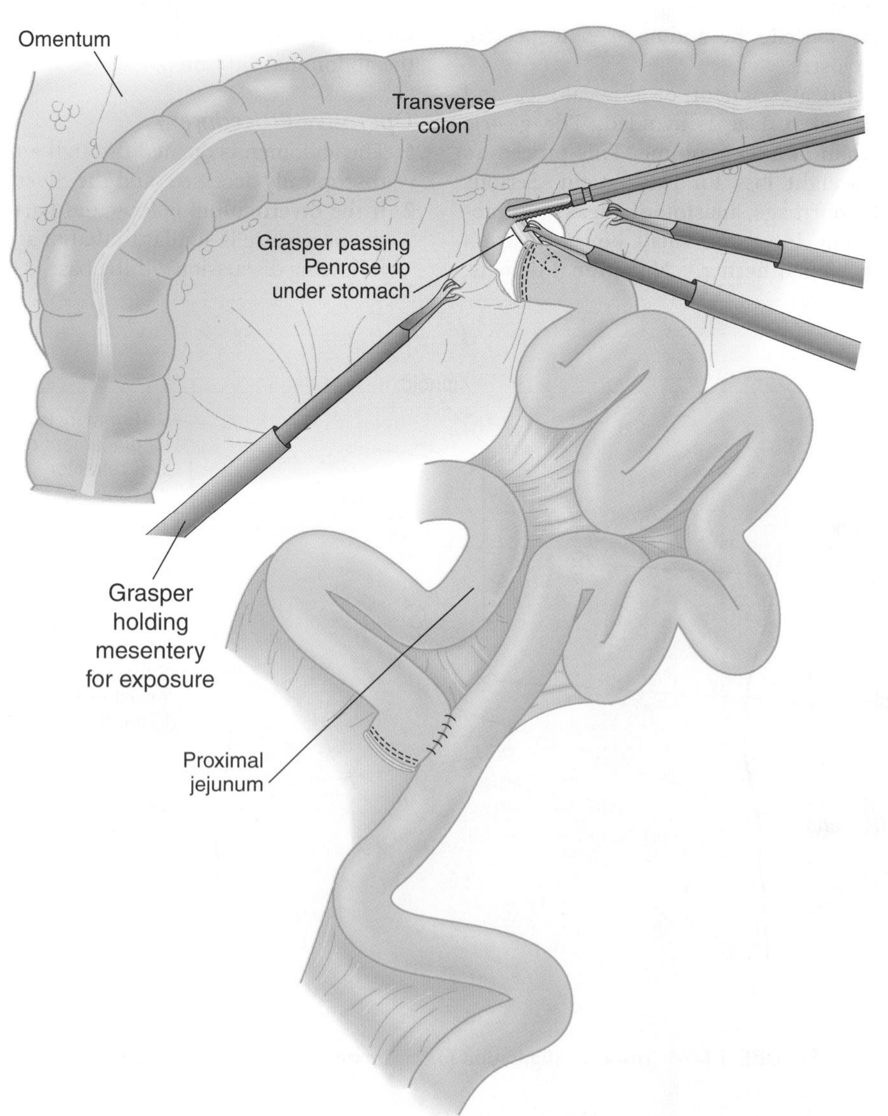


**FIGURE 11-26** Passing the Roux limb into a retrocolic and retrogastric position.

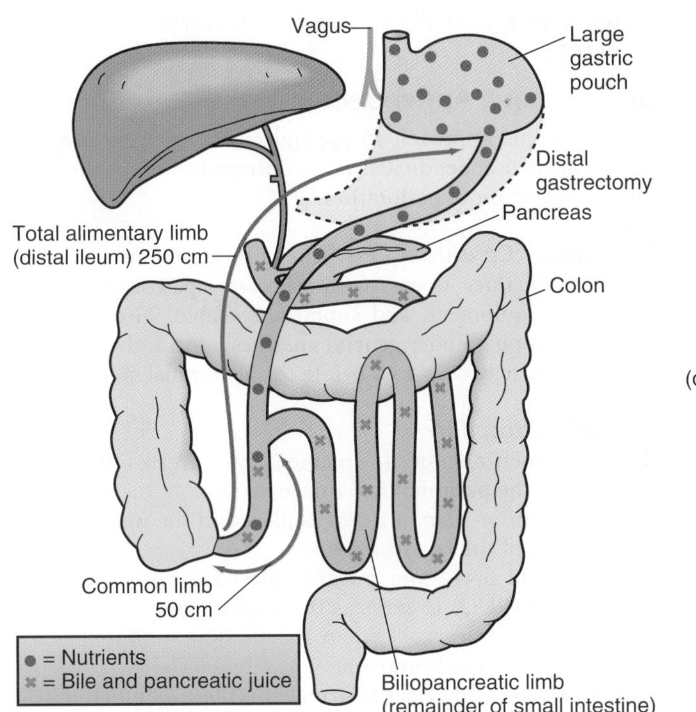


**FIGURE 11-27** Configuration of the biliopancreatic diversion (BPD), which is transection of the stomach with anastomosis of the duodenum to the distal ileum. In this malabsorptive procedure, the pancreatic enzymes and bile enter near the ileum, allowing nutrients to pass from the stomach to the distal ileum without being digested. Weight loss occurs because of the partial gastrectomy, which restricts intake, and a shortened alimentary canal, which causes malabsorption.

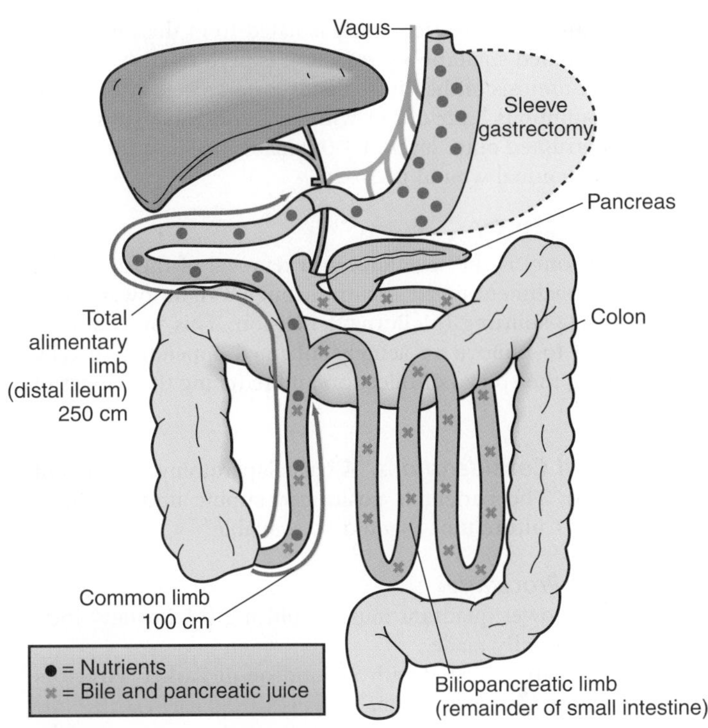


**FIGURE 11-28** Configuration of the duodenal switch, which leaves a larger portion of the stomach intact, including the pyloric valve. This helps in alleviating dumping syndrome.

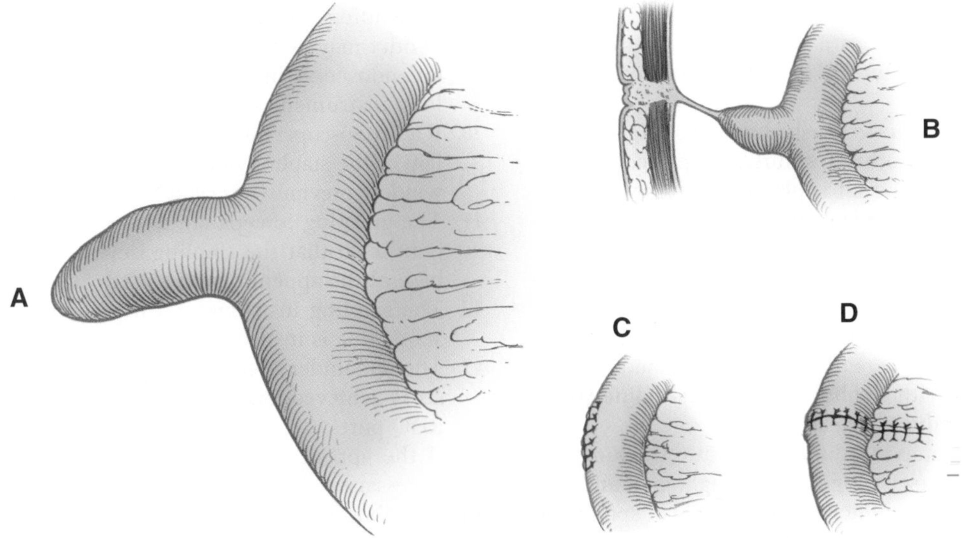


**FIGURE 11-29** **A,** The most common nonpathologic appearance of Meckel's diverticulum arises from the antimesenteric border of the distal ileum. **B,** A persistent fibrous band of tissue connects the apex of the diverticulum to the anterior abdominal wall at the umbilicus. **C,** The suture line of a local Meckel's diverticulectomy. **D,** Completed ileoileal anastomosis after excision of 1 to 2 cm of ileum on each side of a Meckel's diverticulum.

containing the diverticulum is isolated from the mesentery and a limited small bowel resection is performed.
3. An anastomosis of the divided ends is completed with an inner continuous layer of 3-0 synthetic absorbable suture and an interrupted outer layer of 4-0 nonabsorbable sutures.
4. The abdominal wound is closed.

## Appendectomy

Appendectomy is the severance and removal of the appendix from its attachment to the cecum through a right lower quadrant muscle-splitting (McBurney) incision. This procedure is performed to remove an acutely inflamed appendix, thereby controlling the spread of infection and reducing the danger of peritonitis.

***Procedural Considerations.*** A basic laparotomy instrument set is used. The patient is positioned supine under general anesthesia. Culture tubes should be available.

### *Operative Procedure*

1. A right lower quadrant muscle-splitting (McBurney) incision is usually made.
2. Muscles are retracted with Richardson or Parker retractors to expose the peritoneum.
3. The peritoneum is grasped with tissue forceps or an Allis forceps, and a small incision is made with a scalpel using a #15 blade.
4. A culture sample may be taken.
5. The incision is completed with a Metzenbaum scissors.
6. The mesoappendix is grasped near the tip with a Babcock forceps or a hemostat for gentle traction.
7. The mesoappendix is dissected from the appendiceal wall and ligated with 3-0 nonabsorbable suture. If a suture ligature is required, 2-0 synthetic absorbable suture on an atraumatic GI needle is preferred.
8. The appendix is elevated as a purse-string suture of 2-0 synthetic absorbable suture is placed in the cecal wall at the appendiceal base.
9. The base of the appendix is crushed with a straight hemostat, a 3-0 synthetic absorbable suture tie is placed over the crushed area, and a hemostat is placed above the ligature.
10. A basin is provided for the specimen and discarded instruments that have come into contact with GI mucosa.
11. Protective gauze sponges are placed over the cecum around the base of the appendix.
12. The appendix is amputated between the clamp and synthetic absorbable suture with a scalpel. Sometimes the stump is swabbed with alcohol or povidone-iodine (Betadine) solution to reduce bacterial flora.
13. The appendiceal stump may be inverted into the lumen of the cecum as the purse-string suture is tightened and tied by means of a fine straight hemostat and a small sponge on a holder. Soiled instruments are discarded into the basin.
14. If the appendix has ruptured, copious amounts of warm fluids are used to irrigate the peritoneal cavity. A drain may be inserted down to the appendiceal bed to allow continuous drainage. Deeper layers are closed, leaving the subcutaneous tissue and skin open. The wound may then be packed open with moist fine-mesh gauze to heal by secondary intention. (This packing method may be used in any case in which bowel contamination or abscess formation is present. It allows clean healing and prevents pocketing of pus.)

## Laparoscopic Appendectomy

A laparoscopic approach to appendectomy may be used for uncomplicated appendicitis. It is contraindicated in the presence or suspicion of perforation.[28]

***Procedural Considerations.*** The procedure involves the placement of three trocars with standard laparoscopic instrumentation, equipment, and supplies available. The patient is positioned supine under general anesthesia. An indwelling urinary catheter may be placed before the abdominal skin prep.

### *Operative Procedure*

1. Pneumoperitoneum is obtained by a Verres needle or through the periumbilical trocar.
2. An 11-mm or 12-mm trocar is placed in the umbilicus for insertion of the laparoscope.
3. An 11-mm or 12-mm trocar is placed in the right upper quadrant (RUQ) to serve as the working port.
4. The 5-mm trocar placed in the midline suprapubic site serves as the traction trocar.
5. A laparoscopic Babcock instrument is inserted into the RUQ trocar to grasp the cecum and retract it toward the liver.
6. The appendix is grasped at its tip by a grasping forceps that has been inserted through the suprapubic trocar and is held in an upward position.
7. The Babcock forceps is removed, and a dissecting instrument is inserted through the RUQ trocar to create a mesenteric window in the mesoappendix.
8. Dissection is performed in proximity to the appendix, beginning directly under the base and progressing to a 1-cm to 2-cm length.
9. Depending on the surgeon's preferred technique, the appendix may be transected in several different ways: (a) by an endoscopic linear stapling instrument, (b) by a ligating loop instrument, or (c) by a suturing instrument.
10. If an endoscopic linear stapling instrument is used, the lower jaw of the stapling device is passed through the mesenteric window previously created by way of the RUQ trocar.
11. The grasping forceps are used to rotate the tip of the appendix so that the stapling device can be snugged to the base of the appendix and closed.
12. The stapling instrument is fired and withdrawn, and the staple line is inspected.
13. The remainder of the mesoappendix is dissected, hemostasis is achieved, and the appendix is removed through the RUQ port.
14. If the appendix is too thick, a specimen pouch may be necessary to facilitate its extraction.
15. The abdomen is irrigated, the irrigation fluid is aspirated with a suction and irrigation device, and then the abdomen is deflated.
16. Trocar sites are closed and dressed or closed with skin bonding sealer.

## Resection of the Small Intestine

Resection of the small intestine involves excision of the diseased intestine through an abdominal incision and frequently includes some type of bowel reanastomosis. It is performed to remove tumors, a gangrenous portion of the intestine caused by strangulation from bands of adhesions, intestinal obstruction, areas of ulceration and bleeding as in Crohn's disease, a herniation of the intestine, or a volvulus.

***Procedural Considerations.*** A laparotomy set and a GI instrument set are required. Linear stapling instruments should be available. The patient is positioned supine under general anesthesia. The anesthesia provider inserts a nasogastric tube after intubation. An indwelling urinary catheter is inserted before the abdominal skin prep. Small bowel procedures are also safely and effectively accomplished through the laparoscopic approach.

#### *Operative Procedure*

1. The abdominal wall is incised through a midline incision and retracted.
2. The peritoneal cavity is explored and protected with moist warm saline packs.
3. Intestinal clamps are placed above and below the diseased segment of the small bowel and mesentery.
4. The involved area is removed with a linear stapling instrument such as a GIA, an electrosurgical blade, or a scalpel.
5. The continuity of the GI tract is established by an end-to-end, end-to-side, or side-to-side anastomosis.
6. The wound is closed and dressed.

An alternative approach to a traditional suture anastomosis is the use of a mechanical stapling device. The device allows the surgeon to perform an end-to-end, end-to-side, or side-to-side anastomosis. An enterotomy is made close to the anastomosis site. The stapler is inserted, and the distal bowel is secured between the anvil and the head of the stapler. The anvil is then inserted into the proximal loop of bowel and secured to the center rod. The gap is closed, and the stapler is fired. The stapler is extracted through the enterotomy. The integrity of the anastomosis is verified, and the enterotomy is closed with sutures.

## Ileostomy

Ileostomy is the formation of a temporary or permanent opening into the ileum. This procedure is indicated in the presence of an extensive lesion to reduce large bowel activity, often called *bowel rest,* by means of a temporary fecal diversion to the outside of the body, or as a permanent fecal diversion in total colectomy. The patient is site-marked before surgery and anesthesia by the WOCN (see Box 11-1).

***Procedural Considerations.*** A laparotomy set, a GI instrument set, and linear stapling instruments are required. The patient is positioned supine under general anesthesia. The anesthesia provider inserts a nasogastric tube after intubation. An indwelling urinary catheter is inserted before the abdominal skin prep. An ostomy appliance for the stoma should be available.

#### *Operative Procedure*

1. Through a midline incision, the peritoneal cavity is explored and the pathologic condition is determined.
2. The ileum is mobilized with a Metzenbaum scissors and hemostatic clamps.
3. The mesentery is clamped, divided, and ligated with 3-0 nonabsorbable sutures at the proposed site, usually about 15 cm from the ileocecal junction.
4. Two intestinal clamps are placed on the bowel, and the ileum is divided with a scalpel or linear stapling instrument (GIA) between the two clamps.
5. The distal end of the ileum is closed with 2-0 synthetic absorbable suture on a taper needle if a stapling device has not been used.
6. The proximal end is brought out to the skin through an opening on the right side and is held in place by clamps, making sure that the ileum is not overstretched or its blood supply compromised.
7. The mesentery of the ileum is sutured to the parietal wall to eliminate a potential internal hernia.
8. The abdomen is then closed.
9. The stoma is sutured to the skin after the ileum is everted to form a protective cover over the exposed ileal serosa.
10. A disposable ostomy appliance is placed over the stoma to collect small bowel contents.

An alternative to a conventional ileostomy for selected patients is the Kock pouch, or continent ileostomy. The internal pouch is created from a segment of small intestine with an outlet to the skin. When functioning properly, the stoma and pouch are continent and do not continually drain stool. A catheter is inserted into the stoma three or four times daily to evacuate the contents. This procedure eliminates the need for an external appliance.

## Intestinal Transplantation

Small bowel transplantation may be indicated for patients with intestinal failure caused by short gut syndrome as a result of extensive resections necessitated by Crohn's disease, necrotizing enterocolitis, mesenteric thrombosis, atresias, volvulus, trauma, dysmotility, or congenital enteropathy. Intestinal failure leads to malabsorption and malnutrition, preventing the bowel from meeting the body's nutrient and fluid requirements. Approximately 10 to 20 cm of small intestine with an ileocecal valve, or 40 cm without an ileocecal valve, is minimally required to maintain nutritional status.[2,17] Patients with short gut syndrome require TPN to sustain life. A critical indication for intestinal transplant arises when they can no longer receive TPN because of clotting of major veins, frequent IV line sepsis, episodes of dehydration despite TPN and IV fluids, and TPN-induced liver failure.[36] Intestinal transplantation may also include the liver in the presence of impending progressive end-stage liver disease. The perioperative time frame, beginning with immunosuppression, surgery, transition from parenteral to enteral feedings, and the long recovery process, may be 6 months and poses many physical and emotional challenges to the patient and family. Despite these challenges, refinements in surgical technique and patient selection, coupled with advances in immunosuppression protocols, have contributed to significant improvements in patient survival rates.

***Procedural Considerations.*** The transplant surgeon does the final visual inspection and assessment of the donor organ. The allowable cold ischemic time of the donor intestine (allograft intestine) is approximately 12 hours.[3] The patient is positioned supine and anesthetized with general endotracheal anesthesia. Arterial and multiple venous lines are inserted. Nasogastric tube, urinary catheter, and full physiologic monitoring are indicated.

*Operative Procedure*

1. The incision is made along previous incision lines, or a vertical midline approach is used.
2. The superior mesenteric artery of the donor organ is anastomosed to the recipient's infrarenal aorta.
3. Venous drainage of the donor organ is established by connecting the superior mesenteric vein to the portal vein if the patient has no liver disease or signs of portal hypertension.
4. Reperfusion begins with the release of the venous flow when the clamps are opened.
5. Bleeding sites are identified and ligated or coagulated.
6. The arterial clamp is released.
7. The continuity of the intestine is restored after the vascular supply is established.
8. Proximal anastomosis joins the donor jejunum to the recipient stomach, duodenum, or proximal jejunum.
9. Distal ileum is anastomosed side-to-side with the remaining colon.
10. A distal loop ileostomy is created for later endoscopic evaluation and intestinal biopsies.
11. The intact intestine is inspected, hemostasis is verified, and the abdomen is closed.

## SURGERY OF THE COLON

### Laparoscopic Colectomy

Resection of a segment of bowel and anastomosis can be accomplished using laparoscopic techniques. Laparoscopic colectomy requires advanced laparoscopic skills on the part of the operative surgeon.[48] The advantages of laparoscopic colectomy include the reduction of morbidity associated with open techniques (e.g., postoperative ileus), decreased postoperative pain, more rapid return to normal activities, shorter length of stay, and improved cosmesis. Laparoscopic colectomy is indicated for obstruction and benign tumors of the large bowel.

***Procedural Considerations.*** Depending on the intended segment of bowel to be resected, the patient is initially positioned supine or in a modified lithotomy for access to the rectum for end-to-end anastomosis. Pneumatic compression stockings are applied to minimize the risk of DVT. The patient is secured with restraining straps to support and maintain position during steep position changes during the procedure. A bean bag device, secured to the OR bed, may be used. A nasogastric tube and urethral catheter are inserted before the abdominal skin prep. Laparotomy instrumentation, mechanical stapling devices, and endostapling devices should be readily available. To assist the surgeon in accurately identifying the segment of bowel to be resected, a colonoscope may be used preoperatively or during the laparoscopic procedure to tattoo the lesion with India ink.

*Operative Procedure (Right Hemicolectomy)*

1. Pneumoperitoneum is established at 10 to 12 mm Hg, and the 10-mm umbilical trocar is placed after a supraumbilical cutdown. Alternatively, a 12-mm Hasson trocar may be inserted through the rectus muscle and into the abdominal cavity by way of a small incision in the left upper quadrant, 3 to 4 cm below the costal margin.
2. Usually two 10- or 12-mm trocars are placed in locations dependent on the anatomic segment of colon that will be resected; 5-mm ports may be placed at sites where stomas might be created in the conventional open procedure.
3. After the patient is moved into Trendelenburg position, with rotation to the left, dissecting scissors are inserted as well as a grasper. The peritoneum along the cecum is incised as are the appendiceal and terminal ileal attachments. The bowel is then bluntly dissected from the retroperitoneum, the ureter identified, and the colon mobilized as necessary for resection of the diseased segment. A mesenteric window is created, and the mesenteric artery and vein and right colic vessels are identified and clipped.
4. A multifire endoscopic linear stapling device (GIA) is positioned over the segment of bowel and fired to both transect and staple the segment.
5. Unless an end-to-end anastomosis can be performed, as in a low sigmoid or rectal resection, a small incision is made over the area of the abdomen that will provide access to the segments for anastomosis.
6. The segment of bowel to be resected is grasped and brought through the small laparotomy incision and transected, and anastomosis is performed by the surgeon's preferred manner (either with staples or with sutures).
7. The anastomosed bowel is returned to the peritoneal cavity, and the cavity is irrigated and inspected for hemostasis and drained by suction. The cannulas are removed, port sites closed, and the skin closed with a subcuticular absorbable suture. Skin tapes (Steri-Strips) are then applied.

### Colostomy

Colostomy is the mobilization of a loop of colon through a right rectus incision to expose the transverse colon. A left rectus incision can also be made to expose the descending sigmoid colon. The layers of the wound beneath or around the colostomy are subsequently closed. A colostomy is performed to treat an obstruction in the sigmoid colon resulting from a malignant lesion. Another possible indication for this procedure is advanced inflammation or trauma that has caused distention or obstruction of the proximal portion of the colon. A temporary colostomy is often done to decompress the bowel or to divert bowel contents (bowel rest) to promote healing (Figure 11-30).

***Procedural Considerations.*** A laparotomy set and a GI instrument set are required. Linear stapling instruments may be used. Stoma appliances are required. These items may include a colostomy rod, rubber tubing, or a loop ostomy bridge. The patient will be site-marked by the WOCN before surgery. The patient is positioned supine under general anesthesia. The anesthesia provider inserts a nasogastric tube after intubation. An indwelling urinary catheter is inserted before the abdominal skin prep.

*Operative Procedure*

FIRST-STAGE LOOP COLOSTOMY

1. The abdomen is opened, and the wound edges are protected and retracted.
2. The peritoneal cavity is opened and walled off with moist laparotomy packs, and appropriate retractors are inserted.
3. A small opening is made in the mesentery near the bowel with curved hemostats and a Metzenbaum scissors.
4. A piece of tubing or Penrose drain is passed around the colon, and the two ends are held with a hemostat to maintain gentle traction.

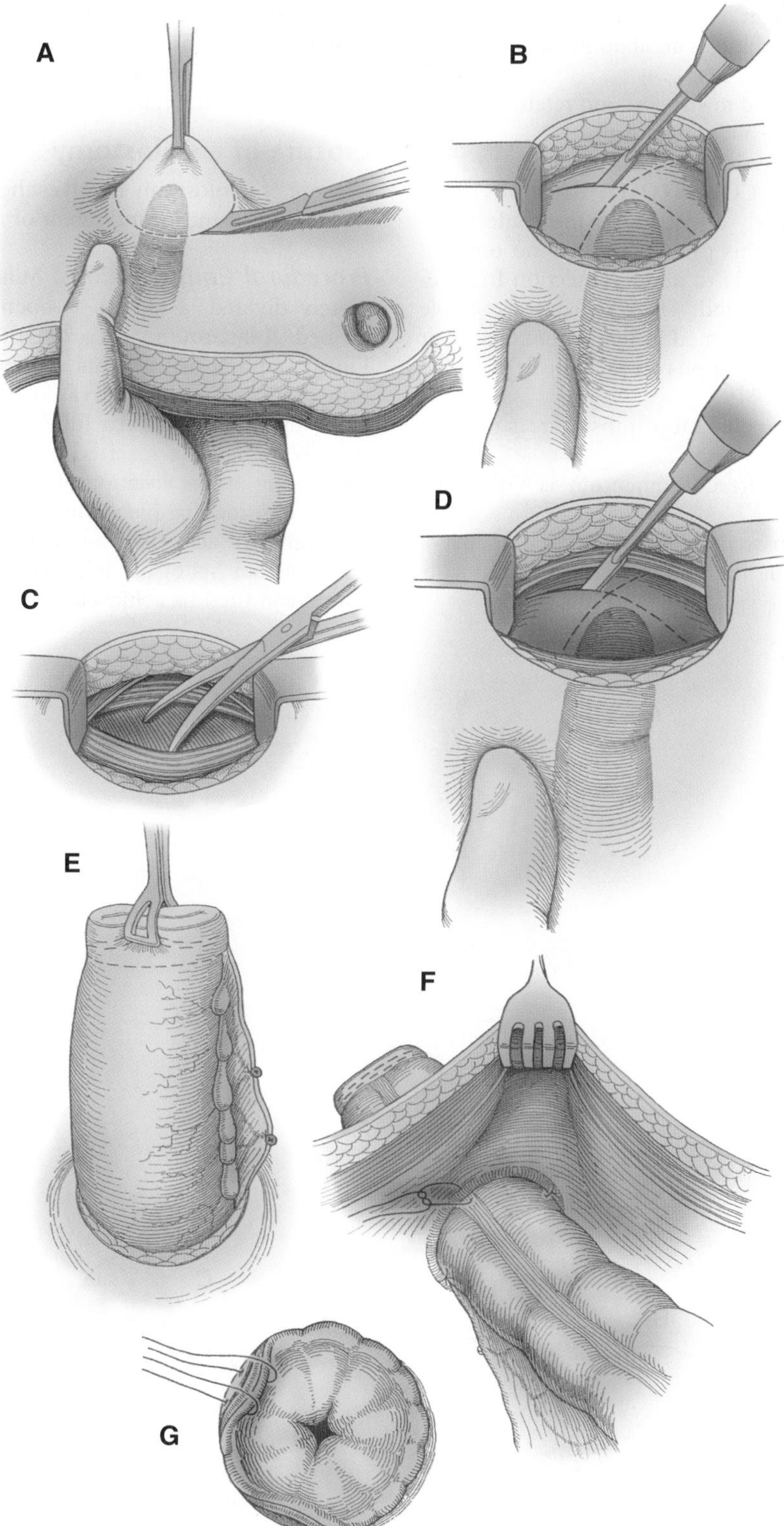


FIGURE 11-30 Construction of a colostomy through the anterior abdominal wall. **A**, A core of subcutaneous tissue is removed after making a circular skin incision with a #10 blade and using an electrosurgical pencil to dissect down to the anterior fascia. **B**, Muscle fibers are split. **C**, Tissues are dissected to the posterior layers, and, **D**, the peritoneum is opened. **E**, The colon is delivered through the abdominal wall so that it extends 2 to 3 cm beyond the skin surface. **F**, The bowel is tacked internally to the peritoneal defect. **G**, Four sutures are placed in each quadrant, incorporating the full-thickness cut end of the colon, the serosal surface approximately 1 to 2 cm below the open end of the colon, and up to the dermis. Additional sutures are used to mature the stoma, which refers to the procedure of everting the mucosa to create a stable opening through which feces can be evacuated.

5. The loop of colon is brought out through an incision made on the left side of the midline. The abdominal incision is closed.
6. A loop ostomy bridge is used to support and retain the loop of colon in position on the abdominal wall.
7. The loop of intestine is dressed with petrolatum gauze.

SECOND-STAGE LOOP COLOSTOMY. After 48 hours the loop of colon is completely opened with the blade tip of an electrosurgical pencil. By this time, if there is no tension, healing has advanced sufficiently to allow protection from feces contamination onto the wound. This procedure is simple and painless and is usually performed in the patient's room or in a treatment room. An ostomy appliance is applied.

TRANSVERSE COLOSTOMY

1. A short incision, vertical or preferably transverse, is made to reach the transverse colon.
2. A loop of transverse colon, freed of omentum, is withdrawn (Figure 11-31).
3. A loop ostomy bridge is passed through an avascular area of the mesocolon, preventing the loop from returning to the peritoneal cavity.
4. A mushroom catheter, which is held in place with a purse-string suture, brings about immediate decompression.

The bowel is opened 24 to 36 hours later, and the bridge may be removed in about 7 to 10 days.

## Closure of a Colostomy

Closure of a colostomy involves the reestablishment of internal intestinal continuity and repair of the abdominal wall.

***Procedural Considerations.*** When the loop has been completely divided, a closed or open anastomosis may be performed. A laparotomy set and GI instrument set are required. Linear stapling instruments may be used. The patient is positioned supine under general anesthesia. The anesthesia provider inserts a nasogastric tube after intubation. An indwelling urinary catheter is inserted before the abdominal skin prep. Depending on the location of the bowel to be reanastomosed, the patient may be placed in low lithotomy position to facilitate transanal access for a circular stapling device. An end-to-end anastomosis of the left colon or ileal pouch to the rectal stump can then be achieved.

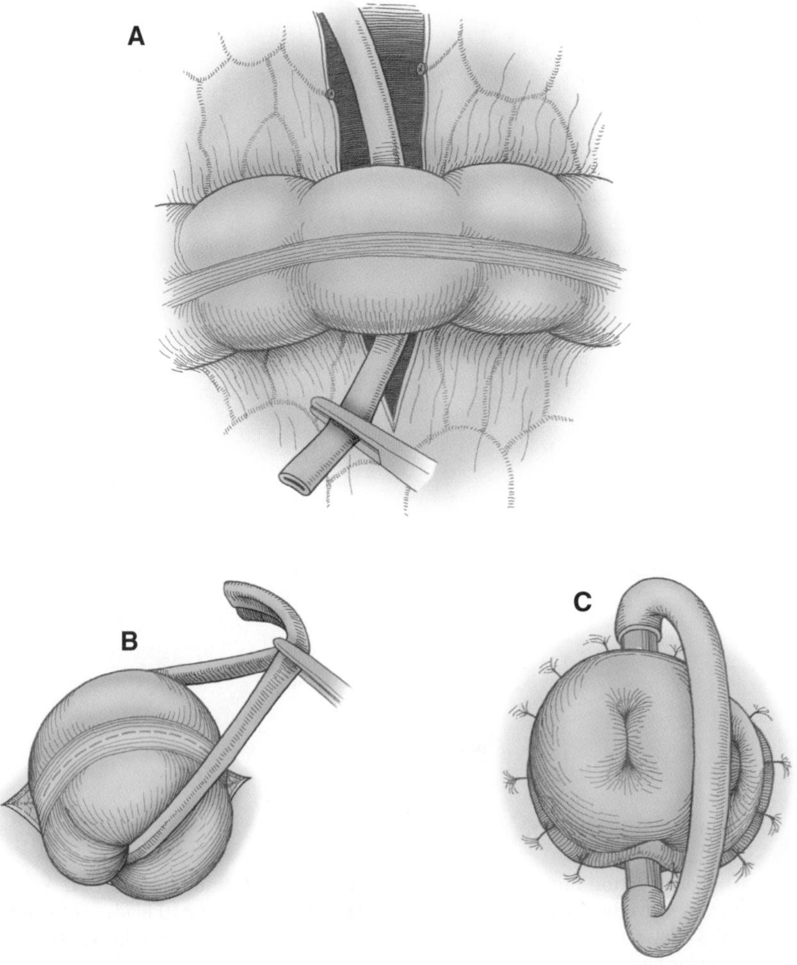


FIGURE 11-31 Transverse loop colostomy. **A,** The mesentery adjacent to the colon is taken down so that a Penrose drain may be passed beneath the colon. **B,** The colon is pulled through the transverse incision and opened longitudinally along the taeniae. **C,** An apparatus or rod is placed underneath the stoma; sutures are used to mature the colostomy. The rod can be removed after the seventh postoperative day.

*Operative Procedure*

1. A circumferential incision is made around the colostomy to free the skin margin.
2. Moist packs, a scalpel with a #10 blade, a Metzenbaum scissors, and Crile hemostats are used as the layers of the abdominal wall are identified and dissected free.
3. An end-to-end anastomosis is completed in two layers—the inner with 3-0 synthetic absorbable suture and the outer with 3-0 nonabsorbable suture on an intestinal needle, using interrupted sutures. Alternatively, a surgical stapling device may be used.
4. The abdominal wound is closed in layers. A dressing is applied.

The surgeon may elect to leave the subcutaneous tissue and skin open. In this instance the wound is packed and permitted to heal by secondary intention.

## Right Hemicolectomy and Ileocolostomy

Right hemicolectomy and ileocolostomy involve the resection of the right half of the colon—including a portion of the transverse colon, the ascending colon, and the cecum—and a segment of the terminal ileum and mesentery (Figure 11-32, *A*). An end-to-end, side-to-side, or end-to-side anastomosis is done between the transverse colon and the ileum. A right hemicolectomy and ileocolostomy are performed to remove a malignant lesion of the right colon and in some cases to remove inflammatory lesions involving the ileum, cecum, or ascending colon.

***Procedural Considerations.*** When a side-to-side anastomosis is carried out, the transected stumps of the ileum and the transverse colon are closed before the anastomosis is done. It is completed between the side portions of the ileum and the transverse colon. A side-to-side anastomosis can also be performed by inserting the GIA stapler into both colon segments and firing the device. The stumps are then closed using a TA linear stapling device.

When an end-to-end anastomosis is performed, the layers of the transected stumps of the ileum and the transverse colon are sutured together. Circular linear stapling devices, such as an EEA, may be used for anastomosis.

A laparotomy set and a GI instrument set are required. The patient is positioned supine under general anesthesia. The anesthesia provider inserts a nasogastric tube after intubation. An indwelling urinary catheter is inserted before the abdominal skin prep.

*Operative Procedure*

1. The abdomen is opened, and the peritoneal cavity is retracted and packed with warm moist sponges.
2. The mesentery of the transverse colon and the terminal ileum is incised at the points where the resection is to be done.
3. Moist packs are placed to isolate the viscera to be resected. A Metzenbaum scissors, hemostats, and 3-0 nonabsorbable ligatures are used to clamp, cut, and ligate mesentery vessels.
4. The lateral peritoneal fold along the lateral side of the right colon is incised, and the right colon is mobilized medially. Metzenbaum scissors, hemostats, and sponges on holders are used.
5. The ureter and duodenum are carefully identified.
6. The same procedure is carried out on the terminal ileum. The mesenteric vessels are clamped and ligated with 2-0 nonabsorbable ligatures.
7. The operative field is prepared for anastomosis (bowel technique).
8. Intestinal clamps are placed on the transverse colon and ileum.
9. Division is completed with a scalpel, and the specimen is removed.
10. An end-to-end anastomosis is completed between the severed ends of the terminal ileum and the transverse colon.
11. Instruments and supplies that have come into contact with bowel mucosa are discarded.
12. The mesentery and posterior peritoneum are closed with interrupted 3-0 nonabsorbable sutures.
13. The abdominal wound is closed. A dressing is applied.

## Transverse Colectomy

Transverse colectomy is excision of the transverse colon through an upper midline or transverse incision (Figure 11-32, *C* and *D*). Bowel integrity is reestablished by an end-to-end anastomosis. A transverse colectomy is performed for malignant lesions of the transverse colon. A more radical procedure may be required when the lesion has perforated the greater curvature of the stomach. If the entire lesion is resectable, a partial gastrectomy may also be performed.

***Procedural Considerations.*** A laparotomy set and a GI instrument set are required. Linear stapling instruments and a self-retaining retractor system should be available. The patient is positioned supine under general anesthesia. The anesthesia provider inserts a nasogastric tube after intubation. An indwelling urinary catheter is inserted before the abdominal skin prep.

*Operative Procedure*

1. The abdomen is opened, and the peritoneal cavity is explored to determine the extent of the pathologic area.
2. Moist packs are used to wall off surrounding structures to expose the hepatic and splenic flexures of the colon.
3. The colon is mobilized by incising the lateral peritoneum on either side and transecting the transverse mesocolon. Hemostats, Metzenbaum scissors, and 3-0 nonabsorbable ligatures are used.
4. The operative field is prepared for resection by placing towels or laparotomy sponges around the colon to isolate any contamination from the lumen of the bowel.
5. Two intestinal resection clamps are applied.
6. Transection is completed with a scalpel or mechanical linear stapling device.
7. An end-to-end or side-to-side anastomosis is completed.
8. Contaminated articles are isolated (bowel technique).
9. Approximation of mesentery and lateral peritoneum is completed with 3-0 nonabsorbable sutures.
10. The abdominal wound is closed. Retention sutures may be used.
11. The wound is dressed.

## Anterior Resection of the Sigmoid Colon and Rectosigmoidostomy

Anterior resection of the sigmoid colon and rectosigmoidostomy involve the removal of the lower sigmoid and rectosigmoid portions of the rectum (Figure 11-32, *E*). This is usually done through a laparotomy incision, and an end-to-end anastomosis is completed. This operation is selected to treat lesions

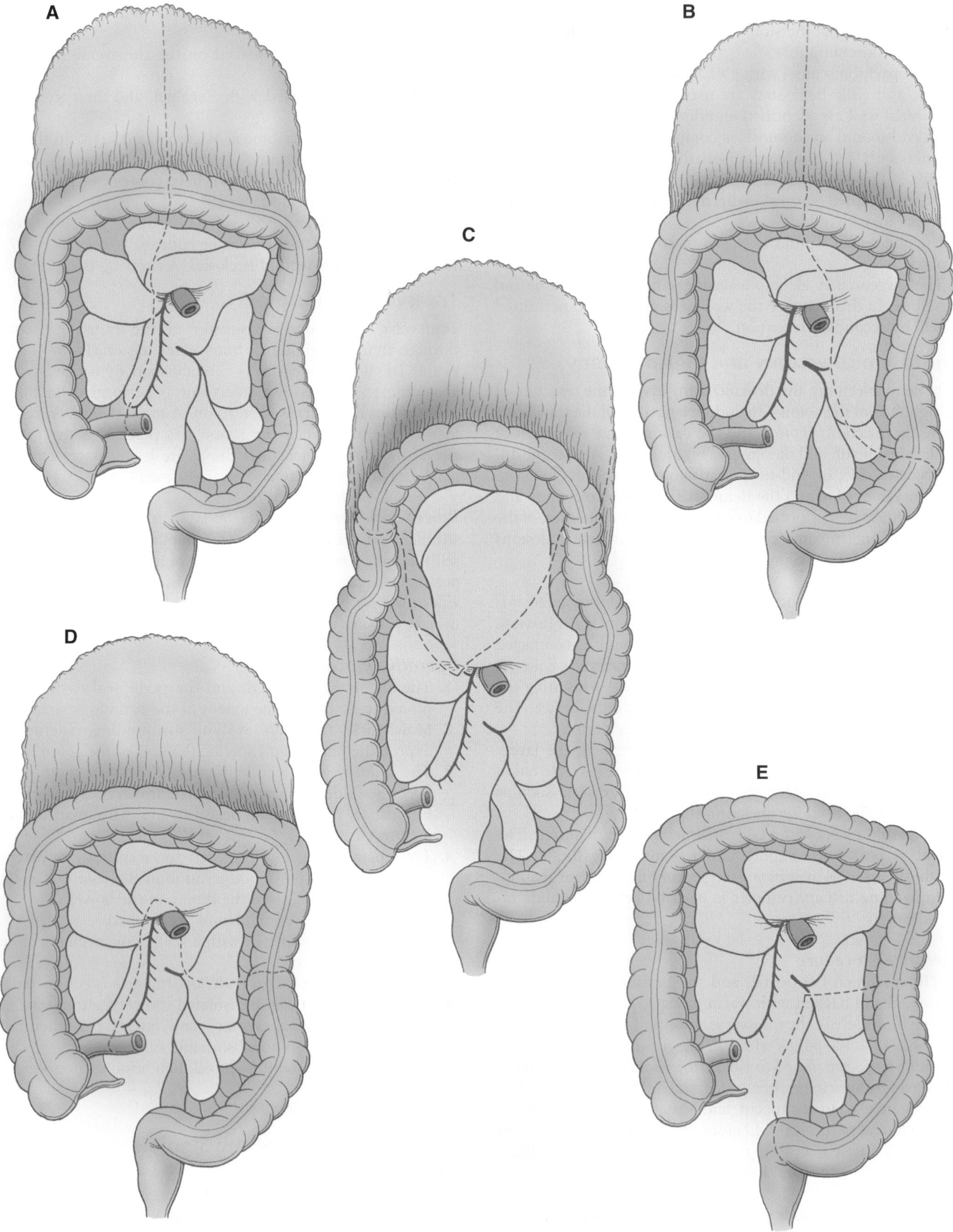


FIGURE 11-32 The resection lines for various types of colon resection. **A,** Right hemicolectomy and ileocolostomy. **B,** Left hemicolectomy. **C** and **D,** Transverse colectomy. **E,** Anterior resection of sigmoid colon and rectosigmoidostomy.

in the lower portion of the sigmoid and rectum that can be excised with a wide margin of safety and still retain sufficient tissues with adequate blood supply for a viable rectosigmoid end-to-end anastomosis.

***Procedural Considerations.*** A laparotomy set and a GI instrument set are required. Linear stapling instruments as well as the end-to-end curved mechanical stapling instruments (EEA) are used. Long instruments for dissecting into the pelvis may be necessary. A rigid sigmoidoscope is used before patient preparation and after the anastomosis. A self-retaining retractor set is required. The patient is placed in a modified lithotomy position with legs extended in stirrups. An indwelling urinary catheter is inserted before the abdominal and perineal preps.

If there is an assisting surgeon, a table with a basic minor set and rectal instruments should be available to facilitate the end-to-end stapling of the anastomosis. Cross-contamination from the table of instruments used on the patient's rectum to the table with the laparotomy instruments is prevented. A table with laparotomy closure instruments may be the surgeon's preference. In this case, only laparotomy instruments are required.

Identification of the ureters during extensive deep abdominal procedures may be achieved by preoperative placement of ureteral catheters by a transurethral approach. If the tumor is believed to involve the ureters, a urologist will place ureteral stents cystoscopically in the OR before the abdominal prep begins.

### Operative Procedure

1. The abdomen is entered through a laparotomy incision.
2. The peritoneal cavity is explored for metastasis and resectability of the lesion.
3. Before the colon is mobilized, the tumor-bearing segment is isolated by ligatures to the lymphovenous drainage (i.e., provided that these structures are accessible).
4. A loop of sigmoid colon is elevated as the small intestines are walled off with moist packs; retractors are placed.
5. The peritoneum on the left side of the colon is incised with a long scalpel, scissors, hemostats, and sponge forceps.
6. Traction sutures (2-0 nonabsorbable) may be used as the peritoneum is reflected.
7. Bleeding vessels are ligated with 2-0 or 3-0 nonabsorbable ligatures.
8. The pelvic peritoneum is exposed and dissected free to form the left side of the reconstructed pelvic floor. Long dissecting instruments are used.
9. Vessels are ligated with 30-inch nonabsorbable ligatures.
10. Extreme care must be exercised throughout to protect the ureters from injury.
11. The sigmoid colon is turned toward the left, and incision and dissection of the peritoneum are performed on the right side of the pelvis.
12. The two incisions are then curved and joined in front of the rectum.
13. The rectum is freed anteriorly and posteriorly from the adjacent structures.
14. The sigmoid colon is clamped with intestinal clamps after mobilization of the proximal portion. A right-angled intestinal clamp or a reticulating linear stapling device may be used to clamp the distal portion of the rectosigmoid colon.
15. As the sigmoid colon is divided distally to the clamp, the transected rectal edges are grasped with Allis or Ochsner forceps and the rectal opening is exposed.
16. The diseased portion is removed, and the soiled instruments are discarded into a separate basin.
17. Continuity is established by an end-to-end anastomosis of the proximal colon and the rectum using a curved mechanical stapling instrument (EEA) (Figure 11-33).
18. "Donuts" of tissue removed from the EEA stapling device are examined closely for thickness and continuity and then sent as separate specimens to the pathology laboratory.
19. The assisting surgeon passes a rigid sigmoidoscope into the lumen of the bowel transanally.
20. Warm irrigating solution is poured into the peritoneal cavity, and the lumen of the bowel is insufflated.
21. The surgeon observes for air leak from the anastomosis and oversews the site if indicated.
22. The pelvic floor is reperitonealized, and drains may be placed.
23. The abdominal wound is closed in the routine manner, and a dressing is applied.

## Abdominoperineal Resection

Abdominoperineal resection (APR), also called a *Miles resection,* is the mobilization and division of a diseased segment of the lower bowel through a midline incision. The proximal end of bowel is exteriorized through a separate stab wound as a colostomy. The distal end is pushed into the hollow of the sacrum and removed through the perineal route (Figure 11-34). An abdominoperineal resection is performed for malignant lesions and inflammatory diseases of the lower sigmoid colon, rectum, and anus that are too low for the use of EEA stapling devices.

***Procedural Considerations.*** The choice of patient position depends on the surgeon. Some surgeons prefer to start with the patient in the supine position and move the patient to the lithotomy position for the perineal portion of the operation. Others initially place the patient in a modified lithotomy position; thus surgery may be performed simultaneously by two teams, which may require two scrub persons with two different setups. An indwelling catheter is inserted into the urinary bladder after induction. The anesthesia provider inserts a nasogastric tube after intubation. A GI instrument set and an ostomy appliance are required for the abdominal portion of the procedure. A perineal set is used for the rectal portion of the procedure. Identification of the ureters during extensive deep abdominal procedures may be achieved by the preoperative placement of ureteral stents using the transurethral approach.

### Operative Procedure

1. A midline incision is made.
2. After thorough exploration of the abdominal cavity and inspection of the colon, the surgeon determines the extent of the lesion and probable surgical outcome. If a resection is indicated, the sigmoid colon is retracted to the right side.
3. The peritoneum on the left of the mesocolon is divided.
4. The incision into the peritoneum is made opposite the main branches of the inferior mesenteric vessels and extended into the pelvis and around anterior to the rectum.

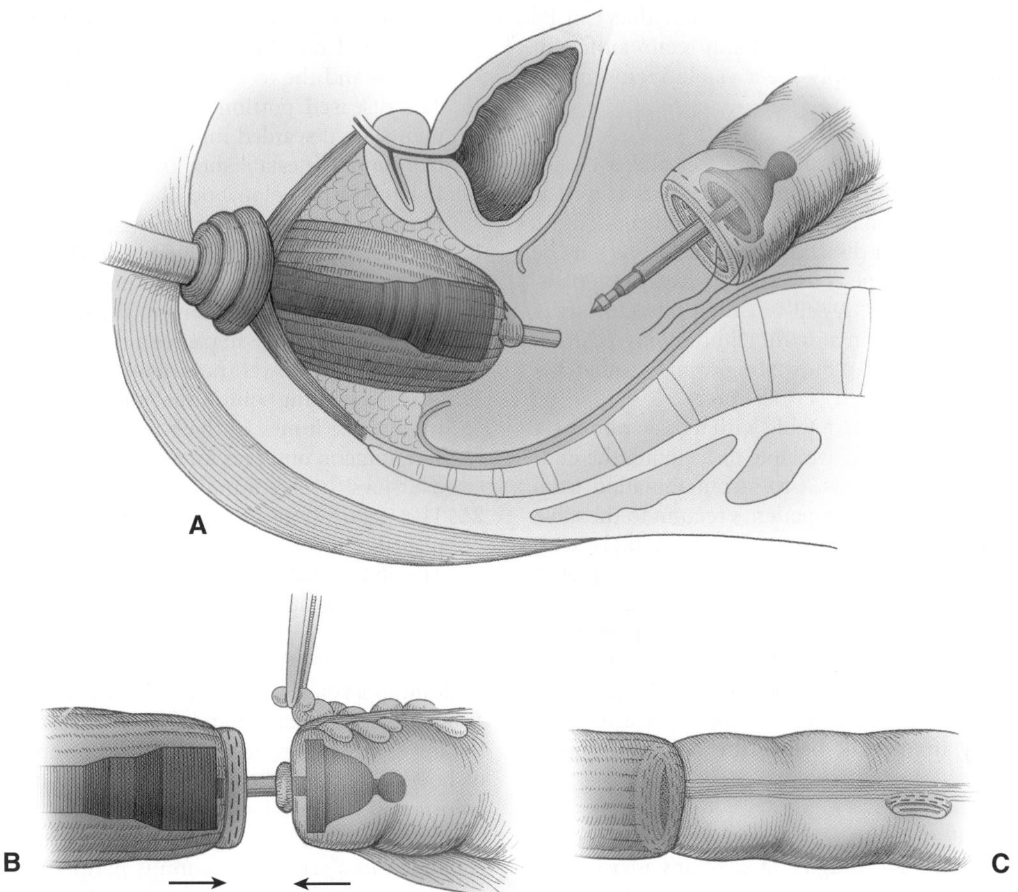


**FIGURE 11-33** EEA stapling device, used to perform low anterior anastomosis. **A,** Stapler is introduced into anus, and the anvil is placed into the proximal colon loop. **B,** EEA is advanced to level of the anvil, and the EEA is closed and fired. **C,** Circular double-staggered row of staples joins bowel; simultaneously, circular blade in instrument cuts stoma. Instrument is gently removed. The resulting anastomosis is illustrated with bowel wall transparent to depict reconstruction.

5. The pelvic peritoneum is mobilized by blunt dissection to form the left side of the new pelvic floor and permit early visualization of the left ureter.
6. The peritoneum is incised on the right side until the incision connects with that made on the left.
7. The right ureter is identified and protected.
8. The blood supply of the portion of intestine to be removed is isolated and ligated. Care must be taken not to damage the left colic artery, which will supply the blood to the colostomy.
9. The mesentery is tied to permit greater exposure in the operative field.
10. The surgeon frees the rectum, usually as low as the sacrococcygeal junction. Care is taken to avoid injury to the presacral nerves, which could result in sexual and bladder dysfunction.
11. After the bowel is freed, the distal segment is transected with a linear stapling instrument (Figure 11-34, *B*).
12. The proximal margin of resection is examined and transected. The bowel and mesentery are removed from the abdominal cavity.
13. The surgeon prepares the permanent colostomy by extending the stump through the abdominal wall. The colostomy will be "matured" (sutured externally to the abdominal wall tissues so that the mucosa is everted into a raised and secured ostomy) after abdominal closure.
14. The combined excision and perineal dissection are initiated when the lesion is determined to be resectable.
15. To prevent contamination, the anus is often closed with a purse-string suture.
16. An incision is made around the anus in an elliptic manner outside the sphincter muscles with a generous margin of perianal skin.
17. The anus is grasped with an Allis or Ochsner forceps and tipped upward to enable its attachment to the coccyx to be severed more readily.
18. Electrodissection is used. The levator ani muscle is exposed; while the finger of the surgeon is held beneath it, it is divided as far from the rectum as possible.
19. All bleeding points are clamped and tied. The Foley catheter allows the surgeon to get as close to the bladder as possible without damaging it.
20. After the anococcygeal raphe is divided, the surgeon's hand is thrust up into the hollow sacrum to free the rectum by blunt dissection, grasp the upper end of the distal fragment, and deliver the stump through the perineum.

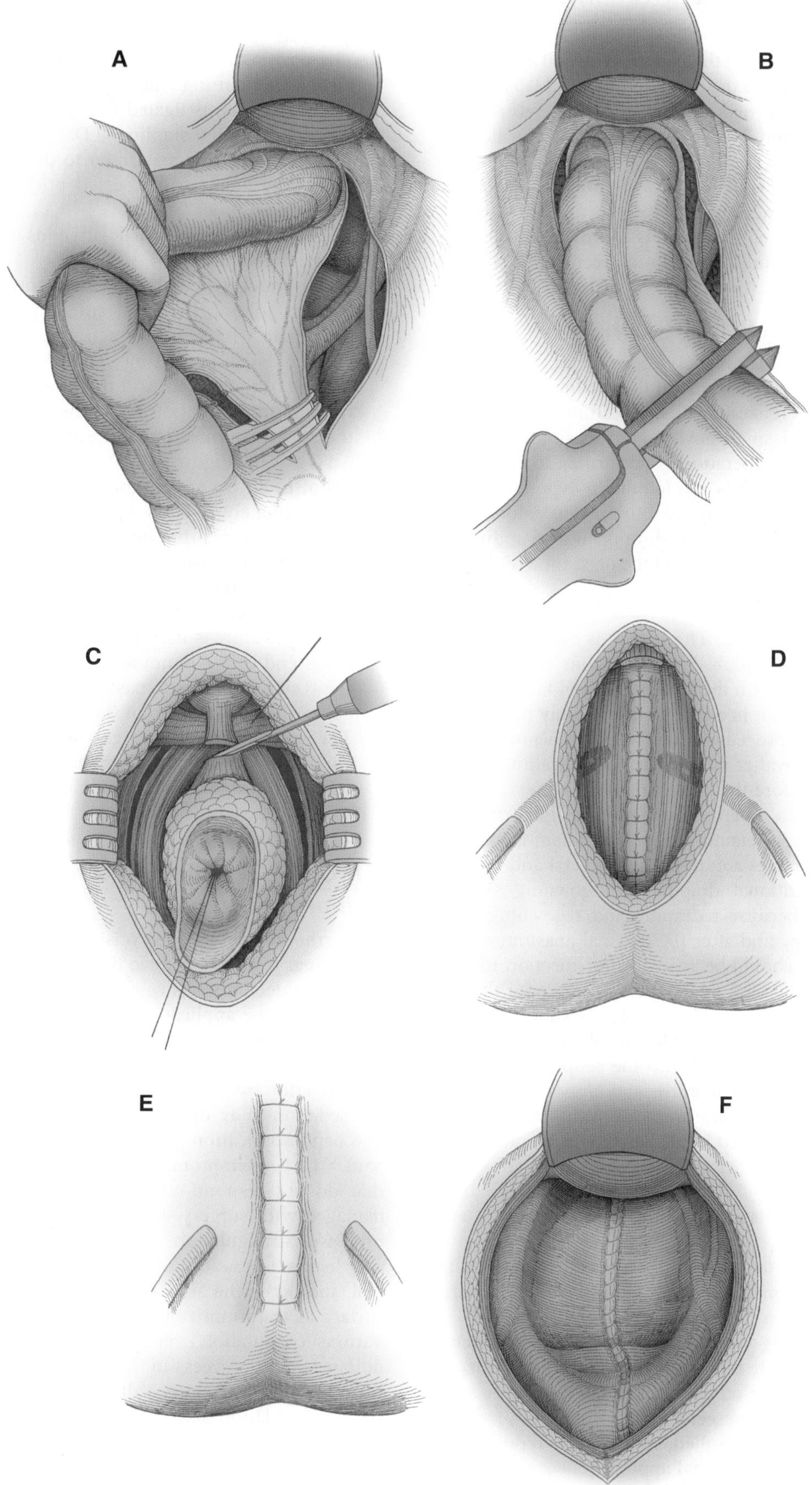


**FIGURE 11-34** Abdominoperineal resection for cancer of the rectum. **A,** The sigmoid colon is deflected to the right to complete the rectosigmoid peritoneal detachment. **B,** The distal sigmoid is transected to allow for better access to mobilize the rectum from the sacrum. **C,** The rectal stump is excised from the perineal approach. **D,** Drains are placed and brought through stab wounds; the levator tissues are reapproximated with 2-0 synthetic absorbable sutures. **E,** The perineal skin is closed. **F,** The pelvic peritoneal floor is closed from the abdominal approach.

21. Drains may be placed into the pelvic cavity and exteriorized through stab wounds in the buttocks (Figure 11-34, *D*).
22. The surgeon is regowned and gloved before returning to the abdominal wound. When all bleeding is controlled, the incision is closed.

If two teams are not available for synchronous excision of the perineum, the perineal portion of the operation is performed after the abdominal resection is complete. In this case, the abdomen is closed and the remaining rectosigmoid stump is excised perineally.

## Ileoanal Endorectal Pull-Through

Ileoanal endorectal pull-through is the removal of the entire colon and the proximal two thirds of the rectum. It includes a mucosectomy of the remaining distal rectum, creation of a pouch from the distal small bowel, and anastomosis of the pouch to the anus. The operation is performed to relieve the symptoms of ulcerative colitis and familial polyposis (e.g., diarrhea, pain, cramping, bleeding) and to prevent colon cancer in high-risk individuals. This procedure is an anal sphincter–saving operation that is done to avoid the need for a traditional ileostomy.

***Procedural Considerations.*** The patient is usually placed in a modified lithotomy position. Some surgeons prefer to perform the mucosectomy with the patient in a jackknife position and then place the patient in a modified lithotomy position for the remainder of the procedure. The anesthesia provider inserts a nasogastric tube after intubation. An indwelling urinary catheter is inserted before the abdominal skin prep.

A GI instrument set, a perineal set, and rectal instrumentation are required. A self-retaining retractor system is an asset. Separate instrument tables are used for the rectal and abdominal approaches. Additional draping and gowning supplies should be available because redraping and regowning occur after the mucosectomy and after the ileoanal anastomosis. An epinephrine solution should be available for injection into the submucosal tissue, proximal to the anus, to separate the mucosa from the muscularis layer. A proctoscope should be available; this may be used at the conclusion of the procedure to check for leaks. (Air is pumped into the scope, which is inserted in the anus. The surgeon at the abdominal site looks for air bubbles. If there are none, the anastomosis has no leaks.) An ileostomy appliance is applied immediately postoperatively.

### *Operative Procedure*

1. The anal canal is dilated and inspected through an anoscope.
2. Starting at the dentate line (the anorectal junction), the epinephrine solution is injected circumferentially, separating the mucosa from the muscularis layer.
3. The mucosectomy is then performed by making a circular incision at the dentate line, cutting only through mucosa.
4. The mucosa is peeled off the muscularis tissue for a distance of 2 to 8 cm and resected.
5. When all bleeding is controlled, the patient is repositioned, if necessary, for the abdominal approach.
6. A midline incision is made, and the abdomen is explored.
7. The entire large intestine from the ileocecal junction through the upper two thirds of the rectum is freed and immobilized. All vessels are ligated.
8. The terminal ileum is separated from the cecum using a mechanical cutting and stapling device (GIA).
9. The mesocolon is ligated using suture ligatures or a ligating, dividing, and stapling (LDS) instrument.
10. The rectum is resected down to the level of the mucosectomy. The colon and resected portion of the rectum are removed en bloc.
11. The pouch is created. Most surgeons use either the J pouch or the S pouch.
12. The J pouch (Figure 11-35) is created at the terminal ileum by folding two adjacent loops of small bowel, approximately 10 to 15 cm each, parallel with each other and anastomosing them using a GIA. An opening is made at the bottom of the pouch, and the pouch is pulled through the rectal stump. The bottom of the pouch is anastomosed to the anus with interrupted absorbable sutures.
13. An S pouch (Figure 11-36) is created by aligning the distal ileum in an S configuration with each of the three limbs approximately 10 cm in length. The most distal 2 cm of the ileum is not incorporated into the pouch but is preserved for the anastomosis to the anus. The three limbs are manually incised and anastomosed to create a pouch. Mucosal tissue is approximated with absorbable suture, and nonabsorbable suture is used for the serosal layer. The preserved distal end of the ileum and the pouch are pulled through the rectal stump and anastomosed to the anus. This completes the anal portion of the procedure.
14. The scrub team changes gowns and gloves, redrapes, and completes the abdominal procedure by creating a loop ileostomy through the abdominal wall, on a previously designated site.

# SURGERY OF THE RECTUM

## Hemorrhoidectomy

Hemorrhoidectomy is the excision and ligation of dilated veins in the anal region to relieve discomfort and control bleeding. Hemorrhoidectomy has essentially become an outpatient procedure with the application of sclerotherapy, heater probe coagulation, monopolar or bipolar coagulation, laser, and infrared energy coagulation. The most popular therapy is rubber band ligation, which can be done through an anoscope without sedation in an office or endoscopy setting. Typically only one band application is done per session to avoid sepsis and pain.[32] Larger symptomatic external and internal hemorrhoids that do not respond to conservative medical treatment are managed with surgery. This patient is at risk for hemorrhoid prolapse, strangulation, thrombosis, and possible ulceration and fistula formation. Surgical treatment aims to coagulate, seal, and excise the hemorrhoid, leaving sufficient anal mucosa surface as to minimize pain and prevent stenosis or stricture. Various coagulation, vaporization, and tissue-welding technologies offer successful outcomes. Radiofrequency tissue/fusion energy (LigaSure, Valley Lab, Inc.) is a unique form of electrocoagulation that provides hemostasis and sealing by fusing the collagen in the vessel walls. A specific stapling device may also be used (stapled hemorrhoidectomy).

***Procedural Considerations.*** Preoperative anal dilation aids in exposing the vessels and contributes to the patient's comfort in the immediate postoperative period. Many sur-

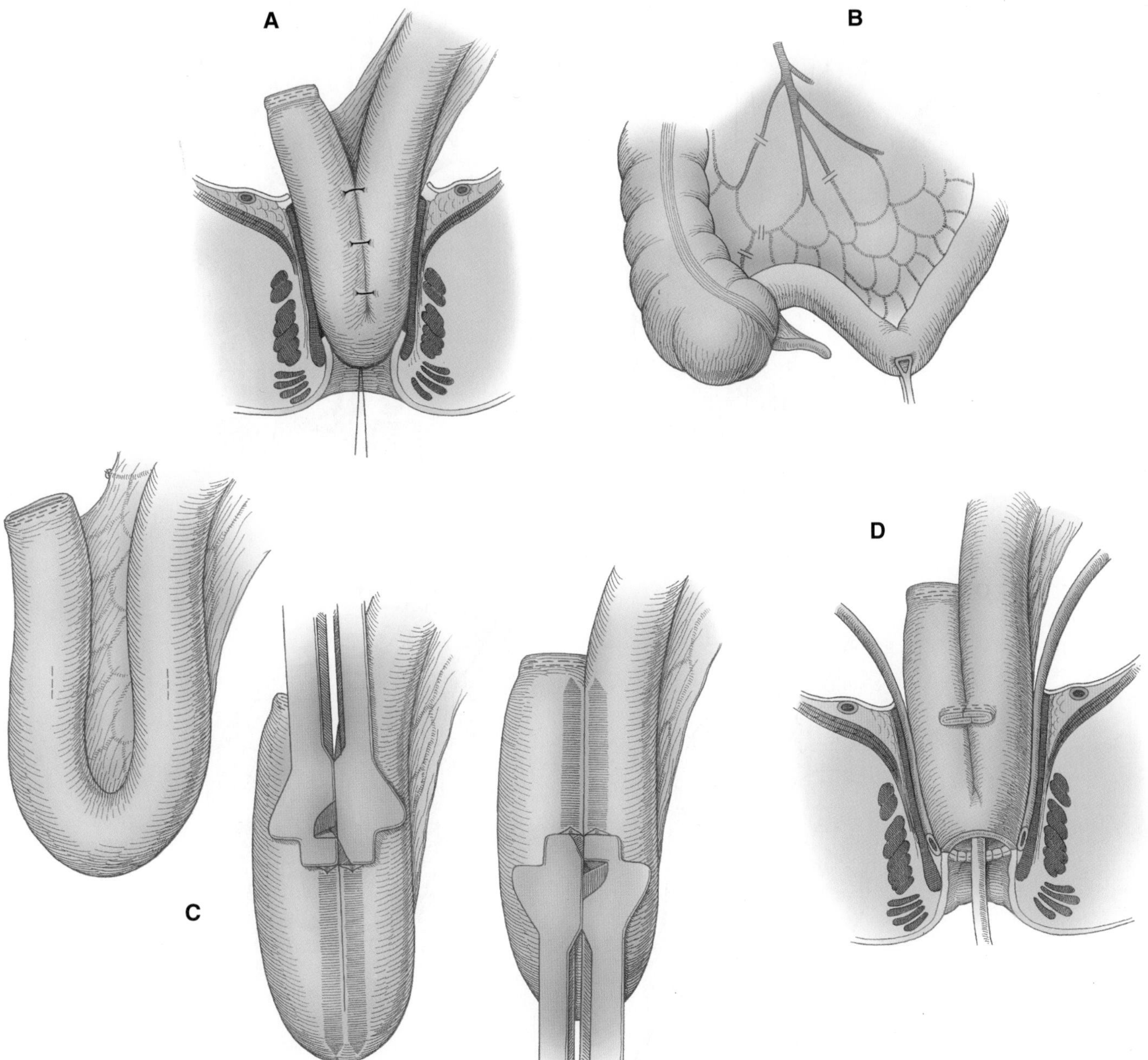


FIGURE 11-35 J pouch for ileoanal endorectal pull-through. **A,** The J pouch is created at terminal ileum by folding two adjacent loops of small bowel, approximately 10 to 15 cm each, parallel to each other. **B,** Mesenteric vascular arcades may need to be divided to provide adequate length for anal anastomosis. **C,** The two loops are anastomosed using a mechanical cutting and stapling device (GIA). **D,** Opening is made at bottom of pouch, and pouch is pulled through rectal stump. Bottom of pouch is anastomosed to anus.

geons prefer to precede the operation with a sigmoidoscopy. Spinal, caudal, epidural, or local anesthesia may be used. The patient is usually placed in the lithotomy or jackknife position. Postoperative complications may include hemorrhage, pain, constipation, fecal impaction, infection, and urinary retention.

### *Operative Procedure*

1. The anal canal is dilated and inspected through an anoscope.
2. Four Allis forceps are applied several centimeters from the anal margin to expose the anus.
3. The base of the hemorrhoid and tissue are grasped with Allis forceps and held.
4. An intestinal suture of 2-0 synthetic absorbable suture is placed and tied at the proximal end of the hemorrhoid, and a Buie pile forceps is applied across the base and above the proposed incision line.
5. Excision is completed with a scalpel. Coagulation and excision may also be done with monopolar or bipolar electrosur-

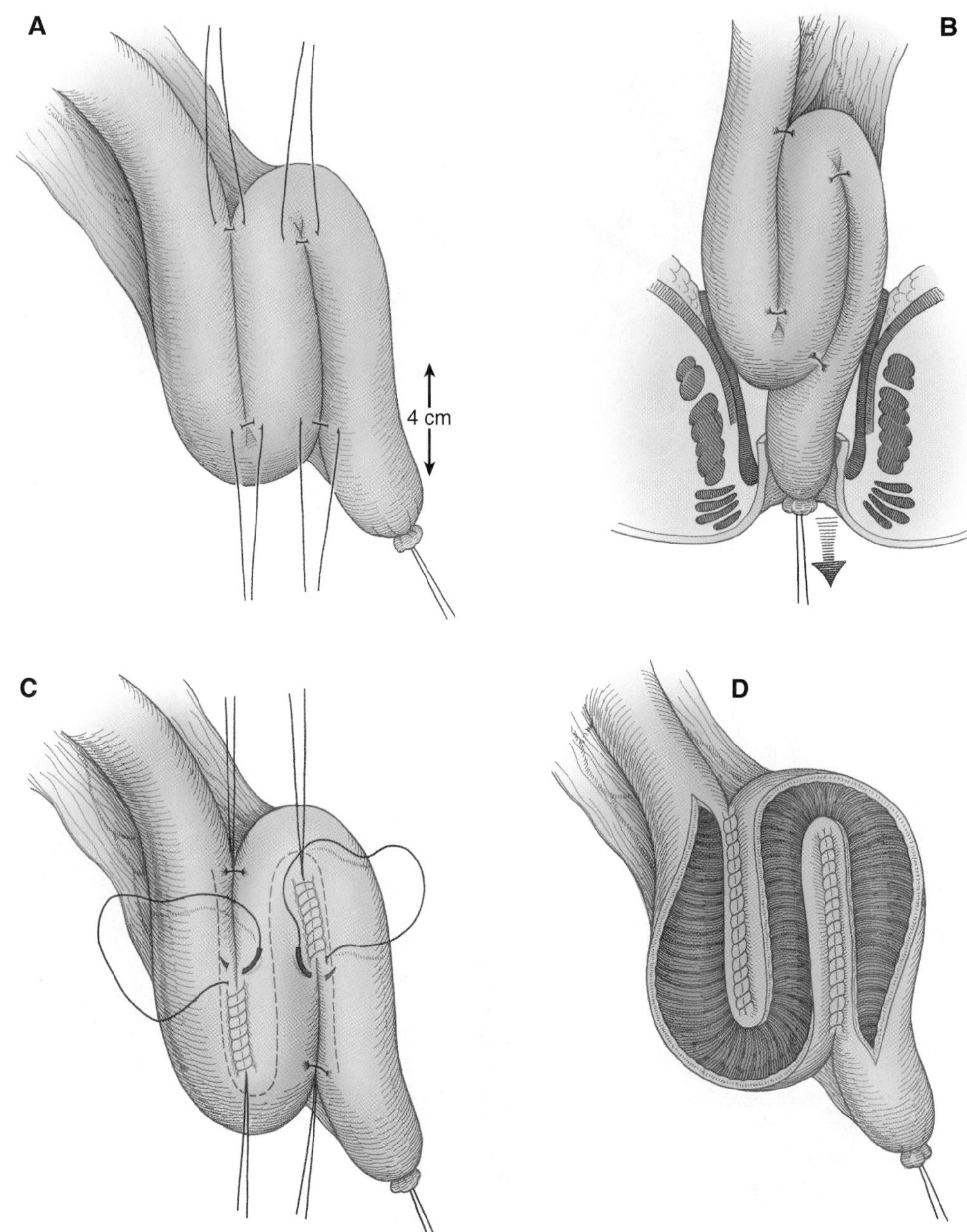


FIGURE 11-36 S pouch for ileoanal endorectal pull-through. **A,** Pouch is created by aligning distal ileum in S configuration with each limb (three in total) approximately 12 cm in length. **B,** The length is measured before anastomosis begins. **C,** Three limbs are incised and anastomosed to create pouch. **D,** Incision is made as illustrated.

gery, laser vaporization, infrared energy, radiofrequency fusion/ligation, cryotherapy, or even heater probe coagulation. Care is directed toward preserving the rectal sphincter.

6. Loosely placed continuous sutures are placed over the Buie forceps. The suture is tightened as the forceps are removed, and the suture ends are tied.
7. Traction may be maintained as hemostatic forceps are applied and dissection is completed segmentally.
8. Suture ligatures of 2-0 synthetic absorbable suture are used as each hemostat is removed.
9. Remaining hemorrhoids are excised in a similar manner.
10. Petrolatum gauze packing may be placed in the anal canal. A dressing is applied.

## Excision of Anal Fissure and Lateral Sphincterotomy

Excision of an anal fissure or ulcer is considered when the lesion is chronic and not healed after medical therapy. The most common surgical treatment is the partial lateral internal sphincterotomy.

*Procedural Considerations.* A minor instrument set and rectal instruments are required. The patient is placed in the lithotomy or jackknife position.

### *Operative Procedure*

1. A small incision is made along the intersphincteric groove.

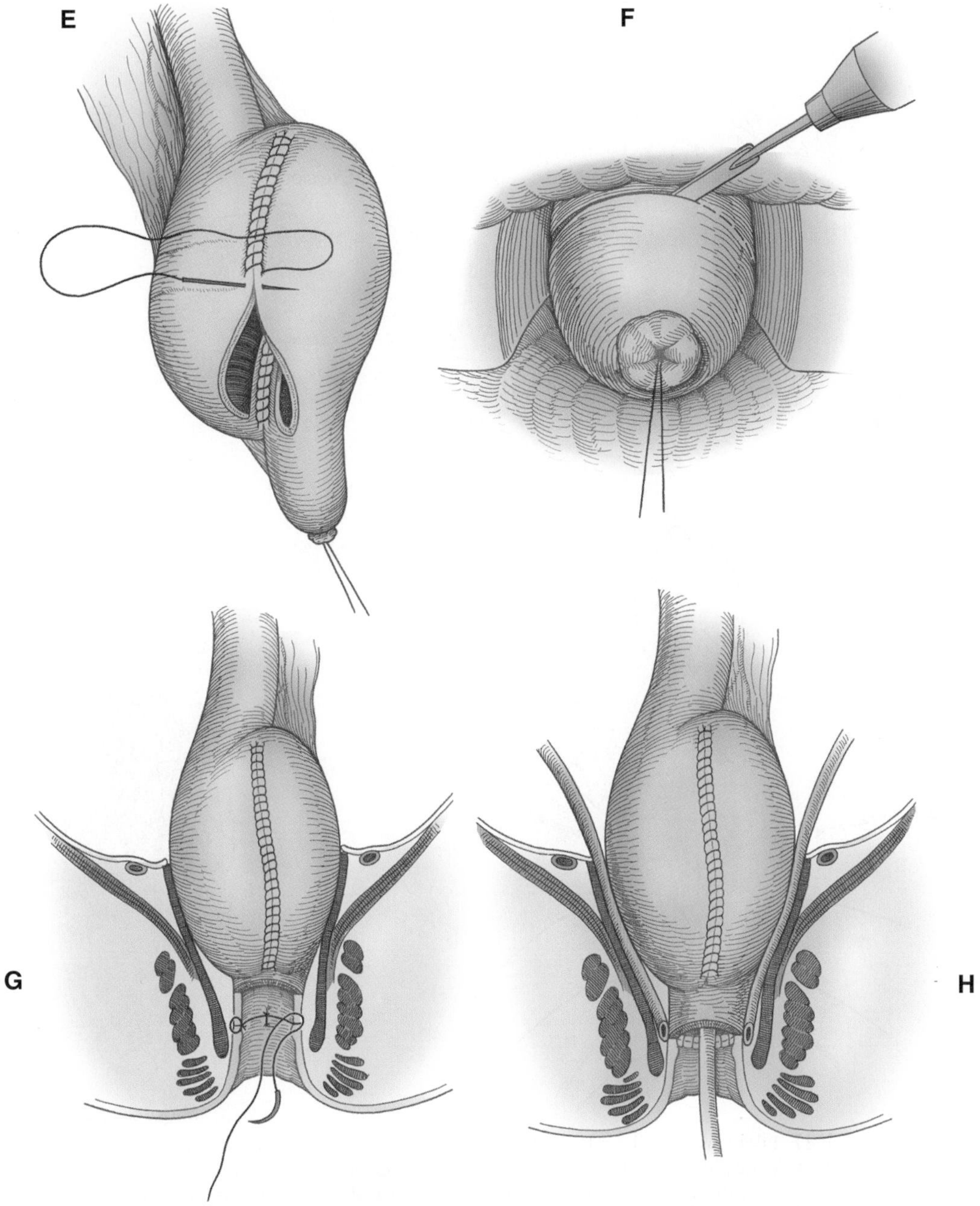


**FIGURE 11-36, cont'd** **E,** The pouch is closed using suture for the formation of the reservoir. **F,** Distal ends of ileum and pouch are pulled through the rectal stump, and the lower outflow tract is trimmed. **G,** With 3-0 absorbable sutures, the outflow tract is anastomosed to the anus at the dentate line. **H,** Drain in place in the lumen of the newly created ileoanal-rectal canal.

2. The constricting band of tissue is released by elevating the mucosa and underlying internal sphincter.[32]
3. A drain or packing is inserted and a dressing applied.

## Excision of Pilonidal Cyst and Sinus

Excision of a pilonidal cyst and sinus is removal of the cyst with sinus tracts from the intergluteal fold on the posterior surface of the lower sacrum (Figure 11-37). A pilonidal cyst and sinus, which may have a congenital origin, rarely become symptomatic until the individual reaches adulthood, most commonly in young men. Inflammatory reaction varies from a mild, irritating, draining sinus tract to a painful acute abscess with secondary recurrences. Treatment consists of drainage in the acute stage and total surgical excision during remission.

The excision of the cyst and sinus tracts must be complete to prevent recurrence. The defect resulting from recurrences may become too large for primary closure. In this case the wound is left open to heal by granulation.

***Procedural Considerations.*** A minor set and rectal instruments are required, as well as methylene blue, a 10- or 20-ml syringe, and a blunt-tipped needle. The patient is placed in the

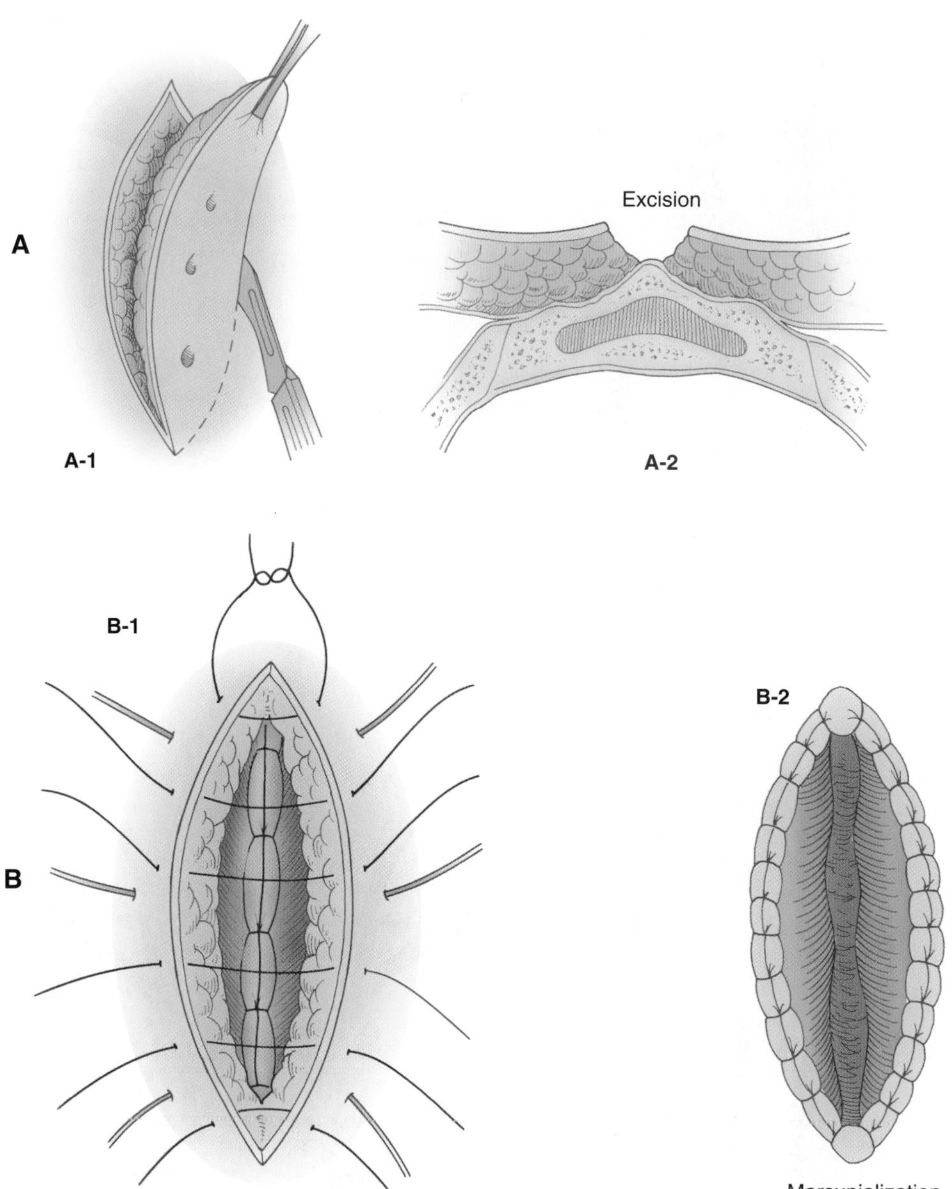


FIGURE 11-37 Pilonidal cyst. The pilonidal sinus tract is identified with injection of methylene blue into the tract. **A,** Wide elliptic incision *(A-1)* is made to include all the subcutaneous tracts and tissue to the fascia overlying the sacrum and coccyx *(A-2)*. **B,** Closure of the wound can be primary *(B-1)* or secondary *(B-2)*.

jackknife position with the buttocks taped open laterally and secured to the sides of the OR bed. Hair must be clipped in the operative area before skin prep.

### *Operative Procedure*

1. The sinus tracts are identified with probes and an incision made over the probe.
2. The tract is marked by injecting methylene blue with a blunt needle.
3. An elliptic incision is made down to the fascia.
4. A curette is used to remove granulation tissue.
5. Excision of cyst and sinus tracts is completed. Bleeding is controlled.
6. If the wound is to be left open, it is packed and a pressure dressing is applied.
7. If the wound is closed, 2-0 nonabsorbable sutures are used for stay sutures on the deeper tissue and fine nonabsorbable suture is used on the skin.

## REFERENCES


1. American Cancer Society: *Cancer facts and figures 2005*, Atlanta, 2005, The Society.
2. Anderson D and others: Intestinal transplantation in pediatric patients: a nursing challenge. I. Evaluation for intestinal transplant, *Gastroenterology Nursing* 23(1):3-9, 2000.
3. Anderson D and others: Intestinal transplantation in pediatric patients: a nursing challenge. II. Intestinal transplantation and the immediate postoperative period, *Gastroenterology Nursing* 23(5): 201-209, 2000.

4. Association of periOperative Registered Nurses: AORN bariatric surgery guidelines. In *AORN standards, recommended practices, and guidelines,* Denver, Colo, 2005, The Association.
5. Ballantyne GH: The pitfalls of laparoscopic surgery: challenges for robotics and telerobotic surgery, *Surgical Laparoscopic and Endoscopic Percutaneous Technology* 12(1):1-3, 2002.
6. Beyea SC: *Perioperative nursing data set*, ed 2, Denver, 2002, Association of periOperative Registered Nurses.
7. Bickley LS: *Bates' guide to physical assessment and history taking*, ed 8, Philadelphia, 2003, Lippincott Williams & Wilkins.
8. Birn CS: Endoscopic ultrasound reveals GI tract secrets, *Nursing Spectrum* 17:5-17, 2005.
9. Blackwood HS: Help your patient downsize with bariatric surgery, *Med Surg Insider*, Fall 2005.
10. Bowers S: All about tubes: your guide to enteral feeding devices, *Nursing* 30(12):41-47, 2000.
11. Carmel JE, Goldberg MJ: Preoperative and postoperative management. In Colwell JC and others: *Fecal and urinary diversions: management principles*, St Louis, 2004, Mosby.
12. Carpenito-Moyet LJ: *Nursing diagnosis: application to practice*, ed 10, Philadelphia, 2004, Lippincott Williams & Wilkins.
13. Cohen BJ, Wood DL: *Memmler's the human body in health and disease*, ed 9, Philadelphia, 2000, Lippincott Williams & Wilkins.
14. Cox JA and others: Treating benign colon disorders using laparoscopic colectomy, *AORN Journal* 73(2):377-398, 2001.
15. Ewing DR and others: Robots in the operating room—the history, *Seminars in Laparoscopic Surgery* 11(2):63-72, 2004.
16. Ferzli GS, Fingerhut A: Trocar placement for laparoscopic abdominal procedures: a simple standardized method, *Journal of the American College of Surgeons* 198(1):163-172, 2003.
17. Gerber DA: Intestinal transplantation, *Medscape Transplantation Clinical Management Modules, Online, 2001*. Accessed May 19, 2005, online: www.medscape.com/Medscape/transplantation/ClinicalMgmt/CM.v09/pnt-CM.v09.h.
18. Goldsmith H, Herman L: Endoluminal gastroplication: a new therapeutic endoscopic procedure for gastroesophageal reflux disease, *Gastroenterology Nurse* 25(1):15-19, 2002.
19. Gomez G: Emerging technology in surgery: informatics, electronics and robotics. In Townsend CM and others, editors: *Sabiston textbook of surgery*, ed 17, Philadelphia, 2004, Saunders.
20. Hemminger LL, Wolfsen HC: Photodynamic therapy for Barrett's esophagus and high grade dysplasia, *Gastroenterology Nursing* 25(4):139-141, 2002.
21. Hollander D: Intestinal permeability in health and disease. In Kirsner JB: *Inflammatory bowel disease,* ed 5, Philadelphia, 2000, Saunders.
22. Hong D and others: Laparoscopic vs. open resection for colorectal carcinoma, *Diseases of the Colon and Rectum* 44(1):10-19, 2001.
23. Jefferson University Medical Center: "Pilcam" enables Jefferson Physicians to diagnose diseases of esophagus without using endoscope, 2005. Accessed June 16, 2005, on-line: www.healthorbit.ca/NewsDetail.asp?opt=1&nltid=107130605.
24. Kuhls DA and others: Reconsidering abdominal incisions, *Surgical Rounds,* June 2000.
25. Kwon RS and others: Gastrointestinal cancer imaging: deeper than the eye can see, *Gastroenterology* 128:1538-1553, 2005.
26. Lee JM and others: Enduring effects of thoracoscopic Heller myotomy for treating achalasia, *World Journal of Surgery* 28:55-58, 2004.
27. Lewis BS: Obscure gastrointestinal bleeding. In Ginsberg GG and others, editors: *Clinical gastrointestinal endoscopy*, Philadelphia, 2005, Saunders.
28. McConnell EA: Appendicitis: what a pain! *Nursing* 31(8):321-323, 2001.
29. McCormick DG: Stretta procedure for the treatment of gastroesophageal reflux disease, *Gastroenterology Nursing* 27(1):22-28, 2004.
30. Meyers WC: Device facilitates hand-assisted laparoscopy for complex procedures, *Annals of Surgery* 231:715-723, 2000.
31. Milson J and others: Prospective randomized trial comparing laparoscopic vs. conventional surgery for refractory ileocolic Crohn's disease, *Diseases of the Colon and Rectum* 44(1):1-9, 2001.
32. Nelson H: Anus. In Townsend CM and others, editors: *Sabiston textbook of surgery*, ed 17, Philadelphia, 2004, Saunders.
33. Onderdonk AB: Intestinal microflora and inflammatory bowel disease. In Kirsner JB: *Inflammatory bowel disease,* ed 5, Philadelphia, 2000, Saunders.
34. Ransohoff DF: Colon cancer screening in 2005—status and challenges, *Gastroenterology* 128:1685-1695, 2005.
35. Reeves AL: Endoscopic mucosal resection, *Gastroenterology Nursing* 23(5):215-220, 2000.
36. Regueiro MD, Abu-Elmagd KM: Small bowel transplantation for Crohn's disease, *Foundation Focus: the Magazine of CCFA,* Spring/Summer 2001.
37. Reiland KE: GI surgery patient outcomes influenced by nutrition, *AORN Journal* 71(1):199-204, 2000.
38. Rubin M: Wireless capsule endoscopy: beyond bleeding. Presentation to New York Society of Gastrointestinal endoscopy 27th annual New York Course, December 17, 2003.
39. Rush University Medical Center: Patients swallow "camera-in-a-pill" to help doctors check for diseases of esophagus, GERD, 2005. Accessed April 21, 2005, on-line: www.healthorbit=107130605, www.healthorbit=105180405.
40. Rothstein RI: Gastroesophageal reflux. In Townsend CM and others, editors: *Sabiston textbook of surgery*, ed 17, Philadelphia, 2004, Saunders.
41. Schirmer BD: Morbid obesity. In Townsend CM and others, editors: *Sabiston textbook of surgery*, ed 17, St. Louis, 2004, Saunders.
42. Society of Gastroenterology Nurses and Associates: *Gastroenterology nursing: a core curriculum*, ed 3, Philadelphia, 2003, Lippincott Williams and Wilkins.
43. Society of Gastroenterology Nurses and Associates: *Manual of gastrointestinal procedures,* ed 5, Philadelphia, 2004, Lippincott Williams & Wilkins.
44. Sunada K and others: Clinical outcomes of enteroscopy using the double balloon method for strictures of the small intestine, *World Journal of Gastroenterology* 11(7):1087-1089, 2005.
45. Tortora GJ, Grabowski SR: *Principles of anatomy and physiology,* ed 9, New York, 2000, John Wiley & Sons.
46. Wang KK: Endoscopic therapy for superficial esophageal carcinomas. In Ginsberg GG and others, editors: *Clinical gastrointestinal endoscopy*, St. Louis, 2005, Saunders.
47. Weber PA and others: Telerobotic-assisted laparoscopic right and sigmoid colectomies for benign disease, *Diseases of the Colon and Rectum* 45(12):1695-1696, 2002.
48. Young-Fadok TM, Nelson H: Laparoscopic right colectomy, *Diseases of the Colon and Rectum* 43(2):267-273, 2000.
49. Yu M: M2A capsule endoscopy: a breakthrough diagnostic tool for small intestinal imaging, *Gastroenterology Nursing* 25(1):25-27, 2002.
50. Zwischenberger JB and others: Esophagus. In Townsend CM and others, editors: *Sabiston textbook of surgery*, ed 17, St Louis, 2004, Saunders.

CHAPTER 12

# Surgery of the Liver, Biliary Tract, Pancreas, and Spleen

JANICE A. NEIL

A pathologic condition in the liver, biliary tract, pancreas, or spleen often requires surgical intervention. These organs are highly vascular and control many metabolic and immune functions of the body. Surgical intervention may be indicated for infection, cystic anomalies, congenital anomalies, metabolic diseases, trauma (see Chapter 31), or malignancy. Approximately 57,400 new cases of malignancy of the pancreas, gallbladder, or extrahepatic biliary tract are diagnosed each year, and the prognosis for these is poor.[23]

In the past decade, surgeries of the liver and biliary tract have become more advanced as research and new technology have permitted more complete diagnosis of pathologic conditions involving this complex organ and portal system. A resection of the liver for carcinoma has achieved a recognized role for cure or substantial palliation with safety and low morbidity.

Cholecystectomy is the most common nonemergency abdominal operation performed. In the United States more than 700,000 cholecystectomies are performed each year. It is one of the most frequently performed inpatient procedures in the United States.[8] Laparoscopic cholecystectomy has become the gold standard surgical intervention for the treatment of cholecystitis. Since the early 1990s, laparoscopic cholecystectomy, as compared with an open-incision cholecystectomy, has yielded advantages of reduced trauma to tissues as well as a significant reduction in the length of postoperative recovery. Approximately 94% of cholecystectomies are elective surgeries, and 6% are emergencies.[18] Laparoscopic cholecystectomy procedures were the precursor to the evolution of numerous abdominal procedures now being performed or assisted through the laparoscope.

New diagnostic technology and the intraoperative use of ultrasonography, biliary endoscopy, and radiography have enabled surgeons to better treat diseases of the biliary tract. Solid organ transplantation (History box), such as with the liver, pancreas, and kidneys, has become common as a means of treatment for primary hepatic tumors, end-stage liver disease, and insulin-deficient diabetes. Liver transplant procedures have evolved and can be entire organ transplants or living-related organ donations.

This chapter contains information pertaining to the most common open and minimally invasive procedures performed on the liver, biliary tract, pancreas, and spleen.

## Surgical Anatomy

The liver is in the right upper quadrant of the abdominal cavity, beneath the dome of the diaphragm and directly above the stomach, duodenum, and hepatic flexure of the colon. The external covering, known as *Glisson's capsule,* is composed of dense connective tissue. The visceral peritoneum extends over the entire surface of the liver, except at the point of posterior attachment to the diaphragm. This connective tissue branches at the porta hepatis into a network of septa that extends into an intrahepatic network of support for the more than 1 million hepatic lobules. The porta hepatis is located on the inferior surface of the liver and is the location of entry and exit for the major vessels, ducts, and nerves. The arterial blood supply is maintained by the hepatic artery, and venous blood from the stomach, intestines, spleen, and pancreas is carried to the liver by the portal vein and its branches (Figure 12-1). The hepatic venous system returns blood to the heart by way of the inferior vena cava.

The lobules are the functional units of the liver. Each lobule contains a portal triad that consists of a hepatic duct, a hepatic portal vein branch, and a branch of the hepatic artery, nerves, and lymphatics. A central vein is located in the center of each lobule and provides for venous drainage into the hepatic veins.

The lobules also contain hepatic cords, hepatic sinusoids, and bile canaliculi. The hepatic cords comprise numerous columns of hepatocytes—the functional cells of the liver. The hepatic sinusoids are the blood channels that communicate among the columns of hepatocytes. The sinusoids have a thin epithelial lining composed primarily of Kupffer's cells—phagocytic cells that engulf bacteria and toxins. The sinusoids drain into the central vein.

Bile is manufactured by the hepatocytes. The bile canaliculi are tiny bile capillary vessels that communicate among the columns of hepatocytes. The bile canaliculi collect bile and transport it to the bile ducts in the portal triad of each lobule, and subsequently it flows into the hepatic ducts at the porta hepatis. These ducts join immediately to form one common hepatic duct that merges with the cystic duct from the gallbladder to form the common bile duct (Figure 12-2). The common bile duct opens into the duodenum in an area called the *ampulla,* or *papilla of Vater,* located about 7.5 cm below the pyloric opening from the stomach.

## HISTORY

### Solid Organ Transplant

In the eighteenth century, researchers were experimenting with solid organ transplants on animals and humans. The science evolved after many trials and failures. In the past 2 decades, important medical breakthroughs, such as surgical technique, tissue typing, and the use of immunosuppressant drugs, have permitted more success in the viability of the organs and a longer survival rate for transplant recipients. The following is a summarized timeline of significant "firsts" and milestones in the evolution of solid organ transplant surgery.

**1954** The first successful kidney transplant.
Dr. Joseph E. Murray, Brigham & Women's Hospital, Boston, Massachusetts.

**1966** The first simultaneous pancreas/kidney transplant.
Dr. Richard Lillehei, William Kelly, University of Minnesota, Minneapolis.

**1967** The first successful liver transplant.
Dr. Thomas Starzl, University of Colorado Health Sciences Center, Denver.

**1968** The first isolated pancreas transplant.
Dr. Richard Lillehei, University of Minnesota, Minneapolis.

**1968** The first successful heart transplant.
Dr. Norman Shumway, Stanford University Hospital, Stanford, California.

**1981** The first successful heart/lung transplant.
Dr. Bruce Reitz, Stanford University, Stanford, California.

**1983** The first successful lung transplant.
Dr. Joel Cooper, Toronto Lung Transplant Group, Toronto General Hospital, Canada.

**1986** The first successful double-lung transplant.
Dr. Joel Cooper, Toronto Lung Transplant Group, Toronto General Hospital, Canada.

**1989** The first living-related liver transplant.
Dr. Christoph Broelsch, University of Chicago Medical Center, Chicago, Illinois.

**1990** The first successful living-related lung transplant.
Dr. Vaughn A. Starnes, Stanford University Medical Center, Stanford, California.

**1992** The first baboon-to-human liver transplant.
The University of Pittsburgh Medical Center, Pittsburgh, Pennsylvania.

**1992** The first pig-to-human liver transplant.
Cedars-Sinai Medical Center, Los Angeles, California.

**1993** The first successful living-related lung lobes transplant (one from each of the recipient's parents).
University of Southern California, Los Angeles.

**2002** The first uterus transplant took place in Saudi Arabia. The transplanted organ remained viable for 99 days. The intent of the transplant is to make childbirth possible for women who have undergone hysterectomies; the transplant would be temporary—the uterus would be removed once the baby was born to prevent ongoing administration of antirejection drugs.

Modified from *History of transplantation.* Accessed February 18, 2006, on-line: www.transweb.org/reference/timeline/historytable.htm; *Saudi surgeons perform first uterus transplant,* 2002. Accessed February 18, 2006 on-line: www.nytimes.com/2002/03/07/health/07UTER.html?pagewatned_print&position_top; www.unos.org/data/default.asp?display=liver&displayType=internationalData.

Bile contains bile salts, which facilitate digestion and absorption, and various waste products. The liver is essential in the metabolism of carbohydrates, proteins, and fats. It metabolizes nutrients into glycogen stores for regulation of blood glucose levels and energy sources for the brain and body functions.

The liver plays several important roles in the blood-clotting mechanism. It is the organ that synthesizes plasma proteins, excluding gamma globulins but including prothrombin and fibrinogen. Vitamin K, a co-factor to the synthesis of prothrombin, is absorbed by the metabolism of fats in the intestinal tract as a result of bile formation by the liver. Patients with liver disease may have altered blood-coagulation abilities.

The liver also synthesizes lipoproteins and cholesterol. Cholesterol is an essential component of the blood plasma. It serves as a precursor for bile salts, steroid hormones, plasma membranes, and other specialized molecules. A diet high in cholesterol reduces the amount that must be synthesized by the liver. When the diet is deficient in cholesterol, the liver increases synthesis to maintain the levels necessary for the production of the vital chemical molecules.

The liver also serves in the metabolic alteration of foreign molecules or biotransformation of chemicals. The microsomal enzyme system (MES) plays a major role in the body's response to foreign chemicals, such as pollutants, drugs, and alcohol. Patients with liver disease may have an altered response to chemical substances. This consideration is most important in the induction and management of general anesthesia for patients with liver disorders.

The gallbladder, which lies in a sulcus on the undersurface of the right lobe of the liver, terminates in the cystic duct (Figure 12-3). This ductal system provides a channel for the flow of bile to the gallbladder, where it becomes highly concentrated during the storage period. The liver daily produces approximately 600 to 1000 ml of bile. The gallbladder's average storage capacity is 40 to 70 ml. As food, especially fats, is ingested, the duodenal cells release cholecystokinin. The musculature of the gallbladder contracts, forcing bile into the cystic duct and through the common duct. As the sphincter of Oddi in the ampulla of Vater relaxes, bile pours forth, flowing into the duodenum to aid in digestion by emulsification of fats. The gallbladder receives its blood supply from the cystic artery—a branch of the hepatic artery. The triangle of Calot contains the cystic artery (and possibly the right hepatic artery); it is an anatomic landmark in surgical removal of the gallbladder. Its boundaries may be remembered as the *3 Cs:* Cystic duct, Common hepatic duct, and Cystic artery.[6] Innervation for the gallbladder and biliary tree is controlled by the autonomic nervous system. The parasympathetic innervation stimulates contraction, whereas sympathetic innervation inhibits contraction.

The pancreas (see Figure 12-3) is a fixed structure lying transversely behind the stomach in the upper abdomen. The head of the pancreas is fixed to the curve of the duodenum. Blood is supplied to the pancreas and the duodenum by way of the celiac axis and the superior mesenteric artery (Figure 12-4). The body of the pancreas lies across the vertebrae and over the superior mesenteric artery and vein. The tail of the pancreas extends to the hilum of the spleen. In total, the pancreas extends approximately 25 cm. The pancreatic secretions, containing digestive enzymes, are collected in the pancreatic duct, or duct of Wirsung, which unites with the common bile duct

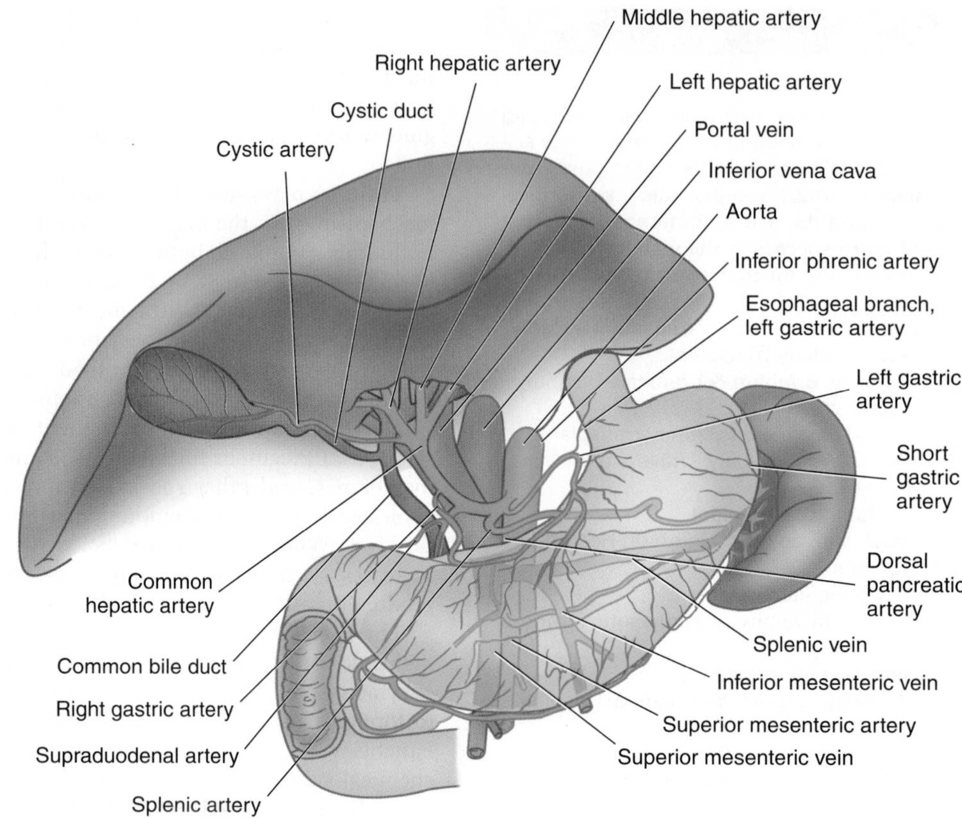


**FIGURE 12-1** Intricate relationships of the arterial and venous blood supply of the liver, gallbladder, pancreas, spleen, and the biliary ductal system.

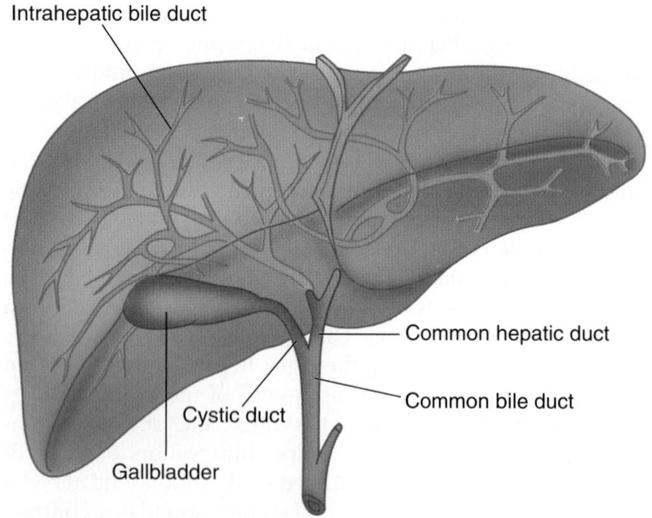


**FIGURE 12-2** Biliary system can be divided into three anatomic areas: the intrahepatic bile duct, the extrahepatic bile duct (common hepatic and common bile ducts), and the gallbladder and cystic duct.

to enter the duodenum about 7.5 cm below the pylorus. The dilated junction of the two ducts at the point of entry forms the ampulla of Vater.

The pancreas also contains groups of cells, called *islets,* or *islands, of Langerhans,* that secrete hormones into the blood capillaries instead of into the duct. These hormones are insulin and glucagon, and both are involved in carbohydrate metabolism.

The spleen (Figure 12-5) is in the upper left abdominal cavity, with full protection provided by the tenth, eleventh, and twelfth ribs; the lateral surface is directly beneath the dome of the diaphragm. The anterior medial surface is in proximity to the cardiac end of the stomach and the splenic flexure of the colon. The spleen is covered with peritoneum that forms supporting ligaments. The splenic artery, a branch of the celiac axis, furnishes the arterial blood supply. The splenic vein drains into the portal system.

The spleen has many functions. Among them are the defense of the body by phagocytosis of microorganisms, formation of nongranular leukocytes and plasma cells, and phagocytosis of damaged red blood cells. It also acts as a blood reservoir.

# *Perioperative Nursing Considerations*

## Assessment

The patient with hepatobiliary disease may have extreme jaundice, urticaria, petechiae, lethargy, and irritability. Depending on the extent of the disease, bleeding and coagulation times may be increased and the platelet count decreased, contributing to intraoperative concerns with achieving hemostasis. A thorough nursing history is necessary for proper assessment of the health status of patients with dysfunctions of the hepatobiliary system, the pancreas, or the spleen. Assessment should include data pertaining to the patient's history of chronic dis-

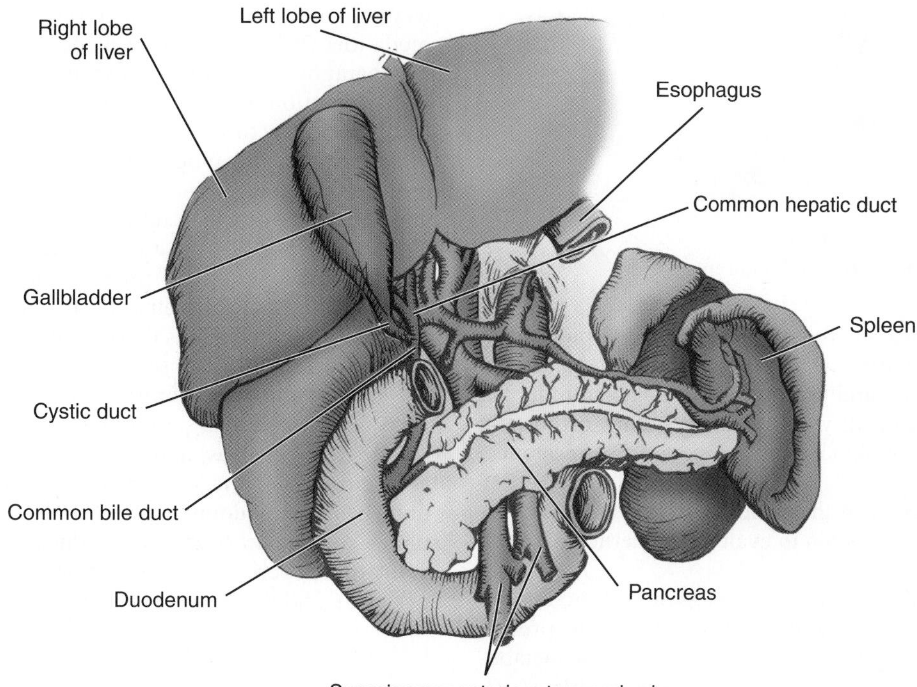


**FIGURE 12-3** Gallbladder and surrounding anatomy.

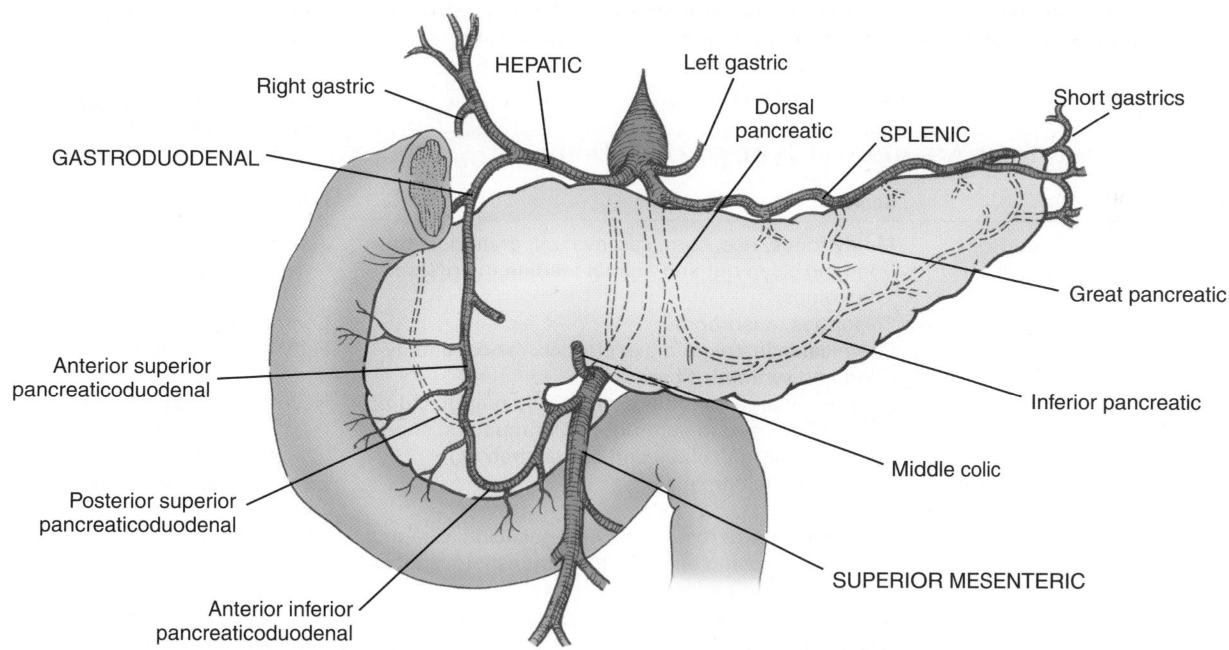


**FIGURE 12-4** Arterial supply to the pancreas arises from the celiac axis (hepatic and splenic arteries) and the superior mesenteric artery. The blood supply to the head of the gland is by way of the pancreaticoduodenal (anterior and posterior) arcades, which arise from the gastroduodenal artery (superior) and superior mesenteric arteries (inferior).

ease, current medication use, perception of his or her disease, comfort status, nutritional status, fluid and electrolyte balance, bowel and elimination patterns, energy level and independence, and exposure to toxins. Many industrial compounds are toxic to the liver (Table 12-1).

Establishing an objective database for a person with hepatobiliary or pancreatic dysfunction requires a comprehensive patient assessment. Particular attention should be directed toward observing for characteristic signs of organ dysfunction. Increased abdominal girth and distention, palmar erythema,

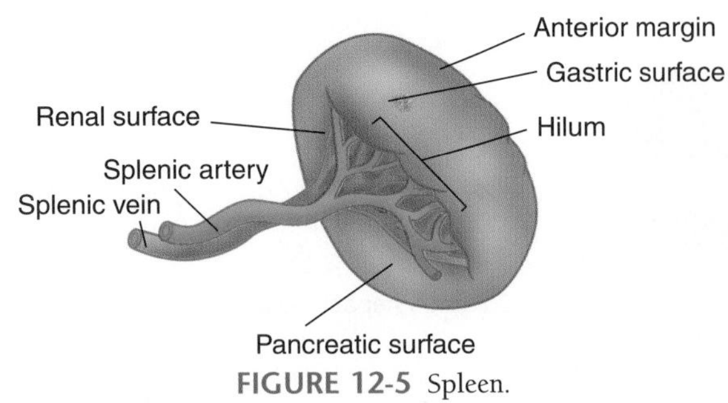

FIGURE 12-5 Spleen.

distended periumbilical veins, hemorrhagic areas, spider nevi, muscle wasting, and dry mucous membranes are a few of the characteristic signs and symptoms. Vascular volume can be assessed by monitoring vital signs, including orthostatic changes, assessment of skin turgor, temperature, appearance, and weight gain or loss.

Physical examination of the patient's abdomen should include palpation and percussion to evaluate tenderness, ascites, and organ enlargement.

The common laboratory tests to assess liver function are those that provide an evaluation of fat metabolism, protein metabolism, blood coagulation properties, bilirubin metabolism, and antigens and antibodies of hepatitis (Table 12-2). Common tests of pancreatic function can be found in Table 12-3. Radiographic studies commonly used to evaluate function of the liver, pancreas, and spleen include abdominal examination, upper gastrointestinal (GI) series, ultrasound studies, computerized tomography (CT) scan, radioisotope scanning, nuclear magnetic resonance imaging (MRI), angiography, cholecystography, and cholangiography. State-of-the-art imaging modalities include contrast-enhanced MRI, MR cholangiopancreatography (MRCP), endoscopic ultrasound (EUS), and high-resolution, thin-section spiral CT for imaging pancreatic and biliary structures.[14]

Endoscopy and biopsy are more invasive diagnostic procedures that may be used in evaluation of the liver, pancreas, and spleen. Endoscopic retrograde cholangiopancreatography (ERCP) (Figure 12-6) is a procedure that allows for direct visualization of the biliary tract, the injection of radiographic dye into the ductal system, and biopsy when indicated (Best Practice).[25] Percutaneous transhepatic cholangiography (PTC) involves percutaneous insertion of a long flexible needle into a bile duct of the liver. Contrast medium is injected, and serial x-ray examination is performed. Arteriography of the liver, biliary tree, pancreas, and spleen is accomplished by femoral arteriotomy and the placement of a catheter into the celiac branch of the abdominal aorta under fluoroscopic visualization. Contrast medium is then injected, and serial x-ray examination is performed as the vessels are visualized during the perfusion and drainage phases.

## Nursing Diagnosis

After a thorough review of the nursing assessment, nursing diagnoses are formulated. Nursing diagnoses related to the care of patients undergoing surgery of the liver, biliary tract, pancreas, or spleen might include the following:

- Anxiety related to impending surgical procedure, perioperative events, and surgical outcome

**TABLE 12-1**

### Common Hepatotoxic Agents and Type of Liver Damage

| Toxic Agent | Source | Liver Damage |
|---|---|---|
| Aflatoxin B | Moldy foods, rice, corn, cassava, oil, grain dust (during bin clean out and animal feeding in enclosed buildings) | Jaundice, fatty liver, hepatocellular carcinoma, thromboses |
| *Amanita phalloides* | Poisonous mushrooms | Centrolobular and massive necrosis |
| Benzene | Chemical industry, to make plastics, resins, and nylon and synthetic fibers | Fatty liver, cirrhosis |
| Beryllium | From x-ray tube and fluorescent lamp manufacture; alloys are used in automobiles, computers, sports equipment (golf clubs and bicycle frames) | Necrosis and granulomas |
| Boron, cadmium, nickel, chromium, copper | From gold melting, plating | Liver damage, rise in liver enzymes |
| Carbon tetrachloride | Propellants for aerosol cans, as a pesticide, cleaning fluid, degreasing agent, fire extinguishers, spot removers (now banned) | Centrolobular necrosis |
| Kerosene | From fuel handling | Liver damage, rise in liver enzymes |
| Lead | Environment | Steatosis, hepatitis |
| Pesticides | Polyvinyl chloride, farming industry | Steatosis, angiosarcoma (liver tumors) |
| Phosphorus | From poisons and firecrackers | Fatty liver, necrosis, fibrosis |
| Toluene, xylene | Occurs naturally in crude oil | Fatty liver, fibrosis |
| Vinyl chloride | Used to make polyvinyl chloride (plastics); also named PVC | Angiosarcoma (liver tumors), fibrosis |

Modified from Orfei L: *Toxic liver injury,* 2005. Accessed February 15, 2006, on-line: www.meddean.luc.edu/lumen/MedEd/orfpath/toxicinjury.htm; *Levels and distribution of aflatoxin B1 in grain dust,* 2002. Accessed February 15, 2006, on-line: www.cdc.gov/nasd/docs/d001301-d001400/d001376/d001376.html; *ToxFaqs for benzene,* 2004. Accessed February 15, 2006, on-line: www.atsdr.cdc.gov/tfacts3.html; *ToxFaqs for beryllium,* 2004. Accessed February 15, 2006, on-line: www.atsdr.cdc.gov/tfacts4.html; *ToxFaqs for carbon tetrachloride,* 2004. Accessed February 15, 2006, on-line: www.atsdr.cdc.gov/tfacts30.html; *Liquid fuel,* 2004. Accessed February 15, 2006, on-line: www.fireworks.com/liquid.html; *ToxFaqs for toluene,* 2004. Accessed February 15, 2006, on-line: www.atsdr.cdc.gov/tfacts56.html; *ToxFaqs for vinyl chloride,* 2004. Accessed February 15, 2006, on-line: www.atsdr.cdc.gov/tfacts20.html.

**TABLE 12-2**

## Liver Battery (Liver Function Studies)

| Test Name | Normal Values |
|---|---|
| **SERUM ENZYMES** | |
| Alkaline phosphatase (ALP) | 30-120 units/L. Elevated levels with biliary obstruction, cholestatic hepatitis, liver disease. |
| Aspartate aminotransferase (AST; previously SGOT) | 0-35 units/L. Elevated levels with hepatocellular injury, necrosis. |
| Alanine aminotransferase (ALT; previously SGPT) | 4-36 units/L. Elevated levels with liver damage, acute hepatitis; the ratio of AST/ALT usually is higher in liver necrosis and acute hepatitis and lower in cirrhosis, chronic hepatitis, cancer of the liver. |
| Lactate dehydrogenase (LDH) | 100-190 units/L (normal value may differ with method). Elevated levels in liver disease, untreated pernicious anemia, acute myocardial infarction, renal disease, muscle disease, malignant tumors. |
| 5-Nucleotidase | 0-1.6 units at 37°C. Elevated levels may indicate hepatobiliary disease. |
| Leucine aminopeptidase (LAP) | Males: 80-200 units/ml. Females: 75-185 units/ml. Elevated in liver necrosis and cancer, extrahepatic biliary obstruction (stones), viral hepatitis. |
| Gamma-glutamyl transferase (GGT), gamma glutamic transpeptidase (GGTP) | Adults 45 yr or older: 8-38 units/L; below 45 yr: 5-27 units/L. Newborns: 5× higher than adults. Elevated levels in cirrhosis, acute and chronic liver necrosis, alcoholism, acute and chronic hepatitis, liver cancer.<br>Enzyme produced by the bile ducts. Reflects rare forms of liver disease. Medications commonly cause GGT to be elevated. Liver toxins such as alcohol can cause increases in GGT. |
| Alpha-fetoprotein | <15 ng/ml. Elevated in cirrhosis, hepatitis. May indicate liver metastases from another cancer source. |
| Mitochondrial antibodies | The presence of these antibodies can indicate primary biliary cirrhosis, chronic active hepatitis, certain other autoimmune disorders. |
| **BILIRUBIN METABOLISM** | |
| Serum bilirubin | |
| Indirect (unconjugated) | 0.2-0.8 mg/dl. Elevated levels with hemolysis (lysis of red blood cells) and severe liver damage. |
| Direct and total (conjugated) | Total: 0.3-1.0 mg/dl. Direct: 0.1-0.3 mg/dl. Newborn: 1.0-12.0mg/dl. Elevated levels are seen with intrahepatic or extrahepatic obstruction. |
| Urine bilirubin | Negative: 0.02 mg/dl. Bilirubin in the urine may be seen with hepatic disease or biliary obstruction; only conjugated bilirubin spills into the urine because unconjugated bilirubin is bound to albumin in the serum and thus cannot pass the glomerular membrane. |
| Urine urobilinogen | Random: negative or <1.0 Ehrlich units. 2 hr: 0.3-1.0 Ehrlich units.<br>24 hr: 0.5-4.0 Ehrlich units. Increased levels are seen with hemolytic processes, shunting of portal blood flow. |
| Fecal urobilinogen | 50-300 mg/24 hr. Reduced levels cause clay-colored stools and are seen in biliary obstruction. |
| Ammonia | Adult: 10-80 mcg/dl. Elevated levels may be seen with liver dysfunction, hepatic failure, or heart failure. |
| **SERUM PROTEINS** | |
| Albumin | 3.5-5.0 g/dl. Decreased levels seen in liver disease. |
| Globulin | Reduced levels are seen with hepatocellular injury test of specific proteins:<br>Serum globulin: 2.3-3.4 g/dl<br>Immunoglobulin M (IgM) component: 75-300 mg/dl<br>IgG component: 650-1850 mg/dl<br>IgA component: 90-350 mg/dl |
| Total | Albumin + Globulin: 6.4-8.3 g/dl. Decreased levels may be seen with hepatocellular injury. |
| Albumin/globulin (A/G) ratio | >1.0 (Albumin ÷ Globulin). Low ratio in liver disease. |
| Transferrin | 215-365 mg/dl. Reduced levels may be seen with liver damage; increased levels may be seen with iron deficiency. |
| **BLOOD-CLOTTING FUNCTIONS** | |
| Prothrombin time (PT) | 11-12.5 sec, or 90%-100% of control. Increased levels may be seen with chronic liver disease (e.g., cirrhosis) or vitamin K deficiency. |
| Partial thromboplastin (PTT) | Activated partial thromboplastin time (APTT): 30-40 sec. PTT: 60-70 sec. Increased levels may be seen with severe liver disease or heparin therapy. |
| International normalized ratio (INR) | Oral coagulant therapy: 1.5-3.5 INR. Test used to monitor therapy for patients receiving warfarin sodium (Coumadin) therapy. More consistent measure than PT. |

Modified from *Liver disease. Common liver function tests,* 2005. Accessed February 15, 2006, on-line: www.umm.edu/liver/tests.htm; Pagana KD, Pagana TJ: *Mosby's diagnostic and laboratory test reference,* St Louis, 2005, Mosby; *Serum globulin electrophoresis,* 2005. Accessed February 15, 2006, on-line: www.nlm.nih.gov/medlineplus/ency/article/003544.htm.

**TABLE 12-3**

## Tests of Pancreatic Function

| Test Name | Normal Values |
|---|---|
| Serum amylase | 60-120 units/dl (Somogyi method). Elevated levels are seen with acute exacerbation of chronic pancreatitis, ampulla of Vater obstruction, pancreatic duct obstruction, pancreatic cancer, acute pancreatitis, and pancreatic trauma. |
| Serum lipase | 0-10 units/L. Elevated levels are seen with pancreatic carcinoma, pancreatic trauma, and pancreatitis. |
| Urine amylase | 0-5000 Somogyi units/24 hr. 6.5-48.1 units/hr (SI units). Elevated levels are the same as for serum amylase. |
| Secretin test | Volume: 95-235 ml/hr. Assessment of exocrine secretory ability of the pancreas for carcinoma, ductal obstruction, or chronic pancreatitis. Low volume may indicate obstruction. |

Modified from Chernecky CC, Berger BJ: *Laboratory tests and diagnostic procedures,* ed 3, Philadelphia, 2001, Saunders; Pagana KD, Pagana TJ. *Mosby's diagnostic and laboratory test reference,* St Louis, 2005, Mosby.

A

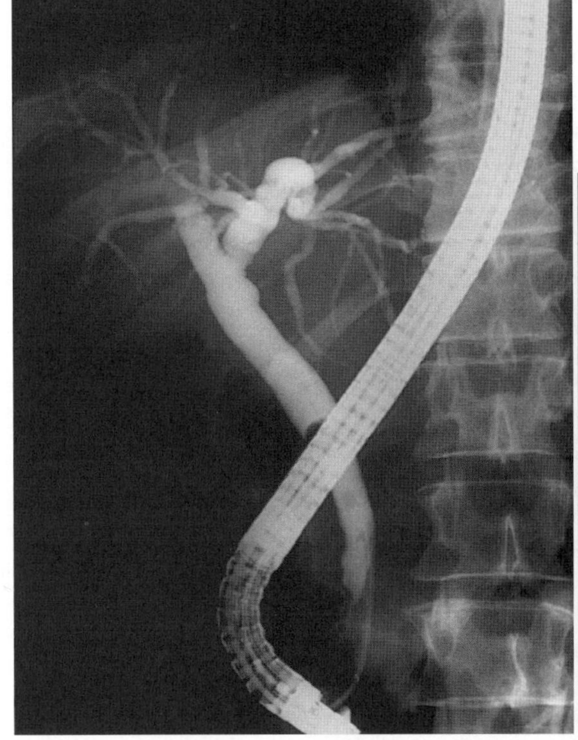

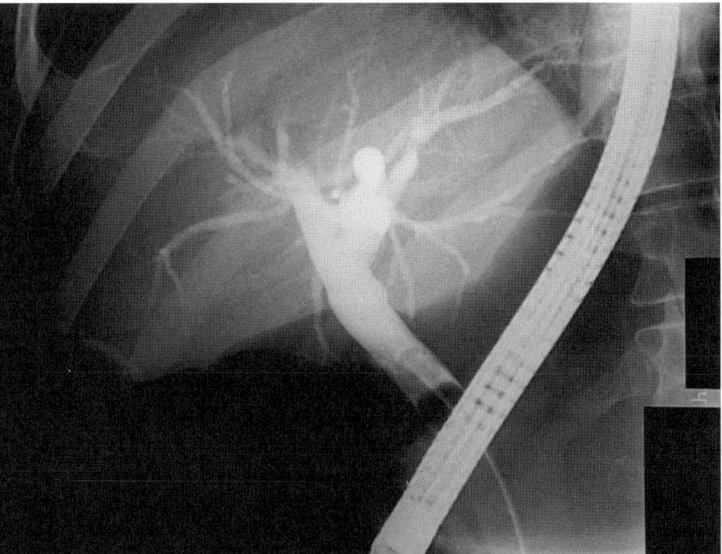

B

**FIGURE 12-6** **A,** Endoscopic retrograde cholangiopancreatography demonstrates several calculi within the distal common bile duct. **B,** Stone removal with a Fogarty catheter.

- Risk for Imbalanced Fluid Volume
- Risk for Hypothermia related to exposure of body surface or abdominal cavity and effects of anesthesia on thermoregulation
- Risk for Infection related to organ systems involved (portions of the GI tract)
- Risk for Perioperative Positioning Injury
- Risk for Impaired Skin Integrity related to invasion of body structures, disruption of skin surface
- Risk for Acute Pain related to surgical procedure[1]

## Outcome Identification

Statements regarding desired outcomes reflect the nursing diagnoses identified for a patient population. Nursing diagnoses are individualized according to cultural, ethnic, religious, and spiritual values, as well as an individual patient's status. From these are derived the outcomes the perioperative nurse wishes to achieve. The best outcome statement has specific criteria by which the perioperative nurse intends to measure whether the outcome has been met. These criteria are more significant when they are established in partnership with the patient. Not all outcomes will be planned with the patient, but ones relating to nursing diagnoses such as anxiety and coping can and should reflect the patient's participation. Outcomes identified for the selected nursing diagnoses could be stated as follows:

- The patient will verbalize management of anxiety and ability to cope, demonstrate knowledge of his or her psychologic responses to the planned procedure, and indicate an understanding of the planned sequence of perioperative events.

## BEST PRACTICE

The Agency for Healthcare Research and Quality (AHRQ) conducts evidence reports on a number of topics. Because an estimated 6 per 100,000 Americans experience common bile duct stones each year, part of this evidence report focused on patients with known or suspected common bile duct stones. The topic of interest was the diagnostic performance of endoscopic retrograde cholangiopancreatography (ERCP) in comparison with alternatives of endoscopic ultrasound (EUS), magnetic resonance cholangiopancreatography (MRCP), computed tomography cholangiography (CTC), or surgical management. The methodology included a comprehensive literature search from which studies were selected for inclusion in a meta-analysis. A number of strict criteria guided study selection. The quality of the evidence in the studies was then further assessed and rated as "good," "fair," or "poor." The evidence suggested the following:

- EUS is similar to ERCP in detecting common bile duct stones.
- MRCP has a degree of concordance with ERCP that results in sensitivities and specificities greater than 90% in most studies.
- Concordance of CTC with ERCP is lower (around 80%).
- Laparoscopic common bile duct exploration may be better than ERCP strategies to manage cholecystectomy patients with the least resource use.
- Definitive surgery with cholecystectomy prevents long-term complications at acceptable short-term morbidity when compared with sphincterotomy alone in high-risk patients with suspected common bile duct stones.
- Endoscopic treatment of acute cholangitis reduces short-term morbidity when compared with emergency surgery.
- The single risk factors most commonly assessed to predict presence of common bile duct stones were clinical jaundice or elevated bilirubin, liver function tests, and ultrasound findings of a dilated common bile duct.

Modified from U.S. Department of Health and Human Services, Public Health Service: *Endoscopic retrograde cholangiopancreatography,* Washington, DC, 2002, Agency for Healthcare Quality and Research, Evidence Report/Technology Assessment no. 50.

- The patient will maintain fluid volume equilibrium throughout the operative procedure.
- The patient will evidence an intraoperative core body temperature of 35.5°C to 37.2°C (96°F to 99°F).
- The patient will be free of clinical signs and symptoms of surgical site infection (SSI).
- The patient will maintain baseline neuromuscular function and intact skin at positional pressure sites.
- The patient will demonstrate understanding of the plan to heal the incision site.
- The patient will report that the pain management regimen relieves pain to a satisfactory level.[1]

## Planning

Planning for the care of the patient having surgery of the liver, biliary tract, pancreas, or spleen requires assimilation of knowledge of the anatomy and subsequent physiologic complications that may occur with surgical interruption of tissues. Principles of safe surgical positioning, maintenance of asepsis, prevention of biologic and electrical hazards, and provision of proper instrumentation and equipment are a few constituents of the plan of care.

A review of the nursing assessment followed by a patient interview provides insight as to the specific needs of the individual patient. The patient's past medical and surgical history as well as age, size, and nutritional status will assist the perioperative nurse in developing an effective plan of care. A typical plan of care for a patient undergoing surgery of the liver, biliary tract, pancreas, or spleen follows.

## Implementation

Patients having surgery of the liver, biliary tract, pancreas, or spleen are usually given general anesthesia. The following pertinent factors should be considered in caring for these patients.

***Universal Protocol.*** The Joint Commission on Accreditation of Healthcare Organizations (JCAHO) requires that the "wrong site, wrong procedure, wrong person" prevention protocol be

## SAMPLE PLAN OF CARE

### NURSING DIAGNOSIS

**Anxiety** related to impending surgical procedure, perioperative events, and surgical outcome

### OUTCOME

The patient will verbalize management of anxiety and ability to cope, demonstrate knowledge of his or her psychologic responses to the planned procedure, and indicate an understanding of the planned sequence of perioperative events.

### INTERVENTIONS

- Greet the patient positively; determine the name he or she prefers to be called.
- Introduce the patient to the operating room (OR) team.
- Avoid hasty movements or gestures of indecision.
- Speak slowly and clearly when addressing the patient, and use terminology the patient can understand.
- Offer emotional reassurance through touch, assisting the patient to a position of comfort on the OR bed and offering warm blankets.
- Classify the patient's level of anxiety (mild, moderate, severe) by asking the patient and observing signs of anxiety (e.g., clenching/unclenching hands, crying, tremors).
- Determine the patient's personally effective coping mechanisms, and facilitate the use of these.
- Identify the patient's special concerns, values, and wishes concerning his or her care.
- Provide explanations of perioperative events; encourage questions.

### NURSING DIAGNOSIS

**Risk for Imbalanced Fluid Volume**

### OUTCOME

Patient will maintain fluid volume equilibrium throughout surgical procedure.

### INTERVENTIONS

- Review orders for blood and blood products; have these available in close-by, refrigerated storage for timely access.

*Continued*

## SAMPLE PLAN OF CARE

### INTERVENTIONS—CONT'D

- Measure, communicate, and record estimated or real fluid volume loss throughout surgical procedure.
- Anticipate and communicate to blood bank personnel the potential need for additional blood and blood products.
- Collaborate with anesthesia provider in fluid replacement therapies.
- Check laboratory values intraoperatively; monitor and note deviations in study results.

### NURSING DIAGNOSIS

**Risk for Hypothermia** related to exposure of body surface or abdominal cavity and effects of anesthesia on thermoregulation

### OUTCOME

The patient will evidence an intraoperative core body temperature of 35.5°C to 37.2°C (96°F to 99°F).

### INTERVENTIONS

- Ask the patient if he or she is cold.
- Adjust room temperature and humidity to accommodate preservation of body temperature.
- Provide warm blankets on transfer to OR bed.
- Expose only that part of the body necessary for the surgical prep; cover all other body surfaces to maintain body heat.
- Provide warm irrigation solutions, ensuring temperature is below 105°F (40.5°C.)
- Collaborate with anesthesia provider in warming intravenous (IV) fluids and blood and blood products before infusion.
- Use forced-air warming system for supporting body temperature maintenance.
- Monitor body temperature to evaluate response to thermoregulation measures.

### NURSING DIAGNOSIS

**Risk for Infection** related to organ systems involved (portions of the gastrointestinal tract)

### OUTCOME

The patient will be free of clinical signs and symptoms of surgical site infection.

### INTERVENTIONS

- Implement aseptic technique; communicate and correct breaks in asepsis.
- Ensure that preoperative antibiotics are administered as ordered; prophylactic antibiotics should be administered 1 hour before the incision. Follow guidelines for safe medication practices.
- Contain and confine contaminants appropriately.
- Ensure that all sterilization procedures have been properly observed.
- Ensure that the integrity of sterile supply packaging is intact before dispensing items to the sterile field.
- Perform skin preparation with antimicrobial agent of choice (institutional protocol).
- Implement measures to prevent cross-contamination.
- Initiate traffic control and environmental measures, which reduce risk for infection.
- Use aseptic technique in applying dressings to surgical sites.
- Correctly classify wound according to established wound classification system.
- Manage culture specimen collection according to institutional policy.

### NURSING DIAGNOSIS

**Risk for Perioperative Positioning Injury**

### OUTCOME

The patient will maintain baseline neuromuscular function and intact skin at positional pressure sites.

### INTERVENTIONS

- Identify any physiologic alterations or mobility limitations that may affect procedure-specific positioning.
- Implement measures to prevent shearing forces during patient transfer to and from OR bed and during positional changes.
- Ensure that all positioning equipment is clean and functioning properly.
- Ensure patient is in optimal anatomic alignment after induction of anesthesia.
- Adequately pad all bony prominences and vulnerable neurovascular areas.
- Secure limbs with safety strap to ensure position is maintained and to prevent limb from falling from positioning device (as appropriate to procedure-specific position).
- Ensure safe and proper placement of electrosurgical dispersive pad.
- Verify correct position during time out.
- Ensure that no weight or stress is placed on body parts and structures during the surgical intervention.
- Check protective padding and safety restraints after all positional changes.

### NURSING DIAGNOSIS

**Risk for Impaired Skin Integrity** related to invasion of body structures, disruption of skin surface

### OUTCOME

The patient will regain integrity of skin surface.

### INTERVENTIONS (POSTOPERATIVE)

- Monitor incision site for color, redness, swelling, warmth, and pain.
- Avoid positioning patient on incision site.
- Individualize plan according to patient's skin condition, needs, and preferences.
- Monitor incision edges for intactness, bleeding, and drainage.
- Maintain a moist wound healing environment that is balanced with the need to absorb exudate.

### NURSING DIAGNOSIS

**Risk for Acute Pain** related to surgical procedure

### OUTCOME

The patient will report that the pain management regimen relieves pain to a satisfactory level, using a pain assessment scale.

### INTERVENTIONS (POSTOPERATIVE)

- Review use of a pain scale with the patient and family before surgery.
- Identify cultural and value components related to pain.
- Provide patient and family with information on pain management.
- Determine whether the patient is experiencing pain at the time of the initial postoperative assessment.
- Assess and document intensity and location of pain.
- Assume pain is present and treat as ordered.
- Use a preventative approach to keep pain at or below an acceptable level.

carried out before each surgical procedure.[24] This protocol involves the following principles:

- Wrong site, wrong procedure, wrong person surgery can and must be prevented.
- Active involvement and effective communication among all members of the surgical team are required.
- The patient (to the extent possible) should be involved in the process.
- Consistent implementation is necessary.
- The protocol is flexible to allow for implementation with adaptation to patient needs.
- Site marking should focus on operative and other invasive procedures involving right/left distinction (laterality) and multiple structures or multiple levels.
- The protocol is adaptable to all procedures that expose patients to the risk for harm.

The implementation of the Universal Protocol should occur using the following steps:

1. Preoperative verification process
   - Relevant documents and studies should be available before the start of the procedure and should be consistent with each other; with the patient's expectations; and with the team's understanding of the intended patient, procedure, site, and, as applicable, any implants, special equipment or positioning needs, availability of ordered blood/blood products, and so on. Missing information or discrepancies must be addressed before starting the procedure. This begins an ongoing process of information gathering and verification.
   - The consent should have the correct site and procedure documented.
   - The surgical posting should match the procedure.
   - The patient (or the patient's representative) should know and be able to state what the procedure and site of surgery are before receiving sedation.
2. Marking the operative site
   - This is intended to unambiguously identify the intended site of incision/insertion. For procedures with right/left, multiple structures, or multiple levels, the site must be marked with a mark that is visible after the patient has been prepped and draped. Special marking pens are available for this process.
   - The physician performing the procedure marks the site with "yes" or his or her initials. Check marks or *X*s are not appropriate.
3. "Time out" immediately before starting the procedure
   - The final verification of the correct patient, procedure, site, surgical position, and, if applicable, implants, and other required special items occurs before the incision is made. At this time, it should also be verified that any flammable prep solutions have dried (see Chapter 2 for a full discussion of fire safety and prep solutions).
   - Active communication among all members of the surgical/procedure team must be consistently initiated by a designated member of the team (usually the registered nurse). This must be conducted in a "fail-safe" mode; that is, the procedure may not be started until any questions or concerns are resolved (this is also referred to as a *hard stop*).
   - The time out procedure must be documented on the patient record.

***Positioning the Patient.*** For biliary surgery, the patient is placed in a supine position. The surgeon may request a small positioning aid placed under the lower right side of the thorax. This elevates the lower rib cage to provide better exposure and access to the viscera in the right upper quadrant of the abdomen. Alternatively, a lateral tilt of the operating room (OR) bed may be used in combination with reverse Trendelenburg for procedures such as laparoscopic cholecystectomy.

Positioning the patient for laparoscopic procedures requires the perioperative nurse to exercise caution when applying the safety straps. Because of the potential for the patient to be placed in a severe side tilt or reverse Trendelenburg position, the safety or restraining straps must be placed securely but not too tightly. Attention is given to proper alignment of the patient's body and extremities; padded footboards are applied to prevent the patient from slipping. Areas of pressure in the select surgical position (see Chapter 5) and bony prominences are padded well to prevent interruption of circulation and pressure injury to tissues and neurovascular structures. This precaution is especially important with diabetic, circulatory-impaired, immunocompromised, and elderly patients. Close monitoring of the patient is essential during positional changes, especially in laparoscopic procedures because of the decreased lighting in the room.

When an operative cholangiogram is anticipated, the perioperative nurse must ensure that the OR bed has been equipped and positioned so that C-arm image intensification can be efficiently accomplished. Radiation-protection devices for the surgical team and patient should be available.

***Thermoregulation.*** The risks of intraoperative hypothermia have been well documented (see Chapters 4 and 9). When laparotomy is performed, patients are at further risk for hypothermia. To prevent unplanned hypothermia, the perioperative nurse ensures that measures are taken to maintain body temperature in the operating room.[5] The environmental temperature and humidity are set to prevent body heat loss caused by evaporation and convection. A forced-air warming blanket placed over the patient's upper body, head, and neck assists in maintenance of body temperature. Minimizing body exposure to ambient air and the use of warm irrigating solutions also support thermoregulation for the patient. The temperature of irrigating fluids should be below 105°F (40.5°C) and recorded on the operative record.[22] A blood- and fluid-warming device may be used by the anesthesia provider to deliver intravenous (IV) fluids at a temperature higher than room air temperature (see Chapter 4). The anesthesia provider commonly monitors the patient's core temperature by use of an esophageal temperature probe when the duration and complexity of the surgical procedure place the patient at risk for hypothermia. Additional comfort measures, such as using warm blankets before and after surgery, demonstrate caring and concern for the patient.

***Application of Sequential Compression Device.*** Patients undergoing lengthy surgical procedures may be at risk for venous dilation and blood pooling in the lower extremities. This may predispose the surgical patient to development of deep venous thrombosis (DVT) in the postoperative period. Sequential compression devices (SCDs) are frequently applied in the OR before commencing lengthy surgical procedures.[3]

***Draping the Patient.*** After the abdominal prep, time must be allowed for the prep solution to dry and vapors to dissipate. This is an essential patient safety precaution when flammable prep solutions are used in conjunction with electrosurgery (or other ignition sources, such as a laser). Sterile towels are then arranged to accommodate the intended incision. A sterile drape sheet may be placed over the patient's lower torso, and a laparotomy sheet then is placed to provide a wide sterile field and cover all exposed body surfaces except the incisional site.

***Instrumentation.*** Instrumentation for surgeries of the liver, biliary tract, spleen, and pancreas, if performed through a laparotomy incision, includes a basic laparotomy set, biliary probes and forceps for dilating and exploring the ducts of the pancreas and biliary tract, vascular clamps, GI clamps, and ligating clips of all sizes with appliers; linear stapling instruments also should be available. A self-retaining system such as the Bookwalter retractor set (Figure 12-7) enhances exposure for the surgeon and allows optimal safe retraction of tissues and excellent exposure of the abdominal viscera. In addition, a flexible choledochoscope, Cavitron ultrasound suction aspirator (CUSA), intraoperative ultrasound, laser, argon beam coagulator, harmonic scalpel, and electrosurgical unit may be required to perform certain procedures on the hepatobiliary system.

The basic instrumentation and equipment for minimally invasive surgical (MIS) procedures consist of two high-density monitors, an insufflation unit, electrosurgical unit, light source, camera, and 0-degree and 30-degree telescopes in 10-mm and 5-mm sizes; a printer may be optional. An ultrasonic dissecting unit is often used with MIS procedures. Trocars and sleeves are available in reusable, disposable, and resposable designs. Trocars and sleeves are now commonly designed to accommodate 10-mm to 5-mm instruments and 12-mm to 5-mm accessories and instruments. Scissors and shears, dissecting forceps, atraumatic grasping forceps, hooks, Babcock clamps, retractors, needles, suturing devices, pouches, suction-irrigating devices, and mechanical stapling devices are designed to assist the surgeon in MIS procedures.

Thrombin, Gelfoam, Surgicel, Avitene, and other chemical hemostatic agents (Surgical Pharmacology) should be available in the OR suite. Radiographic dye, supplies, and radiation-protection devices will be required if intraoperative radiography or angiography is planned as part of the procedure.

***Drainage Materials.*** Tubes and catheters must be in optimal condition and suitable for the areas to be drained. If a defective drain is used, a free fragment may remain in the wound on removal of the tube. Thus the scrub person should note the

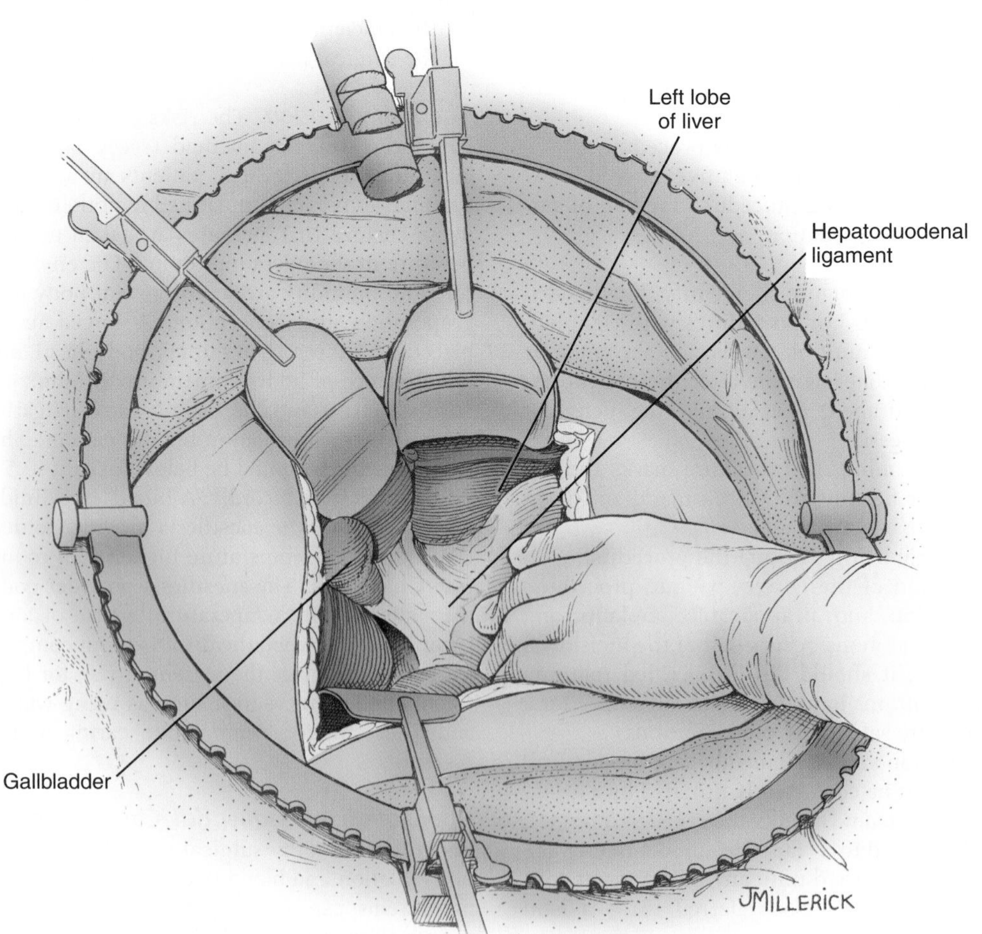


**FIGURE 12-7** Bookwalter self-retaining retractor in place to provide optimal exposure to the abdominal viscera.

SURGICAL PHARMACOLOGY

## Chemical Hemostatic Agents

| Agent | Chemical Composition | Actions | Perioperative Precautions |
|---|---|---|---|
| Absorbable gelatin: powder or compressed forms (Gelfoam) | Purified porcine gelatin, beaten, dried, and heat sterilized | On areas of capillary bleeding, deposits fibrin forming a clot. Absorbs 45× its own weight. | Dipped in warm saline or soaked in thrombin. Must be squeezed to remove air. |
| Absorbable collagen (Collastat, Superstat, Helistat, Lyostypt) | Bovine collagen origin | Collagen activates coagulation mechanism, aggregation of platelets. | Must be kept dry and applied with dry gloves. Do not use in infected areas or in pooled blood. |
| Microfibrillar collagen (Avitene, Instat) | Hydrochloric acid salt of purified bovine corium collagen | Adhesion of platelets and prompt fibrin deposition. | Applied dry. Firm pressure against the bleeding surface. |
| Oxidized cellulose (Surgicel, Surgicel Nu-Knit) | Absorbable oxidation product of cellulose | On contact with blood, clot forms. Increases in size and forms a gel. Absorbs 10× its own weight | Applied dry; may be sutured in place. |
| Oxytocin | Synthetic pituitary hormone | Injected directly into uterine muscle during cesarean birth to cause contraction after delivery of baby and placenta. Prevents uterine hemorrhage. | Also may be given intravenously to induce labor. |
| Phenol and alcohol | Chemical compounds used to cauterize tissue across the lumen of the appendix | Phenol coagulates proteins, and alcohol 95% neutralizes the phenol. | Phenol is caustic and may cause severe burns. |
| Epinephrine (Adrenalin) | Adrenal hormone | Powerful vasoconstrictor—prolongs action of local anesthetics to decrease bleeding. | Gelatin sponges may be soaked in 1:1000 epinephrine—especially useful in ear and microsurgical procedures. |
| Tannic acid | Powder from astringent plant | Used on nose and throat mucous membranes to stop capillary bleeding. | Also used in dental procedures. |
| Silver nitrate | Crystals of silver nitrate compound mixed with silver chloride and molded on to applicator sticks. | Astringent and antimicrobial. Seals areas of surgical incisions. | May also be used in the treatment of burns. |
| Thrombin | Enzyme extracted from bovine blood | Accelerates coagulation of blood. Unites rapidly with fibrin to form a clot. | May be used topically as a dry powder or as a solution that gelatin sponges are dipped in. May also be sprayed on. Topical use only. Loses potency after 3 hr. |

Modified from Phillips NF: *Berry and Kohn's operating room technique,* ed 10, St Louis, 2004, Mosby.

condition of all drainage materials and should test them for patency before they are placed in the patient.

Soft rubber or latex tissue drains may be used after an open cholecystectomy or a choledochostomy. Verify that the patient does not have a latex allergy before using these devices and substitute nonlatex drains if necessary (Box 12-1 presents guidelines for latex-allergic patients). A latex rubber T-tube drain of suitable size is prepared by the surgeon after the duct has been explored. The center of the crossbar is notched opposite the junction of the vertical limb so that its ends will bend more readily during removal. The ends are beveled and tailored to fit the duct.

Drains are usually exteriorized through separate stab wounds and anchored to skin edges to prevent their retraction. The perioperative nurse should document the types of drains and reservoirs inserted during the operative procedure; depending on institutional protocol, these may be identified with an applied label. All drains and their locations should be included in the perioperative nurse's hand-off report to the nursing unit to which the patient is transferred postoperatively.

***Aseptic Considerations.*** When the common duct is opened or an anastomosis is established between a duct and other parts of the alimentary tract, it may be the institution's policy or the surgeon's preference to isolate contaminated instruments and materials from the remainder of the operative field, as described for GI surgery. The wound should be classified according to a standard system; any procedure in which the alimentary tract is entered under controlled conditions and without unusual contamination is considered a *clean contaminated wound.* If there is gross spillage, the wound is classified

BOX 12-1

**Latex Sensitivity and Allergy Guidelines**

Natural rubber latex allergy can be a serious and life-threatening condition. Health care workers and others who have experienced repeated exposure to latex can develop latex sensitivity or allergy. The following is a list of guidelines that should be instituted in persons with suspected or known latex sensitivity or allergy:

- Identify the patient's risk factors and report them to the operating room (OR) team. Those at high risk include persons with the following:
  - Myelomeningocele
  - Multiple surgeries, particularly if begun in early infancy
  - A positive serum latex antibody test
  - Occupational exposure to latex products, particularly powdered products
  - Allergy to bananas, kiwi, avocado, stone fruits, raw potato, tomato, papaya, chestnuts
  - History of hives or itching after incidental exposure: condom use, dental or other procedures
- Patient with known latex sensitivity should be scheduled as the first procedure of the day if facility is not latex-safe.
- When possible, anesthesia and the operating room should be notified 24 to 48 hours in advance.
- Notify health care providers in other areas of the patient's latex sensitivity status.
- Plan for a latex-safe environment of care:
  - Remove all latex products from the room unless no alternative exists.
  - Obtain a latex-free cart from the designated area.
  - Place a latex precaution card on the OR door.
  - Look for the signs and symptoms of latex reaction: contact rash, wheezing, bronchospasm, chest pain or tightness.

Modified from AORN: *2006 Standards, recommended practices, and guidelines with official AORN statements,* 2006 ed, Denver, Colo, 2006, Association of periOperative Registered Nurses (AORN).

as *contaminated.* Proper wound classification is considered an important predictor of postoperative SSI.[11]

***Blood Products.*** During the preoperative verification process, the perioperative nurse should ascertain the type and amount of blood and blood products requested and available for the patient as well as ensuring that a consent for transfusion was signed by the patient. Constant, ongoing evaluation of blood loss is communicated to the anesthesia provider and surgical team during the procedure. When additional blood or blood products are required, the perioperative nurse communicates with blood bank personnel so that additional required blood products are readily available and carries out the required steps in verifying blood/blood products with the anesthesia provider before transfusion.

Autologous blood or donor-directed blood products may be used in elective procedures involving the liver, pancreas, spleen, and biliary tract. Cell-saver devices may be used when the potential for contamination of the blood from bile or bowel does not exist.

## Evaluation

Evaluation of the patient after surgery includes examination of all skin surfaces and comparison with the preoperative assessment data. Abdominal drains, chest drainage systems, urinary drainage systems, and peripheral infusion lines are assessed for patency. Fluid volume use and loss are documented and communicated appropriately. A thorough report of the patient's history, preoperative assessment, intraoperative events, and postoperative evaluation is communicated to the postanesthesia care unit (PACU) or surgical intensive care unit (SICU) nurse during the hand-off report.

The evaluation of patient status can be phrased as outcome statements such as the following:

- The patient verbalized management of anxiety and ability to cope, expressed knowledge of his or her psychologic responses to the planned procedure, and indicated an understanding of the sequence of perioperative events.
- The patient maintained equilibrium in fluid volume; hematocrit remained in the expected range; vital signs were stable.
- The patient's intraoperative core body temperature remained consistently in the 35.5°C to 37.2°C (96°F to 99°F) range.
- The patient's surgical incision was dressed aseptically and was dry and intact. There will be no clinical signs or symptoms of infection.
- At the conclusion of the surgical procedure, skin surfaces were clean, intact, and free of reddened areas; adequate capillary filling was noted after blanching of tissues. The patient had palpable pulses in all distal extremities and showed no evidence of diminished neuromuscular function.
- The patient will be able to perform activities of recovery with acceptable levels of pain.

## Patient and Family Education and Discharge Planning

The length of time and complexity of recovery will vary greatly for patients undergoing surgical intervention for disorders of the liver, pancreas, spleen, or biliary tract.[10] Laparoscopic cholecystectomy may be performed on an ambulatory surgery basis with extended recovery and observation of 6 to 8 hours. In contrast, patients undergoing liver transplantation or resection may require extensive recovery that includes a stay in the intensive care unit.

Patients undergoing laparotomy for surgical intervention of the liver, pancreas, spleen, or biliary tract may have varying degrees of postoperative edema, decreased GI peristalsis, and alterations in tissue oxygenation and lymphatic drainage, depending on the amount of manipulation, resection, and trauma to the normal anatomic structures of these viscera. General anesthesia is commonly administered to the patient undergoing surgical intervention for disorders of the liver, pancreas, spleen, or biliary tract. Smooth muscle relaxation is imperative for most major abdominal viscera interventions. The patient will usually experience decreased peristalsis for 2 to 5 days after laparotomy. A nasogastric tube or gastrostomy tube is inserted during the surgical event to evacuate the large volumes of gastric juices. Diet is introduced only after bowel sounds return. The patient may experience nausea and vomiting if food or oral fluid is introduced too early for the GI system to function with normal absorption and motility.

Coughing and deep breathing are important for the patient recovering from general anesthesia and abdominal surgery. Splinting of the abdominal muscles and the use of an incentive spirometer will assist the patient in postoperative coughing and deep-breathing initiatives. Early ambulation will assist the patient in regaining overall muscle tone and preventing DVT in the lower extremities.

Pain management is a very important factor in the patient's recovery and discharge planning. For most patients undergoing abdominal surgery, patient-controlled analgesia (PCA) or epidural analgesia may be used for better and more consistent control of pain and discomfort in the first 1 to 3 postoperative days of hospital recovery (see Chapter 9). Narcotics may, however, add to the length of time at which normal bowel peristalsis returns, so their use is monitored closely after the third postoperative day.

General discharge instructions for the patient undergoing surgery for disorders of the liver, pancreas, spleen, or biliary tract may include the following:

- Keep incisional area clean and dry.
- Swelling inside the GI tract may produce a feeling of tightness; this should dissipate in 6 to 8 weeks.
- Solid foods should be added to the diet gradually. Chew solid foods well, and avoid gulping or eating fast or swallowing large, bulky portions.
- Avoid carbonated beverages for 3 to 4 weeks to help prevent gas bloating.
- Plan small, frequent meals because the feeling of fullness will come quickly.
- Increase exercise gradually to return to activities of daily living. Exercise regularly.
- Make an appointment for follow-up care with the surgeon.

In addition to such general information, surgical patients and their family or caregiver should receive surgery-specific special instructions. Any medications the patient will be taking after discharge should be reviewed, explaining the purpose, dosage, schedule, and route of administration, as well as any side effects to be reported to the physician or nurse. Part of discharge planning and family education includes the provision of both verbal and written instructions, with phone numbers of those to call if questions arise.[9] For most patients, a health care provider should be notified if any of the following develop:

- Persistent fever (38.3°C [101°F] or higher)
- Bleeding
- Increased abdominal swelling or pain
- Chills
- Persistent cough or shortness of breath
- Purulent drainage from incision sites

Follow-up care may also require providing referrals for home care (or other) services.

# Surgical Interventions

## SURGERY OF THE BILIARY TRACT

### Cholecystectomy (Open Approach)

Cholecystectomy is removal of the gallbladder. It is performed for the treatment of diseases such as acute or chronic inflammation (cholecystitis) or stones (cholelithiasis) (Box 12-2). Most of these procedures can be completed laparoscopically. The few contraindications to the laparoscopic approach include uncontrolled coagulopathy or severe chronic obstructive pulmonary disease (COPD) or heart failure (HF)—these patients may not be able to tolerate the pneumoperitoneum required in laparoscopy. If the surgeon is unable to identify all the anatomic structures during a laparoscopic approach, conversion to an open procedure then becomes necessary.

***Procedural Considerations.*** A basic laparotomy set and biliary instruments are used when cholecystectomy is performed through an open abdominal incision. The patient is positioned supine and usually receives general anesthesia. After the patient is intubated, the anesthesia provider inserts a nasogastric tube. Antibiotic prophylaxis may be prescribed to be administered in the immediate preoperative period. When an operative cholangiogram is anticipated, the perioperative nurse must ensure that the OR bed has been equipped and positioned so that C-arm image intensification can be efficiently accomplished. Radiation-protection devices for the surgical team and patient should be available.

#### *Operative Procedure*

1. The abdominal cavity is opened through a right subcostal or upper midline incision.
2. Hemostasis of capillary vessels is achieved with electrocoagulation. Larger vessels are clamped with hemostats and tied with suture material.
3. Retractors and laparotomy packs are placed as the abdominal cavity is carefully examined.
4. The common duct is palpated for evidence of stones, and the pathologic conditions are determined.
5. Harrington, Deaver, or automatic retractors, such as an upper-hand or Gomez retractor, are placed to provide exposure. Long tissue forceps and suction are used to manipulate tissues. The surrounding organs are walled off from the gallbladder region by moistened laparotomy packs and deep retractors.
6. To facilitate gentle traction, Pean forceps are usually placed on the body of the gallbladder (Figure 12-8, *A*).
7. The peritoneal fold overlying the junction of the cystic and common duct is incised with a #7 knife handle and a #15 blade, long Metzenbaum scissors, and forceps. Suction is available, and bleeding points are clamped and ligated or electrocoagulated.
8. Adhesions are separated by blunt dissection with small, round, dry dissector sponges; sponges on holders; and blunt right-angled clamps.
9. Dissection is continued to expose the neck of the gallbladder, the cystic artery, and the cystic duct. Lateral traction on the gallbladder neck allows incision of the peritoneum overlying the triangle of Calot.
10. Dissection is continued to expose the cystic artery as it enters the wall of the gallbladder.
11. On complete exposure and visualization of the branches, the cystic artery is doubly ligated with silk or clamped with ligating clips and divided (Figure 12-8, *B*).
12. Occasionally a third ligature or clip may be used. If the cystic artery has more than one branch, each is ligated and divided separately.
13. Abnormalities of the arterial and ductal anatomy are common (Figure 12-9), and the surgeon and assistant work with meticulous care to identify these structures.
14. The true junction of the cystic duct with the common bile duct is visualized.

BOX 12-2

**Overview of Cholelithiasis and Cholecystitis**

**OVERVIEW**

The two most common diseases of the biliary tree are *cholelithiasis* (stone formation in the gallbladder) and *cholecystitis* (inflammation of the gallbladder). These conditions may occur alone but usually occur simultaneously. Gallstones are becoming more common in the United States, affecting an estimated 20 million adults. Cholecystectomy is one of the most common surgeries performed. Gallstones are usually found in individuals older than 20 years, with a high incidence in Pima and Chippewa people, white women, and African Americans.

Clinical conditions that may predispose to gallstones include diabetes, obesity, cirrhosis, ileal disease or resection, cancer of the gallbladder, and pancreatitis. Cholecystitis usually results from obstruction of the cystic duct from gallstones (acute calculous cholecystitis); however, in a few patients, it results from stasis, bacteria, or sepsis (acute acalculous cholecystitis).

**PATHOPHYSIOLOGY**

The pathophysiology of gallstones depends largely on the following factors: the type of stone, the stone's location within the ductal system, and whether the occurrence is acute or chronic. Gallstones are classified as (1) cholesterol stones, (2) pigment stones, and (3) mixed stones. Cholesterol stones are the most common type and occur most often in women. Pigment stones are present in approximately 30% of those presenting with gallbladder disorders. They consist primarily of calcium bilirubinate. Mixed stones are a combination of pigment and cholesterol stones. The exact cause of gallstone formation is unclear. Contributing factors may include the following:

- *Supersaturation of bile with cholesterol.* Bile is composed mainly of water, with other components including cholesterol, bile salts, and pigments. Cholesterol alone is insoluble in water; it must be combined with other components (e.g., bile salts) to remain in solution. When bile salts are insufficient to maintain cholesterol in solution, cholesterol crystals form.
- *Bile stasis.* This occurs when the gallbladder has not contracted normally in response to a meal and the bile is stagnant and then becomes thick and concentrated. This occurs in patients receiving total parenteral nutrition (TPN) for a prolonged period. Approximately 50% of these patients develop "sludge" (a mucous gel composed of calcium bilirubinate and cholesterol crystals) in the gallbladder by week 6 of TPN therapy. Gallstones frequently occur during periods of fasting or dieting, during which there is a lack of stimulus for the gallbladder to contract.
  - *Nucleation.* A nucleus (nidus) is formed of agents such as bacteria, bile, pigments, cellular debris, and calcium salts. Additional substances aggregate around this nucleus, forming a stone.
  - *Genetics* may be a factor, as evidenced by increased prevalence in Pima and Chippewa people.

Some stones may form and pass through the ducts without causing clinical manifestations (asymptomatic cholelithiasis). Symptomatic cholelithiasis occurs when stones intermittently become lodged in the cystic duct, causing biliary colic (episodic pain in the right upper quadrant or epigastric area). The pain usually occurs after meals, especially high-fat meals, as a result of increased intraluminal pressure when the gallbladder attempts to contract to release bile (a normal response to food entering the duodenum) against the obstructing stone.

Cholecystitis develops as stones become impacted within the cystic duct, causing unyielding obstruction, edema, distention, and inflammation of the gallbladder. In chronic cholecystitis, gallstones remain, causing recurrent obstructions and producing changes in the gallbladder wall from recurrent edema and inflammation. The muscular coat becomes fibrous, and the gallbladder functions less effectively.

**COMPLICATIONS**

Edema and distention of the gallbladder walls decrease blood supply, resulting in patchy areas of necrosis and gangrene. Perforation of these areas can then occur. Bile leakage through these perforations into the peritoneum results in peritonitis. Abscess formation may occur if secretions from the ruptured gallbladder are confined by omentum or other adjacent organs (e.g., colon, stomach, duodenum, pancreas).

Stone migration from the gallbladder to the common bile duct (CBD) may cause cholangitis (acute CBD inflammation). The presence of gallstones in the CBD is called choledocholithiasis. CBD stones are a major source of morbidity in patients with symptomatic gallstone disease. Stone migration to the ampulla of Vater can cause pancreatitis.

From George-Gay B, Chernecky CC: *Clinical medical-surgical nursing: a decision-making reference,* Philadelphia, 2002, Saunders.

15. The cystic duct is identified and carefully dissected down to its junction with the hepatic duct.
16. Any stones in the cystic duct are milked back into the gallbladder, and a tie is placed around the proximal part of the cystic duct.
17. If necessary, a cholangiogram is performed at this time (see "Intraoperative Cholangiogram" procedure). If a cholangiogram is not done, the cystic duct is doubly ligated and divided (Figure 12-8, *C*). A transfixion suture of fine absorbable suture may be used on the stump of the cystic duct near the common bile duct.
18. The gallbladder is then dissected from the liver bed, working upward to the fundus, and removed (Figure 12-8, *D*).
19. If the anatomy cannot be clearly identified, working from the fundus downward to the neck of the gallbladder may be necessary to make the ductal and vascular anatomy easier to identify.
20. All bleeding is controlled; reperitonealization of the liver bed, if indicated, is accomplished with interrupted or continuous fine absorbable intestinal sutures.
21. A closed suction drain may be inserted near the cystic duct stump. The free end of the drain is exteriorized through a stab wound in the lateral abdominal wall.
22. The wound is closed in layers and a dressing applied.

## Intraoperative Cholangiogram

An intraoperative cholangiogram is usually performed with both open and laparoscopic cholecystectomy to visualize the common bile duct and the hepatic ductal branches and to assess patency of the common bile duct. The procedure is under-

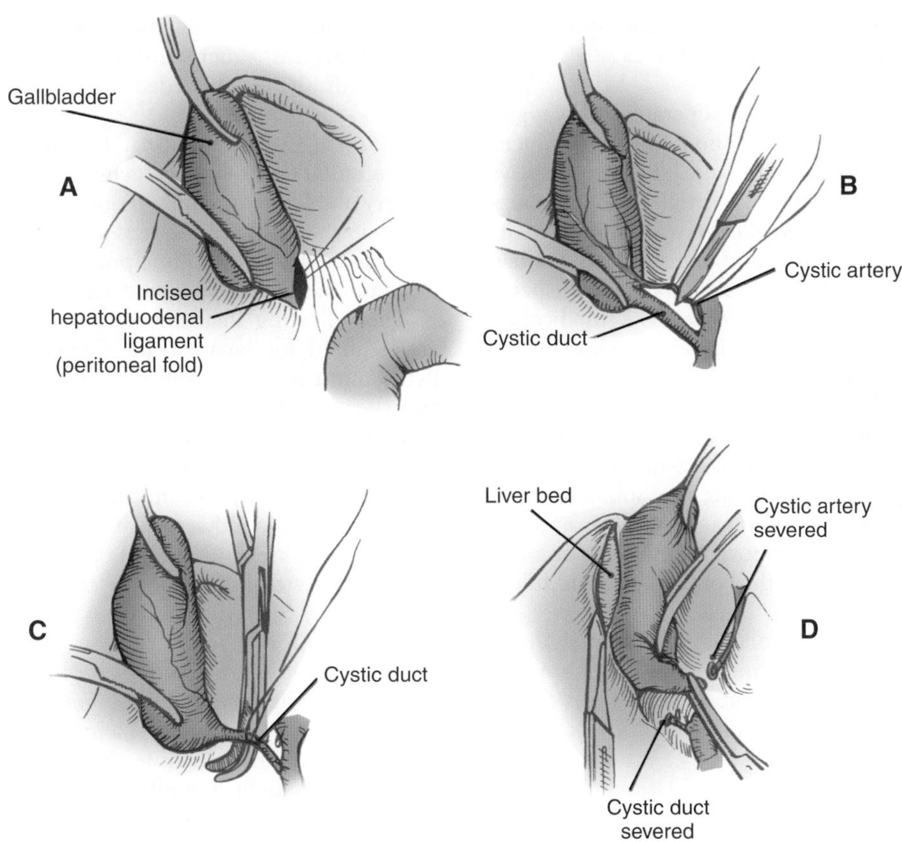


**FIGURE 12-8** Cholecystectomy. **A,** With Pean forceps in place, gentle traction is maintained as peritoneum over the triangle of Calot is incised. **B,** Cystic artery is clearly visualized, doubly ligated, and divided. **C,** Cystic duct is carefully dissected and identified before forceps and ligatures are applied. **D,** Dissection of gallbladder from liver bed is completed.

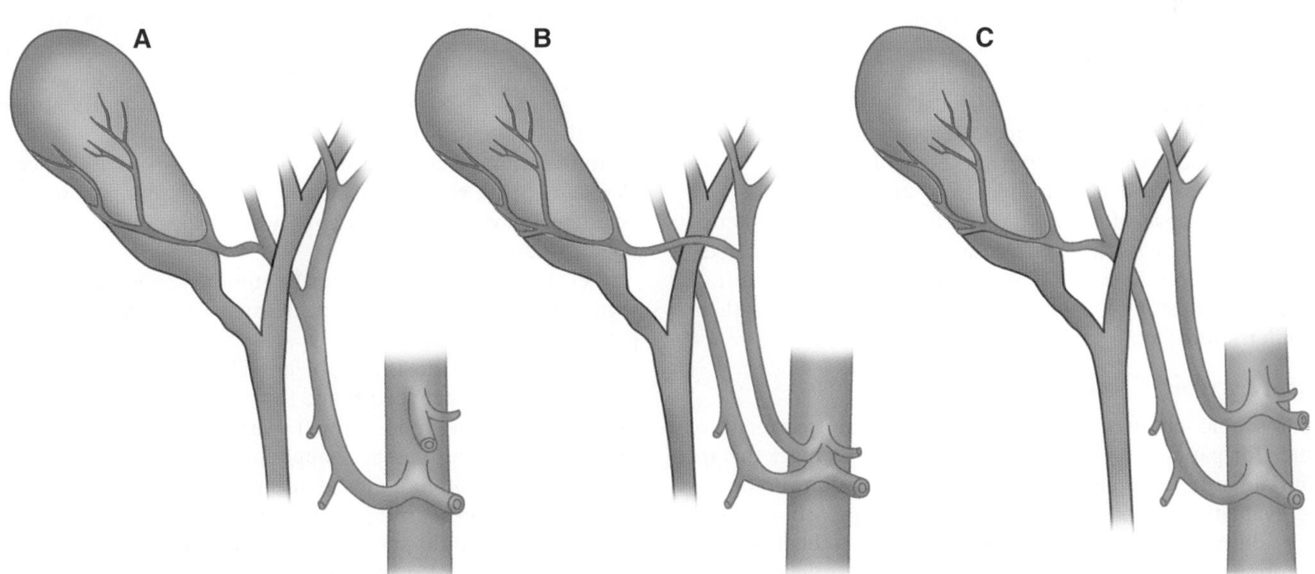


**FIGURE 12-9** Arterial blood supply of the liver and biliary system is quite variable. **A,** The most common anatomic arrangement is a cystic artery arising from the right hepatic artery. **B,** A dual hepatic blood supply is found in 15% to 20% of patients, with the right hepatic artery arising from the superior mesenteric artery in a significant number of patients, as in **C.**

taken during open cholecystectomy, and radiation-protection devices are used for the patient and surgical team.

***Procedural Considerations.*** An intraoperative cholangiogram requires fluoroscopy to visualize the filling of the ducts. Before the patient's arrival in the OR suite, the perioperative nurse ensures that a radiolucent bed is available or prepares the OR bed with an image-intensification attachment. The perioperative nurse should ensure that the patient has not had previous allergic reactions to the x-ray medium before dispensing the pharmaceutic agent to the sterile field. Medication safety protocols should be followed for dispensing and labeling all medications on and off the sterile field. Protection such as x-ray aprons or leaded shields should be readily available for all members of the surgical team and the patient. Because the patient's abdomen remains open while the x-ray equipment is positioned directly over the operative site, appropriate draping to maintain asepsis is necessary. Radiopaque sponges and any unnecessary instrumentation are removed from the abdominal site to avoid obscuring the view of the contrast medium filling the ducts.

The scrub person prepares a cholangiocath by attaching a stop cock with a 20-ml syringe of saline and a 20-ml syringe of contrast medium to the Luer-Lok ports. All air bubbles are removed because they might be misinterpreted as gall duct stones on the x-ray film.

### *Intraoperative Procedure*

1. The cholangiocath is irrigated with saline before and during its insertion into the cystic and common bile ducts.
2. The cholangiocath is inserted into the duct using an atraumatic grasping forceps. Irrigation during insertion facilitates dilation and reduces trauma to the ductal lumen.
3. The cholangiocath is anchored in the lumen of the common bile duct by the surgeon's preferred method. The more common methods are applying a Ligaclip proximal to the insertion site, tying or suturing the catheter in place, or using a ring-jawed holding clamp, such as a Swenson clamp, that has been designed specifically for this purpose.
4. With placement of the cholangiocath confirmed and anchored, all radiopaque sponges, instruments, and obstructing equipment are removed from the field.
5. The surgical field is draped with a sterile drape sheet to maintain asepsis of the wound and field. The image-intensifier equipment (C-arm) is positioned, as the surgeon redirects the stop cock to allow for injection of the contrast medium. If stones are found, the surgeon removes them under fluoroscopic guidance.

## Laparoscopic Cholecystectomy

Laparoscopic cholecystectomy is the surgical treatment of choice for patients with gallbladder disease who meet the appropriate criteria for safe laparoscopic intervention. Preoperative evaluation of patients having laparoscopic cholecystectomy differs little from that for patients scheduled for laparotomy. For patients with a history of peptic ulcer disease, a flexible esophagogastroduodenoscopy (EGD) may be performed to rule out existing disease. For patients with suspected ductal stones, a preliminary ERCP or other diagnostic evaluation is often done. A laparoscopic procedure always has the potential to be converted to a laparotomy—a potential the patient should be informed about before the surgical procedure. Laparotomy instrumentation and supplies should be readily available in the OR if needed.

***Procedural Considerations.*** Patients are generally admitted to the ambulatory surgery center (ASC) on the morning of surgery and will commonly require less than a 24-hour stay or admission to an extended recovery unit (ERU). General anesthesia is used, and antibiotic prophylaxis may be prescribed to be administered in the immediate preoperative period.

The following instrumentation, supplies, and equipment are required for laparoscopic cholecystectomy: laparoscope, two 5-mm trocars and sheaths, two 10-mm or 11-mm trocars and sheaths (trocar size depends on surgeon preference and may vary), a #7 knife handle with a #11 blade, multiple clip appliers, blunt grasping forceps (an assortment of alligator, Babcock, and spatula), and laparoscopic scissors. A laparoscopic video unit and secondary "slave" monitor, laparoscopic camera and control unit, light source, $CO_2$ tank and insufflation unit, electrosurgical unit, electrosurgical suction-irrigator (disposable), filtered insufflation tubing (disposable), and a pressure bag for IV saline 0.9% are items commonly used by the surgeon. Instrumentation and supplies for laparoscopic common bile duct exploration should also be available in the room. This may include a balloon-tipped Fogarty catheter; wire baskets; a small, flexible choledochoscope; dilators; and a T-tube. The patient is positioned supine with the usual comfort and safety measures observed. A Foley catheter (for bladder decompression) and a nasogastric tube (for decompression of the stomach) will be inserted. The patient is then placed in a reverse Trendelenburg position of 10 to 20 degrees.

Pneumoperitoneum may be accomplished using the open technique, sometimes termed the *Hasson technique.* A small incision is made above the umbilicus into the peritoneal cavity. A blunt-tipped cannula (Hasson) with a gas-tight sleeve is inserted, and then insufflation takes place. This approach is used for patients who have had a prior abdominal incision near the umbilicus or for those who have the potential for intraperitoneal adhesions. The Hasson technique may also involve the use of sutures placed on either side of the sleeve to anchor and hold the sleeve in place.

In the closed technique, a special hollow insufflation needle (Verres) with a retractable cutting sheath is inserted into the peritoneal cavity through a supraumbilical incision and used for insufflation.

$CO_2$ is the gas of choice for pneumoperitoneum. Gas flow is initiated at 1 to 2 liters/min. Because $CO_2$ diffuses into the patient's bloodstream during laparoscopy, elevated $CO_2$ levels and respiratory acidosis may occur. The intraabdominal pressure is normally between 8 and 10 mm Hg and is commonly used as an indicator for proper Verres needle placement by the surgeon. If the pressure gauge indicates a higher pressure, the needle may be in a closed space such as fat, be buried in the omentum, or be in the lumen of the intestine. The perioperative nurse should set the insufflation unit to a maximum pressure of 15 mm Hg. When intraabdominal pressure reaches 15 mm Hg, the flow will stop. Pressure higher than 15 mm Hg may result in bradycardia or a change in blood pressure or may force a gas embolus into an exposed blood vessel during the operative procedure. Most insufflation units are equipped with an alarm mechanism to alert the operative team if the intraabdominal pressure is exceeded. The surgeon may frequently ask what the pressure reading is, as may the anesthesia provider.

### *Operative Procedure*

1. A small skin incision is made in the folds of the umbilicus with a #11 blade on a #7 knife handle.
2. Pneumoperitoneum is accomplished by two options. The first option is to place a Verres needle percutaneously through the umbilicus into the peritoneal cavity, and insufflation is performed with $CO_2$ gas before the introduction of the trocar. When 3 to 4 liters of gas have been infused and the abdomen is rounded, the insufflation needle is removed and the trocar is inserted. The second technique requires the surgeon to grasp the abdominal flesh and pull upward as the trocar and sheath are placed through the umbilicus at an angle so as to avoid visceral puncture. The insufflation tubing is then attached to the port on the sleeve, and insufflation commences as in the Hasson technique.
3. An 11-mm trocar is inserted through the supraumbilical incision; this becomes the umbilical port.
4. The laparoscope with attached video camera is inserted through the umbilical port, and the peritoneal cavity is examined. The surgeon usually stands on the left side of the patient while the first assistant stands on the right. Video monitors are positioned at eye level at both the right and left sides of the operative field. The patient is then placed in a 30-degree, reverse Trendelenburg position and tilted slightly to the left.
5. Three additional trocars are inserted into the peritoneal cavity under direct visualization of the laparoscopic view (Figure 12-10). Most surgeons use a second 11-mm trocar placed subxiphoid and two 5-mm trocars placed subcostally in the right upper quadrant, in the midclavicular and anterior axillary lines.[2]
6. Blunt grasping forceps are inserted through the 5-mm port.
7. The gallbladder is retracted cephalad (Figure 12-11, *A*), elevating the inferior edge of the liver and exposing the gallbladder and cystic duct. The medial 5-mm port is used to grasp the infundibulum, retract it laterally, and expose the triangle.
8. An intraoperative cholangiogram may be performed by placing a hemoclip proximally on the cystic duct, incising its anterior surface, and passing the cholangiogram catheter into the duct. Once the cholangiogram is completed, two clips are placed distally on the cystic duct and it is divided (Figure 12-11, *B*).

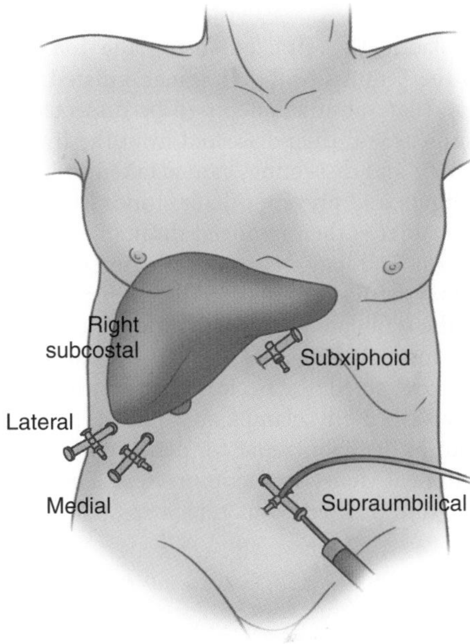


**FIGURE 12-10** Trocar placement for laparoscopic cholecystectomy.

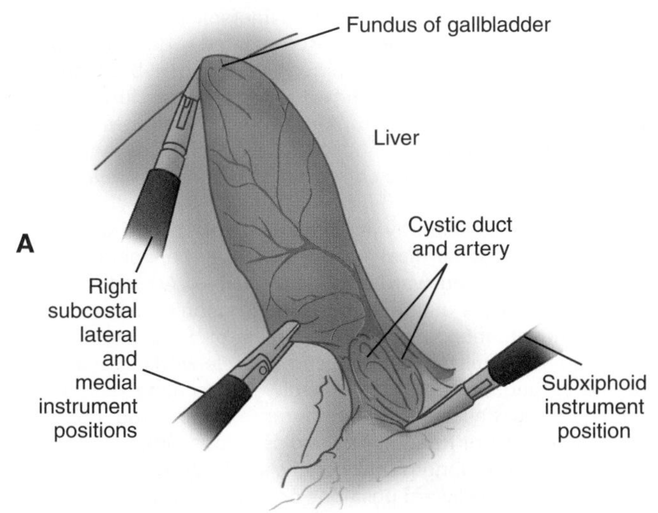


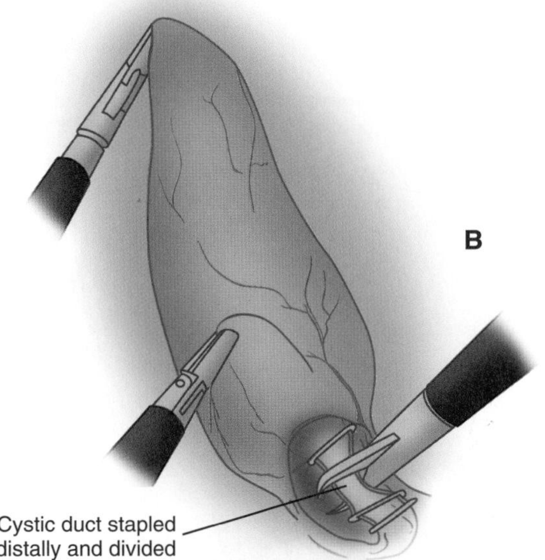


**FIGURE 12-11** **A,** The gallbladder is retracted cephalad (using the grasper on the fundus) and laterally at the infundibulum. The peritoneum overlying the gallbladder infundibulum and neck and cystic duct is divided bluntly, exposing the cystic duct. **B,** Once the gallbladder cystic duct junction has been clearly identified, clips are placed proximally and distally on the duct and it is sharply divided.

9. The cystic artery is then identified and dissected free, hemoclips are placed, and the artery is divided. The use of a disposable, preloaded, multiple-clip applier assists in the placement of ligating clips in a more efficient manner than a singly loaded, reusable applier. A pretied suture loop may be used if the surgeon desires.
10. Attention is then given to dissection of the gallbladder from the liver. This is often accomplished by use of electrosurgery. The electrosurgical instrument (active electrode) may have a channel through which suction can be applied. This is particularly useful in evacuating the smoke plume during the procedure. Some disposable instruments permit suction, electrocoagulation, and irrigation through the same instrument.
11. The gallbladder is retracted, using the forceps inserted through the 5-mm sheaths. It is manipulated to allow the medial and lateral attachments to be dissected by way of electrosurgery and then dissected from the liver bed. During grasping and dissecting, care is taken to keep the gallbladder intact and prevent bile or stones from spilling.
12. The gallbladder is then removed through the supraumbilical port. An Endobag or similar specimen-containing accessory may be used to secure the gallbladder for extraction, or the gallbladder may be brought out through the umbilical incision (Figure 12-12). If the gallbladder is too large to be extracted, the neck is brought above the surface of the incision, Kelly clamps are applied, and bile is suctioned out of the gallbladder for decompression.
13. The peritoneal cavity is decompressed. The stab wounds are closed and dressed with Steri-Strips.

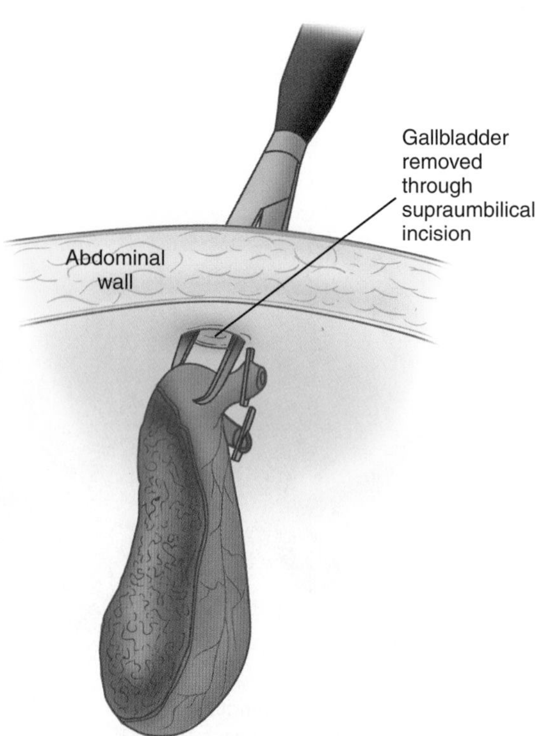


**FIGURE 12-12** The gallbladder being removed through the supraumbilical incision.

## Robotic-Assisted Laparoscopic Cholecystectomy

***Procedural Considerations.*** Robotic surgery is becoming more and more prevalent in operative laparoscopic procedures. It has enabled surgeons to perform more advanced and complex procedures. For this type of surgery, two robotic arms with laparoscopic instruments and cameras are controlled by the surgeon sitting at a console. Many laparoscopic instruments have been developed to facilitate the performance of abdominal procedures. These include a bladeless trocar to minimize injury on entry and the ultrasonic shear to facilitate laparoscopic dissection with hemostasis. An endoscopic stapler and suture device may be used to facilitate intracorporeal anastomosis and knot-tying techniques.[19] Laparoscopic cholecystectomy was one of the first procedures to prove the applicability of surgical robots in general surgery[7] (Research Highlight). For cholecystectomies, operative times have been reported as slightly longer because of the setup of the equipment, but the clinical outcomes are equivalent. The view of the ductal anatomy is subjectively superior with robotic surgery because of the magnified

### RESEARCH HIGHLIGHT

#### Robot-Assisted Laparoscopic Cholecystectomy

Laparoscopic cholecystectomy has been the gold standard since 1987. Robots were first used in surgery in the mid-1990s. With the current robotic systems, the surgeon sits at an operative console with three-dimensional imaging and handheld controls. Movement of the controls follows the movement of the tip of the instrument.

The Mayo Clinic in Scottsdale, Arizona reviewed all robotically assisted laparoscopic cholecystectomies from October 2002 to July 2003. The Zeus Robotic Surgical System was used to dissect the cystic duct and artery, and the surgical assistant at the operating table placed the clips on the cystic duct and artery. The gallbladder was dissected from the liver with the robot. Cholangiocatheters were inserted into the cystic duct with the robotic instruments. Nineteen patients underwent the procedure. Sixteen were completed robotically. Conversions to laparoscopic techniques were done because of malfunctioning instruments; however, open procedures were not necessary. The mean setup time was 28.1 minutes (range 7 to 51 minutes). The mean hospital stay was 0.9 days (range 0 to 2 days). There were no complications or injuries related to the use of the robot.

Often cholecystectomy is the initial robotically assisted procedure to test surgical robots because the operation is technically straightforward and reproducible. Advantages of surgical robots are elimination of the surgeon's tremor, scaling of movements, increased degrees of freedom, three-dimensional visualization, and a comfortable working position for the surgeon, sitting at a console. The scaling of movements makes delicate dissection more exact, and the increased degrees of freedom make dissections simpler. Sitting at the console is ergonomically beneficial. The surgeon does not have to assume awkward positions or reach over assistants.

Telesurgery, the performance of surgery from a distant site using robotics, may lead to procedures being performed worldwide from remote sites.

Modified from Miller DW and others: Robot-assisted laparoscopic cholecystectomy: initial Mayo Clinic Scottsdale experience, *Mayo Clinic Proceedings* 79(9):1132-1136, 2004.

three-dimensional picture. The rate of bile duct injury is slightly higher with laparoscopic surgery; thus robotic usage may translate into reduction of this problem.[12]

The da Vinci Surgical System (Intuitive Surgical Inc., Sunnyvale, Ca.) and the Zeus Robotic Surgical System (Computer Motion, Inc., Goleta, Ca.) are robotic systems used for minimally invasive laparoscopic surgery. The Automated Endoscopic System for Optimal Positioning (AESOP) can be trained to recognize the surgeon's voice.[13] A CT scan can also be imported in to the console so the surgeon can perform preoperative planning and surgical rehearsal of the procedure.[12] It is possible to perform telesurgery—the complete separation of the surgeon from the operative field. Transcontinental cholecystectomies have occurred between Strasbourg, France and New York City.[7] It may be possible in the future for surgeons to perform surgeries at remote sites; the patient can be at one location and the surgeon at another. Assistants at the surgical field would still be necessary, however. For advantages and myths about robotic surgery see Box 12-3 and Table 12-4.

BOX 12-3

### Advantages of Robot-Assisted Surgery for the Patient and Surgeon

**ADVANTAGES FOR THE PATIENT**

Smaller incisions
Decreased postoperative pain
Shorter length of hospital stay
Reduced blood loss
Reduced tissue trauma and inflammatory response to surgery
Improved cosmetic result
Faster return to work

**ADVANTAGES FOR THE SURGEON**

Better visualization (higher magnification)
Hand tremor eliminated, allowing great precision
A three-dimensional video image of the operative field; view of ductal anatomy enhanced
Robotic "wrist" more flexible than human wrist, improving maneuverability around organs and vessels
Movements can be reduced, allowing complex technical tasks
Better ergonomic environment (sitting at a console), better levels of concentration
Less need for assistants

Modified from Purkayastha S and others: Robotic surgery: a review, *Hospital Medicine* 65(3):153-159, 2004.

## Cholecystostomy (Open Procedure)

Cholecystostomy is establishment of an opening into the gallbladder to permit drainage of the organ and removal of stones. This procedure is usually selected for patients with acute gallbladder disease and advanced medical problems who cannot tolerate general anesthesia or more extensive surgery. Ultrasound-guided percutaneous cholecystostomy has become an accepted procedure for patients who are not good candidates for surgery. In the rare situation where interventional radiology is not available, an open procedure may be done, which is described here.

***Procedural Considerations.*** A large Toomey syringe (50 ml) or an Asepto syringe may be needed for irrigation purposes. If a local anesthetic is used, the anesthetic agent, syringes, and needles are necessary; protocols for safe medication administration and labeling of all medications/solutions on and off the sterile field must be followed. Specified drainage tubes or catheters should be available. The patient is positioned supine. Although many surgeons prefer the right subcostal incision, cholecystostomy procedures are often performed as emergencies and a quicker midline or transverse incision may be used. Instrumentation includes a basic laparotomy set and a gallbladder set.

### *Operative Procedure*

1. After incision into the abdominal cavity, the gallbladder is isolated by retraction of the surrounding viscera.
2. The fundus of the gallbladder is grasped with an Allis or Babcock forceps, and the proposed opening is encircled by means of an absorbable purse-string suture, leaving the ends long.
3. To protect the abdominal cavity from contamination, the gallbladder is isolated with moistened laparotomy packs. Suction is available.
4. An incision is made into the gallbladder for insertion of a trocar with sheath.
5. Within the purse-string suture the gallbladder contents are aspirated by means of suction tubing attached to the trocar sheath.

TABLE 12-4

### Myths About Robotic Surgery

| Myth | Reality |
|---|---|
| Robots do all the work. | The surgeon manages the robot system from a console away from the operative field. |
| Robotic surgery is better than conventional surgery. | Currently the surgical outcomes are comparable. |
| Robotic arms function just like a surgeon's hands. | Robotic arms are better than human hands—steadier and more precise, with no tremor and smaller hand movements. However, hand dexterity is missing—human hand can move 20 ways, robotic arm can move 4 ways. |
| Robots make surgery simpler, faster, or less expensive. | System setup time can be lengthy. Some surgeries take longer to perform with robotic system. |
| Robotic surgery has been a big disappointment. | Robotic surgery is constantly being changed and improved. Developing technology has significant implications for the future of surgery. |

Modified from 5 Myths about robotic surgery, *The Cleveland Clinic Heart Advisor* 7(5):4-5, 2004.

6. As the contents are aspirated, culture specimens are taken. The contaminated trocar and sheath are removed and isolated in a discard basin.
7. The opening into the gallbladder can be enlarged with Metzenbaum scissors; gallstones are removed with malleable scoops and stone forceps.
8. Irrigating the gallbladder with isotonic saline solution is necessary to remove small stones, grit, or pastelike material. A syringe with a catheter or an Asepto syringe may be used for irrigation.
9. Remaining contaminated instruments are placed into the discard basin.
10. A drainage tube is inserted into the gallbladder opening. The purse-string suture is tightened around the catheter, with care taken not to occlude it.
11. A second purse-string suture or separate mattress sutures may be used to secure the gallbladder to the peritoneum and the posterior rectus fascia.
12. The free end of the catheter or tube is exteriorized through a stab wound and then anchored to the skin edges, as described for cholecystectomy.
13. Drainage of the abdominal cavity is established with the exterior ends of each drain secured.
14. The wound is closed in layers, as described for laparotomy, and dressings are applied at the incision and drain sites.

## Open Common Bile Duct Exploration

With the advent of endoscopic, percutaneous, and laparoscopic techniques to remove gallstones, open exploration of the common bile duct is performed much less commonly. When these newer methods are not available, when they are not possible because of prior surgery, or when an open operation is otherwise necessary, open common bile duct exploration becomes necessary.

***Procedural Considerations.*** The patient is positioned supine under general anesthesia. The anesthesia provider inserts a nasogastric tube after intubation. An indwelling urinary catheter may be inserted before the abdominal skin prep.

Instrumentation includes a basic laparotomy set with the addition of gallbladder instruments. T-tubes of assorted sizes should be available. Intraoperative cholangiography will most likely be used to confirm that all stones have been removed; radiation-protection devices for the patient and surgical team are required. Culture tubes are needed. Soft rubber catheters for irrigation, balloon-tipped catheters such as a biliary Fogarty catheter, stone baskets, and the surgeon's preference for cholangiocath should be available, as well as choledochoscopes (flexible and rigid). The use of the choledochoscope requires the following:

- Choledochoscope with accessories: biopsy forceps, stone-grasping forceps, and a sheath that can be used to direct other instruments into various portions of the biliary tract
- Video camera and viewing screen
- Light cord
- 0.9% Normal saline (1000-ml bag)
- Sterile IV tubing
- Pressure bag
- Light source for the choledochoscope

Distending the common duct is necessary for better visualization and is accomplished by irrigating the duct with copious amounts of sterile saline. A pressure bag is placed around an IV bag of 0.9% saline, and pressure to 300 mm Hg is applied. Sterile tubing is then passed from the sterile field and attached to the saline bag. The scrub person attaches the distal end of the sterile IV tubing directly to the irrigating stop cock on the scope.

### *Operative Procedure*

1. The abdomen is opened through a subcostal incision or midline incision.
2. If the gallbladder has not been previously removed, it is exposed and removed or retracted by means of laparotomy packs and retractors.
3. The common duct may be identified by means of an aspirating syringe and fine-gauge needle to make certain that the suspected duct is not a blood vessel.
4. Culture specimens may be obtained.
5. Two fine traction sutures are placed in the wall of the duct, below the entrance of the cystic duct.
6. The common duct region is walled off with moistened laparotomy packs and narrow-blade retractors. A discard basin for contaminated instruments is placed at the lower end of the operative field; a suction apparatus is made ready for immediate use.
7. A longitudinal incision is made in the common duct (Figure 12-13), between the traction sutures, with a long #3 knife handle and a #15 or #11 blade.
8. Constant suction is maintained with a Yankauer suction tube to keep the field free from oozing bile as the incision is enlarged with Potts angled or Metzenbaum scissors.
9. Additional stay sutures may be applied to the ductal opening.
10. Visible stones are removed with gallstone forceps, after which exploration of the duct is begun with small, malleable scoops proximal and then distal to the opening.
11. Probing is continued as stones are removed from both the common and hepatic ducts. Isotonic saline solution in an Asepto syringe and a soft, small-lumen catheter or a balloon-tipped catheter are used to facilitate the removal of small stones and debris as well as to demonstrate patency of the common bile duct through to the duodenum.
12. The flexible and rigid choledochoscopes are both useful for identifying additional stones. The scope is inserted into the common duct, which is then flushed with saline. After visualizing the duct to ensure that no stones remain, a T-tube is placed in the common bile duct, and the choledochotomy is closed around the tube. A completion cholangiogram is then performed to be certain all stones have been removed.
13. The wound is closed in layers; the T-tube is carefully anchored to the skin, and dressings are applied. Sterile tubing is used to connect the T-tube to a small drainage container or bag.

## Cholecystoduodenostomy and Cholecystojejunostomy

Cholecystoduodenostomy and cholecystojejunostomy are the establishment of continuity by creating an anastomosis between the gallbladder and duodenum or the gallbladder and jejunum to relieve an obstruction in the distal end of the common duct. An obstruction in the biliary system may be caused

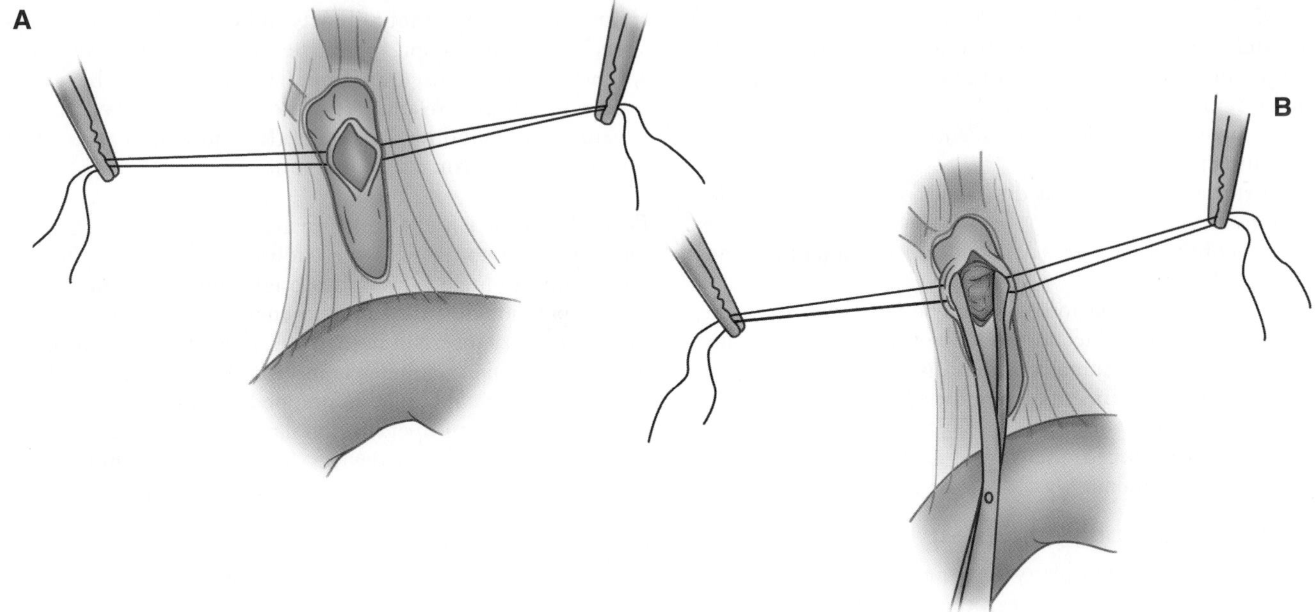


FIGURE 12-13 **A,** During choledochotomy, the common bile duct is opened longitudinally between two traction sutures. **B,** Any stones in the duct can then be extracted with stone forceps or removed by irrigation of the duct with saline solution.

by a tumor of the ducts involving the head of the pancreas or the ampulla of Vater, the presence of an inflammatory lesion, a stricture of the common duct, or the presence of stones.

***Procedural Considerations.*** Instrumentation includes a basic laparotomy set; gallbladder instruments with two Doyen intestinal forceps, curved with guards, or similar nontraumatic holding forceps; and a self-retaining retractor system. Fluoroscopy should be anticipated. Radiation-protection devices for the patient and surgical team should be available. The patient is positioned supine under general anesthesia. The anesthesia provider inserts a nasogastric tube after intubation. An indwelling urinary catheter is inserted before abdominal skin preparation.

### *Operative Procedure*

1. The abdomen is opened, the gallbladder is exposed, the contents are aspirated, and the pathologic condition is confirmed, as described for cholecystostomy.
2. The anastomosis site is prepared, posterior serosal silk sutures are placed, and open anastomosis is performed.
3. The surgical technique for anastomosis of the gallbladder to the duodenum or loop of jejunum is usually performed as a two-layer anastomosis.
4. The serosa of the duodenum or loop of jejunum is sutured to the full thickness of the fundus of the gallbladder.
5. A 1-cm to 1.5-cm opening is made into the small bowel and gallbladder in corresponding positions. GI technique is instituted.
6. Interrupted fine monofilament (5-0 or 4-0) sutures are then placed around the entire circumference.
7. Contaminated instruments are placed into the discard basin, and the operative field is prepared for closure.
8. A drain may be introduced; the wound is closed in layers, and dressings are applied.

## Choledochoduodenostomy and Choledochojejunostomy

Choledochoduodenostomy is anastomosis between the common duct and the duodenum, and choledochojejunostomy is anastomosis between the duct and the jejunum. These procedures may be necessary in postcholecystectomy patients to circumvent an obstructive lesion and reestablish the flow of bile into the intestinal tract.

***Procedural Considerations.*** Surgical approaches are similar to those for choledochostomy and cholecystojejunostomy. The patient is positioned supine under general anesthesia. The anesthesia provider inserts a nasogastric tube after intubation. An indwelling urinary catheter is inserted before abdominal skin preparation.

Instrumentation and supplies necessary for this procedure include a basic laparotomy set with the addition of gallbladder instruments, a self-retaining retractor system, linear stapling devices, T-tubes in varying sizes; a Silastic biliary stent should be available as should magnifying loupes. Fluoroscopy should be anticipated; radiation-protection devices will then be required for the patient and surgical team.

### *Operative Procedure*

CHOLEDOCHODUODENOSTOMY

1. The abdomen is opened through a midline incision.
2. The common duct and duodenum are exposed.
3. The common duct is identified and dissected free, using forceps and Metzenbaum scissors.
4. The common duct and duodenum are approximated, either side-to-side or the end of the common duct to the side of the duodenum, and an anastomosis is established.
5. An intraluminal catheter is inserted.
6. The wound is closed in layers, and dressings are applied.

CHOLEDOCHOJEJUNOSTOMY

1. The abdomen is opened through a midline incision.
2. The jejunum is mobilized, and the common duct is identified and opened (Figure 12-14, *A*).
3. Anastomosis is established between the common duct and the transected jejunum.
4. A catheter is introduced, as described for cholecystoduodenostomy.
5. Jejunal continuity is reestablished by jejunojejunostomy (Figure 12-14, *B*).
6. As an alternative, anastomosis may be fashioned from the end of the severed duct to the side of a loop of jejunum, with a side-to-side jejunal anastomosis.
7. Contaminated instruments are removed from the operative field.
8. A drain is exteriorized, the wound is closed in layers, and dressings are applied.

## Transduodenal Sphincteroplasty

Transduodenal sphincteroplasty is a method of achieving a choledochoduodenostomy between the distal end of the common duct and the side of the duodenum. The sphincters normally affecting the distal common and pancreatic ducts are rendered functionless because the stoma is noncontractile and remains permanently open. Indication for transduodenal sphincteroplasty includes sphincter of Oddi dysfunction—a poorly defined clinical syndrome that is characterized by pain characteristic of biliary colic and recurrent acute pancreatitis.[2] There may be a structural or functional abnormality of the sphincter, with or without fibrosis and elevated sphincter pressures. Both endoscopic sphincterotomy and transduodenal sphincteroplasty with transampullary septectomy have been used with similar results. The procedure described has the advantage of including division of the transampullary septum, thus promoting pancreatic duct drainage.

***Procedural Considerations.*** Instrumentation is as described for choledochotomy, with the addition of a GI set, since the duodenum is entered through a longitudinal incision. The patient is positioned supine under general anesthesia. The anesthesia provider inserts a nasogastric tube after intubation. An indwelling urinary catheter is inserted before abdominal skin preparation. The abdomen is prepped from nipple line to pubis. Supplies for an operative cholangiogram are necessary as are radiation-protection devices for the patient and surgical team.

### *Operative Procedure*

1. A right subcostal or midline incision is made, and the biliary tract is exposed.
2. All structures are inspected, and the normal configuration is established before any structure is tied, clamped, or divided during biliary tract dissection.
3. Operative cholangiography is then performed by placing a cholangiocath through a small incision made with a #11 blade into the cystic duct.
4. If the gallbladder is present, cholecystectomy is performed.

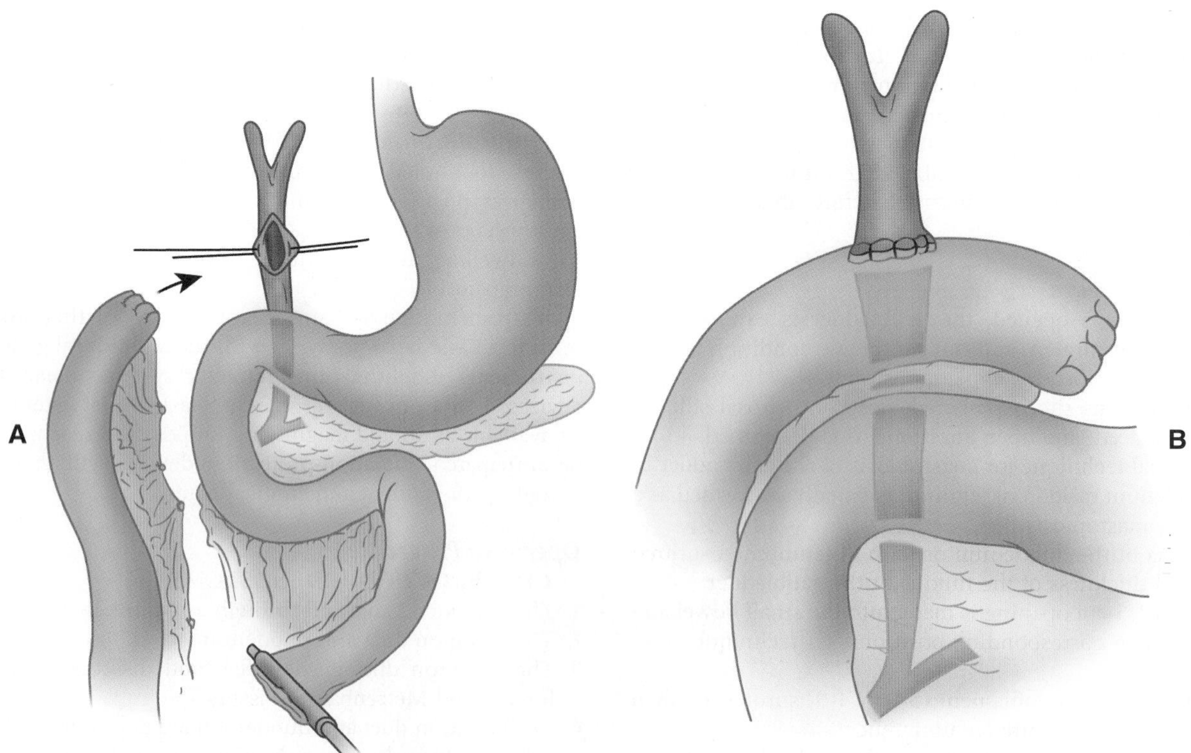


FIGURE 12-14 Choledochojejunostomy. **A,** The divided end of the jejunum is closed, and an end-to-side choledochojejunostomy is made in two layers to the jejunum. **B,** A jejunojejunostomy completes the operative procedure.

5. The duodenum is mobilized by dividing the peritoneal reflection that covers the lateral portion of the second part of the duodenum and holds it in place.
6. The common duct is incised longitudinally between two stay sutures and explored.
7. Any residual stones are removed. Duodenotomy is performed with a longitudinal incision, and the papilla of Vater is located (Figure 12-15, *A*).
8. The sphincter of Oddi is divided at the 11 o'clock position with angled Potts scissors, and the ductal mucosa is sutured to the duodenal mucosa with a fine monofilament synthetic absorbable suture on a small needle (Figure 12-15, *B*).
9. The duodenum is then closed in two layers.
10. The common bile duct is joined to the apex of the mobilized duodenum in a two-layer anastomosis.
11. A T-tube may be inserted to splint the anastomosis (Figure 12-15, *C*).
12. The abdominal cavity is closed.

## SURGERY OF THE PANCREAS

### Drainage or Excision of Pancreatic Cysts (Open Method)

Pancreatic pseudocysts are localized collections of pancreatic secretions in a cystic structure. The preferred operative therapy in patients with uncomplicated pseudocysts is internal drainage by one of three options: cystojejunostomy (use of a defunctionalized Roux-en-Y jejunal limb) (Figure 12-16); cystogastrostomy (drainage into the stomach); or cystoduodenostomy (drainage into the duodenum).[23] Cystogastrostomy is a faster and technically less difficult procedure and is used when the cyst is adherent to the posterior wall of the stomach. Cystojejunostomy is the most versatile drainage procedure. Cystoduodenostomy is used in selected cases, depending on cyst location, but has limited utility.

***Procedural Considerations.*** The patient is positioned supine under general anesthesia. The anesthesia provider inserts a nasogastric tube after intubation. An indwelling urinary catheter is inserted before abdominal skin preparation. Instrumentation and supplies necessary for this procedure include a basic laparotomy set, gallbladder instruments, a GI set, and a self-retaining retractor system.

#### *Operative Procedure*

1. A midline incision is made into the abdomen.
2. A self-retaining retractor system is used to expose the pancreatic area.
3. The pancreatic cyst is examined, and the area is isolated with moist packs.
4. Internal drainage may be accomplished by an incision into the anterior wall of the stomach, directly opposite the cyst if it adheres to the posterior wall, thereby providing drainage through the GI tract.
5. A fistula is established between the anterior wall of the cyst and the posterior wall of the stomach. Many surgeons prefer an anastomosis between the cyst and a Roux-en-Y loop of jejunum or into the duodenum directly, depending on the location of the cyst (see Figure 12-16).
6. The anterior gastrotomy is closed, and the wound closure is completed.

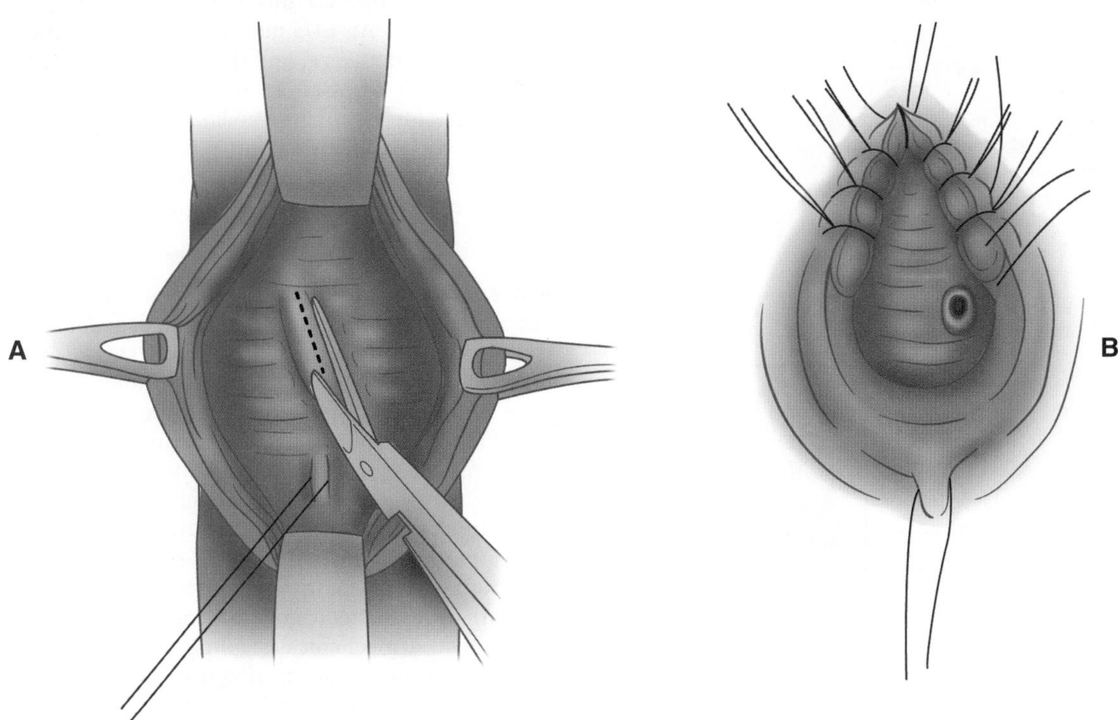


**FIGURE 12-15** Transduodenal sphincteroplasty. **A,** The duodenum is opened longitudinally. **B,** The sphincter of Oddi is divided at 11 o'clock with angled Potts scissors, and the ductal mucosa is then sutured to the duodenal mucosa with 4-0 absorbable suture. The duodenum is then closed longitudinally in two layers.

*Continued*

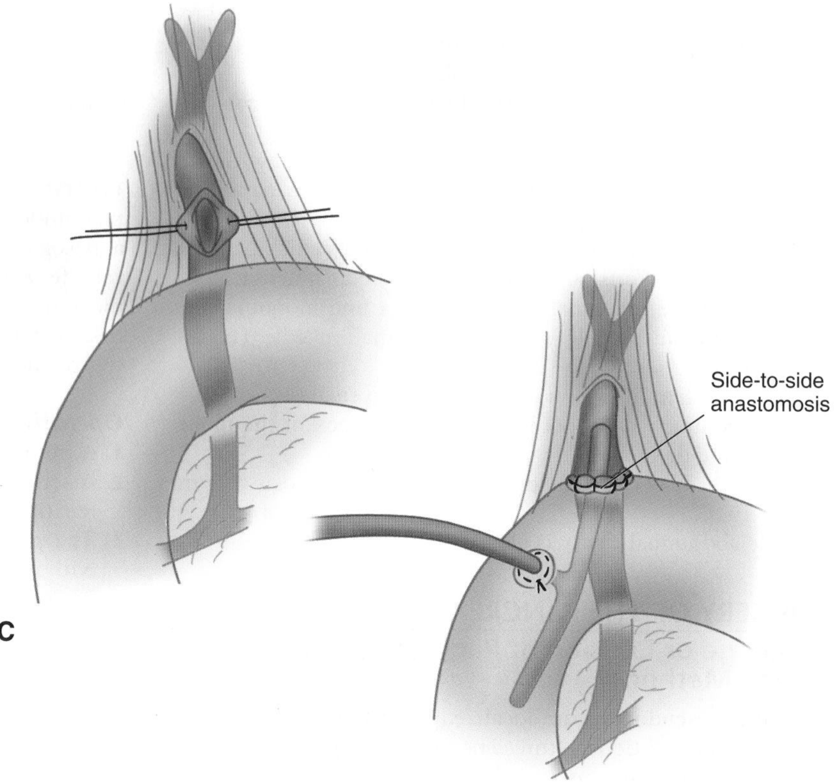


**FIGURE 12-15, cont'd** Transduodenal sphincteroplasty. **C**, Choledochoduodenostomy. The common bile duct is joined to the apex of the mobilized duodenum in a two-layer anastomosis. A T-tube is placed to stent the anastomosis, with the external stem of the tube brought out through the bile duct or through the wall of the duodenum.

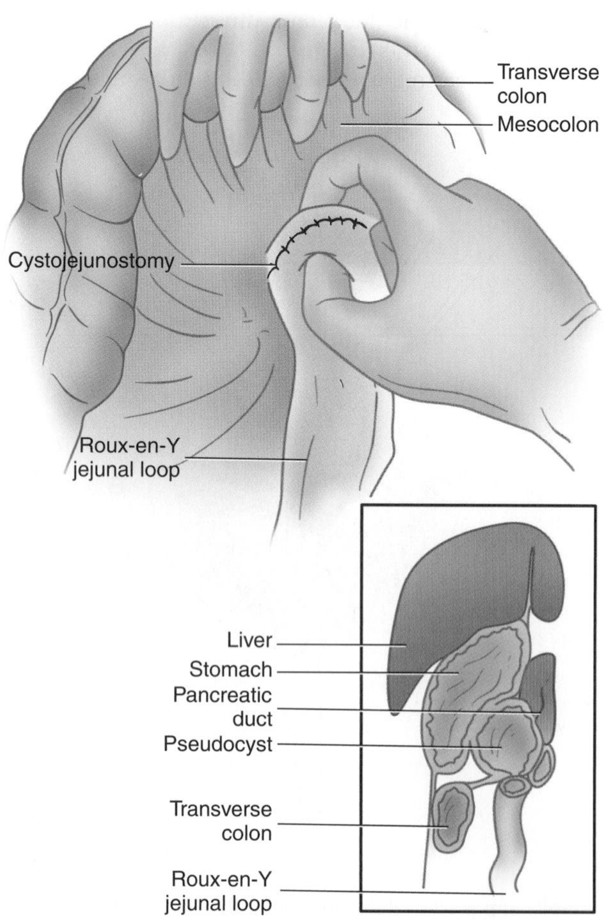


**FIGURE 12-16** Internal drainage of a pancreatic pseudocyst by Roux-en-Y cystojejunostomy through the base of the transverse mesocolon.

## Laparoscopic Pancreatic Cyst–Gastrostomy

Laparoscopic techniques have enabled surgeons to perform internal drainage procedures for pancreatic pseudocysts by way of laparoscopy. CT imaging is used to diagnose a pancreatic pseudocyst. An EUS may also provide additional information. The location, size, and thickness of the wall of the pseudocyst are all assessed to determine the most appropriate procedure for drainage—a laparoscopic pancreatic cyst–gastrostomy versus a Roux-en-Y pancreatic cystojejunostomy. Endoscopic drainage of pseudocysts may also be done in centers where endoscopists are experienced in percutaneous drainage techniques.[14]

***Procedural Considerations.*** General anesthesia by means of endotracheal intubation is administered, and a nasogastric tube is inserted. The patient is positioned supine, with arms extended to the side on armboards. Vulnerable neurovascular sites and positional pressure points are padded and protected. The following equipment and instrumentation are needed: a 30-degree telescope (10 mm or 5 mm); a video camera; two high-density video monitors; a high-flow insufflator with $CO_2$ tank; an electrosurgical unit; two trocar ports (12.5 mm); two trocar ports (5 mm); an endodissecting instrument (5 mm), or atraumatic grasping forceps (5 mm); endoshears/scissors (5 mm) with electrocoagulation connection; an endo-Babcock instrument; a mechanical stapling device; a 10-mm endoclip applier; a 10-mm endosuturing instrument (optional); 2-0 suture material, 7-inch length (optional); an electrocoagulation hook; a long 5-mm laparoscopic needle; and an endoretractor.

### *Operative Procedure*

1. Pneumoperitoneum is created, and the trocars are inserted by way of port sites as illustrated in Figure 12-17.

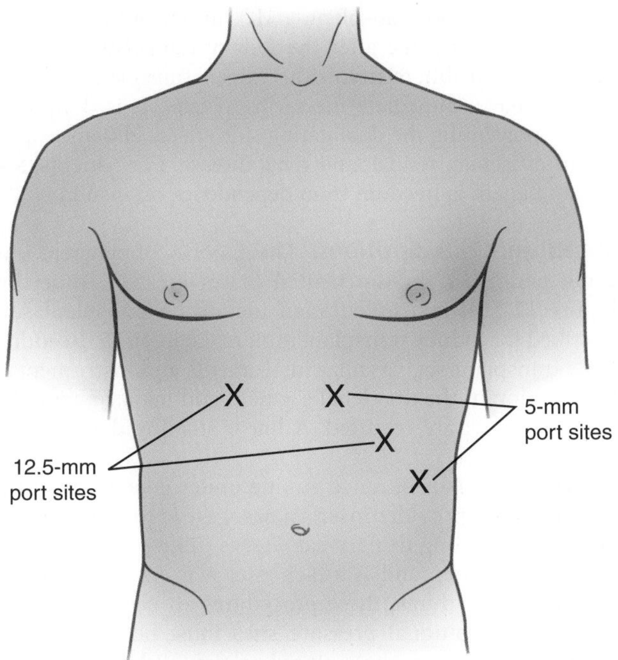


**FIGURE 12-17** Port sites for trocar placement in laparoscopic pancreatic cyst–gastrostomy.

2. The pancreatic pseudocyst is located by entering the lesser sac by way of the greater curvature. Hemostasis is achieved by using the endoclip applier. An endostapling device (GIA type) with vascular cartridges is used for dissection of the greater curvature.
3. The surgeon will assess the site for entry into the stomach. An endoretractor may be used to retract the left hepatic lobe upward.
4. Using electrodissection, an incision, centered between the lesser and greater curvatures, is made on the anterior wall of the stomach and then extended.
5. A long laparoscopic aspiration needle is inserted into the intraabdominal and gastric cavity. The camera is advanced to visualize the posterior wall of the stomach.
6. The needle is inserted into the cyst, and its presence is confirmed by aspiration.
7. A small incision is made into the cyst and the pancreatic fluid aspirated.
8. The endostapling device is inserted into the gastric cavity. The smaller jaw of this instrument is inserted into the pseudocyst. The stapling device is closed with great precaution. It is important that the anastomosis not be under tension. The stapling device is fired, and the anastomosis is checked for integrity. An endosuturing instrument is used to close any defects in the anastomotic line.
9. A nasogastric tube is inserted and directed into the pseudocyst.
10. The two edges of the anterior wall gastrostomy are approximated using endograsping forceps (atraumatic) or an endodissecting instrument. The gastrostomy is then closed using an endostapling device (thoracic abdominal [TA] type).
11. A drain is placed next to the gastrostomy.
12. The abdomen is deflated, the trocar ports are removed, and the sites are closed and dressed.

## Robotic-Assisted Laparoscopic Pancreatic Procedures

***Procedural Considerations.*** Pancreatic lesions can be resected with robotic-assisted laparoscopy. Pancreaticojejunostomy may be performed following an open pancreaticoduodenectomy.[12] Computer-assisted robotic surgery may be used for resection, drainage, and manipulation and reconstruction of the pancreatic duct. Precise tissue manipulation and three-dimensional imaging allow for better surgical approaches for reconstruction of the pancreatic or common bile ducts than open techniques.[17]

## Pancreaticoduodenectomy (Whipple Procedure)

Tumors arise from the exocrine glands (95%) and endocrine glands (5%) in the pancreas. Ductal adenocarcinoma constitutes 80% of all pancreatic tumors. Most tumors begin in the head of the exocrine gland, obstruct the bile duct, and extend to the duodenum, intestines, and spine. Spread occurs to regional lymph nodes, and common metastatic sites include the liver and lungs. Because symptoms occur late in the disease, prognosis is often poor. Pancreaticoduodenectomy is the removal of the head of the pancreas, the entire duodenum, a portion of the jejunum, the distal third of the stomach, and the lower half of the common bile duct, with the reestablishment of continuity of the biliary, pancreatic, and GI tract systems.

***Procedural Considerations.*** A basic laparotomy set, a GI instrument set, a self-retaining retractor system (e.g., Bookwalter), linear stapling devices, and appropriate drains and catheters are used for this procedure. The perioperative nurse should ensure that ordered blood and blood products are available. Pancreaticoduodenectomy may take 5 to 6 hours and the transfusion of many units of blood or blood products. The patient is positioned supine under general anesthesia. Attention is paid to padding positional pressure points with gel pads or using a pressure-reducing OR bed mattress. SCDs are applied as well as a forced-air warming device and other measures to prevent hypothermia. The anesthesia provider inserts a nasogastric tube after intubation. An indwelling urinary catheter is inserted before abdominal preparation. The abdomen is prepped from nipple line to midthigh.

### *Operative Procedure*

1. The abdomen is entered through an upper transverse, bilateral subcostal, or long paramedian incision. Resectability is assessed, exploring for hepatic metastases, serosal implants of tumor, and lymph node metastases. If these are outside the zone of resection, the disease is unresectable.
2. Laparotomy packs and retractors are used to expose the operative site and protect vital structures.
3. The duodenum is mobilized using the Kocher maneuver (incision of peritoneal reflection lateral to the second portion of the duodenum) with Metzenbaum scissors and subsequent blunt dissection of loose areolar tissue.
4. Mobilization of the duodenum continues, and bleeding vessels are ligated with silk.
5. The gastrocolic ligament and the gastrohepatic omentum are divided between curved forceps and are ligated or transfixed.

6. The gastroduodenal and right gastric arteries are clamped, divided, and ligated.
7. The prepyloric area of the stomach is mobilized.
8. The operative field is prepared for open anastomosis by isolating the area with laparotomy sponges.
9. By placing two long Allen or Payr clamps near the midportion of the stomach, the transection is completed.
10. The duodenum is reflected, the common duct is divided, and the hepatic end is marked or tagged for later anastomosis.
11. The jejunum is clamped with two Allen forceps, and the duodenojejunal flexure is divided.
12. The pancreas is divided, and the duct is carefully identified.
13. Further mobilization of the duodenum and division of the inferior pancreaticoduodenal artery are done to permit complete removal of the specimen.
14. The most common reconstructive technique anastomoses the pancreas to the jejunum first, followed by the bile duct and the duodenum (Figure 12-18).
15. Drains may be placed, and the abdomen is closed. An abdominal dressing is applied.

## Pancreatic Transplantation

Pancreatic transplantation is the implantation of a pancreas from a donor into a recipient for patients with type 1 (formerly known as juvenile-onset) diabetes. Options for pancreatic transplant include a pancreas transplant alone (PTA), which is undertaken with patients with functioning kidneys; a simultaneous pancreas-kidney transplant (SPK), because severe diabetes is often associated with chronic renal failure; or a pancreas transplant after a kidney transplant (PAK), in which the pancreas is transplanted sometime after the kidney transplant. Pancreatic transplantation differs from other organ transplants in that it does not have immediate life-saving results. It is done in the hope of preventing the debilitating side effects of diabetes, such as cardiovascular, retinal, and renal disease. For patients, a significant benefit is freedom from dependence on insulin.

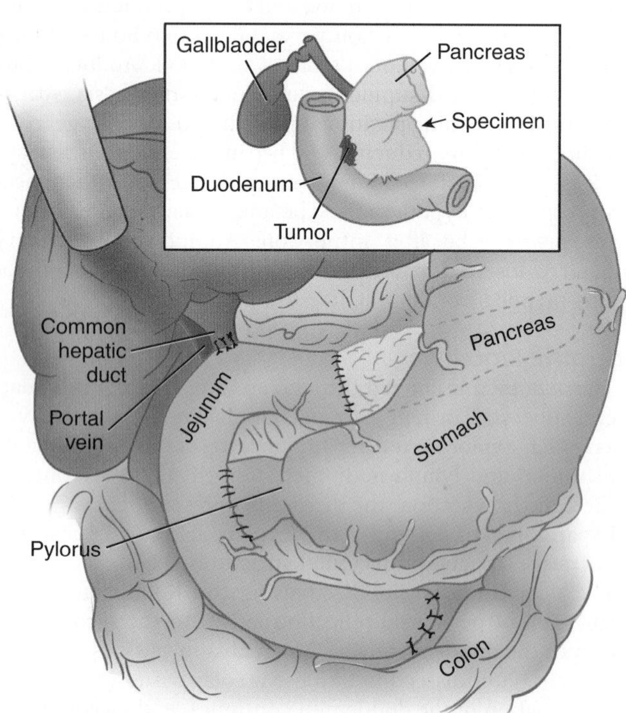


FIGURE 12-18 Illustration of a pylorus-preserving pancreaticoduodenectomy and the subsequent reconstruction. The inset at the top depicts the resected specimen. The jejunal limb is brought through and sutured to the transverse mesocolon.

***Procedural Considerations.*** The majority of pancreas transplants performed in the United States are SPK procedures (Figure 12-19). Instrumentation includes a transplant set as described for kidney transplantation in Chapter 15. In addition to the transplant set, vascular instruments and instruments for the resection of the duodenal segment and management of the pancreatic duct are required. A linear stapling device may be used.

The patient is positioned supine under general anesthesia. The anesthesia provider inserts a nasogastric tube after intubation. An indwelling urinary catheter is inserted before the abdominal skin prep and is attached to a urometer. Like other transplant procedures, these procedures are lengthy, lasting 5 to 7 hours. Positional pressure sites must be padded and a pressure-reducing mattress placed on the OR bed. Because the patient has diabetes, considerations of maintaining skin and tissue integrity are paramount. SCDs will likely be used. Blood and blood products will be ordered, and their availability must be verified. Blood-warming devices, a forced-air warming device, warmed irrigating solution ($<$40.5°C [$<$105°F]), and other measures are implemented to maintain normothermia. Communication between and among team members is essential in all transplant surgery. The patient is transferred to an intensive care unit on completion of the procedure. Measures to reduce both patient and family anxiety are part of all transplant programs. At-home rehabilitation is a gradual process, and social services and other resources are part of the transplant team. The patient will be taking immunosuppressive drugs indefinitely. The verification process for organ transplant as now set forth by the United Network for Organ Sharing (UNOS) must be followed to ensure that the organs of the donor and the recipient are compatible (Patient Safety).

### *Operative Procedure*

1. The whole-organ pancreatic transplantation procedure is performed through an oblique incision opposite the side of the renal transplant in the lower abdominal quadrant. A midline incision may also be used for pancreatic transplant.
2. The external iliac artery and vein are skeletonized, and lymphatics are tied off with 4-0 nonabsorbable ligatures.
3. The external iliac vein is clamped with noncrushing vascular clamps, and a #11 blade is used to make a venotomy.
4. The venotomy incision is extended with Potts scissors.
5. An end-to-side anastomosis of the donor portal vein to the recipient's external iliac vein is performed with four double-armed 5-0 polypropylene sutures.
6. The external iliac artery is then clamped, and an aortic punch is used to make an arteriotomy.
7. An end-to-side anastomosis of the recipient's external iliac artery with the donor aortic patch containing the origin of the superior mesenteric artery and the celiac axis is performed with four double-armed 6-0 polypropylene sutures.

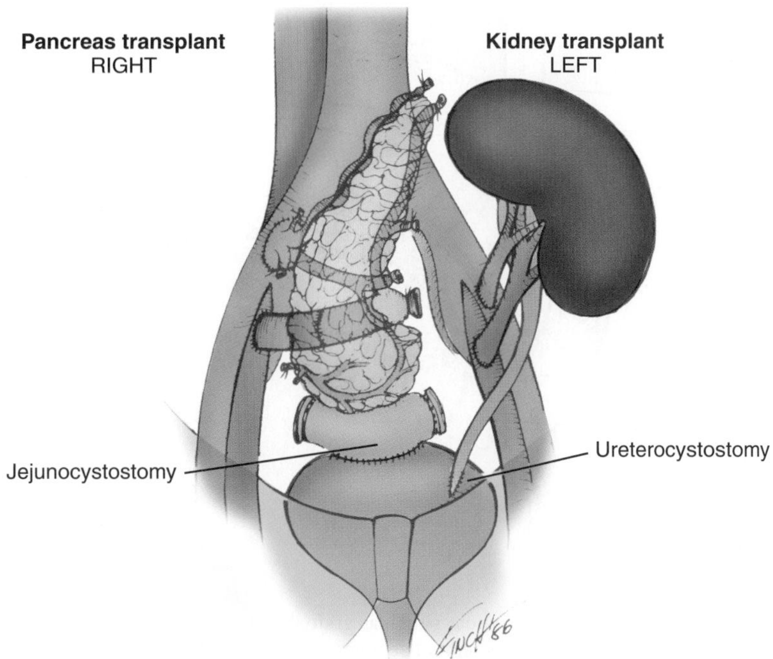


FIGURE 12-19 Whole-pancreas transplantation with simultaneous or serial kidney transplantation illustrating the position of the two donor grafts in the recipient.

## PATIENT SAFETY

### Transplant of Donor Organs/Tissues: Example of Procedure for Establishing Identity and Matching Donor with Recipient

To ensure identity and match the deceased organ donor's organs/tissues between donor and recipient before the surgical procedure, a process of nine checkpoints are implemented.

Before the patient enters the OR the following occur:

1. Once a transplant has been posted, Preliminary Transplant Crossmatch reports are faxed from the human leukocyte antigen (HLA) lab to the OR where the transplant is to occur. The blood bank will fax ABO reports.
2. The OR charge nurse will verify the posted recipient's preliminary transplant crossmatch report and the ABO report.
3. The organ will arrive at the OR.
4. The circulating nurse will apply an addressograph label to the box with the organ.
5. The circulating nurse and another registered nurse will together do the following:
   a. Verify the tag on the organ with the Preliminary Transplant Crossmatch Report to ensure the following match:
      i. Recorded ABO type of the recipient is the same or is compatible with the recorded ABO type of the donor.
      ii. The UNOS (United Network for Organ Sharing) number on the organ is the same as the UNOS number on the Preliminary Transplant Crossmatch Report.
   b. The patient is identified using the usual hospital policy.
   c. The two nurses sign the Transplant Verification form.

In the OR the following occur:

6. Preliminary anatomic checks are done by the surgeon. The transplant surgeon verifies that the UNOS number on the Preliminary Transplant Crossmatch Report is the same as the UNOS number on either the organ container or the paperwork provided and verifies the compatibility of the organ and the patient by ABO blood type. The transplant surgeon signs the Transplant Verification form.
7. Once the patient is taken into the OR, a time out is taken with the OR team according to OR policy and procedure.
8. The Kidney Transplant Verification form and Preliminary Transplant Crossmatch Report are a permanent part of the patient's medical record.
9. The Transplant Verification form (deceased donor) is attached to the record.

Modified from *UNOS Policy 3.1.4.1: ABO verification prior to transplant,* 2005. Accessed February 22, 2006, on-line: www.unos.org/PoliciesandBylaws/policies/docs/policy_3.doc.

8. Management of the pancreatic duct is then performed, according to the type of en bloc procedure performed.
9. Various enteric procedures for drainage of pancreatic duct secretions have been performed with whole-organ transplants en bloc with a segment of duodenum and the spleen. They include cutaneous jejunostomy, drainage into an ileal loop, and duodenojejunostomy with an end-to-end or side-to-side anastomosis. Direct grafting of the pancreatic duct into the enteric or urinary system is also performed for management of exocrine secretions. Surgical procedures include pancreaticojejunostomy with an established Roux-en-Y loop of jejunum (Figure 12-20), pancreaticoductoureterostomy, and pancreaticocystostomy. The whole-organ pancreas transplant may also be performed as pancreaticoduodenal transplantation or a pancreaticoduodenal-splenic transplantation.

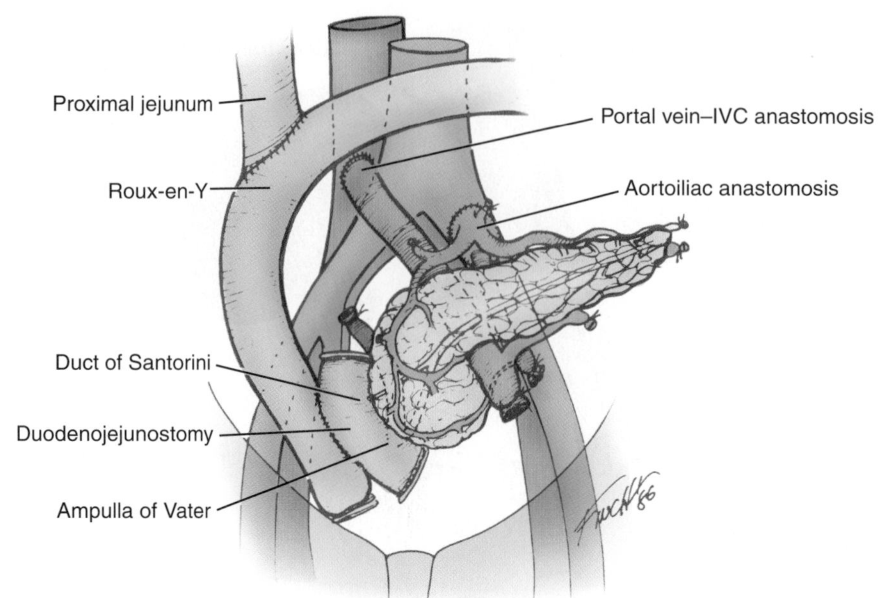


FIGURE 12-20 Enteric drainage of a whole-pancreas graft showing a side-to-side anastomosis of the donor duodenal patch and the recipient's jejunal segment of a Roux-en-Y. *IVC,* inferior vena cava.

## SURGERY OF THE LIVER

### Drainage of Abscess

Abscesses of the liver occur primarily by spread of bacteria or other organisms through the portal system, a direct route after trauma, the biliary tract, the hepatic artery in generalized septicemia, or direct extension from a subdiaphragmatic or subhepatic abscess. Although rare in the United States, amebic abscess is encountered. This cyst (hydatid) contains larvae of the tapeworm *Echinococcus granulosus,* whose eggs are carried from the intestinal tract to the liver by way of the portal circulation. Pharmacologic therapy with either antibiotics or amebicidal agents is usually initiated. In most instances, percutaneous drainage is effective and safe in the drainage of hepatic abscesses. However, open procedures may be required, often by way of the transperitoneal route. This approach permits inspection of the abdominal cavity for the underlying source.

***Procedural Considerations.*** A basic laparotomy set is used. Biliary instrumentation, drainage materials, and aerobic and anaerobic culture tubes should be available. The patient is positioned supine under general anesthesia. The anesthesia provider inserts a nasogastric tube after intubation. An indwelling urinary catheter may be inserted before the abdominal skin prep.

#### *Operative Procedure*

1. The incision preferred by many surgeons is the transperitoneal route; however, the surgical approach may be modified according to location of the abscess (e.g., in a high posterior abscess, where the transpleural approach may be selected).
2. The abdomen is opened as described for laparotomy, and abdominal inspection is carried out.
3. The abscess is mobilized and evacuated; cultures are obtained.
4. Surgical drains are placed, and the wound is closed.

### Hepatic Resection

The liver is divided into the left lobe and the right lobe, with the caudate lobe lying in the dorsal segment. Resection of the liver is undertaken for many primary tumors, benign conditions (e.g., hepatolithiasis), and metastatic tumors. Surgeons at major liver centers approach hepatic resection in three ways. The *anatomic* approach is based on the premise that malignant cells distribute along the portal venous segmental supply. In the *enucleation* approach, specific benign lesions with limited chance of local invasion are removed. The third approach, the *nonanatomic,* includes resections appropriate for a pathologic process in which a limited margin is acceptable, such as in tumor debulking.

***Procedural Considerations.*** Supplies and equipment should be available for thermoregulation, electrosurgery, measurement of portal pressure, and replacement of blood loss. In major liver centers, intraoperative ultrasound (to guide vessel isolation and minimize vascular occlusion), the argon beam coagulator, and the CUSA are required. Special blunt needles for suturing liver tissue are also necessary. Instruments used are a laparotomy set, biliary instruments, vascular instruments, noncrushing liver clamps, a self-retaining retractor, and a surgical stapler.

The patient is placed in the supine position. The anesthesia provider will insert a nasogastric tube after induction of general anesthesia and intubation. An indwelling urinary catheter is inserted before abdominal skin preparation. The abdomen is prepped from nipple line to midthigh. A right subcostal incision is often used, with the ability to extend with a left subcostal if necessary. In some instances, a median sternotomy or right thoracotomy incision is required; chest instruments are then necessary. Liver sutures, absorbable or nonabsorbable, according to surgeon's preference, vessel loops, and umbilical tapes should be available on the sterile field.

Hemostatic material, such as Gelfoam, Surgicel, or Avitene, and absorbable collagen sheets should be readily available when the resection is begun.

The surgeon may use various methods to remove liver tissue. The CUSA allows the surgeon to dissect tissue using ultrasonic waves incorporated with fluid and suction. The ultrasonic waves cut through liver tissue, emulsifying it and diluting the tissue with fluid so that it can be suctioned away. The electrosurgical pencil uses electrical current to cut through and desiccate liver tissue. Finger-fracture of the liver tissue is performed by applying digital pressure against the parenchyma to fracture the tissue.

### *Operative Procedure*

1. Through a right subcostal incision, the abdominal cavity is opened and examined.
2. Pathologic condition is determined, and resectability is evaluated.
3. Moist laparotomy packs are inserted, and a self-retaining retractor is placed.
4. Intraoperative ultrasonography (US) is performed to assess all segments of the liver (Figure 12-21). Ultrasound-guided, digital intraparenchymal isolation of vessels is also used during resection.
5. Lymph nodes in the porta hepatis and along the gastrohepatic ligament are then assessed by palpation to determine extrahepatic metastasis.
6. The intended resection line is scored with an electrosurgical pencil with blade tip, and coagulation is set at the surgeon's preferred setting (Figure 12-22).

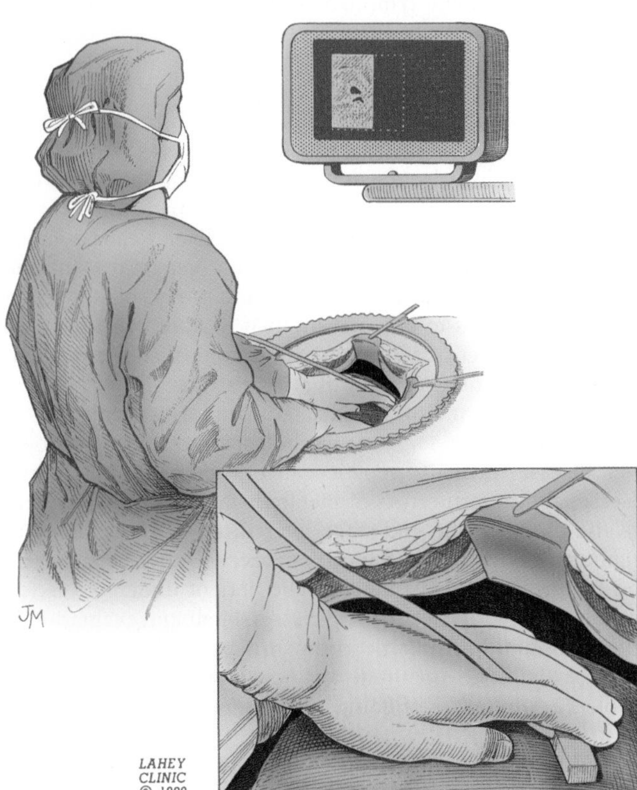


**FIGURE 12-21** Use of intraoperative ultrasound using a 7-MHz T-probe to permit assessment of the liver.

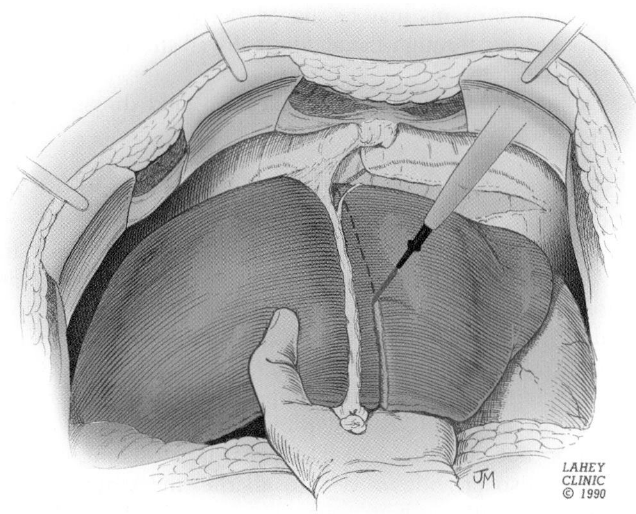


**FIGURE 12-22** Use of electrosurgical pencil with blade tip to score the line of resection on the surface of the liver.

7. The liver parenchyma is then delicately resected using the CUSA handpiece (Figure 12-23).
8. Use of the CUSA handpiece continues for dissection through the parenchyma.
9. Electrosurgical charring of surfaces or use of the argon beam coagulator is intermittent.
10. Once the portion of the liver is resected, the remaining liver resection margins are assessed for bleeding and bile leakage.
11. A laparotomy sponge may be placed against the transected surface for several minutes. The laparotomy sponge is gently rolled from the surface, which is then examined for bile leakage.
12. Areas may then be oversewn with 2-0 or 3-0 absorbable suture, or an intended layer of eschar is applied using electrocoagulation or the argon beam coagulator.

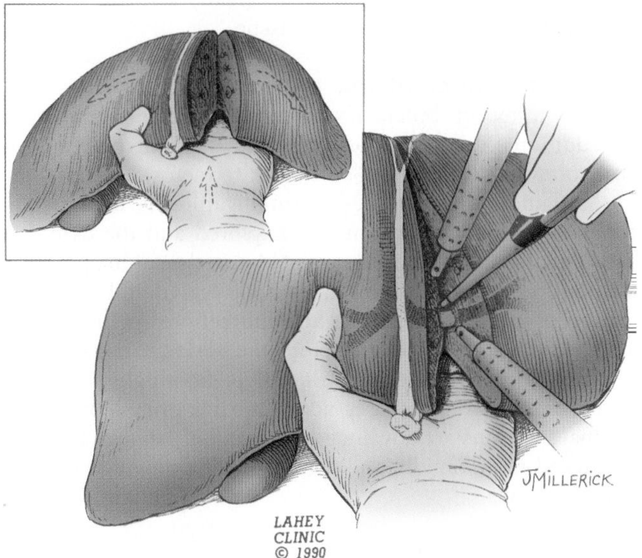


**FIGURE 12-23** Use of the Cavitron ultrasonic surgical aspirator (CUSA) handpiece to dissect through the hepatic parenchyma.

13. Abdominal drains may be placed along the liver bed and brought out through the abdominal wall through separate stab wounds.
14. The abdominal wound is then closed, and dressings are applied.

## Robotic-Assisted Laparoscopic Hepatic Surgery

***Procedural Considerations.*** Liver procedures using a robotic-assisted approach have already been performed in the United States. For example, a right hepatectomy was performed, removing approximately 60% of the liver using the da Vinci Surgical System.[12] The benefits associated with robotic technology include less blood loss, faster recovery, less scarring, and reduced postoperative pain. The robot extends the surgeon's skills by providing a 360-degree range of motion not possible with traditional laparoscopic instruments. It also provides access to all the fine structures of the liver and allows better visualization of delicate blood vessels.[16]

## Radioimmunoguided Surgery

Radioimmunoguided surgery (RIGS) is a technique used intraoperatively to detect cancer that may not be readily detected by inspection or palpation. This technique has been found useful in determining safe margins of resection for metastatic colon cancer and extrahepatic disease and occult tumor in patients with rising serum carcinoembryonic antigen (CEA) levels.

About 2 to 3 weeks before surgery, patients receive an IV injection of radiolabeled monoclonal antibody, which binds reactive antigen on or near the surface of tumor cells. The antigen-antibody bond keeps minute amounts of radioactivity, or gamma emissions, localized in tumor tissue. An intraoperatively used, handheld gamma ray–detecting probe connected to a microcomputer emits an audible signal when the radioactive waves hit the crystal in the distal end of the probe. The Neoprobe instrument gives a digital reading as well as an audible pitch that rises or falls when placed on the gamma ray–emitting tissue. This advance in the intraoperative detection of adenocarcinoma and metastases can greatly assist in decision making and resection of diseased tissue.

***Procedural Considerations.*** Instrumentation includes a basic laparotomy set, biliary instruments, vascular instruments, and additional items such as long clamps and a self-retaining retractor system (e.g., the Bookwalter retractor). Minimal suture (2-0 and 3-0 silk ties, 2-0 suture ligature) is added to the sterile field until the abdomen is explored and the extent of disease is assessed. The patient is placed in the supine position. The anesthesia provider will insert a nasogastric tube after induction of general anesthesia and intubation. An indwelling urinary catheter is inserted before the abdominal prep. The abdomen is prepped from nipple line to midthigh. A midline abdominal incision provides access to the liver. Vertical abdominal incisions are advantageous because they can be made and closed more rapidly and permit better exposure of all abdominal organs.

***Operative Procedure.***

1. A midline abdominal incision is made from the xiphoid process to the pubis.
2. Intraoperative scanning of the liver and abdominal viscera is performed using the probe.
3. The digital readings as well as the anatomic structures being scanned are recorded.
4. Great care is taken to scan mesenteric, pelvic, and periaortic lymph nodes individually.
5. The liver is scanned, and areas emitting strong-pitched tones are marked with a sterile marking pen. A very distinct change in pitch may be noted on liver tissue within a 2-cm to 3-cm radius of the tumor site.
6. Intraoperative ultrasonography and a review of the CT and MRI scans of the patient's liver are used to further confirm the liver lesions.
7. Margins for resection are drawn using an electrosurgical knife on a blend mode.
8. Resection of the lesion may be segmental, circumferential, or lobar.
9. After each resection, the margins of healthy liver tissue adjacent to the resection site are scanned and readings are recorded. This procedure continues until all tissue emitting high gamma-ray waves has been resected.
10. Specimens are sent to the pathology laboratory for further pathologic and histologic analysis. The perioperative nurse greatly enhances the correlation of pathologic diagnosis with the intraoperative RIGS findings by specifically and accurately identifying the tissue specimens.
11. The surgeon determines the best plan of treatment for the patient based on the information obtained from intraoperative assessment of the extent of the patient's disease. Resection of RIGS-positive tissue may result in an extensive retroperitoneal lymphadenectomy, liver resection, gastrohepatic ligament lymphadenectomy, or the resection of colon, uterus, or bladder.

## Liver Transplantation

Liver transplantation is the implantation of a liver from a donor into a recipient. The total procedure involves retrieving, or procuring, the liver from a donor, transporting the donor liver to the recipient's hospital, performing a hepatectomy on the recipient, and then implanting the donor liver. Reanastomoses are then undertaken of the suprahepatic vena cava, infrahepatic vena cava, portal vein, and hepatic artery; biliary reconstruction with end-to-end anastomosis of donor and recipient common bile ducts; or Roux-en-Y anastomosis if the recipient bile duct is absent as a result of biliary atresia.

Liver transplantation is indicated for patients with chronic hepatocellular disease, chronic cholestatic disease, metabolic liver disease, primary hepatic cancer, acute fulminant liver disease, and inborn errors of metabolism. When malignancies are the cause of the end-stage liver disease, the right upper quadrant may be radiated intraoperatively—after hepatectomy and before the transplantation. The patient undergoes extensive physiologic and psychologic assessment and evaluation by physicians and transplant coordinators before being placed on a donor list. The potential for postoperative complications (Table 12-5) requires ongoing evaluation.

***Procedural Considerations.*** Successful transplantation requires the cooperative efforts of the organ-procurement agency and the staffs of the donor and recipient hospitals. Usually two members of the surgical team from the recipient's hospital

**TABLE 12-5**

## Assessment and Prevention of Common Postoperative Complications Associated with Liver Transplants

| Assessment | Prevention |
|---|---|
| **ACUTE GRAFT REJECTION** | |
| Occurs from the fourth to tenth postoperative day.<br>Manifested by tachycardia, fever, right upper quadrant (RUQ) or flank pain, diminished bile drainage or change in bile color, or increased jaundice.<br>Laboratory changes include increased levels of serum bilirubin, transaminases, and alkaline phosphatase and prolonged prothrombin time. | Prophylaxis with immunosuppressant agents, such as cyclosporine.<br>Early diagnosis to treat with more potent antirejection drugs, such as muromonab-CD3 (Orthoclone OKT3).<br>Antibiotic prophylaxis. |
| **INFECTION** | |
| Can occur at any time during recovery.<br>Manifested by fever or excessive, foul-smelling drainage (urine, wound, or bile); other indicators depend on the location and the type of infection. | Early diagnosis and treatment with organism-specific anti-infective agents.<br>Frequent cultures of tubes, lines, and drainage.<br>Early removal of invasive line.<br>Good hand hygiene. |
| **HEPATIC COMPLICATIONS (BILE LEAKAGE, ABSCESS FORMATION, HEPATIC THROMBOSIS)** | |
| Manifested by decreased bile drainage, increased RUQ abdominal pain with distention and guarding, nausea or vomiting, increased jaundice, and clay-colored stools.<br>Laboratory changes include increased levels of serum bilirubin and transaminases. | Keep the T-tube in a dependent position and secure to patient; empty frequently, recording quality and quantity of drainage.<br>Report manifestations to the physician immediately.<br>May necessitate surgical intervention. |
| **ACUTE RENAL FAILURE** | |
| Caused by hypotension, antibiotics, cyclosporine, acute liver failure, or hypothermia.<br>Indicators of hypothermia include shivering, hyperventilation, increased cardiac output, vasoconstriction, and alkalemia.<br>Early indicators of renal failure include changes in urinary output, increased blood urea nitrogen (BUN) and creatinine levels, and electrolyte imbalance. | Monitor all drug levels with nephrotoxic side effects.<br>Prevent hypotension.<br>Observe for early signs of renal failure, and report them immediately to the physician. |

Modified from Ignatavicius DD, Workman ML: *Medical surgical nursing: critical thinking for collaborative care,* ed 4, Philadelphia, 2002, Saunders.

travel to the donor's hospital to procure the donated liver. Multiple transplant teams may arrive at the donor hospital to procure the various organs available and viable for transplantation. UNOS policies dictate a detailed system for checking and re-checking organs for transplantation. This system ensures that organs of the donor and recipient are compatible (see Patient Safety). These policies must be strictly adhered to before any transplant can take place.

PREPARING THE OPERATING ROOM FOR THE DONOR. The donor operating room is set up for a major laparotomy procedure. Basic instrumentation and equipment include a basic laparotomy set, cardiovascular instruments, power sternal saw, and nephrectomy instruments. A sterile, draped, medium-size instrument table is needed for preparation of the liver away from the main sterile operative field and instrument tables. The procurement team provides special Collins solution for flushing the organs, sterile plastic containers and ice chests for organs, and in situ flush tubing. The liver is generally placed in two Lahey bags immediately after procurement. A common practice is to procure the heart and kidneys as well as the liver; other organs, tissues, and bone may also be procured.

PREPARING THE OPERATING ROOM FOR THE RECIPIENT. Each transplantation surgeon has preferred instruments, supplies, and sutures. In general, the following are needed in the recipient's operating room: a basic laparotomy set, a cardiovascular instrument set, an assortment of T-tubes, a slush unit or means of providing iced lactated Ringer's solution, two electrosurgical units, a forced-air warming device, a temperature probe, IV volumetric pumps on stands, two blood warmers or water baths, an indwelling urinary catheter, an insertion tray, and a urometer. The argon beam coagulator may be used and should be available. A defibrillator is always located in the room with sterile external paddles available.[15]

Large-bore cannulas for IV monitoring and fluid or blood replacement lines are placed in addition to an arterial line and a central venous line.

Two surgeon headlights and light sources will be necessary to augment visualization of the abdominal site. A venovenous bypass system may be used to support peripheral blood flow. Extra drape sheets, table covers, gowns, towels, gloves, sponges, and laparotomy pads, cold IV Ringer's solution, sterile IV administration set for flushing the new liver, umbilical tape, booties, and vessel loops should be available to support the many steps of the transplantation procedure.

A cart containing sutures and the numerous other small items should be set up and placed in the room for each procedure. This practice eliminates the need for the circulating nurse to leave the patient and surgical team to obtain extra supplies.

The procedure requires a bilateral subcostal incision with possible midline extension and removal of the xiphoid. The right side of the chest may be entered to provide more exposure when needed.

The procedure for liver transplantation is a three-part process: retrieval of the donor organ, hepatectomy, and implantation of the donor liver. It is a lengthy procedure that takes many hours.The following aspects of implementing a plan of care deserve special attention.

**Patient Positioning.** The patient is placed in the supine position with knees slightly flexed and padded. Accurate body alignment is essential. A gel pad that is the length of the OR bed or a pressure-reducing OR bed mattress should be used, with attention paid to all potential pressure areas. Heel protectors are applied. The safety strap is placed over the lower part of the thighs and secured. A forced-air warming blanket is applied over the upper body, neck, and head to assist in maintaining the patient's temperature. Fluid warmers will be used to warm the blood products and IV solutions that will be infused during the procedure. SCDs are placed on the patient's legs. An indwelling urinary catheter is inserted after induction of anesthesia.

**Skin Preparation.** The patient is prepped from the neck to midthigh, bedline to bedline. Prep solution should not pool at the bedline or wet the sheets on the OR bed. Fire safety precautions for prep solutions must be followed.

**Blood Loss and Replacement.** Blood loss may be extensive, and replacement must be timely. The perioperative nurse should confirm that blood products are available at the beginning of the procedure; these include 10 units each of packed red blood cells (RBCs) and fresh frozen plasma (FFP), and 1 unit of pooled donor platelets. The perioperative nurse should collaborate with the anesthesia provider during the insertion of peripheral and arterial lines. An autologous cell-saver device may be used to assist in blood replacement by way of autotransfusion.

**Intraoperative Laboratory Testing.** It is possible that as many as 50 blood specimens will be drawn for analysis during the procedure. This blood must be recorded on the blood-loss record and calculated into replacement needs. The specimens are delivered to the laboratory immediately. A telephone in the OR is useful for receiving and reading back critical test results/reports directly from the laboratory. Safety precautions in collection of specimens must be initiated.

**Length of Procedure.** Procedures may last from 6 to 20 hours. Special attention must be directed toward maintaining the integrity of the sterile environment from the standpoint of time and the number of people moving in and out of the room.

**Communication with Family.** Frequent reports to the family are important. Family members usually are knowledgeable about liver function tests and laboratory values and want this information in addition to reports on the condition of their loved one. One person should be assigned in advance to make regular contacts with family and support persons. The UNOS team often works closely with the donor's and recipient's families and can be instrumental in communicating with the families.

**COMMUNICATION AMONG TEAMS.** The perioperative nurse ensures that communication occurs among teams. Coordination among the procurement team, anesthesia team, and surgical teams is essential for a successful transplantation procedure. Perioperative nursing responsibilities also include monitoring and communicating blood-loss volume in suction canisters and on sponges, the availability of blood and blood products, laboratory results, time of organ arrival, ischemic time, and other events as they unfold in preparation for and during the transplant procedure.

### *Operative Procedure*

1. Bilateral subcostal incisions are made with a midline incision extended toward the umbilicus.
2. Initial dissection of the underlying tissues is achieved with electrosurgery and suture ligatures.
3. Isolation of all hilar structures and dissection to mobilize the lobes of the native liver are performed.
4. The retrohepatic vena cava is skeletonized, as are the hepatic artery, portal vein, common bile duct, and inferior vena cava.
5. The donor liver is examined.
6. Preparations may be made at this time for venovenous bypass using an extracorporeal assist device if the patient is unstable.
7. The infrahepatic vena cava and the suprahepatic vena cava are clamped, as are the portal vein, the hepatic artery, and the common bile duct.
8. Native hepatectomy is then performed.
9. The donor liver is placed in the right upper abdomen, and revascularization of the donor organ begins with end-to-end anastomoses in the vena cava and portal vein, with double-armed fine vascular suture (Research Highlight).
10. At this point, the clamps on the portal vein, suprahepatic vena cava, and infrahepatic vena cava are released slowly and blood flow through the vena cava and portal vein is restored.
11. The anastomosis sites are then checked for leaks.
12. If it was used, venovenous bypass is discontinued and the cannulation sites are closed.
13. The postrevascularization phase focuses on achieving hemostasis. Complete hemostasis may require extensive time

## RESEARCH HIGHLIGHT

### Liver Transplant Technique Option

Although first described in 1993 by a French surgeon, the approach to liver transplantation technique in this study was not well researched until studies by two American surgeons at the Ohio State University Medical Center. In usual liver transplant procedures, the entire liver is removed from the recipient and the donor liver placed, with end-to-end inferior vena cava anastomoses above and below the liver. In large patients, these anastomoses are technically challenging. With this newer technique, instead of removing the entire liver, including the vena cava behind it, the liver is removed off of the inferior vena cava, leaving the inferior vena cava intact. In this method, operating time is reduced close to 1 hour and blood transfusion requirements reduced by approximately 25%. In this study of 140 patients, survival outcomes were comparable to those obtained with the traditional method.

Modified from *New liver transplantation technique reduces time and transfusion requirements.* Accessed November 12, 2001, on-line: surgery.medscape.com/reuters/prof/2001/11/11.05/20011102clin015.html.

at this point. Bleeding may be exacerbated by a fibrinolytic episode associated with the reperfusion of the donor organ. The liver is monitored for a change in color from dusky to pink. An intraoperative Doppler may be used to confirm patency of the blood supply.

14. The anastomosis of the hepatic artery is then commenced, followed by bile duct reconstruction. This varies with the status of the recipient's biliary tract. If biliary atresia is the cause of the patient's end-stage liver disease, choledochoenterostomy into a Roux-en-Y loop of jejunum is performed (Figure 12-24).
15. The anastomoses are then checked for leaks.
16. Drains are placed behind and in front of the liver and brought through the skin. The abdomen is then closed.

## Donor Hepatectomy

Donor hepatectomy is performed for procurement of a healthy liver for transplant into a patient who has end-stage liver failure. This procedure occurs only after the donor patient has been determined to be brain dead and family consent for organ donation has been obtained. Donor hepatectomy can be performed at any hospital. Organ procurement agencies arrange contact with transplant centers when a viable organ donor has been identified. Candidates for liver transplantations are placed on a national-network waiting list and are matched according to urgency of need, blood type, and body size.

***Procedural Considerations.*** Once the liver transplant candidate has been identified, the procurement team from that transplant center travels to the institution where the organ donor is hospitalized. If multiple organs are being donated, surgeons from several transplant centers may arrive to procure the organs they will be transplanting at their respective centers.

The procedure for procurement of multiple organs may differ according to the transplant centers represented. Most commonly, the systemic cooling of the donor's body temperature is started before the procurement of the heart. Cannulation sites may also vary according to which organs are procured.

The perioperative nurses at the donor hospital are responsible for supplying a basic laparotomy setup with instrumentation to open the sternum. Basic vascular clamps are also required for clamping the major vascular structures. Cold lactated Ringer's solution for parenteral infusion and cold Ringer's solution for irrigation are usually used in large amounts.

### *Operative Procedure*

1. The donor patient is positioned supine on the OR bed. The skin area from neck to midthigh is prepped and draped.
2. A midline incision is made from the suprasternal notch to the pubis.
3. A subcostal incision is performed bilaterally on the abdomen for better exposure of the abdominal viscera.
4. Retractors are placed to provide optimal exposure of the organs that will be procured.
5. The aorta and vena cava, superior and inferior to the liver and kidneys, are skeletonized by dissection and ligation of the lymphatics and smaller vasculatures.
6. The porta hepatis is dissected; the superior mesenteric artery and celiac trunk are then dissected and delicately exposed as close to the aorta as is convenient.
7. The superior mesenteric vein is dissected and prepared for cannulation. The donor is heparinized and systemically cooled.
8. If the heart is to be procured, procurement takes place at this time.
9. Further cooling and flushing of the pancreas, liver, and kidneys are achieved by cannulation and infusion of cold lactated Ringer's solution through the inferior vena cava just superior to the bifurcation.
10. One to two liters of lactated Ringer's solution are infused before the organs have been properly cooled.
11. The liver, pancreas, spleen, and a segment of the duodenum harboring the pancreatic duct are procured en bloc by placing clamps on the suprahepatic and infrahepatic venae cavae.

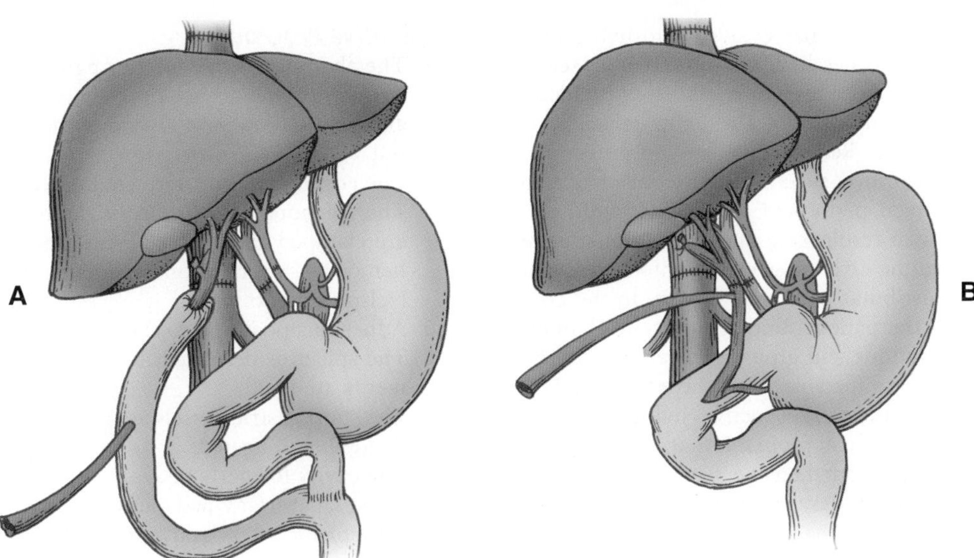


**FIGURE 12-24** Completed orthotopic liver transplant with Roux-en-Y biliary reconstruction, **A**, and end-to-end anastomosis of the donor-to-recipient common bile ducts, **B**.

12. The suprahepatic vena cava is transected with a surrounding cuff of diaphragm intact.
13. The infrahepatic vena cava is transected above the level of the renal veins.
14. The celiac axis is detached from the aorta with an aortic patch or taken with a full aortic circumference.
15. The duodenal segment is procured, using a linear stapling device at opposite ends of the segment.
16. The en bloc organs are taken to a back table for further dissection and ligation to separate the liver from the en bloc pancreas, spleen, and duodenal segment graft. Meanwhile, other members of the procurement team continue working to free the kidneys and ureters if they are to be taken.
17. The liver is placed in a basin of very cold Ringer's solution, double-bagged in sterile Lahey bags, and placed in an ice chest for transport to the recipient's hospital.
18. The kidneys are placed in sterile cassettes and mechanically perfused.
19. The pancreatic en bloc graft is also placed in a basin of cold Ringer's solution, bagged, and transported in a thermal chest of ice.
20. The abdomen is closed with a single layer of size 1 or 0 nonabsorbable suture.
21. Drapes are removed, and the donor patient is cleaned and washed. Tubes and infusion lines are tied off or clamped. Sometimes family members of the donor patient request to view the body after organ donation. This factor may be important in helping them face the loss of their loved one. The perioperative nurse can assist them in their grieving process by providing them with a quiet and private environment in which to say good-bye to their family member. Removing the donor patient's body from the OR where the surgical procedure took place is best. The perioperative nurse should make sure that the donor patient is covered with a warm blanket and then should stay with family members to support them.
22. The donor patient is then transported by stretcher to the morgue.

### Living-Related Liver Transplantation

Just as kidney transplantation has evolved into living-related donor possibilities, so too has liver transplantation (see History box). The capacity of the liver to regenerate provided the scientific basis for development of the living-related donor transplantation procedure. Reduced-size and split-liver transplants have been performed successfully. Reduced-size liver transplantation has been performed for infants, children, or very small adults. Initial results of reduced-size and split-liver transplantations from the early pioneering centers were disappointing. This was attributable, at least in part, to the critical clinical condition of the patients undergoing transplantation. Improvements in technique and growing experience have led to satisfactory results comparable with those obtained with whole-organ transplantation. Prospective living donors are thoroughly evaluated, with a protocol that includes blood group compatibility, a comprehensive history and physical examination, laboratory studies, psychosocial evaluation, independent advocate opinion, anatomic compatibility, review of candidacy with the donor, and presentation to a selection committee.[20] As cloning, biogenetic engineering, and other technologic advances increase the possibilities for organ transplants, society will need to deal with ongoing debates of ethical dilemmas surrounding them.

## SURGERY OF THE SPLEEN

### Splenectomy (Open Approach)

Splenectomy is removal of the spleen. It is usually performed for trauma to the spleen, for specific malignant conditions (Hodgkin's disease and non-Hodgkin's lymphomas; hairy cell, chronic lymphocytic, and chronic myelogenous leukemias); for hemolytic jaundice or splenic anemia; for idiopathic thrombocytopenia purpura; or for tumors, cysts, or splenomegaly. Another indication for splenectomy is accidental injury to the spleen during vagotomy or other gastric procedures or operations involving mobilization of the splenic flexure of the colon. If accessory spleens are present, they are also removed because they are capable of perpetuating hypersplenic function. In most instances, patients evaluated for elective splenectomy are considered candidates for laparoscopic splenectomy. Contraindications to the laparoscopic procedure include severe portal hypertension, uncorrectable coagulopathy, severe ascites, extreme splenomegaly, and most traumatic injuries to the spleen. For these patients, an open approach is required.

***Procedural Considerations.*** Massive splenomegaly may occasionally require a thoracoabdominal approach. Abdominal suction apparatus should be available throughout all splenectomies. A cell saver may be requested.

Instrumentation is as described for a basic laparotomy, plus two large, right-angled pedicle clamps, long instruments, and hemostatic materials or devices. The patient is placed in the supine position. The anesthesia provider will insert a nasogastric tube after induction of general anesthesia and intubation. An indwelling urinary catheter is inserted before the abdominal prep. The abdomen is prepped from nipple line to midthigh. A midline abdominal incision provides access to the spleen. Vertical abdominal incisions are advantageous because they can be made and closed more rapidly and permit better exposure of all abdominal organs.

#### *Operative Procedure*

1. The abdomen is opened through the selected incision.
2. Retractors are placed over moistened laparotomy packs, and gentle retraction is employed as exploration is carried out.
3. The costal margin is retracted upward.
4. The splenorenal, splenocolic, and gastrosplenic ligaments are clamped and divided with long dressing forceps, long hemostats, sponges on holders, and long Metzenbaum or Nelson scissors.
5. Adhesions posterior to the spleen are freed.
6. The spleen is delivered into the wound after these attachments are freed.
7. The short gastric vessels are now easily identified, clamped, divided, and ligated.
8. The cavity formerly occupied by the spleen is packed with moist laparotomy pads, if necessary.
9. The splenic artery and vein are dissected free with fine dissecting scissors and forceps.
10. The artery is clamped and doubly ligated with silk. The artery is ligated first and then the vein; such ligation permits

disengorgement of blood from the spleen and facilitation of the return of venous blood to the circulatory system.

11. The splenic vein is clamped, divided, and ligated.
12. The specimen is removed; all bleeding vessels are controlled. The wound is closed in layers, as described for laparotomy, and dressings are applied.
13. Drainage is usually required only if many adhesions to the diaphragm were divided or if significant clotting abnormalities exist.

## Laparoscopic Splenectomy

Indications for laparoscopic splenectomy are the same as with open procedures, with the exception of the contraindications noted in the discussion of open splenectomy.

***Procedural Considerations.*** General anesthesia is administered. A nasogastric tube and indwelling urinary catheter are inserted, and SCDs are applied to the lower extremities. The patient usually is positioned in a right lateral decubitus position, with the OR bed flexed and the kidney rest raised to increase the distance between the lower rib and iliac crest. The anterior abdomen is brought close to the edge of the OR bed. A beanbag device may be used. Safety restraints must be placed, especially in anticipation of a possible slight backward tilt of the patient (supine position or modified lithotomy may also be used). The surgeon stands on the right side of the patient as does the scrub person, and the assistants stand to the left.

Instrumentation and equipment include a 30-degree telescope (10-mm or 5-mm); a camera (triple-chip or single-chip); a high-flow insufflator with $CO_2$ tank; a high-resolution monitor (second monitor optional for assistant); a printer (optional); a Surgineedle or Verres needle; four 12-mm trocars (trocar size depends on surgeon preference—some surgeons substitute one or two of the 12-mm trocars with 5-mm trocars or even 3-mm trocars); endoshears/scissors; an endodissecting forceps or endograsper (atraumatic); an endoretractor; an endoclip applier; a linear stapling device (GIA type) with vascular cartridges, an endoretrieval pouch; and a suction-irrigation system. As with other laparoscopic procedures, instruments and supplies should be available if the need arises to convert to an open approach.

### *Operative Procedure*[4]

1. Local anesthetic may be injected into the skin at the midpoint of the anterior costal margin. The first trocar is placed under direct visualization, and a symmetric 12– to 15–mm Hg pneumoperitoneum is created.
2. The laparoscope is inserted through the port, and the camera is placed.
3. The stomach is retracted to expose the spleen. A thorough search is made for any accessory spleens; if an accessory spleen (or spleens) is found, it is removed immediately because it is more difficult to relocate after the primary spleen has been removed.[21]
4. Initial dissection is begun by mobilizing the splenic flexure of the colon.
5. The splenocolic ligament is divided using sharp dissection, mobilizing the inferior pole of the spleen. The spleen is now retracted cephalad, taking care not to rupture the splenic capsule during retraction.
6. The lateral peritoneal attachments of the spleen are then incised using either sharp dissection or ultrasonic endoshears.
7. The lesser sac is entered along the medial border of the spleen.
8. With the spleen elevated, the short gastric vessels and main vascular pedicle are visualized. The tail of the pancreas is also visualized and avoided.
9. The short gastric vessels are divided by means of an ultrasonic dissector, endoclips, or an endovascular stapling device.
10. After the short gastric vessels have been divided, the splenic pedicle is carefully dissected from both the medial and lateral aspects.
11. After the artery and vein are dissected, the vessels are divided by application of the endovascular stapler. Multiple vascular branches may be encountered, and each is taken individually if necessary.
12. The spleen is now devascularized and ready for entrapment.
13. To remove the spleen, an Endobag is introduced through one of the trocar sites (usually the left lateral site).
14. The bag is opened, and the spleen is placed into it. The drawstring is grasped and the bag closed, leaving only the superior pole attachments, which are now divided.
15. The open end of the bag is brought outside the abdomen through the supraumbilical port or epigastric trocar site. The spleen is then morcellated and removed in fragments.
16. The laparoscope is reinserted, and the splenic bed is assessed for hemostasis.
17. If necessary, a drain is placed in the intraabdominal cavity, the abdomen is deflated, and the trocars are removed.
18. The trocar sites are then closed.

## REFERENCES


1. Ackley BJ, Ladwig GB: *Nursing diagnosis handbook,* ed 7, St Louis, 2006, Mosby.
2. Ahrendt SA, Pitt HA: Biliary tract. In Townsend CM and others: *Sabiston textbook of surgery,* ed 17, Philadelphia, 2004, Saunders.
3. Baas LS and others: Cardiovascular care. In *Illustrated manual of nursing practice,* ed 3, Philadelphia, 2002, Lippincott Williams & Wilkins.
4. Beuchamp RD and others: Spleen. In Townsend CM and others: *Sabiston textbook of surgery,* ed 17, Philadelphia, 2004, Saunders.
5. Beyea SC: The ideal state for perioperative nursing, *AORN Journal* 73(5):897-901, 2001.
6. Blackbourne LH: *Surgical recall,* ed 2, Philadelphia, 1998, Lippincott Williams & Wilkins.
7. Bodner J and others: Long-term follow-up after robotic cholecystectomy, *American Surgeon* 71(4):281-288, 2005.
8. Buechner J: *Trends in cholecystectomies,* 2002. Accessed February 16, 2006, on-line: www.health.ri.gov/publications/hpb9707.pdf.
9. Canobbio MM: *Mosby's handbook of patient teaching,* ed 3, St Louis, 2006, Mosby.
10. Fakhry SM and others: Postoperative management. In Souba WW and others: *ACS surgery: principles & practice,* New York, 2006, WebMD.
11. Gruendemann BJ, Mangum SS: *Infection prevention in surgical settings,* Philadelphia, 2001, Saunders.
12. Hanley EJ, Talamini MA: Robotic abdominal surgery, *American Journal of Surgery* 188(4A, Suppl):19S-26S, 2004.

13. Jacobsen G and others: Robotic surgery update, *Surgical Endoscopy* 18(8):1186-1191, 2004.
14. Lo SK: *Pancreatic and biliary endoscopy: a clinical update from the 8th Annual International Symposium on Pancreatic and Biliary Endoscopy,* January 26-28, 2001. Accessed February 16, 2006, on-line: www.medscape.com/viewarticle/407973.
15. McKenney E: Liver transplants, *Advance for Nurses* 3(2):19-20, 2001.
16. *Medical center performs first robotic complex liver surgery,* 2005. Accessed, February 16, 2006, on-line: www://uillinoismedcenter.org/content.cfm?contentid=1117
17. Melvin WS: Minimally invasive pancreatic surgery, *American Journal of Surgery* 186(3):274-278, 2003.
18. Miroshnik M and others: Biliary tract injury in laparoscopic cholecystectomy: results of a single unit, *Australian and New Zealand Journal of Surgery* 72(12):867-870, 2002.
19. Nguyen NT and others: Application of robotics in general surgery: initial experience, *American Surgeon* 70(10):914-917, 2004.
20. Patt CH, Thuluvath PJ: Adult living donor transplantation. *Medscape Gastroenterology*. Accessed Febuary 16, 2006 online: www.medscape.com/viewarticle/458740?src=search
21. Poulin EC and others: Laparoscopic splenectomy. In Wilmore DW and others: *ACS surgery: principles & practice,* New York, 2002, WebMD.
22. *Standards, recommended practices, and guidelines with official AORN statements*, 2005 ed, Denver, 2005, Association of periOperative Registered Nurses (AORN).
23. Steer ML: Exocrine pancreas. In Townsend CM and others: *Sabiston textbook of surgery,* ed 17, Philadelphia, 2004, Saunders.
24. *Universal protocol for preventing wrong site wrong procedure, wrong person surgery*. accessed February 16, 2006, on-line: www.jcaho.org/accredited+organizations/patient+safety/universal+protocol/wss_universal+protocol.htm.
25. U.S. Department of Health and Human Services, Public Health Service: *Endoscopic retrograde cholangiopancreatography,* Washington, DC, 2002, Agency for Healthcare Quality and Research, Evidence Report/Technology Assessment no. 50.

CHAPTER 13

# *Repair of Hernias*

MICHELLE SLOAN

*NO DISEASE OF the body, belonging to the province of the surgeon, requires in its treatment, a better combination of accurate, anatomical knowledge with surgical skill than hernia in all its varieties.*

SIR ASTLEY PASTON COOPER, 1804

A hernia is an abnormal protrusion of a peritoneum-lined sac through the musculoaponeurotic covering of the abdomen. The word *hernia* is a Latin term that means "rupture" of a portion of a structure. Descriptions of hernia reduction date back to Hammurabi of Babylon and the Egyptian papyrus (History box). Weakness of the abdominal wall, congenital or acquired, results in the inability to contain the visceral contents of the abdominal cavity within their normal confines. More than 700,000 surgical procedures are performed each year to repair congenital hernia defects; nearly 75% of all acquired hernias occur in the inguinal region. Of these, about 50% of hernias are indirect inguinal hernias and 24% are direct inguinal hernias. Incisional and ventral hernias account for approximately 10% of all hernias; as the frequency and magnitude of abdominal surgeries have increased in recent years, so has the incidence of incisional hernia. Femoral hernias account for 3%, and unusual hernias account for the remaining 5% to 10%.

Most hernias occur in males. The most common hernia in males and females is the indirect inguinal hernia. Femoral hernias occur much more frequently in females, and only 2% of females will develop inguinal hernias in their lifetime. Also, hernias occur more commonly on the right side than on the left. Herniorrhaphy is one of the most common operative procedures performed and is the preferred treatment when a defect is detected.

Hernias have a tremendous economic significance in the United States. The number of workdays lost is substantial. The trend toward ambulatory surgery for hernia repair is one of many attempts to provide cost-effective health care that also leads to patient satisfaction.

A hernia can occur in several places in the abdominal wall, with protrusion of a portion of the parietal peritoneum and often a part of the intestine. The weak places or intervals in the abdominal aponeurosis are (1) the inguinal canals, (2) the femoral rings, and (3) the umbilicus. Any number of conditions causing increased pressure within the abdomen can contribute to the formation of a hernia. Contributing factors to hernia formation include age, gender, previous surgery, obesity, nutritional state, and pulmonary and cardiac disease. Loss of tissue turgor occurs with aging and in chronic debilitating diseases. Current evidence suggests that adult male inguinal hernias are likely associated with impaired collagen metabolism and weakening of the fibroconnective tissue of the groin.[9] Smoking has also been noted as a contributing factor to hernia formation (Research Highlight).[13] A successful herniorrhaphy is measured by the percentage of recurrence, the number of complications, total costs, and return to normal activities of daily living.

## *Surgical Anatomy*

A hernia is a sac lined by peritoneum that protrudes through a defect in the layers of the abdominal wall. Generally, a hernia mass is composed of covering tissues, a peritoneal sac, and any contained viscera. Hernias may be acquired or congenital.

Depending on their location, hernias are classified as direct inguinal, indirect inguinal, femoral, umbilical, incisional, or epigastric (Figure 13-1). Hernias in any of these groups are either reducible or nonreducible; that is, the contents of the hernia sac either can be returned to the normal intraabdominal position or are trapped in the extraabdominal sac (incarcerated). The conditions preventing the return of the hernia contents to the abdomen can result from (1) adhesions between the contents of the sac and the inner lining of the sac, (2) adhesions among the contents of the sac, or (3) narrowing of the neck of the sac. Patients with incarcerated hernias may have signs of intestinal obstruction, such as vomiting, abdominal pain, and distention. The greatest danger of an incarcerated hernia is that it may become strangulated. In a strangulated hernia, the blood supply of the trapped sac contents becomes compromised and eventually the sac contents necrose. When bowel is strangulated in such a hernia, resection of necrotic bowel, in addition to the repair of the hernia defect, becomes necessary.

### Inguinal Hernias

The anterolateral abdominal wall consists of an arrangement of muscles, fascial layers, and muscular aponeuroses lined interiorly by peritoneum and exteriorly by skin (Figure 13-2). The abdominal wall in the groin area is composed of two groups of these structures: a superficial group (Scarpa fascia, external and internal oblique muscles, and their aponeuroses) and a deep group (internal oblique muscle, transversalis fascia, and peritoneum).

Essential to an understanding of inguinal hernia repair is an appreciation of the central role of the transversalis fascia as the major supporting structure of the posterior inguinal floor. The inguinal canal, which contains the spermatic cord and associ-

## HISTORY

### History of Hernia Repairs

Groin hernias were originally documented 3500 years ago, with surgical intervention starting approximately 1500 years after that. Before the intervention of surgical repair of the hernia, external supports called *trusses* were used to contain hernias that protruded from the body. A brief chronology of some of the events that laid the foundation for modern hernia repair is presented below.

| | |
|---|---|
| **2800 BC** | Herodotus reported that physicians specialized in treating hernia. |
| **1700 BC** | Hammurabi described hernia reduction. |
| **400 BC** | Hippocrates described hernia as a tear in the abdomen. |
| **200 BC** | Galen described anatomy of the abdominal wall. |
| **AD 100** | Celsus described clinical signs to differentiate a hernia from a hydrocele. |
| **1559** | Maupassius performed the first surgical intervention to correct a strangulated hernia. |
| **1724** | Heister described direct hernias. |
| **1814** | Scarpa described sliding hernias. |
| **1881** | Lucas-Championniere laid the basis for the most important inguinal hernia repair procedure—reinforcing the posterior wall of the inguinal canal and narrowing the internal inguinal ring. |
| **1887** | Bassini introduced his repair that sutured together the conjoined tendon and the inguinal ligament up to the inguinal ring; he is considered the father of modern-day hernia surgery. |
| **1898** | Lotheissen modified the Bassini repair, recommending the oblique internus and transversus abdominis muscles be attached to the Cooper ligament. (Cooper was the first to describe the superior pubic ligament, although he never used it to surgically repair a groin hernia.) |
| **1918** | Nursing textbook listed instruments for femoral, inguinal, umbilical, and ventral herniorrhaphy. |
| **1940** | Shouldice introduced multilayer closure; founded Shouldice Hospital near Toronto. Local anesthesia was used; patients walked to and from the operating room. |
| **1942** | McVay again described Lotheissen repair; it became known as the *McVay/Cooper repair.* |
| **1958** | Usher introduced use of "Marlex" mesh for repair of both primary and recurrent hernias, describing it as "tension-eliminating." |
| **1971** | Nursing textbook described the Gallie method, in which fascia lata is removed from the thigh and stitched around the hernial orifice. |
| **1982** | Ger performed the first laparoscopic herniorrhaphy. |

## RESEARCH HIGHLIGHT

### Possible Link Between Hernia Development and Smoking

While practicing with the Veterans' Administration in the early 1960s, R.C. Read, MD, performed an inguinal hernia repair on a 27-year-old male patient. At the time of surgery it was noted that he had a direct inguinal hernia and not the expected indirect hernia. The hernia had presented as groin pain and had developed during weight lifting. He had none of the known risk factors for hernia development but was a heavy smoker. Consequently, a research study was undertaken to examine samples of rectus sheath in other veterans undergoing hernia repair. Biochemical analysis revealed a collagen defect; further analysis identified damaged fibroblasts. The predominant common factor in the study cohort of veterans was that they were heavy smokers. The study suggested that hernia formation was the result of a disease process in which fibroblasts were impaired, with disarray of collagen fibers similar to that found in other disease states, including emphysema, $\alpha$1-antitrypsin deficiency, osteogenesis imperfecta, hereditary hyperextensibility, scurvy, varicose veins, and nicotine intoxication. By the 1980s, evidence was presented that the increased serum proteolytic activity was typical of the increased levels of polymorphonuclear leukocytes primed by the lung inflammation caused by smoking. Similar findings have also been found in patients with aortic aneurysm.

Modified from Read RC: Inguinal herniation in the adult, defect or disease: a surgeon's odyssey, *Pioneers in Hernia Surgery* 8:296-299, 2004.

ated structures in males and the round ligament in females, is approximately 4 cm long and takes an oblique course parallel to the groin crease. The inguinal canal is covered by the aponeurosis of the external abdominal oblique muscle, which forms a roof (Figure 13-3). A thickened lower border of the external oblique aponeurosis forms the inguinal (Poupart) ligament, which runs from the anterior superior iliac spine to the pubic tubercle.[14] Structures that traverse the inguinal canal enter it from the abdomen by the internal ring, a natural opening in the transversalis fascia, and exit by the external ring, an opening in the external oblique aponeurosis, to go to either the testis or the labium. If the external oblique aponeurosis is opened and the cord or round ligament is mobilized, the floor of the inguinal canal is exposed. The posterior inguinal floor is the structure that becomes defective and is susceptible to indirect, direct, or femoral hernias.

The key component of the important posterior inguinal floor is the transversalis muscle of the abdomen and its associated aponeurosis and fascia. The posterior inguinal floor can be divided into two areas. The superior lateral area represents the internal ring, whereas the inferior medial area represents the attachment of the transversalis aponeurosis and fascia to the Cooper ligament (iliopectineal line). The Cooper ligament is the site of the insertion of the transversalis aponeurosis along the superior ramus from the symphysis pubis laterally to the femoral sheath. The inguinal portion of the transversalis fascia arises from the iliopsoas fascia and not from the inguinal ligament.

Medially and superiorly the transversalis muscle becomes aponeurotic and fuses with the aponeurosis of the internal oblique muscle to form anterior and posterior rectus sheaths. As the symphysis pubis is approached, the contributions from the internal oblique muscle become fewer and fewer. At the pubic tubercle and behind the spermatic cord or round ligament, the internal oblique muscle makes no contribution and the posterior inguinal wall (floor of the inguinal canal) is composed solely of aponeurosis and fascia of the transversalis muscle.

None of the three groin hernias (direct and indirect inguinal hernias and femoral hernia) develops in the presence of a strong transversus abdominis layer and in the absence of per-

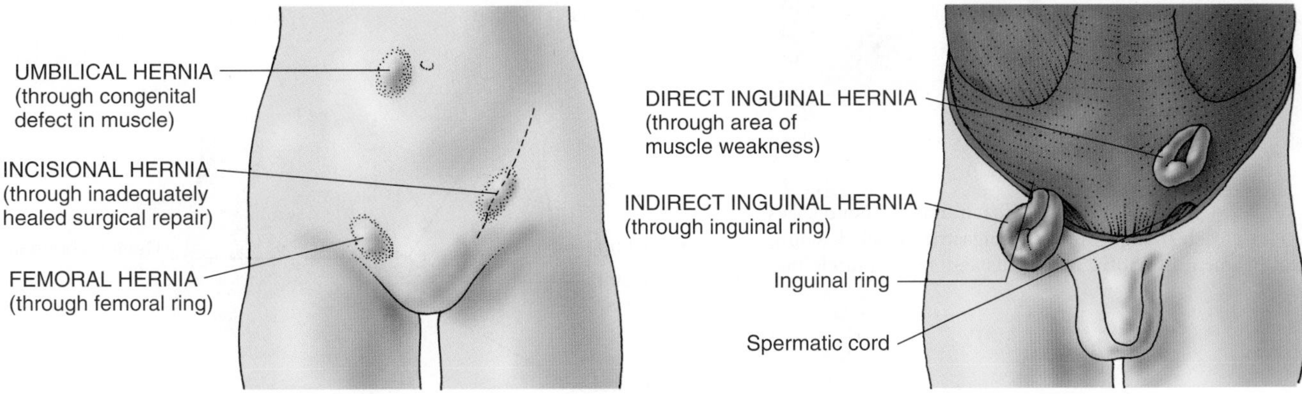


**FIGURE 13-1** Types of abdominal hernias.

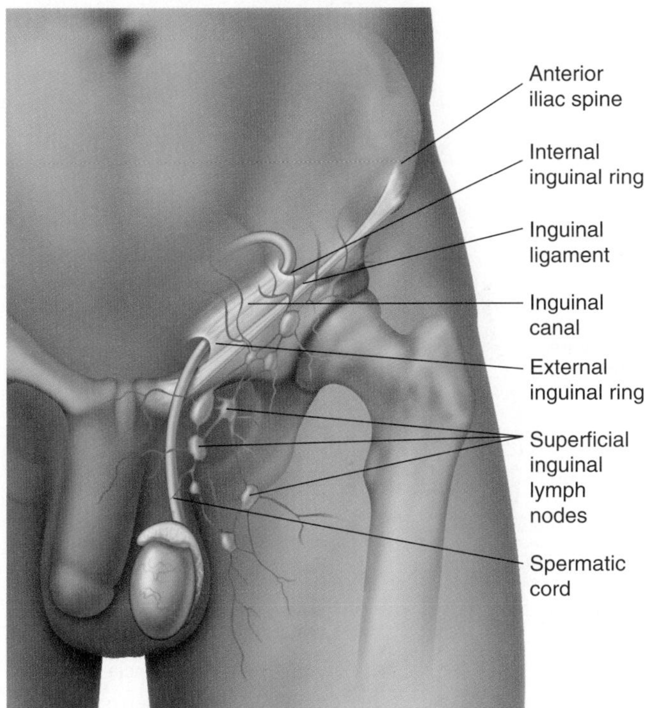


**FIGURE 13-2** Structures of the inguinal area.

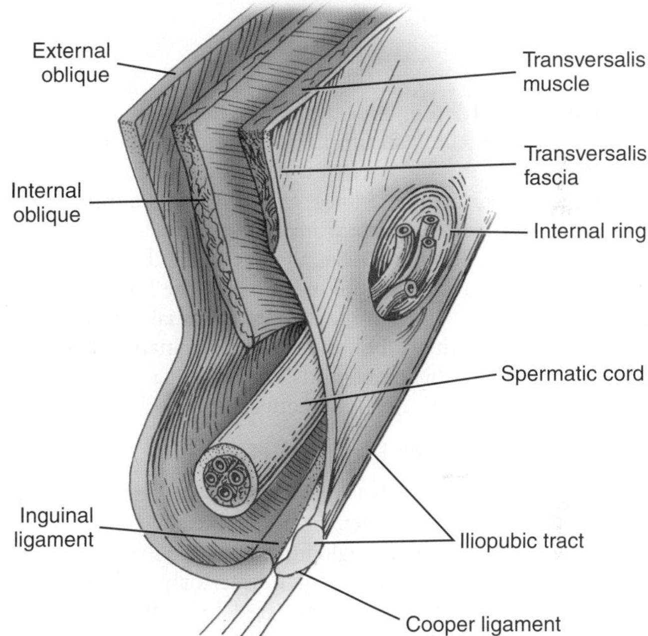


**FIGURE 13-3** Right inguinal region, parasagittal section. Roof of inguinal canal is formed by external oblique aponeurosis, and floor is formed by transversalis aponeurosis and fascia.

sistent stress on the connective tissue layers. When a weakening or a tear in the aponeurosis of the transversus abdominis and the transversalis fascia occurs, the potential for development of a direct inguinal hernia is established.

## Femoral Hernias

When the transversus abdominis aponeurosis and its fascia are only narrowly attached to the Cooper ligament, a femoral hernia may develop. This results in an enlarged femoral ring and canal, which allows for the prominence of the iliofemoral vessels, resulting in femoral herniation.[10]

The walls of the femoral sheath are formed anteriorly and medially from the transversalis fascia, posteriorly from the pectineus and psoas fascia, and laterally from the iliaca fascia. The pelvis ostium consists of a relatively fixed rim of bone and connective tissue: anteriorly and medially the iliopubic tract, posteriorly the superior ramus, and laterally the iliopectineal arch.

The femoral sheath is subdivided into three compartments. The lateral compartment contains the femoral artery, and the intermediate compartment contains the femoral vein. The medial compartment is the smallest and constitutes the femoral canal, which is formed anteriorly and medially by the iliopubic tract. This opening is bound laterally by the iliofemoral vessels and posteriorly by the superior pubic ramus and pectineus fascia. Superiorly, laterally, and inferiorly the fossa is formed by the falciform margin of the fascia lata.

## Abdominal Hernias

The anterior abdominal wall is composed of external abdominal oblique muscles attached to a thick sheath of connective tissue called the *rectus sheath*. The linea alba extends superi-

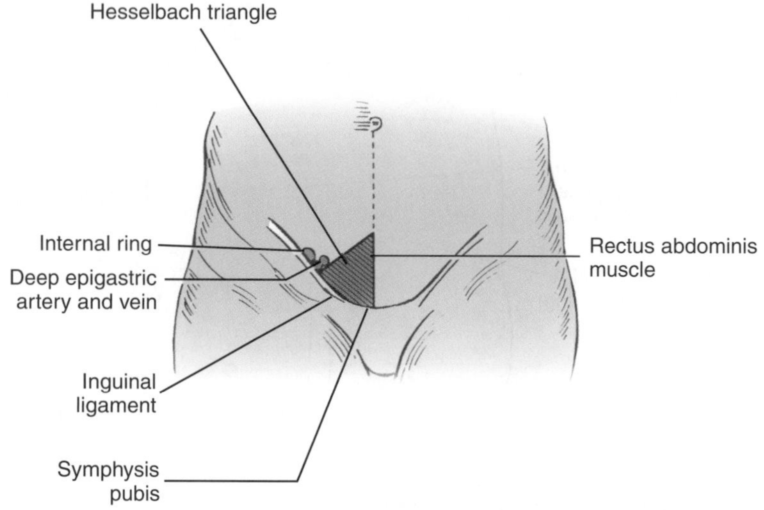


FIGURE 13-4 Schema of the Hesselbach triangle. Boundaries of the Hesselbach triangle are deep epigastric vessels laterally, inguinal ligament inferiorly, and rectus abdominis muscle medially.

orly and inferiorly from above the xiphoid process to the pubis. Beneath the rectus sheath lies the rectus abdominis muscles, laterally to the right and left of the linea alba. Lateral to the rectus abdominis is the linea semilunaris. The transversus abdominis muscles originate from the seventh to the twelfth costal cartilages, lumbar fascia, iliac crest, and the inguinal ligament and insert on the xiphoid process, the linea alba, and the pubic tubercle. The third layer of abdominal wall includes the internal abdominal oblique muscles originating from the iliac crest, inguinal ligament, and lumbar fascia and inserting on the tenth to twelfth ribs and rectus sheath.

## Direct and Indirect Inguinal Hernias

The deep epigastric vessels (inferior epigastric) arise from the external iliac vessels and enter the inguinal canal just proximal to the internal ring. The triangle formed by the deep epigastric vessels laterally, the inguinal ligament inferiorly, and the rectus abdominis muscles medially is referred to as the *Hesselbach triangle* (Figure 13-4).

Hernias that occur within the Hesselbach triangle are called *direct inguinal hernias*. Indirect inguinal hernias occur laterally to the deep epigastric vessels. Both direct and indirect hernias represent attenuations or tears in the transversalis fascia (Figure 13-5).

Direct hernias protrude into the inguinal canal but not into the cord and therefore rarely into the scrotum. Direct inguinal hernias usually result from heavy lifting or other strenuous activities. Indirect hernias leave the abdominal cavity at the internal inguinal ring and pass with the cord structures down the inguinal canal. Consequently the indirect hernia sac may be found in the scrotum. Indirect hernias may be either congenital, representing a persistence of the processus vaginalis, or acquired. In a congenital hernia, the hernia sac has a small neck, is thin-walled, and is closely bound to the cord structures. In an acquired indirect hernia, the neck is wide and the sac is both short and thick-walled. When both direct and indirect hernias are present, the defect is called a *pantaloon hernia* after the French word for "pants," which this situation suggests.

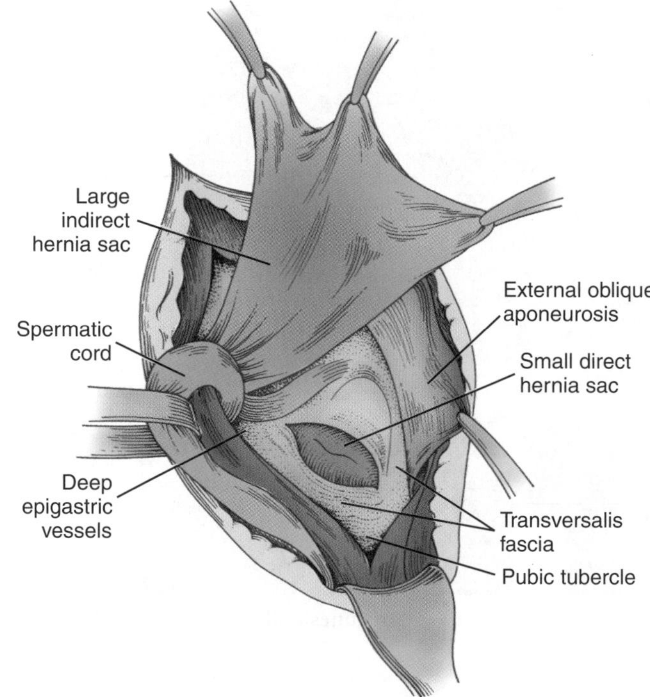


FIGURE 13-5 Defect in transversalis fascia, medial to deep epigastric vessels, gives rise to direct hernia. Defect lateral to deep epigastric vessels results in indirect hernia.

# *Perioperative Nursing Considerations*

## Assessment

A thorough assessment of the patient with a hernia begins with the history of previous surgeries related to the herniated area. Information relating to a familial history of hernias, the patient's nutritional status, when the symptoms occurred, a history of obesity, increased intraabdominal pressure, chronic cough, constipation, benign prostatic hypertrophy, intestinal obstruction, colon malignancy, and, for women, pregnancy should be obtained. A list of the patient's current medications should be collected, as well as a history of chronic illness and allergies, including latex allergies (because a Penrose drain may be used during the procedure). The patient's occupation and physical activities should also be determined.

Pain is often a notable symptom for the patient; it may be described as a burning sensation. An accurate description of the type and degree of pain is included in the assessment. Patients often describe the feeling of a foreign body, or mass, at the hernia site. This may appear on arising in the morning and disappear while sleeping.

The diagnosis of hernias should be accompanied by a clinical physical examination. Palpation of the herniated area reveals the contents of the hernia sac. Fingertip palpation allows the nurse to feel the edges of the external ring or abdominal wall. Having the patient stand and cough or prolonged strain during the examination also assists in the evaluation of the herniated area. If a definitive diagnosis is not confirmed, ultrasonic scanning and imaging techniques (e.g., computerized tomography [CT], herniography, standard radiography) may be employed.

In some patients, a hernia may cause no symptoms; its only sign may be a swelling or protrusion in a restricted area of the abdominal wall. If the hernia is unilateral, the patient notes the lack of a protrusion on the other side in comparison. The area may be visible when the patient stands or coughs and may disappear on reclining. Femoral hernias can be difficult to diagnose and may resemble an enlarged lymph node.

Preoperative testing for a hernia repair facilitates safe and efficient perioperative care. Baseline data are obtained by a complete blood count. Patients older than 40 years may need an electrocardiogram (ECG) and chest radiograph. Patients with a history of more complex medical problems must be fully evaluated with appropriate laboratory tests.

## Nursing Diagnosis

Nursing diagnoses related to the care of the patient undergoing hernia surgery might include the following:

- Activity Intolerance related to pain
- Risk for Urinary Retention
- Risk for Ineffective Tissue Perfusion of the scrotal area
- Deficient Knowledge related to disease process (hernia) and convalescence

## Outcome Identification

Outcome measurement and management are important parts of perioperative nursing care.[15] Outcomes identified for the selected nursing diagnoses could be stated as follows:

- The patient will return to previous level of activity.
- The patient will not experience urinary retention.
- The patient will be free of or manage scrotal edema.
- The patient and family or significant others will verbalize knowledge regarding disease process (hernia) and convalescence.

## Planning

The perioperative nurse formulates a plan of care for the patient undergoing herniorrhaphy by assimilating knowledge pertaining to the anatomy involved and principles of asepsis. Instrumentation, draping, and positioning for the patient's surgery depend on the type of hernia and repair to be performed—for example, open versus laparoscopic.

A Sample Plan of Care for a patient having surgery for repair of a hernia is shown on p. 398.

## Implementation

The patient may undergo general anesthesia, spinal or epidural block, regional anesthesia with sedation, or local anesthesia with sedation. Routine monitoring equipment, such as a three-lead or five-lead ECG, oxygen-saturation monitor, and blood pressure cuff, is used for a hernia repair. An intravenous (IV) line is inserted for fluid replacement and medication administration. The surgical site is marked as part of the preoperative verification process and rechecked during the time out.

The patient is usually positioned supine (see Chapter 5) with basic prepping and draping procedures followed (see Chapter 3). As with any surgical procedure, the prep solution must dry before the start of the surgical procedure as part of fire safety measures. To maintain the patient's dignity and modesty, expose only the part of the patient's body necessary for antimicrobial skin preparation.[4] Instruments used for herniorrhaphies are those found in standard laparotomy sets, laparoscopy sets, or minor sets.

A self-retaining retractor, such as a Weitlaner, facilitates the separation of tissue layers. A moistened Penrose drain is used to retract the spermatic cord structures for better exposure. Because the peritoneal cavity may be entered in this procedure, sponge, sharp, and instrument counts are performed.

With a sliding hernia or an incarcerated hernia, the possibility of having to enter the peritoneal cavity must be considered. If the hernia is strangulated, necrotic bowel must be resected and instruments for doing a bowel anastomosis must be ready. For this procedure, antibiotics may be added to the irrigation to prevent an infection.

Repair of an inguinal hernia includes approximation of the transversalis fascia with a heavy nonabsorbable type of suture; mesh may also be used. With some indirect hernias, only 2 or 3 sutures may be necessary. In other cases, however, up to 10 sutures in succession may be needed. Scarpa fascia is approximated with absorbable sutures, and the skin is closed by one of several methods. Several types of prosthetic mesh are available to support hernia repair.

A laparoscopic hernia repair is technically similar to an open laparotomy, but the instrumentation includes laparoscopic equipment. There is always a possibility that a laparoscopy may become a laparotomy, and instrumentation for this change in procedure must always be available.

## Evaluation

Evaluation of the patient having repair of a hernia should include examination of all skin surfaces to assess variances with the preoperative assessment data. The patient should awaken from general anesthesia, if it is used, in a reasonable amount of time without exhibiting signs of anxiety or extreme disorientation. Extubation should be timely to avoid stress on the repaired hernia site. The evaluation of the patient's status can be phrased in outcome statements such as the following:

- The patient will return to previous level of activity.
- The patient will not experience urinary retention or scrotal edema.

## SAMPLE PLAN OF CARE

**NURSING DIAGNOSIS**
**Activity Intolerance** related to pain

**OUTCOME**
The patient will return to previous level of activity.

**INTERVENTIONS**
- Determine the patient's baseline activity level.
- Encourage early postoperative ambulation.
- Instruct the patient to use prescribed pain medications before physical activity and as needed.
- Advise the patient to gradually increase activity as tolerated.
- Explain anticipated postoperative activity recommendations and limitations (Patient and Family Education).

**NURSING DIAGNOSIS**
**Risk for Urinary Retention**

**OUTCOME**
The patient will not experience urinary retention.

**INTERVENTIONS**
- Encourage patient to void before surgery.
- Monitor and record intake and output status.
- Assess postoperatively bladder for signs of urinary retention (palpable bladder or patient discomfort).
- Encourage and assist patient with early ambulation.
- Maintain adequate oral fluid intake without nausea or vomiting before discontinuing IV fluids.
- Catheterize the patient if urinary retention occurs.

**NURSING DIAGNOSIS**
**Risk for Ineffective Tissue Perfusion** of the scrotal area causing scrotal edema and ecchymosis

**OUTCOME**
The patient will not experience any scrotal edema or ecchymosis.

**INTERVENTIONS**
- Discuss the possibility of swelling and ecchymosis during preoperative assessment.
- Apply scrotal support intraoperatively.
- Assess scrotum for evidence of swelling, ecchymosis, and redness.
- Apply ice packs as prescribed.
- Elevate the scrotum on a soft pillow to prevent or control swelling.
- Reassure the patient, and instruct him on the importance of wearing the scrotal support.
- Reassure the patient that the swelling and ecchymosis will subside.

**NURSING DIAGNOSIS**
**Deficient Knowledge** related to disease process (hernia) and convalescence

**OUTCOME**
The patient and family or significant others will verbalize an understanding of the disease process (hernia) and convalescence.

**INTERVENTIONS**
- Review possible contributing factors (as individualized for type of hernia and specific patient) to hernia formation.
- Discuss postoperative pain-management strategies during recovery at home.
- Describe and verify patient understanding of surgical site or incision care and reportable signs and symptoms (temperature, wound redness, tenderness at incision site, swelling, drainage). Use language such as "Can you tell me, in your own words, how you will take care of this at home and when you should call your doctor?"
- Determine patient's dietary habits; discuss importance of fiber (fruits, vegetables, grains) to prevent constipation.
- Provide written discharge instructions. Review these with patient and family or significant others to validate understanding.
- Provide opportunity for "teach back" (Patient Safety) by the patient or family. Have them repeat discharge instructions in their own words.
- Allow time for questions; provide (or reinforce) answers and clarification.
- Verify that patient has or knows how to schedule follow-up appointment.

- The patient will remain free of or manage scrotal edema.
- The patient and family or significant others will verbalize understanding of hernia and recommendations for convalescence and will be able to describe possible complications (infection, seroma formation, hematoma, or postoperative neuralgia) that are to be reported to the physician.

The perioperative nurse gives a hand-off report to the postanesthesia care unit (PACU) nurse pertaining to relevant events and patient status during the operative procedure.

Urinary retention may occur after a herniorrhaphy, and measures must be taken to prevent overdistention of the bladder. Early ambulation is encouraged to facilitate resumption of bladder and bowel functions. If the bowel has been resected because of strangulation, a nasogastric tube and suction may be required to reduce the incidence of postoperative vomiting and distention with subsequent strain on the suture line.

## Patient and Family Education and Discharge Planning

Greater involvement of patients in their care increases the likelihood of achieving the best outcomes and simultaneously supports a quality-improved, cost-conscious environment. For the hernia patient to assume such responsibilities, plans for patient and family education along with plans for discharge and home recovery need to be designed. Options such as open or laparoscopic repair techniques, surgical and recovery times, analgesic requirements, complication rates, and times for return to full activity become part of informed consent (Patient Safety). Once the patient and surgeon have decided on the surgical approach, the perioperative nursing responsibilities for teaching the patient initial postoperative management strategies become crucial. Preferably, discharge planning is begun before admission. This becomes increasingly important because hernia repair is commonly performed as an ambulatory procedure. Anticipated postoperative care, including incision care, incisional splinting as appropriate to the repair approach, and the importance of early ambulation and deep breathing, is reviewed. Pain management is important as a part of discharge planning; frequently, surgical patients report inadequate pain management during their postoperative recovery and convalescence. The Patient and Family Education box presents specific home care requirements. Perioperative nurses may also participate in the development of critical paths for specific diagnoses or surgical procedures such as hernia repair; these have the goals of reducing patient complication rates, controlling resource utilization, decreasing errors, and enhancing patient education and satisfaction.

## PATIENT AND FAMILY EDUCATION

### Home Care for the Hernia Patient

**HOME CARE**

- Give the patient and the caregiver *verbal* and *written* instructions. Provide them with the name and telephone number of a physician or nurse to call if questions arise.
- General information
  - Review any explanation about the procedure and specific follow-up care.
  - Explain and discuss the development of hernias, causes or contributing factors, care and treatment, and prevention.
- Wound/incision care
  - Discuss and demonstrate proper wound management and dressing changes: procedures, frequency, and signs to report.
- Warning signs
  - Stress the importance of seeking emergency care if bleeding from the incision or wound dehiscence with exposure of deep wound tissue occurs.
  - Review the signs and symptoms that should be reported to a physician or nurse.
    - Infection: fever, pain, edema, erythema, warmth, purulent drainage, foul odor from the incision
    - Abdominal distention, nausea, vomiting
    - Separation of wound edges
    - Hernia recurrence: firm, tender, globular, irreducible swelling in the groin or midabdomen
- Special instructions
  - Apply and demonstrate to the male patient scrotal support or ice packs to decrease scrotal edema and discomfort.
  - Assist the patient in obtaining appropriate supplies, such as sterile dressings.
  - Advise patient with diabetes that optimal glucose control promotes wound healing.
- Medications
  - Explain the purpose, dosage, schedule, and route of administration of any prescribed drugs, as well as side effects to report to a physician or nurse.
    - Analgesics
    - Stool softeners
    - Laxatives
- Activity
  - Encourage the patient to discuss allowances and limitations with respect to occupation, recreation, or activities.
  - Instruct the patient to avoid coughing, straining, stretching, constipation, heavy lifting (>10 lb), strenuous exercise, and sports for 6 weeks.
  - Demonstrate splinting the incision manually or with a pillow during coughing, sneezing, or hiccups.
  - Stress the importance of activity restrictions and splinting the incision for up to 6 weeks after surgery.
  - Demonstrate proper body mechanics for moving and lifting.
  - Advise returning to work in 2 weeks for desk work and 6 weeks for heavy labor.
  - Advise that sexual activity should be avoided for several weeks to avoid strain on the incision and discomfort to the scrotum, if edematous.
- Diet
  - Advise the patient to plan a high-fiber diet to help prevent constipation; provide the patient with a list of high-fiber foods.
  - Advise the patient to drink plenty of fluids, up to 2 to 3 liters per day, unless contraindicated.
  - Stress the importance of weight loss if the patient is obese.

**ALTERNATIVE THERAPY**

- Advise patient to avoid yoga exercises for 6 weeks postoperatively.
- Advise patient and family to refrain from applying lotions and creams to the incision until wound edges are completely closed and healed.
- Discuss strategies for pain management, including music therapy and guided imagery, to minimize use of narcotics, which can cause constipation.

**ELDER CARE**

- The older adult may be at greater risk for delayed wound healing because of preexisting cardiac disease or nutritional deficits.
- Vitamin supplements may promote wound healing, if not contraindicated.

**PSYCHOSOCIAL CARE**

- Encourage the verbalization of fears and concerns about altered sexual function secondary to impaired blood supply to the vas deferens.
- Encourage active participation in plan of care.

**FOLLOW-UP CARE**

- Stress the importance of regular follow-up visits. Make sure the patient has the necessary names and telephone numbers.
- Stress the importance of smoking cessation to eliminate the smoker's cough as a contributing factor to hernia development.

**REFERRAL**

- Provide information and refer the patient to community resources for weight loss and smoking cessation, if indicated.

From Canobbio MM: *Mosby's handbook of patient teaching,* ed 3, St Louis, 2006, Mosby.

PATIENT SAFETY

**Surgical Consent and "Teaching Back"**

The National Quality Forum (NQF) has identified Safe Practice 10 for informed consent, recommending that each patient (or legal surrogate) be asked to "teach back" what he or she has been told during the informed consent discussion. Elements of Safe Practice 10 include the following:

- Physicians, nurses, and interpreters, along with others who communicate with the patient in the informed consent process, should use "teach back" strategies.
- Patients should be able to explain, in everyday words and in their primary language, the following:
  - Diagnosis or health problem
  - Name, type, and general nature of treatment or procedure
  - Its risks, benefits, and alternatives

"Teach back" should occur well before the day of surgery, whenever possible, so that patients have time to think about their options and make informed choices. "Teach back" assists the surgeon and perioperative nurse in gauging how well patients understand and whether informed consent was really given.

Modified from Wu HW and others: *Improving patient safety through informed consent for patients with limited health literacy,* Washington, DC, 2005, National Quality Forum.

# *Surgical Interventions*

## SURGERY FOR REPAIR OF GROIN HERNIAS

### Repair of Inguinal Hernias

Several operative procedures for repair of inguinal hernias are currently used. Approaches that reestablish the integrity of the transversalis fascia and simultaneously reestablish and strengthen the posterior inguinal floor are favored. A surgical repair in which transversalis fascia is sewn to the Poupart ligament accomplishes this goal.

***Procedural Considerations.*** The patient is in the supine position for abdominal wall and inguinal or femoral hernia repairs. The patient's skin surface area from above the umbilicus to midthigh is exposed, prepped with antimicrobial solutions, and draped with sterile drapes. A sterile drape should be placed under the scrotum if it becomes necessary to enter the scrotum.

#### *Operative Procedures*

**MCVAY, OR COOPER LIGAMENT, REPAIR.** A McVay, or Cooper ligament, repair approximates transversalis fascia superior to the inferior insertion of the transversalis fascia along the Cooper ligament. It is accompanied by a relaxing incision to reduce tension on the suture line.

1. A transverse suprainguinal skinfold incision is made; some surgeons prefer an oblique incision, made parallel to the inguinal ligament, ending two fingerbreadths lateral to the pubic tubercle (Figure 13-6).
2. The incision is carried through the superficial and deep (Scarpa) fascia to the external oblique aponeurosis. Hemostasis is maintained with fine ties or electrocoagulation.
3. The external oblique aponeurosis is opened by way of a small incision over the inguinal canal, lateral to the inguinal ring, in the direction of its fibers, to the external ring. The aponeurotic flaps are reflected back along the iliohypogastric and ilioinguinal nerves, which are identified and preserved from injury (see Figure 13-6). The ilioinguinal nerve is a sensory nerve that innervates the medial thigh and the scrotum.
4. The cremaster muscles that form an envelope around the spermatic cord and represent the continuation of the internal oblique muscles are opened, and the cord is exposed. The medial fibrous portion of the internal oblique is called the *conjoined tendon.*
5. The cord and surrounding structures are dissected and freed circumferentially from the canal, and a moistened Penrose drain is often used to gently retract the vessels and vas deferens. The cord is then examined for an indirect hernia, the sac of which is located adjacent to the cord; the sac originates from the internal ring lateral to the inferior epigastric vessels and is initially adherent to the cord.
6. If an indirect sac is identified, it is carefully dissected away from the cord until the neck of the hernia is clearly delineated (Figure 13-7).
7. The sac is opened, and any abdominal contents are returned to the peritoneal cavity.
8. A suture ligature or purse-string suture is placed high in the neck of the sac, and the excess peritoneum of the hernia is excised. The ligated stump quickly retracts into the peritoneal cavity. (If the sac is long, the distal segment may be splayed open and left in place.) The inguinal floor is then inspected for evidence of a direct hernia. If only a direct sac is present, usually no resection of the hernia is done because the sac easily returns to the abdominal cavity.
9. If transversalis fascia is present on both sides of the hernia defect, it is sutured together or a piece of mesh is interposed (Figure 13-8). Suturing begins at the pubic tubercle and continues laterally to the internal ring. If the inferior transversalis fascia is weak or not present, the superior portion is sutured to the Cooper ligament, the site of insertion of the transversalis fascia. In this case, suturing again begins at the pubic tubercle and is continued laterally along the Cooper ligament to the medial border of the femoral sheath, where a transition stitch is placed. The repair is then carried laterally, approximating transversalis fascia to inguinal ligament (Figure 13-9).
10. When the transversalis fascia is pulled down to the Cooper ligament, a relaxing incision in the rectus sheath is sometimes necessary to relieve excess tension. Essentially this incision is 5 to 7 cm long in the anterior rectus sheath. The incision begins immediately above the pubic crest, approximately 1 cm from the midline, and extends cephalad, following the line of fusion of the external oblique aponeurosis with the rectus sheath. The posterior rectus sheath

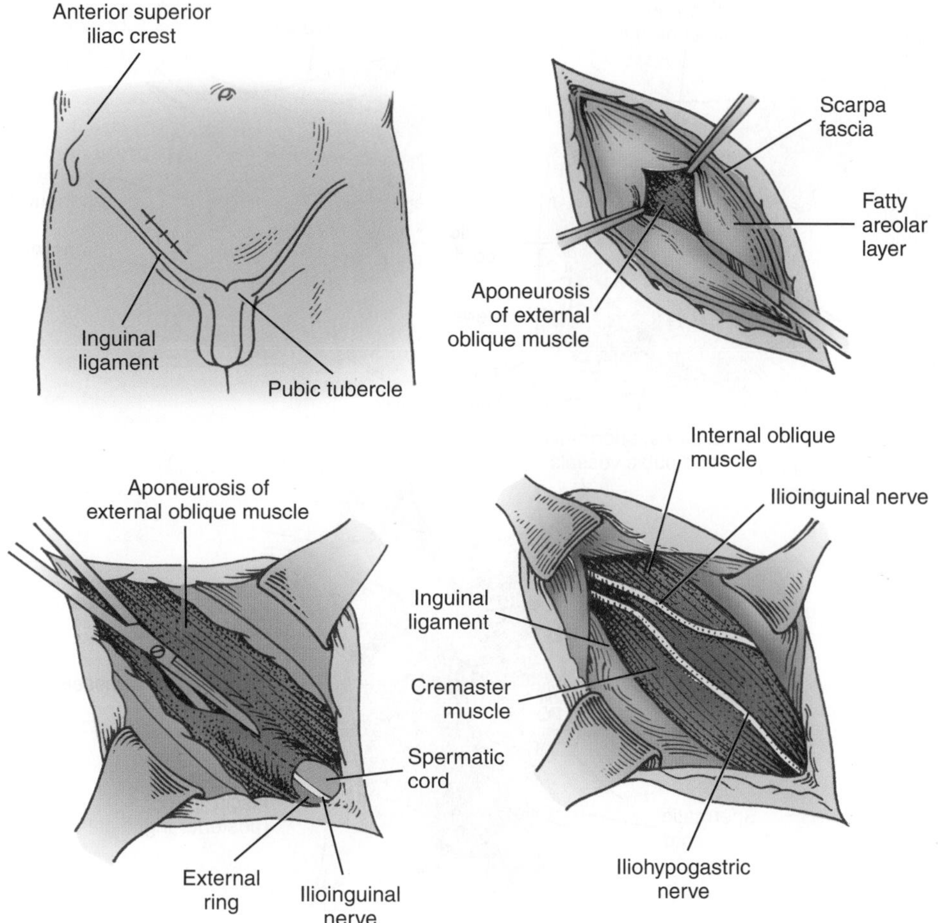


**FIGURE 13-6** Skin incision with division of superficial muscle and fascial layers.

and the rectus muscle itself guard against later herniation at the point where the relaxing incision is made. If too much tension makes direct approximation undesirable, a synthetic surgical mesh may be sutured in place as the new inguinal floor ("tension-free" mesh repair). The caudad edge of the mesh is sutured to the shelving edge of the inguinal ligament, the cephalad edge sutured to the conjoined tendon, and the lateral edge of the mesh split to accommodate the spermatic cord.[8]

11. After the integrity of the posterior inguinal floor has been reestablished, the cremaster muscles are reapproximated around the cord. Repair is completed with the approximation of the external oblique aponeurosis, the Scarpa fascia, and the skin.

BASSINI REPAIR. The Bassini repair was introduced in 1887 and was formerly the standard of repair. In this procedure the conjoined tendon and the shelving edge of the inguinal ligament are sutured together up to the internal ring.[3] The major difference with this repair is that the superior transversalis fascia is sutured to the inguinal ligament with no attempt made to approximate it to the inferior portion of the transversalis fascia or Cooper ligament (pectineal ligament). Critics of this procedure claim that it is not anatomic because layers that originally are not one (transversalis fascia and inguinal ligament) now are approximated. Nonetheless, this repair has been used successfully by many surgeons.

SHOULDICE REPAIR. More than 250,000 hernias have been repaired at the Shouldice hospital in Ontario, Canada, with a recurrence rate of less than 1%. In the Shouldice repair a double layer of transversalis fascia is sutured to the inguinal ligament. It is reinforced by a layer of internal oblique muscle and conjoined tendon approximated to the undersurface of the fascia of the external oblique.

MESH-PLUG REPAIR. The mesh-plug technique has been recommended for the treatment of primary and recurrent direct and indirect inguinal hernias. The various hernia types as classified by Gilbert have a corresponding relationship to the use of mesh plugs.[7] Types I, II, and III are indirect hernias. Type I is characterized by a tight internal ring through which any size peritoneal sac can pass. The sac, when surgically reduced, is held within the abdominal cavity by the intact internal ring. Type II hernias have a moderately enlarged internal ring, 4 cm or smaller. Type III hernias have a patulous internal ring larger than 4 cm. In this type, the sac can have a sliding component that impinges on the direct space. Type IV and type V hernias are direct hernias. In type IV hernias, the defect involves virtually the entire floor of the inguinal canal. Type V is a diverticular defect of the floor and is generally in a suprapubic position, resembling a punched-out recurrent hernia. Type VI includes components of both indirect and direct hernias. Femoral hernias are classified as type VII.

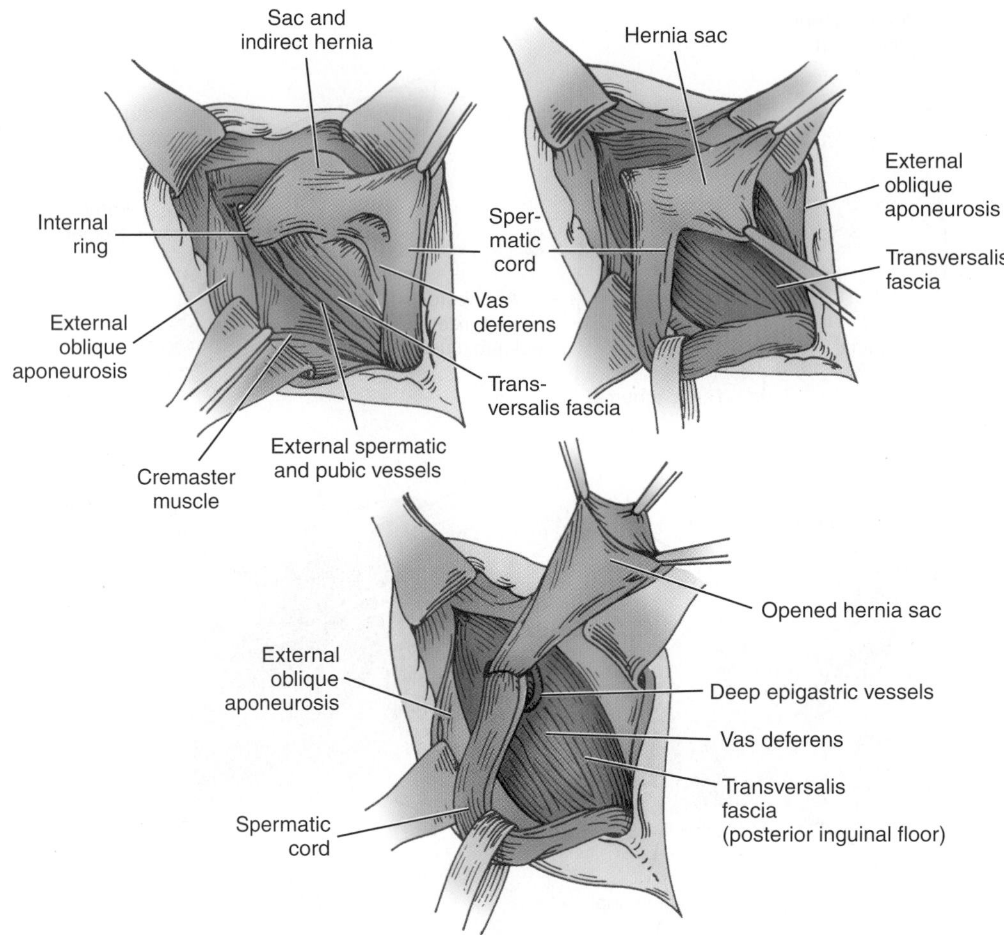


**FIGURE 13-7** Indirect hernia sac is identified along with cord structures and dissected away from cord. Neck of hernia sac is clearly delineated, and sac is opened to check for abdominal contents.

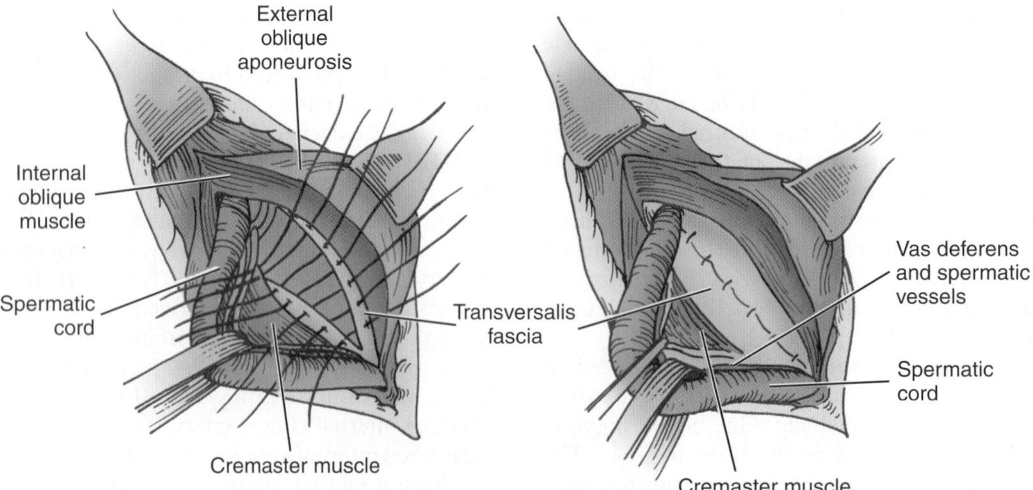


**FIGURE 13-8** Transversalis fascia on either side of large hernia defect is approximated.

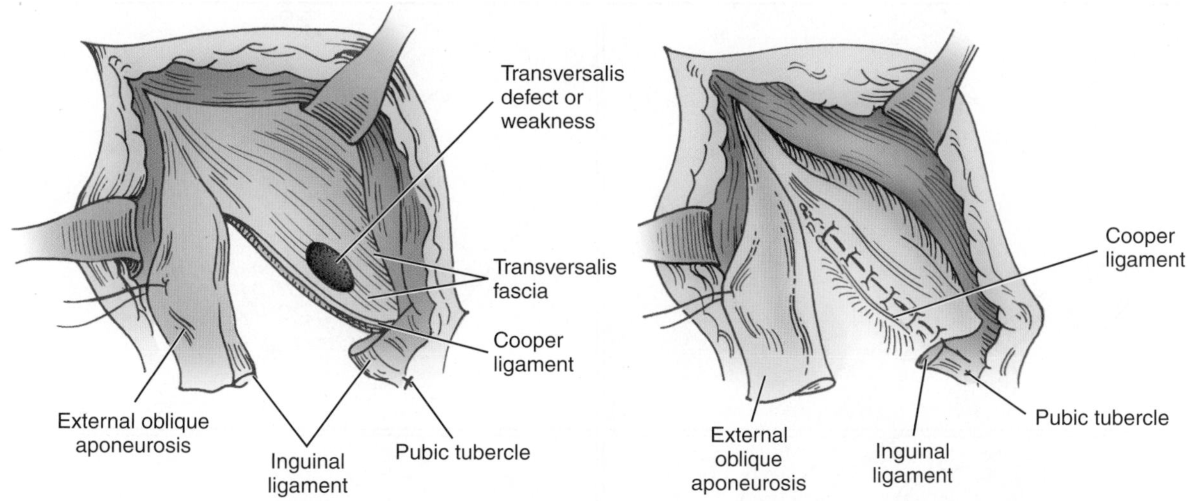


**FIGURE 13-9** Defect in transversalis fascia repaired by approximation of fascia to Cooper ligament.

Regardless of the hernia type, the mesh-plug technique is performed on an ambulatory basis, through a small incision. Repair of inguinal hernias with the mesh-plug technique has provided significant advantages when compared with conventional suture technique. A plug repair requires less overall dissection, has a decreased chance of nerve injury, and ensures a tension-free hernioplasty. These factors increase patient comfort, speed rehabilitation, and contribute to a very low recurrence rate.

**Surgical Technique Using the PerFix Plug**

1. An oblique incision, 6 cm in length, is made, and the external oblique fascia is opened through the external ring. Exposure is obtained by use of a self-retaining retractor (e.g., a Beckmann); a handheld retractor such as a Gouley may also be required. Hemostasis is usually achieved with the use of electrocoagulation.
2. The spermatic cord is mobilized, as previously described in the McVay repair. The ilioinguinal and genital femoral nerves are identified and preserved. The medial external oblique fascia is separated from the underlying transversus abdominis aponeurosis with a sweeping motion of the index finger.
3. An indirect sac and any lipoma of the cord are dissected free (Figure 13-10, *A*). The sac and lipoma are allowed to drop back through the internal ring and into the abdominal cavity. Rarely is the sac opened except for incarcerated hernias.
4. Using the Gilbert classification, the internal ring is sized and the tapered end of the mesh plug is inserted through the internal ring and positioned just beneath the crura. The plug is designed such that its fluted outer layer, combined with its inside configuration of eight mesh petals, maintains its overall contour while allowing it to conform tension-free to the configuration of the internal ring (Figure 13-10, *B*).
5. *Repair of indirect hernias.* Type I indirect hernias require 1 or 2 synthetic absorbable sutures; in types II and III hernias, more sutures are required because of the increased size of the internal ring.
6. *Repair of direct hernias.* In direct hernias, the fusiform or saccular defect is circumscribed near its base with an electrosurgical device and the hernia is reduced, providing a surrounding margin of intact tissue for securing the plug. The plug is then inserted through the floor of the defect (Figure 13-10, *C*). With types IV and V (direct) hernias, the mesh plug is routinely secured with up to 10 interrupted synthetic absorbable sutures. Where there are both indirect and direct hernias (type VI), two mesh plugs may be needed. Type VII defects are treated similarly with mesh plugs.
7. *Repair of femoral hernias.* In femoral hernias, a small or medium-size plug is secured in position after the sac has been reduced.
8. In most types of mesh-plug hernia repairs, a second piece of flat mesh is used for reinforcement. The piece is cut to match the shape of the inguinal canal and then placed without sutures on the anterior surface of the posterior wall of the inguinal canal. The proximal portion is split to provide an opening for the spermatic cord, and the mesh tails are brought together with sutures to form a new internal ring (Figure 13-10, *D*).
9. With the spermatic cord structures placed on top of this flat mesh, the external oblique fascia is reapproximated over the structures with a running synthetic nonabsorbable suture.
10. An interrupted suture of a similar size is used to bring the subcutaneous tissue together, and the skin is closed with a subcuticular stitch.

**LAPAROSCOPIC HERNIA REPAIRS.** Ger was the first surgeon to perform a laparoscopic herniorrhaphy. In 1982 he described a laparoscopic transabdominal hernia approach. Variations in techniques for laparoscopic hernia repair continue to develop as surgeons gain experience with these procedures.

Three techniques are used today for laparoscopic herniorrhaphy. These are the transabdominal preperitoneal patch (TAPP) repair, the totally extraperitoneal patch (TEP) repair, and the intraperitoneal onlay mesh (IPOM) repair. The differ-

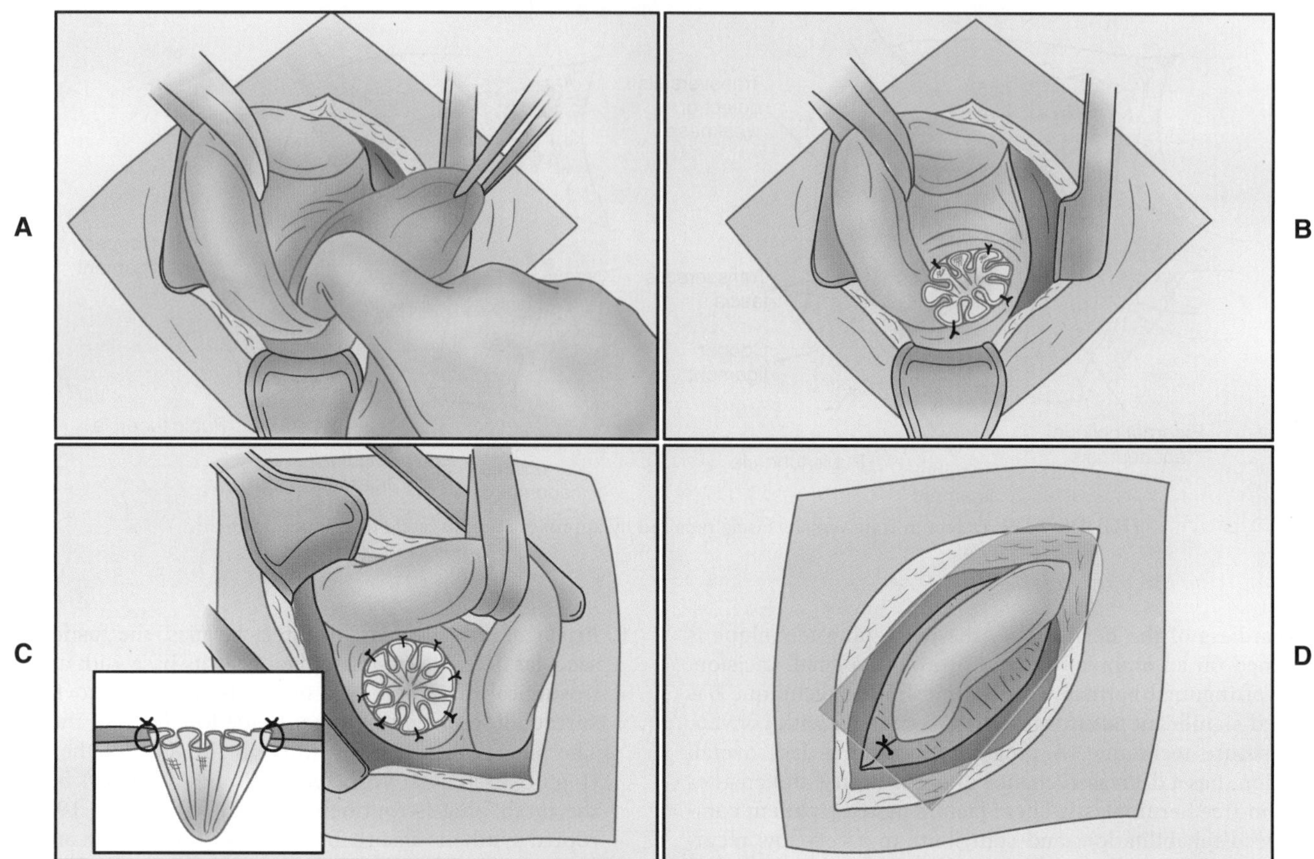


**FIGURE 13-10** Mesh-plug repair using the PerFix Plug. **A,** The hernia sac is dissected free of the cord structure to the level of the internal ring. **B,** Typically, a large plug is used. Some of the internal petals may be removed if the plug is too bulky. **C,** Large or extra-large PerFix Plug is inserted. The plug should not be stretched to fill the defect. Typically, 8 to 10 sutures are used. **D,** Sutureless onlay patch. The tails of the onlay patch are taken around the cord and sutured together. The onlay patch is not sutured to the floor of the inguinal canal.

## RESEARCH HIGHLIGHT

### Comparison of Types of Hernia Repair[11]

This study was done to determine whether laparoscopic methods are more effective and cost-effective than open mesh methods of inguinal hernia repair. A secondary analysis was an exploration of whether laparoscopic transabdominal preperitoneal patch (TAPP) repair was more effective and cost-effective than laparoscopic totally extraperitoneal patch (TEP) repair. Laparoscopic repair was associated with a faster return to usual activities and less persisting pain and numbness. There also appeared to be fewer cases of wound or superficial infection and hematoma. However, operation times were longer, and there appears to be a higher rate of serious complications (e.g., bowel, bladder, and vascular injuries). Mesh infection is very uncommon, with similar rates noted among the surgical approaches. There is no apparent difference in the rate of hernia recurrence. The increased adoption of laparoscopic techniques may allow patients to return to usual activities faster. Economic savings in the form of fewer days of work missed and reduced worker's compensation have been reported.

Modified from McCormack K and others: Laparoscopic surgery for inguinal hernia repair: systematic review of effectiveness and economic evaluation, *Health Technology Assessment* 9(1):218, 2005.

ence between TAPP and TEP is the manner in which access is gained to the preperitoneal space. The TAPP uses intraperitoneal trocars and the creation of a peritoneal flap over the posterior inguinal region. TEP provides access to the preperitoneal space without entering the peritoneal cavity (Research Highlight).

Studies indicating long-term postoperative hernia recurrence and complication rates with these approaches vary. The average recurrence rate for TAPP ranges from 2% to 7%; for TEP it approximates 1.8%.[1] Although recurrence rates are decreasing, postoperative pain has been recognized as a major complication (Best Practice).[6] A laparoscopic hernia repair allegedly has the advantages of a quicker return to normal activity and some reduction of postoperative adhesions related to the minimal dissection required. A recent analysis of postoperative pain and paresthesia associated with laparoscopic hernia repair revealed that most patients experience minimal immediate postoperative pain and, after postoperative day 1, have little or no need for analgesics.[5] The American Hernia Society recommends that laparoscopic inguinal hernia repair be undertaken when recurrent and bilateral hernias are present.[8] In general, the procedure requires the placement of operative cameras and ports, identification of the inguinal floor, removal of an indirect hernia sac, mesh to fit around the spermatic cord and form a new inguinal floor, and port closure.[10]

## BEST PRACTICE

### Assessing Postoperative Pain in Hernia Patients

As rates of hernia recurrence have been reduced, particularly with the use of mesh, chronic postoperative pain is emerging as a major complication that requires investigation. The incidence of some degree of long-term groin pain after surgery was as high as 53% in a review of inguinal herniorrhaphy studies between 1987 and 2000. Chronic pain was noted without regard to the type of repair performed and was most likely a consequence of scarring, reaction to prosthetic material, or incorporation of a nerve in staples of suture material during the repair. Careful consideration must be given to determine whether the postoperative pain is the same as or different from the pain that brought the hernia to the attention of the surgeon initially. Of the various diagnostic procedures, magnetic resonance imaging (MRI) has been proven to be the most successful tool to assist the surgeon in differentiating among muscle tears, osteitis pubis, bursitis, a stress fracture, or a strain in the adductor muscle complex.

Modified from Fitzgibbons RJ and others: What's new in ACS surgery—open hernia repair. In *ACS surgery: principles & practice,* 2003. Accessed July 25, 2005, on-line: www.medscape.com/viewarticle/463738.

**Operative Procedure—Totally Extraperitoneal Patch (TEP) Approach** (Figure 13-11)

1. An infraumbilical incision is made. The anterior rectus sheath is incised and the ipsilateral rectus abdominis muscle is retracted laterally.
2. With blunt dissection, a space is created beneath the rectus.
3. A dissecting balloon is inserted deep to the posterior rectus sheath, advanced to the pubic symphysis, and inflated under direct laparoscopic vision.
4. The space is opened and insufflated, and additional trocars are placed.
5. Using a 30-degree telescope, the inferior epigastric vessels and lower portion of the rectus sheath are identified and retracted anteriorly.
6. The Cooper ligament is cleared from the pubic symphysis medially to the level of the external iliac vein.
7. The iliopubic tract is identified. Care is taken to avoid injury to the femoral branch of the genitofemoral nerve and the lateral femoral cutaneous nerve.
8. Lateral dissection is carried out to the anterior superior iliac.
9. The spermatic cord is skeletonized.
10. A *direct hernia sac* is gently reduced by retraction if it has not already been reduced by balloon expansion of the peritoneal space. A *small indirect sac* is mobilized from the spermatic cord and reduced into the peritoneal cavity. *A large sac* may be divided with electrocoagulation near the internal ring. The proximal peritoneal sac is closed with a loop ligature to prevent pneumoperitoneum from occurring. A piece of polypropylene mesh is inserted, unfolded to cover the direct, indirect, and femoral spaces and rest over the cord structures, and carefully secured with a tacking stapler.

**REPAIR OF INGUINAL HERNIAS IN FEMALES.** Regardless of the specific technique used, the initial approach to the repair of a hernia in the female is the same as that used in the male. After the cremaster muscles are opened to expose the round ligament, variations that may be encountered include the following: (1) with the sac exposed and cleared from the round ligament, the round ligament and accompanying vessels are dissected free from the inguinal floor to the labium; (2) at the labium the round ligament is clamped, ligated, and divided; (3) the sac at the internal ring is opened, checked to be sure that no abdominal contents are present, and ligated at its neck, together with the round ligament and associated vessels; or (4) the sac distal to the ligature is removed with the distal round ligament, while the ligated stump retracts promptly into the abdomen. The remainder of the repair is the same as that previously described.

**REPAIR OF FEMORAL HERNIAS.** A femoral hernia protrudes from the groin below the inguinal ligament into the thigh (Figure 13-12). In its most obvious form, a femoral hernia is an inflamed, tender mass below the inguinal ligament. Unfortunately, the presentation is frequently more subtle and the diagnosis is completely missed or confused with enlarged inguinal lymph nodes, a psoas muscle abscess, a saphenous varix, a lipoma, or an indirect or direct inguinal hernia. The defect is usually small and frequently nonreducible. Femoral hernias are highly likely to become incarcerated and strangulated; elective repair is clearly indicated unless serious contraindications to surgery exist.

**Operative Procedure.** The general approach is surgical treatment to free the tightly bound hernia, closely examine the contents of the hernia for ischemic change, and repair the hernia defect. The principles for repair of this type of hernia are the same as those described for inguinal herniorrhaphies. Ultimately, the defect must be obliterated. Repair of a femoral hernia requires approximating the aponeurotic margins of the femoral canal. The sutures are placed through the iliopubic tract superiorly and through the Cooper ligament and pectineus fascia inferiorly. Care is taken to not compromise the femoral artery and vein.

**PREPERITONEAL (PROPERITONEAL) REPAIR—OPEN APPROACH.** Preperitoneal (properitoneal) repair also is based on the essential role of the transversalis fascia in the cause and subsequent correction of a hernia. This repair is suitable for direct, indirect, and femoral hernias. It is particularly applicable in dealing with recurrent hernias and bilateral hernias, because exposure is obtained by operating through virgin surgical fields rather than through previous scars.

**Operative Procedure**

1. A transverse incision is made 2 cm above the symphysis pubis, through the rectus abdominis muscle on the affected side (Figure 13-13, *A*).
2. The wound is deepened by cutting the external oblique, internal oblique, and transversalis muscles.
3. The transversalis fascia is then cut, and the preperitoneal space is entered. This is the proper plane of dissection for the remainder of the operation.
4. Retraction on the lower side of the incision reveals the posterior inguinal wall and the hernia defect.

Variations in the procedure are performed for different types of hernias.

1. If the hernia is direct, it can be reduced easily and the superior edge of the hernia defect (the transversalis fascia) is sutured to the iliopubic tract (origin of the transversalis fascia) (Figure 13-13, *B*).

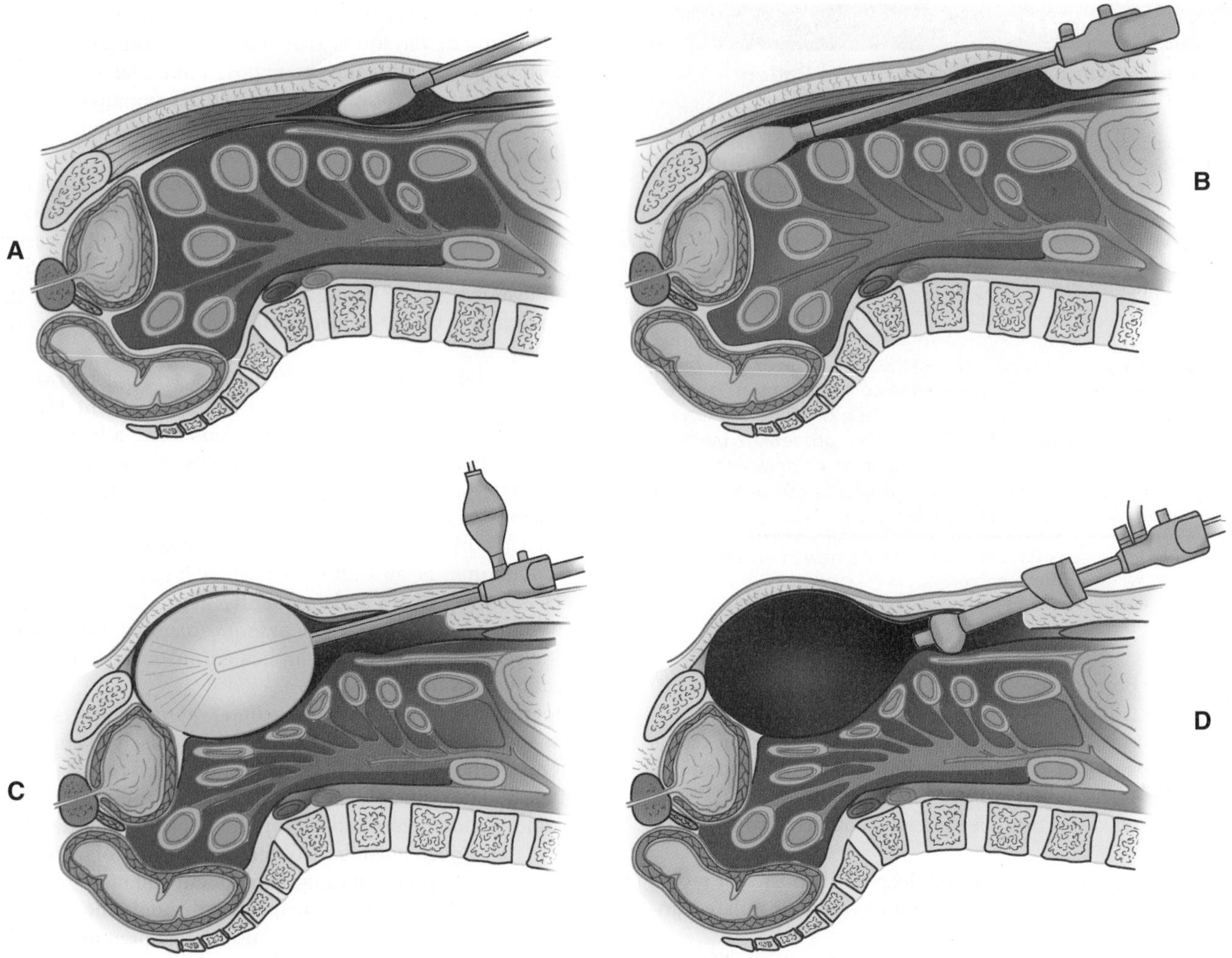

**FIGURE 13-11** The totally extraperitoneal patch (TEP) laparoscopic hernia repair. **A,** The TEP approach for laparoscopic hernia repair is demonstrated. Access to the posterior rectus sheath is gained in the periumbilical region. A balloon dissector is placed on the anterior surface of the posterior rectus sheath. **B,** The balloon dissector is advanced to the posterior surface of the pubis in the preperitoneal space. **C,** The balloon is inflated, thereby creating an optical cavity. **D,** The optical cavity is insufflated by carbon dioxide, and the posterior surface of the inguinal floor is dissected.

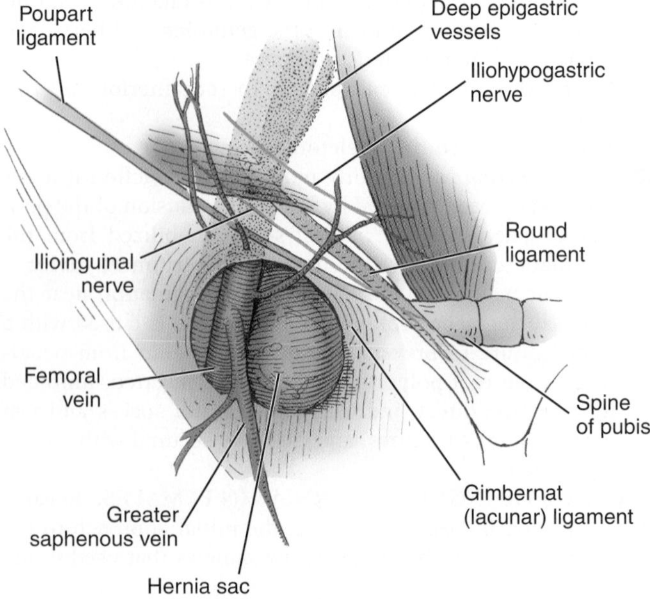


**FIGURE 13-12** Bulge from femoral hernia occurring below inguinal ligament.

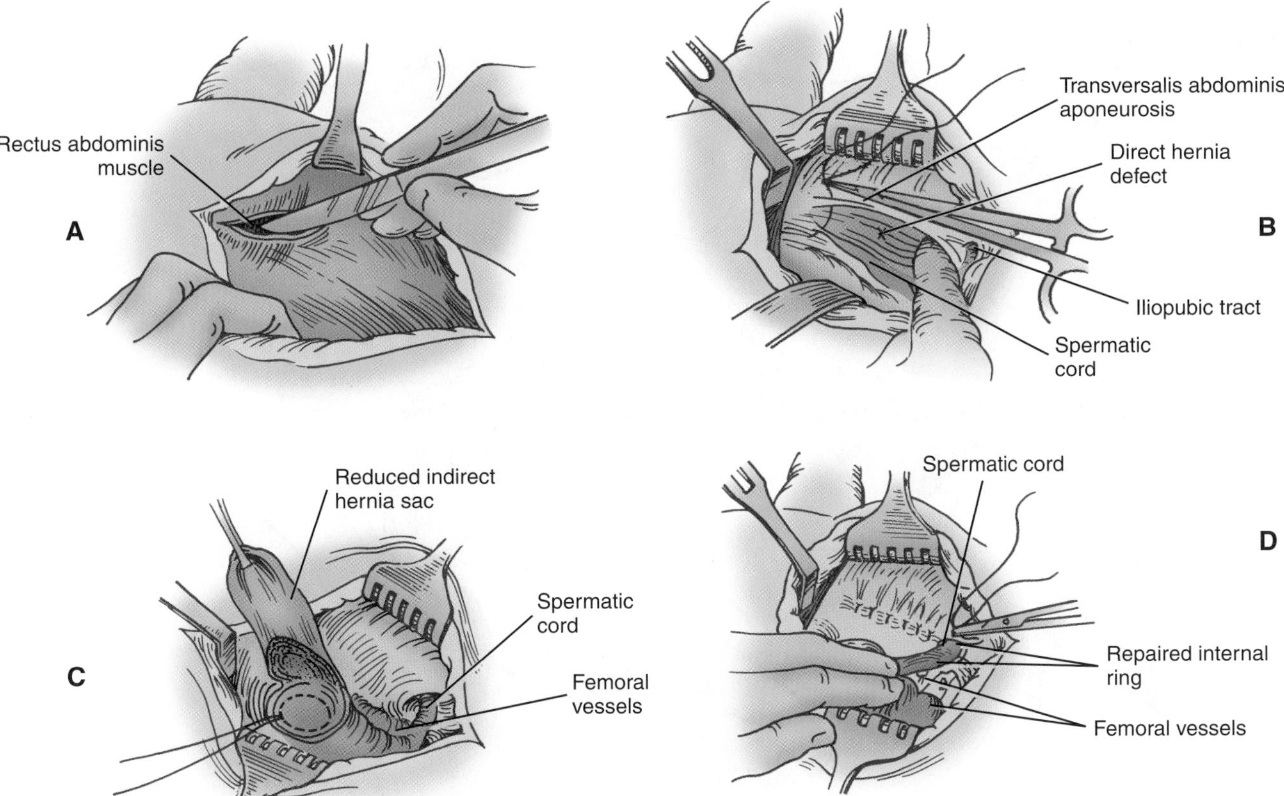


**FIGURE 13-13** Preperitoneal repair. **A,** Skin incision starts 2 cm above symphysis pubis and is extended through external oblique, internal oblique, and transversalis muscles. **B,** With finger in direct hernia defect, the surgeon sutures transversalis abdominis aponeurosis to iliopubic tract. **C,** In case of indirect defect, the sac is reduced and then excised, with high ligation being achieved by use of a purse-string suture. **D,** Internal ring is tightened after transversus abdominis aponeurosis has been approximated to iliopubic tract.

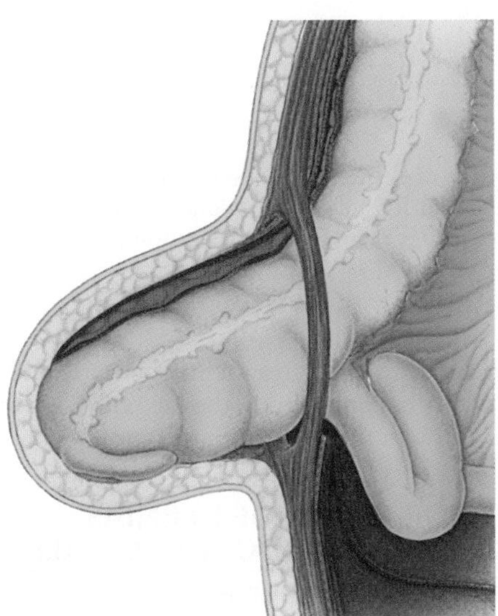

**FIGURE 13-14** Sliding hernia.

2. In an indirect hernia, the sac is gently retracted from the inguinal canal. A purse-string suture is placed around the peritoneal defect as the sac is excised (Figure 13-13, *C*). The lateral aspect of the internal abdominal ring is closed, and the posterior wall is reinforced as with the direct hernia.
3. In repair of a femoral hernia, the sac is again reduced by traction. After the sac is inspected for contents, a high ligation is performed. As it approaches the Cooper ligament, the defect in the posterior inguinal floor is clearly identified and is repaired by direct approximation (Figure 13-13, *D*).

After repair of any of the aforementioned hernias, the preperitoneal space is irrigated with saline solution and the appropriate layers are approximated.

**REPAIR OF SLIDING HERNIAS.** Direct or indirect hernias may occur as sliding hernias. A sliding inguinal hernia occurs when the wall of a viscus forms a portion of the wall of the hernia. The most common sliding hernias involve the bladder in direct hernias, the sigmoid colon in left indirect hernias, and the cecum in right indirect inguinal hernias (Figure 13-14). This hernia must be recognized early in the repair because attempts at surgical removal of the entire sac will injure the sliding viscus.

**Operative Procedure.** All operations designed to repair sliding hernias adhere to the basic principle of repairing the defect in the transversalis fascia. To free the bowel from the sac, the following steps must be taken:

1. The sac is opened in an area where no bowel is present and is excised medially and laterally to a point at which the bowel can be mobilized (Figure 13-15).
2. The lateral and medial peritoneal margins are approximated.
3. The bowel is reduced to the peritoneal cavity, and high ligation of the sac is performed.

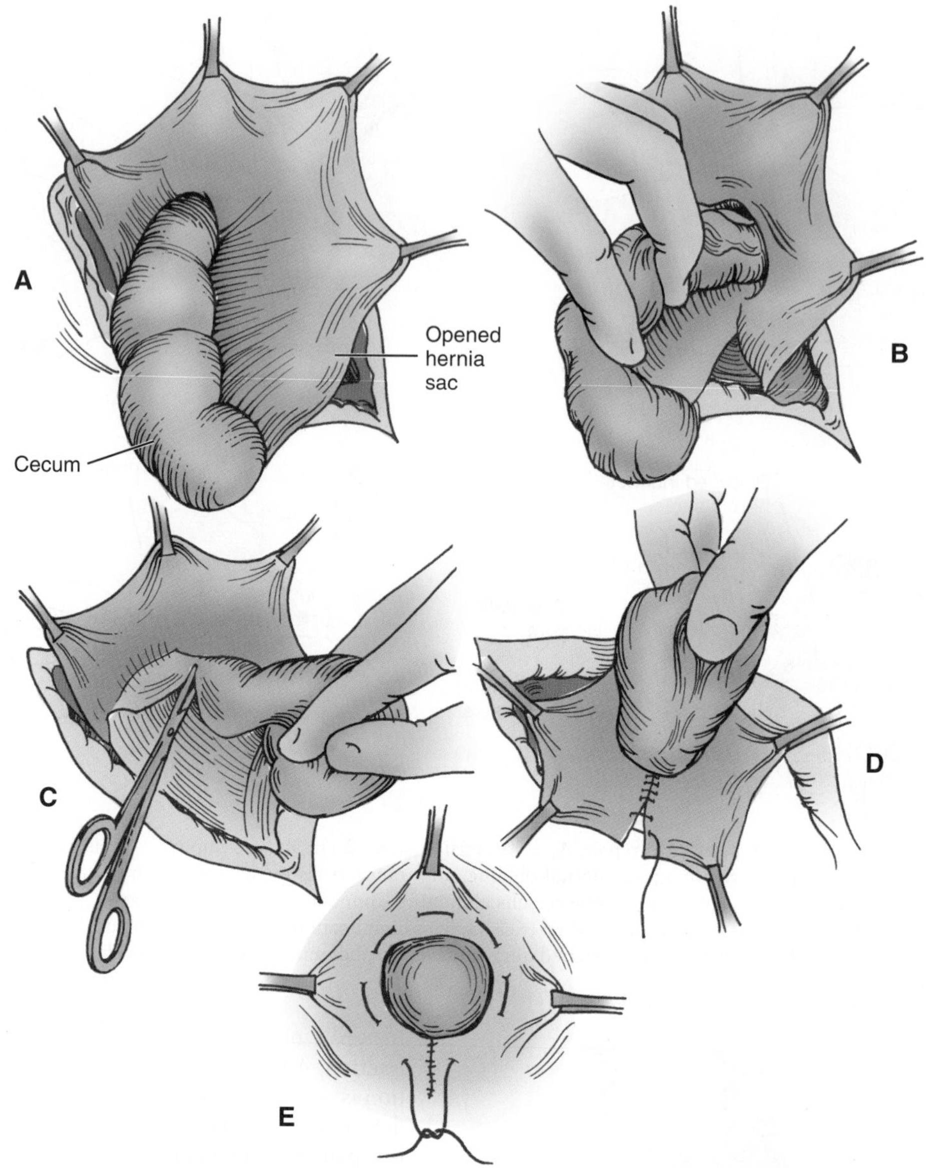


**FIGURE 13-15** Right sliding hernia. **A,** Cecum forms posterior wall of hernia sac. **B,** Peritoneum is excised medially **(C)** and laterally **(D)** to allow mobilization of cecum for subsequent reduction to peritoneal cavity. Lateral and medial margins are approximated. **E,** After reduction, high ligation is accomplished using purse-string suture.

4. Repair of the transversalis fascia is done by one of the methods previously described.

LITTRE HERNIA, MAYDL HERNIA, AND RICHTER HERNIA. An inguinal hernia containing a Meckel diverticulum is called a *Littre hernia,* and one containing two loops of bowel is called a *Maydl hernia.* A special type of strangulated hernia is a *Richter hernia* (Figure 13-16). In this hernia, only a part of the circumference of the bowel is incarcerated or strangulated in the hernia. Frequently it is described as a knuckle of bowel that becomes trapped and ischemic. Because initially a very small area is necrotic, diagnosis may be delayed. A Richter hernia most frequently occurs in femoral hernias because of the small size and sharp, relatively inflexible nature of the fascial ring in this area. A strangulated Richter hernia may be reduced spontaneously, and the gangrenous piece of intestine may be overlooked at the time of operation. Most commonly, the distal ileum is involved in a Richter hernia; however, omentum is frequently encountered in the sac. The favored approach for repair is through the preperitoneal space.

## SURGERY FOR REPAIR OF HERNIAS OF THE ANTERIOR ABDOMINAL WALL

### Ventral or Incisional Hernias

Ventral hernias can appear either spontaneously or after previous operations. Spontaneously occurring ventral hernias include epigastric and umbilical hernias. Postoperative ventral hernias, called *incisional hernias,* appear more frequently when the original incision was T shaped or a vertical midline. Operations that involve a potential for contamination, such as that for acute perforated ulcer or other perforated abdominal viscera, or wounds that become infected are more prone to developing

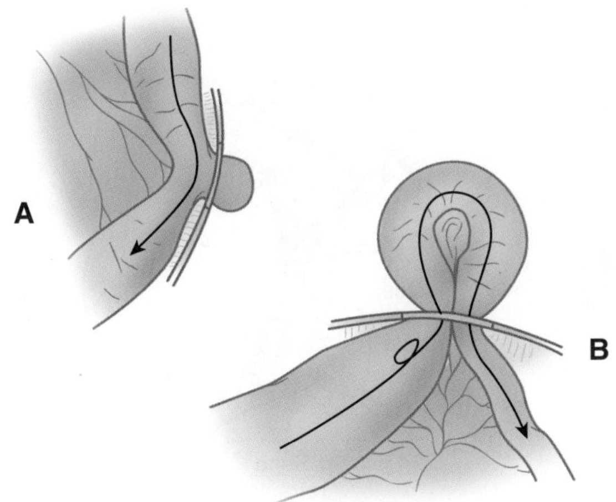


**FIGURE 13-16** **A,** Richter hernia. Only a portion of bowel passes through hernial ring; arrow indicates that bowel need not be obstructed mechanically even with strangulation. **B,** Incarcerated hernia. Distended bowel in hernia cannot return to abdomen through narrow fascial defect.

subsequent ventral hernias. Patients taking steroids, diagnosed with chronic obstructive pulmonary disease (COPD), or with a poor nutritional state with resulting hypoproteinemia are predisposed to ventral hernia formation. Finally, faulty surgical technique, such as the choice of inappropriate suture materials, may result in the ultimate appearance of a ventral hernia.

Several methods have been developed for repairing ventral hernias. If all layers of the abdominal wall are easily identified, anatomic layer-by-layer repair may be done. Frequently a type of overlap method for repair is employed. Vertical and transverse overlap procedures are referred to as *vest-over-pants repair.* For large defects, in which approximation of tissue would result in closure with excessive tension or would cause either circulatory or respiratory compromise, synthetic materials such as surgical mesh or patches are employed.

When a very large fascial defect is present, a technique that extrapolates on the principles of tissue expansion may be used. A Tenckhoff catheter is placed percutaneously into the peritoneal cavity. Gradual expansion of the abdominal fascia is accomplished by insufflation of the abdomen with 1 to 2 liters of nitrous oxide gas, similar to the procedure for laparoscopy. The patient's vital signs are monitored during and after the insufflation procedure, which may be performed on a nursing unit or possibly in an outpatient clinical setting. The graduated expansion of the tissues sometimes allows for primary closure of the defect without the use of synthetic mesh or a patch.

## Umbilical Hernias

Umbilical hernias are extraperitoneal and occur as small fascial defects under the umbilicus. They are common in children and frequently disappear spontaneously by 2 years of age. If the defect persists, a simple approximation of the overlying fascia is all that is necessary for repair. (See Chapter 29 for a description of hernia repair in children.) In adults, umbilical hernias represent a defect in the linea alba just above the umbilicus. These hernias tend to occur more frequently in obese people, making diagnosis more difficult. Umbilical hernias are potentially dangerous because they have small necks and frequently become incarcerated. Surgical repair is indicated for all adults with both symptomatic and asymptomatic umbilical hernias.

## Epigastric Hernias

Epigastric hernias are protrusions of fat through defects in the abdominal wall between the xiphoid process and the umbilicus. Patients with epigastric hernias can have nausea, vague abdominal pain, or epigastric pain similar to that observed with cholecystitis or duodenal ulcers. Surgical repair of epigastric hernias is simple and very successful.

## Spigelian Hernias

The linea semilunaris, often referred to as the *Spigelius line,* marks the transition from muscle to aponeurosis in the transversus abdominis muscle. The area of aponeurosis that lies between the linea semilunaris and the lateral edge of the rectus muscle is referred to as the *spigelian zone.* Protrusion of a peritoneal sac, preperitoneal fat, or other abdominal viscera through a congenital or acquired defect in this area is called a *spigelian hernia.* It is usually located between the different muscle layers of the abdominal wall. For this reason the spigelian hernia may be referred to as an *interstitial* or *intramuscular hernia.*

Spigelian hernias are uncommon and are generally difficult to diagnose. Ultrasonic scanning has improved the diagnosis of such intramural hernias. When ultrasonic scanning is not conclusive, CT can better visualize the hernia orifice.

## Interparietal Hernias

An interparietal hernia lies between the layers of the abdominal wall. These hernias may be classified by dividing them into those that present with ventral swelling and those without ventral swelling. Diagnosis is often made during an exploratory laparotomy for symptoms of intestinal obstruction.

Repair follows the same procedure as that done for a strangulated hernia. The sac contents are closely examined for ischemia, the sac is resected, and the defect is repaired.

## Synthetic Mesh and Patch Repairs

An ideal prosthetic mesh should not be physically modified by tissue fluids; be chemically inert, noncarcinogenic, and nonallergenic; resist mechanical strain; be permeable, allowing tissue ingrowth; and be pliable.[7] Synthetic meshes, such as Mersilene, Marlex, Prolene, and Dacron, have been particularly helpful in repairing recurrent or large ventral hernias. Closure of the defect is obtained with minimal or no tension on the suture line. These synthetic materials are strong and durable, promoting fibrovascular growth within their pores, which lends extra strength to the repair. Single-dose antibiotic prophylaxis may be used to reduce wound infection rates with prosthetic hernia repair.[16] Some studies show that, although routine use of prophylactic antibiotics is not recommended for open nonimplant herniorrhaphy, there is little direct clinical evidence on which to base recommendations when implantable mesh is used.[12]

A major criticism of synthetic meshes is that, as with any foreign-body implant, the risk of infection is increased.

Another synthetic material, the Gore-Tex patch, has become popular for the reconstruction of abdominal wall defects and repair of soft tissue. Gore-Tex soft-tissue patches come in both 1-cm and 2-cm thicknesses. Impregnation of Gore-Tex patches with an antimicrobial agent has been associated with reduced incidence of infection. Gore-Tex is, however, very expensive, and surgical services departments should evaluate products such as surgical mesh with consideration to its performance, cost, effect on quality patient care, and value analysis.[2]

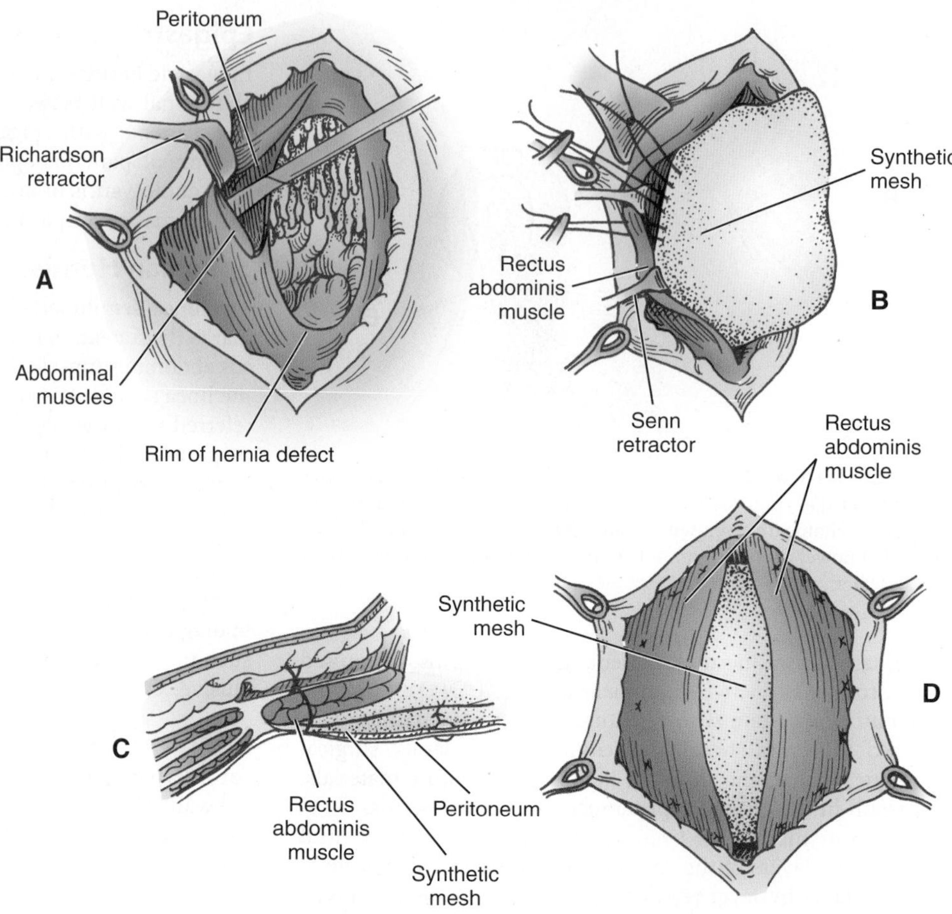


**FIGURE 13-17** Use of mesh in hernia repair. After layers of abdominal wall surrounding ventral hernia are identified **(A)**, mesh is inserted between rectus and peritoneum **(B)**. **C,** Mesh is sutured into place on one side. **D,** With moderate tension, mesh is inserted between appropriate layers on opposite side and is sutured into place.

Essential to the use of mesh or patch in a hernia repair are the identification and cleaning of tissue planes to which the mesh or patch will be attached (Figure 13-17, *A*). In a ventral hernia, the peritoneum is dissected from the undersurface of the rectus abdominis muscle and the mesh or patch is placed between the peritoneum and the rectus (Figure 13-17, *B*). After the mesh or patch is positioned, it is sutured in place on one side, using the synthetic suture material compatible with the type of mesh or patch employed (Figure 13-17, *C*).

At this point the peritoneum can be closed, if possible. If the peritoneum cannot be closed, mesh or patch can be placed directly over the omentum. The mesh or patch is then placed and sutured to the other side of the defect, with moderate tension maintained (Figure 13-17, *D*). If possible, the mesh or patch is then covered with a fascial or muscular layer before the subcutaneous fat and skin are closed. Closed-wound drainage catheters may be placed in the wound, and antibiotics are frequently used prophylactically. Using mesh or patch to repair inguinal hernias is based on the same principles used for closing ventral hernias. With inguinal hernias, the mesh or patch is sutured to transversalis fascia on both sides of the defect.

## REFERENCES


1. Advances in hernia repair. Presented March 13-15, 2001, Dallas, Tex, CR Bard, Inc.
2. Association of periOperative Registered Nurses: Recommended practices for product selection in perioperative practice settings. In *AORN standards, recommended practices, and guidelines,* Denver, Colo, 2005, The Association, pp. 433-435.
3. Bascom J: Inguinal hernia. In Harken AH, Moore EE, editors: *Abernathy's surgical secrets,* ed 5, Philadelphia, 2004, Hanley & Belfus.
4. Beyea SC: *Perioperative nursing data set,* Denver, 2000, Association of periOperative Registered Nurses (AORN).
5. Feldman L and others: What's new in ACS surgery—laparoscopic and open herniorrhaphy compared. In ACS surgery principles and practices, June 2005. Accessed June 17, 2006, online: www.medscape.com/viewarticle/506634.
6. Fitzgibbons RJ and others: What's new in ACS surgery—open hernia repair. In *ACS surgery: principles and practice,* 2003. Accessed July 25, 2005, on-line: www.medscape.com/viewarticle/463738.
7. Gilbert AI and others: *Inguinal hernia: anatomy and management*. Accessed February 23, 2006, on-line: www.surgery.medscape.com/viewarticle/414075.
8. Hwang KO: *Surgery cue cards,* Philadelphia, 2001, Davis.
9. LaFrance R: *Ask the experts: inguinal hernias and physical strain.* Accessed February 23, 2006, on-line: surgery.medscape.com/viewprogram/357.
10. Lawrence PF: *Essentials of general surgery,* ed 3, Philadelphia, 2000, Lippincott Williams & Wilkins.
11. McCormack K and others: Laparoscopic surgery for inguinal hernia repair: systematic review of effectiveness and economic evaluation, *Health Technology Assessment* 9(1):218, 2005.
12. Perez AR and others: A randomized, double-blind, placebo-controlled trial to determine effectiveness of antibiotic prophylaxis for tension-free mesh herniorrhaphy, *Journal of American College of Surgeons* 200(3):393-397, 2005.
13. Read RC: Inguinal herniation in the adult, defect or disease: a surgeon's odyssey, *Pioneers in Hernia Surgery* 8:296-299, 2004.
14. Tortora GJ, Grabowsky SR: *Principles of anatomy and physiology,* ed 9, New York, 2000, John Wiley & Sons.
15. Wojner AW: *Outcomes management: applications to clinical practice,* St Louis, 2001, Mosby.
16. Yerdel MA and others: Ampicillin reduces hernia repair wound infection rate, *Annals of Surgery* 233:26-33, 2001.

CHAPTER 14

# Gynecologic and Obstetric Surgery

DONNA R. McEWEN

Whereas changes in science and technology have impacted every area in medicine over the past century, changes in the specialty of women's health have had enormous influence over the way women live. At some point in their lives, many women face the prospect of surgery. Surgical procedures on the structures of the female reproductive system are performed for diagnostic or therapeutic purposes, for conditions such as abnormal bleeding from the reproductive organs, for suspected malignant or benign neoplasms, and for infertility. Procedures are done also to remove or repair weakened anatomic structures. Recent statistics show the majority of surgical procedures performed in the United States were performed on females.[13] A holistic approach with sensitivity to the special needs of this population is an essential component of perioperative care.

## Surgical Anatomy

The female reproductive organs and their relationships are shown in Figures 14-1 and 14-2. The adult female structures associated with the process of reproduction are the external organs (vulva), the associated ligaments and muscles, the soft tissues and contents of the pelvic cavity, and the bony pelvis.

### FEMALE EXTERNAL GENITAL ORGANS (VULVA)

The external organs, referred to collectively as the *vulva,* include the mons pubis, the labia majora and labia minora, the clitoris, the vestibular glands, the vaginal vestibule, the vaginal opening, and the urethral opening (Figure 14-3).

The mons pubis is a mound of adipose tissue covered by skin and, after puberty, by hair. It is situated over the anterior surface of the symphysis pubis.

The labia majora are two folds of adipose tissue covered with skin that extend downward and backward from the mons pubis. Varying in appearance according to the amount of adipose tissue, they unite below and behind to form the posterior commissure and in front to form the anterior commissure. The labia minora are the two hairless, flat, delicate folds of skin that lie within the labia majora. Each labium splits into lateral and medial parts. The lateral part forms the prepuce of the clitoris, and the medial part forms the frenulum. The posterior folds of the labia are united by a delicate fold extending between them. This forms the fossa navicularis.

The clitoris is the homologue of the penis in the male. It hangs free and terminates in a rounded glans (small, sensitive vascular body). Unlike the penis, the clitoris does not contain the urethra. The vaginal vestibule is a smooth area surrounded by the labia minora, with the clitoris at its apex and the fossa navicularis at its base. It contains openings for the urethra and the vagina.

The urethra, which is about 4 cm long, is close to the anterior vaginal wall and connects the bladder with the urethral meatus. Two small paraurethral ducts, which are commonly known as *Skene ducts,* lie on either side of the urethral meatus and drain the *Skene glands.*

The vaginal opening lies below the urethral meatus. The hymen surrounds the vaginal opening and may be circular, crescentic, or fimbriated.

Bartholin glands and ducts are located on each side of the lower end of the vagina. These narrow ducts open into the vaginal orifice on the inner aspects of the labia minora. The glands secrete mucus and can become infected or inflamed.

### PELVIC CAVITY

#### Uterus

The uterus (from the Greek word *hysteria*) is a pear-shaped organ situated in the pelvic cavity between the bladder and the rectum. It gains much of its support from its direct attachment to the vagina and from indirect attachments to nearby structures, such as the rectum and pelvic diaphragm. The uterus is supported on each side by the broad, round, cardinal, and uterosacral ligaments and levator ani muscles. The upper lateral points, the uterine cornua, receive the fallopian tubes. The fundus of the uterus is the upper rounded portion situated above the level of the tubal openings and just below the pelvic brim. Below, the body, or corpus, of the uterus joins the cervix. The corpus is separated from the cervix by a slight constriction (canal) called the *isthmus.* The cervix lies at the level of the ischial spines. The body of the uterus communicates with the cervical canal at the internal orifice, called the *internal os.* The constriction (canal) ends at the vaginal portion of the cervix at the external orifice, called the *external os.* The external os varies in appearance and may be oval, round, slitlike, or everted.

The uterine body has three layers: (1) the outer peritoneal, or serous, layer, which is a reflection of the pelvic peritoneum; (2) the myometrium, or muscular layer, which houses involuntary muscles, nerves, blood vessels, and lymphatics; and (3) the endometrium, or mucosal layer, which lines the cavity of the uterus.

#### Fallopian Tubes (Oviducts)

The Greek word *salpinx,* meaning "trumpet" or "tube," is used to refer to the fallopian tubes (Figure 14-4). The tubes are paired and consist of a musculomembranous channel about 10 to 13 cm long, forming the canals through which the ova are conveyed to the uterus from the ovaries. The outer surfaces of the tubes are covered by peritoneum. The inner layers are com-

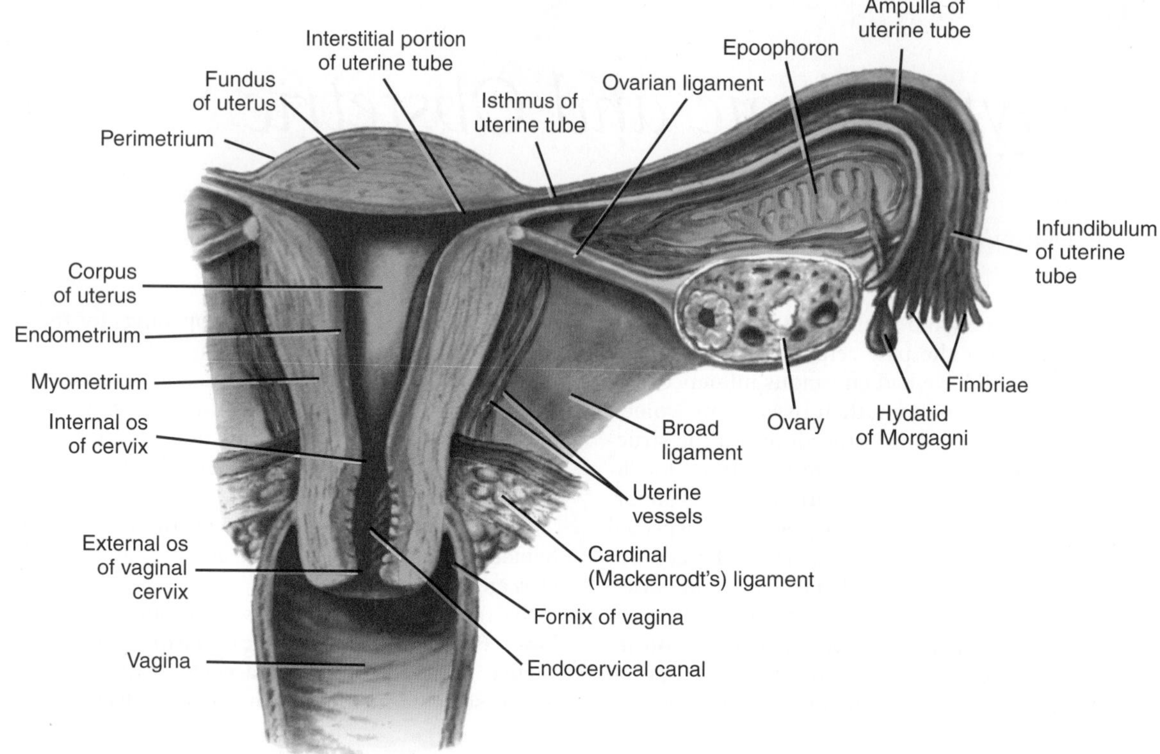


FIGURE 14-1 Female reproductive organs.

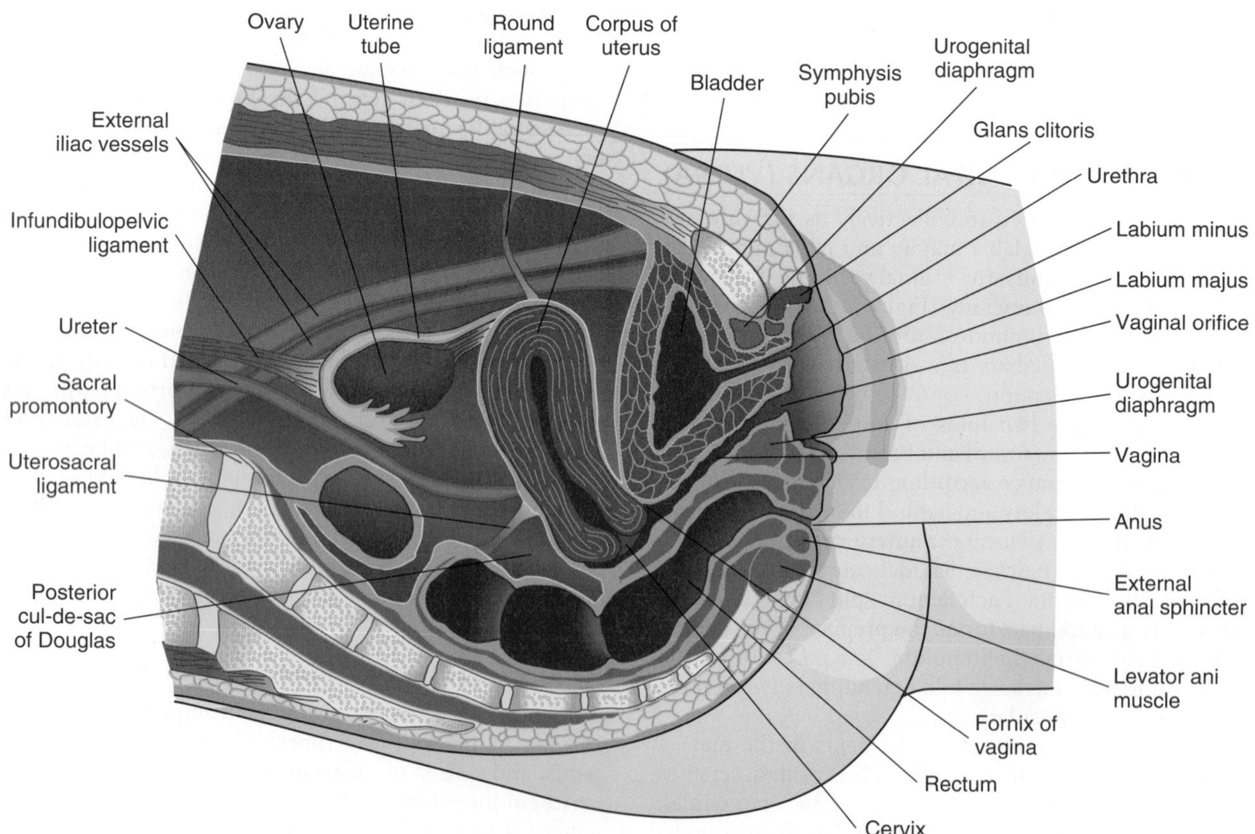


FIGURE 14-2 Female pelvic organs as viewed in midsagittal section.

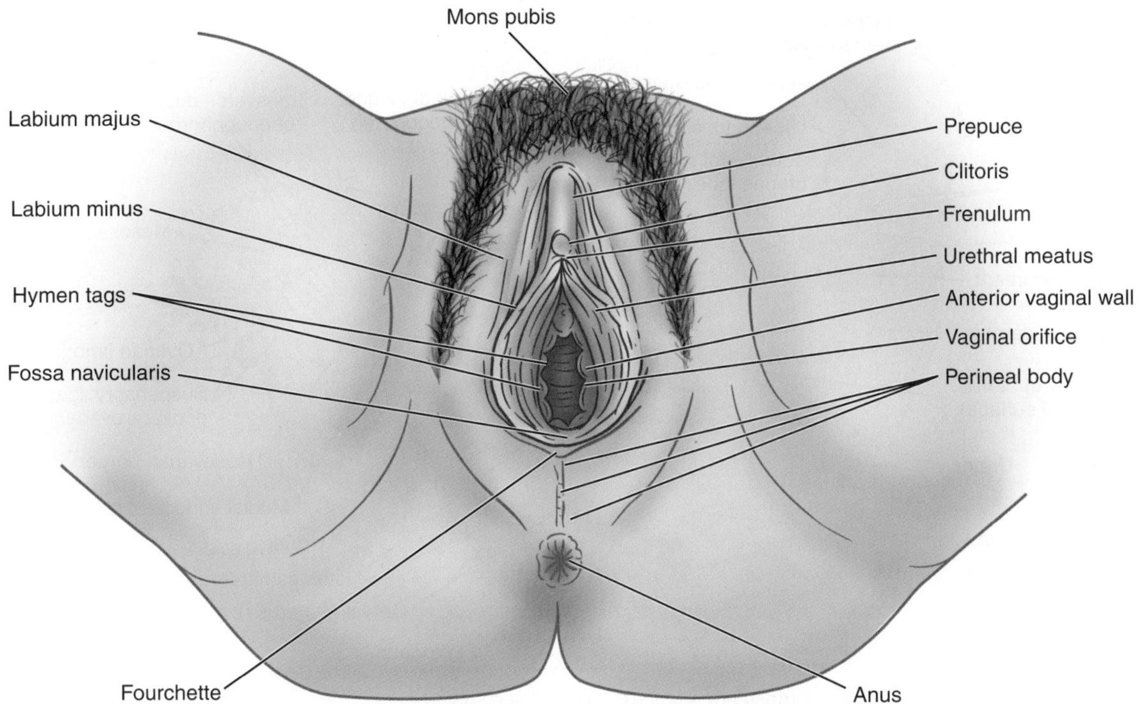


**FIGURE 14-3** The structures of the external genitalia that are collectively called the *vulva*.

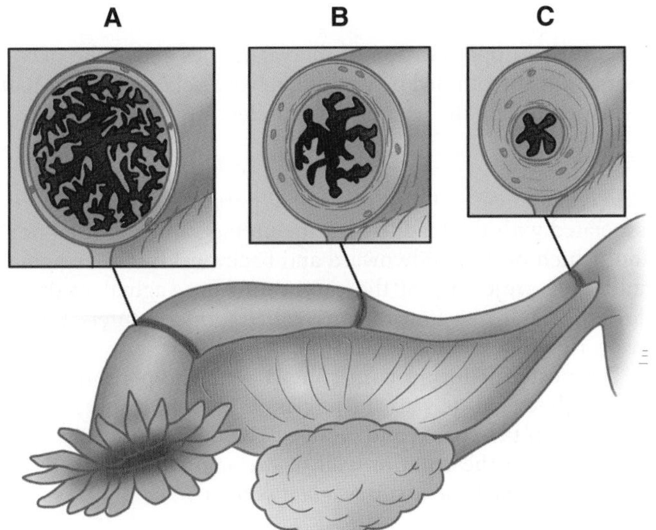


**FIGURE 14-4** The longitudinal folds of the fallopian tube seen in cross section. **A,** Infundibulum. **B,** Ampulla. **C,** Isthmus.

posed of muscular tissue lined with ciliated epithelium. Each tube receives its blood supply from the branches of the uterine and ovarian arteries and has four parts. The infundibulum is trumpet-shaped, opens into the abdominal cavity, and has fingerlike projections called *fimbriae.* The ampulla forms more than half of the tube and is thin-walled and tortuous. The isthmus is cylindric and forms approximately one third of the tube. The remainder of the tube is the uterine portion. Measuring approximately 1 cm in length, it passes through the wall of the uterus.

It has been theorized that the transfer of the ova from the ruptured follicles into the uterus is accomplished through vascular changes that occur with contraction of the smooth muscle fibers of the tube. The peristaltic action of the muscular layer and the ciliary movement propel the ova toward the uterus.

The right tube and ovary are in close relationship to the cecum and appendix; the left tube and ovary are situated near the sigmoid flexure. The fallopian tubes are also in proximity to the ureters.

## Ovaries

The ovaries are situated on each side of the uterus. The ovaries and tubes are collectively known as the *adnexa.* Each ovary lies within a depression (ovarian fossa) on the lateral wall of the pelvic cavity and above the broad ligament (see Figure 14-1). The anterior border of each ovary is attached to the posterior layer of the broad ligament by a peritoneal fold (mesovarium) and is suspended by the ovarian ligament.

The ovaries are small, almond-shaped organs composed of an outer layer, known as the *cortex,* and an inner vascular layer, known as the *medulla.* The medulla consists of connective tissue containing nerves, blood vessels, and lymph vessels. The ovary is covered by epithelium, not peritoneum. The cortex contains ovarian (graafian) follicles in different stages of maturity. After ovulation, the corpus luteum arises from the graafian follicle that expelled the ovum.

The ovaries are homologous with the testes of the male. They produce ova after puberty and also function as endocrine glands, producing hormones such as estrogen, secreted by the ovarian follicles. Estrogen controls the development of the secondary sexual characteristics and initiates growth of the lining of the uterus during the menstrual cycle. Progesterone, which is secreted by the corpus luteum, is essential for the implantation of the fertilized ovum and for the development of the embryo.

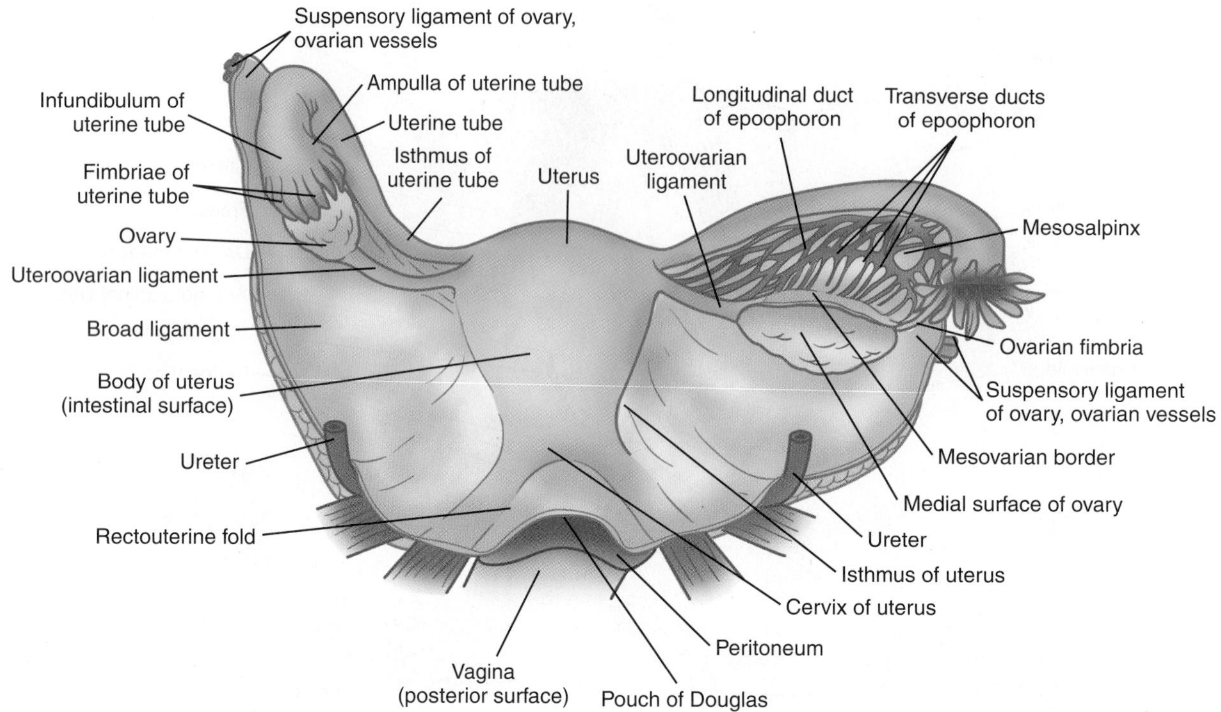


**FIGURE 14-5** Schema of the broad ligament, posterior view. Note the many structures contained within the broad ligament. Note the posterior aspect of the rectouterine fold, called the *cul-de-sac,* or *pouch, of Douglas.*

### Ligaments of the Uterus

The uterine ligaments are the broad, round, cardinal, and uterosacral ligaments (Figure 14-5).

The pelvic peritoneum extends laterally, downward, and posteriorly from each side of the uterus. A double fold of pelvic peritoneum forms the layers of the broad ligament, enclosing the uterus. These layers separate to cover the floor and sides of the pelvis. The fallopian tube is situated within the free border of the broad ligament. The free margin of the upper division of the broad ligament, lying immediately below the fallopian tube, is termed the *mesosalpinx.* The ovary lies behind the broad ligament.

Round ligaments are fibromuscular bands attached to the uterus. Each round ligament passes forward and laterally between the layers of the broad ligament to enter the deep inguinal ring.

Cardinal ligaments are composed of connective tissue with smooth muscle fibers and provide strong support for the uterus.

Uterosacral ligaments are a posterior continuation of the peritoneal tissue. The ligaments pass posteriorly to the sacrum on either side of the rectum.

### Vagina

The vagina is a rugated musculomembranous tube. It carries the menstrual blood from the uterus, serves as the organ for sexual intercourse, and is the terminal portion of the birth canal. The anterior wall measures 6 to 8 cm in length and the posterior wall 7 to 10 cm (see Figures 14-1 and 14-2). The anterior wall of the vagina is in proximity to the bladder and urethra. The lower posterior wall is anteriorly adjacent to the rectum. The upper portion of the vagina lies above the pelvic floor and is surrounded by visceral pelvic fascia. The lower half is surrounded by the levator ani muscles.

### Cervix

The cervix consists of a supravaginal portion, which is closely associated with the bladder and the ureters, and a vaginal portion, which projects downward and backward into the vaginal vault. The projection of the cervix into the vaginal vault divides the vault into four regions, called *fornices:* anterior, posterior, right lateral, and left lateral.

The posterior fornix is in contact with the peritoneum of the pouch, or cul-de-sac, of Douglas. The rectovaginal septum lies between the vagina and rectum. The dense connective tissue separating the anterior wall of the vagina from the distal urethra is termed the *urethrovaginal septum.*

## BONY PELVIS

The Latin word *pelvis* means "basin." The pelvis is that portion of the trunk below and behind the abdomen. The bony pelvis is composed of the ilium, symphysis pubis, ischium, sacrum, and coccyx. The so-called *pelvic brim* divides the abdominal false portion, located above the arcuate line, from the true portion of the pelvis, located below this line. The bony pelvis accommodates the growing fetus during pregnancy and the birth process.

The true pelvis may be considered to have three parts: inlet, cavity, and outlet. The muscles lining the pelvis facilitate movement of the thighs, give form to the pelvic cavity, and provide a firm elastic lining to the bony pelvic framework. All organs located in the pelvis are covered by pelvic fascia, which is extremely important in the maintenance of normal strength in the pelvic floor.

The fascia covering the muscles is usually dense and firm, whereas that covering organs is often thin and elastic. The nerves, blood vessels, and ureters coursing through the anatomic structures are closely associated with muscular and fascial structures.

## PELVIC FLOOR

The pelvic floor acts as a supportive sling for the pelvic contents. The pelvic fascia may be divided into three general groups: parietal, diaphragmatic, and visceral. The parietal pelvic fascia covers the muscles of the true pelvic wall and perineum. The diaphragmatic fascia covers both sides of the pelvic diaphragm, which is made up of the levator ani and coccygeal muscles. The visceral fascia is thin and flexible and covers the pelvic organs. The floor of the pelvis, known as the *pelvic diaphragm*, gives support to the abdominal pelvic viscera in this region. It consists of the levator ani and coccygeal muscles with their respective fascial coverings; it separates the pelvic cavity from the perineum.

The levator ani muscles, varying in thickness and strength, may be divided into three parts: the iliococcygeal, the pubococcygeal, and the puborectal muscles. The fibers of the levator ani muscles blend with the muscle fibers of the rectum and vagina. The pubovaginal fibers of the pubococcygeal portion of the levator ani muscles, lying directly below the urinary bladder, are involved in the control of micturition. The pubococcygeal fibers of the levator ani muscles control and pull the coccyx forward and assist in the closure of the pelvic outlet. The fibers pull the rectum, vagina, and bladder neck upward toward the symphysis pubis in an effort to close the pelvic outlet and are responsible for the flexure at the anorectal junction. Relaxation of the fibers during defecation permits a straightening at this junction. During parturition, the action of the levator ani muscles directs the fetal head into the lower part of the passageway.

### Vascular, Nerve, and Lymphatic Supply of the Reproductive System

The blood supply of the female pelvis is derived from the internal iliac branches of the common iliac artery and is supplemented by the ovarian, superior rectal, and median sacral arteries—branches of the aorta.

The nerve supply of the female pelvis comes from the autonomic nerves, which enter the pelvis in the superior hypogastric plexus (presacral nerve). The lymphatics of the female pelvis either follow the course of the vessels to the iliac and preaortic nodes or empty into the inguinal glands (Figure 14-6).

# *Perioperative Nursing Considerations*

### Assessment

The provision of quality perioperative nursing care depends on thorough assessment and planning. Data about the gynecologic patient are gathered through the review of systems, physical examination, nursing and medical histories, and diagnostic test results in the patient record (Table 14-1).

Application of interpersonal communication techniques is vital during nursing assessment. The interview may be conducted on the patient care unit or in the holding area of the surgical suite. Privacy must be maintained to facilitate discus-

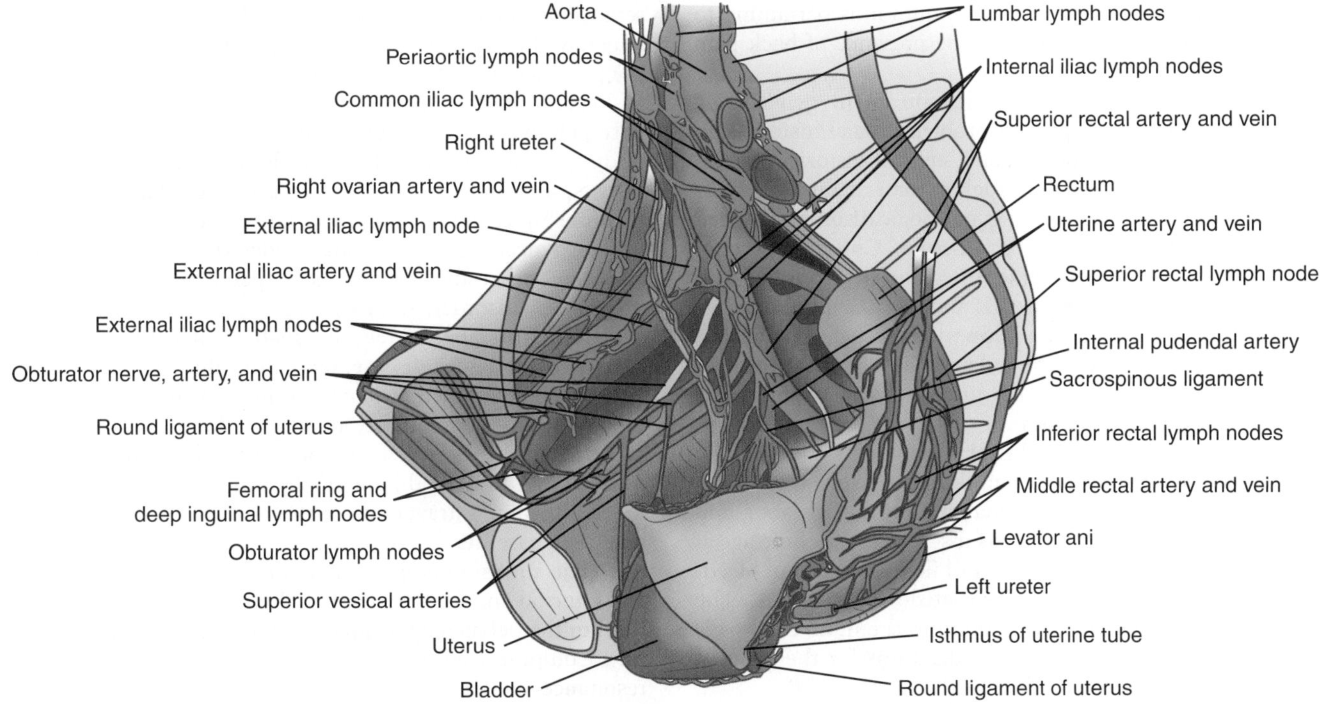


**FIGURE 14-6** A lateral view of the female pelvis demonstrating the extensive lymphatic network. Note that most of the lymphatic channels follow the courses of the major vessels.

**TABLE 14-1**

## Common Laboratory Studies Used in the Reproductive Assessment

| Test | Normal Range for Adults | Significance of Abnormal Findings |
|---|---|---|
| Follicle-stimulating hormone (FSH) (follitropin) | Follicular phase, 1.37-9.9 milliinternational units/ml<br>Midcycle, 6.17-17.2 milliinternational units/ml<br>Luteal phase, 1.09-9.2 milliinternational units/ml<br>Postmenopause, 19.3-100.6 milliinternational units/ml | Decreased levels indicate possible infertility, anorexia nervosa, neoplasm<br>Elevations indicate possible Turner syndrome |
| Luteinizing hormone (LH) | Follicular phase, 1.68-15 milliinternational units/ml<br>Midcycle, 21.9-56.6 milliinternational units/ml<br>Luteal phase, 0.61-16.3 milliinternational units/ml<br>Postmenopause, 14.2-52.3 milliinternational units/ml | Decreased levels indicate possible infertility, anovulation<br>Increased levels indicate possible ovarian failure, Turner syndrome |
| Prolactin | 0-20 ng/ml; 20-400 ng/ml in pregnancy | Increased levels indicate possible galactorrhea, pituitary tumor, disease of hypothalamus or pituitary gland, hypothyroidism |
| Estradiol | Follicular phase, 20-350 pg/ml<br>Midcycle, 150-750 pg/ml<br>Luteal phase, 30-450 pg/ml<br>Postmenopause, ≤20 pg/ml | Increased levels indicate normal pregnancy, precocious puberty, ovarian tumor<br>Decreased levels indicate failing pregnancy, Turner syndrome, menopause, anorexia nervosa |
| Progesterone | Follicular phase, <50 ng/dl<br>Luteal phase, 300-2500 ng/dl<br>Postmenopause, <40 ng/dl | Increased levels indicate possible ovarian luteal cysts<br>Decreased levels indicate possible inadequate luteal phase, amenorrhea |
| Testosterone | <1 ng/dl | Increased levels indicate possible adrenal neoplasm, polycystic ovaries, ovarian tumors, trophoblastic tumors, idiopathic hirsutism |

Modified from Lowdermilk DL: Assessment of the reproductive system. In Ignatavicius DD, Workman ML: *Medical-surgical nursing: critical thinking for collaborative care,* ed 5, Philadelphia, 2006, Saunders.

sion. Questions about reproduction and gynecologic history may embarrass the patient. Open-ended questions, progressing from general to specific, are incorporated throughout this process. For example, the perioperative nurse may initially inquire about the patient's understanding of the surgical intervention to be performed and then proceed to questions pertaining to intraoperative positioning, such as the presence of back pain and limitations in joint mobility.

The assessment includes identification of the gynecologic patient's chief complaint, present problem, social history, sexual history, and relevant medical and surgical histories. A family history includes information such as maternal use of diethylstilbestrol and deaths related to gynecologic disorders, cancer, hypertension, diabetes, and heart disease. Cultural, psychologic, and religious beliefs are identified and incorporated into the plan of care. Throughout this process the perioperative nurse must remain open and supportive to help establish a trusting therapeutic relationship. These factors can greatly affect the patient's perception of her intended surgery and play a major role in patient outcomes.

The gynecologic patient's history includes a chronologic listing of each pregnancy with length of gestation, type of delivery, complications during pregnancy, duration of labor, and fetal weight. The menstrual cycle is discussed to include age at onset, length of each cycle, amount of flow, duration of bleeding, and pain or discomfort associated with menses. The amount of flow is described in relation to the number of pads and tampons used. Additional considerations for the gynecologic assessment are noted in Box 14-1.

A medication history is taken, including use of analgesics, oral contraceptives, estrogen therapy, diuretics, antihypertensives, and cardiac medications. Medication frequency, dosage, and duration of use are noted.

Gynecologic disorders may be associated with urinary problems. Stress incontinence or loss of urine while coughing, sneezing, or laughing should be identified. Pain or burning sensations on urination are noted. The gynecologic patient may have urologic studies ordered preoperatively, especially in the presence of uterine prolapse.

Results of the physical examination are reviewed by the perioperative nurse. Baseline vital signs; height; weight; and findings from assessment of the thyroid, chest, heart, lungs, breasts, abdomen, pelvis, and rectum are analyzed for their relationship to planning intraoperative care.

The gynecologic patient may undergo numerous diagnostic studies. The studies performed depend on the gynecologic problem or disorder. A laparoscopy may be performed for diagnostic or therapeutic reasons, such as infertility, pelvic pain, pelvic inflammatory disease, ova retrieval for in vitro fertilization (IVF), lysis of adhesions, evaluation of pelvic mass, removal of ectopic pregnancy, or sterilization.

Gynecologic surgery is performed in proximity to the kidneys, ureters, and bladder and may warrant preoperative studies such as an intravenous pyelogram (IVP) to establish an anatomic baseline.

Pelvic ultrasonography helps diagnose ectopic pregnancy and adnexal and uterine disease. Uterine fibroids and blood or fluid in the pelvis may be identified by means of ultrasonography. Computerized tomography (CT) scanning and magnetic resonance imaging (MRI) may be used in evaluation of the patient with suspected malignancy in the retroperitoneal lymph nodes or bone.

BOX 14-1

## Focused Assessment for Gynecologic Patients

**GYNECOLOGIC HISTORY**
- Prior Papanicolaou (Pap) smears and results
- Prior abnormal Pap smears, how treated, follow-up
- Recent gynecologic procedures
- Past gynecologic procedures or surgery (e.g., tubal ligation, hysterectomy, oophorectomy, laparoscopy, cryosurgery, conization)
- Sexually transmitted infections (STIs)
- Pelvic inflammatory disease
- Vaginal infections
- Cancer of reproductive organs

**MENSTRUAL HISTORY**
- Age at menarche
- Date of last normal menstrual period: first day of last cycle
- Number of days in cycle and regularity of cycle
- Character of flow: amount (number of pads/tampons used in 24 hours), duration, presence, and size of clots
- Dysmenorrhea: characteristics, duration, frequency (occurs with each cycle?), relief measures
- Intermenstrual bleeding or spotting: amount, duration, frequency, timing in relation to phase of cycle
- Intermenstrual pain: severity, duration, timing, association with ovulation

**ABNORMAL BLEEDING**
- Character: shortened interval between periods (<19-21 days), lengthened interval between periods (>37 days), amenorrhea, prolonged menses (>7 days), bleeding between periods
- Change in flow: nature of change, number of pads/tampons used in 24 hours (tampons/pads soaked?), presence of clots
- Associated symptoms: pain, cramping, abdominal distention, pelvic fullness, change in bowel habits, weight loss or gain
- Medications: prescription or nonprescription; oral contraceptives

**PAIN**
- Sequence: date and time of onset, sudden versus gradual onset, course since onset, duration, recurrence
- Character: specific location, type, and intensity of pain
- Associated symptoms: vaginal discharge or bleeding, gastrointestinal symptoms, abdominal distention or tenderness, pelvic fullness
- Association with menstrual cycle: timing, location, duration, changes
- Relationship to body functions and activities: voiding, eating, defecation, flatus, exercise, walking up stairs, bending, stretching, sexual activity
- Aggravating or relieving factors
- Previous medical care for this problem
- Efforts to treat
- Medications: prescription or nonprescription

**VAGINAL DISCHARGE**
- Character, amount, color, odor, consistency, changes in characteristics
- Occurrence: acute or chronic
- Douching habits
- Clothing habits: use of cotton or ventilated underwear and pantyhose, tight pants or jeans
- Presence of discharge or symptoms in sexual partner
- Use of condoms
- Associated symptoms: itching; tender, inflamed, or bleeding external tissues; dyspareunia; dysuria or burning on urination; abdominal pain or cramping; pelvic fullness
- Efforts to treat: antifungal vaginal cream
- Medications: prescription or nonprescription; oral contraceptives; antibiotics

**SEXUAL HISTORY**
- Sexual activity: number of current and previous partners; number of their partners; gender of partner or partners
- Method of contraception: current and past; satisfaction with
- Use of barrier protection for STIs
- Prior STIs

**OBSTETRIC HISTORY**
- G: **g**ravida: total number of pregnancies
- T: number of **t**erm pregnancies
- P: number of **p**reterm pregnancies
- A: number of **a**bortions, spontaneous or induced
- L: number of **l**iving children
- Complications of pregnancy, delivery, abortion, or with fetus or neonate
- Duration of labor, fetal weight
- Diabetes (gestational)

**INFERTILITY**
- Length of time attempting pregnancy, sexual activity pattern, knowledge of fertile period in menstrual cycle
- Abnormalities of vagina, cervix, uterus, fallopian tubes, ovaries
- Contributing factors: stress, nutrition, chemical substances
- Factors relating to partner's fertility
- Diagnostic evaluation to date

**MENOPAUSAL HISTORY**
- Age at menopause or currently experiencing
- Associated symptoms: menstrual changes, mood changes, tension, hot flashes
- Postmenopausal bleeding
- Birth control measures during menopause
- General feelings about menopause: self-image, effect on intimate relationships
- Mother's experience with menopause
- Medications: hormone replacement therapy (HRT), related side effects, breast tenderness, bloating, vaginal bleeding, other medications—prescription or nonprescription, including herbal remedies

Modified from Seidel HM and others: *Mosby's guide to physical examination,* ed 5, St Louis, 2003, Mosby.

The gynecologic patient may have a hysterosalpingogram preoperatively to identify abnormalities in the uterine cavity and occlusions in the tubal folds. This diagnostic tool is useful in detecting potential reasons for infertility.

A colposcopy, with colpomicroscopy, is often performed in the physician's office. This examination is indicated for the patient with an abnormal Papanicolaou (Pap) smear suggestive of dysplasia. It identifies cellular abnormalities that may involve the vulva, vagina, or cervix and helps identify areas of dysplasia and carcinoma in situ. Endocervical curette samples may be obtained during the colposcopic procedure to rule out invasive carcinoma or to detect early adenocarcinoma.

*Gynecologic Carcinoma.* Gynecologic cancers commonly occur in the endometrium, the cervix, the ovaries, or the vagina. Less common sites are the vulva and fallopian tubes. Risk factors associated with the development of these cancers are noted in Table 14-2.

Endometrial cancer is the most common gynecologic cancer and is responsible for approximately 40,880 new cases of cancer each year in the United States (Figure 14-7). Patients with this type of cancer may be asymptomatic, or they may experience postmenopausal bleeding as their primary symptom.[2]

Cervical cancer is the third most common cause of death related to gynecologic cancers. In its early, preinvasive stage, cervical cancer may be asymptomatic or associated with painless vaginal spotting or bleeding. During the early preinvasive stage, the disease may be described as dysplasia. From dysplasia, the disease progresses to carcinoma in situ (CIS). Preinvasive cancers may also be designated as cervical intraepithelial neoplasia (CIN) and classed according to severity[2,17]:

CIN 1: Mild
CIN 2: Moderate
CIN 3: Severe, to carcinoma in situ (Figure 14-8)

Ovarian cancer is often accompanied by symptoms attributable to other disease processes (Research Highlight). It is the leading cause of death from gynecologic malignancies. These

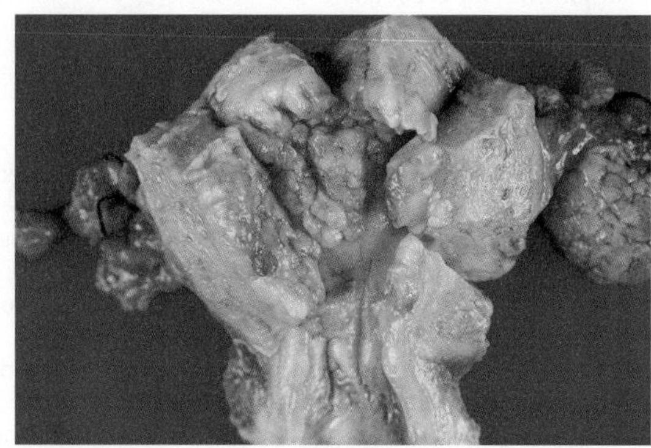

FIGURE 14-7 Endometrial cancer on posterior wall of uterus.

**TABLE 14-2**

**Risk Factors for Cancers of the Reproductive System**

| Risk Factor | Endometrial Cancer | Cervical Cancer | Ovarian Cancer | Vulvar Cancer | Vaginal Cancer | Fallopian Tube Cancer |
|---|---|---|---|---|---|---|
| Age | 50-65 yr | CIS: 30-40 yr<br>Invasive: 40-60 yr | Infrequent before 35 yr, range usually is 40-65 yr | After 40 yr; peak is 60-70 yr | Most after 50 yr; adenocarcinoma: 14-30 yr | Most after 50 yr; range is 18-80 yr |
| Family history | Increased risk | — | Increased risk | — | DES exposure in utero | — |
| Personal history | Diabetes, hypertension | — | Breast, bowel, or endometrial cancer | Cervical cancer, diabetes, vulvar disease | Vulvar or cervical cancer | Ovarian or uterine cancer, infertility |
| Race | Caucasian | African American, Native American | Caucasian | — | — | — |
| Mother's age at delivery | — | <18 yr | >30 yr | — | — | — |
| Body size | Obese | — | — | Possibly obese | — | — |
| Parity | Nulliparity | Multiparity | Nulliparity | — | Multiparity | Nulliparity |
| Estrogen use | Prolonged use >3 yr after menopause | Possibly long-term birth control pill use | — | — | — | — |
| Smoking | Possibly increased risk | Possibly double the risk | — | — | — | — |
| Infection (STI) | — | Possibly STI (herpes simplex virus type 2 or papillomavirus infection) | — | Possibly STI (papillomavirus infection) | STI (herpes simplex virus type 2 or papillomavirus infection) | PID, chronic salpingitis |

Modified from Novak K, Ignatavicius DD: Interventions for clients with gynecologic problems. In Ignatavicius DD, Workman ML: *Medical-surgical nursing: critical thinking for collaborative care,* ed 5, Philadelphia, 2006, Saunders.
*CIS,* Carcinoma in situ; *DES,* diethylstilbestrol; *STI,* sexually transmitted infections; *PID,* pelvic inflammatory disease.

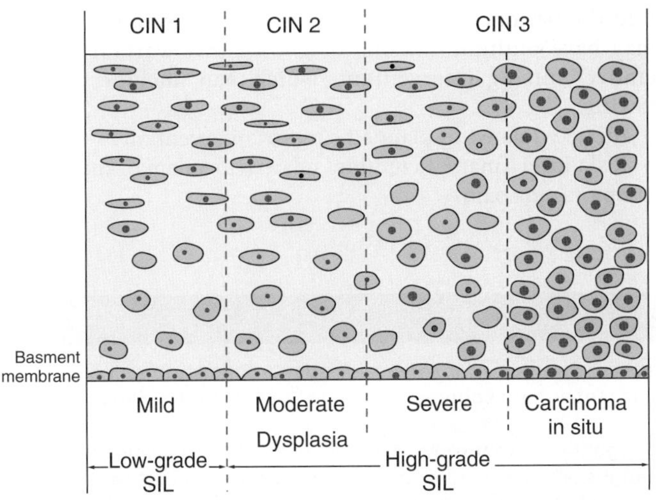


**FIGURE 14-8** Diagram of cervical epithelium showing progressive changes and various terms used. *SIL*, Squamous intraepithelium lesion.

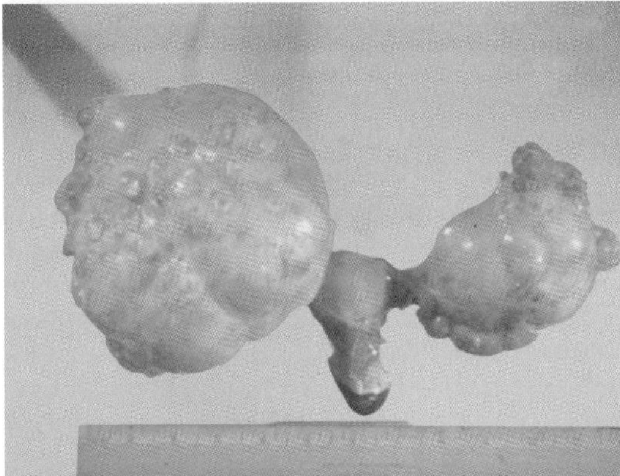

**FIGURE 14-9** Bilateral ovarian carcinoma.

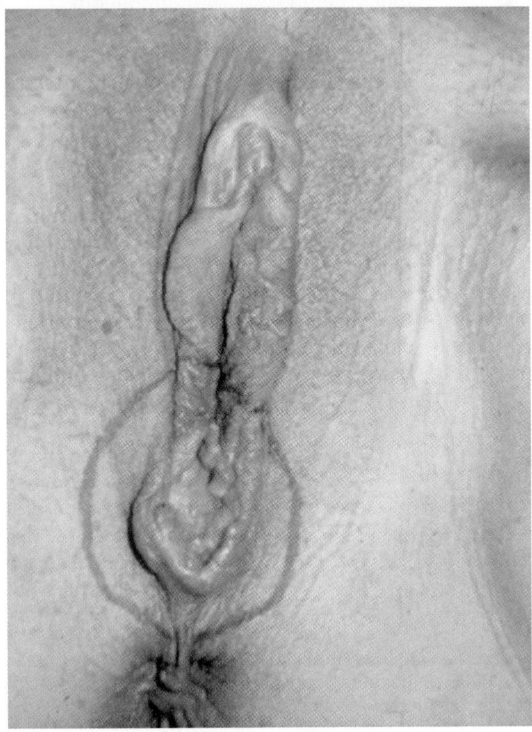

**FIGURE 14-10** Vulvar/perineal carcinoma.

## RESEARCH HIGHLIGHT

### Diagnosing Ovarian Cancer

The poor prognosis associated with ovarian cancer is generally related to the high incidence of metastatic lesions at the time of pathologic diagnosis. Traditionally this disease has been difficult to diagnose because the symptoms the woman reports may mimic other conditions. Previous studies have demonstrated that women who are eventually diagnosed with ovarian cancer do report symptoms, and research is ongoing to explore and quantify symptom reporting.

This study sought to define "target symptoms" in a group of 1,985 women aged 68 years or older. The study compared these women with two control groups. Claims records were obtained and the diagnosis and procedure codes analyzed. The target symptoms associated with ovarian cancer were abdominal pain, abdominal swelling, gastrointestinal symptoms, and pelvic pain. The researchers also aimed to determine the length of time between target symptoms and diagnosis, the types of tests used for evaluation, and if there was evidence that an earlier clinical diagnosis could have been made.

During the 1 to 3 months before the cancer was diagnosed almost half of the patients studied (47.5%) showed at least one target symptom. The most frequent target symptom experienced was abdominal pain, followed by abdominal swelling, gastrointestinal symptoms, and pelvic pain. Further analysis showed abdominal swelling symptoms were present 10 to 12 months before diagnosis and abdominal pain symptoms were present 7 to 9 months before diagnosis. The most frequent testing used in the diagnostic period was abdominal imaging followed by pelvic imaging and CA-125 testing.

Based on their findings, the authors recommend that women presenting with target symptoms be given a differential diagnosis of ovarian cancer. The authors note that while abdominal imaging is probably sufficient to diagnose advanced or metastatic ovarian cancer, in instances where the woman's target symptom is not diagnosed by other means, pelvic imaging and CA-125 testing may be of more use in diagnosis of the disease while it is still early and confined to the pelvis.

Modified from Smith LH and others: Ovarian cancer: can we make the clinical diagnosis earlier? *Cancer* 104(7):1398-1407, 2005.

tumors are generally epithelial in nature and are associated with a poor prognosis (Figure 14-9). They spread directly to other organs in the pelvic space and distally to the lymphatics, or they seed into the peritoneum.[2]

Vulvar cancer (Figure 14-10) represents the fourth most common gynecologic cancer and is typically slow-growing. It appears most often in women in their middle 60s to 70s. In younger women, the incidence is often linked to genital warts (condylomata acuminata) caused by human papillomavirus (HPV). Symptoms include irritation and itching in the perineal area or nonhealing lesions.[2,17]

Vaginal cancer ranks fifth of gynecologic cancers, causing fewer than 1000 deaths per year.[2] This form of cancer is rare as a primary diagnosis and is usually an extension of cervical, endometrial, or vulvar cancers. It is generally asymptomatic in the early stages and may be accompanied by pain, foul-smelling discharge, painless bleeding, pruritus, and urinary symptoms in the later stages.[17]

Fallopian tube cancer is very rare, with an incidence of less than 1%. It is seen primarily as a metastasis from ovarian and endometrial cancers.[17]

## Nursing Diagnosis

Perioperative nursing care is a planned process that is implemented to ensure safe, quality patient outcomes. Nursing diagnoses are formulated after reviewing the patient record and conducting a patient assessment. All significant data collected are reviewed and prioritized and then incorporated into the perioperative plan of care. The gynecologic patient may have multiple nursing diagnoses that warrant perioperative nursing intervention, which may include the following:

- Anxiety related to planned surgical intervention
- Risk for Urinary Retention related to edema, anesthesia, opioids, or pain

### SURGICAL PHARMACOLOGY

### Medication Safety and Pharmacology

Part of safe perioperative patient care focuses on safe medication practice. Strategies for safe medication administration include standardization of medication labeling both on and off the surgical field, separating sound-alike and look-alike medications, and minimizing distractions.

In addition to practicing the "five rights," (right patient, right drug, right time, right route, right dose) for the medications he or she administers, the perioperative nurse must be familiar with medications administered to the patient by others (i.e., anesthesia care providers, surgeons, etc.). Many of the medications used in gynecologic and obstetric surgery are unique to the specialty or have unique uses within the specialty. The perioperative nurse must be familiar with how these medications work, dosage ranges, adverse reactions, and nursing implications to be able to constantly modify the patient's plan of care as needed throughout the perioperative period.

**Oxytocics:** Medications that increase motor activity within the uterus by hormonal stimulation or direct stimulation on the smooth muscles, usually resulting in uterine contractions. Used intraoperatively and postoperatively.

| Medication | Perioperative Uses | Actions | Dosage/ Administration | Adverse Reactions | Nursing Considerations |
|---|---|---|---|---|---|
| Oxytocin (Pitocin) | Postabortion bleeding, postpartum bleeding, improvement of uterine contractility after cesarean delivery | Acts on uterine myofibril activity | Given IV only 10-40 units per liter of fluid | Hypertonicity with tearing of the uterus | Monitor BP; assess for continued bleeding; monitor fundal response to drug. |
| Methylergonovine maleate (Methergine) | Postabortion bleeding, postpartum bleeding | Ergot alkaline that causes vasospasm of the coronary arteries and directly stimulates uterine muscle | May be given PO, IM, or IV; most frequent route in OR is IM; IM/IV dose is 0.2 mg; may be repeated q2-4hr for no more than a total of five doses | Nausea; cramping; vomiting; dizziness; diaphoresis; bradycardia; chest pain; tachycardia; pale, cool, and blotchy skin; facial swelling; increased uterine pain | Monitor BP; assess for continued bleeding; monitor fundal response to drug. Use cautiously in patients with heart disease, hepatitis, or renal insufficiency because of vasoconstrictive effect. Assess extremities for color, warmth, movement and pain. |
| Dinoprostone (Cervidil) | Postabortion bleeding, postpartum bleeding | Prostaglandin that directly acts on the myometrium causing softening of the cervix; causes myometrial contractions in the gravid uterus | May be administered as an endocervical gel, vaginal insert, or vaginal suppository | Vomiting, nausea, bradycardia, chills/shivering, diarrhea | Keep frozen and bring to room temperature just before use. Use caution when handling to prevent skin contact. Have the patient remain supine for 15-30 min after administration. Be prepared to treat nausea. Monitor BP; assess for continued bleeding; monitor fundal response to drug. |

Modified from Hodgson BB, Kizior RJ: *Saunders nursing drug handbook 2006,* St Louis, 2006, Saunders; Hodgson BB, Kizior RJ: *Mosby's 2006 drug consult for nurses,* St Louis, 2006, Mosby; Lexi-Comp Online. Accessed November 1, 2005, on-line: www.crlonline.com/crlsql/servlet/crlonline; Wanzer LJ: Perioperative initiatives for medication safety, *AORN Journal* 82(4):663-666, 2005; Zhang J et al: A comparison of medical management with misoprostol and surgical management for early pregnancy failure, *New England Journal of Medicine* 353:761-769, 2005.

## SURGICAL PHARMACOLOGY

### Medication Safety and Pharmacology—cont'd

**Tocolytics:** Medications that decrease uterine contractility. Most commonly used in the perioperative setting during fetal surgery or in surgical procedures on pregnant females. May also be used in the postanesthesia care unit.

| Medication | Perioperative Uses | Actions | Dosage/ Administration | Adverse Reactions | Nursing Considerations |
|---|---|---|---|---|---|
| Ritodrine (Yutopar) | Prevention of preterm labor | Beta-adrenergic that inhibits uterine activity by relaxing smooth uterine muscle tissue | May be given PO or IV; IV dose is 0.05-0.1 mg/min | Shortness of breath, tachypnea, tachycardia, palpitations, chest pain, fluid retention, hypotension, nausea, vomiting | Monitor vital signs closely; be prepared to treat nausea. Have propranolol available to reverse cardiovascular effects. |
| Terbutaline (Brethine) | Prevention of preterm labor | Adrenergic agonist that stimulates beta-adrenergic receptors resulting in relaxation of uterine smooth muscle | May be given PO, subcutaneously, or IV; usual IV dose is 2.5-10 mcg/min; may increase gradually q15-20 min up to 17.5-30 mcg/min; PO dose is 2.5-10 mg q4-6hr | Tremors, anxiety, nervousness, drowsiness, headache, nausea, heartburn, dizziness; flushing and weakness | May decrease serum potassium levels. Assess baseline maternal heart rate and fetal heart rate. Provide emotional support to help ease anxiety. |
| Magnesium sulfate | Prevention of preterm labor, prevention/ treatment of convulsions caused by pregnancy-induced hypertension (preeclampsia/ eclampsia) | Relaxes smooth muscle of the uterus; blocks neuromuscular transmission to produce seizure control | Loading dose of 4-6 g diluted in 100 ml of IV fluid, given over 30-60 min; maintenance dose is 2-4 g/hr | Reduced respiratory rate, decreased reflexes, decreased heart rate, hypotension, sedation | Test patellar reflexes before giving drug to determine baseline. Suppressed patellar reflexes may be sign of impending respiratory arrest. Monitor vital signs.<br>Maintain accurate I&O.<br>Ensure calcium gluconate is available to reverse magnesium sulfate toxicity. |

**Antimetabolites:** Medications that interrupt cell division. May be given intraoperatively or postoperatively.

| Medication | Perioperative Uses | Actions | Dosage/ Administration | Adverse Reactions | Nursing Considerations |
|---|---|---|---|---|---|
| Methotrexate | Used in ectopic pregnancy and hydatidiform mole surgery to eradicate any remaining trophoblastic cells | Inhibits RNA and DNA and protein synthesis in rapidly dividing cells | PO, IM, IV<br>Most commonly given IM in perioperative setting (15-30 mg) | Nausea, vomiting, stomatitis, dizziness, blurred vision, photophobia, hepatotoxicity, nephrotoxicity | Encourage patient to maintain scrupulous oral hygiene; be prepared to treat nausea and vomiting. Review good handwashing practices with patient. Discuss the need for weekly repeated lab studies to monitor hCG levels 2-8 wk after procedure. |

*Continued*

## SURGICAL PHARMACOLOGY

### Medication Safety and Pharmacology—cont'd

**Miscellaneous Agents**

| Medication | Perioperative Uses | Actions | Dosage/ Administration | Adverse Reactions | Nursing Considerations |
|---|---|---|---|---|---|
| Misoprostol (Cytotec) | Used for cervical ripening, may be used instead of dilation and evacuation (D&E) for missed or incomplete abortion (off-label use) | Synthetic prostaglandin that acts directly on the uterine muscle | Oral, rectal, or intravaginal, available in 100- to 200-mcg tablets; oral dose for missed abortion: 600 mcg; cervical ripening: intravaginal, 25 mcg (¼ of 100-mcg tablet) 2-3 hr before procedure | Diarrhea, abdominal pain; headache, nausea, uterine rupture | May increase the effect of oxytocin. *Do not confuse* with similarly named drugs Cytoxan and metoprolol. Not approved by FDA for use in cervical ripening or missed/incomplete abortion but endorsed by ACOG. Should not be used in patients with prior cesarean delivery. |
| Estrogen cream (Estrace cream) | Lubricant for vaginal packing | Increased synthesis of RNA, DNA, protein in tissues; reduces release of gonadotropin hormone from the hypothalamus, reduces FSH and LH from the pituitary gland | Topical cream, 0.1 mg/g, intravaginally | Local irritation, vaginal discharge | Assess preoperatively for any sensitivity to topical estrogens. Do not use excessive amount of cream. Cream will liquefy from patient's body heat and may soil bedding. |
| Miconazole nitrate cream (Monistat) | Lubricant for vaginal packing, treatment of vulvovaginal candidiasis | Inhibits synthesis of ergosterol (an important component of fungal cell formation) | 2% Topical cream intravaginally | Local irritation, vaginal discharge | Assess preoperatively for any sensitivity to antifungals. Do not use excessive amount of cream. Cream will liquefy from patient's body heat and may soil bedding. |
| Sulfathiazole/sulfacetamide/ sulfabenzamide cream (Triple Sulfa) | Lubricant for vaginal packing, treatment of *Gardnerella* vaginitis | Exerts bacteriostatic action by competitive antagonism of PABA (a component of folic acid synthesis) | Topical cream used intravaginally; concentration: sulfathiazole 3.42%, sulfacetamide 2.86%, and sulfabenzamide, 3.7% | Local irritation, vaginal discharge, Stevens-Johnson syndrome | Assess preoperatively for any sensitivity to sulfa medications or derivatives. Do not use excessive amount of cream. Cream will liquefy from patient's body heat and may soil bedding. |
| Vasopressin (Pitressin) | Injected directly into the uterus to decrease bleeding during hysterectomy | Causes vasoconstriction through direct stimulation of smooth muscle; pituitary hormone | 20 units/ml to be diluted in injectable saline as directed by surgeon | Diaphoresis, circumoral pallor, wheezing, allergic reactions | Potential for confusion related to name. *Do not confuse* Pitressin with Pitocin! Monitor vital signs. Verify dilution with surgeon. |
| Methylene blue | Indicator dye: intraoperative hysterosalpingogram, used to test patency of ureters | Converts ferrous iron to methemoglobin | 0.1%-0.2% ml/kg given IV push, slowly | Hypertension, dizziness, staining of skin, discoloration of urine or stool | Warn patient about urine and stool discoloration. Methylene blue stains can be removed with mild bleach solution. |

*ACOG*, American College of Obstetricians and Gynecologists; *BP*, blood pressure; *DNA*, deoxyribonucleic acid; *FDA*, Food and Drug Administration; *FSH*, follicle-stimulating hormone; *hCG*, human chorionic gonadotropin; *I&O*, intake and output; *IM*, intramuscular; *IV*, intravascular; *LH*, luteinizing hormone; *OR*, operating room; *PO*, by mouth; *RNA*, ribonucleic acid.

- Risk for Infection at the surgical site related to operative or other invasive procedures
- Disturbed Body Image related to surgery
- Risk for Perioperative Positioning Injury

## Outcome Identification

Outcomes identified for the selected nursing diagnoses could be stated as the following:

- The patient will verbalize reduced or controlled anxiety.
- The patient will maintain or regain normal patterns of urinary elimination.
- The patient will remain free from surgical site infection.
- The patient will acknowledge feelings regarding her body image (as applicable).
- The patient will be free from injury related to surgical positioning.

## Planning

Planning enables the perioperative nurse to provide patient care in an organized and individualized manner. Planning involves preparation for both the psychosocial and physiologic needs of the gynecologic patient. Part of planning efficient and effective patient care is the gathering of the required equipment and supplies, positioning accessories, devices, and adjuncts requisite to the specific gynecologic surgical intervention. For example, if the gynecologic patient is undergoing a lengthy surgical intervention, the perioperative nurse will plan to have a forced-air warming device, pressure-reducing positioning devices, antiembolic stockings, and sequential compression devices (SCDs) available. These actions will help maintain the patient's body temperature, promote skin integrity, and prevent venous stasis. Similar nursing interventions that will help the gynecologic patient reach the desired outcomes are identified for each patient. Examples of interventions for the gynecologic patient are shown in the Sample Plan of Care on p. 424.

## Implementation

During implementation of the plan of care, the perioperative nurse performs the identified nursing interventions. Part of implementation includes gathering the appropriate instruments and patient care supplies, positioning the patient on the operating room (OR) bed, antimicrobial skin preparation, insertion of urinary catheters, draping, creation and maintenance of a sterile field, initiation of safety measures, and patient monitoring. Data continue to be collected, the plan of care is adjusted as required and documented, and reports are given to relief personnel, ensuring continuity of the patient's plan of care.

***Instrumentation.*** A basic vaginal instrument set is required for vaginal and vulvar surgery. A basic abdominal gynecologic instrument set is required for abdominal gynecologic surgery. Surgeons' instrument preferences may vary, and instrument lists described in this chapter are not meant to be all-inclusive.

For most abdominal gynecologic procedures, a dilation and curettage (D&C) set should be available.

***Positioning.*** Principles and methods of patient positioning for different types of surgical procedures are described in Chapter 5. Stirrups for the lithotomy position may support only the patient's feet (canvas, fabric, or gel-pad ankle straps) or may cradle and support the thighs, popliteal spaces, and lower legs. Padded cradle stirrups promote maintenance of skin integrity and assist in preventing nerve injury. Patient positions may be modified based on the surgical procedure and surgeon's preference. The patient is placed in the lithotomy position for most vaginal and vulvar surgery. Careful attention must be focused on placing the patient in the lithotomy position to prevent injury and vascular changes. The legs must be raised and lowered simultaneously. For abdominal gynecologic surgery, the Trendelenburg position may be used. Some surgeons use the low lithotomy position with the Trendelenburg position for abdominal oncology procedures to facilitate access to pelvic and paraaortic nodes. Patients placed in the Trendelenburg position for prolonged gynecologic procedures are at increased cardiovascular risk because of decreased pulmonary compliance and functional residual capacity (FRC).[10] Care should be taken to protect all patients from integumentary, musculoskeletal, and nerve injury while ensuring adequate circulatory, renal, and respiratory functions.

Because pelvic and vaginal procedures involve manipulation of the ureters, bladder, and urethra, indwelling urinary drainage is frequently established before or during surgery with an indwelling urethral catheter or a suprapubic cystostomy catheter, depending on the type of procedure. The size of sutures, needles, and drains also varies, depending on the surgical procedure, surgeon preference, and patient needs.

***Prepping.*** Skin preparation and routine draping procedures are described in Chapter 3. Care must be taken not to cross-contaminate when prepping multiple areas, such as for an abdominal hysterectomy. The abdomen is prepped before the vaginal prep begins. The vaginal prep setup should be separate from the abdominal prep setup. Attention should be paid while performing vaginal preps on patients who have been experiencing vaginal bleeding and may have clots in the vaginal vault. The clots and any gross blood on the thighs or vulva should be removed before beginning the prep to allow full contact of the prepping solution.

***Examination Under Anesthesia (EUA).*** Many physicians will perform a pelvic examination after the patient is anesthetized and positioned. The perioperative nurse should anticipate this examination and ensure that nonsterile gloves and an appropriate lubricant are available. Culture specimens (e.g., gonococcal, chlamydial, trichomonal) and a Pap smear may be obtained during the examination.

***Dressings, Drains, and Packing.*** Various dressings are used in gynecologic surgery and may range from simple (e.g., Band-Aids, Steri-Strips) to complex (e.g., multilayer gauze, ostomy appliances, binders). Perineal pads are used after vaginal surgery.

Closed and open drains are used. A Penrose drain may be inserted in the vaginal cuff after hysterectomy. Indwelling and suprapubic catheters are also commonly employed in gynecologic surgery. All drains and catheters should be secured for patient comfort and to avoid dislodgment.

Packing may be used in fistulas or other created cavities. It is frequently used to support and stent the vagina, to absorb postoperative drainage, or to aid in hemostasis. Products used

## SAMPLE PLAN OF CARE

**NURSING DIAGNOSIS**

**Anxiety** related to planned surgical intervention

**OUTCOME**

The patient will verbalize reduced or controlled anxiety.

**INTERVENTIONS**

- Determine the patient's previous experience with surgery and her level of knowledge related to the current planned surgical intervention.
- Assess the patient's level of anxiety and physical reactions to anxiety (e.g., tachycardia, tachypnea, nonverbal expressions of anxiety); classify her anxiety as low, moderate, or high.
- Use presence and touch (if welcome) to communicate comfort and caring.
- Provide time for and encourage expression of concerns or clarification of needs.
- Explore coping skills previously used by the patient to relieve anxiety (e.g., relaxation, deep breathing, imagery); reinforce these skills; and facilitate their use.
- Explain the sequence of perioperative nursing activities and procedures, using nonmedical terms and clear, concise speech.
- Minimize environmental stimuli and noise.
- If conducive to anxiety reduction, provide patient with a means to listen to music in the preoperative period and intraoperatively, as applicable.

**NURSING DIAGNOSIS**

**Risk for Urinary Retention** related to edema, anesthesia, opioids, or pain

**OUTCOME**

The patient will maintain or regain normal patterns of urinary elimination.

**INTERVENTIONS**

- Before surgery, explain that an indwelling catheter will be inserted (if applicable).
- Insert indwelling catheter using aseptic technique.
- Secure tubing to prevent inadvertent stretching or stress on catheter.
- Document size of catheter inserted.
- Keep drainage bag below the level of the bladder.
- Observe and document the color and amount of urine; report abnormalities.
- Check patency of catheter and drainage system whenever patient is repositioned.
- Discuss with the patient the importance of adequate postoperative fluid intake and early ambulation.
- Review elements of catheter care, management of drainage system, catheter removal, and signs and symptoms of urinary tract infection.
- Clarify any misconceptions that the patient may have.
- Encourage the patient to verbalize feelings and concerns regarding inability to void postoperatively, presence of indwelling catheter, and catheter removal.

**NURSING DIAGNOSIS**

**Risk for Infection** at the surgical site related to operative or other invasive procedures

**OUTCOME**

The patient will remain free from surgical site infection.

**INTERVENTIONS**

- Administer and document antibiotic prophylaxis as prescribed. Follow safe practices for all medication administered.
- Initiate measures to warm patient and maintain normothermia.
- Prepare surgical site with an antiseptic solution; document skin condition at surgical site and solution used.
- Apply dressing to surgical site before sterile drapes are removed to prevent contamination of incision.
- Follow Standard Precautions and infection prevention and control practices.
- Maintain aseptic technique, and monitor members of the surgical team for breaks in technique.
- Correctly classify surgical wound at end of procedure.
- Document the presence, location, and type of any drains inserted during surgical intervention.
- Review with patient signs and symptoms of infection at surgical site:
  - Redness
  - Swelling
  - Warmth
  - Tenderness
  - Pain
  - Discuss the importance of proper handwashing techniques when changing dressings at surgical site, as applicable.

**NURSING DIAGNOSIS**

**Disturbed Body Image** related to surgery

**OUTCOME**

The patient will acknowledge feelings regarding her body image (as applicable).

**INTERVENTIONS**

- Determine the patient's expectations of her planned surgery.
- Correct unrealistic perceptions of the planned surgical intervention (as appropriate).
- Encourage the patient to express feelings about her diagnosis and surgery and how she believes it will affect her body image; clarify any misconceptions.
- Acknowledge denial, anger, or depression as normal feelings when adjusting to changes in body image or function.
- Determine the influence of cultural beliefs, norms, and values on the patient's body image.
- Maintain the patient's privacy.
- Demonstrate empathy and positive regard.
- Reinforce information provided by other health care team members.

**NURSING DIAGNOSIS**

**Risk for Perioperative Positioning Injury**

**OUTCOME**

The patient will be free from injury related to surgical positioning.

**INTERVENTIONS**

- Note and document any preexisting patient considerations (e.g., nutritional status, weight, preoperative chemotherapy, limitations in mobility or range of motion, neurovascular impairments) that place the patient at risk for positioning injury.
- Use adequate numbers of personnel to transfer and position the patient.
- Secure the patient to the operating room (OR) bed without friction or pressure at restraining straps.
- Assess and document condition of dependent skin areas.
- Use pressure-reducing positioning devices.
- Pad and protect bony prominences and dependent pressure sites.
- Maintain proper body alignment.
- Provide support stockings or antiembolic device, such as sequential compression devices (SCDs), as indicated.
- Reassess padding and protection during any positional changes.

for vaginal packing can include narrow fine-mesh gauze in various yardage, iodoform packing, and Kerlix. Vaginal packing is usually moistened with saline or coated with antibiotic or antifungal cream before insertion. Packing must be placed with care to avoid distention of the vault and compression of its vasculature.

## Evaluation

During evaluation the perioperative nurse determines whether the patient met the established outcomes. Some outcomes can be reached during the preoperative and intraoperative phases of care; they are evaluated before the patient's discharge from the operating room. Others require ongoing monitoring and measurement in the postoperative phase; these are denoted by the word "will" to indicate their ongoing nature. Part of the perioperative nursing report to the postanesthesia care unit (PACU) or ambulatory recovery should include the outcomes of the nursing plan of care. They can be phrased as follows:

- The patient's anxiety was reduced; she verbalized concerns and used personally effective coping strategies.
- Urinary elimination patterns were maintained; urinary output was adequate; and catheter patency was maintained.
- The patient's skin integrity was maintained; she verbalized understanding of the signs and symptoms of infection to report to her physician and acknowledged measures to prevent infection (e.g., handwashing).
- The patient will effectively cope with her disturbance in body image; questions will continue to be answered and misconceptions clarified.
- There was no evidence of injury related to surgical positioning; range of motion and neurovascular status were consistent with preoperative levels.

## Patient and Family Education and Discharge Planning

Patient and family education, along with discharge planning, is a priority perioperative nursing activity. No longer is this a nursing intervention that is begun after the patient is admitted to an acute care setting. Many gynecologic surgical procedures are performed on an ambulatory basis, and for those that require an inpatient admission, length of stay continues to decrease. Thus patient education and discharge planning often begin before any admission, be it ambulatory or inpatient. Regardless of the gynecologic procedure performed, the perioperative nurse should begin patient and family education with necessary postoperative care information. The goal of this information is to restore normal body function and may include areas such as early ambulation, prevention of respiratory complications, incision care, anticipated postoperative discomfort, managing postoperative pain, restrictions in activity, diet, and any other concerns the patient has. Areas such as progression of activities, emotional and physical issues, sexual activity, general nutritional needs, and health maintenance guide the education process. Gynecologic patients should also be provided specific information regarding signs and symptoms to report, especially in relation to vaginal bleeding and the surgical site, along with restrictions related to douching and vaginal penetration (tampons or sexual intercourse). With the growth in same-day surgery, many types of hysterectomies, some myomectomies, and even laparotomies are now same-day, or 23-hour–stay procedures. Simple, clear information and instructions such as those presented in the Patient and Family Education box are helpful to enhance patient learning and retention.

### PATIENT AND FAMILY EDUCATION
### Gynecologic Surgery

Whenever possible, provide the patient and her caregiver with *verbal* and *written* instructions. Provide them with the phone number of the physician to call if questions arise. Use visual aids to enhance instruction. Encourage the patient to verbalize any concerns she may have regarding her condition and surgery. Misconceptions about the outcome of gynecologic surgery are common. Patients may believe that undergoing a hysterectomy will cause depression, nervousness, mental instability, weight gain, wrinkles, masculinity, and hirsutism. Provide education to correct any misconceptions, and discuss any other concerns, such as fear of death, cancer, loss of femininity and childbearing ability; pain; and changes in sexuality. Education points for common gynecologic procedures are as follows.

**DILATION AND CURETTAGE OF THE UTERUS**

- Take your temperature once each day for the next 2 days; if your oral temperature is more than 37.7°C (100°F), call the clinic or your physician.
- Avoid sexual intercourse, tub baths, and the use of tampons for 2 weeks to allow healing and prevent infection.
- Slight bleeding is normal. However, if bleeding is as heavy as during your normal menstrual period or if it lasts longer than 2 weeks, call your physician.
- Use a heating pad or hot water bottle to relieve abdominal cramping if it occurs.
- If procedure was performed for miscarriage, add the following:
  - Mood swings and depression are common after pregnancy loss. It can be helpful to talk to friends, family, or clergy about your loss.
  - Support groups may be helpful in the recovery period.
  - Attempts at subsequent pregnancy should be postponed until indicated by your physician.

**ENDOMETRIAL ABLATION**

- Spotting and vaginal drainage are normal for several days after the procedure.
- Use a heating pad or hot water bottle to relieve abdominal cramping if it occurs.
- You can return to your normal activities within 2 to 3 days.
- Avoid sexual intercourse, tub baths, and the use of tampons for 2 weeks to allow healing and prevent infection.

**FIBROID EMBOLIZATION**

- Eat a normal diet including fluids and fiber.
- Avoid straining during a bowel movement.

Modified from Canobbio MM: *Mosby's handbook of patient teaching,* ed 3, St Louis, 2006, Mosby; Lowdermilk DL: Structural disorders and neoplasms of the reproductive system. In Lowdermilk DL, Perry SE: *Maternity and women's health care,* ed 8, St Louis, 2004, Mosby; Novak K, Ignatavicius DD: Interventions for clients with gynecologic problems. In Ignatavicius DD, Workman ML: *Medical-surgical nursing: critical thinking for collaborative care,* ed 5, Philadelphia, 2006, Saunders.

*Continued*

## PATIENT AND FAMILY EDUCATION

### Gynecologic Surgery—cont'd

**FIBROID EMBOLIZATION—cont'd**

- Monitor your puncture site (groin) for any excessive swelling or redness. Slight bruising may occur, but a large area of bruising or tenderness should be reported to your physician.
- Call your physician if you have any abnormal or foul-smelling vaginal discharge.
- Do not use tampons, douche, or have vaginal intercourse for at least 4 weeks or as long as directed by your physician.

**VULVECTOMY**

- Avoid sexual activity for 4 to 6 weeks or as long as directed by your physician.
- Rest frequently.
- Avoid crossing your legs and sitting or standing for long periods.
- Avoid tight, constricting clothing, and wear cotton underwear.
- Keep your perineal area clean and dry. Wash perineum after each elimination, and pat dry.
- Report any swelling, redness, unusual tenderness, drainage, or foul odor of incision site to your physician.
- Eat a well-balanced diet to promote healing.
- Elevate legs periodically to prevent pelvic congestion.

**HYSTERECTOMY**

- You will no longer have a period, although you may have some vaginal discharge after you go home.
- Eat foods high in protein, iron, and vitamin C to aid tissue healing; include foods with high fiber content, and drink six to eight glasses of water daily.
- Rest when tired; resume activities as comfort level permits. Avoid vigorous exercise and heavy lifting for 6 weeks. Avoid sitting for long periods. Resume driving when comfort allows or on advice from your physician.
- Avoid tub baths, intercourse, and douching until after your follow-up examination.
- When vaginal intercourse is resumed, use water-based lubricants to decrease discomfort.
- Report the following symptoms to your physician: vaginal bleeding, gastrointestinal changes, persistent postoperative symptoms (e.g., cramping, distention, change in bowel habits), and signs of wound infection (e.g., redness, swelling, heat, or pain at the incision site).
- Avoid activities that increase pelvic congestion (e.g., dancing, horseback riding, sitting for long periods) until allowed to resume by your physician.
- If your ovaries were removed you may experience symptoms of menopause, including hot flashes, night sweats, and vaginal dryness.
- Estrogen replacement therapy may be prescribed.

## LASERS IN GYNECOLOGIC SURGERY

The carbon dioxide ($CO_2$), neodymium:yttrium-aluminum-garnet (Nd:YAG), and argon lasers are used in gynecology to treat extrauterine disease such as pelvic endometriosis, cervical dysplasia, condylomata acuminata, pelvic adhesive disease, and premalignant diseases of the vulva and vagina. Lasers are generally used in conjunction with the colposcope and operating microscope, or the laparoscope. A laser plume evacuator or suction system is necessary to remove smoke and fumes from the operative field.[3] All accessories and instrumentation used should be laser safe, secure, and tested or examined for working order before use. Safety precautions must be implemented by the OR team when the laser is used (see Chapter 7).

# *Surgical Interventions*

## VULVAR SURGERY

A variety of malignant and nonmalignant conditions may affect the vulva. Nonmalignant lesions are generally excised. The treatment of early malignant disease of the vulva is accomplished by a skinning technique, local wide excision, or, for more multicentric or extensive lesions, simple or radical vulvectomy. Vulvar surgery may also be indicated in the treatment of vestibulitis and vestibulodynia.

### Excision of Condylomata Acuminata

Vulvar/perineal condylomata are caused by the human papillomavirus (HPV) (Figure 14-11) and may be transmitted sexually. Often these warty lesions will extend into the vaginal vault and may be aggravated by hormonal changes in pregnancy. Depending on the strain of the virus, the condition may be benign or associated with dysplasia and malignancy. Surgical treatment ranges from desiccation of the lesions with electrocoagulation to sharp excision or eradication through use of the laser. Surgical intervention is based on the type and extent of the lesions.

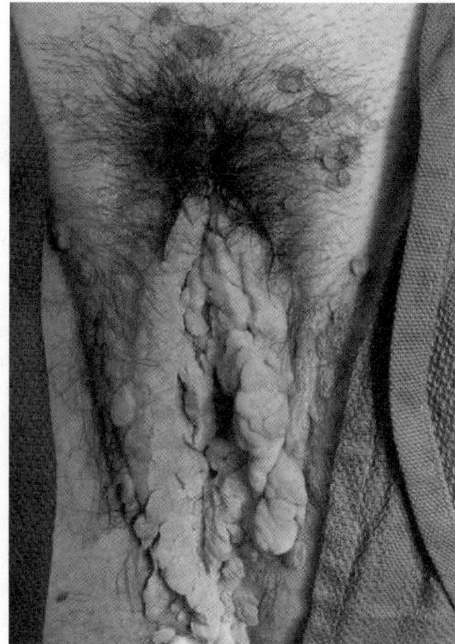

**FIGURE 14-11** Condylomata acuminata.

## Simple Vulvectomy

Simple vulvectomy is removal of the labia majora and labia minora, possibly but not preferably the glans clitoris, and occasionally tissue from the perianal area. A simple vulvectomy is usually done to treat carcinoma in situ of the vulva when it is multicentric. Occasionally a vulvectomy is necessary for the treatment of either leukoplakia or intractable pruritus, especially when a skinning procedure is impractical or has failed.

***Procedural Considerations.*** The basic vaginal instrument set is required, plus an electrosurgical unit (ESU), if desired. The patient is positioned in lithotomy.

### *Operative Procedure*

1. The affected skin is incised, usually starting anteriorly above the clitoris. The incision is continued laterally to the labia majora, to the midline of the perineum, and around the anus, if it is involved. A knife, hemostats, gauze sponges on sponge-holding forceps, tissue forceps, and Allis forceps are needed. Bleeding vessels are clamped and electrocoagulated or ligated.
2. Periurethral and perivaginal incisions are made. Bleeding of this vascular area can be controlled by means of Kelly or Crile hemostats and electrocoagulation. Ligation of blood vessels should be minimal. Allis-Adair forceps are used for holding diseased tissues.
3. All skin and subcutaneous tissues are undermined and mobilized with curved dissecting scissors, tissue forceps, Allis forceps, and sponges on holding forceps.
4. The wound is closed, usually by simple bilateral Z-plasty. In some cases, skin is excised around the anus to accomplish a sliding skin flap.
5. Closed-wound drainage catheters may be placed in the dependent areas, an indwelling urinary catheter is inserted, and vaginal gauze packing may be placed in the vagina. Dressings are applied.

## Skinning Vulvectomy

Skinning vulvectomy is the simple removal of the external skin from the affected area, which has been previously identified with a stain such as toluidine blue. The purpose of this procedure is to preserve the underlying structures of the external genitalia. A skinning procedure may be done to treat leukoplakia, intractable pruritus, or other types of skin lesions, such as kraurosis, vitiligo, and chronic venereal granulomas.

***Procedural Considerations.*** The instrumentation required and patient position are as described for simple vulvectomy.

***Operative Procedure.*** The external skin is simply excised from the affected area (Figure 14-12, *A*).

## Radical Vulvectomy and Groin Lymphadenectomy

Radical vulvectomy and groin lymphadenectomy are the en bloc dissection of the following structures: a large segment of skin from the abdomen and groin, the labia majora, the labia minora, the clitoris, the mons veneris, and terminal portions of the urethra, vagina, and other vulvar organs, as well as the superficial and deep inguinal nodes, portions of the round ligaments, portions of the saphenous veins, and the lesion itself. It also involves reconstruction of the vaginal walls and pelvic floor and closure of the abdominal wounds. Full-thickness pinch or split-thickness grafts may be placed if the denuded area of the vulva appears too large for normal granulation. A plastic surgeon may immediately complete skin grafts or rotation flaps to cover defects (see Chapter 24).

Radical vulvectomy and groin lymphadenectomy involve abdominoperineal dissection and groin dissection, which may be performed as a one- or two-stage operation. When performed as a one-stage operation, it is optimally done by a four-person team. The skin prep is extensive, including the abdomen and thighs; if a skin graft will be done, the donor site will also need to be prepped.

***Procedural Considerations.*** The patient lies supine and may be placed in the Trendelenburg and low lithotomy positions, as required for the various stages. The skin prep includes the abdomen, vulva, and thighs. An indwelling urinary catheter is often inserted to act as a urethral marker and to prevent postoperative urethral trauma. As in other radical surgery, the perioperative nurse should be prepared to measure blood loss and anticipate procedures to combat shock.

For radical vulvectomy, the basic vaginal instrument set is required, with the addition of assorted sizes of Richardson

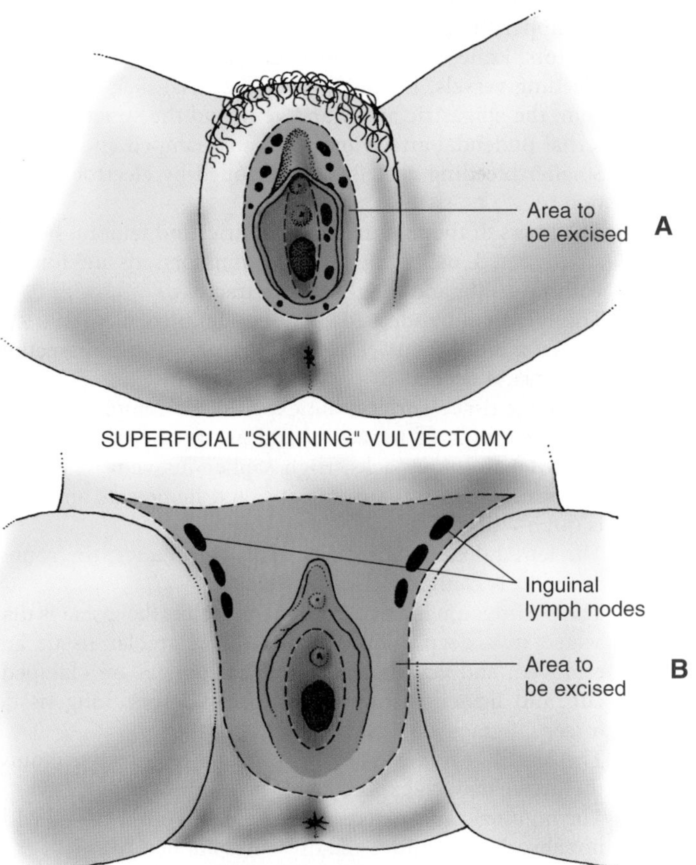


**FIGURE 14-12** Outline of incisions used for, **A**, superficial skinning vulvectomy and, **B**, radical vulvectomy.

retractors, Richardson appendectomy retractors, Volkmann rake retractors, skin hooks, and closed-wound drainage systems.

For groin lymphadenectomy, the basic abdominal gynecologic instrument set is required, with the addition of Schnidt tonsil forceps, Kantrowitz thoracic clamps, ligating clips and appliers, and closed-wound drainage systems.

### *Operative Procedures*

RADICAL VULVECTOMY

1. The skin incisions of the abdomen and thigh join with those for vulvectomy. The incisions in the vulva encircle the urethra.
2. In the vulvar dissection, terminal portions of the urethra and vagina, the mons veneris, the clitoris, the frenulum, the prepuce of the clitoris, Bartholin and Skene glands, and fascial coverings of the vulva are removed with the specimen (Figure 14-12, *B*).
2. Reconstruction of the vaginal walls and the pelvic floor is completed.
4. An indwelling urinary catheter is inserted, closed-wound drainage catheters are placed in the denuded area, and pressure dressings are applied.

GROIN LYMPHADENECTOMY

1. The first skin incision is made on the side opposite the primary lesion. The end of the incised skin is grasped with Allis forceps. The incision is carried down to the aponeuroses of the external oblique muscle.
2. The fascia over the inguinal ligament and the fascia lata of the upper thigh are exposed, separated, and freed with retractors, knife, scissors, hemostats, and sponges.
3. Bleeding vessels, including the superficial iliac artery and vein, the epigastric artery and vein, and the superficial external pudendal artery and vein, are clamped and ligated. Smaller bleeding vessels are controlled by electrocoagulation.
4. The fibers of the inguinal, hypogastric, and femoral nerves are resected using Metzenbaum scissors, tissue forceps without teeth, and long-bladed retractors.
5. The lymphatic node beds may be identified with silk sutures or metal clips. Fine, long, sharp tissue dissection scissors are needed.
6. The large tissue surfaces are exposed for complete dissection by means of retractors and are protected by warm, moist laparotomy packs. High saphenous vein ligation is performed with scissors, forceps, and hemostats and then is doubly tied.
7. The femoral canal is cleaned of its lymphatics; the round ligament is clamped, cut, and ligated.
8. The peritoneum is freed from the muscles; the fascia is dissected free; deep lymphatic nodes and areolar tissue are removed; and vessels and their attachments are clamped, cut, and ligated, using long curved scissors, long tissue forceps, hemostats, and ligatures.
9. The lesion is removed. In deep pelvic lymphadenectomy, the ureter may be exposed and the area drained.
10. The inguinal canal is reconstructed, the wound closed with nonabsorbable suture, and dressings applied.
11. An indwelling urethral catheter is inserted before the patient is transferred to the PACU.

## Vestibulectomy and Vestibuloplasty

Vestibulodynia is defined as severe pain or burning on vestibular touch or attempted vaginal entry or tenderness localized within the vulvar vestibule. It is often associated with erythema of varying degrees (vestibulitis).[21] Surgical intervention is often successful in relieving the symptoms associated with the condition (Research Highlight).

***Procedural Considerations.*** The instrumentation required and patient position are as described for simple vulvectomy. Before the administration of the anesthetic agent, the patient identifies the painful areas of the vestibule in response to pressure from a cotton-tipped applicator.

***Operative Procedure.*** For vestibulectomy, the vulvar area identified by the patient is excised with a #15 blade, taking care to avoid injury to the urethra. The mucosa of the hymen is removed, and the mucosa and subcutaneous tissue are closed with interrupted absorbable suture. For vestibuloplasty, the procedure is the same but closure is accomplished by advancing a vaginal flap and suturing it to the excision line.

## RESEARCH HIGHLIGHT

### Modified Vulvar Vestibulectomy in the Treatment of Vulvar Vestibulitis

Vulvar vestibulitis is a condition that causes women to experience vulvar pain and dyspareunia (painful intercourse). This condition may be treated medically or surgically. Surgical treatments include vestibuloplasty, vestibulectomy and modified vestibulectomy, vestibuloplasty, and perineoplasty. The etiology of the condition is unclear.

This study examined the effectiveness of the modified vestibulectomy procedure as treatment for vulvar vestibulitis. The modified vestibuloplasty procedure offers the advantages of reduced tissue loss, shorter operative time, and simplified technique compared with other surgical procedures for this condition. Fifty-nine patients underwent modified vulvar vestibulectomy, and 53 were available for follow-up. The patients were interviewed at 4 to 8 weeks after surgery and again at 6 months after surgery. Response to the surgery was measured as complete if the patient was able to undertake sexual intercourse without any pain or discomfort; partial if the patient had some discomfort with intercourse; and as no response if no or minimal improvement was noted.

From the group of 53 women, 73.6% reported a complete response, 13.2% had a partial response, and 13.2% had no response.

Because the etiology of vestibulitis is not known, the extent of surgical excision is also not easily defined. Although this study used a small sampling and was not randomized, it provides important information for women with this condition. The modified vestibulectomy is less invasive than other vestibulitis procedures and may be associated with less postoperative morbidity. Additional studies are required to substantiate the effectiveness of this technique.

Modified from Lavy Y et al: Modified vulvar vestibulectomy: simple and effective surgery for the treatment of vulvar vestibulitis, *European Journal of Obstetrics, Gynecology, and Reproductive Biology* 120:91-95, 2005.

## GYNECOLOGIC SURGERY USING VAGINAL APPROACH

### Plastic Reconstructive Repair of the Vagina (Anterior and Posterior Repair; Colporrhaphy)

A vaginal repair is done to correct a cystocele or a rectocele and to reestablish the support of the anterior and posterior vaginal walls, restoring the bladder and rectum to their normal positions.

A cystocele is a herniation of the bladder that causes the anterior vaginal wall to bulge downward (Figure 14-13). A defect in the anterior vaginal wall is usually caused by obstetric or surgical trauma, advanced age, or an inherent weakness. A large protrusion may cause a sensation of pressure in the vagina or present a mass at or through the introitus; it may also cause voiding difficulties.

A rectocele is formed by a protrusion of the anterior rectal wall (posterior vaginal wall) into the vagina. In general, the anterior rectal wall forms a bulging mass beneath the posterior vaginal mucosa (Figure 14-14). As the mass pushes downward into the lower vaginal canal, the rectum may be torn from the fascial and muscular attachments of the urogenital diaphragm and the pelvic wall. The levator ani muscles become stretched or torn. The patient may present with a mass protruding into the vagina, difficulty in evacuating the lower bowel, hemorrhoids, and a feeling of pressure.

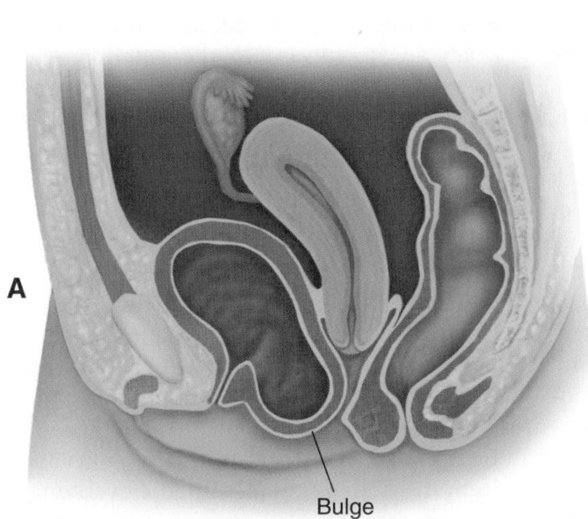


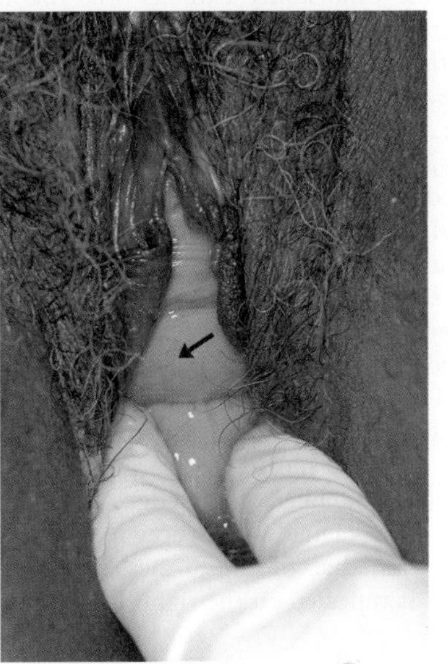


**FIGURE 14-13** **A,** Cystocele resulting from unrepaired tears of muscles of pelvic floor and those under bladder, usually resulting from childbirth, surgical trauma, advanced age, or inherent weakness. **B,** Cystocele.

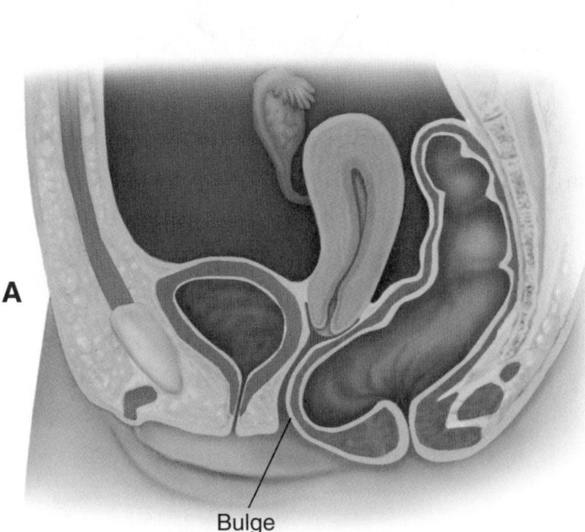


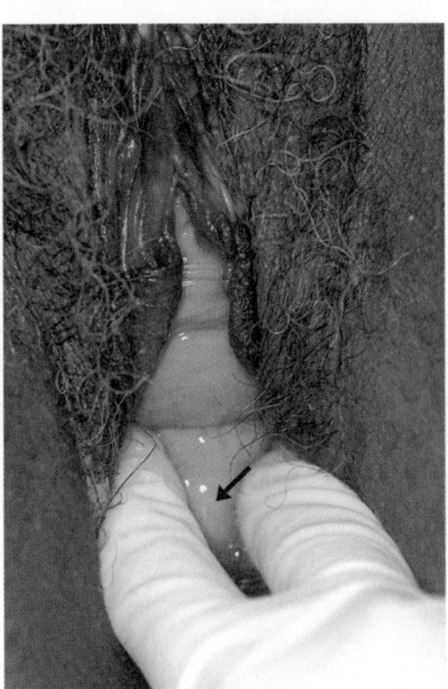


**FIGURE 14-14** **A,** Rectocele resulting from unrepaired tears of muscles of pelvic floor and those under bladder, usually resulting from childbirth, surgical trauma, advanced age, or inherent weakness. **B,** Rectocele.

An enterocele is a herniation of the cul-de-sac of Douglas and almost always contains loops of the small intestine. An enterocele herniates into a weakened area between the anterior and posterior vaginal walls.

***Procedural Considerations.*** The basic vaginal instrument set is required. A D&C may be done in conjunction with the repair. Vaginal retractors are used for exposure. The labia may be sewn back if the exposure is inadequate.

### *Operative Procedures*

CYSTOCELE REPAIR

1. The bladder may be drained, or an indwelling urinary catheter or suprapubic cystostomy catheter may be inserted (surgeon's preference). Areolar tissue between the bladder and vagina at the bladder reflection is exposed. The full thickness of the vaginal wall is separated up to the bladder neck by a knife, curved scissors, tissue forceps, Allis-Adair or Allis forceps, and gauze sponges. Bleeding vessels are clamped and tied with ligatures or electrocoagulated.
2. The urethra and bladder neck are mobilized with a knife, gauze sponges, and curved scissors.
3. Sutures are placed adjacent to the urethra and bladder neck in such a manner that, after they have been tied, the bladder neck and the posterior urethrovesical angle are narrowed (Figure 14-15, *A*).
4. The connective tissue on the lateral aspects of the cervix is sutured into the cervix to shorten the cardinal ligaments.
5. Allis-Adair forceps are applied to the edges of the incision, and the left flap of the vaginal wall is drawn across the midline. Edges are trimmed according to the size of the cystocele. This process is repeated on the right flap of the vaginal incision.
6. The anterior vaginal wall is closed in a manner resulting in reconstruction of an anterior vaginal fornix (Figure 14-15, *B*).

RECTOCELE REPAIR

1. Allis forceps are placed posteriorly at the mucocutaneous junction on each side, at the hymenal ring, and just above the anus (Figure 14-16, *A*).
2. Skin and mucosa are incised and dissected from the muscles beneath with a knife, tissue forceps, curved scissors, and gauze sponges.
3. Allis-Adair forceps are placed on the posterior vaginal wall, scar tissue (from obstetric trauma) is removed, and dissection is continued to the posterior vaginal fornix and laterally, depending on the size of the rectocele (Figure 14-16, *A* and *B*).
4. The perineum is denuded by sharp dissection, and the trimming of the posterior vaginal wall is carried out with Allis forceps and curved scissors (Figure 14-16, *C*).
5. The rectal wall proximal to the puborectal muscle is strengthened by placement of sutures.
6. Bleeding is controlled, and the vaginal wall is closed from above, downward to the anterior edge of the puborectal muscle. The rectocele is repaired from the posterior fornix to the perineal body. Remains of the transverse perineal and bulbocavernosus muscles are used to build up the perineum. The anterior edge of the levator ani muscle may be approximated (Figure 14-16, *D*).
7. The mucosa and skin are trimmed, and the remaining closure is performed with interrupted sutures.
8. The vagina may be packed with 2-inch vaginal gauze packing to which antibiotic or antifungal cream may be added. An indwelling urinary catheter or suprapubic cystostomy catheter is inserted, according to the surgeon's preference.

ENTEROCELE REPAIR. The procedure is illustrated in Figure 14-17. The peritoneal sac must be carefully dissected from the underlying rectum, the overlying bladder, or both, so that the peritoneal tissues are completely freed from the surrounding structures. The sac is opened to establish true iden-

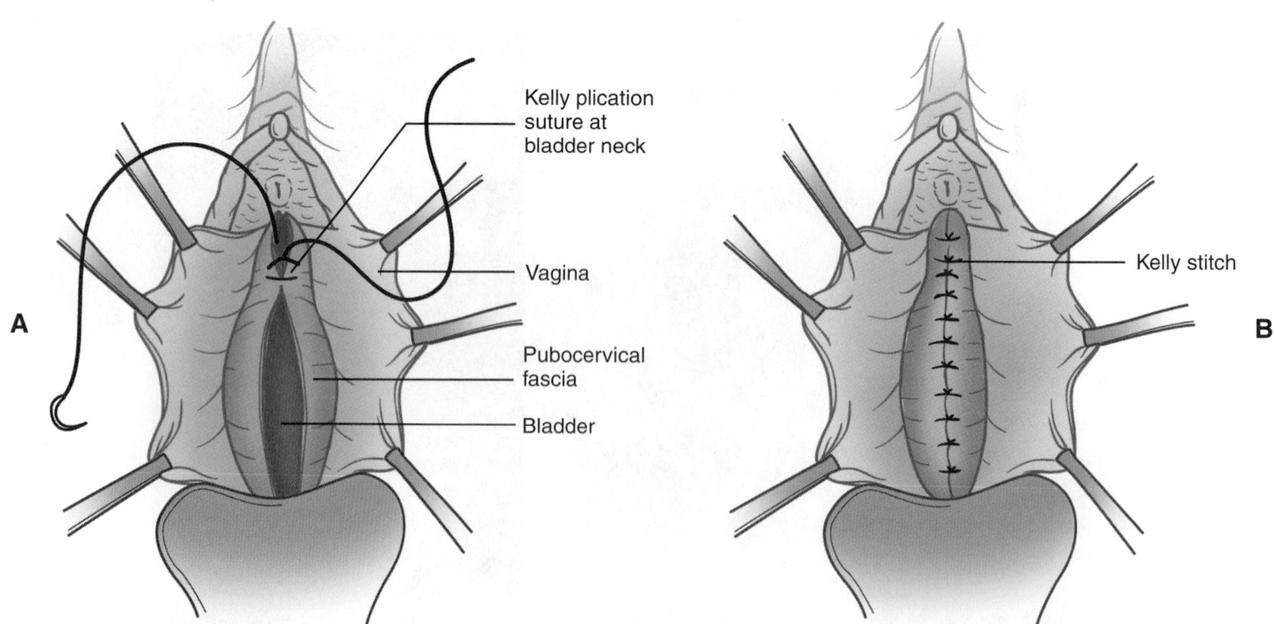


FIGURE 14-15 Cystocele repair. **A,** The placement of a Kelly stitch in the pubocervical fascia at the junction of the urethra with the bladder neck. **B,** The repair of the cystocele as the pubocervical fascia is sutured. Thus the cystocele is plicated.

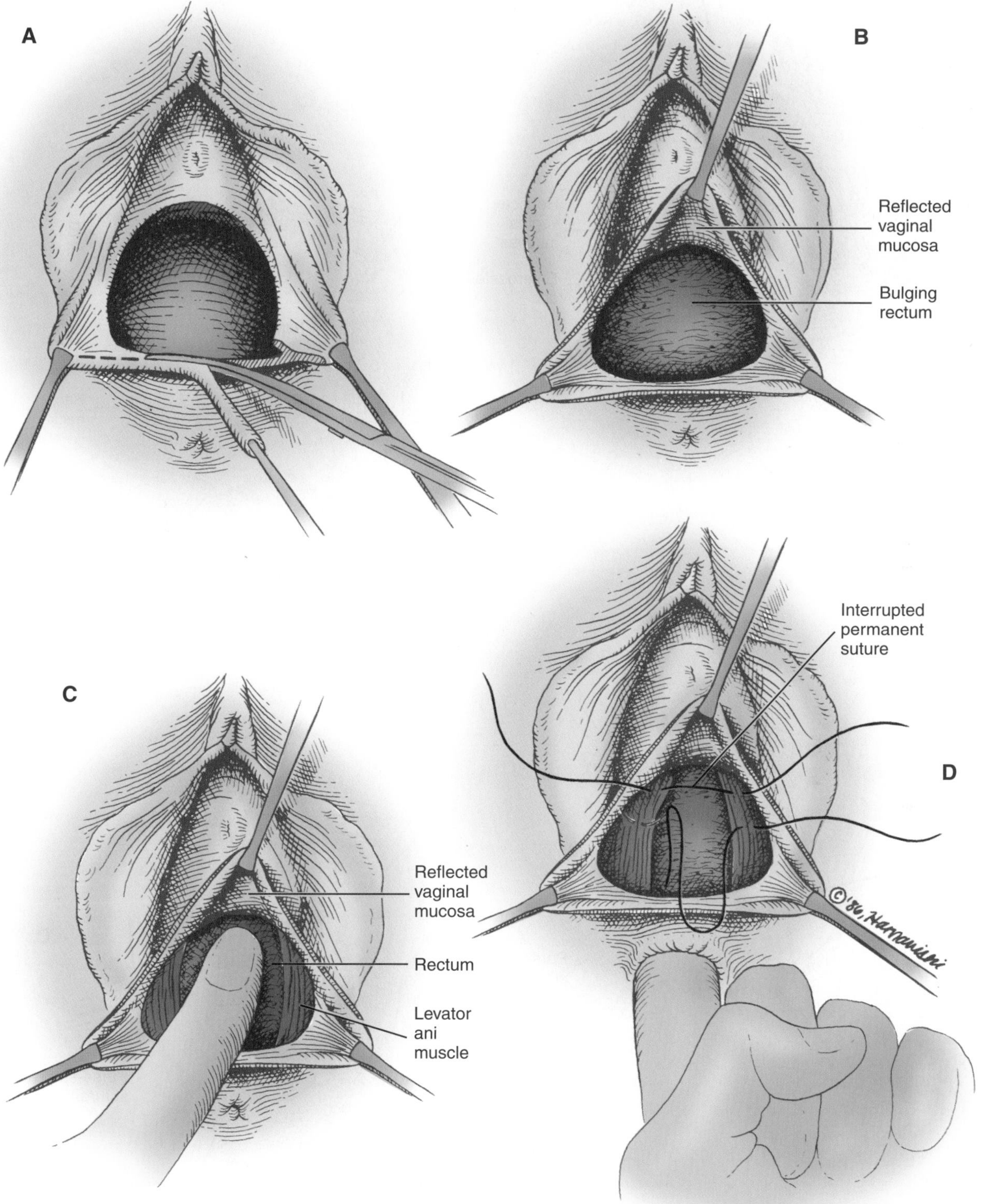


**FIGURE 14-16** Rectocele repair. **A,** Placement of Allis clamps at margins of perineal incision; perineal incision is being made. **B,** Reflected vaginal mucosa with rectum bulging. **C,** Depression of rectum identifying margins of levator ani muscle. **D,** Placement of sutures in perirectal tissue and levator ani bundles.

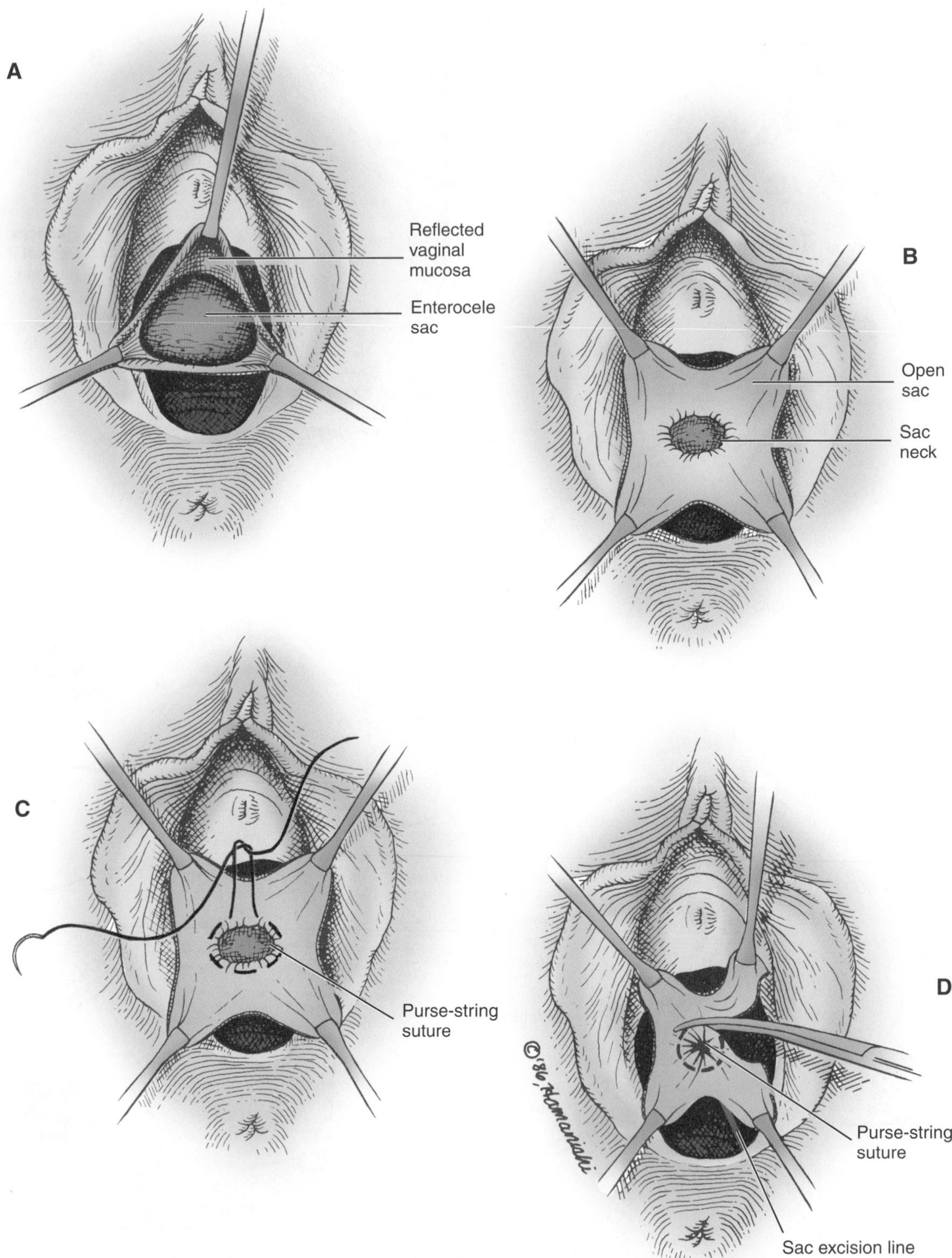


FIGURE 14-17 Enterocele repair. **A,** Appearance of enterocele sac with vaginal wall reflected. **B,** Appearance of open enterocele sac with sac neck identified. **C,** Placement of purse-string suture at neck of enterocele sac. **D,** Excision of enterocele sac.

tification and is then closed as high as possible by permanent purse-string sutures. The portion of peritoneal tissue distal to the purse-string ties is then excised, and the area is reinforced locally by transverse suture closures of whatever supportive tissues may be available. This technique is used to prevent recurrence.

**PERINEAL REPAIR.** The procedure is illustrated in Figure 14-18.

**VESICOVAGINAL FISTULA REPAIR.** A vesicovaginal fistula (a communication between the urinary bladder and the vagina) is repaired by free dissection of the mucosal tissue of the anterior vaginal wall, closing of the fistula tract, and repair of the fascial attachments between the bladder and vagina, with establishment of urinary drainage. Fistulas vary in size from a small opening that permits only slight leakage of urine into the vagina to a large opening that permits all urine to pass into the vagina (Figure 14-19). They may result from radiation therapy, radical surgery for the management of pelvic cancer, chronic ulceration of the vaginal structures, penetrating wounds, or obstetric trauma.

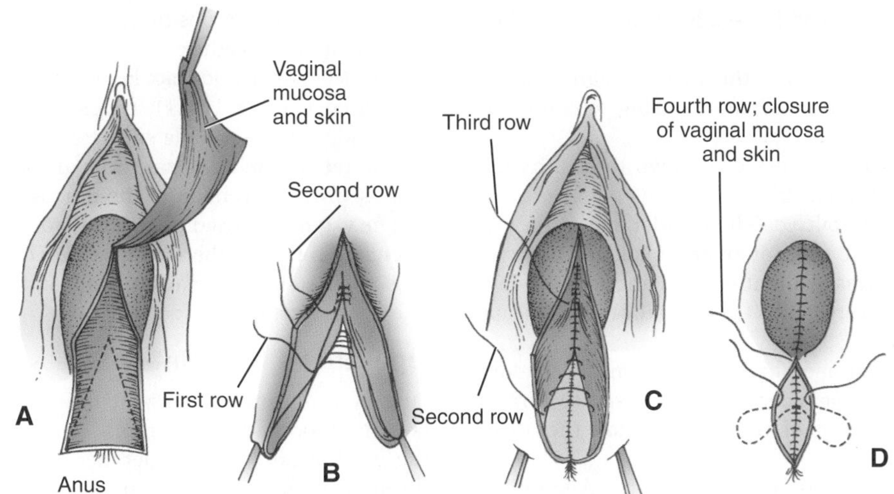


**FIGURE 14-18** Repair of complete lacerations of the perineum. **A,** Lower margins of incision. **B,** Placement of first and second rows of sutures. **C,** Second and third rows of sutures. **D,** Fourth row of sutures.

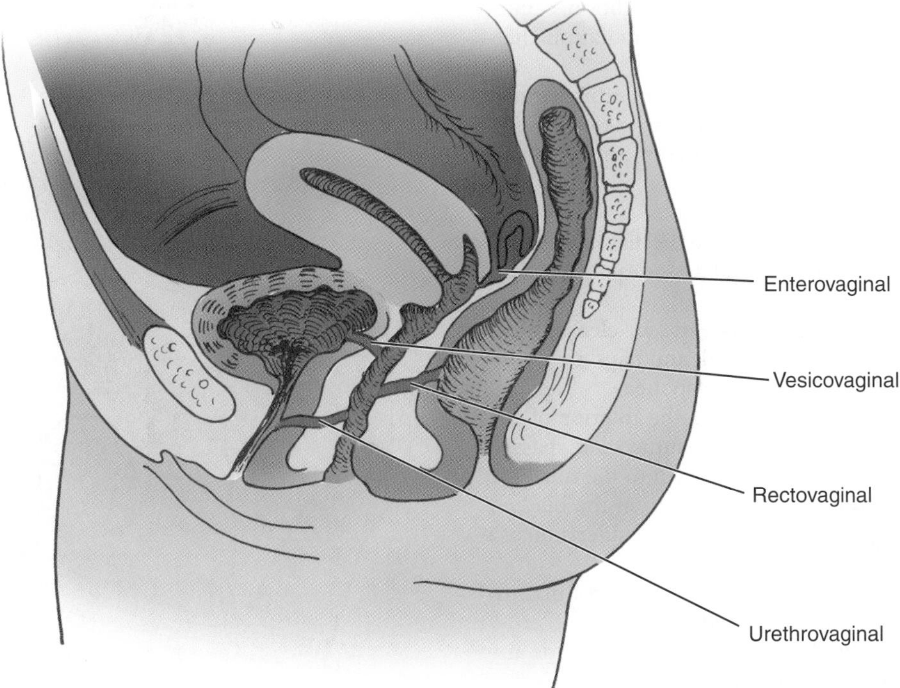


**FIGURE 14-19** Genital fistulas may present as communications between the urethra, bladder, one of the ureters, or the bowel and some part of the genital tract. Two of the most common types are urethrovaginal and vesicovaginal, both of which empty into the vaginal canal.

**Vesicovaginal Fistula Repair (Transperitoneal Approach)**

***Procedural Considerations.*** In the presence of a high vesicovaginal fistula, a suprapubic incision is used. The opening from the bladder into the vagina is closed, and the fascial attachments are repaired.

The patient is placed in slight Trendelenburg position. Ureteral catheters may be inserted just before surgery (see Chapter 15). An abdominal gynecologic instrument set is required. The vagina is cleansed and may be packed with moist gauze saturated with an antibiotic or antimicrobial solution before prepping the abdominal site.

*Operative Procedure*

1. A midline abdominal incision is usually made, as described for laparotomy.
2. The fistulous tract is identified; the vaginal vault and the adjacent adherent bladder are separated using scissors, forceps, and sponges.
3. The vesicovaginal septum is dissected down to healthy tissue beyond the site of the fistula.
4. The fistulous tract is mobilized. The bladder site of the fistula is inverted into the interior of the bladder with two rows of inverting sutures. The muscularis and mucosa layers of the vagina are inverted into the vaginal vault by means of two rows of sutures.
5. Flaps of peritoneum are mobilized, both from the bladder and from the adjacent vaginal vault, and closed to form a new vesicovaginal reflection of peritoneum below the site of the old fistulous tract.
6. The wound is closed in layers, as for laparotomy. Abdominal dressings are applied. An indwelling urinary catheter is inserted.

**URETHROVAGINAL FISTULA REPAIR (VAGINAL APPROACH).** A urethrovaginal fistula (a communication between the urethra and the vagina) usually causes constant incontinence or difficulty in retaining urine. This condition occurs after damage to the anterior wall and bladder, radiation therapy, or parturition.

**Procedural Considerations.** The basic vaginal instrument set is required, with the addition of Kelly fistula scissors, dressing forceps, probes, skin hooks, Frazier suction tips, urethral catheters, and sterile water for irrigation.

**Operative Procedure**

1. After traction sutures are placed about the fistulous tract, the tissues are grasped with Allis-Adair forceps and plain tissue forceps.
2. The scar tissue around the fistula is excised; cleavage between the bladder and vagina is located, and flaps are mobilized using scissors, forceps, and gauze sponges.
3. The bladder mucosa is inverted toward the interior of the bladder with interrupted sutures. The sutures are passed through the muscularis of the bladder down to the mucosa.
4. A second layer of inverting sutures is placed in the bladder and tied, thereby completely inverting the bladder mucosa toward the interior.
5. The vaginal wall is closed with interrupted sutures in a direction opposite the closure of the bladder wall.
6. The bladder is distended with sterile saline to determine any leaks. An indwelling urinary catheter is inserted.

**URETEROVAGINAL FISTULA.** A ureterovaginal fistula (a communication between the distal ureter and the vagina) develops as a result of injury to the ureter. In some cases, reimplantation of the ureter in the bladder or ureterostomy may be done.

**RECTOVAGINAL FISTULA REPAIR (VAGINAL APPROACH).** Rectovaginal fistula repair by the vaginal approach includes repair of the perineum, fascia, and muscle-supporting structures between the rectum and vagina, thereby closing the fistula formed between the rectum and the vagina (Figure 14-20). In the presence of a large rectovaginal fistula, as in patients who have incurable cancer, a colostomy may be performed (see Chapter 11).

**Procedural Considerations.** The basic vaginal instrument set is required for a rectovaginal fistula repair. The patient is placed in lithotomy position.

**Operative Procedure**

1. The scar tissue and tract between the rectum and vagina are excised (Figure 14-21); edges of fresh tissue are approximated with absorbable sutures.
2. The rectum and vaginal walls are mobilized; the rectum is closed with inversion of the mucosa into the rectal canal.
3. The vagina is closed transversely or in a sagittal plane different from that of the rectal canal. The vaginal mucosal layer is inverted into the vaginal wall; an indwelling urinary catheter is inserted.

## Operations for Urinary Stress Incontinence

Surgery for urinary stress incontinence entails repair of the fascial supports and the pubococcygeal muscle surrounding the urethra and the bladder neck. This repair is performed through either a vaginal or an abdominal approach.

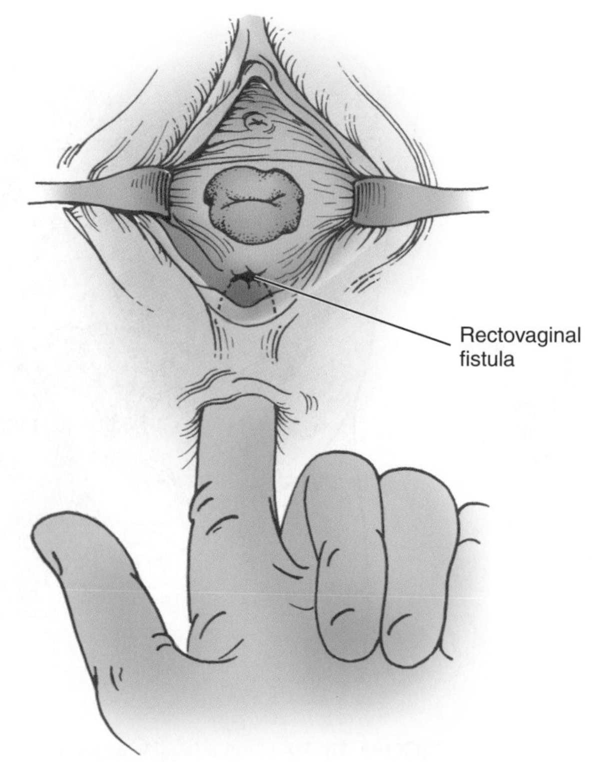


**FIGURE 14-20** Rectovaginal fistula. Examiner's finger puts tension on rectovaginal septum.

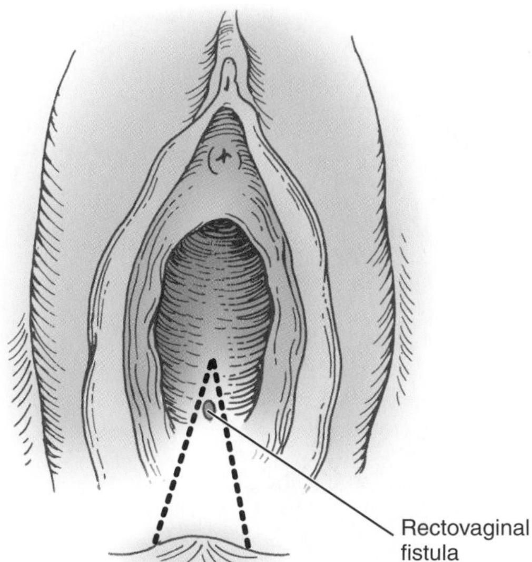


**FIGURE 14-21** Repair of rectovaginal fistulas of all types is essentially the same as shown here. Portion of scar tissue to be excised is included within dotted lines; repair is as described for complete lacerations of perineum (see Figure 14-18).

The proper operative approach for the treatment of stress incontinence must be selected specifically for each patient. Normal micturition depends on a finely coordinated group of voluntary and involuntary movements. As a result of volitional impulses, voiding may be inhibited or stopped by the intrinsic muscles of the bladder neck and proximal urethra and the puborectalis division of the levator ani muscle (see Chapter 15).

The type of operation selected depends on the severity of stress incontinence, the extent of the condition causing it, the patient's ability to use the anatomic mechanism for voluntary inhibition of urination, and any operations that have previously been performed. States of stress incontinence are classified in relation to frequency and degree of incontinence, the presence of other diseases, and the function of the pubococcygeal muscle (levator ani).

Previous pelvic procedures may have resulted in scarring and distortion, with displacement of the bladder neck. Conditions such as uterine prolapse, cystocele, urethrocele, cystourethrocele, or urogenital fistulas after radiation therapy may be associated with stress incontinence.

The desired outcome of any operation for urinary stress incontinence is to improve the performance of a dislodged or dysfunctional vesical neck, to restore normal urethral length, and to tighten and restore the anterior urethral vesical angle.

### *Operative Procedures*

VAGINAL APPROACH

1. An indwelling urinary catheter or suprapubic cystostomy catheter is inserted, according to the surgeon's preference. The posterior vaginal wall is retracted, and an incision is made through the anterior vaginal wall down to the urethra and bladder.
2. The vaginal wall is dissected from the bladder and urethra; the neck of the bladder is sutured together. The wound is closed as described for anterior vaginal wall repair.

VESICOURETHRAL SUSPENSION. The Marshall-Marchetti-Krantz procedure is fully described in Chapter 15. Basic steps of the procedure follow:

1. The space of Retzius is entered through a suprapubic abdominal incision, and the bladder and urethra are freed from the underlying structures.
2. Mattress sutures are inserted through the peravaginal fascia on either side of the vesicourethral angle area and preferably at a right angle to the long axis of the urethra and bladder. These are then passed through the central portion of the undersurface of the symphysis pubis under direct vision. The application of the sutures to the peravaginal connective tissue is done with the surgeon's hand in the vagina to ensure that the suture material is not passed through the vaginal mucosa.
3. The wound is closed and may be drained if the vascularity of the area warrants. An abdominal dressing is applied.

## Construction of a Vagina

Two basic approaches are used for repairing or overcoming a congenital or surgical defect of the vagina: obtaining a skin graft, which is applied to a mold and placed in the area of vaginal reconstruction; or making a simple opening in the area of vaginal reconstruction and placing a mold to permit spontaneous epithelialization of the area.

***Procedural Considerations.*** For a skin graft, the plastic surgery instrument set (see Chapter 24) is required, with the addition of a dermatome, marking pen, and nonadherent gauze dressing. For vaginal construction, the basic vaginal instrument set is required, with the addition of iris scissors, skin hooks, a vaginal mold, Halsted mosquito hemostats, and a ruler.

### *Operative Procedure*

1. The skin graft is taken from the abdomen or anterior area of the thigh. The donor site is dressed in the routine manner with nonadherent gauze and a pressure dressing.
2. The skin graft is kept in a moist gauze sponge until it is ready to be used.
3. A vaginal orifice is created by sharp dissection. Great care must be taken to prevent damage to the rectum and bladder. A mold is used to apply the donor skin or simply to hold the dissected area open to permit spontaneous epithelialization (Figure 14-22).

## Trachelorrhaphy

Trachelorrhaphy is removal of torn surfaces of the anterior and posterior cervical lips and reconstruction of the cervical canal. It is performed to treat deep lacerations of a cervix that is relatively free from infection.

***Procedural Considerations.*** The basic vaginal instrument set is required, plus the ESU and a conization loop electrode, if desired. An indwelling urinary catheter may be inserted into the bladder, depending on the surgeon's preference.

### *Operative Procedure*

1. The labia may be retracted with Allis-Adair tissue forceps or sutures. The cervix is grasped with a tenaculum.
2. The infected tissue of the exocervix is denuded with a knife. The flaps are undermined by means of a knife and curved

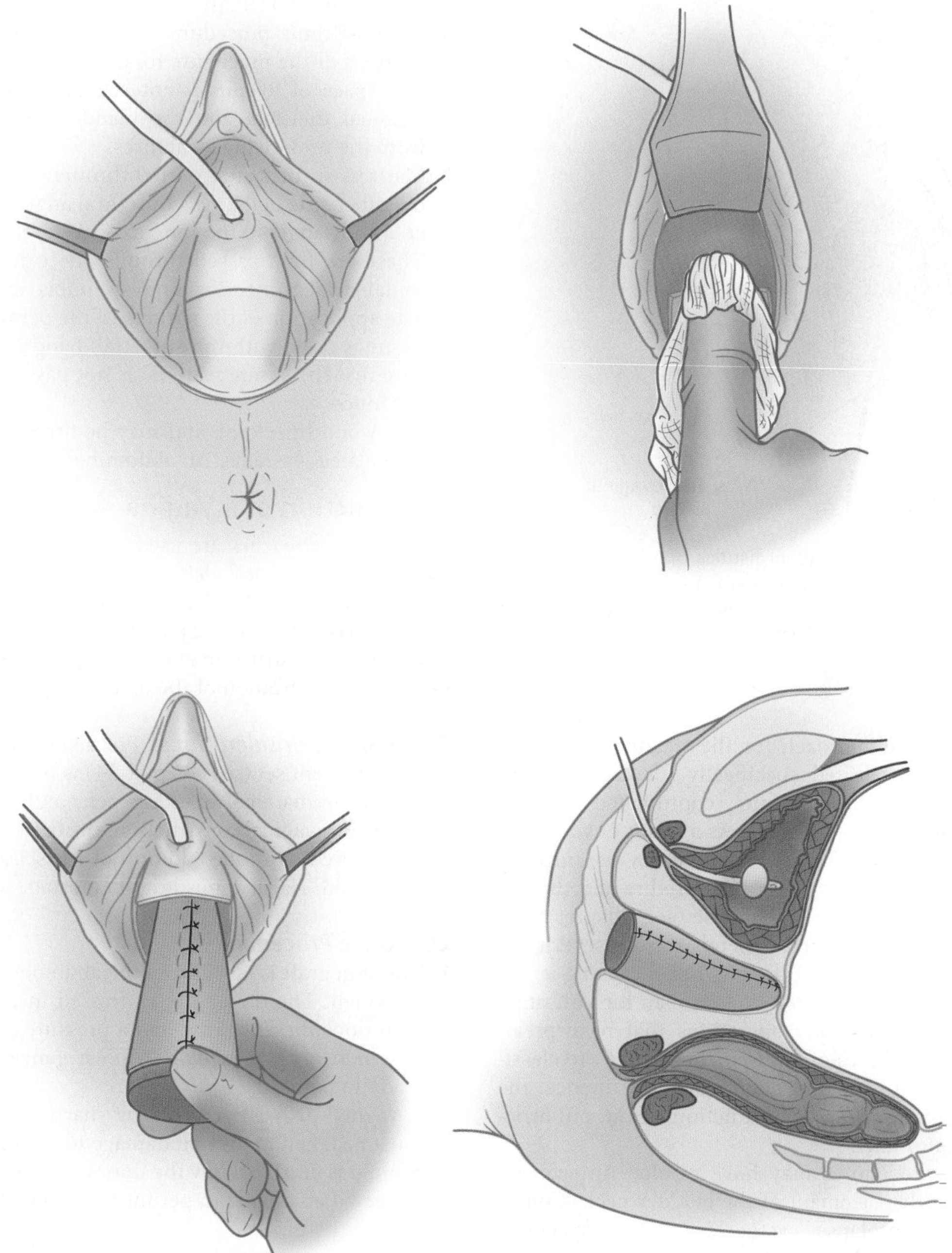

**FIGURE 14-22** Vaginal reconstruction using split-thickness skin graft.

scissors. Bleeding vessels are clamped and ligated. The mucosa is dissected from the cervix.

3. A small distal portion of the cervical canal is coned with a knife or a loop electrode to remove infected tissue. Bleeding vessels are clamped and ligated.
4. The denuded and coned areas are covered by transversely suturing the mucosal flaps of the exocervix, using interrupted sutures. Tissue forceps, hemostats, and gauze sponges are needed. The sutures are placed in such a manner that the fibromuscular tissue of the cervix is included, thereby eliminating dead space, where a hematoma may form, and providing a complete reconstructed cervical canal.
5. A vaginal pack may be inserted. A perineal pad is applied.

## Dilation of the Cervix and Curettage (D&C)

D&C is done either for diagnostic purposes or as a form of therapy for a variety of pelvic conditions, such as incomplete abortion, therapeutic abortion, abnormal uterine bleeding, or primary dysmenorrhea. D&C may also be performed when carcinoma of the endometrium is suspected, in the study of infertility, before amputation of the cervix, or before surgery for a prolapsed uterus.

***Procedural Considerations.*** In D&C, instruments are introduced through the vagina for the purpose of dilating the cervix. Dilation of the cervix can also take place by inserting laminaria tents into the cervical os before surgery; these tents are removed immediately before the procedure.

### Operative Procedure

1. A Jackson or Auvard weighted speculum is placed posteriorly in the vagina. A Sims or Deaver retractor is placed anteriorly to expose the cervix. The anterior lip of the cervix is grasped with a tenaculum (Figure 14-23).
2. The direction of the cervical canal and the depth of the uterine cavity are determined by means of a blunt probe or graduated uterine sound.
3. The cervix is gradually dilated by means of graduated Hegar or Hank dilators and possibly a Goodell uterine dilator.
4. Exploration for pedunculated polyps or myomas may be done with a polyp forcep.
5. The interior of the cervical canal and the cavity of the uterus are curetted to obtain either a fractional or a routine specimen. For specific identification of the site of specimens, the endocervix is scraped with the curette first, and the specimen is separated from the curetted matter of the uterine endometrium. In a routine curettage, all curetted matter is sent together for identification of tissue cells.
6. Fragments of endometrium or other dislodged tissues may be removed with warm, moist gauze sponges on sponge-holding forceps or with a teaspoon and are then collected on Telfa.
7. Multiple punch biopsies of the cervical circumference (at the 3, 6, 9, and 12 o'clock positions) may be taken with a Gaylor biopsy forceps to supplement the diagnostic studies.
8. Retractors are withdrawn; iodoform or plain gauze packing may be inserted into the uterus, using dressing forceps. The tenaculum is removed from the cervix. A vaginal pack may be inserted. A perineal pad is applied.

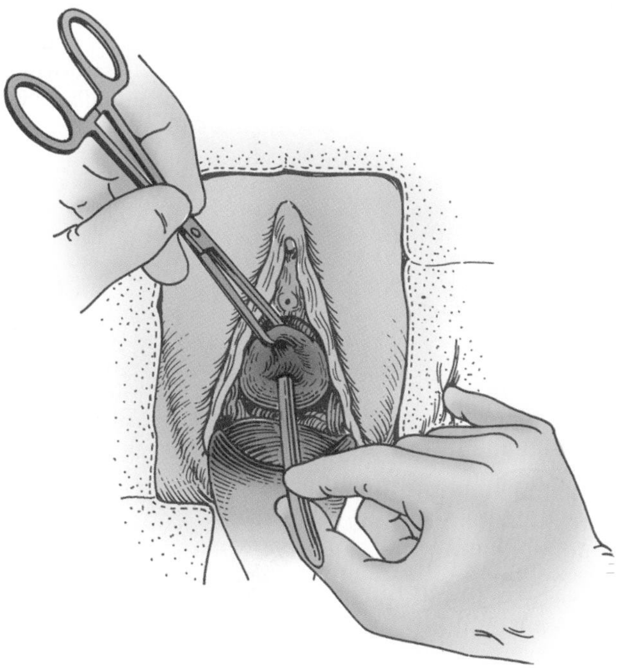

**FIGURE 14-23** Dilation of cervix and curettage. Vaginal wall retracted; cervix held by tenaculum; cervix dilated with dilator. Uterine cavity curetted with sharp curettes.

## Suction Curettage

Suction curettage is vacuum aspiration of the uterine contents. Aspiration has proved to be a safe and effective method for early termination of pregnancy and for use in missed and incomplete spontaneous abortions. Advantages are smaller dilation of the cervix, less damage to the uterus, less blood loss, less chance of uterine perforation, and reduced danger of infection. Laminaria tents may be inserted approximately 4 to 24 hours before suction curettage to dilate the cervix; they are removed before the surgical prep begins. Suction curettage is the treatment of choice for benign gestational trophoblastic neoplasia, more commonly known as hydatidiform mole. Hydatidiform mole is a condition that arises from fertilization by the sperm in a defective egg that has no nucleus or fertilization of the egg by two sperm. This results in the synthesis of material that is termed a mole and consists of multiple fluid-filled vesicles resembling a cluster of grapes (Figure 14-24).

***Procedural Considerations.*** The instrumentation required includes the D&C set, with the addition of one set of Pratt, Hawkin, or Hank uterine dilators, placenta forceps, urethral catheter, sterile cannulas, aspirator tubing, a vacuum aspirator unit, and oxytocic drugs.

### Operative Procedure

1. The cervix is exposed with an Auvard weighted speculum and an anterior retractor; it is then grasped with a sharp tenaculum and is drawn toward the introitus.
2. The cervix can be further dilated, allowing 1 mm of cannula diameter for each week of pregnancy.
3. The appropriate-size cannula is inserted into the uterus until the sac is encountered. The suction is turned on with immediate disruption and aspiration of the contents. Continued gentle motion of the cannula removes the uterine

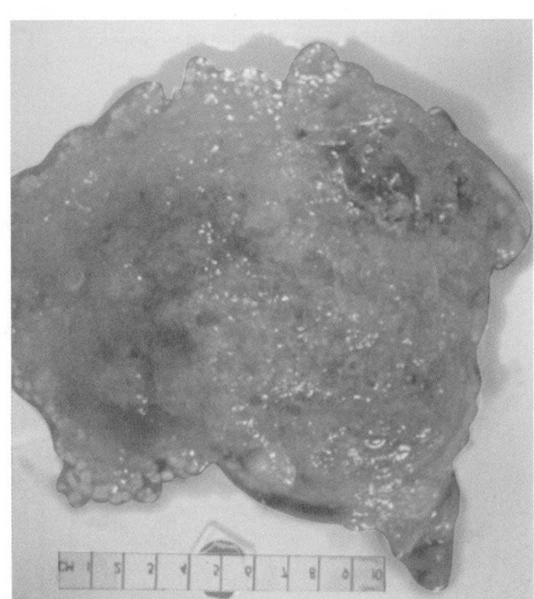

**FIGURE 14-24** Hydatidiform mole. Note vesicles have appearance of grapes.

contents (Figure 14-25). Use of uterine curettes may supplement suction in removing the entire uterine contents.
4. Retractors and tenaculum are removed.
5. A perineal pad is applied.

The specimen is removed from the suction bottle and sent for pathologic examination.

## Removal of Pedunculated Cervical Myomas (Cervical Polyps)

Cervical polyps (small pedunculated lesions) stem from the endocervical canal and consist almost entirely of columnar epithelium with or without squamous metaplasia. They may vary in size and are soft, red, and friable. Bleeding may result from the slightest trauma. Pedunculated lesions may be removed by the snare method or by dissection from the cervical canal with a knife, cold-knife conization, or resectoscope. Usually the surgeon performs an endometrial and endocervical curettage, and a cytologic smear is taken.

*Procedural Considerations.* A D&C set, a tonsil snare with medium-size snare wire, glass slides, the ESU, and a blade electrode or resectoscope are required.

### Operative Procedure

1. The anterior lip of the cervix is grasped with a Jacobs vulsellum or a tenaculum. The canal is sounded and dilated either to visualize or palpate the base of the pedicle.
2. If the pedicle of the tumor is thin, a tonsil snare may be placed over the body of the tumor, permitting the snare to crush the base of the tumor and to control bleeding. If the tumor is large, its base is dissected out with a knife. Bleeding may be controlled by the use of warm, moist gauze sponges with or without electrocoagulation. A resectoscope with the use of electrosurgery may be used to dissect the tumor.
3. Iodoform or plain gauze packing may be introduced into the cervical os. The tenaculum is removed from the cervix, and the retractors are withdrawn. A vaginal pack may be inserted for hemostasis. A perineal pad is applied.

## Conization and Biopsy of the Cervix

Conization and biopsy of the cervix are generally performed for the diagnosis or treatment of cervical dysplasia. The procedure may be initiated with colposcopy and punch biopsy, followed by electrocoagulation, cryosurgery, cold-knife cone biopsy, loop electrosurgical excision cone (LEEC), or laser excisional cone.

*Procedural Considerations.* The instruments required include a D&C set along with an ESU or laser, conization electrical loop, and ball-tipped electrode, depending on the procedure.

### Operative Procedure

1. The posterior vaginal wall is retracted by a speculum and the anterior vaginal wall by lateral retractors. The outer portions of the cervix are grasped with a tenaculum, and the cervix is drawn toward the introitus. Cystic areas of the cervix may be treated with a needle electrode or laser. Endometrial biopsy may be done (Figure 14-26, *A*). Bleeding points are coagulated or lased.
2. The electrode is passed into the cervical canal, and the diseased tissue is treated. Ferrous subsulfate (Monsel's solution) may be used for hemostasis.
3. The electrical loop (Figure 14-26, *B* and *C*) or the laser may be used to remove the diseased tissue and obtain a histologic specimen, which is sent to the pathology laboratory for examination.
4. If a wide conization is performed, the cervix may be sutured and vaginal packing may be used. An indwelling urinary catheter may be inserted. A perineal pad is applied.

## Cesium Applicator Insertion for Cervical and Endometrial Malignancy

Cesium has generally replaced radium insertions for treatment of malignancy of the cervix and endometrium.

*Procedural Considerations.* The patient is brought to the OR for insertion of the applicators. The bladder is drained with an indwelling urinary catheter. The catheter balloon is inflated with

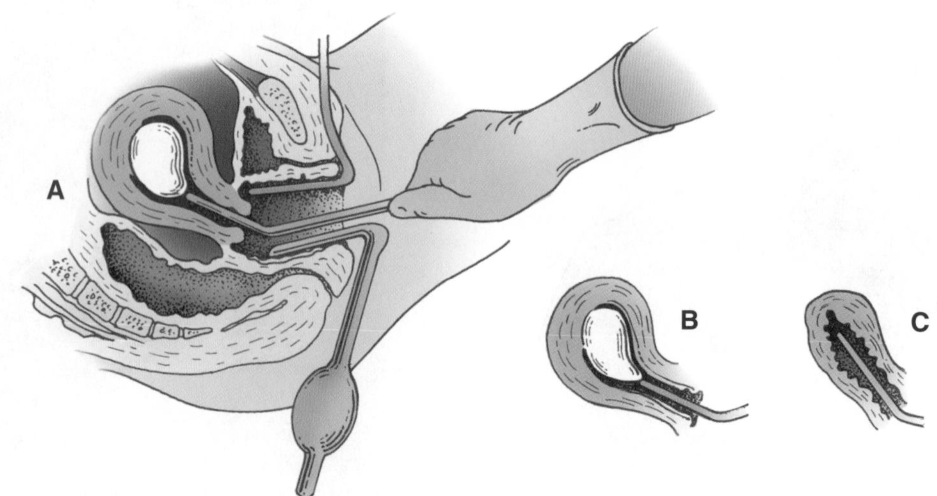


FIGURE 14-25 Suction curettage. **A,** Insertion of cannula. **B,** Gentle suction motion to aspirate contents. **C,** Uterine contents evacuated.

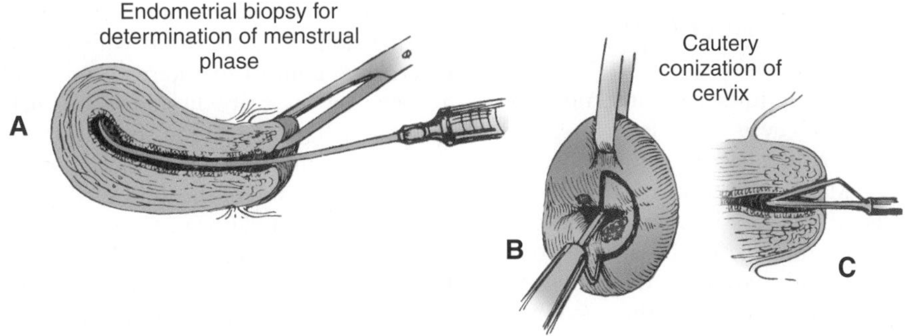


**FIGURE 14-26** **A,** Endometrial biopsy technique. **B** and **C,** Methods of treating cervical conditions or obtaining specimens for diagnostic tests.

a radiopaque medium for radiographic visualization after insertion of the cesium. An indwelling rectal marker is also placed by the surgeon for radiographic visualization. Various types of cesium applicators may be used according to the surgeon's preference and the area of malignancy (Figure 14-27). The cesium is loaded into the applicators later in the radiation department or in the patient's room under controlled conditions, in which all personnel are monitored by use of a dosimeter.

***Interstitial Therapy.*** Cesium needles are available in various lengths with small diameters for insertion into the tissue surrounding the cervix (Figure 14-28). They are inserted vaginally with a needle applicator and are used as a supplement to intravaginal or intrauterine sources. To facilitate removal, the needles have wires or threads attached to their distal ends.

## Posterior Colpotomy (Culdotomy)

Posterior colpotomy (culdotomy) is an incision through the vagina and peritoneum into the cul-de-sac. Posterior colpotomy can be performed to carry out definitive operative procedures: various kinds of tubal ligations, aspiration or the removal of ovarian cysts, the occasional management of an ectopic pregnancy, and exploratory diagnostic operative procedures.

***Procedural Considerations.*** The basic vaginal instrument set is required, with the addition of a 15-gauge needle, syringe, culture tubes, and drains. An abdominal gynecologic instrument set should be available in case laparotomy is indicated.

### *Operative Procedure*

1. A transverse incision is made through the posterior vaginal wall with curved scissors. This incision is carried into the peritoneum, behind the cervix at the superior point of the posterior fornix.
2. Allis forceps are used to facilitate exposure, and hemostasis is obtained by placing a number of sutures into the corners or angles of the wound.
3. The posterior vaginal wall is held open with a weighted retractor.
4. In case of infection in the cul-de-sac, the opening is enlarged enough to permit drainage from the cul-de-sac. The cavity is explored; drains may be inserted.
5. Bleeding of the vaginal wall is controlled by sutures. The peritoneum and the vaginal mucosa are closed with a continuous suture. Vaginal packing and an indwelling urinary catheter may be inserted. A perineal pad is applied.

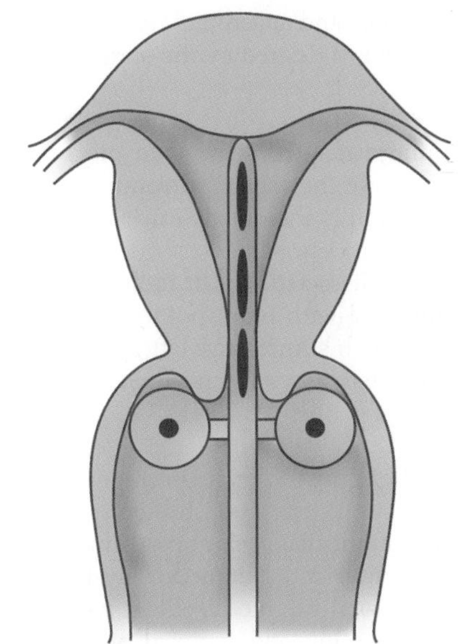

**FIGURE 14-27** Intracavitary implant. Applicator in place in uterus.

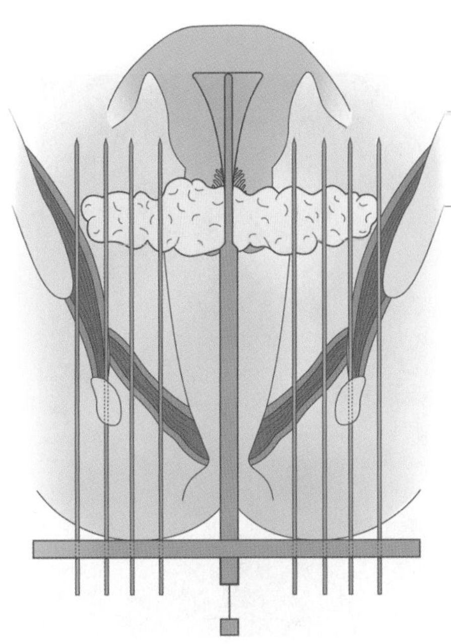

**FIGURE 14-28** Interstitial intracavitary implant.

## Marsupialization of Bartholin Duct Cyst or Abscess

A cyst in a Bartholin gland usually follows acute infection and is treated by marsupialization. Such cysts result from retention of glandular secretions caused by blockage somewhere in the duct system (Figure 14-29). Marsupialization of a Bartholin duct cyst or abscess entails removal or incision of the cyst through the vaginal outlet and drainage of the area. In true marsupialization the cyst is surgically exteriorized by resecting the anterior wall and suturing the cut edges of the remaining cyst to the adjacent edges of the skin.

*Procedural Considerations.* The basic vaginal instrument set is required, with the addition of a 15-gauge needle, syringe, culture tubes (aerobic and anaerobic), iodoform or plain gauze packing, and a drain, if desired by the surgeon.

### *Operative Procedure*

1. The labia minora may be sutured to the perineal skin on each side to expose the vaginal introitus.
2. An elliptic incision is then made into the mucosa, which is distended over the cyst.
3. The cyst wall is dissected, and if indicated, removal of the gland is completed with blunt-pointed scissors. The tissue may be everted with sutures and left open. A drain or packing may be inserted, and a perineal pad is applied.

## Hysteroscopy

Hysteroscopy is the endoscopic visualization of the uterine cavity and tubal orifices. A fiberoptic hysteroscope is introduced vaginally and aids in the diagnosis and treatment of intrauterine disease. The common indications for hysteroscopy include evaluation of abnormal uterine bleeding, with possible endometrial ablation, location and removal of "lost" intrauterine devices (IUDs), evaluation of infertility, diagnosis and surgical treatment of intrauterine adhesions, verification of submucous leiomyomas or endometrial polyps, resection of uterine septa or submucous leiomyomas, and tubal sterilization. Laparoscopy may be done in association with hysteroscopy to assess the external contour of the uterus. Contraindications to either diagnostic or operative hysteroscopy include pelvic infection, cervical malignancy, and in some instances, heavy bleeding.

A significant potential complication related to hysteroscopy is the intravasation of the fluid used to distend the uterine cavity. Intravasation can lead to hyponatremia. Signs and symptoms of hyponatremia may include bradycardia, hypertension followed by hypotension, nausea, vomiting, headache, visual disturbances, agitation, confusion, and lethargy. The perioperative nurse is responsible for accurately monitoring fluid intake and output during hysteroscopy. Monitoring may be manual (i.e., calculating the difference between inflow and outflow) or may be automatically calculated on commercially available hysteroscopy pumps. Discrepancies of more than 1500 ml must be communicated to the surgeon and the anesthesia provider.[24]

*Procedural Considerations.* The instrumentation required includes a D&C set, with the addition of a hysteroscopy set (Figure 14-30), 50-ml syringes, polyethylene tubing, fiberoptic light source, the ESU or laser, hysteroscopic insufflator, pressure-infusion pump, and a video camera and monitor.

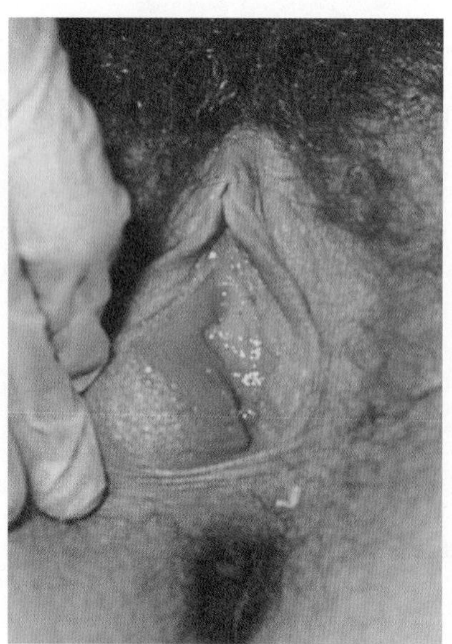

FIGURE 14-29 Bartholin abscess.

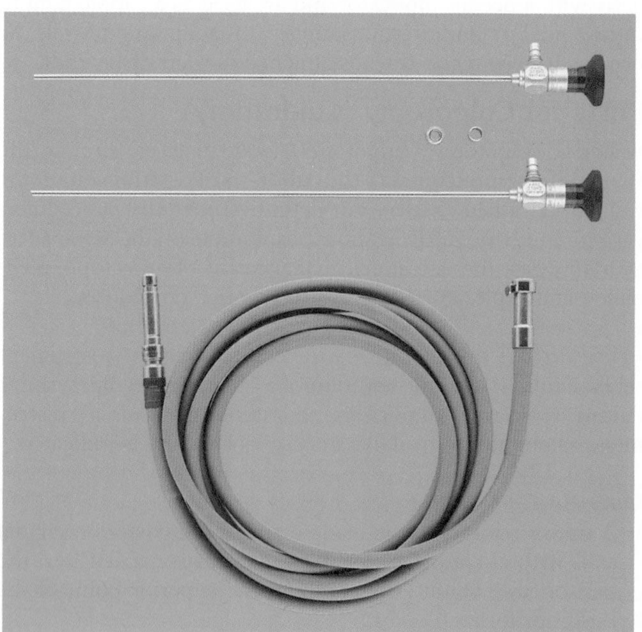



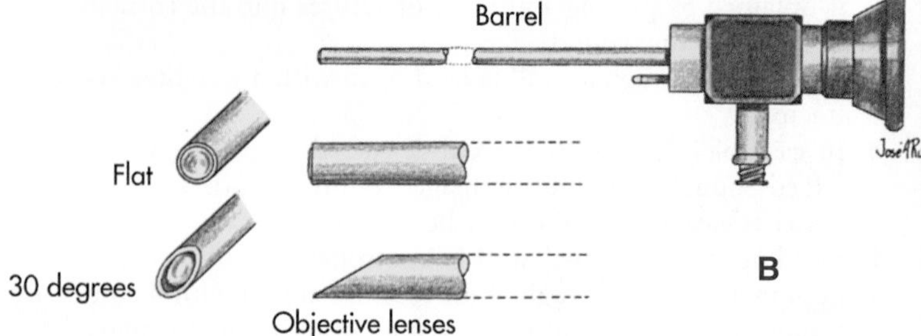



FIGURE 14-30 Instruments for hysteroscopy.

### *Operative Procedure*

1. The cervix is exposed with an Auvard weighted speculum and an anterior retractor; the anterior lip of the cervix is grasped with a tenaculum and is drawn toward the introitus.
2. The direction of the cervical canal and the depth of the uterine cavity are determined by means of a graduated uterine sound.
3. The endocervical canal is dilated by means of graduated Hegar or Hank uterine dilators to 6, 7, or 8 mm, depending on the size of the hysteroscope.
4. A self-retaining vacuum cannula with obturator may be placed into contact with the cervix. The cannula is firmly applied to the cervix by vacuum created with a negative pressure.
5. The obturator is withdrawn, and the hysteroscope is introduced to the level of the internal cervical os.
6. To achieve satisfactory visualization and sustained intrauterine pressure, the uterine cavity must be distended with one of the following media: 32% dextran 70 in dextrose (Hyskon), dextrose 5% in water ($D_5W$), sorbitol, mannitol, saline (normal saline solution [NSS]), sterile water, or by $CO_2$ gas insufflation. Because air or gas used for uterine insufflation may result in air or gas embolism, $CO_2$ pressures must be monitored closely. Injection of liquid media may be under continuous pressure from a 50-ml syringe or delivered by means of a pressure-controlled fluid-infusion (hysteroscopic) pump into the irrigating channel of the hysteroscope. When the syringe is used, care must be taken to prevent air bubbles, which distort the view or could lead to air embolism. Uterine distention with $D_5W$ may be achieved by inserting a 500-ml plastic bag containing the medium into an intravenous pressure infusor or the infusion pump. The fluid runs freely through polyethylene tubing through the channel of the hysteroscope.
7. Exploration of the uterine cavity is begun. A video camera monitor may be used to enhance visibility for the OR team, and the procedure may be videotaped for record keeping and reevaluation.
8. Ancillary instruments, such as rigid and flexible biopsy forceps, scissors, grasping forceps, insulated coagulation electrodes, resectoscope with "rollerball" electrode, laser fiber tips, and tubal occlusive devices, may be introduced for intrauterine manipulation or surgical intervention through the operating channel of the hysteroscope.
9. On completion of the procedure, the hysteroscope is withdrawn and the self-retaining vacuum cannula is removed.

If Hyskon is used for uterine distention, the instruments must be rinsed immediately and cleaned in hot water, because dextran has a tendency to harden and is difficult to remove if permitted to dry.

## Endometrial Ablation

Endometrial ablation is performed to treat abnormal uterine bleeding. The overall goal of endometrial ablation is to create amenorrhea or to reduce menstrual bleeding to a normal, tolerable flow for the patient. It may be an alternative to hysterectomy in some patients with chronic menorrhagia. The procedure is performed through the hysteroscope with the use of energy from either the laser or the ESU.

The Nd:YAG laser destroys the endometrium and results in scarring of the uterine lining. It is often the laser of choice for this procedure because of its ability to penetrate deep into the tissue, resulting in greater tissue destruction. The Nd:YAG, argon, and potassium titanyl phosphate (KTP) 532 lasers may be used hysteroscopically.

The two endometrial ablation techniques when the Nd:YAG laser is used are *blanching* and *dragging*. In the blanching technique, the tip of the laser fiber is held away from tissue. In the dragging technique, the laser fiber tip is in direct contact with the endometrium. The endometrial lining is treated from the fundus to approximately 4 cm above the external cervical os. Air or gas is not used in cooling the laser fiber because of the risk of air or gas embolism. Because of the systemic effects of fluid absorption through open capillaries, Hyskon is not generally used as an irrigant for endometrial laser ablation.

A specially designed diode laser may also be used for endometrial ablation. The diode laser utilizes a disposable handset that emits laser beams through three separate parallel panels. The handset conforms to the shape of the uterus and delivers energy in all directions to destroy the tissue in the fundus and cornua, away from the cervical opening. A hysteroscopy may be performed at the conclusion of the therapy to evaluate the results.

Electrical energy delivered through an adapted urologic resectoscope, using continuous-flow irrigation, either coagulates or resects the endometrium. Endometrial ablation with the use of a resectoscope, with a rollerball electrode attached, is not an option for a patient who desires to remain fertile. When using the resectoscope, often Hyskon is chosen as the distending medium because it is electrolyte-free and compatible with electrosurgery.

Reported complications associated with endometrial ablation using the Nd:YAG laser and electrosurgery include hemorrhage, fluid overload, uterine perforation, recurrent bleeding, injury to bowel and bladder, cervical lacerations, and rupture of a fallopian tube.

General anesthesia is usually administered, although endometrial ablation can be performed using a local anesthetic. The patient is placed in the lithotomy position, and all potential pressure points are padded. If the Nd:YAG laser is to be used, all laser safety precautions for the patient and the OR team are followed (see Chapter 7). If electrosurgery is being used for the procedure, an electrosurgical dispersive pad is applied. The length of the procedure is typically less than that for a hysterectomy. Therefore the patient requires less anesthetic and may be discharged the same day, provided that her condition remains stable.

***Balloon Endometrial Ablation.*** Endometrial ablation may also be accomplished using balloon therapy. The action of balloon therapy is thermal. The uterine balloon catheter conforms to the internal uterine contour and contains a heating element. Suction curettage is performed before the therapy to provide maximal balloon contact with the uterine lining. The cervix is dilated to 5 mm, and the balloon catheter is inserted in the uterus until the tip touches the fundus. The balloon is inflated with sterile $D_5W$ to a pressure of 160 to 180 mm Hg. The solution is heated to a temperature of 86.6°C (188°F) and maintained for 8 to 10 minutes. The procedure may be performed as an ambulatory surgical procedure and does not require hysteroscopy.[25]

### Vaginal Hysterectomy

Vaginal hysterectomy is removal of the uterus through an incision made in the vaginal wall and the pelvic cavity (History box). Contraindications to a vaginal approach are (1) a large uterine tumor, (2) a pelvic malignancy, and (3) the possibility of missing metastatic disease that might be present if malignancy is suspected.

***Procedural Considerations.*** The instrumentation includes the basic vaginal instrument set with the addition of two 22-gauge needles and two 10-ml syringes. An abdominal gynecologic instrument set should be available in case laparotomy is indicated. To facilitate dissection and decrease bleeding, the vaginal walls may be infiltrated with normal saline or a local anesthetic (vasoconstrictors are optional). The patient is placed in lithotomy position.

#### HISTORY

Women undergoing vaginal hysterectomy in the 1900s did so without the benefit of technology available today. The woman was admitted to the hospital several days in advance of the planned surgical procedure. Vigorous bowel preparation and thrice-daily douches with caustic solutions were a routine preoperative preparation, as was the removal of all hair from the abdomen and genitalia.

On the day of surgery, the perioperative nurse was responsible for administering a douche before bringing the patient into the operating room (OR). After positioning the patient for the procedure, the nurse used green soap to cleanse the vulva and vaginal canal, followed by a rinse of saline and a douche of 10% creolin. The creolin was followed by an additional douche of corrosive sublimate in a 1:2000 concentration in sterile water. Using a glass catheter, the nurse ensured the patient's bladder was empty before the start of the procedure.

During the vaginal hysterectomy, the surgeon controlled the patient's bleeding with clamps or ligatures. After the uterus was removed, as many as six clamps, which were equipped with detachable handles, were left in place for hemostasis. The clamps were surrounded with a roll of iodoform gauze extending up into the vagina. A retention catheter was placed in the bladder at the end of the procedure. The catheter would be used in the postoperative period for bladder irrigations.

Before the patient returned to consciousness, the nurse tied the patient's legs together with a broad towel to prevent strain on the clamps and any ligatures that had been placed. The towel was not removed until the patient regained consciousness and was able to cooperate.

The patient was transported back to her room, with the clamps in place, experiencing considerable pain. Two days after the procedure, the perioperative nurse accompanied the surgeon to the patient's room to assist with the removal and retrieval of the clamps. The previously placed gauze packing was removed. The surgeon reattached the handles to the clamps and began removal, using a rocking motion, starting with the uppermost clamp. As the clamps were released, pieces of tissue would adhere, causing great discomfort for the patient. The nurse assisted the surgeon with repacking the patient's vagina with gauze and then returned the clamps, which were coated with rust, tissue, and secretions, to the instrument room.

The patient was allowed to sit up in bed 2 days after the clamps were removed; she was lifted to a chair on the fourth day, and began to ambulate on the fifth or sixth day.

Modified from Fowler R: *The operating room and the patient,* ed 3, St Louis, 1913, Mosby; Haubold HA: *Preparatory and after treatment in operative cases,* New York, 1910, D Appleton.

#### *Operative Procedure*

1. The labia may be retracted with sutures. A vaginal retractor is inserted to retract the vaginal wall.
2. A Jacobs vulsellum, tenaculum, or suture ligature is placed through the cervical lips to permit traction on the cervix.
3. The vaginal wall is incised with a knife anteriorly through the full thickness of the wall (Figure 14-31, *A*). The bladder is freed from the anterior surface of the cervix by sharp and blunt dissection. The bladder is then elevated to expose the peritoneum of the anterior cul-de-sac, which is entered by sharp dissection (Figure 14-31, *B*).
4. The peritoneum of the posterior cul-de-sac is identified and incised.
5. The uterosacral ligaments containing blood vessels are clamped, cut, and ligated (Figure 14-31, *C* and *D*). The ends of the ligatures are left long and are tagged with a clamp.
6. The uterus is drawn downward, and the bladder is held aside with retractors and moist, small laparotomy packs.
7. The cardinal ligament on each side is clamped, cut, and ligated. The uterine arteries are doubly clamped, cut, and ligated.
8. The fundus is delivered with the aid of a uterine tenaculum.
9. When the ovaries are to be left, the round ligament, the uteroovarian ligament, and the fallopian tube on each side are clamped together (Figure 14-31, *E*) and cut and the uterus is removed. These pedicles are then ligated.
10. The peritoneum between the rectum and vagina is approximated with a continuous suture. The retroperitoneal obliteration of the cul-de-sac is accomplished by passing sutures from the vaginal wall through the infundibulopelvic ligament and round ligament, through the cardinal ligament, and out the vaginal wall. The sutures are tied on the vaginal aspect of the new vault (Figure 14-31, *F* and *G*). The round, cardinal, and uterosacral ligaments may be individually approximated for additional support.
11. Any existing cystocele and rectocele and the perineum are repaired. In the presence of prolapse, reconstruction of the pelvic floor may be required.
12. An indwelling urethral or suprapubic catheter is usually inserted. The vagina may be packed, and a drain may be inserted. A perineal pad is applied.

## GYNECOLOGIC SURGERY USING ABDOMINAL APPROACH

### Laparoscopy

Laparoscopy is the endoscopic visualization of the peritoneal cavity through the anterior abdominal wall after the establishment of a pneumoperitoneum. It is used to investigate and diagnose the causes of abdominal and pelvic pain and infertility and to evaluate pelvic masses. Ancillary procedures such as adhesiolysis, fulguration of endometriotic implants, aspiration of cysts, biopsy of tissue, aspiration of peritoneal fluid for cyto-

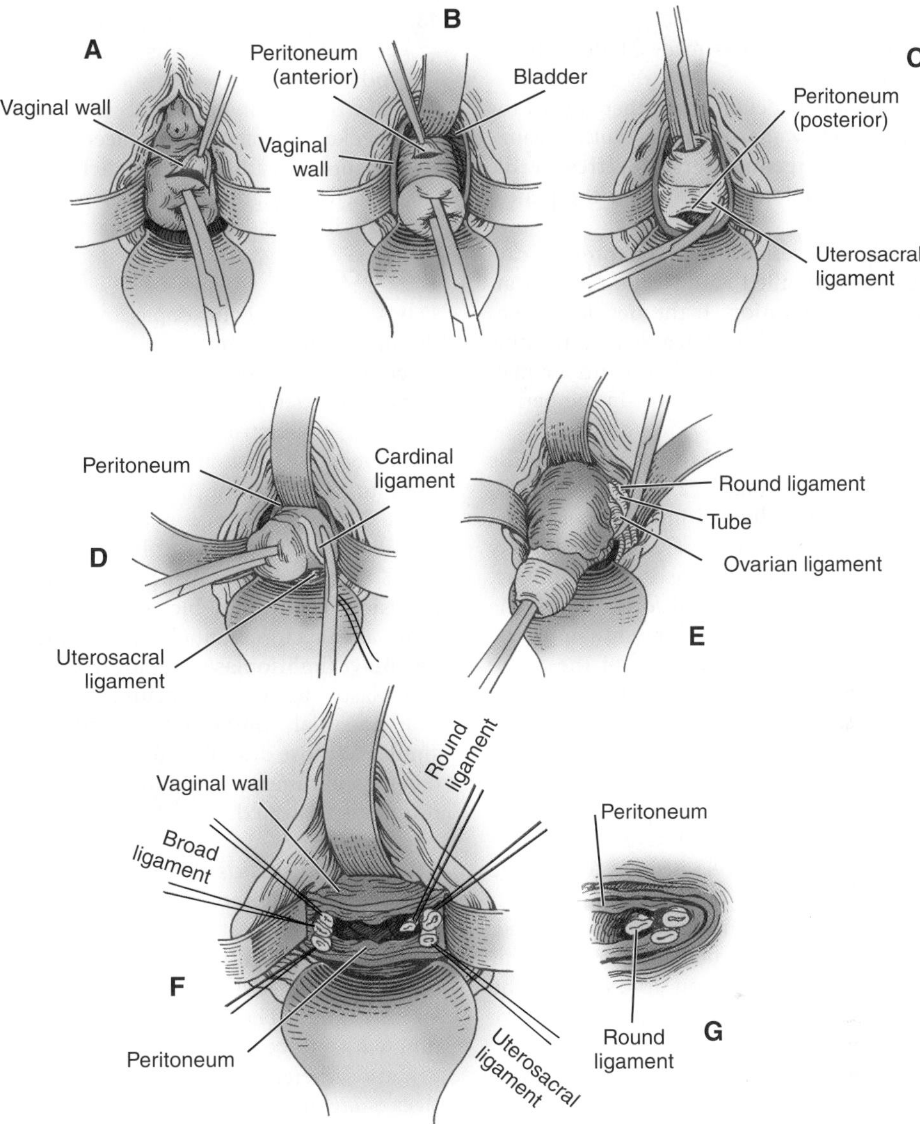


FIGURE 14-31 Vaginal hysterectomy. **A,** Incision of vaginal wall around cervix. Anterior vaginal wall slightly elevated. **B,** Deaver retractor on each side; one Deaver retractor under bladder. Peritoneum opened. **C,** Posterior cul-de-sac opened. Heaney clamp applied to left uterosacral ligament. **D,** Left uterosacral ligament cut and tied. Clamp applied to left cardinal ligament. **E,** Clamp applied to ovarian ligament, round ligament, and fallopian tube. **F,** Uterosacral ligament, broad ligament, and round ligament shown in their respective normal positions. **G,** Peritoneum closed and cardinal broad ligament and uterosacral ligaments reattached to angle of vagina. Left uterosacral and broad ligaments anchored.

logic study, and tubal sterilization may be performed. Laparoscopy also can be used for oocyte retrieval for IVF procedures. Lasers and electrosurgery may be used with the laparoscope.

***Procedural Considerations.*** A general or local anesthetic is administered. The patient is placed in lithotomy position. The abdomen, perineum, and vagina are prepped. The abdomen and perineum are then draped for a combined procedure. Specially designed drapes with openings for the umbilical and perineal areas may be used. The bladder should be emptied.

A D&C may be done with laparoscopic procedures when indicated. After the cervix is exposed and the position and depth of the uterus are confirmed, a uterine manipulator or dilator may be introduced into the cervix to manipulate the uterus during the laparoscopy so that the surgeon has better visibility. If chromotubation to evaluate the patency of the fallopian tubes will be performed during the laparoscopy, an intrauterine cannula is placed in the cervical canal at the time of D&C.

The usual instrumentation for the vaginal portion of the procedure includes a D&C set, with the addition of a uterine manipulator, intrauterine cannula, diluted methylene blue or indigo carmine solution, and a syringe.

An abdominal gynecologic instrument set should be readily available in the event that a laparotomy is indicated.

### Operative Procedure

1. A small incision (0.7 to 1.2 cm) is made at the inferior margin of the umbilicus.
2. Elevating the skin with a towel clamp on either side of the umbilicus or grasping below the umbilicus with a gauze sponge for traction, the surgeon inserts a Verres needle through the layers of the abdominal wall into the peritoneal cavity.
3. Once the Verres needle is inserted into the peritoneal cavity, a 10-ml syringe partially filled with sterile saline is attached to the needle for aspiration. If the needle has entered a blood vessel, blood is aspirated. If a loop of intestine or the stomach has been entered, bowel contents or malodorous gas is aspirated. If the needle is free in the peritoneal cavity, nothing is aspirated.
4. A plastic or Silastic tubing is attached to the Verres needle and the gas insufflator. Approximately 2 to 3 liters of $CO_2$ or nitrous oxide gas is then delivered into the peritoneal cavity to achieve pneumoperitoneum. $CO_2$ is commonly used as the insufflation medium because it is nontoxic, highly soluble in blood, and rapidly absorbed from the peritoneal cavity. The intraabdominal pressure must be closely monitored to prevent overdistention of the abdomen and to ensure free passage of gas into the peritoneal cavity.
5. After insufflation is completed, the Verres needle is withdrawn.
6. The trocar covered by the trocar sleeve is inserted through the abdominal wall into the peritoneal cavity. The angle taken by the trocar is approximately 45 degrees toward the concavity of the pelvis. The plastic or Silastic tubing is attached to the trocar sleeve, and insufflation is resumed. Some surgeons prefer a direct trocar-insertion technique or open laparoscopy technique of Hasson to establish the pneumoperitoneum through the valve of the trocar sleeve rather than through a Verres needle.
7. With the trocar sleeve in place, the trocar is withdrawn and the laparoscope is introduced.
8. Visualization of the pelvis and lower abdomen and the visceral contents is begun. If the lens of the laparoscope becomes foggy, application of a commercially available defogger solution may control the problem. Alternatively, the surgeon may touch the lens to a loop of intestine to clear it. Before use, warming the tip of the scope in warm saline or towels may prevent fogging of the distal lens.
9. The patient is placed in the Trendelenburg position.
10. The video camera is attached to the scope to aid in the OR team's visualization, and the procedure may be recorded for future reference. If an ancillary instrument such as biopsy forceps or bipolar forceps is needed, a second trocar with sleeve is inserted under direct laparoscopic visualization through an incision made suprapubically.
11. To test for tubal patency, diluted methylene blue or indigo carmine solution is injected through the intrauterine cannula into the cervical canal. If the fallopian tubes are patent, dye can be seen at the fimbriated ends.
12. On completion of the intraabdominal procedure, the laparoscope is withdrawn and the insufflated gas is allowed to escape from the trocar sleeve or by suction. The trocar sleeve is removed.
13. Application of skin clips or subcuticular closure of the primary skin incision is followed by placement of a Band-Aid or Steri-Strip.
14. The uterine manipulator is removed, and the cervix is checked for bleeding. If bleeding is present, pressure may be applied with a sponge stick or a suture ligature may be passed through the bleeding portion.
15. A perineal pad is applied.

## Pelviscopy

Pelviscopy is an endoscopic approach to pelvic and intraabdominal examination or surgery. It differs from operative laparoscopy in two ways: (1) a 10-mm pelviscope with a 30-degree angle replaces the standard 7-mm laparoscope with a 0-degree angle; (2) the instrumentation used is capable of intraabdominal hemostasis and suturing. A 30-degree–angle telescope is used to visualize the intrapelvic and intraabdominal structures. The field of vision is wide, and the size, depth, and mobility of the organs can be assessed throughout the procedure. Procedures performed through the pelviscope include adhesiolysis, ovarian biopsy, ovarian cystectomy, oophorectomy, adnexectomy, enucleation of intramural myomas, appendectomy, fimbrioplasty, removal of ectopic tubal pregnancy, tuboplasty, uterosacral neurectomy, and lymphadenectomy. The potential complications associated with pelviscopy are similar to those described for laparoscopy. An abdominal gynecologic instrument set should be readily available in case laparotomy is indicated.

***Procedural Considerations.*** Many of the procedural considerations for pelviscopy are similar to those associated with laparoscopy. The patient may be typed and crossmatched for blood preoperatively, as for ectopic pregnancy. If the pelviscopic surgery is elective, autologous blood donation may be an alternative. The patient may be placed in the supine position, with a forced-air warming blanket in place. An indwelling urinary catheter is inserted, and antiembolic stockings or SCD sleeves are applied. Bony prominences are padded, and a dispersive electrosurgical pad is applied. In the instance of possible ectopic pregnancy, D&C may be performed to rule out an intrauterine pregnancy. Usually two or three puncture sites are established for the necessary accessory instrumentation.

The surgeon and assistants manipulate instruments through trocar sheaths, as described with laparoscopy. The OR team uses the video monitors placed on opposite sides of the OR bed for visualization. Accessory instruments used with the pelviscope include dissecting forceps, grasping forceps, scissors, sponge holders, needle holders, suture forceps, knot tiers, appendix extractors, suction manipulators, fulgurating electrodes, laser probes, and applicators for loop ligature. A tissue morcellator may be used to slowly fragment the tissue; the tissue is then loaded into the barrel of the morcellator for removal. Endocoagulation and endoligation may be used. Intraabdominal ligation is accomplished using loops of synthetic and natural suture materials.

## Ectopic Tubal Pregnancy

Ectopic pregnancy is defined as any gestation developing outside of the endometrial cavity. Risk factors for developing an ectopic pregnancy include use of intrauterine devices (i.e., IUDs) for contraception, pelvic inflammatory disease, tubal ligation, in vitro fertilization, and previous ectopic pregnancy. Although the fallopian tube is the most common site for ectopic pregnancies (occurring in up to 95% of all cases), they can develop in the cervix or broad ligament; in a previous cesarean section scar (myotomy), they can develop in the ovary and the peritoneal cavity.[9,11,27] Women who experience ectopic pregnancy generally present with abdominal pain, abnormal vaginal bleeding, and a palpable adnexal mass. Diagnosis is confirmed through human chorionic gonadotrophin (hCG) levels and the absence of a gestational sac on ultrasound. A serious complication of ectopic pregnancy is tubal rupture and hemorrhage (Figure 14-32). The ultrasound is also useful in identifying free fluid in the peritoneal cavity.[22] Ruptured ectopic pregnancy is considered a surgical emergency and is associated with severe abdominal pain, tachycardia, and hypotension. The woman with a ruptured ectopic pregnancy may also experience shoulder pain because of irritation of the phrenic nerve from the hemoperitoneum. Ectopic pregnancy may be treated medically with methotrexate or surgically through salpingostomy, segmental resection, fimbrial expression, and salpingectomy (Figure 14-33). Methotrexate destroys rapidly dividing cells and is often given in conjunction with the surgical procedure to destroy any residual trophoblastic cells that might remain.[11] Laparoscopic and/or ultrasound-guided application of methotrexate to the extrauterine gestational sac may also be used as an alternative therapy.[26]

***Pelviscopic Salpingostomy.*** Pelviscopic salpingostomy may be used in the treatment of unruptured ampulla gestations.

OPERATIVE PROCEDURE

1. After successful pelviscopic entry, the distal end of the fallopian tube is mobilized and the adhesiolysis is completed. Grasping forceps are placed on either side of the fallopian tube, and gentle traction is applied.
2. Before making an incision, coagulation of the serial vessels on both sides of the anticipated incision may be performed. A dilute solution of vasopressin may also be injected into the mesenteric margin to avoid excessive bleeding (Figure 14-34).
3. A single incision is made with scissors from the mesenteric to the antimesenteric side of the fallopian tube, where the products of conception are exposed.
4. The tissue is removed gently with forceps while constant irrigation is maintained with an isotonic solution (Figure 14-35). Vigorous evacuation is avoided so that the highly vascular underlying interstitial layer is not disturbed.

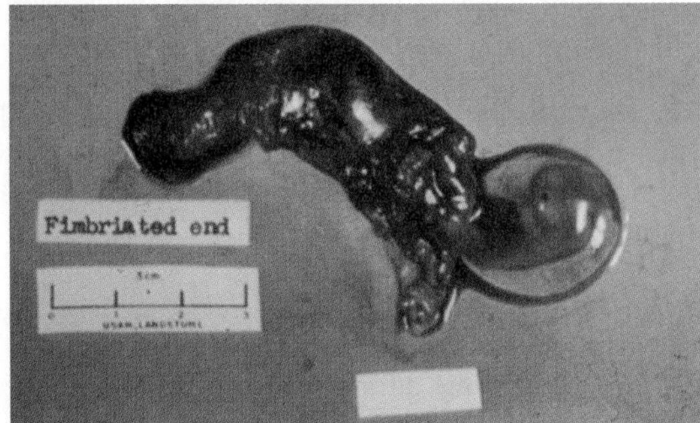
Fimbriated end

FIGURE 14-32 Ruptured ectopic pregnancy with fetus in sac.

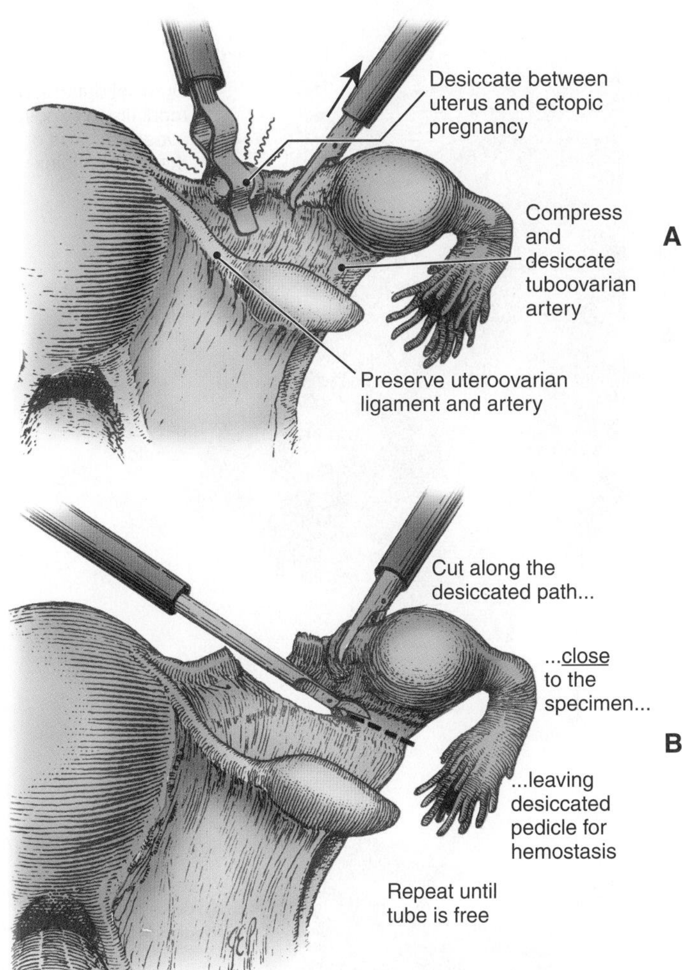
Desiccate between uterus and ectopic pregnancy
Compress and desiccate tuboovarian artery
A
Preserve uteroovarian ligament and artery
Cut along the desiccated path...
...close to the specimen...
B
...leaving desiccated pedicle for hemostasis
Repeat until tube is free

FIGURE 14-33 **A,** Electrodesiccation of the proximal fallopian tube during salpingectomy. **B,** Excision of the fallopian tube.

5. Small bleeding vessels can be ligated with a fine, nonreactive suture. Simple traumatic compression of bleeding margins will also promote hemostasis. Mesosalpingeal vessel ligation may be performed.
6. The tubal incision may be closed by second intention or, as in the instance of salpingotomy, the incision may be closed in one or two layers, with 6-0 interrupted sutures. On completion, the pelviscope and instrumentation are removed. The insufflated gas is permitted to escape from the trocar sleeves. Trocar sleeves are then removed. Application of skin clips or subcuticular closure of the primary skin incisions is followed by placement of Band-Aids, Steri-Strips, or dressings.

## Ovarian Cystectomy

Ovarian cystectomy is frequently performed by means of pelviscopic surgery.

### *Operative Procedure*

1. After successful pelviscopic entry, adhesiolysis is achieved.
2. On entry, peritoneal washings for cell block are obtained, if indicated.
3. The ovarian cyst is mobilized, and the cortex is grasped with a biopsy instrument.

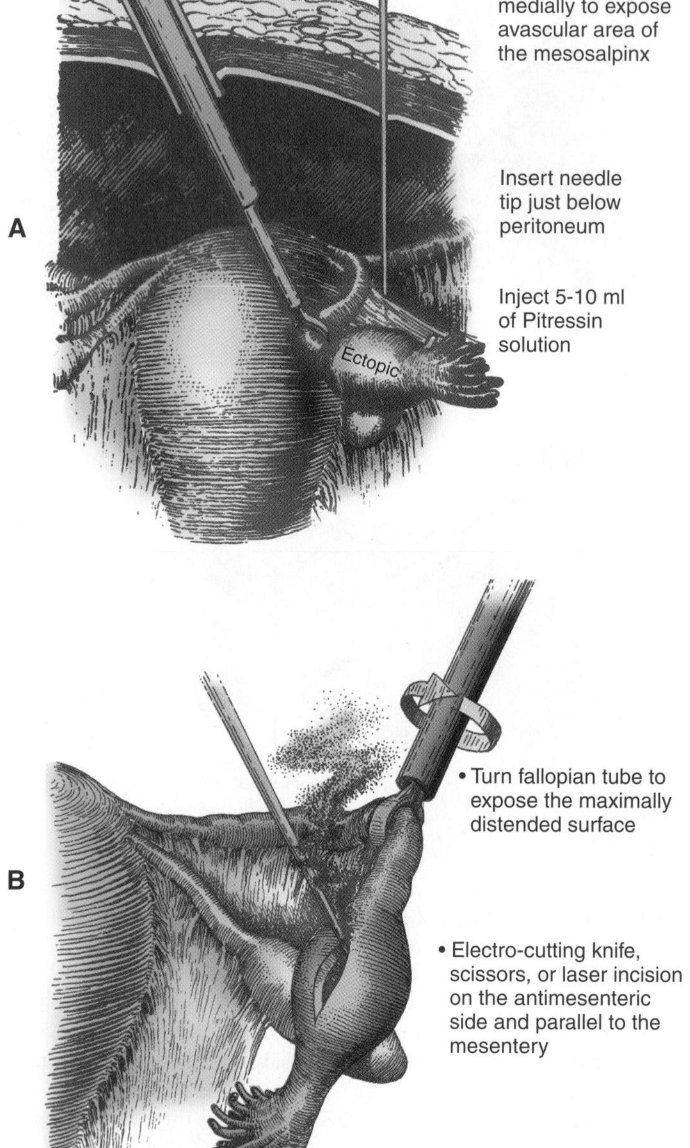
A
Draw fallopian tube medially to expose avascular area of the mesosalpinx
Insert needle tip just below peritoneum
Inject 5-10 ml of Pitressin solution
Ectopic
B
• Turn fallopian tube to expose the maximally distended surface
• Electro-cutting knife, scissors, or laser incision on the antimesenteric side and parallel to the mesentery

**FIGURE 14-34** Salpingostomy. **A,** Injection of vasopressin into mesosalpinx. **B,** Incision made into fallopian tube.

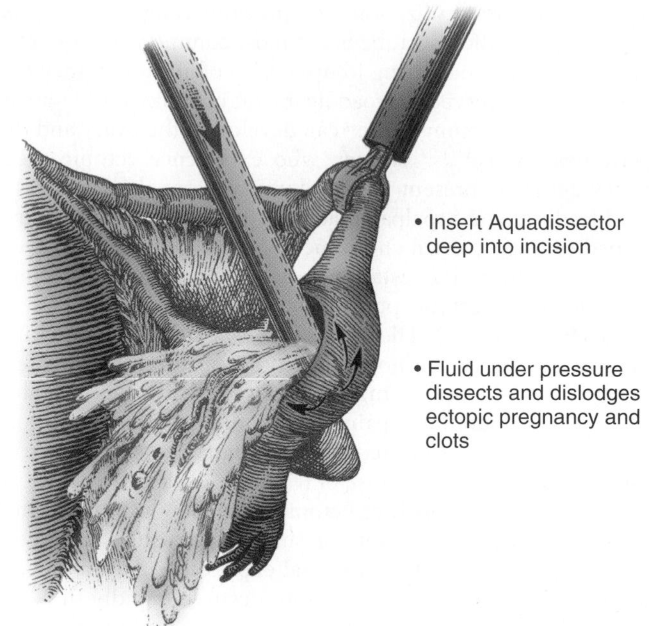
• Insert Aquadissector deep into incision
• Fluid under pressure dissects and dislodges ectopic pregnancy and clots

**FIGURE 14-35** Hydrodissection used to separate ectopic pregnancy from fallopian tube during salpingostomy.

4. The cortex is then incised by scissors or laser, exposing the cyst wall.
5. The incision is then enlarged with scissors, and pressurized hydrodissection is used to separate the cyst from the ovarian stroma.
6. The cyst is dissected and may be removed intact by a culdotomy incision, or the cyst may be opened, evacuated, thoroughly cleaned by lavage with the hydrodissector, and then removed.
7. If the cyst is opened intraperitoneally, the patient should be taken out of the Trendelenburg position while the fluid is removed and the pelvis is cleaned by lavage.
8. Arterial bleeders are identified and desiccated.
9. The ovary usually does not require suturing; however, if the edges gape widely, they may be loosely approximated with interrupted 4-0 synthetic absorbable suture.
10. On completion, the pelviscope and accessory instrumentation are removed. The insufflated gas is permitted to escape from the trocar sleeves. Trocar sleeves are then removed.
11. Application of skin clips or a subcuticular closure of the primary skin incisions is followed by placement of Band-Aids, Steri-Strips, or dressings.

## Laparoscopic-Assisted Vaginal Hysterectomy

Laparoscopic-assisted vaginal hysterectomy (LAVH) or pelviscope-assisted vaginal hysterectomy (PAVH) offers an alternative to total abdominal hysterectomy (TAH) and vaginal hysterectomy (VH). The patient does not have the large abdominal incision, hospital stay, and long recovery period that occur with a TAH. LAVH may be associated with less pain than VH or TAH. Patients who are not candidates for traditional VH may be candidates for LAVH.

The surgeon uses laparoscopy to visualize the pelvis and thereby determine whether disease is present. This is not possible with traditional vaginal hysterectomy. Conditions leading to LAVH include postmenopausal bleeding, pelvic pain, uterine leiomyomas, and adnexal masses. Indications for LAVH may be absence of genital prolapse, required adnexectomy, history of abdominopelvic surgery, salpingitis or endometriosis, lymphadenectomy, and endometrial cancer.

***Procedural Considerations.*** Procedural considerations and accessory instrumentation and approach are similar to those used in other pelviscopic surgical procedures. The patient is placed in the low lithotomy position with attention to positioning interventions to protect the patient from injury.

***Operative Procedure.*** The operative procedure may include the following:

1. Hydrodissection of the broad ligament
2. Desiccation of round and infundibulopelvic ligaments with bipolar coagulation
3. Dissection of the broad ligaments
4. Freeing of the urinary bladder from the lower uterine segment
5. Opening of the vaginal vault with endoscopic scissors or monopolar electrode and removal of the uterus vaginally

## Total Abdominal Hysterectomy (TAH)

TAH is removal of the entire uterus, including the corpus and the cervix. When TAH is combined with bilateral salpingo-oophorectomy, the procedure is commonly termed *panhysterectomy* or *complete hysterectomy.* TAH may be performed for symptomatic pelvic relaxation or prolapse, pain associated with pelvic congestion, pelvic inflammatory disease, endometriosis, recurrent ovarian cysts, fibroids (myomas), bleeding with no apparent cause in postmenopausal women, adenomyosis, or dysfunctional uterine bleeding (Best Practice). TAH, usually with bilateral salpingo-oophorectomy, is also indicated in malignancy, premalignant states, and conditions of high risk for development or recurrence of malignancy. The procedure can also be used to accomplish sterilization. Approximately 588,000 hysterectomies are performed each year in the United States.[13]

***Procedural Considerations.*** Before the abdominal skin prep, an internal vaginal prep is done, ensuring contact of the prep solution with the cervix. An indwelling urinary drainage cath-

## BEST PRACTICE

Hysterectomy is the most common non–pregnancy-related major surgery performed on women in the United States. It is widely accepted as appropriate treatment for cancer and various noncancerous conditions, such as pain, discomfort, uterine bleeding, emotional distress, and related symptoms. Although hysterectomy can alleviate uterine problems, less-invasive treatments are available. Alternatives to hysterectomy recommended by the Agency for Healthcare Research and Quality (AHRQ) are noted in the table below.

| | | Pharmacologic Therapies | | |
|---|---|---|---|---|
| **Condition** | **Conservative Surgery** | **Hormonal** | **Nonhormonal** | **Other Strategies** |
| Fibroids | Myomectomy<br>Endometrial ablation | GnRH agonists with add-back therapy<br>Oral contraceptives<br>RU-486 (experimental)<br>Gestrinone (experimental) | NSAIDs | Watchful waiting |
| Endometriosis | Adhesiolysis<br>Excision or endometrial ablation<br>Resection or cul-de-sac obliteration<br>Nerve blocks<br>Uterosacral nerve ablation | GnRH agonists with add-back therapy<br>Danazol<br>Progestins<br>Oral contraceptives<br>Tamoxifen (experimental)<br>RU-486 (experimental) | NSAIDs<br>Analgesics<br>Anxiolytics | Watchful waiting<br>Biofeedback<br>Hypnosis<br>Acupuncture<br>Life-style modifications (nutrition/exercise) |
| Prolapse | Colporrhaphy<br>Laparoscopic or vaginal suspension techniques | Estrogen | | Watchful waiting<br>Kegel exercises<br>Pessaries<br>Electrical stimulation<br>Urethral beads<br>Periurethral injections (e.g., of fat, silicone) |
| Dysfunctional bleeding | Dilation and curettage<br>Endometrial ablation | Progestins<br>Estrogens<br>Oral contraceptives<br>Danazol<br>Prostaglandin inhibitors<br>GnRH agonists<br>Antifibrinolytic agents<br>Luteinizing hormone agonists | | Watchful waiting<br>Antidepressants |
| Chronic pelvic pain | Adhesiolysis<br>Nerve blocks<br>Denervation procedure<br>Uterosacral nerve ablation | Danazol<br>GnRh agonists with add-back therapy<br>Oral contraceptives<br>Medroxyprogesterone acetate | NSAIDs<br>Analgesics<br>Nerve blocks<br>Narcotics | Watchful waiting<br>Counseling<br>Biofeedback<br>Relaxation techniques<br>Trigger-point injections<br>Acupuncture<br>Psychotropics<br>Antidepressants<br>Physical therapy |

Modified from *Common uterine conditions: options for treatment.* AHCPR Publication No. 98-0003, Rockville, Md, December 1997, Agency for Health Care Policy and Research, Accessed October 15, 2005, on-line: www.ahrq.gov/consumer/uterine1.htm.
*GnRH,* Gonadotropin-releasing hormone; *NSAID,* nonsteroidal antiinflammatory drug.

eter is inserted to provide constant bladder drainage during the operation. The supine position, modified during the procedure with the Trendelenburg position, is used. Instrumentation includes the abdominal gynecologic set. Provisions are made to remove those instruments used in separating the cervix from the vagina from the surgical field, thereby avoiding vaginal contamination of the pelvis.

### *Operative Procedure*

1. In an obese patient or for exploration of the upper abdominal cavity, a left rectus or midline incision may be made. For simple hysterectomy, a Pfannenstiel incision may be used. The abdominal layers and the peritoneum are opened as described for laparotomy.
2. As the peritoneal cavity is opened, the patient is usually placed in the Trendelenburg position to provide better visualization of the pelvic organs.
3. Vasopressin may be injected into the uterus. The round ligament is grasped with forceps, clamped, and ligated with sutures on long needle holders. Pedicles are cut with a knife or Metzenbaum scissors; sutures are tagged with a hemostat to be used as traction later. This procedure is done on both sides (Figure 14-36, *A*).
4. The layer of the broad ligament close to the uterus is separated on each side using blunt dissection. Bleeding vessels are clamped and ligated, and a moist laparotomy pack is inserted behind the flap. The fallopian tube and the utero-ovarian ligaments are doubly clamped together, incised, and doubly tied with suture ligatures (Figure 14-36, *B*).
5. The uterus is pulled forward to expose the posterior sheath of the broad ligament, which is incised with a knife or Metzenbaum scissors. Ureters are identified. The uterine vessels and uterosacral ligaments are doubly clamped, divided by sharp dissection at the level of the internal os, and ligated with suture ligatures (Figure 14-36, *C*).
6. The severed uterine vessels are bluntly dissected away from the cervix on each side with the aid of sponges on sponge-holding forceps, scissors, and tissue forceps.
7. The bladder is separated from the cervix and upper vagina with sharp and blunt dissection assisted by sponges on sponge-holding forceps. The bladder may be retracted with a moist laparotomy pack and a retractor with an angular blade. The vaginal vault is incised close to the cervix with a knife or scissors (Figure 14-36, *D*).
8. The anterior lip of the cervix is grasped with an Allis, Kocher, or tenaculum forceps. With scissors, the cervix is dissected and amputated from the vagina. The uterus is removed. Potentially contaminated instruments used on the cervix and vagina are placed into a discard basin and removed from the field (including sponge-holding forceps and suction). Bleeding is controlled with hemostats and sutures.
9. The vaginal vault is reconstructed with interrupted sutures. Angle sutures anchor all three connective tissue ligaments to the vaginal vault. The pedicles, fallopian tubes, and ovarian ligaments are left free of the vault.
10. The vaginal mucosa is approximated with a continuous suture on a long needle holder. The muscular coat of the vagina may be closed with figure-of-eight sutures to make the vault of the vagina firm and provide resistance against prolapse. A drain may be placed in the vagina.
11. The peritoneum is closed over the bladder, vaginal vault, and rectum (Figure 14-36, *E*). The laparotomy packs are removed, and the omentum is drawn over the bowel.
12. The abdominal wound is closed as described for laparotomy closure (see Chapter 11).
13. Abdominal dressings and a perineal pad are applied.

## Abdominal Myomectomy

Uterine fibroids are benign tumors that arise from the muscular wall of the uterus (Figure 14-37). They may also be located in the endometrium, or the subserosal surface of the uterus. On occasion, they may become pedunculated and extend into the cervical canal. Rarely, a subserosal fibroid may pedunculate and migrate to become a parasitic fibroid attached to the omentum or mesentery. Another term for uterine fibroids is *uterine leiomyomas*. Abdominal myomectomy is removal of fibromyomas, or fibroid tumors, by carefully separating each fibroid from the uterine wall and its blood supply. Myomectomy is usually done in young women who have symptoms that indicate the presence of tumors and who wish to preserve their potential fertility. Uterine fibroids may cause pelvic pain and pressure or dysfunctional uterine bleeding, and they are a leading cause of infertility. Fibroids are more common in African American women and become more common during the later reproductive years.[20] Myomectomy may be performed as a prophylactic measure with other abdominopelvic surgery.

***Procedural Considerations.*** The basic abdominal gynecologic instrument set and ESU are required. A laser may also be used.

### *Operative Procedure*

1. The patient is prepped as described for abdominal hysterectomy. A midline or Pfannenstiel incision is used, and the uterus is exposed.
2. To contract the musculature of the uterine wall, a suitable drug may be injected into the fundus.
3. The fibroid tumor is grasped with a tenaculum. The broad ligament may be opened with curved hemostats and Metzenbaum scissors to determine the course of the ureter or to free the bladder.
4. Each tumor is shelled out of its bed, using blunt and sharp instruments, or the laser. Bleeding vessels are clamped and ligated or electrocoagulated.
5. The uterus is reconstructed with interrupted or continuous sutures.
6. The perimetrium is closed over the operative site, and the abdominal wound is closed.

## Uterine Fibroid Embolization

Uterine fibroid embolization (UFE) is an alternate treatment for fibroids that blocks the blood vessels supplying nutrients and oxygen to the tumors. The blockage causes the fibroid muscle cells to degenerate and form scar tissue, which causes the fibroids to shrink. The greatest period of shrinkage occurs in the first 6 months following the procedure with an additional 42% to 82% shrinkage over the next 6 months.[14] This procedure appeals to many women because of its minimally invasive nature and ability to be performed in the outpatient setting. The main complication associated with the procedure

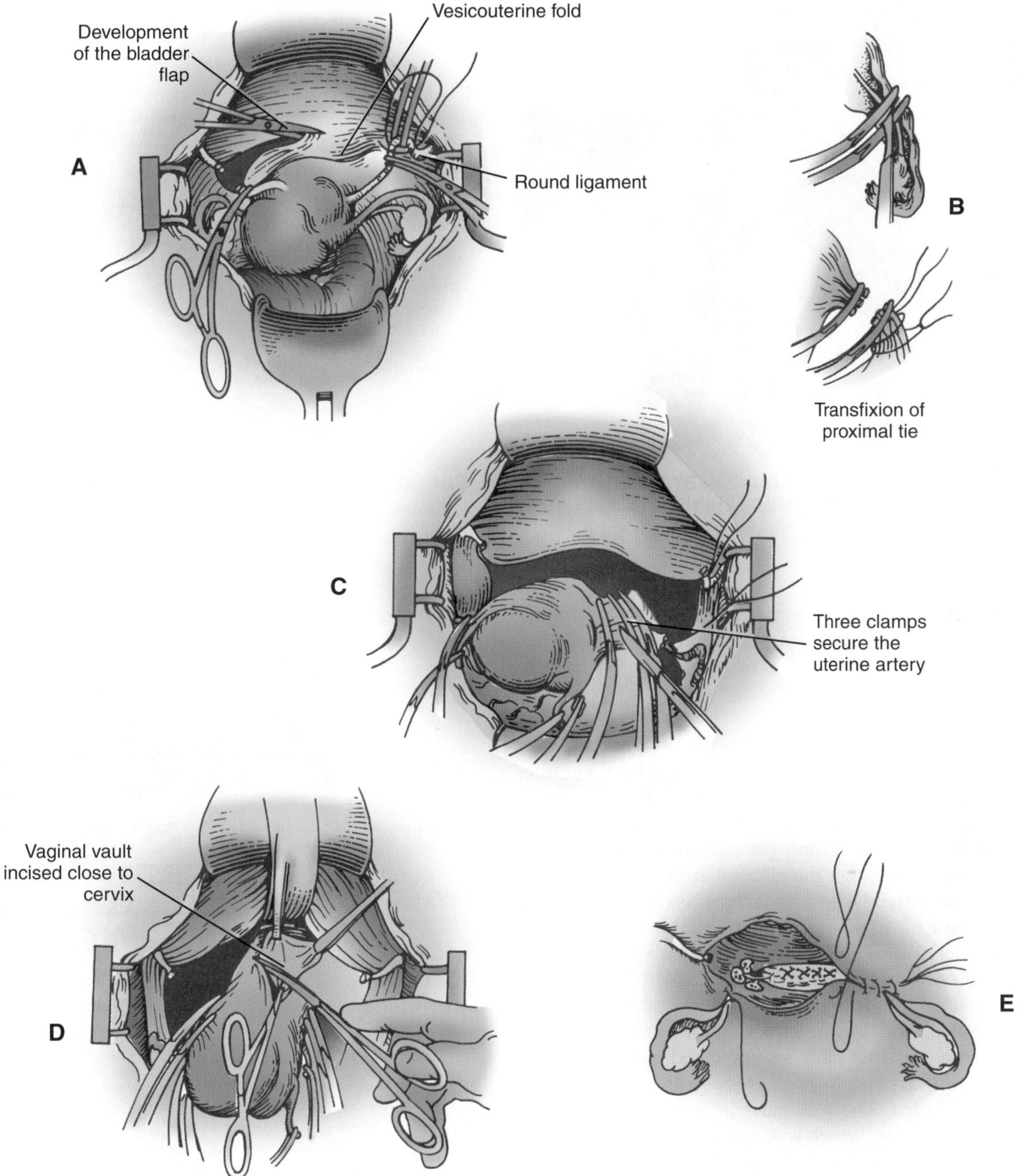


**FIGURE 14-36** Abdominal hysterectomy for single fibroid uterus. **A,** Peritoneum retracted with self-retaining retractors, and organs protected with laparotomy packs saturated in warm normal saline solution. Transverse incision made through uterine peritoneum and carried to each side of uterine attachments of round ligaments. Bleeding vessels clamped and ligated. Round ligament grasped, ligated, and cut. **B,** Tube and ovarian ligaments clamped, cut, and sutured. **C,** Uterus pulled forward, posterior sheath of broad ligaments divided, and uterine artery and veins secured by three heavy curved clamps. Pedicle divided, leaving two hemostats on proximal pedicle. **D,** Bladder separated from cervix and upper vagina. Vaginal vault opened and grasped with Allis forceps. Allis forceps placed on anterior lip of cervix, and dissection of cervix carried out to complete its amputation from vagina. **E,** Three connective tissue thickenings anchored to vaginal vault, vaginal mucosa approximated, and vault closed. As shown, peritoneum closed with continuous suture.

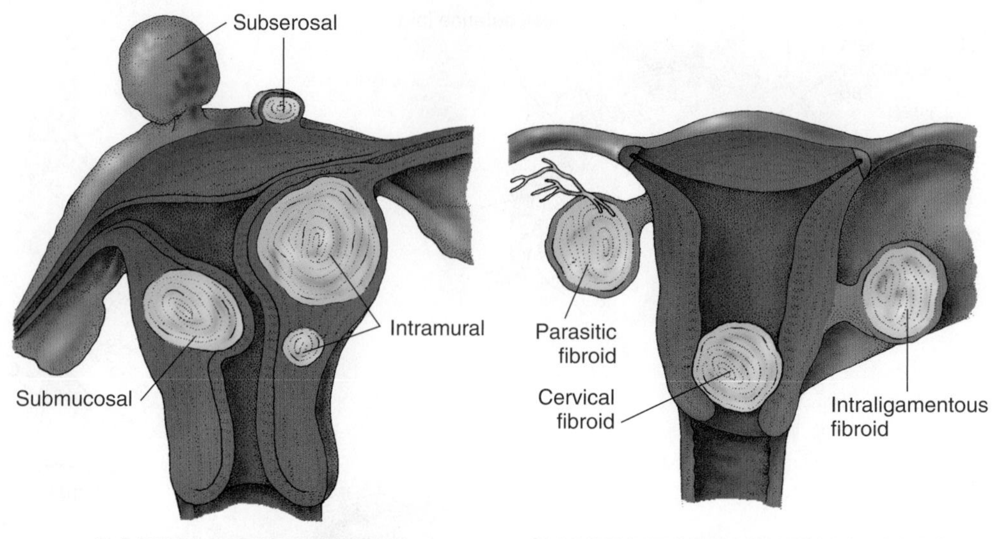


**FIGURE 14-37** Classification of uterine leiomyomas.

is postembolization syndrome, occurring in 2% to 10% of patients. Postembolization syndrome is characterized by pelvic pain, low-grade fever, vomiting, loss of appetite, and malaise in the first 48 hours after UFE.[4]

***Operative Procedure.*** The procedure is performed under fluoroscopic guidance using spinal anesthesia or local anesthesia supplemented with moderate sedation. A femoral artery sheath is inserted, and arteriography of the pelvic vasculature is performed by injecting radiologic contrast through a 5-Fr catheter as it passes through the femoral artery to the iliac artery to the uterine artery. An embolic agent is injected through the catheter until no more proximal arterial flow or reflux of contrast material is noted. Commonly used embolic agents are gelatin sponge, nonspheric polyvinyl alcohol (PVA) particles, and trisacryl gelatine microspheres. Gelfoam pledgets are cut into strips, rolled, and loaded into a nozzle of a syringe for injection. Nonspheric PVA particles are mixed with equal parts of saline and contrast and injected through the catheter until the vessel is occluded. The PVA particle size ranges from 350 microns to 700 microns, which is comparable in size to a grain of sand. Trisacryl microspheres are smaller than PVA particles at 700 microns to 900 microns.[16] Collateral circulation maintains the blood supply to the myometrium. The particles remain inert in the vessel.

## Radical Hysterectomy (Wertheim)

Radical hysterectomy is en bloc dissection and wide removal of the uterus, tubes, ovaries, supporting ligaments, and upper vagina, together with careful removal of all recognizable lymph nodes in the pelvis (Figure 14-38). Extensive dissection of the ureters and of the bladder is also involved.

Radical hysterectomy is performed for gynecologic malignancy. Abdominal exploration determines lymph node involvement. With no lymph node involvement, a wide-cuff hysterectomy is performed. The uterus, tubes, and ovaries, together with most of the parametrial tissues and the upper portion of the vagina, are dissected en bloc. Dissection of the ureters from the paracervical structures takes place so that the ligaments supporting the uterus and vagina can be removed.

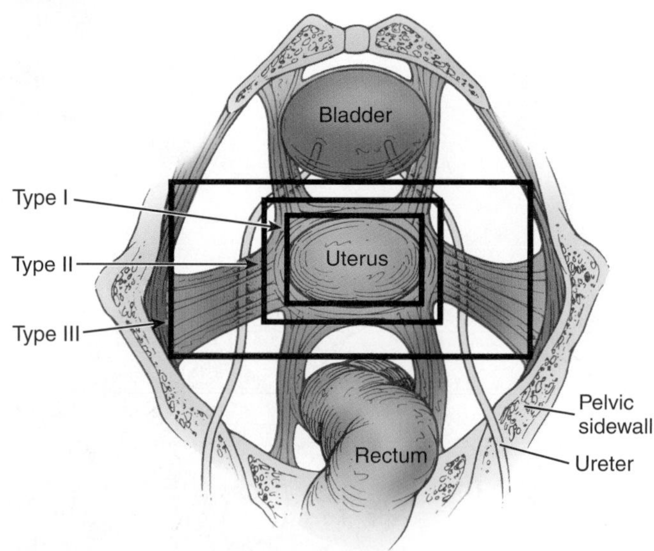


**FIGURE 14-38** Different types of hysterectomy: type I—simple hysterectomy; type II—modified radical hysterectomy; type III—radical hysterectomy.

***Procedural Considerations.*** Careful estimation of blood loss and calculation of urinary output are needed throughout the operative procedure. The patient is prepped as described for TAH. An indwelling urinary catheter is inserted. The basic abdominal gynecologic instrument set is required, with the addition of long and deep instruments and a self-retaining retractor.

### *Operative Procedure*

1. The skin is incised, and the abdominal layers are opened, as described for laparotomy.

2. The peritoneum is cut at its reflection on the anterior surface of the uterus between the round ligaments (Figure 14-39, *A*). By blunt dissection, the bladder surface is freed from the cervix and vagina.
3. The right round and infundibulopelvic ligaments are clamped, cut with a knife or Metzenbaum scissors, and ligated with sutures to expose the external iliac artery. The ureter is identified and retracted with a vein retractor (Figure 14-39, *B*).
4. The lymph and areolar tissues are dissected from the iliac artery, obturator fossa, and ureter with Lahey forceps, Kitner sponges, and Metzenbaum scissors. A complete lymph gland dissection removes the tissue from the Cloquet node to the bifurcation of the iliac arteries bilaterally. The uterine artery and vein are clamped, cut, and doubly ligated.
5. The uterus is elevated, the cul-de-sac is opened (Figure 14-39, *C*), and the uterosacral and cardinal ligaments are clamped, cut with scissors, and doubly ligated with suture ligatures. The pararectal and paravesical areolar tissues are dissected free to skeletonize the upper vagina, and the paraurethral tissues are removed as near to the pelvic walls as possible.
6. The upper third of the vagina is cross-clamped with Heaney forceps (Figure 14-39, *D*) and divided using a long knife handle and #20 blade. The uterus and surrounding tissues are removed. Electrocoagulation is used to minimize venous oozing from small venules and capillaries. Lowering the head of the OR bed 15 degrees is also helpful in reducing the oozing of blood and serum.
7. The vagina is sutured with a running locked stitch, and closed wound drainage is provided from above (Figure 14-39, *E*). The pelvis is peritonealized with a continuous suture.
8. The abdominal wound is closed (retention sutures may be used) and dressed in the usual manner. Vaginal packing and drains may be used. A suprapubic indwelling catheter may be placed to assist in preventing postoperative bladder spasm and for bladder drainage if the patient is unable to void after removal of the urethral catheter.
9. A perineal pad is applied.

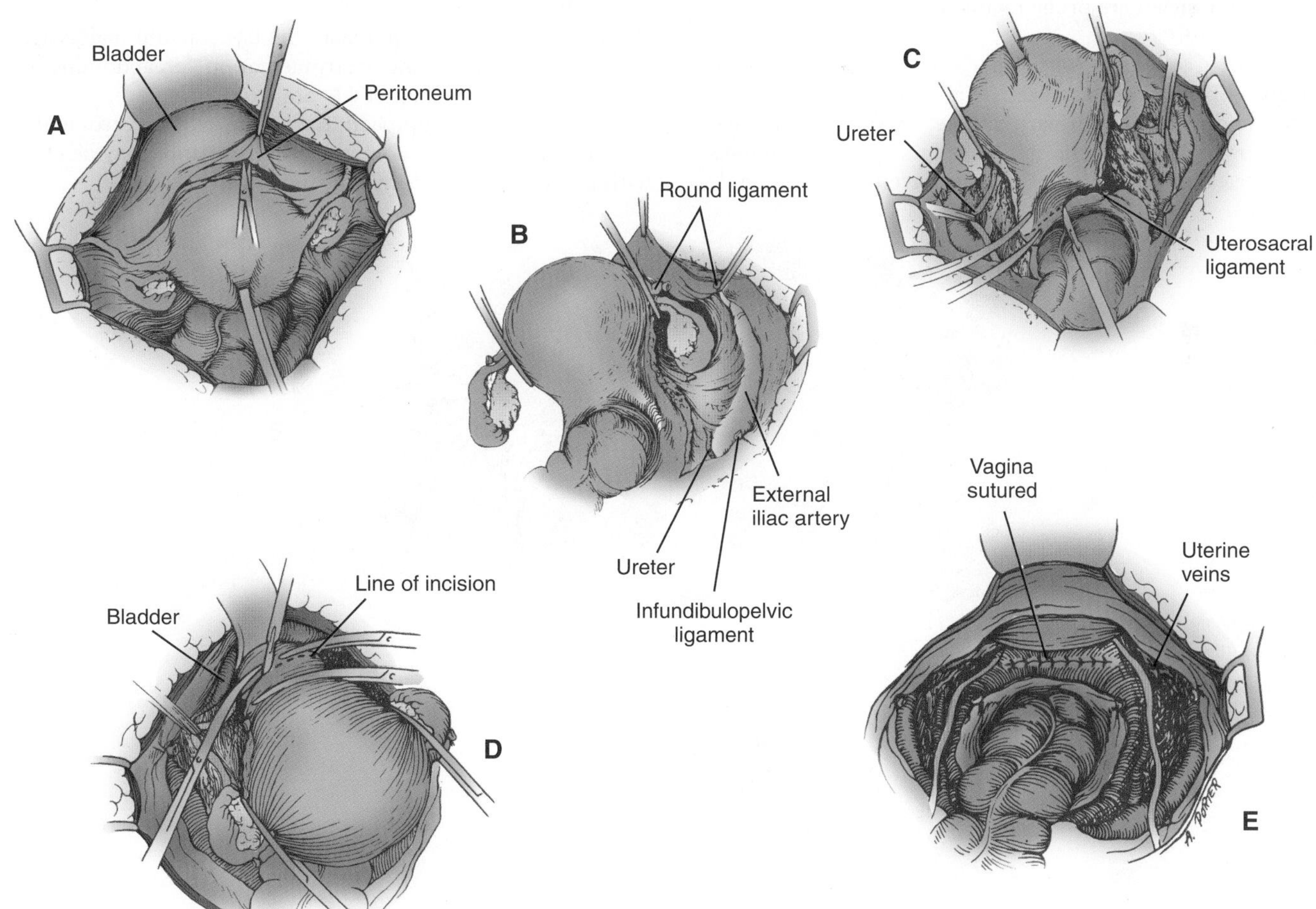


**FIGURE 14-39** Wertheim radical hysterectomy. **A**, With upward traction applied on uterus, peritoneum is incised from round ligament to round ligament. **B**, Right round and infundibulopelvic ligaments are ligated and cut, thus exposing right external iliac artery. **C**, Uterus is held upward and forward, exposing cul-de-sac, which is incised as shown by dotted line. **D**, After dissection is completed, vagina is doubly clamped preparatory to transection, after which entire specimen is lifted out en masse. **E**, Vagina is closed. Peritoneum remains to be reperitonealized.

## Pelvic Exenteration

Pelvic exenteration is the en bloc removal of the rectum, the distal sigmoid colon, the urinary bladder and the distal ureters, the internal iliac vessels and their lateral branches, all pelvic reproductive organs and lymph nodes, and the entire pelvic floor with the accompanying pelvic peritoneum, levator muscles, and perineum. A partial exenteration, either anterior or posterior, may be performed, depending on the origin of the carcinoma and the extent of local tissue invasion (Figure 14-40).

Pelvic exenteration is the preferred treatment for recurrent or persistent carcinoma of the cervix after radiation therapy. Advanced or recurrent vaginal, vulvar, or occasionally endometrial and rectal carcinomas are often amenable to exenteration.[12] Exenteration is considered only after a thorough investigation of the patient and disease status to determine if there is a reasonable chance of cure and of return to a productive life.

The need to create urinary and bowel diversions must also be considered, together with the patient's ability to cope with these diversions postoperatively. Plastic surgery may be required for creation of a neovagina. Psychologic preparation and support of the patient and family by the perioperative nurse and physician are prime requisites.

***Procedural Considerations.*** The bowel is cleansed preoperatively with antibiotics and cathartics or enemas. A nasogastric tube and indwelling urinary catheter are inserted before or during surgery. Antiembolic stockings or sequential compression sleeves are placed on both legs. A forced-air warming device is applied to maintain body temperature, and all fluids are warmed. Cardiac and central venous pressure monitoring is maintained throughout the procedure.

Utmost care must be taken in positioning the patient because of the duration of surgery. Strict attention should be paid to the knees, hips, and lower back to prevent vascular and nerve damage. The patient is placed in the supine position with legs abducted in the ski position (lower extremities resting on a well-padded plantar surface rather than on the heel or popliteal area) or elevated in a modified lithotomy position to allow access to the perineum without disruptive position changes. Skin prepping includes the abdomen, thighs, perineum, and internal vaginal vault.

The circulating nurse and scrub person must be alert to fluid and blood loss. Irrigation solutions must be accurately measured, laparotomy packs must be weighed to assess blood volume loss, and the anesthesia provider and surgical team must be apprised of the measurements.

When the colon is transected or ureteral drainage is diverted into a segment of the ileum the gastrointestinal technique as described in Chapter 11 should be followed.

Separate instrument setups are required for the abdominal and perineal approaches. Extra drapes, gowns, and gloves should be available.

For the abdominal approach, the basic abdominal gynecologic instrument set and instrumentation for abdominoperineal resection (see Chapter 11) are required.

For the perineal approach, the basic vaginal instrument set is required. To prevent contamination, the anus may be closed with a purse-string suture.

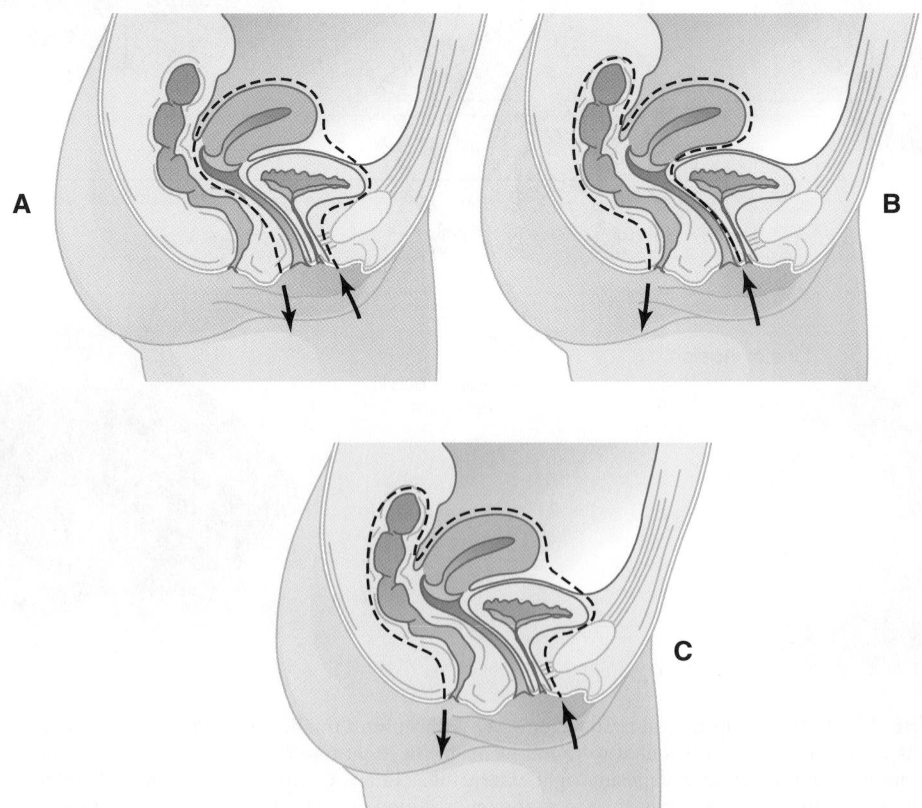


**FIGURE 14-40** Organs removed in pelvic exenteration. **A,** Anterior exenteration. **B,** Posterior exenteration. **C,** Total pelvic exenteration.

### Operative Procedure

1. A long midline incision from the symphysis pubis to the umbilicus is made, and the abdomen is opened in the usual manner. A second incision within the perineum encircling the vestibule and anus is also made.
2. The peritoneal cavity is explored for metastasis to the liver, the nodes of the celiac axis, the superior mesenteric artery, and the paraaortic tissues.
3. The pelvis is explored, and the peritoneum along the brim of the pelvis is examined for lymph node involvement. Frozen sections may be indicated. The obturator fossa and the region of the uterosacral ligaments are explored. When findings at exploration are negative, retractors are placed and the small bowel is packed off with moist laparotomy packs (Figure 14-41).
4. The sigmoid mesocolon is freed and sectioned by means of intestinal clamps and a scalpel or a stapling device. The proximal end is exteriorized through an opening in the left side of the abdomen; an intestinal clamp is left across the lumen until later, when the permanent colostomy will be secured to the skin.
5. The remaining sigmoid mesentery is clamped with Rochester-Pean forceps, cut, and ligated down to and including the superior hemorrhoidal vessels. Long instruments and sutures are used to reach the deep pelvic structures.
6. The distal sigmoid colon is closed with an inverting suture. The sigmoid colon and rectum are freed from the sacrococcygeal area by blunt and sharp dissection.
7. The lateral pelvic peritoneum is cut along the iliac vessels; the ovarian vessels and round ligaments on each side are clamped with Rochester-Pean forceps, cut, and doubly ligated.
8. The peritoneum is incised over the dome of the bladder with a long knife and Metzenbaum scissors, and the blad-

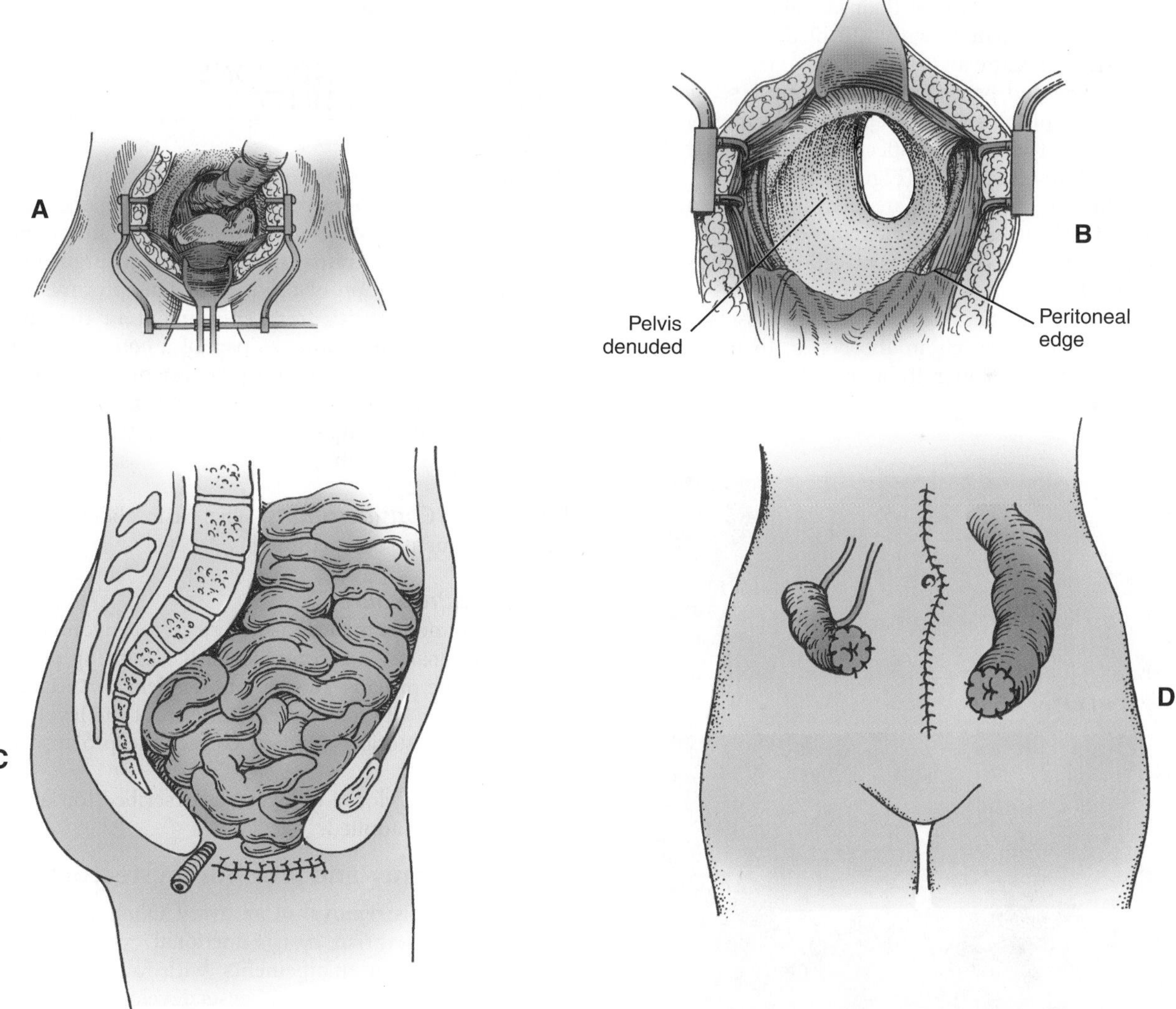


FIGURE 14-41 Pelvic exenteration. **A**, Pelvic viscera in situ as viewed from operating surgeon's vantage point after retractors are placed and small bowel is packed off. **B**, Empty pelvis after dissection of paravesical and paravaginal tissues and removal of specimen en bloc. **C**, Sagittal view of small bowel above pelvic defect. Perineal packing or drain may be used. **D**, After closure of abdominal wall, colostomy and ileostomy stomas are sutured to skin edges.

der is separated from the symphysis pubis down to the urethra.

9. The ureters are identified and divided 2 to 3 cm below the brim of the pelvis. The proximal end is left open to allow urinary drainage, whereas the distal end is ligated.
10. The hypogastric artery, the internal iliac vein, and the superior and inferior gluteal vessels are exposed, clamped with hemostats, doubly ligated, and cut. The external iliac vein is retracted to allow evacuation of the contents of the obturator fossa, leaving the obturator nerve intact. Care must be taken in dissection not to damage the sacral plexus and sciatic nerve.
11. The internal pudendal vessels are isolated, ligated with transfixion sutures, and cut. The remaining soft-tissue attachments of the pelvis are clamped and cut. Steps 10 and 11 are then performed on the opposite side.
12. The perineum is incised by an elliptic incision that includes the clitoris and anus. The ischiorectal fat is incised up to the area of the levator muscle.
13. The coccygeal attachment of the rectum is severed. The levator muscles are severed at their lateral attachments by using a long knife handle with #20 blade; hemostasis is maintained by pressure and traction.
14. The paravesical and paravaginal tissues are resected from the periosteum of the symphysis pubis and superior pubic rami by means of a knife. The specimen is completely freed and removed from the pelvis (Figure 14-42).
15. After residual bleeding vessels are identified and controlled by transfixing ligatures, the subcutaneous tissue is closed by interrupted sutures. A drain is placed in the wound, and the skin is closed.
16. In the abdomen, further residual bleeding vessels are controlled. Packs may be left in the pelvis, to be removed through the perineum after 48 hours.

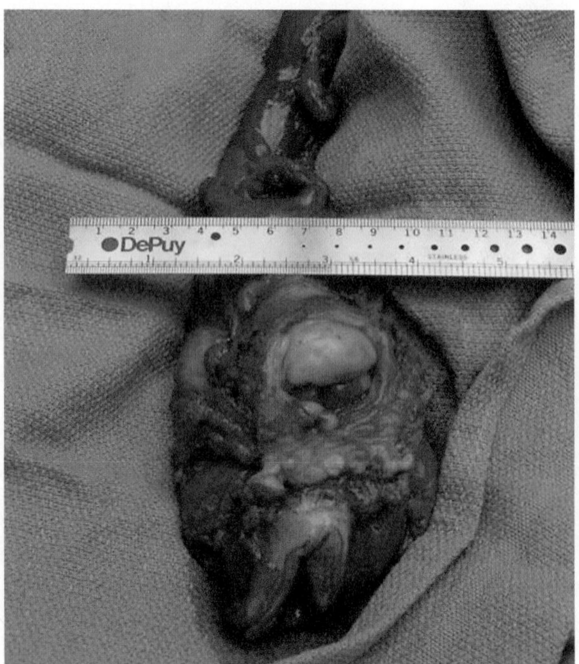


FIGURE 14-42 Pelvic exenteration specimen.

17. The ileal segment is then fashioned, and the ureters are anatomized to it. The external stoma is placed on the right side of the abdomen.
18. A jejunostomy catheter is inserted into the proximal jejunum to aid in postoperative bowel decompression. It is connected to the bowel with a purse-string suture and brought out to the skin, where it is sutured in place.
19. A gastrostomy tube is placed into the stomach in the same manner.
20. Hemostasis is checked. The small intestine is carefully repositioned into the pelvis. Packs and retractors are removed.
21. The peritoneum, rectus muscles, and fascial sheaths are closed with interrupted figure-of-eight sutures. The skin is closed with interrupted sutures.
22. The colostomy stoma is prepared by removing the intestinal clamp from the sigmoid colon, opening the colon, and suturing the stoma to the skin edges.

The abdominal wound and tube sites are dressed in the usual manner. Drainage devices are applied to the colostomy and ileostomy stomas.

## SURGERY FOR CONDITIONS THAT AFFECT FERTILITY

### Uterine Suspension

Uterine suspension is shortening of the ligaments of the uterus and positioning them retroperitoneally. The ligaments are then sutured bilaterally to the undersurface of the abdominal fascia in the corners of the transverse incision to ensure maintenance of an anterior position of the uterus. This prevents the fallopian tubes and ovaries from entrapment in the cul-de-sac. Uterine suspension is done as part of a conservative surgical treatment of pelvic inflammatory disease or endometriosis, for patients who require lysis of extensive pelvic adhesions, for the correction of the symptoms of uterine retroversion, and for uterine prolapse in young women.

***Procedural Considerations.*** The basic abdominal gynecologic instrument set is required.

#### *Operative Procedure*

1. The abdomen is opened as described for myomectomy.
2. The suspension is accomplished. If it is being done to correct uterine prolapse, a strip of Mersilene material is placed retroperitoneally to elevate the uterus at the level of the internal os posteriorly and to correct the prolapse into the vagina.
3. The wound is closed in layers, as described for laparotomy.
4. Dressings are applied.

### Oophorectomy and Oophorocystectomy

Oophorectomy is removal of an ovary. Oophorocystectomy is removal of an ovarian cyst. Functional cysts constitute the majority of ovarian enlargements, with follicular cysts being the most common. Functional cysts develop in the corpus luteum. Benign cystic teratomas, also known as dermoid cysts, are very common and are composed of ectodermal tissues (sweat glands, hair follicles, and teeth) (Figure 14-43). Other tissues found in dermoid cysts include adult brain, bronchus, thyroid, cartilage, bone, and intestinal cells.[20] Ovarian epithe-

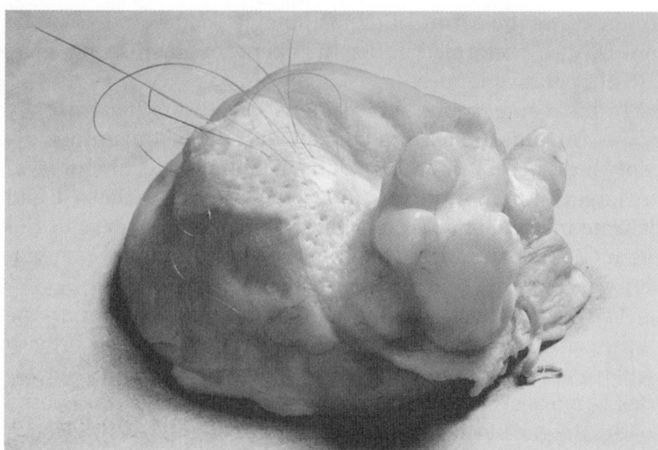

FIGURE 14-43 Dermoid cyst.

lial tumors, serous cystadenomas, and pseudomucinous cystadenomas are prone to malignant change.

The choice of operation depends on the patient's age and symptoms, findings during physical examination, and direct examination of the adnexa during exploration. If the ovarian tumor is recognized as benign, only the visibly diseased portions of the adnexa are removed. In the presence of dermoid, follicular, and corpus luteum cysts, the cyst is usually enucleated and most of the ovarian parenchyma is preserved. In tubal pregnancy, the ectopic pregnancy may be removed from the tube or the pregnant fallopian tube may be removed and, in some instances, the ovary.

*Procedural Considerations.* The basic abdominal gynecologic instrument set is required, with the addition of a trocar and cannula, suction tubing, 10-ml syringe, and 21-gauge needle.

### Operative Procedure

1. The abdominal cavity is opened as described for laparotomy.
2. a. For *removal of a large ovarian cyst,* a purse-string suture may be placed into the cyst wall and a trocar introduced in its center; the suture is tightened around the trocar as the fluid is aspirated. The trocar is removed, and the purse-string suture is tied. All normal ovarian tissue is preserved.
   b. For *removal of a smaller ovarian cyst,* a clamp is placed at the base of the cyst and the cyst is excised. The wound in the ovary is closed with absorbable suture (Figure 14-44).
   c. For *removal of a dermoid cyst,* the field is protected with laparotomy packs because the cystic contents produce irritation if they are spilled into the peritoneal cavity. An incision is made along the base of the cyst between the wall and normal ovarian tissue. The cystic wall is dissected away. The ovary is closed with interrupted or continuous sutures.
   d. For *decortication of the enlarged ovary and wedge resection,* a large segment of the ovarian cortex opposite the hilum is removed. The cysts are punctured with a needle point and collapsed. A wedge of ovarian stroma, extending deep into the hilum, is resected with a small knife; the cortex of the ovary is closed with interrupted or continuous sutures.
3. To prevent prolapse of the tube into the cul-de-sac, the tube may be sutured to the posterior sheath of the broad ligament.
4. The abdominal wound is closed as described for laparotomy, and dressings are applied.

## Salpingo-Oophorectomy

Salpingo-oophorectomy is removal of a fallopian tube and all or part of the associated ovary. Unilateral salpingo-oophorectomy may be done to cure chronic salpingo-oophoritis, for ectopic tubal gestation, or for certain disease conditions of the adnexa or large adnexal cysts. If both tubes and ovaries are diseased, they are removed with total hysterectomy.

*Procedural Considerations.* The basic abdominal gynecologic instrument set is required.

### Operative Procedure

1. The abdominal cavity is opened as described for laparotomy.
2. The affected tube is grasped with Allis or Babcock forceps. The infundibulopelvic ligament is clamped with hemostats, cut, and ligated.
3. The mesosalpinx is grasped with hemostats and divided with the suspensory ligament of the ovary.

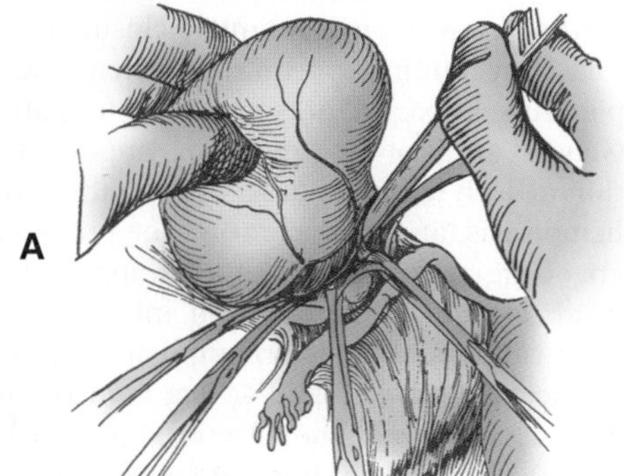


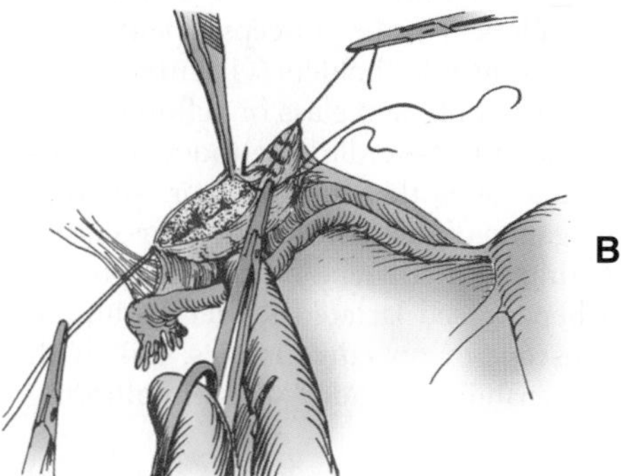


FIGURE 14-44 Resection of small cyst from ovary. **A,** Incision made around ovary near junction of cyst wall and normal ovarian tissue. Knife handle is convenient instrument for shelling out cyst. **B,** Wound in ovary closed.

4. The cornual attachment of the tube is excised with a knife or curved scissors. Bleeding vessels are clamped and ligated.
5. The edges of the broad ligament are peritonealized from the uterine horn to the infundibulopelvic ligament as described for total hysterectomy.
6. The wound is closed as described for laparotomy, and dressings are applied.

## Microscopic Reconstructive Surgery of the Fallopian Tube

The obstructed portion of a fallopian tube may be removed and the tube reconstructed to create patency of the remaining portion of the tube to promote the possibility of fertilization. Reconstructive surgery of the tube, broadly called *tuboplasty,* includes reanastomosis, salpingoneostomy, fimbrioplasty, and lysis of adhesions.

The development of microsurgical techniques has advanced surgical reconstruction of fallopian tubes. Microsurgical techniques may be used with minilaparotomy or laparoscopy or both. Microsurgical tubal anastomosis permits atraumatic, accurate alignment of fallopian tube segments. After surgery the fallopian tubes are shorter in length yet remain normal in other aspects. The laser may be adapted to the operating microscope, or the freehand approach may be used in tubal reconstructive surgery.

***Procedural Considerations.*** The patient is placed in the supine position. The vagina is prepped as described previously. An indwelling urinary catheter is inserted into the bladder. A Kahn, Calvin, Rubin, Hui, or Humi cannula or a pediatric Foley catheter may be placed into the uterine cavity for intraoperative chromotubation with diluted methylene blue or indigo carmine solution. Intraoperative chromotubation can also be achieved by applying a Buxton uterine clamp around the lower segment of the uterus and inserting an Angiocath catheter through the fundus into the cavity. A vaginal pack may be inserted to help elevate the uterus.

The basic abdominal gynecologic instrument set is required, with the addition of iris scissors (1 curved and 1 straight), Adson forceps without teeth, Halsted mosquito hemostats, a set of Bowman lacrimal probes, Webster needle holders, Frazier suction tip, Kirschner retractor (if desired), and a Buxton uterine clamp (if desired).

Basic microsurgical instruments include microscissors (1 curved and 1 straight), bayonet microscissors, jeweler's forceps, microforceps, fallopian tube forceps, petit-point mosquito hemostats, micro-needle holders (1 curved and 1 straight), ball-tipped nerve hook, and glass or Teflon rods.

Accessory items include micro-needle electrodes, electrosurgical pencil, bipolar forceps with cord, irrigator, syringes and blunt needles for irrigation of the tissues, plastic or Silastic tubing and connectors, diluted methylene blue or indigo carmine solution, diluted heparinized lactated Ringer's solution, microscope drape, microscope or operative loupes, ESU with monopolar and bipolar capabilities, and a video monitoring system (if desired).

***Operative Procedure.*** Operative procedures for correction of postsurgical tubal occlusion are usually performed under the operating microscope. Other reconstructive procedures vary according to the nature of the pathologic condition of the tube and may be performed under the operating microscope or by use of operative loupes.

In microsurgery the surgeon must make sure that virtually no instruments are used in contact with the fallopian tube except those necessary to carry out the surgical technique. Microsurgery for infertility requires the use of specialized and delicate instruments. Each of these instruments is designed to permit gentle, atraumatic handling of tissues and prevent abrasions, lacerations, and vascular damage.

The tissues must be continually irrigated to prevent drying of the serosal surfaces. Lactated Ringer's solution alone or with heparin added may be used as the irrigating solution. Meticulous hemostasis is required in microsurgery. Irrigation is used to identify the bleeders. Hemostasis can be achieved by electrocoagulation with a micro-needle electrode or very fine bipolar forceps. When a $CO_2$ laser beam is used, the smoke from laser vaporization should be evacuated to prevent carbon deposits on the tissue.

## Tubal Ligation

Tubal ligation is interruption of fallopian tube continuity, resulting in sterilization of the patient. In general, the indication for sterilization depends entirely on the desire of the patient. Certain medical indications and concern for the psychosocial needs of the patient are factors, and occasionally an obstetric indication exists, such as inherited fetal deformity. However, at least in the United States, sterilization is entirely a voluntary procedure. Depending on state law, a sterilization permit may have to be signed by the husband. Thorough presurgical counseling is needed for the patient and her husband or significant other because this procedure is not predictably reversible. Approximately 1% of sterilized women seek reversals as a result of sterilization performed at an early age, death of a child, or remarriage.[1] Patients may elect to have the procedure performed on an ambulatory surgery basis at a time that is convenient for them.

Tubal ligation may be performed during or soon after delivery. This timing usually does not delay the normal discharge time for the patient. An objection to this practice is that the danger of hemorrhage still exists soon after delivery. With a vaginal delivery, tubal ligation is done on the first or second postpartum day. If a cesarean delivery is done, the tubes may be ligated at that time.

***Operative Procedures.*** Many surgical methods and techniques are available for tubal ligation. The objective of each method is to achieve complete closure of the fallopian tube so that conception is prevented. When a segment of each fallopian tube is excised, it is preserved for pathologic examination. General surgical considerations are directed to excising a section of each fallopian tube, ligating the severed ends, achieving hemostasis, and incorporating the proximal stump within layers of the mesosalpinx. Another approach, involving insertion of an expandable spring coil into the fallopian tube to mechanically block it, is accomplished hysteroscopically via the transcervical route. The device is made from titanium, stainless steel, nickel, and Dacron fibers. Ultimately the device provides an inflammatory response and fibrosis of the intramural tubal lumen over a 3-month period.[27]

LAPAROSCOPIC TUBAL OCCLUSION

1. Operative approach is the same as that for laparoscopy.

2. An accessory suprapubic incision may be made for the occluding instrument.
3. Sterilization may take place by thermal coagulation or by placement of a spring clip or Silastic band after the tube has been identified and isolated in the grasping forceps.
   a. Bipolar coagulation occurs when electrical current passes only through the tube from prong to prong (Figure 14-45). At least 3 cm of the tube is destroyed, which therefore prevents spontaneous recanalization. It has been recommended that the tube be grasped at least 2 to 3 cm away from the uterocornual junction at the time of this procedure so that a stump of isthmus remains to absorb the intrauterine fluid under pressure and minimize fistula formation, which could result in an ectopic pregnancy for the patient in the future.
   b. The *spring clip* occludes the isthmus of the tube by two plastic jaws (Figure 14-46, *A* and *B*). The tube is compressed by a stainless-steel spring that presses the jaws together. Spring-clip application requires careful surgical technique to ensure that the clip is completely across the isthmus of the tube (Figure 14-46, *C*). Some surgeons apply two spring clips positioned close together on each tube when using this approach.
   c. With a *Silastic band,* the tube is drawn 1.5 cm into a 0.5-cm diameter metal cylinder, which destroys approximately 3 cm of the tube (Figure 14-47, *A*). A Silastic ring stretched on the outside of the cylinder is released to form an occlusion (Figure 14-47, *B*). Over time, about 3 cm of the constricted tube undergoes necrosis and the tubes separate (Figure 14-47, *C*).

MINILAPAROTOMY APPROACH

1. A 2-cm transverse incision is made above the pubic hairline.
2. A large bivalved speculum may be placed through the incision and into the peritoneal cavity. The large Graves bivalve speculum serves as a small abdominal retractor and permits easy access to the tubes.
3. Spring clips or Silastic bands can be applied, or the original Pomeroy method of ligation can be carried out. The Pomeroy technique provides a tissue specimen of each tube. Suture material is tied around each tube, and a section of tube is removed. Over time, the tubes pull apart, destroying the passage between the ovary and the uterus.

TRANSCERVICAL APPROACH (ESSURE)

1. The operative approach is the same as for hysteroscopy.
2. The uterus is distended, and the ostia are visualized.
3. The spring device (Figure 14-48) is placed on the tip of the plastic carrier provided in the kit and inserted through the hysteroscope's channel.
4. The device is guided to the tubal ostium, and the handle for the carrying device is stabilized.
5. The device is released from the plastic carrier, and the coil is deployed as the handle is retracted (Figure 14-49).
6. The surgeon counts the number of coils trailing into the uterine cavity. There should be 3 to 8 visible coils (Figure 14-50).
7. The sequence is repeated for the remaining fallopian tube.

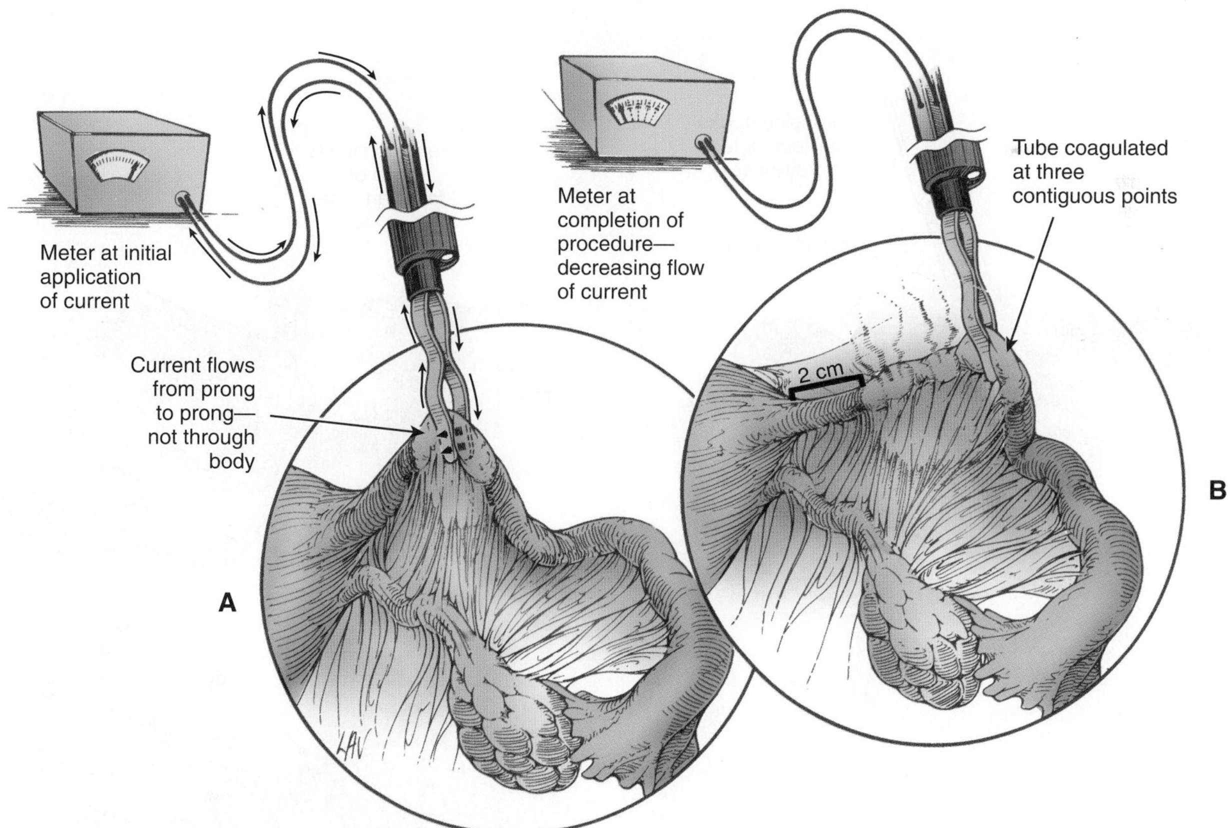


FIGURE 14-45 Bipolar coagulation. **A,** Current passes only through the tube from prong to prong of the forceps. **B,** Three contiguous burns are needed to prevent spontaneous recanalization. The end point for coagulation is tissue desiccation, at which point current ceases to flow through the dry, nonconducting tube. A meter on the generator to monitor current flow is therefore necessary.

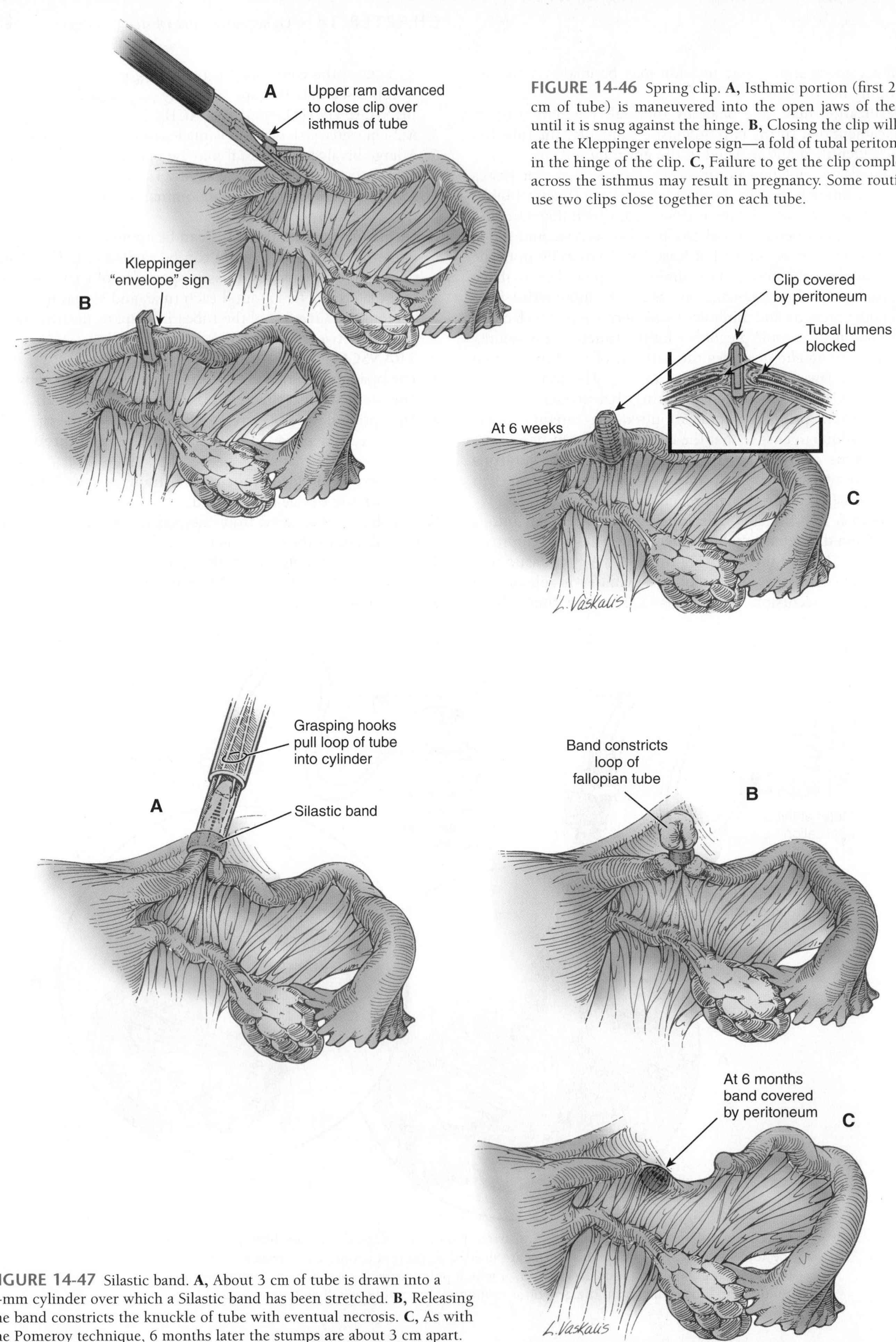


**FIGURE 14-46** Spring clip. **A,** Isthmic portion (first 2 to 3 cm of tube) is maneuvered into the open jaws of the clip until it is snug against the hinge. **B,** Closing the clip will create the Kleppinger envelope sign—a fold of tubal peritoneum in the hinge of the clip. **C,** Failure to get the clip completely across the isthmus may result in pregnancy. Some routinely use two clips close together on each tube.

**FIGURE 14-47** Silastic band. **A,** About 3 cm of tube is drawn into a 5-mm cylinder over which a Silastic band has been stretched. **B,** Releasing the band constricts the knuckle of tube with eventual necrosis. **C,** As with the Pomeroy technique, 6 months later the stumps are about 3 cm apart.

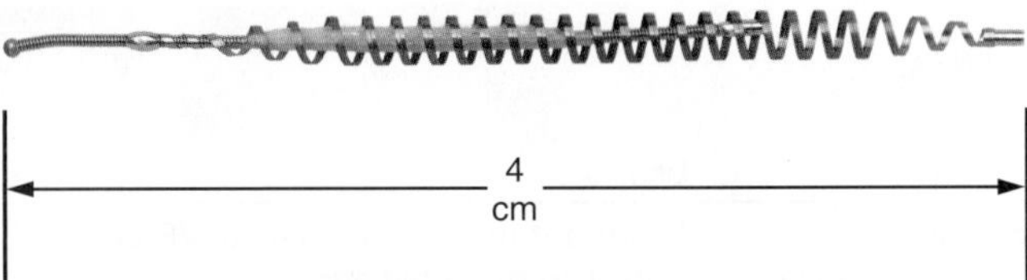


FIGURE 14-48 Essure implant.

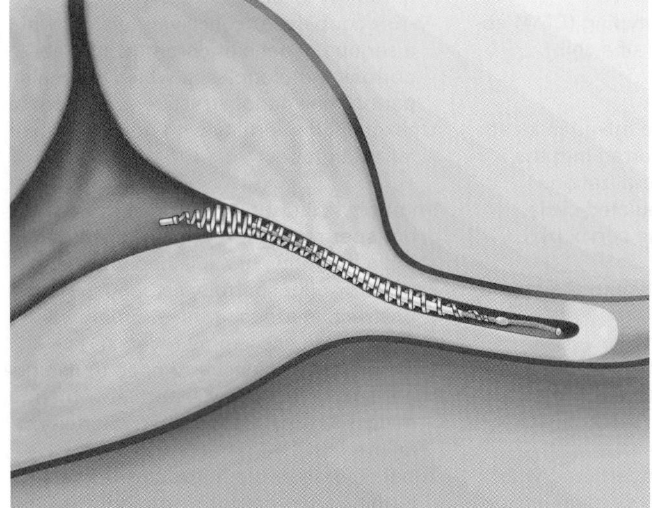

FIGURE 14-49 Essure device placed in fallopian tube.

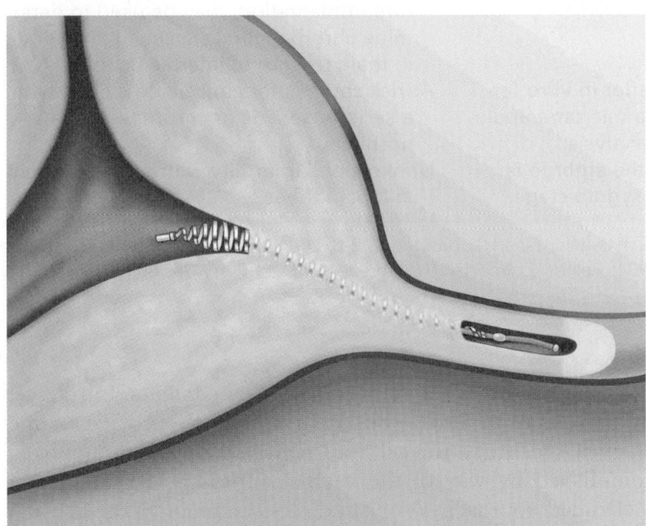

FIGURE 14-50 Essure device after carrier detached. Note coils in uterine cavity.

## ASSISTED REPRODUCTIVE THERAPIES FOR INFERTILITY

Infertility is a condition that affects approximately 10% of reproductive-age couples. Infertility implies subfertility—a prolonged time to conceive—as opposed to sterility, which means inability to conceive.[23] Infertility is referred to as primary when it occurs without a prior pregnancy and secondary if it occurs after a successful conception.[19] Facing infertility is an emotionally stressful process for both partners. Treatment of infertility is multidimensional and may involve medical as well as surgical interventions. Often by the time a woman presents in the perioperative setting for a procedure related to infertility, she and her partner have undergone many months or years of testing and medical interventions. Individuals with infertility use various coping strategies, and the perioperative nurse needs to be aware of these in providing supportive care.

Eighty percent of couples that do not have fertility issues achieve conception within 1 year. A couple is considered infertile if they have not conceived after attempting for 1 year.[19] Both partners undergo extensive testing to identify possible organic or functional causes for their infertility. Identifiable conditions contributing to infertility are attributed to the female partner in 37% of couples, the male partner in 8% to 30% of couples, and both partners in 20% to 35% of couples.[7] Table 14-3 lists common infertility factors.

The term *assisted reproductive therapies (ARTs)* refers to the multiple options couples may select to assist them in the reproduction process. ARTs are described briefly in Table 14-4. Techniques for ART have evolved over time with the majority of interventions conducted in the physician's office. The use of ARTs has made it possible for women to successfully conceive and have children into their 40s (Research Highlight).

## OBSTETRIC SURGERY

Providing safe nursing care for the perioperative patient is the goal of every registered nurse. The interventions necessary to reach that goal intensify in the pregnant woman who presents for surgery. The team is now faced with the challenge of caring for at least two patients, the mother and her child.

Maternal changes in pregnancy increase as the gestation progresses and include hormonal fluctuations, mechanical changes to the viscera related to the enlarging uterus, increased metabolic and oxygen demands, and hemodynamic changes. The fetus also has unique metabolic and hemodynamic needs that must be considered. Hazards of performing surgery on the pregnant patient include fetal loss, fetal asphyxia, premature labor, premature rupture of the membranes, and thromboembolic events. Many medications used in the perioperative setting cross into the placental circulation on administration to the mother.[6]

**TABLE 14-3**

**Common Infertility Factors**

| Factor | Incidence (%) | Investigative Intervention |
|---|---|---|
| Male-coital | 40 | Semen analysis<br>Postcoital test |
| Ovulatory | 15-20 | Urinary luteinizing hormone (self-test)<br>Serum progesterone<br>Endometrial biopsy |
| Cervical | 5 | Postcoital test |
| Uterine-tubal | 30 | Hysterosalpingogram<br>Laparoscopy |
| Peritoneal | 40 | Laparoscopy |

Modified from Meldrum DR: Infertility and assisted reproductive technologies. In Hacker NF and others, editors: *Essentials of obstetrics and gynecology*, ed 4, Philadelphia, 2004, Saunders.

**TABLE 14-4**

**Assisted Reproductive Technologies**

| Technology | Description | Use |
|---|---|---|
| Assisted hatching (AH) | The zona pellucida is micromanipulated chemically or mechanically to allow the embryo to hatch and attach to the uterine wall. | Recurrent miscarriage, failed IVF, advanced maternal age |
| Embryo transfer (ET) | Follows in vitro fertilization. The fertilized ovum is implanted in the woman's uterus. Typically three embryos are transferred. | Tubal disease or blockage, endometriosis, unexplained infertility, cervical factors, immunity issues |
| Multicolor fluorescence in situ hybridization (FISH) | Laboratory technique to screen for karyotyping (DNA) abnormalities. Can determine the gender of a cell. | At-risk couples for conceiving a child with a serious genetic or chromosomal abnormality or couples in which the male partner has nonobstructive azoospermia |
| Gamete intrafallopian transfer (GIFT) | Oocytes are retrieved from the ovary and mixed in a catheter with sperm. The solution is transferred into the fimbriated end of the tube for in situ fertilization. | Unexplained infertility with normal, patent fallopian tubes |
| Intracervical insemination (ICI) | Performed during a natural cycle or stimulated cycle. Sperm are placed inside the neck of the cervix by means of a catheter and syringe. | Immunity issues, desire or need to use donor sperm in otherwise fertile woman, male infertility, unexplained infertility |
| Intracytoplasmic sperm injection (ICSI) | Selection of single sperm injected directly into the egg to achieve fertilization. | Failed IVF, oligospermia, asthenospermia, obstructive azoospermia, immunity issues, failed vasectomy reversal |
| Intrauterine insemination (IUI) | Similar to ICI; performed during a natural cycle or stimulated cycle. Sperm are placed inside uterus by means of a catheter and syringe. | Immunity issues, desire or need to use donor sperm in otherwise fertile woman, male infertility, unexplained infertility; failure of ICI |
| In vitro fertilization (IVF) | Oocytes are retrieved from the ovary and fertilized with sperm in the laboratory and allowed to develop into embryos. Embryos are then transferred to the woman using a variety of techniques. | Tubal disease or blockage, severe male infertility, endometriosis, immunity issues, unexplained fertility, cervical factors |
| Polymerase chain reaction (PCR) | Genetic screening technique. | Used for genetic screening of embryos before implantation; may be used to determine chromosomal causes of infertility in male partner of infertile couples |
| Preimplantation genetic diagnosis (PGD) | Screening for genetic defects. On day 3 after in vitro fertilization, a biopsy is performed using a micromanipulator to remove a single blastomere for analysis. | At-risk couples for conceiving a child with a serious genetic or chromosomal abnormality |
| Zygote intrafallopian transfer (ZIFT) | In vitro fertilization is accomplished and the embryo is placed in the fallopian tube during the zygote stage. | Unexplained infertility with normal, patent fallopian tubes |

Modified from Boyle KE and others: Assisted reproductive technology in the new millennium: part 1, *Urology* 63:2-6, 2004; Boyle KE and others: Assisted reproductive technology in the new millennium: part 2, *Urology* 63:217-224, 2004; Raines C: Infertility. In Lowdermilk DL, Perry SE, editors: *Maternity and women's health care,* ed 8, St Louis, 2004, Mosby.

Special considerations for the obstetric surgical patient include continuous monitoring of the fetal heart rate, rapid induction for general anesthesia, and preparation for the possible use of tocolytics (e.g., medications to decrease uterine activity) to prevent labor. Ready access to neonatal resuscitative drugs and equipment should be established when performing surgery on pregnant women in the second trimester and beyond. If permitted by the surgical approach, the pregnant woman should be positioned with a lateral tilt or with a wedge or pillow under her right hip to provide uterine displacement and relieve pressure on the maternal vena cava. This maneuver promotes blood flow to the placenta.

## Cervical Cerclage

Incompetence of the cervix is a condition characterized by habitual midtrimester spontaneous miscarriages. The condition is characterized by shortening of the length of the cervix (observed on ultrasound) and occasional funneling of the cervix. Surgical intervention is designed to prevent cervical dilation that results in the release of uterine contents. Introduced by Shirodkar in 1951, the cervical cerclage provides a mechanical closure to the cervix. Cerclage is most commonly accomplished by way of the vaginal approach (Shirodkar and McDonald approaches) or, much less commonly, the abdominal or laparoscopic approach.[15] The Shirodkar technique involves the *submucosal* placement of a purse-string type of ligature of Mersilene, Dacron tape, heavy nylon suture, or plastic-covered braided-steel suture at the level of the internal os to close it.[11] The McDonald cerclage uses a secured tie or tape placed horizontally and vertically across the cervix. The vaginal cerclage is generally removed in an office procedure when the woman reaches the thirty-seventh week of gestation, or the child may be delivered by cesarean.

***Procedural Considerations—Vaginal Approach.*** Gentle vaginal preparation is carried out. The instrumentation includes the basic vaginal instrument set, with the addition of right and left Deschamps ligature carriers, trocar needles, su-

## RESEARCH HIGHLIGHT

### Rewinding the Biologic Clock

A continuing trend in the field of obstetric medicine is the frequency with which women delay conception and childbirth. It is not uncommon for women to wait until their 40s to begin trying to attempt pregnancy. In these situations, it may take longer to conceive because of decreased oocyte production as a natural element of advancing maturity and the increased incidence in chromosomal abnormalities preventing conception or causing spontaneous abortion. When a woman encounters difficulties she may turn to assisted reproductive technology (ART) for answers and assistance.

This retrospective study sought to determine the age-based chance of achieving a live birth with ART using the woman's own oocytes. A secondary goal was to determine if success rates in this group had plateaued or improved compared with previous studies.

The researchers reviewed data for 1263 women ranging in age from 40 to 48.8 years with a mean age of 42.1 years across 2705 ART cycles. They also examined the etiology of infertility in a subset of 830 women whose first ART cycle took place at the age of 40 years or older.

The overall live birth rate per cycle for all women who initiated an ART cycle at age 40 years or above was 9.7%. A younger age at cycle start was associated with an increased live birth rate. Live birth rates were significantly higher at age 40 years than at any other age cycle start between 41 and 43 years. In reviewing causes of infertility in the subset group, 40% were attributed to unexplained infertility. This rate is higher than the overall rate of unexplained infertility in all patients undergoing ART.

Contributing to the low live birth rate for the study group was the rate of pregnancy loss. The study noted a 44% loss rate in women aged 40 years and older. Loss rates rose with each year a woman aged, to more than 70% at age 44 years.

The study also examined factors such as the number of ART cycles, number of embryos retrieved and implanted, number of embryos in reserve for repeat cycles, and the role of follicle-stimulating hormone (FSH) levels as it related to pregnancy outcomes. Predictors of success included younger age, increased numbers of embryos for implantation, excess embryos to cryopreserve for future attempts, more than one fetal heartbeat on initial ultrasound, and low FSH levels.

The researchers concluded that there was a reasonable chance of pregnancy (>5%) up until the end of the forty-third year. Although pregnancy success with ART is documented up until age 44 years and beyond, the rate of success falls below 3% at 44 years and well below 1% within ages 45 and 46 years.

Modified from Klipstein S et al: One last chance for pregnancy: a review of 2705 in vitro fertilization cycles initiated in women age 40 years and above, *Fertility and Sterility* 84(2):435-445, 2005.

tures for the internal os, and the surgeon's preference for closure of the mucosal incisions.

### Operative Procedure (Shirodkar/McDonald)

1. Anterior and posterior vaginal retractors are placed, and the cervix is pulled down with smooth ovum or sponge-holding forceps. With smooth tissue forceps and dissecting scissors, the mucosa over the anterior cervix is opened to permit the bladder to be pushed back (Figure 14-51).
2. The cervix is lifted, and the posterior vaginal mucosa is similarly incised at the level of the peritoneal reflection. The corners of the anterior and posterior incisions are bilaterally approximated in the area of the lateral mucosa with curved tonsil or Allis forceps.
3. The prepared ligature is placed at the desired level by passage of the material through the approximated tissue and is drawn tight posteriorly to close the cervix. The suture material for the ligature is then tied. It is not necessary to suture the ligature to the underlying tissues. The suture material used for this ligation is 5-mm Dacron or Mersilene tape. The anterior and posterior mucosal incisions are usually closed with 2-0 absorbable suture to complete the procedure.
4. The McDonald cerclage is performed in a similar manner, using the same instrumentation, supplies, and preparation. The suture is not buried in the submucosa in the McDonald technique (Figure 14-52).

***Procedural Considerations—Abdominal Approach.*** The transabdominal cerclage is reserved for select women who have a cervix that is so short or damaged that the vaginal approach is not feasible.[5] A vaginal and abdominal prep is performed. A Foley catheter may be placed to ensure the urinary bladder remains decompressed. A basic vaginal set and an abdominal set are needed for instrumentation. Sutures used for the transabdominal cerclage are identical to those used in the vaginal approach.

### Operative Procedure—Abdominal Approach

1. The abdomen is opened and the viscera retracted. The Trendelenburg position may be used to facilitate exposure.
2. The suture material or tape is placed around the uterine isthmus medial to the uterine vessels and fixed to the anterior isthmus, to Mackenrodt's ligaments, and to the insertions of the uterosacral ligaments.
3. The abdominal wound is closed as described for laparotomy closure (see Chapter 11).
4. Abdominal dressings and a perineal pad are applied.

***Procedural Considerations—Laparoscopic Approach.*** The laparoscopic approach may be associated with decreased postoperative pain and morbidity compared with the laparotomy approach. Standard laparoscopic equipment commonly used in gynecologic procedures is required.

### Operative Procedure—Laparoscopic Approach

1. The laparoscopic camera and ports are placed for a standard laparoscopic approach, and pneumoperitoneum is established.
2. The bladder peritoneum is opened at the level of the uterine isthmus.
3. A window is created through the broad ligament medially to the uterine vessels at the level of the internal os.
4. A strip of polypropylene mesh is placed retroperitoneally through the window circumferentially around the isthmus above the cardinal and sacrouterine ligaments.
5. The mesh is anchored with a nonabsorbable suture.
6. The laparoscopic instruments are removed, and the wounds are closed.

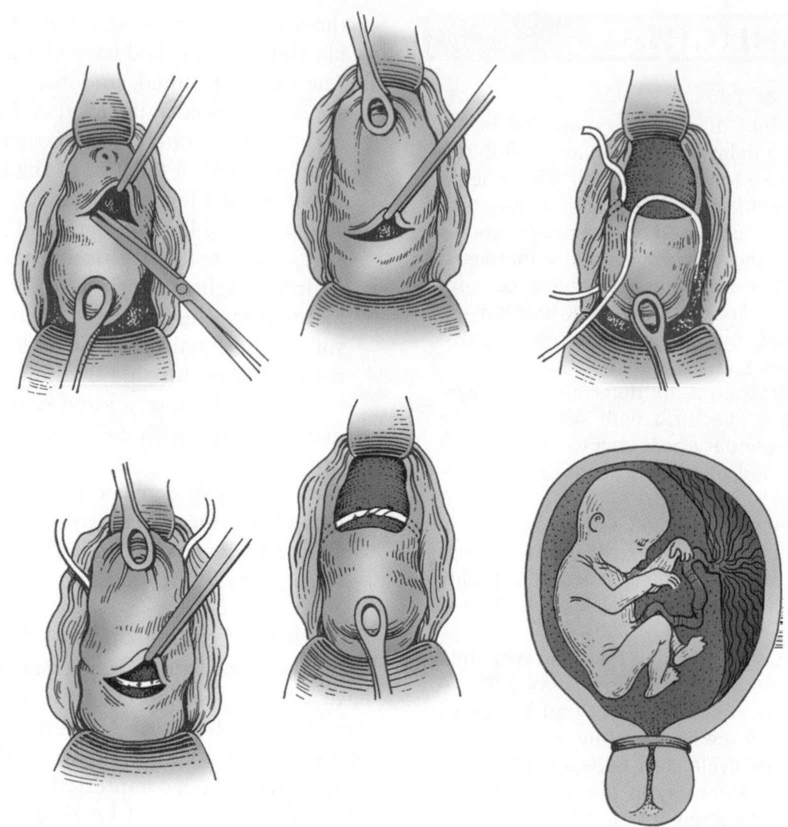

FIGURE 14-51 Principles of Shirodkar operation for treatment of incompetent internal cervical os during pregnancy.

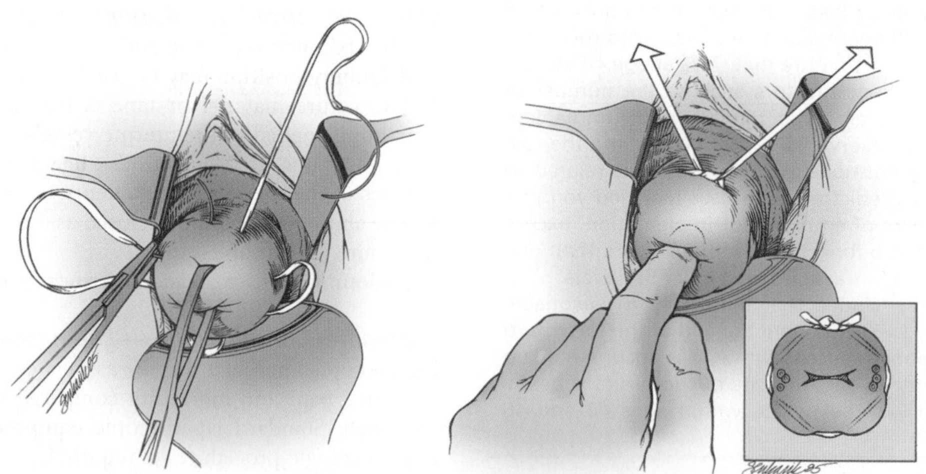

FIGURE 14-52 McDonald cerclage.

## ABDOMINAL SURGERY DURING PREGNANCY

The incidence of the immediate need for abdominal surgery occurs as frequently among pregnant women as among non-pregnant women of childbearing ages. Diagnosis of the abdominal problems in the pregnant woman is challenging because of the enlarged uterus and displaced organs. Mild leukocytosis and increased levels of alkaline phosphatase and amylase are normal during pregnancy and may also indicate surgical intraperitoneal processes. Abnormally high or rising laboratory values should be noted. X-ray evaluation is contraindicated in most instances during pregnancy.[18]

Laparotomy or laparoscopy may be required for conditions such as appendicitis and intestinal obstruction. Appendicitis is the most common nonobstetric surgical condition that complicates pregnancy and occurs with equal frequency in each of the trimesters and the postpartum period in approximately 1 in every 2000 pregnancies.[18]

### Fetal Surgery

Developments in prenatal diagnosis have progressed to the point where clinicians may consider the fetus to be the patient. Serious congenital anomaly is diagnosable by ultrasonography, alpha-fetoprotein specimen, amniocentesis, chorionic villi sampling, or percutaneous umbilical blood sampling. When an anomaly is identified, a multidisciplinary team reviews the mother's complete medical history and prenatal ultrasonograms.

Depending on the anomaly and the immediate danger posed to the fetus, the family will be counseled on their options. If no treatment is available and the condition is fatal, the family may elect to terminate the pregnancy if it is earlier than 24 weeks of gestation or may choose to carry the fetus to term. If postnatal correction is possible, the family may consider terminating the pregnancy or may continue the pregnancy with monitoring, hoping for successful correction after delivery. Lethal and nonlethal anomalies may be treated with prenatal surgery. If a family elects this option, both the mother and fetus are evaluated to determine if they will be acceptable surgical candidates. Fetal surgery was previously confined to treatment of anomalies that would result in fetal death before term or during the immediate postnatal period, but it now includes treatment of nonlethal conditions in selected cases. Conditions treated by fetal surgery include congenital diaphragmatic hernia (Figure 14-53), congenital cystic adenomatoid malformation, bronchopulmonary sequestration, obstructive uropathy, sacrococcygeal teratomas (Figure 14-54), twin-to-twin transfusion syndrome, thoracic lesions, twin reversed arterial perfusion syndrome, monochorionic twins, discordant twins, and myelomeningocele (Figure 14-55).[8]

Fetal surgery may be accomplished by way of laparotomy and hysterotomy or, in some instances, with endoscopic techniques.[8]

Postoperatively, preterm labor is of great concern, and uterine contractions, fetal heart rate, and fetal electrocardiogram (ECG) are closely assessed. Tocolytic medications are titrated to control uterine contractions. The mother is educated in self-monitoring of uterine contractions, and tocolytic therapy is continued on an outpatient basis. Frequent fetal ultrasonic scans are performed postoperatively to monitor fetal growth, amniotic fluid volume, and the adequacy of the surgical repair. Fetal surgery may also place the mother at risk for uterine rupture in subsequent pregnancies (Research Highlight).

## Cesarean Birth

Cesarean birth, also referred to as *cesarean section* or *C-section,* is delivery of the fetus or fetuses through abdominal (laparotomy) and uterine (hysterotomy) incisions. In general, cesarean birth is employed whenever further delay in delivery may seriously compromise the fetus, the mother, or both, and vaginal delivery cannot be safely accomplished. In recent years the use of cesarean birth has increased as a result of fetal monitoring, fetal scalp blood sampling for pH determination, and the wide-

Perfusion scope
Ultrasound
Balloon inflated
Balloon detached

**FIGURE 14-53** Fetal surgery for congenital diaphragmatic hernia. The trachea is isolated in preparation of hemoclip placement.

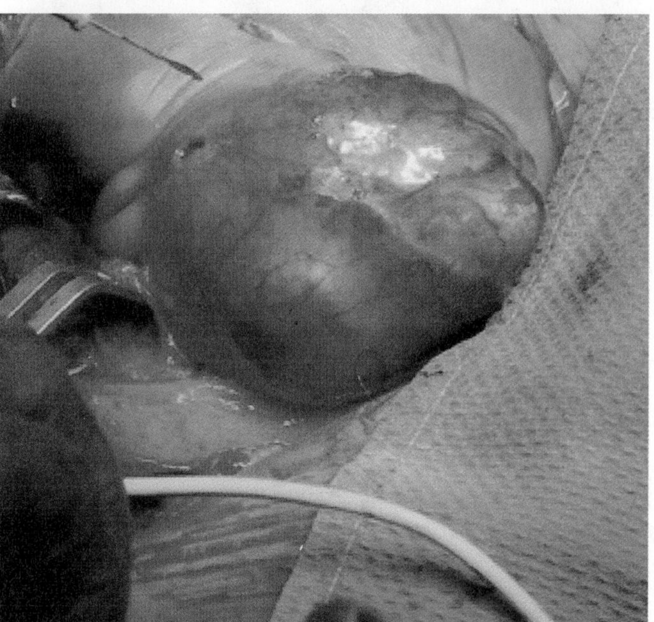


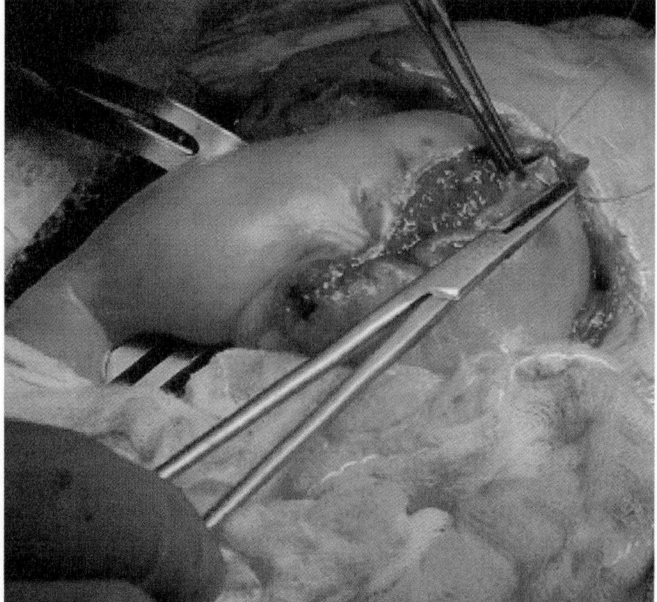


**FIGURE 14-54** **A,** Start of fetal resection of a sacrococcygeal teratoma at 21 weeks of gestation. **B,** Closure of the defect.

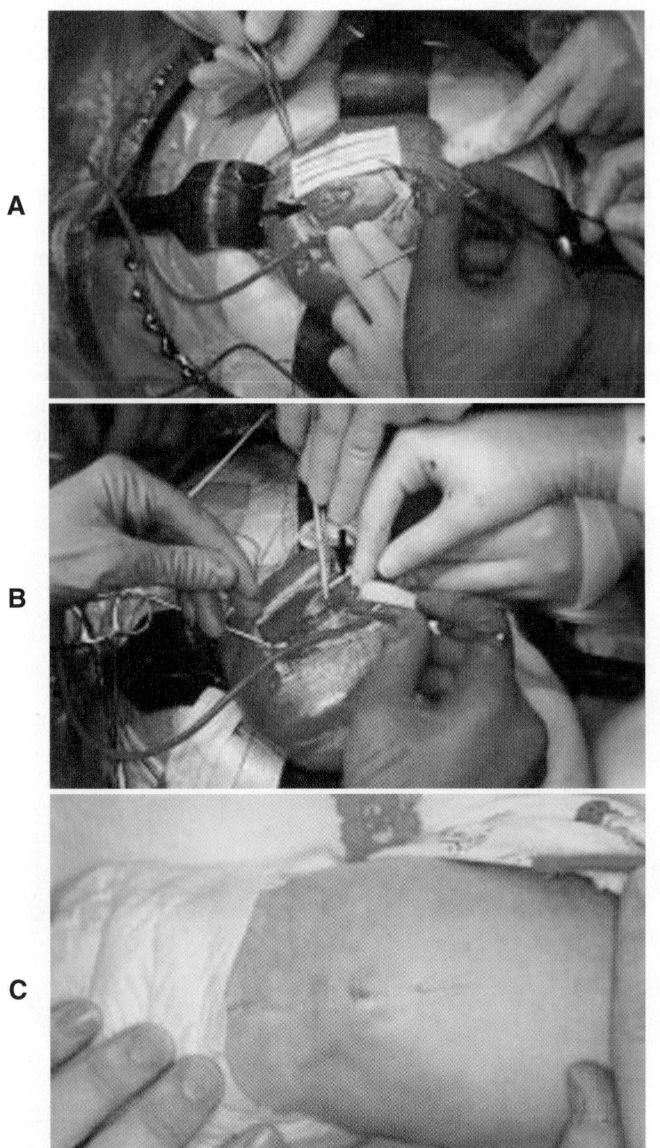


FIGURE 14-55 **A,** Myelomeningocele. **B,** Uterus is opened over defect. **C,** Myelomeningocele repair completed appearance of the delivery.

## RESEARCH HIGHLIGHT

### Fetal Surgery and Outcomes in Subsequent Pregnancies

Fetal surgery carries documented risks for both the mother and the fetus. The effect of fetal surgery on subsequent pregnancies is not well documented in the literature. However, the risks of previous uterine surgery (i.e., hysterotomy) are well known. The hysterotomy used in maternal-fetal surgery may affect placental attachment in subsequent pregnancies, resulting in a spontaneous abortion or placenta accreta.

This retrospective study sought to evaluate the reproductive outcomes of subsequent pregnancies in women after fetal surgery. The study focused on 83 women who had undergone fetal-maternal surgery for nonlethal myelomeningocele (52 procedures), lethal lung malformation/fetal hydrops (14 procedures), congenital diaphragmatic hernia (13 procedures), and lethal sacrococcygeal teratoma/fetal hydrops (4 procedures). Data were collected by means of a questionnaire that the participants completed. Fifty-five women completed and returned the questionnaire.

A subset of the data focused on participants who experienced subsequent pregnancies and focused on any complications related to those pregnancies. Thirty-four women successfully conceived and delivered. Within this group, 12 women experienced adverse outcomes (uterine problems, uterine rupture/dehiscence, cesarean hysterectomy, preterm labor, preterm delivery, pregnancy-induced hypertension, miscarriage, issues with postdelivery lung maturity, and congenital anomalies). The highest adverse outcome was uterine dehiscence (12%), followed by uterine rupture (6%) and cesarean hysterectomy (3%). The authors note that the uterine rupture rate is similar to that seen in classic cesarean deliveries.

Modified from Wilson RD and others: Reproductive outcomes after pregnancy complicated by maternal-fetal surgery, *American Journal of Obstetrics and Gynecology* 191:1430-1436, 2005.

spread emphasis on recognition of actual or suspected impairment of fetal well-being if delivery were delayed or vaginal delivery attempted. Reasons for cesarean birth include failure to progress, malposition and malpresentation, cephalopelvic disproportion, abruptio placentae, toxemia, fetal distress, uterine dysfunction, placenta previa, prolapsed cord, previous pelvic surgery, cervical dystocia, active herpes progenitalis, and diabetes. Multiple pregnancy may also be an indication for cesarean delivery.

Cesarean delivery is ranked as the second most frequently performed major surgical operation in the United States. Approximately 20% of all births are cesarean deliveries. Rates have decreased slightly because of increased use of labor trials and vaginal birth after cesarean birth (VBAC) in selected patients.[13]

Cesarean delivery may take place in the obstetric labor and delivery suite or in the OR suite. Patients about to undergo cesarean birth need careful assessment and emotional support. Because cesarean birth frequently involves emergency situations, the mother may express grave concern for the infant's well-being. If the mother has participated in childbirth classes, she may believe that she has failed in some way. The perioperative nurse must be aware of the psychologic as well as physiologic needs of this patient population. Mothers may choose to remain awake under regional anesthesia; the mother's birthing partner may be permitted to accompany and support her in the OR and witness the birth (based on hospital policy). The birthing partner may need the perioperative nurse's assistance in preparing for the delivery by washing hands and donning scrub attire or a protective gown. The perioperative nurse may need to reassure and encourage the birthing partner to coach and lend support to the mother during this intensely stressful time. The birthing partner can be included in the bonding process that is initiated at birth. The mother, if awake and stable, is shown and encouraged to hold the infant. The perioperative nurse promotes a positive family-oriented experience.

If the cesarean delivery is performed as an emergency, the family-oriented approach may not be feasible. In this emergency situation, the mother's support persons need to be directed to the surgical waiting area, where information will be communicated regarding the condition of the mother and infant. Support persons may then be able to accompany the infant as he or she is transferred to the nursery.

***Procedural Considerations.*** The patient should be in a supine position with elevation of the right side to displace the uterus and prevent aortocaval compression. Bony prominences are padded, and the patient is positioned in good body alignment with a safety strap above the knees. It may be necessary to assist the anesthesia team with the administration of regional anesthetia before placing the patient in the supine position. Throughout this process, maternal vital signs and fetal heart tones are monitored and recorded per institutional protocol.

If a general anesthetic is to be employed, all preparations, including skin prep, bladder drainage, draping, suction connection, counts, and gowning and gloving of all scrubbed personnel, are done before induction. In many hospitals, health care providers qualified to deliver newborn care and resuscitation are in attendance for the delivery. A radiant warmer and resuscitative equipment for immediate postdelivery care of the infant are available in the OR because these infants are considered to be at risk until there is evidence of physiologic stability.

The skin is prepped as for abdominal surgery. The vagina is not prepped. An indwelling urinary catheter is inserted. Instrumentation includes the basic abdominal gynecologic set, with the addition of Lister bandage scissors, Foerster sponge-holding (ring) forceps, Pennington forceps, cord clamps, DeLee retractor, delivery forceps, a head extractor (if desired), laboratory tubes for cord blood, a drain (optional), and a bulb syringe.

### *Operative Procedure*

1. An infraumbilical vertical incision or lower transverse Pfannenstiel incision is made. The incision should be long enough to allow the infant to be delivered without difficulty but no longer. Therefore the length of the incision varies with the estimated size of the fetus.
2. The abdominal wall is opened in layers. The rectus and pyramidalis muscles are separated in the midline by sharp and blunt dissection to expose the underlying transversalis fascia and peritoneum.
3. The peritoneum is elevated with two Crile hemostats about 2 cm apart. The peritoneum between the two clamps is palpated to rule out the inclusion of bowel, omentum, or bladder. The peritoneum is opened, and the abdominal cavity is entered.
4. Bleeding sites anywhere in the abdominal incision may be clamped but not ligated until later, unless the clamps obstruct exposure. When the patient is under general anesthesia, speed is important to prevent an anesthetized infant. Electrocoagulation may be used at this point to stop bleeding, especially if the patient is awake and under regional anesthesia.
5. The uterus is quickly but carefully palpated to determine the size and presenting part of the fetus as well as the direction and degree of rotation of the uterus.
6. The reflection of the peritoneum (serosa) above the upper margin of the bladder and overlying the anterior lower uterine segment is gently separated by sharp and blunt dissection.
7. The developed bladder flap is held downward beneath the symphysis with a bladder retractor such as the DeLee.
8. The uterus is opened with a knife through the lower uterine segment about 2 cm above the bladder flap. Once the uterus is opened, the incision can be extended by cutting laterally with a large bandage scissors or by simply spreading the incision by means of lateral pressure applied with each index finger when the lower uterine segment is thin.
9. The presenting membranes are incised. Suction is imperative here, and many surgeons prefer no suction tip (only the large open end of the suction tubing) during the expulsion and suctioning of amniotic fluid.
10. All retractors are removed. The fetal head is gently elevated, either manually or by use of obstetric forceps, through the incision, aided by transabdominal fundal pressure (Figure 14-56) to help expel the fetus.
11. As soon as the head is delivered, a bulb syringe or aspirator tip is used to aspirate the exposed nares and mouth to minimize aspiration of amniotic fluid and its contents.
12. Oxytocin (20 units per liter of fluid or as directed by the physician) may be administered intravenously as soon as the shoulders are delivered (or after delivery of the infant), so that the uterus contracts. This use of oxytocin minimizes blood loss.
13. On delivery of the entire infant, the cord is clamped and cut (Figure 14-57) and the infant is given to the member

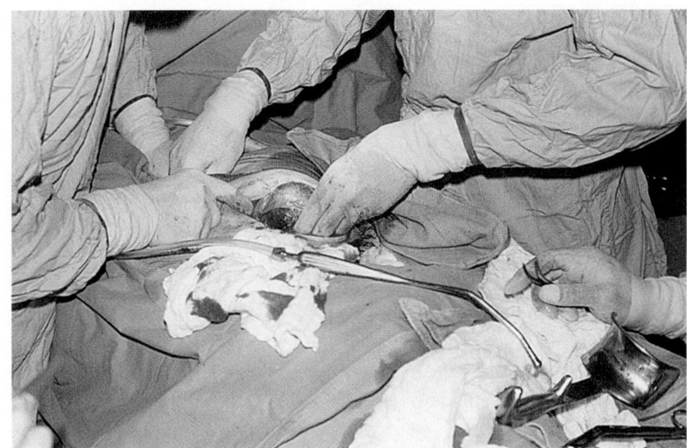

**FIGURE 14-56** Fundal pressure applied. Infant's head emerging from hysterotomy.

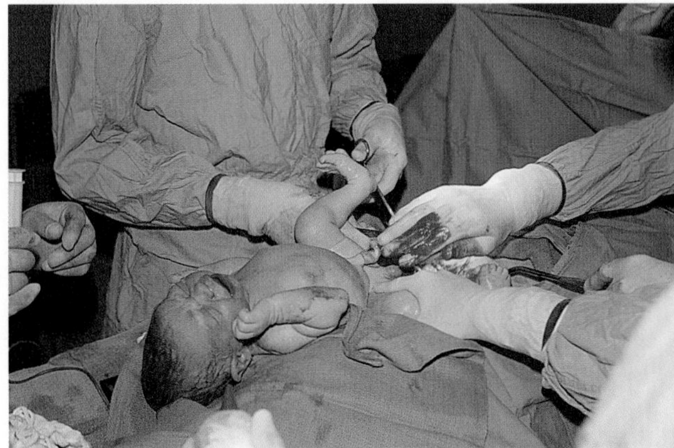

**FIGURE 14-57** Cord clamped in preparation for passing infant off field.

of the team who is responsible for resuscitation efforts as needed. A sterile gown or sheet should be provided to the individual receiving the infant to avoid any break in aseptic technique and to maintain Standard Precautions during transfer of the infant.

14. The edges of the uterine incision are promptly clamped with Pean forceps, ring forceps, or Pennington clamps.
15. The placenta is delivered and placed in a large receptacle provided from the back table. Fundal massage or manual removal may be employed to hasten delivery of the placenta and reduce bleeding.
16. One or two separate layers of suture may be used to close the uterine incision.
17. After determination that there is no further bleeding after closure of the uterine incision, the cut edges of the serosa overlying the uterus and bladder are approximated with a continuous suture.
18. Any blood, blood clots, vernix, and amniotic fluid in the pelvis and peritoneal cavity are removed. The fallopian tubes and ovaries are also inspected. Tubal ligation may be carried out at this point.
19. The peritoneum and each abdominal layer are closed.
20. After the wound is closed, the fundus is massaged and any clots are expressed from the vagina.
21. The abdominal dressing and a perineal pad are applied.

## REFERENCES


1. ACOG practice bulletin: clinical management guidelines for obstetrician-gynecologists, *Obstetrics Gynecology*, Number 46,102(3):647-658, 2003.
2. American Cancer Society: *Cancer facts and figures 2005*, Atlanta, 2005, The Society.
3. *AORN standards, recommended practices, and guidelines*, Denver, Colo, 2004, The Association of periOperative Registered Nurses.
4. Baakdah H, Tulandi T: Uterine fibroid embolization, *Clinical Obstetrics & Gynecology* 48(2):361-368, 2005.
5. Besio M, Oyarzun E: Transabdominal cervicoisthmic cerclage, *International Journal of Gynaecology and Obstetrics* 88:318-320, 2005.
6. Birnbach DJ, Browne I: Anesthesia for obstetrics. In Miller RD: *Miller's anesthesia*, ed 6, Philadelphia, 2005, Churchill Livingstone.
7. Boyle KE and others: Assisted reproductive technology in the new millennium: Part 1. *Urology* 63:2-6, 2004.
8. Cortes RA, Farmer DK: Recent advances in fetal surgery, *Seminars in Perinatology* 28(3):199-211, 2004.
9. Dialani V, Levine D: Ectopic pregnancy: a review, *Ultrasound Quarterly* 20(3):105-117, 2004.
10. Faust RJ and others: Patient positioning. In Miller RD: *Miller's anesthesia*, ed 6, Philadelphia, 2005, Churchill Livingstone.
11. Genovese SK: Antepartal hemorrhagic disorders. In Lowdermilk DL, Perry SE, editors: *Maternity and women's health care*, ed 8, St Louis, 2004, Mosby.
12. Hacker NF: Cervical dysplasia and cancer. In Hacker NF and others, editors: *Essentials of obstetrics and gynecology*, ed 4, Philadelphia, 2004, Saunders.
13. H-CUPnet: Statistics for US community hospital stays, principle procedure based on clinical classifications software, 2003. Accessed October 12, 2005, on-line: www.hcup.ahrq.gov.
14. Helmberger TK and others: Embolization of uterine fibroids, *Abdominal Imaging* 29:267-277, 2004.
15. Kjollesdal M and others: Laparoscopic cervico-uterine cerclage using polypropylene mesh for treatment of cervical incompetence, *Acta Obstetricia et Gynecologica Scandinavica* 84:823-824, 2005.
16. Lampmann LE and others: Uterine fibroids: targeted embolization, an update on technique, *Abdominal Imaging* 29:128-131, 2004.
17. Lowdermilk DL: Structural disorders and neoplasms of the reproductive system. In Lowdermilk DL, Perry SE, editors: *Maternity and women's health care*, ed 8, St Louis, 2004, Mosby.
18. McAteer J: Medical-surgical problems in pregnancy. In Lowdermilk DL, Perry SE, editors: *Maternity and women's health care*, ed 8, St Louis, 2004, Mosby.
19. Meldrum DR: Infertility and assisted reproductive technologies. In Hacker NF and others, editors: *Essentials of obstetrics and gynecology*, ed 4, Philadelphia, 2004, Saunders.
20. Moore GJ, Nelson AL: Congenital anomalies and benign conditions of the ovaries and fallopian tubes. In Hacker NF and others, editors: *Essentials of obstetrics and gynecology*, ed 4, Philadelphia, 2004, Saunders.
21. Munday P, Buchan A: Vulval vestibulitis, *BMJ* 328:1214-1215, 2004.
22. Nelson AL and others: Ectopic pregnancy. In Hacker NF and others, editors: *Essentials of obstetrics and gynecology*, ed 4, Philadelphia, 2004, Saunders.
23. Raines C: Infertility. In Lowdermilk DL, Perry SE, editors: *Maternity and women's health care*, ed 8, St Louis, 2004, Mosby.
24. Schafer M and others: Isotonic fluid absorption during hysteroscopy resulting in severe hyperchloremic acidosis, *Anesthesiology* 103(1): 203-204, 2005.
25. Shirk GJ: Minimally invasive surgery for ablation of the endometrium, *Clinical Obstetrics and Gynecology* 48(2):325-326, 2005.
26. Sowter MC, Farquhar CM: Ectopic pregnancy: an update, *Current Opinion in Obstetrics and Gynecology* 16:289-283, 2004.
27. Ubeda A and others: Essure: a new device for hysteroscopic tubal sterilization in an outpatient setting, *Fertility and Sterility* 82(1): 196-199, 2004.

CHAPTER 15

# Genitourinary Surgery

GRATIA M. NAGLE

Advances in genitourinary surgery, with the use of robotics, laparoscopic techniques, cryotherapy, brachytherapy, lasers, ultrasonography, lithotriptors, innovative diagnostic measures, and minimally invasive surgical approaches, have expanded treatment options. As urologic surgery becomes more complex and far more precise, the perioperative urology nurse has challenges in maintaining up-to-date knowledge, documented competence, and new technical skills. More procedures are being done on an ambulatory or short-stay basis, allowing limited time for patient and family education and discharge planning. The success of surgical intervention and patient outcomes depends greatly on the perioperative nurse's ability and knowledge in designing, developing, and implementing a perioperative plan of care.[47]

## Surgical Anatomy

The normal genitourinary system includes one pair of kidneys, two ureters, the urinary bladder, the urethra, and the prostate gland in the male.[49] Also considered essential to the genitourinary system are the adrenal glands, male reproductive organs, and the female urogynecologic system.

Urine is excreted by the kidneys and conveyed to the bladder through the ureters. Urine is stored in the bladder, which serves as a reservoir until its full capacity (350 to 700 ml) is reached, and is eliminated from the body by way of the urethra. Normal urinary output ranges from 0.5 to 1.0 ml/kg of body weight per hour for the average adult.

### Kidneys

The kidneys are located in the retroperitoneal space along the lateral borders of the psoas muscle, one on each side of the vertebral column at the level of the twelfth thoracic to the third lumbar vertebrae. Usually the right kidney is several centimeters lower than the left because the liver rests above and anterior to the right kidney (Figure 15-1).

Each kidney is surrounded by a mass of fatty and loose areolar tissue known as *pararenal fat*. A capsule enclosing the renal space is known as the *fascia renalis*. This is composed of *Gerota's fascia* (anterior renal fascia) and *Zuckerkandl's fascia* (posterior renal fascia). These structures help keep the kidneys in their normal anatomic position. The anterior and posterior relationships of the kidneys are shown in Figure 15-2.

On the medial side of each kidney is a concave area known as the *hilum*, through which the renal artery and vein enter and leave. The renal pelvis, a funnel-shaped structure that lies within the kidney and posterior to the renal vascular pedicle, divides into several branches called *calyces* (Figure 15-3). When surgery is indicated in these structures, a posterior flank approach is preferred. When surgery for removal of a mass is anticipated, a transabdominal or thoracoabdominal incision may be chosen.

The kidneys are highly vascular organs that process approximately one fifth of the entire volume of blood at any one time. The blood supply to the kidney is conveyed through the renal artery (a large branch of the aorta) and leaves through the renal vein. On entering the kidney, the renal artery divides into anterior and posterior sections. These undergo further division into interlobular arteries from which smaller afferent branches pass to the glomeruli. Efferent arterioles in the glomeruli then pass to the tubules of the nephron. Renal arteriography performed preoperatively helps identify the patient's renal vascular anatomy when renal hypertension[24,56] and horseshoe kidney are suspected and as part of the routine workup before renal transplantation.

The renal lymphatic supply originates beneath the capsule of the kidney and empties into the lumbar lymph nodes at the junction of the renal vascular pedicle and aorta. The nerves of the autonomic (involuntary) nervous system come from the lumbar sympathetic trunk and from the vagus. Removal of the nerve pathways does not impair renal function. The renal artery and vein with their accompanying nerves and lymphatics are referred to as the *pedicle* of the kidney.

### Adrenal Glands

The adrenal glands lie retroperitoneally beneath the diaphragm, capping the medial aspects of the superior pole of each kidney. On the right side, the gland is triangular and adjacent to the inferior vena cava; on the left side, it is a rounded, crescent-shaped gland posterior to the stomach and pancreas. Each adrenal gland has a medulla, which secretes epinephrine (adrenaline), and a cortex, which secretes steroids and hormones. Secretions from the adrenal cortex are influenced by the activity of the pituitary gland. The adrenal glands are liberally supplied with arterial branches from the inferior phrenic and renal arteries and from the aorta. Venous drainage is accomplished on the right side by the inferior vena cava and on the left by the left renal vein. The lymphatic system accompanies the suprarenal vein and drains into the lumbar lymph nodes.

### Ureters

Each ureter is a continuation of the renal pelvis. The ureter extends in a smooth S curve from the renal pelvis to the base of the bladder. It is approximately 25 to 30 cm long and 4 to 5 mm in diameter in the adult. This fibromuscular cylindric tube is lined by transitional epithelium (urothelium) and lies

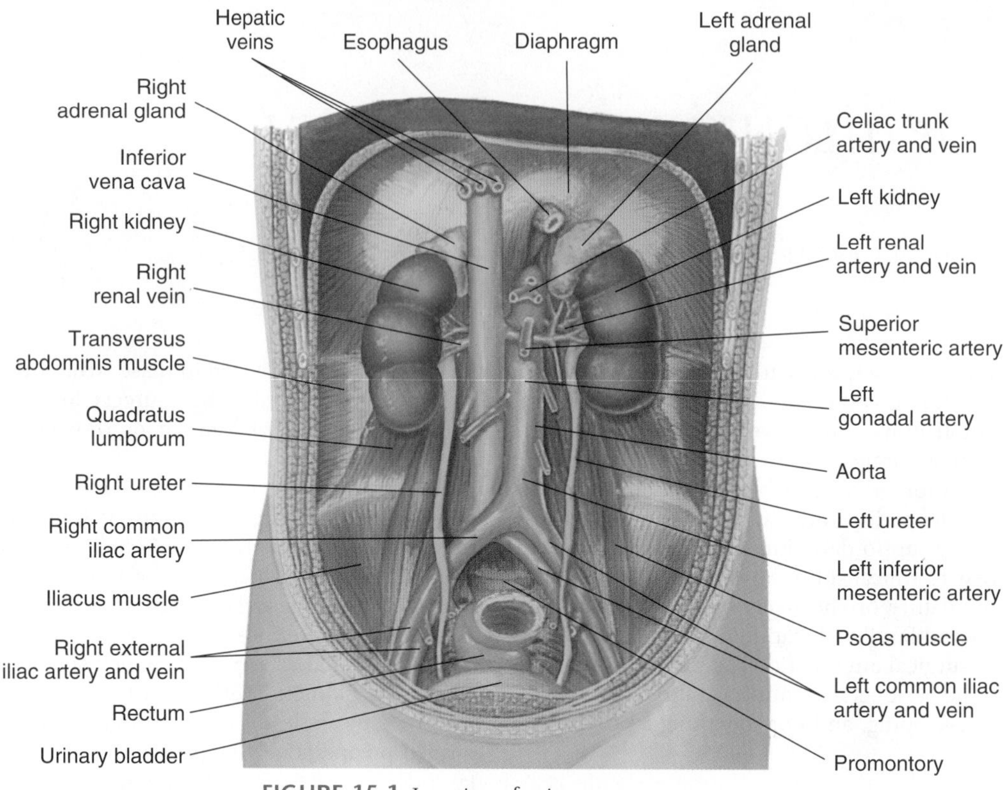


**FIGURE 15-1** Location of urinary system organs.

on the psoas muscle, passing medially to the sacroiliac joints and laterally to the ischial spines. As urine accumulates in the renal pelvis, slight distention initiates a wave of muscular contractions. This peristaltic activity continues down the ureter, propelling urine into the bladder.

The ureter has three areas of narrowing where calculi may become lodged and pose a potential problem with pain and obstruction: (1) the ureteropelvic junction (UPJ), (2) the crossing of the ureter over the external iliac vessels, and (3) the ureterovesical junction (UVJ) (Figure 15-4). Urine may sometimes cause calculi to be washed down the ureter to produce severe ureteral colic. Of all renal calculi, 90% are spontaneously passed into the bladder. However, if they become lodged in the ureter, an extracorporeal shock-wave lithotripsy (ESWL), ureteroscopy for stone manipulation, laser lithotripsy, or ureterolithotomy may be indicated. During pelvic or intestinal surgery, ureteral catheters or stents are often inserted to facilitate positive identification of the ureters and reduce the potential for severing or ligating them. These stents are frequently removed at the conclusion of the surgery, although some surgeons prefer to leave them in place through the early recovery period.

## Urinary Bladder

The adult urinary bladder is a hollow, muscular viscus that acts as a reservoir for urine until micturition (voiding) occurs. It has an outer adventitial and inner urothelial layer. The trigone, a triangular area, forms the base of the bladder. The three corners of the trigone correspond to the orifices of the ureters and the bladder neck (opening of the urethra) (Figure 15-5). The ureteral orifices, on the proximal trigone at the interureteric ridge, are 2.5 cm apart. The bladder neck (internal sphincter) is formed from converging detrusor muscle fibers of the bladder wall that pass distally to form the smooth musculature of the urethra. Physiologically, the bladder fills with urine and expands into the abdominal cavity. The extraperitoneal location is advantageous because a suprapubic (above the pubic arch) incision may be performed without violating the peritoneum and potentially causing intraperitoneal complications.

The main arterial supply of the bladder comprises the superior, middle, and inferior vesical arteries. These vessels are derived from the internal iliac (hypogastric) artery, the obturator and inferior gluteal arteries, and in females the uterine and vaginal arteries. The bladder has a rich venous supply that drains into the internal iliac (hypogastric) vein. The lymphatic system is served by the vesical, external and internal iliac, and common iliac lymph nodes.

The bladder's size, position, and relation to the bowel, rectum, and reproductive organs vary according to the bladder's distention. In a female the vagina lies dorsal to the base of the bladder and parallel to the urethra (Figure 15-6). In a male the prostate gland is interposed between the bladder neck and the urethra (Figure 15-7). These anatomic relationships influence the symptoms that a patient experiences preoperatively and are important landmarks during pelvic surgery.

The process of bladder evacuation appears to be initiated by nerve cells from the sacral division of the autonomic nervous system. These sacral reflex centers are controlled by higher voluntary centers in the brain. Stimulation of the sacral centers results in contraction of the bladder muscles and relaxation of the bladder outlet sphincters. Muscles inside and adjacent to the urethral wall and from the pelvic floor maintain closure of the sphincters of the bladder, thus enabling continence.

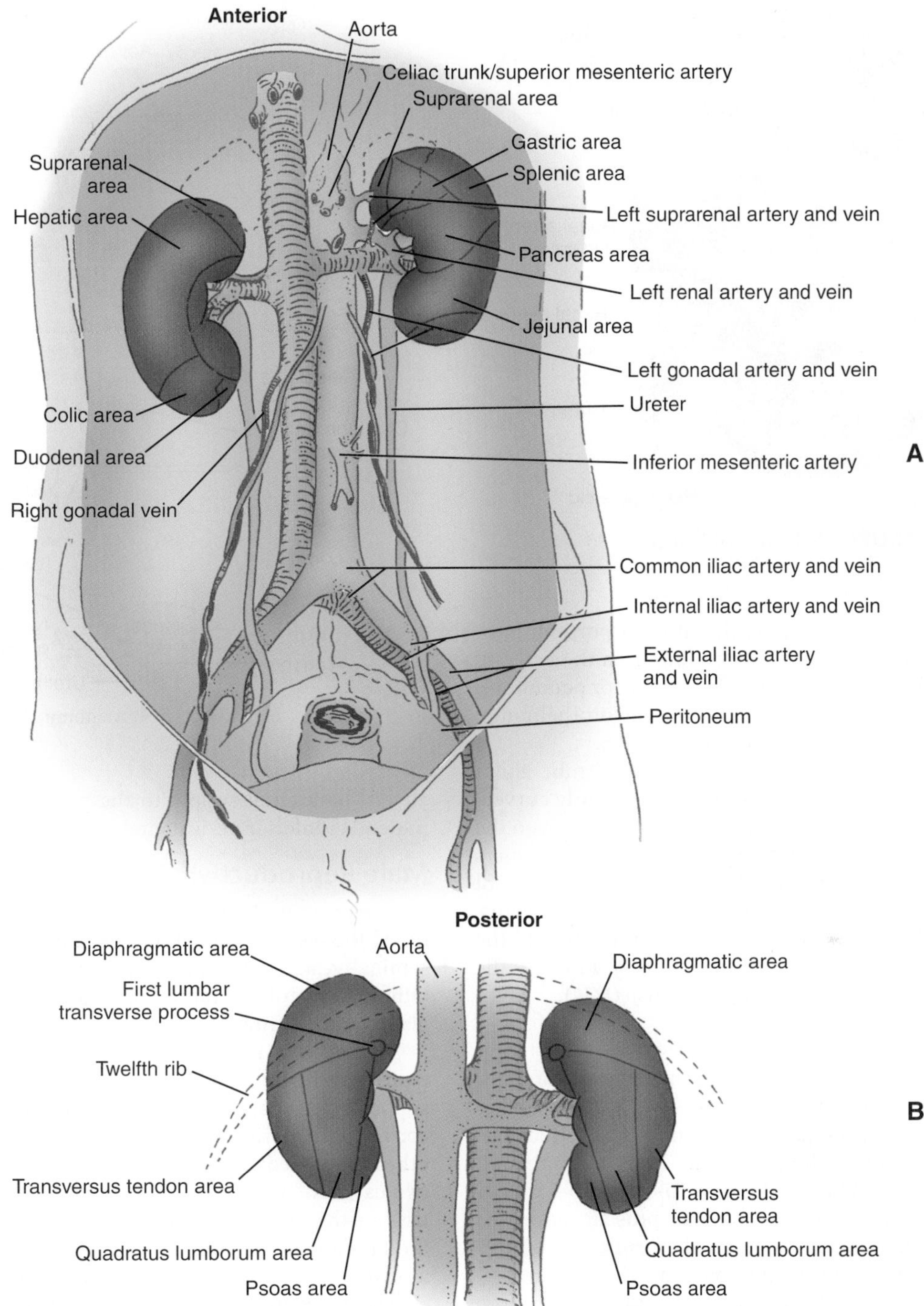


**FIGURE 15-2** **A,** Blood supply of kidneys and relationship of kidneys and ureters to the main arteries and veins and the intraperitoneal organs. **B,** Relationship of the kidneys and ureters to the spinal column.

## Urethra

The male urethra, normally 20 to 25 cm long, extends from the bladder neck to the tip of the penis and varies in diameter from 7 to 10 mm. It is divided into two portions: the proximal (sphincteric) urethra and the distal (conduit or anterior) urethra, both of which undergo further subdivision. The proximal urethra is commonly referred to as the *posterior urethra,* where it is elevated by the verumontanum, extending from the bladder neck through the prostate and the membranous portion. Within the posterior urethra lie the prostatic and membranous portions (see Figure 15-5). As the urethra exits the prostate and crosses the pelvic (urogenital) diaphragm, it is called the *membranous urethra.* The distal urethra, commonly called the *anterior urethra,* is subdivided into the bulbar, pendulous (penile), and glandular urethras. The bulbar urethra is the area most prone to urethral strictures in the male. The prostatic urethra is approximately 3 cm long and is the widest portion of the urethra. On the floor of the prostatic urethra is the verumontanum, which contains the openings of the ejaculatory

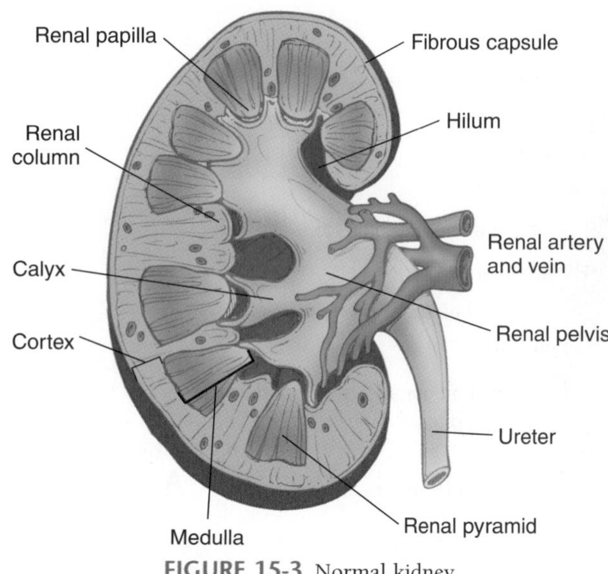


FIGURE 15-3 Normal kidney.

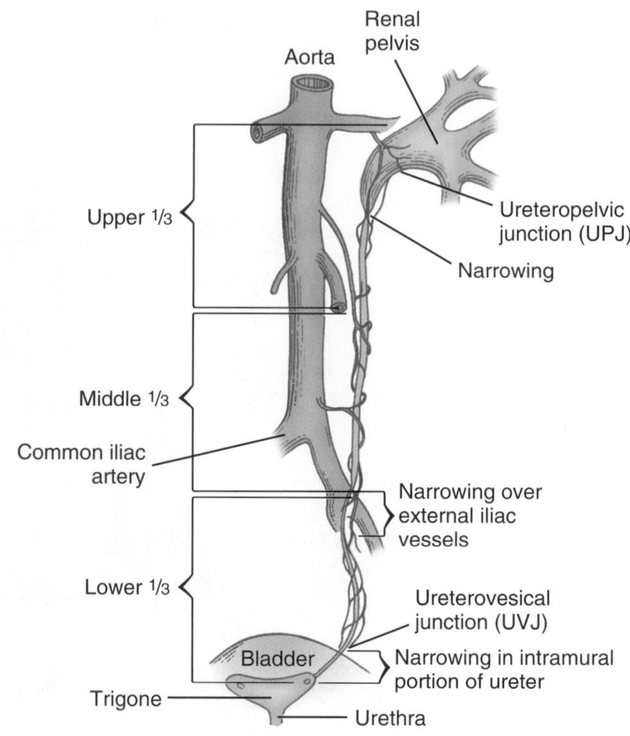


FIGURE 15-4 Anatomy of ureter.

ducts. The membranous urethra is the shortest portion, measuring approximately 2.5 cm and extending from the external sphincter to the apex of the prostate. The penile, or pendulous, urethra lies within the corpus spongiosum. The urothelium of the urethra is continuous with that of the bladder.

The female urethra is a narrow, membranous tube about 3 to 5 cm in length and 6 to 8 mm in diameter. Slightly curved, it lies behind and beneath the symphysis pubis, anterior to the vagina. It passes through the internal and external sphincters and the urogenital diaphragm. The periurethral glands of Skene open on the floor of the urethra just inside the meatus. Because the female urethra is so short and in proximity to the anal and vaginal areas, microorganisms find easy access to the bladder and can cause urinary tract infections (UTIs).

## Prostate Gland

The prostate gland is a donut-shaped organ composed of fibromuscular and glandular components. It is located at the base of the bladder neck and completely surrounds the urethra. The gland is about 4 cm at the base, is about 2 cm in depth, and normally weighs 20 to 30 g (see Figures 15-5 and 15-7).

The four glandular regions within the prostate have two major zones (the peripheral zone and the central zone) and two minor zones (the transitional zone and the periurethral zone). Many clinicians still prefer to divide the prostate into the intraurethral lobe (right and left lateral) and the extraurethral lobe (posterior and median). The posterior lobe is readily palpable during rectal examination and prone to cancerous degeneration. Benign prostatic hyperplasia (BPH, often referred to as hypertrophy) generally occurs in the transitional zone (intraurethral lobe).

Behind the prostatic capsule is a fibrous sheath known as the *true prostatic capsule,* which separates the prostate gland and the seminal vesicles from the rectum. This fascia is an important landmark during perineal prostatectomy.

The lobes of the prostate gland secrete highly alkaline fluid that dilutes the testicular secretion as it is excreted from the ejaculatory ducts. These secretions are believed to be essential to the passage of spermatozoa and helpful in keeping them alive. The arterial supply to the prostate is derived from the pudendal, inferior vesical, and hemorrhoidal arteries.

## Male Reproductive Organs

The male reproductive organs include several paired structures: the testes, epididymides, seminal ducts (vasa deferens), seminal vesicles, ejaculatory ducts, and bulbourethral glands. Other organs of the reproductive tract are the penis, prostate gland, and urethra.

The *scrotum* is located behind and below the base of the penis and in front of the anus. Each loose sac contains and supports a testis, an epididymis, and some of the spermatic cord. The two sides of the scrotum are separated from each other by a median raphe (septum). Within the scrotum are two cavities, or sacs, that are lined with smooth, glistening tissue—the tunica vaginalis. Normally, a small amount of clear fluid is contained in the tunica vaginalis. The condition known as *hydrocele* is an abnormal accumulation of this fluid.

The *testes* manufacture the spermatozoa and also contain specialized Leydig's cells that produce the male hormone *testosterone.* Each testis consists of many tubules in which the sperm are formed, surrounded by dense capsules of connective tissue. The tubules coalesce and continue into the adjacent epididymis, where the sperm mature and are stored. At the upper pole of the testis is the appendix testis, a small body that may be pedunculated (stalked) or sessile (flat).

The *epididymis* is a long, convoluted duct located along the posterolateral surface of the testis. It is closely attached to the testicle by fibrous tissue and secretes seminal fluid, which gives the sperm a liquid medium in which to migrate. The vas deferens (ductus deferens, seminal duct) is a distal continuation of the epididymis as it enters the prostate gland and conveys the sperm to the seminal vesicle.

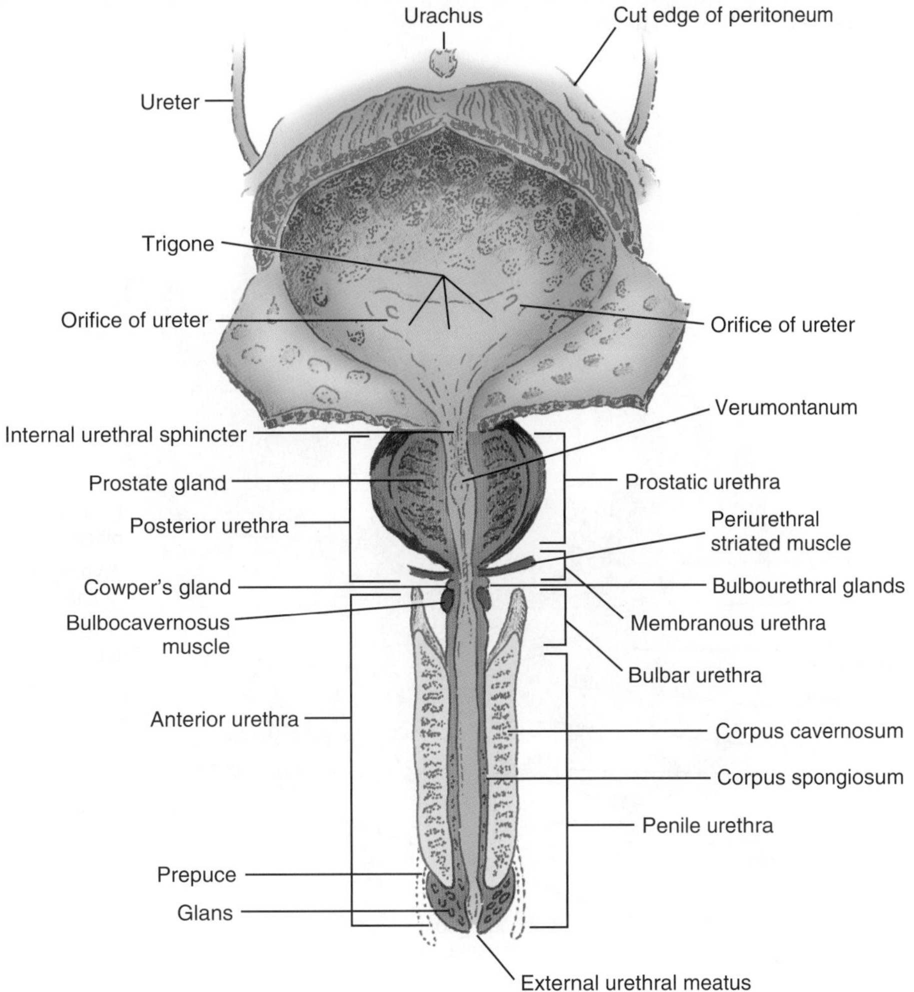


**FIGURE 15-5** Anatomy of male urinary bladder, prostate gland, and urethra.

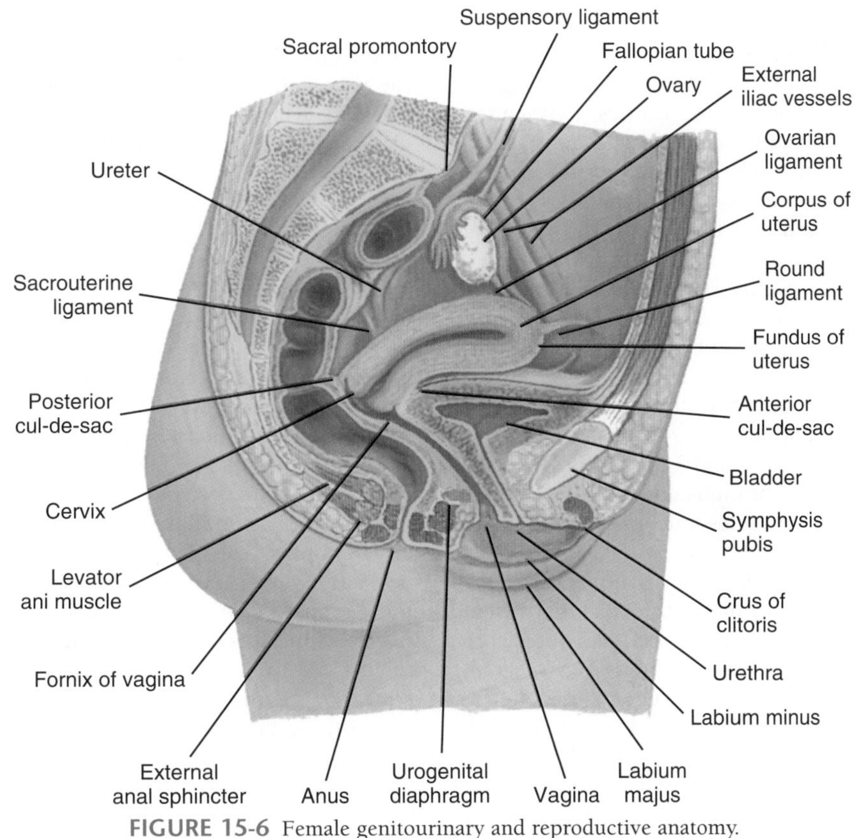


**FIGURE 15-6** Female genitourinary and reproductive anatomy.

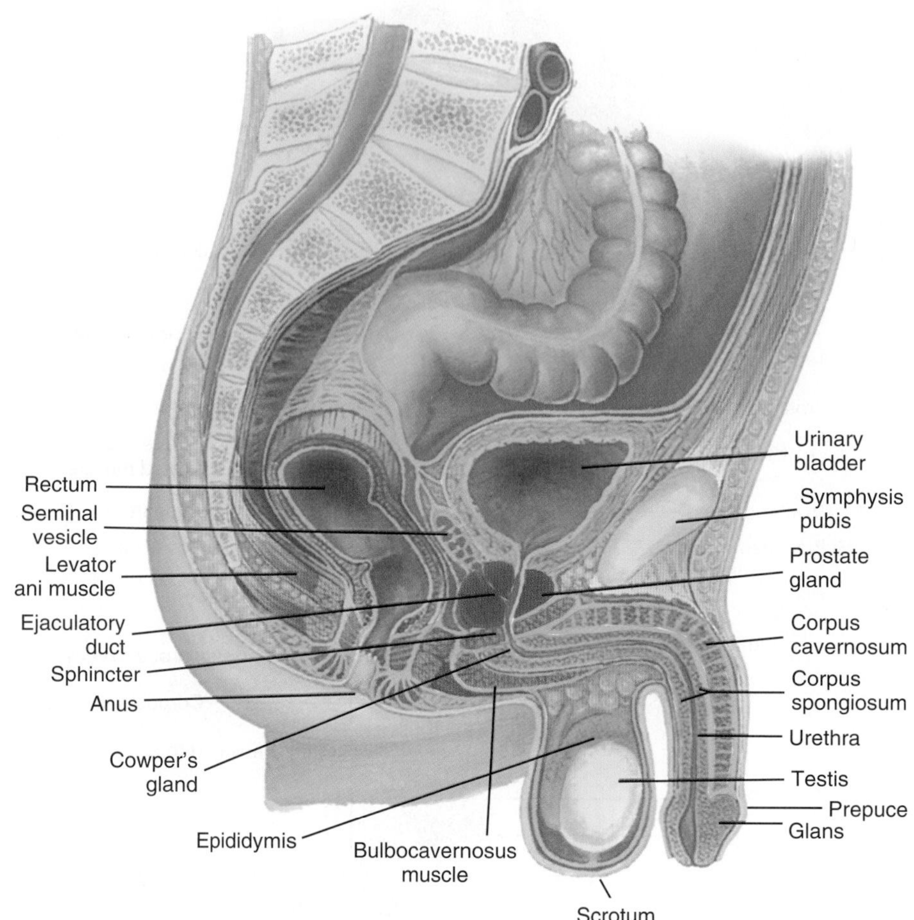


**FIGURE 15-7** Male genitourinary and reproductive anatomy.

The *vas deferens* extends from the epididymis into the abdomen and lies within the spermatic cord in the inguinal region. The spermatic cord also contains veins, arteries, lymphatics, nerves, and surrounding connective tissue (cremaster muscle), which give support to the testes. The terminal portion of each vas deferens is called the *ejaculatory duct;* it passes between the lobes of the prostate gland and opens into the posterior urethra.

The *accessory reproductive glands* include the seminal vesicles, prostate gland, and bulbourethral gland. The seminal vesicles unite with the vas deferens on either side, are situated behind the bladder, and produce protein and fructose for the nutrition of the sperm cell. Sperm and prostatic fluid are discharged at the time of ejaculation.

*Cowper's glands* (bulbourethral glands) are located on each side at the juncture of the membranous and bulbar urethras. Each gland, by way of its duct, empties mucous secretions into the urethra.

The *penis* is suspended from the pubic symphysis by the suspensory ligaments. The penis contains three distinct vascular, spongelike bodies surrounding the urethra: two outer bodies called the *right corpus cavernosum* and *left corpus cavernosum* and an inner body, the *corpus spongiosum urethrae.* These tissues contain a network of vascular channels that fill with blood during erection (see Figure 15-5). At the distal end of the penis, the skin is doubly folded to form the prepuce, or foreskin, which serves as a covering for the glans penis. The glans penis contains the urethral orifice.

## *Perioperative Nursing Considerations*

### Assessment

Patients entering a hospital or ambulatory surgery unit for genitourinary surgery exhibit many emotions and reactions, including fear, embarrassment, helplessness, hostility, anger, and grief. To most, a successful surgical outcome is of prime importance. The urology patient population varies from infants with congenital anomalies to elderly people with physiologic impairments. Because of the dramatic increase in same-day admissions and ambulatory surgeries, the nursing staff must prepare to meet patients' specific needs, from preoperative teaching to postoperative home care. The families of patients need to be involved in this preparation process. Patient education begins in the urologist's office. Communication between the office and perioperative nursing staff allows continuity of care and increases the efficiency and effectiveness of surgical procedures.[58]

In addition to routine admission information, urologic and cardiac histories are usually obtained. This information includes but is not limited to vital signs, allergies (including latex), the patient's primary problem, history of the present illness, nature of symptoms, and limitations imposed by the disease condition. All data pertinent to the proposed operative procedure should be reviewed. Nursing observation should include the patient's general physical appearance as well as nonverbal behaviors, such as restlessness, which may indicate discomfort or anxiety. Any limitations in mobility or sensory deficits should be noted.[33] Urologic procedures frequently require positions that create unusual stress for the patient, both anatomic and physiologic.[17] Assessment provides the perioperative nurse with data adequate to support preoperative planning, intraoperative implementation, and postoperative evaluation.[4,41,58,59]

Many urologic surgical interventions require the patient to be in a flank position, causing compression of the vena cava and dependent lung.[6] In addition, large amounts of irrigating fluids are frequently used intraoperatively. For these reasons, a current cardiac and electrolyte status should be available for review. Studies that have been done preoperatively may include serum and urine electrolytes, blood glucose, blood urea nitrogen (BUN), urinalysis and urine cultures (Table 15-1), cardiac enzymes, complete blood count (CBC), prothrombin time (PT) and partial thromboplastin time (PTT), blood chemistry profiles (see Table 15-1), electrocardiogram (ECG), and chest x-ray examination.[23,58] The medical history, including a list of medications and any infectious processes or chronic diseases, should be reviewed. Specific genitourinary studies can be found in the patient's medical record. They may encompass all or some of the following: computerized tomography (CT) scans, magnetic resonance imaging (MRI), bone and Dexa Scans, positron emission tomography (PET), Prostascint scans, intravenous (IV) pyelograms or urograms (IVPs, IVUs), genitourinary flat plate (KUB [kidney, ureter, bladder]), urinary flow studies, fluoroscopic examinations (angiography, cavernosography), prostate-specific antigen (PSA), and ultrasonography. After the medical record is reviewed, assessment information is compiled, perioperative nursing diagnoses are identified, and the perioperative plan of care is formulated.[47]

**TABLE 15-1**

**Common Preoperative Laboratory Analyses for Patients with Genitourinary Disorders**

| Laboratory Studies | Normal Range (Adult Values) |
|---|---|
| **COAGULATION PROFILES** | |
| Bleeding time | 1-9 min |
| Partial thromboplastin time (PTT) | 60-70 sec |
| Platelet count | 150,000-400,000/mm$^3$ |
| Prothrombin time (PT) | 11-12.5 sec |
| **FERTILITY PROFILES (MALE)** | |
| Follicle-stimulating hormone (FSH) | 1-15 milliinternational units/ml |
| Luteinizing hormone (LH) | 7-24 milliinternational units/ml |
| Testosterone (total) | 300-1000 ng/dl |
| Sperm count | 50-200 million/ml, 0%-80% motile |
| **HEMATOLOGY VALUES (LOW: FEMALE; HIGH: MALE)** | |
| Hematocrit (Hct) | 37%-52% |
| Hemoglobin (Hgb) | 12-18 g/dl |
| Red blood cells (RBCs) | 4.2-6.1 million/mm$^3$ |
| White blood cells (WBCs) | 5000-10,000 million/mm$^3$ |
| **SERUM PROFILES (LOW: FEMALE; HIGH: MALE)** | |
| Bicarbonate | 21-28 mEq/liter ($HCO_3$) |
| Blood urea nitrogen (BUN) | 10-20 mg/dl |
| Calcium ($Ca^{++}$) | 9-10.5 mg/dl |
| Chloride ($Cl^-$) | 90-106 mEq/liter |
| Cholesterol | <200 mg/dl |
| HDL (high-density lipids) | Male <45 mg/dl; Female: <55 mg/dl |
| LDL (low-density lipids) | 60-180 mg/dl |
| VLDL (triglycerides) | 25%-50% |
| **SERUM PROFILES (LOW: FEMALE; HIGH: MALE)—cont'd** | |
| Creatinine | 0.5 – 1.2 mg/dl |
| Glucose (blood sugar) | 70-105 mg/dl |
| Osmolality | 285-295 mOsm/kg $H_2O$ |
| Potassium ($K^+$) | 3.5-5 mEq/liter |
| Phosphorus (P) | 3-4.5 mg/dl |
| Prostate-specific antigen (PSA) | <4 ng/dl |
| Prostatic acid phosphatase (PAP) | 0.013-0.63 unit/liter |
| Protein | 6.4-8.3 g/dl |
| Sodium ($Na^+$) | 136-145 mEq/liter |
| Uric acid | 2.7-8.5 mg/dl |
| **URINE PROFILES (VALUES NOT LISTED SHOULD BE NEGATIVE)** | |
| Calcium ($Ca^{++}$) | 4.5-5.6 mg/day |
| Chloride ($Cl^-$) | 110-250 mEq/liter/day |
| Creatinine | 88-137 ml/min |
| Glucose (24 hr) | 50-300 mg/day (<0.5g/day) |
| Hyaline casts | Occasional |
| Osmolality (random) | 50-1400 mOsm/kg $H_2O$ |
| Phosphorus | 0.4-1.3 g/24 hr |
| Potassium ($K^+$) | 25-100 mEq/liter/day |
| Protein | 0-8 mg/dl |
| Red blood cells (RBCs) | 0-2 cells |
| Sodium ($Na^+$) | 40-220 mEq/liter/day |
| Uric acid | 250-750 mg/day |
| White blood cells (WBCs) | 0-4 per lower field |
| pH | 4.6-8 (average: 6) |
| Specific gravity | 1.005-1.030 |

Data from Pagana K, Pagana T: *Mosby's diagnostic and laboratory test reference,* ed 7, St Louis, 2005, Mosby; Tanagho EA, McAninch JW: *Smith's general urology,* ed 16, New York, 2003, McGraw-Hill.

## Nursing Diagnosis

Nursing diagnoses related to the care of patients undergoing genitourinary surgery might include the following[27]:

- Anxiety
- Risk for Perioperative Positioning Injury[17,47]
- Risk for Impaired Urinary Elimination
- Risk for Deficient Fluid Volume
- Risk for Impaired Gas Exchange
- Fear of Sexual Dysfunction

## Outcome Identification

Outcomes identified for the selected nursing diagnoses could be stated as follows[59]:

- The patient will verbalize an acceptable anxiety level to the perioperative nurse.
- The patient will be free from injury related to the surgical position.
- The patient will demonstrate or regain a normal pattern of urinary elimination.
- The patient will maintain adequate fluid volume and electrolyte balance.
- The patient will maintain adequate oxygen supply and alveolar ventilation.
- The patient will discuss fears and concerns regarding sexual function.

## Planning

Plans of care are the organizing framework for perioperative nursing activities, wherein nursing interventions are clinical processes in a quality health outcome model.[47,59] Frequently the urology patient presents a complex medical picture. Any alterations in the patient's physical, mental, or emotional status may greatly influence both the surgical and the postoperative course. A review of the patient's record; communication with the patient or family; recognition of specific psychosocial, cultural, ethnic, and spiritual needs of the patient and family; and knowledge gained from other members of the patient care team are all used to formulate the nursing database. A typical plan of care for a patient undergoing genitourinary surgery is found on p. 475.

## Implementation

Implementation begins during the patient interview. Information that is concise and simply presented enhances the final surgical outcome. Meeting the patient's emotional needs is a nursing priority. A calm patient retains more information and is cognitively and emotionally more receptive to perioperative teaching. Explanations of what to expect throughout the operative period allay fears and nurture confidence in the nursing care provided, assisting patients to minimize the effect of the surgical experience on their coping ability and to be emotionally comfortable. Perioperative nursing care requires not only the collection of pertinent patient data but also the coordination of numerous supplies and equipment to support the smooth implementation of the plan of care.

***Patient Safety.*** It is the responsibility of the perioperative nurse to follow institutional protocols for ensuring correct patient, correct procedure, and correct site surgery. Such a protocol includes proper patient identification, proper operative site identification, proper procedure identification, and proper medication identification. All wrong-site, wrong-procedure, and wrong-patient surgery occurrences are considered sentinel events by the Joint Commission on Accreditation of Healthcare Organizations (JCAHO). In addition, the Association of periOperative Registered Nurses (AORN) has established guidelines for ensuring correct medication administration.[4]

To fulfill these requirements preoperative verification, surgical site marking, and time out processes must occur for every surgical procedure. What the patient expresses as the intended surgical procedure is compared with what is documented on the operative permit and other items, such as the operating room (OR) schedule. Patient identification is achieved by also asking the patient to state his or her full name and birth date. This information is compared with the patient identification bracelet. Documentation of the processes implemented is completed on the designated institutional form or forms.

The surgical site is marked with a permanent nontoxic marking pen. The patient should be involved in this process. A standard policy needs to be developed within the particular facility as to how marking will be accomplished for urologic, endoscopic, and abdominal procedures, particularly when they involve laterality. This mark should be clearly visible following prepping and draping.

"Time out" is a pause in the activity that occurs before the start or incision on all procedures. The entire team stops to verbally confirm the patient's identity, verify the position, state and agree on the procedure and surgical site, and review that all implants and necessary equipment are available and ready (Patient Safety). This process is documented according to hospital policy.

When medications are used intraoperatively the containers should always be marked with the medication and dose (refer to Chapter 2 for a full discussion of medication safety). Verbal verification of the medication and dosage should take place when passing the drug in its administration device to the surgeon. Local anesthetics that contain epinephrine should be used with caution in urology. Many urologic interventions involve "end-organs," for example, the scrotum, testicles, and penis. The use of epinephrine in these areas can result in an ischemic situation and should be avoided.

***Positioning.*** Thorough understanding of the urologic OR bed and its functions is essential for optimum patient positioning. The position in which the patient is placed for surgery is determined by the particular operation to be performed. For urologic operative procedures, the patient may be placed in the lateral, supine, prone, or lithotomy position. Any of these positions may be exaggerated to give optimum access to the organ involved, particularly in radical surgery of the prostate and bladder. Considerable care must be taken to ensure that the patient's position does not interfere with respiration or circulation.[6] It is essential to avoid displacement of the joints and undue tension on neurovascular bundles or ligaments.[17] A patient positioned laterally (flank position) for renal surgery has the spine extended for greater access to the retroperitoneal space. Padding and stabilized support with gel pads, pillows, sandbags, and straps should be available for precise anatomic positioning and safety (see Chapter 5). When an electrosurgi-

## SAMPLE PLAN OF CARE

**NURSING DIAGNOSIS**

**Anxiety**

**OUTCOME**

The patient will verbalize an acceptable anxiety level to the perioperative nurse.

**INTERVENTIONS**

- Provide an accepting and supportive environment.
- Use touch (as appropriate) to convey caring and support.
- Encourage expression of feelings.
- Promote feelings of self-worth.
- Provide comfort measures (warm blankets, pillow).
- Facilitate or assist patient in using personally effective coping strategies (relaxation, deep breathing, music, imagery).
- Maintain patient privacy.
- Encourage participation of patient and family in plan of care.

**NURSING DIAGNOSIS**

**Risk for Perioperative Positioning Injury**

**OUTCOME**

The patient will be free from injury related to the surgical position.

**INTERVENTIONS**

- Maintain proper body alignment.
- Assess range of motion and musculoskeletal, peripheral vascular, and cardiovascular status preoperatively.
- Pad all bony prominences.
- Avoid compression of vulnerable nerves and neurovascular bundles.
- Secure patient to operating room (OR) bed without friction or pressure.
- Provide support stockings or sequential compression devices (SCDs) as indicated.
- Initiate measures to warm patient and maintain normothermia.

**NURSING DIAGNOSIS**

**Risk for Impaired Urinary Elimination**

**OUTCOME**

The patient will demonstrate or regain a normal pattern of urinary elimination.

**INTERVENTIONS**

- Include catheter care and measures to facilitate voiding after catheter removal as part of preoperative patient and family education and discharge planning.
- Instruct patient in importance of any postoperative antibiotic or anticholinergic therapy.
- Follow aseptic technique during catheter insertion and connection to drainage device.
- Maintain closed urinary drainage system.
- Note amount, color, and character of urine; report abnormalities.
- Keep drainage tubing and collection device below the level of the patient's bladder.
- Keep urine draining freely; avoid kinks in tubing.
- Check patency of catheter after all position changes.
- Secure drainage tubing to patient to prevent pulling or retraction during transfer.
- Assess bladder for distention.
- Provide patient with information/referral on preventing recurrent urinary tract infection (UTI).

**NURSING DIAGNOSIS**

**Risk for Deficient Fluid Volume**

**OUTCOME**

The patient will maintain adequate fluid volume and electrolyte balance.

**INTERVENTIONS**

- Provide appropriate intravenous (IV) solutions, volumetric pumps, and fluid warmers.
- Monitor patency of all IV lines.
- Record volume of IV and irrigating fluids instilled.
- Monitor electrocardiogram (ECG), vital signs, and cardiopulmonary status as appropriate.
- Monitor blood loss and volume replacement.
- Monitor urinary output, and note color; report output less than 30 ml/hr and changes in color or clarity.
- Collaborate with anesthesia provider in monitoring serum electrolyte status.
- Monitor pH and specific gravity of urine as appropriate.

**NURSING DIAGNOSIS**

**Risk for Impaired Gas Exchange**

**OUTCOME**

Patient will maintain adequate oxygen supply and alveolar ventilation.

**INTERVENTIONS**

- Review breathing exercises and use of incentive spirometer with patient preoperatively.
- Position patient to provide maximum lung perfusion; have positioning devices available; check that these are clean and functioning properly.
- Assist anesthesia provider in applying cardiac monitor leads, blood pressure cuff, and pulse oximeter.
- Collaborate with anesthesia provider in monitoring ventilation or perfusion.
- Administer oxygen as required; assist with intubation and maintenance of airway during positioning.
- Assist with collection of arterial blood gases; report results promptly.

**NURSING DIAGNOSIS**

**Fear of Sexual Dysfunction**

**OUTCOME**

The patient will discuss fears and concerns regarding sexual function.

**INTERVENTIONS**

- Clarify patient's understanding of risks and benefits of surgical procedure.
- Provide an open, accepting environment for the patient to discus potentially embarrassing issues.
- Maintain patient privacy and dignity.
- Consider making a referral for patient to discuss options available to achieve sexual function postoperatively.

## PATIENT SAFETY

### Improving Teamwork to Reduce Errors

Publication of the 1999 Institute of Medicine report focused attention on medical errors and the critical importance of patient safety. Reducing errors, such as wrong-person, wrong-procedure or wrong-site surgery, requires, in part, human solutions, such as improving teamwork and communication in the OR team. Interdisciplinary teamwork is especially important in the so-called high-risk areas in hospitals, such as the OR. Perioperative nurses have long believed that a team approach to patient care reduces errors. Effective teamwork in perioperative patient care consists of knowledge, attitudes, and skills. Developing sustainable efforts to improve teamwork requires thoughtful application. Interventions focused on changing the behavior of team members must first take into account their attitudes. Subsequently, skills and knowledge are assessed, and a training program can be designed to improve teamwork. The benefits of improved teamwork are well exemplified in the time out process, which aims to enhance effectiveness, increase efficiency, and lower the possibility of error. Preoperative verification processes and the time out result in fewer errors because these processes are planned by each institution and standardized through use of the Universal Protocol of the Joint Commission. Each member of the OR team knows his or her own responsibilities as well as those of teammates; members look out for each other and note errors before they happen; and members trust one another's judgments and concerns. Teamwork during preoperative verification and the time out allows proper integration and execution of clinical activities, gives caregivers increased control over their work environment, and provides a safety net against error. As more is learned about improving safety and reducing risks, OR teams are adding elements to the time out, including the need to verify that alcohol-based prep solutions have not pooled and that they have completely dried before draping the patient.

Modified from Kaissi A and others: Measuring teamwork and patient safety attitudes of high-risk areas, *Nursing Economics* 21(5):211-218, 2003; Rajnish P and others: Fires in the operating room and intensive care unit: awareness is the key to protection, *Anesthesia & Analgesia* 102:172-174, 2006.

cal unit (ESU) is to be used, care must be taken that the patient does not contact metal parts of the OR bed.

In some procedures involving stones of the kidneys or ureters, intraoperative fluoroscopy may be required. When fluoroscopy (C-arm) is to be employed, the patient must be placed on an OR bed compatible with its use. Whenever possible, the patient should be protected from undue radiation exposure to the thyroid and chest areas by the use of small leaded shields. In urologic procedures it generally is not feasible to shield the reproductive organs.

***Aseptic Techniques and Safety Measures.*** Prevention of infection is an important nursing goal in the care of the genitourinary patient. It is, however, seldom possible to confirm freedom from infection intraoperatively or immediately postoperatively. Aseptic techniques must be carefully maintained and monitored. Skin preparation and draping procedures (see Chapter 3) vary, depending on the surgery to be performed and institutional protocols. Special care must be taken when cleansing the perineal area to avoid contamination from the rectum to the urethra.[20] Prepping solutions should be applied with downward strokes and the sponge discarded once it has contacted the inner vaginal or anal areas. Transurethral passage of instruments and catheters requires meticulous technique to prevent retrograde infections of the urinary tract, which account for close to 40% of all nosocomial infections.

Visualization of the bladder during transurethral procedures is often enhanced by darkening the room. Provision should be made for proper adjustments to lighting. ESUs and fiberoptic light systems are common adjuncts in urologic surgery. The staff must be familiar with the manufacturer's safety precautions and recommendations during their use.

***Use of Irrigating Fluids.*** When the bladder is entered, sterile distilled irrigating fluid is administered to distend it for effective visualization. Commercially prepared sterile irrigation solutions with appropriate closed administration sets are highly recommended. Such closed systems prevent the inherent risks of cross-contamination. Large volumes of irrigating solutions are frequently used, particularly during more extensive endoscopic procedures. When these solutions are at the room temperature of the OR, they are cold compared with the patient's internal body temperature and can cause hypothermia. Solution-warming units are available commercially and are a useful tool to help decrease this risk. The drawback to these units may be that the warmth delays clotting, thus increasing the risk of blood loss.

Commercially prepared sterile irrigation solutions are available in collapsible bags and rigid plastic containers, both of which have the same advantage: neither depends on air, and each may be hung in series, thus providing continuous irrigation without interruption. Air bubbles, a problem that distorts visibility during the procedure, are eliminated with these systems.

For simple observation cystoscopy, retrograde pyelography, and simple bladder tumor fulgurations, sterile distilled water may be used without complication. However, during transurethral resection of the prostate (TURP), venous sinuses may be opened and varying amounts of irrigant are invariably absorbed into the bloodstream. Studies indicate that the use of distilled water during TURP may result in hemolysis of erythrocytes and possible renal failure. Other important complications include dilutional hyponatremia and cardiac decompensation.

Therefore a clear, nonelectrolytic and isosmotic solution should be used. The most widely used urologic irrigating fluids are 3% sorbitol, an isomer of mannitol, and 1.5% glycine, an aminoacetic solution. In dilute solutions, sorbitol and glycine have many properties that make them particularly useful for irrigation during transurethral prostatectomy. At slightly hypotonic concentrations, they do not produce hemolysis. However, if too much intravasation occurs with glycine, an encephalitic state can result from the ammonia produced (Surgical Pharmacology). Because the solutions are nonelectrolytic, they do not cause dispersion of high-frequency cur-

## Agents Used in Urologic Surgery

| Category | Dose/Route | Purpose/Action | Adverse Reactions | Contraindications (C)/ Precautions (P) |
|---|---|---|---|---|
| **BULKING AGENTS** | | | | |
| 1. Contigen<br>2. Durasphere EXP | Transurethral, periurethral injection | Correct UH, ISD, SUI | 1. Swelling, urinary retention<br>2. Local tissue infarction/necrosis, vascular occlusion, embolus | **C:** 1. Sensitivity to bovine products; 1 and 2. Acute cystitis, urethritis, other genitourinary infection<br>**P:** Avoid injection into blood vessel |
| **IRRIGANTS** | | | | |
| 1. Glycine (monocarboxylic amino acid)<br>2. Sorbitol (nonelectrolytic isosmotic, hypotonic aminoacetic)<br>3. Water<br>4. NS | 1. 1.5%, 3-5 liters, intravesical<br>2. 3%, 3-5 liters, intravesical<br>3. Distilled, 3-5 liters, intravesical<br>4. 0.9%, 3-5 liters, intravesical | 1. No hemolysis or dispersion of electrocurrent<br>2. Isomer of mannitol, no hemolysis or dispersion of electrocurrent<br>3. Irrigant, lyse cancer cells<br>4. Physiologic irrigant | 1. Increased ammonia production, encephalitic reaction, biosynthesis of heme, blurred vision, CNS disturbances<br>2. None<br>3. Hyponatremia, hemolysis of erythrocytes<br>4. Hypernatremia | **C:** 1. Clozapine usage; 3. Avoid with TURP; 4. Not for use with electrosurgery<br>**P:** 1. Use with caution in diabetic patients; patients with liver disease, inhibitory neurotransmitter; 3. Intravasation can lead to dilutional hyponatremia, cardiac decompensation, and renal failure; 4. Disperses electrocurrent |
| **IONIC RADIOPAQUE CONTRAST AGENTS (HIGH OSMOLAR)** | | | | |
| 1. Conray-60<br>2. Hypaque-50<br>3. Renografin-60 | 30 ml half strength; intraurethral, intraureteral, intravesical, intrarenal | Retrograde pyelography, renal arteriography, retrograde cystourethrography | Asthmatic response, rash, lactic acidosis, anaphylaxis | **C:** Iodine-seafood allergy, severe renal disease, dehydration<br>**P:** Metformin usage |
| **NONIONIC RADIOPAQUE CONTRAST AGENTS (LOW OSMOLAR)** | | | | |
| 1. Omnipaque-300<br>2. Optiray-320 | 30 ml half strength; intraurethral, intraureteral, intravesical, intrarenal | Retrograde pyelography, renal arteriography, retrograde cystourethrography | Back pain, dizziness, headache, diarrhea | **C:** Anuria, pregnancy, dehydration, severe renal and/or hepatic disease, serum creatinine >3 mg/dl<br>**P:** Reduced clearance with renal disease, consider pretreatment with steroids; metformin usage |
| **STERILANT** | | | | |
| Glutaraldehyde (Cidex) | 14 or 28 days | Disinfectant | Inhalation hazard | **P:** Toxicity with inhalation of fumes, toxic to tissues when not rinsed from item properly |
| **INJECTABLES** | | | | |
| 1. Indigo carmine<br>2. Phenylephrine (Neo-Synephrine)<br>3. Papaverine<br>4. Vasopressin (Pitressin) | 1. 40 mg, IV or local<br>2. 0.05% (5 mg), subcutaneous<br>3. 30 mg/ml, 2 ml in solution, intercavernosal<br>4. 20 units/ml: 2 ml (40 units) in solution, local | 1. Colorize urine, vessels<br>2. Vasoconstriction for priapism<br>3. Vasodilation, antispasmodic<br>4. Vasoconstriction | 1. Bradycardia, hypertension<br>2. Hypertension, reflex bradycardia<br>3. Dizziness, dysrhythmia, hypotension, flushing, hypothermia<br>4. Water intoxication, dizziness, headache, pallor | **C:** 2. Hypertension; 3. AV block, pregnancy; 4. Uremia, coronary artery disease, hypertension<br>**P:** 1. Moderately reduces $Spo_2$; 2. Decreased renal blood flow; 3. Depressed AV or intraventricular conduction, physiologic antagonist; 4. Tenesmus, tremors, cramps, abdominal pain, hyponatremia, retards absorption of local anesthetics |
| **TOPICAL** | | | | |
| Methylene blue | 1 ml/100+ ml NS, topical | Colorize tissues, vessels | Hypertension, dizziness, headache, anemia, diaphoresis | **C:** Severe renal disease, hemolytic anemia<br>**P:** Destroys erythrocytes, methemoglobinuria |
| **OTHER** | | | | |
| B&O Supprette (belladonna/opium) | 16.2 mg/30 mg, rectal | Prevent/decrease bladder/ureteral spasm | Constipation, decreased sweating | **C:** Hemorrhage with cardiovascular instability, paralytic ileus, respiratory depression, toxin-mediated diarrhea, pseudomembranous enterocolitis<br>**P:** MAOs, agents that affect GI motility, select narcotics |

*AV,* Atrioventricular; *CNS,* central nervous system; *GI,* gastrointestinal; *ISD,* intrinsic sphincter dysfunction; *IV,* intravenous; *MAO,* monoamine oxidase; *NS,* normal saline; *$Spo_2$,* SUI, stress urinary incontinence; *TURP,* transurethral prostatectomy; *UH,* urethral hypermobility.

rent with consequent loss of electrosurgical cutting capacity, as occurs with normal saline.

During ureteropyeloscopy, sterile normal saline is the irrigant of choice unless electrosurgery is to be employed. This solution most closely approximates a physiologic solution—an important factor if perforation and extravasation of fluid into the retroperitoneum occur. If electrosurgery is required, as with a TURP, 3% sorbitol or 1.5% glycine should be used.

Thorough knowledge of the potential hazards encountered intraoperatively during transurethral surgery is extremely important. Although complications are more prevalent in the postoperative stage, close observation during the intraoperative period is essential. Signs and symptoms such as sudden restlessness, apprehension, irritability, confusion, nausea, slow pulse, seizures, dysrhythmias, and rising blood pressure may be suggestive of TURP syndrome, a severe hyponatremia caused by systemic absorption of irrigating fluid used during surgery.[6,11,25,41] Minimum amounts of fluids should be given and urine output carefully monitored. Irrigation fluid should be under as little pressure as possible and the bladder emptied before it reaches full capacity to prevent intravesical pressure. During ureteropyeloscopy it is frequently necessary to use a pressure bag to ensure adequate visualization of the upper urinary tract. Serum electrolyte values should be obtained, and if a low serum sodium value is reported, hypertonic sodium chloride is administered by means of a slow IV drip, often on a volumetric pump. IV diuretics such as furosemide (Lasix) may be required to prevent possible pulmonary edema associated with the administration of hypertonic saline. If the patient's reaction is severe, surgery may have to be terminated.

***Endoscopic and Ancillary Equipment.*** Cystoscopic and ancillary equipment often varies from one institution to another. Therefore it is valuable to have a reference manual or Kardex system that illustrates and describes in detail the required instrumentation for each specific procedure.

The basic cystoscopy tray should include instruments and accessory items that are routinely used for all cystoscopy procedures. If ureteral catheterization is planned, catheterizing telescopes or an Albarrán bridge, which can be packaged and sterilized separately, may be easily added to the basic cystoscopy setup. Instruments for transurethral surgery and other special procedures may be wrapped, sterilized, and placed on separate trays so that they are available on request. This concept minimizes handling of the delicate lensed instruments and ultimately reduces costly repairs.

Cystoscopic procedures frequently require additional instrumentation. Instruments of various types and sizes, such as a visual obturator, biopsy forceps, urethral sounds, Phillips filiforms and followers, and Ellik evacuators, are available as prepackaged, sterile, disposable items. The reusable products may also be packaged separately and sterilized.

***Urethral and Ureteral Catheters.*** A variety of urethral and ureteral catheters are designed for specific procedures. Ureteral catheters are manufactured of polyurethane material and are graduated so that the urologist may determine the exact distance the catheter has been inserted into the ureter (Figure 15-8, *A*). Most manufacturers provide sterile disposable catheters wrapped in peel-open packages to allow aseptic handling during ureteral insertion. Some indications for the use of ureteral catheters are to (1) perform retrograde pyelography, (2) identify the ureters during pelvic or intestinal surgery, and (3) bypass partial or complete obstruction that may be present as a result of ureteral tumors, calculi, or strictures. Not uncommonly it is necessary to insert a ureteral stent in a pregnant female because of hydronephrosis or obstructing calculi.

The most commonly used catheters include the open-ended, whistle tip, cone tip, and olive tip. When a retrograde ureterogram is indicated, a cone-tipped ureteral catheter may be helpful in occluding the ureteral orifice to accomplish the x-ray study effectively. When a ureteral catheter is left indwelling, a special adapter (Figure 15-8, *B*) may be connected to the end of the ureteral catheter to facilitate connection to a closed urinary drainage system. A small slit may also be created in the Foley catheter, and the distal end of the ureteral catheter can be slipped into it and taped in place.

Indwelling double-pigtail or double-J stents are available and are passed cystoscopically to reside within the ureter (Figure 15-9). When the guidewire is removed from the core of the stent, a proximal and distal J or "pigtail" forms in the tubing to retain the stents. Many of these stents have a nonabsorbable suture attached to the distal end, which extends through the urethral meatus. A suture may be easily tied to the distal end of those that do not. The surgeon can then remove the stent in the office setting postoperatively without needing to perform a cystoscopy.

Urethral catheters have a multitude of functions as stents, as drainage tubes, and in diagnostic studies in the OR. They are generally divided into two categories—plain and indwelling (retention)—and range in different French (Fr) sizes, most commonly 10 through 30. The Foley catheter is the most fre-

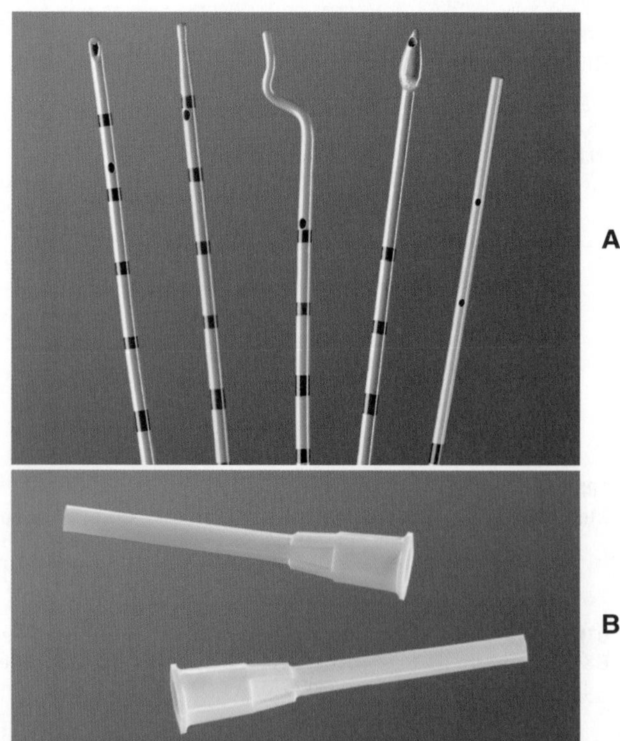


FIGURE 15-8 **A,** Ureteral catheters. **B,** Adapters.

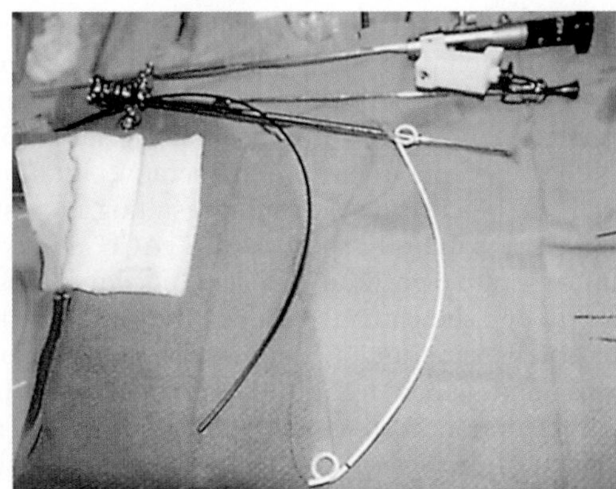

**FIGURE 15-9** Double-pigtail stent set.

quently used retention catheter and is manufactured with a variety of balloon sizes, tip styles, lengths, and eye arrangements.

After transurethral prostatic surgery, a three-way Foley catheter with a 30-ml balloon capacity may be left indwelling. This type of catheter is preferred because it facilitates continuous bladder irrigation (CBI), and the large balloon aids in achieving hemostasis in the prostatic bed. The urologist may apply light traction on the Foley catheter with a leg strap, adhesive catheter anchor, tape, or the FoleyGoalie (Figure 15-10). This traction causes pressure against the bladder neck and aids in hemostasis (Figure 15-11). The FoleyGoalie is designed to prevent traumatic catheter removal in men. It is a cylindric device of helically arranged fibers that fits over the catheter and penis, Velcros to the base of the penis, and tapes to the catheter (Figure 15-12). If force is applied to pull out the catheter, the device tightens around the penis and catheter holding it in position. When the force is released the FoleyGoalie loosens.

A hematuria catheter, a three-way Foley specifically for patients with excessive clot formation, is also available. This catheter is reinforced with a stretch spiral wire within the catheter lining that permits vigorous aspiration without fear of lumen collapse.

Diagnostic studies performed in the cystoscopy suite may require special catheters for specific studies. A Davis or Trattner triple-lumen double-balloon urethrographic catheter or any of a variety of urodynamic catheters may be used to diagnose lesions of the female urethra, such as urethral strictures, diverticula, and fistulas. To accomplish female urethrography, the catheter is inserted through the urethra into the bladder; the two balloons on the catheter are inflated, one in the bladder and one at the external urethral orifice, effectively isolating the urethra. Contrast medium is injected to visualize the entire urethra.

Another type of self-retaining catheter frequently used in the OR is a Pezzer, also known as a *mushroom* catheter (Figure 15-13, *A*). It may be straight or angulated with a large single channel and a preformed tip in the shape of a mushroom. The flexible mushroom tip helps keep the catheter in place. This catheter is used primarily for suprapubic bladder drainage, often for poor-risk patients who have uremia, neurogenic bladder syndrome, or possibly long-standing urinary retention. The catheter is inserted into the bladder through a midline or small transverse abdominal wall incision and secured to the

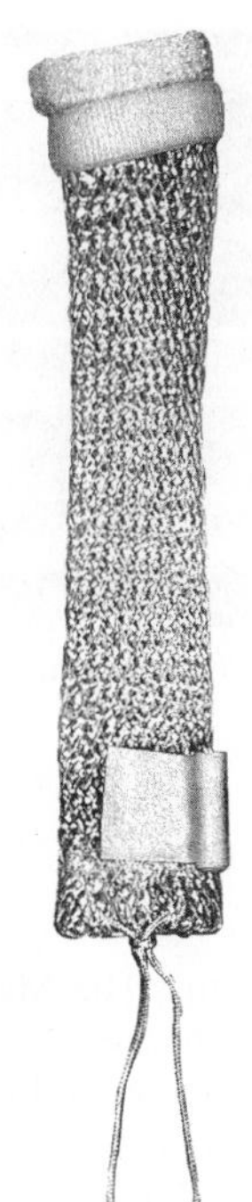

**FIGURE 15-10** FoleyGoalie.

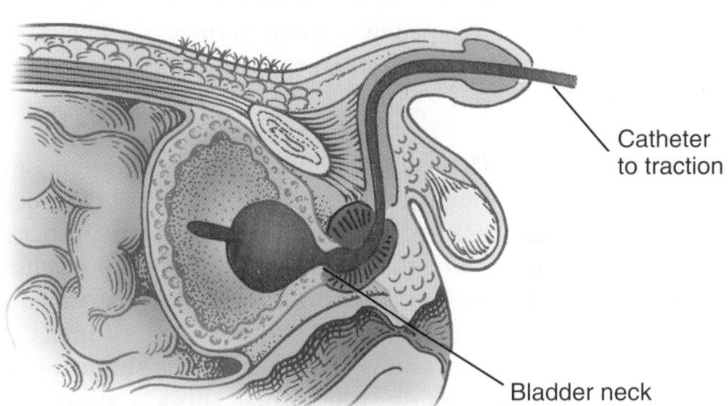


**FIGURE 15-11** Balloon of Foley catheter inflated to size that prevents catheter from being pulled into prostatic fossa.

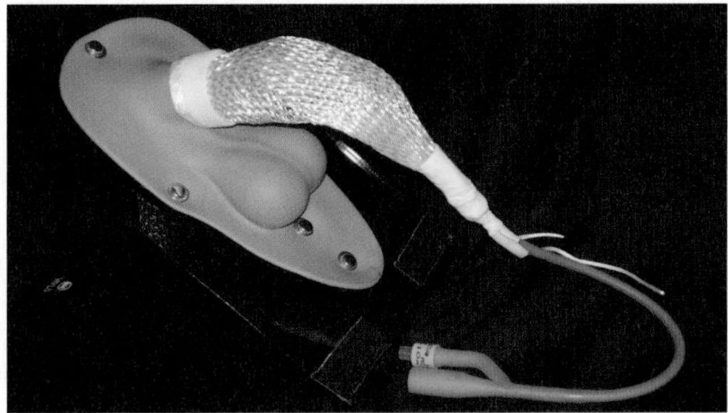

**FIGURE 15-12** Attaching FoleyGoalie to catheter and penis; Velcro at base of penis, drawstring and Velcro at distal end of device to allow tightening in place.

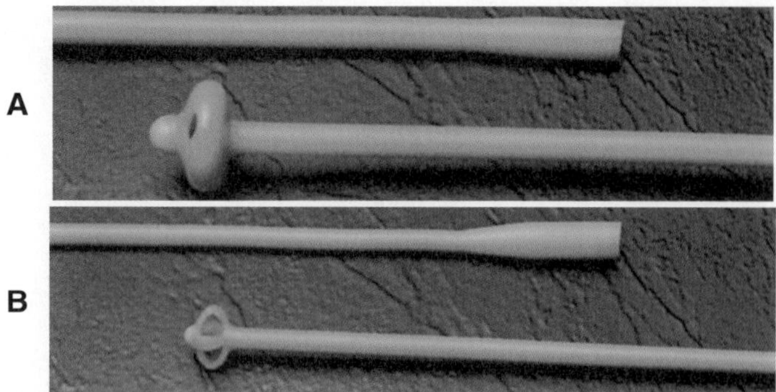


FIGURE 15-13 **A,** Pezzer (mushroom) catheter. **B,** Malecot (bat-winged) four-winged catheter.

abdomen with suture or tape. The Malecot four-winged catheter, often used as a nephrostomy tube to provide temporary or permanent diversion of urine after kidney surgery and when renal tissue needs to be restored, may also be used for suprapubic drainage (Figure 15-13, *B*). A Foley catheter of preferred size is frequently chosen for either purpose. Nephrostomy tube replacement is accomplished by introducing the catheter into the surgical tract with a straight catheter guide and securing it in place with a suture or a nephrostomy retention disk that is one size smaller than the nephrostomy tube being used. The flanges of the disk are taped or sutured to the skin. The use of other variations of urethral catheters is described throughout the chapter.

***Photography in Urology.*** The use of photographic and video imaging equipment in urologic surgery serves to document the patient's disease, the progress of a disease process, and long-term follow-up study. It is also an important teaching resource. Video equipment adapts to endoscopic instrumentation and has the capability of projecting an enhanced image on a television monitor, permitting members of the surgical team to observe and learn during the actual surgical procedure. Other visual aids, such as slides and photographs, are used in teaching, as visual references in publication, and as documentation in patient records.

When any form of photography or video imaging is used, the patient's privacy must be ensured and an informed consent should be obtained. Special release forms should also be signed preoperatively by the patient for any videotapes or photographs to be used in teaching or publications.

## Evaluation

Before the patient is taken to the postanesthesia care unit (PACU) or observation unit, his or her general condition is evaluated. The skin is assessed, and bony prominences, prepped and draped areas, and areas contacted by the attachment of ancillary equipment are observed for signs of pressure, irritation, or other changes from the preoperative status. Ancillary attachments include but are not limited to the ESU dispersive pad and ECG lead pads. Because many urology patients are nutritionally deficient and consequently have friable tissue, the trend has been to minimize the use of tape and to coat the skin with a protective sealant before the use of tapes.

Many urology patients are discharged to the PACU with drains inserted, including urethral, ureteral, suprapubic, and wound drains. Local anesthesia may have been used for either primary analgesia or postoperative pain management (preemptive analgesia); preoperative or intraoperative infiltration of the surgical site blocks sensory input, resulting in postoperative analgesia. A hand-off report to the PACU nurse should include intraoperative position, problems encountered specific to the patient, and the patient's preoperative physical status as well as comprehension and anxiety levels. Documentation of medications administered from the sterile field or by the perioperative nurse intraoperatively should include time of administration, medication, dosage, site and route of administration, and who performed the application or injection. Drains should be documented as to size and type, insertion site, time and date of insertion, type of collection device, who performed the insertion, and character of drainage. When several drains are in place, additional labeling on the collection devices is beneficial. Any postoperative observations before or during transport should be recorded. Evaluation should also address whether the patient met the identified outcomes related to specific nursing diagnoses in the perioperative nursing plan of care.[41] Attainment of identified desired outcomes, included in the documentation and report to the PACU, may be phrased as follows[47,59]:

- The patient verbalized an acceptable anxiety level to the perioperative nurse.
- The patient had no evidence of positional injury; neurovascular status was consistent with preoperative level, and skin integrity was intact.
- The patient maintained patency of the urinary catheter with no signs of blockage or retention. Urinary output remained within normal limits. The patient should void without difficulty after catheter removal.
- The patient had no evidence or signs of fluid volume or electrolyte imbalance; vital signs were stable, arterial blood gases were within normal limits, and urinary output was maintained at acceptable levels.
- The patient maintained adequate gas exchange; lung expansion and $O_2$ saturation were satisfactory.
- The patient discussed fears and concerns regarding sexual function.

## Patient and Family Education and Discharge Planning

Patient and family education and preparation for discharge allow perioperative nurses to plan for the urologic surgery patient's care across a continuum. General guidelines for preoperative education are presented in Box 15-1. Information provided should be presented in language the patient can understand (lay terms) and clarified with the patient by having the patient repeat back in his or her own words information provided. When possible and with the patient's approval, family members or others who will serve as caregivers should be included in the educational process at the outset. Institutions may find it helpful to inventory the patient education materials available for select surgical procedures. An example of patient education for home care after nephrectomy is presented in the Patient and Family Education box.

Discharge instructions should be printed and include community resources and support groups as appropriate for the

BOX 15-1

## Teaching: Preoperative

**DEFINITION**

Assisting a patient to understand and mentally prepare for surgery and the postoperative recovery period

**ACTIVITIES**

1. Inform the patient and family/significant others of the scheduled date, time, location of surgery, and how long the surgery is expected to last.
2. Determine the patient's previous surgical experiences and level of knowledge related to surgery.
3. Appraise the patient's level of anxiety relating to surgery; determine what the patient considers an acceptable anxiety level.
4. Provide time for the patient to ask questions and discuss concerns.
5. Describe the preoperative routines (e.g., anesthesia, diet, bowel preparation, tests/labs, voiding, skin preparation, IV therapy, clothing, family waiting area, transportation to operating room), as appropriate.
6. Describe any preoperative medications, the effects these will have on the patient, the rationale for using them, and when they will be administered.
7. Inform the family/significant others of the location of the surgical waiting area.
8. Provide information on what will be heard, smelled, seen, tasted, or felt during the preoperative and intraoperative phases of care.
9. Discuss pain management strategies and the use of pain rating scales.
10. Explain the purpose of frequent postoperative assessments.
11. Describe postoperative routines/equipment (e.g., medications, respiratory treatments, tubes, machines, support hose, surgical dressings, ambulation, diet, family visitation), and explain their purpose.
12. Reinforce information provided by other health care members as appropriate.
13. Determine the patient's expectations of the surgery.
14. Correct unrealistic expectations of the surgery as appropriate.
15. Instruct the patient to use coping techniques directed at controlling specific aspects of the experience (e.g., relaxation, imagery) as appropriate.
16. Include the family/significant others as appropriate.

Modified from Johnson M and others: *NANDA, NOC and NIC linkages*, ed 2, St Louis, 2006, Mosby.

PATIENT AND FAMILY EDUCATION

## Home Care Education for the Nephrectomy Patient

Give the patient and the caregiver both verbal and written instructions. Provide them with the name and telephone number of a physician or nurse to call if questions arise. At the end of reviewing home care instructions, have the patient or family member repeat back, in his or her own words, information provided.

**GENERAL INFORMATION**

- Review the purpose and explain the type of procedure performed: partial or total nephrectomy.

**WOUND/INCISION CARE**

- Instruct the patient on caring for the incision and changing the dressing:
  - Wash hands.
  - Inspect the incision for signs of infection.
  - Cleanse the area with an antiseptic agent.
  - If there is no evidence of drainage, leave the site open to the air. Otherwise, cover the incision with sterile gauze squares held in place with tape.
- Teach the patient how to care for the nephrostomy tube, if present.

**SPECIAL INSTRUCTIONS**

- Inform the patient that showering and bathing may be resumed as recommended by the physician.
- Explain how to measure urine output as indicated.

**WARNING SIGNS**

- Review the signs and symptoms that should be reported to a physician or nurse:
- Infection: incision red, warm to touch, painful, with increased or purulent drainage (define)
- Urinary tract infection: fever, chills, hematuria ("blood in urine"), flank pain, sudden increase in urinary output

**ACTIVITY**

- Discuss the need to exercise to tolerance and to plan frequent rest periods. Explain that fatigue is common.
- Encourage the patient to discuss allowances and limitations with respect to occupation, recreation, and activities.
- Tell the patient to avoid heavy lifting (>10 lb) for at least 6 weeks.
- Advise the patient to avoid contact sports (e.g., wrestling, football) that could endanger the remaining kidney.

**DIET**

- Inform the patient that a regular diet can be followed unless there are restrictions related to the underlying reason for nephrectomy.
- Encourage the patient to drink 8 to 10 glasses of fluids per day unless restrictions of the underlying disease apply. Half of these should be fruit juices (to maintain electrolyte balance).

**FOLLOW-UP CARE**

- Stress the importance of regular follow-up visits. Make sure the patient has the necessary names and telephone numbers.

Modified from Canobbio MM: *Mosby's handbook of patient teaching*, ed 3, St Louis, 2006, Mosby.

surgical intervention and the patient's diagnosis. These too should be presented in easily understood terms, reviewed, and confirmed by having the patient repeat back in his or her own words information provided. Any requisite skills that the patient or family will be responsible for should be demonstrated, with return demonstrations as time permits. Perioperative nurses may find it helpful to involve institutional resource persons or departments such as the social services department in developing information related to home care services, durable medical equipment, and transfers to aftercare facilities other than home (skilled nursing center, rehabilitation facility, other long-term care facility). Patients and their families need preparation for mastering information and tasks that need to be performed. The goal of such interdisciplinary discharge planning is to provide information for the patient that is comprehensive and easy to use. This is part of perioperative nursing's ethical and professional responsibility to patients; it also meets the JCAHO requirements of providing consistent patient and family education (see Chapter 10).

# *Surgical Interventions*

## INTERVENTIONAL URORADIOLOGY

Many procedures that were once reserved for the OR are now being performed in the radiology department by specialists in uroradiology. As technology advances, procedures performed in the radiology department become a more common event. Those procedures include but are not limited to cystoscopy with stent placement, IV urogram, retrograde pyelogram, percutaneous antegrade stent placement and nephroscopic radiography, and ultrasound procedures with percutaneous access. The latter may be done to drain an abscess, place a catheter or stent, or simply to introduce contrast material for direct fluoroscopic examination. Renal artery hypertension and stenosis may be treated successfully through new and advanced uroradiology methods, such as percutaneously placing stents in stenotic renal arteries (Figure 15-14).[24,56]

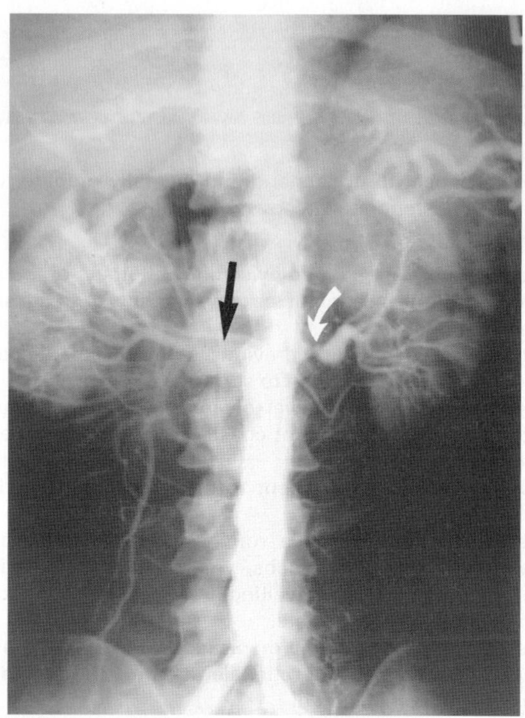

**FIGURE 15-14** Bilateral renal artery stenosis. Severe stenosis of the right renal artery *(straight arrow)* is difficult to see because the artery overlies the vertebral body. The left renal artery stenosis is easier to identify *(curved arrow)*.

## DIAGNOSTIC AND ENDOSCOPIC PROCEDURES

### Cystoscopy

Cystoscopy is an endoscopic examination of the lower urinary tract, including visual inspection of the interior of the urethra, the bladder, and the ureteral orifices. In a male patient, special attention is given to the examination of the verumontanum (which contains the ejaculatory duct), the bladder neck, and the median and lateral lobes of the prostate. In a female patient, the urethra, bladder neck, and bladder are examined.

Cystoscopy is an important diagnostic tool that provides the urologist with valuable information concerning the patient's urologic condition (History box). Indications for cystoscopy include hematuria, urinary retention, urinary tract infection, cystitis, tumors, fistulas, vesical calculus disease, and urinary incontinence. Urinary incontinence in postmenopausal women may be related to estrogen deprivation.

***Procedural Considerations.*** Once in the OR, before entering the cystoscopy suite, all patients should be greeted by name and identified by their identification bracelet and number. The perioperative nurse should check the chart for operative consent and pertinent laboratory reports; IVPs and any other diagnostic x-ray studies ordered preoperatively should also be available for review. Customarily, the patient voids immediately before transport to the OR. The time of urination and the output volume should be documented for ruling out residual urine in the bladder.

After the patient is placed on the cystoscopy bed, correct positioning requires optimum relaxation of muscles of the legs and perineum. Proper positioning is a vital consideration for patient safety and comfort. Allen and Yellow Fin stirrups are boot-style stirrups that support the foot and calf. These have thick gel padding within the stirrup and provide optimum patient comfort and protection, relieving pressure on the popliteal space. They are especially beneficial for the patient who has limited hip mobility and altered peripheral circulatory status. Bilateral pedal pulses should be assessed preoperatively and postoperatively when using any stirrups. Stirrups should be adjusted carefully to avoid undue pressure on the calf. If knee crutches are employed, the curve of the yoke suspension should flow outward from the perineum, as the patient's legs do. Padding the knee crutches reduces pressure on the popliteal areas. If sling stirrups that support only the feet are employed, the post should be padded and positioned to prevent pressure on the peroneal nerve. Special pads are designed for use with both of these stirrups. Arms should be supinated and extended on bilateral padded armboards at no more than a 90-degree angle. If hands are tucked, care must be taken to prevent injury to the fingers (see Chapter 5).

After the patient is properly positioned, the bed may be tilted so that the patient's head is slightly higher than the buttocks to allow the prep solution to drain into the collecting pan.

## HISTORY

### How Cystoscopy Began

The blueprint for all other endoscopes is the cystoscope. In 1805 Philip Bozzini of Germany lit the way with his *Lichtleiter*, a primitive prototype of what we now know as the cystoscope. In 1872 British scientist John Tindell established the principle of internal light reflection inside glass rods. Then in 1877, Maximilian Nitze (the father of the cystoscope), in collaboration with Austrian manufacturer Joseph Leiter, turned Bozzini's prototype into the first direct-vision *kystoskop* for viewing the interior of the bladder, urethra, and larynx. This consisted of an incandescent platinum wire loop that fluoresced the bladder from the inside while magnifying the image externally through a system of lenses.

American physicians, in the meantime, worked with a German immigrant named Reinhold Wappler, who by the 1900s became known as a superior endoscope innovator. Endoscopic devices finally began to gain widespread popularity when Thomas A. Edison developed the incandescent lamp. Through miniaturization a low-amperage mignon bulb was created from his lamp, allowing for simple, manageable, and low-cost cystoscopes to be produced.

Heinrich Lamm of Germany confirmed in 1930 that optical fibers could transmit images. But it was not until the mid-1950s that fiberoptics entered the scene, replacing these mignon bulbs with glass-fiber bundles. In 1954, fiberoptics became practical when British physicist Harold H. Hopkins produced the first usable system. A suggestion by a Dutch optics professor, Abraham van Heel, to coat the optic fibers with a transparent sheath led to unlocking the key to continuous illumination. This coating protected the fibers and prevented light from "leaking" out.

The contributions of Hopkins and van Heel became the inspirations behind the first fiberoptic gastroscope in 1957 and the first ureteroscope in 1960. Also in 1960, Hopkins introduced a refinement of his original technology, the "rod lens" rigid endoscope. This was created by combining air with long ground-up pieces of glass into an optical surface. In 1967 this method was applied to the cystoscope, thus replacing the previous prisms, mirrors, and lenses.

The 1980s brought the marriage of fibers and lenses into co-axial fiberoptic bundles through which one package of strands carried light and another returned images. These allowed increased flexibility and maneuverability without image distortion. Today endoscopy is so refined that visualization and treatment are achieved with flexible pencil-size tipped cystoscopes, ureteroscopes, and laparoscopes working through spearlike channeled sheaths and trocars.

Modified from Engel RM: Philipp Bozzini—the father of endoscopy, *Journal of Endourology* 17(10):859-862; Oct. 2003; Wm. P. Didusch Center for Urologic History of the American Urological Association, Linthicum, Md. Accessed February 3, 2006, on-line: www.auanet.org/museum/content/collections/scopeurology/cystoscopes.cfm.

Pooling of solutions beneath the patient may cause skin reaction and chemical irritation, as well as the potential for burns if an ESU is used. If the cystoscopic procedure requires the use of an ESU, the dispersive pad is placed on the patient in direct contact with the skin as close to the operative site as practical and accessible to the circulating nurse; the pad is usually placed on the upper thigh. When placing the ESU pad, it is important to avoid hairy areas, bony prominences, scar tissue, and proximity to prosthetic metal implants or pacemakers.

After properly positioning the patient, the nurse or urologist dons gloves and preps the entire pubic area, including the scrotum and perineum, with an antimicrobial solution. A disposable drape sheet with a sterile screen material incorporated into it is a standard part of the cystoscopy drape pack. The patient is draped to ensure that aseptic technique is maintained during the urologic procedure. If a general or spinal anesthetic is required, it is administered before prepping and draping. If a local anesthetic is preferred, it is instilled into the urethra of the male patient after prepping and draping but before instrumentation. For a female patient, a cotton applicator that has been dipped into the anesthetic solution is placed in the urethral meatus. Usually, viscous lidocaine (Xylocaine), 1% or 2%, is used. If the patient is allergic to lidocaine, instillation of 50 to 60 ml of lubricant accompanied by anesthesia-monitored sedation is often adequate to afford painless access to the urethra and bladder. The patient should be informed that a sensation of pressure is to be expected.

The basic cystoscopy setup requires a cystoscopy pack, a sterile gown or apron, sterile gloves, a fiberoptic light source, a prep cup and solution, gauze sponges, the cystourethroscope (Figure 15-15), a short bridge and fiberoptic light cord, lateral and Foroblique telescopes, a Luer-Lok stop cock, irrigation tubing and sterile water irrigant, and water-soluble lubricant. Additional items that should be sterile and available include a calibrated container to measure residual urine, test tubes with screw tops for urine specimens, an Albarrán bridge and rubber catheter nipples or adapters, a medicine glass for dye, anesthetic solution, disposable 10-ml and 20-ml syringes, medication labels and a marking pen, a penile clamp (to occlude male urethra after local anesthetic is instilled), contrast material, an ESU, a patient dispersive pad, and a Bugbee electrode.

The flexible cystoscope (Figure 15-16) is used for patients with obstructive symptoms resulting from prostatic hyperplasia and rigid prostatic urethra. In addition, the flexible cystoscope can be used for patients who cannot assume a lithotomy position, such as those with spinal cord injuries or severe arthritis. Flexible cystoscopy may be accomplished with the use of a local anesthetic. It affords the patient a higher degree of

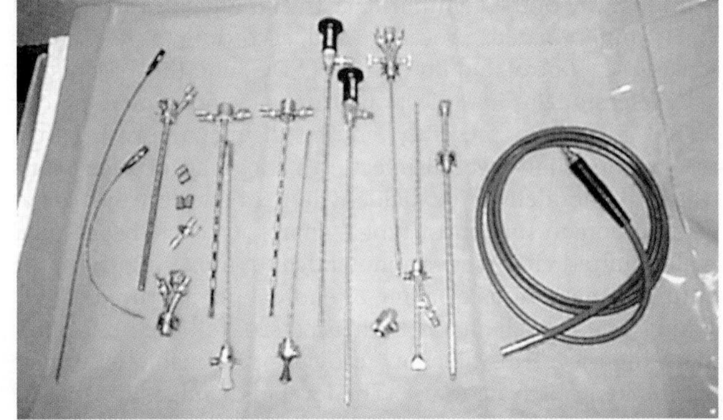

**FIGURE 15-15** Basic instruments for cystoscopy, catheterization, cauterization, and retrograde ureteral pyelography (add ureteral catheter of choice). *Left to right,* Bugbee electrodes, single-horn Albarrán deflecting bridge, nipple adapters, stop cock, short double-horn bridge, 23-Fr and 17-Fr Foroblique cystourethroscopes and sheaths, 30-degree and 70-degree telescopes, double-horn Albarrán deflecting bridge, single-horn examining bridge, visual obturator, and fiberoptic cable.

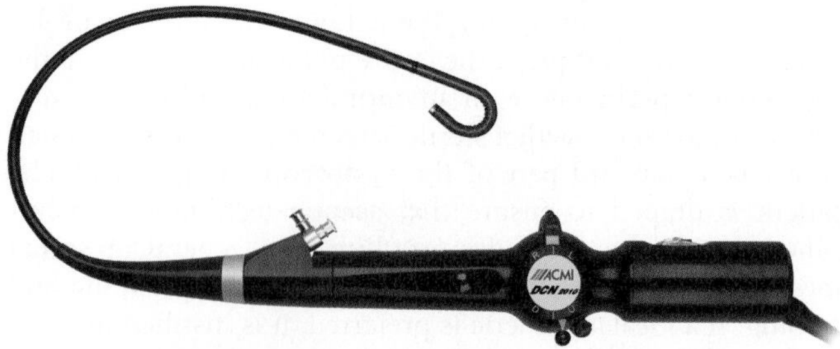


FIGURE 15-16 Flexible cystoscope.

comfort, is less traumatic to the urethra, and can be performed in the patient's bed on the nursing unit.

Cleaning, sterilization, disinfection, and maintenance of endoscopic equipment are important procedures in the care of fiberoptic lensed instruments. Ultimately this process reduces costly repairs and ensures the availability of properly functioning instruments.

Protective padding should be placed on the countertop and on the bottom of the sink in the instrument decontamination area to prevent possible damage to lensed telescopes. After each surgical procedure, components of each cystoscopic set should be disassembled and washed in a solution of warm water and germicidal detergent with enzymatic action (breaks down proteins). All stop cocks and sheaths should be cleaned thoroughly with a soft brush to remove blood, dried lubricant jelly, or other debris. Instruments should then be thoroughly rinsed in warm water, placed on protective padding, and allowed to dry. Although warm water is appropriate for washing the instrumentation, lensed instruments should not be allowed to soak in warm water for too long. Lengthy soaking can cause the seals to loosen, which allows water to leak into the scope and results in cloudiness and bubbles. All moving parts must be individually evaluated for mobility. A lubricating, instrument milk solution may be applied as required. The patency of all outlets must be maintained to ensure proper sterilization or disinfection. Fiberoptic light cords must not be tangled, twisted, or sharply angulated because the fibers inside the cord are easily broken.

Endoscopy of the genitourinary tract is considered a class II (clean-contaminated) procedure and, according to the Centers for Disease Control and Prevention (CDC) and the Association for Professionals in Infection Control and Epidemiology (APIC) guidelines, presently requires disinfection rather than sterilization. High-level disinfection with an agent such as activated glutaraldehyde or dialdehyde that can destroy vegetative microorganisms, most fungal spores, tubercle bacilli, and small nonlipid viruses is recommended. In most situations, the routine of meticulous cleaning of endoscopic instruments and making sure that all channels are accessed, followed by appropriate high-level disinfection, provides reasonable assurance that the items are safe to use. The level of disinfection is based on the contact time, temperature, and concentration of the active ingredients of the disinfectant, as well as the nature of microbial contamination.

Many institutions are, however, treating endoscopic interventions as sterile procedures because the sterilization of instruments provides the greatest assurance that the risk of infections transmitted by contaminated instruments has been eliminated (see Chapter 3). Some options available include glutaraldehyde (Cidex) solution, hydrogen peroxide solution (Sporox), an automated peracetic acid unit (Steris), an ETO (ethylene oxide, "gas") sterilizer, a hydrogen peroxide and plasma sterilizing unit (Sterrad), and high-vacuum or gravity steam autoclaving for those components that may be sterilized in this manner. The manufacturer's recommendations should always be followed. If soaking is chosen the lid should remain on the soaking container when not in use; masks should be worn when in direct contact with the fumes. It is also imperative that the instrumentation be thoroughly rinsed in sterile distilled water after removal from soaking solution and before use. Cidex residue remaining in the channels or on the lens can result in chemical burns for the patient and the surgeon (see Surgical Pharmacology box). For sterilization or disinfection, instruments should be assembled on a covered tray and protected with padding. Because the lens system is delicate and costly, a plastic covering available from some manufacturers may be used to protect the lens. Various instrument manufacturers provide sterilization containers for endoscopy equipment and have written recommendations for the cleaning, sterilization, and disinfection of their equipment.

Stone removal, bladder biopsy, and bladder fulguration may be accomplished by using special cystoscopic accessories, such as the Hendrickson-Bigelow lithotrite, which crushes large bladder calculi. This procedure is called a *litholapaxy.* Lowsley forceps, Wappler rigid cup forceps, and flexible foreign body forceps may also be employed. Bladder fulguration requires the use of flexible-stem electrodes available in various French sizes and tip configurations such as the ball, cone, dome, and bayonet.

### Operative Procedure

1. After the urologist has scrubbed, gowned, and gloved, the fiberoptic light cord is connected to the light source and tested for proper intensity.
2. The irrigating system is set up, and if required, the high-frequency cord is connected to an electrosurgical unit.
3. The cystourethroscope is lubricated and introduced into the urethra, the obturator is withdrawn, and the bladder is drained. Residual urine may be measured at this time if the patient voided before the examination. The specimen may be saved for cultures or cytologic studies.
4. The cystourethroscope is connected to the irrigating system, and the telescope is inserted and locked in place. If the patient is awake, telling him or her to try to urinate also helps facilitate passage of the scope. The urologist controls the rate of flow and volume of fluid by adjusting the stop cock on the scope. If difficulty is encountered during insertion, the visual obturator may be used to introduce the scope under direct vision. This accessory is constructed to smooth the fenestrated edges of the cystourethroscope. It requires the use of the telescope for direct vision and permits irrigation during introduction.
5. For retrograde ureteral catheterization and pyelography, ureteral catheters are passed through the cystoscope sheath and directed by the Albarrán bridge deflector through the ureteral orifice and into the ureter. A radiopaque substance (e.g., nonionic, low-osmolar agents Omnipaque-300 and Optiray-320, or ionic high-osmolar Renografin-60 and Hypaque-50) is injected (see Surgical Pharmacology box). Fluoroscopic imaging is used to outline the entire upper urinary collecting system.

## Periurethral-Transurethral Injection of Bulking Agents

Collagen injection is an ambulatory surgery procedure achievable with the patient under local anesthesia with or without sedation. Collagen (Contigen) is a live bovine dermal natural protein and is prepackaged in a sterile syringe containing the collagen material. Injection needles available are an 8-inch, 23-gauge, noncoring needle for transurethral use or a 5-inch, 22-gauge needle for periurethral insertion. Female patients with intrinsic sphincter deficiency (ISD) demonstrated by urodynamic evaluation and male patients (usually after prostatectomy) with incontinence lasting more than 1 year may benefit from this procedure. Other indications for collagen injection include urethral hypermobility (UH), stress urinary incontinence (SUI) secondary to previous stricture treatment, trauma, or myelodysplasia.[13, 43]

Durasphere is a bulking product consisting of pyrolytic, carbon-coated beads within a water-based viscous medium.[8] Needles for instillation include a 1.5-inch spinal-tip subcutaneous needle and a 15-inch spinal-tip transurethral needle. It is designed to treat women with SUI secondary to documented ISD. Durasphere is not absorbed as readily as collagen and may provide a more durable effect. Men have been successfully treated with Durasphere, but this indication has not yet received U.S. Food and Drug Administration (FDA) approval.

***Procedural Considerations.*** Collagen must be kept under refrigeration and the FDA guidelines for its use and documentation followed. Durasphere requires no refrigeration. Patients selected for collagen injection must be skin-tested with collagen 1 month before periurethral injection. The patient receiving Durasphere does not require skin testing. A urine culture and sensitivity will be done approximately 10 days preoperatively. It is optimal to use a video system for the procedure. A basic cystoscopy set is required. The patient will usually be in lithotomy position.

### *Operative Procedure*

1. Urethral anesthetic is instilled, and a perineal block of 1% or 2% lidocaine may be injected. Cystoscopic examination is performed before the bulking agent is injected to rule out any associated findings. It is recommended that the irrigation be instilled by use of a pressure bag to minimize extravasation of the material by increasing the intraurethral pressure.
2. The injection needle provided by the manufacturer is introduced through the cystoscope and the tip placed transurethrally, below the urethral mucosa, just distal to the bladder neck. In the female the shorter needle may also be employed for periurethral introduction. Positioning of the needle tip is accomplished when the surgeon sees the indentation of the urethra by the tip while manipulating the needle.
3. The material is injected until the urothelium coapts in the midline, approximating the appearance of lateral lobe enlargement of the prostate. It may not be possible to achieve coaptation of the urothelium during the first injection; however, it may be possible to do so with subsequent injections, once the pockets established originally have congealed and become compact.

## Transurethral Ureteropyeloscopy

Transurethral ureteropyeloscopy is an endoscopic examination of the ureters and renal pelvis. The use of rigid or flexible ureteroscopes or ureteropyeloscopes provides the opportunity to diagnose filling defects in the ureter and renal pelvis, congenital anomalies (Figure 15-17), hematuria, ureteral obstruction, and damage from trauma. Manipulation, fragmentation, basketing of ureteral and renal calculi, and retrieval of foreign bodies are possible with transurethral ureteropyeloscopy. ESWL, electrohydraulic lithotripsy (EHL), sonic lithotripsy, or laser lithotripsy may accompany the procedure. It may also be used to manage residual sludge and *Steinstrasse* (German for "street of stones") after these treatments. ESWL and EHL are addressed in more detail on p. 541.

Ureteral strictures may be treated transurethrally, and biopsies of tumors of the ureter and renal pelvis are performed under direct visualization. Internal ureteral stents may also be inserted for ureteral patency. These range in size from 3 Fr to 8.5 Fr and are available in single-J, double-J, and pigtail configurations.

***Procedural Considerations.*** The setup is similar to that for a cystoscopy with the addition of a rigid or flexible ureteroscope system (Figure 15-18). A critical factor in this procedure is allowing enough time for careful dilation of the ureter under C-arm fluoroscopy. The flexible ureteroscope has gained popularity because of its inherent tip mobility, which provides a more panoramic view of the entire circumference of the ureter. The perioperative nurse must be prepared to tilt the radiolucent operative bed at head and foot and laterally, as well as raise the bed.

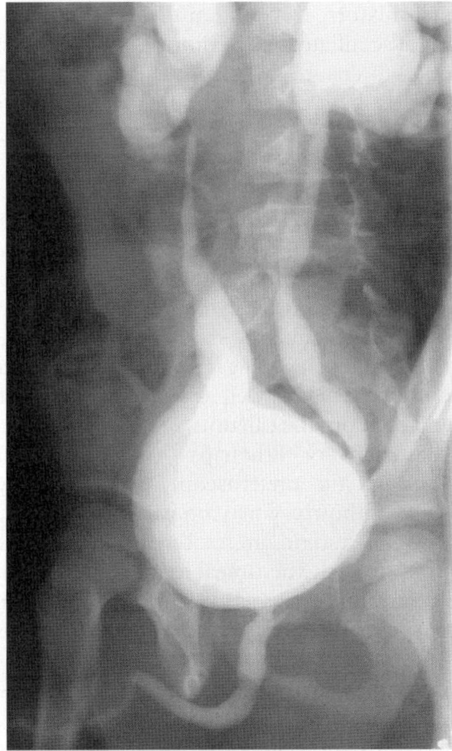

**FIGURE 15-17** Grade 5 bilateral ureteral reflux.

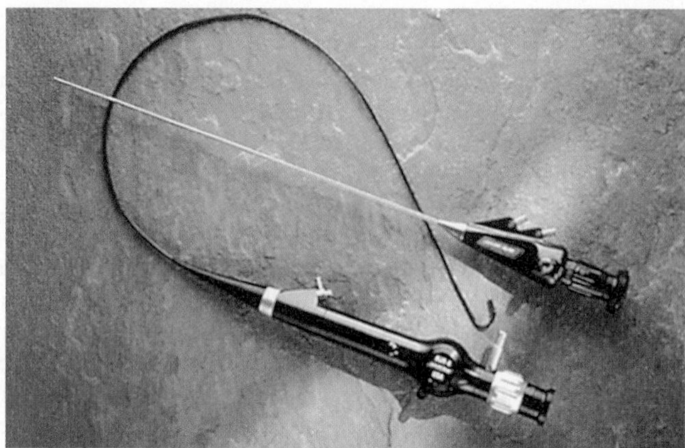

**FIGURE 15-18** Flexible ureteropyeloscope and rigid ureteropyeloscope.

In addition to the standard cystoscopy setup, the following items should be available: a rigid or flexible ureteroscope, ureteral dilators of graduated sizes and styles, size 3-Fr to 5-Fr ureteral stone baskets of various styles, a ureteral grasping forceps, biopsy forceps, snare, scissors, catheters of various styles and sizes, stents, guidewires, balloon dilators, and radiographic contrast material. Patient allergies should be checked before the use of radiographic contrast material.

#### *Operative Procedure*

1. Once the ureteropyeloscope has been inserted, access to the ureter is gained with a guidewire passed under fluoroscopic control. The ureter is irrigated as the guidewire is advanced. The assistance of a scrub person to hold the wire on slight tension will allow for a smoother course of operation.
2. The ureter is dilated to 10 Fr to 12 Fr with a balloon dilator or co-axial dilators. If a balloon dilator is chosen, the balloon should be inflated with contrast material, using a pressure syringe to ensure that it not exceed the maximum allowable atmosphere (ATM) pressure (burst pressure).
3. A working guidewire to be used as a safety wire is placed in addition to the initial guidewire.
4. The ureteroscope is passed over the working guidewire; and biopsy of suspicious lesions, diagnostic pyeloscopy, and ureteroscopy are performed. The characteristics of calculi are observed to determine the best treatment approach. Urine may be obtained for cytologic and microbiologic examination. If a calculus is small enough to be delivered through the ureter, it is engaged in a retrieval basket and removed under visual as well as fluoroscopic control. If, after ureteral dilation, the calculus does not appear to be small enough for delivery, lithotripsy (fragmentation) is performed through the ureteroscope, or ESWL may be performed later. Lithotripsy may be performed with the ultrasonic (through a rigid ureteroscope) or electrohydraulic lithotriptors or with the tuneable pulse-dyed or holmium: yttrium-aluminum-garnet (Ho:YAG) lasers. Appropriate laser precautions must be enforced. Chapter 7 discusses laser safety issues in more depth.
5. After the completion of the procedure, the ureter is assessed for integrity (perforation or laceration) with retrograde pyelography. A ureteral stent is placed over the remaining safety guidewire, and the guidewire is removed.

## SURGERY OF THE PENIS AND THE URETHRA

### Laser Ablation of Condylomas and Penile Carcinoma

Laser ablation of condylomas or penile cancer is the eradication of diseased tissue by means of a laser beam. Laser therapy has been determined to be effective for condylomas and penile cancers that are refractory to other treatments. One of the major advantages of the laser is that heat is distributed evenly to the tissue underlying the lesion. When any laser is being used, precautions appropriate to that system must be initiated (see Chapter 7).

***Procedural Considerations.*** Laser treatment may be performed successfully with local infiltration of an anesthetic. A U-shaped, craterlike lesion of predetermined depth with a 2-mm radius can be created. A power setting ranging from 2 to 20 watts (W) on continuous or super-pulse mode is commonly used. With laser ablation, less edema and necrosis occur, fibrosis is minimized, and rapid healing is facilitated. The argon, $CO_2$, potassium-titanyl-phosphate (KTP), and neodymium (Nd):YAG lasers are all suitable for this therapeutic application.

#### *Operative Procedure*

1. The operator moves the beam transversely across the tissue and then in a crosshatch matrix, thereby treating all perimeters of the lesion. Periodically the area should be wiped with a sponge moistened in acetic acid (5% vinegar). This treatment causes diseased tissue to stand out and allows therapy to deeper layers.
2. Postoperatively the affected areas may be coated with an antibiotic ointment. Wounds are generally left uncovered. A mild oral pain medication is usually adequate for postoperative discomfort.

### Circumcision

Circumcision is the excision of the foreskin (prepuce) of the glans penis. Circumcision in adult males is performed for the relief of phimosis, a condition in which the orifice of the prepuce is stenosed or too narrow to permit easy retraction behind the glans. Another condition that may require circumcision is balanoposthitis, an inflamed glans and mucous membrane with purulent discharge. Circumcision may also be done to prevent recurrent paraphimosis, a condition in which the prepuce cannot be reduced easily from a retracted position. (See Chapter 29 for pediatric considerations during circumcision.)

***Procedural Considerations.*** The patient is placed in the supine position. A plastic or minor instrument set and a local anesthetic with IV sedation is sufficient. The ESU should be available.

#### *Operative Procedure*

1. If the prepuce is adherent, a probe or hemostat may be used to break up adhesions. The prepuce is clamped in the dorsal midline and incised toward the coronal margin (Figure 15-19, A), leaving about 5 cm of coronal mucosa intact.
2. A similar procedure is performed ventrally. The two incisions are then joined circumferentially. Alternatively, a superficial circumferential incision is made in the skin with a

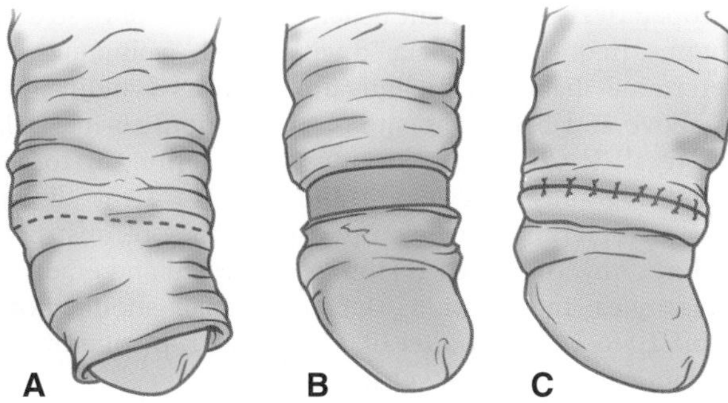

FIGURE 15-19 Circumcision.

scalpel at the level of the coronal sulcus and the mucosa at the base of the glans.
3. The redundant skin is undermined between the circumferential incisions and removed as a complete cuff (Figure 15-19, *B*).
4. Bleeding vessels are coagulated or clamped with mosquito hemostats and tied with fine absorbable ligatures.
5. Before closure, the area may be cleansed with an appropriate antiseptic solution.
6. The raw edges of the skin incision are approximated to a coronal cuff of mucosal prepuce, generally with 4-0 or 5-0 absorbable sutures on atraumatic, plastic cutting, or fine gastrointestinal (GI) needles (Figure 15-19, *C*).
7. The wound is usually dressed with petrolatum gauze.

## Excision of Urethral Caruncle

A urethral caruncle is a benign lesion or inflammatory prolapse of the external urinary meatus in the female. Excision entails the removal of these papillary or sessile tumors from the urethra.

***Procedural Considerations.*** The patient is placed in the lithotomy position. A minor or plastic set, an ESU, and a local anesthetic are used. A urethral catheter of an appropriate size may be required if the distal urethral prolapse is severe.

### *Operative Procedure*

1. With a small, fine-tipped Metzenbaum or plastic scissors, the tumor is exposed and excised within a wedge of ventral urethral tissue.
2. Figure-of-eight 4-0 absorbable sutures at the edge of the incision are usually sufficient to achieve good hemostasis.

## Urethral Meatotomy

Urethral meatotomy is an incisional enlargement of the external urethral meatus to relieve congenital or acquired stenosis or stricture at the external meatus.

***Procedural Considerations.*** A male patient is placed in the supine position. Prepping and draping are as described for urethral catheterization. For a female patient, the lithotomy position is used. Local anesthesia is generally employed. A plastic instrument set is required.

### *Operative Procedure*

1. A straight hemostat is placed on the ventral surface of the meatus.
2. An incision is made along the frenulum to enlarge the opening and overcome the stricture. Bleeding vessels are clamped and ligated with fine absorbable sutures.
3. The mucosal layer is sutured to the skin with fine absorbable sutures. A dressing of petrolatum gauze may be applied.

## Urethral Dilation and Internal Urethrotomy

Urethral dilation and internal urethrotomy entail the gradual dilation and lysis of a urethral stricture to provide relief of distal lower urinary tract obstruction. Urethral strictures or narrowing of the urethra may be caused by a congenital malformation that is usually found at the external urinary meatus. Infection or trauma may also contribute to stricture of the membranous and pendulous urethra. Urethral stricture disease may be treated by periodic dilation with Phillips filiforms and followers, Van Buren sounds, or balloon dilation catheters.

***Procedural Considerations.*** The male patient may be placed in a supine position for routine urethral dilation and in the lithotomy position for other procedures. Prepping and draping are as required for male catheterization. A local anesthetic such as viscous 2% lidocaine (Xylocaine) is used. The female patient is placed in the lithotomy position. Local anesthesia is achieved either (1) by placing cotton-tipped applicators, which have been dipped into the local anesthetic, into the urethral opening or (2) by using a urethral syringe to instill the local anesthetic. Female urethral dilation is performed with short, straight metal dilators or with hollow McCarthy dilators. The latter allow a urine specimen to be obtained.

In addition to a cystoscopy setup, required instrumentation includes urethrotomes (Figure 15-20), the resectoscope working element with sheath, obturator, and cold knives, urethral dilators, Phillips filiforms and followers, Van Buren sounds, and a silicone Foley catheter. Before use, the filiforms and followers should be carefully inspected for damaged or weak points, particularly around the scored-threaded end.

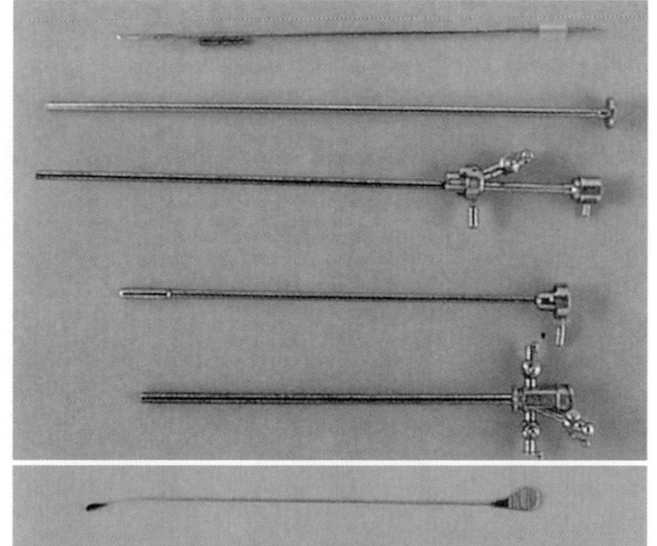

FIGURE 15-20 **A,** Optical internal urethrotome. **B,** Otis urethrotome.

### Operative Procedures

GRADUAL DILATION

1. In a male patient, the urethra is lubricated and anesthetized with a viscous anesthetic that is instilled into the urethra with a urethral or Uro-Jet syringe. A penile clamp occludes the penile urethra at the coronal sulcus and keeps the anesthetic within the urethra.
2. Phillips filiforms of various tips and sizes are introduced first in an attempt to pass an instrument beyond the urethral stricture. Followers of increasing size are connected to the filiforms and passed through the strictured portion of the urethra, stretching the scarred area (Figure 15-21, *A*).
3. Slow dilation is also achieved with a small catheter or follower left in the urethra. It leads to softening of the stricture over the course of several days.

INTERNAL URETHROTOMY

1. The assembled visualizing urethrotome is inserted under direct vision into the urethra.
2. When necessary, a filiform or ureteral catheter is fed into the catheterizing channel to help identify the patent portion of the urethra.
3. The urethrotome is advanced to the desired position, and the blade is used to incise the urethral scar. The normal urethra is incised 1 cm proximally and distally beyond the stricture to achieve optimum results.
4. A silicone Foley catheter is usually left in place for 3 to 5 days after surgery.

## Urethroplasty

Urethroplasty is reconstructive surgery of the urethra for strictures, urethral fractures, or narrowing of the urethral lumen that are congenital, inflammatory, or traumatic in origin. Urethral grafts are generally required and may include free skin grafts and mobilized vascular flaps. There are many combinations of these procedures, and in all of them some type of temporary urinary diversion may be used, depending on the location and severity of the condition.

Preoperatively, the patient usually complains of obstructive symptoms, frequently associated with a UTI. Techniques used to determine diagnosis include urodynamics (voiding pressures above and below the site of obstruction), urinary flow cytometry, IVU to rule out an upper tract lesion, cystoscopy, and urethrography. The length and density of the diseased urethra are determined to plan the appropriate reconstructive procedure. Any associated UTI must be treated and eradicated before surgical intervention. Definitive repair should not be done for 10 to 12 weeks after diagnostic instrumentation until the inflammatory reaction subsides.

***Procedural Considerations.*** The patient is placed in the exaggerated lithotomy position. Routine prepping and draping procedures are employed with precautions for isolating the anus (e.g., the use of an impervious plastic adherent drape). The setup includes a minor instrument set with fine plastic instruments for dissection and plastic repair. Strictures may be located deep, requiring fiberoptic lighting. An ESU may be required.

### Operative Procedures

JOHANSON URETHROPLASTY. The Johanson urethroplasty is a two-stage procedure to repair and reconstruct the urethra for severe urethral stricture disease. Approximately 3 months after the first stage, if the operative site is healing and the patient is voiding adequately, a second-stage procedure is performed. Vascularized flaps of preputial or penile skin may be mobilized to the ventrum by leaving them attached to the outer surface of the prepuce or as an island flap. One modification is the transverse preputial island flap neourethra with glans channel positioning for the meatus. Preputial skin is preferred because of its rich reliable blood supply and non–hair-bearing characteristics.

First Stage

1. An inverted U incision is made in the perineum from the inner borders of the ischial tuberosities up to and including the base of the scrotum.

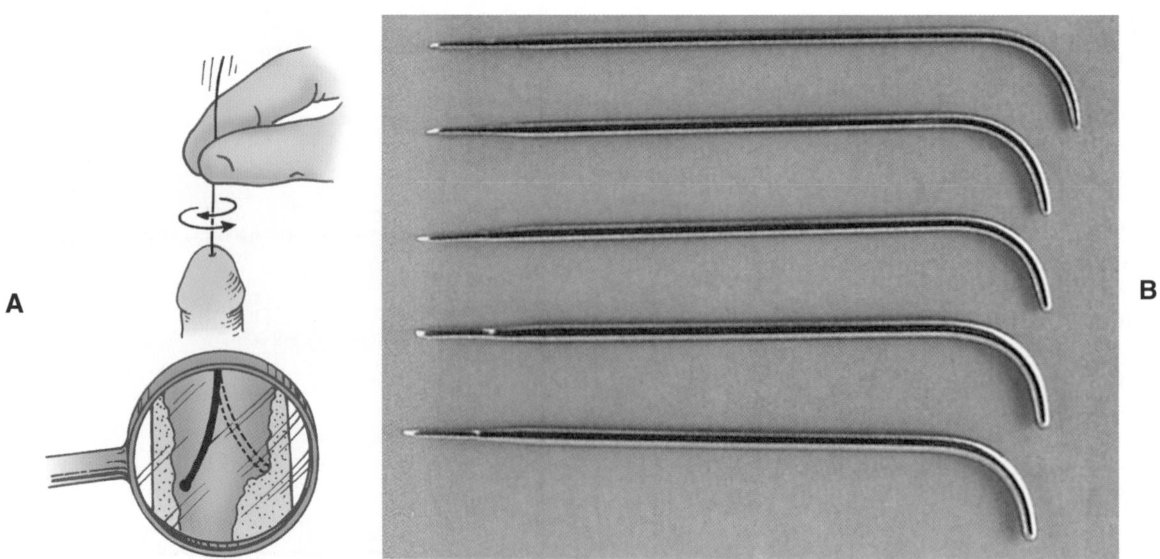


FIGURE 15-21 **A,** Method of using coudé-tipped bougie for passing stricture. **B,** Variety of urethral sounds (dilators).

2. A Van Buren sound is passed into the urethra up to the stricture (Figure 15-21, *B*). The bulbocavernosus muscle is dissected and retracted laterally.
3. An incision is made in the urethra over the strictured area and is extended in each direction at least 1 cm beyond the diseased area. The abnormal scar tissue is excised or simply incised, because scrotal skin ultimately increases the lumen.
4. A 28-Fr sound is passed through both the proximal and the distal urethral lumens to rule out further stricture.
5. The remaining urethral mucosa is sutured to the scrotal skin with 4-0 absorbable sutures.
6. A cystotomy tube to divert the urinary stream may be left indwelling and removed in 5 to 7 days.

**Second Stage (Mobilized Vascular Flap)**

1. A red rubber catheter is temporarily inserted into the bladder through the proximal urethral stoma.
2. The penoscrotal skin is incised longitudinally, adjacent to the urethra.
3. A new urethra is constructed by developing the ventral preputial skin that is dissected free and fanned out. The rectangle of skin is rolled into the neourethra and measured.
4. A channel is sharply created on the ventral aspect of the glans, in a plane just above the corpora.
5. The glans tissue is removed, forming a groove approximately 14 Fr in diameter.
6. Layers of subcutaneous tissue are dissected free from the dorsal penile skin to create an island flap that is spiraled to the ventrum. The flaps are brought together in the midline and closed with a continuous or interrupted 4-0 absorbable suture.
7. The neourethra is anastomosed proximally to the urethra and carried to the tip of the glans.
8. The dorsal penile flaps are transposed laterally to the midline, and excess skin is excised.
9. Closure is with 4-0 absorbable interrupted mattress sutures around the glans and down the penile shaft. A bulky pressure dressing is applied.
10. Suprapubic cystostomy drainage is an option, but a urethral catheter usually suffices.

HORTON-DEVINE URETHROPLASTY (URETHRAL PATCH GRAFT). Urethral patch graft is a one-stage operative procedure that incorporates a free skin graft to correct a urethral stricture. Free skin grafts should be at full thickness. Because the free graft must be revascularized, it is important that it have a perfect skin cover of well-vascularized dorsal, preputial, penile skin.

1. A 17-Fr panendoscope is passed into the posterior urethra, and a 20-Fr urethral dilator is passed into the posterior urethra.
2. A perineal vertical midline incision is made into the urethral lumen. The panendoscope is reinserted, and the incision is examined to determine if it crossed the stricture.
3. The defect is measured, and a circumferential incision is made on the posterior penile shaft to harvest an oval piece of skin the size of the defect.
4. The epidermal side of the graft is defatted, and 4-0 absorbable sutures are placed at the apex and base.
5. The apex is sutured into position at the proximal and distal ends of the stricture with the epidermal side toward the urethral lumen.
6. The graft is anastomosed proximally to the urethra with the suture line of the graft next to the corpus. The middle glans dart is fixed to the corpus. The graft is formed into a neourethra over a Silastic stenting catheter.
7. The panendoscope is again inserted, and the urethra is irrigated to check for suture-line leaks.
8. A Foley or fenestrated catheter is inserted to serve as a stent.
9. The corpus spongiosum is approximated and closed over the patched area as a separate layer with interrupted 3-0 absorbable sutures. Subcutaneous 4-0 absorbable sutures are placed.
10. The skin and the graft site are closed with interrupted 4-0 sutures.
11. A suprapubic catheter is inserted to divert urine for healing. Petrolatum gauze is wrapped around the penis and covered with gauze sponges and fluffed dressings. A scrotal supporter is applied to provide support and pressure.

## Penectomy

Penectomy is the partial or total removal of a cancerous penis. The procedure selected depends on the extent of involvement and disease stage. Invasive penile cancer not suited for irradiation because of its size, depth, or location is best dealt with by penectomy. Excision of a 2-cm gross tumor margin is adequate for local management. Partial penectomy may afford a sufficient length for directable and upright urination. At least 3 cm of viable proximal shaft is necessary for consideration of a partial penectomy. If the residual stump is inadequate in length, detachment and mobilization of the suspensory ligaments may be an option in selected patients. A total penectomy is generally required when tumor margins are beyond a 2-cm retrievable length from the penoscrotal junction.

Options are available to limit the extent of the disfiguring surgery previously indicated for penile cancer. Chemotherapy agents, often combined with irradiation, are proving effective in shrinking penile carcinomas that would have previously mandated radical penectomy. Bleomycin, usually combined with irradiation, is showing great success in patients with known metastasis. Methotrexate is another effective agent. A third therapy involves the use of cisplatin.

Reconstruction is possible after penectomy. Evaluation must take into account sexual, urinary, and cosmetic factors. Extensive or proximally invasive lesions that include the scrotum, perineum, abdominal wall, and pubis necessitate emasculation as well as expanded resection of involved tissues.

***Procedural Considerations.*** The setup necessary is similar to that for any inguinal surgery, with the addition of a medium Penrose drain for use as a tourniquet.

### *Operative Procedures*

PARTIAL PENECTOMY

1. The lesion is excluded by a towel attached to the planned amputation line. A penile tourniquet is applied at the base (Figure 15-22, *A*).
2. After circumferential skin incision, the cavernous bodies are divided to the urethra with a 2-cm gross margin (Figure 15-22, *B*).
3. Dorsal vessels are ligated, margins of the tunica albuginea are approximated, and the urethra is dissected proximally and distally (spatulated) to obtain a 1-cm redundant flap (Figure 15-22, *C*).

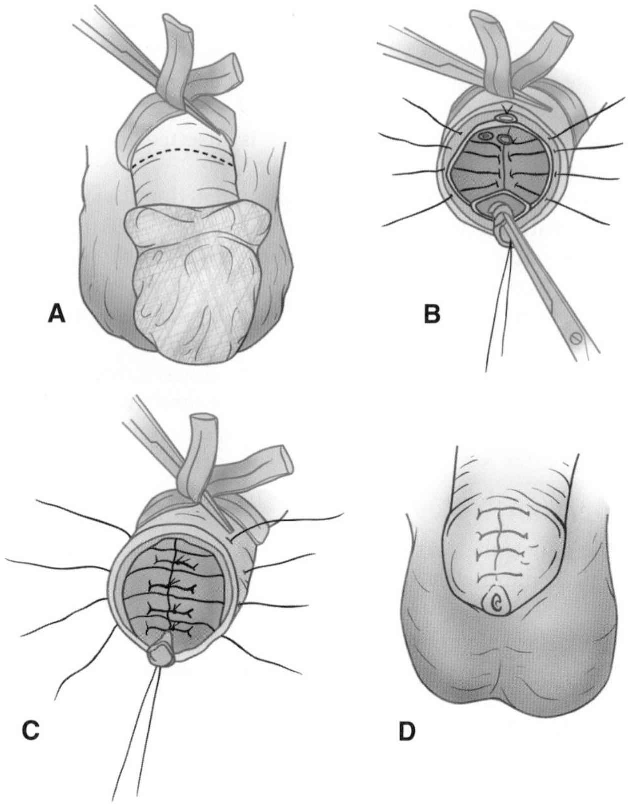


FIGURE 15-22 Partial penectomy.

4. Without sacrificing the tumor margin, the urethra is then divided. Interrupted sutures are placed on the opposite margins of the tunica albuginea to secure the corpora. The tourniquet is removed, and hemostasis is achieved.
5. After the dorsal urethrotomy, a skin-to-urethra anastomosis is performed. The redundant skin flap is then dorsally approximated (Figure 15-22, *D*).
6. A small urinary catheter is inserted, and a nonadherent dressing is applied. They are generally removed in 3 or 4 days.

TOTAL PENECTOMY

1. A vertical elliptic incision is made around the penile base (Figure 15-23, *A*).
2. The distal urethra and its ventral traction are divided through an incision in Buck's fascia, mobilizing the urethra and aiding its dissection, which extends from the corpora to the bulbar region.
3. The corpora are then separated and ligated (Figure 15-23, *B*). The suspensory ligaments and dorsal vessels are divided as corporal dissection is carried out.
4. The urethra is transected from the corpora (Figure 15-23, *C*).
5. An ellipse of skin approximately 1 cm in size is taken from the perineal area. A tunnel is fashioned in the perineal subcutaneous layer of tissue. A traction suture through the tunnel, at the penile base, aids dissection for transposition of the urethra to the perineum (Figure 15-23, *D*).
6. The urethra is grasped with forceps and transferred to the perineum. The urethra is spatulated, and a skin-to-urethra anastomosis is performed through a buttonhole incision in the perineum (Figure 15-23, *E*).
7. The primary incision is closed horizontally, elevating the scrotum away from the urethral opening (Figure 15-23, *F*).
8. An indwelling urinary catheter is inserted, and the wound is covered with a nonadherent dressing.

## Penile Implant

A penile prosthesis is implanted for treatment of organic sexual impotence. Sexual impotence may be caused by (1) diabetes mellitus, (2) priapism, (3) Peyronie's disease, (4) penile trauma, (5) pelvic surgery, (6) neurologic disease (in selected cases), (7) vascular disease, (8) hypertension, and (9) idiopathic impotence (in carefully screened patients). The penile implant serves as a stent to enable vaginal penetration for sexual intercourse. Penile implants are available as malleable one-piece devices, self-contained inflatable devices, and two- and three-piece devices. The procedure described for the inflatable penile implant is for the three-piece device.

***Procedural Considerations.*** Spinal or general anesthesia is required. The patient is placed in either the supine or lithotomy position. A 5- to 10-minute skin prep is usually performed before draping is carried out. To prevent urethral injury and potential urinary retention, a 14-Fr or 16-Fr Foley catheter may be inserted to identify the urethra intraoperatively. The ESU may be required. A local anesthetic of 0.5% plain bupivacaine (Marcaine) or 1% etidocaine may be injected at the beginning of the procedure into the incisional sites. Often, a penile block, composed of 0.9% saline (150 ml):1% plain lidocaine (50 ml):30 mg/ml papaverine (2 ml), is instilled intraoperatively before the incision into the corpus cavernosum. This enables the surgeon to evaluate erectile size and provides some postoperative pain management.

A separate sterile Mayo stand or small table covered with a plastic drape is set up for some types of implants. It is recommended that the implants not be in contact with paper or cloth that may shed fiber particles.

The instrument setup includes a minor set with fine instruments, plus Hegar dilators, the penile prosthesis of choice (Figure 15-24), the Furlow inserter, closing tool, the assembly tool for clamping connectors (Figure 15-25, *A*), and the connectors of choice (Figure 15-25, *B*). Medications needed in the operative field include 50 ml of 1% lidocaine, 150 ml of injectable 0.9% normal saline, 1 ml of methylene blue (optional by surgeon preference), 2 ml of papaverine, 50 ml of 0.5% bupivacaine (Marcaine) or 1% etidocaine (Duranest), 50,000 units of bacitracin, and 80 mg of kanamycin. Medication safety practices must be implemented for all medications on the sterile field.

A serious risk with a penile implant is infection. Infection rates for first-time implantation are low at 1%, but the rate can rise to as high as 18% with reimplantation procedures. Because of the high risk of infection, models that have been irradiated and embedded with minocycline hydrochloride and rifampin (Inhibizone) are now available.[2] The sterile team should be double-gloved throughout the procedure. Some surgeons coat their hands with Betadine (povidone-iodine complex) just before donning sterile gloves. A 5-minute antimicrobial prep of the operative area is critical in reducing skin flora. The anus should be isolated in the perineal approach. Intraoperatively and before insertion of the implant components, a prophylactic antibiotic irrigant of bacitracin and kanamycin in normal saline is used on the implants without Inhibizone and in the insertion sites. Systemic antibiotics may also be required. As with any implant procedure, it is vital to maintain an environment conducive to infection prevention. Traffic in and out of the room should be minimized.

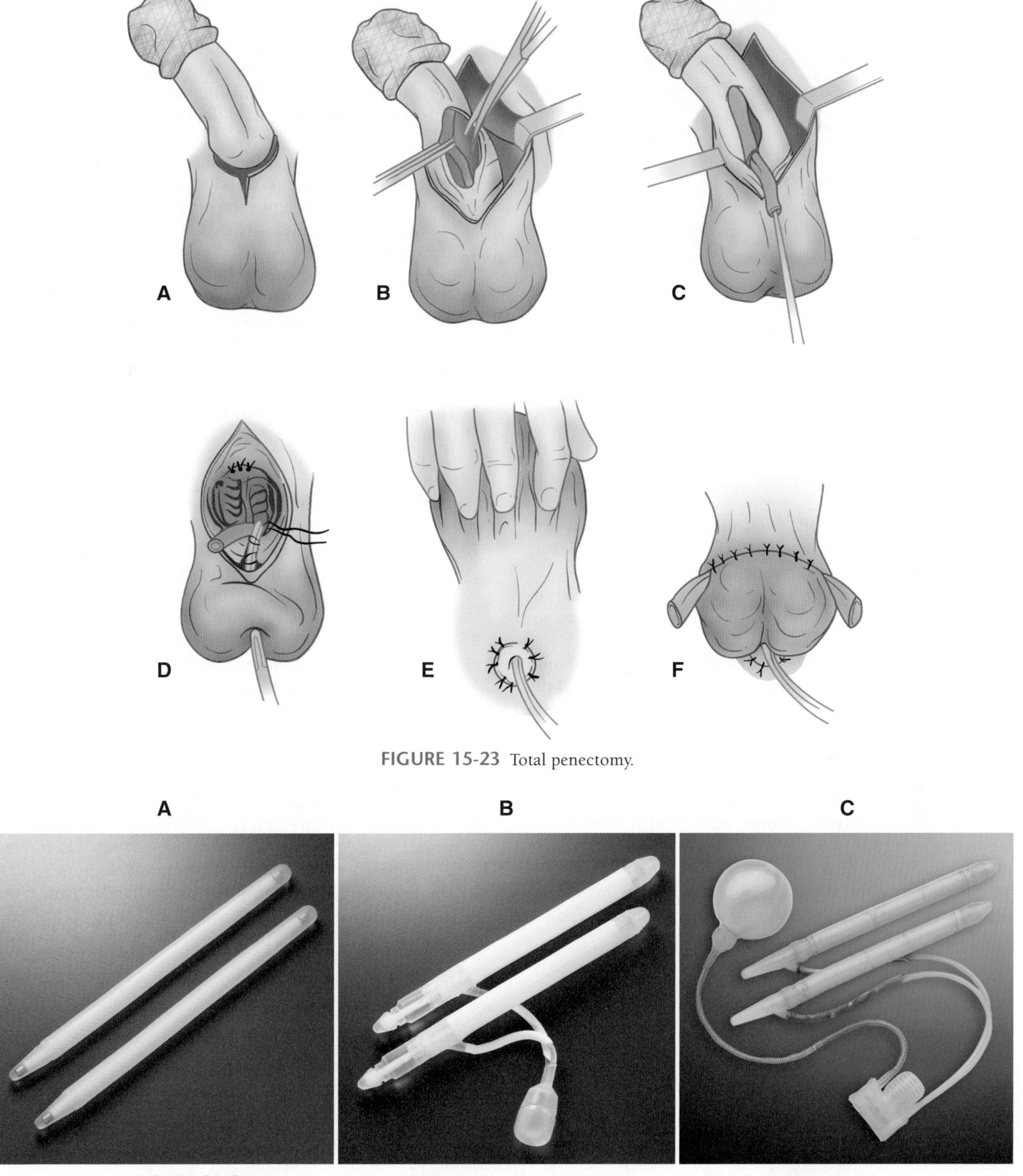


**FIGURE 15-23** Total penectomy.

**FIGURE 15-24** **A,** AMS malleable 650 penile prosthesis. **B,** AMS Ambicor inflatable two-piece penile prosthesis. **C,** AMS tactile inflatable penile prosthesis, three-piece with rifampin (Inhibizone).

It is recommended that the implants with Inhibizone not be soaked in any solution before implantation because this may cause the antibiotic component to break down. The area to be implanted may be irrigated with antibiotic solution, and the implant itself may be dipped in a sterile solution of 0.9% normal saline to assist with insertion if desired. Prophylactic antibiotic protocols remain the same.

### *Operative Procedures*

#### IMPLANTATION OF NONINFLATABLE (SEMIRIGID) PROSTHESIS

1. A 14-Fr or 16-Fr Foley catheter is inserted and attached to a drainage collection device to be maintained within the sterile field. The amount and color of urine are noted. It is

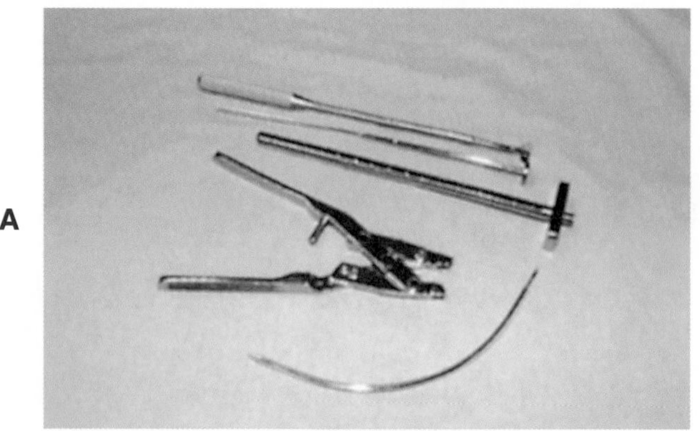


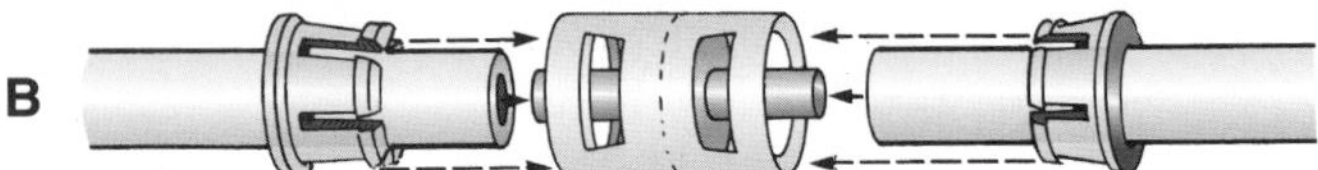


**FIGURE 15-25** **A,** *Top to bottom,* Closing tool, Furlow inserter, assembly tool, tubing passer. **B,** Quik-connectors.

best to leave the Foley in place intraoperatively to assist in identifying the urethra.

2. A midline incision is made from the base of the penis into the scrotum for approximately 3 cm. Some surgeons may choose a suprapubic or dorsal penile approach.
3. The tunica albuginea is incised over the most proximal portion of the corpora in a longitudinal manner, and stay sutures are placed.
4. The corpora are dilated proximally and distally with 7-mm to 14-mm Hegar's dilators, depending on the diameter of the implant chosen. The corpora are dilated to 1 mm more than the implant size. Care is taken to not perforate the urethra.
5. Measurements of the entire corporal length are taken with the Furlow inserter or sizing instrument.
6. After placement of the closure sutures, the prostheses are inserted into the corpora. Proper placement is evident immediately by a change in the configuration of the penis with no buckling of the glans.
7. The tunica albuginea is then closed with the previously placed 2-0 absorbable continuous suture; 3-0 or 4-0 absorbable interrupted sutures are used for skin closure.
8. Petrolatum gauze or 2-inch Kling tube gauze may be used for the dressing.

**IMPLANTATION OF INFLATABLE PROSTHESIS**

1. A 14- or 16-Fr Foley catheter is inserted, attached to a drainage collection device, and maintained within the sterile field. This is to identify and retract the urethra out of the operative field.
2. A midline incision is made from the base of the penis into the scrotum for approximately 3 cm (Figure 15-26, *A*).
3. The tunica albuginea of each corpus is incised in the most proximal portion, and stay sutures are placed.
4. The corpora are dilated distally and proximally with 7-mm to 14-mm Hegar dilators. Dilation should be 1 mm more than the diameter of the chosen implant. The 700CX implant is 12 mm at its widest point. When this is used the dilation at the distal end should be 13 mm. The proximal end, however, should be 14 mm to accommodate the input tubing.
5. The Furlow inserter is used for measuring the entire corporal length.
6. Corporal sutures of 2-0 absorbable material are placed along the tunica incision and tagged. Some surgeons prefer to place these sutures last and employ the closing tool to prevent puncture of the cylinders.
7. The cylinders are packaged with attached traction sutures of 4-0 Tevdek at the distal end. These are placed through the eye of a 2½-inch Keith needle, and the needle is slid into the groove of the Furlow inserter.
8. The Furlow inserter is guided along the corporal tunnel, and the plunger is pushed to release the Keith needle, which punctures the glans (Figure 15-26, *B*).
9. The needle is grasped with a heavy hemostat and pulled through the glans, allowing the cylinders to slide to the channel opening. The Furlow inserter is removed, and the cylinder is inserted and guided to its proper position beneath the glans penis (Figure 15-26, *C*).
10. If necessary, rear tip extenders are added to the proximal end of the cylinder. The proximal end is positioned in the crus.
11. The procedure is repeated on the other side.
12. The external inguinal ring is palpated and a path bluntly created. Dissecting scissors are used to separate the transversalis fascia on the inguinal floor. If the new Ambicor

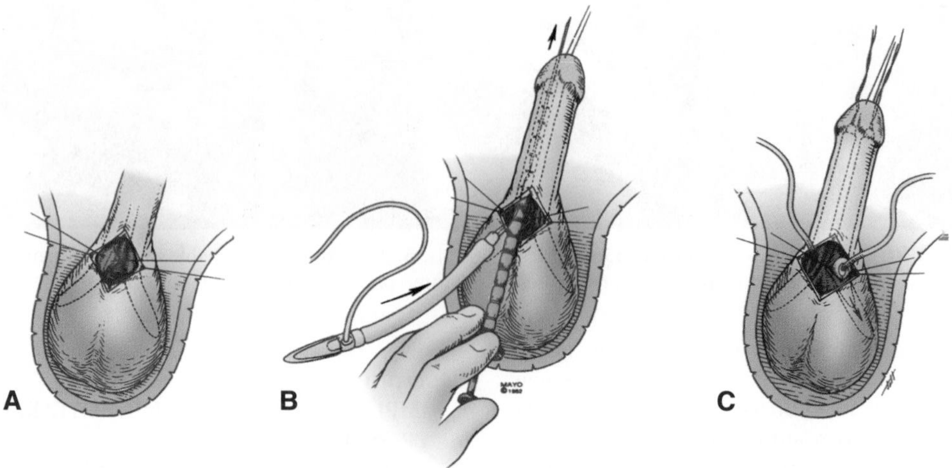


**FIGURE 15-26** Penoscrotal approach for inflatable penile implant.

implant with self-contained reservoir is being placed, steps 12 through 14 are eliminated.

13. The perivesical space is enlarged to allow palpation of the Cooper ligament. The reservoir is then positioned into the perivesical space.
14. The reservoir is filled with 65-ml or 100-ml of saline solution (dependent on the reservoir size selected) and pulled against the floor of Hesselbach's triangle.
15. The pump is then placed into the most dependent portion of the scrotum. It is generally positioned on the patient's dominant side. The space is created by blunt dissection lateral to the testicle.
16. The rods and reservoir tubings are connected to the pump with the connectors of choice, using the assembly tool to clamp them in place, and tested for inflation and deflation.
17. The tunica of the scrotum is closed over the pump with a running stitch of 3-0 absorbable suture.
18. The prosthetic device is left in a partially inflated position to reduce bleeding and promote healing for 24 hours postoperatively (Figures 15-27 and 15-28). (Following this

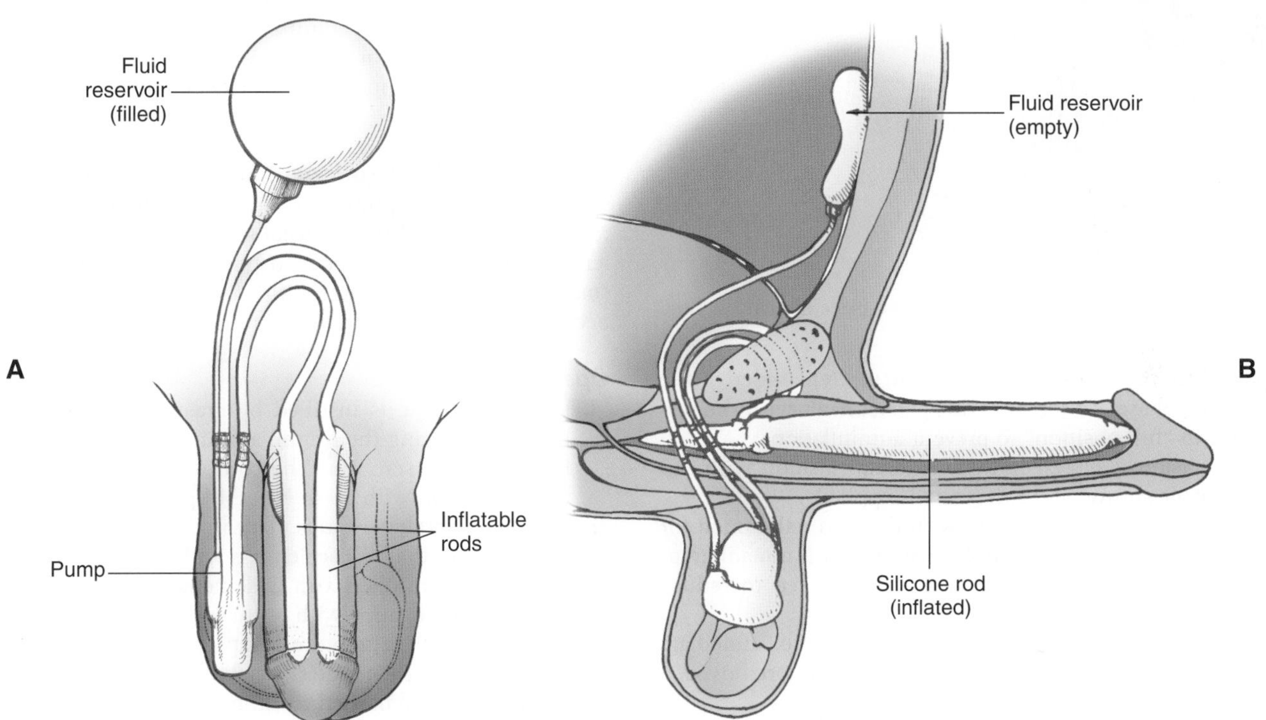


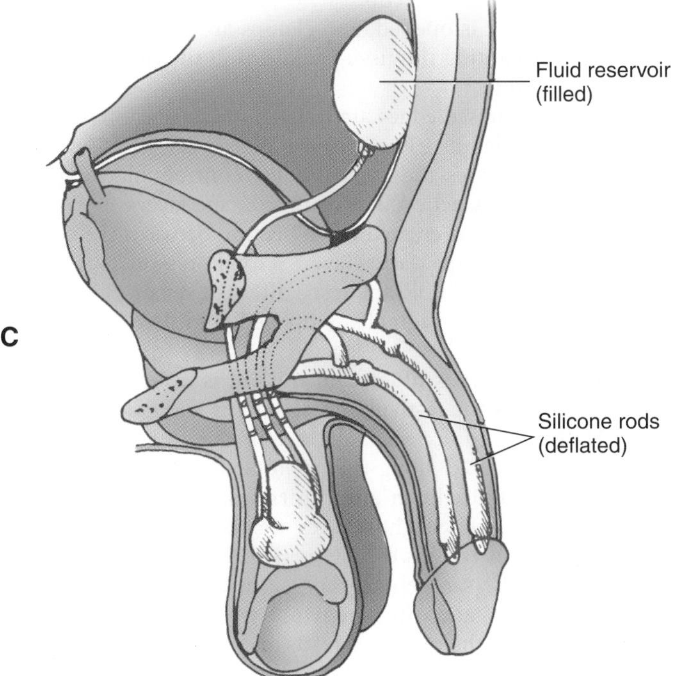


**FIGURE 15-27** AMS inflatable 700CX penile prosthesis. **A,** Frontal view. **B,** Sagittal view—penis in erect position. **C,** Sagittal view—penis in flaccid position.

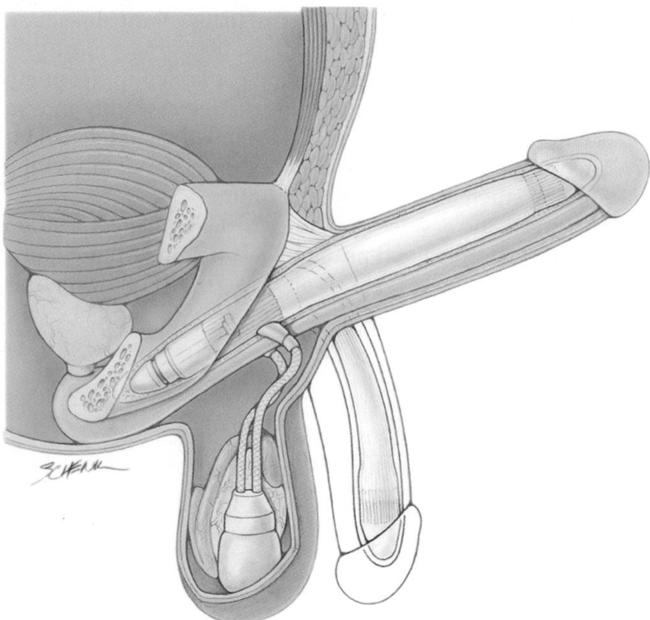

FIGURE 15-28 AMS Ambicor inflatable two-piece implant, sagittal view.

period the implants are deflated for the remainder of the "healing phase" so the reservoir pocket heals with the reservoir in "full position" to prevent autoinflation.)

19. The incision is closed in a subcuticular fashion with 4-0 absorbable suture, and a dressing is applied.
20. The penis is positioned flush with the lower abdomen for patient comfort. Mesh pants are useful as a nonadherent support dressing. An ice pack may be applied to reduce swelling.
21. The Foley catheter is left in place during the immediate 24-hour postoperative period and then usually removed.

## Deep Dorsal and Emissary Vein Ligation

Undertaken for vascular compromise–related impotence, this procedure entails the ligation or elimination of the penile deep dorsal vein and its tributaries. Care is taken to avoid damage to the arteries and nerves lying alongside the deep dorsal vein. A common cause of erectile dysfunction in patients with organic impotence is vascular compromise. Before surgical intervention is undertaken, a definitive diagnosis of a corporal leak is made through dynamic infusion cavernosometry and cavernosography. Diagnostic results may indicate failure-to-store or failure-to-fill impotence. Patients with vascular compromise in a given anatomic region tend to be compromised elsewhere as well. Many are diabetic or hypertensive. Because of this, the perioperative nurse must exercise great care in positioning the patient to prevent further damage to the patient's altered tissue perfusion. The cavernous and crural veins are suture-ligated. All circumflex and emissary branches are ligated or coagulated. The suspensory ligament is detached, and the entire deep and accessory dorsal vein is removed.

## Revascularization of the Penile Arteries

The relationship of focal arterial occlusive disease to sexual dysfunction has prompted efforts to rectify the resulting impotence. Reconstructive surgery has been attempted in patients who demonstrate correctable vascular disease in the large arteries. The most widely attempted repairs are end-to-end and end-to-side microscopic anastomoses of the distal inferior epigastric artery to the proximal deep dorsal artery near the pubic level, below the rectus muscle and Buck's fascia. Paramedian and infrapubic incisions are made, and the arteries are freed and tunneled. This procedure requires both urologic and vascular surgeons.

# SURGERY OF THE SCROTUM AND TESTICLES

## Hydrocelectomy

A hydrocele is an abnormal accumulation of fluid within the scrotum. The fluid is contained within the tunica vaginalis. Excessive secretion or accumulation of hydrocele fluid may be the result of infection or trauma. A hydrocelectomy is the excision of the tunica vaginalis of the testis to remove the enlarged, fluid-filled sac.

***Procedural Considerations.*** The patient is placed in the supine position. Prepping and draping of the patient include routine cleansing of the external genitalia and draping with a fenestrated sheet. A minor instrument set is required, plus a small drain, a 30-ml syringe with a 20-gauge, 2-inch aspirating needle, and a suspensory dressing.

### *Operative Procedure*

1. Local anesthetic is instilled by grasping the cord in one hand and placing the thumb and index finger of the other hand over the scrotum. The cord is infiltrated at the base of the scrotum with 10 to 15 ml of plain lidocaine 1%.
2. An anterolateral incision is made in the stretched skin of the scrotum over the hydrocele mass with a #10 or #15 blade.
3. Bleeding is controlled with Crile hemostats, electrocoagulation, or vessel ligation with 3-0 absorbable ligatures. Stretching the skin of the scrotum compresses the scrotal vessels.
4. An incision is then made between the blood vessels. The fascial layers are incised to expose the tunica vaginalis.
5. The hydrocele is dissected free with fine scissors, forceps, and blunt dissection.
6. The sac is opened, and clamps are placed on each side incorporating the tissue adjacent to the tunica vaginalis and the skin.
7. The incised edges are everted under tension with the Martius clamps. The tension placed by the Martius clamp compresses the incised edge, controls bleeding, and prevents dissection between the tissue layers.
8. A pouch is created by dissecting between the tunica vaginalis and the dartos layer. Scrotal pressure is released. This pouch will hold the testis after the repair.
9. The tunica vaginalis is opened, and the fluid contents are evacuated.
10. The testis is lifted, and the sac is inverted so that it surrounds the testicular attachments and epididymis.
11. Excess tunica vaginalis may be excised. The tunica edges are sutured along the peritoneal surface with 3-0 absorbable suture in an interrupted fashion to the juncture of the testis. Six to eight sutures are placed around the circumference of the testis (Figure 15-29). Some surgeons elect to sew the sac behind the spermatic cord in an interrupted fashion, and others may choose a continuous radial stitch around the posterior testis and epididymis.
12. The testis is replaced into the scrotum.

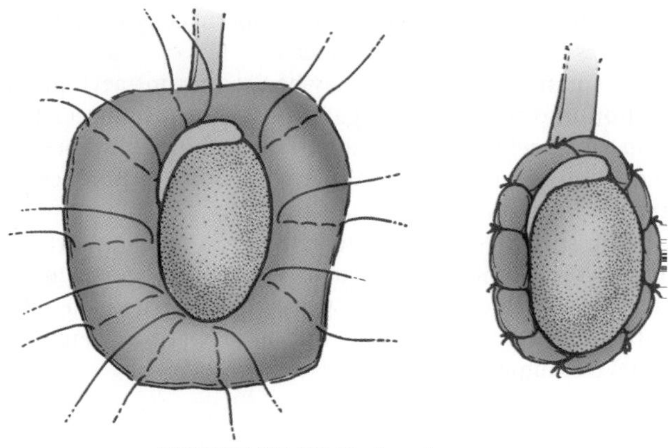

**FIGURE 15-29** Hydrocelectomy.

13. A drain may be placed into the scrotum and brought out through a stab wound in its most dependent portion. The drain is loosely sutured to the external scrotal wall to prevent migration.
14. The scrotal incision may be closed with 3-0 absorbable sutures in a full-thickness continuous manner or in layers with 3-0 and 4-0 continuous absorbable sutures.
15. A fluff compression dressing contained in a scrotal support or mesh underwear aids in reducing postoperative scrotal edema.

## Vasectomy

A vasectomy is the excision of a section of the vas deferens. The operation may be performed selectively as a permanent method of sterilization and also before prostatectomy to prevent possible postoperative epididymitis. Because of the serious implications of permanent sterilization, particular attention must be paid to acquiring informed consent. Although studies have raised the question of a correlation between prostate cancer and vasectomy, a definitive causal relationship has not been established.

The patient having elective sterilization for birth control is encouraged to return to the office setting for sperm-count analysis. Generally, two successive negative counts are sufficient to indicate that sterility has been achieved. Elective vasectomies are frequently performed in the office setting.

***Procedural Considerations.*** The patient usually lies in the supine position. Local anesthesia is used. A minor instrument set and scrotal suspensory are needed.

### *Operative Procedure*

NO-SCALPEL APPROACH. The no-scalpel technique was devised in China and has five fundamental principles:

1. Fixation of the vas deferens without entering the scrotal skin
2. Performance under direct vision to prevent damage from blind sharp scrotal penetration
3. Simplified instrumentation
4. Decreased operative time by simplification of the procedure
5. Elimination of an incision or use of a scalpel

The procedure is as follows:

1. The right vas deferens is fixed under the scrotal skin with three fingers.
2. With the local syringe and needle, a small wheal is raised in the median raphe of the scrotum. The needle is advanced along the vas toward the external inguinal ring. Plain lidocaine 1% or 2%, 10 ml, is injected into the perivasal region.
3. The procedure is repeated on the left side. Pressure is applied to the wheal site to minimize edema.
4. Once adequate anesthesia is accomplished, the right vas is again fixed with three fingers.
5. A vas ring clamp is applied over the scrotal skin, encircling the vas. Lifting the clamp upward, the skin over the vas is stretched as thin as possible, leaving minimal tissue between the vas and the clamp.
6. The ring clamp is locked in place, and the scrotal skin cephalad to the clamp is stretched with an index finger.
7. The skin is punctured, with the inner prong of the pointed dissecting hemostat, directly into the vas deferens. Both prongs of the dissecting hemostat are placed into the puncture site and spread directly on top of the vas.
8. When the surface of the vas is visualized, one prong is used to penetrate the vas itself. The vas is brought out of the wound by twisting the hemostat 180 degrees.
9. The ring clamp is moved to directly encircle the vasal tissue. The vas may then be divided and occluded by intraluminal electrocoagulation, clips, or suture ligation. Fascia should be placed between the severed ends of the vas.
10. The procedure is repeated on the left side. It is usually possible to place the ring clamp around the left vas through the initial entry site. Sutures are not necessary.
11. After ensuring that there is no bleeding, antibiotic ointment, pressure dressings, and a scrotal support are applied.

## Vasovasostomy

Vasovasostomy is the surgical reanastomosis of the vas deferens, using the operative microscope. The number of vasal reanastomosis procedures has increased dramatically. Reanastomosis may often alleviate chronic testicular pain, a not infrequent complication after vasectomy. In addition, a significant number of men who have had a vasectomy want to regain their fertility. A precise reconnection can be performed with the use of a microscope and a modified two-layer anastomosis. Success rates vary from 40% to 70%. When there are no longer two viable segments of vas deferens, a similar procedure, the epididymovasostomy, may be performed. This involves anastomosis of a vas deferens to a segment of the epididymis. Postoperative precautions include no lifting or ejaculation for a minimum of 2 weeks. The sperm count and viability of sperm are rechecked at 3- and 6-month intervals.

***Procedural Considerations.*** A minor instrument set is required, with the addition of selected microsurgical instruments and sutures. The procedure is frequently done under monitored anesthesia care with local injection of 0.5% plain bupivacaine (Marcaine) and 1% lidocaine in a 50:50 ratio.

### *Operative Procedure*

1. After the vas deferens has been located by external manipulation, a vertical scrotal incision is made.
2. The testicle, epididymis, and vas are displaced from the scrotum. The vasectomy site is identified, and the scarred area is excised.

3. The proximal end of the vas deferens is cut back until fluid is expressed. Fluid is collected on a glass slide and examined for the presence of live sperm. Surgery continues even if results for sperm are negative unless an epididymal obstruction exists.
4. The distal end of the vas is resected until a normal lumen is visible.
5. The distal and proximal lumens are then dilated.
6. The two portions of the vas are placed in an approximator clip with background material placed underneath. Six stitches of 10-0 nonabsorbable microsuture are placed in the inner layer. The proximal end is sutured through the serosa to the mucosa, and the distal end is sutured through the mucosa to the serosa (Figure 15-30).
7. A second layer of 8 to 10 stitches of 9-0 nonabsorbable suture is placed without penetrating the lumen of the vas.
8. The incision is closed in two layers with interrupted 3-0 and 4-0 absorbable sutures.
9. Gauze sponges and a suspensory support are placed on the patient to provide a pressure dressing.

## Microscopic Epididymal Sperm Aspiration

Microscopic epididymal sperm aspiration (MESA) requires the availability of an in vitro fertilization team so that the aspirated sperm may be immediately processed and used for the selected in vitro technique or frozen for later use. The procedure must be timed according to the partner's cycle of ovulation. Ova are aspirated as an office procedure just before MESA is performed.

MESA should be done using the micropipette technique. The tip of a 250- to 350-micrometer (μm) pipette is inserted into an epididymal tubule to retrieve sperm cells without contamination by red blood cells. After aspiration, the fluid is given to the in vitro fertilization team to process the sperm cells. Processing involves washing debris from the cells, retrieving the most active cells from the sample, and removing any red blood cells, if possible. This is critical because red blood cells significantly interfere with sperm cell function.

After the sperm cells are aspirated, the epididymal tubule is closed using microscopic technique. If adequate numbers of sperm cells can be obtained from one testis, the other side may be aspirated to add to the sperm bank if this is desirable. It may be necessary to aspirate sperm cells from the rete testis (tubules between the testicles and the epididymal head that carry cells to the head of the epididymis) if sperm cells are not found in tubules closer to the vas deferens.

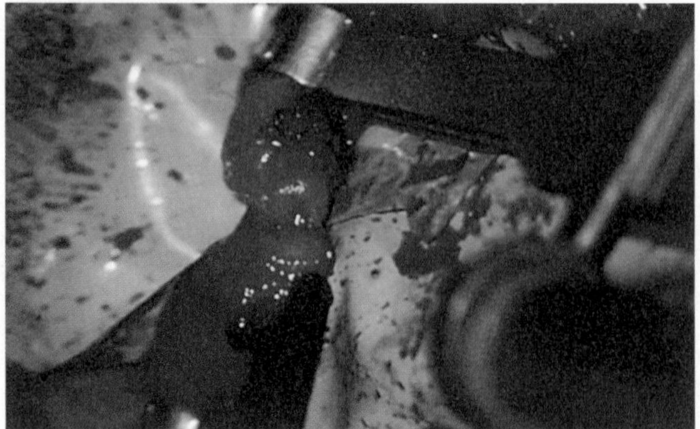

**FIGURE 15-30** The two portions of the vas in approximator clip with background material as the proximal end is sutured through the serosa to the mucosa with 10-0 nylon.

The sperm cells retrieved may be used for intracytoplasmic injection into the partner's egg (ICSI), the most successful of the in vitro techniques available. This technique is not as dependent on the quality of the sperm as earlier techniques of in vitro fertilization.

Using sperm cells from the epididymis and intracytoplasmic injection techniques, pregnancy rates may approach 50%. It may be possible to retrieve sperm cells by percutaneous aspiration of the testis, but the numbers of sperm cells retrieved by this technique are not as high as with MESA.

## Epididymectomy

An epididymectomy is the excision of the epididymis from the testis. Epididymectomy is rarely performed, usually only as a last-choice treatment for degenerative cystic disease, chronic infection, and intractable pain of the epididymis.

***Procedural Considerations.*** The patient is placed in the supine position with the legs slightly abducted. A general, spinal, or regional anesthetic is required. Setup is as described for hydrocelectomy, plus an ESU, if desired.

### *Operative Procedure*

1. An anterolateral incision is made over the testis in the scrotum to expose the tunica vaginalis. The tunica is incised to expose the testis and overlying epididymis.
2. An incision is made along the superior head of the epididymis, which is then sharply dissected from the testis. A portion of the vas deferens may also be excised.
3. Bleeding is controlled by electrocoagulation and absorbable ties.
4. The skin wound is closed with 4-0 absorbable sutures.
5. A small drain may be left intrascrotally for 24 to 48 hours.

## Spermatocelectomy

Spermatocelectomy is removal of a spermatocele—a lobulated intrascrotal cystic mass attached to the superior head of the epididymis. It is usually caused by an obstruction of the tubular system that conveys the sperm. This complication after vasectomy is not infrequent and does not exhibit itself immediately.

***Procedural Considerations.*** The setup for a spermatocelectomy is as described for a hydrocelectomy, plus a microscope and slides, if desired.

### *Operative Procedure*

1. The mass is approached through a scrotal incision as described for hydrocelectomy.
2. The structures of the testis and spermatic cord are identified, and the cystic structure is dissected free.
3. Bleeding is controlled with electrocoagulation.
4. The wound is closed and dressed as described for hydrocelectomy.

## Varicocelectomy

A varicocelectomy is the high ligation of the gonadal veins of the testes. Varicocelectomy is done to reduce venous backflow of blood into the venous plexus around the testes and to improve spermatogenesis.[30] When surgery for this condition was originally devised, the veins of the pampiniform plexus were ligated and divided individually.

Varicoceles occur more frequently on the left side because the gonadal vein of the left testis unites retroperitoneally with the renal vein at a 90-degree angle and is consequently under greater backpressure. As a result of this unusual backpressure, the pampiniform plexus of the spermatic cord becomes tortuous and engorged, resembling a bag of worms.

***Procedural Considerations.*** The setup for inguinal varicocelectomy is as described for an inguinal hernia repair (see Chapter 13). A microscope may be employed to better visualize the vessels involved.[30]

***Operative Procedure.*** The incision may be through a suprainguinal approach or an oblique inguinal approach over the external inguinal ring.

1. The structures of the spermatic cord are identified, and the vessels are dissected free from the vas deferens.
2. The abnormal dilated veins in the inguinal canal are clamped and ligated. The redundant portions are excised. A drain may be placed.
3. The incision is closed in layers.

## Testicular Biopsy

A biopsy of the testicle involves a wedge excision of suspicious tissue for diagnostic confirmation. Men experiencing infertility who are azoospermatic or oligospermatic with normal or minimally elevated follicle-stimulating hormone may be evaluated through this means. Biopsy may also be performed to obtain sperm cells for in vitro fertilization techniques.

***Procedural Considerations.*** If required, hair may be removed from the scrotum, which is then aseptically cleansed. General, regional, or spinal anesthesia may be selected. A minor instrument set is used. Special fixatives, such as Bouin or Zenker solution, must be available when pathologic confirmation is required. If retrieval of sperm cells is planned the biopsy specimen should be placed in a small amount of saline, kept warm, and taken immediately to the fertility laboratory for aspiration of cells. Formalin destroys the germinal epithelium and should not be used.

### *Operative Procedure*

1. The scrotum is held firmly on its posterior aspect. This causes the skin on the anterior aspect to stretch tightly over the incisional site, forcing the epididymis to remain posterior and allowing the scrotal skin to part without retraction.
2. A 1-cm to 2-cm vertical incision is made, with care taken to avoid injury to the epididymis.
3. The incision is continued to the tunica vaginalis. As the tunica is incised, there should be a normal efflux of clear fluid.
4. Absorbable 4-0 stay sutures are placed in the tunica vaginalis. Two more are placed in the tunica albuginea.
5. A small ellipse of tunica with its tubules is resected with a scalpel in a shaving action, using no-touch technique. The tissue is placed in the fixative or sent to the histology department as a fresh specimen.
6. The wound is closed in three layers with 3-0 and 4-0 absorbable suture.
7. Gauze sponges and fluffed dressings are placed over and around the scrotum. A suspensory support is applied to provide pressure and support.

## Orchiectomy

An orchiectomy is the removal of the testis or testes. Removal of both testes is castration and renders the patient sterile and deficient in the hormone *testosterone,* which is responsible for development of secondary sexual characteristics and potency. This operation, like vasectomy, has legal implications that require attention to acquiring informed consent for surgery. Bilateral orchiectomy is usually performed to control symptomatic metastatic carcinoma of the prostate gland. A unilateral orchiectomy is indicated because of testicular cancer, trauma, or infection. Testicular implants are available for cosmetic purposes. These must be ordered preoperatively based on preoperative measurements for size. This procedure has recently been approached through laparoscopic techniques, usually in conjunction with laparoscopic herniorrhaphy.

***Procedural Considerations.*** The patient is placed in the supine position and draped according to established procedure. A minor instrument setup is required.

### *Operative Procedures*

SCROTAL APPROACH

1. For benign conditions the incision is made over the anterolateral surface of the midportion of the scrotum.
2. The skin incision is carried through the subcutaneous and fascial layers through the tunica vaginalis, exposing the testicle.
3. Retractors are placed, and bleeding vessels are clamped and tied.
4. The spermatic cord is divided into two or three vascular bundles. Each vascular bundle is doubly clamped, cut, and ligated, first with 0 absorbable suture ligature and then with a proximal free 0 absorbable tie.
5. The vas is separately ligated with a 0 absorbable tie. The testis is removed.

INGUINAL APPROACH

1. For malignant conditions the incision is begun just above the internal ring, extending downward and inward over the inguinal canal to the external inguinal ring.
2. The inguinal canal is exposed, and the spermatic cord is dissected free, cross-clamped, and divided into vascular bundles at the internal ring.
3. Gentle forward traction is applied to the cord, which is dissected from its bed.
4. The testis is everted into the wound from the scrotum and excised.
5. Bleeding is controlled with electrocoagulation. A small drain may be placed in the empty hemiscrotum if desired.
6. The external oblique fascia is reapproximated with 2-0 absorbable interrupted sutures.
7. Subcutaneous tissue, including Scarpa fascia, is closed with 4-0 absorbable sutures.
8. The skin is reapproximated with surgical staples or 4-0 subcuticular sutures.

## Radical Lymphadenectomy (Retroperitoneal Lymph Node Dissection)

Radical lymphadenectomy is a bilateral resection of retroperitoneal lymph nodes. Dissection usually includes lymph nodes, channels, and fat around both renal pedicles, the vena cava, and the aorta, including the bifurcation of the aorta. Lymph node dissection is performed for treatment of nonseminomatous testicular tumors. The procedure is performed after radical inguinal orchiectomy.

***Procedural Considerations.*** The patient is placed in the supine position. If the dissection is unilateral, the patient is supine with the operative side tilted upward. Routine skin preparation from nipples to midthigh and draping procedures are carried out. Long fine dissection instruments along with basic laparotomy instruments are required.

Although this procedure may be performed laparoscopically with successful outcomes,[1] this approach has not yet become standard of practice because of its technical difficulty.

### Operative Procedure

1. A midline abdominal incision is made from the xiphoid process to the symphysis pubis.
2. The abdominal contents are explored to determine the degree of gross nodal involvement. The colon is either packed within the abdominal cavity or mobilized and kept moist outside the abdomen.
3. The posterior peritoneum is opened between the aorta and the vena cava.
4. Using blunt and sharp dissection, the lymphatic structures and fat are removed en bloc from around both renal pedicles, the vena cava, and the aorta from above the renal hilum to beyond the bifurcation of the iliac vessels on the side of the original testicular neoplasm.
5. The spermatic vessels of the affected side are removed down to and including the stump of the previous orchiectomy.
6. The inferior mesenteric artery may be sacrificed if technically necessary, but the superior mesenteric artery is not disturbed.
7. The ureter on the affected side is skeletonized to remove any perilymphatic tissue.
8. If reperitonealization is desired, the posterior peritoneum is closed with a 2-0 absorbable continuous suture.
9. The viscera are repositioned into the abdominal cavity, and the wound is closed, usually without placement of a drain.

## SURGERY OF THE PROSTATE GLAND

Glandular hyperplasia of the prostatic urethra usually manifests itself after 50 years of age. Prostatic enlargement may occur in one or more lobes of the prostate but most frequently occurs in the lateral or median lobes. Progressive growth of the hyperplastic gland compresses the remaining normal prostatic tissue, forming what is called a *surgical capsule*. The growth of adenomatous tissue slowly encroaches on the prostatic urethral lumen, causing obstruction of urinary outflow. Symptoms of prostate cancer may mimic those of BPH.

Prostatic enlargement may be benign or malignant. In BPH only the periurethral adenomatous portion of the gland is removed. Operable prostatic malignancy requires radical prostatectomy, which includes removal of the entire prostate gland and the seminal vesicles.

A blood sample is drawn to determine the PSA level, followed by a digital rectal examination (DRE). The blood is often drawn first, since manipulation of the gland has been known to alter the efficacy of the PSA test (Best Practice). The PSA test is considered a valuable tool for early detection of carcinoma of the prostate, but if used alone, it will miss 20% to 30% of all prostate cancers. If the test value is elevated, the patient is at risk for carcinoma of the prostate; a PSA value above 10 ng/ml is highly suggestive of prostatic carcinoma. Clinical evaluation and an elevated PSA usually indicate the need for a transrectal ultrasound needle biopsy to confirm the diagnosis (see Best Practice). When the results of the biopsy are positive for malignancy, a bone scan and skeletal survey are necessary to rule out metastasis. A more precise blood study, the free total PSA (PSA II), has proved to be quite accurate in delineating those patients at increased risk for prostate cancer. An older blood study, which is still being used, is the prostatic acid phosphatase (PAP) level. When elevated, it usually indicates that the tumor has extended beyond the prostatic capsule.

In an attempt to provide cost-effective, curative treatment with a low morbidity, treatment protocols that provide alternatives to the open-surgery approach have been developed. A thorough workup procedure includes a DRE, free and total serum PSA II, bone scans, CT and MRI scans of the pelvis, and transrectal, ultrasonically guided biopsies with histologic grading of the malignancy.[23] After these evaluations, select patients with well-differentiated or moderately differentiated lesions may be candidates for transperineal, ultrasonically guided implantation of radium seeds (brachytherapy) or cryoablation of the prostate (cryotherapy) (see Best Practice).

Three open surgical approaches are possible in removing the benign hyperplastic obstructive prostate gland: retropubic prostatectomy, suprapubic prostatectomy, and perineal prostatectomy. Of these, the one most commonly employed is the suprapubic prostatectomy. All open prostatectomies hold the risk for loss of sexual potency.

TURP is the endoscopic (closed) surgical approach that has been traditionally performed on patients. Alternative modalities that have had moderate to good success in the treatment of BPH are photoselective vaporization of the prostate (PVP),[18,19,32,48] interstitial laser coagulation of the prostate (ILC),[26] transurethral incision of the prostate (TUIP), transurethral laser incision of the prostate (TULIP),[26] holmium laser enucleation of the prostate (HoLep),[35] and holmium laser ablation of the prostate (HoLap).[34] A visual laser ablation of the prostate (VLAP) was originally performed with the Nd: YAG laser but may now also be accomplished with the holmium laser. Proper laser protocol must be followed for the type of laser being employed. The standard TUIP procedure involves the use of electrosurgery only. Transurethral microwave therapy (TUMT) is another alternative that is performed as an office procedure.

If the prostate gland is cancerous, a radical retropubic or radical perineal prostatectomy, in conjunction with open or laparoscopic pelvic lymph node dissection, is performed. Many patients desire to retain sexual function. The surgeon may attempt to save the neurovascular bundles in what is termed a *nerve-sparing approach*. The site and size of the prostatic lesion, however, often determine if this can be achieved successfully and without undue risk to the patient.

Several factors must be considered to determine the best route for removal of the prostatic obstruction: the age and medical condition of the patient, the size of the gland and location of the pathologic condition, and the presence of associated medical disease.

## Prostatic Core Needle Biopsy

Needle biopsy of the prostate is indicated for patients in whom prostatic cancer is clinically suspected. It may be accomplished transrectally with a needle designed for this purpose or transperineally.

***Procedural Considerations.*** Needle biopsy of the prostate has the risk of both intraoperative and postoperative bleeding. A cystoscopic examination may accompany a needle biopsy. Most needle biopsies are performed in the office or ultrasound department.

The most significant potential complication of a biopsy is systemic infection. This risk can be decreased with antibiotic coverage before and after the procedure and bowel cleansing before the examination. The patient is given antibiotic therapy 24 hours before the procedure and is advised to use a Fleet enema 2 to 3 hours before the test is performed. Before the examination, an antiseptic solution mixed with a viscous local anesthetic often is instilled into the rectum and allowed to coat the tissues for 5 to 15 minutes. Local anesthetic may also be injected into the prostate and seminal vesicles transrectally with a 22-gauge, 22-cm injection needle through the needle guide on the transducer.

### *Operative Procedures*

TRANSRECTAL, ULTRASONICALLY GUIDED BIOPSY. Transrectal, ultrasonically guided biopsy commonly is performed in the urologist's office using a high-frequency transrectal ultrasound transducer to assess the prostate gland. The size, volume, and shape of the prostate may be assessed in addition to the likelihood of the presence of a malignancy. Biopsy specimens of suspicious areas or lesions may be obtained with a needle passed across the rectal wall, with the aid of ultrasound guidance. The needle penetrates the rectal mucosa with a core biopsy system. Color-flow imaging may also be used to help identify areas that are likely invaded with prostatic carcinoma or have acute and chronic inflammation. Highly vascular areas carry a greater probability of harboring a carcinoma. A full bladder helps delineate the base of the prostate.

The prostate is visualized in three dimensions, allowing more accurate localization of abnormalities and extent of disease. For the axial view, the transrectal transducer is placed deeply into the rectum, just proximal to the seminal vesicles, to about 10 cm above the anal verge. Here the vas deferens may be distinguished. The transducer is slowly withdrawn to the level of the base of the gland, enabling visualization of the inner gland. Seminal vesicles are seen in cross section. To evaluate the prostate in the sagittal planes, the probe may be rotated clockwise or counterclockwise (Figure 15-31). A series of 12 biopsy specimens is generally taken with a disposable "core biopsy" needle. These are taken from the right and left medial and lateral apices, the right and left midline, and the right and left medial and lateral bases. Lesions as small as 2 to 3 mm are visible with this procedure.

TRANSPERINEAL APPROACH. The patient is placed in the lithotomy or lateral position. The procedure may be performed with the patient under general, regional, or local anesthesia. The examining finger is inserted into the rectum and the induration identified. The needle is inserted through the perineal skin and guided ahead until the tip is against the lesion. The biopsy specimen is taken in the same fashion as described for the transrectal approach. Some surgeons may incise

## BEST PRACTICE

### Diagnosing and Managing Prostate Cancer

Early detection is important in the diagnosis and management of prostate cancer. Information relating to a patient's profile in initiating the algorithm (see p. 500) includes the following.

**RISK FACTORS**

1. Age: After 50 years old, the risk increases rapidly, with the incidence at 75 years old 30% more than at 50 years old. Although the lifetime risk for prostate cancer is 12%, it accounts for 27% of all cancer in men and 13% of cancer-related deaths.
2. Race: African American men are at 30% higher risk, and at an earlier age, than men of other ethnicities.
3. Diet: High dietary fat is associated with a greater risk for developing cancer.
4. Family history: risk is increased for men who have first-degree relatives with prostate cancer.

**CANDIDATES FOR EARLY DETECTION**

1. Men 50 years old or older with a life expectancy of 10 years or longer. A man older than 50 years has a 20% risk of prostate cancer if his prostate-specific antigen (PSA) is between 4 and 10 ng/dl.
2. Men 40 years old or older with a family history of prostate cancer or African American ethnicity.

**DIAGNOSTIC MEASURES USED IN COMBINATION FOR EARLY DETECTION**

1. Digital rectal examination (DRE)
2. Serum PSA*
3. Biopsy if indicated (three of four men undergoing biopsy will not have cancer)

Modified from American Urological Association, Inc (AUA): Prostate-specific antigen (PSA) best practice policy, *Oncology* 14(2). Accessed February 2002, on-line: www.cancernetwork.com/journals/oncology; Eastham JA: Variations of serum prostate-specific antigen levels: an evaluation of year-to-year fluctuations, *JAMA: The Journal of the American Medical Association* 289:2695-2700, 2003; Partin AW and others: Contemporary update of prostate cancer staging nomograms (Partin tables) for the new millennium, *Urology* 58(6):843-848; Dec. 2001; PSA scale/Partin table, 2003, UAB Health System. Accessed June 2005; on-line: http://www.health.uab.edu/kirklin.

*When total PSA is more than 4 ng/dl, a free prostatic antigen is useful in predicting the likelihood of cancer. PSA is a glycoprotein produced by both normal and cancerous prostate tissue; one component binds to plasma protein, and the other is in a free state. Patients with prostate cancer tend to have lower free/total ratios and men with benign prostatic hyperplasia (BPH) have high free/total ratios. Of men who have prostate cancers currently detected, 75% have abnormal PSAs. Consideration of 30 days of antibiotic therapy followed by repeat PSA before proceeding with biopsy is valid under certain conditions.

*Continued*

## BEST PRACTICE

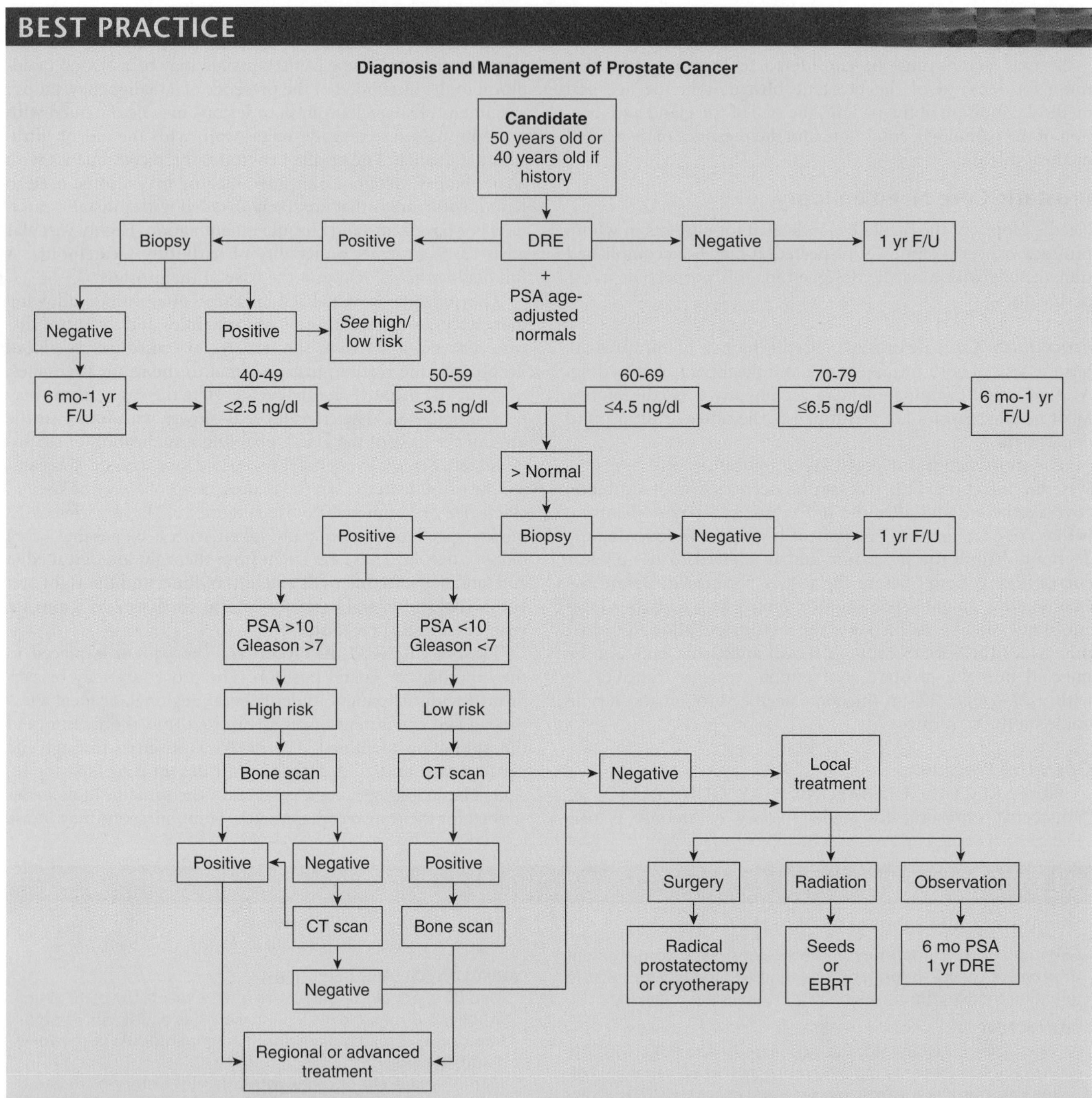


Algorithm modified from Antenor JAV and others: Relationship between initial prostate specific antigen level and subsequent prostate cancer detection in a longitudinal screening study, *Journal of Urology* 172(1):90-93, 2004; Albertsen PC and others: Twenty-year outcomes following conservative management of clinically localized prostate cancer, *JAMA: The Journal of the American Medical Association* 293:2095-2101, 2005; Sang JM, Marshburn J: Clinical practice guidelines for prostate cancer, *Cancer Control: Journal of the Moffitt Cancer Center* 3(6):526-530, 1996. Accessed June 2005, on-line: www.moffitt.usf.edu; Thompson IM and others: Operating characteristics of prostate-specific antigen in men with an initial PSA level of 3.0 ng/ml or lower, *JAMA: The Journal of the American Medical Association* 294:66-70, 2005.

*CT,* Computed tomography; *DRE,* digital rectal examination; *EBRT,* external beam radiation therapy; *F/U,* follow-up; *ng/dl,* nanograms/deciliter; *PSA,* prostate-specific antigen.

the site with the #11 or #15 scalpel and place a 4-0 absorbable closing suture.

Another transperineal approach is to perform template biopsies with ultrasound guidance, utilizing the brachytherapy (seed implant) template. The patient is placed in the lithotomy position, and the scrotum is secured toward the abdomen with a transparent adhesive dressing. The brachytherapy grid, template fixation device, and probe with cradle are positioned adjacent to the perineum. The perineum is prepped and draped according to facility protocol. The prostate is measured and total volume

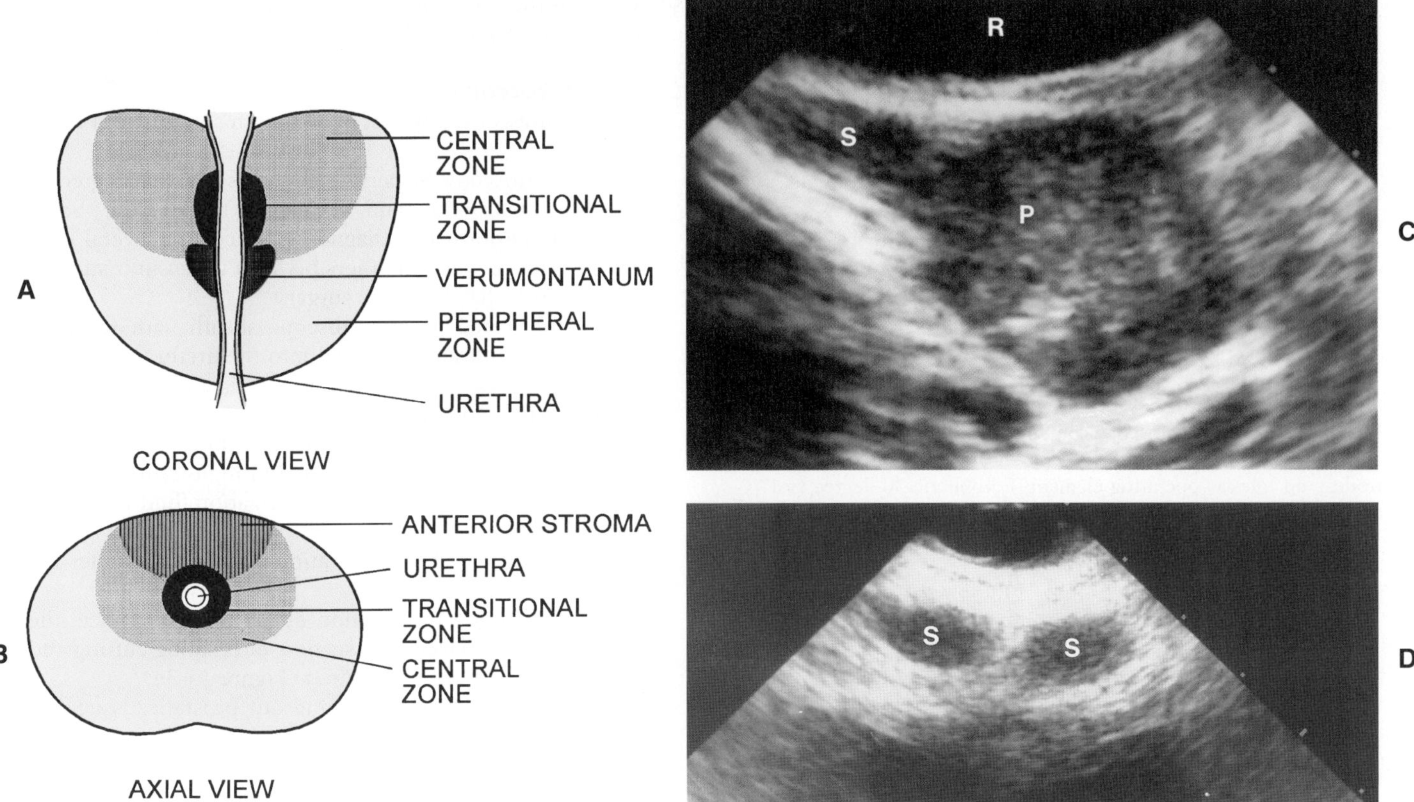


**FIGURE 15-31** Schematic drawing of zonal anatomy of the prostate (*nonshaded area* is peripheral zone). **A,** Coronal view. **B,** Axial view and transrectal ultrasound views of prostate during biopsy. **C,** Sagittal image showing prostate *(P)*, seminal vesicles *(S)*, and rectum *(R)*. **D,** Transverse image of seminal vesicles *(S)*.

calculated using the ultrasonic transrectal transducer. Biopsies are then obtained transperineally through the template grid.

## Transurethral Resection of the Prostate Gland

In transurethral resection of the prostate gland, a resectoscope is passed into the bladder through the urethra and successive pieces of tissue are resected from around the bladder neck and the lobes of the prostate gland, leaving the capsule intact. The resectoscope uses a stabilized cutting loop to resect tissue and coagulate blood vessels by means of electric current. The electric current that powers the electrode is supplied by a high-frequency ESU. The current settings are specified by the urologist, who activates the cutting or coagulating current with a foot pedal during the course of the procedure.

TURP is one surgical method of treating benign obstructive enlargement of the prostate gland. Several factors influence the surgical approach: size of the gland and location of the pathologic condition, age and condition of the patient, and presence of associated diseases.

***Procedural Considerations.*** The instrument setup for TURP is as described for cystoscopy with additional necessary instruments. The four principal types of resectoscopes are McCarthy, Nesbit, Iglesias, and Baumrucker. Adult resectoscopes range in size from 24 Fr to 28 Fr and have the following components: Foroblique telescope, operating element, cutting loops, and postresectoscope sheaths and obturators (Figure 15-32). A TURP requires a resectoscope (multiple working elements); a Foroblique telescope as well as a backup telescope; stabilized or unstabilized cutting loops; a postresectoscope sheath with its corresponding articulated obturator; a high-frequency cord; a short bridge; a Toomey syringe or the Ellik or Urovac evacuator; Van Buren sounds; a 22-Fr or 24-Fr, 30-ml, three-way Foley catheter; a disposable urologic drape with rectal sheath; and a system for continuous bladder irrigation and urinary drainage. Supplementary instruments include a resectoscope adapter and a lateral telescope.

The continuous-flow resectoscope (CFR) (Figure 15-33) has unique components that include an outlet stop cock to which a suction tube is attached, an inflow tube on the inner sheath, and outflow holes on the outer sheath. These features enable the urologist to resect tissue without interruption to empty the bladder, as must be done with the standard resectoscope. In addition to the CFR, which replaces the standard resectoscope, the setup includes thick-walled Silastic suction tubing and a continuous-flow pump. The continuous-flow technique decreases intravesical pressure on the bladder during the procedure, provides a clearer field of vision because of the constant inflow and outflow of irrigant, reduces the operating time because the resection process need not be interrupted to evacuate the bladder, and provides a "still" bladder for the resection of bladder tumors.

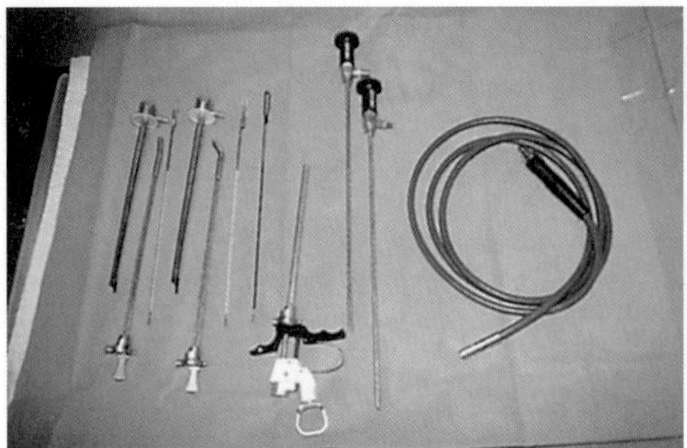

**FIGURE 15-32** Resectoscope components: 24-Fr and 26-Fr Timberlake obturators and postresectoscope sheaths with fulgurating electrodes and Iglesias operating element, Foroblique 30-degree and 70-degree telescopes, and fiberoptic cable.

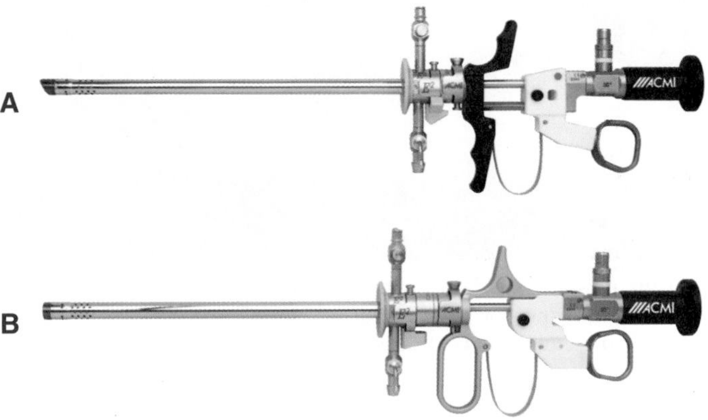


**FIGURE 15-33** **A,** Continuous-flow resectoscope (CFR). **B,** Vista CFR bipolar resectoscope.

A continuous flow of isotonic and nonelectrolytic irrigating fluid is necessary to ensure transmission of electrical current and clear visualization throughout surgery. Irrigating solution such as 3% sorbitol or 1.5% glycine, 3 to 5 liters, may be connected in tandem to provide a constant flow. Warming units, available for these solutions, help to eliminate the hypothermia often experienced when large amounts of cold irrigants are employed. On the other hand, when solutions are warm, the patient may show a tendency to bleed more. At all times perioperative nursing personnel must be alert to replace the irrigation solution as required.

During transurethral prostatic surgery, return of irrigation fluid must be monitored because intravasation and absorption of fluid into open prostatic venous sinuses or bladder perforation may occur. The perioperative nurse should be aware of the early signs and symptoms and measures employed to remedy these complications.[11,25,41] The patient usually experiences significant respiratory changes and abdominal discomfort. Other important observations are rigidity and swelling of the lower abdomen, coupled with changes in sensorium. If extravasation of irrigating fluid is evident, the surgical procedure is discontinued and a cystogram is obtained immediately to determine if bladder perforation has occurred. Insertion of a Foley catheter is generally all that is necessary to control the situation. In the rare instance of a major perforation, surgical closure may be accomplished through a cystotomy incision.

### *Operative Procedure*

1. The urethra is usually first dilated with sounds from 20 Fr to 30 Fr.
2. Cystourethroscopy is performed to assess the degree of prostatic obstruction and to inspect the bladder. Some urologists perform this diagnostic procedure several days before surgery, whereas others perform the examination in the OR immediately before surgery.
3. A well-lubricated postresectoscope sheath with its fitted Timberlake obturator is passed into the urethra.
4. The Timberlake obturator is removed, and the working element (resectoscope), assembled with the Foroblique telescope and cutting loop, is inserted through the sheath.
5. The irrigation tubing, light cord, and high-frequency cord are appropriately connected, and irrigation fluid is allowed to fill the bladder.
6. Initial inspection of the prostatic urethra and bladder trigone is carried out.
7. After determining the location of the ureteral orifice, the urologist initiates electrodissection, alternating cutting and coagulating currents as required (Figure 15-34).
8. The bladder is drained, washing out prostatic tissue and small blood clots. At times it is necessary to employ the Ellik evacuator to remove resected prostatic tissue. To do this the urologist must remove the working element of the resectoscope. The nozzle of the evacuator is fitted onto the resectoscope sheath, and by manual pulsatile pressure the bladder contents are removed. An Ellik or Urovac evacuator or Toomey syringe should be readily available for manual irrigation. Fluid may be drawn from the irrigant directly into the resectoscope sheath through the already attached tubing.
9. When the resection is completed, the prostatic fossa is inspected to ensure that all bleeding points have been coagulated.
10. The resectoscope is then removed, and a Foley catheter (22-Fr or 24-Fr, two-way or three-way, 30-ml balloon) is inserted into the bladder for urinary drainage. The balloon is inflated (Figure 15-35, *A*), pulled gently in traction against the bladder neck, and secured, to help control venous bleeding (Figure 15-35, *B*). The Foley balloon must not be inflated within the prostatic fossa (Figure 15-35, *C*), where it may cause excessive bleeding from the resected prostatic capsule. If desired, continuous irrigation with gravity drainage is initiated, with normal saline as the bladder irrigant instead of sorbitol or glycine. A 3-liter to 4-liter urinary drainage system is suggested to avoid frequent emptying of the drainage bag.
11. When VLAP, TUIP, or TULIP is performed, the surgeon may choose to place a standard 18-Fr Foley with a 5-ml or 30-ml balloon connected to straight drainage. If irrigation is required postoperatively, it is then performed manually with sterile solution and a Toomey syringe.

## Transurethral Incision of the Prostate

TUIP is a procedure in which the prostate is incised at the 5 and 7 o'clock positions to provide relief of obstruction, with results similar to those provided by a complete transurethral

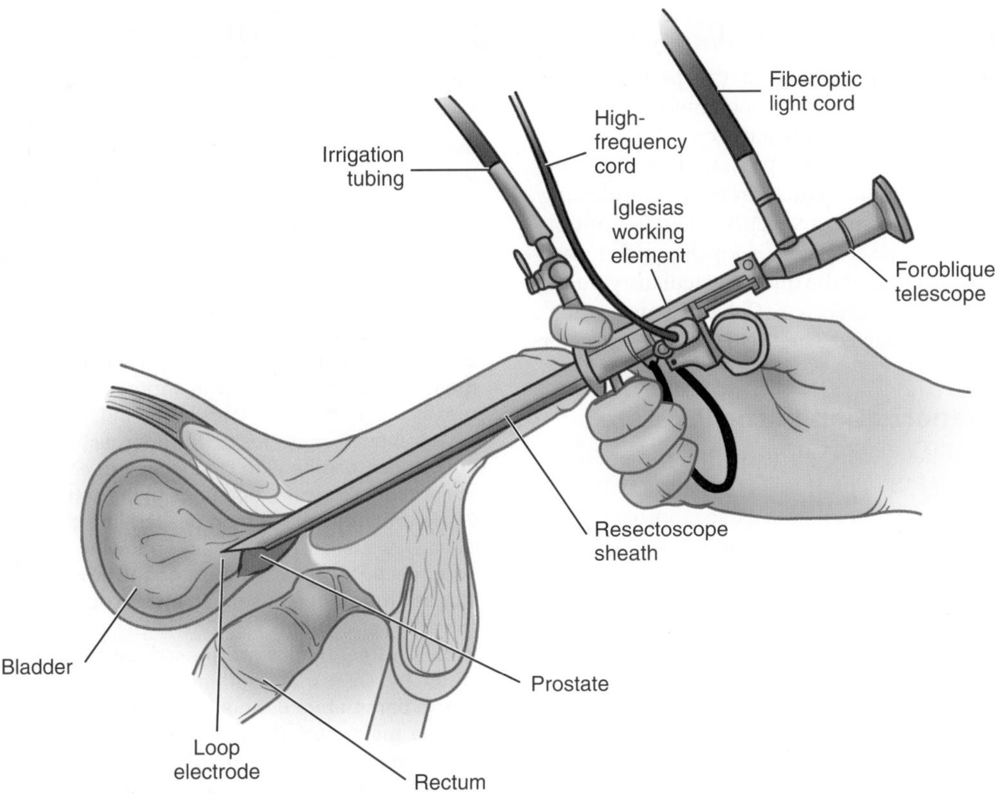


**FIGURE 15-34** Sectional view illustrating removal of portion of hypertrophied middle lobe of prostate gland with Iglesias resectoscope.

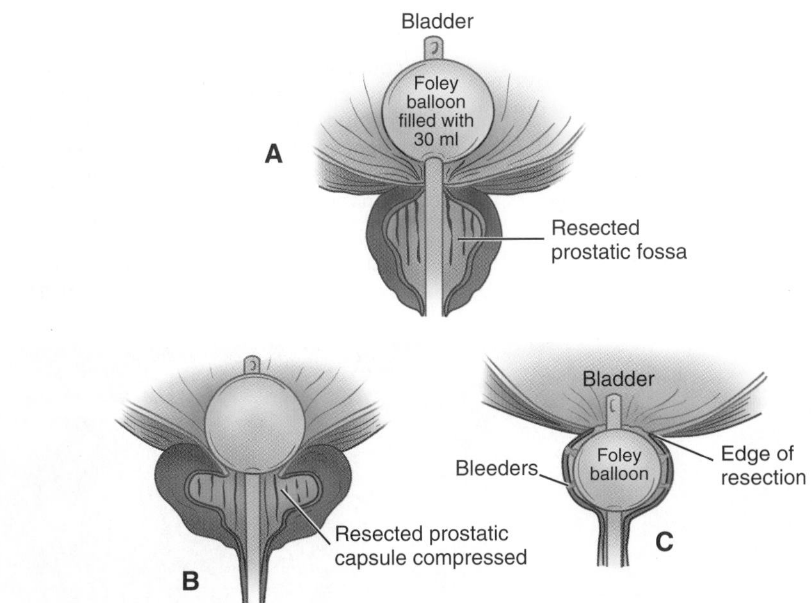


**FIGURE 15-35** **A** and **B**, Proper position for Foley catheter with inflated balloon beyond prostatic capsule. **C**, Improper position.

resection but with a lower incidence of bladder neck contracture and retrograde ejaculation. The shorter operative time inherent with the procedure minimizes fluid absorption and may decrease postoperative pulmonary and cardiovascular complications. The procedure may be performed with cold or hot knives as well as the standard resectoscope, or laser fiber (TULIP).[26] This procedure is appropriate for sexually active patients with moderate to small obstructive prostates without a significant middle-lobe component. One major disadvantage is the potential for missing occult prostatic cancer. Despite this, some clinicians view this as an underused, feasible form of treatment.

## Transurethral Incision of the Ejaculatory Ducts

Transurethral incision of the ejaculatory ducts is performed for the relief of obstructed ejaculatory ducts, a common condition in men with chronic prostatitis and prostatic calculi (Research Highlight). Symptoms closely mimic prostatodynia and include aching in the perineal and genital areas with no lasting or significant improvement from conservative therapy (antibiotics and analgesics). The resectoscope loop is guided with transrectal ultrasound imaging to the dilated ejaculatory ducts, and the obstructed ducts are resected. Calculi may be fragmented if necessary and removed (Figure 15-36). A catheter generally is not needed.

## Photoselective Vaporization of the Prostate

The KTP laser is now being used to treat BPH or prostatic enlargement. *Green-light PVP* is photoselective vaporization of the prostate and a new minimally invasive approach performed on an outpatient basis. The approach is the same as with other endoscopic techniques. This is the first procedure to challenge the "gold standard": TURP.[18] A noncontact laser fiber is used to heat the prostate tissue and rapidly vaporize it to a penetration depth of 0.8 mm with minimal to no blood loss. Vaporization occurs from within the tissues where the collagen matrix eventually bursts as a result of the vapor buildup. The laser is operated in a continuous wave mode and induces a coagulation zone of only 1 to 2 mm in thickness. This prevents the excessive sloughing of necrotic tissue. The patient may not always need a Foley catheter following the procedure.

## Interstitial Laser Coagulation of the Prostate (Indigo)

Interstitial laser coagulation (ILC) with the Indigo laser is a minimally invasive procedure for treatment of urinary outflow obstruction secondary to BPH.[26] It is indicated for men older than 50 years with a median or lateral prostatic lobe volume of 20 to 85 ml. Designed for those men who wish to minimize the risk for incontinence and impotence found with conventional TURP, this procedure is now performed in the office setting about 80% of the time.

## RESEARCH HIGHLIGHT

### Treatment of Seminal Vesicle Stones

Seminal vesicle stones frequently present with hematospermia, testicular or perineal pain, painful ejaculation, and infertility. Diagnosis is confirmed by means of radiologic (x-ray and magnetic resonance imaging [MRI]) and ultrasound examination. The condition usually occurs within seminal cysts in men older than 40 years old and is often accompanied by seminal vesiculitis. In a study by Yang and others 16.2% of patients presenting with hematospermia had seminal vesicle calculi.

Open vesiculectomy and transurethral resection of the ejaculatory ducts have been the traditional methods of treatment for removal. A newer approach, endoscopic stone removal through the utricular opening, is a viable alternative that prevents organ loss. The approach, described by Ozgok and others, begins with cystoscopy to confirm the location of the prostatic utricular openings to the seminal ducts. A flexible 6.9-Fr ureteroscope is then passed into the utricular orifice to directly visualize the stones. Following this, a rigid, 15.5-Fr ureteroscope is inserted through the now dilated openings. All stones are removed using an endoscopic grasper. An indwelling urethral catheter remains in place for 1 week postoperatively and antibiotics are prescribed for 10 days. In the case study by Ozgok and others, the patient exhibited normal sperm parameters 6 months postoperatively.

The major reason for removal of the seminal vesicle is a secondary pathologic condition. All the open methods employed carry certain caveats with them and require a significant incision to access the seminal vesicle. Recent methods by means of endoscopy and laparoscopy may overcome some of the obstacles presented with the open techniques. In the study presented, a cystoscope was used because of the already enlarged utricular openings. In a patient who has not previously been treated, a 5-Fr ureteroscope with a working channel could be successfully used. Expertise in unroofing the ejaculatory ducts and transurethral resection is necessary for the method. One risk is postoperative urinary reflux and consequent epididymitis, however. Despite the inherent risk of postoperative sequelae, this is a viable, less invasive alternative to standard therapies.

Modified from Ozgok Y and others: Endoscopic seminal vesicle stone removal, *Urology* 65(3), 2005; Yang SC and others: Transutricular seminal vesiculoscopy, *Journal of Endourology* 16:343-345, 2002.

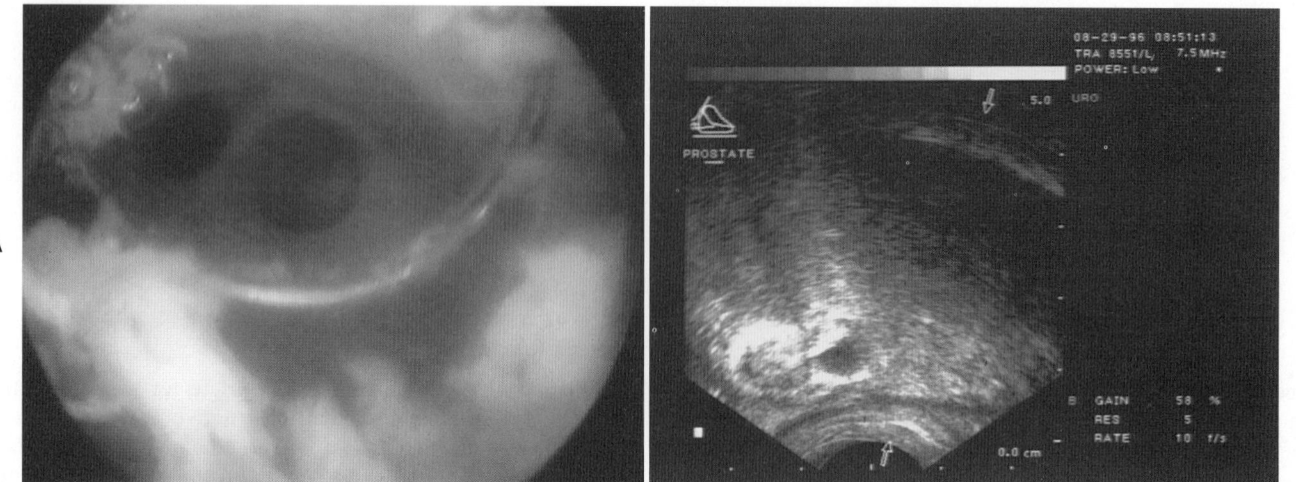


**FIGURE 15-36** **A,** Dilated seminal vesicle (ejaculatory duct) with resectoscope loop approaching. **B,** Resectoscope loop entering dilated seminal vesicle (ejaculatory duct).

The procedure is contraindicated for the treatment of prostate cancer and for those patients who had previous brachytherapy with radioactive seeds. However, some physicians may elect to perform ILC before brachytherapy (or cryotherapy) in the hopes of minimizing, if not relieving, the postoperative voiding symptoms associated with these more definitive treatments.

*Procedural Considerations.* The patient is placed in the lithotomy position and prepped as for cystoscopy. An optional local anesthetic with oral or monitored IV sedation is generally adequate. Oral sedation is used more commonly with the office-based procedure; if the surgery takes place in the hospital or ambulatory center, monitored IV sedation may be used. An ultrasound machine with transrectal capability is often used to measure the size of the prostate gland and determine the appropriate number of laser applications (sticks). Some surgeons choose to measure by cystoscopy alone.

The setup includes a 17-Fr or 23-Fr panendoscope and 30-degree fiberoptic lens, ultrasound and transrectal transducer, and the Indigo laser machine with laser fiber (Figure 15-37). The fiber has graduated black depth markings used to guide placement into the prostate gland. The laser machine automatically times each "stick" for 2 minutes, 30 seconds.

*Operative Procedure*

1. The transrectal transducer is inserted, and the prostatic volume is measured. (This may have been performed as an office procedure preoperatively.) Local anesthetic may be injected through the transducer guide pin with an 8-inch spinal needle or with the 8-inch Collagen injection needle if ultrasound is not employed.
2. Cystoscopy is performed, and the prostatic urethra is evaluated.
3. The laser fiber is introduced through the panendoscope and passed into the lateral lobe of the prostate gland through the urethral wall to the desired depth.
4. This is repeated one to three times on each side, depending on the measured prostatic volume.
5. A TUIP may be performed utilizing the bare-tip fiber (Figure 15-38).
6. A 16-Fr or 18-Fr urethral catheter is inserted and connected to straight drainage. A 16-Fr suprapubic Foley catheter may also be employed and attached to irrigation or drainage.

### Transurethral Microwave Therapy/ Transurethral Needle Ablation

TUMT is a minimally invasive method of applying heat to the prostate gland for the relief of the symptoms associated with BPH and bladder-outlet obstruction. TUMT maintains temperatures in the urethra, sphincter, and rectum at a level that is physiologically safe while heating the tissue deep within the transitional zone of the prostate. A water-cooled catheter is combined with microwave radiation to the lobes of the prostate. This treatment is an office-based procedure.

Transurethral needle ablation (TUNA) is also a minimally invasive office procedure for the treatment of BPH of the median and lateral lobes. This technique delivers radiofrequency (RF) energy through two electrodes that are embedded in a special urethral catheter. Specific target areas of the prostate are thermally ablated by the RF energy and combined inductive heating of water molecules, leaving the urethra and the remainder of the prostate intact.

### Simple Retropubic Prostatectomy

Simple retropubic prostatectomy is the enucleation of hypertrophic prostatic tissue through an incision in the anterior prostatic capsule by an extravesical approach. The retropubic approach offers excellent exposure of the prostate bed and vesical neck and readily controllable intraoperative and postoperative bleeding.

A preoperative bowel prep and antibiotic therapy are the standard of care for all open prostatectomies.

*Procedural Considerations.* The patient is placed in a slight Trendelenburg position with the pelvis elevated and the legs slightly abducted. Routine skin prep is carried out. Electrocoagulation is usually employed. Although the draping proce-

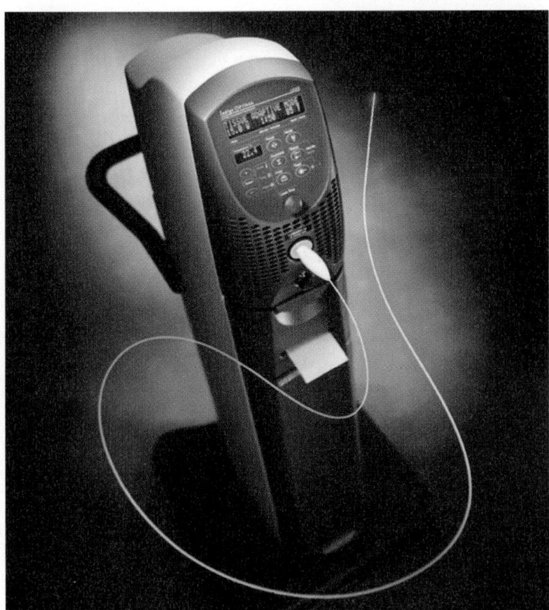

**FIGURE 15-37** Indigo Optima Laser unit with diffuser-tip fiber.

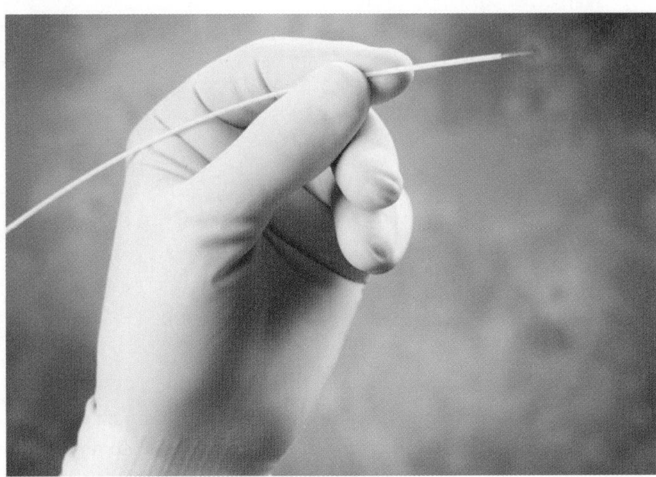

**FIGURE 15-38** Indigo bare-tip laser fiber.

dure must conform to individual OR policies, the following procedure is suggested for draping the patient:

1. The first towel, with a cuff, is placed under the scrotum.
2. The next three towels are placed around the lower abdominal incision site, followed by a sterile laparotomy sheet.
3. A fifth towel, folded in half, is placed over the penis and scrotum below the retropubic incision site and secured with two nonperforating towel clamps.

The instrument setup includes a basic laparotomy set and bladder and prostatic instruments (Figures 15-39 and 15-40). The following supplies should be readily available: Jackson-Pratt drains; water-soluble lubricant; Toomey and Asepto syringes; urinary drainage system; 20-Fr, 5-ml Foley catheter; 22-Fr or 24-Fr, 30-ml Foley catheter; 10-ml and 30-ml syringes, and a self-retaining retractor such as the adjustable Omni-Tract Surgical UO400 Urology Retractor System (Figure 15-41).

### *Operative Procedure*

1. A 20-Fr or 22-Fr Foley catheter with 30-ml balloon is inserted into the urethra and through the bladder neck and inflated within the bladder. This is clamped and maintained within the sterile field. Frequently, a three-way catheter is used for continuous bladder irrigation.
2. Through a Pfannenstiel or low vertical midline incision, the anterior rectus sheath is incised along with portions of the internal and external oblique muscles.
3. The rectus abdominis muscles are retracted laterally to expose the space of Retzius.
4. After placement of traction sutures, the anterior portion of the prostatic capsule is incised transversely (Figure 15-42, *A*).
5. The prostatic adenoma may be dissected or finger-enucleated from the surgical capsule (Figure 15-42, *B*).
6. Care is taken to place hemostatic sutures at the 5 and 7 o'clock positions, encompassing the vesical neck and prostatic capsule, to ligate the primary blood supply to the prostate. Other bleeding points within the capsule may be suture-ligated with 2-0 absorbable sutures.
7. The prostatic capsule incision is closed with either a continuous or an interrupted 0 absorbable suture (Figure 15-42, *C*).
8. A drain is placed in the space of Retzius and brought out through the fascia and skin through a separate stab incision.

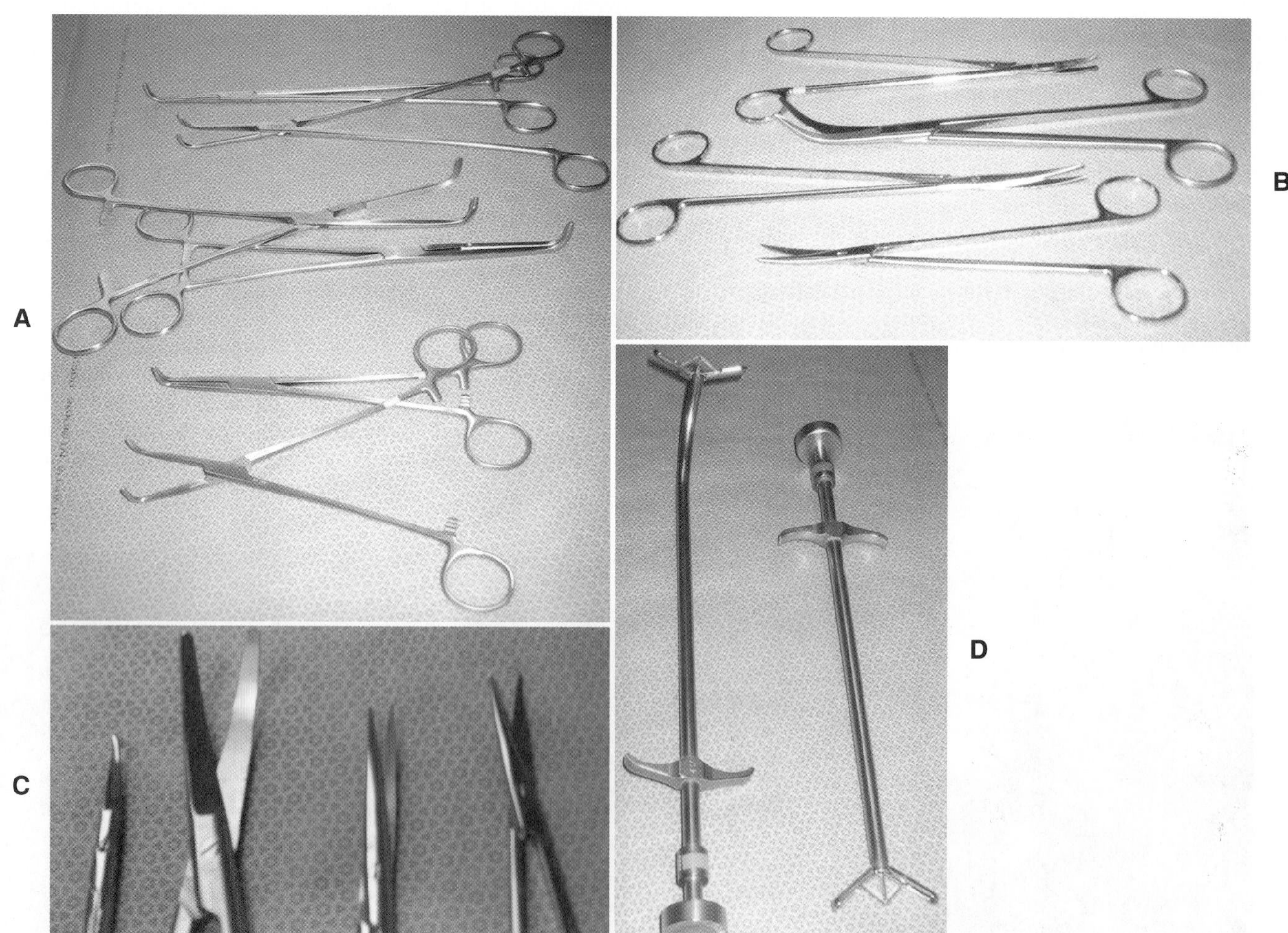


**FIGURE 15-39** **A,** Right-angle (Mixter) clamps in various tip lengths. **B,** Scissors *(top to bottom):* Strully, curved Jorgenson, long sharp-tip Metzenbaum, standard sharp-tip Metzenbaum. **C,** Same scissor tips, *left to right.* **D,** Curved and straight Lowsley tractors in open position.

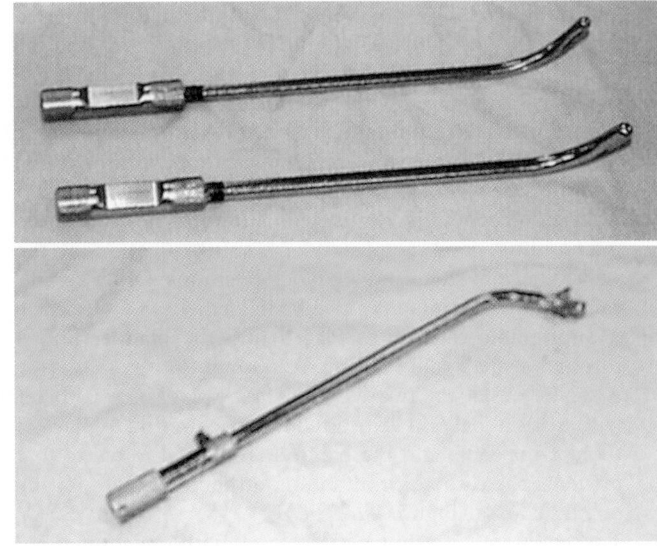

FIGURE 15-40 **A,** Urethral suture guides. **B,** Roth grip-tip urethral suture guide.

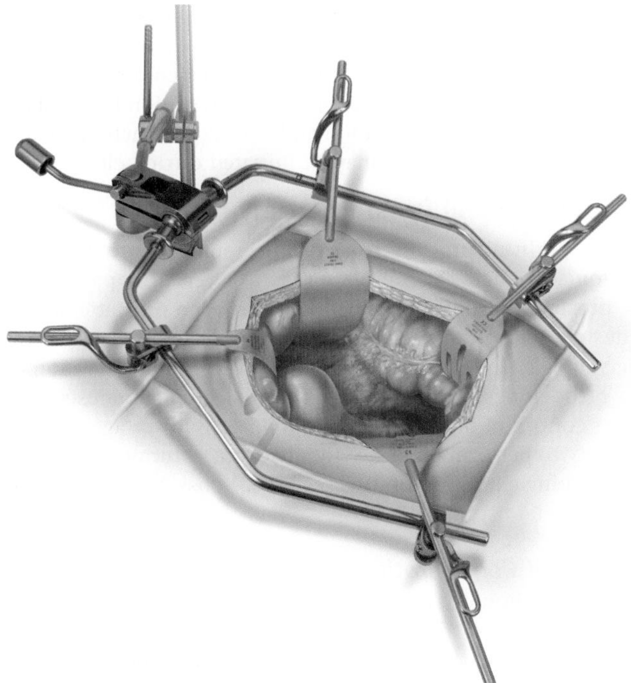

FIGURE 15-41 Adjustable Omni-Tract Surgical UO400 Urology Retractor System.

9. The abdominal incision is then closed in layers, and the wound is dressed.
10. If continuous bladder irrigation is to be used, normal saline solution irrigation is initiated through a 3-liter closed irrigation system.

## Suprapubic Prostatectomy

Suprapubic prostatectomy is the removal, through a transvesical approach, of benign periurethral glandular tissue obstructing the outlet of the urinary tract. A low midline, or Pfannenstiel, incision may be used. One advantage of the suprapubic approach is that it allows access for surgical correction of any existing bladder condition such as vesical calculi or vesical diverticula. Control of bleeding is a major consideration in any prostatectomy and is one disadvantage of the suprapubic approach. Because the prostate is located beneath the symphysis pubis, ligation of bleeding capsular vessels is difficult. However, control of hemorrhage and replacement of blood loss, coupled with skilled perioperative nursing care and early mobilization of the patient, have greatly minimized complications.

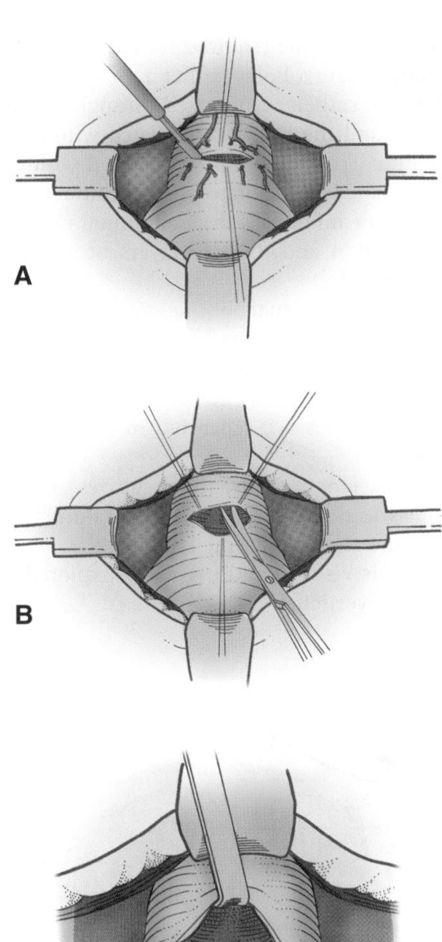

FIGURE 15-42 Retropubic prostatectomy.

***Procedural Considerations.*** Spinal, epidural, or general anesthesia may be selected for anesthesia for patients having a suprapubic prostatectomy, depending on their medical condition. The patient is placed in a slight Trendelenburg position with the umbilicus elevated and the legs slightly abducted. Skin prep, draping, and instrumentation are as described for retropubic prostatectomy.

***Operative Procedure.*** Bilateral vasectomy may be performed to decrease the postoperative incidence of epididymoorchitis.

A meatotomy may also be required if the penile meatus is too small to accommodate a Foley catheter.

1. A 20-Fr Foley catheter is inserted through the urethra into the bladder, and the bladder is inflated with a preferred irrigating fluid. The catheter is maintained within the sterile field. This maneuver facilitates identification of the bladder.
2. A transverse or midline lower abdominal incision is made through the skin and the two layers of superficial fascia (Figure 15-43, *A*).
3. The external and internal oblique muscles are cut along the lines of the original incision.
4. Bleeding vessels are clamped, coagulated, or tied with fine absorbable ties.
5. The rectus muscles are separated in the midline and retracted laterally.
6. After the placement of traction sutures, the bladder is opened at the dome with a scalpel. Liquid contents are aspirated, and the bladder incision is enlarged.
7. The bladder is visually and manually explored for calculi, a tumor, or diverticula.

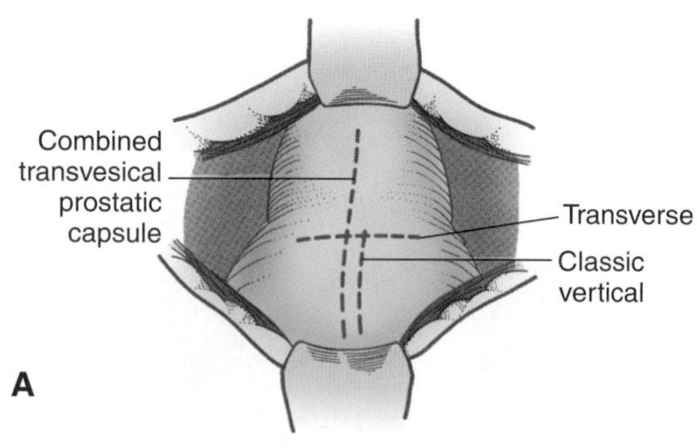


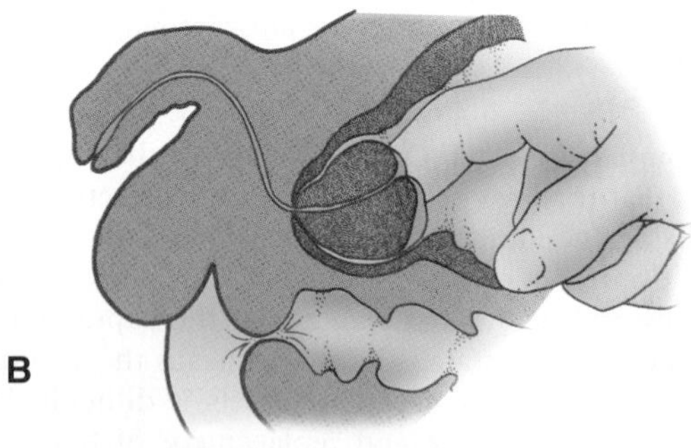


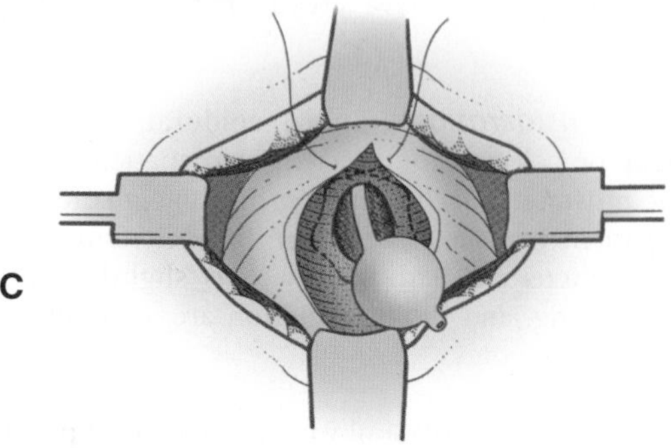


**FIGURE 15-43** Suprapubic prostatectomy.

8. The tip of the index finger of the operating hand is inserted through the vesical neck into the prostatic urethra, and the adenomatous tissue is enucleated (Figure 15-43, *B*). If difficulty is experienced with the enucleation, a finger may be placed into the rectum to elevate the prostate gland. Aseptic technique is maintained during enucleation with the use of a sterile second glove on the hand used in the rectum.
9. After enucleation is completed, attention is directed to maintaining good hemostasis by suture ligation of the vesical neck at the 5 and 7 o'clock positions. Other significant bleeding points may also be ligated.
10. A suprapubic catheter is placed into the bladder lumen through a small stab incision.
11. A 22-Fr or 24-Fr, two-way or three-way Foley catheter with a 30-ml balloon is inserted into the urethra in place of the original one, and the balloon is inflated to a size that prevents the catheter from falling or being pulled into the prostatic fossa (Figure 15-43, *C*).
12. The cystotomy incision is then closed with interrupted 2-0 absorbable sutures.
13. A drain is left along the cystotomy incision, brought out through a separate stab wound, and secured to the skin with a silk suture.
14. The muscles, fascia, and subcutaneous tissues are closed in layers, and a dressing is applied.
15. Normal saline irrigation solution may be connected to the Foley catheter to provide continuous irrigation to the bladder to reduce clot formation and maintain catheter patency. Continuous irrigation may be initiated during closure.

## Simple Perineal Prostatectomy

Simple perineal prostatectomy is the removal of a prostatic adenoma through a perineal approach. A perineal approach to the prostate gland is most suitable when open prostatic biopsy is desired and, after receipt of pathologic confirmation, radical excision is to follow. Other advantages include preservation of the bladder neck, improved urethrovesical anastomosis, and easier control of bleeding. Some surgical disadvantages are (1) inability to perform biopsy of the iliac and obturator nodes for determining extension of disease and (2) possible formation of urethrorectal fistulas.

***Procedural Considerations.*** The patient is placed in an exaggerated lithotomy position with the legs above the level of the pelvis (Figure 15-44). A bolster beneath the sacrum allows the perineum to be as parallel to the OR bed as possible, with the buttocks extending several inches over the bed edge.[6] Stirrups should be well padded to protect the popliteal fossa. Sequential compression stockings are recommended to assist peripheral vascular flow. The patient is often placed in a steep Trendelenburg position. Well-padded shoulder braces, placed over the acromial processes in a manner to prevent stretch or pressure injury, may be required to prevent the patient from sliding upward on the bed. It is preferable if these can be avoided. Routine skin preparation is carried out and includes an interior rectal prep. Special draping is as follows:

1. A towel folded in half is placed over the pubic area.
2. Two towels with a cuff are placed on either side of the perineum.
3. Two leggings, with points down, are placed over the legs.
4. One impervious drape is placed over the anus.

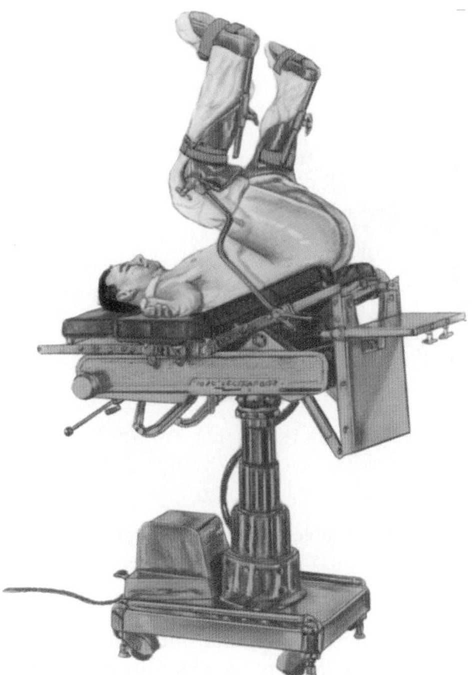

**FIGURE 15-44** Exaggerated lithotomy position for perineal prostatectomy.

5. A large sheet fully opened with a large cuff is placed across from one stirrup to the other and secured by towel clamps.
6. A laparotomy sheet follows, with the short end to the floor.

The instrument setup is as described for suprapubic prostatectomy, omitting abdominal self-retaining retractors and adding straight and curved Lowsley tractors (Figure 15-45), Roux retractors, Jackson retractors with short and long blades, Doyen vaginal retractors, Young retractor, perineal prostatic retractors (Figure 15-46), Sauerbruch retractors, and a narrow and wide self-retaining perineal retractor, such as the Thompson retractor or the Omni-Tract Surgical UO100 Pelvic Retractor System (Figure 15-47).

### Operative Procedure

1. A curved Lowsley tractor is placed through the urethra into the bladder and held back by the surgical assistant, causing the prostate to be pushed down toward the perineum.
2. An inverted U-shaped incision is made from one ischial tuberosity to another, curving just anteriorly to the anus (Figure 15-48, *A*).
3. Three Martius or Allis clamps are secured to the posterior edge of the incision and retracted downward, over the anal drape.
4. Subcutaneous bleeders are clamped with straight mosquitoes and coagulated or tied with 3-0 absorbable ligatures.
5. The central tendon is isolated, clamped, and cut distally to the external anal sphincter (Figure 15-48, *B*).
6. The rectourethral muscle is incised and pushed downward from the central tendon.
7. The levator ani muscle is exposed and retracted laterally (Figure 15-48, *C*).
8. The prostate gland is exposed. Biopsy of the prostate may be performed for pathologic confirmation. If the results are negative, the prostatic adenoma is removed. If the frozen section reveals malignancy, a radical prostatectomy may be done at this time.
9. If simple enucleation is to be performed, the prostatic capsule is incised and the Lowsley tractor is removed (Figure 15-48, *D*).
10. The urethra is divided, and the Young prostatic retractor is inserted.
11. The blades are opened, drawing the prostate down, and the adenoma is manually enucleated from the surgical capsule.
12. A 22-Fr Foley catheter with a 30-ml balloon is inserted through the urethra into the bladder.

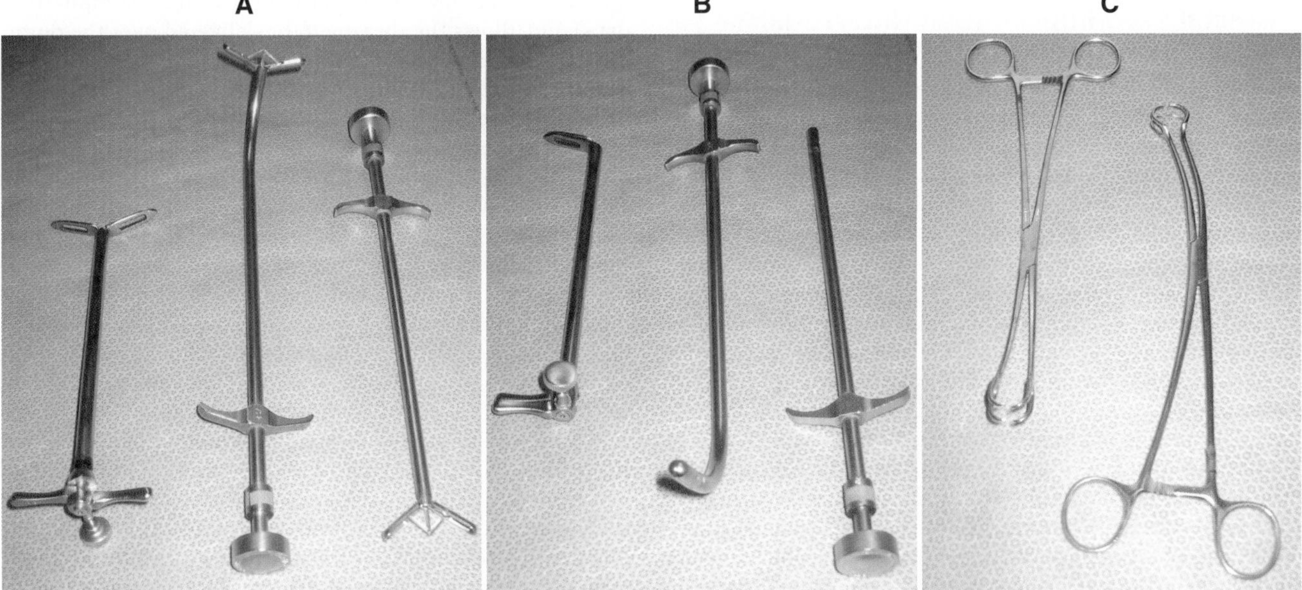


**FIGURE 15-45** Young, curved Lowsley, and straight Lowsley "tractors" in open **(A)** and closed **(B)** positions. **C,** Curved double-prong prostate clamps.

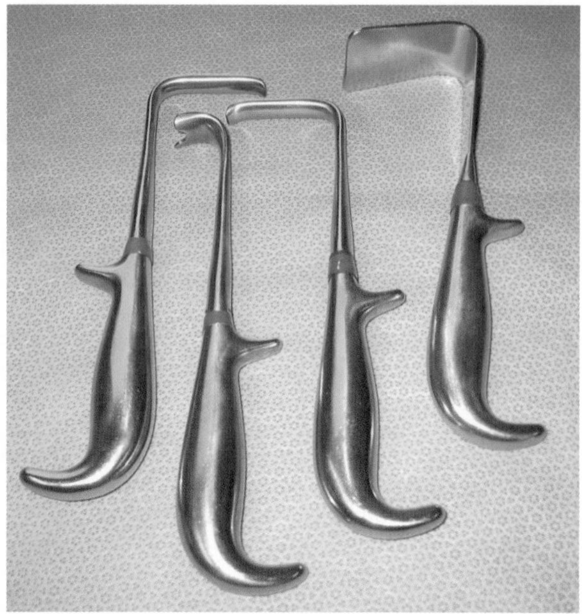

**FIGURE 15-46** Lateral, bulb, and anterior perineal prostatectomy retractors.

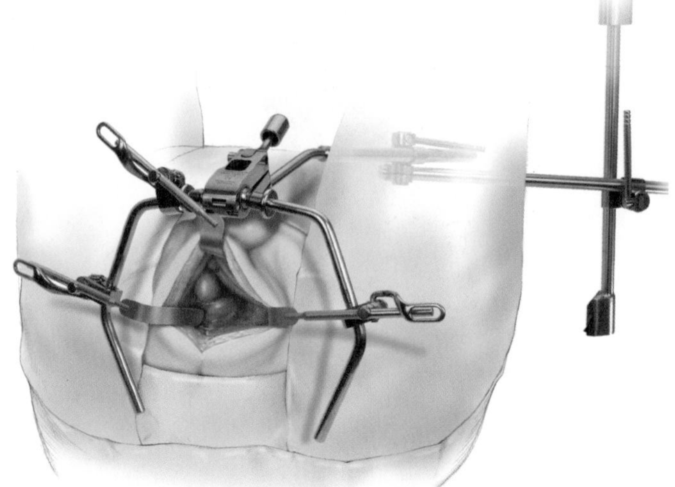

**FIGURE 15-47** Adjustable Omni-Tract Surgical UO100 Pelvic Retractor System.

13. Bleeding is controlled at the 5 and 7 o'clock positions.
14. The capsulotomy incision is repaired with a continuous 2-0 absorbable suture (Figure 15-48, *E*).
15. A drain is left in place at the level of the capsulotomy incision.
16. The subcutaneous tissue is reapproximated with 3-0 absorbable suture.
17. The skin incision is reapproximated with 4-0 absorbable subcutaneous sutures.
18. The wound is dressed according to the surgeon's preference and taped or held with a supportive device, such as mesh pants. A vasectomy may be performed before the prostatectomy.

## Transrectal Seed Implantation (Interstitial Radiotherapy with Brachytherapy)

Brachytherapy of the prostate gland is one procedure that validates the necessity of a collaborative, multidisciplinary approach to patient care. The radiation oncologist and medical physicist, in addition to the urologist, are vital to an optimum outcome from the initial planning stage throughout the postoperative surveillance. Preplanning is required to determine the dose of each seed, the spacing necessary between each seed, and the number of seeds required. A template plan is developed preoperatively by using the ultrasound and the probe-anchoring equipment to measure and map the appropriate seed sites within the prostate. This may be accomplished in the surgeon's office, radiology department, or oncology clinic. The implant plan is finalized at the time of surgery.

The facility that offers this treatment must be licensed for "Group 6" with the radioactive materials licensing department of their respective state. Six-year follow-up examinations from multiple institutions indicate a disease-free interval and survival equivalent to the results of radical prostatectomy. If seed implantation is indicated as an adjunct to radiation therapy, it should be performed 3 to 4 weeks after the radiation treatment.

During percutaneous implantation of iodine-125 or palladium-103 seeds, the patient is positioned in the lithotomy position. The prostate is visualized with transrectal ultrasonic imaging, and the midportion of the prostate is located on a transverse image. This location becomes an index for positioning the axial ultrasound plane at the base of the prostate. Approximately 2 to 3 hours should be allowed from start to completion. The procedure is amenable to outpatient management using regional or general anesthesia.

Iodine seeds are commercially available in titanium-encased rods that absorb the electrons. These seeds may be obtained embedded in an absorbable suture that allows them to remain positioned appropriately in relation to themselves and their location within the prostate and minimizes the risk of seed migration. Palladium seeds, not presently available prethreaded, are plated onto a graphite pellet. The pellets are loaded into titanium tubes with a lead marker. The half-life of iodine-125 (60 days) is longer than that of palladium-103 (17 days) and allows the therapy to be delivered over the duration of tumor cell replication, altering the ability of the tumor cells to multiply. Palladium-103 affords a larger dose of radiation in a shorter time interval to more rapidly growing tumors than iodine-125 does.

***Procedural Considerations.*** Percutaneous implantation of radioactive seeds allows the delivery of significantly higher doses of radiotherapy to the prostate than external beam therapy provides. The radius of penetration around each seed is only 5 mm, thus sparing adjacent organs. The typical radiation dose that can be delivered by external beam may be 6500 centigrays (cGy), whereas the dose that can be delivered with implantation of seeds alone is in the range of 12,000 to 16,000 cGy. The patient will be receiving hormone therapy, to shrink the prostate gland, for 3 months before implantation, and some will undergo radiation therapy before implantation. Patients with stage A or stage B prostate cancer are appropriate candidates, and selection is not influenced by a rise in the PSA, biopsy specimens indicative of further involvement, or age.

Intraoperatively there is the danger of implantation into the bladder; implantation too close to the urethra resulting in post-

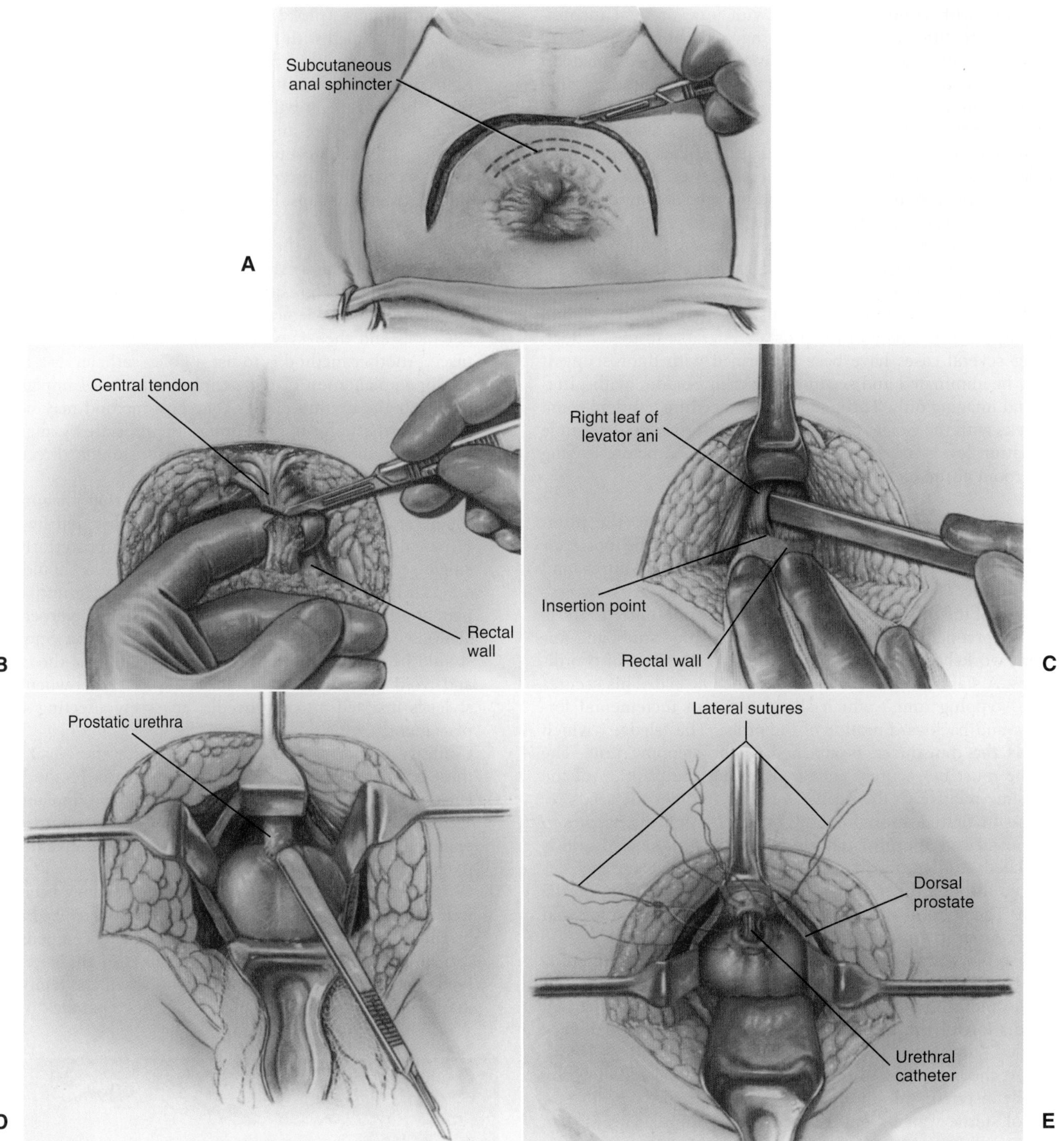


**FIGURE 15-48** Simple perineal prostatectomy.

operative urethral stricture; implantation into the perineum if the needles are withdrawn too quickly; and implantation into the neurovascular bundle, because the anterior venous plexus is not distinguishable from the prostate on CT scan. There is also the chance of migration of seeds, placed just outside the periphery of the gland and in the periprostatic plexus, to the lung. The patient should be cautioned to avoid extended contact with and keep a 6-foot distance from children and pregnant females for 2 months. Urine must be strained, and any seeds expelled should be retrieved and returned to the oncologist. Body wastes are not considered hazardous, however.

Bleeding from the percutaneous sites is minimal, but postoperative ecchymosis of the perineum is to be expected. Other postoperative complications that may occur in the first 12 months include acute cystitis, prostatitis, and urinary retention. After 12 months, chronic prostatitis with cystitis, urethral stricture with contracture, stress with urge or total incontinence, proctitis, and impotence have been documented.[54] Some patients have required posttreatment TURP, bladder-neck incision, suprapubic catheter insertion, or urethral dilation to alleviate the just-mentioned conditions. Less commonly, interventions such as laparotomy, colostomy, and urinary diversion have been necessary. Patients are generally able to void 24 to 48 hours after implantation. The patient is placed in the lithotomy position and prepped and draped as for cystoscopy. The scrotum must be secured cephalad to allow a clear operating field. This may be accomplished with a traction stitch placed through the lateral edges of the scrotum and anchored to the groin region.

Initially, C-arm fluoroscopy is used to judge the position of the needle at the base of the prostate referable to the bladder. After several cases have been performed with fluoroscopy, it may be eliminated and seeding may then be done with ultrasound imaging only. Throughout the procedure, random room checks with the Geiger counter will be performed to determine radiation levels. All personnel will be scanned before leaving the room at the end of the procedure.

***Operative Procedure.*** Before seeding is begun, the ultrasound transducer must be positioned so that the posterior margin of the prostate is parallel to the axis of the ultrasound transducer. The direction of seed insertion and the transverse images of the prostate must have a similar appearance to those on the preoperative volume study. The volume study and implant worksheet are used for continual verification of coordinates. A stabilizer bar is attached to the OR bed. This secures the "stepping unit," which allows a 5-mm incremental forward-and-backward motion of the probe. The "sledge," which holds the transducer, is attached to the stepping unit. The probe must be securely anchored so that the position of the prostate relative to the needles used to implant the seeds remains unaltered throughout the procedure. For the needles to be positioned appropriately, the template with labeled grid is attached to the transrectal transducer so that the needles placed through the probe grid match the grid locations on the plan. The volume of the apex of the gland is drawn somewhat larger on the plan. The grid is labeled alphabetically *Aa, Bb, Cc,* and so on, with the center of the prostate corresponding to *D* on the grid. The plan is designed to avoid the urethra, bladder neck, and rectum to prevent urethrorectal fistula formation, irradiation of the bladder, and scarring at the bladder neck level.

1. At the beginning of the procedure a urethral catheter may be inserted to drain the bladder and to refill it with 150 ml of sterile water. Contrast medium for fluoroscopy is then instilled to more clearly delineate the bladder neck. Alternatively, a cystoscopy may be performed, the bladder drained, and an open-ended ureteral catheter placed to instill contrast material; the catheter is then removed. Ureteral catheters may also be inserted and left in situ during the implantation.
2. The urethral catheter is removed during implantation of seeds to avoid placement of seeds close to the urethra. The catheter causes the tissue surrounding the urethra to be compressed, and if attempts are made to implant seeds into this compressed tissue, penetration of the catheter and urethra may occur.
3. The transducer (probe) is covered with a sterile probe cover that is filled with 15 ml of sterile water to remove the artifact. Filling with too much fluid will change the configuration of the prostate and alter the anatomic presentation. The transducer will be aimed with the tip toward the floor at a 20-degree angle (Figure 15-49). The posterior wall of the prostate must be far enough away from the probe so that the posterior row of seeds is placed just inside the posterior capsule. Seeds are implanted by means of loaded needles placed into the prostate according to the template plan, with the midline seeds placed slightly off center to avoid the urethra.
4. Stabilization of the prostate may be achieved with stabilization needles placed laterally to the center into the right and left lobes and then moved once the anterior seeds are in place. Another method is to use a Foley catheter as a tractor for implantation of the periphery and until implantation near the urethra occurs. The best method may be to overcompensate for the rotation of the prostate by angling or turning the needle slightly opposite to the direction desired.
5. The most anterior seeds are placed first so that imaging of the anterior portion of the gland is not obscured by the ultrasonic shadows created by seeds placed posteriorly. If single seeds are used, the bevel of the needle should be sealed with bone wax to keep the seed in place until implantation. If strands are used, Anusol-HC (hydrocortisone) is used to seal the bevel before implantation. Strands should be cut cleanly with electrosurgery to seal the ends and avoid frayed ends, which may be split further when the stylet is inserted into the needle, adversely affecting seed placement.
6. Contrary to normal needle insertion with the bevel up, these needles are placed into the prostate with the solid, or back, side up. Every effort is extended to avoid implanting seeds into the bladder or too close to the urethra, to prevent necrosis, which causes significant postoperative irritative symptoms.
7. When placing the anterior seeds, the needle may become lodged in the pubic bone. The needle tip is visualized as a bright echo, and the angle may be altered to compensate for the bone. Alternatively, the placement of the anterior seeds may be postponed until the end when the template may be dropped down, the probe positioned parallel to the

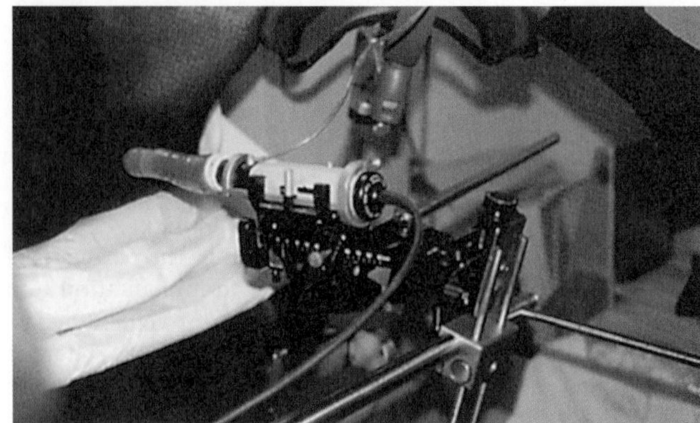

FIGURE 15-49 Transducer on stepping unit and slide, aimed toward floor at 20-degree angle.

pubic arch, and the needles inserted past the anterior portion into the prostate. During implantation, measurements can be taken from the hub of the needles to the template to check the location of the needle tips, since this distance should not change and ensures positioning of the first seeds at the base of the prostate. The distance, in centimeters, from the needle hub to the needle trocar is equal to the number of seeds in each needle.

8. The needle is inserted beyond the desired site and then retracted. The bladder wall can generally be felt with the needle tip, and insertion should just enter the wall but not pass through it. The first seed will then determine where the balance will lie because the seeds will fall into a plane that follows the first seed in a specific needle. The target volume is greater than the actual volume of the prostate so the capsular edge of the prostate and just beyond are also subjected to seed penetration (Figure 15-50). These peripherally placed seeds have a higher energy and may also have a greater tendency for migration if the tissue is not dense enough to hold the seed in place.
9. The base of the prostate is also slightly overimplanted.
10. Cystoscopy is carried out at the end of the treatment so that seeds protruding into the urethra or left in the bladder may be removed.
11. A Foley catheter is placed and left for 24 to 48 hours.

## Transrectal Cryosurgical Ablation of the Prostate Gland

Cryoablation of the prostate is a feasible, less invasive option for patients with prostate cancer. The continence rates 1 year postoperatively are more than 99%, making this an attractive alternative to conventional therapy.[45] Definitive results regarding postcryoablation erectile dysfunction are still not available but may be a significant consideration for the sexually active patient because the recovery rate is anticipated to range between 30% and 50%. Five-year statistics indicate equivalent results compared with those of surgery. Of 382 patients treated, 80% had normal prostate biopsy specimens and 50% had PSA levels less than 1 ng/dl. All the other therapeutic options remain open to the patient, including repeat cryosurgery, radiation therapy, hormone therapy, observation, or surgery. Recurrence of an elevated PSA and abnormal biopsy specimen after cryosurgery prompt additional therapy. A prior TURP may increase the difficulty but is not a contraindication. Patients with extensive local tumor that does not allow for adequate visualization of disease extension or poses increased risk to the ureters, bladder, or rectum, if fully encompassed by freezing, may not be candidates for cryoablation.

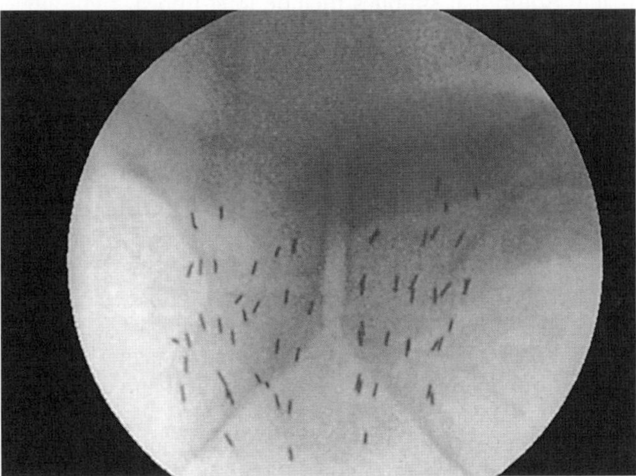

FIGURE 15-50 C-arm view of completed seed implant.

During this procedure, five 3-mm probes are inserted percutaneously into the prostate. Liquid nitrogen is then circulated through the probes to freeze the gland. This causes cell destruction and cell membrane rupture during thawing. A suprapubic catheter is inserted to allow urinary drainage and trials of voiding until prostatic swelling has subsided enough to allow micturition to occur (approximately 14 days). The freezing process may be extended beyond the prostatic capsule, potentially eradicating extracapsular extension. The purpose is to eradicate locally recurrent cancer and cure disease. The procedure may kill diverse populations of cancer cells, including chemoresistant and androgen-resistant forms.

***Procedural Considerations.*** The patient is positioned in the lithotomy position (low or exaggerated by surgeon preference). The procedure averages about 2 hours. Alternating compression stockings and Allen boot stirrups, or well-padded candy-cane stirrups, are employed. The perineum is shaved, prepped with an antimicrobial solution, and draped as for cystoscopy. Patients treated with cryosurgery are generally admitted to the hospital after the procedure and discharged the following morning unless bleeding, fever, or anesthetic complications prevent their discharge.

### *Operative Procedure*

1. A cystoscopic examination is carried out to assess the external sphincter, prostatic urethra, bladder neck, and bladder (trigone in particular).
2. The bladder is filled with sterile irrigant to facilitate percutaneous insertion of a Cope suprapubic catheter.
3. An 18-gauge needle with trocar is inserted suprapubically into the bladder. The trocar is removed, allowing passage of the 0.038-gauge guidewire through the needle.
4. The tract is progressively dilated with 6-Fr to 12-Fr fascial dilators.
5. The catheter is placed into the bladder dome to reduce bladder spasms and is connected to drainage.
6. A trocar with cannula is inserted into the bladder through a 1-cm suprapubic incision placed between the pubis and the suprapubic catheter.
7. Cystoscopic evaluation is performed to assess puncture site and bladder integrity, the trocar is removed, and irrigation tubing is passed through the cannula, into the bladder, and out the urethra under cystoscopic guidance. This tubing is attached to sterile water irrigant that is circulated through a solution warmer and irrigation pump system to raise the urethral temperature during the freezing process (Figure 15-51).
8. The scrotum is tethered to the lower outer abdominal wall using a 3-0 silk stay suture.
9. A Bookwalter retractor is attached to the OR bed, with the oval ring extending over the patient's genitalia.
10. Transrectal ultrasonography is carried out and the volume of the prostate calculated. The anatomy of the bladder

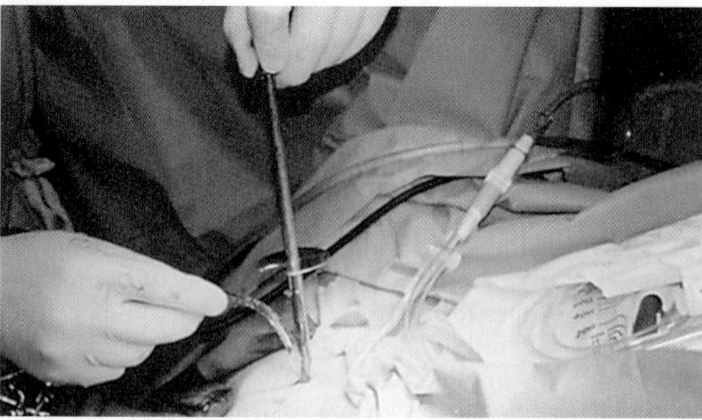

FIGURE 15-51 Trocar is removed from the cannula as suprapubic tubing is passed.

neck, trigone, seminal vesicles, and urogenital diaphragm is noted.

11. Five 18-gauge needles with trocar obturators are inserted into the prostate at the 10, 2, 4, 6, and 8 o'clock positions with their tips placed within 5 mm of the upper extent (base) of the prostate (Figure 15-52).
12. As each needle is inserted, the trocars are removed and 0.038-gauge, J-tipped guidewires are inserted.
13. Once all wires are in place, fascial-sleeved dilators are used to create tracts into the prostate. A stab wound may be necessary initially to allow entrance of the dilators.
14. The dilators are removed, leaving the sleeves in situ for placement of the cryoprobes.
15. Each sleeve is irrigated with saline to confirm its position before placement of the cryoprobes.
16. The cryoprobes are inserted, and the cryotechnician is instructed to "stick all probes." This will cause the probes to adhere to the prostate so that they will be stabilized. Elastic straps (leg straps) may be used to support the probes, attaching them to the ring of the retractor.
17. Freezing is begun through the anterior probes, followed by complete freezing to the prostate-rectal border, to a freeze temperature of −180°C. The freezing process is begun at the anterior aspect of the gland so that the border of the freeze zone may be observed on ultrasonography as it progresses posteriorly. Care is taken to avoid freezing the rectal wall and bladder neck and below the pelvic floor. Some surgeons place thermocouples into the prostate to determine the exact freeze temperature.
18. Ultrasound examination is performed on the apex of the gland to assess for residual unfrozen tissue. The probes are thawed and withdrawn 1 to 2 cm.
19. When the probes have been repositioned, the remaining apical tissue is frozen.
20. After all tissue has been frozen, the procedure is terminated by removing the cryoprobes once they have been "unstuck" (thawed).
21. The warming tubing is removed, and its insertion site and all cryoprobe sites are closed with absorbable 3-0 suture on a cuticular needle.
22. An 18-Fr, 5-ml Foley catheter is inserted and connected to straight drainage if the urine is bloody. The catheter may be removed the following morning.

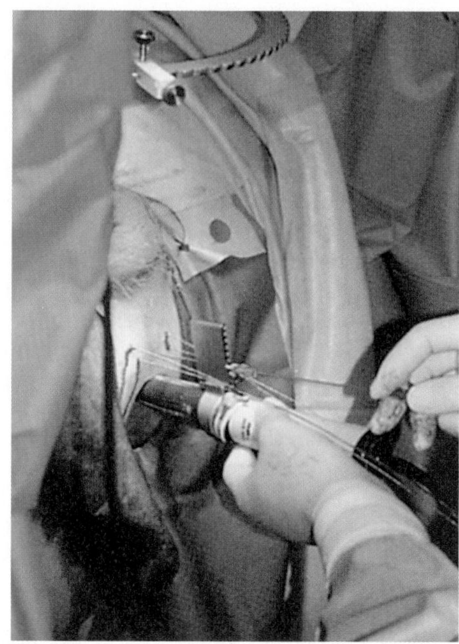

FIGURE 15-52 Placing fifth trocar needle in perineum.

## Nerve-Sparing Radical Retropubic Prostatectomy with Pelvic Lymphadenectomy

Radical prostatectomy is the treatment preferred for patients with organ-confined carcinoma of the prostate. This procedure involves removal of the entire gland, its capsule, and the seminal vesicles. Until recently the risk of impotence was extremely high after this approach. Now, with careful anatomic consideration, the posterolateral neurovascular bundles, supplying the corpora cavernosa, may be spared for erectile potency in many patients.[39,55] Urinary incontinence is generally not the threat it used to be. Those with tumors confined in the prostatic capsule are the best candidates. Often, however, in the presence of more advanced tumor extension, one of the bundles may still be spared, allowing the chance for potency.

***Procedural Considerations.*** Patient preparation and basic surgical instrumentation are as for the simple retropubic approach. Additional supplies include long-tipped, right-angled clamps, urethral suture guides (see Figure 15-40), a Bookwalter or Wishbone (UO400) retractor (see Figure 15-41), long Martius clamps, straight and right-angled clip appliers and clips, and right-angled scissors.

### *Operative Procedure*

1. After insertion of a 20-Fr or 22-Fr Foley catheter, a vertical midline lower abdominal extraperitoneal incision is made.
2. A bilateral pelvic lymphadenectomy is performed, removing the external iliac, obturator, and hypogastric nodes en bloc. This is done primarily for tumor staging. Theories differ on whether to proceed with radical surgery if nodal packets reveal metastatic disease.
3. The puboprostatic ligaments are exposed, and the endopelvic fascia is incised on each side of the gland to the puboprostatic ligaments (Figure 15-53, *A*). Right-angled scis-

sors are employed to divide the puboprostatic ligaments. The dorsal vein complex is easily subject to injury, and excessive venous bleeding may occur during this phase of the procedure. The perioperative nurse needs to be alert to this potential complication.

4. A plane is developed between the lateral prostatic border and the levator ani muscles with sharp and blunt dissection. Once visualized, the muscle is dissected laterally to the urogenital diaphragm.
5. Collateral veins originating from the levator ani muscle and running laterally to the puboprostatic ligaments are ligated and divided to free the apex of the prostate. The perioperative nurse may hear the surgeon refer to these tributaries as the *veins of Kelley.*
6. The dorsal venous complex, supplying the penis, is carefully retracted medially. Once a plane is developed, the venous complex is separated from the urethra with a long-tipped, right-angled clamp. The venous complex is tied off

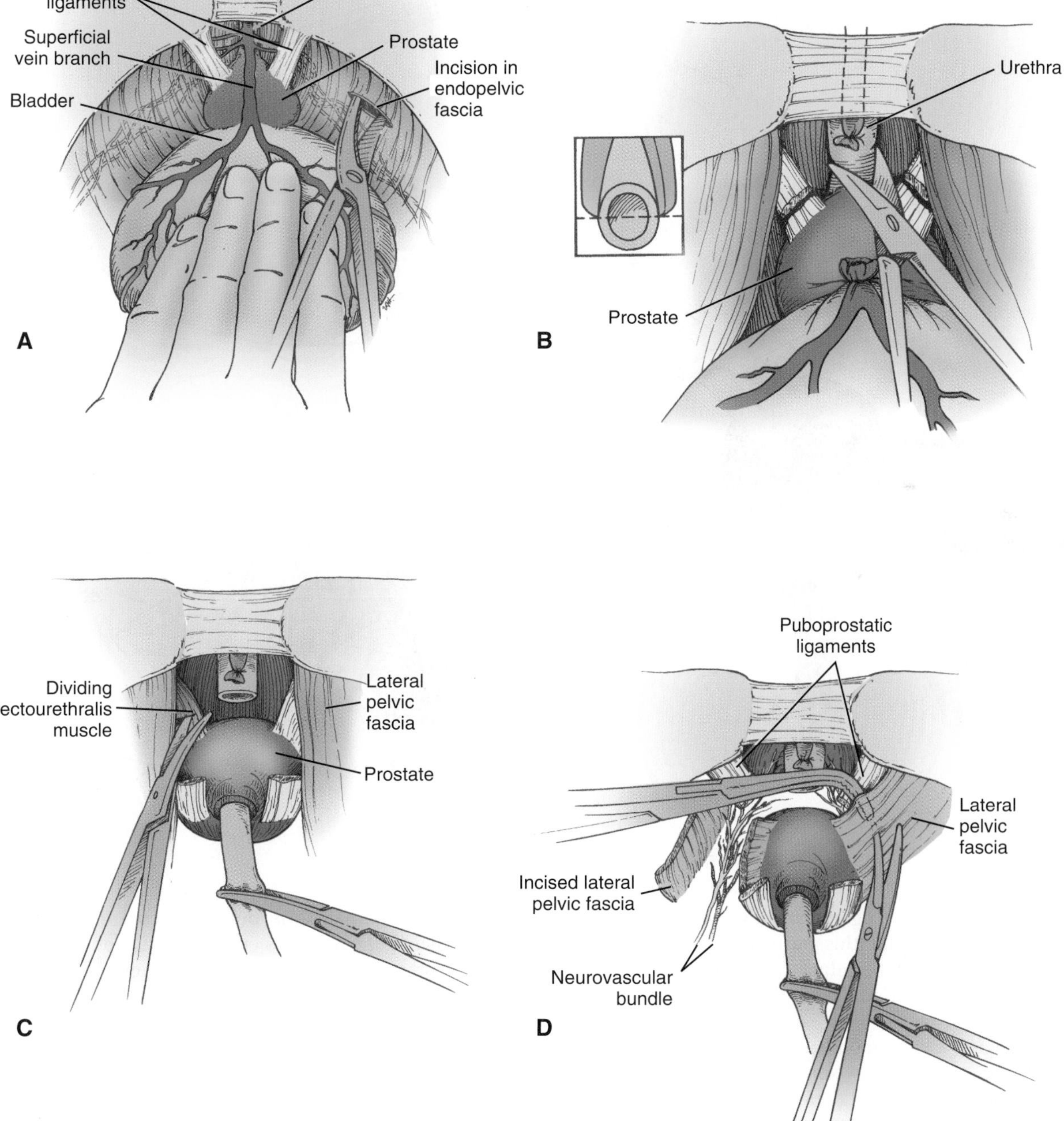


**FIGURE 15-53** Radical retropubic prostatectomy.

*Continued*

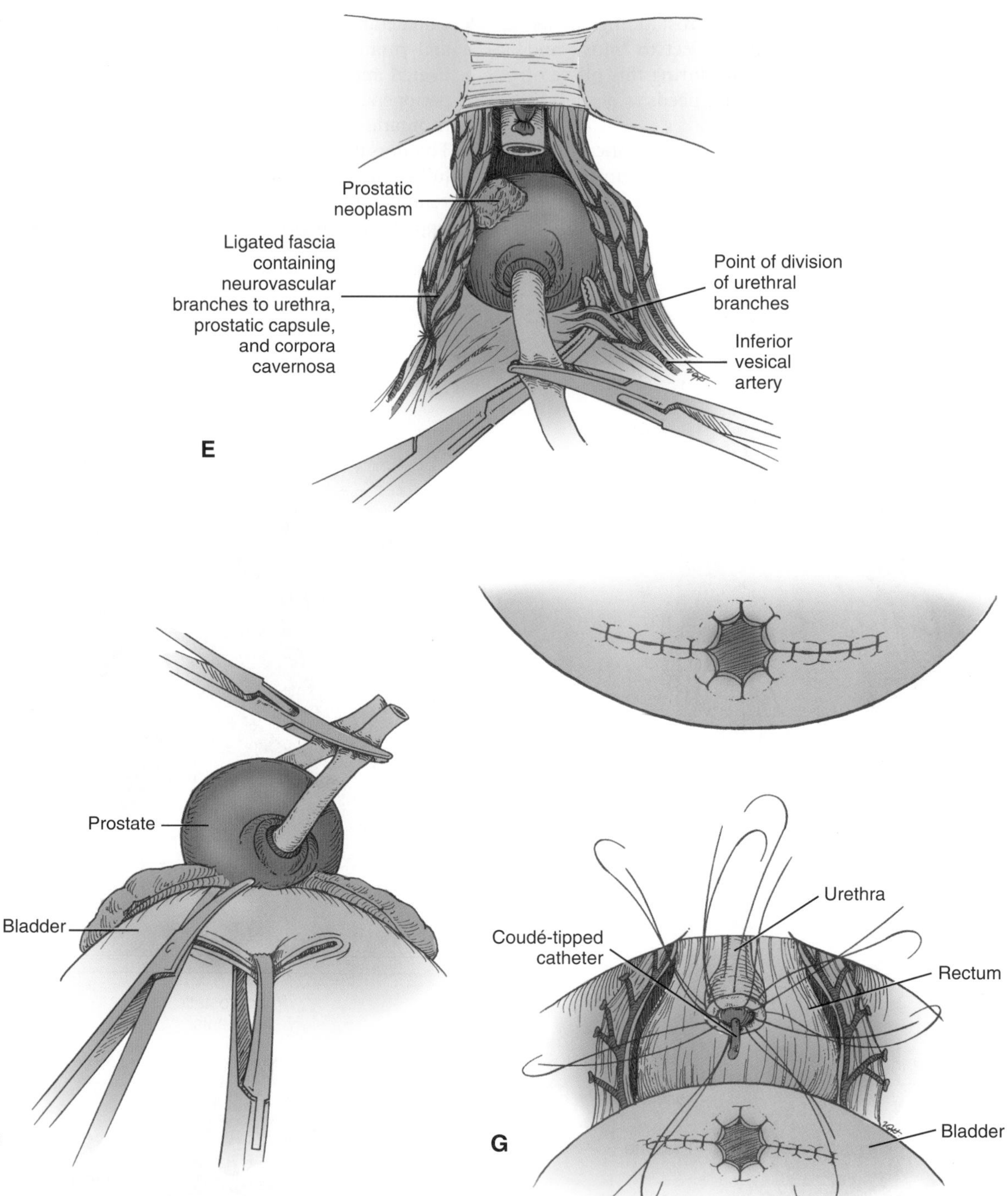


**FIGURE 15-53, cont'd.** Radical retropubic prostatectomy.

with 0 or 2-0 absorbable ligatures. Some surgeons opt to use a stapler designed for this purpose. The complex is then transected with a #15 scalpel. Backbleeding, from the vessels onto the anterior surface of the prostate, is suture-ligated.

7. The right-angled clamp mobilizes the urethra from the rectourethralis muscle between the two neurovascular bundles, avoiding damage to them.
8. A Penrose drain or vessel loop is passed around the urethra, and it is elevated and divided with a long-handled scissors or scalpel (Figure 15-53, *B*). The catheter is clamped proximally and pulled upward through the urethral incision, where it is cut and held cephalad.
9. The posterior urethra is transected (Figure 15-53, *B*).
10. The rectourethralis fibers are dissected free from and medial to the neurovascular bundles (Figure 15-53, *C* and *D*).
11. Enucleation of the prostate, division of the bladder neck, and clip ligation of the seminal vesicles follow (Figure 15-53, *E* and *F*).
12. Once bleeding is controlled, the urethral suture guide is inserted in place of the Foley and six 2-0 absorbable sutures on a ⅝ curved needle are placed inside to outside on

the distal urethral segment. These are tagged and left uncut to be anastomosed to the bladder neck (Figure 15-53, *G*).

13. The bladder neck is trimmed and everted, and a rosebud stoma is fashioned. The sutures are placed from the urethra to a corresponding position on the bladder neck. When all are placed, they are brought together in single fashion and tied.
14. Closure is as for simple retropubic prostatectomy. Continuous postoperative irrigation is rarely used. A 22-Fr, 30-ml Foley catheter is inserted and placed to gentle traction, and dressings are applied.

## Radical (Total) Perineal Prostatectomy

Patient preparation and instrumentation are the same as for simple perineal prostatectomy. The radical approach is accompanied by laparoscopic or low abdominal lymph node dissection, if not previously performed as a separate procedure. Currently, laparoscopy is performed more frequently than the standard incisional approach. Supplies needed for laparoscopy include standard laparoscopic instrumentation, three 10-mm trocars, one 5-mm trocar, an insufflation needle, a video camera unit, and $CO_2$ insufflation supplies.

***Procedural Considerations.*** Two operative setups are necessary. Most commonly, laparoscopy precedes prostatectomy. The patient is in the supine position for the laparoscopy, with the area of the umbilicus slightly elevated. Sequential compressive stockings and preoperative Foley catheterization are necessary. Instruments should be available in the operating room to do an open procedure if necessary. Lymph nodes are sent for frozen section, primarily for tumor staging. Theories differ about proceeding if abnormal nodes are discovered.

### *Operative Procedures*

LAPAROSCOPIC LYMPH NODE DISSECTION

1. After initial instillation of $CO_2$ gas through the umbilical needle, 10-mm trocars are placed at the 12 o'clock (umbilicus), 3 o'clock, and 9 o'clock positions.
2. A 5-mm trocar is placed at the 6 o'clock position.
3. The placement of the last three trocars is observed with the laparoscope.
4. The peritoneum is grasped over the vas deferens, and an incision is made with scissors. The vas is identified, clipped or coagulated, and divided.
5. The peritoneal dissection is continued laterally and cephalad to the sigmoid colon on the left and the ascending colon on the right.
6. After identification of the spermatic cord structures, iliac vessels, ureters, and psoas muscle, the incision is extended to the pubic ramus.
7. The Cloquet node is identified and freed from under the external iliac vein.
8. Dissection continues until the obturator nerve is isolated.
9. At the level of the bifurcation of the common iliac vein, the large lymph channel is located and removed. Endoclips or scissor-coagulation may be employed. Clips offer a lower risk of postoperative lymphocele.
10. In a similar fashion, the tissue overlying the external iliac artery is removed.
11. The procedure is repeated on the opposite side.
12. Trocars are removed once hemostasis has been achieved. Each trocar is removed under direct observation with the laparoscope, to allow for identification of inner abdominal wall bleeding sites.
13. After evacuation of the gas from the abdomen, the fascia layers are closed at the 12, 3, and 9 o'clock positions.
14. The skin is then closed with 4-0 absorbable subcuticular sutures. The wounds are dressed with Steri-Strips, Telfa, and Tegaderm.
15. The patient is then repositioned and prepared for radical perineal prostatectomy.

RADICAL PERINEAL PROSTATECTOMY. Surgical approach is as for simple perineal prostatectomy (Figure 15-54).

1. A layer of subcutaneous fascia is incised, and a space is developed within the ischial rectal fossa (Figure 15-55, *A*).

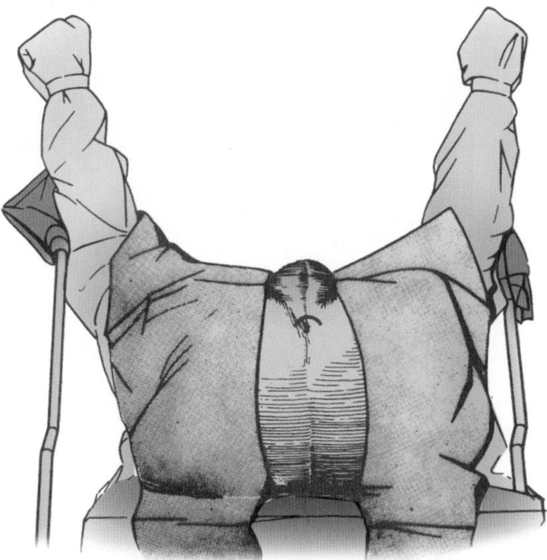

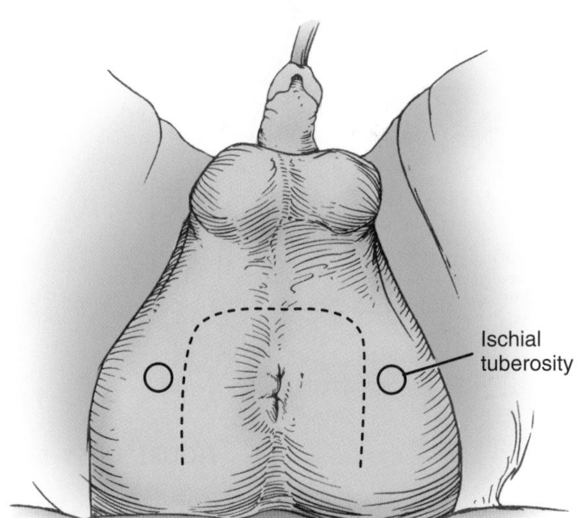


FIGURE 15-54 Radical perineal prostatectomy, draping and incision.

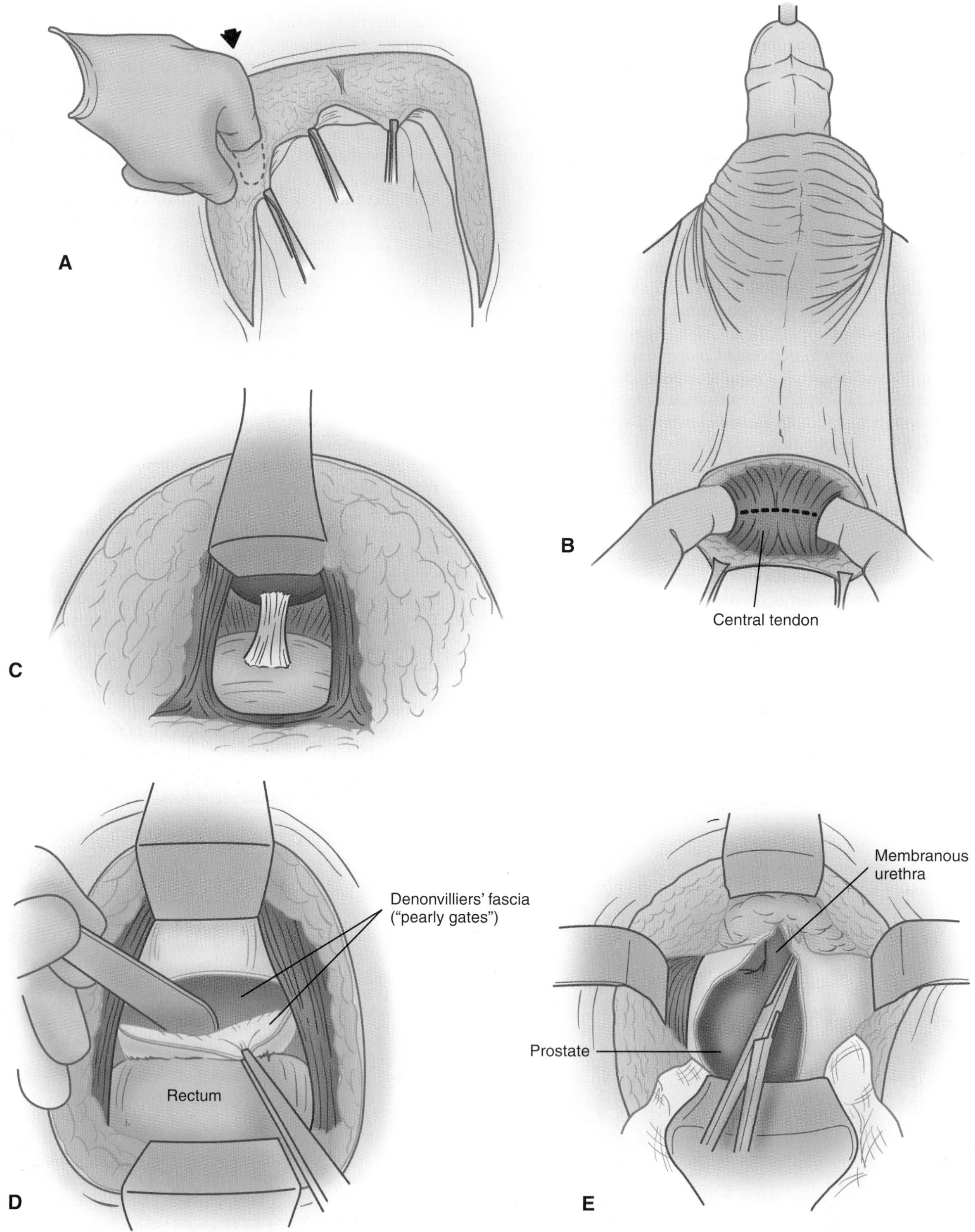


FIGURE 15-55 Radical perineal prostatectomy.

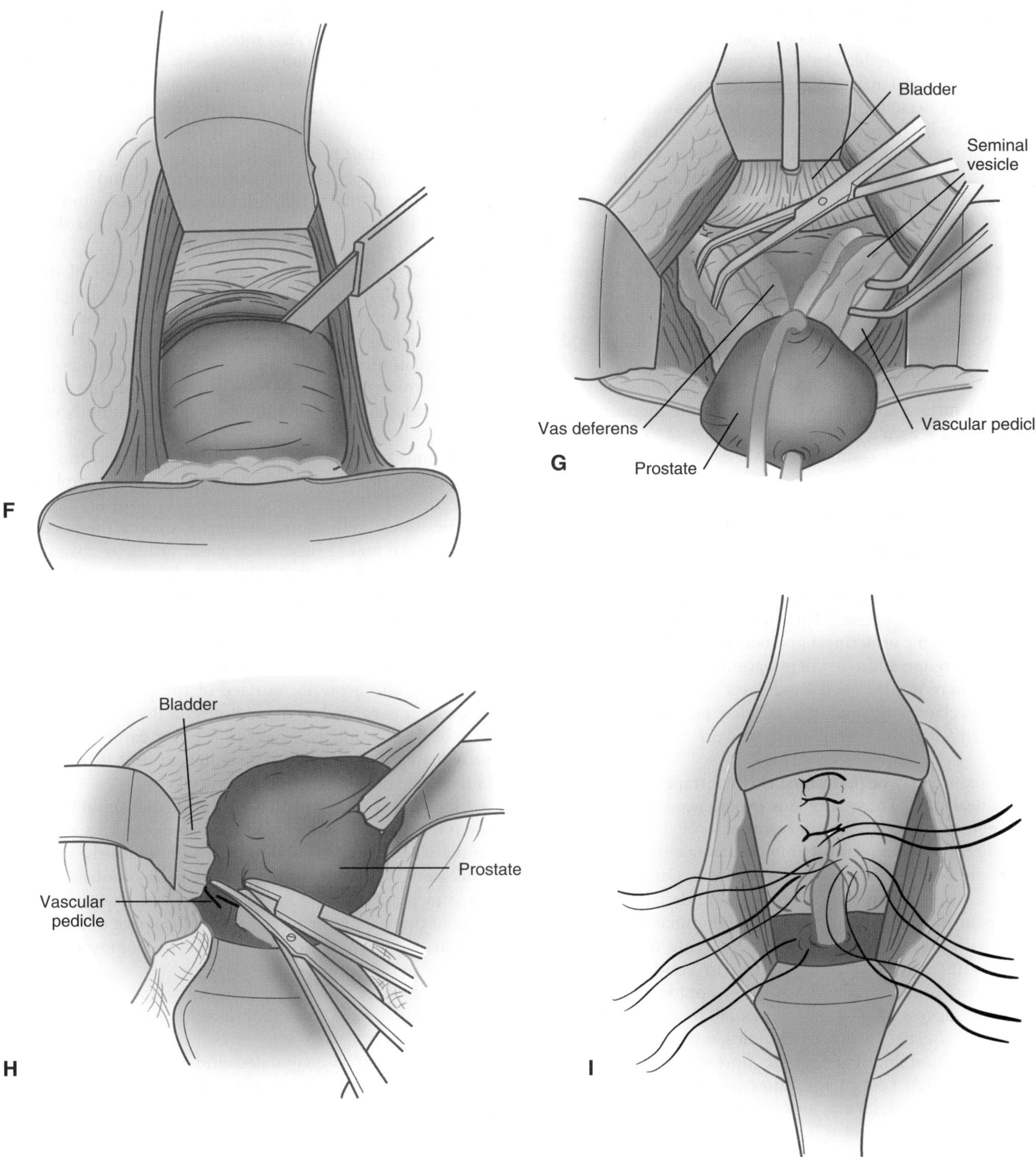


**FIGURE 15-55, cont'd.** Radical perineal prostatectomy.

2. The central tendon is incised, permitting dissection to be carried out beneath the triangle formed by the superficial external anal sphincter (Figure 15-55, *B*).
3. The sphincter is retracted cephalad, and the recto-urethralis is visualized (Figure 15-55, *C*).
4. The true prostatic capsule is exposed by incision of the overlying fascia (Figure 15-55, *D*).
5. After dissection of the periprostatic fascia unilaterally, a right-angled clamp is passed around the membranous urethra and the urethra is sharply incised (Figure 15-55, *E*).
6. The posterior bladder neck is severed, and the bladder is retracted superiorly (Figure 15-55, *F*).
7. A plane is then developed between the anterior bladder and the posterior prostate and seminal vesicles (Figure 15-55, *G*).

8. The vascular pedicles are identified at the 5 and 7 o'clock positions, incised, and divided (Figure 15-55, *H*).
9. Before closure of the bladder neck, vest sutures of 0 or 2-0 absorbable material may be placed in a mattress fashion in the open bladder neck at the 2 and 10 o'clock positions and left long for later lateral perineal placement (Figure 15-55, *I*).
10. Once reanastomosis is accomplished, these vest sutures are crossed and brought through the perineal body laterally and parallel to the urethra, anterior to the incision, and secured either just beneath the skin or to the skin with suture buttons.
11. After placement of the Foley catheter, the urethra is reanastomosed to the bladder neck with four to six 2-0 absorbable sutures and placed at the 2, 4, 8, and 10 o'clock positions. Some surgeons opt to place sutures at the 6 and 12 o'clock positions as well.
12. A drain of the surgeon's preference is placed anteriorly to the rectal surface and drawn out through the incision line or through a separate stab wound.
13. Final closure and dressings are as described in the simple procedure.

## Laparoscopic Radical Prostatectomy

A laparoscopic approach to removal of the cancerous prostate gland was initially performed at the Cleveland Clinic.[12] Although it is too early to predict long-term effects, results to date appear to have promise.[39] Patient selection is the same as for radical retropubic or perineal prostatectomy. Those patients who have undergone androgen deprivation, radiation, or perineal surgery may not be good candidates for the procedure, however. Cleveland surgeons indicate that patients return to normal activity within 2 weeks and to work activity within 3 weeks.

The procedure may be performed either intraperitoneally or extraperitoneally.[21,40] Those surgeons experienced in the technique are able to complete the intervention in 2½ to 3½ hours, but this procedure has a relatively high learning curve and may initially require 6 to 8 hours of surgical time. One-year data indicate a faster recovery, less blood loss, and decreased postoperative pain than with the traditional abdominal retropubic approach, with hospital stays ranging from 1½ to 6 days. Preliminary results suggest that the return to continence and sexual potency is comparable with other approaches. Some practitioners suggest that retaining sexual potency is more likely because the neurovascular bundles may be visualized under magnification and therefore are more readily preserved. Because of the high cost of the numerous disposable items needed, many institutions may opt to not offer this approach to their patients.

***Procedural Considerations.*** Generally no bowel prep is performed preoperatively. The morning of surgery IV administration of a third-generation cephalosporin and 2500 units of low–molecular weight subcutaneous heparin are the standard treatment.

The patient is positioned in low lithotomy with his arms at the sides. The abdomen, entire perineal area, and the upper and inner thigh region are prepped. This entire area is draped open, and separate leggings are employed. The patient is placed in the Trendelenburg position with the video monitor positioned between the legs. A Foley catheter is inserted into the urethra and attached to drainage. The laparoscope may be connected to a voice-activated robot.

Heparin is given once daily for 2 weeks postoperatively. The drain and Foley catheter are generally removed on the third postoperative day, and the patient is discharged.

### *Operative Procedure*

1. A subumbilical incision is made, and the insufflation needle is inserted into the abdominal cavity. Once an internal pressure of 15 mm Hg of $CO_2$ is achieved the needle is removed and replaced with a 10-mm trocar.
2. The laparoscope is used to inspect the interior of the abdominal wall. A second incision is then created at McBurney point, a 10-mm trocar is inserted, and the $CO_2$ line is moved and reattached to this port to prevent fogging of the lens.
3. Three small incisions are made for 5-mm trocar placement: one inferolateral to McBurney point, one in the left iliac fossa, and the third midline between the umbilicus and pubis.
4. If a lymph node dissection is to be performed this is accomplished first as described in laparoscopic lymph node dissection.
5. The peritoneal reflection is incised to expose the vas deferens and seminal vesicles. The vasal artery is coagulated, and the vas is transected bilaterally. The seminal vesicles are transected bilaterally and well mobilized.
6. Denonvilliers' fascia is incised longitudinally close to the ampulla of the vas and seminal vesicles and placed on mild traction. Once the prerectal fat is visible, inferior blunt dissection to the posterior surface of the prostate is begun. Dissection is carried to the rectourethralis muscle.
7. The bladder is filled through the Foley catheter with approximately 120 ml of sterile saline to pull it posteriorly and help identify the bladder contours.
8. An incision is made medial to the medial umbilical ligament for the initiation of bladder dissection. This is carried to the vas and up the abdominal wall anteriorly and caudally until contact is made with the pubic ramus.
9. The urachus is divided in the midline and dissected to the level of the symphysis pubis, across the space of Retzius. A bipolar or monopolar dissector is often employed for this purpose.
10. After the bladder is freed anteriorly and laterally, it is manually emptied of its contents with a suction or syringe device.
11. The dorsal vein is coagulated and incised. The fascia of Zuckerkandl (fat) covering the prostate is resected or pushed laterally cephalad. The periprostatic space is entered, and the endopelvic fascia is incised on its line of reflection.
12. The puboprostatic ligaments are incised to allow dissection of the dorsal venous complex. This is accomplished with a curved monopolar or bipolar scissors. The vessels surrounding the dorsal venous complex are electrocoagulated with bipolar forceps and then ligated with 2-0 absorbable ligature passed from one side to the other.
13. A plane between the bladder neck and prostate is then developed with sharp and blunt dissection. The anterior wall of the urethra is incised, and the Foley catheter is deflated and pulled into the operative field. The lateral and posterior urethral walls are then incised.

14. The posterior bladder neck is finally incised and the retrovesical space entered. The prostatic pedicles are bilaterally electrocoagulated with bipolar forceps.
15. A lateral incision is made to expose and preserve the neurovascular bundles on each side. They are dissected free of the prostatic base to the entrance of the pelvic floor and posterolateral to the urethra.
16. The dorsal vein complex is transected and retracted anteriorly to expose the anterior urethral wall. A knife is used to cut across the anterior urethra, and a urethral suture guide is pushed through the urethrotomy into the pelvis. The posterior wall is then transected.
17. The prostate is retracted superiorly and the remaining attachments freed.
18. The urethrovesical anastomosis is made with interrupted 3-0 absorbable sutures using two needle holders. Once all sutures are placed and tied, the Foley is reinserted and the bladder filled to check the patency of the anastomosis.
19. A specimen collection bag is passed through the second port at McBurney point and opened. The prostate is placed in the sac, the sac is closed, and the string is cut. The port is removed and the string to the sac is placed on the abdomen outside the port, a mosquito clamp is attached to the end, and the port is reinserted.
20. Abdominal pressure is lowered to 5 mm Hg, and peritoneal incisions are left open. A drain is placed in the pelvis through the lower left port and sutured to the skin. The abdominal muscles are split, and the specimen is extracted after removal of the trocar. All trocars are then removed and the incisions closed in a routine manner.

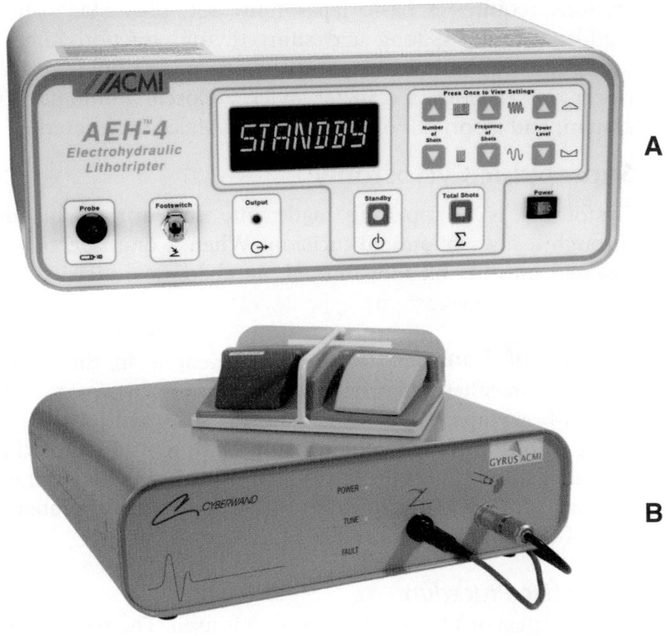


**FIGURE 15-56** **A,** Electrohydraulic lithotriptor. **B,** Ultrasonic lithotriptor.

## SURGERY OF THE BLADDER

Operations on the urinary bladder may be performed through an open abdominal incision or a transurethral route. In the past, special transurethral instruments such as the lithotrite were commonly used to crush vesical calculi manually. The electrohydraulic lithotriptor fragments the stone within the bladder by using an electric current to initiate shock waves (Figure 15-56, *A*).

Ultrasonic lithotripsy is another procedure used in the management of vesical calculi. Ultrasound waves are transmitted through a hollow metal probe (Sonotrode), which creates vibration at the tip. When applied to the surface of a calculus, the vibrating tip drills and fragments the calculus. This mechanical disintegration is continued until the stone is reduced to small fragments that are evacuated by suction through the hollow center of the probe (Figure 15-56, *B*). The holmium:YAG laser (Ho:YAG) has more recently been employed successfully in the fragmentation of bladder calculi (Figure 15-57).

Stones may also be removed from the bladder through a suprapubic incision (cystolithotomy). Bladder tumors, diverticula, congenital defects, or trauma may necessitate an open abdominal approach. A thorough diagnostic workup and endoscopic examination help to determine the appropriate surgical approach to be employed. Radical procedures, such as total cystectomy, are performed for the treatment of invasive carcinoma of the bladder and require permanent urinary diversion.

For most open-bladder surgery the patient is placed in the supine position with a bolster under the pelvis. The Trendelenburg position may be desired because this position tilts the head down and allows the viscera to fall cephalad. This allows excellent exposure of the pelvic organs, including the bladder. The patient is draped as described for routine suprapubic prostatectomy, using a disposable impermeable drape that is placed immediately below the bladder incision. A catheter may be inserted into the urethra and the bladder distended with sterile saline at the start of surgery for easy identification. The ESU may be required. The instrument setup for open-bladder op-

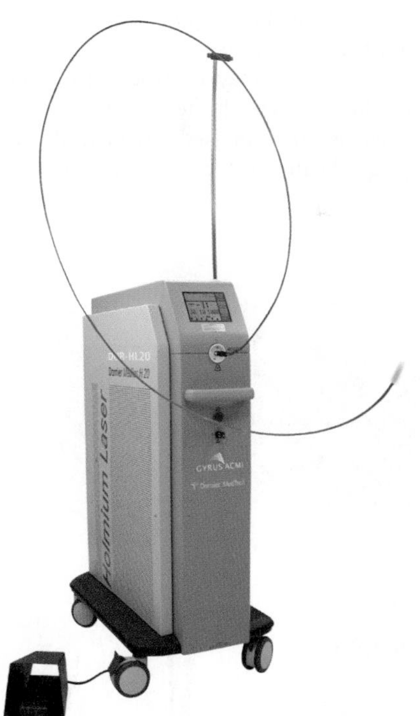


**FIGURE 15-57** Holmium laser unit.

erations requires a basic laparotomy set, plus Mason-Judd bladder retractors, long and short thyroid traction forceps, retropubic needle holders (or other long needle holders), one trocar, vessel loops, a catheter stylet, a closed-wound suction system, and assorted Foley, Pezzer, and Malecot catheters.

## Suprapubic Cystostomy

Cystotomy is an opening made into the urinary bladder through a low abdominal incision. When a drainage tube is inserted into the bladder through an abdominal incision, the procedure is a cystostomy.

***Procedural Considerations.*** The patient is in the supine position. Anesthesia may be general, spinal, or local with sedation. A basic laparotomy set is generally sufficient for the procedure. Foley catheters ranging from 22 Fr to 30 Fr should be available, as well as Malecot suprapubic catheters and a drainage bag. Frequently, a flexible cystoscopy is incorporated as part of the procedure.

### *Operative Procedure*

1. A vertical or Pfannenstiel incision is used. The rectus fascia is divided in the midline (Figure 15-58, *A*).
2. The bladder is distended with saline solution that is instilled with an Asepto syringe through a catheter.
3. The dome of the bladder is then dissected free with Metzenbaum scissors and blunt dissection (Figure 15-58, *B*).
4. The wall of the bladder is grasped on either side of the midline with Martius forceps (Figure 15-58, *C*).
5. Two traction sutures may be placed through the bladder wall and held with straight hemostats.
6. The bladder is then incised downward with a scalpel. Bleeding vessels in the bladder wall are clamped and ligated.

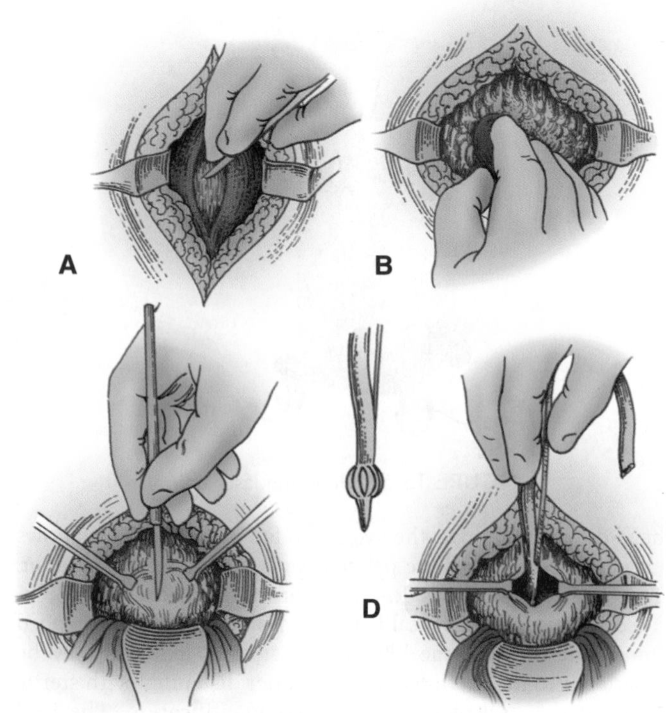


**FIGURE 15-58** Suprapubic cystostomy.

7. The bladder contents are aspirated with a suction device.
8. The bladder opening may be extended if the bladder is to be explored for diverticula or calculi.
9. A large-size Malecot or Pezzer catheter is introduced into the bladder (Figure 15-58, *D*).
10. The incision is closed snugly about the catheter with absorbable sutures to render the closure watertight about the cystostomy tube.
11. The muscle, fascia, and subcutaneous tissue are closed with absorbable suture.
12. The skin is closed with staples or suture.
13. The cystostomy tube is secured to the skin with a 0 or 2-0 nonabsorbable suture to prevent it from being inadvertently dislodged from the bladder. A drain such as a Jackson-Pratt may be left in the prevesical space.
14. The wound is dressed, and the cystostomy tube is connected to a straight urinary drainage system.

## Transurethral Resection of Bladder Tumors

Bladder lesions may be removed using a standard resectoscope, working element, loop, and a Foroblique telescope, which is passed through the urethra into the bladder. A 24-Fr cystoscope sheath with a catheterizing bridge and biopsy forceps may be used to remove bladder tumors located at the very top or dome of the bladder (Figure 15-59). Transitional cell carcinoma of the bladder is one of the most difficult lesions to track because it can occur wherever there is transitional cell lining of the urinary tract. Bladder cancer has a tendency to recur in other areas of the bladder, even after complete resection of the original lesion.

Usually the surgeon removes not only the bladder lesion but also a portion of the bladder muscle underlying the lesion so that the pathologist can determine if any tumor has invaded the muscle. Random biopsy specimens of the normal bladder lining are also taken to ascertain if microscopic transitional cell carcinoma in situ is present. Lesions that deeply invade the muscle must be treated with an open surgical procedure, such as a partial cystectomy or total cystectomy.

The resection technique, setup, and preparation of the patient are virtually the same as for TURP. A general, spinal, or regional anesthetic is administered. A retrograde pyelogram may be done to check for lesions existing in the upper urinary tract.

Sterile water is recommended as an irrigating solution in transurethral resection of bladder tumors. Because few vessels are uncovered during this short resection procedure, water absorption with hemolysis and systemic complications such as hyponatremia do not occur. In addition, cancer cells released during the procedure tend to absorb water, causing them to rupture and lyse rather than remain viable and capable of implanting themselves into the raw surface of the bladder created by the surgery. When the procedure is completed, a large catheter, usually a 24 Fr, is passed into the bladder and connected to drainage.

## Transurethral Laser Ablation of Bladder Tumors

The neodymium (Nd):YAG or holmium (Ho):YAG laser may be used to destroy small recurrent bladder tumors and to coagulate the tumor bed of larger bladder tumors resected with an electrosurgical loop. A powerful, highly focused beam of light in the near-infrared range is transmitted to the tumor site

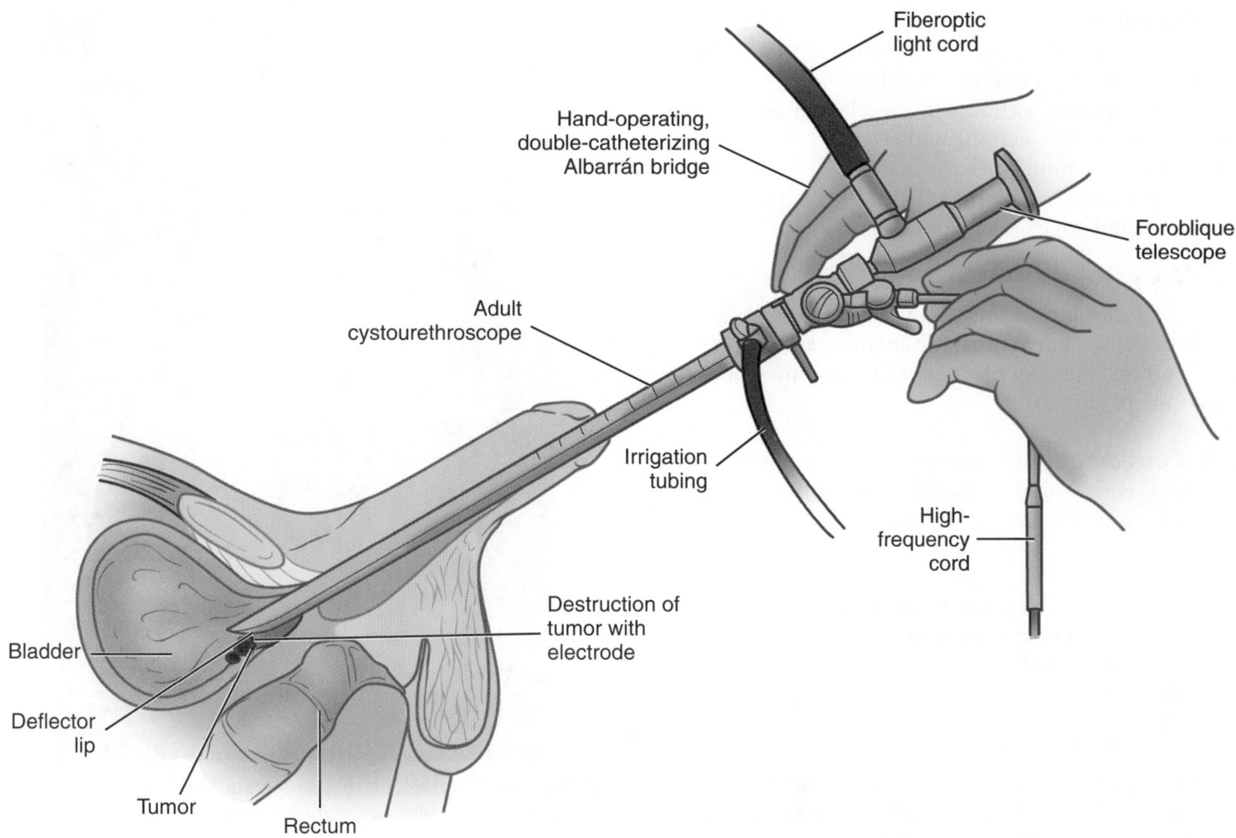


**FIGURE 15-59** Bladder fulguration.

through a flexible glass fiber. This laser fiber is passed through the catheter channel of a cystoscope, and the fiber is directed by a deflecting laser bridge (Figure 15-60). The advantages of a laser in the eradication of bladder tumors are as follows: (1) bleeding is minimized, (2) only sedation is required, (3) the operating time is shortened, (4) there is minimal damage to healthy tissue, and (5) postoperative drainage of the bladder by a urethral catheter is not needed.

## Alternatives to Surgery for Superficial Bladder Cancer

Patients with various types of cancer may be treated in the urology office setting with various therapeutic modalities. These measures may be initiated instead of surgery or as an adjunct to surgery. Instillations are aimed at eradicating existing disease, reducing tumor recurrence and progression, and improving overall patient survival.[31]

Patients with bladder cancer that has been staged as Ta, carcinoma in situ (CIS), and T1 may be treated with intravesical, antineoplastic chemotherapy agents such as *thiotepa, mitomycin C* (Mutamycin), *doxorubicin* (Adriamycin), and *etoglucid* (Epodyl). Chemotherapy has become the treatment of choice for low-risk patients. Analysis of data shows a long-term reduction in recurrence of 6%.

Immunotherapy with TheraCys or Tice *bacille Calmette-Guérin (BCG)* is used to treat patients considered to have high-risk tumors. BCG, through an unknown mechanism, strengthens the body's immune reaction to cancer and is considered the most effective therapy for recurrent and residual bladder cancer. Currently the complete response rate of BCG is 84% if protocol is followed. *Interferon alfa-2b* has a response rate of 47% in CIS and 25% with papillary carcinomas and a recurrence rate of 28% but has not been specifically approved for superficial bladder cancer.

Combination chemotherapy and immunotherapy have become standard treatment for patients with metastatic transitional cell carcinoma. BCG has been combined with *mitomycin C* and with *interferon alfa-2b*. The latter combination has been highly effective, rescuing approximately 60% of those who failed with BCG alone.[31]

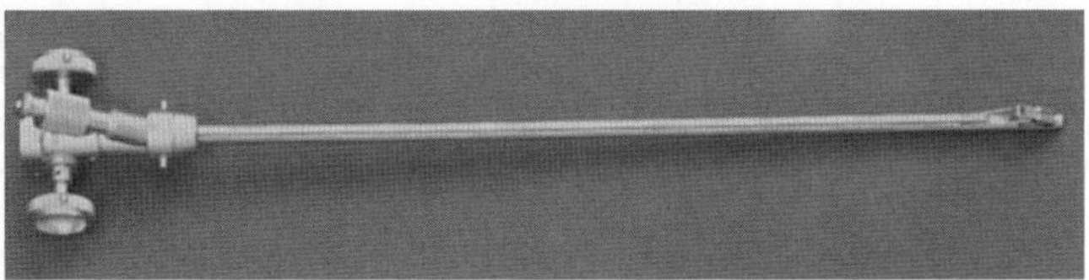

**FIGURE 15-60** Resectoscope laser bridge.

## Trocar Cystostomy

Trocar cystostomy consists of draining the bladder by puncture with a needle or trocar and inserting a catheter.

***Procedural Considerations.*** A minor instrument set along with a metal probe and grooved director, an Anthony suction tube and tubing, and trocar catheters or a prepackaged cystostomy kit are required. Local anesthesia may be used.

### *Operative Procedure*

1. The skin at the site of the puncture is nicked with a scalpel, and the trocar is inserted into the bladder.
2. The trocar obturator is withdrawn, the bladder is drained through the trocar by suction, and a catheter is passed through the trocar cannula into the bladder.
3. The cannula is carefully withdrawn, and the catheter is sutured to the wound edges. The wound is dressed.

## Suprapubic Cystolithotomy

Suprapubic cystolithotomy is the removal of calculi from the bladder. Obstructions, such as prostatic enlargement or foreign bodies, are common causes of bladder calculi and may be corrected at the time of surgery.

***Procedural Considerations.*** Instruments for open-bladder operations along with Millin T-shaped stone forceps, Millin capsule forceps, and Lewkowitz lithotomy forceps are required.

***Operative Procedure.*** The surgical approach is similar to that described for suprapubic cystotomy. When the bladder is opened, calculi are identified and extracted. If indicated, bladder outlet obstruction is repaired.

## Repair of Vesical Fistulas

Vesical fistulas occurring between the bladder and the intestines or vagina may be repaired surgically.[42,46] *Vesicointestinal fistulas* may be caused by ulcerative colitis, diverticulitis, or neoplasms of the colon or rectum. *Vesicovaginal fistulas* may be a complication of radiotherapy for cervical cancer, endoscopic procedures involving surgery of the trigone or vesical neck, obstetric injuries, and hysterectomies.

***Procedural Considerations.*** The instrument setup is as described for open-bladder operations. Intestinal instruments (Chapter 11) are necessary for vesicointestinal fistulas. For vesicovaginal fistulas, vaginal preparation and a colporrhaphy set (Chapter 14) with colostomy or ileostomy instruments are used. Sequential compression devices (SCDs) are applied.

Vesicointestinal fistulas are more common than vesicovaginal fistulas. Of the intestinal fistulas, the sigmoid colon is most often involved (Figure 15-61). A colostomy proximal to the fistula may be performed to protect the repaired segment of bowel. The communicating area of bladder and bowel is totally resected. Generally, an end-to-end bowel resection is performed after excision of the involved intestinal segment. The bladder is then repaired in three layers.

If the fistula is at the dome of the bladder, the approach will be transperitoneal, transvesical, or a combination of the two. If the fistula is in the trigone of the bladder, a vaginal approach may be employed. A suprapubic tube is usually left in the bladder.

### *Operative Procedures*

VESICOVAGINAL FISTULA REPAIR—VAGINAL APPROACH

1. With the patient in the lithotomy or supine position, a suprapubic catheter is inserted, clamped, and connected to closed drainage.
2. The patient is placed in the hyperflexed lithotomy position or Kraske position (jackknife).

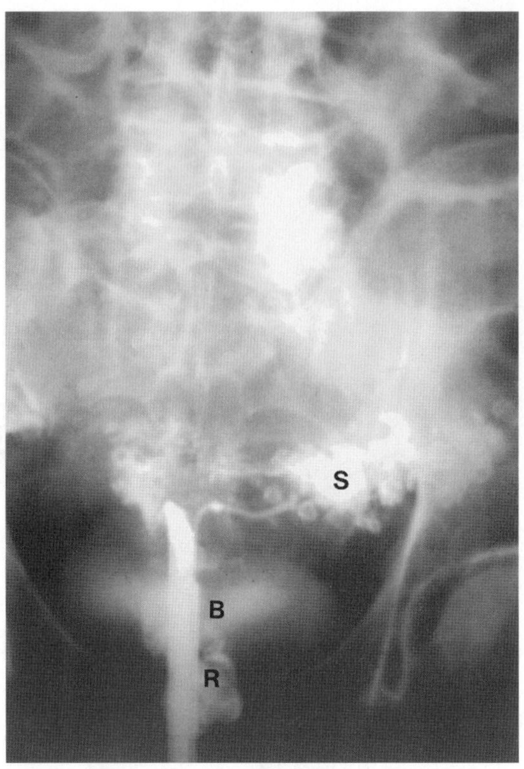


**FIGURE 15-61** Vesicoenteric fistulogram (cystogram) showing contrast material in bladder *(B)*, sigmoid colon *(S)* and rectum *(R)*.

3. The vagina and external genitalia are prepped.
4. The area is draped with a lithotomy or laparotomy sheet. If the intended position is Kraske, separate draping material and instrumentation are set up for the suprapubic catheter insertion with the patient supine. The catheter is secured, and the patient is turned for the procedure.
5. The labia are sutured to the outer groin or inner thigh for retraction and visualization.
6. A weighted vaginal retractor is placed posteriorly, and the defect is examined. A relaxing vaginal incision may be necessary at the 5 or 7 o'clock position.
7. A 4-Fr ureteral catheter is inserted through the fistula, and the tract is dilated to admit an 8-Fr balloon catheter. The balloon is inflated, and the catheter is used as a tractor.
8. The area is infiltrated with vasopressin (Pitressin) solution.
9. The vaginal mucosa and perivesical fascia around the defect are incised, well outside the scarred tissue.
10. Two planes are developed—one between the mucosa and fascia and one between the fascia and the bladder wall—with fine scissors, forceps, and gauze (Kittner) dissectors.
11. The bladder wall is freed from the vaginal wall.
12. The vesical defect is grasped with Martius clamps, the scarred edges are everted, and then the defect is closed vertically with interrupted 3-0 absorbable sutures after removal of the catheter previously placed. In some instances, a labial pedicle or full-thickness flap (Martius flap) may be placed between the vesical closure and the vaginal closure (Figure 15-62). This prevents suture-line stress and overlay and removes the need for a relaxing incision. Larger fistulas that do not adequately reapproximate may necessitate a vascularized muscle flap to reinforce closure.

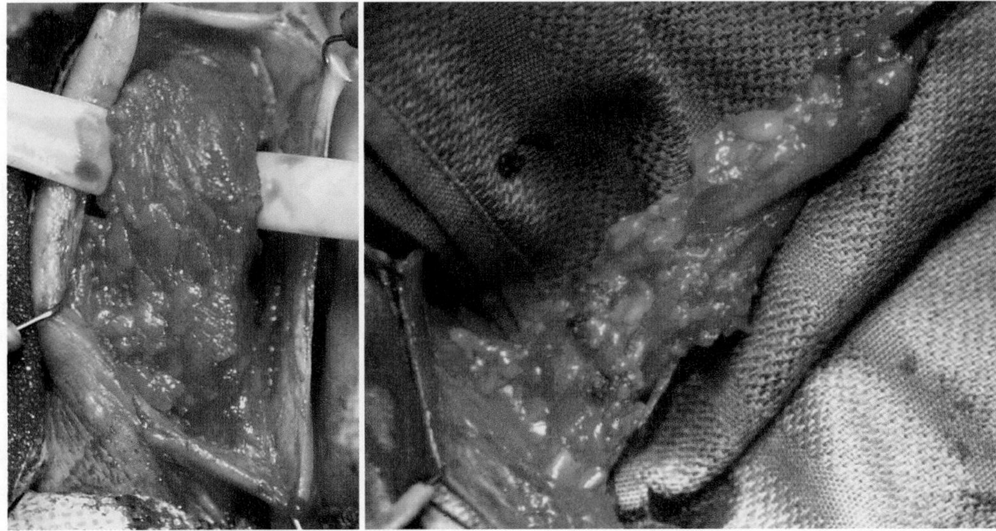

**FIGURE 15-62** Creation of Martius flap.

13. The perivesical fascia and vaginal mucosa are approximated separately with transverse interrupted 3-0 absorbable sutures. A one-sided ellipse of vaginal mucosa may be excised to offset the closure.
14. Alternatively, an inverted-U incision may provide more exposure than other incisions and result in a posterior flap that completely covers the site of the defect.
15. The suprapubic catheter is unclamped, the labial stitches are removed, and the vagina is loosely packed.

VESICOVAGINAL FISTULA—TRANSPERITONEAL (TRANSVESICAL) APPROACH

1. The patient is placed in the low lithotomy and moderate Trendelenburg position. Both the perineum and the abdomen are prepped and draped appropriately. A laparoscopy pack works well for this approach.
2. Ureteral catheters are inserted endoscopically, and a 16-Fr Foley catheter is placed in the bladder and clamped.
3. A tight gauze pack or vaginal ball is placed into the vagina.
4. A vertical midline or Pfannenstiel incision is made.
5. The peritoneum is incised and bluntly dissected from the dome of the bladder.
6. The small bowel is packed cephalad.
7. Stay sutures of 2-0 absorbable material are placed in the bladder dome, and the bladder is opened.
8. The bladder wall and overlying peritoneum are divided down to the fistula. Stay sutures are placed periodically to serve as tractors for bladder elevation.
9. The peritoneum is incised transversely at the level of the fistula, forming a pedicle flap.
10. The vagina and bladder are separated widely on each side of the fistula. An assistant places upward pressure on the vaginal ball or pack to facilitate dissection.
11. As the fistula is exposed, it is excised until completely removed. A probe may be used to localize it, if small, or an 8-Fr balloon catheter may be inserted and used for traction during dissection.
12. The bladder and vagina are freed from each other until there is enough mobility for separate closures.
13. The vagina is then closed, without tension, with inverting 2-0 or 3-0 interrupted sutures in two layers.
14. The peritoneal flap is swung into the defect and sutured in place for reperitonealization. A long, attached peritoneal or free peritoneal pedicle flap may be needed for reperitonealization. Alternatively, the omentum may be brought from behind the right side of the colon for an omental graft. A vascularized muscle flap may be placed for fistulas resulting from radiation necrosis.
15. A 22-Fr Malecot catheter and a wound drain are inserted and pulled through separate stab wounds in the abdomen.
16. The ureteral catheters are removed, and the bladder mucosa and submucosa are closed in separate layers with 2-0 or 3-0 absorbable suture in a running fashion.
17. The muscularis and adventitia are externally approximated with interrupted 3-0 sutures.
18. The wound is closed in layers.
19. Dressings are applied, the Foley is unclamped, the rubber ball or gauze pack is removed, and the vagina is loosely repacked.

VESICOSIGMOID FISTULA REPAIR—ABDOMINAL APPROACH

1. With the patient in the Trendelenburg position, a 20-Fr or 22-Fr, 5-ml Foley catheter is inserted and the bladder filled with 100 ml of sterile water. Once the patient is prepped and draped as for laparotomy, a midline, or paramedian, and transperitoneal incisions are made.
2. The abdomen is explored, and contents are examined.
3. The descending colon and sigmoid colon are mobilized by incising along the fascia fusion line of Toldt.
4. The involved loop of colon is identified. If a walled-off inflammatory mass is found, a transverse colostomy may be performed and a two-stage intervention considered.
5. The fistulous tract is separated by blunt finger dissection.
6. A probe is inserted to determine the extent of involvement.
7. The defects in the bladder and bowel are debrided to obtain healthy tissue. Large inflammatory masses require a colon resection.

8. The bladder is closed in two layers with a 3-0 absorbable submucosal running stitch and a 2-0 absorbable interrupted muscularis and adventitial stitch.
9. The edges of the bowel defect are trimmed to reach normal tissue, and stay sutures are placed on each side.
10. The cavity is pulled transversely, and the mucosa and submucosa are closed in one pass with a Connell stitch of 3-0 chromic catgut.
11. The muscularis and serosa are approximated and closed in one pass with 4-0 silk Lembert sutures.
12. The abdomen is irrigated with 2000 ml of sterile saline with an attempt to reach all areas.
13. A sump-style drain is placed intraperitoneally, and a Penrose or small Jackson-Pratt drain is placed suprapubically, exiting through separate stab wounds.
14. The abdomen is closed in layers in the conventional manner. If a colostomy was performed, it is opened for fecal diversion and the appropriate appliance applied.
15. Gauze and bulky absorbable dressings are applied and secured; Montgomery straps may be used.

## Vesicourethral (Marshall-Marchetti-Krantz) Suspension

A Marshall-Marchetti-Krantz suspension is performed for the correction of stress incontinence caused by an abnormal urethrovesical angle. The intent of the Marshall-Marchetti-Krantz operation is to bring the bladder and urethra into the pelvis by suturing paraurethral vaginal tissue to the back of the symphysis pubis. A modification of this technique is the Burch procedure. The approach mimics the Marshall-Marchetti-Krantz until placement of the buttressing sutures. Instead of attempting difficult periosteal sutures, the surgeon places nonabsorbable size 0 sutures into the Cooper ligament from each side of the bladder neck. The Burch is technically easier, and long-term results are fairly equivalent.

A large percentage of patients with stress incontinence are obese and have diabetes. It is important to evaluate for these conditions and prepare for proper patient management (i.e., positioning concerns relating to peripheral vascular circulation and pressure points, skin breakdown, risk for infection, wound healing).

***Procedural Considerations.*** The patient is usually placed in a moderate Trendelenburg position, frog-legged, with supports under each knee to allow for intraoperative vaginal manipulation. Abdominal and vaginal preps are required. A Foley catheter is inserted at the beginning of surgery. This procedure is combined with an abdominal hysterectomy. Both the surgeon and assistant double-glove for vaginal manipulation. Basic laparotomy and abdominal hysterectomy instruments (see Chapter 14), if needed, are used. Postoperatively, the patient commonly has a vaginal pack, a urethral catheter with or without a suprapubic catheter, and possibly a wound drain.

### *Operative Procedure*

1. A Foley catheter is inserted into the bladder through the urethra.
2. A suprapubic transverse incision is made to expose the prevesical space of Retzius.
3. The bladder retractor is positioned with small, moist laparotomy pads in place.
4. The bladder and urethra are freed from the posterior surface of the rectus muscle and symphysis pubis by gentle blunt manipulation.
5. The assistant places two fingers into the vagina, lifting the urethra upward against the symphysis pubis to facilitate ease of repair of the periurethral musculofascial structures.
6. A heavy, nonabsorbable atraumatic suture on a Heaney needle holder is placed through the supporting fascia of the vaginal wall on each side of the urethra. The suture is passed through the symphysis pubis, providing support to the urethra and bladder neck. Generally, a row of three heavy, nonabsorbable sutures is placed on each side of the urethra, the most proximal being located just at the vesical neck.
7. The area is drained, and the wound is closed in layers and dressed.
8. The vagina may be packed with 2-inch packing, which is removed after 24 to 36 hours.
9. The Foley catheter is connected to a closed urinary drainage system.

## TVT Sling (Tension-Free Vaginal Tape)

Tension-free vaginal tape may be used for the correction of female incontinence.[13,22,42] The tape is composed of polypropylene mesh (Figure 15-63) encased in a plastic sleeve that has a center slit and is secured to a large, curved trocar needle at each end. A T-shaped introducer is attached to these needles for passage of the sling material. The mesh is passed through the pelvic tissue and positioned under the urethra, creating a supportive sling. Unlike other corrective procedures for incontinence, no screws, anchors, or internal sutures are required.

A TVT sling is indicated for women diagnosed with urethral hypermobility, intrinsic sphincter deficiency, and pure stress incontinence caused by pelvic floor relaxation. It will not correct urge incontinence, although it may be used in women with combination stress and urge incontinence. This patient will need to have her urge incontinence controlled in another manner. It appears to be a viable option for the overweight and older female and for women who have had previous corrective measures that failed (Research Highlight). It is not recommended for younger women who are pregnant or intend to become pregnant. Other contraindications include patients with intrinsic bleeding problems or who are receiving anticoagulant therapy. Risks include bladder perforation, perforation of pelvic viscera adherent to the pubis, retropubic hemorrhage and hematoma formation, infection, and urinary retention.

***Procedural Considerations.*** After IV sedation the patient is placed in the lithotomy position. The procedure takes about

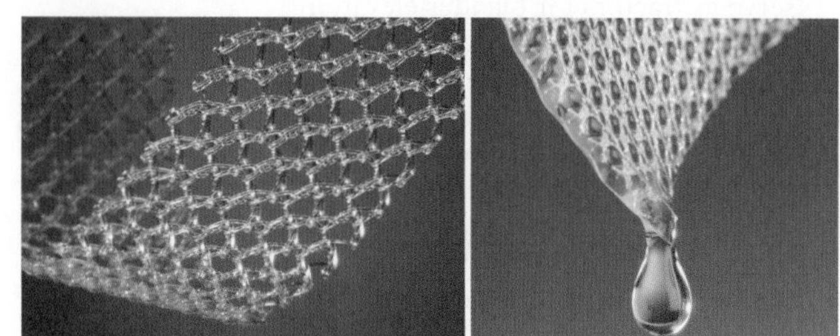


FIGURE 15-63 **A,** Uretex self-anchoring urethral support system. **B,** Pelvitex polypropylene mesh.

## RESEARCH HIGHLIGHT

### TVT Sling Candidates

Urinary incontinence affects the quality of life in women worldwide. Prevalence rates range from 4.5% to 53%, peaking in midlife at 30% to 40%. This increases steadily with aging to a prevalence of 30% to 50%. Stress urinary incontinence (SUI) accounts for about 50% of all incontinent women. In the older woman, however, a mix of urge and stress incontinence is predominant. In addition, impaired bladder emptying in older women, as a result of detrusor instability or bladder outlet obstruction, often accompanies incontinence.

Tension-free vaginal tape (TVT) has gained popularity worldwide as a minimally invasive surgical technique for the treatment of SUI. However, age-related medical conditions could adversely affect the outcome. This study compared the efficacy and safety of TVT in elderly women (older than 70 years of age) and TVT in younger women (ages 35 to 69 years).

Women with SUI only were treated with TVT repair alone. Those with urogenital prolapse in addition to SUI (67%) were treated with TVT and vaginal prolapse repair. Early postoperative observation involved evaluation and documentation of surgery-related and age-related morbidity. Patients were evaluated at 1-, 3-, 6-, and 12-month intervals with a repeat video urodynamic (VUD) study at 3 months postoperatively. Surgical safety and efficacy were compared between the two groups. Outcome measurements included postoperative morbidity, persistence of urge incontinence or de novo (new-onset) urge incontinence, postoperative SUI, and voiding dysfunction.

The incidence of postoperative fever, urinary tract infection (UTI), hematoma, and blood loss was similar in both age-groups. TVT-related complications were also similar in both groups with the exception that fewer bladder perforations occurred in the elderly group. Only one elderly patient failed to resume spontaneous voiding within the first postoperative month. She was successfully treated with tape excision and urethrolysis. The incidence of tape erosion in the two groups was also similar.

Long-term follow-up revealed similar outcomes with SUI and urge incontinence. The incidence of de novo urge incontinence proved to be significantly more common in the elderly group (18% versus 4%).

This study confirmed that TVT is associated with a good outcome for all age-groups. Serious age-related complications (6 of 157 patients) occurred in the elderly group who had TVT in addition to prolapse repair. Only one patient in the younger group of concomitant repair developed a serious complication.

Modified from Gordon D and others: Tension-free vaginal tape in the elderly: is it a safe procedure? *Urology* 65(3):479-492, 2005.

30 minutes and may be performed using local anesthesia with monitored sedation. Vaginal packing and a postoperative Foley catheter are usually not necessary. Cystoscopy is performed before, during, and at the end of the procedure. Local anesthesia is administered into the abdominal wall muscle and fascia lateral to the midline and just above the symphysis pubis bilaterally, and suburethrally into the retropubic space bilaterally. Approximately 3 to 4 minutes should be allowed for the anesthetic to take effect; cystoscopy may be performed during this time. Vasopressin (Pitressin) is commonly added to the anesthetic to help control bleeding. A Foley catheter with stylet in place is used to retract the bladder away from the midline to allow passage of the TVT needle.

### *Operative Procedure*

1. A 16-Fr or 18 -Fr Foley catheter is inserted to drain the bladder.
2. Local anesthetic is injected through the skin and into the muscle and fascia lateral to the midline and just above the symphysis pubis, bilaterally.
3. Local anesthetic is injected suburethrally into the anterior vaginal mucosa to the retropubic space, bilaterally.
4. Cystoscopy is performed to confirm integrity of the bladder wall, urethral patency and length, and location of the ureters.
5. Two incisions, 0.5 to 1 cm in length, are made in the abdominal skin over each injection site.
6. A weighted speculum is placed in the vagina, and the anterior vaginal mucosa is grasped with two Allis clamps and placed on moderate tension.
7. A 1.5-cm incision is made into the anterior vaginal mucosa, 1 cm to the right of the external meatus, with a #10 or #15 scalpel.
8. Blunt Metzenbaum scissors are used to dissect suburethrally and periurethrally to the level of the endopelvic fascia.
9. The rigid stylet is inserted into the Foley catheter, and the catheter is placed into the bladder.
10. The bladder neck and urethra are deflected away to allow passage of the first needle by holding the Foley with its stylet against the inner ipsilateral thigh. An Allis or hemostat may be placed in the center of the sling material to prevent twisting of the mesh or its sleeve.
11. After attaching the introducer, the first needle is passed 1 cm lateral to the urethra with the curve of the needle in the palm of the surgeon's hand. The needle penetrates the urogenital diaphragm behind the symphysis pubis.
12. Two fingers of the other hand are placed over the skin incision, the needle is pushed through the retropubic space, and the introducer is removed. The needle is guided up to partially protrude through the abdominal wall.
13. Before the trocar needle is extracted and removed, the Foley is removed and cystoscopy is performed. When bladder integrity has been confirmed, the first needle may be brought out through the abdominal wall, cut from the sling material, and a hemostat attached to the mesh and sleeve.
14. The procedure is then repeated on the other side with the Foley directed toward the ipsilateral inner thigh during insertion and passage of the needle.
15. Once the tape is in place, an 8-Fr Hegar dilator is positioned between the tape and the urethra for tension testing. The patient is asked to cough, and the tape is adjusted until there is no leak or only a few drops of fluid are lost during coughing. The plastic sleeves are then removed by pulling them up through the abdominal incisions. The excess mesh that protrudes is cut at the skin surface.
16. The vaginal mucosa is closed with a running stitch of 2-0 chromic suture. Steri-Strips or skin sutures are used to close the abdominal incisions.
17. A perineal pad may be placed to absorb any vaginal bleeding. Abdominal dressings are applied at the surgeon's discretion.

## Transvaginal Sling with Bone Anchor

Indications and contraindications for this procedure are the same as with the TVT sling procedure. In addition, the patient with severe osteoporosis may not be a good candidate for this technique because the bone anchors may not get incorporated into the pubic bone properly.

Risks with this technique include bladder perforation, inadequate fixation of the bone anchor (this generally requires abandoning the method and using a different type of sling approach), urinary retention, pain, osteitis pubis or osteomyelitis of the pubic bone, and recurrent incontinence.

***Procedural Considerations.*** After IV sedation the patient is placed in the lithotomy position. The procedure takes about 30 minutes and may be performed using local anesthesia with monitored sedation. A vaginal packing and postoperative suprapubic Foley catheter are usually placed. Cystoscopy is performed before, during, and at the end of the procedure. Local anesthesia is administered into the abdominal wall muscle and fascia lateral to the midline and just above the symphysis pubis bilaterally, and suburethrally into the retropubic space bilaterally. Approximately 3 to 4 minutes should be allowed for the anesthetic to take effect; cystoscopy may be performed during this time.

A formal incision may not be necessary for this procedure. The bone anchors may be drilled into the pubic bone through the vaginal wall (Figure 15-64).[9,42,57] A tunnel is created under the vaginal wall, and the sling material is passed through the tunnel to the opposite side (Figure 15-65). The sling material may be cadaveric fascia or polypropylene mesh. A small retropubic entry wound is created, and the Prolene sutures attached to the bone anchor are tied against the pubic bone suprapubically.

### *Operative Procedure*

1. Before beginning the procedure the bone screw with preloaded #1 Prolene suture is loaded onto the bone drill. A plastic cover fits over the screw, protecting the patient during insertion.
2. A Foley catheter is inserted, the bladder drained, and the catheter clamped.
3. Allis clamps are placed and pulled gently upward expose the anterior vaginal wall.
4. Tension is put on the Prolene stitch that protrudes through the handle of the bone drill. The drill is inserted into the vagina in a line parallel to the plane of the symphysis pubis, and the drill head is held against the pubic bone.
5. Insertion is complete when the Prolene stitch stops rotating. Fixation of the screw is tested with a gentle downward tug on the suture. The bone screws should lie lateral to the symphysis pubis in the posterior midthird of the pubic bone.
6. The Foley is opened and drained. If the urine is bloody a cystoscopy is performed. Some surgeons choose to routinely perform cystoscopy after each screw insertion to evaluate bladder patency.
7. A right-angle clamp is employed to follow the tunnel of the Prolene suture upward. A small puncture is created in the urethropelvic ligament to allow passage of the sling material into the retropubic space.
8. A 2-cm tunnel is then established between the midurethra and bladder neck, behind the vaginal wall.
9. The sling material is perforated with a Keith needle, and the Prolene is passed through the eye of the needle. The suture is then transferred to the sling material. This is done twice on each end of the material.
10. The material is passed through the tunnel.
11. Following cystoscopy, steps 4 through 6 are repeated on the contralateral vaginal wall. The Prolene sutures are tied individually so that the material lies in close proximity to the pubic bone.
12. The vagina is sutured on each side with a single stitch of absorbable 2-0 sutures.
13. A vaginal pack soaked in antibiotic or estrogen cream is inserted. The Foley catheter is drained and attached to a closed drainage system.

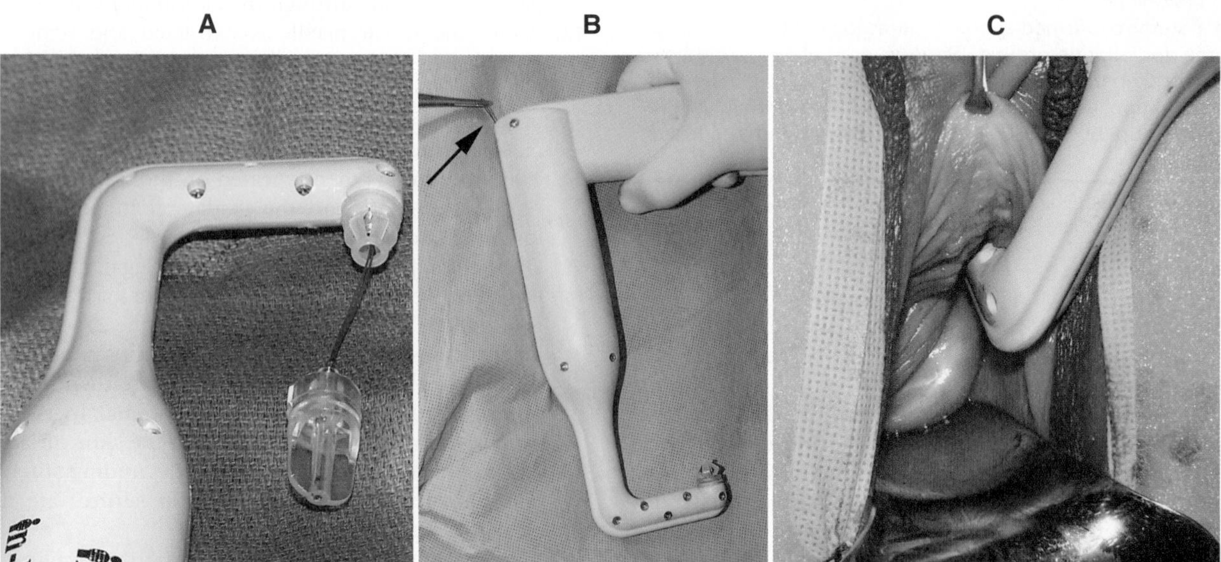


**FIGURE 15-64 A,** Bone anchor on bone drill with #1 Prolene. **B,** Bone drill ready, Prolene extends out handle. **C,** Bone drill in place.

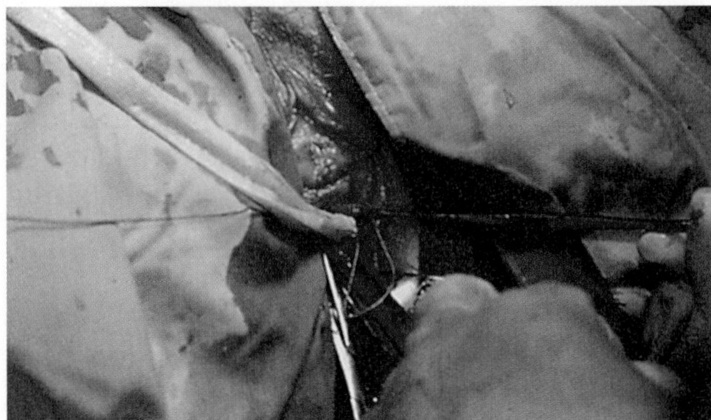

**FIGURE 15-65** Fascia lata graft being placed for suburethral sling procedure.

## Implantation of InterStim Sacral Nerve Stimulator (Neuromodulator)

The InterStim System is indicated for the treatment of urinary urge incontinence, urinary retention, and significant urgency-frequency in patients who have failed or could not tolerate other measures.[10,37] Before implantation, a period of test stimulation that may last from 3 to 7 days is carried out. If the patient fails to achieve an appropriate response during this test period, he or she may not be a candidate for the procedure. Patients who are unable to operate the neurostimulator should not be considered for this treatment.

Some precautions must be taken by the patient who has had this device implanted. MRI studies are not recommended. Caution should be taken and the device turned off if electrocoagulation will be employed during any future surgery the patient might undergo. Female patients should be instructed to carry their purses on the opposite side of the implant. The use of a magnet could turn the device off.

***Procedural Considerations.*** Preoperative antibiotics may be administered. The patient is placed in the prone position with a 30-degree flexion at the hips. Pillows may be placed under the patient's abdomen to support the lumbar area and decrease lordosis. Pillows are also placed under the ankles to elevate the feet and prevent pressure on the toes.

C-arm fluoroscopy is employed to visualize sacral landmarks and verify lead position intraoperatively. Although general anesthesia may be employed, monitored sedation with local anesthetic is preferable so that the patient may verbally respond to nerve stimuli during the procedure. It is suggested that no IV muscle relaxants be administered, because this will affect the physiologic response to the stimulator. If electrocoagulation is needed, a bipolar system should be employed, because unipolar current could potentially travel into the sacral foramen. The patient is typically discharged from the hospital on the same day.

The sacral area, buttocks, and perineum are prepped with the solution contained in the InterStim kit. The test stimulation ground pad is approximately 5 to 8 cm in size and is affixed to the patient's heel. An alternative to this placement is the calf or skin below the rib cage or iliac crest. This will be attached by a test stimulation cable to the external stimulator. The patient is draped to expose the entire buttock area so that responses to nerve stimulation may be assessed. The feet and lower legs are also exposed to allow visualization of muscle response.

The sacral outline and S3 foramen are located and identified with a sterile marking pen. The posterior iliac spine, coccygeal tip, and midline should also be marked. To do this the upper border of the greater sciatic notch is palpated. The S3 sacral foramen is approximately one finger breadth from the midline whereas the S2 and S4 foramina are one finger breadth above and below S3. The sacral crest corresponds to S4, and the S3 foramen is 9 cm above the coccygeal tip and 2 cm from the midline.

### *Operative Procedure*

TINED LEAD TECHNIQUE—STAGED PROCEDURE. The foramen needle is used to identify the position of the electrode desired. Stimulation is now performed to elicit a bellows response (flattening of the perineum) and flexion of the great toe. This confirms that the needle is in the S3 foramen.

1. The guidewire is inserted into the foramen needle.
2. A 5-mm stab wound is created for the lead introducer.
3. The lead introducer, consisting of dilator and sheath, is slid over the guidewire and advanced into the foramen. The depth marker on the directional guide is aligned with the top of the dilator.
4. The dilator is then removed, and the sheath remains in place.
5. The tined lead, with its stylet (Figure 15-66), is inserted and passed through the sheath until the second white marker is aligned with the back of the sheath. The four electrodes on the lead are now exposed and visible on fluoroscopy.
6. Nerve responses are again assessed at this time by connecting the mini-J hook on the patient cable to the uninsulated

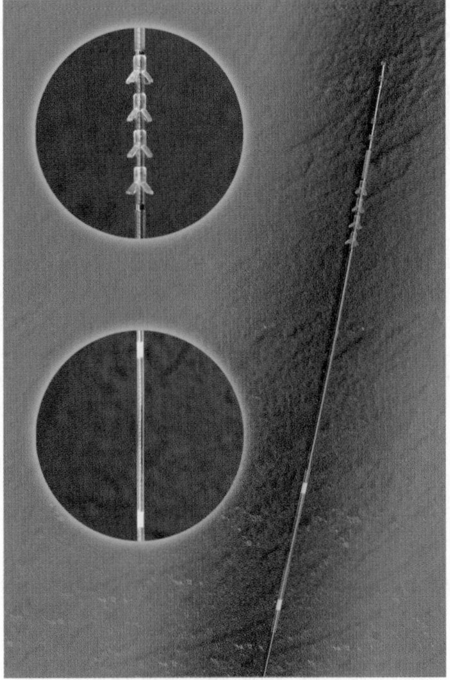

**FIGURE 15-66** InterStim tined lead.

section of the foramen needle. The electrodes are numbered zero to three, and the connector contacts on the needle correspond to these numbers. Beginning at the distal tip of the needle, all four electrodes are tested. The lead is repositioned according to the verbalized and visualized responses of the patient. The foramen producing the best results is chosen.

7. Once the electrodes are in optimal position the lead body proximal to the sheath is held in place and the sheath is slowly backed out of the wound. This is often accomplished under live fluoroscopy.
8. As the sheath is withdrawn the tines on the lead open, anchoring it in place.
9. A tunnel is now created for the subcutaneous neurostimulator generator pocket by means of the same incision. Placement is in the upper buttock below the beltline.
10. A pocket is created with the bipolar ESU. The pocket depth should not be greater than 4 cm to avoid interference with programming and shifting of the neurostimulator. The ideal pocket is 3 to 5 cm below the superior iliac crest and lateral to the outer sacral edge.
11. The tunneling tool with its metal tip and plastic tube is used to develop the tunnel from the lead to the intended pocket. Once tunneling is achieved the metal tip is removed and the tool is withdrawn, leaving the plastic tubing in place. The proximal lead end is then fed through the tubing to the pocket, and the tubing is removed. The protective boot is placed over the end of the lead. Leads may be placed bilaterally at the surgeon's discretion.
12. The percutaneous extension is then tunneled from the eventual generator site to the opposite posterior iliac side and exits the skin. This is then attached to the external device.
13. The incisions at all wound sites are closed. The wounds are dressed with small gauze and Tegaderm.

If the patient has a good response (50% or greater decrease in symptoms), then the area of generator site is extended in a second stage and the generator is connected to the lead (Figures 15-67 and 15-68). The percutaneous extension is pulled out through the other side and taken away from the field.

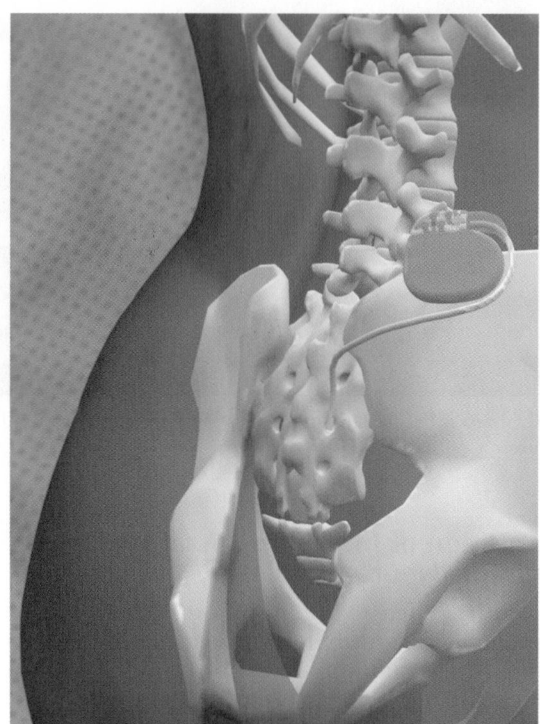

**FIGURE 15-67** Graphic placement of InterStim.

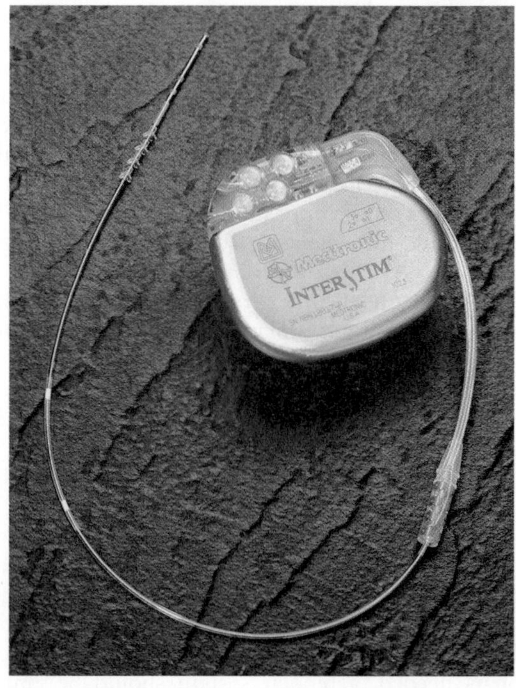


**FIGURE 15-68** InterStim implant.

## Male Sling

In the past few years, sling procedures have also been performed on the male patient. This has mixed success but warrants a brief overview. Using cadaveric dermis, fascia lata, or pericardium, a triangular sling is placed with three infrapubic bone screws under the bulbous urethra, bilaterally. This is accomplished through a midline perineal incision to the level of the scrotum. The sling is anchored by six screws that are placed into the inner portion of the descending ramus just below the symphysis pubis. The incidence of urgency postoperatively is presently higher in men than in women, but this is certainly a promising option versus the artificial urinary sphincter.[2,52]

## Bladder Augmentation

Augmentation enterocystoplasty is a procedure employed to surgically enlarge the bladder capacity. The segment of bowel used is re-formed into a semispheric shape to decrease peristaltic contractions and anastomosed to the opened bladder dome. The result is a low-pressure reservoir that provides improved bladder capacity and urinary compliance. Almost all segments of bowel as well as the stomach have been employed for bladder augmentation. Selection depends on anatomic factors, functional characteristics, and the surgeon's preference. In some cases, ureteral reimplantation or associated bladder-outlet procedures are incorporated in a one-stage procedure.

A wide range of conditions that were previously treated with urinary diversion may now be successfully managed with this technique. Indications include reflex incontinence unresponsive to medical management, detrusor hyperactivity with compromised bladder function, chronically contracted bladder resulting from radiation or repeated infections, and neuropathic bladder combined with recurrent urinary tract infections or compromised renal function.

Postoperatively, intermittent catheterization and bladder irrigations may be necessary. The patient must be able and willing to learn and perform these and must be accepting of this alteration in life-style.

***Procedural Considerations.*** The patient is placed in the supine position under general or regional anesthesia. The female patient may be in a frog-leg or lithotomy position, particularly if access to the perineum is necessary. A nasogastric tube is frequently inserted after induction. The entire abdomen and genitalia are prepped and draped. A Foley catheter is inserted into the sterile field, and the bladder is filled to capacity once the abdomen has been entered. Basic laparotomy and intestinal instruments are required.

### *Operative Procedure*

1. A supraumbilical to symphysis midline abdominal incision is made.
2. The peritoneal cavity is exposed using a Bookwalter or similar retractor.
3. The intestines and stomach are examined, and the appropriate segment for reconstruction is chosen (Figure 15-69, *A*).
4. A sagittal bladder incision is made from 2 cm cephalad to the bladder neck anteriorly across the anterior bladder wall, the peritonealized dome surface, and the posterior bladder wall to 2 cm above the posterior interureteric ridge. This causes the bladder to be bivalved in a clam-shaped design.
5. Traction sutures are placed bilaterally along the bladder incision.

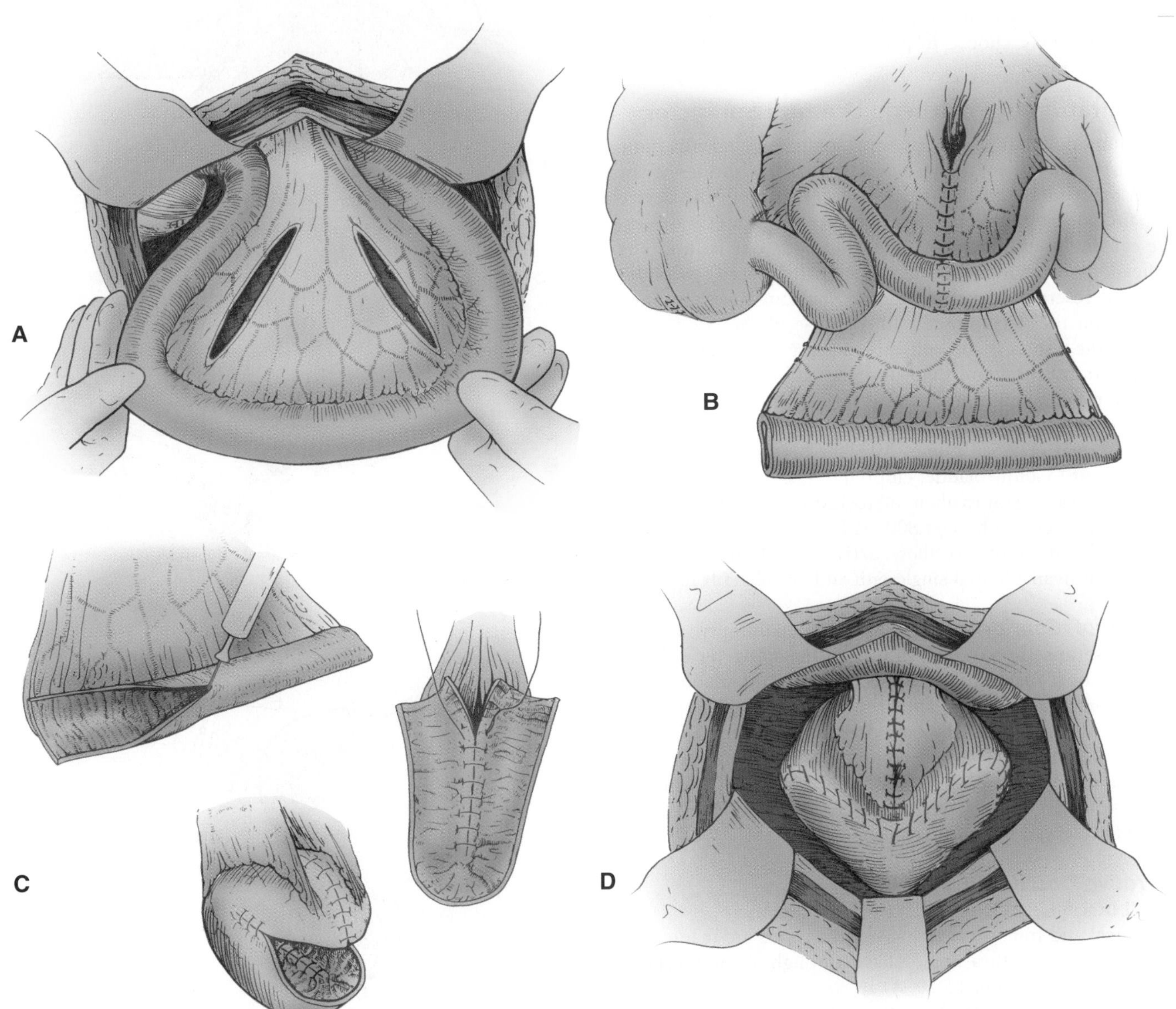


**FIGURE 15-69** Ileocystoplasty for bladder augmentation.

6. The length of the incision is measured to correlate with the corresponding segment of bowel or stomach. Average length required is 25 cm.
7. The segment to be used is mobilized, and the mesentery is closed cephalad so that the segment is on the retroperitoneum. The segment is left attached to its mesentery to maintain blood supply (Figure 15-69, *B*).
8. The isolated segment is opened, trimmed, and detubularized. It is then doubly folded and sutured to form a cup patch (Figure 15-69, *C*).
9. Anastomosis is accomplished with a running, intermittent locking, absorbable suture, beginning at the posterior apex and running up each side.
10. With one third of the attachment complete, sutures are placed at the anterior apex and run bilaterally to meet cephalad (Figure 15-69, *D*).
11. Integrity of the anastomosis is checked by again filling the bladder and observing for leaks.
12. Abdominal closure is performed, and dressings are applied. The nasogastric tube stays in place for 3 postoperative days. The Foley catheter will remain for 7 to 14 days. Some surgeons may choose to place a suprapubic catheter instead of a Foley.

## Implantation of Prosthetic Urethral Sphincter

Implantation of a prosthetic urethral sphincter is usually done as a last measure for patients with stress incontinence for which other modalities have failed. Problems with the device have included foreign-body reaction, persistent urethral pressure causing urethral erosion, and fluid hydraulic failure. The artificial sphincter unit has an abdominally placed, pressure-regulated reservoir that maintains a constant predetermined pressure on the periurethral cuff. Because of the connection between the reservoir and cuff, any increase in intraabdominal pressure transmits more fluid into the cuff. This connection allows for a compensatory increase in urethral resistance during coughing or straining.[2]

The scrotal or labial pump shifts the fluid into the cuff to the reservoir to allow bladder emptying. The fluid reenters the cuff through a resistor in about 60 to 120 seconds. The locking button in the AMS Sphincter 800 artificial sphincter unit traps fluid in the reservoir to allow activation of the cuff. The sphincter is available in a single-cuff and double-cuff model.

***Procedural Considerations.*** Standard laparotomy and lithotomy setups are required, as well as the sphincter components, contrast material diluted according to the manufacturer's recommendations, and an antibiotic solution. The patient is placed in a modified lithotomy position.

Stricture disease is more commonly found in the male population, and the most common cuff placement is around the bulbous urethra. Bladder neck placement of the cuff is generally reserved only for females.

### *Operative Procedure*

BULBOUS URETHRAL CUFF

1. Perineal and transverse suprapubic incisions are made.
2. The bulbous urethra is mobilized through a midline perineal incision (Figure 15-70, *A*).
3. A 2-cm space is created beneath the bulbocavernous muscle and around the bulbous urethra.
4. The cuff, tab end first, is placed around the bulbous urethra (Figure 15-70, *B*).
5. The reservoir is placed beneath the rectus muscle through the suprapubic incision (Figure 15-70, *C*).
6. The pump is attached to the tubing passer (see Figure 15-25, A), introduced through the suprapubic incision and transferred to the scrotum through a subcutaneous tunnel created between the two incisions. The reservoir, cuff, and pump are connected and filled with contrast material or injectable saline to the appropriate volume (Figure 15-71).

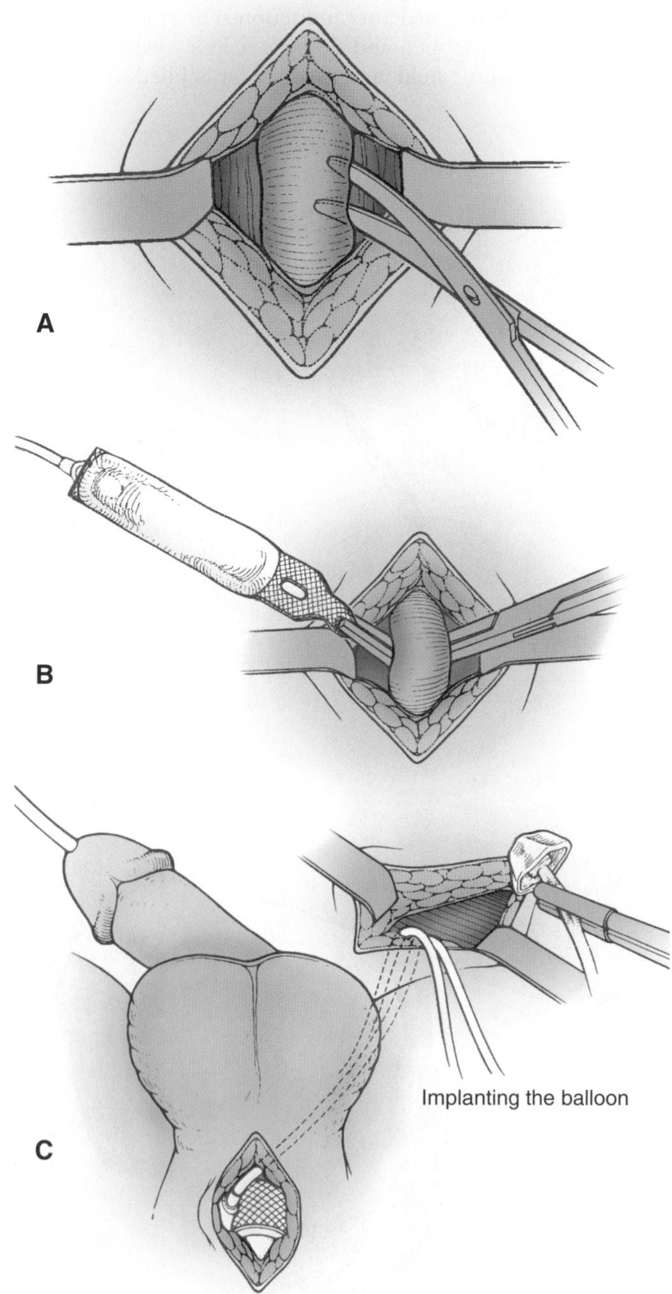


**FIGURE 15-70** Implantation of artificial urinary sphincter.

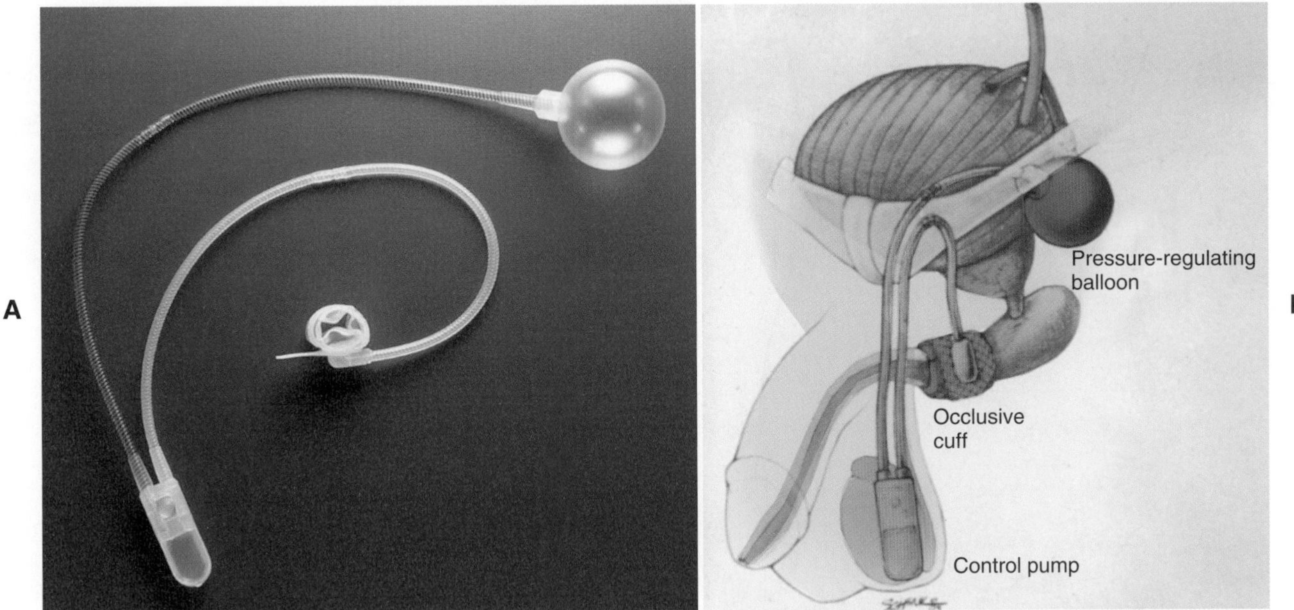


FIGURE 15-71 **A,** AMS 800 single-cuff artificial urinary sphincter. **B,** Final placement of artificial urinary sphincter.

7. The wound is closed and dressed with gauze sponges. A urethral catheter is usually not inserted.

## Radical Cystectomy with Pelvic Lymphadenectomy

Cystectomy is the total excision of the urinary bladder and adjacent structures along with pelvic lymph nodes. Cystectomy is a surgical consideration when a vesical malignancy has invaded the muscular wall of the bladder or when frequent recurrences of widespread papillary tumors do not respond to endoscopic or chemotherapeutic management. The patient should be medically able to withstand surgery with the expectation of reasonable longevity. Total cystectomy necessitates permanent urinary diversion into an ileal or colonic conduit. In a male patient, the prostate gland, seminal vesicles, and distal ureters are removed with the bladder and its peritoneal surface. In a female patient, the bladder, urethra, distal ureters, uterus, cervix, and proximal third of the vagina are removed.

***Procedural Considerations.*** The patient is placed in the supine position. Instruments are as described for major abdominal procedures. For a male patient, if the prostate and seminal vesicles are to be removed, prostatectomy instruments should be added. For a female patient, vaginal and abdominal hysterectomy as well as plastic surgery instruments should be added (see Chapters 14 and 24).

***Operative Procedure.*** A midline incision from the epigastrium to the symphysis pubis, curving to the left of the umbilicus, is generally used.

1. The peritoneal cavity is entered above the umbilicus. The entire urachal remnant is clamped, divided, and tied off with heavy silk ligatures (Figure 15-72, *A*). It will be removed en bloc with the bladder.
2. The bladder dome is lifted at its peritoneal surface, and dissection proceeds laterally on either side with ligation of the major vesical arteries to the level of the vas deferens or round ligament (Figure 15-72, *B*).
3. The vas deferens is divided, and the urethra is cut at the level of the pelvic diaphragm.
4. The ureters are identified and traced to the bladder. Care is taken to preserve the adventitial tissue (Figure 15-72, *C*).
5. Abdominal exploration and pelvic lymphadenectomy with frozen sections are performed to rule out metastatic disease.
6. In the *male* patient, the bladder is then retracted to expose the endopelvic fascia and puboprostatic ligaments. The prostate, dorsal venous complex, and seminal vesicles are dissected free, as described for a radical retropubic prostatectomy (Figure 15-72, *D*). These will be removed in continuity with the bladder.
7. In the *female* patient, the broad ligament is bilaterally incised posterior to the fallopian tube and ovary to the level of the posterior vagina to be removed en bloc with the bladder (Figure 15-72, *E*). The endopelvic fascia is incised at the bladder neck to expose the proximal urethra. The vagina is then incised along the lateral walls to the level of the proximal urethra and bladder neck. The anterior vaginal wall is incised in a U fashion to circumscribe the urethra (Figure 15-72, *F*). The vagina is reconstructed.
8. The surgical specimen consists of the bladder, distal ureters, prostate, seminal vesicles, and distal vas in the male and the uterus, fallopian tubes, and ovaries in the female and is removed en bloc.
9. The urethra is ligated with absorbable suture. If urethrectomy is indicated, this is done en bloc with the bladder.
10. Lap pads are placed in the denuded pelvis, and pressure is applied to reduce blood loss from oozing.

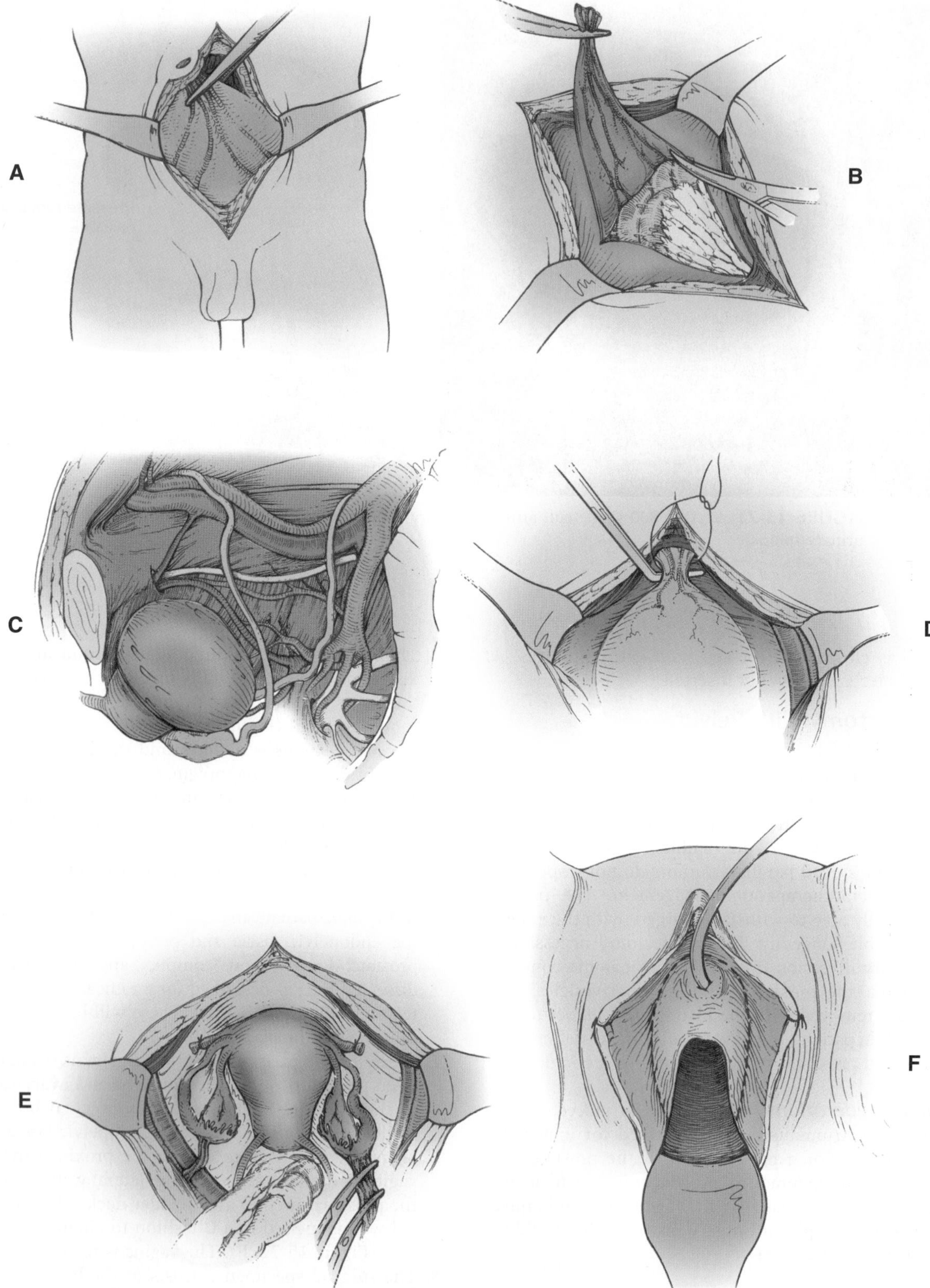


FIGURE 15-72 **A,** The urachal remnant is identified and divided just below the umbilicus. **B,** The peritoneum is divided laterally to the umbilical ligaments to the level of the vas deferens or round ligament. **C,** The ureter crossing the bifurcation of the iliac vessels is identified. **D,** Right-angled clamp is passed beneath the dorsal venous complex, anterior to the membranous urethra. **E,** In female patients the ovaries, fallopian tubes, and uterus are removed en bloc with the bladder and anterior vaginal wall. **F,** U-shaped incision is made on the anterior vagina to circumscribe the urethra.

11. Urinary diversion is accomplished by means of an isolated ileal or colonic conduit, an orthotopic diversion, or a continent urinary diversion.

## Bladder Substitution (Substitution Cystoplasty)

The ideal candidate for a bladder replacement after cystectomy for carcinoma is a patient with a normal urethra; a proximally located, well-differentiated bladder tumor; absence of carcinoma in situ; and proof, in the male patient, that the prostatic urethra is free of disease. High-dose radiation offers appreciable risks for postoperative complications and is contraindicated with enterourethral anastomosis. A discussion of techniques to create a neobladder follows.

***Right Colocystoplasty.*** Depending on the extent of involvement, the right side of the colon may be used to replace the bladder, the bladder and prostatic urethra, or the bladder and prostate with a direct enteric-to-proximal bulbar urethral anastomosis. This procedure has become more functionally effective with the use of intermittent self-catheterization and selective implantation of a prosthetic urinary sphincter.

***Ileocecal Bladder Substitution.*** The ileum has been used as a reservoir to restore urinary continuity because it possesses a low intraluminal pressure. However, the short mesentery does not always permit the bowel to reach the urethra and results are not consistently successful. There have been significant incidences of recurrent carcinoma, renal damage, incontinence, postoperative strictures, fistula, hypokalemia, anemia, suture-line breakdown, and stone formation. Although most patients attain daytime urinary control, approximately 30% still have problems with enuresis. Deterioration of the upper urinary tract as a result of infection and obstruction has historically been a significant risk with this procedure, and therefore ileocecal substitution is met with mixed reactions and recommendations.

***Sigmoidocystoplasty.*** Because of the sigmoid colon's ease of construction, bladder proximity, decreased obstruction from mucus, and large capacity, it has been more appealing to many surgeons in their attempt to create a new bladder. More efficient emptying with a larger reservoir capacity seems to occur with a sigmoid replacement. Results yield higher intraluminal pressures, more effective urinary flow rates, and less nocturnal incontinence than with ileal segments.

***Ileoascending Bladder Substitution.*** In an effort to improve the intestinal reservoir's capacity and antirefluxing effectiveness, the use of the ascending colon as a continent reservoir was introduced. This technique has several anatomic advantages over other methods of bladder replacement. The segment used can include the hepatic flexure and proximal transverse colon. A large-capacity reservoir is obtained, and colonic incision or tailoring is not required to achieve an appropriate shape. It easily reaches any site within the pelvis and can be anastomosed directly to the urethra without tension.

***Orthotopic Ileocolic Neobladder.*** A bladder substitution using the right colon and ileum has shown remarkable effectiveness.[36] "Le bag" continent diversion technique was developed specifically for orthotopic bladder replacement. Bladder substitution relies on meticulous dissection of the prostatic apex with preservation of the urinary sphincter and neurovascular bundles, as well as a watertight urethral anastomosis. Most patients have achieved a high degree of daytime continence and a minimum of nocturnal enuresis. Short-term complications encountered include bleeding, infection, urinary extravasation, bladder perforation, urethral stricture, fistula formation, urinoma, and small bowel obstruction. Long-term problems include chronic constipation or diarrhea, compromised enterohepatic circulation, vitamin $B_{12}$ deficiency, and urinary incontinence in a small percentage of patients.

Considerations influencing patient selection include age, general health, and fitness for extensive, complicated surgery. Contraindications include previous radiation therapy, bowel disease (diverticulosis, Crohn's disease, colitis), and other major medical problems. Preoperative urethral biopsy specimens are frequently taken to rule out tumor or cellular atypia in the urethra, which would prevent this particular intervention.

PROCEDURAL CONSIDERATIONS. The patient is placed in the supine position. SCDs are applied before the induction of anesthesia. A cystectomy and prostatectomy or hysterectomy (female) are performed. Major deep intestinal, bladder, and prostate or hysterectomy instruments, as well as a large self-retaining retractor, are needed.

OPERATIVE PROCEDURE

1. After cystoprostatectomy, the right side of the colon is reflected medially along the mesentery to the hepatic flexure. The distal ileum that is to be used in the neobladder is inspected.
2. The small bowel is divided and laid in an S shape, and stay sutures of 2-0 or 3-0 absorbable material are placed.
3. The posterior walls are sewn from inside to outside with running 3-0 absorbable suture.
4. A seromuscular wedge of the dependent cecum is excised, and the mucosa is everted with 4-0 absorbable sutures to form a bladder neck.
5. The left ureter is brought retroperitoneally under the sigmoid mesentery, a submucosal tunnel is created, and the ureters are reimplanted through the colonic wall. Anastomosis is done from the interior of the pouch.
6. Anchor sutures of 3-0 or 4-0 silk are placed at the outer entry point. The wall of the colon is anchored to the psoas muscle with 3-0 or 4-0 silk to prevent migration of the neobladder.
7. Ureteral stents are placed and brought out through the colonic segment and a separate abdominal stab wound, along with a catheter to serve as a suprapubic tube.
8. Sutures of 2-0 absorbable material are placed around the urethral stump and tagged.
9. A Foley catheter is inserted into the urethra in a retrograde manner, and the urethra is anastomosed to the neobladder at the point of the new bladder neck.
10. The neobladder is closed in an intestinal fashion or with a GI stapler in a side-to-side anastomosis. Wound drains are placed, the bladder filled to test for leaks, and the wound closed.

## Cutaneous Urinary Diversions

***Ileal Conduit.*** The ileal conduit is the classic method by which the urine flow is diverted to an isolated loop of bowel. One end of the isolated loop is brought out through the skin so that the urine can be collected in a drainage bag, which is intermittently emptied. The stoma site should be carefully selected preoperatively by the surgeon and enterostomal therapist. The selected site, usually in the right lower quadrant of the abdomen, above the beltline, is marked with a fine needle dipped in methylene blue to prevent erasure during skin preparation. The goal is to create a round, protruding stoma without wrinkles in the skin, to prevent urine leakage under the collecting device. Puckering of the skin around the stoma is minimized by using a subcuticular technique when the surgeon is suturing the stoma in place. The candidate for ileal diversion must have a retrievable ureter at least 1 cm in diameter with a thick, well-vascularized wall. The patient must be able to care for the appliance. Conditions amenable to diversion include neurogenic bladder, interstitial cystitis, and bladder carcinoma. Cystectomy may be performed before or after this procedure, depending on the patient's diagnosis. In cases that do not involve bladder cancer, a surgeon may choose to leave the bladder in situ rather than subject a debilitated patient to further surgery. In certain cases of extensive bladder carcinoma, the surgeon may elect to treat the patient with radiation in an attempt to decrease the size of the tumor and "sterilize" the regional lymph nodes before performing cystectomy.

PROCEDURAL CONSIDERATIONS. The patient is placed in the supine position. Abdominal and GI instruments are required. A cystectomy, prostatectomy, or hysterectomy may also be done at the time of the surgery. Endostapling devices, with absorbable staples, should be available.

OPERATIVE PROCEDURE

1. The bladder is decompressed with a catheter.
2. The abdomen is entered through a midline abdominal incision. A self-retaining abdominal retractor is placed to exclude the viscera from the region of dissection.
3. The ureters are identified and severed approximately 2.5 cm from the bladder.
4. A retroperitoneal tunnel is made so that the left ureter lies close to the right ureter.
5. The distal ileum and mesentery are inspected to identify the bowel's blood supply.
6. A drain is passed through the mesentery, midway between the two main arterial arcades adjacent to the ileum at the proximal and distal ends of the selected segment. This segment usually makes up 15 to 20 cm of the terminal ileum, a few centimeters from the ileocecal valve. The ileocecal artery is preserved to maintain adequate circulation to the isolated ileal segment.
7. The peritoneum is incised over the proposed line of division of the mesentery.
8. Intestinal clamps are placed across the ileum, and the bowel is divided flush with the clamps.
9. Using GI technique (see Chapter 11), the proximal end of the isolated ileal segment is closed first with a layer of absorbable sutures and then with a second layer of interrupted 2-0 nonabsorbable sutures.
10. The proximal and distal segments of ileum are reanastomosed end-to-end in two layers.
11. The mesenteric incision is closed with interrupted nonabsorbable sutures.
12. The closed proximal end of the conduit segment is fixed to the posterior peritoneum.
13. The ureters are implanted in the ileal segment, using fine instruments and 4-0 absorbable ureteral sutures on atraumatic needles.
14. The peritoneum and muscle of the abdominal wall lateral to the original incision are separated by blunt dissection.
15. The abdominal opening for the stoma is made, and the distal opening of the ileal conduit is then drawn through a fenestration in the muscle, fascia, and skin.
16. The ileum is fixed to the fascia with 2-0 sutures. A rosebud stoma is constructed as the ileum is sutured to the skin using subcuticular stitches (Figure 15-73).
17. Ureteral stents are usually left in the stoma, and a urinary collecting pouch is placed over the rosebud stoma to collect urine.
18. The wound is drained with two Jackson-Pratt drains. The abdominal incision is closed and the skin reapproximated.

## Continent Urinary Diversions

The Kock pouch, the right colocystoplasty, and the Camey version of the ileocystoplasty have been modified for anastomosis to a urethral stump or the prostatic capsule, resulting in effective continent bladder replacement. All continent urinary diversions create an easily catheterized stoma and a nonrefluxing ureteral anastomosis. Different parts of the bowel and the stomach have been used as continent reservoirs. The choice of the antireflux mechanism depends on the implantation site. The stoma does not require an appliance; therefore the site may be placed below the beltline or bikini line, making it able to be catheterized when the patient is sitting. It may be anastomosed to the proximal urethra, thus forming an orthotopic bladder.

### *Ileal Reservoir (Kock Pouch)*

PROCEDURAL CONSIDERATIONS. A continent reservoir formed into a U configuration is constructed of a section of ileum proximal to the ileocecal valve. The legs of the U are

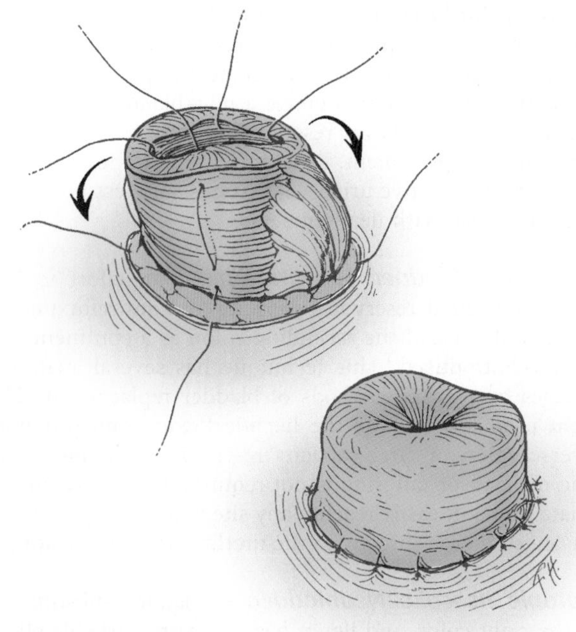

FIGURE 15-73 Rosebud suture technique for stoma.

sewn together at the antimesenteric border. The intestine is opened adjacent to the antimesenteric border, and the back wall of the pouch is reinforced with absorbable suture.

Continence is achieved by the valve mechanism with the nipple valve attached to the skin. Nipple valves are created proximally and distally by intussusception of the bowel into the reservoir cavity. Once the nipples are fixed to the sidewall of the reservoir with absorbable suture or polyglycolic staples, the anterior wall is closed. The ureters are anastomosed to the afferent limb of the pouch, preventing reflux. The efferent limb is drawn through the stoma site and anchored to the abdominal wall fascia.

OPERATIVE PROCEDURE

1. The mesentery is divided and suture- or staple-ligated along the avascular plane between the superior mesenteric artery and the ileocolic artery.
2. The bowel is divided, and four segments are measured and marked with silk suture tags. These segments will serve as the efferent conduit, the pouch, and the afferent limb.
3. A portion of the proximal ileum is resected and discarded along with a wedge of mesentery. Suction is passed down the lumen to clear any fecal material or mucus.
4. The proximal end is closed with suture or stapled.
5. The segment to be employed is spread out in a U-shaped fashion. The sides are sewn together with 3-0 absorbable suture in a running fashion or connected using a GI endostapler.
6. The bowel is incised with electrosurgery laterally to the suture in the two loops. The medial edges are oversewn with 3-0 or 4-0 silk.
7. The mesentery is cleared on the limb segments, and the lumens are intussuscepted into the open pouch.
8. Marlex mesh is used to serve as a strut to prevent peristomal herniation and to fix the base of the efferent nipple to the abdominal wall, facilitating catheterization. The TA or similar endostapler is used to form each nipple and to attach the nipples to the back wall of the pouch.
9. An 8-Fr stenting catheter is placed inside the nipple of the efferent conduit to prevent making the collar too tight.
10. The limbs are secured with 3-0 or 4-0 silk suture.
11. The pouch is closed with sutures or the endostapler.
12. The ureters are anastomosed, as described in the "Ileal Conduit" discussion, to the afferent limb.
13. A small stoma site is prepared, as described in the "Ileal Conduit" discussion. A catheter of choice is placed in the stoma for postoperative care. Stents may be placed in the ureters for the immediate postoperative period. This will necessitate initial placement of an ileostomy appliance until all systems are functioning.
14. A drain is placed, which exits through a separate stab wound.
15. The wound is closed. Retention sutures may be employed. Bulky absorbent dressings are applied; Montgomery straps may be used.

### *Indiana Pouch*

**PROCEDURAL CONSIDERATIONS.** The Indiana pouch technique is a modification of the original ileocecal diversion. A continent reservoir is constructed of the right side of the colon, which may include the ileum and cecum, the ileocecal valve, and ascending colon. Surgery proceeds as for any diversionary procedure. The ileocecal valve is reinforced with nonabsorbable suture. Two rows of nonabsorbable suture are used to then imbricate the ileal segment, which serves as a limb that can be catheterized once it is brought to the skin level as a stoma. The cecal segment is detubularized by incising along the taenia and anastomosing the distal edge horizontally to the proximal portion. Intussusception of the ileocecal valve into the cecum and narrowing of the ileal segment attached to the skin allow for continence.

OPERATIVE PROCEDURE

1. The large bowel is split down the antimesenteric border for approximately three fourths of its length.
2. The U-shaped defect is closed.
3. The terminal ileum is sutured along its length over a small Robinson catheter in an intestinal fashion.
4. The pouch is filled with 400 ml of saline, and a larger catheter is placed to determine ability to be catheterized.
5. The ureters are tunneled into the cecum through its taenia and then tacked to the outer bowel wall. The cecum is secured to the pelvic wall. Ureteral stents may be placed.
6. The pouch is secured to the abdominal wall.
7. The stomal site is prepared as described in the "Ileal Conduit" discussion.
8. A 22-Fr Malecot drain is placed in the reservoir to drain the cecostomy, exiting through a separate stab wound.

## SURGERY OF THE URETERS AND KIDNEYS

Stones, infections, and tumors are the most common causes of urinary tract obstruction, necessitating surgery to prevent renal obstruction and subsequent renal failure. Obstruction may also result from congenital malformations or previous operations on the urinary tract (Figure 15-74).

Although the causes of many kidney stones are obscure, certain conditions, such as obstruction, stasis, and imbalance of metabolism, predispose to their formation. Stones consist of various elements: calcium oxalate, calcium phosphate, magnesium ammonium phosphate, uric acid, calcium carbonate, and cystine. An increase in the concentration of any of these can cause tiny crystals to form; as these clump together, they begin to form a stone. Stones removed during surgery are subjected to chemical analysis. These specimens should be submitted in a dry jar. Fixative agents such as formalin should not be used.

Stones in the renal pelvis may fall into the ureteropelvic junction and obstruct the flow of urine. However, stones less than 3 cm in diameter may also pass down the ureter and lodge at a more distal location. A stone may remain in a renal calyx and continue to enlarge, eventually filling the entire renal collecting system (staghorn calculus). Diverticula may form and harbor stones that can be difficult to reach and treat.[29] Hydroureteronephrosis, infection, and destruction of renal parenchyma frequently result from unrelieved obstruction.

Hypothermia is useful in renal stone surgery as a means of prolonging the safe period of renal ischemia. Several methods enable renal cooling: ice slush or cold saline solution, surface cooling coils, perfusion of cold solutions through the renal artery, or a variation of these basic techniques, such as perfusion of the renal pelvis with saline that has been cooled by a coil immersed in ice slush.

A refrigeration unit "slush machine" that produces sterile slush provides a cost-effective, time-saving alternative to the

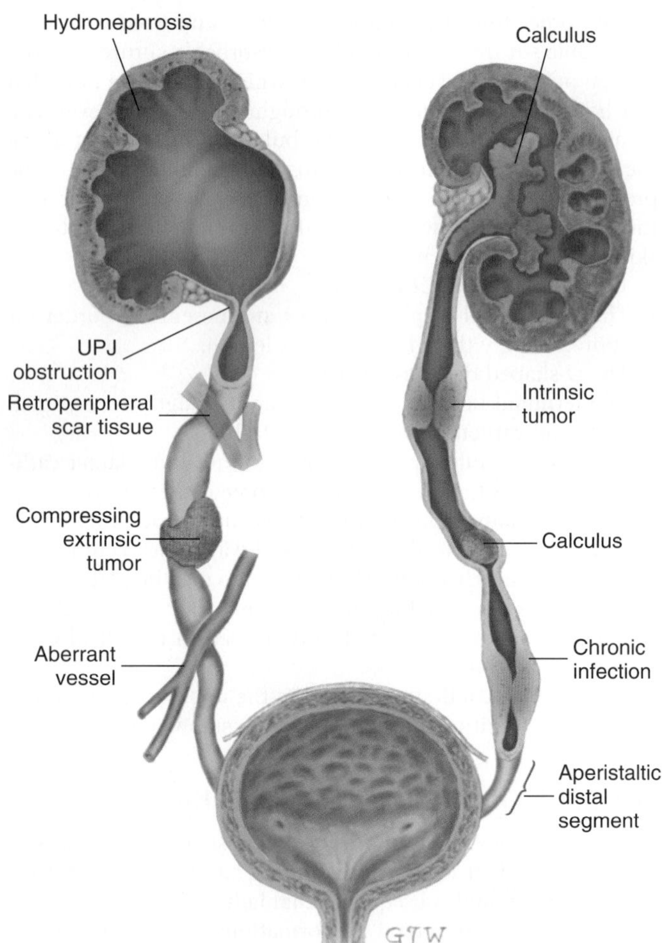


**FIGURE 15-74** Some common causes of urinary tract obstruction. *UPJ,* ureteropelvic junction.

other methods of slush preparation. Commercially synthesized ultrafiltrate of sterile plasma in liter bottles is also available for use as the slush. Saline slush for renal surgery may also be manually prepared in several ways. Sterile Mason jars are filled with sterile normal saline solution and doubly wrapped in sterile plastic bags. Each bag is individually wrapped and secured with a twist tie. The Mason jars are placed in a bucket of ice, to which 2 pints of isopropyl alcohol (isopropanol) and two boxes of salt are added, and mixed for 2 to 3 hours. When the saline is ready for use, the circulating nurse removes the wrapped Mason jar from the ice, opens the plastic bags by sterile technique, and presents the Mason jar to the scrub nurse. The scrub person shakes the contents of the Mason jar to cause crystallization of the saline. The slush is removed from the Mason jar with a sterile spoon. Alternatively, a rigid plastic container of 1000 ml of normal saline or lactated Ringer's solution may be placed on its side in a freezer several hours before surgery. To prevent the solution from solidifying, the container should be rotated one-half turn every 20 to 30 minutes. Sterile slush may then be poured directly into a sterile basin as required.

The surgical approach in renal surgery depends on the patient's condition, the amount of exposure needed, and the surgical procedure to be performed. There are three principal surgical approaches to the kidney. The simple *flank,* or *transabdominal,* incision is most frequently used and may include removal of the eleventh or twelfth rib. The incision begins at the posterior axillary line and parallels the course of the twelfth rib. It extends forward and slightly downward between the iliac crest and the thorax. For the *lumbar* incision, the patient may be initially positioned supine and then rotated to lateral and slightly forward over protective bolsters with the operative side up. This effectively places the flank in an oblique position, causing the abdominal viscera to fall away from the operative incision, and affords an excellent approach to the renal pedicle. Alternatively, the patient may be placed prone with bolsters under the affected side to provide elevation. The *thoracoabdominal* exposure is employed primarily for large upper-pole renal neoplasms. The tenth and eleventh ribs are usually removed, and the chest cavity is opened, collapsing the lung. The leaves of the diaphragm are separated to expose the kidney. A large retractor, such as a Finochietto, and chest drains are required.

## Surgery of the Ureter

*Ureterostomy* (ureterotomy) is opening the ureter for continued drainage from it into another body part. Cutaneous ureterostomy is diversion of the flow of urine from the kidney, through the ureter, away from the bladder, and onto the skin of the lower abdomen. A suitable urinary collecting device is then placed over the ureteral stoma.

*Ureterectomy* is complete removal of the ureter. This procedure is generally employed in collecting system tumors and includes nephrectomy and the excision of a cuff of bladder.

*Ureteroureterostomy* is segmental resection of a diseased portion of the ureter and reconstruction in continuity of the two normal segments.

*Ureteroenterostomy* is diversion of the ureter into a segment of the ileum (ureteroileostomy, or more commonly, ileal urinary conduit) or into the sigmoid colon (ureterosigmoidostomy). Ureteroneocystostomy (ureterovesical anastomosis) is division of the distal ureter from the bladder and reimplantation of the ureter into the bladder with a submucosal tunnel.

Reconstructive operations may be indicated because of a pathologic condition of the bladder or lower ureter that interferes with normal drainage. Conditions requiring urinary diversion or reconstruction of the urinary tract include malignancy, cystitis, stricture, trauma, and congenital ureterovesical reflux. Invasive vesical malignancy requiring surgical removal of the bladder necessitates urinary diversion.

Ureterocutaneous transplant, ureterosigmoid anastomosis, and ileal conduit are urinary diversionary procedures performed when the bladder is no longer functioning as a proper urine reservoir. Etiologic factors causing irreparable vesical dysfunction are chronic inflammation, interstitial cystitis, neurogenic bladder, exstrophy, trauma, tumor, and infiltrative disease (amyloidosis). Ureterolithotomy is incision into the ureter and removal of an obstructing calculus.

***Procedural Considerations.*** The site of the incision and position of the patient depend on the nature of the proposed surgery. The patient may be placed in the supine position for abdominal surgery, in the modified Trendelenburg position for low abdominal or pelvic surgery, or in the lateral position for high or mid ureteral obstructing calculi (see Figure 5-24, p. 156). The arms should be supinated when on armboards; in lateral position the upper arm is placed on an overbed armboard such as the Allen lateral arm support and the lower arm is supinated on a padded armboard. The kidney rest should lie just under the dependent iliac crest.

Instruments include the nephrectomy set, plus plastic instrumentation for pyeloplasty. Additional instruments may be required, depending on the type of operation and the surgical approach used.

### *Operative Procedures*

URETERAL REIMPLANTATION

1. The ureter is exposed through an incision determined by the location of the pathologic condition. A ureteral catheter, passed retrograde, may be used to facilitate identification and isolation of the ureter.
2. The ureter is dissected free with long forceps and scissors, picked up with the fine traction sutures, freed from the surrounding tissues, and severed at the desired level.
3. The distal end of the ureter is ligated, and the proximal stoma is transferred to the site of anastomosis. The anastomosis is accomplished with fine dissection instruments and fine atraumatic sutures.
4. A soft splinting stent is usually left in place until healing has taken place and free drainage is ensured. The wound is closed in layers and dressings applied.

URETEROCUTANEOUS TRANSPLANT (ANASTOMOSIS). The surgical approach is the same as that for a low ureterolithotomy.

1. The ureter is divided as far distally as possible.
2. The severed ureter is passed retroperitoneally through the lower abdominal wall and sutured to the skin with an absorbable everting suture of 4-0 on an atraumatic needle to form a stoma. The ureter is handled gently with plastic instruments, fixation forceps, and iris scissors.
3. A small Silastic stenting catheter is passed up into the ureter and left in place for 48 to 72 hours, as ureteral edema subsides. The patient requires a urine-collecting device after surgery.

URETEROSIGMOID ANASTOMOSIS

1. The peritoneal cavity is entered through a lower left paramedian incision.
2. The major portion of the large bowel is protected with moist packs.
3. Deep retractors are placed, and with long forceps and scissors the posterior peritoneum is incised.
4. The ureters are identified, divided close to the bladder, mobilized, and brought through the posterior peritoneal incision to lie near the sigmoid. Traction sutures and smooth tissue forceps are used to handle the ureters.
5. The sigmoid colon is mobilized to prevent tension on the ureteroenteric anastomosis.
6. The sigmoid colon is sutured with 3-0 nonabsorbable material to the pelvic peritoneum at a point where the ureter falls easily on the bowel.
7. Using a scalpel with a #15 blade, the surgeon makes an incision into the taenia of the sigmoid down to the mucosal layer. The edges of the taenia are undermined to create two parallel flaps.
8. The ureter is laid on the bowel mucosa, and a small slit is made through the mucosa into the lumen of the colon.
9. With fixation forceps and iris scissors, the ureter is beveled to lie flat in the tunica incision.
10. The distal ureter is anchored to the bowel mucosa with 4-0 absorbable ureteral sutures on atraumatic needles. The other ureter is anastomosed in the same manner in a position slightly above the first.
11. The tunicae are then loosely reapproximated over the ureter with 4-0 absorbable sutures, creating an antireflux anastomosis.
12. The posterior peritoneum is closed with absorbable sutures. Drains are brought out retroperitoneally. The incision is closed and dressings applied.

### *Ureterolithotomy*

PROCEDURAL CONSIDERATIONS. A KUB x-ray examination should be done immediately before surgery to determine the exact location of the stone. The surgeon may also schedule a cystoscopic examination preoperatively and may attempt to remove the stone endoscopically. The location of the stone determines the surgical approach. A stone high in the ureter requires a flank incision with possible removal of the twelfth rib; a more distal ureteral stone requires a lower abdominal incision.

OPERATIVE PROCEDURE

1. After exposure of the ureter, the stone may be kept stationary with Babcock clamps or vessel loops applied above and below it.
2. With a #15 blade, an incision in the ureter is made directly over the stone, which may be easily removed with a Randall stone forceps.
3. A 10-Fr catheter is passed proximally up and distally down the ureter while irrigating with saline to check for ureteral patency and to dislodge any remaining stone fragments.
4. The ureter is closed with 4-0 or 5-0 absorbable sutures. All stones should be placed in dry receptacles and sent to the chemistry laboratory for analysis.

## Surgery of the Kidney

See Box 15-2 for terms pertaining to kidney surgery.

**BOX 15-2**

**Terms Pertaining to Kidney Surgery**

| | |
|---|---|
| **Nephrostomy** | Creation of an opening into the kidney to maintain temporary or permanent urinary drainage. A nephrostomy is used to correct an obstruction of the urinary tract and to conserve and permit physiologic functioning of renal tissue. It is also used to provide permanent urinary drainage when a ureter is obstructed or for temporary urinary drainage immediately after a plastic repair on the kidney. |
| **Nephrotomy** | Incision into the kidney, usually over a collecting system containing a calculus. |
| **Pyelolithotomy** | Removal of a calculus through an opening in the renal pelvis. |
| **Pyelostomy** | Making an opening in the renal pelvis for temporarily or permanently diverting the flow of urine. |
| **Pyelotomy** | Incision into the renal pelvis used as an access to stones in the renal pelvis or collecting system. |

***Procedural Considerations.*** Patient preparation and instrument setup are as described for ureteral surgery.

### *Operative Procedures*

PYELOTOMY AND PYELOSTOMY

1. The pelvis of the kidney is incised with a small scalpel blade. Fine traction sutures may be placed at the edges of the incision for gentle retraction while the pelvis and calyces are explored.
2. In pyelostomy a small Malecot or Foley catheter is placed through the incision into the renal pelvis. Pyelotomy is used only for very short periods of renal drainage because tubes tend to be dislodged easily from the renal pelvis.

NEPHROSTOMY

1. A curved clamp or stone forceps is passed through a pyelotomy incision into the renal pelvis and then out through the substance of the renal parenchyma through a lower pole minor calyx.
2. The tip of a Malecot, Foley, or Pezzer catheter is drawn into the renal pelvis, and the pyelotomy incision is sutured closed.
3. The distal end of the nephrostomy tube is brought out through a separate stab incision in the flank.
4. A drain is placed at the level of the pyelotomy incision, and the wound is closed.

PYELOLITHOTOMY AND NEPHROLITHOTOMY

1. The renal pelvis is opened (Figure 15-75, *A*), and the pelvic calculus is gently removed.
2. The pelvis and collecting systems are thoroughly irrigated with saline using an Asepto syringe to dislodge and remove any small remaining stones from the kidney.
3. Nephrolithotomy or extended pyelolithotomy is employed when stones are locked in the calyceal system and cannot be removed through a pyelotomy incision. In such cases, the renal parenchyma above the stone is incised and the stone removed. In many instances, such a situation is associated with a calyceal diverticulum (Figure 15-75, *B*).
4. After the stone is removed, the collecting system is closed and the renal cortex reapproximated with deep hemostatic 2-0 absorbable sutures.
5. A nephroscope is sometimes used to localize and remove calyceal stones. The nephroscope is also useful with staghorn calculi to remove residual fragments in the pelvic portion of the calculus.
6. An incision in the renal pelvis may be closed with 4-0 absorbable atraumatic sutures.
7. The renal fossa is drained and closed, as for nephrectomy. Reinforced absorbent dressings are useful because some urinary leakage occurs for 3 to 4 days after surgery.

PERCUTANEOUS NEPHROLITHOTOMY. Percutaneous nephrolithotomy facilitates the removal or disintegration of renal stones using a rigid or flexible nephroscope (Figure 15-76) passed through a percutaneous nephrostomy tract. Accessory instrumentation, such as the ultrasound wand (sonotrode), electrohydraulic lithotriptor probe, laser fiber, stone basket, and stone grasper, is passed through the lumen of the nephroscope.

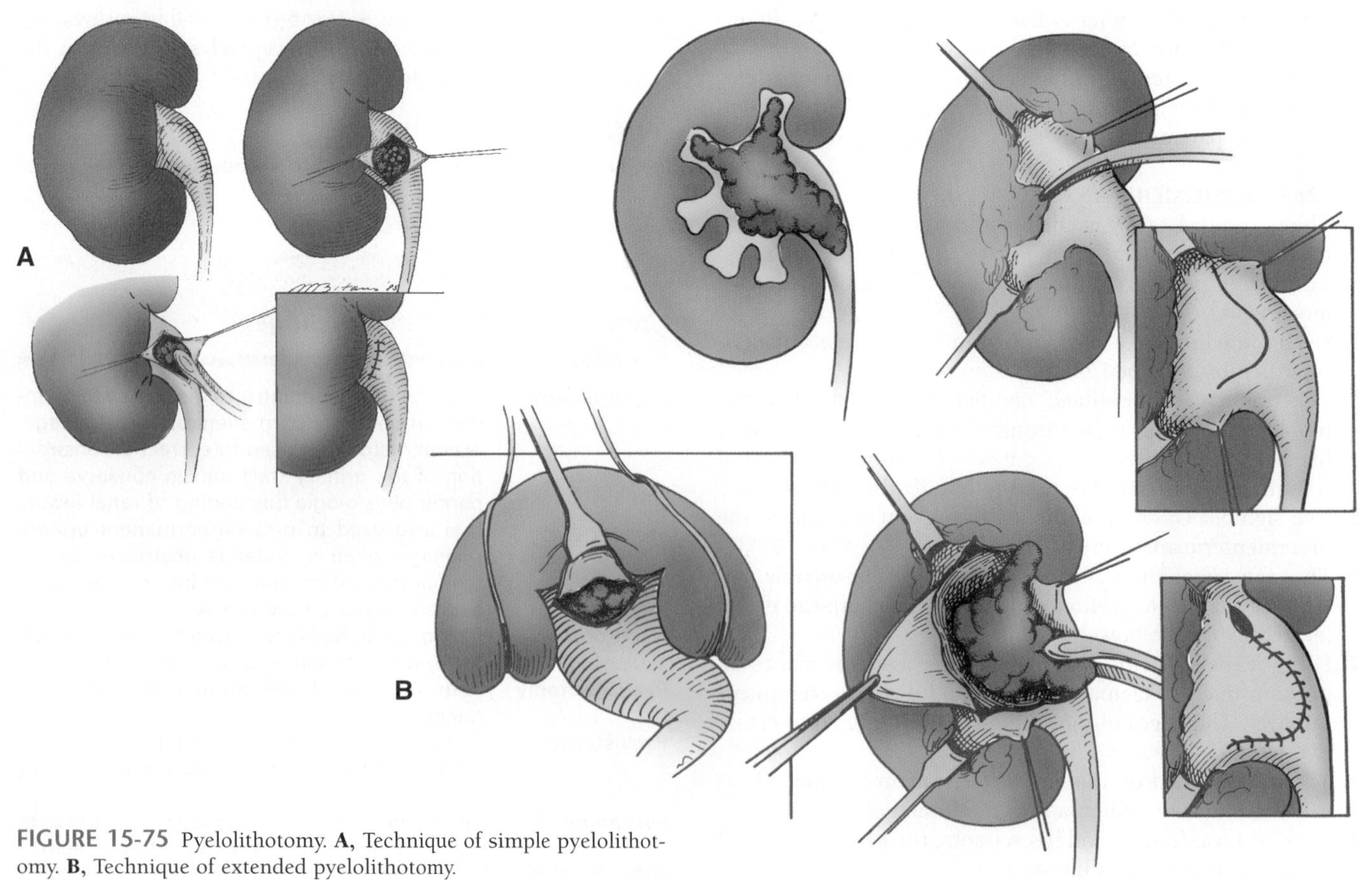


FIGURE 15-75 Pyelolithotomy. **A,** Technique of simple pyelolithotomy. **B,** Technique of extended pyelolithotomy.

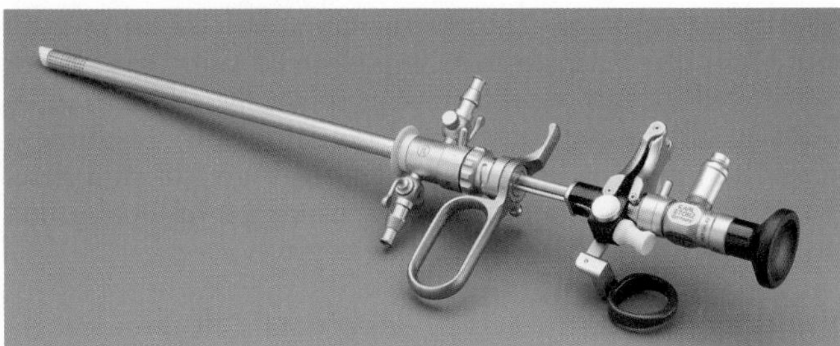

**FIGURE 15-76** Kuntz laser working element.

Ideally, the patient is in good health and not obese and the calculus is no larger than 1 cm in diameter, free-floating, radiopaque, and solitary. However, advances in technology complemented by the experience gained by the uroradiology team have allowed patients with more complex problems to be managed in this manner. The patient may or may not have had previous renal surgery or stone recurrence and may have an established nephrostomy tract.

Creation of the nephrostomy tract and removal of the stone can be accomplished by three different methods. Proper placement of the nephrostomy wire can decrease the operating time significantly. In the *one-step procedure,* creation of the nephrostomy tract, tract dilation, and stone removal are completed in a single session.[28] This method is generally preferred unless there are contraindications. In the *immediate two-step procedure,* the radiologist places the nephrostomy tube under radiographic guidance and the urologist removes the stone later the same day or the next morning. The second step is usually done in the OR with general anesthesia. In the *delayed two-step procedure,* the nephrostomy tract is established with the patient under local anesthesia. The patient is discharged the following day with a 22-Fr or 24-Fr nephrostomy tube connected to drainage. The patient is readmitted to the hospital 5 to 7 days later for the percutaneous removal of the stone with the patient under general anesthesia.

Of basic concern during the operative phase are the patient's position and body temperature, the potential for sudden and rapid blood loss, the type of anesthesia, medications required during surgery, and catheter management during and after the procedure. The patient's position, which may be prone or up to 30 degrees prone-oblique, and the draping procedure depend on whether the surgery is done in the radiology department or the OR and the type of x-ray equipment that will be used.

***Extracorporeal Shock-Wave Lithotripsy.*** ESWL units use water-filled cushions adjacent to the kidney area. An x-ray image intensifier with two monitors is used to visualize the kidney stone at the focal point of the shock wave. After every 100 shocks, fluoroscopy is used to locate remaining stone particles. Adjustments are made, and the patient is repositioned before further treatments. ESWL is often used with percutaneous nephrolithotomy and transurethral ureteropyeloscopy if the patient does not pass the gravel.

Stones that are treated with ESWL are fragmented by the energy focused on the stone with the lithotriptor. The shock waves are administered over a time that can vary from 30 minutes to 2 hours. Shock waves reverberate inside the stone causing fragmentation, with ultimate complete or partial destruction of the calculus. The amount of destruction depends on the number and energy of the shock waves delivered and the hardness of the stone. This technique is effective because shock waves can be transmitted and focused through tissue without loss of energy. A loud, reverberating, popping sound occurs each time a wave pulse is activated. It is advisable that earplugs be worn.

The requirement for anesthesia is determined by the power of the shock wave, the area of shock-wave entry at the skin level, and the size of the shock-wave focal point. The summation of shock waves used during the procedure can cause pain at the skin level. Typically, general, spinal, or local anesthesia is used with the older lithotriptors, such as the HM-3. Modern versions allow for lithotripsy with only IV sedation, oral sedation, or a transcutaneous electrical nerve stimulator (TENS) unit.

The use of a stent before ESWL depends on the patient and the character of the stone or stones. It should be predetermined that the urine culture is negative. Studies show that complication rates decrease if a stent is used with a stone larger than 1.5 cm. A stent placed before ESWL tends to decrease the need for ancillary interventions, reduces overall complications, and assists in proper positioning for ESWL by delineating the ureteral anatomy and the precise stone location. On the other hand, those patients who tend to readily form stones may demonstrate calcification of the ureteral stent in a relatively short time. Without a stent, the risk of silent renal obstruction resulting in loss of kidney function, obstruction of the ureter, nephritis, and sepsis is increased.

Complications related to ESWL are attributable to the cavitation effects of treatment and are proportional to the number of shocks. The ability of the kidney's tubular cells to survive shock waves is related to the number of shock waves to which the kidney is exposed and not to the energy level. The overall mortality for ESWL is 0.02%. Gross hematuria is seen almost universally, resolves in 12 to 48 hours, and is believed to be attributable to parenchymal edema that spontaneously heals within 1 week. Subcapsular or perirenal hematoma caused by perinephric fluid collections is seen in 15% to 30% of cases. The incidence appears to be higher in the hypertensive patient. Subcapsular hematoma may resolve in 6 weeks or may take up to 6 months, whereas perirenal hematoma will be relieved usually in a matter of days. Fewer than 1% of patients have demonstrated cardiac dysrhythmias, myocardial infarction, pulmonary contusion, pancreatitis, or splenic rupture. Renal colic has been exhibited in fewer than 25% of patients, obstructive pyelonephritis in 2% to 6%, and sepsis in 0.5%. Impairment of renal function may be seen in patients with solitary kidneys. Iliac artery and vein thromboses have been reported with lithotripsy for ureteral stones. The majority of lithotripsy patients will demonstrate little or no long-term morbidity.

***Laser Lithotripsy.*** Laser lithotripsy has become an exciting alternative to ESWL and EHL. The Ho:YAG (holmium:yttrium-aluminum-garnet), tunable pulse-dyed (coumarin), Er:YAG (erbium:yttrium-aliminum-garnet), the tunable Alexandrite (a chromium doped mineral) or the Q-switched Nd:YAG (neodymium:yttrium-aluminum-garnet) laser systems have the ability to disintegrate stones without damaging soft tissue.[28] The technique may be used during a ureteropyeloscopy or nephroscopy or to manage ureteral stones instead of performing a ureterolithotomy. When the laser probe is discharged in direct contact with the calculus, plasma (ionized gas) coats the stone's surface. This plasma expands with repeated firings, creating a shock wave that fractures the stone. Normal saline is used for continuous irrigation throughout the procedure. It is not necessary to immobilize the calculus. All persons in the room wear laser goggles, and all laser precautions apply (see Chapter 7).

***Dismembered Pyeloplasty.*** *Pyeloplasty* is revision or plastic reconstruction of the renal pelvis. Pyeloplasty is performed to create a better anatomic relationship between the renal pelvis and the proximal ureter and to allow proper urinary drainage from the kidney to the bladder.[50,51] A temporary nephrostomy is often included to protect the plastic reconstruction of the ureteropelvic junction (UPJ). Tissue healing usually occurs in 10 to 12 days, and the nephrostomy tube is removed once ureteral patency is demonstrated. *Ureteroplasty* is reconstruction of the ureter distal to the UPJ. A *dismembered pyeloplasty* is the combined correction of the redundant renal pelvis and resection of a stenotic portion of the UPJ.

PROCEDURAL CONSIDERATIONS. The instrument setup is as described for nephrectomy, plus fine plastic and vascular instrumentation and Randall stone forceps. A ureteral stent and red rubber catheters will also be employed. The patient is generally in the lateral position.

OPERATIVE PROCEDURE

Open Approach

1. The kidney and upper ureter are exposed through a supracostal flank incision.
2. Gerota's fascia is entered, and the renal pelvis and ureter are freed while the kidney is rotated medially.
3. The ureter is freed and stabilized with a vessel loop below the level of the UPJ.
4. A 4-0 stay suture is placed in the tip of the ureter, and the ureter is incised, trimmed, and shaped to the desired contour with fine forceps and scissors.
5. Anchoring sutures of 4-0 material are placed for traction during reconstruction of the renal pelvis. A diamond-shaped incision is made into the renal pelvis, and the tissue is removed. The Y-V-plasty technique may be followed. It converts a Y-shaped surgical incision of the renal pelvis into a V by drawing the apex of the arms of the Y to the foot of the Y with absorbable sutures.
6. Sutures are placed at each end of the refashioned renal pelvis, passed to the ureteral stoma, and tagged. The pelvis is irrigated free of clots. The sutures are run in a continuous manner, creating the anastomosis.
7. A Silastic tubing may be used to stent the repaired pelvis until adequate healing has occurred. A nephrostomy tube is also placed within the pelvis to divert urine safely while the edema in the area of the repair resolves.
8. Gerota's fascia is closed over the repair.
9. A drain is placed where the pelvis was reconstructed, and the surgical incision is closed in layers.

Laparoscopic Approach. UPJ obstruction has recently joined the rank of surgeries that may be treated laparoscopically.[14,44,50] Generally, a standard transperitoneal approach is used. The patient may be placed supine with a lateral tilt or in lateral decubitus and the bed rotated to access the ports.

After placement of four trocars as in laparoscopic nephrectomy (described on pp. 543-544), the proximal ureters and renal pelvis are freed. The obstruction at the UPJ is excised, and a spatulated anastomosis is performed using running or interrupted sutures. A ureteral stent is usually left in place.

Decreased postoperative pain and shorter hospitalization make this approach appealing. A higher degree of skill is required for this technique, however, making it an option that has not become standard treatment as yet.

***Nephroureterectomy—Open Approach.*** Nephroureterectomy is removal of a kidney and its entire ureter. This procedure is indicated for hydroureteronephrosis of such a degree that reconstructive repair is impossible. It is also employed for collecting system tumors of the kidney and ureter.

PROCEDURAL CONSIDERATIONS. Open nephroureterectomy requires an extension of the incision anteriorly with the patient positioned semilaterally and fully prepped and draped for the surgeon to access the flank and lower abdomen. Only one instrument set is required, but a second skin-prep setup and set of sterile drapes may be necessary. An alternative to open nephroureterectomy is laparoscopic nephroureterectomy.

OPERATIVE PROCEDURE

1. The patient is placed in a lateral position.
2. The kidney and upper ureter are exposed, and nephrectomy is performed as described below. The kidney may be placed in a plastic bag to prevent possible spillage of tumor cells.
3. The ureter is mobilized as far distally as possible. The OR bed is adjusted so that surgery on the lower ureter may proceed. The lower ureter and bladder are identified and mobilized.
4. The ureter and a small cuff of the bladder are removed in continuity, and the bladder is repaired with a single layer of 2-0 absorbable interrupted sutures. The ureter and cuff of bladder are pulled superiorly, and the intact kidney and ureter are removed.
5. An 18-Fr or 20-Fr Foley catheter is left in the bladder, and a drain is placed behind the bladder. The incision is closed in layers.

***Nephrectomy—Open Approach.*** Nephrectomy is the surgical removal of a kidney. It is performed as a means of definitive therapy for many renal problems, such as congenital UPJ obstruction with severe hydronephrosis, renal tumor, renal trauma, calculus disease with infection, cortical abscess, pyelonephrosis, and renovascular hypertension.

In routine renal surgery the patient is placed in the lateral position with the dependent iliac crest over the kidney rest. The operative flank is uppermost, with the patient's back brought to the edge of the OR bed. The upper arm is supported on an overhead arm support, and the lower arm is supinated on a padded armboard. It may be flexed slightly at the elbow and angled cephalad to promote better access to the flank. The patient's legs are positioned by placing a pillow between them and flexing the lower leg at the knee. The upper leg remains extended. The kidney rest is then raised, and when the desired bed flexion is achieved, 3-inch adhesive tape is used to stabilize the patient throughout surgery. Routine skin preparation and draping procedures are carried out.

PROCEDURAL CONSIDERATIONS. The nephrectomy setup includes a routine laparotomy setup; kidney instruments (Figure 15-77); a variety of red rubber, Malecot, or Pezzer

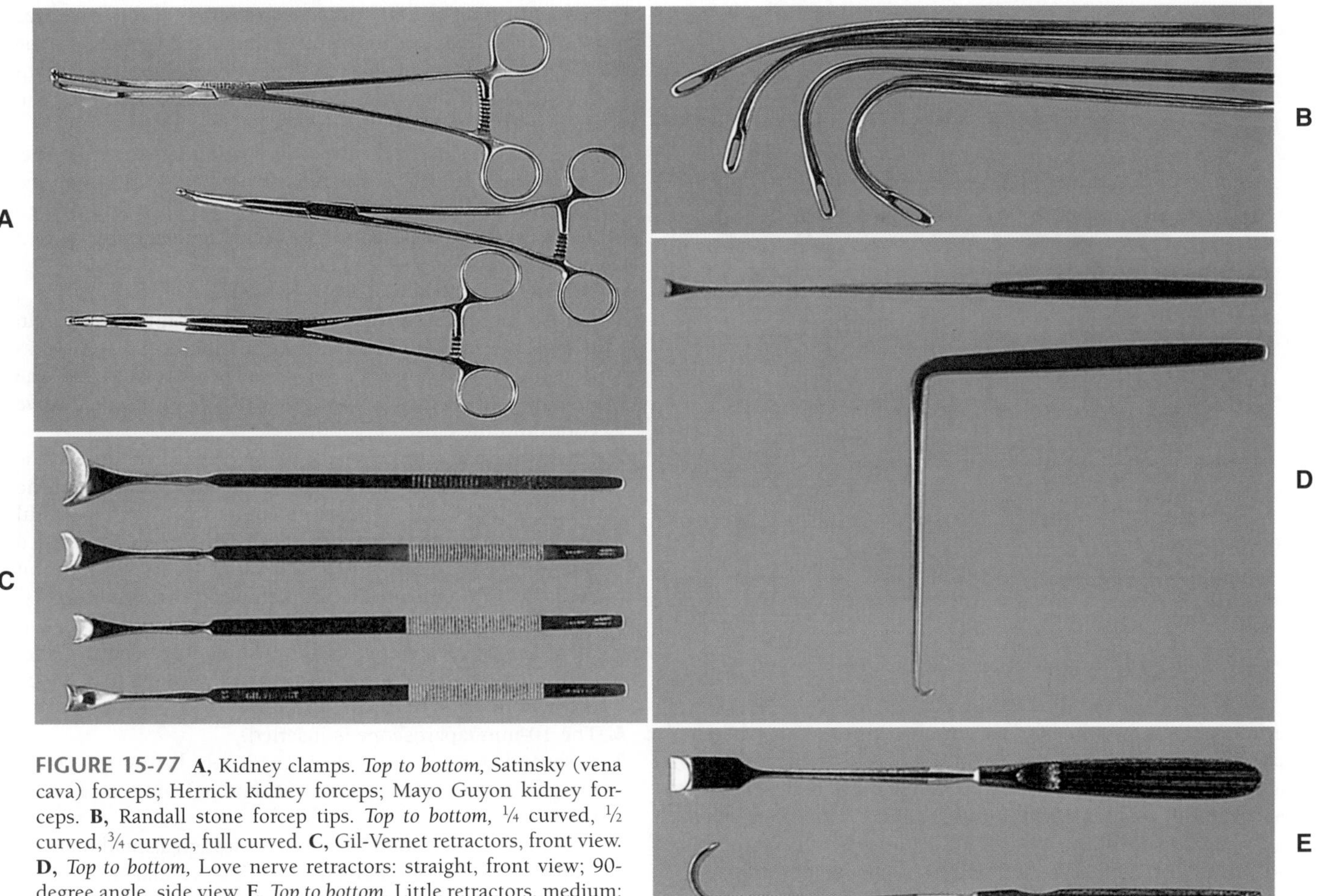


FIGURE 15-77 **A,** Kidney clamps. *Top to bottom,* Satinsky (vena cava) forceps; Herrick kidney forceps; Mayo Guyon kidney forceps. **B,** Randall stone forcep tips. *Top to bottom,* ¼ curved, ½ curved, ¾ curved, full curved. **C,** Gil-Vernet retractors, front view. **D,** *Top to bottom,* Love nerve retractors: straight, front view; 90-degree angle, side view. **E,** *Top to bottom,* Little retractors, medium: front view, side view.

catheters; a wound drainage system; and vessel loops. In certain nephrectomies the chest or the GI tract may be opened. If the chest is opened, appropriate instruments and postoperative chest drains are needed. Rib resection requires the addition of a Finochietto rib retractor, a large Matson costal periosteotome, an Alexander costal periosteotome, right and left Doyen rib raspatories, a Bethune rib cutter, a double-action duckbill rongeur, a Bailey rib approximator, and a Langenbeck periosteal elevator. When the GI tract is opened, GI technique is used for the anastomosis.

OPERATIVE PROCEDURE

1. The incision is carried through the skin, fat, and fascia. Bleeding vessels are clamped and ligated.
2. The external oblique, internal oblique, and transversalis muscles are sequentially exposed and incised in the direction of the initial skin incision.
3. If necessary, a rib or ribs (eleventh or twelfth) may be resected to provide better access to the kidney. The periosteum is stripped with an Alexander costal periosteotome and Doyen rib raspatory. A scalpel and heavy scissors are used to cut through the lumbocostal ligaments. The rib is grasped with an Ochsner clamp and cut with rib shears, removing the portion necessary to expose the kidney. Gerota's fascia is identified and incised with Metzenbaum scissors.
4. The incision is extended, and the kidney and perirenal fat are exposed by blunt and sharp dissection. All perirenal fat that is removed during surgery may be saved in a small basin of normal saline for later use as a bolster to stop bleeding.
5. The ureter is identified, separated from its adjacent structures, doubly clamped, divided, and ligated with absorbable 0 material.
6. The kidney pedicle containing the major blood vessels is isolated and doubly clamped; each vessel is triply ligated with heavy nonabsorbable ties. Each vessel is then severed, leaving two ligatures on the pedicle, and the kidney is removed (Figure 15-78).
7. The renal fossa is explored for bleeding, and necessary hemostasis is achieved. The fossa is then irrigated with normal saline, and the irrigant is removed by suction.
8. The fascia and muscles are closed in layers with interrupted absorbable sutures. Retention sutures may be used in obese or chronically ill patients in whom wound healing may be delayed.
9. The skin edges are approximated with sutures or skin staples, and the dressing is applied.

***Laparoscopic Nephrectomy.*** The approach for laparoscopic nephrectomy may be transabdominal (transperitoneal), extra-

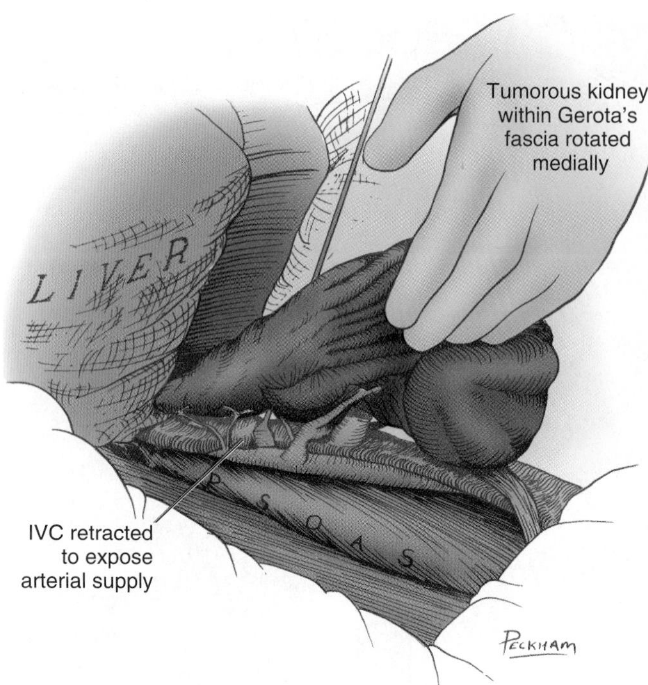


**FIGURE 15-78** Nephrectomy. *IVC,* inferior vena cava.

peritoneal (retroperitoneal),[15] or intraperitoneal. Transabdominal is the most common approach. Indications for laparoscopy are generally for benign disease, although more radical surgeries have been accomplished in this manner. A full mechanical antibiotic bowel prep is prescribed. Although surgery time is longer (an average of 3½ to 5 hours), postoperative recovery, analgesia requirements, and total hospital stay are lessened. The procedure always includes cystoscopy with placement of a renal balloon catheter, a ureteral catheter, and a Foley urethral catheter under C-arm fluoroscopy. Indigo carmine may be injected into the skin overlying the renal pelvis.

The patient is initially placed on a beanbag in the supine position. A standard laparoscopy instrument and equipment setup that includes three 5-mm trocars, an insufflation needle, and two 10-mm to 12-mm trocars is used. Cystoscopic and ureteroscopic supplies will be needed, as well as an 0.035-gauge Bentson guidewire, an occlusion balloon catheter, an 0.035-gauge Amplatz stiff guidewire, a 16-Fr Foley catheter and drainage bag, Indigo carmine, an irrigator/aspirator, a 1-liter bag of saline, a 1-liter pressure bag (to pressurize the irrigant to 250 mm Hg), a #12 or #11 knife blade, 10-mm clip appliers, the entrapment sack, and tissue morcellator. An open setup should always be available in the event laparoscopy is unsuccessful.

**PROCEDURAL CONSIDERATIONS.** After endotracheal intubation and placement of SCDs, a nasogastric tube and ESU dispersive pad are placed. The patient is prepped and draped as for laparotomy. Use of a draping pack with four large adherent drape sheets, instead of a standard laparotomy sheet, affords better access for the port sites.

The patient may be placed in lateral decubitus position on a deflated beanbag positioner at the outset or turned after endoscopic intervention. Ensuring that the patient is adequately secured to the OR bed is critical.[6] Before prepping the patient, the bed is tilted laterally to afford a central abdominal access. The patient is prepped and draped, and access of the first three ports is achieved. Before insertion of the remaining trocars, the bed is returned to its normal configuration so that the patient is again in lateral decubitus position. The kidney rest is then elevated, and the operation continues.

Some surgeons begin the procedure with the patient supine. The contralateral arm is padded with thick foam from the shoulder to the fingertips. The patient is prepped and draped for thoracoabdominal surgery. Extra draping materials are used when the patient is repositioned.

**OPERATIVE PROCEDURE**

1. Access is gained to the peritoneal cavity through a 1-cm transverse, subumbilical, stab-wound incision. After elevation of the anterior abdominal wall with towel clips, the insufflation needle is inserted with the stop cock valve control in the closed position.
2. Once the insufflation needle is in place, sterile saline is dropped into the lumen of the needle and the valve of the needle is opened. If the saline enters freely (a successful test), the abdominal cavity is inflated with $CO_2$ until a pressure of 15 to 20 mm Hg is obtained. If saline does not enter freely, it indicates improper placement of the needle.
3. A nick is made in the rectus fascia with the knife blade, and the 10-mm trocar replaces the insufflation needle. Towel clips are again used on each side of the incision to stabilize the abdominal wall during insertion.
4. The 10-mm laparoscope is inserted.
5. A second incision is made immediately below the costal margin in the midclavicular line, and a 10-mm to 12-mm trocar is inserted.
6. The third trocar, 5-mm, is inserted through a small incision 2 cm below the umbilicus in the midclavicular line.
7. The last two 5-mm trocars are placed, one in the anterior axillary line level with the umbilicus and one subcostal in the anterior axillary line. All trocars are then withdrawn until 2 to 3 cm of each sheath protrudes into the abdomen. Polypropylene (Prolene) suture may be used to secure the side arm ports to the patient's skin. Each trocar site is laparoscopically inspected after trocar insertion to identify any bleeding or perforation. On occasion, it may be necessary to extend the incision for trocar insertion.
8. The ascending or descending colon is completely mobilized with electrosurgical scissors and deflected medially. The retroperitoneum is opened.
9. Through gentle motion of the ureteral catheter, the ureter is identified and dissected. A Babcock forceps is clamped around the dissected ureter for retraction.
10. The ureter is dissected until the lower pole of the kidney is visualized. Any veins encountered are clipped twice proximally and twice distally. The kidney is cleared of surrounding tissue and freed laterally and superiorly. Gerota's fascia is entered to free the adrenal gland and exclude it from the dissection.
11. The renal artery and vein are identified and cleared to create a 360-degree window around each vessel. The clip applier is inserted through the 10-mm to 12-mm port. Two clips are placed on the specimen side, and three clips are placed on the stump side of both the artery and vein, which are then sharply incised.
12. Two pairs of clips are placed proximally and distally on the ureter, which is sharply incised. The specimen end is

grasped, and the kidney is moved into the upper abdominal quadrant (Figure 15-79).

13. The entrapment sac is introduced through the 10-mm to 12-mm port. The bottom of the sac is pulled into the abdomen with graspers until the neck of the sac clears the end of the port and is then unfurled.
14. The sac is opened, and the ureteral stump with attached kidney is placed inside. The drawstrings are pulled tight, closing the mouth of the sac.
15. The patient is returned to the supine position by tilting the OR bed, and the sac strings are extracted through the umbilical port. Under laparoscopic observation, the port is removed and the neck of the sac is brought to lie on the abdominal surface. The tissue morcellator is inserted into the sac, and the kidney is morcellated under suction in a clockwise fashion.
16. The abdominal cavity is exited with laparoscopic observation of each trocar site, during and after removal, to ensure that hemostasis has been achieved. Fascial layers at the 12-mm trocar sites are closed with 2-0 or 3-0 absorbable suture in a figure-of-eight pattern.
17. Subcuticular closure of 4-0 absorbable suture is done on all port sites. Steri-Strips, Telfa, and Tegaderm complete the dressings.

The nasogastric tube is removed in the OR, and the Foley catheter is removed on the first postoperative day. Oral intake may begin 6 hours postoperatively. The SCDs are removed when the patient is ambulatory. Most patients leave the hospital in 4 days, return to work in approximately 2 weeks, and achieve full convalescence in 3 weeks.

***Heminephrectomy.*** Heminephrectomy is removal of a portion of the kidney. It is usually indicated for conditions involving the lower or upper pole of the kidney, such as calculus disease, or trauma limited to one pole of a kidney. In rare instances in which a patient has only one kidney, such surgery may be used for renal neoplasms to avoid the need for dialysis and subsequent renal transplantation.

PROCEDURAL CONSIDERATIONS. The setup is as described for nephrectomy with the addition of vascular and bulldog clamps.

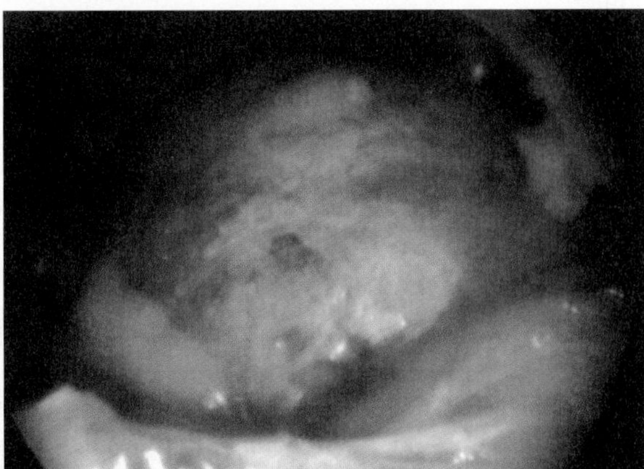

**FIGURE 15-79** Interior view of exposing right kidney laparoscopically.

OPERATIVE PROCEDURE

1. The kidney and its pedicle should be completely mobilized as described for nephrectomy. The main vessels may be temporarily occluded for only 20 to 30 minutes, after which progressive renal damage may occur. Local hypothermia may be indicated to prolong ischemic operating time.
2. The renal capsule is incised and stripped back.
3. A wedge of kidney tissue containing the diseased or damaged cortex is excised. Interlobar fat or arcuate and interlobular arteries are clamped with Hopkins clamps and suture-ligated with 4-0 absorbable suture on urologic needles.
4. The open collecting system is reapproximated with a continuous 4-0 suture.
5. Perirenal fat is placed in the area in which tissue was excised, and the renal parenchyma is reapproximated with horizontal mattress sutures.
6. If possible, the renal capsule is reapproximated with a continuous 2-0 suture.

***Radical Nephrectomy.*** Radical nephrectomy is excision of the kidney, perirenal fat, adrenal gland, Gerota's capsule (fascia), and contiguous periaortic lymph nodes. This procedure is performed for parenchymal renal neoplasms. In the open approach, a lumbar, transthoracic, or transabdominal approach to the kidney is used, depending on the size and location of the lesion. The transthoracic or transabdominal approach is preferred because the blood vessels of the kidney can be more easily reached and ligated before the tumor is mobilized, decreasing the possibility of tumor embolization into the bloodstream. For the laparoscopic approach a retroperitoneal or transperitoneal approach may be employed.[16]

PROCEDURAL CONSIDERATIONS. The setups are as described for open nephrectomy and laparoscopic nephrectomy.

OPERATIVE PROCEDURE. In general, the procedure is as described for nephrectomy with two exceptions: (1) the renal pedicle is ligated before the kidney is mobilized, and (2) Gerota's capsule is not incised but is removed en bloc with the kidney. Involved lymph nodes surrounding the renal pedicle are excised. A chest tube is inserted if the transthoracic approach is used.

## Kidney Transplant

Kidney transplant entails transplantation of a living-related or cadaveric donor kidney into the recipient's iliac fossa (Figure 15-80). It is performed in an effort to restore renal function and thus maintain life in a patient who has end-stage renal disease.[53]

***Transplant from a Living Donor.*** The kidney donor must be in good health. ABO (blood typing) and histocompatibility (human leukocyte antigen [HLA] tissue typing) along with a negative white cell (lymphocyte) crossmatch determine donor-recipient compatibility. It is not necessary to match the Rh factor. Once the donor has been chosen, a complete workup that includes history, physical examination, chest x-ray examination, ECG, CBC, BUN and creatinine values, blood chemistry profiles, coagulation studies, and viral titers is done. Renal function is assessed with three creatinine clearances, urinalysis, and urine cultures followed by IVP and excretory urography. A flush aortogram assesses the vascular anatomy, and re-

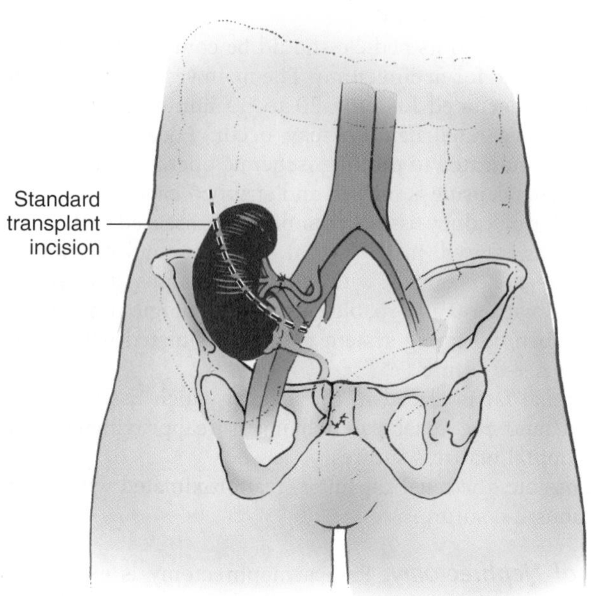


FIGURE 15-80 Transplanted kidney in recipient's iliac fossa.

nal angiography pinpoints the kidney of choice while ruling out the presence of renal lesions. A kidney with a single renal artery is preferred, but kidneys with double and triple arteries may be used if necessary. If there is a family history of diabetes, a 5-hour glucose tolerance test is also performed.[7,53,58]

The ideal living donor is an identical twin, although any immediate family member (usually a sibling or parent) may be a donor. The donor is given an IV solution of 1000 ml of 5% dextrose in lactated Ringer's on the evening before nephrectomy. This is followed with 500 ml of 5% dextrose in water over the next 10 to 12 hours. The morning of surgery, about 45 minutes before transport to the operating room, 12.5 g of mannitol is administered to ensure diuresis during the induction of anesthesia.

**PROCEDURAL CONSIDERATIONS.** Two adjacent operating rooms are prepared for the procedures; surgery on the donor and surgery on the recipient proceed simultaneously.

Usually the right kidney is chosen for removal because of its smaller size, leaving the donor patient with the left and larger kidney. An indwelling Foley catheter is inserted, and a nasogastric tube is placed. Two IV lines are required. The patient is placed on a beanbag positioning device and moved into the left lateral decubitus position following endotracheal intubation. The lower arm is positioned extended outward on a well-padded armboard at a right angle to the torso; the upper arm is positioned on an elevated lateral armboard. The sternum and anterior superior iliac spine are brought near the edge of the OR bed. A pillow is placed between the patient's legs, and the ankles and feet are appropriately padded. The bed is flexed to 30 degrees, and the upper portion is angled downward to approximately 140 degrees. The skin is prepped from midchest to midthigh and draped to expose the flank area.

Required instruments and equipment are identical to those for a nephrectomy plus an IV pole and supplies for the sterile perfusion table. These include electrolyte solution (in iced basin until needed), two IV extension tubes, a kidney basin with cold (4°C) IV saline solution, a three-way stop cock, an 18-gauge needle catheter, mosquito hemostats, vascular forceps, Metzenbaum scissors, suture scissors, and Kelly hemostats.

An electrolyte solution of Ringer's lactate that contains procaine and heparin may be used to perfuse the harvested kidney. A more common perfusion is CUW (Chelex-treated University of Wisconsin) solution. It contains hydroxyethyl starch, providing a better metabolic substrate for organ metabolism.

Collins or Sachs solution may be used to perfuse cadaveric kidneys after harvest but should never be used to perfuse a kidney from a living donor because of the potential effect of elevated potassium in the recipient from residual perfusate in the kidney.

**OPERATIVE PROCEDURE**

**Open Approach**

1. The donor nephrectomy procedure is as described for nephrectomy; however, the ureter and renal vein and artery require meticulous dissection.
2. Maximum length of the ureter is achieved by dividing it at or below the pelvic rim if possible. To preserve adequate ureteral vascularization, the surgeon is cautious not to skeletonize the ureter.
3. Particular care is taken to remove the maximum length of the renal vein and artery. To obtain the maximum length of the right renal vein sometimes requires partial occlusion of the inferior vena cava with a Satinsky clamp and dissection of a portion of the inferior vena cava. This is done after the ureter has been freed.
4. Repair of the inferior vena cava is made with a continuous 4-0 or 5-0 vascular suture.
5. Five minutes before the surgeon clamps the renal vessels, 5000 units of heparin sodium and 12.5 g of mannitol are systemically administered to the patient to prevent intravascular clotting and maximize diuresis.
6. Immediately after the kidney is removed from the donor, 50 mg of protamine sulfate is given intravenously to reverse the heparinization.
7. Furosemide, mannitol, and IV fluids are administered to the donor to maintain adequate urinary output from the donor's remaining kidney.
8. Gentle handling of the kidney is essential. Team members must prevent undue traction on the vascular pedicle, which may induce vasospasm and reduce perfusion of the kidney.
9. To reduce warm ischemia time, the surgeon double-clamps the vein and the artery, excises the kidney, and immediately places it in cold saline solution on a sterile back table, where the kidney is flushed with the designated electrolyte solution. Warm ischemia time (from the clamping of renal vessels to a point at which the kidney is perfused with cold electrolyte solution) should be kept to a minimum to prevent acute tubular necrosis and to maintain maximum renal function after transplantation.
10. Mosquito clamps and fine vascular forceps are used to expose the renal artery to permit insertion of a needle catheter, such as a Medicut. The cold electrolyte solution passes through the IV tubing and the needle catheter, flushing any remaining donor's blood from the kidney. This also decreases the kidney's metabolic rate by lowering its temperature. Flushing time is usually 2 to 5 minutes.

11. After flushing, trimming the vessels of adventitia may be necessary to facilitate the vascular anastomosis to the recipient's iliac vessels.
12. The kidney, in cold saline solution, is covered with sterile drapes and taken by the surgeon to the room in which the recipient's iliac vessels have been exposed.
13. Wound closure for the donor is as described for nephrectomy.

**Laparoscopic Approach.** Five trocars are used (four trocars if the left kidney is chosen). Generally the operating trocar is 12-mm, the second and third trocars are 10-mm, and the last two trocars are 5-mm. Instruments required include the following: four 5-mm fenestrated graspers, 5-mm straight and curved dissecting scissors, a coagulating hook, a bipolar grasper, ultrasonic scissors, two 5-mm curved graspers and a 10-mm curved grasper, two needle holders, a clip applier, a vascular stapler, and an atraumatic retrieval bag without a system for opening and closing it and a minimal opening of 15 cm. In addition, the standard open setup needs to be ready with open vascular instrumentation, a smooth perfusion tip, sterile IV tubing, and sterile ice for ex vivo perfusion.[7]

1. The first 12-mm trocar is introduced through an open technique at a level 2 to 5 cm cephalad to McBurney point to allow access to the superior pole and as far caudad as possible so the renal vein may be divided parallel to the vena cava.
2. The second 10-mm trocar is inserted in the periumbilical position about 3 cm lateral and cephalad to the umbilicus. This will be used for the laparoscope.
3. The third 10-mm trocar is placed 6 to 8 cm cephalad to the second trocar.
4. A 5-mm trocar is inserted into the flank at the convex border of the kidney.
5. The final 5-mm trocar is placed below the xiphoid process to the left of the round ligament.
6. The OR bed is rotated vertically, and the small intestine and omentum are pushed into the inferior pelvic cavity.
7. Beginning at the foramen of Winslow, the subhepatic parietal peritoneum is incised and followed by division of the triangular ligament of the liver. Grasping forceps are placed posterior to the liver and used to retract the right lobe ventrally.
8. The pericolic gutter is incised by beginning at the cecal base, extending to the hepatic flexure and ending at the duodenum.
9. The duodenum is then freed of its attachments to the mesenteric root. The entire length of the subhepatic vena cava is exposed to the level of the iliac bifurcation.
10. The renal vein is identified and a vessel loop placed around it. Dissection of the right border of the subhepatic vena cava is carried out along the entire length. The right gonadal vein is clipped and divided at its caval origin.
11. A vessel loop is then passed around the right renal artery.
12. The ureter lies anterior to the iliac vessels. It is located, controlled with a vessel loop, and dissected caudad to cephalad also removing areolar tissue. Once dissection reaches the inferior pole of the kidney, Gerota's fascia is incised and dissection continues to the renal parenchyma.
13. Pararenal fat is removed and a dissection plane is created against the renal capsule. When the anterior surface of the kidney has been freed the superior pole is separated from the adrenal gland.
14. Dissection is now directed to the inferior renal pole to free the kidney posteriorly from pararenal fat. Once free it is rotated ventrally to expose the vessels already marked with the vessel loops. The vessels are circumferentially dissected, and the kidney is freed.
15. Attention is now directed at the ureter. It is clipped distally and divided at its bifurcation with the iliac vessels. Copious diuresis generally occurs at this point.
16. A 6-cm incision is made just above the pubic symphysis. The aponeurosis is transversely divided, and the rectus abdominis muscles are retracted.
17. The retrieval bag is introduced directly into the peritoneal cavity. It is placed around the kidney and held firmly without obstructing the vessels.
18. The grasper that has been placed in the suprapubic area is used to keep the retrieval bag closed and exert enough traction on the renal vessels to promote maximum length.
19. The renal side of the renal artery is left open while one or two clips are applied on the aortic side. This is divided in two steps to ensure occlusion.
20. The vein is divided with a vascular stapler, bringing along a small cuff of the vena cava to add extra length.
21. The suprapubic peritoneal opening is widened manually, allowing the kidney to be extracted. It is immediately perfused on ice with 4°C CUW solution. Vessels are individually perfused. The volume corresponds to about 300 ml. This continues until the outflow from the vein becomes completely transparent.[7]
22. The peritoneum is irrigated and bleeding points controlled. A drain may be inserted into the peritoneal space for a short period of time postoperatively.
23. The wounds are sutured and dressings applied.

***Transplant from a Cadaveric Donor.*** The ideal cadaveric donor is young, free from infection and cancer, normotensive until a short time before death, and under hospital observation several hours before death. Permission to harvest the donor kidney must be obtained from the family and the medical examiner after brain death has been unequivocally established. Awareness of existing state legislation in this complex area is advisable.

The donor is completely evaluated. The medical history is reviewed for any possible contraindications, such as chronic disease, ongoing systemic infection, IV drug abuse, malignancy, heart or lung disease, trauma to the donor organ, and the presence of human immunodeficiency virus (HIV). Laboratory studies include blood typing, urinalysis, urine and blood cultures, BUN, serum creatinine, CBC, hepatitis B antigen evaluation, VDRL for presence of venereal disease, and p24 antigen capture assay for the presence of HIV antigen. Evaluation of arterial blood gases, electrolyte values, and liver enzymes is also necessary. Because of improvements in medical therapy, the only absolute contraindications to organ donation are HIV and metastasis.

Preoperative management of the cadaver donor is vital to the success of the transplant. Organ perfusion, oxygenation, and hydration must be maintained. Arterial blood gas (ABG) evaluation determines ventilatory support, and dopamine may be administered if fluids alone are not able to maintain an adequate systolic blood pressure. Urine output is monitored, and antibiotics may be administered to combat and prevent infection.

**PROCEDURAL CONSIDERATIONS.** After brain death has been established, the donor is taken to the OR with respiratory and cardiac function maintained mechanically. The donor is placed in the supine position and is prepared for a laparotomy. Anticoagulant and alpha-adrenergic receptor blocking agents are administered systemically during the procedure. Adequate renal perfusion and function are maintained with IV fluids and diuretics.

Instruments and equipment are the same as for nephrectomy, with the addition of Metzenbaum scissors, suture scissors, vascular forceps, DeBakey forceps, Dean hemostatic forceps, mosquito hemostats, DeBakey clamps, angled clip appliers with medium and large clips, bulldog clamps, vascular clamps, Deaver retractors, Harrington splanchnic retractors, vascular needle holders, a sternal saw or Lebsche knife and mallet, umbilical tapes, electrolyte solution (lactated Ringer's, Sachs, or Collins), cold packing in an iced basin until needed, an IV pole, IV extension tubes, a kidney basin with cold (4°C) IV saline solution, a three-way stop cock, an 18-gauge needle catheter, a centimeter ruler, the perfusion machine or kidney transplantation equipment, and ice.

OPERATIVE PROCEDURE

1. A midline incision is made from the xiphoid process to the symphysis pubis with bilateral supraumbilical transverse extensions through the skin, subcutaneous layer, fascia, and muscle.
2. Hemostasis is obtained with clamps, ties, suture ligatures, and electrocoagulation.
3. The kidney, renal vessels, and ureter are carefully dissected with Metzenbaum scissors, DeBakey forceps, and Dean hemostatic forceps.
4. Heparin sodium, 15,000 units, is given intravenously 5 to 10 minutes before the renal vessels are clamped.
5. The usual method of resection is en bloc resection (harvesting of donor kidneys) (Figure 15-81), which involves the removal of sections of the inferior vena cava and aorta with both kidneys in continuity.
6. An incision is made along the route of the small bowel mesentery up to the esophageal hiatus.
7. The entire GI tract, spleen, and inferior portion of the pancreas are mobilized by dividing the celiac axis and the superior mesenteric artery, exposing the entire retroperitoneal region.
8. The inferior vena cava and aorta are clamped below the renal vessels with vascular clamps, and the vessels are divided.
9. Lumbar tributaries are secured with metal clips and are divided.
10. The kidneys and ureters are freed from their surrounding soft tissues.
11. The ureters are divided distally at the pelvic brim.
12. The suprarenal aorta and inferior vena cava are clamped and divided at the level of the diaphragm, close to the bifurcation.
13. The vessels and kidney are severed and the aorta and vena cava ligated.
14. After removal of the kidneys, immediate perfusion with cold (4°C) CUW or electrolyte solution is carried out. The kidneys are placed in a container of cold saline solution and surrounded by saline slush in an insulated carrier or placed on a hypothermic pulsatile perfusion machine for transport. While kidney perfusion is begun, the abdominal lymph nodes and spleen are removed for use in tissue typing.
15. The incision is closed with interrupted sutures, and artificial life-support systems are terminated. The perioperative nurse cares for the patient's body, preserving privacy, dignity, and humanity at the patient's death.

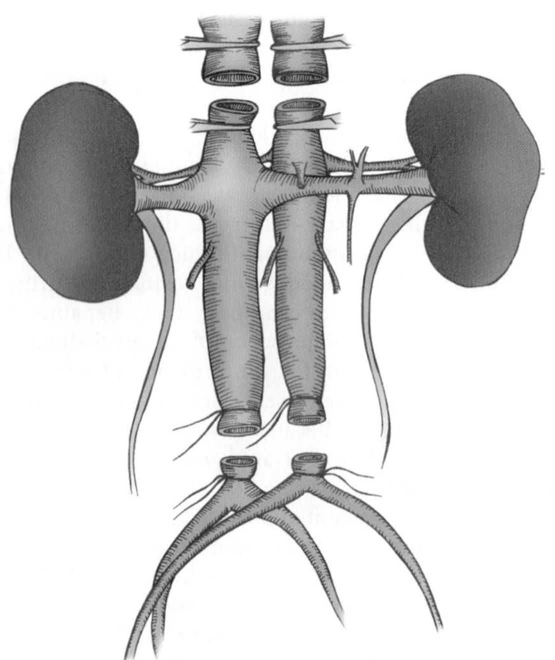

**FIGURE 15-81** En bloc resection.

***Transplant Recipient.*** Each potential recipient is judged individually in regard to kidney transplantation. Most persons younger than 55 years are acceptable; older patients are less tolerant of postoperative complications. Contraindications for renal transplantation include (1) systemic disease that precludes major surgery, (2) oxalosis (a metabolic disorder), (3) a positive HLA cytotoxic antibody screen, and (4) active cancer. If required, a patient may need to undergo bilateral nephrectomy before renal transplantation for uncontrollable hypertension, for kidney infections, or for reflux when there is a significant history of infections.[5] Occasionally a large polycystic kidney may need to be removed to create a space for the new kidney. Splenectomy may be performed at this time to improve leukopenia and enhance the effects of myelosuppressive and immunosuppressive drugs.

The transplant recipient requires optimal nutritional support and adequate dialysis. All potential sources of infection must be treated. Most commonly these include teeth, bladder, nasal sinuses, and skin. The patient may need a short hemodialysis to control fluid overload or electrolyte imbalances. A repeat cytotoxic crossmatch with fresh serum specimens should follow hemodialysis. Preoperative antibiotics are commonly administered. Other important diagnostic tools for preoperative evaluation are chest x-ray examination, abdominal ultrasonography, voiding cystourethrography, liver function studies, hematologic assays, and serum values for screening hepatitis, HIV, and viral diseases.

PROCEDURAL CONSIDERATIONS. The patient is placed in the supine position. A Foley catheter with an attached Silastic stenting catheter is inserted into the bladder by sterile technique. From 50 to 75 ml of antibiotic solution is instilled into the bladder through a sterile, catheter-tipped syringe, allowed to remain for 20 minutes, and drained. The patient is prepped from nipples to knees and draped.

OPERATIVE PROCEDURE

1. A curved right lower quadrant incision is made through the skin, subcutaneous layer, fascia, and muscle.
2. Bleeding is controlled with clamps, ties, and electrocoagulation.
3. The inferior epigastric vessels are divided between suture ligatures.
4. Retroperitoneal dissection is performed by mobilizing the peritoneum superiorly and medially.
5. A Balfour self-retaining retractor is placed in the wound for exposure, and a wide Deaver retractor used to reflect the peritoneum superiorly and medially.
6. With the use of Metzenbaum scissors and DeBakey forceps, dissection is made along the entire length of the hypogastric artery and the external and common iliac arteries to the bifurcation of the aorta, continuing down the internal iliac artery.
7. The internal iliac artery is ligated distally and divided, with proximal control maintained by a vascular clamp.
8. The iliac vein may be dissected free by ligating and dividing the internal iliac venous branches with 3-0 nonabsorbable sutures or ligating clips. More commonly, only the hypogastric artery and that portion of iliac vein to be anastomosed are dissected free.
9. The donor kidney is brought into the operative field and placed in cold (4°C) IV saline solution.
10. Mosquito hemostats, 4-inch DeBakey forceps, and curved and straight fine scissors are used to make the necessary alterations on the donor kidney vessels to facilitate the anastomoses.
11. The donor kidney is returned to the cold IV saline solution until the time of the anastomosis.
12. Two angled DeBakey vascular clamps are placed on the internal iliac vein.
13. A #11 blade is used to make a 1-cm incision in the iliac vein between the clamps.
14. The vessel is rinsed with heparin sodium solution (10 units/ml) in the Asepto syringe.
15. Angled Potts scissors are used to extend the incision to accommodate the donor renal vein.
16. The donor kidney is placed in a 3-in by 10-inch, cold saline-soaked stockinette, with the renal vessels leaving from a hole in the side. Use of the stockinette prevents direct contact with the kidney and therefore trauma.
17. The renal vein is anastomosed to the side of the recipient's iliac vein with 5-0 double-armed vascular sutures.
18. In like manner the renal artery is anastomosed end to end with the proximal portion of the internal iliac artery using 5-0 vascular sutures.
19. The vessels are irrigated proximally and distally with heparin sodium solution by using the 10-ml syringe attached to the Medicut catheter before placing the final sutures.
20. The stockinette is removed for adequate visualization of the entire kidney. The angled DeBakey clamps are removed from the venous vessels, and the anastomosis is checked for leakage.
21. The clamps on the internal iliac artery are then released, and the anastomosis is checked.
22. Meticulous inspection is made of the hilum and surface of the kidney for bleeding and infarction.
23. Diuretics are administered intravenously as needed.
24. Attention is then directed to the ureter and bladder.
25. Two long Martius forceps are used to grasp the anterior bladder wall.
26. Using a scalpel with a #10 knife blade, a 4-cm incision is made anteriorly.
27. Two narrow Harrington retractors and one narrow Deaver retractor are inserted into the bladder for exposure.
28. The ureter is passed through the bladder wall and tunneled suburothelially for 2 to 2.5 cm.
29. The spatulated end of the ureter is then sutured into the bladder urothelium with four to six 4-0 or 5-0 atraumatic absorbable sutures, creating a ureteroneocystostomy.
30. A 5-Fr pediatric infant feeding tube is passed through the ureteroneocystostomy, up to the renal pelvis, and out through the urethra with the Foley catheter. This stenting catheter will remain in place for 36 to 48 hours to ensure ureteral patency during a period in which ureteral edema may occur.
31. Retractors are removed, and the bladder is closed in three layers.
32. Continuous 4-0 absorbable suture is used for urothelial closure and interrupted 2-0 absorbable suture for closure of bladder muscles.
33. An imbricating layer of 2-0 nonabsorbable material is used to bury the suture line.
34. The bladder is irrigated with an antibiotic solution to check for leaks.
35. The renal anastomoses are again checked for bleeding.
36. Three metal clips are placed on the superior, inferior, and lateral aspects of the kidney to radiographically measure renal size and determine postoperative swelling.
37. Retractors are removed from the incision.
38. Closed wound suction drains are inserted into the wound, brought through the skin laterally, and secured with 2-0 nonabsorbable suture on a cutting needle.
39. Muscle and fascial layers are closed with a single layer of 0 nonabsorbable sutures on a large atraumatic needle.
40. The subcutaneous layer is closed with 3-0 absorbable sutures on an atraumatic needle.
41. Skin closure is accomplished with skin staples, and dressings are applied.
42. The bladder is irrigated with 50 to 75 ml of antibiotic solution to prevent infection and free any blood clots.

## Adrenalectomy

Adrenalectomy is partial or total excision of one or both adrenal glands. It may be performed for several reasons: hypersecretion of adrenal hormones; neoplasms of the adrenal gland; secondary treatment of neoplasms elsewhere in the body that depend on adrenal hormonal secretions, such as carcinoma of the prostate and breast; and pheochromocytoma.

Care of the patient with pheochromocytoma carries with it particular concerns for the perioperative nurse. These patients are subject to extreme elevations in blood pressure, often accompanied by tachycardia, and hypovolemic states that can induce vascular collapse. If an adrenal tumor is being excised, early ligation of the adrenal vein is crucial in avoiding a sudden blood pressure elevation from the manipulation of the gland. After tumor removal there will be a rapid drop in blood pressure that can be minimized by maintenance of blood volume and administration of norepinephrine. With bilateral adrenalectomy, cortisone replacement will be instituted.

***Procedural Considerations.*** For unilateral adrenalectomy, the patient may be placed in the lateral or supine position depending on the intended approach. If both glands are to be removed the supine or prone position is selected. The prone position is especially useful for a known disorder, such as aldosteronism, localized benign lesions, and solitary adenomas of Cushing disease, and for debilitated patients with an advanced neoplasm.

The setup for a lateral approach is like that described for nephrectomy, including rib resection instruments, vascular instruments, and vessel clips and appliers. The setup for an abdominal approach is like that described for laparotomy, including vascular instruments, extra-long scissors, tissue forceps, Rochester-Pean forceps, Mixter forceps, and needle holders. Penrose tubing is needed for retraction. Vessel clips and appliers also may be needed, as well as various sizes of nonabsorbable braided sutures.

The setup for the posterior approach is like that described for the lateral approach. The patient is placed prone in a 35-degree jackknife position with the kidney rest under the inferior margin of the anterior rib cage. Both arms should be carefully extended cephalad with adequate support under each shoulder.

Laparoscopic adrenalectomy has recently become the treatment of choice.[3,38]

### *Operative Procedures*

LAPAROSCOPIC APPROACH

1. A 1.5-cm incision is made at the tip of the twelfth rib. The thoracolumbar fascia is entered by blunt dissection, and the 12-mm balloon dissector is placed behind Gerota's fascia and along the anterior axillary line. The balloon is inflated with 800 ml of saline, and the laparoscope is used to confirm balloon placement.
2. The operating balloon trocar is then placed in this position.
3. Two 10-mm trocars are inserted on each side of the initial trocar, along the costal margin, in the anterior and posterior axillary line.
4. The fourth trocar is placed along the posterior costal margin.
5. Dissection begins near the renal hilum, incising into Gerota's fascia.
6. Adrenal arteries are identified, clipped, and divided.
7. The anterior, lateral aspect of the gland is freed from the upper pole of the kidney.
8. The adrenal vein is clipped and divided.
9. The posterior, superior, and anterior surfaces of the adrenal gland are sequentially mobilized. A fan retractor is employed to retract the pancreas and spleen, or pancreas and liver, depending on which side the gland is being excised.
10. The adrenal branches of the inferior phrenic vessels and any accessory vessels are clipped and divided. The gland is removed through the original port using a retrieval sac. Hemostasis is achieved. The trocars are then sequentially removed, the incisions closed, and dressings applied.

LATERAL APPROACH

1. A flank, thoracolumbar, or transthoracic incision is performed as described for nephrectomy.
2. The rib underlying the chosen approach is resected or deflected for optimum exposure of the upper pole of the kidney.
3. Entry is between the eleventh and twelfth ribs in a flank approach, the tenth and eleventh ribs in a thoracolumbar approach, and the ninth and tenth ribs in a transthoracic approach.
4. An opening is made with scissors through the transverse fascia.
5. The pleura and diaphragm are protected with moist packs, and Gerota's capsule is incised to expose the kidney and adrenal gland.
6. The gland is identified and dissected free from the upper pole of the kidney by scissors and Babcock forceps.
7. The blood supply of the gland is identified, clamped or clipped, and divided. Bleeding vessels are ligated.
8. To release the gland, the left adrenal vein, a branch of the left renal vein, is separated by clamping and cutting. The right adrenal vein, a tributary of the vena cava, is also divided. Fine vascular sutures may be required to repair inadvertent injury to the vena cava.
9. When hemostasis has been ensured, the wound is closed sequentially in layers: muscle, fascia, subcutaneous tissue, and skin, and dressings are applied.

ABDOMINAL APPROACH

1. The abdominal wall is incised with an upper abdominal incision, and the peritoneal cavity is opened and explored.
2. Bleeding vessels are clamped and ligated.
3. The abdominal wound is retracted, and the surrounding organs are protected with moist laparotomy packs.
4. The retroperitoneal area near the diaphragm is opened on the left side, exposing the renal fascia.
5. The renal fascia is opened to reveal the left kidney and adrenal gland.
6. The adrenal gland is freed from the kidney by sharp and blunt dissection, and all bleeding vessels are clamped and ligated with 3-0 nonabsorbable sutures.
7. After all bleeding is controlled, the kidney is gently replaced in the renal fascia, which is closed with interrupted 0 absorbable sutures.
8. The peritoneum is closed over the left kidney and renal fascia.
9. The abdominal retractors are rearranged to give access to the peritoneum over the right kidney and adrenal gland. Care must be taken to prevent trauma to the liver.
10. The same procedure is repeated on the right side, taking care to clamp and ligate the short adrenal vein.
11. The abdomen is inspected for bleeding vessels, which are clamped and ligated.
12. The wound is closed and dressings applied.

POSTERIOR APPROACH

1. An incision is made over the eleventh or twelfth rib.
2. The periosteum is elevated, avoiding the nerve and vessels on the inferior margin.

3. The diaphragm and pleura are displaced superiorly, and the appropriate rib is resected.
4. Hemostasis is maintained with electrocoagulation.
5. Gerota's fascia is incised, and through sharp and blunt dissection the posterior aspect of the upper pole of the kidney is exposed.
6. The upper pole is mobilized, and a padded retractor is placed to deflect the kidney downward for the approach to the adrenal gland.
7. The suprarenal fat is meticulously dissected.
8. Vessel clips are used for control of smaller vessels.
9. Dissection continues superiorly, laterally, and inferiorly while the integrity of the hilum of the adrenal gland is maintained.
10. With right-angled clamps, the adrenal vein and artery are freed, divided, and ligated with 0 or 2-0 braided nonabsorbable ties.
11. Babcock clamps are employed for manipulation and removal of the adrenal gland.
12. Bleeding is controlled, and the wound is inspected for injury to renal structures.
13. Gerota's fascia is closed with interrupted absorbable sutures.
14. The wound is closed and dressings applied.

## REFERENCES


1. Allaf ME and others: Laparoscopic retroperitoneal lymph node dissection: duplication of open technique, *Urology* 65(3):575-577, 2005.
2. American Medical Systems: Erectile Dysfunction, 2005. Accessed July 2005, on-line: www.americanmedicalsystems.com/professional/medical_solutions.html.
3. Arca MJ, Gagner M: *Laparoscopic adrenalectomy*, 2005. Accessed July 2005, on-line: (American Gastrointestinal and Endoscopic Surgeons) www.sages.com/primarycare/adrenalectomy.html.
4. Association of periOperative Registered Nurses: *AORN standards, recommended practices, and guidelines,* Denver 2006, The Association.
5. Bakoletti SA and others: *Calcium channel blockers as the treatment of choice for hypertension in renal transplant recipients: fact or fiction*. Accessed July 2005, on-line: www.medscape.com.
6. Barash PG and others: *Clinical anesthesia*, ed 4, Philadelphia, 2001, Lippincott Williams & Wilkins, p. 653.
7. Bettschart V, Mosimann F: *Laparoscopic living donor nephrectomy for kidney transplantation,* 2005. Accessed Aug. 2005, on-line: (World Electronic Book of Surgery) www.websurg.com.
8. Boston Scientific: *Durasphere EXP injectable bulking agent*, 2005. Accessed Aug. 2005, on-line: www.bostonscientific.com/med_specialty/deviceDetail.
9. Boston Scientific: *Precision-twist transvaginal anchor system*, 2005. Accessed Aug. 2005, on-line: www.bostonscientific.com.
10. Buback D: The use of neuromodulation for treatment of urinary incontinence, *AORN Journal* 73(1):176-190, 2001.
11. Chambers A: Transurethral resection syndrome: it does not have to be a mystery, *AORN Journal* 75(1):155-169, 2002.
12. Cleveland Clinic, Cleveland, Ohio: *A minimally invasive approach to prostate cancer,* 2002. Accessed June 2005, on-line: www.clevelandclinic.org/misc/ surgical/urology/prostateCancer.htm.
13. CR Bard, Inc: *Continence overview*, Covington, Ga, 2004. Accessed July 2005, on-line: www.bardurological.com.
14. Eden C: *Extraperitoneal laparoscopic pyeloplasty*, 2005. Accessed Aug. 2005, on-line: www.websurg.com.
15. Eden C: *Extraperitoneal simple nephrectomy*, 2005. Accessed June 2005, on-line: www.websurb.com.
16. Galli B and others: Laparoscopic radical nephrectomy in renal cell carcinoma, *Urologic Nursing* 25(2):83-86, 2005.
17. Goodman T: Pressure damage in surgery, *Advance for Nurses* 7(15): 39-40, 2005.
18. *Greenlight laser instead of TUR for benign prostate adenoma.* Accessed Sept. 2005, on-line: www.germanmedicine.net/en/infogreenlight.html.
19. Greenlight PVP: *Prostate laser surgery*. Accessed Sept. 2005, on-line: www.laserscope.com/surgical/consumers/greenlight.html.
20. Gruendemann BJ, Mangum SS: *Infection prevention in surgical settings*, Philadelphia, 2001, Saunders.
21. Guillonneau B and others: *Laparoscopic radical prostatectomy*, 2005. Accessed, June 2005 on-line: www.computermotion.com.
22. Gynecare TVT: *Tension-free support for incontinence,* 2005. Accessed July 2005, on-line: www.gynecare.com.
23. Hanson KA: Diagnostic tests and tools in the evaluation of urologic disease. II, *Urologic Nursing* 23(6):405-415, 2003.
24. Marinara S: *Current controversies in the management of hypertension in patients with chronic kidney disease*. Accessed November 2004, on-line: www.medscape.com.
25. Herminie JJ: Transurethral resection of the prostate syndrome, *Seminars in Perioperative Nursing* 10(1):43-46, 2001.
26. *Indigo laser system for BPH*, 2005. Accessed Aug. 2005, on-line: www.indigomedical.com.
27. Johnson M and others: *NANDA, NOC and NIC linkages*, ed 2, St Louis, 2006, Mosby.
28. Jou YC and others: Percutaneous nephrolithotomy with holmium: yttrium-aluminum-garnet laser and fiber guider—report of 349 cases, *Urology* 65(3):454-458, 2005.
29. Kim SC and others: Percutaneous nephrolithotomy for caliceal diverticular calculi: a novel single stage approach, *Journal of Urology* 173:1194-1198, 2005.
30. Ku JH and others: Benefits of microsurgical repair of adolescent varicocele: comparison of semen parameters in fertile and infertile adults with varicocele, *Urology* 65(3):554-558, 2005.
31. Lamm DL and others: Bladder cancer: current optimal intravesical treatment, *Urologic Nursing* 25(5):323-332, 2005.
32. Laserscope: *KTP vs. holmium-greenlight PVP treatment for BPH*. Accessed Sept. 2005, on-line: www.laserscope.com/surgical/professionals/holmium.html.
33. LeBlond RF and others: *DeGowin's diagnostic examination*, New York, 2004, McGraw-Hill.
34. Lumenis Surgical: *BPH HoLap*, 2005. Accessed Sept. 2005, on-line: www.surgical.lumenis.com/wt/content/bph_holap.
35. Lumenis Surgical: *BPH HoLep*, 2005. Accessed Sept. 2005, on-line: www.surgical.lumenis.com/wt/content/bph_holep.
36. Mathews SD, Courts NF: Orthotopic neobladder surgery, *American Journal of Nursing* 101(7):24AA-24GG, 2001.
37. Medtronic: *InterStim therapy for bladder control*, 2005. Accessed June 2005, on-line: www.medtronic.com/neuro/interstim/tined_lead.html.
38. Micali S and others: Reviews in endourology, laparoscopic adrenal surgery: new frontiers, *Journal of Endourology* 19(3):272-278, 2005.
39. Namiki S: Recovery of quality of life in year after laparoscopic or retropubic radical prostatectomy: a multi-institutional longitudinal study, *Urology* 65(3):517-523, 2005.
40. Piechaud T, Gaston R: *Laparoscopic radical prostatectomy: transperitoneal approach*, 2005. Accessed June 2005, on-line: websurg.com.
41. Quinn DM, Schick L: *Perianesthesia nursing core curriculum*, Philadelphia, 2004, Saunders.
42. Raz S: *Atlas of transvaginal surgery*, ed 2, Philadelphia, 2002, Saunders.
43. The Regence Group: *Periurethral bulking agents for the treatment of urinary incontinence*. Accessed October 5, 2004, on-line: www.regence.com/trgmedpol/surgery/sur33.html.
44. Saussine C: *Laparoscopic intraperitoneal pyeloplasty*, 2005. Accessed June 2005, on-line: www.websurg.com.
45. Shinohara K: Prostate cancer: cryotherapy, *Urology Clinics of North America* 30(4):725-736, 2003.
46. Stanton SL, Monga AK: *Clinical urogynaecology*, ed 2, London, 2000, Churchill Livingstone.

47. Swearingen P: *All-in-one care planning resource*, St Louis, 2004, Mosby.
48. Tertzakian G and others: *PVP (photo-selective vaporization of the prostate) also known as Greenlight PV, laser prostatectomy, laser TURP: a new advance in laser prostate surgery and an alternative to prostate surgery (TURP) for enlarged prostate*, 2005. Accessed Sept. 2005, on-line: www.ocurology.com/PVP.html.
49. Thibodeau GA, Patton KT: *Structure and function of the body*, ed 12, St Louis, 2004, Mosby.
50. Turk IA and others: Laparoscopic dismembered pyeloplasty—the method of choice in the presence of an enlarged renal pelvis and crossing vessels, *European Urology* 42(3):268-275, 2002.
51. Turk TM and others: *Pyeloplasty*, 2005. Accessed June 2005, on-line: www.emedicine.com/med/topic3059.htm#section~introduction.
52. Ullrich NFE, Comiter CV: The male sling for stress urinary incontinence: 24 month follow-up with questionnaire based assessment, *Journal of Urology* 172(1):207-209, 2004.
53. Wallace MA: What is new with renal transplantation, *AORN Journal* 77(5):945-965, 2003.
54. Ward-Smith P and others: Quality of life among men treated with brachytherapy for prostate cancer, *Urologic Nursing* 24(2):95-99, 2004.
55. Willener R, Hantikainen V: Individual quality of life following radical prostatectomy in men with prostate cancer, *Urologic Nursing* 25(2): 88-1000, 2005.
56. Williamson MR, Smith AY: *Fundamentals of uroradiology*, Philadelphia, 2000, Saunders, pp. 75-77.
57. Wilson WJ, Winters JC: Is there still a place for the pubovaginal sling at the bladder neck in the era of the midurethral sling? *Current Urology Reports* 6:335-339, 2005. Accessed Sept. 2005, on-line: www.current-reports.com/home_journal.cfm?JournalID=UR.
58. Winkelman C: Assessment of the renal/urinary system. In Ignatavicius DD, Workman ML: *Medical-surgical nursing: critical thinking for collaborative care,* ed 5, Philadelphia, 2006, Elsevier Saunders.
59. Wojner AW: *Outcomes management: applications to clinical practice,* St Louis, 2001, Mosby.

CHAPTER 16

# Thyroid and Parathyroid Surgery

JANE C. ROTHROCK

The first documented thyroid surgery occurred in the twelfth century (History box), and today operative procedures continue to be performed on the thyroid gland for various underlying causes. Surgical strategies range from lobectomy and isthmectomy for papillary microcarcinomas (lesions smaller than 1 cm) to near-total or total thyroidectomies for symptomatic multinodular goiters.[4] In 1925 Felix Mandl did the first successful surgery for primary hyperparathyroidism in Vienna.[16] Since then, technologic advances have added new approaches to thyroid and parathyroid surgery, such as minimally invasive surgery (MIS) techniques.

This chapter discusses the structure and function of the thyroid and parathyroid glands. Nursing considerations are presented, including assessment, nursing diagnosis, outcome identification, planning, implementation, and evaluation. A Sample Plan of Care is provided on p. 559. Patient and family education and discharge planning are covered, and sample home care information is provided. Surgical interventions include definitions, reasons, procedural considerations, and procedural steps for thyroid, thyroglossal duct, and parathyroid surgery.

## Surgical Anatomy

### Thyroid Gland

The thyroid gland (Figure 16-1) is a highly vascular organ situated in the anterior portion of the neck, deep to the paired strap muscles. It consists of right and left lobes united by a middle portion, the isthmus, and it weighs approximately 20 g. The isthmus is situated near the base of the neck, between the second and fourth tracheal rings, and the lobes lie beside the larynx and trachea. The pyramidal lobe, a long, thin projection of thyroid tissue protruding cephalad from the isthmus, is found in about 80% of patients at surgery; it is the vestige of the embryonic thyroglossal duct.

Blood supply to the thyroid is from the superior thyroid artery, which originates from the external carotid artery, and the inferior thyroid artery, which originates from the thyrocervical trunk of the subclavian artery. The points at which these two arteries enter the thyroid gland are referred to as "poles" of the thyroid and are important anatomic landmarks during surgery. The thyroid gland is drained by three pairs of veins (superior, middle, and inferior thyroid veins). Occasionally a single thyroid artery (thyroidea ima) may come directly from the arch of the aorta or the innominate artery and rise in front of the trachea to enter the midline of the gland inferiorly.

The recurrent laryngeal nerve, which is a branch of the vagus nerve, innervates the intrinsic muscles of the larynx. The right recurrent laryngeal nerve loops under the subclavian artery ascending in an oblique direction lateral to the tracheoesophageal groove. The recurrent laryngeal nerve contains both motor and sensory fibers. The motor component innervates the abductor muscles of the true vocal cords. The sensory component supplies sensation to the larynx below the vocal cords. During surgery, care is taken to identify and protect this nerve. Immediate hoarseness occurs if the nerve is divided on one side. If the recurrent nerve is injured bilaterally, acute paralysis of both vocal cords may obstruct the airway and require emergency tracheotomy because of adduction of the true vocal cords. Injury to the external branch of the superior laryngeal nerve, which innervates the cricothyroid muscle, results in difficulty shouting or singing high notes.

The thyroid gland produces three hormones: thyroxine ($T_4$) and triiodothyronine ($T_3$), together known as the *thyroid hormones (TH)*, and calcitonin. $T_3$ and $T_4$ cannot be synthesized without iodine. Calcitonin increases calcium storage in the bone and decreases blood calcium levels. The thyroid hormones' primary function is to regulate energy metabolism; they also play an important role in growth and development. Thyroid-stimulating hormone (TSH) is synthesized by the anterior pituitary, which stimulates the production and release of thyroid hormones and the uptake of iodide.

### Parathyroid Gland

The parathyroid glands usually consist of four small, red-brown to yellow, flat, ovoid masses.[7] The upper pair of glands lies in proximity to the posterior portion of the superior pole of the thyroid; the lower pair usually (approximately 60%) lies near the posterior lateral aspect of the lower pole of the thyroid (Figure 16-2, *A*). Ectopic parathyroid glands, more common in the inferior parathyroid glands, may be found in the superior mediastinum, especially within the thymus and as low as the pericardium (Figure 16-2, *B*). Each parathyroid gland measures approximately 3 mm × 3 mm × 3 mm and generally weighs less than 50 mg. The upper glands are generally smaller than the lower ones. Both the upper and lower parathyroid glands receive their blood supply from the inferior thyroid artery.

The parathyroid gland secretes parathyroid hormone (PTH) and is an antagonist to calcitonin. Both PTH and calcitonin work together to maintain calcium homeostasis by increasing calcium removal from storage in bone and increasing absorption of calcium by the intestines, thereby increasing the blood calcium levels.

## HISTORY

Since 2700 BC, long before the thyroid gland was identified, goiters (from Latin *gutter* for "throat") have been described. Europeans living 2000 years ago, especially those living in the Alps, noted a swelling in the neck and called it *bronchocele,* ancient Greek for "tracheal out-pouching." It was thousands of years later when it was recognized by Hieronymus Fabricius ab Aquapendente in 1619 that goiters arose from the thyroid gland.

With the Italian Renaissance period came the expansion of inquiry into the human body. During this time, the thyroid gland was identified. Around the year 1500 Leonardo da Vinci depicted the gland, and in 1543 Vesalius called the thyroid gland the "laryngeal glands." Leonardo da Vinci's drawings portrayed the thyroid as two separate glands on either side of the larynx. Thomas Wharton, because of his 1656 publication *Adenographia,* is credited for replacing the term "laryngeal gland" with the term "thyroid gland" (Greek *thyreoeides,* "shield shaped").

Thyroid surgery was first described in 1170 by Roger Frugardi. Thyroid surgery was hazardous, with mortality rates of more than 40%. High mortality rates continued until the 1800s, when increased knowledge and advances in general anesthesia, antisepsis, and hemostasis had been attained.

In the 1800s, two of the most notable thyroid surgeons—C.A. Theodor Billroth (1829 to 1894) and Emil Theodor Kocher (1841 to 1917)—revolutionized the treatment of thyroid diseases. Despite Billroth's earlier success with thyroidectomies, Kocher is regarded as the father of thyroid surgery. Kocher performed more than 2000 thyroid surgeries in the late 1800s, with only a 4.5% mortality rate; he received the Nobel prize in 1909 for advances in this field. In 1914 Kendall isolated the hormone *thyroxine* ($T_4$). Since 1941, thyroidectomy as treatment of thyroid mass (goiter) has become less frequent because of the use of radioactive iodine (RAI) and antithyroid drugs, which reduce the activity of the thyroid gland.

Modified from Kaplan EL: Thyroid and parathyroid. In Schwartz SI and others, editors: *Principles of surgery,* ed 6, New York, 1994, McGraw-Hill; Sadler GP and others: Thyroid and parathyroid. In Schwartz SI and others, editors: *Principles of surgery,* ed 7, New York, 1999, McGraw-Hill; Sawin CT: The heritage of the thyroid. In Braverman LE, Utiger RD, editors: *Werner and Ingbar's the thyroid: a fundamental and clinical text,* ed 7, Philadelphia, 1996, Lippincott-Raven; Yousem DM, Scheff AM: Thyroid and parathyroid. In Som PM, Curtin AD, editors: *Head and neck imaging,* ed 3, St Louis, 1996, Mosby.

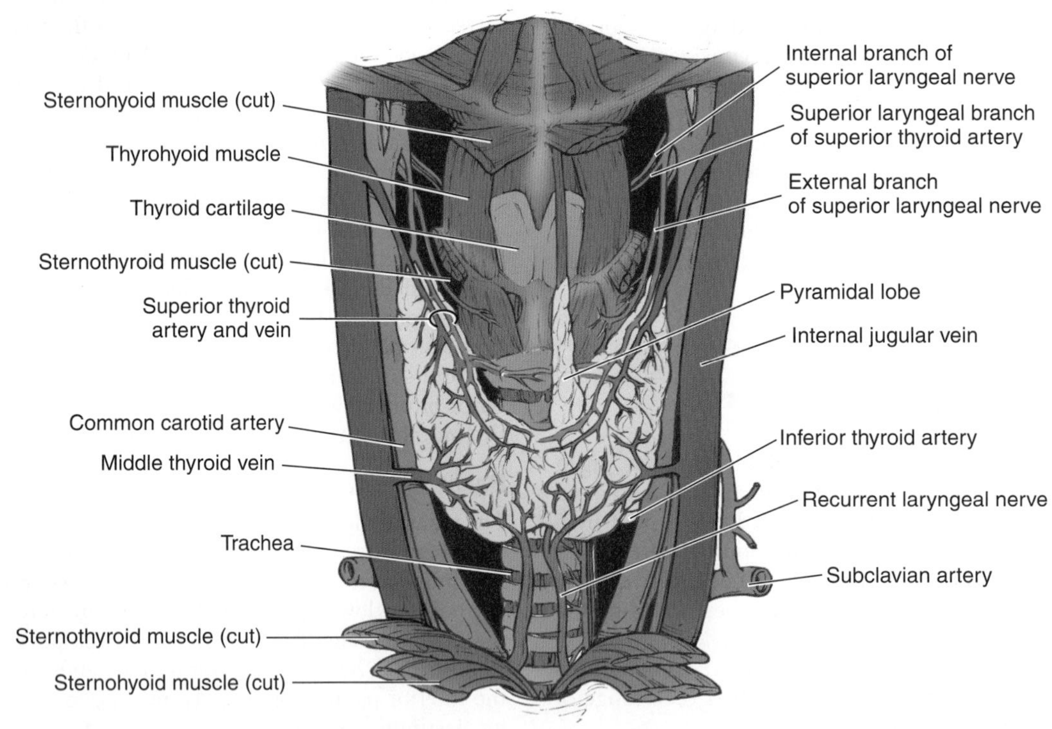


**FIGURE 16-1** The thyroid gland.

# *Perioperative Nursing Considerations*

## Assessment

Preoperatively, the patient with hyperthyroidism most likely has undergone appropriate drug therapy that has returned the thyroid hormone levels and metabolic state to normal.[5] Nonetheless, the perioperative nurse should assess the patient for the presence of any symptoms that may relate to accelerated metabolism (Box 16-1). The patient's baseline vital signs should be noted for an abnormally elevated resting pulse, elevated systolic blood pressure, and cardiac symptoms, such as palpitations or atrial fibrillation. Atrial fibrillation is the most common cardiac complication of hyperthyroidism.[6] For this reason, the perioperative nurse should review the patient's medication history to determine if anticoagulation medication

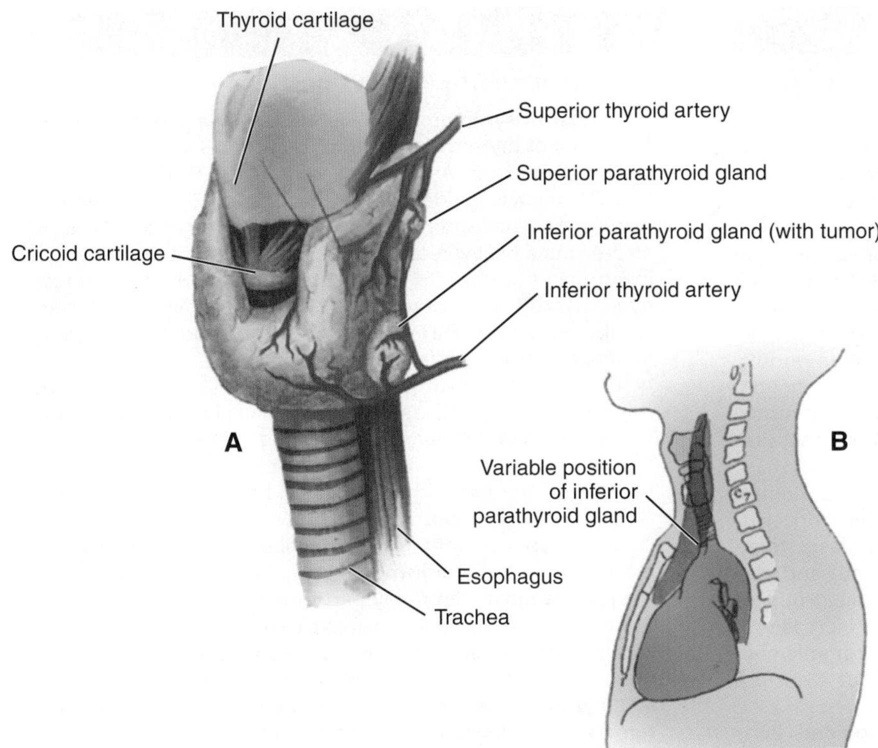


**FIGURE 16-2** **A,** Thyroid and parathyroid glands. Note their relation to each other and to the trachea. **B,** Note the shaded area for varied locations of inferior parathyroid glands.

**BOX 16-1**

### Common Symptoms and Signs of Thyroid Dysfunction

**HYPOTHYROIDISM**
Fatigue
Weight gain
Cold intolerance
Hair dryness or loss
Dry skin
Depression
Hoarse voice
Poor concentration
Muscle stiffness and pain
Edema
Bradycardia
Constipation
Menstrual irregularity (especially heavy menses)
Infertility

**HYPERTHYROIDISM**
Vision changes
Emotional liability, mood changes
Irritability
Exercise intolerance
Fatigue
Weight loss
Heat intolerance
Increased sweating
Nervousness
Insomnia
Tremor
Muscle weakness
Dyspnea
Palpitations
Tachycardia and atrial tachydysrhythmias
Frequent bowel movements
Menstrual irregularity (oligomenorrhea; infertility)

Modified from Roberts CG, Ladenson PW: Hypothyroidism, *Lancet* 363(9411):793-803, 2004; Surks MI and others: Subclinical thyroid disease: scientific review and guidelines for diagnosis and management, *JAMA: The Journal of the American Medical Association* 291(2):228-238, 2004.

is being taken. The patient's cardiac and respiratory rate, muscle strength, elimination patterns, history of weight loss and heat intolerance, and emotional status should be noted. The patient may be anxious about the disease state and the success of surgery and may express concern regarding surgery in the area of the neck and its cosmetic results (Research Highlight). Patients who are concerned about body image should have the opportunity to discuss these issues with the perioperative nurse. Skin integrity should be determined; patients with hyperthyroidism may have finely textured skin and edema in the lower extremities, placing them at risk for skin breakdown. Although complications are infrequent, the most common ones specific to thyroid surgery are hypoparathyroidism and injury to the recurrent laryngeal nerve. Preoperative assessment of the patient's voice quality should therefore be noted.

In addition to clinical signs and symptoms, results of diagnostic tests should be reviewed. Tests performed most commonly before thyroid surgery include measurements of TSH, $T_3$, and $T_4$; radioisotope or ultrasonic scans; and a current electrocardiogram (ECG). Adult normal ranges for several of the tests just mentioned are as follows[13]:

- TSH: 0.35 to 5.5 microinternational units/ml
- $T_3$: (25 to 50 years old) 75 to 220 ng/dl; (older than 50 years old) 40 to 180 ng/dl
- $T_4$: (males) 4 to 12 mcg/dl; (females) 5 to 12 mcg/dl; (older than 60 years) 5 to 11 mcg/dl

Thyroid function tests are interpreted in light of the patient's clinical presentation. They complement the findings of the physical examination. The single best test to measure the thyroid status in a given person is a TSH assay (Best Practice).

***Thyroid Assessment.*** In addition to palpation of the thyroid gland for size, contour, consistency, nodes, fixation, and bruits,[10] scans are used to elucidate thyroid anatomy.

**THYROID ISOTOPE SCAN (THYROID SCINTIGRAPHY).** A thyroid nodule, the most common endocrine problem in the United States, is any abnormal growth of thy-

## RESEARCH HIGHLIGHT

### Laser Thermocoagulation for Benign Thyroid Nodules

In this study, 30 women who had solitary, solid, benign thyroid nodules declined surgical treatment. They all had concerns about the appearance of their neck or about symptoms of compression from the nodule. This study was undertaken to compare the effects of laser-induced thermocoagulation on nodule size and symptoms versus no treatment. A laser fiber was inserted into the nodule with the patient under local anesthesia, with ultrasound guidance. Treatment resulted in an irregular, enlarging echogenic area within the benign nodule. Data regarding nodule volume, as measured by ultrasound, and ratings of cosmetic appearance and pressure symptoms were assessed at baseline and then at 1 and 6 months after treatment.

At baseline, the women in the treatment and control groups had similar ages, frequency of cosmetic concerns, pressure symptoms, and nodule volume. In the laser treatment group, nodule volume decreased at 1 month and at 6 months, with a median decrease of 44%. In the group of women who had no treatment, nodule volume increased a median of 9% over the same 6-month period. Cosmetic concerns decreased in the laser treatment group but were unchanged in the control group.

The researchers conclude that ultrasound-guided laser thermocoagulation decreases cosmetic symptoms and the size of the thyroid nodule and is well tolerated.

Modified from Dosing H and others: Effect of ultrasound-guided interstitial laser photocoagulation on benign solitary cold thyroid nodules—a randomized study, *European Journal of Endocrinology* 152:341-345, 2005.

roid cells. Most nodules are discovered during routine physical examination, since they rarely produce symptoms. Imaging of the normal thyroid with radionuclide agents shows normal size, shape, position, and function of the thyroid, with no areas of decreased or increased uptake. Nodules that are *hot* demonstrate an increased uptake of radionuclide agent; this may indicate a benign adenoma or localized toxic goiter. *Cold* nodules are hypofunctioning or nonfunctioning and may indicate a cyst, nonfunctioning adenoma or goiter, lymphoma, localized area of thyroiditis, or carcinoma. Two commonly used agents in thyroid imaging are radioactive iodine and technetium 99m–pertechnetate ($^{99m}TcO_4^-$).

**ULTRASONIC SCAN.** Ultrasonic scans are useful for determining the size and number of nodules within the thyroid as well as for monitoring size progression during follow-up. Ultrasonography is also helpful in facilitating accurate needle placement and sampling the target nodule during a fine needle aspiration.[11]

**FINE NEEDLE ASPIRATION.** Performing a fine needle aspiration (FNA) is the most useful diagnostic tool currently available in the management of thyroid nodules. The procedure is performed in the surgeon's office. Several samples are usually taken from various parts of the nodule. Pathologic examination of fine needle biopsy specimens reveals a benign nodule (70% of biopsies), a nondiagnostic or inadequate biopsy (15%), a suspicious nodule (10%), or a malignancy (5%).[15] A suspicious nodule usually implies the finding of a follicular neoplasm, which can be either benign or malignant, and requires removal in order to be fully evaluated histologically by the pathologist to make the correct diagnosis. The number of patients undergoing thyroid surgery has been reduced and the incidence of malignancy in the resected specimens has increased with the use of FNA.[11]

Patient education for the FNA should include the following:

- The patient will be lying down for the procedure and may expect coldness on the neck from the prepping solution.
- Local anesthesia may or may not be used.

## BEST PRACTICE

### Screening for Thyroid Dysfunction

A number of symptoms and signs are well-established manifestations of thyroid dysfunction (see Box 16-1).

The American Association of Clinical Endocrinologists (AACE) practice guidelines for the diagnostic evaluation of hyperthyroidism and hypothyroidism recommend TSH assay as the single best screening test. Hyperthyroidism results in a lower-than-normal TSH level (suppressed TSH). To diagnose hyperthyroidism accurately, TSH assay sensitivity, the lowest reliably measured TSH concentration, must be 0.02 milliinternational units/liter or less.

In most outpatient clinical situations, serum TSH is the most sensitive test for detecting mild (subclinical) thyroid hormone excess or deficiency. An elevated serum TSH concentration is present in both overt and mild (subclinical) hypothyroidism. In the latter, the free thyroid hormone ($fT_3$ and $fT_4$) levels are, by definition, normal.

Three types of treatment are available for Graves' disease, a type of hyperthyroidism. Surgery, frequently performed in the past, is most commonly performed when it co-exists with thyroid cancer. Surgeons well-experienced in thyroid surgery should perform the intervention, because potential complications include hypoparathyroidism and vocal cord paralysis. Antithyroid drugs are prescribed to achieve a remission, but remission rates are variable and relapses frequent. Radioactive iodine is currently the treatment of choice. Most treated patients require lifelong thyroid replacement therapy.

Hypothyroidism results from undersecretion of thyroid hormone. In the United States, hypothyroidism affects close to 11 million people each year; the most common cause of primary hypothyroidism is chronic autoimmune thyroiditis (Hashimoto's disease). The most valuable laboratory test is a sensitive measurement of TSH level. Clinical hypothyroidism is treated with levothyroxine replacement therapy. The AACE supports treating subclinical hypothyroidism if TSH levels are greater than 10 microunits/ml or if TSH levels are between 5 and 10 microunits/ml in conjunction with goiter or positive antibodies or both.

Serum TSH measurement is the single most reliable test to diagnose all common forms of hypothyroidism and hyperthyroidism, with a high sensitivity (98%) and specificity (92%).

Modified from American Association of Clinical Endocrinologists: Medical guidelines for clinical practice for the evaluation and treatment of hyperthyroidism and hypothyroidism, *Endocrine Practice* 8(6):457-469, 2002; Mauk KL: Rooting out hypothyroidism in the elderly, *Nursing 2005* 35(12):65-66, 2005; Screening for thyroid disease: recommendation statement, U.S. Preventive Services Task Force, January 20, 2004, 140(2):125-127, 2004.
*$fT_3$,* Free triiodothyronine; *$fT_4$,* free thyroxine; *TSH,* thyroid-stimulating hormone.

- Once the prick of the needle is felt, no talking, swallowing, or moving is allowed.

FNA may be an emotionally stressful procedure for the patient. Vials of ammonia should be kept in the room in case the patient feels faint. Lowering the head (as in the Trendelenburg position or sitting with the head down) is also important in treating vasovagal syncope. Postprocedure education should include (1) the need to refrain from using aspirin or aspirin-containing medications or nonsteroidal antiinflammatory drugs (NSAIDs) for the next 24 hours and (2) to expect to have a half-dollar–size bruise at the FNA site. There are no restrictions on food or activity.

Preoperative patient education for patients undergoing a partial or total thyroidectomy should include an explanation of perioperative events, discussion of the incision site, type of dressing to be used, and explanation of any drains, if their use is anticipated. Discussion of pain and pain management therapy should also be covered. Patients may also be told that there are various ways of protecting their eyesight during surgery, and if ointment is used, they can expect temporary blurred vision when they first open their eyes. If sequential compression devices (SCDs) are to be used for prophylaxis of deep vein thrombosis (DVT), an explanation of their use and sensation should be included. The patient should also be encouraged to slowly flex and extend the neck early in the postoperative period. (See "Patient and Family Education and Discharge Planning" later in this chapter for further discussion of patient education.)

***Parathyroid Assessment.*** An elevation of serum PTH in association with hypercalcemia is diagnostic of hyperparathyroidism in most cases. PTH normal levels are between 10 and 65 pg/ml (the value varies with laboratory); serum ionized calcium (4.5 to 5.6 mg/dl) is usually measured at the same time.[13] The causes of primary hyperparathyroidism are single adenoma (80% to 85%), four gland hyperplasia (10% to 15%), and rarely parathyroid carcinoma (less than 1%). Preoperative localization studies with parathyroid sestamibi scan (Figure 16-3) or high-resolution ultrasonography can identify parathyroid adenomas with high sensitivity (70% to 80%). Sensitivities decrease significantly for hyperplasia (less than 50%).

Hyperparathyroidism causes an increase in the level of serum calcium and a decrease in the level of serum phosphate. Nursing diagnoses and care planning will be based on these imbalances and on the severity of the associated symptoms. Some patients are asymptomatic; others have symptoms that manifest themselves as disturbances in the central nervous system or cardiovascular, renal, gastrointestinal, or musculoskeletal system (Box 16-2).

Assessment should include determining whether the patient is apathetic or emotionally irritable; whether there is muscle weakness and atrophy, back or joint pain, nausea, vomiting, constipation, peptic ulcer disease, or cardiac dysrhythmia; or whether there is renal damage, stones, or disease.[3] If any of these signs or symptoms are present, the plan of care should be adjusted. Otherwise, perioperative patient education and nursing management of the patient undergoing parathyroidectomy are essentially the same as those for thyroidectomy. In the early postoperative period for both thyroidectomy and parathyroidectomy, the patient should be closely observed for any signs of hypocalcemia. The serum calcium level reaches its lowest in 48 to 72 hours and returns to normal within the following 2 to 3 days. Symptoms include numbness and tingling of extremities and around the lips. Hyperactive tendon reflexes and a positive Chvostek sign (tapping on the facial nerve elicits contraction of facial muscles) can be demonstrated on physical examination. Tetany may develop and is exhibited by carpopedal spasms, tonic-clonic convulsions, and laryngeal stridor, which can be fatal.

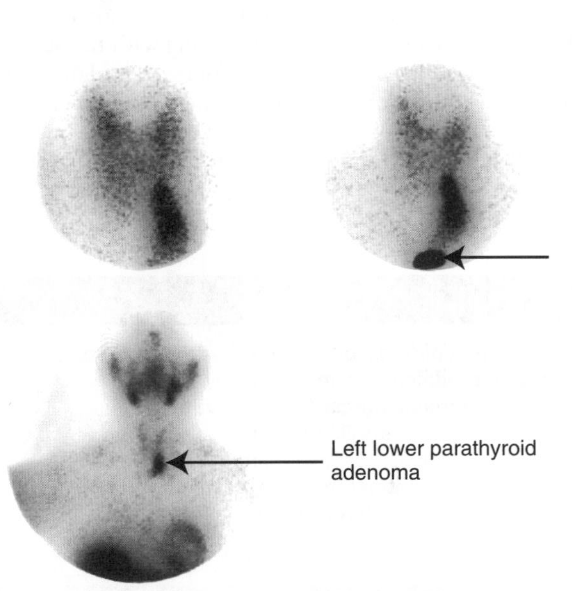


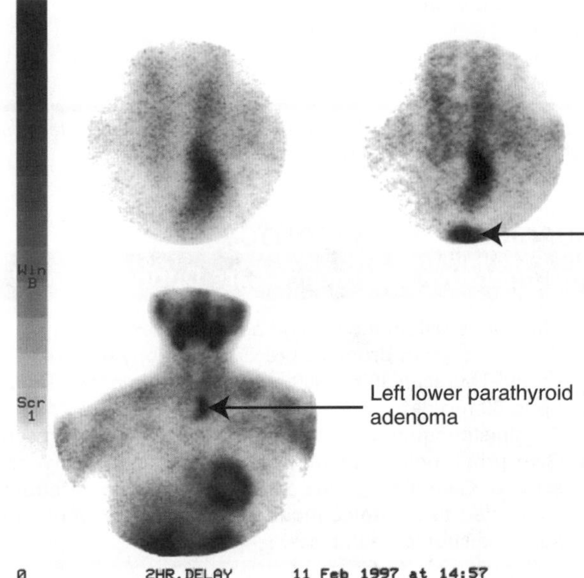


**FIGURE 16-3** Sestamibi scan, showing a left lower adenoma at arrow.

BOX 16-2

### Parathyroid Dysfunction

**HYPERPARATHYROIDISM**

**Definition**

Overactivity of one or more of the parathyroid glands; excessive secretion of parathyroid hormone causes an increase in calcium (hypercalcemia)

**Signs and Symptoms**

Polyuria, polydipsia, kidney stones
Abdominal pain, constipation, nausea, anorexia
Fractures of ribs, spine
Joint or back pain
Depression, paranoia, mood swings
Muscle weakness and atrophy

**Complications**

Cardiac dysrhythmias, cardiac failure
Gastric ulcer
Skeletal problems: pathologic fractures
Renal disorders: kidney stones, urinary tract infections, renal failure
Pancreatitis
Stupor/coma

**HYPOPARATHYROIDISM**

**Definition**

Deficiency of parathyroid hormone, which is necessary to maintain normal levels of serum calcium; may occur as a result of radiation therapy for head and neck cancer or as a postoperative complication from thyroid or parathyroid surgery[12]; symptoms are related to reduced calcium levels (hypocalcemia)

**Signs and Symptoms**

Personality disturbances: anxiety, depression, irritability
Tetany: muscle cramps, spasms (hands, face, feet); paresthesias: numbness and tingling (around mouth, lips, and tongue)
Dry, scaly skin; brittle nails; thin, patchy hair
Week tooth enamel/dental caries
Cataracts

**Complications**

Cardiac dysrhythmias
Seizures
Psychoses
Cardiac arrest

Modified from Canobbio MM: *Mosby's handbook of patient teaching,* ed 3, St Louis, 2006, pp. 446-447, 466.

## Nursing Diagnosis

Nursing diagnoses related to the care of patients undergoing thyroid and parathyroid surgery might include the following:

- Impaired Swallowing related to mechanical obstruction (enlarged thyroid preoperatively; edema or hematoma postoperatively)
- Ineffective Thermoregulation related to altered metabolic rate
- Disturbed Body Image related to surgical scar in prominent location
- Ineffective Airway Clearance related to obstruction (enlarged thyroid preoperatively; edema or hematoma postoperatively) or bilateral recurrent laryngeal nerve injury
- Impaired Gas Exchange related to postoperative bleeding or swelling or inability to move secretions

## Outcome Identification

Outcomes identified for the selected nursing diagnoses could be stated as follows:

- The patient will maintain normal swallowing.
- The patient will maintain normal body temperature.
- The patient will verbalize decreased disturbance in feelings related to body image.
- The patient will maintain a patent airway.
- The patient will maintain effective gas exchange.

## Planning

If a patient scheduled for thyroid surgery is not at optimal weight, the perioperative nurse should consider the patient at high risk for pressure ulcer development and plan on padding pressure areas to prevent skin and tissue damage. Intraoperatively, warm saline should be provided for irrigation. Because a potential problem for patients with hyperthyroidism is thyroid storm (thyrotoxic crisis), the perioperative nurse must be prepared to respond quickly. Thyroid storm can occur in patients who have been partially controlled or whose hyperthyroidism is untreated. Thyrotoxic crisis can be precipitated by a stressful event, such as surgery. By planning a quiet, calm atmosphere and helping the patient relax, the perioperative nurse can reduce the risk of thyroid storm. Collaborating with the surgical and anesthesia team, the perioperative nurse can plan for appropriate interventions to assist in reducing body temperature and heart rate, provide oxygen and intravenous solutions, and administer medications as prescribed in the event thyrotoxic crisis occurs (Surgical Pharmacology).

SURGICAL PHARMACOLOGY

### Postoperative Emergency Care During Thyroid Storm

- Maintain a patent airway and adequate ventilation.
- Give antithyroid drugs as prescribed: propylthiouracil (PTU, Propyl-Thyracil), 300 to 900 mg/day; methimazole (Tapazole), up to 60 mg/day.
- Administer sodium iodide solution, 2 g/day IV as prescribed.
- Give propranolol (Inderal, Detensol), 1 to 3 mg IV as prescribed. Give slowly over 3 minutes; the patient should be connected to a cardiac monitor, and a central venous pressure line should be in place.
- Give glucocorticoids as prescribed: hydrocortisone, 100 to 500 mg/day; prednisone, 4 to 60 mg/day IV or IM.
- Monitor continuously for cardiac dysrhythmias.
- Monitor vital signs every 30 minutes.
- Provide comfort measures, including a cooling blanket.
- Give nonsalicylate antipyretics as prescribed.
- Correct dehydration with normal saline infusions.

Modified from Workman LM: Interventions for clients with problems of the thyroid and parathyroid glands. In Ignatavicius DD, Workman ML, *Medical-surgical nursing: critical thinking for collaborative care,* ed 5, Philadelphia, 2006, Saunders.
*IM,* Intramuscularly; *IV,* intravenously.

A typical plan of care for a patient undergoing thyroid and parathyroid surgery follows.

## Implementation

***Positioning.*** Proper patient positioning on the operating room (OR) bed is crucial for optimal exposure of the thyroid gland. The patient is positioned supine, with some surgeons preferring a beach chair position. Hyperextension of the neck is required for maximal exposure. A circular headrest will provide proper support, keep the head straight, and prevent postoperative headache and aggravation of prior neck problems. Alternatively, a shoulder roll may be used. To protect the ulnar nerve, the elbows should be padded when tucking the arms in at the sides. All pressure points should be padded, especially in the patient who is not at optimal weight. Reduction of venous congestion can be accomplished by a 30-degree reverse-Trendelenburg tilt of the OR bed.[4]

***Skin Preparation.*** The operative area, including the chin and anterior neck region, lateral surfaces of the neck from the earlobes down to the outer aspects of the shoulder, and upper anterior chest region to the nipples, is prepped with an antimicrobial solution. Appropriate precautions must be taken to prevent the solution from pooling under the neck or in the axillary area. Pooled solutions present the risk for a surgical fire. Any bed sheets that become soaked with a flammable prep solution should be removed from the OR. The patient is draped with sterile towels and a fenestrated sheet. A sterile towel or lap sponge may be placed on each side of the neck to prevent pooling of blood under the neck during surgery. If lap sponges are used, they should be noted on the count sheet to avoid confusion in accounting for all counted items.

The surgeon marks the incision site with a marking pen or with the pressure of a full-length fine silk tie to help ensure a

### SAMPLE PLAN OF CARE

**NURSING DIAGNOSIS**

**Impaired Swallowing** related to mechanical obstruction (enlarged thyroid preoperatively; edema postoperatively)

**OUTCOME**

Patient will maintain normal swallowing.

**INTERVENTIONS**

- Keep suction line and suction catheter connected and ready until patient is discharged from OR.
- Monitor for and report difficulty in swallowing during emergence from anesthesia or transport to PACU.
- Gently suction oropharyngeal secretions as required.
- Keep vein open postoperatively until patient can swallow without difficulty.

**NURSING DIAGNOSIS**

**Ineffective Thermoregulation** related to altered metabolic rate

**OUTCOME**

Patient's body temperature will be maintained within normal range.

**INTERVENTIONS**

- Monitor patient's temperature; report abnormalities.
- Provide light covers if temperature is elevated or patient states that he or she is warm.
- Change linens preoperatively and postoperatively if wet from perspiration.
- Avoid using plasticized drapes.

**NURSING DIAGNOSIS**

**Disturbed Body Image** related to surgical scar

**OUTCOME**

Patient will verbalize decreased disturbance in feelings related to body image.

**INTERVENTIONS**

- Explain that incision is made in natural fold of skin.
- Explain how techniques used for surgical closure minimize scarring.
- Instruct patient in postoperative turning measures that decrease strain on suture line.
- Suggest that jewelry, scarves, and certain necklines can be used to cover scar until normal fading occurs.

**NURSING DIAGNOSIS**

**Ineffective Airway Clearance** related to obstruction secondary to enlarged thyroid (preoperatively), edema (postoperatively), or bilateral recurrent laryngeal nerve injury

**OUTCOME**

Patient's airway will remain patent.

**INTERVENTIONS**

- Position patient so that enlarged gland does not obstruct airway. Head of transport vehicle may need to be elevated preoperatively.
- Assist anesthesia personnel during induction.
- Monitor respiratory rate and signs of respiratory distress (stridor, wheezing, dyspnea, labored respirations).
- If distress occurs because of recurrent laryngeal nerve injury, a tracheotomy may be required. Have oxygen, suctioning equipment, and a tracheotomy tray available.
- Observe neck dressing and behind neck area for signs of edema or bleeding (postoperatively). Urgent intubation for airway protection and reexploration in the OR can be lifesaving.

**NURSING DIAGNOSIS**

**Impaired Gas Exchange** related to postoperative bleeding or swelling, bilateral recurrent laryngeal nerve surgical injury, or inability to move secretions

**OUTCOME**

Patient's gas exchange will remain effective.

**INTERVENTIONS**

- Monitor respiratory status and results of pulse oximetry.
- If patient is extubated in OR, be prepared to assist anesthesia personnel; closely observe for respiratory stridor or respiratory obstruction (recurrent laryngeal malfunction). Tracheotomy may be required; oxygen, suctioning equipment, and a tracheotomy tray should be available.
- Assess color of nailbeds.
- Monitor surgical site for swelling and bleeding.
- Suction patient as required to remove secretions.
- Monitor patency of surgical drain and amount/nature of drainage in collection device.
- Instruction in coughing and deep breathing should include supporting the neck; placing both hands behind the neck when coughing reduces strain on the suture line.

*OR,* Operating room; *PACU,* postanesthesia care unit.

BOX 16-3

### Home Care After a Thyroidectomy

**HOME CARE**

- Give both the patient and the caregiver *verbal* and *written* instructions. Provide them with the name and telephone number of a physician or nurse to call if questions arise.
- Explain and discuss with the patient whether the procedure was subtotal or total thyroidectomy.
- Wound/incision care
  - Teach the patient to keep the surgical site clean and dry.
  - Teach methods to conceal the surgical site without affecting healing. Suggest loosely buttoned collars, high-neck blouses, jewelry, or scarves.
  - Explain that the paper strip over the wound will peal off in 7 to 10 days; when the ends curl up, it may be removed.
  - Inform the patient that lotion may soften the healing scar and improve its appearance (if approved by the physician).
- Warning signs: review the signs and symptoms that should be reported to a physician or nurse.
  - General: respiratory distress, bleeding
  - Wound infection: redness, warmth, swelling, persistent drainage from site, purulent exudates
  - Total thyroidectomy: signs and symptoms of hypothyroidism: intolerance to cold; decreased body temperature; dry, rough, or scaly skin; puffy face, hands, and feet; periorbital edema; decreased blood pressure; bradycardia; nonspecific fatigue, weakness; decreased exercise tolerance; weight gain; constipation; anorexia; delayed deep tendon reflexes; muscle aches and joint stiffness; speech changes (slowed, slurred, monotonous); somnolence, lethargy; impaired memory, inattentiveness, slow cognition; loss of initiative; paranoia, depression, agitation; decreased libido; female: decreased or missed menstrual cycles; abdominal distention
  - Parathyroid damage: signs of hypocalcemia: numbness, tingling, twitching, spasm, tetany
- Medications
  - Explain the purpose, dosage, schedule, and route of administration of any prescribed drugs, as well as side effects to report to a physician or nurse.
  - Discuss the importance of not taking over-the-counter medications without checking with a physician or nurse.
  - If the patient has had a total thyroidectomy, explain the importance of taking thyroid replacement medication regularly.
  - If the patient has parathyroid damage, explain the need for calcium supplements.
- Activity
  - Encourage the patient to discuss allowances and limitations with respect to occupation, recreation, and activities.
  - Teach prescribed head and neck exercises: flexion, lateral movement, hyperextension.
  - Teach the importance of a balance between activity and rest.
- Diet
  - Discuss the need to maintain a well-balanced diet.

**FOLLOW-UP CARE**

- Stress the importance of regular follow-up visits to monitor thyroid levels: thyroid-stimulating hormone (TSH), thyroxine ($T_4$). Make sure the patient has the necessary names and telephone numbers.

Modified from Canobbio MM: *Mosby's handbook of patient teaching,* ed 3, St Louis, 2006, pp. 469, 754-755.

wound line that blends with the patient's neck creases and skin lines.

## Evaluation

Evaluation of intraoperative interventions determines effectiveness of positioning aids and pressure-relief devices, drip towels to collect excess prep solutions, and other interventions based on the patient's special needs. The hand-off report to the postanesthesia care unit (PACU) personnel includes the surgical procedure, anesthesia given, location of drain if any, dressing used, condition of skin postoperatively, and any other information specific to the patient's nursing diagnoses. Documentation is according to hospital protocol. It should reflect achievement of patient outcomes related to planned interventions; these should also be included in the hand-off nursing report to PACU personnel. Outcomes identified for the selected nursing diagnoses could be stated as follows:

- The patient maintained normal swallowing.
- The patient maintained normal body temperature.
- The patient verbalized decreased disturbance in feelings related to body image.
- The patient maintained a patent airway; there was no edema or hematoma at the surgical site or signs of respiratory distress.
- The patient maintained adequate gas exchange; $O_2$ saturation remained normal. The patient was extubated without incident.

## Patient and Family Education and Discharge Planning

Patient education and discharge planning should include any family members, significant others, or even friends who will be helping the patient at home. Written discharge instructions should be provided (Box 16-3) and orally reviewed, with clarification of information and correction of misperceptions. The name and telephone number of the physician or nurse to call with questions should be included, as should information regarding a follow-up office appointment (if that is available). General information, such as the name of the thyroid or parathyroid procedure and any changes that will occur as a result of the surgery, should be explained. Included with signs and symptoms to report are those of hypocalcemia (see Box 16-2). If hypocalcemia occurs, it usually manifests itself 1 or 2 days after surgery.[1] The patient should note and report any numbness or tingling around the lips or extremities, twitching, or spasms. Time should also be spent discovering the patient's concerns, anxieties, thoughts, and feelings. Education begins with the perioperative nursing assessment and continues through discharge and perhaps even home care.

# *Surgical Interventions*

## UNILATERAL THYROID LOBECTOMY, SUBTOTAL LOBECTOMY, BILATERAL SUBTOTAL LOBECTOMY, NEAR-TOTAL THYROIDECTOMY, AND TOTAL THYROIDECTOMY

*Unilateral thyroid lobectomy* is removal of one thyroid lobe with division at the isthmus. *Subtotal lobectomy* is a lobectomy that spares the posterior capsule and a portion of the adjacent thyroid tissue. *Bilateral subtotal thyroidectomy* is removal of both lobes of the thyroid in the fashion stated for subtotal thyroidectomy. *Near-total thyroidectomy* is a total lobectomy with contralateral subtotal thyroidectomy. *Total thyroidectomy* is removal of both lobes of the thyroid and attempted removal of all thyroid tissue present. The purpose of the surgical intervention relates to the patient's medical diagnosis. For patients with cancer of the thyroid, total thyroidectomy is the desired surgical treatment[2,14] followed by iodine-131 remnant ablation. Patients are then prescribed thyroid hormone suppression therapy and monitored by physical examination, laboratory studies (serum thyroid function and thyroglobulin levels), and scans.

Graves' disease, the most common cause of hyperthyroidism, is associated with diffuse, bilateral enlargement of the thyroid gland. Surgery is not the first line of treatment for Graves' disease in the United States but is reserved for those patients who fail medical therapy (antithyroid drugs and radioactive iodine) or have a contraindication to medical therapy. Hashimoto's thyroiditis is believed to be an autoimmune disease, and nontender enlargement of the gland occurs. Surgery is performed to relieve tracheal obstruction. Nontoxic nodular goiter does not produce an excess of hormones and is noninflammatory in character; thyroid tissue proliferates in an apparent attempt to produce the minimal hormonal requirement. Surgery may be indicated to relieve tracheal or esophageal obstruction or to rule out a malignant nodule of the thyroid gland. Total thyroidectomy may be done for malignant tumors.

Minimally invasive video-assisted neck surgery (VANS) has been described in the surgical literature, and surgeons have begun to adapt this technology for surgery of the thyroid gland. Figures 16-4 and 16-5 illustrate one technique used in video-assisted MIS performed on the thyroid gland.

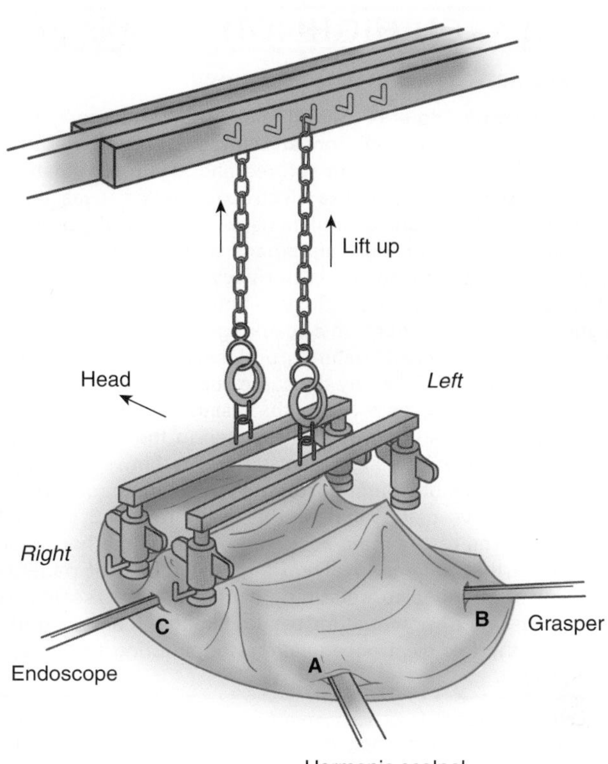


**FIGURE 16-5** Schema of the anterior neck-lift method. The main incision is made depending on tumor size at the chest wall below the clavicle *(A)*. The other two 0.5-cm incisions are made; one is at the same site of the opposite side of the chest wall *(B)*, and the other is at the lateral neck of tumor side *(C)*.

## Procedural Considerations

The patient is positioned supine, as previously described. A drape pack with a fenestrated sheet is required, along with a set of thyroid instruments that is added to the basic instrument set. The electrosurgical unit, dissector sponges, and a small drain (optional) are commonly used. A headlight for the surgeon and assistant may be required. The patient is prepped from the chin to the upper chest, using safety precautions for fire prevention (see Chapter 2 for a discussion of fire prevention strategies in surgical settings). The harmonic scalpel (Research Highlight) or LigaSure Precise may also be utilized.

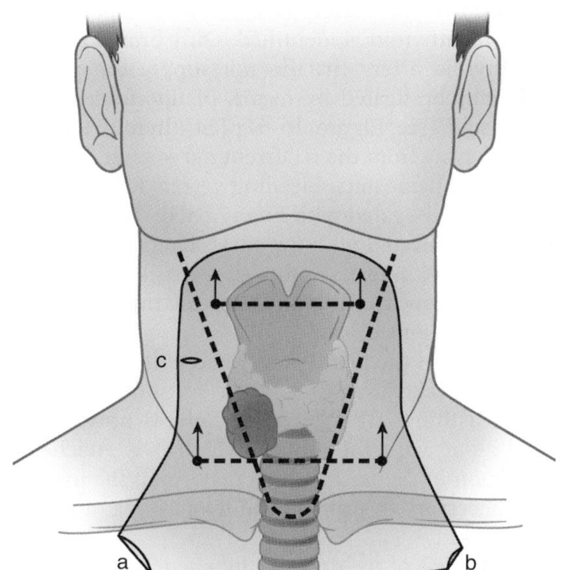


**FIGURE 16-4** The schema of the anterior neck area. Two horizontally inserted pieces of Kirschner wire are indicated by dotted lines and are lifted up, as indicated by arrows. The layer under the platysma is indicated by oblique lines.

## Operative Procedure

Figure 16-6 provides an overview of safe thyroidectomy principles.

1. A transverse incision (slightly curved and symmetric) parallel to the normal skin lines of the neck (skin crease) is made through the skin and first layer of the cervical fascia and platysma muscle, approximately 2 cm above the sternoclavicular junction.
2. An upper skin flap is undermined to the level of the thyroid notch of the thyroid cartilage; double skin hooks are placed on the dermis and retracted anteriorly and superiorly to facilitate dissection. A lower flap is then undermined to the sternoclavicular joint. A knife, fine curved scissors, tissue forceps, and gauze sponges are used to undermine the flaps. Bleeding vessels are clamped with hemostats and ligated with fine nonabsorbable sutures. Lateral retraction with a vein retractor or Army-Navy retractor helps identify the plane for dissection.
3. Flaps may be held away from the wound with stay sutures inserted through the cervical fascia and platysma muscle or by one of the various self-retaining retractors.

## RESEARCH HIGHLIGHT

### Ultrasonic Scalpel in Thyroidectomy

Thyroidectomy requires careful dissection and meticulous hemostasis to protect adjacent structures. Common methods of achieving hemostasis are sutures and electrocoagulation. The harmonic scalpel, unlike electrocoagulation, uses ultrasonic energy to cut and coagulate tissue, theoretically producing less potential for thermal damage to adjacent tissue and structures. The purpose of this study was to evaluate this and other potential advantages. Sixty patients were randomly assigned to either the harmonic scalpel group (study group) or electrocoagulation and ligature group (control group). All procedures were performed by the same surgeon.

Outcome measures revealed that using the harmonic scalpel reduced operating time and resulted in the use of fewer sutures. There was no significant difference between groups in intraoperative bleeding, postoperative bleeding, or reports of postoperative pain. Whereas this study revealed reduced operating time as the main advantage of using the harmonic scalpel, further studies involving larger numbers of patients were recommended to determine if the harmonic scalpel is safer, in terms of potential for tissue damage, than the traditional method of electrocoagulation and suturing to achieve hemostasis.

Modified from Allen G: Evidence for practice: ultrasonic scalpel use versus electrocoagulation in thyroidectomy, *AORN Journal* 82(1):117-118, 2005.

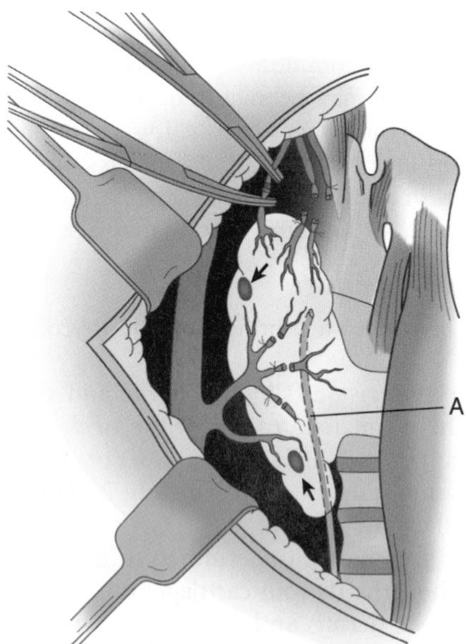


**FIGURE 16-6** Safe thyroid principles emphasize the following: division of all branch vessels on the capsule of the thyroid with fine mosquito hemostats to prevent injury to the superior laryngeal nerve in detaching the superior thyroid artery and to prevent injury to the parathyroid glands in detaching the inferior thyroid artery; mobilization of parathyroid glands by medial-to-lateral dissection *(arrows)* to preserve their vascular pedicle; constant awareness of the location of the recurrent laryngeal nerve *(A)*, especially near its penetration into the larynx.

4. The fascia in the midline is incised between the strap (sternohyoid and sternothyroid) muscles with a knife. The sternocleidomastoid muscle may be retracted with a loop retractor. Ordinarily it is not necessary to divide the strap muscles; however, the strap muscles may be divided between clamps should additional exposure be required, such as with a very large gland, using Mastin muscle clamps, Kocher clamps, or hemostats and a knife. The divided muscles are retracted from the operative site with retractors, thereby exposing the diseased lobe.
5. The inferior and middle thyroid veins are clamped, divided with Metzenbaum scissors, and ligated with fine nonabsorbable sutures.
6. The lobe is rotated medially, and loose areolar tissue is divided posteriorly and medially toward the tracheoesophageal sulcus with hemostats and Metzenbaum scissors. Small sponges are used for blunt dissection. Bleeding is controlled by hemostats and ligatures, as well as by electrosurgery; the bipolar electrosurgical unit (ESU) may be used. The recurrent laryngeal nerve, which enters the cricothyroid muscle at the level of the cricoid cartilage, is identified and carefully preserved. Electrocoagulation should not be used in the vicinity of the recurrent or superior laryngeal nerve because the spread of the current could damage the nerve. Nerve integrity monitoring systems (NIMSs) are helpful in identifying the branches of the laryngeal nerve.
7. The thyroid lobe is pulled downward, a Lahey goiter or polar retractor is inserted as necessary, and the avascular tissue between the trachea and upper pole of the thyroid is dissected by means of Metzenbaum scissors.
8. The superior thyroid artery is secured with two or three curved hemostats or right-angle clamps; the artery is ligated, divided, and then transfixed with nonabsorbable sutures. Care is taken here to not injure the superior laryngeal nerve. The upper parathyroid gland is often identified at this time.
9. The inferior thyroid artery is identified and preserved. The inferior parathyroid is identified. Only branches of the inferior thyroid artery that do not supply the parathyroid glands may be ligated by means of fine forceps, sutures, and scissors (see Figure 16-6). The thyroid lobe is then dissected away from the recurrent nerve with Metzenbaum scissors and hemostats. Bleeding vessels are clamped with hemostats and ligated with fine nonabsorbable sutures.
10. The lobe is elevated with Babcock clamps; it is freed from the trachea with fine scissors, forceps, knife, and hemostats. The fibrous bands attached to the trachea and cricoid cartilage are divided.
11. The isthmus of the gland is elevated with fine forceps and divided between hemostats with scissors, removing the lobe and isthmus. If a pyramidal lobe is present, it is removed along with the lobe to which it is attached to its termination in the neck, which may reach the hyoid bone. If it is necessary to transect the hyoid bone, a small bone cutter is used.
12. The cut surface of the opposite lobe requires careful hemostasis. Interrupted sutures may be used for this purpose, as well as to reapproximate it to the pretracheal fascia.
13. The strap muscles, if severed, are reapproximated with fine interrupted absorbable or nonabsorbable sutures. If neces-

sary, a drain may be inserted into the thyroid bed and brought out through the midline. Some surgeons prefer to drain the wound laterally through the sternocleidomastoid muscle and the lateral extremity of the incision in the belief that this produces better healing and cosmetic results.
14. The edges of the platysma muscle are reapproximated. The skin edges are then reapproximated with subcuticular fine absorbable sutures.
15. Wound closure tapes (e.g., Steri-Strips) are applied to the wound edges, and gauze dressings, if required, are placed on the wound with minimal tape.

## SUBSTERNAL OR INTRATHORACIC THYROIDECTOMY

Extensions of enlarging goiters into the substernal and intrathoracic regions may occur. They may cause tracheal and esophageal obstruction, in which case they are usually excised surgically. Longer instruments are sometimes required. Splitting the sternum is rarely necessary because access to the substernal part of the gland is usually satisfactory through the standard collar incision used in thyroid surgery.[8]

## THYROGLOSSAL DUCT CYSTECTOMY

The thyroglossal duct cyst is the most common congenital cyst found in the neck. Although a thyroglossal duct cyst may be found in patients of any age, 50% usually occur before 20 years of age and about 70% are seen by 30 years of age. The thyroglossal duct is an embryonic structure arising from the descent of the thyroid gland into the anterior portion of the neck. When present in an adult, it exists as a pretracheal cystic pouch attached to the hyoid bone, with or without a sinus tract to the base of the tongue at the foramen cecum (Figure 16-7). Thyroglossal duct cystectomy requires complete excision of the cyst in continuity with its tract, the central portion of the hyoid bone, and the tissue above the hyoid bone extending to the base of the tongue[17] to avoid recurrent cystic formation and to prevent infections.

### Procedural Considerations

The perioperative nursing assessment should be appropriate to the patient's age because the patient is frequently a child or teenager (see Chapter 29 for a detailed discussion of the younger patient's needs). Reassurance and information regarding the procedure should be given. The patient is positioned supine, with the neck supported in extension. Bone instruments will be needed in addition to the basic instrument set.

### Operative Procedure

1. After the head is extended and the chin is elevated, a transverse incision is made between the hyoid bone and the thyroid cartilage through the subcutaneous tissue.
2. The platysma muscle is incised, and the flaps are raised as described for thyroidectomy.
3. The strap (sternohyoid and sternothyroid) muscles are separated in the midline.
4. Sharp dissection and blunt dissection are used to mobilize the cyst and duct, up to the attachment to the hyoid bone. The hyoid bone is transected twice, removing the center section with bone-cutting forceps, and the segment of bone and cyst is freed from adjacent structures.
5. The duct is traced superiorly through or near the hyoid up to the musculature of the tongue and removed completely.

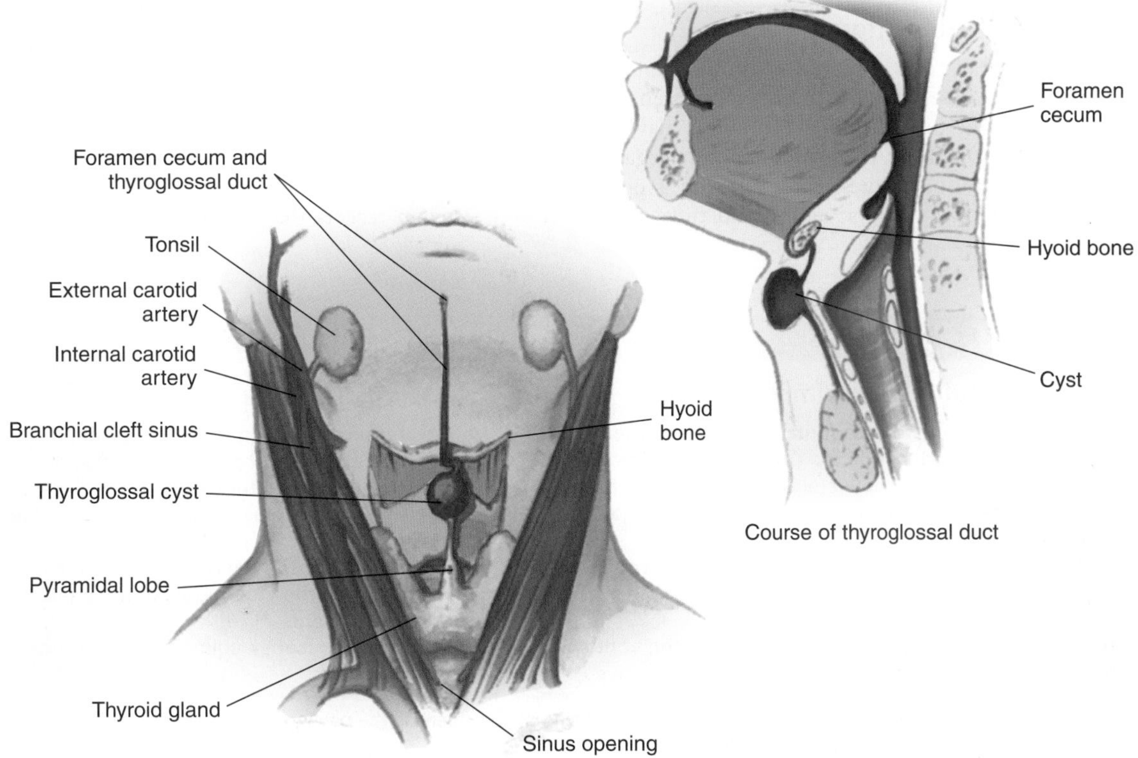


**FIGURE 16-7** Thyroglossal cyst showing both anterior and lateral views.

(Methylene blue dye injection is used occasionally to visualize the whole tract.)

6. The cyst is removed. The strap muscles are closed with interrupted fine nonabsorbable sutures. A drain may be placed. The skin is closed with subcuticular fine absorbable sutures.

## PARATHYROIDECTOMY

Parathyroidectomy is excision of one or more parathyroid glands. Normal or atrophic glands are generally not removed. The presence of adenomas (hypersecreting neoplasms), hyperplasia, or carcinomas requires surgical excision. For carcinomas, resection of the ipsilateral thyroid lobe and lymph nodes is essential, although metastasis may also occur by way of the bloodstream. Any residual parathyroid cancer may secrete parathormone, causing hypercalcemia and its attendant problems.

The gold standard for parathyroidectomy remains a bilateral neck exploration with biopsy of all four glands to confirm the presence of adenoma or hyperplasia. Often, the diagnosis of an adenoma can be made by gross inspection of the glands by the surgeon but is confirmed histologically by the pathologist.

A variety of minimally invasive techniques have evolved over the last decade. The most popular technique is the focused or minimally open approach. A localization study with sestamibi scan or ultrasound is required to identify the offending adenoma. A small 2-cm incision is made in the neck based on the localization studies. Blood samples are drawn before, during, and after the operation to measure parathyroid hormone levels to confirm an appropriate decrease in levels after the adenoma is removed. This minimally invasive technique cannot be used for hyperplasia. Hyperplasia requires removal of three and one half glands through a bilateral neck exploration.

### Procedural Considerations

During the bilateral neck exploration multiple biopsies are often performed to determine the presence or absence of parathyroid tissue. Numerous specimen containers may be necessary (Patient Safety). Check with the surgeon in regard to any preoperative localization studies. If the surgeon is performing a focused parathyroidectomy, several blood tubes will be required to measure parathyroid levels intraoperatively. Have mediastinotomy instruments available if necessary (see Chapter 25). The patient is positioned, prepped, and draped as described for thyroidectomy. Hemoclips should be available. Some surgeons may perform this procedure using a minimally invasive approach with intraoperative parathyroid hormone assays to determine if the gland removed was the cause of hypersecretion.[9] Instrumentation and accessory equipment will then be required.

### Operative Procedure

See the discussion of the approach to the thyroid gland on p. 561.

Classically, with the thyroid gland visible, bilateral neck exploration of the "normal" locations of the four parathyroid glands is conducted. Meticulous hemostasis by means of mosquito hemostats and fine ligatures is a prerequisite to location and identification of these small glands.

The thyroid gland is gently rotated anteriorly to provide access to the posterior thyroid sulcus, where the parathyroid glands are almost always found. Identification of the parathyroid vascular pedicle as it leaves either the superior thyroid artery or inferior thyroid artery is a means of locating both the inferior and superior glands. Metzenbaum scissors, mosquito hemostats, and gauze dissector (Kittner or peanut) sponges are used in the dissection.

Attention is directed toward the posterior lateral surface of the thyroid lobe or just beneath the lower thyroid pole, where the lower parathyroid glands are frequently found. Finding the vascular pedicle from the inferior thyroid artery may aid in identification (Figure 16-8). Occasionally the lower pair is found in the thymic capsule or tissue, in which case a portion of the thymus is resected. A mediastinotomy is indicated for only a small percentage of patients. Thoracoscopy (see Chapter 25) is also a successful minimally invasive technique that may be used to remove parathyroid tumors situated deep in the mediastinum.

If one of the parathyroid glands shows evidence of disease, an effort is made to find other glands on the same side to ensure that they are free of disease. When found, biopsy of these glands is performed, using a marker such as a hemoclip. The surgeon resects the diseased gland by clamping the vascular

#### PATIENT SAFETY

**Handling Multiple Specimens**

The perioperative nurse has accountability for specimen collection, identification, and handling. During parathyroidectomy, multiple specimens may be collected. To accurately identify and safely manage these specimens, the perioperative nurse should do the following:

- Verify specimen collection and handling needs with the surgeon. This should occur before the procedure start and may be part of the time out.
- Have available an adequate number of specimen containers, labels, laboratory forms, and appropriate preservative.
- Communicate with the pathology department the nature of the procedure and anticipated specimens. Plan for direct communication methods about specimens between the surgeon and pathologist or plan for a read-back or repeat-back of findings with the pathologist.
- Use Standard Transmission-Based Precautions.
- Arrange for timely transport of the specimens to the pathology department.
- Document specimen collection according to institutional protocol.

Modified from AORN recommended practices for the care and handling of specimens in the perioperative environment. In *AORN standards, guidelines, and recommended practices,* Denver, 2006, The Association.

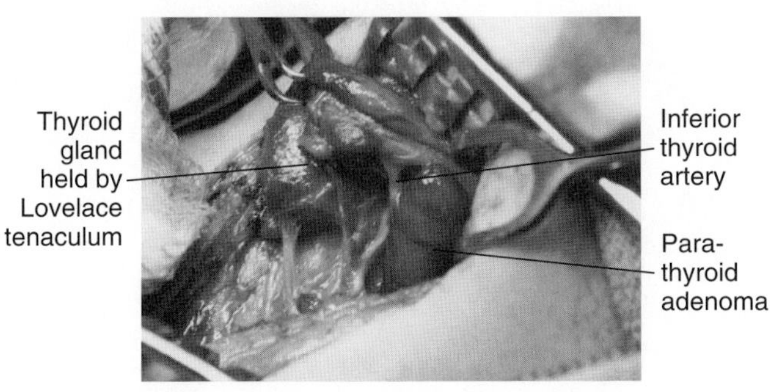


**FIGURE 16-8** Left lower parathyroid adenoma. Note the relationship between the adenoma and the inferior thyroid artery.

pedicle with mosquito hemostats, dividing with small scissors or knife, and ligating with a fine nonabsorbable suture. The question of how much parathyroid tissue to remove is controversial and relates to whether single or multiple glands are involved, regardless of their size and appearance. One gland must remain to prevent hypocalcemia and its complications. A current concept or alternative for multiple gland involvement is to excise all four glands, transplanting a portion of one in an accessible site, such as the neck or forearm, for later removal if hypercalcemia recurs. This eliminates reexploration and potential injury to the recurrent laryngeal nerve.

The neck region is explored for aberrant parathyroid tissue, which is also resected (see Figure 16-2, *B*).

The remainder of the operation is the same as that described for the thyroid gland.

## REFERENCES

1. Bellantone R and others: Is routine supplemental therapy (calcium and vitamin D) useful after total thyroidectomy? *Surgery* 132: 1109-1113, 2002.
2. Burman KD: Advances in thyroid cancer treatment, *Medscape Diabetes & Endocrinology* 7(1), 2005. Accessed January 5, 2005, online: www.medscape.com.
3. Canobbio MM: *Mosby's handbook of patient teaching,* ed 3, St Louis, 2006, Mosby.
4. Efron G: Thyroid cancer. In Cameron JL, editor: *Current surgical therapy,* ed 7, St Louis, 2001, Mosby.
5. Elberling TV and others: Impaired health-related quality of life in Graves' disease: a prospective study, *European Journal of Endocrinology* 151:549-555, 2004.
6. Frost L and others: Hyperthyroidism and risk of atrial fibrillation or flutter: a population-based study, *Archives of Internal Medicine* 164:1675-1678, 2004.
7. Gauger PG, Doherty GM: Parathyroid gland. In Townsend CM, editor: *Sabiston textbook of surgery,* ed 17, Philadelphia, 2004, Saunders.
8. Hedayati N, McHenry CR: The clinical presentation and operative management of nodular and diffuse substernal thyroid disease, *The American Surgeon* 68:245-251, 2002.
9. Howe JR: Minimally invasive parathyroid surgery, *Surgical Clinics of North America* 80(5):1399-1426, 2000.
10. Jarvis C: *Physical examination and health assessment,* ed 4, Philadelphia, 2004, Saunders.
11. Kukora JS and others: Thyroid nodule. In Cameron JL, editor: *Current surgical therapy,* ed 7, St Louis, 2001, Mosby.
12. Mercado G and others: Hypothyroidism: a frequent event after radiotherapy and after radiotherapy with chemotherapy for patients with head and neck cancer, *Cancer* 92:2892-2897, 2001.
13. Pagana KD, Pagana TJ: *Mosby's diagnostic and laboratory test reference,* ed 7, St Louis, 2005, Mosby.
14. Sarkar SD, Savitch I: Management of thyroid cancer, *Applied Radiology* 33(11):34-45, 2004.
15. *Thyroid nodules.* American Thyroid Association, 2005. Accessed December 13, 2005, on-line: www.thyroid.org.
16. Udelsman R and others: One hundred consecutive minimally invasive parathyroid explorations, *Annals of Surgery* 232(3):331-339, 2000.
17. Warner BW: Pediatric surgery. In Townsend CM, editor: *Sabiston textbook of surgery,* ed 17, Philadelphia, 2004, Saunders.

CHAPTER 17

# Breast Surgery

JANE C. ROTHROCK

Most surgical procedures on the breast are performed to establish a definitive diagnosis or to treat breast cancer. Changing hormone levels from puberty throughout the remainder of life affect breast tissue in its physical and microscopic characteristics. In association with these changes, numerous aberrations and tumors can occur.

The possibility of and actual occurrence of breast changes, either benign or malignant, are some of the most emotionally upsetting health problems confronting women. Breast cancer is the most common cancer in women, accounting for nearly one of every three cancers diagnosed. The probability of developing breast cancer increases with age. Estimates predict that one in eight women in the United States will develop breast cancer during her life. If the cancer is detected early, there is a 97% 5-year survival rate. Breast cancer risk is increased if a woman's mother, sister, or daughter has had breast cancer, especially if the cancer developed before menopause. An early menarche before 12 years of age and a late natural menopause after 50 years of age are associated with a slight increased risk for developing breast cancer. Further, a woman who has had cancer in one breast is at increased risk for another cancer in the other breast.[17] Heightened public awareness, an increased number of women practicing self-examination, and the early detection of breast masses by mammography have started to slow the annual increase in breast cancer mortality.

Reconstructive surgery of the breast is discussed in Chapter 24.

## Surgical Anatomy

The breasts are bilateral mammary glands that lie on the pectoralis major fascia of the anterior chest wall. They are surrounded by a layer of fat and are encased in an envelope of skin. The breasts extend from the second to the sixth rib and horizontally from the lateral edge of the sternum to the anterior axillary line. The largest part of the mammary gland rests on the connective tissue of the pectoralis major muscle and laterally on the serratus anterior (upper outer quadrant of the breast), with a normal globular contour occurring as a result of the fascial support (Cooper ligaments). An elongation of mammary tissue normally extends laterally on the pectoralis major toward the axilla and is known as the *tail of Spence* (Figure 17-1).

Each breast is made up of 12 to 20 glandular lobes that are separated by connective tissue. Each lobe drains by a single lactiferous duct that opens on the nipple. The nipple, located at about the fourth intercostal space, forms a conical projection into which the ducts open independently of each other on the surface. A pigmented circular area called the *areola* surrounds the nipple. Smooth muscle fibers of the areola contract to allow for nipple projection.

Three major arterial systems (Figure 17-2) generously supply the mammary glands with blood. The main sources are branches of the internal mammary and the lateral branches of the anterior aortic intercostal arteries, all of which form an extensive network of anastomoses over the breast. A third source is the pectoral branch, deriving from a branch of the axillary artery. The veins that mainly drain the breasts follow the course of the arteries. The superficial veins frequently become dilated during pregnancy.

The lymph drainage system generally follows the course of the vessels. The lymphatics drain into two main areas represented by the axillary nodes and the internal thoracic chain of nodes (Figure 17-3). The internal thoracic nodes are few but are responsible for most of the lymph drainage from the inner half of the breast. Thus one can see how the lymph system could be a channel for the spread of malignant disease from the breast to associated areas of the chest wall or to the axilla.

The sensory nerve supply is mainly from the anterior cutaneous branches of the upper intercostal nerves, the third and fourth branches of the cervical plexus, and the lateral cutaneous branches of the intercostal nerves.

Occasionally, developmental errors of the breast occur. Additional nipples or extramammary tissue in the axilla or over the upper abdomen may be present. The preferred treatment of these supernumerary structures is excision. Absence of one or both nipples may also occur and may be associated with absence of the underlying pectoral muscle and chest wall. The mammary glands are affected by three types of physiologic changes: (1) those related to growth and development, (2) those related to the menstrual cycle, and (3) those related to pregnancy and lactation. The mammary glands are present at birth in both males and females. Hormonal stimulation, however, produces the development and function of these glands in females. Estrogen promotes growth of the ductal structures, whereas progesterone promotes lobular development.

### BENIGN LESIONS OF THE BREAST

A fibroadenoma, affecting primarily women younger than 30 years, is usually a solitary nodule (Table 17-1). These masses are small, painless lesions that are well delineated and relatively mobile. They are solid and round, grow very slowly, and are discovered generally by accident.

*Fibrocystic change in the breast* is an all-encompassing term used to describe many different breast changes. This descriptive

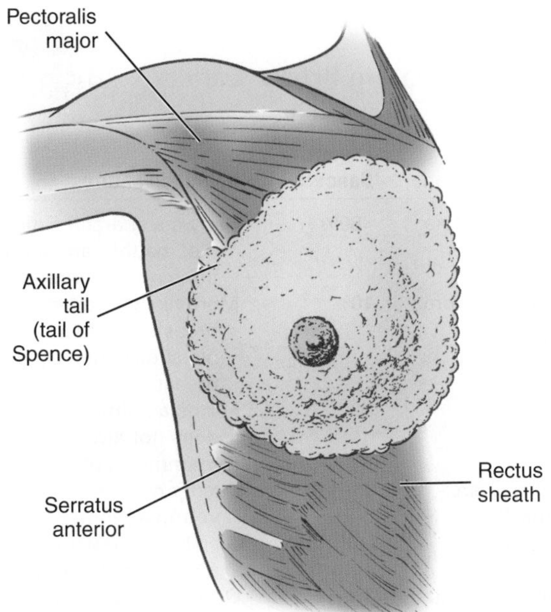


FIGURE 17-1 Normal distribution of mammary tissue of adult female breast.

term should be discouraged and the more specific diagnosis used. Examples of benign lesions that are generally considered in this category are multiple lesions of fibrous disease, intraductal papillomas, cysts, and solid masses. These changes affect almost all women at some time in their lives. Frequently pain is present, which calls attention to the problem. Pain, fluctuations in size, and multiple lesions are common features that help differentiate these generally benign lesions from cancer.

Nipple discharge is more commonly associated with benign lesions than with cancer. A postmenopausal woman who has some duct ectasia or who has borne children can manually produce nipple discharge. Discharge is usually significant only if it is spontaneous and persistent. Chronic unilateral nipple discharge, especially if bloody, should prompt an investigation for occult carcinoma.

## BREAST CANCER

Breast cancer affects primarily women, although it can occur in the mammary gland of men. Until it can be prevented, early detection is the greatest hope for cure. All women should practice monthly self-examination to detect palpable lesions, and they should immediately report any changes or masses to a physician. External physical changes, such as dimpling of the skin, can also indicate the presence of a benign or malignant pathologic process. The older the patient, the more likely it is that a mass is malignant. The most common form of breast cancer is infiltrating ductal carcinoma (Table 17-2).

The cause of breast cancer is still unknown. Many factors, including environmental, dietary,[18] and familial influences, have been suggested as contributors to its development (Table 17-3). The previously held belief that breast cancer spreads by direct extension from the initial site in the breast to adjacent lymph nodes may not always be correct. Breast cancer may be

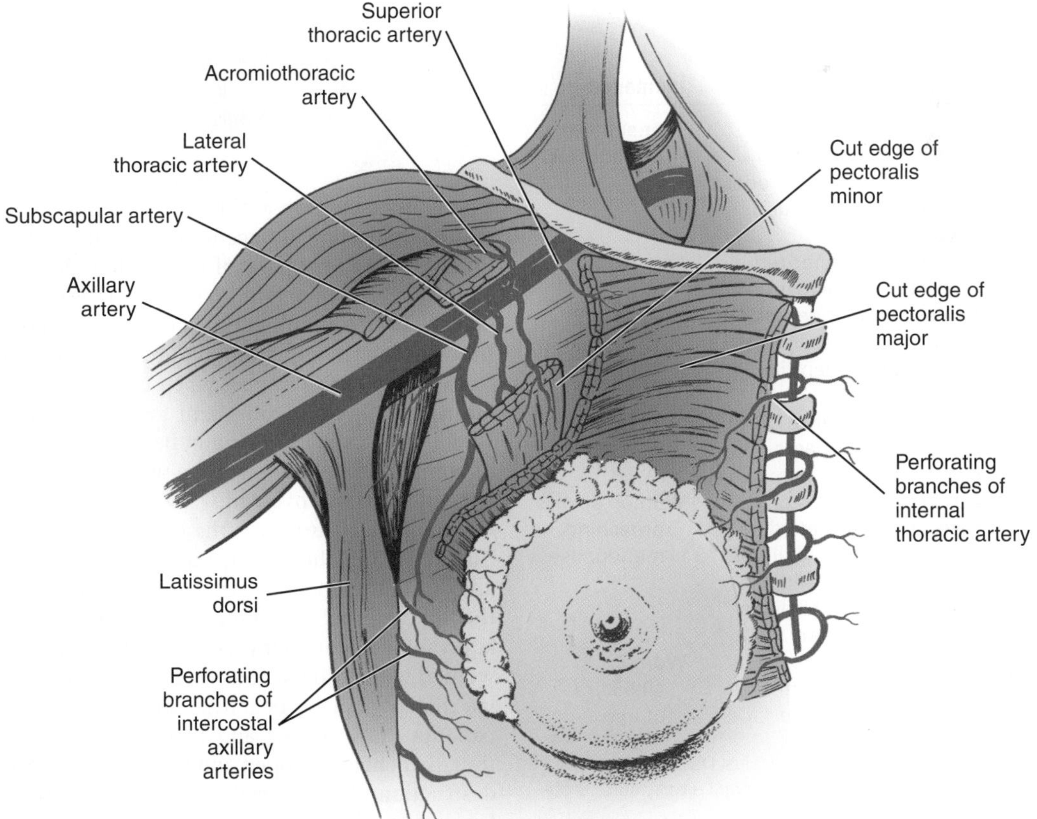


FIGURE 17-2 Normal arterial blood supply of the breast.

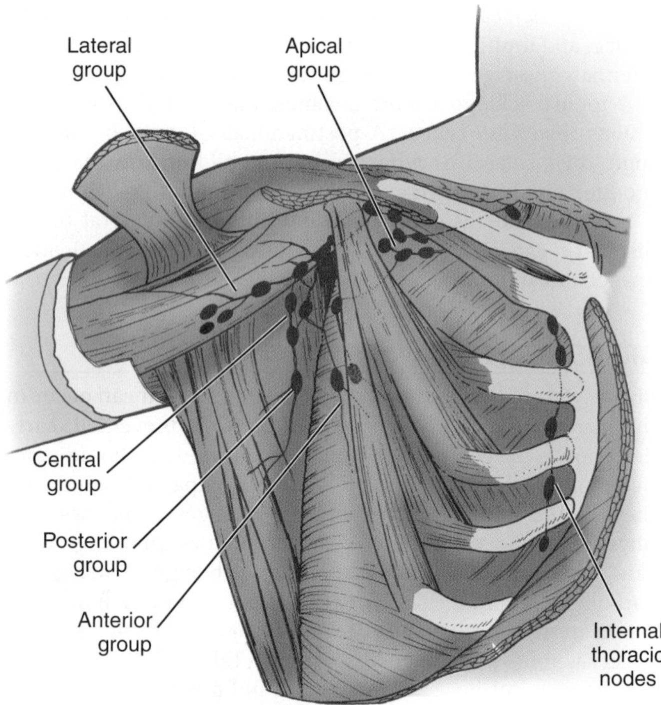


FIGURE 17-3 Distribution of axillary and thoracic lymph nodes.

**TABLE 17-1**

## Typical Presentation of Benign Breast Disorders

| Breast Disorder | Description | Incidence |
|---|---|---|
| Fibroadenoma | Most common benign lesion; solid mass of connective tissue that is unattached to the surrounding tissue | Teenage years into the 30s |
| Fibrocystic breast disease (FBD) | *First stage:* characterized by premenstrual bilateral fullness and tenderness<br>*Second stage:* presence of bilateral, multicentric nodules<br>*Third stage:* presence of microscopic and macroscopic cysts | Late teens and 20s |
| Ductal ectasia | Hard, irregular mass or masses with nipple discharge, enlarged axillary nodes, redness, and edema; difficult to distinguish from cancer | Women approaching menopause |
| Intraductal ectasia | Mass in duct that results in nipple discharge; mass is usually not palpable | Women 40-55 yr of age |

Data from National Cancer Institute. In Ignatavicius DD, Workman ML: *Medical-surgical nursing: critical thinking for collaborative care*, ed 5, Philadelphia, 2006, Saunders.

**TABLE 17-2**

## Types of Invasive Breast Cancer

| Breast Cancer Type | Percent of Breast Cancers | Specific Features |
|---|---|---|
| Ductal carcinoma | ≈80% | Shows a characteristic "spicule" pattern and calcifications on mammography |
| Lobular carcinoma | 10% | More likely to affect both breasts and to have multiple sites within each breast<br>Forms a palpable lump but does not always show on mammography |
| Medullary carcinoma | 1%-5% | Occurs more frequently in younger women, especially those who are *BRCA1* or *BRCA2* positive |
| Colloid (mucinous) carcinoma | 1%-6% | Occurs more frequently in older women<br>Soft and slow-growing, may be hard to distinguish from cysts or benign breast disease on palpation or mammography<br>Good prognosis |
| Inflammatory carcinoma | >1% | Rapidly growing, often with metastasis present at diagnosis<br>First manifestations are breast skin edema and redness |

Data from Cotran R and others: *Robbins pathologic basis of disease*, ed 6, Philadelphia, 1999, Saunders. In Ignatavicius DD, Workman ML: *Medical-surgical nursing: critical thinking for collaborative care*, ed 5, Philadelphia, 2006, Saunders.

a systemic condition at the time of diagnosis. Distant metastases may have already occurred without adjacent lymph node involvement at the time of its palpable detection. This theory could explain why radical breast surgery of the past, which involved removal of the affected breast and all axillary and thoracic lymph nodes, did not greatly lower mortality. Survival from breast cancer is best when detected early, reducing axillary lymph node involvement and improving long-term survival. Tumor size can usually be correlated with involvement of lymph nodes. The larger the tumor, the more likely it is that lymph nodes are involved.

Less radical surgery is the treatment of choice today. Surgical excision of the tumor, the use of radiation therapy alone, and a combination of surgery, chemotherapy, and radiation therapy have become the recommended treatment. The use of adjuvant chemotherapy is recommended for premenopausal women with axillary-node metastasis. Studies show that similar therapy can be beneficial in node-negative breast cancer patients. New studies and new therapeutic options are continually being developed and tested. Laser treatment for in situ destruction of tumor cells may someday replace lumpectomy. Clinical trials using accelerated partial breast irradiation

**TABLE 17-3**

## Risk Factors for Breast Cancer

| Factor | Degree of Risk | Comments |
|---|---|---|
| Female gender | Increased | Ninety-nine percent of all breast cancers occur in women. |
| History of a previous breast cancer | Increased | The risk of developing a cancer in the opposite breast is five times greater than for the average population at risk. |
| Age >40 yr | Increased | Incidence increases with age and peaks in the fifth decade. |
| Menstrual history (early menstruation, late menopause, or both) | Increased | The risk of breast cancer rises as the interval between menarche and menopause increases. Women who undergo bilateral oophorectomy before age 35 yr have only 40% of the risk of breast cancer compared with women who undergo natural menopause. |
| Reproductive history (nulliparity or first child born after age 30 yr) | Increased | Childless women have an increased risk, as do women who bear their first child near or after age 30 yr. |
| Family history (mother, sister, or both) | Increased | Risk increases three or more times if the mother or a sister has had breast cancer and is further increased if the relative was younger than 40 yr of age, if the cancer was bilateral, or if the relative also developed ovarian cancer. |
| Diet | Controversial | Animal data and descriptive epidemiology of breast cancer incidence strongly suggest an association of dietary factors, specifically a high-fat diet, with an increased risk of breast cancer. The association is stronger if the patient is also obese. |
| Alcohol | Unknown | A suggested small increase in risk with moderate alcohol consumption has been reported, although limitations in methodology have been cited and results require confirmation. |
| Obesity | Controversial | Weight, obesity (especially increased abdominal fat), increased body mass, insulin resistance, and hyperglycemia have been reported to be associated with an increased risk for breast cancer. |
| Ionizing radiation | Increased | Women who received frequent low-level radiation exposure to the thorax demonstrated an increased risk, especially if the exposure occurred during periods of rapid breast formation. |
| Benign breast disease | None | Fibrocystic breast disease is not associated with breast cancer. However, biopsy-proven atypical hyperplasia is associated with an increased risk. |
| Oral contraceptives | None | There is no evidence that suggests a causal relationship between oral contraceptives and the incidence of and survival from breast cancer. |
| Exogenous (external) hormones | Controversial | Several studies report no link with replacement hormones and breast cancer, and those studies that do show a link appear to identify only subsets of patients at risk: those who have taken replacement estrogens for more than 5 yr and those who have taken large cumulative doses. |

Modified from McPherson CM and others: ABC of breast disease: breast cancer—epidemiology, risk factors, and genetics, *BMJ* 321(9):624-628, 2000. In Ignatavicius DD, Workman ML: *Medical-surgical nursing: critical thinking for collaborative care*, ed 5, Philadelphia, 2006, Saunders.

(APBI), in which only the tumor site and not the entire breast are radiated, may reduce radiation treatment therapies from the traditional 6-week treatment period to one of 5 to 10 days.[24] Minimally invasive cryoablation technology for freezing and destroying benign breast tumors was approved by the U.S. Food and Drug Administration (FDA) in 2001.[10] Investigation has also begun using magnetic resonance imaging (MRI)–guided ultrasound (focused ultrasound therapy) as another alternative for breast cancer surgery. The perioperative nurse should refer to the Evolve website for ongoing updates regarding treatment modalities and their success rates.

## SCREENING TECHNOLOGIES

Imaging methodologies, such as mammography and ultrasonography, have helped in the detection of breast masses too small for clinical detection.[3] The American Cancer Society recommends a clinical breast exam by a physician every 3 years for women aged 20 to 39 years and a clinical breast exam and a mammogram every year for women 40 years and older (Table 17-4). There is a lack of agreement regarding the value of annual screening mammograms in women younger than 40 years without the evidence of definite risk factors or family history of breast or ovarian cancer, which may suggest hereditary carcinoma syndrome.[13]

The most common screening mechanism for occult and palpable lesions is x-ray (film-screen) mammography (Figure 17-4). In mammography the entire breast is visualized when x-ray beams are directed in several planes through the breast. Mammograms can detect abnormal-appearing densities, irregular or spiculated margins, microcalcifications, and clusters of calcium deposits that are clinically nonpalpable. These masses may be only 3 to 10 mm in diameter. Often, previous mammograms are used for comparison. The increasingly wide-

**TABLE 17-4**

**American Cancer Society Breast Cancer Screening Guidelines for Asymptomatic Women***

| Age | Screening Activity |
|---|---|
| 20-39 yr | Breast self-examination (BSE) monthly<br>Clinical breast examination (CBE) every 3 yr |
| 40 yr and older | BSE monthly<br>CBE annually<br>Screening mammography (two views of each breast) annually |

Data from American Cancer Society: *Cancer prevention and early detection. Facts and figures—2003.* Report no. 8600.03, Atlanta, 2003, American Cancer Society. In Ignatavicius DN, Workman ML: *Medical-surgical nursing: critical thinking for collaborative care*, ed 5, Philadelphia, 2006, Saunders.

*Asymptomatic women who are identified to be at higher risk need to have an individualized screening plan that may differ from these guidelines.

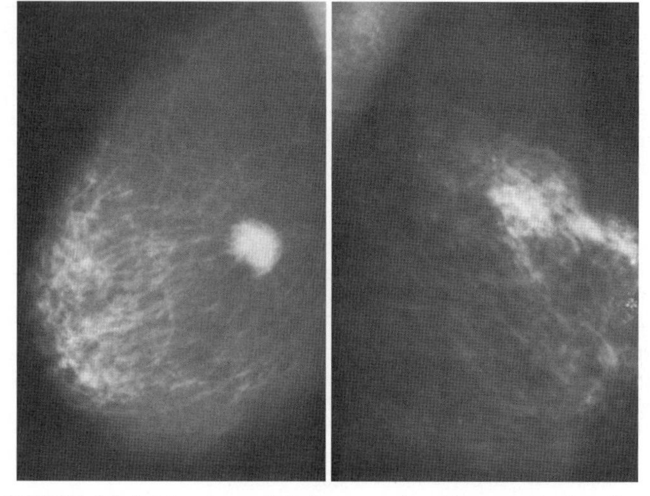


FIGURE 17-4 Mammographic features of malignancy. **A,** A stellate mass. The combination of a density, surrounding spicules, and distortion of the breast architecture strongly suggests a malignancy in this mammogram. **B,** Clustered microcalcifications. Fine, irregular, and branching forms suggest malignancy in this mammogram. Fine calcifications, less than 0.5 mm in size, are more often associated with cancer than are larger, coarse calcifications.

spread use of mammography has led to identification of more nonpalpable breast masses, and 15% to 30% of such lesions prove to be malignant.[16] The accuracy of mammography depends on careful x-ray technique and breast size, structure, and density. Radiation dosage varies with individuals and techniques. As a result of improvement in radiologic techniques, the radiation exposure in a mammogram is very low. The benefits of this screening mechanism far outweigh the minute risks of radiation exposure. Advances in computer-assisted detection (CAD) allow the computer to analyze the mammogram, placing asterisks and triangles on small potential problem areas, which are then reviewed by a radiologist.

In some instances, such as when the lesion is too small to palpate, mammograms are done immediately before surgery. The lesion, previously detected by mammogram, is localized by the insertion of a needle or needles or a wire within a needle. The wire is placed within the suspect area, and the distal end is left on the outside of the skin. The needle may be left in place or removed after insertion of the wire (Figure 17-5). Once the suspect area is identified by the wire localization, the needle or wire is taped in place and the patient is sent to the operating room for surgical biopsy. Wire localization and surgical biopsy occur on the same day. After the biopsy, the specimen is sent to the radiology department for mammography validation of the correct surgical excision of the questionable breast tissue before the pathology examination.

Digital mammography takes an electronic image of the breast and stores it directly in a computer. Digital mammography uses less radiation than film mammography and allows improvement in image storage and transmission because images can be stored and sent electronically. Radiologists also can use software to help interpret digital mammograms. One of the obstacles to greater use of digital mammography is its cost, with digital systems currently costing approximately 1.5 to 4 times more than film systems. Digital screening mammograms are more accurate than film-screening mammograms, with a 70% detection rate compared with film screens at 55%. The groups of woman most likely to benefit from digital screening include women younger than 50 years, with dense breast tissue, and who are premenopausal and perimenopausal.[9,23]

Ultrasonography differentiates between solid and cystic lesions (History box). As a screening methodology, its sensitivity and specificity are less definitive than mammography is. This technique can be useful with dense or dysplastic breasts and in pregnant or lactating women. However, a method that uses the patient's own clotted blood, which is injected near nonpalpable breast abnormalities identified on MRI, allows ultrasonic-guided biopsy. MRI is another technique used as an adjunct to mammography in the detection of breast lesions. Breast MRI can image dense breast tissue, which shows poorly with conventional mammography. In addition, scar tissue does not obscure visualization of tissue as it may with conventional mammography.

Molecular breast imaging (MBI) involves the injection of short-lived radiotracer, which is taken in by breast tissue and preferentially by breast tumors. A gamma camera is used to pick up the isotope signal and image the breast. In a small initial trial, the MBI was highly accurate in identifying lesions previously confirmed by mammography and ultrasound as

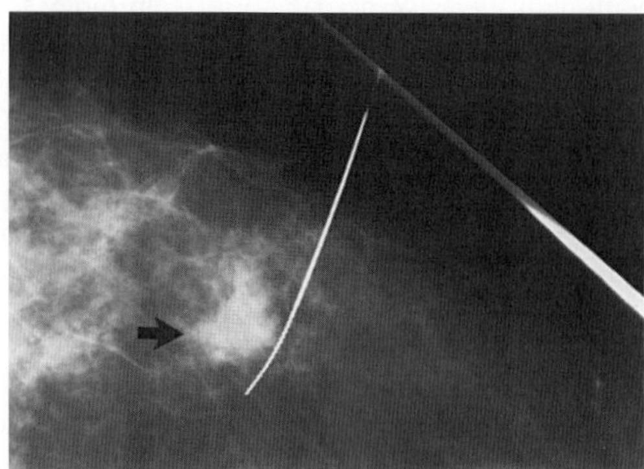

FIGURE 17-5 Mammogram section. Craniocaudad view of breast. Arrow indicates breast lesion localized by wire before surgical excision.

## HISTORY

Research on ways to make cancer surgery less invasive has intensified in recent years. One method uses focused ultrasound to beam into the breast tumor, emitting bursts of heat to "cook" the tumor and destroy the tissue, all without a surgical scar. The pilot study required participants to undergo a regular lumpectomy to determine if the tumor is destroyed and if the tissue margins are free of cancer cells. It will be years before the true efficacy of this therapy is fully determined. Clearly, ultrasonography has become an important modality in diagnosing and treating many conditions. Its potential for diagnostics was recognized in the 1930s, when attempts were made to use ultrasound in the diagnosis of brain tumors. It was not until the 1970s, however, that the early work on diagnostic imaging came to fruition. Technologic advances resulted in smaller, more user-friendly, and yet sophisticated equipment that produced detailed and useful images. It was the confluence of physics, physiology, medicine, engineering, and research that finally produced an imaging modality that has become a term commonly understood by most of the public.

The first basis for ultrasonography was the development of SONAR (sound navigation and ranging); this was pioneered in 1838, when attempts were undertaken to map the ocean floor to lay telegraph lines. In 1877 Strutt published the *Theory of Sound,* which became the foundation for the science of ultrasound. In medicine, physicians began studying the effects of ultrasound in the 1930s. Working with engineers, the medical applications of ultrasound were studied by general surgeons, gynecologists, cardiologists, and neurologists. Today, this high-frequency radiant energy has multiple applications; it has progressed such that ultrasound-directed biopsy of breast lesions is a common office procedure for general surgeons. Advances in ultrasound technology have resulted in a renewed interest in fine needle and core biopsy tissue sampling as alternatives to open biopsies, holding forth the promise of minimally disfiguring surgical procedures of the breast.

Modified from Neergaard L: *Using ultrasound to battle cancer,* 2000. Accessed October 30, 2000, on-line: dailynews.yahoo.com/h/ap/20001030/hl/cooking_cancer_ 1.html; Rozycki GS: Ultrasonography: surgical applications. In Wilmore DW and others, editors: *ACS surgery: principles & practice,* New York, 2002, WebMD.

well as detecting lesions missed by both other techniques. Further research will be required before MBI becomes a standard for detecting small tumors.[5]

Deoxyribonucleic acid (DNA)–based genetic testing for breast cancer–associated genes *(BRCA)* is not recommended in women without family histories that suggest risk for *BRCA1* or *BRCA2* mutations. However, if a woman is at high risk (determined by three first- or second-degree relatives with breast cancer) for harmful *BRCA* mutations, it is recommended that she be referred for genetic counseling and evaluated for testing.[20] In these women, increased surveillance, chemoprevention, or prophylactic surgery may decrease risk for breast and ovarian cancers.[25]

## DIAGNOSTIC TECHNIQUES

Once a mass has been identified, the physician has a variety of techniques available to establish a diagnosis. During a fine needle aspiration biopsy (FNAB), the physician anesthetizes a small area of the breast with lidocaine. A 22- or 25-gauge needle attached to a 20-ml syringe is inserted into the mass, and a small amount of the contents is aspirated. Cytologic examination of the aspirate can assist in microscopic evaluation of the mass. FNAB yields more diagnostic accuracy if the physician has been thoroughly trained in the technique. A multicenter study examined results for 6282 women who underwent needle biopsy (55%), open surgical biopsy (42%), or another test (3%) for initial evaluation of breast cancer. Of the 3481 women who underwent needle biopsy, 23% required breast reexcision (more than one surgical operation on breast parenchyma) compared with 92% of the 2650 women who underwent surgical biopsy, further suggesting that using needle biopsy for the initial evaluation of breast cancer is preferable to surgical biopsy.[8]

Ultrasound-guided FNAB, a newer technique, may be used before a sentinel node biopsy to determine whether breast cancer has spread to lymph nodes.[21]

Advances in instrumentation technology now allow for the biopsy and removal of mammographic densities that are up to 20 mm in size. This system combines digital stereotactic imaging and minimally invasive instruments to locate and remove tissues for diagnosis. The patient is assessed preoperatively for neck or back problems. In addition, the patient should not be receiving anticoagulant therapy. Masses located near the patient's areola, high in the axilla, or near the chest wall are not appropriate for this technique.

The patient is placed on a specially designed table (Figure 17-6) in the prone position with the affected breast through the table's 10-inch aperture to the work area below. The patient's head is turned away from the physician. Padding is placed under the patient's bony prominences to improve the patient's comfort. When the suspicious area in the breast is located through stereotactic imaging, its coordinates are transferred to the table's automated instrument. After preparing the skin with an antiseptic solution while the patient is under local anesthesia, the physician makes a small incision in the breast. The disposable biopsy device is available in a variety of sizes and consists of a localization needle, cannula, blade, and coagulation adapter. The physician positions the disposable device to remove the identified tissue. Additional biopsies can be made if indicated, and coagulation can be used if necessary. A titanium vessel clip can be placed at the base of the biopsy specimen as a point of reference for future evaluations. A postoperative dressing is then applied to the area. The benefits to the patient include small incisions for cosmetic results and decreased disfigurement, shortened time between detection and diagnosis, and elimination of the need for more involved surgical intervention.

## SURGICAL TREATMENT OPTIONS

Surgical treatment ranges from minimally invasive breast biopsy, lumpectomy, or the wide excision of the tumor mass to modified radical mastectomy involving the breast and axillary lymph nodes. The goal of surgery is removal of the cancerous mass with a margin of normal tissue and a good cosmetic result. When a specimen of breast tissue is sent to the laboratory, it is rolled in special ink to identify the margins. The pathologist evaluates these margins on all sides of the tumor for malignant cells. If a margin is positive, it indicates that malignant

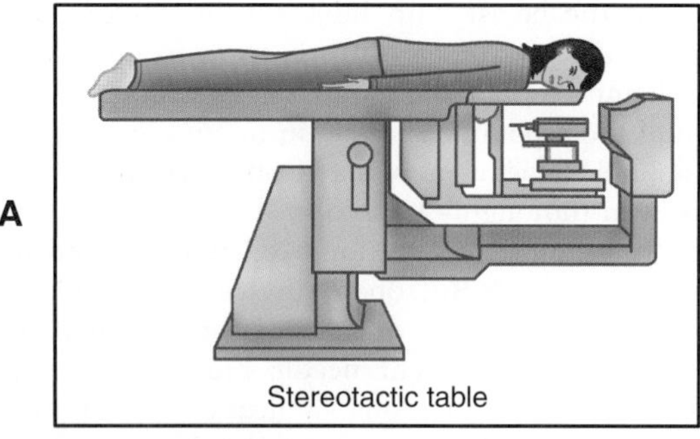


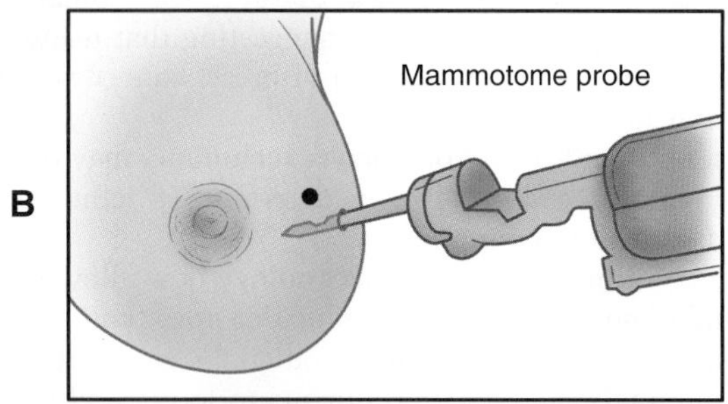


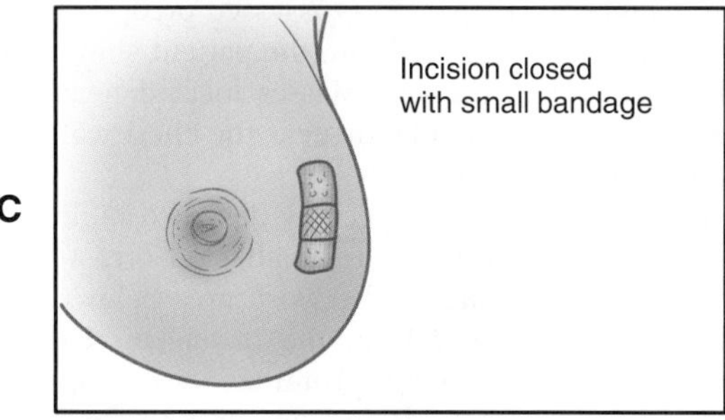


**FIGURE 17-6** **A,** In stereotactic procedures, patients lie facedown on a special table. The woman's breast protrudes through a hole in the table's surface, where it is lightly compressed and immobilized while a computer produces detailed images of the abnormality. **B,** Once the biopsy area has been located and mapped, the Mammotome probe is inserted through a small ¼-inch incision in the breast, where it gently vacuums, cuts, and removes breast tissue samples. **C,** The incision is then closed with a small adhesive bandage.

## RESEARCH HIGHLIGHT

### Benign Breast Biopsy with Atypical Cells

A breast biopsy that comes back benign is reassuring to most women, but about one third are still at a significantly higher risk of breast cancer and need to discuss their options, according to findings from a large study reported in 2005. Every year, about 1 million women who have a worrisome lump or suspicious mammogram undergo a biopsy that is reported as benign. However, it has long been known that certain cell growth patterns are ominous, even though technically not malignant. This is especially of concern about the degree of risk conferred by certain patterns and whether a family history of breast cancer intensifies the risk.

This large and rigorous study identified more than 9000 women who had benign biopsies at the Mayo Clinic in Rochester, Minn., between 1967 and 1991. The biopsy tissue was reanalyzed using current expert guidelines to classify it. The women were observed for an average of 15 years, during which they developed 707 cases of breast cancer. Their rates of cancer were compared with those from a state cancer registry.

About two thirds of the women had benign growths composed of nonproliferative cells, which were not rapidly dividing. These women had a tiny increase in risk, not enough to warrant extra measures to try to reduce it. Thirty percent of the women had proliferative growths, with rapidly multiplying cells; they had an 88% greater chance of later developing cancer. The smallest subgroup—about 4% of the women—had the most worrisome growths, made up of abnormal-shaped, fast-dividing cells. These women had a 324% greater risk of developing cancer.

Contrary to the results in previous studies, a family history of cancer did not have a significant effect on risk, even for the women with abnormal cells (atypia). However, for women diagnosed with atypia before age 45 years, the risk quadrupled.

A benign biopsy that reveals fast-growing or abnormal growth warrants a discussion of risk and options. Putting that risk in perspective is important. The study found that 6 out of 100 women diagnosed with nonproliferative breast changes would be expected to develop breast cancer within 15 years—not substantially different from the 5 out of 100 women in the general population. But the rate jumps to 10 out of 100 for women with fast-dividing breast cells and to 19 out of 100 for women with atypia. These women, in addition to routine screening, may be recommended to follow-up with ultrasound, magnetic resonance imaging (MRI), or other supplemental screening procedures.

Modified from Hartmann LC and others: Benign breast disease and the risk of breast cancer, *New England Journal of Medicine* 353(3):229-237, 2005.

cells may remain in the breast. Additional surgery is usually required until the margin contains only normal tissue.[8] The choice of operation depends on the size and site of the mass, the characteristics of the cells (Research Highlight), the stage of the disease, and the patient's choice. A breast cancer diagnosis is usually staged to measure the extent of the disease and to classify patients for possible treatment modalities (Figure 17-7). The TNM (T = tumor; N = node; M = metastasis) classification has been adopted as a mechanism to clinically stage this disease. The results of staging are used in designing a specific treatment plan. Radiation therapy, chemotherapy, or hormonal therapy may be used with surgery or as alternative treatment methods.

Tumors excised at surgery are evaluated for their estrogen-binding and progestin-binding abilities.

Techniques have been developed to determine the ability of breast cancer to bind with estrogen and progestins. This positive binding capability identifies the patient with a hormone-dependent tumor (Figure 17-8). It is estimated that about two thirds of all breast cancers are positive for estrogen binding, and the majority of these tumors are also positive for progestins. The presence of these receptor sites is conducive to hormone manipulation, with the goal of preventing breast cancer cells from receiving stimulation from estrogen. The use of antiestrogen tamoxifen, in addition to surgery and chemotherapy, increases disease-free survival in premenopausal women with positive binding for estrogen.

Another therapy can be offered by aromatase inhibitors (AIs). These may be nonsteroidal, such as anastrozole and letrozole. Aromatase inhibitors are only effective in postmeno-

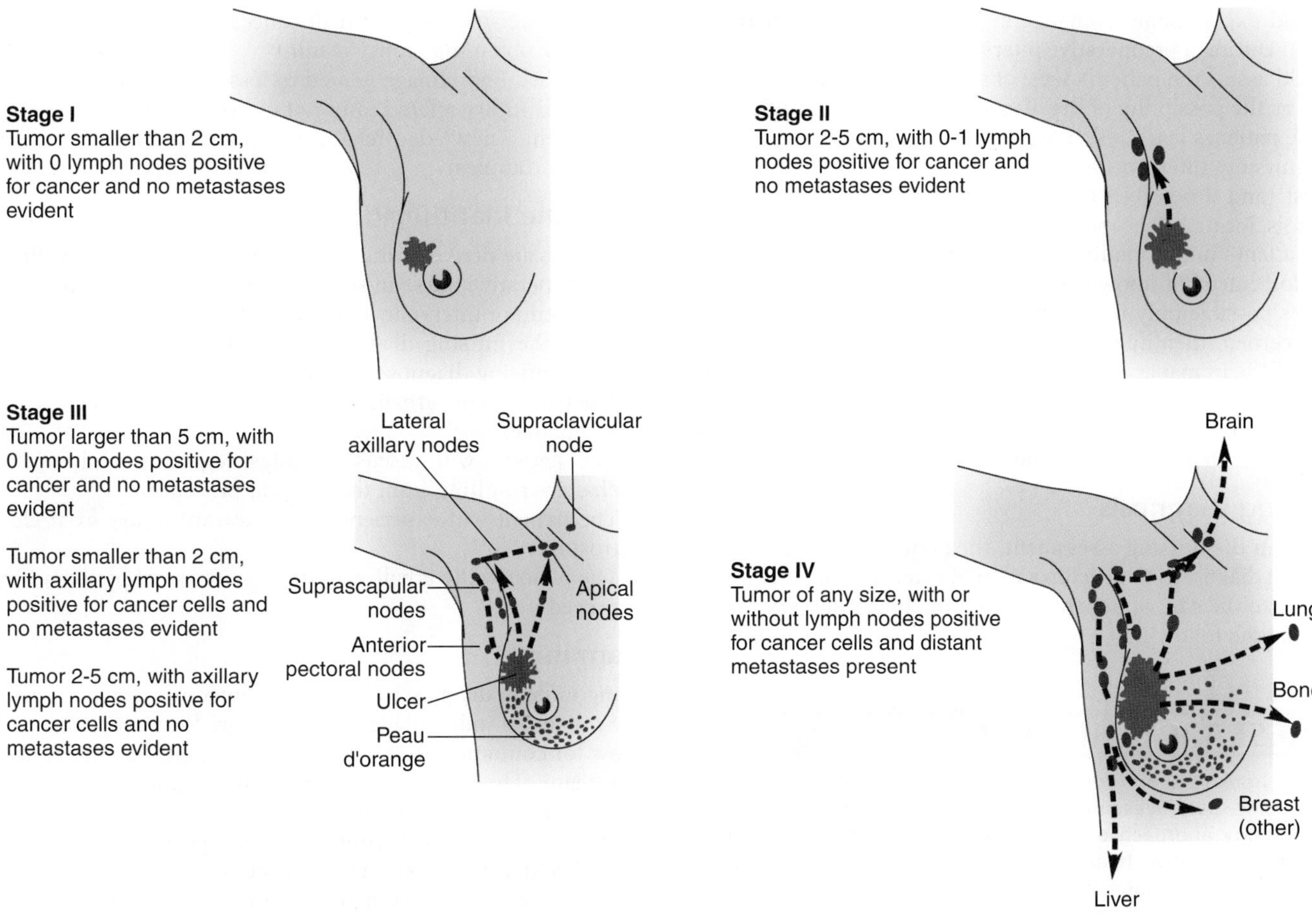

Stage I
Tumor smaller than 2 cm, with 0 lymph nodes positive for cancer and no metastases evident
Stage II
Tumor 2-5 cm, with 0-1 lymph nodes positive for cancer and no metastases evident
Stage III
Tumor larger than 5 cm, with 0 lymph nodes positive for cancer and no metastases evident
Tumor smaller than 2 cm, with axillary lymph nodes positive for cancer cells and no metastases evident
Tumor 2-5 cm, with axillary lymph nodes positive for cancer cells and no metastases evident
Lateral axillary nodes
Supraclavicular node
Suprascapular nodes
Apical nodes
Anterior pectoral nodes
Ulcer
Peau d'orange
Stage IV
Tumor of any size, with or without lymph nodes positive for cancer cells and distant metastases present
Brain
Lungs
Bone
Breast (other)
Liver

**FIGURE 17-7** Staging of breast cancer.

Estrogen
Receptors
Receptor dimers
Gene transcription
XXXXXXXXXXXXXXX
Progesterone receptor
Other genes

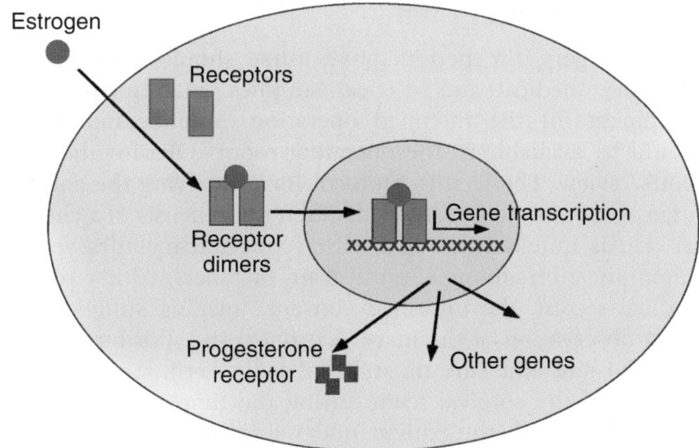

**FIGURE 17-8** Physiology of estrogen and the estrogen receptor, shown schematically. Estrogen binds to estrogen receptors, translocates to the nucleus of the cell, and interacts with cellular deoxyribonucleic acid (DNA). This interaction results in the transcription of estrogen-responsive genes, such as the receptor for progesterone. In addition, other genes are induced by the estrogen receptors that influence cell growth and differentiation.

pausal women. They appear to work better than tamoxifen on certain breast cancers, with fewer side effects. A large study found that anastrozole may prevent 70% to 80% of the most common breast cancer tumors that occur in postmenopausal women; this was compared with 50% for tamoxifen.[22] A new class of parenteral hormone therapy, estrogen receptor (ER) down-regulators (e.g., fulvestrant [Faslodex]), is available for the treatment of metastatic breast cancer.[19]

Some of the most promising data reported in recent years for advanced breast cancer has involved HER-2 (human epidermal growth factor receptor 2), a cellular proto-oncogene coding for a transmembrane receptor. Agents such as trastuzumab (Herceptin) to target HER-2 were first approved for treatment of metastatic HER-2–positive breast cancer in 1998. More recent research indicates that women with early-stage HER-2–positive cancer who received trastuzumab after surgery, and combined with standard chemotherapy agents, had a significant reduction in risk of recurrence.[4] Research and understanding of the immune system, the development of methods to evaluate aspects of the immune response, and the ongoing development of monoclonal antibodies are transforming the field of immunotherapy and breast cancer treatment.

# *Perioperative Nursing Considerations*

## Assessment

A patient undergoing breast surgery can be extremely apprehensive about the possibilities of having a malignancy, losing a body part, facing a negative reaction from her spouse and family, and experiencing a change in self-image (Research Highlight). During a preoperative interview the perioperative nurse should assess the patient's level of anxiety and possible causes, such as the possibility of the diagnosis of cancer. Identification of the patient's fears and concerns helps in planning appropriate nursing interventions. The patient should identify the breast (and if possible, the quadrant of the breast) where the mass is located. The perioperative nurse should also assess the patient's understanding of the proposed surgical procedure. Reinforcement of knowledge or correction of misunderstandings is possible only if the patient's current level of knowledge is discerned. Identifying the patient's psychologic support system will help manage anxiety during the patient's stay and enhance the discharge planning process. If the patient has lost a relative or close friend to breast cancer, her coping mechanisms may be affected because of memories of that loss.

## Nursing Diagnosis

Based on the nursing assessment, the perioperative nurse uses nursing diagnoses to develop a plan of care. Nursing diagnoses related to the care of patients undergoing breast surgery might include the following:

- Anxiety related to the fear of cancer, the surgical intervention, or obtaining biopsy results[6]
- Disturbed Body Image related to loss of body part
- Risk for Injury related to use of electrosurgery
- Deficient Knowledge related to unfamiliarity with perioperative routines

## RESEARCH HIGHLIGHT

In his book *Healing From the Heart,* Dr. Mehmet Oz, a highly respected cardiovascular surgeon, describes the value of mind-body approaches to healing the human body. By integrating alternative healing into the mainstream of Western medicine, he suggests that health care professionals can provide a more natural way of healing and restoring health—a way that helps patients help themselves heal. In this study, women with breast cancer were interviewed about how they coped with their illness. It is generally accepted that survivors of breast cancer confront fears of recurrence, alterations in their family life, challenges to their feelings of sexuality and their body image, side effects of fatigue and discomfort, financial strain, and feelings of loss and anger. In recent years, nurse researchers have recommended that studies focus not only on negative consequences and impact but also on strengths and ways of effective coping. Through interviews with breast cancer survivors, four phases of transforming personal tragedy into something positive were uncovered. *Encountering darkness* involved pain, wondering "Why me?," depression, confusion, and crying. The second phase, *converting the darkness,* involved acceptance—realizing that some questions were unanswerable and choosing to live beyond the questions. By beginning to set priorities, such as spending time with family and friends, breast cancer survivors began to see the light. In this phase, the question was "Where do I go from here?" While *encountering the light,* they began to enjoy each day, adopting an attitude of getting on with their lives and placing value on their time. In the fourth phase, *reflecting the light,* they were more sensitive to the needs of others, typified by their involvement in cancer survivor organizations and activities.

Perioperative nurses can assist their breast cancer patients by supporting them through psychospiritual pain that is necessary for the transformation of attributing positive meaning to illness and urging them to go beyond "Why me?"

Modified from Oz M: *Healing from the heart,* New York, 1999, Plume Printing; Taylor EJ: Transformation of tragedy among women surviving breast cancer, *Oncology Nursing Forum* 27(5):781-788, 2000.

## Outcome Identification

Outcomes are derived from the nursing diagnoses. They direct the perioperative nurse in selecting nursing interventions that will prevent, or intervene in, the actual or high-risk areas identified in the nursing diagnoses. Outcomes identified for the selected nursing diagnoses could be stated as follows:

- The patient will verbalize a level of anxiety that is personally acceptable.
- The patient will discuss feelings regarding body image changes resulting from the surgical procedure.
- The patient will experience no untoward injury from electrosurgery.
- The patient will verbalize an understanding of perioperative procedures.

## Planning

Using nursing diagnoses and desired outcomes, the perioperative nurse can individualize a plan of care for each patient and allow for communication with other colleagues on the patient care team. The plan of care for a patient undergoing breast surgery can include nursing interventions that allow the patient freedom to express concerns, have specific questions answered, and discuss breast reconstruction options, as appropriate. The Sample Plan of Care on p. 575 shows such an example. As part of planning patient care, priorities are established and a method of ensuring continuity of care ensured.

## Implementation

Before surgery, the perioperative nurse should procure the necessary medical and surgical supplies, instruments, and equipment for the intended operation. Mammogram films should be available in the operating room (OR) for the surgeon's review. The facility protocol for identifying the correct surgical site should be followed. Often this consists of a checklist that is initiated during the time out and includes verbal communication among surgical team members, review of the medical record, the informed consent, imaging studies, and direct observation of the marked surgical site. For breast surgery, the site and side must be verbally verified with each member of the surgical team during the time out.[1] A breast biopsy done with the patient under local anesthesia will require local anesthetics, adjunct sedation, and monitoring equipment (electrocardiogram [ECG], pulse oximeter, blood pressure apparatus). Patient allergies should be re-reviewed to avoid allergic or toxic reactions to local anesthetics. For a mastectomy, extra sponges and instrumentation are often needed. An electrosurgical unit (ESU) or a surgical laser is used to provide both hemostasis and tissue dissection. The incision site is usually drained postoperatively with a closed-wound suction device. Ensuring the availability of supplies before the procedure allows the nurse to remain with, provide support to, monitor, and observe the patient.

During the intraoperative phase, the patient is placed on the OR bed in a supine position with the operative side near the

## SAMPLE PLAN OF CARE

### NURSING DIAGNOSIS

**Anxiety** related to fear of cancer, the surgical intervention, or obtaining biopsy results

### OUTCOME

The patient will verbalize a level of anxiety that is personally acceptable.

### INTERVENTIONS

- Encourage questions, and allow time for the verbalization of fears and anxieties.
- Review the surgeon's explanation of the planned procedure and the reason for it (as appropriate).
- Assess verbal and nonverbal signs of anxiety.
- Provide emotional support and comfort measures (warm blankets, touch as appropriate).
- Maintain quiet, calm environment.
- Demonstrate warmth and acceptance of the patient's anxiety.
- Determine the patient's personally effective coping techniques (or recommend some), such as relaxation, rhythmic breathing, or guided imagery. Support the patient in using these.
- Record patient's reactions.

### NURSING DIAGNOSIS

**Disturbed Body Image** related to loss of body part

### OUTCOME

The patient will discuss feelings regarding body image changes resulting from the surgical procedure.

### INTERVENTIONS

- Allow patient to discuss concerns about her sexual attractiveness and perceived loss of femininity.
- Promote an environment of support, respect, and comfort.
- Discuss available resources and options (external prosthesis, alternatives in garments and dress, reconstructive surgery, as appropriate). Make referrals to nurse on discharge unit or community agency as indicated.
- Maintain patient's privacy.
- Encourage a visit by a *Reach to Recovery* volunteer (as applicable).

### NURSING DIAGNOSIS

**Risk for Injury** related to use of electrosurgery

### OUTCOME

The patient will experience no untoward injury from electrosurgery.

### INTERVENTIONS

- Position the dispersive pad as close to the operative site as possible.
- Select a site that is clean and dry, with good muscle mass; note and document the condition of the skin at the selected site.
- Protect pad from fluids and contact with metal objects.
- Turn electrosurgical unit on after dispersive pad and active electrode are connected.
- Set power setting as low as possible to achieve desired effect.
- Use holster for active electrode on the sterile field.
- Check dispersive pad contact and all connections after changes in position or requests to increase power.
- Evaluate and document the condition of the skin on removal of the dispersive pad.

### NURSING DIAGNOSIS

**Deficient Knowledge** related to unfamiliarity with perioperative routines

### OUTCOME

The patient will verbalize understanding of perioperative procedures.

### INTERVENTIONS

- Assess the patient's experience with previous surgical procedures.
- Review the need for correct-site surgery verification protocols.
- Explain that the skin will be cleansed with antiseptic solution at the surgical site and that solution may feel cold.
- Provide clear and concise explanations of all nursing interventions.
- Explain roles of the health care team members.
- Encourage questions.
- Describe the types of dressings and equipment that may be used postoperatively. If lymph node dissection is performed, describe the presence of incisional drains.

edge of the bed. The arm on the involved side is carefully extended on a padded armboard at no greater than 90 degrees to prevent brachial plexus injury. Depending on the location of the lesion and the planned surgery, a small pad can be placed under the operative side to facilitate exposure of the incision area. Positioning the OR bed in slight Fowler position with a lateral tilt away from the surgeon can also facilitate exposure.

Skin preparation depends on the location of the lesion and the surgery intended. Before skin preparation, any body jewelry, such as a nipple ring, must be removed and the area thoroughly cleaned before the surgical skin prep. Skin prep solutions vary, depending on the surgeon's preference. For a breast biopsy, the area prepped is usually the affected breast and the immediate surrounding skin. For a mastectomy, the area prepped can extend from above the clavicle to the umbilicus and from the opposite nipple to the bed line of the operative side, including the axilla, and possibly the upper arm on the operative side. Some surgeons caution against vigorous scrubbing of the surgical site to prevent possible seeding of cancer cells from the main mass. The surgeon may request that only an antiseptic solution be applied to the breast.

Surgical draping should allow exposure of the affected breast. For a mastectomy, the arm on the operative side should be draped free, using a stockinette and drapes that allow free movement of the associated arm to facilitate access to the axilla. If a breast biopsy is to be immediately followed by a modified radical mastectomy, the surgeon may prefer to repeat the skin prep and surgical draping before proceeding with the definitive surgery.

During implementation of the plan of care, the perioperative nurse continues to collect data, continuously reassesses the patient's needs and the needs of the surgical team, initiates nursing interventions, and documents all care delivered. Formats for documenting perioperative patient care vary from institution to institution. However, documentation of patient problems and nursing interventions addressing these problems is essential. For the patient undergoing breast surgery, consideration should be given to documenting the patient's level of anxiety, the surgical position and accessory positioning devices used, the time out, the location of the electrosurgical dispersive pad, unit settings and identification number, results of perioperative monitoring, medications administered by the perioperative nurse or from the sterile field, specimens collected, and any drains inserted into the surgical wound.

### Evaluation

Evaluation of the patient before discharge from the operating room includes both general observation parameters important for every surgical patient and specific evaluation of the goals of the plan of care. The patient's skin at dependent pressure sites, skin prep sites, and the dispersive pad placement site should be assessed and any change in skin integrity documented. The hand-off report to the nurse in the postanesthesia care unit (PACU) should include any unusual events or patient problems during surgery, the incorporation of any drains in the wound, and the achievement of identified patient outcomes. These outcomes, based on the nursing diagnoses selected, should be a part of documentation as well as the nursing report. Outcomes identified for the selected nursing diagnoses could be stated as follows:

- The patient verbalized an acceptable level of anxiety; she communicated her specific anxieties, her facial and body structures were relaxed, and her vital signs remained within a normal range.
- The patient discussed feelings regarding possible body image changes resulting from the surgical procedure; her coping strategies were reviewed and supported during the procedure.
- The patient experienced no untoward injury from electrosurgery; there were no skin changes at the site of the dispersive pad.
- The patient verbalized an understanding of perioperative procedures; she cooperated with requests and was provided with ongoing explanations.

### Patient and Family Education and Discharge Planning

Discharge planning should begin as soon as the patient is informed of the necessity for surgery or when the nurse first meets the patient. According to the extent of the anticipated surgery, information about appropriate exercises to enhance recovery, prosthetic devices, reconstruction options, and available community support groups should be explained to the patient. The perioperative nurse provides or reinforces information based on clinical nursing judgment and the patient's desire for information, readiness to learn, and anxiety level.

The patient is often discharged within hours or the day after the surgery. The patient and other caregivers need to be instructed regarding aseptic wound care, how to care for the closed-wound suction drain (if present), and pain management. Possible signs of complications should be included, along with instructions regarding when and how to notify the physician. Postoperative exercises need to be taught to the patient to facilitate her return to normal activities. Homecare may be necessary and should be coordinated with the physician and the patient. A follow-up telephone call to the patient can help the nurse assess the patient's ability to cope with her diagnosis and surgery. Box 17-1 provides a sample of discharge information for home care for the patient undergoing breast surgery.

# *Surgical Interventions*

## BIOPSY OF BREAST TISSUE

Biopsy of breast tissue is removal of suspicious tissue for pathology examination. In a *core needle biopsy (CNB)*, a disposable, cutting-type needle is introduced and advanced into the breast mass to entrap a core or plug of tissue. The needle is withdrawn, and the tissue specimen is sent to a pathologist for diagnostic examination. CNB may also be performed with a vacuum-assisted core biopsy (VACB) device.[14] In an *incisional biopsy*, a portion of the mass is surgically excised using a curved incision line. The tissue is sent for pathology examination. Alternatively, a percutaneous device may be used. These deliver large, intact samples under radiographic guidance. These devices are used for benign lesions.[14] In an *excisional biopsy*, the entire tumor mass is excised from adjacent tissue for examination as with incisional biopsy. Less invasive methods of diagnosing and treating image-detected breast cancer are recommended (Best Practice).

### Procedural Considerations

The biopsy procedure is usually performed with the patient under local anesthesia or local anesthesia with intravenous (IV) conscious sedation. Perioperative staff should be sensitive to the fact that the patient may be alert during the procedure and use caution with pathology reports called over a speaker phone. Pathology reports, especially if they are malignant, should be discussed when the patient is fully awake and has a support system available. A minor instrument set is used. The short delay between biopsy and further treatment has not been shown to adversely affect survival. However, when an extensive surgical procedure is anticipated in conjunction with the biopsy or when multiple lesions are to be excised and the amount of local anesthetic would exceed the maximum safe dose, general anesthesia is administered. In the instance of anticipated extensive surgery based on pathology results, the patient must have preoperatively given informed consent to proceed with the more definitive surgery.

### Operative Procedure—Open Breast Biopsy

1. An incision in the direction of the skin lines (curvilinear) or along the border of the areola is made over the tumor mass. The circumareolar incision gives the best cosmetic effect. If the lesion is located in an extremely lateral or medial site, a radial incision may be used.
2. Gentle traction is applied to the mass with holding forceps. If the lesion is small, the entire mass and an edge of normal tissue are removed by sharp dissection. If a large lesion is present, a small incisional biopsy of the main mass is done. The specimen should not be placed into a formalin solution if a frozen section is to be done at the time of surgery. Exposure to formalin prevents this type of pathology examination. The specimen may be marked with a sterile marker as to its orientation in the breast and/or may be placed on a sterile towel that is marked with a sterile marker to orient the specimen (Patient Safety). This assists the surgeon in

BOX 17-1

## Discharge Instructions and Home Care for Breast Surgery Patients

**HOME CARE**

- Give both the patient and the caregiver *verbal* and *written* instructions. Provide them with the name and telephone number of a physician or nurse to call if questions arise. Use visual aids to assist in instruction.
- General information
  - Review explanation of the disease, the surgical procedure performed, and adjuvant therapy to be carried out.
  - Explain that if the axillary nodes were removed, the affected arm may swell and is less able to fight infection. Discuss measures to prevent lymphedema:
- Exercise arm daily (provide specific exercises).
- Report loss of shoulder or joint mobility.
- When healing is complete, begin strengthening and stretching exercises.
- Wound/incision care (select applicable education based on surgical procedure performed)
  - Teach the patient how to care for the skin at the site of surgery.
    Advise the patient that there may be a dry gauze dressing over the incision site and the drain site.
    Provide information regarding dressing changes, amount of fluid leakage at drain site that is normal, when to change soiled drain-site dressing, and what to report to a physician or nurse (including emptying and measuring drain reservoir).
    Discuss numbness in the area of surgery and typical sensations (heaviness, tingling, "pins and needles"). These are likely to resolve by 1 year.
  - For modified radical mastectomy:
    Teach the patient to change the dressing, assess appearance of the incision and drain site, empty the drainage container, and record the amount and character of drainage.
    Caution the patient not to abduct the affected arm or elbow above the shoulder until drains are removed.
    Instruct the patient to report any redness or drainage around the drain.
    Instruct the patient to avoid use of deodorants or antiperspirants until stitches and drains have been removed from the axilla and the wound has healed. If no drain is present, the patient may shower.
    Caution the patient not to allow injections, placing of intravenous lines, drawing of blood, or taking of blood pressure in the affected arm if axillary dissection was done.
    Instruct the patient to avoid wearing constricting clothing or jewelry on the affected arm and to carry her handbag on the unaffected arm if axillary dissection was done.
    Discuss the types of temporary and permanent prostheses available; assist with referral as needed.
    Advise the patient not to use an external prosthesis or bra pad until swelling has subsided and healing of the incision is complete. Tell her to check with a physician or nurse before using a prosthesis.
    Discuss the types of reconstruction available.
    Stress the importance of continuing breast self-examination and mammography of the unaffected breast.
- Warning signs
  - Review the signs and symptoms that should be reported to a physician or nurse:
    Swelling of arm
    Drainage from incision, excessive drainage or blood in drainage unit, difficulty keeping container flat
    Infection: redness, purulent drainage, pain, incision warm to touch
- Medications
  - Explain the purpose, dosage, schedule, and route of administration of any prescribed drugs, as well as side effects to report to a physician or nurse.
  - Discuss alternative methods of postoperative pain management: visualization, guided imagery, meditation, relaxation, biofeedback, music, other personally effective techniques.
- Activity
  - Encourage discussion of allowances and limitations with respect to occupation, recreational sports, or activities.
  - Encourage resumption of self-care activities (feeding, combing hair) and activities of daily living as tolerated.
  - Explain that sexual activity may be resumed when desired. The partner should use a position that does not place pressure on the chest wall.
  - Discuss the need to continue postmastectomy exercises to regain full range of motion (as applicable).

**FOLLOW-UP CARE**

- Stress the importance of regular follow-up visits. Make sure the patient has the necessary names and telephone numbers.
- Prepare the patient for adjuvant therapies: hormone therapy, chemotherapy (see Research Highlight, p. 578), radiation therapy.

**PSYCHOSOCIAL CARE**

- Encourage verbalization about feelings and fears regarding diagnosis, adjunctive therapy, actual and perceived changes in body image and sexuality.
- Encourage patient and family to seek individual or group counseling to reduce emotional stress and help with effective coping.

**REFERRALS**

- Provide referrals for home health services and social services as indicated.
- Assist the patient to obtain referral services and contact support groups, such as the American Cancer Society's *Reach to Recovery* program, to cope with alterations in body image and other concerns.

Modified from Canobbio MM: *Mosby's handbook of patient teaching,* ed 3, St Louis, 2006, Mosby.

reexcision if the pathologist finds positive margins on the specimen. The tissue specimen is examined by a frozen section to determine immediate diagnosis while the patient is still anesthetized. If a 48-hour permanent section is required for a definitive diagnosis, the patient must be scheduled at a later time for any further surgery that may be necessary.

3. If the lesion is benign, hemostasis is checked and the subcutaneous breast tissue of the wound is approximated with an absorbable suture. The skin is closed with fine sutures or skin staples, and a firm pressure dressing is applied.
4. If the lesion is malignant, the incision is tightly closed with a continuous locking suture on a cutting needle.

## RESEARCH HIGHLIGHT

### Symptoms Experienced by Breast Cancer Patients Undergoing Adjuvant Chemotherapy

Symptom distress derives from an individual's perception and response to symptoms. This study explored symptoms and the distress from them in 20 women with breast cancer undergoing surgery and current chemotherapy protocols. The subjects were asked to tell their story, and transcripts were analyzed to determine common themes. Study findings confirmed that women experienced symptoms congruent with the type of treatment they were receiving. For example, fatigue and various ways of coping with it were commonly reported. For patients undergoing surgical lumpectomy or mastectomy, postprocedure pain was minimal compared with experiences of numbness, which caused great distress. Body image disturbance was frequently reported, even with lumpectomy. Nausea associated with chemotherapy was described as intense. Hair loss, although anticipated, was handled differently by the subjects. Some took control and shaved their heads when hair loss began, viewing this action as a "badge of honor." Other side effects of certain chemotherapy agents were unpleasant (loss of taste) or severe in their distress, such as intense bone and joint pain and numbness and tingling.

Symptoms varied in affecting functioning in daily activities and return to work. Cognitive changes were especially distressing, since memory loss, inability to concentrate, and inability to focus were experienced in varying degrees. Some women referred to this as "chemo brain" and found it to be a significant issue.

Perioperative nurses need to be aware of the symptoms associated with various treatment modalities. Part of patient and family education strategies should include informing women about to start chemotherapy about anticipating these symptoms and how to deal with them effectively. Patients and their families should be encouraged to share symptom experiences and distress throughout treatment so that plans for managing symptoms can be created and/or modified. Listening carefully to the patient can assist the perioperative nurse in offering strategies or referrals to ultimately improve the quality of the patient's life during treatment.

Modified from Boehmke MM, Dickerson SS: Symptom, symptom experiences, and symptom distress encountered by women with breast cancer undergoing current treatment modalities, *Cancer Nursing* 28(5):382-389, 2005.

## BEST PRACTICE

In 2005, an International Consensus Conference met to review implications of new and ongoing investigations in diagnosing and treating breast cancer. As a result of this conference, recommendations were developed regarding diagnosis and treatment of image-detected breast cancers. Some of the Consensus Conference recommendations include the following:

- Mammography is currently the only imaging modality that should be used routinely to screen patients for breast cancer
- Data support the use of magnetic resonance imaging (MRI) screening for younger patients at high risk of breast cancer because of the presence of *BRCA1* or *BRCA2* mutation or strong family/personal history of breast cancer or in clarifying the results of mammography, ultrasound, or clinical exam.
- If an abnormal axillary node is detected, confirmation of malignant involvement by ultrasound-guided core biopsy or fine needle aspiration biopsy (FNAB) should be done (minimally invasive breast biopsy). For microcalcifications, vacuum-assisted needle biopsy is preferred over conventional needle biopsy because of greater accuracy and more complete tissue removal.
- Minimally invasive breast biopsy is the optimal initial tissue-acquisition method and procedure of choice for image-detected abnormalities. It should be performed before definitive treatment in every possible case.
- Sentinel lymph node (SLN) biopsy is the preferred method of axillary nodal staging for clinically node-negative, image-detected breast cancers. This less-invasive alternative to axillary dissection provides suitable accuracy but a much lower risk of complications, particularly lymphedema.
- Until randomized trials comparing accelerated partial breast irradiation (APBI) with whole breast radiation therapy are completed, APBI should be performed as part of a clinical trial.
- Breast surgical fellowships should include oncoplastic techniques (combination of oncologic surgical principles with plastic surgical techniques).
- Patients should undergo careful history and physical examination after diagnosis of image-detected invasive cancer.

Modified from Silverstein MJ and others: Image-detected breast cancer—state of the art diagnosis and treatment, *Journal of the American College of Surgeons* 201(4):586-597, 2005.

5. If a more extensive operation is required, it may be performed immediately. The team members regown and reglove in an attempt to not transfer cancerous cells to healthy tissue; the operative site is again prepped and draped. A separate sterile setup and set of instruments for a more radical procedure are then used.

### Operative Procedure—Open Breast Biopsy with Needle (Wire) Localization

Wire placement is performed by a radiologist before the patient's arrival in the OR. Care should be taken during transfer to the OR bed and gown removal not to dislodge or bump the wire. Similar precautions should be taken during positioning, prepping, and draping the patient.

1. The skin incision is placed as directly as possible over the expected location of the mammographically determined lesion to minimize tunneling through the breast tissue.
2. The dissection is carried out using the wire as a guide.
3. The tissue around the wire is removed en bloc, with the wire, and sent for specimen mammography.
4. The patient is kept on the OR bed with the sterile field maintained until there is confirmation that the lesion has been excised.

## INCISION AND DRAINAGE FOR ABSCESS

Incision of an inflamed and suppurative area of the breast is performed for drainage of abscess. Breast abscesses occur most frequently during the first 4 weeks of breastfeeding. Staphylococcal or streptococcal organisms enter the breast through abraded or lacerated nipple surfaces or through the lactiferous ducts. Chronic abscesses are rare. Free drainage is required with the association of an abscess around the nipple or in breast tissue.

## PATIENT SAFETY

### Specimen Handling for Excisional Breast Biopsy

Collecting, identifying, and handling surgical specimens constitute a multidisciplinary task that mandates vigilance and attention to detail. Each person in the chain of custody must have correct and verifiable information about the specimen. Mishandling or misidentification of a specimen can lead to an inaccurate or incomplete diagnosis. For specimens obtained for analysis during excisional breast biopsy, safe practices such as the following should be adhered to:

- Two unique identifiers should be used based on the organization's defined unique identifiers.
- A read-back, or write-down/read-back process should be used when identifying the specimen for the pathologist. The surgeon and nurse should confirm specimen source, type of tissue, clinical diagnosis, and pertinent clinical information.
- After an open breast biopsy, the pathologist should receive a specimen labeled to preserve three-dimensional orientation. Margins should be marked with a tissue marker, inked, or tagged with a suture.
- The specimen should be documented on the operative record, pathology request/form, and container. Critical information regarding tissue margins and orientation of the breast tissue, as it relates to anatomy, should also be documented and confirmed by way of read-back verification by the nurse with the operating surgeon.

Modified from AORN recommended practices for the care and handling of specimens in the perioperative environment. In Association of periOperative Registered Nurses: *Standards, recommended practices, and guidelines*, Denver, 2006, The Association; Silverstein MJ and others: Image-detected breast cancer—state of the art diagnosis and treatment, *Journal of the American College of Surgeons* 201(4):586-597, 2005.

### Procedural Considerations

The condition is very painful and may require surgery with the patient under general anesthesia. Instruments are the same as those for a biopsy.

### Operative Procedure

1. Generally, a radial incision extending outward from the nipple or a circumareolar incision is preferred. A short incision into the thoracomammary fold may be used for deep breast abscesses in the lower or outer quadrant.
2. After skin incision, the wound is deepened until pus is encountered.
3. A curved hemostat is directed into the cavity to determine the extent of the abscess. Specimens for aerobic and anaerobic organisms are usually taken for culture.
4. Loculations are broken up by exploring the cavity with the index finger.
5. The opening is enlarged to ensure adequate drainage, the cavity is irrigated with warm saline solution, and bleeding vessels are ligated with absorbable sutures or coagulated.
6. The wound is drained or loosely packed with gauze. Healing occurs by granulation.

## LUMPECTOMY (SEGMENTAL RESECTION)

Lumpectomy is removal of the tumor mass with at least a 2.5-cm margin of surrounding tissue. Lumpectomy, with subsequent radiation therapy, is often the treatment of choice for tumors smaller than 5 cm; it is not an option for patients who have two or more cancer sites that cannot be removed through one incision, those whose surgery will not result in a clean margin, those who have had previous radiation to the affected breast, or those with tumors larger than 5 cm.[12] A lumpectomy combined with an axillary node dissection (Figure 17-9) and irradiation in stage I and stage II breast cancer appears to provide results equal to a more radical procedure. If one or more axillary nodes are involved, chemotherapy also is recommended.

### Procedural Considerations

In patients with large breasts, increased bleeding may occur, requiring additional hemostatic clamps.

### Operative Procedure

The procedure is as described for excisional biopsy.

## SENTINEL LYMPH NODE BIOPSY

Identification and microscopic examination of the sentinel lymph nodes (SLNs), the first lymph nodes along the lymphatic channel from the primary tumor site, will help determine the need for additional or more extensive surgeries and treatments and potentially adverse outcomes for the patient[11,15] (see Best Practice). The sentinel node is not located in the same site in every patient. This procedure helps to focus pathology attention in more detail on a small amount of tissue to determine the evidence of micrometastatic disease. Patients with histologically negative lymph nodes can have a greater likelihood of survival than patients with metastatic lymph nodes. Evidence of a positive node requires an axillary node dissection and adjunct therapy. Complications of SLN biopsy include risk of allergic reactions to the blue dye (1%), rare instances of sensory or motor nerve damage, and, with internal mammary node biopsy, risk of pneumothorax. If this occurs, the surgeon may request a red rubber catheter. This is inserted through a stab incision and removed after administration of a positive breath by the anesthesia provider.[17]

### Procedural Considerations

The procedure for an SLN biopsy is similar to that for a breast biopsy. Sentinel node identification is accomplished by an injection of either isosulfan blue dye (vital blue) or a radiocolloid (technetium 99 [$^{99m}$Tc]), a gamma-emitting material. Isosulfan blue is contraindicated in patients with a known hypersensitivity to the dye; careful patient monitoring and observation are mandatory, and a crash cart should be available in the instance of severe anaphylactic reaction (Surgical Pharmacology). The procedure is coordinated with the staff of the nuclear medicine department and requires the use of a handheld detector like a Geiger counter if technetium is used. In addition to the minor instrument set, if isosulfan blue is to be used, a 5-ml syringe, a 25-gauge needle, an alcohol wipe, and the dye are required. For technetium, the gamma tracer probe, counter, and sterile sleeve for the probe are required. Multiple specimen containers should be on hand along with pathology request forms. The surgeon

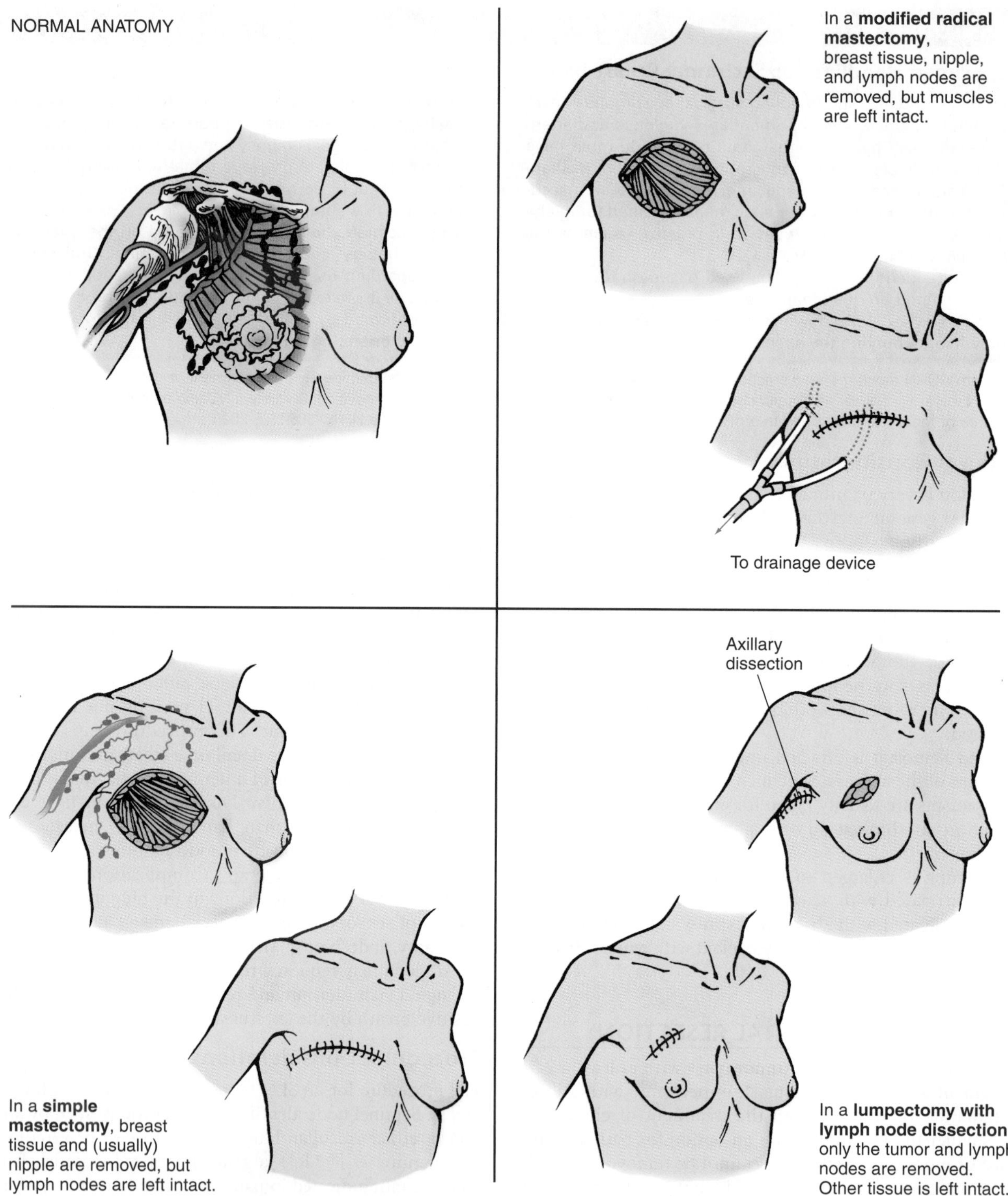

NORMAL ANATOMY
In a **modified radical mastectomy**, breast tissue, nipple, and lymph nodes are removed, but muscles are left intact.
To drainage device
In a **simple mastectomy**, breast tissue and (usually) nipple are removed, but lymph nodes are left intact.
Axillary dissection
In a **lumpectomy with lymph node dissection,** only the tumor and lymph nodes are removed. Other tissue is left intact.


**FIGURE 17-9** Surgical management of breast cancer.

may request that each specimen be numbered on the specimen container and the pathology request form.

## Operative Procedure—Using Isosulfan Blue Dye

1. Dye injection may be subareolar, or dye may be injected into the area of the breast mass that has been exposed as part of a breast biopsy.
2. After identification of the tumor mass, the surgeon injects the dye directly into the tumor mass or the previous biopsy site (peritumoral injection).
3. This may be followed by a 5-minute massage based on the "Rule of 5s"—5 ml of dye is injected at 5 sites fanning over a 5-cm diameter, followed by a 5-minute massage approximately 5 minutes before axillary dissection.[7]

**SURGICAL PHARMACOLOGY**

**Preventing Allergic Reaction in Sentinel Lymph Node Biopsy With Isosulfan Blue**

In 2005, the Association of periOperative Registered Nurses (AORN) developed a Safe Medication Administration Tool Kit. Data linked to the tool kit's importance included the following:

- A study from the Institute of Medicine (IOM) reported that 44,000 to 98,000 people die each year from medical accidents, costing from $17 billion to $29 billion for preventable adverse medical events.
- According to the U.S. Food and Drug Administration (FDA), more than 770,000 patients are injured by medication errors each year.
- The IOM reported that adverse events in surgery account for 20% of the errors in health care, whereas medication errors make up about 16% of all medical adverse events.

Isosulfan blue (Lymphazurin), a dye commonly used in SLN biopsies, contains a sulfite derivative that may cause a potentially life-threatening allergic reaction. Before the procedure starts, patients should be queried regarding allergies to sulfa drugs. Lymphazurin 1% (isosulfan blue) has demonstrated a 1.5% *incidence* of adverse reactions. All the reactions were of an *allergic* type. Localized swelling at the site of administration and mild pruritus of hands, abdomen, and neck have been reported within several minutes following administration of this drug.

Reports of mild to severe reactions have appeared in the literature for compounds similar to isosulfan blue. Severe reactions may be manifested by edema of the face and glottis, respiratory distress, or shock; such reactions may prove fatal unless promptly controlled by emergency measures such as maintenance of a clear airway and immediate use of oxygen and resuscitative drugs. Like other sensitivity phenomena, severe reactions are more likely to occur in patients with a personal or family history of bronchial asthma, allergies to sulfa drugs, or previous reactions to triphenylmethane dyes.

Modified from Association of periOperative Registered Nurses: *Safe medication administration tool kit,* Denver, 2005, The Association; Dye may cause allergic reaction, *AORN Management Connections* 1(8):14, 2005.

4. The sentinel nodes stained with the blue dye are identified and excised.
5. The nodes are sent to the pathology department for examination.
6. Based on the results, the surgeon proceeds with the planned surgery or may elect breast conservation.

## Operative Procedure—Using Technetium

1. The patient's tumor or previous biopsy site is injected with a small amount of radioactive material in the nuclear medicine department on the morning of surgery.
2. This may be followed by the "Rule of 6s"—6 ml of radiocolloid at 6 sites fanning out over a 6-cm diameter followed by a 5- to 6-minute massage before axillary exploration.[7]
3. A handheld detector is passed over the top of the patient's chest to identify the area of the sentinel node through a positive reading. The probe may also be used with the addition of a sterile sleeve during excisional biopsy. Isosulfan blue dye may be used in conjunction with the technetium during a procedure to enhance the visibility of the nodes.
4. The surgeon marks the skin with a skin scribe to indicate the reactive area.
5. The area is prepped, and the surgeon proceeds with the planned procedure for excisional biopsy.

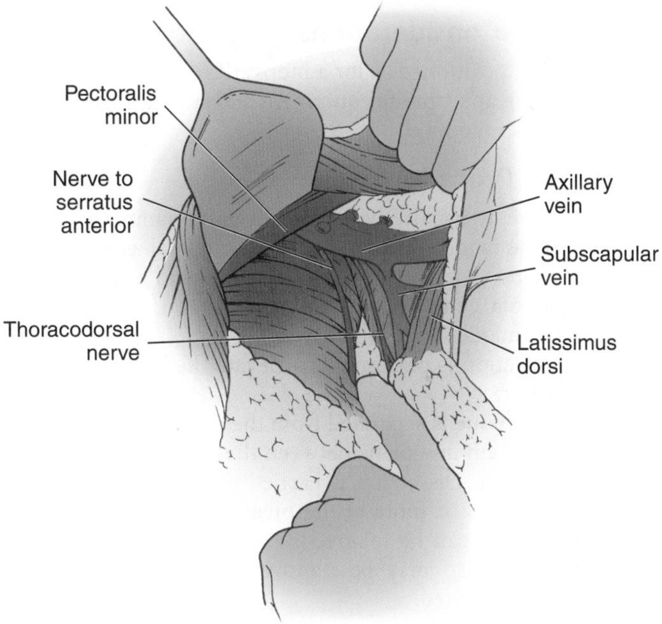

**FIGURE 17-10** Axillary dissection.

## AXILLARY NODE DISSECTION

Axillary node dissection (Figure 17-10) is the removal of the axillary nodes through an incision in the axilla following determination that the sentinel node is malignant. An axillary dissection is usually done through an incision separate from that for other breast operations. The removal and examination of the axillary nodes allow staging (see Table 17-2) of the disease. Adjunct treatment can be more accurately planned when the pathologic stage is determined.

### Procedural Considerations

The patient is placed supine on the OR bed with the operative side near the bed edge. The arm on the operative side is extended to less than 90 degrees on an armboard. The skin is prepped and draped as previously described.

### Operative Procedure

1. An incision is made slightly posterior and parallel to the upper lateral border of the pectoralis major muscle or transversely across the axilla.
2. The fascia is incised over the pectoralis muscle. The pectoralis minor muscle is exposed. Major blood and lymphatic vessels are clamped and ligated. The use of electrosurgery is avoided around the axillary vessels and nerves to reduce the risk of inadvertent injury and subsequent impaired muscle function.
3. The tissue over the axillary vein is incised.

4. The lymph nodes between the pectoralis major and pectoralis minor muscles are removed. Care is taken not to injure the medial and lateral nerves of the pectoralis major muscle.
5. The axillary fat and lymph nodes are freed from the axillary vein and chest wall. The long thoracic nerve is identified along the chest wall near the axillary vein, and the thoracodorsal nerve posteriorly is dissected free from the specimen.
6. The fat and nodes are removed. The incision is closed with sutures and staples, and a dressing is applied. A suction drain is usually placed through a separate stab incision for lymphatic drainage.

## SUBCUTANEOUS MASTECTOMY (ADENOMAMMECTOMY)

Subcutaneous mastectomy is removal of all breast tissue with the overlying skin and nipple left intact. This procedure is recommended for patients who have central tumors of noninvasive origin, chronic cystic mastitis, hyperplastic duct changes, or multiple fibroadenomas or who have undergone several previous biopsies. Breast reconstruction may be undertaken at the time of mastectomy or at a later date if desired.

### Procedural Considerations

The patient is positioned as for a biopsy. If reconstruction is to be undertaken, appropriate equipment and supplies (see Chapter 24) are also required.

### Operative Procedure

1. An incision is usually begun in the inframammary crease and may be made on the medial or the lateral aspect of the breast. Some surgeons initially remove and preserve the nipple areola complex by employing lateral extensions of wide circumareolar incisions.
2. Blunt dissection is performed to elevate the breast from the pectoral fascia.
3. The breast tissue is separated from the skin with an attempt made to remain in a plane between the subcutaneous tissue and the breast. Dissection is carried out toward the axilla. With care, 90% or more of the breast tissue, including the tail of Spence, can be removed. Some lymph nodes in the axillary area also may be removed. Bleeding vessels are clamped and ligated.
4. If a preoperative decision was made for immediate reconstruction, that procedure follows at this time. Provided that the subareolar tissue shows no signs of tumor, as verified by a pathologist, the salvaged areolar complex is placed on a de-epithelialized dermal bed.
5. A closed-wound suction catheter typically is inserted. The wound is closed, and a light pressure dressing is applied.

## SIMPLE MASTECTOMY

Simple mastectomy is removal of the entire involved breast without lymph node dissection (see Figure 17-9). A simple mastectomy is performed to remove extensive benign disease, if malignancy is believed to be confined only to the breast tissue, or as a palliative measure to remove an ulcerated advanced malignancy.

### Procedural Considerations

The patient is positioned as for a biopsy.

### Operative Procedure

1. Through a transverse elliptic incision (Figure 17-11, *A*), using a knife and curved scissors, the skin edges are freed from the fascia. Bleeding vessels are clamped with hemostats and ligated with sutures or electrocoagulated.
2. The skin edges of the wound can be protected with warm, moist laparotomy pads; the breast tissue is grasped with Allis forceps and is dissected free from the underlying pectoral fascia with curved scissors and a knife.
3. The tumor and all breast tissue are removed. Bleeding vessels are clamped and ligated or electrocoagulated.
4. A closed-wound drainage catheter is inserted and anchored to the skin with a fine suture. The wound is closed with fine sutures or staples; a dressing is applied.

## MODIFIED RADICAL MASTECTOMY

Modified radical mastectomy is performed after a tissue biopsy with a positive diagnosis of malignancy and involves removal of the involved breast and all axillary contents (all three levels of nodes—axillary, pectoral, and superior apical) (see Figure 17-9). The underlying pectoral muscles are not removed before or after removal of axillary nodes. A modified radical mastectomy is done to remove the involved area with the hope of decreasing the spread of the malignancy. This surgery's elliptic incision with lateral extension toward the axilla gives a good cosmetic result for plastic surgery reconstruction[2] (see Chapter 24), provides good arm movement because the pectoralis muscles are not removed, and usually does not require a skin graft.

### Procedural Considerations

The patient is placed supine on the operating room bed with the operative side near the bed edge. The arm on the operative side is extended to less than 90 degrees on a padded armboard. The skin is prepped and draped as previously described. Tissue removed during surgery will be submitted for microscopic analysis to further classify it (type, tumor size, grade, invasion, lymphocytic response, clean margin size). Additional analysis such as hormone receptor status (estrogen and progesterone positive or negative) and HER-2/neu (human epidermal growth factor receptor 2) expression may also be performed. This information assists the oncologist in planning subsequent adjuvant therapies.[12]

### Operative Procedure

1. An oblique elliptic incision with a lateral extension toward the axilla is made through the subcutaneous tissue (see Figure 17-11, *A*). The bleeding points are controlled with hemostats and ligatures or electrocoagulation.
2. The skin is undercut in all directions to the limits of the dissection by means of a #3 knife handle with a #10 blade and curved scissors. Knife blades need to be changed frequently to ensure precise dissection.
3. The margins of the skin flaps are covered with warm, moist laparotomy pads and held away with retractors. The fascia and breast are resected from the pectoralis major muscle (Figure 17-11, *B*) starting near the clavicle and extending down to the midportion of the sternum. The pectoralis muscle is left intact.
4. The intercostal arteries and veins are clamped and ligated.

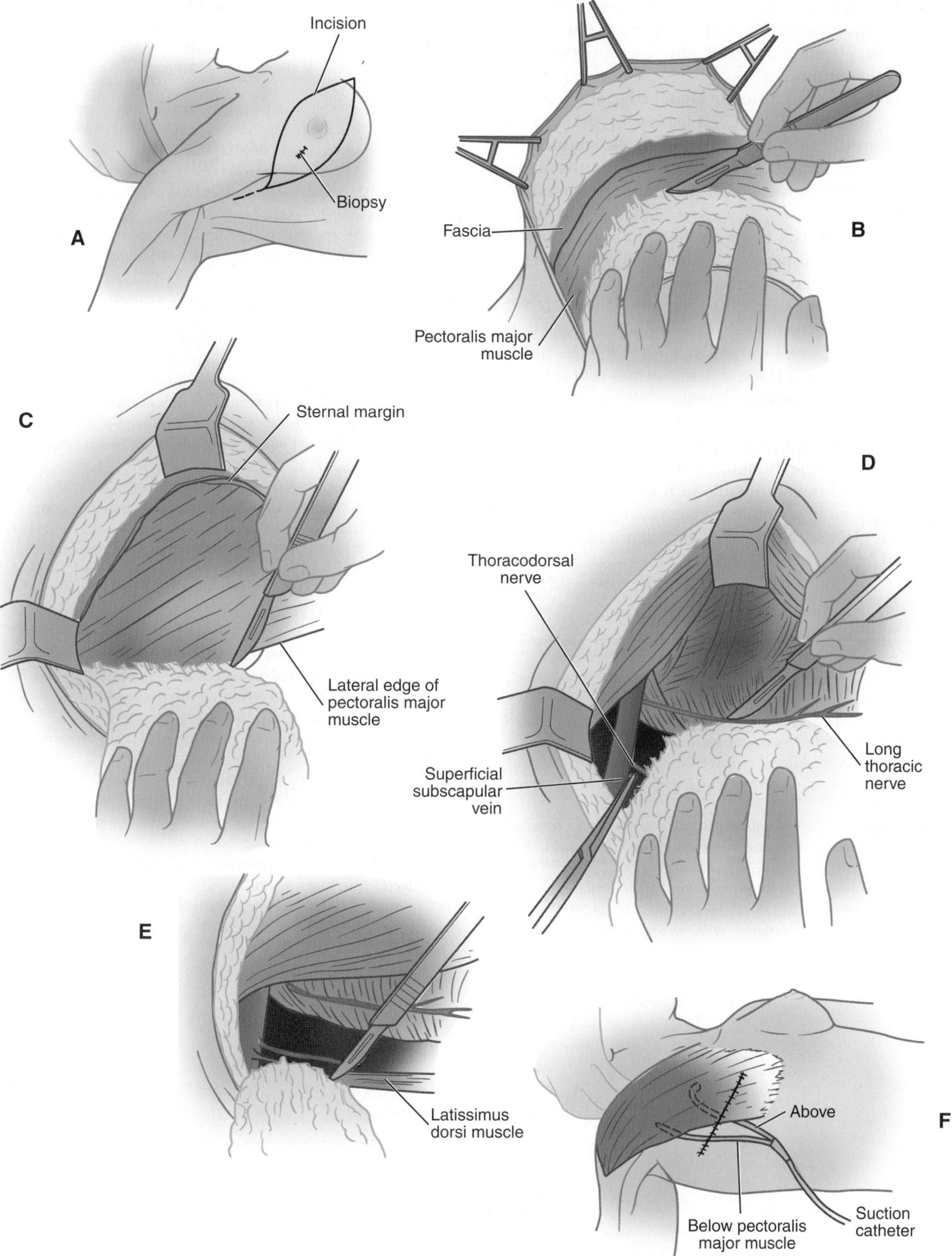


FIGURE 17-11 Modified radical mastectomy. **A,** Lines of incision. **B,** Resection of breast from lateral edge of pectoralis major muscle. **C,** Dissection of breast from lateral edge of pectoralis major muscle. **D,** Thoracodorsal and long thoracic nerves identified. **E,** Resection from latissimus dorsi muscle. **F,** Incision is closed, and drains are placed.

5. The axillary flap is retracted for a complete dissection of the axilla. Careful attention is directed to preventing injury to the axillary vein and medial and lateral nerves of the pectoralis major muscle.
6. The fascia is dissected from the lateral edge of the pectoralis muscle (Figure 17-11, *C*). Ligation of the vessels is performed in the axilla and adjacent to the sternum. The fascia is then dissected from the serratus anterior muscle. The thoracic and thoracodorsal nerves are preserved (Figure 17-11, *D*).
7. The breast and axillary fascia are freed from the latissimus dorsi muscle and suspensory ligaments (Figure 17-11, *E*). The specimen is then passed off the field.
8. The surgical area is inspected for bleeding sites, which are ligated and electrocoagulated. The wound is irrigated with normal saline. Closed-wound suction catheters are inserted into the wound through stab wounds and secured to the skin with a nonabsorbable suture on a cutting needle (Figure 17-11, *F*).
9. A few absorbable sutures may be used in the subcutaneous tissue to approximate the skin edges. The incision is closed with interrupted nonabsorbable sutures or staples.
10. The dressing can be a simple gauze dressing, a bulky dressing held in place by a Surgi-Bra, or a gauze or elastic bandage wrap.

## REFERENCES


1. Association of periOperative Registered Nurses: *AORN standards, recommended practices, and guidelines,* Denver, 2006, The Association.
2. Barclay L: Breast implants do not appear to decrease survival after mastectomy for breast cancer, *Medscape Medical News.* Accessed December 30, 2004, on-line: www.medscape.com.
3. Berry DA and others: Effects of screening and adjuvant therapy on mortality from breast cancer, *New England Journal of Medicine* 353:1784-1792, 2005.
4. *Breast cancer drug hailed—treatment found to curb relapses from tumor.* Accessed October 20, 2005, on-line: www.boston.com/yourlife/health/women/articles/2005/10/20/breast_cancer_drug.
5. Brem RF: The future of breast cancer diagnosis: molecular breast imaging, *Mayo Clinic Proceedings* 80(1):17-18, 2005.
6. Chappy SL: Women's experience with breast biopsy, *AORN Journal* 80(4):885-901, 2004.
7. Cox CE and others: Postinjection massage increases sensitivity of sentinel lymph node biopsy, *Journal of the American College of Surgeons* 192:9-16, 2001.
8. Dell DD: Spread the word about breast cancer, *Nursing 2005* 35(10):56-63, 2005.
9. *Digital vs. film mammography in the Digital Imaging Screening Trial (DMIST).* Accessed January 12, 2006, on-line: www.nci.nih.gov/newscenter/pressreleases/DMISTQandA.
10. *FDA OKs Irvine firm's breast tumor treatment,* 2001. Accessed October 17, 2001, on-line: www.latimes.com/templates/misc/printstory.jsp?slug/la%2D000082772oct17.
11. Harlow SP and others: Lymphatic mapping and sentinel node biopsy, *What's New in ACS Surgery.* Accessed January 17, 2005, on-line: www.acssurgery.com.
12. Holmes SR: Current protocols for managing breast cancer, *Nursing Spectrum* 13(7):22-23, 2004.
13. Hughes KS and others: Family history common in women with breast or ovarian cancer, on-line journal *Cancer,* accessed September 26, 2005, on-line: www.medscape.com/viewarticle/518752.
14. Kass RB, Souba WW: Minimally invasive breast biopsy, *What's New in ACS Surgery.* Accessed August 30, 2004, on-line: www.acssurgery.com.
15. Kellar SJ: Sentinel lymph node biopsy for breast cancer, *AORN Journal* 74(2):197-201, 2001.
16. Lind DS, Souba WW: Breast procedures, *What's New in ACS Surgery.* Accessed March 7, 2004, on-line: www.acssurgery.com.
17. Lind DS and others: Breast complaints, *What's New in ACS Surgery.* Accessed June 6, 2004, on-line: www.acssurgery.com.
18. Low fat diet and regular exercise may reduce risk of breast cancer. In Summary of ASCO 2005 meeting, *Journal of Clinical Oncology* 21(1):190-205, 2006.
19. Lynn JM: Breast tumors, *Advance for Nurses* 6(7):48, 2004.
20. Nelson HD and others: Genetic risk assessment and BRCA mutation testing for breast and ovarian cancer susceptibility—systemic evidence review for the U.S. Preventive Service Task Force, *Annals of Internal Medicine* 143:362-369, 2005.
21. New biopsy technique reduces need for surgery, *AORN Journal* 81(4):870, 2005.
22. Newer drug outperforms tamoxifen, *Nursing 2005* 35(2):30, 2005.
23. Pisano ED and others: Diagnostic performance of digital versus film mammography for breast cancer screening, *New England Journal of Medicine* 353:1773-1783, 2005.
24. *Radiation therapy in treating women who have undergone surgery for ductal carcinoma in situ or Stage I or Stage II breast cancer.* Accessed January 12, 2006, on-line: www.clinicaltrials.gov.
25. Veitz AL: Breast cancer and genetic testing, *Advance for Nurses* 7(16):24-26, 2005.

CHAPTER 18

# Ophthalmic Surgery

SARAH C. SMITH

Years ago, ophthalmic surgery was confined mainly to the eyelids and intracapsular cataract extraction, for which bed rest, a prolonged hospital stay, and thick "cataract" glasses were required (History box). Since that time, newer innovations use lasers to reshape the cornea, topical anesthesia and no-stitch techniques with foldable and injectable intraocular lenses (IOLs) for cataract extraction, and fiberoptics and microsurgical technology for vitreoretinal procedures. Advances in surgical techniques and improved anesthetics, along with increasing pressures to contain health care costs, have created another major change in the management of patients who undergo ophthalmic surgery. Except for a small percentage of patients who have complex procedures or medical problems that contraindicate early discharge, today eye surgery is done on an ambulatory basis.

The perioperative nurse who cares for ophthalmic patients must combine the art and science of nursing with up-to-date knowledge and highly proficient technologic skills. The perioperative nursing team coordinates preoperative patient preparation, intraoperative interventions, and discharge planning in a very limited time period. The success of the surgical intervention depends, to a degree, on the knowledge and skill of those team members as they develop and implement a perioperative plan of care. The increasing emphasis on shorter stays, even in ambulatory settings, and the demand for providing quality care with a more cost-effective approach to using resources present the challenges of constant change and new technology, as well as the challenge of finding ways to decrease labor and supply costs.[11] Such challenges are opportunities for perioperative nurses to reevaluate established protocols and seek research- and evidence-based practices when faced with new ideas (e.g., patients wearing their street clothes and shoes during eye surgery).

## Surgical Anatomy

A working knowledge of the anatomic structures involved in ophthalmic surgery is necessary to facilitate selection of instrumentation, supplies, and equipment for the procedure. The surgical team must also use this knowledge to understand the surgeon's plan of treatment and prepare the patient accordingly.

### Bony Orbit

The two orbital cavities are situated on either side of the midvertical line of the skull between the cranium and the skeleton of the face. Above each orbit are the anterior cranial fossa and the frontal sinus; medially, the nasal cavity; below, the maxillary sinus; and laterally, from behind forward, the middle cranial and temporal fossae.

The seven bones that form the orbit are the maxilla, palatine, frontal, sphenoid, zygomatic, ethmoid, and lacrimal bones (Figure 18-1). The margins of the bony orbit may be divided into four continuous parts: supraorbital, lateral, infraorbital, and medial.

Each orbit is in the shape of an irregular, four-sided pyramid, with its base at the front of the skull and its axis pointing posteromedially toward the apex. The periosteum of the orbital walls is continuous with the dura mater. The orbit contains the globe, orbital fat, extraocular muscles, nerves, blood vessels, and part of the lacrimal apparatus. The orbit also acts as a distribution center for certain vessels and nerves that supply the facial areas around the orbital aperture.

### Lacrimal Apparatus

The lacrimal apparatus consists of the lacrimal gland and its ducts, the lacrimal passages, the lacrimal canaliculi and sac, and the nasolacrimal duct. The lacrimal gland produces tears and secretes them through a series of ducts into the conjunctival sac. The tears then make their way inward to the puncta, from which they are conducted by the canaliculi to the lacrimal sac and finally pass into the nasolacrimal duct (Figure 18-2). When the lacrimal glands secrete too profusely, the normal drainage process becomes insufficient and overflow tearing results.

### Conjunctiva and Eyelids

The conjunctiva is a thin, transparent mucous membrane divided into a palpebral and a bulbar part (Figure 18-3). The palpebral portion lines the back surface of the eyelids and contains the openings (puncta) of the lacrimal canaliculi, which establish a passageway between the conjunctival sac and the inferior meatus of the nose. The bulbar part of the conjunctiva lines the front surface of the globe, allowing the sclera, or white of the eye, to show through. The central portion of the bulbar conjunctiva is continuous at the limbus with the anterior epithelium of the cornea.

The conjunctiva forms a sac (conjunctival sac) that is open in front. The opening, called the *palpebral fissure,* is located between the margins of the two eyelids. When the eye is closed, the fissure becomes a mere slit and the cornea is completely covered by the upper eyelid.

The eyelids are two movable musculofibrous folds in front of each orbit that protect the globe and the eye from light. The upper eyelid is more mobile and larger than the lower. The upper and lower lids meet at the medial and lateral angles (canthi) of the eye. The eyelids are closed by the orbicularis

## HISTORY

Although the history of cataract surgery is hundreds of years old, an 1879 manual of surgery described four ways of removing the lens. At that time, the author suggested the von Graefe operation for lens extraction. In this procedure, the incision was made just within the corneal margin, a piece of iris removed, the capsule torn, and the lens pressed out. Regarding patient recovery, it was noted that "if all goes well, the wound is healed by the end of a week or 10 days, but the eye will require protection and rest for a considerable time. The patient should not be allowed to use the glass, which will be necessary for accurate vision, for at least 3 months."

In the 1950s, both eyes were patched and postoperative activity was extremely restricted. Patients were lifted off the operating room (OR) bed with special lifts and remained flat in bed with the head immobilized with sandbags for up to 10 days. They required total care—bed baths, catheterization if unable to void in a reclining position, feeding of liquids and soft foods, daily dressing changes, and a cleansing enema on the third or fourth postoperative day. Nurses played a paramount role in the care of these patients.

Cataract surgery evolved from a form of extracapsular extraction (using pressure on the eye from below with a metal spoon) to intracapsular extraction. Both these methods required the patient to wear thick "cataract glasses" to correct his or her vision. There was a definite need to find a substitute for the crystalline lens that would take the place of these cumbersome and unattractive glasses. The development of intraocular lenses was attributed to observations of World War II fighter pilots with retained fragments of plastic in their eyes. Surgeons noted no foreign-body reaction to these plastic pieces from the shattered aircraft windows. With the development of operative microscopes, finer sutures, and anterior chamber intraocular lenses (IOLs), cataract surgery continued to evolve. Extracapsular techniques with posterior chamber IOLs were eventually developed, progressing to the present use of phacoemulsification; topical anesthesia; small, clear cornea incisions; and foldable IOLs.

Throughout this evolution, perioperative nurses have provided care, acted as patient advocates, and served as the guardians of sterile techniques. As the cataract procedure evolved, postoperative restrictions were lessened, the hospital stay was shortened to 1 day, and then the procedure became an ambulatory surgery procedure. Perioperative nurses continue to influence patient outcomes with preoperative patient and family education; implementation of safe, efficient, and effective care; discharge planning; and postoperative evaluation of achievement of desired outcomes.

Modified from Clarke WF: *A manual of the practice of surgery,* New York, 1879, William Wood & Co.

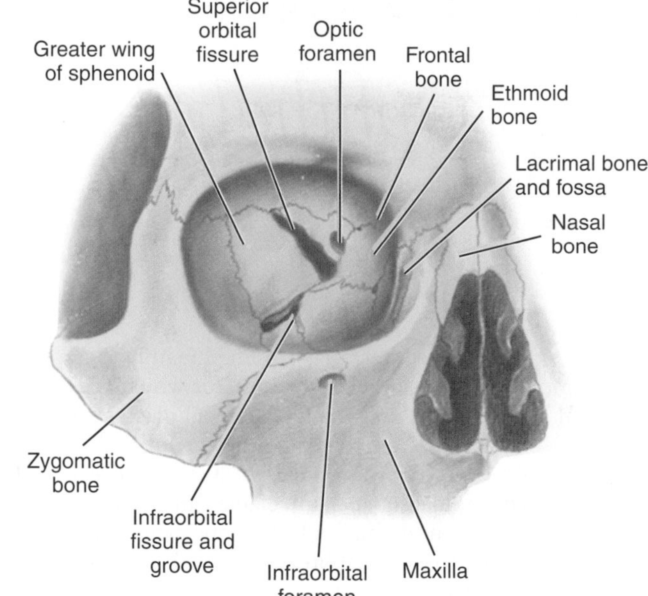


**FIGURE 18-1** Bony orbital cavity.

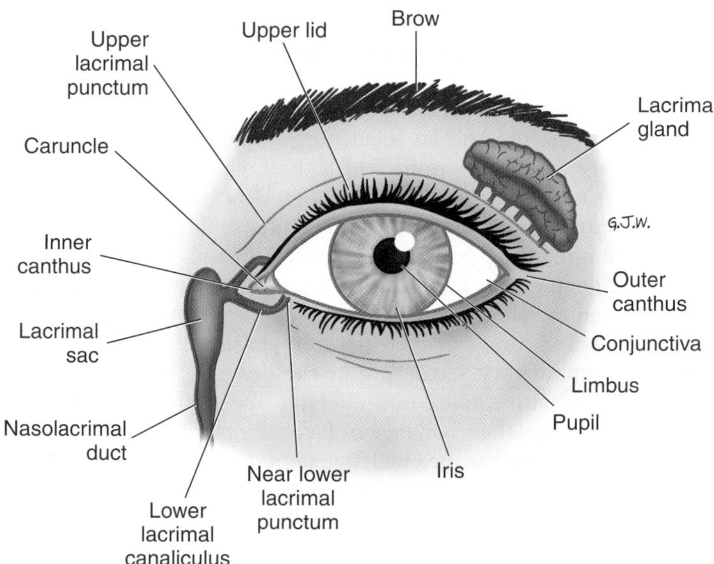


**FIGURE 18-2** Lacrimal apparatus, external view.

oculi muscle, a circular muscle that acts as a sphincter. When the fibers contract, the eyes close. The upper lid is opened by the levator muscle, which is innervated by the third cranial nerve, as well as by relaxation of the orbicular muscle.

Each eyelid consists of several layers. From front to back these are the skin, subcutaneous tissue that contains the lymphatics, and muscles. Dense fibrous tissue, called *tarsal cartilage,* forms the framework of the lids. The tarsus is anchored to the walls of the orbit by the medial and lateral palpebral ligaments.

The free margins of each eyelid possess two or three rows of hairs called *cilia,* or *eyelashes.* Posterior to the lashes is a row of glandular orifices of the meibomian glands. Near the medial edges the free margin of each eyelid presents an opening called the *punctum lacrimale.* The eyelids distribute all lacrimal secretions, thereby keeping the cornea moist and washing away any dust.

## Muscles

The extrinsic ocular muscles of the eyeball are the four rectus and two oblique muscles (see Figure 18-3). These six striated muscles are inserted into the sclera by tendons. Except for the inferior oblique muscle, they arise from the back of the orbit. All the muscles are supplied by cranial nerves: third (oculomotor), fourth (trochlear), and sixth (abducens). The muscles work in pairs. Movements of the eyes are brought about by an increase in the tone of one set of muscles and a decrease in the

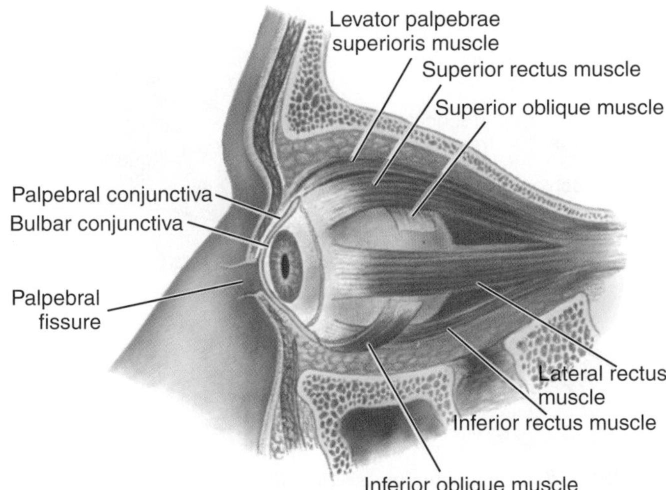


**FIGURE 18-3** Diagrammatic section of orbit. Medial rectus is located on nasal side of globe.

tone of the antagonistic muscles. According to the position of the rectus muscles on the eyes, they are referred to as the *superior rectus, inferior rectus, medial rectus,* and *lateral rectus.* The oblique muscles insert on the back of the eye and are designated the *superior oblique* and *inferior oblique.*

## Globe

The eyeball (globe) is supported in the orbital cavity on a cushion of fat and fascia. It is composed of three layers surrounding a fluid-filled center and occupies less than one third of the orbit. The external, corneoscleral layer is fibrous and protects the other two; the middle, vascular pigmented layer comprises the iris, ciliary body, and choroid; and the internal layer is the sensory retina. The fluid contents, which give the eye its globular shape, are aqueous humor (anterior to the lens) and vitreous humor (posterior to the lens). The lens, suspended behind the pupillary opening of the iris, and the cornea, combined with the aqueous and vitreous humor, form the refractive media of the eye (Figure 18-4).

***External Layer (Corneoscleral).*** The *cornea* is the anterior, transparent, avascular part of the external layer. It is crescent-shaped and joins the sclera at a transitional zone called the *limbus.* The cornea serves as a window through which light rays pass to the retina. The branches of the ophthalmic division of the fifth cranial nerve supply the cornea.

The cornea is composed of five layers: the epithelium, Bowman's membrane, the stroma, Descemet's membrane, and the endothelium (Figure 18-5). The epithelium consists of five constantly renewing cell layers and many nerve endings, which account for corneal sensitivity. Bowman's membrane is composed of connective tissue fibers and forms a barrier to trauma and infection. If damaged, it does not regenerate and a permanent scar is left. The stroma accounts for 90% of the corneal thickness and is composed of multiple lamellar fibers. Descemet's membrane is a thin layer between the endothelial layer of the cornea and the substantia propria. This membrane may become inflamed (descemetitis) or may protrude (descemetocele). The endothelium is a single layer of hexagonal cells that do not regenerate. These cells are responsible for the proper state of dehydration (deturgescence) that keeps the cornea clear. Damage to these cells causes corneal edema and loss of transparency.

The *sclera* is the posterior, opaque part of the external layer. A portion of the sclera can be seen through the conjunctiva as the white of the eye. The sclera is made up of collagenous fibers loosely connected with fascia, which receives the tendons of the muscles of the globe. The sclera is pierced by the ciliary

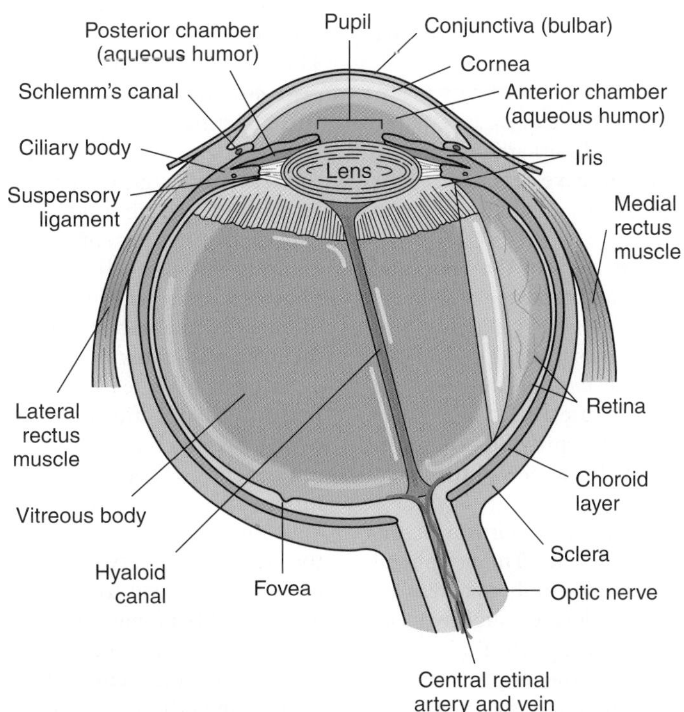


**FIGURE 18-4** Horizontal section through left globe.

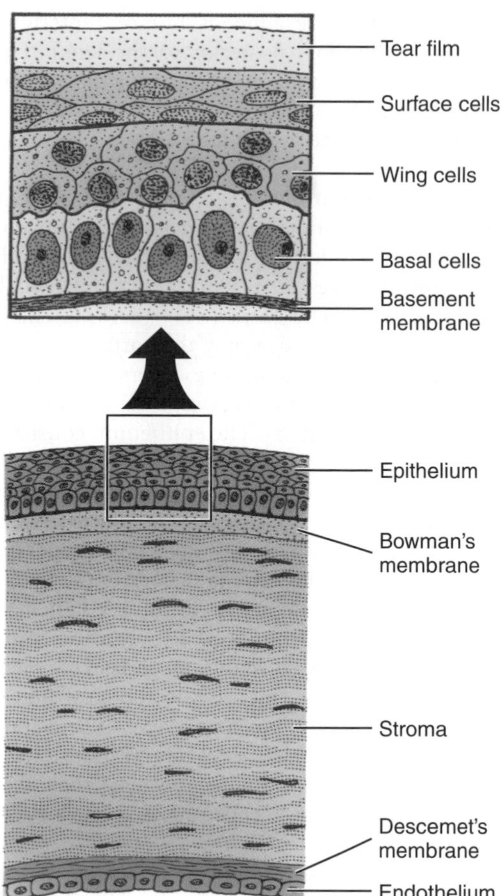


**FIGURE 18-5** Cornea is composed of five layers: the epithelium, Bowman's membrane, stroma, Descemet's membrane, and endothelium. *Inset*, Layers of epithelium.

arteries and nerves and posteriorly by the optic nerve (see Figure 18-4).

***Middle Layer.*** The middle covering of the eye comprises the choroid, ciliary body, and iris from behind forward (see Figure 18-4). The choroid contains many blood vessels and is the main source of nourishment of the receptor cell and pigment epithelial layer of the retina.

The *ciliary body* consists of an extension of the choroidal blood vessels, a mass of muscle tissue, and an extension of the neuroepithelium of the retina (Figure 18-6). It extends 6 to 6.5 mm from the root of the iris to the ora serrata. The anterior 2 mm of the ciliary body is called the *pars plicata,* and the posterior 4 to 5 mm is the *pars plana* (Figure 18-7). The ciliary muscle affects accommodation. The neuroepithelium is secretory in nature and is responsible for the formation of the aqueous humor.

The *iris,* a thin membrane, is the anterior portion of the middle layer and is situated in front of the lens. The peripheral border of the iris is attached to the ciliary body, whereas its central border is free. The iris aperture is located slightly nasal to its center, known as the *pupil* (see Figure 18-4). The iris divides the space between the cornea and the lens into an anterior and a posterior chamber. Both chambers are filled with aqueous humor.

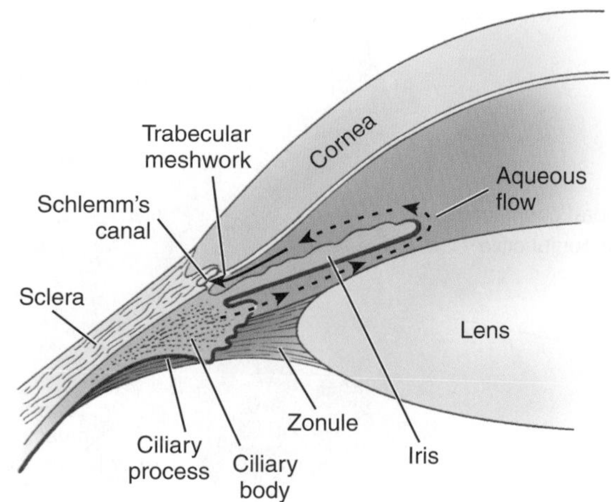


**FIGURE 18-6** Diagrammatic section of anterior chamber, ciliary body, and aqueous circulation.

The iris with its many striations regulates the amount of light entering the eye and assists in obtaining clear images. The iris moves by means of smooth muscle fibers within the connective tissue. The sphincter pupillae muscle contracts the pupil, and the dilator pupillae dilates it. As more light strikes the eye, the sphincter constricts the pupil.

***Internal Layer.*** The innermost layer, sometimes called the *nervous covering,* is the retina, a thin, transparent membrane extending from the ora serrata to the optic disc (Figure 18-8). This network of nerve cells and fibers receives images of external objects and transfers the impression through the optic nerve, optic tracts, lateral geniculate body, and optic radiations to the occipital lobe of the cerebrum. The nerve fibers from the retina converge to become the optic nerve, which enters the eyeball almost at its posterior point, slightly to the inner side. The point at which the nerve enters the eyeball is called the *optic disc.* In field testing, this is the anatomic blind spot.

The retina is composed of many layers. The pigment epithelium is a single layer of epithelial cells on the external side of the retina through which oxygen and other nutrients are diffused from the choroid. The other nine layers of the retina consist of photoreceptor cells (rods and cones) and sensory neurons (bipolar cells and ganglion cells) (Figure 18-9). The photoreceptors within the retina respond to light energy and initiate the neural response, which is eventually interpreted in the occipital cortex.

The macula lutea shows as a yellow spot in the center of the retina located 2 mm from the optic disc. The fovea centralis, which is a pit consisting of a layer of closely packed cone cells in the center of the macula, is responsible for the highest resolution and central vision.

An inverted image of the object being viewed is focused on the retina. The nerve fibers, leaving the retina by way of the optic nerve, travel to the lateral geniculate body of the thalamus. The fibers, nasal to the fovea, cross in the optic chiasma to go to the contralateral geniculate body. Thus all fibers composing the same half of the visual field project to the same geniculate body, from which fibers project to the ipsilateral occipital cortex for interpretation (Figure 18-10).

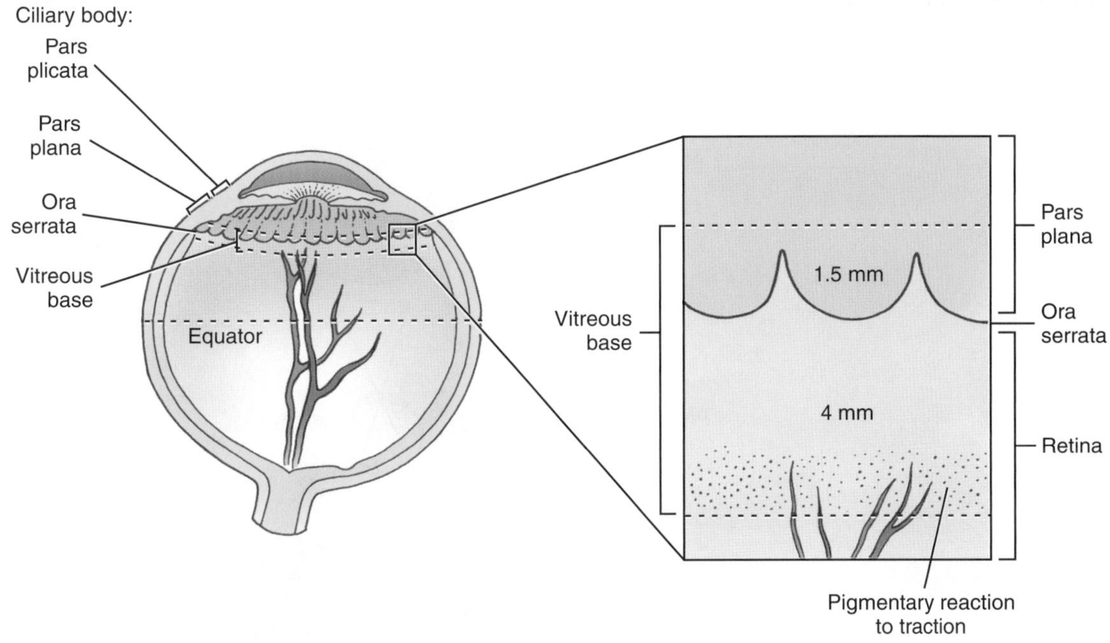


**FIGURE 18-7** Location of the pars plicata, the pars plana, and the ora serrata.

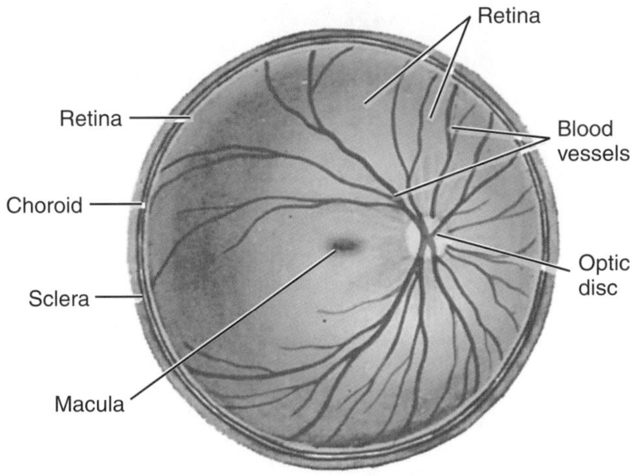

**FIGURE 18-8** Normal fundus of eye seen through ophthalmoscope.

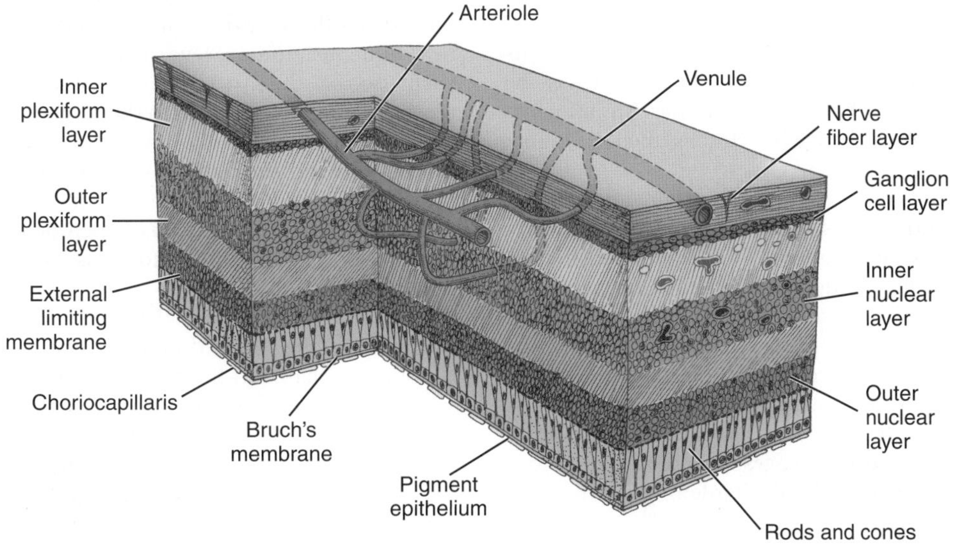

**FIGURE 18-9** Retinal layers. Retinal arterioles provide two major capillary layers in retina: one in nerve fiber layer and one in inner nuclear layer. In general, diseases affecting primarily arteries, such as vascular hypertension, involve capillary network in nerve fiber layer, whereas predominantly venous diseases, such as diabetes mellitus, involve layer of capillaries in inner nuclear layer. Outer receptors, together with their cell bodies in outer nuclear layer and portion of outer plexiform layer, are nurtured by choriocapillaris of the choroid. Both systems are necessary to the function of the retina.

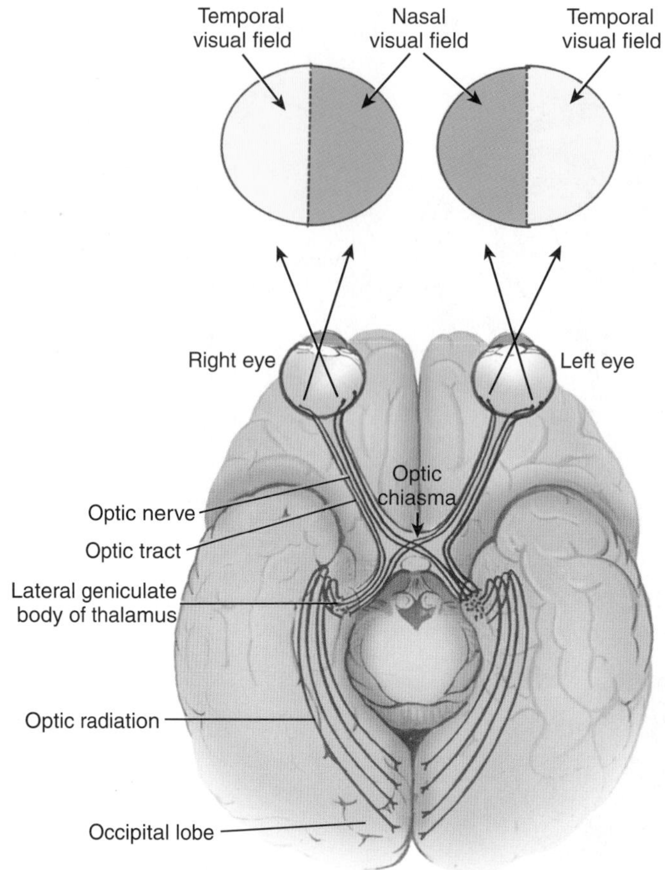


**FIGURE 18-10** Visual pathways. Note structures that compose each pathway: optic nerve, optic chiasma, lateral geniculate body of thalamus, optic radiations, and visual cortex of occipital lobe. Fibers from nasal portion of each retina cross over to opposite side at optic chiasma, hence terminating in lateral geniculate body of opposite side. Location of lesion in visual pathway determines resulting visual defect. For example, destruction of an optic nerve produces permanent blindness in same eye, and pressure on optic chiasma (e.g., by pituitary tumor) produces bitemporal hemianopsia, or more simply blindness in both temporal visual fields, because it destroys fibers from nasal sides of both retinas.

## Refractive Apparatus

The refractive apparatus consists of the cornea, the aqueous humor, the lens, and the vitreous body. The cornea has the greatest refractive power of the ocular structures. Variations in the curvature of the cornea change its refractive power (Figure 18-11).

The lens of the eye is biconvex and has a diameter of 1 cm. It is suspended behind the iris and connected to the ciliary body by zonular fibers (see Figure 18-6). A rounded border, the equator, separates its anterior and posterior surfaces. The crystalline lens does not shed cells. As it grows, the cells are compressed and harden. The lens can expand and retract by means of the zonular fibers (accommodation); this accommodative power is lost with the aging process, as the lens loses its elasticity when the cells harden. This visual defect, known as *presbyopia,* usually occurs between ages 40 and 45 years and is corrected with bifocals. Eventually the hardening causes opacity of the lens—a cataract.

The vitreous body is a glasslike, transparent, gelatinous mass composed of 99% water and 1% collagen and hyaluronic acid. It fills the posterior four fifths of the eyeball and is adherent to the retina at the vitreous base.

The eye functions similarly to a camera. Light rays from an object pass through the system of refractory devices—the cornea, aqueous humor, lens, and vitreous—and are refracted (bent) so that the rays strike the retina.[6] For information to be received correctly and sent to the cerebral cortex, all structures must function together to focus the light rays. The lens must be able to bend the light waves correctly and bring an object into clear focus. Refractive errors, or errors in focusing ability, occur when the cornea is misshapen or when the lens cannot appropriately change shape to focus images.[20]

## Nerve and Blood Supply

The optic nerve (second cranial nerve) extends between the posterior eyeball and the optic chiasma. This nerve carries visual impulses, as well as the sensations of pain, touch, and temperature, from the eye and its surrounding structures to the brain. The third cranial nerve (oculomotor) is the primary motor nerve to all rectus muscles except the lateral rectus, which is innervated by the sixth cranial nerve (abducens). The fourth cranial nerve (trochlear) innervates the superior oblique muscle. This motor nerve supply to the extraocular muscles is easy to remember using a pseudo formula of LR6(SO4)3—lateral rectus by the sixth cranial nerve (abducens), superior oblique

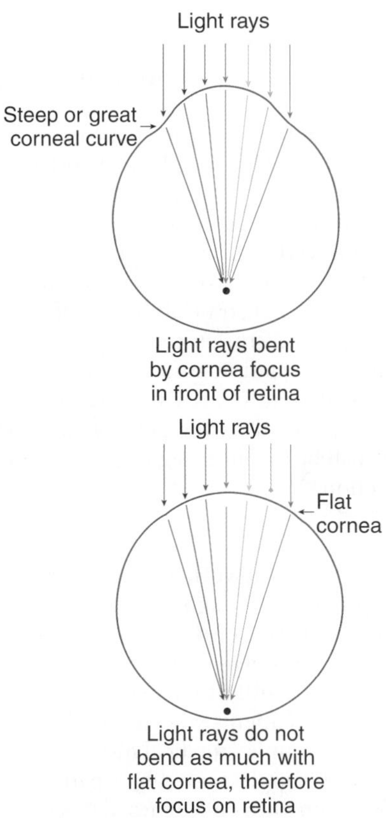
Light rays
Steep or great corneal curve
Light rays bent by cornea focus in front of retina
Light rays
Flat cornea
Light rays do not bend as much with flat cornea, therefore focus on retina

**FIGURE 18-11** Variations in the curvature of the cornea change its refractive power.

by the fourth cranial nerve (trochlear), and the remainder of the extraocular muscles by branches of the third cranial nerve (oculomotor).

Injection of local anesthetic into the lateral adipose compartment from an inferior temporal needle insertion blocks the nasociliary, lacrimal, frontal, supraorbital, and supratrochlear branches of the ophthalmic division of the trigeminal nerve and infraorbital branch of the maxillary division.

The ophthalmic artery, the main arterial supply to the orbit and globe, is a branch of the internal carotid artery. It divides into branches supplying the globe, muscles, and eyelids. The central retinal artery and central retinal vein travel through the optic nerve and provide an independent circulation for the inner retina.

# *Perioperative Nursing Considerations*

## Assessment

Patients scheduled for eye surgery exhibit many emotions and reactions. Of prime concern to most is the success of the surgical procedure. Patients undergoing eye surgery vary from infants with congenital conditions to elderly patients whose conditions result from the aging process. Perioperative nursing, based on a caring process, should focus on providing assurance, delivering information in terms that are understandable, performing patient care activities with skill, being respectful of the patient's feelings and needs, and including the patient in planning his or her care whenever possible.[22]

The perioperative nursing staff must be prepared to meet the specific needs of each patient and family, collaborate and communicate effectively for continuity of patient care, and prepare the patient for home care. Preparation is begun in the physician's office or clinic. Communication with the physician's office staff to coordinate patient preparation and teaching and to collate preoperative test results increases the efficiency and effectiveness of preoperative procedures. Preoperative phone calls to the patient are used to provide needed information concerning the day of surgery and sometimes are used to obtain initial preoperative assessment.

Most patients are admitted through an ambulatory admission area adjacent to the surgical suites. On admission, a staff member should fully orient the patient to the physical surroundings. Constant description and reinforcement are important to visually impaired patients. Approaching the patient from the unaffected side increases the patient's independence and decreases the possibility of startling the patient.

The assessment is designed to collect and disseminate pertinent information and must be carried out in a comprehensive, yet efficient, manner. A standard set of parameters should provide enough information to facilitate appropriate care in the event of an emergency. Physiologic information (e.g., height, weight, vital signs), psychosocial factors (e.g., support systems, fears, anxiety), and environmental, education, and self-care needs are assessed. The general health history includes current medication therapy and whether the patient has brought medications along. Because ocular problems may be directly related to other diseases, the medical history is very important. Additional discharge planning factors are also explored.

Data may be collected from family or significant others or directly from physicians or their office staff. All information should be documented so that it is readily available to others. An ocular history, which includes the patient's primary problem, history of the present condition, symptoms, and visual limitations, is collected. An external examination of the eye, including lids, lashes, conjunctiva, and lacrimal apparatus, should be performed to detect any deviations from normal. The corneal reflex should be tested and the cornea inspected for superficial irregularities. Pupil size and contour, as well as pupillary reaction, both direct and consensual, should be noted. Anterior chamber depth should be checked with oblique illumination to alert staff members to the potential for angle closure with dilation of the pupil. When a light is shined from the side of the pupil, if the entire iris is illuminated, the anterior chamber depth is normal; however, when half of the iris is in shadow, the anterior chamber is considered to be shallow.

The function of the extraocular muscles should be determined. Movement should be synchronous, and visual lines should meet on a fixed object. Documentation of this examination must be descriptive, accurate, and concise. It is of value later in assessing the outcome of the procedure. The following observations should be obtained or confirmed during assessment:

- General appearance of the eye (edema, asymmetry, redness, condition of conjunctiva, sclera, and skin around eyes)
- Symptoms of irritation (itching, burning)
- Position of eyelids (opened and closed), condition of upper and lower lid surfaces, eyelid spasm

- Visual acuity, pupillary dilation (note whether pupils are equal, round, reactive to light, and accommodative), visual fields
- Extraocular muscle movement
- Drainage from eye
- Vital signs
- Restlessness, discomfort, anxiety
- Limitations in mobility
- Presence of prosthesis
- Current and significant past medical problems (eye disease, diabetes, cardiovascular disease, hypertension, allergies)
- Current medication history, including anticoagulants, analgesics, herbs, and nutritional supplements

***Laboratory Studies.*** The results of laboratory studies that were performed should be reviewed during the assessment. Deviations from normal should be noted, documented, and reported.

- Blood glucose (70 to 105 mg/dl): increase in normal range after age 50 years; may be higher or lower depending on intake; critical levels are less than 50 or more than 400 mg/dl in adult males and less than 40 or more than 400 mg/dl in adult females[13]
- Serum potassium (adults, including elders: 3.5 to 5 mEq/L) and other electrolytes (calcium: total 9 to 10.5 mg/dl, ionized 4.5 to 5.6 mg/dl; sodium: 136 to 145 mEq/L)[13]
- Serum enzymes and other blood work (hemoglobin: males 14 to 18 g/dl, females 12 to 16 g/dl, elderly values slightly decreased; hematocrit: males 42% to 52%, females 37% to 47%, elderly values slightly decreased)[13]
- Coagulation studies (bleeding time: 1 to 9 minutes, critical value more than 12 minutes; prothrombin time [pro-time, PT]: 11.0 to 12.5 seconds, critical value more than 20 seconds; activated partial thromboplastin time [APTT]: 30 to 40 seconds, critical value more than 70 seconds; partial thromboplastin time [PTT]: 60 to 70 seconds, critical value more than 100 seconds)[13]

***Electrocardiogram and Chest X-ray Examination.*** In older adults, chest x-ray examination and an electrocardiogram (ECG) may be prescribed; if so, these reports should be on the patient's record. The older adult is more predisposed to respiratory infection from less elastic alveoli, decreased heart size unless there is enlargement associated with hypertension or heart disease, and ECG changes secondary to cellular alteration, conduction system fibrosis, and neurogenic changes.

After the assessment information has been compiled, nursing diagnoses are identified and the plan of care for the entire perioperative period is developed.

## Nursing Diagnosis

Nursing diagnoses related to the care of patients undergoing ophthalmic surgery might include the following:

- Deficient Knowledge related to diagnosis, surgical intervention, and home care management
- Anxiety related to vision loss, surgical intervention, awake status during surgical intervention, and surgical outcome
- Disturbed Sensory Perception related to visual impairment, surgical intervention, and patching of operative eye or both eyes
- Acute Pain related to increased intraocular pressure and surgical intervention
- Risk for Infection related to surgical intervention

## Outcome Identification

Outcomes identified for the selected nursing diagnoses could be stated as follows:

- The patient, family, or significant others will verbalize knowledge of the diagnosis, planned surgical intervention, medication management, and requirements for home care maintenance before discharge.
- The patient will verbalize an acceptable level of anxiety and use personally effective coping mechanisms.
- The patient will demonstrate ability to safely adapt to visual sensory perception disturbances.[21]
- The patient will remain comfortable during surgical intervention and will identify activities that increase intraocular pressure to be avoided during postoperative period.
- The patient will be free from signs and symptoms of postoperative infection.

## Planning

Plans of care are the framework for organizing activities in the perioperative period. Although ophthalmic surgery is often perceived as minor because of the small incision site and because many procedures generally are not lengthy, the perioperative nurse must be fully prepared for potential complications or emergencies. Patients who are admitted for ophthalmic surgery often have complex medical histories. After a review of the patient's record, supplemented by a patient or family interview or collaboration with colleagues, data collected are incorporated into a perioperative plan of care. A typical plan of care for a patient undergoing ophthalmic surgery follows (p. 593).

## Implementation

***Managing and Monitoring Patient Safety Needs.*** Because many ophthalmic procedures are performed with local anesthesia, the circulating nurse or an additional perioperative nurse must be prepared to monitor the patient and provide supportive care. Reassurance is especially important for patients who are awake. Ophthalmic patients, like other surgical patients, have increased sensitivity to noise and activities within the room. The room should be kept quiet and peaceful to decrease anxiety and increase cooperation, thereby reducing the need for heavy sedation.

Both the scrub person and the circulating nurse must also manage additional patient safety needs. Foreign substances must not be introduced intraocularly. Lint-free drapes should be used to create the sterile field. If powder-free gloves are not used, gloved hands must be wiped with moistened gauze sponges to remove starch powder particles before the procedure begins. Gloved hands should not touch the portion of an instrument used in an intraocular wound, and debris should be cleansed from instruments with cellulose sponges. The entire surgical team must be knowledgeable about their roles and be prepared to function quickly in the event of a complication or emergency.

Members of the perioperative nursing team have several important responsibilities in the preparation of the room and the equipment. Technologic advances in ophthalmic surgery require that perioperative nurses be familiar with equipment and check each piece carefully before the patient arrives in the operating room. The availability of specially ordered implants or prostheses needs to be checked to prevent delay or cancellation of the procedure. Scrupulous attention to aseptic technique

## SAMPLE PLAN OF CARE

**NURSING DIAGNOSIS**

**Deficient Knowledge** related to diagnosis, surgical intervention, and home care management

**OUTCOME**

The patient, family, or significant others will verbalize knowledge of the diagnosis, planned surgical intervention, medication management, and requirements for home care maintenance before discharge.

**INTERVENTIONS**

- Review the surgeon's explanation of the procedure and the reason for it.
- Determine the patient's understanding of the diagnosis, the planned intervention, and the type of anesthesia to be administered.
- Clarify misconceptions and provide additional explanations (refer to appropriate member of health care team as needed).
- Explain sequence of perioperative events and what to expect in terms that the patient can understand. If topical anesthetic is planned, advise the patient to expect to be asked to keep eyes open and to look up or down.
- Review postoperative limitations to self-care activities.
- Provide and review written instructions (in large letters) and diagrams regarding medications, including specific techniques for instilling eyedrops and ophthalmic medications; applying compresses (as necessary); and applying appropriate eye patch, dressing, or protective shield.
- Demonstrate and supervise patient or family practice with prescribed self-care activities (e.g., instillation of medications).

**NURSING DIAGNOSIS**

**Anxiety** related to vision loss, surgical intervention, awake status during surgical intervention, and surgical outcome

**OUTCOME**

The patient will verbalize an acceptable level of anxiety and use personally effective coping mechanisms.

**INTERVENTIONS**

- Allow the patient time to verbalize concerns.
- Assist the patient in identifying sources of anxiety.
- Help the patient identify existing personal strengths and external resources; reinforce personally effective coping mechanisms.
- Encourage independence by having the patient participate in his or her plan of care; involve patient in identifying diversional activities.
- Observe the patient's facial expressions, body posture, and vital signs.
- Broadly classify the patient's level of anxiety, based on nursing observation (low, moderate, high).
- Offer comfort measures (e.g., warm blankets, a pillow for under knees).
- Provide emotional support; reinforce information the patient has been previously given.
- Use touch (as appropriate) to communicate reassurance.
- Control environmental stimuli in the operating room.

**NURSING DIAGNOSIS**

**Disturbed Sensory Perception** related to visual impairment, surgical intervention, and patching of operative eye or both eyes

**OUTCOME**

The patient will demonstrate ability to safely adapt to visually disturbed sensory perception.

**INTERVENTIONS**

- Introduce self and other team members so that patient can recognize voices.
- Familiarize and orient patient to immediate surroundings; continuously reorient patient.
- Approach patient from unaffected side.
- Offer reassurance, explanations, and understanding.
- Before discharge, review and have the patient repeat back in his or her own words safety measures to prevent falls and other injuries.
- Make referral to appropriate agency if home assistance is required.

**NURSING DIAGNOSIS**

**Acute Pain** related to increased intraocular pressure and surgical intervention

**OUTCOME**

The patient will remain comfortable during surgical intervention as determined by response on a verbal pain scale.

**INTERVENTIONS**

- Instruct patient to verbalize pain during procedure under local anesthesia or sedation; use a verbal pain rating scale.
- Observe for physical signs of pain, such as facial grimacing, groaning, muscle tightening, or changes in vital signs.
- If using local anesthesia, alert physician to any patient reports of significant pain from the injection or signs of toxicity (e.g., tinnitus, tingling around the mouth).
- During procedure, make sure patient understands what is happening (e.g., stinging or pressure from local anesthetic injection) and how long it will last.
- Monitor the presence of or an increase in eye pain, pain around orbit, blurred vision, reddened eye, abdominal pain, nausea, vomiting, neurologic changes, and changes in visual fields; initiate appropriate action.
- Instruct the patient to refrain from excessive exertion, such as crying, coughing, straining, overlifting, bending, rubbing the eyes, and blowing the nose postoperatively.
- Discuss other methods to promote patient comfort, such as music, guided imagery, relaxation techniques.

**NURSING DIAGNOSIS**

**Risk for Infection** related to surgical intervention

**OUTCOME**

The patient will be free from signs and symptoms of surgical site infection.

**INTERVENTIONS**

- Preoperatively, document whether the patient has a preexisting infection, is immunocompromised, or has other conditions that compromise resistance to infection.
- Maintain an aseptic perioperative environment.
- Adhere to good handwashing practices.
- Determine and record the wound classification.
- Postoperatively, monitor vital signs, fluid balance, and presence of pain.
- Instruct the patient and family in self-care, including postoperative antibiotic therapy if prescribed.
- Teach the patient and family to wash hands before the instillation of any ophthalmic medications.
- Instruct the patient and family to watch for redness, pain, swelling, drainage, and changes in visual acuity postoperatively and to report these problems promptly to the physician.

and perioperative nursing interventions designed for safety and comfort of the patient is of prime importance. The duties of the perioperative nursing team include the following:

1. Identifying the patient by name; seeking the patient's cooperation and confidence by speaking softly, distinctly, and confidently; and endeavoring to keep the patient reassured and relaxed by staying close by and establishing contact by touch.
2. Checking the patient's name on the wristband with the name on the chart and surgical schedule and orally confirming it with the patient or a family member. The patient or family member should also state which eye is being operated on and which procedure is being performed.
3. Reviewing the surgical consent, surgeon's preoperative orders, and operating room (OR) schedule to determine if the correct operative eye has been prepared (including verification of operative eye using the word "right" or "left [abbreviations are not accepted], marking of operative site, and dilation, if appropriate) and other procedures have been carried out according to facility policies on correct-site surgery. Such a policy may require that, before the administration of eyedrops or medication, the nurse asks the awake patient which eye is being operated on. If there is any discrepancy among the patient's response, the informed consent, the physician's orders, ophthalmic history, and exam, the discrepancy is corrected during the preoperative verification process. Immediately before the incision, this information is re-confirmed during the time out.[2]
4. Preparing the surgical microscope and ensuring that all the necessary attachments are ready.
5. Preparing the OR bed or ophthalmology stretcher and ensuring that all the necessary attachments are ready. An ophthalmology stretcher is a special transport gurney tapered at one end to allow the surgeon close access to the patient's head. The patient remains on the ophthalmology stretcher throughout the procedure; it may also be used preoperatively and postoperatively. Because patients may receive hyperosmotic drugs, which induce diuresis, have urinals, bedpans, and sterile catheters available.
6. Starting an intravenous (IV) drip or inserting a heparin lock, placing the blood pressure cuff and pulse oximeter, recording the baseline blood pressure and heart rate, and attaching the cardiac monitor according to facility policy. When the patient is not managed with monitored anesthesia care (MAC), an oxygen cannula should be available for administration of oxygen if needed.
7. Observing laser safety precautions.
8. Documenting care including recording of implants and lot numbers.

***Safety Measures in Administering Medications.*** Medications used in the perioperative period are extremely important to the outcome of the procedure and the safety of the patient. Drugs for diagnosing and treating eye disorders are potent. One error could result in total, irreversible blindness (see Chapter 2 for a discussion of medication safety).

The patient's medical and ocular histories determine the selection of an appropriate ophthalmic agent. This information should be included in the patient's initial assessment. The perioperative nurse needs to be aware that mydriatic and cycloplegic eyedrops are contraindicated in narrow-angle glaucoma.

The following established protocols for medication administration greatly reduce the possibility of medication errors:

1. The perioperative nurse must be knowledgeable about the specific medication ordered, including purpose, strength, action, duration, adverse reactions, route of administration, and contraindications.
2. The medication label must be checked for name, strength, and expiration date during preparation and before medication administration. This precaution is especially important because many ophthalmic drugs are distributed in single-dose units that closely resemble one another.
3. The patient must be positively identified, and the site of the administration must be clearly translated from the physician's orders. Abbreviations should not be used. The words "right eye," "left eye," or "both eyes" should be used in writing orders.
4. The precise dosage of medication must be given at its scheduled time to enhance its effectiveness.
5. Handwashing between patients when administering eyedrops is imperative, and Standard Precautions should be followed.
6. All solutions on and off the sterile field must be clearly labeled, and intraocular solutions must be separated from those not used intraocularly.

***Instillation of Eyedrops.*** There is a growing trend to use pledgets to administer preoperative eyedrops (e.g., mydriatics, cycloplegic drugs) after the administration of local anesthetic drops. When this method is used, the perioperative nurse soaks the pledgets in the prescribed medication in a sterile cup. After waiting a few minutes for the local anesthetic drops to take effect, a sterile forceps is used to place the medication-soaked pledget in the cul-de-sac of the operative eye. The pledget stays in the eye for 10 to 15 minutes. Institutions should have standardized pledget medication regimens.

When eyedrops are administered using a dropper, the perioperative nurse should wash his or her hands and wear gloves, maintaining Standard Precautions. The patient may be supine or sitting, with the head tilted back slightly. The patient should be requested to look upward and the lower eyelid gently pulled open to expose the lower conjunctival sac (Figure 18-12). The prescribed number of drops is then administered without touching the tip of the dropper to the eye or the nurse's fingers.[9] Avoid placing eyedrops directly onto the cornea. The natural blink-

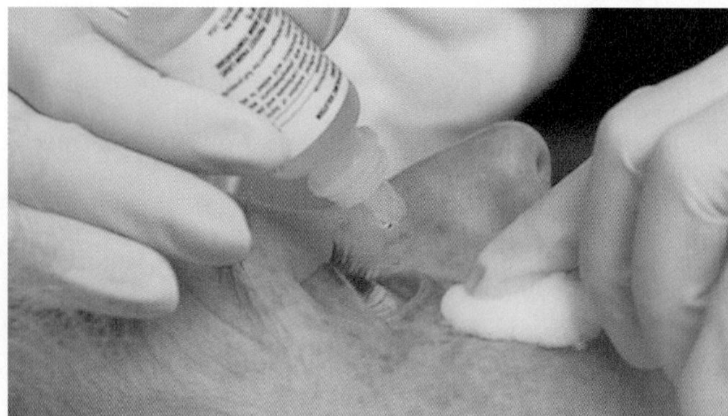

**FIGURE 18-12** Proper position of head for instillation of eyedrops. Gentle retraction of lower lid is necessary for drop to be placed in lower conjunctival sac.

ing of the lids distributes the drug evenly onto the eye surface. When anesthetic eyedrops are instilled for topical anesthesia, they are placed on the cornea and the patient is instructed to keep the eye closed to avoid the drop's drying effect on the cornea.

After instillation of a systemic drug, such as atropine, hold light finger pressure over the lacrimal duct for 1 minute to prevent absorption into the circulatory system. When a toxic drug is instilled, the inner corners of the eyelids should be dried of excessive fluid with a tissue or clean cotton ball after each drop to minimize systemic absorption of the drug.

The patient should be made aware of the expected effect of each medication to be able to evaluate its effectiveness, detect signs and symptoms of adverse reactions, and know when to notify the perioperative personnel concerning problems. The patient should also be well informed of the special considerations associated with specific medications so that appropriate safety precautions can be taken. An example is protection of the cornea after application of a topical anesthetic.

***Ophthalmic Pharmacology.*** Numerous medications are used during ophthalmic surgery. See the Surgical Pharmacology table for the purpose and description of each.

### *Anesthesia*

**GENERAL ANESTHESIA.** Youth, deafness, language barriers, dementia, severe anxiety, specific systemic diseases, known sensitivity to local anesthetics, and long duration of the operative procedure are among the conditions that may dictate use of general anesthesia.

**LOCAL ANESTHESIA.** Local anesthesia or MAC is used for most eye surgery. Consideration must be given to the patient's age, systemic condition, and discharge plan in determining whether to use preoperative sedation, such as sublingual midazolam hydrochloride (Versed). Intraoperative sedation, when indicated, may be prescribed and managed by either the anesthesia provider or surgeon. The perioperative nurse, however, is often accountable for monitoring the patient's response to the sedation and the local anesthetic in the perioperative period.

The circulating nurse assembles the sterile local anesthesia setup as required by the surgeon before the patient enters the operating room, checking to ensure correct medications, proper concentrations and dosages, and needles and syringes of appropriate sizes and gauges. Local anesthetics should not be mixed far in advance of the time of intended use, because they may deteriorate, producing a reduced effect for the patient. The addition of epinephrine prolongs the duration of action of most local anesthetics.

**Administration Methods of Local Anesthesia.** The *topical method* of local anesthesia has gained popularity for cataract-extraction procedures. A combination of anesthetic eyedrops is instilled into the eye and may be supplemented with infiltration anesthetic into the anterior chamber. Selection of patients for the topical method requires that they can cooperate and follow verbal commands to keep their eyes open and look up or down. Conditions that render the patient a poor candidate for topical anesthesia include inability to tolerate eyedrops, Alzheimer's disease, extreme anxiety, and communication problems (e.g., language barriers, hearing impairment, auditory aphasia).

The *infiltration method* involves the surgeon injecting the anesthetic solution beneath the skin, beneath the conjunctiva (subconjunctival), or into Tenon's capsule, depending on the type of surgery (Best Practice).

The most common technique for regional anesthesia in eye surgery is a *peribulbar block*. The anesthetic is injected around the soft tissue of the globe after the needle is directed to the floor (inferior) or roof (superior) of the orbit (Figure 18-13).

*Retrobulbar block* is injection of anesthetic solution into the base of the eyelids at the level of the orbital margins or behind the eyeball to block the ciliary ganglion and nerves (Figure 18-14). For eyelid repairs, the solution is injected through the upper or lower lid. For operations on the lacrimal apparatus, the anesthetic is injected at the level of the anterior ethmoidal foramen to anesthetize the internal and external nasal nerves. Retrobulbar injection is usually performed 10 to 15 minutes before surgery to produce temporary paralysis of the extraocular muscles. Potential risks of retrobulbar injection are hemorrhage, ptosis, conjunctival or eyelid bruising, globe penetration, optic nerve damage, central vein and artery occlusion, and brainstem anesthesia and death.[8]

***Positioning.*** Positioning the patient for ophthalmic surgery generally requires additional devices for stabilizing the head, protecting bony prominences, and providing appropriate alignment to prevent peripheral neurovascular injury. The ophthalmology stretcher, which is a combination transport device and OR bed, is often used for convenience and comfort as the surgical bed. This special bed, with a tapered head end, allows for closer access to the patient's face and eliminates several transfers for the patient. The perioperative nurse positions the patient with a foam donut or headrest under the head and a pillow under the knees; he or she pads the arms before securing them at the patient's side.

The safety needs of the patient are related to age, size, and risk factors for discomfort. If patients are to be sedated, ask them if they are comfortable and reassure them that there are ways to make them more comfortable. Some elderly patients prefer not to discuss their discomfort for fear of being bothersome.

In addition, because most ocular surgery is carried out with the use of a microscope, a special wrist rest is used to stabilize the surgeon's hands and may include a perforated tubing or bar to provide oxygen under the drapes. This should be attached to the bed and secured approximately 2.5 cm below the lateral canthus before the patient is draped. The wrist rest may be placed unilaterally or may encircle the head. A 2.5-cm strip of nonallergenic tape may be placed over the patient's forehead (avoiding the eyebrows) and secured to the operative bed to prevent movement of the head.

***Prepping.*** The operative site is prepped under aseptic conditions, usually after the anesthetic is administered. A sterile prep tray containing sterile normal saline solution, irrigation bulb, basins, gauze sponges, cotton-tipped applicators, towels, and antimicrobial skin disinfectant is prepared.

If eyelashes are clipped, it is done before the skin prep. A thin film of water-soluble lubricant is smoothed over the cutting surfaces of a curved eyelash scissors so that the free lashes adhere to the blades rather than fall into the eyes or onto the face.

## SURGICAL PHARMACOLOGY

### Medications Used During Ophthalmic Surgery

| Drug/Name | Purpose/Description |
|---|---|
| **MYDRIATICS** | |
| Phenylephrine (Neo-Synephrine, Mydfrin), 2.5%, 10% | Mydriasis (dilates the pupil but permits focusing), used for objective examination of the retina, testing of refraction, easier removal of lens; used alone or with a cycloplegic |
| **CYCLOPLEGICS** | |
| Tropicamide (Mydriacyl), 1% | Cycloplegia (paralysis of accommodation; inhibits focusing); dilates the pupil; anticholinergic, used for examination of fundus, refraction |
| Atropine, 1% | Anticholinergic, dilates pupil, inhibits focusing; potent, long duration (7-14 days) |
| Cyclopentolate (Cyclogyl), 1%, 2% | Anticholinergic, dilates pupil, inhibits focusing |
| Scopolamine hydrobromide (Isopto-Hyoscine), 0.25% | Anticholinergic, dilates pupil, inhibits focusing |
| Homatropine hydrobromide (Isopto Homatropine), 2%, 5% | Anticholinergic, dilates pupil, inhibits focusing |
| Epinephrine (1:1000) preservative free (PF) | Dilates the pupil; added to bottles of balanced salt solution for irrigation to maintain pupil dilation during cataract or vitrectomy procedure |
| **MIOTICS** | |
| Carbachol (Miostat), 0.01% | Potent cholinergic, constricts pupil, used intraocularly during anterior segment surgery |
| Carbachol (Isopto Carbachol), 0.75%, 1.5%, 2.25%, 3% | Potent cholinergic, constricts pupil, used topically for lowering intraocular pressure in glaucoma |
| Acetylcholine chloride (Miochol-E), 1% | Cholinergic, rapidly constricts pupil, used intraocularly during anterior segment surgery; reconstitute immediately before using |
| Pilocarpine hydrochloride, 1%, 4% | Cholinergic, constricts pupil, used topically for lowering intraocular pressure in glaucoma |
| **TOPICAL ANESTHETICS** | |
| Tetracaine hydrochloride (Pontocaine), 0.5% | *Onset:* 5-20 sec; *duration of action:* 10-20 min |
| Proparacaine hydrochloride (Ophthaine), 0.5% | *Onset:* 5-20 sec; *duration of action:* 10-20 min |
| **INJECTABLE ANESTHETICS** | |
| Lidocaine (Xylocaine), 1%, 2%, 4% | *Onset:* 4-6 min; *duration of action:* 40-60 min, 120 min with epinephrine |
| Methylparaben free (MPF) | Preservative free; adjunct to topical anesthesia |
| Bupivacaine (Marcaine, Sensorcaine), 0.25%, 0.50%, 0.75% | *Onset:* 5-11 min; *duration of action:* 480-720 min with epinephrine; often used in 0.75% combination with lidocaine for blocks |
| Mepivacaine (Carbocaine), 1%, 2% | *Onset:* 3-5 min; *duration of action:* 120 min; duration of action greater with epinephrine |
| Etidocaine (Duranest), 1% | *Onset:* 3 min; *duration of action:* 300-600 min |
| **ADDITIVES TO LOCAL ANESTHETICS** | |
| Epinephrine 1:50,000-1:200,000 | Combined with injectable local anesthetics to prolong anesthesia and reduce bleeding |
| Hyaluronidase | Enzyme mixed with anesthetics (75 units/10 ml) to increase diffusion of anesthetic through tissue, improving the effectiveness of the block; contraindicated if skin inflammation or malignancy present |
| **VISCOELASTICS** | |
| Sodium hyaluronate (Healon, Amvisc, Provisc, Vitrax) in a sterile syringe assembly with blunt-tipped cannula | Lubricant and support; maintains separation between tissues to protect the endothelium and maintain the anterior chamber intraocularly; removed from anterior chamber to prevent postoperative increase in pressure; should be refrigerated (except Vitrax); allow 30 min to warm to room temperature |
| Sodium chondroitin–sodium hyaluronate (Viscoat) in a sterile syringe assembly with blunt-tipped cannula | Maintains a deep chamber for anterior segment procedures, protects epithelium of cornea, and enhances visualization; may be used to coat intraocular lens before implantation; should be refrigerated |
| Duovisc | Packages of separate syringes of Provisc and Viscoat in the same box |
| **VISCOADHERENTS** | |
| Hydroxypropyl methylcellulose 2% (Occucoat) in a sterile syringe assembly with blunt-tipped cannula | Maintains a deep chamber for anterior segment procedures, protects epithelium of cornea, and may be used to coat intraocular lens before implantation; removed from anterior chamber at end of procedure; stored at room temperature |
| Hydroxyethylcellulose (Gonioscopic Prism Solution) | Bonds gonioscopic prisms to the eye; stored at room temperature |
| Hydroxypropyl methylcellulose 2.5% (Goniosol) | Bonds gonioscopic prisms to the eye; stored at room temperature |

## SURGICAL PHARMACOLOGY

### Medications Used During Ophthalmic Surgery—cont'd

| Drug/Name | Purpose/Description |
|---|---|
| **IRRIGANTS** | |
| Balanced salt solution (BSS, Endosol) | Used to keep cornea moist during surgery; also used as internal irrigant into anterior or posterior segment |
| Balanced salt solution enriched with bicarbonate, dextrose, and glutathione (BSS Plus, Endosol Extra) | Used as internal irrigant into anterior or posterior segment; need to reconstitute immediately before use by addition of part I to part II with transfer device |
| **HYPEROSMOTIC AGENTS** | |
| Mannitol (Osmitrol) | Intravenous (IV) osmotic diuretic; increases the osmolarity of the plasma, causing osmotic pressure gradient to pull free fluid from the eye to the plasma and reduces the intraocular pressure |
| Glycerin (Osmoglyn, Glyrol) | Oral osmotic diuretic given in chilled juice or cola; increases the osmolarity of the plasma, causing osmotic pressure gradient to pull free fluid from the eye to the plasma and reduces the intraocular pressure |
| **ANTIINFLAMMATORY AGENTS** | |
| Betamethasone sodium phosphate and betamethasone acetate suspension (Celestone) | Glucocorticoid; injected subconjunctivally after surgery for prophylaxis; also used to treat severe allergic and inflammatory conditions |
| Dexamethasone (Decadron) | Adrenocortical steroid; injected subconjunctivally after surgery for prophylaxis; also used to treat severe allergic and inflammatory conditions and intraocularly for endophthalmitis |
| Methylprednisolone acetate suspension (Depo-Medrol) | Glucocorticoid; injected subconjunctivally after surgery for prophylaxis; also used to treat severe allergic and inflammatory conditions |
| **ANTIINFECTIVES** | |
| Polymyxin B/bacitracin (Polysporin ointment) | Topically to treat superficial ocular infections of the conjunctiva or cornea; prophylactically after surgery |
| Polymyxin B/neomycin/bacitracin (Neosporin ointment) | Topical treatment of superficial infections of the external eye; prophylactically after surgery; potential hypersensitivity to neomycin |
| Neomycin and polymyxin B sulfates and dexamethasone (Maxitrol ointment or suspension) | Topical treatment of steroid-responsive inflammatory ocular conditions or bacterial infections of the external eye; potential hypersensitivity to neomycin |
| Tobramycin/dexamethasone (TobraDex) | Topical treatment or prevention of superficial infections of the external part of eye; also has antiinflammatory properties |
| Cefazolin (Ancef, Kefzol) | Prophylactically injected subconjunctivally after procedure; also topically, intraocularly, and systemically for endophthalmitis |
| Gentamicin sulfate (Garamycin) | Prophylactically injected subconjunctivally after procedure; also topically, subconjunctivally, and intraocularly for endophthalmitis |
| Ceftazidime (Fortaz, Tazicef, Tazadime) | Injected subconjunctivally and intraocularly for treatment of endophthalmitis |
| **MISCELLANEOUS** | |
| Cocaine, 1%-4% | Topical use, never injected; used on cornea to loosen epithelium before debridement and on nasal packing to reduce congestion of mucosa |
| 5-Fluorouracil (5-FU) | Antimetabolite used topically to inhibit scar formation in glaucoma-filtering procedures; handle and discard in compliance with Occupational Safety and Health Administration (OSHA) and facility policies for safe use of antineoplastics |
| Mitomycin (Mutamycin) | Antimetabolite used topically to inhibit scar formation in glaucoma-filtering procedures and pterygium excision; handle and discard in compliance with OSHA and facility policies for safe use of antineoplastics |
| Tissue plasminogen activator (TPA) (Activase) | Thrombolytic agent; to treat fibrin formation in postvitrectomy patients; lysis of clots on retina |
| Fluorescein | Yellowish green fluorescence of this IV diagnostic aid is used in fluorescein angiography to diagnose retinal disorder; topical stain—fluorescein strip temporarily stains the cornea yellow-green in areas of denuded corneal epithelium |
| Timolol maleate (Timoptic) | Beta-adrenergic receptor blocking agent; treatment of elevated intraocular pressure in ocular hypertension or open-angle glaucoma |
| Acetazolamide sodium (Diamox) | Carbonic anhydrase inhibitor; given IV to decrease the secretion of aqueous humor and results in a drop in intraocular pressure; diuretic effect |
| Dextrose, 50% | Added to BSS, Endosol, BSS Plus, or Endosol Extra for diabetic patients during intraocular procedures |

## BEST PRACTICE

### Comparison of Regional Blocks in Cataract Surgery

Evidence-based medicine (EBM) and evidence-based nursing (EBN) deemphasize practice based on tradition and instead stress the use of research findings, other sources of credible data, and/or the consensus of national or local experts. Cataract surgery is the highest-volume surgical procedure performed on Medicare beneficiaries. Carried out almost exclusively as an ambulatory surgical procedure, it usually involves the administration of a local anesthetic and may be accompanied by systemic sedation administered by an anesthesia provider. One of the principal objectives of this evidence report was to summarize published literature on the risks and benefits associated with the use of one form of regional anesthesia rather than another. Some of the findings from the review of 122 published studies were as follows:

- *Globe akinesia (control of ocular movement):* Evidence indicated no difference between peribulbar and retrobulbar blocks. Although there was not enough evidence to compare subconjunctival/sub-Tenon's block with retrobulbar and peribulbar blocks, all three techniques appeared to produce adequate akinesia.
- *Pain of block administration:* Moderate evidence suggested that subconjunctival/sub-Tenon's block was less painful than retrobulbar blocks and weak evidence suggested that peribulbar injection was slightly less painful than retrobulbar injection.
- *Pain control during surgery:* All of the major techniques yielded good or excellent intraoperative pain control during cataract surgery.
- *Specific agents used:* All agents reported had high rates of excellent pain control. There was not enough evidence to analyze whether some agents produced better pain control than others.

Modified from *Anesthesia management during cataract surgery. Summary, Evidence Report/Technology Assessment: number 16, anesthesia management during cataract surgery.* AHRQ Publication No. 00-E015, August 2000. Accessed February 20, 2006, on-line: www.ahrq.gov/clinic/epcsums/anestsum/htm; Hasnain-Wynia R: Is evidence-based medicine patient-centered and is patient-centered care evidence-based? *Health Services Research* 41(1):1-8, 2006.

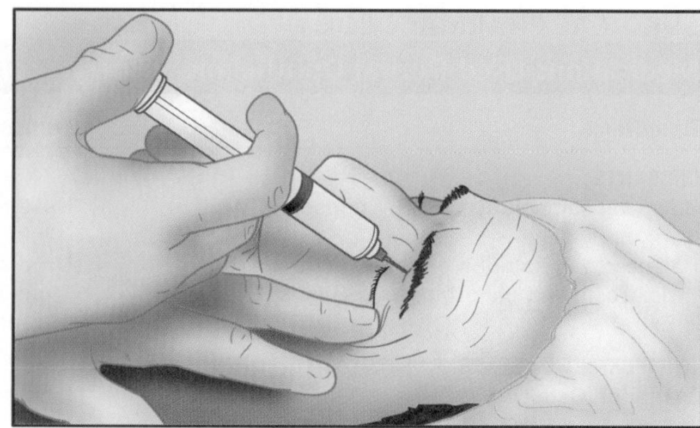

**FIGURE 18-13** Peribulbar anesthesia.

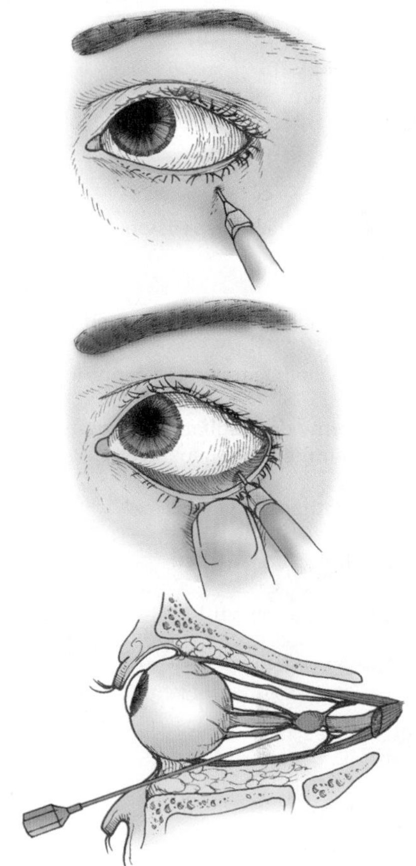

**FIGURE 18-14** Retrobulbar block.

As part of the prep, some surgeons use drops of 5% povidone-iodine complex solution on the conjunctiva to remove surface microbes. One or two drops of the 5% povidone-iodine solution is placed onto the eye surface before the prep of the face and eyelids and then rinsed from the eye with normal saline.

Eye preparation includes cleansing the eyelids of the operative eye or eyes, lid margins, lashes, eyebrows, and surrounding skin with an appropriate antimicrobial solution. Only the necessary amount of prep solution should be used, and it should be allowed to dry completely before draping or activation of an ignition source, such as a laser, eye cautery, or the electrosurgical unit (ESU).[10] Povidone-iodine solution may be contraindicated in some patients who have allergic reactions to topical iodine preparations. For these patients, hexachlorophene can be used, but avoid getting it in the eye and flush the eye with saline. Chlorhexidine gluconate is not used, because it is very toxic to the eye.

To clean the lid margins, evert the lids and clean with cotton-tipped applicators moistened with antimicrobial skin disinfectant. Prevent the solution from entering the patient's eyes and ears. The eye or eyes are then irrigated with normal saline solution using an irrigating bulb. The skin is dried so the drape will adhere. When toxic chemicals or small particles of foreign matter must be removed, the eye surface and conjunctival sac are thoroughly flushed with tepid sterile normal saline solution using an irrigation bulb or an Asepto syringe.

***Draping.*** Special concerns for eye surgery draping include water repellence, eliminating lint and fiber particles, and providing adequate air exchange for patients receiving local anesthetics. A cardboard bridge that adheres to the sides of the patient's face may be used to support the drape above the patient's mouth and nose. To avoid placing handpieces on top of patients, a Mayo stand may be placed above the patient and incorporated into the draping process. The use of a one-piece disposable drape, with a self-adherent, fenestrated plastic section for the eye, eliminates the need to lift the patient's head during draping and facilitates drape removal at the end of the procedure. The eyelids may be separated when applying the self-adherent plastic eye drape to keep the eyelashes out of the operative eye. A fluid drainage bag with wicking strip may also be adhered to the plastic eye drape.

In an alternative method, the head is draped with a half-sheet and two towels, a large sheet is used to cover the patient and OR bed, and a fenestrated plastic eye drape is placed over the operative site.

***Instrumentation.*** Basic eye instruments are shown in Figure 18-15. Additional instruments, depending on the type of procedure, can be added to the basic instrument set. Special surface finishes are used to reduce light reflection. Instruments are designed with round handles for smoother motion and rotation under the microscope. The instruments to be placed on the Mayo stand and the order of their use can also be listed on the preference card or computerized picklist.

A variety of ophthalmic forceps are designed for specific use with different tissues of the eye. Fixation forceps, used to hold tissue firmly in place or provide traction before incision, have an angled tooth that overlaps for secure fixation. Suturing forceps, used to pick up wound edges for dissection or suturing, are single-toothed forceps with the tooth at a right angle to the shank of the forceps. Tying forceps have a flat platform for holding suture as it is tied. The tips of the most commonly used forceps are illustrated in Figure 18-16.

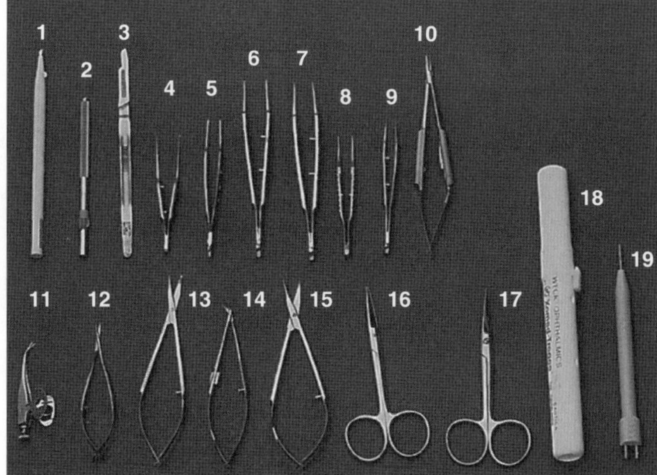


FIGURE 18-15 Basic eye instrument setup. *1,* Super blade (disposable); *2,* Beaver knife handle; *3,* #9 Bard-Parker knife handle; *4,* Colibri corneal forceps; *5,* Bishop-Harmon suturing forceps; *6,* Castroviejo suturing forceps, 0.5 mm; *7,* Castroviejo suturing forceps, 0.12 mm; *8,* Castroviejo tying forceps; *9,* Kelman-McPherson suturing forceps; *10,* Harper needle holder; *11,* Barraquer iris scissors; *12,* Vannas iridocapsulotomy scissors; *13,* Westcott tenotomy scissors; *14,* Castroviejo corneal scissors; *15,* Westcott stitch scissors; *16,* Knapp strabismus scissors; *17,* iris scissors; *18,* eye cautery, disposable; *19,* bipolar eraser-tip eye cautery, disposable.

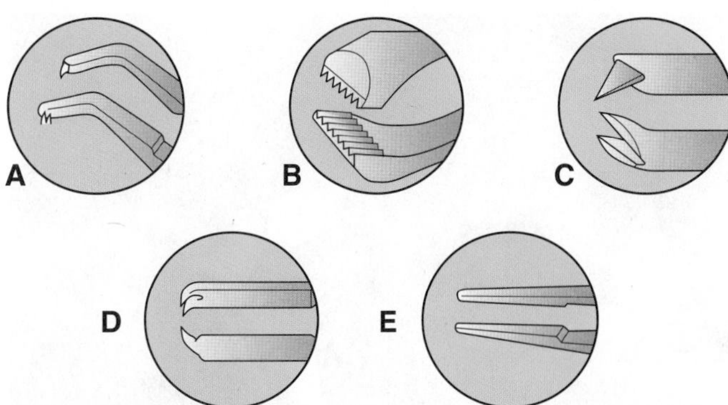


FIGURE 18-16 Close-up of tips of forceps. **A,** Colibri forceps. **B** and **C,** Fixation forceps. **D,** Suturing forceps. **E,** Tying forceps.

CARE AND HANDLING. To maintain the quality and precision of all ophthalmic instruments, including microsurgical instruments, strict criteria for care and handling must be followed. Storage cases protect instrument tips and cutting surfaces. The instruments should be inspected under magnification when purchased and before and after each use, observing for burrs on tips, nicks on cutting surfaces, and alignment of jaws. Eye instruments should be cleaned during use with non-fibrous sponges to avoid damaging delicate instrument tips. Personnel handling instruments should know the name and purpose of each instrument. Tissue can be damaged by the use of an inappropriate instrument, and instruments can be damaged by inappropriate use. After use, the instruments should be cleaned, thoroughly dried, and terminally sterilized before storage in protective containers.

It is recommended that microsurgical instruments undergo ultrasonic cleaning with distilled water and an appropriate enzymatic cleansing agent. They can be individually handheld or immersed together in the ultrasonic cleaner as long as they are not touching each other. Instruments should be rinsed with distilled water and thoroughly dried. A hot air blower (never a towel) should be used for drying instruments. Instrument lubricant should not be used on irrigating cannulas because residue can be introduced into the eye and cause damage.

In addition to basic care and handling, a routine preventive maintenance program should be established for sharpening, realigning, and adjusting the precision eye instruments. Keeping an instrument in good repair is much less expensive than buying a new one.

***Operating Microscope.*** The operating or surgical microscope is employed in many types of surgical procedures. For ophthalmology it is an integral part of the surgery. Because of the demand for use of the operating microscope and its special adaptations, perioperative nurses must understand the basic principles of operation and care of this important piece of surgical equipment.

MICROSCOPE COMPONENTS. Generally, the surgical microscope comprises two parts—the microscope and the suspension system. The principal part of the microscope is the optical system, which has several subparts: the eyepieces, binocular tube, magnification changer, objective lens, and illumination system (Figure 18-17). To facilitate understanding of the functions of the operating microscope, a few basic optical principles are defined and explained.

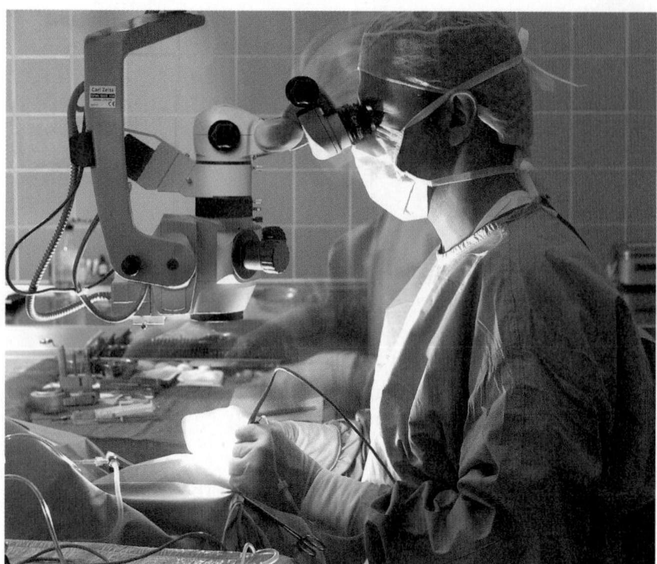

**FIGURE 18-17** Surgical microscope.

Surgical microscopes are stereoscopic and feature the ability for the user to adjust the level of magnification. Viewing the surgical image starts with the binoculars. Binoculars are two telescopes mounted side by side that give stereoscopic vision (three-dimensional). The length of the binoculars is condensed by the use of prisms.

The eyepieces, or oculars, which fit into the binocular tubes, are the lens combinations through which a surgeon views the microsurgical field. Eyepieces are interchangeable and are available in different magnifying powers, such as 10×, 12.5×, 16×, and 20×. To focus the microscope, the user sets the spheric diopter adjustment on the oculars to correspond to his or her individual eyeglass correction and works without eyeglasses. Users who have astigmatism should wear their eyeglasses and set the oculars at zero.

The binocular tubes permit the distance between the oculars to be adjusted to fit the pupillary distance of the user (the distance between the pupils of the user's eyes), ensuring stereoscopic vision.

The objective lens is attached to the bottom of the microscope, usually by a threaded mount, and the working distance is the distance between the objective lens and the operative field. The working distance determines the focal length of the objective. Longer focal lengths, such as 400 mm, are commonly employed in neurosurgery. Procedures with shorter working distances and needing less magnification for a relatively large surgical field, such as an ophthalmic procedure, might require a 12.5× eyepiece and a 175-mm or 200-mm objective lens.

Illumination is the source of light used to view an object. The microscope illuminator is the light source used to throw light downward to illuminate the surgical area. The most common type of microscope illumination is co-axial illumination. Light from the illuminator bulb is routed near the viewing axis of the microscope and projected down through the objective lens. This type of illumination provides a bright circular spot that is uniformly illuminated, often referred to as *homogeneous*, even in deep and narrow wounds. Co-axial light can be transferred through a fiberoptic cable or from an incandescent bulb housed near the objective lens of the microscope. The big advantage of fiberoptic illumination is the ability to place the light source and generated heat away from the surgical field. The light that is transmitted through the fiberoptics is then a so-called *cold light*.

Magnification is the process by which the apparent size of an image is increased. Magnification of an image is increased when the object is moved closer to the eye or when optical aids, such as telescopes, binoculars, or microscopes, are used to increase the image size on the retina without reducing the eye-to-object distance. The amount of image increase becomes the magnification value of the optical aid. The objective lens, magnification changer, binocular tube length, and eyepieces influence the microscope's magnification. Two types of magnification changers used on surgical microscopes are (1) the *revolving telescope* type, in which miniature telescopes of differing powers are rotated into position by means of knobs on the microscope body and (2) the *zoom* type, which is a motorized system of shifting lens elements to vary the magnification, operated with a hand switch or foot control. These principal parts are integrated in or attached to the microscope body.

MICROSCOPE ACCESSORIES. The use of microscope accessories varies according to requirements of the procedure and the surgeon's preferences. On the upper portion of the microscope body is a ring-dovetail receptacle for attaching accessories. One of the most common accessories is a beam splitter, which fits into the receptacle, permitting the attachment of binocular and monocular observation tubes and documentation accessories, such as cameras and video equipment. A beam splitter has two-way mirrors or prisms that divert or split the optical image in several directions. With use of a beam splitter, 50% or less of available light is usually diverted away from the surgeon's oculars. However, the human eye is usually versatile enough to adjust to lower light levels. Adequate lighting is essential for photographic systems, which may in some instances of older microscope systems require a beam splitter that diverts as much as 70% of the available light. Some accessories that attach to the operating microscope may include a video camera, a laser shutter, and a wide-angle viewing system. The individual manufacturers of these accessories will provide information on installation and care of these devices. Wide-angle viewing systems may have lenses that require specific care and sterilization to keep them in proper working order.

MOVEMENT AND MOUNTING OF THE MICROSCOPE. The X-Y coupling, located above the entire optical system and contained in a casing, enables the operator to move the microscope body horizontally and accurately over the operative field. The microscope body is mounted onto the yoke, the connecting carrier arm, which in most cases attaches to the X-Y coupling and then to the articulated arm. The articulated arm is part of the suspension system, which can be either a floor stand or ceiling-mounted. Each suspension system can offer manual or motorized features for various functions such as gross positioning, focus, and magnification (zoom).

CARE AND MAINTENANCE. Proper care and maintenance of the operating microscope are essential to ensure optimal function and durability of this sophisticated, expensive piece of equipment. The procedures are as follows:

1. Inspecting and cleaning of all external lens surfaces before use

2. Checking all power controls including illumination intensity, magnification changer, focus, and X-Y coupling to ensure proper functioning before use
3. Determining the particular procedure in advance and checking the needed accessories, such as the correct objective lens, beam splitter, cameras, observer tubes, filters, shutters, wide-angle viewing system
4. Cleaning and covering after use

CARE OF OPTICS. Before and after each procedure all external lens surfaces should be cleaned and inspected for damage. The objective lens frequently needs cleaning as a result of dried splash marks of balanced salt solution (BSS). Scratched or damaged optical systems must be repaired or replaced.

The following procedure is used for cleaning lens surfaces:

1. Loose particles (lint or dust) are removed with a soft, clean camera lens brush or with air from a bulb syringe. When a bulb syringe is used, the bulb is held about 1 cm from the surface and squeezed briskly, directing the air toward the lens surface.
2. Blood, water, and irrigating solutions are removed with a cotton-tipped applicator or cotton ball moistened with distilled water. A circular motion is used, beginning at the center of the optic and working toward the outer edge (lens paper also may be used). The surface is dried with a cotton-tipped applicator or cotton ball in the same manner.
3. Oil or fingerprints are removed with a cleaning solvent of commercially prepared lens-cleaning solution or with 50% denatured alcohol. The lens is wiped with a lightly moistened cotton-tipped applicator or cotton ball in a circular motion. The process is repeated until the surface is clean and free from streaks.

Solvents should be used sparingly. Excessive fluid may destroy the cemented surfaces of the lens or plastic mounts if used.

CLEANING. The external surfaces of the microscope should be cleansed after use and before storage. The cleaning procedures are as follows:

1. The external surfaces are washed with a clean, damp cloth moistened with a mild soap or disinfecting solution.
2. The surfaces are wiped dry with a lint-free cloth.
3. The function of each moving part is inspected during the cleaning process. The coupling joints can be greased with petroleum jelly if necessary. The lamp cable should be free from kinks. A new bulb should be used for each procedure expected to take longer than 4 hours to complete. It is good practice to have a spare bulb on hand at all times. Fiberoptic cables are cleaned with cotton-tipped applicators.
4. The microscope arms are moved to the lowest position. The locks on the arm are loosened, and the ocular systems are moved in toward the base.
5. Dust caps are placed over the eyepieces and a dust cover over the microscope head. The microscope is ready for storage.

Proper care and preventive maintenance add years of service to an operating microscope. Checking the microscope before use and being knowledgeable about proper function of the microscope and its accessories are responsibilities of the perioperative nurse.

***Ophthalmic Sutures.*** Sutures used in ophthalmic surgery are very fine and range in size from 4-0 to 10-0. Handling and arming these sutures can be a challenge for the perioperative nurse with uncorrected presbyopia. Fine eye sutures produce minimum reaction and discomfort for the patient. They should be handled as little as possible to avoid weakening and fraying. Surgical gut and collagen suture, which is packaged in solution, should be rinsed before use to prevent introducing irritants into the eye. Ophthalmic needles also are very delicate and must be handled with extreme care. Before use, needles must be inspected for evidence of burrs.

***Ophthalmic Dressings.*** Advances in cataract procedures have altered the usual postoperative dressing of ophthalmic ointment, an eye pad, and a protective shield. Collagen corneal shields that are rehydrated in an antiinfective-antiinflammatory solution may be all that is used as a dressing. With some topical anesthetics and clear corneal incisions, no dressings are needed. The type of dressing, if one is used, depends on the procedure.

At the completion of the operation, the operative eye area is cleansed with saline sponges. After plastic procedures on the lids or lacrimal ducts, antibiotic ointment may be thinly spread over the skin and eyelashes to prevent adhesion of the bandage.

The initial dressing is a sterile eye pad secured with nonallergenic tape (Figure 18-18). After intraocular operations, when external pressure on the eyes might be harmful, the initial dressing is covered with a protecting, perforated aluminum plate or another variety of eye shield.

A pressure bandage may be used when a compression effect is desired. A gauze roller bandage is applied over the initial dressing, encircling the head.

## Evaluation

Before the patient is transported to the postanesthesia care unit (PACU) or observation unit, his or her general condition is evaluated. The general appearance of the skin is assessed, with areas around the face and bony prominences noted for redness and other changes from the preoperative condition.

If the procedure was lengthy and osmotics were given, the patient may be catheterized while still anesthetized or given a bedpan if awake. A hand-off report to the receiving nurse in the PACU or observation area should include postoperative positioning requirements, potential problems specific to the patient, and preoperative anxiety level and use of coping mechanisms. Some patients have one or both eyes patched, and disturbed sensory perception should be noted. Documentation of all postoperative observations is important.

Evaluation should address whether the patient met the desired perioperative nursing outcomes; the patient's responses may be documented as outcome statements. The following examples are based on the nursing diagnoses identified in the plan of care:

- The patient, family, or significant others verbalized knowledge regarding the diagnosis, planned intervention, medication management, and requirements for home care maintenance.
- The patient verbalized an acceptable level of anxiety and used coping mechanisms that were effective.
- The patient safely adapted to visual disturbed sensory perception.
- The patient remained comfortable during the intervention as determined by response on a verbal pain scale.

**Nonpressure Eye Patch**

1. Assemble the equipment:
   - Eye patch
   - Skin preparation pad
   - Nonallergenic paper tape
2. Explain the procedure to the patient.
3. Wash your hands.
4. Apply a skin preparation pad to the patient's forehead and cheek.
5. Instruct the patient to close both eyes gently.
6. Place a patch over the closed eyelid.

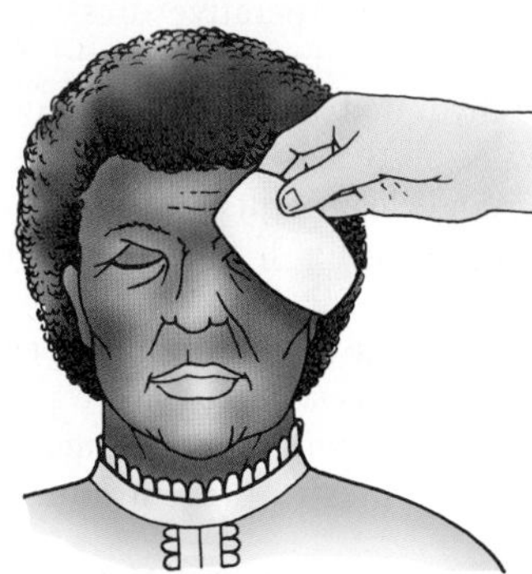

7. Apply tape from the cheek to the middle of the forehead in a diagonal line.

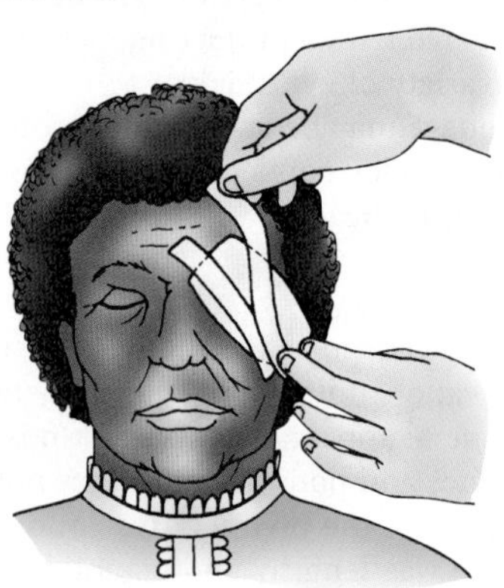

8. Cover the patch with overlapping pieces of tape.

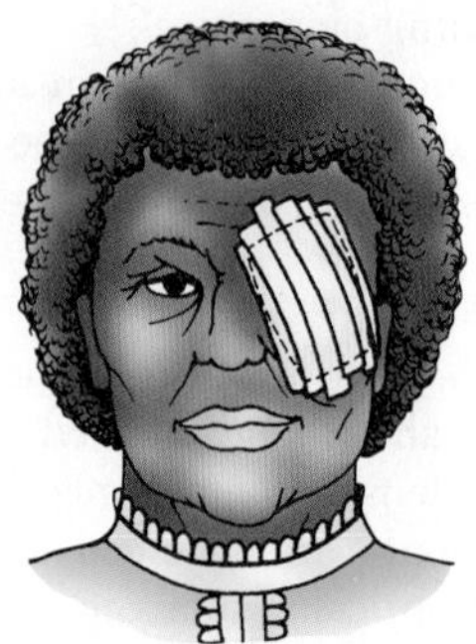

**Pressure Eye Patch**

1. Assemble the equipment:
   - Two eye patches for each eye requiring treatment
   - Skin preparation pad
   - Nonallergenic paper tape

2-5. Follow corresponding steps under Nonpressure Eye Patch.

6. Fold one eye patch in half, place it over the closed eyelid, and apply a second eye patch (unfolded) over the folded one.

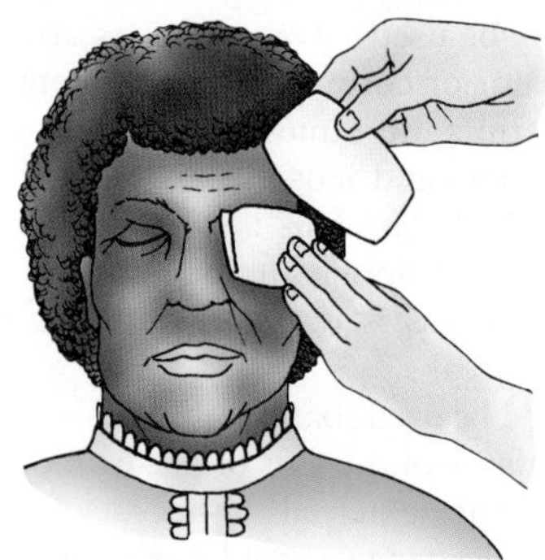

7, 8. Follow corresponding steps under Nonpressure Eye Patch.

FIGURE 18-18 Application of an eye patch.

- The patient will remain free from signs and symptoms of surgical site infection.

## Patient and Family Education and Discharge Planning

Implementation of the plan of care actually begins during the patient interview. Planning to meet the patient's educational needs should play an equal role with meeting other needs. Verbal review and reinforcement of information initially provided in the physician's office ensure consistency in teaching. Written material and audiovisual media (closed circuit television, videocassettes, photos, and patient information Internet websites) may be used to enhance patient education programs but do not eliminate the need for direct interchange with patients and feedback from them.

Family members or friends should be included to add support and increase understanding of the planned surgery. The loss of sight produces the same staged coping behaviors of grieving that move the individual from denial to acceptance. Thorough preoperative preparation of the patient and in most cases the family, who will assist with care at home in the postoperative period (Patient and Family Education), plays a vital role in the successful outcome of the surgical procedure.

Patient and family education for the patient undergoing ophthalmic surgery should include the following:

- Purpose and desired results of preoperative eyedrops and sedation
- Explanation of what to expect from the anesthetic
- Activities and routines of the intraoperative period
- What to expect immediately after surgery
- Designated driver after procedures using sedation
- Verbal and written instructions for use of eyedrops and other medications
- Any limitations on activities (bending, lifting, eye rubbing, special positioning)
- Wound care, protective sunglasses

PATIENT AND FAMILY EDUCATION

**Discharge Instructions and Home Care After Cataract Surgery**

**HOME CARE**

- Give both the patient and the caregiver *verbal* and *written* instructions. Provide them with the name and telephone number of a physician or nurse to call if questions arise.
- Advise the patient to avoid squeezing the eyelids shut or touching the eyes postoperatively; encourage elderly patients to wear glasses during the day to avoid rubbing the eyes.
- Warning signs: Review the signs and symptoms that should be reported to a physician or nurse.
  - Increased intraocular pressure: sudden onset of eye pain, photophobia, sudden decrease in vision, sudden severe headache
  - Infection: redness and watering of eyes, swelling, blurred vision, pain
- Special instructions
  - Discuss the need to wear an eye shield at night for 2 to 6 weeks to avoid eye injury.
  - Warn that depth perception may be lost and that 50% of peripheral vision will be lost because of the eye patch.
  - Review safety precautions, especially with elderly patients.
    - Instruct the patient to avoid falls by turning the head fully to the affected side to view objects.
    - Advise the patient to use up-and-down head movements to judge stairs and oncoming objects and to move slowly.
  - Discuss the need to wear dark glasses during the day to avoid pupil constriction and glare, since the eye is sensitive to light after surgery.
  - If the patient had cataract surgery without a lens implant, warn that vision will be diminished in one or both eyes until prescription eyeglasses or contact lenses are obtained (in about 4 to 8 weeks).
  - If the patient is receiving eyeglasses, explain that images will be magnified 30%, peripheral vision will be impaired and distorted, and lenses will be bifocal or trifocal. Review safety precautions.
    - Advise the patient to turn head side to side to see peripherally.
    - Advise the patient to judge distances when descending stairs or viewing oncoming objects.
  - If the patient is receiving contact lenses, explain that images will be magnified 7% to 10%, peripheral vision will be intact, and reading glasses may also be prescribed.
  - Review the care, insertion, and removal of lenses. Advise the patient of the importance of routine appointments with the physician for removal, cleansing, and reinsertion of extended-wear lenses.
  - If the patient is receiving an intraocular lens implant, explain that the lens implant aids in focusing but that glasses will be prescribed for close vision in 8 to 12 weeks; there will be no loss in depth perception.
- Medications
  - Review the name, purpose, dosage, schedule, and route of administration of all prescribed drugs, how and how long to continue taking the prescribed medication, as well as side effects to report to a physician or nurse.
  - Review the correct procedure for instilling eyedrops and ointments and applying an eye shield (without touching or applying pressure on the eyeball) to avoid self-inflicted injury.
  - Advise the patient to avoid over-the-counter medications, eyedrops, or ointments without checking with the physician.
  - Encourage the patient to share the list of medications with all providers of care, including primary care and specialist physicians, nurses, pharmacists, and other caregivers.
- Activity
  - Explain the need to avoid activities that can increase intraocular pressure: heavy lifting, straining with elimination, bending over at the waist, coughing, vomiting.
  - Instruct the patient to take medications for nausea and constipation as ordered.
  - Instruct the patient to avoid sleeping on the operative side.
  - Explain the need to avoid any strenuous exercise for 6 weeks; tell the patient to check with the physician before resuming occupational or recreational activities.
  - Explain that it will be necessary to adjust to mild magnification when performing daily activities.

**FOLLOW-UP CARE**

- Stress the importance of regular follow-up visits. Make sure the patient has the necessary names and telephone numbers.

Modified from Canobbio MM: *Mosby's handbook of patient teaching,* St Louis, 2006, Mosby, pp. 212-215; Using medication reconciliation to prevent errors, *Joint Commission Sentinel Event Alert,* Issue 35, January 23, 2006.

- Signs and symptoms of complications
- Follow-up postoperative phone calls from the ambulatory surgery center, as applicable
- Who to call with questions or concerns
- Follow-up appointments

# *Surgical Interventions*

## SURGERY OF THE EYELIDS

The oculoplastic procedures performed on the eyelids are for treatment of chalazion, entropion, ectropion, dermatochalasis, ptosis repair, excisional biopsy, excision of eyelid tumors and reconstruction of the eyelid, and repair of traumatic injuries.

### Removal of Chalazion

Removal of a chalazion is the incision and curettage of a chronic granulomatous inflammation of one or more of the meibomian glands in the tarsal plate of the eyelid.

***Procedural Considerations.*** This procedure is most commonly done with the patient under local anesthesia. The incisional approach depends on the location of the major portion of the chalazion. If the chalazion is located anterior to the tarsal plate, an external or transcutaneous incision may be used. If the majority of the chalazion is located on the conjunctival side of the tarsal plate, the transconjunctival approach is used (Figure 18-19).

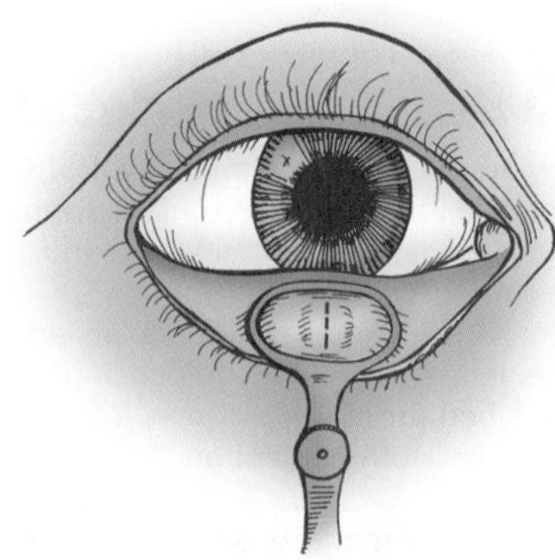

FIGURE 18-19 Transconjunctival approach. Clamp everts eyelid during surgery for chalazion. Viscous contents of chalazion will be removed with curette.

### Operative Procedure (Transconjunctival Approach)

1. The affected lid is everted with a chalazion clamp to expose the chalazion.
2. A vertical incision is made on the inner lid surface with a sharp blade; the small lesion is curetted, or the granuloma is excised.
3. The wound is left open for drainage. Bleeding is controlled with the eye cautery, and the eye is patched.

## Repair of Entropion

Entropion (turning inward of the lower lid margin) seldom occurs in persons younger than 40 years. The turned-in eyelashes and skin of the lower lid rub against the corneal surface and cause irritation, which leads to breaks in the integrity of the corneal surface. The most common type is *involutional entropion* resulting from lid laxity and degeneration of facial attachments between the pretarsal muscle and the tarsus, which permits the pretarsal muscle to override the lid margin during contraction. *Cicatricial entropion* is attributable to contraction of either the upper or the lower tarsus and its conjunctiva, turning in the lashes (trichiasis) so that they rub on the cornea.

***Procedural Considerations.*** The causes of entropion vary, and corrective procedures also vary depending on the pathologic process. Local anesthetic is typically used, and antiinfective ointment is applied postoperatively.

### Operative Procedures

BLEPHAROPLASTY OF LOWER LID FOR INVOLUTIONAL ENTROPION

1. Local anesthetic is injected into the lower lid through the conjunctiva using an angled needle.
2. The skin is marked, and an incision is made in the lateral canthus.
3. The orbicularis is dissected off the orbital septum.
4. The skin excision is extended across the lower lid.
5. The orbital septum is incised to expose fat pockets.
6. Extra fat is removed, and hemostasis is achieved.
7. An incision is made into the lateral canthus, and the lower lid is pulled laterally and shortened to correct entropion.
8. The tarsus is reattached to the lateral canthal tendon, and the lower lid fascia is reattached to the orbicularis.
9. The excess skin is pulled up, marked, and excised.
10. The skin incisions are closed.

WIES PROCEDURE FOR CICATRICIAL ENTROPION

1. A marking pen is used to draw a parallel line 4 mm below the lower lid margin; the local anesthetic is then injected.
2. A double-armed 4-0 nonabsorbable retraction suture is passed through the conjunctiva and lower lid 4 mm from the lateral canthus and 4 mm from the medial canthus.
3. A lid plate retractor is placed behind the lower lid as it is pulled up with the traction suture. The surgeon uses a #15 blade to make the skin incision on the marked line.
4. The lid plate retractor is placed in front of the lid, and the lower lid is everted using the traction suture. The conjunctiva is incised with the #15 blade.
5. A full-thickness blepharotomy is extended laterally and medially with scissors.
6. One end of the double-armed 4-0 suture is passed through the conjunctiva and lower lid tendons and between the orbicularis and tarsus on the medial aspect of the lower lid. This process is repeated approximately 4 mm laterally with the other end of the 4-0 suture.
7. Six mattress sutures are placed and tied to evert the lower lid (Figure 18-20).
8. Excess skin is excised, and the skin incision is closed with 7-0 nonabsorbable sutures.

## Repair of Ectropion

Ectropion (sagging and eversion of the lower lid), usually bilateral, is common in older persons (Figure 18-21). Ectropion may be caused by the relaxation of the orbicular muscle and canthal tendons. Symptoms are tearing, conjunctival infection, irritation, and inadequate corneal protection leading to injury to the cornea. Surgery is indicated when facial paralysis is permanent or when scarring follows lacerations, lesions, or penetrating injuries and the cornea becomes exposed, resulting in ulceration and photophobia.

***Procedural Considerations.*** The causes of ectropion vary, and corrective procedures also vary depending on the pathologic process. Local anesthetic is typically used, and antiinfective ointment and ice compresses are applied postoperatively.

### Operative Procedure

LATERAL CANTHAL SLING PROCEDURE. One method of correction for ectropion is the lateral canthal sling procedure (Figure 18-22), which repositions and tightens the lower lid in a horizontal direction.

1. The lateral canthus is incised, and a strip of tarsus and lateral canthal tendon is isolated.
2. The tarsal/tendon strip is sutured to the periosteum along the inner surface of the lateral wall of the orbit, thereby tightening the lid and correcting the ectropion.

## Plastic Repair for Dermatochalasis

Dermatochalasis is a condition of drooping skin and herniated fat of upper and lower lids that causes the skin of the upper eyelids to hang down over the palpebral fissure, sometimes obscuring vision. It may occur in older persons who have lost normal elasticity in the skin of their upper lids or in persons who have persistent angioneurotic edema with stretching of the skin of the eyelids. If ptosis is present, it accentuates the condition.

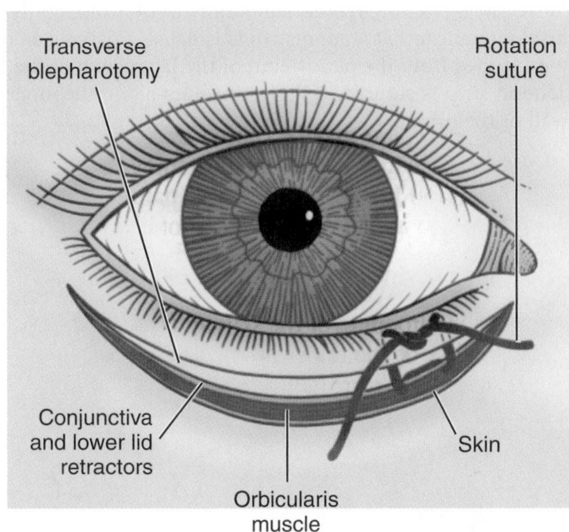


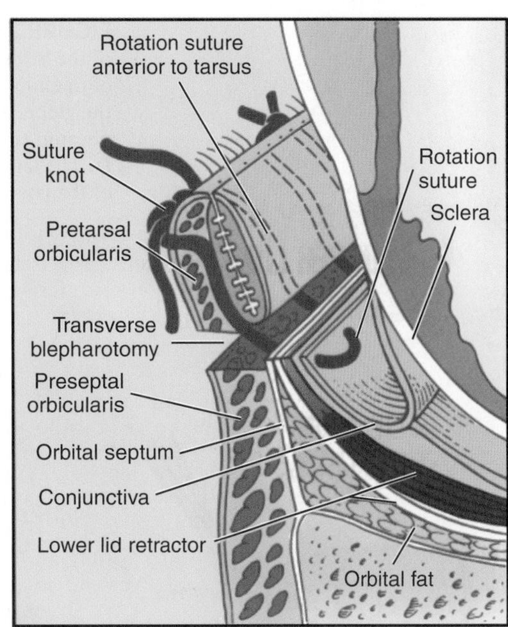


**FIGURE 18-20** Wies procedure for entropion. Placement of an everting mattress suture across a transverse blepharotomy.

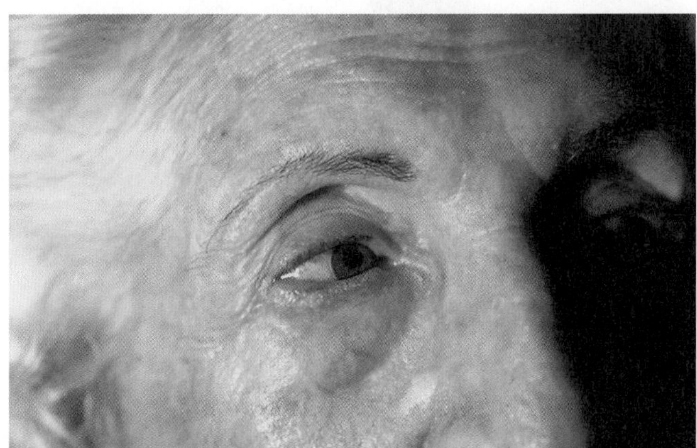

**FIGURE 18-21** Ectropion, or eyelid eversion (turning out of lid), is most commonly caused by relaxation of eyelid framework.

***Procedural Considerations.*** Dermatochalasis is corrected with blepharoplasty of the redundant skin of the upper or lower eyelid or both eyelids. A segment of skin and fat is removed. In the lower lid, a transconjunctival excision that leaves no external incision may be performed. Brow droop, or ptosis, may also be corrected alone or in combination with blepharoplasty to correct dermatochalasis. Procedures for correcting brow ptosis include direct brow lift, coronal brow lift, and endoscopic brow lift.

### *Operative Procedures*

BLEPHAROPLASTY OF UPPER LID FOR DERMATOCHALASIS

1. The amount of skin to be excised in the upper lid is marked above the lid crease, and local anesthetic is injected.
2. With a constant stretch applied to the skin of the upper lid, the incision is made along the predrawn lines.
3. The skin between the marked lines is excised, the orbicularis between the incision edges is excised, and hemostasis is achieved.
4. The septum is incised in a buttonhole fashion; finger pressure is applied on the globe; and bulging fat is clamped, cut, and cauterized.
5. If fat is found in the temporal pocket, it may contain a prolapsed lacrimal gland. The lacrimal gland should be resuspended with 5-0 nonabsorbable suture.
6. The lid crease is re-formed by suturing the lower skin muscle incision line to the levator at the upper edge of the tarsus.
7. The skin can be closed with 6-0 nonabsorbable suture in a continuous running fashion.

TRANSCONJUNCTIVAL BLEPHAROPLASTY OF LOWER LID

1. Local anesthetic is injected into the lower lid through the conjunctiva using an angled needle.
2. Finger pressure is placed on the upper lid while the lower lid is being retracted to expose the conjunctiva of the inferior cul-de-sac.
3. The conjunctiva is incised to expose the fat pockets. Prolapsed fat is clamped and removed, and hemostasis is achieved.

## Surgery for Unilateral or Bilateral Ptosis

Ptosis is true drooping of the upper lid and may be congenital or acquired. In congenital ptosis there usually is developmental weakness of the levator muscle. The condition frequently occurs unilaterally and may be accompanied by weakness of the superior rectus muscle.[7] The child often compensates by raising the eyebrow or tilting the head upward.

Acquired ptosis can be (1) neurogenic or myogenic or (2) involutional, which is manifested by a gradual stretching or dehiscence of the levator aponeurosis. The eyelid crease may be high or absent.

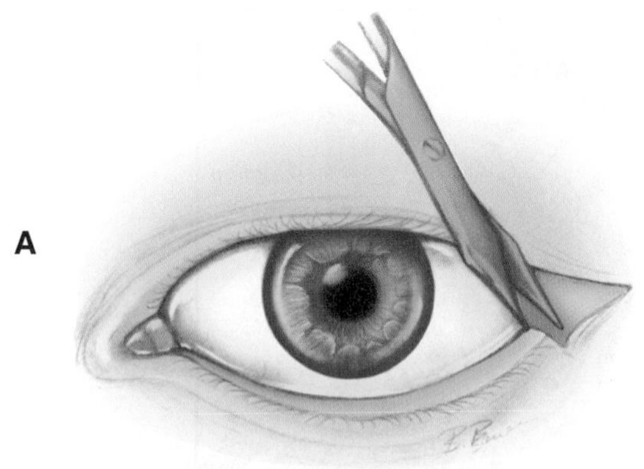

FIGURE 18-22 Lateral canthal sling procedure for ectropion. **A,** A cantholysis of the lower arm of the lateral canthal tendon is performed. **B,** Horizontal laxity of the lid is relieved by stretching the lid temporally until it fits tightly against the globe. A tarsal lateral canthal tendon strip is isolated. **C,** Using a cotton applicator, tissue is cleaned from the periosteum of the lateral rim of the orbit. **D,** The tarsal tendon strip is sutured to the periosteum along the inner surface of the lateral wall of the orbit.

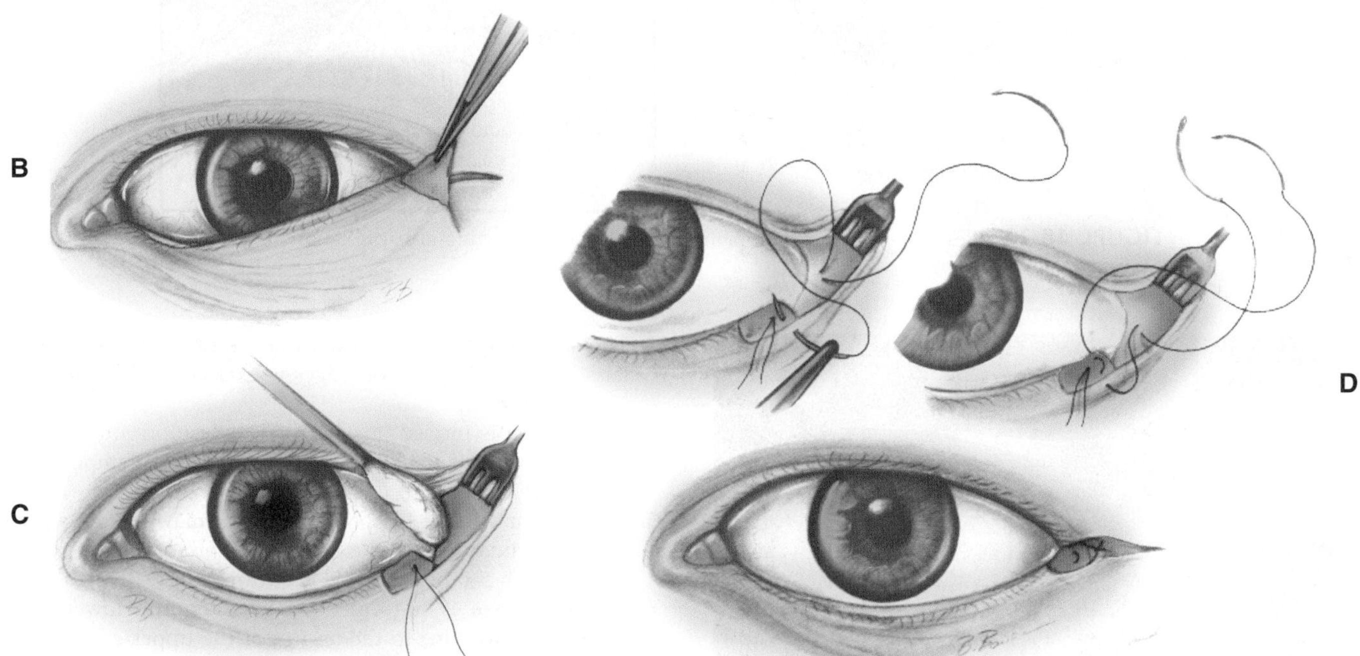

***Procedural Considerations.*** The objective of ptosis surgery is to achieve a good cosmetic result and restore function with elevation of the lid. The many surgical procedures that have been devised are directed at the levator aponeurosis, the frontalis muscles, or the levator-Müller muscle complex. These muscles are the elevating forces of the upper lids. Some of the commonly used procedures are levator aponeurosis repair, frontalis suspension, and posterior Müller muscle–conjunctival resection. Local or general anesthesia can be used. Local anesthesia may be preferred so that required adjustments can be made with the patient's cooperation. Frontalis suspension uses fascia lata or synthetic materials. Harvesting fascia lata requires an additional incision in the leg.

### *Operative Procedures*

LEVATOR APONEUROSIS REPAIR

1. The existing or potential eyelid crease is marked. With the skin of the upper lid held taut, the skin incision is made (Figure 18-23).
2. An incision is made through the orbicularis. The orbicularis is dissected off the orbital septum and the levator aponeurosis anterior to the tarsus.
3. The aponeurosis is incised across the tarsus and dissected off the orbicularis. The levator is reattached to the tarsus with interrupted 6-0 suture.
4. If the patient is awake, he or she is asked to look forward and the sutures are adjusted as needed.
5. The pretarsal orbicularis is sutured to the aponeurosis to reconstruct the lid crease.
6. The skin incision is closed with a running 6-0 nonabsorbable suture.

FRONTALIS SUSPENSION

1. The upper lid is marked, one incision is made in the lid crease, and two incisions are made above the eyebrow (Figure 18-24, *A* and *B*).
2. A lid plate is placed behind the upper lid, the tarsus is exposed, and the suspension material (fascia graft or a synthetic implant) is secured to the tarsus with nonabsorbable sutures (Figure 18-24, *C*).
3. Using a Wright needle, the suspension material is passed away from the globe deeply into the orbital septum and out through one eyebrow incision (Figure 18-24, *D*).
4. The remaining end of the suspension material is passed in the same manner.

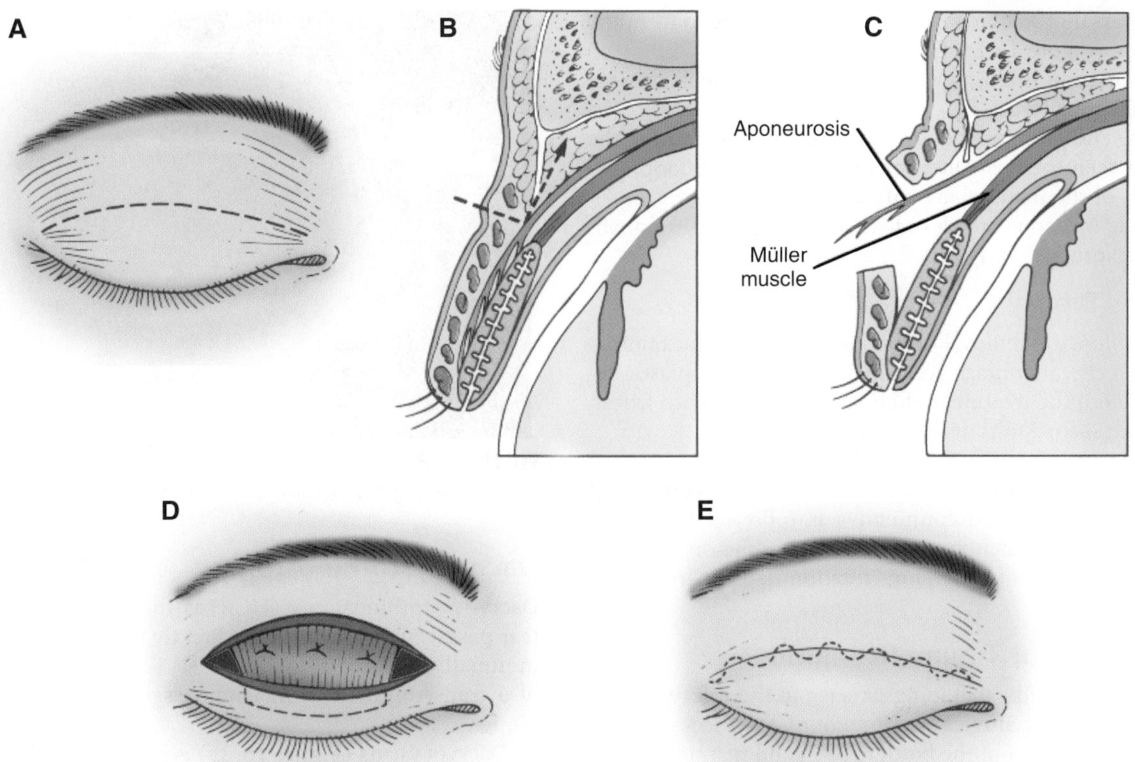


FIGURE 18-23 Levator aponeurosis repair for ptosis. **A,** Eyelid crease is marked. **B,** Skin incision is made, and the orbicularis and orbital septum are divided while dissection proceeds toward the orbital rim. **C,** The anterior surface of the tarsus is exposed, and the aponeurosis is separated from the Müller muscle. **D,** The aponeurosis is reattached to the tarsus with partial-thickness permanent sutures. Lid contour and position are adjusted. **E,** The eyelid crease is created by suturing the pretarsal orbicularis muscle to the aponeurosis, and the skin is closed.

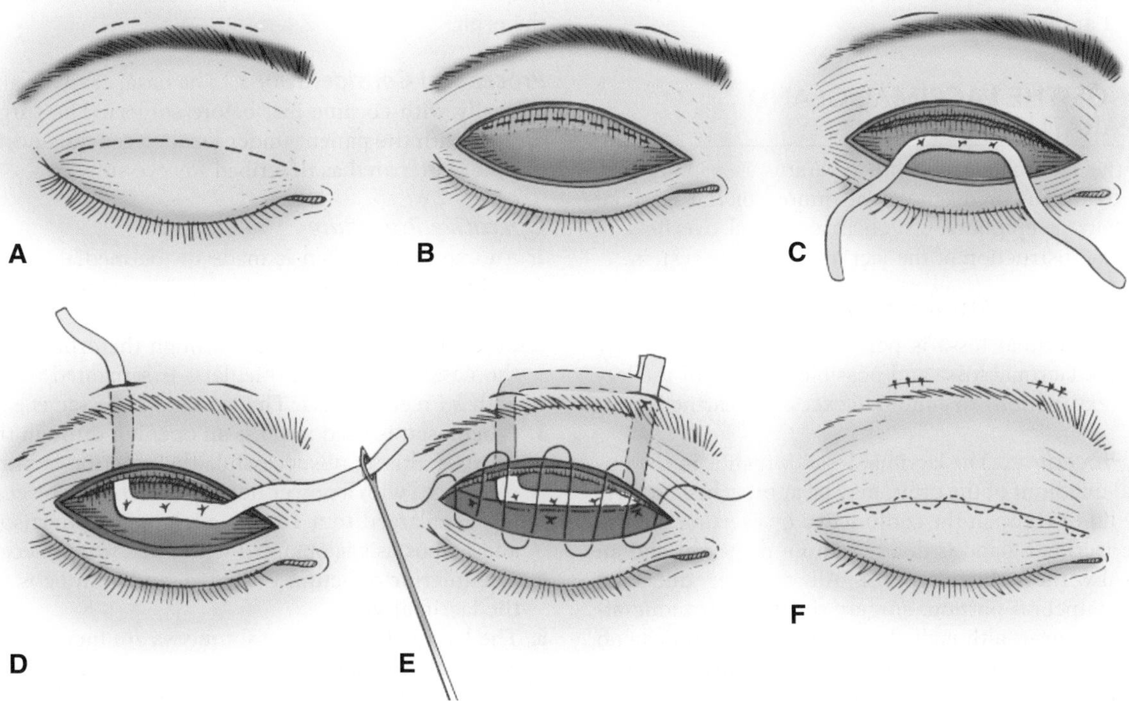


FIGURE 18-24 Frontalis suspension for ptosis. One method used to suspend the eyelid from the brow.

5. The pretarsal orbicularis is sutured to the tarsus to form the lid crease (Figure 18-24, *E*).
6. The lid incision is closed with a running 6-0 nonabsorbable suture (Figure 18-24, *F*).
7. The long end of the suspension material is passed under the skin between the brow incisions to complete the loop, and the ends of the material are sutured together.
8. The brow incisions are closed with interrupted 6-0 nonabsorbable suture.

### Excisional Biopsy

Excisional biopsy is removal of lesions for diagnostic examination. Basal cell carcinomas account for 95% of neoplastic lesions of the lid; the treatment of choice is excision with frozen section analysis or Mohs' technique.

***Operative Procedure.*** Through-and-through excision of skin, muscle, tarsus, and conjunctiva is followed by careful structural closure of anatomic spaces. Depending on the type, extent, and location of the lesion, rotation flaps or free grafts may be necessary.

### Plastic Repair for Traumatic Injuries

Lacerations of the lids, including damage to the inferior canaliculus, are repaired surgically. Paramount for success is the careful approximation of the borders of the lid margin and the ends of a torn canaliculus.

***Operative Procedure.*** Lacerations of the lid margin are closed with a 6-0 silk suture to align the gray line of the lid that lies between the lash follicles and the orifices of the meibomian glands. Once this anatomic line has been approximated, all other sutures are placed, maintaining the approximation. If the canaliculus has been lacerated, the lacrimal drainage system is intubated with a silicone tube and the canaliculus and lid are reconstructed around the tube.

## SURGERY OF THE LACRIMAL GLAND AND APPARATUS

Surgery of the lacrimal gland and apparatus is usually performed for treatment or diagnosis of tumors of the lacrimal fossa or to correct epiphora, which is abnormal overflow of tears related to obstruction of the lacrimal drainage system.

### Surgery of the Lacrimal Fossa

Surgery of the lacrimal fossa is performed for biopsy of any structure in the lacrimal fossa and possible removal of the lacrimal gland (extirpation) to eliminate excessive tearing.

***Operative Procedure.*** The lacrimal fossa, which is in the upper temporal quadrant of the orbit, may be approached directly through the lid or through the conjunctiva by everting the upper lid. The lacrimal gland is divided into a palpebral and an orbital part by the orbital septum. All drainage ducts go through the palpebral portion; surgery on this part alone affects tearing because, although the orbital part is intact, no access to the eye is available. Routine surgical closure procedures are followed.

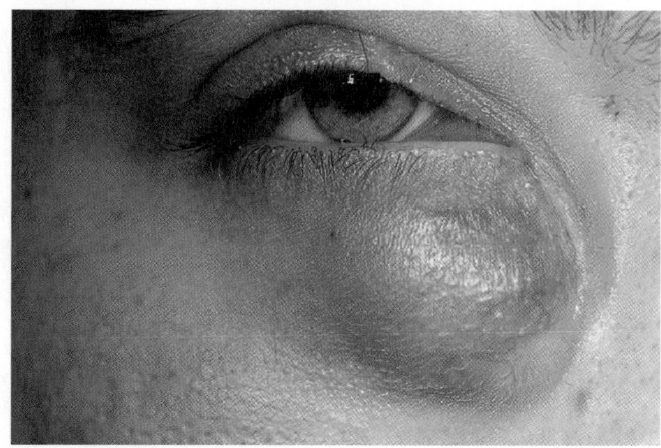

**FIGURE 18-25** Chronic infection of lacrimal sac (dacryocystitis) causes swelling of inner lower corner of eye socket.

### Dacryocystorhinostomy

Dacryocystorhinostomy (DCR) is the establishment of a new tear passageway for drainage directly into the nasal cavity. The minimally invasive approach to DCR surgery includes the use of a transconjunctival incision, lasers, and endoscopic techniques.

Dacryocystitis (Figure 18-25) is an infection in the lacrimal sac and its mucous membranes that extends to the surrounding connective tissue and results in a localized cellulitis. Chronic dacryocystitis in adults requires DCR because of resistant obstruction of the nasolacrimal duct related to infection, dacryolith (calculus in the duct), or trauma.

DCR is also performed when the lower canaliculus is patent but the tear duct is blocked, causing epiphora (abnormal overflow of tears) that the patient cannot tolerate. This deformity frequently follows a malunited fracture of the medial wall of the orbit.

***Procedural Considerations.*** The nasal cavity is anesthetized topically with cocaine just before surgery. The surgery is performed with the patient under local or general anesthesia. The patient is prepared as described for eye surgery.

***Operative Procedure***

1. An external incision is made in the medial canthal area or inside the nose when an internal approach is used (Figure 18-26).
2. Blunt dissection is carried through the orbicularis down to the nasal bone. The orbicularis is separated from the bone with a Freer elevator. The lacrimal fossa sac is exposed.
3. A hemostat is used to press an opening through the lacrimal bone. If this is unsuccessful, the anterior lacrimal crest is perforated with a power burr or mallet and chisel. The opening is enlarged to a 10-mm circle with a Kerrison rongeur, and hemostasis is obtained with bone wax if necessary.
4. The inferior punctum is dilated, and a probe is passed into the lacrimal sac.
5. The lacrimal sac and nasal mucosa are incised with H flaps. The posterior nasal mucous membrane flap is sutured to the posterior lacrimal sac flap with 4-0 absorbable sutures.

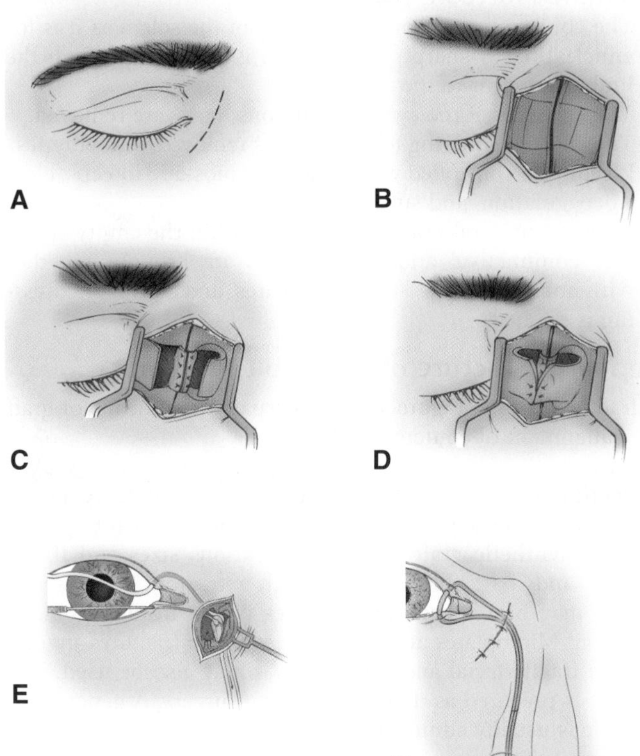


FIGURE 18-26 Dacryocystorhinostomy. **A,** Skin incision for dacryocystorhinostomy or dacryocystectomy. **B,** Lacrimal sac and lacrimal bone exposed. Opening made in lacrimal bone and lacrimal crest. **C,** Posterior flap of wall of sac sutured to posterior flap of nasal mucosa. **D,** Anterior flap of wall of sac sutured to anterior flap of nasal mucosa. (Drawing is somewhat distorted for visualization of relative positions.) **E,** Canaliculi are intubated with Silastic tubes. **F,** Tubes are secured to lateral nasal wall and allowed to slide back into nose.

6. The first end of the wire stylet of a Silastic lacrimal duct intubation set is passed through the upper canaliculus, through the opening, and out through the nose. The other end is passed in the same fashion through the lower canaliculus.
7. The anterior nasal mucous membrane flap is sutured to the anterior lacrimal sac flap with 4-0 absorbable sutures to create a bridge over the Silastic tubing. The tubing remains in place until the sutures become absorbed, thereby acting as a stent about which epithelial union between the lacrimal and nasal mucosa can occur.
8. The orbicularis is closed with 6-0 absorbable sutures. Skin margins are approximated and closed with nonabsorbable 6-0 sutures. Antiinfective ointment is applied to the incision.
9. The wire stylets are cut off the Silastic tubing, and the ends of the tubing are tied together. The tubing is sutured to the lateral nasal wall with 6-0 nonabsorbable suture. The tubing is cut so that it retracts into the nostril. An absorbent sponge may be taped under the nostrils.

## SURGERY OF THE GLOBE AND ORBIT

Surgery of the globe (eyeball) and orbit is usually performed because of trauma. Rupture of the eyeball may be direct at the site of injury or, more frequently, indirect from an increase in intraocular pressure that causes the wall of the eyeball to tear at weaker points, such as the limbus. When the intraocular contents have become so deranged that useful function is prohibited or the blind eye becomes painful, removal of the eye contents (evisceration procedure) or of the entire eyeball (enucleation) is indicated. If either procedure is required, an inert globe or a coralline hydroxyapatite (coral) implant may be inserted as a space filler and to aid in the movement of a prosthesis (artificial eye) (Figure 18-27).

Fractures of the walls of the orbit may be caused by direct blows or by extension of a fracture line from adjacent bones. Isolated orbital floor, or blowout, fractures usually occur after injury to the region of the eye by an object the size of an apple or an adult's fist. Orbital contents herniate into the maxillary sinus, and the inferior rectus or inferior oblique muscle may become incarcerated at the fracture site (Figure 18-28). A Caldwell-Luc antrostomy may be done with reduction of the fracture from below, or the fracture site may be approached directly through the lower lid along the orbital floor; the prolapsed tissue is reduced, the orbital floor is reduced, and the orbital floor defect is bridged with bone grafts, molded metal implants, or plastic material.

### Enucleation

Enucleation is removal of the entire eyeball, usually with the insertion of a round implant into the socket to replace the globe. Hydroxyapatite sphere implants are coralline or synthetic and have gained popularity as the sphere of choice after enucleation and evisceration. Hydroxyapatite, a lightweight, coral-like implant, may be used as the foundation for a prosthetic eye because its porous structure encourages fibrovascular ingrowth. The hydroxyapatite implant is wrapped in human donor sclera or Silastic sheeting before insertion into the

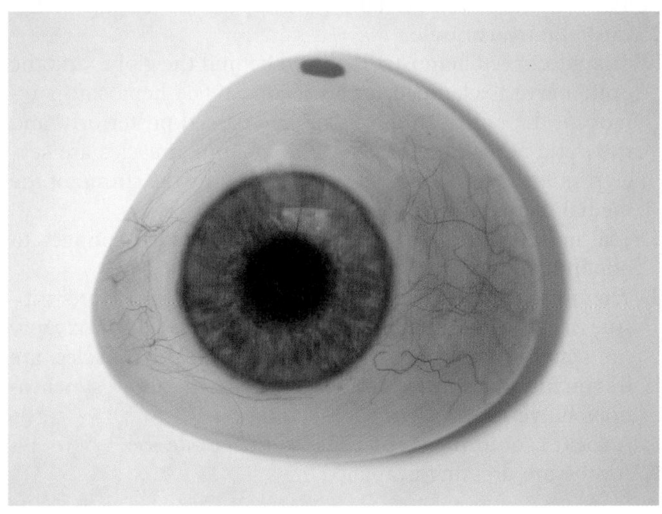

FIGURE 18-27 Artificial eye.

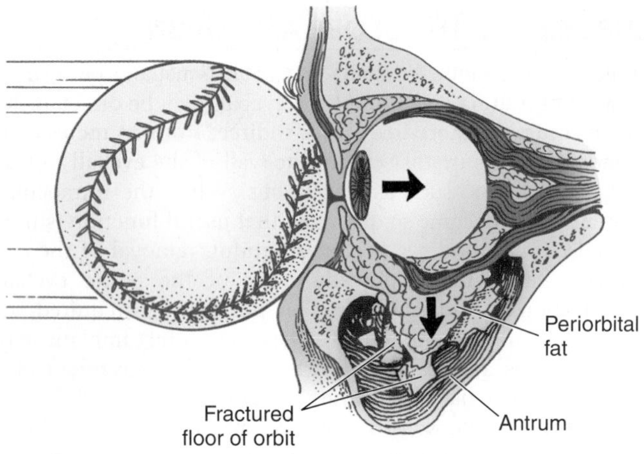


FIGURE 18-28 Ball has struck rim of orbit and has pressed orbital contents backward, displacing fragments of bone into maxillary sinus. Inferior rectus muscle is incarcerated in fracture. Inferior oblique muscle may also be involved.

orbital space. New porous polyethylene implants have the advantage of allowing the rectus muscles to be sutured directly to the implant, thus eliminating the wrapping and expense of donor sclera.[18]

### *Operative Procedure*

1. A speculum retractor is introduced into the palpebral fissure.
2. The conjunctiva is divided around the cornea with sharp and blunt dissection.
3. The medial, lateral, inferior, and superior rectus muscles are divided, leaving a stump of medial rectus muscle. If a coralline hydroxyapatite implant with donor sclera will be used, the four rectus muscles and two oblique muscles are identified and secured with 6-0 nonabsorbable suture (to be used to reattach muscles to cut-out areas in donor sclera) before the muscles are divided.
4. The globe is separated from Tenon's capsule with blunt-pointed curved scissors, retractors, hemostats, and forceps. The eye is rotated laterally by grasping the stump of the medial rectus muscle.
5. A large, curved hemostat is passed behind the globe, and the optic nerve is clamped for 60 seconds. The hemostat is removed, the enucleation scissors are passed posteriorly, and the optic nerve is transected. The oblique muscles are severed as the eye is lifted out of the socket by the stump of the medial rectus muscle.
6. The muscle cone is packed with saline-soaked sponges to obtain hemostasis.
7. The muscle cone is filled with an implant, and Tenon's capsule and the conjunctiva are carefully closed. Hydroxyapatite spheres, with donor sclera to reattach the muscles, are frequently placed for later use, which will allow synchronous movement.
8. A socket conformer is placed into the cul-de-sac.
9. A pressure dressing is applied.

## Evisceration

Evisceration is removal of the contents of the eye, leaving intact the sclera and the attached muscles.

### *Operative Procedure*

1. The conjunctiva is not separated from the sclera as it is for enucleation. A sharp-pointed knife is inserted through the limbus anterior to the iris.
2. The contents of the eye (iris, vitreous, lens) are removed.
3. The choroid adhering to the sclera is removed with curettes.
4. Bleeding is controlled with delicate hemostatic forceps, electrocoagulation, and sutures.
5. A plastic or coral implant is placed within the empty shell.
6. The conjunctival and scleral edges are brought together with nonabsorbable 4-0 or 5-0 sutures, and a pressure dressing is applied.

## Repair of Fracture of the Orbit (Blowout)

A fractured orbit (Figure 18-29) is repaired by means of graft or realignment of contents of the orbit.

***Procedural Considerations.*** The setup is as for dacryocystorhinostomy, plus a graft set (for implantation of an autogenous graft or synthetic graft materials of various sizes and thicknesses) and a flexible, narrow-width retractor. Interosseous wiring may be required for fractures of the frontozygomatic junction. Microplates and screws to stabilize fractures involving the fragile facial and orbital bones may also be used. The patient is prepared as described for eye surgery. A general anesthetic is usually administered.

### *Operative Procedure*

1. The maximum ocular rotation is tested by exerting traction with a forceps on the tendon of the inferior rectus muscle to determine if the inferior muscle sling is trapped in the fracture.
2. To distribute tension over the lower lid and stretch the orbicular muscle, a traction suture is inserted through the lower lid margin.
3. With a #3 knife handle and #15 blade, the lower lid is incised in the lid fold above the orbital rim.
4. The skin is separated from the orbicular muscle, and the orbital septum is identified by blunt dissection. Dissection

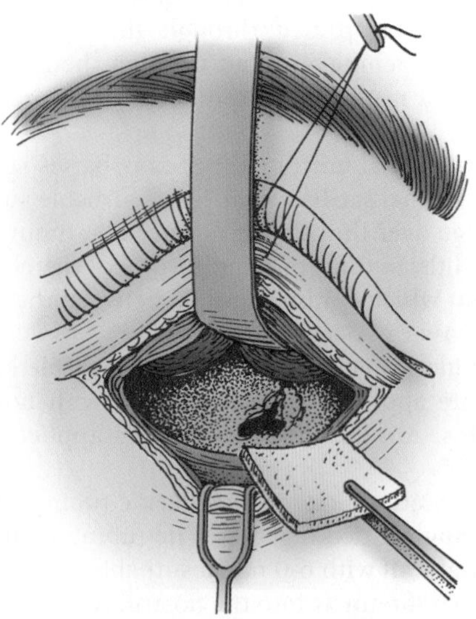

FIGURE 18-29 Stippled area shows blowout fracture site. Autogenous graft from iliac crest is held by forceps ready to be placed over fracture site. Graft usually does not require suturing.

is continued down to the periosteum of the orbital rim by means of scissors, loop retractors, elevators, and forceps.

5. The periosteum of the orbital rim is incised with a #15 blade. With periosteal elevators, the floor of the orbit is exposed and explored. When the fracture site is identified, bone spicules (needle-shaped bone fragments) are removed and the herniated contents are freed from the maxillary antrum. The contents of the orbit are elevated by means of narrow-width, flexible retractors. A 4-0 traction suture is placed around the tendon of the inferior rectus muscle.
6. An autogenous graft is taken from the iliac crest, or an alloplastic material of proper size is used to repair the bony defect. The material may or may not be anchored to the orbital rim by wire sutures.
7. The periosteum is carefully closed with 4-0 absorbable sutures.
8. The skin is closed with 6-0 nonabsorbable sutures, and a pressure dressing is applied.

## Exenteration

Exenteration is removal of the entire orbital contents, including periosteum, for certain malignancies of the globe or orbit. The procedure may also include removal of the external structures of the eyelids.

***Procedural Considerations.*** Considerations are as described for fracture of the orbit. General anesthesia is usually administered.

### *Operative Procedure*

1. Depending on circumstances, exenteration of the eye may include the removal of the lids. An incision is made down to the orbital rim, through the periosteum, and around the entire orbit.
2. With periosteal elevators, the periosteum is freed from the orbital walls and the apex of the orbit.
3. The optic nerve is clamped, and the entire contents of the orbit are removed en bloc.
4. Hemostasis is obtained using electrocoagulation and bone wax.
5. A skin graft or temporal muscle implant may be used to fill the orbital cavity, or the patient may be fitted with an oculofacial prosthesis 2 months postoperatively. If a graft is not placed, iodoform gauze is used to fill the cavity, a pressure dressing is put in place, and the cavity is allowed to granulate.

## Myectomy

Myectomy is a method of weakening the action of a muscle for V-pattern strabismus or superior oblique palsy. This may be done as an excision (resection) of the inferior oblique muscle or as a complete severance of a muscle, such as an inferior oblique myectomy.

### *Operative Procedure*

1. A traction suture is placed at the limbus, and the globe is pulled upward to expose the muscle site.
2. An opening is made into the conjunctiva and Tenon's capsule, and the involved muscle is isolated, lifted, and spread with two muscle hooks.
3. Myectomy of the inferior oblique muscle is performed by placing two straight hemostats across the muscle belly and excising the isolated strip of muscle close to the hemostats. The ends of the muscle are cauterized and released. Because of the peculiar anatomy of this muscle, lateral discontinuity weakens but does not paralyze it.
4. The edges of the conjunctiva are lifted with forceps, and the incision is closed with interrupted absorbable sutures.

## Tuck

A tuck is a method of shortening a muscle and thus strengthening it for patients with superior oblique palsy and torsional diplopia. Tucking is performed primarily on the superior oblique muscle tendon.

### *Operative Procedure*

1. A traction suture is placed at the limbus, and the globe is pulled downward to expose the tendon site. An opening is made in the conjunctiva and Tenon's capsule, medial to the superior rectus muscle.
2. A lid retractor is inserted into the incision to hold back the conjunctiva and Tenon's capsule. The superior rectus muscle is retracted out of the way with muscle hooks.
3. The Jameson muscle hook is passed posteriorly into the orbit, and the superior oblique muscle tendon is hooked and brought into the incision.
4. The tendon is elevated and doubled, like looping a rope, and a double-armed nonabsorbable suture is passed through the base of the loop, effectively shortening the muscle.
5. The tip of the loop is sutured to the sclera, laterally to the superior rectus muscle.
6. The edges of the conjunctiva are lifted with forceps, and the incision is closed with interrupted absorbable sutures.

# SURGERY OF THE CONJUNCTIVA

The conjunctiva of the eye is a transparent and elastic membrane that lines the inner surface of the eyelids and covers the sclera. Lacerations caused by injury as well as deficits resulting from excision of tumors, cysts, nevi, or pterygia can usually be repaired by simple undermining and suturing.

## Pterygium Excision

A pterygium is a fleshy, triangular encroachment of conjunctiva onto the peripheral area of the cornea. Because pterygia tend to recur, surgery is delayed until vision is affected by encroachment on the visual axis.

***Operative Procedure.*** The major steps in the McReynolds technique are illustrated in Figure 18-30. A pterygium can also be excised totally and the limbus treated with an eye cautery or electrocoagulation. The conjunctiva can then be closed, or the sclera can be left bare.

Surgery may be combined with beta-radiation, application of mitomycin, conjunctiva autologous grafts, and lamellar corneal grafts.

## Excisional Biopsy

Any suspect lesion of the conjunctiva can be removed by simple elliptic excision and sent for pathology examination. The conjunctiva may or may not be closed, depending on the surgeon's particular technique.

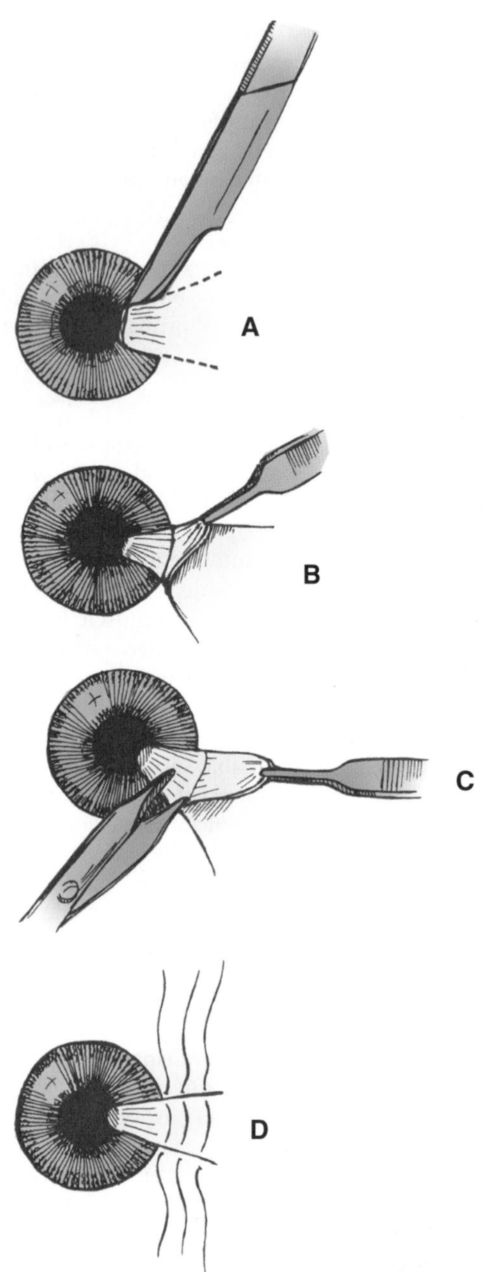


**FIGURE 18-30** McReynolds technique for pterygium excision. **A,** Cornea around head of pterygium is incised. **B,** Pterygium flap is dissected upward, leaving clear cornea. **C,** Lower margin of pterygium is dissected, and whole pterygium is freed from sclera. **D,** Sutures are placed for closure of conjunctiva.

## SURGERY OF THE CORNEA

Surgery of the cornea is indicated for a variety of conditions in which cosmetic, therapeutic, restorative, and refractive outcomes are desired.

### Repair of Lacerations

Corneal lacerations may be closed with direct appositional suturing with 10-0 suture viewed through an operating microscope or with a tissue adhesive, such as cyanoacrylate monomers. The sterile tissue adhesive is applied to well-dried tissue that has been properly oriented anatomically. It polymerizes and seals the wound on contact with the tissue.

Culture specimens are usually obtained at the time of surgery. Antibiotics are injected subconjunctivally before the dressing is applied.

### Corneal Transplantation (Keratoplasty)

A corneal transplantation (keratoplasty) is performed when the patient's cornea is thickened or opacified by disease and degeneration. The transparency of the cornea may be impaired as a result of scars, infection (bacterial, fungal, or viral), thermal or chemical burns, Fuch's dystrophy, or keratoconus (abnormal steepening). Corneal transplantation, in which corneal tissue from one human eye is grafted to another, is done to improve vision when the retina and optic nerve are functioning properly. Because the cornea is tissue that lacks blood vessels, it can be transplanted with less rejection and at a 90% success rate. Keratoplasty may be performed as a lamellar (partial-thickness) graft or a penetrating (full-thickness) graft.

Phototherapeutic keratectomy (PTK) procedures use excimer laser ablation to remove superficial corneal lesions and smooth the corneal surface. PTK can be used on conditions that would require corneal transplant and may delay or replace the occurrence of penetrating keratoplasty in some cases.

***Procurement of Corneas.*** The eye bank may be a central community agency or may be owned and operated by a hospital. Eye banks help coordinate the procurement of eyes from recently deceased persons under the Eye Bank Association of America (EBAA) guidelines. Persons 2 to 70 years of age can be eye donors, and poor eyesight or cataracts do not matter. The donor's family, medical, and social histories are reviewed. It is not necessary to do antigen matching as with other tissue or organ transplants, but blood serum tests for human immunodeficiency virus (HIV) and hepatitis B virus are performed on the donor. Donor eyes are removed within 6 hours of death in accordance with legal regulations. Tissue, such as a cornea, must be recovered, processed, and transplanted in controlled surgical environments.[3] If the donor eye is unsuitable for the cornea to be transplanted, the eye can be used for research or education.

Many individuals have signed donor cards or eye-donor designation on their drivers' licenses. A special consent form is required and should be signed by the authorized next of kin and by a hospital representative designated by institutional policy. Federal regulations require hospitals to report all deaths and imminent deaths to organ procurement organizations. With the collaboration of hospitals, organ procurement organizations, and eye and tissue banks, the family of every potential donor is informed about the option to donate organs or tissues.

The enucleations may be done in the hospital morgue or emergency department under aseptic conditions. The procured cornea is placed in Optisol GS sterile buffered tissue culture medium within 12 hours of death and transplanted within 3 to 7 days. Optisol GS sterile buffered tissue culture medium contains polypeptides, dextran, and antibiotics (gentamicin and streptomycin) and can preserve a donor cornea for 14 days under refrigeration. It is best if corneal transplantation is performed in 2 or 3 days because the cornea may become boggy from constant exposure to the tissue culture solution.

***Procedural Considerations.*** Postmortem preparation includes elevating the donor's head with a pillow to minimize edema in the face or near the eye. The eyes are irrigated and lightly taped closed to avoid pressure on the eye. A small ice pack may be applied to the forehead or over the eyes if the donor is not in a refrigerated morgue within 1 hour of death.

For the procurement procedure, the eyes are washed and irrigated in the routine manner of preparation for eye surgery. The sterile field, drapes, and instruments are essentially the same as those for an enucleation on a living patient.

### *Operative Procedures*

1. Eye specimen jars are labeled for right and left eyes.
2. The speculum is inserted, and after routine enucleation the donated eye is placed with the cornea up and secured in a metal eye cage or on gauze in the sterile specimen jar.
3. The eye sockets are packed with cotton, and the lids are closed.
4. Specimen jars are sealed with tape and labeled with the donor's name or identification number, time of death, time of enucleation, and date. The jars are placed on wet ice in an insulated carrier and transported to the eye bank. The entire cornea with a scleral rim will be placed in Optisol GS before transplant.

PENETRATING KERATOPLASTY

1. The eye speculum is put in place, and superior rectus and inferior rectus bridle sutures are placed if a Flieringa ring is not to be used. If a ring is used, it is sutured in place with four 5-0 sutures (Figure 18-31).
2. A corneoscleral button that has been refrigerated and stored in tissue culture medium (Optisol GS) is removed from its container.
3. The corneoscleral button is placed epithelial (outside) surface down on a sterile Teflon block. The corneal trephine is then used as a punch, and the donor button is pressed out centrally. A drop of Optisol GS may be used to cover the donor button until it is implanted.
4. The section of cornea removed from the recipient's eye is usually 0.25 mm in diameter smaller than the graft taken from the donor's eye. The button is excised with a handheld trephine or a disposable suction trephine.
5. Peripheral iridectomies or iridotomies may be performed at this time at the surgeon's discretion, or a cataract extraction with IOL implantation may also be performed if the lens is opaque.
6. The graft is placed into the opening of the recipient's eye and anchored in place by means of four single-armed sutures placed at the four cardinal meridians, viewed through an operating microscope. Some surgeons preplace sutures in the graft. The graft is sutured to the host with either continuous or interrupted 10-0 nonabsorbable sutures.
7. Air or sodium hyaluronate (Healon) may be injected into the anterior chamber of the recipient's eye to keep the iris from adhering to the suture line. Mydriatic or miotic solutions are used at the surgeon's discretion.
8. A subconjunctival injection of antibiotic solution or a topical application of antibiotic drops may be used at the completion of the procedure. Antibiotic ointment is applied, followed by an eye pad and a protective shield.

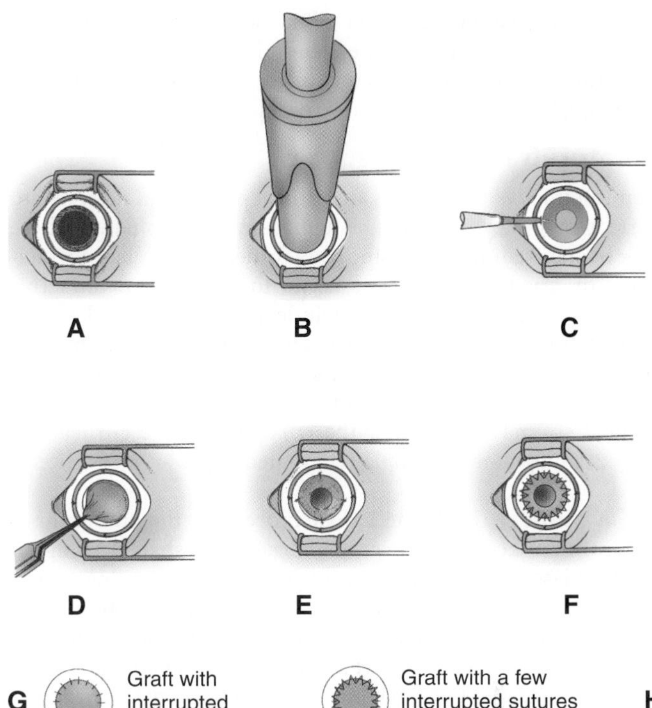


**FIGURE 18-31** Corneal transplantation. **A,** Eye of patient who will undergo corneal transplantation. Flieringa fixation ring is sutured in place with 5-0 nonabsorbable sutures. **B,** Corneal trephine is placed on recipient cornea, and partial penetration is made approximately three fourths through stroma. **C,** Anterior chamber is entered through groove, and the remainder of button is excised with right and left corneal micro scissors. **D,** Corneal button is removed. **E,** Donor cornea graft is sutured in place with four sutures. **F,** Donor cornea graft is sutured in place with interrupted or continuous 10-0 nonabsorbable suture (**G** and **H**).

LAMELLAR KERATOPLASTY

1. The eye speculum and superior rectus and inferior rectus bridle sutures are placed if needed.
2. The eye from the eye bank is removed from its container and washed in balanced salt solution.
3. The eye is wrapped in a surgical dressing. A groove is made at the desired depth in the cornea with the trephine. The Castroviejo keratome is set at the desired depth, and the lamellar sheet of cornea is removed and placed into a Petri dish.
4. The recipient cornea is grooved with the same trephine to the appropriate depth. Using the operating microscope, the surgeon performs a lamellar resection, that is, removes the anterior part of the cornea at a predetermined depth with a Gill knife, Beaver knife blade #64, or other corneal splitter.
5. The donor tissue is sutured in place with a continuous 10-0 nonabsorbable suture.
6. A mydriatic agent and subconjunctival or topical antibiotics may be used.
7. The eye is patched.

***Deep Lamellar Endothelial Keratoplasty.*** Deep lamellar endothelial keratoplasty (DLEK) is an emerging technique. It consists of replacing the endothelium without transplanting the cornea to restore vision. This technique offers the potential for highly predictable corneal power for extended periods without the astigmatism that often occurs with penetrating keratoplasty. The transplanted endothelium is inserted into host through a small incision rather than an open-sky approach, greatly reducing the risk of infection.

## Keratorefractive Procedures

Keratorefractive procedures are corneal procedures designed to correct myopia, hyperopia, astigmatism, and aphakia. These procedures require reshaping the cornea with relaxing incisions or cryolathing corneal tissue to change the refractive power of the cornea. They include photorefractive keratectomy (PRK), which uses the excimer laser to treat myopia (nearsightedness), and laser-assisted in-situ keratomileusis (LASIK), which uses the excimer laser for photoablation of the corneal stroma bed to alter the curvature of the cornea and correct myopia or hyperopia (farsightedness).[19]

***LASIK Surgery.*** With the LASIK procedure, the curvature of the front surface of the eye, the cornea, is reshaped using an excimer laser.[16] The purpose is to permit the individual to see well at a distance without glasses. For nearsighted patients the central curvature of the cornea is flattened. To flatten the cornea, stromal tissue is removed from the center of the cornea (Figure 18-32, *A*). For farsighted patients the central curvature of the cornea is steepened. To steepen the cornea, stromal tissue is removed from the periphery of the cornea, leaving the center untreated (Figure 18-32, *B*).

**PROCEDURAL CONSIDERATIONS.** An extensive preoperative evaluation is necessary to be sure that the patient is a candidate for the LASIK procedure. Before surgery, a topical antibiotic and topical anesthetic are placed in the patient's eye. If the patient has astigmatism, he or she is taken to a slit lamp and a mark is made on the conjunctivae to assist in the correction of the astigmatism. Circular corneal markers (3 mm and 4 mm) may be used.

OPERATIVE PROCEDURE

1. The patient lies down, and a locking lid speculum is placed in position. The patient's head position is adjusted to account for the astigmatism.
2. The cornea is marked to assist in the placement of the "corneal cap" after the procedure. A suction device is placed on the eye to immobilize it.
3. A microkeratome (Hansatome, ACS, Moria, Amadeus) is used to create a lamellar keratectomy of 0.130 to 0.180 microns in thickness. This piece of cornea is reflected out of the way with a flat cornea spatula, and the laser treatment is applied to the base of the lamellar keratectomy.
4. The corneal cap is replaced on the stromal bed using a Slade irrigating cannula on a 3-ml syringe with saline. The corneal cap is permitted to dry for several minutes. The corneal cap stays in position because of capillary attraction.
5. Antibiotic drops and nonsteroidal antiinflammatory drops are placed in the eye. A goggle is placed over the eye to prevent slippage of the corneal cap for the next 24 hours.

***LASEK Surgery.*** Laser epithelial keratomileusis (LASEK) is similar to PRK, because the procedure is performed on the surface of the cornea. After numbing the eye with topical anesthetic drops, the surgeon loosens the epithelium with a diluted alcohol solution and pushes it aside. A laser is then used to treat the corneal surface, similar to PRK and LASIK procedures. The epithelial flap is then returned to its original posi-

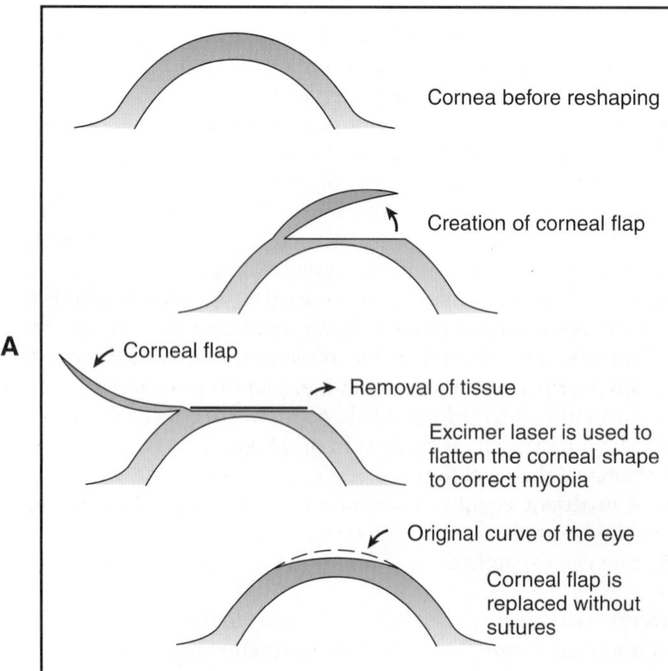


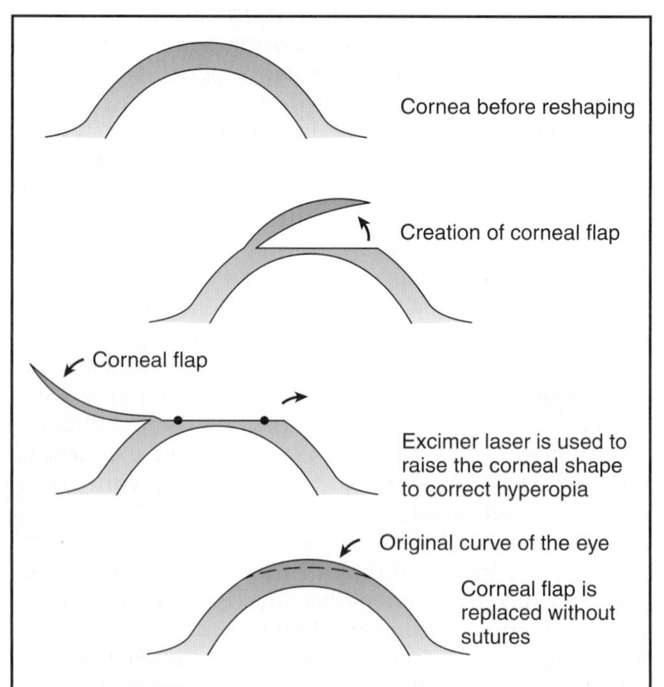


**FIGURE 18-32** Laser-assisted in-situ keratomileusis (LASIK) surgery. **A,** Diagram of LASIK correction for nearsightedness. **B,** Diagram of LASIK correction for farsightedness.

tion, and a bandage contact lens is placed for the duration of the healing process, which may last several days.

## SURGERY OF THE LENS

### Cataract Extraction

A cataract (from the Greek word meaning "waterfall") extraction is removal of the opaque lens from the interior of the eye.[5] The lens consists of 65% water, 35% protein, and a trace of other body minerals. The disorders of the lens are opacification and dislocation, resulting in blurred vision without pain or inflammation. Cataracts (opacification) vary in degree of density, size, and location and are usually caused by aging or trauma.

The intracapsular cataract extraction (ICCE) method of cataract removal consists of removing the lens within its capsule with a cryoprobe and is rarely performed today except in the event of a dislocated lens. Because ICCE is not frequently used, the medication alpha-chymotrypsin (Catarase, Chymar), which is an enzyme that acts on the zonules of the lens, will not be immediately available. If an ICCE is scheduled, the medication and a cataract cryoprobe need to be procured.

In the extracapsular method, the anterior portion of the capsule is first ruptured and removed and the lens cortex and nucleus are expressed from the eye, leaving the posterior capsule behind. Restoration of functional vision is necessary after removal of the crystalline lens (aphakia). Contact lenses can be used to correct aphakia. They offer an excellent option for visual correction and can be used for monocular aphakia.

***Intraocular Lens.*** The most commonly used option for visual correction after lens removal is the implantation of an IOL during the surgical procedure. IOLs offer many advantages to patients. They are used for monocular aphakic correction. Rehabilitation times for patients are shortened.

The newer generation IOLs are made of silicone or acrylic resin.[17] Foldable and injectable designs and new implantation techniques challenge perioperative nursing personnel to keep abreast of constant changes in techniques for IOL implantations. Posterior chamber lenses (PCLs) can be implanted only when the cataract was removed by extracapsular cataract extraction (ECCE). This is the most physiologic position for an artificial lens and is now the most common method of lens extraction. Anterior chamber lenses (ACLs) are used after ICCE and for secondary lens implantation.

IOLs are available in various diopter powers. The necessary power is determined by measuring the curvature of the patient's cornea (keratometry) and the axial length (length from cornea to retina). A mathematical formula is then used to calculate the correct lens power. IOLs are also available in bifocal and multifocal types.

In recent years sutureless cataract techniques have become increasingly popular because of rapid visual rehabilitation. Clear cornea microincisions with the use of topical anesthesia and insertion of foldable IOLs have produced even better visual results with the opportunity to fully correct refractive errors (Research Highlight).

***Procedural Considerations.*** Instrumentation varies with surgeon's preference but usually includes forceps to insert the lens and lens haptics and a hook to aid in rotating and positioning the lens (Figure 18-33). Perioperative nursing person-

#### RESEARCH HIGHLIGHT

**Photolysis Laser Technology**

Cataract surgery is one of the most frequently performed surgical procedures in the United States. Although today's standard of cataract surgery performed by phacoemulsification with insertion of a foldable intraocular lens (IOL) implant is one of the safest and most efficient surgical procedures, interest is ongoing in finding techniques for even smaller incisions and for eventually performing an endocapsular cataract extraction. This type of procedure would leave the lens capsule intact and allow the potential for an injectable substance that would be used instead of IOLs as replacement for the crystalline lens. A clinical study of 1000 consecutive cataract surgeries with the photolysis Q-switched neodymium:yttrium-aluminum-garnet (Nd:YAG) laser and implantation of a foldable posterior chamber IOL was conducted at 12 international clinical sites. Mean values for visual acuity improvement ranged from 20/70.2 to 20/24.4. Mean photolysis time was 2.15 minutes for up to +1 nuclear sclerosis; 4.8 minutes for up to +2 nuclear sclerosis; and 9.8 minutes for up to +3 nuclear sclerosis. Minor complications occurred in 18 cases. These results suggest that photolysis laser technology may be a safe, effective alternative for laser cataract extraction and that it is possible to perform cataract extraction with IOL implantation with incisions less than 2 mm.

Modified from Kanellopoulos AJ and the Photolysis Investigative Group: Laser cataract surgery: a prospective clinical evaluation of 1000 consecutive laser cataract procedures using the Dodick photolysis Nd:YAG system, *Ophthalmology* 108(4):649-653, 2001.

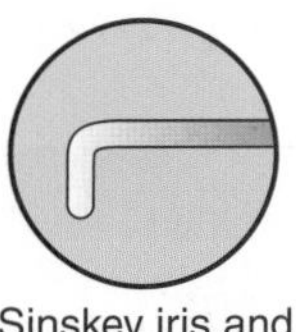
Sinskey iris and IOL hook

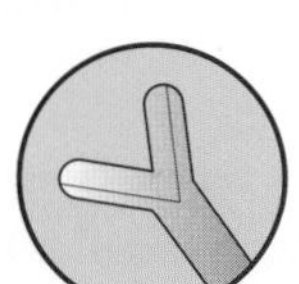
Bechert nucleus rotator

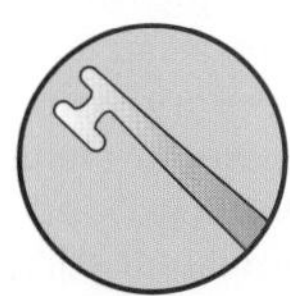
Kuglen push-pull hook

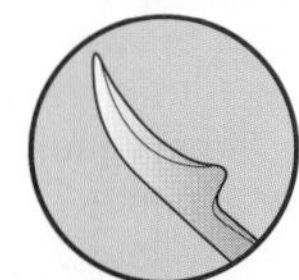
Bechert-Hoffer nucleus rotator

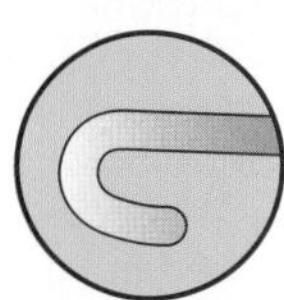
Maumenee iris hook

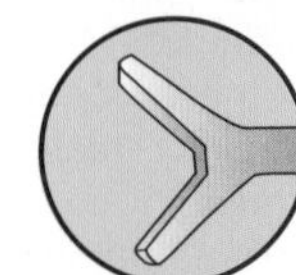
Osher "Y" hook

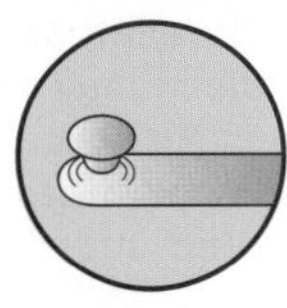
Graether collar button

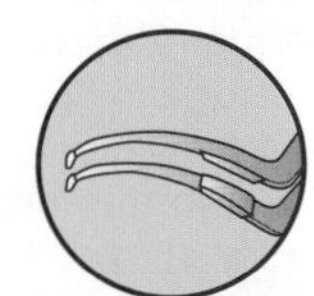
Lehner-Utrata capsulorrhexis forceps

**FIGURE 18-33** Close-up of tips of micro instruments used in phacoemulsification procedures and for inserting intraocular lenses (IOLs).

nel must be familiar with institutional policies pertaining to IOLs and their use (Patient Safety).

**EXTRACAPSULAR METHOD WITH PHACOEMULSIFICATION.** Over the past years numerous microsurgical techniques have been developed for lens removal through a small self-sealing incision and most recently through a clear cornea incision. ECCE with phacoemulsification is still performed, especially with very mature or hard cataracts, and may be performed in combination with trabeculectomy for patients with glaucoma.

Basically, each technique involves opening the lens capsule and using a phacoemulsification unit with irrigation and aspiration (I/A). The ultrasonic energy of phacoemulsification fragments the hard lens material, which can then be aspirated from the eye. All perioperative personnel using specialized instruments and equipment must have thorough knowledge of the operation as well as problems that may be encountered and actions to correct them.

**Operative Procedure**

1. After a superior rectus bridle suture is placed, a small limbus-based flap is dissected superiorly (Figure 18-34).
2. The surgical limbus is cleaned by sharp dissection with a Beaver knife blade. Hemostasis is obtained with the eye cautery.
3. A 3-mm incision is made into the eye with either a keratome or a sharp microknife.
4. The lens capsule is opened with capsulorrhexis forceps or a cystotome. The anterior chamber may be kept formed with air or an irrigating solution.
5. The lens nucleus is loosened from the cortex with the cystotome or a blunt cyclodialysis spatula.
6. The ultrasonic handpiece is checked by the physician for appropriate vacuum control. *This check should be made before any handpiece is introduced into the eye.*
7. The ultrasonic handpiece is introduced into the eye. The following modes are operational with the foot pedal under the surgeon's control: irrigation alone; irrigation and aspiration; phacoemulsification; and irrigation, aspiration, and phacoemulsification. Some machines also have an anterior vitrector. As the surgeon manipulates the handpiece and operates the foot pedal to emulsify the lens nucleus, the perioperative nurse is responsible for operating the console controls and monitoring the function of the instrument.
8. When the lens nucleus has been emulsified and removed, the lens cortex is removed with the I/A handpiece.
9. If a foldable IOL is to be implanted, a keratome is used to widen the incision to 3.2 mm and the lens is folded and inserted. If a rigid IOL is to be implanted, the wound is extended to 5.1 mm to accommodate the lens diameter. Acetylcholine may be introduced to constrict the pupil.
10. A peripheral iridectomy may be performed.
11. The corneoscleral wound is closed with a 10-0 nonabsorbable suture.
12. The conjunctival flap is closed with a suture or using bipolar electrocoagulation.
13. An eye pad and shield are applied.

**TOPICAL CLEAR CORNEAL CATARACT PROCEDURE.** Developments with the use of topical anesthetics, new

## PATIENT SAFETY

### Preventing Wrong IOL Placement

Although rare, insertion of an incorrect intraocular lens (IOL) in cataract surgery can occur. The IOL can be the wrong power, wrong size, or wrong type. Any of these errors can lead to postoperative refractive errors and less satisfactory vision for the patient. The surgeon is ultimately responsible for ensuring that the correct lens is placed at the time of surgery. Good communication is essential among the surgeon/assistant surgeon and operating room (OR) personnel. Although a number of potential errors can lead to the placement of a wrong IOL, mistakes in the OR can be minimized by observing the following suggested protocol for safety:

- Check the lens power against the medical record in the OR.
- The correct lens should be in the OR before sedation/anesthesia.
- Perform a final verification of the IOL power and diopter before incision or before IOL insertion against the IOL Calculation Report.
- The ophthalmic history and exam and form that contains keratometry and axial length, primary and alternate lens or lenses for each patient should be available in the OR.
- If at all possible, there should only be one IOL measurement per eye on the form. If the computerized IOL measurement program allows, measurements for the left and right eyes should be printed on separate forms.
- The surgeon or assistant surgeon should select the primary and alternate IOL or IOLs before the start of the procedure. The surgeon verifies the IOL number, diopter, optic, A-constant, and length against the IOL Calculation Report form, documentation, or patient medical record.
- Before incision or when the surgeon requests the IOL, the circulating nurse shows the IOL box to the surgeon. The surgeon and circulating RN verify the IOL model, power, and other calculation information, patient identification, and operative eye against the IOL Calculation Report.
- The circulating nurse then repeats this procedure with the scrub person (i.e., shows the IOL box and verbally states the model number and lens power).
- The scrub person verbally states the model number and lens power as he or she passes the lens to the surgeon for implantation.
- The surgeon may elect to perform visual inspection of the IOL under the microscope for appropriateness and any lens defect or deposit.
- If there is a discrepancy, the surgeon reviews the IOL Calculation Report or ophthalmic history and exam or designated institute form.
- The circulating nurse puts the IOL labels on the IOL card and operative record/patient chart right after the surgeon implants the IOL. He or she documents the IOL verification procedure in the patient record.

Modified from American Academy of Ophthalmology: *Patient safety bulletin number 2.* Accessed February 8, 2006, on-line: www.aao.org/aao/education/library/safety.

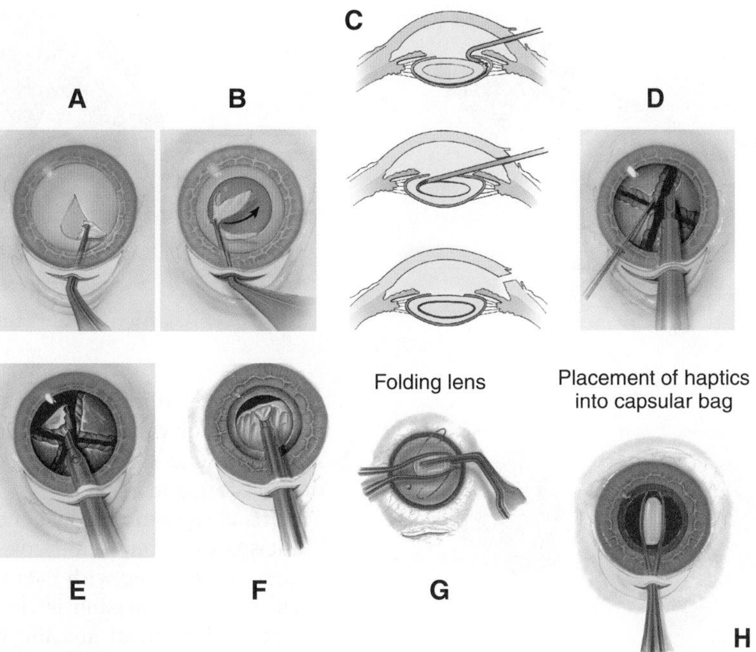


FIGURE 18-34 Cataract extraction with phacoemulsification. **A** and **B**, Capsulorrhexis is performed on anterior capsule of lens. **C**, The nucleus of the lens is loosened by hydrodissection. **D**, The nucleus of the lens is "cracked" into four quadrants and, **E**, removed with phacoemulsification. **F**, The irrigation and aspiration (I/A) handpiece is used to strip the remaining cortex from the capsule. **G**, The intraocular lens (IOL) is folded. **H**, The IOL is placed into the capsular bag.

materials for foldable IOLs, and diamond knives for self-sealing or no-stitch wounds led to clear cornea incisions and new techniques for phacoemulsification and lens implantation for cataracts. Clear cornea microincisions create the opportunity for full correction of refractive errors during the surgical procedure.

Topical anesthesia replaces retrobulbar anesthesia for cataract surgery, and because the patient can fixate, this allows for refractive surgical techniques. Patients must be able to hear and follow directions to cooperate with verbal instructions to fixate on the microscope light. Various medications and protocols are used for administering topical anesthesia before cataract surgery.

A typical protocol is as follows. A drop of topical tetracaine 0.5% is placed into the operative eye before the patient enters the operating room. The patient is instructed to keep this eye closed to prevent the cornea from drying out. As the patient is being positioned, another drop of tetracaine is given. An armrest is positioned on the operative side, and the patient's head and microscope are adjusted. The patient is instructed to look at the light of the microscope and told where to fixate. If the patient cannot open his or her eye, a facial nerve block should be considered. If the patient cannot fixate on the light at all, a retrobulbar block should be considered.

**Operative Procedure**

1. A speculum that sits over the nose and has no attachment temporally is placed in the eye.
2. A stab incision is made at 5 o'clock in a left eye or at 11 o'clock if the right eye into the anterior chamber. A 1-mm–wide incision is desirable.
3. One ml of unpreserved lidocaine is slowly injected into the anterior chamber through a 30-gauge cannula using a tuberculin syringe.
4. A viscoelastic material is injected into the anterior chamber to deepen the chamber and widen the pupil.
5. A space of 3 mm is marked on the cornea temporally with a caliper. A vertical incision of 0.3-mm to 4.0-mm depth is made with a trifacet diamond knife.
6. A diamond keratome is used to make a stepped incision into the anterior chamber 2.6 mm in length on the endothelial surface of the cornea (Figure 18-35, *A*).
7. A capsulotomy and capsulorrhexis are performed with a capsulorrhexis forceps (Figure 18-35, *B*).
8. Hydrodissection and hydrodelineation are carried out with a 30-gauge cannula and saline (Figure 18-35, *C*).
9. A phacoemulsification tip is placed into the eye and used to sculpt the nucleus.
10. Using a cyclodialysis spatula at 5 o'clock in the left eye or at 11 o'clock if the right eye the nucleus is divided into quadrants with the phacoemulsification tip and removed from the eye (Figure 18-35, *D*).
11. An I/A tip is placed into the eye and used to remove the remaining cortical material (Figure 18-35, *E*).
12. A Kratz scratcher is used to polish the posterior capsule.
13. Viscoelastic material is placed into the capsular bag to inflate it.
14. A steel keratome is used to widen the incision to 3.2 mm.
15. A posterior chamber IOL is folded and placed into the eye with forceps or an injector and into the capsular bag (Figure 18-35, *F* and *G*). The IOL is positioned with a Sinsky hook or other positioning tip.
16. An I/A tip is used to remove the remaining viscoelastic material. Using saline through a 30-gauge cannula, the anterior chamber is repressurized. Leaking of the wound can be stopped by hydrating the wound edges. Occasionally a 10-0 nylon suture is necessary.

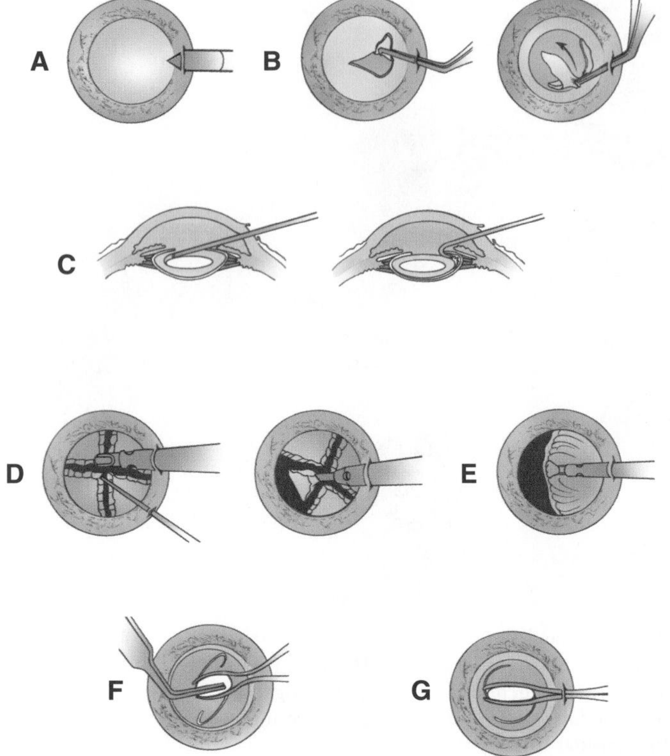


FIGURE 18-35 Clear cornea cataract extraction. **A,** A 2.6-mm incision is made into the cornea. **B,** Capsulorrhexis is performed on anterior capsule of lens. **C,** Nucleus of lens is loosened by hydrodissection. **D,** Nucleus of lens is "cracked" into four quadrants and removed with phacoemulsification. **E,** Irrigation and aspiration (I/A) handpiece is used to strip the remaining cortex from the capsule. **F,** Intraocular lens (IOL) is folded. **G,** IOL is placed into the capsular bag.

17. Timoptic (timolol) 0.5% drops and TobraDex (tobramycin and dexamethasone) drops or Ocuflox (ofloxacin) drops are placed on the eye. The eye is not patched.

## SURGERY FOR GLAUCOMA

### Iridectomy

Peripheral iridectomy is removal of a section of iris tissue (Figure 18-36). Peripheral iridectomy is usually performed as part of a trabeculectomy procedure or may be performed when laser iridotomy is not feasible because of cloudy cornea or uveitis. Peripheral iridectomy is done in the treatment of acute, subacute, or chronic angle-closure glaucoma when extensive peripheral anterior synechiae have not formed. This operation is performed to reestablish communication between the posterior and anterior chambers, thus relieving pupillary block and permitting the iris root to drop away from the trabecular meshwork to reestablish the outflow of aqueous fluid through Schlemm's canal.

#### *Operative Procedure*

1. The speculum is introduced. The globe is fixed with a 4-0 traction suture passed under the superior rectus and fastened to the drape with a hemostat.

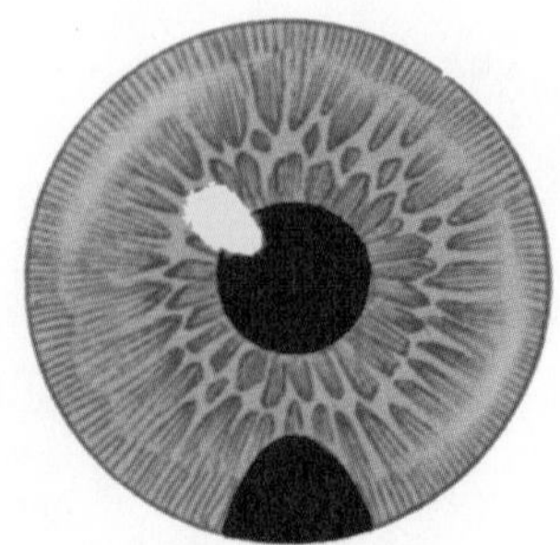

FIGURE 18-36 Peripheral iridectomy.

2. A small beveled incision is made at the superior limbus, or a perpendicular incision is made in the clear cornea.
3. The peripheral iris is grasped with forceps, pulled through the incision, and excised.
4. The iris is repositioned by gently stroking the cornea with a blunt spatula or muscle hook. The iris can also be repositioned by irrigating with balanced salt solution.
5. A clear corneal incision is closed with 10-0 nonabsorbable suture, and a limbal incision is closed with absorbable suture. Subconjunctival antibiotics may be administered, and an eye pad is applied.

### Trabeculectomy

The term *trabeculectomy* is a misnomer because it implies that part of the trabecular meshwork is removed during surgery. Trabeculectomy is a filtering procedure accomplished by incising a conjunctival flap and a scleral flap, creating a fistula, performing an iridectomy, and creating the filtering bleb. Trabeculectomy is often combined with cataract removal (phacoemulsification) and insertion of an IOL.

***Procedural Considerations.*** Adjunctive medical therapy to decrease postoperative fibrosis includes application of an antimetabolite-soaked sponge (5-fluorouracil [5-FU] or mitomycin C) placed under the conjunctival flap. Because 5-FU and mitomycin C are antimetabolites, nursing precautions for handling hazardous waste must be carried out.[3] The circulating nurse must wear gloves while drawing up the antimetabolite from the vial to transfer to the operative field. All items used with the medication should be disposed of as hazardous waste. Instruments that come into contact with antimetabolites should be washed separately.

#### *Operative Procedure*

1. Incisions are made into the conjunctiva and Tenon's capsule, dissection is done, and a conjunctival–Tenon's capsule flap is created. Hemostasis is obtained with bipolar coagulation (Figure 18-37).
2. If antimetabolite is to be used, it is applied to the sclera before any incision into the sclera. A small piece of sponge is saturated in the antimetabolite (5-FU or mitomycin C) and placed between the conjunctival–Tenon's capsule flap and the sclera. The sponge is left in place for 3 to 5 minutes, and then the site is irrigated vigorously with copious amounts of BSS.
3. A partial-thickness scleral flap is incised. The flap can be square or triangular.
4. The scleral flap is retracted, and an incision is made into and through the limbus into the anterior chamber with the tip of

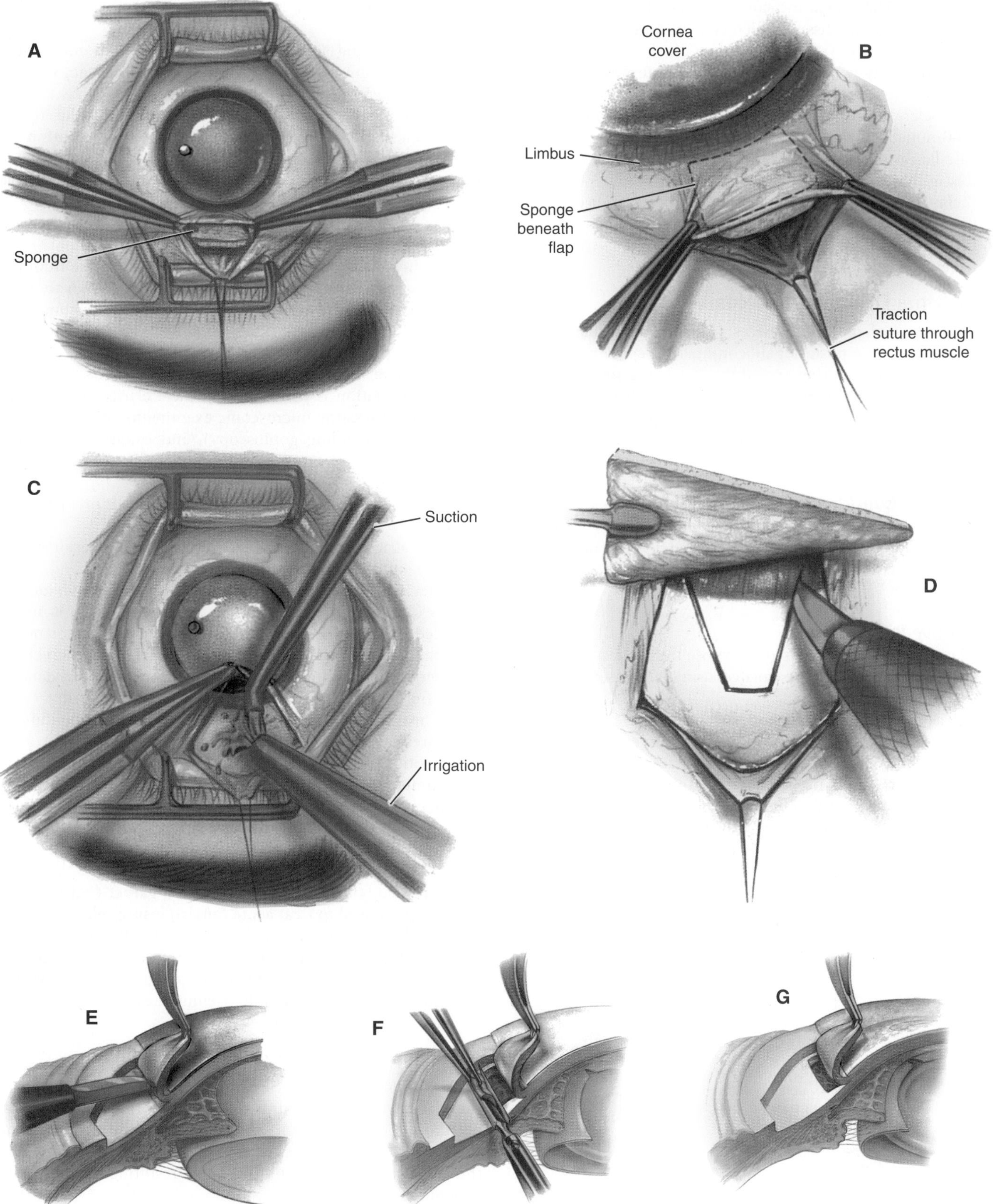


FIGURE 18-37 Trabeculectomy. **A,** Sponge soaked in antimetabolite is placed on sclera and, **B,** held in place for 3 to 5 minutes. **C,** Area is thoroughly irrigated. **D,** Scleral flap is formed. **E,** Incision is made into anterior chamber. **F** and **G,** Fistula is created by removing a flap of limbal tissue.

the blade. The limbal incision is extended to a rectangular flap of deep limbal tissue, which is then excised to create the fistula.
5. An iridectomy is performed. The eye cautery is applied to bleeding sites and to the ciliary processes.
6. The scleral flap is replaced and sutured with interrupted 10-0 nonabsorbable sutures. The conjunctival–Tenon's capsule flap is closed with a running suture, and the conjunctiva is closed.
7. BSS is injected through a cannula into the anterior chamber to deepen the anterior chamber and elevate the conjunctival bleb.
8. An eye pad and shield are applied.

## Glaucoma Drainage Devices

Several types of drainage devices (Figure 18-38) have been implanted into the posterior subconjunctival space with varying success when filtering procedures have been unsuccessful. These include the Molteno implant, Krupin valve, Ahmed device, Baerveldt device, and Schocket implant.[4] Complications have been reduced through modifications in design and technique.

***Procedural Considerations.*** The glaucoma drainage device may be soaked in an antibiotic solution, and the pericardium or patch graft will also need to be hydrated or soaked.[7] The drainage device and graft are documented as implants per facility procedure.

### *Operative Procedure*

1. The conjunctiva is incised to expose the sclera.
2. Two rectus muscles are isolated using silk ties as traction sutures.
3. Measurements are made for placement of the plate of the device. The plate is then sutured to the sclera.
4. After the patency of the device is checked, an occluding suture is inserted into the drainage tube.
5. With a needle, a tunnel is created into the anterior chamber for the tube and paracentesis tract.
6. The tube is trimmed and inserted into the anterior chamber. The tube is sutured to the sclera with 9-0 nonabsorbable suture.

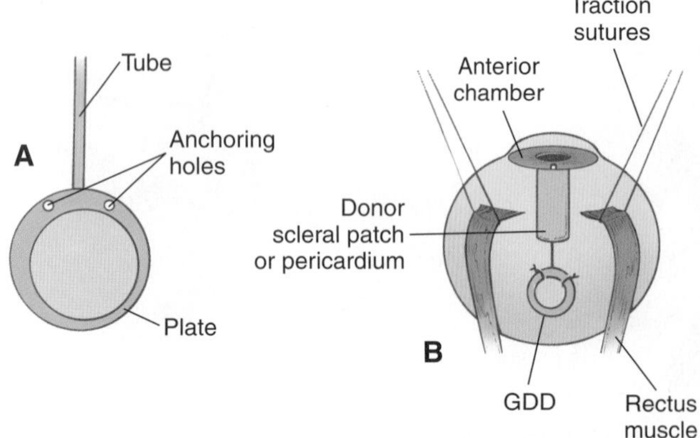


**FIGURE 18-38** Glaucoma drainage devices (GDDs). **A,** Components of GDD. **B,** GDD in place. Tip of drainage tube in anterior chamber. Donor scleral patch or pericardium covering tube from plate to edge of cornea.

7. The tube is covered with patch graft of donor sclera or pericardium.
8. The occluding suture is passed through Tenon's capsule and the conjunctiva into the inferior cul-de-sac, secured with absorbable suture, and trimmed.
9. Traction sutures are removed from around the rectus muscles, and the conjunctiva is closed with a continuous 7-0 absorbable suture.
10. Antiinfective agents are injected subconjunctivally. The eye is dressed with an eye pad and shield.

## Goniotomy

Goniotomy is the opening of a congenital membrane from the iris surface to Schwalbe line, allowing aqueous humor to reach the trabecular meshwork in cases of congenital glaucoma.

### *Operative Procedure*

1. The patient is anesthetized without intubation.
2. An examination is performed. Corneal clarity and size, intraocular pressure, microscopic examination of the anterior segment (including gonioscopy), and examination of the posterior pole of the eye (especially the optic disc) are recorded.
3. The patient is intubated, if indicated, and prepped and draped.
4. A pediatric eye speculum and superior and inferior rectus bridle sutures are placed.
5. Under microscopic control with an appropriate goniotomy lens (gonioprism) in place, the goniotomy knife is introduced through the temporal limbus. The anterior chamber is maintained with viscoelastic material. The membrane covering the iris and angle structures is cut without damaging the trabecular meshwork. The knife is removed.
6. BSS may be used to re-form the anterior chamber, and a suture may be used to close the incision.
7. A miotic (pilocarpine) may be used topically. Antiinfective-antiinflammatory ointment is used.
8. The eye is dressed with an eye pad and protective shield.

# LASER THERAPY AND PHOTOCOAGULATION

Argon or neodymium:yttrium-aluminum-garnet (Nd:YAG) laser therapy is used to treat acute (angle-closure) glaucoma and open-angle glaucoma. Laser therapy is a fairly uncomplicated ambulatory procedure in which a slit lamp is used for delivery of the laser beam. Laser treatment of glaucoma is a noninvasive procedure and, if successful, may eliminate the need for more invasive surgical procedures.

## Laser Trabeculoplasty

Laser trabeculoplasty is treatment for open-angle glaucoma by the placement of laser burns in the posterior part of the trabecula, anterior to the scleral spur, to cause the surface of the trabecular meshwork to contract. This theoretically pulls open the adjacent intertrabecular spaces, resulting in increased aqueous outflow.

***Procedural Considerations.*** Preoperative sedation is usually unnecessary. A topical anesthetic such as proparacaine is used. Intraocular pressure is measured preoperatively. Laser safety precautions are initiated.

*Operative Procedure*

1. One or two proparacaine (Ophthaine) drops are instilled in the operative eye.
2. The patient is positioned at the laser slit lamp (Figure 18-39).
3. A three-mirror Goldmann lens is placed, allowing visualization of the chamber angle and retraction of the eyelid. The perioperative nurse assists in this placement.
4. A landmark is selected as a starting point, and laser treatment is begun, with a 50-mm spot size applied for 0.1 second at 850 milliwatt (mW) power. Light-pigmented tissue requires more power, whereas dark-pigmented tissue requires less power. The laser "burns" are placed into the anterior portion of the functional trabecular meshwork, pigmented zone, to yield about 20 burns in each quadrant for a total of 70 to 90 burns. The power should be titrated to the threshold of whitening or tiny bubble formation.
5. One hour after completion of the treatment, the intraocular pressure is measured and topical prednisolone or dexamethasone drops instilled.
6. The procedure may be performed in two treatment segments rather than completed in one.

## Laser Iridotomy

Laser iridotomy is the placement of penetrating argon or Nd:YAG laser burns in the peripheral part of the iris to create an opening, allowing aqueous humor to flow from the posterior chamber into the anterior chamber and out through Schlemm's canal to treat angle-closure glaucoma.

***Procedural Considerations.*** The operative considerations are as for laser trabeculoplasty. With an argon laser, the duration of exposure will need to be adjusted depending on the color of the iris (0.5 second for blue, 0.1 second for medium brown, and 0.05 second for dark brown). This procedure is more effectively done with a Nd:YAG laser. Similar operative procedures apply, but power is in millijoules (mJ) and there is no spot size.

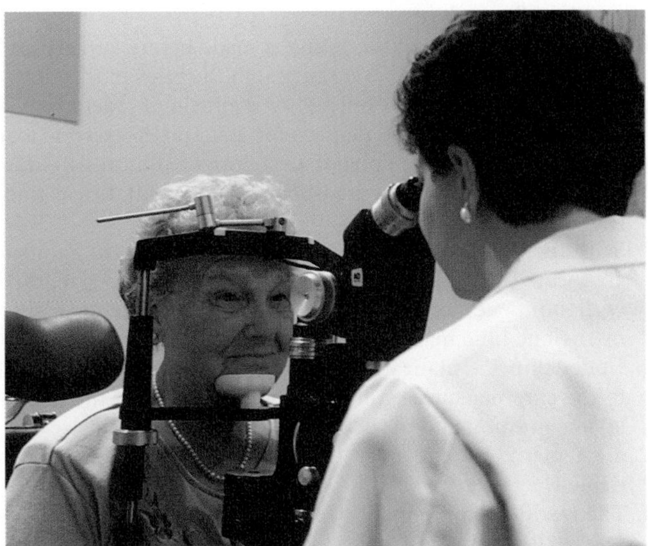

FIGURE 18-39 Patient positioned at laser slit lamp.

*Operative Procedure*

1. Topical anesthetic drops of proparacaine or an equivalent are instilled.
2. The patient is positioned at the laser slit lamp.
3. The Abraham lens is placed into the operative eye.
4. An iris crypt or "thin" area of iris is selected.
5. Initial burns are placed in a circle to put the iris on a stretch using 200-mm spot size for 0.1 second at 200- to 300-mW power. (Usually six to eight burns accomplish this.)
6. Penetrating burns are placed as needed to make an adequate opening (usually 10 to 30 applications) using 50-mm spot size for 0.1 to 0.2 second at 600- to 1000-mW power.
7. Prednisolone or dexamethasone eyedrops are instilled into the operative eye.

## Laser Cyclophotocoagulation

Cyclophotocoagulation (CPC) is performed with a thermal diode or the Nd:YAG laser. Using a combination of topical and retrobulbar anesthesia, the laser is applied through a fiberoptic probe to the sclera over the ciliary processes. Approximately 60 degrees is treated in a single session. The goal of treatment is to lower intraocular pressure by direct destruction to the aqueous ciliary processes. The patient returns several weeks after treatment for reassessment of intraocular pressure. If needed, another 60 degrees may be treated to further decrease intraocular pressure (IOP). Adequate control is usually achieved with one or more treatments.

## Laser Photocoagulation

In addition to intraocular photocoagulation with argon laser or cryocoagulation used during vitrectomy procedures, argon laser photocoagulation can be delivered through a slit lamp to the retina as a noninvasive, ambulatory procedure. This is done to treat flat retinal holes or tears, sites of potential pathologic conditions, and vascular proliferative diseases, such as diabetic retinopathy and the "wet" form of macular degeneration.

*Operative Procedures*

ARGON LASER TREATMENT

1. The patient's pupil is dilated, and a retrobulbar anesthetic may be used.
2. Proparacaine drops are instilled into the operative eye.
3. A three-mirror Goldmann or similar lens, which has been lubricated, is placed on the cornea, and the patient is positioned at the laser slit lamp.
4. The proper spot size, power setting, and duration of exposure are set.
5. Laser burns are placed in the prescribed areas.
6. The patient's eye is irrigated with physiologic saline solution to remove the viscous lens lubricant.
7. The eye is patched as necessary.

Nd:YAG LASER TREATMENT. An Nd:YAG laser is also used for lysis of vitreous strands or bands and to open opaque posterior capsules. The procedure is similar to argon laser treatment in its delivery through a slit lamp. A Peyman lens for a specific depth is selected and used in place of the Goldmann lens when cutting vitreous strands. No lens or anesthetic is needed to open posterior capsules. The patient is positioned at the laser slit lamp, and pulsed laser applications using 1 to 3 mJ of power are used to open the posterior capsule.

### Photodynamic Therapy

Photodynamic therapy (PDT) is a combination of systemically injecting the light-activating drug *verteporfin* and then exposing the affected retina to a low-beam diode laser. This two-step process is used to treat the "wet" type of age-related macular degeneration (AMD).[14] Photodynamic therapy allows selective destruction of target vessels without harming the overlying sensory retinal and retinal pigment epithelium. Research continues in refining treatment options for "wet" AMD (Research Highlight).

***Procedural Considerations.*** Patient assessment for PDT also focuses on porphyrin allergies, hypersensitivity to sunlight, liver disease, or pregnancy. Verteporfin is prepared based on the patient's body surface area, so height and weight are accurately assessed. Verteporfin is reconstituted, protected from light, and given as an IV infusion. Preparation includes checks of the laser and timing of the infusion with the readiness of the laser. The patient is instructed to wear protective glasses and to avoid postoperative exposure of eye and skin to any bright light (sunlight or halogen indoor light) for at least 5 days.[15]

***Operative Procedure.*** Laser light is applied 15 minutes after the start of the infusion or approximately 5 minutes after verteporfin infusion is completed. The laser light is provided by a diode laser through a fiberoptic and a slit-lamp biomicroscope for a period of 83 seconds.[15]

#### RESEARCH HIGHLIGHT

**Age-Related Macular Degeneration (AMD)**

Age-related macular degeneration (AMD) is a disease that accounts for more than 60% of legal blindness in persons older than 60 years. In the "wet" form of AMD, choroidal neovascular membranes affect the area around the fovea. Damage to the outer retinal layers often leads to permanent loss of vision. Laser treatment of the macula may also have poor visual outcomes. In recent times, ophthalmic scientists have delved into the possibility of trying to treat wet macular degeneration by inhibiting the growth of the new blood vessels. This group of drugs is referred to as antiangiogenics. They are used in other diseases where the formation of new blood vessels in response to disease creates a worse scenario.

This study was designed to assess the vision benefits of treatment of early wet macular degeneration (AMD) with an antiangiogenic drug. The hypothesis was that by slowing or stopping the growth of abnormal new blood vessels, vision loss could be slowed or stopped. Baseline characteristics of clinical trial subjects were well balanced. Subjects were randomly selected to receive 0.3 mg of pegaptanib or sham injections intravitreally every 6 weeks for 54 weeks. This was compared with a third group who received usual care. Subjects in the treated group lost less vision and remained more stable. In fact, subjects in the usual care group were 10 times more likely to have severe vision loss, established as losing 15 or more letters on the visual acuity chart.

Modified from Gonzales CR: Enhanced efficacy associated with early treatment of neovascular age-related macular degeneration with pegaptanib sodium: an exploratory analysis, *VEGF Inhibition Study in Ocular Neovascularization (V.I.S.I.O.N.) Clinical Trial Group Retina* 25(7):815-827, 2005.

## SURGERY FOR RETINAL DETACHMENT

Retinal detachment is a separation of the neural retinal layer from the pigmented epithelium layer of the retina. Retinal detachment may occur because of the presence of intraocular neoplasms originating in the retina or choroid (exudative type) or, more commonly, as a result of retinal tears or holes associated with injury, degeneration, or vitreous contraction.

Retinal detachment usually causes the sudden onset of the appearance of floating spots before the eye, resulting from freeing of pigment or blood cells in the vitreous. The vitreous humor of the eye is a gelatinous liquid possessing an ultrastructure of fine protein fibers in a network arrangement, with some attachment to the retina. Fluid from the vitreous cavity seeps through the retinal tears and progressively detaches the retinal components. The part of the retina that has separated from its nutritional source becomes damaged and relatively nonfunctional. Prompt treatment of retinal detachment is aimed at preventing permanent loss of central vision.

### Scleral Buckling

***Procedural Considerations.*** In the treatment of retinal detachment, the aim is to return the retina to its normal anatomic position. Repair is done from outside the globe. The purpose of the scleral buckling procedure for retinal detachment is to cause an intrusion or push into the eye at the site of the pathologic cause. Treatment by diathermy or cryotherapy causes an inflammatory reaction that leads to a permanent adhesion between the detached retina and underlying structures. The surgery also involves sealing off the area in which the tear or hole is located and may include drainage of the subretinal fluid.

The procedure may be performed using general anesthesia or MAC with local blocks. The scleral buckling may be done using episcleral (working outside of the sclera) technique or by scleral dissection (making a partial-thickness incision into the sclera and creating flaps to expose the underlying tissue). Both techniques may use drainage of subretinal fluid, encircling bands, diathermy, light coagulation, or cryotherapy. Cryosurgery or light coagulation may be used alone or in combination with a buckling procedure.

***Operative Procedure***

1. A detailed drawing of the retina is made before surgery and is displayed in the operating suite. On the basis of this drawing, the conjunctiva is opened to a previously determined extent, for example, 90 degrees for a simple horseshoe tear or 360 degrees for an aphakic detachment (Figure 18-40).
2. The four rectus muscles are isolated using 0 silk ties as traction sutures.
3. With the indirect ophthalmoscope, the detachment and tear are located under direct visualization and the site is marked with nonpenetrating diathermy by indentation or with a methylene blue marking pen.
4. Under direct visualization, the retinal cryoprobe is applied to the external surface of the globe in the area of the pathologic condition and the area is treated. An ice ball is seen to form in the proper areas until the entire lesion has been treated.
5. The buckling component of the procedure secures explants (e.g., silicone bands, sponges, plates, tires) to the sclera. Nonabsorbable sutures (4-0 or 5-0) are set into the sclera

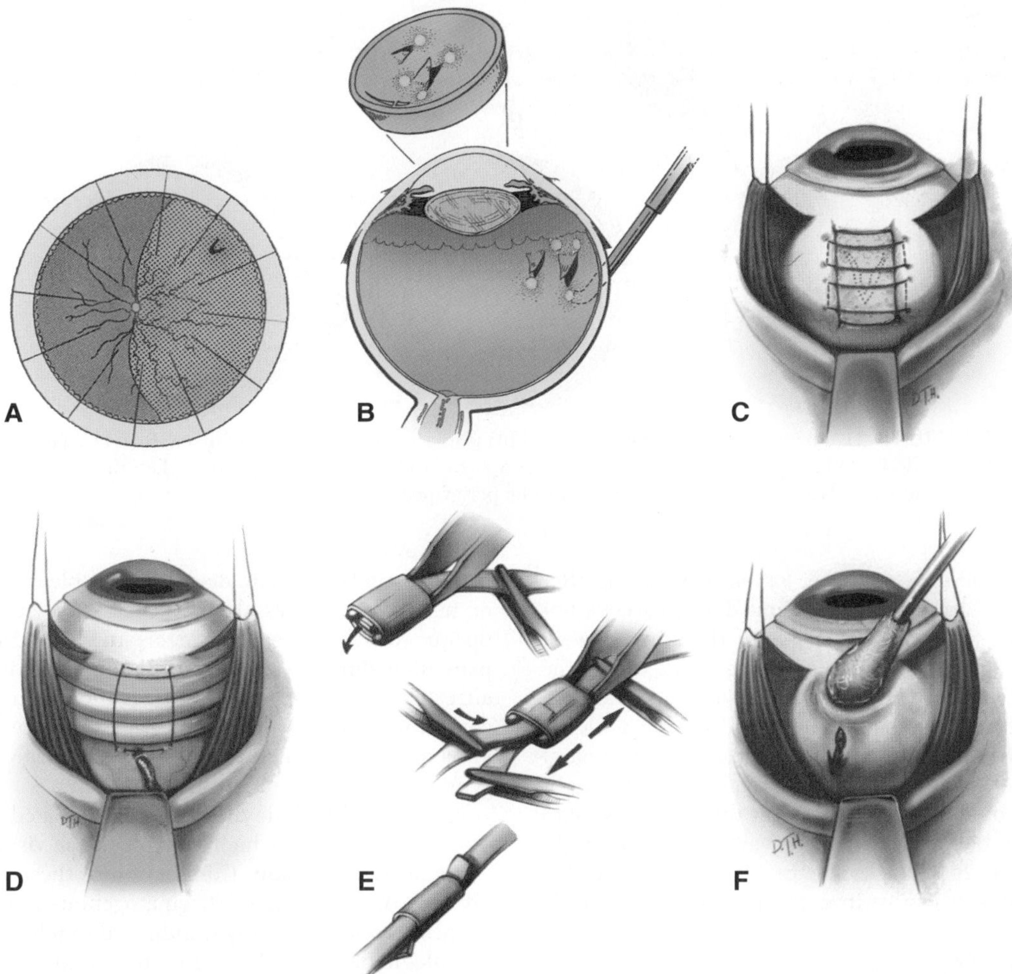


FIGURE 18-40 Scleral buckling operation for treatment of retinal detachment. **A,** Diagram of retina showing detachment of retina of temporal half of left eye, with retinal tear at equator of globe at 1:30 o'clock position. **B,** Examination of fundus by means of ophthalmoscope and handheld lens and depression of sclera with diathermy electrode. Surgeon visualizes field and places electrode beneath retinal tear; burn mark is made on sclera at site of retinal tear with diathermy electrode. **C,** A sponge is sutured in place over treated site of retinal tear. **D,** Band and tire are used to encircle the eye. **E,** Placement of Watzke silicone sleeve is one method to secure edges of encircling band. **F,** Small incision is made through sclera, and choroid is finely incised to allow subretinal fluid to drain.

surrounding the lesion and tied over silicone sponges, causing the outer shell of the eye to be pushed toward the elevated retina.

6. If an encircling band is to be used, mattress sutures are placed into the sclera in four quadrants. A silicone band is passed 360 degrees around the eye under the sutures and the rectus muscles. The sutures are tied, and a self-holding Watzke sleeve is applied to the band to maintain a predetermined circumference. This causes a 360-degree constriction of the outer coats into the eye.
7. If drainage of subretinal fluid is desired, under direct visualization an area is chosen in which a significant fluid level exists under the retina, and a diathermy mark is made on the sclera. The sclera is split to the choroid, and a small amount of diathermy is applied to the choroid bed. A 6-0 or 7-0 absorbable suture is placed at the proposed drainage site. A needle or blade is then used to puncture the choroid into the subretinal space to permit drainage of fluid. The preplaced suture is tied.
8. Air or replacement fluids may be introduced into the eye after the drainage of subretinal fluid. This is usually done through the pars plana under direct visualization.
9. The traction sutures are removed from around the muscles. The conjunctiva is closed with a 7-0 absorbable suture. A subconjunctival injection of an antibiotic, steroid, or both may be given, and an eye pad is applied.

## Retinopexy

Pneumatic retinopexy (Figure 18-41) is the intraocular injection of a bubble of air or therapeutic gases to press against retinal breaks and allow the detached retinal breaks to approximate the pigment epithelium. Retinopexy may be used in combination with scleral buckling and posterior vitrectomy; it may be performed as part of an ambulatory procedure for treatment of certain retinal detachments using laser photocoagulation with injection of the gas bubble followed by specific postoperative positioning. The gases are drawn through a Millipore 0.22-micron filter and may be mixed with filtered air so

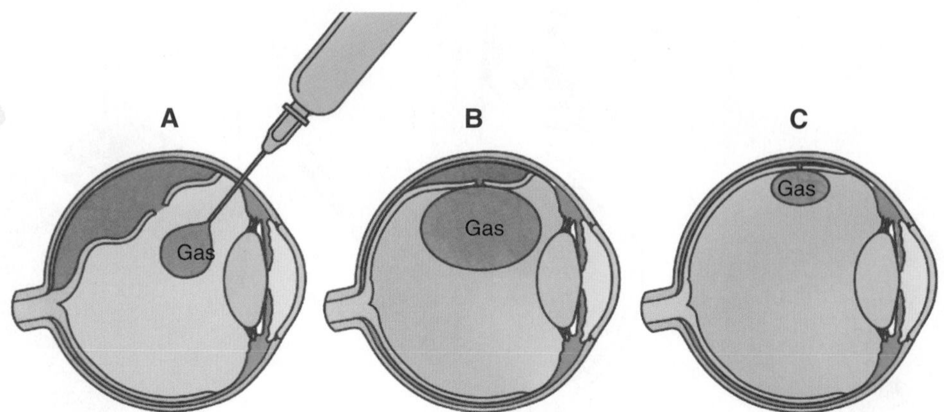


**FIGURE 18-41** Pneumatic retinopexy. **A,** Gas bubble is injected through the pars plana. **B** and **C,** The bubble closes and supports the retinal break. After a 7- to 10-day healing period and when the retina is back in place, laser surgery or cryotherapy can be performed to seal the break.

that the concentration may be varied. Patient positioning after retinopexy is often face down for several days to weeks but may include tilting the head to one side or the other as well. The gas bubble is a ratio mixture of gas and air. The higher the concentration of gas to air, the longer the bubble remains in the eye before being "absorbed." The head position is determined by the location of the retinal tear/hole. For example if the retinal tear/hole is located superior temporal in the right eye, the patient would be instructed to tilt the head down and to the left, so the bubble will float upward and to the right where the tear/hole is located. The larger the tear/hole, the longer the bubble needs to be in contact with the area to be reattached.

Sulfur hexafluoride gas ($SF_6$) is colorless, odorless, and nontoxic. It increases 2.5 times in volume within 48 hours after injection by drawing other gases, specifically nitrogen and oxygen, from the surrounding tissues. A 1-mm bubble will diffuse from the eye in 7 to 10 days.[2]

Perfluoropropane gas ($C_3F_8$) is colorless, odorless, and nontoxic. It quadruples its volume within 48 hours after injection. A 1-mm bubble will diffuse from the eye in 30 to 50 days.[1]

Because $SF_6$ and $C_3F_8$ are expandable gases, certain precautions are required. Patients are given a wristband to wear that states what kind of gas bubble is in their eye and when it was instilled. If they would require surgery, they need to alert the anesthesia provider of the presence of the gas bubble. The use of nitrous oxide can rapidly equilibrate with the gas, expand, and raise the pressure in the eye. Patients are instructed to avoid air travel until the gas bubble is completely resolved or decreased to a level of 5% of the vitreous volume. Cabin pressurization in air travel will cause severe enlargement of the gas bubble with an increase in intraocular pressure and eye pain. Car or train travel to high elevations should also be avoided unless the change in altitude is done gradually.[1]

## VITRECTOMY

*Vitrectomy* is narrowly defined as removal of all or part of the vitreous gel (body). In the broader clinical sense of the term, it also includes the cutting and removal of fibrotic membranes, removal of epiretinal membranes, and electrocoagulation of bleeding vessels. In its normal state, the vitreous gel of the eye is transparent. In certain disease states, bleeding from damaged or newly formed vessels may cause the vitreous to become opaque, which may severely decrease vision. In addition to the patient's inability to see, the ophthalmologist is unable to visualize the retina and therefore treat the underlying pathologic condition before permanent damage can occur. In these cases, vitrectomy is indicated to allow the patient to see and the surgeon to institute treatment if indicated.

Certain ophthalmic diseases are associated with the formation of membranes, which may block the visual axis and may cause decreased vision. Contraction of these membranes may produce traction-type or rhegmatogenous retinal detachment. In these cases, vitrectomy is indicated to relieve the underlying pathologic processes leading to decreased vision.

### Anterior Segment Vitrectomy

The main indications for vitrectomy in the anterior segment are as follows:

- Vitreous loss during cataract extraction
- Opacities in the anterior segment
- Complications associated with vitreous in the anterior chamber
- Miscellaneous causes, such as hyphema, pupillary membranes, and residual soft lens material

***Procedural Considerations.*** The procedure varies according to the location of the pathologic condition (anterior or posterior segments), the instrumentation available, and the surgeon's preference. A pathologic condition in the anterior segment can be approached through a limbal incision, as in lens extraction with vitreous loss; through "open sky," after trephine incision for penetrating keratoplasty; or through the pars plana. Most phacoemulsification equipment has a vitrector that can be quickly attached if needed.

#### *Operative Procedures*

ANTERIOR VITRECTOMY FOR ACCIDENTAL VITREOUS LOSS DURING CATARACT EXTRACTION

1. A vitreous cutter is placed into the eye through the cataract wound. Infusion may be through the handpiece or a separate cannula and infusion line (Figure 18-42, *A*).

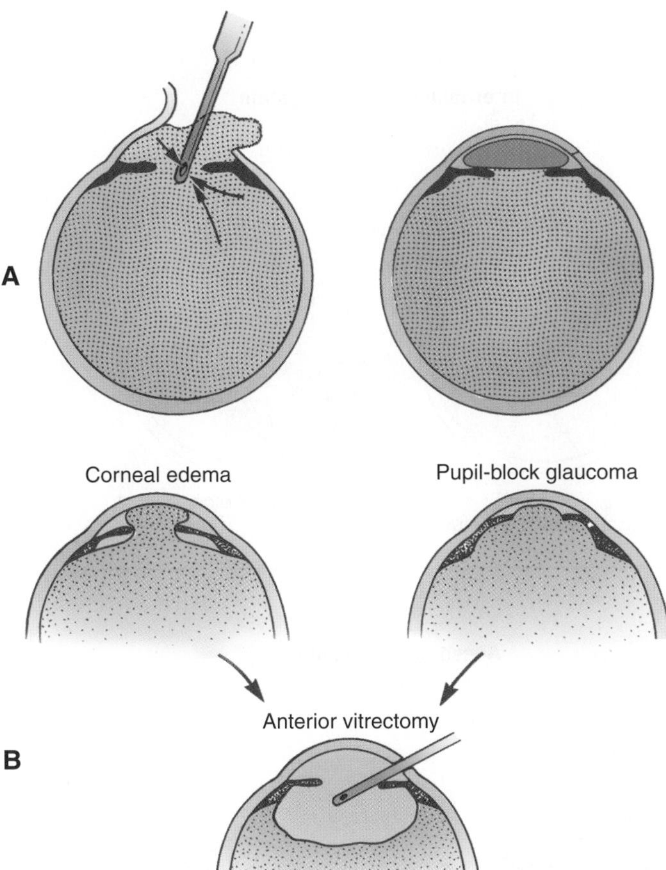


FIGURE 18-42 **A,** Diagram of management of vitreous loss at time of cataract extraction. **B,** Anterior vitrectomy procedure for complications of vitreous in anterior chamber.

2. The cutter is placed in the middle of the pupil, posterior to the iris, and enough vitreous is removed to ensure that no vitreous remains in the anterior chamber and that the iris has fallen back into its normal position.
3. The pupil is constricted with acetylcholine. The anterior chamber may be re-formed with BSS.
4. The procedure is completed as for a lens extraction.

ANTERIOR VITRECTOMY FOR ANTERIOR SEGMENT OPACITIES, HYPHEMA, PUPILLARY MEMBRANES, AND RESIDUAL SOFT LENS MATERIAL

1. Appropriate fixation sutures or a lid speculum is placed (Figure 18-42, *B*).
2. An incision is made at the limbus either through clear cornea or under a conjunctival flap. One to three incisions are made, depending on the vitreous cutter chosen and the technique.
3. If a multifunction probe is not used, an infusion cannula is placed into one incision and the vitreous cutter into another. A third incision may be used for an accessory instrument. The vitreous, blood, or other material is removed.
4. The incisions are closed, and the eye is patched.

## Posterior Segment Vitrectomy

A pathologic condition in the posterior segment is usually approached through the pars plana. The main indications for posterior segment vitrectomy through the pars plana are as follows:

- Vitreous opacities of long standing
- Advanced diabetic eye disease
- Severe intraocular trauma
- Retained foreign bodies
- Proliferative vitreoretinopathy
- Retinal detachment from giant tears
- Endophthalmitis
- Diagnostic vitreous biopsy

***Procedural Considerations.*** Vitrectomy of the posterior segment is a microsurgical procedure requiring a viewing system (operating microscope with an X-Y coupling, zoom lens, and fine focus), contact lens system or noncontact wide-angle viewing system (Biom), an illumination system, a cutting-suction-infusion system, and accessory instruments (Figure 18-43).

Another option to a sew-on lens is the use of a noncontact panoramic wide-angle viewing system (Figure 18-43, *A*). This system allows a wide, noncontact view of the macula and is mounted to the microscope and swings out of the way for extraocular phases of the vitrectomy. Other advantages are that it provides a good view under air, eliminates the time needed to sew on a lens, and does not require an assistant to hold the lens. The eye may be rotated freely to view the extreme periphery. The image is inverted by a manual knob, foot pedal, or hand control.

The infusion system consists of a 500-ml bottle of buffered BSS, such as BSS Plus or Endosol Extra, a standard IV administration set, and an infusion needle or sleeve. The level of intraocular pressure can be varied by elevating or lowering the infusion bottle in relation to the patient's eye.

The suction and cutting systems vary in sophistication and technology. All cutters engage tissue into a port and then cut it by the shearing action between the edges of a moving and a nonmoving part. Guillotine cutters have a linear, to-and-fro action, whereas reciprocating or oscillating cutters rotate in a clockwise-counterclockwise fashion. Suction is operated with a pump controlled by a foot switch to maintain the level of aspiration. The cutter may be part of a single-use multifunction handpiece.

An endolaser or indirect laser delivery system is usually available for photocoagulation. Illumination for vitrectomy is *external,* using the operating microscope for anterior segment vitrectomy; and *internal,* using a fiberoptic light pipe (endoilluminator) for posterior segment vitrectomy. A special light pipe (cannonball) that illuminates a wider area is needed if a wide-angle viewing system is used on the microscope.

Replacement of the vitreous with air is facilitated with a special air-exchange unit. Other substances for intraocular tamponade are liquid perfluorocarbons, silicone oil, perfluoropropane gas ($C_3F_8$), and sulfur hexafluoride gas ($SF_6$). (See p. 624 for precautions.) A fibrin patch may be used in the case of a macular hole. Topical thrombin and a sample of the patient's plasma are needed for this procedure.

Accessory instruments usually have a 20-gauge diameter so that they can be interchanged throughout the procedure. Several accessory instruments may be used for pars plana vitrectomy, depending on the extent of the procedure. Micro hooks, picks, and subretinal forceps and scissors (Figure 18-44) are used for dissection, peeling, and removal of membranes. These instruments can be manually operated with a thumb control or run with compressed air from the automated vitrectomy console.

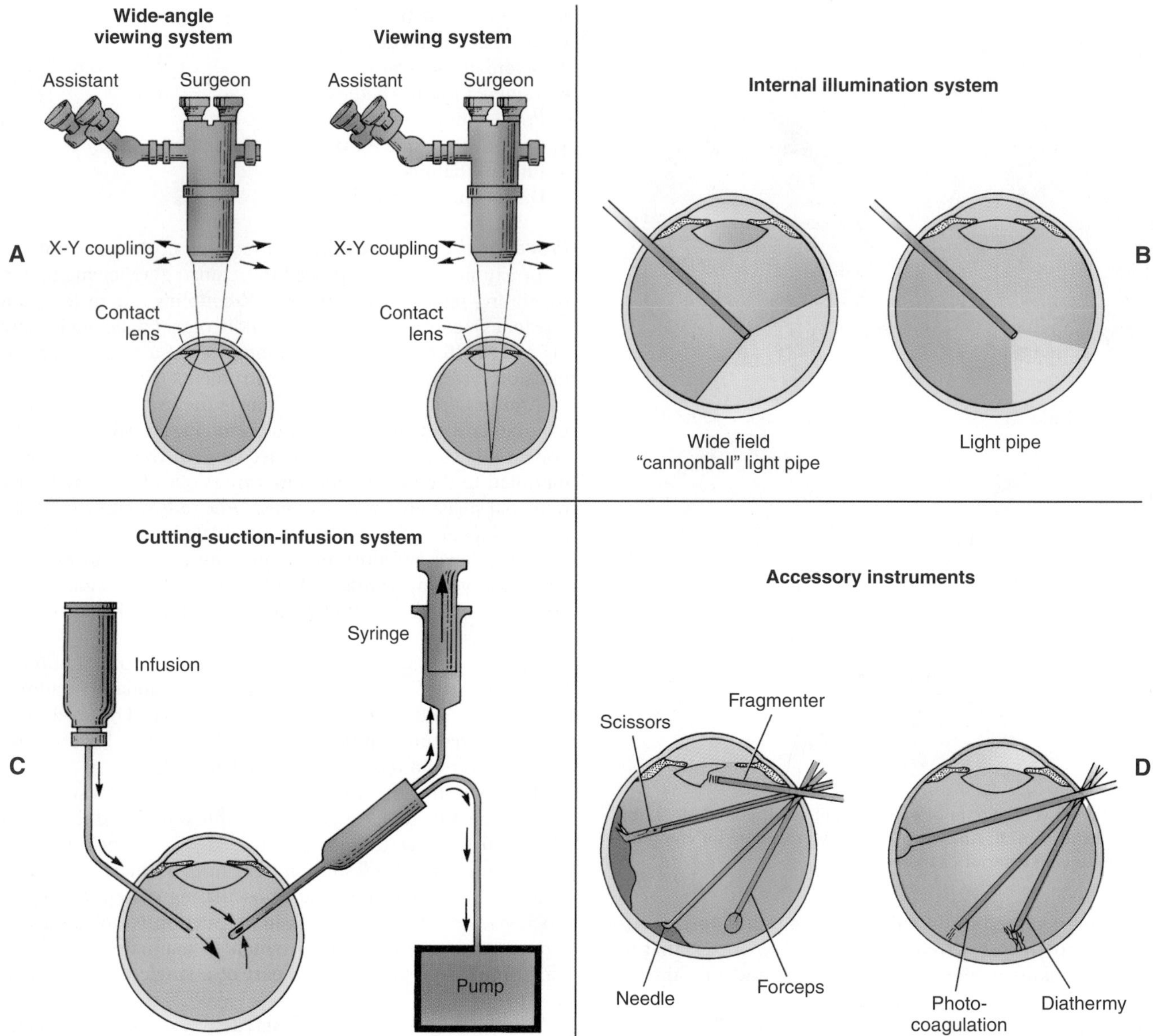


**FIGURE 18-43** Vitrectomy procedures require the following: **A,** Wide-angle viewing system with X-Y coupling. **B,** Internal illumination system. **C,** Cutting-suction-infusion system. **D,** Accessory instruments.

Foreign-body microforceps and various magnetic devices are used to retrieve foreign objects of glass, metal, or other substances. An intraocular cryoprobe for cryocoagulation directly on the retina surface can be attached to the cryotherapy device. Flute needles or disposable soft-tipped cannulas are handheld or attached to an extrusion or aspiration line for evacuating pools of blood or for fluid-gas exchange.

To prepare for a vitrectomy procedure, the perioperative nurse must know the location of the problem, how the surgeon plans to address the problem (route of entry into the eye—anterior or posterior, "open sky" or closed), instrumentation to be used, and anticipated extent and length of the procedure. Instrument and equipment functioning should be thoroughly checked before the patient is brought into the operating room. When a lens extraction procedure is planned, vitrectomy instrumentation should be ready in the event of accidental vitreous loss. When preparing for pars plana vitrectomy in the posterior segment, the perioperative nurse must be aware that a combined scleral buckling procedure may be necessary.

In the case of giant retinal tears, $C_3F_8$, $SF_6$, liquid perfluorocarbons, and silicone oil are used to provide retinal tamponade. These techniques allow repositioning and tamponade of the retina without the need for extremely awkward and uncomfortable positioning that was previously mandated.

Liquid perfluorocarbons such as perfluorooctane (PFO), being heavier than BSS, will allow the retina to be pushed posteriorly and so are used as a tamponade to reduce a giant retinal tear. The liquid is then removed from the posterior segment. Silicone oil is a highly viscous oil with a high surface tension that mechanically limits fibrovascular proliferation. Silicone oil may cause increased intraocular pressure and secondary glaucoma.[12] The oil may be left in place, but it is recommended that it be removed within 1 year if the retina is reattached and stable.

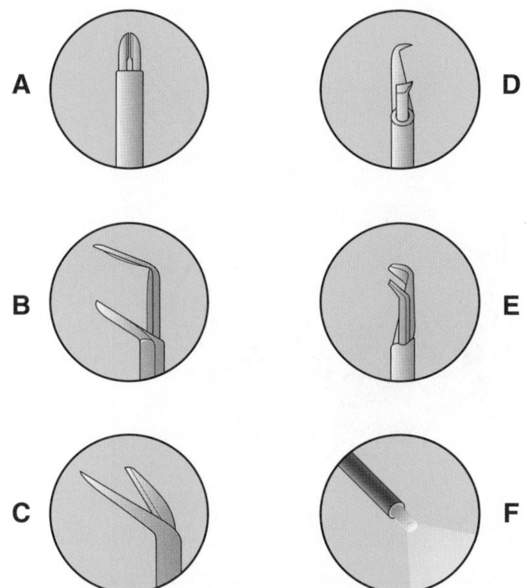


FIGURE 18-44 Tips of micro instruments used in vitrectomy procedures. **A** and **B**, Peeling forceps. **C**, Horizontal scissors. **D**, Vertical scissors. **E**, Membrane peeler and cutter (MPC). **F**, Lighted pick.

Vitrectomy procedures vary in length from less than 1 hour to more than 3 hours. When a long procedure is anticipated, care must be taken to protect the patient's skin and reduce pressure areas. A foam mattress pad, heel and elbow protectors, and elasticized stockings may be used. When the patient is positioned for vitrectomy, the head should be higher than the heart, the cheeks higher than the forehead, and the neck extended. A wrist support may be placed around the patient's head to support the surgeon's wrist during manipulation of the intraocular instruments.

While draping, the perioperative nurse should provide for removal of infusion fluid from the operative field and should take care to protect electrical foot switches from fluid damage.

### *Operative Procedure*

#### PARS PLANA VITRECTOMY

1. A lid speculum is placed, and the conjunctiva is incised. The rectus muscles may be isolated, and 0 silk fixation sutures are placed (Figure 18-45).
2. The infusion line is sutured in place with a purse-string suture. The line is checked to ensure proper placement.
3. Three incisions are made through the pars plana: one for infusion, one for endoillumination, and one for a vitreous

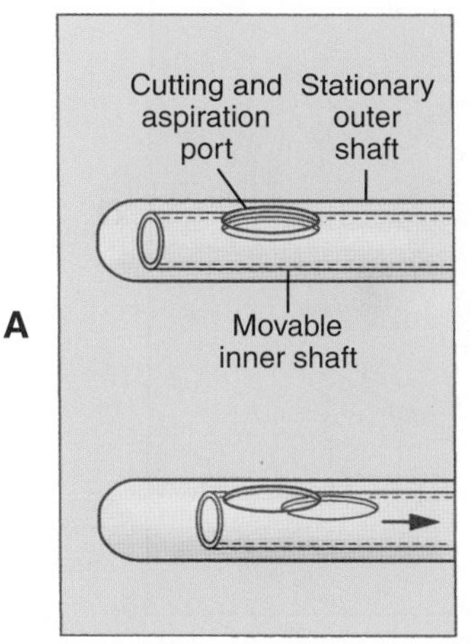


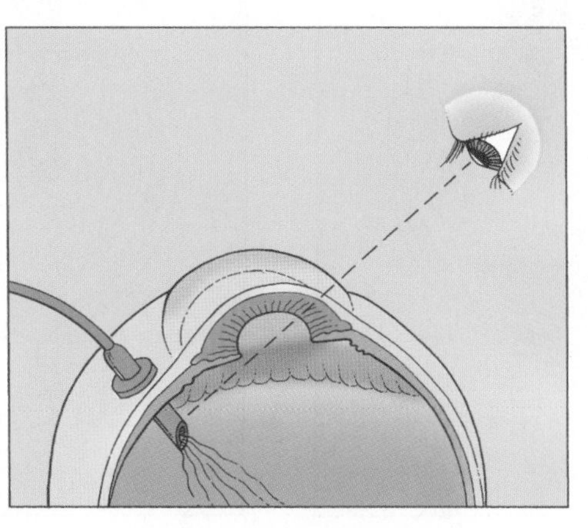


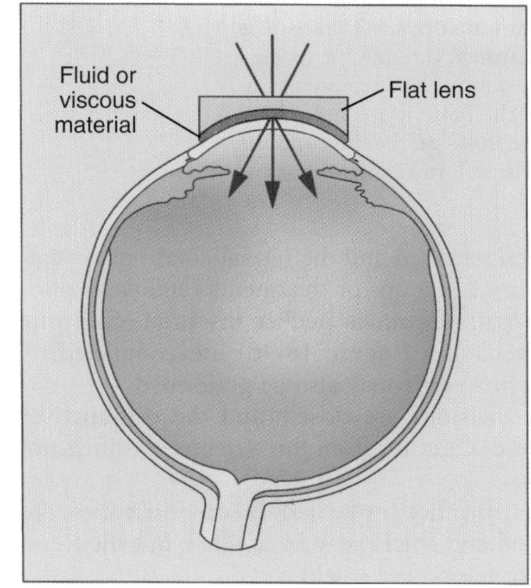


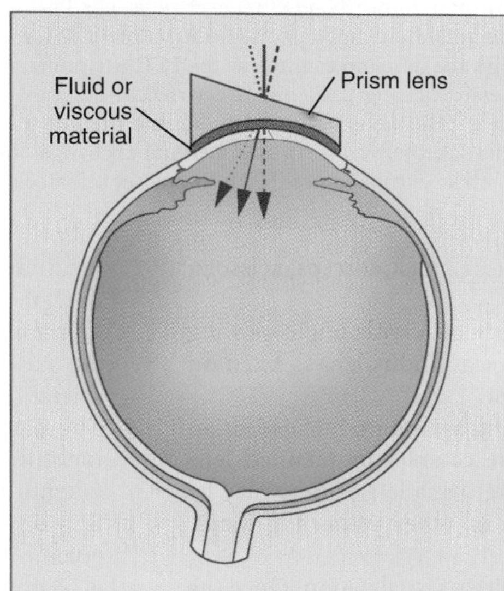


FIGURE 18-45 Essential components for vitrectomy. **A**, Vitrector probe with its cutting/aspirating port close to the tip of the intraocular portion of the handpiece. **B**, Infusion cannula, placed in pars plana, is viewed for correct position. **C**, Flat contact lens, resting on cushion of fluid or viscoelastic material on the cornea, is used for viewing posterior half of the vitreous cavity and retina. **D**, Prism contact lens used for viewing anterior structures in the vitreous cavity.

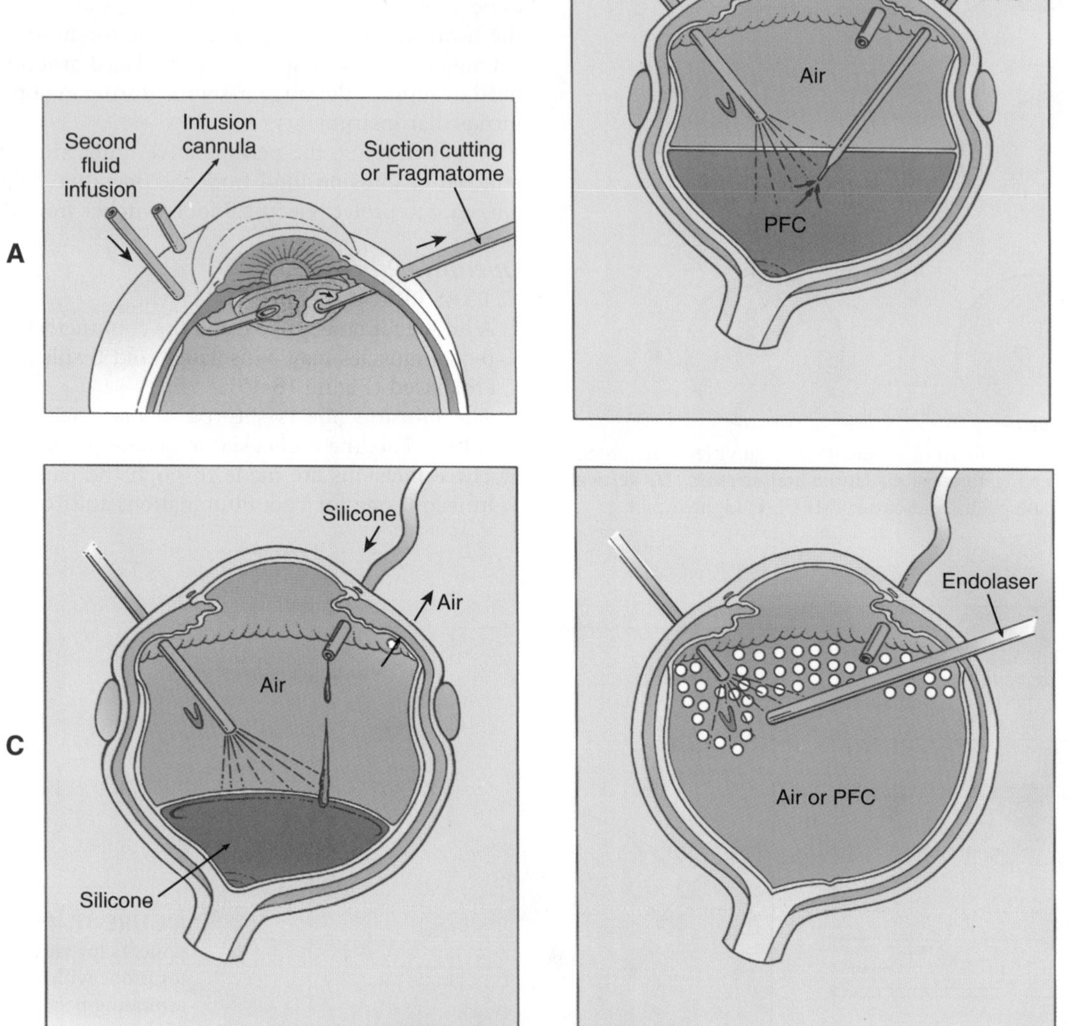


**FIGURE 18-46** Procedures done with vitrectomy. **A,** Pars plana lensectomy performed with a second infusion line. **B,** Air/perfluorocarbon (PFC) exchange. The PFC has been placed in the vitreous cavity for removal of subretinal fluid and anatomic reattachment of the retina. Air under positive pressure is then placed through the infusion cannula as the PFC is simultaneously extruded through the tapered needle. **C,** Silicone/air exchange. Silicone is inserted through the infusion cannula as a temporary intraocular tamponade. Silicone is heavier than air and fills the globe from the bottom up, and the air escapes through the sclerotomy site. In silicone/fluid exchange, the silicone floats on the fluid and the fluid is removed with an extrusion needle. **D,** Endolaser photocoagulation is performed after the retina is back in place.

cutter or other instrumentation (e.g., pick, forceps, scissors, laser probe, extrusion needle).

4. The operating microscope is aligned. A wide-angle viewing system is swung into position, or a fundus lens is fixed on the anterior surface of the cornea.
5. The infusion rate, cutting rate, and aspiration rate are set on the machine console. If a dense cataract or retained lens material blocks the view of the retina, a lensectomy may be performed with a Fragmatome or other ultrasonic handpiece at this time.
6. The vitreous is removed under direct visualization. Once the medium has been removed and the retinal condition visualized, the necessary injections or treatments (endolaser photocoagulation, repair of macular pucker, insertion of silicone oil, gas-fluid exchange) (Figure 18-46) are completed. A scleral buckling procedure may also be performed.
7. The pars plana incisions are closed, and the conjunctival incision is sutured. Cultures from the vitreous washings are taken if necessary.
8. Subconjunctival injections of steroids or antibiotics are given. An eye pad and shield may be applied, but the trend is to not patch or use an eye shield.

## REFERENCES


1. Alcon Laboratories: *Tamponade products: product inserts C3F8 and SF6, PDF files.* Accessed August 13, 2001, on-line: www.alconlabs.com/us/aj/products/surgical_vitreo/A252_VitTamponade.jhtml.
2. American Academy of Ophthalmology: *Patient safety bulletin number 1. Suggestions for a checklist to verify the operative eye, developed by the AAO quality of care secretariat in collaboration with ASORN and AAEEH,* March 2001. Accessed February 6, 2006, on-line: www.aao.org/aao/education/library/safety.
3. Association of periOperative Registered Nurses: *AORN standards, recommended practices and guidelines*, Denver, 2005, The Association.
4. Duffy TS: No end in sight: the nurse's role in ensuring a holistic approach in the care of a patient undergoing a drainage implant for end-stage glaucoma, *INSIGHT* 25(3):88-91, 2000.
5. Glynn-Milley C: Outlook positive for today's cataract patients, *Nursing Spectrum* 14(9):15-17, 2005.
6. Herlihy B, Maebius NK: *The human body in health and illness*, ed 2, Philadelphia, 2003, Saunders.
7. Ho-Shing D: Treating glaucoma with drainage devices and pericardial grafts, *AORN Journal* 71(6):1237-1251, 2000.
8. Hutchisson B, Nicoladis CB: Topical anesthesia: a new approach to cataract surgery, *AORN Journal* 74(3):340-350, 2001.
9. Lilley LL and others: *Pharmacology and the nursing process*, ed 4, St Louis, 2005, Mosby.
10. Lypson ML and others: Preventing surgical fires: who needs to be educated? *Joint Commission Journal on Quality and Patient Safety* 31(9): 522-527, 2005.
11. OR Benchmarks: Benchmarking study for cataract extraction, *OR Manager* 17(2):24, 2001.
12. Orticio LP: Silicone oil-induced secondary glaucoma: a case study, *INSIGHT* 25(2):44-49, 2000.
13. Pagana KD, Pagana TJ: *Diagnostic and laboratory test reference,* ed 7, St Louis, 2005, Mosby.
14. Porter T, Nesbitt P: Psychosocial implications of clinical trials on patients with age-related macular degeneration and pathologic myopia as seen in the photodynamic therapy trials, *INSIGHT* 26(2):40-43, 2001.
15. Rich D and others: Photodynamic therapy: the nurse's role, *INSIGHT* 26(2):44-48, 2001.
16. Steefel L: Eye-openers on refractive surgery, *Nursing Spectrum* 15(2): 22-23, 2005.
17. Steefel L: Eye-opening facts about cataracts, *Nursing Spectrum* 14(5):14-15, 2005.
18. Ticho BH, Dreger V: Enucleation: indications, methods, and prosthetic options, *INSIGHT* 25(1):23-26, 2000.
19. Wilson TS: LASIK surgery, *AORN Journal* 71(5):963-983, 2000.
20. Wold GH: *Basic geriatric nursing*, ed 3, St Louis, 2004, Mosby.
21. Workman ML: Interventions for clients with eye and vision problems. In Ignatavicius DD, Workman ML: *Medical-surgical nursing: critical thinking for collaborative care*, Philadelphia, 2006, Saunders.
22. Wu Y and others: Caring behaviors inventory, *Nursing Research* 55(1):18-25, 2006.

CHAPTER 19

# Otologic Surgery

DONNA R. McEWEN

Hearing is the sense by which sounds are appreciated. Referred to as the "watchdog of the senses," hearing is the last sense to disappear when one falls asleep and the first to return when one awakens. The word *auditory* refers to the sense of hearing and comes from the Latin word *audire,* which means "to hear." The physical nature of sound results from the compression and rarefaction of pressure waves and moving molecules, but the sensations humans actually experience are the product of complex mechanical, electrical, and psychologic interactions in the ear and central nervous system. The study of the ear and its diseases is known as *otology,* derived from the Greek word *aaotos,* which means "ear." *Position sense* refers to the orientation of the head in space and the movement of the body through space, its balance, and equilibrium.

The basic principles applied to all operations on the ear and temporal bone include the necessity for maintaining aseptic technique; the use of the operating microscope; the development of specialized instrumentation; and the use of preoperative sedation, anesthesia, and antibiotic therapy.

The success of surgical restoration of useful hearing is attributed to new concepts and techniques, the types of approaches to gain access to the temporal region, and improvements in the design of and materials used in implantable prosthetic devices. Better understanding of the anatomy and physiology of the ear has allowed the surgeon to perform reconstructive surgeries to improve the patient's hearing and equilibrium and to have greater control of diseases in the middle ear and mastoid. Procedures to correct conductive hearing loss resulting from conductive apparatus abnormalities may include a stapedectomy and partial or total ossicular replacement surgery. Surgical treatment for sensorineural hearing loss, or Meniere's disease, can be offered to patients who experience intolerable tinnitus or the disabling effects of vertigo. Cochlear implants and implantable hearing aids have brought new hope for deaf patients. These technologic advancements have contributed to decreased otologic complications, shortened hospital stays, and improved outcomes for patients.

## Surgical Anatomy

### External, Middle, and Inner Ear

The ear is a sensory organ that functions in the identification, localization, and interpretation of sound as well as in the maintenance of equilibrium. Anatomically, it is divided into the external ear, middle ear, and inner ear (Figure 19-1).

The *external ear,* including the auricle (or pinna) and external auditory canal, is composed of cartilage covered with skin. The auricles, which are fixed in position and lie close to the head, are responsible for concentrating sound waves and conducting them into the external auditory canal. Both ears provide stereophonic hearing for judging the direction of sound, whereas the shape of the auricles helps differentiate sounds coming from directly behind from those sounds arriving directly in front (Figure 19-2).

The external auditory canal, an S-shaped pathway leading to the middle ear, is approximately 2.5 cm in length in adults and shelters the tympanic membrane. Its skeleton of bone and cartilage is covered with very thin, sensitive skin. The canal lining is protected and lubricated with cerumen, a waxy substance secreted by sebaceous glands in the distal third of the canal. Cerumen helps to trap foreign material and reduces bacterial levels in the outer ear.

Located at the end of the external auditory canal is the *tympanic membrane* (eardrum). It is a thin, fibrous membrane covered with skin on its lateral aspect; medially it is covered with mucous membrane that is continuous with the lining of the middle ear.

The *middle ear* is filled with air, which comes from the nasopharynx through the eustachian tube. Posteriorly the middle ear communicates with the mastoid air cells of the temporal bone. The mucous membrane of the middle ear is continuous with that of the pharynx and the mastoid cells, making it possible for infection to travel to the middle ear (otitis media) and mastoid cells (mastoiditis). The eustachian tube serves to aerate the air-filled spaces of the temporal bone and to equalize pressure in the middle ear with atmospheric pressure. It will open during yawning, sneezing, or swallowing and remains closed when the pressure is greater outside.

A chain of three tiny, movable bones (ossicles) extends across the middle ear cavity and conducts vibrations (airborne sound waves) from the tympanic membrane across the middle ear into the oval window and the fluid-filled inner ear.

The *malleus* (hammer) consists of a head, neck, handle, and short process (Figure 19-3). The handle and short process are attached to the undersurface of the eardrum and join it to the incus. The *incus* (anvil) consists of a body and long and short processes (see Figure 19-3). The long crus of the incus is attached to the stapes, which is the third, innermost bone. The *stapes* (stirrup) consists of a head, neck, anterior and posterior crura, and a footplate that fits into the oval window (see Figure 19-3). The movable joints between these bones contribute to a lever system converting the transmission of vibrations from air to the fluid of the inner ear.

The inner ear is protected from loud noise by two small muscles. The *tensor tympani* muscle draws the drum inward to increase tension, thus restricting its ability to vibrate. The *stapedius* muscle pulls the stapes away from the oval window, reducing the intensity and potentially damaging vibrations pass-

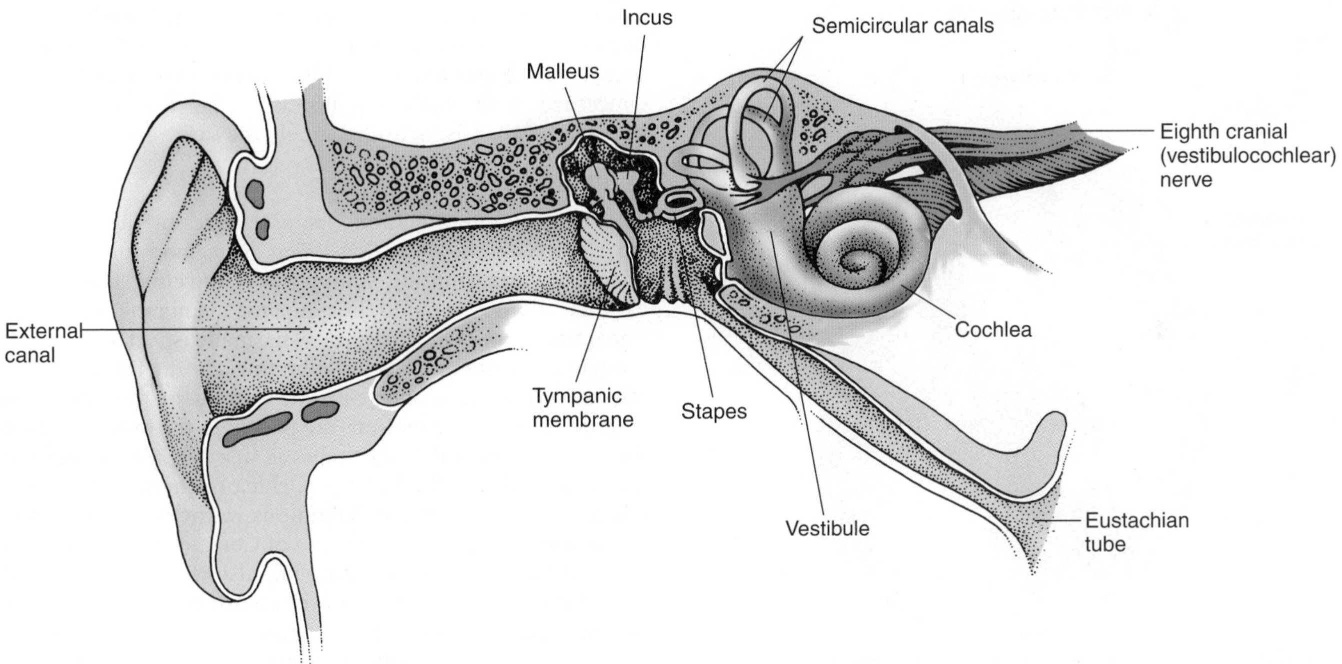


FIGURE 19-1 Anatomic structures of external ear, middle ear, and inner ear.

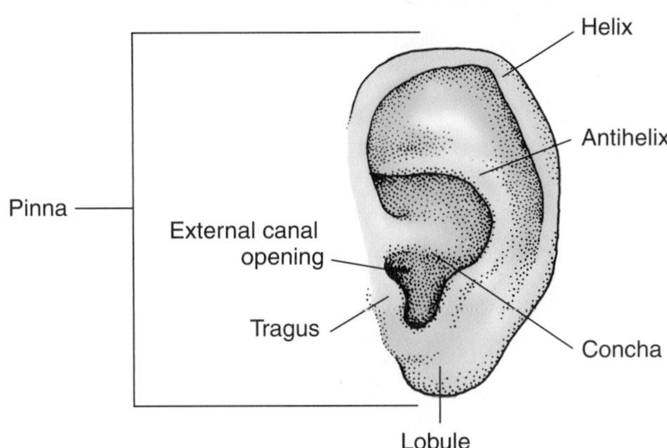


FIGURE 19-2 Anatomic structures of external ear.

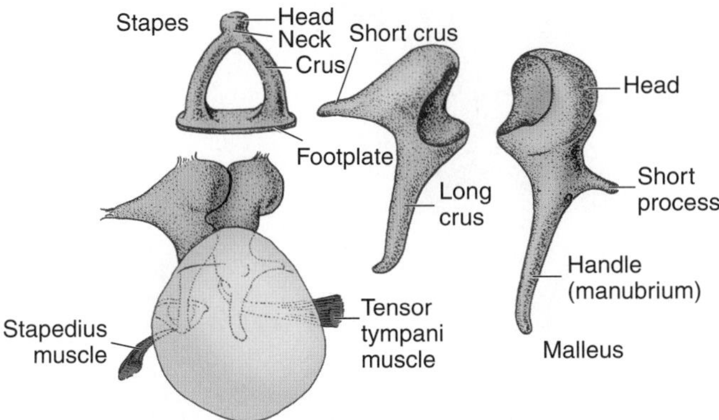


FIGURE 19-3 Articulated ossicles of right middle ear.

ing through the ossicles into the inner ear. The middle ear and mastoid are supplied with blood from the branches of the internal and external carotid artery systems.

The *inner ear* is a membranous, curved cavity located in the petrous portion of the temporal bone containing receptors for hearing and balance. It consists of a bony labyrinth filled with a watery fluid (perilymph) that surrounds and bathes a membranous labyrinth. Perilymph serves as a protective cushion to the end organ of hearing. The three divisions of the bony labyrinth are the cochlea, the vestibule, and the semicircular canals.

Within the membranous labyrinth lie four structures: the cochlear duct, the utricle, the saccule, and the semicircular ducts. A second fluid (endolymph) bathes and nourishes the sensory cells contained within the membranous labyrinth.

## Cochlea

The cochlea has a tubular shape resembling a snail shell. It is divided into three compartments: the scala vestibuli, which is associated with the oval window; the scala tympani, which is associated with the round window; and the cochlear duct. Both the scala vestibuli and scala tympani are filled with perilymph, whereas the cochlear duct contains endolymph. On the basilar membrane of the cochlea lies the organ of Corti—the neural end organ for hearing. From its neuroepithelium project thousands of hair cells that are set into motion by vibrations passing through the ossicles and oval window to the perilymph. The hair cells convert mechanical energy of wave movement from vibration in the perilymph into electrochemical impulses. The inner ear is connected to the brain through the vestibulocochlear nerve (eighth cranial nerve).

## Vestibular Labyrinth

The vestibular labyrinth is composed of the utricle, the saccule, and three semicircular canals referred to as the *lateral, superior,* and *posterior canals.* They are positioned at right angles to one

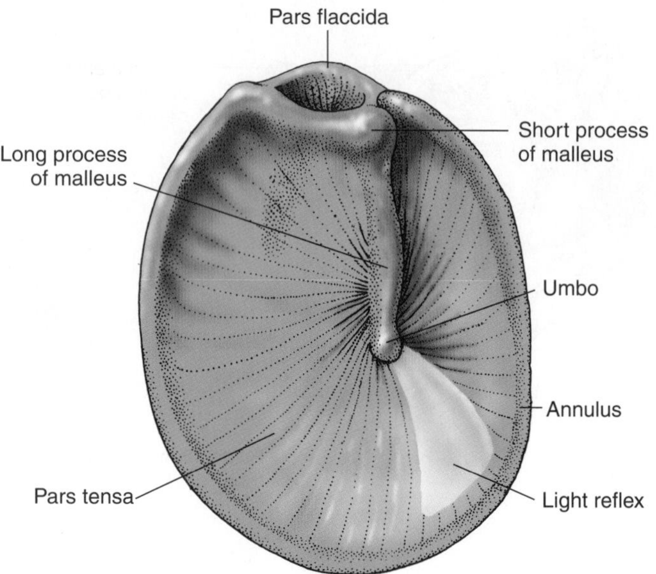


**FIGURE 19-4** Structural landmarks of tympanic membrane.

another so that any movement of the head will excite at least one of the semicircular canals. The maculae of the utricle and saccule of the vestibular labyrinth are gravity-oriented and are concerned with static equilibrium. The internal auditory branches of the basilar artery supply the inner ear.

## Hearing

Hearing is an interpretation of sound waves by the brain. The auricle serves as a sound-localizing device and functions as a conduit by transmitting sound waves traveling through the external auditory canal to the tympanic membrane. This vibration initiates ossicular motion. The malleus, attached to the tympanic membrane, begins vibrating, as do the incus and stapes, which are attached to the malleus on the other side (Figure 19-4). The vibrations are passed to the oval window of the inner ear in which the stapes is inserted. From here they travel through the fluid of the cochlea to the round window, where they are dissipated. Vibrations in the membrane cause the delicate hair cells of the organ of Corti to strike against the tectorial membrane, stimulating impulses in the sensory endings of the auditory division of the eighth cranial nerve. These impulses are transmitted to the temporal lobe of the brain for interpretation. Sound vibrations may also be transmitted by bone directly to the inner ear. A cross section of the external, middle, and inner ear in relation to other structures of the head and face is shown in Figure 19-5.

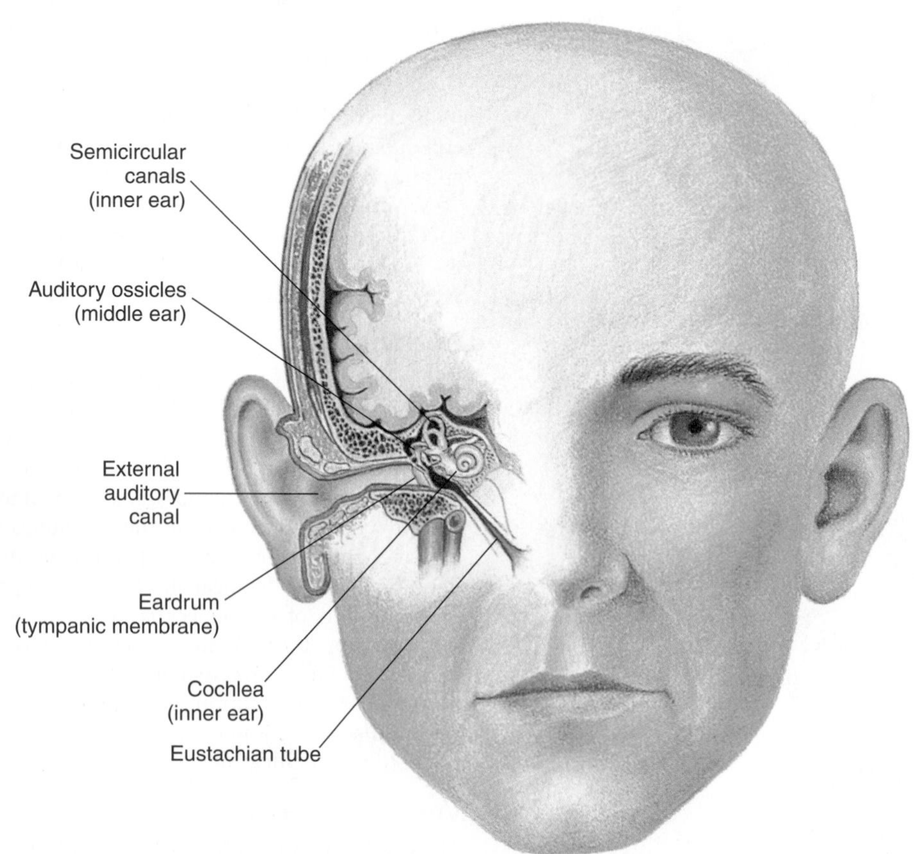


**FIGURE 19-5** Cross section of external, middle, and inner ear in relation to other structures of head and face.

## Equilibrium

The three semicircular canals each contain a sense organ (crista). These sense organs respond to fluid movement in the endolymph, which sets up impulses in the vestibular branch of the acoustic nerve. Cristae are stimulated by sudden movements, such as turning the head. Linear accelerations are detected by another set of specialized balance organs in the inner ear. The utricle and saccule each have a mat of sensory cells weighted with tiny stones called *otoconia*. The weight of these stones constantly orients us to the direction of gravity. Their inertia gives information about linear accelerations. The combined signals from the cristae of the semicircular canals and the sensory cells of the utricle and saccule provide a sense of orientation in space.

## Facial Nerve

The facial nerve is encased in the temporal bone and is the longest bony enclosure of a nerve in the human body. Its path through the bone and its intracranial and extracranial relationship determine its vulnerability to disease and the particular symptoms of whatever segment of the nerve is involved. This bony enclosure also subjects the facial nerve to injury from swelling and injury to the temporal bone.

The facial nerve enters the internal auditory meatus above the cochlear nerve and travels through the internal auditory canal, passing through the labyrinthine portion of the temporal bone to the geniculate ganglion, where it turns sharply and passes superior to the oval window. It then turns inferiorly through the mastoid and exits through the stylomastoid foramen. There are three primary branches of the facial nerve in the temporal bone: the greater superficial petrosal nerve controls lacrimation; the stapedial branch controls the stapedius muscle; and the chorda tympani nerve carries taste to the anterior two thirds of the tongue.

# *Perioperative Nursing Considerations*

## Assessment

It is estimated that 28 million Americans have a hearing loss severe enough to cause problems with communication. This number is expected to increase as the population ages.[5] Hearing loss may be classified as conductive, sensorineural, or mixed (Table 19-1). Familiarity with hearing loss and related otologic conditions is essential for effective patient assessment. Assessment is a systematic and intentional process of collecting and interpreting data concerning a patient's health history and status with otologic dysfunctions. Information obtained helps to develop nursing diagnoses, which direct nursing plans, interventions, and evaluation. The assessment should include a review of the following:

1. The presenting complaint (listening to what brings the patient to the hospital often provides clues to fears and psychologic factors that will need attention)
2. Symptoms of vertigo or dizziness
   a. Description of the attack, time of onset, frequency, duration, and relation to a positional change of the head and neck; to-and-fro movements versus rotary motion—a room spinning around the patient or the patient rotating
   b. Associated symptoms—the presence of ataxia, nausea, vomiting with or without tinnitus, hearing loss, distortion of hearing, fullness or pressure in the ear, visual changes, unsteadiness, loss of balance, or falling
3. Symptoms of impaired hearing (in one or both ears)
   a. Mode of onset—instant (may indicate a vascular disruption) or over a few hours or days (may indicate viral infection); and progression (slow or gradual, fluctuations of hearing, influenced by illnesses)

**TABLE 19-1**

**Types of Hearing Loss**

| Classification | Definition | Causes |
|---|---|---|
| Conductive | Loss of hearing acuity resulting from failure to conduct sound from the external ear to the middle ear | Blockage of the external canal with cerumen or foreign bodies<br>Edema<br>Trauma<br>Infection<br>Tympanic perforation<br>Otosclerosis |
| Sensorineural | Loss of hearing acuity resulting from a failure to conduct sound to the inner ear (cochlea or acoustic nerve) | Ototoxic medications<br>Exposure to loud noise<br>Trauma<br>Meniere's disease<br>Tumor<br>Presbycusis<br>Infectious disease (measles, mumps, meningitis) |
| Mixed | Loss of hearing acuity resulting from a combination of conductive and sensorineural factors | Develops secondary to either conductive or sensorineural loss (e.g., patient with presbycusis and impacted cerumen) |

b. Behavioral changes—no reaction to loud noises, inattention, and reliance on gestures
c. Adaptive responses—lip reading, sign language, written communication, physical disability that interferes with adaptation, such as difficulty operating a hearing aid
d. Speech preference—soft or loud, monotonous tone or erratic volume
e. Optimal hearing—on the telephone, in quiet or noisy environment, using a hearing aid
f. Effect of hearing loss on daily life—inability to hear traffic, alarms, telephone, conversation, television

4. History of earache
   a. Onset, duration, pain, fever, discharge (serous, mucoid, purulent, sanguineous)
   b. Concurrent upper respiratory tract infection, frequent swimming, head trauma, related complaints in the mouth, teeth, sinuses, or throat
   c. Associated symptoms—reduced hearing, ringing in the ear, vertigo
   d. Method of ear cleaning
5. Medical history, age, frequency of ear problems during childhood, previous medical or surgical therapy, trauma to head, physical limitations, such as arthritis and neck and back problems
6. Ototoxic drugs taken, including salicylates, aminoglycosides, furosemide, streptomycin, quinine, and ethacrynic acid
7. Family history—hearing problems, hearing loss, or Meniere's disease
8. Environmental factors and exposure to loud, continuous noise (factory, airport, loud music, power equipment, machinery)
9. External ear examination, including size, shape, symmetry, landmarks, color, position, and presence of deformities, lesions, and nodules
10. Facial or abducens nerve involvement—inability to look downward, nystagmus, facial asymmetry, and facial paresis

In addition to standard office diagnostic procedures performed by the surgeon, several other tests may be performed on the patient before arrival in the operating room (OR). Study results of most significance to the perioperative team that should be available in the OR may include the following.

***Audiogram.*** The audiogram determines whether the patient has normal hearing, conductive hearing loss, or sensorineural hearing loss. Two types of audiometric testing are performed on patients with suspected hearing loss, as described below.

*Pure-tone audiometry* is a technique that presents a single-frequency tone to patients through a headphone and is performed in each ear. The intensity of the tone is then varied until the lowest audible intensity in decibels (dB) is measured. It determines the degree of hearing impairment by evaluating air-conduction and bone-conduction thresholds. Air-conduction thresholds are a measure of the entire auditory system, whereas bone-conduction thresholds are a measure of the perceptive mechanism of the ear (cochlea and auditory nerve). In normal hearing and in pure sensorineural hearing loss, air- and bone-conduction thresholds are equal. In conductive hearing loss, bone-conduction scores are essentially normal and slightly better than air-conduction scores. In mixed hearing loss, air- and bone-conduction scores are lower but with less bone-conduction loss.

*Speech audiometry* evaluates the patient's ability to hear, understand, and distinguish phonetic elements of speech. Higher scores reflect excellent speech-discrimination ability and are seen in normal hearing, pure conductive loss, and some cochlear losses. Patients who have a cochlear sensory hearing loss often demonstrate reduced scores on this test, even when the verbal stimuli are presented well within their audible range.[7]

Pure-tone and speech audiometry testing is performed preoperatively and up to 6 weeks postoperatively.

***Magnetic Resonance Imaging.*** Magnetic resonance imaging (MRI) is an imaging modality using powerful magnetic and radiofrequency waves to reproduce cross-sectional images of the human body without exposing the patient to ionizing radiation. On an MRI scan, fat and fluid produce high-intensity signals, which appear as bright areas, whereas bone and air (as in the normal mastoid) emit weak signals and appear as darkened areas on the scan. Abnormal tissue and fluid caused by infection, trauma, and tumors within the external auditory canal, middle ear, and mastoid are identified by abnormally high intensity signals. MRI is more sensitive than computed tomography (CT) for early identification of changes in pathologic conditions of the temporal bone; however, it is unable to detect the exact location and extent of the abnormality and involvement of bony structures (e.g., the ossicles). MRI may be contraindicated for patients with implantable metal objects, such as inner ear implants or cranial plating, since the magnet could move the implant, causing injury to the patient. Today, many implantable prostheses are manufactured using nonmagnetic materials, but careful assessment of the patient for any implanted metallic device is advised before the MRI.

***Computed Tomography.*** CT scans are x-ray studies that visualize structures by producing serial sections in various planes. They use computers to measure small x-ray absorption differentials not recognizable by direct recording on x-ray films. This enables the radiologist to manipulate factors that produce the image to optimize visualization of bone, soft tissue, and adjacent intracranial and extracranial pathologic conditions. Intravenous (IV) injection of iodine contrast agents produces visual enhancement of some anatomic structures and pathologic tissues, including highly vascularized tumors. CT is the study of choice to assess intratemporal bone pathologic conditions by showing the relationship of mass to ossicles and other bony structures of the ear and for postoperative evaluation of the ear. However, if a lesion extends outside the confines of the temporal bone, MRI defines involvement of intracranial and extracranial spaces more precisely than CT.

## Nursing Diagnosis

Nursing diagnoses related to the care of patients undergoing otologic surgery might include the following:

- Disturbed Sensory Perception
- Anxiety
- Risk for Injury
- Risk for Impaired Skin Integrity
- Acute Pain

## Outcome Identification

Outcomes identified for the selected nursing diagnoses could be stated as follows:

- The patient will demonstrate improved self-expression and decreased frustration with communication.
- The patient will be able to identify factors that cause anxiety and verbalize an ability to cope.
- The patient will be free from injury.
- The patient will maintain skin integrity.
- The patient will communicate adequate pain control.

## Planning

The development of a plan of care is based on the preoperative assessment, nursing diagnoses, expected outcomes, and the surgery being performed. Hearing deficits may increase patient anxiety. Thus effective communication techniques are essential when providing explanations and information to the patient (Best Practice). The perioperative nurse should determine the best way to communicate with the patient and use the institution's hearing-impaired services for patients requiring assistance (Patient Safety). Information given to the patient should be reinforced as needed throughout the perioperative experience. The OR environment must be quiet and free of any loud noise. Intraoperative noises generated from suction, electrosurgical units (ESUs), and other equipment should be explained to the patient before use, thus avoiding startling the patient and adversely affecting the success of the surgery. Patients receiving local anesthesia need to remain still during the procedure, so providing for comfort measures becomes especially important. The room temperature should be regulated at a comfortable setting, and the patient should be adequately covered to maintain normal body temperature.

A typical plan of care for a patient undergoing otologic surgery is on p. 637.

### BEST PRACTICE

#### Strategies for Communicating with a Hearing-Impaired Patient

Hearing deficits in patients must be considered when performing assessment, planning and implementing interventions, and providing education. Preexisting and postoperative hearing deficits can present a communication challenge for patients, their families, and perioperative nurses. Recommended strategies for communicating with a hearing-impaired patient include the following:

- Position yourself directly in front of the patient. Most people who have hearing loss rely heavily on seeing the speaker's face.
- Ensure that the room is well lighted, making sure the light is shining at the speaker and not in the eyes of the patient.
- Get the patient's attention before beginning to speak.
- If one ear is better than the other, move closer to the less-affected side.
- Speak clearly and slowly.
- Do not shout. Shouting raises the frequency of sound and makes understanding more difficult.
- Try not to mumble or lower the sound intensity of words at the end of sentences.
- Decrease background noise as much as possible; turn off medical equipment alarms if possible when attempting communication with the patient.
- Do not chew gum and speak at the same time.
- Keep hands and other objects away from your mouth and the speaker's mouth when talking to the patient.
- When family members are present, speak directly to the patient. Do not refer to the patient in the third person.
- Minimize distractions.
- Rephrase rather than repeat—the patient may not have understood a particular word or phrase.
- Have the patient repeat back, in his or her own words, your statements and the speaker's statements to assess understanding.
- Use appropriate hand motions.
- Write messages on paper if the patient is able to read.

Modified from Martin J: Interventions for clients with ear and hearing problems. In Ignatavicius DD, Workman ML, editors: *Medical-surgical nursing: critical thinking for collaborative care,* ed 5, Philadelphia, 2006, Saunders; Palmer CV, Ortmann A: Hearing loss and hearing aids, *Neurology Clinics* 23:901-918, 2005.

## Implementation

The following nursing interventions should be instituted for the otologic patient:

1. Use the institutional verification process immediately before surgery to identify the correct surgical site. This should include verifying the operative side and site with the patient or family and confirmation through review of the medical record, informed consent, diagnostic test reports, and other members of the surgical team during the time out.
2. Verify that the patient has maintained nothing-by-mouth (NPO) status and that requested laboratory studies are on the medical record.
3. When in the OR, provide calm, careful, and comforting nursing measures to reduce the patient's anxiety. Allow the patient time to comply with requests, and explain the sequence of perioperative events.
4. If the patient uses a hearing aid, it should be worn to surgery and then properly removed at the time of or after anesthesia induction. Prescription eyewear should be brought into the OR because patients may require them to assist in lip reading when instructions and procedures are explained. If local anesthesia is used, the hearing aid in the unaffected ear should remain in place. Disposition of the hearing aid must be documented.
5. Patients with impaired hearing acuity need to be protected from injury. The environment should be controlled, because excess stimulation interferes with the patient's ability to hear and comply with instructions and explanations. If hearing loss is uncompensated, a pad of paper and pencil may be used as a means of communication.
6. For the patient receiving a local anesthetic, carefully review with the patient the need to remain immobile during the procedure. Explain perioperative monitoring devices and accessories (e.g., ESU, drills) that may be used if the patient will be awake.
7. If the patient has local anesthesia, the perioperative nurse may monitor him or her during stapedectomy or tympanoplasty procedures and should follow institutional protocol for monitoring parameters and documentation.
8. Remain with the patient throughout the induction phase of anesthesia.

## PATIENT SAFETY

### Effective Communication with Patients Who Are Deaf or Hard of Hearing

Effective communication between the patient and the health care team is a cornerstone of patient safety. Failure to communicate or ineffective communication has wide-ranging effects, from patient anxiety, to lack of understanding about informed consent, misdiagnosis, and improper treatment, to not following preoperative/postoperative instructions. The responsibility for effective communication is greater when dealing with patients who are deaf or hard of hearing.

Health care providers are obligated under the Americans with Disabilities Act (ADA) to provide effective means for communication for patients' family members and hospital visitors who are deaf or hard of hearing.

The person with the hearing disability is best qualified to determine which aids or services will be needed to ensure effective communication. The perioperative nurse should be familiar with available technologies and interpretative services to assist the hard of hearing or deaf patient.

Technologies and other terminology relating to the deaf and hard of hearing community are included in the glossary within this box. Considerations regarding the use of interpreters and assistive technology include the following:

- Planning in advance whenever possible to avoid delays in obtaining necessary assistive devices or interpreters and minimizing patient anxiety
- Recognizing that assistive devices or interpretive services may also be needed for deaf or hard of hearing parents or guardians of minors (or adults) who participate in the patient's care and give informed consent for medical treatment
- Informing the entire health care team of the patient's hearing disability and interpretive services to be used
- Using a qualified interpreter who is familiar with the specialized vocabulary or medical terms and concepts; using a family member as an interpreter may compromise patient confidentiality or lead to undue cultural influence or coercion, so this situation should be avoided
- Adapting written materials (i.e., consent forms, discharge instructions) as necessary; including visual information such as symbols, pictures, or diagrams may help understanding as will using active versus passive voice
- Assessing the comprehension of the information communicated by encouraging questions and soliciting feedback

#### Glossary of Terms Relating to Deafness and Hearing Loss

**American Sign Language (ASL):** A manual language that uses the hands, facial expression, and body movements for expression and is visually received

**Assisted listening (AL) device:** A device, such as a hearing aid or cochlear implant, that assists a person to receive auditory information, usually designed for a specific situation

**Audiologically deaf:** A term used to describe the fact of being deaf from a physical or audiologic perspective; term normally used in contrast to the term *culturally deaf*

**Computer-assisted real-time transcription (CART):** A service in which an operator types what is said into a computer that displays the typed words on a screen; the same technology used for closed captioning television

**Cued speech interpreter:** An interpreter who uses hand cues and codes to represent each speech sound

**Culturally deaf (CD):** A person who generally became deaf before acquiring spoken language or shortly thereafter and uses American Sign Language (or another native sign language) as his or her primary language

**Deaf:** When written with a lowercase *d* the word "deaf" refers to the inability to hear; when written with an uppercase *D*, the word "Deaf" refers to culturally Deaf people

**Deaf community:** a term that is usually interpreted broadly to include all persons who have or are interested in hearing loss

**Hard of hearing (HOH):** A person with significant hearing loss but still able to function in the hearing world, possibly with AL devices

**Late deafened (LD):** a person who has lost the ability to understand speech through the ear, originating after the acquisition of spoken language in a person raised in the hearing community

**Oral deaf (OD):** A person who was born deaf or became deaf before the acquisition of language and who relies on oral communication rather than sign language

**Oral hearing loss:** A term that includes all people with hearing loss who prefer spoken English as their primary means of communication; this includes HOH, LD, and OD

**Oral interpreters:** Specially trained individuals who articulate speech silently and clearly, sometimes rephrasing words and phrases to give higher visibility on the lips; natural body language and gestures may also be used

**Sign language interpreters:** Individuals trained in a visually interactive language that uses a combination of hand motions, body gestures, and facial expressions; there are several different types of sign language; American Sign Language (ASL) and Signed English are commonly used in the United States and Canada, whereas other countries have differing versions of sign language

**Signed English:** A form of communication in which signs are used in exact English word order, with some additional signs for conventions such as the "ing," "ment," and "ly" word endings; also known as *Signing Exact English,* or SEE; SEE is often used in a classroom setting where sentence structure is being emphasized

**TDD:** Telecommunications device for the deaf; this term, as opposed to TTY, is normally used by HOH and LD people

**Text telephone:** A device that allows text communication over standard telephone equipment

**TTY:** Teletype; this term, as opposed to TDD, is normally used by CD people

Modified from *ADA business brief, communicating with people who are deaf or hard of hearing in hospital settings.* Accessed December 5, 2005, on-line: www.usdoj.gov/crt/ada/hsopcombr.htm; *Are doctors required to provide interpreters for medical visits and other medical-related situations.* Accessed December 5, 2005, on-line: www.scadservices.org/SCIRT/ada%20medical.htm; *New to hearing loss.* Accessed December 5, 2005, on-line: www.hearinglossweb.com/Misc/glossary.htm.

## SAMPLE PLAN OF CARE

**NURSING DIAGNOSIS**
**Disturbed Sensory Perception**

**OUTCOME**
The patient will demonstrate improved self-expression and decreased frustration with communication.

**INTERVENTIONS**
- Assess degree of hearing impairment.
- Allow patient to wear hearing aid to the OR.
- Identify a method by which patient can communicate basic needs if and when the hearing aid needs to be removed.
- Maintain a quiet surgical environment.
- Speak slowly and deliberately into the dominant ear.
- Reorient patient as needed, and provide frequent explanations and reassurance.
- Provide interpreters (i.e., sign language interpreter, oral interpreter, cued speech interpreter, etc.) as needed to facilitate communication.

**NURSING DIAGNOSIS**
**Anxiety**

**OUTCOME**
The patient will be able to identify factors that cause anxiety and verbalize an ability to cope.

**INTERVENTIONS**
- Describe anticipated perioperative events.
- Validate sources of anxiety; provide factual information in response to these.
- Observe for expressions of distress (e.g., clenched fists, crying, facial tension, restlessness).
- Introduce staff at time of admission to OR.
- Prevent unnecessary body exposure during transfer, positioning, and skin preparation.
- Give simple, concise directions.
- Control extraneous noise and other external stimuli.
- Determine personally effective coping methods, and support these.
- Reinforce preoperative education.

**NURSING DIAGNOSIS**
**Risk for Injury**

**OUTCOME**
The patient will be free from injury.

**INTERVENTIONS**
- Note that patient is deaf or hard of hearing on a separate wristband.
- Leave patient's hearing aid or aids in place until after induction of anesthesia.
- Speak slowly, clearly, and deliberately to patient, and confirm that patient has heard and understood communication.
- Provide adequate assistance during transfer to and from OR bed and while positioning takes place.
- Complete all transfer and positioning maneuvers slowly.
- Identify physical limitations, and position or support patient accordingly to provide optimal comfort during the procedure.
- Control excess stimulation and noise level in OR.
- Assess for vertigo and tinnitus.

**NURSING DIAGNOSIS**
**Risk for Impaired Skin Integrity**

**OUTCOME**
The patient will maintain skin integrity.

**INTERVENTIONS**
- Determine whether the patient has any limitations in mobility, implants, or problems with range of motion.
- Secure, prepare, and apply additional positioning devices as required for planned surgical procedure.
- Use appropriate padding at positional pressure sites; document condition of skin at pressure sites before and at conclusion of procedure.
- Use clippers or razor carefully if hair removal is required.
- Apply SCDs according to manufacturer's recommendations.
- Prevent skin irritation from antimicrobial agents used for skin preparation; verify absence of allergy to prep solution; prevent pooling of solution. Allow prep solution to dry before application of drapes.
- Implement protective measures to prevent skin or tissue injury caused by thermal injury (use of the ESU, laser, other electrical equipment).

**NURSING DIAGNOSIS**
**Acute Pain**

**OUTCOME**
The patient will communicate adequate pain control.

**INTERVENTIONS**
- Assess location, intensity, and frequency of pain; select a pain rating scale appropriate to age.
- Identify any allergies, idiosyncrasies, or sensitivities to medication before administration.
- Administer analgesics, sedatives, and narcotics as prescribed; monitor and document medications administered, dose, route, time, and response.
- Observe for signs of pain, such as grimacing, clenching of teeth, or groaning.
- Assist with nonpharmacologic management of pain, such as distraction, imagery, or music (as appropriate and according to patient preference).

*ESU,* Electrosurgical unit; *OR,* operating room; *SCDs,* sequential compression devices.

9. Secure the patient's hair within a disposable surgical hat. Clipping or shaving the hair near the incision site may be indicated, depending on the surgical approach. Skin preparation should be carried out carefully to protect the eyes and prevent pooling of solution.
10. Thermal warming blankets, forced-air-warming units, and warm IV and irrigating solutions assist in maintaining normothermia. Warm irrigation is essential during local procedures to reduce the risk of inducing dizziness.
11. Sequential compression devices (SCDs) may be used to decrease the risk of deep venous thrombosis (DVT) and pulmonary embolism (PE) during long surgical procedures, such as acoustic neuroma resection.
12. Document the serial number and lot numbers of otologic implants according to institutional policy.
13. If a laser is used, initiate and document laser safety precautions (see Chapter 7).

***Preoperative Room Preparation.*** Before the patient enters the OR, equipment and supplies for the scheduled procedure should be gathered. A well-organized surgical environment can significantly reduce anesthesia time and enable the perioperative nurse to spend more time attending to the preoperative and intraoperative needs of the patient. Planning includes identifying equipment, instrumentation, furniture, and positioning accessories necessary to perform the surgery. Such equipment may include the operating microscope, video system, monopolar and bipolar ESUs, suction, nerve-integrity monitors, specialty instrument kits, prosthetic devices, drill and irrigation accessories, and the laser. An otologic specialty storage cart centrally houses assorted prostheses, drill burrs and accessories, backup ear instrumentation, ear drapes, and dressing and packing materials.

***Positioning.*** Proper patient positioning is essential for adequate surgical exposure during otologic surgery. Based on the design of microscope and OR bed used, the patient may be placed on the bed in the reverse position—with the patient's head at the foot of the bed. This position facilitates proper placement of a microscope mounted on a floor stand and allows adequate space for the surgeon and assistant to be positioned on sitting stools near the surgical site. Before the patient is transferred to the OR bed, the bed should be prepared with the mattress taped securely to its frame to prevent the mattress from sliding during lateral rotation of the bed.

The patient should be in a supine position with the operative side as close to the edge of the OR bed as possible, with the head turned and the operative ear upward. This positioning gives the surgeon access in viewing all areas of the middle ear and mastoid. One or more safety/ restraining belts are used to secure the patient on the OR bed to ensure safety when turning or rotating the bed. During some procedures, such as myringotomy with the patient under local anesthesia, the patient's head may be secured in position by placing tape across the head and attaching it to the frame of the OR bed or by an attendant holding the patient's head firmly in position. For other procedures, the patient's head may be immobilized and supported on a foam headrest. A donut-shaped foam head support helps to immobilize the head and permits easy adjustment of the angle while the operating microscope is being used.

To protect the nonoperative ear, the perioperative nurse should ensure that it is in the center of the donut hole and that the headrest does not cause any pressure on the ear. The dependent arm on the nonoperative side must also be well padded and properly positioned to minimize pressure injury from the weight of the patient when the OR bed is rotated laterally to optimize surgical access. Special consideration must be given when the patient's head is positioned for surgery, especially under general anesthesia. Extremes in neck extension and head torsion can cause injury to the brachial plexus or cervical spine. If the patient has a neck or back disorder caused by arthritis or other conditions, special padding or supports must be provided. Other options to assist in patient positioning are determined by the otologic procedure to be performed and by the surgeon's preference. They may include ophthalmic headrests with a crescent-shaped pad, a padded horseshoe-shaped headrest, and a headrest with skull pins such as the Mayfield, which is used in certain neurotology procedures.

Positioning of the surgeon is equally important to the success of the surgery. The surgeon's chair should be positioned at a height and distance that allows comfortable access to the operative site. The use of hydraulic or electric chairs enables the surgeon to adjust the position to meet these needs.

***Anesthesia.*** The infiltration of a local anesthetic agent (local anesthesia) and the use of general anesthesia each have advantages during ear surgery. Local anesthesia allows hearing to be tested on the adult patient and may result in slightly less bleeding with some procedures. General anesthesia provides better airway control and allows the patient to remain still throughout the procedure, thereby making it technically easier to perform.

Local anesthesia combined with closely monitored conscious sedation is often employed for surgery in the premeatal region and for stapedectomy and uncomplicated middle ear procedures of less than 2 hours' duration. Conscious sedation should render the patient calm, comfortable, cooperative, and able to understand and communicate. Patients should not be overmedicated to the point of demonstrating obtunded reflexes or being out of touch with their surroundings (see Chapter 4 for a full discussion of conscious sedation). General anesthesia requires particular attention to preserving the facial nerve, extremes in head positioning, possible air emboli, the control of bleeding, and the effects of nitrous oxide in the middle ear.

**NITROUS OXIDE AND THE MIDDLE EAR.** The middle ear and paranasal sinuses are normal body air cavities and consist of open, nonventilated spaces. The middle ear cavity is vented periodically when the eustachian tube opens. During general anesthesia, inhaled nitrous oxide diffuses into the middle ear space through the capillaries of the middle ear mucosa. This results in increased middle ear pressure. Rapid increases in middle ear pressure proportional to inhaled levels of nitrous oxide and abnormal eustachian tube function may cause nausea, vomiting, and rupture of the tympanic membrane in susceptible patients. This includes patients having previous ear surgery, otitis media, sinusitis, upper respiratory infections, enlarged adenoids, or other disorders of the nasopharynx.

When nitrous oxide is discontinued, the gas is rapidly reabsorbed and strong negative pressure in the middle ear may occur. This negative pressure may result in nausea, vomiting, serous otitis, hemotympanum, disarticulation of the stapes, and impaired hearing. Some practitioners believe the use of nitrous oxide as an anesthetic inhalation agent is hazardous to hearing in patients who have undergone previous reconstructive middle ear surgery.[3]

***Preparation of the Operative Site.*** Many otologic procedures require hair removal. Clipping is preferred because shaving may injure the skin and increase the risk of infection. Proper skin preparation combined with adequate isolation draping techniques helps lower infection rates and facilitates postoperative dressing of the ear. Postaural and endaural incisions extending upward from the meatus require hair to be clipped 2 inches in front, above, and behind the ear. Under hair may be clipped, whereas the top hair is maintained for postoperative image enhancement. Plastic adhesive drapes may be applied to the clipped area to ensure that the surgical field is free from hair.

A povidone-iodine solution is generally used (unless the patient is allergic to iodine) to prep the exposed auricle and the periauricular skin. The meatus is cleansed with cotton applicators if there is no hole in the eardrum. If requested by the surgeon, the external ear canal is irrigated with the prepping solution. The face may be prepped on the operative side to permit observation of facial nerve stimulation.

***Facial Nerve Monitoring.*** Audible facial nerve monitors are used intraoperatively during procedures in which the facial nerve is at risk. The purpose of this monitoring technique is to assist in the early identification of the nerve, to increase the possibility of its preservation by minimizing trauma, and to assess its integrity after dissection.[9] Electrodes are placed into the facial muscles before draping the patient. Consultation and communication with the anesthesia provider are essential because the use of muscle relaxants and long-term paralyzing agents must be avoided. Facial nerve monitoring is used during acoustic neuroma and mastoid surgery (Figure 19-6).

***Draping.*** Barrier draping minimizes the risk of postoperative infection. Draping technique is based on the surgeon's preference. For major otologic procedures, plastic adhesive drapes are applied around the ear to keep the patient's hair out of the surgical field. Sterile, plastic, aperture drapes may be placed over the surgical site with the ear exposed through the opening. The surgeon may elect to expose a portion of the face on the affected side to observe facial movement.

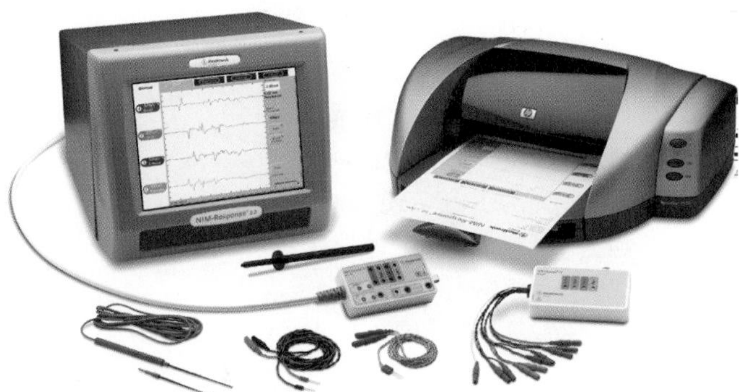

FIGURE 19-6 Nerve integrity monitor system for intraoperative facial nerve monitoring.

Three or four towels are draped over the aperture drape around the ear and may be secured with towel clips. A fenestrated drape is unfolded over the patient, with the opening centered over the operative site. An alternative method is the use of a split sheet with the split end secured at the base of the ear and the open flaps wrapped around the patient's head. Disposable drapes with adhesive backing may be used to secure the sheet to the patient.

During mastoid surgery and for resections of acoustic tumors, fluid-collection pouches may be attached to the drape. These pouches will catch fluid runoff when drilling and irrigation are planned. The operating microscope is draped to extend the sterile field (Figure 19-7).

Special consideration must be given to the selection of draping material used during ear surgery and to the technique for removing powder from surgical gloves. Powder and lint cling to gloves and can be transferred to instruments and introduced into the ear. They act as a foreign body in the wound, causing the formation of granulomas in the middle and inner ear and may contribute to irreversible hearing loss. Therefore gloves worn by the surgical team should be rinsed to remove powder and lint. Lint-free drapes should be used.

***Surgical Microscope.*** The complexity of ear surgery is partly attributable to the location of the delicate, bony anatomic structures contained within a confined operative area. The surgical microscope is often used to provide illumination and magnification. Several kinds of surgical microscopes (Figure 19-8) with different attachments are available for otologic surgery. The microscope may be floor- or ceiling-mounted. Optimal light for an otologic microscope is provided by a xenon or halogen light source. Numerous types of monocular and binocular heads are available for the microscope. These heads may be fixed in a straight or angled plane, or they may be designed to be adjustable in an inclinable plane. For operations through an ear speculum, the microscope provides direct light and permits the surgeon to select a magnification of 6, 10, 16, 25, or 40. A common eyepiece magnification for an otologic microscope is 12.5, and a usual objective (lens) is a 250 or 300 focal length (f). The total magnification is determined by multiply-

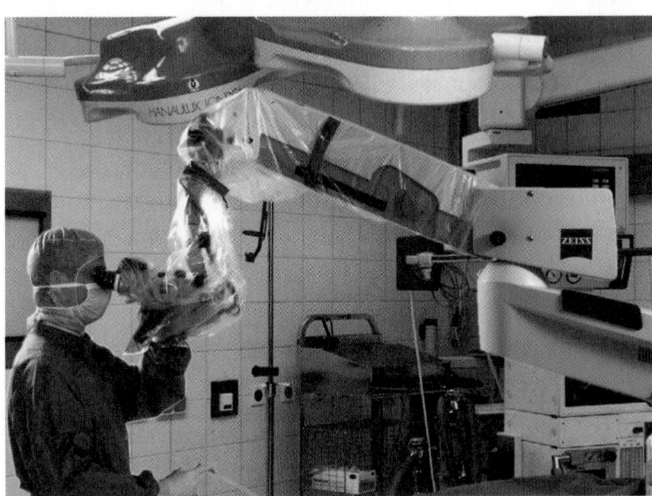


FIGURE 19-7 Draped microscope for otologic surgery.

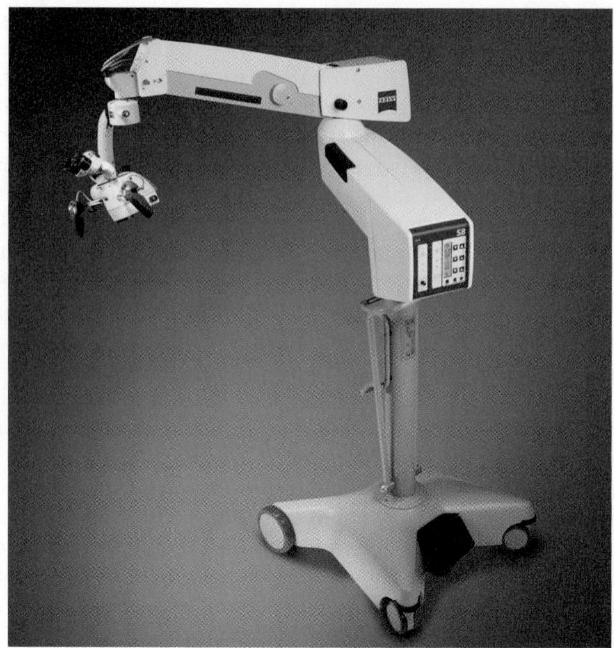

**FIGURE 19-8** Operating microscope used during various otologic procedures. Lens system allows magnification of 6 to 40 without change in distance between microscope and ear. Xenon light provides excellent visualization.

ing the magnification of the eyepiece times that of the microscope body times that of the objective. The type of head and objective selected is based on the surgeon's preference. Microscopes, equipped with a variable distance feature, allow the surgeon to adjust the focal length from 200 mm to 400 mm without changing the lens objective. Video equipment may be attached to the microscope, which allows other team members to follow the procedure and to anticipate the necessary instrumentation. Before lenses are put into the microscope, they should be checked to ensure that they are free from lint, dust, fingerprints, and soil. The surgeon adjusts the microscope before it is draped for surgery and manipulates it during the procedure. The microscope is draped with a sterile cover. It is necessary to keep the drape material away from the light source fan of the microscope. Doing so will allow cool air to continue to circulate and will avoid overheating of the fan, which could prematurely burn out the lamp and possibly cause a fire. When micromanipulators are secured to transmit laser energy to tissue through the operating microscope, special microscope laser drapes must be used. These drapes have an opening in the plastic at the base of the micromanipulator covering the objective, allowing laser energy to pass through the opening of the drape without risk of burning the drape.

Care should be taken when removing the drapes from the microscope to avoid discarding the eyepieces with the drapes or dropping them on the floor. Eyepieces have been lost or damaged in this manner, necessitating costly repair or replacement.

When the microscope is not in use, it should be kept in a locked, upright position and stored in an area that is away from traffic, free from dust, and properly ventilated. Ideally, a set of eyepieces should be left in the scope to prevent the inside of the scope from becoming dusty. The microscope may also be covered with either a protective cover or a plastic bag.

***Care and Handling of Otologic Instruments.*** The basic principles of care, handling, and sterilization of instruments are discussed in Chapter 3. To prevent damage, delicate microinstruments should be handled individually and should not be allowed to come into contact with each other. They should be washed, rinsed, and dried individually. Soft-bristled brushes can be used to clean the instruments, and care should be taken to prevent damage to their delicate tips. Preoperatively, instruments should be closely inspected to ensure that they are in good working order. Fine tympanoplasty and stapedectomy instrumentation should be kept in special storage and sterilization trays (Figure 19-9). These trays help separate instruments, aid in quick identification, protect the instruments from damage, and facilitate handling during surgery (Figure 19-10). When arranging instruments in the trays, one should consider grouping like items together, such as knives, elevators, hoes, and hooks. Numbering and color-coded taping of the instruments and the tray help maintain the order of the instruments and help the scrub person quickly identify and deliver the instrument to the surgeon.

***Drills and Burrs.*** A power drill and assorted rotating burrs are essential for middle ear surgery. They are used for the removal of cortical, or hard, cellular bone. Many drills are commercially available that are pneumatically or electrically driven. Pneumatic drills must have high torque (power) and more than 20,000 revolutions per minute (rpm) (speed). Electrically powered drills are believed by some surgeons to offer equal torque but better control of the drill tip. The two types of electric drills are those with the motor in the handpiece and those with a separate power supply. The drill may be fitted with either a straight or angled handpiece (Figure 19-11). A selection of burrs including assorted sizes of round cutting burrs and diamond polishing burrs should be available.

A diamond burr cuts slowly and pushes soft tissue away rather then tearing into it; it is commonly used around vital structures. It has been known to help control bleeding from bone by pushing the vessel down into its channel and filling the channel with bone dust.

Cutting burrs assist in quickly removing bone from areas not close to vital structures. The grooves or teeth of burrs must be clean of bone dust. Bone-cutting burrs tend to clog more easily than coarse-toothed burrs. A sterile wire brush may be used to keep burrs clean intraoperatively. Bone dust must be prevented from settling in areas such as those in stapedectomy,

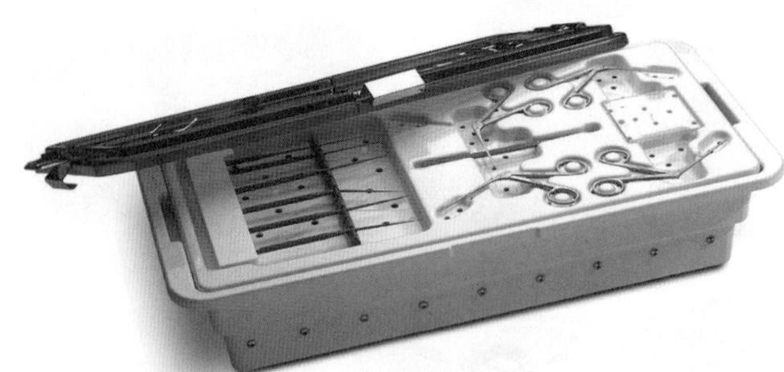

**FIGURE 19-9** Microsurgical middle ear instruments in protective rack, which separates the instruments from one another. The delicacy of these instruments requires protection of tips.

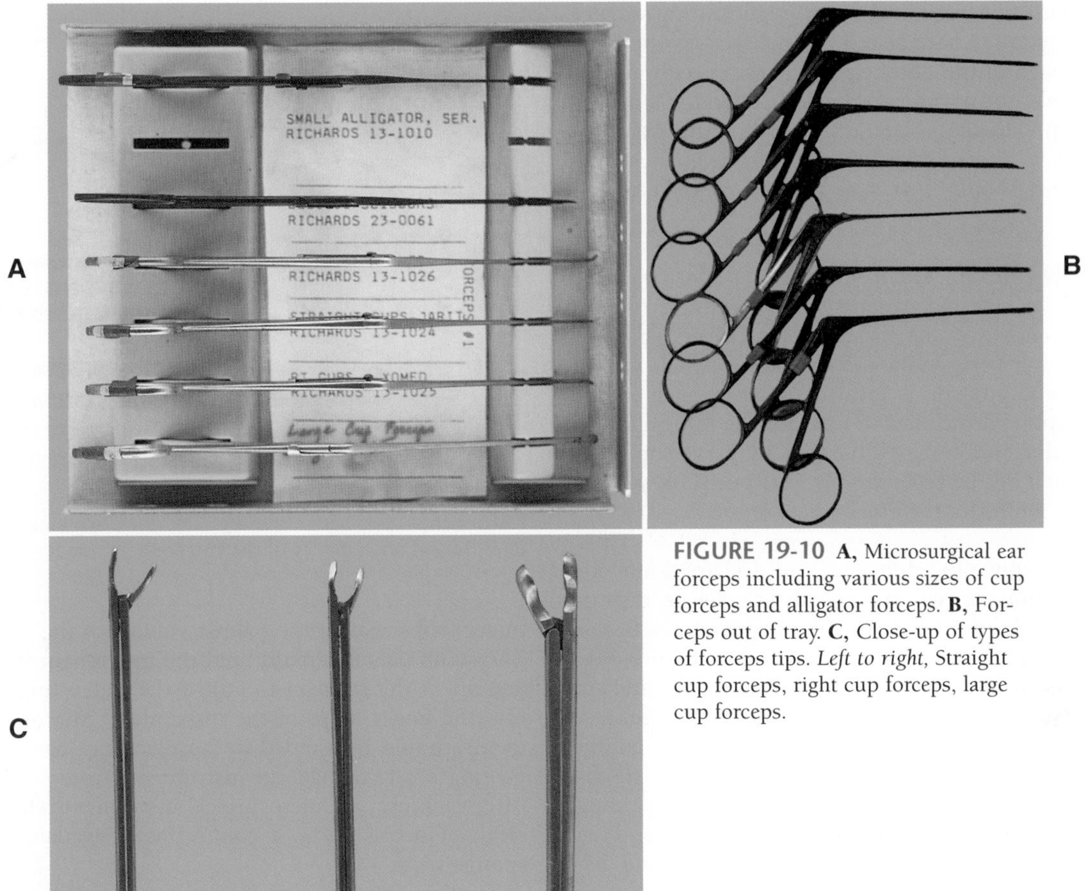


**FIGURE 19-10** **A,** Microsurgical ear forceps including various sizes of cup forceps and alligator forceps. **B,** Forceps out of tray. **C,** Close-up of types of forceps tips. *Left to right,* Straight cup forceps, right cup forceps, large cup forceps.

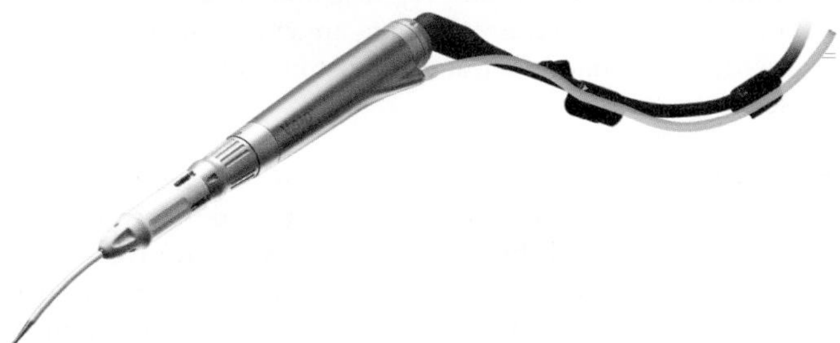

**FIGURE 19-11** Surgical drill handpiece with irrigation tubing.

tympanoplasty, endolymphatic sac, or fenestration surgery. A sterile field continuously flooded with irrigation solution helps to lessen clogging of the burr and washes away bone dust.

***Irrigation and Suctioning of the Operative Field.*** Adequate irrigation and suction ensure visibility of the operative field while clearing it of bone dust, blood, and bacteria from chronically infected ears. Irrigation solutions include warm saline or lactated Ringer's solution and may be delivered to the sterile field by means of bulb syringes or suction irrigators or through sterile IV tubing connected to irrigation ports on the handpiece of selected drill systems. Some surgeons prefer to have the scrub person irrigate as they suction and drill; others choose a suction irrigator, allowing them to control the flow and direction of the irrigation as they drill and suction away debris.

Multiple suction tips should be available in sizes ranging from 18 gauge through 26 gauge. They are designed to allow the operator's thumb to control and vary the degree of suction. Small-gauge suction tips clog frequently, especially during drilling of bone, and must be routinely flushed throughout the procedure to ensure patency.

***Bone Curettes.*** Bone curettes are used for the removal of soft cellular bone. Whenever possible, larger curettes are preferred because they decrease the risk to dura, sinus wall, and facial nerve. Sharp curettes are safer, cut with less pressure, and are more effective than dull curettes. They should be held so that the cutting edge is in full view and not obscured by the hand.

***Specula and Holder.*** A universal ear speculum holder fits into the sliding bar clamp of the OR bed and remains adjustable and flexible until locked in a semirigid position. This allows the surgeon's hands to remain free. A work table containing several wells with a transparent wheel-like cover may be used to safely store prosthesis, ossicles, and ear packing. The work table may be secured to the lower portion of the speculum holder or used separately.

Ear specula are designed with a nonreflective finish to reduce glare generated by the operating microscope's bright halogen lamp. This finish minimizes eye fatigue during surgery and reduces reflection of laser beams during laser-assisted procedures. The design of the distal tip of the ear speculum may be oval and beveled or round and nonbeveled and is a matter of the surgeon's preference. The largest speculum that fits comfortably into the ear should be used to achieve the greatest area of visualization. It should not cause pain or pressure in the bony canal.

***Needles and Syringes for Local Anesthesia.*** Local anesthesia is preferred for selected patients and procedures. In the absence of inflammation, the mastoid bone lacks sensation except for the outer periosteum and to a lesser extent within the tympanum and antrum. A local anesthetic consisting of lidocaine with epinephrine may be used for the infiltration of the skin and periosteum to block the sensory nerve supply. A 27-gauge, 1½-inch needle secured to a 3-ml Luer-Lok syringe may be used to administer the block injection.

***Knives.*** Myringotomy procedures require a sharp knife for making incisions into the tympanic membrane. Sterile, disposable, single-use blades are supplied with integrated handles or as single blades that may be secured into reusable handles. Myringotomy blades are spear-, lancet-, and sickle-shaped and are a matter of the surgeon's preference. Disposable myringotomy kits containing a speculum, blade, suction tip, and ventilation-tube inserter are available. For stapes surgery, right and left circumferential knives are designed for various uses, including making the primary incision, elevating the periosteum and the fibrous annulus, separating the incudostapedial joint, and dissecting or resecting scar tissue or the stapedial tendon.

***Scissors.*** In addition to Mayo and Metzenbaum scissors, which may be used for general dissection purposes, delicate finger-loop scissors with angular blades or crossover blades (Bellucci or Jacobsen type) are used in middle ear operations to incise and divide the stapedial tendon or scar tissue bands.

***Dissecting Forceps.*** In radical mastoidectomy and tympanoplasty, several types of smooth and serrated alligator forceps are needed for manipulation within the canal and the middle ear (Figure 19-12).

***Instrumentation Features.*** Like ear specula, instruments used in the path of the operating microscope may have an ebony glare-reducing finish. Handles of assorted knives and dissectors may be flat, hexagonal, or round for better gripping or handling during surgery (see Figure 19-12). The shaft of these instruments may be straight, angled, or bayonet.

Sterile instruments should be passed in a manner that allows the surgeon to remain focused on the operative site and not forced to turn away from the microscope. Middle ear instruments should be passed with the tips pointing downward. Slight pressure is used when the scrub person is placing it into the web of the surgeon's hand between the thumb and index finger (as one would place a pencil ready for use). The surgeon senses the instrument and is able to close the fingertips on the instrument without needing to visualize it. The scrub person passes the middle ear forceps (scissors and crimpers) by holding onto the shaft of the instrument just above the finger loops and delivers the forceps by providing slight pressure of the finger loops against the palmar surface of the surgeon's hand. The scrub person should hold the instrument in this position and allow the surgeon to adjust the index finger and thumb into the finger loops of the instrument. Microsurgical instruments should be handed on an exchange basis, thereby preventing costly damage to instruments from inadvertent falls. After each use, all microsurgical instruments should be wiped clean of debris using a commercially available foam-rubber sponge wipe.

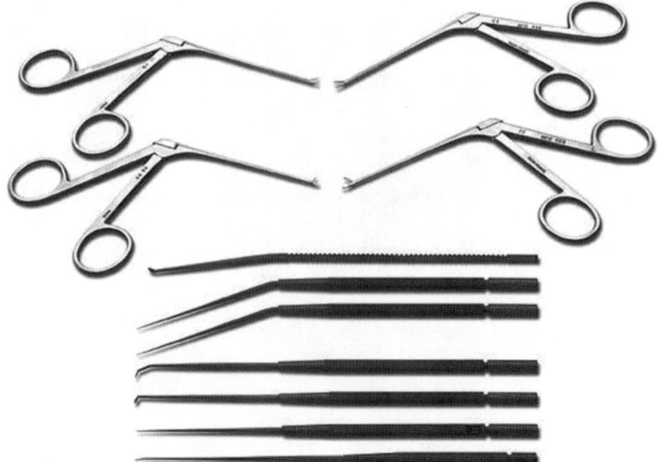

**FIGURE 19-12** Microsurgical dissecting forceps and picks. Angled instruments offer better views of the operative area than nonangled ones do and are a matter of the surgeon's preference.

Suction tips are passed in the same fashion as the middle ear instruments and should be irrigated clean after each use with a control syringe filled with water.

A universal set of ear surgery instruments can be used for all middle ear procedures. When an endaural approach is required, only endaural retractors must be added to the universal set.

***Hemostasis.*** Intraoperative management of bleeding is critical so as not to compromise surgical exposure. Methods may include infiltration of the skin and underlying soft tissue with lidocaine-containing epinephrine. For transcanal approaches, slow ooze can be controlled with small pieces of cotton, pledgets, MeroGel (esterified hyaluronic acid), or Gelfoam material soaked in epinephrine and left in place. To control bleeding from bony surfaces as in mastoid surgery, the application of bone wax may be necessary. However, bone wax is considered to be a foreign body, and absorbable substances are preferred. MeroGel and synthetic collagen sponges moistened with thrombin will stop venous bleeding and can be left in the wound. Blood vessels in the skin, subcutaneous tissue, and lateral wall should be coagulated with a monopolar ESU, but deeper vessels, especially those adjacent to the facial nerve, should be coagulated using a bipolar unit.

***Lasers.*** The ability of laser energy to precisely vaporize tissue without vibratory movements makes microscopic laser surgery an attractive modality for otologic surgery. Lasers assist in vaporization of scar tissue, granulomas, and cholesteatomas without damaging surrounding tissue. They have also been used to divide the vestibular nerve on patients with severe vertigo. During acoustic tumor surgery, the $CO_2$ laser offers a significant advantage in debulking of tumors. The surgery is less traumatic because laser vaporization eliminates much of the tugging and pulling necessary with conventional techniques.

During stapedectomy, laser energy may be used to create (drill) a hole in the footplate of the stapes for insertion of a prosthesis or to vaporize the stapedial tendon. Ideal laser energy should be completely absorbed by the footplate and should not heat the perilymph or damage the inner ear.[6] The carbon dioxide ($CO_2$) laser has ideal tissue properties for stapedectomy and its revision. It has limited tissue penetration and is completely absorbed by the stapes footplate without significant scatter. The laser stapedotomy offers improved postoperative hearing results while reducing postoperative dizziness and sensorineural hearing loss.

$CO_2$, potassium titanyl phosphate (KTP), and erbium: yttrium-aluminum-garnet (Er:YAG) lasers can be secured to the operating microscope and laser energy delivered to the tissue by means of a micromanipulator. Laser energy is delivered directly to tissue by fiberoptic probes, which can be navigated around obstructing structures.

KTP and Er:YAG lasers have ideal optical properties and provide precise focus, whereas the optical properties of the $CO_2$ laser must be routinely aligned and preoperative "test firing" must be performed before every procedure to ensure that the beam is co-axial and parfocal.

Laser safety in otologic laser surgery includes draping wet towels around the surgical field and having a basin of sterile water and a syringe on the field to extinguish a possible fire. Smoke must be evacuated to remove vaporized tissue because the plume can contain carcinogens such as nitrosamines, toxic by-products (benzene, formaldehyde, acrolein), and viral deoxyribonucleic acid (DNA).[10] The laser should be placed in a standby mode when not in use. Documentation of laser settings, as well as patient and personnel safety measures, is recorded per institution standards (see Chapter 7).

### Evaluation

Perioperative nursing care should be evaluated at the completion of the procedure before the patient is transported to the postanesthesia care unit (PACU) or ambulatory recovery area. If the patient has had a local anesthetic, the nurse will have had the opportunity to evaluate care on an ongoing basis, communicating with the patient throughout the procedure.

Potential surgical complications include hearing loss, altered taste, and injury to the facial nerve. Evaluation of facial nerve function is routinely performed and requires the patient's cooperation in smiling, closing the eye, and wrinkling the nose on the operative side. If facial palsy is observed and not resolved within 2 hours of the procedure, it may be caused by surgical trauma.

During evaluation, the perioperative nurse determines if the patient met the outcomes in the plan of care. Some outcomes can be reached during the preoperative and intraoperative phases of care; they are evaluated before the patient's discharge from the OR. Others require ongoing monitoring and measurement in the postoperative phase. Part of the hand-off report to the PACU or nursing unit should include the outcomes of care provided:

- The patient expressed himself or herself effectively and with minimal frustration; his or her hearing aid remained in place until after induction of anesthesia and was then sent to the PACU.
- The patient identified factors that caused anxiety and verbalized effective coping; frequent explanations were provided, which assisted in coping with an unknown environment.
- The patient was free from injury; skin preparation produced no rashes or irritated skin.
- The patient's skin integrity was maintained; there were no reddened or bruised areas at pressure sites.
- The patient communicated adequate pain management using a pain scale.

### Patient and Family Education and Discharge Planning

Visual teaching aids, teaching brochures, and written discharge instructions provide the patient with knowledge of the surgery and what to expect during the postoperative period. Many patients undergoing otologic surgery present with an existing hearing deficit. By the day of discharge, patients and family members should have a thorough knowledge and understanding of what to expect during the postoperative recuperation period. Specific instructions based on the type of surgery performed must be reviewed with the patient, focusing on important areas, such as management of pain and discomfort, restricted activity levels, and observing for signs of infection. General instructions for otologic surgery are detailed in the Patient and Family Education box on p. 644.

# *Surgical Interventions*

## INCISIONAL APPROACHES

The majority of otologic procedures are performed either through the ear canal or from behind the ear. Incisions through the ear canal include endaural and transcanal approaches. The postauricular approach is made through an incision from behind the ear.

### Endaural Approach

The endaural incision is made in two steps, using a Lempert triangular knife or a #15 blade. The first incision is made from the superior meatal wall about 1 cm in from the outer edge of the meatus and extends down the posterior meatal wall to the edge of the conchal cartilage. The second incision on the superior meatal wall extends upward to a point halfway between the meatus and upper edge of the auricle. This approach offers direct access to the external auditory meatus and tympanic membrane and may be used for meatoplasty, canalplasty, selected tympanic membrane perforations, and stapes surgery.

### Transcanal Approach

The transcanal approach is used for those procedures that are limited to the mesotympanum, hypotympanum, and tympanic membrane. The incision involves a superiorly based tympanomeatal flap through the ear canal and involves making a semilunar canal skin incision just lateral to the tympanic membrane. For exposure, the skin, fibrous annulus, and tympanic membrane are elevated as a unit. Posterior tympanomeatal flaps may be used in stapedectomy, labyrinthectomy, myringoplasty, tumor biopsy, ossiculoplasty, and removal of glomus

**PATIENT AND FAMILY EDUCATION**

**Patient Education After Otologic Surgery**

The nurse should provide the patient with the following information:

- Keep the ear canal dry for 10 to 21 days postoperatively for all stapes and middle ear surgery and for up to 3 months after mastoid surgery.
- Do not lie on the operative side for the first 24 hours postoperatively.
- Elevate the head of the bed 30 degrees for the first 24 hours.
- Antibiotics, analgesics, and antiemetics may be prescribed for the postoperative period.
- Hearing may be diminished during the immediate postoperative period. It is temporary, and usually hearing improves gradually. This may be attributable to full packing of the ear at the completion of surgery.
- Vertigo may occur postoperatively. Assistance may be needed to get out of bed. Moving slowly and smoothly may alleviate these sensations. If symptoms persist or are severe, call your physician; antimotion medication may be prescribed.
- To prevent possible dislodgment of a graft or prosthesis, do the following:
  - Refrain from heavy lifting, straining, or strenuous exercise.
  - Avoid rapidly moving the head, bouncing, or bending over for 3 weeks.
  - Exercise caution when coughing or blowing nose; open both the nose and mouth if sneezing is unavoidable.
  - Avoid drinking through a straw.
- Restricted activities include the following:
  - Do not drive for the first postoperative week.
  - Do not swim or dive for the first month after surgery. Depending on the procedure performed, longer restrictions may apply.
  - Air travel is not advised for 1 to 4 weeks postoperatively. This depends on the type of surgery performed and the surgeon's preference.
- The physician should be immediately consulted for any of the following:
  - An upper respiratory tract infection
  - Any other change in physical status
  - Foul-smelling drainage from the affected ear
  - Increasing pain from the affected ear
  - Fever
  - Bleeding or a discharge of clear fluid from the ear or nose
  - Vertigo

Modified from Martin J: Interventions for clients with ear and hearing problems. In Ignatavicius DD, Workman ML, editors: *Medical-surgical nursing: critical thinking for collaborative care,* ed 5, Philadelphia, 2006, Saunders.

tympanicum tumors. Congenital cholesteatomas are best approached by superior tympanomeatal flaps, whereas perforations of the tympanic membrane may be accessed through an inferior tympanomeatal flap.[1]

### Postauricular Approach

The postauricular incision is made behind the ear as the surgeon follows the curve of the posterior auricular fold, providing wide-field exposure and a versatile and adaptable incision. It is used to expose the mastoid process for simple mastoidectomy and for surgery on the endolymphatic sac, internal auditory meatus, and, on occasion, tympanoplasty and radical mastoid procedures.

The middle fossa approach represents a neurosurgical incision for access to the middle cranial region. Above the ear and at the level of the zygomatic arch, skin and subcutaneous tissue incisions are made and bleeding is controlled with electrocoagulation. The temporalis fascia and muscle are incised and retracted using self-retaining retractors. After the squamous portion of the temporal bone is exposed, a standard craniectomy is performed. The middle fossa approach may be used for small acoustic tumor excision and vestibular nerve sections.

A postaural incision may be used to expose the mastoid process. It follows the curve of the postaural fold, beginning at the upper attachment of the auricle and continuing behind the postaural fold downward to the tip of the mastoid process.

For stapes surgery, a circumferential incision is made in the posterior half of the canal, starting at the inferior aspect of the annulus and ending posterior to the short process of the malleus.

For myringotomy, a circumferential (posteroinferior) incision is made. It provides for wide drainage and removal of pus or fluid under pressure from the middle ear.

## OTOLOGIC PROCEDURES

### Myringotomy

Myringotomy is the incision of the pars tensa of the tympanic membrane, the aspiration of fluid under pressure in the tympanum, and often the subsequent placement of small, hollow, pressure equalization tubes (PETs) (also known as *tympanostomy* or *myringotomy tubes*). It is indicated for acute otitis media in the presence of an exudate that has not responded to antibiotic therapy. Serous otitis media is the most commonly diagnosed bacterial illness in children in the United States, with 50% of all children having an episode by their first birthday and 80% having one by their third birthday.[2] The majority of children with serous otitis media have spontaneous resolution. Hearing loss is the main concern when fluid is present in the middle ear. If left untreated, hearing loss can affect language development and intelligent quotient (IQ) level. If the fluid persists more than 8 to 12 weeks and is accompanied by hearing loss, the removal of the fluid and placement of ventilating tubes in the eardrum are necessary.

Otitis media, although primarily a pediatric problem, may be seen in adults. Tympanic fibrosis is common in adults and is a result of repeated infections that occurred in childhood. Acute otitis media is a collection of infected pus in the middle ear. The patient may have severe pain and bulging of the tympanic membrane (Figure 19-13). Failure to respond to oral

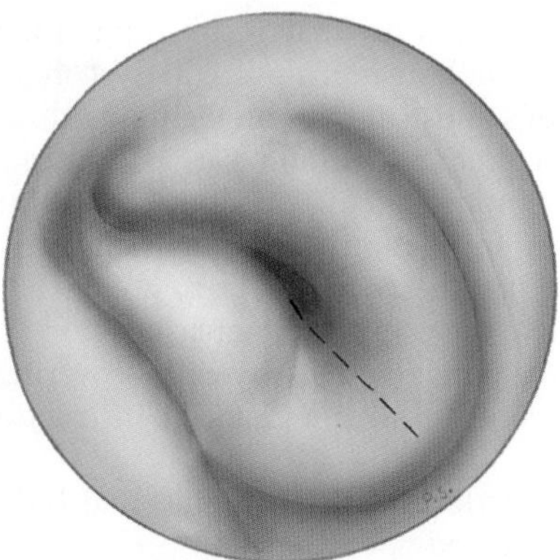

FIGURE 19-13 In purulent otitis media, pus under pressure pushes eardrum outward, resulting in bulging tympanic membrane. *Dotted line,* Radial myringotomy incision.

antibiotics and analgesics or other complications, such as facial nerve paralysis or labyrinthitis, may require a myringotomy. By release of the pus or fluid, hearing is restored and the infection can be controlled. The procedure may be performed for chronic serous otitis media in which the presence of fluid in the middle ear produces a hearing loss. Frequently, tubes are inserted into the tympanic membrane (Figure 19-14) to allow ventilation of the middle ear. Myringotomy tubes may be used for the treatment of colds and fluid in the ear on a short-term basis (a few months), on an intermediate basis (6 to 18 months), and in long-term treatment (years) for chronic situations. Tubes may also be placed in patients undergoing hyperbaric therapy to prevent ear pain and tympanic rupture while in the hyperbaric chamber. Care must be taken to avoid getting water in the ears while the tubes are in place. Myringotomy is usually performed on an ambulatory surgery basis. A recent alternative to tube placement is $CO_2$ laser–assisted myringotomy, in which the laser energy is used to create a precise hole in the tympanic membrane. This remains open for 4 to 6 weeks. Laser-assisted myringotomy is done under topical anesthesia and may be performed in the physician's office (Research Highlight).

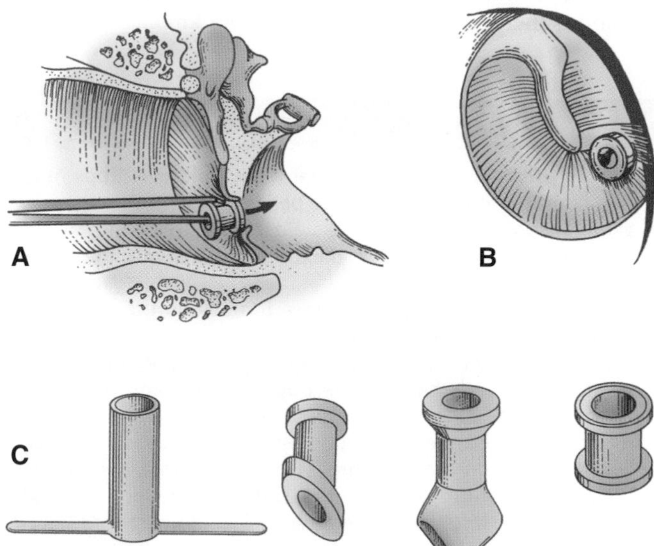


FIGURE 19-14 **A,** Tube (placed on end of alligator forceps) being inserted into tympanic membrane. **B,** Tube in place. **C,** Several types of plastic tubes that may be inserted into tympanic membrane. Purpose of tubes is to aerate middle ear and reduce middle ear infections.

***Procedural Considerations.*** Myringotomy with tube placement is considered a clean procedure. In adult patients, the procedure may be performed using topical anesthesia. Pediatric patients generally require general anesthesia. The surgeon may wear gown and gloves or gloves only, depending on the policy related to Standard Precautions at the institution in which the procedure is performed. The instrument setup includes a myringotomy knife and disposable blade, assorted sizes of aural specula, ear curettes, suction tip and tubing, a delicate Hartmann forceps, metal aural applicators, a Rosen needle, a culture tube if cultures are to be taken, and myringotomy tubes (as applicable). Several types of disposable myringotomy tubes are available for implantation, depending on the length of time the surgeon wishes the tube to remain in place (see Figure 19-14). Once the tube falls out, the tympanic membrane incision usually heals.

## RESEARCH HIGHLIGHT

### Laser Myringotomy for Otitis Media

When watchful waiting and antibiotics fail to effectively treat otitis media with effusion (OME), surgical intervention is often indicated. Insertion of ventilation tubes by means of myringotomy is one of the most frequently performed operations on children. Laser myringotomy is an established treatment for OME. Researchers in this study sought to determine if laser myringotomy (without the insertion of ventilation tubes) was more effective than myringotomy with the insertion of ventilation tubes.

This randomized study examined 208 children with OME. At the time of surgical intervention, conventional "cold knife" myringotomy with ventilation tube insertion was performed on one ear and laser myringotomy using the $CO_2$ laser was performed on the other ear. Assignment of the side for laser myringotomy or tube insertion was made randomly by computer-generated lists to ensure equal distribution between left and right ears. Postoperative follow-up to monitor closure of the laser perforation was undertaken weekly with the first 90 children in the study to establish a baseline. Following closure of the perforation, monitoring continued on a monthly basis for 6 months.

The main outcome variable was the absence of effusion or otorrhea documented by binocular otoscopy. Presence of otorrhea or effusion was considered a failure. The mean time of laser closure was 2.38 weeks, and mean tube extrusion time was 3.88 months. At the 6-month follow-up, an effusion-free middle ear was observed in 39.1% of laser myringotomy sides and in 70.7% of the myringotomy with ventilation tube sides.

The researchers concluded that although laser myringotomy is gaining in popularity because it can often be performed in the physician's office, the higher recurrence rate of effusion has to be weighed against the success of the ventilation tube that carries the need for general anesthesia.

Modified from Koopman JP and others: Laser myringotomy versus ventilation tubes in children with otitis media with effusion: a randomized trial, *Laryngoscope* 114:844-849, 2004.

### Operative Procedure

1. With the head and microscope in position, the aural speculum is inserted into the ear canal. The external canal is cleaned of excess cerumen using a wire loop curette. With a sharp myringotomy knife, a small, curved or radial incision is made in the anterior inferior quadrant of the pars tensa (see Figure 19-13).
2. A culture may be taken to determine the type of organism present. Pus and fluid are suctioned from the middle ear.
3. A tube may be inserted into the incision with alligator forceps or a tube inserter. Care should be taken to consult the manufacturer's directions for handling the tube.
4. Antibiotic drops may be instilled after positioning the tube (Surgical Pharmacology).
5. A cotton ball may be placed in the external canal at the end of the procedure.

## Tympanoplasty

Tympanoplasty is the surgical repair of the tympanic membrane and the tympanum and the reconstruction of the ossicular chain. It is indicated for conductive hearing losses caused by perforation of the tympanic membrane as a result of trauma or infection; for ossicular discontinuity; for chronic or recurrent otitis media; for progressive hearing loss; and for the inability to safely bathe or participate in water activities as a result of perforation of the tympanic membrane with or without hearing loss.

Perforation of the eardrum (tympanic membrane) is the most common serious ear injury necessitating surgical intervention. Perforations may result from (1) direct injury (e.g., cotton applicators, pencil), (2) blow to the ear, (3) tears from temporal bone fractures, and (4) lightning injury. Early diagnosis is the key to proper management.

Conductive hearing loss is caused by an obstruction in the external canal or middle ear, which impedes the passage of sound waves to the inner ear. It may be attributable to disease of the middle ear or tympanic membrane. Occasionally the tympanic membrane does not heal after myringotomy.

Ossicular discontinuity may result from chronic otitis media, trauma, or cholesteatoma—a skin cyst that erodes bone. Various methods and materials are being used in constructing a closed, air-contained middle ear cavity and restoring a sound-pressure transforming action. Among these materials are homografts and Teflon, Plastipore, silicone, hydroxyapatite, and metal prostheses.

There are five types of tympanoplasties:

1. Repairing the tympanic membrane by covering the perforation in the eardrum with a graft; reconstruction extends to the malleus
2. Closing the perforation with a graft and building the eardrum onto the body of the incus
3. Positioning the graft against the head of the stapes when the malleus and incus are missing
4. Securing the graft to the mobile footplate of the stapes when all ossicles are missing
5. Securing the graft to the oval window when the footplate of the stapes is immobile

***Procedural Considerations.*** The ear is prepped and draped as previously described. An endaural or postauricular approach may be used. Both approaches provide similar functional results. The procedure most often is performed with the patient under local anesthesia.

### Operative Procedure

1. a. When an *endaural approach* is used, the ear speculum is introduced into the external meatus of the ear canal, and the microscope is brought into place. The surgeon injects local anesthetic into the external meatus and external auditory canal and postauricularly, using a 1-ml or 3-ml syringe. Lidocaine (Xylocaine) with epinephrine is generally used unless the patient's general medical condition necessitates a substitute. The purpose of the injection of local anesthetic is twofold: to make the operation painless and to reduce the amount of bleeding. A tympanomeatal incision is then made using a sharp, round knife.

### SURGICAL PHARMACOLOGY

#### Perioperative Use of Cortisporin

Cortisporin ear drops are commonly administered in the intraoperative setting following surgical procedures. The solution may also be used to soak foam pledgets.

**DRUG**

Cortisporin Otic Suspension (neomycin, bacitracin, polymyxin B, hydrocortisone)

**DOSE**

**Children:** 3 or 4 drops into the affected ear TID
**Adults:** 4 drops into the affected ear TID

**ADVERSE REACTIONS**

Itching, pain, stinging, burning, ototoxicity

**NURSING CONSIDERATIONS**

- Gather the solution to be administered.
- Check the label to ensure correct drug, dosage, and expiration date.
- Ensure drops are at room temperature. Cold ear drops may be uncomfortable for the awake patient.
- When dispensing to the sterile field, do the following:
  - Verify the drug, dosage, and expiration date with the scrub person.
  - Using sterile technique dispense the solution to a labeled container on the sterile field.
- When administering to the patient, do the following:
  - Tilt the patient's head in the opposite direction of the affected ear.
  - Instill the prescribed number of drops toward the ear canal, not directly on the eardrum. (Tip: To promote the correct placement of drops in children pull the auricle down and posterior; in adults pull the auricle up and posterior.)

Modified from Hodgson BB, Kizior RJ: *Mosby's 2006 drug consult for nurses,* St Louis, 2006, Mosby; *Lexi-Comp.* Accessed December 1, 2005, on-line: www.crlonline.com/crlsql/servlet/crlonline.
*TID,* Three times daily.

b. When a *postauricular approach* is used, the surgeon injects local anesthetic (lidocaine with epinephrine) postauricularly, using a 3-ml or 5-ml syringe. An ear speculum is introduced, and the microscope is brought into place. The surgeon injects local anesthetic into the external auditory canal using a 1-ml syringe. The microscope head is moved from directly over the patient's ear. The skin incision is made behind the fold of the ear with a #15 knife blade. Bleeding vessels are coagulated. An incision is then made into the periosteum down to the bone, and the periosteum is elevated from behind the incision with a Lempert elevator.

c. During the *transcanal approach,* the surgeon uses a 27-gauge angled needle to inject the four quadrants of the fibrocartilaginous canal with a 1% or 2% lidocaine solution with 1:100,000 epinephrine. An endaural speculum gently compresses the tissue edema resulting from the injection and assists in the placement of a speculum within the confines of the bony canal. A 30-gauge needle is used to inject the skin of the bony canal. Two canal incisions are made with a roller knife or other sharp knife. The posterior tympanomeatal flap is made superior and posterior to the lateral process of the malleus and ends laterally on the midpoint of the posterior canal wall. The inferior incision extends from the inferior canal wall to the superior incision. The skin is elevated to the tympanic annulus, subcutaneous tissue at the tympanomastoid suture is dissected, and bleeding is controlled before the middle ear is reached.

2. At this point the temporalis fascia is usually harvested to provide the graft material for the repair of the tympanic membrane. Lidocaine with epinephrine may be injected under the fascia to separate it from the temporalis muscle. A narrow Shambaugh elevator or duckbill elevator is used to separate the fascia. Small, sharp scissors or a knife blade serves to remove the amount of fascia needed. The fascia is trimmed of excess tissue with small, sharp scissors and either laid flat or molded onto an ear speculum. Some surgeons prefer to thin the fascia by using a House Gelfoam press. The fascia is then set aside to dry while the tympanic membrane is prepared.
3. The canal skin may be elevated from the canal with a duckbill elevator, Rosen needle, gimmick, or similar microinstrument, or it may be removed, depending on the size and location of the tympanic membrane perforation.
4. The edges of the tympanic membrane are prepared for the graft by removing all epithelium from the drum surrounding the perforation, usually with a sickle knife, Rosen needle, 45- or 90-degree pick, or cup forceps.
5. If an edge of the perforation or tympanic membrane cannot be visualized because of the bony canal, the surgeon uses a microcurette or drill to remove the overhang of bone.
6. The middle ear is explored with a pick or similar instrument, and any epithelium present is removed with an alligator, or cup forceps. The ossicular chain is tested for mobility. Each ossicle is inspected to ensure that it is intact and mobile.
7. If the malleus or incus is diseased or eroded, it may be removed and replaced with a partial ossicular replacement prosthesis (PORP). Ossicles that are removed may be reshaped with the aid of a drill and small burr and replaced. If all ossicles are diseased or eroded, they may be removed and replaced with a total ossicular replacement prosthesis (TORP). This step is accomplished with microinstrumentation, such as Bellucci scissors, cup forceps, malleus nipper, incudostapedial joint knife, sickle knife, picks, and Rosen needle.
8. The surgeon prepares the graft for insertion. The edges are trimmed with a #15 knife blade or sharp scissors. The surgical site is suctioned with a microsuction device. Hemostasis may be achieved by applying very small, epinephrine-soaked Gelfoam balls with an alligator forceps. Radiopaque microcottonoids are available for use in hemostasis if necessary.
9. Different tissues, such as temporalis fascia, or loose connective tissue, tragus perichondrium, and vein grafts, have been used for a tympanoplasty procedure. The most common tissue used is temporalis fascia. Most surgeons prefer to use autograft tissue, although homograft tympanic membranes have also been used. The risk of transmission of infectious disease has reduced homograft use. For easier manipulation, the graft may be dipped in water or saline before its insertion with alligator forceps. A gimmick, sickle knife, pick, Rosen needle, or similar microinstrument is used to position the graft into place. Small pledgets of absorbable gelatin sponge may be packed around the graft to ensure support and position. Some surgeons prefer to pack the middle ear before the graft insertion to provide support.
10. The external ear canal is packed with MeroGel; moistened, absorbable, gelatin sponge pledgets; or antibiotic ointment.
11. The incision is closed with suture of the surgeon's preference.
12. A pressure dressing consisting of fluffed gauze placed around the ear and an elastic gauze wrapped around the affected ear and the head may be applied for the first 24 hours to prevent dislodgment of the new graft.

## Mastoidectomy

Mastoidectomy is the removal of diseased bone of the mastoid process and mastoid space. Before the introduction of antibiotic therapy, mastoidectomy was commonly performed for infection (History box). Although occasionally still performed for eradication of infection, it is more frequently performed in the treatment of cholesteatoma. Cholesteatoma is the result of accumulation of squamous epithelium and its products in the middle ear and mastoid. It occasionally forms a cystlike mass. As it expands, it is destructive to the middle ear and mastoid. As a result, the diseased bone (ossicles and mastoid bone) must be removed to prevent recurrence of the cholesteatoma.

There are three types of mastoidectomy. A *simple mastoidectomy* is removal of the diseased bone of the mastoid, but the ossicles, eardrum, and canal wall are left intact. This procedure is performed to eradicate chronic infections unresponsive to antibiotics or to remove cholesteatoma. The surgeon uses facial nerve monitoring to preserve the facial nerve.

A *modified radical mastoidectomy* is removal of the diseased bone of the mastoid along with some of the ossicles and the canal wall. The eardrum and some of the ossicles remain, leaving a mechanism for the patient to hear. A canal wall-up mastoidectomy is similar to the modified mastoidectomy without taking down the canal wall.

A *radical mastoidectomy* is removal of the canal wall along with the ossicles and tympanic membrane. It is rarely performed except for unresectable disease. With either the modi-

## HISTORY

Mastoiditis was a frequent otologic diagnosis associated with a high morbidity until the mid-1930s, when antibiotics were introduced. A common complication of mastoiditis was brain abscess. Before 1935, most cases of mastoiditis were treated surgically with a cortical mastoidectomy, performed with a gouge and hammer. The nurse had multiple responsibilities throughout the perioperative period. Many mastoidectomies were emergency procedures and occasionally were performed in the patient's home or, in the case of a brain abscess, at the patient's bedside. Hospitalized patients required extensive preparation before the surgery. Preoperatively, the nurse would wash the patient's hair, part it to create a forelock (later used to cover the scar), and braid it on the unaffected side. After the hair braiding, collodion strips (a single layer of gauze painted with collodion) were folded diagonally near the edge of the anticipated incision and adhered to the skin with additional collodion. With the waterproof strips in place, the nurse would prep the patient's skin by scrubbing the surfaces thoroughly and cleaning the auricle with toothpick swabs dipped in alcohol. The toothpick swabs were made before the prep by dipping the end of the toothpick into water and winding absorbent cotton around the tip until it was of the desired size. After ensuring the skin prep was complete, the nurse would assist the physician in preparing the local anesthetic used for most procedures. A mixture of 1⁄12 grain of heroin and 1⁄150 grain of atropine was given by intramuscular injection. During the hour required for the preoperative medication to take effect, the nurse assisted the physician with the preparation of additional local anesthetic—sterile Novocain (procaine hydrochloride) with 3 or 4 drops of adrenaline added. The operation was accomplished very quickly, and the wound was left open. Postoperatively, patients were very ill and required attentive nursing care. The wound was left dressed for 4 or 5 days unless something necessitated removal of the dressing. At the first dressing change, the wound was irrigated and repacked with iodoform gauze saturated in alum solution to promote granulation. Dressings were then changed daily until the wound had healed by granulation. With the introduction of sulfonamides in 1935 and penicillin in 1944, the need for mastoidectomy became radically reduced.

Modified from Atkinson DT: *Handbook of eye, ear, nose and throat diseases,* New York, 1927, Vail-Ballou; Denison A: *A textbook of eye, ear, nose and throat nursing,* New York, 1934, MacMillan; House HP: Otitis media: a comparative study of the results obtained in therapy before and after the introduction of sulfonamide compounds, *Archives of Otolaryngology—Head and Neck Surgery* 43:371-378, 1946; Turner AL: *Diseases of the nose, throat and ear for practitioners and students,* London, 1927, John Wright and Sons.

fied radical or radical mastoidectomy, a meatoplasty is performed to enlarge the ear canal opening. This facilitates cleaning the mastoid bowl that has been created.

***Procedural Considerations.*** General anesthesia is usually selected, but local anesthesia can be used. The patient is prepped and draped as for a tympanoplasty. An endaural or postauricular incision may be used (Figure 19-15), but most surgeons believe that the postauricular incision offers better exposure to all areas of the mastoid and middle ear. A drill is used to remove diseased bone and tissue.

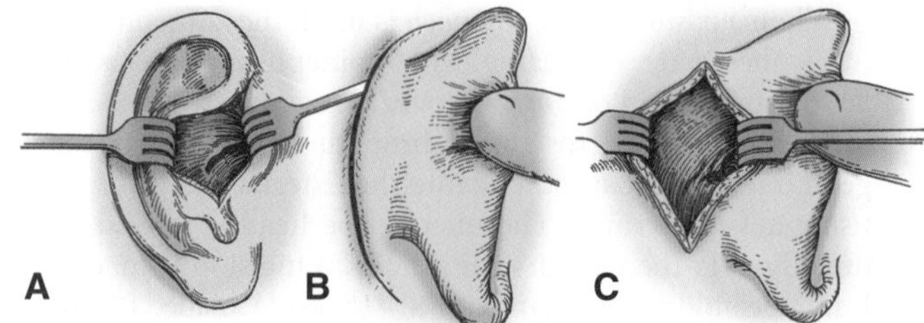


FIGURE 19-15 Mastoidectomy incision. **A,** Endaural. **B,** Postauricular. **C,** Postauricular incision retracted.

### *Operative Procedure*

**Steps 1 through 6 are as for tympanoplasty.**

7. The mastoid bone is drilled initially with a large cutting burr, usually under direct vision. As the mastoid cavity is created, the scrub person should be able to anticipate changes needed in burr size. Once the vital structures have been identified, diseased bone is usually removed from them by use of diamond burrs of the appropriate size. The surgeon may interrupt drilling to explore areas of the mastoid with a pick, Rosen needle, mastoid searcher, or other microinstrument to identify surrounding structures.
8. On completion of the mastoidectomy, the surgeon focuses on the middle ear. Diseased ossicles are removed, middle ear mucosa is inspected and removed if necessary, and all evidence of cholesteatoma is removed. Depending on the extent of the disease and the reliability that the patient will be available for follow-up study, the surgeon then reconstructs the ossicular chain or prepares the cavity created by a radical mastoidectomy. Some surgeons do not reconstruct at the time of mastoidectomy but observe the patient for a specified time. If cholesteatoma does not recur during that period, the patient receives a reconstructive procedure to restore hearing.
9. The mastoid cavity and middle ear may be packed with absorbable gelatin sponge or MeroGel. The external auditory canal may be packed with MeroGel, absorbable gelatin sponge, or antibiotic ointment.
10. The incision is closed and a pressure dressing applied, consisting of fluffed gauze around the ear and plain or elastic gauze wrapped around the head and affected ear, and kept in place for the first 24 hours.

## Stapedectomy

Stapedectomy is removal of the stapes for treatment of otosclerosis and replacement with a prosthesis to restore ossicular continuity and alleviate conductive hearing loss. Otosclerosis is the overgrowth of bone around the stapes footplate, resulting in immobility of the footplate. Sound waves cannot be transmitted adequately through the oval window and round window to be changed into electrochemical impulses in the cochlea.

There are two types of procedures for replacing the immobile stapes. In *stapedotomy,* the footplate of the stapes is not removed; only the superstructure is removed. A hole is made in the stapes footplate, and the prosthesis is secured laterally to the long process of the incus and positioned medially over the hole created in the footplate. In *stapedectomy,* the entire stapes (superstructure and footplate) is removed, a graft is placed over the oval window, and a prosthesis is attached laterally to the long process of the incus and positioned medially on the graft over the oval window. The procedure may be performed with the patient under monitored anesthesia care (MAC) or local anesthesia for adults, enabling the surgeon to test hearing before the conclusion of the surgery. Children, who may find it difficult to remain immobile during the procedure, are often given a general anesthetic.

***Procedural Considerations.*** Various materials are used as the prosthesis for the stapes; the most common are stainless steel and Teflon. The types of prostheses (Figure 19-16) include the following:

- The *Robinson (bucket-handle)* type of prosthesis has a metal stem designed to fit under the lenticular process of the incus. The footplate must be removed and the oval window sealed with a tissue graft before the implant can be inserted. Advantages include easy insertion with no required crimping; the prosthesis is self-centered and sits in the center of the oval window after insertion.
- The *Shea* Teflon prosthesis attaches to the long process of the incus. It can be used with total footplate removal or small fenestra techniques. The prosthesis measures from the undersurface of the long process of the incus to the footplate, plus 0.5 mm. The Teflon ring is opened and secured onto the incus. Because of the memory of Teflon, the prosthesis is said to be self-crimping (the ring closes without crimping). The position of the prosthesis is adjustable.
- The *Fisch-McGee* type of stainless steel and Teflon pistons has a malleable ribbon crook connected to a metal or Teflon stem. The crook is secured to the long process of the incus and crimped into position. It is measured from the undersurface of the incus to the footplate and is easy to attach and crimp into position.

The prosthesis of choice is determined by the surgeon. The scrub person must be aware of each step in the procedure and hand the instruments to the surgeon expediently. Because the oval window is left uncovered, some perilymph may leak from the inner ear into the middle ear. This leak subjects the patient to the possible complication of a sensorineural hearing loss postoperatively or, more seriously, a "dead ear."

Microsuction tips (18- to 26-gauge) are used in this procedure because large suction tips may suction perilymph from the oval window as well as promote bleeding in the middle ear. After the incision and reflection of the flap, footplate hooks are used because the tips on picks are too large and long and may cause damage rather than assist in the procedure.

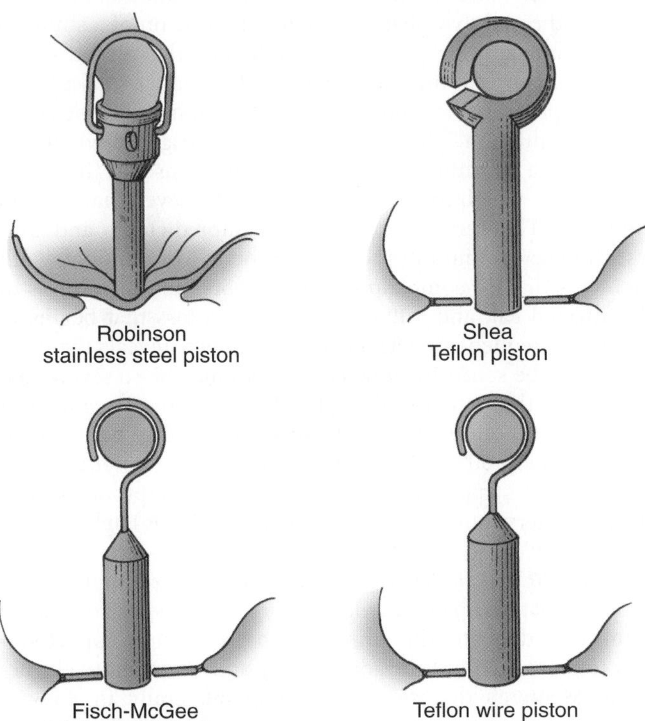


**FIGURE 19-16** Stapedectomy prostheses. *Top left,* Prostheses used after the footplate has been removed. *Top right and bottom,* Footplate had been "drilled" to accept a prefabricated piston precisely.

## *Operative Procedures*

### STAPEDECTOMY

1. A temporalis fascia, fat, perichondrium, or vein graft may be harvested before the procedure to cover the oval window. Depending on the surgeon's graft preference, the ear, hand, or a portion of the abdomen may be prepped for the graft.
2. The ear speculum is introduced, and the microscope is brought into position. The ear canal is cleansed of wax and debris and may be gently washed with physiologic irrigating solution and suctioned with microsuction tip.
3. The surgeon injects lidocaine with epinephrine into the ear canal.
4. An ear speculum is inserted, the tympanomeatal flap is created (using a flap knife, roller knife, or sickle knife), and the tympanic membrane is reflected forward (using duckbill elevators or a drum elevator), exposing the middle ear.
5. If visualization of the ossicles is inadequate because of the overhang of bone, the surgeon may use microcurettes or a drill to remove enough bone to allow proper visualization. Attempts to save the chorda tympani nerve are made because it controls taste from the anterior two thirds of the tongue. If this nerve obstructs the view of the stapes, it may on rare occasion be sacrificed for exposure.
6. The surgeon may measure the distance from the incus to the stapes footplate at this time or after the removal of the stapes. It is accomplished with a depth gauge and done to ensure the proper fit of the prosthesis.
7. The incudostapedial joint is disarticulated to allow fracture and subsequent removal of the stapes, usually accomplished through the use of a House or Guilford-Wright joint knife or by a laser ($CO_2$, Er:YAG, or KTP).
8. Both crura of the stapes are treated with a laser or fractured laterally, usually with a footplate pick or Rosen needle, and the superstructure is removed with alligator forceps. The surgeon may take this opportunity to ensure hemostasis, using tiny sponges soaked in epinephrine along with a microsuction tip. The laser helps coagulate middle ear vessels, thus improving hemostasis.
9. An opening is created in the footplate with a laser or a sharp footplate pick. If the footplate is extremely thick, a microdrill may be used. If a stapedectomy is to be carried

out, each half of the footplate is removed using a Hough hoe, footplate pick, or footplate hook.

10. The oval window is inspected, and the graft is placed over the oval window with alligator forceps or a pick. The edges of the graft are smoothed and positioned with a Hough hoe, pick, or gimmick.
11. The prosthesis is passed on alligator forceps to the surgeon and then introduced into the middle ear with the shaft of the prosthesis resting against the oval window graft.
12. The wire is positioned over the long process of the incus (Figure 19-17) using picks, Hough hoes, or footplate hooks. Once it is in proper position, the surgeon crimps the wire onto the long process of the incus to ensure its attachment.
13. The surgeon may test the patient's hearing by softly whispering to the patient (if the procedure is performed with the patient under local anesthesia) or by touching the malleus with a pick and observing for mobility of the malleus, incus, and stapes prosthesis (if performed with the patient under general anesthesia).
14. Tiny squares of moistened, compressed gelatin sponge may then be placed around the base of the prosthesis to ensure its stability. Alligator forceps, picks, a gimmick, and similar instruments may be used for this step.
15. The tympanomeatal flap is returned to its original location, using a drum elevator, duckbill elevator, or Rosen needle. The external ear canal may be packed with an antibiotic gel or ointment or a moistened, compressed gelatin sponge.
16. Cotton is placed in the concha of the ear, and a Band-Aid or small dressing is usually applied to the graft site.

STAPEDOTOMY. The stapedotomy procedure is similar to stapedectomy but has these differences:

1. No graft is taken before the procedure.
2. The footplate is not removed. A hole is made in the footplate, using the $CO_2$, Er:YAG, or KTP laser or drill bits of increasing size. The prosthesis is inserted when the perforation in the footplate is the appropriate size.
3. After positioning and crimping of the prosthesis, either a moistened, compressed gelatin sponge or a few drops of the patient's blood may be placed around the junction of the prosthesis and the footplate to ensure stability of the prosthesis.

## Ossicular Chain Reconstruction

Ossicular reconstruction may be required for long-standing recurrent ear infections. It is commonly performed for the replacement of the incus portion of the ossicular chain. There are many surgical techniques for ossicular reconstruction.

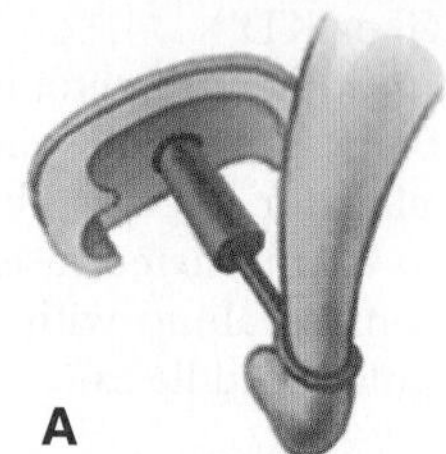


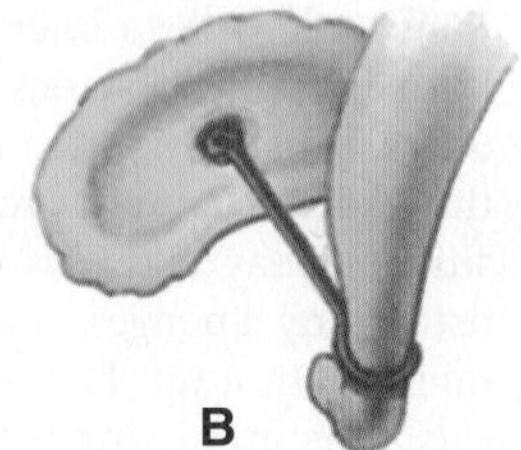


FIGURE 19-17 **A,** Placement of wire piston firmly crimped about incus. **B,** Total stapedectomy after placement of perichondrium over oval window. Wire loop prosthesis is crimped and placed against oval window membrane.

Natural and synthetic prosthetic materials are available for ossicular reconstruction or replacement. The autologous ossicle (incus or head of malleus) taken from the patient's ear is the prosthesis of choice. Preserved homologous ossicles are less popular than in the past because of the risk (albeit very low) of transmission of infectious disease.

A PORP is indicated if an ossicle is not available. A TORP is indicated for difficult major columella reconstruction.

Alloplastic materials for partial and total ossicular reconstruction prostheses are available. Hydroxyapatite is used in many prostheses because its mineral content is very similar to that of bone and it is well tolerated by the middle ear, thereby decreasing extrusion rates. Because it is brittle, it is often combined with other materials to make it more easily trimmed for a precise fit in the middle ear. Regardless of the type of prosthesis used, the surgeon must sculpt it to bridge the ossicular gap by simulating the ossicular configuration and preserving the lever mechanism of the middle ear.

***Procedural Considerations.*** *Minor columella* is a term that refers to an ossiculoplasty with a strut from the head of the stapes to the tympanic membrane (or graft) or manubrium. *Major columella* refers to a strut extending from the footplate to the tympanic membrane (or graft) or manubrium. The patient is prepped and draped as for stapedectomy.

***Operative Procedure.*** The procedural steps are similar to those for stapedectomy except that the stapes footplate is not removed or opened.

## Endolymphatic Sac Decompression or Shunt

An endolymphatic shunt procedure is the creation of an opening into the endolymphatic sac and the insertion of a shunt to allow drainage of excess endolymph into the cerebrospinal fluid (CSF) or into the mastoid cavity. In Meniere's disease the endolymphatic sac cannot resorb endolymph, resulting in an overaccumulation. This surplus leads to vertigo, in which patients feel a spinning sensation. Movement usually increases the vertigo, which may be accompanied by severe nausea and vomiting. The vertigo attacks occur unpredictably and may last from several minutes to several hours. Most patients with Meniere's disease complain of tinnitus, pressure or fullness in the affected ear, and a fluctuating hearing loss that begins in the lower frequencies. Diagnostic audiometry reveals the hearing loss to be sensorineural. The vertigo may be so severe that it disrupts the patient's life-style. With a medical regimen of tranquilizers, diuretics, vasodilators, and a low-sodium diet, approximately 60% to 80% of patients are able to adequately control their symptoms.[12] For those whose symptoms persist, surgical intervention is recommended (Research Highlight).

***Procedural Considerations.*** Preoperative assessment should confirm that the patient's electrolyte levels (especially potassium) are adequate; this provides a basis for the support system to be carried out intraoperatively and postoperatively. Because Meniere's disease may develop bilaterally in 45% of patients, conservative therapy is often employed.[14] The patient is prepped and draped as for a mastoidectomy.

***Operative Procedure***

Steps 1 through 7 are as for mastoidectomy.

## RESEARCH HIGHLIGHT

### Controlling Vertigo in Meniere's Disease

Vertigo can be a frustrating and disabling consequence of Meniere's disease. When dietary and diuretic treatment fails to provide relief and vertigo becomes intractable, treatments such as the instillation of ototoxic medications into the middle ear to eliminate vestibular hair cells (thereby reducing the episodes of vertigo) may be a nonsurgical option for some patients. This retrospective study sought to determine if the intratympanic injection of dexamethasone was effective in long-term control of vertigo. Researchers reviewed the charts of 34 patients with intractable Meniere's disease who were given intratympanic injections of dexamethasone over a 4-week period and evaluated control of vertigo over a 2-year period. Forty-seven percent of the patients in the study achieved control with one or more courses of intratympanic dexamethasone. A single injection only produced long-term control in 8 of the 34 patients.

This study demonstrated that although some patients did have good results with intratympanic dexamethasone as a means of controlling their vertigo, the treatment did not produce long-term results in the study population. Multiple courses of treatment, combined with other therapies, are required to provide relief for this debilitating condition.

Modified from Barrs DM: Intratympanic injections of dexamethasone for long term control of vertigo, *Laryngoscope* 114(11):1910-1914, 2004.

8. Drilling with a diamond burr over the posterior fossa dura is continued until the endolymphatic sac is identified.
9. An incision is made into the lateral wall of the sac with a microknife, such as a sickle, Beaver blade, or Ziegler. An incision is then made through the medial wall, exposing the subarachnoid space.
10. A shunt (commercially prepared tube, Silastic tubing, or Silastic sheeting) is inserted with microforceps and manipulated into place, using microinstruments, such as a Rosen needle, fine pick, or gimmick. When the shunt is designed to drain into the mastoid, only the lateral wall of the sac is incised.
11. The incision is closed and a pressure dressing applied to the affected ear.

## Labyrinthectomy

Labyrinthectomy is a procedure that destroys the vestibular and auditory function of the labyrinth to relieve severe vertigo. The procedure is usually performed when the disease is unilateral, a shunt has been ineffective, and the affected ear has severe or total loss of hearing. Because the inner ear is destroyed, the patient may be very dizzy for several days until the brainstem begins to compensate for the destroyed labyrinth. The operation also leaves the ear deaf.

***Procedural Considerations.*** This procedure may be performed by way of the transcanal or transmastoid approach. The patient is prepped and draped as described for tympanoplasty.

### *Operative Procedures*

TRANSCANAL APPROACH

1. Through a tympanomeatal flap, with the chorda tympani nerve preserved, the incudostapedial joint is separated and the stapedial tendon is sectioned.
2. The incus and stapes are disarticulated and removed.
3. A right-angled hook is inserted into the vestibule, and all neuroepithelium (the contents) is removed.
4. The open vestibule is filled with Gelfoam soaked in streptomycin to ensure destruction of all nerve elements. The tympanomeatal flap is returned to its original position and a pressure dressing applied.

TRANSMASTOID APPROACH

1. Through a postauricular incision, a simple mastoidectomy is performed.
2. The vertical segment of the facial nerve is identified, and the incus is disarticulated and removed.
3. The horizontal, posterior, and superior semicircular canals are drilled away. The neuroepithelium is completely removed from the ampullae of the three semicircular canals.
4. The external auditory canal may be packed with absorbable gelatin sponge or a rosebud pack as described for the tympanoplasty procedure.
5. The incision is closed in layers. An external pressure dressing of elastic gauze is applied.

## Vestibular Neurectomy

Vestibular neurectomy is the cutting of the vestibular portion of the eighth cranial nerve (acoustic nerve) with the cochlear portion left intact. It may be performed for a unilateral ear disorder, including classic Meniere's disease, recurrent vestibular neuronitis, traumatic labyrinthitis, or vestibular Meniere's disease. It may also be performed when attacks of vertigo severely affect a patient's life-style. Vestibular neurectomy is performed when a patient has adequate hearing and a labyrinthectomy is not indicated.

***Procedural Considerations.*** The patient's abdomen or lateral aspect of the thigh is prepped and draped for the purpose of obtaining fat or a segment of muscle and fascia to be used for obliteration of the mastoid cavity at the end of the procedure. If the abdomen is used, most surgeons prefer to take fat from the left side to avoid future confusion with an appendectomy scar. Setups for the graft and neurectomy procedure are separate to avoid cross-contamination. The graft may be taken before the procedure or after the vestibular nerve has been transected, depending on the surgeon's preference. The patient is prepped and draped as for tympanoplasty. The procedure may be done through a transcochlear, translabyrinthine, middle fossa, retrolabyrinthine, or retrosigmoid approach.

### *Operative Procedures*

TRANSCOCHLEAR APPROACH

1. A postauricular incision is made, and the posterior external auditory canal is incised. A large tympanomeatal flap is elevated to expose the middle ear structures.
2. A bony canaloplasty is created, and the round window and facial nerve are identified. The incus, stapes, and promontory bone are removed. The utricle is removed, using a 3-mm right-angled pick.
3. The posteroinferior aspect of the internal auditory canal is skeletonized (the process of removing soft tissue to clearly define the bony or skeletal anatomy), the transverse crest is removed, and the superior vestibular nerve is identified.
4. The middle turn of the cochlea is opened anteriorly to assist with cochlear nerve identification.

5. The modiolus is opened, and CSF flows freely and provides irrigation during the drilling. Bone is removed to expose the superior vestibular nerve before it enters the internal auditory canal.
6. The dura is opened, and the cochlear nerve is transected at the modiolus. The facial nerve lies anterior to, superior to, and beneath the vestibular nerve and is identified by electrical stimulation.
7. After a cleavage plane is found between the facial and superior vestibular nerves, the vestibular fibers are transected, using caution to avoid stretching the facial nerve.
8. A free temporalis muscle and fascia graft obliterate the opening in the internal auditory canal.
9. The flap is returned to its position over the muscle and secured in place by packing the ear for 2 weeks.

TRANSLABYRINTHINE APPROACH

1. A postauricular incision is made, and a simple mastoidectomy is performed.
2. The sigmoid sinus is identified and skeletonized.
3. The attic is opened and the incus extracted. The bone over the posterior fossa and endolymphatic sac is removed. The vertical portion of the facial nerve is identified.
4. A bony labyrinthectomy is performed, and the semicircular canals are removed. The endolymphatic duct is followed into the vestibule of the internal auditory canal.
5. The bone is removed, skeletonizing the dura of the internal auditory canal from the vestibule to the porus acusticus. Half of the circumference of the internal auditory canal provides good exposure to perform the eighth-nerve section safely.
6. The petrosal facial nerve, superior vestibular nerve, and the vertical crest (Bill's bar) are identified at the superior aspect of the internal auditory canal. The superior vestibular nerve lies more superficially and distally in the bone than the facial nerve.
7. A sharp sickle knife is used to incise the dura of the internal auditory canal, and the superior vestibular nerve is transected in its bony canal and dissected from the facial nerve. The inferior vestibular nerve and cochlear nerve are bisected.
8. Harvested abdominal adipose tissue is used to obliterate the mastoid defect.
9. The attic and the antrum are sealed with bone wax. The wound is closed, and a mastoid dressing is applied and remains intact for 48 hours.

RETROLABYRINTHINE APPROACH

1. Lidocaine with or without epinephrine is injected subcutaneously, using a 3-ml or 5-ml syringe.
2. A retrolabyrinthine U-shaped incision is made slightly posterior to the area of the postauricular incision used in other otologic surgery.
3. An incision is made in the mastoid muscles with a #10 or #15 blade. The muscles are elevated with a Lempert, Joseph, or similar elevator.
4. A self-retaining retractor is inserted after the muscles and periosteum are elevated.
5. The surgeon begins drilling, usually with a large cutting burr, and continues until a complete mastoidectomy is performed. The sigmoid sinus and posterior and inferior semicircular canals are skeletonized with a diamond burr. The posterior fossa bone is removed to expose the posterior fossa dura. During the drilling process, burr sizes and types (cutting and diamond) may be changed as vital structures are identified. The scrub person must ensure that irrigation and suction are adequate. The surgeon may pause during the drilling to verify vital structures with a microinstrument, such as a Rosen needle, gimmick, pick, or searcher.
6. The posterior fossa dura is incised with a sickle or Ziegler microknife. Hemostasis may be achieved by the use of bipolar forceps; a moistened, absorbable gelatin sponge covered by a cottonoid; or Surgicel. Cottonoids, Surgicel, and gelatin sponge may be loaded onto bayonet forceps before the forceps are placed into the surgeon's hand or may be introduced into the field by the scrub person with the use of bayonet forceps while the surgeon controls another bayonet forceps.
7. As exploration and dissection of the cochleovestibular nerve are carried out, cottonoids may be used to cover vital structures. The vestibular portion of the eighth cranial (acoustic) nerve is identified by the surgeon and transected with microscissors or a microknife.
8. Hemostasis is achieved by the methods mentioned in step 6.
9. The dural incision is closed, usually with 4-0 silk or nylon on a very small needle.
10. Fat from the abdomen or fascia and muscle from the lateral aspect of the thigh are packed over the closed dural incision, the skin incision is closed, and a pressure dressing is applied.

## Facial Nerve Decompression

Facial nerve decompression is a procedure designed to identify and relieve an area of compression of the facial nerve. The most common form of facial paralysis is Bell's palsy. It provokes more controversy regarding proper management than any other disorder of the facial nerve. The cause is unknown, although clinical and laboratory evidence indicates a virus of the herpes simplex group may be involved. The patient experiences multiple problems, such as decreased tearing, inability to close the affected eye, and drooping of the affected corner of the mouth with pooling of oral secretions. Preoperatively, ointments protect the eye and the eyelid is taped closed, or an adhesive bubble is placed over the eye to trap moisture. This protection is continued into the postoperative period unless a tarsorrhaphy (suturing the eyelid closed) is performed intraoperatively. The patient is taught to place food at the back of the tongue on the unaffected side to assist in mastication. Tilting the head to the unaffected side while eating decreases the pooling of oral secretions and drooling. The patient must be taught proper mouth care because the pooling of oral secretions may lead to dental caries or gingivitis. This regimen is continued until the nerve manifests its regeneration by the return of facial movement. The facial nerve may be decompressed by a translabyrinthine approach when trauma has destroyed hearing and caused facial nerve paralysis. The narrowest segment of the bony canal compressing the facial nerve is deep in the temporal bone and may also be accessed through the middle cranial fossa approach when hearing is to be preserved. Both approaches may be useful under selected circumstances.

### *Transmastoid, Translabyrinthine Approach*

PROCEDURAL CONSIDERATIONS. The patient is prepped and draped as described for tympanoplasty. Neurologic intensive care is required for the first 24 hours.

OPERATIVE PROCEDURE

**Steps 1 through 7 are as for mastoidectomy.**

8. After complete mastoidectomy, the dissection is carried out by the use of cutting and diamond burrs until the internal auditory canal and the posterior fossa bone are removed.
9. The bone immediately over the facial nerve is removed by the use of nerve excavators and picks.
10. The facial nerve sheath is incised with a facial nerve knife, neurectomy knife, sickle knife, neurectomy scissors, or micropicks. The incision and decompression are carried out from the stylomastoid foramen to the brainstem.
11. Hemostasis is achieved by the use of moistened, absorbable gelatin sponge; cottonoids; Surgicel; bipolar forceps; or a combination of these.
12. The incision is closed and a pressure dressing of elastic gauze applied.

### *Middle Cranial Fossa Approach*

PROCEDURAL CONSIDERATIONS. The patient's hair is shaved almost to the midline on the affected side. Povidone-iodine solution generally is used for the prep, which includes the portion of the head that has been shaved, the affected side of the face, and the neck. Lidocaine with or without epinephrine usually is injected subcutaneously above the ear to assist in hemostasis.

OPERATIVE PROCEDURE

1. The temporalis muscle is incised and elevated with a Lempert, Shambaugh, or similar elevator.
2. Hemostasis is achieved by clamping and tying vessels or by electrocoagulation.
3. A square of bone is drilled from the temporal bone to expose the middle cranial fossa dura. (The bone is saved for replacement at the end of the procedure.)
4. A self-retaining retractor with a blade for retraction of the middle fossa (e.g., Fisch middle fossa retractor, House-Urban retractor) is inserted.
5. The microscope is brought into place, and the dura is elevated from the floor of the middle fossa with a Freer elevator, a gimmick, or similar instruments.
6. Once hemostasis is achieved and the blade is inserted over the dura to expose the middle fossa, drilling may proceed.
7. When the bone becomes quite thin, the surgeon may remove the remaining bone with excavators to avoid damaging the nerve sheath.
8. The facial nerve sheath is incised with a facial nerve knife, neurectomy knife, neurectomy scissors, or microknife.
9. The retractor is removed when hemostasis is achieved, and the bone flap is replaced.
10. The temporalis muscle is approximated and sutured, the incision closed, and a pressure dressing applied.

• • •

Damage to the facial nerve from trauma, infection, or tumors may be treated surgically by these approaches. Facial nerve grafting requires the use of a separate setup for obtaining a nerve for grafting and microinstruments as well as microsutures (e.g., sizes 8-0 to 11-0) for the nerve graft.

## Removal of Acoustic Neuroma (Vestibular Schwannoma)

Acoustic neuromas arise from the Schwann cells of the vestibular portion of the eighth cranial (acoustic) nerve and are therefore more appropriately termed *vestibular schwannomas*. These tumors are benign but may grow to a size that produces symptoms of cerebellar and brainstem origin. Bilateral vestibular schwannomas are a common finding in patients with neurofibromatosis type 2 (NF2).[4]

Most patients experience unilateral tinnitus and hearing loss—the main symptoms of a possible acoustic neuroma. However, depending on the rate and direction of tumor growth, signs and symptoms may include hearing loss, tinnitus, vertigo, headaches, double vision, diplopia, decreased corneal reflex, decreased blink reflex, impaired taste, reduced lacrimation, facial paralysis, diminished gag reflex, vocal cord paralysis, atrophy or fasciculation of the tongue, weakness of the sternocleidomastoid and trapezius muscles, disturbance in balance and gait, hydrocephalus, lethargy, confusion, drowsiness, and coma.

Several centers have developed great expertise in acoustic neuroma surgery, which requires the combined team of an otologist and a neurosurgeon.

***Procedural Considerations.*** The translabyrinthine approach for the removal of an acoustic tumor reduces mortality and morbidity and offers a good chance of saving the facial nerve if the tumor has not directly invaded it. The patient should be informed about the presence of a Foley catheter, arterial line, temperature probe, shaved head, and graft-site incision. The patient's hair is shaved to the midline of the affected side. Some patients prefer to have the entire head shaved to facilitate wearing a wig. This option should be presented preoperatively to enable the patient to make a decision before surgery. The patient is prepped and draped as described for labyrinthectomy. Lidocaine with or without epinephrine may be injected subcutaneously behind the ear. A facial nerve monitor is routinely used in the excision of cerebellopontine angle tumors. An SCD is used intraoperatively and for the first 24 to 48 hours postoperatively or until the patient is ambulatory to decrease the risk of DVT and PE.

### *Operative Procedure*

1. A postauricular incision is made slightly longer and wider than the incision for mastoidectomy. The periosteum is elevated from the mastoid bone with a Lempert, Shambaugh, or similar elevator.
2. Self-retaining retractors are inserted, and the cortical mastoidectomy is begun with a large cutting burr.
3. The microscope is brought into position, and the attic is opened to visualize the ossicles. The sigmoid sinus, middle fossa dura, and superior petrosal sinus are left with a thin covering of bone. The semicircular canals are exposed. The incus is removed with alligator forceps or cup forceps and suction.
4. The semicircular canals are excised with the drill. The utricle and saccule are removed, and the aqueduct of the vestibule is drilled out.
5. Nerve excavators, Fisch dissectors, or picks are then used to remove the remainder of bone from the dura of the internal meatus, posterior fossa, middle fossa, and petrosal angle.

The wedge of bone between the facial and superior vestibular nerves (Bill's bar) is removed.
6. The dura is opened with microscissors or a dura knife. Dissection of the tumor ensues with a gimmick, Freer microelevator, microinstrument, and bipolar forceps (with or without suction). Hemostasis is achieved with a moistened, absorbable gelatin sponge; cottonoids; Surgicel; or a bipolar coagulator.
7. The tumor is removed by the use of pituitary cup forceps, long alligator forceps, and similar instruments.
8. Graft material is obtained to pack the mastoid cavity created from the drilling. It may be fat, fascia, or muscle. The packing is performed meticulously to avoid a CSF leak.
9. The wound is closed and a thick pressure dressing applied.

## ASSISTIVE HEARING DEVICES

A variety of assistive devices are available to patients with hearing loss, including phone amplifiers, closed captioning broadcasts, Telecommunication Device for the Deaf (TDD), and electronic devices, such as hearing aids. Technology has evolved tremendously in the field of otology, enabling surgeons to use surgically implantable devices in the treatment of hearing loss. These devices have greatly benefited the recipients, allowing some to distinguish sounds for the first time. Research continues in this field to develop applications for conditions previously considered untreatable and to refine and improve existing technology.

### Cochlear Implantation

Technologic advances have given the deaf patient new hope in the area of cochlear implantation. The device is implanted in the cochlea, with the receiver resting in the mastoid (Figure 19-18). As the device receives sound through the receiver, it emits electrical impulses through the transmitter into the cochlea and along the acoustic nerve. These impulses are interpreted as sound in the temporal cortex of the cerebrum. The patient must be taught to interpret these sounds through extensive training. Adult candidates for cochlear implantation generally possess the following characteristics: (1) severe or profound hearing loss with pure-tone average of 70-dB hearing loss, (2) use of appropriately fitting hearing aids or a trial with amplification, (3) aided scores on open-set sentence tests of less than 50%, (4) no evidence of central auditory lesions or lack of an auditory nerve, and (5) no evidence of contraindications for surgery in general.[15] Pediatric candidates (1) are 12 months through 17 years of age, (2) have profound sensorineural hearing loss, (3) experience minimal benefit from hearing aids, (4) have no evidence of central auditory lesions or lack of an auditory nerve, and (5) have no evidence of contraindications to surgery.[15] Appropriate auditory training and psychologic counseling are needed after appropriate selection of candidates.

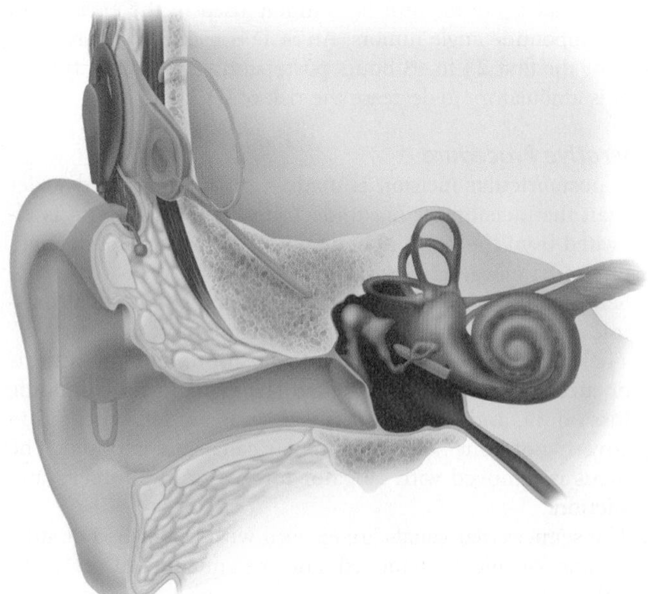

**FIGURE 19-18** Cochlear implant system. Sound is transformed into electrical signal in speech processor. Signal is transmitted from external to internal induction coil, which is connected to electrode implanted near cochlear nerve.

#### *Operative Procedure*

1. A U-shaped or inverted J–shaped incision is made, creating a skin flap well behind the mastoid. The flap, including the temporalis muscle, is elevated, exposing the underlying bone. The site of the internal receiver is identified, and with a special drill a circular depression in the squamous portion of the temporal bone is made to house the receiver.
2. A mastoidectomy is performed with preservation of the bony ear canal and opening of the facial recess.
3. The internal receiver is secured in the depressed area in the temporal bone, and the intracochlear electrode is introduced through the facial recess and through a cochleostomy into the cochlea. It is secured in place with a piece of temporalis fascia.
4. The wound is closed. The patient is observed for 4 to 6 weeks until the wound is completely healed. Then the external signal processor is fitted and programmed (Figure 19-19). This allows transmission of an electrical signal, picked up at an ear-level microphone and processed in a microprocessor worn on the body.

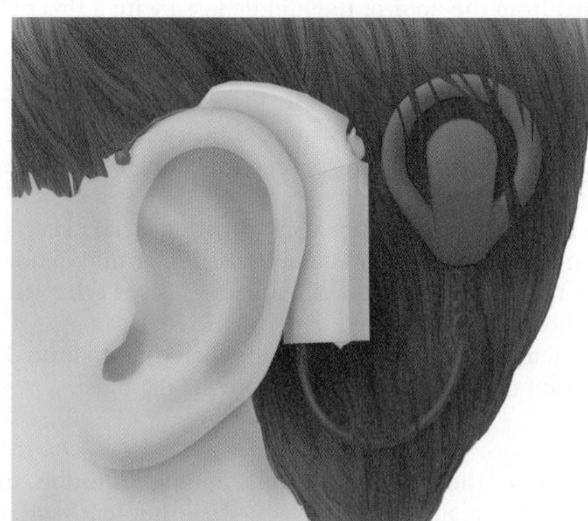

**FIGURE 19-19** Cochlear implant external sound processor in place.

## Implantable Hearing Aids

Conventional hearing aids transmit sound using air conduction and bone conduction. Traditional bone-conduction hearing aids are external and secured to the head with a spring device. Their design makes them uncomfortable and obtrusive, causing headaches and skin abrasions. The quality of sound is inferior, and they often require a higher battery consumption. Air-conduction devices use an ear mold that fits into the ear canal. These devices may be contraindicated for patients with physical abnormalities that prevent the insertion of the ear mold into the canal and for those who have chronic eczema, ear drainage, or inflammation in the ear canal. Implantable hearing devices are designed for patients with moderate to severe conductive and sensorineural hearing loss (unilateral or bilateral). Ideally, implantable hearing devices should improve sound quality, provide comfort, improve appearance, and reduce the risk of chronic ear infections. Surgical implantation of hearing devices may be performed on an ambulatory basis using local anesthesia or general anesthesia. The device is usually implanted in the ear with the best cochlear function.

***Bone-Anchored Hearing Aids.*** Conventional bone-conduction hearing aids transmit sound vibrations transcutaneously to the skull, bypassing a diseased or impaired external or middle ear and going directly to the cochlea. Disadvantages to using traditional bone-conduction hearing aids include discomfort, poor sound quality, poor aesthetics, and shifting of the transducer, which affects speech recognition.[11]

The bone-anchored hearing aid (BAHA by Entific, Goteborg, Sweden) eliminates many of the disadvantages associated with traditional external bone-conduction hearing aids. It is designed for patients 5 years of age and older with moderate to severe conductive hearing loss (unilateral or bilateral) caused by congenital malformations but who maintain good cochlear function (down to 45-dB hearing loss [HL]) and for patients with otitis media, cholesteatoma, otosclerosis, microtia, and canal atresia who are unable to benefit from conventional amplification. The BAHA system consists of a conventional microphone and amplifier, a specially designed transducer, and a coupling device to attach the device to the skin-penetrating and bone-anchored implant[8] (Figure 19-20). The area behind the ear is prepped and draped, and the implant site is marked. It is important to ensure that the hearing aid does not touch the pinna, which may cause acoustic feedback. A semicircular incision is made around the proposed fixture site. A titanium fixture is permanently implanted (tapped) into the mastoid bone, and a permanent skin penetration is made with a titanium snap coupler (Figures 19-21 and 19-22). A sound processor is fitted and adjusted to the patient's hearing loss 3 to 6 months after the implantation, depending on the age of the patient and ensuring the osseointegration process has taken place[13] (Figure 19-23).

***Semi-Implantable Hearing Aids.*** Semi-implantable hearing aids are used in the middle ear and provide sound through direct stimulation of the ossicles; they allow for comfort because the external ear canal remains open. They consist of a microphone speech processor connected to a transmitter with an external coil that transmits electrical energy transcutaneously to an internal device (Figure 19-24). The internal device consists of an internal receiving coil con-

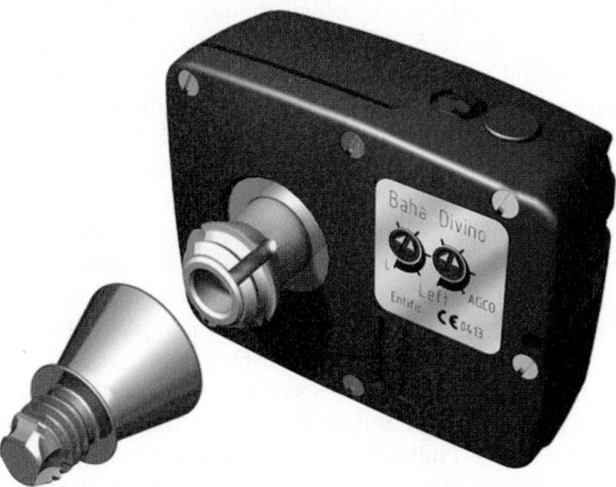


**FIGURE 19-20** Bone-anchored hearing aid (BAHA) components. *Top to bottom,* External processor, abutment, fixture.

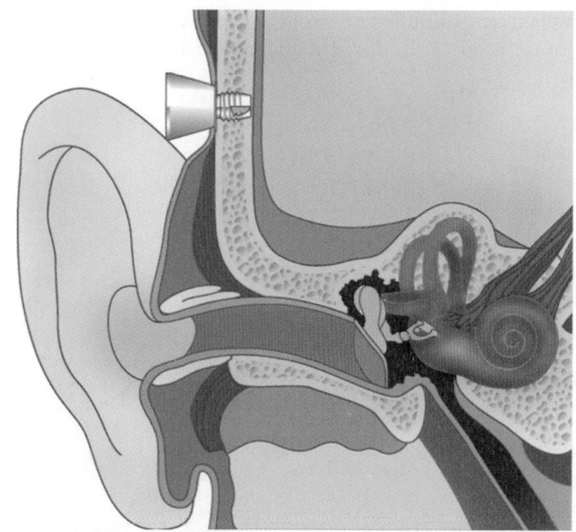

**FIGURE 19-21** Cross section showing fixture and abutment.

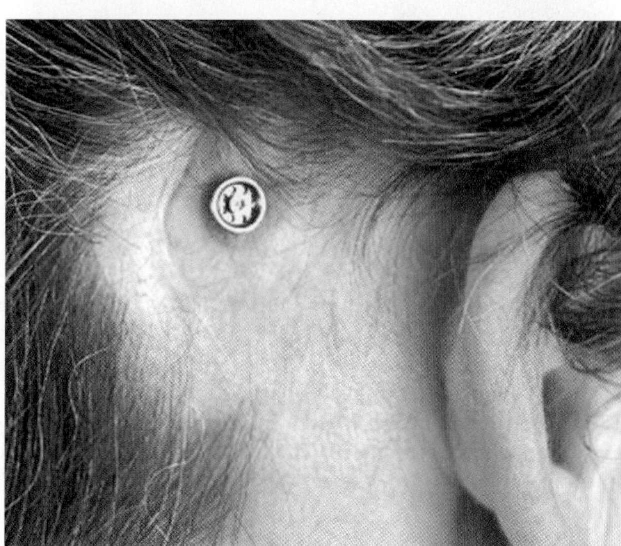

**FIGURE 19-22** Bone-anchored hearing aid (BAHA) abutment.

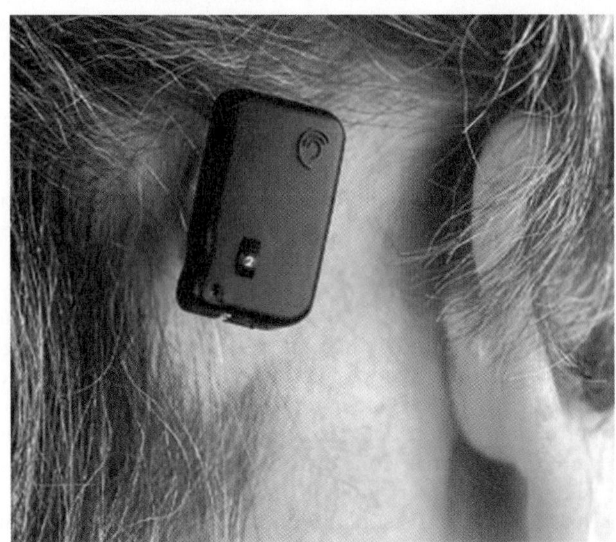

FIGURE 19-23 Patient with implanted bone-anchored hearing aid. The implant is positioned to avoid contact with the pinna, which could cause acoustic feedback if the device is driven at maximum output.

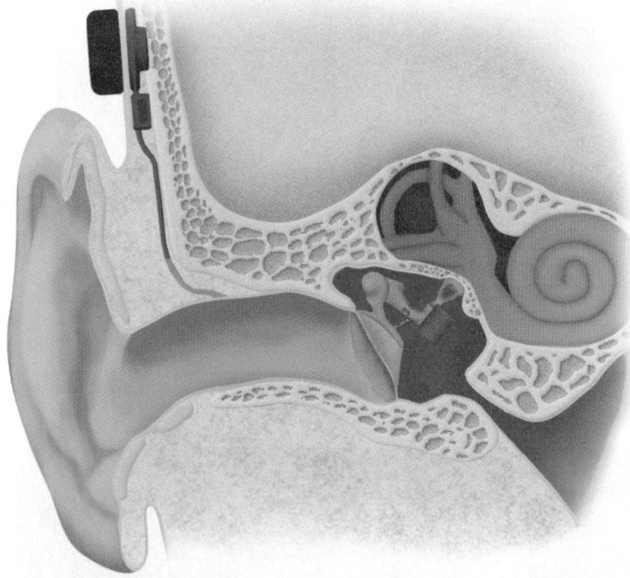

FIGURE 19-24 Semi-implantable hearing aid system. Audio processor, internal receiver, conductor link, floating mass transducer.

nected to a receiver, which provides electrical energy to a mechanical driver connected to the ossicular chain (Figure 19-25). The driver vibrates the ossicles, mimicking the normal vibrations that occur as a result of acoustic sound input.[13] The internal receiver is implanted in the temporal bone, and the driver is attached to the incus. The external processor is fitted approximately 3 to 6 weeks after the surgery.

• • •

Research is ongoing in the development of semi-implantable and fully implantable hearing devices.

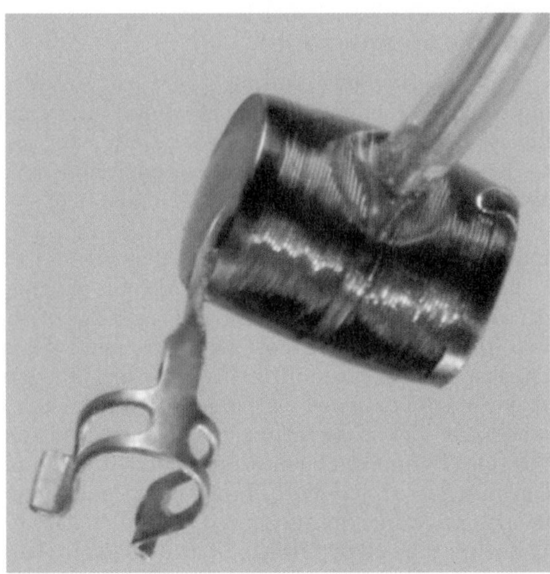

FIGURE 19-25 Mechanical driver (Floating Mass Transducer). Clip attaches to the incus.

## REFERENCES


1. Chole RA, Suddath HH: Chronic otitis media, mastoiditis and petrositis. In Cummings CW and others, editors: *Otolaryngology: head and neck surgery*, ed 4, Philadelphia, 2005, Mosby.
2. Cook K: *Otitis media.* Accessed January 3, 2006, on-line: www.emedicine.com/EMERG/topic351.htm.
3. Donlon JV and others: Anesthesia for eye, ear, nose, and throat surgery. In Miller RD, editor: *Miller's anesthesia,* ed 6, Philadelphia, 2005, Churchill Livingstone.
4. Gantz BJ, Meyer TA: Auditory brainstem implants. In Cummings CW and others, editors: *Otolaryngology: head and neck surgery,* ed 4, Philadelphia, 2005, Mosby.
5. *Hearing, ear infections and deafness.* Accessed January 3, 2006, on-line: www.nidcd.nih.gov/health/statistics/hearing.asp.
6. House JW, Cunningham CD: Otosclerosis. In Cummings CW and others, editors: *Otolaryngology: head and neck surgery*, ed 4, Philadelphia, 2005, Mosby.
7. Kileny PR, Zwolon TA: Diagnostic and rehabilitative audiology. In Cummings CW and others, editors: *Otolaryngology: head and neck surgery,* ed 4, Philadelphia, 2005, Mosby.
8. Koch DB and others: Bioengineering solutions for hearing loss and related disorders. *Otolaryngologic Clinics of North America* 38(2): 255-272, 2005.
9. Mahlan ME and others: Neurologic monitoring. In Miller RD, editor: *Miller's anesthesia*, ed 6, Philadelphia, 2005, Churchill Livingstone.
10. Ossoff RH and others: Laser surgery, basic principles and safety considerations. In Cummings CW and others, editors: *Otolaryngology: head and neck surgery*, ed 4, Philadelphia, 2005, Mosby.
11. Palmer CV, Ortmann A: Hearing loss and hearing aids, *Neurologic Clinics* 23:901-918, 2005.
12. Ruckenstein M: Otology/neurology. In Ruckenstein M: *Comprehensive review of otorhinolaryngology,* Philadelphia, 2004, Saunders.
13. Santina CC, Lustig LR: Surgically implantable hearing aids. In Cummings CW and others, editors: *Otolaryngology: head and neck surgery*, ed 4, Philadelphia, 2005, Mosby.
14. Schessel DA and others: Meniere's disease and other peripheral disorders. In Cummings CW and others, editors: *Otolaryngology: head and neck surgery,* ed 4, Philadelphia, 2005, Mosby.
15. Wackym PA and others: Patient evaluation and device selection in cochlear implantation. In Cummings CW and others, editors: *Otolaryngology: head and neck surgery,* ed 4, Philadelphia, 2005, Mosby.

CHAPTER 20

# Rhinologic and Sinus Surgery

CHARLOTTE L. GUGLIELMI AND THERESA M. JASSET

Rhinologic surgery is performed to treat internal and external malformations and injuries to the nose. Sinus procedures are performed to treat disease processes of the sinuses. The surgical goal of these types of procedures is to ensure effective functioning of the respiratory system.

Sinus surgery has changed significantly during the past several decades, primarily because of the evolution and refinement of endoscopic sinus surgery (ESS). As with other surgical procedures that are now being done endoscopically, successful sinus surgery can be accomplished in a less-invasive manner in an ambulatory setting. Continued advances in radiologic techniques, especially tomography, allow for the identification of even subtle pathophysiologic changes that can be safely addressed in a surgical setting. Sinus endoscopy has moved from a once diagnostic procedure to a therapeutic surgical intervention that can be offered to patients who have sinus disease.

## Surgical Anatomy

The nose is covered with skin and is supported internally by bone and cartilage. The two external nares provide openings through which air can enter and leave the nasal cavity. These openings contain internal hairs that help prevent coarse particles that are sometimes carried by air from entering the nose.

The nose is divided into the prominent external portion and the internal portion known as the *nasal cavity* (Figure 20-1). The chief purpose of the nose is to prepare air for use in the lungs.

The external nose projects from the face. The nasal bones and the frontal process of the maxillae form the upper portion of the external nose, and the lower portion is formed by a group of nasal cartilages and connective tissue covered with skin (Figure 20-2). The nostrils and the tip of the nose are shaped by the major alar cartilages. The nares are separated by the columella, which is formed by the lower margin of the septal cartilage, the medial parts of the major alar cartilages, and the anterior nasal spine, all of which are covered by skin. The nasal cavity is a hollow space behind the nose that is divided medially into right and left portions by the nasal septum.

The nasal septum is composed of three structures: the nasal cartilage, the perpendicular plate of the ethmoid bone, and the vomer bone. The septum is covered by mucous membrane on either side. The mucous membrane contains blood vessels and mucus-secreting cells; the rich blood supply warms and moistens the air while the sticky mucus traps dust, pollen, and other small particles.[7] A deviated or fractured septum may be repaired surgically by mobilization of the fracture or removal of the deformed cartilage or bone.

The internal portion, or nasal cavity, is divided by the nasal septum into two parts at its midline. The nasal cavity communicates with the outside by its external openings, called the *nares.* The nares open into the nasopharynx through the choanae. The nasal cavity is also associated with each ear by means of the eustachian tube and with the paranasal sinuses (frontal, maxillary, ethmoidal, sphenoidal) through their respective orifices (meatuses). The nasal cavity also communicates with the conjunctivae through the nasolacrimal duct. The nasal cavity is separated from the lingual cavity by the hard palate and soft palate (see Figure 20-1) and from the cranial cavity by the ethmoid bone. It is held together by periosteal covering over bone and by perichondrium, which extends over the cartilages. The turbinate bones of the nasal structure are arranged one above the other, separated by grooves and meatuses. These act as drainage passages of the accessory sinuses and are known as the *sphenoethmoidal recesses* and the *superior, middle,* and *inferior meatuses,* respectively (Figure 20-3).

The nasal sinuses serve as air spaces and communicate with the nasal cavity through the meatuses. Anteriorly, on each side of the skull, the frontal sinus, the anterior ethmoidal sinus, and the maxillary sinus (antrum of Highmore) drain into the middle meatus; posteriorly, the ethmoidal and the sphenoidal sinuses drain into the superior meatus and the sphenoethmoidal recess. A passageway for the flow of air is provided by the irregular air spaces between these structures. Because of their shape, the air is forced to flow in thin air waves.

The sensory nerve supply of the nasal cavity is derived from the trigeminal nerve. The nose and sinuses receive their blood supply (Figure 20-4) from the branches of the internal maxillary, anterior ethmoid, sphenopalatine, nasopalatine, pharyngeal, and posterior ethmoid arteries. Masses of communicating veins lie below the epithelial layer of the turbinate bones, and the veins just beneath the skin anastomose freely. Dilation of the superficial veins may cause the turbinate tissue to swell, whereas contraction of these vessels may cause the tissue to shrink.

## Perioperative Nursing Considerations

### Assessment

The primary areas of focused assessment of the surgical patient include the patient's history, results of preoperative diagnostic studies, risk factors that pose the potential for surgical problems, the patient's experience with previous surgery, and his or her coping resources.[11] As with any surgical procedure, the patient's and family's understanding and cooperation are im-

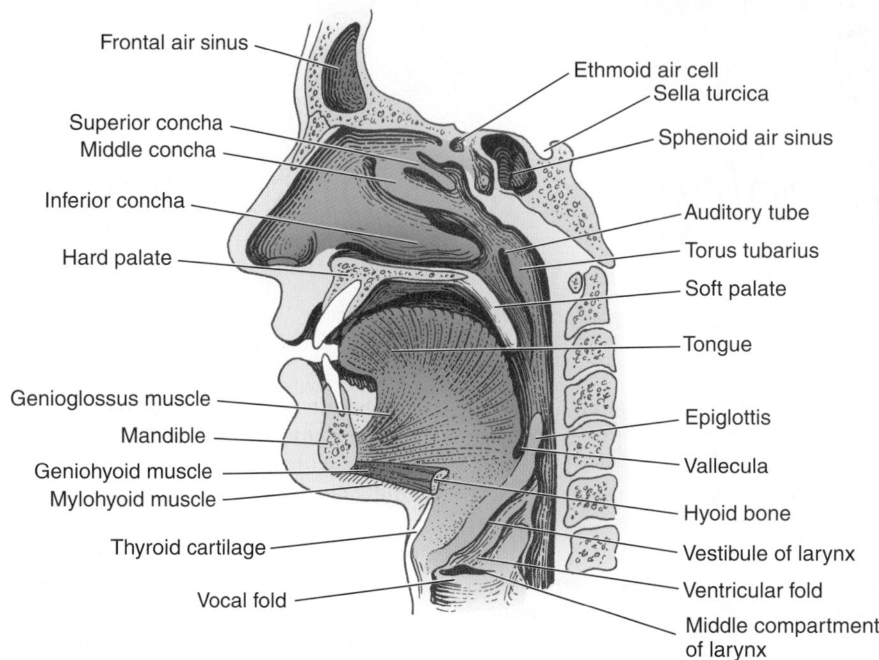


**FIGURE 20-1** Sagittal section of face and neck.

**FIGURE 20-2** Nasal bony framework. *1,* Nasal bone; *2,* frontal bone; *3,* lacrimal bone; *4,* maxillary bone; *5,* upper lateral cartilage; *6,* nasal septum; *7,* lower lateral cartilage, lateral crus; *8,* lower lateral cartilage, medial crus; *9,* sesamoid cartilage; *10,* fibrofatty tissue.

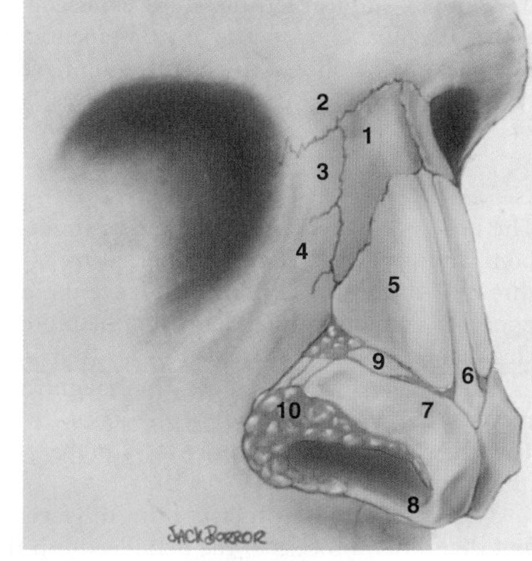


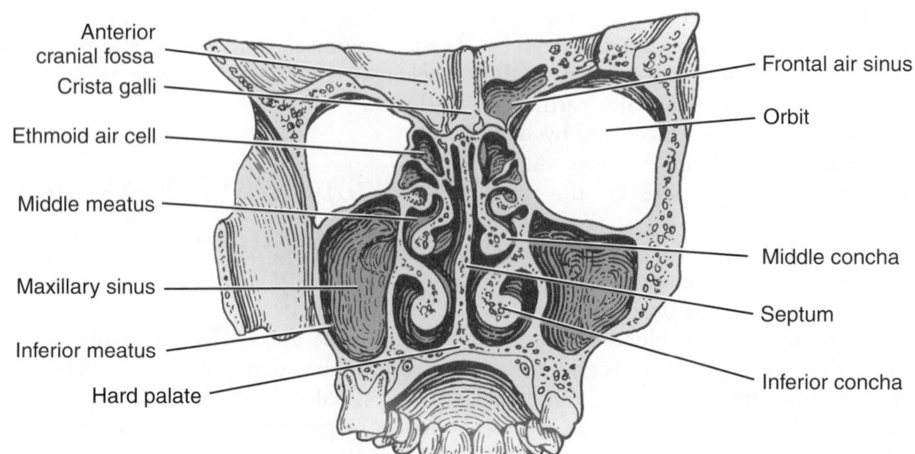


**FIGURE 20-3** Vertical section through nose. Plane of section passes slightly obliquely through left first molar tooth and behind second right premolar tooth. Posterior wall of right frontal sinus removed.

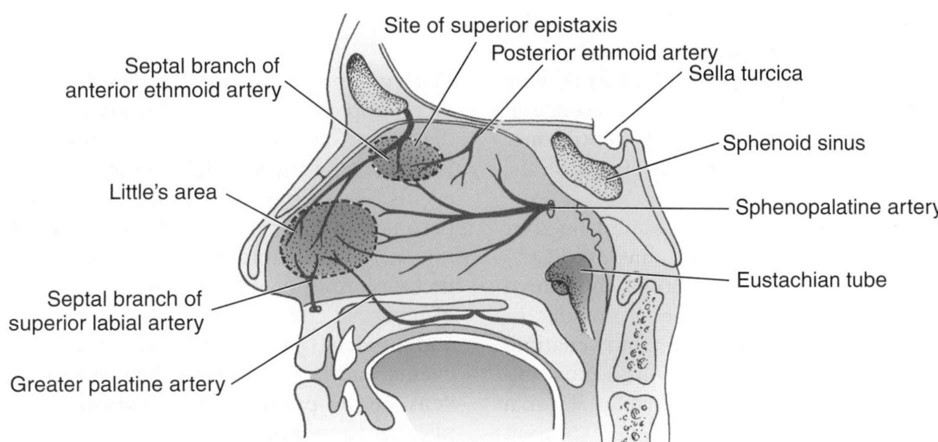


**FIGURE 20-4** Arteries of nasal septum.

portant. The purpose and nature of the nasal and sinus procedures must be explained in a manner that is understandable, with respect for cultural beliefs, values, and customs.[8] Before the day of surgery, the surgeon will have discussed the indications, purpose, sequence, and risks of the proposed procedure. In anticipation of the fact that in many situations the patient is a conscious participant in the procedure, he or she should also be informed about the sedative effects of the preoperative medications. Although drowsy, patients will still be aware that their nose is being operated on but they will not feel pain. Preoperative assessment and education must include a clearly outlined plan of pain management (Best Practice). Patients should also be informed that they will be awake enough to expectorate if necessary and that they should indicate to the surgical team if they do not feel well, are experiencing pain, or become nauseated. The surgeon's postoperative protocol should be explained. Depending on the type of anesthesia planned, a preanesthetic evaluation will have been conducted by an anesthesia provider, who determines risk factors that affect the planned anesthesia technique and evaluates the patient's health status to determine if further tests or consultations are required. Communication regarding patient management issues among the surgeon, anesthesia provider, and perioperative nurse optimizes safe and effective patient care and minimizes perioperative morbidity as well as surgical delays or cancellations.[2,9,13]

A nursing preoperative assessment is usually obtained by a nurse either in person during scheduled preoperative evaluation or by telephone before the day of surgery. The perioperative nurse caring for the patient in the operating room (OR)

## BEST PRACTICE

### Pain Assessment

In 2001, the Joint Commission established standards for pain management. The underpinning element of these standards is the patient's right to appropriate assessment and management of pain. Among other things, the standards also call for education of patients and families regarding pain management, after consideration of their personal, cultural, spiritual, and ethnic beliefs. Expected outcomes in pain management and comfort, which may help patients heal more quickly and have improved outcomes, were researched to develop the following clinical guidelines:

**PREOPERATIVE PAIN ASSESSMENT**

- Patient states an understanding of plan of care and priority of individual needs.
- Patient states understanding of pain intensity scale, comfort scale, and pain relief/comfort goals.
- Patient states understanding of methods to communicate pain levels to the provider during the operative phase of care (patients receiving local or managed anesthesia care).

**POSTANESTHESIA PHASE I**

- Patient maintains hemodynamic stability, including respiratory/cardiac status and level of consciousness.
- Patient states achievement of pain relief/comfort treatment goals.
- Patient shows effective use of at least one nonpharmacologic method.
- Patient verbalizes evidence of receding pain level and increased comfort with pharmacologic and nonpharmacologic interventions.

**POSTANESTHESIA PHASE II/III**

- Patient states acceptable level of pain relief and comfort with movement or activity at time of transfer or discharge to home.
- Patient verbalizes understanding of discharge instruction plans (specific drug, frequency of administration, potential side effects of medication, potential drug interactions, precautions or limitations when taking drugs, name and telephone number of the physician/resource to contact with emergencies or problems).
- Patient states understanding or shows effective use of nonpharmacologic methods.
- Patient states achievement of pain/comfort treatment goals and level of satisfaction with pain relief and comfort management in the perianesthesia setting.

Modified from *ASPAN (American Society of PeriAnesthesia Nurses) pain and comfort guidelines.* Accessed February 8, 2006, on-line: www.aspan.org/painandcomfort.htm; Kolcaba K: *Comfort theory and practice: a vision for holistic health care and research,* New York, 2003, Springer Publishing; Leddy KM, Wolosin RJ: Patient satisfaction with pain control during hospitalization, *Joint Commission Journal on Quality and Patient Safety* 31(9):507-513, 2005.

should review this assessment as well as the physician's evaluation in preparation for caring for the patient. The assessment immediately preceding the procedure should include vital signs, allergies, nothing-by-mouth (NPO) status, presence of preexisting pain, skin condition, sensory deficits, central nervous system (CNS) problems, and the mental status of the patient.

Anesthetic choices include local anesthetics administered by the surgeon with a monitoring nurse who is trained in airway management and the safe administration of drugs, monitored anesthesia care (MAC) delivered by an anesthesia provider, or general anesthesia. When intravenous (IV) conscious sedation/analgesia is used, the monitoring perioperative nurse must follow established institutional protocols (see Chapter 4 for a discussion of IV conscious sedation/analgesia). The evolution of new short-acting anesthetic agents employed in the ambulatory setting has improved the safety and efficiency of care for those patients who have a surgical procedure while under general anesthesia and who return home on the same day.

Close attention should be paid to any known allergies or past drug reactions experienced by the patient, especially if related to administration of local anesthetics.[7] The patient's account of previous dental experiences with local anesthetics can provide a clue as to how the patient will respond to the anesthetic agents. Cardiac status should be noted because many surgeons use epinephrine as an additive to the local anesthetic. The epinephrine acts as a vasoconstrictor and reduces the blood loss, which should be minimal, during surgery. The epinephrine effect may contribute to cardiac dysrhythmias and an increased potential for cardiac arrest. In addition, cocaine is often administered topically intranasally to achieve vasoconstriction and to afford the awake patient more comfort during the injection of local anesthesia. Respiratory patterns and any respiratory conditions, such as asthma, should also be noted. These and other medications commonly used in rhinologic and sinus surgery are described in the Surgical Pharmacology box.

## Nursing Diagnosis

A nursing diagnosis is a decision about a patient problem or need that requires and is amenable to nursing intervention. Problems and needs may be identified by the perioperative nurse, the patient, or the patient's family or significant others, focusing attention on a physical or behavioral response that currently exists or one at risk for developing. Nursing diagnoses related to the care of patients undergoing rhinologic or sinus surgery might include the following:

- Risk for Ineffective Breathing Pattern
- Acute Pain
- Disturbed Sensory Perception
- Anxiety

## Outcome Identification

Outcomes identified for the selected nursing diagnoses could be stated as follows:

- The patient will demonstrate effective breathing patterns.
- The patient will demonstrate effective coping with the physical and psychologic effects of pain during administration of local anesthesia.
- The patient will verbalize understanding of the anticipated postoperative alteration in the senses of smell and taste.
- The patient's anxiety will be reduced or controlled.

## Planning

Planning the patient's care is based on the preoperative assessment, application of critical thinking skills, identified nursing diagnoses, and expected outcomes, as well as the nurse's knowledge of the scheduled surgical procedure and associated events. Development of a meaningful plan of care enables the perioperative nurse to effectively meet the patient's needs during the surgical intervention. Perioperative nursing priorities include provision for the patient's physical safety; prevention of potential complications; the alleviation of discomfort, pain, and anxiety; provision of information about perioperative events; and facilitation of effective and efficient surgical interventions by preparing the environment with necessary supplies and equipment.

Supplies necessary to ensure comfort of the patient in a supine position should be obtained. These usually include a foam headrest, a pillow for under the knees, and warm blankets. Foam padding should be available to assist in positioning the arms if they are going to be placed at the side. The placement of IV lines in the arm that is to be tucked at the side should be avoided, but in cases where this is not avoidable, patency of those lines must be ensured. Specific equipment needs for endoscopic procedures are discussed later in this chapter.

Preparation of the OR includes checking the availability and functional capacity of suction, the surgeon's headlight and light source, and the electrosurgical unit (ESU). It is essential that the x-ray view box is in working order and appropriately located so that scans may be easily viewed by the surgeon during the procedure. In video-assisted cases, the camera should be checked, the printer should be set up as preferred by the surgeon, and an adequate supply of paper should be available. In procedures in which the perioperative nurse functions as the primary patient monitor, equipment such as oxygen-saturation monitor, blood pressure monitor, electrocardiogram (ECG) monitor, and oxygen delivery system should be checked before the procedure.

Because local anesthesia is frequently used for nasal surgical procedures, the nurse must be prepared to react quickly to signs of allergic reactions or toxic symptoms. Symptoms of adverse drug reactions include changes in skin, such as rash or itching; restlessness; unexplained anxiety or fearfulness; diaphoresis; and complaints of blurred vision, tinnitus, dizziness, nausea, palpitations, disturbed respiration, pallor or flushing, and syncope. Emergency drugs, suction apparatus, and resuscitation equipment including a defibrillator should be readily available. In the awake patient, intraoperative pain can serve an important warning function that contributes greatly to the avoidance of injury to the roof of the ethmoid, the orbit, and the optic nerve.

A typical plan of care for a patient undergoing rhinologic or sinus surgery is given on p. 662.

Several principles of nursing care are basic to nasal surgery. The information in the Patient and Family Education box on p. 663 should be reviewed with patients and their families.

## Implementation

Patient positioning for nasal cases is supine. A standard headrest may be used to maintain the head in normal position. The entire bed is turned 90 degrees to allow the right-handed sur-

## SURGICAL PHARMACOLOGY

### Medications Commonly Used in Rhinologic and Sinus Surgery

| Category | Dose/Route/ Mechanism | Purpose/Action | Adverse Reactions | Contraindications (C)/ Precautions (P) |
|---|---|---|---|---|
| **LOCAL ANESTHETICS** | | | | |
| Lidocaine, 1% or 0.5% | Local injection | Blocks pain and temperature fibers, used as medium to dilute epinephrine | Cardiovascular, hypotension, confusion, dizziness, headache, somnolence, tremor, injection site pain, cardiac arrest, cardiac dysrhythmia, seizure | **C:** Hypersensitivity to amide locals<br>**P:** CHF, bradycardia, hypovolemia, liver disease, renal impairment |
| Cocaine | 4% topical swab, packing instilled into a cavity or spray | Local anesthetic (also used as a vasoconstrictor) | CNS depression, CNS stimulation, anxiety, tachydysrhythmia, seizures; may interact with cannabis, promethazine (Phenerzine), and St. John's wort | **C:** Hypersensitivity to cocaine products<br>**P:** Acutely ill patients, children, used with caution on severely traumatized mucosa or when sepsis is present in the area of intended application |
| **VASOCONSTRICTORS** | | | | |
| Oxymetazoline hydrochloride (Afrin Nasal Spray, Neo-Synephrine 12 Hr, Nasacon) | 0.05% nasal spray | Nasal decongestant used for vasoconstriction | Headache, insomnia, nervousness, nasal congestion, rebound congestion, nasal mucosa dry, nasal stinging/ burning, sneezing, cardiac dysrhythmia, hypertension, tachydysrhythmias | **C:** Hypersensitivity to oxymetazoline or other adrenergic agents, narrow angle glaucoma<br>**P:** Cardiovascular disease, concurrent MAOI or tricyclic depressant therapy, diabetes, hypertension, prostatic enlargement, thyroid disease |
| Epinephrine | 1:100,000–1:200,000 | Used for vasoconstriction | Palpitations, tachydysrhythmia, body pale and sweating symptoms, nausea and vomiting, asthenia, dizziness, headache, tremor, pain in eye, anxiety, apprehension, nervousness, dyspnea, cardiac dysrhythmia, hypertensive crisis, pulmonary edema | **C:** Hypersensitivity to epinephrine products, narrow angle glaucoma (ophthalmic form) within 2 wk of MAOI (inhalational form)<br>**P:** Cerebrovascular insufficiency, diabetes, geriatrics, heart disease, coronary insufficiency, hypertension, thyroid disease, pregnancy |
| **ANTIBIOTICS** | | | | |
| Mupirocin (Nasal Bactroban) | 2% topical | Antibacterial and lubricant for nasal packing | Dermatologic, nasal stinging and burning, disorder of taste, headache | **C:** Hypersensitivity to mupirocin products<br>**P:** Prolonged use may result in overgrowth of nonsusceptible organisms including fungae; not intended for open wounds or mucous membranes |
| Bacitracin | Topical ointment, 500 units/g | Antibacterial, antibiotic | Swelling, contact dermatitis, pruritus | **C:** Hypersensitivity to bacitracin products<br>**P:** Prolonged use may result in overgrowth of nonsusceptible organisms; not intended for open wounds or mucous membranes |
| **STEROIDS** | | | | |
| Triamcinolone acetonide (Aristocort, Kenalog) | Topical | Used topically to lubricate packs or expand packing | Hypertension, atrophic condition of skin | **C:** Hypersensitivity to triamcinolone acetonide; local, viral, fungal, or bacterial infections<br>**P:** Hypertension, hypothyroidism, pregnancy |

 MICROMEDEX® Healthcare Series, vol. 127, expires March 2006, accessed February 8, 2006; Skidmore-Roth L; *Mosby's drug guide for nurses,* ed 6, St Louis, 2005, Mosby.

*CHF,* Congestive heart failure; *CNS,* central nervous system; *MAOI,* monoamine oxidase inhibitor.

## SAMPLE PLAN OF CARE

**NURSING DIAGNOSIS**

**Risk for Ineffective Breathing Pattern**

**OUTCOME**

The patient will demonstrate effective breathing patterns.

**INTERVENTIONS**

- Assess respiratory status and breathing pattern. Monitor respiratory rate, rhythm, and depth and oxygen saturation (pulse oximetry). Maintain oxygen saturation at greater than 90%. Report any variances from normal.
- Note any restlessness, apprehension, agitation, lethargy, or repeated swallowing. Use a penlight to examine the throat for bleeding. Notify the surgeon if bleeding is present.[12]
- Have emergency medications and airway equipment available.
- Elevate head of the bed (to decrease edema, which can interfere with breathing).
- Apply ice compresses (to increase vasoconstriction, thereby decreasing edema).
- Increase humidification with a bedside humidifier or a humidified facemask.
- Explain to patient and family that packing will interfere with ability to breathe through the nose.
- Review mouth breathing with patient and family.
- Encourage increased frequency of oral hygiene with patient and family.

**NURSING DIAGNOSIS**

**Acute Pain**

**OUTCOME**

The patient will demonstrate effective coping with the physical and psychologic effects of pain during administration of local anesthetic.

**INTERVENTIONS**

- Review with patient normal coping mechanisms that are personally effective; support and encourage these during surgical intervention. As appropriate, consider nonpharmacologic measures, such as guided imagery, music, and relaxation exercises.[6]
- Describe the anticipated sequence of perioperative events.
- Explain that some initial discomfort (e.g., pinprick followed by slight burning and then numbness) may be felt during the administration of local anesthetic.
- Inform the patient before the injection of local anesthetic; provide support and reassurance; evaluate patient response.
- Observe for, document, and report any changes in the patient's vital signs (blood pressure, heart rate and rhythm, respiratory rate, oxygen saturation), skin condition, and mental status.
- Be aware of the maximum recommended dosage of local anesthetics (see Chapter 4), and be alert for signs of allergic reactions or toxic responses.
- Ask the patient whether he or she is experiencing any pain; communicate the presence of pain sensation to the surgeon.
- Administer sedation or analgesics as ordered by the surgeon. Describe the purpose and expected response to the medication administered. Document medications administered (see Patient Safety).
- Verify with the patient that desired response has been achieved.

**NURSING DIAGNOSIS**

**Disturbed Sensory Perception**

**OUTCOME**

The patient will verbalize understanding of the anticipated postoperative alteration in the senses of smell and taste.

**INTERVENTIONS**

- Explain to the patient and family that a "mustache" dressing and packing will be in place postoperatively and will interfere with the sense of smell.
- Inform the patient and family that the sense of taste will also be altered, such as with having a head cold.
- Assure the patient and family that these alterations are usually temporary.
- Encourage the patient to maintain proper dietary intake even if the food does not smell or taste as it should.
- Encourage frequent mouth care; rinse with water or half hydrogen peroxide and half normal saline.

**NURSING DIAGNOSIS**

**Anxiety**

**OUTCOME**

The patient's anxiety will be reduced or controlled.

**INTERVENTIONS**

- Following the protocol in place, inform the patient and family what to expect on the day of surgery and the environment of care (preoperative area, operating room [OR], postanesthesia care unit [PACU]).
- Introduce members of the surgical staff. Explain activities performed by the nursing staff in simple language the patient can understand.
- Assure the patient that he or she will be informed before any procedure is done.
- Provide time for the patient and family to express fears and concerns. Provide factual, accurate information.
- Note expressions of distress and anxiety.
- Prevent unnecessary body exposure during transfer and positioning.
- Control external stimuli and noise levels.

geon to work from the patient's right side, and the right arm is tucked in at the patient's side. The arm should be padded as necessary when tucked to prevent nerve injury. Depending on the procedure, the left arm may be maintained by the anesthesia provider and usually has the IV line placed in it for easier access. The anesthesia provider and equipment will be to the patient's left as well. Alternatively, a modified "beach chair" position can be used for these procedures. The scrub person may stand at the patient's head or down near the patient's waist next to the surgeon's right arm. A Mayo stand can be set up either at the head of the bed off to the side or positioned over the patient's chest, depending on where the scrub person is standing. Video equipment should be set up at the patient's head if applicable. Safety straps should always be used. Adjustments to positioning should be made to meet the needs of left-handed surgeons.

### PATIENT AND FAMILY EDUCATION

### Principles of Care Basic to Nasal Surgery

1. Some discomfort may occur during the initial administration of a local anesthetic. If the surgeon uses a topical anesthetic (usually cocaine) as the first phase of anesthesia, it is applied to the nose with cottonoids or applicators. The patient may find the applicators or packing uncomfortable or may have the urge to sneeze. These sensations will disappear as the anesthetic takes effect. The injection may cause momentary discomfort, and a burning sensation may occur as the anesthetic is injected. If the patient expresses difficulty in breathing, the nurse should encourage slow, deep breaths through the mouth and continually provide reassurance to allay the patient's anxiety. If the surgeon uses epinephrine with the local agent, the resulting weak, quivering feeling and increased heart rate are effects of the epinephrine and disappear after a few minutes. To prepare the patient in advance, the nurse may liken this to the experiences a patient may have had in the dentist's office. The patient's cardiac status should be noted at this time.
2. Certain procedures may be performed on entry to the preoperative holding area or the operating room in accordance with institutional policies, such as insertion of intravenous lines and application of monitoring devices. Attempts should be made to allow the patient to continue to be supported by his or her family or significant others as long as possible before the patient is admitted to the operating room (OR).
3. During the surgical procedure, the awake patient feels the surgeon working and may feel pressure at some point but should not feel pain. The patient should let the perioperative nurse and surgeon know if any discomfort is felt during the procedure, and more anesthetic can be given. There may be occasions during the procedure in which the patient is unable to speak to communicate with the circulating nurse. The circulating nurse and the patient should discuss this during the preoperative assessment to agree on a mechanism to communicate when unable to speak. A gesture as simple as raising the hand nearest to the nurse monitoring the patient may be appropriate.
4. After surgery, the head of the bed is elevated to facilitate breathing and promote drainage.
5. A nasal pack will probably be inserted, and there may be some difficulty in swallowing. When the patient attempts to swallow, a sucking action occurs in the throat because the packing does not allow air passage through the nose, thereby creating a partial vacuum.
6. Some bruising and swelling can be expected after surgery, but it will gradually subside.
7. Forceful nose blowing must be avoided for a time to prevent movement of the rearranged nasal structures. If necessary to clear nasal passages, the patient should sniff.
8. The sense of smell is diminished for a time after surgery but gradually returns.
9. Some numbness may be noted postoperatively but gradually disappears.
10. A moderate amount of discomfort should be expected after surgery; analgesics are often prescribed, and the patient should be encouraged to take medication for pain. The perioperative nurse may encourage patients to take pain medication for pain higher than 3 on a 10-point scale.[10] Discharge instructions should include clear direction about the management of pain and include steps and contact information for follow-up if needed. The perioperative nurse should emphasize clear, concise information regarding the name of the medication, frequency of administration, potential side effects, actions to take to prevent or ameliorate these, and precautions to follow. These instructions should be provided in both verbal and written form.[4]
11. The procedure for changing the mustache dressing (or drip pad) that is in place postoperatively to absorb any drainage should be reviewed with the patient and family. This is usually a folded 2-inch × 2-inch gauze pad placed under the nose and secured by tape. Blood-tinged secretions in the nasopharynx are normal in the first few hours after the procedure.
12. Potential complications of bleeding, cerebrospinal fluid leak, and visual or tear duct problems should be reviewed with the patient or family.

***Local Anesthesia.*** As discussed in the assessment section, rhinologic and sinus surgery can be done with various routes of anesthetic delivery. Safe administration of medication is essential for achieving optimal outcomes (Patient Safety). Two types of medications are commonly used in rhinologic and sinus surgery. The first is a local anesthetic used to block the patient's pain and temperature fibers. Lidocaine, often used for local anesthesia, is frequently combined with epinephrine. A concentration of 1:200,000 provides maximum vasoconstriction, but some surgeons prefer a concentration of 1:100,000. Cocaine 4% topical solution is the second medication that is used commonly. It too is a good vasoconstrictor but has the added benefit of anesthetic properties. Some surgeons use a nasal decongestant instead of cocaine for nasal vasoconstriction. These decongestants do not produce some of the cardiac effects seen with cocaine. Because nasal and sinus surgeries are performed in such a confined space, vasoconstriction becomes crucial for appropriate visualization of the surgical field. Hypertension can increase bleeding despite vasoconstrictive agents used and may need to be managed medically by the anesthesia provider intraoperatively if the visual field becomes compromised and surgery is impaired.

The surgeon usually packs the nose with the vasoconstrictive solution before prepping and draping, to allow time for the vasoconstrictive properties to work. A separate prep table, which includes a labeled container of the vasoconstrictor solution, x-ray–detectable cottonoids (usually ½ inch × 3 inches with attached strings), bayonet forceps, and a small nasal speculum, should be prepared for this purpose. These cottonoids should always be counted before and at the end of the procedure. (If a cottonoid is placed extremely posterior along the nasal floor, it can slide past the palate and be swallowed by the patient.) The cottonoids are left in place. Some surgeons will also inject local anesthetic at this time, but others may wait to inject at the time of surgery. Maximum vasoconstriction occurs in approximately 10 to 12 minutes after the administration of epinephrine. If a local anesthetic is to be injected next, the prep table should also include a 10-ml Luer-Lok syringe, appropriate-size needle (usually 25 gauge, 1½ inch), and labeled lidocaine (0.5% to 2%, according to surgeon's pref-

## PATIENT SAFETY

### Guidelines for Safe Medication Administration

Numerous medications of varying strengths and dosages, and many of them clear solutions, are used in rhinologic and sinus surgery. The safe delivery of medication to patients during operative procedures is an essential aspect of reducing significant risks and preventing harm. In both the scrub and circulating roles meticulous adherence to guidelines and clear communication among caregivers is essential.

As the circulating nurse, do the following:

1. Verify absence of patient allergy or sensitivity to all prescribed medications and irrigation solutions.
2. Check the solution/medication twice for the following:
   a. Correct medication
   b. Correct dosage/concentration of medication
   c. Sterility
   d. Expiration date
3. State the name of the medication, dose, concentration, and expiration and/or irrigating solution name and expiration to the scrub person when delivering to the field. If there is no designated scrub person, the circulating nurse should verify the medication visually and verbally with the licensed professional performing the procedure.
4. When multiple medications are to be delivered to the sterile field, complete the preparation for administration, delivery to the sterile field, and labeling before another medication is prepared.
5. Medications will be delivered to the sterile field using one of the following techniques:
   a. Opening a sterile, labeled bottle from a sterile Steri-pak and placing directly on the sterile field
   b. Using a vial decanter to dispense the medication into a labeled container on the sterile field
   c. Drawing up the medication with a blunt-fill needle and syringe and delivering to a labeled container on the sterile field
6. When delivering a medication using a syringe or vial decanter, pour into a receptacle close to table edge; pour entire contents of bottle onto the sterile field in a steady stream to avoid splashing.
7. Medication bottles/vials are to be retained in the room until the end of the case for later identification if necessary.
8. Document all medications used. Include the name of medication, dose, route, and person administering the drug on the Perioperative Documentation record. Name of drug must be written in entirety. No medication abbreviations may be used.
9. Document topical ointments used on the incision site as part of the dressing under "dressing."
10. At shift change or break relief, all medications on and off the sterile field and their labels should be noted and verified concurrently by entering and exiting staff. Report is to include the amount of medication that has been administered at the time the change is being made.

As the scrub person, do the following:

1. Prepare containers to accept medications from the circulating nurse.
2. Visually and verbally confirm the name of the medication, the dose, the volume, and the expiration date with the circulating nurse before he or she dispenses the medication to the sterile field.
3. Verify with the circulating nurse the presence of allergies.
4. Label all containers and syringes, using sterile labels and marking pen, immediately after a medication/irrigating solution is dispensed to the sterile field. Include the full name of the medicati on, dosage, and concentration.
5. When passing the medication to the licensed professional performing the procedure, visually and verbally verify the medication, strength, and dose with that practitioner by reading the medication label aloud as the drug is handed to the surgeon or designee.
6. At shift change or break relief, all medications on and off the sterile field and their labels should be noted and verified concurrently by entering and exiting staff. Report is to include the amount of medication that has been administered at the time the change is being made.
7. Keep all sterile medication bottles/vials on the sterile field until the end of the case for later identification if necessary.
8. At the conclusion of the procedure communicate to the circulating nurse the dosage of medication that was delivered by the surgeon.
9. At the conclusion of the procedure, transfer any controlled substances to the circulating nurse for disposition per medical center policy.

Modified from *Beth Israel Deaconess Medical Center perioperative services manual #PSM 200-220. Delivery and administration of intraoperative medications and solution,* Boston, 2004.

erence). Additional syringes, needles, and labeled local anesthetic solution should be available on the sterile field for additional administration intraoperatively. Additional labeled cocaine solution and cottonoids should be available on the sterile field as well. The circulating nurse, monitoring nurse, or anesthesia provider should observe any changes in the vital signs of the patient. Documentation should follow institutional policy for recording intraoperative medications administered.[1]

***Prepping and Draping.*** Prepping of the nose and face may or may not be done, depending on the surgical procedure and institutional policy. The intranasal area is considered "dirty" and not possible to prep as effectively as other surgical sites, such as an abdomen. Some surgeons cleanse the nose and face with povidone-iodine solution or other topical surgical antiseptic solution, such as hexylresorcinol 1%. The surgical field is maintained in sterile fashion, and these procedures usually have a "clean contaminated" wound classification (see Chapter 3).

Draping is done as for most head and neck cases. A small sheet with a towel on top of it is placed under the patient's head, and the towel is secured around the hairline with a towel clip. A split sheet is then placed around the head. It is good practice to place a towel over the endotracheal (ET) tube if one is in place to prevent the adhesive portion of the split sheet from sticking to the ET tube and inadvertently pulling on the tube once the procedure is completed and drapes are removed. Except during certain endoscopic procedures, the patient's eyes should be covered with moist gauze or towels if the patient is awake or taped closed if the patent is under general anesthesia to protect them from nasal drainage or injury from instruments.

***Instrumentation and Equipment.*** A headlight is worn for local and topical administration of medications before draping. If the planned procedure is endoscopic, the headlight will not be necessary after that point. Headlights will be required for septoplasty and rhinoplasty procedures. A standard ESU should be available but is usually not required in endoscopic procedures.

Specimen cups, labels, and a marking pen should be available on the sterile field because often several specimens are obtained. Institutional procedure for correct patient and specimen identification should be followed.[1]

Postoperative care of the instruments used in nasal surgery follows the general care regimen of all other surgical instruments. Chisels, gouges, and other cutting instruments should be inspected carefully for any nicks and dullness and repaired as needed. Rasps and files should be thoroughly cleaned and all bone debris removed. Special attention should be given to suction tips. Sinus endoscopes should be cleaned and sterilized according to institutional protocols. Sinus instruments should be handled carefully because of their delicate nature. They should be in good working order and should open and close easily to grasp and release delicate nasal and sinus tissue. Lenses on headlights used during the procedure should be checked for cleanliness and cleaned according to the manufacturer's instructions.

## Evaluation

At the conclusion of the procedure, the patient should be assessed postoperatively for any difficulties in breathing. Nasal packing inhibits breathing; however, the patient should be able to breathe normally through the mouth. Skin integrity at positional pressure sites and the ESU dispersive electrode site should be assessed and documented. The amount of drainage present on the mustache dressing should be noted. Repeated swallowing should be noted, because this may indicate posterior nasal bleeding. The head of the postanesthesia care unit (PACU) bed should be elevated before transport to the unit. A hand-off report of the patient's status and special needs should be given to the PACU nurse. Goals of the nursing plan of care are reviewed; an evaluation of outcomes as identified in the assessment phase may be communicated and documented as follows:

- The patient demonstrated effective breathing patterns. Respiratory rate and depth were within normal limits, and the respiratory pattern appeared effective with no cyanosis or other signs of hypoxia.
- The patient's anxiety was reduced or controlled. The patient acknowledged feeling anxious, reported a reduction in anxiety to a manageable level, and appeared relaxed.
- The patient demonstrated effective coping with the physical and psychologic effects of pain during the administration of local anesthesia. Vital signs remained stable, there were no ECG or CNS changes, and the patient tolerated the discomfort of injection and understood the effects of loss of feeling and sensation.
- The patient verbalized understanding of anticipated postoperative alteration in the senses of smell and taste.

## Patient and Family Education and Discharge Planning

Discharge teaching and planning for postdischarge activities and needs are essential for the patient and family to successfully cope with the postoperative recovery period. These may be initiated by the perioperative nurse. Key education points for discharge instructions for surgical patients include information about medications, activity restrictions, dietary instructions, surgical or anesthesia side effects, possible complications and the pertinent signs and symptoms of these, as well as information related to postdischarge care and follow-up care. Printed information should be reviewed with the patient, and the patient should repeat back the key points that are essential to a successful recovery.[4] Patients and families should be made aware of the following activities, restrictions, and precautions as they relate to rhinologic or sinus surgery:

1. When the patient goes home, the head should be elevated during the day in either a sitting position or reclining chair. During sleep, pillows should be used.
2. If a nasal pack is in place, the patient may have some difficulty swallowing. When the patient attempts to swallow, a sucking action occurs in the throat because the packing does not allow air to pass through the nose, thereby creating a partial vacuum.
3. The patient should be encouraged to breathe through the mouth until the packing is removed. Frequent oral hygiene measures should be encouraged. For the first few days after the packing is removed, forceful coughing or straining at bowel movements should be avoided; laxatives or stool softeners may be prescribed.
4. The patient should be made aware of the temporary nature of nasal and periorbital edema and discoloration and numbness in the nasal tip and upper lip. Edema and discoloration may persist for several weeks.
5. Forceful nose blowing must be avoided to prevent movement of the rearranged nasal structures. If necessary to clear nasal passages, the patient should sniff. If a sneeze is unavoidable, the mouth should be opened.
6. The sense of smell is diminished for a time after surgery but gradually returns.
7. A moderate amount of discomfort should be expected after surgery; an analgesic is prescribed, and the patient should be encouraged to take it. Aspirin and nonsteroidal antiinflammatory drugs (NSAIDs) are usually avoided to prevent the possibility of bleeding.[12]
8. The procedure for changing the mustache dressing that may be in place postoperatively to absorb any drainage should be reviewed with the patient and family. Blood-tinged secretions on the dressing may persist for 1 or 2 days.
9. Signs and symptoms such as bleeding, visual or tear duct problems, respiratory difficulty, an elevated temperature, or vertigo should be reported to the physician or other appropriate health care provider (e.g., the nurse practitioner).
10. Patients should avoid smoking or exposure to other noxious fumes that could irritate the nasal passages or nasal mucosa.
11. Use of a humidifier or normal saline nasal spray may help keep nasal passages and mucosa moist.
12. Lifting heavy objects and excessive straining should be avoided.

# Surgical Interventions

## RHINOLOGIC SURGERY

Procedures that involve both internal and external nasal reconstruction can be done with local anesthesia, usually supplemented with IV sedation and analgesia. If the patient is particularly apprehensive or anxious, general anesthesia may be more appropriate.

### Nasoseptoplasty or Submucous Resection of the Septum (SMR)

A nasoseptoplasty is straightening of either the cartilaginous or osseous portions of the septum that lie between the flaps of the mucous membrane and the perichondrium. When the nasal septum is deformed, fractured, or injured, normal respiratory and nasal function may be impaired, interfering with airflow and sinus drainage. Deviations of the septum involving cartilage, bony parts (spurs), or both may block the meatus and compress the middle turbinate on that side, thereby resulting in an obstruction of the sinus opening. Septal deviations tend to produce sinus disease and nasal polyps.

The objective of the septoplasty is to establish an adequate partition between the left and right nasal cavities, thereby providing a clear airway through both the internal and external cavities of the nose.

***Procedural Considerations.*** The setup is as described in the general preparation for nasal surgery. In most cases, the surgeon will opt to wear a headlight to improve visualization of the intranasal structures.

#### *Operative Procedure*

1. The nostril is opened with a nasal speculum. An incision is made through the mucoperichondrium of the septum with a knife having a #15 blade. The tissues are separated and elevated with a Freer elevator (Figure 20-5).
2. The cartilage is incised with a knife, and the mucous membrane is elevated with a septal elevator; deviated cartilage and bony, thickened structures are trimmed or removed with a septum punch and a nasal cutting forceps.
3. The bony septal spurs are trimmed by means of a punch forceps or chisel, gouge, and mallet. Suction is used to expose the field. Bleeding is controlled by insertion of additional cottonoids soaked with a topical hemostatic agent.
4. The perpendicular plate of the ethmoid as well as the vomer may be removed by means of a suitable septum-cutting forceps.
5. The incision may be sutured with 4-0 absorbable atraumatic suture on a small, straight needle.
6. Nostrils are packed with gauze impregnated with antibiotic ointment to keep the septal flaps in a midline position. Nasal splints made of plastic or Silastic may also be used to prevent adhesions and maintain the septum. Some surgeons use mattress sutures to provide a patent airway while maintaining support for the septum. The face is cleansed, and a mustache dressing (i.e., a 2-inch × 2-inch gauze folded and placed below the nose and secured with tape across the face or bridge of the nose) may be applied. A small ice bag (e.g., a surgical glove filled with ice) may be applied to the nose.

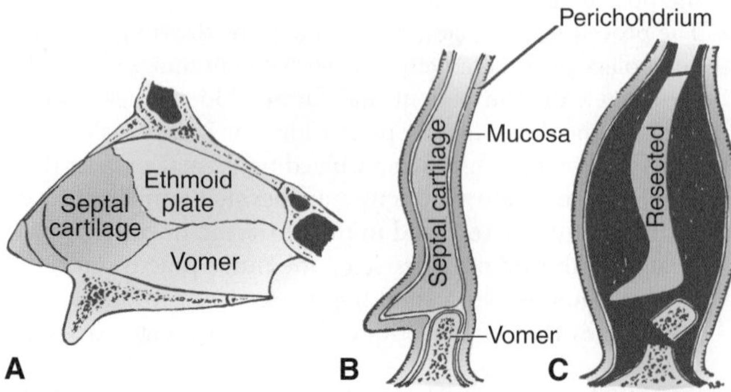


**FIGURE 20-5** **A,** Primary components of septum. Incision line is for Killian type of submucous resection. **B,** Septum with deviated cartilage and spur at junction of vomer and septal cartilage. **C,** Resection of obstructive parts after careful elevation of mucoperichondrium and mucoperiosteum.

### Corrective Rhinoplasty

A corrective rhinoplasty is removal of the hump, narrowing and shortening of the nose, and reconstruction of the tip of the nose. It is considered an elective cosmetic procedure. Often it is done in combination with a septoplasty so that there is only one anesthetic and recovery period for the patient. Procedures may be scheduled so that a plastic surgeon performs the rhinoplasty after the otorhinolaryngologist completes the septoplasty, but many otorhinolaryngologists are trained to perform the rhinoplasty procedure as well.

***Procedural Considerations.*** The patient is prepped and positioned for nasal surgery. Rhinoplasty can be performed internally, where all the incisions are within the nasal cavity, or as an external procedure, where the incision is on the skin across the bases of the nasal columella (Figure 20-6). This incision allows for the reflection of the columellar nasal tip flap, providing exposure of the underlying bony and cartilaginous structures.

#### *Operative Procedure*

1. A hemitransfixion incision is made through the skin of one nostril with a knife having a #15 blade. A nasal speculum, sponges, and skin hooks are used for exposure.
2. The skin of the nose is undermined by elevators, knives, and scissors. The periosteum and perichondrium are freed with elevators and a periosteal dissector.
3. The nasal bones may be fractured (controlled fracturing) with a straight or curved osteotome or a saw. The upper lateral cartilage may be trimmed with a #15 blade or a small

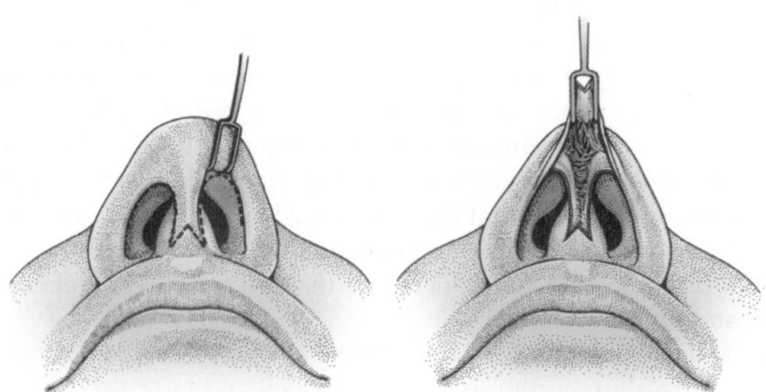

**FIGURE 20-6** Surgical technique of external rhinoplasty.

plastic scissors. The dorsal hump can be taken down with an osteotome or rasped. A cartilaginous hump can be taken down with a #15 blade. The septal cartilage may be resected by a cutting forceps, such as the Jansen-Middleton. Bony spurs can be taken down with a mallet and osteotome.[3] The field is cleared by suctioning.

4. The edges of the cartilage are trimmed with scissors or a #15 blade.
5. To prevent or control infection or the formation of a hematoma, blood is suctioned from the nose and the wound is cleansed. A drainage port is often made in the mucoperichondrial flap to allow for drainage.
6. The cartilage and bones are molded into proper position. The hemitransfixion incision is sutured with absorbable suture. Dressings with a pressure splint are applied. A mustache dressing and ice packs to the nose may be applied as previously described. The head of the bed should be elevated postoperatively. According to the surgeon's preference, iced gauze may be applied to the periorbital area to reduce postoperative bruising and swelling.

## Repair of Nasal Fracture

The nose is the structure most susceptible to trauma because it is seated midface. The paired nasal bones are thin and project like a tent on the frontal process of the maxilla. If the trauma is caused by a direct frontal blow, usually both nasal bones are fractured, displaced outward, and depressed into the ethmoid sinus (see Figure 20-3) and the septal cartilages become displaced.

***Procedural Considerations.*** Repair of nasal fractures can be performed in either an ambulatory or inpatient setting. Simple nasal fractures often can be managed with topical and local anesthesia. However, as with most nasal procedures, if the patient is significantly anxious, general anesthesia may be necessary. Topical and local anesthetics are used even with a general anesthetic to provide vasoconstriction and enhance visualization for the procedure. The patient is prepped and positioned for nasal surgery.

### *Operative Procedure*

1. The nose is packed with nasal cottonoids saturated with a hemostatic agent, and the local anesthetic is injected. When epinephrine is used, 10 minutes is the optimum time to wait for the effects of the hemostatic agent. This period of time will vary with other agents.
2. A Boies elevator is inserted into the nostril, and the nasal bones are elevated and molded into place by external manipulation (Figure 20-7).
3. Nasal packing or intranasal splints may be used to stabilize the reduction because sometimes the bony fragments tend to return to a depressed status.

## Treatment of Epistaxis

The treatment of patients with epistaxis dates back more than 2 centuries (History box). Patients with nasal bleeding usually control the problem themselves with direct pressure application. When their efforts fail, they seek help from their own physician or an emergency department. When more conservative measures (which involve vasoconstrictive agents and nasal packing) taken in the emergency department fail, surgical intervention becomes necessary. Most epistaxis can be treated

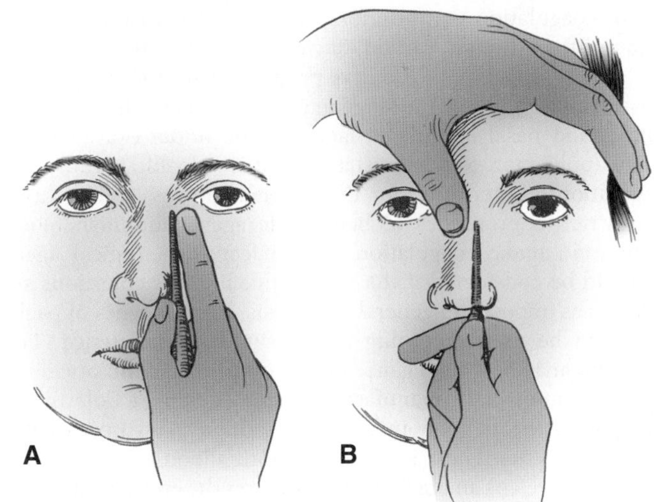


FIGURE 20-7 Reduction of nasal fracture. **A,** Boies elevator is placed along lateral wall of nose to point below nasofrontal angle. Distance to ala is marked with thumb. **B,** Elevator is then placed under depressed nasal bone, lifting it into position; opposite thumb carefully exerts downward pressure on elevated contralateral bone.

## HISTORY

It is well accepted that today's current management of epistaxis is based on sound principles. However, one of the earliest references to the treatment of epistaxis was noted to be more than 2500 years ago. A review from those ancient times onward reveals not only some curious methods for epistaxis treatment but also evidence that many of the procedures we perform today would have been understood by our ancient forebears.

Hippocrates, in the fourth century BC, recommended the application of cold towels to the shaven head for prolonged bleeding. However, he also recommended nasal packing in selected cases and described the use of wool soaked in oil figs as an anterior pack. In the Middle Ages, "mummia" was used as a local application to treat epistaxis. Mummia is derived from resins that were used for embalming Egyptian mummies because they were believed to have therapeutic effects. As a prelude to contemporary management, evidence in medical literature dating back to 1760 suggests that cautery was directly applied to the bleeding vessel. Early nineteenth century medical practitioners used the idea of applying continuous pressure to the area with the use of a dried pig intestine filled with water as an intranasal balloon. In 1879, Clarke, assistant surgeon at Charing Cross Hospital in London, noted that epistaxis may depend on plethora and congestion or result from an operation or injury. He recommended elevation of the head, bathing the nose in cold water or laying a bag of ice on the forehead, and then having the patient snuff powdered matico or gall nuts. He further suggested injecting styptic solution (alum or the perchloride of iron) into the nostril and plugging it with strips of lint. For posterior plugging in cases where other measures failed, he described arming a catheter, or an elastic bougie, with a fine twine, passing it along the floor of the nose, introducing a pharyngeal forceps, and pulling one end out of the mouth. A small roll of lint was then attached and pulled through the nasal end, thus plugging the posterior nares behind the soft palate. Both ends were secured, and the plug was allowed to remain in place for 2 days.

Modified from Clarke WF: *A manual of the practice of surgery,* New York, 1879, William Wood & Co; Pothula V, Alderson D: Historical article: nothing new under the sun: the management of epistaxis, *Journal of Laryngology and Otolaryngology* 112(4):331-334, 1998.

with coagulation or posterior packing, but occasionally ligation of the ethmoid, carotid, or maxillary artery is necessary.

The basic actions to achieve proper visualization apply: the use of a headlight by the surgeon; suction to clear the operative field; and nasal specula to facilitate the initial examination. The application of a hemostatic agent is valuable because coagulation is often used for the problematic vessel. The vasoconstrictive properties of hemostatic agents diminish blood flow and make coagulation more effective. A topical agent should be considered if the anesthetic choice is conscious sedation as opposed to general anesthesia. Various types of packing can be used according to the surgeon's preference. The packing may be 1-inch gauze impregnated with antibiotic ointment, commercially manufactured nasal packing, a Foley catheter with the balloon inflated, or balloon pressure catheter tubes or stents. These have an exterior balloon along the tube length as well as an anchoring balloon on the end. The anchoring balloon is first inflated to keep the tubes in place, and then the pressure balloons are inflated to compress bleeding vessels. If packing is used, it is placed directly against the bleeding site. Posterior nasal packing is placed by inserting a red rubber catheter through the nostril; the proximal end of the catheter is pulled through the oral cavity with a Kelly clamp (while the distal end remains extending from the nostril). The strings of the posterior pack, which has been coated with antibiotic ointment, are attached to the proximal end of the catheter, and the catheter is withdrawn through the nose to position the pack in the nasal pharynx. Anterior nasal packing is placed into both nares. The posterior pack is untied from the catheter, and the strings are tied over a tonsil sponge to secure the packing.

## SINUS SURGERY

Sinusitis may be acute or chronic. It is caused by bacteria and fungi and may be associated with anatomic abnormalities of the nose, such as a deviated septum. Medical management of acute sinusitis involves a course of appropriate antibiotic therapy. If a patient does not respond to medical treatment and the symptoms persist, surgical drainage of the sinuses is necessary. Sinus procedures can be performed intranasally with or without the aid of endoscopes and video or through an open approach determined by which sinus cavity is involved. Generally, surgical treatment involves endoscopy to create a nasal window in acute maxillary sinusitis; a Caldwell-Luc procedure for chronic maxillary sinusitis; ethmoidectomy for ethmoid or sphenoidal sinusitis; and creation of an osteoplastic flap to drain the frontal sinus.

The field of ESS has expanded as surgeons' experience with it has increased and technology and instrumentation has improved. Procedures performed endoscopically decrease trauma to normal structures and reduce morbidity. Less trauma means a shortened healing process for the patient. Many procedures that were once done with an open approach are now performed endoscopically and are considered safer because they are performed under direct visualization by means of an endoscope.

The following sections are discussed with the understanding that they are more commonly performed endoscopically but may be done with an open approach as necessary.

### Endoscopic Sinus Surgery

ESS involves the endoscopic resection of inflammatory and anatomic defects of the sinuses. Because of the anatomic relationship to multiple systems, this procedure has many risks, which should be incorporated into the informed consent process[5] (Research Highlight). It is considered to be technically demanding surgery, and techniques vary significantly. It is also referred to as *functional endoscopic sinus surgery* (FESS) because it provides a more physiologic type of drainage by reducing trauma to normal tissues. It is performed using direct endoscopic visualization. Many surgeons prefer the endoscope to be attached to a video monitor as in many other endoscopic procedures, but some prefer to look directly through the eyepiece. The operative instruments are introduced into the nose alongside the endoscope.

The purpose of ESS is to ensure adequate ventilation and restore mucociliary clearance in the sinuses. If there is contact between the mucosa and the sinus, mucociliary clearance is inhibited and secretions are retained in the sinus. This predisposes the patient to sinus infections.

Sinusitis can be either recurrent acute or chronic. Chronic sinusitis can be caused by anatomic deformities that require correction. Often the patient will first require a septoplasty to correct a deviated septum and allow access to the sinuses. Chronic sinusitis can also be caused by an allergy history, and contributing factors may include immunologic abnormalities, fluctuations in hormones, and environmental factors. Patients who are considered candidates for ESS undergo an office endo-

#### RESEARCH HIGHLIGHT

**Communicating Risks of FESS During the Informed Consent Process**

Functional endoscopic sinus surgery (FESS) is one of the most common surgical procedures performed by otolaryngologists in the United States. Because the anatomic relationship of the sinus subjects the patient to potential risks, patients must have the information to make informed decisions about their care. The purpose of this study was to analyze how otolaryngologists define the material risks of FESS and to identify what practicing surgeons are communicating as material risks to patients during the informed consent process. The study defines informed consent as "the process of explaining a procedure and its risks, benefits and alternative treatments before instituting therapy." In the United States the requirements for informed consent are controlled at the state level. The following method was employed. Surveys were mailed to 1000 members of the American Academy of Otolaryngology–Head and Neck Surgery. The sample was taken from a list of members that was divided into six regions by geography; 166 members were selected randomly from each region. Three hundred forty-six surveys were returned, eleven of which were not valid. About 1% of respondents thought that a 1% incidence of a complication warrants that it be included in the informed consent process. Nineteen percent of respondents used their own experience when informing patients about the risks of surgery, 37.5% used published data, and 35% used both. Whereas countries such as Great Britain have numeric standards for including incidence of risks and complications in the consent process, there are no such standards in the United States. The study also demonstrated variability in the potential complications that are discussed by surgeons. As a result of their research, the authors recommend creation of a more standardized consent to enhance communication and appropriate communication of significant risks.

Modified from Wolf J and others: Informed consent in functional endoscopic sinus surgery, *Laryngoscope* 112:774-777, 2002.

scopic examination preoperatively when none of the sinus cavities are opened but merely explored for diagnostic purposes. Patients also have a preoperative computed tomography (CT) scan to determine the specific areas affected by the sinusitis. These CT scans should be available in the OR and will be referred to by the surgeon during the surgery (Figure 20-8).

***Procedural Considerations.*** ESS instruments enable the surgeon to view the patient's anatomy as well as to remove diseased or problematic tissues that are interfering with the sinus cavity functioning and drainage processes. The surgery can be performed with the patient under general anesthesia or MAC, depending on the surgeon's and patient's preference.

The endoscopes used in sinus surgery are much like endoscopes used in other procedures. They are 4 to 5 mm in diameter and have different directions of view: 0, 30, 70, 90, or 120 degrees. Depending on which sinus the surgeon is planning to work in, the appropriate lens will be requested. Often if work is to be done in several sinus cavities, the surgeon may change lenses intraoperatively to obtain the optimal view in each cavity.

The setup for ESS is the same as the setup for nasal surgery in terms of prepping, draping, and positioning. The instruments required are the basic nasal set, video equipment including monitor, and light source with the appropriate light cord adapted to the type of endoscope used. In addition to endoscopes, other instruments that may be used in ESS include endoscopic suction tips and suction elevators, biopsy forceps, forceps for retracting and cutting/excising tissue, and scissors.

The room setup is described for nasal procedures and includes the video equipment, which is located at the head of the bed. The surgeon operates from the right side of the patient and may sit during the procedure. If so, the surgeon's legs must be able to fit under the OR bed at the level of the patient's neck; to prevent fatigue, the surgeon's elbows may rest on the armrest of the chair or on a table placed nearby.

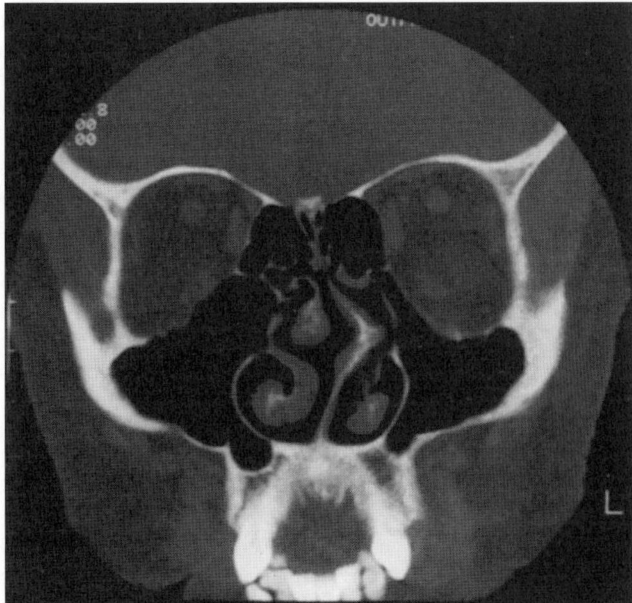

FIGURE 20-8 Computed tomography (CT) scan of maxillary and ethmoid sinuses. Note septal deviation, maxillary sinus ostia, turbinates, and ocular muscles.

To avoid possible injury, instruments should be passed to the surgeon in the closed position and never over the patient's face. They should be passed smoothly and carefully so that the surgeon's eyes do not leave the endoscope or video monitor and to limit distractions. Some surgeons will request a suction-irrigation device that provides visualization of the sinus recesses by allowing simultaneous suction and irrigation of the operative field.

An antifog solution can be used to treat the lens of the endoscope. The solution should not be wiped off the lens; it should be left on in a thin layer.

Another consideration that is crucial to a successful outcome in ESS is to maintain the integrity of the patient's periorbital cavities. The patient's eyes must be visible to the surgeon at all times to avoid injury to the orbit or to immediately recognize injury if it occurs. The surgeon will monitor for movement of the eyeball or appearance of an intraorbital hematoma.

Encroachment of the orbit can be recognized if yellow tissue is seen because orbital fat is yellow in color. This finding should be communicated immediately to the surgeon. Another good technique is for the scrub person to place all tissue removed by the surgeon into a small labeled container of normal saline or lactated Ringer's solution on the surgical field. If any of the tissue "floats," the surgeon should be notified immediately. The surgeon will push the tissue in question with an instrument and rotate it a few times to release any small air bubbles that may be trapped in it, which could be causing it to float. If this is the case, the tissue will then sink to the bottom of the container and be considered diseased tissue which needs to be removed. However, any tissue that continues to float naturally is presumed to be fat or brain tissue. In this case, it is presumed that the orbit has been encroached, and the situation is treated as a potentially serious complication.

### Operative Procedure

1. The surgeon applies topical anesthetic and administers the local anesthesia.
2. The lens of the endoscope is treated with antifog solution before the endoscope is introduced into the nose.
3. The natural ostium of the maxillary sinus is enlarged to provide physiologic drainage through the middle meatus (see Figure 20-3).
4. The diseased tissue is visualized through the endoscope, and straight or angled forceps are used to remove it (Figure 20-9).
5. If an anterior ethmoidectomy is indicated, the endoscope is inserted into the ostial meatal complex and the ethmoidectomy is performed.
6. Because of the small incision made, no sutures are required.
7. Absorbable gelatin film may or may not be placed into the patient's middle meatus to maintain patency and reduce stenosis (Research Highlight). If used, it is rolled into a cylindric splint and set in place with bayonet forceps. An antibiotic ointment may be applied to the splint first, according to the surgeon's preference. The gel splints dissolve gradually, or they may be removed with irrigation.
8. A mustache dressing is applied.

## Computer-Assisted Endoscopic Sinus Surgery

Before the introduction of computer-assisted ESS, surgeons could rely only on direct visualization of the actual operative field, which they combined with their previous surgical experience and their own ability to mentally translate data from the

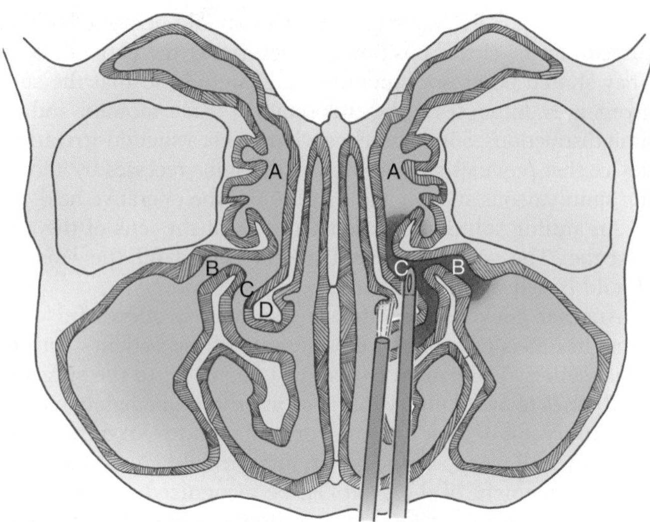


**FIGURE 20-9** Surgery is performed using endoscope and forceps by intranasal approach. Diseased tissue is being removed from shaded areas depicting ethmoid sinus area *(A)*, maxillary sinus ostia *(B)*, and middle meatus *(C)*. *(D)*, Middle turbinate is unaffected.

## RESEARCH HIGHLIGHT

### The Use of Packing or Local Hemostatic Agents in Endoscopic Sinus Surgery

This study was aimed at evaluating the routine use of packing or local hemostatic agents in endoscopic sinus surgery (ESS). Chronic rhinosinusitis is one of the most common health problems in Western countries. ESS has replaced conventional surgical procedures because of its higher success rate; low incidence of complications; and advances in instruments, technology, and imaging. One hundred consecutive patients were analyzed. Three patients were eliminated from the cohort, leaving 97 patients, male and female, aged 16 to 86 years, with varying medical histories. Fifty-six percent of procedures were conducted with the patient under general anesthesia, and 44% were done with local anesthesia (no image-guided navigation system). No patient under local anesthesia had to be converted to general anesthesia. Blood loss was less than 30 ml in 85% of patients, and packing or a hemostatic agent was not used in 92% of patients. No cases of postoperative bleeding complications occurred, and no "no-packing" patient required packing between the end of the procedure and discharge. Packing is commonly used in conjunction with these procedures, and patients often report the removal of packing to be more stressful than the initial surgery. Procedures in this study were completed utilizing usual operating techniques with no additional measures taken to minimize bleeding. The results of the study supported the results of a previous study by the same investigators stating that most ESS procedures can be managed without packing or other hemostatic agents. Local anesthesia, application of local vasoconstrictors, and careful operative techniques minimize the need for packing, thus reducing patient discomfort, postoperative complications, and cost of surgery.

Modified from Eliashar R and others: Packing in endoscopic sinus surgery: is it really required? *Otolaryngology—Head and Neck Surgery* 134:276-279, 2006.

patient's two-dimensional CT scan to determine their location within the patient's sinuses. Computer-assisted ESS combines the use of computerized planning tools and intraoperative navigation systems with endoscopic techniques. The operative field is more clearly defined and the patient's risk of surgical complications is reduced compared with such surgery without the aid of a computer.

With the use of a navigational system, the surgical procedure can also be viewed on a computer monitor by the rest of the surgical team. Attending surgeons are able to "supervise" the resident during the procedure because they can see exactly where the instruments are positioned in the sinuses and provide direction as indicated. It is also very helpful for the nursing staff to be able to follow the progress of the procedure.

Navigational systems are especially useful in revision sinus surgery, in which the familiar anatomy of the sinuses has been altered by previous surgery and the typical landmarks of the sinuses are now changed. Unfortunately, because of the nature of sinus disease itself in terms of allergic tendencies and mucous membrane irritation that are often chronic conditions, sinus disease can recur. Some patients may decide that their symptoms have recurred to the troublesome point where they elect to come in for surgery more than once. From a safety standpoint and to reduce the risk of a revision surgery, many surgeons will not attempt a revision sinus procedure without having an image-guided system available.

Several navigational systems are available, and many of these systems have applications for different types of surgeries, so the initial expense of the machine itself can be defrayed if it is shared with different surgical specialties, such as neurosurgery. Also, technical components to facilitating this type of sinus surgery must be mastered by the perioperative nursing staff, who must develop competence in system setup, transfer of the CT scan data into the system, and maintenance procedures.

## Microdebriders

The introduction of powered instrumentation in FESS further enhanced this highly effective surgical treatment of chronic sinusitis. The microdebrider is a powered instrument that functions much like an arthroscopic joint shaver (see Chapter 22) but is much smaller. It consists of a powered rotary shaving device whose mechanism is to pull tissue (whether it is blood, bone, or soft tissue) through a small window by means of suction and then remove the tissue with internal rotating blades. The tissue is removed from the instrument through the suction tubing attached at the end; therefore the working instrument does not have to be removed from the operative field to clear the tissue. Microdebriders are used in extensive bony dissection of the sinuses. They can be used in various sinus procedures, including ethmoidectomy, maxillary antrostomy, sphenoidotomy, and frontal recess dissections. The internal rotating blades are disposable and come in many sizes and varieties of cutting edges depending on what area of the sinus is involved and what type of tissue is being removed (burrs are good for diseased bony tissue while cutting edges are helpful to morcelate a polyp). Many models of microdebriders have continuous irrigation lines that help decrease clogging of the lines as the diseased sinus tissue can be thick and will obstruct the small bores of the blades.

Microdebriders facilitate greater surgical precision by increasing the visual field. The patient's postoperative recovery time is shortened because of decreased trauma to the tissues as a result of reduced bleeding.

Several rhinologic and sinus procedures may be accomplished by either internal (with or without endoscopic assistance) or external approaches. The following procedures fit into this category.

## Frontal Sinus Trephination

Frontal sinus trephination is the creation of a hole in the frontal sinus to drain pus or fluid accumulation. It is performed to treat the signs and symptoms of frontal sinusitis, which may include fever and headaches. A catheter may be surgically sewn into place at the incision site of the opening made into the affected frontal sinus; this serves as a drain and medium with which to irrigate the sinus until the disease resolves.

***Procedural Considerations.*** The patient's face is prepped according to the surgeon's preference. The head is draped as in nasal procedures. Local anesthesia may be injected in the skin under the eyebrow. Culture tubes should be available as should drainage catheters.

### *Operative Procedure*

1. The incision is made medially below the eyebrow, along the same contour of the brow (Figure 20-10).
2. The periosteum is elevated from the bone, and a small diamond or cutting burr is used to drill a hole into the sinus.
3. Cultures may be taken of any pus present in the sinus, followed by irrigation.
4. A large Silastic or Teflon tube or appropriate-size catheter may be placed through the incision into the sinus.
5. The incision is closed with suture of the surgeon's preference.
6. A small dressing is usually applied to absorb drainage from the incision and catheter.

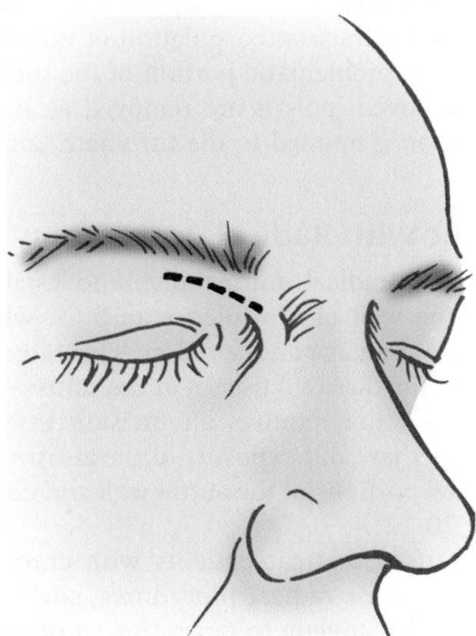

**FIGURE 20-10** Incision to expose ethmoidal and frontal sinuses. Resulting scar is almost invisible.

## Frontal Sinus Operation (External Approach)—Trephination and Obliteration

A frontal sinus operation involves making an incision through the anterior wall of the floor of the frontal sinus for removal of diseased tissue, cleansing the sinus cavity, and drainage. In acute frontal sinusitis, patients experience persistent headaches and edema of the upper eyelid. As with other types of sinus problems, when conservative medical management of these symptoms fails, surgical treatment may be indicated. Drainage of the frontal sinus may be achieved through a simple frontal sinus trephination alone. If chronic suppuration with repeated acute attacks of frontal sinusitis persists, further surgery may be performed to remove the diseased lining of the sinus and reconstruct the nasofrontal duct to provide the necessary drainage.

***Procedural Considerations.*** The setup is as for nasal surgery with the addition of a power saw with oscillating blade, frontal rasps, blunt nerve hook, straight fine Cushing forceps, Adson tissue forceps, dural hooks, and Raney clip appliers and clips.

General anesthesia is used. The surgical approach depends on the preference of the surgeon and the patient. If a coronal incision is to be made, the hair should be shaved from the hairline to slightly past the crown of the head. If a brow incision is to be made, no shaving is necessary. Fat may be harvested from the abdomen for subsequent use in obliterating the sinus space.

The patient's eyes are protected during the procedure, and the head and face are prepped according to the surgeon's preference.

### *Operative Procedure*

1. a. When a coronal approach is used, the incision is made in the scalp skin from ear to ear, well behind the hairline. The edges of the skin are compressed by the application of Raney clips. The flap is reflected to expose the upper portion of the nose, thus exposing the anterior sinus.
   b. When a brow approach is used, the incision is made in the superior margin of the eyebrow or eyebrows, hemostasis is obtained, and the flap is elevated to expose the anterior sinus wall.
2. A template (steam-sterilized radiologic outline of the frontal sinus) is placed over the sinus and marked on the pericranium with a marking pen.
3. The pericranium is elevated.
4. An oscillating saw is used to cut through the overlying frontal sinus. An elevator may be used to free the bone from the sinus.
5. The mucosa of the sinus is removed in its entirety through the use of elevators and a drill.
6. Absorbable gelatin sponge or a fat graft taken from the abdomen is placed in the sinus to obliterate the space.
7. The bone flap is replaced, and the pericranium is repositioned and sutured.
8. The skin incision is closed with suture of the surgeon's preference.
9. A pressure dressing of elastic gauze is applied for 48 to 72 hours.

Potential postoperative complications include osteomyelitis, meningitis, cerebrospinal fluid leak, abscess, and stenosis of the nasofrontal duct.

## Ethmoidectomy

Ethmoid sinus surgery is usually performed to treat chronic inflammatory sinus disease or polyps that are caused by allergies. An ethmoidectomy is the removal of the diseased portion of the middle turbinate, ethmoid cells, and diseased tissue in the nasal fossa, reducing the many-celled ethmoid labyrinth into one large cavity to ensure adequate drainage and aeration. It can be accomplished by three approaches: intranasal (the endoscopic approach is most common), external, or transantral.

***Procedural Considerations and Operative Procedure.*** The setup for the intranasal approach is the same as that for a nasal setup, along with endoscopic sinus equipment. The external approach is as described for frontal sinus trephination. The transantral approach is described in the Caldwell-Luc procedure presented below.

## Sphenoidotomy

A sphenoidotomy is the creation of an opening into one or both of the sphenoidal sinuses. It can be performed by either the intranasal route or through an external approach as described for the frontal sinus operation. Sphenoidotomies are often done with ethmoidectomies because once the ethmoid labyrinth is removed, the surgeon has excellent access to the sphenoidal sinuses. These procedures are typically done endoscopically.

***Procedural Considerations and Operative Procedure.*** For the intranasal route, the setup and operative procedure are as described for intranasal surgery, often with endoscopic sinus equipment. Additional instruments that may be required are long sphenoid curettes, antrum rasps, and antrum punches. The external approach is as described for frontal sinus surgery.

## Nasal Polypectomy

A nasal polypectomy is the removal of polyps from the nasal cavity (Figure 20-11). Nasal polyps are benign grapelike clusters of mucous membrane and connective tissue. When the polyps become large, they obstruct the free passage of air, make breathing difficult, and also cause a change in speech quality. Nasal polypectomies are often performed with other sinus procedures that also require removal of diseased tissue and are done endoscopically. Because of the viscous nature of polyps, microdebriders are particularly helpful in these cases as they can greatly shorten surgical time by their mechanism of morcelating the polyp and removing it by immediate suctioning while controlling bleeding as opposed to each polyp being manually extracted with an instrument in small pieces.

***Procedural Considerations and Operative Procedure.*** Nasal polypectomy setup is as for any intranasal procedure, with the addition of endoscopic equipment. Additional instruments may include a nasal polyp snare if a microdebrider is not used. Packing is according to the surgeon's preference.

## Turbinectomy and Outfracture Coagulation of Turbinates

*Anterior inferior turbinectomy* is removal of the anterior end of the inferior turbinate. *Inferior turbinectomy* is removal of the greater part of the lower border of the hypertrophied inferior turbinate. *Anterior middle turbinectomy* is removal of the anterior end of the middle turbinate body. In all cases, turbinectomy may include removal of any existing nasal polyps. Turbinectomies are often performed endoscopically with other sinus procedures.

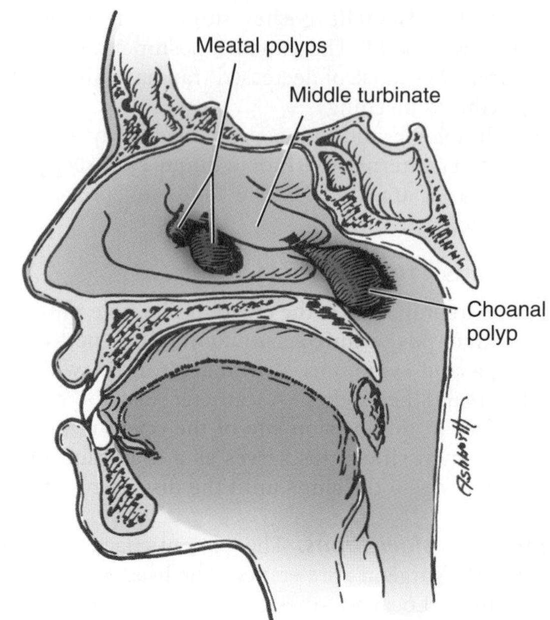


FIGURE 20-11 Nasal polyps. A choanal polyp is usually single and originates in maxillary sinus; however, most polyps are found in middle meatus.

Outfracture of the turbinates is similar to turbinectomy except that the turbinate is infractured and then outfractured by the use of a septal displacer or Boies elevator. A turbinate needle designed to deliver unipolar electrocoagulation may be used on the turbinate to reduce the potential for recurring hypertrophy. These procedures are performed to provide adequate ventilation and drainage as well as to relieve pressure against the floor of the nose.

***Procedural Considerations and Operative Procedure.*** Turbinectomies and outfracture coagulation of turbinates require a nasal setup. The problematic portion of the turbinate is amputated and removed, polyps are removed as indicated, and electrocoagulation is applied to the turbinates after fracturing is completed.

## Caldwell-Luc with Radical Antrostomy

The purpose of a radical antrostomy is to establish a large opening into the wall of the inferior meatus, which ensures adequate gravity drainage and aeration. This large opening allows removal of the diseased tissues in the sinuses under direct vision. The procedure requires an incision into the canine fossa of the upper jaw and exposure of the antrum for removal of bony diseased portions of the antral wall and contents of the sinus (Figure 20-12).

ESS can be used to treat patients with chronic sinusitis, obviating the need for radical procedures, such as Caldwell-Luc. ESS allows the surgeon to target the ostiomeatal complex (OMC) in the anterior ethmoid sinus region, where thickened and diseased tissue often blocks the OMC. Obstruction in this

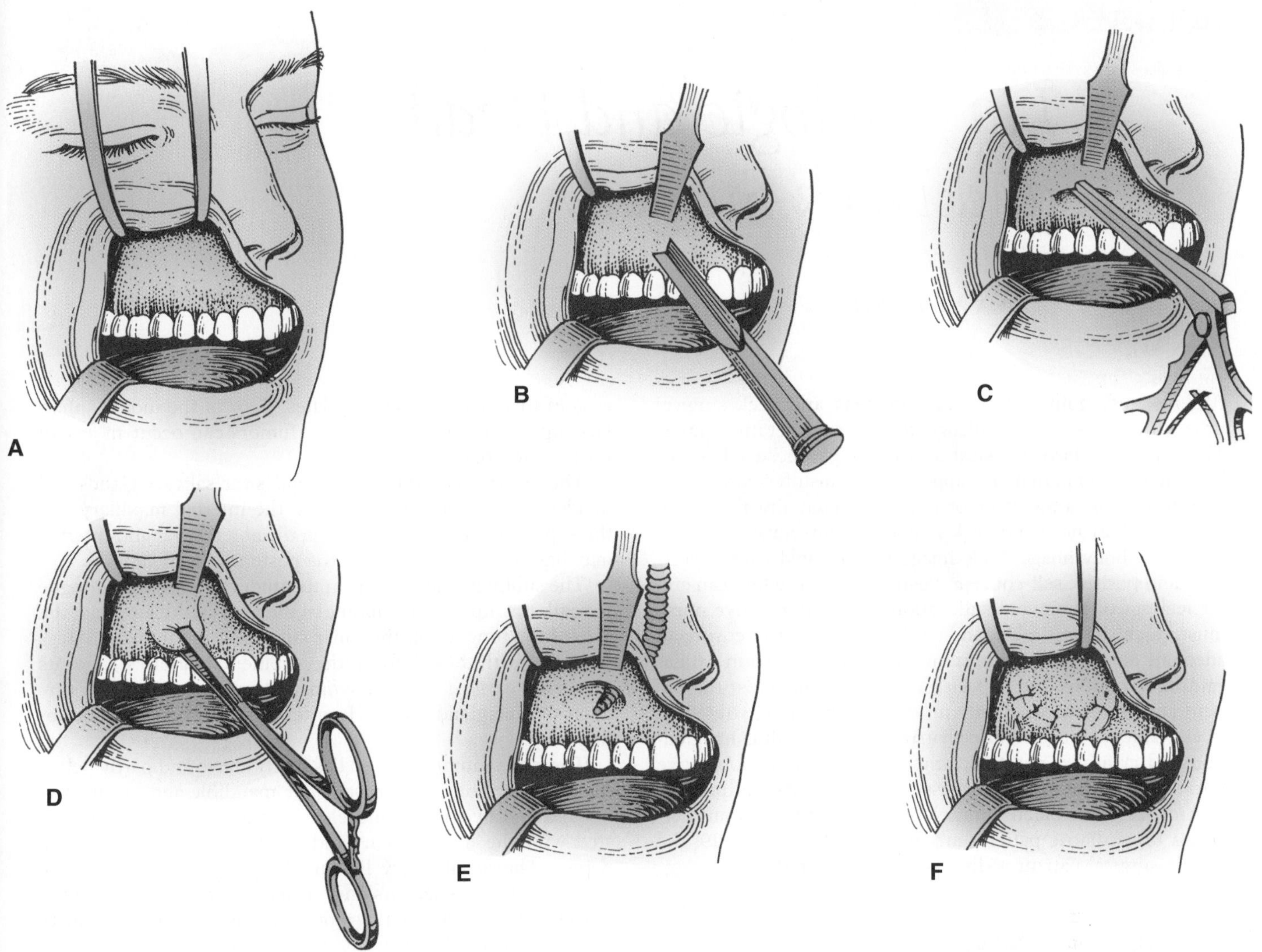


**FIGURE 20-12** Caldwell-Luc operation. **A,** Incision. **B,** Flap retracted and perforation made in canine fossa. **C,** Perforation enlarged with Kerrison rongeur. **D,** Removal of diseased antral membrane. **E,** Rasp used to make nasoantral window. **F,** Incision closed.

area leads to subsequent infection in the maxillary, frontal, and sphenoidal sinuses. ESS permits removal of only the diseased tissue; recovery is more rapid, with minimal and usually temporary effects on the patient's appearance.

## REFERENCES


1. Association of periOperative Registered Nurses: *AORN standards, recommended practices, and guidelines,* Denver, 2006, The Association.
2. Brancato VC: Improving nurse-physician collaboration, *The Pennsylvania Nurse* 60(1):23, 2005.
3. Burns JL, Blackwell SJ: Plastic surgery. In Townsend CM and others: *Sabiston textbook of surgery,* ed 17, Philadelphia, 2004, Saunders.
4. Canobbio MM: *Mosby's handbook of patient teaching,* ed 3, St Louis, 2006, Mosby.
5. Harkreader H, Hogan MA: *Fundamentals of nursing—caring and clinical judgment,* ed 2, St Louis, 2004, Saunders.
6. Hawke M: A potpourri of pain relief, *Nursing Spectrum* 15(2):10-11, 2005.
7. Herlihy B, Maebius NK: *The human body in health and illness,* ed 2, St Louis, 2003, Saunders.
8. Lilley LL and others: *Pharmacology and the nursing process,* ed 4, St Louis, 2005, Mosby.
9. Manojlovich M: Linking the practice environment to nurses' job satisfaction through nurse-physician communication, *Journal of Nursing Scholarship* 37(4):367-373, 2005.
10. Pasero C, McCaffery M: Pain control: comfort-function goals, *American Journal of Nursing* 104(9):77-81, 2004.
11. Potter PA, Perry AG: *Fundamentals of nursing,* ed 6, St Louis, 2005, Mosby.
12. Workman ML: Interventions for clients with noninfectious upper respiratory problems. In Ignatavicius DD, Workman ML, editors: *Medical-surgical nursing: critical thinking for collaborative care,* ed 5, St Louis, 2006, Saunders.
13. Ziolkowski L, Strzyzewski N: Perianesthesia assessment: foundation of care, *Journal of PeriAnesthesia Nursing* 16(6):359-370, 2001.

CHAPTER 21

# Laryngologic and Head and Neck Surgery

DONNA R. McEWEN

Patients undergoing laryngologic or head and neck surgical procedures present a challenge to the perioperative nurse. These patients have physical as well as psychosocial needs. They may be experiencing upper airway insufficiency on arrival in the operating room or have an altered airway postoperatively. Many head and neck surgery patients must cope with an altered body image. Body image is associated with appearance and positive self-concept. Postoperative bleeding can create feelings of panic and suffocation. The perioperative nurse must quickly assess, plan, and implement actions to ensure an adequate airway as well as reassure the patient, explain patient care interventions and expected outcomes, and assist the patient and the patient's family in identifying coping strategies. These patients range from pediatric to geriatric; thus imagination and creativity are vital components of the perioperative nurse's armamentarium in assessing the patient's comprehension of the anticipated surgical procedure. Special considerations for pediatric patients are discussed in Chapter 29; the elderly surgical patient is discussed in Chapter 30.

## Surgical Anatomy

The throat includes the structures of the neck in front of the vertebral column; these are the mouth, tongue, pharynx, tonsils, larynx, and trachea.

### Oral Cavity

The mouth is formed by the cheeks, the hard palate, the soft palate, and the tongue. It extends from the lips to the anterior pillars of the throat. The portion of the mouth outside the teeth is the buccal cavity, and that on the inner side of the teeth is the lingual cavity. The hard palate and the soft palate form the upper and posterior boundaries of the oral cavity. The hard palate is formed by the maxilla and palatine bones. The soft palate is an arch-shaped muscular partition between the oropharynx and the nasopharynx. The soft palate emerges from the posterior border of the hard palate to form the uvula, a fingerlike, movable projection. The uvula joins the base of the tongue anteriorly and the pharynx posteriorly.

***Salivary Glands.*** The salivary glands consist of three paired glands: the sublingual, the submandibular, and the parotid. They communicate with the mouth and produce saliva, which serves to moisten the mouth and initiate digestion of carbohydrates. The salivary glands consist of tissues found in the mucosa of the cheeks, tongue, palates, floor of the mouth, pharynx, lips, and paranasal sinuses. Tumors can occur in any of these structures.

The external carotid artery supplies the salivary glands and divides into its terminal branches: the internal maxillary and the superficial temporal. The superficial temporal and internal maxillary veins unite to form the posterior facial vein.

The sublingual gland lies on the undersurface of the tongue beneath the mucous membrane in the floor of the mouth at the side of the tongue, on the inner surface of the mandible. It is supplied with blood from the submental arteries, and its nerves are derived from the sympathetic nerves. The many tiny ducts of each gland separately enter the oral cavity on the sublingual fold.

The submandibular gland lies partly above and partly below the posterior half of the base of the mandible and on the mylohyoid and hyoglossus muscles. This gland is closely associated with the lingual veins and the lingual and hypoglossal nerves. The facial artery lies on the posterior border of the gland. Its duct (Wharton's duct) runs superficially beneath the mucosa of the floor of the mouth and enters the oral cavity behind the central incisors.

The parotid gland, the largest of the salivary glands, lies below the zygomatic arch in front of the mastoid process and behind the ramus of the mandible. This gland is enclosed in fascia, attached to surrounding muscles, and divided into two parts—a superficial and a deep portion—by means of the facial nerve. The parotid duct (Stensen's duct) pierces the buccal pad of fat and the buccinator muscle, finally opening into the oral cavity opposite the crown of the upper second molar tooth. The superficial temporal artery and small branches of the external carotid artery arise in the parotid gland behind the neck of the mandible. Because of the facial nerve's location, injury to it is a risk from any surgical procedure involving the parotid gland area.

### Pharynx

The pharynx, extending from the posterior portion of the nose to the esophagus and larynx, serves as a channel for both the digestive and respiratory systems. Approximately 13 cm long, it lies anterior to the cervical vertebrae and posterior to the nasal and oral cavities. The food and air passages cross each other in the pharynx, a funnel-shaped structure that is wider above and narrower below. It is composed of muscular and fibrous layers and is lined with mucous membrane. It is associated above with the sphenoidal sinus and the basilar part of the occipital bone, and it joins the esophagus below. Seven cavities communicate with the pharynx: the two nasal cavities, the two tympanic cavities, the mouth, the larynx, and the esophagus. Infection can spread from the pharynx to the middle ear through the eustachian tube. The pharynx comprises three groups of constrictor muscles. Each muscle fits within the one below, and each inserts posteriorly in the median line with its mate from the opposite side. The constrictor muscles provide constriction of the pharynx for swallowing. Between the origins of the constrictor muscle groups are so-called *intervals,* through which ligaments, nerves, and arteries pass. The recurrent laryngeal nerve is closely associated with the lower portion of the pharynx. The pharynx is divided anatomically into three sections: the nasopharynx, the oropharynx, and the hypopharynx.

***Nasopharynx.*** The nasopharynx lies posterior to the nasal cavity and extends over the soft palate. It communicates with the oropharynx through the pharyngeal isthmus, which is closed by muscular action during swallowing.

***Oropharynx.*** The oropharynx lies posterior to the oral cavity and extends from the soft palate to the level of the hyoid bone. The tonsils are situated one on each side of the oropharynx, lodged in a tonsillar fossa that is attached to folds of membrane-containing muscle. One pair, the palatine tonsils (a pair of oval structures), are the only lymphatic organs covered with stratified squamous epithelium. These tonsils may become inflamed (tonsillitis). The lateral surface of each tonsil is usually covered with a fibrous capsule. The anterior and posterior tonsillar pillars join to form a triangular fossa, with the posterior lateral aspects of the tongue at its base. The lingual tonsils are lodged in each fossa. The adenoids, or pharyngeal tonsils, are suspended from the roof of the nasopharynx and consist of an accumulation of lymphoid tissue.

The arteries of the tonsils enter the upper and lower poles. The tonsils are supplied with blood by tonsillar branches of the ascending palatine branch of the facial artery (branch of the external carotid artery). The external carotid artery on each side lies behind and lateral to each tonsil. The nerves supplying the tonsils are derived from the middle and posterior palatine branches of the maxillary and glossopharyngeal nerves.

***Hypopharynx.*** The hypopharynx extends from the hyoid bone and empties into the esophagus posteriorly and the larynx anteriorly.

## Larynx and Associated Structures

***Larynx.*** The larynx lies in the midline of the neck and is supported by cartilage. It is situated between the trachea and the root of the tongue, at the upper front part of the neck. The location of the larynx between the gastrointestinal (GI) and respiratory systems is strategic in protecting the airway during swallowing and breathing. The larynx has three main functions: as a passageway for air, as a valve for closing off air passages from the digestive system and the pharynx, and as a voice box on which sound and speech depend to a degree.

The larynx is a cartilaginous box situated in front of the fourth, fifth, and sixth cervical vertebrae. The upper portion of the larynx is continuous with the pharynx above, and its lower portion joins the trachea. The skeletal structure provides for patency of the enclosed airway. The complex muscle action and arrangement of tissues within the structure provide for closure of the lumen for protection against trauma and entrance of foreign bodies and for speech.

***Laryngeal Cartilages.*** The skeletal framework of the larynx consists of cartilages and membranes. Of the nine separate cartilages, three are single and six are arranged in pairs. The main cartilages of the larynx include the thyroid, the cricoid, the epiglottis, two arytenoid, two corniculate, and two cuneiform. The thyroid cartilage, or Adam's apple, forms the anterior portion of the voice box. The cricoid cartilage is a complete cartilaginous ring that resembles a signet ring and rests beneath the thyroid cartilage and supports the airway (Figure 21-1). The epiglottis is a slightly curled, leaf-shaped, elastic, fibrous membrane. It is prolonged below into a slender process, attached in the midline to the upper border of the thyroid cartilage. The epiglottis helps to protect the larynx during deglutition. When the cricothyroid muscle contracts, it pulls the thyroid cartilage and the cricoid cartilage, thereby tightening the vocal cords and, if unopposed, closing the glottis. The arytenoid cartilages, which rest above the signet-ring portion of the cricoid cartilage, support the posterior portion of the true vocal cords.

***Laryngeal Ligaments.*** The extrinsic ligaments of the larynx are those connecting (1) the thyroid cartilage and epiglottis with the hyoid bone and (2) the cricoid cartilage with the trachea (Figure 21-2). The intrinsic ligaments of the larynx are those connecting several cartilages of the organ to each other. They are considered the elastic membrane of the larynx.

The mucous lining of the larynx blends with fibrous tissue to form two folds on each side of the larynx. The upper set is known as the *false cords.* The lower set is called the *true vocal cords* because they are concerned primarily with the speaking voice and protection of the lower respiratory channels against the invasion of food and foreign bodies. The region of the larynx at the true vocal cord level is called the *glottis,* a triangular space between the vocal cords. During swallowing, the rising action of the muscular larynx, the closure of the glottis, and the doorlike action of the epiglottis all serve to guide food and fluid into the esophagus.

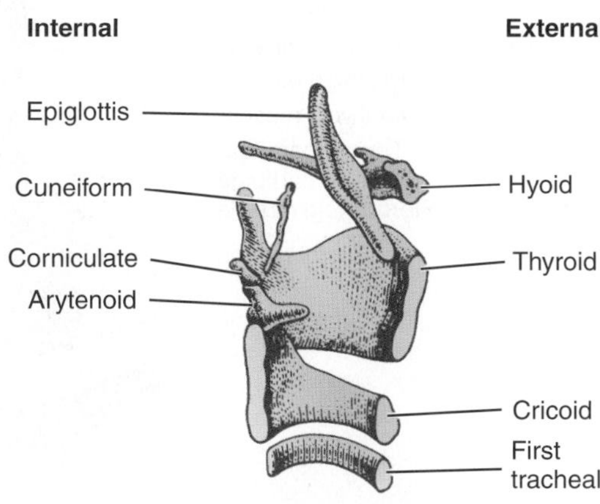


**FIGURE 21-1** Skeletal framework of larynx.

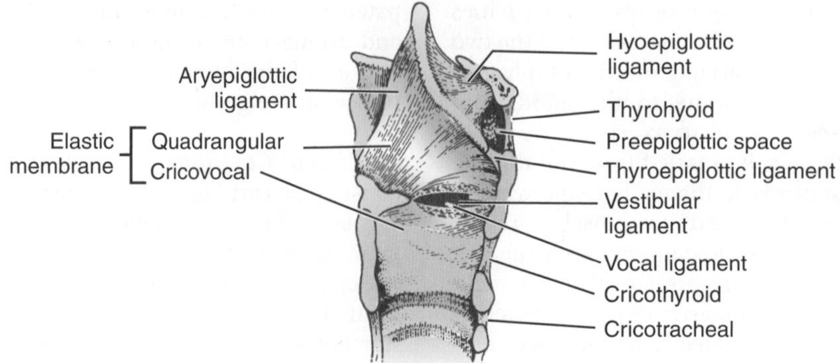


**FIGURE 21-2** Ligaments of larynx.

***Laryngeal Muscles.*** The laryngeal muscles perform two distinct functions: the extrinsic muscles (Figure 21-3) regulate the degree of tension on the vocal cords, and the intrinsic muscles open and close the glottis. The spoken voice also depends on the sphincter action of the soft palate, tongue, and lips. The muscle action of the larynx permits the glottis to close either voluntarily or involuntarily by reflex action. The closure of the inlet by this mechanism protects the respiratory passages. The closure of the glottis and the action of the vocal cords are precisely coordinated to produce the voice. The recurrent laryngeal nerve branch of the vagus is the important motor nerve of the intrinsic muscles of the larynx. The sensory nerve, which is derived from the branches of the superior laryngeal nerve, supplies the mucous membrane of the larynx. The larynx derives its blood supply from the branches of the external carotid and the subclavian arteries.

***Trachea.*** The trachea, a cartilaginous tube about 15 cm in length and 2 to 2.5 cm in diameter, begins in the neck and extends from the lower part of the larynx, on a level with the sixth cervical vertebra, to the upper border of the fifth thoracic vertebra. The tube descends anteriorly to the esophagus, enters the superior mediastinum, and divides into right and left main bronchi. The trachea is composed of a series of C-shaped rings of hyaline cartilage. The posterior surface of the trachea is flattened rather than round because the cartilaginous rings are incomplete. The carina is a ridge on the inside of the bifurcation of the trachea. It is a landmark during bronchoscopy and separates the upper end of the right main branches from the upper end of the left main branches of the bronchi. The carina is heavily innervated and can produce severe bronchospasm and coughing when stimulated. Branches from the arch of the aorta—the brachiocephalic (innominate) and left common carotid arteries—are in close relation to the trachea. The cervical portion of the trachea is related anteriorly to the sternohyoid and sternothyroid muscles and to the isthmus of the thyroid gland.

## General Structures of the Neck

A layer of deep cervical fascia surrounds the neck like a collar and is attached to the trapezius and sternocleidomastoid muscles. The sternocleidomastoid muscle extends from the

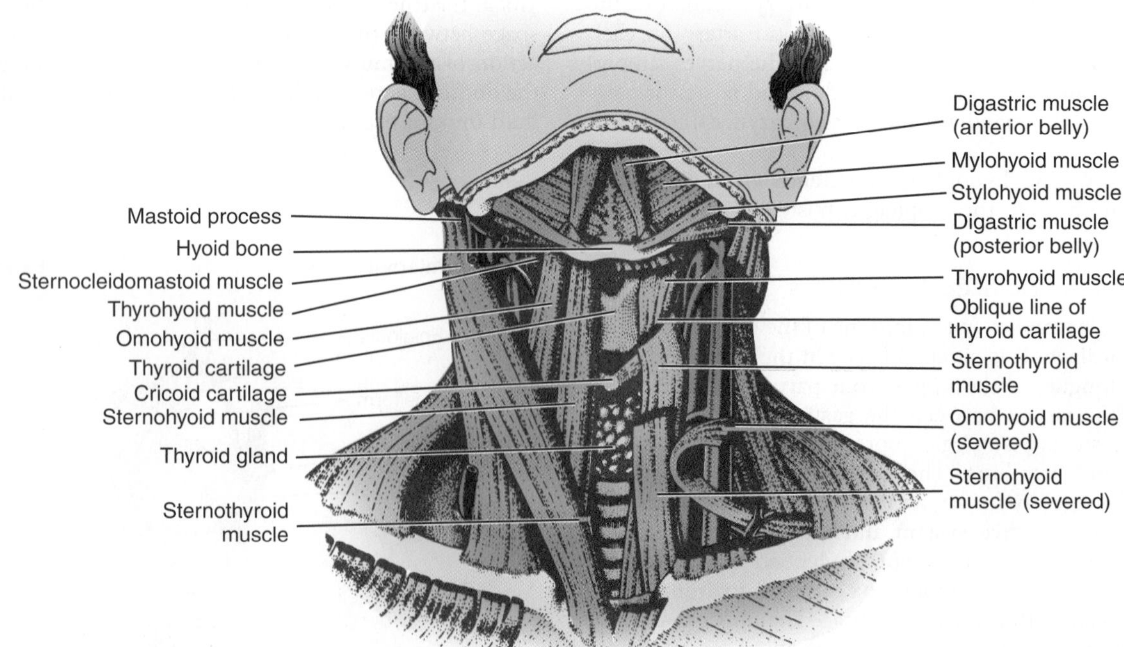


**FIGURE 21-3** Extrinsic muscles of larynx.

upper part of the sternum and medial third of the clavicle to the mastoid process. The trapezius muscle extends from the scapula, the lateral third of the clavicle, and the vertebrae to the occipital prominence. The relationship of these muscles to each other and to the adjacent bone creates triangles used as anatomic landmarks.

The pretracheal fascia of the neck lies deep in the strap muscles (sternothyroid, sternohyoid, and omohyoid) and partially encloses the thyroid gland, trachea, and larynx. The pretracheal fascia is pierced by the thyroid vessels. It fuses with the front of the carotid sheath on the deep surface of the sternocleidomastoid muscle. The carotid sheath consists of a network of areolar tissue surrounding the carotid arteries and vagus nerve.

Laterally the carotid sheath is fused with the fascia on the deep surface of the sternocleidomastoid muscle; anteriorly it is fused with the middle cervical fascia along the lateral border of the sternothyroid muscle. Lying between the floor and roof of this triangular formation of muscles are the lymph glands and the accessory nerve. Arteries and nerves traverse and pierce this triangle.

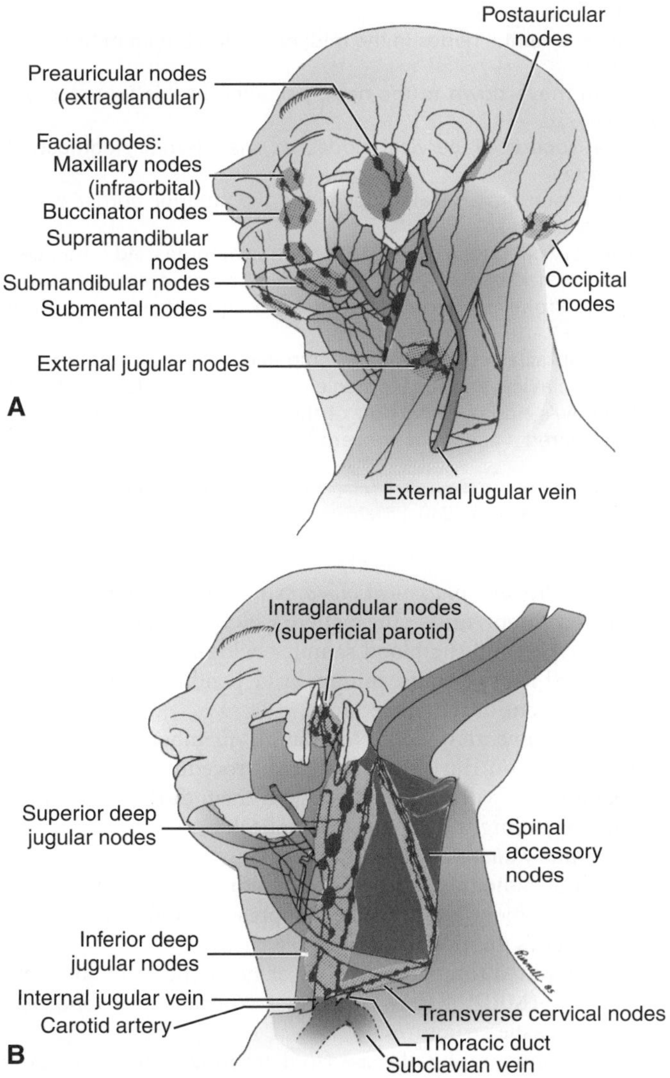

***Lymphatic System of the Neck.*** The lymphatic system serves both immunologic and circulatory functions. Interstitial fluid, which may contain bacteria, viruses, or tumor cells, is returned to the blood circulation through the lymphatic channels. As the lymph nodes trap the foreign matter, the nodes may become enlarged, infected, or the focus of metastatic cancer.[8] The lymphatic drainage of the neck can be divided into superficial and deep nodes (Figure 21-4). The nasal cavity, the paranasal sinuses, and the pharynx drain into the retropharyngeal nodes. The mouth, lips, and external nose are drained by the submandibular nodes. The lymphatics of the tip and lateral aspects of the tongue drain to the submental nodes, and the posterior tongue lymphatics drain to cervical nodes.



**FIGURE 21-4** Lymphatic drainage of neck. **A,** Superficial cervical and facial nodal drainage patterns. **B,** Deep cervical lymphatic drainage patterns. Note that sternocleidomastoid muscle is reflected.

# Perioperative Nursing Considerations

## Assessment

The nursing history must be thorough, including the patient's symptoms, health history, and definite and questionable risk factors, such as sun exposure, tobacco use, ethanol use, previous radiation therapy, family history of carcinoma, and the patient's dental history. In addition to reviewing the nursing history and findings from physical assessment of the neck (Box 21-1), specific factors that should be reviewed include the following:

- *Respiratory status.* Observe and note the quality and character of respirations; observe and note the quality and character of the voice—hoarseness, "hot potato" voice, or hyponasal speech; inspiratory stridor, expiratory stridor, hemoptysis, or dyspnea; a lesion in the oral cavity, nasopharynx, or larynx; bleeding from the oral cavity or nasopharynx. Note any history of chronic obstructive pulmonary disease (COPD).
- *Nutritional status.* Note weight loss and over what length of time. The patient may be nutritionally depleted from dysphagia, tumor, chemotherapy, or radiation therapy.
- *Circulatory status.* Observe and note pedal pulses and color of the nailbeds, especially in children, elderly patients, and patients in respiratory distress. Note preoperative vital signs compared with vital signs on admission to the patient care unit; note the presence of antiembolism stockings (the perioperative nurse should ensure proper fit of these stockings when checking pedal pulses).
- *Infection.* Note the temperature, color, and turgor of the skin over the affected site; note any lesions and their characteristics.
- *Dentition.* Observe dentures and their fit, lesions, loose teeth, persistent bad breath, and poor oral hygiene.
- *Emotional status and anxiety level.* Observe for restlessness, poor eye contact, facial tension, increased perspiration. Note the area around the patient's eyes for signs of crying (edema, redness).
- *Pain.* Observe location and character, odynophagia, sore throat, facial pain, otalgia; note preoperative medications and the time they were administered.

BOX 21-1

## Review of Physical Assessment of the Neck

**INSPECTION**

Inspect the neck in the usual anatomic position, in slight hyperextension, and as the patient swallows. Look for bilateral symmetry of the sternocleidomastoid and trapezius muscles, alignment of the trachea, the landmarks of the anterior and posterior triangles, and any subtle fullness at the base of the neck. Note any apparent masses, webbing, excess skinfolds, unusual shortness, or asymmetry. Observe for any distention of the jugular vein or prominence of the carotid arteries.

Webbing, excessive posterior cervical skin, and an unusually short neck may be associated with chromosomal anomalies. The transverse portion of the omohyoid muscle in the posterior triangle can sometimes be mistaken for a mass. Noticeable edema of the neck is associated with local infections. A mass filling the base of the neck or visible thyroid tissue that glides upward when the patient swallows may indicate an enlarged thyroid.

Evaluate range of motion by asking the patient to flex, extend, rotate, and laterally turn the head and neck. Movement should be smooth and painless and should not cause dizziness.

**PALPATION**

The ability to palpate and identify structures in the neck varies with the patient's habitus. It is more difficult to examine a short, thick, muscular neck than a long, slender one.

Palpate the trachea for midline position. Place a thumb along each side of the trachea in the lower portion of the neck. Compare the space between the trachea and the sternocleidomastoid muscle on each side. An unequal space indicates displacement of the trachea from the midline and may be associated with a mass or pathologic condition in the chest.

Identify the hyoid bone and the thyroid and cricoid cartilages. They should be smooth and nontender and should move under your finger when the patient swallows. On palpation, the cartilaginous rings of the trachea in the lower portion of the neck should be distinct and nontender.

With the patient's neck extended, position the index finger and thumb of one hand on each side of the trachea below the thyroid isthmus. A downward tugging sensation, synchronous with the pulse, is evidence of tracheal tugging, suggestive of the presence of an aortic aneurysm.

**LYMPH NODES**

Palpate the entire neck lightly for nodes. The anterior border of the sternocleidomastoid muscle is the dividing line for the anterior and posterior triangles of the neck and serves as a useful landmark in describing location. Bending the patient's head slightly forward or to the side will ease taut tissues and allow better accessibility for palpation.

Feel for nodes in the following six-step sequence:

1. The occipital nodes at the base of the skull
2. The postauricular nodes located superficially over the mastoid process
3. The preauricular nodes just in front of the ear
4. The parotid and retropharyngeal (tonsillar) nodes at the angle of the mandible
5. The submaxillary nodes halfway between the angle and the tip of the mandible
6. The submental nodes in the midline behind the tip of the mandible

Then move down to the neck, palpating in this four-step sequence:

1. The superficial cervical nodes at the sternocleidomastoid muscle
2. The posterior cervical nodes along the anterior border of the trapezius muscle
3. The cervical nodes deep to the sternocleidomastoid (The deep cervical nodes may be difficult to feel if you press too vigorously. Probe gently with your thumb and fingers around the muscle.)
4. The supraclavicular areas, probing deeply in the angle formed by the clavicle and the sternocleidomastoid muscle, the area of Virchow's nodes (Detection of these nodes should always be considered a cause for concern.)

From Seidel HM and others: *Mosby's guide to physical examination,* ed 5, St Louis, 2003, Mosby, pp. 240, 261-262.

- *Musculoskeletal system.* Observe problems in range of motion in all four extremities; note joint replacements, back or neck stiffness or pain, trismus.
- *Allergies.* Note allergic reactions to medications, foods, or latex.
- *Medication history.* Note medications taken by the patient for the presenting condition and any other diagnosed medical condition. Medications should include prescription medications, over-the-counter medications, vitamins, herbals, nutraceuticals, and others. Ensure key participants in the patient's care are aware of the medication history (Patient Safety).
- *Patient's knowledge and understanding of the surgical procedure.* Note questions and provide answers, or ask surgeon to clarify information for the patient. Review equipment and care (e.g., suctioning) that will be part of the postoperative regimen.
- *Presence of a mass.* Note the length of time the mass has been evident; note if the size of the mass decreased after antibiotic therapy; note a fixed mass versus a mobile mass; note cranial nerve palsies involving VII, IX, X, XI, and XII.
- *Availability of replacement blood.* Note if the patient has designated donor units (the patient's blood usually will have been typed and the blood samples held or typed and crossmatched for two units, minimally, depending on the anticipated extent of the procedure).
- *Patient's support system.* Note family members' names and their location during the surgical procedure, and explain that a nurse will be in contact with them during the procedure regarding the patient (as applicable).
- *Laboratory and diagnostic studies.*
  - Chest radiograph (to rule out mediastinal or pulmonary involvement and tracheal compression and to assess the patient's pulmonary status)
  - Computed tomography (CT) or magnetic resonance imaging (MRI) of neck (to delineate normal and abnormal soft tissue structures)
  - Ultrasonography of mass (to determine solid versus cystic mass)
  - Electrocardiogram (ECG)
  - Complete blood count (CBC)

## PATIENT SAFETY

### Medication Reconciliation

A National Patient Safety Goal (NPSG) established by the Joint Commission is to "accurately and completely reconcile medications across the continuum of care." Reconciliation of medication information can prevent prescribing errors, such as duplicate prescriptions, incompatible medications, and overprescribing. Whether undergoing an inpatient or outpatient procedure, the patient entering the perioperative setting may be at risk for medication errors because of decreased communication with the patient's primary care physician or other treating specialists. In ambulatory surgery, perioperative nurses typically review the patient's medication history in the preoperative period and then review medications again in the postoperative/discharge phase. Nurses can positively impact patient safety and reduce the risk for prescribing errors by following medication safety practices, using medication reconciliation processes, and implementing these risk reduction strategies:

- Collect a current home medication list (including dose and frequency along with allergies, drug intolerance information, and immunization history) for each patient on admission.
- Validate the home medication list with the patient whenever possible; a family member, significant other, or surrogate decision maker may be involved.
- Have the home medication list available for the physician whenever writing orders; place the reconciling form in a consistent highly visible location within the patient chart.
- Assign primary responsibility for collecting the home list to someone with sufficient expertise, within a context of shared accountability.
- Assign responsibility for comparing admission orders with the home medication list; identifying discrepancies, interactions, and so on; and reconciling variances to someone with sufficient expertise.
- Reconcile medications within specified time frames (within 24 hours of admission; shorter time frames for high-risk drugs, potentially serious dosage variances, and/or upcoming administration times).
- On discharge from the ambulatory surgery setting, in addition to communicating the updated medication list to the next provider of care during the hand-off report, provide the patient with the complete list of medications that he or she will be taking after discharge as well as instructions on how and how long to continue taking newly prescribed medications. Encourage the patient to carry the list and share it with any providers of care, including primary care and specialist physicians, nurses, pharmacists, and other caregivers.
- Adopt a standardized form to use for collecting the home medication list and for reconciling the variances (includes both electronic and paper-based forms).
- Develop clear policies and procedures for each step in the reconciliation process.
- Provide access to drug information and pharmacist advice at each step in the reconciliation process.
- Provide orientation and ongoing education on procedures for reconciling medications to all health care providers.
- Provide feedback and ongoing monitoring.

Modified from Joint Commission on Accreditation of Healthcare Organizations: *Sentinel Event Alert, Issue 35—January 26, 2006* (updated February 9, 2006). Accessed March 30, 2006, on-line: www.jcaho.org/about+us/news+letters/sentinel+event+alert/sea_35.htm.

Red blood cell (RBC) count (may be increased with dehydration or decreased with dietary deficiencies)
*Male:* 4.7 to 6.1 million/mm$^3$
*Female:* 4.2 to 5.4 million/mm$^3$
*Child:* 4 to 5.5 million/mm$^3$

Hemoglobin (values for the elderly may be slightly decreased; may be increased with dehydration, congestive heart failure [CHF], or COPD; may be decreased with cancer, nutritional deficiency, or severe hemorrhage)
*Male:* 14 to 18 g/dl
*Female:* 12 to 16 g/dl
*Child:* 10 to 15.5 g/dl

Hematocrit (may be increased with trauma or dehydration; may be decreased with hyperthyroidism, cirrhosis, hemorrhage, malnutrition, dietary deficiency, or in the elderly)
*Male:* 42% to 52%
*Female:* 37% to 47%
*Child:* 32% to 44%

White blood cell (WBC) count (may be increased with infection, trauma, stress, tissue necrosis, and inflammatory process; may be decreased with dietary disease, autoimmune disease, and overwhelming infections)
*Adult:* 5000 to 10,000/mm$^3$
*Child 2 years old and younger:* 6200 to 17,000/mm$^3$

Platelet count: 150,000 to 400,000/mm$^3$ (may be increased with malignant disorders, polycythemia vera, postsplenectomy syndrome, rheumatoid arthritis, iron deficiency anemia; may be decreased with hemorrhage, liver disease, kidney disease, or systemic lupus erythematosus [SLE])[7]

- Urinalysis (observe glucose level; if positive, check blood glucose level)
- Prothrombin time (PT), partial thromboplastin time (PTT), and activated partial thromboplastin time (APTT)
  PT: 11 to 12.5 seconds (may be increased with cirrhosis, hepatitis, vitamin K deficiency, salicylate intoxication, or disseminated intravascular coagulation [DIC])
  PTT: 60 to 70 seconds
  APTT: 30 to 40 seconds (may be increased with clotting factor deficiencies, biliary obstruction, hepatocellular diseases, vitamin K deficiency, or DIC; may be decreased with early stages of DIC or extensive cancer)[7]
- Blood chemistry analysis
  Chloride—adult and elderly: 98 to 106 mEq/L (may be increased with dehydration, kidney dysfunction, or anemia; may be decreased with CHF, diuretic therapy, or hypokalemia)
  Potassium—adult and elderly: 3.5 to 5 mEq/L (may be increased with acute or chronic renal failure; may be decreased with diuretic therapy, diarrhea, vomiting, or insulin, glucose, or calcium administration)
  Blood urea nitrogen (BUN)—adult: 10 to 20 mg/dl (elderly may be slightly higher; may be increased with renal disease, CHF, or dehydration; may be decreased with liver failure, overhydration, or malnutrition)[7]

- If the thyroid gland is suspect, the following tests may be indicated:
  - Serum calcium levels (to determine parathyroid function)—adult: 9 to 10.5 mg/dl
  - Serum calcitonin (to assess potential for medullary carcinoma)
  - Thyroid scan (to assess presence of "cold" nodule, which is often indicative of carcinoma)
  - Thyroid antibody tests (may show decreased levels in carcinoma): titer less than 1:100
  - Serum thyroxine ($T_4$): *male,* 4 to 12 mcg/dl; *female,* 5 to 12 mcg/dl
  - Thyroid-stimulating hormone (TSH): 2 to 10 milliunits/ml
  - Triiodothyronine uptake, resin (T3RU): *20 to 50 years,* 75 to 220 ng/dl; *older than 50 years,* 40 to 180 ng/dl[7]

To decrease the patient's apprehension, the perioperative nurse should explain the operating room (OR) environment and the perioperative routines and their sequence. Warm blankets, thermal drapes, reassurance, and a quiet environment should be provided to ensure that the patient is comfortable, calm, and warm before the surgical experience. Keeping the patient warm is both a part of the "caring" of perioperative nursing and a physiologic intervention to prevent unplanned hypothermia during or after surgery.

## Nursing Diagnosis

Nursing diagnoses related to the care of patients undergoing laryngologic or head and neck surgery might include the following:

- Impaired Gas Exchange
- Anxiety
- Risk for Infection
- Disturbed Body Image
- Impaired Verbal Communication

## Outcome Identification

Outcome identification and measurement are processes that allow perioperative nurses to demonstrate that their care makes a difference. By including patient-perceived dimensions, such as physical, social, and role function; mental health; coping ability; satisfaction with care; and overall perceptions of health, perioperative nurses are more likely to capture the contributions of their nursing interventions, analyze them, and subsequently improve them.

Outcomes identified for the selected nursing diagnoses could be stated as follows:

- The patient will experience adequate gas exchange.
- The patient will demonstrate effective coping skills and a decreased level of anxiety.
- The patient will be free from infection at the surgical site.
- The patient will experience a sense of self-worth and self-respect.
- The patient will establish an effective communication method with staff and family.

## Planning

Development of a meaningful plan of care is essential in meeting the needs of patients undergoing laryngologic or head and neck surgery. A typical plan of care for a patient undergoing laryngologic and head and neck surgery is shown on p. 681.

## Implementation

The patient with a malignant neck mass seldom undergoes surgical excision of the neck mass as a primary procedure. Endoscopic evaluation may be the initial surgical procedure unless the primary lesion is clearly delineated.

***Positioning.*** Routine positioning of the laryngologic or head and neck surgical patient involves placement of the patient in a supine position on the OR bed. A shoulder roll may be used for hyperextension of the neck. The headrest should allow easy movement of the head from side to side yet should maintain support. The extremities are well padded at pressure points and at major nerves. A pillow should be placed under the thighs and the legs should be slightly angled to decrease pressure on the patient's back; this positioning should be carried out before the patient is anesthetized to ensure comfort, with the exceptions of placement of the shoulder roll and hyperextension of the neck.

***Prepping.*** Removal of hair intraoperatively depends on the site of surgery and the anticipated extensiveness of the surgical intervention. Parotid surgery may require hair removal from just below the temple to a line even with or slightly behind the pinna of the ear. Head and neck surgeries may require removal of hair on the chest to the nipple area on both sides.

Laryngeal procedures for benign lesions do not usually involve preparation of the skin because of the intraoral approach. Head and neck procedures may involve extensive skin preparation and usually include the entire area from the chin to the nipples; it may also include a donor skin graft site if a defect or large flap coverage is anticipated. Some surgeons prefer the patient's face to be included in the prep, depending on the type of surgery anticipated and the site of the lesion. Povidone-iodine scrub and solution are generally used for prepping of the skin. If a flap may be raised to reconstruct a defect, saline should be available to remove the discoloration from the skin to allow the surgeon to check for flap viability.

***Draping.*** As with prepping, draping of the patient for a laryngeal procedure for a benign lesion (intraoral approach) is minimal, with the primary focus being protection of the patient's eyes and face. This may be accomplished by (1) placing ointment in the patient's eyes, (2) taping the eyelids closed with a nonabrasive, nonirritating tape, (3) applying moist padding over the tape (if use of a laser is anticipated), and (4) placing self-adhering eye pads over the moistened pads. A head drape may be placed over the patient's face to expose only the lips and chin.

Draping for head and neck procedures often varies according to surgeon preference. If the preference is to have the patient's face exposed, a commercially prepared head drape may be used. If unavailable, a head drape can be made by using a sterile sheet folded in half with a sterile towel on the innermost side to wrap the patient's hair. A towel clamp or sterile tape can secure the head drape in place. If penetrating towel clamps are used, care must be taken not to pierce the patient's skin. Towels can be opened fully, crushed, and placed into the space at both sides of the patient's neck and shoulder area to prevent contact with the unsterile OR bed linen during the procedure. The area of the endotracheal tube may be isolated by a self-adherent,

## SAMPLE PLAN OF CARE

**NURSING DIAGNOSIS**

**Impaired Gas Exchange** caused by airway obstruction, glottic resection, secretions, and edema

**OUTCOME**

The patient will experience adequate gas exchange.

**INTERVENTIONS**

- Check blood pressure (BP), rate and quality of respirations, rate and quality of pulse, and apical pulse preoperatively.
- Auscultate chest for breath sounds preoperatively.
- Elevate head of bed 30 degrees or higher as tolerated preoperatively and intraoperatively.
- Check arterial blood gases if obtained.
- Monitor oxygen saturation perioperatively.
- Administer steroids as ordered.
- Monitor preoperatively for and report signs of impaired gas exchange, such as stridor, confusion, hypoxia, restlessness, and irritability.
- Provide equipment, instruments, and supplies for a tracheotomy and tracheostomy.

**NURSING DIAGNOSIS**

**Anxiety**

**OUTCOME**

The patient will demonstrate effective coping skills and a decreased level of anxiety.

**INTERVENTIONS**

- Assess patient's level of anxiety (alertness, ability to comprehend, ability to perform activities of daily living [ADLs]).
- Maintain calm and safe environment.
- Assist patient in identifying possible sources of stress.
- Allow patient to ventilate and ask questions. Assess patient for desire for preoperative visit by persons with altered communication methods.

**NURSING DIAGNOSIS**

**Risk for Infection**

**OUTCOME**

The patient will be free from infection at the surgical site.

**INTERVENTIONS**

- Check temperature and white blood cell (WBC) count preoperatively.
- Check temperature, color, and turgor of skin at operative site.
- Check for lesions in proximity to surgical site.
- Check patient's nutritional status.
- Ensure sterile environment during surgical procedure.
- Monitor traffic patterns during surgical procedure.
- Monitor blood loss and fluid replacement during surgical procedure.
- Ensure that initial dressing is dry and clean.
- Administer antibiotics as prescribed.

**NURSING DIAGNOSIS**

**Disturbed Body Image**

**OUTCOME**

The patient will experience a sense of self-worth and self-respect.

**INTERVENTIONS**

- Encourage patient to verbalize feelings and self-perceived changes related to health status and surgical procedure.
- Involve family or significant others in initial communication with patient.
- Encourage patient to ask questions.
- Discuss referrals for support groups.

**NURSING DIAGNOSIS**

**Impaired Verbal Communication**

**OUTCOME**

The patient will establish an effective communication method with staff and family.

**INTERVENTIONS**

- Agree on a method of communication preoperatively to be used postoperatively. Suggestions include the following:
  - Writing with a pen or pencil and paper, or using an erasable slate
  - Hand signals or signs, body expressions
  - Picture board
- Provide assurance and support postoperatively as speech pathologist initiates speech training.
- Collaborate with surgeon in determining patient's ability to learn esophageal speech.
- Consult with surgeon regarding prosthetic voice restoration.
- Place intravenous (IV) lines in nondominant hand.

clear drape. Sterile towels are used to drape the neck, shoulder, and chest areas. An impervious drape is used to cover the patient from the chest to the foot of the operating room bed. A split sheet may then be used to drape over the towels and body drape. Commercially prepared split sheets have adhesive backing along the split that facilitates adherence to the area to be draped and decreases slippage with subsequent contamination resulting from manipulation of the head during the surgical procedure.

***Instrumentation.*** The instrumentation used in laryngologic surgery is quite specific and is discussed with each surgical intervention. Head and neck instrumentation combines general surgical instruments and procedure-specific instruments.

Intraoral, laryngeal, and mandibular procedures require the addition of periosteal elevators (e.g., Joseph, Freer, Cleoid), cartilage scissors, bone cutters, rongeurs (e.g., Lempert, Adson), oral or mouth retractors, tracheal hooks, a tracheal spreader, and saws. Although a Gigli saw and handles may be used on rare occasions, the sagittal saw is standard. Saws are either nitrogen powered, battery powered, or electric. A dermatome may be used if skin grafting of surgical defects or flap reconstruction is anticipated. In the case of large reconstructive surfaces, a skin mesher may be used to extend the skin graft.

***Equipment.*** Equipment that may be used in head and neck surgery includes an electrosurgical unit (ESU) (both monopolar and bipolar), a forced-air–warming unit or other device to maintain normothermia, and headlights (both fiberoptic and nonfiberoptic). Lasers used in head and neck and laryngeal surgery include the carbon dioxide ($CO_2$) and neodymium: yttrium-aluminum-garnet (Nd:YAG) lasers, depending on the location and type of lesion.

The evolution of microvascular free flap surgery for head and neck reconstruction has added a host of equipment to ensure the success of the surgical procedure and the safety of the patient. This equipment includes a surgical microscope (where the assistant may work at a 180-degree angle from the surgeon), a Doppler unit (to determine the viability of blood vessels), an electromyographic nerve monitor (to determine the location and quality of nerves), and a demagnetizer (to treat microsurgical instruments).

Safety in head and neck surgery is primarily patient related, except when lasers are used, which warrant both patient and staff safety precautions (see Chapter 2 for a discussion of laser safety). All equipment should be checked before use to ensure that it is in proper working condition. Visual inspection should ensure that all equipment is clean. Headlights, in particular, should be inspected for blood before and after each use. Guidelines for between-use processing of the various endoscopes used are essential in preventing inadequate disinfection. Guidelines established by the Association for Practitioners in Infection Control and Epidemiology (APIC) recommend immediate, thorough manual cleaning with an enzymatic cleaner, followed by complete immersion in a high-level disinfectant or use of an automated processing system.[6] See Chapter 3 for a discussion of the care and handling of endoscopic instruments and accessory items.

***Medications.*** Medications used in laryngeal surgery are targeted at providing anesthesia and decreasing bleeding and edema in the airway (Surgical Pharmacology). Typical medications include the following:

- Steroids are sometimes given intraoperatively and postoperatively and may be given preoperatively in the presence of edema or airway obstruction.
- Epinephrine, phenylephrine hydrochloride, or cocaine may be placed topically when vocal cord lesions are excised manually or biopsy specimens are taken to identify a primary tumor site.
- Lidocaine (Xylocaine) is often instilled into the trachea to decrease coughing immediately before insertion of a tracheostomy tube.

Antibiotics are also used in head and neck surgery. They are given primarily intravenously; however, an antibiotic may also be added to irrigating solutions.

***Monitoring Considerations.*** Intraoperative monitoring of the patient includes assessment of the circulatory, metabolic, urinary, respiratory, and musculoskeletal systems at regular intervals. Assessment of fluid volume is a collaborative effort. Blood loss and urinary output are communicated to anesthesia personnel. The perioperative nurse participates in the administration of fluid replacement therapy, assists in maintaining patency of lines, provides in-line blood and solution warmers, and notes the patient's response. Pedal pulses and pressure points should be checked without disturbing the surgical field or team. Additional methods of monitoring include pulse oximetry and blood pressure (BP) readings, as well as the following:

- *Arterial line.* Detects sudden changes in BP and serves as a vehicle to obtain blood samples for partial pressure of oxygen ($PO_2$) and partial pressure of carbon dioxide ($PCO_2$) levels.
- *Foley catheter.* Monitors the patient's urinary function; especially important for the elderly or debilitated patient.
- *Temperature monitoring.* Usually by a rectal probe or an endotracheal tube probe to monitor core temperature.
- *Esophageal stethoscope.* Usually contraindicated in laryngeal procedures because of the interruption of the esophagus or structures adjacent to the esophagus, but it may be used in other head and neck procedures.
- *Computerized anesthesia-monitoring system.* Standardized method of ensuring the safety of the patient while the anesthetic is being administered (see Chapter 4).

Perioperative nurses should be familiar with monitoring equipment, collaborate in interpreting results, and remain responsive to implementing collaborative interventions based on those results.

## Evaluation

Postoperative evaluation includes reassessing potential patient problems identified in the preoperative assessment as well as assessing the ESU dispersive pad site, surgical incision, dressing, drains, respiratory status, skin turgor, core temperature, and color of the head and extremities. Preoperative assessment findings, intraoperative changes in the patient's condition, and the postoperative evaluation must be documented and communicated during the hand-off report to ensure continuity of care and patient safety. The hand-off report should also include relevant nursing diagnoses and outcomes of care. Some nursing diagnoses may have already been resolved; others are ongoing and require continued planning and intervention during the patient's recovery from anesthesia and postoperative rehabilitation. A complete hand-off report allows the postanesthesia care unit (PACU) or intensive care unit (ICU) nurse to detect significant changes in the patient's condition in an early stage. Special considerations should also be included, such as the necessity for flexion of the neck to avoid disruption of the suture line of the trachea in a patient who has undergone tracheal resection. Based on the nursing diagnoses selected for the patient undergoing laryngologic or head and neck surgery, the hand-off report might include the following outcome statements:

- The patient's gas exchange remained adequate; respiratory rate and skin color were satisfactory.
- The patient demonstrated effective coping skills and a decreased level of anxiety and communicated needs and concerns.
- The patient will not exhibit signs of surgical site infection (ongoing); temperature will remain normal, and the surgical incision will heal without erythema, odor, or drainage at the site.
- The patient verbalized feelings regarding disturbances in body image, interacted positively with perioperative staff, maintained eye contact, and identified personally effective coping strategies.
- The patient is able to communicate effectively (ongoing) and use alternative method (specify) of communication.

## Patient and Family Education and Discharge Planning

Patient and family education is an important component of the age-appropriate and culturally sensitive care provided by perioperative nurses. Part of patient education is ensuring continuity of care by means of reports and referrals, coordinating the patient's care across settings and among various caregivers,

## SURGICAL PHARMACOLOGY

### Topical Medication and Administration

Topically applied medications are frequently used in laryngologic and head and neck surgical procedures. These medications may be used as adjuncts to locally injected anesthetics or to exert vasoconstrictive actions in the surgical field. The table below highlights commonly used topical medications. All provide anesthesia by inhibiting the conduction of nerve impulses from sensory nerves.

Topical medications used in this specialty may be administered by anesthesia care providers in the preoperative area or in the operating room (OR), by the surgeon conducting the procedure, or by the perioperative nurse. All medications must be clearly labeled and medication safety precautions followed.

Medications in this category inhibit the gag reflex and suppress coughing. The patient should be reminded not to eat, drink, or chew gum for at least 1 hour after the procedure or until cleared by the physician; return of the gag reflex should be determined before discharge from the postanesthesia care unit (PACU).

| Medication | Perioperative Uses | Dosage/Administration | Adverse Reactions | Nursing Considerations |
|---|---|---|---|---|
| Lidocaine hydrochloride: 4% solution, 2% viscous solution | 4% solution may be dripped on the vocal cords with Abraham cannula; viscous solution may be used to eliminate gag reflex in preparation for endoscopic laryngologic and adjunctive procedures performed with patient under local or monitored anesthesia care | 1-5 ml; peaks in 2-5 min, lasts 15-45 min | High doses may cause cardiac dysrhythmias, minor burning and stinging of the mouth and throat on initial contact | Provide patient with an emesis basin to expectorate any secretions. Patient may be instructed to gargle or swish with viscous solution to numb oral cavity in preparation for introducing Abraham cannula with 4% solution. |
| Cocaine hydrochloride: 4% solution, 10% solution | May be applied directly to vocal cords or other laryngeal structures on pledgets to promote vasoconstriction | Dose is dependent on the area to be anesthesized, tissue vascularity, technique and patient tolerance. Peaks in 1-5 min, lasts 30-60 min | Cardiac dysrhythmias, restlessness, increased pulse and respirations | Vasoconstrictive action is due to increase in norepinephrine at postsynaptic receptor sites. Rate of absorption is decreased by pledgets. Ensure solution is clearly labeled on surgical field and all pledgets are reconciled in the sponge count. |
| Tetracaine (Pontocaine) | 2% solution used to anesthetize oral cavity | 0.25%-0.5% by nebulization or direct application. Should not exceed 20 mg. Peaks in 3-8 min, lasts 30-60 min | Pain, redness, irritation on initial contact | Solution must be refrigerated. Frequently given by way of an atomizer. |
| Benzocaine/ Tetracaine (Cetacaine) | Available in gel, liquid, and spray | Dose is dependent on the area to be anesthesized, tissue vascularity, technique and patient tolerance. Peaks in 30 sec, lasts 30-60 min | Dry mouth, dizziness | Spray is given by way of metered applicator; 1- to 2-sec spray is approximately 200 mg/sec. Should not be used over prolonged periods. |
| Benzocaine | Available in 20% gel and 20% spray | Dose is dependent on the area to be anesthesized, tissue vascularity, technique and patient tolerance. Peaks in less than 5 min, lasts 15 min | Dry mouth, dizziness | Spray delivers 180-200 mg/sec when container is full, 60-80 mg/sec when inverted. |

Modified from Dimmitt P: A review of topical anesthetics and decongestants, *ORL Head & Neck Nursing* 23(2):21-24, 2005; Hodgson BB, Kizior RJ: *Saunders nursing drug handbook 2006,* St Louis, 2006, Saunders; Hodgson BB, Kizior RJ: *Mosby's 2006 drug consult for nurses,* St Louis, 2006, Mosby.

## BEST PRACTICE

### Care of Patients with Stomatitis

It is not infrequent for patients undergoing chemotherapy or radiation therapy to develop stomatitis (often referred to by the patient as "canker sores"). Stomatitis is characterized by painful single or multiple ulcerations of the oral mucosa. These may bleed, become infected, and interfere with nutrition. Perioperative nurses can assist their patients in coping with this disorder by encouraging careful oral hygiene, which enhances debridement of the lesions and helps prevent superinfections. Frequent oral care also promotes a sense of well-being. Pain management through the use of prescribed analgesics, many of which are orally or topically applied, is an important nursing intervention, because pain is commonly present throughout the outbreak of stomatitis.

- Encourage the patient to perform oral hygiene after each meal or as often as needed.
- Tell the patient to increase mouth care to every 2 hours for uncontrolled stomatitis.
- Advise the patient to use a soft toothbrush, Toothette, or gauze for oral care.
- Encourage frequent rinsing of the mouth with hydrogen peroxide, warm saline, sodium bicarbonate (baking soda) solution, or a combination of these solutions.
- Educate the patient to avoid commercial mouthwashes and lemon-glycerin swabs.
- Review with the patient the selection of soft, bland, and nonacidic foods.
- Instruct the patient on the use and application of topical analgesics and anesthetics as ordered by the physician.

Modified from Dietzen KK: Interventions for clients with oral cavity problems. In Ignatavicius DD, Workman ML, editors: *Medical surgical nursing: critical thinking for collaborative care,* ed 5, Philadelphia, 2006, Saunders.

managing information, and communicating effectively with colleagues, patients, and patients' families.

Preoperative patient education includes preparing the patient for alterations in body image and function. Altered methods of communication must be discussed before disruption of oral or laryngeal function, allowing the patient the opportunity to practice before speech is disrupted. The presence of edema, drains, nasogastric tube, Foley catheter, dressings, and altered mobility must be discussed. The OR environment and presence of equipment should be described to the patient preoperatively to keep anxiety at a minimum. Dietary preferences and eating habits should be discussed to effectively develop a postoperative nutritional plan. Any special considerations for surgical positioning should be discussed before surgery to prevent injury or postoperative discomfort.

Postoperative patient education for laryngologic and head and neck surgery includes interventions to keep the airway clear and patent (turning, coughing, deep breathing; providing a humidified environment; monitoring sputum; tracheostomy care), maintenance of adequate nutritional status to promote healing (dietary consultation; monitoring intake and weight; eating small, multiple meals and snacks), wound care (incision site care, oral hygiene, symptoms indicative of infection or potential wound breakdown), medications, pain management, activity limitations, potential complications, postoperative course, additional therapies (Best Practice) and coping mechanisms to avoid alcohol and tobacco use, as well as the patient's altered body image. Recommended content for patient and family education and discharge planning is included in "Procedural Considerations" for select surgical interventions discussed in the following sections.

# *Surgical Interventions*

## SURGERY OF THE ORAL CAVITY AND PHARYNX

The oral cavity is susceptible to both benign and malignant lesions, in part because of environmental risk factors. Oral malignancies may be initiated after exposure to a carcinogen, the most important one being tobacco use. The American Cancer Society estimates about 29,370 new cases of oral cavity and oropharyngeal cancer were diagnosed in the United States during 2005. Incidence rates are more than twice as high in men as in women and are greatest in men who are older than 50 years. For all stages combined, about 85% of persons with oral cavity and pharynx cancer survive 1 year after diagnosis. The 5-year and 10-year relative survival rates are 59% and 44%, respectively.[1]

Benign or malignant lesions of the tongue, floor of the mouth, alveolar ridge, buccal mucosa, or tonsillar area are excised. Benign or small malignant tumors of the oral cavity may be excised without neck dissection. In the presence of tongue cancer without evidence of metastasis, a prophylactic neck dissection may be performed in an effort to control a cancerous growth in the upper jugular lymphatic chain of the neck.

In the treatment of carcinoma of the floor of the mouth with involvement of the mandible, a portion of the tongue is removed in a combined operation—a radical neck dissection and a composite resection of both the mandible and the tongue. When the primary intraoral lesion is confined to the tongue, a neck dissection and a hemiglossectomy are performed without resection of the mandible. In the presence of a lesion of the tonsil or an extensive lesion at the base of the tongue with pharyngeal wall involvement, a resection of the ascending ramus of the mandible is necessary and portions of the base of the tongue, pharyngeal wall, and soft palate are removed to secure an adequate margin of normal tissue around the lesion. Colloquially, these operations may be referred to as the "commando procedure." The designation of "commando" became popular in the 1940s after courageous allied commando raids. The patients who submitted to the procedure were seen as very courageous; thus the term "commando procedure" was coined. Several years later, the term was changed to *composite resection,* but the derivation "commando" may still be used to describe the procedure.

Psychologic preparation of the patient is extremely important because these procedures may be done for a minor lesion in the oral cavity or may be the first stage of much more extensive surgery in the head and neck area. A supportive and accepting family is important to the patient because of the possibility of disfigurement after surgery.

### Procedural Considerations

The patient is placed in a supine position with shoulders elevated. Generally, endotracheal anesthesia is used and a pharyngeal pack of moist gauze may be inserted in the mouth. Instruments and supplies vary, depending on the surgical intervention.

### Operative Procedure

Although the procedure may be scheduled as a local excision, frequently lesions of the oral cavity require more extensive excision. The setup should be designed to include the instruments for a neck dissection, or they should be readily available. For some tumors of the oral cavity, a tracheostomy is performed to ensure a patent airway after surgery. A laser may be used to excise locally confined lesions of the oral cavity.

## SALIVARY GLAND SURGERY

Disorders of the salivary glands typically fall into three categories: inflammatory, obstructive, and neoplastic. Inflammatory conditions, such as bacterial or viral infections, can lead to salivary gland abscesses and ductal stone formation. Obstructive conditions can be a secondary consequence of inflammatory processes. Masses of the salivary glands may be benign or malignant, and 70% of them occur in the parotid gland. Three fourths of these parotid masses are benign.[3] Perioperative nurses will facilitate surgical care for patients experiencing any of these conditions.

### Excision of the Submandibular Gland

Excision of the submandibular gland is performed to remove mixed tumors and multiple calculi associated with extensive chronic inflammation. An incision is made below and parallel to the mandible and extending to beneath the chin to remove the gland and tumor.

***Procedural Considerations.*** The patient is placed on the OR bed in a supine position, with the affected side uppermost, and is prepped as for neck surgery. The instruments include a minor neck dissection setup. A set of lacrimal probes should also be added to the instrument setup if exploration of the submandibular (Wharton's) duct is necessary during surgery. The circulating nurse must ensure that no local anesthetic is delivered to the sterile field if identification of major nerves is anticipated. A nerve stimulator and bipolar ESU may be requested.

#### *Operative Procedure*

1. A small skin incision is made below and parallel to the mandible, extending forward to beneath the chin (Figure 21-5, *A*). The platysma is incised with scissors; the skin flaps and undersurface of the platysma and cervical fascia covering the gland are undermined with fine hooks, tissue forceps, and Metzenbaum scissors (Figure 21-5, *B*).
2. The mandibular branch of the facial nerve is retracted away with a small loop retractor or nerve hook.
3. The submandibular gland is elevated from the mylohyoid muscle (Figure 21-5, *C*). The edge of the muscle is retracted anteriorly to expose the lingual veins and nerve and the hypoglossal nerve, which is identified and preserved.
4. The gland is freed by blunt dissection, and the submandibular duct is clamped, ligated, and divided with care to prevent injury to the lingual nerve.
5. The facial artery is clamped, ligated, and divided. The submandibular gland is removed (Figure 21-5, *D*).
6. The wound is closed with interrupted absorbable sutures. The skin edges are approximated with nonabsorbable sutures. A drain is inserted into the submandibular bed and secured to the skin. Dressings are applied.

### Parotidectomy

Parotidectomy may be performed to treat recurrent parotiditis, but it is more commonly performed as part of the management of parotid gland tumors. In parotidectomy for tumor removal, the tumor and a portion of or the entire parotid gland are removed through a curved incision in the upper neck, in front of the ear lobe, or through a Y type of incision on both sides of the ear and below the angle of the mandible. Even when a mass in the parotid gland is benign, the closeness of the facial nerve makes removing the entire mass surgically challenging (Figure 21-6). The facial nerve exits the stylomastoid foramen, enters the substance of the salivary gland, and then bifurcates into the temporofacial and cervicofacial branches, variably communicating with the gland. These branches then further divide into the temporal, zygomatic, buccal, and marginal mandibular and cervical branches near the edge of the parotid. The gland is divided artificially into a *superficial* and a *deep* lobe according to its relationship to the facial nerve. The possibility of damaging the facial nerve (resulting in facial nerve weakness or paralysis) during the dissection of the gland should be considered carefully by all patients contemplating parotidectomy. In addition, they should understand that a more radical procedure might be required if a malignant tumor is discovered to involve adjacent structures.

***Procedural Considerations.*** The patient is placed on the OR bed in a supine position with the entire affected side of the face uppermost. The entire side of the face, the mouth, the outer canthus of the eye, the ear, and the forehead are prepped and left exposed.

The instrument setup is a neck dissection set. A nerve stimulator or nerve integrity monitor should be available. A set of lacrimal probes should be included in the setup if exploration of the ductal system of the parotid is necessary during the course of surgery. Bipolar ESU may also be required.

#### *Operative Procedure*

1. The incision (Figure 21-7) may extend from the posterior angle of the zygoma downward in front of the tragus of the ear and behind the lobule of the ear backward; the incision continues over the mastoid process and then downward and forward on the neck parallel to and below the body of the mandible. (A chin incision may also be used.) Bleeding vessels are controlled by hemostats and fine ligatures or by electrocoagulation.
2. With fine-toothed tissue forceps and scissors, the skin flaps are elevated as described for thyroidectomy (see Chapter 16) and retracted by means of silk sutures fastened to clamps.
3. The upper portion of the sternocleidomastoid muscle is exposed and retracted, the auricular nerve is identified, and the lower part of the parotid gland is elevated with curved hemostats.
4. The superficial temporal artery and vein and external jugular vein are identified by means of blunt dissection. The parotid tissue is dissected from the cartilage of the ear and the tympanic plate of the temporal bone. The temporal, zygomatic, mandibular, and cervical branches of the facial nerve are identified and preserved.

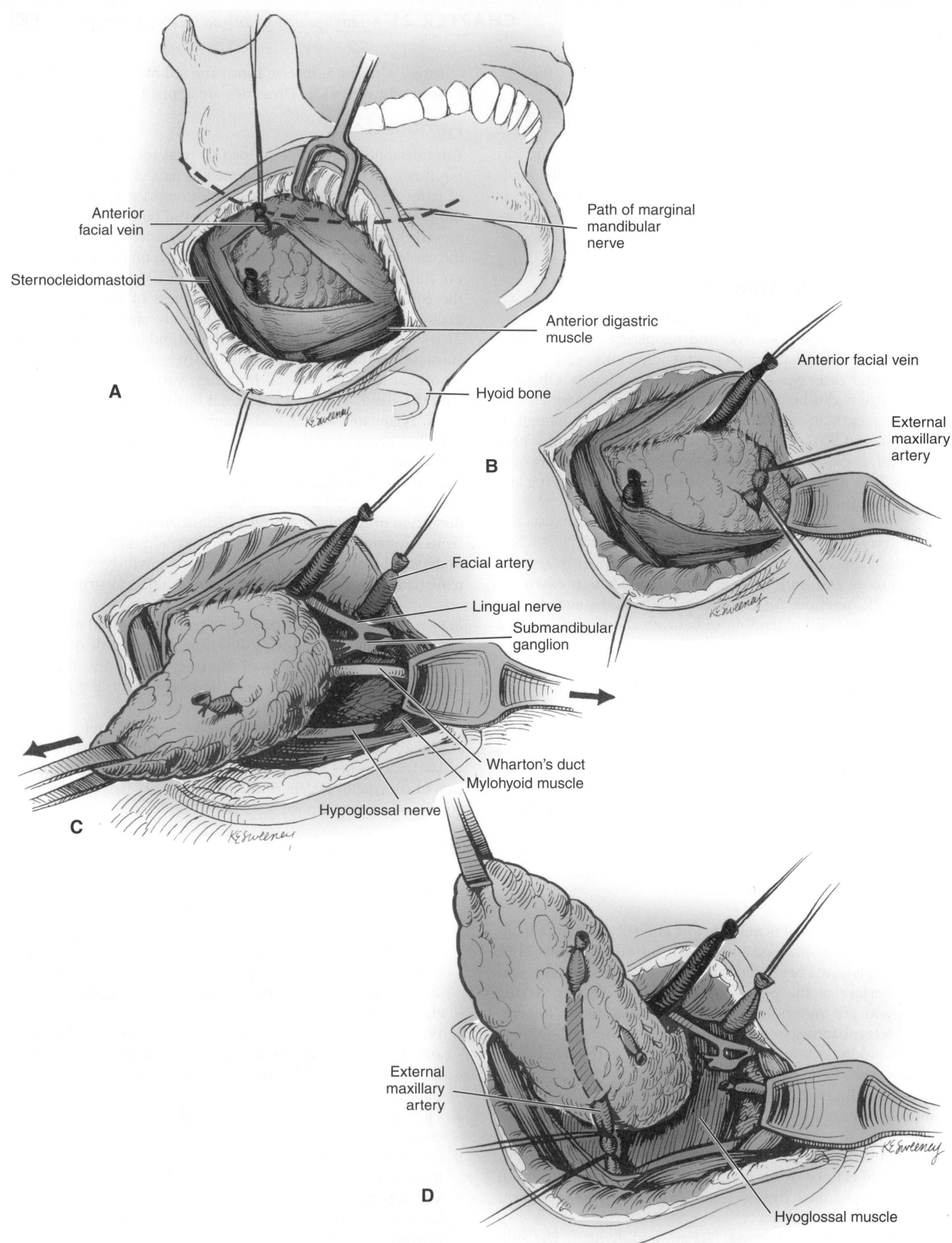


**FIGURE 21-5** Excision of submandibular gland. **A,** Submandibular incision made in a natural skin crease 3 to 4 cm inferior to mandible. Marginal mandibular nerve generally lies just superficial to anterior facial vein. **B,** External maxillary artery is identified on submandibular gland. **C,** Mylohyoid muscle is retracted anteriorly and submandibular gland posteriorly. This exposes lingual nerve, submandibular ganglion, and Wharton's duct. **D,** Hypoglossal nerve, running between hypoglossal and mylohyoid muscles. External maxillary artery must be divided a second time.

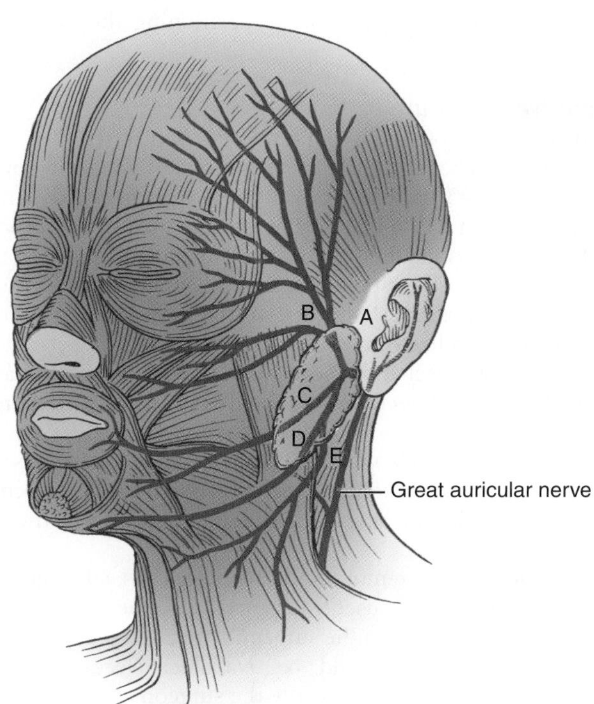


FIGURE 21-6 Branches of facial nerve. *A,* Temporal; *B,* zygomatic; *C,* buccal; *D,* mandibular; *E,* cervical.

5. a. The *superficial portion* of the parotid gland containing the tumor is removed. In some cases the entire superficial portion is removed, followed by ligation and division of the parotid duct.
   b. When the *deep portion* of the parotid gland must be removed, the facial nerve is retracted upward and outward and then the parotid tissue is removed from beneath the nerve. Kocher retractors are used to retract the mandible. The external carotid artery is identified. In many cases the internal maxillary and superficial temporal arteries are clamped, ligated, and divided.
6. The wound is closed in layers with absorbable suture. A small drain is inserted, the skin is closed with fine nonabsorbable suture, and a pressure dressing is applied.

## Uvulopalatopharyngoplasty

Uvulopalatopharyngoplasty (UPPP) is performed primarily to relieve obstructive sleep apnea (OSA) and snoring (Figure 21-8). Two or more of the following indications are reason to perform the operation:

- An $O_2$ saturation that drops below 80
- Apnea index worse than 20
- Significant daytime sleepiness
- Heroic snoring, producing social or marital problems
- Cardiac dysrhythmias, other than tachycardia or bradycardia, during sleep

***Procedural Considerations.*** A tracheostomy may be performed with UPPP because of postoperative edema with subsequent risk of airway obstruction. The tracheostomy tube is removed and the incision is closed when the danger of postoperative edema and bleeding has passed. Because some of these

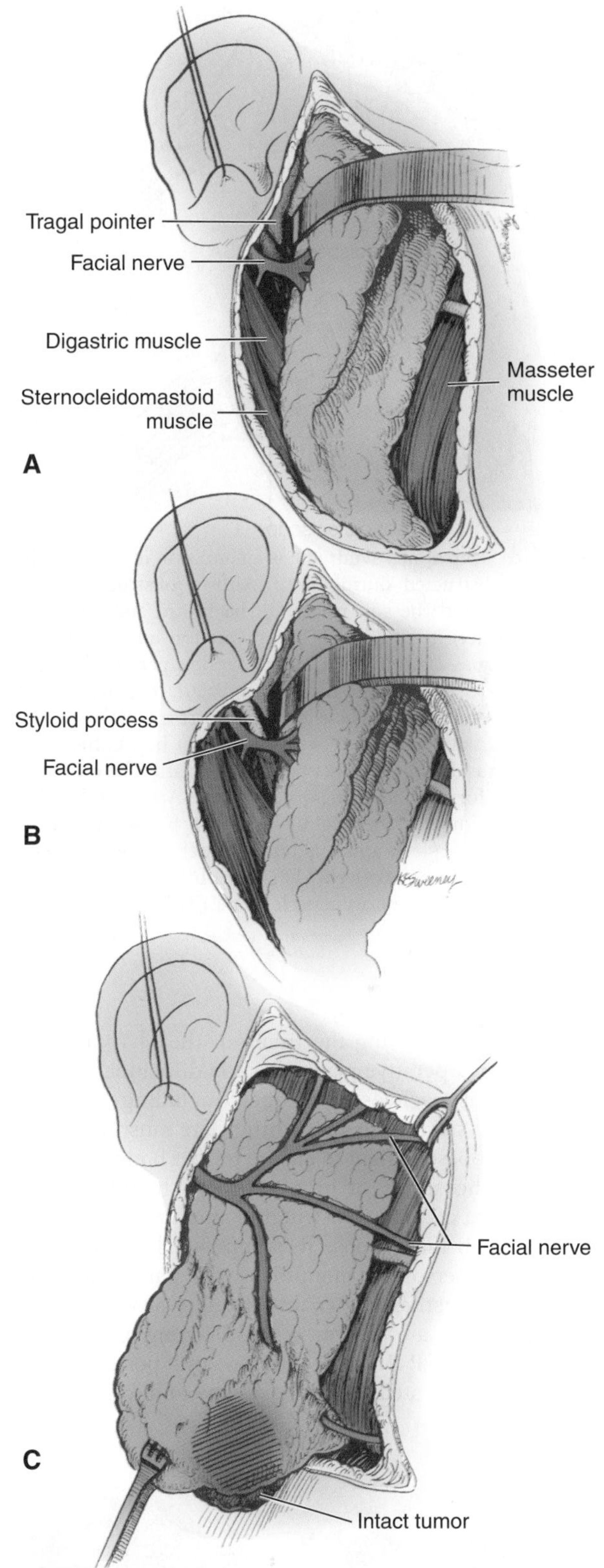


FIGURE 21-7 Operative technique for parotidectomy. **A,** Blunt dissection of parotid gland from external auditory canal cartilage exposes tragal pointer. Facial nerve lies approximately 1 cm deep and slightly anteroinferior to pointer and 6 to 8 mm deep to tympanomastoid suture line. **B,** Facial nerve exits stylomastoid foramen to run anteriorly between styloid process and attachment of digastric muscle to digastric ridge. **C,** Nearly completed process with tumor within intact superficial parotidectomy specimen.

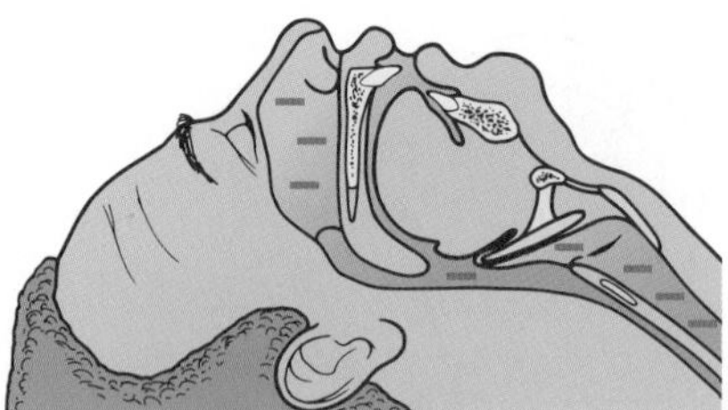


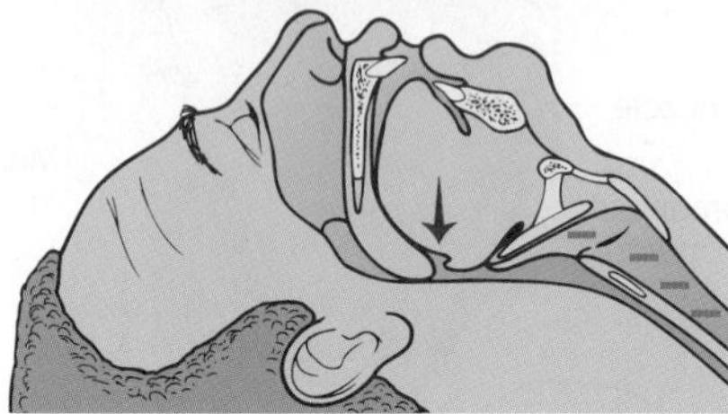


**FIGURE 21-8** Sleep apnea syndrome is a condition in which airflow is temporarily obstructed during sleep. Airflow obstruction occurs when the tongue and the soft palate fall backward and partially or completely obstruct the pharynx. The obstruction may last from 10 seconds to as long as 2 minutes. During the apneic period, the patient experiences severe hypoxemia (decreased $Pa{O_2}$), hypercapnia (increased $Pa{CO_2}$), and acidosis. These changes interrupt sleep and cause the patient to partially awaken. When the patient begins to awaken, the tone of the muscles of the upper airway increases. The tongue and soft palate move forward, and the airway opens. Apnea and arousals occur repeatedly during the night, separated by several normal breaths. The cause of sleep apnea is not definitely known. However, three factors appear to be involved: (1) shape of the upper airway, (2) neural control of the respiratory muscles, and (3) hormonal balance. *OSA,* obstructive sleep apnea.

patients are obese (causing the tissue of the pharynx to sag during sleep), preoperative planning should include obtaining an assortment of tracheostomy tubes, including extra long tubes, before the start of the procedure. Care must be taken in positioning the obese patient to ensure proper body alignment. Emergency tracheostomy or bronchoscopy should be anticipated in the event of airway obstruction after anesthesia induction. The surgeon may choose to administer local anesthesia with anesthesia personnel monitoring the patient and then induce general anesthesia after an adequate airway is established. If the tonsils are present, a tonsillectomy is performed along with the UPPP. Instrumentation and positioning are similar to those discussed for tracheostomy and tonsillectomy, with special attention to properly positioning the obese patient.

### *Operative Procedure*

1. The mouth gag (usually self-retaining) is inserted.
2. The tissue to be resected may be outlined by an electrosurgical blade. A #3 knife handle with a #15 blade or a #7 knife handle with a #12 blade may be used to make the incision. The incision is made in the soft palate and anteriorly to the tonsillar pillar (if the patient has not previously had a tonsillectomy) or posteriorly to the tonsillar pillars (if the patient has had a tonsillectomy) (Figure 21-9).
3. The tissue is resected by means of Metzenbaum scissors and long forceps with teeth or by a hand-controlled electrosurgical pencil.
4. Larger blood vessels may be clamped until the tissue is removed, or a suction coagulator or hand-controlled electrosurgical pencil may be used to obtain hemostasis as the tissue is excised.
5. Once the tissue is removed and hemostasis is achieved, absorbable sutures are used to approximate the edges of the mucosa. Depending on the surgeon's preference, 2-0 and 3-0 absorbable suture should be available. Needle holders should be long enough to allow the surgeon ease in delivering the atraumatic needle to the edges of the mucosa.
6. The oral cavity should be rinsed of blood and debris and the incision inspected before the patient is transferred from the OR.

Care should be taken when inspecting the incision in the postoperative period not to disturb the incision with a tongue blade, if one is used to provide access for inspection. The patient must not use a straw for fluid intake because it might disturb the suture line. Gentle oral cavity rinsing is recommended several times daily to decrease the chance of postoperative infection and to increase patient comfort.

## LARYNGEAL SURGERY

Laryngeal surgery may be performed for diagnostic reasons or as a means of treatment for both benign and malignant conditions. This type of surgery involves both endoscopic and traditional "open" approaches and always has the potential to alter the patient's ability to communicate verbally in the postoperative period. As is the case with oral cavity malignancies, cancerous lesions within the laryngeal structures are often attributed to environmental factors, such as tobacco and alcohol use (Figure 21-10). Benign conditions, such as vocal cord polyps and nodules, are often treated with laryngeal surgery.

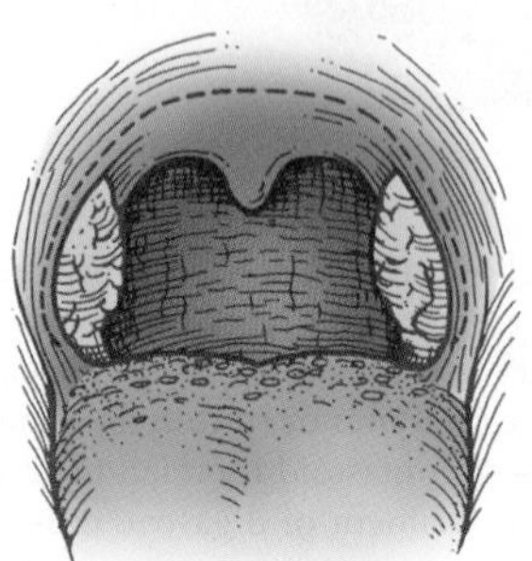
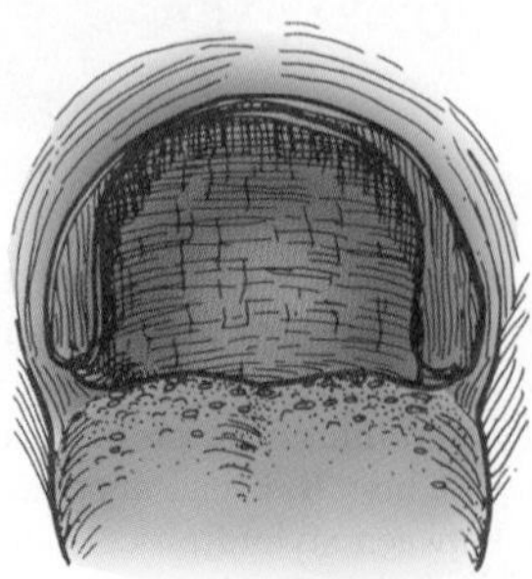
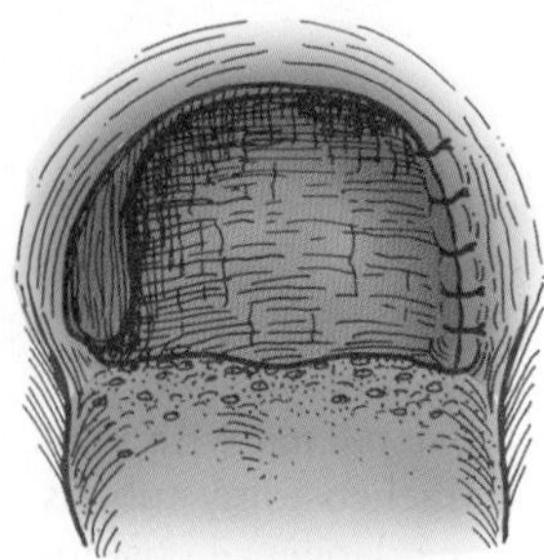
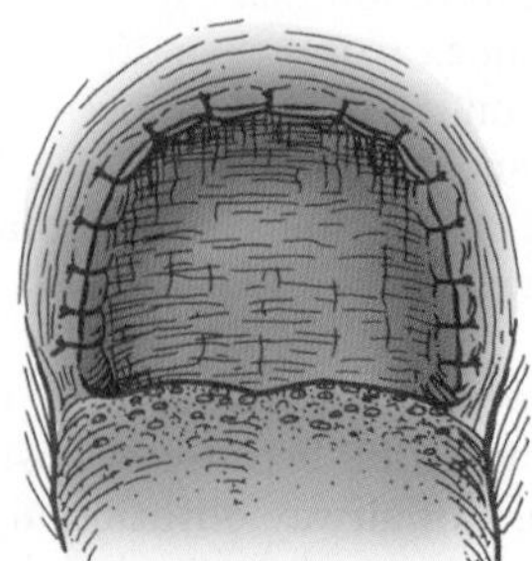

**FIGURE 21-9** Technique of palatopharyngoplasty as advocated by Simmons and associates.

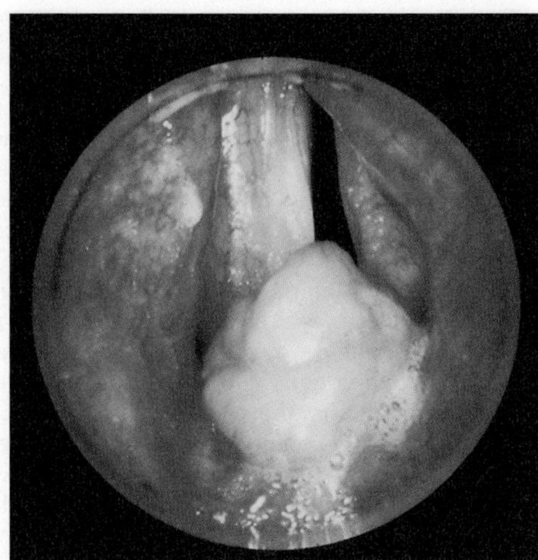

**FIGURE 21-10** Large granular tumor on the true cord.

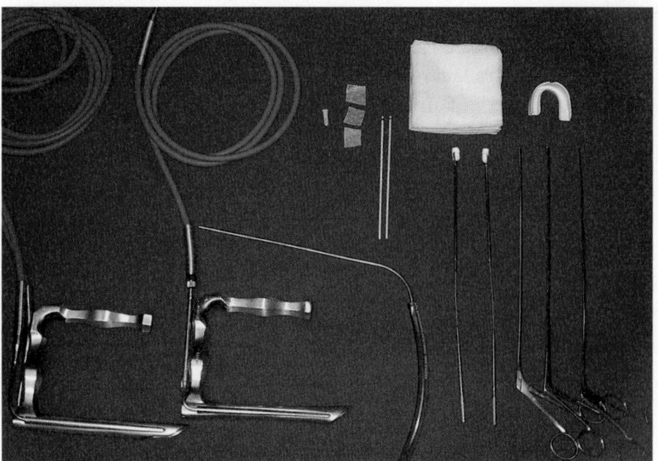

**FIGURE 21-11** Instrument setup for direct laryngoscopy includes Jako and Dedo laryngoscopes, laryngeal suction, assorted laryngeal forceps, and sponge carriers.

## Endoscopic Procedures

***Laryngoscopy.*** Laryngoscopy is direct visual examination of the interior of the larynx by means of a rigid, lighted speculum known as a *laryngoscope* (Figure 21-11) to obtain a specimen of tissue or secretions for pathologic examination. Vocal cord visualization may also be accomplished in the office setting with a flexible, fiberoptic nasopharyngoscope.

PROCEDURAL CONSIDERATIONS. Most rigid laryngoscopies are performed with the patient under general anesthesia. If the patient is unable to tolerate general anesthesia, a local or topical anesthetic of lidocaine (Xylocaine), tetracaine (Pontocaine), cocaine, or benzocaine/tetracaine (Cetacaine) will be administered. The patient should be sufficiently relaxed by reassurance and by pharmacologic preparation if the procedure is performed with the patient under local anesthesia. Sedatives may be administered before surgery. Immediate preoperative assessment should include the presence of any dental appliances and loose teeth and the condition of dental work. Any stiffness or immobility of the neck or shoulders should be evaluated. Respiratory problems such as asthma must receive careful attention. The patient should be cautioned about not eating or drinking after surgery until the gag reflex has returned and swallowing occurs without difficulty.

The setup includes the following:

- Labels for all medications and solutions used in the sterile field
- Local anesthesia setup
- Gauze sponges, 4 × 4 inches
- Laryngeal mirror
- Cotton balls
- Small cup of hot water (to warm the laryngeal mirror so that it does not fog when inserted into the mouth to view the vocal cords) or an antifog solution
- Emesis basin
- Syringe, 5 ml; and Abraham cannula
- Medication cup
- Jackson laryngeal application forceps
- Cetacaine spray, with angulated tip, or other topical anesthetic for the oral mucosa
- Instrument setup
  - 1 laryngoscope (surgeon's choice)
  - 2 laryngeal suction tubes
  - 1 light carrier, fiberoptic
  - 2 laryngeal biopsy forceps, 1 straight and 1 up-biting
  - 2 sponge-carrier forceps with extra sponges
  - 1 tooth guard
  - 1 fiberoptic light cord
  - Zero-degree telescope: may be requested for close visualization or attached to the camera for photographs of specific areas
  - 1 laryngeal probe: may be used to retract tissue or assess mobility of tissue

Accessory items include suction tubing, a specimen container, a basin with sterile saline, gauze sponges, sterile towels, and gloves.

If the surgeon wishes to perform a suspension laryngoscopy, a self-retaining laryngoscope holder is added to the instrument table, as well as microlaryngeal instruments, which include scissors, cup forceps, and alligator forceps. A special platform may be mounted onto the OR bed or a Mayo stand may be placed above the patient's chest and over the OR bed to provide a place for the laryngoscope holder to rest. The surgeon normally uses the operating microscope with a 400-mm lens during suspension laryngoscopy. The patient is placed in a supine position to facilitate visualization of the vocal cords. A shoulder roll should be available if slight hyperextension of the neck is necessary to assist in visualization of the larynx.

OPERATIVE PROCEDURE

1. Moist gauze pads or tape should be put over the patient's eyes to protect them from the instrumentation and to prevent injury and irritation from secretions during the procedure. The head may also be wrapped in a sterile towel. A sterile drape may be used to cover the patient. A tooth guard or moist 4-inch × 4-inch gauze sponge is placed to protect the patient's teeth.
2. The spatula end of the laryngoscope is introduced into the right side of the patient's mouth and directed toward the

midline; then the dorsum of the tongue is elevated so that the epiglottis is exposed.
3. The patient's head is first tipped backward and then lifted upward as the laryngoscope is advanced into the larynx.
4. The larynx is examined, a biopsy is taken, secretions are aspirated, and bleeding is controlled.
5. The patient's face is cleansed.

Laryngoscopy instrumentation should remain set up in the room until the patient is transferred because the equipment may be needed if the patient experiences laryngospasm postoperatively.

***Microlaryngoscopy.*** Microlaryngoscopy facilitates improved diagnosis and allows the laryngologist to view with relative ease areas that previously were inaccessible or difficult to visualize. It may also be used for minor surgery of the larynx, especially for the removal of polyps or nodules on the vocal cords (Figure 21-12). Intralaryngeal surgery using the laryngoscope is often referred to as *phonosurgery.* Instrumentation may vary according to surgeon preference. Research is currently under way to determine the feasibility of using robotics for laryngeal surgery (Research Highlight).

PROCEDURAL CONSIDERATIONS. If the procedure is done to remove polyps or nodules from the vocal cords, the patient must be cautioned to observe complete voice rest or to whisper postoperatively. The patient should be provided with a pencil and paper or erasable slate to aid in communication. The patient's restriction on speaking should be noted on the nursing plan of care and on the front of the chart.

The basic instrument setup for laryngoscopy is used. Microlaryngeal instruments are added to the setup and include the following (Figure 21-13):

- Self-retaining laryngoscope holder
- Jako microlaryngeal grasping forceps
- Jako microlaryngeal cup forceps, straight and up-biting cups
- Jako microlaryngeal scissors, straight, angled, and up-biting
- Jako microlaryngeal knives, straight and curved
- Laryngeal probe
- Microlaryngeal mirror
- Open-ended microlaryngeal suction tube
- Laryngoscope (dual light channel)

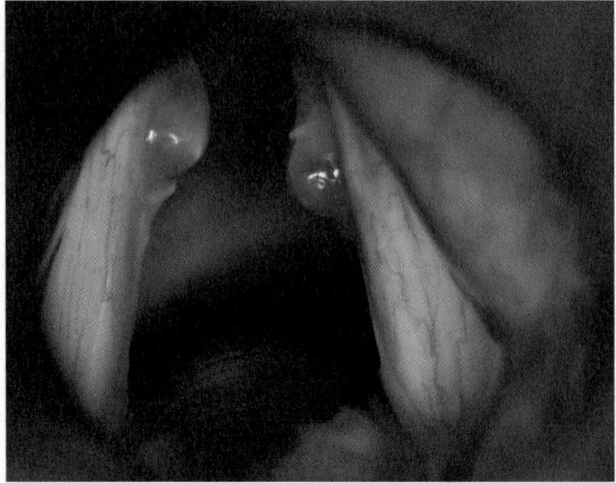

**FIGURE 21-12** Unilateral left vocal cord nodule.

## RESEARCH HIGHLIGHT

### Using Robots in Laryngologic Surgery

Surgical robots are gaining popularity in abdominal and thoracic surgery. Robotic technology offers the advantage of improved optics and increased instrument manipulation and also decreases the impact of human tremor on surgical technique.

This study sought to determine the feasibility of using surgical robots in microlaryngeal surgery. Researchers used an airway mannequin to help determine the optimal setup for robot-assisted microlaryngeal surgery. They experimented with different combinations of laryngoscopes, retractors, and other instruments used in conjunction with the surgical robot to determine the best system to visualize the larynx of the airway mannequin. Researchers carefully documented the relationship of the operating room (OR) bed, robot, camera, and instrumentation to determine the optimal setup for robotic assistance. They determined the best setup was to rotate the bed 30 degrees relative to the base of the robot to allow use of three of the robotic arms through the mouth into the larynx. This setup differs from conventional robotic surgery, where the patient is perpendicular to the robot.

Using the 30-degree rotation and a McIvor mouth gag, the researchers were able to manipulate the mannequin's epiglottis, arytenoids, cartilages, and vocal folds. The setup was tested with and without an endotracheal tube in place; the endotracheal tube did not hamper access to the field. Other advantages to the robotic approach include improved endolaryngeal suturing, which is normally very challenging with conventional instrumentation. An obstacle identified was the lack of availability of suction instruments.

Further study into this technology is needed, but early results indicate the feasibility of using these techniques in microlaryngeal and pharyngeal surgery. The application of robot-assisted surgery in other areas of head and neck surgery may require new instrument development.

Modified from Hockstein NG and others: Robotic microlaryngeal surgery: a technical feasibility study using the daVinci surgical robot and an airway mannequin, *Laryngoscope* 115:780-785, 2005.

The aforementioned instruments are 22 cm long to allow use with the microscope, being long enough to keep the surgeon's hands out of the visual field. The microscope is used. The head is adjusted to allow visualization of the larynx. The surgeon usually adjusts the microscope. The microscope lens should have a 400-mm focal length. Focal length is the distance from the lens to the operative area and is the point at which the field can be clearly viewed through the microscope. Beyond this point the field becomes fuzzy. The 400-mm lens gives the surgeon a 40-cm focal length, or working distance.

***Carbon Dioxide Laser Surgery of the Larynx.*** Laryngologists often use the $CO_2$ laser to treat lesions of the larynx and vocal cords. This laser is efficient and has a high power output. It uses a combination of $CO_2$, nitrogen, and helium gases that becomes energized to a high degree by an electric current. As the energy level subsides, light beams are produced and are reflected off the mirror-lined walls of the laser tube. These beams eventually form a single beam of light that has a high intensity in the ultraviolet range and is therefore invisible to the eye. For this reason, a red beam from a helium-neon laser

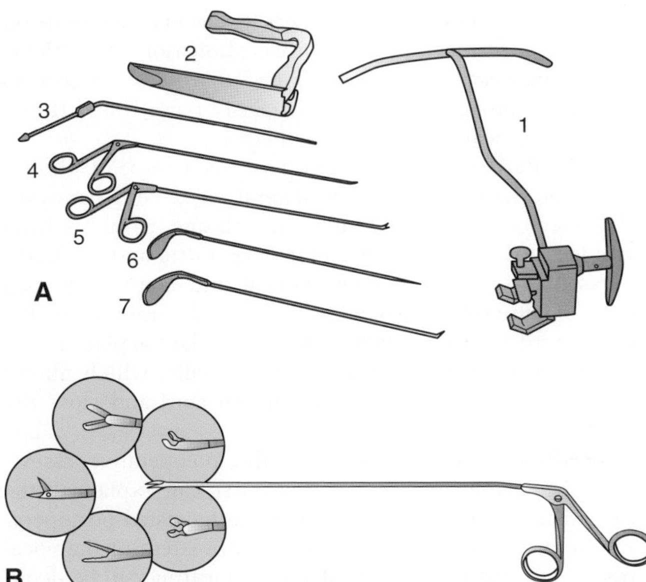


**FIGURE 21-13** Jako microlaryngeal instrumentation. **A,** Basic setup for microlaryngoscopy. *1,* Lewy self-retaining laryngoscope holder; *2,* Jako laryngoscope; *3,* suction tube; *4,* grasping forceps; *5,* cup forceps; *6,* probe; *7,* mirror. **B,** Close-up view of working ends of instruments.

is added to the $CO_2$ beam so that it can be properly aimed at the affected tissue. The beam destroys tissue at a precise point with minimal destruction of the surrounding tissue. It is especially useful in surgeries such as removal of webs in the larynx, vocal cord papillomas, and carcinoma in situ of the larynx, as well as benign endobronchial lesions.

PROCEDURAL CONSIDERATIONS. The basic setup for laryngoscopy and microlaryngoscopy is used. All instrumentation used for laser laryngoscopy should be ebonized. General anesthesia is usually given. The operating microscope with a 400-mm lens is used, with the laser micromanipulator attached to the microscope head. The manufacturer's instructions for attaching it must be followed. The beam should also be tested for proper working order before use on the patient. Signal lights on the console become illuminated if any malfunction occurs in the equipment or if the gas supply is low. Extreme care should be used when handling this delicate piece of equipment. A smoke evacuator should be used to remove the laser plume—a smokelike steam rising from the impact site; high-filtration laser masks should be worn by personnel. Where minimal plume is generated, a central wall suction with an in-line filter may be used for plume evacuation.[2] All other laser precautions apply (see Chapter 3).

## Adjunctive Procedures

Although the following procedures do not technically involve the larynx, they are often performed by otorhinolaryngologists in conjunction with laryngeal surgery and are of particular use in the diagnostic arena.

***Bronchoscopy.*** The trachea, bronchi, and lungs are visualized directly with a rigid or flexible bronchoscope that has a fiberoptic lighting system. A rigid scope gives a larger viewing area, whereas a flexible scope is easily inserted into the patient and manipulated. Bronchoscopy is fully described in Chapter 25. The Nd:YAG laser may be used for lesions of the trachea or bronchi, depending on the type of lesion. Most diagnostic bronchoscopies are performed with use of topical anesthesia and conscious sedation, requiring careful patient monitoring by the perioperative nurse.

***Esophagoscopy.*** Esophagoscopy is the direct visualization of the esophagus and the cardia of the stomach. This procedure is used to observe the area for extension of tumor, to remove tissue and secretions for study, or to observe for primary tumor site.

PROCEDURAL CONSIDERATIONS. Esophagoscopy facilitates the diagnosis of esophageal carcinoma, diverticula, hiatal hernia, stricture, benign stenosis, and varices. Patients with suspected obstruction, symptoms of bleeding, or regurgitation may require endoscopy. The Nd:YAG laser may be used in the treatment of some of these lesions. Esophagoscopy may also be used for therapeutic manipulations, such as removal of a foreign body or insertion of an esophageal bougie.

The setup includes the following:

- Esophagoscopes of desired type, size, and length (Figures 21-14 and 21-15)
- Suction tubing
- Fiberoptic light source and light cords
- Bougies, if desired
- Forceps of desired type and length
- Specimen containers
- Water-soluble lubricating jelly
- Gauze sponges
- Basin with sterile saline
- Suction tips (with velvet-eyed tips to avoid suctioning the mucosa of the esophagus into the tip)

OPERATIVE PROCEDURE

1. The fiberoptic light carrier is inserted into the esophagoscope and the fiberoptic light cord attached. A thin layer of lubricant is applied to the scope. The scope is passed into the mouth. The tongue, epiglottis, laryngeal inlet, and cricopharyngeal lumen are identified. If necessary, a person holding the patient's head may be required to tip the head

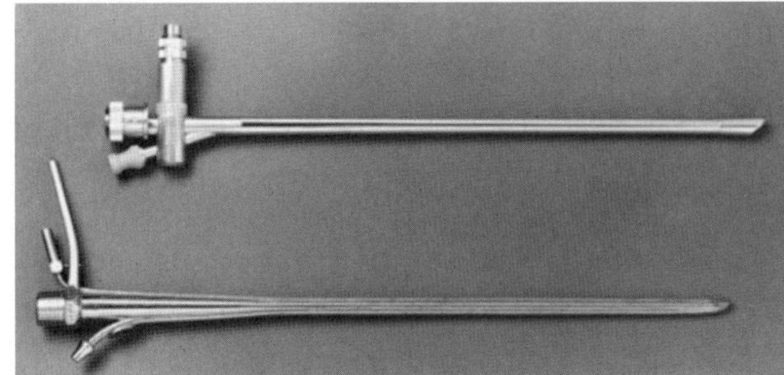

**FIGURE 21-14** Pediatric and adult esophagoscopes.

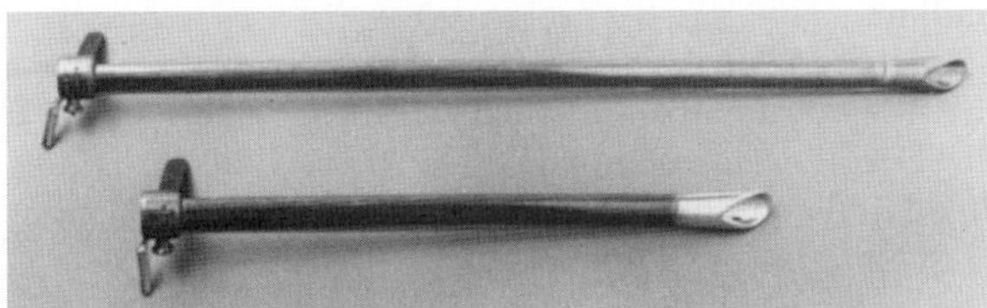

**FIGURE 21-15** Jesberg adult esophagoscopes.

backward while extending the neck anteriorly. Usually the esophagoscope is passed to the right side of the tongue, and the patient's head is turned slightly to the left.

2. When the scope has passed the inferior constrictors, the patient's head is moved in various directions so that all areas of the esophageal wall may be examined.
3. Specimens of secretions from the esophageal lumen may be obtained with an aspirating tube and suctioning apparatus. In some cases, saline may be injected through the esophagoscope's aspirating channel and the fluid is withdrawn immediately for histologic study. A tissue biopsy may be taken. After biopsy, the area is assessed for bleeding and the esophagoscope is then removed.

***Triple Endoscopy.*** When laryngoscopy, bronchoscopy, and esophagoscopy are performed in a single session on a patient, the procedure is termed *triple endoscopy* or *panendoscopy.* The order in which the procedures are performed depends on the surgeon's preference. The purpose of triple endoscopy is usually diagnostic. While inspecting for a malignancy, the surgeon views the structures, takes specimens for biopsy, and possibly makes smears or washings of the suspect areas. For any of the aforementioned endoscopy procedures, all equipment or instrumentation should be set up and be in working order (i.e., light carriers in place; light cables connected and working). Instrumentation to be used through the various scopes (i.e., suction tips, telescopes, biopsy forceps) should be checked for appropriate length. Specimens taken during endoscopic procedures should be labeled and removed from the table as soon as possible. In some instances, it may be helpful to indicate on the label that the specimens are microscopic.

## Open Laryngeal Procedures

***Laryngofissure.*** Laryngofissure is an opening of the larynx for exploratory, excisional, or reconstructive procedures that cannot be accomplished endoscopically.

PROCEDURAL CONSIDERATIONS. A laryngofissure may be performed when access to the intrinsic larynx is necessary. The thyroid cartilages are split in the midline, and the true vocal cords and false vocal cords are incised at the midline anteriorly. A neck dissection instrument set is required, plus an oscillating power saw.

OPERATIVE PROCEDURE

1. A tracheotomy is performed, and an endotracheal tube is inserted. A general anesthetic is administered.
2. A transverse incision is made through the skin and first layer of the cervical fascia and platysma muscles, approximately 2 cm above the sternoclavicular junction or in the normal skin crease. The upper skin flap is undermined to the level of the cricoid cartilage, and the lower flap is undermined to the sternoclavicular joint.
3. Bleeding vessels are clamped with mosquito hemostats and ligated. The strap muscles are elevated and incised in the midline.
4. The thyroid cartilages are cut with an oscillating saw, and the true vocal cords are visualized through an incision into the cricothyroid membrane. The true vocal cords are divided in the midline (anterior commissure), and the interior of the larynx is exposed.
5. The tracheostomy tube must be left in place after surgery to ensure an airway.

***Phonosurgery.*** Phonosurgery refers to various operations on the laryngeal framework to improve phonation for patients with communication disorders.[4] Type I thyroplasty is used to change or improve the voice. Thyroplasty types II and III are used to alter vocal cord tension and voice pitch.

THYROPLASTY. Type I thyroplasty is a form of phonosurgery for the treatment of unilateral vocal cord paralysis, which may be caused by trauma, neoplasms, paralysis from thyroidectomy, paralysis after extensive aortic and mediastinal vascular surgery, and mechanical and central nervous system dysfunctions. A window is created surgically in the thyroid cartilage, into which a silicone implant is placed. The implant pushes the paralyzed cord medially, which allows the moving cord to touch the paralyzed cord and close the opening.

**Procedural Considerations.** As the preoperative assessment is being done, the circulating nurse can explain to the patient that his or her voice will need to be rested postoperatively in an effort to minimize edema and stress of the vocal cords. An alternative method of communicating can be determined, such as writing.

The procedure is done with the patient under monitored local anesthesia to allow the patient to speak during surgery. This allows the surgeon to evaluate the quality of the patient's voice in an effort to attain the best result.

**Operative Procedure**

1. The patient is positioned on the OR bed in a semisitting position. A laryngoscopy is done by means of a flexible fiberoptic laryngoscope.
2. As the patient is asked to speak, the surgeon is determining the extent of approximation of the vocal cords as well as the patient's breath control. After a thorough evaluation, the patient is then prepped and draped.
3. A local anesthetic is injected into the surgical site. A horizontal incision is made at the middle level of the thyroid ala. Gelpi retractors are used to maintain exposure as dissection to the thyroid cartilage is completed. Measurements for the placement of the window are taken and marked with a marking pencil. A #15 blade is used to create a window in the thyroid cartilage. In some cases, a power drill with a cutting burr may be used. A periosteal elevator may be used to displace the vocal cords during phonation in an effort to determine voice quality.
4. When voice quality is satisfactory, the implant is placed into the window. Final laryngoscopy is done to view approximation of the vocal cords with the implant in place. The incision is then closed, and a dressing is applied.

***Partial Laryngectomy.*** Partial laryngectomy is removal of a portion of the larynx. It is done to remove superficial neoplasms that are confined to one vocal cord or to remove a tumor extending up into the ventricle on the anterior commissure or a short distance below the cord. A cancer confined to the intrinsic larynx (Figure 21-16, *A*) is generally a low-grade malignancy and tends to remain localized for long periods. The patient should be prepared for an altered voice quality postoperatively as well as for the possibility of total laryngectomy if the tumor proves too extensive for partial resection. General guidelines for patient education and homecare teaching for laryngectomy patients are presented in the Patient and Family Education box on p. 694.

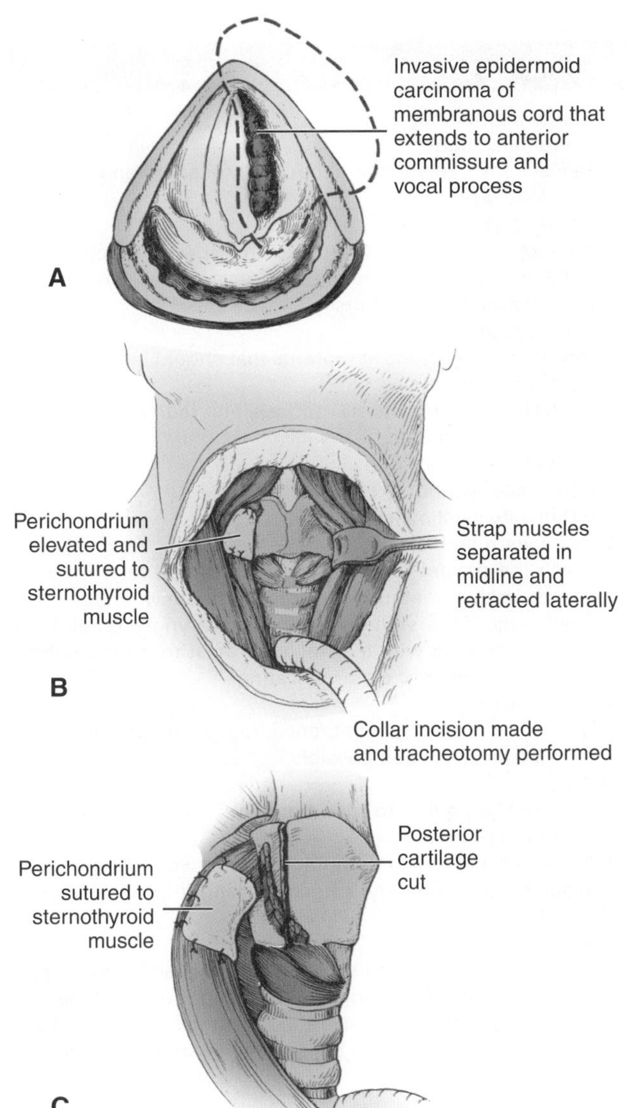


**FIGURE 21-16** Standard hemilaryngectomy. **A**, Broken lines outline full extent of resection in standard hemilaryngectomy for invasive epidermoid carcinoma of membranous cord that extends to anterior commissure and vocal process. **B**, Neck flap is elevated after collar incision is made and tracheotomy is performed. Strap muscles are separated in midline and retracted laterally. On side of lesion, perichondrium is elevated and its attachment to sternothyroid muscle is maintained. **C**, External perichondrium is sutured to overlying sternothyroid muscle and is retracted laterally to expose posterior border of thyroid cartilage so that posterior cartilage cut can be made approximately 5 mm from edge.

PROCEDURAL CONSIDERATIONS. The patient is placed in the supine position. The operative site is prepped and draped as described for thyroidectomy (see Chapter 16) or for the head and neck procedure. The setup for partial laryngectomy includes a neck dissection setup, Freer or Cottle periosteal elevator, oscillating saw, tracheostomy tubes, and an ESU.

OPERATIVE PROCEDURE

1. A tracheostomy is performed as described on page 697 and an endotracheal tube is inserted.
2. A vertical incision or a thyroid incision with elevation of a flap may be employed (Figure 21-16, *B*).
3. The sternothyroid muscles are separated in the midline and retracted by means of Green retractors.
4. The fascial covering over the thyroid cartilage is incised with a knife, and with a Freer periosteal elevator the perichondrium is elevated from the cartilage on the side of the tumor.
5. The thyroid cartilage is divided longitudinally in the midline by means of an oscillating saw.
6. The cartilages are retracted, and the cricothyroid membrane is incised with a knife. A blunt-nosed laryngeal scissor is introduced between the vocal cords to divide the mucosa of the anterior wall of the glottis.
7. The divided cartilages are retracted to expose the interior of the larynx. A small, moist gauze pack may be placed in the trachea to prevent aspiration of blood or mucus. A small amount of a topical anesthetic may be applied to the larynx to prevent laryngeal muscular spasm. The extent of the intrinsic laryngeal tumor is determined.
8. With a small periosteal elevator, the mucosa on the involved side of the larynx is freed; the false cord and mucosal layer of the region are lifted by means of a periosteal elevator and hooks. The involved cord is excised with straight scissors (Figure 21-16, *C*).
9. In some cases the thyroid cartilage may be removed with a knife and straight scissors. Bleeding is controlled with hemostats, fine absorbable ligatures and sutures, and electrocoagulation.
10. The gauze pack is removed from the trachea. The perichondrium is approximated with 2-0 absorbable sutures. The strap muscles are approximated in the midline with 2-0 absorbable sutures. The platysma and the skin edges are approximated separately with fine nonabsorbable sutures.
11. Dressings are applied to the wound and around the tube. A tracheolaryngeal tube is left in place and removed at a later date when the airway is adequate.

***Supraglottic Laryngectomy.*** Supraglottic laryngectomy (Figure 21-17) is excision of the laryngeal structures above the true vocal cords, hyoid bone, epiglottis, and false vocal cords.

PROCEDURAL CONSIDERATIONS. Supraglottic laryngectomy is indicated in cancer of the epiglottis and false vocal cords. It is designed to remove the cancer yet preserve the phonatory, respiratory, and sphincteric functions of the larynx. A neck dissection is almost always performed. The patient will have to undergo swallowing therapy postoperatively to learn how to decrease the incidence of aspiration. The instrument setup is as described for neck dissection.

OPERATIVE PROCEDURE. The procedure is similar to that described for partial laryngectomy except for the use of an oscillating saw.

***Total Laryngectomy.*** Total laryngectomy is complete removal of the cartilaginous larynx, the hyoid bone, and the strap muscles connected to the larynx and possible removal of the preepiglottic space with the lesion (History box). A wide-field laryngectomy is done when there is a loss of mobility of the cords and to treat cancer of the extrinsic larynx and hypopharynx (Figure 21-18). Malignant tumors of the extrinsic

## PATIENT AND FAMILY EDUCATION

### Patient Education and Home Care Teaching for Partial and Total Laryngectomy

**PREPROCEDURAL TEACHING**

Review the physician's explanation of the procedure and the reason for it; encourage the patient to ask questions and to discuss any fears or anxieties. Discuss the need for informed consent for surgery and anesthesia.

**REVIEW OF PREPROCEDURAL CARE**

- Inform the patient that the skin will be cleansed with bactericidal soap or antiseptic solutions to remove bacteria.
- Discuss preprocedural tests: complete blood count and urinalysis to check for infection and bleeding.
- Tell the patient that nothing-by-mouth (NPO) status must be maintained from midnight of the night before surgery.
- Provide preparatory instruction in suctioning (oral and tracheal) and wound care.
- Teach the patient to do own tube feedings.
- Review the use of a Magic Slate, paper and pencil, flash cards, or a communication board.
- Prepare the patient for permanent loss of speech if total laryngectomy is to be performed.
- Have a speech therapist visit the patient to discuss and plan for alternative means of speech.

**REVIEW OF POSTPROCEDURAL CARE**

- Explain that the patient will be in the high-Fowler position to lessen edema, improve coughing and deep breathing, ease suctioning, and provide comfort.
- Explain that the patient will be given mechanical ventilation by a tracheostomy tube and that suctioning will be done frequently to maintain a clear airway for breathing.
- Discuss the importance of frequent deep breathing and coughing.
- Demonstrate the use of intermittent positive-pressure breathing devices and ultrasonic nebulization treatments.
- Explain the presence of pressure dressings and neck drainage tubes. Discuss the use of a nasogastric tube to assist with feedings (bolus or continuous drip, based on patient's tolerance).
- Explain that swallowing and speech rehabilitation will begin soon after surgery, with the need based on the type and extent of surgery.

**SIDE EFFECTS AND COMPLICATIONS**

- Hemorrhage
- Airway obstruction
- Infection
- Thoracic duct leakage
- Nerve injury

**HOME CARE**

Give both the patient and the caregiver *verbal* and *written* instructions. Provide them with the name and telephone number of a physician or nurse to call if questions arise. Use visual aids to assist in instruction.

- General information
  - Review any explanation about the procedure and any specific follow-up care.
- Wound or incision care
  - Instruct the patient and caregiver to inspect the incision site daily and to change the dressing using sterile supplies as demonstrated by the nurse.
- Warning signs
  - Review the signs and symptoms that should be reported to a physician or nurse.
    - Infection of the stoma or incision: redness, drainage, pain, warm to touch
    - Fever
    - Dyspnea without exertion
    - Difficulty swallowing
- Special instructions
  - Teach the patient to avoid voice strain and to whisper or use alternative methods of communication when the voice needs rest. If the voice is gone (total laryngectomy), have the patient work with a speech therapist to develop an alternative method of communicating.
- Medications
  - Review pain management, encouraging the patient to use mild analgesics when possible.
- Activity
  - Remind the patient to plan frequent rest periods to avoid shortness of breath.
  - Assist the patient to begin self-care as soon as possible, including tracheostomy care and taking food and fluids by mouth.
- Diet
  - Plan a diet with the patient and caregivers that will avoid the possibility of choking or aspirating. For example, the patient may initially receive tube feedings and progress to soft foods and liquids as the swallowing reflex returns.

**FOLLOW-UP CARE**

Stress the importance of regular follow-up visits. Make sure the patient has the necessary names and telephone numbers.

**PSYCHOSOCIAL CARE**

Encourage questions and verbalization of fears and anxieties regarding possible loss of the voice.

**REFERRALS**

Assist the patient to obtain referral services, supplies, and information about support groups from the Lost Cord Club/International Association of Laryngectomies, sponsored by the American Cancer Society. Arrange a reconstructive surgery consultation as needed.

Modified from Canobbio MM: *Mosby's handbook of patient teaching,* ed 3, St Louis, 2006, Mosby.

larynx are more anaplastic and tend to metastasize. When laryngeal carcinoma involves more than the true cords, a prophylactic (preventive) radical neck dissection is done to remove the lymphatics.

Laryngectomy presents many psychologic problems. The loss of voice that follows total laryngectomy is traumatic for the patient and family. The patient may be taught to talk by using either his or her esophageal voice or an artificial larynx. The esophageal voice is produced by the air contained in the esophagus rather than by that in the trachea. Speech requires a sounding air column. With instruction and practice, the patient is able to control the swallowing of air into the esophagus and reintroduction of this air into the mouth with phonation. The sounding air column is then transformed into speech by means of the lips, tongue, and teeth. A tracheoesophageal fistula facilitates insertion of a Blom-Singer duckbill prosthesis

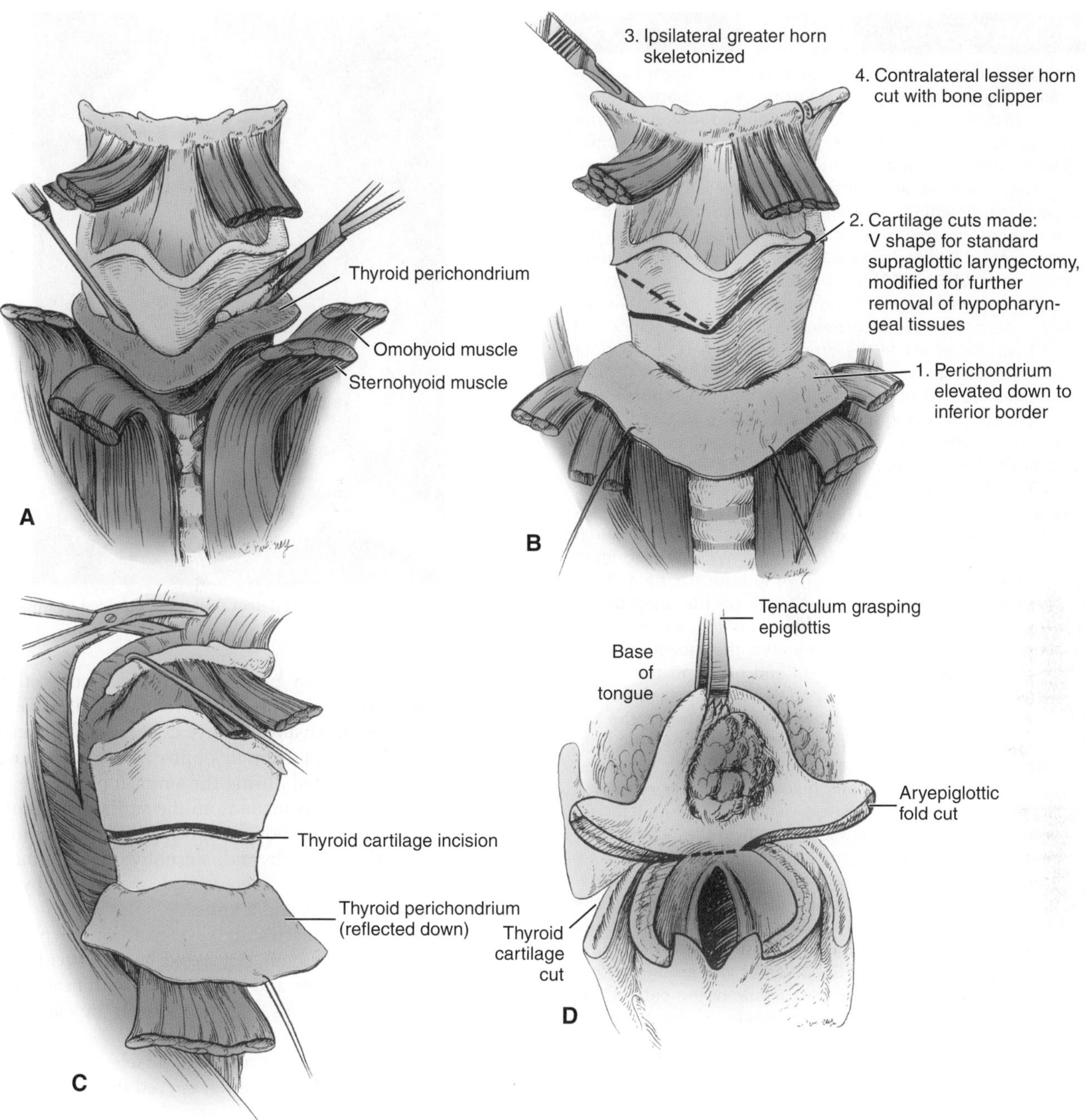


FIGURE 21-17 Supraglottic laryngectomy. **A,** Strap muscles are cut just above thyroid cartilage, and thyroid perichondrium is incised along superior border of thyroid cartilage. Thyroid cartilage perichondrium is carefully elevated and dissected inferiorly by first using a "peanut" (gauze dissector) and then a Freer elevator. **B,** Thyroid cartilage perichondrium elevation is completed down to inferior border, and then cartilage cuts are made. V shape is outlined for standard supraglottic laryngectomy. This may be modified for further removal of hypopharyngeal tissues according to size of lesion. Ipsilateral greater horn is skeletonized, and contralateral lesser horn is cut with bone clipper. **C,** Piriform fossa and vallecula are then entered on side of lesion, while greater horn of hyoid bone is retracted for exposure. **D,** Epiglottis is grasped with tenaculum, and scissors are used to cut through aryepiglottic fold in front of arytenoid and down into ventricle. Once both supraglottic cuts have been made through aryepiglottic folds, intervening tissues are cut to join up with thyroid cartilage cuts.

for the purpose of speech (Figure 21-19, *A*). This fistula may be created during the initial surgical procedure or at a later date when healing has occurred (Figure 21-19, *B*).

Because the stump of the trachea is brought out to the skin of the neck to form a permanent stoma, all the patient's breathing is done directly into the trachea and no longer through the nose and mouth. The nose no longer moistens this air. Drying and crusting of the tracheal secretions occur. Humidification may be provided when the opening is covered with a moist gauze compress. The patient will be anxious to know about

## HISTORY

By the 1920s, laryngectomy as a treatment for laryngeal cancer was being performed with good results. A perioperative nurse of that era preparing for a laryngectomy procedure faced very different challenges from those of today's practitioner. The surgery was done with the patient under basal anesthesia supplemented with local anesthesia infiltration. The nurse was responsible for preparing the tribromoethyl alcohol (Avertin) solution, which was administered rectally before the procedure. Avertin was dissolved in distilled water with Congo red solution at 38.8°C (102°F). Occasionally, Avertin was administered in the patient's room to "steel" the patient for surgery if he or she was extremely apprehensive. Once the optimal hypnotic effect of the drug was reached, the patient was transported to the operating room (OR). Several days before the scheduled procedure, the perioperative nurse was responsible for preparing a special cannula to be used in the prevention of aspiration in the nonintubated patient. The nurse sterilized a sponge by soaking it in 25% alcohol solution for 2 to 3 days. Immediately before the patient's arrival in the OR suite, the nurse removed the sponge from the alcohol solution and squeezed it dry. Next the nurse securely fastened it to a previously boiled silver tracheostomy tube and then dipped it into a 10% ether solution of iodoform. The sponge was again squeezed dry and introduced by the surgeon by way of a standard tracheotomy incision. After the modified cannula was in place for 5 to 10 minutes, the moisture in the trachea caused the sponge to swell and block off the larynx above. The surgery commenced, and the larynx was removed. Neck dissection was not performed. Postoperatively, the patient was transferred directly from the OR to the nursing unit, where he or she was positioned prone in bed with his or her head turned to one side on a stiff pillow. The patient remained prone until the drainage ceased—usually a few hours later. As the drainage subsided, the nurse would turn the patient over to a low-Fowler position with the head slightly elevated to facilitate breathing. An oxygen tank was nearby in case the patient turned cyanotic. Eight hours after the procedure, the modified tracheostomy cannula was taken out, the sponge was accounted for, and the physician inserted a standard unmodified tracheostomy tube. Sensitive to the emotional impact of the surgery and the complex needs of the patient, the nurse generally provided one-on-one care in the first few postoperative days.

Modified from Scott RJE, editor: *Pocket clycopedia of nursing,* New York, 1923, Macmillan; Atkinson DT: *Outline of ear, nose, and throat surgery,* New York, 1929, Vail-Ballou.

postoperative voice quality, which depends on the specific procedure performed. Table 21-1 lists surgical procedures and associated predictions of postoperative voice qualities.

**PROCEDURAL CONSIDERATIONS.** The patient is placed on the OR bed in a supine position with the neck extended and shoulders elevated by a shoulder roll or folded sheet. A general anesthetic is administered. An effective suction apparatus is essential. The proposed operative site, including the anterior neck region, the lateral surfaces of the neck down to the outer aspects of the shoulders, and the upper anterior chest region, is prepped and draped in the usual manner. The instrument setup is a neck dissection set.

**OPERATIVE PROCEDURE**

1. A tracheostomy may be performed initially to control the airway, or it may be incorporated into the procedure, depending on surgeon preference. If the tracheostomy is performed initially, a cuffed, wire-reinforced, flexible endotracheal tube will ensure effective delivery of the anesthetic and give the surgical team flexibility as the larynx and trachea are manipulated during the surgical procedure.
2. A midline incision is made from the suprasternal notch to just above the hyoid bone. Skin flaps are undermined on each side. The sternothyroid, sternohyoid, and omohyoid muscles (strap muscles) on each side are divided by means of curved hemostats and a knife.
3. The suprahyoid muscles are severed from the portion of the hyoid to be divided. The hyoid bone is divided at the junction of its middle and lateral thirds with heavy scissors or bone-cutting forceps. Bleeding vessels are clamped and ligated.
4. The superior laryngeal nerve and vessels are exposed and ligated on each side with long, curved fine hemostats and fine ligatures.
5. The isthmus of the thyroid gland is divided between hemostats. Each portion of the thyroid gland is dissected from the trachea with Metzenbaum scissors and fine tissue forceps. The superior pole of the thyroid is retracted. The superior thyroid vessels are freed from the larynx by sharp dissection.
6. The larynx is rotated. The inferior pharyngeal constrictor muscle is severed from its attachment to the thyroid cartilage on each side.
7. The endotracheal tube is removed. The trachea is transected just below the cricoid cartilage over a Kelly or Crile hemostat previously inserted between the trachea and esophagus. The upper resected portion of the trachea and the cricoid cartilage are held upward with Lahey forceps. A balloon-cuffed, wire-reinforced endotracheal tube with a Murphy eye is inserted into the distal portion of the trachea.

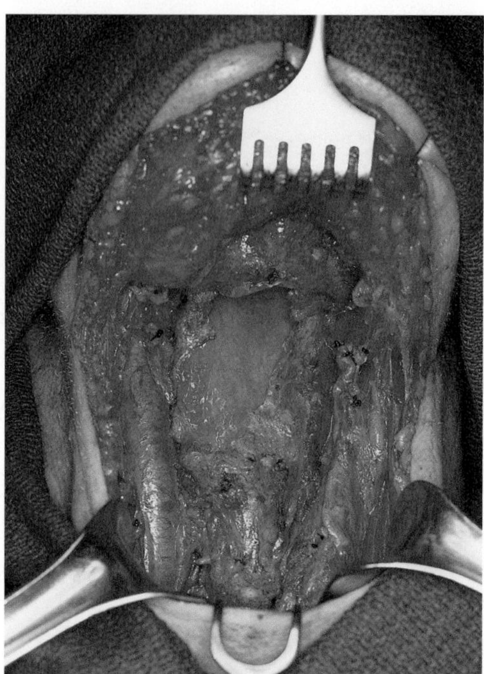

**FIGURE 21-18** Wide field defect following removal of the larynx.

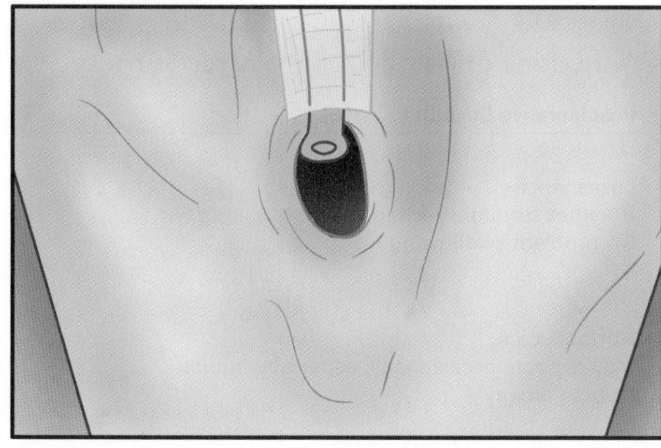


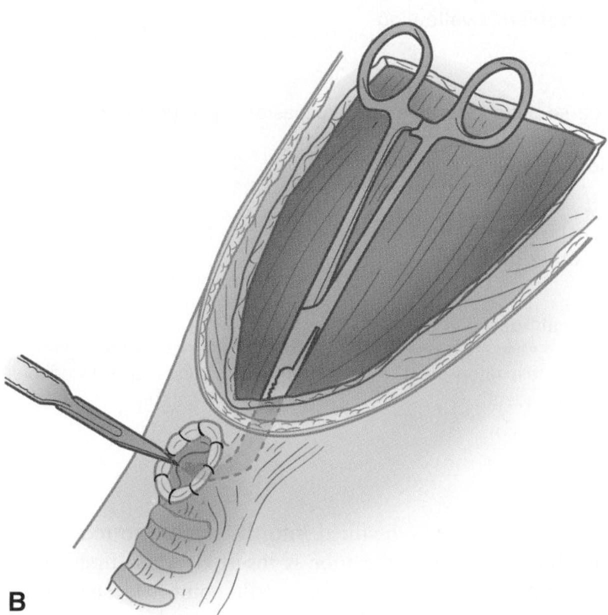


**FIGURE 21-19** Artificial larynx to facilitate speaking. **A,** Speech valve in place. **B,** Primary tracheoesophageal puncture technique. Note preliminary repair of stoma to allow accurate positioning of puncture site before pharyngeal closure. Feeding tube (14 Fr) is inserted through puncture down esophagus to the stomach.

8. The larynx is freed from the cervical esophagus and attachments by sharp and blunt dissection. A moist pack is placed around the endotracheal tube to help prevent leakage of blood into the trachea.
9. The pharynx is entered. In most cancers of the intrinsic larynx, the pharynx is entered above the epiglottis. The mucous membrane incision is extended along either side of the epiglottis; the remaining portion of the pharynx and cervical esophagus is dissected well away from the tumor by means of fine-toothed tissue forceps, Metzenbaum scissors, knife, and fine hemostats. The specimen is removed en bloc.
10. A nasal feeding tube is inserted through one naris into the esophagus; closure of the hypopharyngeal and esophageal defect is begun with continuous inverting fine 3-0 absorbable sutures. The nasal tube is guided down past the pharyngeal suture line.
11. The pharyngeal suture line is reinforced with interrupted sutures; the suprahyoid muscles are approximated to the cut edges of the inferior constrictor muscles.
12. The diameter of the tracheal stoma is increased by means of a knife and heavy scissors. The two portions of the thyroid behind the tracheal opening are approximated with interrupted nonabsorbable sutures, thereby obliterating dead space posterior to the upper portion of the trachea.
13. A closed wound-drainage system is used, and the suction drains are appropriately placed.
14. The edges of the deep cervical fascia and the platysma are closed separately.
15. A laryngectomy tube of desired size is inserted into the tracheal stoma; a pressure dressing may be applied to the wound and neck, although some surgeons prefer leaving the wound without dressings to observe the skin flaps. (A cuffed tracheostomy tube may be inserted for 24 to 48 hours postoperatively until edema subsides; then it is replaced with a laryngectomy tube.)

## NECK SURGERY

### Tracheostomy

Tracheostomy is the opening of the trachea and the insertion of a cannula through a midline incision in the neck, below the cricoid cartilage. A tracheostomy may be permanent or temporary. It is used as an emergency procedure to treat upper respiratory tract obstruction, which can be caused by bilateral vocal cord paralysis, inflammatory swelling, or edema caused by trauma or allergic reaction or neoplasms. It is also used as a prophylactic measure in the presence of chronic lung disease, in extensive composite resections where massive upper airway edema is anticipated, and for sleep apnea in which an obstruction could occur. A prophylactic tracheostomy is performed at the time of surgery to permit easy and frequent aspiration of the tracheobronchial tree secretions and diminish the dead space that exists from the opening of the mouth down to the supraclavicular region. The creation of a new clearance (tracheostomy) nearer to the functional areas in the lung provides for a greater volume of air for the patient with a partly destroyed lung. Anesthesia may be maintained through a prophylactic tracheostomy.

The patient's psychologic status should be carefully evaluated because of the altered body image, which may be either temporary or permanent, depending on the disease entity involved. Tracheostomy care should be explained carefully and thoroughly so that the patient will understand why it must be done so frequently, especially the suctioning of the tube. Reinforcement should be given about the ability to communicate with others by means of a pencil and paper or message board. As recovery progresses, the patient can be shown how to occlude the opening of the tube for brief periods to be able to speak a few words; the patient also can be taught to master tracheostomy self-care (Patient and Family Education). If a tracheostomy tube with a disposable inner cannula is inserted, the circulating nurse must ensure that the patient has replacement cannulas in the event occlusion or blockage occurs in the immediate postoperative period.

***Procedural Considerations.*** Before tracheostomy tube cuffs are inserted, they should be tested for air leaks by inflating and then deflating the balloon. The patient is placed in a supine

**TABLE 21-1**

## Surgical Procedures for Laryngeal Carcinomas and Predictions of Vocal Quality After Surgery

| Structures Removed | Structures Left | Postoperative Condition |
|---|---|---|
| **TOTAL LARYNGECTOMY** | | |
| Hyoid bone<br>Entire larynx (epiglottis, false cords, true cords)<br>Cricoid cartilage<br>Two or three rings of trachea | Tongue<br>Pharyngeal walls<br>Lower trachea | Loses voice<br>Breathes through tracheostoma<br>No problem swallowing |
| **SUPRAGLOTTIC OR HORIZONTAL LARYNGECTOMY** | | |
| Hyoid bone<br>Epiglottis<br>False vocal cords | True vocal cords<br>Cricoid cartilage<br>Trachea | Normal voice<br>May aspirate occasionally, especially liquids<br>Normal airway |
| **VERTICAL LARYNGECTOMY (OR HEMILARYNGECTOMY)** | | |
| One true vocal cord<br>One false cord<br>Arytenoid<br>Half thyroid cartilage | Epiglottis<br>One false cord<br>One true vocal cord<br>Cricoid | Hoarse but serviceable voice<br>Normal airway<br>No problem swallowing |
| **LARYNGOFISSURE AND PARTIAL LARYNGECTOMY** | | |
| One vocal cord | All other structures | Hoarse but serviceable voice; occasionally almost normal voice<br>No airway problem<br>No swallowing problem |
| **TRANSORAL CORDECTOMY** | | |
| Portion or all of one vocal cord | All other structures | May have a normal/hoarse voice<br>No other problems |
| **LASER SURGERY** | | |
| Tumor only removed | All other structures | Normal/hoarse voice |

From Workman ML: Interventions for clients with noninfectious problems of the upper respiratory tract. In Ignatavicius DD, Workman ML, editors: *Medical surgical nursing: critical thinking for collaborative care,* ed 5, Philadelphia, 2006, Saunders.

position, with the shoulders raised by a small rolled sheet to slightly hyperextend the neck and head. The neck is prepped, and sterile drapes are applied. A soft suction catheter should be available on the sterile field for suctioning after the tube is inserted.

### *Operative Procedure*

1. A local anesthetic may be injected into the tracheotomy site before the incision is made. A vertical or transverse incision may be used. A vertical incision is made with a #10, #15, or #11 blade in the midline about midway between the cricoid cartilage and the suprasternal notch. With this incision there is less risk of damage to nerves and vessels and less bleeding. When a transverse incision is made, it extends approximately one fingerbreadth above the suprasternal notch parallel to it and from the anterior border of one sternocleidomastoid muscle to the opposite side. Soft tissues and muscle are divided, using blunt and sharp dissection. The isthmus of the thyroid gland that joins both lobes of the gland in the midline over the trachea is either (1) retracted cephalad or caudad or (2) divided; this exposes the underlying tracheal rings—usually the second and third (Figure 21-20, *A*). In some cases, two curved clamps may be inserted through this incision across the isthmus and the isthmus is transected (Figure 21-20, *B*). The transected ends of the isthmus are oversewn or suture-ligated with absorbable sutures.
2. Lidocaine 4% may be instilled into the trachea to reduce the coughing reflex when the tube is inserted. Air is first drawn into a syringe to ensure that the needle point is located in the lumen. With a knife and #15 blade or a tracheal punch, a transverse incision is made in the trachea directly across the two tracheal rings. (Some surgeons prefer to make an H-shaped or T-shaped cut.) The cricoid cartilage is elevated with a hook (Figure 21-20, *C*) or 2-0 monofilament retraction suture.
3. With the stoma spread, a tracheostomy tube with the obturator in place is inserted into the trachea (Figure 21-20, *D*), the obturator is quickly removed, and the trachea is suctioned with a soft catheter to remove blood and mucus from the airway.
4. The wound edges are lightly approximated with nonabsorbable 2-0 sutures, or the wound edges are allowed to fall together around the tube. One or two skin sutures are inserted above the tube. The lower angle of the wound may be left open for drainage.
5. The tracheostomy tube is held in place with tapes tied with a square knot; the knot should be positioned on the side of the neck. The inner cannula is then inserted. A gauze dressing split around the tube is applied to the wound.

An additional tracheostomy tube of the same size and the obturator should be kept with the patient at all times, in the event the tube becomes dislodged or plugged with secretions. This practice expedites changing the tracheostomy tube with minimal potential for complications to the patient.

PATIENT AND FAMILY EDUCATION

## Patient Education Guide for Tracheostomy

The nurse should provide the patient with the following instructions:

1. Bacteria can easily enter the tracheostomy. To avoid infection, always wash your hands before touching your tracheostomy.
2. Observe the stoma daily for any signs of redness, swelling, or drainage.
3. Clean the stoma twice each day using a clean, damp face cloth; do not use soap.
4. A thin coat of petrolatum may be applied to the skin around the stoma; be careful not to let any enter the stoma.
5. Avoid dust, smoke, aerosol sprays, perfumes, car exhaust, powder, and raking leaves. Particles from any of these may enter directly into your tracheostomy. If you must be exposed to any of these agents, cover your tracheostomy with a piece of cotton cloth.
6. Vacuum instead of sweeping. Use damp cloths or mops rather than dry ones.
7. Wear a stoma covering to warm and filter the inspired air, especially in cold weather. A variety of clothing and accessories can be worn by men and women over the stoma covering. High-neck sweaters, turtlenecks, and scarves work well. They should fit loosely around the neck, so that there is always easy access to the stoma and breathing is not obstructed.
8. Cover your tracheostomy, not your nose and mouth, when coughing or sneezing.
9. Do not use tissues or cotton-tipped applicators near the stoma because pieces of these materials may break off and enter the tracheostomy.
10. Additional humidification of the air, especially during the winter when rooms are heated, helps keep secretions moist enough to be removed by coughing. Commercially available vaporizers or humidifiers may be used. The water ($H_2O$) in the vaporizer should be changed daily and the vaporizer cleaned with soapy water at least twice weekly. Alternatively, a pan of water can be kept on the stove or radiator. The water should be changed daily. Moist gauze may be used for a stoma cover, rather than the piece of cotton cloth.
11. When taking a bath or shower, stand on a nonskid bath mat because a fall could cause water to be splashed into your tracheostomy.
12. When showering, adjust the shower head so that the water is directed to a level on your body below your tracheostomy.
13. Be sure to cover your tracheostomy with your hand or with a commercially available shower guard while rinsing your head.
14. While shaving or having a haircut, wear a protective covering and a towel over the stoma to prevent dust and hair particles from entering. Use of an electric razor when shaving the face is suggested to avoid the chance of getting lather into the stoma.
15. Avoid wearing clothing with small ornaments, such as sequins or small buttons, near the neckline. Women should avoid wearing necklaces with small individual parts (e.g., pearls).
16. Clean mouth and teeth at least three times daily. Use mouthwash often because the ability to detect mouth odor is lessened.
17. Purchase and wear a Medic-Alert tag indicating that you have a tracheostomy. Accompanying instructions should address what to do if the tracheostomy becomes obstructed or in the event of a cardiopulmonary arrest.
18. No change in sleep habits is required. You will be able to breathe easily, even with blankets covering your tracheostomy.
19. If your tracheostomy tube has an inner cannula, clean it daily and as needed with a solution of equal parts of hydrogen peroxide and water. Rinse the cannula thoroughly under running water before reinserting it.
20. Change the twill tape holding your tracheostomy in place when needed. Secure the new tape in place before removing the old tape.
21. Suction the tracheostomy using clean technique as needed.
22. Carry some means of communication with you (e.g., pad and pencil, Magic Slate).
23. Do not smoke or use tobacco products. Avoid passive smoke.

Modified from Canobbio MM: *Handbook of patient teaching,* ed 3, St Louis, 2006, Mosby.

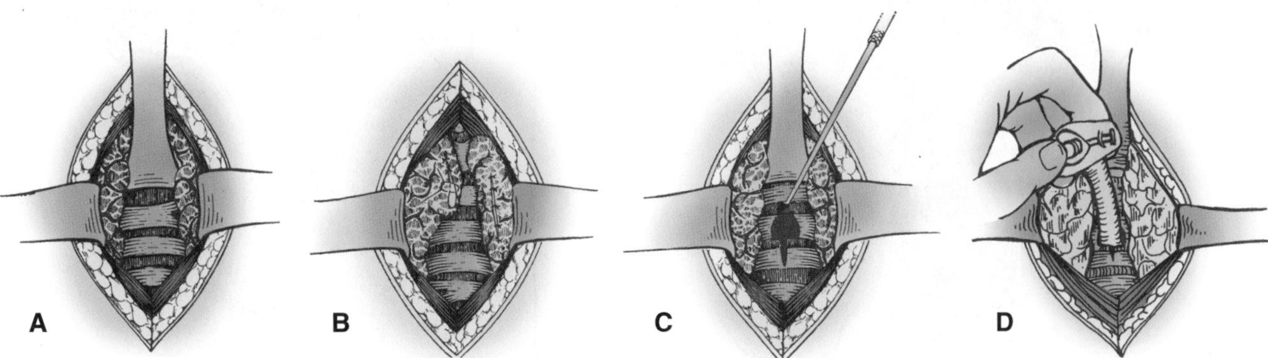


FIGURE 21-20 Operative technique for elective tracheostomy. **A,** Retractor exposing trachea by drawing isthmus of thyroid upward. **B,** Alternative method to that shown in A. Isthmus of thyroid is divided to expose trachea. **C,** Two tracheal rings are cut, and upper ring is partially resected. Tracheal hook pulls trachea from depth of wound nearer surface. **D,** Insertion of tube.

## Radical Neck Dissection

In a radical neck dissection, the tumor, all soft tissue from the inferior aspect of the mandible to the midline of the neck to the clavicle end posterior to the trapezius muscle, and lymph nodes are removed en bloc from the affected side of the neck.[5] This procedure is done to remove the tumor and metastatic cervical nodes present in malignant lesions as well as all non-vital structures of the neck (Figure 21-21, *A*). Metastasis occurs through the lymphatic channels by way of the bloodstream. Diseases of the oral cavity, lips, and thyroid gland may spread slowly to the neck. Radical neck surgery is done in the presence of cervical node metastasis from a cancer of the head and neck that has a reasonable chance of being controlled.

A prophylactic neck dissection implies elective radical neck surgery when there is no clinical evidence of metastatic cancer in the cervical lymph nodes.

***Procedural Considerations.*** The patient is placed on the OR bed in a supine position. General endotracheal anesthesia is induced before the patient is positioned for surgery. A shoulder roll may be placed to slightly hyperextend the neck with the head slightly turned to the contralateral side. The head of the bed may be slightly elevated to reduce venous bleeding.

During the operation the anesthesia provider works behind a sterile barrier at the patient's unaffected side. The preoperative skin prep is extensive, including the neck, lower face, and upper chest. The patient's neck is draped so as to leave a wide operative field. On rare occasions, a dermal graft is harvested to cover and protect the carotid artery (as when a patient has received extensive previous radiation therapy). If this is the case, the thigh area is also prepped and draped with sterile towels in readiness for obtaining a dermal graft before closure of the neck wound. It is usually more convenient to use the thigh on the same side as the neck dissection. Patient and family education includes tracheostomy care (if applicable), pain management, care of the surgical incision, reportable signs and symptoms, healthful behaviors, and review of physical therapy exercises.

### *Operative Procedure*

1. One of several types of incisions may be used, including the Y-shaped, H-shaped, or trifurcate incision (Figure 21-22), all of which aim for complete lymphadenectomy while preserving good, viable skin flaps.
2. The upper curved incision is made through the skin and platysma with a knife, tissue forceps, and fine hemostats; ligatures are used for bleeding vessels. The upper flap is retracted; then the vertical portion of the incision is made, and the skin flaps are retracted anteriorly and posteriorly with retractors. The anterior margin of the trapezius muscle is exposed by means of curved scissors. The flaps are retracted to expose the entire lateral aspect of the neck. Branches of the jugular veins are clamped, ligated, and divided.
3. The sternal and clavicular attachments of the sternocleidomastoid muscle are clamped with curved Pean forceps and then divided with a knife. The superficial layer of deep fascia is incised. The omohyoid muscle is severed between clamps just above its scapular attachment.
4. By sharp and blunt dissection, the carotid sheath is opened. The internal jugular vein is isolated by blunt dissection and then doubly clamped, doubly ligated with medium silk, and divided with Metzenbaum scissors. A transfixion suture is placed on the lower end of the vein.
5. The common carotid artery and vagus nerve are identified and protected. The fatty areolar tissue and fascia are dissected away using Metzenbaum scissors and fine tissue

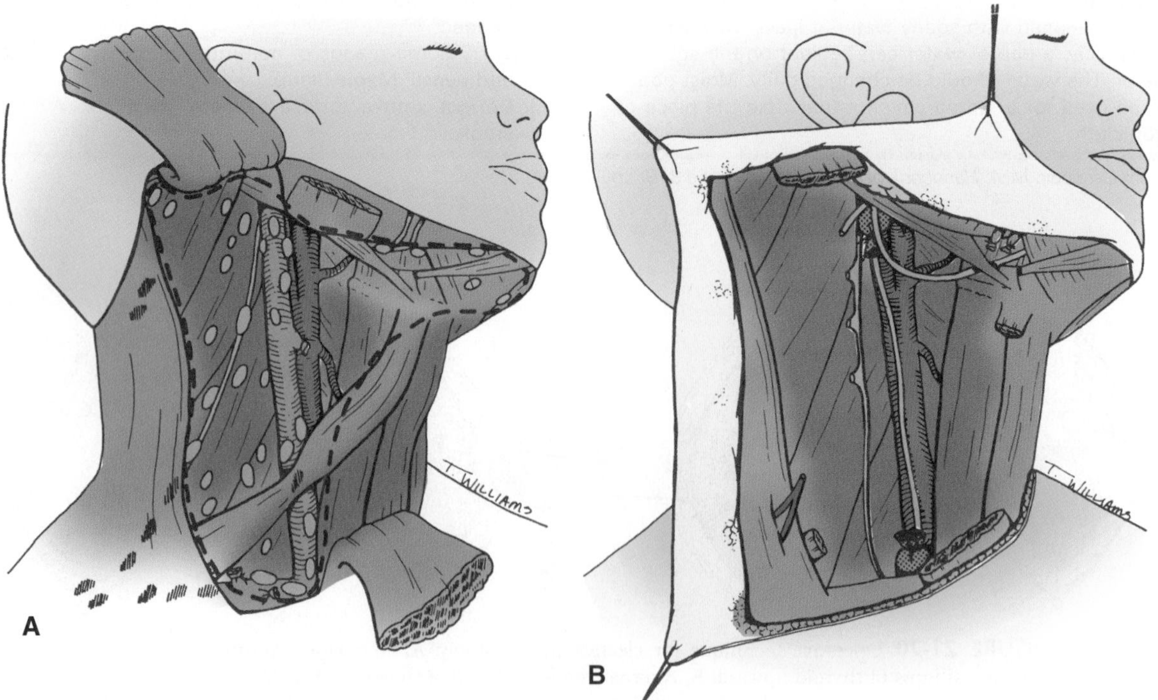


**FIGURE 21-21** Radical neck dissection. **A,** Diagram of extent of operation. **B,** Diagram of operation.

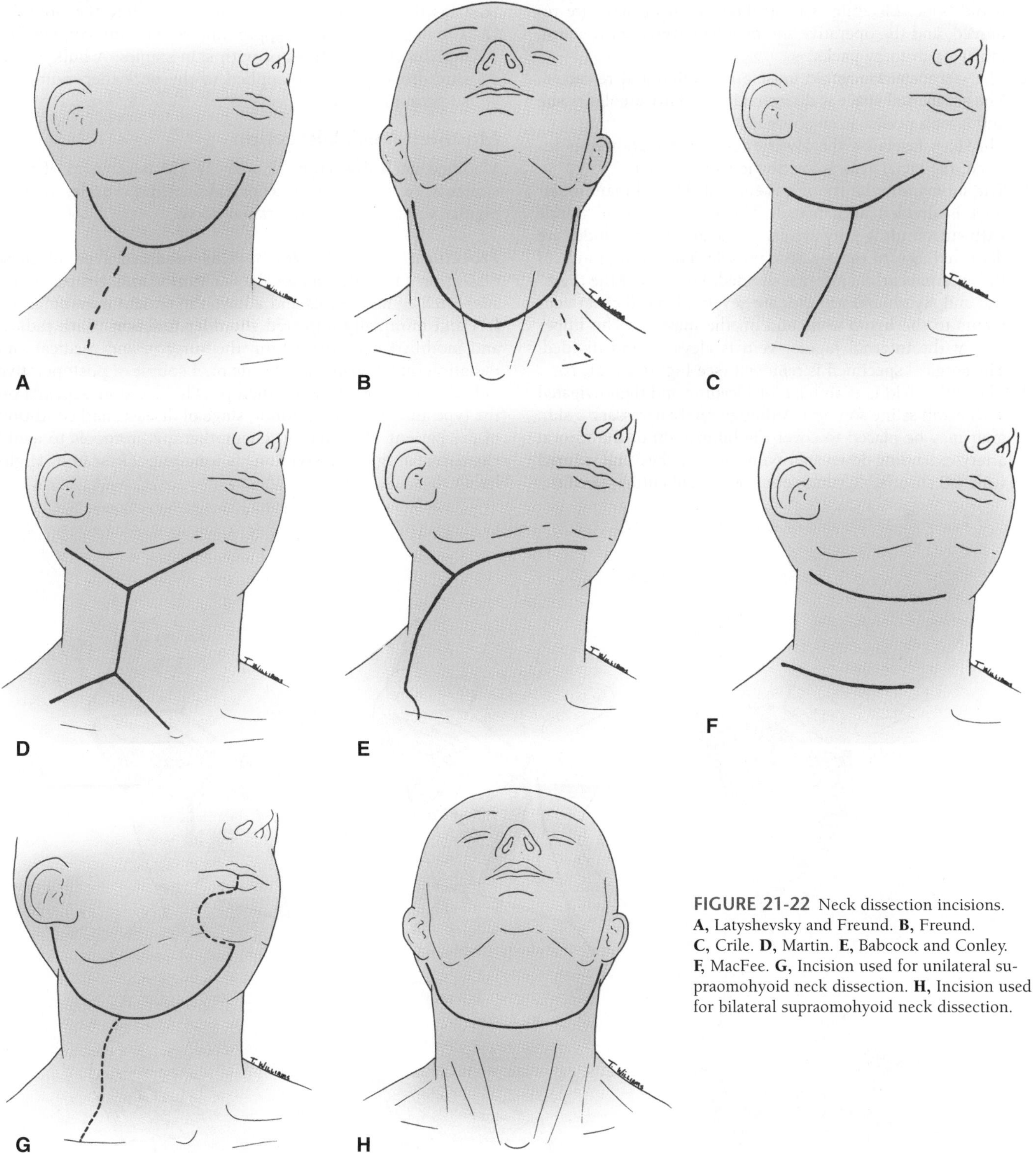

FIGURE 21-22 Neck dissection incisions. **A,** Latyshevsky and Freund. **B,** Freund. **C,** Crile. **D,** Martin. **E,** Babcock and Conley. **F,** MacFee. **G,** Incision used for unilateral supraomohyoid neck dissection. **H,** Incision used for bilateral supraomohyoid neck dissection.

forceps. Branches of the thyrocervical artery are clamped, divided, and ligated.

6. The tissues and fascia of the posterior triangle are dissected, beginning at the anterior margin of the trapezius muscle and continuing near the brachial plexus and the levator scapulae and scalene muscles. During the dissection, branches of the cervical and suprascapular arteries are clamped, ligated, and divided.
7. The anterior portion of the block dissection is completed. The omohyoid muscle is severed at its attachment to the

hyoid bone. Bleeding is controlled. All hemostats are removed, and the operative site may be covered with warm, moist laparotomy packs.

8. The sternocleidomastoid muscle is severed and retracted. The submental space is dissected free of fatty areolar tissue and lymph nodes, from above downward.
9. The deep fascia on the lower edge of the mandible is incised; the facial vessels are divided and ligated.
10. The submandibular triangle is entered. The submandibular duct is divided and ligated. The submandibular glands with surrounding fatty areolar tissue and lymph nodes are dissected toward the digastric muscle. The facial branch of the external carotid artery is divided. Portions of the digastric and stylohyoid muscles are severed from their attachments to the hyoid bone and on the mastoid. The upper end of the internal jugular vein is elevated and divided. The surgical specimen is removed (see Figure 21-21, *B*).
11. The entire field is examined for bleeding and then irrigated with warm saline solution. Although rarely necessary, a skin graft may be placed to cover the bifurcation of the carotid artery, extending down approximately 4 inches, and sutured with 4-0 absorbable suture on a very small cutting needle.
12. Closed wound-suction drains are placed into the wound.
13. The flaps are carefully approximated with interrupted fine nonabsorbable sutures or with skin staples. A bulky pressure dressing may be applied to the neck, depending on surgeon preference.

## Modified Neck Dissection

Modified neck dissection (Figure 21-23) is removal of neck contents, except for the sternocleidomastoid muscle, internal jugular vein, and eleventh cranial nerve.

***Procedural Considerations.*** This modified type of neck dissection facilitates removal of a tumor and lymph nodes suspected of metastases and allows the patient a minimal defect and minimally impaired shoulder function. With radical and modified neck dissection, the surgeon and medical and radiation oncologists may decide on a course of postoperative radiation therapy or chemotherapy. The decision depends on the type and location of tumor, stage of disease, and condition of the patient. Research on chemotherapy protocols to avoid extensive surgical dissection is ongoing (Research Highlight).

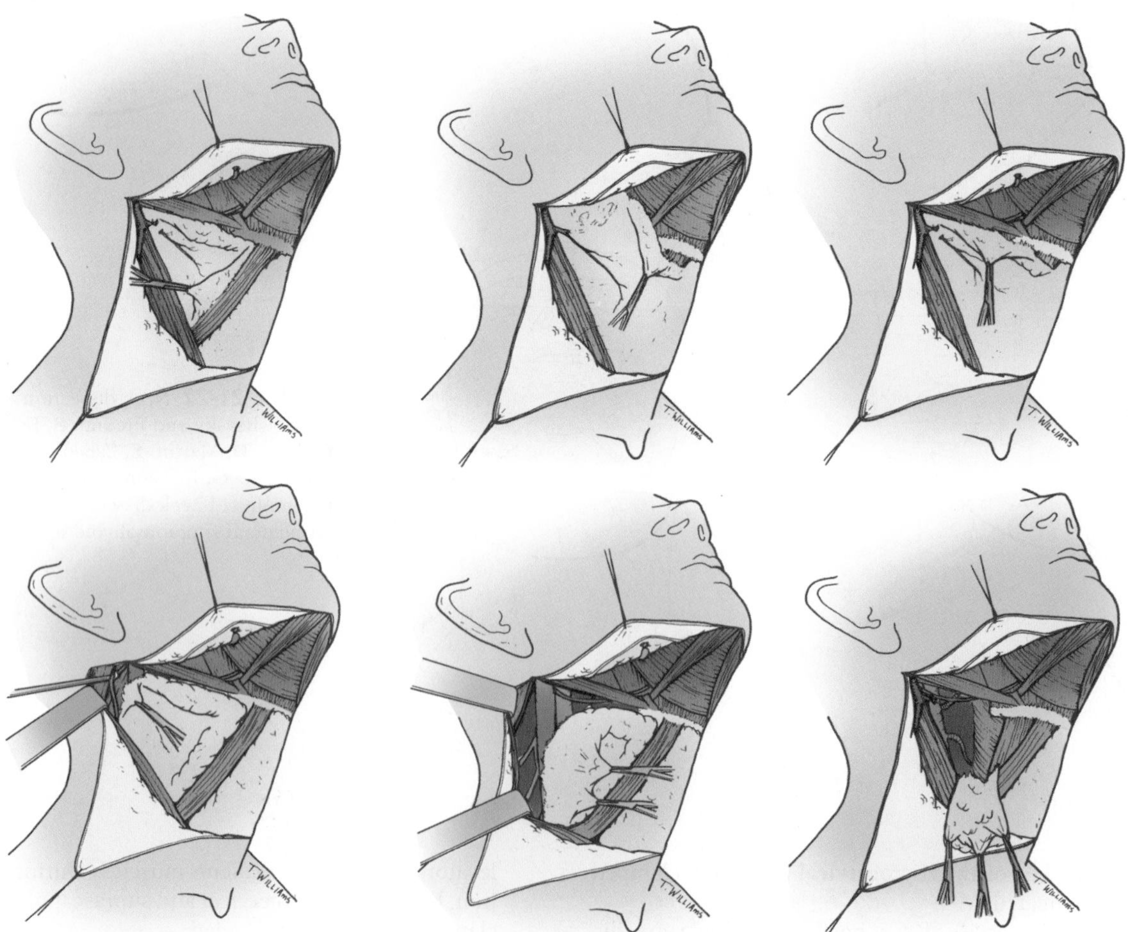

**FIGURE 21-23** Steps of modified radical neck dissection with preservation of spinal accessory nerve, internal jugular vein, and sternocleidomastoid muscle.

## RESEARCH HIGHLIGHT

### Preserving the Voice in Advanced Vocal Cord Cancer

Losing the ability to speak is a devastating consequence of many surgical procedures for laryngeal cancer. This study sought to determine if using chemotherapy and radiation instead of surgery in advanced laryngeal cancer had any impact on survival rates.

Researchers studied 547 patients with advanced cancer of the larynx. They divided the patients into three groups: one group received only radiation therapy, the second group underwent chemotherapy followed by radiation, and the third group had radiation and chemotherapy together.

Patients were observed for an average of 4 years after treatment. Analysis of the data showed that both the chemotherapy-based protocols suppressed distant metastasis and resulted in better disease-free survival than radiation alone. Within the chemotherapy/radiation group, 88% of the patients were able to avoid surgery and retain their ability to speak; 75% of patients in the chemotherapy followed by radiation group were able to avoid surgery, and 70% of those in the radiation-alone group did not require surgery.

Recurrence rates were lowest in the groups that received chemotherapy, at 8% to 9%. The group that had radiation alone had a recurrence rate of 16%.

The overall survival rate in this study was the same in all three groups. This treatment may be a feasible option for patients with later-stage cancers who wish to preserve their voice.

Modified from Forastiere AA and others: Concurrent chemotherapy and radiotherapy for organ preservation in advanced laryngeal cancer, *New England Journal of Medicine* 22(349):2019-2028, 2003.

## RECONSTRUCTIVE PROCEDURES

Head and neck surgical procedures to remove malignant tumors are reconstructed depending on the surgical defect. The wound may be closed primarily, or local flaps and split-thickness skin grafts (as for facial and intraoral defects) or full-thickness skin grafts (as for nasal and facial defects) may be used. Regional flaps (e.g., pectoralis major musculocutaneous flap), microvascular tissue transfer (e.g., radial forearm flap, free jejunal flap, rectus abdominis flap), or microvascular osteocutaneous flaps (e.g., iliac crest flap) may be used to restore function as well as cover defects. Combinations of these grafts and flaps are often necessary when large defects are created. Skin grafts and flaps are discussed in Chapter 24.

If microvascular flaps are used, surgical and anesthesia time is extended significantly; since veins and arteries are microscopically connected, nerve grafts may be used, and bone must be connected with the use of plates and screws.

The use of a Doppler unit (intraoperatively and postoperatively) and thorough nursing assessment skills are paramount in detecting occlusions or spasms of the vessels and subsequent survival of the transplanted flap.

## REFERENCES


1. American Cancer Society: *Cancer facts and figures 2005*, Atlanta, 2005, The Society.
2. Association of periOperative Registered Nurses: Recommended practices for laser safety in practice settings. In *Standards, recommended practices, and guidelines*, Denver, Colo, 2004, The Association.
3. Elluru RG, Kumar M: Physiology of the salivary glands. In Cummings CW and others, editors: *Otolaryngology: head and neck surgery*, ed 4, St Louis, 2005, Mosby.
4. Flint PW, Cummings CW: Medialization thyroplasty. In Cummings CW and others, editors: *Otolaryngology: head and neck surgery*, ed 4, St Louis, 2005, Mosby.
5. Montgomery WW, Varvares MA: Surgery of the neck. In Montgomery WW, editor: *Surgery of the larynx, trachea, esophagus and neck*, Philadelphia, 2002, Saunders.
6. National Guideline Clearinghouse: *APIC guideline for selection and use of disinfectants*. Accessed January 29, 2006, on-line: www.guideline.gov.
7. Pagana KD, Pagana TJ: *Mosby's diagnostic and laboratory test reference*, ed 7, St Louis, 2005, Mosby.
8. Seidel HM and others: *Mosby's guide to physical examination*, ed 5, St Louis, 2003, Mosby.

CHAPTER 22

# Orthopedic Surgery

BARBARA BOWEN

The word *orthopédie* is derived from the Greek *orthos*, meaning "straight," and *paideia*, meaning "rearing of children." It was first used by Nicholas Andry in 1741 in the title for a book dealing with the prevention and correction of skeletal deformities in children. Orthopedic surgery has been defined by the American Association of Orthopaedic Surgeons' Board of Orthopaedic Surgery as "the medical specialty that includes the investigation, preservation and restoration of the form and function of the extremities, the spine, and associated musculoskeletal structures by medical, surgical and physical means."[1]

Orthopedic surgery is an ever-changing field that is a challenge for the perioperative nurse. Technologic advances in the multitude of systems and hardware used have resulted in improved treatment of orthopedic disorders. In addition to understanding anatomic and physiologic responses, the perioperative nurse should have a general understanding of the concepts and purposes of these systems to provide the most safe and efficient care. Knowledge of the principles of bone fixation and healing and the relationship of bone and soft tissues will provide a strong basis to ensure continued understanding of the care required for the orthopedic patient.

## Surgical Anatomy

### Anatomic Structures

The 206 bones of the body form the appendicular or axial framework that supports soft tissues, provides storage areas and reservoirs for minerals, and serves as a site for formation of blood cells (Figure 22-1). The skeletal system is composed of varied elements, including bone, muscle, and associated structures.

Bone remains in a constant state of formation and resorption, preventing development of excessive thickness or thinness. These processes are related to individual metabolism and absorption of calcium, vitamin D, and phosphorus. Levels of minerals affect disease processes, causing bone changes. A layer of connective tissue called *periosteum* covers all bone.

Muscles are masses of tissue that cover bones and provide movement to the skeletal system. Muscles interact with nerves, minerals, skin, and other connective tissue to contract and extend. Individual muscles are short or long and vary in diameter, depending on their position on a specific bone.

Ligaments, tendons, and cartilage also form the skeletal structures. Ligaments are bands of dense connective tissue that hold bone to bone. They provide stability to a joint by encircling or holding ends of bone in place. Tendons are tough, long strands of fibers that form the ends of muscles. They transmit forces to bone or cartilage without being damaged. Cartilage is a layer of elastic, resilient supporting tissue found at the ends of the bones. It forms a cap over the bone end to protect and support the bone during weight-bearing activities and provides a smooth gliding surface for joint movement. Cartilage is aneural (without nerves), alymphatic (without lymph tissue), avascular (without blood vessels), and high in water content. The lack of vascularity and loss of water from cartilage during a lifetime are causes of resulting degenerative disease, such as arthritis. Weight bearing and joint movements keep cartilage from becoming thin or damaged and help prevent degenerative conditions.

Joints are articulations where bones are joined to one another or where two surfaces of bones come together. Joints are classified by the type of material between them or according to movement. Material between joints is fibrous, cartilaginous, or synovial. The type of movement is synarthrotic (immovable), amphiarthrotic (slightly movable), or diarthrotic (freely movable). Synarthrotic joints are connected by fibrous tissue or ligaments (e.g., the suture type of joints holding the bones of the skull; connections between two bones, such as the radius and ulna). Amphiarthrotic joints are connected by cartilage. Joints of this type include the symphysis pubis, intervertebral joints, and manubriosternal joint. The majority of joints are diarthrotic; these are the only joints with one or more ranges of motion. These joints are lined with a synovial membrane and are called *synovial joints*. Examples include the knee, cervical vertebrae 1 and 2 (C1 and C2), the radius articulating on the wrist bones, the hip, and the shoulder.

The two types of bone tissue are *cortical* and *cancellous*. Cortical bone is the hard bone forming the outer shell—the main supporting tissue. Cancellous bone is soft and spongy—located at the iliac crest, tibia, sternum, and ends of long bones. It contains the red bone marrow for hematopoiesis.

Bones are divided according to their shape: long, short, flat, irregular, and round (Figure 22-2). Long bones are present in the limbs and consist of a shaft and two ends; the ends generally flare out, are covered with articular cartilage, and provide a surface for articulation and musculotendinous attachment. Short bones, such as the carpals and tarsals (in the wrist and midfoot area), are present where the structure is strong but limited movement is required. Flat bones are the scapula, the sternum, and the pelvic girdle. Irregular bones are found in the skull and vertebral column. Round, or sesamoid, bones (resembling a sesame seed) are found within tendons. The patella is a large sesamoid bone; however, most are small, such as the two found on the head of the first metatarsal, which form the "ball" of the foot.

Long bones consist of a shaft (diaphysis) and two ends (epiphyses). The shaft is composed of compact bone. The

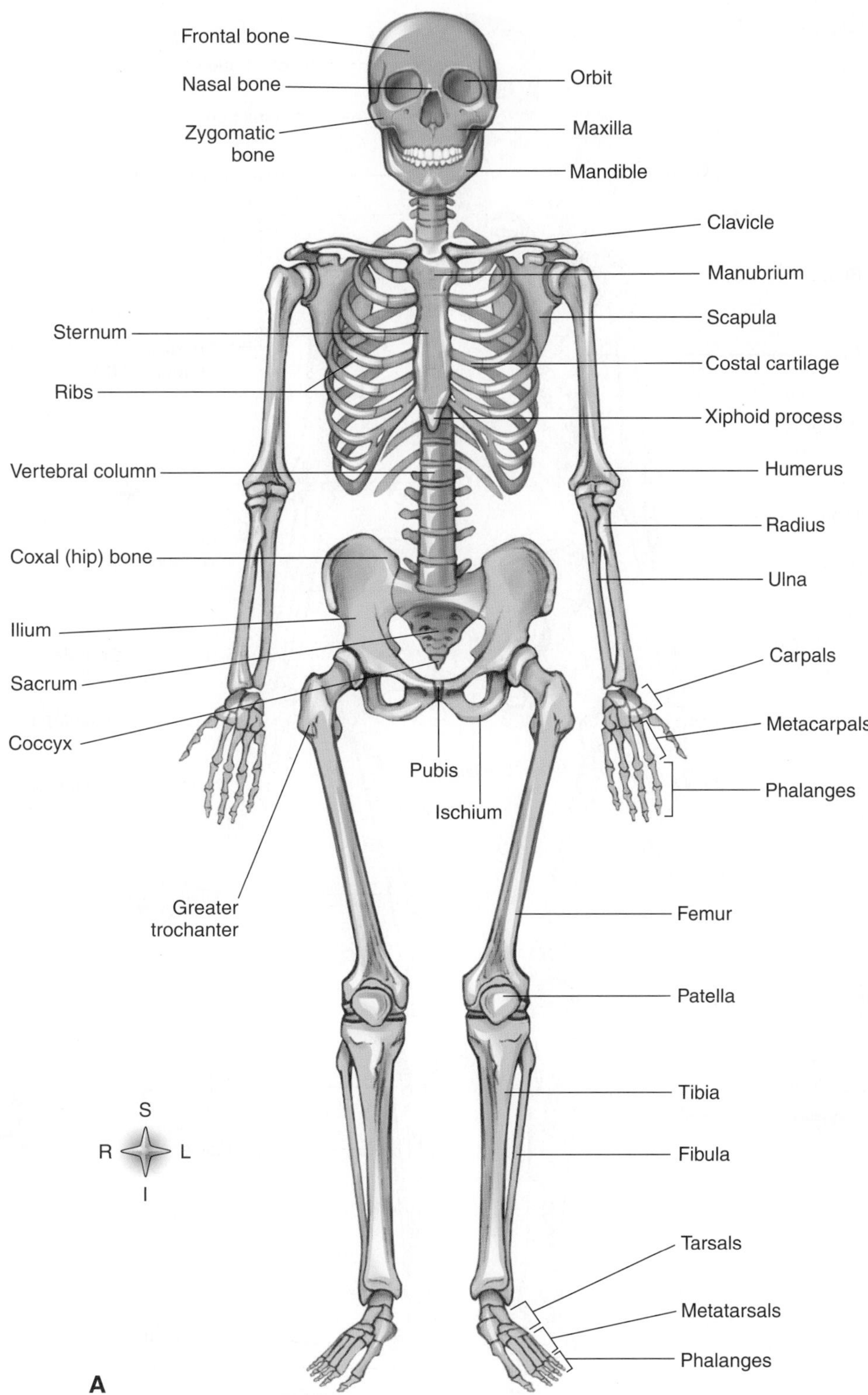


**FIGURE 22-1** **A,** Anterior view of the skeleton.

*Continued*

epiphyses flare out and consist of cancellous bone. They are covered by cartilage, which provides a cushion and offers protection during weight bearing and movement. Until skeletal maturity, a line of cartilage called the *epiphyseal plate* separates the epiphysis from the diaphysis. Fractures in this region by children can be devastating because they often lead to malformation and permanent limb shortening.

Trabeculae are located within cancellous bone and consist of an interconnecting network of bone oriented along the lines of stress. These structures are important for weight bearing, providing strength to withstand stress placed on the bone. The periosteum is a thin, outer covering of bone containing nutrient arteries for nourishment of bone cells. Disruption of these periosteal vessels after bone trauma can influence the ability of

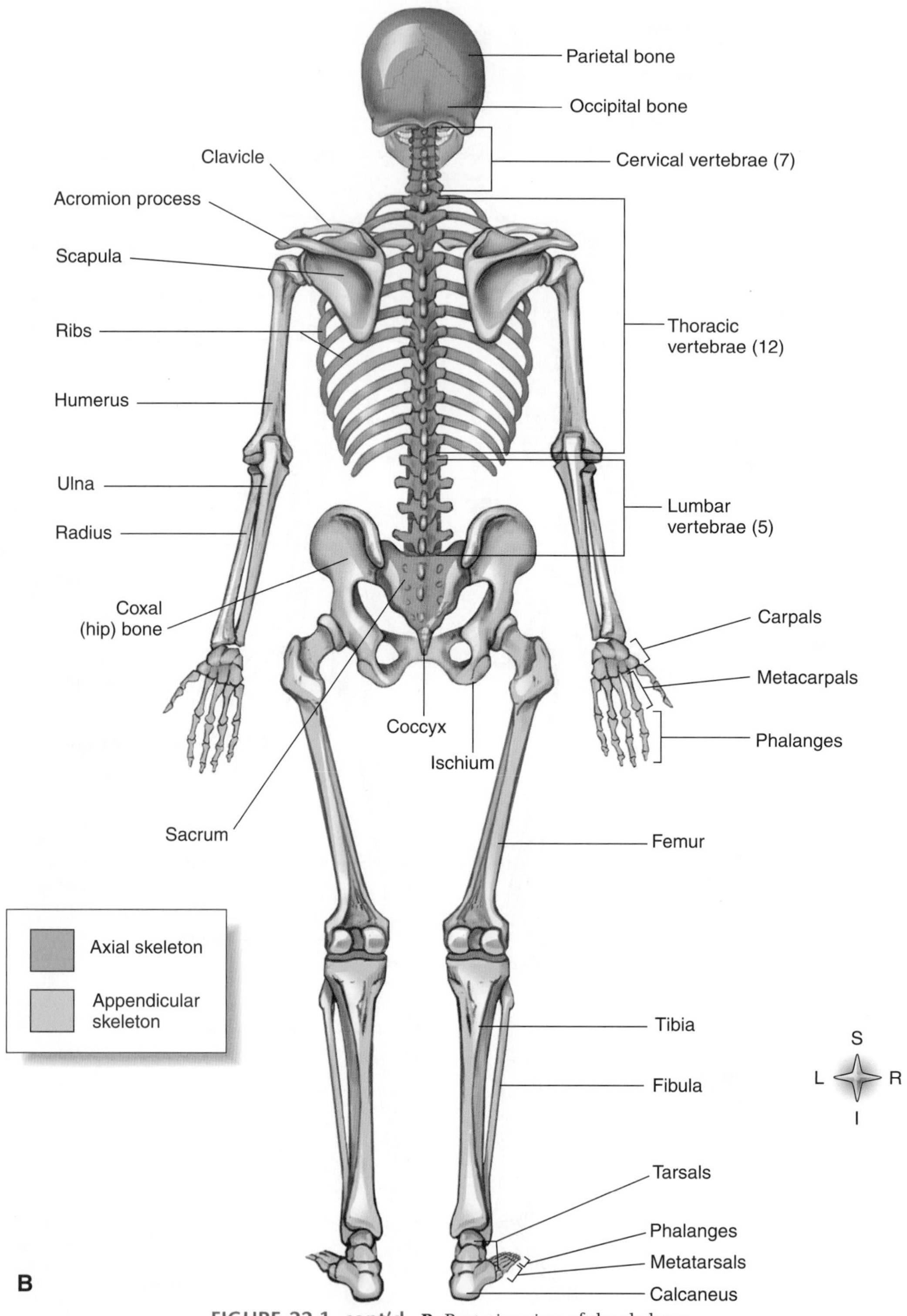


**FIGURE 22-1, cont'd.** **B,** Posterior view of the skeleton.

bone to heal. The haversian system consists of thousands of microscopic units found in the cortical bone. These units of matrix cells, canals, and conduits allow flow of nutrients and facilitate calcium absorption.

## Vertebrae

Vertebrae form the longitudinal axis of the skeleton. The vertebral bodies are connected by several cartilaginous joints, which enable the vertebrae to flex, extend, or rotate while being held together. Intervertebral disks and ligaments connect the bodies of adjacent vertebrae. The ligamenta flava bind the laminae of adjacent vertebrae together. Other ligaments connect the spinous processes and vertebral bodies.

Seven cervical vertebrae form the skeletal framework of the neck. Twelve thoracic vertebrae support the thoracic region, and five lumbar vertebrae support the small of the back. Below the lumbar vertebrae lie the sacrum and coccyx. Each of these

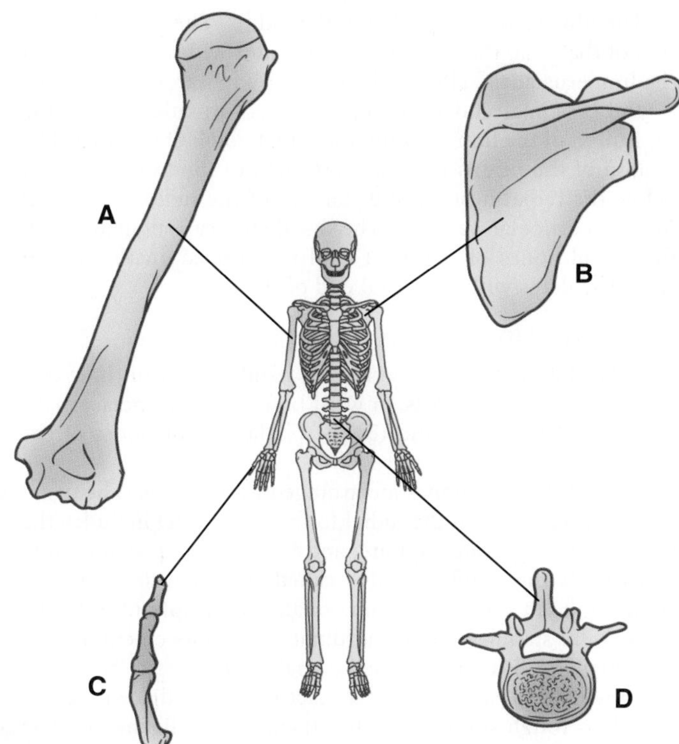


FIGURE 22-2 Types of bones, as examples. **A,** Long bones (humerus). **B,** Flat bones (scapula). **C,** Short bones (phalanx). **D,** Irregular bones (vertebra).

bones is composed of fused vertebrae—five for the sacrum and four for the coccyx.

The vertebral column is curved. After birth, there is a continuous posterior convexity. As development occurs, secondary posterior concavities develop in the cervical and lumbar regions, resulting in improved balance.

Each area of the vertebral column has specific bony structures. General features include a body (except the first two cervical vertebrae) on the anterior part. The posterior portion of the vertebrae consists of a neural arch formed by pedicles and laminae and the spinous and transverse processes.

## Shoulder and Upper Extremity

The clavicle, which is a long, doubly curved bone, serves as a prop for the shoulder and holds it away from the chest wall. The clavicle rests almost horizontally at the upper and anterior part of the thorax, above the first rib. It articulates medially with the manubrium of the sternum and laterally with the acromion of the scapula; it is tethered to the underlying coracoid process of the scapula by the coracoclavicular ligaments.

The scapula (shoulder blade) is a flat, triangular bone that forms the posterior part of the shoulder girdle, lying superior and posterior to the upper chest. The glenoid cavity on the lateral side of the scapula provides a socket for the humerus (the bone of the upper arm). The acromion process articulates with the clavicle medially. The scapula is attached to the thorax by muscles.

The shoulder (pectoral) girdle consists of the glenohumeral, sternoclavicular, and acromioclavicular (AC) joints (Figure 22-3). The glenohumeral joint has a multidirectional range of motion, whereas the latter two joints have limited motion. The AC joint, located at the top of the shoulder, is the articulation between the outer end of the clavicle and a flattened articular facet situated on the inner border of the acromion. The muscles immediately surrounding the shoulder joint are the supraspinatus, infraspinatus, teres minor, and subscapularis muscles; together they are referred to as the *rotator cuff*. These muscles stabilize the shoulder joint, whereas the powerful deltoid, pectoralis major, teres major, and latissimus dorsi muscles move the entire arm. Shoulder girdle strength and stability are maintained by the soft tissue integrity—not

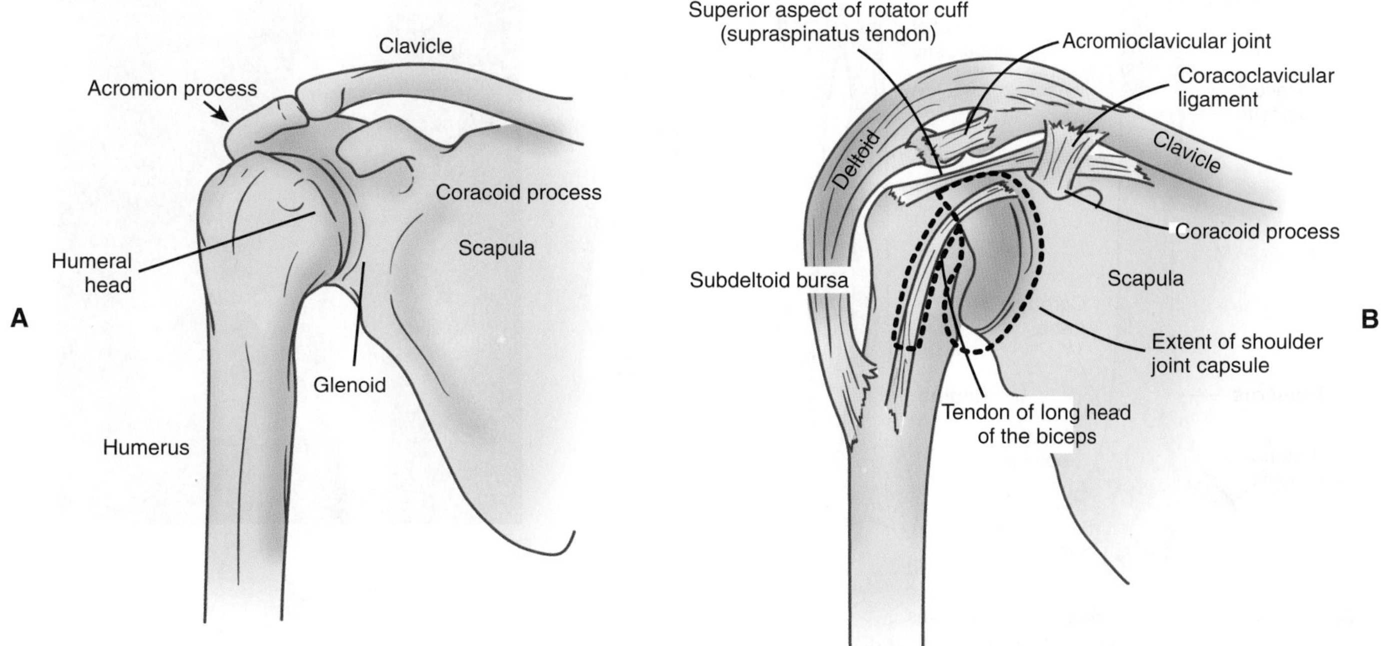


FIGURE 22-3 Shoulder. **A,** Joint showing anterior view. **B,** Girdle showing articulations.

the bony structures. A pathologic condition in this area can be the result of bone, soft tissue, or combined injury.

The humerus is the longest and largest bone of the upper extremity. It is composed of a shaft and two ends. The proximal end, or head, has two projections—the greater and lesser tuberosities (Figure 22-4). The circumference of the articular surface of the humerus is constricted and is termed the *anatomic neck*. The anatomic neck marks the attachment to the capsule of the shoulder joint. The constriction below the tuberosities is called the *surgical neck* and is the site of most fractures.

The greater tuberosity is situated at the lateral aspect of the humeral head. Its upper surface has three impressions where the supraspinous, infraspinous, and teres minor tendons insert. The lesser tuberosity is situated in the anterior neck and has an impression for the insertion of the tendon of the subscapular muscle. The attachment sites for the rotator cuff, the tuberosities, are separated from each other by a deep groove (bicipital groove), in which lies the tendon of the long head of the biceps muscle of the arm. The tendon of the pectoralis major inserts on the lateral margin of the bicipital groove, and the latissimus dorsi and teres major insert on the medial margin.

The distal humerus flattens and ends in a broad articular surface. The surface is divided into the medial and lateral condyles, which are separated by a slight ridge. On the lateral condyle, the rounded articular surface is called the *capitulum,* which articulates with the head of the radius. On the medial condyle, the articular surface is termed the *trochlea,* which articulates with the ulna.

The ulna is located medial to the radius. The proximal portion of the ulna, the olecranon, articulates with the trochlea of the humerus at the elbow. The radius rotates around the ulna. At the proximal end is the head, which articulates with the capitulum of the humerus and the radial notch of the ulna. The tendon of the biceps muscle is attached to the tuberosity just below the radial head. The distal end of the radius is divided into two articular surfaces. The distal surface articulates with the carpal bones of the wrist, and the surface on the medial side articulates with the distal end of the ulna.

## Wrist and Hand

The skeletal bones of the wrist and hand consist of three distinct parts: (1) the carpals, or wrist bones; (2) the metacarpals, or bones of the palm; and (3) the phalanges, or bones of the digits (Figure 22-5).

The eight carpal bones are arranged in two rows. The distal row, proceeding from the radial to the ulnar side, includes the trapezium, trapezoid, capitate, and hamate; the proximal row consists of the scaphoid (also called the *navicular*), lunate, triquetrum, and pisiform. Functionally, the scaphoid links the rows as it stabilizes and coordinates the movement of the proximal and distal rows. Each carpal bone consists of several smooth articular surfaces for contact with the adjacent bones, as well as rough surfaces for the attachment of ligaments. The five metacarpal bones (long bones) are situated in the palm. Proximally they articulate with the distal row of carpal bones, and distally the head of each metacarpal articulates with its proper phalanx. The heads of the metacarpals form the knuckles. The phalanges, or fingers, consist of 14 bones in each

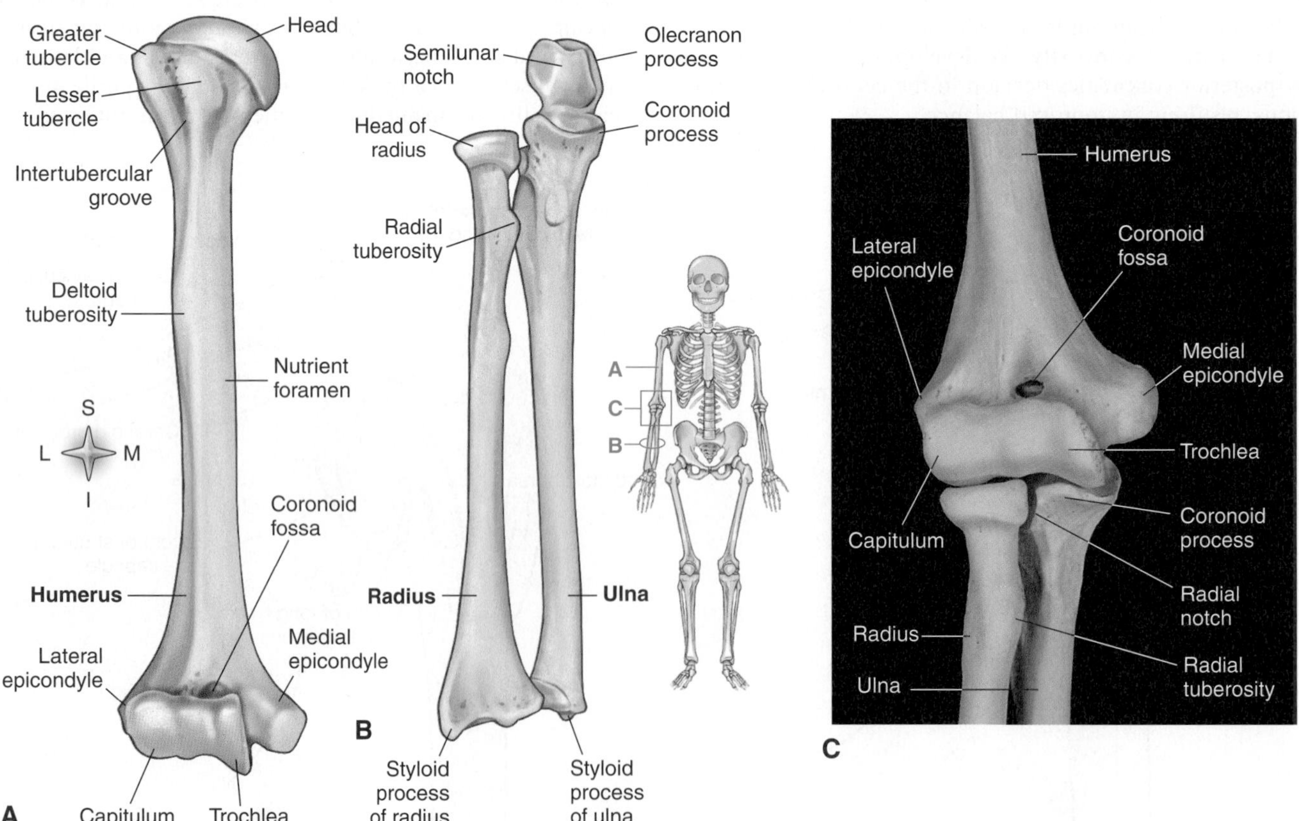


FIGURE 22-4 Bones of the arm, anterior view, showing the humerus, radius, and ulna.

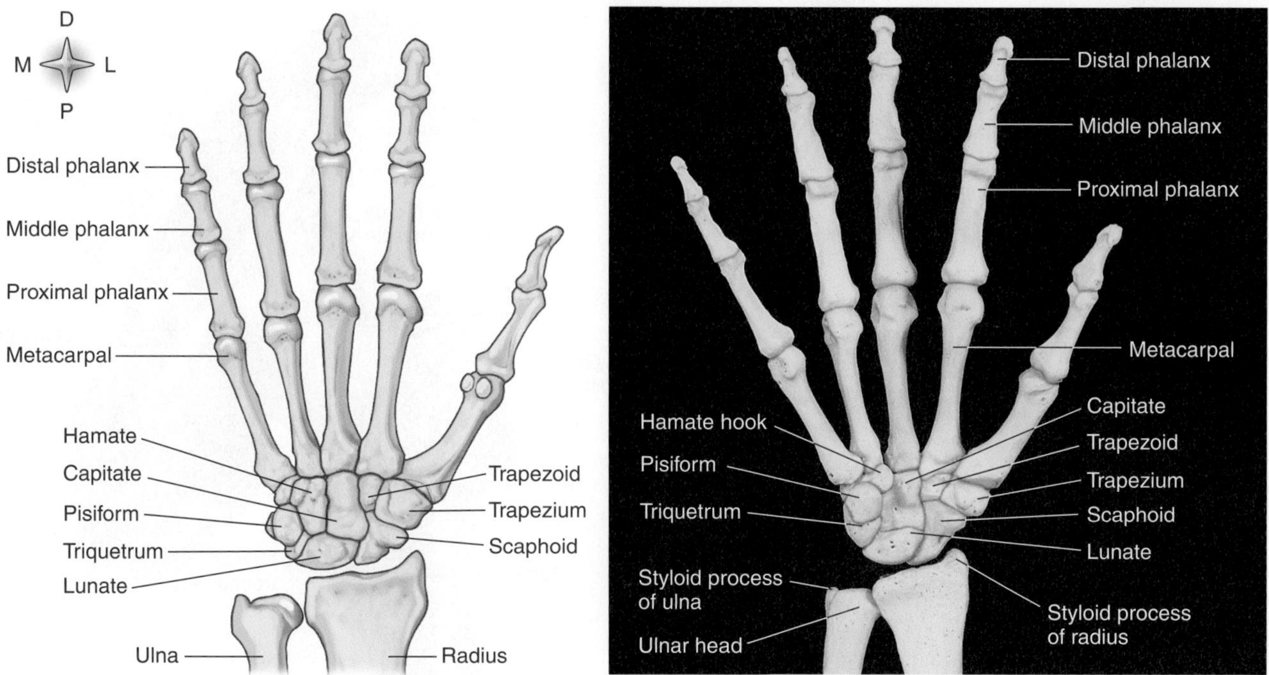


**FIGURE 22-5** Bones of the wrist and hand, palmar view.

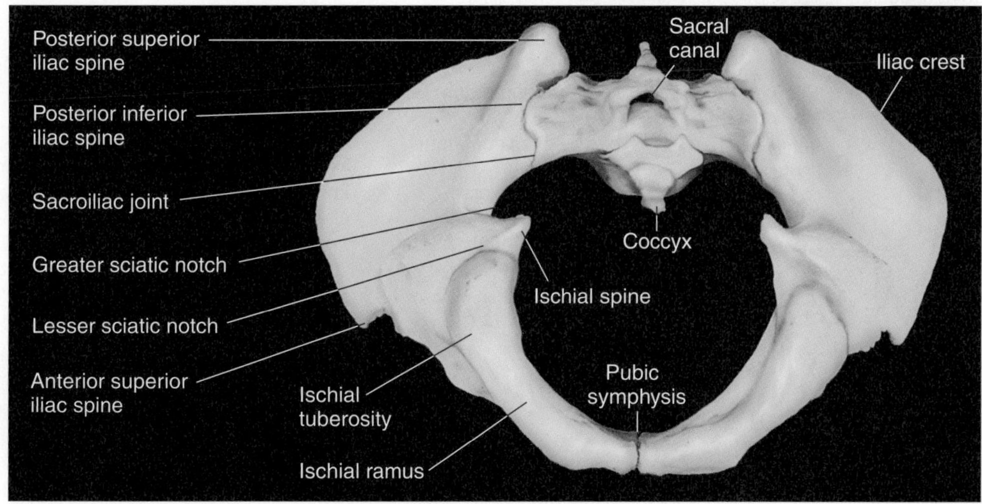


**FIGURE 22-6** Pelvis, superior view.

hand—two in the thumb and three in each finger. Each phalanx consists of a shaft and two ends.

## Pelvis, Hip, and Femur

The pelvis (Figure 22-6) is a stable circular base that supports the trunk and forms an attachment for the lower extremities. It is a massive, irregular bone created by the fusion of three separate bones. The largest and uppermost of the three bones is the ilium, the strongest and lowermost is the ischium, and the anterior-most is the pubis. Together these are termed the *os coxae,* or innominate bone.

The acetabular portion of the innominate bone and the proximal end of the femur (Figure 22-7) form the hip—a ball-and-socket joint. The hip joint is surrounded by a capsule, ligaments, and muscles that provide stability. The iliofemoral ligament connects the ilium with the femur anteriorly and superiorly, and the ischiofemoral and pubofemoral ligaments attach the ischium and pubis to the femur, respectively. The acetabulum is a deep, round cavity that articulates with the head of the femur. The proximal end of the femur consists of the femoral head and neck, the upper portion of the shaft, and the greater and lesser trochanters (Figure 22-8).

The greater trochanter is a broad process that protrudes from the outer, upper portion of the shaft and projects upward from the junction of the superior border of the neck with the

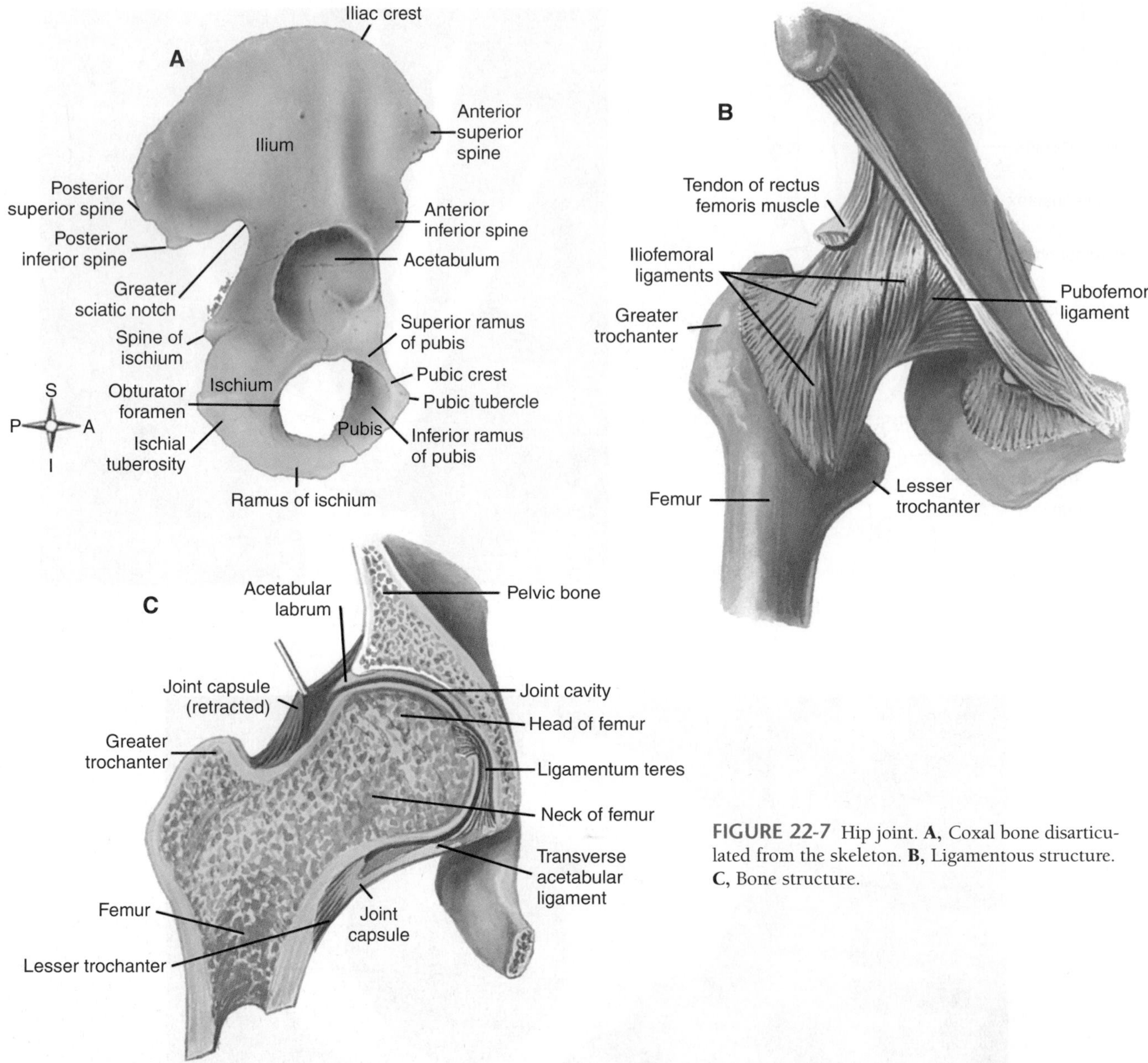


FIGURE 22-7 Hip joint. **A,** Coxal bone disarticulated from the skeleton. **B,** Ligamentous structure. **C,** Bone structure.

outer surface of the shaft. It serves as a point of insertion for the abductor and short rotator muscles of the hip.

The lesser trochanter is a conical process projecting from the posterior and inferior portion of the base of the neck of the femur at its junction with the shaft. It serves as a point of insertion for the iliopsoas muscle. The lower end of the femur terminates in the two condyles. Anteriorly, the condyles are separated from one another by a smooth depression, called the *intercondylar,* or *patellar, groove,* forming an articulating surface for the patella. Posteriorly, they project slightly, and the space between them forms the intercondylar fossa—a supporting structure for neurovascular structures.

The upper or condylar end of the tibia presents an articular surface corresponding with those of the femoral condyles. The articular surface of the two tibial condyles forms two facets, which are deepened by the semilunar cartilage into fossae for the femoral condyles.

## Knee, Tibia, and Fibula

The knee joint (Figure 22-9) consists of two articulations. One articulation is between each condyle of the femur and the tibial plateau; the other is between the patella and the femur. These areas are subject to degenerative changes, often requiring reconstructive surgery. The bones of the knee joint are connected by extraarticular and intraarticular structures. The extraarticular attachments consist of the joint capsule, multiple muscular attachments, and two collateral ligaments. The intraarticular ligaments consist of the two cruciate ligaments and the attachments of the menisci.

The patella, or kneecap, is anterior to the knee joint in the intercondylar groove, or trochlea, of the distal femur. It is a sesamoid bone contained within the quadriceps tendon. The anterior surface of the patella is united with the patellar tendon as the tendon originates and inserts above and below the knee

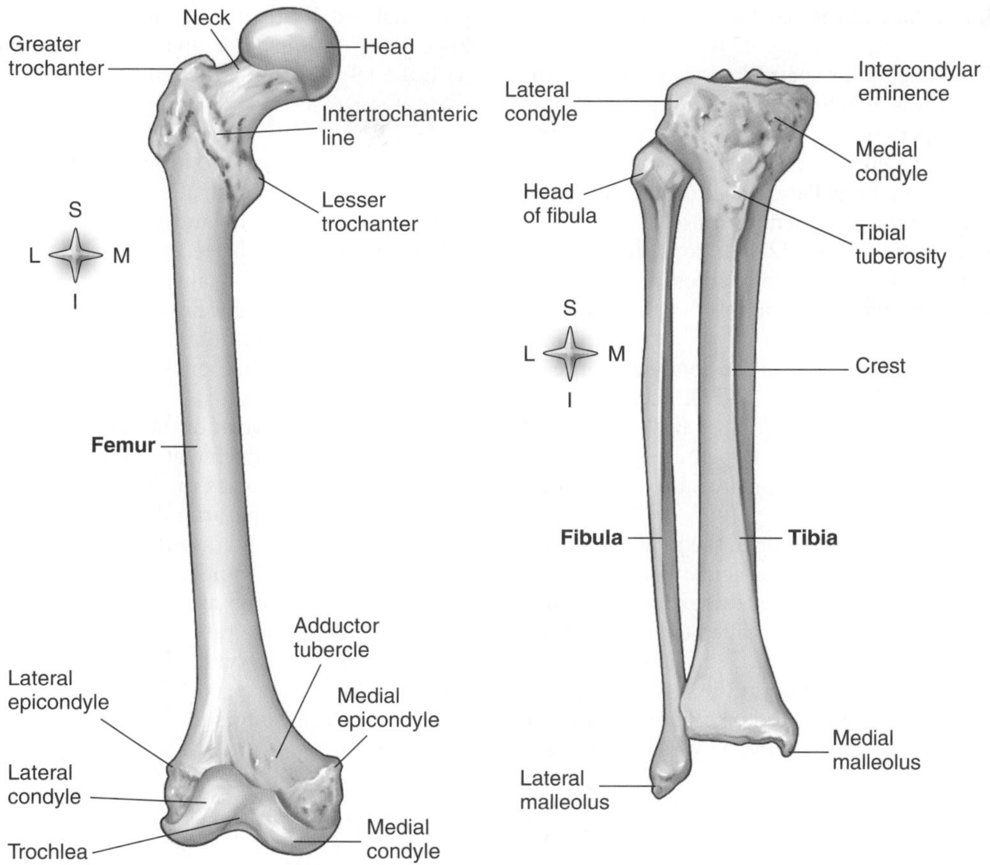


**FIGURE 22-8** Bones of the upper and lower leg.

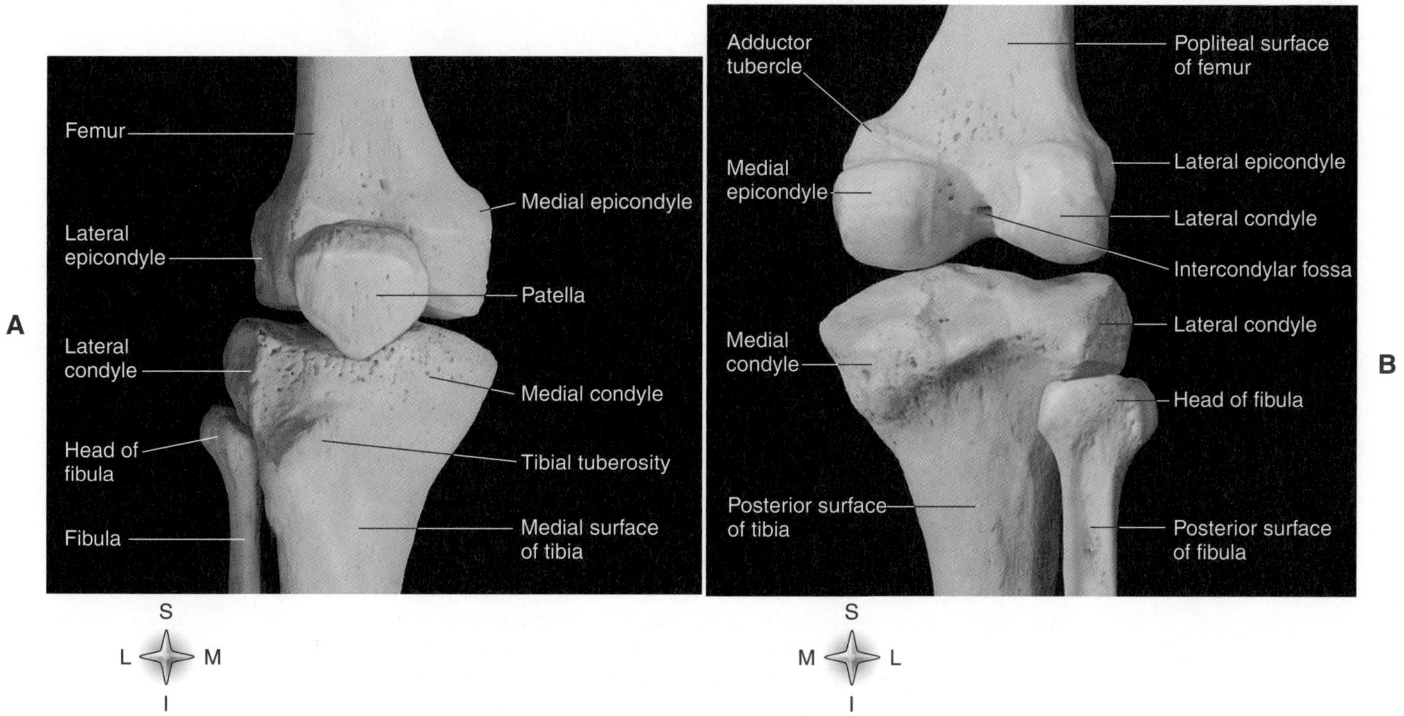

**FIGURE 22-9** Bones of the knee showing the tibia and fibula. **A,** Anterior aspect, **B,** Posterior aspect.

joint. The posterior surface of the patella articulates with the femur.

The capsule of the knee joint is attached proximally to the femoral condyles, and it is attached distally to the condyles of the tibia and to the upper end of the fibula. The capsule is reinforced in front by the patellar and quadriceps tendon, on the sides by the medial and lateral collateral ligaments, and posteriorly by the popliteus and gastrocnemius muscles.

The cruciate ligaments (Figure 22-10), consisting of two fibrous bands, extend from the intercondylar fossa of the femur to attachments anterior and posterior on the intercondylar surface of the tibia.

The menisci are interposed between the condyles of the femur and those of the tibia (see Figure 22-10). Each meniscus is attached to the joint capsule. The ends of the cartilage are attached to the tibia in the middle of its upper articular surface. These structures are almost totally avascular, and degenerative changes are usually permanent.

Synovial membrane lines the capsule of the joint and covers the infrapatellar fat pad, parts of the cruciate ligaments, and portions of the bone. The portion of the knee joint cavity that extends upward in front of the femur is called the *suprapatellar pouch,* or *bursa* (Figure 22-11).

The tibia is the larger and stronger of the lower leg bones. The fibula is smaller and located more laterally, articulating at the proximal end with the lateral condyle of the tibia. The proximal end of the tibia articulates with the femur to form the knee joint. Distally the tibia articulates with the fibula and with the talus, forming the ankle joint.

## Ankle and Foot

The ankle is a hinge joint, formed by the distal end of the tibia and fibula and the proximal end of the talus. The tibia (medial and posterior malleoli) and fibula (lateral malleolus) form a mortise (notch) for the reception of the upper surface of the talus and its facets. The talus is an irregular bone consisting of a body, neck, and head. The bones are connected by ligaments, which spread out from the malleoli to attach to the talus, calcaneus, and navicular bones (Figure 22-12). A thin capsule surrounds the joint.

The bony framework of the foot (Figure 22-13) comprises seven tarsal bones, five metatarsal bones, and fourteen phalanges. The calcaneus forms the heel and gives support to the talus. The cuboid bone articulates proximally and posteriorly with the calcaneus and distally with the fourth and fifth metatarsals and the third cuneiform bones.

The navicular bone articulates with the cuneiform bones, which lie side by side just anterior to it. The metatarsal bones articulate proximally with the tarsal bones and distally with the bases of the first phalanges of the corresponding toes. There are two phalanges for the great toe and three for each of the other toes.

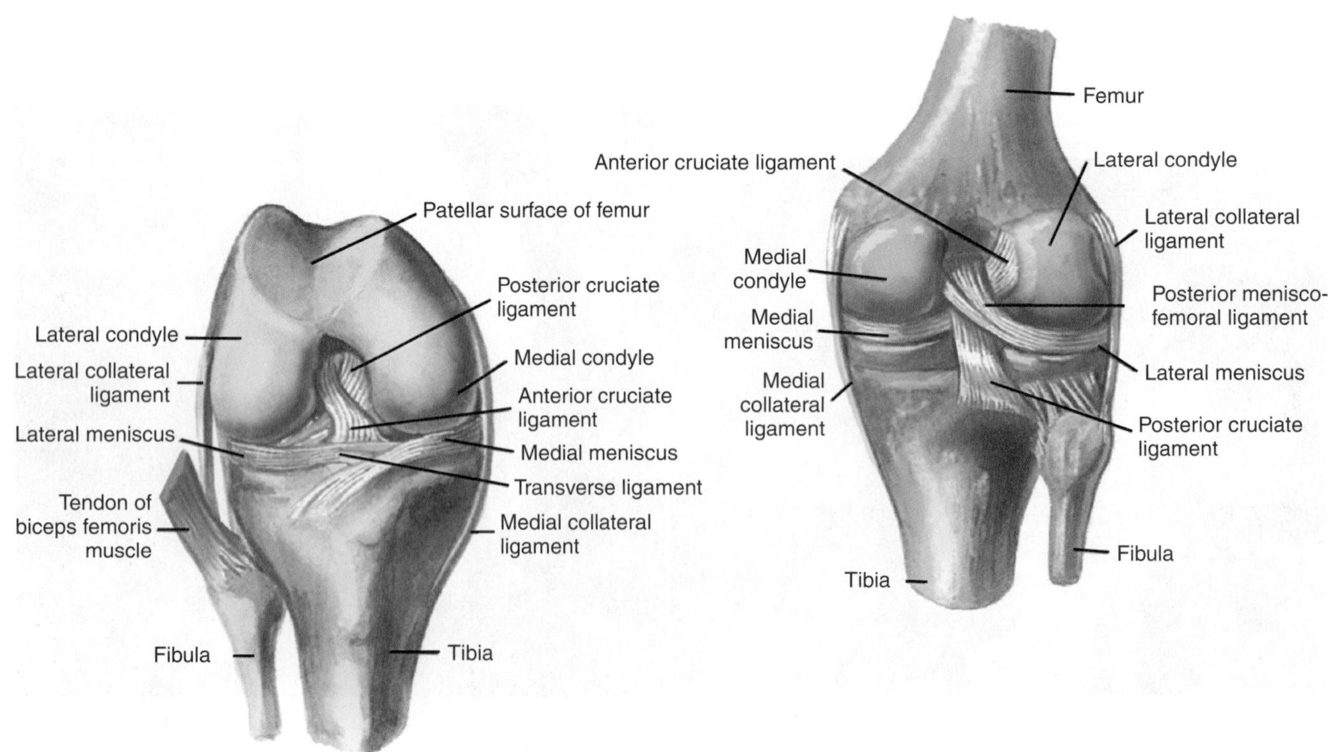


**FIGURE 22-10** Bony structures of the knee joint.

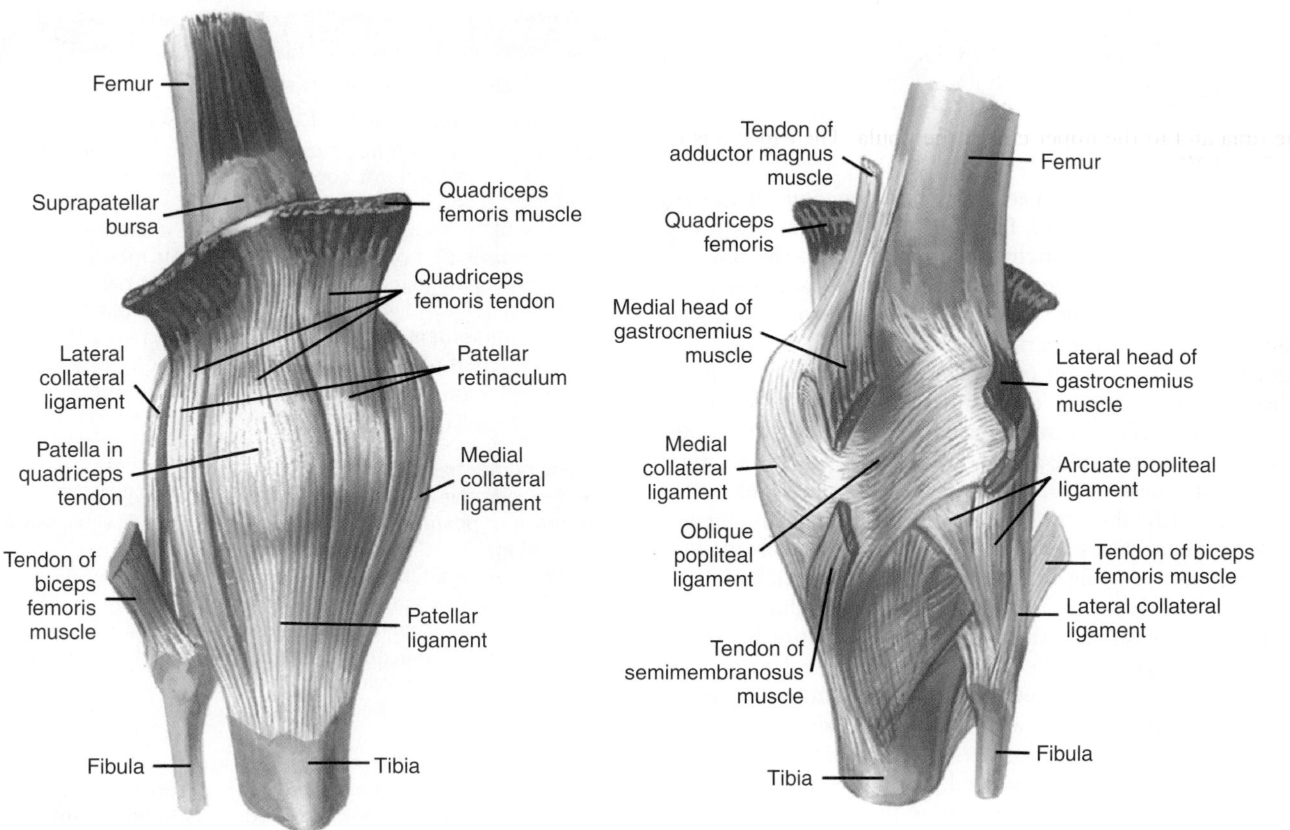


FIGURE 22-11 Superficial aspect of the knee joint.

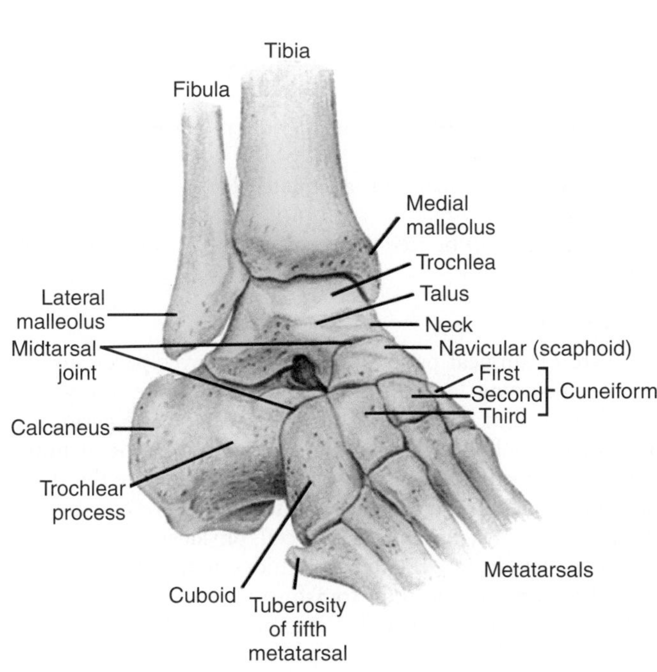


FIGURE 22-12 Anatomy of the ankle.

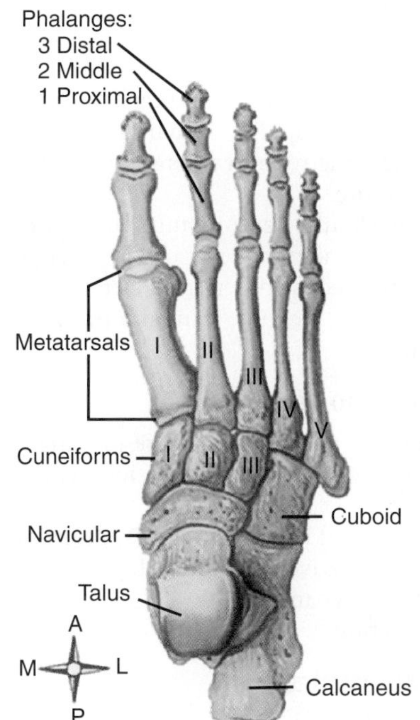


FIGURE 22-13 Bones of the foot viewed from above.

# *Perioperative Nursing Considerations*

## Assessment

Assessment of the orthopedic patient is ongoing, beginning with initial patient contact. Familiarity with orthopedic procedures and anticipated patient outcomes improves the ability to gather appropriate information and complete the nursing process. Obtaining patient-specific information from the physician also enhances the perioperative nursing assessment. The signed operative consent provides information to confirm the scheduled procedure or procedures and verify the operative site and side.[15] The consent is usually obtained before admission to the surgery suite and should be reviewed for accuracy and completeness. Additional measures that should be undertaken to verify the correct operative side and site include marking the surgical site and having the patient involved in the marking process; using a verification checklist (which includes documents such as the medical record, x-ray films, imaging studies); using verbal verification by the patient of his or her identity, surgical site/side, and planned surgical procedure; confirming this information during the time out by each member of the surgical team; and monitoring safe site protocol compliance with these procedures (Best Practice).

The patient record is reviewed, noting relevant aspects of the history and physical examination; the nature of the problem and its onset; and results of radiographic studies, laboratory data, and other findings. The nursing history is reviewed to determine physical, psychosocial, cultural, spiritual, and other needs. The patient should be assessed for range of motion, neurovascular status, and general condition. The patient's understanding of the surgical procedure and postoperative rehabilitation is determined, and patient education is begun.

Assessment information helps determine specific needs related to surgical positioning, skin preparation, equipment, instrumentation, and supplies. Environmental safety is also considered, including room temperature, traffic flow, lighting, and personnel attire.

Information should be communicated with surgical and anesthesia team members and persons in other disciplines. The information collected helps the perioperative nurse plan and coordinate activities, facilitate a smooth transition, and reduce operative time.

## Nursing Diagnosis

Nursing diagnoses related to the care of patients undergoing orthopedic surgery might include the following:

- Anxiety
- Risk for Peripheral Neurovascular Dysfunction
- Risk for Perioperative Positioning Injury
- Impaired Gas Exchange
- Risk for Infection

## Outcome Identification

Outcomes identified for the selected nursing diagnoses could be stated as follows:

- The patient will verbalize concerns and apprehension related to surgery and recovery.
- The patient will be free from peripheral neurovascular dysfunction.
- The patient will be free from perioperative positioning injury.
- The patient will maintain adequate ventilation and oxygen exchange.
- The patient will be free from postoperative surgical site infection.

## BEST PRACTICE

### Safe Site Protocol for Spine Surgery

The Joint Commission's Universal Protocol for correct patient, procedure, and surgical side and site, as well as the AORN Position Statement on correct site surgery both emphasize verification and marking of the surgical site (or invasive procedure site), especially when it involves laterality, levels, or multiples. As part of this process, protocols are used to verify the correct patient, correct procedure, correct patient position, and availability of necessary equipment, implants, imaging studies/equipment, or other special requirements. These protocols are part of the preoperative verification process as well as the time out before the start of the surgical procedure.

For surgery of the spine and other procedures involving level, such as the ribs, a recommended protocol may involve these additional steps:

- Preoperative skin marking of the spinal procedure site: anterior or posterior, and general level (e.g., cervical, thoracic, lumbar)
- Preoperative films/images: present in the operating room (OR) or procedure room
- The time out: includes patient identity (using two unique identifiers); procedure to be performed; correct patient position; correct procedure side, level, or site; and presence of necessary implants, imaging, equipment, or other special requirements
- If there are any discrepancies by any members of the surgical team the spinal procedure will not proceed until the institution's reconciliation procedure is initiated; the results of the reconciliation should be documented
- Intraoperatively: imaging with opaque instruments marking the specific bony landmarks is taken and compared with the preoperative films/images by the surgeon performing the procedure

Modified from Institute for Clinical Systems Improvement: *Health care protocol—safe site protocol for all invasive, high-risk, or surgical procedures,* January 2006. Accessed February 20, 2006, on-line: www/icsi.org.

## Planning

The care of surgical patients undergoing any type of surgery requires planning for routine procedures that are always followed, as well as anticipating the unexpected. The perioperative nurse should be consistent and systematic in the planning process to expedite actual steps required to facilitate the surgical procedure. Care of the orthopedic patient presents unique challenges because of the psychosocial, physical, and technical aspects of patient care. Planning includes attention to environmental factors, positioning, transfusion supplies, equipment, and instrument needs, in addition to practices that will prevent complications.

The optimal environment is comfortable for the patient and surgical team. The patient should feel relaxed and secure enough to allow the surgical team to become his or her advocates during the procedure. Physical preparation of the environment changes with individual patients. At the time the procedure is posted in the operating room (OR), traffic flow is considered to determine room location. The temperature is selected for the procedure with consideration given to the patient's age and general health, attire worn by the operative personnel (body exhaust suits), or use of polymethylmethacrylate (PMMA) (bone cement). Temperature should be monitored for all but very brief surgical procedures, such as those lasting less than 30 minutes. To maintain normothermia, the perioperative nurse might consider using warm cotton blankets preoperatively; warming the ambient room temperature, warming intravenous fluids, and warming the skin surface with a forced-air–warming device intraoperatively; and reapplication of warm cotton blankets at the end of the surgical procedure.

Equipment and instrumentation needed for the procedure are planned before the patient's arrival in the OR; orthopedic procedures may vary significantly because of the patient's physical condition or age. It may be necessary to communicate with the manufacturer's representative to facilitate obtaining items needed for the procedure. It is common for health care industry representatives to bring requisite orthopedic instruments to the OR or to act as a product resource regarding new equipment. However, industry representatives must comply with all institutional policies defining requirements and procedures and restrictions that govern their presence in the OR.[4]

Procedural information should be reviewed to plan positioning (Patient Safety) and protective measures. Aseptic technique is essential in the perioperative environment and should be considered a priority when caring for the orthopedic patient. Osteomyelitis is an infection of the bone that can go unrecognized for a long time and requires expensive, intensive treatment. Osteomyelitis can lead to severe bone loss and possible loss of a limb. Preventive measures, including administration of antibiotics within 60 minutes of making the incision, have been demonstrated to be efficacious in preventing surgical site infection.

OR equipment such as defibrillators and resuscitative equipment must always be available, functional, and familiar to staff. This includes supplies needed for emergency treatment of a patient condition, such as malignant hyperthermia or unanticipated blood loss. All medications and solutions along with their containers should be labeled both on and off the surgical field. Equipment alarms should be activated with appropriate settings and should be sufficiently audible. Orthopedic procedures may also require a change in the plan of care in the event of a fracture, damage to vascular integrity, or changes in the patient's condition, requiring an understanding of methods and equipment needed to manage these situations.

The nursing process requires continual reassessment and modifications. An effective plan entails communication, creating a culture that supports patient safety,[3] creation of an optimal environment, and effective use of human and physical resources. A typical plan of care for a patient undergoing orthopedic surgery begins on p. 716.

## Implementation

Implementing care for the orthopedic surgical patient requires an understanding of anatomic, physiologic, psychologic, cultural, spiritual, and technical patient needs. Orthopedic surgical procedures demand special equipment, instruments, and psychomotor skills that differ from those required by other specialties. Implementation includes an understanding of the procedures, patient needs, perioperative practices, and perioperative nursing interventions to protect the patient while delivering care.

Explanations about the intraoperative phase, including the anticipated sequence of events, personnel, environment, required positioning, and procedures such as administration of regional anesthetic and application of the tourniquet, should be reviewed with the patient. The patient may be alert during the procedure; therefore noise from power equipment and activities that will occur should be explained. Immobilization devices, such as splints, casts, braces, and drains, should also be explained.

## PATIENT SAFETY

### Perioperative Visual Loss Associated with Spine Surgery

Postoperative visual loss is considered a sentinel event under the Joint Commission's existing definition. Any unanticipated postoperative blindness is reviewable under the sentinel event policy. Since 1999, the Postoperative Visual Loss Registry has studied and investigated cases of perioperative ischemic optic neuropathy. Of the 130 reported cases of postoperative visual loss, 95 were in patients having spine surgery. In 2004, the American Society of Anesthesiologists (ASA) released a Practice Advisory for perioperative visual loss associated with spine surgery. Possible risks that may be associated with postoperative visual loss include preoperative anemia, hypertension, carotid artery disease, smoking, and obesity. Visual loss has also been associated with long surgical procedures and substantial intraoperative blood loss.

The ASA Practice Advisory notes the following:

- Some patients undergoing spine surgery in the prone position under general anesthesia have an increased risk for developing perioperative visual loss. They include patients undergoing prolonged procedures, having substantial blood loss, or both.
- High-risk patients should be positioned so that their heads are level with or higher than their hearts when possible.
- The patient's head should remain in a neutral forward position.
- Colloids along with crystalloids should be used to maintain intravascular volume in patients who have substantial blood loss.

Perioperative nurses can play a major role in managing postoperative visual loss by assessing the patient for changes in vision as soon as they can. Even if the patient is intubated, the perioperative nurse can determine if the patient can see how many fingers the nurse is holding up. If there is a visual loss noted, an ophthalmologist should be consulted.

Modified from Kostka J: Professionals grapple with causes of post-op blindness, *AORN Management Connections* 1(12):10-11, 2005.

## SAMPLE PLAN OF CARE

### NURSING DIAGNOSIS
**Anxiety**

### OUTCOME
The patient will verbalize concerns and apprehension related to surgery and recovery.

### INTERVENTIONS
- Encourage verbalization of feelings, expression of fear, and questions about procedure, anticipated outcome, postoperative rehabilitation, pain management, and home care/self-care requirements.
- Explain anticipated routine activities (diagnostic studies, operating room [OR] environment, preoperative holding area, postanesthesia care unit [PACU]), and encourage questions.
- Encourage patient and family participation in decision-making activities related to discharge planning.
- Demonstrate respect, and attend to patient's individual needs and those of the family or significant others.
- Remain with patient; ensure other personnel are introduced.
- Provide comforting and caring, for example, through the use of warm blankets, touch, hand holding.
- Discuss any other concerns with the patient and family, and initiate appropriate referrals.

### NURSING DIAGNOSIS
**Risk for Peripheral Neurovascular Dysfunction**

### OUTCOME
The patient will be free from peripheral neurovascular dysfunction.

### INTERVENTIONS
- Complete and document a preoperative neurovascular assessment including skin color and temperature, pulses, motor strength and movement, and sensation; reassess and document at procedure conclusion.
- Position in proper body alignment, considering range of motion or any limitations in mobility.
- Protect vulnerable neurovascular structures and prevent pressure by properly padding bony prominences and pressure points.
- For the brachial plexus, pad the elbow, avoid excessive abduction, secure arm gently on locked armboard.
- For the radial nerve, pad the wrist and secure it gently on an armboard or at the patient's side.
- For the medial or ulnar nerves, pad and tuck the arm carefully at the patient's side or on an armboard.
- For the peroneal nerve, place a pillow at the knee (but not under it), support the lower extremities, and use restraining straps such that they are not tight and do not compress the knee.
- For the tibial nerve, keep equipment off the lower extremities.
- Apply pneumatic tourniquet correctly, observing, verifying, and documenting pressure settings and tourniquet inflation time.
- Provide padding (air mattress or gel pads) when long surgical times are expected or patients are predisposed to peripheral vascular compromise.
- Anticipate patient's and surgical team's needs to minimize surgical time.

### NURSING DIAGNOSIS
**Risk for Perioperative Positioning Injury**

### OUTCOME
The patient will be free from perioperative positioning injury.

### INTERVENTIONS
- Assess range of motion; identify joints at risk for injury caused by immobilization, pain, trauma, or arthritic or other disease processes.
- Position arthritic joints carefully to prevent strain.
- Observe and document condition of patient's skin before transfer to the OR bed and again at conclusion of procedure.
- Use proper lifting and transfer techniques when transferring the patient to and from the OR bed to prevent shearing forces on skin.
- Keep sheets on OR bed dry and wrinkle-free.
- Ensure that personnel with knowledge of the patient's condition and equipment are available to supervise and assist with transfer of the patient.
- Use proper restraint devices to protect patients from falls or movement of the extremities.
- Avoid extending or flexing extremities beyond range of motion when there is resistance.
- Protect skin in dependent areas from pooling of solutions.
- Use positioning devices, such as pillows, to maintain position; use a small head pillow under the head if head and neck are normally bent slightly forward.
- Pad all dependent pressure sites; provide extra padding for patients with decreased circulation.
- Protect vulnerable neurovascular areas from compression.

### NURSING DIAGNOSIS
**Impaired Gas Exchange**

### OUTCOME
The patient will maintain adequate ventilation and oxygen exchange.

### INTERVENTIONS
- Review preoperative evaluation of the patient's pulmonary status.
- Assist anesthesia provider in airway management.
- Ensure full chest excursion when positioning, particularly in the lateral and prone positions.
- Collaborate with anesthesia provider in monitoring vital signs, oxygen saturation, ventilation, cardiac rhythm, and blood loss.
- Complete a vascular assessment (pulse, sensation, movement, temperature, and color check) preoperatively, and compare with postoperative status.

### NURSING DIAGNOSIS
**Risk for Infection**

### OUTCOME
The patient will be free from postoperative surgical site infection.

### INTERVENTIONS
- Modify the plan of care for high-risk patients as determined by assessment results.
- Confirm that the patient has complied with preoperative skin cleansing (as appropriate).
- Implement strict aseptic practices for skin prep, draping the patient and equipment, opening supplies and equipment for the procedure, removing hair (as necessary), and controlling traffic patterns in the operating room.
- Prepare for pulsatile lavage or irrigation (as needed).
- Initiate antibiotic therapy preoperatively and/or intraoperatively per physician's orders; check for medication allergies before antibiotic administration.
- Implement procedure-specific activities, such as using body exhaust systems and pulsatile lavage.
- Anticipate equipment needs, and check equipment function; implement safety precautions when using equipment.
- Sterilize instruments according to policy and procedure and the manufacturer's guidelines.
- Handle implants according to manufacturer's recommendations.

***Positioning and Positioning Aids.*** The orthopedic patient requires proper positioning on the OR bed or specialty bed to provide adequate exposure of the operative area, maintain body alignment, minimize strain or pressure on nerves and muscles, allow for optimal respiratory and circulatory function, and provide adequate stabilization of the body. Selection of position depends on several factors, including the type of procedure, location of the injury or lesion, and surgeon's preference. Guidelines for placing the patient in the supine or recumbent position are followed (see Chapter 5), with modifications to facilitate the specific orthopedic procedure.

Procedures performed in lateral, prone, or modified positions require use of positioning aids and devices to support these positions. Patients undergoing surgical procedures risk neuromuscular and skin injury. Preoperative assessment should be thorough to plan the position, taking into consideration the prevention of neurovascular compromise, impaired chest excursion, and the danger of falls. The safety strap does not always provide adequate security, and other methods of securing the patient on the OR bed may need to be implemented. The surgeon is responsible for selecting the position and ensuring that adequate exposure can be obtained. The perioperative staff must understand the meaning of terms such as *flexion, extension, abduction,* and *adduction* when positioning the patient. The staff must also be thoroughly familiar with the function of the orthopedic surgical bed and its various attachments (e.g., the leg attachment for arthroscopy, the three-point positioner for lateral position, and positioning devices for shoulder procedures).

Many orthopedic operations require a device for holding the extremities. Various holders are available for both upper and lower extremities. Positioners used intraoperatively can be sterilized for the procedure, resulting in the ability to reposition as needed throughout the procedure. These types of positioners include the shoulder positioner (Figure 22-14), Alvarado foot holder (Figure 22-15), and ankle distractor (Figure 22-16). Many other orthopedic positioning devices are also available.

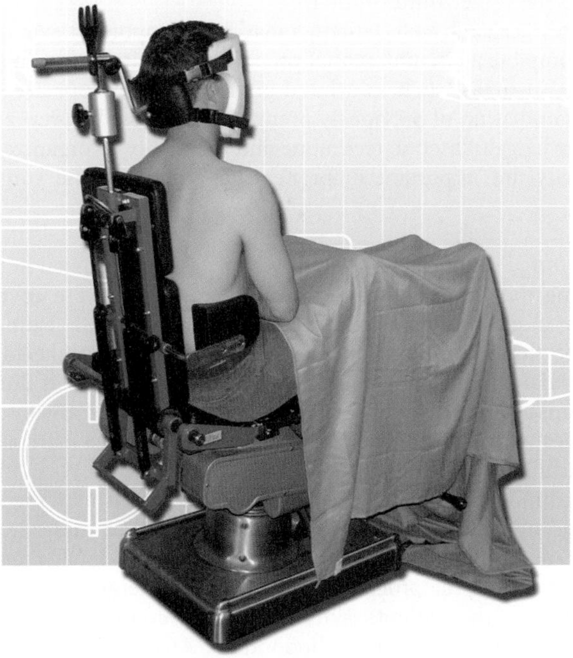

**FIGURE 22-14** Shoulder positioner allows distraction of the joint for visualization.

The lateral position is sometimes used for a total hip arthroplasty. Padded anterior and posterior supports may be positioned at the umbilicus and lumbar regions, respectively, to hold the patient in the lateral position. A vacuum beanbag can also achieve this position. Pressure points on the lateral area of the skull, ear, axilla, hip, knee, and ankle should be adequately padded. The feet are placed in the neutral position to prevent excessive plantar flexion or dorsiflexion. A conscientious effort

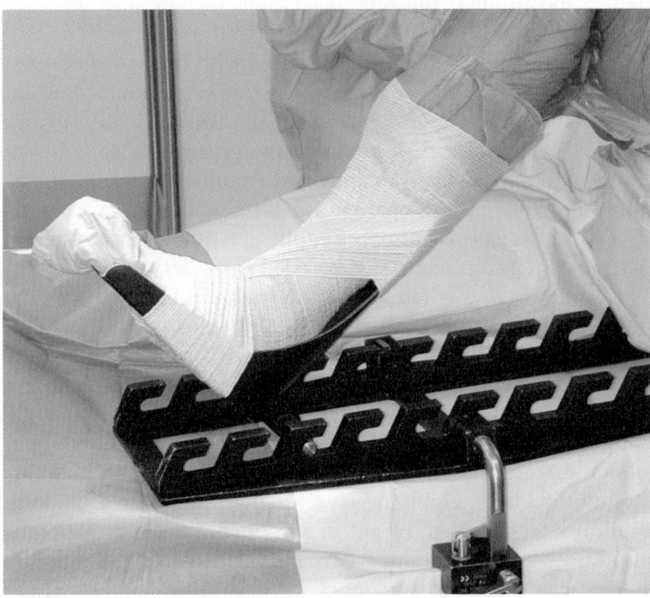

**FIGURE 22-15** Alvarado foot holder used during total joint procedures to position the extremity for exposure.

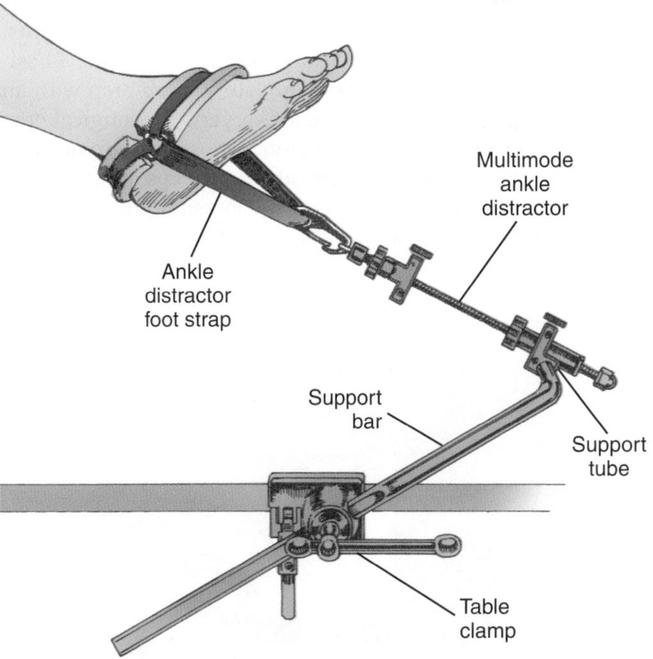


**FIGURE 22-16** Ankle distractor, noninvasive, for distraction of the joint and visualization.

should be made by the surgical team to avoid leaning on the patient during the procedure.

The patient is positioned prone for surgery on the posterior aspect of the body, including the back; posterior portion of the shoulder, arms, and legs; and Achilles tendon; and for posterior iliac bone graft harvesting. This position presents a challenge for the anesthesia team to monitor and manage the airway because of the potential for impaired chest excursion and gas exchange. Extremities need to be brought through a normal range of motion when transferring and positioning into the prone position. Vascular integrity is always assessed before the patient is moved into position and reassessed after the patient is positioned; the quality of pulses, extremity warmth, and capillary refill should be noted.

The prone position is often attained with the use of adjunctive frames, such as the Wilson, Hastings, Canadian, Relton-Hall, Collard saddle, or Andrews, or the Andrews bed (Figure 22-17). Each frame has qualities that meet the patient's or physician's needs. The Hastings and Andrews frames and Andrews bed maintain the patient in a modified knee-chest position. The frames require assembly and are labor intensive when positioning; some can be used only with certain beds. The Andrews bed is similar to the frame but has the attachments built in and is used exclusively for this position.

On an OR fracture bed (Figure 22-18), generally used for femoral neck and shaft fixation, the patient is placed in supine or lateral position to allow exposure of the surgical site while maintaining alignment. The legs are positioned on outriggers, allowing access by the image intensifier to obtain multiple radiographic views. Applying or releasing traction can be done to reduce the fracture or aid in intramedullary surgical techniques. Like all positioning devices, the fracture bed must be set up by experienced personnel and padded adequately. There are several moving parts, which can lead to injury if not operated properly.

***Surgical Prep.*** A primary concern in orthopedic surgery is the prevention of infection. The orthopedic surgical prep must be meticulously carried out using aseptic technique. Physicians often instruct patients to complete a scrub prep with an antimicrobial agent before arrival for surgery. The surgical prep for the orthopedic patient may include preoperative removal of hair from the surgical site. Surgical shave preps contribute to the possibility of infection caused by abrasion and cutting of the skin. If hair removal from the incisional site is ordered, it should occur immediately before surgery, using clippers or a depilatory. If a razor is required, the site should be lathered with soap before shaving. Trauma patients require precautions during the skin prep to prevent further injury caused by solution contact with membranes or injury to the bone and soft tissue from movement.

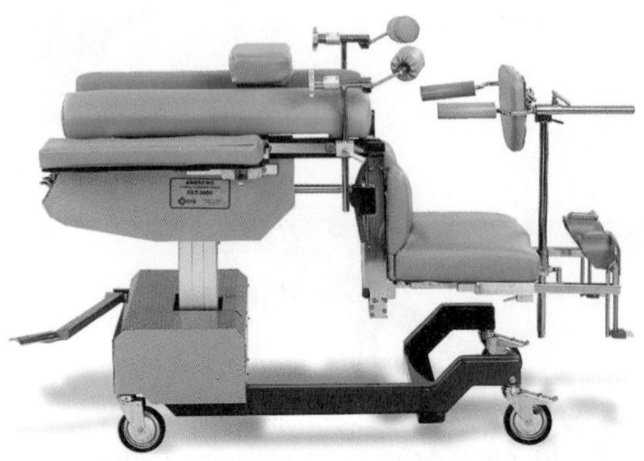

FIGURE 22-17 Andrews bed used for prone positioning.

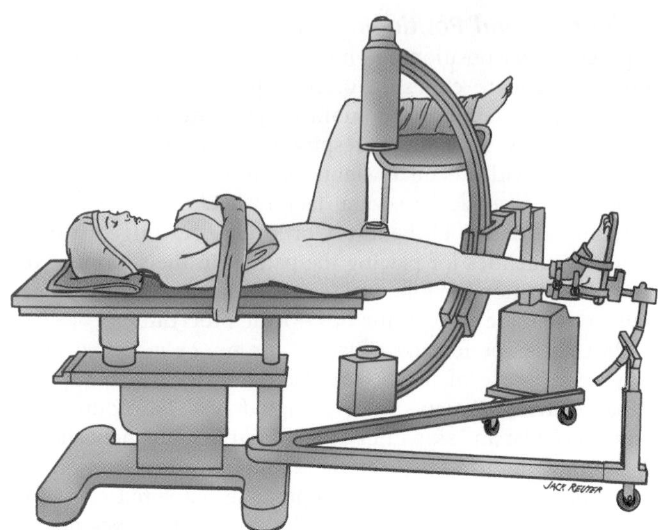

FIGURE 22-18 Patient positioned on the orthopedic fracture bed for femoral neck, femoral shaft, or tibial fixation, with image intensifier in position.

Skin preparation is performed to remove microorganisms from the operative site. The site should be prepped with a broad-spectrum antimicrobial agent. The prep proceeds from the incision site to the periphery. Pooling of the prep solution beneath the patient or tourniquet must be avoided. Prep solutions should be allowed to dry before draping; this is a fire safety precaution and may be included in the time out. The groin and anal areas should be isolated when the surgical site is on the upper third of the leg.

Devices such as leg stirrups may help support an extremity to complete a circumferential prep. When multiple extremities or other areas, such as a bone graft site, are prepped, cross-contamination of previously prepped areas must be prevented. Knowledge of aseptic technique and the ability to organize the activity are important in proper preparation of the surgical site.

***Draping.*** Application of sterile drapes is the final step in preparing the patient for the operation. Extremities are covered with a cloth or water-impervious stockinette—a cylindric drape that is rolled up the arm or leg. Impervious sheets are essential when large amounts of fluid are used, such as during arthroscopy and wound irrigation. Prefabricated disposable drapes with fenestrations for the upper and lower extremities are available.

Antimicrobial incise drapes can be used to isolate the surrounding area from the incisional site. Many of these drapes contain iodophor-impregnated adhesive, which slowly releases iodine during the procedure, inhibiting proliferation of organisms from the patient's skin.[14] They are contraindicated for patients with an allergy to iodophors. An alcohol skin wipe may be done before placement of the antimicrobial incise drape.

***Equipment and Supplies.*** Orthopedic operating rooms require a variety of special equipment and accessories in addition to routine operating room equipment. Nitrogen-powered, battery-powered, and electrically powered equipment, video systems, pneumatic tourniquets, laminar airflow systems, x-ray equipment, lasers, and special orthopedic tables are included in the operative armamentarium. Manufacturers' pamphlets with illustrations and directions on equipment use and sterilization should be readily available for reference.

RADIOGRAPHIC INTERVENTION. Radiographic intervention is widely used in orthopedic surgery (History box). Many procedures require portable x-ray or fluoroscopy machines. Fluoroscopy, also known as *image intensification* or *C-arm,* allows the team to view the progression of the procedure, confirming fracture reduction or intramedullary reaming of the humerus, femur, or tibia. An x-ray technician operates radiographic equipment. An understanding of equipment placement, function, and safety precautions is necessary. The perioperative nurse is responsible for communicating with the radiology personnel concerning the procedure, aseptic technique, and traffic flow in the operating room. X-ray cassettes brought onto the sterile field are draped with a sterile plastic cover. Lead aprons and thyroid shields are to be worn by all personnel in proximity to the x-ray equipment, and personnel should be monitored for exposure to radiation. Measures should be taken to protect patients from direct and indirect radiation exposure, and these should be documented on the perioperative nursing record.

PNEUMATIC TOURNIQUETS. Pneumatic tourniquets are frequently used for procedures involving the extremities (Figure 22-19). A tourniquet is a cylindric bladder inflated by compressed gas or ambient air. It applies circumferential pressure on arterial and venous circulation, which results in a relatively bloodless surgical field; this promotes visualization of structures during the procedure. Limb exsanguination is achieved by elevating the limb or by wrapping it, distally to proximally, with an Ace or Esmarch rubber bandage before tourniquet inflation. The majority of tourniquets used today are run by a microprocessor for regulation of pressure and time setting, providing both auditory and visual feedback for the user.

Tourniquet safety should be a priority; the surgical team should understand recommended parameters and precautions. Safety guidelines for the use of tourniquets include preventive measures and evaluation.[5] Preoperative assessment of the patient includes determining contraindications for use, including compartment syndrome, McArdle syndrome, hypertension, or other vascular problems. If the tourniquet must be used for patients with these conditions, specific guidelines must be observed.

Before application, the tourniquet equipment should be checked for proper function. Inflation pressures are established based on the systolic blood pressure, age of the patient, and circumference of the extremity. Duration of tourniquet inflation should be kept to a minimum. It is recommended in the average, healthy 50-year-old person to apply continuous tourniquet pressure less than 1 hour on the upper extremity and less than 2 hours on the thigh. Tourniquet pressure should not exceed the recommended maximum cuff pressure limits of 300 to 350 mm Hg for the thigh and 250 to 300 mm Hg for the arm and the lower leg. The interval between inflation and deflation should be 5 minutes for every 30 minutes of tourniquet ischemia to minimize effects on muscle and nerves.[19]

## HISTORY

As humans became more aware of injuries and how to treat them, certain people in each culture accepted the responsibility and honor of healing. In some tribal cultures, that person was a medicine man, or bonesetter. Neolithic people may have had fractures splinted—probably with bark and sticks. Other tribes used clay, soaked strips of rawhide, and linen. Hippocrates described using a wooden rack to treat a fracture of the femur and using techniques such as traction and counter-traction. However, bone healing as we know it today depended much on the development of imaging techniques.

The era of medical imaging began with the publication of *De Humani Corporis Fabrica* in 1543 by Andreas Vesalius. This comprehensive, detailed, and accurate set of anatomic illustrations set new standards in the art of medical observational science and research. Through direct observation, Vesalius conveyed his knowledge of the anatomy of the human body. These works were undisputed and stood the test of time until 1895, when Wilhelm Konrad Roentgen accidentally discovered x-rays (roentgenograms). Composed of high-energy electrons, x-rays are absorbed in varying degrees by structures in the body, based on their density and mass. The image is produced in two dimensions on photographic film and allows for indirect observation through noninvasive technique. For the next 70 years, x-rays stood as the standard in medical imaging until computerized axial tomography, or CAT scan, was introduced in 1972 by Godfrey Hounsfield. Detailed images of the body could be created by directing narrow x-ray beams at various angles. This was the first technique that incorporated computers into medical imaging. Since then, medical imaging has dramatically expanded, facilitating the surgical team's understanding of anatomy, physiology, and pathophysiology.

Modified from Gray JE, Orton CG: Medical physics: some recollections in diagnostic x-ray imaging and therapeutic radiology, *Radiology* 217(3): 619-625, 2000.

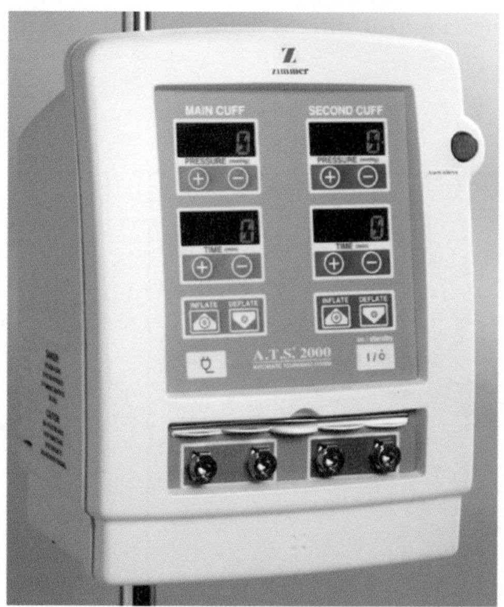


**FIGURE 22-19** Pneumatic gauge.

The tourniquet should be placed on the extremity without compression on bony structures and superficial neurovascular structures. The cuff should be positioned as high as possible without pinching skinfolds. Webril or stockinette is wrapped around the extremity and kept free of wrinkles and gatherings beneath the cuff. Cuffs should overlap a minimum of 3 inches and a maximum of 6 inches; excess overlap can pinch skinfolds. A tourniquet cuff that is too short can loosen after inflation. Care must be taken to ensure that the line from the air supply to the cuff is not kinked.

Tourniquet equipment should be checked periodically and serviced when problems arise. Injury from tourniquets may result from inadequate precautions, faulty preparation, or use of inaccurate equipment. The gauges and other related equipment should be checked with commercially available test equipment. Patient evaluation requires assessment of the extremity (skin color, temperature, pulses, movement, sensation) after removal of the tourniquet. Abnormal findings need to be reported to the surgeon and documented.

**TRACTION.** Traction is used preoperatively, intraoperatively, or postoperatively for prevention or reduction of muscle spasm, immobilization of a joint or body part, reduction of a fracture or dislocation, and treatment of a joint disorder. Traction alignment must be constant.

Various traction techniques can be used, including manual, skin, and skeletal (Figure 22-20). In manual traction, the hands provide the forces pulling on the bone being realigned. Skin traction uses strips of tape, digital straps, moleskin, or an elastic bandage applied directly to the skin. Common forms of skin traction are Buck's extension and Russell traction. Skeletal traction applies forces directly to the bone, using pins. Manual and skin traction can be applied in the emergency room or patient room, whereas skeletal traction is applied preoperatively in the emergency room or in the OR.

Skeletal traction is often used in conjunction with the OR fracture bed, using the traction attachment to aid in reduction of a long bone fracture. Postoperatively the patient may be confined to bed with balanced skeletal traction using a Thomas splint (Figure 22-21) and a Pearson attachment. Some cervical spine fractures or injuries may require Crutchfield or Gardner-Wells tongs inserted directly into the skull to stabilize the vertebrae and reduce spinal cord damage or further injury. Application of skeletal traction requires the use of sterile supplies, including a traction bow, pins, and drill.

Traction frames are placed immediately on the postoperative bed to accommodate traction. Nursing care of the patient in traction should include ensuring that the traction is continuous and skin tapes or skeletal pins are secured. Neurovascular status should be checked routinely, including skin color, pulse, temperature, and sensation. Changes from baseline or normal value must be reported. Supplies and frames should be available and assembled before transferring the patient to the postoperative bed.

**POSTOPERATIVE IMMOBILIZATION.** Postoperative immobilization may require use of a cast, splint, or other supplies designed for the specific anatomic part. A cast is a common method of immobilizing a fractured bone during healing. The forces of distraction, rotation, and malalignment can be overcome with the application of a cast. Closed reduction with a cast may be an option, thus minimizing the disadvantages and complications of open reduction, such as infection and tissue damage.

Casting is accomplished primarily with plaster or synthetic materials such as fiberglass. Plaster is less expensive, with a greater weight/strength ratio (it requires a greater weight of plaster to produce the same strength of fiberglass). Plaster casts may be burdensome if the casts are too heavy. They are routinely used as the primary cast after surgical procedures and are replaced later with a lighter fiberglass cast to promote patient mobility.

Casting material sets up and hardens rapidly once activated with water, and such a property necessitates that it be prepared with all necessary materials. Webril or stockinette should be applied to the extremity before the cast is applied to protect the skin from thermal injury while the plaster sets, as well as to protect the skin from undue abrasion and pressure. The plaster must be prepared, applied, and handled carefully and safely.

Figure 22-22 shows types of casts. A short arm cast is applied from below the elbow to the metacarpal heads after wrist fractures. A long arm cast is carried from the axilla to the metacarpal heads, immobilizing forearm or elbow fractures. The short leg cast is applied from the tibial tuberosity to the meta-

A

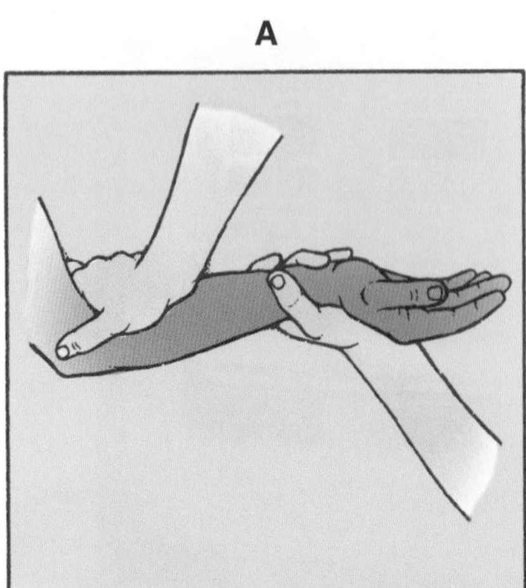

B

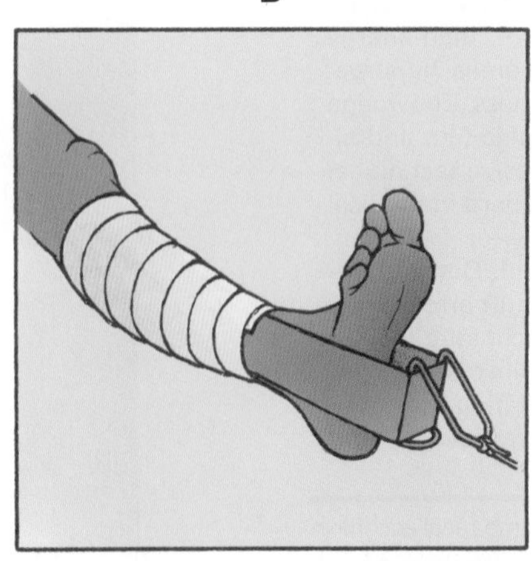

C

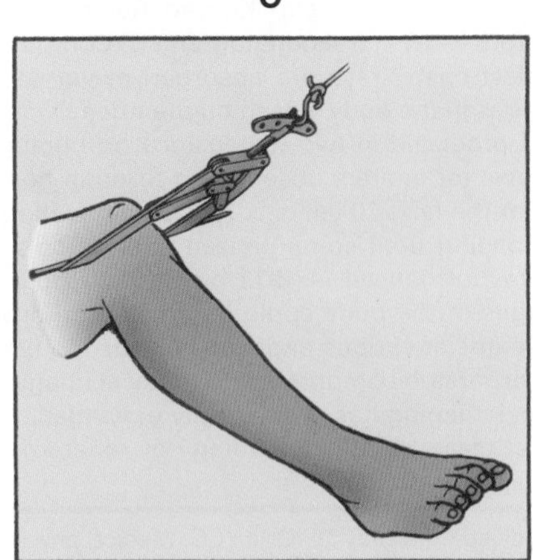

**FIGURE 22-20** Traction techniques. **A,** Manual. **B,** Skin. **C,** Skeletal.

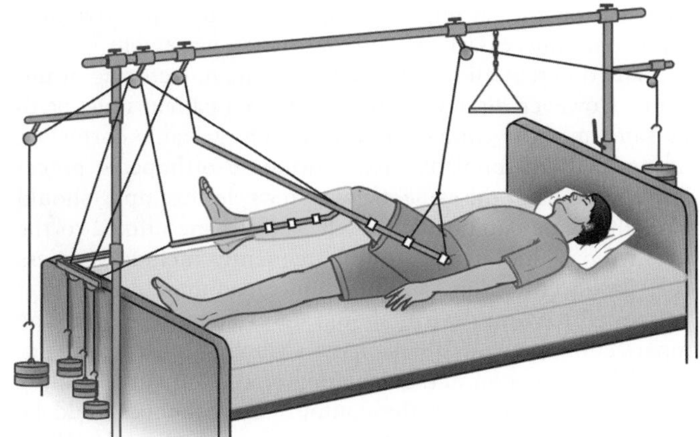

**FIGURE 22-21** Thomas splint balanced suspension.

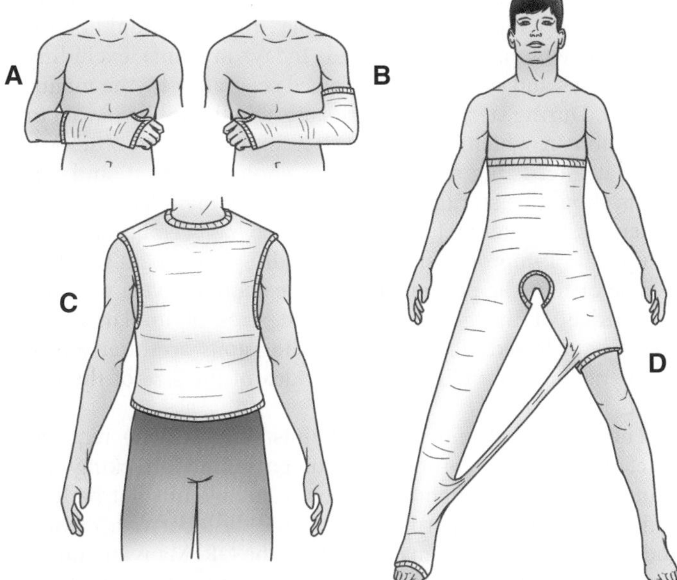


**FIGURE 22-22** Types of casts. **A,** Short arm cast. **B,** Long arm cast. **C,** Plaster body jacket cast. **D,** One and one half hip spica cast.

tarsal heads to immobilize the ankle and foot. The long leg cast is used for fractures involving the femur, tibia, or fibula or for complicated ankle fractures. The femoral cast brace is used in the treatment of femoral shaft fractures. A snug-fitting thigh cast and short leg cast are hinged at the knee joint. The cast brace is generally used after 4 to 6 weeks of skeletal traction after initiation of callus formation at the fracture site. A cylinder cast incorporates the leg from the groin to the ankle and is applied when complete knee immobilization is required. This is often required after surgery involving soft tissue reconstruction around the knee.

The hip spica cast is used when complete leg immobilization is desired. The trunk, affected side, and unaffected side may all be incorporated into the cast. Spinal immobilization is accomplished with a body jacket.

Splints are also employed for postoperative immobilization but are not circumferential and allow for swelling and closer observation of the surgical site.

Another immobilization device is the abduction pillow, used after total joint replacement. This prevents leg adduction, internal rotation, and hip flexion, which could cause dislocation of the hip. Further discussion of this and other devices is included in "Surgical Interventions," p. 728.

**LASERS.** Laser application has been increasing in the field of orthopedics. Their use mandates safety precautions, certification, patient consent, and protective attire (see Chapter 7 for a full discussion of lasers and laser safety). Laser types include carbon dioxide, holmium:yttrium-aluminum-garnet (Ho:YAG), neodymium:YAG (Nd:YAG), potassium titanyl phosphate (KTP), erbium:YAG (Er:YAG), and excimer. Laser technique differs for use on bone, muscle, tendon, and cartilage. Lasers have been used successfully for osteotomy, revision arthroplasty (removal of PMMA), nerve and tendon repair, arthroscopy, and diskectomy.

**AIRFLOW CONTROL.** Airflow control in the orthopedic operating room is critical to prevent introduction of microorganisms. Surgical site infections may result from airborne bacteria or transient bacteria from the patient or surgical team.[5] Laminar airflow is a system designed to provide highly filtered air and continuous air exchange for reducing airborne bacteria. Body exhaust suits are also used as a defense against airborne bacteria (Figure 22-23). Aseptic practices, sterile technique, and conscientious behaviors in operating rooms using conventional airflow can be used to maintain low rates of surgical site infections. The addition of other protective measures should be weighed to determine the benefit and outcome.[14]

**POSTOPERATIVE MANAGEMENT.** Postoperative patient management is planned during the preoperative period. Special equipment may include continuous passive motion (CPM) machines, pain management devices and techniques, compression devices, and blood salvage. CPM machines (Figure 22-24) stimulate the healing effect on articular tissues, including car-

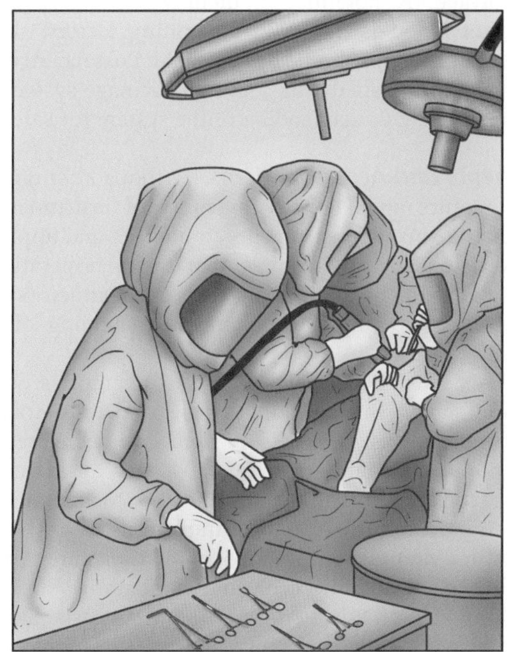

**FIGURE 22-23** Laminar airflow with body exhaust system.

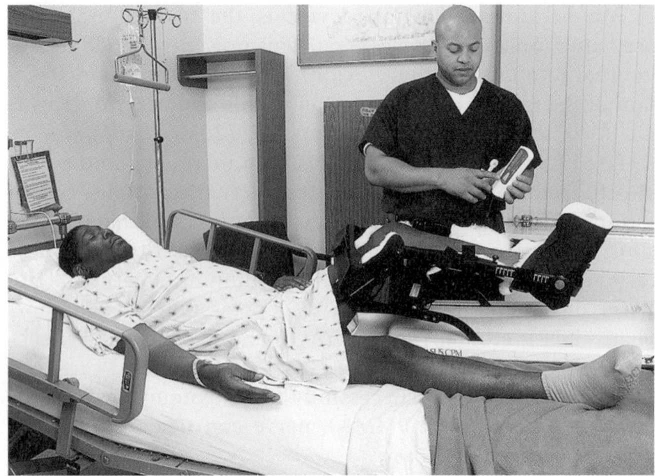

**FIGURE 22-24** Continuous passive motion (CPM) machine used for passive range of motion.

tilage, tendon, and ligaments, without interfering with healing incisions over the moving joint. The benefits of CPM include inhibition of adhesion formation and joint stiffness, decreased pain and swelling, early functional range of motion, and decreased effects of immobilization. The device is applied early in the postoperative period.

Pain management may include insertion of an epidural catheter or use of a patient-controlled analgesia (PCA) pump. The PCA pump administers a predetermined intravenous dose of the prescribed pain medication. It allows continuous infusion of analgesic as well as bolus administration when the patient feels it is necessary. The advantages include rapid pain relief, increased patient satisfaction, and, often, less use of medication than with traditional intramuscular analgesic.

Management of fluid and electrolyte balance may include use of intraoperative autologous transfusion or postoperative blood salvage. A potential problem with salvage of large amounts of blood is depletion of clotting factors; therefore coagulation problems should be identified. Postoperative blood salvage is accomplished with a closed-drainage system. It requires a complete understanding of the system for safe use.

***Instruments and Accessory Items.*** Orthopedic surgical procedures require an extensive inventory of instruments and implants and specific instruments to implant and apply hardware. Revision surgery requires that the perioperative staff be prepared with the appropriate tools and extractors needed to remove an old implant and an understanding of equipment use.

**IMPLANT INVENTORIES.** Implant inventories comprise plates and screws, intramedullary nails and rods, total joint implants, and a host of accessory items. Surgeon preference, patient population, and equipment cost are considered when selecting stock items. These items must be stocked in a timely fashion to prepare for consecutive implant use.

Inventory should be organized by manufacturers, type of implants (e.g., total hip, knee), and comparative sizes. Some may be provided on a loaner or consignment basis. Staff must be familiar with the varied types and refer to manufacturer's information pertaining to each implant. Practices should ensure that the correct implant is opened on the operative field to prevent unnecessary expense or error in placement.

Many different alloys are used in the manufacturing of implants. However, all devices implanted in a patient must be of the same metallic composition to prevent galvanic corrosion; internal fixation implants used during an orthopedic procedure should be of the same metal. Screws, for example, should be of the same composition as the metal plate affixed to the bone. Alloys that are used most frequently include stainless steel, cobalt-chromium, and titanium-vanadium-aluminum.

Internal fixation devices should never be reused. Resulting imperfections, such as abrasions or scratches, increase the potential for corrosion and weakening of the implant. Bending implants to conform to the contour of the bone should be avoided whenever possible to prevent loss of strength. When bending is necessary, the proper bending press should be used. Once an implant is bent, it should not be reshaped or straightened; doing so may weaken the implant.

Orthopedic equipment and implants require special care, storage, and handling. When possible, implants should be individually wrapped and processed. Today's implants, excluding some plates and screws, are packaged separately by the manufacturer. During sterilization, implants should not be placed in a position in which knocking or bumping might occur. Appropriate sterilizing cases and trays should be used, and implants should be sterilized according to the manufacturer's instructions. An internal fixation device that has become damaged as a result of improper storage or handling must be discarded.

The orthopedic perioperative nurse should have a working knowledge of the general types and sizes of implants that might be selected. Templates of radiographs are often made preoperatively, providing a general idea of the size of the implants needed.

The U.S. Food and Drug Administration (FDA) requires strict guidelines in properly documenting and tracking implant devices. Documentation should include but not be limited to the patient's permanent record, the operative record, and an implant registry maintained by the OR. Many manufacturers now include mailers to return information to the company for data collection. Information to be recorded includes the lot and serial numbers of those implants used and the manufacturer, size, type, and anatomic position of the implants.

**ORTHOPEDIC INSTRUMENTATION.** Orthopedic instrumentation varies from very small to large instruments. Some procedures require multiple instrument containers (sets). Organization of instrument sets for multiple uses prevents the need for duplication and requires thoughtful consideration of anatomic and physiologic needs. When preparing for a procedure, the perioperative nurse should open the minimum of instruments yet be prepared for unexpected or untoward events. Careful planning and preparation of instrumentation ensure efficient use of time and equipment.

Instruments that do not function properly (as a result of dullness, poor adjustment, lack of lubrication, damage, improper fit, or incomplete cleaning) are primary sources of complaints and problems in the operating room. Instrument maintenance is vital to ensure availability for the procedure and ease in completion. Instruments should be used for the intended purpose during the procedure. Movable parts should be lubricated after each cleaning and checked for cracks or damage after each use. The perioperative nurse is responsible for instrument maintenance and familiarity with sterilization and packaging procedures.

The following basic bone instrument sets should be available in the orthopedic OR. Soft tissue instrument sets appropriate for the size of the anatomic site are used for procedures not requiring bone instruments or in addition to the sets. Additional instruments and special equipment are mentioned in "Surgical Interventions," p. 728.

- *Incision hip set:* total hip arthroplasty or fractures of the neck and proximal femur
- *Total knee set:* total knee arthroplasty or supracondylar and distal femoral fractures
- *Shoulder set:* shoulder arthroplasty and other shoulder procedures
- *Large bone set:* bone work on the large bones, including hip, knee, upper arm, and elbow
- *Extremity or small bone set:* bone work on the hand or foot
- *Fusion or bone graft instruments:* additional instruments necessary for an autograft

POWERED SURGICAL INSTRUMENTS. Powered surgical instruments (Figure 22-25) used in the OR have eliminated the need for many hand-operated tools, thereby reducing operative time and improving technical results. They are available as air-driven, battery-driven, or electrically driven equipment. Fingertip control provides the surgeon speed and power. Variable-speed saws, drills, and reamers offer wide flexibility. Power equipment has a safety control that prevents inadvertent activation; this should be engaged when passing the instrument to the surgeon or assistant. Powered instruments should not be rested on the patient when they are not in use.

It is important to follow the manufacturer's recommended cleaning, sterilizing, and lubricating instructions. With proper care, powered surgical instruments have a long life span and many uses.

SUTURE MATERIAL. Suture material requires increased tensile strength and minimal degradability for the select type of tissue. Tendons and ligaments are fibrous, avascular tissues, resulting in a slower healing process than that in tissues rich in blood supply. Absorbable suture may be used for sewing tendon or ligaments to bone. Nonabsorbable sutures, including polyester and surgical steel, are also used. For various ligament replacement grafts, a harvested tendon may be customized with multiple strands of suture material, increasing tensile strength and length of time until fibrous union occurs.

POLYMETHYLMETHACRYLATE. PMMA (bone cement) is an acrylic, cementlike substance composed of a liquid methylmethacrylate monomer and a powder methylmethacrylate-styrene co-polymer. The powder component is 10% barium sulfate, U.S. Pharmacopoeia (USP), which provides radiopacity to the finished product. The liquid monomer is highly flammable, and the OR should be properly ventilated. Caution should be exercised during mixing of the two components to prevent excessive exposure of OR personnel to the vapors of the monomer. This exposure can cause irritation of the respiratory tract and eyes. Personnel in a room where methylmethacrylate is being mixed should not wear soft contact lenses. Many special hoods and mixing devices are available to minimize staff exposure to the fumes.

Adverse patient reactions with PMMA include transitory hypotension, cardiac arrest, cerebrovascular accident, pulmonary embolus, thrombophlebitis, and hypersensitivity reaction. Cardiac arrest and death, although uncommon, have resulted after insertion of bone cement. Adverse reactions have been attributed to a combination of factors, including a rise in intramedullary canal pressure causing embolic phenomena, a possible chemical and blood reaction causing sudden hypotension, and certain preexisting patient conditions. More research is needed to discover the exact cause of adverse reactions. Patient care should include collaborating with the anesthesia

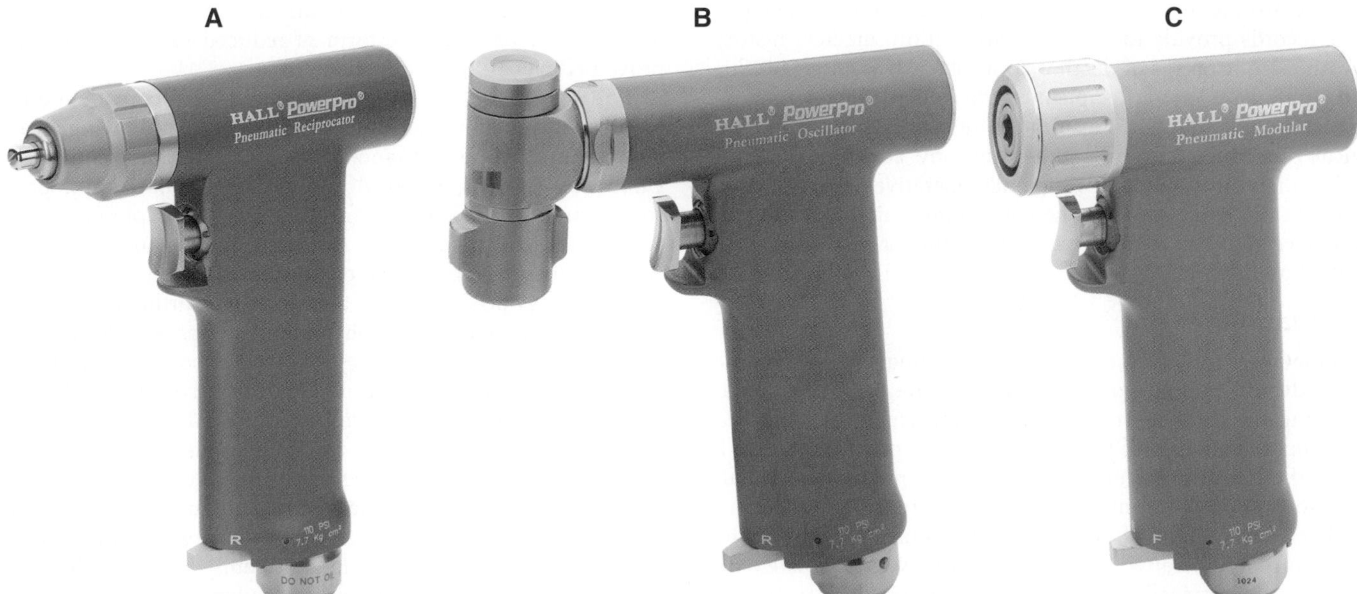


**FIGURE 22-25** Pneumatic-powered surgical instruments for large bone procedures. **A,** Reciprocating saw. **B,** Oscillating saw. **C,** Single-trigger modular handpiece.

provider before insertion of PMMA and then monitoring for side effects after insertion.

***Medications.*** Antibiotics, hemostatics, and antibacterial agents are used commonly. Antibiotics are delivered both intravenously and locally in irrigation solutions. Common antibiotics used in the irrigation include polymyxin and bacitracin. Irrigation may also be delivered using pulsatile lavage, with antibiotics added to the solution. Hemostatic agents may include bone wax, Gelfoam, thrombin, Avitene, and the DynaStat hemostat. DynaStat is a liquid, sprayable hemostatic consisting of collagen, thrombin, the patient's own platelets, and fibrinogen. Antibacterial ointments are impregnated in gauze dressing (Xeroform) or applied before the application of the dressing. Other medications used during orthopedic procedures include steroids, local anesthetics, and normal saline. Local anesthetics are often injected near the end of the surgical procedure to minimize postoperative pain.[16]

***Protective Measures.*** Orthopedic procedures require caution as a result of the use of fluids for irrigation or bloody procedures. Personnel protective measures include handling items (blades, sharp instruments, bone) cautiously to prevent inadvertent punctures or cuts and wearing protective masks, eyewear, or a face shield as well as protective attire, including gowns and boots. Sharp bone edges are a hazard and can puncture gloves and skin. Double-gloving or use of protective gloves should be employed to protect the patient and personnel.

***Bone Banking.*** The American Association of Tissue Banks (AATB) accredits and periodically inspects bone-banking programs to ensure that specific standards are followed in the retrieval, processing, storage, and distribution of bone allografts.[2] Allografts are frozen until use. Vacuum-sealed freezers are monitored with an alarm. When requested for a procedure, the bone allograft is delivered to the field, slightly thawed, cultured, and washed with an antibiotic solution. Banked bone is available in many shapes of cortical and cancellous tissue.

Records are maintained on both donors and recipients. Donor records provide the donor identification, medical history (with circumstances of death if applicable), laboratory results, and graft description. Recipient records include recipient identification, surgeon and organization implanting the graft, surgical procedure, culture results, and any adverse reactions. Like other implants, the recipient's operative record should include the name of the bone bank from which the allograft was received, type of allograft, tissue number, and expiration date if applicable.

## Evaluation

Evaluation is an ongoing process, occurring throughout the procedure. The perioperative nurse evaluates the patient, considering the nursing diagnosis and achievement of identified outcomes. This part of the nursing process provides feedback as to the effectiveness of the plan, its implementation, and alterations needed for improving patient care. Was the patient protected from peripheral neurovascular injury? Was he or she free from perioperative positioning injury? Was adequate oxygenation maintained? Does the patient have more questions pertaining to recovery and rehabilitation? The answers will dictate whether there is a need to maintain or modify the plan. The evaluation information is shared with the nurse caring for this patient postoperatively to provide continuity of care.

The following sample outcome statements apply to evaluating care of the orthopedic patient when using the nursing diagnoses identified earlier in this chapter:

- The patient verbalized fears and feelings and indicated that anxiety and apprehension were lessened.
- The patient was free from peripheral neurovascular dysfunction on discharge to the postoperative area as evidenced by presence of pulses, warmth of the extremity, good capillary refill, and intact movement and sensation.
- The patient was free from injury related to perioperative positioning as evidenced by maintenance of skin integrity and absence of reddened areas.
- The patient maintained adequate ventilation and perfusion as evidenced by blood gases, arterial saturation, and vital signs within normal limits.
- The patient was free from surgical site infection as evidenced by temperature within normal limits and a clean and dry incision site.

## Patient and Family Education and Discharge Planning

Discharge planning and patient education should be initiated when the health care provider evaluates the patient for surgery. It should continue when the patient comes into contact with the health care system and should involve a multidisciplinary approach.[24] One method of planning the overall care from preadmission to discharge is to place a patient on a clinical guideline based on "best practice"—a multidisciplinary case management tool. "Best practices" define the expected processes of care and are, in essence, strategies of care to encourage physicians and other health providers who care for the same surgical patient population to agree with each other on a sequence of common interventions.[26] Included with the clinical guideline on the patient's medical record is a set of orders that mirrors the guideline and allows the physician to make minor changes to the protocol. Receiving feedback from all disciplines involved in the patient's care and discharge planning reaps benefits in the form of reduced variance and improved efficiency, outcomes, and costs.[13]

For the patient undergoing orthopedic surgery, patient and family education and discharge planning in the following areas are essential: wound care and dressing changes, pain control,[18] wound assessment, physical and occupational therapy, personal care, housekeeping, mobility, nutrition, prescriptions other than pain medication, extended anticoagulant therapy (for patients undergoing hip or knee arthroplasty see Surgical Pharmacology box), donning and doffing of orthopedic appliances, and follow-up with a physician. Information concerning these content areas should be described, discussed, and reinforced with written instructions. Perioperative nurses should ensure that the patient and family understand the instructions, have the opportunity to demonstrate a requisite skill if that is part of home care and convalescence, and allow time for questions and concerns. A sample of written educational material that might be provided to the orthopedic surgical patient with a cast is presented in the Patient and Family Education box on p. 725. Relevant content for devising patient and family educational material on pain management at home is presented in the Patient and Family Education box on p. 726-727.

## SURGICAL PHARMACOLOGY

### Anticoagulation Therapy

Venous thromboembolism (VTE), including deep vein thrombosis (DVT) and pulmonary thromboembolism (PE), is one of the most common preventable causes of hospital death. More than 900,000 Americans experience a DVT each year, and 500,000 of these persons develop PE, which causes some 300,000 deaths. Analysis of related data has suggested that fewer than 50% of patients diagnosed and hospitalized with DVT had received prophylaxis. In 2003, recognizing that the incidence of DVT/VTE was a significant patient safety issue, the National Quality Forum (NQF) endorsed Safe Practice 17: *Evaluate each patient upon admission, and regularly thereafter, for the risk of developing DVT/VTE. Utilize clinically appropriate methods to prevent DVT/VTE,* and Safe Practice 18: *Utilize dedicated anticoagulation services that facilitate coordinated care management.*

In addition, the Surgical Care Improvement Project (SCIP) targeted DVT as a key area for improvement in surgical patient care. SCIP is a national partnership of organizations committed to improving the safety of surgical care through the reduction of postoperative complications, with a goal of reducing the incidence of surgical complications nationally by 25% by the year 2010. SCIP identified two process measures in the reduction of VTE: (1) that surgery patients have the appropriate VTE prophylaxis ordered and (2) that it be administered within 24 hours before their surgery or within 24 hours after it.

More than 50% of major orthopedic procedures are complicated by DVT, and up to 30% by PE, if prophylactic treatment is not instituted. DVTs in the perioperative period involve several components, including venous stasis, acquired hypercoagulable state, endothelial injury, and the positioning of the limb intraoperatively. Despite the well-established efficacy and safety of preventive measures, studies show that prophylaxis is often underused or used inappropriately. Both low-dose unfractionated heparin (LDUH) and low–molecular-weight heparin (LMWH) have similar efficacy in DVT and PE prevention.

Some common drugs used to prevent DVT and their mechanisms of action are as follows:

Ardeparin—LMWH, prevents conversion of fibrinogen to fibrin and prothrombin to thrombin by enhancing inhibitory effects of antithrombin III; used for preventing DVT after total knee arthroplasty (TKA)

Danaparoid—glycosaminoglycan, prevents conversion of fibrinogen to fibrin and prothrombin to thrombin by enhancing inhibitory effects of antithrombin III; used for DVT prevention in total hip replacement or hip fracture surgery

Desirudin (Iprivask)—thrombin inhibitor, prevents thrombin resulting in prolongation of clotting time; used for DVT prophylaxis in hip replacement surgery

Enoxaparin (Lovenox)—LMWH, prevents conversion of fibrinogen to fibrin and prothrombin to thrombin by enhancing inhibitory effects of antithrombin III and produces higher ratio of anti–factor Xa to anti–factor IIa; used for prevention of DVT and PE in hip and knee replacement surgery

Heparin (Calcilean, Calciparine, Hepalean, heparin sodium, Heparin Leo, Heparin Lock, Hep-Lock)—anticoagulant and antithrombotic, prevents conversion of fibrinogen to fibrin and prothrombin to thrombin by enhancing inhibitory effects of antithrombin III; used for prevention of DVT and PE

Warfarin (Coumadin, Sofarin, warfarin sodium, Warfilone Sodium)—anticoagulant, interferes with blood clotting by indirect means, depresses hepatic synthesis of vitamin K–dependent coagulation factors (II, VII, IX, X); DVT and PE prevention

Patient education should include the reason for DVT prophylaxis, the name (both generic and trade) of the drug, dosage, time of administration, and side effects. Because bleeding is a dangerous complication, signs and symptoms of both minor bleeding and major bleeding should be reviewed. Patients should receive both oral and written information along with the name of a physician or nurse to call if complications or questions arise.

Modified from Canobbio MM: *Mosby's handbook of patient teaching,* ed 3, St Louis, 2006, Mosby; SCIP: A national quality partnership. Accessed April 12, 2006, on-line: www.medqic.org/scip/scip_homepage.html; Skidmore-Roth L: *Mosby's drug guide for nurses,* St Louis, 2005, Mosby.

## PATIENT AND FAMILY EDUCATION

### Casts

**EXPLANATION OF THE CAST**

The cast is only one of several devices used to promote the healing of broken bones. Surgeons also use traction and pins, or a combination of these three, to help heal broken bones. The cast has the advantage of being less expensive, requiring little care on your part, and allowing you to move around. The cast also encloses and immobilizes the broken bone and injured soft tissues to prevent movement that could cause further injury and to keep the bone in place for proper healing. Your cast may be made of plaster or of a synthetic material, such as fiberglass. Although the plaster cast is heavy, the surgeon can mold a plaster cast more easily for a close fit over severe injuries. The synthetic cast is lightweight and easier to move around.

**CAST CARE**

- Keep a plaster cast dry; cover it or wrap it in a plastic bag when bathing or going out in the rain or snow.
- For a fiberglass (or other synthetic) cast, your surgeon may permit immersion in water if there are no surgical wounds under the cast.
- Maintain good skin care around your cast. However, do not do the following:
  - Insert objects, such as a coat hanger, under your cast.
  - Put any creams, lotions, or powder inside the cast.

**THINGS TO WATCH FOR AND REPORT TO YOUR SURGEON OR NURSE**

The skin under your cast will feel warm at first because of the setting process. However, warm areas on the cast later on may indicate infection, and you should notify your surgeon or nurse at once.

You should watch for increased pain or soreness under the cast, particularly around a bony prominence such as the wrist or ankle that is not relieved by repositioning the body. Check the skin color and temperature periodically. When the tip of a finger or the big toe that extends from the cast is squeezed until it is white, the pink color should return within 4 to 6 seconds. If skin color does not return within 4 to 6 seconds or if the skin is red, blue, white, or otherwise discolored, notify your physician. If fingers or toes are cool, cover them. If they do not warm up in 20 minutes, call your physician. Call your physician immediately if any of these other symptoms occur:

- An increase in swelling and pain. Some swelling is common at first. Your surgeon may have advised you to elevate your cast after it was applied. Your cast should feel snug for the first 48 hours. If it continues to feel too snug and causes pain and swelling, call your surgeon.
- A tingling or burning sensation.
- An inability to move muscles around the cast.
- A foul odor detected around the edges of the cast.
- Any drainage that may show through the cast.
- Any cracks or breaks in the cast.
- Marked loosening of the cast, allowing the parts inside the cast to move fairly easily.

Modified from Canobbio MM: *Mosby's handbook of patient teaching,* ed 3, St Louis, 2006, Mosby.

PATIENT AND FAMILY EDUCATION

## Content on Educating the Patient and Family on Pain Management at Home

Give the patient and the caregiver both *verbal* and *written* instructions. After reviewing instructions, have the patient or caregiver "repeat back" the instructions in his or her own words. Provide the patient or caregiver with the name and telephone number of a physician or nurse to call if questions arise.

**GENERAL INFORMATION**

- Explain the relationship of pain to the disease process. Assist the patient to understand the source of pain.

**SPECIAL INSTRUCTIONS**

- Assist the patient to identify factors or actions that trigger pain, such as activity, movements, and temperature extremes.
- Discuss past effective and ineffective pain relief measures and their effects, such as sleepiness, lethargy, and decreased energy or sexual activity.
- Assist the patient to localize and describe the intensity of pain using a scale (e.g., 0 to 10, with 0 meaning absence of pain and 10 meaning intense pain) and to identify any alleviating or aggravating factors.
- Encourage use of a log to record pain rating and effectiveness of management strategies.
- Discuss alternative strategies patients can use to relieve pain without taking prescribed drugs, and explain that these techniques may also augment the effect of pain medication (see "Pain Management Techniques").
  - *Sensory interventions: massage*—to relax muscular tension and increase local circulation; *range-of-motion exercises* (passive, assistive, or active)—to relax muscles, improve circulation, and prevent pain related to stiffness and immobility; *cold application*—used initially to decrease tissue injury response (swelling) and decrease pain; *heat application*—used after cold to aid in clearance of tissue toxins and mobilize fluids; *transcutaneous electrical nerve stimulation* (TENS)—pocket-size, battery-operated device used to send mild continuous electrical impulses through the skin by means of electrodes placed on the body
  - *Emotional interventions to increase pain threshold by controlling or reducing anxiety, fatigue, or depression: prevention or control of anxiety*—to reduce muscle tension and increase pain tolerance through relaxation exercises and slow, controlled breathing; *promotion of self-control*—to reduce feelings of helplessness and lack of control that contribute to anxiety and pain; *pacing of activities*
  - *Cognitive interventions: distraction*—focus on something unrelated to pain (e.g., conversing, watching television or videos, listening to music); *humor; guided imagery*—use of images to alter a physical or emotional state, promote relaxation, and decrease pain sensation
- Discuss the need to identify body positions of comfort; encourage attention to proper posture and body alignment. Advise the patient to immobilize or rest the affected area.
- Tell the patient to relieve pressure areas by turning or using pressure-reduction devices, such as an air-fluidized support system.

**PAIN MANAGEMENT TECHNIQUES**

- *Relaxation:* relieves pain by easing muscle tension. This can also help you feel less tired and nervous and help other pain-relieving methods work better.
- How to relax:
  - Sit or lie down in a quiet place. Be sure you are comfortable. Do not cross your legs or arms. Take a deep breath, and tense your muscles (you may tense up your whole body or concentrate on one set of muscles at a time, such as your facial muscles or those in your arms and hands).
  - Hold your breath, and keep your muscles tense. Release your breath and your muscles at the same time. Let your body go limp (repeat for other muscle areas if you are concentrating on one set at a time).
  - You can add imagery or music to help you relax. Relaxation tapes are available from your health care agency or local music store.
  - Do not be discouraged if relaxation does not help immediately. Practice the relaxation technique for at least 2 weeks before you give it up. If you find that it aggravates your pain, try another method.
- *Imagery:* involves using your imagination to create mental scenes that use all your senses: sight, sound, touch, smell, and taste. You can imagine exotic locations or revisit one of your favorite places. You can create stories and characters to add to your scenes. Imagery can take your mind off your fear, boredom, and pain.
- How to use imagery:
  - Close your eyes. A few moments of the relaxation techniques (see above) will help your body and mind prepare for imagery. Let your mind begin forming its image. The following is an example of imagery: Imagine that you are at the seashore. You are sitting in the wet sand; the afternoon sun is warm on your shoulders. The ocean rolls into the shore in gentle waves, and the water laps teasingly at your toes. A hungry pair of seagulls cries overhead and takes swift, darting dives at a dog that is scavenging along the shore. Your tension lessens with each wave that touches your toes and retreats. You close your eyes and take a deep, slow breath of air. You are completely relaxed. Stay on the beach as long as you like. To end the image, count to three and open your eyes. Resume your regular activities slowly.
- *Distraction:* any activity that takes your mind off your pain and focuses your attention elsewhere. Doing crafts, reading a book, watching television, or listening to music through headphones can distract your mind. Distraction works well when you are waiting for drugs to take effect or if you have brief bouts of pain. Sometimes people can take their minds off their pain for long periods, especially if the pain is mild.
- *Skin stimulation:* used to block pain sensation in the nerves. Pressure, massage, hot and cold applications, rubbing, and mild electrical current are all ways to stimulate the skin. If you are having radiation therapy, consult your physician before applying any skin stimulation. You can do the stimulation at the site of the pain, near it, or on the side opposite the pain. For example, stimulating the left wrist when the right wrist is in pain can actually ease the pain in the right wrist.
- How to use skin stimulation:
  - *Pressure:* using your entire hand, the heel of your hand, your thumb, your knuckles, or both hands, apply pressure for at least 15 seconds at the point where you feel pain. Keep trying spots around the painful area if you find no

Modified from Canobbio MM: *Mosby's handbook of patient teaching,* ed 3, St Louis, 2006, Mosby.

## PATIENT AND FAMILY EDUCATION

### Content on Educating the Patient and Family on Pain Management at Home—cont'd

relief the first time. You may extend the time you apply pressure to 1 minute.

- *Massage:* you or someone else can perform the slow, circular motions of massage. The feet, back, neck, and scalp can be massaged to relieve tension and pain anywhere in the body. Some people prefer to use oils or lotions during the massage. If deep massage is too uncomfortable, try light stroking. Do not massage red, raw, or broken skin.
- *Heat and cold:* some people prefer cold; others prefer heat. Use whichever works better for you. A convenient way to use cold is to freeze gel-filled packs and wrap them in towels. Ice cubes can also be used. Heat can be applied with a heating pad; hot, moist towels; or a hot water bottle; or by taking a hot bath. Be careful not to burn your skin with water that is too hot or to go to sleep with a heating pad on. Do not expose your skin to intense cold for long periods.

◆ *TENS:* can be used to eliminate or ease pain. A TENS unit is a pocket-size, battery-operated device that provides a mild, continuous electrical current through the skin by the use of two to four electrodes taped to the skin. Lead wires connect the electrodes to the device. It is this mild electrical current that blocks or modifies the pain messages and replaces them with a buzzing, tingling sensation. TENS is also thought to stimulate the body's production of endorphin, a natural pain reliever.

◆ Discuss the use of TENS. Explain that the mild electrical current blocks or modifies pain messages before they reach the brain and replaces them with a buzzing or tingling sensation. Inform the patient that TENS may stimulate the body's production of endorphin, a natural pain reliever. Instruct the patient in the use and home care of the TENS unit:
- Apply a thin coat of gel over each entire electrode.
- Place the electrodes securely on the skin with tape.
- Place the electrodes close to the site of pain.
- Turn the intensity knob until a slight tingling or buzzing sensation is felt on the skin. Increase the intensity if the pain is still felt, or decrease the intensity if the tingling sensation causes discomfort.
- Turn the TENS unit off before removing it.
- Wipe the electrodes with an alcohol and water mixture after removing them from the skin.
- Do not allow the unit to get wet. If it does get wet, allow it to dry thoroughly before using it again.
- Replace the electrodes if the adhesive surface separates from the backing or if they no longer adhere firmly to the skin.
- Replace the battery pack or recharge as needed. If there is no tingling sensation when the intensity is turned up, the batteries are weakening.
- Use hypoallergenic tape to secure the electrodes to prevent redness or rash, cleanse the skin well after removing the electrodes, and apply lotion to the placement sites.

**MEDICATIONS**

◆ Explain the purpose, dosage, schedule, and route of administration of any prescribed drugs, as well as side effects to report to a physician or nurse. Be sure the patient or caregiver knows the name of the medication.

◆ Give the patient general guidelines for the use of pain medication.

◆ Explain that a variety of pain relief measures may be necessary for some types of pain.

◆ Instruct the patient to use pain relief measures before pain becomes severe.

◆ Encourage the patient to try a pain relief measure at least twice before abandoning it as ineffective.

◆ Urge the patient to keep trying to relieve the pain and not to become discouraged.

◆ Discuss the use of non-narcotic analgesics:
- Inform the patient that non-narcotic analgesics include acetaminophen, aspirin, and nonsteroidal antiinflammatory drugs, such as ibuprofen, indomethacin, and naproxen.
- Explain that these medications are generally well tolerated but have the potential to cause gastrointestinal ulceration, renal and hepatic toxic effects, and inhibition of platelet aggregation.
- Tell the patient that if the non-narcotic does not have a therapeutic effect initially, the dosage should be increased before another type of drug is tried.

◆ Discuss the use of narcotics, which are indicated for severe postoperative pain or intractable pain such as that associated with cancer:
- Inform the patient that narcotics include morphine, hydromorphone, and methadone and that these may be administered by intravenous drip, intrathecally, or epidurally to enhance the analgesic effect.
- Explain that fixed dosage schedules with adequate doses for pain relief provide more constant blood levels and predictable pain relief. Suggest that additional doses may be needed for breakthrough pain.
- Discuss the side effects of narcotic analgesics: constipation, vomiting, and respiratory and central nervous system depression.

◆ Discuss and demonstrate the use of equipment for administering pain relief medications:
- External and implantable pumps for intravenous, epidural, and intrathecal administration of narcotic analgesics
- Patient-controlled analgesia (PCA), particularly for the management of acute pain such as postoperative pain
- Continuous subcutaneous infusion with an ambulatory infusion pump

◆ Discuss the treatment for side effects of narcotics. For example, constipation requires the use of laxatives and stool softeners (e.g., senna [Senokot]).

# Surgical Interventions

## BONE GRAFTING

Bone grafting may be used (1) to fill cavities after removal of large amounts of bone that might result in instability, (2) to fill bony defects, and (3) to promote union of fractures at the time of open reduction. The type of graft used depends on the location of the fracture or defect, the condition of the bone, and the amount of bone loss as a result of injury. Bone graft may be used for procedures involving revision of joints if there is significant bone loss caused by resorption or mechanical destruction after removal of bone cement.

The bone graft may be the patient's own bone (autogenous in origin and referred to as *autograft*) or bone obtained from a tissue bank (homogeneous in origin but referred to as *allograft*). Autografts are often harvested from the iliac crest, where there is cortical and cancellous bone. Various harvesting techniques are used. Struts of cortical bone from the iliac crest can be fashioned to the desired shape and used in areas needing structural strength. The amount of cancellous bone is plentiful. It is used to promote bone growth in areas of defect. Local bone graft material may be taken from the site of injury. Allografts are used when bone is not available from the patient because of the lack of sufficient quantity or because a secondary procedure is undesirable for the patient.

### Procedural Considerations

Cancellous grafts may be taken from the ilium, olecranon, or distal radius; cortical grafts may be taken from the tibia, fibula, iliac crest, or ribs. When the recipient site of an autogenous graft is diseased, instruments used for the recipient site must be separated from donor graft site instruments. The operating team must change their gowns and gloves to take the bone graft and again follow the procedure to prevent cross-contamination. The patient is positioned to allow exposure to the surgical site. A sandbag may be placed beneath the area for easier access.

The instrumentation for taking a bone graft includes soft tissue instruments and a bone graft set. Grafts may be harvested with hand instruments, power tools such as an oscillating saw, or high-speed tools such as the Midas Rex. Power tools may be necessary if a uniformly shaped graft is needed to fill a defect. Because hemostasis is sometimes difficult to achieve as a result of the vascular nature of bone, wound drains may be desirable.

### Operative Procedure

***Harvest of Bone Graft.*** A cancellous bone graft consists of spongy bone usually taken from the anterior or posterior crest of the ilium. A cortical bone graft, consisting of hard, dense bone, is removed from the crest of the ilium or the tibia. The location of the crest of the ilium is subcutaneous, allowing exposure without difficulty.

1. An incision is made along the border of the iliac crest, and the muscles on the outer table of the ilium are stripped, elevated, and retracted.
2. Strips of the iliac crest can be removed with an osteotome or oscillating saw.
3. A cortical window may also be made in the outer table, and cancellous bone chips may be obtained with curettes or gouges.
4. A drain may be inserted. The wound is closed in layers, and a pressure dressing is applied.

## ELECTRICAL STIMULATION

The healing process in bone involves several stages (Figure 22-26). When a bone is damaged, such as during a surgical procedure or fracture, bleeding occurs. The amount of extravasated blood depends on the vascularity of the fracture site. The blood exudate infiltrates the surrounding area, where a clot is formed. Fibroblasts invade the hematoma and form a fibrin meshwork.

As osteoblasts invade the fibrin meshwork, blood vessels develop to build collagen. After several days, calcium deposits may form in the granulation tissue. These deposits eventually form new bone, known as *callus*. Within the callus, cartilage cells develop a temporary semirigid tissue that helps stabilize the bone fragments. The callus is immature bone that is remodeled by new connective tissue cells (osteoblasts) of the periosteum and the inner membrane of the bone cavity. Through this process, mature bone is formed, excess callus is resorbed, and trabecular bone is laid down.

After several months, depending on the age and physical condition of the individual, the bone becomes firmly united, although the ossification process is not yet completed. Complete union of the fractured bone or joint is determined by means of clinical and radiologic examination.

Healing of bone is classified by degree. *Delayed union* signifies that healing has not occurred within the average time. The average time depends on many factors, and delayed unions must not be considered nonunion until the healing process has ceased without bony union. *Malunion* signifies that the fracture has united with deformity sufficient to cause impairment of the function or a significant angulation of the extremity. *Nonunion* signifies that the process of healing has ended without

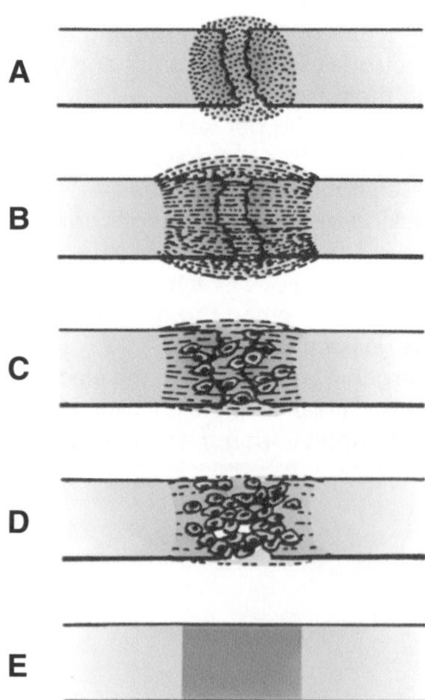


**FIGURE 22-26** Bone-healing process. **A,** Hematoma formation. **B,** Fibrin network formation. **C,** Invasion of osteoblasts. **D,** Callus formation. **E,** Remodeling.

producing bony union; in this case, electrical stimulation may be used.

Electrical stimulation is artificially applied electrical current that induces or influences osteogenesis. Various types of stimulators (Figure 22-27) are available for treatment of nonunion, including invasive (implantable), semi-invasive (percutaneous), and noninvasive (capacitance coupling). The bone stimulator of choice depends on the patient, pathologic condition, and the physician's comfort with the device.

The bone-growth stimulator is used in patients with high risk of nonunion. It can be used to provide electrical stimulation for treatment of nonunion, delayed union, congenital pseudarthrosis, and bone defects. It may be used with or without internal fixation devices, external fixation devices, or bone grafting. Patients who have undergone previous surgery, who have sustained significant tissue loss, or in whom bone grafting is contraindicated are candidates. Electrical stimulation requires long periods of immobilization of the site. This prolonged immobilization may impede rehabilitation.

### Procedural Considerations

Instructions for implanting and components selected vary according to the type. The position of the patient depends on the implant site.

In addition to the implant of the surgeon's choice and the implant-specific instrumentation, a soft tissue set is used. Curettes, osteotomes, or bone rasps are used for bony debridement and to scarify the donor bed. Power drills with drill bits may be necessary to create access through the bone for the electrical leads.

### Operative Procedure

1. The surgical site is exposed and debrided as necessary. A stimulator may be implanted after the surgical procedure.
2. A slot is fashioned spanning the nonunion site.
3. A second incision is made about 8 to 10 cm from the first one and dissected. Before the generator is implanted, hemostasis must be achieved. The use of electrosurgical equipment may interfere with function of the bone-growth stimulator.
4. A subcutaneous channel for the cathode is created, using blunt or mechanical dissection.
5. The long cathode lead is guided through the channel.
6. The generator is carefully implanted near the skin surface. The generator should be inserted into soft tissue—not against bone or metal fixation devices; it should not create a bulge beneath the skin.

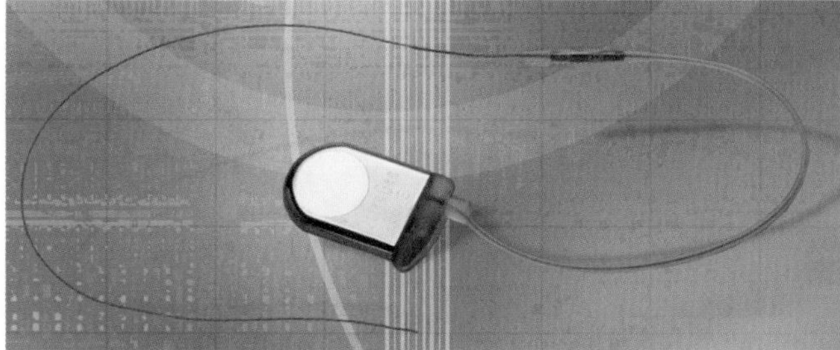

FIGURE 22-27 Bone-growth stimulator used after procedures to induce bone formation.

7. The electrical coils are placed in the prepared bone slot in equal lengths above and below the fracture site.
8. Cancellous bone grafts are placed between the coils if large bony defects are being treated.
9. Routine closure of the subcutaneous and skin tissue is carried out.

Once union has occurred (5 to 6 months), the generator is removed. The stimulator can be removed using local anesthesia with minimal instrumentation.

## FRACTURES AND DISLOCATIONS

A fracture is a break in the continuity of a bone. The care of fractured bones or dislocation of a joint is complicated when there is trauma to the soft tissues, including muscles, nerves, ligaments, and blood vessels. Bone diseases, which can increase the risk of a fracture, can be metabolic, infectious, or degenerative. Metabolic diseases are disorders of bone remodeling. The most common are osteoporosis, osteomalacia, and Paget's disease, all of which may result in bone fractures. The most common infectious process is osteomyelitis. Degenerative musculoskeletal conditions are associated with aging. Osteoarthritis is the most common degenerative change.

Osteoporosis is one of the most common and serious of bone diseases. More than 1 million fractures occurring each year are attributed to osteoporosis; 40% are vertebral fractures, 20% are femoral (hip) fractures, 15% are distal forearm fractures, and 25% are assorted other types of fractures.[10]

Osteoporosis is characterized by excessive loss of calcified matrix, bone mineral, and collagenous fibers, causing a reduction of total bone mass. Decreasing levels of estrogen and testosterone in the older adult result in reduced new bone growth and maintenance of existing bone. Inadequate intake of calcium or vitamin D; lack of weight-bearing activities, exercise, and physical activity; smoking; and caffeine intake are other contributing factors. Osteoporotic bone is porous, brittle, and fragile, fracturing easily under stress. This results in susceptibility to spontaneous fractures and pathologic curvature of the spine.

Osteomalacia is a metabolic bone disease characterized by inadequate mineralization of bone as a result of vitamin D deficiency, which leads to a reduced absorption of calcium and phosphorus. Risk factors for development of osteomalacia include malabsorption problems, vitamin D and calcium deficiencies, chronic renal failure, and inadequate exposure to sunlight. Medical treatment includes dietary supplements and exposure to sunlight.

Paget's disease is a disorder affecting older adults. It is characterized by proliferation of osteoclasts and compensatory increased osteoblastic activity, resulting in rapid, disorganized bone remodeling. The bones are weak and poorly constructed.

### Types of Fractures

Fractures are classified into two main groups: closed fractures and open or compound fractures. *Closed fractures* are those in which there is no communication between the bone fragments and the skin surface. *Incomplete closed fractures* are those in which the whole thickness of the bone is not broken but is bent or buckled, such as in greenstick fractures, which commonly occur in prepubertal children. *Open fractures* exist when the break in the bone communicates with a wound in the skin. These fractures are usually considered contaminated, requiring measures to control potential infection.

The many varieties of fracture architecture (Figure 22-28) include (1) transverse fracture, in which the fracture line runs at a right angle to the longitudinal axis of the bone; (2) longitudinal fracture, which runs along the length of the bone; (3) oblique fracture and spiral fracture, in which bone is twisted apart (similar except that oblique is shorter than spiral); (4) comminuted fracture, in which the bone fragments splinter into more than two pieces; (5) compression fracture, in which one fragment is driven into the other end and is relatively fixed in that position; and (6) pathologic fracture, in which a bone will fracture easily because it is weakened by disease. A fracture in the shaft of a long bone is described as being in the proximal, middle, or distal third or at the junction of one of these two divisions. A fracture of one of the bony prominences of the end of a long bone is described as a fracture of that prominence by name. Examples include a fracture of the olecranon, medial malleolus, or lateral condyle of the femur.

An epiphyseal separation occurs when a fracture passes through or lies within the growth plate of a bone. When this occurs in a child with immature bone, retardation of limb length and growth may occur. These injuries require immediate and expert treatment.

An avulsion fracture results in a ligamentous attachment remaining intact on a separated bone fragment. This may occur after joint dislocation or rotational injury, such as the femoral condyle separating from the tibial plateau. A dislocation (luxation) is a complete displacement of one articular surface from another. This injury can disrupt neurovascular structures, requiring immediate attention. A subluxation is a partial dislocation, often indicated by ligamentous instability.

## Principles of Treatment

The purpose of fracture treatment is to reestablish the length, shape, and alignment of the fractured bones or joints and restore anatomic function. Acute fracture treatment is necessary to alleviate neurovascular compromise. The surgical team should consider the following principles when providing care for the patient: (1) the patient's extremity or fracture site must be handled gently; (2) initial general medical treatment must be provided; (3) equipment and personnel must be readily available to treat impending or existing shock and to control hemorrhage; (4) aseptic technique must be maintained; (5) positioning must allow adequate circulatory and respira-

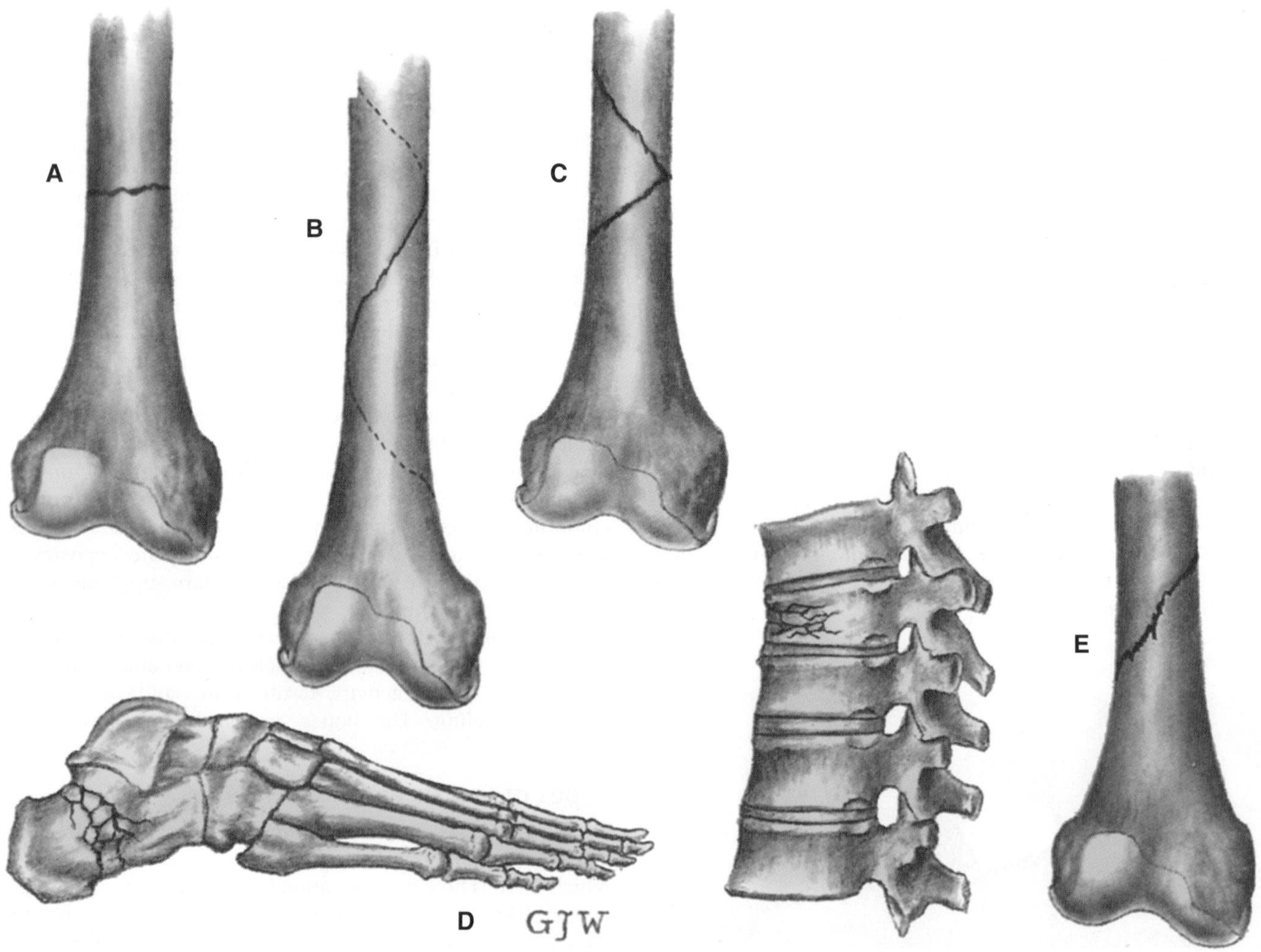


**FIGURE 22-28** Fracture types, which may be open or closed. **A,** Transverse. **B,** Longitudinal or spiral. **C,** Comminuted. **D,** Compression. **E,** Oblique.

tory function with adequate exposure; and (6) patient comfort must be considered.

The primary goal in treatment of an upper extremity fracture is to preserve mobility and restore range of motion, enabling the individual to perform skilled and delicate work. In fractures of a lower extremity, the objectives of surgery are to restore alignment and length and provide stability of the extremity for weight bearing.

In the presence of open fractures involving soft tissues, several associated conditions may arise, including (1) secondary hemorrhage, (2) infection, (3) severe damage to soft tissues, (4) damage to blood vessels and nerves, and (5) Volkmann's contracture (ischemic paralysis).

## Basic Treatment Techniques

***Closed Reduction.*** Fractures may be treated by closed reduction—manipulating the fragments into position without incising the skin. This is the treatment of choice when possible to decrease the opportunity for infection, improve results (including bone union of the fracture), and minimize the recovery period. Significant bone comminution, periosteal damage, or soft tissue entrapped within the fracture site may result in complications.

PROCEDURAL CONSIDERATIONS. The choice of anesthesia depends on the site of fracture and the patient's condition. A closed reduction can be performed with (1) infiltration of local anesthetic agent into the fracture site (hematoma block), (2) intravenous regional anesthesia (Bier block), (3) regional or spinal nerve block, or (4) general anesthesia. Closed reduction may take place before an open procedure to reduce the fracture site. Skeletal traction may also be applied to the fracture site (Figure 22-29), requiring a surgical skin prep and application of drapes. The appropriate casting or brace materials should be readily available to prevent loss of fracture reduction. Supplies should be available in the event it is necessary to open the fracture site and apply fixation.

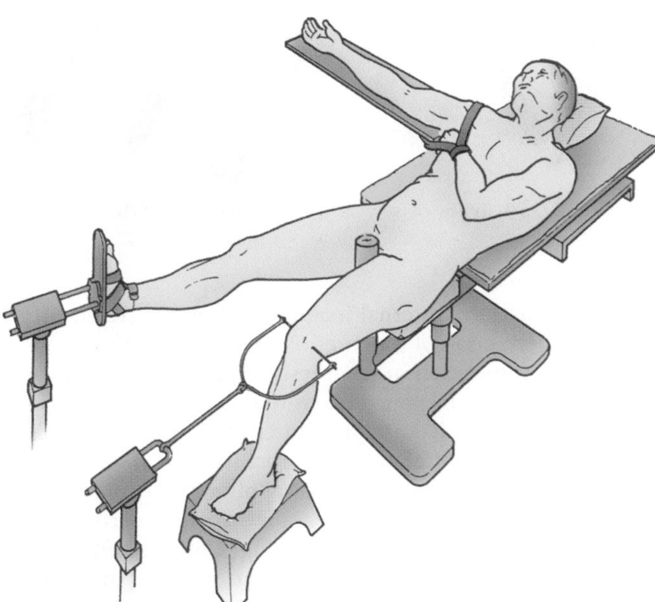

**FIGURE 22-29** Application of skeletal traction with the patient positioned supine on the operating room (OR) fracture bed.

OPERATIVE PROCEDURE. The fragments are manipulated into alignment by the surgeon, using manual traction. Reduction is confirmed using radiography (x-ray or fluoroscopy). After the fracture is reduced, it is immobilized with casting material or bracing technique.

***External Fixation.*** External fixation of fractures provides rigid fixation and reduction with the ability to manage severe soft tissue wounds. Because of the increased chance of infection in patients with an open fracture, external fixation is often the preferred treatment. Advantages of external fixation include the absence of casting material, fracture stabilization at a distance from the injury site, ability to perform subsequent procedures such as skin grafts or vascularized grafts, minimal joint interference, early mobilization, and the ability to use internal fixation or other skeleton-fixation devices at the same time or sequentially.

Indications for external fixation include (1) severe open fractures, (2) highly comminuted closed fractures, (3) arthrodesis, (4) infected joints, (5) infected nonunion, (6) fracture stabilization to protect arterial or nerve anastomoses, (7) major alignment and length deficits, (8) congenital deformities, and (9) static contractures. External fixation provides a bridge between fracture reduction and insertion of an internal fixator such as an intramedullary nail, allowing time for vascular recovery. Internal fixation can take place at a later date.

Many improvements have been made in the design and articulations of external fixation devices. The fixators can be applied to most anatomic sites. The available external fixators vary greatly in design; however, all contain three main components: (1) bone-anchoring devices (threaded pins, Kirschner wires), (2) longitudinal supporting devices (threaded or smooth rods), and (3) connecting elements (clamps and partial or full rings). Improvements have resulted in the use of lightweight and stronger materials, which are radiopaque, for use as connecting rods. The radiopaque feature prevents postoperative radiographic interference when viewing the fracture site for progress in healing.

The Ilizarov device uses principles of tension-stress and distraction to correct bone defects and limb-length discrepancies. It is not routinely used for acute fracture fixation; however, the principles and technique are similar. Limb length may be adjusted with gradual bone distraction of bone ends, stimulating new bone formation.

PROCEDURAL CONSIDERATIONS. External fixators are applied using sterile technique with the patient under general or regional anesthesia. Radiographic imaging ensures fracture reduction after closed manipulation; it also ensures proper pin placement. Because the incision site is small to allow introduction of pins, a soft tissue set appropriate to the site will be necessary. Many different external fixators are available for use. Some examples are shown in Figures 22-30 to 22-33. Irrigation and debridement at the fracture site and surrounding soft tissue may be necessary if soft tissue is damaged, so pulsatile lavage with 3000 ml normal saline solution should be available. A power drill will be used at the pin sites, and a periosteal elevator should be available for blunt or sharp dissection. An appropriate-size pin cutter should also be available to shorten the pins if the need arises. The dressing consists of an antibacterial ointment, antibiotic-impregnated gauze, or Telfa with gauze overwrap.

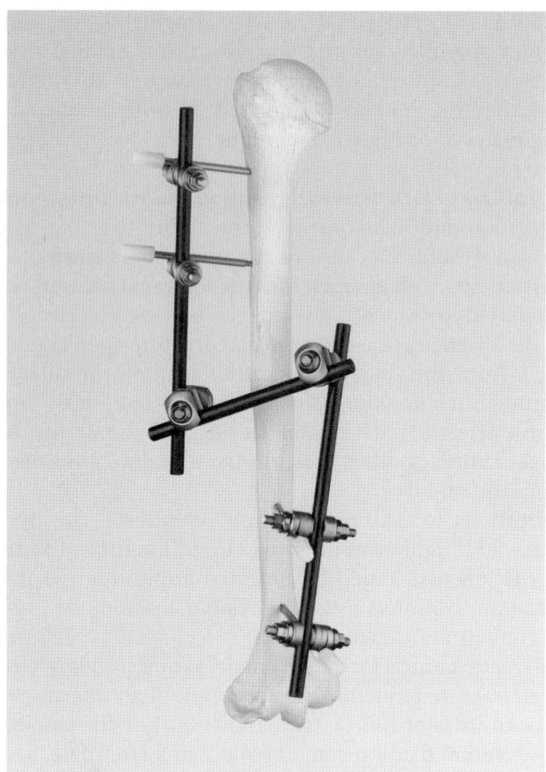

FIGURE 22-30 Synthes external fixator.

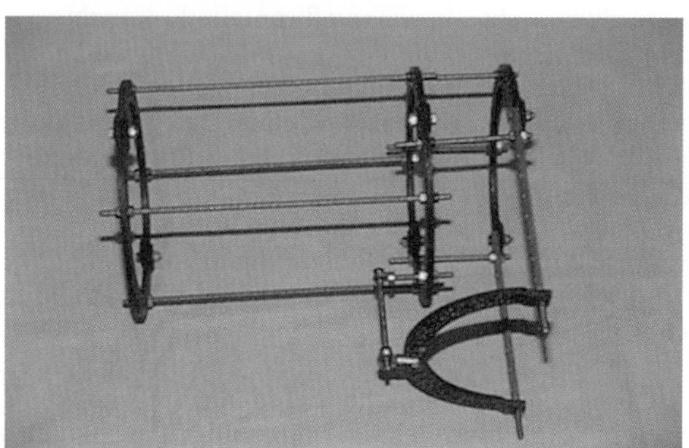

FIGURE 22-31 Ilizarov tibial external fixator.

OPERATIVE PROCEDURE

1. The fracture is reduced manually.
2. The skin is incised over an area free from neurovascular structures.
3. Blunt dissection to the bone or with the elevator may be necessary.
4. A drill sheath is used to protect surrounding soft tissue while predrilling the cortex.
5. Hand drilling or low-speed power drilling is used to insert the half pins above and below the fracture.
6. Universal joints are slipped over the pins and joined with a connecting rod.
7. The frame is tightened using the appropriate wrenches.
8. Radiography or fluoroscopy is used to confirm reduction and alignment.
9. Dressings are applied to the pin sites.

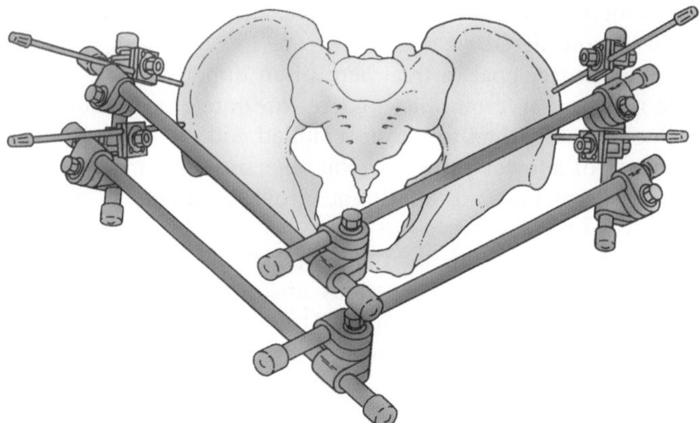

FIGURE 22-32 AO/ASIF pelvic external fixator, double frame using tube-to-tube clamps.

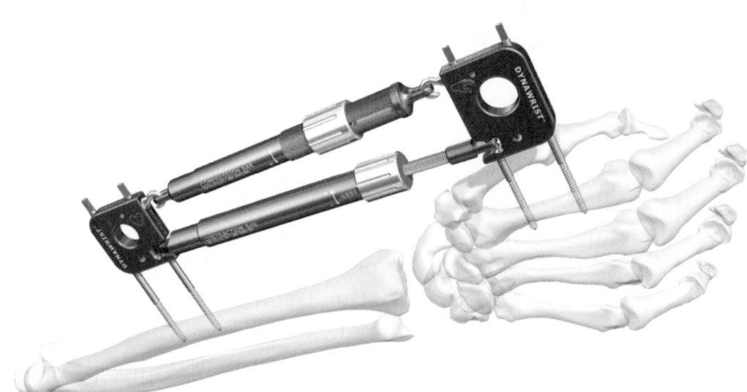


FIGURE 22-33 Dynawrist dynamic wrist external fixator.

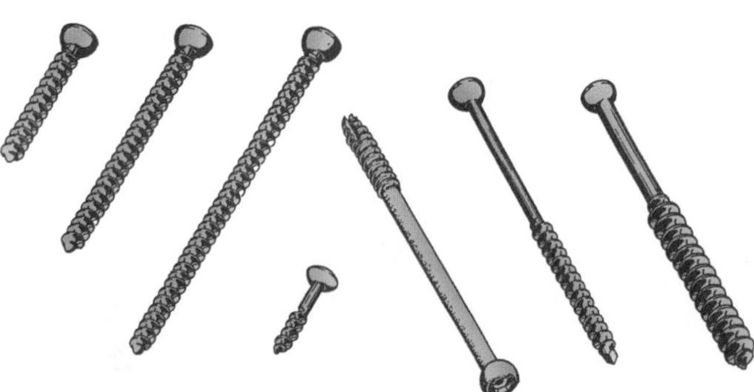

FIGURE 22-34 Types of screws used for fixation with or without plating systems.

***Internal Fixation.*** Internal fixation is often the treatment of choice for correction of fractures of long bones or those in the hip region. Application of compression plates and screws and insertion of pins, intramedullary rods, nails, or wiring are methods of internal fixation. Fractures of most anatomic parts in adults can be repaired using internal fixation.

Many principles and techniques apply when using internal fixation. Types of screws (Figure 22-34) include cortical, cancellous, lag, pretapped, and self-tapping. Cortical bone screws have threads that are closer together and narrower than other types of threads. These threads run along the entire length of the screw and transfix bone, gaining purchase (grab) of bone cortex.

Cancellous bone screws feature threads that are broader and farther apart than those of cortical screws. Cancellous screws are used in cancellous bone, which is less dense than cortical bone; the bone accumulates within the threads to provide the purchase for fixation. Like cortical screws, cancellous screws can traverse fracture sites and hold plates onto bone. The screw threads do not completely traverse the bone through the opposite cortex. Cancellous screws are commonly used when fractures occur at the condylar ends of the shaft.

Plating of a fracture may occur with or without dynamic compression (Figure 22-35). Dynamic compression uses screw and plate configurations to apply forces through the fracture site. Semitubular plates are less rigid and do not have the ability to produce dynamic compression. This type of plate is used in the forearm and fibula, where weight bearing, which could break the plate, is not a factor.

**CLOSED METHOD.** Fractures may also be reduced using closed reduction methods of manipulation and traction and then aligned with percutaneous insertion of pins, intramedullary nails, or rods. Pins can be placed percutaneously (Figure 22-36) to fix fractures involving the digits, wrist, elbow, and foot. A rod or nail is placed percutaneously (Figure 22-37) in a large bone such as the humerus or femur. Closed reduction is, however, a misnomer, since small openings in the soft tissue and bone are made to facilitate introduction of the devices. These incisions are considerably smaller than those created when repairing the fracture using open reduction. The advantages of closed reduction over open reduction and internal fixa-

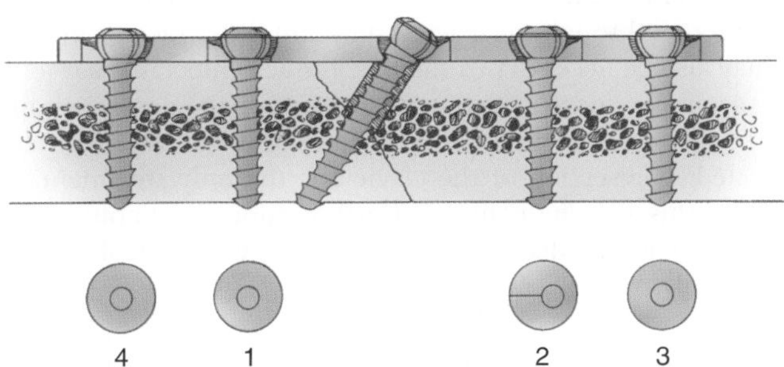


**FIGURE 22-35** Plating a closed forearm fracture using dynamic compression showing final position of the screw insertion.

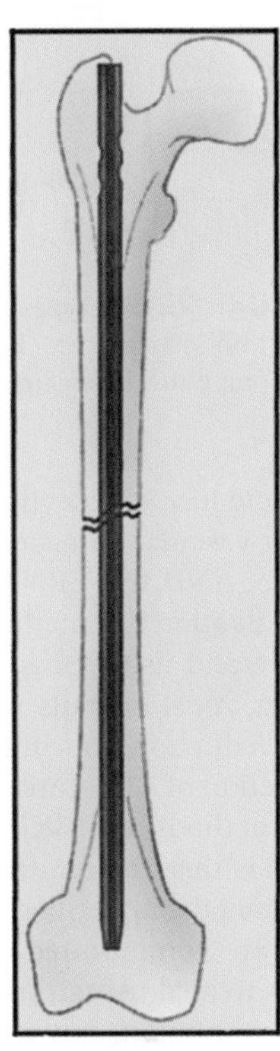

**FIGURE 22-37** Rod placement for femoral fracture.

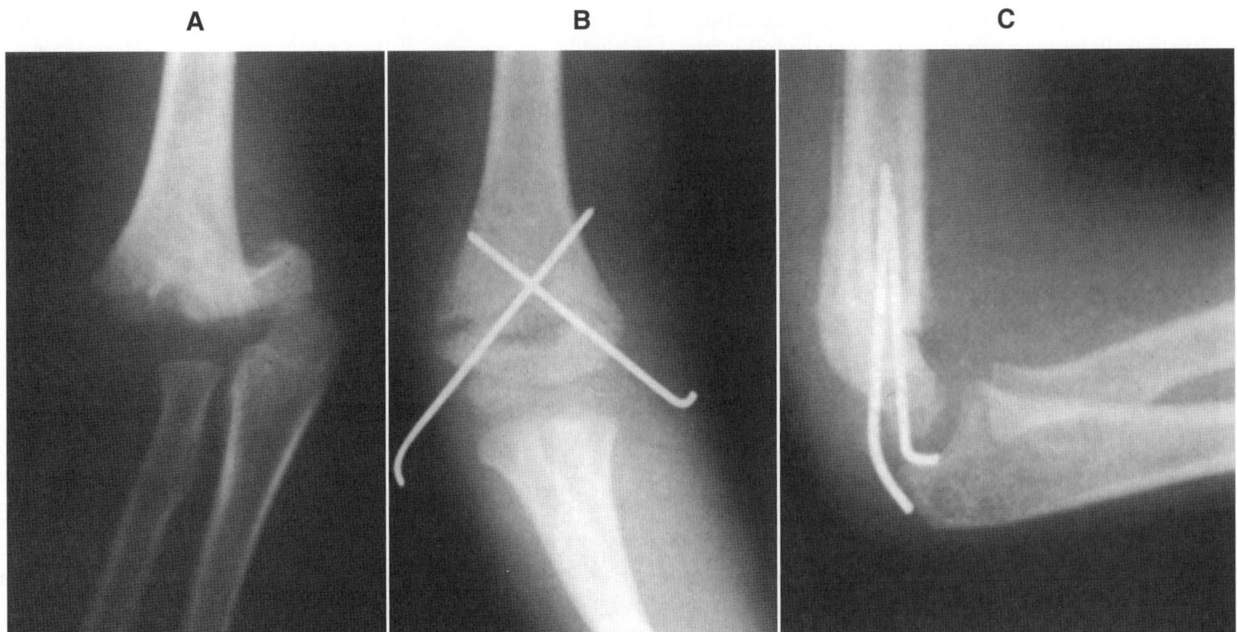


**FIGURE 22-36** Percutaneous pinning of a supracondylar fracture. **A,** Severely displaced supracondylar fracture. **B** and **C,** Treated by closed reduction and percutaneous pinning.

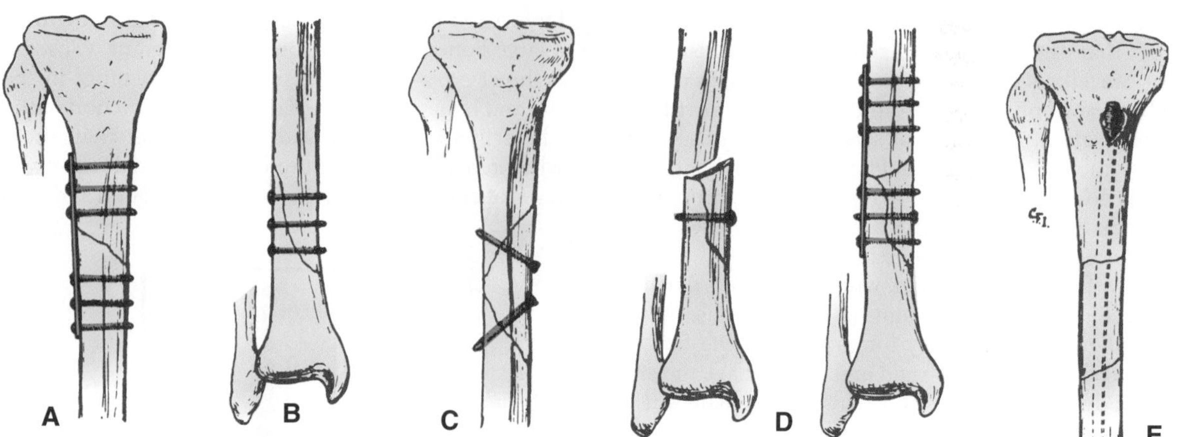


FIGURE 22-38 Types of internal fixation for fracture repair. **A,** Plate and screws for transverse or short oblique fracture. **B,** Transfixion screws for long oblique or spiral fractures. **C,** Transfixion screws for long butterfly fragment. **D,** Fixation for short butterfly fragment. **E,** Medullary fixation.

tion are (1) a lower incidence of infection and (2) absence of additional soft tissue or vascular damage.

**OPEN REDUCTION AND INTERNAL FIXATION.** Open reduction and internal fixation is a method of providing exposure of the fracture site and using pins, wire, screws, a plate and screw combination, rods, or nails to correct the fracture (Figure 22-38). Open reduction and internal fixation is used when satisfactory reduction of a fracture cannot be obtained or maintained by closed methods and skeletal traction is not indicated. The advantage is that anatomic alignment of the fracture can usually be obtained and verified through direct observation. Fractures that are comminuted or difficult to reduce can be more effectively treated using this technique. The incidence of infection and nonunion, however, is increased when the wound is opened.

The procedure varies for each anatomic site, using the principles for specific fixation devices. Several procedures described in the text identify steps for completion of open reduction and internal fixation. Reference examples include the following:

- *Pin fixation:* application of a unilateral frame
- *Wire fixation:* reduction of patellar fracture, tension banding of the olecranon
- *Screw fixation:* correction of scaphoid fractures
- *Plate and screw fixation:* repair of the comminuted distal humeral fracture
- *Rod or nail fixation:* correction of fractures of the shaft of the humerus, femoral shaft, or tibial shaft

## SURGERY OF THE SHOULDER

### Correction of Acromioclavicular Joint Separation

Acromioclavicular joint separation (Figure 22-39), a common occupational and athletic injury, results from a force applied downward, most commonly from a fall, directly to the top of the shoulder. The ligamentous support of the distal clavicle in the form of the coracoclavicular, coracoacromial, and acromioclavicular ligaments is disrupted. The result is either a posterior or superior displacement of the lateral end of the clavicle.

The purpose of surgery in an acutely injured patient is to reestablish the proper relationship between the clavicle and the acromion, thereby reducing long-term shoulder pain and increasing function. This is done by replacing the coracoclavicular ligaments with heavy suture or Mersilene tape or by inserting a screw through the clavicle and into the coracoid process. It may also be necessary to stabilize the acromioclavicular joint by placing a smooth Steinmann pin across the acromion and into the clavicle. Sometimes the distal end of the clavicle is also resected. If resection of the clavicle is the only treatment required, this may be completed arthroscopically. Shoulder arthroscopy is detailed in the "Arthroscopy of the Shoulder" section of "Arthroscopy," p. 789.

***Procedural Considerations.*** The patient is placed in the supine or semisitting position with a sandbag or folded sheet under the affected shoulder. The shoulder is positioned slightly off the OR bed (Figure 22-40) to allow full range of motion, or if mobility of the arm is unnecessary, a shoulder positioner is used (see Figure 22-14). The head is turned to the opposite side, taking care not to apply too much stretch to the nerves of the brachial plexus. The extremity is draped with a stockinette to the midhumeral level.

A soft tissue set and bone instrumentation specific for the shoulder (Figure 22-41) are required. Depending on the technique used, bone screws and their instrumentation, free-cutting needles, bone-anchoring devices, and power instruments may be necessary.

#### *Operative Procedure*

CORACOCLAVICULAR SUTURE FIXATION

1. A curved incision is made to expose the acromioclavicular joint, the distal end of the clavicle, and the coracoid process.
2. The acromioclavicular joint is exposed, and any loose fragments or debris is removed.
3. Mattress sutures are placed in the ruptured coracoclavicular ligaments but not tied.
4. Drill holes are made in the clavicle above the coracoid in the anteroposterior (AP) plane.
5. A #5 nonabsorbable suture is placed beneath the base of the coracoid and superiorly through the two holes in the clavicle. With the joint reduced, the sutures are tied.

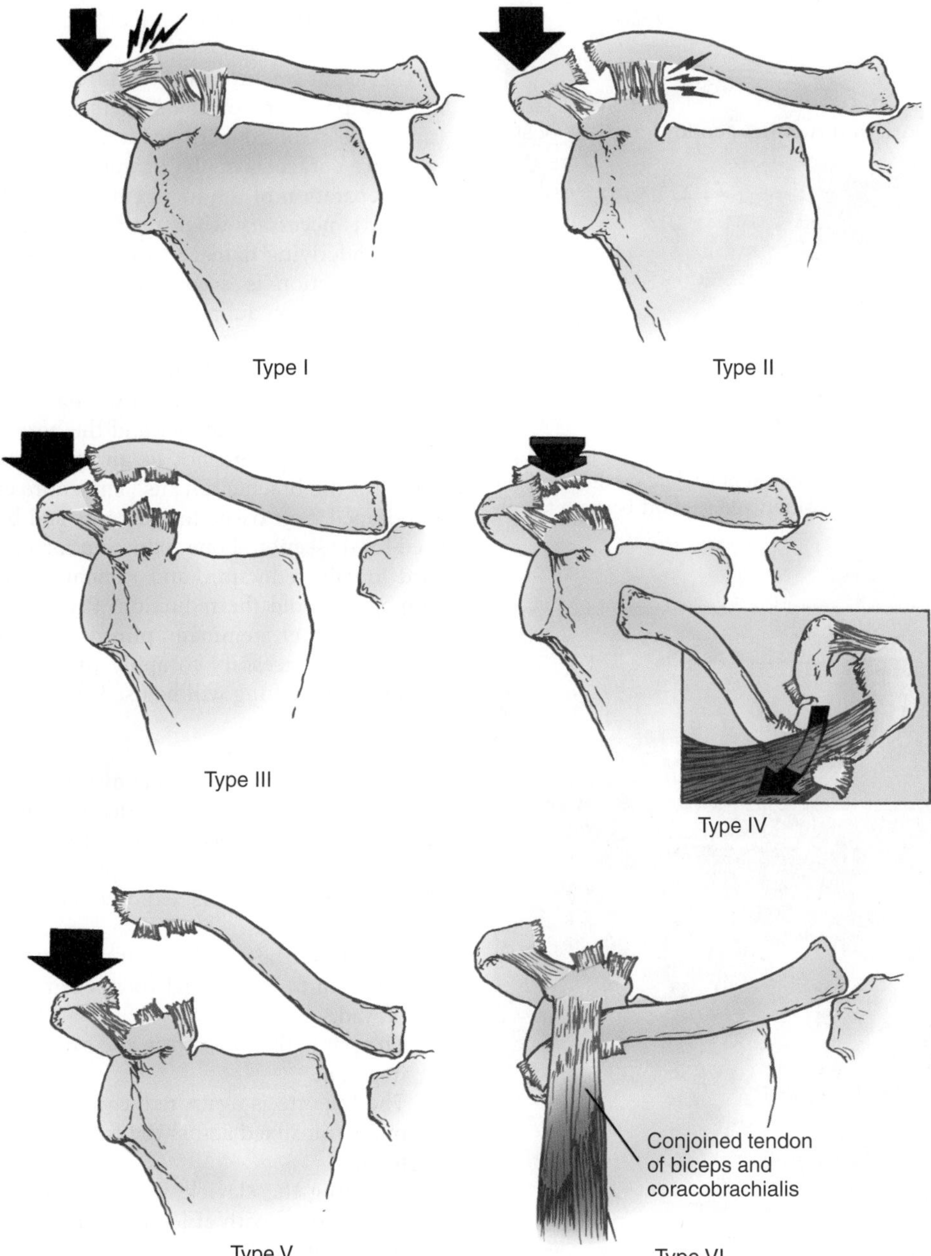


**FIGURE 22-39** Classification of acromioclavicular injuries. *Type I,* Neither acromioclavicular nor coracoclavicular ligaments are disrupted. *Type II,* Acromioclavicular ligament is disrupted, and coracoclavicular ligament is intact. *Type III,* Both ligaments are disrupted. *Type IV,* Ligaments are disrupted, and distal end of clavicle is displaced posteriorly into or through trapezius muscle. *Type V,* Ligaments and muscle attachments are disrupted, and clavicle and acromion are widely separated. *Type VI,* Ligaments are disrupted, and distal clavicle is dislocated inferior to coracoid process and posterior to biceps and coracobrachialis tendons.

6. If instability is still a concern, small Kirschner wires can be placed across the acromioclavicular joint, through the lateral border of the acromion. The ends of the wires are bent 90 degrees at the lateral border to prevent proximal migration.
7. The sutures previously placed in the coracoclavicular ligaments are then tied.
8. The acromioclavicular joint capsule and the origins of the deltoid and trapezius muscles are repaired.
9. A sling-and-swathe bandage is then applied to the extremity.

## Correction of Sternoclavicular Dislocation

Traumatic dislocation of the sternoclavicular joint usually occurs from an indirect blow on the anterior shoulder while the arm is abducted. The clavicle most frequently is displaced anteriorly, but posterior or retrosternal dislocations can occur. Posterior dislocation can be more severe because injury to the trachea, esophagus, thoracic duct, and large vessels of the mediastinum is possible. Except in severe cases, dislocation of the

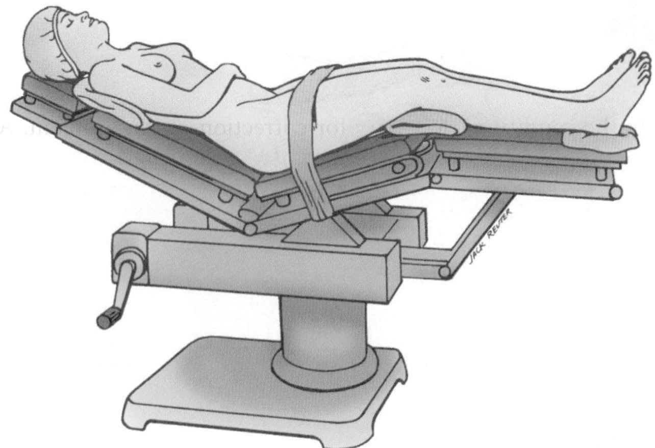

FIGURE 22-40 Positioning for a surgical procedure on the shoulder with the patient in a semisitting position and support beneath the affected shoulder.

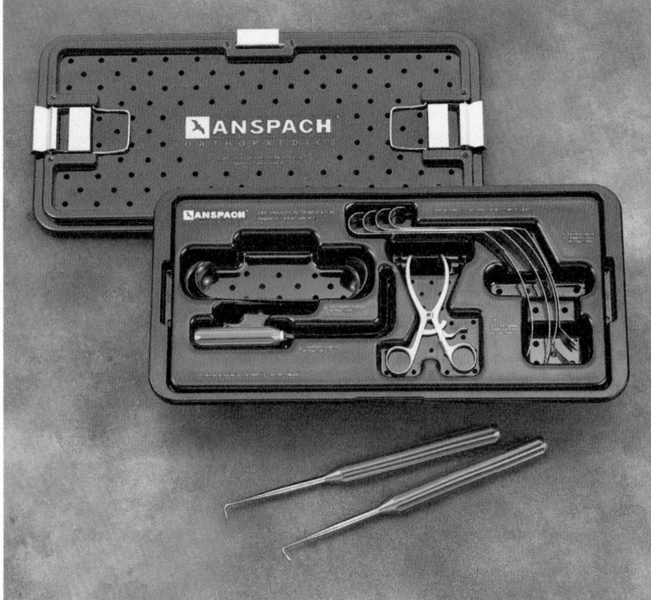


FIGURE 22-41 Shoulder instrumentation set including humeral head retractors, glenoid neck retractor, modified Gelpi retractors, Goulet retractors, conjoined tendon retractor, subscapularis retractor, and glenoid awl.

sternoclavicular joint is treated nonoperatively with manual traction and immobilization bandages.

## Clavicular Fracture

Fractures of the clavicle are some of the most common bony injuries. These injuries rarely require surgical intervention. Approximately 94% of clavicular fractures are the result of a direct blow on the clavicle. The most common site of clavicular fractures is the middle-third portion of the bone, mainly at the middle- and outer-third junction.

Clavicular fractures are usually treated by immobilization in a figure-of-eight splint. The chances of nonunion are greatly increased when open reduction is used for a clavicular fracture. The outcome may result in a bony prominence, which may be disturbing to the patient; the overriding fragments are resorbed with time.

Clavicular fractures may require open reduction and internal fixation after nonunion, neurovascular compromise that cannot be resolved with reduction, distal clavicular fracture with torn coracoclavicular ligaments in the adult, or persistent wide separation of the fragments with soft tissue entrapment. Surgery is necessary when the fracture is displaced enough to cause underlying damage to the vessels and brachial plexus. Open reduction is accomplished with a tubular plate and screws or intramedullary pin fixation.

***Procedural Considerations.*** The patient is placed in the supine or semisitting position with a sandbag or folded sheet under the affected shoulder and the head turned to the opposite side, taking care not to apply too much stretch to the nerves of the brachial plexus. The entire extremity is prepped and draped. Soft tissue instruments and bone instruments are used for dissection. Bone reduction forceps and clamps will be used to gain reduction, and Kirschner wires may be used to temporarily hold the reduction. Permanent reduction will be held with either Steinmann pins or plate and screws. A power drill will be necessary to apply these. In the case of a nonunion, bone grafting will be used.

### *Operative Procedure*

1. A 2.5-cm incision is made over the fracture site. The incision may need to be extended for comminuted fractures.
2. Dissection is carried down to the clavicle, taking care not to strip periosteum or disrupt vessels or nerves.
3. The fracture site is exposed and reduced using bone-holding forceps.
4. If pinning the clavicle is to be done, a Steinmann pin is passed into the medial fragment medullary canal and removed.
5. The pin is then passed in the same manner into the distal fragment.
6. The fracture is again reduced, and a threaded Steinmann pin is transfixed across the fracture site through both fragments.
7. If plating the clavicle is to be done, a small semitubular plate is used with at least two screw holes on each side of the fracture site.
8. The periosteum must be stripped off the clavicle sparingly but sufficiently so that a plate can be applied to the anterior surface.
9. Extreme care must be taken when drilling screw holes to avoid damage to the subclavian vein and thoracic contents.
10. After closure, an immobilization sling is applied.

## Correction of Rotator Cuff Tear

Most rotator cuff tears occur through the insertion of the tendinous fibers of the supraspinatus muscle that attaches onto the greater tuberosity of the proximal humerus. In severe tears, the remaining tendons of the cuff, the subscapularis, infraspinatus, and teres minor, may also be involved. Supraspinatus syndrome, also known as *impingement syndrome,* can involve multiple pathologic conditions, such as calcium deposits, bicipital tendonitis, subacromial bursitis, tenosynovitis, and other nonarticular lesions along with a cuff tear. The approach to diagnosis and treatment is similar for both.

Partial rotator cuff tears and impingement usually affect people in the middle decades of life or later and are often attributable to a long-term degenerative process. Complete tears of the rotator cuff occur after accidental injury of younger patients, such as pitchers and football quarterbacks. Patients with rotator cuff tears may not be able to initiate abduction of the shoulder because the stabilizing forces of the ruptured tendons on the humeral head are lost. Many rotator cuff tears can be treated conservatively with physical therapy and nonsteroidal antiinflammatory drugs (NSAIDs).

A variety of procedures may be performed for these conditions when conservative treatment is unsuccessful. Methods of repair depend on the size and shape of the tear. The common goal is to restore joint stability, alleviate pain, and allow the patient to return to normal activities. In some instances a significant reduction in preinjury activity may be permanent.

***Procedural Considerations.*** If surgery is necessary, the patient is placed in the supine or semisitting position with a sandbag or folded towel under the affected shoulder. The head is turned to the opposite side, taking care to avoid undue stretch to the brachial plexus. A shoulder positioner can be used if intraoperative mobility of the arm is not a factor. In addition to a bone set and a soft tissue set, shoulder instruments will be required. The remaining equipment needs will depend on the severity of the tear. Minor tears may require no more than heavy nonabsorbable suture. Major tears will require a power drill and burr and possibly a microsagittal saw. Fixation may be gained with bone-anchoring devices. Free needles will be necessary if these are used.

#### *Operative Procedure*

1. An anterosuperior deltoid incision is made.
2. The coracoacromial ligament is divided at the acromial attachment.
3. A subacromioplasty (resection of the undersurface of the acromion) is completed. This is also primary treatment for impingement syndrome.
4. Small, simple tears can be repaired by suturing the torn edges with heavy nonabsorbable sutures.
5. Massive tears may require attaching the torn edges to the greater tuberosity using bone-anchoring devices.
6. If the defect cannot be bridged, a flap from the subscapularis tendon can be transposed and sutured to the supraspinatus and infraspinatus muscles.
7. If impingement is involved or solely the cause of a rotator pathologic condition, other measures involving the same approach are taken.
8. Calcium deposits encased in tendon are excised to alleviate mechanical obstruction, or acromioplasty is performed.
9. After closure, a sling is applied.

Patients with small tears may begin motion on the third to fourth postoperative day. Larger tears may require immobilization for 2 to 8 weeks.

### Correction of Recurrent Anterior Dislocation of the Shoulder

The anterior fibers of the shoulder capsule are stretched and weakened as a result of frequent dislocations of the shoulder joint. More than 150 operations or modifications have been devised to treat recurrent anterior dislocation. The goals are to (1) prevent recurrence, (2) prevent surgical complications, (3) prevent creation of arthritic changes, (4) maintain joint motion, and (5) correct the problem. The surgeon selects the procedure appropriate for the patient's condition that will satisfy the conditions necessary for correction of the problem. A stapling procedure was once common treatment of recurrent dislocation, but it has been replaced by other accepted procedures.

***Procedural Considerations.*** The patient is placed in the supine or semisitting position with a sandbag or folded sheet under the shoulder. The arm is draped free so that the extremity can be manipulated. An anterior curved incision or a longitudinal incision in the anterior axillary fold is made over the shoulder joint. A soft tissue set and a bone set will be required, as well as a set of instruments specific to shoulder surgery, power drill and burr, bone-anchoring devices, and free needles.

#### *Operative Procedures*

BANKART PROCEDURE. For the Bankart procedure (Figure 22-42), the scapula is not elevated with a sandbag or folded sheet. The attenuated anterior capsule is reattached to the rim of the glenoid fossa with heavy sutures. The glenoid fossa rim is decorticated with a curette to provide a raw surface to which the capsule is attached. Special instruments designed for the Bankart procedure, such as the curved awl and humeral head retractor, facilitate the surgery, although the capsule may be attached with bone anchors, obviating the use of the awl. If the coracoid process is to be removed to obtain better operative exposure, a drill, bone screws, and washer should be available for reattachment. Postoperatively the extremity is immobilized in a sling or shoulder immobilizer. Shoulder motion is begun at 3 days postoperatively, and the patient may return to contact sports or heavy labor after approximately 6 months.

PUTTI-PLATT PROCEDURE. The steps of the Putti-Platt procedure are similar to those of the Bankart procedure in that the joint capsule is sutured to the glenoid rim. In addition, the

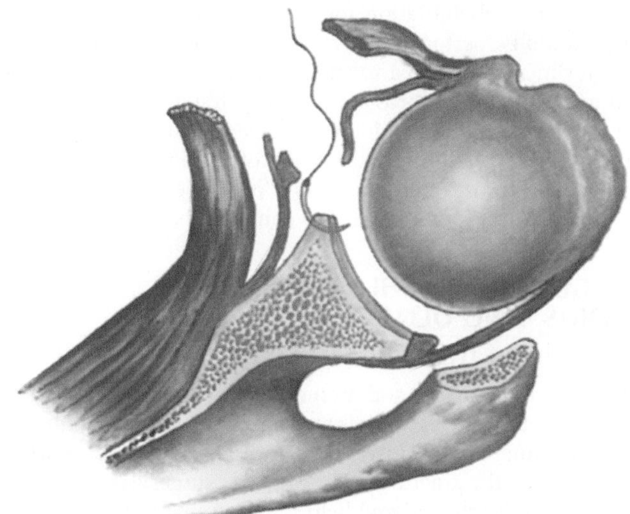

FIGURE 22-42 Bankart procedure for restoration of shoulder stability. Holes are made in the rim of the glenoid, and the free lateral margin of the capsule is sutured to the rim of the glenoid. The medial margin of the capsule is sutured to the lateral surface.

Putti-Platt procedure requires the lateral advancement of the subscapularis. This produces a barrier against dislocation of the shoulder. This procedure is rarely useful when the anterior capsular mechanism is of poor quality.

The subscapularis tendon is divided 2.5 cm medially to its insertion. The glenoid and humeral head are inspected using palpation to assess osteochondral changes. The lateral portion of the subscapularis is sutured to the anterior glenoid rim. The medial portion of the subscapularis is sutured to the rotator cuff at the greater tuberosity. The layers of the shoulder joint are imbricated (overlapped), a technique used often in soft tissue reconstruction. The incision is closed, and a shoulder immobilizer is applied. This is worn for approximately 3 weeks. External rotation of the arm should be avoided immediately after the repair.

**BRISTOW PROCEDURE.** In the Bristow procedure, the coracoid process, along with the attached muscles, is detached and inserted onto the neck of the glenoid cavity, where it is attached with a screw through the subscapularis muscle. This stabilizes the anterior joint capsule and prevents recurrent dislocation. A Bristow procedure is considered an appropriate alternative when the anterior capsular mechanism is of poor quality. Disadvantages of this procedure are (1) internal rotation contracture, (2) inattention to labrum or capsule disorders, (3) potential for injury to the musculocutaneous nerve, (4) reduction of internal rotation power by shortening of the subscapularis muscle, (5) possible limitation of external rotation, (6) possible penetration of the screw into the articular surface of the glenoid, and (7) later development of early joint disease of the shoulder.

### Correction of Humeral Head Fracture

Comminuted fractures of the humeral head (Figure 22-43) with displacement may require open reduction and internal fixation with screws or pins or closed reduction with a humeral nail or rod. However, if the fracture is badly comminuted, a prosthetic replacement is indicated. Traumatic or degenerative arthritic shoulder joints may be so painful or dysfunctional that a total shoulder joint replacement is necessary.

Extensive rehabilitation for the shoulder is required. Surgery should be performed as soon as possible. Delay can allow time for increasing scar formation, contracture of the muscles, and increasing osteoporosis of the bone fragments. The shoulder is the most difficult joint in the body to rehabilitate because it has (1) the greatest range of motion, (2) a second space beneath the acromion that must be mobilized, and (3) many muscles that enter into complex movements.

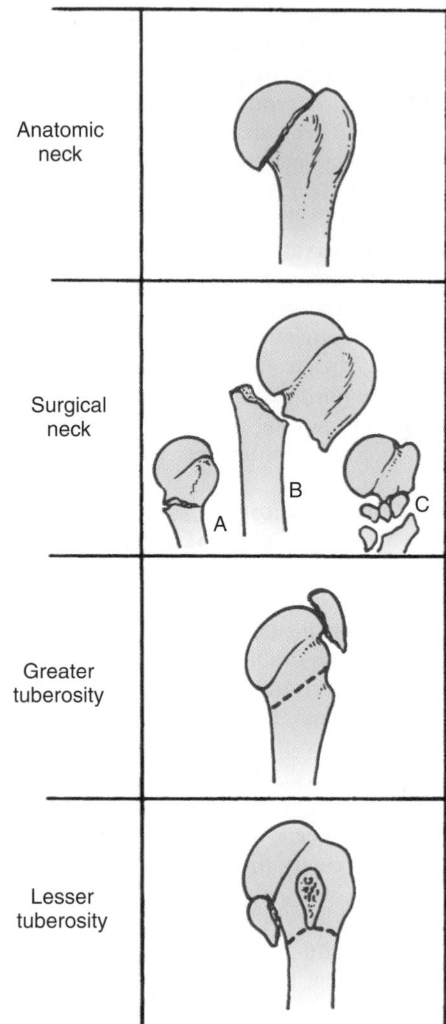


**FIGURE 22-43** Fractures and fracture-dislocations relate to the pattern of displacement. Fractures can occur in two, three, or four parts.

## SURGERY OF THE HUMERUS, RADIUS, AND ULNA

### Fractures of the Humeral Shaft

Closed manipulation and immobilization usually reduce a fractured humerus as well as minimize the risk of nonunion and infection. When closed reduction is impossible or when nonunion of the fracture has occurred, surgery is indicated. The fracture is reduced and held with intramedullary fixation, a compression plate, a lag screw, or a rigid locking nail, with distal and proximal bone screws that will transfix the rod within the canal. This last device can control rotation of the fracture fragments and prevent distraction at the fracture site (Figure 22-44). Multiple flexible nails may be used if more rigid nails are not available. Bone graft may be used, depending on both the extent of the fracture and the length of time since injury. Compression plating of shaft fractures is usually reserved for supracondylar involvement or when other treatment has failed.

***Procedural Considerations.*** The patient is positioned supine with the body near the edge of the bed to facilitate moving the extremity. The extremity is prepped and draped from the middle of the chest to below the elbow. Fluoroscopy and permanent radiographs are required to ensure proper alignment, reduction, and placement of implants. A radiolucent table improves imaging ability.

A soft tissue set and a large bone set are required. In addition, the intramedullary fixation device of choice and the required instruments for its insertion will be needed. PMMA may be used in the case of pathologic fractures. Instruments that are required for harvesting bone graft might be needed as

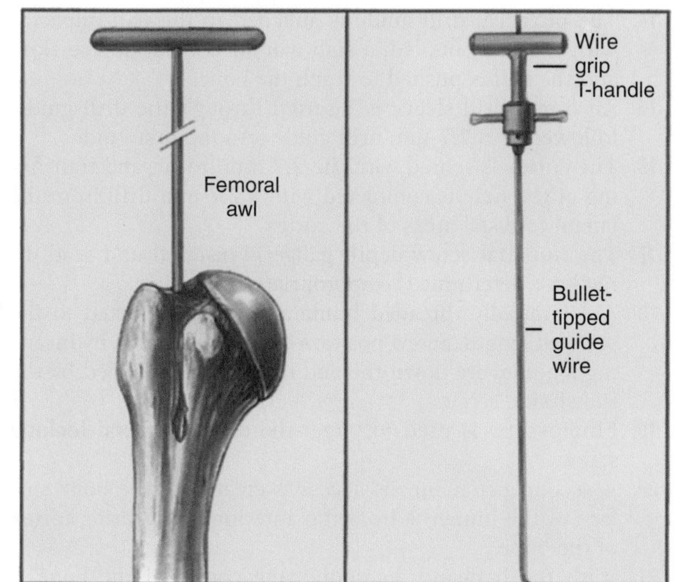


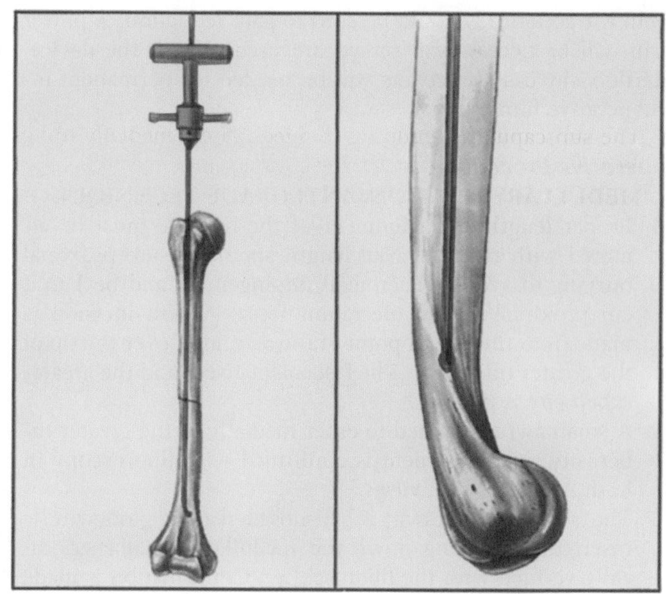


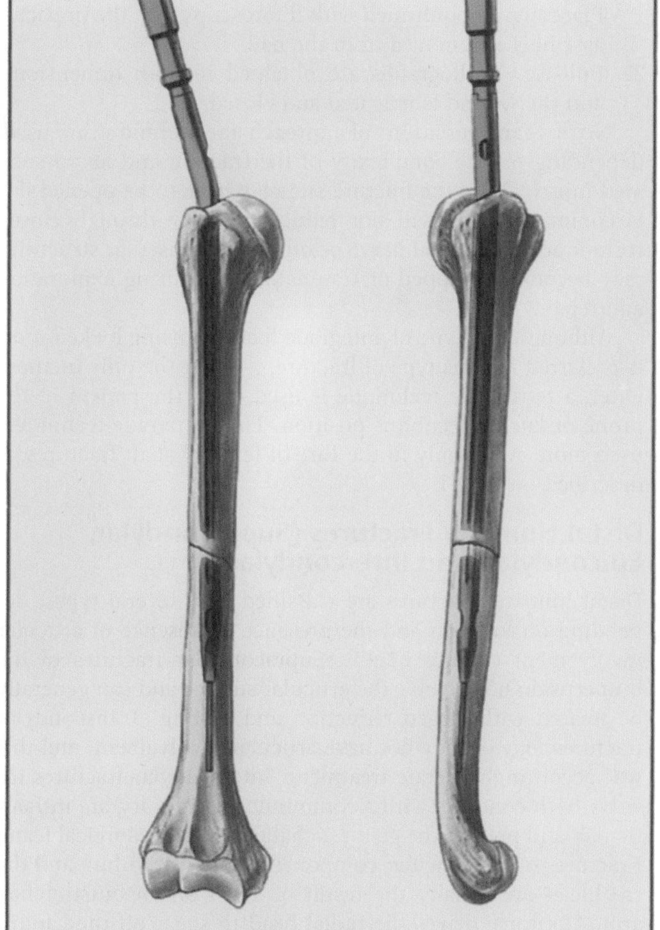


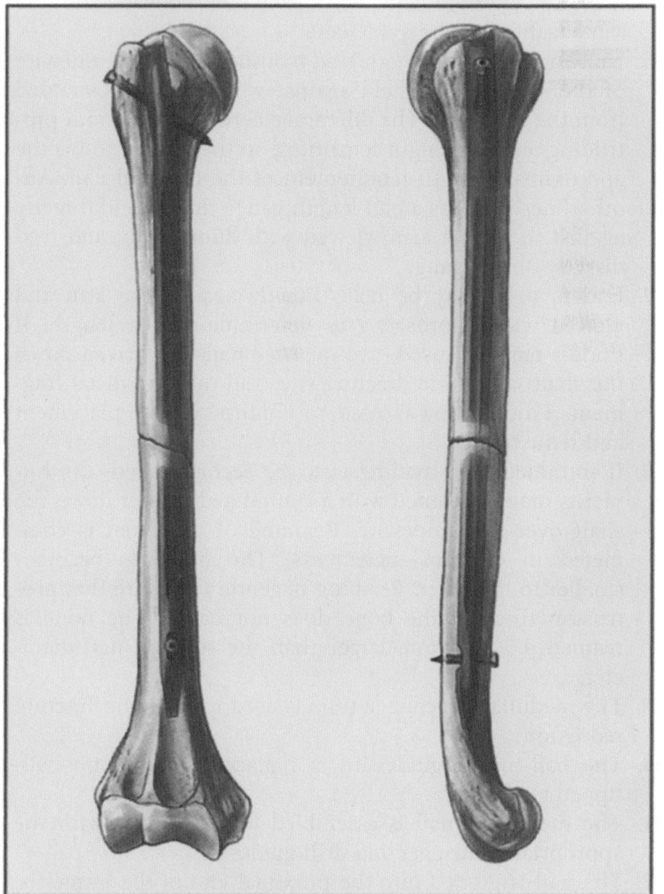


**FIGURE 22-44** Placement of the humeral rigid locking nail with distal and proximal screws. **A,** After incision and exposure, a femoral awl is used to make an entry portal. **B,** Guidewire is advanced into the center of the epicondylar region. **C,** After reaming, the nail is advanced over the fracture site and seated. **D,** Proximal and distal locking takes place after the correct screw placement is determined.

well. A traction tray could be used to gain reduction. A power drill will be necessary if screws are used to lock the device. Sterile x-ray cassette covers will be needed for permanent intraoperative films.

### *Operative Procedure*

MEDULLARY FIXATION: ANTEGRADE TECHNIQUE

1. Proper length and alignment of the fracture must be attained with traction. Nail length should ensure proximal burying to avoid subacromial impingement and be 1 to 2 cm proximal to the olecranon fossa. A skin incision is made from the lateral point of the acromion over the tip of the greater tuberosity. The fascia is incised, and the greater tuberosity is palpated.
2. A small awl is inserted to enter medially to the greater tuberosity, and placement is confirmed with fluoroscopy in both AP and lateral views.
3. The awl is withdrawn; a ball-nosed reamer guidewire is inserted, advancing down the medullary canal (periodically verified with the fluoroscopy). Confirmation is made with each step to ensure that the wires, reamers, or implant has not fractured through the cortex along the shaft.
4. The guidewire is advanced to within 1 to 2 cm of the olecranon fossa, avoiding distraction or shortening.
5. If Enders nails are being used, each one is advanced in the same fashion as the guidewire.
6. Nail length can be determined by using a second guidewire of the same length held against what remains extended from the humerus. The difference between the length protruding and the length remaining on the second rod is the approximate length requirement of the humeral nail. Another method uses a nail-length gauge that is held directly against the upper arm, viewed with fluoroscopy, and read directly on the gauge.
7. Enders nails may be held directly against the arm and viewed with fluoroscopy to determine proper length. If Enders nails are used, two or three nails are driven down the shaft, across the fracture site, and into the distal fragment. Fluoroscopy is used to confirm proper placement and reduction.
8. If intramedullary nailing is to be accomplished, the humerus may be reamed with a cannulated reamer down the shaft over the guidewire. Reaming of the canal is completed in 0.5-mm increments. The humerus becomes smaller in diameter. Reaming is gentle to ensure that protrusion through the bone does not occur. The bone is reamed 0.5 to 1 mm larger than the selected nail diameter.
9. The medullary exchange tube is used to maintain fracture reduction.
10. The ball-tipped guidewire is replaced with a non–ball-tipped guidewire.
11. The medullary nail is assembled for impaction with the appropriate outrigger and drill guides.
12. The nail is guided into the proximal end of the humerus, and the humeral nail driver is used to impact the nail within the canal. Care must be taken to avoid splitting the humerus or creating a supracondylar fracture by wedging the tip of the nail.
13. As the nail approaches and crosses the fracture site, manual reduction must be maintained.
14. The proximal drill guide is attached to the nail impactor with the nail coupled; a stab wound is made in the skin, and the nail is pushed to reach the bone.
15. An 8-mm drill sleeve is inserted through the drill guide, followed by a 2.7-mm drill guide into the first guide.
16. The cortex is scored with the 2.7-mm trocar, and transfixing of the hole is completed with a 2.7-mm drill from the lateral to distal areas of the cortex.
17. The humeral screw-depth gauge is inserted and read directly to determine the appropriate screw size.
18. A 4-mm fully threaded humeral screw is inserted to the selected length. Screw position can be confirmed by inserting a guidewire down the end of the nail, impeded by the transfixing screw.
19. Fluoroscopy is used to target the distal humeral locking screw.
20. A second percutaneous access is created to the bone surface of the humerus from the anterior to posterior cortex of the bone.
21. With the freehand technique, the cortex of the bone is scored followed by insertion of the 8-mm handheld drill sleeve and the 2.7-mm drill bit.
22. The selected size of humeral screw is gauged and inserted. Placement is confirmed with fluoroscopy, and the impactor assembly is removed from the nail.
23. Full-view radiographs are obtained in both dimensions, and the wound is irrigated and closed.

NOTE: Many variations of approach and technique are used, depending on the complexity of the fracture and any associated injury. Often the fracture site may have to be opened if it is comminuted or will not reduce properly through closed techniques. The radial nerve or other neurovascular structures may become entrapped or traumatized, requiring exploration and repair.

Although this type of antegrade fixation, using locked rods, is preferred for this type of fracture, it is not the only method. Often a retrograde technique is used, with the patient in the prone or lateral decubitus position. The retrograde technique, used more commonly in the care of femoral shaft fractures, is described on p. 751.

## Distal Humeral Fractures (Supracondylar, Epicondylar, and Intercondylar)

Distal humeral fractures are classified into several types, depending on location and the presence or absence of articular involvement (Figure 22-45). Supracondylar fractures of the humerus do not involve the articular surface and can generally be treated with closed reduction and casting. Transcondylar fractures may or may not have articular involvement, and this will accordingly dictate treatment. Intercondylar fractures involve both condyles with a comminution of injury, are intraarticular, and present the greatest challenge for the surgical team. Fractures of the articular components—the capitulum and the trochlea—are usually the result of a fall on an outstretched arm. The force drives the radial head to shear off the capitulum, producing an intraarticular fragment. The lateral or medial condyles and epicondyles are also subject to fracture by various mechanisms.

Patients may present with a single isolated fracture or any combination just mentioned. Neurovascular and other soft tissue trauma is considered in selecting the type of reduction and

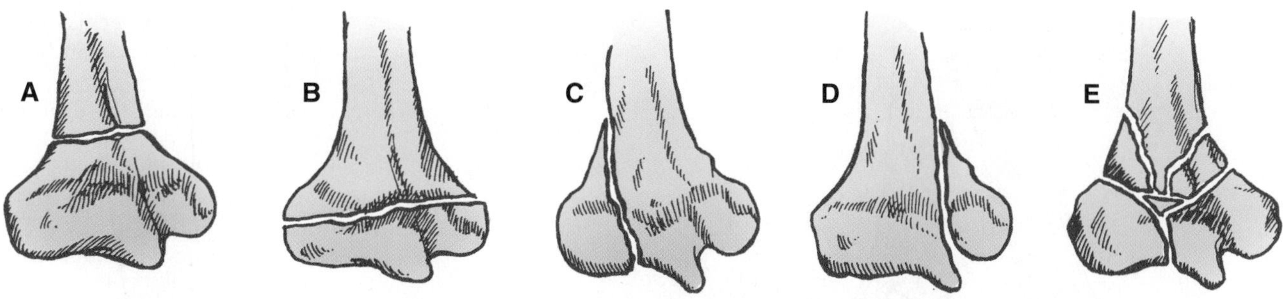


FIGURE 22-45 Classification of distal humeral fractures. **A,** Supracondylar. **B,** Transcondylar. **C,** Lateral condyle with trochlea. **D,** Medial condyle. **E,** Intercondylar with comminution.

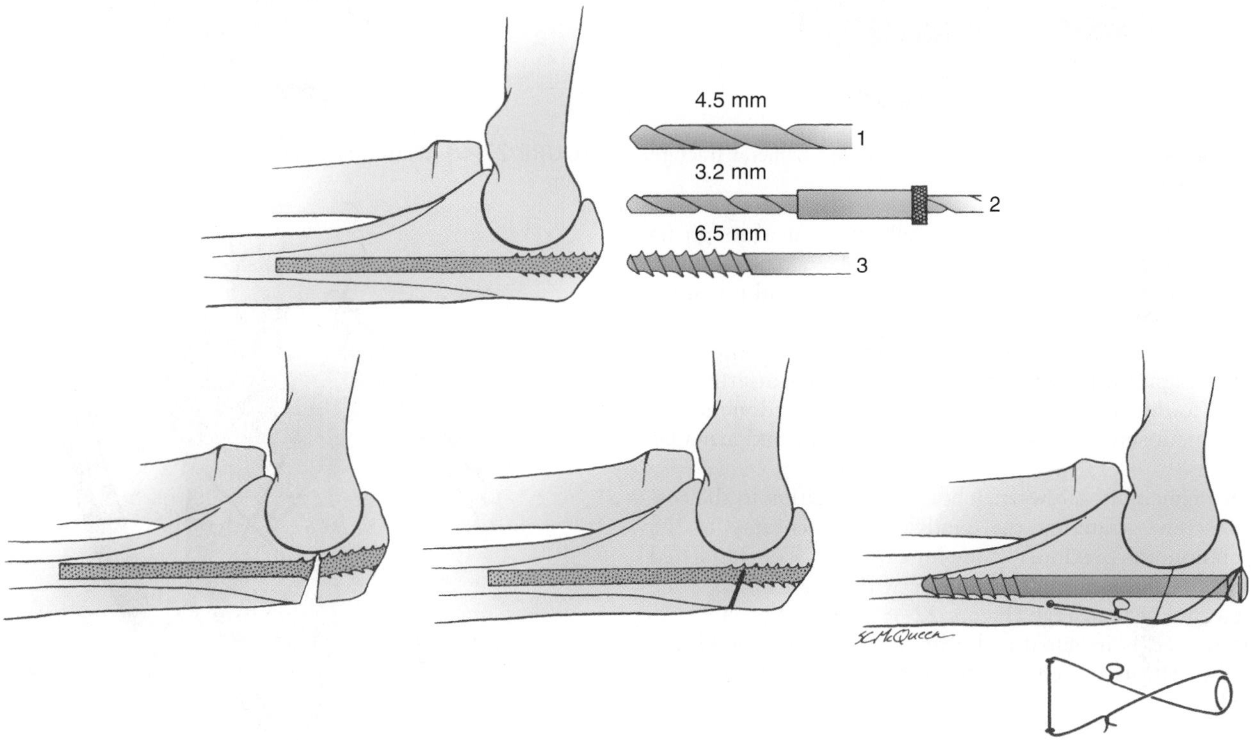


FIGURE 22-46 Osteotomy of the olecranon with placement of a lag screw and tension band wire fixation.

fixation. Screws, pins, a variety of different plates, and dynamic compression technique can be used for internal fixation. Certain fixation techniques of the distal portion of the humerus may require an osteotomy of the olecranon (proximal ulna) to properly align and affix hardware (Figure 22-46). The general goals of treating these injuries are to (1) maintain neurovascular integrity, (2) restore normal joint articulation, (3) preserve motion of the joint, and (4) correct other soft tissue injuries.

***Procedural Considerations.*** Regional anesthesia can be used for procedures on the distal end of the humerus. Bone graft harvesting may require use of general anesthesia. The patient may be prone with the elbow flexed over a small table, supine with the arm over the chest, supine with the arm on a hand table, or in the lateral position. A tourniquet is placed before the surgical prep and inflated during surgery as needed.

A soft tissue set, a large bone set, and a bone graft set are needed, in addition to a compression set, bone-holding clamps, reconstruction plates, and smooth Kirschner wires. A power drill and Kirschner wire driver will be needed to apply the hardware.

### *Operative Procedure*

#### COMMINUTED DISTAL HUMERAL FRACTURE (FIGURE 22-47)

1. An incision is made over the distal humeral fracture site.
2. The fracture is exposed and reduced using bone reduction clamps and temporary small smooth Kirschner wires, driving them across the fracture site with the power drill.
3. A cancellous bone screw is placed using drill and tap to transfix from one condyle to the other. Care must be taken not to violate the joint surface with the threads of the screw.
4. Kirschner wires are removed if reduction is maintained.
5. A one-third tubular or reconstruction plate is contoured to the shape of the distal humeral fracture and applied to bridge the fracture fragments.
6. Throughout the entire procedure, the articular surface is periodically inspected to ensure integrity. The plates are

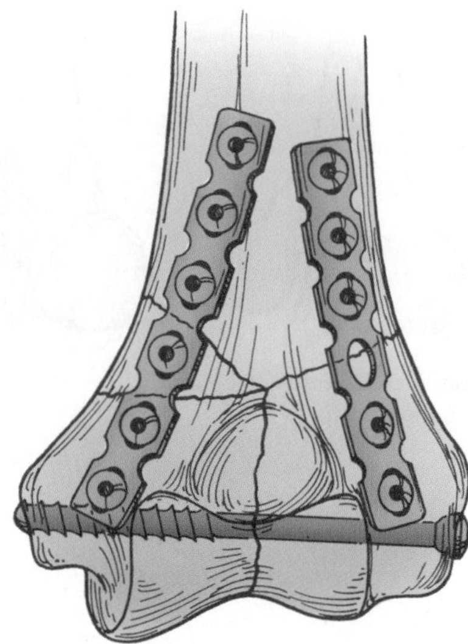

FIGURE 22-47 Repair of the distal comminuted humeral fracture with 3.5-mm reconstruction plates.

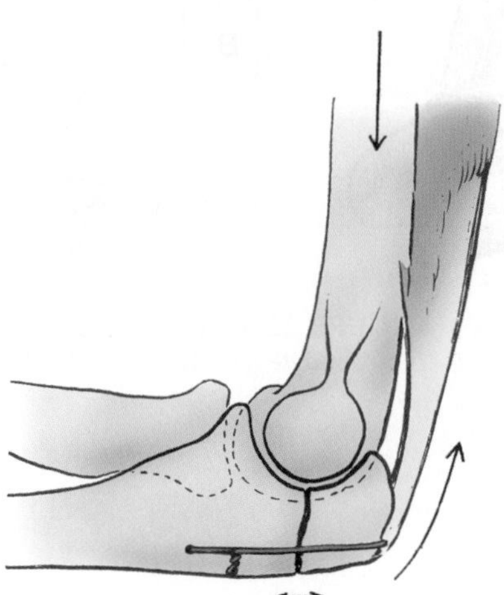

FIGURE 22-48 Tension band technique used for repair of the olecranon.

held in place by hand while the elbow is put through its range of motion. The plates should not encroach on the olecranon or coronoid fossa (distal end of the ulna), since this will limit flexion and extension of the arm.

7. The bone is drilled and tapped from one cortex to the other with the appropriate drill and tap. The screw is inserted and seated to the bone surface on the plate. This is done for all subsequent screws, observing the fracture site and articular surface.
8. Interfragmentary screws may be used in addition to the cortical screws spanning the condyles. If osteotomy of the olecranon was previously done for exposure, it is reattached using the tension band technique with a cancellous bone screw and heavy-gauge (Figure 22-48) (18 or 20) wire.
9. The wound is irrigated and a drain placed as needed; the incision site is closed. A long arm posterior splint is applied.

## Olecranon Fracture

If the olecranon fracture fragment is small, it may be excised and the triceps tendon reattached to the ulnar shaft. This does not result in loss of stability of the elbow joint. However, larger fragments must be reduced and held with internal fixation. Osteotomy of the olecranon is often done electively for surgical exposure (see previous section) and repaired in the same fashion as for a traumatic fracture.

***Procedural Considerations.*** The patient is placed in the prone position with the arm on an armboard or hand table. A soft tissue set, a bone set, AO/ASIF instrumentation (AO/ASIF is the abbreviation for Swiss Association of Osteosynthesis/Association for the Study of Internal Fixation), heavy stainless steel wire (16 and 18 gauge in long lengths), a wire tightener, Kirschner wires, bone-reduction clamps, a power drill, and Kirschner wire driver will be needed.

### *Operative Procedure*

TENSION BANDING (FIGURE 22-49)

1. An incision is made over the olecranon, and the fracture is exposed.

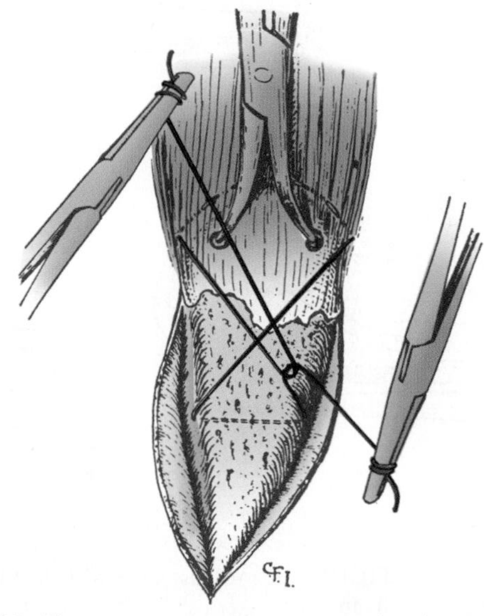

FIGURE 22-49 Operative procedure: tension banding with stainless steel wire passed through drill holes; figure-of-eight adds stability to the fracture.

2. A drill hole is made in the distal fragment traversing the bone.
3. Stainless steel wire is passed through the drilled holes, crossed over, and pulled toward the tip of the olecranon.
4. After using the drill and tap, a cancellous bone screw is used to attach the proximal fragment to the distal, stopping short of totally seating the screw.
5. The wire is pulled and looped around the exposed shaft of the screw while reduction is maintained manually or by using a reduction clamp. The wire can be tightened using the wire tightener. Two smooth Steinmann pins, bent over the exposed portion to hook the loop of wire, can substitute for the cancellous screws.
6. The remaining screw is threaded into the bone; the fracture site is observed for opposition.
7. The wound is irrigated and closed. Drains are generally not necessary. A long arm posterior splint is placed.

NOTE: Using this technique requires early active motion of the arm. Compression of the fracture site is achieved by placing the elbow through its range of motion and applying force by the hardware.

## Transposition of the Ulnar Nerve

Transposition of the ulnar nerve involves freeing the nerve from a groove at the back of the medial epicondyle of the humerus and bringing it to the front of the condyle. The ulnar nerve is frequently divided or damaged after fracture or wounds to the elbow caused by trauma. Dislocation of the elbow may also cause ulnar nerve damage. Late traumatic neuritis may occur after an old injury, resulting in stretching of the ulnar nerve. The hand appears atrophied, and sensory loss is high. In severe cases, a clawhand deformity develops.

***Procedural Considerations.*** The patient is placed in supine position with the extremity slightly flexed on a hand table or over the chest. A tourniquet is applied to the upper arm, and the entire arm (fingers to tourniquet) is prepped and draped. A soft tissue set is required. Bone instruments may be required.

### *Operative Procedure*

1. An incision is made on the lateral aspect of the elbow near the epicondyle.
2. The fascia and the flexor carpi ulnaris muscle are divided.
3. The ulnar nerve is freed, and the medial intermuscular septum is dissected.
4. The nerve is then drawn anteriorly and placed deep into the brachialis flexor muscle origin.
5. The wound is irrigated and closed. A drain is not necessary. A short arm posterior splint is applied to the elbow postoperatively.

## Excision of the Head of the Radius

Fractures of the radial head can be displaced or nondisplaced, segmental, or comminuted.[8] Complications can arise when treatment is delayed, causing limitation of motion, pain, and posttraumatic arthritis. A congruous radial head is essential for proper rotation of the forearm at the elbow. Consequently, in an adult it is necessary to excise the radial head if a severely comminuted fracture with angulation interferes with rotation. The radial head should never be excised in children. The outcome for the patient undergoing radial head excision may result in some permanent loss of pronation and supination of the forearm. Noncomminuted fractures that are easily reduced can be treated using closed reduction and casting.

***Procedural Considerations.*** The patient is supine with the arm over the chest or on a hand table. A tourniquet is applied. A soft tissue set, a small bone set, and an oscillating microsaw with blades are needed.

### *Operative Procedure*

1. An incision is made on the shaft of the radius from 5 cm distal to the radial head extending proximally over the lateral humeral condyle.
2. Dissection is continued between the extensor carpi ulnaris and extensor digitorum muscles onto the joint capsule.
3. With the head and neck of the radius exposed through the joint capsule, the joint is irrigated to clear bone debris and blood clots.
4. The radial head is then excised just proximal to the radial tuberosity, taking care to remove all periosteum and limit new bone formation. The remaining annular ligament is also excised. The fragments of the radial head should be saved and readily available so that they may be reassembled to ensure that all have been retrieved.
5. The wound is closed, and a long arm posterior splint is applied with the elbow at 90 degrees.

## Fractures of the Proximal Third of the Ulna with Radial Head Dislocation (Monteggia)

The Monteggia type of fracture presents with a proximal ulnar fracture and dislocation of the radial head. The fracture is rarely treated with open reduction in children. The open technique is often used to treat adults. A direct blow to the ulnar aspect or a fall while the arm is hyperextended produces this type of injury. If the open reduction approach is chosen, closed reduction of the radial dislocation is attempted and often is successful. At times the annular ligament may prevent reduction of the radial head dislocation, and open reduction becomes necessary. Deforming forces of the forearm vary, depending on the location of the fracture in relation to the insertion of muscles. These forces are often encountered when treating forearm injuries. The Dynamic Compression technique uses compression plates that are stockier and stronger than the semitubular plates mentioned earlier for distal humeral fractures. They are used to plate shaft fractures, where stress forces on the shaft are greater and stronger plates are required.

***Procedural Considerations.*** The patient is placed in the supine position with or without a hand table. A tourniquet is applied and inflated as needed. A soft tissue set and a large bone set are required, as well as bone-reduction clamps and bone-grasping forceps, AO/ASIF instrumentation, plates and screws, and a power drill.

### *Operative Procedure*

FIXATION WITH DYNAMIC COMPRESSION PLATE (FIGURE 22-50)

1. The radial head dislocation is reduced using a closed technique.
2. An incision is made; the ulnar fracture site is dissected.
3. The periosteum is stripped, and the fragments are reapproximated using bone-reduction and grasping forceps.
4. The bone is assessed for placement of a small- or large-fragment dynamic compression plate (DCP), with at least three screw holes proximal and three distal to the fracture site.
5. A concentric (neutral) hole is drilled into the ulna (through one of the screw holes on the plate) to the opposite cortex.
6. After the hole is gauged, the selected size of screw is inserted, with purchase of the opposite cortex ensured. A second screw is inserted on the opposite fragment in the neutral position.
7. On either side of the fracture site, an eccentric (loading) hole is drilled in the same fashion to the opposite cortex. The hole is gauged and tapped, and the screw is inserted.

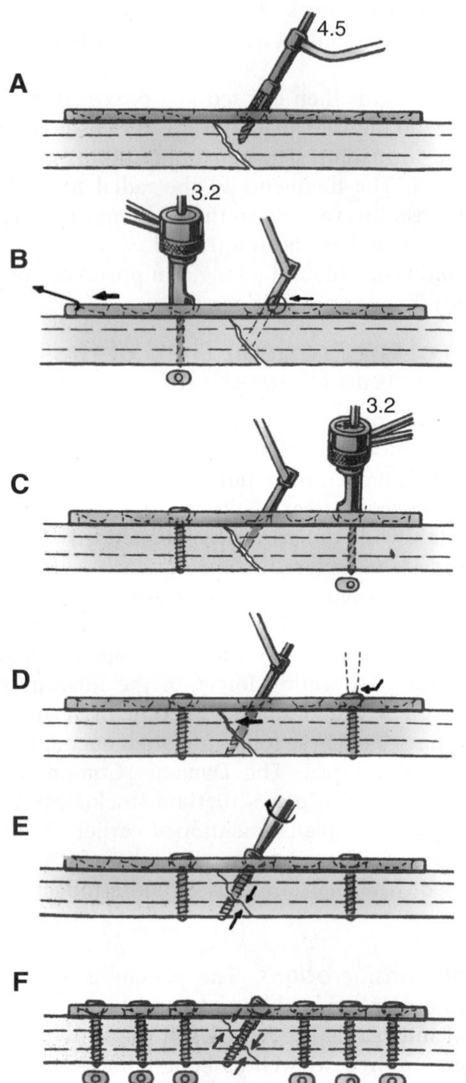


FIGURE 22-50 Fixation with dynamic compression plate. **A,** Gliding hole with drill bit. **B,** Fracture is reduced, drill sleeve is inserted, the fracture is drawn together, a hole is drilled, and a screw is inserted in the neutral position to correct the fracture. **C** and **D,** One screw is inserted in load position (eccentric) into the other fragment; as the screw is tightened, axial compression is generated. **E,** Lag screw inserted across the fracture site. **F,** Remaining screws inserted in the neutral position.

8. The selected screw is entered eccentrically into the plate. As the screw seeks the center of the screw hole while riding the bevel of the screw hole, it compresses the fracture site. This screw should be tightened down, and the other screws should be slightly loosened.
9. The fracture site is now visualized as the action of the screw in the plate compresses the fracture site.
10. The remaining bone screws are inserted following the same procedure.
11. The wound is irrigated and closed; a drain may or may not be inserted.
12. A long arm posterior splint is placed with the arm in 110 to 120 degrees of flexion.

### Correction of Colles Fracture with External Fixation

Colles fracture is a dorsally angulated fracture of the distal end of the radius. Most of these fractures can be managed successfully with closed reduction and immobilization, but external fixation is especially useful in the case of a comminuted intraarticular fracture. Internal fixation is indicated when the distal end of the radius is severely comminuted and displaced. In these cases, Kirschner wires are used for internal fixation.[10]

***Procedural Considerations.*** The patient is in the supine position with the arm extended on a hand table and may require traction by means of finger traps. A soft tissue set and a small bone set are required, along with a power drill, small elevator, and the external fixation device of choice. Fluoroscopy is necessary.

#### *Operative Procedure*

1. Small incisions are made, and two pins are placed through the second metacarpal—one at the base and the other distalward a distance equal to the span between the openings in the fixator.
2. Two pins are placed in the radius 8 cm from the styloid.
3. Pin placement is confirmed in both the AP and lateral views.
4. A frame is constructed to incorporate all four pins.
5. Reduction of the fracture is obtained, and the frame is secured.
6. Postreduction films are obtained to check alignment and pin position.

## SURGERY OF THE HAND

Hand surgery has become highly specialized. The orthopedic perioperative nurse encounters numerous procedures for treating bone, soft tissue, or both. Many of the techniques and principles used to treat large bone defects are used in the treatment of hand injuries. Hand procedures range from carpal tunnel release to complex digit reimplantation.

Tourniquets and regional anesthetics are often used for hand surgery. The OR team usually sits down at a hand table but may move to areas such as the iliac crest for bone grafting. The instruments for hand surgery are common to orthopedics but on a smaller scale. Many instruments and reconstruction systems have been developed primarily for hand surgery. Air- or battery-powered drills and saws are frequently used. The surgery often requires the use of eye loupes (glasses for magnification) or the microscope.

### Carpal Tunnel Release

Carpal tunnel syndrome results from entrapment of the median nerve on the volar surface of the wrist; it is caused by thickened synovium, trauma, or aberrant muscles. Carpal tunnel syndrome is frequently seen in patients with rheumatoid synovitis or malaligned Colles' fracture and is associated with obesity, Raynaud's disease, pregnancy, and occupational injuries. The symptoms are pain, numbness, tingling of the fingers, and weakness of the intrinsic thumb muscles. These symptoms are usually reversible after the flexor retinaculum is incised so that the compressed median nerve is relieved. Carpal tunnel release may be completed endoscopically or by open incision.

***Procedural Considerations.*** The patient is placed in the supine position with the arm extended on a hand table. A tourniquet is applied to the forearm or upper arm. A hand set is required. The endoscopic approach requires use of specialized equipment.

#### *Operative Procedure—Open Approach*

1. A curvilinear, longitudinal volar incision is made from the proximal side of the palm, paralleling the thenar crease and extending to the crease of the wrist across the wrist joint.
2. The deep transverse carpal ligament is divided, taking care to avoid damage to the median nerve.
3. At this point the release is completed.
4. If indicated, a tenosynovectomy is completed.
5. The wound is closed, and a compression dressing and volar splint are applied.

### Excision of Ganglions

A ganglion is a cystic lesion arising from a joint capsule or tendon sheath and containing glassy, clear fluid. Ganglions are most common on the dorsum of the wrist, palm of the hand, and dorsolateral aspect of the foot. Ganglions appear as firm masses that vary in size. They may resolve spontaneously but occasionally require excision because of discomfort or cosmetic reasons.

***Procedural Considerations.*** The patient is supine with the arm extended on a hand table, and a tourniquet is applied. A hand set is required.

#### *Operative Procedure*

1. A transverse incision is made over the ganglion.
2. The ganglion is excised with a rim of normal joint capsule or tendon sheath at its base.
3. The wound is irrigated and closed, and a pressure dressing is applied. A plaster splint may also be applied to immobilize the affected joint.

### Fractures of Carpal Bones

Most fractures of the carpal bones are treated by closed reduction and immobilization. However, it is occasionally necessary to operate on a fracture because of acute instability, delayed union, or nonunion. The scaphoid is the most commonly fractured carpal bone. Internal fixation is accomplished with Kirschner wires, small compression screws, or minifragment compression plates and screws. A bone graft from the distal end of the radius or olecranon may be taken.

For displaced or unstable scaphoid fractures, the Herbert bone screw (Figure 22-51) has several advantages: (1) strong internal fixation, (2) compression at the fracture site with reversed threads at each end of the screw, and (3) reduced time required for external immobilization.

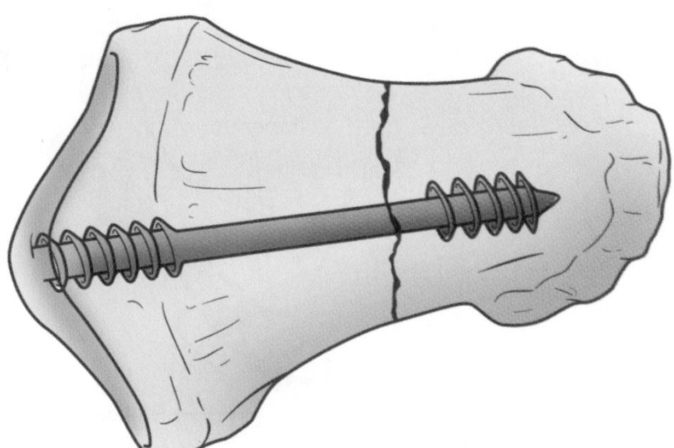

**FIGURE 22-51** Herbert bone screw placement.

***Procedural Considerations.*** The patient is supine with the arm extended on a hand table. A tourniquet is applied and fluoroscopy should be available. A soft tissue set and a small bone or hand set are required in addition to the Herbert screw set. If a minifragment compression set is used, a power drill and smooth Kirschner wires will also be needed. A bone graft set should also be available.

#### *Operative Procedure* (Figure 22-52)

1. A longitudinal skin incision is made over the palmar surface of the wrist.
2. The superficial palmar branch of the radial artery is ligated and divided.
3. The flexor carpi radialis tendon sheath is incised and retracted to expose the capsule of the wrist.
4. The capsule is entered, and the scaphoid fracture is identified and inspected to determine the need for bone grafting.
5. The fracture is reduced by manipulation and temporarily held with small Kirschner wires.
6. The scaphoid fracture is reduced and held with the Herbert jig.
7. A short drill bit and then a long drill bit are inserted to create a channel for the screw.
8. The Herbert screw is then inserted and turned until it is seated within the scaphoid.
9. Bone graft is placed around the fracture site if needed. (The loss of significant bone can often be corrected by fashioning a strut of bone from graft.)
10. The wound is irrigated and closed.
11. A splint is applied with a thumb spica or long arm cast incorporating the thumb.

## SURGERY OF THE HIP AND LOWER EXTREMITY

### Fractures of the Acetabulum

Fractures of the acetabulum usually result from high-energy injuries such as motor vehicle accidents and falls with a landing on the extended extremities. The fracture is directly related to the force transmitted to the femoral head through the greater trochanter or lower extremity. Management of these fractures can often present the orthopedic team with a complex and challenging task. Indications for internal fixation of acetabular fractures include (1) greater than 2 mm of displacement, (2) presence of intraarticular loose bodies, (3) inability to reduce under closed methods, (4) unstable fractures of the posterior acetabular wall, and (5) open fractures. Internal fixation is usually delayed 3 to 10 days to allow time for the patient to be evaluated and clinically stabilized. Until internal

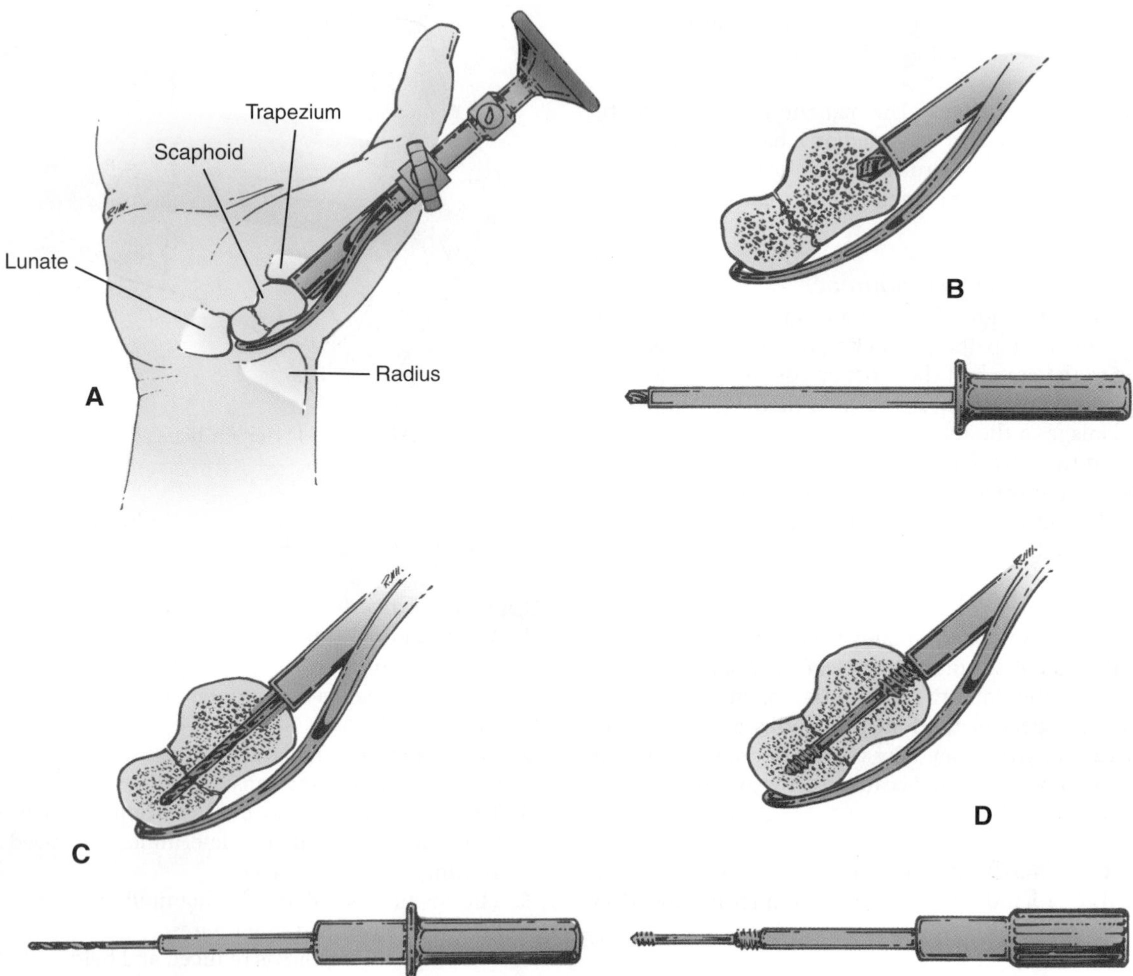


FIGURE 22-52 Repair of the scaphoid. **A,** Fracture site is exposed. **B,** Alignment guide reduces the fracture and guides all subsequent instrumentation. **C,** The screw hole is drilled by hand, and the tap is inserted. **D,** The Herbert bone screw is inserted through the drill guide.

fixation is undertaken, the fracture is reduced by means of closed methods and the patient is maintained in skeletal traction. General anesthesia may be required for closed reduction and placement of skeletal traction when the acetabular fracture is severely displaced or dislocated. The fractures are divided into five basic groups: fractures of the posterior wall, posterior column, anterior wall, and anterior column and transverse fractures (Figure 22-53). Internal fixation is accomplished with reconstruction plates and screws, total hip replacement with bone grafting (see "Total Hip Replacement," p. 766), or fusion if the fracture cannot be reduced.

***Procedural Considerations.*** The surgical approach depends on the type and area of the fracture and the surgeon's preference. The patient is placed on a fracture or standard OR bed in the lateral or supine position. General anesthesia is usually administered, but the procedure can be performed solely with a regional block or concurrent epidural infusion. Procedures of this magnitude can be lengthy and involve considerable blood loss. Appropriate measures should be taken to avoid complications attributable to these factors. The room should remain warm, the patient protected from pressure injury, and red blood cell–salvaging techniques employed.

A soft tissue set, large bone and acetabular instruments, pelvic reduction clamps, reconstruction plates and screws (both 3.5 and 4.5 mm), plate-bending irons, and a femoral distractor will be necessary. A total hip set should be available. Also needed are Kirschner wires and Steinmann pins, large-fragment bone screws, pulsatile lavage supplies, and power drill and reamer. Fluoroscopy may be used for this procedure.

### *Operative Procedure*

POSTEROLATERAL APPROACH

1. A lateral incision is made over the acetabular fracture site.
2. The joint is opened and the femur dislocated from the acetabulum.
3. Self-retaining or handheld hip retractors are used to maintain exposure of the acetabulum.
4. Femoral distraction or osteotomy of the trochanter may be used to improve visualization and access to the fracture.
5. The fracture is reduced using bone clamps, forceps, and a ball spike.
6. Reduction is accomplished in gradual steps using Kirschner wires to hold the fragments temporarily in place.
7. Reconstruction plates are fitted and contoured to the fracture site and secured with screws.

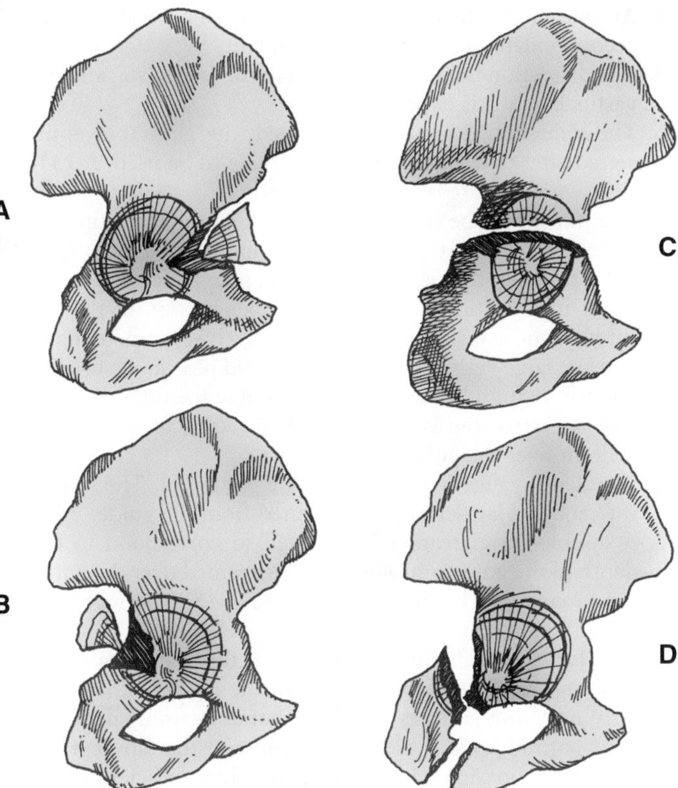


FIGURE 22-53 Acetabular fractures. **A,** Anterior wall. **B,** Posterior wall. **C,** Transverse. **D,** Posterior column.

8. Long cancellous lag screw fixation is also used to provide interfragmentary compression, particularly in column fractures.
9. Bone graft may be needed for additional fixation. A femoral head allograft technique is sometimes used, in which the allograft is mushroomed to create a new acetabulum.
10. The wound is irrigated with antibiotic solution delivered by pulsatile lavage, ensuring the articular surfaces are free from loose bodies.
11. The wound is closed, drains are inserted, and pressure dressings are applied.

The leg is maintained in abduction and external rotation with traction. Once the fracture is stabilized, traction is no longer necessary.

NOTE: If there is associated traumatic dislocation of the hip with the acetabular fracture, the dislocation should be treated promptly. The dislocation should be reduced as soon as possible and skeletal traction inserted if needed to maintain reduction. Acetabular fractures often accompany femoral shaft fractures, which also need to be treated concurrently with the surgeon's desired method (see "Femoral Shaft Fractures: Internal Fixation," p. 751).

## Hip Fractures

Hip fractures are classified by anatomic location and can be categorized as femoral neck fractures, intertrochanteric fractures, and subtrochanteric fractures (Figure 22-54), and these can each be subclassified. Fracture-dislocations also have a classification system and treatment protocol. Fractures of the greater or lesser trochanters alone are less common and can usually be treated nonoperatively.

Femoral neck fractures and intertrochanteric fractures commonly require open reduction and internal fixation. Neck fractures are more common in women because of several factors, including osteoporosis. Most elderly patients require a comprehensive preoperative medical evaluation to define and treat anesthetic risks.[22] However, efforts should be made to correct the fracture as soon as possible to avoid complications related to immobility, skin pressure, pulmonary congestion, and thrombophlebitis. Avascular necrosis and degenerative changes can occur as a result of diminished blood supply to the femoral head, resulting in irreversible changes. Buck's traction may be placed preoperatively to reduce discomfort from muscle spasm caused by overriding of fracture fragments.

Manipulation, reduction, and internal fixation of these fractures are greatly facilitated by use of the OR fracture bed, which also permits adequate radiographic examination to determine placement of the internal fixation.

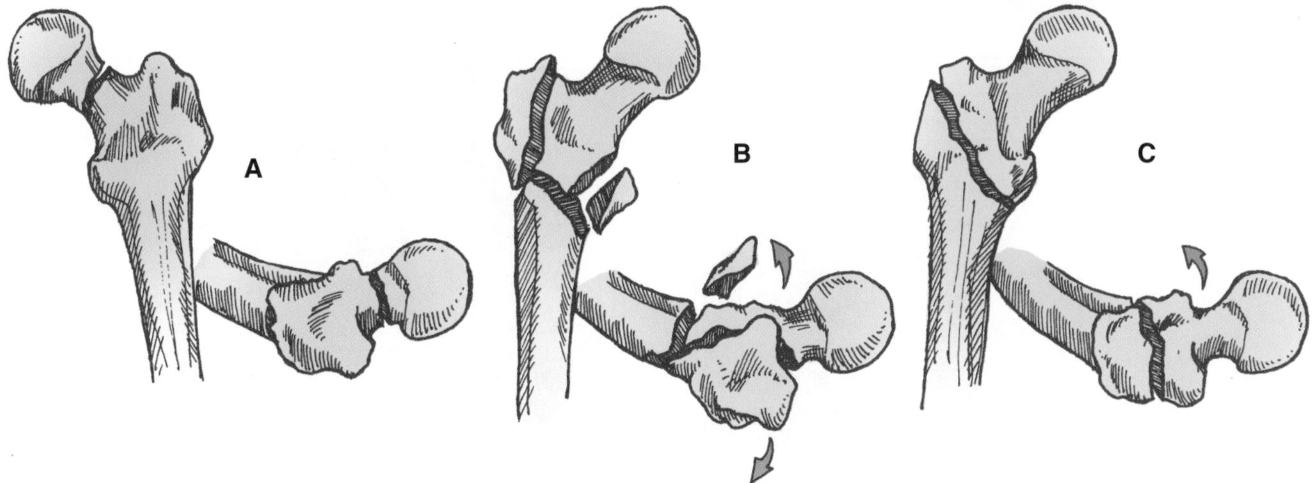


FIGURE 22-54 Proximal femur fractures. **A,** Midcervical. **B,** Comminuted subtrochanteric. **C,** Intertrochanteric.

***Intertrochanteric Fractures.*** Intertrochanteric fractures occur most frequently in older patients. The fractures usually unite without difficulty. However, because the lower extremity is externally rotated at the fracture site, internal fixation is necessary to prevent malunion. Internal fixation allows patients to be mobilized earlier, thereby decreasing mortality and morbidity.

**PROCEDURAL CONSIDERATIONS.** The patient is placed in the supine position on the OR fracture bed, and the fracture is reduced by manipulating the extremity and then confirming with fluoroscopy. Various internal fixation devices, including Ambi, Freelock, Dynamic Hip Screw (DHS), and medullary fixation may be used. Success of the procedure is determined by bone quality, fragment configuration, ability to reduce adequately, implant design, and implant-insertion technique. Intraoperative blood loss is minimized because the hip joint is not opened.

A soft tissue set and a large bone set are required in addition to the compression hip screw instrumentation and implants, bone-reduction and plate-holding clamps, and a power drill and reamer.

**OPERATIVE PROCEDURE**

**Freelock Compression Plate and Lag Screw (Figure 22-55)**

1. The fracture is reduced by closed reduction, and reduction is maintained by adjusting the table traction.
2. Reduction is checked in both the AP and lateral views with fluoroscopy.
3. An incision is made from the greater trochanter distally to accommodate the length of the implant.
4. The dissection is completed through the fascia lata, and the vastus lateralis is exposed.
5. The reduction is visually confirmed; the guide pin is inserted after determining the angle plate to be used. A 135-degree angle plate is commonly used.
6. The pin should be centralized in the femoral head approximately 1 cm short of the femoral articular surface. Care must be taken to not enter the joint space, since this might result in arthritic changes. Further penetration of the pin through the acetabulum and into the pelvis can potentially damage large vessels or bowel. A second pin can be used to control rotation in high neck or unstable fractures.
7. The lateral cortex is opened with the conical cannulated drill bit over the guide pin.
8. The depth gauge is placed over the guide pin. The size of the required lag screw is determined from the guide.
9. A double-barrel reamer is adjusted to correspond to the depth of the guide pin. The cortex is reamed over the guide pin to create a channel for the lag screw and barrel of the compression plate.
10. The lag screw channel is tapped to the full distance of reaming to allow proper seating of the lag screw, particularly in young patients with firm bone. Reaming depth of osteoporotic bone is reduced 5 mm, and the tap depth is reduced approximately 1 to 2 cm to allow sufficient screw purchase.

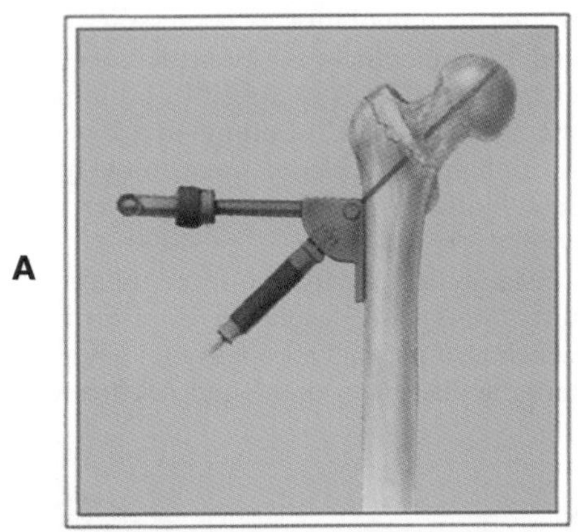


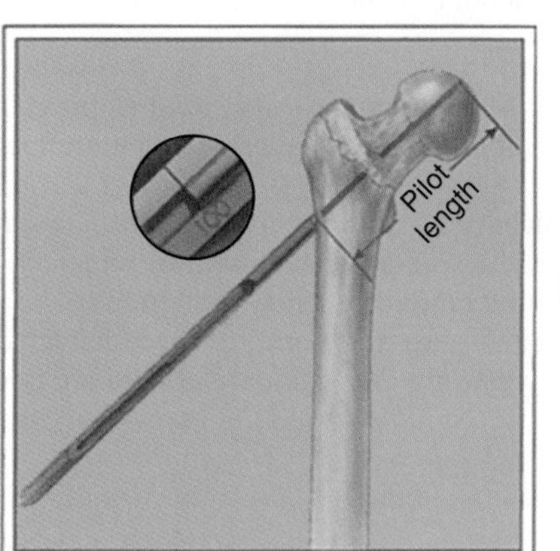


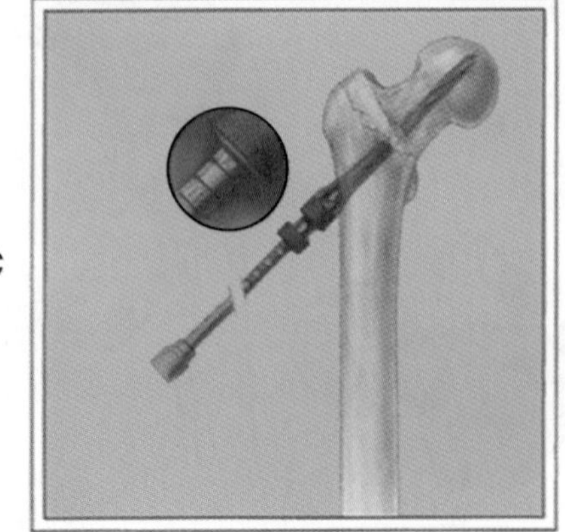


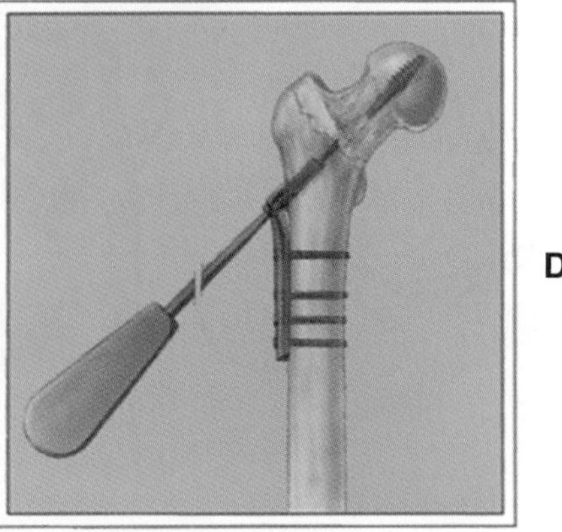


**FIGURE 22-55** Intertrochanteric fracture repair with compression plate. **A,** Guide pin is inserted. **B,** Depth of guide is measured. **C,** Lag screw channel is reamed. **D,** Tube/plate is applied, and lag screw is inserted.

11. The plate angle can be confirmed with a trial; the implants (plate and lag screw) are then delivered to the back table.
12. The plate, lag screw, and insertion wrench with centering sleeve are assembled. A screw stabilizer is passed through the center of the insertion wrench and threaded into the lag screw.
13. The entire assembly is placed over the guide pin, and the lag screw is advanced to the desired depth, with periodic verification with fluoroscopy. Penetration of the lag screw through the femoral articular surface must be avoided.
14. The insertion wrench is disassembled, and the barrel of the compression plate is placed over the lag screw. The barrel of the plate should fully cover the lag screw. The plate is seated on the lateral femoral shaft.
15. The plate is secured to the shaft of the femur with plate-holding forceps. The guide pin is removed. At this point, traction can be released to allow compression of the fracture site.
16. Screw holes are made using the drill guide and a 3.5-mm drill bit. The length is determined, and cortical screws are inserted through the screw hole on the plate with sufficient purchase on the opposite cortex of the shaft. The top screw hole on the plate can accept a 6.5-mm cancellous screw, which can be angled for better purchase in comminuted fractures.
17. Traction is released if not done previously. A compression screw is inserted into the barrel of the screw and threaded into the back of the lag screw, compressing the fracture site. The compression screw exerts a powerful force. The amount of compression applied should correlate with the quality of the bone.
18. The wound is irrigated and closed. Two suction drains may be inserted during closure.

Weight bearing may begin as early as the first postoperative day, depending on reduction and quality of bone.

NOTE: Many of the same techniques and principles of long bone fracture fixation are used in treatment of various types of hip fractures. The different screw types, dynamic compression, and lag screw effect are described throughout the chapter.

***Femoral Neck Fractures: Internal Fixation.*** Anatomic reduction is necessary before internal fixation of femoral neck fractures because of the high incidence of associated complications, such as nonunion and avascular necrosis of the femoral head. The degree of displacement, tamponade pressure from intracapsular bleeding, and delays in reduction and fixation can affect the blood supply to the femoral head. These factors contribute to death of the femoral head and failed fixation. Growing children may sustain fractures through the epiphyseal growth plate (slipped capital femoral epiphysis). These injuries are treated by reduction and internal fixation of the femoral head, similar to the procedures used in the adult. The Garden and AO nomenclature are the most popular classifications for grading the fractures. Pins of various designs, such as Knowles and Hagie pins and universal cannulated screws (Figure 22-56), are used for fixation (Figure 22-57). In cases of severe comminution or avascular necrosis of the femoral head, the patient may require a prosthetic replacement (see "Total Joint Arthroplasty," p. 765).

**PROCEDURAL CONSIDERATIONS.** The patient is placed on the OR fracture bed under general or regional anesthesia (spinal or epidural). Slight traction and external rotation are adjusted on the affected side. A soft tissue set and a large bone set are required, as well as the fixation device of choice with instrumentation, Kirschner wires, Cobra retractors, a power drill, and fluoroscopy.

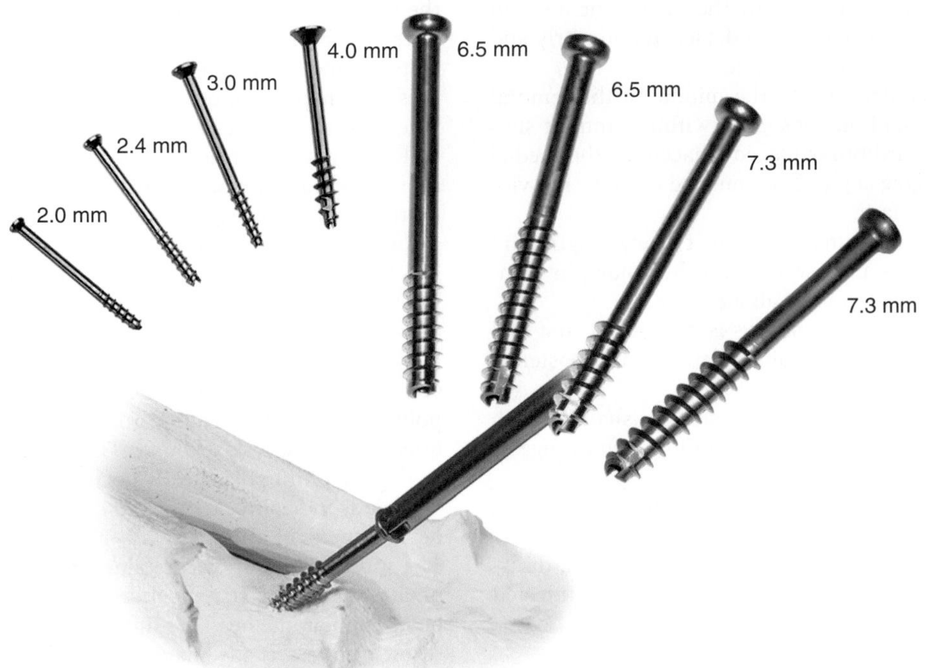


FIGURE 22-56 Cannulated screw system.

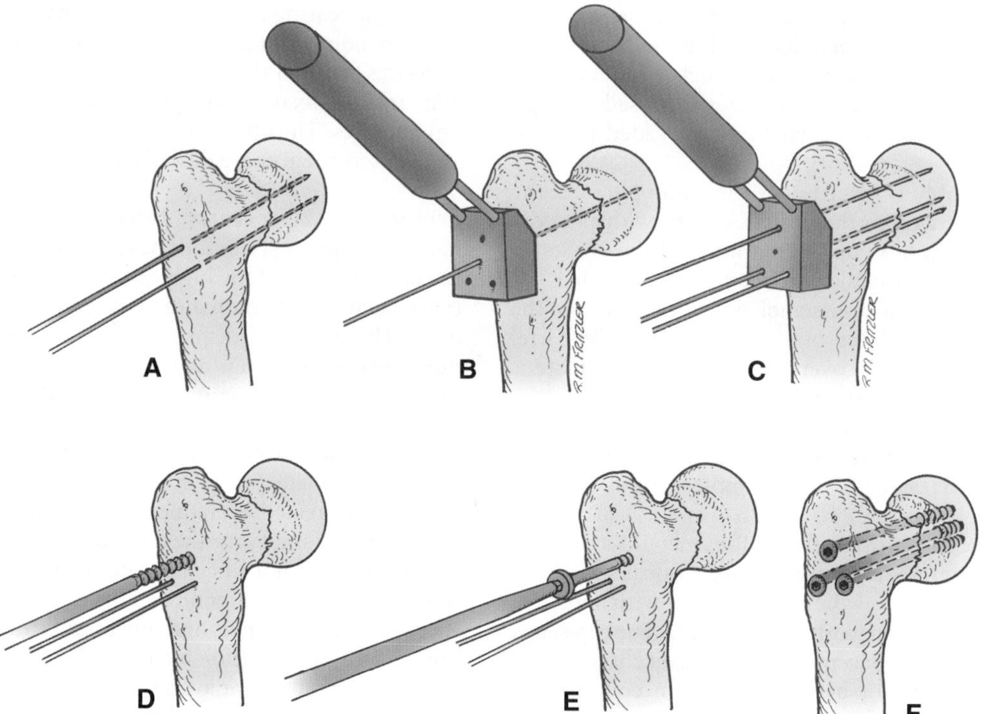


FIGURE 22-57 Internal fixation with cannulated screws (AO technique). **A,** Guidewire parallel to anteversion wire. **B,** Guidewire placed over positioning wire through diamond-patterned positioning holes. **C,** Guidewire placed through each outer triangle of holes. **D,** Cannulated tap passed over guidewire to tap near cortex. **E,** Large cannulated screw inserted over guidewire. **F,** Remaining screws inserted in same manner.

OPERATIVE PROCEDURE

**Cannulated Screw Fixation for Nondisplaced Femoral Neck Fractures**

1. The fracture is exposed through a 5-cm lateral incision over the greater trochanter.
2. The dissection is carried through the subcutaneous and fascial layers; the vastus lateralis is detached anteriorly and retracted, exposing the femoral neck.
3. Two guide pins are driven into the middle of the femoral head, one anterior and one posterior, within 5 mm of subchondral bone; a third pin is placed adjacent to the medial cortex at a 135-degree angle. Care must be taken to not violate the articular surface.
4. The guide pins are measured for correct screw length, and the cannulated screws are inserted over the guide pin without applying compression until all are seated.
5. Compression of the anterior screws is completed first and the posterior screws last to avoid collapse of the posterior aspect of the neck.
6. Traction is released, and the fracture site is visualized with fluoroscopy while the hip is rotated through a full range of motion.
7. Radiographs are taken to verify the position of the screws; the wound is irrigated and closed.

NOTE: Screw protrusion into the joint space can be disastrous to the articular surface. Radiopaque dye can be injected to rule out communication with the joint.

***Femoral Head Prosthetic Replacement: Unipolar and Bipolar Implants.*** With the development of current cement fixation techniques and the evolution of the modular bipolar and monopolar design, the use of fixed endoprostheses such as the Austin-Moore and Thompson designs declined. During the early 1980s the bipolar system in conjunction with a cemented femoral stem became popular. Bipolar endoprostheses (Figure 22-58) were introduced to reduce the shear stresses affecting the acetabular surface, decreasing the motion and friction between the prosthetic head and the acetabulum that is seen with conventional (unipolar) endoprostheses. A femoral head prosthesis is snapped into a rotating polyethylene-lined cup that, when inserted, moves as one unit. Friction occurs between the ball and plastic instead of between the head and the acetabulum. This was a revolutionary design in the mechanics of hip motion and stresses. Current data, however, have some surgeons and engineers reevaluating the use of bipolar prostheses. It is believed that bipolar motion subsides after fibrous growth has taken place, allowing for only unipolar motion. There have also been reports of bone resorption and subsequent prosthetic loosening in cases in which bipolar prostheses were used. Researchers are evaluating evidence of metallic head wear of the polyethylene cup, creating microscopic debris with a subsequent chemical lysis of bone. Thus there has been resurgence in the use of unipolar heads for femoral head replacement.

Trends in health care toward cost reduction precipitated the development of the *diagnosis-related group (DRG) prosthesis.* The modular design was retained, allowing for different combinations of head size, neck length, and stem size. Instead of being bipolar, the head is solid, or unipolar, and the stem is the result of a less costly manufacturing process. The most cost-effective prosthesis is still the original Austin-Moore design, which may be selected for those patients whose life expectancy is short and who have a minimal level of activity. If major de-

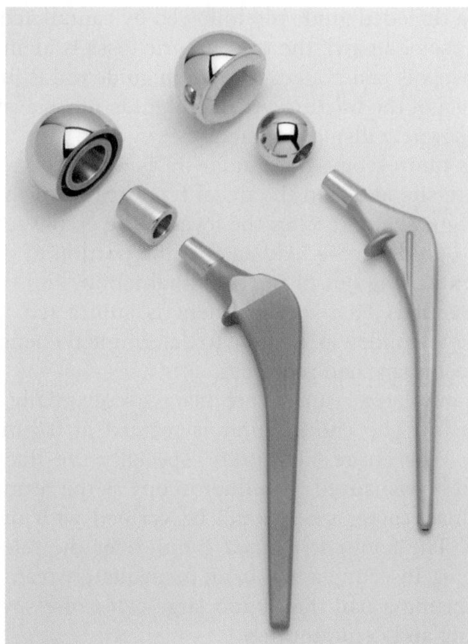

**FIGURE 22-58** Modular bipolar endoprosthesis.

ficiencies in the acetabular side of the joint are present, a total joint arthroplasty may be performed. In deciding between the hemiarthroplasty and total hip reconstruction, the patient's medical condition, age, and level of activity must be considered.

Current biomaterials, methods of fixation (cemented versus uncemented), prosthetic life, and modular components allow conversion of a hemiarthroplasty (reconstruction of one side of the joint) to a total hip arthroplasty, provided that the femoral component is adequately fixed. Depending on the patient condition, the acetabulum may eventually require arthroplasty as a result of degenerative changes. Improved technology and surgical technique have increased the life span of implanted components. The portion of the implant that articulates within the acetabulum can be removed and replaced with a smaller femoral head. The acetabulum is then prepared for prosthetic implantation by various means of fixation. The ability to convert from hemiarthroplasty to total arthroplasty considerably reduces the amount of surgery required.

**PROCEDURAL CONSIDERATIONS.** The patient is placed in the lateral position after the administration of general or regional anesthetic. The prep is done from the umbilicus down to and including the foot. Instrumentation for total hip replacement should be available but not opened until inspection of the resected joint is completed to determine if a total arthroplasty is required.

The soft tissue and the large bone sets are required, as well as the endoprosthesis instruments, trials, and implants. A power reciprocating (see Figure 22-25) or sagittal saw may be necessary. Templates or a caliper will be used to measure the size of the femoral head. Bone cement and the supplies for preparing and inserting it should also be available.

OPERATIVE PROCEDURE

**Modular Austin-Moore Endoprosthesis.** Both posterior and anterior approaches can be made to the hip to place an endoprosthesis. The posterior approach is quicker and generally involves less blood loss, but detractors suggest that there is a higher dislocation rate and a greater chance of infection because of the proximity of the incision to the anus. Although both approaches are widely used, the posterior approach is described as follows:

1. A linear incision is made from 5 cm below the posteroinferior iliac spine toward the posterior aspect of the greater trochanter and distally along the posterior aspect of the proximal femur for 7 mm.
2. The capsule is entered, and the femoral head is removed and gauged with the template. Fragments that may be loose in the acetabulum or attached to the ligamentum teres are removed.
3. A trial cup is inserted into the acetabulum, and axial compression is applied while clearance of lateral motion is checked.
4. The femoral neck is fashioned to achieve an accurate prosthetic fit.
5. A punch is then used to open the medullary canal from the femoral neck. The intramedullary canal is reamed and rasped to accommodate the prosthesis.
6. Once the canal is prepared, the prosthesis of choice is inserted with or without bone cement.
7. A unipolar or bipolar assembly is snapped onto the neck of the femoral stem. The height of the head determines the neck length and is selected after trial reduction.
8. The hip is reduced, and closure is accomplished in layers over suction drains.

***Femoral Shaft Fractures: Internal Fixation.*** Fractures involving the femoral shaft are very common in today's orthopedic operating room. Prolonged immobility, with its attendant complications, and disability can result if femoral shaft fractures are not managed appropriately. The femur is the largest principal load-bearing bone in the body. Fractures of the femoral shaft can be surgically treated with several available techniques. Considerations for treatment are type and location of fracture (location on shaft), the number of segments involved, the degree of comminution (Figure 22-59), and the activity level of the patient. Femoral shaft fractures are often associated with ipsilateral (same-side) trochanteric or condylar fractures. Pathologic fractures often occur in this region.

Possible treatment methods for femoral shaft fractures are closed reduction, skeletal traction, and femoral cast bracing. External fixation has limited utility when fractures associated with surgical site infection or neurovascular compromise are treated, but it may serve temporarily until such time that internal fixation can be performed. Although plates and screws are used for femoral shaft fractures, their use has been widely disputed. Complications such as bent or broken plates, re-fractures, and deep surgical site infections have been reported. Intramedullary (IM) fixation devices have become the preferred method of treatment. IM nails and rods increase the load sharing of the bone, making the implant less likely to fracture. Bone healing requires a load across the fracture site to promote osteosynthesis and prevent re-fracture. The open or closed method of intramedullary nailing can be used with locked and nonlocked nails. Closed methods of intramedullary fixation often minimize exposure of the surgical site and surgical time, resulting in less opportunity for infection.

Intramedullary nail and rod designs vary: (1) flexible nails such as the Rusch or Enders type, (2) standard rods such as the Sampson and AO rods, and (3) interlocking nails (see "Frac-

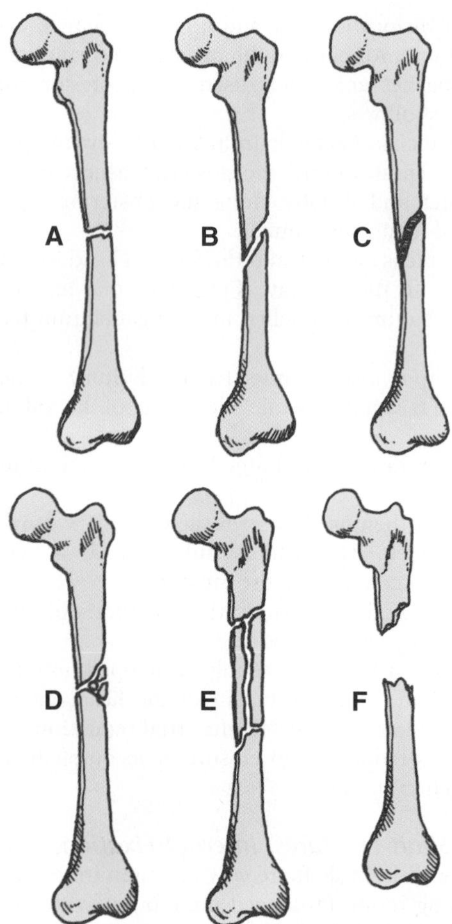


FIGURE 22-59 Femoral shaft fractures. **A,** Transverse. **B,** Oblique. **C,** Spiral. **D,** Comminuted. **E,** Longitudinal split. **F,** Complete bone loss.

tures of the Humeral Shaft, p. 738) such as the Grosse-Kempf and Russell-Taylor varieties. Closed reduction and intramedullary nailing with or without locking screws have become the method against which other methods are measured. Incidences of scarring, blood loss, and infection are all favorable. Fracture hematoma remains intact at the fracture site, which is important in bone healing, and the rate of bone union is increased.

PROCEDURAL CONSIDERATIONS. General or epidural anesthetics are used. The patient is placed on the OR fracture bed in the supine position, traction applied, and the fracture manually reduced and confirmed with fluoroscopy. If the fracture is profoundly unstable, care must be taken during manipulation to prevent neurovascular complications. For open IM fixation, extra retractors and bone instruments may be required. For a percutaneous reduction, a soft tissue set and a large bone set are required in addition to the IM nail implants and associated instruments, a power reamer and drill, and long guidewires for reamers. This procedure requires the use of fluoroscopy. A skeletal traction tray with Steinmann pins may be necessary.

OPERATIVE PROCEDURE

**Russell-Taylor Rod with or without Locking Screws**

1. An incision is made over the tip of the greater trochanter and continued proximally and medially for 6 to 8 cm. The fascia of the gluteus is incised, and the piriformis fossa is palpated.
2. With a threaded guide pin followed by cannulated reamers or by use of an awl, the trochanteric fossa is identified and the cortex is penetrated. A 3.2-mm guide rod is inserted to the level of the fracture. A curved guide pin is available for more severely displaced fractures.
3. Under fluoroscopy, the guidewire is advanced across the fracture site and into the distal fragment until the ball tip of the guidewire reaches the level of the epiphyseal scar. A second guidewire is held against the portion of the guidewire extending out of the proximal femur, and the length is measured. That measurement is subtracted from 900 mm (total guidewire length) to determine the length of the intramedullary nail required.
4. The cannulated reamers are placed sequentially over the guidewire. The entire femur is reamed at 0.5-mm increments. The entire shaft, and especially the fracture site, should be visualized with fluoroscopy as the reamers pass.
5. The final reamer size should be verified with the reamer gauge. The femur is reamed 1 mm over the selected nail diameter. Inserting a nail in an inadequately reamed femur or inserting a nail that is too large can cause severe bone splitting and comminution.
6. The proximal screw guide/slap hammer is assembled onto the nail. The nail is oriented to match the curve of the femur.
7. Using the handle of the inserter, the rotation of the nail is controlled and the nail is driven into the femur. The nail is fully seated when the proximal screw guide is flush with the greater trochanter. The inserter is disengaged from the slap hammer.
8. Using the power drill and correct drill sleeves, a 4.8-mm hole is drilled through both cortexes and the depth is measured directly off the bit.
9. Through the appropriate drill sleeve, a 6.4-mm self-tapping locking screw is inserted and the drill sleeve is removed.
10. By fluoroscopy, the distal screw holes are confirmed as perfect circles on the screen. The distal targeting device is mounted on the nail, followed by the left or right adapter block. The adapter block is adjusted until the calibration reads the length of the nail. The cross hairs are aligned in the adapter to the holes in the distal nail, with confirmation by fluoroscopy.
11. An incision is made through the adapter block over the distal femur to the lateral cortex. Following the same steps as those for placing the proximal screw, one or two distal locking screws are inserted. There are various freehand techniques for inserting distal locking screws.

## SURGERY OF THE LOWER LEG (DISTAL FEMUR, TIBIA, AND FIBULA)

Many procedures on the lower leg use the same principles of fracture fixation already mentioned. Meticulous detail is required to ensure proper alignment and optimal surgical results for the patient. As in the hip, fractures around the knee require secure fixation to allow bone healing, preserve motion, and provide joint mobility as early as possible. Fracture treatment for the various described injuries is based on location and the pattern of fracture. Methods of fixation for the distal end of the femur and proximal end of the tibia include pins, wire, compression plates, intramedullary nails, supracondylar plates, and cannulated screws. Multiple-trauma patients with one or a combination of fractures may require more than one method of fixation. Open reduction and internal fixation must ensure anatomic restoration of the joint surface and rigid fixation and allow early motion of the knee joint.

Most operations on the knee are performed with the patient in the supine position and the leg prepped and draped from the groin to the middle of the calf or including the entire foot. It is occasionally necessary for the surgeon to operate with the foot of the OR bed dropped and the patient's knee flexed to 90 degrees. Consequently it is important to position the patient so that the knee is at a break in the bed; if it is necessary, the lower leg can then be flexed at the knee during the operation. A tourniquet is often used.

## Femoral Condyle and Tibial Plateau Fractures

The joint surfaces are often involved with fractures of the distal end of the femur and proximal end of the tibia. Anatomic alignment of the articular surfaces is necessary to provide joint stability and decrease the chance of posttraumatic arthritis. Nonunion is the most common complication in supracondylar fractures, leading to failure of surgery. As with humeral head and hip fractures, it is important that the articular surfaces are reopposed as close as possible to avoid future degenerative changes. Unfortunately, these often cannot be avoided, and patients with this type of injury often face future joint arthroplasty and replacement (see "Total Joint Arthroplasty," p. 765).

Distal femoral fractures result in varying degrees of comminution. Condylar fractures can be unicondylar or bicondylar, with separation of both condyles (Figure 22-60). Type A fractures are extraarticular. Type B are single condyle fractures in the sagittal or coronal planes, whereas type C fractures are T and Y configurations. Type C fractures have varying degrees of shaft and condylar comminution, presenting the greatest challenge to treat.

Simple, nondisplaced distal femoral fractures can be treated with closed reduction and immobilization by casting if anatomic reduction is achieved. Nondisplaced, extraarticular fractures can be treated with a hinged cast brace. Comminuted fractures in this region can also be treated in this manner if shortening and angulation are minimal. Traction can be used initially to augment this type of treatment. Distal femoral fractures are treated with open reduction if distal tibial traction and manipulation attempts fail. Flexible nails, locking intramedullary nails, blade plates, condylar compression screws, and condylar buttress plates are accepted methods of treating condylar fractures. Attention must be given to the attachment of the cruciate ligaments, which originate in the condylar notch and may require fixation of a partial or full disruption as a result of the injury to the knee (see "Ruptured Anterior Cruciate Repair," p. 758).

Tibial plateau fractures historically have been attributed to bumper or fender injuries, but a variety of falls or other traumas frequently are the cause. Compression force of the distal end of the femur on the tibia produces the various types of plateau fractures. Commonly this occurs from abduction of the tibia while the foot is planted, driving the lateral femoral condyle into the lateral tibial plateau (also called the *condyle*). Several authors have developed classification systems based on fracture and dislocation patterns. The general theme of these fracture classifications and examples of their treatment can be summarized by the following types (Figure 22-61): (1) pure cleavage, unicondylar fracture, (2) cleavage fracture combined with local depression, (3) pure central depression, (4) medial condylar wedge with depression or comminution, (5) bicondylar but with continuity of diaphysis and metaphysis, and (6) comminution with dissociation of metaphysis from diaphysis. Fractures of the tibial plateau are often associated with dislocation, which may spontaneously reduce at the time of trauma.

Special attention must be given to the possibility of neurovascular insult, which must be addressed immediately. Elevation and fixation of the depressed fracture are the focus for treatment of plateau fractures. As with distal femoral fractures, the articular surfaces and cruciate insertion require reapproximation and fixation. Repair to the menisci and ligaments should occur simultaneously to prevent knee instability.

Blade plates, buttress plates, and cannulated screws are all methods by which fractures of the tibial plateau are fixed. Severe fractures are treated using multiple buttress plates and screws (Figure 22-62). Bone graft from the iliac crest and fibular head autograft are often used when there is a significant amount of bone lost to comminution with proximal tibial fractures.

## Supracondylar Fractures of the Femur

Fractures of the distal femur in the multiple-trauma patient are treated early to promote rapid ambulation, which decreases complications caused by immobility. In an effort to deliver quick fracture reduction and stabilization, many orthopedic trauma systems have been developed. Often these are the same systems used in daily orthopedic procedures with modifications to expedite implantation and fixation. Some of the intramedullary devices do not require reaming.

***Procedural Considerations.*** Initial stabilization of the patient may immediately precede the nailing procedure. Often other team members are attending to treatment of other systems. The perioperative nurse is challenged to control traffic, coordinate team efforts, and protect the patient from increased risk of infection by the inadvertent contamination of instruments and implants. The patient is placed in the supine position under general or regional anesthesia. If possible, the patient is positioned on the OR fracture bed; if not, a radiolucent OR bed is used. A pneumatic tourniquet may be applied as high up on the femur as possible, taking care to protect the genitals during placement. The nail can be inserted using the closed or open technique.

The soft tissue set and large bone set are required, as well as the intramedullary supracondylar nail implant (Figure 22-63) and the instruments necessary for its insertion. A power drill, guidewires, intramedullary rod set, and fluoroscopy will also be needed. In addition, Steinmann pins, Kirschner wires, bone reduction clamps, and a bone graft set should be available. Occasionally a primary total knee arthroplasty will be performed, and the appropriate instruments should be available should that possibility exist.

### *Operative Procedures*

#### INTERCONDYLAR FRACTURE OF THE FEMUR, T TYPE (AIM SUPRACONDYLAR INTRAMEDULLARY NAIL)

1. A standard midline skin incision with parapatellar arthrotomy is used. Depending on the degree of intraarticular extension, the incision may be as small as 1 inch or involve

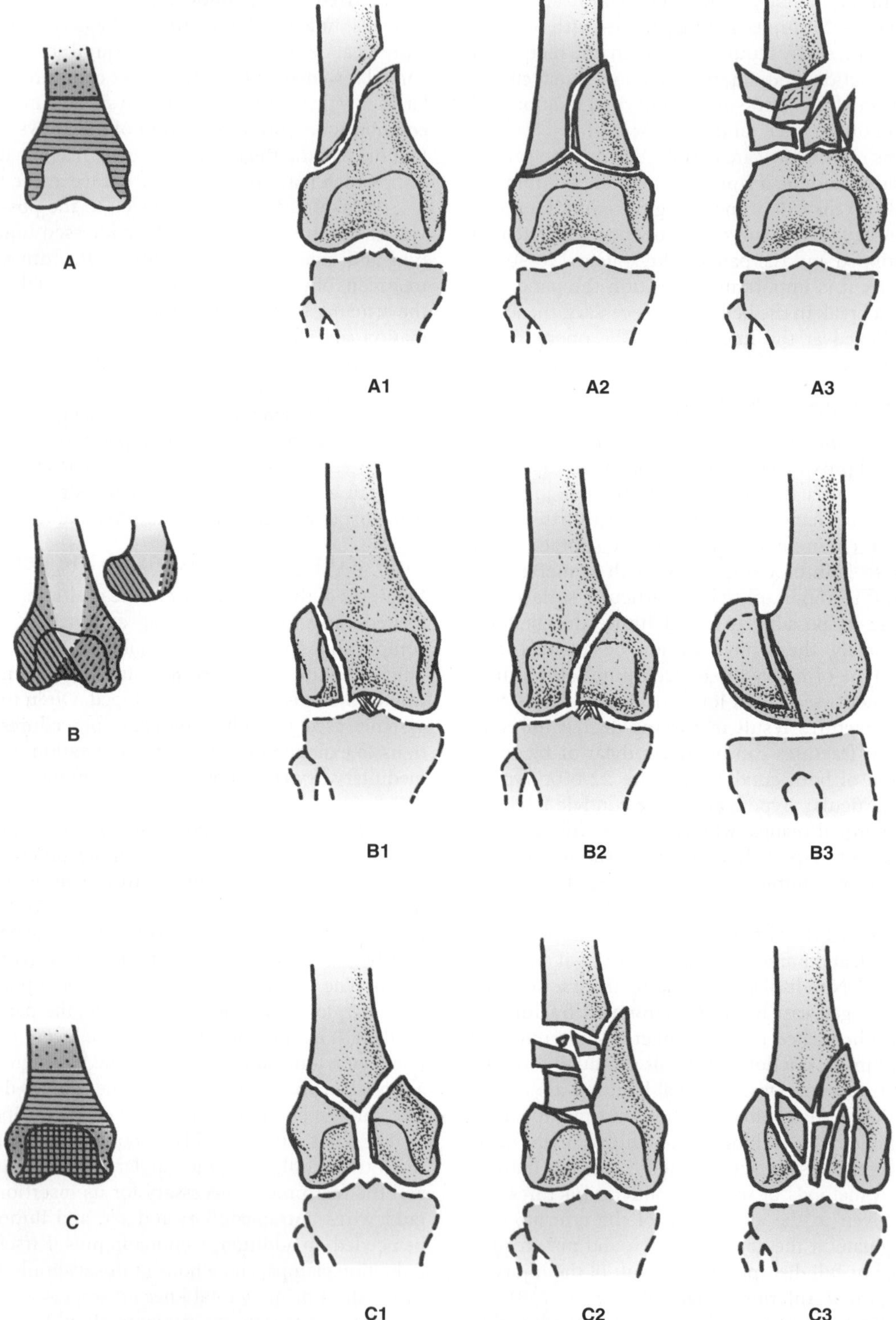


**FIGURE 22-60** Classification of fractures of distal femur described by Müller and associates.

lateral eversion of the patella to gain visualization of the entire joint.

2. Articular fractures should be anatomically reduced and secured with 6.5-mm or 8.0-mm cannulated screws placed in the anterior and posterior aspect of the condyles to allow adequate space for the placement of the nail.
3. An entry hole is made with an awl into the femoral canal just anterior to the femoral insertion of the posterior cruciate ligament. Care is taken to ensure anatomic alignment of the condyles to avoid varus or valgus femoral alignment.
4. The hole is enlarged with the nonadjustable step reamer to accept the largest diameter of the chosen nail. Further ream-

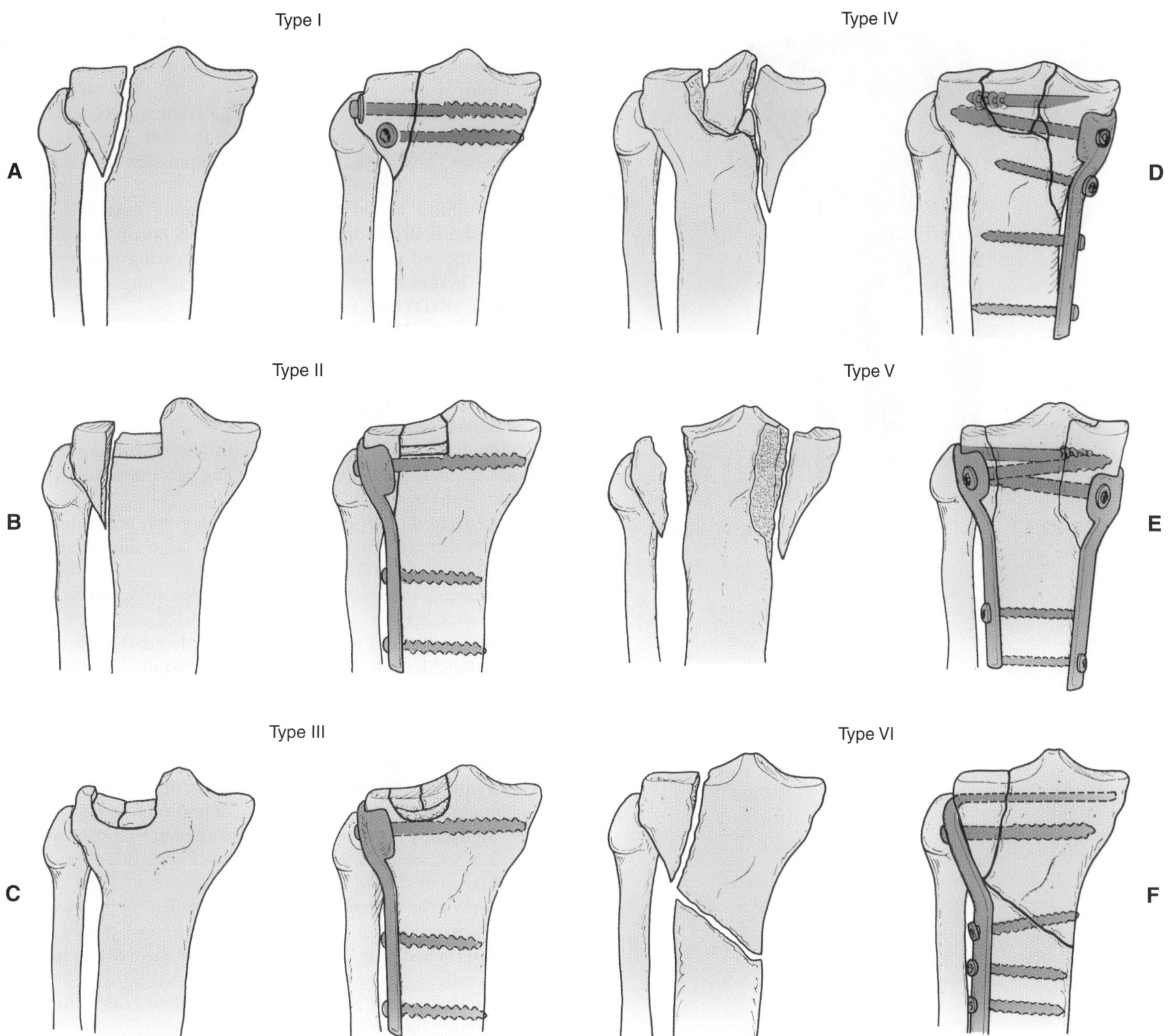


**FIGURE 22-61** Classification of fractures of the tibial plateau. **A,** *Type I.* Pure cleavage fracture. **B,** *Type II.* Cleavage combined with depression. Reduction requires elevation of fragments with bone grafting of resultant hole in metaphysis. Wedge is lagged on lateral aspect of cortex protected with buttress plate. **C,** *Type III.* Pure central depression. There is no lateral wedge. Depression may also be anterior or posterior or involve whole plateau. After elevation of depression and bone grafting, lateral aspect of cortex is best protected with buttress plate. **D,** *Type IV.* Medial condyle is either split off as wedge, or it may be crumbled and depressed, which is characteristic of older patients with osteoporosis (not illustrated). **E,** *Type V.* Note continuity of metaphysis and diaphysis. In internal fixation, both sides must be protected with buttress plates. **F,** *Type VI.* Essence of this fracture is fracture line that dissociates metaphysis from diaphysis. Fracture pattern of condyles is variable, and all types can occur. If both condyles are involved, proximal tibia should be buttressed on both sides.

ing of the canal is necessary only in the case of nonunion, when the canal is reamed 0.5 to 1 mm over the size of the selected nail.

5. The selected nail is attached to the screw-targeting jig, which is then locked into place by the jig adapter. Before the nail is inserted, the alignment of the jig and nail holes is carefully checked by inserting the sheath and trocar through the selected holes by hand.
6. The nail is placed in the prepared canal and advanced retrograde either by hand or with gentle blows of a mallet on the jig adapter. The nail should be countersunk approximately 3 to 5 mm below the articular surface.

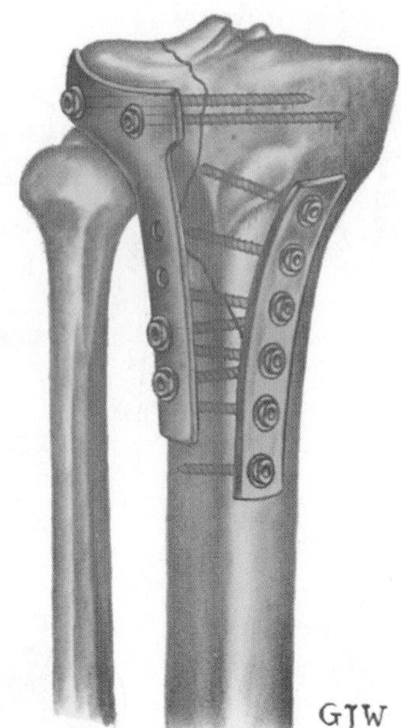


FIGURE 22-62 Severe fractures are treated by use of multiple buttress plates and screws.

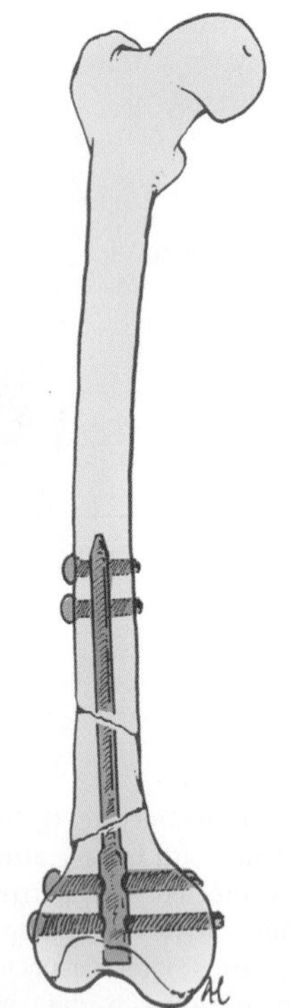

FIGURE 22-63 Supracondylar nail.

7. The screws may then be placed using the targeting jig and sheath and trocar assembly. A small lateral incision is made, and the sheath and trocar are advanced to the femoral cortex. A 5.3-mm drill bit is advanced through the medial cortex, and the length is measured from the calibrated drill bit or by use of a depth gauge. The appropriate 6.5-mm cortical screw is inserted, and the process is repeated for placement of the second screw.
8. Proximal locking of the nail is then performed in a similar fashion, taking care to use the appropriate holes in the targeting jig for the length of nail inserted. The 3.8-mm drill bit and 4.5-mm self-tapping screws are used to fill these holes after femoral rotation and alignment are confirmed with fluoroscopy.
9. The jig adapter and screw-targeting jig are removed, and an end cap is placed into the distal end of the nail. The wounds are irrigated and closed in layers. A compression dressing is applied.

Range-of-motion and muscle-strengthening exercises are begun on the first postoperative day. Care is taken to protect against varus and valgus stresses. Weight bearing is discouraged until there is radiographic evidence of healing.

SUPRACONDYLAR FRACTURE (COMPRESSION PLATE)

1. The lateral area of the distal end of the femur is exposed above and below the knee joint.
2. The fracture site is reduced, and multiple Kirschner wires are inserted to ensure fixation.
3. A calibrated Steinmann pin is placed transversely across the condyles parallel to the joint line. The pin must stop 8 to 10 mm short of the medial cortex.
4. The length of the lag screw is gauged when it is read directly on the calibrated Steinmann pin, and adjustable double reamers are used to ream to this depth.
5. A lag screw is inserted across the condyles, followed by the compression screw.
6. The plate is secured and attached to the femoral shaft with cortical bone screws. The repair is visualized by fluoroscopy.
7. The incision site is irrigated and closed. A knee immobilizer is placed.

MEDIAL AND LATERAL Y-TYPE TIBIAL PLATEAU FRACTURES

1. A long anterolateral incision is made, starting 2.5 cm above the superolateral aspect of the patella and tendon and proceeding distally around the patella to the anterior aspect of the tibia just below the tibial tuberosity. The distal end of the tibial shaft should be exposed.
2. The level of the prepatellar bursa is identified. Blunt dissection beneath the skin is used, and the proximal end of the tibia is retracted to expose it from midline medially to midline laterally.
3. The patellar tendon is detached with a tibial bone plug to expose both the medial and lateral articular surfaces. The articular surface is reconstructed using temporary Kirschner wires. A contoured T-plate is attached to the medial aspect of the tibia using cancellous screws in the proximal portion and cortical screws in the distal portion. A smaller T-plate is inserted on the lateral side and secured in the same manner. The Kirschner wires are removed. Care should be taken to see that the screws do not interfere with each other as they traverse from opposite sides of the tibia.
4. The patellar tendon is reattached using a 6.5-mm cancellous screw through the bone plug.
5. The wound is closed and immobilized at 30 degrees with a posterior splint.

## Patellectomy and Reduction of Fractures of the Patella

Patellectomy was a frequently performed procedure until the early 1970s. It is possible to excise a portion of the patella (for comminuted fracture) or the entire patella (for painful degenerative arthritis) without significantly affecting ordinary activities. However, patellectomy has been shown to significantly reduce power of extension as the joint extends, which is the most important function of the knee. Other complications associated with patellectomy are (1) slow return of quadriceps mechanism strength, (2) quadriceps muscle atrophy, and (3) loss of knee protection from the patella. Removal of the entire patella may result in relative lengthening of the knee extensor mechanism, which necessitates imbrication of the quadriceps tendon at the time of operation to prevent a lag in knee extension. Patellectomy should be performed only when comminution is extensive and reconstruction of the articular surface of the patella is not possible.

If the fracture consists of two large fragments that can be anatomically reduced, fixation is accomplished with a tension band, a circumferential loop technique, or bone screws. Tension band wiring produces compression forces across the fracture site and results in earlier union and immediate mobility of the knee.

***Procedural Considerations.*** The patient is supine. The tourniquet is applied, and the leg is prepped and draped. A soft tissue set and a bone set are required, along with a power drill and bits, bone-reduction clamps, 18-gauge wire, heavy needle holders, and a wire tightener.

### *Operative Procedure*

1. A transverse curved incision is made over the patella.
2. Dissection is carried down to expose the surface of the patella, the quadriceps, and the patellar tendons.
3. The joint is irrigated, and the fracture is reduced with bone-reduction clamps.
4. One length of wire is passed around the insertion of the patellar tendon and then around the quadriceps tendon. A second wire is passed more superficially through the bone fragments.
5. The fracture is overcorrected, and the wire is tightened with the wire tightener. In flexing the knee or contracting the quadriceps, the condyles press against the patellar fragments, producing compression at the fracture site.

## Correction of Recurrent Dislocation of the Patella

Recurrent dislocation of the patella can be the result of violent initial dislocation or more commonly from underlying anatomic abnormalities. The underlying condition causes an abnormal excursion of the extensor mechanism over the femoral condyles. Dynamic forces, such as the vastus lateralis, and static forces, such as arising from the shape of the patella, tend to displace the patella laterally. Dislocations occur when there are extreme displacing forces combined with internal rotation of the femur and flexion of the knee. If untreated, patellar dislocations will deteriorate the knee by causing abnormal patellofemoral articulation, chondromalacia, and meniscal tears.

Conservative treatment aimed at quadriceps strengthening may be indicated in some patients. Numerous operations have been designed to realign the knee extensor mechanism. All the procedures include incising the lateral quadriceps tendon and shifting the insertion of the patellar tendon medially or distally to the original insertion of the tibia.

***Procedural Considerations.*** The patient is positioned supine. The tourniquet is applied, and the leg is prepped and draped. A soft tissue set and a bone set are required, along with a large-fragment screw set, a power drill, a microsagittal saw (Figure 22-64), and osteotomes.

### *Operative Procedure*

#### PATELLAR REALIGNMENT (ELMSLIE-TRILLAT) (FIGURE 22-65)

1. A lateral parapatellar incision is made beginning proximally to the patellar pole, laterally around the patella, and extending to 2 cm distally and just laterally to the tibial tuberosity.
2. A skin flap is developed and retracted medially to expose the capsule. A medial arthrotomy is completed, the joint is inspected, and any pathologic condition present is repaired.

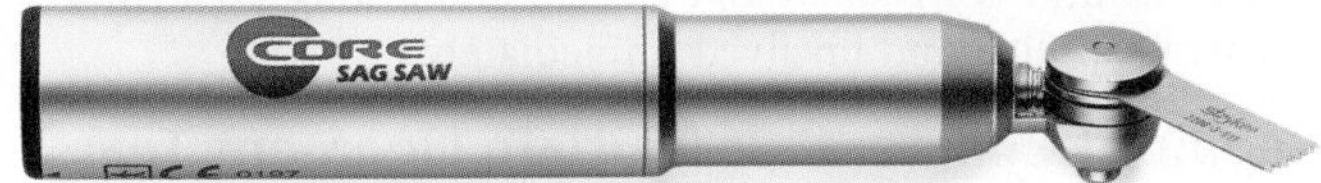


**FIGURE 22-64** Microsagittal saw.

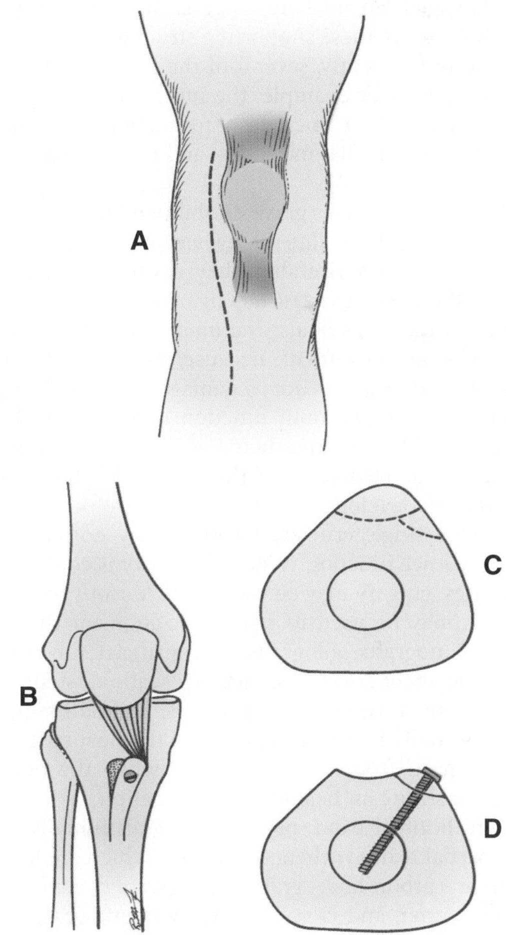


**FIGURE 22-65** Elmslie-Trillat procedure as modified by Cox. **A,** Skin incision. **B,** Completed procedure. **C,** Cross section of tibia at level of tibial tuberosity to show bone cuts made to free tuberosity in center and to create new bed for transposed tuberosity to right. **D,** Cross section of tuberosity fixed with screw in new location anteromedially. Screw should not penetrate posterior aspect of cortex.

3. The lateral retinaculum is released from the vastus lateralis proximally and the patellar tendon distally.
4. With a ½-inch osteotome, the tibial tuberosity is scored medially and laterally, just below the fat pad and under the patella.
5. The osteotomy is continued using a microsagittal saw distally for 4 to 6 cm, leaving the periosteum hinged at the distal-most part of the osteotomy.
6. The entire segment, with patellar tendon attached, is displaced medially and held in place by hand while putting the knee through a range of motion. Tracking of the patella on the femoral groove is completed by systematically moving the knee medially in increments.
7. A cancellous bone bed is prepared at the point of reattachment of the tibial tuberosity.
8. The tuberosity is displaced medially, and a 6.5-mm cancellous bone screw is placed.
9. The wound is irrigated and closed, and a long leg cylinder cast is applied and bivalved immediately.

## Repair of Collateral or Cruciate Ligament Tears

The stability of the knee depends on the integrity of the cruciate and collateral ligaments. If any of these supporting structures is damaged, an unstable knee is likely unless properly repaired. Injuries to these supporting structures are usually not isolated. More frequently, several of the ligaments are injured at the same time. For example, the injury commonly referred to as the "terrible triad" includes a torn anterior cruciate ligament (ACL), torn medial meniscus, and torn medial collateral ligament.

The knee demonstrates grave disability with major ligamentous disruption. The *collateral ligaments* reinforce the knee capsule medially and laterally. They resist varus and valgus stresses on the knee. The *cruciate ligaments* control AP stability. Along with the ligaments, the muscle groups stabilize the joint and control movement. Because muscle strength is the first line of defense for the knee, damage is repaired to protect the ligaments. For optimum function of the joint, damaged structures should be reconstructed as close as possible to the original anatomic structures. If the knee is left untreated, osteoarthritis will develop.

Injury to a single cruciate ligament may not significantly compromise knee function. When the injury is combined with other injuries, surgery may be warranted. Various types of ligament grafts may be used to replace or augment the cruciate ligaments. Autografts, allografts, and artificial substitutes are available. Ligament substitutes act as a scaffold, stent, or augmentation of the torn cruciate ligaments. Scaffolds support the soft tissue initially to allow ingrowth of the host tissue. Stents protect the joint from excessive stress while the permanent ligament substitute is healing. Augmentation, as by the patient's own iliotibial band, protects the graft initially after repair of a partial tear. Synthetic ligaments, which are less popular, include carbon-fiber grafts, polyglycolic acid material, Dacron, polyester, and Gore-Tex. All synthetic grafts are subject to mechanical failure from weakening with fragmentation and synovitis. These are recommended for salvage procedures only when conventional reconstruction has failed and when other autogenous tissue is unavailable for substitution. Biologic materials from animals, such as bovine xenografts, are also available for ligament substitution, although they are subject to increased risk of infection, synovitis, and rejection. Homogeneous allografts are the substitute of choice for knee reconstruction when no autogenous graft is available from the patient. Disadvantages of homogeneous allografts include long-term weakening, possible rejection, and the possibility of infectious disease transfer.

Autogenous tissues are currently the substitute of choice, with the middle third of the patellar tendon and a block of patella being the most reliable. To minimize necrosis and maintain graft strength, the fat pad with its blood supply may be preserved along with the patellar tendon. Using this graft and other soft tissue autografts, the cruciate-deficient knee can be reconstructed arthroscopically (see "Arthroscopy," p. 784). A combination of a torn ACL, medial meniscus, and medial collateral ligament often indicates the need for an open procedure (arthrotomy). When reconstructing the cruciate ligament, it is important to have the graft biomechanically correct to maintain proper function. Many devices and systems are used to provide placement assistance and gauge appropriate graft tension. These devices are used either separately or in some combination. Though the variations are many, the principles are the same.

***Procedural Considerations.*** The patient is placed in the supine position with a tourniquet applied to the upper area of the thigh. A surgical prep is done from the upper area of the thigh down to and including the foot. Soft tissue instruments, arthroscopy instruments, ACL reconstruction instruments, Steinmann pins, reconstruction guides (Figure 22-66), and a tension isometer are required. A power drill, microsagittal saw, and burrs are essential. The fixation device of choice should also be available. Meniscal repair instruments should be in the room.

### *Operative Procedure*

**RUPTURED ANTERIOR CRUCIATE REPAIR.** An examination under anesthesia (EUA) is performed immediately after induction, when the ligaments are completely lax, to evaluate the severity of the injury.

1. A straight midline or slightly medial incision is made across the knee.

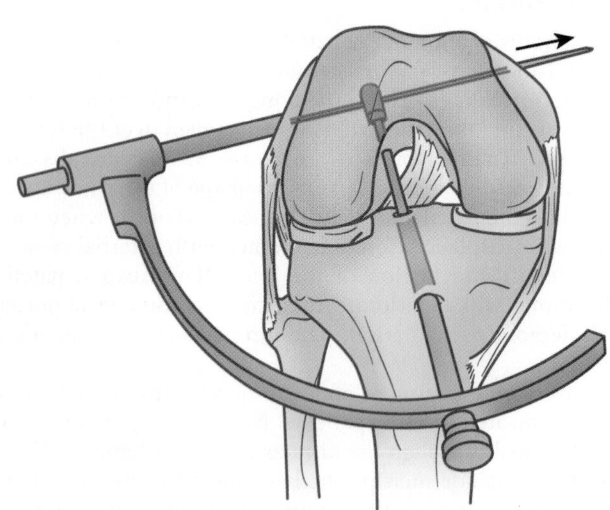

**FIGURE 22-66** Reconstruction guide used for ligament repair.

2. Meniscus tears in the vascular zone (peripheral) are repaired with arthroscopic meniscal repair instruments or cutting needles with a heavy absorbable suture to repair the meniscofemoral and meniscotibial ligaments. If the meniscus is not repairable, partial meniscectomy is performed.
3. The middle third of the patellar tendon with patellar and tibial bone plugs is harvested using a power saw and osteotome.
4. A notchplasty is then performed, debriding and smoothing the lateral intercondylar wall with a burr and curette.
5. The femoral and tibial osseous tunnels are developed using the ligament guide to pass guidewires from the lateral area of the femoral condyle and tibial tubercle into the intercondylar notch at isometric points near the anatomic attachment site of the ACL.
6. The pins are then overdrilled with cannulated drills as close to the size of the patellar tendon graft as possible. The tunnels are smoothed with a curette.
7. Sutures are placed through drill holes at both ends of the graft to pass the graft through the tunnels.
8. Once the graft is passed through the femoral and tibial osseous tunnels, it is fixed at both ends with interference screws, staples, or polyethylene buttons.
9. The medial collateral ligament and posterior oblique ligament are then individually repaired at their insertion sites with bone screws and spiked washers.
10. Additional extraarticular repair is done if necessary.
11. The wound is closed over intraarticular and subcutaneous drains, and a locking knee brace or knee immobilizer is applied.

## Popliteal (Baker's) Cyst Excision

Baker's cysts occur in joints, frequently affecting the popliteal fossa. Baker's cysts are often painful and can become very large, especially when associated with rheumatoid arthritis. Cysts in the popliteal fossa occur without a precipitating cause in children; in adults they often indicate an intraarticular disease process, such as rheumatoid arthritis, or a torn meniscus.

***Procedural Considerations.*** In contrast to many other operative procedures on the knee, the patient is placed in the prone position. A soft tissue set and a bone set are required.

### *Operative Procedure*

1. An oblique incision is made in the popliteal area over the mass.
2. The deep fascia is divided to expose the mass.
3. The cyst is then freed by blunt dissection and clamped at its attachment to the joint capsule.
4. The cyst is divided, and the pedicle is inverted and closed.
5. After the mass has been removed, the wound is irrigated and closed.

Postoperatively, the knee may be immobilized in extension with a posterior splint.

## Fractures of the Tibial Shaft

The location of the tibia results in frequent exposure to injury. Open fractures are more common in the tibia than in other major bones because one third of its surface is subcutaneous. Tibial shaft fractures are difficult to treat. The blood supply to the tibia is more precarious than that of other long bones because of its lack of enclosure by heavy muscle. The presence of hinge joints at the knee and ankle allows no adjustment for rotational deformity after fracture, so special care is required to correct for rotation during reduction and fixation. Rotational deformities are often seen. Delayed union, nonunion, and infection are fairly common complications. Arguments can be made that closed reduction and casting provide excellent healing without significant complications, but this treatment can require casting for 6 months or more. Arguments can also be made for surgical reduction and internal fixation. This treatment approach generally allows for earlier weight bearing and a shortened period of casting; however, the rate of complications is higher.

In general, torsional fractures seem to heal better and are more amenable to treatment than transverse fractures. It is theorized that twisting injuries cause less damage to endosteal vessels than transverse fractures do, in which periosteum and endosteal vessels are torn circumferentially. The important prognostic indicators for tibial fractures are as follows: (1) the amount of initial displacement, (2) the degree of comminution, (3) the presence or absence of infection, and (4) the severity of soft tissue injury, excluding infection. As a rule, high-energy fractures, such as those caused by auto accidents or crushing injury, have a much worse prognosis than low-energy fractures, such as those caused by falls on ice or skiing accidents.

Because of the increase in intramedullary tibial nailings without a significant increase in infections arising from them, external fixation of open tibial shaft fractures is less commonly done. However, in the presence of gross contamination, severe soft tissue and vascular injury, bone infection, and delayed treatment, external fixation is the treatment of choice. The Ilizarov external fixation device is indicated when bone loss is significant and limb lengthening is required. Plate and screw fixation is another method in which tibial shaft fractures can be treated, although infection and nonunion of tibial shaft fractures are twice as likely with this method. Plate and screw fixation is indicated when intraarticular fragments of the knee and ankle are associated with the injury. Closed intramedullary nailing is the treatment of choice in tibial shaft fractures because infection is less likely to occur and the periosteal blood supply is preserved. Static locking nails (locking both proximal and distal ends of the nail) are indicated for fractures with comminution, bone loss, and lengthening osteotomies. Dynamic locking nails (locking the end closest to the fracture site) are indicated for proximal or distal tibial fractures, nonunions, and malunions. Locking tibial nails include the Russell-Taylor and the Grosse-Kempf tibial nail.

The key to successful treatment of open tibial fractures, as in all open fractures, is meticulous and systematic debridement of all foreign matter and devitalized tissue. Care should be taken to minimize devascularization when reducing and fixing the fracture. Systemic antibiotics and those delivered by pulsatile lavage help reduce the chance of infection.

***Procedural Considerations.*** The patient is usually given general or regional anesthesia while still on the hospital bed or in the transport vehicle and then transferred to the OR fracture bed. The patient is then positioned supine with the affected hip flexed approximately 45 degrees and the knee at 90 degrees. This provides a horizontal orientation of the tibia. Using a calcaneal traction pin or table foot holder, traction is applied and rotational alignment obtained. After rotational alignment is obtained, a tourniquet is applied and the leg is prepped and draped. Some surgeons prefer to use a standard OR bed, breaking it at the knee. This obviates the need to insert the calcaneal traction pin and allows for easier maneuvering of the tibia during insertion of the locking screws.

A soft tissue set and a large bone set are required, in addition to the intramedullary nail and insertion instruments of choice. A power drill and reamer-driver will be needed to use the necessary intramedullary reamers (Figure 22-67). Fluoroscopy will be needed as well. If open plating is being considered, the plates of choice and the large-fragment screws need to be available as well as bone-reduction clamps.

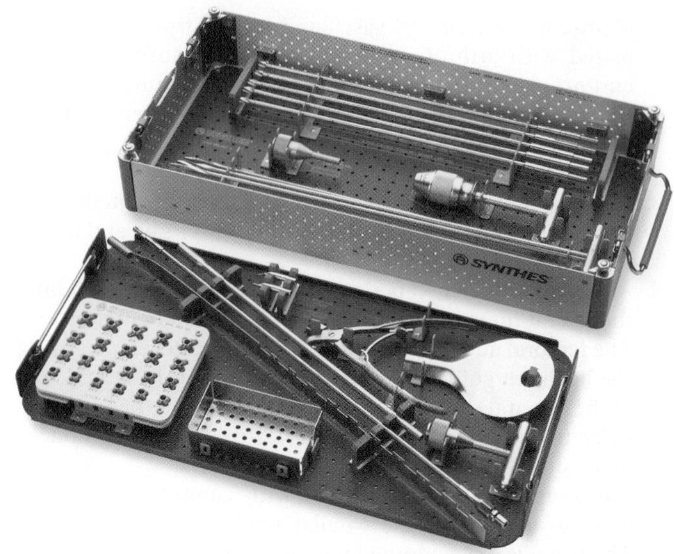


FIGURE 22-67 Intramedullary flexible reamer system.

### *Operative Procedures*

#### CLOSED OR OPEN TIBIAL INTRAMEDULLARY NAILING (FIGURE 22-68)

1. If the open technique is required, the fracture site is exposed, reduced, and irrigated as necessary. Focus is then turned toward the nailing procedure.
2. A 5-cm incision is made medial to the patellar tendon to just below the tibial tuberosity.
3. Using a curved awl, the medullary canal is opened just proximal to the tibial tuberosity.
4. A guide rod (3.2 mm) is inserted into the shaft of the tibia down to the fracture site. The proximal fragment is reduced distally and the guide rod advanced into the distal fragment. Rod types include the straight guide rod for simple fractures, a curved guide rod for the displaced type, and a cutting tip for an obstructed canal.
5. The length of the required nail is determined by the guide rod method (see "Operative Procedure" under "Femoral Shaft Fractures: Internal Fixation," p. 751) or by using the nail-length gauge and confirming with fluoroscopy.
6. With cannulated reamers over the guide rods, the entire tibia is reamed 1 mm greater than the nail to be inserted. Inserting a nail too large for the canal can have a detrimental effect.
7. The driver, proximal drill, guide, and hexagonal bolt are assembled onto the tibial nail.
8. The nail is inserted over the guide rod and, with a mallet, driven down the proximal fragment to enter the distal fragment, crossing the fracture site. The nail is not fully seated.
9. The guide rod is removed to prevent incarceration, and complete seating of the nail is performed. The proximal tip of the nail should be flush with the tibial entry site.
10. Proximal locking is accomplished with the corresponding drill and tap through the proximal drill guide for 5-mm cortical bone screws.
11. Distal screws are inserted using the distal targeting device or the freehand technique. The 5-mm cortical bone screws are inserted, traversing the tibia through the tibial nail.
12. The wounds are irrigated. If bone graft is to be used, it is placed around the fracture site and the layers are closed. Dressings are applied, and a cast or splint for immobilization may be applied.

Dynamization, or removal of either the proximal or the distal screws, may take place after 3 months for fractures that are stable but lack callus. Dynamization produces compressive forces at the fracture, thereby promoting osteogenesis.

#### TIBIAL DYNAMIC COMPRESSION PLATING

1. A longitudinal incision is made (to accommodate the selected plate) lateral to the tibial crest to expose the fracture site.
2. The periosteum is stripped only enough for application of the plate. Circumferential stripping can diminish blood supply.
3. The fracture is reduced, and a plate is placed across the fracture site and secured with bone- and plate-holding forceps. The plate may have to be contoured with a handheld or plate-bending press.
4. Using the neutral drill guide, a 3.2-mm bicortical hole is drilled into the plate screw hole close to the fracture site, gauged, and tapped to 4.5 mm. The first bone screw is inserted, ensuring purchase of the screw on the opposite cortex.
5. Using the load drill guide (eccentric), the second hole is drilled next to the fracture line in the opposite fragment. Drill and tap are accomplished as in the previous step. As the screw enters the bone, it will seek the center of the screw hole (the screw is eccentric, and the screw hole is beveled). The fracture site is brought under compression as the screw seats into the hole.
6. The wounds are irrigated. If bone graft is to be used, it is placed around the fracture site and the layers are closed. Dressings are applied, and a cast or splint for immobilization may be applied.

## SURGERY OF THE ANKLE AND FOOT

### Ankle Fractures

Ankle fractures include fractures of the medial malleolus (tibia), lateral malleolus (fibula), and posterior malleolus (posterior aspect of the articular surface of the distal end of the tibia). They may or may not be associated with ligamentous injury. Ankle fractures can be classified in anatomic lines as

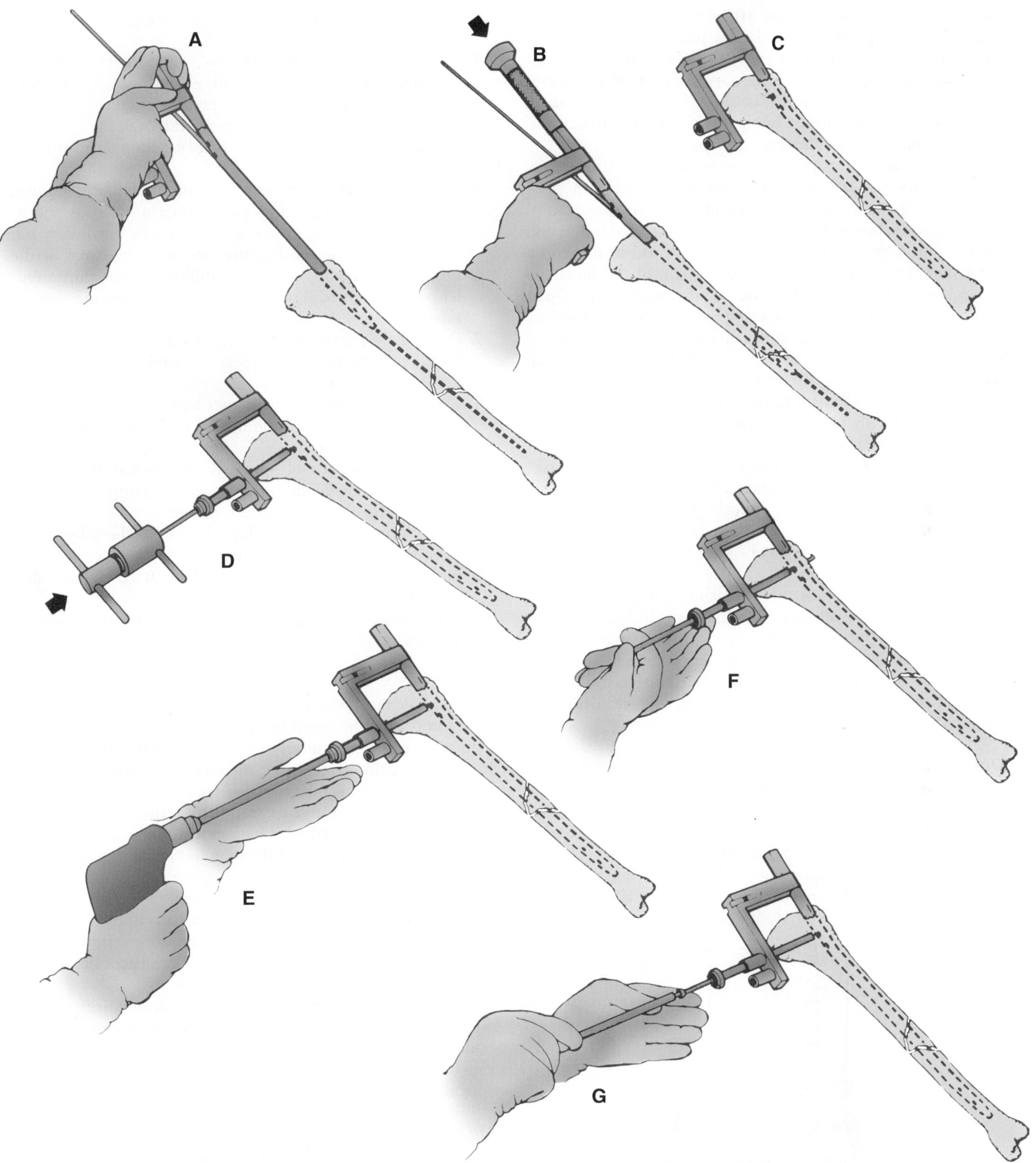


**FIGURE 22-68** Tibial intramedullary nailing. **A,** Attachment of nail to proximal drill guide. **B,** Driving nail over guide rod. **C,** Final seating of nail with its tip flush with tibial entry portal. **D,** For proximal interlocking, cortex is dimpled. **E,** Depth measurements are made. **F,** Locking screw length is confirmed. **G,** Self-tapping screw is inserted through drill sleeve.

unimalleolar, bimalleolar, and trimalleolar. Because medial malleolar and posterior malleolar fractures involve the distal weight-bearing articular surface of the tibia, open reduction and anatomic alignment are necessary. Fixation of the lateral malleolus is also important because it forms the ankle mortise—the socket formed by the distal tibia and fibula into which the body of the talus fits.

Anatomic reduction prevents the occurrence of degenerative joint disease. Displaced fractures are treated with pins, malleolar or bone screws, or plates and screws (Figure 22-69). Bimalleolar fractures can be treated with closed reduction and casting, but approximately 10% of these go on to develop a nonunion. The lateral malleolus (distal end of the fibula) is important for lateral and rotational stability of the joint. Open reduction and internal fixation using Steinmann pins or screws placed obliquely into the tibia is a common technique. Lateral malleolar fractures can be fixed with the cancellous lag technique—overdrilling the first fragment and allowing compression of the fragments. Fracture of the lateral malleolus can also be treated with a Rush rod, inserted through the fragment and into the fibular canal. Trimalleolar fractures require surgery more than the other varieties of fractures do. The posterior lip of the articulating surface of the tibia is usually involved and needs to be anatomically reduced to minimize degenerative changes. Cannulated screws can provide efficient reduction of a posterior fragment.

***Procedural Considerations.*** The patient is placed in the supine position. The affected leg is prepped and draped after application of a pneumatic tourniquet. If the lateral ankle is involved, a padded sandbag is placed beneath the hip to internally rotate it. A soft tissue set; a small bone set; a small-fragment set with plates, screws, and pins; a power drill; and bone-reduction clamps are required.

### *Operative Procedure*

TRIMALLEOLAR FRACTURE

1. Incisions are made medially and laterally across the ankle.
2. The posterior malleolar fracture is exposed and reduced with bone-holding clamps and manipulation.
3. The fracture is temporarily held in reduction with two Kirschner wires inserted above the anterior tibial lip and directed anteriorly to posteriorly, engaging both fragments.
4. A drill hole is made anteriorly to posteriorly through both fragments. After measuring with a depth gauge, a malleolar, small cancellous, or other preferred screw is inserted through the fracture. The wires are removed.
5. The lateral malleolar fracture is then manipulated into reduction.
6. If the fracture is oblique and not comminuted, it is reduced with one or two lag screws placed anteriorly to posteriorly. If the fracture is transverse, a long screw or medullary pin is inserted across the fracture line into the canal of the proximal fragment. A small semitubular or one third tubular plate is applied if the fracture occurs above the syndesmosis.
7. Once the posterior and lateral malleolar fractures have been fixed, the medial malleolar fracture is finally reduced using bone clamps.
8. The reduction is held with two Kirschner wires while a hole is drilled through the medial malleolus into the metaphysis of the tibia.
9. Appropriate length of screw is determined by a depth gauge; then a malleolar screw is inserted across the fracture site. The Kirschner wires are removed.
10. If rotational stability is needed, an additional smaller screw or compression wiring is added.
11. Intraoperative radiographs are taken in AP, lateral, and mortise views.
12. The wounds are irrigated and closed, and a short or long leg cast or splint is applied.

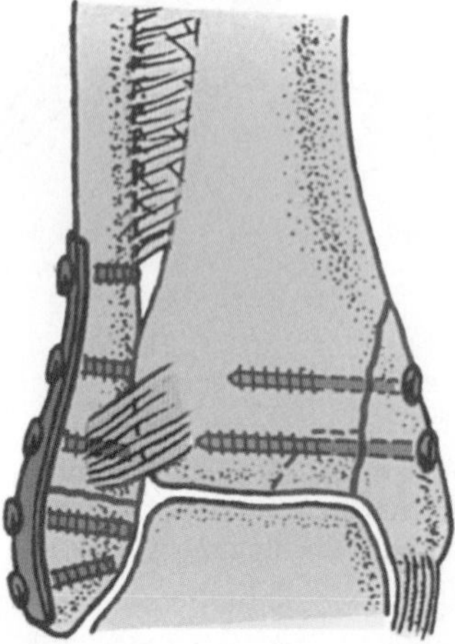

FIGURE 22-69 Plate-screw placement for lateral malleolar fragment repair using one third tubular plate.

## Triple Arthrodesis

The talocalcaneal (subtalar), talonavicular, and calcaneocuboid joints must be fused in patients with pronounced inversion or eversion deformities of the foot. Such deformities occur in clubfoot, poliomyelitis, and rheumatoid arthritis. Occasionally this operation is necessary for patients who have pain resulting from degenerative or traumatic arthritis, such as that occurring after intraarticular fractures of the calcaneus. Triple arthrodesis limits motion of the foot and ankle to plantar flexion and dorsiflexion.

***Procedural Considerations.*** The patient is placed in the supine position. The surgical prep is carried out from midcalf down to and including the foot. The iliac crest area should also be prepped if bone grafting is anticipated.

A soft tissue set; a small bone set; a power saw, drill, or rasp; a bone graft set; and the AO compression plates and screws or bone staples to hold the fusion are required. Kirschner wires can be used to provide temporary fixation. A small lamina spreader is helpful in providing exposure.

### *Operative Procedure*

1. An anterior or anterolateral approach is used.
2. The subtalar and calcaneocuboid joints are exposed, as well as the lateral portion of the talonavicular joint.
3. The capsules of the talonavicular, calcaneocuboid, and subtalar joints are incised circumferentially to obtain as much mobility as possible. If this release allows the foot to be placed into a normal position, removal of large bony wedges is not required.

4. An osteotome, power saw, or power rasp is used to remove the articular surfaces of the calcaneocuboid joint, the subtalar joint, and the talonavicular joint. The small lamina spreader is used to expose these surfaces. Care is taken to save all bone removed for later use in the fusion.
5. The removed bone is cut into small pieces to be used for bone grafting. If the quantity is insufficient, graft is harvested from the anterior ilium. Most of the bone is placed around the talonavicular joint and in the depth of the sinus tarsi.
6. Smooth Steinmann pins, staples, or screws are used for internal fixation.
7. The wound is closed over a suction drain. A short leg cast or splint is applied.

## Bunionectomy

A bunion (hallux valgus) is a soft tissue or bony mass at the medial side of the first metatarsal head. It is associated with a valgus deformity of the great toe (Figure 22-70). A bunion is caused by a basic structural defect of the foot, which predisposes to the development of this deformity. Ill-fitting shoes accentuate the situation and speed the development of bunions. Bunions are 40 times more common in women because of shoe styles, including high heels and pointed toes. Other factors that may contribute to this deformity are heredity, flatfeet, foot pronation, longer first toe, muscle imbalance, and inflammatory disturbances of the feet.

Symptoms include pain on the dorsomedial aspect of the first metatarsal head or directly over the medial exostosis, swelling of the big toe, painful plantar callus, and plantar keratosis. Discomfort to the entire foot occurs as the forefoot becomes more fatigued and symptomatic, with pain radiating to the leg and knee.

Hallux valgus is treated with a variety of surgical procedures (Figure 22-71). All these procedures remove the exostosis and attempt to realign the great toe by removal of bone, transfer of tendons, osteotomy of the first metatarsal shaft, or appropriate imbrication of soft tissue.

The goals of surgery are correction of the deformity (cosmesis), resection of the abnormal bony components (reconstruction), and normal or near-normal range of motion (function).

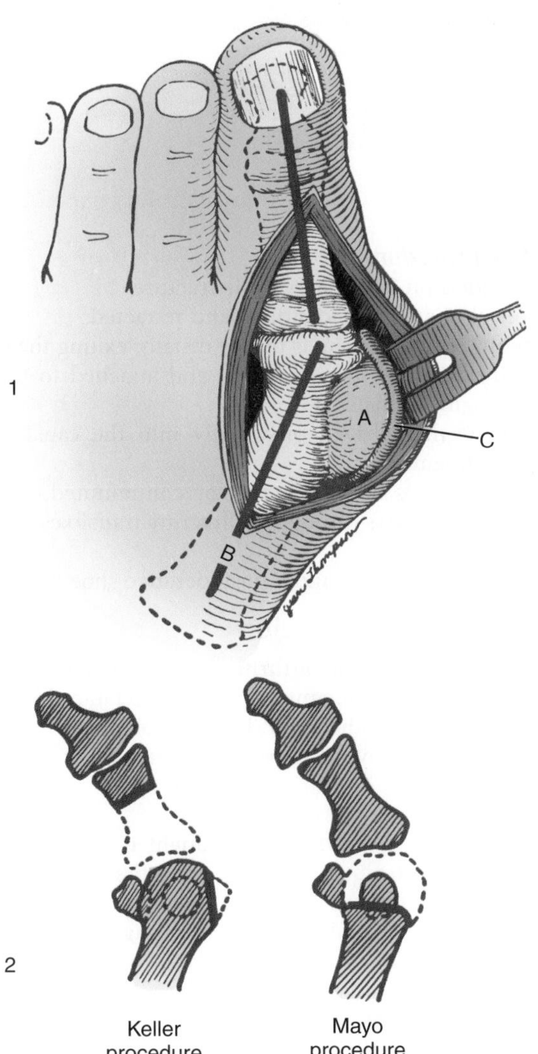


**FIGURE 22-70** Bunionectomy. *1*, Bunion. *A*, Exostosis of metatarsal head; *B*, hallux valgus deformity; *C*, overlying bursa. *2*, Operations for hallux valgus.

***Procedural Considerations.*** The patient is given general or regional anesthesia, and a tourniquet is applied. The foot and leg are prepped and then draped using a sterile stockinette.

A soft tissue set, a small bone set, Kirschner wires, a power wire driver, and a microsagittal saw are required.

### *Operative Procedure*

KELLER PROCEDURE

1. A midline, straight, medial incision is made, beginning at the neck of the proximal phalanx and extended proximally.
2. Dissection is carried down through the joint capsule. A flap incision is made to expose the underlying hypertrophic bone found at the dorsomedial aspect of the first metatarsal head.
3. All soft tissue attachments are removed from the base of the proximal phalanx.
4. The proximal third of the proximal phalanx is resected with a power-oscillating saw.
5. Proper alignment of the toe is maintained as one or two 0.062-inch Kirschner wires are placed in the center of the medullary canal of the phalanx and then driven into the metatarsal head, neck, and shaft.
6. The wound is then irrigated and closed, and a bandage is applied to maintain the toe in the correct position.
7. Postoperative convalescence requires a minimum of 6 weeks.

## Correction of Hammer Toe Deformity

The term *hammer toe* is most often used to describe an abnormal flexion posture of the proximal interphalangeal joint of one of the four lesser toes. This deformity causes painful calluses to develop on the dorsal joints of the four lesser toes, since the cocked-up digits rub against the shoes. Incising the long extensor tendon to the toes and fusing the proximal interphalangeal joint treat the deformities. A smooth Kirschner wire is frequently used to stabilize the fusion and position the toe properly during the postoperative period.

***Procedural Considerations.*** The patient is placed in the supine position, and the tourniquet is applied. The foot is prepped and draped. A soft tissue set, a small bone set, Kirschner wires, and a power wire driver are required.

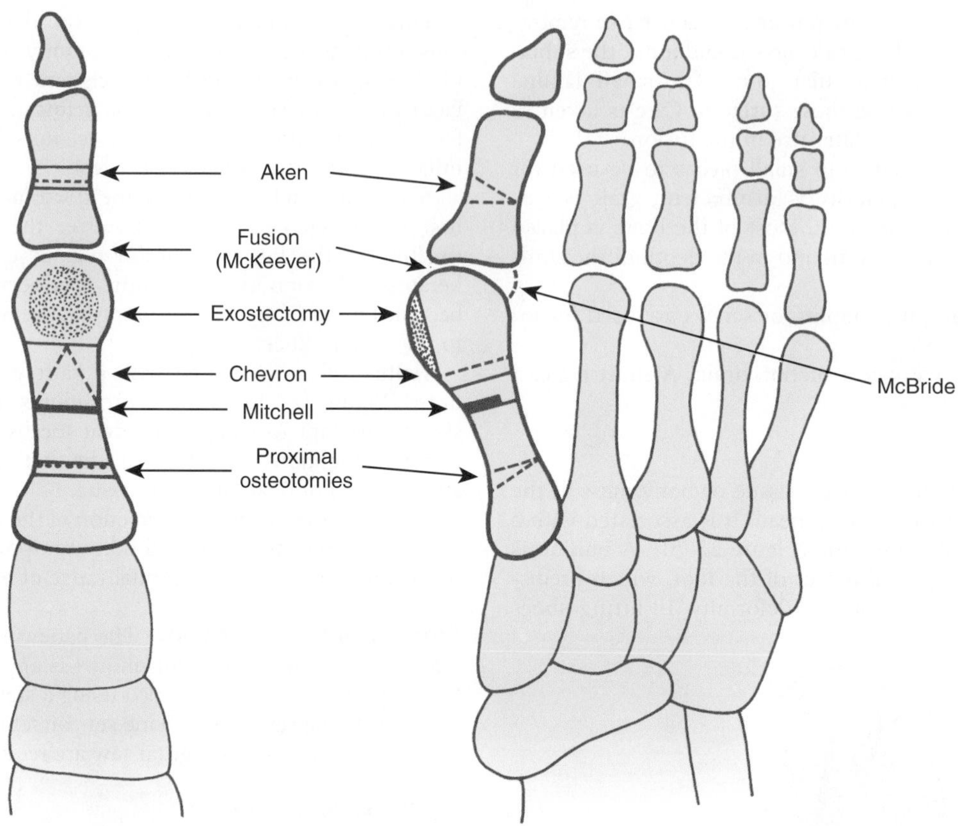


FIGURE 22-71 Types of bunionectomies.

*Operative Procedure*

1. An elliptic incision over the proximal interphalangeal joint that measures 5 to 6 mm wide and has a 2-mm or 3-mm lateral extension on either side is made.
2. The capsular tissue of the distal third of the proximal phalanx and proximal interphalangeal joint is entered to expose the defect completely.
3. A small rongeur or microsaw is used to resect the distal third portion of the proximal phalanx. Once the capital fragment is excised, the remaining portion of the distal proximal phalanx is debrided with a rongeur or rasp.
4. Digital alignment can be maintained with small Kirschner wires.
5. The wounds are irrigated and closed, and a sterile dressing and orthopedic shoe are applied for postoperative recovery.

## Metatarsal Fractures

Metatarsal fractures occur in various sites. These fractures have a reduced healing potential because metatarsals consist mainly of cortical bone, which lacks vascularity. Treatment is determined by the extent of the fracture—the greater the displacement, the greater the need for reduction. In general, transverse and short, oblique, midshaft fractures of the metatarsals are internally fixed because of their instability and displacement. Pins, wires, screws, and plates are used for internal fixation of metatarsal fractures. The simplest method is Kirschner wire fixation.

***Procedural Considerations.*** The patient is placed in the supine position, a tourniquet is applied, and the foot is prepped and draped. A soft tissue set, a small bone set, Kirschner wires, and a power wire driver are required.

*Operative Procedure*

1. A small incision is made over the fracture.
2. The distal fragment is identified and retracted.
3. A smooth Kirschner wire is driven distally, exiting the skin.
4. The wire driver is then switched and attached to the end protruding from the skin.
5. The pin is then driven proximally into the canal of the proximal fragment.
6. If the fracture is more complex or comminuted, crossing two Kirschner wires through the fracture transfixes the fracture site.
7. The incision is closed, and a postoperative shoe is applied.

## Metatarsal Head Resection

Patients with rheumatoid arthritis frequently have dorsally dislocated toes and prominent and painful metatarsal heads on the plantar surfaces of their feet. Excision of all the metatarsal heads commonly relieves the pain and corrects an associated bunion deformity.

***Procedural Considerations.*** The patient is placed in a supine position, a tourniquet is applied, and the foot is prepped and draped. A soft tissue set, a small bone set, Kirschner wires, a power wire driver, and a power microsagittal saw are required.

*Operative Procedure*

CLAYTON TECHNIQUE

1. A transverse plantar incision is made, and tissue is dissected to the metatarsal heads.
2. All metatarsal heads and half the proximal phalanges are removed with the microsagittal saw.

3. The extensor tendons are transected and not repaired.
4. The skin is closed, and a dressing and postoperative shoe are applied.

## PELVIC FRACTURE AND DISRUPTION

Patients with multiple trauma often present with multiple fractures that can be life threatening. Complications of pelvic fractures include injury not only to major vessels and nerves but also to major visceral organs, such as the intestines, bladder, and urethra. Factors influencing mortality include associated visceral injury, hemorrhage, and head injury.

Pelvic fracture classification is divided into three main groups (Table 22-1). *Type A fractures* are stable, without ring involvement (A1) or minimally displaced fractures of the ring (A2). *Type B fractures* are rotationally unstable and vertically stable and are also subclassified: B1 is an open book fracture, B2 has ipsilateral compression, and B3 has contralateral compression. *Type C fractures* are both rotationally and vertically unstable: C1 is unilateral, C2 is bilateral, and C3 is associated with the acetabulum. Radiographic films, computed tomography (CT) scan, and magnetic resonance imaging (MRI) all prove useful in determining the type and appropriate treatment for pelvic trauma.

Treatment is based on classification and may include closed manipulation and reduction or internal and external fixation. Internal and external fixation can be used concurrently in the treatment of some pelvic fractures.

Type A fractures are stable and can be treated nonoperatively. Type B1 fractures may be treated with external fixation or anterior plate fixation. Type C fractures usually require open procedures to fix the fractures with plates and screws and reduce sacral disruptions with transiliac rods or screws. Type C fractures may be treated with external fixation when the patient is hemodynamically unstable and a quicker, simpler procedure is prudent.

External fixation is the most widely recommended treatment for type B fractures of the pelvis. A technique similar to that of external fixation of extremity fractures is done in the OR with anesthesia and sterile conditions. If external fixation is to be used, the earlier it is attempted, the greater chance of success.

### Procedural Considerations

This procedure is often done during other emergent and trauma resuscitative efforts. The patient's entire pelvic area is prepped and draped. A pelvic skeleton in the room may help the team visualize maneuvers and pin placement to be attempted to complete the reduction. A soft tissue set is needed in addition to the external fixator of choice and the instruments for its insertion, including a power drill.

### Operative Procedure

#### *AO External Fixation*

1. The pelvic disruption is reduced manually and confirmed radiographically. It may be impossible to completely reduce the disruption without skeletal traction using a distal femoral pin. If required, this is inserted under sterile conditions.
2. Kirschner wires are inserted percutaneously to determine the position of the pin placement, taking into consideration the inward and downward crest slope.

**TABLE 22-1**

**Classification of Pelvic Injuries**

| | |
|---|---|
| Type A | Stable<br>A1—Fractures of the pelvis not involving the ring<br>A2—Stable, minimally displaced fractures of the ring |
| Type B | Rotationally unstable, vertically stable<br>B1—Open book<br>B2—Lateral compression: ipsilateral<br>B3—Lateral compression: contralateral (bucket handle) |
| Type C | Rotationally and vertically unstable<br>C1—Unilateral<br>C2—Bilateral<br>C3—Associated with an acetabular fracture |

3. Parallel rows of pins are placed into the anterior iliac crest area. This is done by drilling the outer cortex and placing 5-mm half pins medially and distally. The pins should enter cancellous bone between the outer and inner tables of ilium.
4. Three universal frames are placed over the pins as close to the skin as possible for maximum rigidity.
5. Optimal reduction of the fracture is visualized using radiography. The crossbar is applied, and compression and distraction maneuvers are used to maintain the reduction.
6. The crossbar is removed, and connecting rods are applied with couplers.
7. The crossbar is reattached, and the joints of the frame are tightened.
8. The pin sites of tented skin are released. The wounds are dressed with iodine ointment and gauze.
9. The frames are left in place generally for 8 to 12 weeks.

## TOTAL JOINT ARTHROPLASTY

Arthroplasty of the joints is performed to restore motion of the joint and function to the muscles and ligaments. It is indicated in individuals with a painful, disabling arthritic joint that is no longer responsive to conservative therapy. The procedure is generally reserved for those with a less active life-style. The younger patient, very active older person, or laborer may better be served with a reconstructive procedure such as arthrodesis or osteotomy. Many total hip and knee replacements are done each year. Improvements in implant design, materials, and fixation techniques are ongoing, as is research on enhancing soft and hard tissue healing.[12]

The classic combination of metal on polyethylene is the mainstay of joint implants. Metals used in hip and knee implants include *cobalt-chromium* (weight-bearing femoral head) and *titanium* (stems of hips and tibial components). The acetabulum and tibial articulating surfaces continue to be substituted with *ultra-high-molecular-weight polyethylene* (UHMWPE), which provides superior wear characteristics. Other designs have emerged in total hip arthroplasty, including metal on metal and the use of ceramic femoral heads.

At one time it was thought that bone cement was the weak link in the longevity of a joint implant because of a relatively high rate of loosening of cement-fixed implants, especially in younger, more active patients. In response to this belief, alternative methods of fixation have been developed. One method involves the application of a precoat of PMMA to the femoral stem to enhance prosthesis–to–cement mantle bonding. Another method involves the attachment of a porous metal surface to parts of the femoral stem and the entire outer surface of the acetabular component. Most of the porous surfaces are composed of multiple layers sintered in place, creating interconnecting, open pores among the various particles. This allows for the ingrowth of bone to occur, ultimately anchoring the prosthesis in place. "Porous coating" was an attempt to eradicate what was termed *cement disease*—a lysis of bone around the prosthesis causing early loosening. It is now believed that this condition is caused by "wear debris"—particulate matter being shed from metal-to-polyethylene interfaces—and not necessarily from the effects of PMMA.

Bone cement, or PMMA, is an area that has received considerable attention in the search for optimal bone-to-implant fixation. Cement seems to exhibit various degrees of porosity depending on mixing methods and cement pressurization within the canal. Bone cement must prevent motion at the implant interface. Porosity can lead to fatigue and fracture, which ultimately can lead to implant loosening. PMMA, chemically similar to Plexiglas, has barium sulfate added to it to make it possible to assess distribution and changes at a later time. Local tissue effects of PMMA may include (1) tissue protein coagulation caused by polymerization, (2) bone necrosis caused by occlusion of nutrient metaphyseal arteries, and (3) cytotoxic and lipotoxic effects of nonpolymerized monomer.

Despite the high rate of success of total joint implantation over the years, there are numerous potential complications. They are generally divided into medical complications, mechanical complications, and infections. Medical complications include but are not limited to cardiac dysrhythmias, myocardial infarction, hemorrhage, and pulmonary emboli. Mechanical complications are implant breakage, loosening, and wear. Infection in the patient with a total joint implant is a catastrophic complication that usually requires additional surgery and prolonged hospitalization.

Most surgeons recommend the routine use of antibiotics in primary and revision joint arthroplasty. Antibiotic coverage is initiated preoperatively, continued during lengthy procedures, and administered for 24 to 48 hours postoperatively. Pulsatile lavage systems are used to keep tissues moist, remove debris, and dilute bacteria that may be present. Additional antibiotics are added to the physiologic saline solutions used for irrigation and to PMMA; however, data do not conclusively support or dispute this practice.

## Total Hip Replacement

Total hip replacement (arthroplasty) is a common orthopedic procedure performed on patients with hip pain caused by degenerative joint disease or rheumatoid arthritis. A total hip replacement can be cemented, noncemented, or hybrid. Hybrids involve cementing one component, usually the femoral stem, and then inserting a metal-backed, porous-coated acetabular component in a press-fit state. Hybrid arthroplasty is a controversial procedure for two reasons. The first relates to research that demonstrates that wear debris is increased with the larger metal-to-polyethylene interface present in the metal-backed, porous-coated acetabular component. The second relates to cost. The metal-backed, porous-coated acetabular component is significantly more expensive than the all-polyethylene component. Consequently, patient selection is very important in determining which type of component is best.

The primary function of the femoral component is the replacement of the femoral head and femoral neck after resection. The femoral head should ultimately sit where it reproduces the center of rotation of the hip. The neck length is variable and is built into several different heights of femoral heads that are eventually seated onto the Morse taper of the femoral stem. The version (implant rotation within the canal) is very important; too much anteversion or retroversion leaves the hip prone to dislocation. The normal position of the proximal femur is in 10 to 15 degrees of anteversion.

Femoral stems can be collarless or have collars that sit down on the resected femur. Collars will produce forces on the bone and may be desired in cases of osteoporotic bone, where bone genesis may be diminished because of the disease process.

Acetabular cups have also presented challenges in trying to maintain fixation within the socket. When cement techniques of the 1970s were used, femoral loosening plateaued about 5 years after surgery. Wear properties of the ultra-high-molecular-weight polyethylene are also a concern. For this and other reasons associated with component failure, the idea of modularity was developed. Modular components, such as a polyethylene cup that snaps into a metal acetabular shell, greatly decrease the amount of surgery needed in the case of some revisions. In the case of excessive cup wear or a short femoral neck, surgery is minimized with the ability to exchange the modular components without removing the implants fixed to the bone.

Acetabular cups come with a textured back for cement fixation and may have standoff pegs to allow an appropriate cement mantle. Noncemented cups usually are porous-coated and may have screw holes present to aid in anchoring the less-than-stable cup. The presence of screw holes in an acetabular component is another controversial issue. Some believe that more wear debris is created with micromotion between the screw head and the cup as well as between the uneven surface of the screw and the polyethylene liner.

Prostheses are available for every patient's needs. Modular hip systems allow the orthopedic surgeon to choose from an array of interchangeable components that have been developed. Various femoral head sizes (22, 26, 28, and 32 mm) are available to maintain proper center of rotation. Acetabular cups may be snap fit, low profile, or deep profile, which adds additional thickness to the medial wall, where bone loss may be significant.

With modular systems, unipolar or bipolar cups are also an option when the acetabular articular surface is relatively normal. The unipolar and bipolar cups with appropriate head sizes are designed to fit on various modular system stems.

Custom prostheses or revision and extra-long stems are available when bone loss is significant. These implants are employed in cases of revision where fixation is needed farther down the femoral canal or in oncologic cases where tumor and corresponding bone have been resected.

Young, active individuals with strong, healthy bones are ideal candidates for noncemented total hip replacement arthroplasties. Elderly patients with osteoporosis and poor-quality bone are usually candidates for cemented components because their bones may lack the compressive strength to support weight-bearing forces.

***Hip Reconstruction (Cemented).*** Numerous implants are available for total hip implantation. Many of the implants can be used for the same surgical indications, and one implant may not function any better than another, provided that all other conditions and techniques are the same. The instruments required to implant any one device cannot be used for another. It is very important to ensure that all the instrumentation is available during the preoperative verification process and time out.

PMMA adheres to the polyethylene and metal but not to the bone. It fills the cavity and interstices of the bone and forms a mechanical bond. PMMA is manufactured as a liquid monomer and a powder and is mixed under sterile conditions by the scrub person in the OR at the time of implantation. It usually takes 10 to 12 minutes to harden. Because of the potentially harmful effects of PMMA fumes to the nasal epithelium, an exhaust system should be used during the mixing process.

**PROCEDURAL CONSIDERATIONS.** The patient is positioned in the lateral decubitus position and secured in place with anterior and posterior bolsters. This position is essential to ensure correct anatomic placement of the acetabular cup. Bony prominences should be adequately padded. The skin prep is completed from the level of the umbilicus down to and including the foot; then the patient is draped. The radiographs are overlaid with the implant templates.

A soft tissue set and a large bone set are required. In addition, the total hip implants and corresponding instrumentation, acetabular reamers, hip retractor set, power reamer-driver and saw, and pulse lavage with a 3-L bag of normal saline solution (Figure 22-72) will be needed. If PMMA is used, femoral canal suction wicks, a cement restrictor and its inserter, and PMMA and supplies used to mix it will be needed (Figure 22-73). If a trochanteric osteotomy is performed, the equipment of choice for its reattachment will be required.

Revision of total hip arthroplasties requires the same instrumentation as for cemented total hip in addition to cement removal instrumentation, fluoroscopy, and the revision implants and their corresponding instrumentation.

**OPERATIVE PROCEDURE**

**Cemented Modular Hip System, Anterior Approach**

1. An incision is made 2.5 cm distal and lateral to the anterosuperior iliac spine and curved distally and posteriorly over the lateral aspect of the greater trochanter and lateral surface of the femoral shaft to 5 cm distal to the base of the trochanter.
2. The tensor fasciae latae are divided over the greater trochanter, and this is carried distally to the extent of the incision. Dissection is carried proximally between the interval of the gluteus medius and the tensor fasciae latae muscles.
3. The anterior fibers of the gluteus medius tendon are tagged and detached from the trochanter. The capsule is incised longitudinally along the anterosuperior surface of the femoral neck. In the distal part of the incision, the origin of the vastus lateralis may be either reflected distally or split longitudinally to expose the base of the trochanter and proximal part of the femoral shaft.
4. Once a capsulotomy is performed, the hip can be dislocated. Adduction and external rotation will present the femoral head anteriorly into the surgical site.
5. The femoral osteotomy guide is placed over the lateral femur. This identifies the point on the femoral neck where the osteotomy should be made. Some femoral osteotomy guides also gauge the neck length required. The level is marked, and a femoral osteotomy is carried out with either an oscillating or a reciprocating saw.
6. The femur is retracted to expose the acetabulum, allow completion of the capsulotomy, and expose the bony rim of the entire acetabulum.
7. The acetabulum is inspected, any osteophytes are removed, and articular cartilage is reamed with bone-conserving reamers in a circumferential manner. The smallest reamer is

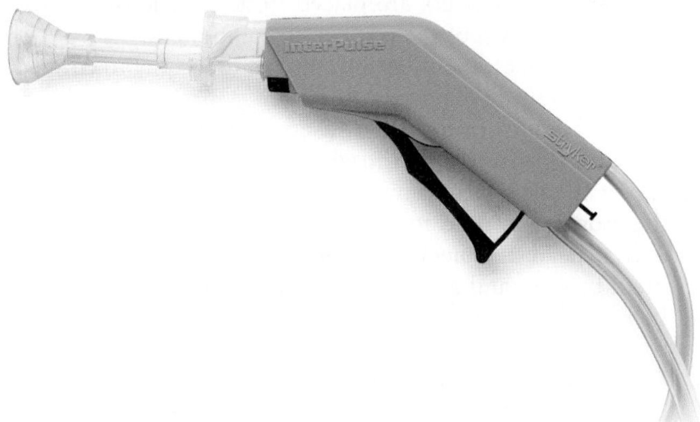


FIGURE 22-72 Pulse lavage used for pressurized irrigation when one is irrigating surgical wounds, debriding bone during a joint replacement, debriding open fractures or physically induced wounds, irrigating soft tissue injuries, or irrigating contaminated wounds.

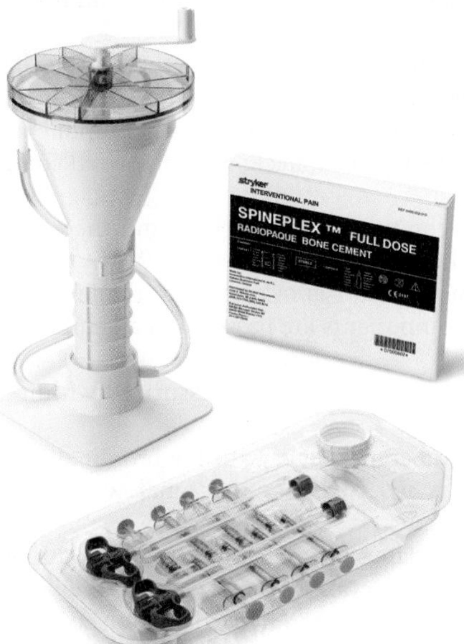


FIGURE 22-73 Polymethylmethacrylate and supplies for mixing and delivery in the canal.

progressed in a graduated method 1 or 2 mm at a time until the cartilage is reamed down to expose osteochondral bone. A hemispheric shape and bleeding bone should result.

8. Remaining soft tissue is curetted from the floor of the acetabulum, and cystic areas are filled with cancellous bone from the femoral canal and packed with a bone tamp. Any other bone grafting of major bony defects is accomplished using the fixation method of choice (bone screws).
9. Several 6-mm holes are drilled into the floor of the acetabulum, aimed into the ilium, ischium, and pubis. Holes are undercut using curettes. These prepared holes act as anchoring areas for the bone cement.
10. Trial acetabular components are placed on the positioning device and positioned in the socket. The cup is assessed for size, position within the socket, and the relationship of the component compared with the bony margins of the acetabulum.
11. The prepared acetabular socket is lavaged, dried with wicks, and filled with cement that has been injected and pressurized with an injection gun. The acetabular shell component is positioned and held motionless until the cement polymerizes. Extruded cement is trimmed from around the edge of the component. A polyethylene insert is later snapped into the shell.
12. A sponge is placed in the acetabulum to protect the component from bone debris and subsequent cement as attention is turned to the femur.
13. Dropping the foot toward the floor and internally rotating and pushing the leg proximally exposes the proximal femur. The femoral canal is accessed using a box osteotome or trochanteric reamer followed by the T-handle canal reamer.
14. Beginning with the smallest broach, the proximal femoral canal is alternately impacted and extracted. Progressively larger broaches are used to crush and remove cancellous bone until cortical bone is reached. A broach that is not advancing should not be used. This could result in shattering the femur.
15. With the final broach seated to the desired depth in the canal, the neck is prepared with a calcar reamer. The broach remains as the femoral trial component along with the various-size head, neck, and offset trial components are placed.
16. The trial component is removed, and the canal is lavaged and brushed to accommodate the PMMA.
17. A cement restrictor is inserted into the femoral canal. The femoral components are passed and assembled on the back table.
18. The cement is injected and pressurized within the femoral canal.
19. The femoral component, with the proximal and distal centralizers, is inserted into the canal with or without the femoral head.
20. The appropriate size of femoral head is positioned onto the stem, and reduction is carried out. The joint is taken through a range of motion to check for positioning, stability, and the limit to which dislocation occurs.
21. Depending on the surgeon and the surgical approach, the greater trochanter may or may not have been removed for exposure of the hip joint. If removed, it is reattached with 18-gauge wire or a cable grip system.
22. The wound is closed in layers over suction drains. The skin is closed with staples, and a sterile dressing is applied to provide compression to the wound.
23. An abduction pillow or splint is placed between the patient's legs postoperatively if stability of the joint is of concern.

***Hip Reconstruction (Noncemented).*** Fixation with a noncemented prosthesis is initially accomplished by a tight fit and intimate contact of the implants within bone of substantial strength. As with all prosthetic designs, it is essential to fill the medullary canal and wedge the prosthesis in as tightly as possible to provide temporary press-fit fixation. These prostheses closely follow normal anatomic shape. Only the instrumentation corresponding to the implant should be used. Precise machining of the femoral canal must be ensured. Acetabular components are usually press-fitted, but many systems provide holes for screw fixation if stability of the prosthesis is in doubt. Sufficient time is then allowed for the cancellous bone to heal by growing into the porous portions of the prosthesis.

The healing process requires the same amount of time as a long bone cortical fracture (approximately 3 months). Extreme caution is taken postoperatively to protect the operative hip from excessive compression, rotation, and shear stresses.

**PROCEDURAL CONSIDERATIONS.** The position and incision are the same as for the total hip replacement (cemented). The radiographs and implant templates are placed on the view box.

OPERATIVE PROCEDURE

**Noncemented Anatomic Medullary Locking (AML) Hip System** (Figure 22-74)

1. After the incision is made, the capsule is entered and the femoral head is dislocated.
2. A pilot hole is established in the trochanteric fossa as an intramedullary reference point.
3. The intramedullary canal is then reamed in a progressive manner with fully fluted rigid reamers.
4. A femoral neck osteotomy is achieved by positioning an osteotomy template along the axis of the femur and cutting at the level of the collar.
5. Attention is directed to the acetabulum, which is cleared of soft tissue and reamed with hemispheric reamers.
6. Trial acetabular sizers are placed to determine the correct position and size of the prosthetic component.
7. A hollow osteotome is used in the femoral canal to connect the pilot hole to the osteotomy site.
8. Femoral broaches are then inserted to enlarge the intramedullary space for trial insertion.
9. A power calcar planer may be placed over the trunnion of the broach and used to contour the femoral neck.
10. A trial head and neck component is positioned onto the fitted broach, and a trial reduction is carried out.
11. If trial reduction is satisfactory, all trial components are removed.
12. The appropriate size of acetabular component is inserted into the acetabulum, and a polyethylene insert is locked into place.
13. The femoral component is placed into the canal, and the modular head is seated on the trunnion.
14. Reduction of the hip is followed by standard closure with drains.

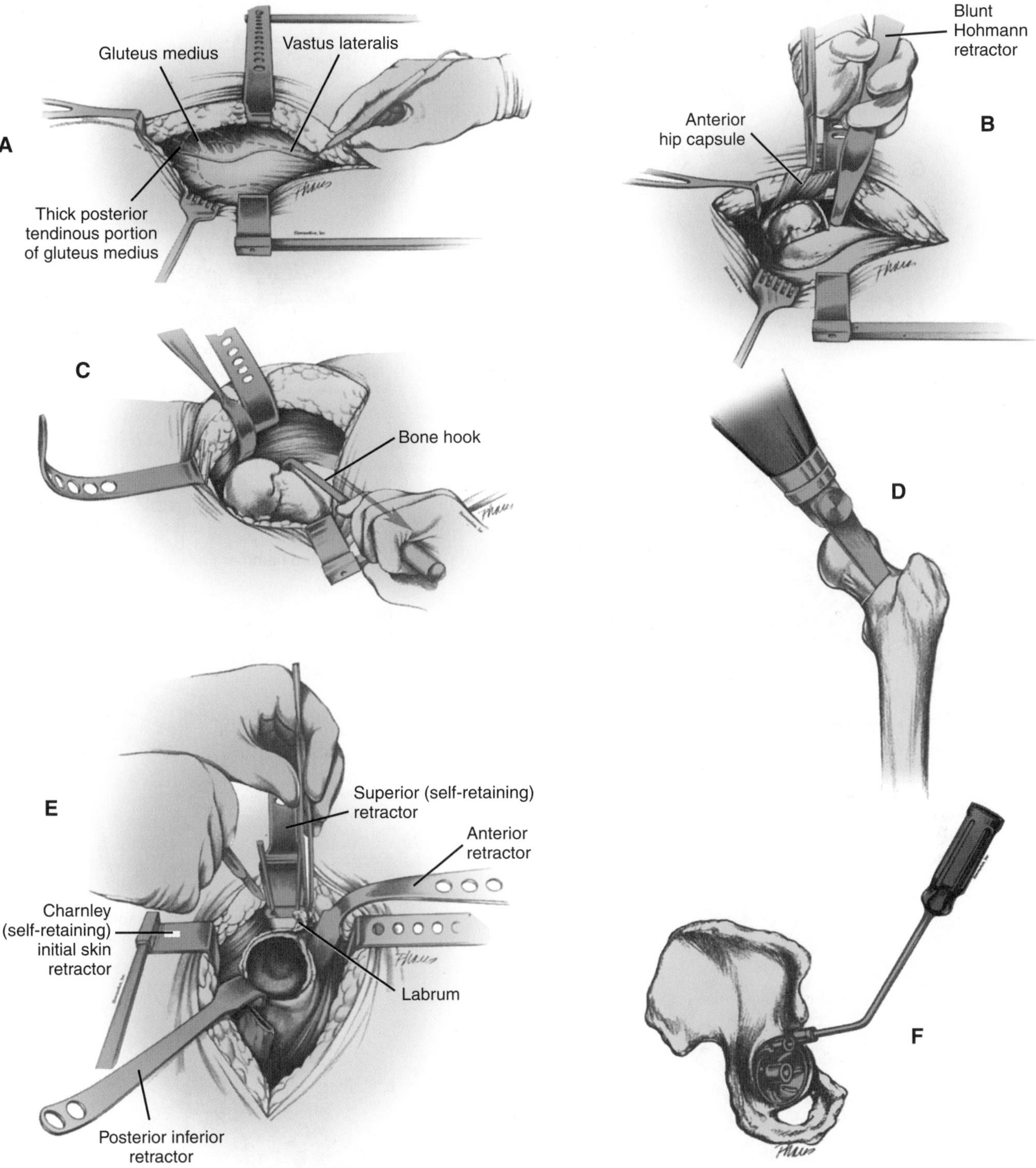


**FIGURE 22-74** Noncemented hip reconstruction. **A,** After the incision, the Charnley retractor is placed, the fascia lata is incised, and the gluteus minimus is detached. **B,** An anterior capsulotomy is completed. **C,** The hip is flexed, adducted, and externally rotated to dislocate from the acetabulum. **D,** The femoral neck is cut by use of an oscillating saw blade. **E,** The rim of the acetabulum is debrided of labrum, redundant capsule, and marginal osteophytes. **F,** The acetabulum is reamed; after reaming, the appropriate drill guide is inserted into the acetabulum.

*Continued*

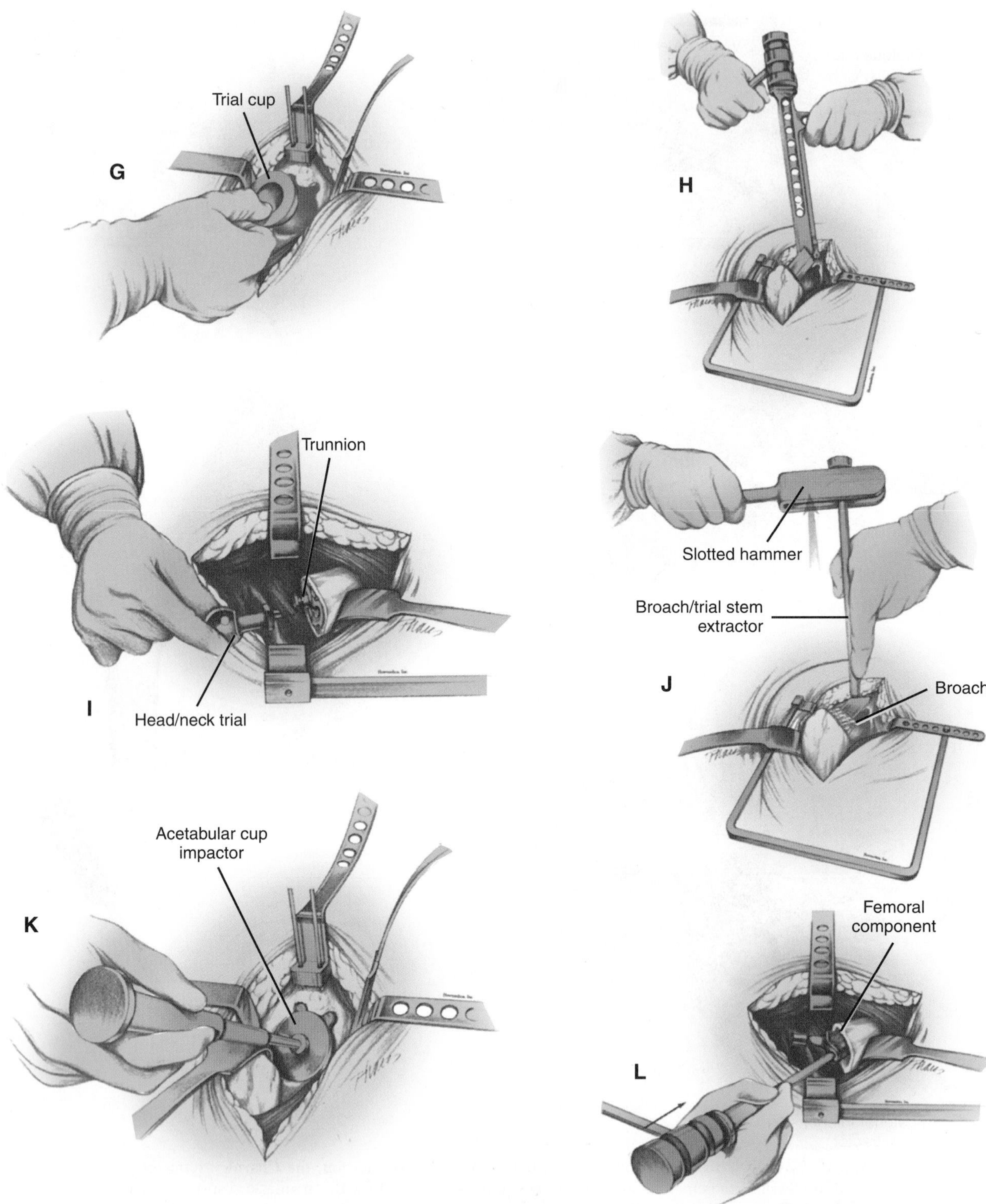


**FIGURE 22-74, cont'd.** **G,** After drilling the holes for the acetabular fixation pegs, the trial acetabular cup is inserted. **H,** The proximal wedge of cancellous bone is removed, and the appropriate size of femoral broach is introduced down the axis of the femoral canal. **I,** The trial head is placed on the broach trunnion of trial reduction. **J,** With the slotted hammer, the femoral broach is extracted; the trial acetabular cup is removed. **K,** Acetabular fixation pegs are seated, the acetabular cup is introduced, and the component is seated. **L,** The femoral canal is irrigated with pulsatile lavage and dried with suction and sponges; the femoral canal is plugged and filled with methylmethacrylate; the femoral component is inserted.

*Continued*

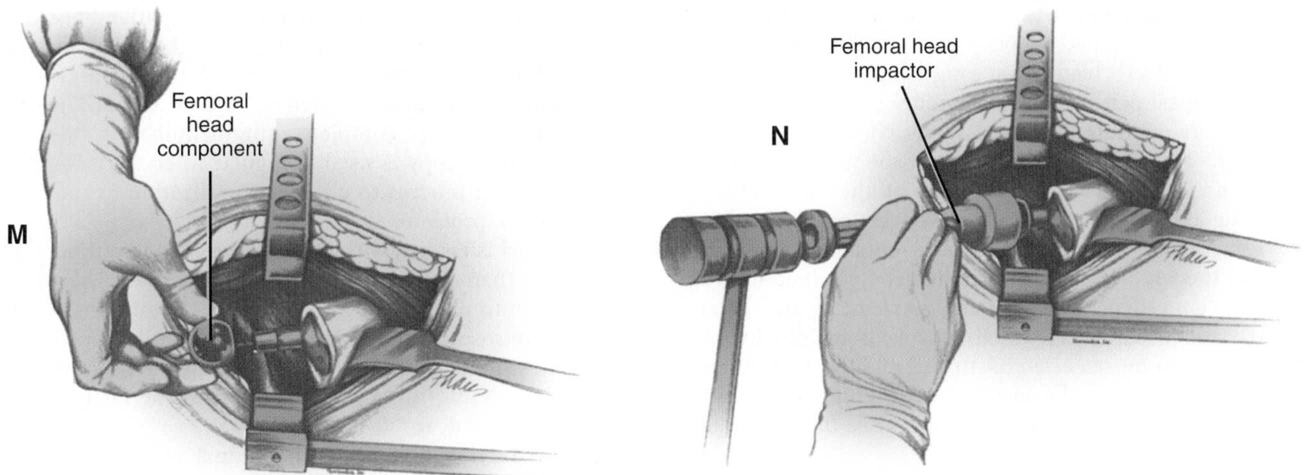


FIGURE 22-74, cont'd. **M,** The femoral head component is placed on the trunnion. **N,** The femoral head is impacted, the femur is reduced, and the wound is irrigated before closure.

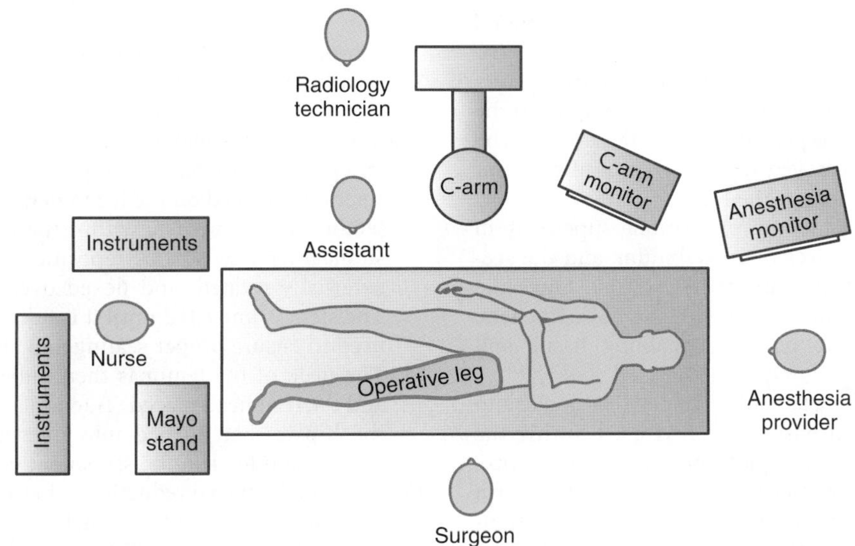


FIGURE 22-75 Illustration of room setup, including positioning of C-arm and monitor, for minimally invasive total hip arthroplasty (THA).

15. Abduction of the hip is maintained postoperatively with a foam abduction pillow if necessary.

***Minimally Invasive Total Hip Arthroplasty.*** Minimally invasive total hip arthroplasty (MITHA) has resulted in minimized scarring, reduced patient morbidity, a shortened hospitalization period, and an accelerated rehabilitation process.[9] MITHA can be performed with a single or double incision (described here). For a single incision, the patient is placed in a lateral position; the patient is supine for a double-incision procedure.[17] With two-incision MITHA, the acetabular and femoral components are inserted through two small incisions, one anterolateral and one posterolateral, each approximately 2 inches long.[7] The technique spares the muscles and tendons around the hip.

PROCEDURAL CONSIDERATIONS. As with any joint replacement, templates of the x-rays preoperatively are recommended. A regular OR bed with x-ray capability is used. The perioperative nurse should alert the radiology department that fluoroscopy (often referred to in the OR as the C-arm) will be used. Equipment should be arranged carefully (Figure 22-75). The patient is positioned supine with a small bolster placed under the pelvis on the operative side. The patient's entire hip, from above the waist to the ankle, is then prepped and draped in the usual fashion. The time out includes confirmation of the correct patient, site, side, procedure, position, and implants.

OPERATIVE PROCEDURE (VERSYS HIP SYSTEM)

1. The C-arm is used to define the femoral neck. The anterior incision is made first directly over the femoral neck from the base of the femoral head. A Weitlaner retractor, DeBakey forceps, and electrocoagulation will be used. The lateral femoral cutaneous nerve is identified and located, then carefully retracted along with the sartorius with an Army-Navy retractor. A second retractor is used for the tensor fasciae latae laterally. This exposes the lateral border of the rectus femoris.

2. The lateral femoral vessels are coagulated. The Army-Navy retractors are extended deeper as the rectus femoris is dissected with a #10 blade on a long handle. A long-tipped electrosurgical pencil (active electrode) may also be used.
3. The femoral capsule is incised, along with the fat pad. A Cobb elevator is used to move the tissue medially underneath the rectus muscles and laterally off the femoral neck, allowing exposure of the capsule over the femoral neck.
4. Two curved lit retractors are placed outside the capsule around the femoral neck, perpendicular to it. If additional leverage is needed, retractor handle extenders may be attached and used. The femoral capsule is incised in line with the femoral neck lateral to the midline to facilitate future placement of the head of the femoral prosthesis. Sutures can be used to retract the capsule so that the femoral head and neck are clearly visible.
5. Fluoroscopy may then be used to verify osteotomy position. Using the oscillating saw, a high femoral neck cut is made. A straight, 4-cm osteotome completes the cut. A second cut is then made, and a threaded Steinman pin is inserted to remove the small wafer of bone. This allows enough room for the surgeon to make the final femoral neck cut.
6. Fluoroscopy is used to check the angle and length of resection. It is important for the surgical team to help keep the leg in neutral position, especially during these cuts. The femoral head is then removed while the surgical assistant is applying gentle traction on the leg.
7. Three lit anterior retractors are placed: one superiorly in the line of the incision, over the acetabulum, and the second and third at 90-degree angles to the first. Once the acetabulum is exposed, dissection with the ESU, Kochers, and forceps are used to remove remaining tissue and synovium.
8. Reaming starts with the acetabular reamer that is close to the template size. C-arm visualization is used during the reaming. Once reaming is completed to the acceptable size, the trial components are placed to determine fit. C-arm images are used to confirm location and size. The positioning bolster is removed at this time. The appropriate-size cup and liner are then chosen. The acetabular component is then seated using the offset shell inserter, retractors are removed, and the cup is impacted into place. Multiple images are taken to check the placement and position of the cup while impacting. The inserter is then removed. If screws are used, a drill, screws, drill guide, depth gauge, and flexible screwdriver will be required. Once the cup and screws are in place, their position is again checked with fluoroscopy. The liner is inserted.
9. The second incision is found by direct palpation. The nonoperative leg is adducted. The operative leg is fully adducted, externally rotated, and flexed over the nonoperative leg. Location is verified by fluoroscopy. A stab wound is made in the posterior lateral buttock and extended to 1.5 to 3 cm as needed. A self-retaining Weitlaner retractor is used to retract the gluteus maximus and subcutaneous fat. Long Mayo scissors spread the tissue along the co-axial pathway to the piriformis fossa. The scissors are advanced into the canal in the closed position, then opened, and then slowly backed out of the wound in the opened position, repeating as necessary to clear a good pathway.
10. Downward pressure is applied to the operative knee to elevate the trochanter. The tissue protector is inserted. Reaming the femoral canal begins with the lateral reamers. All reamers should be inserted in the locked position. Once lateral reaming is complete, intramedullary reamers are used. Fluoroscopy is used at regular intervals throughout the reaming process to ensure centralization in the canal. The tissue protector is then removed.
11. The canal is rasped, with the initial rasp two to three times smaller than the template size of the canal. The rasp is tapped into place until fully seated; its position is verified with fluoroscopy. The canal is rasped until proper sizing and positioning are obtained. The C-arm is used to check the final depth, fill, and positioning of the rasp with the apex of the calcar.
12. Trial reduction is done with the final rasp in place. The provisional head is placed on the rasp, and the hip is reduced by providing longitudinal traction and internal rotation. The hip is put through a full range of motion. Fluoroscopy can assess the levels of the lesser trochanters to check possible leg length discrepancies. Once trial reduction is complete, the rasp is removed by way of a posterior exit and the head through the anterior incision.
13. Two lit anterior retractors are placed in the posterior incision to keep the tissue away from the stem as it is placed in the femoral canal. Once the implant is through the skin and properly rotated, the implant driver is attached. Gentle traction is placed on the leg in neutral abduction. Once the femoral component is within the capsule of the hip, the surgical leg needs to be repositioned; it is fully adducted, externally rotated, and flexed over the nonoperative leg. The stem is impacted until it is fully seated. Fluoroscopy is used to ensure proper seating and alignment.
14. The neck of the femur is then pulled through the wound and the trial head placed. Traction is placed on the hip, and the hip is then turned into internal rotation. Range-of-motion and leg length assessment is then done.
15. After the final trial reduction is performed, the hip is dislocated in order to put the final head in place. Hip dislocation is done using a dull bone hook and external rotation of the hip. Two sutures are placed in the capsule: one medially and the other laterally. This is done before the head is reduced to prevent the capsule from invaginating posteriorly. The prosthetic head can then be seated and impacted. Again gentle traction and internal rotation are used to reduce the hip. A final range-of-motion and leg length assessment is performed.
16. Both incisions are irrigated with antibiotic irrigation. A local anesthetic such as bupivacaine (Marcaine) may be infiltrated into the incision, the two previously placed sutures tied, and additional sutures placed to fully close the capsule. A drain may be placed.

## Total Knee Replacement

Total knee replacement (arthroplasty) is a surgical procedure designed to replace the worn surfaces of the knee joint. Patients with severe destruction of the knee joint resulting from degenerative rheumatoid or traumatic arthritis or destruction of only the medial or lateral compartments of the knee joint as a result of extreme varus or valgus deformity complain of pain and instability (Research Highlight). Arthroplasty of the knee has been successful in relieving these symptoms. Success depends on patient selection, component design, surgical technique, and rehabilitation (Research Highlight).

The challenge of finding the optimal knee implant is in reproducing the complicated range of motion of the knee. Motion of the knee occurs in three planes: flexion and extension, abduction and adduction, and rotation. Designs of total knees should allow preservation of the normal ligaments whenever possible while providing soft tissue balance when necessary to maintain stability.

Total knee implants may be classified into three different categories, according to the portions of the knee to be replaced. *Unicompartmental* implants are used to replace just one opposing articular surface (medial or lateral) of the femur and tibia. These implants, however, lost popularity as a result of biomechanical and technical pitfalls. *Bicompartmental* designs, mentioned only to demonstrate the progression of total knee design, replaced both the medial and lateral surfaces of the femur and tibia. Most of the total knee replacements completed today are *tricompartmental* implants, which replace not only the opposing femorotibial joint but also the patellofemoral joint.

The tricompartmental knees are further divided into three categories (Figure 22-76). *Unconstrained* prostheses have very little constraint built in between the femoral and tibial components and depend on the integrity of soft tissues to provide stability of the reconstructed joint. Where there is significant deformity and the need for soft tissue release, the surgeon may decide to use a *semiconstrained* prosthesis, which lends itself to more inherent stability necessitated by ligamentous deficiency.

*Fully constrained* prostheses are linked together with pure hinges, rotating hinges, and nonhinged designs. They are used in the presence of considerable bone loss, instability, deformity, and revision surgery where bone loss has been significant. Fully constrained prostheses do not provide a normal range of motion, and such a lack leads to excessive wear and implant loosening and breakage.

Methods of fixation of total knee implants include both cemented and noncemented techniques. The noncemented variety encompasses both porous bony ingrowth and press-fit designs. The choice of implant and method of fixation depend on the predisposition of the bone, the patient's age and activity level, and the surgeon's comfort with a particular technique. Previous designs did not retain the posterior cruciate ligament, which possibly led to increased joint instability. Newer designs allow the posterior cruciate to be retained. Some surgeons believe that the retention of the posterior cruciate ligament dictates the need for absolute ligament balancing beyond what may be possible in the reconstructed knee.

In the interest of more cost-effective use of medical resources, new designs have been developed for the less-active patient with a shorter expected life span. The femoral compo-

## RESEARCH HIGHLIGHT

### Cartilage Paste Grafting for Arthritic Knees

Degenerative changes in the cartilage of the knee result in loss of motion, joint effusion, and deformity. Surgical procedures such as cartilage debridement, penetrating subchondral bone to stimulate marrow, and cartilage resurfacing and regrowth with autologous osteochondral transplant have been used with inconsistent results. None of the procedures are indicated for patients who have significant arthritic knee changes.

Cartilage paste grafting is an arthroscopic procedure involving the formation of an osteocartilaginous paste from the intercondylar notch and injecting it into the chondral defect. The paste is believed to improve the vascular flow to the area and stimulate normal cartilage growth. In this study, 145 patients with a confirmed full-thickness chondral fracture in the knee, classified as Outerbridge grade IV, underwent treatment with a cartilage paste graft; 125 patients were considered a clinical success, based on significant improvement in pain, functioning, and activity measures ($p < .001$). Of 66 patients undergoing second-look arthroscopy, 63.6% demonstrated evidence of replacement of their articular surface and 27.3% developed areas of cartilage that were indistinguishable from normal.

Based on the results of their longitudinal study, the authors concluded that the procedure offers excellent, long-lasting pain relief and restored function for patients with painful chondral lesions in arthritic knees.

Modified from Stone KR and others: Cartilage paste grafting may be cost-effective, long-lasting for arthritic knees, *Journal of Arthroscopy* 22: 291-299, 2006.

## RESEARCH HIGHLIGHT

### Total Knee Replacement: A Consensus Statement

Total knee replacement (TKR) often represents a final attempt to alleviate painful primary osteoarthritis. The benefits of TKR in restoring mobility and relieving discomfort have been confirmed. More than 300,000 of these procedures are done each year, and 90% of patients have improvement in pain, function, and quality of life. Perioperative mortality is low at 0.5%, and deep wound infections occur in fewer than 1% of patients. A panel convened by the National Institutes of Health reviewed 20 years of follow-up data on patients who underwent TKR, noting the following:

- Candidates for elective TKR have radiographic evidence of joint damage, pain not relieved by lesser means, diminished quality of life, and realistic goals and expectations.
- Relative contraindications include morbid obesity, severe peripheral vascular disease, and neurologic impairment.
- Rheumatoid arthritis, diabetes, obesity, and use of corticosteroids are associated with wound and deep-tissue infections.
- Both the volume of procedures performed by the individual surgeon and the hospital are related to better outcomes.
- Proper alignment of the prosthesis is crucial to minimize loosening, which is the main factor requiring a surgical revision.
- Goals of revision surgery include restoration of alignment, restoration of joint line and space, and achievement of stable implant fixation.
- Use of ultra clean–air operating rooms (ORs) and whole-body exhaust ventilated suits is supported by some data but not universally adopted because of lingering uncertainty about their impact.
- TKR is considered a high-risk procedure for the development of venous thromboembolism (VTE).

Modified from *NIH Consensus Development Conference on Total Knee Replacement.* Accessed April 12, 2006, on-line: www.consensus.nih.gov/2003/2003TotalKneeReplacement; Rankin EA, Thomas CM: *Orthopedic surgery update: what's new in total joint replacement.* Presented at the 2006 AORN Congress, Washington, DC, March 20, 2006.

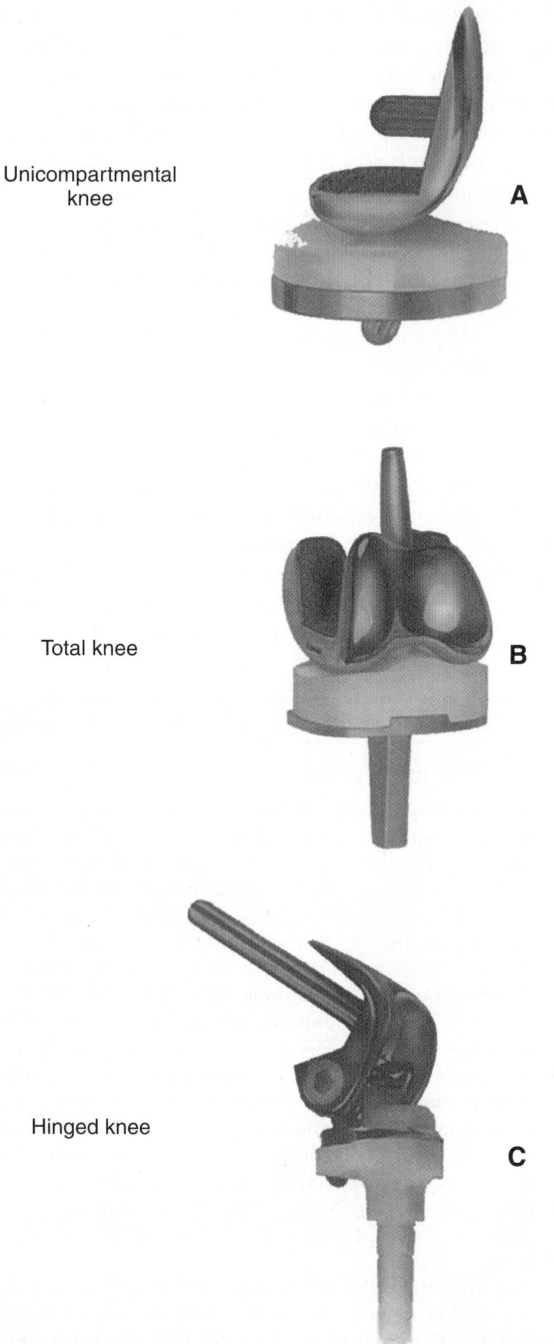


FIGURE 22-76 Knee arthroplasty implants. **A,** Unconstrained hinge. **B,** Semiconstrained hinge. **C,** Fully constrained hinge.

nent design is a symmetric design that can be used on either the left or the right knee. The tibial component is composed entirely of UHMWPE, thereby lowering manufacturing costs. Both components are placed with the use of PMMA.

***Procedural Considerations.*** The patient is placed in the supine position. A tourniquet is applied to the upper thigh. The surgical prep is completed. A soft tissue set and a large bone set; the total knee instruments, trials, and implants of choice; a power drill and saw; PMMA and cement supplies; and a pulse lavage will be required.

### *Operative Procedure*

#### NEXGEN TOTAL KNEE REPLACEMENT (FIGURE 22-77)

1. With the knee slightly flexed, a straight midline incision is made from 3 to 4 inches above the patella, ending at the patellar tubercle.
2. The capsule is entered medially. After a median parapatellar incision is made, Kochers are placed on both lateral and medial sides of the capsule, and then the patella is reflected laterally to expose the entire tibiofemoral joint.
3. Hypertrophic synovium, a portion of the infrapatellar fat pad, is excised using a toothed forceps and knife or the ESU, and then the osteophytes are removed using a rongeur. This allows easy access to the medial, lateral, and intercondylar spaces and to facilitate soft tissue releases, should the need arise.
4. The knee is flexed to 90 degrees, and Hohmann retractors are placed deep to the collateral ligaments and anterior to the posterior capsule as well as laterally to the patella to protect these structures during resection of the proximal tibia. A Richardson retractor is placed medially to protect the medial collateral ligament (MCL).
5. The distal cutting alignment guide is positioned extramedullary and parallel to the proximal tibial spine. Proper rotational alignment is established by positioning the appropriate malleoli wings parallel to the transmalleolar axis. The alignment rod is proximally placed just slightly lateral to the tibial tubercle.
6. The osteotomy saw is then used to resect the proximal portion of the tibia. The distal cutting guide is removed. Alignment is checked with a Gerber guide (spacer block with the alignment rod) by placing the guide on the tibia. This checks the tibial cut for valgus alignment. The tibia is then sized with templates.
7. Before proceeding further, the surgeon ensures that the extremity can be brought into normal mediolateral (ML) alignment in extension. If not, additional soft tissue balancing is performed until the normal mechanical axis is obtained.
8. The AP cutting guide is then used to size the femur. The guide yoke is attached to the AP block, and the yoke is slipped under the muscle anteriorly on the periosteum. The middle nail is hammered into place, while pressing down on the guide yoke. Then by pulling up on the yoke, the valgus alignment is achieved such that it is square with the tibial cut. The block is then nailed into place with two pins.
9. With the AP femoral guide in place, right-angle retractors are positioned to protect the MCL and lateral collateral ligament (LCL). The anterior and posterior portions of the femur are resected. The tibial and femoral cuts are checked for balance and size at the same time with a tibial block.
10. Once the flexion balance is determined, the distal femoral cutting block is set. The tensor, placed in flexion, is then slowly brought out into extension. Tension is placed on the extension gap by dialing between 30 to 40 pounds of pressure on the tensor. The amount of pressure dialed up on the tensor is based on the patient's size and tightness of the ligaments. The distal cutting jig is then placed in the tensor. Once the jig is secured, the two pin holes are drilled and the tensor removed. The distal cutting guide is then

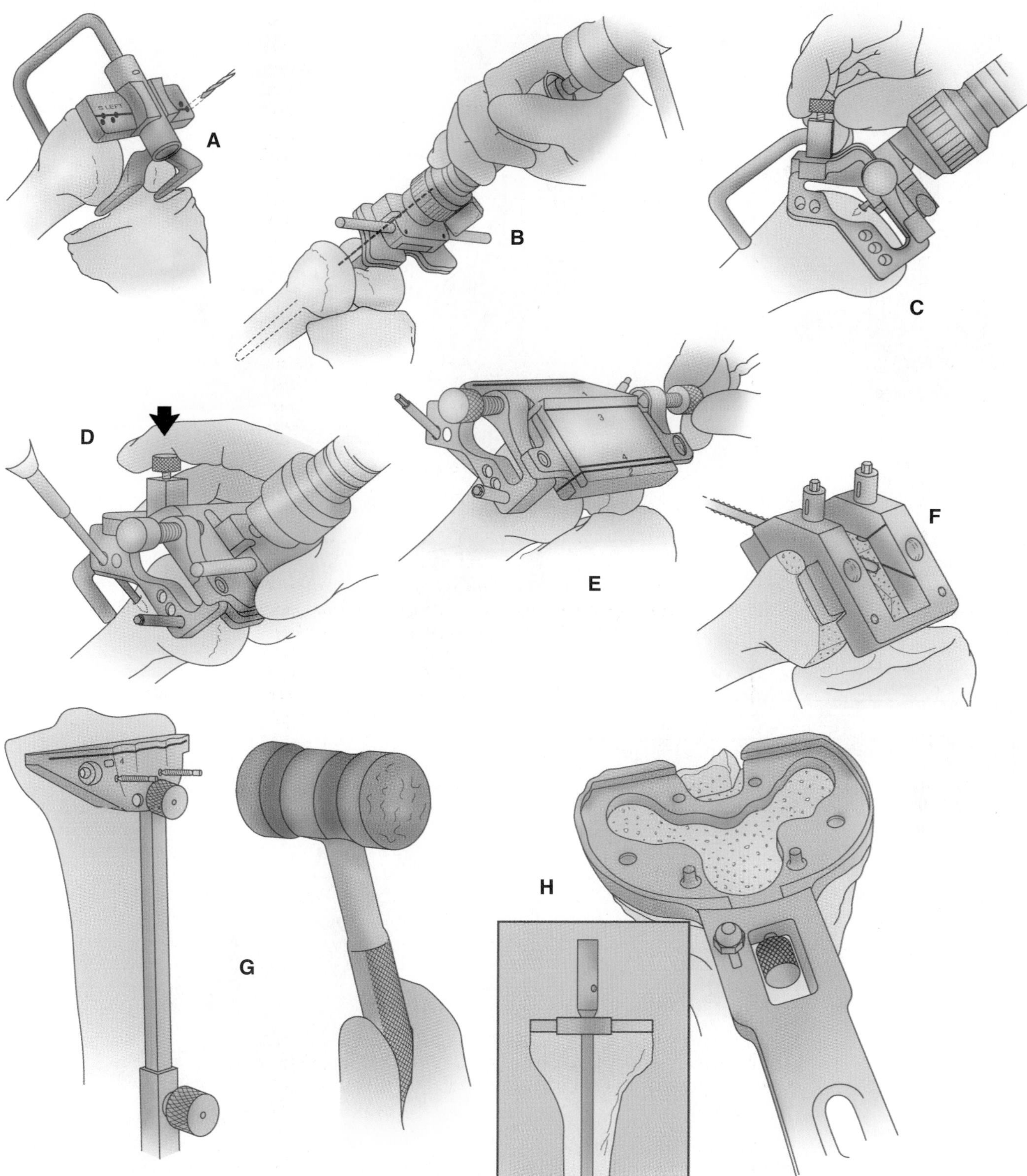


**FIGURE 22-77** Total knee implant, instrumentation, and procedure. **A,** After exposure of the intercondylar notch, the femoral sizer is placed at the distal end of the femur. **B,** After the femoral canal is reamed, the femoral intramedullary alignment guide is inserted and passed up the medullary canal. **C,** Correct rotational alignment is maintained; the anterior femoral cutting guide is attached to the femoral intramedullary alignment guide. **D,** The femoral cutting guide is mounted in place. **E,** The femur is resected. **F,** Femoral cuts are completed. **G,** The tibial alignment guide is placed and secured; the tibia is resected. **H,** The tibia is sized.

*Continued*

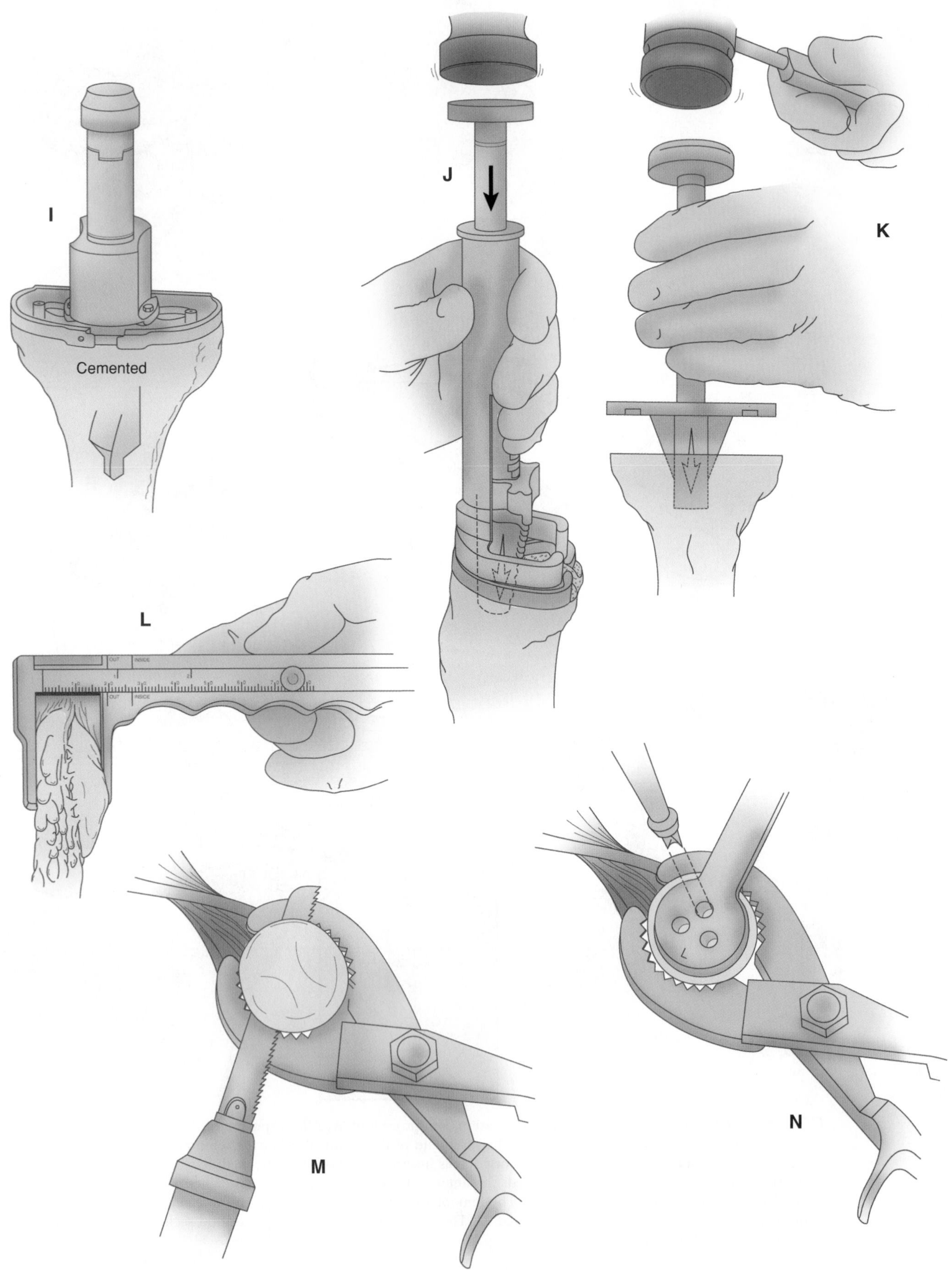


**FIGURE 22-77, cont'd.** **I,** The tibia is reamed. **J,** The tibia is impacted. **K,** The tibial trial is inserted. **L,** The patella is measured. **M,** The patella is sized. **N,** The patella is drilled.

placed in the exact two pin holes made by the distal cutting jig. The knee is then flexed, and the distal portion of the femur is resected.

11. The appropriate spacer block is then used to ensure equal tension in flexion and extension.
12. The knee is placed in flexion; the femoral notch and chamfer guide is centered between the epicondyles and impacted until fully seated. Three anterior fixation pins secure the guide to the femur. Two ¼-inch holes are drilled into the distal end of the femur, and the anterior and posterior chamfers are cut with the oscillating saw. The box osteotome is used to make the notch cut from the proximal end of the finishing guide. A power saw is used to resect the posterior femoral condyle remnants to ensure adequate flexion clearance. The femoral trial is then positioned.
13. The tibial size is reassessed using the tibial templates. The selected tibial template is then positioned rotationally and drilled, and the appropriate-size centering punch is used to cut through the subchondral bone. The tibial trial is then placed.
14. The patella is first measured. Then two towel clips are placed onto the distal and proximal portions of the patella tendon, and the appropriate resection is performed. The patellar template is placed over the resected surface, and the cruciate channels are created using the patellar drill through the slots in the template.
15. A trial reduction is performed. If this reduction proves satisfactory with regard to alignment and ligament laxity, trial components are removed, bone surfaces are irrigated with a pulsatile lavage, and the permanent components are placed. These can be inserted without bone cement, with bone cement, or with a combination of both.
16. Drains are placed in the joint depending on the surgeon's preference. The joint is closed in the usual fashion, and a compression dressing is applied to the leg. The tourniquet can be released before closure or after the dressing has been applied.

Aftercare consists of rapid mobilization and strengthening, with a target discharge of 3 to 4 days postoperatively.

### *Stryker Navigation Total Knee Arthroplasty*

PROCEDURAL CONSIDERATIONS (FIGURE 22-78). During the surgical approach, the company representative will be initializing (setting up) the Smart Tools instrumentation with the scrub person. Health care industry representatives can provide valuable technical support to the perioperative team.[4] Integration of surgical instrumentation and computers results in the ability to build a customized, digital map of the patient's anatomy and navigate the surgical instruments according to this map.[27] Successfully executed steps are marked with a blue checkmark and are graphically visualized. Proper setup is achieved when all Smart Tools are shown inside the camera's working space.

A tourniquet, foot holder, and ESU are required. An indwelling Foley catheter is inserted, and antibiotics and heparin will usually be ordered.

OPERATIVE PROCEDURE

1. The capsule is entered medially. After a median parapatellar incision is made, Kochers are placed on both lateral and medial sides of the capsule, and then the patella is reflected laterally to expose the entire tibiofemoral joint.

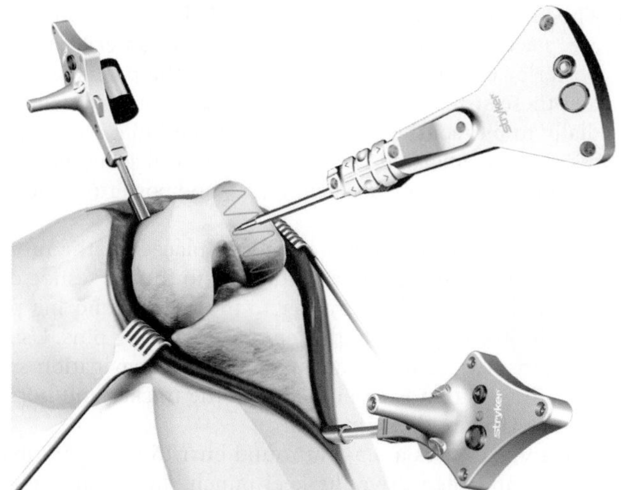


**FIGURE 22-78** Stryker Navigation Tracking Equipment.

2. Using electrodissection at the anterior tibia, raising the medial flap is started.
3. With a finger to retract medially, the tibial anchoring pin is placed (self-tapping screws) at the distal aspect of the exposure. Drilling is then undertaken from the anterior to posterior tibial cortex using a 3.2-mm drill bit parallel to the joint line and rotated approximately 30 degrees medially.
4. Using a depth gauge, the surgeon rounds off to the size larger than measured (pins are available in 5-mm increments).
5. The pin is placed on a T-handle for the surgeon to manually screw in the anchoring pin.
6. For the femoral anchoring pin, the surgeon next drills from the anterior to posterior femoral cortex, measures with a depth gauge, rounds up to the next larger size, and inserts the pin with a T-handle.
7. The blue tracker (B = bottom) is attached to the tibial pin and the green tracker to the femoral pin. Trackers should be placed so they are facing the camera attached to the navigation system.
8. The femoral head is registered. The hip is placed at 0 to 20 degrees of flexion and then at 45 degrees of flexion. As the leg is rotated, the LED locations yield a set of data points relative to the size of the femoral head.
9. The distal femur is then registered. The medial and lateral condyles, the center of the knee, and the AP axis of the knee are digitalized to identify the articulating surfaces.
10. The proximal tibia is then registered. The center of the tibia, AP axis, and medial and lateral tibial plateaus are traced in a similar fashion to the femur, which identifies the slope of the tibia.
11. The knee is brought through range of motion from full extension to full flexion. This kinematic datum is calculated and then recorded. Once data are recorded, the trackers are removed.
12. Hypertrophic synovium and a portion of the infrapatellar fat pad are excised using a toothed forceps and knife or ESU; the osteophytes are removed using a rongeur. This allows easy access to the medial, lateral, and intercondylar spaces and facilitates soft tissue releases, should the need arise.

13. The knee is flexed to 90 degrees, and Hohmann retractors are placed to the MCL and immediately anterior to the posterior capsule as well as laterally to the patella to protect these structures. A Richardson retractor is placed medially to protect the MCL. A Kocher and knife are used to resect the medial and lateral menisci as well as remnants of the anterior cruciate ligament (ACL) and posterior cruciate ligament (PCL).
14. The navigated tibial cutting guide is placed on the proximal tibia. A cutting guide is attached to the horseshoe device and then the blue tracker to the tibial anchoring pin and the green tracker to the femoral anchoring pins. Using two pins, the guide is anchored. With the navigation system, the position is confirmed, and the tracker and horseshoe device are then removed.
15. The surgeon uses a 5.5-mm round burr to open the tibial surface and then drive the keel punch slightly anteriorly. The guide and pins are then removed.
16. The horseshoe device is placed with the opening posterior on the distal femur with two pins. The distal femoral cutting guide is attached to the device, and the blue tracker is attached to the blue anchoring pins. Finally, the green tracker is attached to the femoral anchoring pins.
17. The surgeon manipulates the cutting guide to the distal femur. The first pin is driven into the guide and adjusted, and then the second and third pins are placed. The horseshoe and pins are removed. The saw is flushed with the cutting guide, the green top is attached, and the blue Gurba guide set on the tibial surface to check the cuts.
18. The femoral 4-in-1 cutting guide is placed, and the pin is placed and cut with the saw. The LCL and MCL are protected with a finger or right angle retractors and the pins removed.
19. The Booth retractor is then placed over tibia. After the notch guide and pin are placed, the tibia is cut to an appropriate depth, using a saw as well as chamfer cuts. The pins and guide are then removed.
20. Next, the patella is measured; then two towel clips are placed onto the distal and proximal portions of patella tendon, and the appropriate resection is performed. The patellar template is placed over the resected surface, and the cruciate channels are created using the patellar drill through the slots in the template.
21. Trial components are placed, trackers attached, and the knee brought through a full range of motion. The trials and anchoring pins are then removed.
22. PMMA is prepared. Bone surfaces are irrigated with a pulsatile lavage, and the permanent components are placed. These can be inserted without bone cement, with bone cement, or using a combination of both.
23. Drains are placed in the joint depending on the surgeon's preference. The joint is closed in the usual fashion, and a compression dressing is applied to the leg. The tourniquet can be released before closure or after the dressing has been applied.

Aftercare consists of rapid mobilization and strengthening, with a target discharge of 3 to 4 days postoperatively.

***Total Knee Revision Arthroplasty.*** Total joint revision can be very demanding and complicated surgery. Attention to detail, anticipation, and preparation are essential. Important patient information includes the preoperative x-rays, bone scan, laboratory results (including aspiration results), and physical findings.

**PROCEDURAL CONSIDERATIONS.** The patient is placed in supine position with a footrest for the affected leg. An OR bed with x-ray capability is used. Following the administration of anesthesia, an EUA is done. Although one of the most difficult aspects of revision surgery is that there is no clear-cut sequence of events, it is best, if possible, to approach revision surgery using the same logical sequence for each procedure. This allows all members of the surgical team to anticipate the steps in the procedure and the needs of the patient. Antibiotics are held, usually at the surgeon's request, to allow for one final attempt to recover an organism if infection is present. Tissue and fluid cultures are obtained when the initial incision is made through the capsule and into the joint space. Once the cultures are obtained, antibiotics are given.

Instrumentation includes a basic knee set, primary total knee instrumentation and trials (in case only one portion of the prosthesis is revised); revision instrumentation to extract the components and cement; instrumentation and trials for the revision components; cementing system and extra cement (usually double the amount of cement used in a primary total knee arthroplasty); and power equipment including saw, reamer, and burrs.

**OPERATIVE PROCEDURE.** The previous skin incision is usually used. This maintains adequate blood flow to the skin. The skin is marked to reapproximate the skin edges after surgery. A tourniquet is used after determining that there are no contraindications based on the patient's medical and surgical history.

1. Using a #10 blade, a skin incision is made through the scar from the original surgery.
2. With heavy tooth forceps and knife, the skin is undermined on each side of the incision; this allows the skin to be more easily closed at the end of the procedure.
3. Once at the capsule, a clean #10 blade is used to make a medial parapatellar incision into the joint. A Kocher is placed on the medial side of the capsule, and a towel clip is placed laterally, immediate to the patella, to aid with eversion.
4. Both tissue and fluid cultures are taken. Antibiotics are then administered by the anesthesia provider.
5. Using heavy tooth forceps or a Kocher, a synovectomy is performed with a knife or electrodissection. A clean dissection is needed to allow visualization of the bone prosthesis interface and to remove any synovitis caused by poly debris or metalosis.
6. The medial ligament, stripped during the original surgery, is peeled cleanly away with a periosteal elevator.
7. The knee is dislocated with posterior placement of a Hohmann retractor immediately behind the tibia. A second Hohmann retractor is placed laterally to the patella and LCL. Medially, a Richardson retractor provides protection of the MCL.
8. If possible, the poly tibia insert is removed at this time to allow better visualization and an increased work space.
9. Using an osteotomy saw with a small blade, the surgeon will proceed to remove the tibial plate at the bone-prosthesis interface. If the saw is unable to complete the cuts, ¼- or ½-inch curved osteotomes may be used to get to the pos-

terior lateral corner. Cement is then removed from the canal using a Kocher, ¼-inch straight osteotome, chisels, mallet, and curettes. If the cement is deep, a heavy toothed alligator forceps may be required.

10. Once the tibia and cement are removed, the tibia surface is recut using an osteotomy saw and alignment guide. Sometimes, the tibia is completely revised before the next step. If so, the tibial template, pins, mallet, and punch will be needed.
11. With the patella everted, a Booth retractor is placed under the femur. Using a ½-inch curved osteotome and mallet, the femoral component is removed. A ¼-inch curved osteotome may be required if there are metal pegs at the distal end on the femoral component or at the posterior edge of the prosthesis. Once both sides of the prosthesis are loosened, it should fall off. If not, a femoral distractor will be used.
12. Any remaining cement is removed using osteotomes, chisels, or the saw. Any cement in the canal will be removed with a Kocher or alligator forcep.
13. Next the posterior capsule is addressed. With the leg in extension, a lamina spreader is placed between the femur and tibia. Using curettes and a rongeur, the scar on the posterior capsule is removed to improve postoperative range of motion.
14. Once the capsule is released, attention is turned to rebuilding the femur. This is done by using a series of guides and trial components.
15. Augmentation of both tibia and femur components can be done using either metal augments or bone grafting. Balance between the femur and tibia is obtained first in flexion and then in extension.
16. The last component to be revised is the patella. Two towel clips are placed, distal and proximal on either side of the patella, and the button is removed, using a large-blade osteotomy saw. All poly buttons can be readily removed by this method. However, a metal-backed patella requires the additional use of a ¼-inch osteotome. Any remaining cement is removed from holes with a curette or 6.0 mm burr on a drill. The patella will be recut using a large-blade osteotomy saw.
17. The guide is placed on the patella, and the drill is used for new holes. The trial button is placed, the patella inverted, and the knee placed through a range of motion.
18. All components are removed, and the knee is irrigated with antibiotic solution using pulsatile lavage. The bone edges are dried with suction and clean sponges. This is done while the cement is being mixed.
19. Components can be cemented all at once or in stages, depending on the surgeon's preference.
20. The femur is usually cemented first. The Booth retractor is placed under the femur, and cement is put on the posterior phalanges of the femoral component and then on the distal edges of the bone. The component is placed on the end of the femur and impacted with impactor and mallet. The cement is removed using glue knives anteriorly, laterally, and medially. Posterior glue is removed using curettes. The Booth retractor is then removed.
21. Hohmann retractors are placed posteriorly and laterally; a Richardson retractor can be placed medially if necessary. Cement is then placed on the tibia surface and on the tip of the tibial stem. The tibial component is then placed and impacted. Remaining cement is removed using glue knives or bayonet forceps. The retractors are removed, and the knee is relocated.
22. Cement is put on the patella in the predrilled holes as well as on the patella button itself. The button is placed on the patella and held with a patella clamp. Remaining cement is again removed using glue knife or bayonets.
23. Drains are used at the discretion of the surgeon, and the wound is closed.

## Total Shoulder Arthroplasty

Physically induced or accidental injury or degenerative arthritis may necessitate prosthetic replacement of the shoulder joint. The procedure may be a hemiarthroplasty with reconstruction of the humeral side or total arthroplasty with replacement of the humeral head and glenoid (Figure 22-79).

***Procedural Considerations.*** The patient is placed in a 30-degree semisitting position with the arm draped free on a padded armboard and the shoulder hanging slightly off the OR bed to allow movement through the entire range of motion. The head is supported to avoid neck extension. A pad is placed beneath the scapula.

A soft tissue set and a large bone set; shoulder instruments; PMMA and cement supplies; the implants with associated instrumentation and trials; a power drill, reamer, and saw; and a pulsatile lavage system will be needed.

### *Operative Procedure*

NEER TOTAL SHOULDER ARTHROPLASTY (FIGURE 22-80)

1. A 16-cm incision is made from the midacromion distally along the deltopectoral groove.
2. The cephalic vein is identified, and the deltopectoral groove is opened and retracted.
3. The deltoid attachment may be removed if the patient is large or muscular, which may affect rehabilitation.
4. The long head of the biceps is identified as the landmark between the tuberosities and rotator interval.
5. The subscapularis is elevated from the underlying capsule and is divided 2 cm medially to the bicipital groove, and a stay suture is placed.
6. The subscapularis is retracted medially with the lesser tuberosity, thereby exposing the joint and associated structures.
7. The capsule is exposed by elevation. An elevator is placed beneath the capsule to protect the axillary nerve. The long head of the biceps is left undisturbed and free in its groove so that it will continue to function as a depressor of the head after surgery.
8. After external rotation, the fractured humeral head is removed. The incision site is irrigated to remove blood and clots from the joint.
9. The proximal humeral shaft is examined to select the appropriately sized stem, available in various lengths and diameters.
10. Marginal osteophytes are trimmed.
11. The glenoid is inspected for integrity and sized for a prosthesis if it is to be replaced.
12. A central hole for a prosthesis fit is made into the glenoid with a high-speed burr and curette.

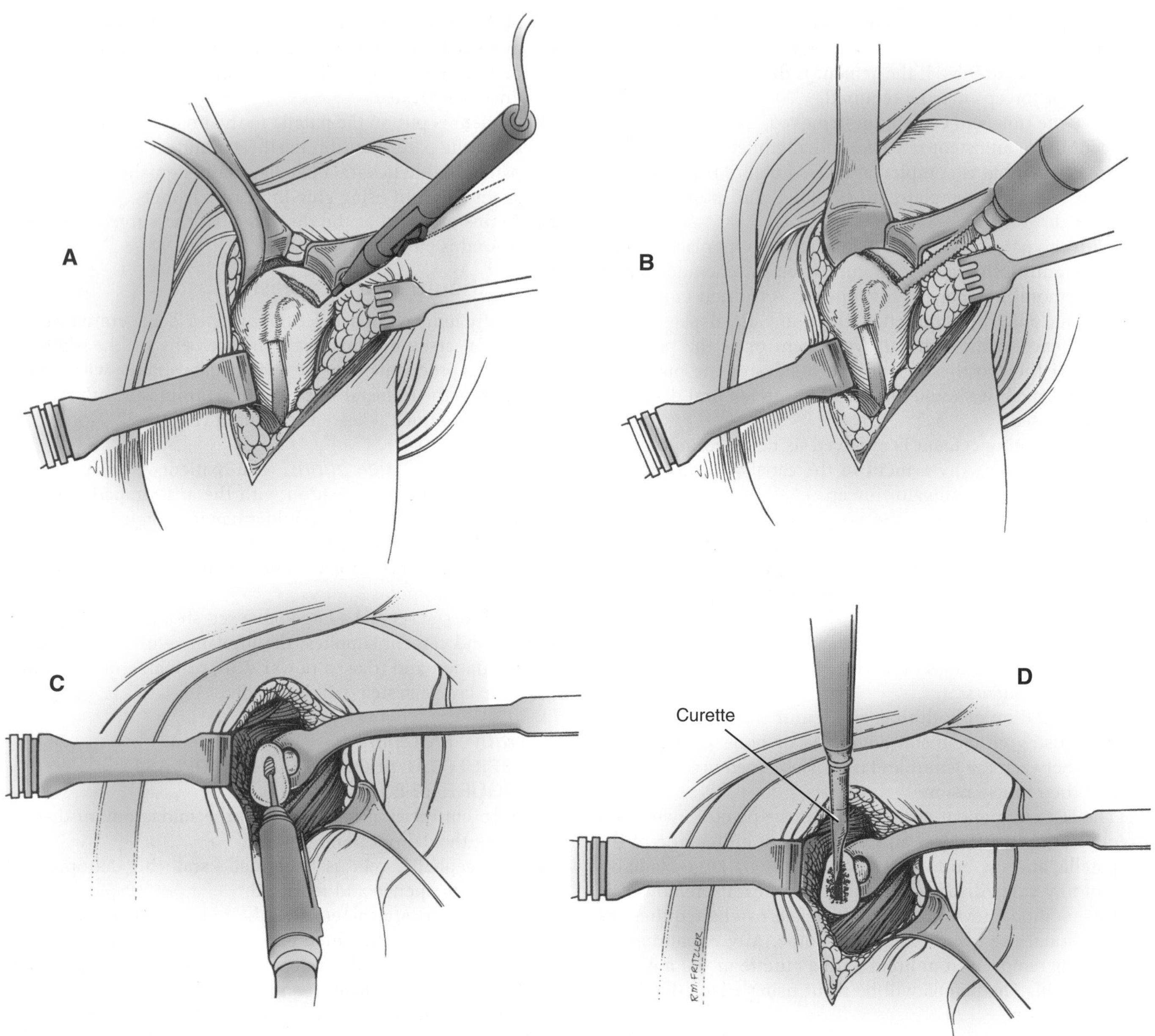


FIGURE 22-79 Total shoulder arthroplasty. **A,** The patient is positioned, and a deltopectoral incision is made to release the capsule. **B,** The humeral head is removed with a reciprocating saw. **C,** After exposure of the glenoid, a fenestration for the glenoid component is made. **D,** The glenoid bow is curetted.

*Continued*

13. Stem diameter and length are estimated to check the prosthesis for fit. The largest stem diameter possible is used.
14. With the shaft held forward and upward, the intramedullary canal is located with a long curette. A 1/4-, 3/8-, or 1/2-inch drill bit is selected to correspond to the diameter of the canal; depending on the prosthesis stem length, 5 or 6 inches down the medullary canal is drilled. Final preparation of the shaft is accomplished with the appropriately sized tapered reamer.
15. A heavy-gauge nonabsorbable suture is passed through holes that have been drilled on the tuberosities. The length of the rotator cuff is checked by pulling the tuberosities distal to the collar of the prosthesis.
16. Neck length and stability of the joint are determined before final impaction of the prosthesis.
17. A check for 35- to 40-degree retroversion is done by palpating the epicondyles at the elbow.
18. The implant is seated on the calcar with a driver and mallet, with its articular surface protected with a moist sponge. Just before final seating, further trimming of high spots with an osteotome or high-speed burr may be required. PMMA is used except in young patients, in whom a firm press-fit can be achieved.
19. Wires or sutures are passed through the holes in the neck of the prosthesis, reducing the tuberosities beneath the collar, and are secured. If wires are used, they are buried in drill holes in the bone.
20. The shoulder is reduced. The interval of the rotator cuff is closed and the biceps tendon reattached if previously detached.

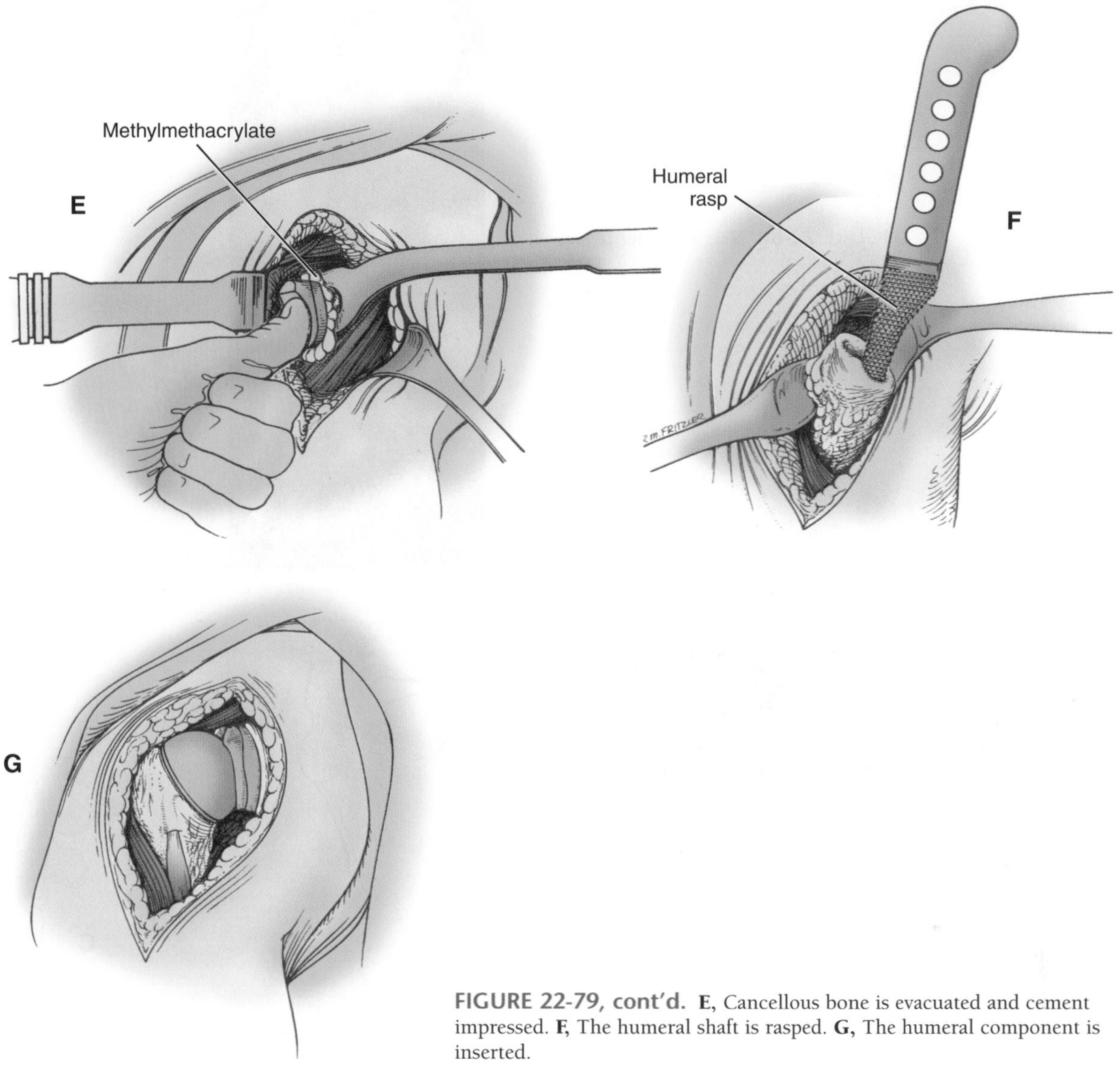


FIGURE 22-79, cont'd. **E,** Cancellous bone is evacuated and cement impressed. **F,** The humeral shaft is rasped. **G,** The humeral component is inserted.

21. The joint is irrigated as each compartment and layer is closed.
22. A closed-drainage system is inserted between cuff and deltoid, avoiding contact of the drainage tubes with the axillary artery. Routine closure is accomplished.
23. Dressings are placed between the body and the arm. A shoulder immobilizer is applied.

Passive range-of-motion machines may be used for patients prone to adhesion or contracture. Pendulum and gentle exercise are permitted at 10 days.

## Total Elbow Arthroplasty

Total elbow replacement (Figure 22-81) is indicated for patients with traumatic lesions or excessive bone loss from rheumatic or degenerative arthritis, resulting in elbow instability and pain or bilateral elbow ankylosis. Arthroplasty of the elbow is not as prevalent as arthroplasty of the shoulder, knee, or hip. The design of implants and methods of fixation for postoperative stability have presented challenges that have been overcome in arthroplasty of other joints but remain a challenge in elbow arthroplasty. Postoperative stability of the elbow implant depends largely on the soft tissues surrounding the joint. There are devices that provide more constraint for the patient with significant soft tissue laxity or loss of bone stock. The Coonrad-Morrey, Tri-Axial, and Pritchard-Walker are just a few of the total elbow prostheses available.

The prosthesis may be used with or without PMMA, depending on the quality of the diseased bone and the design of the implant. If PMMA is not employed, bone grafting with local bone that has been resected may be used to help seat the ulnar component snugly and achieve adequate bony contact against the porous coating of the metal ulnar component. After elbow arthroplasty, patients with degenerative arthritis generally have better results than those with injury.

***Procedural Considerations.*** The patient is in the supine or semi-Fowler position with the arm over the chest. A tourniquet is applied and can be inflated if needed. The arm is prepped from shoulder to fingers and draped. A soft tissue set and a small bone set; the total elbow implants and instruments; a power saw, drill, and burr; an awl; heavy-gauge wire; and a wire tightener will be needed. PMMA and cement supplies as

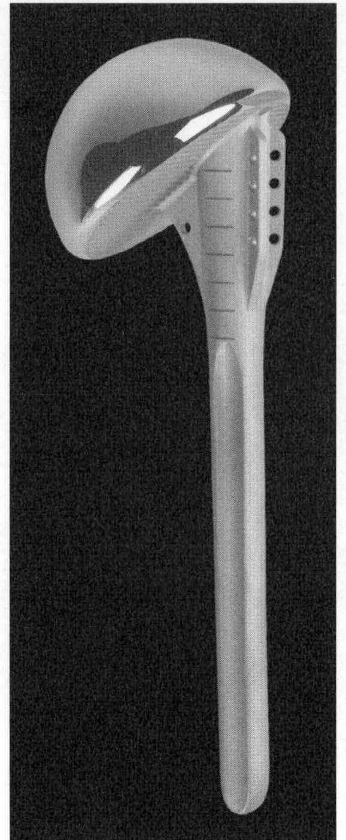

**FIGURE 22-80** Neer shoulder prosthesis.

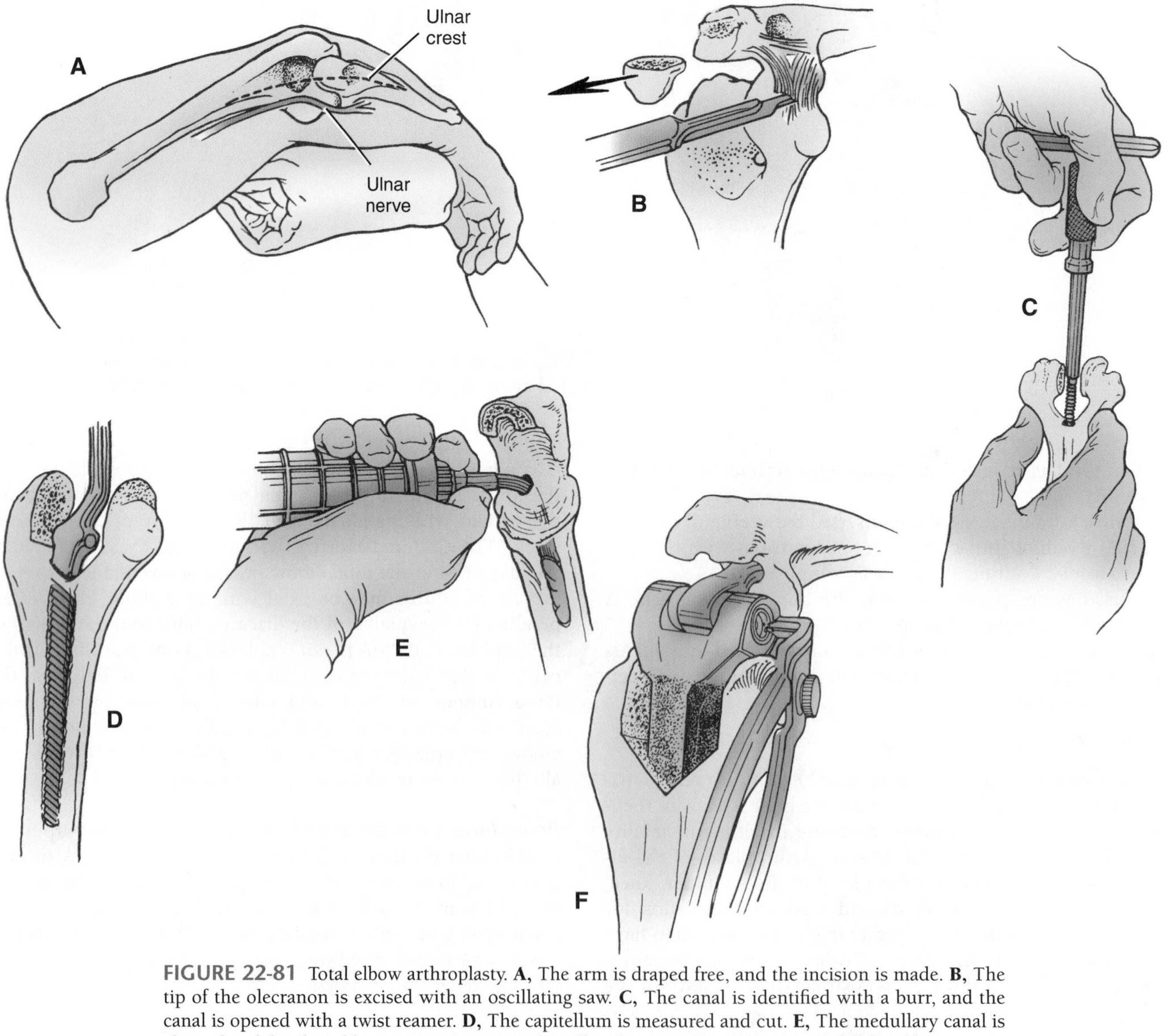

**FIGURE 22-81** Total elbow arthroplasty. **A,** The arm is draped free, and the incision is made. **B,** The tip of the olecranon is excised with an oscillating saw. **C,** The canal is identified with a burr, and the canal is opened with a twist reamer. **D,** The capitellum is measured and cut. **E,** The medullary canal is cleaned and dried, and bone cement is inserted. **F,** The ulnar prosthesis is inserted, followed by cementing and inserting of the humeral components.

well as a pulsatile lavage system are required if the prosthesis is placed with the use of PMMA.

### *Operative Procedure*

1. The limb is exsanguinated, and the tourniquet is inflated to the desired pressure.
2. A midline posterior incision is made, protecting the ulnar nerve.
3. The triceps mechanism is elevated in continuity with the periosteum, and the elbow joint is explored.
4. The distal end of the humerus, proximal end of the ulna, and radial head are explored, preserving the collateral ligaments.
5. The midportion of the trochlea is removed to allow access to the distal end of the humerus; the medullary canal is opened with a high-speed burr, and the canal is entered with a twist hand reamer.
6. The distal end of the humerus is notched with the appropriate cutting guide.
7. A high-speed burr is used to drill through subchondral bone to allow access to the medullary canal of the ulna and serially ream the canal.
8. After the humerus and ulna have been prepared for insertion of the trial prosthesis, the elbow is evaluated for flexion and extension. Bony adjustments are made where necessary.
9. The canals are cleaned of all bone fragments by irrigating with pulsatile antibiotic lavage.
10. The canal is dried before implant insertion, and the preparation is checked before the cement is mixed to ensure that the correct size of component is available.
11. The cement is inserted into the canals followed by the prosthesis. Flexion and extension of the elbow are avoided until the cement has hardened.
12. Any bone graft that may be required is secured with wire or pins.
13. The tourniquet is deflated, and hemostasis is achieved.
14. The triceps mechanism is repaired. The incision site is irrigated and closed. A drain may be inserted.
15. A long arm posterior splint is applied with the elbow at 90 degrees.

## Total Ankle Joint Replacement

Long-term results for total ankle arthroplasty, especially in the young population, are extremely poor. The procedure is reserved for older or more sedentary patients, especially those with subtalar or midtarsal arthritis. Ankle arthrodesis should be considered first in joint reconstruction. Indications for total ankle arthroplasty include (1) failed arthrodesis, (2) bilateral ankle arthritis when arthrodesis has already been performed on one ankle, (3) after talectomy because of avascular necrosis, and (4) revision of a previous arthroplasty. Total ankle replacement prostheses are made of high-density polyethylene and metal components.

***Procedural Considerations.*** The patient is positioned supine with the tourniquet placed. The leg is prepped and draped. A soft tissue set, a small bone set, the total ankle joint replacement instrumentation and implants, a power drill and saw, a pulsatile lavage system, and PMMA cement and supplies will be necessary.

### *Operative Procedure (Figure 22-82)*

1. An anterior incision is made over the ankle joint.
2. Exposure of the tibiotalar joint and talus dome is achieved by dissection.
3. Once the center of the talus is identified and marked, a sizing template is used to mark the tibia.
4. A 1-inch–wide by $3/8$-inch–deep defect is made using the air drill. Anchoring holes can be made in the tibia. The template is positioned in the defect while the foot is distracted.
5. The talus is marked, and a $1/2$-inch–deep by $3/16$-inch groove is made with a reciprocating saw to accommodate the talar component.
6. A trial fit is carried out to ensure that the talar unit is in the center of the talus and that the tibial unit is parallel to the plane of the floor, both centered over the dome of the talus.

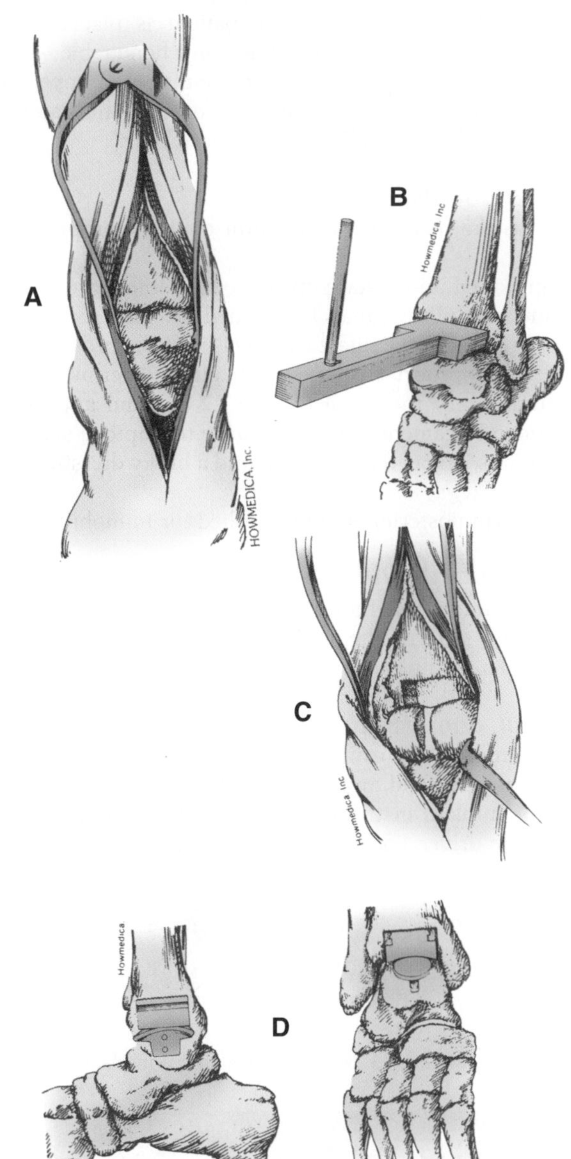


**FIGURE 22-82** Total ankle arthroplasty. **A,** An anterior incision is made, and the tibiotalar joint and talus dome are exposed. **B,** The sizing template is used to mark the tibia. **C,** An air drill is used to create a defect, and anchoring holes are prepared. **D,** Trial reduction is completed, and the talar and tibial components are cemented into place.

7. Once trial reduction is complete, the talar and tibial components are cemented into place.
8. The ankle joint is irrigated and closed, a drain inserted, and a posterior splint applied.

## Metacarpal Arthroplasty

Metacarpal joint replacement is most often performed in patients who have pain or a disabling deformity associated with rheumatoid or degenerative arthritis of the metacarpophalangeal or interphalangeal joints. The results of rheumatoid reconstructive surgery are generally good, and pain can be eliminated and joint alignment and joint stability restored in the majority of patients. The greatest problems after surgery are weakness of grasp and pinch and progression of the disease in adjacent joints.

***Procedural Considerations.*** The patient is placed in the supine position with the arm extended on a hand table. A tourniquet is applied, and the entire extremity is prepped and draped. A hand set, instrumentation for implants, and implants are required, as well as a high-speed burr.

### *Operative Procedure*

1. Incisions are made on the dorsum of the appropriate fingers.
2. The proximal and distal portions of the joints are excised, and intramedullary canals are reamed.
3. Sizers are used to facilitate a correct fit of the prosthesis.
4. Once the appropriately sized implant is determined, it is positioned into the canal (Figure 22-83) and appropriate tendon and ligament repairs are made to improve stability.
5. The joint is irrigated and closed, and a bulky dressing is applied.
6. A short arm posterior splint is applied for immobilization.

## Metatarsal Arthroplasty

Silastic implantation is indicated in the treatment of deformities associated with rheumatoid arthritis, hallux valgus, hallux rigidus, and a painful or unstable joint.

***Procedural Considerations.*** The patient is placed in the supine position. A tourniquet is applied, and the entire extremity is prepped and draped. A small bone set is required, as well as the implant instruments and implants (Figure 22-84), a power wire driver, and the microsagittal saw.

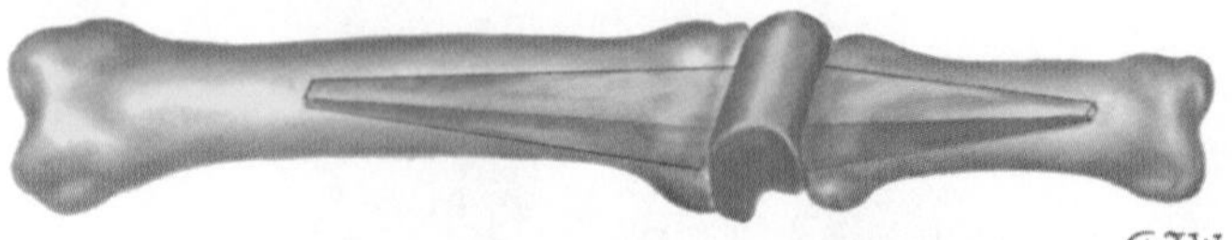


**FIGURE 22-83** Metacarpophalangeal implant.

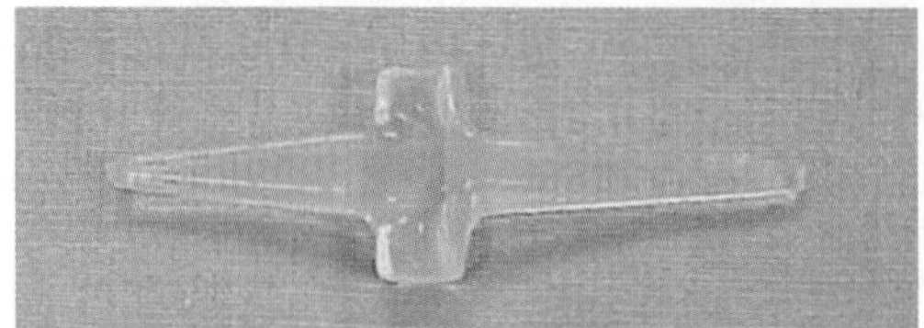

**FIGURE 22-84** Silastic implant for finger joint.

### *Operative Procedure*

1. The incision is made over the appropriate joints.
2. Resection of the proximal phalanx with removal of exostosis of the metatarsal head is carried out.
3. The medullary canal is reamed, and trial implants are fitted.
4. The appropriately sized metatarsal implant is determined and seated.
5. The wound is irrigated and closed.
6. A bulky compression dressing and orthopedic shoe are applied for early ambulation.

# ARTHROSCOPY

Progress and development of arthroscopy and arthroscopic procedures have changed the approach, diagnosis, and treatment of many joint ailments. Arthroscopic techniques require skill and accomplishment in identifying three-dimensional relationships. The advantages of arthroscopic surgery surpass the disadvantages. Among the advantages are (1) decreased recovery and rehabilitation time; (2) smaller incisions; (3) less inflammatory response; (4) less postoperative pain, scar, and extensor disruption; (5) reduced complications; (6) reduced hospital stay and cost; and (7) easier, more rapid surgical procedures.

Disadvantages usually relate to the size and delicacy of the instruments. Maneuverability within a joint may be difficult and produce scuffing and scoring of the articular surfaces.

Improvements in scope and camera systems, sharper scope optics, and miniaturization have made operative arthroscopy a logical extension of diagnostic arthroscopy.[23] Surgical arthroscopy has also been aided with development of numerous second puncture instruments and devices to repair and excise defects. There are a multitude of motorized shaving and abrader systems. Irrigation systems provide regulated distention of the knee joint by infusing normal saline or lactated Ringer's solution. These systems may function by gravity flow or are mechanized with microprocessors built in to monitor joint pressures and adjust accordingly. Lasers and ESUs can be used in tandem with arthroscopic equipment. Integrated video systems can record and store still and video images on film, tape, or floppy disk for education and documentation.

Arthroscopy is commonly performed on the knee, shoulder, and wrist. It is used less often in the elbow, hip, and ankle. Many corrective procedures that previously required an arthrotomy or other open procedure can be completed with the assistance of the arthroscope.

Arthroscopic equipment has certain requirements for care and handling. Fiberoptics, lenses, and cameras are heat-sensitive, requiring consideration for sterilization. Temperatures and moisture generated by steam autoclaves can damage materials used in video equipment or deteriorate the sealant, making the moisture accessible to the lens. Alternatives to steam sterilization for this equipment are ethylene oxide, cold sterilization, and high-level disinfection. Each requires consideration of patient care options for consistency. Equipment must be soaked according to the manufacturer's instruction, followed by complete rinsing and immersion in sterile water to prevent chemical burns.[5] Cold-water sterilizing machines, which use bactericidal and sporicidal agents, can also be used to sterilize heat-sensitive equipment.

Scopes, lenses, and fiberoptic cords should be handled carefully, and cords should never be kinked or twisted. When cables are mishandled, gradual deterioration and fiber breakage occur in them and light cannot be transmitted. When stored, the cords should be loosely coiled or hung.

Two types of arthroscopy may be performed. *Diagnostic arthroscopy* is for patients whose diagnosis cannot be determined by history or physical examination or whose CT or MRI findings are insufficient to warrant surgical exploration. Diagnostic arthroscopy may be performed before an anticipated arthrotomy, and surgical treatment may be modified on the basis of the findings of the arthroscopic examination. *Operative arthroscopy* is for patients presenting with an intraarticular abnormality or ligamentous injury.

## Arthroscopy of the Knee

The knee is the joint in which arthroscopy lends itself to the greatest number of diagnostic and surgical procedures. Arthroscopic surgery of the knee is indicated for diagnostic viewing, synovial biopsies, removal of loose bodies, resection of plicae, shaving of the patella, synovectomy, partial meniscectomy, meniscus repair, and ACL reconstruction. Anesthesia for knee arthroscopy may be general, spinal, or local. Tourniquets are often placed on the thigh but are inflated only if bleeding obscures the view. If there are no contraindications, an epinephrine solution may be injected at the portal sites or diluted into the distention fluid.

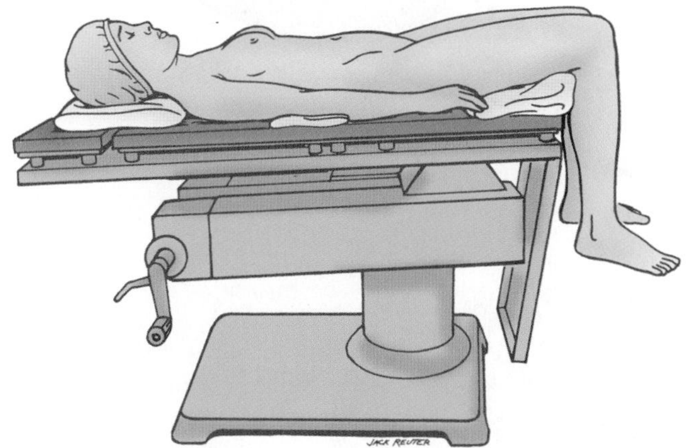

FIGURE 22-85 Positioning for a knee arthroscopy to enhance visualization.

***Procedural Considerations.*** The patient is placed in the supine position on a standard OR bed. The surgeon may perform EUA before the patient is placed in position for the arthroscopy. The foot end of the bed may be flexed 90 degrees (Figure 22-85). A lateral post can be attached to the bed at the level of the midthigh. This post can provide a method of counter-traction to open the medial side of the joint, providing better visualization of structures. After the leg is prepped, the entire extremity is draped to allow complete range of motion and manipulation of the knee joint. The procedure requires specialized equipment for fluid collection and personnel protection.

Instruments and equipment needed for an arthroscopy depend on whether it will be diagnostic or operative. Diagnostic arthroscopy instruments needed include arthroscopy instrumentation (Figure 22-86); arthroscopes of 30 and 70 degrees; video with camera, light source, and peripheral equipment (Figure 22-87); an arthroscopy pump and tubing (Figure 22-88); inflow and egress cannulas (Figure 22-89); 3-L bags of normal saline or lactated Ringer's solution; and a spinal needle. Operative arthroscopy instruments depend on the procedure planned. Arthroscopic powered shavers and abraders (Figure 22-90) are almost universally used. Instruments specific for ACL reconstruction or meniscal repair will be needed if those procedures are planned.

### *Operative Procedures*

DIAGNOSTIC ARTHROSCOPY

1. The anteromedial and anterolateral joint lines and portal positions are marked with a skin marker.
2. The skin areas for portal placement are infiltrated with 1% lidocaine with 1:200,000 epinephrine. If the knee has an

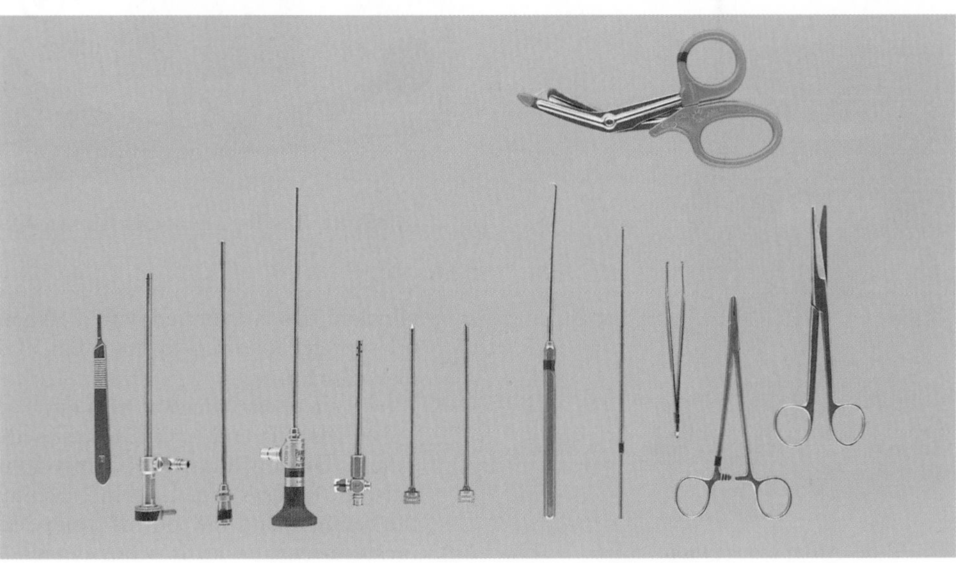

FIGURE 22-86 Arthroscopy instrumentation.

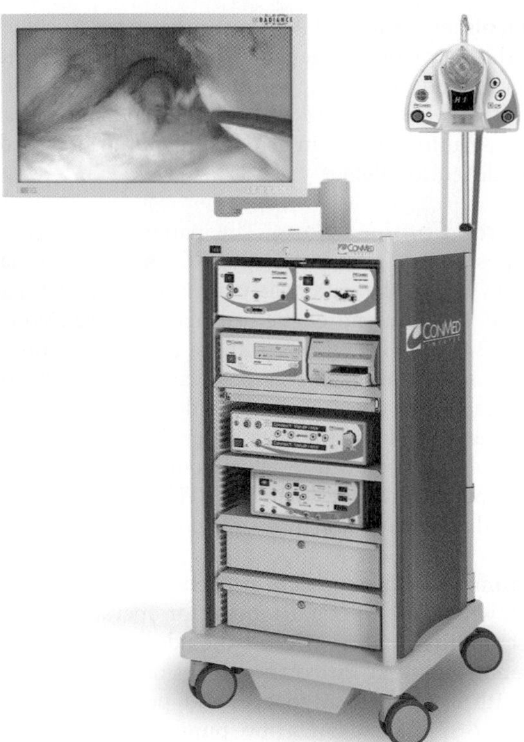


FIGURE 22-87 Arthroscopy tower with video monitor, light source, camera, and shaver system.

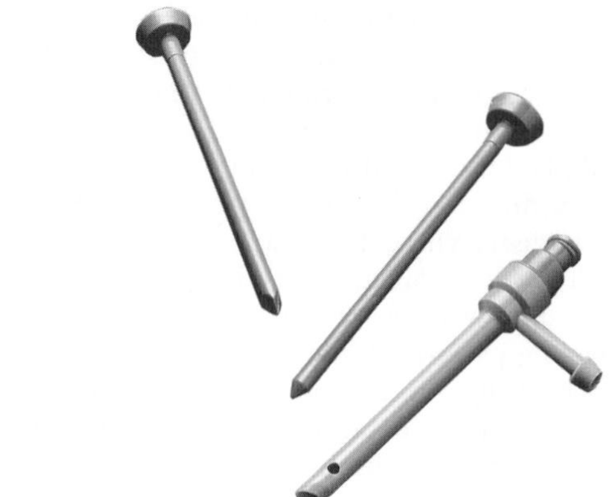

FIGURE 22-89 Cannulas.

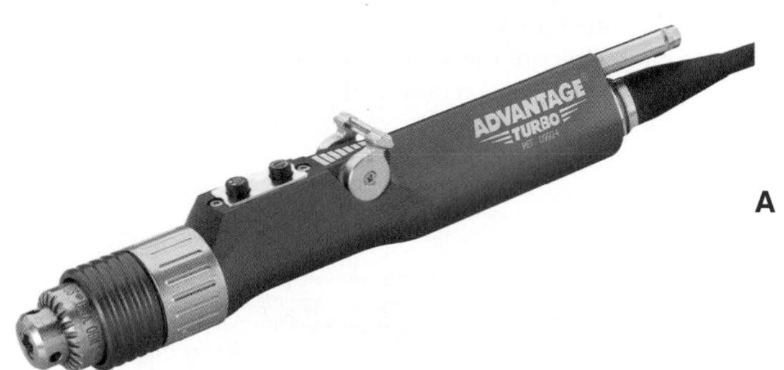


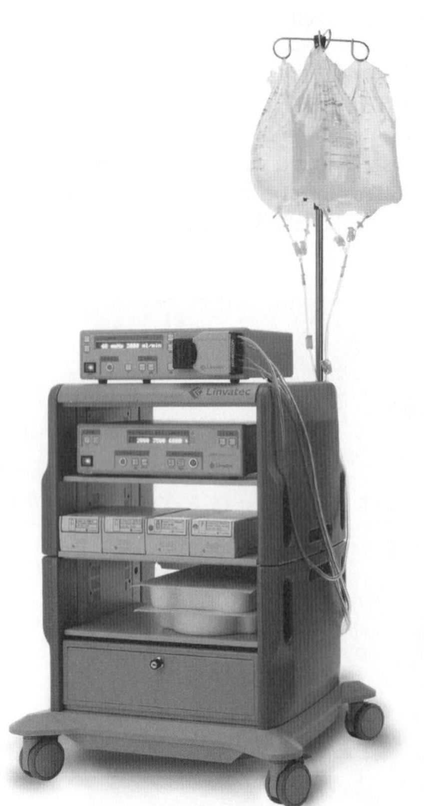


FIGURE 22-88 Arthroscopy pump.

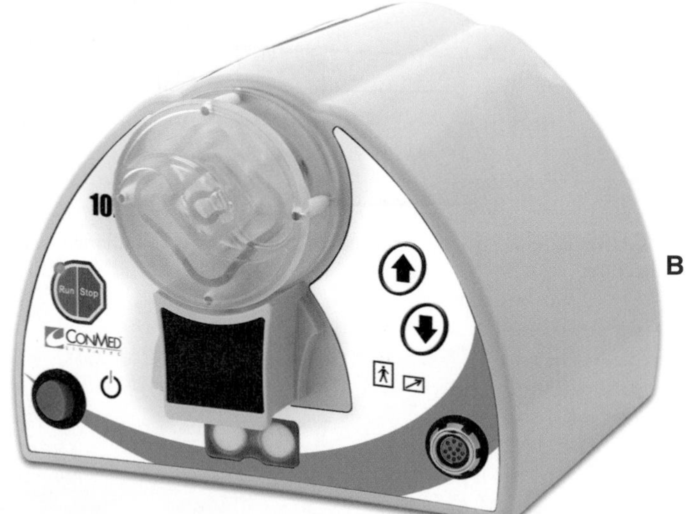


FIGURE 22-90 Arthroscopic shaver, **A,** with console, **B.**

effusion, this is aspirated with a 16-gauge needle on a 60-ml syringe, followed by injection of a small amount of distending fluid.

3. After a small stab incision with a #11 knife blade, the irrigation cannula and trocar are inserted into the lateral suprapatellar pouch near the superior pole of the patella. Lactated Ringer's or normal saline solution is connected to the cannula, and the joint is distended using gravity or a pressure-sensitive arthroscopy pump.

4. A stab incision is then made anterolaterally or anteromedially 2 to 3 mm above the tibial plateau or patellar tendon at the joint line. A sharp trocar and sheath are inserted through the stab wound and just through the capsule.
5. A blunt trocar is used to pass the sheath into the knee joint. The trocar is removed, and a 30-degree scope is inserted into the sheath. The light source and video camera are connected to the scope.
6. The inflow may remain in the suprapatellar area, and the egress tubing is connected to the arthroscope, or the position may be reversed.
7. A spinal needle can be introduced under direct vision to determine the best angle for an opposite portal for insertion of probes and operative instruments. The cruciates and menisci are probed to determine integrity and tears.
8. The scope is moved to the opposite portal to allow a complete examination to be performed.
9. The joint is irrigated periodically and at the end of the procedure to maintain good visualization and clear the joint of blood and tissue fragments.
10. The portals are closed with nylon or undyed Vicryl suture and ½-inch Steri-Strips.
11. Bupivacaine (Marcaine) 0.25%, 30 ml, with epinephrine 1:200,000 may be injected intraarticularly to minimize bleeding and postoperative pain.
12. Gauze dressing, Webril, and 4-inch and 6-inch elastic bandages are applied.

**OPERATIVE ARTHROSCOPY.** Operative arthroscopy includes procedures for resection of synovial plica, patellar debridement, excision of meniscal tears, partial or total meniscectomy, lateral retinacular release, removal of loose bodies, abrasion or drilling of osteochondral defects, synovectomy, treatment of osteochondritis dissecans, meniscal repairs, and ACL reconstruction.

**Arthroscopic Resection and Repair of Meniscal Tear.** Menisci are important structures in the knee joint that distribute load across the joint and provide capsular stability. A tear in the meniscus is the most common knee injury requiring arthroscopic surgery (Figure 22-91). Although both menisci can sustain tears, the medial meniscus is injured much more frequently than the lateral one.

Treatment of meniscus tears is aimed at preserving the structures. Some minor tears heal with cast immobilization, but some persist and cause symptoms. In these more severe cases, surgical intervention is necessary. A partial or complete meniscectomy may be necessary to alleviate troublesome symptoms such as locking, pain, and swelling (Figure 22-92). Partial meniscectomy is preferred, leaving a peripheral rim to share load bearing and stabilize the knee. Complete meniscectomy removes all of this load-bearing protection and also reduces knee stability. The goal is to leave an intact, balanced rim.

Arthroscopic meniscal repair is widely accepted as the standard of care. Arthroscopy provides better exposure than an arthrotomy does and enables the surgeon to approach the meniscus from the inner margin, where most tears begin. Suture repair is appropriate for meniscal tears occurring in the vascular zone (outer 10% to 25%), which heal predictably with repair and immobilization.

*Operative Procedure*

1. Steps 1 to 9 of the diagnostic arthroscopy procedure are repeated.
2. Working and scope portals are determined. The lateral bucket handle tear is identified, displaced, and reduced with a probe.
3. The attachment of the anterior horn of the meniscus is cut with a hook knife and clamped with a grasper.
4. An accessory portal is determined with a spinal needle.
5. Traction and twisting motions are maintained on the meniscal horn to present a better edge to divide the remainder of the tear. Various scissors or push knives can be used to complete resection.
6. The motorized shaver is used to trim any frayed edges of the meniscus.
7. Limited debridement of chronic tears is completed to clean the edges.
8. When the medial meniscus is to be sutured, a cannula is placed next to the inner edge of the tear. Two long meniscal-stitching needles with synthetic absorbable suture are inserted into the cannula, through the meniscus, across the tear, and through the capsule.
9. The needle tips are felt beneath the skin, and a small incision is made to pull the suture out of the joint.
10. The sutures are tied over the capsule. Positioning the cannula enables either horizontal or vertical sutures to be placed.
11. After completing partial meniscectomy or suture repair, the joint is thoroughly irrigated.
12. The incisions are closed, and the knee is lightly dressed and wrapped with Webril and elastic bandages.

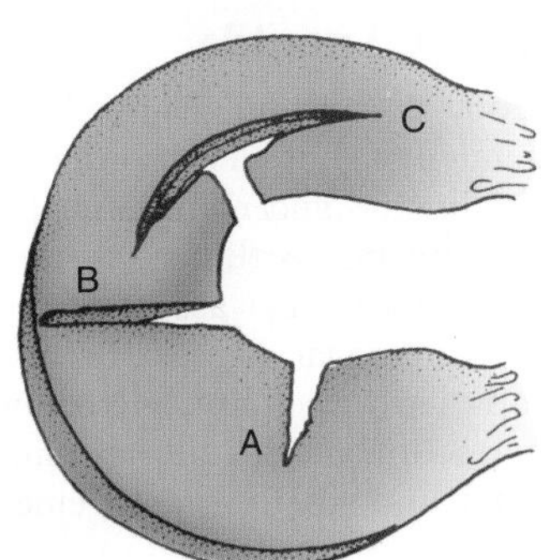


**FIGURE 22-91** Meniscal tear. *A,* Incomplete. *B,* Complete. *C,* Incomplete longitudinal.

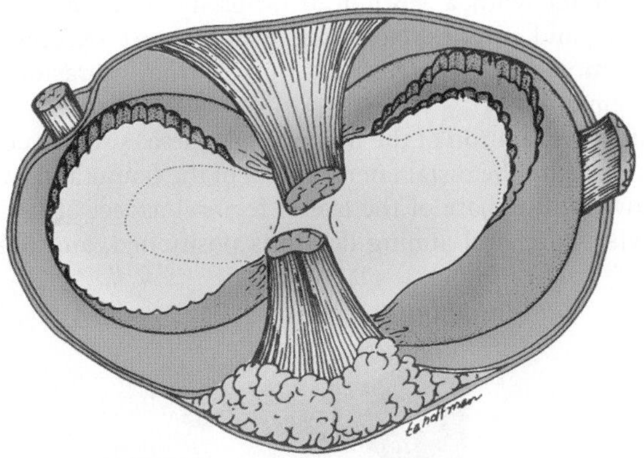

**FIGURE 22-92** Lateral and medial meniscal excision.

**Arthroscopic Anterior Cruciate Ligament Repair.** The ACL is an important stabilizing structure of the knee and is the most frequently torn ligament. Injury is usually a result of simultaneous anterior and rotational stresses. Candidates for ACL reconstruction are active individuals with instability that is sufficient to interfere with their activities and that has failed to respond to bracing, rehabilitation, exercises, and other nonoperative treatment methods. The selected treatment method depends on the classification and severity of the tear, the experience and preference of the surgeon, and whether a previous repair has failed.

ACL reconstruction may be intraarticular, extraarticular, or a combination of both. Arthroscopic repair causes less patellar pain and decreased disturbance of extensor mechanisms and therefore is becoming the treatment of choice if there is no other significant capsular instability or gross disruption of the knee joint.

ACL repair most often involves replacement of the ligament with a substitute. Substitutes include autografts, allografts, and synthetic ligaments. Autografts are currently the method of choice, with a free central-third patellar tendon graft attached to patellar and tibial bone blocks used most often. The semitendinosus tendon and iliotibial band are sometimes used instead. Autografts may be used alone or augmented, although synthetic augmentation devices have fallen out of favor because of the development of chronic synovitis.

*Procedural Considerations.* Instrumentation for an ACL repair includes all instruments required for an operative arthroscopy. In addition, an ACL reconstruction guide system, fixation device of choice (bone screws, staples, spiked washers, or interference screws), bone tunnel plugs (Figure 22-93), a power drill, and microsagittal saw will be needed. If the surgeon believes that isometric placement of the graft is important, a tension isometer will be needed, as well as a system for finding that intraarticular position.

*Operative Procedure: Patellar Tendon Graft*

1. An EUA is performed immediately after induction to further evaluate the stability of the knee.
2. A diagnostic arthroscopy is then carried out through the standard anteromedial and anterolateral portals.
3. Any meniscal tears or other intraarticular injuries are treated before attending to the ligament.
4. The remaining ACL tissue is debrided with a full-radius resector.
5. A notchplasty is then performed, widening the intercondylar notch with a 4.5-mm arthroplasty burr, rasp, osteotome, and curettes. Notchplasty aids in arthroscopic visualization and protects the graft from abrasion and amputation.
6. After preparation of the intercondylar area, a small incision is made on the distal lateral aspect of the femur and carried down to the flare of the lateral femoral aspect of the condyle. A femoral aiming device is positioned, and a guide pin is inserted from the femoral site into the posterosuperior region of the intercondylar notch at an isometric point (Figure 22-94). Another small incision is made anteriorly, below the knee and medial to the tibial tubercle.
7. The tibial aiming device is positioned, and a guide pin is inserted from the anterior tibial incision into the intercondylar notch, anterior and medial to the center of the tibial anatomic attachment site of the ACL.
8. The pins are then replaced with a heavy suture passing through the femoral and tibial pin sites.
9. Isometric placement of the guide pins is checked with a tensioning device that is attached to the heavy suture. The knee is put through a range of motion to determine correct isometric measurement.
10. Once isometric positioning is determined, a longitudinal skin incision is made medial to the midline near the patellar tendon.
11. The central-third portion of the patellar tendon with tibial and patellar bone plugs is harvested with a mini-saw and osteotome. The graft is sized to the appropriate width, usually 10 to 12 mm, using sizing tubes (Figure 22-95).
12. Heavy nonabsorbable suture is placed through drill holes made at each end of the graft in the bone plugs (Figure 22-96).
13. The guide pins are then reinserted and overdrilled with cannulas that are close in width to the prepared graft. Overdrilling establishes the tunnels so that they are in the center of the previous insertion sites of the ACL.
14. The femoral and tibial osseous tunnels are smoothed with curettes, a rasp, or an abrader. If the tunnels are made before the graft is harvested, they are temporarily occluded with bone tunnel plugs to minimize fluid extravasation.
15. Both ends of the graft are fixed with a barbed staple, bone screw with washer, interference screw, or ligament button (Figure 22-97).
16. The incisions and joint are irrigated and closed.
17. A hinged knee brace may be applied over the dressing. The brace allows 10 to 90 degrees of motion.

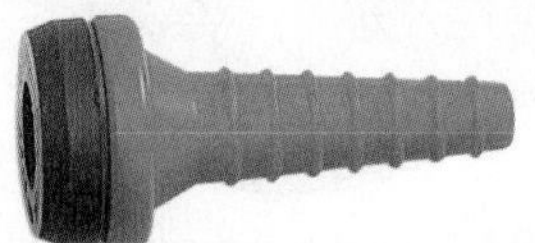

FIGURE 22-93 Example of a bone tunnel plug.

**Arthroscopic Posterior Cruciate Ligament Repair.** Surgical procedures for tears of the PCL are considered if significant disabling instability has occurred. Patients usually return to adequate function without operative treatment. The arthroscopic procedure for repair of the PCL is similar to the technique used to repair the ACL, except that isometric placement is posterior within the joint and the femoral attachment is proximal to the medial epicondyle.

## Arthroscopy of the Shoulder

Shoulder arthroscopy is a useful diagnostic and therapeutic tool in the management of shoulder disorders. It is particularly beneficial in the evaluation and management of patients with chronic shoulder problems. Arthroscopy provides extensive visualization of the intraarticular aspect of the shoulder joint and is performed for removal of loose bodies; lysis of adhesions; synovial biopsy; synovectomy; bursectomy; stabilization of dislocations; correction of glenoid labrum, biceps tendon, and rotator cuff tears; and relief of impingement syndrome.

*Procedural Considerations.* The patient may be placed in the lateral position or in a sitting position using a "beach chair" positioner. The lateral position is maintained using a

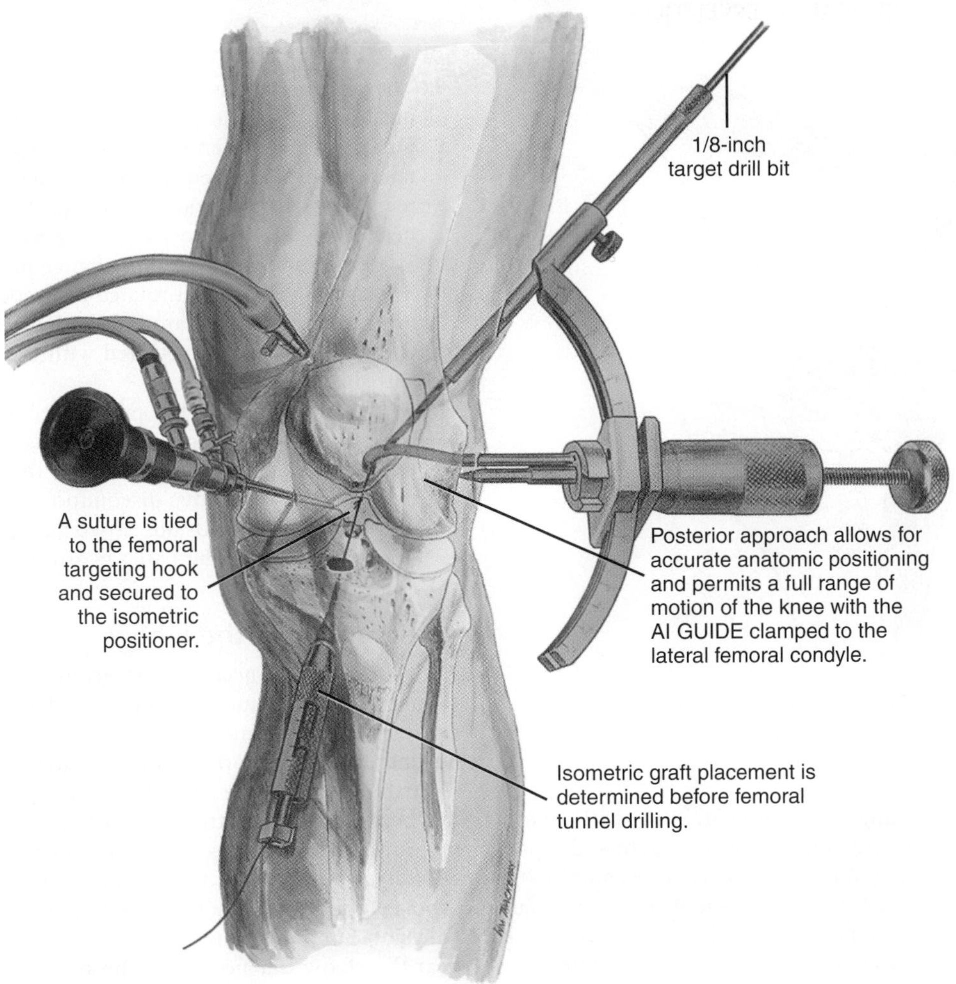
1/8-inch
target drill bit
A suture is tied
to the femoral
targeting hook
and secured to
the isometric
positioner.
Posterior approach allows for
accurate anatomic positioning
and permits a full range of
motion of the knee with the
AI GUIDE clamped to the
lateral femoral condyle.
Isometric graft placement is
determined before femoral
tunnel drilling.

**FIGURE 22-94** Femoral aiming device positioned for anterior cruciate ligament reconstruction.

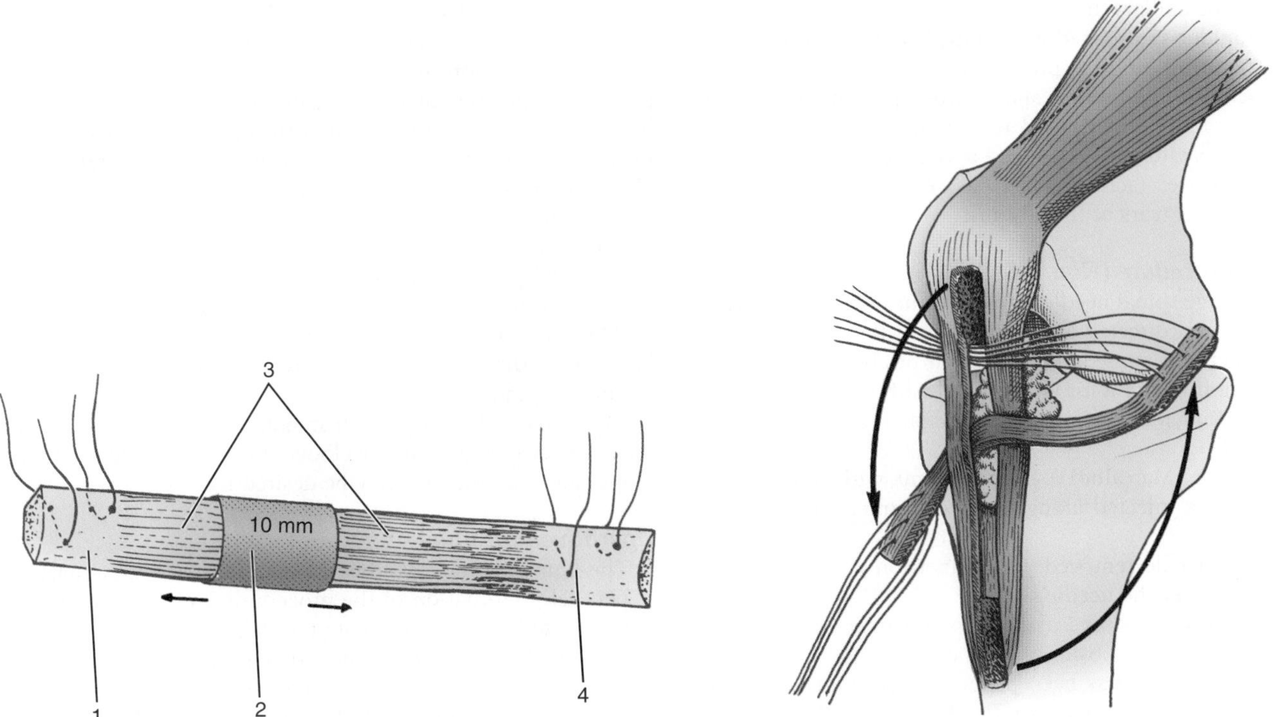
3
10 mm
1
2
4

**FIGURE 22-95** Sizing tubes are used to determine the minimum diameter of tunnel necessary for passage of the graft.

**FIGURE 22-96** Three drill holes are placed into each bone block of the patellar graft, and a heavy suture is placed into each drill hole.

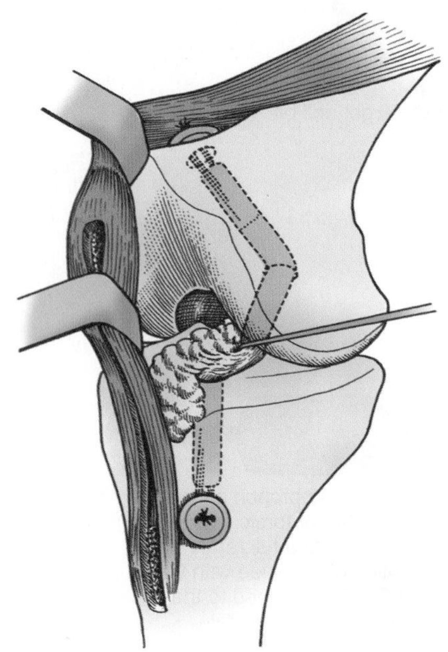

FIGURE 22-97 A patellar tendon graft is affixed by tying of sutures over bone buttons at the tibial and femoral drill holes.

vacuum beanbag positioning device or lateral rolls with a kidney rest. Three-inch adhesive tape is secured across the patient's hips. Proper padding of the uninvolved axilla and lower extremity is important to prevent soft tissue or neurovascular problems. The affected extremity is placed in a shoulder suspension system, and Buck's traction or a Velcro immobilizer is applied to the forearm to achieve adequate distraction to the glenohumeral joint. The extremity is abducted 40 to 60 degrees and forward-flexed 10 to 20 degrees, with 5- to 15-pound weights placed on the pulley system. Weight may be added to further distract the glenohumeral joint, taking care not to overstretch the axillary artery.

The shoulder is prepped and draped free, permitting full range of motion during the procedure.

The operative instruments and arthroscope commonly used for the knee may also be used in the shoulder, plus an 18-gauge needle, switching sticks, and a Wissinger rod. A variety of fixation devices (screws and tacks) can be used to repair bony defects and tears of the labrum.

### *Operative Procedure (Figure 22-98)*

1. An 18-gauge spinal needle is inserted through the posterior soft spot and directed anteriorly toward the coracoid process, where the surgeon's index finger has been positioned.
2. The glenohumeral joint is distended with normal saline or lactated Ringer's solution. This facilitates entry of the arthroscope.
3. Bupivacaine (Marcaine) 0.25%, 2 to 3 ml, with epinephrine 1:200,000 is injected along the needle track to minimize bleeding.
4. With the needle removed, a stab incision is made with a #11 blade over the needle site.
5. The arthroscope sleeve and sharp trocar are then introduced through the posterior joint capsule.
6. Once the capsule has been penetrated, a blunt obturator replaces the sharp trocar to enter the joint.
7. The arthroscope is inserted and attached to inflow and outflow tubing, the video camera, and the light source.
8. Operative instruments are placed through an anterior portal that is established laterally to the coracoid process by using a Wissinger rod. A third portal can be established near the anterior portal or supraspinous fossa portal. Switching sticks are used to change portals.
9. The arm is moved and rotated as needed to visualize various structures in and around the joint.
10. Glenoid tears can be repaired with the insertion of an absorbable fixation tack.
11. At the conclusion of the procedure, the joint is irrigated. The surgeon may inject a long-acting local anesthetic into the joint and subacromial space through the portal to minimize postoperative discomfort.
12. The puncture wounds are closed and dressed with a sterile 4 × 4 gauze pad. The patient's arm is placed in a sling for recovery.

## Arthroscopy of the Elbow

The elbow joint is accessible to arthroscopic examination, although it requires more attention to detail than the knee because instruments must be placed through deeper muscle layers and close to important neurovascular structures.

Arthroscopy of the elbow, both diagnostic and operative, has become fairly routine. Indications for its use include extraction of loose bodies, evaluation or debridement of osteochondritis dissecans of the capitulum and radial head, partial synovectomy in rheumatoid disease, debridement and lysis of adhesions of posttraumatic or degenerative processes at or near the elbow, diagnosis of a chronically painful elbow when the diagnosis is obscure, and evaluation of fractures of the capitulum, radial head, or olecranon.

***Procedural Considerations.*** General anesthesia is preferred to local anesthesia because it affords complete comfort to the patient and provides total muscle relaxation.

The patient is placed in either supine or prone position. In the supine position, the forearm is flexed on an armboard or placed in a prefabricated wrist gauntlet connected to an overhead pulley device and tied off at the end of the OR bed. This provides excellent access to both the medial and lateral aspects of the elbow, allows the forearm to be freely pronated and supinated, and places the important neurovascular structures in the antecubital fossa at maximum relaxation.

A tourniquet is routinely used for hemostasis. The entire arm, including the hand, is prepped and draped.

The three portals most commonly used for diagnostic and operative arthroscopy of the elbow are the anterolateral, anteromedial, and posterolateral.

Operative arthroscopy instruments commonly used for the knee may also be used in the elbow. However, smaller-diameter scopes and instruments may be desired instead.

### *Operative Procedure*

1. The bony anatomic landmarks are outlined with a marking pen before initiation of the procedure. Lateral structures to be marked and identified are the radial head and the lateral epicondyle. The medial epicondyle is also marked.
2. An 18-gauge needle is inserted anteriorly to the radial head from the lateral side, and the joint is distended.

3. Once joint distention has been achieved with approximately 15 to 30 ml of lactated Ringer's or normal saline solution, a stab wound incision is made with a #11 blade, and the sharp trocar with cannula is inserted through the joint capsule.
4. The sharp trocar is replaced with the blunt obturator to provide safe entry of the cannula into the joint.
5. The scope replaces the blunt obturator and is attached to the video and light source.
6. A second portal and third portal are established anteromedially and posterolaterally for triangulation. With the patient's elbow flexed to 90 degrees and adequate distention maintained at the time of insertion of the instruments, the neurovascular structures are displaced anteriorly. This provides a greater area above the medial and lateral humeral epicondyles in which to insert the various instruments.
7. Outflow and inflow are controlled by alternating the valve on the scope or using a separate 18-gauge needle with drainage tubing.
8. After diagnostic and operative procedures have been completed, the joint is irrigated, the puncture sites are sutured, and a compression dressing is applied with Webril and elastic bandages.

## Arthroscopy of the Ankle

The talocalcaneal articulations are complex and play an important role in the movements of inversion and eversion of the foot. The subtalar joints function as a single unit, but anatomically they are divided into anterior and posterior joints. The surgeon and perioperative nurse must be familiar with the extraarticular anatomy of the ankle to prevent neural or vascular damage.

Indications for ankle arthroscopy include osteochondral fragments or loose bodies, persistent ankle pain after trauma and despite adequate conservative treatment, biopsy, posttraumatic arthritis of the ankle joint, unstable ankle before lateral ligamentous reconstruction, and osteochondritis dissecans of the talus.

***Procedural Considerations.*** General anesthesia is preferable because manipulation and distraction of the joint to obtain adequate arthroscopic viewing require muscle relaxation. The position of the patient is based on the surgeon's preference. The patient may be supine with the knee flexed approximately 70 degrees or supine with a sandbag under the buttock of the

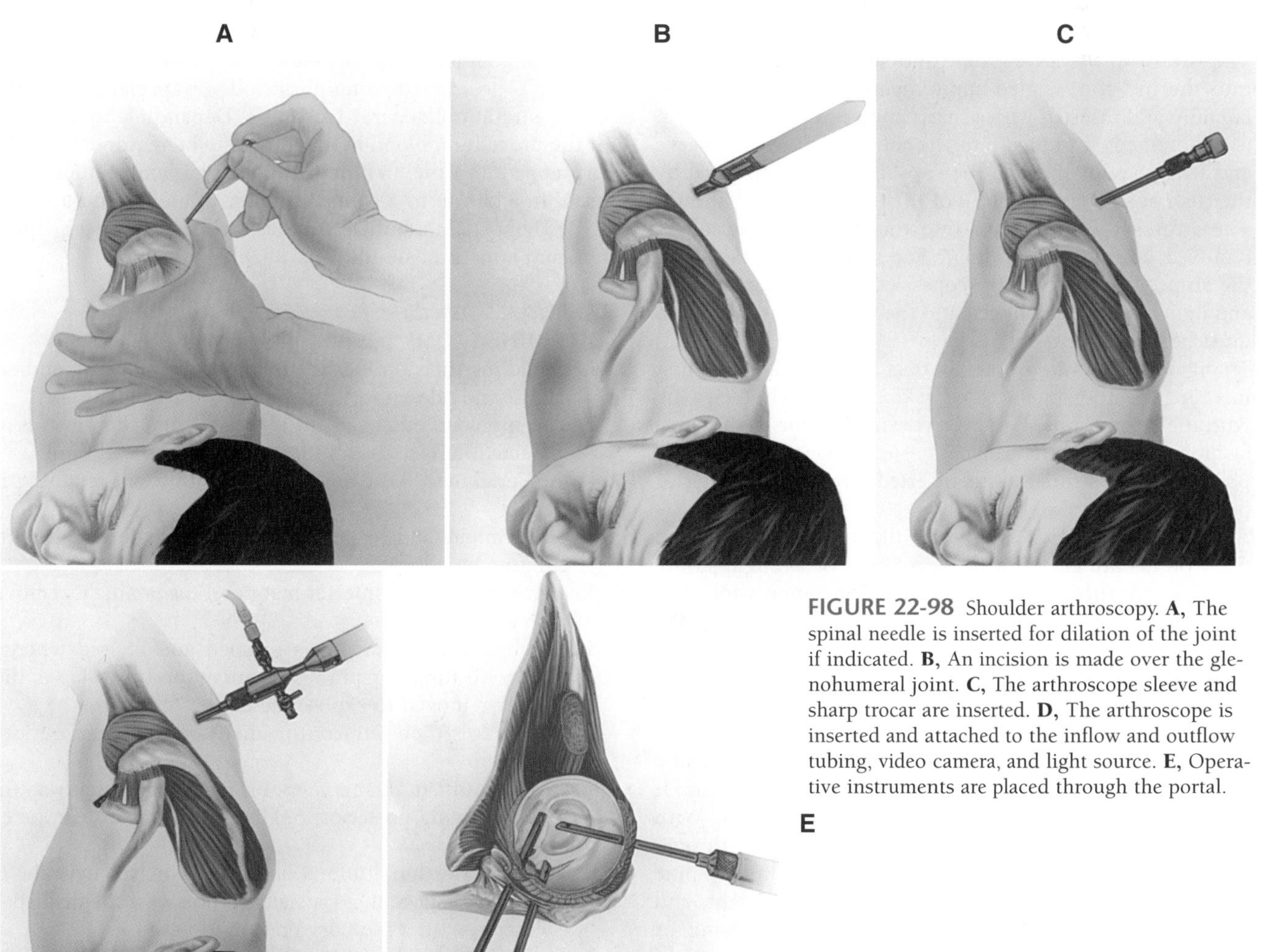


**FIGURE 22-98** Shoulder arthroscopy. **A,** The spinal needle is inserted for dilation of the joint if indicated. **B,** An incision is made over the glenohumeral joint. **C,** The arthroscope sleeve and sharp trocar are inserted. **D,** The arthroscope is inserted and attached to the inflow and outflow tubing, video camera, and light source. **E,** Operative instruments are placed through the portal.

operative side. Ankle and thigh holders may be used; when better posterior visualization is necessary, a distractor may be used to increase the space between the tibia and talus. A tourniquet is placed around the upper thigh but is not used unless excessive bleeding, uncontrolled by irrigation, is encountered. Routine skin prepping and draping are done. Miniaturized instruments and needle scopes for the ankle are used.

### Operative Procedure

1. The important extraarticular anatomic structures are outlined on the skin, using a sterile marking pen.
2. The ankle joint is then examined, using the anterolateral portal. The anteromedial joint line is palpated, and an 18-gauge, 1½-inch needle is inserted into the joint.
3. Sterile plastic extension tubing is attached to the needle, and a 50-ml plastic Luer-Lok syringe filled with normal saline is connected to the tubing to distend the joint. Approximately 15 to 20 ml is needed.
4. After intraarticular injection is confirmed by the ease with which the saline can be injected and by palpation of the joint as it is distended, a small incision is made with a #11 blade over the site of the anterolateral portal.
5. A hemostat is then inserted and used to dissect to the capsule.
6. The sheath of the arthroscope and sharp trocar are placed into the incision, angled approximately 30 to 45 degrees laterally, and inserted with a sharp plunge as joint distention is maintained. Entrance into the joint is felt as the sleeve and trocar "pop" through the capsule and is confirmed by the rush of saline on removal of the trocar from the sheath.
7. The arthroscope is inserted into the sheath, the needle is removed, and the plastic tubing and syringe are attached to the stopcock on the arthroscope sleeve. The video camera and light source are connected to the scope. Joint distention must be maintained.
8. Triangulation through other portals is easily done by first inserting the 18-gauge needle for localization while viewing with the arthroscope. Posterior viewing is done in the same fashion except that the patient is usually placed in the prone position and instruments are inserted through the posterior portals.
9. After the procedure is completed, the joint is irrigated and the wounds are closed with Steri-Strips or a single suture and covered with a dressing and short leg compression elastic wrap.

## SURGERY OF THE SPINAL COLUMN

### Treatment of Back Pain

Back pain is a natural result of degenerative and arthritic change, punctuated by protrusion or rupture of a disk. It gradually progresses but may also disappear gradually. With aging, a degenerative disk-space narrowing or facet arthropathy begins to appear radiologically. The lower lumbar spine carries the burden of the body, holds a person upright, and returns the body to the vertical position from sitting, lying, or a bent-over position. Degenerative changes, ruptured disk, and facet arthropathy develop at the lowest two limb segments, where the greatest weight, torsion, and shearing stress occur. It sometimes extends into the upper and middle spine.

Cervical-spine degenerative disk narrowing also develops most often at the two lowest cervical spaces, which are also the levels of greatest stress resulting from movement of the head and neck. Sometimes lumbar or cervical degenerative changes develop early from excessive repetitive movements or injury.

Epidural steroid injections, electrodes, stimulators, braces, or traction may treat back pain. A natural recovery may result after 6 or 7 days of intense pain, subsiding between 6 weeks and 4 months. Motor and sensory deficits usually disappear with resolution of pain. The ability to recover without surgery depends on fragment size and compression on the nerve root. Neural compression remains the major indication for disk excision.

Spinal fusion is a consideration, usually for patients with demonstrable posttraumatic, postsurgical, rheumatoid, infectious, or neoplastic instability.

***Procedural Considerations.*** After assessment, the patient-specific plan of care is implemented. Radiographs are obtained. Bilateral pulses are assessed in the extremities. Elastic wraps or sequential compression devices (SCDs) may be placed. Range of motion is assessed, particularly of the arms, because of the need for the extended prone position. The patient is positioned prone to eliminate lordosis, reduce venous congestion, and keep the abdomen free. A Foley catheter may be placed. The patient is positioned using chest rolls or special frames after administration of general anesthesia. Depending on the extent of the procedure, blood availability may be required. The skin is prepped and the area draped. A spinal laminectomy set is used, in addition to a spinal retractor of choice and a bipolar ESU. Hemostatic adjuncts such as Gelfoam, Surgicel, thrombin, and bone wax should be available.

### Operative Procedure

#### LAMINECTOMY

1. A midline incision is made over the affected disk and carried sharply down to the supraspinous ligament.
2. The supraspinous ligament is incised, and the muscles are dissected subperiosteally from the spines and laminae of the vertebrae. These are retracted with a self-retaining retractor.
3. The laminae and ligamentum flavum are denuded with a curette.
4. A small part of the inferior margin of the lamina is removed with a rongeur.
5. The ligamentum flavum is grasped and incised where it fuses with the interspinous ligament, and this flap is then sharply removed to expose the dura.
6. The dura is then retracted medially, and the nerve root is identified.
7. Once identified, the nerve root is retracted medially so that the underlying posterior longitudinal ligament can be exposed.
8. The posterior longitudinal ligament is incised over the intervertebral space in a cruciate fashion, and the disk space is entered with a pituitary grasping forceps.
9. The disk material is systematically removed, taking care not to exceed the distance to the anterior annulus. A complete search for additional fragments of nucleus pulposus, both inside and outside the disk space, is then carried out.

10. All cotton pledgets are removed and counted, and residual bleeding is controlled with bipolar coagulation.
11. The wound is closed routinely with absorbable sutures in the supraspinous ligament and subcutaneous tissue. Various nonabsorbable sutures or staples are used for skin closure.

## Pedicle Fixation of the Spine

Pedicle screw fixation (Figure 22-99) is a method of surgical fixation of the spinal column. Screw fixation was initially used in an attempt to avoid postoperative external immobilization and prolonged bed rest. Pedicle screw fixation has been used most often in degenerative processes, particularly iatrogenic instability after decompression, degenerative and isthmic spondylolisthesis, and diskogenic disease. It is also indicated for tumor, trauma, degenerative spinal disorders, postoperative hypermobility, and infection.

Three basic approaches for fixation have been described as the procedure has evolved. Each has improved on the first, based on anatomic placement of the screw. Positioning and placement of the screw within the spine are established after direct visualization of the pedicle.

***Procedural Considerations.*** After the administration of general anesthesia, the patient is positioned prone. The skin is prepped, and drapes are applied. A spinal laminectomy set is used in addition to the instrumentation and implants of choice, a spinal retractor, power equipment such as a high-speed motorized hand tool, and hemostatic adjuncts such as Gelfoam, thrombin, and bone wax. A bone graft set will be needed to harvest graft from the iliac crest.

### *Operative Procedure*

1. A standard midline incision is made. The laminectomy procedure is followed.
2. The areas of the pedicles to be fixated are located using external landmarks.
3. The posterior cortical wall at the entrance site is removed using a high-speed burr.
4. A Penfield dissector is used to identify the entrance hole through the pedicle.
5. A gearshift probe is inserted to identify the path into the vertebral body.
6. The hole is tapped (5.5-mm tap) and widened.
7. The screw is placed. Guidelines for screw sizes are 7 mm for S1, L5, and L4; 6.25 mm for L3 and L2; 5.5 mm for L1 and T12.
8. A posterolateral graft is performed, using graft strips from the iliac crest.
9. The plate or rod is contoured to approximate the patient's physiologic lordosis. The longitudinal device is locked onto the screws in the appropriate position.
10. A screw-plate system may require use of the oblique and transverse washers between the screw head and plate to provide a flush fit at the screw-plate interface.
11. The foramina are checked for patency before closure. The excess portion of the screw is cut close to the upper locking device.
12. A suction drain is placed; the wound is closed in layers.

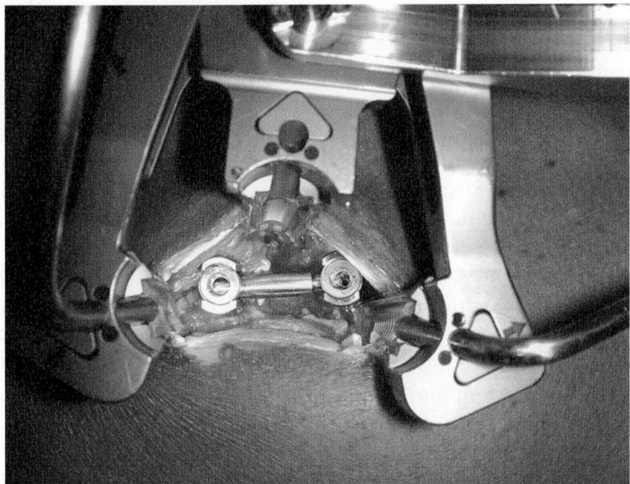

FIGURE 22-99 Pedicle screw placement using the MaXcess retractor and SpheRx fixation system by NuVasive, Inc., San Diego, CA.

## Treatment of Scoliosis

Scoliosis is a three-dimensional deformity (Figure 22-100) with lateral deviation of the spinal column from the midline; it may include rotation or deformity of the vertebrae. Types are congenital, juvenile, adolescent, and adult. School screening programs provide quick and simple detection. For effective treatment of scoliosis, early detection is critical.

The prevalence of scoliosis in the general population ranges from 2% to 4%.[20] Scoliosis can be idiopathic (80% of the time) or congenital and may result from muscular or neurologic diseases or unequal leg lengths.[28] Numerous posterior and anterior segmental spinal instrumentation systems are available for the treatment of idiopathic scoliosis. As a consequence, fixation strategies are more complex than they were with Harrington instrumentation. The newer systems provide better sagittal control and more stable fixation, allowing quicker mobilization of the patient. On thin patients, however, the bulk of these implants may be a problem.[6,28]

***Posterior Spinal Fusion with Harrington Rods.*** Posterior spinal fusion is most frequently performed in adolescence,[25] when the laterally deviated curve is still flexible. Harrington rods are internal splints that help maintain the spine as straight as possible until the vertebral body fusion has become solid.

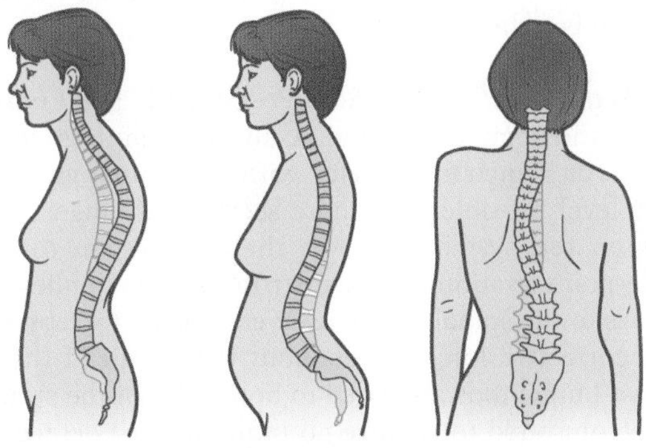

FIGURE 22-100 Scoliotic deformity.

Distraction rods are placed on the concave side of the curve, and compression rods are placed on the convex side. On the convex side of the curve, three to eight hooks are inserted in the transverse processes of the vertebrae and pulled together with a threaded rod. In this way the scoliotic deformity can be corrected as much as the flexibility of the spine allows.

The posterior elements of the vertebrae are denuded of soft tissue, and the bone graft is added. Blood loss can be expected, and an accurate record of the loss must be maintained. After surgery the patient is placed in an immobilizing jacket.

Some disadvantages of the Harrington rod system over other systems are that there is only end-point fixation, rod breakage is increased, fixation is less, sagittal plane curves are difficult to manage, distraction for correction is not always desired, and the patient is required to wear a postoperative cast or brace. Other systems have evolved from the Harrington rods that are used for correction of some scoliotic deformities. It remains a feasible treatment of idiopathic scoliosis.

PROCEDURAL CONSIDERATIONS. The patient is placed in the prone position on a frame or with rolls under the chest and abdomen to facilitate respiration. Before the procedure begins, an x-ray cassette is placed under the patient so that a radiograph for accurate identification of the vertebrae to be fused can be taken during the operation. A single straight longitudinal incision is made down the midline of the back. Because of the amount of bleeding, the skin and subcutaneous tissues are often infiltrated with a vasoconstricting solution, such as epinephrine.

Basic spinal instrumentation and bone graft instruments are required, plus the Harrington rod instrumentation. A large pin cutter, designed to cut large pins but provided with a small end so that it will fit in the wound, should be available.

OPERATIVE PROCEDURE

1. The appropriate hooks are selected and inserted. A Harrington distraction rod of appropriate length is inserted through the two proximal self-adjusting hooks, which have been placed under the laminae.
2. A rod clamp is clamped onto the Harrington rod just below the hook, and a single regular spreader is used to obtain the first inch of distraction.
3. The Bobechko spreader is used to span over the first hook, closest to the smooth part of the rod, to apply distraction force on the most proximal hook.
4. Two C locking rings are inserted around the first ratchet immediately below the hook to prevent dislodgment of the hooks. The excessive length of protruding rod above the most proximal hook is cut off with a rod cutter. The compression is tightened.

***Luque Segmental Spinal Rod Procedure.*** The Luque segmental method employs smooth, L-shaped, stainless steel rods, usually $^{3}/_{16}$ or $^{1}/_{4}$ inch in diameter, with sublaminar wires placed at every level possible. It is more secure and longer than the Harrington rod system and was the first system to employ multiple-point fixation. Luque instrumentation applies corrective forces to the spinal segments at each level, thereby spreading the corrective forces throughout the length of the deformity. Two Luque rods are wired to both sides of the spine. The rods are contoured to achieve no more than 10 degrees of increased correction beyond that exhibited on preoperative x-ray study.

PROCEDURAL CONSIDERATIONS. The patient is placed in the prone position on a frame or with rolls under the chest and abdomen to facilitate respiration. Patient care is provided (see "Laminectomy," p. 792), including assessment of pulses. A straight midline incision is made in the back. Because of the amount of bleeding, the skin and subcutaneous tissues are often infiltrated with a vasoconstricting solution, such as epinephrine. Basic spinal instrumentation is required. In addition, Luque rods and instrumentation, a wire tightener and cutter, and bone graft instruments will be needed.

OPERATIVE PROCEDURE

1. The ligamentum flavum is detached, exposing the neural canal.
2. Doubled stainless steel suture wire is passed under the lamina. The wire loop is cut later to form two wires at each level.
3. Total bilateral facetectomies are made, forming posterolateral troughs for subsequent bone grafts.
4. Wedge osteotomies may be necessary in severe immobile curves to avoid stretching the spinal cord during correction.
5. The wire loop is cut, resulting in two separate wires at each level.
6. The L bend is secured to the base of the spinous process to prevent rod migration.
7. Initial placement of the convex rod is made.
8. Initial placement of the concave rod is made.
9. Transverse wiring is done to add increased stability to the system.
10. Stabilization of the lumbosacral joint is corrected by bending the rods distally to form sacral bars.

***Cotrel-Dubousset System Procedure.*** The Cotrel-Dubousset system (Figure 22-101) provides three-dimensional correction of spinal deformities without sublaminar wiring and neurologic risks. This instrumentation permits distraction, compression, and derotation. The scoliotic curve is corrected by derotation and, at the same time, restores the normal sagittal contours. In addition to correction of scoliosis, the Cotrel-Dubousset system can be applied to correct kyphosis or lordosis and to stabilize and rebuild the spine after tumor resection or after injury. No external support is necessary. The Cotrel-Dubousset system has no ratchets or notches. It consists of metallic rods with diamond crosscut patterns on which hooks and screws can be positioned in any position, level, or degree of rotation. The rod is held in the open hooks with blockers. The rods are then interlocked by means of devices for transverse traction. The Cotrel-Dubousset system was the forerunner to the systems used today, such as the Texas Scottish Rite Hospital (TSRH) system and the Isola system.

PROCEDURAL CONSIDERATIONS. The patient is placed in the prone position under general anesthesia. Patient assessment and precautions for the prone position are initiated. Basic spinal instrumentation is required in addition to the Cotrel-Dubousset system and instrumentation and instruments used for harvesting bone graft.

OPERATIVE PROCEDURE

1. Closed hooks are inserted at both ends of the surgical site, and open hooks are inserted at various levels in between.
2. Decortication and facet excision are done at the remaining interposed vertebral levels for rod placement.

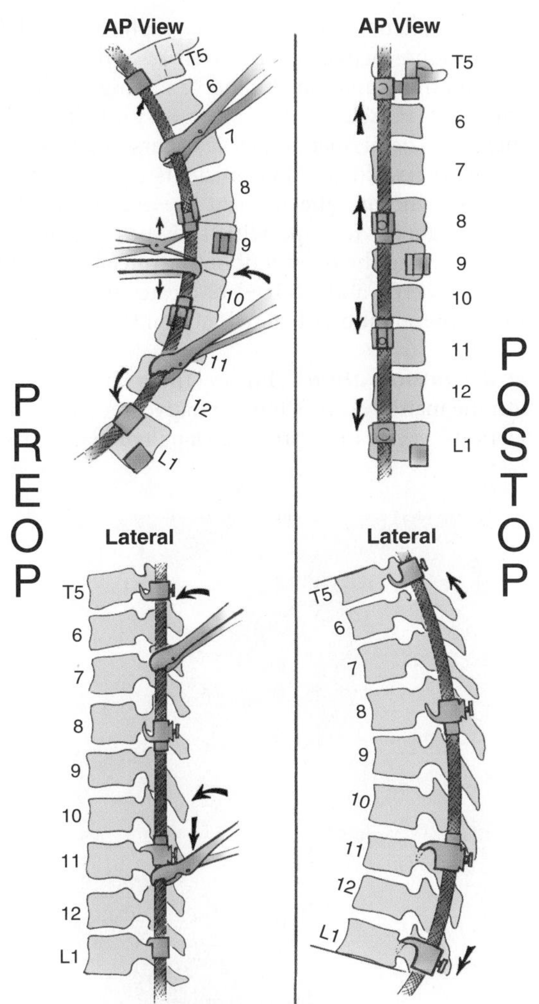


FIGURE 22-101 Cotrel-Dubousset system, representing rotation of rods.

3. Bone graft is placed in the areas that will be under the rod.
4. The appropriate concave rod is bent to shape for sagittal-plane correction and manipulated into the end hooks.
5. Stabilization along the length is achieved with blockers that anchor the rod into the open hooks.
6. The spine is then derotated using the rod holders. The frontal-plane scoliosis curve becomes the sagittal-plane kyphosis.
7. Hooks are reseated for secure fixation.
8. To correct kyphosis, the convex rod is then bent to shape and seated.
9. Once the rods are placed, applying the device for transverse traction (DTT), usually near the ends of the rods, completes stabilization.
10. Remaining bone graft is then applied to the fusion area.

***Texas Scottish Rite Hospital (TSRH) Crosslink System.*** The TSRH crosslink system (Figure 22-102) is a multicomponent stainless steel implant used to lock spinal rods together rigidly. Locking the rods increases construction stiffness and prevents rod migration. The system was originally designed for the Luque segmental system to prevent migration between the rods and wires before complete fusion occurred. By rigidly crosslinking the rods, loss of scoliotic correction was reduced. This system can also be used with the Harrington and Cotrel-Dubousset systems. Crosslinks are indicated when the rigidity of a spinal system alone is not sufficient to generate fusion in a reasonable amount of time.

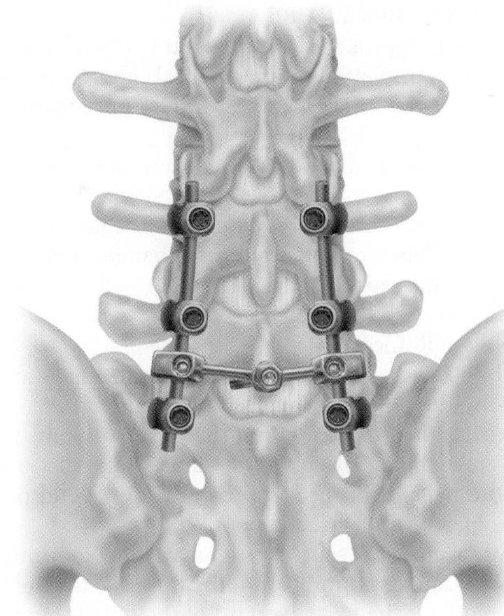

FIGURE 22-102 Texas Scottish Rite Hospital (TSRH) system.

PROCEDURAL CONSIDERATIONS. The patient is placed under general anesthesia and positioned prone. The skin is prepped, and drapes are applied. A spinal laminectomy set is used. Instrumentation and implants of choice, a spinal retractor, and power equipment such as a high-speed handheld tool will be necessary. Hemostatic adjuncts such as Gelfoam, thrombin, Oxycel, and bone wax should be available.

OPERATIVE PROCEDURE

1. Eyebolts are placed on the spinal rods before the rods are implanted.
2. The rods are secured with hooks or wires, depending on the system used.
3. Once the rods are positioned, cross plates of varying widths accommodating different rod-to-rod distances are bolted in place between the rods and nuts.

***Anterior Spinal Fusion with Isola Instrumentation.*** Isola instrumentation involves screw fixation into each vertebral body, complete disk excision and grafting, and segmental connection of the vertebral bodies. A semirigid rod connects the segments. The Isola anterior instrumentation is indicated in idiopathic scoliosis patients, approximately 10 to 30 years of age, with thoracolumbar or upper lumbar curves of 40 to 65 degrees.[28]

PROCEDURAL CONSIDERATIONS. The patient is positioned in a lateral decubitus position so that posteroanterior and lateral intraoperative radiographs can be taken. The usual anesthetic and positioning precautions are necessary. The anesthetic technique should provide incomplete pharmacologic paralysis, allowing for intraoperative neurophysiologic monitoring. In addition to a major soft tissue set and laminectomy set, the Isola instrumentation and implants, a vascular set, and power equipment will be needed.

OPERATIVE PROCEDURE

1. The spine is approached through a transthoracic retroperitoneal (or retropleural retroperitoneal) approach, resecting the rib two vertebral levels above the upper instrumented vertebrae.
2. The sympathetic chain is mobilized laterally with the psoas.
3. The segmental vessels are temporarily occluded and, provided that there are no monitoring changes, ligated.
4. The disks are exposed to the far side to allow a full annulectomy. The bodies, however, are not exposed much beyond the midline.
5. A full 360-degree diskectomy and annulectomy are done, exposing the posterior longitudinal ligament.
6. Screws are then placed within the vertebral body, with the end screws being placed first. Care is taken to place the longitudinal axis of the screw parallel to the end plate and at the apex of the vertebral body.
7. Screw placement is started with an awl and continued with a 5.5-mm tap, continuing until the tip just exits the far side of the cortex. The first one third of the hole is tapped with a 7.0-mm tap, and a 7.0-mm closed top screw with a washer is inserted. The screw must protrude through the opposite cortex by a thread or two. The same process is then repeated at the lower end vertebra.
8. A rod of proper length is cut and contoured to re-create the sagittal-plane angular position of the normal spine. It is then positioned in the end vertebra and used as a guide to locate the entry point for the intermediate screws.
9. Open-ended intermediate screws are inserted in a fashion similar to the end screws, taking care that their travel is parallel to the end screws.
10. The rod is back-entered through the upper screw and then the lower screw and seated into the intermediate open screws. The open screws are capped, and the rod is rotated to place the sagittal-plane contour of the rod in the sagittal plane. An intermediate set screw is tightened to secure the new position of the rod.
11. As the remaining screws are tightened about the rod, it is essential that the disk spaces be opened completely. A Cobb elevator can be used to pry the disk space open.
12. Rib corticocancellous autograft is used to completely fill the disk spaces. This is done using the tenth rib (the usual site of entry), the twelfth rib taken from inside the chest, and the eighth rib taken from outside the chest.
13. The disk spaces are compressed to provide anterior column load sharing. Care should be taken to ensure that the set screws are visited at least twice for the end-closed connections and three times for the center-capped connections.
14. Closure is in the standard manner, using chest tubes if the chest has been entered or a retropleural Hemovac if a retropleural retroperitoneal exposure has been done.
15. Aftercare consists of an overnight intensive care stay with the patient sitting out of bed the next morning. A cast or brace is used at the physician's discretion. Activities are restricted for 6 to 12 months, until there is clear indication of graft incorporation.

## Artificial Disk Replacement

Degenerative disk disease (DDD) occurs when the intervertebral disk (IVD) is worn because of aging or trauma. Diskogenic back pain results from degeneration of the disk and is confirmed both by patient history and radiographically.[11] The IVD acts as the padding between the vertebrae. Once the IVD is worn out, pain, inflammation, and nerve impingement leading to numbness and muscle weakness can occur. Left untreated, nerve damage can be permanent. DDD occurs in 50% of people older than 40 years of age. Many patients are asymptomatic; however, those who are affected can be severely debilitated, changing their ability to cope with activities of daily living (ADLs) and affecting the quality of life. Artificial disk replacement (Figures 22-103 and 22-104) re-creates the natural disk function with preservation of spinal motion.[21]

***Procedural Considerations.*** Ensure the availability of implants with the manufacturer's representative; reconfirm during the preoperative verification process. Hang templates of x-rays

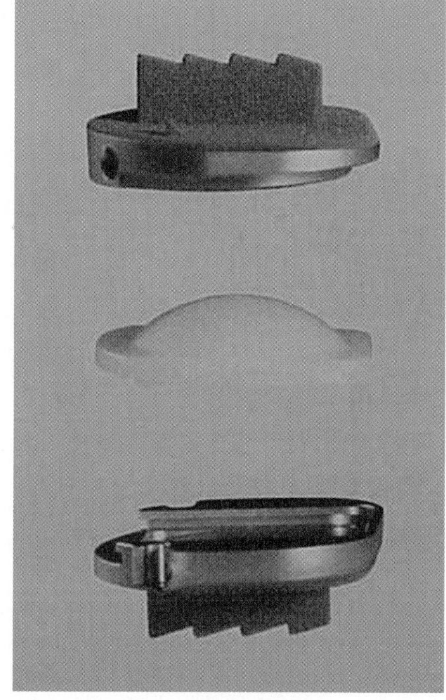

FIGURE 22-103 Three components of the ProDisc.

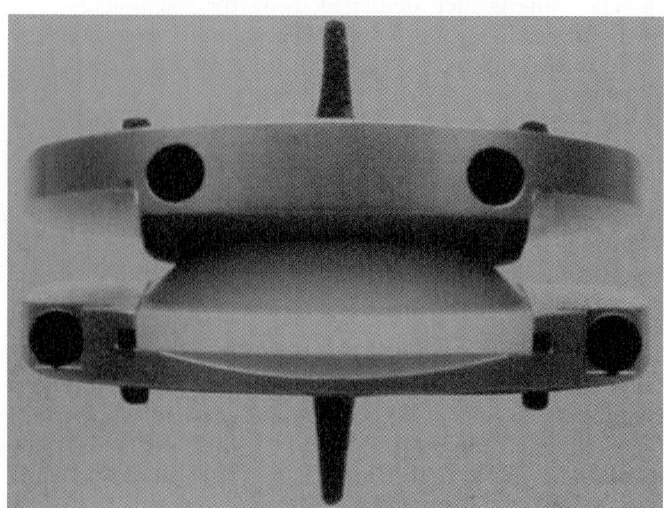

FIGURE 22-104 Assembled ProDisc.

before the procedure on the view box. The cell saver should be available for blood salvaging intraoperatively and postoperatively. The patient is positioned on a Jackson table in the supine position with the right arm draped across the body. A C-arm is used to identify the disk or disks to be replaced in the marked areas. In many institutions, laminar airflow is used.

***Operative Procedure.*** The two general anatomic routes for anterior exposure to the lumbar spine are retroperitoneal and transperitoneal.

The *retroperitoneal approach* can proceed from a variety of incisions, including vertical midline, paramedian, oblique, and transverse. This is determined by both the spinal level and the number of lumbar levels to be exposed. An infraumbilical transverse incision can accommodate most approaches to the L4-5 and/or S1 disk levels, whereas a more obliquely oriented incision is favored for accessing disk levels above L4.

The *transperitoneal route* is not generally used except in extenuating circumstances (e.g., prior extensive retroperitoneal surgery or revisional spine surgery). A midline incision provides direct visualization of the abdominal cavity. Fixed retraction is used to keep small and large bowel out of the field. Trendelenburg position can be used to assist with maintaining exposure. For the L5-S1 level, the peritoneum superficial to the sacral prominence is incised. Vascular structures are identified, and blunt dissection can be used to tease open the area of the facet of the disk. Excessive electrocoagulation should be avoided to decrease the risk of injury to the sympathetic nerves. The middle sacral vessels generally need to be divided to complete the exposure.

Once the exposure is complete the surgeon will use a #3 long handle with a #15 blade to make an incision into the disk body. The diskectomy is completed using a rongeur and curettes to remove remaining disk tissue. Correct sizing is determined using templates. Trial instrumentation is inserted and correct placement is verified with an AP and lateral C-arm view. The trial is centered in the AP plane, and the marker appears as a plus sign aligned with the spinous process. On the lateral x-ray, a hole in the trial represents the center of rotation.

Once correct placement of the trial is verified, the ESU is used to make a mark midline of the superior vertebral body; the trial is then removed. Next, the pilot driver is aligned with the midline ESU mark. The pilot driver that corresponds to the chosen foot print is then carefully impacted to verify the ability to accurately place end plates. During this process, lateral C-arm imaging is used to accurately monitor the depths of the pilot driver. Once the depth is achieved, the slap hammer is used, removing the pilot driver from the disk space. The end plate insertion tips are then attached to the corresponding superior and inferior end plates. The end plates are then carefully inserted into the disk space with the assistance of the guided impactor. The insertion is monitored with fluoroscopy to accurately control the posterior depth and verify the appropriate lordotic angle. With the superior and inferior end plates in place, the disk space is opened using the spreading and insertion forceps. Once the appropriate distraction is achieved, the size on the spacer can be used to select the appropriate core trial. The appropriate core insertion tip is loaded into the core insertion instrument, and the sliding core is inserted between the end plates. The distraction on the spreading forceps is released, allowing the end plates to close around and engage the sliding core. The core insertion instrument is removed and the final position verified using fluoroscopy (Figures 22-105 and 22-106). The wound is irrigated and closed.

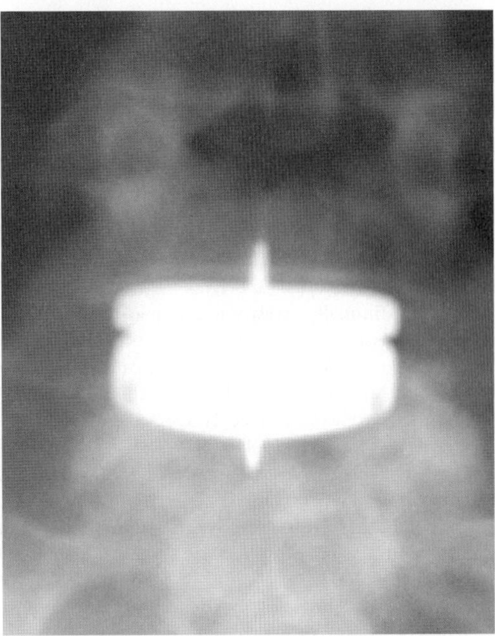

**FIGURE 22-105** Implanted ProDisc.

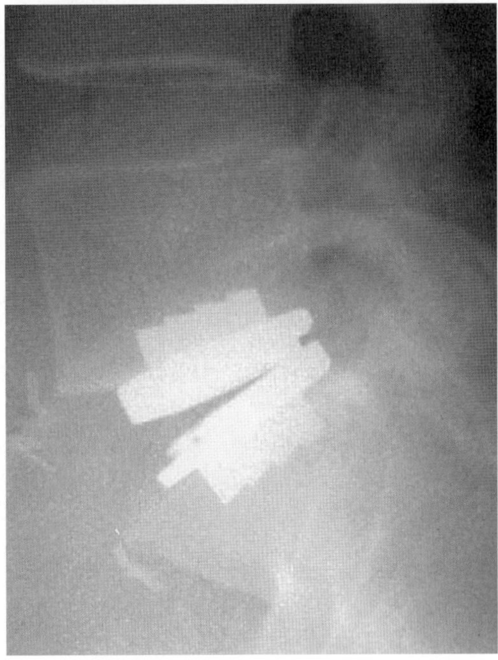

**FIGURE 22-106** Implanted ProDisc with patient bending backward.

## REFERENCES


1. American Association of Orthopaedic Surgeons: Rosemont, Ill, 2005, The Academy.
2. American Association of Tissue Banks: *Standards for tissue banking,* McLean, Va, 2005, The Association.
3. AORN position statement on creating a patient safety culture, *AORN Journal* 83(1):109-110, 2006.

4. AORN position statement on the role of the health care industry representative in the perioperative setting, *AORN Journal* 83(1):115-116, 2006.
5. Association of periOperative Registered Nurses: *AORN standards, recommended practices, and guidelines,* Denver, 2006, The Association.
6. Benli IT and others: Isola spinal instrumentation system for idiopathic scoliosis, *Archives of Orthopaedic Trauma Surgery* 121:17-25, 2001.
7. Berger RA: Taking total hip replacement outpatient, *Outpatient Surgery Magazine* 4(10):50-54, 2003.
8. Broos PL and others: Fractures of the distal radius: current concepts for treatment, *Acta Orthopaedica Belgica* 67(3):211-218, 2001.
9. DeFrancesco J: Minimally invasive total hip arthroplasty, *RN First Assistant Specialty Assembly Newsletter* 11(3):1, 4, 2004.
10. Delmas PD: *Update of diagnosis, evaluation, and treatment of osteoporosis.* Presented at Joint Meeting of the International Bone and Mineral Society and the European Calcified Tissue Society, June 5, 2001.
11. *FDA Center for Device and Radiological Health New Device Approval—Charite™ artificial disc.* Accessed January 24, 2005, on-line: www.fda.gov/cdrh/mda/docs/p040006.html.
12. Floryan KM and others: Intraoperative use of autologous platelet-rich and platelet-poor plasma for orthopedic surgery patients, *AORN Journal* 80(4):668-674, 2004.
13. Grimmer K, Moss J: The development, validity, and application of a new instrument to assess the quality of discharge planning activities from the community perspective, *International Journal of Quality in Health Care* 13(2):109-116, 2001.
14. Gruendemann BJ, Mangum SS: *Infection prevention in surgical settings,* Philadelphia, 2001, Saunders.
15. Guido GW: *Legal and ethical issues in nursing,* ed 3, Upper Saddle River, NJ, 2001, Prentice-Hall.
16. Harby K: *Peri-articular analgesia injection gives significant pain control in total knee replacement.* Accessed March 3, 2005, on-line: www.medscape.com/viewarticle/500446.
17. Hohler SF: Minimally invasive total hip arthroplasty, *AORN Journal* 79(6):1244-1258, 2004.
18. *JCAHO, AMA, and NCQA to focus on measuring effectiveness of appropriate pain management.* Accessed January 18, 2002, on-line: www.jcaho.org/tip/j_online0102.html.
19. Kleinert HE and others: Hand surgery. In Townsend CM, editor: *Sabiston's textbook of surgery,* ed 16, Philadelphia, 2001, Saunders.
20. LaMontagne LL and others: Adolescent scoliosis: effects of corrective surgery, cognitive-behavioral interventions, and age on activity outcomes, *Applied Nursing Research* 17(3):168-177, 2004.
21. Mathias JM: Technology trends: new artificial disc has learning curve, payment issues, *OR Manager* 21(1):1, 16-18, 2005.
22. McGinn T and others: *Decreasing mortality for patients undergoing hip fracture surgery, Joint Commission International Center for Patient Safety.* Accessed December 2, 2005, on-line: www.jcipatientsafety.org/show.asp?durki=11521.
23. Meltzer B: Arthroscopy equipment update, *Outpatient Surgery Magazine* 5(4):73-75, 2004.
24. Nickel JT and others: Discharging older patients from home care: who decides and when? *Caring* 20(7):44-49, 2001.
25. Reamy BV, Slakey JB: Adolescent idiopathic scoliosis: review and current concepts, *American Family Physician* 64(1):32, 34-35, 2001.
26. Stetler CB: Updating the Stetler model of research utilization to facilitate evidence-based practice, *Nursing Outlook* 49:272-279, 2001.
27. Swank ML, Lehnert IE: Orthopedic personnel roles in the OR for computer-assisted total knee arthroplasty, *AORN Journal* 82(4):631-643, 2005.
28. Wiggins GC and others: Management of complex pediatric and adolescent spinal deformity, *Journal of Neurosurgery* 95:17-24, 2001.

CHAPTER 23

# Neurosurgery

DIANE L. FERRARA

Neurosurgery is possibly the most diverse, complex, and challenging specialty in surgery. Brain surgery is performed for head injury, tumors, vascular disorders, hydrocephalus, epilepsy, and Parkinson's disease. Neurosurgery also treats disorders of the spine from trauma and fractures, spinal cord injury, spinal stenosis, spinal tumors, and disk disease. In addition, neurosurgeons treat peripheral nerve disorders, carotid artery disease, chronic pain, and pediatric disorders. Advancements in the highly technical field of neurosurgery are constant.

Perioperative nurses and surgical technologists who care for neurosurgical patients are challenged by the need to have a working knowledge of neuroanatomy, function, and clinical presentations of the many neurologic conditions that require surgical interventions. Understanding the surgical procedure to be performed allows the perioperative nurse to anticipate and respond to the intraoperative needs of the patient and neurosurgical team, as well as to surgical complications as they arise. Given the range and complexity of today's neurosurgical interventions an understanding of highly sophisticated equipment and instrumentation is necessary. Like all patients undergoing surgery, the neurosurgical patient is often vulnerable secondary to the presenting pathologic condition. For perioperative personnel to deliver sensitive, humanistic care in this highly technical environment, they must recognize and appreciate the individual's emotional and spiritual state, whether it is manifested by fear, pain, or grief. Reaching out and making the human connection allay the fear, moderate the pain, and facilitate the patient's grieving process. Information in this chapter will assist those working in neurosurgery to give optimal patient care.

## Surgical Anatomy

The nervous system is the most complex and least understood of body systems. It is divided structurally into the central nervous system (CNS) consisting of the brain and spinal cord and the peripheral nervous system (PNS), which encompasses every neurologic structure outside the CNS, including the cranial and spinal nerves. The brain and spinal cord are protected by the skull and vertebral columns, respectively. The cranial nerves originate within the brain and emerge through openings in the skull to run peripherally. The spinal nerves that emerge from the spinal cord through the vertebral foramina also run peripherally.

The nervous system is divided functionally into a voluntary system and an autonomic, or involuntary, system. It provides a means of communication for the rest of the body. The functions of all body systems depend, in part, on nervous system function. In turn, the nervous system depends directly on circulatory system function for life-sustaining glucose and oxygen. Nervous system functions include motor and sensory functions, orientation, coordination, conceptual thought, emotion, memory, and reflex response.

Nervous system tissue is composed of vast amounts of neurons and far more neuroglial cells. Neurons are intercommunicating nerve cells that encode, conduct, and transmit information to other neurons, muscle, and glandular tissue (Figure 23-1). They are composed of a body or soma with branches or extensions, called dendrites and axons, that communicate with other cells at synapses. Dendrites are short branches that conduct impulses toward the soma. Cell bodies and dendrites are mostly confined to areas of gray matter in the CNS. Axons are long branches, often encased in a white myelin sheath, that conduct away from the soma. Axons pass into bundles of nerve fibers that tend to form tracts or pathways and are referred to as white matter (see Figure 23-11 on p. 805).[21] Tracts that cross midline to create a communication pathway from each side of the body to the opposite side of the brain are called commissures. Neuroglial cells support the neurons by creating and maintaining an appropriate environment in which neurons can operate efficiently.[21] Glial cells include astrocytes, oligodendrocytes, ependymal cells, and microglia. The mutation of these cells can form a glioma, one of the more common brain tumors.

This chapter divides the nervous system into logical divisions within the framework of neurosurgical techniques. The brain and adjacent structures include the cranial nerves of the PNS, which are commonly encountered during brain surgery. Discussion of the spine and spinal cord includes the adjacent spinal nerves and the disks and ligaments that support the spine. Surgically significant pathology is incorporated with the normal anatomy of structures.

### BRAIN AND ADJACENT STRUCTURES

#### Scalp

Scalp layers (Figure 23-2) include skin, subcutaneous tissue, galea, and periosteum. Scalp skin is thick. The subcutaneous tissue, which is exceptionally dense, tough, and vascular, is firmly attached to the galea. Most of the blood vessels lie superficial to the galea. The subgaleal space contains loose areolar tissue that permits mobility of the scalp. It is in this bloodless plane that the standard craniotomy scalp flap is created. The pericranium, or outer periosteum of the skull, separates the galea from the cranium.

The arterial supply of the scalp comes from the external carotid artery through the superficial temporal, posterior au-

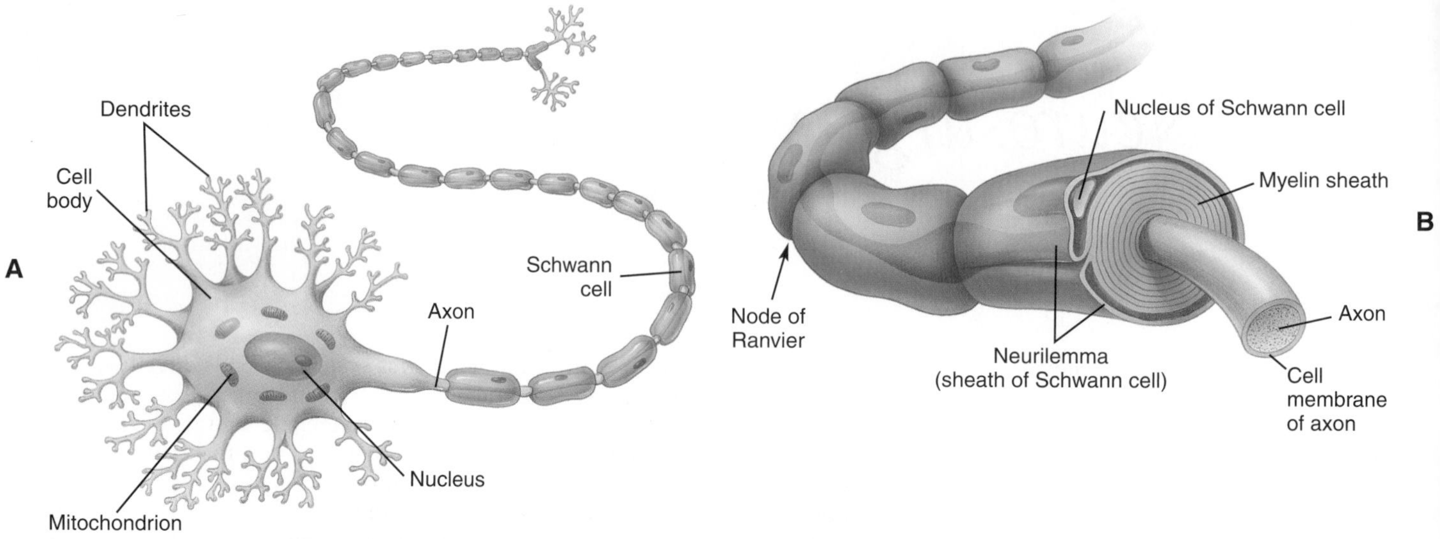

FIGURE 23-1 **A**, Many dendrites carry nerve impulses to the cell body, which then sends the nerve pulses along a single, long axon. Long axons are encased at intervals by a myelin sheath. **B,** A segment of myelinated fiber in cross section, showing myelin sheath composed of several layers of myelin, which insulate the axon.

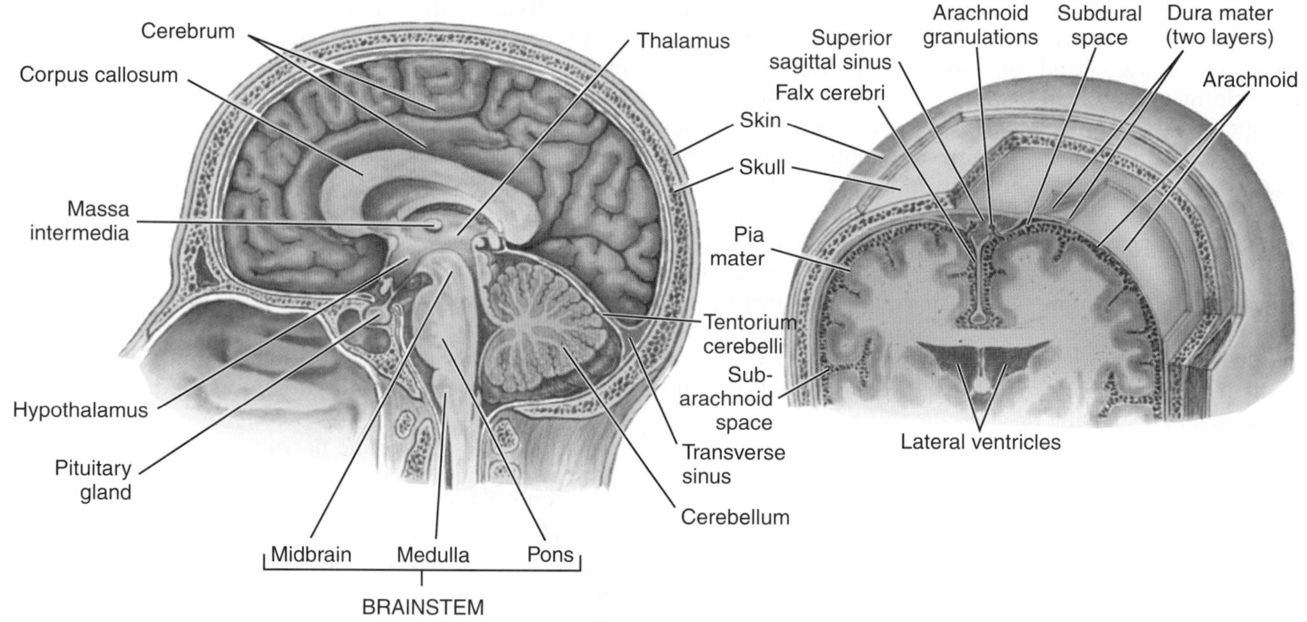


FIGURE 23-2 Scalp is composed of the following layers: skin, subcutaneous tissue, galea, and periosteum of skull. Skull bone has three tables: outer, diploë (or spongy layer), and inner. Dura mater lies beneath skull and completely encapsulates brain. Other structures are identified for reference and are described in text.

ricular, occipital, frontal, and supraorbital branches. Most veins roughly follow the course of the arteries, except the emissary veins, which drain directly through the skull into the intracranial venous sinuses. The scalp, the extracranial arteries, and portions of the dura mater are the only pain-sensitive structures that cover the brain. The brain itself is insensate.

## Skull

The skull provides protection for the brain. It is formed by 28 bones, most of which are paired although some in the median plane are single. Many of the bones are flat bones, consisting of two thin plates of compact bone encasing a spongy layer of cancellous bone containing bone marrow (see Figure 23-2). Infants are born with two fontanelles. These are openings in the skull that are located both anterior and posterior to the parietal bones (Figure 23-3). The posterior fontanelle is generally closed by 2 months and the anterior by about 18 months after birth. The bones of the skull are joined by bony seams called *sutures*. Eight bones form the walls of the cranial cavity, which houses the brain. There are four single bones (frontal, occipital, ethmoid, and sphenoid) and four paired bones (temporal and parietal) (Figure 23-4). The sagittal suture lies in the medial plane and joins the two parietal bones. The coronal suture joins the frontal and parietal bones. The squamous su-

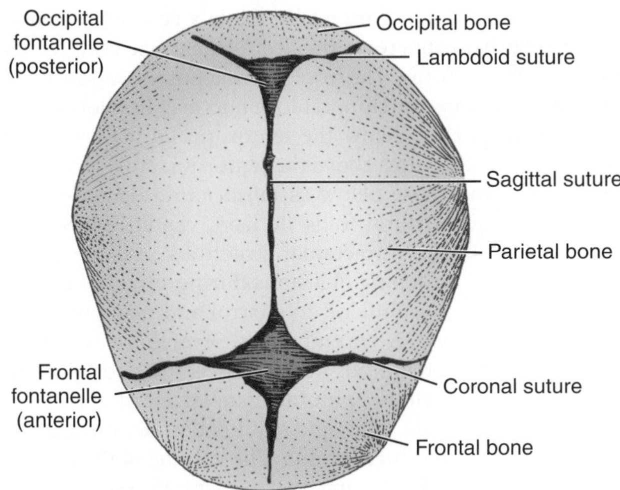


**FIGURE 23-3** Skull at birth viewed from above.

tures border the squamous part of the temporal bones. The lambdoid suture joins the occipital and parietal bones. Skull bones vary in thickness and tend to be thinner where they are covered in muscles, for example, in the temporal and posterior fossae. The skull articulates with the first cervical vertebra to allow for flexion and extension of the skull. The skeletal surface landmarks of the head can be palpated and are commonly used to plan surgical approaches (Figure 23-5).

The interior of the skull is anatomically divided into three cranial fossae: anterior, middle, and posterior (Figure 23-6). The anterior fossa is limited posteriorly by the sphenoid ridge, along which pituitary tumors and aneurysms of the circle of Willis are generally approached. The frontal lobes and olfactory bulbs and tracts lie in the anterior fossa. The temporal lobes lie in the middle fossa, which is shaped like a butterfly. The sella turcica, formed by the sphenoid bone, is the most central part of the middle fossa and houses the pituitary gland. The floor and lateral walls of the middle fossa are shaped from the greater wings of the sphenoid bone and parts of the temporal bone, which house the internal and middle ear structures. The posterior fossa, the largest and deepest fossa, is formed by the occipital, sphenoid, and petrous portions of the temporal bones; the cerebellum and brainstem lie here, as do many cranial nerves. The foramen magnum, the largest opening in the skull, permits the spinal cord to join the brainstem in the posterior fossa. Numerous other openings exist in the base of the skull for passage of arteries, veins, and cranial nerves.

***Skull Fractures.*** The severity of skull fractures depends on the degree of resulting brain injury. Simple skull fractures can be serious if they cross major vascular channels in the skull. If vessels are torn, epidural or subdural hematomas may form. Depressed skull fractures require a surgical procedure to elevate the depressed bone. Open skull fractures should be irrigated copiously and closed to prevent infection. Basilar skull fractures may cause cerebrospinal fluid (CSF) rhinorrhea or otorrhea. A few patients with these CSF leaks require surgical repair if they do not resolve after 2 weeks.

***Deformities of the Cranium.*** Craniosynostosis is the most common pediatric skull deformity seen and treated by the neurosurgeon. The phenomenon is a premature closure or lack of formation of cranial sutures, leading to cosmetic abnormalities, eventual life-threatening intracranial pressure (ICP) increases, and arrested brain development unless diagnostic and surgical interventions ensue. Cranial remodeling is most often undertaken during the first year of life, when brain capacity triples (see Chapter 29).

## Meninges

The brain and spinal cord are completely enveloped by the meninges, which are three membranes that provide support and protection. The meningeal layers from superficial to deep are the dura mater, arachnoid mater, and pia mater (see Figure 23-2). The space superficial to the dura is known as the epidural space. The cranial meninges are located between the skull and the brain.

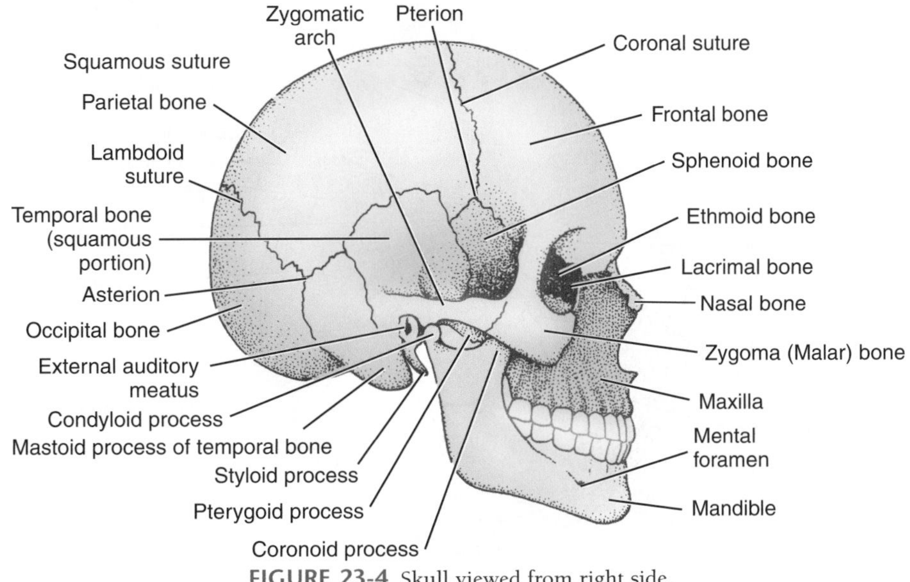


**FIGURE 23-4** Skull viewed from right side.

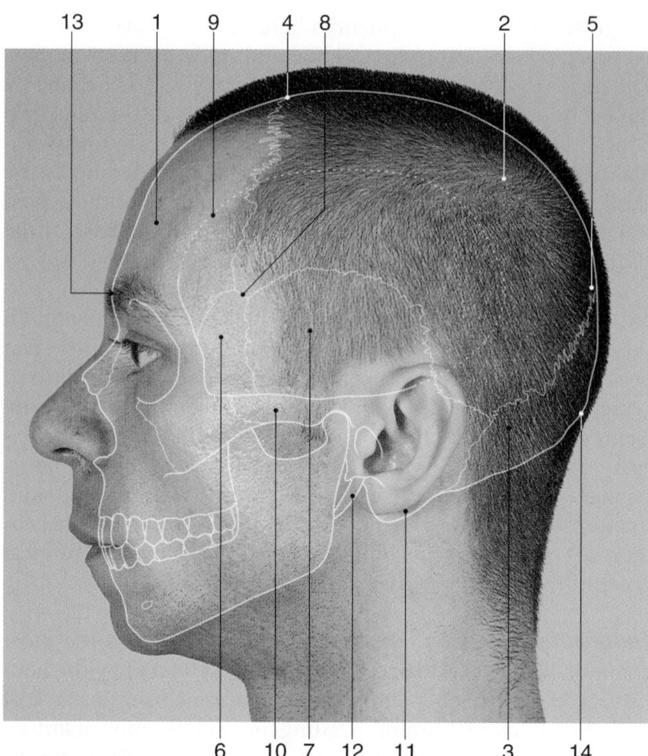


**FIGURE 23-5** Lateral aspect of the head: bones. 1. Frontal. 2. Parietal. 3. Occipital. 4. Bregma (anterior fontanelle). 5. Lambda (posterior fontanelle). 6. Greater wing of sphenoid. 7. Squamous temporal. 8. Pterion. 9. Temporal lines. 10. Zygomatic arch. 11. Mastoid process. 12. Styloid process. 13. Glabella. 14. External occipital protruberance.

The dura mater is a tough, shiny, fibrous membrane that is close to the inner surface of the skull and folds to separate the cranial cavity into compartments. The largest fold is the falx cerebri—an arch-shaped, vertically placed, midline structure separating the right and left cerebral hemispheres (see Figure 23-2). A smaller fold of dura mater, the falx cerebelli, separates the cerebellar hemispheres vertically. A transverse fold, the tentorium cerebelli, forms the roof of the posterior fossa. The tentorium supports the temporal lobe and occipital lobes of the cerebral hemispheres. Below the tentorium lie the cerebellum and brainstem. Structures above the tentorium are referred to as *supratentorial* and those below as *infratentorial* (Figure 23-7). At margins of these dural folds lie large venous sinuses that drain blood from the intracranial structures into the jugular veins. Accidental breaching of a sinus during surgery can cause severe bleeding that is difficult to control and may put the patient at risk for a venous air embolism. Several arteries also lie within the layers of the dura. The largest is the middle meningeal, a source of serious epidural hemorrhage if torn by an overlying skull fracture. The rigid skull makes hemorrhage and swelling in the brain critical events. The volume of the intracranial cavity is fixed. Increasing the intracranial contents by a hemorrhage, tumor, or edema may lead to serious ICP problems. Pressure on brain tissue may cause irreparable damage.

Beneath the dura mater is a transparent membrane called the *arachnoid.* Although the outer layer of arachnoid closely approximates the dura mater, the space between is considered the subdural space. The inner arachnoid layer forms innumerable weblike filaments that bridge to the surface of the brain (see Figure 23-2). The arachnoid passes over the sulci and fissures of the brain, without dipping into them. The arachnoid is separated from the pia mater beneath it by the subarachnoid space, which is filled with CSF that bathes the brain. Around the base of the brain, particularly, this space becomes enlarged to form cisterns. The major intracranial nerves and blood vessels pass through these compartments. Intracranial approaches can be charted in terms of the basal cisterns.

The pia mater, the innermost membrane, closely follows the contours of the surface of the brain into the sulci and fissures. Only the microscopic subpial space separates the pia from the brain. The pia mater has a rich vascular network. Vascular fringes of pia mater project into the ventricles to form the choroid plexus of the ventricles, which produce CSF.

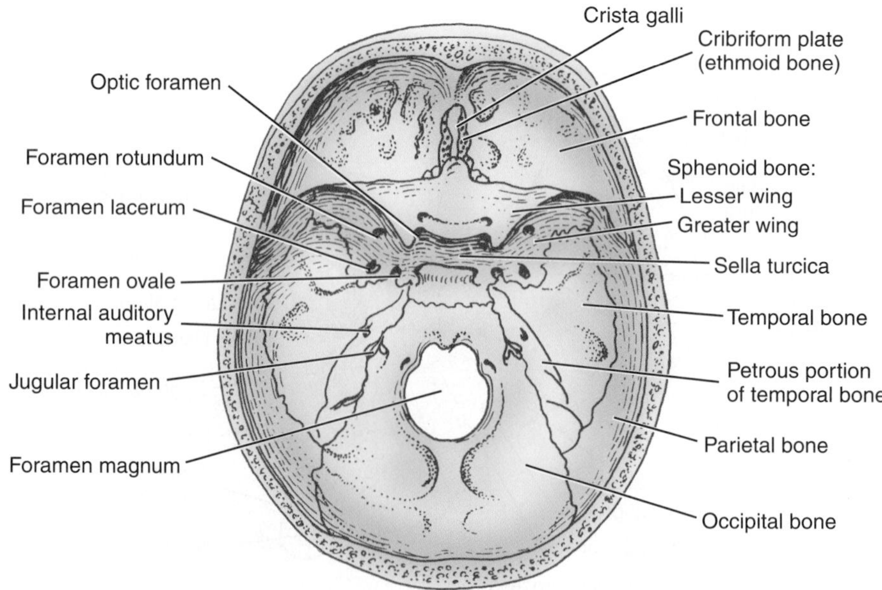


**FIGURE 23-6** Floor of cranial cavity.

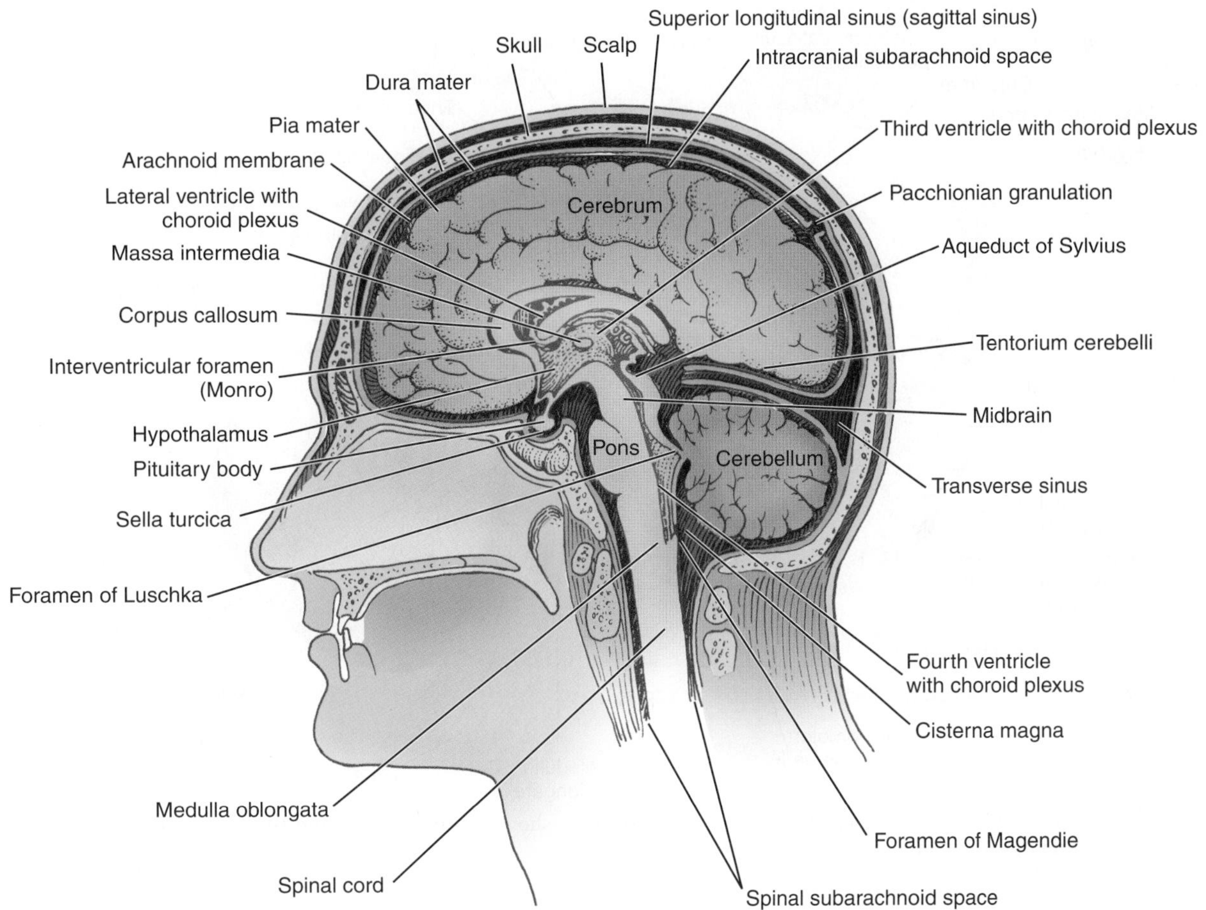


**FIGURE 23-7** Sagittal section of head showing cerebrospinal fluid spaces and their relationship to venous circulation and their principal subdivision of the brain and its coverings.

## Brain

The anatomy of the brain, formally known as the encephalon, can be considered in multiple ways. Based on prenatal development, the principal divisions from rostral (head) to caudal (tail), descending toward the spinal cord, are the forebrain or prosencephalon, the midbrain or mesencephalon, and the hindbrain or rhombencephalon. The rhombencephalon is subdivided into the cerebellum, the medulla oblongata, and the pons. The prosencephalon includes the diencephalon and the telencephalon, or cerebrum. The medulla oblongata, pons, and midbrain are collectively referred to as the brainstem (Figures 23-7 and 23-8).

***Cerebrum.*** The right and the left cerebral hemispheres are the largest parts of the brain and occupy the anterior and middle fossae. Each hemisphere is divided into frontal, parietal, occipital, and temporal lobes. The two hemispheres are separated by the longitudinal fissure and the falx cerebri but remain connected underneath the falx by a large transverse bundle of nerve fibers called the corpus callosum (see Figure 23-8). Each of the cerebral hemispheres controls sensation and motor activity to and receives sensory stimuli from the opposite half of the body.

The convoluted surface of the cerebrum consists of gray matter, called the *cerebral cortex,* which contains the cell bodies of the many nerve pathways of the brain. The underlying white matter contains millions of myelinated nerve axons and is relatively avascular compared with the cortex. The nerve pathways, or fiber tracts, are of three types: (1) commissural fibers, which pass from one cerebral hemisphere to the other; (2) association fibers, which connect regions of gyri and lobes longitudinally within a cerebral hemisphere; and (3) projection fibers, including the great motor and sensory systems, which run vertically to connect the cortical regions with other portions of the CNS.

The surfaces of the hemispheres form convolutions called *gyri* and intervening furrows called *sulci,* which serve as anatomic landmarks. Two sulci of particular anatomic importance during surgery are (1) the lateral sulcus, or sylvian fissure, which divides the temporal lobe from the frontal and parietal lobes, and (2) the central sulcus, or fissure of Rolando, which separates the frontal from the parietal lobe. The central sulcus also separates the motor cortex (precentral gyrus) from the sensory cortex (postcentral gyrus). The motor cortex lies anterior to the central sulcus, and the sensory cortex lies posterior to the central sulcus. Both the motor and sensory cortex can be represented by a topographically organized map called a homunculus that proportionately represents each body part at the area of the gyri that controls it. The diagrams illustrate how the number of neurons corresponds to the degree of motor and sensory control required. For example, areas that need more fine motor control, such as the fingers and face, have a higher concentration of neurons than other areas. Keep in mind that the left motor and

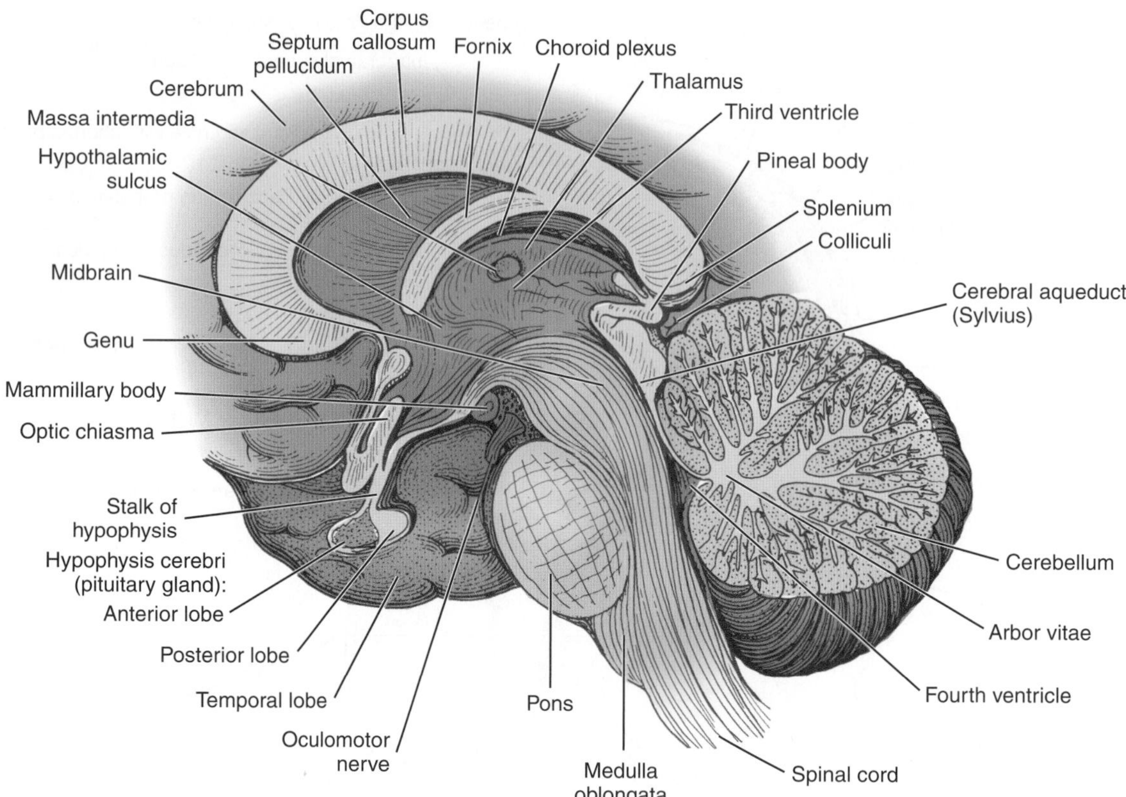


**FIGURE 23-8** Sagittal section through midline of brain showing structures around third ventricle, including corpus callosum, thalamus, and hypothalamus.

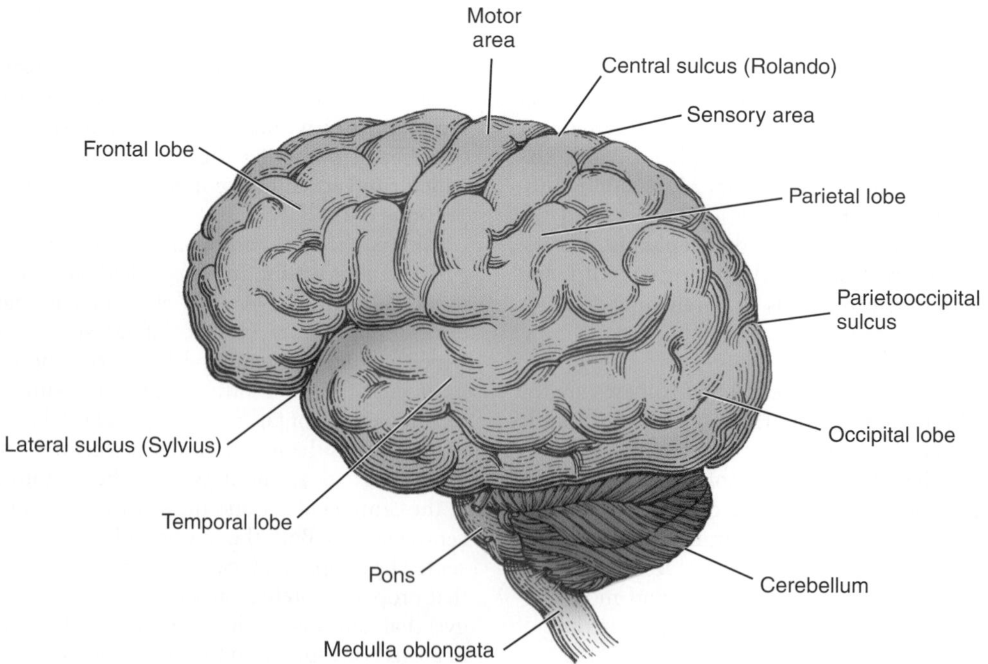


**FIGURE 23-9** Lateral view of cerebral hemisphere (showing lobes and principal fissures), cerebellum, pons, and medulla oblongata.

sensory cortices control the right side of the body and vice versa (Figure 23-9). Destruction of an area of motor cortex results in loss of voluntary motor function on the corresponding area of the opposite side of the body (Figure 23-10).

The frontal lobe is anterior to the central sulcus and controls the higher functions of intellect and abstract reasoning, along with movement, language, and personality. Posterior to the central sulcus is the parietal lobe, extending back to the parietooccipital fissure. This area contains the final receiving and integrating station for sensory impulses, such as pain and touch, from the contralateral side of the body. It is also involved with special relationships and object identification. The occipital lobe lies posterior to the parietooccipital fissure. It receives and integrates visual impulses and registers them as meaningful images (see Figures 23-9 and 23-10).

Inferior to the lateral sulcus, in the middle fossa, is the temporal lobe, which is involved with memory, speech, and smell. Lesions of the left temporal lobe in right-handed persons and in many left-handed persons may affect the comprehension and verbalization of words, resulting in aphasia. The insula (island of Reil) is an area of cortex that lies deep within the lateral sulcus and can be exposed when the upper and lower lips of the fissure are separated. The insula is believed to be involved with smell, taste, touch, and possibly language.

The limbic system consists of large parts of the cortex near the medial wall of the cerebral hemisphere (cingulate and parahippocampal gyri) along with the hippocampus, amygdala, and septum. It is closely and significantly connected with the hypothalamus. It has a diffuse distribution in the brain, and many components of the limbic system have overlapping functions. The hippocampus is critical for learning and memory. The amygdala regulates the perceptive and expressive aspects of emotional and social behavior. The limbic system affects endocrine and autonomic functions of the body, recent memory, emotions, behaviors, and motivational and mood states. Restlessness and hyperactivity may result from lesions of this area.

The basal ganglia are subcortical collections of nuclei (gray matter) that include the caudate nucleus, putamen, and globus pallidus (collectively referred to as the *corpus striatum*), the substantia nigra (which is located in the midbrain), and the subthalamic nucleus (part of the diencephalon). The basal ganglia influence movement and behavior through projections to the thalamus and brainstem and subsequently the cortex (Figure 23-11). The basal ganglia function to promote and support patterns of behavior and movement that are appropriate in a given situation and to inhibit unwanted or inappropriate behavior and movements. Disorders of the basal ganglia are principally characterized by abnormalities of movement, muscle tone, and posture. Damage to these neural components may cause rigidity of the skeletal muscles and various types of spontaneous tremors. Sections of the basal ganglia and thalamus can be selectively destroyed surgically in an effort to relieve the tremors and rigidity associated with multiple sclerosis, Parkinson's disease, various forms of cerebellar degeneration, and late effects of severe brain trauma (Research Highlight).

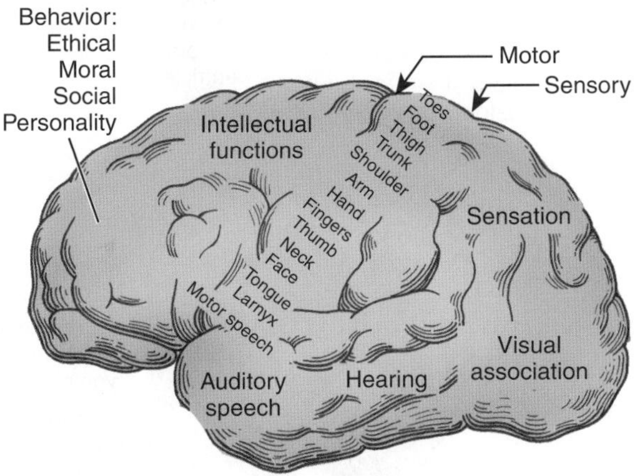


FIGURE 23-10 Principal functional subdivisions of cerebral hemispheres.

***Diencephalon.*** The diencephalon is composed of the thalamus, hypothalamus, epithalamus, and subthalamus and surrounds the third ventricle. The thalamus is the major relay station for incoming sensory stimuli. Except for some olfactory impulse transmission, all sensory information coming into the cerebral hemispheres is relayed through the thalamus. This is also true for motor pathways from the cerebellum and basal ganglia. Because of the central role of the thalamus in perception of body sensations, surgical lesions can be made in it in an attempt to alleviate pain.

Along the floor of the third ventricle is the hypothalamus (see Figure 23-8), which is concerned principally with the autonomic regulation of the body's internal environment and is intimately connected with the pituitary gland. It controls fluid and electrolyte balance, appetite, reproduction, thermoregulation, immune response, and many emotional responses. It influences levels of attention and consciousness. The pituitary gland is suspended from the base of the hypothalamus by the pituitary stalk. It secretes multiple hormones that are regulated by the hypothalamus. A pituitary tumor can result in a

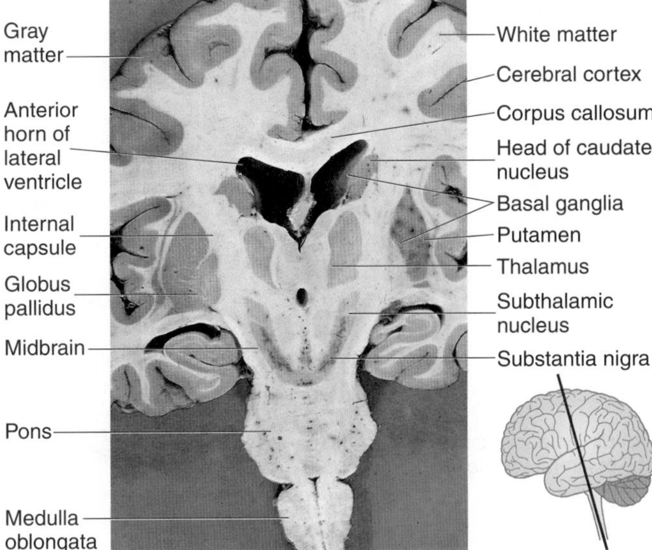


FIGURE 23-11 Oblique coronal section through the cerebral hemisphere and brainstem showing the disposition of gray and white matter, the basal ganglia, and the internal capsule.

## RESEARCH HIGHLIGHT

### Deep Brain Stimulation and Parkinson's Disease

Patients with Parkinson's disease can experience a number of symptoms, many of which are quite disabling. Surgery may be an option for these patients when medical treatment is no longer effective or when the side effects of medication become intolerable.

Deep brain stimulation (DBS) targets the subthalamic nucleus and inactivates it with an implantable electrode. The stimulation blocks the abnormal nerve transmission and results in a decrease in symptoms such as immobility and dyskinesia and may also reduce medication requirements. An advantage of DBS over other surgical treatments for Parkinson's disease (i.e., thalamotomy, pallidotomy, and subthalamotomy) is that the procedure is not destructive to tissue.

Researchers implanted 191 subthalamic stimulator devices in 100 patients and reviewed the results over a 1-year period to determine if this technique resulted in clinical improvement without mortality or major morbidity.

Immobility symptoms were reduced by 69%, and dyskinesia symptoms were reduced by 60%. Medication requirements were reduced by 30%. None of the patients in the study died, and only 26% experienced any morbidity related to the procedure. Postoperative confusion was the most frequent complication associated with DBS and was experienced by 13% of the patients.

The authors reviewed the literature to compare the mortality and morbidity of DBS with pallidotomy and subthalamotomy. Mortality rates for pallidotomy were 1.2%. Morbidity for pallidotomy and subthalamotomy was more than 30% with a rate of permanent morbidity of 13.8%.

Research continues in the field of surgical options for treating Parkinson's disease and other movement disorders. DBS appears to be a promising option with minimal morbidity.

Modified from Goodman RR and others: Operative techniques and morbidity with subthalamic nucleus deep brain stimulation in 100 consecutive patients with advanced Parkinson's disease, *Journal of Neurology, Neurosurgery and Psychiatry* 77:12-17, 2006.

hormonal imbalance. It can also encroach on the optic chiasma, causing vision changes.

The subthalamus is a complex region of nuclear groups and fiber tracts, including the subthalamic nucleus, which is considered with the basal ganglia. The epithalamus consists of multiple nuclei and the pineal gland, an endocrine gland that regulates the circadian rhythm.

***Brainstem.*** The brainstem consists of the midbrain, pons, and medulla oblongata. It is located in the posterior fossa and forms the floor of the fourth ventricle. It is the site of many ascending and descending fiber tracts that allow for communication among the structures of the brain and between the brain and spinal cord. All but two of the twelve cranial nerves attach to the brainstem. The short, stocky portion of the brain, between the cerebral hemispheres and pons, is the midbrain (see Figure 23-7), also referred to as the *mesencephalon.* It is composed of the cerebral peduncles, the substantia nigra, numerous nerve tracts and nuclei, and association centers that control the majority of eye movements. Immediately below the midbrain is the pons, which contains control areas for horizontal eye movement and face movement. The medulla oblongata is continuous with the spinal cord at the foramen magnum. It contains the vital cardiovascular and respiratory regulatory centers (see Figure 23-9). Damage to the brainstem is often devastating and life threatening, because it can affect movement, senses, consciousness, perception, and cognition. Surgery directly on the brainstem is of high risk.

***Cerebellum.*** The cerebellum, which occupies most of the posterior fossa, forms the roof of the fourth ventricle (Figures 23-8 and 23-12). It has two lateral lobes, or hemispheres, and a medial portion, the vermis. The fissures of the cerebellum are small and run transversely. The cerebellum is concerned principally with balance and coordination of movement. It has many complex connections with higher and lower centers and

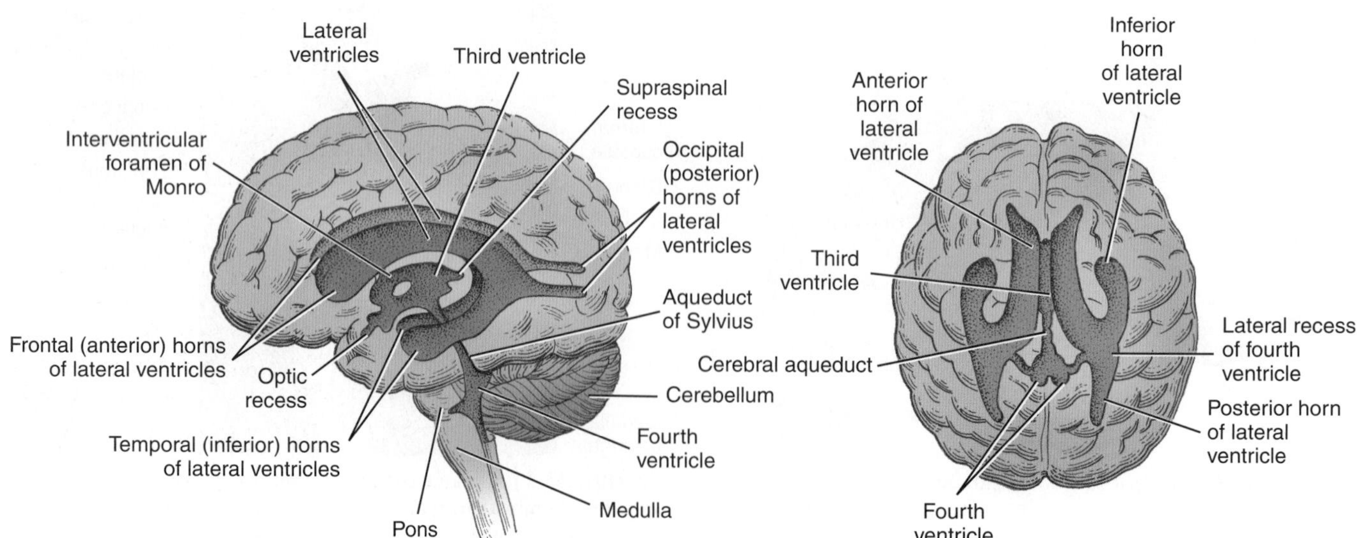


FIGURE 23-12 Ventricular system showing its relationship to various parts of brain.

exerts its influence unilaterally—in contrast to the cerebral hemispheres, which act contralaterally. By splitting the vermis in the exact midline, a satisfactory exposure of tumors that lie in the fourth ventricle is obtained without sacrificing the important cerebellar functions.

***Pathologic Lesions of the Brain.*** Approximately 17,000 new cases of primary intracranial tumors are diagnosed each year in the United States. A similar number of people who have systemic malignancies develop CNS metastasis.[6] Only about 50% of adults with brain tumors are alive 1 year following the diagnosis. Five-year survival rates vary considerably with different tumor types. In children the 5-year survival with a brain tumor is approximately 58%. For adults, 5-year survival is approximately 25%.[6]

Multiple factors are suspected of playing a role in the pathogenesis of intracranial neoplasms. Early diagnosis simplifies surgical treatment because increased ICP and severe neurologic changes are not usually present. Brain tumors are either malignant or benign, depending on the cell type. Primary tumors generally do not resemble the carcinomas and sarcomas found elsewhere in the body and rarely metastasize outside the CNS. Both primary and metastatic tumors of the brain and its membranes are included in the term *intracranial tumors.*

Traditionally, tumors are classified by cell type; however, classification of brain tumors is an evolving process. The widely used World Health Organization (WHO) system lists more than 120 types of brain tumors.[19] Table 23-1 gives the approximate incidence of brain tumors by histologic type. A brief description of a select list of brain tumors follows:

1. *Tumors of intraepithelial tissue* encompass gliomas, tumors believed to originate from neuroglial cells.

   a. Astrocytomas are the most common of all primary brain tumors, accounting for about 80% of gliomas.[6] They usually occur in the cerebellum of children and the cerebrum of adults. They are often cystic and discrete in children and infiltrating and ill defined in adults. Astrocytomas are classified in the WHO system based on the principal cell type and on the degree of anaplasia as grade I to IV, with grade I being the more favorable type of tumor and grade IV being the most malignant. Glioblastoma multiforme (GBM), a grade IV astrocytoma, is an infiltrative, fast-growing, rapidly recurring cerebral tumor that occurs most frequently in the sixth and seventh decade. It is the most common type of primary brain tumor, accounting for about 50% of gliomas.[20] It is one of the few tumors that is capable of invading both cerebral hemispheres by crossing the midline. Areas of necrosis are characteristic. Recent studies have consistently demonstrated the benefits of radical surgical resection. Postoperative radiation therapy significantly improves survival. Even with aggressive multimodality therapy, median survival is less than 1 year and 5-year survival is less than 5%.[20]

   b. Oligodendroglioma, typically found in the cerebral hemispheres, is usually infiltrating but occasionally moderately well defined. It frequently presents in middle age with seizure. It is now believed that the true incidence of oligodendrogliomas is 5% to 15% of gliomas, much higher than previously thought. Therapy usually consists of surgery followed by radiation therapy and chemotherapy.[20]

   c. Ependymoma occurs most frequently in children and is likely to arise in or near the ventricular walls. It commonly occurs in the fourth ventricle, where it abuts or involves vital medullary centers. It also frequently metastasizes into the subarachnoid spaces. This tumor accounts for 3% to 4% of gliomas. Surgical resection followed by radiation therapy is the usual treatment. The 5-year survival rate is 74%.[4]

   d. Medulloblastoma is a fast-growing, rapidly recurring tumor of the vermis of the cerebellum and fourth ventricle that usually occurs in young children. It characteristically metastasizes into the subarachnoid spaces, usually spreading to the base of the brain by this route. It accounts for 15% to 20% of childhood intracranial brain tumors and is the most common malignant pediatric brain tumor.

2. *Tumors of the meninges (meningiomas)* commonly occur in people in the fourth to sixth decades of life.[1] They are usually benign, circumscribed, slow-growing tumors, arising from arachnoid cells with secondary attachment to the dura. Various factors have been implicated in the development of meningiomas (Research Highlight). They typically involve the cortex and bone of the skull with growth. They can be very vascular and may adhere to the dural venous sinuses or major arteries, making their complete removal challenging. However, meningiomas often can be totally surgically removed (see Figure 23-34 on p. 828).
3. *Tumors of the cranial nerves (vestibular schwannomas)* are benign; they usually arise from the neurilemma sheath cells of the vestibular portion of the eighth cranial nerve within the auditory meatus. The term *acoustic neuroma* is a misnomer. These tumors grow slowly to fill the cerebellopontine angle and may indent the brainstem. Presenting symptoms include hearing loss, tinnitus, and disequilibrium.
4. *Hemopoietic neoplasms and lymphomas:* CNS involvement with lymphoma may occur secondarily from a systemic lymphoma or may arise primarily in the CNS.[4] Primary CNS lymphoma constitutes fewer than 2% of primary brain tumors.[6] The main role for surgery is for tumor biopsy. Stereotactic techniques are well suited for these often-deep tumors. The standard treatment after biopsy is radiation therapy, allowing for a median survival of 10 months. Adding chemotherapy can prolong survival.[8]

**TABLE 23-1**

### Approximate Incidence of Brain Tumors by Histologic Type

| Tumor Type | Incidence |
|---|---|
| Metastases | 20%-40% |
| Gliomas | 37.8% |
| Meningiomas | 30.1% |
| Other | 13.9% |
| Nerve sheath and cranial nerve tumors | 8% |
| Pituitary adenomas | 6.3% |

Modified from Central Brain Tumor Registry of the United States (CBTRUS): *Statistical report: primary brain tumors in the United States, 1998-2002,* 2005. Accessed March 27, 2006, on-line: www.cbtrus.org; National Cancer Institute: *Adult brain tumors PDQ treatment.* Accessed March 27, 2006, on-line: www.cancer.gov/cancerinfo/pdq/treatment/adultbrain/healthprofessional/#top.

## RESEARCH HIGHLIGHT

### Risk Factors for the Development of Meningioma

Meningiomas are mostly benign and relatively slow-growing tumors of the central nervous system. The etiology of meningiomas is largely unknown, but some predisposing factors that lead to their development may be trauma, neurofibromatosis type II, chronic virus infection, chromosome 22 aberrations, and female hormones. This study was designed to identify new associations between biologic factors or comorbidities that may represent risk factors for developing meningioma in adult patients.

Researchers performed a retrospective study of 306 patients who were treated for symptomatic cranial and spinal meningioma over a 4-year period. They collected data by way of chart review and sent a questionnaire to the patients. Forty-seven percent of the questionnaires were returned.

Data analysis showed that preexisting diabetes was positively associated with meningioma in both males and females, particularly in age-groups over 40 years for females and over 50 years for males. Arterial hypertension was associated with meningioma in female patients older than 60 years. Some factors, such as rheumatoid arthritis, bronchial asthma, smoking, and obesity, either had a negative factor or were not statistically significant in the development of meningioma.

The authors acknowledge that because many of the comorbidities, such as hypertension or diabetes, frequently occur in middle-aged or elderly people, they could coincide with the peak age for the incidence of meningioma and be mistakenly associated with the disease. Their findings may aid in the identification of specific areas for research and confirmation through other studies.

Modified from Schneider B and others: Predisposing conditions and risk factors for development of symptomatic meningioma in adults, *Cancer Detection and Prevention* 290:440-447, 2005.

5. *Germ cell tumors* occur in the midline (suprasellar and pineal region). Other than benign teratomas, all intracranial germ cell tumors are malignant and may metastasize by way of CSF and systemically. Tumors of the pineal region are very challenging to the neurosurgeon. Open microsurgery, endoscopy, and stereotactic biopsy are surgical options. Pineal region tumors often cause hydrocephalus. An endoscopic third ventriculostomy or a shunting procedure is routinely performed to alleviate the symptoms of hydrocephalus. Radiation therapy, chemotherapy, and radiosurgery are also treatment considerations.
   a. Germinoma is a neoplasm arising from germ cells. Survival with germinomas is much better than with nongerminomatous tumors (teratoma, embryonal cell carcinoma, choriocarcinoma).
   b. Teratoma is a congenital tumor containing embryonic elements.
   c. Embryonal cell carcinoma consists of a highly primitive group of neoplasms that arise in childhood. Predominantly large hemispheric masses involving deep supratentorial structures, these tumors are highly vascular and have poor prognoses. The primitive neuroectodermal tumor (PNET) is one such tumor.
   d. Choriocarcinoma is an extremely rare, very malignant neoplasm.
6. *Cysts and tumorlike lesions* include the following types:
   a. Epidermoid and dermoid cysts are developmental, benign tumors typically located in the suprasellar region.
   b. Colloid cysts are slow-growing benign tumors. They classically occur in the anterior third ventricle, blocking the foramen of Monro and causing obstructive hydrocephalus.
7. *Tumors of the sellar region* include the following types:
   a. Pituitary adenomas can be classified as nonfunctioning or functioning. Nonfunctioning pituitary adenomas account for approximately 30% of pituitary tumors, usually occur in people in the fourth and fifth decades of life, and do not cause clinical hormone hypersecretion. They are typically large and cause hypopituitarism or blindness from regional compression. The usual treatment is endoscopic or microscopic transsphenoidal removal of the tumor (see discussion of transsphenoidal hypophysectomy, p. 854). Following operative decompression, vision improves in approximately 80% of patients.[15] Radiation therapy or stereotactic radiosurgery may also be used. Functioning pituitary adenomas secrete excess quantities of pituitary hormones. The question of medical versus surgical treatment is ever present in the management of this group of patients. Adenomas may be further subdivided into microadenomas, which are less than 1 cm in diameter and usually discovered because of an endocrinopathy, and macroadenomas, which are larger than 1 cm and usually present with compressive effects of the tumor.[15]
      (1) Chromophobe tumors are relatively common in the anterior pituitary glands of adults. They cause compression of the pituitary, adjacent optic chiasma, and hypothalamus. Compression of the hypothalamus may lead to diabetes insipidus.
      (2) Eosinophilic adenomas are secretory, causing an excessive amount of growth hormone in the serum.
      (3) Basophilic adenomas are responsible for the excessive secretion of corticotropic, gonadotropic, and thyrotropic hormones. Acromegaly or, less commonly, Cushing's syndrome may occur and cause the patient to seek help long before the tumor has expanded sufficiently to compromise the optic chiasma.
      (4) Prolactin cell adenoma exhibits considerable differences in clinical presentation, depending on the gender of the patient. In women of reproductive age, the onset of amenorrhea and galactorrhea with associated infertility is an obvious sign. The diagnosis of a prolactinoma is established early in the course. In men, the clinical endocrinal symptoms, which include decreased libido and impotence, are not as conspicuous and initially may be disregarded by the patient. As a result, male patients frequently do not seek medical attention until the tumors are large and have spread beyond the confines of the sella.
   b. Craniopharyngiomas account for 2.5% to 4% of intracranial tumors, with 50% occurring in childhood.[8] They arise from the region of the pituitary stalk and typically contain both solid and cystic components. Calcification above the sella turcica is often seen radiographically. In addition to headache, vertigo, vomiting, and papilledema, diabetes insipidus and visual field changes are common. Although complete surgical removal is often impossible if it adheres to the carotid artery or hypothalamus, a subtotal resection with radiation offers favorable results.

8. Metastatic tumors are the most common brain tumor seen clinically, making up about half of brain tumors. They usually arise from carcinomas, more rarely from sarcomas, and occasionally from melanomas and retinal tumors. The most common sources are lung and breast cancer. The management of brain metastasis is complex and controversial. The current principal options for treatment include whole-brain radiation therapy, surgery, and stereotactic radiosurgery. The most important prognostic variables are the extent of systemic disease and the patient's functional status and age. These factors, along with the size, number, and location of tumors, guide treatment decisions. Median survival only rises from 3 to 6 months with radiation therapy and steroids to 9 to 12 months with surgery and stereotactic radiosurgery.[12]

A brain lesion is diagnosed by history, neurologic examination, diagnostic studies (especially computed tomography [CT] scan and magnetic resonance imaging [MRI]), and biopsy. The manifestations of an intracranial tumor fall into two classes: those resulting from irritation or impairment of function in specific areas of the brain directly affected by the tumor and those resulting from diffuse increased ICP. The most common presentation of brain tumors is progressive neurologic deficit, usually motor weakness. Headache and seizures are also common presenting symptoms.[8]

Large left or bifrontal lobe tumors may cause striking personality changes and depressive symptoms. Lesions in the left frontotemporal region, where motor speech originates, lead to aphasia. Parietal lobe lesions may result in contralateral weakness and sensory changes, along with defects in the perception of objects. Occipital tumors produce hemianoptic visual defects.

Cortical tumors frequently produce focal seizures of diagnostic value. The onset of epileptiform seizures in an adult is often associated with an intracranial neoplasm. Posterior fossa tumors often manifest their presence by blocking the CSF circulation, but they may also destroy cerebellar function, resulting in incoordination, ataxia, scanning speech, and deafness.

Treatment of brain tumors, although based on the characteristics of the tumor, can involve administration of steroids or antiepileptic medications, management of hydrocephalus, surgery, radiosurgery, radiation, and chemotherapy.

The presentation of multiple brain lesions in a patient is of grave concern, and an infective process should be considered along with the possibility of multiple tumors. Stereotactic biopsy of the lesion is most likely to provide a diagnosis. The operative team may be required to employ precautions to prevent the spread of an unknown infective process. Identification of the infective agent and process determines proper treatment.

## Ventricular System and Cerebrospinal Fluid

Within the brain are four communicating cavities, or ventricles, filled with CSF. In the lower medial portion of each cerebral hemisphere lies a large lateral ventricle that resembles a wishbone and is separated anteriorly from its counterpart by a thin septum (see Figure 23-12). Each lateral ventricle has a body and three horns: frontal, occipital, and temporal. Below the bodies of the lateral ventricles is a central cleft, or third ventricle. It communicates anteriorly with the lateral ventricles through the foramen of Monro and posteriorly with the fourth ventricle through the aqueduct of Sylvius—a long, narrow channel passing through the midbrain. The fourth ventricle is a cavity in the posterior fossa, between the cerebellum and the brainstem. In the roof of the fourth ventricle is the foramen of Magendie, an opening into the cisterna magna; at the lateral margins are the two foramina of Luschka, which open into the cisterna pontis. These cisterns are cavities that serve as reservoirs for CSF.

Much of the CSF originates in the choroid plexuses of the ventricles. These are tufted, vascular structures that allow certain fluid elements of the blood to pass through their ependymal linings. The choroid plexus is found along the floor in each lateral ventricle, on the roof of the third ventricle, and in the posterior portion of the fourth ventricle. Most of the fluid is formed in the lateral ventricles and flows through the interventricular foramen of Monro to the third ventricle and through the aqueduct of Sylvius to the fourth ventricle, where it escapes into the subarachnoid space of the basal cisterns through the foramina of Magendie and Luschka. From the basal cisterns the fluid flows around the spinal cord, over the cerebellar lobes, around the medulla and the base of the brain, and over the cerebral hemispheres in the subarachnoid space. The fluid is absorbed into the venous circulation through villi of the arachnoid (pacchionian granulations) into the great dural venous sinuses, particularly the superior sagittal sinus, and by diffusion through perivascular, perineural, and periradicular channels (see Figure 23-7).

Spinal fluid bathes the brain and spinal cord, helps support the weight of the brain, and acts as a cushion for the brain and spinal cord by absorbing some of the force of external trauma. By variation in its volume, it aids in keeping ICP relatively constant. If the brain atrophies, the amount of CSF increases to fill the dead space; if the brain swells, the amount of CSF decreases to compensate for the increase in brain mass. The fluid can carry certain drugs to diseased parts of the brain. It does not, however, play a significant role in supplying nutrition to the structures that it bathes. The total amount of circulating CSF averages 150 ml in the adult. The ventricles contain about 25 ml, and the remaining CSF circulates in the cranial and spinal subarachnoid space. CSF is secreted at a rate of between 21 and 24 ml/hr, or approximately 450 ml/24 hr. This means that in an adult, CSF is turned over about three times each day.[21]

***Pathologic Conditions Related to Cerebrospinal Fluid.*** CSF can be examined by the lab to provide diagnostic information. CSF is most commonly obtained by way of lumbar puncture (LP). Because the subarachnoid space surrounding the brain is freely connected to the subarachnoid space of the spinal cord, any abnormal increase in ICP will be directly reflected as an increase at the lumbar site. Tumors, infection, hydrocephalus, and intracranial bleeding can cause increased intracranial and spinal pressure.[16] LP is contraindicated when ICP is increased from a suspected intracranial mass that is causing neurologic symptoms. In this situation, the sudden reduction in pressure from the release of CSF could cause brain herniation. The ventricular fluid normally has a protein content of 5 to 15 mg/dl, whereas the spinal fluid has 25 to 45 mg/dl. These values may be considerably elevated in pathologic conditions of the CNS. The characteristics of normal spinal fluid are as follows:

- Appearance: clear and colorless
- Pressure: less than 20 cm $H_2O$

- Glucose: 50 to 75 mg/dl, or two thirds of blood glucose
- Chloride: 700 to 750 mg/dl
- Cells: white blood cells (WBCs)—neonate, 0 to 30 cells/μl; 1 to 5 years, 0 to 20 cells/μl; 6 to 18 years, 0 to 10 cells/μl; adult, 0 to 5 cells/μl
- Protein: lumbar, 15 to 45 mg/dl
- Culture: no growth
- Gamma globulin: 3% to12% of total protein[16]

Elevations in CSF pressure can be caused by an expanding mass within the skull, such as a tumor, hemorrhage, or cerebral edema; an increase in formation or decrease in absorption of fluid, as in meningitis, encephalitis, and other febrile conditions; an increase in venous pressure within the skull from an obstruction to normal venous drainage; a blockage of absorption by inflammatory conditions of the arachnoid and perivascular spaces; any mechanical obstruction of the ventricular or subarachnoidal fluid pathways; or decreased absorption of CSF. These pathologic conditions can cause a dangerous increase in ICP, which ultimately could result in brain herniation and death.

The rate of absorption and production of CSF is related to the osmotic and hydrostatic pressure of the blood. Intravenous (IV) injection of hypertonic mannitol, commonly used with a nonosmotic diuretic, can be employed to pull fluid from tissue to the vascular space for excretion by the kidneys, resulting in systemic diuresis and a decrease in ICP.

Hydrocephalus is a condition marked by an excessive accumulation of CSF resulting in dilation of the intracerebral ventricles where CSF is made and circulated. Enlargement of cerebral ventricles is the result of CSF blockage and interruption of CSF circulation or CSF reabsorption. The causes of hydrocephalus are many, including congenital conditions, aqueductal stenosis, tumors or cysts of the ventricular system, subarachnoid hemorrhage (SAH), posterior fossa tumors, or trauma with increased ICP. Noncommunicating (obstructive) hydrocephalus involves an obstruction of CSF pathways. In communicating hydrocephalus, the normal CSF pathways are open; however, there is an abnormality in CSF absorption with increased ICP. Normal pressure hydrocephalus (NPH) is a communicating hydrocephalus that produces a normal pressure on random LP.[8] NPH most commonly develops in the elderly, probably because of abnormal CSF absorption; however, the cause may not be apparent. Symptoms of dementia, unsteady gait, and urinary incontinence are seen with normal pressure and chronic hydrocephalus. Those with acute hydrocephalus present with headache, nausea, vomiting, drowsiness, and papilledema.

The appropriate surgical procedure depends on the precise type of hydrocephalus. Whenever possible, an obstructing lesion that causes hydrocephalus should be surgically removed. For some cases of obstructive hydrocephalus, endoscopic third ventriculostomy may be possible. With endoscopic third ventriculostomy, CSF can be diverted by surgically creating an opening at the floor of the third ventricle, thus eliminating the need for a shunt. However, treatment of hydrocephalus in both the adult and pediatric population is generally by placement of a ventriculoperitoneal (VP) shunt.[23] With acute symptoms, temporary placement of an external ventriculostomy catheter used to measure the ICP and drain CSF may be preferred, thus postponing or eliminating the need for a permanent VP shunt.

## Cerebral Blood Supply

The brain requires 20% more oxygen than any other organ to maintain its high level of metabolic activity. The arterial supply to the brain enters the cranium through the two internal carotid arteries anteriorly and the two vertebral arteries posteriorly. These communicate at the base of the brain through the circle of Willis (Figure 23-13), which ensures continuity of the circulation if any one of the four main channels is interrupted. However, these connections are extremely variable and do not always have functional anastomoses. The main branches for distribution of blood to each hemisphere of the brain from the internal carotid arteries are the anterior and middle cerebral arteries. Each artery nourishes a specific area of the brain (Figures 23-13 and 23-14). The anterior cerebral artery supplies the anterior two thirds of the medial surface and adjacent region over the convexity of the hemisphere, thus including about half of the frontal and parietal lobes. The middle cerebral artery supplies most of the lateral surface of the hemisphere, including half of the frontal, parietal, and temporal lobes. The posterior cerebral artery, which originates off the basilar artery, supplies the occipital lobe and the remaining half of the temporal lobe, principally on the inferior and medial surfaces. The brainstem and cerebellum are supplied by branches of the basilar and vertebral arteries.

The cerebral veins do not parallel the arteries as the veins do in most other parts of the body. The external cortical veins anastomose freely in the pia mater, forming larger cerebral veins, and as such they pierce the arachnoid membrane, cross the subdural space, and empty into the great dural venous sinuses. A subdural hemorrhage after head trauma may arise from disruption of these bridging vessels; an epidural hemorrhage often results from lacerations of the middle meningeal artery—a branch of the external carotid artery that supplies the dura mater. The deep cerebral veins, which drain the interior of the hemispheres, empty principally into the great vein of Galen and the inferior sagittal sinus (Figures 23-15 and 23-16).

The blood transports oxygen, nutrients, and other substances necessary for the proper functioning of living tissue. The needs of the brain for oxygen and glucose are critical. The brain can store only small amounts of oxygen and energy-producing nutrients. Constant flow of blood to the brain must be maintained.

The brain uses oxygen in the metabolism of glucose—the chief source of energy. Protein and fat metabolism plays little part in energy production. In the face of an oxygen deficit, the survival time of CNS tissue is very short. In the face of low blood glucose, CNS function is compromised and unconsciousness results.

Generally, all factors affecting the systemic blood pressure indirectly affect the cerebral circulation. The brain normally receives 20% of the cardiac output. The cerebral blood flow is kept constant by an autoregulation phenomenon such that increases in blood pressure lead to vasoconstriction of cerebral arteries and decreases in blood pressure cause cerebral vasodilation to maintain a relatively constant cerebral blood flow. When the mean arterial pressure falls below 60 mm Hg, the autoregulation mechanism usually fails.

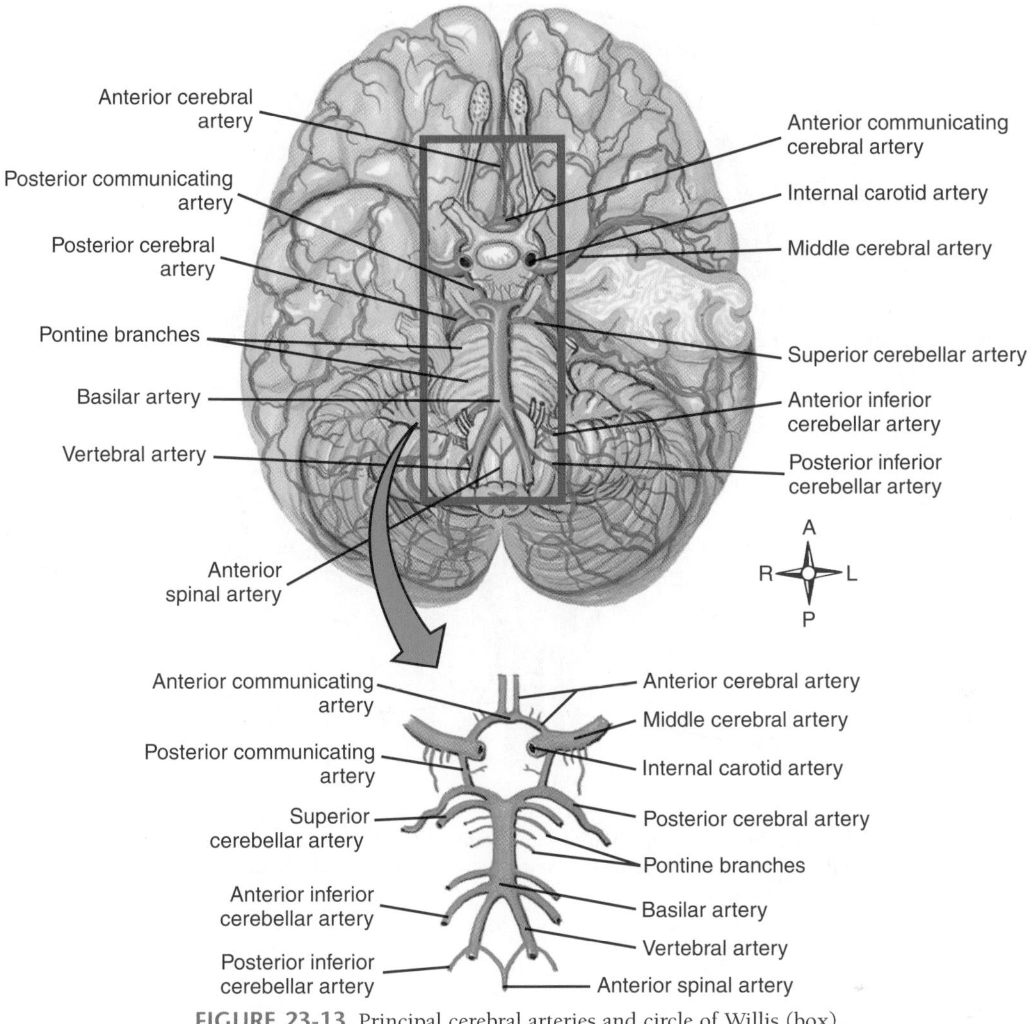


FIGURE 23-13 Principal cerebral arteries and circle of Willis (box).

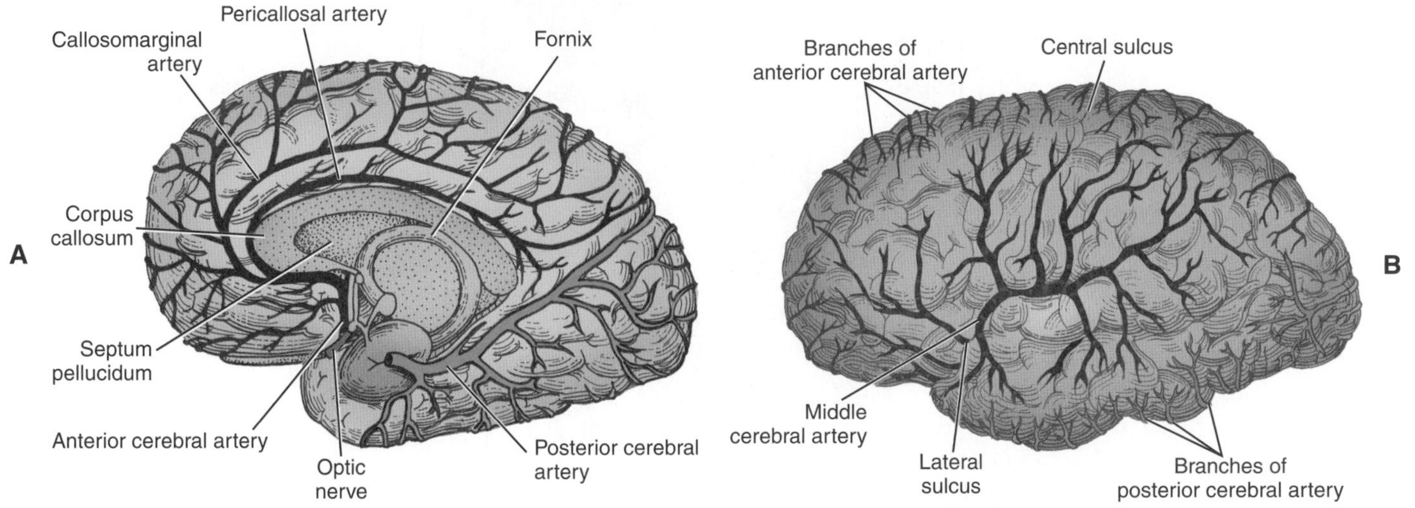


FIGURE 23-14 **A,** Arteries of medial surface of brain. **B,** Arteries of the lateral surface of brain.

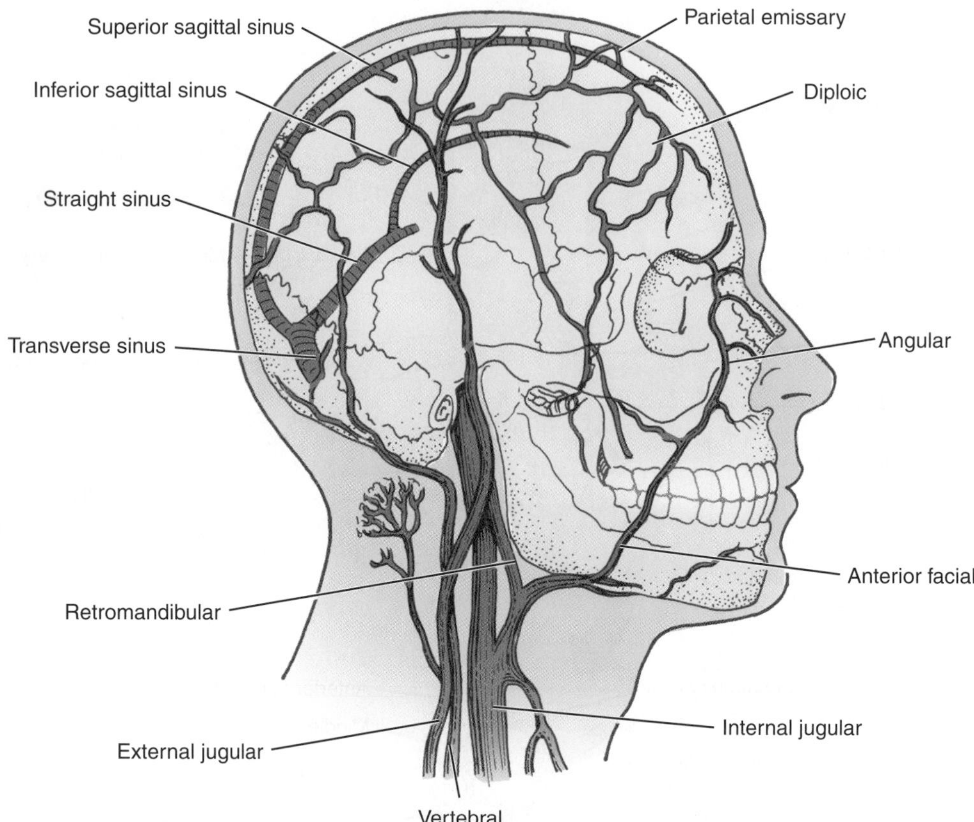


**FIGURE 23-15** Semischematic projection of large veins of head. Deep veins and dural sinuses are projected on skull. Note connection (emissary veins) between superficial and deep veins.

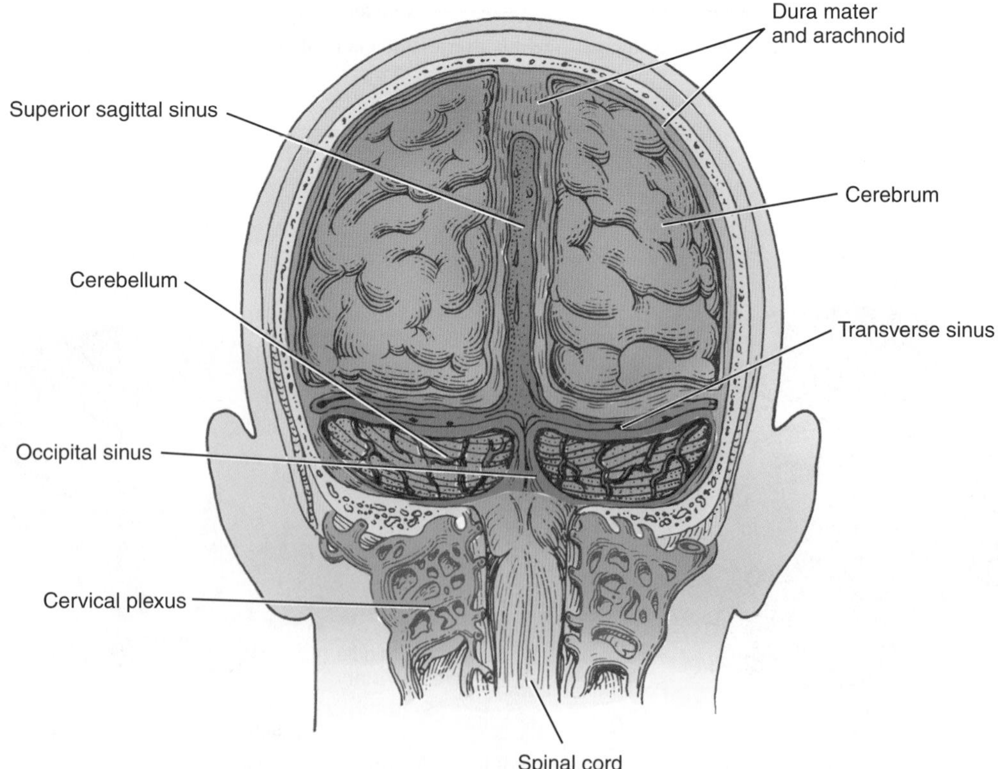


**FIGURE 23-16** Venous sinuses shown in relation to brain and skull.

***Vascular Pathologic Conditions of the Brain.*** Vascular lesions of the brain are most often diagnosed in people who present with acute, spontaneous intracranial hemorrhage.

ANEURYSMS. Aneurysms arise from a complex set of circumstances involving a congenital anatomic predisposition and local or systemic factors that weaken the arterial wall, leading to dilation. The majority of these lesions occur at the branching points of large subarachnoid conducting arteries. The greatest vulnerability to aneurysmal development occurs at points of vessel bifurcation. Acute SAH in this setting can lead to vessel vasospasm (with greatest risk at 4 to 10 days after the SAH), cerebral ischemia, hydrocephalus, increased ICP, diabetes insipidus, syndrome of inappropriate secretion of antidiuretic hormone (SIADH), respiratory failure, brain injury, and risk of rebleeding. The vessels of the circle of Willis are most often implicated, including the posterior communicating artery, anterior communicating artery, middle cerebral artery, carotid artery, posterior inferior cerebellar artery, vertebral artery, and basilar artery. Surgical intervention techniques are based on the characteristics of the aneurysm. Small neck aneurysms may be occluded using coils placed by means of interventional radiology techniques. Aneurysmal clipping by way of a craniotomy approach is most often used to treat broad neck aneurysms.

VASCULAR MALFORMATIONS. Vascular malformations of the CNS are characterized by congenital lesions that have the potential to produce symptoms any time during the life of an individual with the malformation. Types of vascular malformations include arteriovenous malformations (AVMs), cavernous malformations, capillary telangiectasias, and venous malformations. AVMs are complex lesions in which direct shunting of arterial blood to the venous system occurs. The vascular channels are tightly packed and have a propensity to hemorrhage. Capillary telangiectasias are small vascular malformations commonly seen in the pons. They rarely bleed. Cavernous malformations are cystic vascular spaces, similar to capillary telangiectasias but larger and with a tendency to bleed. Venous malformations are the most common type, comprising anomalous veins, a single tortuous vein, or a number of smaller veins joining at a single point. These are considered benign and rarely bleed. Surgical excision of the cavernous malformation and the AVM is recommended.

HEMATOMAS. Hematomas are collections of blood that coagulate to form space-occupying lesions. An intracerebral hemorrhage, the cause of stroke in many hypertensive patients, results in hematoma formation most often in the basal ganglia, subcortical white matter, cerebellum, and brainstem. These hematomas compress vital structures, depress consciousness, and can be catastrophic. They are often inoperable.[8]

Intracranial trauma can cause a shearing of arterial and venous vessels that results in hematoma collections in the epidural and subdural spaces. These space-occupying lesions raise ICP and often result in serious neurologic disruption (Figure 23-17). Epidural hematomas are often the result of a blow to the head causing a tear in the middle meningeal artery, which lies on the dura under the skull. These arterial hemorrhages can be life threatening in that they can cause rapid deterioration in level of consciousness secondary to size of the bleed and brain displacement by the hematoma (Figure 23-18). In contrast to an epidural hematoma, a traumatic subdural hematoma usually results from venous bleeding and collects more slowly. Bridging veins in the subdural space are torn; blood escapes, dissecting a space between the dura and the arachnoid, and collects over one cerebral hemisphere (Figure 23-19). Subdural hematomas may be acute, subacute, or chronic (Figure 23-20). Chronic hematomas can often be evacuated through burr holes, but acute hematomas may require a craniotomy to remove the clot and control bleeding.

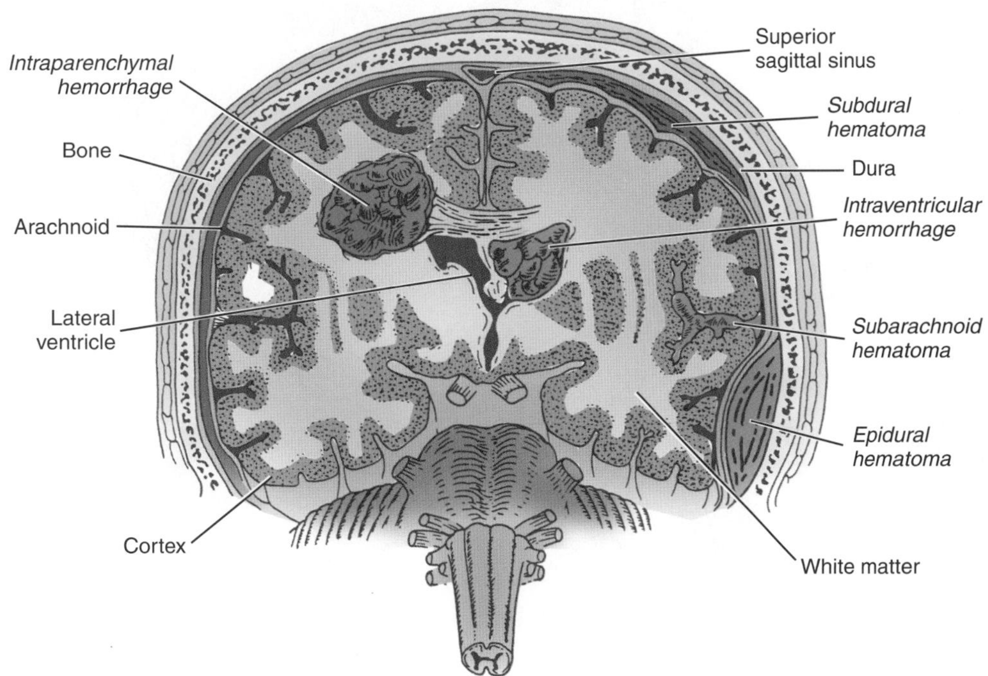


FIGURE 23-17 Types of intracerebral hemorrhage (in italics).

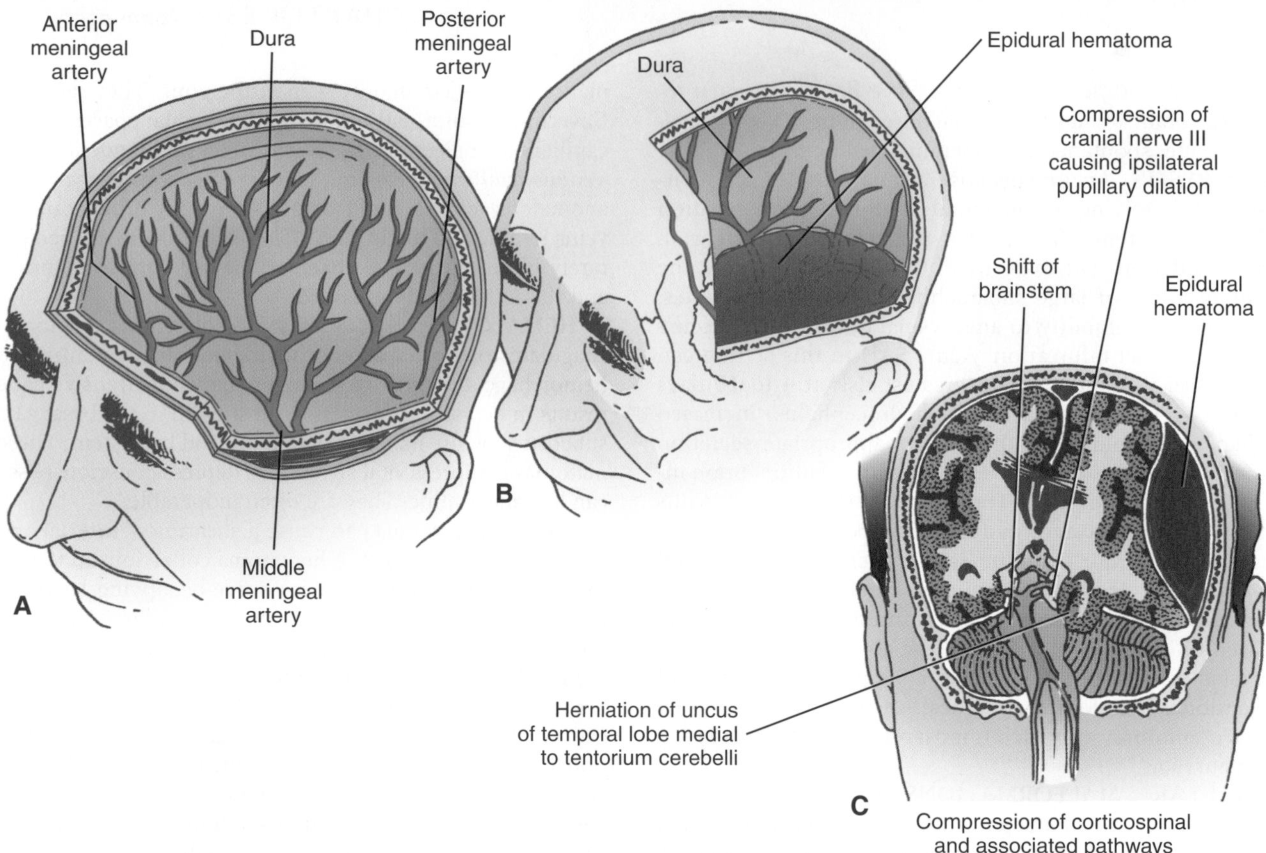


**FIGURE 23-18** Epidural hematoma is typically caused by trauma resulting in laceration of the middle meningeal artery. **A,** The middle meningeal artery. The typical traumatic epidural hematoma is caused by a laceration of this vessel. **B** and **C,** A linear fracture of the squamous portion of the temporal bone has torn the middle meningeal artery, which has resulted in an epidural hematoma.

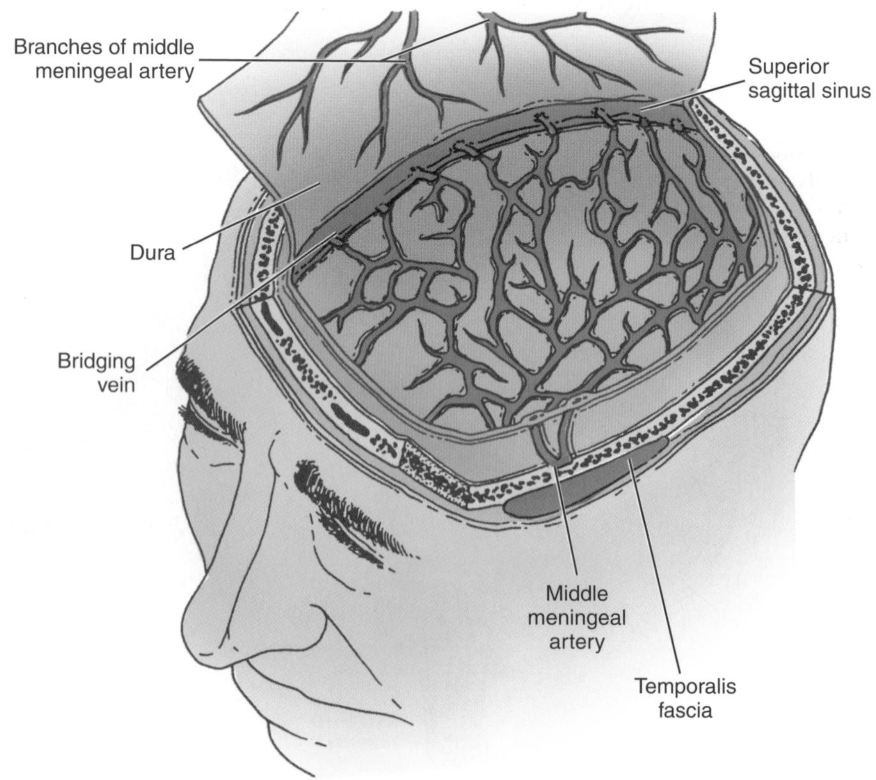


**FIGURE 23-19** Veins are shown extending from the surface of the brain to the superior sagittal sinus. Differential movement of the brain within the skull at the time of injury may tear one or more of these veins, leading to the formation of a subdural hematoma.

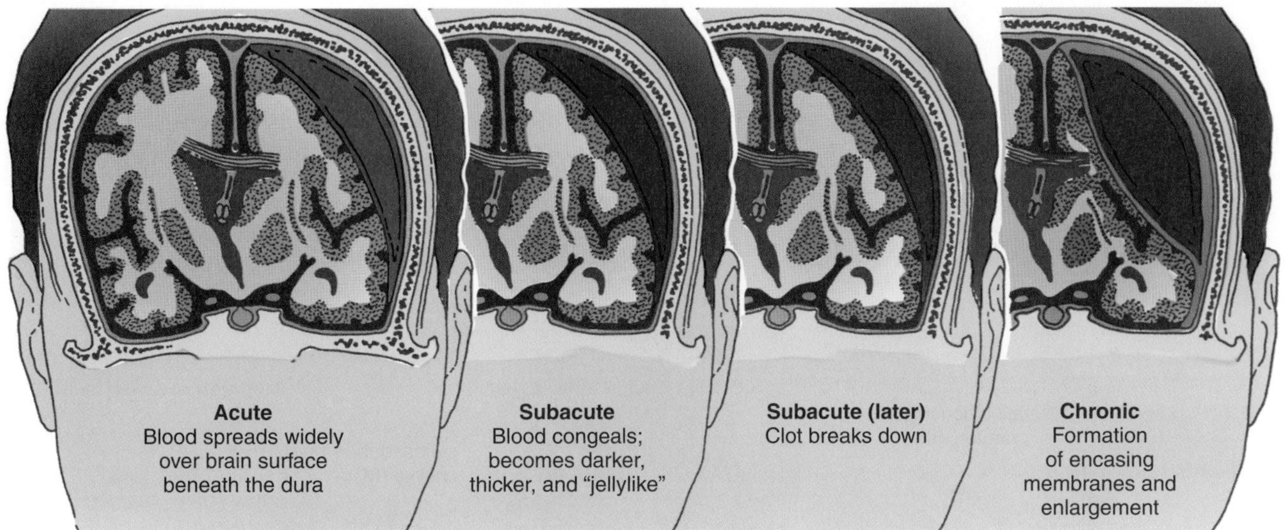
Acute
Blood spreads widely over brain surface beneath the dura
Subacute
Blood congeals; becomes darker, thicker, and "jellylike"
Subacute (later)
Clot breaks down
Chronic
Formation of encasing membranes and enlargement

**FIGURE 23-20** A subdural hematoma is liquid at first and subsequently clots. It is then reabsorbed, or it develops into a chronic subdural hematoma as a thick, vascular, outer membrane and a thin, inner membrane develops around liquefying blood, starting about 2 weeks after injury. The chronic subdural hematoma enlarges as further bleeding occurs within it.

CEREBRAL ISCHEMIA. Any area of the brain can become ischemic from an arterial occlusion or embolization. Symptoms may be gradual or sudden. Intracranial plaques most commonly form at the bifurcation of the internal carotid artery, into the middle and anterior cerebral arteries. In select cases, extracranial-intracranial arterial microanastomosis can be performed. Carotid endarterectomy can be performed for extracranial lesions of the carotid artery (see Chapter 26).

## Cranial Nerves

Twelve pairs of cranial nerves arise within the cranial cavity (Figure 23-21). Although they are part of the PNS, from a surgical standpoint they are considered with the head.

***First Cranial Nerve.*** The olfactory nerve, a fiber tract of the brain, is located under the frontal lobe on the cribriform plate of the ethmoid bone. It transmits the sense of smell. Frontal lobe tumors, fractures of the anterior fossa of the skull, and lesions of the nasal cavity may affect the olfactory nerve.

***Second Cranial Nerve.*** The optic nerve is a fiber tract of the brain. It originates in the ganglion cells of the retina and passes through the optic foramen in the apex of the orbit to reach the optic chiasma. A partial crossing of the fibers occurs there, so the fibers from the nasal half of each retina pass to the opposite side. Posterior to the chiasma, the visual pathway is called the *optic tract*. Still farther back, it becomes the optic radiation. Lesions in various parts of this pathway produce characteristic defects in the visual fields. For example, a lesion near the chiasma usually destroys the temporal vision of each eye (bitemporal hemianopia), whereas a lesion of the occipital lobe produces impairment of vision (homonymous hemianopia), affecting the right or left halves of the visual fields of both eyes.

Lesions that affect the optic nerve and are treated by neurosurgery include primary gliomas of the nerve, pituitary tumors that press on the optic chiasma, and occasionally meningiomas of the optic nerve sheath or in the region of the sella turcica and olfactory groove. The optic nerves and chiasma are best exposed through a frontal craniotomy along the floor of the anterior fossa or through a frontotemporal approach along the sphenoid ridge. Cranial base approaches using an orbital osteotomy or orbital-zygomatic osteotomies improve access and exposure of the optic system.

***Third, Fourth, and Sixth Cranial Nerves.*** The third, fourth, and sixth cranial nerves are three pairs of nerves—the oculomotor, the trochlear, and the abducens, respectively. They are conveniently considered together because they are the motor nerves to the muscles of the eyes. They are affected by many toxic, inflammatory, vascular, and neoplastic lesions. The third nerve may be affected by aneurysms of the posterior communicating artery, and pressure against this nerve accounts for pupillary dilation when temporal lobe (uncal) herniation, resulting from increased ICP, is present.

***Fifth Cranial Nerve.*** The trigeminal nerve has two functions: (1) sensory supply to the forehead, eyes, meninges, face, jaw, teeth, hard palate, buccal mucosa, tongue, nose, nasal mucosa, and maxillary sinus; and (2) motor innervation of the muscles of mastication. The sensory fibers that arise from cells in the trigeminal ganglion travel along the medial wall of the middle cranial fossa and then extend peripherally in three divisions: ophthalmic, maxillary, and mandibular. Behind the ganglion the fibers enter the brainstem by way of the sensory root. The motor root, which originates from cells in the brainstem, follows the course of the larger sensory component (Figure 23-22).

Trigeminal neuralgia (tic douloureux) is characterized by excruciating, piercing paroxysms of pain, affecting one or more of the major peripheral divisions. The recurrent attacks are usually brought on by stimulation of trigger zones present about the face, nares, lips, and teeth. This condition, believed to be caused by a high incidence of vascular compression on the root entry zone of the nerve leading to demyelination, tends to occur unilaterally and in older persons. Medical treat-

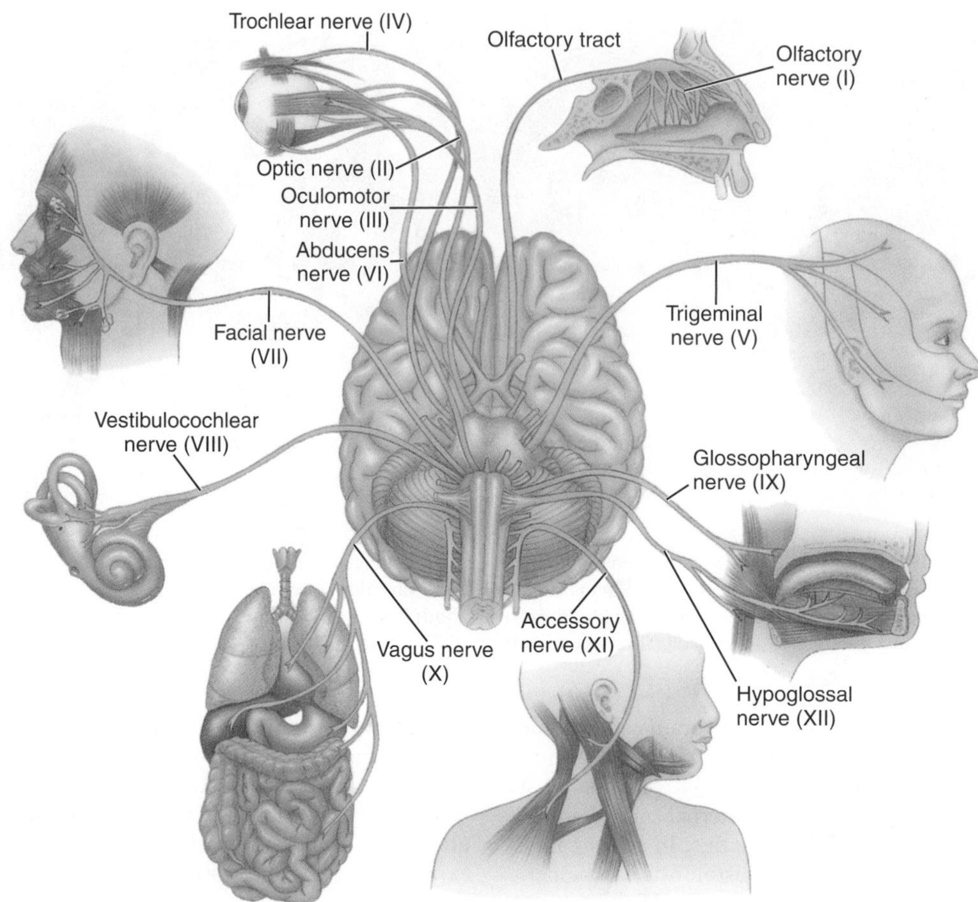


**FIGURE 23-21** Ventral surface of brain showing attachment of cranial nerves.

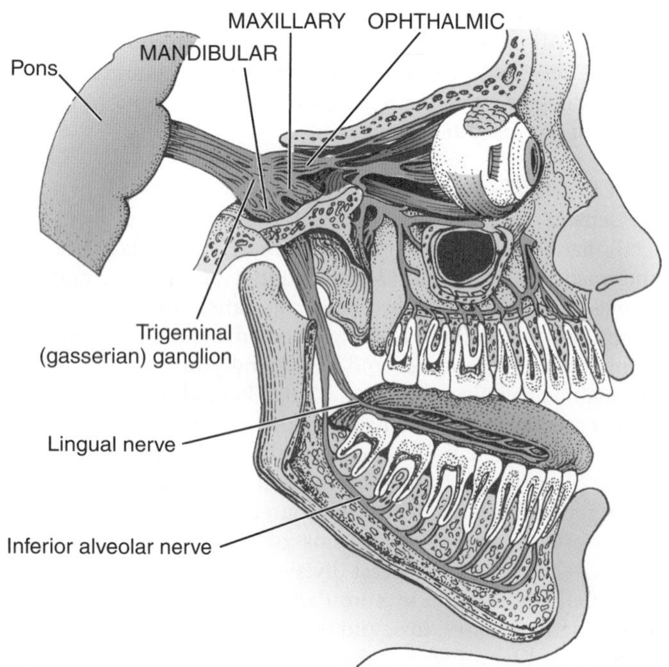


**FIGURE 23-22** Trigeminal (fifth cranial) nerve and its three main divisions.

ment is frequently unsuccessful in the long term. Types of neurosurgical procedures currently recommended for trigeminal neuralgia include percutaneous rhizotomy using glycerol, radiofrequency, or balloon compression; radiosurgery; and microvascular decompression. Microvascular decompression requires a suboccipital craniotomy and is the most invasive of the techniques. However, it is the least destructive and probably the most durable treatment.

***Seventh Cranial Nerve.*** The facial nerve supplies the musculature of the face and taste for the anterior two thirds of the tongue. It originates in the brainstem, passes through the skull with the eighth nerve by way of the internal acoustic meatus, continues along the facial canal, and exits just posterior to the parotid gland. The nerve may be damaged by vestibular schwannomas (e.g., acoustic neuromas), fractures at the base of the skull, mastoid infections, and surgical procedures in the vicinity of the parotid gland.

Bell's palsy, a facial lower motor neuron paralysis, can affect the seventh nerve. It may last for a few weeks to a few months, but recovery usually takes place. When permanent interruption of the nerve occurs, useful operations for restoration of function include spinal accessory–facial and hypoglossal-facial anastomosis. These operations are performed high in the neck behind the parotid gland by use of the operating microscope.

***Eighth Cranial Nerve.*** The acoustic nerve has two parts, both sensory—the cochlear for hearing and the vestibular for balance. The former receives stimuli from the organ of Corti and the latter from the semicircular canals. The major surgical lesion of the eighth nerve is vestibular schwannoma (acoustic neuroma), a histologically benign tumor growing from the nerve sheath at its entrance into the internal auditory meatus. This tumor arises deep in the angle between the cerebellum and pons (cerebellopontine angle). Symptoms may include unilateral deafness, tinnitus, unilateral impairment of cerebellar function, numbness of the face from involvement of the fifth cranial nerve, and, late in the course, papilledema caused by increased ICP. The operative approach is usually through a retrosigmoid craniotomy, exposing the edges of the transverse and sigmoid sinus. The surgeon must take great care to prevent injury to the pons and to preserve the facial nerve. Attempts are made to preserve the acoustic nerve with smaller tumors when hearing preservation is an option.

Meniere's disease is an affliction of the eighth nerve characterized by a recurrent and usually progressive group of symptoms including dizziness and a sensation of fullness or pressure in the ears. When medical measures fail to alleviate the problem, section of the eighth nerve may be a surgical option.

***Ninth Cranial Nerve.*** The glossopharyngeal nerve supplies the sense of taste to the posterior third of the tongue, supplies sensation to the tonsils and pharyngeal region, partially innervates the pharyngeal muscles, and primarily innervates the carotid sinus. Stimulation of the baroreceptors of the carotid sinus causes slowing of the heart, vasodilation, and decreased blood pressure. Its sensory component can be sectioned to treat a hypersensitive carotid sinus, or, along with the fifth nerve, to treat painful malignancies of the face, mouth, and pharynx. The ninth nerve lies near the eighth nerve in the posterior fossa and is exposed in a similar way.

***Tenth Cranial Nerve.*** The vagus nerve has many motor and sensory functions, chief among which are innervation of pharyngeal and laryngeal musculature, control of heart rate, and regulation of acid secretion of the stomach. In neck surgery, the surgeon carefully avoids the recurrent laryngeal branch because its injury results in vocal cord paralysis. In gastric surgery, the surgeon could sever the vagus nerve at the lower end of the esophagus to treat a peptic ulcer. The neurosurgeon may place a vagus nerve stimulator on the left vagus nerve, which is approached through anterior exposure of the neck to treat epilepsy (Research Highlight). The neurosurgeon is also concerned with preventing damage to the vagus nerve during posterior fossa surgery.

***Eleventh Cranial Nerve.*** The spinal accessory nerve is a motor nerve to the sternocleidomastoid and trapezius muscles. To restore mobility to the face, it may be anastomosed to the peripheral end of a damaged facial nerve.

***Twelfth Cranial Nerve.*** The hypoglossal nerve innervates the musculature of the tongue. Its neurosurgical interest is similar to that of the spinal accessory nerve.

Table 23-2 gives the function, origin, structures innervated, and assessment of the cranial nerves.

## RESEARCH HIGHLIGHT

### Vagus Nerve Stimulation for Seizure Disorders

An estimated 1% of the general population has epilepsy. In close to 30% of these patients, epilepsy is intractable to medications, and many others have their seizures controlled at the expense of adverse side effects from pharmacotherapy. Vagus nerve stimulation (VNS) offers an option for pharmacoresistant seizures. The device is approved for use in adults and children over 12 years of age. Stimulation is achieved through an implantable pacemaker–type device that sends electrical impulses to the brain by way of the left vagus nerve.

Research indicates that VNS is safe and well tolerated. A unique feature of the therapy is the ability to decrease seizure frequency over time. A VNS Therapy Patient Outcome Registry was established to track data on seizure control. Registry patients were analyzed as of April 2003. The cohorts analyzed included 2229 patients with 3- and 12-month data and 775 patients with 24-month data. More than half of registry patients had 50% or more seizure reduction at 12 months, and as many as 59% had 50% or more reduction at 24 months. These data are supported through additional research. Researchers performed a retrospective study on 48 patients with intractable partial epilepsy. Mean seizure frequency decreased by 26% after 1 year, 30% after 5 years, and 52% after 12 years with VNS treatment.

Modified from *Long-term seizure control with VNS therapy.* Accessed March 30, 2006, on-line: www.vnstherapy.com/epilepsy/hcp/vnstherapy/seizurecontrol.aspx; Rielo D: Vagus nerve stimulation, January 3, 2006. Accessed March 30, 2006, on-line: www.emedicine.com/NEURO/topic559.htm; Uthman BM and others: Effectiveness of vagus nerve stimulation in epilepsy patients: a 12 year observation, *Neurology* 63(6):1124-1126, 2004.

## SPINE, SPINAL CORD, AND ADJACENT STRUCTURES

### Vertebral Column

The primary roles of the spine are maintaining stability, protecting the neural elements, and allowing range of motion. The vertebral column has four distinct curves: cervical lordosis (a backward bend), thoracic kyphosis (a forward bend), lumbar lordosis, and sacral kyphosis.[7] The spinal column consists of 33 vertebrae: 7 cervical, 12 thoracic, 5 lumbar, 5 sacral (fused as one), and 1 coccygeal which may have 1-3 fused sections (Figure 23-23).

The first cervical vertebra, or atlas, supports the skull. The second cervical vertebra, or axis, can be identified by its odontoid process, a vertical projection extending into the foramen of the atlas like a stick in a hoop. It rests against the anterior tubercle of the first cervical vertebra. Ligaments hold the two together but allow considerable rotational movement. The other cervical, thoracic, and lumbar vertebrae are more alike in structure. Each has a body, an oval block of bone situated anteriorly. An intervertebral disk, a fibrocartilaginous elastic cushion, separates one body from another (Figures 23-24 and 23-25). The spinal cord lies in a canal formed by the vertebral bodies, pedicles, and laminae. Articular surfaces or facets project from the pedicles and form joints with the facets of the vertebrae above and below. Transverse processes extend laterally and serve as hitching posts for muscles and ligaments. Spinous processes extend posteriorly and can be palpated in most people. The vertebrae are held together by multiple liga-

**TABLE 23-2**

## Understanding Cranial Nerves

| Cranial Nerve | Function | Origin | Structures Innervated | Assessment |
|---|---|---|---|---|
| I<br>Olfactory | Sensory | Olfactory bulbs below frontal lobes | Olfactory mucous membranes | Ability to identify familiar odors |
| II<br>Optic | Sensory | Diencephalon | Retina of the eye | Visual acuity<br>Visual fields |
| III<br>Oculomotor | Motor | Midbrain | Medial, superior, and inferior rectus muscles of the eye<br>Inferior oblique eye muscles<br>Sphincter of the iris | Extraocular movements<br>Pupillary reaction to light and accommodation |
| IV<br>Trochlear | Motor | Midbrain | Superior oblique muscle of the eye | Extraocular movements |
| V<br>Trigeminal | Mixed | Pons | *Sensory:* pain, touch, and temperature sensations in the cheeks, jaws, and chin; corneal reflex<br>*Motor:* muscles of mastication | Sensation in the forehead, cheeks, jaw, and chin<br>Mastication |
| VI<br>Abducens | Motor | Pons | Lateral rectus muscle of the eye | Extraocular movement |
| VII<br>Facial | Mixed | Pons | *Sensory:* anterior two thirds of the tongue<br>*Motor:* muscles of the face, forehead, and eye | Taste for anterior two thirds of tongue<br>Movement of the facial muscles (smile)<br>Facial symmetry |
| VIII<br>Acoustic | Sensory | Pons | Cochlear organ of Corti<br>Vestibule and semicircle canals | Hearing acuity<br>Balance |
| IX<br>Glossopharyngeal | Mixed | Medulla | *Sensory:* posterior third of the tongue<br>*Motor:* muscles of the pharynx | Taste for posterior third of the tongue<br>Movement of the pharynx<br>Gag reflex |
| X<br>Vagus | Mixed | Medulla | *Sensory:* skin of external ear and mucous membranes<br>*Motor:* muscles of larynx, pharynx, and esophagus; thoracic and abdominal viscera | Swallowing<br>Movement of the pharynx<br>Gag reflex<br>Cough |
| XI<br>Spinal accessory | Motor | Medulla | Sternocleidomastoid and trapezius muscles | Shoulder shrug<br>Turn head |
| XII<br>Hypoglossal | Motor | Medulla | Tongue | Movement and strength of tongue |

ments and muscles (see Figure 23-25). Motion of the spine occurs at the articular facets and through the elastic intervertebral disks. The intervertebral disks bond the adjacent surfaces of the vertebral bodies. Each disk consists of a fibrous outer annulus that contains the inner nucleus pulposus.

## Spinal Cord

The spinal cord is protected by the bony framework of the spinal column. The dura mater is separated from its bony surroundings by a layer of epidural fat. Beneath the dura mater is the arachnoid, a continuation of the same structure in the head. The subarachnoid space contains CSF. A thin layer of pia mater adheres to the cord, and CSF also circulates from the fourth ventricle into the central canal of the cord.

The spinal cord is a downward prolongation of the brainstem, starting at the upper border of the atlas and ending at the upper border of the second lumbar vertebra (Figure 23-26). The cord is oval in cross section. It is slightly flattened in the anteroposterior diameter. A cross section looks like a gray H surrounded by a white mantle split in the midline, anteriorly and posteriorly, by sulci (Figure 23-27).

The peripheral white matter carries long, myelinated motor and sensory tracts. The central gray matter consists of nerve cell bodies and short, unmyelinated fibers (see Figures 23-26 and 23-27). The principal long pathways are the laterally placed pyramidal tracts, carrying impulses down from the cerebral cortex to the motor neurons of the cord; the dorsal ascending columns, mediating sensations of touch and proprioception; and the anterolaterally placed spinothalamic tracts, carrying pain and temperature sensations to the thalamus—the sensory receiving station of the brain (Figure 23-28).

## Spinal Nerves

At each vertebral level is a pair of spinal nerves, each consisting of an anterior and a posterior root (see Figure 23-27). The anterior, or motor, root contains cell bodies that lie in the

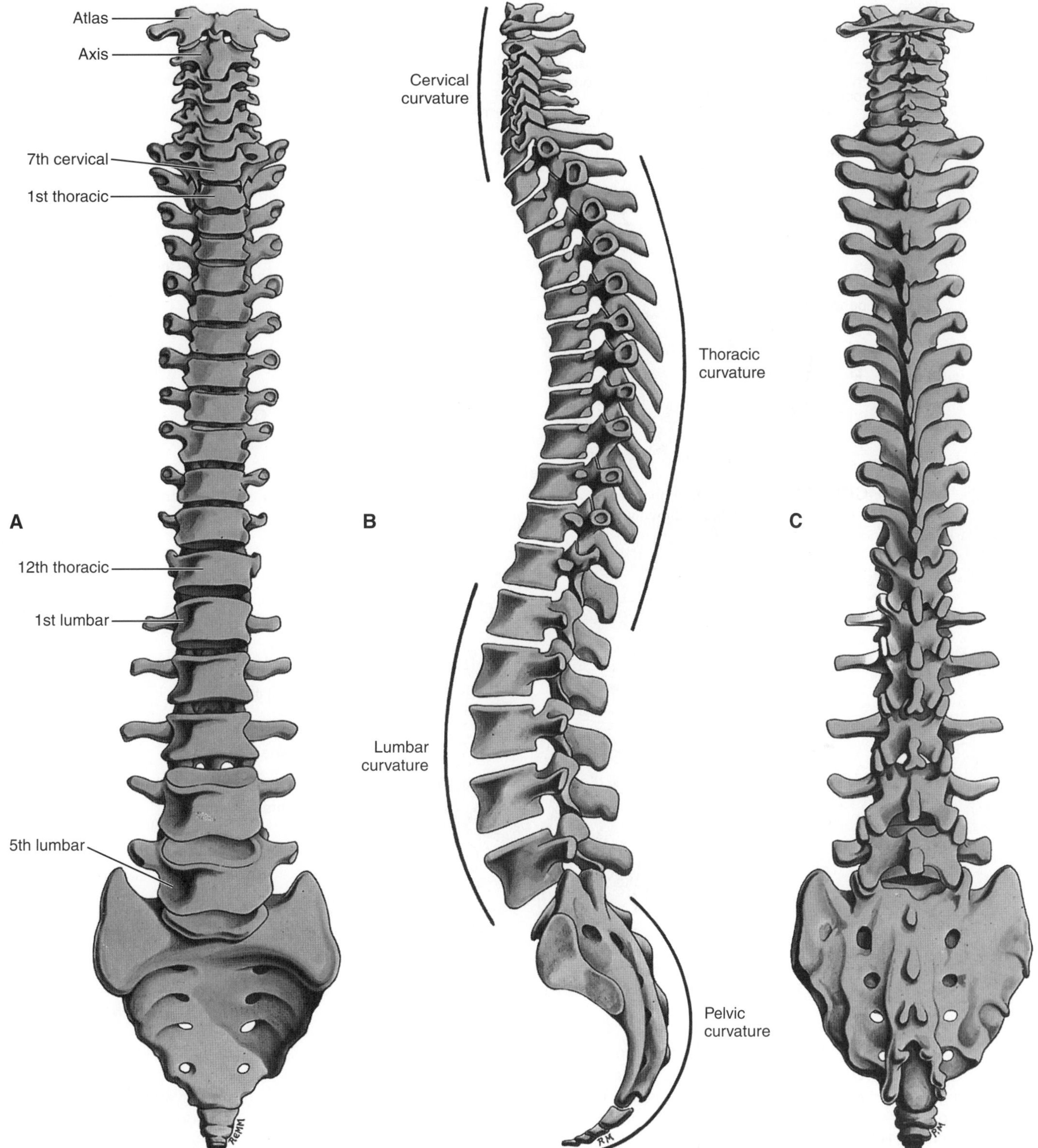


FIGURE 23-23 The vertebral column: **A**, anterior aspect, **B**, lateral aspect, **C,** posterior aspect.

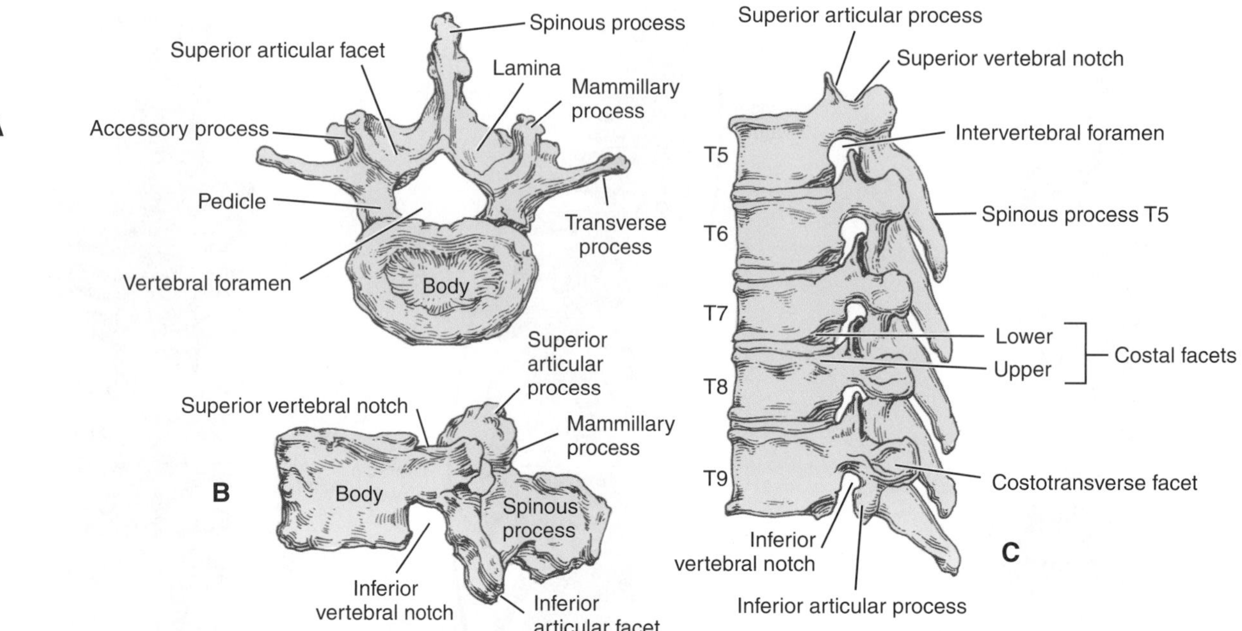


**FIGURE 23-24** **A,** Fourth lumbar vertebra from above. **B,** Fourth lumbar vertebra from side. **C,** Fifth to ninth thoracic vertebrae, showing relationships of various parts.

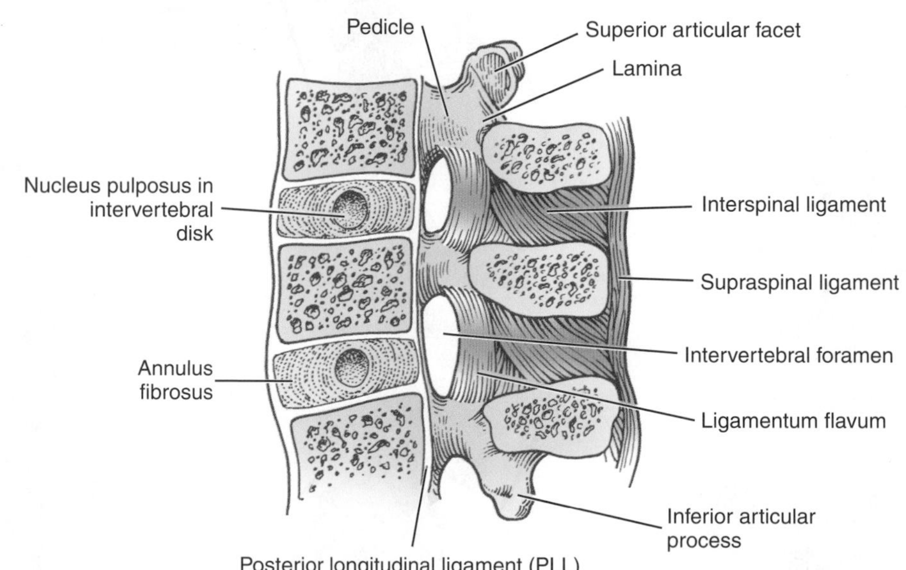


**FIGURE 23-25** Median section through three lumbar vertebrae, showing intervertebral disks (nuclei pulposi).

anterior horn of the spinal gray matter. The posterior, or sensory, root contains cell bodies that lie in the spinal ganglia located in the intervertebral foramina, the opening through which the nerves exit from the spinal canal and emerge from the cord. The cervical nerves pass out horizontally, but at each lower level they take on an increasingly oblique and downward direction. In the lumbar region, the course of the nerves is nearly vertical, forming the cauda equina (see Figure 23-26). The normal segmental sensory distribution is valuable in the anatomic localization of sensory disorders (Figure 23-29).

Dermatomes are bands of skin innervated by a sensory root of a single spinal nerve. Knowledge of these dermatomes aids the practitioner in locating neurologic lesions (Figure 23-30).

## Spinal Vasculature

The vasculature of the spinal cord and vertebral column is a rich, delicate network. The arterial blood supply to the spinal cord arises from the vertebral arteries as the anterior spinal artery and the posterior spinal arteries. These vessels branch and anastomose on both sides of the cord and within the substance of the cord. They also branch into anterior and posterior radicular arteries that form spinal rami as they accompany the spinal nerve roots through the intervertebral foramina.

A series of venous plexuses surround and innervate the spinal cord at each level in the vertebral canal. They anastomose with each other and form the intervertebral veins as they leave through the intervertebral foramina with the spinal

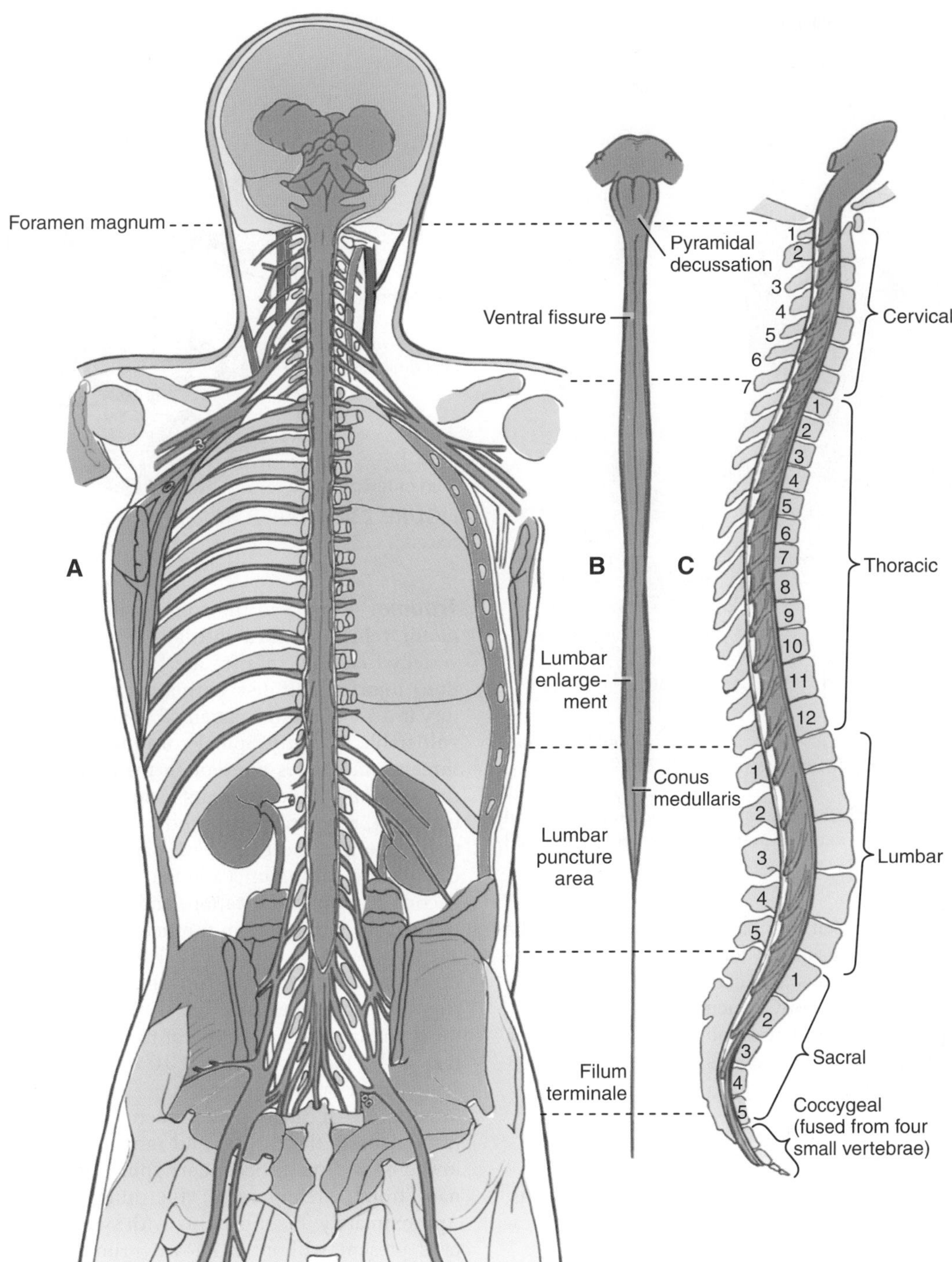


**FIGURE 23-26** Posterior view of brainstem and spinal cord. **A,** Torso dissected from back is shown. Dura mater has been opened and cord exposed. Levels concerned can be easily determined by referring to ribs on left side of thorax. Cord proper terminates opposite body of second lumbar vertebra **(B)** as conus medullaris. **B,** Ventral surface of cord stripped of dura mater and arachnoid. It is symmetric in structure, two halves of which are separated by ventral fissure. This fissure stops at foramen magnum. Caudally, pia mater leaves conus medullaris as glistening thread, or filum terminale. **C,** Cord is exposed from lateral side. Dura mater has been opened. Because cord is shorter than canal and spinal nerves leave through intervertebral foramina, one at a time, lowest portion of canal is occupied only by a bundlelike accumulation of nerve roots—cauda equina. Caudal end of dural sac, enclosing spinal cord and cauda equina, lies somewhere between bodies of first and third sacral vertebrae. Size and position of the three views correspond, and elimination of major vertebral levels is indicated by transverse lines for all three figures.

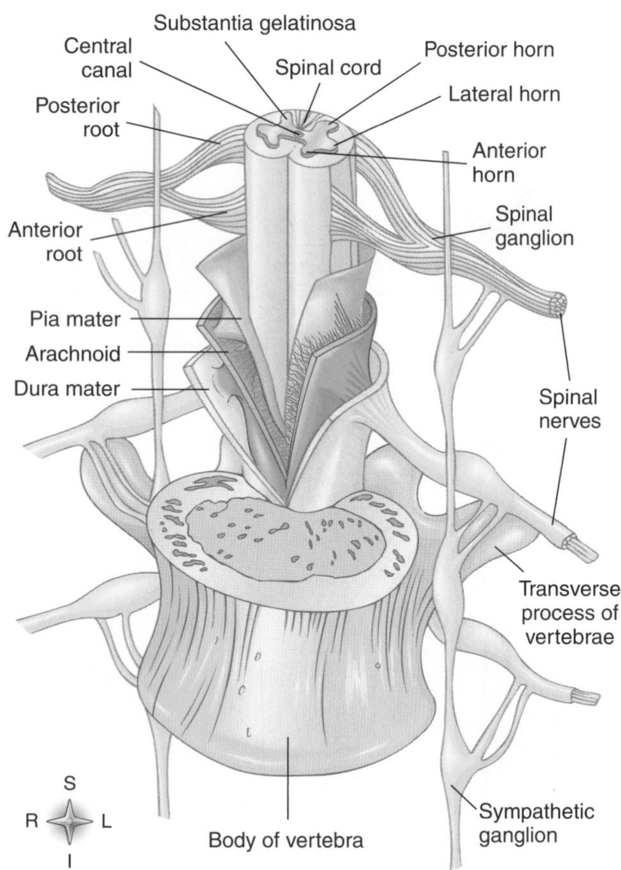


FIGURE 23-27 Spinal cord, showing meninges, formation of spinal nerves, and relationships to vertebra and to sympathetic trunk and ganglia.

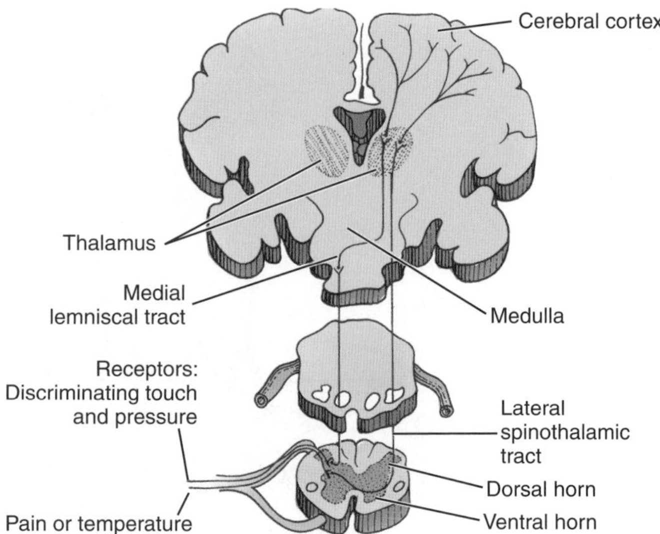


FIGURE 23-28 Lateral spinothalamic and medial lemniscal neural tracts.

nerves to join the intercostal, lumbar, and sacral veins. The lateral longitudinal veins near the foramen magnum empty into the inferior petrosal sinus and cerebellar veins. The venous network innervates the bony structures and musculature as well as the spinal cord and nerve roots. The perioperative nurse considers the possibility of venous bleeding during spinal surgery when planning care.

## Pathologic Lesions of the Spinal Cord and Adjacent Structures

Surgery is performed to correct congenital malformations, traumatic injuries, tumors, abscesses, herniated and degenerative intervertebral disks, and intractable pain.

***Meningocele.*** The most common congenital lesion encountered is a lumbar meningocele, or myelomeningocele—a failure of the union of the vertebral arches during fetal development. The fluid-filled, thin-walled sac often contains neural elements. This fetal anomaly is often diagnosed prenatally and is often seen with other CNS abnormalities, which include hydrocephalus, gyral abnormalities, and Chiari malformation of the hindbrain. The operation consists of excising the sac wall to preserve adhering nerves, closing the dura mater, and reinforcing the closure with fascial flaps swung from the paraspinal muscles. Skin closure without tension is essential for primary healing. Large skin and subcutaneous flaps must occasionally be fashioned to ensure healing.

***Trauma.*** Trauma to the spine is most commonly caused by motor vehicle crashes and falls. The most common types of vertebral column injuries are fractures, subluxation (dislocation) injuries, and disk herniation resulting in neurologic injury in 15% of trauma patients.[13] The cervical spine is the most vulnerable to injury. Spinal cord injury (SCI) occurs in males three to four times more often than females, usually between the ages of 15 and 30 years.[17] Standardized trauma care and transport, early diagnosis, and closed reduction with surgical stabilization as necessary are part of spinal care focused on minimizing cord trauma and maximizing cord recovery. Spinal decompression, stabilization, and traction are all common interventions performed in trauma centers.

***Spine and Spinal Cord Tumors.*** The most frequently occurring tumors of the spine are metastatic, and the spine is the most common site for skeletal metastasis. Although it is estimated that between 5% and 10% of cancer patients develop *symptomatic* spinal metastasis, it is estimated that as many as 50% to 70% of cancer patients actually develop skeletal metastasis.[2] Pain is the earliest and most prominent symptom, followed by weakness. Secondary spinal tumors most often originate from carcinomas of the lung, breast, and prostate. Approximately 9% of patients with symptomatic spinal metastasis present without a known primary cancer.[17] Treatment goals for metastatic tumors of the spine are pain relief and preservation or restoration of neurologic function. Options include radiation, surgery, or a combination of these. Surgery involves both decompression of the spinal cord and nerve roots and stabilization of the spinal column.[17]

Spinal tumors are classified according to location as *extradural* (outside the dura mater) or *intradural* (inside the dura mater). Intradural tumors may be either *extramedullary* (outside the cord) or *intramedullary* (within the cord). Although metastatic tumors may be found in each category, they are usually extradural. Spinal cord tumors account for approximately 15% of CNS tumors.[8] Most primary CNS tumors are benign.

Extradural tumors arise outside the spinal cord in vertebral bodies or epidural tissues. They account for 50% to 60% of

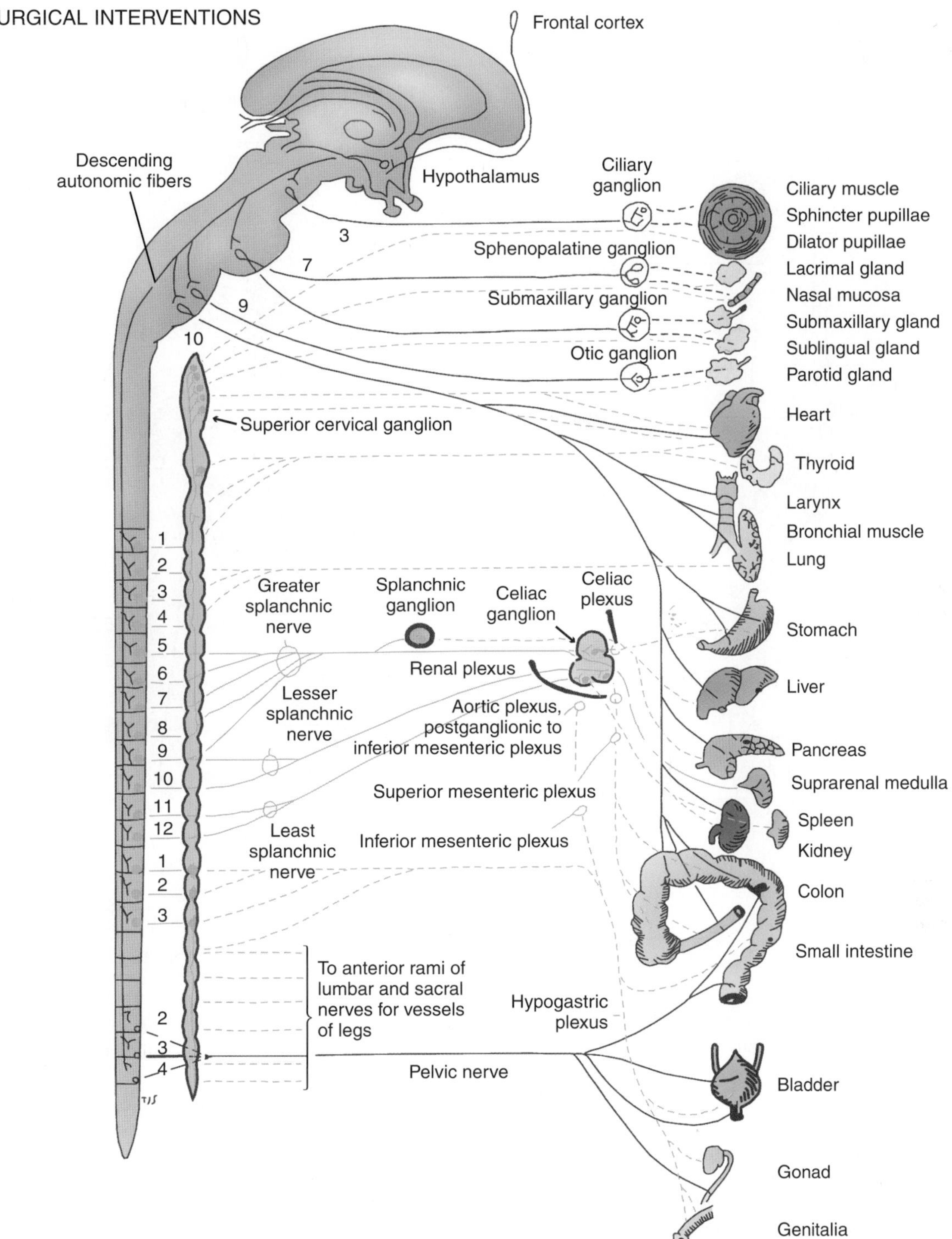


FIGURE 23-29 Sympathetic division of the autonomic nervous system.

spinal cord neoplasms and include sarcomas and carcinomas, which may be metastatic from adjacent structures in or about the vertebrae.[9] Other extradural lesions include lymphomas, lipomas, neurofibromas, chondromas, angiomas, abscesses, and granulomas.

Most intradural tumors are extramedullary and benign and, if diagnosed early before severe neurologic deficits occur, offer an excellent prognosis. They manifest their presence by pain of a radicular nature and various motor and sensory disabilities below their segmental locations. Intradural extramedullary tumors represent 35% to 45% of spinal cord tumors.[9] They are usually benign and originate from the dura mater and arachnoid surrounding the cord and from the root sheaths of spinal nerves. Schwannomas (neuromas) are especially common in the thoracocervical area and may be part of generalized neurofibromatosis. Meningiomas also commonly occur in intradural extramedullary locations. Less frequently, lipomas or other types of tumors are found. Approximately 2% to 7% of spinal cord tu-

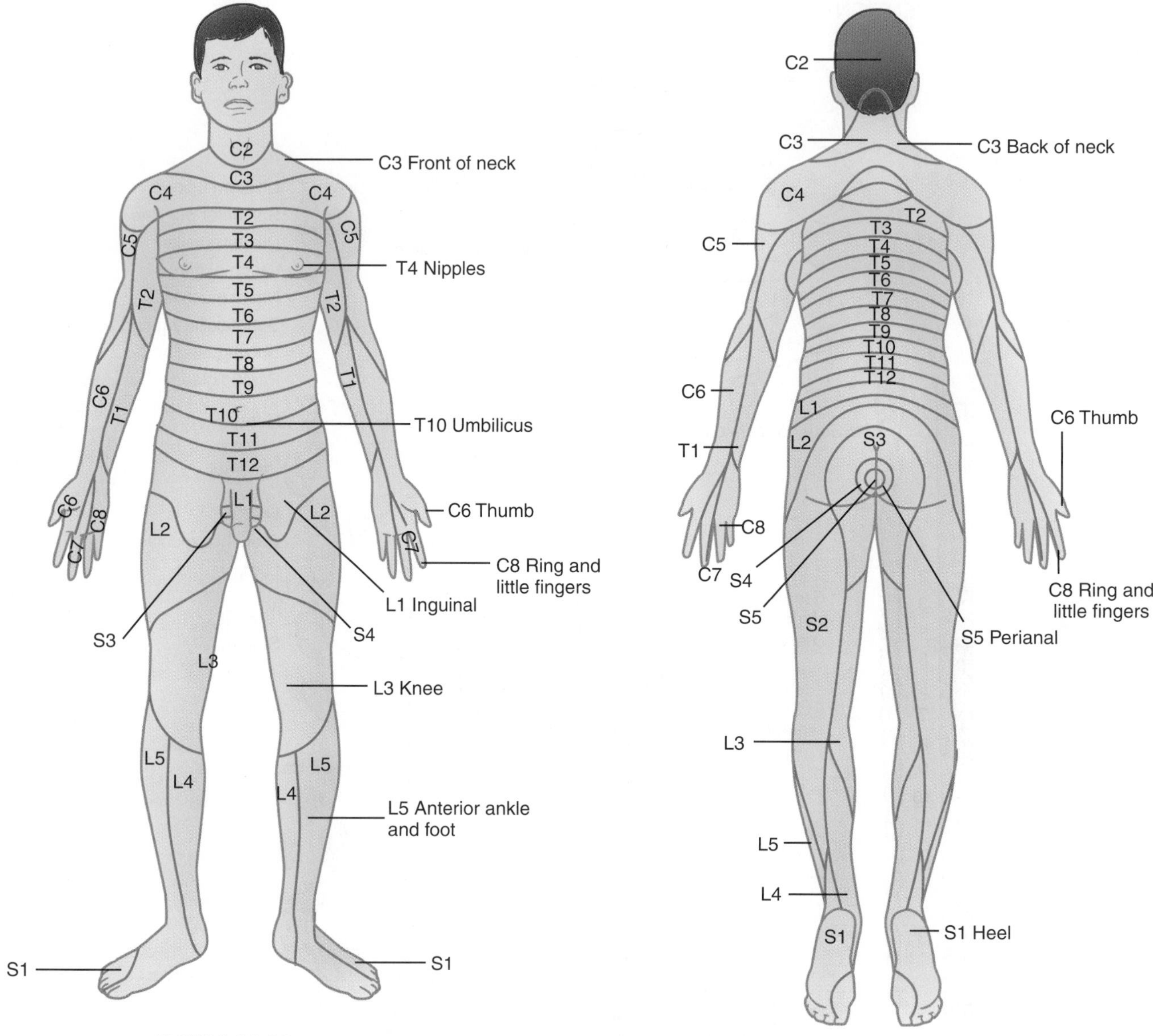


**FIGURE 23-30** Dermatomes innervated by posterior nerve roots and their correlation on the body, anterior and posterior. *C*, Cervical; *T*, thoracic; *L*, lumbar; *S*, sacral.

mors are intradural intramedullary tumors.[9] These tumors infiltrate the cord tissue and are much more difficult to remove than are extramedullary tumors. Of the intramedullary tumors, the most common are ependymomas and astrocytomas.

Cord tumors frequently produce spinal fluid blockage and can be pinpointed accurately with MRI. Intraspinal injection of contrast material (myelography) is another option for diagnosis. Often, a standard laminectomy is used for exposure and removal.

***Spinal Epidural Abscess.*** Spinal epidural abscess can develop from vertebral osteomyelitis, from infection from a distant source that was transferred by the blood, or by direct inoculation from spinal surgery, LP, or epidural administration of anesthetic. Patients who are immunosuppressed are especially at risk for epidural abscesses. Clinical presentation involves spinal and radicular pain and muscle weakness that can progress to paralysis. Epidural abscess is most easily diagnosed by MRI and typically treated with surgical decompression, culture, and irrigation, along with 4 to 8 weeks of IV antibiotic therapy.

***Intervertebral Disk Disease.*** Intervertebral disk disease is the most frequently encountered neurosurgical problem. The axial skeleton bears both the weight of the body and externally applied axial forces while maintaining mobility. Intervertebral disks serve as mechanical buffers that absorb axial loading, bending, and sheer forces. Bipedal posture further stresses the intervertebral disks, leading to degenerative disk disorders. Disk rupture occurs with radial fissuring of the annulus. The nucleus pulposus then escapes, extending to the margin of the annulus and posterior longitudinal ligament. Once the nucleus pulposus protrudes beyond the perimeter of the disk space into the epidural space, it results in nerve root compression and radiculopathy (pain produced by pressure or traction on the nerve roots) (Figures 23-31 and 23-32). Most disk protru-

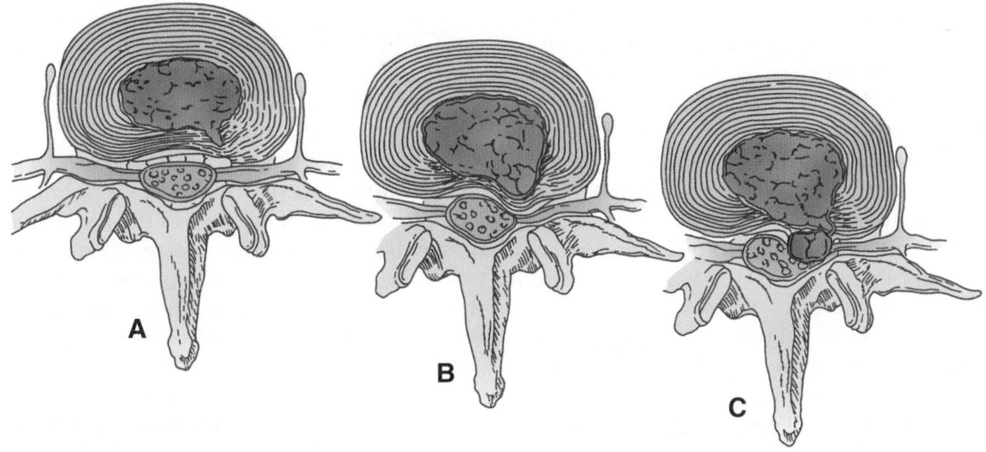


**FIGURE 23-31** Stages in the herniation of an intervertebral disk. **A,** Tearing of the rings of the annulus fibrosus. **B,** Protrusion of the disk against the nerve root. **C,** Extrusion of part of the nucleus pulposus, with further nerve root compression.

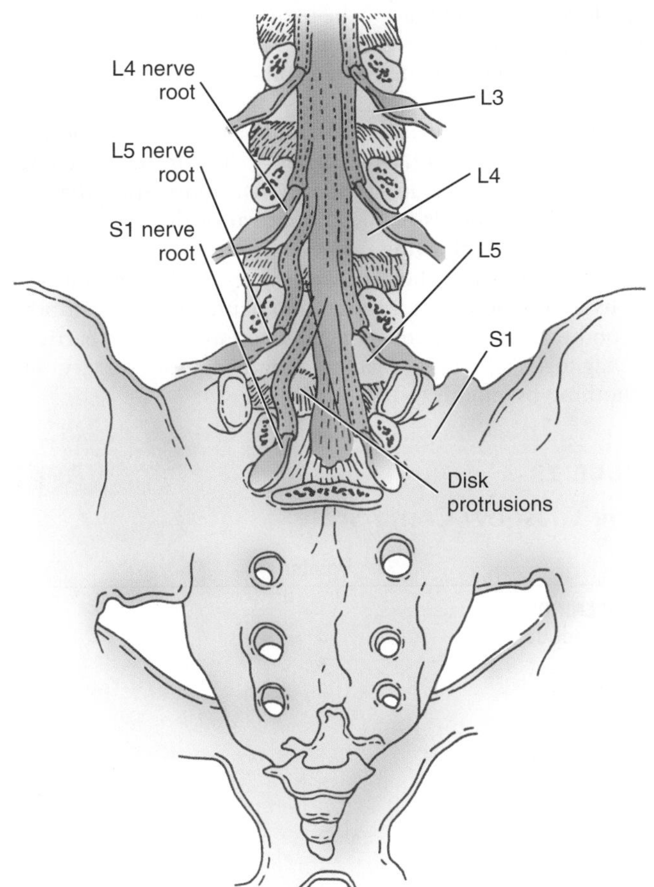


**FIGURE 23-32** Posterior view of the lower lumbar spine. A disk protrusion at L4-5 on the left results in compression of the L5 nerve root where it leaves the dural sac but before it exits from the spinal canal.

sions occur at the L4-L5 and L5-S1 interspaces. Interventions include a medical trial of treatment with steroids, analgesics/narcotics, muscle relaxation, rest, epidural steroid injections, and, in failed cases, laminotomy or laminectomy with diskectomy. In far-lateral disk herniations, percutaneous lumbar diskectomy is often an alternative to laminotomy. This minimally invasive technique gains access to the disk space posterolaterally, using local anesthetic. The disk space is entered by way of a cannula. An aspiration probe may be used to remove the disk matter, or direct removal can be done microscopically or endoscopically.

***Intractable Pain.*** Certain painful spinal lesions, usually of a malignant nature, can be controlled by use of epidural opiates, by use of fentanyl patches, or by temporary or permanent use of a medication pump. Another pain control measure is to divide the pain fibers supplying the affected area. This may be accomplished by sectioning the sensory roots intraspinally (posterior rhizotomy) or by incising the spinothalamic tracts that carry pain and temperature impulses (anterolateral cordotomy). Alternatively, spinal cord stimulation of the affected area can be achieved with the placement of electrodes in the epidural space. A laminectomy for exposure is necessary to perform these surgical procedures.

## Peripheral Nerves

The PNS consists of those structures containing nerve fibers or axons that connect the CNS with motor and sensory, somatic and visceral, end-organs.[8] The PNS includes the cranial nerves (III to XII), the spinal nerves, the autonomic nerves, and the ganglia.

The 31 pairs of spinal nerves are each numbered for the level of the spinal column at which it emerges: cervical one (C1) through eight (C8), thoracic one (T1) through twelve (T12), lumbar one (L1) through five (L5), sacral one (S1) through five (S5), and coccygeal one. The first pair of cervical spine nerves emerges between C1 and the occipital bone. The eighth cervical nerves emerge from the intervertebral foramina between C7 and T1. The first thoracic nerves emerge between T1 and T2.

In the cervical and lumbosacral regions the spinal nerves regroup in a plexiform manner before they form the peripheral nerves of the upper and lower extremities. Those in the thoracic region form cutaneous and intercostal nerves. The principal nerves of the upper plexus include the musculocutaneous, median, ulnar, and radial. Those of the lumbosacral plexus include the obturator, femoral, and sciatic.

Each spinal nerve divides into anterior, posterior, and white rami. Rami are primary divisions of a nerve. Anterior and posterior rami contain voluntary fibers; white rami contain autonomic fibers. Posterior rami further branch into nerves going to the muscles, skin, and posterior surfaces of the head, neck, and trunk. Most anterior rami branch to the skeletal muscles and the skin of extremities and anterior and lateral surfaces. In the process they form plexuses, such as the brachial and sacral plexuses. Spinal nerves contain sensory dendrites and motor axons; some have somatic axons, and some have axons of preganglionic autonomic motor neurons.

The autonomic (involuntary) nervous system consists of all the efferent nerves through which the cardiovascular apparatus, viscera, glands of internal secretion, and peripheral involuntary muscles are innervated (see Figure 23-29). There is a major anatomic difference between the somatic and autonomic nervous systems. In the somatic nervous system an impulse from the brainstem or spinal cord reaches the end-organ through a single neuron. In the autonomic nervous system an impulse passes through two neurons—the first ending in an autonomic ganglion and the second running from the ganglion to the end-organ. Some of the ganglia lie adjacent to the vertebral column to form the sympathetic trunks or chains; others are closely associated with the end-organs.

The preganglionic neurons from the brainstem, which go out along the cranial nerves, and those from the second, third, and fourth sacral segments to the pelvic viscera, end in ganglia in proximity to their end-organs; thus their postganglionic fibers are very short. This is known as the *parasympathetic*, or *craniosacral*, division of the autonomic nervous system. The preganglionic fibers from the thoracic and lumbar spinal cord end in the paravertebral ganglia, making up the sympathetic chain, and their postganglionic fibers are relatively long. This is termed the *sympathetic*, or *thoracolumbar*, division of the autonomic nervous system.

The two divisions are distinct anatomically and physiologically. The chemical substance mediating transmission of impulses at most postganglionic sympathetic nerve endings is *norepinephrine*, and the one at all parasympathetic and preganglionic sympathetic neurons is *acetylcholine*.

The majority of organs have dual innervation—part from the craniosacral division and part from the thoracolumbar division. The functions of these two systems are antagonistic. Together they work to maintain homeostasis. In general, the thoracolumbar division functions as an emergency protection mechanism, always ready to combat physical or psychologic stress. The craniosacral division functions to conserve energy when the body is in a state of relaxation.

Stimuli arising from internal organs or from outside the body traverse visceral and somatic afferent nerve fibers to make reflex connections with preganglionic autonomic neurons in the brainstem and spinal cord. Such stimuli trigger activity of these involuntary systems automatically. When these automatic mechanisms break down or overact, surgery may be indicated. Thoracolumbar sympathectomy was once performed in hypertensive patients to try to decrease blood vessel tone and lower the blood pressure. Vagotomy can be done to decrease acid secretion to the stomach in patients with peptic ulcers. Lumbar sympathectomy is used to relieve vasospastic disorders of the legs. T2 ganglionectomy is done to relieve palmar hyperhydrosis (sweaty palms).

# *Perioperative Nursing Considerations*

## Assessment

***Neurologic Assessment Tools.*** A familiarity with basic neurologic assessment tools gives the nurse the ability to perform a standardized neurologic assessment that can be compared with the patient's previous assessments and easily communicated to other health care professionals. These tools can be used preoperatively to establish a baseline assessment. Postoperatively, they can be used to establish a return to baseline and to assess postoperative neurologic stability. The Glasgow Coma Scale is commonly used to assess patients with brain injury (Table 23-3). Three indicators of cerebral function—eye opening, verbal communication, and motor response to verbal and noxious stimuli—are assessed; and the appropriate number of points for each is assigned and totaled. The best possible score is 15, and the worst possible score is 3. The MRC Scale for Muscle Strength Grading can be used to assess muscle strength in the upper and lower extremities of spinal cord injury patients or patients who are having spine surgery (Table 23-4).

***Preparation for Surgery.*** Communication among the perioperative team is essential for planning care for the neurosurgical patient in the operating room (OR). Information the perioperative nurse needs before the arrival of the patient in the OR includes the following:

- The patient's age, height, weight, level of consciousness, physical disabilities resulting from neuropathologic or other conditions, stability of spine, and communication barriers
- Diagnosis, allergies, medical clearance for surgery, and nothing-by-mouth (NPO) status

**TABLE 23-3**

**The Glasgow Coma Scale**

| | Points |
|---|---|
| **EYE OPENING** | |
| Spontaneous | 4 |
| To speech | 3 |
| To pain | 2 |
| None | 1 |
| **VERBAL COMMUNICATION** | |
| Oriented | 5 |
| Confused conversation | 4 |
| Inappropriate words | 3 |
| Incomprehensible sounds | 2 |
| None | 1 |
| **MOTOR RESPONSE** | |
| Obeys commands | 6 |
| Localizes to pain | 5 |
| Withdraws to pain | 4 |
| Abnormal flexion | 3 |
| Abnormal extension | 2 |
| None | 1 |

Modified from Hausman KA: Assessment of the nervous system. In Ignatavicius DD, Workman ML, editors: *Medical-surgical nursing:critical thinking for collaborative care,* ed 5, St Louis, 2006, Saunders.

**TABLE 23-4**

**Medical Resarch Council Scale for Muscle Strength Grading**

| Grade | Strength |
|---|---|
| 0 | No muscle contraction |
| 1 | Trace of contraction |
| 2 | Active movement with gravity eliminated |
| 3 | Active movement against gravity |
| 4 | Active movement against gravity and resistance |
| 5 | Normal power |

From: Grant GA, Ellenbogen RG: Clinical evaluation of the nervous system. In Rengachary SS, Ellenbogen RG, editors: *Principles of neurosurgery*, ed 2, St. Louis, 2005, Mosby.

- Planned and possible surgical procedures
- Surgical and anesthesia consent signed by the patient or person with power of attorney for medical decisions (if the patient is unable to provide consent)
- Surgical site marked by the surgeon or a representative to designate correct side of head, level of spine, and so on
- Diagnostic and lab studies done and reports needed at the time of operation
- Specific surgical approach and position to be used
- Need for any special equipment, instruments, and supplies
- Amount of blood and blood products (fresh frozen plasma, platelets) ordered and available
- Need for radiologic support, neuromonitoring, intraoperative blood salvage unit, and image guidance
- Planned preliminary procedures, such as carotid ligation, lumbar puncture, placement of lines (IV, central venous, arterial), and Foley catheter insertion
- Verification that all necessary personnel, equipment, and supplies are available
- A focused preoperative neurologic examination should be done as a baseline for postoperative assessment; depending on the pathology and surgery, this may include the following:
  - Mental status (level of consciousness, orientation, behavior, ability to follow commands)
  - Vision, pupil response, extraocular eye movements (EOMs), and hearing
  - Examination of sensation and motor strength of extremities
  - Area and intensity of pain

This information allows the perioperative nurse to properly plan and prepare for the surgery and to ensure the well-being of the patient.

***Diagnostic Procedures.*** Most patients will have undergone diagnostic procedures before arriving in the OR. Radiologic and other diagnostic studies are of great significance to the surgical team. The nurse should ensure that any pertinent radiographic images are available in the OR before the procedure begins. The surgeon can refer to these images to locate the pathologic condition, verify the correct surgical site, and plan the appropriate surgical approach and procedure. Diagnostic studies include the following:

1. *Plain x-rays.* X-rays of the spine can be used initially to identify injury to the spinal column. They are referred to intraoperatively to verify that surgery to the spine is being done at the correct level (Figure 23-33).
2. *CT scan.* A CT scan uses x-ray studies, with or without instilled contrast medium, and computer technology to produce a sequential series of positive images of transverse sections of the brain and spinal cord in which differences in tissue density can be detected and deviations from normal identified. This study remains the criterion standard for evaluation of acute head injury and is considered the first-line screening study.
3. *MRI.* Use of radiofrequency pulses in a powerful magnetic field yields high-resolution images of the human body with no known risk to patients and involves no radiation. Advances in MRI scanning provide enhancement of the scan with the use of gadolinium (contrast medium). A typical MRI study produces views of the brain featured as contiguous slices in three different planes. Axial cuts are from top to bottom. Coronal cuts are from front to back. Sagittal cuts are from side to side. The MRI is the gold standard for the diagnosis of tumors, abscesses, tissue/ligamentous injury, and disk herniation (Figures 23-34 and 23-35).
4. *Stereotactic MRI or CT scan.* Placement of a stereotactic head frame (frame-based system) or fiducials (frameless system) before receiving a CT scan or MRI produces information that is registered into a computer. The goal of stereotactic surgery is to target a point or volume in space precisely by means of a predefined minimally invasive trajectory.[24] The frameless system allows the neurosurgeon to see beyond the actual operative field by using an optical tracking device. This handheld device depicts in three planes on a computer screen where the surgeon is working in the brain relative to deeper structures beyond view.

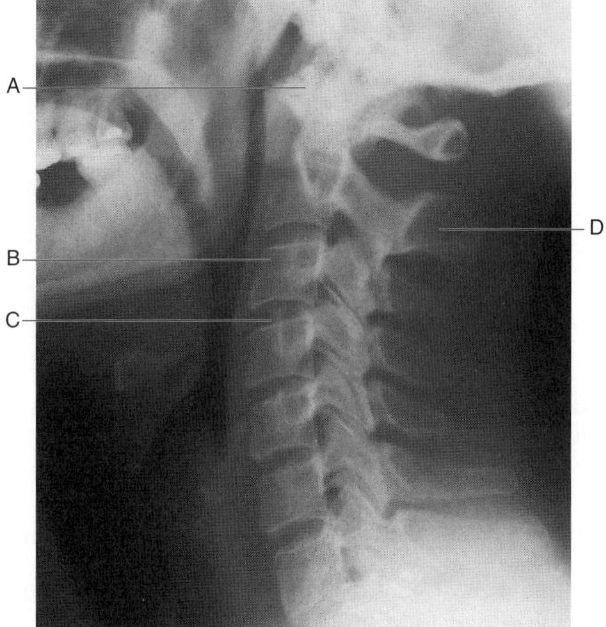


FIGURE 23-33 Lateral x-ray of the cervical spine. **A,** Anterior tubercle of the atlas (C-1) **B,** Cervical body. **C,** Intervertebral disk. **D,** Spinous process of the axis (C-2).

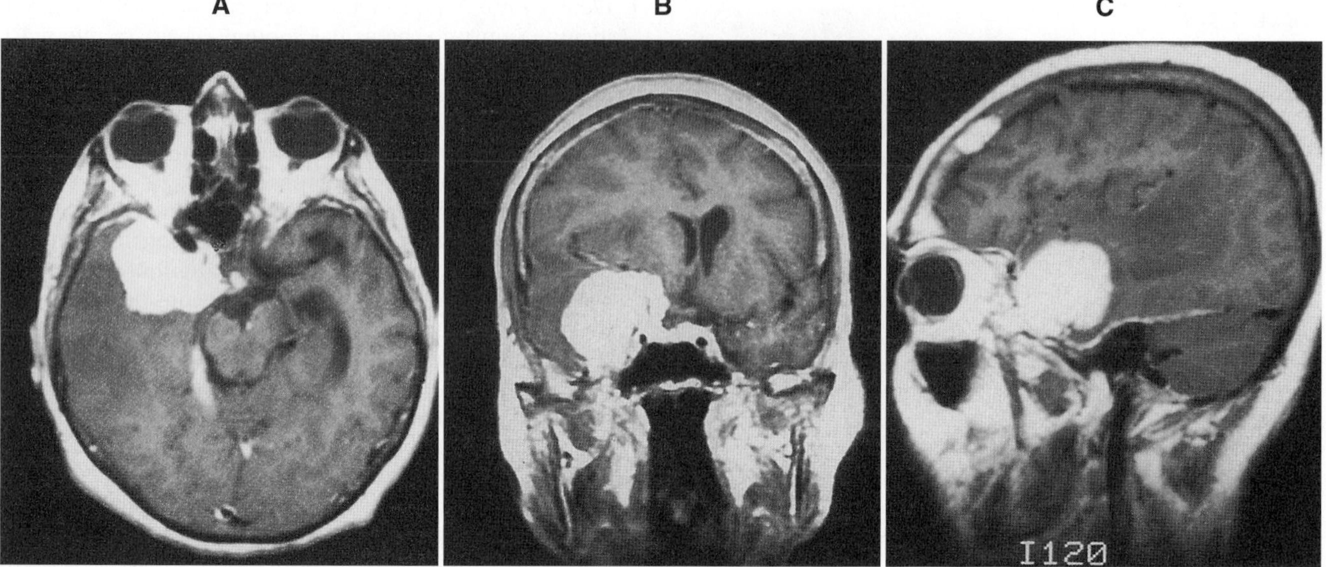


**FIGURE 23-34** Gadolinium-enhanced magnetic resonance image (MRI) of a medial sphenoid wing meningioma in, **A**, axial, **B**, coronal, and **C**, sagittal planes.

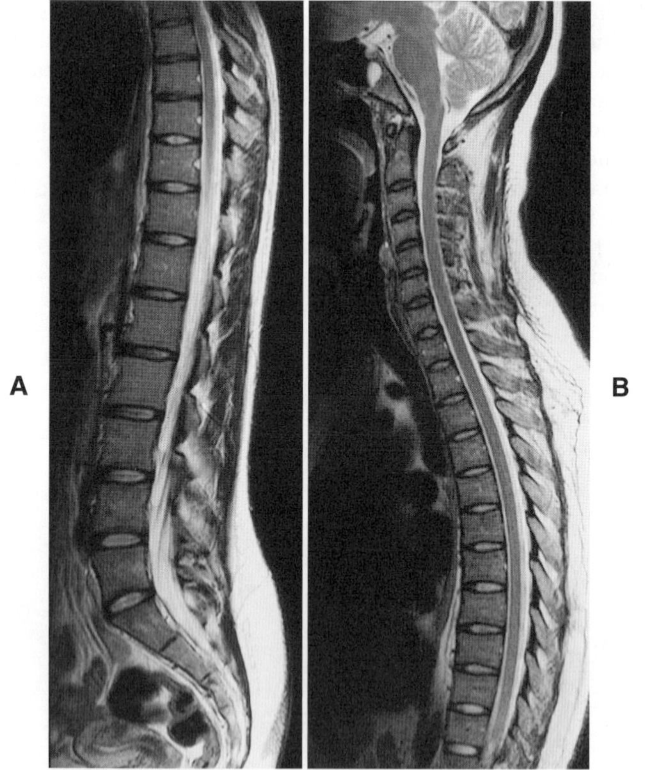


**FIGURE 23-35** Sagittal magnetic resonance image (MRI) of, **A**, thoracolumbar spine and, **B**, cervicothoracic spine.

5. *Magnetic resonance angiography (MRA)*. MRA is a noninvasive means of studying the cerebral vasculature. An MRA study is capable of detecting carotid stenosis, posttraumatic carotid artery dissection, AVMs, and aneurysms.
6. *Angiography (arteriography)*. Injection of contrast medium into the brachial, carotid, vertebral, or femoral arteries is used to study the intracranial blood vessels for size, location, and configuration and to allow diagnosis of space-occupying lesions and vascular abnormalities.
7. *Digital subtraction angiography (DSA)*. DSA is a computerized radiologic procedure. An IV rather than arterial injection is required; a contrast medium injection allows examination of selected arterial circulation. DSA provides an alternative to cerebral angiography for high-risk patients by using computer technology.
8. *Three-dimensional CT angiography.* Contrast-enhanced CT brain scan data are used to generate a three-dimensional image of the intracranial vasculature with minimal risk to the patient.
9. *Stereoscopic display of MRA*. Recent advances in MRI permit high-resolution imaging of blood flow. Projection angiograms can be produced to overcome the tomographic nature of conventional MRI scans. These angiograms are similar to plain x-ray films or digital subtraction angiograms in the demonstration of blood vessels, but the three-dimensional information inherent in them is partially lost in single projections. Stereoscopic image pairs allow the clinician to perceive the relative distance of vessels to one another. MRA permits perception of vascular anatomy in three dimensions.
10. *Myelography.* Contrast medium is injected into the spinal subarachnoid space to demonstrate a defect by radiography.
11. *Ultrasound.* Ultrasound is a noninvasive technique that uses high-frequency sound waves and a computer to create images of blood vessels, tissues, and organs. It is often used to assess the blood flow in the carotid artery. This procedure can be done in or out of the surgical suite. It can be used intraoperatively to localize intradural spinal cord tumors.
12. *Electroencephalogram (EEG)*. An EEG is a procedure that records the brain's continuous electrical activity by means of electrodes placed on the scalp or intraoperatively on the brain.
13. *Evoked potentials (EP)*. Evoked potentials are procedures that record the brain's electrical response to visual, auditory, and sensory stimuli.

14. *Wada's test (intracarotid amobarbital [Amytal] test).* Wada's test can be used before brain surgery to lateralize language, memory, and the dominant hemisphere. It can help in lateralization of seizure focus and assess the ability of the hemisphere with the lesion to maintain memory when isolated.
15. *Lumbar puncture.* A spinal needle is used to gain access to CSF in the subarachnoid space. Opening and closing pressures are measured to determine if there is increased pressure surrounding the brain and spinal cord. This can help diagnose hydrocephalus or a spinal tumor. CSF is sent to the lab to evaluate for blood, infection, malignancy, and other neurologic diseases. LP is contraindicated when an intracranial mass is known or suspected because it can cause herniation of the brain in the presence of increased ICP.

## Nursing Diagnosis

Nursing diagnoses are developed from interpreting and analyzing patient information to determine whether there are specific (actual) or potential (risk for) problems that the perioperative nurse needs to consider in the plan of care.[3] Nursing diagnoses are the basis on which nursing interventions are selected for patients. Neurosurgery patients share common problems that the perioperative nurse should address. Nursing diagnoses related to the care of patients undergoing neurosurgery might include the following:

- Anxiety related to surgery or surgical outcome
- Deficient Knowledge related to diagnostic tests and surgical procedures
- Risk for Ineffective Breathing Pattern related to location of tumor, surgical position, or effects of general anesthesia
- Risk for Hypothermia
- Risk for Perioperative Positioning Injury

## Outcome Identification

Outcomes identified for the selected nursing diagnoses could be stated as follows:

- The patient's anxiety will be reduced or controlled.
- The patient or family will verbalize an understanding of the surgical procedure and postoperative plan of care.
- The patient will maintain effective breathing patterns.
- The patient will remain normothermic.
- The patient will be free from signs and symptoms of positioning injury.

## Planning

Preparation can significantly reduce both anesthesia time and intraoperative time for the patient, as well as physical and psychologic stress for the patient, surgeon, and perioperative nurse. Planning for the patient's care in the OR is based on the results of nursing assessment and the identification of relevant nursing diagnoses. The plan of care then identifies desired outcomes derived from the nursing diagnoses; priorities are set and nursing interventions are designed to assist the patient to reach the desired outcomes. Nursing interventions identified for the patient's plan of care may include reassessment, teaching, counseling, referrals, and specific interventions to assist the patient achieve patient care outcomes. A typical plan of care for a patient undergoing a neurosurgical procedure is given on p. 830.

## Implementation

The perioperative nurse must determine that all personnel, equipment, instrumentation, and supplies necessary for a successful surgery are available. The nurse must use the information obtained through assessment of the patient and communication with the surgical team to provide individualized patient care. Neurosurgical patients vary in age from the very young to the very old. They often have special needs because of conditions such as mental status changes, spinal instability, spinal cord injuries, paralysis, other traumatic injuries, and pain. These conditions need to be considered at all times. Neurosurgery patients who seem to be unconscious may actually be aware of their environment and unable to voice their concerns. The perioperative nurse should always talk to the patient and explain what is happening. Showing compassion and attempting to relieve the fears of the patient and his or her family are essential.

***Equipment.*** Neurosurgical procedures require an extensive amount of equipment. The nurse must analyze the arrangement of the equipment in the OR to ensure that the sterile field is not compromised. Electrical equipment should be placed in proximity to electrical outlets, so that cords are out of high-traffic areas. Monitors should be in comfortable view of the surgeon. A microscope needs a clear path to the surgical field. The surgeon and surgical assistants may require specialized surgical chairs or sitting or standing stools to comfortably perform the surgery.

OPERATING ROOM BED AND ATTACHMENTS. The nurse uses information about the proposed surgical procedure and desired surgical position to gather the proper OR bed, attachments, and positioning devices before the patient arrives in the OR suite. Perioperative nurses must anticipate needs that may arise during the surgery and prepare for them. Is this the right OR bed in the right position with the right attachments? If fluoroscopy will be used, is the base of the OR bed in a position that will accommodate the C-arm? A specialized OR bed, such as a Jackson table or Andrews table or frame, may be required for posterior spine surgery. Skull clamps, skull pins, and tongs are commonly used for craniotomies and posterior cervical spine surgeries to stabilize the head and neck (Figure 23-36). Occasionally, a patient may come to the OR in a halo that was placed for preoperative stabilization of the cervical spine. At least part of the halo will need to be removed so the surgical site can be accessed. Compatible wrenches must be available to accomplish this.

BASIC EQUIPMENT. One special neurosurgical overhead instrument table, such as the Mayfield table (Figure 23-37), or two large Mayo trays can be used along with one back table for neurosurgical procedures. Other basic equipment includes the following: a sequential compression device, a cooling-heating unit, one or two monopolar electrosurgical units (ESUs), a bipolar ESU, and a wall supply or tank of nitrogen with a special pressure gauge for operating air-powered instruments. Usually two suctions are required. Intraoperative blood salvage is used for most spine surgeries, unless infection or malignancy is suspected.

Neurosurgeons usually wear surgical loupes and a fiberoptic headlight, requiring a light source.

OPERATING MICROSCOPE. An operating microscope may be required for surgery on certain areas of the brain, spinal

## SAMPLE PLAN OF CARE

**NURSING DIAGNOSIS**

**Anxiety** related to surgery or surgical outcome

**OUTCOME**

The patient's anxiety will be reduced or controlled.

**INTERVENTIONS**

- Broadly classify intensity of patient's anxiety.
- Determine patient's coping skills.
- Provide listening, reassurance, and information.
- Provide ongoing opportunity for questions or expression of concerns or fears.
- Involve other support systems (e.g., family, friends, social worker, chaplain).
- Assist the patient to use personally effective coping skills.
- Use touch (if welcomed by the patient) and eye contact during communication.

**NURSING DIAGNOSIS**

**Deficient Knowledge** related to diagnostic tests and surgical procedures.

**OUTCOME**

The patient and family will verbalize an understanding of the surgical procedure and postoperative plan of care.

**INTERVENTIONS**

- Determine knowledge level and desire for knowledge.
- Correct misinformation.
- Identify readiness and motivation to learn.
- Provide information regarding tests or surgery.
- Explain perioperative routine, postoperative recovery, and discharge plans.
- Base interventions on patient's needs.

**NURSING DIAGNOSIS**

**Risk for Ineffective Breathing Pattern** related to location of tumor, surgical position, or effects of general anesthesia

**OUTCOME**

The patient will maintain effective breathing patterns.

**INTERVENTIONS**

- Provide appropriate positioning accessories, and assist in their placement.
- Collaborate with anesthesia provider and surgeon during positioning activities relevant to respiratory effectiveness.
- Determine patient's comfort on operating room (OR) bed; provide comfort measures as appropriate.
- Maintain open suction line.
- Observe respiratory rate, depth, and character.
- Encourage deep breaths and coughs.
- Communicate with postanesthesia care unit (PACU) regarding respiratory needs.
- Check airway patency frequently during transport to PACU.

**NURSING DIAGNOSIS**

**Risk for Hypothermia**

**OUTCOME**

The patient will remain normothermic.

**INTERVENTIONS**

- Provide warm ambient OR temperature during surgical intervention.
- Provide warmed intravenous (IV) fluids and blood products.
- Provide body-warming system (e.g., forced warm air) during surgery.
- Keep head covered or wrapped.
- Monitor temperature with anesthesia provider.
- Cover the patient with warm blankets at end of the surgical intervention for transport to PACU.

**NURSING DIAGNOSIS**

**Risk for Perioperative Positioning Injury**

**OUTCOME**

The patient will be free from signs and symptoms of positioning injury.

**INTERVENTIONS**

- Assess patient's physical limitations before positioning; make accommodations.
- Carefully pad and protect all prominences and sites that are vulnerable to neurovascular injury.
- Check all positioning devices for cleanliness, working order, and freedom from sharp edges.
- Collaborate with OR team in placing positioning devices to maintain patient safety.
- Assess patient at completion of surgery for areas of redness, blanching, or bruising.
- Communicate any findings to PACU nursing staff.
- Document findings and follow-up with patient, as applicable.

cord, and peripheral nerves. The operating microscope has revolutionized neurosurgery by providing intense light and up to a 12-fold magnification to areas that previously may have been inoperable or inaccessible. Microsurgery allows for greater surgical precision when operating in close proximity to vital structures and has better surgical results. The perioperative nurse must be able to prepare the microscope for use in neurosurgery, and the surgeon must check it for focal length and focus before scrubbing. Disposable sterile drapes are available for the microscope, as are assistant and observer lenses. Cameras and closed-circuit television monitors are also available for use with the operating microscope.

**ENDOSCOPES.** Surgeons use endoscopes to perform minimally invasive neurosurgery, such as endoscopic biopsy. The endoscope provides illumination and magnification of structures and an extended viewing angle. Perioperative nurses must be prepared to convert from a neuroendovascular procedure to an open procedure if it is determined that the surgery cannot be successfully completed endoscopically. An additional use for endoscopes is in open procedures to see areas that are otherwise visually inaccessible.

**RADIOLOGIC INTERVENTION.** Radiology is commonly used intraoperatively for spine surgery. Typically, a radiology technician will operate the equipment. Lead aprons and thyroid shields must be worn or protective shields must be used by all staff in the OR to protect themselves from radiation exposure. X-rays can be taken to check for proper positioning of the spine and to help the surgeon identify a specific level of the spine. This may be done before incision or after partial exposure of the spinous processes and laminae. In both cases an instrument or needle is used to mark a position on the spine, and an x-ray of the spine is taken. The x-ray enables the surgeon to identify the level of the spine that is marked. The surgeon uses that information to identify the correct surgical

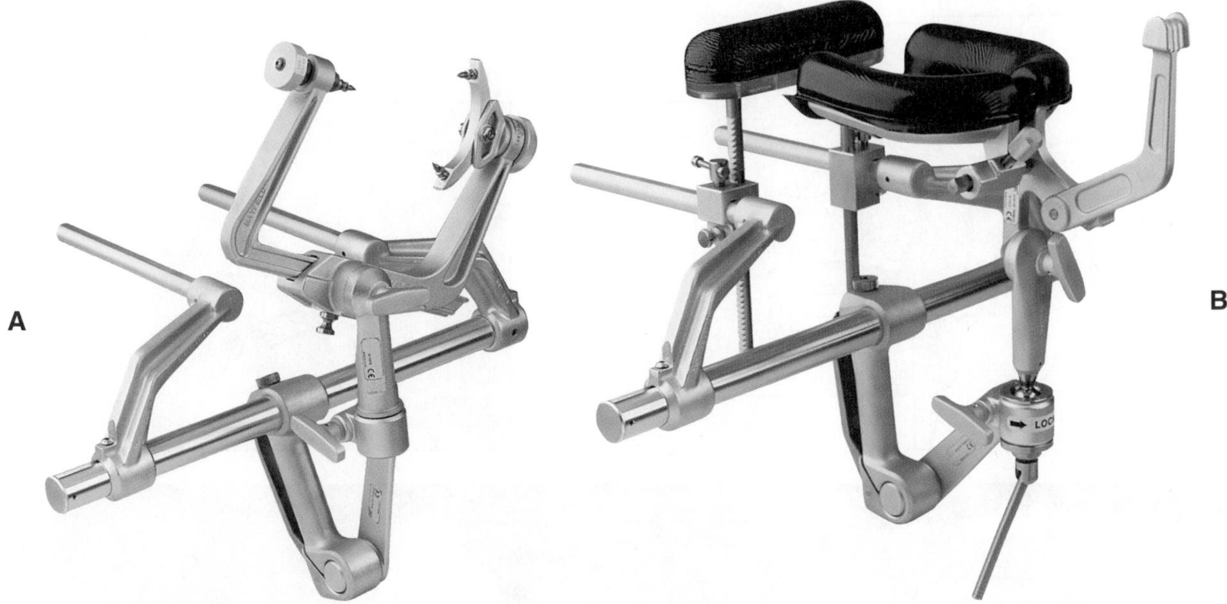


FIGURE 23-36 **A,** Three-pin fixation skull clamp (MAYFIELD) for stabilizing head during neurosurgical procedures. **B,** MAYFIELD horseshoe headrest.

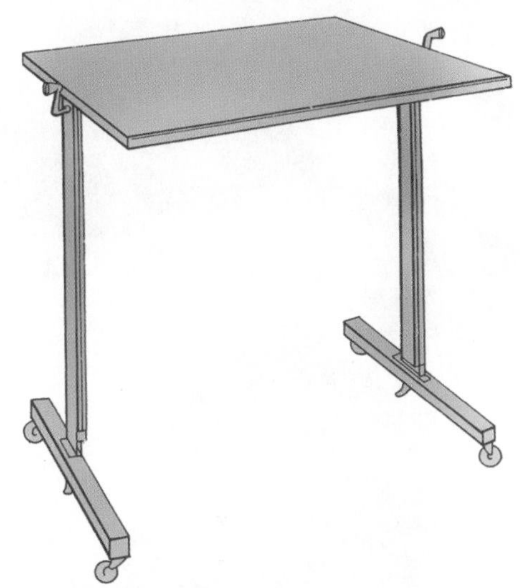

FIGURE 23-37 Mayfield overhead instrument table.

level. A postoperative x-ray is also taken to verify that the surgery was done to the correct level of the spine.

With fluoroscopy, also called direct image intensification, a C-arm (covered with a sterile drape) is used to take a continuous x-ray that is portrayed on a monitor. This gives the surgeon the ability to view the spine and to directly view screws as they are being placed during an instrumented fusion. This ensures that spinal instrumentation for fusion is properly positioned in the correct levels. Fluoroscopy is also used for placement of nerve-stimulator electrodes in brain or spinal areas and stereotactic procedures.

STEREOTACTIC AND IMAGE-GUIDED EQUIPMENT. Stereotactic and image-guided equipment is commonly employed for neurosurgery. Either a frame-based (requiring a head-frame skull attachment, see Figure 23-38) or a frameless system (using fiducials) can be used. Both systems use a computer to register points, based on information obtained from a stereotactic MRI or CT scan done preoperatively, to determine the least traumatic approach to the target (tumor, lesion, ventricle). Both systems have accompanying attachments and instruments that must be available. The frameless image-guided system requires a monitor to display views of the brain or spine in three different planes: axial, coronal, and sagittal (Figure 23-39).

ULTRASONIC ASPIRATOR. An ultrasonic aspirator (CUSA) may be used to emulsify and debulk a tumor with high-frequency sound waves. Various settings allow the surgeon to adjust the instrument to remove firm or calcified lesions, or soft masses. The ultrasonic aspirator provides hemostasis and spares adjacent nerves and vessels as it removes the tumor.

AUDIOVISUAL EQUIPMENT. The use of video cameras, recorders, and television monitors is invaluable to teach staff and enhance understanding of the surgical procedure by perioperative personnel who are otherwise unable to visualize the surgeon's actions directly. By viewing the operative field through the monitor, the experienced scrub person will be able to anticipate the neurosurgeon's next move and will therefore provide better assistance.

INTRAOPERATIVE MONITORING EQUIPMENT. Equipment for intraoperative monitoring, such as EEG, evoked potentials (EPs), ICP, and Dopplers, may also be required.

***Instrumentation, Implants, and Supplies.*** Typically, instrumentation commonly used in neurosurgery is added to basic surgical instrumentation to make neurosurgical-specific trays, such as a basic craniotomy tray or a laminectomy tray. Specialized trays, instruments, or implants can be added based on the surgical procedure.

Powered surgical instruments are commonly used in neurosurgery. Multiple drills, drill bits, and accessories are available.

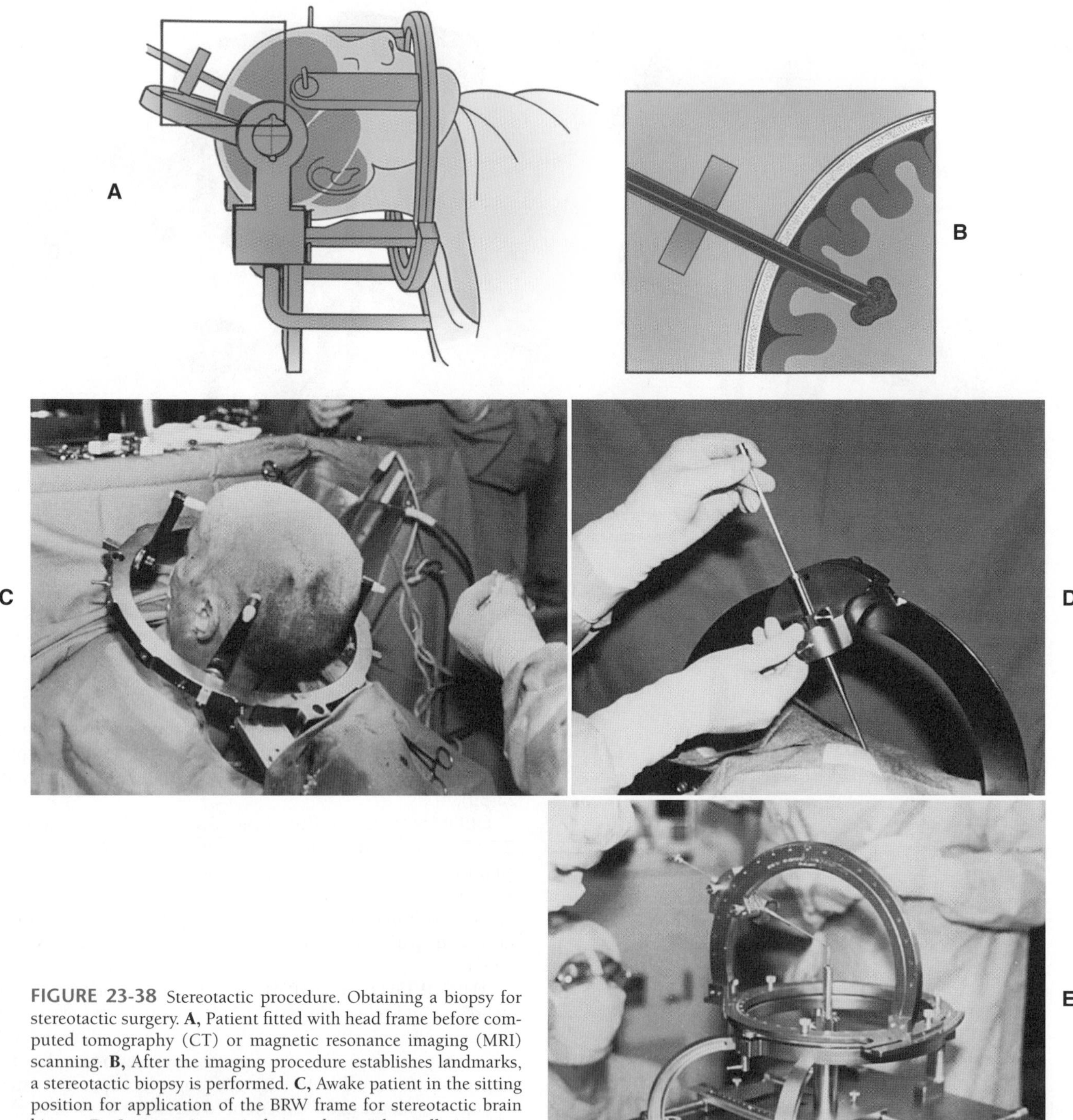


FIGURE 23-38 Stereotactic procedure. Obtaining a biopsy for stereotactic surgery. **A,** Patient fitted with head frame before computed tomography (CT) or magnetic resonance imaging (MRI) scanning. **B,** After the imaging procedure establishes landmarks, a stereotactic biopsy is performed. **C,** Awake patient in the sitting position for application of the BRW frame for stereotactic brain biopsy. **D,** Stereotactic surgical procedure with needle insertion for biopsy. **E,** Stereotactic surgical procedure with arc system placed on phantom base to demonstrate and check accuracy of biopsy needle with *xyz* coordinates for precise depth and angle.

These tools may be powered by air, battery, or electricity and are operated by a hand control or foot pedal. All drills have a safety control that should be engaged at all times the instrument is not in use. The perioperative nurse should monitor the sterile field to ensure that drills and other powered equipment are not left lying on the patient. The use of drills makes bone work easier and reduces operating time. Irrigating the tip of the drill while it is in use prevents overheating of the tissue. By changing drill bits and attachments, different drills can be used to make burr holes, craniotomies, craniectomies, and holes for dural tack-up sutures. They can be used to thin bone for a decompression, to perform decortication for spinal fusion, to harvest hip graft, to shape bone grafts, and to make holes for plating and fixation systems. Examples of specific drills that may be used follow.

The Hall Surgairtome 200 (Figure 23-40) can be used for precision cutting, shaping, and repair of bone. Compressed nitrogen is the power source, as with other air-powered equip-

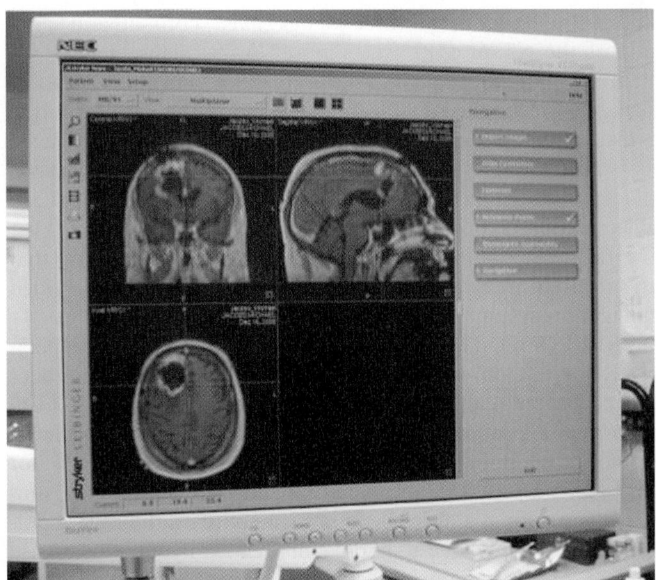


**FIGURE 23-39** Frameless stereotactic image-guided navigation monitor showing the brain with tumor in three planes: coronal *(upper left)*, sagittal *(upper right)*, and axial *(lower left)*.

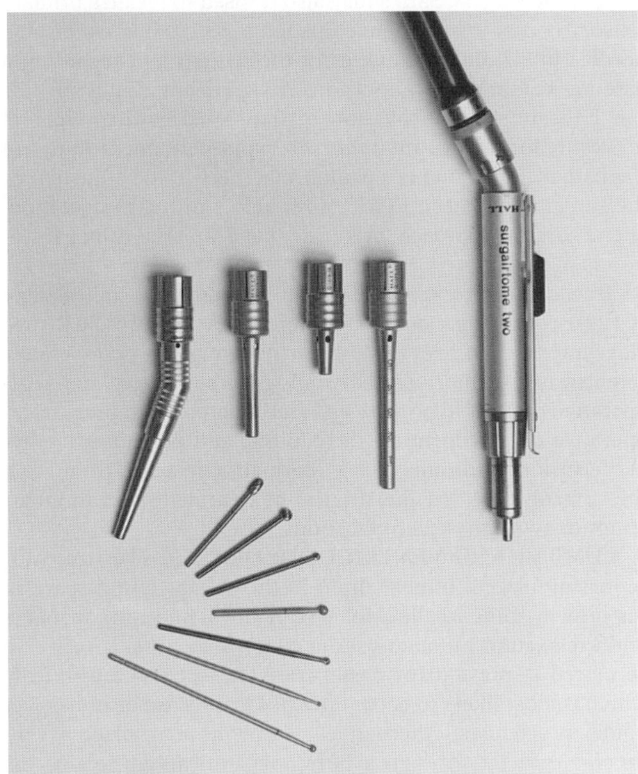


**FIGURE 23-40** Hall Surgairtome 200 with attachments.

ment. The Hall Surgairtome 200 can be used to widen the graft area in anterior fusions and to unroof the auditory canal in eighth cranial nerve surgery. For use in less accessible areas, such as the sphenoidal sinus, pituitary fossa, and vertebral bodies, 20-degree– and 90-degree–angle attachments are available. A range of burrs and guards is available.

The craniotome offers a perforator drive for drilling burr holes. Both 12-mm and 7-mm perforators are available in disposable and reusable forms. The perforator driver attachment can be removed and a saw blade and dura guard attached to adapt the instrument for cutting a craniotomy bone flap. A cranioplasty burr and a skull contour burr as well as guards for each type of burr are available.

Another versatile pneumatic tool is the Midas Rex instrument (Figure 23-41). The variety of disposable cutting tools of this foot pedal–controlled instrument and its attachments provides the neurosurgeon with a versatile bone dissector capable of cutting bone by sawing through it or drilling it away. In addition, large craniotomy flaps can be turned with only a single burr hole. Manufacturers' precautions and instructions must be followed for all powered instruments.

A variety of suction tips, retractors, and retractor systems are required for visualization. A transsphenoidal tray and instruments are required for that specialized approach. Microneurosurgical instruments may be needed for delicate brain or spinal cord surgery. Dural grafts and substitutes may be required to repair the dura. Aneurysm instruments, aneurysm clips, or hemostatic clips may be needed for neurovascular surgery. Titanium plates or wire is used to replace a bone plate after a craniotomy. Spinal instrumentation (plating and fixation systems) may be implanted, and bone grafts and substitutes may be used to promote spinal fusion.

Specific surgeries may require shunts or CSF reservoirs, implantable stimulators or pumps, endoscopes and endoscopic instruments, endovascular instruments, catheters, and coils. These supplies must be available if they are to be placed or implanted during surgery.

The surgical nurse needs to assemble instrumentation with consideration for each individual surgery and according to each individual surgeon's preferences. The instrument list for each procedure and neurosurgeon should be documented, referred to, and frequently updated in collaboration with the surgeon. Specific instruments are referred to in the surgical procedure descriptions that follow.

***Preliminary Procedures.*** A number of procedures or therapeutic measures are performed before the primary surgery begins. It is important that the perioperative nurse anticipate these procedures, understand why they are done, and be prepared to facilitate them.

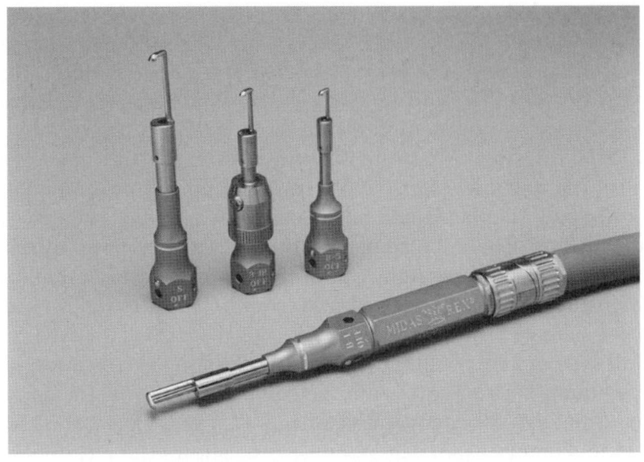

**FIGURE 23-41** Midas Rex drill with attachments.

**ANESTHESIA CONCERNS.** The anesthesia provider collaborates with the surgeon and nurses to provide appropriate care to the patient. The anesthesia provider must be aware of and plan for situations in which the neurosurgery patient may need to be awake during the surgery for intraoperative assessment. Anesthesia agents must be adjusted if intraoperative monitoring of EPs is to be done. If the cervical spine is unstable or unable to extend, endotracheal intubation may need to be done while the patient is awake. The position of the bed in the OR should be communicated to the anesthesia provider. For surgery of the head, the bed may be turned 90 or 180 degrees away from the anesthesia machine to provide comfortable access to the surgical site. Anesthesia providers can prepare by having enough length on their tubing to make the turn while maintaining control of the patient's airway.

Anesthesia for neurosurgery requires sufficient IV access. A central line may be placed if peripheral IV lines are insufficient. Increased risk of an air embolism during surgery exists when the patient is in a sitting position and when a venous sinus may be breeched. A precordial Doppler ultrasound or a pulmonary artery catheter may be placed to monitor for an air embolus. A catheter in the right atrium can be used to remove an air embolus in the heart. An arterial line may be placed for continuous monitoring of blood pressure and for drawing samples for arterial blood gas (ABG) analysis.

Antibiotic prophylaxis is administered within 30 minutes of incision time and continued at the appropriate dose schedule for at least 24 hours. The preoperative antibiotic dose is the most important dose in the prevention of postoperative infection. Generally, a broad-spectrum cephalosporin is the antibiotic drug of choice, but this depends on the needs of the individual patient. In addition, antibiotics such as bacitracin can be added to the irrigation. Preoperative steroids may be given to minimize inflammation and edema when surgery is done involving the brain or spinal cord. Diuretics may be added for brain relaxation during surgery and to decrease ICP. Antiepileptic drugs are typically given when the cerebral cortex is manipulated to prevent seizures. Coagulopathies must be identified and corrected preoperatively.

For all but minor surgeries, a Foley catheter is inserted into the bladder to monitor urinary output during the procedure. It is essential for prolonged procedures, when excessive bleeding is anticipated, or when diuretics are to be given intravenously, so that the bladder does not become distended. A Foley catheter is needed by trauma patients for continuous assessment of kidney function.

**STEREOTACTIC IMAGE-GUIDED NAVIGATION.** To prepare for surgery on the brain, fiducials are placed on bony landmarks or points around the skull before a preoperative MRI or CT scan. Afterward, the fiducials are left in place for entry into the OR. After the patient is asleep and positioned, a skull clamp is placed and an image-guided navigation arm is attached to the skull clamp. This provides a fixed point of reference. The arm should be out of the way of the surgical team to ensure that it will not be inadvertently bumped and moved from its fixed point during surgery, thus disrupting the navigation system and potentially making it useless. The location of the fiducials is registered into the computer, allowing the computer to align the preoperative images (of the CT scan or MRI) to the patient's head. The monitor then shows the location of the navigation probe (which is maneuvered by the surgeon) and its trajectory on all three planes (axial, coronal, and sagittal) of the CT or MRI (see Figure 23-39). This enables the neurosurgeon to plan the approach to the target area and to navigate the surgical area using the navigation probe. After the registration process is complete, the fiducials can be removed so that the area can be prepped for surgery. A sterile sleeve is placed over the navigation arm when draping. The navigation system is used to find the target (tumor, lesion, ventricle) using the least traumatic trajectory. It also helps to ensure that the desired amount of tissue is removed. The image-guided navigation system can also be used for spine surgery.

**NEUROMONITORING.** An EEG can be used intraoperatively to view and record electrical activity by way of electrodes placed on the scalp or directly on the brain. It can be used to identify the location of seizure foci on the brain for possible resection. Nonconvulsive use of EEG monitors is used to monitor for burst suppression during carotid endarterectomy. Burst suppression refers to a decrease in brain activity on the EEG monitor and may be related to hypoxemia-related hypoperfusion.

EPs record the brain's electrical response to visual, auditory, and sensory stimuli. They may be used intraoperatively to monitor hearing during resection of acoustic neuromas or to monitor SSEPs (somatosensory evoked potentials) during some spine surgery. SSEPs may also be used to localize primary sensory cortex in anesthetized patients. SSEPs involve placing needles in significant muscles of the patient and recording a baseline reading before incision. A significant change in EPs can indicate surgical invasion of the spinal cord, peripheral nerves, brainstem, or midbrain. To avoid permanent injury to the patient, the patient's position may need to be adjusted, or the surgeon may need to adjust retractors or instrumentation, alter a surgical approach, or decide that a subtotal tumor resection is necessary.

Transcranial Doppler (TCD) ultrasound is increasingly being used during carotid endarterectomy surgery. TCD provides information relevant to the major causes of perioperative cerebrovascular morbidity, including intraoperative and postoperative emboli, hypoperfusion during cross-clamping, intraoperative or postoperative thrombosis, and postoperative hyperperfusion syndrome. Using information received from TCD, the surgeon can alter the surgical or treatment plan in an attempt to avoid these complications.[14]

**LUMBAR AND VENTRICULAR DRAINS.** The neurosurgeon may place a lumbar drain in the subarachnoid space of the lumbar spine to allow for CSF removal and intraoperative brain relaxation for aneurysm or tumor exposure. It may also be placed to prevent (or postoperatively, to treat) a CSF leak, which is most likely to occur after posterior fossa or transsphenoidal procedures. Alternatively, surgeons may place a ventricular catheter through a burr hole into a ventricle of the brain. In addition to providing the ability to drain CSF, a ventriculostomy provides the most accurate method of monitoring ICP. A transducer-tipped catheter system is a less accurate but less invasive method for monitoring. It does not allow for CSF drainage. With both the lumbar drain and the ventricular catheter, the nurse must ensure that stop cocks and clamps are properly positioned to avoid overdrainage of CSF, which could result in brain herniation. A separate surgical prep and setup are required for placement of these ICP devices.

**CAROTID CUTDOWN.** When excessive intracranial bleeding is a possibility, the neurosurgeon may choose carotid cutdown and temporary ligation or tourniquet placement for occlusion of the carotid arteries during bleeding. Carotid cutdown is a separate surgical procedure and requires a special sterile setup, including drapes and instruments. Procedures that may require such management include intracranial vascular surgery and removal of meningiomas.

***Positioning.*** Many of the basic body positions described in Chapter 5 and their modifications are used in neurosurgery. The perioperative nurse must know the desired position and have the appropriate OR bed, attachments, and supportive positioning devices available. Positioning devices that may be needed include a headrest, pillows, blankets, gel pads, a safety belt, tape, a shoulder roll (supine), an axillary roll (lateral), a beanbag (lateral), and chest rolls (prone).

Specialized neurosurgical headrests and skull clamps are commonly used for craniotomies and posterior cervical spine surgeries to support and stabilize the head and neck. They can be used with any body position. The basic unit of the neurosurgical headrest attaches to the frame of the OR bed after the standard OR bed headpiece has been removed. An articulated arm allows fine adjustments to the position of the head. A horseshoe-shaped headrest may be used. Alternatively, head clamps, skull pins, and tongs that are attached to the neurosurgical headrest bed attachment and provide maximum stability may be required (see Figure 23-36).

Most skull clamps have three sterile pins that are placed in the skull clamp and covered with antibiotic or Betadine (povidone-iodine) ointment. The surgeon or surgeon's assistant places the skull clamps on the patient's head after anesthesia is administered. The surgeon must place the skull clamp strategically in the skull to provide access to the surgical site and to avoid the frontal sinuses, the superficial temporal arteries, and the eyes. The pins on the clamp partially penetrate the outer table of the skull. If the prone position is used, the surgeon will place the skull clamp while the patient is supine. The surgeon supports the patient's head during the position change and adjusts the final head position after the patient is placed prone.

After positional adjustments to the patient's body are complete, the skull clamp (and patient's head) is locked into the articulating arm of the headrest by someone other than the person who is supporting the head. The apparatus is tightened from distal to proximal and double-checked for security. Once the patient's head is locked into place, no positional adjustments can be made to the patient's body without first releasing the head. Not doing so could cause injury to the patient's cervical spine. If necessary, an image-guided navigation arm can be attached to certain skull clamps, and the positions of the fiducials are registered into the system before prepping.

The skull clamp is detached from the basic headrest by loosening the arm from distal to proximal. Finally, while the head is being supported by another person, the skull clamp is loosened, allowing the pins to be released from the skull. Ointment can be applied to the pin sites. Bleeding may occur at the pin sites after the skull clamp is removed. It usually stops with digital pressure, but occasionally a stitch may be required.

The position of the patient's arms must also be considered. For cranial surgery, usually at least one arm is tucked so that the Mayo stand can be positioned over the patient. For cervical spine surgery, both arms are tucked so that the surgical site can be accessed from both sides of the table. For thoracic and lumbar spine surgery, armboards can usually be placed out of the way of the surgeon and radiology equipment.

As always, potential hazards should be identified, and precautions should be taken to prevent them. Sequential compression stockings are applied before induction of anesthesia to prevent deep vein thrombosis (DVT) unless they are contraindicated because of a known DVT. Pressure points must be identified and relieved. Joints must be maintained in functional alignment with no pressure or tension on superficial nerves and vessels. A warming/cooling blanket is applied for temperature control. An occlusive dressing applied over the eyes protects them from chemical burns and corneal abrasions that may occur from solutions used to prep the head. Keeping the head positioned above the heart minimizes bleeding when operating on the head.

Supine position or some modification of it can be used for approaches to the frontal, parietal, and temporal lobes; the anterior cervical spine; and the anterior lumbar spine. Lateral position can be used for an approach to the cerebellopontine angle in the posterior fossa, for anterior thoracic and lumbar spine surgery, and to access the posterior spine. It can be used for lumbar sympathectomies and for placements of nerve stimulators and pumps.

Prone position and modifications of it can be used for access to the posterior spine and for suboccipital and posterior fossa craniotomies. A laminectomy frame or chest rolls are commonly used for prone position. The Jackson table permits access of the C-arm for intraoperative fluoroscopy of the spine. The Andrews table or frame can be used for a modified knee-chest position, which is useful for posterior lumbar spine surgery. The patient's hips and knees are flexed so that the lower body is supported primarily by the knees. The Hicks spinal surgery frame ("butt board") may be used to support this position and allow the abdomen to hang free. The chest is supported on a chest roll. Advantages of this position include decreased bleeding because of the collapse of epidural veins, better exposure resulting from hyperflexion of the spine, absence of pressure on the vena cava, and increased ease of ventilation. Operating time is usually reduced when this position is used. Disadvantages of the knee-chest position include the difficulty of maintaining physical stability on the OR bed, hypotension, and pooling of blood in the lower extremities.

Fowler (sitting) position is used for some craniotomies involving a posterior or occipital approach. Advantages of this position include optimum visibility of the operative field and decreased blood loss because of the lowered arterial and venous pressures. Disadvantages are the potential for orthostatic hypotension and air embolism. In the sitting position the venous pressure in the head and neck may be negative, predisposing the patient to air embolism (Patient Safety). Other potential problems with this position include neck flexion with airway compromise and difficulty in achieving and maintaining functional alignment. Please refer to Chapter 5 for more information on the above-mentioned positions.

***Skin Preparation.*** Prevention of infection is a primary concern in neurosurgery. An antiseptic skin prep is performed by the perioperative nurse, surgeon, resident, or surgical assistant. General principles and precautions cited in Chapter 3 apply to neurosurgical preps. Although studies have shown that shav-

## PATIENT SAFETY

### Preventing and Managing Venous Air Embolism in the Sitting Position

The use of the sitting position is more common in neurosurgical procedures than in other specialties. Patients undergoing posterior fossa, cervical, or supratentorial procedures in the sitting position are at risk for venous air embolism (VAE). VAE is a potentially serious intraoperative condition that may result in significant morbidity and mortality. The incidence of VAE in neurologic procedures performed in the sitting position is 10% to 80% and has a mortality of approximately 1%.

The perioperative nurse partners with the anesthesia provider, neurosurgeon, and scrub person to provide safety for patients during seated neurosurgical procedures. The nurse must be knowledgeable about the factors that contribute to VAE to plan effective and safe patient care.

Common sources of VAE are the major cerebral venous sinuses, in particular the transverse, the sigmoid, and the posterior half of the sagittal sinus, all of which may be noncollapsible because of their dural attachments. Air may also enter through emissary veins, particularly from the suboccipital musculature, the diploic space of the skull, and the cervical epidural veins. VAE is possible anytime there is a negative pressure gradient between the operative site and the right arterial pressure.

**Preventive Measures**

The nurse should anticipate assisting the anesthesia provider with the placement of a pulmonary artery pressure (PAP) catheter, precordial Doppler, and a multiorifice central venous line. The pulmonary artery catheter allows the anesthesiologist to monitor heart pressures; and the right atrial central venous catheter is used to measure right arterial pressure, administer vasoactive medications if needed, and as a means to aspirate air from the right atrium. Depending on availability, transesophageal echocardiography (TEE) may be used to detect VAE. The nurse should collaborate with the anesthesia provider and neurosurgeon to configure the OR to accommodate the TEE equipment. According to the surgeon's preference, the nurse should ensure the patient is wearing compression stockings, sequential compression devices, or elastic Ace bandage wraps on the lower extremities to promote venous return and prevent venous stasis.

**Detection of Venous Air Embolism**

The anesthesia provider will monitor the PAP, Doppler, end-tidal $CO_2$, and TEE (if used). Generally, transient decreases in arterial pressure and end-tidal $CO_2$ not otherwise related to anesthetic administration or surgical condition indicate the presence of VAE. The audible tone of the precordial Doppler changes and turbulence, or "washing-machine" sounds, may indicate early VAE. If VAE is detected or suspected, the nurse must be prepared to assist the surgeon and anesthesia provider to rapidly treat the patient.

**Managing Venous Air Embolism**

Once VAE has been diagnosed, a critical component of treatment is to prevent further air entrainment. The nurse should ensure that sponges and irrigation are available on the sterile field for the surgeon to flood the surgical site with saline and pack the surgical site. These maneuvers will prevent additional air entry while the surgeon tries to locate the source of air. The anesthesia provider is responsible for attempting to aspirate the air by way of the multiorifice right atrial catheter and may administer ephedrine, dobutamine, or norepinephrine to provide inotropic support to the right ventricle. Although changing the patient's position is difficult because of the positioning apparatus, a change to the left lateral decubitus position (right side up) may be indicated to prevent the air in the atrium from moving to the ventricle and causing an air lock.

Modified from Drummond JC, Patel PM: Neurosurgical anesthesia. In Miller RD: *Miller's anesthesia*, ed 6, Philadelphia, 2005, Churchill Livingstone; Goodkin R, Mesiwala A: General principles of operative positioning. In Winn RH: *Youman's neurological surgery*, vol 1, ed 5, Philadelphia, 2004, Saunders; Wong AC, Irwin MG: Large venous air embolism in the sitting position despite monitoring with transoesophageal echocardiography, *Anesthesia* 60:811-813, 2005.

ing the surgical site can contribute to the possibility of infection, usually some hair removal is necessary when operating on the head and posterior cervical spine.

Hair removal from the head causes a disturbance in body image and can be upsetting to patients. A discussion and often a compromise regarding hair removal should take place between the surgeon and patient before the surgery, and an understanding should be reached as to how much hair will be removed. Hair that is removed is the property of the patient. It should be placed in a container, labeled with the patient's name, and kept with the patient after surgery.

Hair removal should be done as close to the time of skin incision as possible to decrease the possibility of surgical site infection. Whenever possible, minimal hair removal is recommended. It is possible to shave a 1- to 2-cm wide area along the length of some craniotomy incisions after parting the hair there. After the minimal shave, the hair can be combed away from the incision and held back with prepping solution or antimicrobial ointment. However, other craniotomies require more extensive hair removal. Electric hair clippers are preferred to razors because they are less irritating and less likely to nick the skin, which would predispose the area to infection. After hair removal, the nurse should inspect the patient's skin carefully for any signs of inflammation or infection. If any such signs are noted, they should be reported to the surgeon immediately. The head and hair surrounding the planned incision can be prepped, even though the hair will be draped out of the operative field.

For surgery on the cervical spine it is possible to secure long hair on top of the head and remove neck hair with clippers to a level even with the top of the ears or to the occipital protuberance. Postoperatively, patients with long hair can comb it down over the shaved area until the hair regrows. Patients undergoing thoracic or lumbar spine surgery may not need to be shaved. If bone graft from the hip will be taken for spinal fusion, that area must be prepped as well as the spinal incision area.

Many neurosurgeons mark the incision line with a marking pen or a marking solution and wooden stick. If a marking solution is used, indigo carmine, gentian violet, or brilliant green is recommended. Methylene blue should never be found in a neurosurgical OR because it produces an inflammatory reaction in CNS tissue. Because the markings tend to wash off during the prep, some surgeons may scratch the scalp along the planned incision with a sharp sterile needle. This increases the risk of infection and should only be done if there is danger of harming the patient by varying from the planned line of incision.

***Draping.*** According to Joint Commission on Accreditation of Healthcare Organizations (JCAHO) recommendations, the surgical team takes a "time out" during the prepping and draping procedures to be sure that everyone is in agreement that the correct surgery is being done to the correct patient in the correct location. The surgical consent is read aloud by the circulating nurse. In neurosurgical procedures, the right or left side of the head and the level of the spine must be specified. The surgical team should also check that the marking (initials) made to the surgical site in the holding area are in the operative field.

Draping for some neurosurgery procedures is complex and requires the cooperation of the surgeon, assistant, and scrub nurse. Four or more towels are placed around the operative site. They may be secured by disposable skin staples, small towel clamps, or silk sutures on a cutting needle.

Draping for a craniotomy is challenging. If a minimal shave was done, an adhesive drape with staples placed around the shaved area near the incision can help to keep hair out of the incision. Towels can be contoured to the prepped area of the head and held in place with staples, leaving the operative site exposed. A craniotomy drape can then be placed over the towels. A sterile drainage bag below the incision will help to catch irrigation and blood and drain it into a suction canister. If a stereotactic head frame is used, be sure that the drapes do not interfere with the head frame attachments.

Prepping out a hip graft incision may need to be done with spinal fusion surgery. Two areas may need to be prepped and squared off with towels, which can be held in place with an adhesive drape. A partially unfolded three fourths drape can be placed between the two planned incision sites before the universal or laparotomy drape is placed. A clamp can be placed over the prepped hip area to positively identify it. The drape can be cut over the prepped area, being sure not to cut an area of the drape that covers a nonsterile area. A second adhesive drape can hold the cut drape in place. Please refer to Chapter 3 for general draping procedures.

***Hemostasis and Visualization.*** A few minutes before making the incision, the surgeon may inject the incision site with a local anesthetic agent, such as lidocaine or bupivacaine (Marcaine). Lidocaine has a more rapid onset and shorter duration than bupivacaine. Along with decreasing the effect of the stimulus of the skin incision, infiltration of the solution will apply pressure within the tissues and decrease bleeding at the time of incision. Using a local anesthetic that also contains epinephrine will constrict blood vessels to further minimize bleeding.

Meticulous hemostasis is particularly important in neurosurgery. Many methods are incorporated to limit blood loss. A major consideration is control of hemorrhage from the highly vascular scalp. Skin edges along the wound are compressed with gauze sponges and fingers during the initial incision. Usually, this is followed by application of disposable scalp clips (Figure 23-42). An automatic clip gun may be used to apply clips to include the galea and skin edge. The clips limit bleeding by applying pressure to the scalp edges. They remain in place until closure. Placement of self-retaining retractors also helps to control bleeding of the scalp.

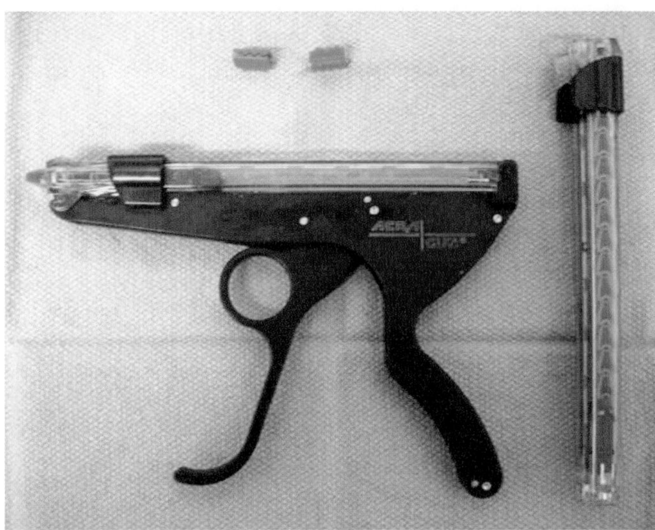

**FIGURE 23-42** Automatic clip gun, with disposable scalp clips and cartridge.

Retraction is required for visualization. Self-retaining retractors such as cerebellar or Gelpi retractors can be used to retract skin, subcutaneous tissue, muscle, or the scalp. Suture can be used to retract the scalp or the dura of the brain or spinal cord. Blunt, malleable retractors are used on brain tissue. Table-mounted self-retaining retractor systems such as the Greenberg help the surgeon to see deep into the brain and may be used with a microscope.

Electrosurgery is routine for neurosurgical procedures. Perioperative nurses must understand the uses and hazards of the ESU and be familiar with the safety measures. Electrocoagulation current seals the blood vessels. To be effective, the electrocoagulating current must contact the vessel in a dry field. For this reason, suctioning is necessary to remove blood as the contact is made between the instrument carrying the current and the bleeding point. A monopolar current is used to cut and coagulate tissue. It can be applied to forceps, a metal suction tip, or another instrument, which acts as a conducting tool. Monopolar electrosurgery is safe to use on the epidermis, dermis, galea, periosteum, muscle, and bone. It is used extensively for exposure of the posterior spine.

Bipolar ESUs provide a completely isolated output with negligible leakage of current between the tips of the forceps, permitting use of electrocoagulating current in proximity to structures where ordinary monopolar electrocoagulation would be hazardous (Figure 23-43). It is safe to use the bipolar ESU to control bleeding on the dura of the brain and spinal cord and near vital nerves and vessels. It can be used to maintain hemostasis and to dissect tissue in the brain. Lactated Ringer's or normal saline solution irrigation is often used during bipolar electrocoagulation to minimize tissue heating, shrinkage, drying, and adherence to the forceps. Some bipolar units have built-in irrigating systems. The use of the bipolar electrocoagulation technique allows hemostasis of almost any size vessel encountered. Vessels as large as the superficial temporal artery,

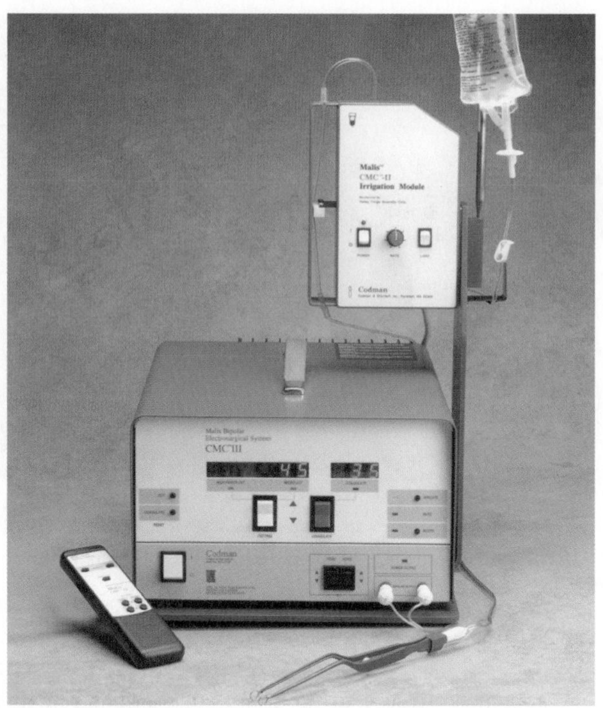


FIGURE 23-43 Malis bipolar coagulator and bipolar cutter, with irrigation module.

as well as those too small for suture or clip ligation, may be coagulated with bipolar units.

Suction is necessary to evacuate blood, CSF, and irrigation solution from the surgical site. Metal suction tips in multiple sizes, such as the Sachs, Frazier, and Adson, are used not only because they keep the wound dry but also because they can conduct electrocoagulation current from a monopolar unit to the bleeding point. Suction applied directly on normal neural tissue may be harmful and is avoided. Instead, a cottonoid patty (described below) may be placed between the suction tip and neural tissue for protection. Suction can be used to aspirate necrotic or traumatized brain tissue or soft brain tumors after a sample has been obtained for pathologic examination. It is also useful in evacuating abscess cavities, removing fluid from a ventricle or the subarachnoid space, holding a solid tumor during its removal, and applying compression to a bleeding vessel.

Bone wax is a hemostatic material that should be available for all cranial and spinal cord operations. Bone wax may be applied with the surgeon's fingertip or with the tip of an instrument such as a Freer or Penfield. The surgeon firmly rubs or packs the wax into the bleeding surfaces of bone. Bone wax is commonly used in burr holes, along the edges of a craniotomy, and on the cut edges of the spine.

Gauze sponges are used to control bleeding before the skull or spinal canal is entered; however, they are coarse and can injure fragile tissues such as the brain and spinal cord. Instead, compressed, absorbent patties made of rayon or cotton (cottonoids) are used to control bleeding beneath the skull and around the spinal cord. Patties are also placed over delicate neural tissue for protection. It is far less traumatic to suction on a patty rather than directly on the tissue. Patties are available in a variety of sizes, both squares and strips, ranging from ¼ inch to 6 inches long and ¼ inch to 1 inch wide (Figure 23-44). A supply of various sizes is typically moistened with irrigation solution or thrombin and offered to the surgeon on a waterproof surface. Patties have x-ray–detectable markers and strings attached and are included in the standard sponge count.

Cotton balls moistened with irrigation solution or thrombin may be used as a temporary pack or tamponade in a bleeding tumor bed after a tumor has been removed. The gentle pressure of the cotton balls along with time and patience on the part of the surgeon may stop bleeding not controllable by other means. Cotton balls also have x-ray–detectable strings and are included in the sponge count.

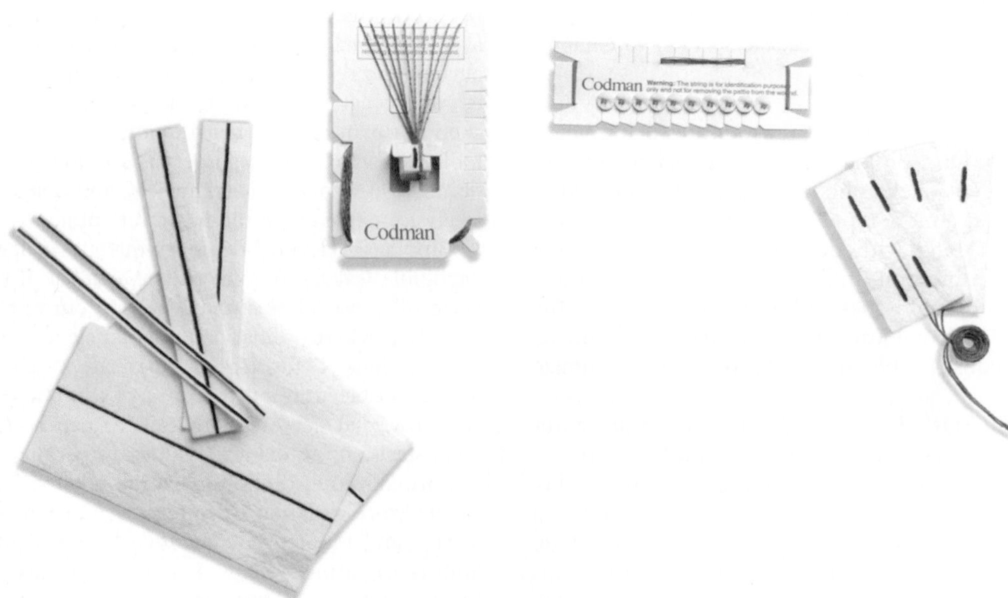


FIGURE 23-44 Cottonoid strips and patties.

A variety of hemostatic clips are available and used by neurosurgeons to occlude both superficial and deep vessels. Unlike clips that were used in the past, hemoclips and Ligaclips are made of an alloy that is compatible with the MRI scanner. The scrub person removes the clips from a special cartridge with the appropriate applicator and passes them to the surgeon for application to a vessel. Such clips enable the surgeon to occlude vessels in areas difficult to reach by other means and to ligate superficial vessels of the brain before cutting them and without destroying any surrounding tissues. Clips are available in a variety of sizes. Numerous types of special clips are used for permanent or temporary occlusion of vessels or an aneurysm neck in the surgical treatment of an intracranial aneurysm (Figure 23-45).

Neurosurgeons almost routinely use certain hemostatic agents in addition to mechanical hemostasis (Surgical Pharmacology). Absorbable gelatin sponge (Gelfoam) can be applied

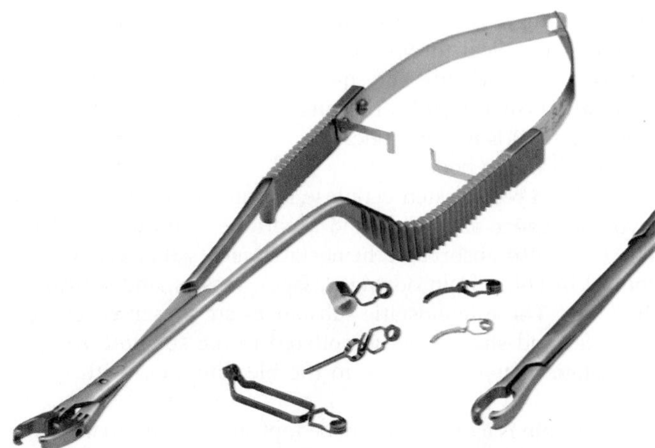

**FIGURE 23-45** Standard aneurysm clips and appliers.

## SURGICAL PHARMACOLOGY

### Hemostatic Agents

Achieving hemostasis in delicate areas can be a challenge for the neurosurgeon. In addition to using meticulous technique to prevent bleeding, topical agents are routinely used as an adjunct to hemostasis. The perioperative nurse must be familiar with the agents used in this setting.

| Agent | Dosage Form | Mechanism of Action | Side Effects | Nursing Considerations |
|---|---|---|---|---|
| Topical thrombin | Powder for reconstitution; packaged with diluent and spray pump, or diluent and spray tip syringe, with diluent only | Catalyzes the conversion of fibrinogen to fibrin | May cause fever or allergic-type reactions | Product is for external use only; must be refrigerated. |
| Gelatin matrix (FloSeal) | Gelatin matrix granules and topical thrombin packaged as a kit with syringes and mixing bowl | Matrix particles form a composite clot that seals the bleeding site, thrombin component converts the fibrinogen in the patient's blood to fibrin | Anemia, atrial fibrillation, infection | Product reaches maximum expansion at approximately 10 min. Excess product should be removed with gentle irrigation. |
| Absorbable gelatin sponge (Gelfoam) | Film, powder, and topical forms | Absorbs and holds blood and fluid within its interstices; exerts physical hemostatic effect | Local infection and abscess formation | Should not be used in the closure of skin incisions since it may interfere with healing of skin edges. Often moistened with saline or topical thrombin before use. |
| Collagen hemostat (Avitene, Helistat, Instat) | Pads, powder, sheets, sponges | When in contact with a bleeding surface, attracts platelets that aggregate into thrombi, initiating the formation of a physiologic platelet plug | Adhesion formation, allergic reaction, foreign-body reaction, inflammation, potentiation of infection | Applied dry. Excess material should be removed. |
| Oxidized regenerated cellulose (Surgicel) | Fibrous, knitted or sheer weave fabric | Allows platelets and aggregates of thrombin and particulate blood elements to cling and form a coagulum that can act as a patch | Encapsulation of fluid, foreign-body reactions | Store at room temperature. |

Modified from LexiComp Online. Accessed April 1, 2006, on-line: www.crlonline.com/crlsql/servlet/crlonline; FloSeal package insert product information. Accessed April 1, 2006, on-line: www.ctsnet.org/baxter/product/931; Gelfoam package insert product information. Accessed April 1, 2006, on-line: www.pfizer.com/pfizer/download/uspi_gelfoam_powder.pdf.

to an oozing surface, either dry or saturated with irrigation solution or topical thrombin. Larger pieces can be cut into a variety of sizes of strips and squares. Gelfoam is often followed by a patty, which enables the surgeon to maneuver and compress it once it is in the surgical site. Gelfoam is absorbable and can be left in the body.

Oxidized regenerated cellulose is available in two forms, a rayonlike gauze (Surgicel) and a cottonlike form (Fibrillar). These are also absorbable hemostatic agents that are used to control bleeding from oozing surfaces, vessels, and sinuses in the brain. These hemostatic substances are presented in various sizes and shapes and are offered to the surgeon dry. The hemostatic material adheres to the bleeding area with gentle pressure.

Thrombin is a drug that can be topically applied to bleeding surfaces to achieve hemostasis. Typically, Gelfoam or patties are saturated with thrombin and placed on the oozing surface. A newer product called FloSeal uses a gelatin matrix to deliver thrombin.

Irrigating the wound helps the surgeon identify active bleeding points and may facilitate hemostasis. Two completely filled bulb or irrigation syringes should always be accessible. A syringe with an angiocatheter tip may be used to deliver irrigation for microsurgery. Many neurosurgeons irrigate surgical wounds with an antibiotic solution before wound closure. The antibiotic is mixed with irrigation solution according to the surgeon's preference so that it is ready for use when needed.

***Suture.*** Required suture will vary according to the surgery, the condition of the wound and patient, and the surgeon's preference. Suture can be used for retraction of the scalp for a craniotomy flap. Dura of the brain and spinal cord may be retracted, tacked up, and closed with braided nylon suture. In general, high tensile strength is needed for closure of the galea of the scalp and the fascia and subcutaneous tissue of the back. Braided, absorbable suture can be used in interrupted stitches to close these layers. Skin may be closed with subcuticular absorbable suture, with either a continuous or interrupted suturing technique using a monofilament, nonabsorbable suture material such as nylon, or with staples. Whatever technique is used for skin closure, skin edges should be everted. A drain may be secured to the skin with a nonabsorbable suture such as nylon. In an environment of infection, monofilament, nonabsorbable suture is preferred.

***Dressings.*** Applying dressings to wounds on the head is challenging, especially if a minimal shave was done. For larger incisions in particular, a head wrap can be the best alternative. It keeps a nonadhering dressing in place over the incision site and provides compression to prevent the formation of a postoperative hematoma. A smaller dressing can sometimes be held in place with a transparent dressing or tape. Applying a liquid adhesive, such as Mastisol, to the skin before application of the dressing can help to hold it in place.

## Evaluation

After the surgical procedure is completed, the patient is transported to the intensive care unit (ICU) or postanesthesia care unit (PACU). A report along with intraoperative documentation is given to the nurse receiving the patient. The identified outcomes from the established nursing diagnoses and interventions are evaluated on an ongoing basis throughout the perioperative period, and adjustments to the plan are made as necessary. Before leaving the OR, postoperative skin integrity is assessed, and a postoperative neurologic assessment is compared with the preoperative assessment. In addition, the patient's outcomes from the identified nursing diagnoses are evaluated. If the outcomes were met, they may be communicated as follows:

- The patient expressed feeling less anxious, coped with perioperative routines adequately, and verbalized an understanding of the planned procedure or procedures.
- The patient or family verbalized knowledge of diagnostic and surgical procedures and had realistic expectations of tests, routines, and postoperative care.
- The patient maintained effective breathing patterns; ventilation was maintained, arterial blood gases were within normal limits, and breath sounds were bilateral.
- The patient will continue to maintain a normal body temperature or undergo rewarming.
- The patient exhibited no signs and symptoms of pressure injury; sensation and motion were the same as preoperative functional levels; and respiratory status and blood pressure were maintained within expected parameters.

## Patient and Family Education and Discharge Planning

Patient and family education is the key to helping the patient return to his or her optimal quality of life. As soon as the need for surgery is identified, a multidimensional education program should begin and include the patient's family. Teaching should address the psychosocial as well as the physiologic aspects of the patient's life. The plan should offer opportunities for the patient to develop new skills, coping mechanisms, and behaviors to adapt to aspects of temporary or permanent neurologic deficit.

Neurosurgery patients may experience a variety of deficits involving vision, hearing, swallowing, speech, motor, sensation, and mental status. Depending on the patient's pathologic condition and surgery, other physicians may observe the patient postoperatively along with the neurosurgeon. Neurologists, ophthalmologists, endocrinologists, cardiologists, radiologists, oncologists, and infectious disease physicians may be involved with managing the medical care of neurosurgery patients. Rehabilitation, physical, occupational, and speech therapists are instrumental in the recovery of neurosurgery patients. They also teach the patients and their families how to cope with temporary and lifelong deficits and how to improve their quality of life. Some patients may benefit from time spent in a rehabilitation facility before returning home. Patients with severe alterations in neurologic function may require long-term care.

The nurse plays an important role in teaching patients and family members how to look for and recognize potential postoperative complications, such as changes in mental status or behavior, progressive weakness, seizure activity, increasing pain, and signs and symptoms of infection. Routine discharge instructions should include information about newly prescribed medications and their potential side effects and treatment options for postoperative and chronic pain. The nurse should also ensure the patient has instructions for the use of cervical collars, braces for spinal stability, and wound dressing changes when applicable.

The entire health care team is responsible for making the transition from the acute care setting to another facility or to home as easy as possible for the patient and family. The patient and family need to be involved in every aspect of the neurosurgery patient's care and should be encouraged to ask questions and voice their concerns and opinions.

# *Surgical Interventions*

## MINIMALLY INVASIVE AND SPECIALIZED NEUROSURGERY TECHNIQUES

### Microneurosurgery

Adaptation of the operating microscope for neurosurgery has resulted in improvement of many neurosurgical procedures and made new procedures possible. For years, neurosurgeons have worn magnifying loupes to see small structures. Loupes usually have a magnification of 2× or 3.5×. The microscope has a variety of magnifications ranging from 6 to 40, providing flexibility and precision. The co-axial illumination overcomes the difficulties of lighting neurosurgical wounds (History box).

Use of the microscope restricts the surgeon's field of vision and mobility; therefore the scrub person and surgical assistant must be proficient. The operative field, unless video monitoring is available, cannot be seen. Surgical personnel must understand the surgical procedure, know the anatomy, know the names and uses of all microinstruments, and be able to place each instrument in the surgeon's hand without delay so that the surgeon will be able to use the instrument without readjusting it. Each time the surgeon must look away and then back to the surgical field, open wound time and anesthesia time are increased while the surgeon becomes reoriented to the field. Therefore the assistance the scrub person gives the surgeon saves time and directly benefits the patient.

Microsurgical instruments have been modified and adapted to the requirements of neurosurgery. These instruments often possess the following characteristics: bayonet shape, so that the surgeon's hand remains outside the line of vision and the beam of the microscope light; finely sprung and fluted grip; long length for access to deep structures; and slender and delicate tips that take up as little space as possible. Microneurosurgical instruments are expensive and delicate. Instructions for handling, cleaning, sterilizing, and storing these instruments should be followed. An instrument that is sprung, bent, dulled, hooked, or in any way damaged must never be handed to a surgeon for use but must be repaired or replaced. Instruments must be kept free from blood and tissue during use because the microscope also magnifies debris on the instruments, occluding the structure the surgeon is about to approach. Very fine microsutures are available.

Microsurgical techniques have been applied to cranial, spinal, and peripheral nerve operations. Some procedures in which microsurgery is of value are posterior fossa explorations, especially for tumors of the fourth ventricle or cerebellopontine angle, and removal of small acoustic neuromas, with resulting preservation of the facial nerve. Small vessel endarterectomy, cerebral arterial bypass, cerebral aneurysm clipping, and excision of AVMs are done under the microscope. Microsurgery also has advantages in the treatment of tumors and AVMs of the spinal cord.

## HISTORY

### Evolution of Surgical Magnification

From 1813 to 1825, English, French, and German opticians attempted to coordinate two monoculars into a single instrument, finally providing the modern binocular, used then as opera glasses. Abbe and Zeiss, circa 1870 to 1880, improved opera glasses with the invention of the binocular roof prism, which enabled greater enlargement of the image without having to deal with the increased length of the optical tube.

In 1886, Westien of Germany, an instrument maker, developed the first surgical loupes for a zoologist interested in performing more accurate dissections. Later, Westien developed binocular loupes for an ophthalmologist. He further adapted magnifying loupes from a stationary device to an instrument to be worn on the head, offering a power of 5× to 6× magnification. These proved impractical because of their weight.

The first teleloupes were developed in 1912. They were the prototype of current surgical loupes, offering a light weight and magnification of 2×. Their initial popularity was appreciated by ophthalmologists, and in 1948 Riechert, initially an ophthalmologist who later became a neurosurgeon, advocated their use during neurosurgical procedures. It is believed that neurosurgeons' use of surgical loupes was more widespread, but they had not published this fact.

Operating microscopes borrowed the technology of optical systems developed for surgical loupes and underwent further development of their optical and mechanical systems between 1921 and 1952. Monocular scopes, first fixed near the head of the patient, evolved to binocular scopes that attached to the operating room (OR) bed and later became freestanding floor mounts. The delayed application of the operating microscope in general surgery has been related to the technical deficiencies of the early microscopes, in that they were unstable, were immobile, and had limited illumination.

In 1952 Littman succeeded in developing a sophisticated, maneuverable microscope for surgical requirements that maintained sharp focus and had a co-axial light system. This prototype was known as the *OPMI 1* and drew the attention of otologic surgeons, ophthalmologic surgeons, and neurosurgeons. The operating microscope has made it possible for neurosurgeons to perform delicate, minimally invasive surgery in anatomic regions requiring magnification and illumination.

### Neuroendoscopy

Neuroendoscopy is a rapidly evolving field of minimally invasive surgery. The endoscope provides illumination and magnification of structures and an extended viewing angle. Brain retraction and manipulation are reduced in endoscopic surgery, resulting in decreased tissue damage.[22] The surgical team must be prepared to convert from a neuroendovascular procedure to an open procedure if it is determined that the surgery cannot be successfully completed endoscopically.

Indications for neuroendoscopic surgery are many. Endoscopic tumor removal or CSF diversion through endoscopic fenestration, such as a third ventriculostomy, can be done for the treatment of hydrocephalus and can eliminate the need for a shunt. Interventricular tumors may be removed endoscopically. In addition, the endoscope can be used to assess adequacy of tumor removal and to identify tumor portions left behind or adherent to vital structures. Stereotactic and image-guided surgery is often used with neuroendoscopy successfully. The endoscope is commonly used in the transsphenoidal approach for pituitary and sellar tumor resection (possibly in collaboration with an otolaryngology surgeon), for microvascular decompression, and for endoscopic biopsy of a lesion. The potential rewards of neuroendoscopy include improved postoperative results, shorter hospitalization times, and fewer postoperative complications.[22]

## Endovascular Procedures

Interventional neuroradiology uses fluoroscopy to insert a percutaneous transfemoral catheter into a vessel in the intracranial circulation that feeds an aneurysm, AVM, vascular occlusion, or tumor with significant blood supply. Embolization of the significant area is done to facilitate surgical resection of the lesion by minimizing potential hemorrhage. In situations where there is a planned sacrifice of a vessel during aneurysm or tumor surgery, a test occlusion may be done to verify that sacrifice of the vessel during surgery would not cause the patient to have a devastating stroke. Endovascular coiling is now considered the definitive treatment for some small neck aneurysms (instead of clipping) (Research Highlight). Endovascular treatment is curative for a small number of AVMs.

## Stereotactic Radiosurgery

In stereotactic radiosurgery, stereotactic localization is coupled with delivery of ionizing radiation to destroy a lesion in the brain. Radiosurgery is technically noninvasive and has a low associated morbidity. The use of radiosurgery has increased, and success of treatment has improved with advancements in neuroimaging (CT and MRI) and computer technology. The goal of radiosurgery is to obliterate a relatively small intracranial target with a high irradiation dose while sparing adjacent and distant tissues. Stereotactic imaging and target localization using CT, MRI, or angiography must be fully integrated with the radiation delivery device to achieve pinpoint localization of the target.[18] Radiosurgical instruments include the Gamma Knife, the Novalis, and the CyberKnife.

Radiosurgery can be used to treat AVMs, tumors, and trigeminal neuralgia. Best results are achieved for lesions smaller than 35 mm. Larger lesions or lesions involving or near cranial nerves can be successfully treated with a fractionated approach where the radiation is precisely delivered in small daily fractions. This technique, called fractionated stereotactic radiotherapy (FSR), has been particularly useful for preserving vision and hearing. Patients with larger lesions often have symptoms of mass effect that are generally not improved with radiosurgery. Radiosurgery and FSR techniques have successfully sterilized a variety of intracranial lesions often with far less morbidity than a surgical approach.

## Stereotactic Procedures

The goal of stereotactic surgery is to target a point or volume in space by way of a predefined minimally invasive trajectory.[24] This is accomplished with coordinate systems that provide a constant frame of reference. Radiographic modalities (CT, MRI) are used to navigate three dimensionally and locate and destroy target structures. Predetermined anatomic landmarks are used as guides.

Originally, special head-fixation devices were developed for stereotactic brain surgery (see Figure 23-38). Over the past decade frameless systems have surpassed frame-based techniques in popularity and versatility. These systems employ fiducial markers that either affix temporarily to the skin or are implanted into the outer table of the skull, thereby eliminating the need to mount a frame on the patient's head. These markers are visible on the imaging modality being used. By registering the physical location of the fiducials on the patient's skull, the corresponding points on the image can be aligned with the operating space.[24]

Both frame-based and frameless stereotactic systems use radiography, fluoroscopy, CT scans, or MRI to permit accurate placement of a probe directed at the target area. The preoperative images are aligned to the patient's head during surgery so that the surgeon has a better idea of what should be treated and what should be left alone.

The many common applications for cranial stereotactic surgery include craniotomies, transsphenoidal approaches, endoscopic surgery, needle biopsies, and therapeutic aspira-

## RESEARCH HIGHLIGHT

### Treatment of Intracranial Aneurysms with Coils

This study sought to determine the effectiveness of using endovascular coils as a method of treating intracranial aneurysms as an alternative to traditional craniotomy with clipping. In this method, a minimally invasive technique is used to deploy a platinum coil to the site of the aneurysm. The coil expands and blocks blood flow to the area, preventing rupture.

In this randomized, multicenter study, researchers enrolled 2143 patients with ruptured intracranial aneurysms and assigned 1070 to undergo neurosurgical clipping and 1083 to have endovascular treatment with platinum coils.

Researchers sought to determine which technique would result in a more favorable clinical outcome based on a modified Rankin scale score. The Rankin scale is a clinical assessment tool where 0 = no symptoms; 1 = no significant disability despite symptoms, able to carry out all usual duties and activities; 2 = slight disability, unable to carry out all previous activities but able to look after own affairs without assistance; 3 = moderate disability requiring some help but able to walk without assistance; 4 = moderately severe disability, unable to walk without assistance and unable to attend to own body needs without assistance; 5 = severe disability, bedridden, incontinent, and requiring constant nurse care and attention; and 6 = dead.

Clinical outcomes were assessed at 2 months and 1 year. Researchers considered a modified Rankin score of 3 to 6 as significant. They found that 23.7% of the patients in the endovascular group and 30.6% of the patients in the surgical group had either died or had a modified Rankin score between 3 and 6 in 1 year. Data also suggested that the long-term risks of further bleeding from the treated aneurysm are low with either therapy (2.4% for the endovascular group and 1% for the surgical group).

For patients with ruptured intracranial aneurysms, endovascular coiling produces better outcomes than surgery in terms of disability at 1 year.

Modified from Molyneux A and others: International subarachnoid aneurysm trial (ISAT) of neurosurgical clipping versus endovascular coiling in 2143 patients with ruptured intracranial aneurysms: a randomised trial, *Lancet* 360(9342):1267-1274, 2002.

tion. It is also used for catheter placement and third ventriculostomy surgery. Spinal stereotactic surgery is used for screw placement and spinal cord lesions. Common target areas for the stereotactic approach include tumors, infectious lesions, vascular malformations, the basal ganglia, the thalamus, and anterolateral spinal tracts. Target areas undergo biopsy or are destroyed by chemical or mechanical means or electrically stimulated to control intractable pain or to treat movement disorders. Stereotactic procedures are also done to place electrodes in various regions of the brain to determine the site of origin of seizures.

***Procedural Considerations.*** As in most image-guided surgery (IGS), carts with a monitor and the computer, along with accessory equipment and supplies, are required. A variety of stereotactic frame systems are on the market. The nurse must be familiar with the system in place at his or her institution. Frameless stereotactic surgery brought about a new era in surgical navigation and information delivery. This technology provides three-dimensional visualization of anatomic features with real-time localization information (see Figure 23-39).

*Operative Procedure*

1. The patient's head is placed into a halo head frame with a stereotactic cage before the surgery (framed stereotaxy). Alternatively, fiducials are placed on the patient's skull (frameless stereotaxy).
2. The patient is then taken for a CT or MRI scan of the brain. The target is identified, and computer coordinates are determined and recorded.
3. The patient is taken to the OR with the frame or fiducials left in place. The stereotactic coordinates are registered or entered into the computer, and the procedure is performed through a burr hole. The stereotactic probe is guided by the computer, directing the surgical approach and trajectory (see Figure 23-38).
4. Hollow cannulas, coagulating electrodes, cryosurgical probes, wire loops, and other lesion-producing or biopsy instruments may be introduced for the destruction of areas in the brain. Temporary and permanent nerve-stimulator electrodes are also introduced to augment the pain-control function of the CNS. These instruments are introduced through a burr hole in the skull.

## SURGICAL APPROACHES TO THE BRAIN

### Burr Holes

A burr hole is the minimum exposure that can be done to gain access to the brain. A small incision is made in the scalp down to the skull. A small self-retaining retractor is placed. The periosteum is retracted using a periosteal elevator. A drill is used to make the appropriate-size burr hole (usually 1 to 2 cm). If necessary, the burr hole can be enlarged using Kerrison rongeurs. The dura is incised, exposing the brain.

Burr holes are necessary for many neurosurgical procedures. They are placed in the skull to remove a localized fluid collection secondary to head trauma that results in an epidural or subdural hematoma. A burr hole is made to gain access to the intracerebral ventricles to place a ventricular catheter to drain obstructed CSF and to measure ICP or to place a ventricular shunting system. Burr holes are placed for many stereotactic procedures, such as stereotactic biopsy or placement of electrodes. Burr holes are also made before turning the bone flap in preparation for a craniotomy procedure.

### Craniotomy

A craniotomy is the removal of a section of the cranium referred to as a bone flap. One or more burr holes are placed, and the dura is dissected away from the cranium. A craniotome with a dura guard attachment is used to cut out a section of the cranium that is removed, exposing an area of the brain. The surgeon replaces the bone flap to its original location and secures it with wire or titanium plates and screws.

Multiple types of craniotomy incisions are used to expose different parts of the brain. Depending on the location of the pathologic condition, a craniotomy may be frontal, parietal, occipital, temporal, or a combination of two or more of these. The pterional craniotomy is an extremely versatile approach to the anterior and middle fossae. It is useful to access lesions of the frontal or temporal lobes near the sylvian fissure or skull base. A craniotomy may be performed to evacuate intracranial hematomas not accessible through a burr hole, to control bleeding, to debulk or resect tumors, to excise or clip vascular lesions, to aspirate abscess formation, and to decompress cranial nerves.

When turning a scalp flap for a craniotomy, the surgeon may peel the scalp back off the pericranium. The surgeon elevates the bone flap with the overlying muscles still attached (osteoplastic) or strips the periosteum off the skull before the bone flap (free flap) is turned. The bone plate may be separated from the soft tissues, removed from the skull, and set aside for replacement at the end of the procedure. It is placed in an antibiotic solution and remains on the sterile field. If the bone is not separated from the soft tissues, it is turned back with the temporal muscle and soft tissues. If intracranial swelling is a major concern or the purpose for the craniotomy, the bone plate may not be replaced. If it is not replaced, it may be frozen in a sterile container according to hospital protocol to be used at a future date.

### Craniectomy

Craniectomy is the permanent removal of a section of the cranium using burrs and rongeurs to enlarge one or more burr holes. The surgeon performs a craniectomy to gain access to the underlying structures. This procedure may be required to remove tumors, hematomas, and infection of the bone. A suboccipital craniectomy, done with the patient in prone or lateral position, allows access to the posterior fossa. Titanium mesh may be used to repair the cranial defect. Craniectomy is also indicated as treatment for craniosynostosis in infants and young children. Severe head injury with increased ICP can be treated with a craniectomy to give the brain room to swell.

### Transsphenoidal Approach

The transsphenoidal route to the pituitary fossa is a less invasive means of removing tumors than the transcranial route. This can be done with a small incision through the nose or through the gingiva under the upper lip. More recently, an endoscope has been used to assist with access through the sphenoid sinus into the pituitary fossa. Tumors of the parasellar region may also be approached using this technique.

## SURGERY OF THE BRAIN AND CRANIUM

### Evacuation of Epidural or Subdural Hematoma

After trauma, decompression of the brain, as well as removal and drainage of blood clots and collections of liquefied blood from above or beneath the dura mater, may be required. The need for hematoma evacuation is primarily determined by a declining neurologic status in the patient. Depending on the severity of the injury, evacuation can be accomplished through burr holes or a craniotomy. If ICP is a major concern, the craniotomy plate may be left off. This gives the brain more room to swell and may prevent brain herniation and death.

#### *Operative Procedure—Burr Hole Placement for Evacuation of Hematoma*

1. A preoperative CT scan is very useful in planning optimal placement of burr holes. At least two linear or small horseshoe incisions are made over the site of the lesion. Two or more burr holes are made.
2. If a blood clot or collection of bloody fluid is found outside or beneath the dura mater, the burr hole can be enlarged with a Kerrison rongeur until adequate exposure is obtained.
3. If the hematoma is subdural, the dura is incised.
4. Clot and fluid are evacuated, and hemostasis is accomplished with electrocoagulation or the use of hemostatic clips.
5. The brain is irrigated using catheters or bulb syringes. Large amounts of irrigating solution are used until the return appears clear.
6. A drain or catheter may be inserted in the subdural or epidural space for postoperative drainage. Additional burr holes can be made as necessary during the course of the procedure to ensure complete evacuation.

### Cranioplasty

Cranioplasty is performed for repair of a skull defect resulting from trauma, malformation, or a surgical procedure. The purpose of cranioplasty is to relieve headache and local tenderness or throbbing, to prevent secondary injury to the underlying brain, and for cosmetic effect.

***Procedural Considerations.*** Repair of a skull defect may be performed acutely in clean cases. In contaminated cases, 6 months should pass before repair is attempted.[5] When a bone plate is removed for control of elevated ICP, it can be repaired following resolution of ICP issues. If the patient's bone plate was frozen under sterile conditions, it could be replaced with microplates and screws.

The most common materials used for cranioplasty include titanium mesh and/or methyl methacrylate. Commercially prepared cranioplastic synthetics that supply the needed chemicals and mixing containers have simplified the procedures of shaping and molding the prosthesis. Sometimes heavy wire mesh is cut to the shape of the defect, and the methyl methacrylate is molded over the mesh.

Recent technologic advancements use CT scans to produce a computer-generated duplication of the defect. A properly sized prosthesis can be produced and sterilized before the surgery. After the defect is exposed, minor adjustments in the shape of the prosthesis can be made with a burr to achieve an optimal fit.

#### *Operative Procedure—Cranioplasty Using Computer-Generated Prosthesis*

1. Typically, the old incision is reopened.
2. Keeping in mind that there is no bony protection between the scalp and the brain, the scalp flap is carefully elevated from underlying scar, dura, and brain.
3. Bone edges are exposed with a curette, and the prosthesis is fitted to the defect using a burr. Debris is irrigated out of the wound.
4. Microplates and screws secure the prosthesis in place.
5. The incision is closed as usual for craniotomy.

#### *Operative Procedure—Cranioplasty Using Cranioplastic Material*

1. A scalp flap is turned, and the bony defect is exposed.
2. The edges of the defect are trimmed, and a ledge is formed to seat the prosthesis.
3. After the bone defect has been prepared so that it is slightly saucerized, the methyl methacrylate is mixed by combining one volume of liquid monomer with one volume of the powdered polymer. When this has formed a doughy mass, it is dropped into a sterile polyethylene bag. The soft plastic is then rolled on a flat surface into the desired shape, leaving the thickness to the approximate depth of the skull edges. A sterile test tube, syringe barrel, or other round object can be used, although a stainless steel roller is preferred because of its weight and ease of use.
4. The soft cranioplastic material in the bag is placed over the skull defect and, through light pressing with the ends of the fingers, is fitted into the missing skull area. Assistants stretch the plastic bag as the surgeon molds the plate into the defect and forms an overlapping bevel edge. This overlapping fringe keeps the plate from falling inside the skull, as the skull saucerization does.
5. When the heat of the chemical reactions begins, the plate is lifted out of the bony wound and removed from the polyethylene bag. Cool saline should be used on the flap while the exothermic reaction takes place.
6. When cool enough to handle, the excess material is trimmed away with bone rongeurs or cut with a saw and placed in the cranial defect.
7. A craniotome is used to smooth the rough spots and bevel the edges so that the plate will blend gradually with the skull.
8. Mixing and fitting the plate take about 7 minutes, as hardening does. Sutures may be used to hold the plate in place, generally at three or more points.

### Ventricular Catheter and Shunt Placement for Hydrocephalus

Hydrocephalus is a condition marked by an excessive accumulation of CSF resulting in dilation of the ventricular system (where CSF is made and circulated) and increased ICP. Conditions that result in the development of hydrocephalus and CSF obstruction in both children and adults include congenital hydrocephalus, spina bifida, tumors, intracranial/intraventricular hemorrhage, aqueductal stenosis, and Chiari malformations. Hydrocephalus is treated by accessing the lateral ventricles for the insertion of a ventricle shunting system. The most commonly used methods to divert CSF from the ventricles are the externalized ventriculostomy catheter and the internalized VP shunt.

Placement of an externalized ventriculostomy catheter requires that a burr hole be made to access either the right or left lateral ventricle. The ventricular catheter is passed into the ventricle. Flow of CSF is verified. The distal end of the catheter is tunneled beneath the scalp, posterior to the burr hole, externalized, and secured to the scalp with suture. The externalized end of the catheter is connected to an external drainage system, which allows for controlled CSF drainage and for ICP measurement. This system has allowed for temporary shunting in patients with elevated ICP and hydrocephalus from any cause. It is an invaluable adjunct in the clinical assessment and management of head trauma with increased ICP.

For more permanent control of hydrocephalus, an internalized ventricular shunt is placed. The type of shunt and the site of insertion are determined by the neurosurgeon. Three approaches for ventricular insertion are frontal, parietal, and occipital. Although the most common drainage site for an internalized shunting system is the peritoneum by way of open dissection or percutaneous trocar, there are other options. If drainage in the peritoneum is inappropriate because of infection or adhesions, other possible distal insertion sites include the right atrium, the pleural cavity, and the gallbladder.[23]

The VP shunt system comprises a ventricular (proximal) catheter, a reservoir, a valve, and a peritoneal (distal) catheter. A unitized shunt has fewer separations and connections. The reservoir, if used, is inserted between the catheter and the valve. Access to the system through the reservoir enables the practitioner to assess the patency of the shunt, to obtain CSF for laboratory analysis, to introduce contrast medium for radiologic studies, and in some specific cases to inject medication into the shunt. The one-way valve system directs flow of CSF out of the ventricular system. Valves come in a variety of different pressure and flow settings. Nonprogrammable valves and shunts are pressure controlled and open to release flow whenever the actual pressure exceeds the pressure that the valve is designed to open (the opening pressure). Some valves are flow controlled and attempt to maintain a constant flow despite pressure changes. A more recent advance is the programmable valve. Programmable valves and shunts allow adjustments to the opening pressure after the shunt is implanted, avoiding surgical procedures to change valves.

***Procedural Considerations—Ventriculoperitoneal Shunt Placement.*** The patient is positioned in a modified supine position using a shoulder roll. The head is turned to the opposite side and supported on a donut. Hair is removed from where the burr hole is to be placed, to behind the ear and down to the neck. The burr hole site must be prepped, along with the neck, chest, and abdomen on the side of the shunt insertion.

The unit should be handled with extreme care. As with all implantable devices, each manufacturer's specific instructions must be followed and care taken to keep the assembly free of lint, powder, or other foreign bodies that could cause a reaction in the patient's tissues. Lubricants are never used. Blood should be kept clear from the lumen of the catheter to prevent clotting and obstruction. The unit is soaked in normal saline and antibiotic solution and primed before implantation. Air trapping in the valve assembly should be avoided. The valve must be properly oriented to facilitate CSF flow from the ventricles to the peritoneum.

The surgeon may use an endoscope or stereotactic image-guided navigation system to locate small ventricles or to fenestrate the septum between ventricles, thus avoiding the necessity to place multiple ventricular catheters. Surgical technique for VP shunt placement is basically the same for adults and children (Figure 23-46).

#### *Operative Procedure—Ventriculoperitoneal Shunt Placement*

1. A horseshoe-shaped incision is made to the right or left of midline, along the papillary line. Skin and periosteum are elevated.
2. Scalp bleeding is controlled, and the skin flap is retracted.
3. A burr hole is placed, and the dura is coagulated and incised. The bipolar ESU is used to electrocoagulate the pia at the catheter insertion site.
4. The ventricular catheter with an introducer is inserted perpendicularly into the lateral ventricle approximately 4.5 cm in the infant and 6.5 cm in the adult. When the ventricle is penetrated, the introducer is removed, CSF flow is verified, and the reservoir and valve are attached and secured with 2-0 silk ties.
5. A subcutaneous tunnel is created from the burr hole to a neck incision, where the peritoneal catheter is then connected.
6. The abdominal incision is made subxiphoid or laterally. The peritoneum is exposed.
7. Further tunneling is performed from the neck to the chest and abdomen, avoiding the nipples and umbilicus. The catheter is passed through the tunneling device to the abdominal incision. After spontaneous distal flow of CSF is verified, the distal end of the peritoneal catheter is passed into the peritoneal cavity, leaving enough length to allow for growth in the child and movement in the adult.
8. The catheter is secured to the peritoneum with a purse-string suture. All incisions are closed, being careful not to puncture the shunt system with a suture needle.

Shunt failure can occur at any time, requiring any single portion of the shunt system or the entire system to be replaced. Obstruction, disconnection, malfunction, and infection are routine causes of shunt failure. Revising a shunt typically involves a troubleshooting process. Therefore it is best to prep and drape the patient to provide access to any and all portions of the shunt system. An infected shunt may be externalized until the infection is treated.

### Craniotomy

***Procedural Considerations.*** Craniotomy is a technique for exposure of the brain to surgically treat intracranial disease. There are multiple types of craniotomy incisions. A key element of these operative approaches is patient positioning, which facilitates exposure, allowing complex procedures to be done through small bony windows with limited dural opening and a minimum of cortex exposure. A skull fixation device provides head stability and allows for rotation, flexion, and extension in the final positioning of the head. If frameless stereotactic image-guided navigation is to be used, registration of fiducials must be done. Careful planning of the incision is imperative for adequate exposure. As a rule, flaps that create a vascular pedicle should be avoided and linear or sigmoid (S-shaped) flaps should be used. This is particularly true for patients with

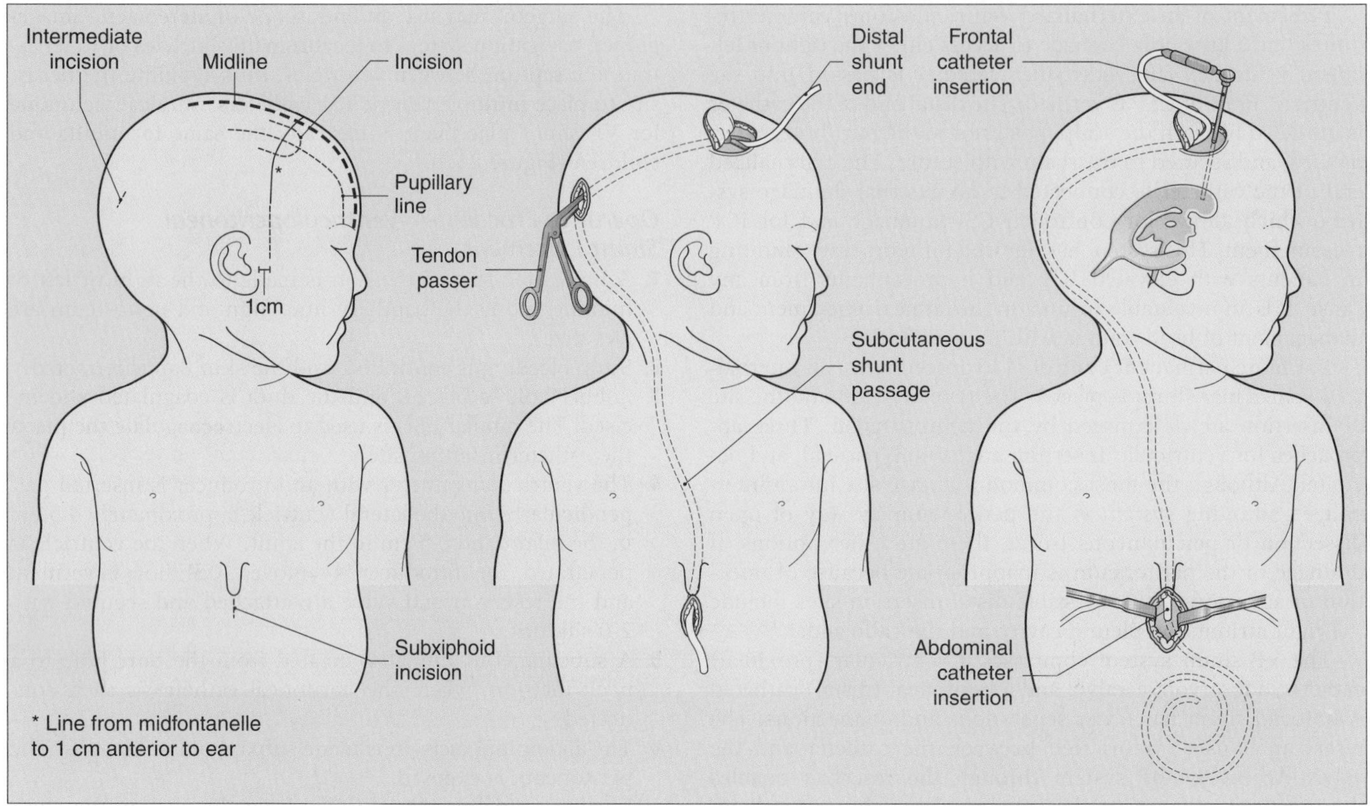


**FIGURE 23-46** Placement of a frontal ventriculoperitoneal (VP) shunt. The technique is similar for adult and pediatric patients. The patient is positioned, and coordinates are marked. The shunt is passed subcutaneously. The ventricular catheter and then the peritoneal catheter are inserted.

malignant brain tumors who will be treated with radiation, steroids, and chemotherapy. A pedicle flap compromises the blood supply to the incision and, with these other treatments, increases the likelihood of wound infection.

### *Operative Procedure—Craniotomy for Tumor Resection*

1. The incision site is infiltrated with local anesthesia with epinephrine.
2. Digital pressure is applied along skin edges as skin is incised through the galea.
3. Raney scalp clips are applied to skin edges, and/or self-retaining retractors are placed. Electrocoagulation of major scalp vessels is done to achieve adequate hemostasis of the scalp.
4. The scalp flap is reflected in the subperiosteal plane with periosteal elevators or with the monopolar device to divide muscle attachments. It is retracted up using devices that may include retractors, towel clips, suture, or rubber bands and supported with a scalp roll.
5. Burr holes are placed exposing the dura and widened using curettes and Kerrison rongeurs. The dura is dissected from the cranium using Woodson, Penfield, or Adson dissectors.
6. The craniotomy is accomplished using a craniotome with footplate attachment as the assistant irrigates to cool the bone. The bone flap is carefully elevated from the dura and placed in irrigating solution on the back table.
7. Bone dust is irrigated away from the wound, and hemostasis is established. Bleeding edges of bone are waxed, and bleeding vessels in the dura are coagulated with the bipolar ESU or occluded with thrombin-soaked gel foam and patties. Hemostatic agents and patties are placed around the craniotomy edges, and dural tacking sutures are placed (and remain permanently to prevent postoperative epidural hematoma formation).
8. After hemostasis is achieved, the dura is opened with a #11 or #15 blade. A dural suture may be placed in the dura before incising it. This tents the dura, ensuring that the surface of the brain is not inadvertently nicked. A Woodson dissector and blade or Metzenbaum scissors are used to extend the dural incision. Bleeding from transected dural vessels can be prevented by cauterizing them with the bipolar ESU before cutting them, or to avoid shrinking of the dura, hemoclips can be placed or vessels can be compressed with a hemostat.
9. A self-retaining retractor system is placed if necessary. Cortical dissection is achieved using the bipolar ESU, microscissors, and suction, and the specific surgical procedure is completed. Samples of tumor are sent for pathologic study if applicable.
10. Hemostasis is established. Irrigation can be used to find bleeding sites in the brain. A resection cavity is lined with Surgicel and filled with irrigation. Valsalva's maneuver can be produced with the ventilator to verify hemostasis.

11. The dura is closed with a 4-0 suture (braided nylon or silk). Gaps in the dura can be repaired using muscle, pericranium, dural substitute, or pericardium. A central dural tacking suture may be placed, and Gelfoam may be placed over the dura.
12. The bone plate is fitted with titanium plates and screws and reconnected to the cranium, or it may be wired into place depending on the surgeon's preference.
13. Muscle/fascia is reapproximated and galea is closed with interrupted absorbable sutures. Skin is closed with suture or staples.

### *Operative Procedure—Pterional Craniotomy*

1. The skin incision for the pterional craniotomy extends from the zygoma to the midline, curving gently just posterior to the hairline (Figure 23-47).
2. The surgeon and the assistant apply digital pressure over folded sponges on both sides of the incision line. The skin and galea are incised in segments, with the length of each segment being equal to that over which the finger pressure is applied. The tissue edges are held with 6-inch toothed forceps as scalp clips are placed on the flap edges. Any remaining active arterial bleeding is controlled by electrocoagulation. If the incision extends into the temporal area, bleeding in the temporal muscle is managed by electrocoagulation, hemostats, tamponade, or suture ligature. Mayo scissors can be used to incise temporal muscle and fascia.
3. The soft tissue is peeled off the periosteum by sharp or blunt dissection or by electrodissection. The scalp flap is turned back over folded sponges and retracted by use of small towel clamps and rubber bands or muscle hooks on rubber bands. In either case, the traction is maintained by securing the rubber band to the drapes with heavy forceps. The flap may be covered with a moist sponge or Telfa strips and a sterile towel. Bleeding is controlled by electrocoagulation (Figure 23-48).
4. When a free bone flap is planned, the muscle and periosteum are incised. Muscle and periosteum are elevated with the skin-galea flap, turned back, and retracted as a unit, as described previously.
5. The periosteum and muscle are incised with a scalpel or electrosurgical knife except at the inferior margins, which are left intact to preserve the blood supply to the bone flap. The periosteum is stripped from the bone at the incision line with a periosteal elevator. Bone wax is used to control bleeding.
6. The scalp edges and muscle are retracted from the bone incision line by a Sachs or Cushing retractor. Two or more burr holes are made (Figure 23-49). A great deal of heat is generated by the friction of the perforator or burr against the bone. The scrub person or assistant must irrigate the drilling site to counteract the heat and remove bone dust, which collects as the holes are made. A large-gauge suction tip is used to remove both irrigating solution and debris from the field. As the inner table is perforated and the dura exposed, tamponade of the burr hole may be done temporarily with bone wax or a cottonoid strip or patty. Each hole is eventually debrided by a #0 or #00 bone curette or small periosteal elevator. The dura mater is freed at the margins with a #3 Adson elevator, #3 Penfield dissector, or right-angle Frazier elevator or similar instrument. The hole is irrigated and suction applied simultaneously. Active bleeding points in the bone are identified, and bone wax is applied.
7. When all burr holes have been made, the dura mater is separated from the bone by a dural separator, such as the Sachs or a #3 Penfield dissector. Dural separation is done to prevent tearing of the dura mater, especially over venous

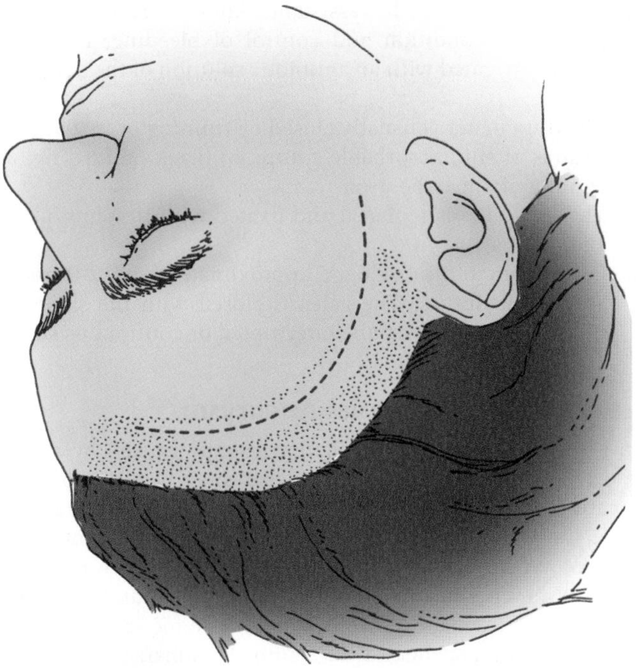

**FIGURE 23-47** The skin incision for a pterional craniotomy.

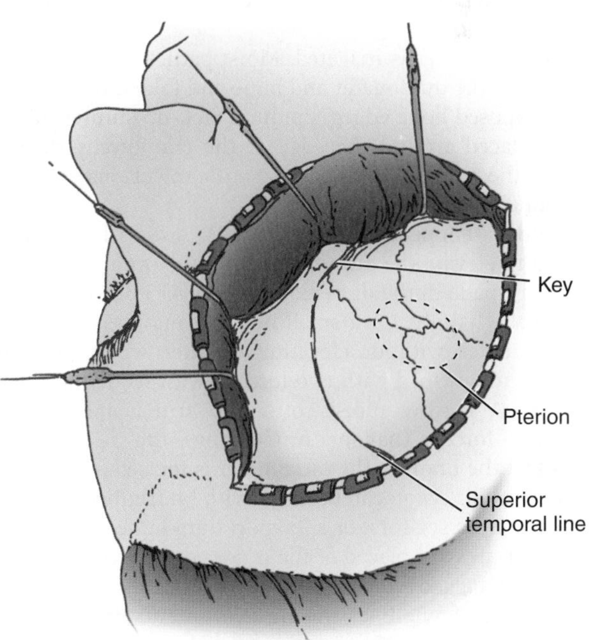


**FIGURE 23-48** A commonly employed means of opening the scalp involves incision of the skin, galea, temporalis fascia, and muscle with reflection of the resultant flap in a single layer.

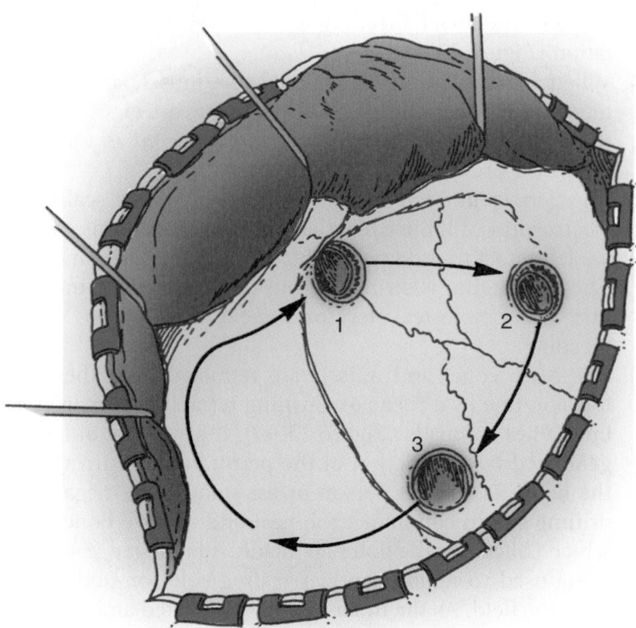


**FIGURE 23-49** The pterion craniotomy is performed with power instruments so that three burr holes are placed. The bone is cut as shown, exposing the frontal and temporal dura and the sphenoid ridge.

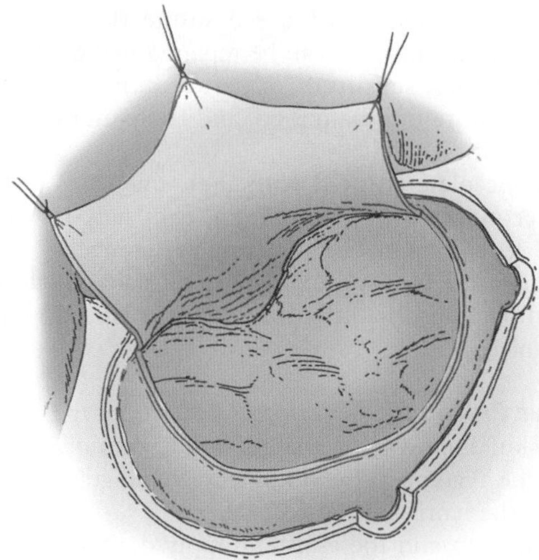

**FIGURE 23-50** The dura is opened and reflected back with stay sutures.

sinuses. An air craniotome or Midas Rex drill can be used for cutting the bone flap. Irrigation and suction are required as the bone flap is cut. Soft tissue edges are retracted with Sachs or Cushing retractors.

8. The bone flap with muscle attached is lifted off the dura mater by two periosteal elevators. Bleeding from the bone is controlled with bone wax. The bone flap is covered with a moist sponge, cottonoid material, or Telfa pads and then a clean sterile towel and is retracted in the same manner as the scalp flap.
9. The dura mater is irrigated. Moist patties may be inserted between the dura mater and bone and folded back to cover the exposed bone edges. Epidural tack-up sutures are usually placed around the edge of the craniotomy defect to close the epidural dead space. Sterile towels may be placed around the operative site.
10. The dura is opened (Figure 23-50). A dura hook may be used to elevate the dura mater from the brain, and a small nick is made in the dura mater with a #15 blade on a #3 or #7 knife handle. Or a small opening may be made in the dura mater without elevating it, after which the dural edges are grasped with two forceps with teeth and are elevated. A narrow, moist cottonoid strip is inserted with smooth forceps (bayonet or Cushing) into the opening to protect the brain as the dura mater is incised and elevated. The dural incision can be made with Metzenbaum scissors, special dura scissors, or a Rayport dura knife. Usually traction sutures are placed at the outer edge of the dura mater and are tagged with small bulldog clamps or mosquito hemostats. Sometimes the tag instruments are attached to the drapes to increase traction and keep tension on them. As the dural veins are approached during dural opening, they are ligated or coagulated before cutting. Ligation is done with hemostatic clips such as Weck hemoclips, McKenzie clips, or Ligaclips. The brain surface is protected by moist cottonoid strips.
11. The surgeon places cottonoid strips and brain retractors, self-retaining (Figure 23-51) and manual, appropriately while working toward visualizing the particular pathologic entity.
12. Brain spoons, Cushing pituitary spoons, Ray curettes as well as pituitary rongeurs, and the CUSA (Cavitron-Ultrasonic Surgical Aspirator) may be needed for tumor removal. Also, a selection of dissectors, Cushing and Gerald forceps, and a bipolar coagulation unit are used. Completely filled irrigating syringes and a full range of moist cottonoid patties and strips must be within easy reach of the surgeon and the assistant. After correction of the pathologic condition and control of bleeding, the brain may be irrigated with an antibiotic solution of the surgeon's choice.
13. The dura mater is usually closed by running or interrupted sutures of silk, absorbable suture, or black braided nylon. Dural grafts may be used.
14. The bone flap is replaced and fixated with titanium plates and screws.
15. Periosteum and muscle are approximated with 2-0 or 3-0 absorbable suture. The galea is closed with the same sutures. Skin closure can be interrupted or continuous suture or skin staples.

## Surgery for Intracranial Aneurysm

An aneurysm is a vascular dilation usually caused by a local defect in the arterial vascular wall, particularly at points of bifurcation (Best Practice). Vessels at risk within the brain involve those of the major circulation within and around the circle of Willis. Aneurysms are believed to arise from a complex set of circumstances involving a congenital anatomic predisposition enhanced by local and systemic factors. Aneurysmal rupture and hemorrhage into the subarachnoid space are frequently the first sign of an aneurysm, resulting in a sudden, severe headache described as "the worst headache ever." Current neurosurgical techniques have made operations on

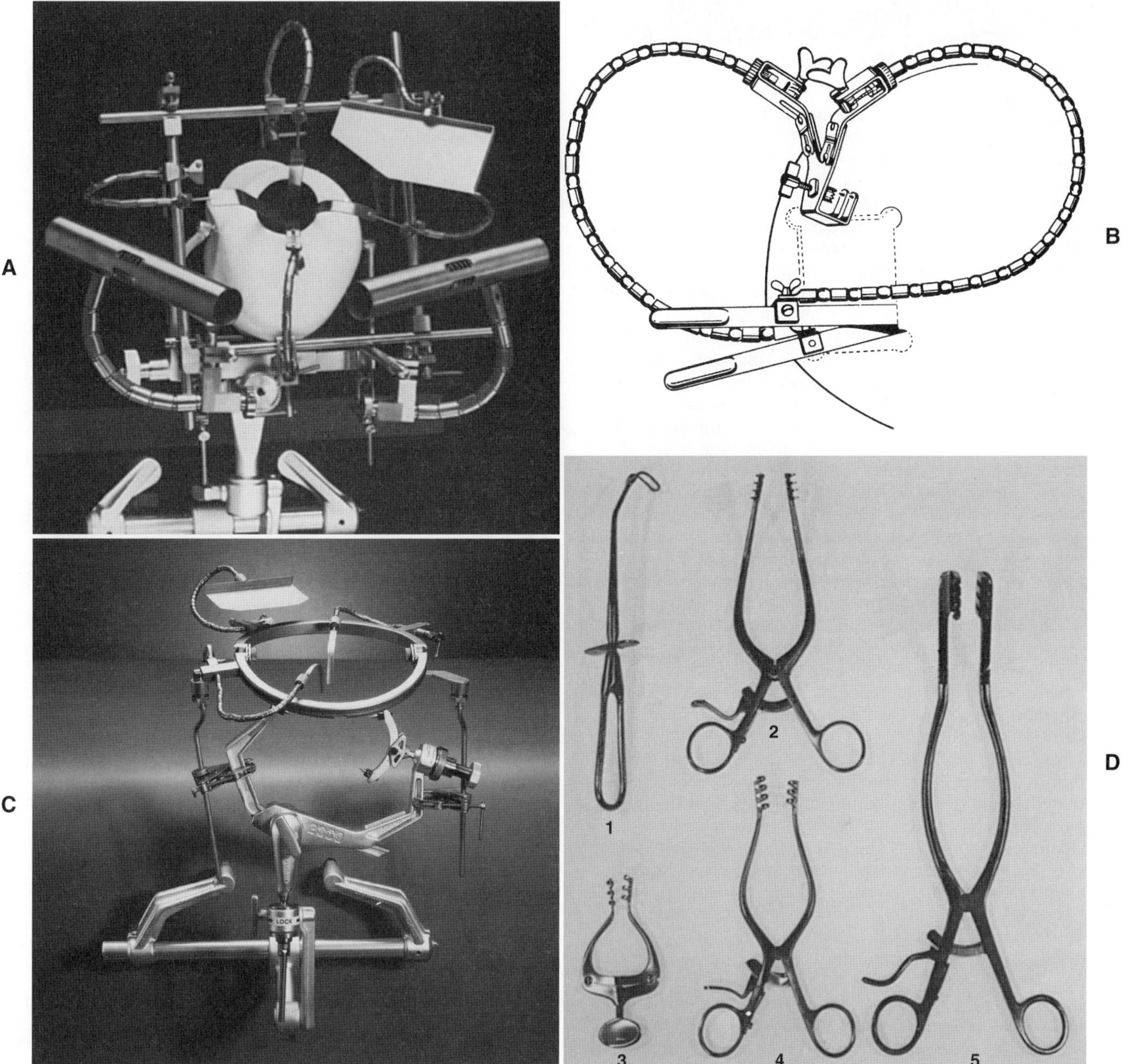


FIGURE 23-51 **A,** Greenberg retractor with blades. **B,** Leyla-Yasargil self-retaining retractor. **C,** Budde halo retractor with attachments. **D,** Retractors: *1,* Cushing subtemporal decompression retractor; *2,* Adson cerebellar retractor; *3,* Jansen mastoid retractor; *4,* Weitlaner retractor; *5,* Beckman laminectomy retractor.

intracranial aneurysms more feasible; however, fewer than 40% of patients with ruptured aneurysm will return to functional life and 30% die before reaching the hospital.[3a] Hemorrhage and the cascade of ensuing cerebral trauma are the greatest hazard of the condition and of the operation. To minimize this, control of blood pressure as well as vascular supply to the region beyond the limits of the lesion may be required. Occasionally, control of the cerebral circulation at the level of the cervical carotid artery is desired. The artery may be exposed and controlled by means of preplaced ligatures or clamps that can be tightened to occlude the vessel if bleeding occurs at the aneurysm site during the operation. This is a separate preliminary surgical procedure.

***Procedural Considerations.*** Aneurysm clips and appliers of the surgeon's choice must be included with the instrumentation. A variety of aneurysm clips are available, and most are spring loaded. Figure 23-45 illustrates a few of the clips and appliers available. Clips may be classified as temporary or permanent, and both must be available with a minimum of two appliers for each type of clip. Temporary clips are commonly used to control giant aneurysms where it may be necessary to

## BEST PRACTICE

### Management of Intracranial Aneurysms

The stroke council of the American Heart Association (AHA) has formulated recommendations for the management of unruptured intracranial aneurysms. These guidelines are intended to serve as a framework for the treatment of and future research on unruptured intracranial aneurysms.

The recommendations are summarized as follows:

- The treatment of small incidental intracavernous aneurysms is not generally indicated. For large symptomatic intracavernous aneurysms, treatment decisions should be individualized on the basis of the patient's age, the severity and progression of symptoms, and treatment alternatives. The higher risk of treatment and shorter life expectancy of older persons must be considered. Observation of older patients with asymptomatic aneurysms is recommended.
- Symptomatic intradural aneurysms of all sizes should be considered for treatment, with relative urgency for the treatment of acutely symptomatic aneurysms.
- Co-existing or remaining aneurysms of all sizes in patients with a history of subarachnoid hemorrhage caused by another treated aneurysm carry a higher risk for future hemorrhage than do similar-sized aneurysms in patients without a history of subarachnoid hemorrhage. In such cases, treatment should be considered. Aneurysms located at the basilar apex carry a relatively high risk of rupture. Treatment decisions must take into account the patient's age and medical and neurologic condition and the relative risks of surgical repair. Periodic computed tomography (CT), magnetic resonance angiography (MRA), or selective contrast angiography should be considered when surgical treatment is not undertaken.
- Treatment of incidental aneurysms measuring less than 10 mm in patients without a history of subarachnoid hemorrhage cannot generally be advocated because the risk of hemorrhage is low in such patients. However, special consideration for treatment should be given if such patients are young. Likewise, treatment should be a consideration for aneurysms that approach 10 mm in diameter, for aneurysms with daughter sac formation and other unique hemodynamic features, and for patients with a family history of aneurysms or aneurysmal subarachnoid hemorrhage. Periodic follow-up imaging should be a consideration if the decision is made to manage the patient conservatively.
- Asymptomatic aneurysms of 10 mm or larger in diameter warrant strong consideration for treatment, taking into account the patient's age and medical condition and the relative risks of treatment.

From Morey SS: Practice guidelines: AHA recommendations for the management of intracranial aneurysms, *American Family Physician* 63(12):2465-2466, 2001. Accessed March 29, 2006, on-line: www.aafp.org/afp/20010615/practice.html.

evacuate clot and debris before permanent occlusion can be accomplished (Figure 23-52). Temporary clips may also be used to establish the best position for the permanent clip. Temporary clips should be discarded after use. Permanent clips are used to occlude the neck of the aneurysm. Aneurysm clips should not be compressed between the fingers. Clips should be compressed only by the surgeon when seated in their appliers. Once a clip has been compressed, it should be discarded. Clips that have been compressed may be sprung and may slip, causing complications such as bleeding or compression of another vessel or a nerve.

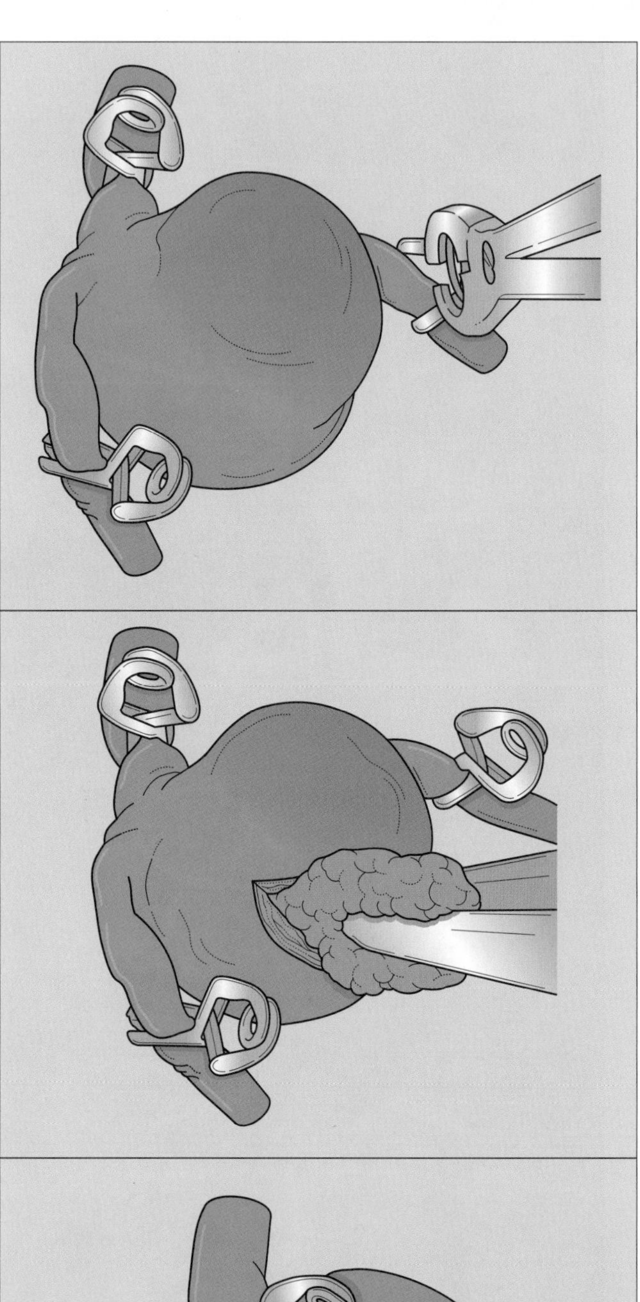


**FIGURE 23-52** Temporary arterial occlusion is often necessary in repairing complex large or giant aneurysms. **A,** Temporary clips are placed on the feeder vessels. **B,** The aneurysm sac is opened to allow evacuation of debris and thrombus. **C,** Permanent clip in place.

The full armamentarium of aneurysm-occlusion tools should be available for the surgeon. Besides clips, fast-setting aneuroplastic resinous material, a piece of temporal muscle, ligature carriers, or any other material requested by the surgeon should be in the room and ready to use. Fine silk ligatures and hemostatic clips, with or without bipolar electrocoagulation of the neck of the aneurysm, have also been used successfully.

A basic craniotomy setup is required in addition to the special items mentioned. Supplementary suction must be immediately available on the field to prevent hemorrhage from obscuring the surgeon's vision if the aneurysm dome ruptures during the operation. A blood salvage unit should be available for reprocessing of blood for replacement when significant blood loss is expected.

Interventional radiology now plays an important role in the management of intracranial aneurysms. Intravascular balloon occlusion and coiling of aneurysms by interventional radiologists are now considerations in the treatment of aneurysms that meet the criteria for endoscopic therapy. The coils, composed of a soft platinum alloy, allow conformability to the dome of the aneurysm. A guide catheter is introduced into the femoral artery under fluoroscopy and advanced from the aorta into the vessel specific to the aneurysm. Coils are first introduced to outline the border of the aneurysm, and then smaller coils are added to fill the center of the aneurysm. Gradually, blood flow will be reduced, allowing the aneurysm to thrombose.[7] Both the neurosurgeon and the radiologist work closely to diagnose and treat these life-threatening anomalies.

### *Operative Procedure—Craniotomy for Aneurysm Clipping*

1. A frontal, pterional, or bifrontal craniotomy may be done to approach an aneurysm in the area of the circle of Willis. The bifrontal approach requires extra scalp clips and hemostatic forceps. All aneurysm instruments preferred by the surgeon must be included.
2. After the dura mater has been opened, a self-retaining brain retractor is placed and the optic nerve and subarachnoid cisterns are exposed. The olfactory nerve may be coagulated and divided with a long scissors for better exposure.
3. The operating microscope is positioned. Microinstruments, including a micropolar bayonet, are used.
4. Bridging veins are coagulated with bipolar electrocoagulating forceps. Irrigation, which may be a part of the bipolar ESU, is necessary during bipolar electrocoagulation.
5. The covering arachnoidal webs are dissected away with microdissectors, hooks, elevators, scissors, knives, forceps, a diamond microknife, and an irrigating bipolar ESU.
6. Careful dissection of the arachnoid and clear visualization of the neck of the aneurysm without rupture of the dome are the aims of the surgeon.
7. The parent arteries are identified and freed so that they can be occluded with a temporary clip if necessary. Other structures, such as the optic chiasma and optic nerves, are identified.
8. As the surgeon works slowly toward the dome and neck of the aneurysm, the patient's blood pressure can be lowered for easier control of hemorrhage, should the aneurysm rupture. If the neck of the aneurysm can be isolated, a clip is placed across it. Clips such as the Sundt-Kees and Heifetz have Teflon linings and can be used to approach the aneurysm from a 180-degree angle to avoid excessive manipulation and traction of the parent vessel, if the neck is on the underside of the vessel. These clips support the vessel and serve as a clip graft.
9. Following clip placement, the surgeon may check the aneurysm sac by puncturing it with a needle to see if the clip pressure is adequate to stop blood flow to the aneurysm or to aspirate the aneurysmal contents.
10. As soon as the aneurysm has been occluded, the blood pressure is returned to normal and the aneurysm site is checked for bleeding. When the surgeon is satisfied that the operative field is dry, wound closure is begun.

## Surgery for Arteriovenous Malformation

An AVM consists of thin-walled vascular channels that connect arteries and veins without the usual intervening capillaries. These vascular lesions may be microscopic or massive. AVMs are rare, affecting only about 300,000 people in the United States.[11] Malformations vary widely in size, area of involvement, and structure. Arteriovenous fistulas may be congenital or may result from trauma or disease. Vascular anomalies may also give rise to subarachnoid or intracerebral hemorrhage or may have extensive irritative effects and cause focal or generalized seizures.

***Procedural Considerations.*** AVMs are difficult to treat successfully. Feeding vessels can be clipped with or without partial removal of the lesion. Total removal, when possible, gives best results. Microsurgical techniques have made total removal without devastating injury to surrounding brain tissue and vessels possible in many cases.

Other methods of treating these malformations include stereotactic radiosurgery with the Gamma Knife. Another method is preoperative embolization, which makes dissection much easier. Surgical glue, such as *N*-butyl cyanoacrylate and tantalum powder, is delivered by means of a catheter into the blood vessels before surgery. During the surgery, the glue is removed along with the AVM. Serial embolization may be performed to reduce the size of the AVM and provide symptom relief when the goal of treatment is not complete obliteration.[11]

### *Operative Procedure—Craniotomy for Arteriovenous Malformation*

1. A supratentorial or infratentorial craniotomy is done, depending on the location of the lesion.
2. The feeding arteries are exposed a distance from the malformation, traced toward it, and then occluded by clipping, electrocoagulation, ligation, or laser beam coagulation.
3. The malformation is dissected out with suction and bayonet forceps. Additional vessels are clipped or coagulated along the way. Usually one or more draining veins are left to be ligated as the last step in the removal. Closure and dressing are as described for craniotomy.

## Craniotomy for Suprasellar and Parasellar Tumors (Pituitary Tumor, Craniopharyngioma, Meningioma, Optic Glioma)

***Procedural Considerations.*** The preferred approach for pituitary tumors and some parasellar tumors is the less invasive transsphenoidal approach. However, for large and complex pituitary and parasellar tumors, a craniotomy may be indicated.

A craniotomy setup is used with these additional pituitary instruments: Ray curettes (ring, sharp); angulated suction tips, right and left; large and small spinal needles, #22 or #24; curettes, small, #0 through #4-0; and a Luer-Lok syringe, 10 ml.

### *Operative Procedure—Craniotomy for Pituitary Tumor Resection*

1. Either a bifrontal or a unilateral incision is made into the frontal or frontotemporal region. Most unilateral approaches are carried out from the right side.
2. Wet brain retractors over moist cottonoids are inserted for exposure of the optic chiasma and the pituitary gland. The frontal and often the temporal lobes are retracted. The olfactory nerve may be coagulated and divided with scissors.
3. A DeMartel, Yasargil, or Greenberg self-retaining retractor is placed to maintain exposure. Aneurysm clips and applicators should be available to control unexpected bleeding from major vessels. The microscope may be moved into place.
4. The tumor capsule is coagulated for hemostasis, incised with a #11 blade on a long knife handle, and removed with a pituitary rongeur or cup forceps.
5. Small stainless steel, copper, or Ray curettes, as well as suction, may be used during tumor removal.
6. A wide clip may be applied to the stalk of the pituitary, which may then be cut distally. A long angulated scissors is especially helpful for this.
7. If the tumor capsule is to be removed, bayonet forceps, cup forceps, nerve hooks, and suction aid in the dissection.
8. Closure and dressing are as described for craniotomy.

Extreme caution must be used in removing fluid from the capsule of a craniopharyngioma because the fluid is extremely irritating and may cause chemical leptomeningitis. Calcified pieces of tumor are dissected and removed in the same manner as the capsule of a pituitary adenoma. This is an extremely difficult procedure because of deposits on the carotid arteries, optic nerves, and optic chiasma. The tumor capsule is often left behind on the hypothalamus to avoid stripping off blood vessels supplying this structure. Many moist cottonoid strips are used to protect the surrounding areas from the cystic contents.

Suprasellar meningiomas usually arise from the tuberculum sellae just anterior to the optic nerves and chiasma. Tumor removal is similar to that of a pituitary adenoma except that the electrosurgical cutting loop may be used to excavate the interior of the tumor. After the tumor has been removed, the site of its attachment to the dura is thoroughly coagulated to prevent recurrence. Other meningiomas arising at the base of the skull are treated by similar techniques.

## Suboccipital Craniectomy for Posterior Fossa Exploration

The posterior occipital bone is perforated and removed using a drill and rongeurs, and the foramen magnum and arch of the atlas are exposed to remove a lesion in the posterior fossa (Figure 23-53). Posterior fossa lesions include lesions in the cerebellum, the fourth ventricle, and the brainstem; posterior fossa meningiomas; and nerve sheath tumors.

***Procedural Considerations.*** Depending on the type and size of the lesion, the exposure may be unilateral or bilateral. The operation may include the removal of the arch of the atlas. This approach gives the surgeon access to the fourth ventricle, the cerebellum, the brainstem, and the cranial nerves.

The prone position with the head of the OR bed elevated is the preferred position, but other positions may also be used. An extra-high instrument table or two Mayo stands and standing stool are necessary for the scrub person.

### *Operative Procedure*

1. Before the initial surgical incision, an occipital burr hole may be made for placement of a ventricular catheter. This can be done as a separate procedure or concurrently with the procedure.
2. The incision may be made from mastoid tip to mastoid tip, in an arch curving upward 2 cm above the external occipital protuberance. Alternatively, a posterior midline incision can be used.
3. Scalp bleeding is controlled, and the skin flap is retracted with the Weitlaner retractors.
4. A periosteal elevator is used to free the muscles, which are then divided with an electrosurgical blade. The incision is deepened. A self-retaining retractor is used. The laminae of the first two or three cervical vertebrae may be exposed.
5. One or more holes are drilled in the occipital bone. The Midas Rex or Anspach drill is used to perform the craniectomy.
6. The dura mater is stripped from the bone. A double-action rongeur, Raney punch, Kerrison punch, or Leksell rongeur is used to enlarge the hole and smooth the edges.
7. Osseous and cerebellar venous bleeding is controlled at each step with bone wax, Gelfoam, and electrocoagulation to prevent air embolism.
8. The dura mater is opened. A small brain spoon or cottonoid strip is used to protect the brain as the initial nick is extended with scalpel or scissors. The dural incision is continued until the cerebellar hemispheres, the vermis, and the cerebellar tonsils can be visualized. Hemostatic clips are used on the dura mater as necessary. Dural traction sutures are placed.
9. The cisterna magna is opened, emptied of spinal fluid, and protected with a cottonoid strip.
10. The cerebellar hemispheres are inspected. Bleeding is controlled with the bipolar coagulator. A needle may be introduced through a small, coagulated incision into the cerebellar hemisphere in an attempt to palpate or tap a deep lesion.
11. Brain retractors over cottonoid strips are placed for exposure. The handle of the retractor must be kept dry to avoid slippage in the surgeon's hand. However, the inserted edge should be wet to prevent damage or tears in the brain surface. These retractors may be positioned in areas that control respiration or other vital functions, so every effort must be made to avoid jarring these instruments in the operative field. When the pathologic entity is identified, a self-retaining retractor may be placed.
12. Long bayonet forceps, bayonet cup forceps, pituitary forceps, suction, and the electrosurgical loop tips may be used to remove the lesion. Clips may be used to aid in hemostasis. A nerve stimulator may be used to identify cranial nerves; EPs for brainstem monitoring are becoming routine practice.

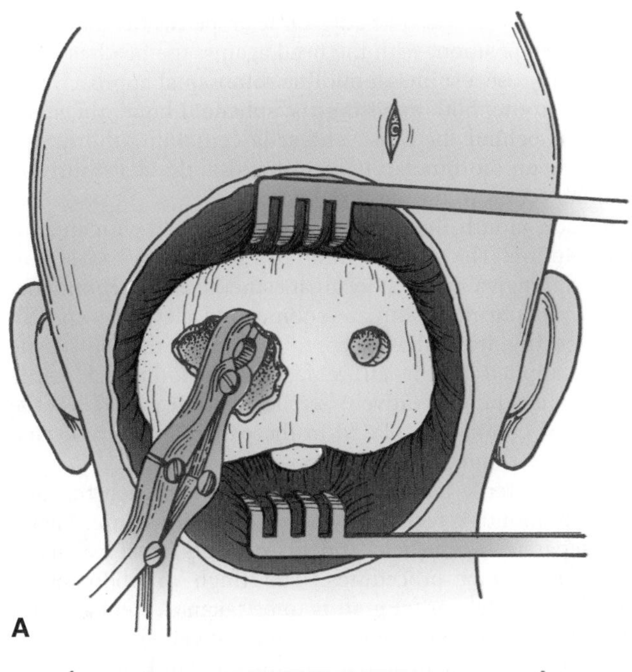


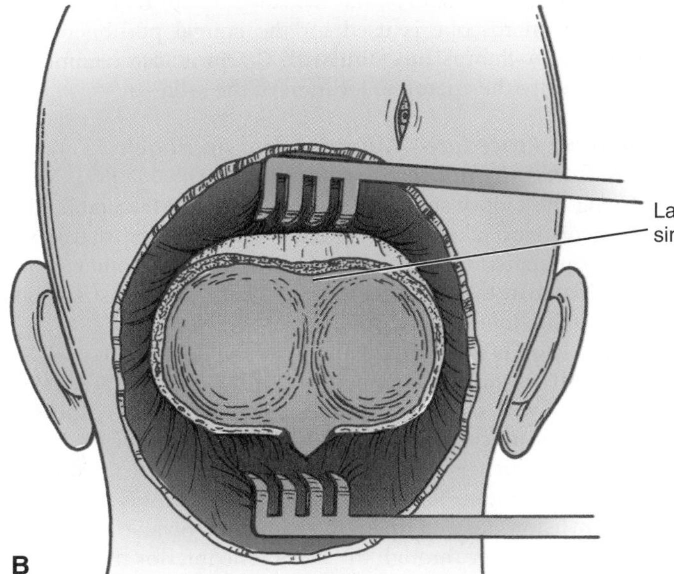


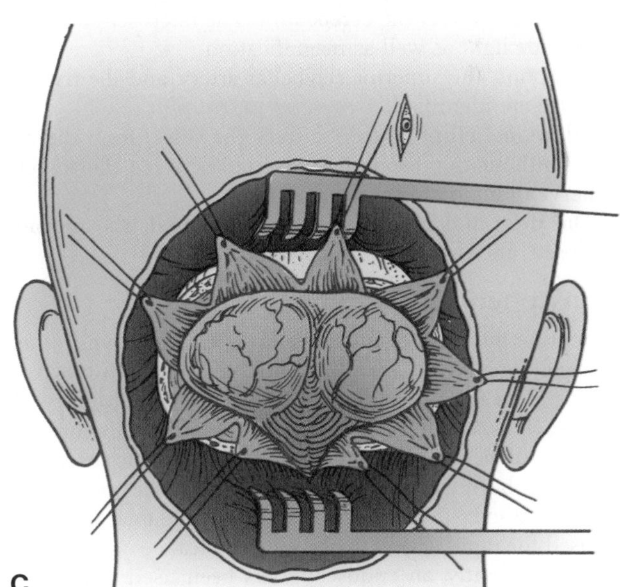


**FIGURE 23-53** Suboccipital craniectomy. **A,** Craniectomy being performed. **B,** Dura exposed. **C,** Dura incised and cerebellum exposed.

13. After the lesion has been removed and bleeding controlled, further checking for adequate hemostasis is required. Venous pressure in the patient's head is increased by the anesthesia provider by generating Valsalva's maneuver.
14. The dura mater may be partially or completely closed. The cranial defect may be repaired with titanium mesh. The muscle, fascia, and skin are closed. A dressing is applied.
15. The patient must remain anesthetized until the supine position is achieved and the prongs of the headrest are removed. Particular attention must be given to the patient's head when these prongs are removed to prevent tearing the scalp or damaging the eyes.

## Retromastoid Craniectomy for Microvascular Decompression of the Trigeminal Nerve

Trigeminal neuralgia (tic douloureux, fifth cranial nerve pain) is a condition characterized by brief, repeated attacks of excruciating, lancinating pain in the face. The etiology of this facial pain is believed to be the compression of the trigeminal nerve at its exit from the pons by an adjacent artery that has elongated over time to become wedged against the nerve, resulting in demyelination. Pain distribution follows one or all of the trigeminal nerve branches. It is characteristically severe, with sudden onset, short duration, and paroxysmal nature. Triggers often precipitate the pain, such as touching the face, chewing, and talking. When pharmacologic measures fail, surgery to decompress the nerve is undertaken. Frequently more than one treatment is necessary during the course of the disease. Newer options include Gamma Knife radiosurgery.

***Procedural Considerations.*** The patient may be placed in the supine, lateral, or sitting position, depending on the surgeon's preference. An endoscope can be used along with the microscope to improve visualization.

### *Operative Procedure*

1. A vertical retromastoid incision is made.
2. The soft tissue is freed from the bone with a periosteal elevator. The bone exposure is maintained with a self-retaining retractor.
3. A burr hole is made, and the dura mater is freed.
4. The burr hole is enlarged with a drill and rongeurs to a diameter of about 2½ inches.
5. With a moist brain retractor, the dura mater overlying the pons and cerebellum is retracted.
6. A self-retaining brain retractor is placed deeper into the wound to retract the cerebellum. The microscope is used to provide light as well as magnification.
7. The pons, the superior cerebellar artery, and the trigeminal nerve are identified.
8. Additional blunt dissection frees the vessel from the nerve. A synthetic microsponge is inserted between the vessel and nerve to maintain the separation.
9. The dura and cranial defect are repaired, the incision is closed, and dressings are applied.

## Transsphenoidal Hypophysectomy

Endocrine pituitary disorders, such as Cushing syndrome, acromegaly, malignant exophthalmos, and hypopituitarism resulting from intrasellar tumors, as well as nonpituitary disorders, such as advanced metastatic carcinoma of the breast and prostate, diabetic retinopathy, and uncontrollable severe diabetes, have been successfully treated by transsphenoidal hypophysectomy (TSH). A transnasal or a sublabial incision can be used for rapid access to the sella turcica.

More recently, an endoscope has been used to assist with access through the sphenoid sinus into the pituitary fossa. ENT (ear, nose, and throat) surgeons can be consulted to assist the neurosurgeon with this approach. The endoscope and instrumentation access the sphenoid sinus by the transnasal route. Endoscopic transsphenoidal surgery eliminates the need for an incision and the need for a microscope. When the sphenoid sinus is reached, instruments and technique are similar to the microsurgical technique. Stereotactic image-guided navigation can also be used with the transsphenoidal technique.

All these approaches produce similar results. Complete extracapsular enucleation of the pituitary in cases of hypophysectomy and possible complete removal of small pituitary tumors, with the remaining normal portion of the gland left intact, can be obtained. Patients are relatively free from pain after surgery. No visible scar remains.

***Procedural Considerations—Microsurgical Approach for Transsphenoidal Hypophysectomy.*** TSH is performed with the patient under general endotracheal anesthesia, combined with a local anesthetic. The surgical team places the patient in a semisitting position, with the head against the headrest. The surgeon may use a subnasal midline rhinoseptal approach or a transnasal route, both exposing the sphenoid bone, the sphenoid sinus behind the bone, and sella containing the tumor. Frequently, an otorhinolaryngologist assists the neurosurgeon in gaining access to the surgical site.

The face, mouth, and nasal cavity are prepped with an antiseptic solution. The surgeon infiltrates the patient's nasal mucosa and gingiva with a local anesthetic agent containing 1:2000 epinephrine to initiate submucosal elevation and diminish oozing from the mucosa. A sterile adhesive plastic drape is applied to the entire face, with additional sterile drapes to ensure a relatively sterile operative field. Sterile sponges (or cotton) are placed in the patient's mouth so that only the upper gum margin is exposed.

Although sterile technique is used, this approach through the nose or mouth is technically not a sterile procedure. Therefore a separate sterile field and instruments must be maintained for adjunct procedures. The thigh or abdomen is prepped if a muscle or fat graft is to be taken. A lumbar drain may be placed preoperatively or postoperatively.

Specialized transsphenoidal instruments are required. The operating microscope is used for the cranial portion of the procedure. A fluoroscopy unit with C-arm is also commonly used to verify the anatomic location of the sella.

### *Operative Procedure—Microsurgical Approach for a Transsphenoidal Hypophysectomy*

1. Using the biopsy setup on a separate small Mayo table, the surgeon may take a small piece of muscle from the previously prepared thigh or a fat graft from the abdomen to be used later in the procedure. This is kept in a moist sponge or soaking in antibiotic solution.
2. An incision is made in the middle of the upper gum margin. The soft tissues of the upper lip and nose are elevated from the bone with an elevator, and the nasal septum is exposed. The nasal mucosa is elevated from either side of the nasal septum, which is flanked by the blades of a Cushing bivalved speculum. The transnasal approach avoids the sublabial incision, instead operating through a bivalve speculum inserted directly through the nares. The inferior third of the anterior cartilaginous septum and osseous vomer are resected, as is the floor of the sphenoidal sinus, exposing the sinus cavity. The floor of the sella turcica can then be identified.
3. The floor is opened with a sphenoidal punch, and the dura mater is incised. The hypophyseal cavity should be opened only in patients undergoing surgery for pituitary adenoma. In these patients, the gland is explored and the tumor is identified and removed.
4. The extracapsular cleavage plane is identified, and the superior surface of the pituitary is dissected until the stalk and the diaphragmatic orifice are found. Cotton pledgets are applied for exposure, hemostasis, and protection of structures.
5. The stalk is sectioned low with a sickle knife, and the lateral posterior and inferior surfaces of the pituitary are dissected with an enucleator.
6. The gland is removed, and the sellar cavity may be packed to prevent CSF leakage. The packing is accomplished with

muscle obtained previously from the thigh or with the fat graft previously obtained from the abdomen or thigh. The floor is reconstructed with cartilage from the nasal septum.

7. Antibiotic powder may be used and nasal packing introduced for 2 days. If a gingiva incision is used, it is closed with suture of the surgeon's preference.
8. Some surgeons prefer to perform this operation by means of a lateral rhinotomy with a transantral-transsphenoidal approach.

## SURGERY OF THE SPINE

Surgery of the spinal column is also discussed in Chapter 22, "Orthopedic Surgery."

### Anterior Cervical Decompression and Fusion

Anterior cervical decompression and fusion (ACDF) are performed to treat cervical disk herniation or cervical spondylosis (degeneration in the spine) with myelopathy (disorder of the spinal cord) or radiculopathy (disorder of the nerve roots). Symptoms include pain in the neck, shoulders, arms, and hands; and upper extremity weakness. An ACDF entails a corpectomy (removal of a vertebral body), diskectomy, and fusion of the vertebral bodies. Bone grafts for the fusion are obtained from the patient's iliac crest (autograft) or from a bone bank (allograft).

***Procedural Considerations.*** Intraoperative fluoroscopy may be employed to confirm the correct surgical site and verify placement of the graft and related hardware. The nurse coordinates the availability of the fluoroscopy equipment and radiology personnel before bringing the patient to the OR.

Awake endoscopic intubation may be required if the patient's neck is unstable or unable to extend. Neurologic monitoring is commonly employed to prevent further injury during surgery. The patient is placed in the supine position, with a small shoulder roll placed horizontally for mild neck extension. The perioperative nurse ensures the patient's arms are tucked, and the hip is elevated for exposure if bone graft is to be taken from the iliac crest (Figure 23-54).

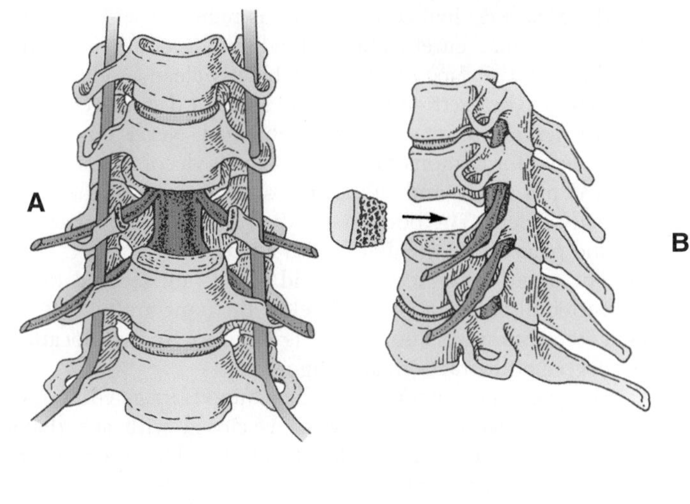


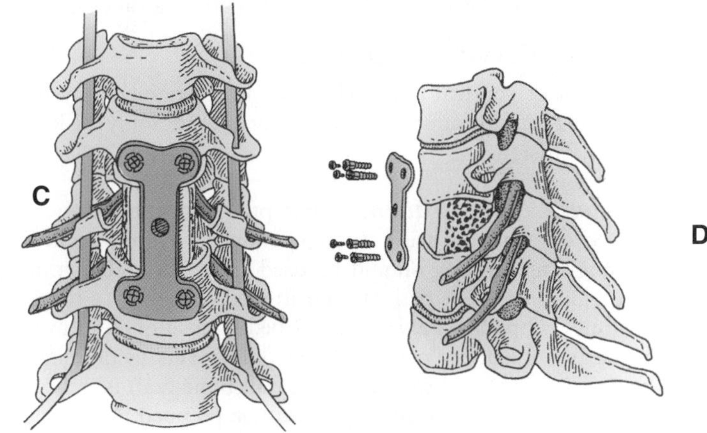


FIGURE 23-54 Anterior cervical decompression and fusion. **A** and **B,** A bone graft from the iliac crest or fashioned from bank bone is tailored to fit the site of corpectomy, resting on the vertebral end plates. **C** and **D,** An anterior spinal plate and screws are secured to the vertebral bodies above and below the spanned segment to stabilize and promote a stable fusion.

#### *Operative Procedure*

1. The surgeon may harvest the iliac crest bone graft before the neck procedure begins, or it may be completed after exposure of the anterior cervical spine. An incision is made over the iliac crest, at least 3 cm posterior to the anterior superior iliac spine. The skin and subcutaneous tissues are retracted with a Weitlaner.
2. Soft tissue is dissected until the crest is reached and exposed.
3. An osteotome or oscillating saw is used to remove the bone graft. The graft is soaked in antibiotic solution and put aside. A separate sponge and sharp count should be initiated for this portion of the procedure. Following verification of a correct count, the wound is irrigated, closed, and covered with a sterile towel.
4. A transverse skin incision is made on one side of the neck, directly over the involved cervical level.
5. A Weitlaner retractor is placed, and the platysma muscle is divided with Metzenbaum scissors and tissue forceps or with the Bovie.
6. The medial edge of the sternocleidomastoid muscle is defined with the scissors by blunt and sharp dissection.
7. A vertical plane of dissection between the carotid artery laterally and the trachea and esophagus medially is created by blunt finger dissection. This plane is held open with retractors.
8. The anterior surface of the spine is identified, and the long muscles of the neck are peeled off the anterior surface of the spine with periosteal elevators or peanut dissectors. Bleeders are coagulated with bipolar forceps.
9. A 20-gauge spinal needle is inserted a short distance into the disk space, and the location is confirmed radiographically.
10. Self-retaining retractors are inserted into the neck incision. Care is used to protect the carotid artery and the esophagus. A combination of sharp and dull blades is used to acquire the best retraction. If a toothed blade is used, the teeth are carefully hooked beneath the long muscle of the neck.
11. A #15 or #11 blade on a #7 knife handle is used to cut into the disk space; a pituitary rongeur is used to remove the disk material, which is saved as a specimen. A vertebral spreader may be inserted into the vertebral space to widen

the area. Residual disk material is removed with the rongeur or small curettes (angled or straight, #0 to #4-0) until the entire surface of both vertebrae is clean. A small burr may also be used until complete anterior decompression of the nerve root or dural sac is obtained. Nerve hooks may be used for demonstration of adequate decompression.
12. A depth gauge and caliper measure the size of the interbody defect. The bone graft is cut to the appropriate size and placed into the defect with a tamp and a mallet.
13. The anterior cervical plate and screws are secured to the vertebral bodies above and below the bone graft.
14. Lateral x-ray or fluoroscopy is done to confirm location, degree of distraction, and alignment.
15. Hemostasis is obtained, and the wound is irrigated. A drain may be placed. The platysma is closed with absorbable suture. A subcuticular closure of the skin is done, and Steri-strips are applied.
16. A cervical collar is placed before the patient awakens.

## Posterior Cervical Approach

The posterior cervical approach is used for laminectomy for decompression, intradural tumor removal, cordotomy, diskectomy, and fusion.[5]

***Procedural Considerations.*** Fiberoptic intubation may be required on a patient with severe spondylosis. Intraoperative neurologic monitoring should be used to detect a change in neurologic status. The patient is positioned prone with a three-pin skull clamp (Mayfield). The OR bed is positioned in mild reverse Trendelenburg position to encourage venous drainage. The patient's arms are tucked. If allograft bone graft is desired for fusion, the posterior iliac spine will be prepped. A cervical collar may be required postoperatively.

### *Operative Procedure*

1. The cervical spinous processes are palpated to plan the incision, and a midline incision is made.
2. Soft tissue dissection is done, and a clamp is placed on the spinous process to verify the correct level with x-ray.
3. Self-retaining retractors help to gain exposure. A subperiosteal dissection is made to the lateral margins of the involved facets using the Bovie, suction, and cervical Cobb elevator.
4. Hemostasis is maintained with bipolar electrocoagulation, Gelfoam, and patties.
5. A laminectomy is performed using a drill, Leksell rongeurs, curettes, a nerve hook, and Kerrison punch rongeurs.
6. Disk is removed with pituitary rongeurs and curettes.
7. If a fusion is required, instrumentation and allograft or autograft may be needed.
8. The wound is irrigated. A drain may be placed.
9. Bupivacaine (Marcaine) may be injected into the paraspinal muscles and subcutaneous tissue for postoperative pain.
10. Absorbable sutures are used to close the fascia and subcutaneous layers. Suture or staples are used for the skin.

## Anterior Thoracic Approach

A transthoracic thalamotomy is done to access the spine for a thoracic diskectomy, burst fracture, osteomyelitis, and metastatic disease.[5] Usually a thoracic surgeon assists the neurosurgeon in obtaining adequate exposure.

***Procedural Considerations.*** The anesthesiologist may need to place a double-lumen endotracheal tube to allow for deflation of the lung for exposure of the higher thoracic levels. Lateral position with a bean bag is preferred. If intraoperative fluoroscopy is necessary, a Jackson table is needed. A bean bag interferes with fluoroscopy. For T1 to T4, a right-sided approach is preferred to avoid the aortic arch and heart. For T5 to T12, a left-sided approach is preferred because the aorta is safer to manipulate than the vena cava.[5] If allograft is desired for fusion, prep the iliac spine.

At times, an anterior thoracic surgery is performed in combination with a posterior thoracic surgery. In this case, the patient is repositioned prone after the completion of the anterior portion of the surgery. The posterior surgical site is prepped and draped, and the posterior portion of the surgery is completed.

### *Operative Procedure*

1. A thoracotomy incision is made, and the latissimus dorsi and other muscles are transected. A rib may be resected with a rib cutter to gain exposure.
2. The parietal pleura is opened, and a thoracotomy retractor is placed. If necessary, the lung is deflated manually.
3. A localization x-ray is done to verify the correct level. The parietal pleura is incised further onto the vertebral body and cleared with blunt dissection. Segmental vessels are ligated as necessary with hemoclips and transected to mobilize the aorta.
4. For diskectomy or decompression, a drill, rongeurs, and curettes may be needed. For spinal fusion, instrumentation and autograft or allograft may be used.
5. The wound is irrigated, and a chest tube is placed. The ribs are reapproximated with a rib approximator and sutured with heavy absorbable suture.
6. The fascia and subcuticular layers are closed.

## Laminectomy

Laminectomy is removal of one or more of the vertebral laminae to expose the spinal canal. Laminectomy, hemilaminectomy, and the interlaminar approach are performed to reach the spinal canal and its adjacent structures to treat compression fracture, dislocation, herniated nucleus pulposus, and cord tumor, as well as for spinal cord stimulation. Section of the spinal nerves, including cordotomy and rhizotomy, requires similar surgical exposure.

***Procedural Considerations.*** Laminectomy is done with the patient in the prone or lateral position. It is performed on the cervical, thoracic, or lumbar spine. Laminectomy instruments include the basic neurosurgical set, the retractor of the surgeon's choice, and an assortment of specialty rongeurs.

### *Operative Procedure—Laminectomy for Spinal Stenosis*

1. A midline vertical incision is made at the operative site.
2. Two self-retaining retractors (Cone, Weitlaner, or Beckman-Adson) are inserted for exposure.
3. The fascia is incised in the midline with Mayo scissors, electrosurgical cutting tip, or a scalpel.
4. Both sides of the spinous processes are exposed by sharp dissection.
5. Correct surgical level is verified by lateral spine x-ray film.

6. The paraspinous muscles and periosteum are stripped off the laminae with sharp periosteal elevators. Dissection with the ESU may be used.
7. As each area is stripped, a gauze sponge is packed around the bony structures with a periosteal elevator to aid in further blunt dissection of muscles from the laminae and to tamponade bleeding.
8. A laminectomy retractor is then placed. A Scoville (with a blade on the tissue side and a slightly shorter hook on the bone side), Tower, Crank, or Adson-Beckman retractor can be used.
9. Cottonoid strips or patties may be placed in the extremes of the field for hemostasis.
10. The spinous processes over the involved area are removed. The bone edges are waxed.
11. The ligamentum flavum is cut with a scalpel, Metzenbaum scissors, or a rongeur. Cottonoid strips or patties are passed through this incision to protect the underlying dura, and a window is cut into the flaval ligament with a #15 blade on a #7 knife handle.
12. Additional ligaments in the lateral gutter of the spinal canal may be removed with a large curette or a Cloward after first protecting the dural sac.
13. Bleeding from the epidural veins is controlled by packing with narrow cottonoid strips and if necessary by careful coagulation with a bipolar bayonet forceps.
14. Various rongeurs are used to remove the laminae after edges are defined with a curette. Bone drills are commonly used to reduce bone down to epidural fat, saving time and wear on the surgeon's hands.
15. Rongeurs—straight and angled, narrow and wide—are used to remove further bony areas until the cord with its dural covering is exposed and decompressed.
16. The nerve roots and extradural space are explored with a blunt nerve hook.
17. If no further stenosis is felt, hemostasis is secured.
18. The cottonoid strips are removed from the epidural space, and the area is further irrigated. All cottonoid strips and patties and retractors are removed, and the wound is closed.

### *Operative Procedure—Laminectomy for Intradural Spinal Cord Tumor*

1. The fascial incision is made in the midline, both sides of the spinous processes are dissected out, and the paraspinous muscles are taken down bilaterally, one side at a time. The level is confirmed with x-ray.
2. One or more Gelpi or Adson-Beckman self-retaining retractors are placed to maintain the bony exposure.
3. A midline laminectomy is performed, and the spinous processes are excised. Various rongeurs (e.g., Leksell, double-action, Cloward) are used to remove the laminae after the edges are defined with a curette. The Midas Rex drill may also be used. The bone edges are waxed for bleeding.
4. The remaining flaval ligament is removed with scissors, scalpel, and Kerrison or Cloward rongeurs. Epidural fat is removed so that the dura mater is fully exposed.
5. A wide, moist cottonoid strip is placed over the superficial soft tissues and muscle down to the bone bordering the exposed dura mater. This provides additional hemostasis.
6. Intraoperative ultrasound may be employed to verify the exact location of the tumor beneath the dura.
7. The dura mater is elevated with a small hook and nicked with a #15 blade. A grooved director is inserted beneath the dura mater, and the dural incision is extended over it using long forceps and fine scissors. Alternatively, the surgeon may lengthen the incision with Metzenbaum scissors. Traction sutures of 4-0 silk or braided nylon on dura needles are placed in the dural edges, and the cord is exposed (Figure 23-55). The operating microscope may be used
8. The cord is explored for the pathologic area. Aspiration through a #22 needle on a plain-tipped syringe may be carried out. Whenever possible, the tumor mass is dissected free and removed using suction, the dissecting scissors, the bipolar forceps, small (pituitary) scoops, curettes, pituitary rongeurs, or an ultrasonic aspirator. Bleeding is controlled

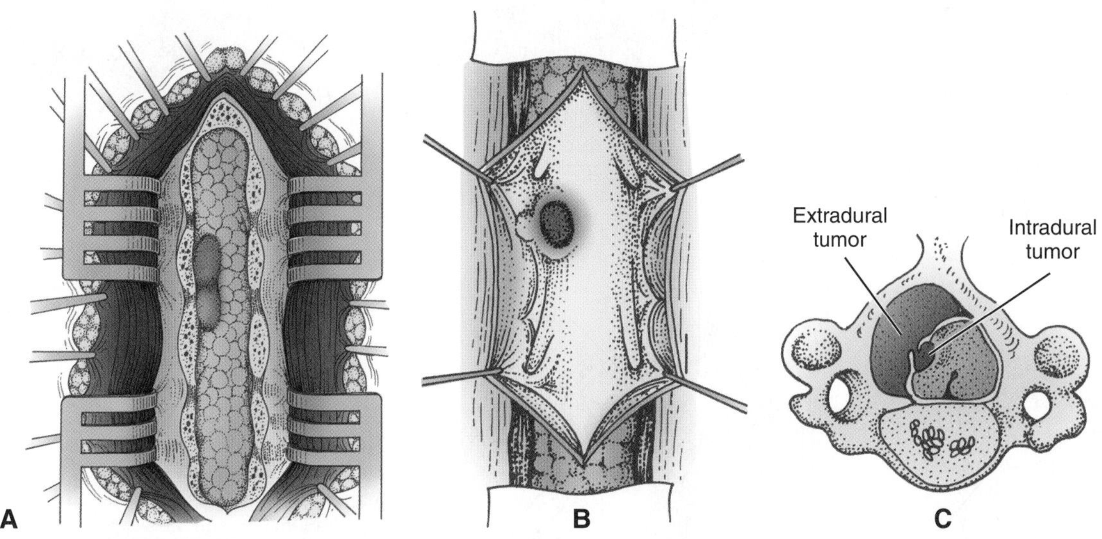


FIGURE 23-55 **A,** Laminectomy completed: dura mater and tumor exposed. **B,** Dura mater incised and retracted, revealing pia arachnoid over spinal cord and part of tumor. **C,** Diagram of cross section of tumor site and location of extradural and intradural pathologic areas.

with moist cottonoids, hemostatic clips, gelatin gauze, and topical hemostatics. Bipolar electrocoagulation is used around the nerves and spinal cord.

9. The wound is irrigated and hemostasis is obtained, being careful to protect the spinal cord.
10. The dura mater is closed with a braided nylon or polytetrafluoroethylene (PTFE) suture.
11. The incision is checked for further bleeding, and the paraspinous muscles are approximated with absorbable suture. The remainder of the wound is closed.

In the case of extradural tumors, invasion of the dura is avoided. Once the dura is opened from a tear or an incision, the neurosurgeon may require that the patient remain flat for 24 hours or longer to allow healing of the dura.

## Laminotomy

Laminotomy is the traditional approach to posterior microdiskectomy at the cervical, thoracic, and lumbar levels. Laminotomy is performed on the symptomatic side with resection of a small portion of the medial facet. The goal of this surgery is the resolution of leg pain with little to no residual back pain and a return to preinjury activity and life-style. In the twenty-first century, patients with herniated lumbar disks will continue to have a range of minimally invasive surgical options, many of which will be performed on an outpatient basis. Some of these newer procedures include nucleoplasty (decompression of a contained herniated disk by ablating and coagulating part of the nucleus), intradiskal electrothermal therapy (IDET), and selective endoscopic diskectomy.[10] Disk replacement is discussed in Chapter 22.

***Procedural Considerations.*** The operating microscope has improved this surgical approach by offering magnification and illumination, which allows for smaller incisions and less tissue dissection. This surgical procedure is associated with less postoperative discomfort and shorter hospital stays. The majority of patients who undergo this procedure can be discharged home on the same day (Figure 23-56).

### *Operative Procedure—Lumbar Laminotomy and Microdiskectomy*

1. With the patient in prone position or modified knee-chest position, a midline skin incision is made, extending from the spinous process above the involved level to the spinous process below. The correct surgical level is confirmed radiographically.
2. Dissection is carried down through the subcutaneous tissue to fascia, which is incised through a paramedian incision on the symptomatic side.
3. Paravertebral muscles are then dissected off the spinous processes and lamina.
4. A self-retaining retractor is placed to provide a visual field.
5. The hemilaminotomy, with a small portion of the medial facet removed, is performed.
6. The ligamentum flavum is incised longitudinally and removed with curettes or rongeurs, exposing the thecal sac.
7. A foraminotomy is then performed to expose and decompress the nerve root.
8. The epidural space is explored with a blunt dissector, nerve hook, dental tool, or Penfield #4.

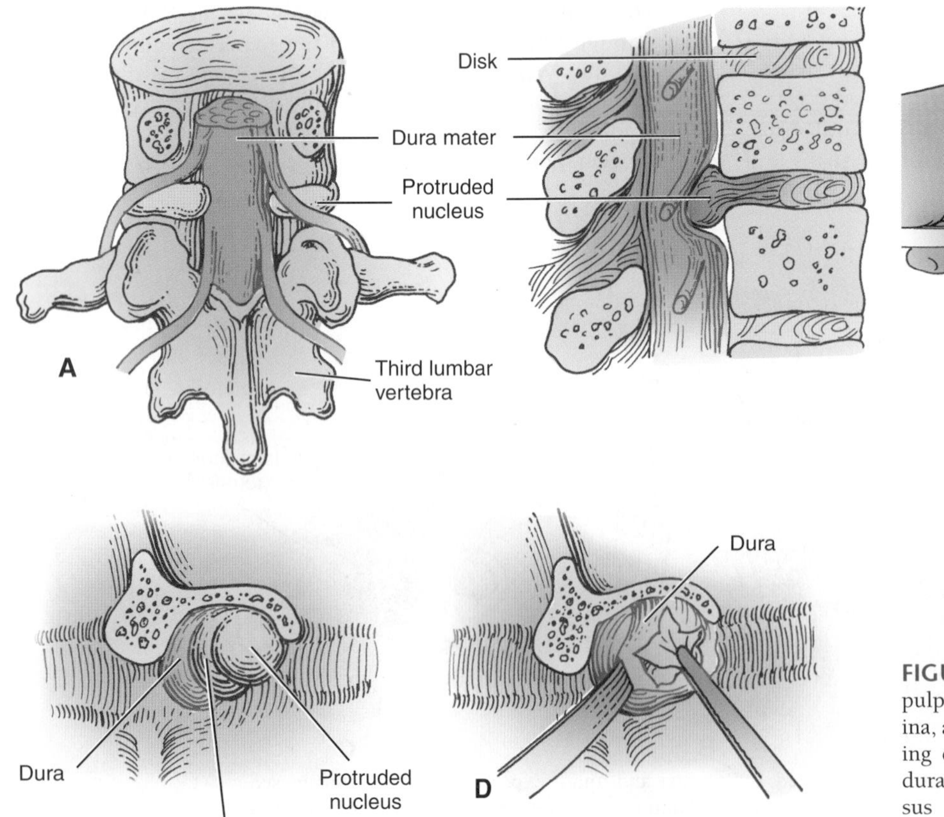


FIGURE 23-56 **A,** Normal and herniated nucleus pulposus (disk). **B,** Window has been made in lamina, and ligament has been incised to expose underlying dura mater and nerve root. **C,** Relationship of dura mater, nerve root, and protruded nucleus pulposus (disk). **D,** Retraction of nerve root over dura mater and removal of disk.

9. The root is then gently retracted medially, exposing the disk bulge or herniation.
10. A window is made in the disk annulus with a #15 blade, and the disk space is entered.
11. Curettes and disk rongeurs are used to remove loose fragments of disk.
12. After diskectomy, the epidural space and the intervertebral foramen are explored with a blunt nerve hook to confirm patency and resolve nerve root pressure.
13. Hemostasis is achieved, and the wound is irrigated generously with saline/antibiotic solution.
14. The wound is then closed in layers.

For cervical or thoracic disks, only the protruding fragment is removed. Limited, if any, exploration of the interspace is performed because attempts at adequate interspace exploration require retraction of the dural sac, which contains the spinal cord at these levels. Such retraction would result in cord injury and paralysis. For a thoracic disk, a costotransversectomy or transthoracic approach is used.

Endoscopic diskectomy for far lateral disk herniations and annular tears has become an applied surgical approach in this subgroup of patients. Endoscopic spine systems have been developed, and further development and evolution of endoscopic equipment will continue to make minimally invasive procedures attractive to both the patient and the neurosurgeon.

Additional spine techniques are covered in Chapter 22.

## CAROTID ARTERY SURGERY

Carotid endarterectomy is discussed in Chapter 26, "Vascular Surgery."

### Carotid Artery Ligation

Carotid artery ligation is performed to occlude the internal carotid artery. It may be done to control anticipated hemorrhage during intracranial surgery for vascular anomalies. A permanent occlusion may be necessary for the control of intracranial hemorrhage or small, repeated strokes from an intracranial lesion.

***Procedural Considerations.*** Special clamps are available for gradual occlusion of the artery. Occlusion may protect the patient from debilitating or fatal intracranial hemorrhage from aneurysm and may be used to treat carotid-cavernous fistula. Only a basic minor instrument set is used.

#### *Operative Procedure*

1. The skin is incised, and a Weitlaner retractor is inserted for exposure.
2. The carotid artery is freed. A small Penrose tubing, umbilical tape, or vessel loop is passed around the vessel for retraction.
3. a. For *temporary* control of the carotid artery (during procedures for very large aneurysms or arteriovenous anomalies), an umbilical tape is passed around the vessel and fixed using the Roper-Rumel tourniquet in such a manner that occlusion can be accomplished immediately if necessary.
   b. For *permanent* occlusion, two heavy silk ligatures are used and the artery may be divided between ligatures. Transfixing suture ligatures may be used as well if the artery is divided.
4. The incision is closed, and a dressing is applied.

### Carotid Surgery for Carotid-Cavernous Fistula

Ligation of the common carotid artery is one mode of surgical treatment for a carotid-cavernous fistula. Another form of surgical treatment is to embolize the fistula. In either case, internal carotid ligation is usually done after satisfactory embolization. In some cases, a frontotemporal craniotomy is also performed and the internal carotid artery is clipped intracranially as well. An interventional radiologist can also perform selective balloon occlusions of these vessels.

## PERIPHERAL NERVE SURGERY

### Sympathectomy

Sympathectomy is excision of a portion of the sympathetic division of the autonomic nervous system. Most sympathectomies are performed on the paravertebral chain and are named for the region resected, such as cervical, thoracolumbar, and lumbar. The periarterial sympathectomy, vagotomy, and presacral neurectomy are other procedures that are occasionally performed on the autonomic system. The principal diseases treated by sympathectomy are vascular disorders of the extremities, intractable pain from certain nerve injuries, chronic abdominal conditions, and hyperhydrosis (overactivity of sweat glands).

The position of the patient depends on the region to be resected. Basic dissecting instruments and the microscope are used. For retropleural and transthoracic approaches, rib-resecting instruments are added. For the thoracic approach, Beckman or Scoville laminectomy retractors and an assortment of handheld retractors, including malleables, Deavers, and Richardsons, are added. For the abdominal approach, Balfour self-retaining retractors are added.

***Cervicothoracic Sympathectomy—Dorsal.*** Dorsal sympathectomy entails removal of the cervicothoracic chain, often from the fourth cervical to the third thoracic ganglion. Sympathetic denervation of the upper extremities and heart may be accomplished by cervicothoracic sympathectomy. The vasospastic phenomenon of Raynaud's disease is relieved by this procedure. It also may be beneficial in relieving intractable angina pectoris.

PROCEDURAL CONSIDERATIONS. For the anterior approach, both the laminectomy set and rib instruments are used, plus deep retractors and a nerve stimulator. The setup for the posterior approach is as for the anterior approach, plus rib-resecting instruments, periosteal elevators, small rib retractors, a firm rubber pad, and OR bed attachments for the posterolateral position.

OPERATIVE PROCEDURE—ANTERIOR APPROACH

1. The patient is placed in a supine position with the head rotated to the opposite side. General endotracheal anesthesia is necessary because puncturing the pleura is a possibility.
2. A transverse incision is made one fingerbreadth above the clavicle, the clavicular head of the sternocleidomastoid muscle is severed, and the deep cervical fascia is divided.
3. The phrenic nerve and the jugular vein are protected, and the anterior scalene muscle is divided to expose and isolate the underlying subclavian artery. One of its branches, the thyroid axis, is ligated and divided.
4. The stellate ganglion, deep against the vertebral body, is brought into view and lifted on a nerve hook. The sympa-

thetic chain is traced upward to the middle cervical ganglion and divided. Deep dissection behind the pleura exposes the upper thoracic ganglia, which are removed to below the third thoracic ganglion. Clips may be placed on the sympathetic nerves before their division.
5. The wound is closed, and dressings are applied.

OPERATIVE PROCEDURE—POSTERIOR APPROACH

1. The patient is placed in the lateral position, and a paravertebral incision is centered over the third rib. The trapezius muscle is divided, and the rhomboid is split in line with its fibers. The third and fourth ribs are isolated extrapleurally, and the posterior 4 to 5 cm is resected. The transverse processes may be removed to provide better exposure.
2. The sympathetic trunk, which lies on the anterolateral aspect of the vertebral body, is reached by carefully reflecting the pleura. The trunk is picked up on a nerve hook, traced up and down, and removed, usually from the stellate ganglion to the fourth thoracic ganglion. Clips may be applied to the nerve before the fibers are severed.
3. A firm rubber tube may be left in the wound during closure. Suctioning apparatus is applied to this tube as the last deep fascial suture is drawn tight; all air is aspirated, and the tube is quickly withdrawn.
4. The subcutaneous tissue and skin edges are closed.

## Nerve Repairs

Peripheral nerve injuries are the most common indication for nerve repair. Nerve tumors are rare in comparison. When the continuity of a nerve is destroyed, function distal to the site of injury is lost. Recovery will occur only if regeneration of nerve axons takes place from the healthy proximal segments. These axons must grow down the axis cylinders of the nerve beyond the injury if they are to reinnervate their end-organs and allow function to return.

When a nerve is divided, the cut ends retract, become scarred, and form neuromas. Regenerating axons from the proximal segment cannot bridge such a gap or penetrate the scar tissue. An unobstructed path down the axis cylinder must be made available if nerves are ever again to move muscles or transmit sensation. All procedures are directed toward obtaining the best possible conditions for regeneration.

***Procedural Considerations.*** A basic dissecting instrument set, microinstruments, a microscope, and a nerve stimulator are used. For lesser procedures such as spinal-accessory-facial anastomosis in the neck, division of the volar carpal ligament for median nerve compression at the wrist, or repair of a small digital nerve, suitable modification may be made. The positioning, skin prep, and draping of the patient depend on the site of the injury. A large area is prepped.

General anesthesia is usually preferred, with the patient positioned for maximum accessibility to the injured nerve. Exposure must be adequate because considerable mobilization of the nerve is often necessary. A dry field may be achieved using a tourniquet on the involved extremity.

### *Operative Procedure*

1. The site of injury is explored, with careful attention to hemostasis. Nerve ends are dissected from surrounding scar tissue, and neuromas are excised. Moist umbilical tapes, vessel loops, or Penrose tubing may be passed about the nerve to handle it more easily and with less trauma.
2. The nerve repair anastomosis is made with multiple fine sutures placed only through the nerve sheath or epineurium (Figure 23-57). Tension at the suture line is eliminated by maneuvers such as freeing up a long length of nerve on either side of the point of injury, transposition of the nerve to shorten its course, appropriate positioning of the extremity with plaster splinting during the postoperative period, and, rarely, use of a nerve graft. Some surgeons apply a cuff of inert material, such as silicone, about the anastomosis.

## Carpal Tunnel Syndrome

Carpal tunnel syndrome is a condition of the hand in which the median nerve is compressed by the transverse carpal ligament or compressed by displacement of the lunate bone or a volar carpal ganglion. Decompression of the nerve is done by removing part of the roof of the fibrous sheath of the ligament or the offending bone or ganglion.

***Procedural Considerations.*** The patient is placed in the supine position with the operative arm extended on a hand table or armboard. Local, regional, or general anesthesia may be used.

### *Operative Procedure*

1. A longitudinal skin incision is made in the thenar palm crease. This runs perpendicular to and stops at the most distal transverse skin crease in the wrist. This incision generally suffices but may be extended into an L or a T.
2. A Weitlaner, mastoid, or self-retaining spring-action retractor is placed.
3. The fibers of the carpal ligament are divided transversely in blunt fashion at the most proximal point of exposure. A hemostat is introduced through this opening in the ligament, pointed distally, and spread. This protects the underlying median nerve. The ligament is divided between the jaws of the hemostat with Mayo or Metzenbaum scissors.
4. The incision is closed with fine sutures, and a bulky dressing is applied, with the fingers visible.

## Ulnar Nerve Transposition at the Elbow

Because of traumatic or anatomic problems, the ulnar nerve may be predisposed to irritation resulting in chronic discomfort. In such instances the position of the nerve can be changed to provide protection and comfort.

***Procedural Considerations.*** The patient is placed in the supine position. The arm may be supported in a functional position, with Webril and elastic bandages to attach it to the anesthesia screen, or it may be left free for the surgeon to manipulate during the procedure. The inner and posterior aspects of the upper and lower arm must be exposed for the operation.

### *Operative Procedure*

1. A long incision is made, and the nerve is dissected free from the surrounding soft tissues with Metzenbaum scissors and hemostatic forceps. Moist umbilical tapes, vessel loops, or Penrose tubing is passed around the freed segment of the nerve to aid in handling it for further dissection until a sat-

**FIGURE 23-57** Nerve repair. **A,** Serial resection of neuroma to healthy nerve fibers. **B,** Placement of sutures in epineurium. **C,** Approximation and tying of sutures.

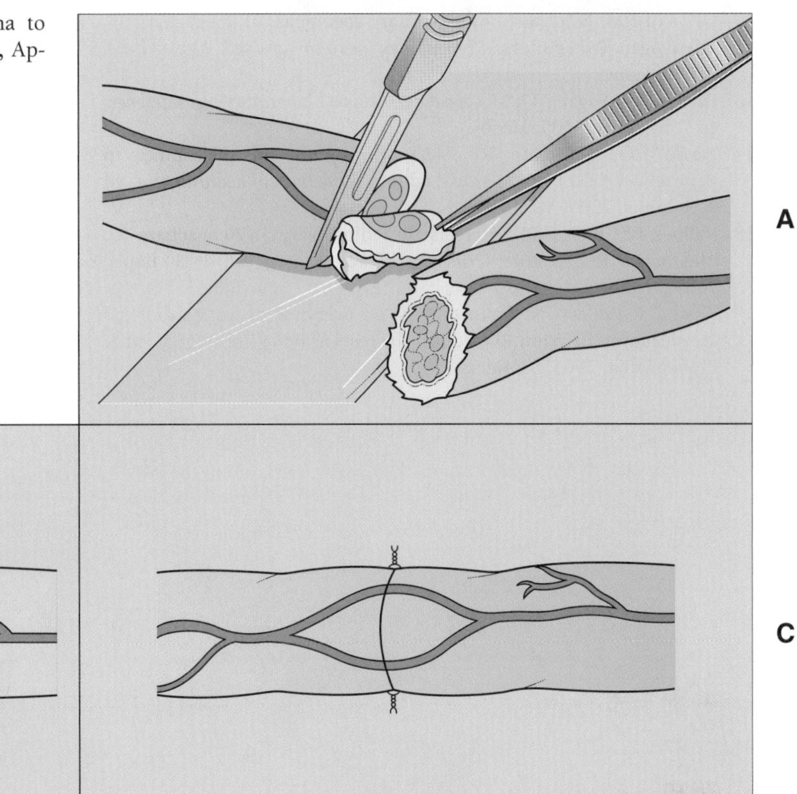


isfactory length of nerve has been freed from above to below the elbow.

2. The muscle and fascia entered by the nerve at each end of the field may be slit with scissors to prevent tethering and kinking at these points after the nerve has been transposed.
3. A fascial flap overlying the medial epicondyle of the humerus is cut and elevated, and the nerve is transposed beneath it.
4. The fascia is then loosely reapproximated to the fascial edge remaining on the epicondyle with 3-0 silk or 2-0 absorbable suture.
5. The wound is closed in layers.

An alternative procedure, medial epicondylectomy, is sometimes performed. In this case the nerve is not dissected out, but the medial epicondyle of the humerus is removed with a rongeur and the residual bone is waxed. The fascia and muscle that are tending to tether or kink the nerve, particularly distally, may be slit with scissors as in the transposition procedure.

## REFERENCES


1. Al-Mefty O, Heth J: Meningiomas. In Rengachary SS, Ellenbogen RG, editors: *Principles of neurosurgery*, ed 2, St Louis, 2005, Mosby.
2. Austin LS and others: Primary and metastatic spinal tumors. In Vaccaro AR, editor: *Spine core knowledge in orthopaedics*, St Louis, 2005, Mosby.
3. Barkauskas VH and others: *Health & physical assessment*, ed 3, St Louis, 2002, Mosby.

3a. Batjer HH, et al: Intracranial aneurysm. In Rengachary SS, Ellenbogen RG, editors: Principles of neurosurgery, ed 2, St Louis, 2005, Mosby.

4. Central Brain Tumor Registry of the United States (CBTRUS): *Statistical report: primary brain tumors in the United States, 1998-2002,* 2005. Accessed March 27, 2006, on-line: www.cbtrus.org.
5. Connolly ES and others: *Fundamentals of operative techniques in neurosurgery*, New York, 2002, Thieme.
6. Doran SE, Thorell WE: Brain tumors: population-based epidemiology, environmental risk factors, and genetic and hereditary syndromes. In Winn RW, editor: *Youman's neurological surgery,* ed 5, Philadelphia, 2004, Saunders.
7. Fisicaro MD and others: Basic anatomy of the cervical, thoracic, lumbar, and sacral spine. In Vaccaro AR, editor: *Spine core knowledge in orthopaedics*, St Louis, 2005, Mosby.
8. Greenberg MS: *Handbook of neurosurgery*, ed 5, New York, 2001, Thieme.
9. Harrop JS: Intradural spinal neoplasms. In Vaccaro AR, editor: *Spine core knowledge in orthopaedics*, St Louis, 2005, Mosby.
10. Lipov E: New outpatient techniques for chronic back pain, *Outpatient Surgery Magazine* 11(10):66-71, 2001.
11. Marshall RS: *Arteriovenous malformations,* October 26, 2004. Accessed March 26, 2006, on-line: www.emedicine.com/NEURO/topic21.htm.
12. McCutcheon IE: Metastatic brain tumors. In Rengachary SS, Ellenbogen RG, editors: *Principles of neurosurgery*, ed 2, St Louis, 2005, Mosby.
13. Mendel E and others: Injuries to the cervical spine. In Vaccaro AR, editor: *Spine core knowledge in orthopaedics*, St Louis, 2005, Mosby.
14. Newell DW, Lam AM: Transcranial doppler ultrasonography. In Winn RW, editor: *Youman's neurological surgery*, ed 5, Philadelphia, 2004, Saunders.

15. Oyesiku NM: Nonfunctioning pituitary adenomas. In Rengachary SS, Ellenbogen RG, editors: *Principles of neurosurgery*, ed 2, St Louis, 2005, Mosby.
16. Pagana KD, Pagana TJ: *Mosby's diagnostic and laboratory test reference*, ed 7, St Louis, 2005, Mosby.
17. Perrin RG, McBroom RJ: Metastatic tumors of the spine. In Rengachary SS, Ellenbogen RG, editors: *Principles of neurosurgery*, ed 2, St Louis, 2005, Mosby.
18. Pollock BE, Brown PD: Stereotactic radiosurgery. In Rengachary SS, Ellenbogen RG, editors: *Principles of neurosurgery*, ed 2, St Louis, 2005, Mosby.
19. Ribalta T, Fuller GN: Brain tumors: an overview of histopathologic classification. In Winn RW, editor: *Youman's neurological surgery*, ed 5, Philadelphia, 2004, Saunders.
20. Sloan AE and others: Gliomas. In Rengachary SS, Ellenbogen RG, editors: *Principles of neurosurgery*, ed 2, St Louis, 2005, Mosby.
21. Standring S: *Gray's anatomy*, ed 39, Edinburgh, 2005, Churchill Livingstone.
22. Teo C, Mobbs R: Neuroendoscopy. In Rengachary SS, Ellenbogen RG, editors: *Principles of neurosurgery*, ed 2, St Louis, 2005, Mosby.
23. Wang P, Avellino AM: Hydrocephalus in children. In Rengachary SS, Ellenbogen RG: *Principles of neurosurgery*, ed 2, St Louis, 2005, Mosby.
24. Zonenshayn M, Rezai A: Stereotactic surgery. In Rengachary SS, Ellenbogen RG, editors: *Principles of neurosurgery*, ed 2, St Louis, 2005, Mosby.

CHAPTER 24

# *Plastic and Reconstructive Surgery*

SUSAN K. CHANDLER

*"WE RESTORE, repair, and make whole those parts which fortune has taken away, not so much that they delight the eyes but that they may buoy up the spirit and help the mind of the beset." So wrote sixteenth century plastic surgeon Gasparo Tagliacozzi hundreds of years ago as he first articulated what today's plastic surgeons attempt to do: provide their patients with the best possible cosmetic as well as functional outcomes following surgery, thus contributing to the patient's body image, self-esteem, and quality of life.*[23]

Few people realize that plastic surgery owes much of its heritage and development to the knowledge gained from the wars of the twentieth century (History box). The word *plastic* is derived from the Greek *plastikos,* which means "to mold, form, or contour." Plastic surgery deals with healing, reconstruction, restoration of function, and correction of disfigurement or scarring resulting from trauma or acquired or congenital lesions and defects. (See Chapter 29 for a discussion of pediatric plastic and reconstructive surgery.)

The field of plastic and reconstructive surgery has advanced rapidly in recent years. Patients who require emergency surgery as well as those undergoing elective cosmetic procedures benefit from innovative and unique technologies and techniques. Experimental reconstructive techniques continue to be developed to afford potential new reconstructive options. There has been a surge in the popularity of cosmetic plastic surgery, no doubt as a result of a decrease in the stigma of cosmetic surgery and heightened consumer awareness achieved through increasing media exposure showcasing dramatic surgical makeovers. Liposuction has been identified as the top aesthetic surgery for both males and females.[3]

## *Surgical Anatomy*

Plastic and reconstructive surgery is not limited either to a single anatomic or biologic system or to a single operative technique. In addition to removing, reducing, enlarging, and recontouring, this specialty includes camouflaging scars into existing skin lines (Figure 24-1) and using a multitude of opportunities the incredible human body offers to borrow (as in skin or muscle flaps), move elsewhere (grafts and reconstruction), or totally recreate (breasts, digits, facial structures). Plastic surgeons are known as the tissue coverage and wound healing experts, and they rely on the basic techniques of surgery and a view of the patient as a whole biopsychosocial being. Microsurgical techniques have been advanced, diverse plastic surgical operations developed, and standard plastic surgical procedures improved, with each contributing to the highly specialized and unique status of plastic and reconstructive surgery today. The aesthetic problems, varieties of acquired defects, diversity of operative techniques, and psychologic responses of patients offer unique learning experiences and challenges for providing perioperative nursing care.

## *Perioperative Nursing Considerations*

The prospect of surgery, even elective, can produce anxiety and fear. Plastic and reconstructive surgery, because it is so often tied to body image and self-esteem, can trigger these emotions when the proposed surgery is associated with potential disfigurement because of disease or trauma. Even a planned (desired) change in body image can be stressful. Many cosmetic patients lack the traditional support system one comes to expect during illness and recuperation because of a desire for confidentiality, making the sensitivity of the perioperative nurse all the more critical.

The nursing process is dynamic, fluid, and complex. The nature of plastic and reconstructive surgery is rarely simple, routine, or predictable, and the nursing care must mirror that fact. It must include thorough and ongoing assessment, the establishment of nursing diagnoses and outcomes, fastidious planning, superior implementation, and thoughtful evaluation. The perioperative nurse's goal is to produce positive, high-quality outcomes in an environment that is safe and nurturing and will facilitate physical and emotional healing. Throughout the process, effective communication is necessary with the patient and his or her family or significant others as well as all members of the perioperative team. Communication is a two-way process that includes verbal and nonverbal messages. Respect for the individual, a nonjudgmental attitude, and effective communication skills are essential ingredients for the perioperative nurse caring for plastic surgery patients.

### Assessment

As part of a holistic assessment, perioperative nurses consider physical and emotional factors of the planned procedure. A comprehensive review of the chart is the first step. The presence of a signed and witnessed informed consent, a systems review and health history, pertinent laboratory and diagnostic data,

## HISTORY

### Origins and Growth of Plastic Surgery

Historically, battlefield combat has been an impetus for the development of new medical and surgical techniques based on the injuries sustained. As battlefield technology and the weapons of war became more sophisticated throughout history, the degree of injury and tissue devastation became more horrific. The trench warfare of World Wars I and II gave rise to a whole new category of facial injuries. Helmets protected combatants' skulls and the trenches offered some protection to the chest, but the face was exposed, and as a result, devastating burns and fractures of the face occurred. Special hospitals were created to address these problems, and even before the United States joined World War I, the Harvard unit sent 35 physicians and surgeons, 3 dentists, and 75 nurses from various medical centers to assist in caring for the wounded. These visionaries were soon developing new techniques and procedures to correct the disfiguring injuries. They were considered the first generation of modern plastic surgeons and helped give much needed respect to the specialty.

Although World War I helped reinvent plastic surgery, the specialty has been identified as long ago as 600 BC, when a Hindu surgeon described using a cheek flap to reconstruct a nose. Another flap technique, this time using the forehead to reconstruct a severed nose, was performed around AD 1000 in India. The Italian surgeon Gasparo Tagliacozzi, also known as the father of plastic surgery, developed still another flap surgery using the upper arm to reconstruct a nose. History tells us that the condition of the nose, whether from war, punishment, or social disease (syphilis), told a story that often was undesirable. This gave way to impetus in the different societies to camouflage the injuries, thus propelling advances in plastic surgery.

Following the end of World War I, plastic surgery turned its attention to the rest of society and concentrated on deformities caused by birth or trauma. Soon, some surgeons began using their talents to improve less than desirable facial features. Fanny Brice underwent a rhinoplasty in her apartment in 1923 in order to change her nose's appearance from "prominent to decorative." In 1924 a New York newspaper ran a contest that would transform the city's homeliest woman into a beauty. Dr. John Howard Crum performed the first face-lift on record in the Grand Ballroom of the Pennsylvania Hotel in New York City in 1931, during which "a pianist accompanied him with appropriate popular tunes, flashbulbs popped, and men and women fainted."

Modified from Feldman E: Before & after: cosmetic surgery was born 2,500 years ago and came of age in the inferno of the western front, *American Heritage* 55(1):60-70, 2004.

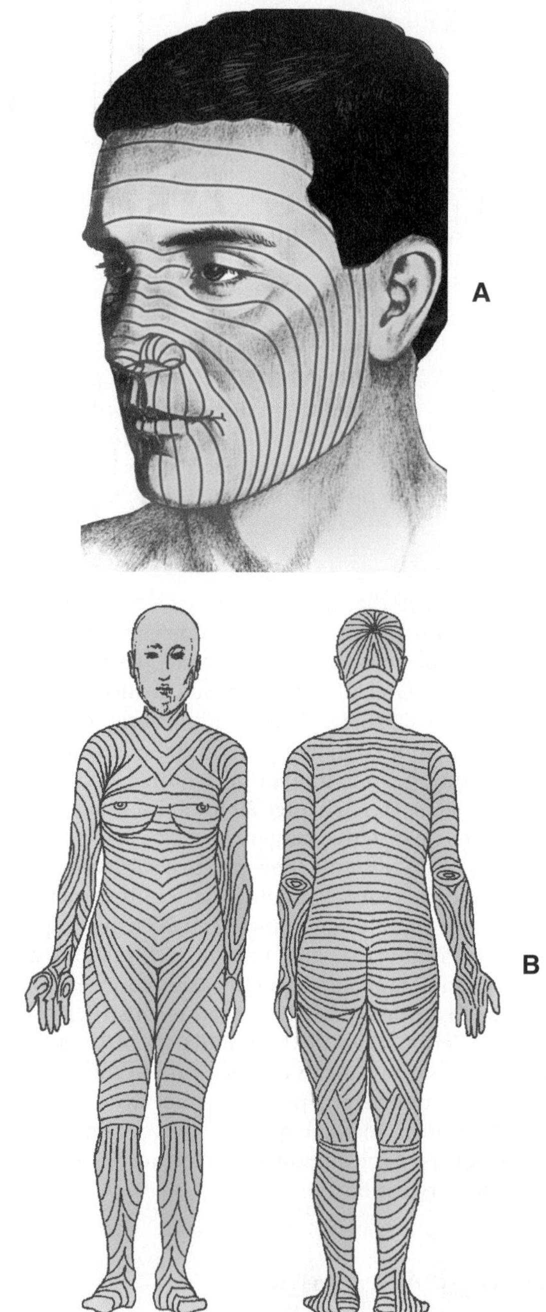


**FIGURE 24-1** The surgeon adheres to several principles when planning skin incisions, one of which is to reduce the amount of tension across the wound, thus minimizing scarring. Elective incisions should preferably parallel relaxed skin tension lines (RSTLs) in the face, **A,** and the body, **B.**

interdisciplinary planning, anesthesia evaluation, and surgical plan will reveal vital information necessary to begin the assessment process. Visual inspection should include overall physical condition, the condition and integrity of the skin, nutritional status, and physical limitations. The next step is the patient interview, which includes checking patient identification, an explanation of the perioperative nursing role, and verifying the patient's understanding of the planned procedure. The perioperative nurse must be skilled in establishing communication quickly in order to create an instant relationship. Greeting the patient by name in a calm, comforting manner, perhaps with a gentle, caring touch (if welcomed by the patient), and maintaining good eye contact will help establish the rapport needed to assess emotional status, body image disturbances, and anxiety level. Asking the patient questions will help reveal any barriers to communication or learning; religious, cultural, or other preferences; mental status; and insight into compliance. Other vital pieces of knowledge the nurse must obtain include the presence of realistic expectations and motivation for surgery, as well as support systems available to the patient.

An important component of the assessment phase of nursing care involves communication with the surgeon and anesthesia provider to determine the need for special equipment, supplies, sutures, or implants. The perioperative nurse should verify the procedure and position and, in the case of multiple procedures on the same patient, identify the planned order of surgeries. The plastic surgeon's office team can be a useful source of information about the patient and the surgery and is often able to offer insight into the psychosocial dimension of the patient.

## Nursing Diagnosis

Nursing diagnoses related to the care of patient undergoing plastic and reconstructive surgery might include the following:

- Disturbed Body Image
- Anxiety related to surgical intervention(s) or outcome
- Deficient Knowledge related to perioperative events
- Risk for Perioperative Positioning Injury
- Risk for Ineffective Tissue Perfusion related to surgical intervention

## Outcome Identification

Nursing diagnoses lead to the formulation of desired or expected patient outcomes. These are desirable and measurable patient states, including biologic or physiologic states; psychologic, cultural, and spiritual aspects; and the knowledge or skills related to these states. As such, the patient outcome indicates progress toward or resolution of the nursing diagnosis. When possible, outcomes should be mutually formulated with the patient, family, and other health care providers. Such formulations should be realistic, involve consideration of the patient's present and potential capabilities and resources, and provide direction for continuity of care, as well as determine satisfaction with that care. Outcomes identified for the selected nursing diagnoses could be stated as follows:

- The patient will acknowledge feelings about altered structure or function.
- The patient will verbalize management of anxiety.
- The patient will verbalize understanding of the perioperative process.
- The patient will be free from signs and symptoms of injury related to surgical positioning.
- The patient's tissue perfusion will be maintained or restored.

## Planning

The perioperative nurse designs a plan of care using critical thinking to integrate knowledge gained from the assessment of the plastic surgical patient with the nursing diagnoses and outcomes that have been identified. The nurse should seek to create and maintain a culture and environment of safety for the patient, the operating room (OR), and all members of the surgical team

### SAMPLE PLAN OF CARE

**NURSING DIAGNOSIS**
**Disturbed Body Image**

**OUTCOME**
The patient will acknowledge feelings about altered structure or function.

**INTERVENTIONS**

- Assist patient to identify and discuss feelings, stressors, and perception of physical deformity.
- Provide environment (e.g., privacy, supportive listening) conducive to expression of feelings.
- Help patient identify significance of culture, religion, gender, and age on perceived changes in body structure or function or image.
- Determine patient's body image expectations and whether expectations are realistic; clarify unrealistic expectations or misconceptions.
- Convey sense of respect for abilities and strengths in coping with problems or concerns.
- Assist patient to separate physical appearance from feelings of personal worth, self-concept, and self-esteem (as appropriate).
- Refer the patient to other health professionals (e.g., clergy, social worker, psychiatric liaison) or support groups as appropriate.

**NURSING DIAGNOSIS**
**Anxiety** related to surgical intervention(s) or outcome

**OUTCOME**
The patient will verbalize management of anxiety.

**INTERVENTIONS**

- Broadly classify the patient's anxiety (mild, moderate, severe).
- Seek to understand the patient's perception of the stressors or stressful situation or event.
- Identify contributing factors.
- Introduce self and other members of the surgical team.
- Explain all perioperative events and any sensations likely to be experienced.
- Determine the patient's normal coping patterns.
- Communicate with the patient in a calm, unhurried, reassuring manner.
- Encourage the patient to ventilate feelings and concerns; listen attentively.
- Reduce distracting stimuli in the perioperative environment.
- If the patient is awake, provide reassurance and information about the progress of the surgery; implement mechanism for family progress reports also.
- Provide comfort measures (e.g., warm blankets, soft music that the patient prefers).
- Use touch as appropriate (e.g., softly stroking the hand).
- Encourage and assist the patient to use personally effective coping strategies (e.g., meditation, guided imagery, relaxation).

**NURSING DIAGNOSIS**
**Deficient Knowledge** related to perioperative events

**OUTCOME**
The patient will verbalize an understanding of the sequence of perioperative events.

**INTERVENTIONS**

- Initiate institution's checklist policy for correct site surgery.
- Verify surgical consent with operating room (OR) schedule and patient's statement of planned surgery.
- Solicit the patient's questions; answer or refer questions as appropriate.
- Explain the sequence of perioperative events and their purpose, as appropriate (e.g., holding area, OR attire, insertion of lines and attachment of monitoring devices, type of anesthesia, postoperative recovery unit, protocols).
- Provide sensory (what the patient will hear and feel, using lay terms) as well as factual procedure-related information.

*Continued*

## SAMPLE PLAN OF CARE—cont'd

- Whenever possible, provide printed material to reinforce patient education (e.g., preoperative routines, explanations of surgical intervention, postoperative management of pain, discharge instructions).

**NURSING DIAGNOSIS**

**Risk for Perioperative Positioning Injury**

**OUTCOME**

The patient will be free from injury related to the surgical position.

**INTERVENTIONS**

- Determine whether the patient has any mobility limitations; adapt surgical position accordingly.
- Assess skin integrity before procedure and document findings.
- When possible, have patient assume surgical position before induction of general anesthesia; observe areas of discomfort, and adapt position accordingly.
- Secure the patient to the OR bed; reapply restraints after positional changes.
- Observe the patient's nutritional status, body height and weight, skin integrity, and adequacy of protective tissue at dependent pressure sites.
- Apply protective padding to OR bed, dependent pressure sites, and vulnerable neurovascular bundles.
- For lengthy procedures, consider the use of a pressure-reducing OR bed mattress.
- When position allows, perform gentle range-of-motion (ROM) exercises.
- Prevent the compression of body parts against one another (e.g., crossed legs), against the hard surface of the OR bed, and against any positioning accessories.
- Maintain the patient in good body alignment; reassess body alignment after positional changes.
- Keep sheets under patient dry and wrinkle-free.
- Provide adequate assistance to safely transfer the patient to and from the OR bed.
- Decrease surgical time by anticipating needs of patient and surgical team.

**NURSING DIAGNOSIS**

**Risk for Ineffective Tissue Perfusion** related to surgical intervention

**OUTCOME**

The patient's tissue perfusion will be maintained or restored.

**INTERVENTIONS**

- Note any sensory or perceptual alterations in the affected body part, and document them.
- Maintain body temperature with the use of warming device or reflective blankets, for example.
- Warm intravenous fluids, blood and blood products, and irrigating fluids.
- Increase the temperature in the operating room as indicated.
- Collaborate with anesthesia provider in monitoring the patient's core temperature.
- Provide intraoperative medications as prescribed for local irrigation (e.g., heparinized saline); label all medications on and off the sterile field, and document their administration.
- Apply compression stockings and antiembolic devices as indicated.
- Monitor tissue perfusion (e.g., by assessing blanching and capillary refill; using Doppler ultrasound), as prescribed, and flap ischemic time; record results.
- Note any swelling, change in color or temperature, or drainage from graft sites before discharge from the OR.
- Provide warm blankets for the patient at the conclusion of the surgical procedure.
- Teach the patient or the family how to care for the incision, including signs and symptoms of infection and graft failure (as applicable).

during the planning process. A typical plan of care for a patient undergoing plastic and reconstructive surgery follows.

## Implementation

The implementation phase begins once the patient has been assessed, nursing diagnoses have been formulated, outcomes have been identified, and planning has been completed. It typically begins with preparation of the room and requires a thorough understanding of the procedure and the special needs of the patient, surgeon, and anesthesia provider. The nurse must continuously monitor and reassess the patient as well as the needs of the perioperative team, implementing and documenting the delivery of care. Constant consideration is given to the safety of the patient and the perioperative environment during this phase.

***Preparation of the Operating Room Suite.*** Before transporting the patient to the OR, the perioperative nurse will assemble all necessary medical and surgical supplies, equipment, suture material, positioning aids, implantable devices, and medications. The nurse is responsible for checking for proper functioning of lights and video equipment, emergency supplies, and adequacy of compressed gases. Depending on the procedure to be performed, the OR bed may need to be configured differently from the standard room setup. The nurse should confirm the position of the bed and any proposed intraoperative changes to the bed or room configuration with the surgeon and anesthesia provider to minimize inefficiencies during the procedure. Plastic and reconstructive surgeons frequently use preoperative photographs of the patient when attempting to restore or modify appearance. These photographs help the surgeon maintain perspective since features may change because of surgical positioning. The nurse should collaborate with the surgeon to determine the best placement of these photographs for intraoperative viewing.

***Equipment and Special Mechanical Devices.*** Essential equipment for any operating room includes a fully functional bed that may be positioned for any number of special needs and also has accessory attachments, such as headrests and aids for extremity positioning. The room must also have well-positioned and numerous electrical outlets, good overhead lighting, suction, mounted x-ray view boxes, and computer terminals for those facilities using electronic medical records. Step stools, tables, chairs, hand tables, and intravenous (IV) poles should be in appropriate supply and accessible. Digital and instant (Polaroid) cameras should also be available for use.

**DERMATOMES.** Dermatomes are used for removing split-thickness skin grafts (STSGs) from donor sites; they are of three basic types: knife, drum, and motor-driven (Figure 24-2). Mineral oil and a tongue blade should be available when STSGs are being obtained.

1. Knife dermatomes
   a. Ferris-Smith: grafts obtained in freehand manner; sterile blades supplied by manufacturer.
   b. Humby (Figure 24-3) or Watson: with adjustable roller to control thickness of graft.
   c. Weck: uses straight razor blades with interchangeable guards (0.008, 0.010, and 0.012 inch) to obtain small grafts; also used for debridement of burn wounds.
2. Drum dermatomes: operate on the principle of fixing outer surface of skin to half of a metal drum and then moving rotating blade back and forth close to surface of the drum to obtain split-thickness skin graft.
   a. Reese: tape containing adhesive is fixed to drum; dermatome cement is applied to skin in thin layer and allowed to dry for 3 minutes; distance between blade and drum (thickness of graft) is adjusted by inserting shim (0.008 to 0.034 inch) adjacent to blade in carrying arm; sterile dermatome tapes, cement, and blades available from manufacturer.

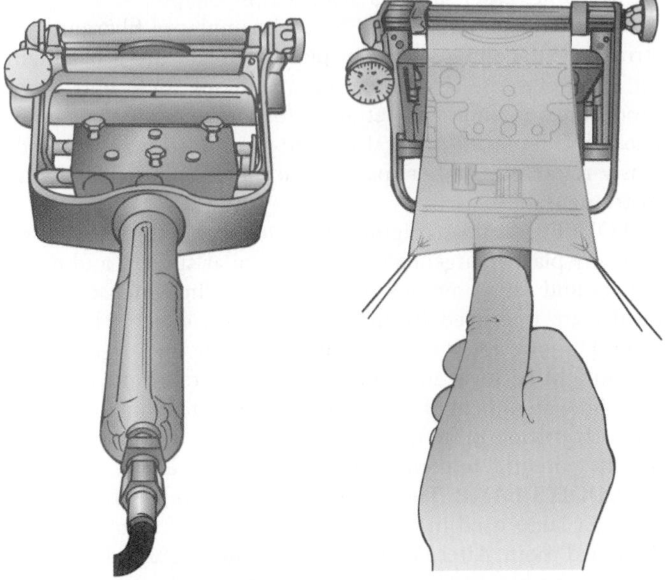

FIGURE 24-2 Powered Brown dermatome.

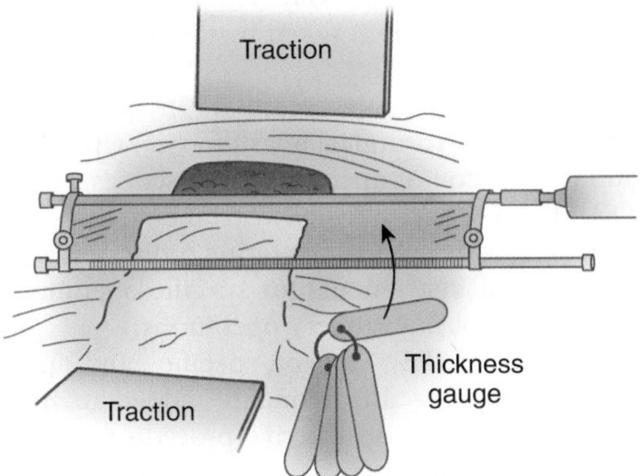


FIGURE 24-3 Harvesting a split-thickness skin graft (STSG) with the Humby knife.

3. Motor-driven dermatomes: graft obtained with knife blade that moves back and forth like the blade of a hair cutter; power supplied by electricity or compressed gas; long, sterile cable serves as drive shaft and runs between dermatome and its power source; motor activated by foot pedal or hand control.
   a. Zimmer dermatome: motor located in handle, sterile blades provided by the manufacturer; consists of four templates (varying in sizes from 1 to 4 inches, determined by size of graft needed) and one screwdriver that secures template on top of the blade; depth of graft desired can be determined by calibrated lever on handle.
   b. Brown dermatome: usually powered by compressed air; sterile blades provided by manufacturer; blade secured in handle with specially designed wrench; depth of graft can be determined by adjusting calibrating knobs on handle; can be steam-sterilized.
   c. Padgett dermatome: motor located in handle; dermatome may be nitrogen-powered or electric; if dermatome is driven by electricity, manufacturer's recommendations must be followed for sterilization; sterile blades also available from the company, and various sizes of templates included; calibration accomplished by adjusting knob on head of dermatome.

Insertion of the knife blade and guards of shims with any dermatome is often done by the surgeon. It is also the surgeon's responsibility to make the final blade adjustment and alignment and to remove the knife blade after obtaining a graft and before perioperative personnel begin any instrument-cleansing procedures. The blade should be disposed of in an appropriate puncture-resistant container.

**SKIN MESHERS.** Several types of skin meshers are available. Each is designed to produce multiple uniform slits in a skin graft, approximately 0.05 inch apart. These multiple apertures in the graft can then expand, permitting the skin graft to stretch and cover a larger area (Figure 24-4). Meshing also facilitates drainage through the graft, preventing fluid accumulation under a graft. The graft is placed on the carrier and passed through the mesher (Figure 24-5). The manufacturer supplies sterile carriers for meshers. They are usually available in several sizes, which determine the expansion ratio of the skin graft.

**PNEUMATIC-POWERED INSTRUMENTS.** Pneumatic-powered instruments use an inert, nonflammable, and explosion-free compressed gas as their power source. The motor may be activated by a foot pedal or hand control. The various attachments should be sterilized as recommended by the manufacturer to prolong instrument life and ensure effective sterilization. The following attachments may be used in plastic surgery:

- Wire driver and bone drill
- Oscillating saw
- Derma-Tattoo (used with reciprocating-saw handpiece)
- Reciprocating saw
- Dermabrader
- Sagittal saw

A pneumatic tourniquet with an inflatable cuff is used in most hand surgery procedures as well as in other upper and lower extremity surgical interventions. The tourniquet is described in Chapter 22.

**BIPOLAR COAGULATION UNIT.** Bipolar electrosurgery is the use of electrical current in which the circuit is completed

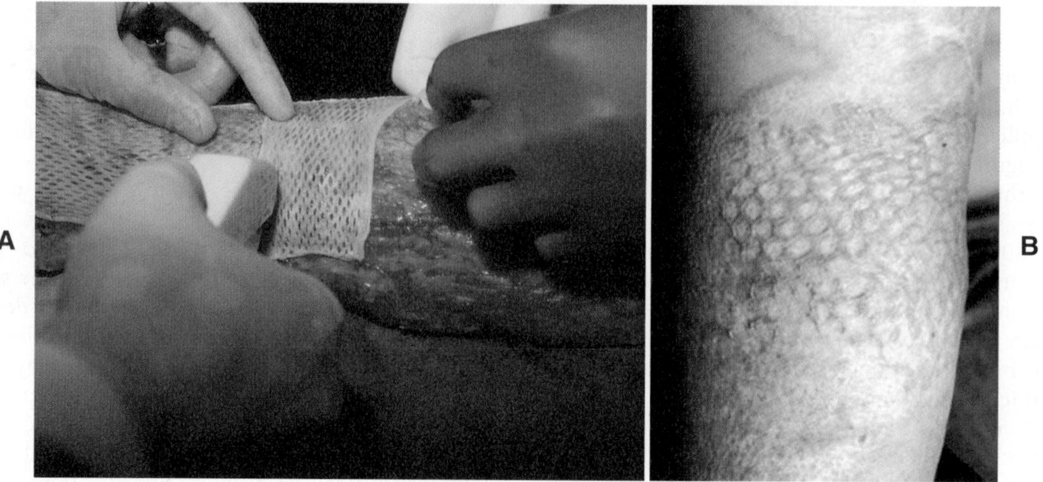


FIGURE 24-4 **A,** Split-thickness skin is meshed and used to cover a marginal wound. Minimal expansion is used, and the holes provide drainage. **B,** Appearance of the graft after healing.

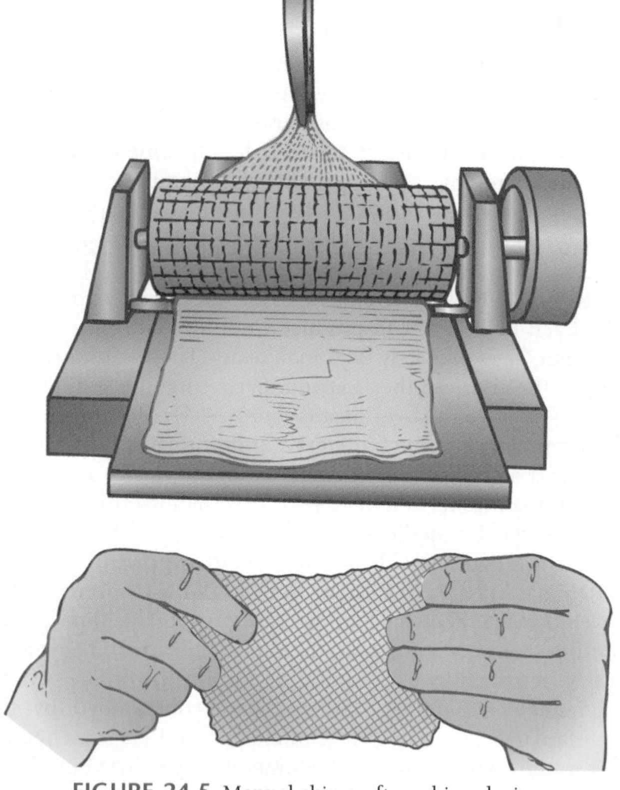

FIGURE 24-5 Manual skin graft meshing device.

by means of two parallel poles located close to one another. One pole is positive; the other is negative. The flow of current is restricted between these two poles, which are usually the tines of the bipolar forceps. Because the poles are so close, low voltages are used to achieve the tissue effect. Because electrical current does not flow through the patient, a return electrode (dispersive pad) is not necessary. This makes bipolar electrosurgery very safe and permits precise coagulation.

LASERS. A variety of lasers are employed for plastic surgical procedures. The perioperative nurse must ensure that the laser safety accessories specific to the type of laser being used are available. Laser safety is discussed in Chapter 7.

FIBEROPTIC INSTRUMENTS. Examples of fiberoptic instrument attachments used in plastic surgery are a headlight for rhinoplasties, augmentation mammoplasties, and other procedures; a mammary retractor for augmentation mammoplasties (Figure 24-6); a rhytidectomy retractor; abdominoplasty retractors; and endoscopic face and forehead fiberoptic instrumentation.

LOUPES. Loupes (Figure 24-7) are magnifying lenses used by many plastic surgeons for microvascular surgery and nerve repairs and for numerous other instances in which cosmetic results are improved by the magnification effect. The nurse should inquire about the use of loupes before the surgeon dons a headlight because adjustments will need to be made to the headlight alignment if the loupes are required in midprocedure. Adjusting or removing the headlight in midprocedure has the potential to contaminate the sterile field.

WOOD'S LAMP. The Wood's lamp (Figure 24-8) is an ultraviolet lamp used in determining viability of skin flaps in a darkened room. After IV injection of 20 ml of 5% sodium fluorescein, the blood vessels appear bright purple (the skin appears yellow). Sodium fluorescein is excreted in the urine, and patients should be informed of this.

ELECTROSURGICAL UNIT. The electrosurgical unit (ESU) and safety precautions taken by the perioperative nurse are described in Chapter 7.

MICROSCOPE. The microscope is frequently used in nerve repairs and microsurgical anastomoses. Chapter 18 provides a full description of operating microscopes.

INSTRUMENTATION. Basic instrument trays are kept available in the plastic surgery operating room. With modification by addition of instruments for specific operations, these trays suffice for all plastic surgery operations.

SPECIAL SUPPLIES. Surgeon-specific and procedure-specific special supplies are frequently added to instrument setups for plastic and reconstructive procedures. These commonly include the following:

- Marking pen or methylene blue
- Ruler

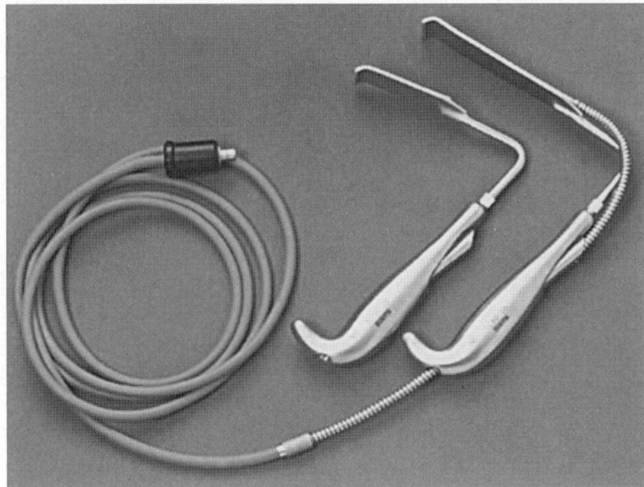

**FIGURE 24-6** Fiberoptic mammary retractors and cord.

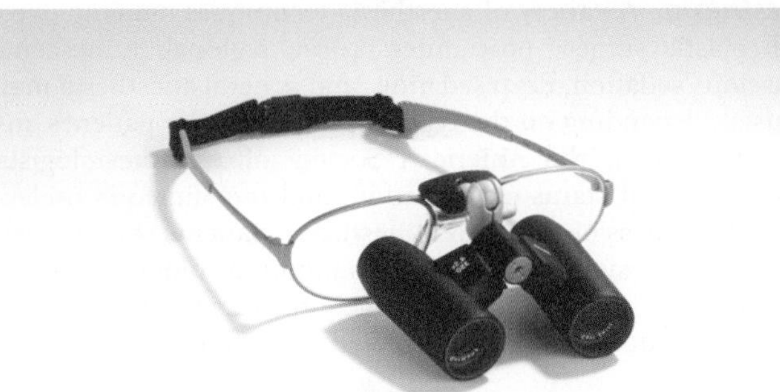

**FIGURE 24-7** Loupes from Carl Zeiss, used for magnification.

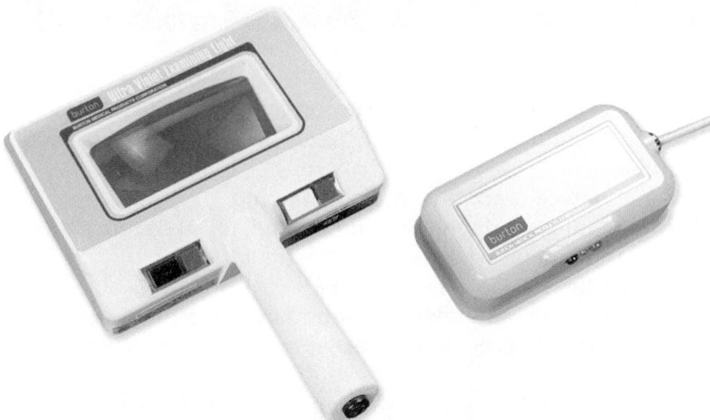


**FIGURE 24-8** Wood's lamp and cord assembly.

- X-ray film, unexposed (for pattern making; this can be steam-sterilized)
- Local anesthetic of choice for injection, with syringes and needles
- ESU, with active electrode (pencil) and tip of choice, with tip cleaner

***Sutures.*** Sutures range from permanent to absorbable and include monofilament and multifilament materials. The perioperative nurse should be a good steward of costly resources and should verify the type and number of sutures needed before opening, as well as needle preference, to prevent waste. Many plastic surgical procedures have multiple techniques, each of which necessitates very specific suture choices.

***Dressings.*** Dressings are an essential part of the operative procedure in plastic surgery and may contribute to the ultimate outcome of the surgical intervention. Dressings are usually applied while the patient is still anesthetized. In general, the dressing should accomplish the following five goals:

1. Immobilize the part.
2. Apply even pressure over the wound.
3. Collect drainage.
4. Provide comfort for the patient.
5. Protect the wound.

Pressure dressings may be used to eliminate dead space, to prevent seroma and hematoma formation, and to prevent third spacing associated with liposuction and reconstructive procedures involving transfer of large muscle or tissue flaps. In some cases pressure can be achieved by the use of catheters or drains placed within the operative site and connected to closed-wound suction devices, such as a Hemovac or Jackson-Pratt. In smaller wounds a butterfly cannula may be inserted into the operative site, with the needle end placed into a red-top tube, such as a blood collection tube, that has a vacuum (evacuated tube).

The perioperative nurse should be familiar with the following common general dressing supplies available in sterile form:

- Nonadherent gauze (e.g., Betadine gauze, Adaptic, NuGauze, Xeroform, Biobrane, Scarlet Red)
- Petrolatum gauze, $\frac{1}{2}$ inch (or other packing material, such as Merocel sponge for nasal packing)
- Telfa
- Fine mesh gauze
- Interface
- Gauze dressing sponges, $4 \times 4$ inches, $2 \times 2$ inches
- Kling, Kerlix fluff, and Kerlix gauze rolls (2, 4, and 6 inches wide)
- Abdominal pads (most commonly used are $5 \times 8$ inches)
- Skin tapes, flesh-colored and regular ($\frac{1}{8}$, $\frac{1}{4}$, $\frac{1}{2}$, and 1 inch wide)
- Cotton sheets and balls
- Webril

Also required are the following:

- Tape (adhesive, plain and waterproof; paper; silk; and foam)
- Benzoin spray or swab
- Ace bandages
- Coban
- Casting supplies (as required for postoperative immobilization)
- Abdominal binders and other postoperative garments
- Slings

In some instances, such as when a free flap is used, nontransparent dressings are avoided so that the flap can be monitored and observed for vascular flow. Compression garments and support devices are also frequently used by plastic surgeons. Proper fit is essential to minimize vascular compromise. Compression garments are typically applied over a light dressing.

***Implant Materials.*** The range of materials available for implantation and augmentation in the specialty of plastic and reconstructive surgery has benefited from ongoing research.

These materials may be classified into four broad categories: metals and alloys, polymers, ceramics, and acellular human and mammalian dermis.[10] Perioperative nurses are responsible for complying with tracking regulations for implantable materials and devices (Patient Safety).

The Incas of Peru (3000 BC) have been credited with using gold and silver to patch the holes they made in skulls after performing trephines.[16] Today, gold, cobalt-chromium, stainless steel, and titanium are commonly used metals and alloys for implantation, especially in craniofacial plating. They are corrosion-resistant, making them highly desirable as long-term implants.

Calcium ceramics may be used as bone graft substitutes. Hydroxyapatite has the ability to osseointegrate with bone.[7] Calcium ceramics are strong and have had long-term use in dentistry. They are silicate-based and chemically similar to osseous bone and teeth.[10]

Polymers (plastic materials) have had the greatest influence on the practice of implantation.[10] They come in various forms: solid, porous, woven, or as an injectable. Examples of solids are silicones, which despite the controversy of the early 1990s remain the most commonly used synthetic implant. Porous implants include Marlex, Proplast, Dacron patches, and Gore-Tex. Meshed polymers are Marlex mesh, Dacron, and Prolene. Polymers can be preformed or molded in situ, such as Cranioplast.[7]

Biologic materials (autogenous grafts) are preferred when available. Autologous human tissue successfully utilized includes fat, solid dermis, and collagen. Human cadavers are used as a source for acellular collagen (Alloderm). This product comes in various sizes of sheeting and must be rehydrated in several steps. An injectable form of cadaver collagen is Cymetra. Nonhuman sources of implantable materials are injectable bovine collagen (Zyderm, Zyplast), animal-based hyaluronic acid compound made from rooster's comb (Hylaform), and nonanimal third-generation hyaluronic acid gel (Restylane).

Implant failure may be directly linked to bacterial contamination; therefore meticulous aseptic technique with minimal handling is essential when using implants of any sort. Most alloplastic implants come presterilized from the manufacturer. When provided unsterile, the standard of care for handling implants is to apply sterile gloves (wiped free of powder with saline), wash the implant with a mild detergent, and rinse thoroughly with saline. After the implant is prepared it should be placed on a lint-free towel to be sterilized according to the manufacturer's recommendations.

***Anesthesia.*** A variety of anesthesia techniques are employed with plastic surgery procedures. Local, regional, tumescent, conscious sedation, deep sedation, and general anesthesia may be used, depending on the type of procedure, the patient's anesthetic history, the American Society of Anesthesiologists (ASA) physical status classification, and the surgeon's preference. Regardless of the type of anesthesia, patients should have baseline vital signs and be fully monitored: blood pressure, heart rate, respirations, cardiac rate and rhythm, oxygen saturation, and end-tidal $CO_2$ if indicated. If local or regional anes-

## PATIENT SAFETY

### Tracking Medical Devices

Popular topics for discussion relating to patient safety often center around the hands-on implementation of patient care. Nurses are cognizant of the importance of positioning, protection of the patient from fire hazards, and maintenance of sterile technique. Less thought may be given to the role of documentation in patient safety. The accurate documentation of perioperative events impacts patient safety, particularly in tracking implantable medical devices.

Tracking of implantable devices is critical to patient safety. The manufacturer of the device must have a mechanism to locate implantable devices after they have been distributed. Devices may be recalled for sterility issues, malfunction, or any event that is found to pose a serious health risk.

The U.S. Food and Drug Administration (FDA) regulates the process of tracking medical devices and directs the tracking of devices whose failure would result in serious, adverse health consequences; devices that are intended to be implanted in the human body for more than 1 year; and devices that are life-sustaining and life-supporting and are used outside a facility such as a hospital, nursing home, or ambulatory surgery center.

Plastic surgeons use a variety of implantable devices, from hardware to breast implants. The perioperative nurse plays an important role in the accurate documentation of these implantable devices for tracking purposes. Information that the nurse typically will gather for tracking purposes includes the following:

- Device identification (i.e., lot, batch, model number, serial number)
- Date of device manufacture and shipping
- Name, address, telephone number, and social security number of the patient who received the device
- Location the device was implanted
- Name, address, and telephone number of the physician who is caring for the patient, if different from the prescribing physician

Patients have the right to refuse to have their devices tracked and may refuse to have their social security number used for tracking. The patient's consent for tracking should be obtained before the procedure. If the patient refuses to have the device tracked, the nurse will document the refusal along with the required product information and report it to the manufacturer.

Under the Safe Medical Device Act, institutions must also report any incident of death or serious injury relating to the use of a medical device. The FDA has classified and identified more than 1700 different devices that must be reported if the device is suspected of causing serious injury or death to an individual. Nurses should work within their institutional policies to report these incidents.

Modified from Beyea SC: Tracking medical devices to ensure patient safety, *AORN Journal* 77(1), 2003; U.S. Food and Drug Administration: *Medical device tracking, guidance for industry and FDA staff.* Accessed February 16, 2006, on-line: www.fda.gov/cdrh/comp/guidance/169.html; U.S. Food and Drug Administration: *Medical device reporting.* Accessed March 18, 2006, on-line: www.fda.gov/cdrh/devadvice/351.html.

thesia is employed without an anesthesia provider, a perioperative nurse should be present whose only function is to monitor and assess the patient.

Injectable anesthetics are frequently used, not only for strictly local cases, but also in conjunction with regional, sedation, and even general anesthesia. Local anesthetics (Xylocaine, Marcaine, Citanest) act by reversibly blocking nerve impulses.[13] When combined with epinephrine, their vasoconstrictive properties allow for less bleeding, slower clearing of the local anesthetic agent, and therefore better visualization of the surgical site. In addition, infiltration of local anesthesia can help define tissue planes through hydrodissection. Use of epinephrine is contraindicated in areas with limited vascularity, such as digits, the penis, nasal tip, and ears. Although true allergic reactions are rare, they are still possible. Central nervous system toxicity is a more frequent occurrence and is dose-related. The nurse must be familiar with the signs and symptoms of toxicity, which are frequently heralded by restlessness. Early symptoms may include light-headedness, dizziness, nystagmus, and numbness of the tongue and lips; these may progress to slurred speech, disorientation, psychosis, muscle twitching, tremors and convulsions, and cardiac arrest.

Topical anesthetics used by the plastic surgeon include tetracaine (Pontocaine) 2% ophthalmic drops (for blepharoplasty or before application of eye shields), EMLA (Eutectic Mixture of Local Anesthetics) for penetration on intact skin (associated with laser surgery), and cocaine 4% for mucous membranes (for rhinoplasty).

Sedation may be light (conscious) or profound (deep). Commonly used agents for sedation include midazolam (Versed), ketamine, fentanyl (Sublimaze), and propofol (Diprivan). Midazolam is a benzodiazepine that provides excellent sedation and amnesia. It will potentiate the respiratory depression from narcotics and is a very mild muscle relaxant. The effects of midazolam can be reversed with flumazenil (Romazicon).

Ketamine, a dissociative anesthetic, is useful in providing pain relief and sedation without the profound respiratory depression associated with other agents. It can cause salivation, hallucinations, tachycardia, and seizures and is usually administered in small dosages following administration of a benzodiazepine. This will decrease the chances of hallucinations, "flashbacks," and seizures.

Fentanyl is a potent narcotic with rapid onset and short duration. As with all narcotics, respiratory depression, sedation, and nausea are common side effects. Respiratory depression (and pain relief) can be rapidly reversed with naloxone.

Propofol is a nonbarbiturate sedative-hypnotic. It can be administered as a bolus and supplemented by infusion. Its rapid onset and offset and amnesic and antiemetic properties make it a mainstay in providing sedation. Propofol does not provide any pain relief so other agents are usually added. It can cause profound respiratory depression and should only be administered in a setting with the equipment and personnel to assist in patient ventilation. For this reason, in many settings only an anesthesia provider is permitted to administer this drug.

***Preoperative Skin Preparation.*** Most surgical interventions require that the operative site and adjacent areas be cleansed before surgery. The physician may prescribe that the patient carry out this treatment before surgery. Special attention is given to the fingernails for patients undergoing hand surgery; to hair for surgery of the head, face, or neck; and to oral hygiene for surgery in or near the mouth. The perioperative nurse should verify with the patient that the prescribed regimens have been carried out. All body jewelry that pierces the skin should be removed before the skin prep. The operative site should be inspected for any rashes, bruises, open sores, cuts, or other skin conditions. Shaving is avoided, if possible, because it creates an access for the entry of bacteria into the operative site. The eyebrows and eyelashes, in particular, are left intact to preserve facial appearance and expression. The surgical site is marked before surgery by the surgeon to designate the correct site and to define landmark areas. Either a povidone-iodine solution, an iodine-alcohol mixture, chlorhexidine gluconate (CHG), or another broad-spectrum agent may be selected for the antimicrobial skin prep. The use of CHG should be avoided around the ears and eyes. It is important to place shields in eyes if prepping the periorbital site or performing an extensive head and neck prep, place plugs in the ear canals, and prevent pooling of the prep agent. The perioperative nurse should query the patient regarding any allergies to antimicrobial agents. If indicated, the plan of care should be changed to avoid the use of these products. When prepping for a skin graft procedure, separate skin prep setups are needed for the graft and donor sites.

***Positioning and Draping.*** The OR bed must be positioned so that remaining space in the room can comfortably accommodate anesthetic equipment, members of the surgical team, instrument tables, and any adjunct equipment (hand table, drills, microscope, laser) to be used. The patient is carefully positioned on the OR bed so that all operative sites may be appropriately exposed and the airway easily observed and accessed.

Before implementing any positioning changes, the perioperative nurse should verify the appropriate placement of the OR bed and the desired patient position. Adequate numbers of personnel and supportive positioning devices must be present. No changes should begin until the anesthesia provider gives permission. Whereas a majority of plastic surgical procedures are performed in the supine position, many also take place with the patient prone or lateral. Liposuction and post-bariatric body contouring procedures may also require repositioning one or more times during surgery. Abdominal procedures may start supine and usually require repositioning to facilitate closure. With each new position should come reassessment and documentation of the position and devices used to stabilize the patient. Chapter 5 reviews patient positioning and appropriate safety measures for the supine, lateral, and prone positions, all of which may be used during plastic surgical patient care.

Correct draping procedures depend on the location of the operative site or sites. Disposable drapes (see Chapter 3) are often used because of their barrier qualities, ease of handling and storage, and versatility in adapting to a variety of plastic surgery procedures. Two of the most frequently used draping techniques in plastic surgery are the head drape and the hand drape. Both of these draping techniques have the goal of providing maximum mobility of the operative part. The head drape includes a fluid-resistant drape that encircles the head and the addition of a drape to cover the remainder of the body.

The following techniques represent methods of obtaining maximum accessibility and sterile coverage for facial surgery:

1. A barrier sheet, folded in half, and two towels are placed beneath the patient's head with the towels uppermost. The folded barrier sheet covers the headrest or head portion of the OR bed. One towel is brought around the patient's head on each side to cover all hair, leaving the entire face (and ears, as necessary) exposed; the towel is then secured with towel clamps. For craniofacial procedures a towel folded lengthwise in quarters may be placed under the head to assist with moving the head from side to side. Two additional towels are then placed diagonally across the neck, just under the chin; they are secured to each other (with towel clamps) in the middle over the neck on each side to the towel around the head. A full sheet is then added to cover the patient from neck to feet.
2. After the head portion of the drape is placed, a split, or U, drape is added to cover the patient from neck to feet.

***Additional Considerations.*** Preparation is a key ingredient in success. Having backup supplies or equipment, sometimes as elementary as an extra bulb for the light source, can mean the difference in a positive outcome for the patient. Occasionally, during the course of a procedure, a flap may become congested and fail, the anatomy may dictate a change in the surgical plan, or perhaps a preselected implant just may not be right. Flexibility, meticulous preparation, and a willingness to improvise and innovate will always serve the perioperative nurse well when working with plastic surgeons.

## Evaluation

During the surgical intervention, the perioperative nurse is constantly evaluating the patient's response to nursing interventions, anesthesia, and the surgery itself. Progress or lack of progress toward the identified patient outcomes is continuously assessed. The results of this ongoing evaluation enable the perioperative nurse to reassess the patient, reorder priorities of patient care, establish new patient outcomes, and revise the perioperative plan of care.

At the conclusion of the surgical intervention the perioperative nurse reviews whether identified patient outcomes have been achieved. The patient's skin integrity is assessed; dressings are applied; and their integrity is established before discharge from the operating room. Any drains or tubes incorporated in the dressing should be noted. Infusion sites are inspected, and the type of infusing solution, flow rate, and amount infused are noted in the patient record. Local anesthetics, sedatives, or other medications received by the patient are similarly documented. The patient's response during the perioperative period is noted; any unusual or untoward responses are reported to the nurse in the recovery unit. The transport vehicle is obtained; any special equipment needed for patient transport is also obtained and checked for proper functioning. Warm blankets may be provided, and the patient is gently moved to the transport vehicle. The patient who is recovering from general anesthesia is placed in a safe position on the vehicle; the awake patient should be assisted to a position of comfort.

The perioperative nurse should give the hand-off report to the nurse in the postanesthesia care unit (PACU). Areas requiring ongoing patient observation should be noted in this report; the patient's preoperative, intraoperative, and immediate postoperative statuses are reported also. Using the Sample Plan of Care introduced earlier in this chapter, the perioperative nurse may give part of the report based on patient outcomes. If they were achieved, they may be stated as follows:

- The patient was able to verbalize his or her feelings about the proposed surgery.
- The patient's anxiety was decreased, and the patient was able to identify and verbalize sources of anxiety.
- The patient expressed understanding of the perioperative process through body language (relaxed expressions and nodding agreement) and verbalization.
- The patient remained free from injury related to the perioperative experience, including positioning.
- The patient exhibited signs of perfusion and sensation that were within normal limits following surgery.

## Patient and Family Education and Discharge Planning

Education of the plastic surgery patient begins at the time of consultation. Anxiety inhibits the retention of information; therefore it is always helpful to have written information or other tools for the patient to refer to, beginning with the preoperative instructions as well as postoperative information. Specifics that should be addressed include pain management (Surgical Pharmacology), self-care, diet, exercise, care of incisions and drains, return to the clinic for follow-up appointments, signs and symptoms of infections or complications, and how to reach the physician in case of an emergency.

Benefits of an effective education intervention are numerous; it serves to decrease anxiety, improves compliance, reduces the incidence of complications, empowers the patient to become an active participant in his or her own care, and maximizes independence, allowing the patient to return to an optimal state of health quicker. Just as the nursing process involves assessing, planning, implementing, and evaluating, so too does the educational plan. The patient's readiness to learn, needs, and styles of learning must be assessed. A teaching plan should be individualized based on the desired outcomes of all parties. The teaching should be implemented with respect to the most effective methods of learning for the individual, taking into account cultural, psychologic, physical, and cognitive limitations. The outcomes should be evaluated in terms of behavior changes that are incorporated into the patient's self-care and return to health.[5]

# *Surgical Interventions*

## Reconstructive Plastic Surgery

Reconstructive plastic surgery seeks to restore or improve function after trauma, disease, infection, congenital anomalies, or acquired defects while trying to approximate an aesthetic appearance.

### REMOVAL OF SKIN CANCERS

More than 1 million skin cancers are diagnosed each year in the United States alone.[21] The three most common skin cancers are basal cell, squamous cell, and melanoma. Basal cells account for approximately 70% of all skin cancers (Figure 24-9). If basal

## SURGICAL PHARMACOLOGY

### Postoperative Pain Medications

A discussion about postoperative pain management is an important component of the patient education process. Patients undergoing plastic surgery procedures have several options available for pain control. The perioperative nurse must be familiar with analgesic medications used in the immediate and discharge phases of postanesthesia recovery to provide safe care and appropriate education to the patient.

**PATIENT-CONTROLLED ANALGESIA**

Depending on the extent and scope of the procedure, patient-controlled analgesia (PCA) may be an effective option in the inpatient setting. PCA is controlled by a special infusion pump that is programmed to administer a calculated intravenous dose of medication when the patient presses a button on the hand control. Opioid analgesics are typically used for PCA.

**LOCAL ANESTHETIC INFUSION SYSTEMS**

An alternative technique for managing postoperative pain is the continuous instillation of local anesthesia to the surgical site by way of multilumen catheters placed intramuscularly or in the subcutaneous tissue.

As the procedure is ending, the surgeon places the catheters in the surgical wound, exiting through the skin. The catheters are attached to a pump that can contain up to 300 ml of local anesthesia. The surgeon or registered nurse first assistant (RNFA) fills the pump reservoir during the intraoperative phase of care, calculating the volume needed based on the anticipated length of time the pump will be in use and volume to be administered per dose. Alternatively, the pump may come prefilled from the pharmacy. A tissue adhesive agent may be used at the exit site to prevent leakage of the local anesthesia. The catheters are secured with Steri-Strips at the exit site and covered with a transparent, occlusive dressing.

The pump enables a continuous infusion of the local anesthetic agent for the desired number of days (usually 2 to 4). A new option for this technique is a device that offers on-demand delivery of local anesthesia by the patient, which features a protective lockout that prevents overdosage. Plastic surgeons routinely use this technique after submuscular augmentation, abdominoplasty, and breast reconstruction.

**NURSING IMPLICATIONS**

Refer to Chapter 4 for information relating to local anesthetics. Commonly used agents include bupivacaine (Marcaine, Sensorcaine), levobupivacaine (Chirocaine), ropivacaine (Naropin), and lidocaine (Xylocaine).

Contraindications for use of the pump include known allergy to local anesthesia, significant kidney or liver disease, insulin-dependent diabetes, a current bacterial infection, or long-term use of local anesthesia. The patient may be sent home with the catheters in place; however, since there is no maintenance once the reservoirs are filled and secured, it is not necessary to use home health nurses. The perioperative nurse should make sure the patient or caregiver has the necessary information to monitor for signs of local anesthesia toxicity: tinnitus, blurred vision, confusion, a metallic taste or numbness of the tongue, or tingling of the fingers or toes.

| Medication | Dosage | Side Effects | Nursing Considerations |
|---|---|---|---|
| Morphine sulfate | Loading dose: 5-10 mg<br>Intermittent bolus: 0.5-3 mg<br>Lockout interval: 5-12 min | Sedation<br>Hypotension<br>Nausea | Monitor for respiratory depression.<br>Initiate deep breathing and coughing exercises.<br>Provide instruction to patient on how to operate the system. |
| Meperidine hydrochloride (Demerol) | Loading dose: 50-100 mg<br>Intermittent bolus: 5-30 mg<br>Lockout interval: 10-20 min | Vomiting<br>Dizziness<br>Diaphoresis<br>Somnolence | Breakthrough pain may be possible as administration ceases when the patient is asleep.<br>Monitor patient's response to patient-controlled analgesia (PCA), and treat oversedation per institutional protocol. |

Modified from Hodgson BB, Kizior RJ: *Mosby's 2006 drug consult for nurses,* St Louis, 2006, Mosby; Kampe S and others: Concept for postoperative analgesia after pedicled TRAM flaps: continuous wound instillation with 0.2% Ropivacaine via multilumen catheters. A report of two cases, *The British Association of Plastic Surgeons* 56:478-483, 2003; Breast PM: Augmentation and abdominoplasty: postoperative management with pain pumps, *Aesthetic Surgery Journal* 25:69-71, 2005; Vinter N and others: Incisional self-administration of Bupivacaine or Ropivacaine provides effective analgesic after inguinal hernia repair, *Canadian Journal of Anesthesia* 49:481-486, 2002; White P and others: Use of a continuous local anesthetic infusion for pain management after median sternotomy, *Anesthesiology* 99(4):918-923, 2003.

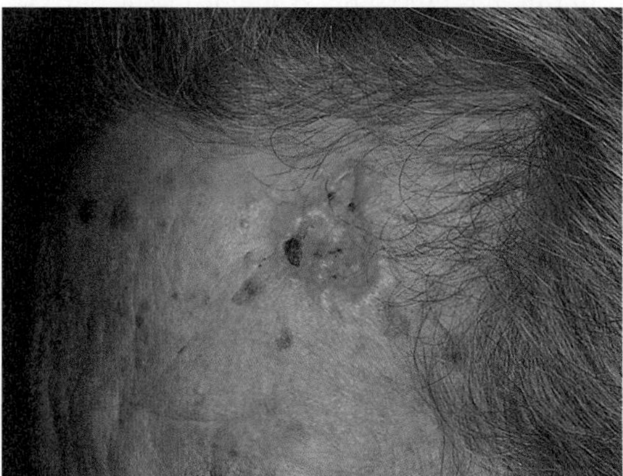

**FIGURE 24-9** Basal cell carcinoma; note the rolled, well-defined margin.

cell cancer is left untreated, it will grow but rarely metastasizes (Box 24-1). Treated early, it may be cured by simple excision and closure (with pathologic diagnosis to ensure disease-free margins). Squamous cell skin cancers are considered more aggressive (Figure 24-10). Surgical treatment is the same as for basal cell carcinomas. Melanoma accounts for the smallest percentage of skin cancers, but it is treated much more aggressively because of its high mortality rate (Figure 24-11). Excision of melanoma may involve sentinel node mapping and excision.[24] Early diagnosis of melanoma is key to successful treatment (Best Practice).

## Procedural Considerations

Consideration must be given to the type of skin cancer to be excised and the anticipated closure. Simple excision and closure with adjacent tissue will be the simplest technique, re-

BOX 24-1

## Important Trends for Skin Cancer

**INCIDENCE**
Approximately 1 million cases per year with the majority being the highly curable basal or squamous cell cancers, accounting for more than 50% of all cancers; not as common is the most serious malignant melanoma, with an estimated 59,580 cases per year.

**MORTALITY**
Total estimated deaths in 2005 were 7700 from malignant melanoma and 10,500 from other skin cancers.

**RISK FACTORS**
- Excessive exposure to ultraviolet radiation from the sun
- Fair complexion
- Occupational exposure to coal tar, pitch, creosote, arsenic compounds, and radium
- Exposure to human papillomavirus and human immunodeficiency virus
- Skin cancer negligible in African Americans because of heavy skin pigmentation

**WARNING SIGNALS**
Any unusual skin conditions, especially a change in the size or color of a mole or other darkly pigmented growth or spot.

**PREVENTION AND EARLY DETECTION**
Avoid sun when ultraviolet light is strongest (e.g., 10:00 AM to 3:00 PM); use sunscreen preparations, especially those containing ingredients such as para-aminobenzoic acid (PABA). Basal and squamous cell cancers often form a pale, waxlike, pearly nodule or a red, scaly, sharply outlined patch; melanomas are usually dark brown or black pigmentation; they start as small molelike growths that increase in size, change color, become ulcerated, and bleed easily from a slight injury.

**TREATMENT**
The four methods of treatment are surgery, electrodesiccation (tissue destruction by heat), radiation therapy, and cryosurgery (tissue destruction by freezing). For malignant melanomas, wide and often deep excisions and removal of nearby lymph nodes are required.

**SURVIVAL**
For basal cell and squamous cell cancers, cure is virtually ensured with early detection and treatment. Malignant melanoma, however, metastasizes quickly; this accounts for a lower 5-year survival rate for Caucasian patients with this disease.

From McCance KL, Huether SE: *Pathophysiology: the biologic basis for disease in adults and children,* ed 5, St Louis, 2006, Mosby.

quires a local plastic tray accompanied by skin markers and the ESU, and usually involves local anesthesia with epinephrine. A simple excision may be performed with the patient under local, sedation, or general anesthesia. If additional procedures will be performed (reconstruction with skin graft, flap, or sentinel node mapping), refer to those sections for additional procedural considerations.

## Operative Procedure—Simple Excision

1. The site is prepped and draped.
2. Local anesthesia is infiltrated.
3. The lesion is curetted or excised and may be sent for frozen section or pathologic diagnosis.

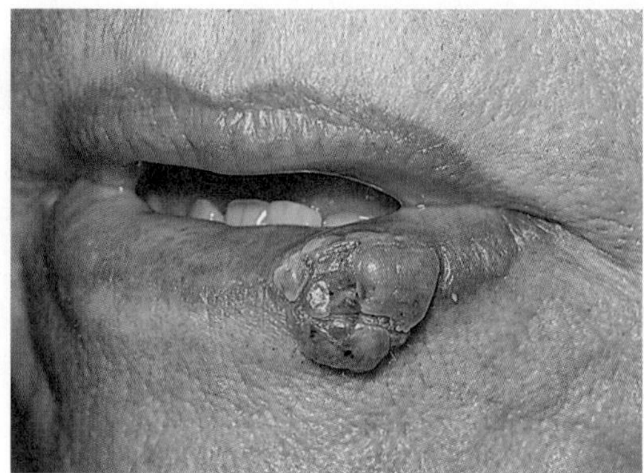

FIGURE 24-10 Squamous cell carcinoma of the lip.

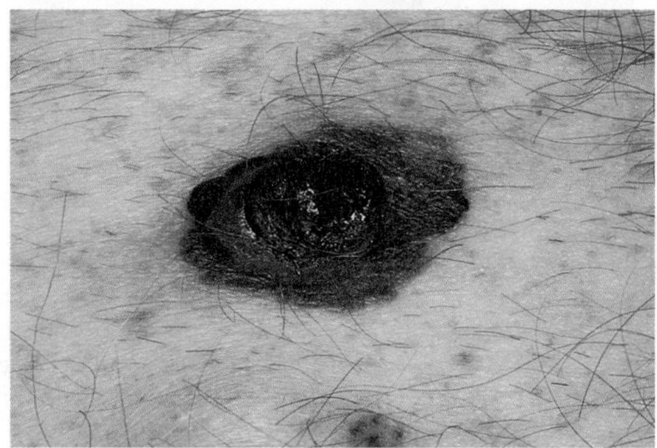

FIGURE 24-11 Malignant melanoma.

4. Hemostasis is obtained.
5. The wound is closed if necessary.

## Mohs' Surgery

Mohs' surgery is a specialized excision used to treat basal and squamous cell skin cancers. The procedure involves excising the lesion layer by layer and examining each layer under the microscope until all the abnormal tissue is removed.

*Procedural Considerations.* Mohs' surgery is usually completed on an ambulatory basis with the patient under local anesthesia. The procedure can be very time consuming to accomplish, but it typically results in the preservation of the surrounding healthy tissue. Because the procedure is lengthy, patient preparation and comfort are essential to facilitate cooperation during the procedure. A minor plastic surgery set is required, along with fine (5-0 or 6-0) suture material.

*Operative Procedure.* Current procedures involve removal of all visible portions of the skin cancer lesion. A horizontal layer of tissue is removed and divided into sections that are color-coded with dyes. A map of the surgical site is then drawn. Frozen sections are immediately prepared and examined microscopically for any remaining tumor. If tumor is found, the location or locations are noted on the map and another layer of tissue is resected. The procedure is repeated as many times as necessary to completely remove the tumor.

## BURN SURGERY

A majority of burns result from exposure to high temperatures, which injures the skin. Flame, scalding, or direct contact with a hot object may cause thermal skin injury. Similar destruction

## BEST PRACTICE

It is estimated that more than 62,190 men and women will be diagnosed with melanoma in 2006, according to the American Cancer Society. The current lifetime risk of developing melanoma is 1 in 63 as compared with 1:1500 in 1935. Half of the melanomas are diagnosed in individuals under the age of 57 years.

Although the exact cause of developing a melanoma is not known, certain risk factors have been identified:

- **Ultraviolet (UV) radiation:** sunlight, tanning beds
- **Moles:** more than 50 = greater risk
- **Fair skin:** fair skin, freckling, red or blond hair
- **Family history:** 10% have a relative with melanoma
- **Immune system compromise:** taking antirejection medications after organ transplantation surgery
- **Age:** increased risk in older adults
- **Gender:** men more than women
- **Previous melanoma:** increased risk for having another melanoma

**PREVENTION**

Limit UV radiation exposure:

1. Wear protective clothing (tight weave) and a hat with a broad brim.
2. Shade is good—avoid too much sunlight; remember that it reflects off water, sand, concrete, and snow.
3. Use sunscreen—SPF 15 or higher; apply 20 to 30 minutes before sun exposure; reapply every 2 hours; protect your lips.
4. Do not forget your eyes—look for sunglasses with 99% UV absorption.
5. Stay away from tanning beds and lamps—more UV exposure; try using self-tanning lotions.
6. Children need sunscreen—their skin is fragile; most damage to skin is acquired before the age of 18 years.
7. Take an inventory—know your moles and what they normally look like so you can detect changes if and when they occur.

**KNOW YOUR A-B-C-Ds**

**A**: Asymmetry—one half of the lesion looks different from the other side.

**B**: Border irregularity—instead of a smooth edge, the border is ragged or irregular.

**C**: Color—the color is usually irregular as well; may have a number of different hues and colors.

**D**: Diameter—lesions larger than 6 mm have a greater chance of being a melanoma.

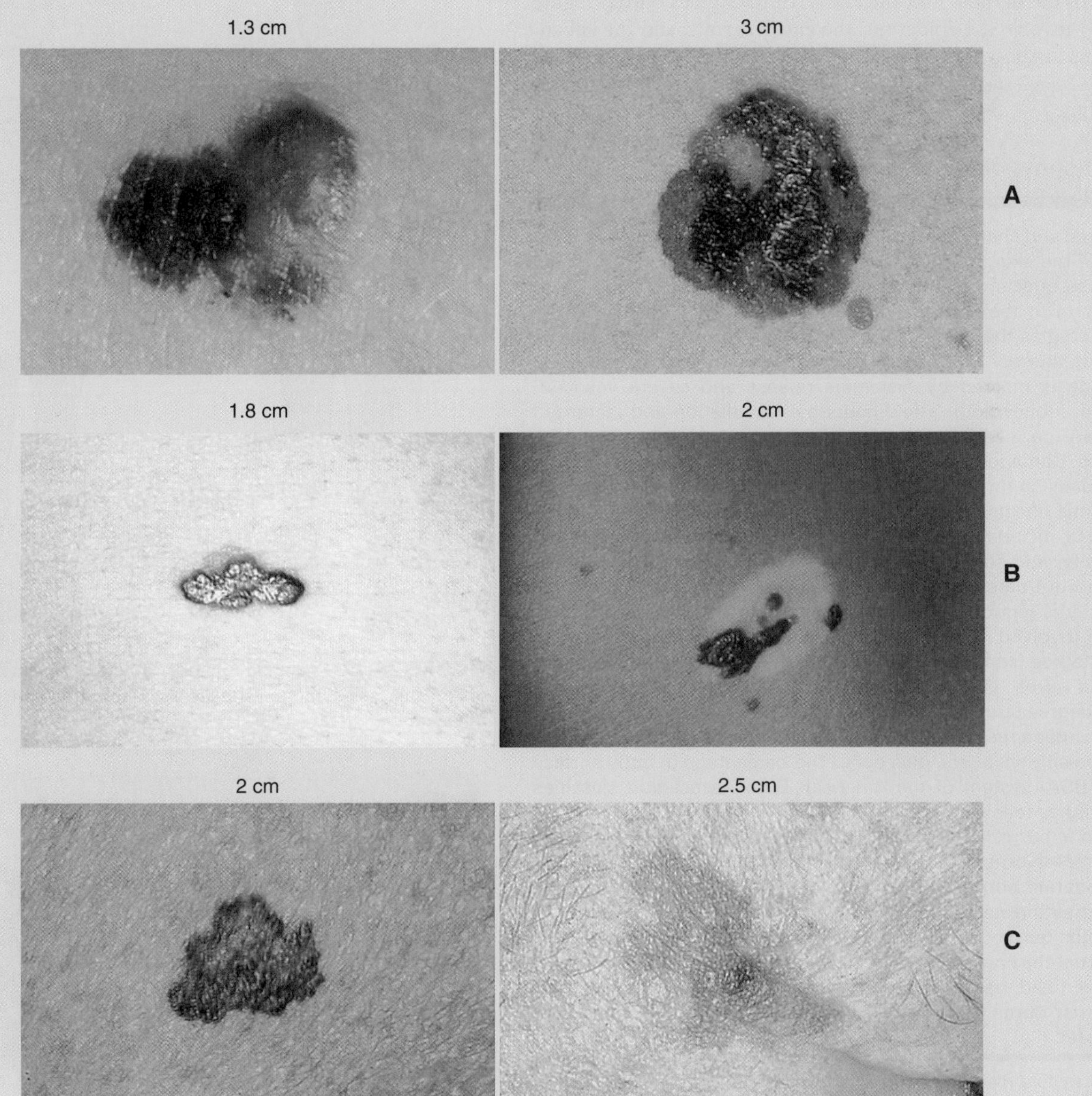


Accessed October 3, 2005, on-line: www.skincarephysicians.com/skincancernet/skin_html.

Malignant melanomas. Note presence of *"ABCDE"* characteristics (*a*symmetry, irregular *b*order, varation in *c*olor, *d*iameter>6mm, *e*nlargement, and elevation.) **A,** Superficial spreading melanoma, **B,** nodular melanomas, **C,** lentigo malignant melanomas of skin can result from contact with chemicals such as acid or alkali or contact with an electrical current. The latter, however, often involves extensive destruction of the underlying tissue and physiologic systems in addition to the skin. Nationwide, more than 2 million burn injuries occur every year.[6]

Intact skin provides protection against the environment for all underlying tissues and organs. It aids in heat regulation, prevents water loss, and is the major barrier against bacterial invasion. The tissue injury resulting from a burn disrupts this normal protective function, resulting in local and systemic effects (Box 24-2). Burn patients are therefore some of the most acutely ill patients brought to the OR. The greater the degree of injury to the skin, expressed in percentage of total body surface area (BSA) and depth of burn, the more severe the injury. One method of measuring BSA is by use of the rule of nines (Figure 24-12).

Partial-thickness (first- and second-degree) burns heal by regeneration of skin from dermal elements that remain intact. First-degree burns involve the epidermis, which appears pink or red; sunburn is usually a first-degree burn. Second-degree burns, also called partial-thickness burns, involve the epidermis and some of the dermis. Full-thickness (third-degree) burns (Figure 24-13) involve the epidermis, the entire dermis, and the subcutaneous tissues; they require skin grafting to heal because no dermal elements remain intact. Both partial- and full-thickness burns may require debridement of necrotic tissue (eschar) before healing can occur by skin regeneration or grafting. Allograft may be used to cover the burned area during the initial healing process (Research Highlight). However, the allograft must be carefully tested for immunodeficiency diseases. Xenograft (e.g., pig skin) may also be used for covering the burned area.

## Procedural Considerations

The essentials of skin grafting are discussed in "Skin and Tissue Grafting," p. 878. This section therefore deals only with the procedure for debridement of burn wounds.

A basic plastic instrument set is required, plus a knife dermatome, an ESU, topical thrombin solution, a pneumatic tourniquet for isolated extremity burns, and a topical antimicrobial agent of choice.

Because patients who have sustained burns are vulnerable to hypothermia from the loss of BSA, the perioperative nurse

### BOX 24-2

### Pathophysiology of Burn Injuries

Thermal and chemical injuries disrupt the normal protective function of the skin, causing local and systemic effects. The extent of these effects depends on the type, duration, and intensity of exposure to the causative agent. With electrical burns, heat is generated as the electrical current passes through body tissues, causing thermal burns along the path taken by the current. Local damage is marked by histamine release and severe vasoconstriction, followed in a few hours by vasodilation and increased capillary permeability, which allows plasma to escape into the wound. Damaged cells swell and platelets and leukocytes aggregate, causing thrombotic ischemia and escalating tissue damage. Systemic effects, which are caused by vascular changes and tissue loss, include hypovolemia, hyperventilation, increased blood viscosity, and suppression of the immune system. The severity of the burn determines the extent of local and systemic effects. Severity is judged by the depth of the burn and the quantity of tissue involved. The depth of the burn is classified by degree. First-degree (superficial) burns affect the epidermis only; second-degree burns (split thickness) affect the epidermis and dermis; third-degree burns (full thickness) affect all skin layers and extend to subcutaneous tissue, muscle, and nerves; fourth-degree burns involve all skin layers, plus bone. The percentage of body surface area (BSA) system of the American Burn Association classifies quantity as follows:

- Minor burn: full-thickness burns over less than 2% of BSA; partial-thickness burns over less than 15% of BSA
- Moderate burns: full-thickness burns over 2% to 10% of BSA; partial-thickness burns over less than 15% to 25% of BSA
- Major burns: full-thickness burns over 10% or more of BSA; partial-thickness burns over 25% or more of BSA; any burn to face, head, hands, feet, or perineum; inhalation and electrical burns; burns complicated by trauma or other disease processes

From Langford RW, Thompson JD: *Mosby's handbook of diseases,* ed 3, St Louis, 2005, Mosby.

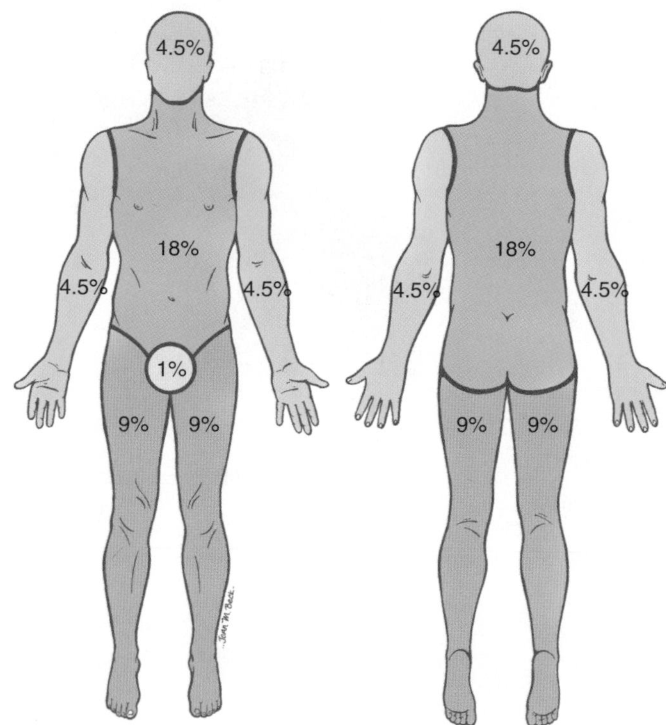


**FIGURE 24-12** The "rule of nines." Dividing the body into 11 areas of 9% each helps one to estimate the amount of skin surface burned in an adult.

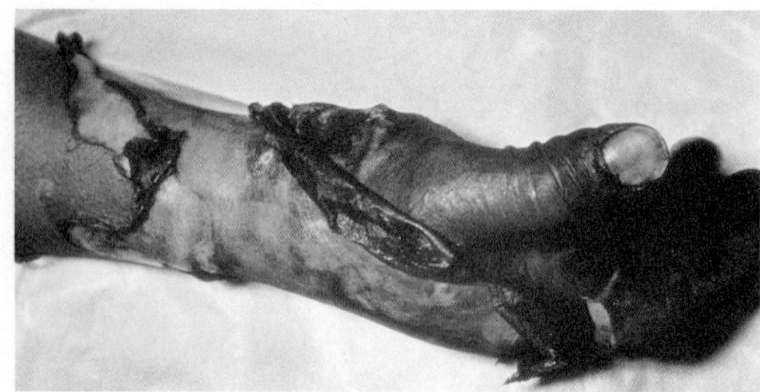

**FIGURE 24-13** Full-thickness thermal injury.

## RESEARCH HIGHLIGHT

### Treating Facial Burns with Allografts

Facial burns are very common, occurring in at least 30% to 50% of minor to moderate burns and more than 50% of major burns. Burns to the face have a clinical and psychologic effect on the victim.

An important factor in scar formation is healing time. The longer a wound stays open, the greater the chance of scarring. This study investigated the use of cadaver skin grafting in deep partial-thickness facial burns in comparison with standard burn care using silver sulfadiazine.

Ten study participants were randomized into two groups. One group received silver sulfadiazine as a treatment, and the other group received early superficial debridement followed by coverage with glycerolized cadaver skin. The outcome measures were time and quality of wound healing and incidence of hypertrophic scarring at 3 and 6 months after the burn.

The group treated with the glycerolized cadaver skin re-epithelialized in 10.5 days while the silver sulfadiazine group took 12.5 days to show re-epithelialization. Scar quality was improved in the allogenic treatment group. At 3 and 6 months, no patients in the allogenic treatment group had significant scarring, whereas two patients in the silver sulfadiazine group developed hypertrophic scars.

A limitation to this study was its small sample size. Replication of the protocol with a larger number of patients is needed to validate the results.

Modified from Horch RA and others: Treatment of second degree facial burns with allografts—preliminary results, *Burns* 31:597-602, 2005.

should ensure the temperature and humidity in the OR are increased and exposure is limited only to the areas related to the planned surgical event. Anesthesia is often induced while the patient is on the burn unit bed; transfer to the OR bed is done carefully and gently, with attention to maintaining the airway. Most burn patients arrive in the OR with dressings covering their wounds. The dressings are removed after the patient has been anesthetized to minimize pain and loss of body heat through the open burn wounds. Throughout the procedure, the temperature in the OR is constantly monitored to prevent hypothermia. The OR team caring for burn patients coordinates activities to prevent any delays in obtaining required equipment or supplies. The perioperative nurse will need to collaborate with the anesthesia provider in determining fluid replacement requirements.

### Operative Procedure

1. Nonviable tissue is excised down to underlying muscle fascia.
2. An alternative method is tangential excision of the burn wound, which is performed with a knife dermatome. This type of excision is usually carried down only to subcutaneous fat, rather than to fascia.
3. Hemostasis is obtained with electrocoagulation or use of topical thrombin solution.
4. Dressings saturated with the topical antimicrobial agent of choice are applied.

Although skin grafting may be done at the time of wound debridement, it is usually performed several days later, particularly in burns that are extensive.

### Cultured Epithelial Autografting (CEA) and Artificial Skin

In the event that the patient has been massively burned (more than 90% of the body surface) or has a wound that would be open for 21 days after injury, the need for coverage is critical. A skin biopsy (about the size of a postage stamp) is taken from the axilla, groin, postauricular area, or sole of the foot. These areas, even in massive burn injuries, are sometimes available. The biopsy tissue is then sent to a specific technologic laboratory, where the full-thickness biopsy tissue is placed in a specially developed culture medium, maintained nutritionally, and allowed to grow. Through the course of 21 days and fastidious care of the cultured skin by the technology laboratory personnel, it can be expected that there will be enough skin to cover the patient's wounds. Another method, artificial skin, was approved in 2001. The bioengineered skin reduces scarring, length of hospital stays, and the number of reconstructive procedures burn patients undergo. In this procedure, cow collagen and a carbohydrate derived from shark cartilage are covered with a thin sheet of silicon, which mimics the outer layer of skin. When placed on a burn wound, it serves as scaffolding for damaged dermis to lay down new collagen in an orderly fashion, resembling normal skin in its appearance. Once the dermal layer has begun to regenerate, the surgeon can remove the flexible top layer and replace it with ultrathin skin grafts.[14]

***Procedural Considerations.*** The previously described considerations for acute burn surgery can be followed. The cultured skin, when ready to be placed on the patient, is transported to the institution in a box that maintains a controlled atmosphere. The cultured skin, which had been placed in individual plastic containers in the atmosphere-controlled box, is positioned on the patient's wound and secured with nylon netting, which is stapled in place; the dressings are applied. The number of cultured skin pieces as well as their location is documented by use of photography and notation on the patient's record.

#### *Operative Procedure*

1. The dressings, Biobrane, or pig skin (if applicable) are removed to expose the burn wound.
2. The cultured skin is applied.
3. The cultured skin is secured with nylon netting, which is stapled in place.
4. Hemostasis is achieved with electrocoagulation and topical hemostatic solutions.
5. The wound is dressed using large pieces of flat gauze, Webril, and Kling wrap.

## DEBRIDEMENT

Debridement is the act of removing dead or devitalized tissue to promote healing. Plastic surgeons use debridement in conjunction with treating injuries, trauma, and infection. Additional information on wound debridement may be found in Chapter 8.

## TREATMENT OF PRESSURE ULCERS

Pressure ulcers result from prolonged compression of soft tissues overlying bony prominences (Figure 24-14). However, whether excessive pressure is sufficient to create an ulcer de-

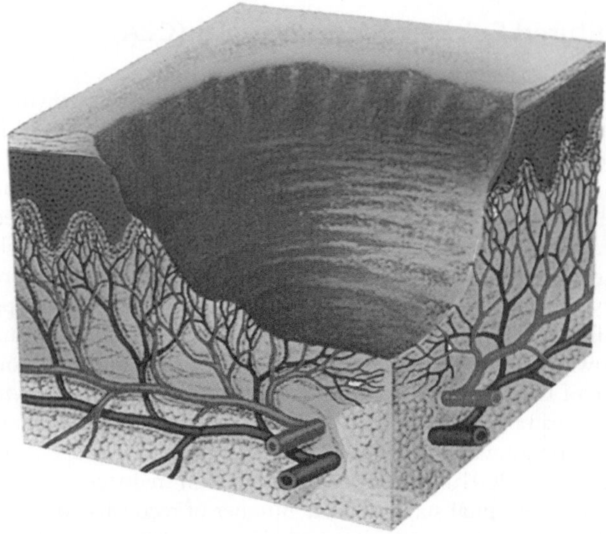

FIGURE 24-14 Pressure ulcers often appear after blood flow to an area slows or is obstructed because of pressure on bony prominences. Infections often follow, since lack of blood flow causes tissue damage or death.

pends on the intensity and duration of the pressure as well as on tissue tolerance. Factors that contribute to pressure ulcer development are immobility, sensory and motor deficits, reduced circulation, anemia, edema, infection, moisture, shearing force, friction, and nutritional debilitation.[8] The most common sites of pressure ulcers are the sacrum, the ischium, the trochanter, the malleolus, and the heel. Surgical interventions for pressure ulcers are usually based on ulcer staging (also referred to as *grading*). In stage I the ulcer involves the epidermis and has soft-tissue swelling that is irregular and ill defined; heat and erythema at the ulcer site are characteristic. A stage II ulcer involves the epidermis and dermis but not the subcutaneous fat. Stage III ulcers show full-thickness skin loss with injury to underlying tissue layers and may contain necrotic material. Thorough debridement is performed, and IV antibiotic therapy is instituted. Although debrided stage III ulcers often heal on their own, surgical excision and closure may be done to prevent a lengthy spontaneous closure, which may result in a weak, unstable scar with resultant recurrence. Stage IV ulcers are the deepest, requiring more radical debridement. Adequate soft-tissue cover may be obtained by either split-thickness or full-thickness skin grafting or tissue flaps (Figure 24-15). Tissue expansion may be used where there is not enough tissue adjacent to the ulcer site to provide flap coverage.

An alternative to the standard surgical approach is the use of the $CO_2$ laser. The laser offers the advantage of minimizing blood loss and possibly reducing infection rates in the presence of gross contamination.

Although many techniques and flaps are surgical options, basic principles apply to all pressure ulcer closure procedures. The following procedure is for an adjacent flap.

### Procedural Considerations

A basic plastic instrument set is required, as well as assorted sizes of osteotomes (straight and curved), a mallet, the Gigli saw and handle, assorted curettes, a Key periosteal elevator, a duck-bill rongeur, bone wax, the dermatome of choice, the ESU, a marking pen, and a closed-wound drainage system. The patient is positioned and draped so that the pressure ulcer, adjacent flap donor site, and a skin graft donor site are well exposed.

### Operative Procedure

1. The area to be excised and the local flap are outlined.
2. The ulcer is excised along with the underlying bony prominence.
3. Large suction catheters are placed into the defect left by excision of the ulcer and beneath the flap.
4. The flap is sutured in place.
5. A split-thickness skin graft generally is used to resurface the flap donor site.
6. A stent dressing is placed over the skin graft, and gauze dressings or a plastic spray dressing is applied over the suture lines of the flap.

## SKIN AND TISSUE GRAFTING

Skin grafting provides an effective way to cover a wound if vascularity is adequate, infection is absent, and hemostasis is achieved. Skin from the donor site is detached from its blood supply and placed in the recipient site, where it develops a new blood supply from the base of the wound. Color match, contour, and durability of the graft are all considerations in selection of an appropriate donor area. Other types of grafts that are available for surgical reconstruction include bone, cartilage, nerve, tendon, and autologous fat grafts.

### Split-Thickness and Full-Thickness Skin Grafts

Skin grafts can be either split-thickness or full-thickness grafts (Figure 24-16). A split-thickness (or partial-thickness) skin graft contains epidermis and only a portion of the dermis of the donor site; it varies from a thin graft to a thick graft. Although this type of graft becomes vascularized more rapidly and the donor site heals more rapidly than a full-thickness graft, it may exhibit postgraft contraction, be minimally resistant to surface trauma, and look the least like normal skin in texture, suppleness, pore pattern, hair growth, and other characteristics. A split-thickness skin graft (STSG) may be meshed; meshed grafts can expand to many times their original size. Meshing allows the graft to be placed on an irregular recipient area; however, its appearance may be aesthetically undesirable. A full-thickness skin graft (FTSG) contains both epidermis and dermis; any remaining subcutaneous tissue is trimmed before the FTSG is applied to the graft site. The advantages of this type of graft are that it causes minimal contracture, can be used in areas of flexion, has a greater ability to withstand trauma, can add tissue where a loss has occurred or where padding is required, and is aesthetically more acceptable than an STSG. The donor site can be closed primarily, leaving a minimal defect.

The donor site for an STSG heals by regeneration of epithelium from dermal elements that remain intact. Therefore only a dressing is placed over this donor site. Because no dermal elements remain when an FTSG is taken, this donor site does not heal spontaneously. It heals either when the wound edges of the donor site are sutured together (primary closure) or when an STSG is applied over it. A scar remains at the donor site of a skin graft. Therefore donor sites that are covered by clothing are generally chosen.

For a graft to survive, the vascularity of the recipient area must be adequate, contact between the graft and recipient bed

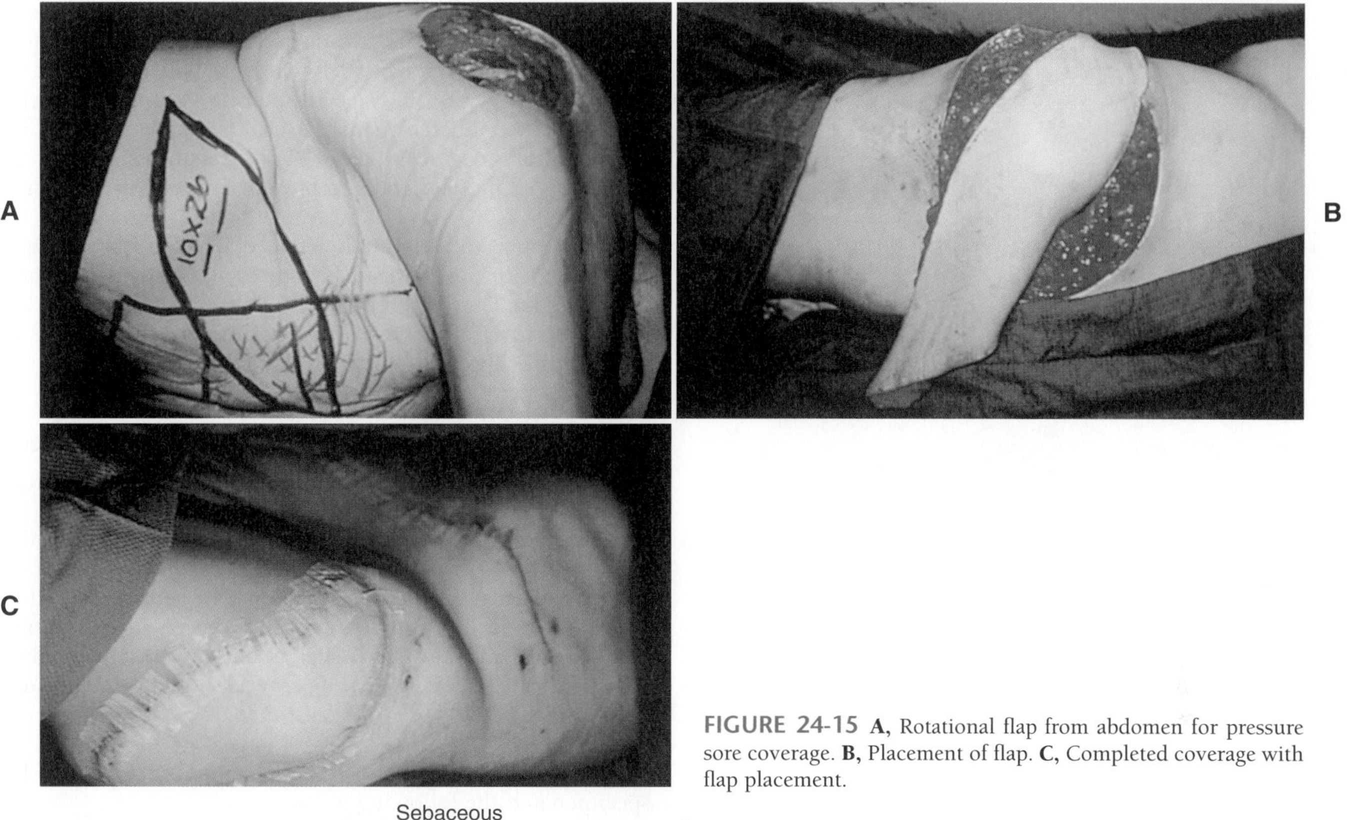


FIGURE 24-15 **A,** Rotational flap from abdomen for pressure sore coverage. **B,** Placement of flap. **C,** Completed coverage with flap placement.

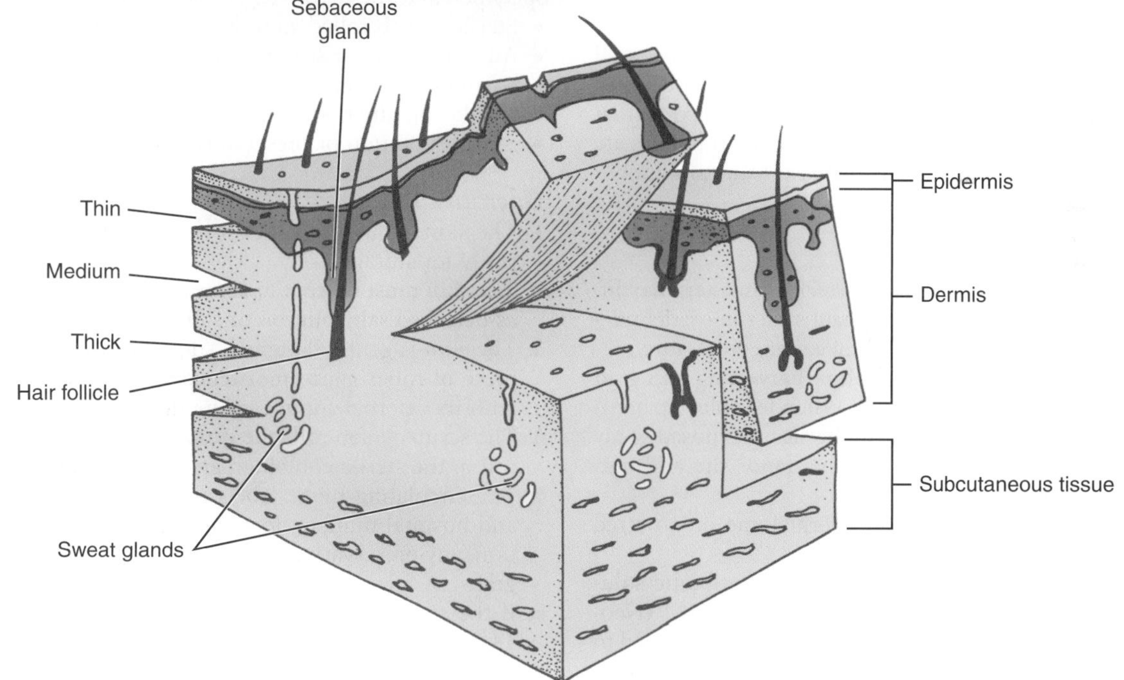


FIGURE 24-16 Split-thickness and full-thickness skin grafts.

must be maintained, and the graft-bed unit must be adequately immobilized.

Color, temperature, signs of infection, blanching of the skin, excessive pain and discomfort, edema, vasoconstriction, and venous congestion should be noted and any change reported to the surgeon.

Any changes should be documented. If the patient is discharged to home after surgery, patient and family education should include reportable signs and symptoms of potential complications.

A stent or tie-over dressing is often placed over a skin graft (Figure 24-17). This exerts even pressure, ensuring good contact between graft and recipient site. It also eliminates potential shearing forces at the graft and recipient site interface that might disrupt new blood vessels growing into the graft.

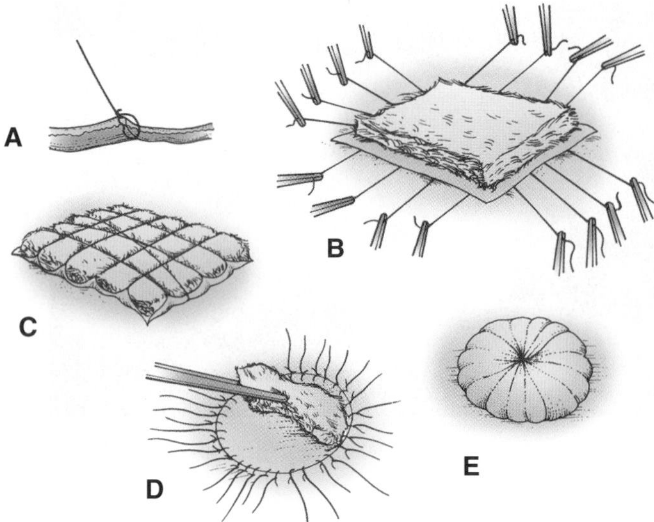


FIGURE 24-17 **A,** Method of fixation of skin graft to edges of wound. **B,** Nonadherent dressing is applied over skin graft and on this a generous pad of acrylic fiber. **C,** Long ends of suture are tied over fiber to produce area of pressure between graft and base. **D,** Similar dressing is applied to circular graft. **E,** Long suture ends are tied over circular graft (often called *stent dressing*).

## Procedural Considerations

A plastic local instrument set is required, with the addition of a dermatome of choice, a skin mesher, a marking pen, and sterile unexposed x-ray film. The patient is positioned so that both donor and recipient sites are well exposed. Both areas are prepped and draped to maintain adequate exposure and mobility, as required.

## Operative Procedure

1. The recipient site is prepared as necessary. This step may involve excision of a benign or malignant skin tumor, debridement of an open wound, or release of a scar contracture.
2. Careful planning and marking before harvesting the graft from the recipient site are essential. When feasible, a pattern of the recipient site is made with sterile unexposed x-ray film. This pattern is transferred to the donor site and outlined with a marking pen.
3. STSGs are harvested with a knife dermatome or powered dermatome of the surgeon's choice.
4. Moist sponges soaked in normal saline, an antibiotic solution, or a solution of 20 mg of phenylephrine HCl (Neo-Synephrine) per 1000 ml of normal saline may be applied to the donor sites to aid hemostasis. A small amount of methylene blue may be placed in the labeled solution of Neo-Synephrine as a marker to further identify it from other solutions on the sterile field. These sponges are removed, and the donor site is covered with Biobrane or OpSite.
5. If the graft is to be meshed, it is now applied to specifically supplied carriers for use with certain skin meshers.
6. A graft that is not immediately applied to the recipient site dries quickly, particularly a meshed graft. Therefore grafts should be kept in moist gauze sponges contained in a small basin to prevent inadvertent loss of the graft. Meshed skin should not be removed from its carrier until it is applied directly to the recipient site. Whether applied as a sheet or meshed, the STSG may be sutured or stapled with a skin stapler. Nonadherent gauze is usually applied as the first layer of dressing over a graft. Moist dressings should be applied to all meshed grafts to prevent desiccation and loss of the graft.
7. Fat adherent to the graft is trimmed. The graft is applied to the recipient site and usually sutured at the edges, and these sutures are left long to tie over a stent dressing. Blood clots beneath the graft are removed by saline irrigation before the dressing is applied.

## Preservation of Skin Grafts

A skin graft may be harvested but not used immediately. Skin can be obtained from the patient on whom it is to be grafted (autograft) or from a living or nonliving donor unrelated to the recipient (allograft). Skin that is obtained for future grafting must be preserved and stored in a safe, controlled environment until it is used. Although description of a general procedure follows, each facility should establish protocols for preserving, maintaining, and storing tissue. Issues of consent, medical contraindications, and screening criteria should be included in these protocols.

***Preservation Procedure.*** The setup should include the skin specimen and the following items:

- Sterile 3-inch rolled gauze
- Adhesive tape for sealing and labeling container
- Basin with isotonic solution
- Sterile container with screw cap
- Storage solution or preservative (as appropriate)

### *Operative Procedure*

1. The skin should be kept on the instrument table until it is ready for storage.
2. The skin must be kept moist with an isotonic solution, such as balanced salt solution or saline, at all times.
3. The skin is gently flattened, smoothed out, and placed on a piece of roller gauze moistened with the isotonic solution, with its external surface facing downward.
4. The scrub person rolls the gauze and skin loosely, places the roll in the sterile container, and secures the cap.
5. The circulating nurse labels the jar with the donor's name and hospital number, location of donor site, date of collection, any preservative used and its concentration, and size of graft.
6. If the surgeon anticipates using the preserved skin within 14 days, it may be stored in a refrigerator at between 1°C and 10°C (34°F and 50°F) until it is used. An alternative method is to place the skin in a tissue medium such as McCoy's; the tissue may then be stored in a refrigerator at between 1°C and 10°C (34°F and 50°F) for 30 days until it is used.

If the surgeon does not anticipate using the skin within 14 days, it can be maintained by one of several long-term storage methods. One method is to place the skin in a cryoprotectant (e.g., ethylene glycol) for 1 to 2 hours at 4°C (39°F), gradually cool the skin to −70°C (−94°F), and then store it in a liquid nitrogen freezer.

## Composite Graft

Composite grafts are composed of skin and underlying tissues that are completely separated from the blood supply of the donor site and transplanted to another area of the body. The survival of a composite graft depends on ingrowth of new blood vessels from the recipient site around the periphery of the graft. Therefore composite grafts are usually small so that no portion of the graft is more than 1 cm from its periphery. An example of compound tissues used as composite grafts is hair transplants, composed of skin, fat, and hair follicles, which are used to treat male pattern baldness. The term *composite* thus indicates a defect that requires a graft be brought to the area to meet more than one type of tissue deficiency.

***Procedural Considerations.*** A plastic local instrument set is required, plus the following:

- Marking pen
- X-ray film, unexposed (sterile)

The patient is positioned, prepped, and draped such that adequate exposure of both donor and recipient sites is achieved.

### *Operative Procedure*

1. The recipient site is prepared by excising tissue, such as a scar or a benign or malignant skin lesion.
2. When feasible, a pattern of the recipient site is made and transferred to the donor site.
3. The composite graft is excised. The donor site is either closed by approximating its skin edges or left unsutured (as in hair transplant donor sites).
4. Meanwhile, the composite graft is kept in a moist sponge until it is sutured to the edges of the recipient site.
5. Dressings of choice are applied to the composite graft and donor site.

## Replacement of Lost or Absent Tissue

When coverage for a defect cannot be achieved through skin grafting plastic surgeons rely on other techniques to replace tissue. Coverage through a tissue flap is a widely used technique that has evolved since its inception in 600 BC.[18] Just as the flap has evolved, other techniques for tissue restoration through biologic engineering have also evolved. Tissue engineering is a rapidly growing field that uses laboratory-grown molecules, cells, tissues, and organs to replace or support the function of defective or injured body parts.[22] Four principal avenues have been explored to make new tissues for biologic replacement: the injection of isolated cell populations, the placement of polymer scaffolds to guide tissue regeneration, the development of encapsulated systems, and the transplantation of cells in polymer matrices.[17] A discussion of flap techniques follows.

## Flaps

The term *flap* refers to tissue that is detached from one area of the body and transferred to the recipient area with either part or all of its original blood supply intact or reestablished (Figure 24-18); thus it has a self-contained vascular system. The base or pedicle of the flap is that portion through which the blood supply enters or exits. Because flaps carry their own blood supply, they generally are used to cover recipient sites that have poor vascularity and full-thickness tissue loss. Flaps are used for reconstruction or wound closure. They are useful for covering exposed bone, tendon, or nerve. They may be used if operating through the wound may be necessary at a later date to repair underlying structures. Flaps containing skin and subcutaneous tissue retain more properties of normal skin and shrink less than skin grafts. Flaps, however, have some disadvantages, such as bulky appearance, failure to match tissue of the recipient site in texture or color, and the possibility of requiring multiple operations and prolonged hospitalization.

Flaps may be classified according to blood supply. *Random pattern flaps* consist of skin and subcutaneous tissue vascularized by random perforators with limited length/width ratio. *Axial pattern flaps* have a well-defined arteriovenous supply along the long axis; they can be comparatively long in relation to width. Flaps may also be classified according to position or how they are rotated after elevation. *Advancement flaps* are cut and advanced to reconstruct a nearby defect. *Transposition flaps* are advanced along an axis that forms an angle to the flap's original position. *Rotation flaps* are similar to transposition flaps but are semicircular and rotate along a greater axis. *Island flaps* of isolated sections of skin and subcutaneous tissue are tunneled beneath the skin to new sites. *Pedicle flaps* were the forerunners of muscle and musculocutaneous flaps. These consist of skin and underlying muscle; they are very mobile and can be rotated into distant defects. *Free flaps* are actually a form of tissue transplantation. Using microvascular techniques, a defined amount of skin, muscle, or bone can be isolated, totally detached, and reattached at the recipient site by microvascular anastomoses between recipient-site blood vessels and the major vessels that supply the flap. The vascular pedicle may contain functional nerves, yielding sensory flaps to provide protective sensation or motor flaps to restore function. Bone and joints may be transplanted as free flaps, as in the case of toe-to-thumb site transfers.

***Procedural Considerations.*** The perioperative nurse should consult with the surgeon in advance of the procedure to determine the donor site and plan for positioning and ordering of the procedure. Generally the surgical site and flap area are marked preoperatively with the patient in a functional position because landmarks and aesthetics are influenced by surgical positioning. If marking is undertaken on the anesthetized and surgically positioned patient, inaccuracies in tissue placement could occur. Flap procedures may involve two teams of surgeons working simultaneously, one raising the flap and closing the resulting defect, the other preparing the site, repositioning the flap in its new site, and, in the case of a free flap, microscopically reanastomosing the blood vessels. For any lengthy procedure, a Foley catheter, sequential compression devices, warming units, and positioning aids that are safe for the skin will be needed. Skin grafts are sometimes used to achieve closure of the flap donor site; if this is needed then add appropriate instrumentation for harvesting a skin graft.

A basic plastic instrument set is required, plus the following:

- ESU
- Marking pen

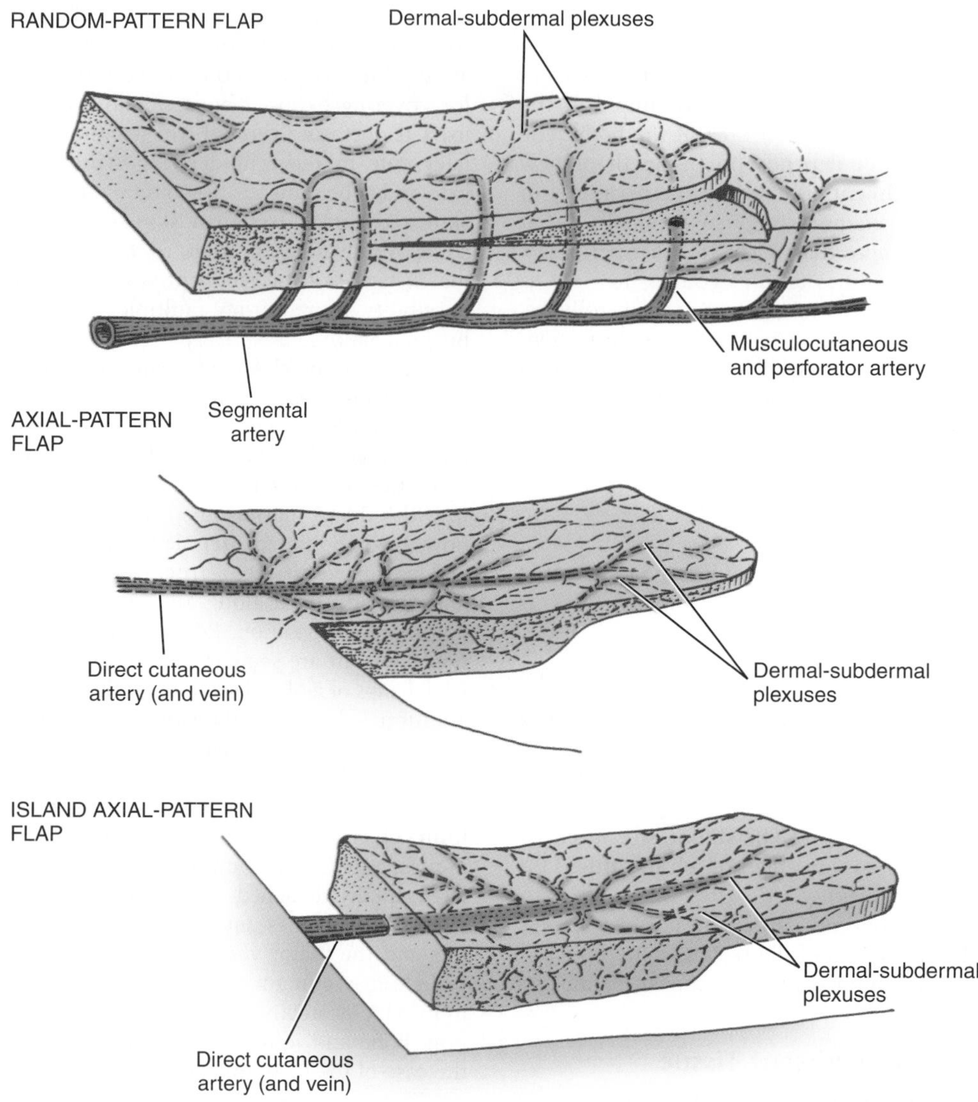


**FIGURE 24-18** Types of flaps. *Top,* Random-pattern flap. A random-pattern skin flap is supplied by a subdermal plexus of small vessels that do not have an axial orientation. *Middle,* Axial-pattern flap. An axial-pattern skin flap is designed parallel to the axis of a known major subcutaneous artery. It can have a greater length/width ratio because its blood supply is more reliable. *Bottom,* Island axial-pattern flap.

- Extra hemostats
- X-ray film, unexposed (sterile)
- Dermatome of choice
- Skin mesher
- Microvascular instruments (as appropriate)

### *Operative Procedure—Advancement, Transpositional, Rotational, Island, and Pedicle Flaps*

1. The recipient site is prepared in the same manner as for a skin graft.
2. When feasible, a pattern of the recipient site is made and transferred to the donor area.
3. The flap is incised, elevated, and transferred to the recipient site.
4. The edges of the flap are sutured to the periphery of the recipient site.
5. The flap donor site is repaired by approximating the skin edges directly or by covering the defect with a skin graft or another flap.
6. Drains are usually placed under flaps.
7. Dressings are applied with particular attention given to immobilization of the flap, which may require stockinette, padding, or plaster of Paris.
8. NOTE: Before a pedicle flap is detached from the donor site, the surgeon may want to determine the adequacy of circulation within the flap. One can check by placing rubber-shod clamps across the base of the pedicle and injecting 20 ml of 5% sodium fluorescein intravenously. After 10 minutes have elapsed, all lights in the OR are turned off and a Wood's lamp is held over the flap to determine the presence or absence of fluorescence within the flap. Fluorescein may be injected locally for the same purpose.

***Operative Procedure—Free Flaps.*** See description of free TRAM flap used in breast reconstruction.

## RECONSTRUCTIVE BREAST SURGERY

The loss of a breast because of cancer may have a devastating effect on a woman. Fortunately, the option of breast reconstruction is available to virtually any woman who loses her breast to cancer.[4] Reconstruction has the ability to offer hope and a return to wholeness and normalcy. Normal, of course, is subjective, and although breasts may be reconstructed, there is a wide range of appearances and results, and it must be stressed that breast reconstruction is not a one-time surgery. Revisions are the rule and not the exception. Techniques and options continue to evolve and improve, and women have many options. Breast reconstruction may be offered at one of many times during this process—initially, at the time of mastectomy; before adjunct therapy or after; or even many years later. The important fact is that each woman and her oncologic status are individual, so the decision for reconstruction must be made according to her desires coupled with her most favorable circumstances. Reconstruction has no known effect on the recurrence of breast cancer.[2] Breast reconstruction options include alloplastic (artificial materials), autogenous (flaps), or a combination of both. Flaps may be pedicle-based or free flaps using microsurgical techniques.

### Breast Reconstruction Using Tissue Expanders

Mastectomy may leave a shortage of skin that prevents creation of a breast mound. For these patients, extra tissue can be created locally with the use of tissue expanders (Figure 24-19). Tissue expansion is a technique used to stretch normal tissue that is adjacent to a defect, mechanically creating redundancy of normal tissue to correct the defect. For breast reconstruction, the expander resembles the shape of a breast prosthesis. The expander has a metal-backed, self-sealing silicone valve at its dome or less often a small, dome-shaped reservoir with a fill tube that is positioned subcutaneously at a distance from the expander but connected to it. Following surgery, the tissue expander is gradually filled with percutaneous injections of normal saline during routine office visits. The expander may be filled as often as weekly, or it may stay until chemotherapy or radiation is completed. Once the tissue expander is filled to the appropriate volume, it may be removed and replaced with a permanent reconstructive mammary prosthesis, either saline or silicone, as an ambulatory surgical procedure. If silicone is chosen, both the surgeon and patient must participate in an adjunct clinical study at this time. Another option is the use of combination tissue expander and breast prosthesis, which remains in place once the desired amount of saline has been sequentially added. The benefit of this prosthesis is the ability to add or remove saline in case an adjustment proves necessary.

***Procedural Considerations.*** A basic plastic set may be used with the addition of fiberoptic breast retractors. Both inframammary folds are marked preoperatively, and both sides of the chest should be prepped and draped. Drains are usually placed to prevent hematoma and seroma formation, the latter of which could cause rotation or malposition of the tissue expander. The breast shape expander is supplied in a sterile package from the manufacturer and is available in a variety of sizes. Meticulous sterile technique is required, and the expander should be handled as little as possible. Positioning is usually supine with both arms extended on armboards. This procedure may be performed immediately following mastectomy or at a later date. If a surgical bra is used, care must be taken that it is not too tight and compromises circulation to the skin flaps.

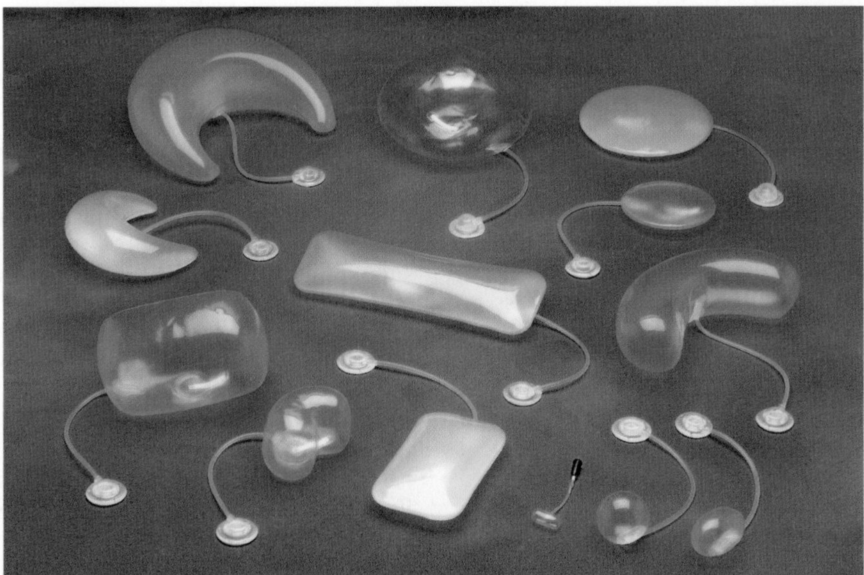

FIGURE 24-19 Tissue expanders are inflatable plastic reservoirs of various shapes and volumes that are implanted under the skin. The skin over the expander is stretched during a period of several weeks as the expander is gradually filled by percutaneous injection of saline into an incorporated part of the remote-fill port. Expanders are useful for breast reconstruction.

### *Operative Procedure*

1. Skin flaps are assessed for adequate blood supply, and then the pectoralis fascia is incised along its lateral border. A submuscular pocket is created for the temporary expander by undermining the muscle over the sternal attachments and down over the lower ribs.
2. The tissue expander is tested before insertion for watertight integrity.
3. After hemostasis is achieved, the expander is checked for integrity and then inserted into the pocket. Muscle coverage is assessed and if adequate, the reservoir is positioned subcutaneously and connected, the wound is closed, and the expander is filled with sterile saline solution until slight blanching of the skin is achieved. The amount is recorded on the patient record.
4. After the desired expansion has occurred, the temporary expander is exchanged for a permanent prosthesis.

## Second-Stage Tissue Expander Breast Reconstruction

Once the tissue expander has been expanded to the desired size the patient is taken back to surgery for the next stage of her breast reconstruction. This is a relatively minor procedure where the tissue expander is deflated and replaced with a permanent mammary prosthesis. At this time, if there is asymmetry of the contralateral breast, surgery may be performed to create bilateral symmetry. The patient may require correction of breast ptosis through mastopexy, with or without the addition of a breast implant, or by performing a reduction mammoplasty on the opposite breast. This procedure is usually performed with the patient under general anesthesia on an outpatient basis.

## Breast Reconstruction Using Myocutaneous Flaps

Flaps are described by the types of tissue they contain, their blood supply, and the method by which they are moved from the donor site to the recipient site. The latissimus dorsi myocutaneous flap is a single-stage reconstruction of the breast after mastectomy. Because the flap consists of skin combined with muscle, it is described as *myocutaneous*. This flap is used when significant tissue deficiency occurs after a mastectomy or when abdominal flap (transverse rectus abdominis myocutaneous [TRAM]) reconstruction is not an option. The latissimus dorsi muscle is a wide, flat muscle extending over the midthoracic portion of the back and inserting into the humerus. Its blood supply comes from the thoracodorsal artery and perforators from the upper lumbar arteries and the intercostal vessels. This rich vascularity allows the surgeon flexibility in orienting and positioning the flap to the pattern of the deficit on the anterior chest wall. Latissimus dorsi flaps are usually used in conjunction with a reconstructive breast prosthesis, in order to create a more natural breast mound.

***Procedural Considerations.*** The donor site of the latissimus dorsi with its skin island, along with the intended recipient site, is marked before surgery with the patient in a sitting position. In the OR, the patient is placed in a lateral position, donor side up with the arm extended and safely supported. Extra padding and positioning aids should be assembled in preparation for the patient's arrival. Once the donor muscle has been mobilized and brought out through the area of defect, the back incision is closed and the patient repositioned supine with the arm extended on an armboard. Instrumentation should include a basic plastic instrument set, fiberoptic breast retractor, vascular instruments, marking pens, suction, long tissue forceps and scissors, and availability of a Doppler probe. The ESU will be required.

### *Operative Procedure*

1. Initially the island of skin is incised transversely across the back, with care being taken so that a bra or bathing suit will cover the resulting scar (Figure 24-20).
2. The muscle, subcuticular fat, and fascia are then freed from the overlying skin by undermining so that part or all of the muscle may be mobilized.
3. The skin island and the muscle are then tunneled under the axilla to the chest wall (Figure 24-20, *C*). The insertion of the muscle on the humerus and accompanying blood vessels are left undisturbed. The latissimus dorsi muscle fills the space left by the missing pectoralis muscle.
4. The island of skin is oriented to the recipient site, and both are sutured into place (Figure 24-20, *D*).
5. A mammary prosthesis is placed under the muscle before suturing to reconstruct the breast mound.
6. The wound is drained by closed-wound suction catheters.
7. The nipple-areola complex may also be reconstructed by sharing the nipple on the unaffected side or by using groin, adjacent tissue, thigh, or auricular tissue. It can be done at the time of reconstruction or at a later date as a minor procedure with the patient under local anesthesia (Figure 24-20, *E*).
8. If a surgical bra is used, care must be taken not to compromise blood supply to the flap.

## Transverse Rectus Abdominis Myocutaneous Flap

TRAM flaps are the most common pedicle-based flaps used for breast reconstruction. The rectus muscle is the broad, wide abdominal muscle that reaches from under the ribs to the pubis, and either one or both sides of the muscle may be used for reconstruction. The blood supply (superior epigastric artery and vein) is carried within the muscle pedicle; it is severed at its most distal origins and pulled up inside the muscle to its new location. Although this procedure has the added benefit of an abdominoplasty, if there is inadequate abdominal tissue the patient may require a small mammary prosthesis.

The several types of TRAM techniques are based on blood supply, but the procedure still follows a basic format. As with other types of breast reconstruction, TRAM flaps may be performed immediately following mastectomy or planned for a later stage in the patient's recuperative phase.

***Procedural Considerations.*** Markings on the patient are made preoperatively with the patient in a standing position. A basic plastic instrument set is used as for the latissimus dorsi flap. The patient is positioned supine with arms extended on armboards. Positioning the patient for this procedure is particularly difficult because of the need to promote closure of the abdominal wound, support circulation to the flap, and protect the patient from injury. The OR bed is often flexed; additional padding of the lower extremities may be required. The skin prep should extend from the lower neck to midthigh.

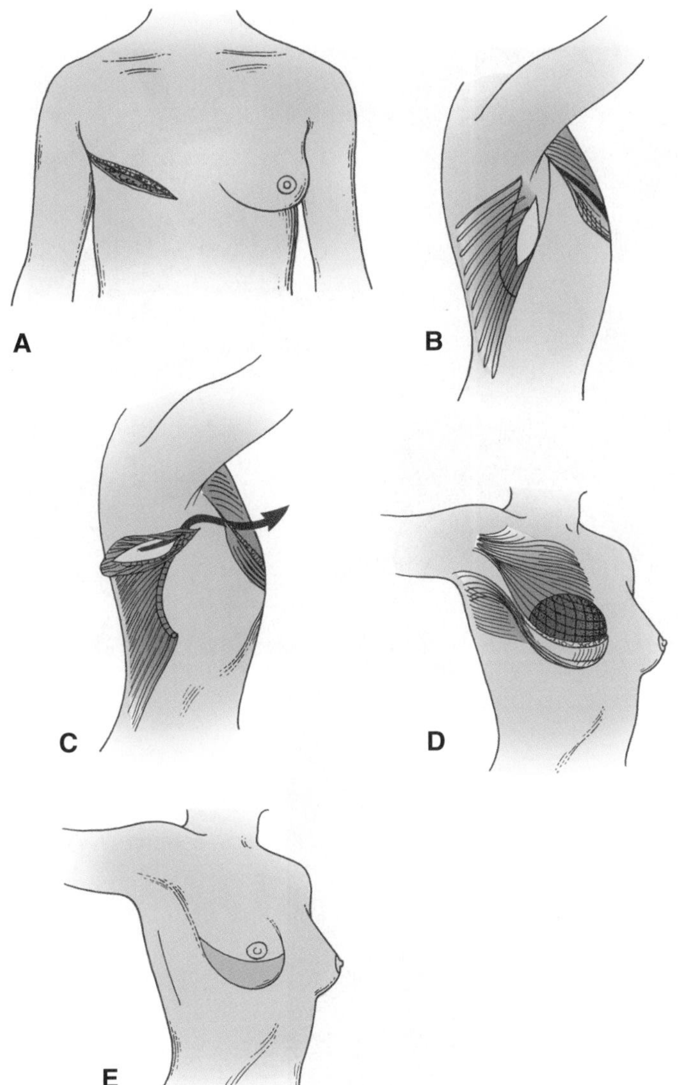


**FIGURE 24-20** Latissimus dorsi flap for reconstruction after mastectomy (see text for procedure).

### *Operative Procedure*

1. The skin from the mastectomy scar is excised and sent for pathologic examination, and the abdominal incision is made. The abdominal flap is dissected with care being taken not to shear the skin and subcutaneous tissue from its underlying muscle attachments (Figure 24-21, *A*).
2. The transverse rectus abdominus muscle is divided from its inferior-most attachment (Figure 24-21, *B*).
3. The flap is rotated and passed through to its new location on the chest wall (Figure 24-21, *C* and *D*) and sutured medially; the thinnest portion of the flap is superior and medial, and the thickest portion is inferior and lateral.
4. Because of the amount of tissue available, an implant is often unnecessary (Figure 24-21, *E*).

## Free Transverse Rectus Abdominis Myocutaneous Flap

The free TRAM flap is indicated when there is concern about the absence of one or both of the rectus muscles following the procedure or the vascularity of the pedicle used in the standard TRAM flap or in the presence of any other factors that may compromise vascularity of the flap. A newer technique of the free TRAM (deep inferior epigastric perforator procedure) has the advantage of not requiring the entire rectus muscle, because only a small portion of the rectus muscle that carries a segment of the deep inferior epigastric perforator vessels is needed to move with the fat and skin to its new location. It is also used when the buttock tissue (superior gluteal perforator flap) is planned to replace the absent breast or breasts.

***Procedural Considerations.*** Care of the patient undergoing a free TRAM procedure is identical to that of patients undergoing pedicle TRAM flaps with the addition of the surgical microscope. Refer to the description for procedural considerations. Two surgical teams may be used, one for harvesting and one for site preparation. Meticulous attention must be paid to positioning and protection from pressure injuries due to the length of the procedure. During the preoperative verification process, the perioperative nurse should check to see if the patient has made preoperative autologous blood donations and that the appropriate blood work has been drawn.

### *Operative Procedure*

1. The site is prepped, and the recipient site blood vessels are identified for anastomosis.
2. The recipient vessels are dissected and isolated.
3. Donor vessels are selected based on pedicle length, and the flap is prepared.
4. Heparin is administered to prevent clotting and vasospasm.
5. Once recipient vessels are ready, the flap is severed.
6. The microscope is positioned in place and draped with a sterile drape.
7. The free flap is transferred to the recipient site, and the blood vessels are anastomosed.
8. The breast mound is shaped and sutured in place.
9. The donor site is closed, covering with a skin graft if necessary.

## Nipple Reconstruction

Although nipple reconstruction can be performed at the time of breast reconstruction or replacement of the tissue expander with a mammary prosthesis, some surgeons prefer to wait and let the new breast tissues "settle" and mature in order to reconstruct the new nipple in the most accurate anatomic position. Generally this may take a minimum of 6 to 8 weeks. Tissue for the new nipple can be recruited locally by raising a flap or by moving in tissue from the groin, buttock crease, auricle, or contralateral nipple. In the absence of areolar skin, the area may be tattooed to create a very pleasing nipple areolar complex (Figure 24-22).

# MICROSURGERY

Microsurgery is a fundamental tool in reconstructive plastic surgery. It allows an almost unlimited choice of reconstructive methods, replacement of lost tissue with similar components, and optimal selection of donor sites with minimal morbidity.[25] Reconstructive microsurgical procedures include but are not limited to replantation of amputated body parts, repair of facial nerves, repair of lacerated nerves and blood vessels, treatment

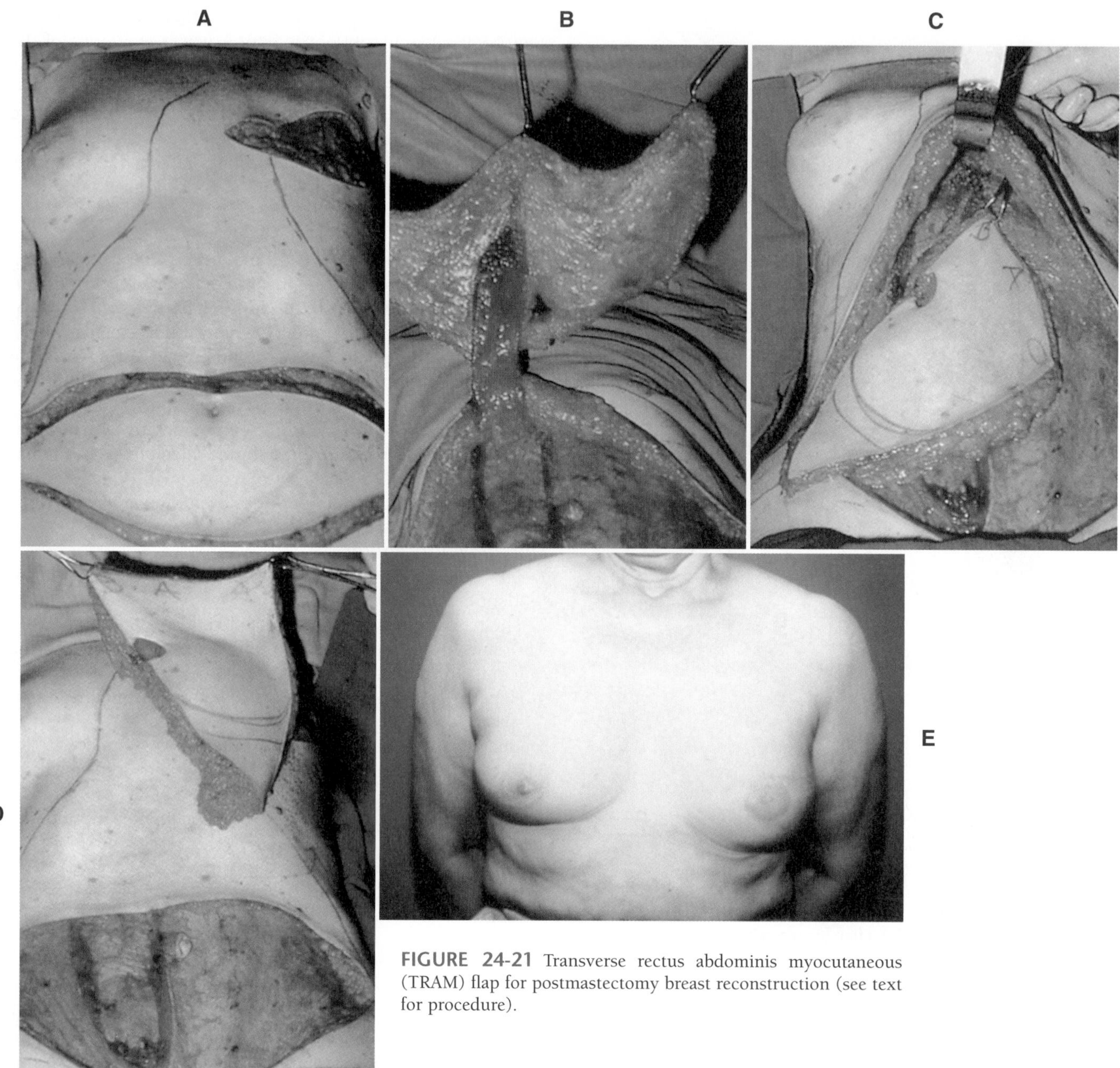


**FIGURE 24-21** Transverse rectus abdominis myocutaneous (TRAM) flap for postmastectomy breast reconstruction (see text for procedure).

of extensive trauma to extremities and hands, reconstruction following removal of extensive cancers, and female to male transsexual reassignment. Today's physicians skilled in microsurgery can successfully anastomose the ends of a vessel measuring less than 1 mm in diameter. The surgeon's use of an operating microscope or loupes for microsurgical procedures depends on the procedure to be performed, condition of the tissue, and personal preference. Endoscopic harvesting of tissues for microsurgical grafting is possible in some circumstances. The success of microsurgery depends on several factors: (1) the individual and collective experiences of the surgical team and the members' ability to work together, relieving each other as necessary during long operations; (2) the surgeon's knowledge of the physiology of the microcirculation; (3) many hours of practice in the laboratory by the surgical team; and (4) the availability of proper microscopes, microvascular instruments, and microvascular suture.

## Replantation of Amputated Body Part

Replantation is an attempt to reattach a completely amputated digit or other body part. Revascularization is the procedure performed on incomplete amputations, when the part remains attached to the body by skin, artery, vein, or nerve. Good candidates for replantation are those with the following amputations: (1) thumb, (2) multiple digits, (3) distal portion of hand at palm level, (4) wrist or forearm, (5) elbow and above the elbow, and (6) almost any body part of a child.

The success of digital replantation depends primarily on the microsurgical repair of one digital artery and two digital veins. Replantation of an amputated part is ideally performed within

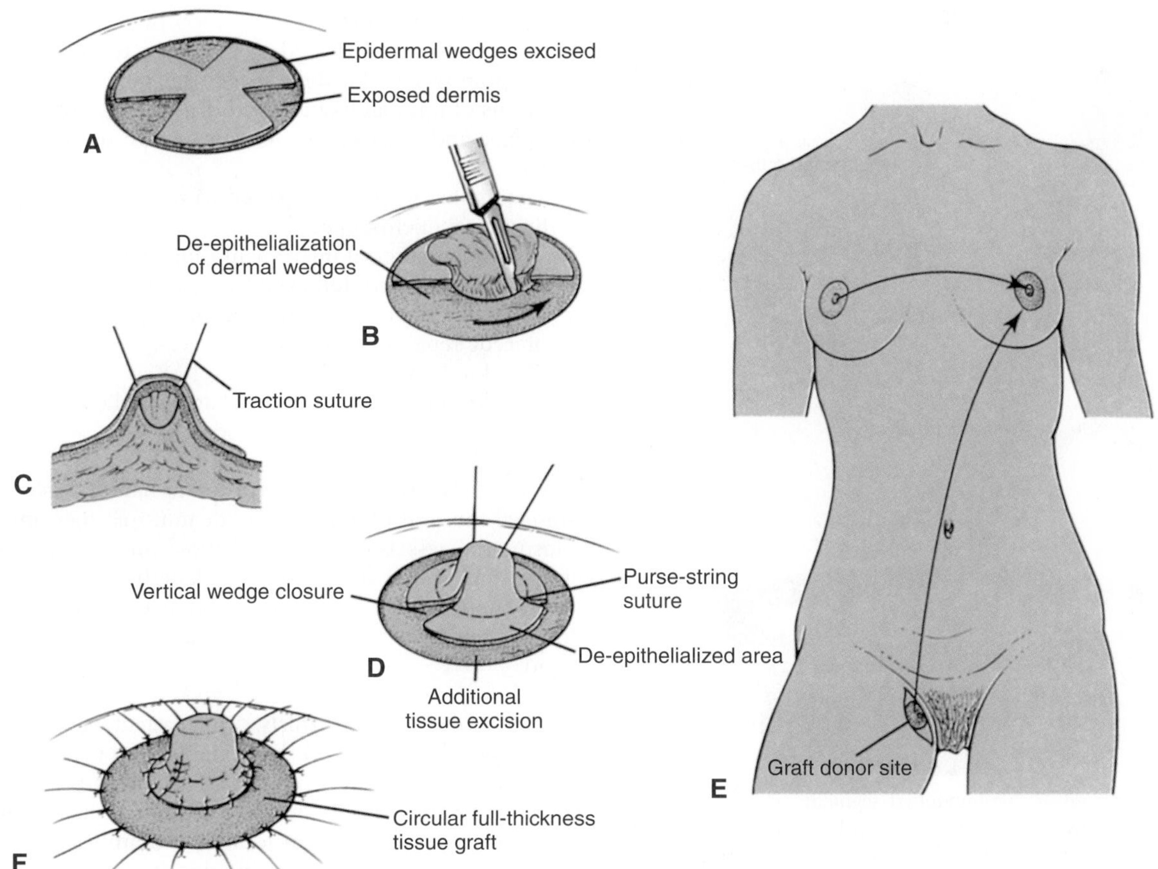


**FIGURE 24-22** **A,** Circumferential demarcation of the nipple periphery with removal of dermal wedges. **B,** Dermal wedges are de-epithelialized from the rim toward the center. **C,** A traction suture is used to elevate the central future nipple tip. **D,** Traction is applied to the future nipple tip as the wedges are approximated to create a permanent projected surface. A purse-string suture is placed, and excess tissue is excised. **E,** Possible full-thickness donor site areolar color match may be found in the labial folds. **F,** The donor graft is measured, cut, and secured to the dermal ring of the neonipple areolar complex.

4 to 6 hours after injury, but success has been reported up to 24 hours after injury if the amputated part has been cooled. Proper care of the amputated body part or parts before surgery is vital to successful replantation (Figure 24-23). The ultimate aim of replantation is the restitution of function beyond that provided by a prosthesis.

***Procedural Considerations.*** A regional anesthetic is usually given to replantation patients if the anticipated length of surgery so permits. Because of the length of these surgeries (12 to 16 hours), positioning is important. The OR bed and armboards should be carefully padded with egg crate–type foam or a gel-filled mattress to support the supine patient. The surgeon may request the room temperature increased before the patient arrives because the warm room will reduce vasoconstriction in the extremities. A warming device, such as warm forced air, is usually applied to maintain the patient's core body temperature. The surgeon usually brings the amputated part to the OR before the patient arrives to ensure ample time for preparation of the amputated part for replantation. The amputated body part should be maintained by wrapping in saline-soaked gauze sponges, placing it in an occlusive bag, and immersing it in a container of iced saline. If radiographs of the amputated body part and amputation site have not been taken before the patient's arrival in the OR the nurse should arrange for these to be taken. Radiographic films are crucial to determine bone trauma and loss.

The hand drape (Figure 24-24), described below, can be applied to either upper or lower extremities, as required by the surgical procedure. Before a hand drape is begun, a pneumatic tourniquet cuff is often applied to the upper arm over padding. The patient is supine on the OR bed, with the affected arm extended and supported on a hand table. While an assistant holds the patient's arm with both hands around the tourniquet cuff, the skin prep solution is applied from fingertips to tourniquet cuff. Care is taken to keep the cuff dry and free of solution. Then two folded barrier sheets are used to cover the hand table. The first sheet is placed with the folded edge nearest the patient (thus forming a cuff). Double-thickness, 4-inch stockinette is used to cover the extremity, and the edge is rolled over the tourniquet. The upper arm and upper half of the body are covered by a folded sheet, with the folded edge placed across the part of the stockinette that covers the tourniquet cuff. A small, nonperforating towel clamp that grasps the edge of the folded top sheet, the stockinette, and the edge of the cuff of the bottom sheet is placed on each side of the arm. This excludes

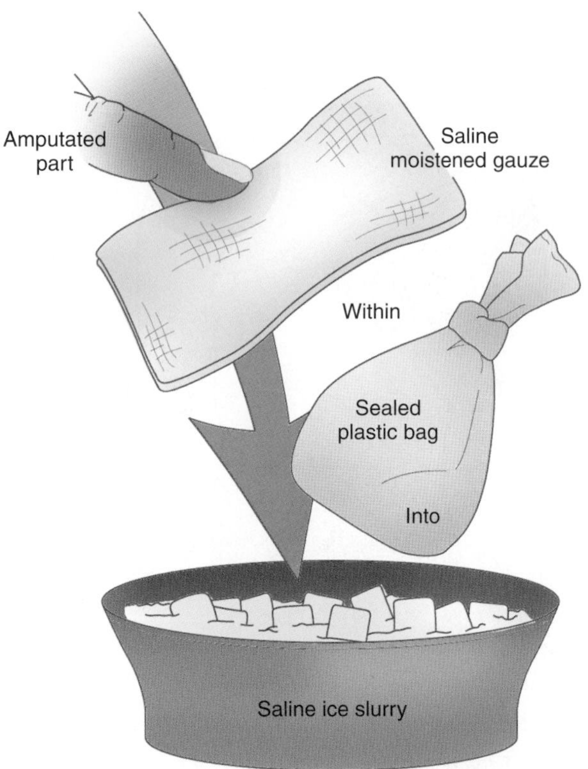


**FIGURE 24-23** Care of the amputated segment, which should be cooled immediately by wrapping it in moist saline gauze, placing it in a sealed plastic bag, and immersing it in an iced saline container.

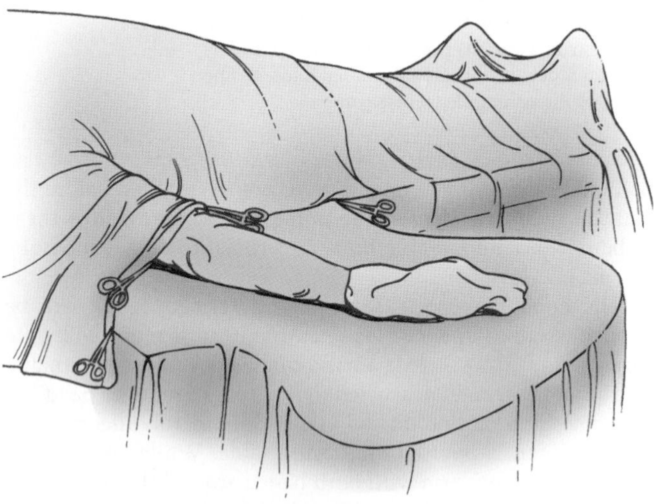

**FIGURE 24-24** Hand drape.

the tourniquet cuff from the sterile field. The remainder of the body is covered with one or two additional sheets. A commercially prepared extremity drape that has an aperture incorporated into the drape may be substituted for the procedure described above.

Instrumentation includes a plastic hand instrument set, microvascular instruments, a Kirschner wire driver, Kirschner wires, an operating microscope, and a bipolar ESU.

### *Operative Procedure*

1. Bone ends are shortened to eliminate tension on vascular anastomoses to be done later; the bone is stabilized by means of internal fixation with Kirschner wires.
2. Flexor and extensor tendon repairs are usually performed next.
3. The digital nerves are repaired with the aid of loupes or the operating microscope.
4. With microsurgical instruments and techniques, two digital veins are repaired, followed by repair of one digital artery. If ischemic time has been prolonged, digital vessel repair may precede repair of tendons and nerves.
5. The skin is sutured.
6. A bulky supportive hand dressing is applied.

## Toe-to-Hand Transfer

The reconstructive procedure of toe-to-hand transfer involves surgical removal of a single toe or multiple toes and anastomosing the vessels of the toes to those on the hand to restore finger and thumb functions. It is lengthy surgery (12 to 16 hours) and entails a two-team approach; one team is at the foot for toe removal, and one team is at the recipient site—the hand.

***Procedural Considerations.*** The patient is placed in the supine position on the OR bed. The patient is put on an anticoagulation regimen during the anastomosis procedure. Two tourniquets are needed—one on the thigh of the operative foot and one on the operative arm. Both extremities are separately prepped and draped. Instrumentation includes a plastic hand set, microvascular instruments, power Kirschner wire driver, and Kirschner wires. Additional equipment includes the operating microscope, two tourniquet power sources, two bipolar ESUs, a marking pen, and an Esmarch bandage.

### *Operative Procedure*

1. The surgeon preparing the hand determines adequate blood flow and vessel location on the thumb site. This may prevent a needless amputation of the toe.
2. Appropriate skin flaps are incised to expose the veins on the dorsum of the hand and clamped with vessel microclips.
3. The radial artery or branches are dissected out and prepared for anastomosis.
4. The flexor and extensor pollicis longus tendons are located and transfixed.
5. The bone at the base of the thumb is prepared for the toe.
6. The nerves to the thumb are dissected out with adequate length for suturing without tension.
7. The toe is circumscribed with a racket-shaped incision (Figure 24-25, *B*), and the veins are isolated through the dorsal aspect and clamped with vessel microclips.
8. The extensor tendon is dissected proximally and transected over the base of the metatarsal.
9. The dorsalis pedis artery is dissected to the digital vessels with ligation of all branches of that vessel to prepare for the anastomosis.
10. On the plantar surface, the digital nerves and flexor tendons are transected at levels of adequate length for anastomosis (Figure 24-25, *C*).
11. The toe is transected at the level previously determined for adequate length of the thumb.

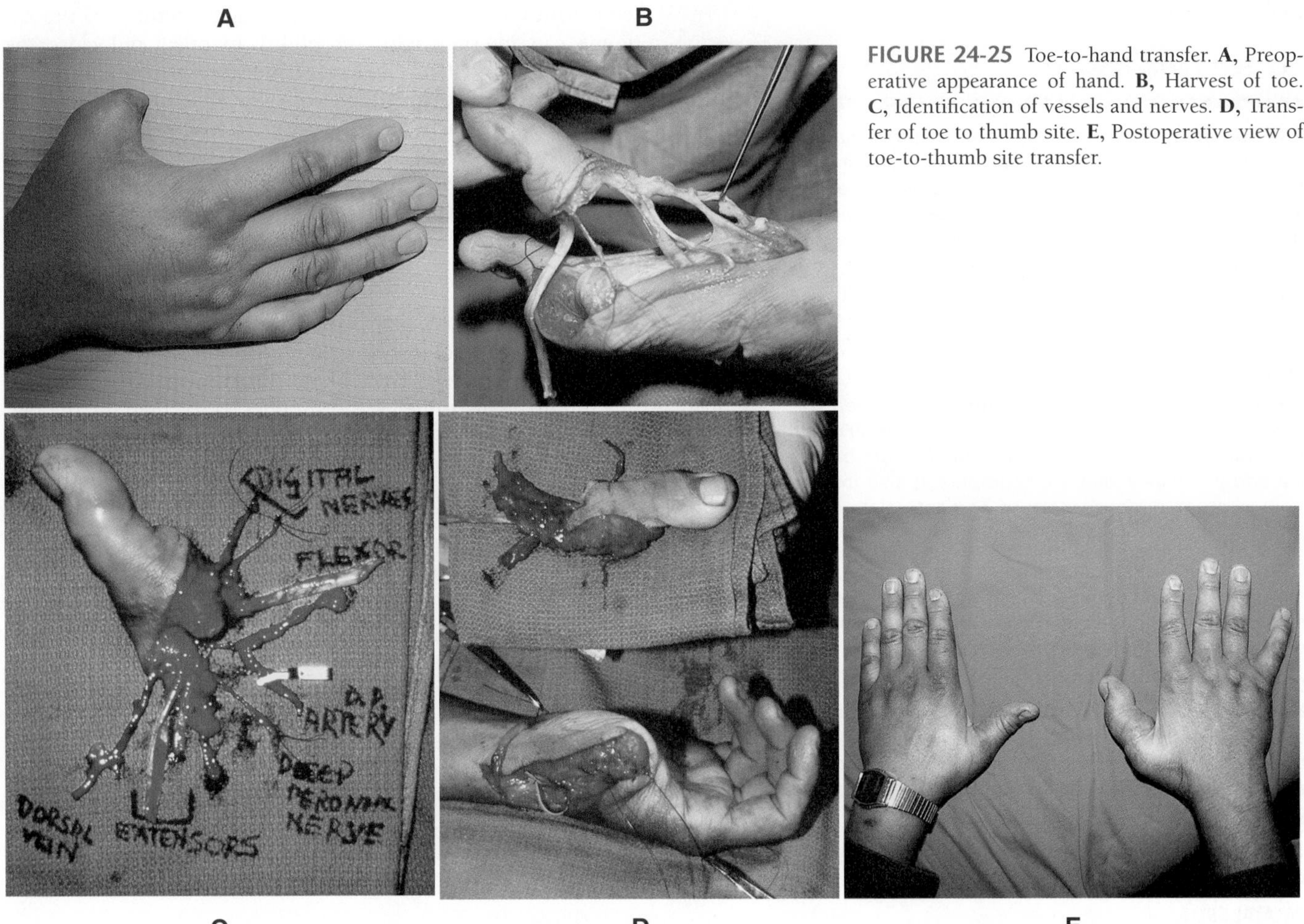


**FIGURE 24-25** Toe-to-hand transfer. **A,** Preoperative appearance of hand. **B,** Harvest of toe. **C,** Identification of vessels and nerves. **D,** Transfer of toe to thumb site. **E,** Postoperative view of toe-to-thumb site transfer.

12. The toe vessels are anastomosed microsurgically to the thumb vessels. The toe is attached to the thumb area by Kirschner wires (Figure 24-25, *D*).

An aesthetic and functionally effective hand can be achieved through this procedure (Figure 24-25, *E*).

## RECONSTRUCTIVE MAXILLOFACIAL SURGERY

The need for maxillofacial surgery results from trauma, disease, or congenital anomaly. Regardless of the cause, the principles are the same: establishment of preinjury/predisease/normal anatomic dental occlusion, anatomic reduction, and stabilization.[9] The technique and approach must be individualized in order to optimize the visual reduction (or reconstruction) of the procedure as well as minimize facial scarring and nerve injury, whether it be a mandibular free flap tissue and bone reconstruction or open reduction and internal fixation of any number and combination of facial fractures. In addition to the midface fractures described in Box 24-3, other common facial fractures include nasal, orbital (blowout) floor, zygomatic, and mandibular fractures.

### Procedural Considerations for Maxillofacial Surgery

The perioperative nurse should ask the surgeon about the precise injuries and the expected surgical treatment plan: open or closed reduction; intraoral or extraoral approach; the order of multiple procedures; need for intraoperative x-rays; and type, number, and sizes of screws and compression plates to be placed if rigid fixation is to be employed. Orbital fractures may require alloplastic implant material. Wire is used less frequently for immobilization because of the greater degree of stability afforded by plating systems. The head should be immobilized and stabilized in a gel-type head ring; the position is almost always supine. Both eyes should be protected, and care must be taken not to displace endotracheal tubes. Instrumentation needs include a plastic surgery set, periosteal elevators, power drill for plating systems, bone hooks, Rowe disimpaction forceps (if maxillary), the ESU, marking pens, and suction. For application of arch bars, the nurse should assemble arch bars, wires, elastics, wire cutters, wire twisters, and dull retractors for good exposure of the teeth.

### Reduction of Nasal Fracture

Usually a closed reduction of the bony nasal fragments is performed by digital and instrumental manipulation. Occasionally an open reduction with interosseous wire fixation of nasal bone fragments is necessary. A nasal fracture may involve a fracture of the nasal bones or cartilage (including the septum). Closed reduction of a nasal fracture is most often performed with the patient under topical and local anesthesia. Procedural considerations and the surgical intervention are described in Chapter 20.

BOX 24-3

### Le Fort Facial Fractures

The Le Fort classification of facial fractures was developed by Rene Le Fort in 1901. Le Fort conducted experiments on cadaver heads to determine if there were patterns of predictable fracture lines, or "linea minoros resistentiae"—weak regions of the bones that were more vulnerable and likely to fracture when met with blunt force trauma. These studies became the basis of today's system for classifying facial fractures of the midface, known as Le Fort I, II, and III, as well as segmental, palatal split, and medial maxillary fractures.

**LE FORT I**
Sometimes called Guerin, after the first surgeon who described this injury pattern, the Le Fort I accounts for 30% to 45% of midface fractures. This is a low horizontal fracture between the maxilla and palatal/alveolar arch complex. It also involves the nasal floor, septum, piriform aperture, and anterolateral maxilla.

**LE FORT II**
One of the most frequent midface injuries, the Le Fort II fracture starts at the nasal bones, crosses the frontal process of the maxilla and lacrimal bones, and goes through the orbital floor, infraorbital rim, and the lateral maxillary sinus wall.

**LE FORT III**
Known as craniofacial dysjunction, Le Fort III fractures are extensive injuries that involve a complete separation of the midface through the skull base. They consist of unilateral or bilateral zygomatic fractures and a Le Fort I or II level fracture.

**SEGMENTAL**
The segmental fracture involves the alveolar ridge. It can be anterior, involving incisors, or posterolateral, involving molars.

**PALATAL SPLIT**
The palatal split fracture begins anteriorly at the incisor space and extends posteriorly. It usually accompanies other midface fractures.

**MEDIAL MAXILLARY**
The impact of a small object striking between the cheek and nose causes the medial maxillary fracture pattern. The frontal process of the maxilla and the nasal bones are involved.

From Frakes MA, Evans T: Evaluation and management of the patient with LeFort facial fractures, *Journal of Trauma Nursing* 11(3):95-101, 2004.

## Reduction of Orbital Floor Fractures

The orbital floor is the eggshell-thin bone on which the eye and periorbital tissues rest. It separates the orbit from the maxillary antrum. Orbital floor fractures usually occur in combination with fractures of the infraorbital rim (maxillary and zygomatic fractures). An isolated depressed orbital floor fracture with an intact infraorbital rim is called a *blowout* fracture. Chapter 18 discusses procedural considerations and surgical repair.

## Reduction of Zygomatic Fractures

Fractures of the zygoma (the cheek or malar bone) are corrected by either closed or open reduction. The two most common types of zygomatic fractures are depressed fractures of the arch and separation at or near the zygomaticofrontal, zygomaticomaxillary, and zygomaticotemporal suture lines, which constitutes a trimalar fracture. Although fractures of the zygoma can interfere with the ability to open and close the mouth properly, their chief consequence is a flattening of the cheek on the involved side, which results from a depressed trimalar or zygomatic arch fracture. Treatment is directed toward elevating the depressed fracture and maintaining the reduction. Closed reduction is the procedure used for treatment of zygomatic arch fractures, whereas most trimalar fractures are reduced by means of open reduction with internal fixation.

***Procedural Considerations.*** A plastic instrument set, a Suraci zygoma hook-elevator, and a jaw hook are required for a closed reduction. A basic plastic instrument set, along with the following instruments and supplies, is required for an open reduction: a Hall II air drill; stainless steel wires (#26, #28, and #30); the Suraci zygoma hook-elevator; a jaw hook; a Kerrison rongeur; two Blair retractors; the bipolar ESU; a marking pen; epinephrine 1:200,000 for injection; and a mini-plating rigid fixation set. The patient is placed in the supine position on the OR bed. The head drape is used.

***Operative Procedure.*** Closed reduction is performed by elevating the depressed fracture with a percutaneous bone hook. Stabilization of a trimalar fracture may then be achieved by inserting a transantral Kirschner wire from the fractured side to the normal side.

The technique of open reduction of a trimalar fracture is as follows:

1. Incisions are marked along the lateral area of the eyebrow and lower eyelid over the zygomaticofrontal suture line and zygomaticomaxillary suture line (infraorbital rim) fractures, respectively.
2. After injection with epinephrine 1:200,000 for hemostasis, incisions are made down to bone, and suture lines are identified and exposed.
3. The depressed zygoma is elevated with a Kelly hemostat or periosteal elevator placed behind the body of the zygoma through the lateral eyebrow incision. Bone hooks placed percutaneously or at the fracture sites may be used instead.
4. Holes are drilled into bone on each side of the fracture lines. Stainless steel wires are passed through the hole and twisted down tightly to maintain the reduction. (Reduction and stabilization of two of the three fractures are sufficient.) Alternative methods of stabilization of the fractures are interosseous wiring of the zygomaticofrontal fracture and placement of a transmural Kirschner wire or stabilization with micro/mini plates and screws.
5. Incisions are closed.
6. An eye-patch dressing may be applied.

## Reduction of Maxillary Fractures

Maxillary fractures are usually classified as follows: (1) Le Fort I, or transverse maxillary, fracture; (2) Le Fort II, or pyramidal maxillary, fracture; and (3) Le Fort III fracture, or craniofacial dysjunction, which includes fractures of both zygomas and the nose (Figure 24-26). A maxillary fracture produces malocclusion, just as a mandibular fracture does. In addition, depending on the severity of the fracture, it may produce considerable deformity of the middle of the face, usually perceived as a flattening or smashed-in appearance.

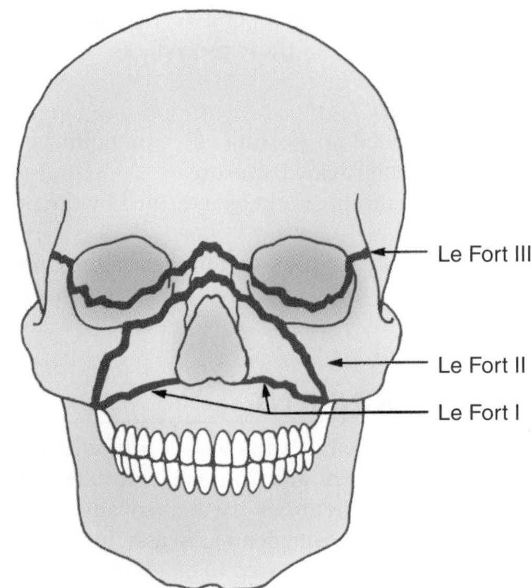


**FIGURE 24-26** Le Fort classification of maxillary fractures.

Closed reduction with intermaxillary fixation suffices for treatment of Le Fort I and some Le Fort II fractures. The more severe Le Fort II and all Le Fort III fractures require open reduction in addition to intermaxillary fixation.

***Procedural Considerations.*** The basic plastic instrument set is required as well as an air drill; stainless steel wires (#25, #26, and #28); a Rowe maxillary forceps, right and left; a Brown fascia needle; polyethylene buttons; a small, foam-rubber pad; a marking pen or methylene blue; the ESU; epinephrine 1:200,000 for injection; periosteal elevators; and a rigid fixation system. A separate Mayo setup for the application of arch bars is required, as described for reduction of mandibular fractures. The patient is placed in the supine position on the OR bed. The head drape is used.

***Operative Procedure.*** Arch bars are applied before or after the open reduction, or they may be the only mode of treatment in closed reduction. In addition to ligating the maxillary arch bar to the teeth, it must also be suspended from stable bones superior to the fractured maxilla (which is unstable). In Le Fort I fractures, suspension may be around both zygomatic arches by passage of percutaneous wires. In Le Fort II and Le Fort III fractures, suspension wires are placed through holes drilled bilaterally into the zygomatic process of the frontal bone. This requires incisions into both lateral eyebrow areas. The following description pertains to open reduction of Le Fort II and Le Fort III fractures:

1. After injection of epinephrine 1:200,000 for hemostasis, bilateral incisions are made to expose the infraorbital rims and zygomaticofrontal suture lines.
2. The Rowe maxillary forceps are applied intranasally and intraorally to disimpact and reduce the maxilla. Holes are drilled into bone on each side of fracture lines along the infraorbital rim (and zygomaticofrontal area for Le Fort III fractures, after reducing the zygomatic fractures).
3. Stainless steel wires are passed through these holes and twisted down tightly to maintain the reduction.
4. Suspension wires are passed from the eyebrow incisions, behind the zygomatic arches, and into the mouth with the Brown fascia needle. A pullout wire is looped through each suspension wire within the eyebrow incision, brought out through the skin near the hairline, and tied down over a polyethylene button and foam-rubber padding. Self-tapping screws, mini compression plates, and bone grafts may also be used, based on the surgeon's preference. Incisions are closed.
5. When indicated, reduction of a nasal fracture is then performed.

## Reduction of Mandibular Fractures

The purpose of treatment for a mandibular fracture is to restore the patient's preinjury dental occlusion. With some types of fractures, a closed reduction with immobilization by means of intermaxillary fixation is sufficient for treatment. With a majority of mandibular fractures, however, an open reduction with wire fixation is necessary, plus supplemental intermaxillary fixation to achieve adequate immobilization for healing.

Intermaxillary fixation is most often accomplished when arch bars are applied to the maxillary and mandibular teeth. Stainless steel wires (#24 or #25) are placed around the necks of the teeth and are ligated around the arch bars to hold the latter in place. Latex bands are attached to the tongs on the maxillary and mandibular arch bars to fix the teeth in occlusion (Figure 24-27). If the patient is edentulous, arch bars are attached to dentures or specially fabricated dental splints. The dentures or splints are held in place by means of wires placed around the mandible (for the mandibular arch bar) and through the nasal spine and around the zygomatic arches (for the maxillary arch bar). Scissors or wire cutters must be sent with the patient to the PACU and the postoperative patient care unit to prevent aspiration if the patient vomits or chokes.

***Procedural Considerations—Open Reduction.*** A basic plastic instrument set, plus the following instruments and supplies, is needed for an open reduction of a fractured mandible: a Hall II air drill, two Dingman bone-holding forceps, a nerve stimulator, a marking pen, stainless steel wires (#24, #26, and #28), the ESU, epinephrine 1:200,000 for injection, and a rigid fixation system.

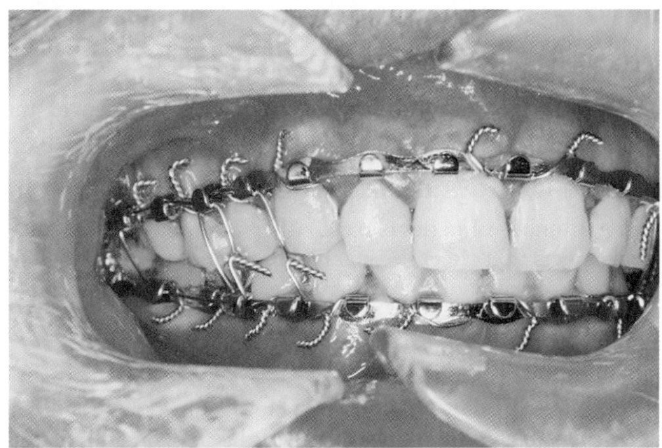

**FIGURE 24-27** Teeth in occlusion with arch bars in place. Tongs on arch bars will accept latex bands, which maintain occlusion for several weeks (wires around tongs are shown).

For the application of arch bars or other types of interdental wiring techniques, a separate Mayo setup with the following instruments and supplies is required: a set of coil arch bars and latex bands; stainless steel wire (#25 or #26); two Mayo-Hegar needle holders, 8 inch; a wire suture scissors, 4¾ inch; a wire twister; a Yankauer suction tube; two Wieder tongue depressors, large and small; six mosquito hemostats, curved, 5¼ inch; a Brown fascia needle (if dentures or splints are used); a Freer septal elevator; and a small drain.

If arch bars are applied before the open reduction is performed, this former setup must be kept completely separate from the instruments used for the open reduction. Because the mouth is a contaminated area, a complete change of gowns, gloves, and drapes is necessary after the intraoral procedure.

The patient is placed in the supine position on the OR bed. The head drape is used.

*Operative Procedure*

1. Arch bars may be applied before or after the open reduction.
2. A line inferior and parallel to the lower border of the mandible at the fracture site is marked, and the area is infiltrated with epinephrine 1:200,000 for hemostasis.
3. The incision is made so that the inferior border of the mandible is exposed. The nerve stimulator may be used to aid in identification of the marginal mandibular branch of the facial nerve in fractures of the posterior body and angle of the mandible.
4. The fracture is reduced by manipulation. Holes are drilled into the mandible on each side of the fracture line with the Hall II air drill while an assistant holds the reduced fracture with the aid of Dingman bone-holding forceps.
5. Stainless steel wire is inserted through the holes and twisted tightly to secure the fracture fragments in anatomic alignment.
6. In the event that rigid fixation is desired with the use of plates and screws, the appropriate drill bit, tap, and depth gauge are chosen. With these items, the proper-size prosthesis is placed and the fracture is approximated, aligned, and placed in anatomic position.
7. A small drain is sometimes placed into the wound, and the wound is closed in layers (periosteum, platysma muscle, and skin).
8. The latex bands may be applied to the arch bars at this time but more frequently are applied later, after the patient is fully awake and reactive.
9. A moderate compression dressing is applied to cover the submandibular wound and drain.

### Elective Orthognathic Surgery

A large number of patients have either acquired or congenital facial defects that affect the maxilla, the mandible, or both. The condition of many of these patients can be improved dramatically with orthodontic care; however, many also require surgical rearrangement of the maxilla or mandible.

***Procedural Considerations.*** Psychosocial and functional deficits are related to abnormalities of the maxilla and mandible. Surgical correction of these defects can improve patients' quality of life. Surgery is usually delayed until an adequate number of permanent teeth are in place for postoperative immobilization. Coordinated preoperative planning is of great importance to the success of these procedures.

*Operative Procedure*

1. Arch bars are applied for postoperative immobilization.
2. Intraoral incisions provide exposure.
3. The maxilla or mandible is cut as indicated by the preoperative workup.
4. Bone is advanced or set back to a predetermined position.
5. Bones are wired in place, with grafts placed in defects as needed.

## GENDER REASSIGNMENT

Transsexualism is defined as the condition in which an individual with chromosomes and internal and external organs normal to one gender identifies psychologically and socially with attributes of the opposite gender. Reassignment of gender by means of surgery is the last step to be taken in treatment of transsexuals. It is performed only after the patient has been treated with hormones of the opposite gender, has experienced a period of cross-gender living, and has had intensive psychiatric evaluation. Most institutions performing this type of surgery have gender-identity teams who evaluate and treat transsexuals. These teams usually include a variety of professionals: psychiatrist, psychologist, endocrinologist, plastic surgeon, urologist, gynecologist, and social worker.

The surgical techniques for assignment of male to female are technically easier. A breast augmentation may be performed if hormone therapy has not sufficiently changed breast size. Construction of the neovagina includes radical penectomy, bilateral orchiectomy, urethroplasty, perineal dissection, creation of a neovaginal vault, vaginoplasty, and vulvoplasty.

The surgical technique for female to male is technically more difficult and requires multiple surgical procedures. Considerations that must be addressed are twofold: the neophallus must be constructed to (1) allow the patient to stand to void and (2) permit stimulation of a sexual partner during intercourse. This may require a radial artery forearm free flap with a later-stage surgical insertion of a penile prosthesis for attaining an erection.

## AESTHETIC SURGERY

Aesthetic surgery may be performed with the patient under general anesthesia or under local anesthesia with conscious sedation. The perioperative nurse must be prepared to monitor the patient during the procedure. Baseline vital signs should be recorded in the operating room record. A blood pressure cuff, pulse oximeter, and cardiac monitor electrodes should be placed. IV fluids should be started. The operating room should be kept quiet and patient privacy protected. Care should be taken to avoid conversation that could be misinterpreted by the patient.

### Scar Revision

Scar revision involves the rearranging or reshaping of an existing scar so that the scar is less noticeable. The simplest form of scar revision is excision of an existing scar and simple resuturing of the wound. This may improve scars that are wide.

The Z-plasty is the most widely used method of scar revision (Figure 24-28). It breaks up linear scars, rearranging them

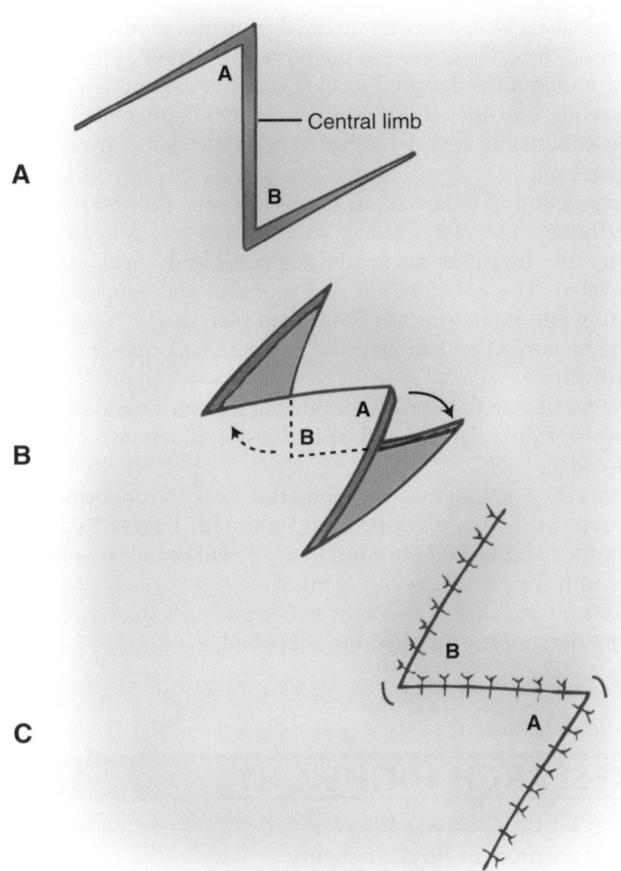


FIGURE 24-28 Z-plasty for scar revision. **A,** The central limb of the Z-plasty is over the scar that needs to be revised. **B,** Two other limbs are incised—each equal in length to the central limb and diverging from it at an equal angle. The flaps are then transposed. **C,** Flaps transposed, and original Z rotated 90 degrees and reversed.

so that the central limb of the Z lies in the same direction as a natural skin line. Scars that are parallel to skin lines are less noticeable than scars that are perpendicular to skin lines. A contracted scar line can also be lengthened with a Z-plasty.

***Procedural Considerations.*** A plastic local instrument set and a marking pen are required. The procedure may be performed with the patient under local or general anesthesia. The patient is positioned, prepped, and draped so that the scar that is to be revised is well exposed.

### *Operative Procedure*

1. The pattern for the planned revision is marked.
2. The scar is excised.
3. The surrounding tissue is undermined, and the wound edges are approximated according to the surgeon's markings.
4. Dressings may or may not be applied.

## Endoscopic Brow Lift

The aging process affects the area above the eyes and brows in several ways. Loss of skin elasticity can cause the appearance of a heavy brow and emphasize hooding of the upper eyelids.

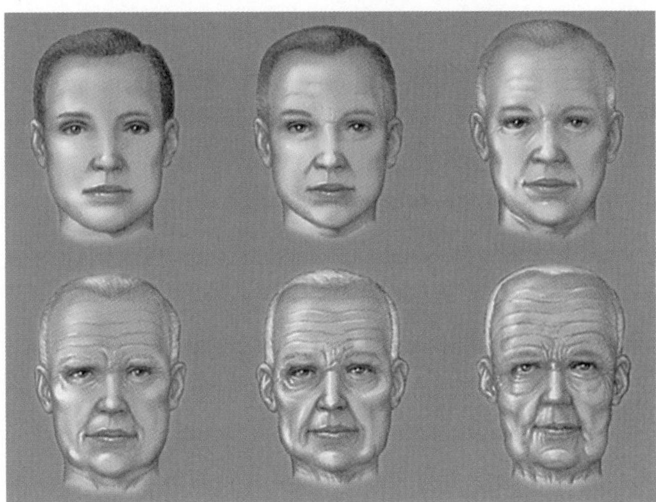

FIGURE 24-29 The sequence of aging.

Repetitive muscle action results in horizontal forehead lines and furrows as well as creases between the brows (Figure 24-29). The goal of endoscopic brow/forehead surgery is to minimize the heaviness of the brow and improve the frown lines of aging, reduce upper eyelid hooding, reposition the eyebrows if necessary, and create a more youthful, refreshed appearance of the forehead and brow area, all through multiple, short incisions in the scalp.

***Procedural Considerations.*** Positioning the patient at the very top of the operating bed is necessary for good utilization and mobility of the endoscopic instruments. For patients with medium to long hair, the hair may be sectioned and tied with sterilized rubber bands to minimize interference with the planned incision. The entire head (scalp, face, ears, and neck) should be prepped and draped with impervious drape material. The eyes should be protected with ointment and shields for the duration of the procedure as well as the ear canals from prep solution pooling. During preparation of the room, perform a check of all endoscopic equipment to ensure it is functioning properly. Endoscopic instrumentation includes elevators, scissors, clamps, needle holders, camera, and light sources. All should be sterilized according to manufacturers' recommendations. Depending on the method of fixation, screws and accompanying instrumentation may be necessary.

### *Operative Procedure*

1. Incision lines and anatomic landmarks are marked.
2. Local anesthesia of preference is injected.
3. Three to five small scalp incisions are placed (one midline and one or two paramedian), and forehead skin is elevated.
4. The endoscope is placed to allow visualization of muscles, vessels, nerves, and tissues.
5. Muscles (corrugator and procerus) and tissues are dissected and redraped to produce a smoother appearance and desired repositioning of brows.
6. Screws are placed in the outer table of the cranium at designated points, and sutures are placed through the galea and tied around screws to facilitate elevation of the brow and forehead.
7. Scalp incisions are stapled or sutured closed.

## Rhytidectomy (Facelift)

As the aging process progresses, the skin of the face and neck becomes loose and redundant. This is particularly noticeable in the "jowl" areas and just beneath the chin. A common misconception is that a facelift involves only the face. Actually, one of the most common complaints of aging is the appearance of the neck and submental skin. The typical facelift treats the face and neck and involves removal and redraping of excess skin of the face and neck once repositioning of the underlying muscle and platysma has been performed. The result is a smooth, rested appearance, without unnatural tightness or distortion of facial features (Figure 24-30). Rather than excising the redundant skin directly, incisions adjacent to or within hairlines are used so that the scars are virtually indiscernible.

***Procedural Considerations.*** The patient is positioned supine with head and shoulders slightly elevated. Attention should be given to safety by using proper positioning to prevent pressure injuries, using sequential compression devices (SCDs), maintaining normothermia, and preventing eye injuries by using shields. An indwelling urinary catheter may be inserted. If conscious sedation is used, an oral or nasal airway is placed and oxygen administered.

Specialized scissors of varying lengths should be available, along with smooth and toothed tissue forceps and various sizes of needle holders. A fiberoptic lighted retractor is standard for facelifts. Since many surgeons have specific instrumentation they desire for this procedure, the nurse should ask before surgery if any instruments were brought and need sterilization, or if they have special requests of facility-owned instruments.

There are numerous techniques for rhytidectomy, and a well-prepared perioperative nurse will ask the surgeon about the specific technique in order to have the appropriate suture material and special needles available (Research Highlight). The underlying superficial muscular aponeurotic system (SMAS) may be repositioned, the cheek may be elevated independently, the midface may be lifted, and there may or may not be accompanying liposuction. Facelift procedures are customized specific to the anatomic needs of the individual patient. The entire head, neck, ears and scalp are prepped and draped.

A

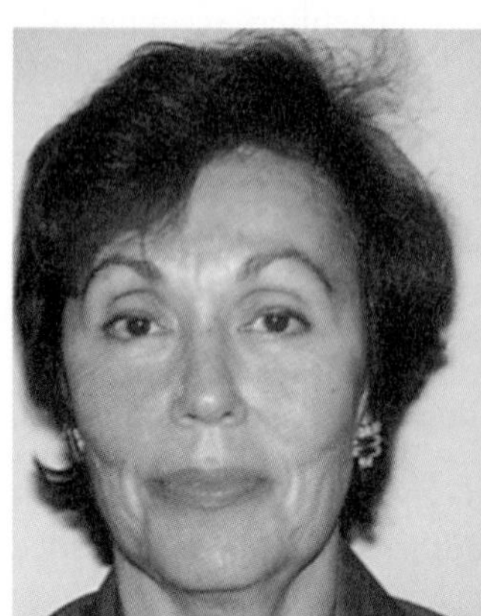

B

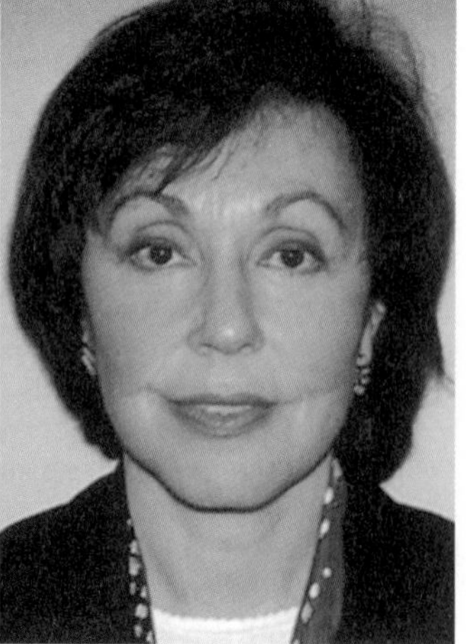

**FIGURE 24-30** **A,** Preoperative and, **B,** postoperative views of 61-year-old patient, 1 year following rhytidectomy.

### *Operative Procedure*

1. Bilateral incision lines are marked from the temporal scalp, around the earlobe, around the posterior margin of the auricula, and into the occipital scalp (Figures 24-31 and 24-32).
2. The incision lines, both temples, cheeks, upper neck, and the submental area are injected with the local anesthetic agent.
3. Liposuction of indicated areas (neck, jowls, cheeks) may be performed.
4. After the incisions are made, temporal and cheek skin is elevated. The SMAS is plicated cephalad and caudally, elevating and tightening the SMAS and platysma.
5. The malar pad is then elevated, repositioned, and anchored with suture.
6. The facial skin flap is then elevated in a superior and slightly posterior direction, tacked, and excess skin trimmed. at the flap edges.
7. Through a submental incision, the neck is undermined, plastysmal bands identified, and plicated. Excess tissue is trimmed and tacked postauricularly. Small drains are placed beneath the skin flaps and secured.
8. Incisions are closed in one or two layers.
9. A moderate pressure dressing is applied.

## RESEARCH HIGHLIGHT

### Using Fibrin Glue for Prevention of Hematoma in Rhytidectomy

Postoperative wound hematoma is a potential complication related to rhytidectomy. The technique of using fibrin glue to reduce postoperative drainage, wound hematomas, and edema and ecchymosis was studied by researchers in a prospective, nonblinded, randomized, and controlled trial with 30 patients. The patients ranged in age from 40 to 72 years old. Risks associated with fibrin glue include potential disease transmission and allergic reactions. The use of the glue adds approximately $500 to the cost of the procedure.

Patients in the study were used as their own controls and were randomized to have the fibrin glue used on one side of their face to provide comparison between the glued and unglued sides during the postoperative period. The researchers sprayed the commercially prepared tissue glue to the subcutaneous plane of the neck and face after placing a drain in the neck just below the border of the mandible. The patients were assessed at 24 hours and again at 8 days after their procedure.

One study participant had a hematoma that required surgical evacuation. In the remaining patients, the mean drainage on the glued side was 26 ml compared with 33.5 ml on the unglued side, but this was not considered to be surgically significant. Scores were assigned to the grade of hematoma, ecchymosis, and edema between the glued and unglued sides, and results indicated there were minimal differences.

Researchers concluded that although fibrin glue may help prevent some but not all hematomas, the added cost and risks associated with its use indicate it should not be used routinely but should be reserved for cases where patients are at significantly higher risk for hematomas.

Modified from Marchac D, Greensmith AL: Early postoperative efficacy of fibrin glue in face lifts: a prospective randomized trial, *Plastic and Reconstructive Surgery* 115(3):911-916, 2005.

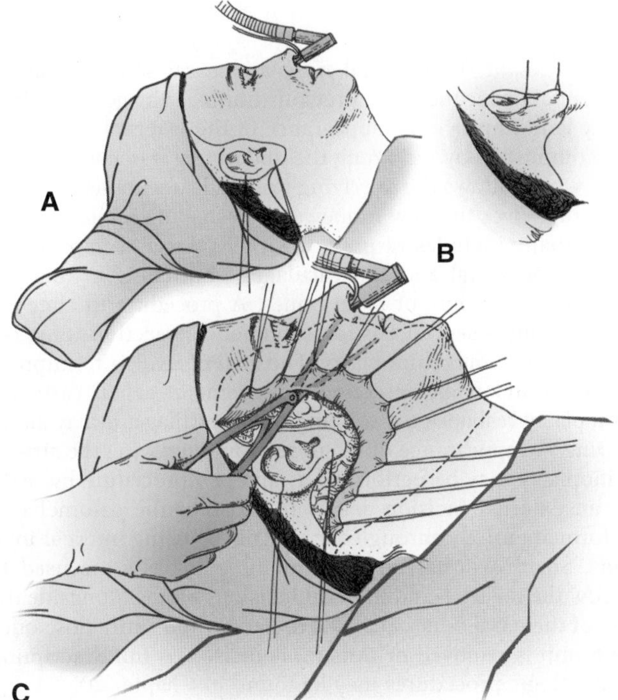


FIGURE 24-31 Rhytidectomy: line of incision and undermining. **A,** Traction sutures of 4-0 silk placed into auricle; temporal incision curved posteriorly for better support of upward pull. **B,** Incision carried under earlobe and then curved posteriorly upward and then caudad toward midline. **C,** Skin undermined almost to nasolabial fold, to area of mental foramen, and to midline of neck as far down as thyroid cartilage. Care is taken to avoid injury to submandibular branches of facial nerve and facial artery.

## Blepharoplasty

The aging process causes a sagging or relaxation of eyelid skin and the orbital septum. As the latter becomes weaker, it allows periorbital fat to bulge. These changes are perceived as baggy eyelids, which give the patient a chronically tired appearance. The goal of blepharoplasty is to improve the patient's appearance by removing excess eyelid skin, removing or repositioning bulging periorbital fat, and tightening and smoothing the muscles under the eye. The upper eyelid skin can be so redundant that it encroaches on the patient's field of vision, and removal of excessive hooding of the upper eyelid skin may even improve peripheral vision. The upper eyelid crease may also be enhanced. Not all patients need removal of skin; for selected individuals, $CO_2$ skin resurfacing may be the procedure of choice to achieve a smoother appearance of the lower eyelid skin. Incisions in the subconjunctival mucosa of the lower lids are sometimes used for this group of patients if resection or repositioning of the periorbital fat is also indicated. Blepharoplasty is often performed with rhytidectomy. Blepharoplasty may be performed on both the upper and lower lids, upper lids only, or lower lids only.

***Procedural Considerations.*** A plastic local instrument set is required. Delicate, short instruments are used, with special attention to scissors (curved Kaye blepharoplasty), fine Adsons with teeth, calipers, and fixation forceps. Webster needle holders are frequently desired. A bipolar coagulation unit may be used. A needle tip for the active electrode may be requested if the monopolar ESU is used (with the monopolar ESU, a lower setting is used. The perioperative nurse should verbally repeat back the settings requested by the surgeon). Blepharoplasty is usually performed with local anesthesia with conscious sedation. The patient is placed in the supine position on the OR bed. The face is prepped, and the head drape is used. Corneal shields may be used to protect the cornea.

### *Operative Procedure—Upper Lids*

1. Lines of incision are marked, and local anesthesia is injected.
2. The incision is placed, and excess skin is removed. Hemostasis is obtained (Figure 24-33, *A* to *C*).
3. The orbicularis oculi muscle is trimmed, and the septum orbitale is identified and incised. Excess periorbital fat is trimmed and coagulated.
4. Upper lid incisions are closed; and the procedure is repeated for the opposite upper lid.
5. Finely crushed ice on moist gauze 4 × 4 pads may be applied to the periorbital region; other means of reducing swelling, such as cold compresses or a mechanical cold

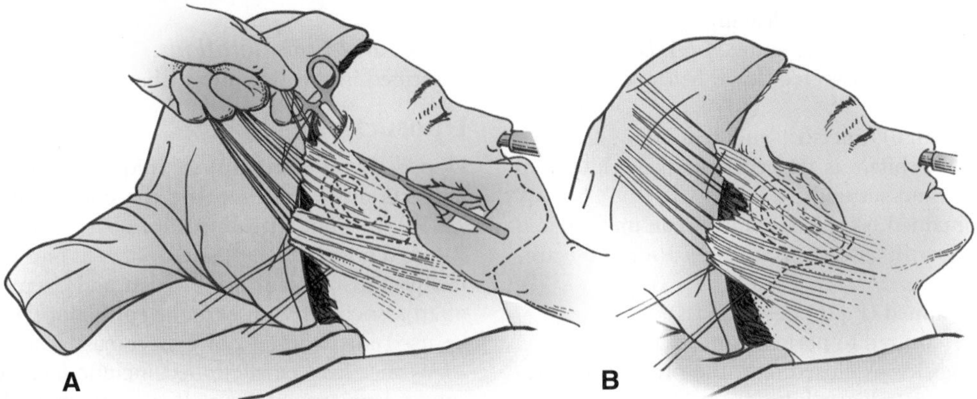


FIGURE 24-32 Rhytidectomy: removal of superfluous skin. **A,** Skin drawn upward to proper degree of tension, and incision made along posterior margin of clamp. **B,** Incision continued upward around posterior margin of auricle and then backward to excise skin specimen.

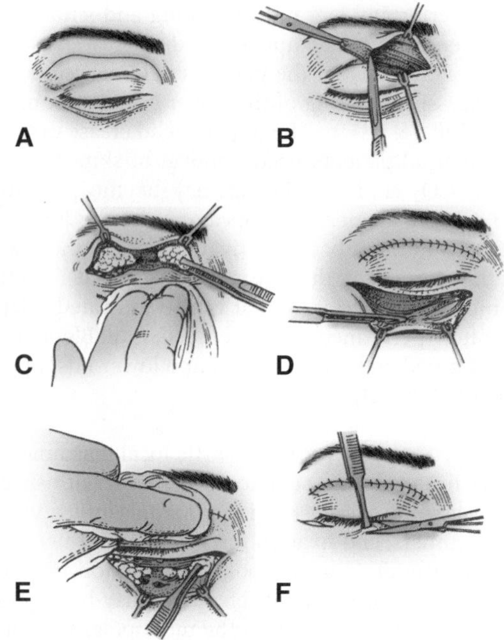


**FIGURE 24-33** Blepharoplasty for baggy eyelids. **A,** Areas of proposed skin excision marked with methylene blue or marking pen. **B,** Strip of skin excised from upper lid; fat pad shining through orbital fascia and orbicular muscle of eye. **C,** Orbital fascia opened in two places (medially and laterally). Pressure on eyeball causes fat pads to bulge. They are eased out meticulously. **D,** Upper lid incision sutured with continuous 6-0 suture material of choice. Orbital muscle fibers are separated from skin. **E,** Orbital fascia opened; fat pads bulge because of digital pressure and are teased out meticulously. **F,** Skin tailored to fit and sutured.

mask, may be similarly applied. Compresses are changed as often as they become warm.

### *Operative Procedure—Lower Lids*

1. Lines of incision are marked, and local anesthesia is injected.
2. A subciliary incision is made and brought out in a natural line in the outer canthal skin.
3. The skin-muscle flap is raised, leaving a 3 mm strip of muscle attached to the tarsus (Figure 24-33, *D*).
4. The skin-muscle flap is dissected down below the level of the orbital rim.
5. The arcus marginalis is incised, and redundant fat with overlying septum orbitale is draped over the orbital rim (Figure 24-33, *E*) and sutured.
6. Hemostasis is obtained. Skin is redraped in an upward and outward fashion with attention to prevention of ectropion.
7. Excess skin is trimmed (Figure 24-33, *F*).
8. Lateral muscle is sutured to periosteum.
9. The lower lid incision is closed, and the procedure is repeated for the opposite lower lid.
10. Compresses are applied as described in the upper lid procedure.

## Rhinoplasty

Deformities of the external nose and nasal septum may be congenital or secondary to previous trauma. The goal of rhinoplasty is to improve the appearance of the external nose. This is accomplished by reshaping the underlying framework of the nose, which allows the overlying skin and subcutaneous tissue to redrape over the new framework. Reshaping the nasal skeleton usually includes rasping down of a dorsal hump, partial excision of lateral and alar cartilages, shortening of the septum, and osteotomy of nasal bones. A procedure to alter the nasal septum—septoplasty, or submucous resection (SMR)—often accompanies rhinoplasty. The goal of SMR is to improve the nasal airway by resecting a segment of septal cartilage. Septoplasty reshapes the existing septal cartilage; it may aid in altering the appearance of the nose or in improving the airway. Rhinoplasty may be performed as an open procedure by making an external incision across the base of the columella or performed entirely through the nostrils by using internal incisions. Small external incisions at the alar bases are used to narrow the nostrils, and internal incisions placed alongside the base of the nasal bones are used to narrow the entire nose once the hump is removed or dorsum is incised. A full description of rhinologic procedures may be found in Chapter 20.

## Laser Surgery

Several different types of lasers are commonly used in plastic and reconstructive surgery. One of the most popular types of laser is the skin resurfacing, or $CO_2$, laser. The laser is attracted to the water in the skin cells and ablates the cells at a predetermined depth. The collagen material is also heated, resulting in smoother and slightly tighter skin. This treatment has virtually replaced dermabrasion, because it is much more consistent in terms of depth of penetration and less dependent on user technique or skill.

Tattoo removal and destruction of vascular lesions, such as facial telangiectasias, spider veins, and hemangiomas, may be achieved with the use of other types of lasers. Whether using lasers for skin resurfacing or tattoo removal procedures, the areas must first be numbed with local anesthesia. Use of sedation depends on the anxiety level of the patient as well as the total surface area to be treated. Vascular lesions may be treated without local anesthesia, although there is some temporary discomfort with each pulse of the laser.

***Procedural Considerations.*** Laser safety and procedures are described in great detail in Chapter 7.

## Liposuction

Liposuction is a surgical technique designed to remove excess deposits of fat and improve the contour of the body (Figure 24-34). It is not a treatment for obesity; rather, the ideal candidate is a normal weight and desires to remove localized fat that has proved resistant despite diet and exercise. Although most often associated with contour correction, liposuction may also be used for treatment of gynecomastia or to remove lipomas. Areas that may be suctioned include face, neck, back, breasts (not a replacement for reduction mammoplasty, only contour correction), waist, abdomen, midriff, flanks, upper arms, hips, medial and lateral thighs, knees, and ankles (Figure 24-35).

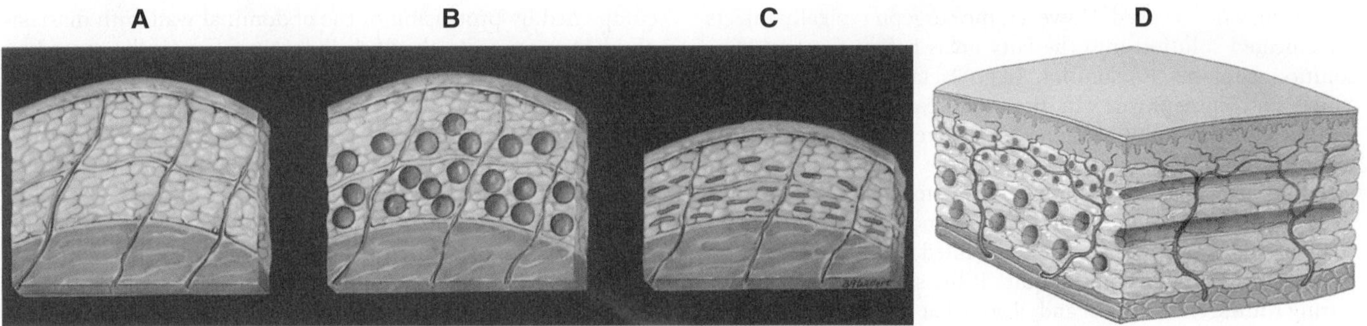


FIGURE 24-34 **A,** Normal appearance of excess fat. **B,** Removal of deep fat by larger-diameter cannulas. **C,** Corrected contour following removal of excess fat by liposuction. **D,** Removal of superficial fat involves using narrower-gauge cannulas.

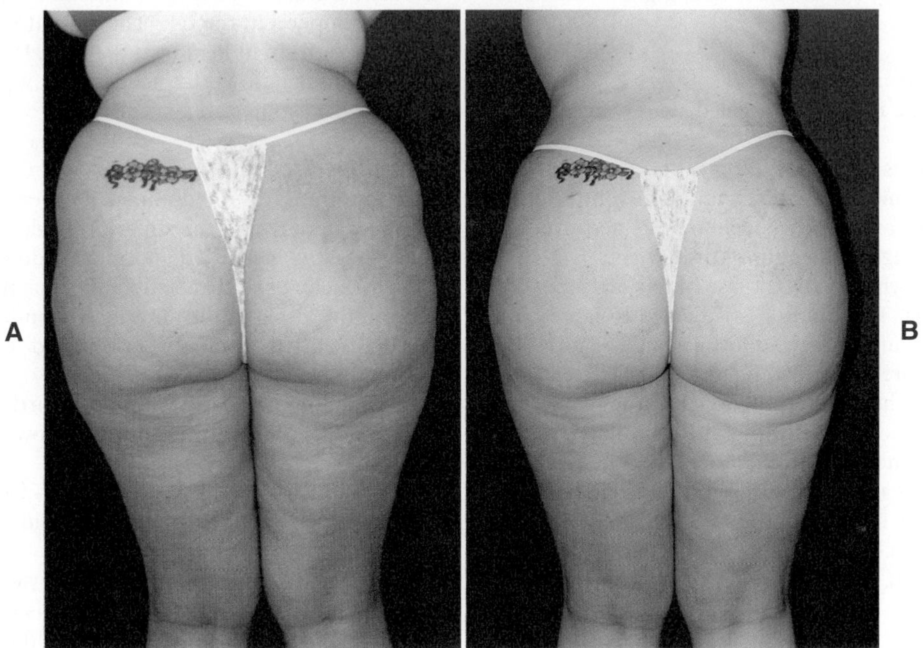


FIGURE 24-35 **A,** Preoperative and, **B,** postoperative appearance after ultrasound-assisted liposuction of posterior flanks, hips, and lateral thighs.

Multiple techniques have been developed to enhance the final results as well as ease the removal of the fat. These techniques are not always used in isolation of each other; rather, some may be combined for the best possible outcome and as a result of the surgeon's preferences. Each procedure has specific equipment needed for that technique and often has highly specific cannulas and other instrumentation. Since multiple areas are usually treated, the nurse should find out the sequence of liposuction the surgeon prefers in order to be prepared for positioning.

***Procedural Considerations.*** Immediate preoperative preparation includes asking the patient to stand while the area of deformity is outlined. Two lines are usually drawn on the skin surface—one delineating the major area of defect and the other placed a short distance outside the first area. These lines make it easier for the plastic surgeon to make a smooth transition toward the normal tissue by adjusting the amount of fat removed from the center to the periphery of the deformity. The patient may remain standing and be prepped circumferentially with a spray bottle of antimicrobial skin solution. The patient's privacy should be protected.

Preoperative patient education should include a discussion of the compression garment, which is typically worn for 2 to 4 weeks postoperatively. Patients should also be informed about the likelihood of the puncture sites leaking tumescent solution during the first 24 hours of the postoperative period. Absorbent dressings are required to minimize soiling of clothing and bedding during this period as well as to maintain the cleanliness of the compression garment.

Depending on the areas targeted for liposuction, draping may require a good deal of innovation. Minimal instrumentation is necessary—knife handle, towel clips, tissue forceps, scissors, clamps, and needle holder are used along with the suction cannulas specific to the proposed liposuction technique. A general anesthetic, IV sedative, or epidural anesthetic may or may not be used. However, the surgeon typically injects a medicated solution into the fatty areas before removal. The solution contains IV solution (e.g., lactated Ringer's), lidocaine, and epinephrine. In the tumescent technique, large volumes of this solution are administered. The "super-wet" technique uses less solution; usually the amount of fluid injected approximates the amount of fat to be removed—thus the name, which refers to the swollen and firm ("tumesced") state of the tissues when they are filled with solution. The perioperative nurse should inquire if the surgeon will be infiltrating tumescent solution and, if so, what ingredients are used for his or her technique. Also, ask whether the surgeon uses internal or external ultrasound (sound waves that liquefy fat) or power-assisted liposuction. One of the newer techniques is the use of Vaser-Assisted LipoSelection, which incorporates thermal energy to liquefy the fat, thus aiding greatly in its removal.

### *Operative Procedure*

1. Stablike incisions are made in concealed areas to access sites to be liposuctioned.
2. Tumescent solution is infused.
3. Depending on technique, at this point either internal or external ultrasound or the Vaser technique is performed at predetermined settings and length of time.
4. Liposuction is performed with the use of various sizes and lengths of cannulas. The cannula is attached to large-bore, firm suction tubing and connected to an aspirating unit. The high vacuum pressure caused by the unit causes the fat cells to emulsify so that they can be suctioned through the vacuum opening near the rounded tip of the cannula. Areas are usually cross-suctioned in order to achieve the best outcomes. Stab wounds may be closed with absorbable suture or left open to drain.
5. The patient's skin is cleaned, and bulky dressings and compression garments are applied.

## Abdominoplasty

Abdominoplasty is particularly useful in improving the appearance (and to a certain extent, function) of persons who have lost a great deal of weight or who suffer from laxity of abdominal skin following pregnancy. Obesity produces distention and stretching of the skin of the abdomen. Weight loss reduces the volume of the underlying fat; however, it does not produce concomitant reduction in the excess surface area of the overlying skin, which results from destruction or insufficiency of elastic fibers in the skin. The rectus abdominis fascia is also stretched in obese patients, and weight loss does not restore its integrity.

There are several versions of the abdominoplasty procedure and the choice of which technique to use depends upon the degree of deformity of the abdominal skin and muscle. All techniques are designed to improve the appearance of the abdomen by tightening the abdominal area (abdominal wall/rectus muscles) and removing excess skin or fullness.

If there is minimal to no laxity of the skin and mostly fullness of the lower abdomen, then a "mini-abdominoplasty" may be indicated. With this technique it is not necessary to relocate or incise the umbilicus and a short incision, resembling a Pfannestiel, may be effectively utilized. However if there is laxity of the peri-umbilical and upper and lower abdominal skin accompanied by protrusion of the abdominal wall with diastasis of the rectus muscle, then full abdominoplasty is the procedure of choice. This version requires relocation of the umbilicus and an incision which stretches from hip to hip. Endoscopic abdominoplasty is another option if only muscle repair (correction of the diastasis deformity or shortening of the rectus muscles) is needed.

***Procedural Considerations.*** A basic plastic instrument set is required, as well as extra retractors and clamping instruments, an ESU, and a marking pen. Frequently tumescent anesthetic solution will be added to minimize bleeding, reduce postoperative discomfort, and aid in dissection. The perioperative nurse should ask the surgeon about the use of tumescent as well as preference for ingredients. A lighted fiberoptic retractor should be available. SCDs or antiembolism hose are usually in place or applied in the OR. The patient is placed in the supine position with slight flexion at the hips. Draping is such that the entire abdomen, lower costal margins, upper thighs, and both anterior iliac spines are exposed.

### *Operative Procedure*

1. A low transverse abdominal incision across both inguinal areas laterally and the superior border of the mons pubis in the midline is marked and incised down to fascia.
2. A large flap of skin and subcutaneous tissue is elevated away from the fascia of the anterior abdominal wall.
3. The umbilicus is circumscribed and left in its normal position.
4. The abdominal flap is elevated further until the xiphoid process of the sternum and the lower costal margins are reached.
5. If diastasis of the rectus abdominis fascia is present, plication is performed from the xiphoid process to the mons pubis.
6. The flap of abdominal skin and subcutaneous tissue is pulled inferiorly, and excess tissue is excised.
7. A small incision is made in the midline of the flap to accommodate the umbilicus, which is then sutured peripherally to the flap.
8. Drains are inserted, followed by closure of the lower abdominal incision in layers.
9. Postoperatively the patient is placed in the hospital bed in high-Fowler position.

## Post–Bariatric Surgery Body Contouring

Successful bariatric surgery produces significant weight loss. The weight loss may result in a trunk that lacks waist and hip definition; ptosis of the mons pubis; and various degrees of skin, fat, and abdominal wall laxity.[1] Upper and lower back rolls accompany the anterior truncal deformities; the buttocks are lower and lack fullness. Upper arms and thighs exhibit similar deformities.

Treatment is aimed at removing the excessive skin and creating a desirable body contour.[15] Most patients are candidates for some form of circumferential recontouring (belt lipectomy) in combination with any number of other recontouring procedures: brachioplasty, thigh lifts, and mastopexy. For the perioperative nurse, these surgeries offer a logistical challenge because of the combination of procedures and positioning required. The malabsorptive effects of the original bariatric surgery may compromise postoperative wound healing after body contouring procedures. The perioperative nurse must be familiar with the complications relating to post–bariatric surgery body contouring to provide comprehensive care for this unique group of patients (Research Highlight).

***Procedural Considerations.*** Any form of body contouring will begin in the preoperative area, where extensive measuring and marking are performed by the plastic surgeon. The nurse should inquire about the ordering of the procedures and positioning if more than one is planned. Sequential compression devices and a Foley catheter should be used once the patient arrives in the OR. During prepping and draping, attempts should be made to preserve the patient's body temperature. Repositioning is a standard part of these procedures. Pressure points should be well padded with appropriate positioning aids to maintain functional alignment and stable positioning. With each repositioning activity, the patient must be reassessed for safety in terms of skin and nerve compression and competence of the grounding pad, Foley catheter, and all monitoring devices.[11] A basic plastic surgery instrument set with additional towel clamps is used. Other supplies include a stapler for skin approximation, multiple drains, and the ESU. The surgeon may choose to use tissue adhesive products in combination with suture material to reduce the incidence of seroma. Compression garments may be applied, but care must be taken not to compromise the vascularity of the skin flaps.

## RESEARCH HIGHLIGHT

### Complications After Total Body Lift

Patients who lose weight after bariatric surgery frequently experience functional and aesthetic issues relating to loose and redundant skin around their torso, abdomen, buttocks, and thighs. Circumferential body lifts (simultaneous abdominoplasty, thigh and buttock lifts) are often used to address post–bariatric surgery body changes. This study sought to define the complications associated with post–bariatric plastic surgery and analyze the surgical techniques used.

Researchers classified patients into three groups based on their body mass index (BMI) at the time of surgery. Type I individuals had a BMI less than 28, type II individuals had a BMI between 28 and 32, and type III individuals had a BMI greater than 32. BMI is a number that shows body weight adjusted for height. The study was performed by means of a retrospective chart review of 200 patients who had undergone circumferential body lifts over a 4-year period.

Type I and many type II patients achieved acceptable aesthetic results. The majority of type II and type III patients had significant functional and aesthetic improvements but were more likely to have complications. The overall complication rate was 50%. The most frequent complications were skin dehiscence and seroma formation at 32.5% and 16.5%. Other complications were skin necrosis, infection, bleeding, deep vein thrombosis, and pulmonary embolus. Fifteen percent of the participants received transfusions to treat postoperative anemia. Within the groups who experienced complications, 18% were smokers. Average length of hospital stay was 2.95 nights (range 0 to 20 days), with heavier patients having longer lengths of stay.

Standard body lifts often involve prepping and draping the patient three times over the course of the procedure. The authors noted fewer complications and better results performing the procedure in one stage, using sterile instrumentation to abduct the lower extremities and sterile sequential compression devices and draping the patient circumferentially above the inframammary fold.

Based on the findings from this study, the authors developed patient selection criteria to maximize safety and reduce complications. Candidates for circumferential body lift should be at a stable weight for several months (ideally at their lowest weight) and have a BMI less than 35 and a baseline hemoglobin of at least 12.

Modified from Nemerofsky R and others: Body lift: an account of 200 consecutive cases in the massive weight loss patient, *Plastic and Reconstructive Surgery* 117(2):414-430, 2006.

***Operative Procedure—Belt Lipectomy.*** Sites addressed are the abdomen including mons pubis, upper and lower back, lateral trunk skin, buttocks, and lateral upper thighs.

1. The patient is positioned, prepped, and draped. Markings are redrawn if necessary.
2. Dilute tumescent solution is infused to aid in hemostasis and facilitate undermining of flaps.
3. Incisions are made and taken down to the level of the fascia, and flaps are elevated to previously marked margins. Liposuction cannulas without vacuum attachments may be used for undermining.
4. Liposuction is used if indicated for contouring only.
5. Muscle plication is performed when indicated.
6. Superficial fascia is approximated and sutured with permanent sutures.
7. Skin flaps are approximated, and excess skin is excised.
8. Drains are inserted and secured with suture.
9. Medical-grade tissue glue is applied, and closure is performed.
10. The patient is repositioned; depending on position at the start of the procedure, this could be lateral decubitus or supine.
11. Similar techniques are used for defects in areas presented by the new position and repeated until all areas are addressed, including relocation of the umbilicus.
12. The patient is cleaned, incisions are dressed, and a garment is applied at the surgeon's preference.
13. The patient is transferred to a stretcher or bed and placed in the flexed position.

## Breast Surgeries

A variety of surgical procedures are available to enhance the aesthetic appearance of the breasts. Patients may choose to enlarge, reduce, and change the position of their breasts. More than 445,000 cosmetic breast surgical procedures were performed by plastic surgeons in 2004.[20]

***Augmentation Mammoplasty.*** Breast augmentation is performed for correction of hypomastia, to correct breast asymmetry, and to recreate the breast after mastectomy. A prosthesis is inserted to enlarge or form the breast mound.

***Breast Implants.*** The two basic types of breast implants are saline-filled and silicone gel–filled. Saline-filled breast implants are approved by the FDA for elective breast augmentation. Silicone gel–filled implants are approved only for use in breast reconstruction and revision and are available only to women who participate in investigational clinical studies.[10] Alternative implants, using soybean oil or organic polymers, such as polysaccharides and water are used in other countries but not approved for use in the United States.[12] Cohesive gel implants are a form of stable implant used outside the United States that are currently being studied in FDA-approved clinical trials (Research Highlight).

Implants are configured into round or tear drop (also known as anatomic) shapes and may have a smooth or textured surface. The surfaces are designed to minimize capsular contracture and migration. The choice to use a round or an anatomic implant is based on the shape and form of the existing breast.

**PROCEDURAL CONSIDERATIONS.** The perioperative nurse should handle the implant according to the manufacturer's recommendations. Handling implants as little as possible assists in efforts to reduce the potential for implant contamination. A basic plastic instrument set is used, plus lighted fiberoptic retractors. The breast implants are packaged in sterile containers from the manufacturer and given to the scrub person when breast size is determined. Breast implants should only be filled with sterile injectable saline using a closed system designed for that purpose. The patient is placed in a supine position. The arms may be extended on armboards to approximately 60 degrees. Alternatively, the hands may be placed over the lower abdomen, the elbows protected with foam padding, and the arms gently secured to the OR bed with adhesive tape. Prepping and draping are carried out in the routine manner to expose the operative site.

## RESEARCH HIGHLIGHT

### Cohesive Gel Breast Implants

Dr. David Kessler, director of the U.S. Food and Drug Administration (FDA), banned the use of silicone breast implants after April 12, 1992. Two million women already had these implants, and Dr. Kessler believed, despite a lack of clinical research, that these women were at risk for developing connective tissues diseases. It was an accepted fact in the surgical implant community that a certain amount of gel bleed occurred through the implant shell and tissue capsule, but it was believed to have no impact on the health of the woman. Subsequent studies have supported this belief scientifically, demonstrating no evidence linking silicone breast implants to autoimmune diseases, such as chronic rheumatoid arthritis, scleroderma, systemic lupus erythematosus, or other connective tissue diseases.

The latest-generation silicone breast implants are cohesive silicone gel implants. Designed to reduce the amount of gel bleed and provide a safer implant if the prosthesis ruptures by maintaining its integrity, it is manufactured by increasing the number of crosslinks among the gel molecules. The prosthesis has a textured silicone elastomer shell and results in a natural-feeling implant with a decreased risk of rippling and a high rate of patient satisfaction. These implants are currently available for patients who qualify for criteria in several adjunct clinical breast implant studies. It is anticipated that they may be released for general aesthetic use in the future.

Modified from Brown M and others: Cohesive silicone gel breast implants in aesthetic and reconstructive breast surgery, *Plastic and Reconstructive Surgery* 11(3):768-79, 2005; Nosé Y: Critical threat to the availability of surgical implant material: lesson to be learned from breast implants, *Artificial Organs* 29(8):595-597, 2005.

**OPERATIVE PROCEDURE.** Augmentation mammoplasty is done through circumareolar, inframammary, axillary, or transumbilical incisions. An open or an endoscopic approach may be used. Depending on the anatomy of the patient and the surgeon's preference, breast implants may be placed subglandularly, subpectorally (Figure 24-36), or biplanar (partial muscle coverage).

**OPERATIVE PROCEDURE—UNFILLED SALINE IMPLANTS**

1. The patient is prepped and draped, and markings are reinforced if necessary.
2. Local anesthesia may be instilled to decrease bleeding and provide analgesia.
3. An incision is made, the pocket is dissected, and hemostasis is achieved.
4. Breast implant sizers (gel or saline) may be inserted to evaluate the size of the pocket and determine the size of the final implant.
5. With the sizers in place, the patient is placed in a 90-degree position to evaluate the appearance from various angles and plan for any adjustments or revisions to the pocket.
6. The sizers are removed, and the pocket is finalized.
7. The implant is dispensed to the field and, if desired by the surgeon, soaked in antibiotic solution.
8. The implant is rolled into a cylindric shape in preparation for insertion.
9. The pocket is irrigated with saline or antibiotic solution.
10. The implant is inserted, unrolled, properly positioned, and inflated with an appropriate amount of saline.
11. The procedure is repeated for the opposite breast.
12. The incision is closed in two layers.
13. The patient is cleaned, and bandages and a surgical bra are applied.

***Capsulotomy.*** Capsule contracture results from an exaggerated scar response to a foreign prosthetic material. All surgical implants undergo some degree of encapsulation, but clinical problems arise when this scar formation becomes excessive.[19] The four grades of capsular contracture range from grade I

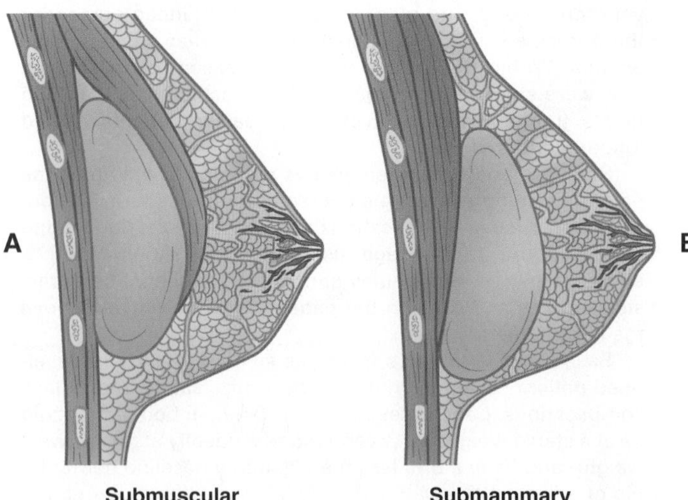


FIGURE 24-36 **A,** Augmentation mammoplasty implant under muscle. **B,** Implant under breast tissue.

(breast is normally soft and looks natural) to grade IV (breast is hard and painful and looks abnormal).[12] Depending on the grade of the contracture, an open capsulotomy may be used to release the constrictive tissue, or a capsulectomy may be indicated to actually remove the tissue.

PROCEDURAL CONSIDERATIONS. The patient is prepared and positioned in the same manner as for breast augmentation. Although patients receive education about capsule contracture as part of the informed consent process for breast augmentation, the actuality of the event may cause emotional distress for the patient. The patient may verbalize disappointment over the results and express fear related to additional postoperative changes in the appearance and functioning of the breast. In addition, the patient now faces the surgical and anesthetic risks associated with a second surgical procedure and may also be struggling with a possible financial burden because these procedures may not be covered by the patient's health plan. An empathetic and understanding approach is paramount to easing the patient's anxiety.

OPERATIVE PROCEDURE

1. The patient is prepped and draped, and markings are reinforced if necessary.
2. An incision is made, and the capsule is exposed.
3. The capsule is scored in multiple areas to achieve the desired release. Depending on the degree of contracture, circumferential incisions may be necessary to release the contracture.
4. If capsulotomy is not effective in releasing the capsule, a partial or full capsulectomy may be required to physically remove all or a portion of the capsule.
   a. The capsule is excised, and the breast implant is removed.
   b. The breast implant may be replaced in the same area, exchanged and replaced, or placed in a new pocket.
5. The site is irrigated with antibiotic solution. Drains are placed if a capsulectomy was performed.
6. The incision is closed in two layers.
7. The patient's skin is cleaned, and dressings are applied.

***Reduction Mammoplasty.*** Reduction mammoplasty is indicated for the patient with gigantomastia or macromastia with resulting back pain, intertrigo, or deep grooving in the shoulders from the bra straps because of the weight of the breasts (Patient and Family Education; Figure 24-37, *A*). The procedure may also be performed to achieve symmetry after a mastectomy on the contralateral side. Excessive breast tissue and its overlying skin are excised, with reconstruction of the breast contour, size, shape, and symmetry (Figure 24-37, *B*).

PROCEDURAL CONSIDERATIONS. A basic plastic instrument set is used with the addition of a "cookie cutter" areola marker or a "keyhole" pattern marker, a marking pen, skin stapler, tape measure, baby Deaver retractors, and two closed-wound suction systems. The ESU and a scale for weighing specimens should also be available, and tissue from each side should be carefully weighed and marked appropriately. The perioperative nurse should ensure the scale is calibrated correctly before weighing any tissue. Numerous blades will be used if de-epithelializing breast skin. If the nipple is removed and placed as a free nipple graft, extra suture will be necessary for tie-over bolsters. There are numerous choices in the reduction mammoplasty technique, and the perioperative nurse should ask the surgeon before opening suture or other supplies.

The patient is placed in a supine position with arms slightly extended on padded armboards. The hips should be positioned at the break in the OR bed so that the patient may be raised to a sitting position if necessary. Standard prepping and draping are done. Care should be taken not to remove the preoperative markings.

OPERATIVE PROCEDURE

The standard reduction mammoplasty procedure is described below. If the surgeon is using the "short scar" technique, the breast tissue is incised and removed according to the technique chosen. The nipple pedicle technique, wherein the nipple is mobilized and secured in a new position, may be chosen, or a free nipple graft may be utilized.

1. The skin to be excised and the new site for the nipple are marked preoperatively with the patient in a sitting position.
2. The skin between the new and the old nipple sites is incised and removed, with the nipple remaining attached to the underlying breast tissue. On patients with very large breasts, the nipples are removed and then reapplied as free grafts when the reduction is complete.

A

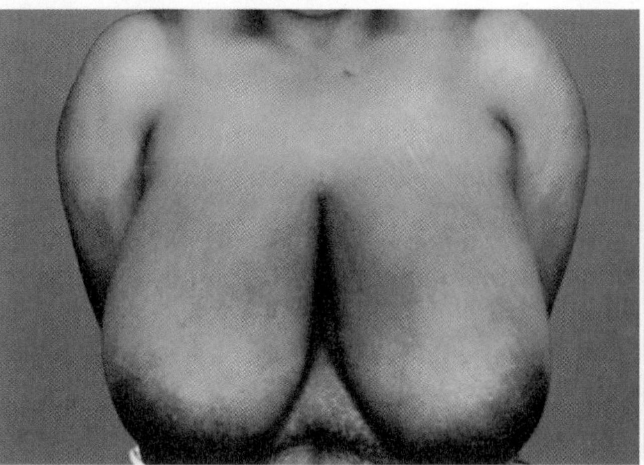

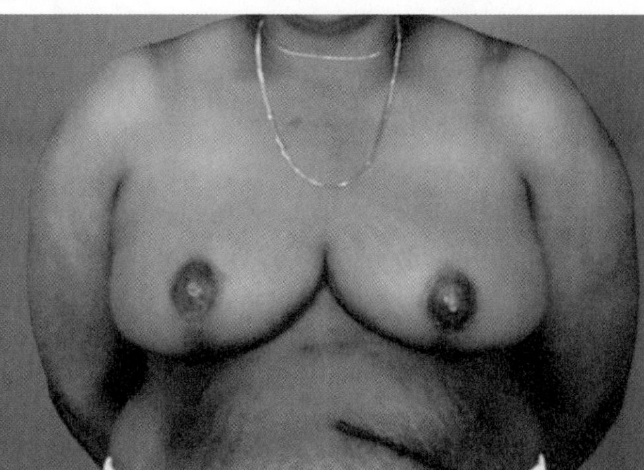

B

**FIGURE 24-37** **A,** Preoperative view of reduction mammoplasty; note grooves in shoulders from bra straps. **B,** Postoperative view.

PATIENT AND FAMILY EDUCATION

## Patient Education for Breast Reduction

**GENERAL INFORMATION**

Women with very large, pendulous breasts (a condition known as macromastia) can experience a number of physical and emotional problems. Macromastia is generally defined as excessive breast size, usually a bra cup size of D or larger. This condition is seen in young girls to middle-aged women. The condition probably is caused by hormonal factors but is also associated with obesity. Often there is a family pattern of large breasts.

**COMMON SIGNS AND SYMPTOMS**

- Breast size that is out of proportion to the torso and larger than the accepted norm
- Upper back and neck pain
- Shoulder pain
- Arm pain
- Breast pain
- Rashes and sometimes infections of the skin under the breasts
- Shoulder grooving from bra straps
- Hyperpigmentation (dark marks) in the bra strap lines
- Difficulty in finding bras or clothing that fits
- Possibly shyness or other personality changes because of appearance and the effects of excessively large breasts

**DIAGNOSIS**

Your surgeon will confirm the diagnosis of macromastia by examining your breasts carefully and relating the findings of your history.

**TREATMENT**

- Women with large breasts have often tried custom bras and weight loss as a way of reducing breast size or adding support. Physical therapy and pain medications may also be used in an effort to relieve symptoms. After trying these methods without success, many women seek surgical help in the form of breast reduction surgery. Technically, breast reduction surgery is known as reduction mammoplasty.
- The best candidates for breast reduction usually have at least two of the symptoms listed in the "Common Signs and Symptoms" category above.
- Breast reduction surgery should be delayed if your breasts are still growing; also, if you are currently gaining or losing weight, you should consider delaying breast reduction until your weight has stabilized.
- The aims of the operation are the following:
  - To remove enough breast tissue to be able to construct a normal-appearing breast mound
  - To reposition the nipple-areola in a suitable position in the "new" breast

There are many operations to reduce large breasts. A common technique is shown in the figures.

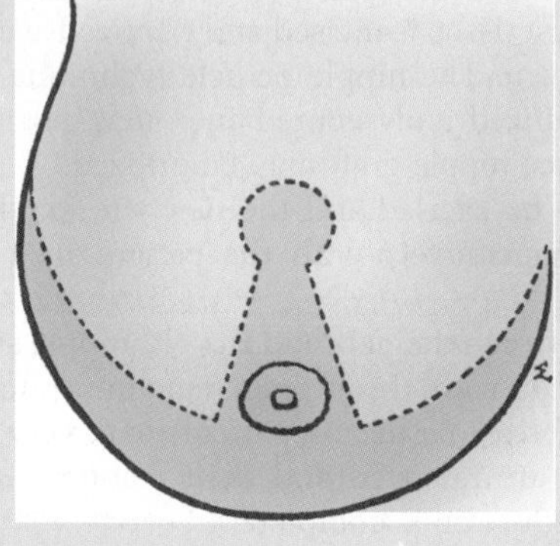

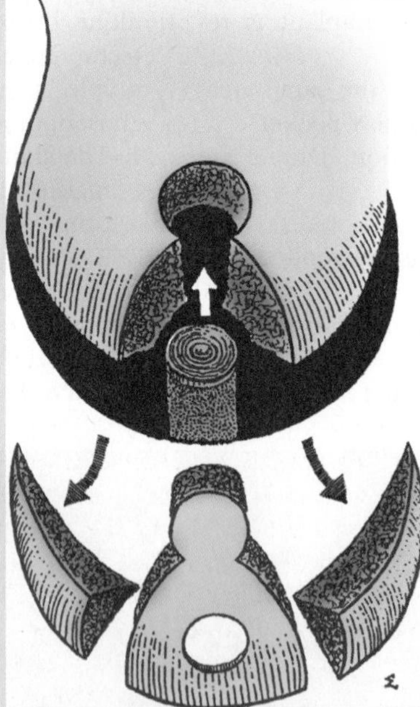

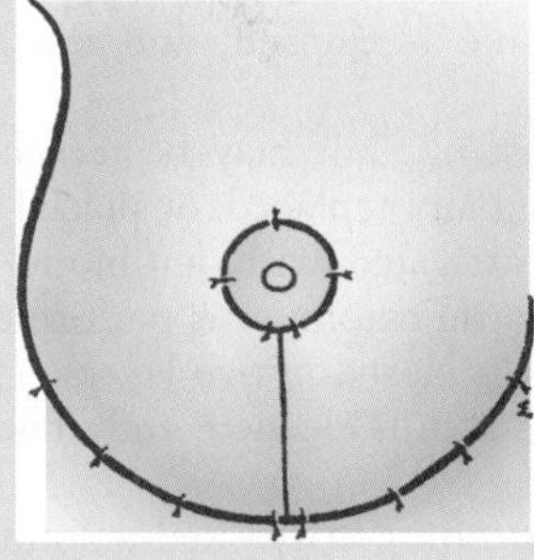

**PREPARING FOR YOUR OPERATION**

- Your surgeon will examine and measure your breasts and will probably photograph you for reference during the surgery and afterward.
- A mammogram may be ordered if you are 35 years or older.
- If you smoke, you should avoid smoking completely for at least 1 month before your surgery. Smoking affects the blood vessels in your skin and can slow your healing.
- Your surgeon may instruct you to avoid taking aspirin, nonsteroidal antiinflammatory drugs (ibuprofen [Motrin]), vitamin E, fenfluramine, or phentermine at least 2 weeks before

Modified from *Consumer's guide to breast reduction.* Accessed March 7, 2006, on-line: www.plasticsurgery.org/public_education/BRAVO-Surgery.cfm; Jones G: Breast reduction. In Mathes SJ, editor: *Plastic surgery,* vol 6, ed 2, Philadelphia, 2006, Saunders.

PATIENT AND FAMILY EDUCATION

**Patient Education for Breast Reduction—cont'd**

your surgery. These substances may interfere with normal blood clotting or with your ability to heal after surgery.
- Before your surgery you may want to do the following:
  - Wash your hair (you will not be able to shower or bathe immediately after surgery).
  - Arrange for temporary care for any house pets that may jump on you.
  - Move your "daily use" items within arm's reach.
  - Fill any prescriptions from your surgeon.
- You should know that the following are common after this operation:
  - The sensation in your nipples probably will be decreased.
  - You may not be able to breast feed.
  - Reading your mammogram may become more difficult for the physician because of the scarring inside the breast.
  - The scars from the operation may be prominent.
- On the day of the operation, the places where the incisions will be made on your breasts and the new position of the nipple-areola will be marked with dissolving ink while you are in a sitting position.
- You may be given medicine that will make you feel drowsy before you are brought to the operating room.

**THE OPERATION**
- Most women have general anesthesia (going to sleep) for breast reduction. Some surgeons may perform the procedure with a local anesthetic and sedation.
- The operation generally takes 3 to 4 hours.

**AFTER YOUR OPERATION**
- You will be taken to a recovery room and observed. When your blood pressure, pulse, and breathing are stable, you will be taken to a regular hospital room.
- You will be wrapped in elastic bandages or a surgical bra over gauze. Small plastic tubes will be coming from the breast incisions and will be connected to small plastic bulbs. They drain any extra fluid that needs to come out.
- Many breast reduction surgeries are done as outpatient procedures, in which case you will go home after you wake up from the anesthesia and your pain is under good control. In some cases you may stay in the hospital after surgery for a short period (1 or 2 days).
- Recovery is different for every patient, but bed rest may only be needed for 1 or 2 days after the procedure. Even in the first 24 to 48 hours after surgery it is important for you to get out of bed and walk around every 2 hours during the day and early evening. Continuous bed rest after surgery may increase your risks for pneumonia or blood clots.
- As with any operation, complications are always possible. With this type of operation, they can include bleeding, infection, delayed wound healing, abnormal scarring, and shape irregularities.

**HOME CARE**

You will want to take it easy at first, but you may walk about as you wish, even climb stairs, but do not overdo things. Avoid heavy exercise, heavy lifting, or stress on the upper body for 1 month. Items that can be helpful as you recover include the following:
- A body or sitting support pillow
- Cordless phone
- Variety of easy-to-cook or precooked meals
- Two or three loose-fitting robes or housedresses with snaps in the front and large pockets
- Slip-on shoes
- Soft sponge for bathing before showering is allowed
- Small containers for drinks (gallon containers are very heavy)
- A listing of your physicians, pharmacy, and caregivers/helpers with telephone contact information. You should call your surgeon if any of the following occurs:
  - Your incisions become red or swollen, or there is drainage from them.
  - You develop a temperature higher than 37.8°C (100°F).
  - You have any questions.

3. The redundant segment of breast tissue inferior to the nipple is excised through an inverted-T incision. Tissue from each breast is weighed and kept separate.
4. The nipple and adjacent tissue are mobilized and sutured in place.
5. The medial and lateral skin edges are approximated in a vertical suture line inferior to the nipple.
6. The inframammary elliptic incision is trimmed and closed transversely. Closed-wound suction catheters may be placed. The wound is dressed.

***Mastopexy.*** Breast ptosis is corrected by moving the nipple to a more normal position and removing excess breast skin (Figure 24-38). With mastopexy surgery there is usually minimal to no removal of breast tissue, although it may be necessary to add a breast implant to achieve the desired result.

PROCEDURAL CONSIDERATIONS. Marking is done before surgery and is key to a good outcome. Positioning is similar to augmentation. Skin incision choices are periareolar only; periareolar combined with a vertical (known as a short scar or vertical mastopexy); the classic inverted T, which adds an inframammary incision to the previous incision; or the horizontal inframammary, which combines the periareolar and inframammary, leaving out the vertical component. Mastopexy may involve reduction of the skin envelope only or combine skin removal with glandular reshaping and placement in a more desirable position.

OPERATIVE PROCEDURE

1. The patient is positioned per the surgeon's preference, prepped, and draped.
2. Incisions are placed; one or more of the following techniques are used:
   a. Excess skin is removed.
   b. The breast cone is reshaped by invagination of lower midbreast tissue.
   c. The lower submammary breast tissue pedicle is advanced below the breast tissue and tacked superiorly to the pectoral muscle.
   d. Lower midbreast tissue is incised and overlapped.
   e. A superiorly based (on nipple areolar complex pedicle) wedge tissue flap is created, turned under, and superiorly attached.

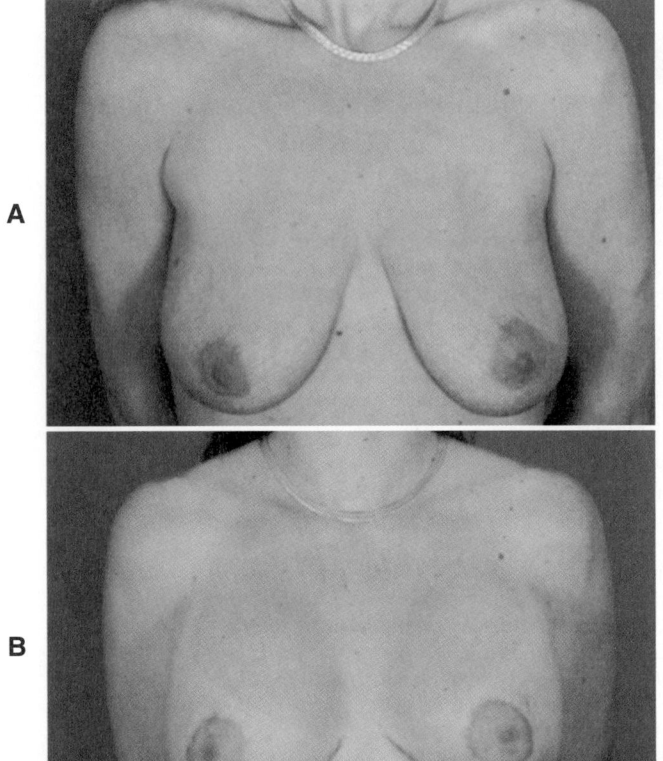


FIGURE 24-38 **A,** Preoperative view. **B,** Postoperative view; ptosis corrected.

f. The upper pole of breast tissue is mobilized and advanced superiorly and tacked to the pectoral muscle fascia.
3. The breast may be sutured entirely at this time or approximated and the same procedure applied to the opposite breast, closing both at the end.
4. The operative area is cleaned, dressings of choice are applied, and a surgical bra is applied.

***Excision of Gynecomastia.*** Gynecomastia is a relatively common pathologic condition that consists of bilateral or unilateral enlargement of the male breast. It occurs primarily during puberty or after the age of 40 years. Although it may be produced by a variety of diseases or be the result of side effects related to certain medications, it is usually related to excessive hormone production or alterations in hormonal balance. It may also be seen in elderly men and in men after excessive use of marijuana. All subareolar fibroglandular tissue is removed, and the resultant defect is surgically closed (Figure 24-39). The patient may be positioned in a supine position or semi-Fowler position, according to the surgeon's preference. Supplies and equipment needed are the same as those for a simple mastectomy, plus a basic plastic instrument set. Because suction-assisted lipectomy (SAL) may be used for contouring, suction cannulas, associated supplies, and an aspirator should also be available. All breast tissue removed should be weighed and then sent for pathologic examination. Although infrequent, men are not immune from breast cancer.

OPERATIVE PROCEDURE

1. Local anesthesia is instilled. A stab wound incision is made for introduction of the liposuction cannula.
2. Liposuction is performed. If satisfactory removal of breast tissue is accomplished, the incision is closed and a compression garment applied.
3. If additional surgery is required, a periareolar incision is made. Through this incision, the fibrous and ductal attach-

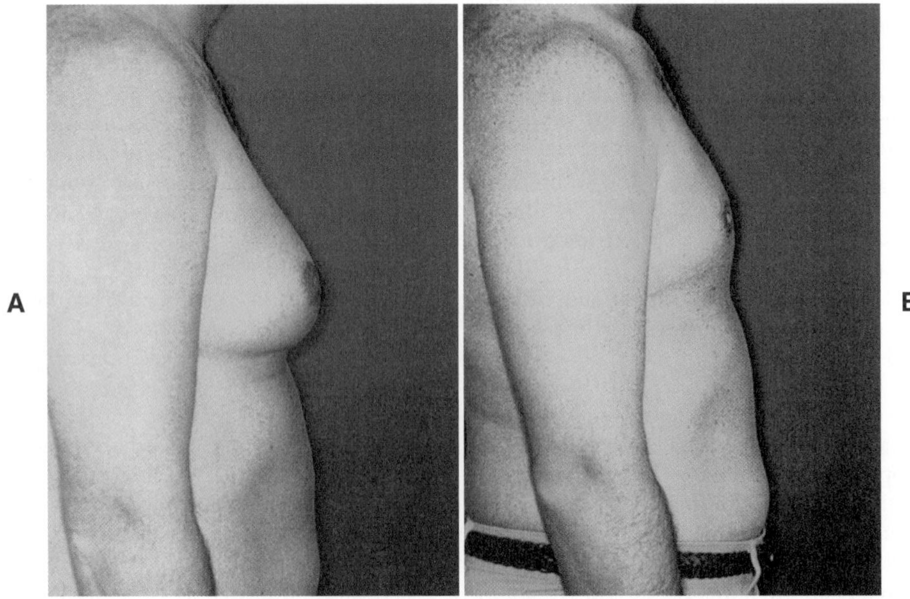


FIGURE 24-39 **A,** Preoperative view of gynecomastia. **B,** Postoperative view after excision of gynecomastia.

ments of the underlying glandular tissue to the nipple are divided.

4. A cuff of fatty tissue is left attached to the underlying nipple surface to protect the blood supply.
5. The breast tissue mass is dissected. Carrying the dissection to the pectoralis fascia is usually necessary to remove the entire mass.
6. Hemostasis is achieved.
7. Closure is performed, the area cleaned, and a compression garment applied.

## REFERENCES


1. Aly AS and others: Truncal body contouring surgery in the massive weight loss patient. In Shestak KC, editor: *Clinics in Plastic Surgery* 31(4), 2004.
2. American Cancer Society: *Breast reconstruction*. Accessed March 27, 2006, on-line: www.cancer.org/docroot/CRI/content/CRI_2_6X_Breast_Reconstruction_After_Mastectomy_5.asp.
3. American Society for Aesthetic Plastic Surgery: *Quick facts*. Accessed March 25, 2006, on-line: www.surgery.org/professional/download/2005 stats.
4. American Society of Plastic Surgeons. Accessed on-line: www.plasticsurgery.org/public_education/procedures/BreastReconstruction.cfm.
5. Bastable S: *Nurse as educator: principles of teaching and learning for nursing practice*, ed 2, Sudbury, Mass, 2003, Jones & Bartlett.
6. *Burn survivor statistics*. Accessed March 5, 2006, on-line: www.burn-survivor.com/burn_statistics.html.
7. Cook TA and others: Soft tissue techniques. In Papel ID and others, editors: *Facial plastic and reconstructive surgery*, ed 2, New York, 2002, Thieme.
8. Cuzzell J, Workman ML: Interventions for clients with skin problems. In Ignatavicius DD, Workman ML, editors: *Medical-surgical nursing: critical thinking for collaborative care,* ed 5, St Louis, 2006, Saunders.
9. Doerr TD, Mathog RH: Le Fort fractures (maxillary fractures). In Papel ID and others, editors: *Facial plastic and reconstructive surgery,* ed 2, New York, 2002, Thieme
10. Dolan R: *Facial, plastic, reconstructive, and trauma surgery*, New York, 2004, Marcel Dekker.
11. Dybec RB: Intraoperative positioning and care of the obese patient, *Plastic Surgical Nursing* 24(3):118-122, 2004.
12. Food and Drug Administration (FDA): *Breast implant consumer handbook*, 2004. Accessed March 25, 2006, on-line: www.fda.gov/chrh/breastimplants/.
13. Hodgson BB, Kizior RJ: *Saunders nursing drug handbook 2006*, St Louis, 2006, Elsevier Saunders.
14. *How Integra template works*. Accessed March 18, 2005, on-line: www.skinhealing.com/5_2_aboutintegra.shtml.
15. Lockwood TE: Maximizing aesthetics in lateral-tension abdominoplasty and body lifts. In Sheshak KC, editor: *Clinics in Plastic Surgery* 31(4), 2004.
16. Marino R, Gonzales-Portillo M: Preconquest Peruvian neurosurgeons: a study of Inca and pre-Columbia trephination and the art of medicine in ancient Peru, *Neurosurgery* 47(4):940-950, 2000.
17. Marler JJ, Upton JJ: Tissue engineering. In Mathes SJ, editor: *Plastic surgery,* vol 1, ed 2, Philadelphia, 2006, Saunders.
18. Mathes SJ, Hansen SL: Flap classifications and applications. In Mathes SJ, editor: *Plastic surgery,* vol 1, ed 2, Philadelphia, 2006, Saunders.
19. Maxwell GP, Hartley RW: Breast augmentation. In Mathes SJ, editor: *Plastic surgery,* vol 1, ed 2, Philadelphia, 2006, Saunders.
20. *National plastic surgery statistics*. Accessed March 2, 2006, on-line: www.plasticsurgery.org/public_education/loader.cfm?url=/commonspot/security/getfile.cfm&PageID=16158.
21. Nicol NH and others: Structure, function and disorders of the integument. In McCance KL, Huether SE: *Pathophysiology: the biologic basis for disease in adults and children*, ed 5, St Louis, 2006, Mosby.
22. *Pittsburgh Tissue Engineering Initiative*. Accessed February 27, 2006, on-line: www.ptei.org.
23. Pruzinsky T and others: Multiple perspectives on the psychology of plastic surgery. In Sarwer DB and others: *Psychological aspects of reconstructive and cosmetic surgery: clinical, empirical, and ethical perspectives*, Philadelphia, 2006, Lippincott, Williams & Wilkins.
24. Rager EL and others: Cutaneous melanoma: update on prevention, screening, diagnosis, and treatment, *American Family Physician* 72(2):269-275, 2005.
25. Wei F, Suominen S: Principles and techniques of microvascular surgery. In Mathes SJ, editor: *Plastic surgery,* vol 1, ed 2, Philadelphia, 2006, Saunders.

CHAPTER 25

# Thoracic Surgery

BRENDA S. GREGORY CRUM

Thoracic surgery, like other specialties, has evolved with the development of surgical techniques and treatments, such as blood transfusion, anesthetic delivery, and screening procedures. During the past 50 years the understanding of pathophysiology and improved techniques has expanded the field of thoracic surgery. The thoracic specialty extends beyond the surgical arena into infectious disease, trauma, and oncology. Improved technology and the determination to treat diseases previously considered untreatable with operative and other invasive procedures continue to improve the recovery rate for patients experiencing thoracic diseases. As the ability to treat thoracic disease has improved, the responsibilities of the perioperative nurse have expanded, resulting in accomplishments throughout the years that have provided an extensive knowledge base and specialized perioperative practitioners.

## Surgical Anatomy

The skeletal framework of the thorax is formed anteriorly by the sternum and costal cartilages, laterally by the 12 pairs of ribs, and posteriorly by the 12 thoracic vertebrae (Figure 25-1). This airtight compartment is enclosed in the root of the neck by Sibson's fascia and is separated from the abdomen by the diaphragm.

The sternum forms the anterior thoracic wall in the midline. It consists of three parts: (1) the upper part, or manubrium; (2) the body, or gladiolus; and (3) the lower cartilage, or xiphoid process. The manubrium articulates with the clavicles and the first two ribs on each side; the gladiolus articulates with the remaining true ribs by separate costal cartilages; and the xiphoid fuses with the gladiolus in early development and is attached to the diaphragm by the substernal ligament.

Normally the lateral walls of the thorax are formed by the 12 pairs of ribs. Posteriorly, each pair of ribs articulates with its corresponding thoracic vertebrae. Anteriorly, the first seven ribs articulate with the sternum. The eighth, ninth, and tenth ribs articulate with the costal cartilages of the rib above; however, the eleventh and twelfth ribs are not fixed to the costal arch (see Figure 25-1).

The muscles of each hemithorax (Figures 25-2 and 25-3) include the 11 external and 11 internal intercostal muscles, which fill the spaces between the ribs. An intercostal artery, vein, and nerve accompany each intercostal muscle. The arteries communicate with the internal thoracic artery anteriorly and arise from the aorta posteriorly. The intercostal veins follow the course of the arteries and communicate with the mammary veins anteriorly and with the azygos and hemiazygos veins posteriorly.

During surgery, great care is taken to prevent injury to the intercostal nerve, which passes forward and alongside the posterior intercostal artery and shares with the superior branch of the artery the intercostal groove on the inferior edge of the corresponding rib. When the nerve must be disturbed, an anesthetic agent may be injected to prevent postoperative pain.

The thoracic outlet is a junction bound anteriorly by the manubrium, anterolaterally by the first ribs, and posteriorly by the first thoracic vertebrae and posterior angles of the first ribs of the space. The great vessels of the head, neck, and arm pass through this space. Compression of these structures causes thoracic outlet syndrome.

The mediastinum is divided into anterior, middle, and posterior compartments. The anterior mediastinum is bound anteriorly by the sternum and posteriorly by the pericardium and great vessels. It contains the thymus gland, lymph nodes, and pericardial fat. The middle mediastinum is bound anteriorly by the pericardium and great vessels and posteriorly by the anterior border of the vertebral bodies. The posterior mediastinum is bound anteriorly by the vertebral bodies and extends posteriorly to the chest wall.

The chest cavity is subdivided into the right and the left pleural cavities, which contain the lungs, separated by the mediastinum, which lies medially between the two pleural membranes. The parietal pleura, the membrane that lines the inner surface of each hemithorax, is adjacent to the inner surfaces of the ribs posteriorly and the mediastinum medially and covers the surface of the diaphragm except at the central portion. Part of the parietal membrane is reflected back at the root of each lung to form a sac around it. This reflection is called the *visceral pleura.* The pleural space holds about 50 ml of pleural fluid, a serous secretion that provides lubrication between these two membranes to minimize friction during inspiration and expiration.[3]

The lungs are the essential organs of respiration. The base of each lung rests on the diaphragm, whereas its apex (upper end) projects into the base of the neck at a level above the first rib. The bronchus, the nerves, the lymphatics, and the pulmonary and bronchial vessels enter and leave the lung on the mediastinal surface in a structure known as the *hilum,* or *root,* of the lung. Deep fissures divide the spongy, porous lung into lobes. The primary bronchi divide and then subdivide into each lobe and eventually become bronchioles. The right lung has an upper, a middle, and a lower lobe; the left lung has only an upper and a lower lobe (Figure 25-4). However, the lungs are similar in that each is composed of 10 major segments (Figure 25-5). Each segment extends to the pleural surface, expanding in volume from its center to its peripheral edges. Each segment also has its own bronchus and branches of the pulmonary artery and vein.

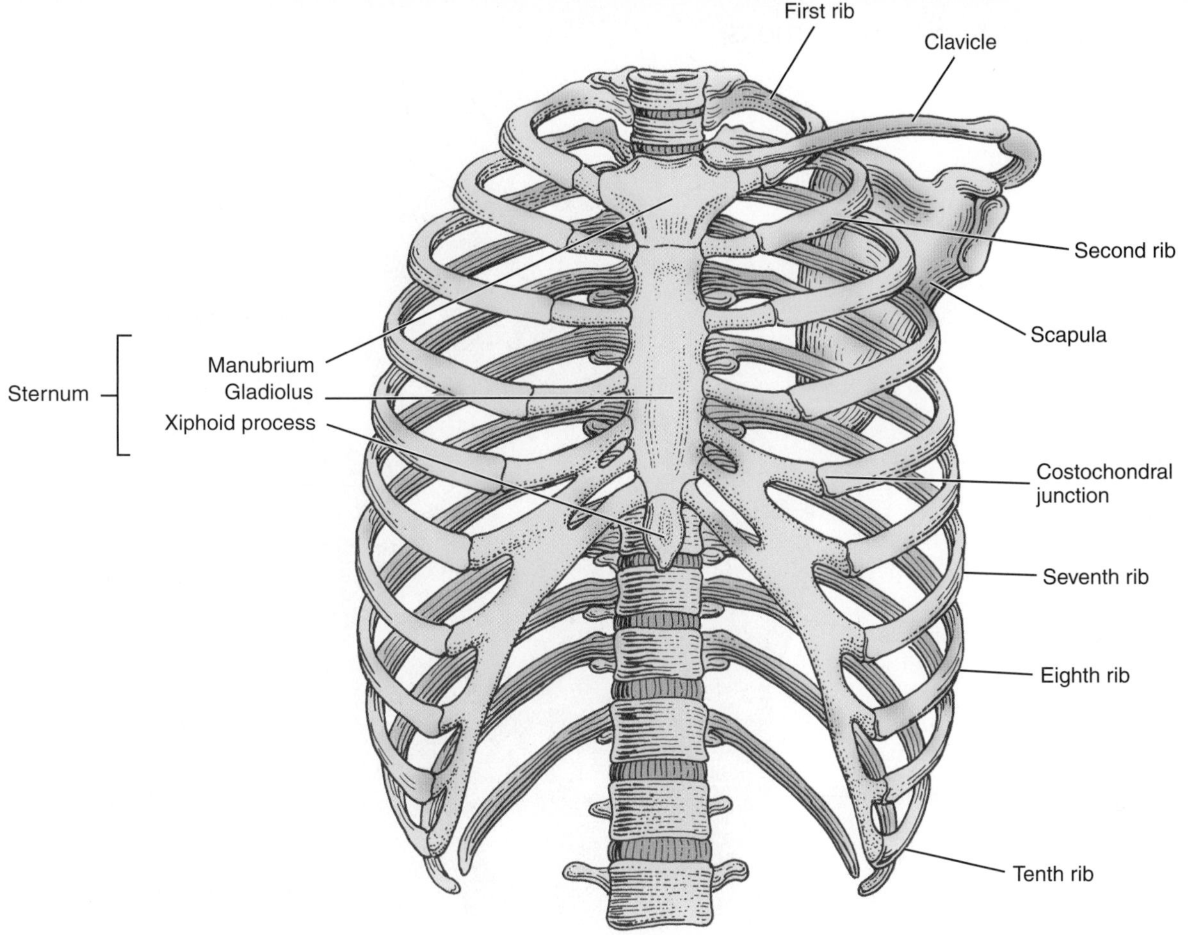


**FIGURE 25-1** Bony thorax.

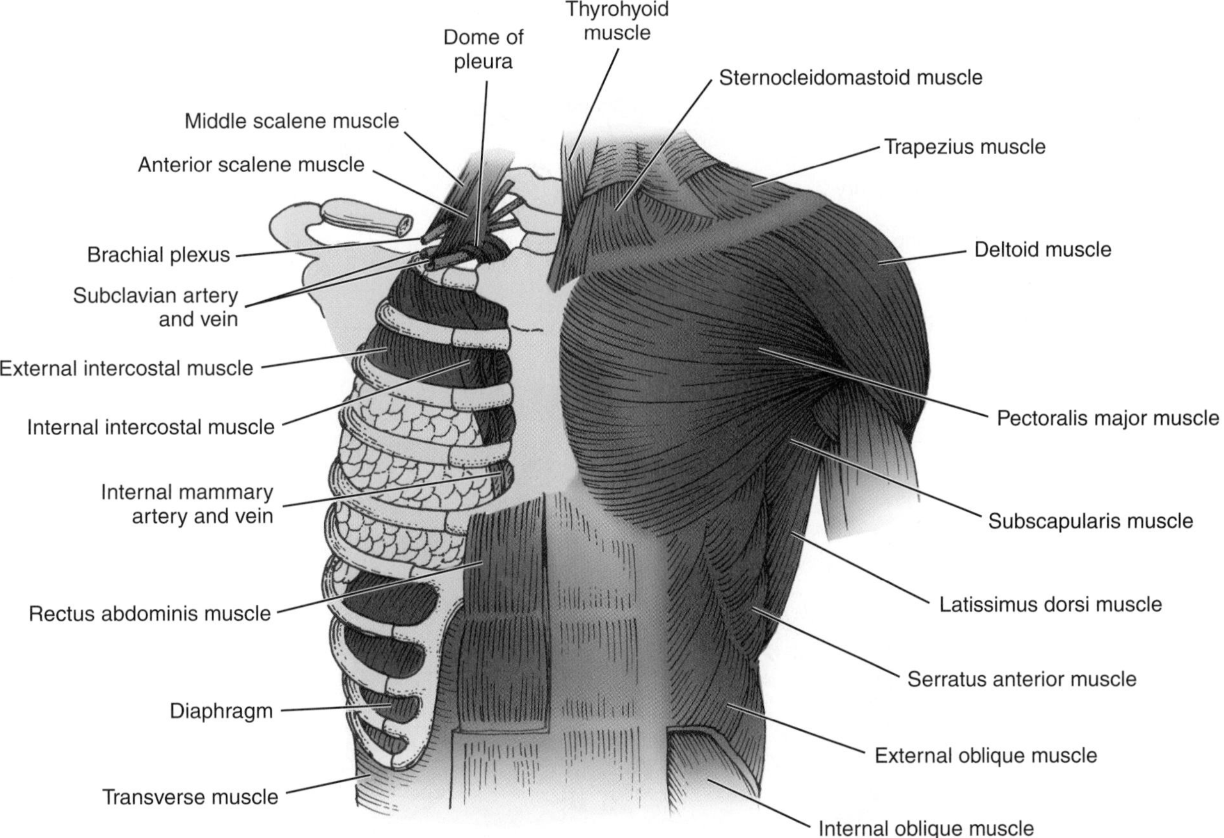


**FIGURE 25-2** Anterior view of thorax and contiguous portions of base of neck and anterior abdominal wall. *Right half,* Superficial layer of muscles and fascia; *left half,* relations of deep muscles of neck and abdomen to rib cage, intercostal muscles, diaphragm, and internal mammary vessels; relations of muscles, nerves, and vessels with first rib; and anterior relations of lung.

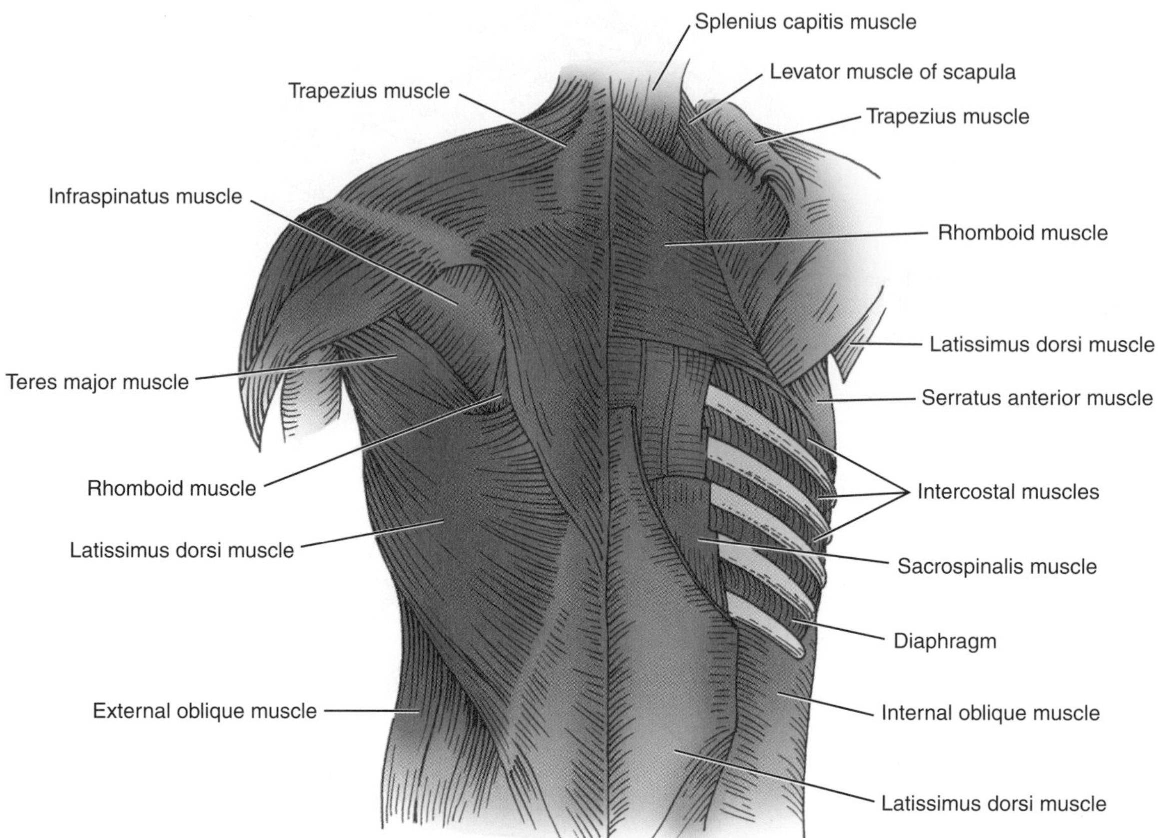


**FIGURE 25-3** Posterior view of thorax and contiguous portions of neck and abdominal wall. *Left half,* Superficial muscles; *right half,* deeper muscles.

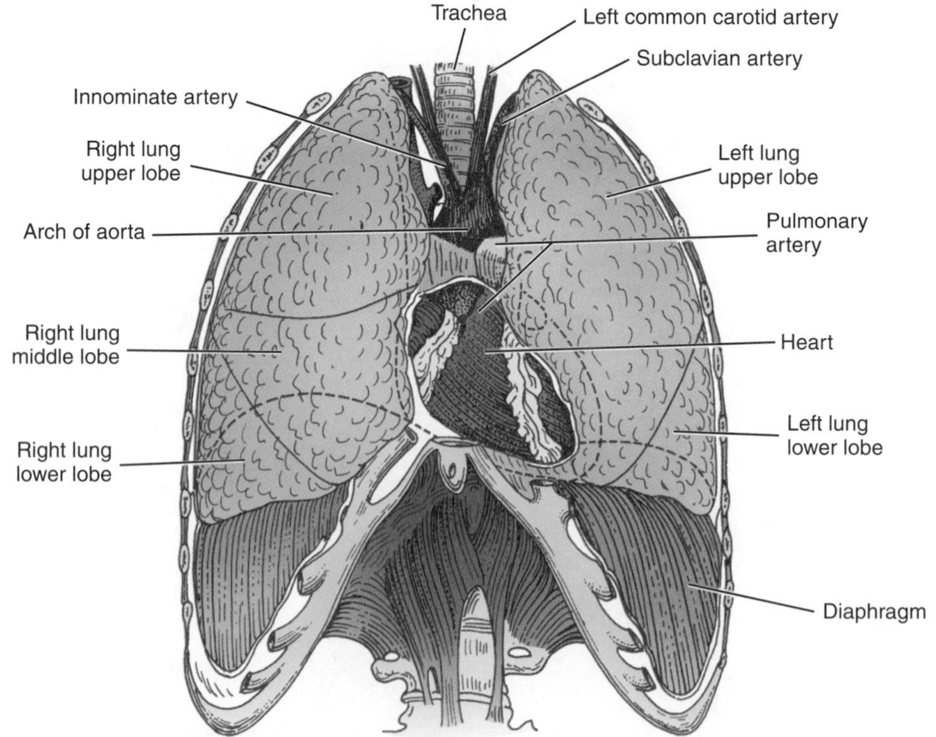


**FIGURE 25-4** Organs of thoracic cavity. Part of pericardium has been removed to expose heart.

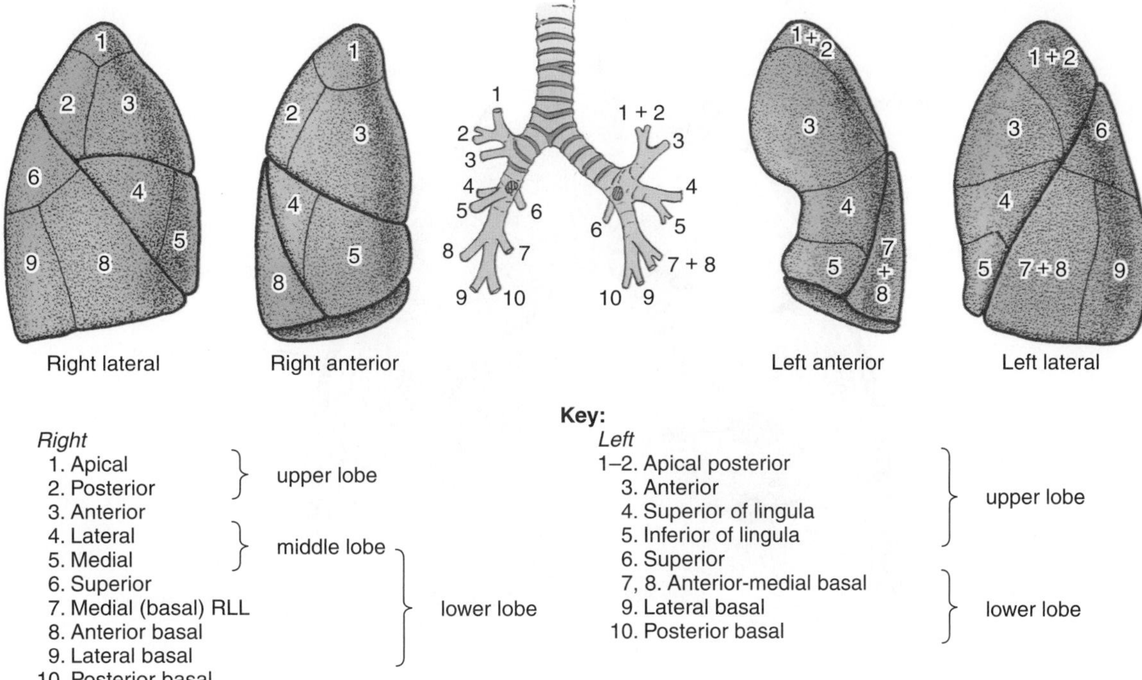


**FIGURE 25-5** Segments of the pulmonary lobes. *RLL,* Right lower lobe.

The bronchial arteries, arising from the aorta, supply nourishment to the lungs. They vary in their number and course. The arrangement may include two branches to the left lung and one branch to the right lung, which later branches into two, or there may be one or two branches for each lung. The pulmonary arteries carry the blood to the pulmonary parenchyma, and the pulmonary veins transport the oxygenated blood to the left atrium.

The nerves of the lungs are a part of the autonomic nervous system (see Chapter 23). They regulate constriction and relaxation of the bronchi and of the blood vessels within the lungs.

Although the thoracic cavity is an airtight space, the lungs receive outside air through the nasal passages, trachea, and bronchi. The main function of the lungs is to exchange carbon dioxide for oxygen. Normally, as the thorax expands, the lungs also expand as air is drawn in; during expiration, the thorax relaxes and the lungs passively contract as air is forced out. Inspiration normally takes place when the intrathoracic pressure is slightly below atmospheric pressure (76 cm Hg, or 760 mm Hg) and when a partial vacuum exists between the parietal and visceral pleural (intrathoracic) surfaces. As the muscles of inspiration contract to enlarge the chest cage, the lungs passively follow the diaphragm and chest wall because of decreased intrathoracic pressure. The acts of inspiration and expiration are the result of air moving in and out of the lung, causing pressure to equalize with that of the atmosphere at the end of expiration (Figure 25-6).

The normal intrapleural pressure varies from −9 to −12 cm $H_2O$ during inspiration and from about −3 to −6 cm $H_2O$ during expiration. The greatest amount of air that can be expired after a maximum inspiration is termed the *vital capacity,* and the volume of gas remaining in the lungs after maximal expiration is *residual volume.* Size, age, gender, and pulmonary disease of the patient influence vital capacity. Any condition that interferes with the normally negative intrapleural pressure affects respiratory function.

# Perioperative Nursing Considerations

## Assessment

During assessment, the perioperative nurse gathers information (patient data) that is important to planning patient care. Signs and symptoms demonstrated by the patient are confirmed by the perioperative nurse during the admission assessment. The perioperative nurse may begin data collection by identifying the patient (Patient Safety) and confirming the correct surgical site. A thorough review of the patient's medical record, including results of the history, physical examination, laboratory tests, other diagnostic workups, and the nursing history and assessment, is critical for subsequent care planning. It is valuable to assess the patient's understanding of the disease process and of the anticipated procedure. The nurse should also assess emotional status, since patients with a possible diagnosis of carcinoma may be highly anxious. A focused assessment of the respiratory system should be included during the physical assessment. The nurse questions the patient or otherwise confirms the presence of an increased frequency of cough, increase in sputum production, recurrent hemoptysis, malaise, shortness of breath, substernal chest discomfort, weight loss, poor appetite, status of nutrition, and hypoxia. The results of the physical examination of the chest should be reviewed; the perioperative nurse may auscultate the chest and confirm the presence of crackles or wheezes on inspiration or expiration, which should be documented on the medical record.

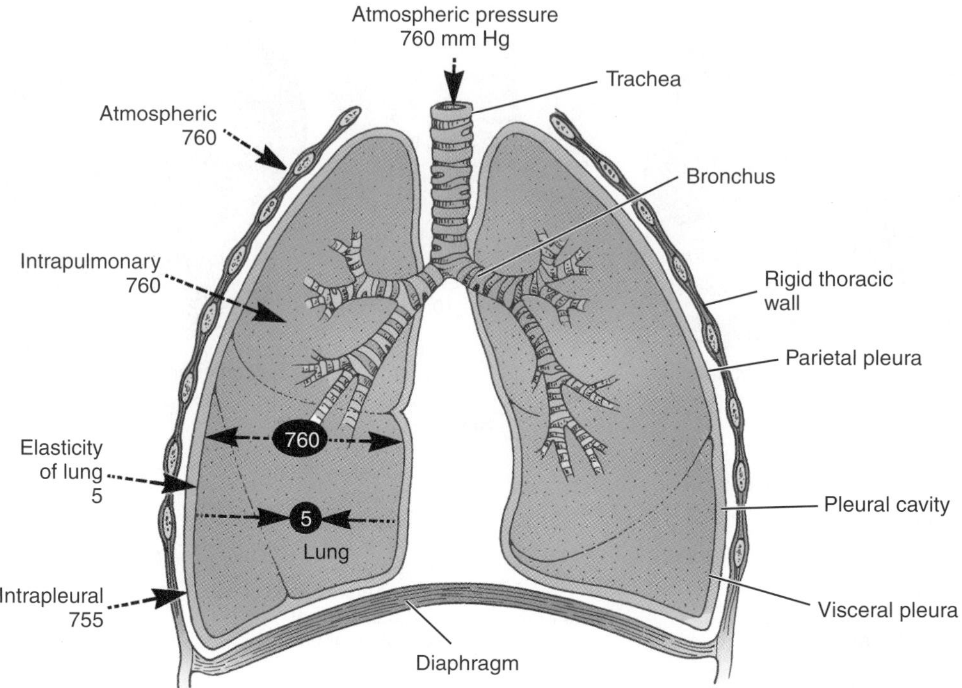


**FIGURE 25-6** Thoracic cavity structures showing intrapulmonary and intrapleural pressures (in mm Hg) with chest wall in resting position.

## PATIENT SAFETY

### Patient Identification

Like the hospital gown, the wrist identification band is a traditional part of the "patient" persona and is linked to the routine of verification before administering medications, treatments, or procedures. When the wristband is present and has correct information, it can be a reliable identifier.

Patients undergoing thoracic procedures are at risk for identification errors because their wristbands are often removed to provide access for starting intravenous (IV) and other invasive monitoring lines or may be inaccessible because of positioning or draping. Correctly identifying the patient is an important Joint Commission National Patient Safety Goal. Research from the Joint Commission found that incorrect patient identification was involved in 13% of surgical errors and 67% of transfusion errors. The nurse must be familiar with the institutional policy regarding patient identification and the methods and procedures used to accomplish it. If a band is removed it should never be retaped in a new location or taped or pinned to the patient's gown. The band that is retaped or repaired may not maintain its integrity. A band pinned to a gown is easily lost if the gown is removed or replaced. The nurse should anticipate that identification bands may need to be removed for access purposes and ensure replacement bands are available. If the patient's arms are not accessible, the nurse should consider placing the new band on the patient's ankle.

Some organizations use color-coded identification bands to indicate allergies, blood type, or do-not-resuscitate (DNR) orders. These color-coded bands can be confused with plastic colored bands that are worn by individuals to show support for a cause. Nurses must be familiar with the color coding used by the institution to avoid misidentification and should encourage patients to remove any personal bracelets.

Technology is available to support the patient identification process. Many identification bands include bar codes that can be read with handheld bar code readers. Bar codes allow nurses to verify identity and capture other important data. A bar code identification band meets the American Hospital Association's guidelines for a tamperproof, nontransferable identification band.

Newer technology uses radiofrequency identification (RFID) systems for accurate patient verification. RFID remotely collects information and stores it on a system consisting of tags (transponders) and readers (interrogators). Microchips inside the tags contain more than 100 times the information of bar codes. The chip can contain patient information such as name, blood type, allergies, and medications.

Regardless of the system used, the perioperative nurse plays a key role in identifying the patient and reinforcing subsequent verification procedures as necessary throughout the surgical experience to provide a safe environment of care.

Modified from Beyea S: Patient identification—a crucial aspect of patient safety—patient safety first, *AORN Journal* 78(3):478-482, 2003; Joint Commission International Center for Patient Safety: *Using identification bands to reduce patient identification errors.* Accessed April 11, 2006, on-line: www.jcipatientsafety.org/show.asp?durki=12346.

The review of diagnostic and laboratory tests may include the chest x-ray films, sputum analysis obtained during bronchoscopy, cytology reports, arterial blood gas (ABG) results, and pulmonary function studies (Table 25-1). Laboratory tests including the complete blood count (CBC) should be within normal limits but can indicate anemia. The chest x-ray film remains an indispensable diagnostic tool and will be needed in the operating room. This film outlines the lesion, if any is present, and defines its shape and space-occupying nature (e.g., tracheal shift). The presence of air in the hilar region, pleural effusion, or atelectasis may also be confirmed by radiologic evidence. Sputum analysis for culture and sensitivity may alert the perioperative nurse to an infectious process; cytologic examination may confirm a malignancy. The patient may have already undergone diagnostic bronchoscopy or mediastinoscopy; if so, the findings for acid-fast bacillus smear, culture, bronchial washing, and bi-

**TABLE 25-1**

**Laboratory Studies and Tests for Assessment of Patients Undergoing Thoracic Procedures**

| Laboratory Study | Normal Results | Significance of Abnormal Findings |
|---|---|---|
| **PERFUSION STUDIES—ARTERIAL BLOOD GASES (ABGs)** | | |
| pH | 7.35-7.45 | Changes indicate metabolic or respiratory acidosis. |
| $Paco_2$ | 35-45 mm Hg | Elevations indicate possible COPD, asthma, pneumonia, anesthetic effects, or use of opioids (respiratory acidosis). Decreased levels indicate hyperventilation/respiratory alkalosis. |
| $HCO_3^-$ | 21-28 mEq/L | Elevations indicate a possible respiratory acidosis as compensation for a primary metabolic alkalosis. Decreased levels indicate a possible respiratory alkalosis as compensation for a primary metabolic acidosis. |
| $Pao_2$ | 80-100 mm Hg | Elevations may indicate possible excessive oxygen administration. Decreased levels indicate possible COPD, asthma, chronic bronchitis, cancer of the bronchi and lungs, respiratory distress syndrome, or any other cause of hypoxia. |
| $O_2$ saturation | 95%-100% | Decreased levels indicate possible impaired ability of hemoglobin to release oxygen to tissues. |
| **COMPLETE BLOOD COUNT** | | |
| RBCs | Male: 4.7-6.1<br>Female: 4.2-5.4 | Elevated levels may be due to the excessive production of erythropoietin, which occurs in response to a hypoxic stimulus, such as COPD. Decreased levels may indicate anemia, hemorrhage, or hemolysis. |
| Hemoglobin | Male: 14.8 g/dl<br>Female: 12-16 g/dl | Same as for RBCs. |
| Hematocrit | Male: 42%-58%<br>Female: 37%-47% | Same as for RBCs. |
| WBCs | 5000-10,000/$mm^3$ | Elevations indicate possible acute bacterial infections or inflammatory conditions (smoking). Decreased levels may indicate overwhelming infection or immunosuppression. |

**Pulmonary Function Tests**

| Test | Purpose |
|---|---|
| FVC (forced vital capacity): records maximum amount of air that can be exhaled in as quickly as possible after maximum inspiration | Provides an indication of respiratory muscle strength and ventilatory reserve. Often reduced in obstructive disease (because of air trapping) and in restrictive disease. |
| $FEV_1$ (forced expiratory volume in 1 sec): records maximum amount of air that can be exhaled in first second of respiration | Effort dependent and declines with age. Reduced in certain obstructive and restrictive disorders. |
| $FEV_1$/FVC: ratio of expiratory volume in 1 sec to FVC | Provides a more sensitive indicator of obstruction to airflow. Ratio is normal or increased in restrictive disease. |
| $FEF_{25\%-75\%}$: records forced expiratory flow over the 25%-75% volume (middle half) of the FVC | This measure provides a more sensitive index of obstruction in the smaller airways. |
| FRC (functional residual capacity): amount of air remaining in lungs after normal expiration | Increased FRC indicates hyperinflation or air trapping, which may result from obstructive disease. |
| TLC (total lung capacity): amount of air remaining in lungs at end of maximum inhalation | Increased TLC indicates air trapping associated with obstructive pulmonary disease. Decreased TLC indicates restrictive disease. |
| RV (residual volume): amount of air remaining in lungs at the end of a full, forced exhalation | RV is increased in obstructive pulmonary disease, such as emphysema. |
| $DL_{co}$ (diffusion capacity of carbon monoxide): reflects surface area of alveolocapillary membrane | $DL_{co}$ is reduced when the alveolocapillary membrane is diminished, such as in emphysema, pulmonary hypertension, and pulmonary fibrosis. |

From Pagana KD, Pagana TJ: *Mosby's diagnostic and laboratory test references,* ed 7, St Louis, 2005, Mosby; Gates CA, Workman ML: Assessment of the respiratory system. In Ignatavicius DD, Workman ML, editors: *Medical-surgical nursing: critical thinking for collaborative care,* ed 5, Philadelphia, 2006, Saunders.

*COPD,* Chronic obstructive pulmonary disease; *$HCO_3^-$;* bicarbonate ion; *$Paco_2$,* partial pressure of arterial carbon dioxide; *$Pao_2$,* partial pressure of arterial oxygen; *RBC,* red blood cell; *WBC,* white blood cell.

opsy should be reviewed. A three-dimensional image reconstruction and display technique—virtual bronchoscopy—may have been undertaken for noninvasive airway evaluation.[6] Pulmonary function tests with a forced expiratory volume in 1 second ($FEV_1$) less than 1.0 L indicate the patient is at extremely high risk for pulmonary complications in the postoperative period. Computed tomography (CT) scans of the chest, as well as of the brain, liver, and abdomen, may reveal the presence or absence of metastasis, pleural calcification, thickening, or plaque; spiral CT detects pulmonary lesions at 1-cm size when the chances of finding stage I lesions might improve outcomes.[12] Radioisotope scans may have been done for similar reasons as the CT. Magnetic resonance imaging (MRI) detects vascular relationships to masses or vascular lesions. Positron emission tomography (PET) is a noninvasive study demonstrated to be highly accurate in diagnosing malignant pulmonary nodules and lymphadenopathy (Research Highlight). The MRI and PET are sometimes performed to rule out metastasis of the lesion. Transbronchial needle aspiration is useful in diagnosing mediastinal lymphadenopathy and staging lung cancer. Ventilation and perfusion studies show the distribution of each function in the lung. These results assist the perioperative nurse in collaborating with the surgical team to maintain effective gas exchange during the surgical intervention. The results are also valuable in predicting postoperative respiratory function and metabolic responses. Patients hospitalized for surgery related to carcinoma may have received chemotherapy or radiation therapy before surgery. Assessment of the skin and the patient's general condition is important in preventing perioperative complications.

The patient's and family's knowledge and understanding of the surgical procedure and expected outcomes should be determined, as well as their willingness to participate in the patient's care and to assist with accomplishing the desired outcomes.[11] Smoking habits and current status (if appropriate) should be assessed to determine the patient's understanding for the need to abstain following surgery.[1] Pain tolerance should be assessed to determine necessary teaching or tools that will assist in achieving positive postoperative outcomes. Patients might be sensitive about smoking history because of the assumed relationship between smoking and lung disease. The nurse should phrase questions in a way that will not result in guilt about smoking habits or assumptions that the diagnosed condition is associated with smoking. Patients undergoing lung transplant may need mental health, behavioral, or social support services either before or after the transplant.

After a general and focused review of the patient's medical record and patient interview, the perioperative nurse formulates nursing diagnoses. These statements reflect problems that will require perioperative nursing intervention, either independently or collaboratively with other members of the surgical team. Nursing diagnoses should be individualized and prioritized for each patient.

## RESEARCH HIGHLIGHT

### Cost of PET Scans in the Diagnosis of Thoracic Malignancy

The discovery of a solitary pulmonary nodule (SPN) on chest x-ray is often the patient's entry point into a malignant disease workup. Approximately one third of SPNs represent primary malignancies, and nearly one quarter are solitary metastases. The SPN workup typically begins with imaging studies, such as computerized tomography (CT). When CT results are not definitive, options may include surgical resection, transbronchial needle biopsy, or watchful waiting. Positron emission tomography (PET) combined with 18-fluorodeoxyglucose (FDG) identifies malignant tumors based on their increased metabolic rate and may be used in selected cases, but it is an expensive test.

This study used a meta-analysis and literature review to determine the accuracy, complications, and cost of diagnostic tests in patients with SPN diagnosed by radiograph. Researchers sorted patients into three groups with low, intermediate, and high probability of malignancy and then analyzed the cost of a variety of diagnostic strategies, including watchful waiting, CT only, CT plus biopsy, CT plus surgery, and FDG-PET. The cost was then analyzed in relation to the quality-adjusted life years (QALYs). The QALY is a measurement of the benefit of a medical intervention based on the number of years of life that is added by the intervention. They determined the cost effectiveness of strategies depended on the pretest possibility of malignancy.

For patients in the low-probability group, strategies that used FDG-PET selectively cost as little as $20,000 per QALY gained. Patients in the high-probability group cost as little as $16,000 for QALY gained, and for patients in the intermediate-probability group, FDG-PET cost more than $220,000 per QALY gained because they were more costly but only marginally more effective than CT-based strategies.

Based on their study, researchers advise that FDG-PET is a cost-effective diagnostic intervention when used selectively in cases where pretest probability and CT findings are discordant or in patients with intermediate pretest probability who are at high risk for surgical complications.

Modified from Gould ML and others: Cost-effectiveness of alternative management strategies for patients with solitary pulmonary nodules, *Annals of Internal Medicine* 138(9):724-735, 2003.

## Nursing Diagnosis

Nursing diagnoses related to the care of patients undergoing thoracic surgery might include the following:

- Impaired Gas Exchange related to surgical intervention
- Risk for Impaired Skin Integrity related to surgical positioning, length of surgical intervention, or use of chemical antimicrobial agents on the skin
- Risk for Imbalanced Fluid Volume related to decreased surface area of the lung for perfusion and to administration of intravenous (IV) fluids during surgery
- Risk for Infection at surgical site related to inadequate secondary defenses (presence of existing disease process) and surgical disruption of tissues
- Impaired Comfort related to pain following surgical intervention.

## Outcome Identification

Outcomes identified for the selected nursing diagnoses could be stated as follows:

- The patient will experience adequate gas exchange during the surgical procedure.
- The patient's skin integrity will be maintained.
- The patient will maintain appropriate fluid balance.
- The patient will be free from postoperative surgical site infection.
- The patient's pain will be monitored and managed.

## Planning

A typical plan of care for a patient undergoing thoracic surgery is included on pp. 913-914.

## Implementation

During implementation of the plan of care, the perioperative nurse is concerned with both preparatory patient considerations (e.g., procedure explanation and teaching for the patient, verification of the patient, surgical procedure and site, positioning, presurgical diagnostic interventions, draping) and the requirements of the surgical intervention (e.g., medication delivery; instrument, equipment, and supply availability). These patient care needs are coordinated with the other nursing interventions identified in the specific patient's plan of care.

***Positioning.*** The type of position used in thoracic surgery is determined by the operative procedure planned. Bronchoscopy is performed in the supine position with a shoulder roll. Thoracotomy can be performed with the patient in one of three common positions: (1) lateral for the posterolateral approach, (2) semilateral for the anterolateral approach (Figure 25-7), and (3) supine for the median sternotomy approach. The

## SAMPLE PLAN OF CARE

**NURSING DIAGNOSIS**

**Impaired Gas Exchange** related to surgical intervention

**OUTCOME**

The patient will experience adequate gas exchange during the surgical procedure.

**INTERVENTIONS**

- Determine the preoperative status of gas exchange by reviewing laboratory results and assessing the patient; report deviations from preoperative laboratory values and patient assessment findings.
- Obtain chest x-ray films for the intraoperative period.
- Verify that a double-lumen endotracheal tube with a soft, inflatable cuff is available for the anesthesia provider.
- Collaborate in obtaining equipment for and monitoring arterial blood gases (ABGs); document results.
- Obtain equipment for and assist with patient preparation for hemodynamic monitoring: electrocardiogram (ECG), $CO_2$ analyzer, pulse oximeter, arterial pressure line, and central venous pressure line; collaborate with the anesthesia provider in evaluating results provided by these monitoring devices during the procedure.
- Apply thermal unit (forced air–warming device or other device as available in institution); check equipment before procedure; monitor and note patient temperature during procedure.
- Collaborate in positioning the patient to provide access to the endotracheal tube, enable efficient ventilatory function, and prevent injury.
- Obtain and label specimens (e.g., ABG, blood count) to be sent to laboratory; document specimens sent, and evaluate results. Report abnormal values to the anesthesia provider and surgical team.

**NURSING DIAGNOSIS**

**Risk for Impaired Skin Integrity** related to surgical positioning, length of surgical intervention, or use of chemical antimicrobial agents on the skin

**OUTCOME**

The patient's skin integrity will be maintained.

**INTERVENTIONS**

- Assess skin integrity and condition of the skin preoperatively. Document findings; and report the presence of any lesions, rashes, cuts, nicks, or reddened areas.
- Determine presence of preexisting conditions that could compromise skin integrity (e.g., age, obesity, diabetes, allergies, radiation therapy).
- Apply principles of positioning for efficient circulatory function for lateral or supine position during the procedure; pad and protect vulnerable neurovascular bundles and dependent pressure areas:
  - *Lateral position:* ear, acromion process, iliac crest, greater trochanter, medial and lateral condyles, malleolus
  - *Supine position:* occiput, scapula, olecranon, sacrum, ischial tuberosity, calcaneus
- Position the patient in the best possible body alignment to allow visualization of the operative field.
- Assess for preexisting conditions (e.g., joint implants, arthritis, restricted movement) to prevent patient injury during positional maneuvers.
- Stabilize the patient in lateral position (e.g., beanbag, sandbag, soft shoulder roll, pillows between knees); check for tape sensitivity if adhesive tape is used. Flex the upper arm slightly (not exceeding 90-degree extension) above the head on a raised, padded armboard or supported on padding.
- Use adequate number of individuals to position the patient for the lateral position.
- Assess the area where the electrosurgical dispersive pad will be placed; clip the area if necessary. Document assessment and pad placement on the intraoperative record.
- If hair must be removed from the operative site, use clippers or a depilatory (check patient sensitivity); shave the patient with wet shave if a razor must be used.
- Prevent pooling of skin prep solutions at the bedline, site of ECG electrodes, and electrosurgical dispersive pad.
- Decrease surgical time by anticipating needs of the patient and surgical team.
- Observe and document skin integrity and condition postoperatively; compare with preoperative status.

**NURSING DIAGNOSIS**

**Risk for Imbalanced Fluid Volume** related to decreased surface area of the lung for perfusion and to administration of intravenous (IV) fluids during surgery

**OUTCOME**

The patient will maintain appropriate fluid balance.

- Insert indwelling urinary catheter; use aseptic technique.
- Position drainage bag off floor, where it is readily observable.
- Monitor urinary output hourly during the procedure; report output less than 30 ml/hr.
- Provide access for administration of IV fluids; assist with fluid administration and insertion of lines. Keep lines protected and patent during positional changes.
- Monitor results of hemodynamic parameters; document and report appropriately.

*Continued*

## SAMPLE PLAN OF CARE

**OUTCOME—cont'd**

- Monitor blood loss during the procedure; document and report appropriately.
- Provide blood (including autologous) or blood products for fluid replacement; assist in replacement therapy and patient monitoring.
- Observe for signs of shock (e.g., hypotension, abnormal ECG); report signs, and initiate corrective nursing actions.
- Observe for signs of excess blood loss (e.g., rapid, weak pulse; rapid respirations; cool, moist skin; early, slight rise in blood pressure); report signs, and initiate corrective nursing actions.
- Observe for signs of fluid excess (e.g., tachycardia, increased blood pressure); report signs, and initiate corrective nursing actions.
- Have available and administer furosemide (Lasix) and other diuretic agents as prescribed; monitor for therapeutic results.

**NURSING DIAGNOSIS**

**Risk for Infection** at surgical site related to inadequate secondary defenses (presence of existing disease process) and surgical disruption of tissues

**OUTCOME**

The patient will be free from surgical site infection.

**INTERVENTIONS**

- Create and maintain a sterile field immediately before use; monitor the sterile field, and take corrective action if breaks in technique occur.
- Administer preoperative antibiotics at least 1 hour before the procedure.
- Do not remove hair preoperatively unless the hair at or around the incision site will interfere with the surgical procedure. If hair must be removed, it should be done immediately before the surgical procedure, preferably using a means other than a razor.
- Practice aseptic technique when opening supplies, moving about the sterile field, catheterizing the patient, inserting IV lines, completing skin preparation, and draping the surgical site.
- Complete skin preparation at the incision site and point of insertion of monitoring lines to decrease microbial contamination. Use an appropriate antiseptic agent, applied in concentric circles moving toward the periphery. The prepped area should be extensive enough to extend the incision or create new incisions or drain sites.
- Monitor traffic patterns; limit the number of persons entering and leaving the operating room.
- Administer prescribed antibiotics for irrigation and IV administration; check for patient allergies; record all medications administered by the perioperative nurse or scrub person at the sterile field.
- Decrease surgical time by anticipating patient and surgical team needs.
- When visible soiling with blood or other body fluids of surfaces or equipment occurs during the procedure, use an Environmental Protection Agency (EPA)–approved hospital disinfectant to wipe the affected area (confine and contain).
- Correctly classify the surgical wound according to the institution's wound classification system on completion of the surgical procedure.
- Using sterile gloves, apply sterile dressings to the surgical site before the drape is removed.

**NURSING DIAGNOSIS**

**Impaired Comfort** related to pain following surgical intervention

**OUTCOME**

The patient's comfort will be assessed, monitored, and managed.

**INTERVENTIONS**

- Teach the pain assessment scale preoperatively.
- Provide education to the patient regarding the physiology of pain and the importance of treating pain before it becomes unmanageable.
- Discuss pain management techniques and options (i.e., oral, intramuscular [IM], IV medications, patient-controlled analgesia [PCA], epidural use, intercostal blocks).
- Assist anesthesia provider in initiating pain control methods (i.e., epidural placement, nerve blocks).
- Assess pain before and following administration of pain medication or use of comfort measures (e.g., repositioning, applying support devices).
- Monitor the effects of pain management strategies and document.
- Assess verbal and nonverbal cues during procedures requiring monitored anesthesia care and administration of local anesthesia.
- Teach pain control methods and medication uses and side effects before discharge.

prone position can also provide access in some procedures (see Chapter 5 for safe positioning interventions). Adequate padding and safe transfer should be implemented to prevent pressure areas.

***Draping.*** Draping may be minimal for bronchoscopic procedures. The principles of draping for other procedures (see Chapter 3) are followed in all other thoracic procedures. Drapes may consist of a fenestrated sheet or single sheets surrounding the incision site. To prevent instruments from falling from the field, a magnetic pad may be placed on the drapes below the incision site when the patient is placed in lateral position. A thermal blanket (forced warm air) is usually placed on the patient before draping to maintain normothermia. Sequential compression devices are often applied also to prevent the development of deep venous thrombosis (DVT).

***Instrumentation.*** Bronchoscopy instruments are designed to directly inspect and observe the larynx, trachea, bronchi, or mediastinum; to remove secretions; to obtain washings or tissue for bacterial and cytologic studies; or to remove tissue. They are also designed to remove foreign bodies. Instrumentation for thoracic surgery includes the laparotomy instrument set (see Chapter 11) and specialty items. Instruments used for a thoracotomy or chest procedure include a combination of delicate and heavy instruments. Stapling equipment com-

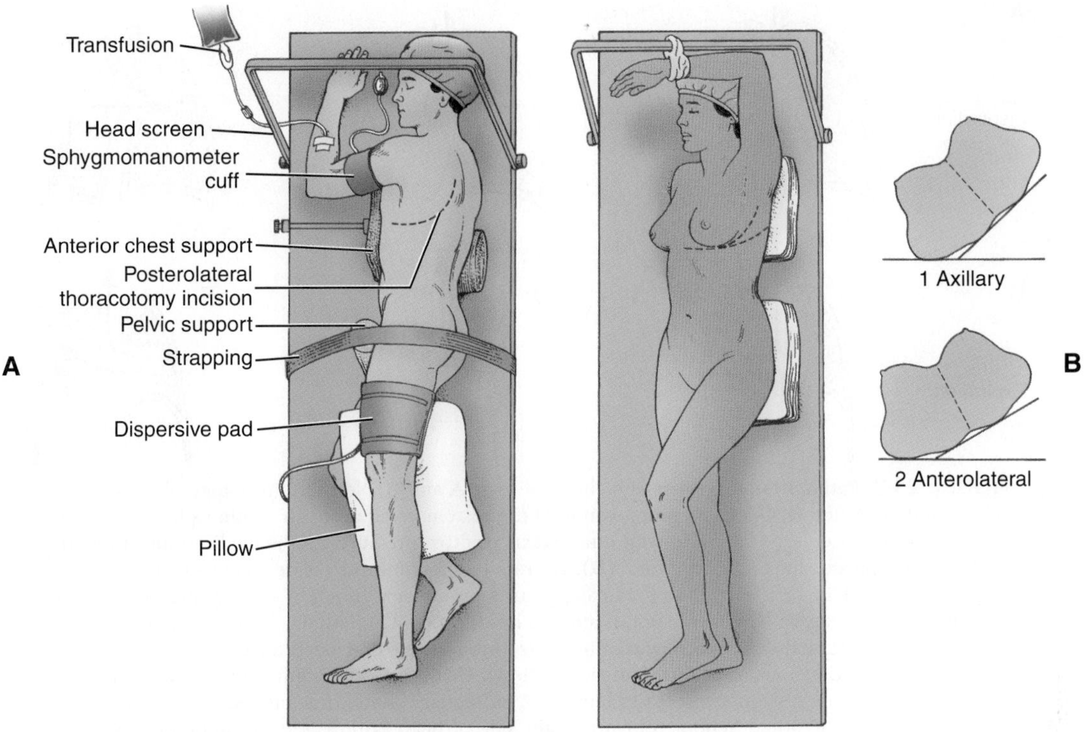


FIGURE 25-7 Positions for thoracotomy incisions. **A,** Lateral position for posterolateral incision. **B,** Semilateral position for axillary or anterolateral position.

monly is used as suturing devices and requires staplers and reload staples of appropriate sizes. The delicate instruments are used to cut tissue and vessels or to clamp tissue in a nontraumatic manner. The heavier instruments are used for bone cutting, dissecting, or retracting. Instrumentation must also be available for hemostasis and suturing of all types of tissue.

Perioperative nursing staff should determine the thoracic surgery arrangement of items on the instrument table and Mayo stand; this arrangement should be an effective standard method that applies principles of work simplification and thorough knowledge of procedures. Lengthy incisions are often required for thoracic procedures; therefore it is critical that the instruments be accounted for before closure.

***Equipment.*** In thoracic surgery, a variety of equipment is used, including a forced air–warming unit, fiberoptic headlights, fiberoptic light sources, video equipment, sequential compression devices, and anesthesia supplies. Double-lumen endotracheal tubes are commonly used for thoracotomies.

The neodymium:yttrium-aluminum-garnet (Nd:YAG) or $CO_2$ laser can be used for treating tracheobronchial lesions with use of a bronchoscope. Obstruction of the mainstem bronchus and trachea caused by benign and malignant lesions can also be effectively treated with laser therapy. Use of laser equipment requires a thorough understanding of the equipment, the safety issues, the responsibilities (see Chapter 7), and the planned surgical procedure.

***Monitoring.*** Monitored anesthesia care, local anesthesia, or topical anesthesia may be used during some bronchoscopic procedures. General anesthesia may also be used for bronchoscopic procedures and is used for other thoracic procedures. Team members work in cooperation to constantly monitor laboratory results (e.g., ABGs), oxygenation, temperature, blood loss, and urine output. Monitoring sequential compression device settings and patient position is also important in providing safe patient care. Results are communicated with other team members and documented for continuity of care.

***Blood Replacement.*** Blood replacement therapy during or after the procedure may be required because of extensive tissue dissection in a highly vascular area. The patient may have autologous blood ordered; however, the diagnosis may prohibit patient donation of his or her own blood. The patient's blood type and amount of blood ordered should be noted before the procedure and its availability confirmed. During the procedure, every effort should be made to control and monitor bleeding. If blood collection or reinfusion systems are used, the manufacturer's instructions and institutional protocols should be followed. Bloodless surgery programs are more common and can prevent the need for allogenic or autologous blood use.[13]

***Chest-Drainage Systems.*** In the presence of restrictive and obstructive pulmonary disease, the lung may not fully expand or contract, causing a reduction in alveolar ventilation with resultant hypoxia. Other conditions that interfere with respiratory function are excessive accumulation of mucus, pleural effusions, a foreign body in a bronchus, closed pneumothorax (simple and tension types), open pneumothorax, hemothorax, and multiple rib injuries that produce paradoxic motion of the thoracic cage, or flail chest (Figure 25-8).

The normal function of the lungs is supported by elasticity and negative intrapleural pressure. Collapse of the normal lung

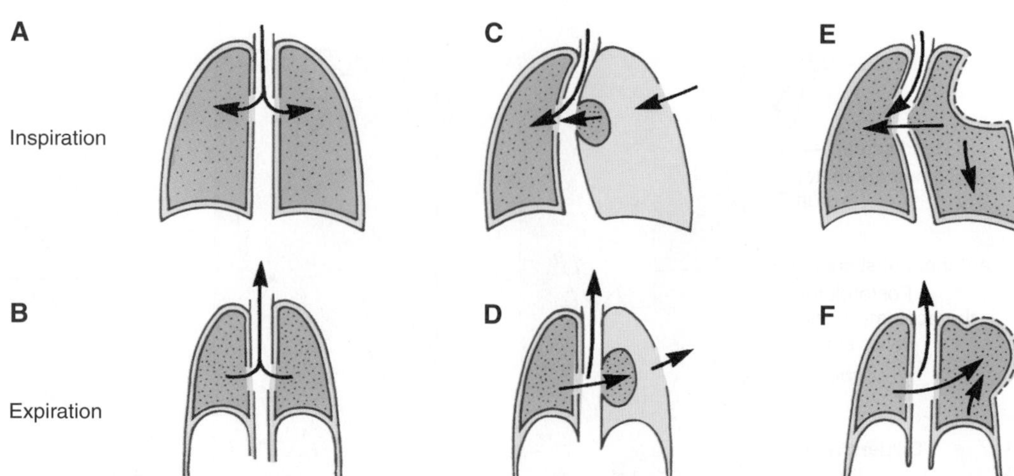


FIGURE 25-8 Pathophysiology of severe chest injuries. **A** and **B,** Normal physiology of inspiration and expiration. **C** and **D,** Open (sucking) wound of thorax. On inspiration, air at atmospheric pressure rushes in through defect **(C),** collapsing lung. Next, positive pressure causes mediastinum to shift, compressing opposite lung. On expiration **(D),** air from lung on uninjured side reenters collapsed lung and is rebreathed in next inspiration. Impaired cardiopulmonary function in presence of sucking wound of chest is caused by (1) collapse of lung on injured side, (2) partial collapse of opposite lung, (3) increased functional dead space caused by rebreathing of unoxygenated air from collapsed lung, and (4) diminished venous return to right side of heart. **E** and **F,** Primary effect of paradoxic motion resulting from flail or stove-in chest is diminution of pulmonary ventilation and extensive rebreathing from one lung to the other. Venous return to right side of heart is impaired. Appropriate treatment requires intubation of trachea and use of volume-limited ventilator.

follows any condition that reduces or eliminates the negative intrapleural pressure if the lung is not adhering to the chest wall. When the pleural space is filled with air, reducing the negative pressure, the lung collapses. This action may cause complete collapse if the pressure within the intrathoracic (pleural) space becomes positive.

A diminished negative pressure or occurrence of actual positive pressure in one pleural space may cause the mediastinum or trachea to shift toward the opposite side. When this happens, not only does the affected lung collapse because of a positive pressure in the pleural space but also the function of the lung on the opposite side may be impaired as a result of compression by the mediastinal shift. Tension pneumothorax can produce serious effects as air continues to escape from the lung into the intrapleural space. The air cannot return to the bronchi to be exhaled, thereby increasing the intrapleural pressure. When a large opening in the chest wall allows direct communication of the pleural space with atmospheric pressure, it may cause death if the mediastinum becomes mobile.

Paradoxic motion of the chest results from severe instability of the chest wall because of multiple and often bilateral rib fractures; with inspiration, partial collapse of the thoracic space occurs. The blunt injury that caused the multiple rib fractures also causes severe contusion of the lung itself. This contusion contributes to impairment of lung function by affecting gas exchange, which may result in severe, life-threatening hypoxia.

One or more chest catheters (tubes) may be inserted for postoperative closed-chest drainage. The chest tubes provide a conduit for drainage of air, blood, and other fluid from the intrapleural or mediastinal space and reestablishment of negative pressure in the intrapleural space. Drainage systems use three mechanisms to drain fluid and air from the pleural cavity: positive expiratory pressure, gravity, and suction. The chest tubes are connected to a sterile water-seal or gravity-drainage system. Water-seal suction may be necessary when a persistent air leak cannot be controlled by drainage alone. Historically a two- or three-bottle system was used to accomplish this.[2] Several compact, disposable units are available that function like the three-bottle system; these units are preferable because they are easier and safer to use. The principles of operation remain the same and can be described more easily using the bottle-system model (Figure 25-9, *A*). The first bottle collects the drainage from the intrapleural space, the second bottle provides the water seal, and the third provides the suction control determined by the level of water. The disposable units have three or four compartments for drainage, water seal, and suction (Figure 25-9, *B*).

If two chest tubes are inserted, they may be attached by a Y connector to a single drainage unit or may be attached individually to two separate units. All connections should be banded or otherwise secured to ensure an intact system (Figure 25-10). The drainage system must be sterile and maintained in a position lower than the patient's body to prevent air and fluid from reentering the chest cavity. Chest tubes are generally removed within 5 to 7 days.

***Documentation.*** Documentation of perioperative care includes a summary of preoperative assessment information that supports formulated nursing diagnoses, nursing interventions, and postoperative evaluation. Documentation for a patient undergoing a thoracotomy specifically addresses patient assessment information related to position of the patient, positioning aids used, medications administered, results of laboratory tests completed, special equipment used, urine output,

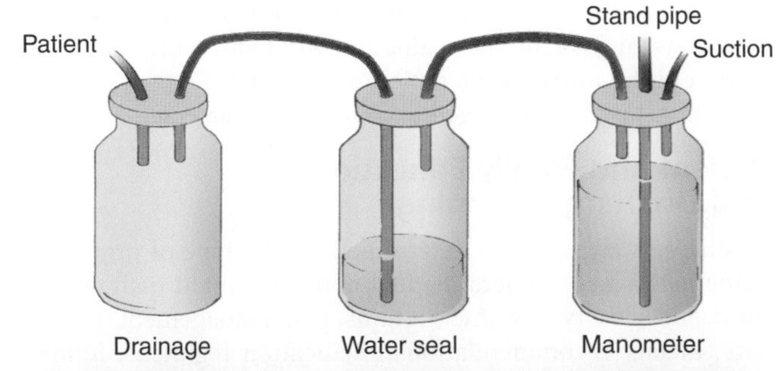


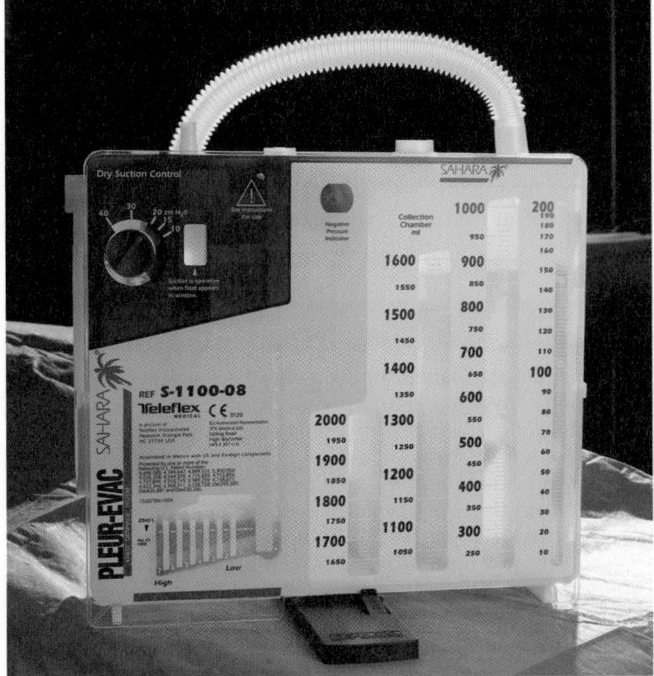


FIGURE 25-9 **A,** Method of draining pleural space, using triple-bottle system as model. **B,** Commercial chest drainage system.

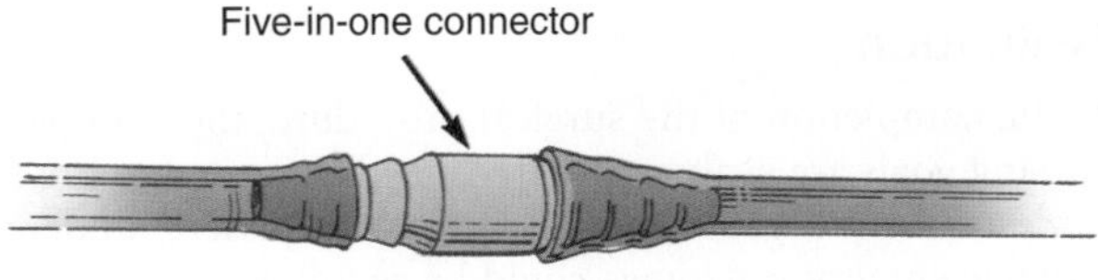


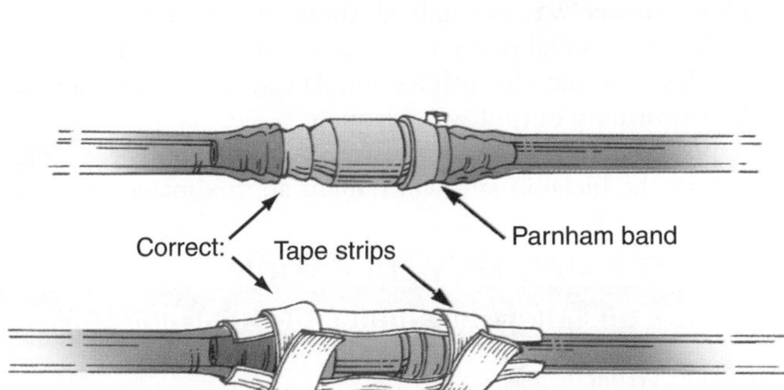


FIGURE 25-10 Method of securing chest tubes after connection to water-seal drainage system.

blood replacement, insertion of chest tubes and drainage systems, and postoperative evaluation of patient care outcomes.

***Transfer Report.*** The patient is transferred from the operating room to the postanesthesia care unit (PACU) after thoracotomy. The report to the PACU nurse is often a collaborative effort of the nurse and anesthesia provider. The perioperative nurse reports the patient's preoperative status, including anxiety level and understanding of the procedure, to assist the PACU nurse in meeting the emotional and educational needs of the patient. A description of the position of the patient during the procedure provides criteria for assessment and evaluation of mobility. Results of immediate postoperative assessment, including skin integrity, location and type of dressing applied, location and type of drains, blood loss, fluid replacement, medications administered, and laboratory results obtained during the procedure, are reported as a baseline control for assessment in the PACU. The PACU nurse must be informed of the procedure performed, particularly if it varies from the anticipated or scheduled procedure. The perioperative care plan should be reviewed and patient outcomes reported.

***Postprocedure Concerns.*** Patients are transferred to the PACU, using care not to dislodge the chest tube, urinary catheter, or monitoring equipment. The endotracheal tube may remain in place to maintain an adequate air exchange. Air exchange and effective ventilation are two immediate needs of the patient after thoracotomy. Chest tubes are connected to suction except for postpneumonectomy procedures. The thoracotomy is considered a painful procedure and, when coupled with muscle injury, affects functional capacity. A postprocedure epidural catheter with an injection of a local anesthetic at the completion of wound closure for pain management should improve the comfort level of the patient as postoperative activities are encouraged.

Fluid volume overload can lead to acute respiratory disease syndrome that can result in death and therefore should be avoided. Monitoring urine output is important, but postthoracotomy patients should be maintained in a state of hydration that does not require a fluid bolus for low urine output.

Patients are often anxious about their limitations, the environment, and the results of the procedure. Patients and families will benefit from preoperative teaching about pain management techniques and use of the institution's pain assessment tool, as well as being allowed to discuss their feelings and needs. Family members should be informed of the patient's status during and as soon as possible after the procedure.

## Evaluation

At the completion of the surgical procedure, the perioperative nursing goals are evaluated. They may be restated as brief outcomes. For the goals identified for the patient undergoing thoracic surgery, outcomes could be as follows:

- The patient's gas exchange was unimpaired; ventilation/perfusion ratios were adequate as evidenced by laboratory results, and vital signs were within normal limits; skin, nailbeds, and mucosa were pink; lung fields were clear bilaterally; and chest excursion was normal.
- The patient's skin integrity was maintained; reddened or discolored skin and other signs of altered tissue perfusion were not present.
- Fluid balance was maintained; there were no fluid excesses or deficits; mental orientation was consistent with preoperative level; serum electrolytes and ABGs were within normal limits; urinary output was adequate.
- A postoperative surgical site infection will not be experienced; the incision site will remain approximated and dry, without redness, drainage, or undue tenderness. (This is a long-term goal, and its evaluation will require the collaboration of the nurse in the patient care unit.)
- Comfort will be managed and pain levels assessed.

## Patient and Family Education and Discharge Planning

Discharge status will be determined by the type of procedure being performed. General patient concerns might include mobility and activity levels/restrictions, pain management, wound care, dietary recommendations, medication regimens, follow-up appointments, and any prescribed outpatient care or referrals. Patients diagnosed with tumors will experience psychosocial concerns. Both the patient and the family need specific instructions for discharge that relate to the specific procedure. These should be reviewed verbally and provided in a written form, with verification of understanding and time for questions and concerns.

After a bronchoscopy, patients will be discharged within hours of the procedure. Their main concerns might be the re-

### PATIENT AND FAMILY EDUCATION

### Patient Education and Home Care Teaching for Oxygen Therapy

**GENERAL INFORMATION**

- Review the physician's order for the type of delivery system and liter flow or percentage of oxygen to be delivered.
- Give the patient and the caregiver both *oral* and *written* instructions. Provide them with the name and telephone number of the physician to call if questions arise. Use visual aids to assist in instruction.

**HOME CARE**

- Explain the purpose for oxygen therapy and how it will be delivered to the patient.
- Warning signs:
  - Review the signs and symptoms that should be reported to the physician:
    - Irregular, shallow, or slow breathing; difficulty in breathing
    - Restlessness or anxiety
    - Tiredness, drowsiness, trouble waking up
    - Persistent headache
    - Slurred speech
    - Confusion, difficulty in concentrating
    - Bluish fingernails or lips
  - Inform the patient about the symptoms of oxygen toxicity:
    - Sore throat
    - Cough
    - Nausea
    - Anxiety
    - Numbness
    - Muscular twitching
    - Chest pain with deep inspiration
  - Special instructions:
    - Assist the patient to obtain a home health care referral for follow-up at home.
    - Explain the importance of maintaining the appropriate flow rate, since high flow rates in patients with chronic obstructive pulmonary disease can suppress the respiratory drive.
    - Teach the patient how to remove and reposition the oxygen equipment to permit wiping and drying the face, blowing the nose, and eating.
    - Instruct the patient on skin care procedures, since prolonged oxygen therapy can cause skin irritation and breakdown, which can provide an additional route for microorganisms. Advise patient to use non–petroleum-based cream on the face, lips, and nostrils to relieve the drying effects of oxygen.
    - Stress the importance of not smoking and not allowing others to smoke near the patient because of the possibility of combustion, fire, or explosion.
    - Ensure that no candles or matches are lit in the immediate area where oxygen is being administered.
    - Explain the necessity of checking all electrical equipment used in the same room as oxygen administration for frayed cords or the potential for sparking to avoid combustion and fire or explosion.
    - Advise the patient to obtain a fire extinguisher and keep it near the oxygen equipment.
  - Activity:
    - Encourage walking and other activities as tolerated. Advise the patient to use a portable oxygen source because continuous oxygen therapy can limit mobility.
    - Suggest that the patient use oxygen, as ordered, during meals, showers, or sexual activities.
  - Alternative therapy:
    - Discuss the use of relaxation techniques to minimize anxiety associated with shortness of breath.

**FOLLOW-UP CARE AND REFERRALS**

- Stress the importance of regular follow-up visits. Make sure the patient has the necessary names and telephone numbers.
- Discuss with the patient and caregiver the need to notify the local fire department and electric and gas utility companies of the presence of oxygen in the home.
- Instruct the patient to keep emergency numbers by the telephone.
- Assist the patient to obtain referral services, supplies, and information about support groups.

From Canobbio MM: *Handbook of patient teaching,* ed 3, St Louis, 2006, Mosby.

sults of biopsy and diagnosis. The patient and family should be aware of the length of time until results will be available and the method used to obtain those results. Patients should also be reminded of the need to rest for 2 to 3 days after the procedure. Side effects might result from medications used for moderate sedation or untoward intraoperative outcomes (e.g., the patient may experience bloody sputum, difficulty breathing). In addition, patients should be reminded that their throats might feel numb 2 to 3 hours after the procedure and difficulty with swallowing will subside.

After a surgical procedure such as thoracoscopy or thoracotomy vigorous pulmonary toilet is encouraged, including use of the spirometer, deep breathing, and turning and coughing every 1 to 2 hours while awake. Patients will ambulate within 4 to 6 hours; length of time until discharge might be a few days to a week or more. Patients who progress without difficulty after a thoracoscopy or thoracotomy will be monitored for drainage from the chest tubes and for pain management or complications. Postoperative air leaks or pulmonary infections will delay discharge from the health care setting.

In-home nursing care is often initiated to monitor oxygen levels, wound care needs, and pain management. The patient may be discharged with supplemental oxygen (Patient and Family Education, p. 918). This will require that the patient be weaned and demonstrate satisfactory ambulatory $SaO_2$ rates of 88% to 90%, which will most likely be supervised by homecare nurses.

# Surgical Interventions

## ENDOSCOPY (DIAGNOSTIC OR THERAPEUTIC)

Endoscopy refers to examination of hollow body organs or cavities with instruments that permit visual inspection of their contents and walls. The endoscopic procedures pertinent to thoracic surgery are bronchoscopy, mediastinoscopy, and thoracoscopy. Each endoscopist has preferences regarding the type of endoscope, positioning of the patient, type of anesthetic, and equipment. Invasive diagnostic or therapeutic measures enhance the decision to pursue surgical intervention by providing information related to the disease process, including histologic characteristics, location of the lesion, and lesion extent. Therapeutic endoscopy provides treatment by removal of the lesion or foreign body.

### Standard Bronchoscopy Using Rigid Bronchoscope

Standard bronchoscopy is the direct visualization of the mucosa of the trachea, the main bronchi and their openings, and most of the segmental bronchi and includes removal of material for microscopic study if necessary.

Bronchoscopy is an integral part of the examination of patients with pulmonary symptoms such as persistent cough or wheezing, hemoptysis, obstruction, and abnormal roentgenographic changes. Common causes of bleeding (hemoptysis) are bronchiectasis, carcinoma, and tuberculosis. Congenital anomalies and suspected presence of a foreign body, especially in infants and children, are responsible for emergency examination of the respiratory tract.

Bronchoscopy is done to determine the presence of a lesion in the tracheobronchial passages, to identify and localize that lesion accurately, and to observe periodically the effects of therapy. It can be completed for dilating structures, debriding tumors, or evacuating clots. In suspected carcinoma, the aspirated secretions obtained by bronchoscopy may contain malignant cells.

***Procedural Considerations.*** Flexible bronchoscopy on an adult patient may be completed with the patient under local (topical) anesthesia or monitored anesthesia care; a child usually receives general anesthesia. Patients undergoing rigid bronchoscopy should be paralyzed and ventilation continued to minimize trauma. The adult patient under local anesthesia may experience discomfort and anxiety. To reduce anxiety, personnel should be introduced, intraoperative activities explained, and reassurance provided to the patient (Patient and Family Education, p. 920). The oral structures, including the teeth and lips, should be assessed for integrity. Loose teeth may require removal before or during the procedure.

IV sedatives or analgesics may be administered during the procedure. See Chapter 4 for perioperative nursing considerations when the patient is receiving local or monitored anesthesia care. The topical (or local) anesthetic setup should include a headlight for visualization, laryngeal mirrors of various sizes, a lingual spatula, sprays with straight and curved cannulas, and anesthetic drugs, as ordered. Other items include the laryngeal syringe with straight and curved cannulas, Jackson cross-action forceps, and the Schindler pharyngeal anesthetizer, if desired. Luer-Lok 10-ml syringes and 20- and 22-gauge needles are needed for transtracheal injection.

The anesthetic drugs frequently used are lidocaine (Xylocaine), procaine (Novocain), and tetracaine (Pontocaine, Cetacaine) with or without epinephrine. Pauses of 3 to 4 minutes are taken between applications of the anesthetic agent to the tongue, palate, and pharynx and then to the larynx and to the trachea. The anesthetic agent is applied by means of a spray or laryngeal syringe with a straight or curved cannula.

Some physicians prefer to have the patient sit upright and gargle with the topical anesthetic mixture, rinse it around in the mouth, and then expectorate it, thereby producing a partial anesthesia of the buccal mucosa and pharynx.

For direct bronchoscopy, a long metal cannula attached to a syringe is generally used to apply the anesthetic agent to the surface of the vocal cords; then the agent is injected through the anesthetized glottis into the trachea. This act causes the patient to produce a sharp, sudden cough. For intrabronchial anesthesia, a portion of the anesthetic agent is introduced through the bronchoscope.

The patient may be positioned either in supine position, with the shoulders elevated on a small roll, gel pad, or a sandbag to gently extend the head and neck, or in the sitting position.

The setup includes the bronchoscope, telescopes of desired types, fiberoptic light cords, and the fiberoptic light source. Each standard scope requires a fiberoptic light carrier, cord, and light source. Duplicates of each, along with the appropriate replacement lightbulbs for the light source, should be available for immediate use. The light source should be tested periodically and immediately before use. To test the fiberoptic light carrier and telescope, the instrument should be held vertically by the ocular end. The endoscope should always be tested immediately before passage into the patient. The light-intensity

PATIENT AND FAMILY EDUCATION

## Patient Education and Teaching for Bronchoscopy with Patient Under Local Anesthesia

**PREPROCEDURAL TEACHING**

- Review the physician's explanation of the procedure and the reason for it; encourage the patient to ask questions and to discuss any fears or anxieties.
- Discuss who will perform the procedure and where it will take place.
- Instruct the patient to have someone available after the procedure to drive the patient home.
- Review the medications that will be used preoperatively (medications to decrease secretions, sedatives) and immediately before the procedure (topical anesthetics). Explain that the topical anesthetic may cause a cold, unpleasant sensation in the throat.
- Explain that the patient will be able to breathe around the bronchoscope.
- Reassure the patient that the nurse will provide emotional support during the procedure.

**POSTPROCEDURAL TEACHING**

- Explain that after the procedure the patient's vital signs will be monitored frequently; discuss the need to maintain nothing-by-mouth (NPO) status until the gag reflex returns.
- Provide explanations about any temporary hoarseness and sore throat. Lozenges and throat gargles can be provided after the gag reflex returns.
- Review the signs and symptoms that should be reported immediately to a physician or nurse:
  - Difficulty breathing
  - Chest pain
  - Inability to swallow
  - Excessive bloody mucus
- Establish a regular routine of deep breathing and ambulation at least every 2 hours; avoid coughing within the first 24 hours following a biopsy.
- Inform the patient that a soft diet may be needed for the first day or until throat pain disappears.
- Explain that extremely hot foods or liquids should be avoided.
- Encourage fluid intake to thin secretions unless contraindicated.
- Discuss the importance of not smoking.

From Canobbio MM: *Handbook of patient teaching,* ed 3, St Louis, 2006, Mosby.

dial should be set at the proper level, as specified by the manufacturer. The light source should be switched on and off to test its function. During a procedure, the light source should be in standby mode whenever it is not in active use.

Other supplies that will be needed are suction tubing, aspirating tubes, specimen collectors, sponge carriers, and the desired type of forceps. The metal sponge carrier consists of two parts: an inner rod, which has two jaws protruding from its distal end; and an outer band, which is screwed down on the inner rod so that a sponge can be held securely within the jaws. Small gauze sponges are used to keep the field dry, remove secretions, and apply a topical anesthetic agent. Cytologic specimen collectors, such as the Clerf or Lukens, are used to hold secretions as they are obtained. Aspirating tubes of different lengths and designs are used to remove secretions and collect material for microscopic examination and culture or cultures. The straight aspirating tube with one or two openings at the distal end is used to remove material from the pharynx, larynx, and esophagus. The curved aspirating tube with a flexible tip is used to remove secretions from the upper and dorsal orifices of the bronchi.

Various types of forceps are designed to remove foreign bodies or tissues for histologic study. Biting-tip forceps may be used to secure tissue for pathologic study. Forceps with jaws that veer laterally at about a 45-degree angle from the instrument's axis permit visualization during the biopsy maneuver. Bronchoesophageal forceps consist of a stylet, a cannula with a handle, a screw, a locknut, and a setscrew. Forceps for laryngeal and bronchial regions are designed to remove tissue specimens. Specimen containers should be ready with the identifying patient information label, as should laboratory slips for specific requests. If brush specimens are collected, slides and alcohol are required.

The standard bronchoscope is a rigid speculum used for visualizing the tracheobronchial tree. The rigid bronchoscope might be selected for biopsy of a large central mass, for removal of a foreign object, or to control hemorrhage during biopsy of a vascular mass. The rigid bronchoscope remains the instrument of choice for removal of foreign bodies in infants and children. A fiberoptic light carrier is inserted into the bronchoscope to illuminate the distal opening. A side channel is incorporated into the bronchoscope to permit aeration of the lungs with oxygen or anesthetic gases. An additional device, the Sanders Venturi system, which is available to the anesthesia provider, provides adequate patient ventilation during bronchoscopies and laryngoscopies.

The endoscopist risks contamination in the presence of communicable diseases. For this reason, the endoscopist and assistants should wear facemasks and eye protection or wear a transparent shield attached to a headband (see Chapter 3 for specific Transmission-Based Precautions). With increasing numbers of patients with tuberculosis, particulate respirators are recommended as protective devices. Aseptic technique is used to prevent cross-contamination.

### *Operative Procedure*

1. The head is placed in position for visualization of the bronchus—to the left when the right main bronchi are inspected and to the right when the left bronchi are inspected. The head is lowered for inspection of the middle lobe.
2. A tooth guard is placed to protect the patient's teeth. The bronchoscope is inserted over the surface of the tongue, usually through the right corner of the mouth. The patient's lip is retracted from the upper teeth with a finger of the endoscopist's left hand. The epiglottis is identified and elevated with the tip of the bronchoscope.
3. The distal end of the scope is passed through the true vocal cords of the larynx, and the upper tracheal rings are viewed. A small amount of anesthetic solution may be sprayed through the tube on the carina of the trachea and into the

bronchus with the bronchial atomizer or spray. The patient's head is moved to the left to obtain a view of the right bronchi. The right-angle telescope is inserted with the light adjusted into the bronchoscope. The optical system should be kept free from precipitated moisture.
4. The segmental bronchial orifices of the upper right lobe bronchi are viewed, and the telescope is removed. Suction and aspirating tubes are introduced to clear the field of vision.
5. The middle lobe branches are inspected by inserting an oblique 45-degree–angle telescope or right-angle telescope and advancing it. The patient's head is lowered to view the right middle lobe or turned to the right to view the left main bronchus.
6. Secretions are aspirated for study. Biopsy forceps are used if indicated; foreign bodies are removed with forceps.
7. The bronchoscope is removed, and the patient's face is cleansed.

Patients who have undergone bronchoscopy under local anesthesia are encouraged to sit on the edge of the operating room (OR) bed before transfer to the stretcher. An emesis basin and sponges should be provided for the patient's use. Assistance and support should be provided to the patient to prevent a fall.

*Postprocedure Concerns.* Patient safety during and after endoscopy under topical anesthesia, local anesthesia, or monitored anesthesia care is a concern attributable to the medications administered. The gag reflex may not return for 2 to 3 hours. The patient may be positioned on his or her side or with the head of the bed elevated to promote drainage of secretions. The patient should be restricted from any oral intake until the gag reflex has returned. During bronchoscopy, particularly with a rigid bronchoscope, teeth could be loosened or oral structures damaged. The lips, teeth, and oral mucosa should be examined to ensure undisturbed integrity. Patients are often anxious to know the results of the procedure, and they benefit from the perioperative nurse's openness and willingness to discuss when results might be available, as well as the patient's feelings and concerns.

## Bronchoscopy Using the Flexible Bronchoscope

Flexible bronchoscopy is performed to view structures that cannot be observed with a rigid scope. Flexible bronchoscopy may be performed in addition to a standard rigid bronchoscopy or as an independent procedure. If performed separately, the patient may remain on the transporting stretcher during the procedure. Flexible bronchoscopy is completed for the same reasons as rigid bronchoscopy. Flexible fiberoptic telescopes permit visualization of the upper, middle, and lower lobe bronchi. They can be passed in patients with a jaw deformity or cervical bone rigidity with less difficulty than the rigid scope. Flexible fiberoptic bronchoscopes are more frequently used, as is video endoscopy.

*Procedural Considerations.* Patient considerations are as described for rigid bronchoscopy. Instruments and equipment used include the flexible bronchoscope, fiberoptic light source, flexible biopsy forceps, flexible brush (optional; if used, slides and alcohol are necessary to collect specimen), labeled specimen collectors, pathology requests, syringe for wash, and suction tubing with collection tube attached to collect the wash specimen.

### *Operative Procedure*

1. The lubricated bronchoscope is passed through the adapter on the endotracheal tube, which is held secure by the anesthesia provider. If the procedure is performed with the patient under local or monitored anesthesia care, the lubricated bronchoscope may be passed nasally.
2. The suction tube is positioned with the specimen collector attached for collection of bronchial washings. When indicated, the suction tubing is connected to the bronchoscope; the container for collection is held securely in an upright position to prevent loss of the specimen through the suction.
3. Approximately 5 ml of saline solution is injected into the channel. Suction is quickly reapplied. This procedure may be repeated.

After completion of the procedure, specimen containers are sent to the laboratory.

### *Care of Endoscopes*

HANDLING INSTRUMENTS. To ensure long life of the optical system of endoscopes, each instrument should be kept straight at all times when not in use. Flexible endoscopes should never be severely bent. Endoscopes should be inspected and tested according to the manufacturer's instructions before they are used in patient care, during the procedure as necessary, after decontamination, and before disinfection or sterilization procedures.

When a telescope is sent for repair, it must be properly packed in a padded instrument case and placed within a padded carton to ensure protection of the lens system during transportation. A direct blow can break the objective window or lenses of telescopic endoscopes. The junction of the flexible and rigid portions of the scope is the most vulnerable point.

During use, the patient might bite down while the flexible portion of the scope is being passed. A specially designed mouthpiece is often used to prevent damage to the scope. The sheath covering the flexible part may become perforated after contact if a mouthpiece is not used. When a new covering is needed, the instrument should be returned to the manufacturer for repair.

PREPARING ENDOSCOPES FOR TERMINAL STORAGE. The manufacturer's procedures for cleaning and terminally disinfecting and sterilizing flexible or rigid endoscopes should be followed. Standard and Transmission-Based Precautions should be used when handling and processing contaminated endoscopes and accessory equipment (see Chapter 3). Usually, both flexible and rigid scopes can be cleaned with enzymatic detergents. A soft brush designed to clean the lumen is used for rigid scopes. After rinsing and drying, both types can be terminally prepared by using a glutaraldehyde solution in a designated endoscope washer or peracetic acid solution sterilization system. Thorough rinsing and drying are required before storage.

CLEANING A TELESCOPIC ENDOSCOPE. The scope is held vertically by its ocular end; it is wiped repeatedly with downward strokes, using gauze sponges or a soft brush saturated with an enzymatic detergent appropriate for use with the telescopic endoscope. Special attention is given to surface joints and crevices that may retain mucus. The scope is then dried thoroughly with clean gauze sponges.

Optical telescopes should never undergo steam sterilization unless specifically designed for autoclave use. Only those sterilizing agents that are recommended by the manufacturer should be used. Sterilization can be achieved by use of chemical agents.

**CLEANING ASPIRATING TUBES AND SPONGE CARRIERS.** Aspirating tubes and sponge carriers are cleaned and flushed with soap and water and are sterilized by steam or gas. Special care must be given to spiral-tipped aspirators. All aspirators with bent or broken tips should be sent to the manufacturer for repair.

The sponge-carrier collar must be unscrewed before it is cleaned. After sterilization, the threads of the carrier are oiled. The carrier is reassembled and stored lying straight.

**CLEANING FORCEPS.** The forceps may be placed in an ultrasonic cleaner. After cleaning, each forceps is taken apart, one at a time, by unscrewing the nut and removing the stylet. All parts are examined carefully, and noncorrosive solvent oil is applied to the joint of the forceps. Each forceps is reassembled and the action tested; then it is stored lying straight with jaws open. Forceps in good condition should have (1) jaws closing together in parallel position; (2) handles touching slightly when the jaws are closed; (3) jaws merging into the cannula when the forceps is closed and protruding widely without expanding the spring when it is open; (4) the end nut, located in the stylet, in place; (5) the side screw tight; and (6) the distal end and jaws' edges smooth on finger examination.

## Mediastinoscopy

Mediastinoscopy is the direct visualization and possible biopsy of lymph nodes or tumors at the tracheobronchial junction, under the carina of the trachea, or on the upper lobe bronchi or subdivisions. Mediastinoscopy may precede an exploratory thoracotomy in known cases of lung carcinoma or may be completed to assist in accurately staging the patient's lymph node status. Patients with positive findings may be treated with radiation or chemotherapy, as indicated. The mediastinoscope is a hollow tube with a fiberoptic light carrier. A fiberoptic light source with a light-intensity dial provides power and control of illumination.

***Procedural Considerations.*** The setup for mediastinoscopy includes a set of instruments for making an incision, cutting, retracting, and suturing similar to those needed for a minor procedure. In addition, the desired type of mediastinoscope, fiberoptic light cords, fiberoptic light source, suction tubing, aspirating tubes, biopsy forceps, electrosurgical unit (ESU), and an 8-inch, 20-gauge endocardiac needle are required. Depending on institutional policy, a thoracotomy tray may be in the OR on standby in the event of uncontrolled bleeding after biopsy.

The patient is given a general anesthetic agent by way of endotracheal intubation and positioned as for a tracheostomy (see Chapter 21).

### *Operative Procedure*

1. A short (approximately 2-cm) transverse incision is made above the suprasternal notch, and the pretracheal fascia is exposed.
2. The pretracheal fascia is incised.
3. Tunneling is accomplished alongside the trachea by blunt (digital) dissection into the mediastinum.
4. The mediastinoscope is introduced under direct vision deep to the fascial plane and advanced along the side of the trachea toward the mediastinum.
5. The scope is manipulated to visualize the tracheal bifurcation, bronchi, aortic arch, and associated lymph nodes.
6. Lymph node tissue is located for biopsy and aspirated with a small-gauge needle and syringe to verify that it is a nonvascular structure.
7. A biopsy forceps is then inserted through the scope, and a tissue specimen is excised. Pressure can be applied to the excision site with a bronchus sponge on a holder. The mediastinum is reinspected for bleeding.
8. The mediastinoscope is withdrawn.
9. Subcutaneous tissue is sutured with absorbable sutures. The skin is approximated and sutured with nonabsorbable material on a small cutting needle.
10. A small dressing is applied.

## Thoracoscopy

The thoracoscope facilitates an endoscopic approach to visualization of the thoracic cavity for diagnosis of pleural disease or treatment of select thoracic conditions. The need for a thoracotomy incision is eliminated. The thoracoscope is used with video equipment, including a monitor and light source. The procedure is often completed with monitored anesthesia care and local anesthetic.

Video-assisted thoracic surgery (VATS) has many benefits, including decreased pain, shortened hospital stay, and reduced morbidity. It can also provide access to the anterior mediastinum with more complete visualization. Its use has been significantly expanded in recent years. Thoracoscopy is indicated for diagnosis of pleural disease or treatment of pleural conditions, such as cysts, blebs, and effusions.[4] Pleurodesis with instillation of talc, tetracycline, or other sclerosing treatment can be accomplished through the thoracoscope (Surgical Pharmacology).[8] VATS is also used for biopsy of mediastinal masses; to perform wedge resections, pericardectomy, and cervical sympathectomy; to obtain hemostasis; and to evacuate blood clots or divide adhesions.

***Procedural Considerations.*** Endoscopic instrumentation and equipment used for a thoracoscopy include 5- and 10-mm telescopes, light cord, camera, graspers, dissectors, scissors, ligators, and endoscopic soft tissue instruments (scissors, hemostats, suction tips, retractors). Accessory equipment for video (television monitors, videocassette recorder, printer, light source for camera and scope, slave television monitor) and insufflation is also used. The patient is positioned supine, semilaterally or laterally, depending on the anatomic structures involved.

### *Operative Procedure*

1. A 2- to 3-cm incision is made between the fifth and seventh intercostal spaces for insertion of the 10- or 12-mm trocar. The 0-degree telescope is inserted to view the site to determine the approach.
2. If the procedure can be completed by thoracoscopy, puncture sites are made for insertion of additional trocars to al-

SURGICAL PHARMACOLOGY

## Agents for Chemical Pleurodesis

Pleurodesis is undertaken as a treatment for malignant pleural effusion and for unresolved spontaneous pneumothorax. A variety of chemical agents are used to cause the layers of pleura to adhere. Adherence of the pleural layers is thought to prevent the accumulation of pleural fluid in the case of pleural effusion and to prevent subsequent pneumothoraces. Commonly used agents for chemical pleurodesis are listed. Other agents may be used according to the surgeon's preference, region, and availability. Perioperative nurses should consult with the surgeon before the procedure to determine the agent used.

| Agent | Mechanism of Action | Dosage | Side Effects | Nursing Considerations |
|---|---|---|---|---|
| Talc | Stimulates mesothelial cells to coordinate an inflammatory response | 5-10 g in 250 ml sodium chloride | Pain, infection, ARDS, pulmonary edema | May be administered as a poudrage, aerosol, or slurry. Facial talc is unsterile, contains asbestos, and requires stringent sterilization technique. Commercially available sterile talc is preferable. |
| Antineoplastics | Chemical pleural irritation and fibrosis of pleural surfaces | Bleomycin: 60 units mixed with 100-200 mg lidocaine | Pain, fever, neutropenia | Antineoplastics require special handling to reduce personal exposure. Nurses should follow hospital policies and procedures for safe medication handling procedures. |
| Cyclines | Indirectly stimulate the pleural macrophages, activating pleural mesothelial cells; low pH initiates an inflammatory reaction, causing fibrosis | Minocycline: 7 mg/kg<br>Doxycycline: 500 mg in 30-50 ml sodium chloride | Pain, fever, hemothorax, neutropenia | Determine if patient is allergic to cycline medications before procedure. |
| Silver nitrate | Coagulates cellular protein to form pleural eschar | 20 ml 0.5% silver nitrate | Pain, fever | Handle with care. Solution stains skin and clothing. |
| Quinacrine | Causes systemic inflammatory response | 500 mg in 200 ml saline | Pain, fever | Not available in the United States or Canada. |
| Iodopovidone | Mechanism of action unknown | 20 ml 10% iodopovidone in 80 ml saline | Severe pain, hypotension | Assess patient for allergies to iodine. |

Modified from Alam I and others: Chemical pleurodesis, an effective symptomatic treatment of malignant pleural effusion, *Journal of Postgraduate Medical Institute* 17(2):194-198, 2003; Chin J and others: Effects of additional minocycline pleurodesis after thoracoscopic procedures for primary spontaneous pneumothorax, *Chest* 125:50-55, 2004; Demmy TL, Nwogu C: Malignant pleural and pericardial effusion: In Selke FW, del Nido PJ, Swanson SJ, editors: *Sabiston & Spencer surgery of the chest*, ed 7, Philadelphia, 2005, Saunders; Dikensoy O, Light RW: Alternative widely available, inexpensive agents for pleurodesis, *Current Opinion in Pulmonary Medicine* 11:340-344, 2005; Kilic D and others: Management of recurrent malignant pleural effusion with chemical pleurodesis, *Surgery Today* 35:634-638, 2005; LexiComp Online. Accessed April 15, 2006, on-line: www.crlonline.com/crlsql/servlet/crlonline.

*ARDS,* Acute respiratory distress syndrome.

low instrument manipulation. The size of trocars and types of instruments vary for the diagnosis.

3. After the selected procedure, a chest tube is inserted through one of the surgical puncture sites and secured to the skin. Trocar sites are closed, and small dressings or adhesive skin tapes are applied.

## Endoscopic Thoracic Sympathectomy

Hyperhidrosis is defined as excessive sweating, usually affecting the palms, axillae, and soles of the feet. It may also affect the face, groin, or legs. Hyperhidrosis affects approximately 2.8% of the general population, with 1.4% of these individuals projected to have axillary hyperhidrosis and 0.5% to have sweating that is intolerable or interferes with daily activities.[5] Familial history of hyperhidrosis is implicated in 65% of cases.[7] Endoscopic thoracic sympathectomy (ETS) is a thoracoscopic intervention used to surgically treat hyperhidrosis. To treat palmar hyperhidrosis, the surgeon interrupts the sympathetic chain at the T2 level. Compensatory sweating, defined as increased sweating in other areas following the procedure, is the most common side effect of this procedure and may occur in 10% to 40% of patients.[7] Many patients who undergo ETS do so on an ambulatory basis or require only an overnight stay. The procedure produces dramatic and immediate results and is associated with a positive outcome for the patient (Research Highlight). ETS may also be used to surgically treat pain syndromes (e.g., complex regional pain syndrome) and Raynaud's syndrome.

## RESEARCH HIGHLIGHT

### Surgical Treatment of Hyperhidrosis

Hyperhidrosis is a socially disabling condition that is characterized by excessive sweating. The symptoms usually begin in childhood or adolescence and may be spontaneous or in response to temperature or emotional changes. Hyperhidrosis can be treated medically with oral medications, botulinum toxin, iontophoresis, and antiperspirants. Although medical interventions may lessen the symptoms of hyperhidrosis, they must be used consistently to manage the condition. For many patients, surgical intervention in the form of video-assisted upper dorsal thoracic sympathectomy offers a viable option resulting in long-term success and in many cases alleviation of the syndrome.

Researchers familiar with the surgical technique sought to determine patient satisfaction and effectiveness of the procedure in a group of 180 patients. The mean age of the patients was 29.2 years old; 33% were male and 67% female. Preoperatively 49% of the patients had palmar sweating only, 7% had axillary only, 24% had palmar and axillary, 16% had face and scalp only, and 69% had plantar hyperhidrosis. Within the study group, familial hyperhidrosis was noted in 57%.

Patient satisfaction with the procedure was assessed at 1 year after surgery. Seventy-eight percent of the patients had experienced compensatory sweating; however, overall satisfaction was 94%. Success rates were 100% in the patients experiencing palmar hyperhidrosis, 98% in axillary hyperhidrosis, 93% in face and scalp hyperhidrosis, and 82% in plantar hyperhidrosis.

Modified from Doolabh N and others: Thorascopic sympathectomy for hyperhidrosis, indications and results, *Annals of Thoracic Surgery* 77: 410-414, 2004.

***Procedural Considerations.*** The patient is positioned supine, and the anesthesia care provider inserts a double-lumen endotracheal tube. Video monitors are placed on each side of the patient to allow the surgeon an unobstructed view from either side, because the procedure is performed bilaterally.

#### *Operative Procedure*

1. The patient's lung is deflated by the anesthesia care provider as directed by the surgeon.
2. A scalpel is used to make a small (2-mm or less) incision between the patient's second and third ribs in the axillary plane.
3. A disposable thoracic port is inserted through the incision, and a small (2- or 5-mm) telescope is inserted through the port.
4. The sympathetic chain is identified at the T2 level, and an endoscopic scissor is used to open the pleura.
5. The nerve is grasped with a bipolar forceps and divided with bipolar electrocoagulation. Alternatively, clips may be applied to the nerve.
6. The port is removed, and a small thoracic catheter is inserted through the incision.
7. The incision is closed, and the lung is reexpanded. As the air is forced out of the pleural cavity, the catheter is removed and wound closure is completed.
8. The procedure is repeated for the opposite side.
9. Adhesive skin tapes are placed over the incision sites.
10. A postoperative chest x-ray film is obtained in the PACU to rule out any residual pneumothorax.

## LUNG SURGERY

### Thoracotomy

Thoracotomy involves an incision in the chest wall through a median sternotomy or a lateral or posterolateral incision for the purpose of operating on the lungs (History box). Thoracotomy may be performed for a variety of benign and malignant conditions. Lung cancer (Figure 25-11) is a common diagnosis associated with thoracotomy. Patients with lung cancer may have specific treatment based on their tumor, node, metastasis (TNM) characteristics. The TNM system defines tumor (T) as the size, location, and spread (pulmonary or extrapulmonary). The designation of nodes (N) refers to spread to a lymph node or group of lymph nodes. Metastasis (M) relates to metastatic tumor activity in distant organs (e.g., brain, liver) (Box 25-1). Staging is based on TNM findings (Figure 25-12). Intraoperative patient care is similar for various thoracotomy procedures, with consideration of the patient's history and disease process, planned procedure, and individualized patient needs. Basic thoracic instrumentation is used and may include a sternal saw and stapling devices. Prep by the anesthesia care provider with careful monitoring of the patient is a priority. Insertion of a double-lumen endotracheal tube, an arterial line for monitoring ABG samples, and a central venous line to ensure patent access for fluids are procedures performed by the anesthesia provider. An epidural catheter may be inserted for intraoperative and postoperative pain management. Patient preparation by the surgical team includes positioning, placement of devices for prevention of complications (e.g., sequential compression stockings, thermal-regulating blanket, electrosurgical dispersive pad), insertion of a urinary catheter, and ongoing evaluation and communication of the patient's status throughout the procedure.

### Pneumonectomy

Pneumonectomy is removal of an entire lung, usually to treat malignant neoplasms. Other reasons for removal include an extensive unilateral bronchiectasis involving the greater part of one lung, drainage of an extensive chronic pulmonary abscess involving portions of one or more lobes, selected benign tumors, and treatment of any extensive unilateral lesion. Other resections are often combined with pneumonectomy, such as resection of mediastinal lymph nodes, resections of portions of the chest wall or diaphragm, and removal of parietal pleura.

***Procedural Considerations.*** The basic thoracic instrumentation is used. The patient is placed in the lateral position for a posterolateral incision.

#### *Operative Procedure*

1. The skin, subcutaneous tissue, and muscle are incised by a scalpel and electrodissection. Hemostasis is attained. If a rib is to be excised, bone instruments are required.
2. The ribs and tissue are protected with moist sponges; the rib retractor is placed (Figure 25-13) and opened slowly and gently.
3. The lung is mobilized when peripheral adhesions are freed, and the pulmonary ligament is divided. Dissection to the hilum of the involved lobe is carried out.
4. The superior pulmonary vein is gently retracted, and the pulmonary artery is dissected.

## HISTORY

As early as 3000 BC, treatments related to the lungs and chest were undertaken as a result of injuries and wounds. It was not until the eighteenth century, however, that physiologic studies and animal experiments included the respiratory system. Several early reports related to trauma, noting that wound closure helped the patient breathe easier. Thus the relationship between respiration and lung function was first established. During World War I, there was increased awareness of the value of immediate closure of chest wounds.

The first thoracic procedure, recorded in 1499, was an unsuccessful excision of a herniation of the lung. From that time, the physiologic effect on the lungs and perceived difficulty entering the chest resulted in hesitancy to perform thoracic procedures. Until the 1880s, the only thoracic procedures performed were to drain empyema and lung abscess or to treat traumatic chest injury. In 1823 the first purposeful resection of a part of the lung for accidental injury was reported by Milton Antony, and in 1861 the French surgeon Péan removed part of a lung for tumor.

Treatment of tuberculosis (TB) also provided an impetus for new developments in thoracic procedures. Thoracoplasty became widely used as a means of collapsing the lungs for treatment of TB, followed by other forms of treatment. In 1907 an article was published describing surgical techniques for access to the thoracic cavity. In 1913 Jacobeus is credited with dividing adhesions with a cautery passed through one cannula while through another he passed a cystoscope-like instrument he called a *thoracoscope.* Student textbooks in the 1920s contained only a short paragraph on cancer of the lung. From that time until the first successful pneumonectomy in 1933, many attempts were made to remove carcinomas, with limited success.

In 1899 the first important article on tumors of the chest wall was written. It summarized case reports of 46 other cases and classified the various tumor types. The first accounts of pulmonary resection were published in 1896, and one of the first cases of cancer of the lung to be reported in the United States was in 1851. Equipment and instrument development also improved the ability to study lung function. Although the bronchoscope was introduced in 1937, it was not used to study chest diseases until later. Using the bronchoscope became more important to remove secretions when Papanicolaou identified the advantages of applying cytologic technique to diagnosis of cancer.

The nursing care of patients with thoracic conditions evolved over time as medical and surgical treatments advanced and technology made new treatments available. Modern-day thoracentesis is generally accomplished using a presterilized disposable kit from a manufacturer. In the 1920s, nurses who assisted with thoracentesis were responsible for acquiring a rubber sheet to protect the bed, sterile sheets to create a sterile field, sterile cotton, a hypodermic syringe and needle, sterile gloves and powder for the physician, and the aspirating set. The aspirating set consisted of a graduated 5- to 8-pint glass bottle with a rubber stopper fitted with a bifurcated metal tube and stop cocks. Rubber tubing with metal connectors was attached to the metal tube, and the sterile aspirating needle was connected to one branch of the tubing. The other branch of the tubing was connected to an exhaust pump. The nurse was responsible for testing the apparatus before the physician arrived, because the apparatus was used instead of a syringe for aspiration. Postprocedure treatment for the patient was described as "the patient must remain quietly in bed, in the recumbent position and no exertion or sudden movements should be allowed. The greatest precautions should be taken to prevent the entrance of infection."

Modified from Meade RH: *History of thoracic surgery,* Springfield, Ill, 1961, Charles C Thomas; Scott RJE: *Pocket cyclopedia of nursing,* New York, 1923, The Macmillan Co.

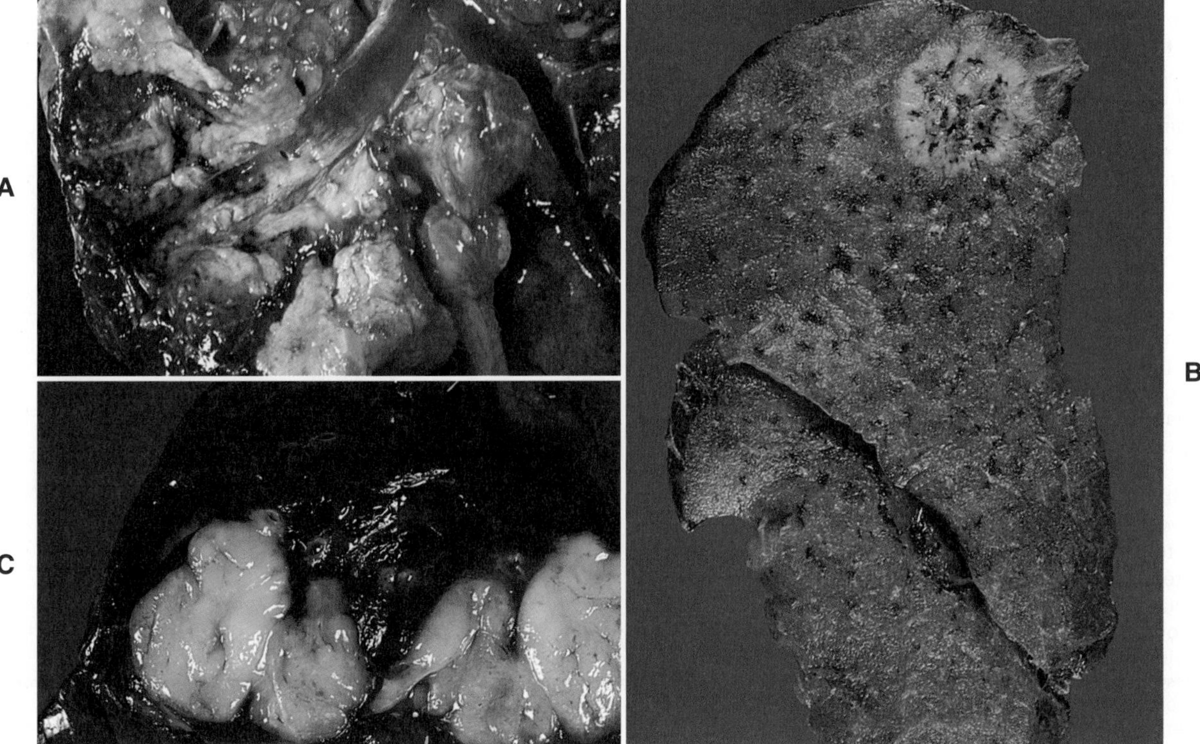


**FIGURE 25-11** Lung cancer. **A,** Squamous cell carcinoma originating from the main bronchus. **B,** Peripheral adenoma. **C,** Small cell carcinoma.

5. The branches of the pulmonary artery and vein of the involved lobe are clamped, doubly ligated, and divided with fine right-angled vascular clamps, scissors, and nonabsorbable suture.
6. The inferior pulmonary vein is exposed by incising the hilar pleura and retracting the lung anteriorly. The inferior pulmonary vein is clamped, doubly ligated, and divided.
7. The bronchus clamp is applied, and the bronchus near the tracheal bifurcation is divided. The stump is closed with atraumatic nonabsorbable mattress sutures or bronchus staples. If staples are applied, the scalpel is used to complete division of the bronchus. The lung is removed from the chest.
8. The pleural space is irrigated with normal saline to check for hemostasis and air leaks during positive-pressure inspiration.
9. A pleural flap is created and sutured over the bronchial stump (other methods of securing the bronchus might be used).
10. Hemostasis is ensured in the pleural space.
11. Chest tubes (28- to 30-Fr) are inserted into the pleural space and brought through a stab wound at the eighth or ninth interspace near the anterior axillary line (Figure 25-14). An upper tube is inserted through a second stab wound if indicated to evaluate leaking air. The tubes are secured with heavy sutures and connected to water-seal drainage after closure of the pleural space.
12. The rib approximator (Figure 25-15) is placed, and closure is begun with interrupted sutures.
13. The muscle, subcutaneous tissue, and skin are closed. Drains are anchored to the chest wall with suture.
14. The dressing is applied.
15. Chest tube connections are secured with Parnham bands or tape and labeled (anterior or posterior).

## Lobectomy

Lobectomy is excision of one or more lobes of the lung. It is performed when the primary tumor is located in a particular lobe or to remove metastatic involvement when the tumor is peripherally located and hilar nodes are not involved. Other conditions affecting the lung and treated by lobectomy might be bronchiectasis; giant emphysematous blebs or bullae; large, centrally located benign tumors; fungal infections; and congenital anomalies.

***Procedural Considerations.*** Basic thoracic instrumentation is used. The patient is placed in a lateral position for a posterolateral approach; the supine position may be used for upper-

**BOX 25-1**

### TNM Definitions and Staging for Lung Cancer

**T—PRIMARY TUMOR**

- **$T_x$** Tumor that cannot be assessed, or malignant cells in sputum or bronchial washings but not visualized by imaging or bronchoscopy.
- **$T_{is}$** Carcinoma in situ.
- **$T_0$** No evidence of primary tumor.
- **$T_1$** A tumor that is 3 cm or less in greatest dimension, surrounded by lung or visceral pleura, and with no evidence of tumor invasion proximal to a lobar bronchus as determined at bronchoscopy
- **$T_2$** A tumor that is either 1: more than 3 cm in greatest dimension or 2: invasive of the visceral pleura or associated with atelectasis or obstructive pneumonitis that extends to the hilar region. At the time of bronchoscopy the proximal extent of the tumor must be within a lobar bronchus or at least 2 cm or more distal to the carina. Any atelectasis or obstructive pneumonitis must not involve the entire lung.
- **$T_3$** A tumor of any size that invades the chest wall (including superior sulcus tumors), diaphragm, the mediastinal pleura, or the pericardium, but not involving the heart, great vessels, trachea, esophagus, or vertebral body. A tumor in the main bronchus within 2 cm of the carina without involving it or associated atelectasis or obstructive pneumonitis of entire lung is also a $T_3$ tumor.
- **$T_4$** A tumor of any size that invades the mediastinum, heart, great vessels, trachea, esophagus, vertebral body, or carina; or presence of malignant pleural or pericardial effusion; or with satellite tumor nodules within the ipsilateral, primary tumor lobe of the lung.

**N—NODAL INVOLVEMENT**

- **$N_x$** Regional lymph nodes cannot be assessed.
- **$N_0$** No metastasis to regional lymph nodes.
- **$N_1$** Metastasis to lymph nodes in the peribronchial or the ipsilateral hilar region or both, including direct extension.
- **$N_2$** Metastasis to ipsilateral mediastinal lymph nodes and subcarinal lymph nodes.
- **$N_3$** Metastasis to contralateral mediastinal lymph nodes, contralateral hilar lymph nodes, or ipsilateral or contralateral scalene or supraclavicular lymph nodes.

**M—DISTANT METASTASIS**

- **$M_x$** Distant metastasis cannot be assessed.
- **$M_0$** No (known) distant metastasis.
- **$M_1$** Distant metastasis present.

| Stage | TNM Subsets |
|---|---|
| 0 | $T_{is}$, $N_0$, $M_0$ |
| IA | $T_1$, $N_0$, $M_0$ |
| IB | $T_2$, $N_0$, $M_0$ |
| IIB | $T_2$, $N_1$, $M_0$ |
| | $T_3$, $N_0$, $M_0$ |
| IIIA | $T_3$, $N_1$, $M_0$ |
| | $T_{1\text{-}3}$, $N_2$, $M_0$ |
| IIIB | $T_4$, $N_{0\text{-}2}$, $M_0$ |
| | Any **T**, $N_3$, $M_0$ |
| IV | Any **T**, any **N**, $M_1$ |

Modified from Mountain CF and others: Lung Cancer: A handbook for staging, imaging and lymph node classification. Accessed May 18, 2006, on-line www.ctsnet..org/book/mountain/RevisedStaging_p.5.html; Selke FW and others, editors: *Sabiston & Spencer surgery of the chest*, ed 7, Philadelphia, 2005, Saunders.

BOX 25-1

**TNM Definitions and Staging for Lung Cancer—cont'd**

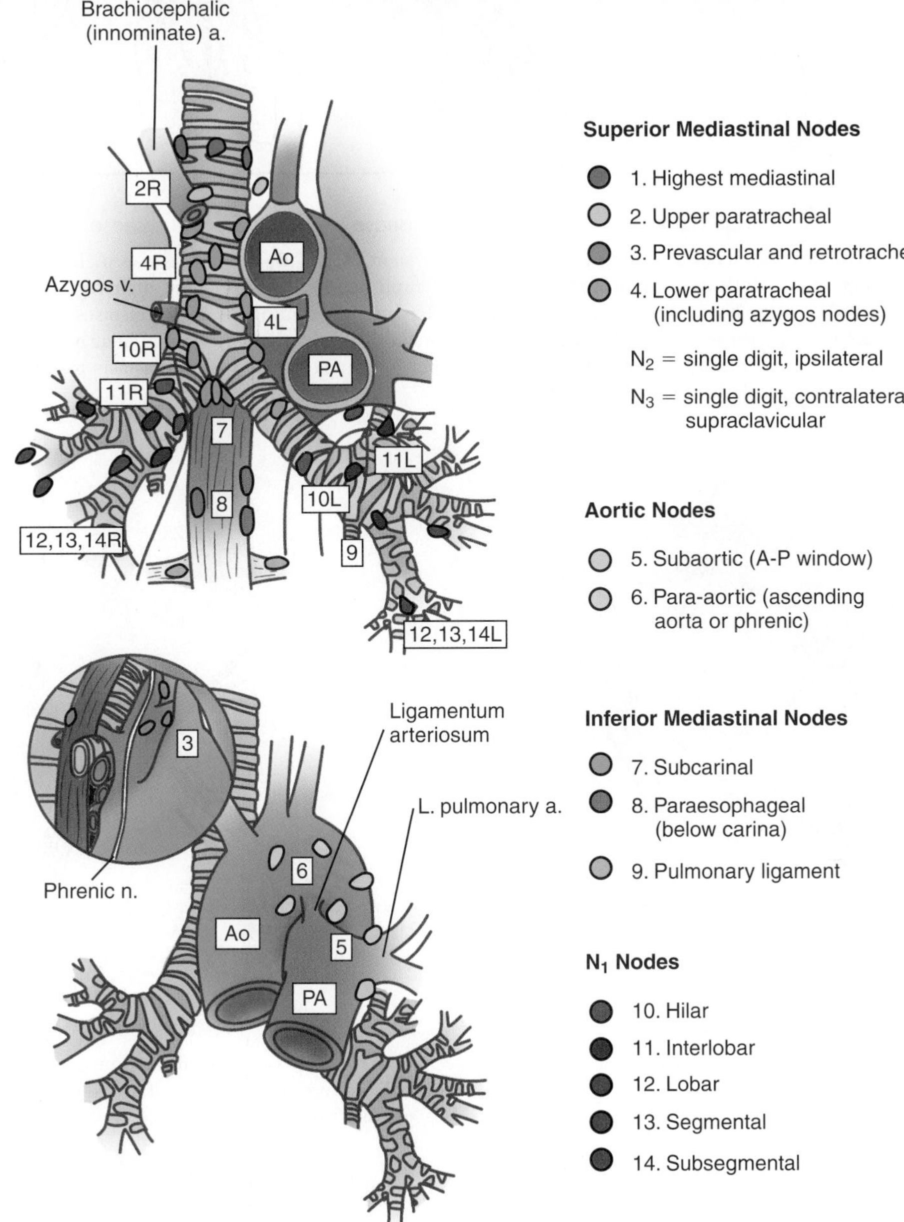


Regional lymph node stations for the staging of non–small cell lung cancer. Mediastinal nodes (i.e., $N_2$ nodes) are depicted by single digits, and intrapulmonary nodes (i.e., $N_1$ nodes) are depicted by two digits.

and middle-lobe resections. The procedure varies with the specific lobe to be removed depending on the anatomic structure. An ESU, sequential compression devices, and a forced air–warming unit to maintain normothermia are often required.

### Operative Procedure

1. The skin, subcutaneous tissue, and muscle are incised using a scalpel and electrodissection. Hemostasis is attained. If a rib is to be excised, bone instruments are required.
2. The ribs and tissue are protected with sponges. The rib retractor is placed and opened slowly and gently.
3. The pleura is entered, and peripheral adhesions are freed with scissors, blunt dissection, or a sponge on a sponge-holding forceps.
4. The hilar pleura is incised and separated.
5. The branches of the pulmonary arteries and veins are isolated, clamped, doubly ligated, and divided with fine, right-angled vascular clamps, scissors, and nonabsorbable suture.

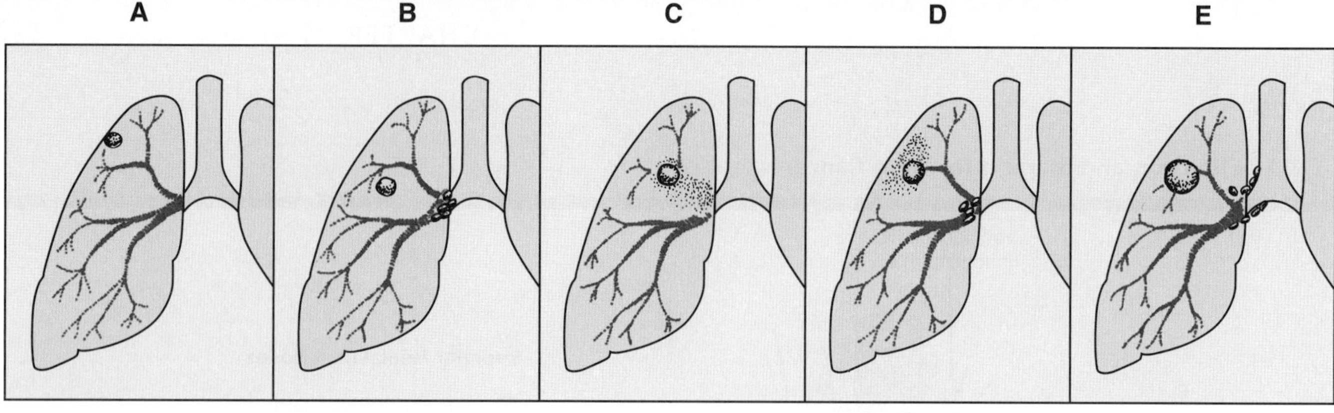


**FIGURE 25-12** Staging of lung cancer by TMN system. **A** and **B**, Stage I disease includes tumors classified as $T_1$ with or without metastasis to the lymph node in the ipsilateral hilar region. **C**, Also included in stage I are tumors classified as $T_2$ but having no nodal or distant metastases. **D**, Stage II disease includes those tumors classified as $T_2$, with metastasis only to the ipsilateral hilar lymph nodes. **E**, Stage III includes all tumors more extensive than $T_2$ or any tumor with metastasis to the lymph nodes in the mediastinum with distant metastasis.

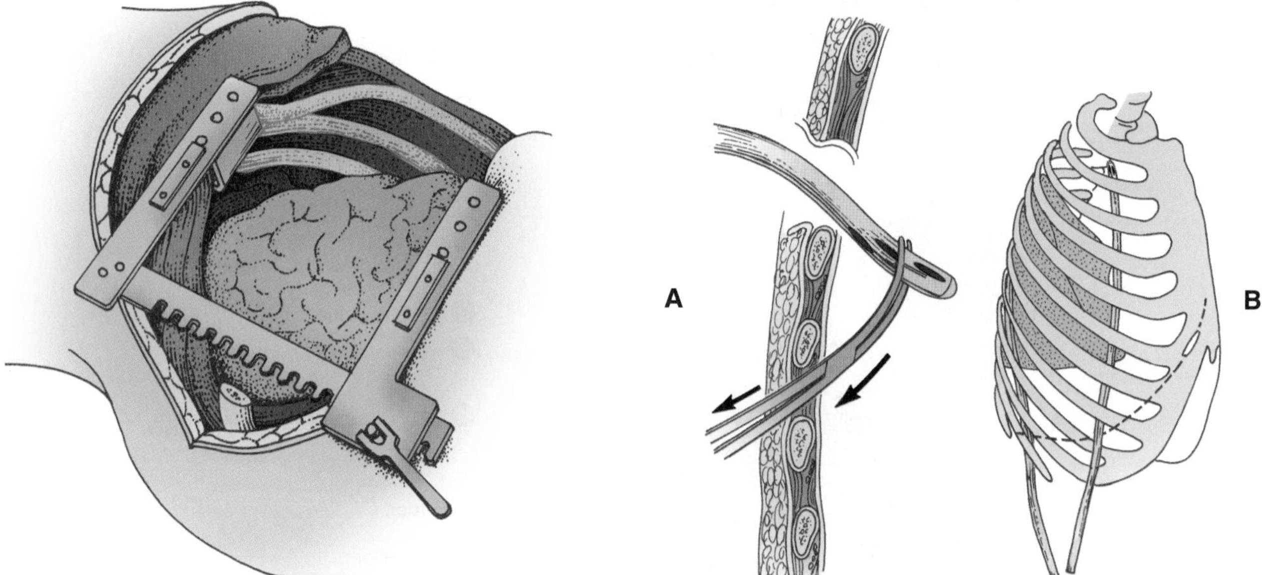


**FIGURE 25-13** Rib retractor placed for thoracotomy.

**FIGURE 25-14** **A**, Introduction of chest drainage tube through a stab wound. **B**, Placement of apical and basal drainage tubes after upper and middle lobectomy.

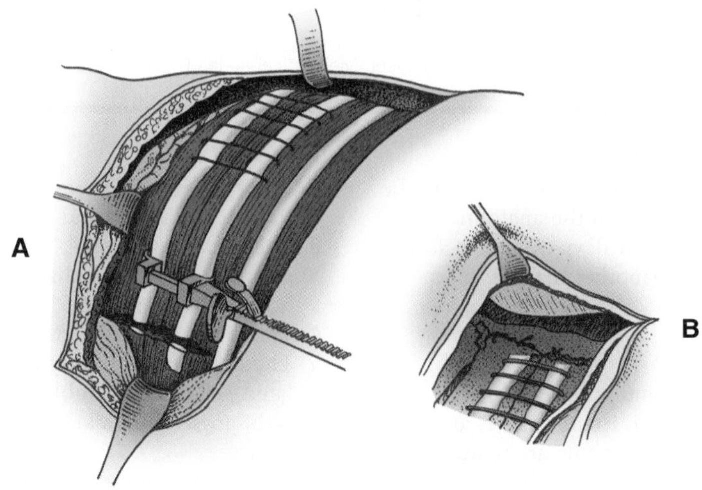


**FIGURE 25-15** **A**, Rib approximator placed for closure of incision. **B**, Heavy-gauge suture used for closure of ribs.

6. The main trunk of the pulmonary artery is identified, as is the fissure between the lobes.
7. The bronchus clamp is applied. The remaining lung is inflated to identify the line of demarcation. The bronchus is divided with a scalpel or heavy scissors.
8. Bronchial secretions are suctioned.
9. The bronchus is closed with atraumatic nonabsorbable mattress sutures or bronchus staples. If staples are applied, the scalpel is used to complete division of the bronchus.
10. Incomplete fissures are divided between hemostats with fine Metzenbaum scissors. Edges may be sutured closed.
11. A pleural flap is created and sutured over the bronchial stump (other methods of securing the bronchus might be used).
12. The pleural cavity is thoroughly irrigated with normal saline, and hemostasis is ensured. The remaining lobes are inflated to check for air leaks, and the degree of expansion of the remaining lobes is assessed.
13. The pleural space is irrigated, and the procedure is completed as for a pneumonectomy.

## Segmental Resection

Segmental resection is removal of one or more anatomic subdivisions of the pulmonary lobe. It conserves healthy, functioning pulmonary tissue by sparing remaining segments. Segmental resection is indicated for any benign lesion with segmental distribution or diseased tissue affecting only one segment of the lung with compromised cardiorespiratory reserve. The most common cause for removal is bronchiectasis. Other conditions requiring removal include chronic, localized inflammation and congenital cysts or blebs.

***Procedural Considerations.*** Basic thoracotomy instrumentation is used. The patient is placed in the lateral position.

### *Operative Procedure*

1. The skin, subcutaneous tissue, and muscle are incised with a scalpel and electrodissection.
2. The parietal pleura is incised with a scalpel and scissors. Adhesions are divided with sharp or blunt dissection.
3. The segmental artery is identified to provide accurate identification of the bronchus of the diseased segment.
4. The segmental pulmonary vein and branches are ligated.
5. The bronchus is clamped with the bronchus clamp, and the remaining lung is inflated. The intersegmental boundary is confirmed, and proper placement of the clamp is ensured.
6. The visceral pleura is incised around the diseased segment, beginning anterior to the hilum and progressing toward the periphery. Exposure is facilitated with malleable or other type of retractors. The intersegmental vessels are clamped with thoracic hemostats and ligated.
7. The segmental bronchus is transected. The stump is closed with atraumatic nonabsorbable mattress sutures or bronchus staples (Figure 25-16).

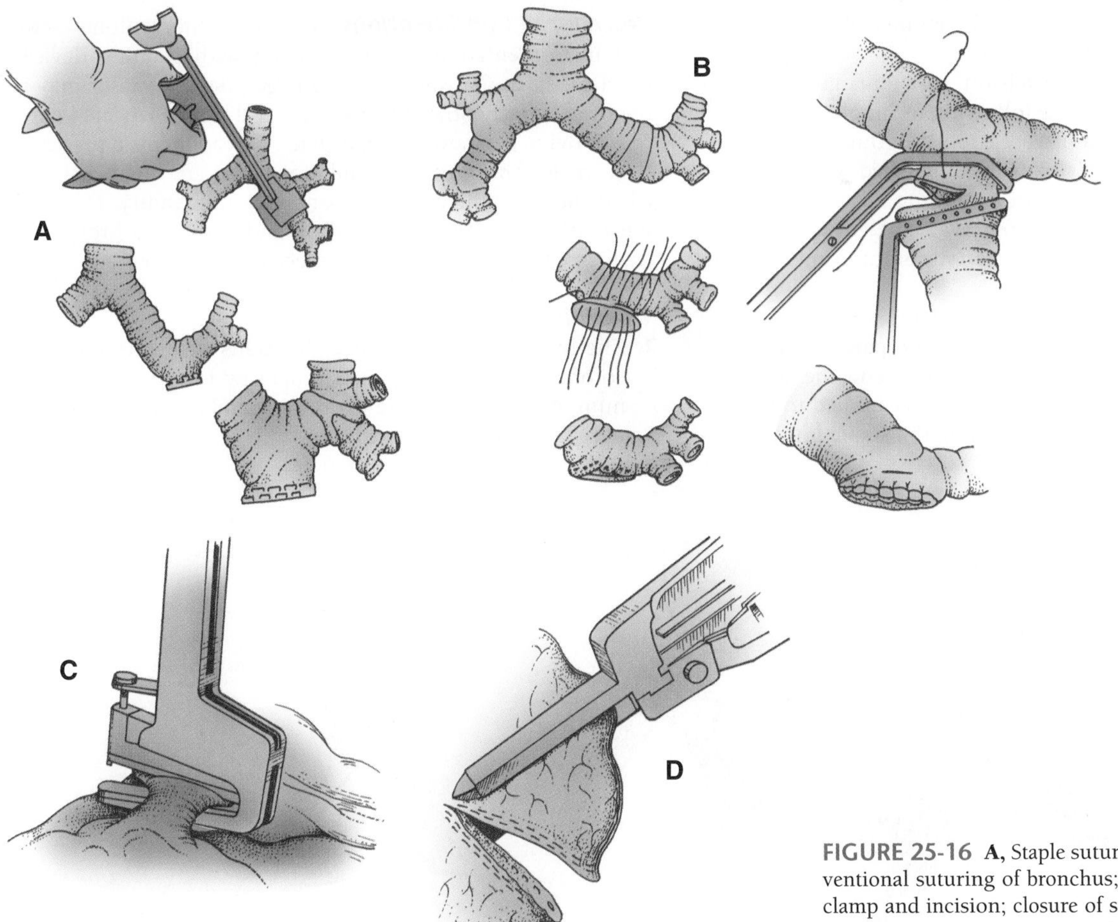


FIGURE 25-16 **A,** Staple suturing of bronchus. **B,** Conventional suturing of bronchus; application of bronchus clamp and incision; closure of stump. **C,** Staple suturing of pulmonary vessels. **D,** Staple suturing of lung tissue (wedge resection or lung biopsy).

8. Dissection is continued to separate segmental surfaces, and vessels are ligated as needed. The segment of the lung is removed.
9. A pleural flap is created and sutured over the bronchial stump (other methods of securing the bronchus may be used).
10. The lung is reinflated and irrigated with normal saline. Bleeding is controlled with ligatures or hemoclips.
11. The procedure is completed as for pneumonectomy.

## Wedge Resection

Wedge resection is removal of a wedge-shaped section of parenchyma that includes the identified lesion, without regard for intersegmental planes. The resection is also used for removal of small, peripherally located benign primary tumors; peripherally located inflammatory disease; and biopsy in chronic diffuse lung disease.

***Procedural Considerations.*** Thoracic instrumentation is used. The patient is positioned to allow access to the operative site with consideration of the area of lung to be resected. An ESU is required.

### *Operative Procedure*

1. The skin, subcutaneous tissue, and muscle are incised using a scalpel and electrodissection.
2. The rib retractor is placed.
3. Bleeding is controlled, and small bronchi are secured with clamps and ligature. Large bronchi are ligated or sutured to prevent persistent air leak.
4. The wedge is outlined for excision, with a margin of normal tissue left, using one of the following techniques:
   a. Long hemostatic clamps are applied in three rows to outline the wedge. Excision is accomplished with a scalpel. The tissue is sutured with a running absorbable suture behind the clamps before removal. The edges of the tissue are oversewn with a continuous or interrupted suture (Figure 25-17).
   b. The lobe is grasped with a lung clamp, and the thoracic stapling instrument is applied to the parenchymal portion of the lung. Staples are applied, and the wedge is excised with the scalpel. Staples are reapplied to the opposite side of the lesion adjoining the staple lines.
5. The specimen is removed. Air leaks are checked by irrigation and inspection. Bleeding is controlled with ligation or hemoclips. The procedure is completed as for pneumonectomy.

## Lung Volume Reduction Surgery

Lung volume reduction surgery (LVRS) is an alternative surgical treatment for patients with chronic pulmonary emphysema (Figure 25-18). The surgery is intended to increase expiratory airflow, maximum exercise capacity, and respiratory muscle strength, thereby relieving dyspnea. The procedure may also be referred to as *lung volume reduction,* or *pneumoplasty.* Candidates for the procedure are those who have progressive, severe dyspnea secondary to pulmonary dysfunction; those whose medical management is ineffective; and those in whom disease distribution is limited to target areas of severity (Best Practice). The two operative approaches for LVRS are median sternotomy and video-assisted thoracic surgery (VATS). Median sternotomy provides excellent bilateral exposure and flexibility, whereas the VATS approach has the advantage of a shorter hospitalization, fewer days of postoperative air leaks, and fewer days on the ventilator.[14] It is standard practice for patients undergoing LVRS to participate in vigorous pulmonary rehabilitation in preparation for surgery. Preoperative pulmonary rehabilitation improves airway clearance and diaphragmatic function, improves tolerance for surgery, and decreases postoperative complications.[15]

***Procedural Considerations.*** The basic thoracotomy setup and instrumentation are used, along with stapling devices, chest tubes, and a water-seal drainage system. A laser may be required, as may other materials for sealing the resected edges (e.g., bovine pericardium, collagen). Positioning is a particular concern for this patient population, who are often malnourished and are at increased risk for positioning injury. The nurse must collaborate with the surgeon and anesthesia provider to ensure optimal positioning practices are implemented.

### *Operative Procedure*

1. The lungs are exposed through a transverse anterior thoracotomy incision using the sternal saw to separate the sternum. Adhesiotomies are performed, and the inferior pulmonary ligaments are incised.

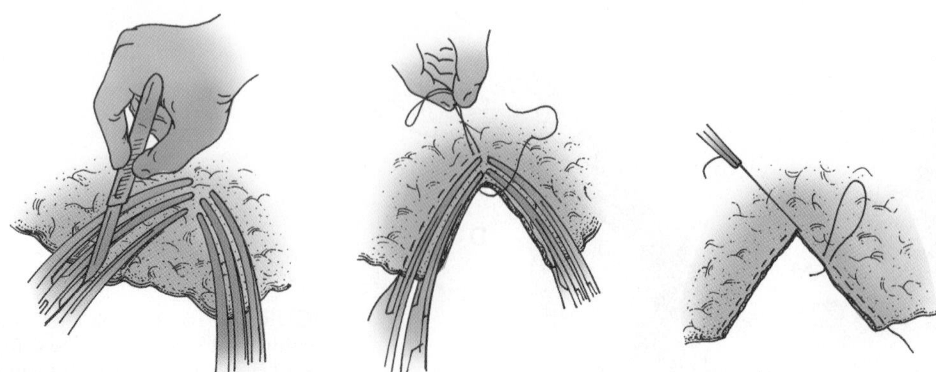

**FIGURE 25-17** Wedge resection. Clamps applied to edge of lung tissue to be excised with scalpel and sutured with a running suture and oversewn.

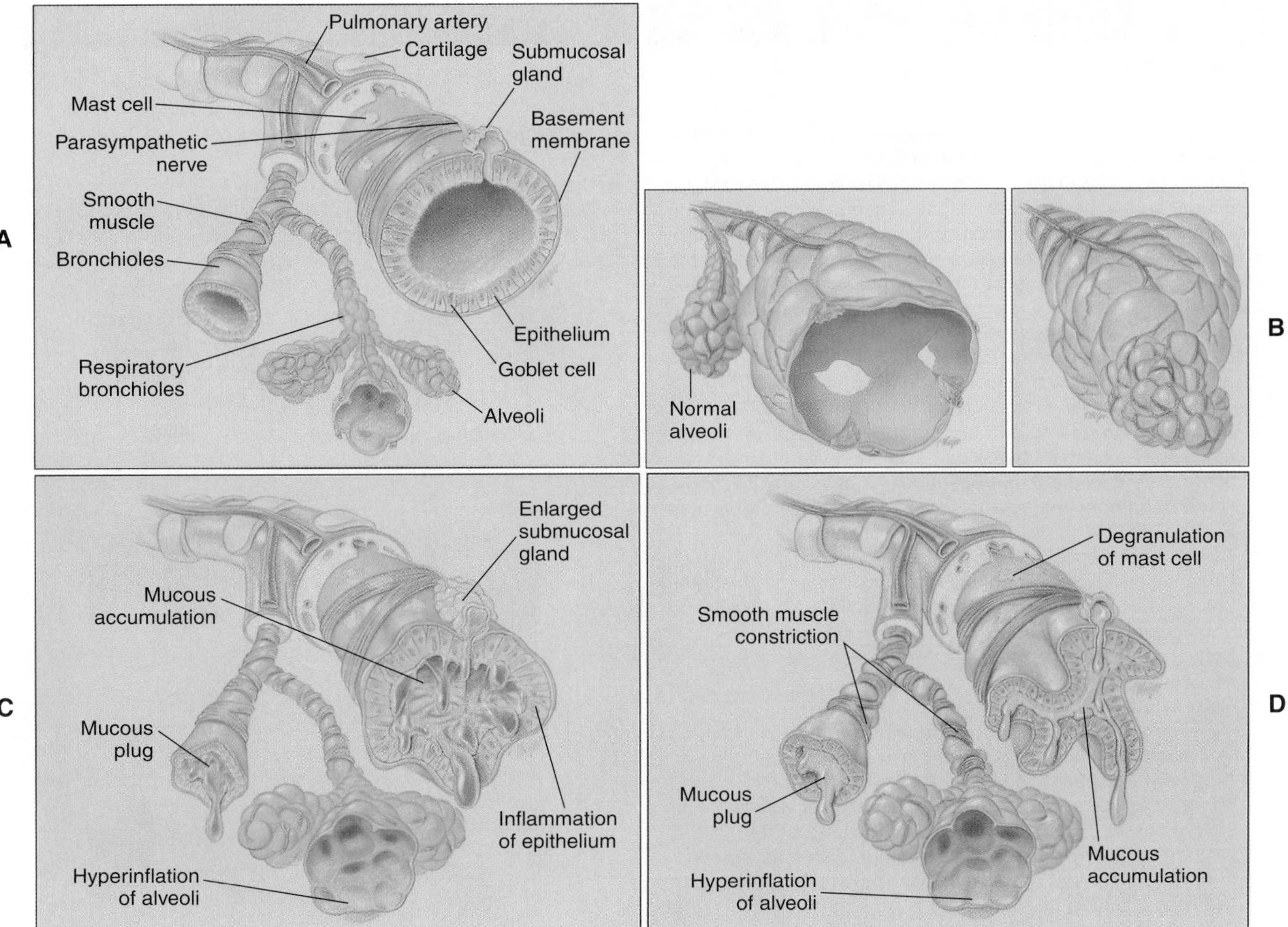


**FIGURE 25-18** Airway obstruction caused by emphysema, chronic bronchitis, and asthma. **A,** The normal lung. **B**, Emphysema enlargement and destruction of alveolar walls with loss of elasticity and trapping of air; *(left)* panlobular emphysema showing abnormal weakening and enlargement of all air spaces distal to the terminal bronchioles (normal alveoli shown for comparison only); *(right)* centrilobular emphysema showing abnormal weakening and enlargement of the respiratory bronchioles in the proximal portion of the acinus. **C,** Chronic bronchitis: inflammation and thickening of mucous membrane with accumulation of mucus and pus leading to obstruction; characterized by cough. **D,** Bronchial asthma: thick mucus, mucosal edema, and smooth muscle spasm causing obstruction of small airways; breathing becomes labored, and expiration is difficult.

2. The lungs are deflated to visualize the portions of the lung where air is trapped in emphysematous lung tissue.
3. A lung-grasping forceps is used to hold the portion of the lung to be excised. A surgical stapling device is lined with bovine pericardium and positioned on either side of the lung. The stapling of emphysematous lung tissue continues, and staple lines are overlapped to prevent air leaks. Other methods of sealing the line of tissue resection include use of a laser (Nd:YAG) or application of alternative buttressing materials, such as collagen.[14]
4. The lung is reinflated to identify air leaks. If air leaks are found, the lung is deflated and the stapling procedure continues.
5. One or two chest tubes are placed into each pleural space. The chest tubes are connected to water-seal drainage systems without suction.
6. The ribs and sternum are reapproximated using stainless steel surgical wire. The muscle layer, subcutaneous tissue, and skin are closed, and dressings are applied.

## Lung Biopsy

Lung biopsy is the resection of a small portion of the lung for diagnosis. The biopsy allows removal of relatively large specimens for microscopic examination of the lung tissue. Indications include (1) failure of closed methods (needle biopsy) for diagnosis and (2) the presence of small, localized lesions that can be removed by biopsy.

***Procedural Considerations.*** In addition to the basic instrument setup, a rib retractor, a lung-grasping forceps, dissecting scissors, a chest tube and water-seal system, and an endostapling device are required. More than one specimen container

## BEST PRACTICE

### Determining Candidates for Lung Volume Reduction Surgery

Although lung volume reduction surgery (LVRS) is considered an effective procedure to treat patients with emphysema, successful outcomes depend on factors such as appropriate patient selection, surgical technique, and experience with performing the procedure. After the reintroduction of LVRS to the medical community in 1995, there was a resurgence of interest in the technique. However, surgical interventions were accompanied by significant morbidity and mortality. As a result, the Health Care Financing Administration (HCFA) organized a clinical trial (the National Emphysema Treatment Trial [NETT]) to identify factors that contribute to successful outcomes. The NETT suggests the following criteria as patient eligibility for LVRS:

- High-resolution computed tomography evidence of moderate to severe bilateral heterogeneous emphysema or moderate to severe bilateral homogeneous emphysema; if emphysema is homogeneous, additional physiologic criteria may be required
- Target zones of poorly perfused lung
- Nonsmoker (tobacco products) for a minimum of 4 months before interview for screening, with willingness to sustain nonsmoking status
- Body mass index below 31.1 kg/m$^2$ (men) or below 32.3 kg/m$^2$ (women)
- No previous laser surgery or LVRS
- No giant bulla (one third or more of the volume of the lung in which the bulla is located)
- No previous coronary artery bypass surgery
- Oxygen requirement of 6 L/min or less to keep saturation at 90% or higher during an oxygen titration assessment
- No cardiac dysrhythmia that, in the judgment of the supervising physician, might pose a risk to the patient during exercise testing or training
- Postbronchodilator total lung capacity (TLC) at 110% or more of predicted
- Postbronchodilator residual volume (RV) at 220% or more of predicted
- Postbronchodilator forced expiratory volume in 1 second ($FEV_1$) at 45% or less of predicted and, if age 70 years or older, postbronchodilator $FEV_1$ at 15% or more of predicted
- $FEV_1$ postbronchodilator increase of 30% or less, or 300 ml or less
- $DL_{CO}$ (lung diffusing capacity for carbon monoxide) at 70% or less of predicted
- Consent for screening and patient registry
- Consent for pulmonary rehabilitation

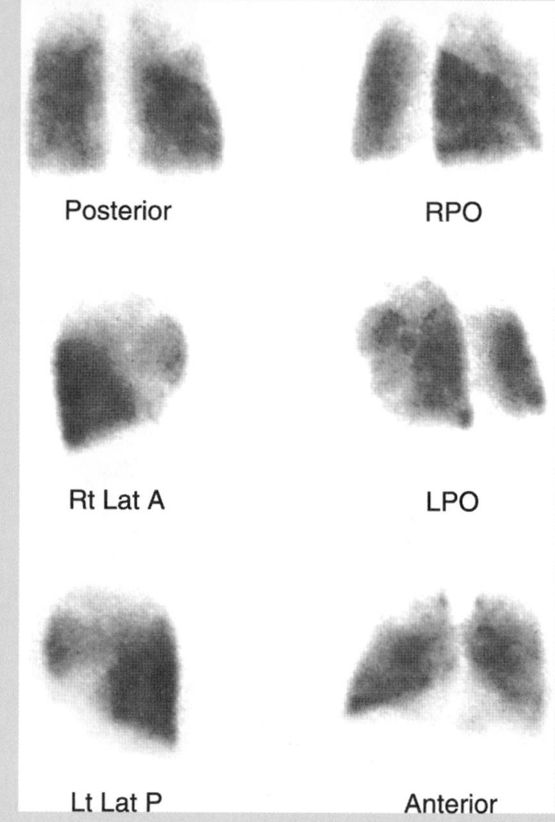


Pulmonary perfusion scintigraphy demonstrating typical upper lobe predominant emphysema that is viewed as the most suitable morphology for lung reduction surgery. (From Selke FW and others, editors: *Sabiston & Spencer surgery of the chest,* ed 7, Philadelphia, 2005, Saunders.)

Modified from Benditt JO: Surgical options for patients with COPD: sorting out the choices, *Respiratory* Care 51(2):173-182, 2006; Meyers BF, Cooper JD: Surgery for emphysema. In Selke FW and others, editors: *Sabiston & Spencer surgery of the chest,* ed 7, Philadelphia, 2005, Saunders.

may be needed. The patient is positioned in a semilateral position for an anterolateral incision.

### *Operative Procedure*

1. A short incision (approximately 5 cm) is made at the fifth intercostal space. The pleura is incised; the ribs are retracted.
2. The lung is secured and pulled out the opening with the Duval lung clamp.
3. Samples from one or more segments of the lung are taken for biopsy with application of a Satinsky clamp or application of staples with a stapling device. The tissue to be removed is excised with a scalpel. After application of the clamp, tissue edges are approximated with absorbable suture.
4. Bleeding is controlled by the application of a moist sponge at the incision site. The area is irrigated and inspected for air leaks.
5. The chest tube (28- to 30-Fr) is inserted and connected to suction.
6. The incision is closed, the chest tube is anchored to the chest wall, and a dressing is applied.

## Decortication

Decortication of the lung is removal of any fibrinous deposit, cancer, or restrictive membrane on the visceral and parietal pleura that interferes with pulmonary ventilatory function. It may also be done in conjunction with a pleurectomy for patients with pleural-based tumors, such as mesothelioma. The procedure results in blood loss and trauma and should be used only if the underlying lung is healthy. The objective is to return the lung to near-normal function.

***Procedural Considerations.*** The basic thoracic instrumentation is used. The patient is placed in a lateral position for a posterolateral incision.

### *Operative Procedure*

1. The skin, subcutaneous tissue, and muscle are incised with a scalpel and electrodissection.
2. A rib, usually the fifth or sixth, is stripped (Figure 25-19) and resected.
3. The ribs and tissue are protected with moist sponges. The rib retractor is placed and slowly and gently opened.
4. Parietal adhesions are divided to the margins of the lung, mediastinal surface, and pericardium with thoracic scissors, forceps, and a moist sponge on sponge-holding forceps.
5. The fibrous membrane is incised and separated from the visceral pleura using blunt and sharp dissection and handling the tissues gently (Figure 25-20). The procedure is completed as for pneumonectomy.

## Drainage of Empyema

The accumulation of pus in the pleural space might be associated with acute or chronic infection. Acute empyema may result from a lung abscess, pneumonia, or infection after thoracotomy. Parapneumonic effusions occur in 20% to 60% of patients hospitalized for bacterial pneumonia; 5% to 10% of these parapneumonic effusions progress to empyema. The mortality of empyema in the elderly and debilitated is 25% to 75%.[9] Empyema (other than a pure tuberculous type) must be drained to prevent fibrothorax, and patients with empyema may require further treatment with decortication. The procedure can be performed with the patient under local anesthesia when the infection is not extensive. Prolonged intrapleural infection results in chronic empyema, which can create additional complications such as mediastinal shift, difficulty in swallowing, respiratory limitations, erosion into the bronchus, and deformity of the chest. Talc poudrage may be the treatment of choice for patients able to tolerate additional procedures and who experience relief of pleural effusion by thoracentesis. Postoperative empyema or empyema occurring in immunosuppressed patients is effectively treated with a rib resection and drainage.

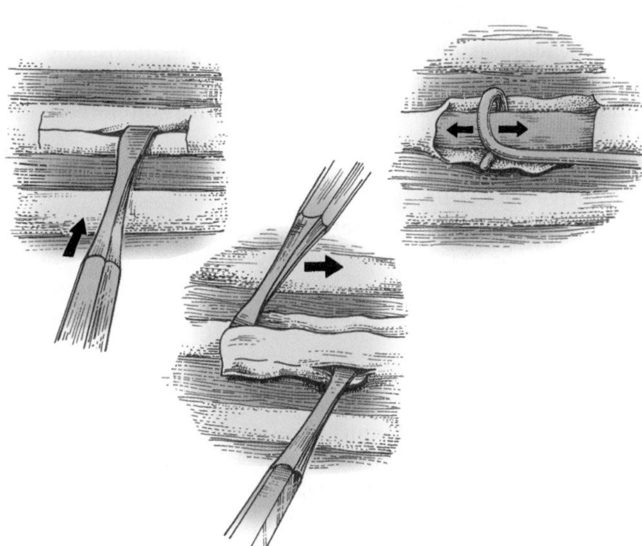

**FIGURE 25-19** Separation of muscles of rib with a periosteal elevator and rib stripper.

***Procedural Considerations.*** If the patient is under general anesthesia, the basic thoracic instrumentation is used. The patient is placed in a lateral position for an anterolateral incision. A catheter for instillation of the sclerosing agent is required. The chest cavity is irrigated profusely during and on completion of the procedure.

### *Operative Procedure*

1. The skin and tissues are incised with a scalpel to expose the affected area of the lung. Suction is used to prevent spillage of drainage from the chest.
2. The adjacent rib is resected, and the intercostal neurovascular bundle is divided.
3. The underlying thickened pleura is incised, and gross pus is evacuated. An inflammatory response might be created by stripping the parietal pleura from the visceral pleura by sharp or blunt dissection.
4. A large-bore catheter (46-Fr) is inserted, and the sclerosing agent is instilled when indicated.
5. The incision site is closed as for other thoracotomy procedures.
6. A dressing is applied.

## Open Thoracostomy (Partial Rib Resection)

Partial rib resection is removal of a portion of selected rib or ribs through an open thoracostomy incision to allow healing and reinflation of an infected lung. The procedure is performed

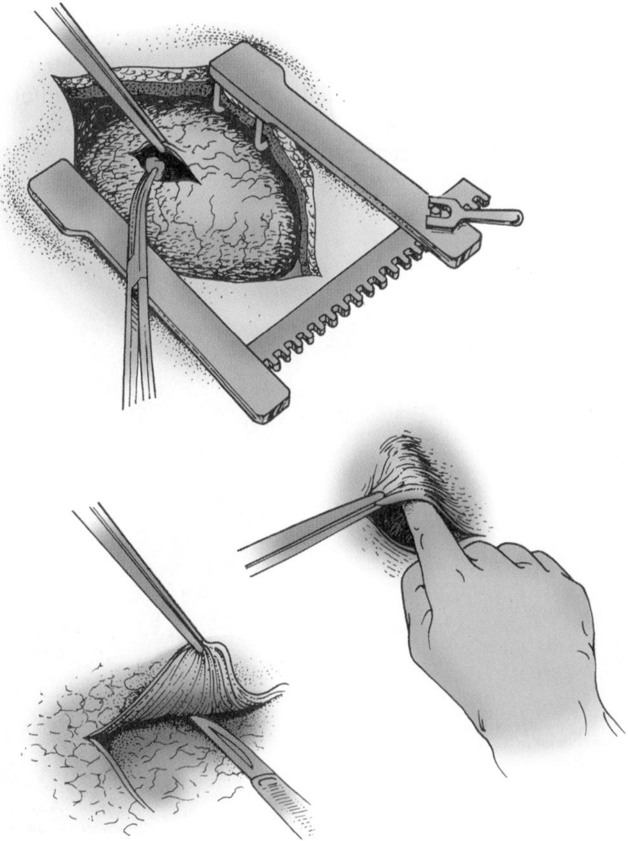

**FIGURE 25-20** Decortication. Methods of separating fibrous membrane from visceral pleura.

for treatment of chronic empyemic lesions to establish a mechanism for continuous drainage.

***Procedural Considerations.*** The basic thoracic instrument set and bone-cutting instruments are used. An ESU, chest tube, and water-seal drainage system are required, as are culture tubes for aerobic and anaerobic laboratory analysis. The patient is placed in a lateral position for a posterolateral incision. The surgical procedure can be completed with the patient under local anesthesia.

### *Operative Procedure*

1. The skin, subcutaneous tissue, and muscle are incised with a scalpel and electrodissection.
2. The rib is resected, and the pleura is incised. Suction is used to control anticipated drainage.
3. Aerobic and anaerobic swabs for culture and sensitivity are obtained. The chest cavity is irrigated.
4. A large chest tube is inserted through the pleural opening. The incision is closed or packed open (depending on the extent of the disease process).
5. The chest tube is secured with a suture of heavy-gauge material on a cutting needle.
6. The chest tube is connected to a water-seal drainage system, and connections are secured.
7. A dressing is applied. A number of layers of dressing may be necessary to absorb drainage.

## Closed Thoracostomy (Intercostal Drainage)

Closed thoracostomy is insertion of a chest catheter through an intercostal space for establishment of closed drainage. The procedure provides continuous aspiration of air, blood, or infectious fluid from the pleural cavity. It is indicated for treatment of spontaneous pneumothorax, traumatic hemothorax, pleural effusion, and acute empyema. Malignant pleural effusions (Figure 25-21) may be managed by drainage and chemical pleurodesis (Research Highlight) by way of the thoracostomy tube.

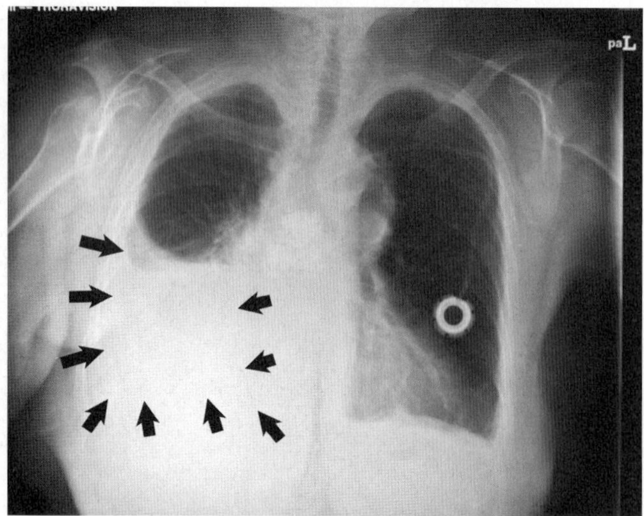


**FIGURE 25-21** Chest x-ray showing large right pleural effusion outlined by arrows.

## RESEARCH HIGHLIGHT

### Treating Malignant Pleural Effusions

Pleural effusion is a common complication of metastatic cancer and occurs in approximately 50% of patients. The condition is characterized by chest pain, tachypnea, dyspnea, coughing, and hiccoughs and can have a significant impact on the patient's quality of life. Effective management of malignant pleural effusion often challenges practitioners.

The treatment for pleural effusion is based on the patient's condition, tumor type, and prior antineoplastic therapy. In patients with smaller effusions, no treatment or percutaneous drainage may be indicated. Patients with larger effusions may be candidates for palliative therapy with pleurodesis.

This review sought to determine the optimal technique for pleurodesis in the treatment of malignant pulmonary effusion and ascertain the most effective sclerosant to be used. Reviewers analyzed the results of 36 randomized clinical trials with 1499 subjects undergoing either tube thoracostomy or thoracoscopic pleurodesis using a variety of sclerosants, such as talc, mitoxantrone, tetracycline, mustine, or bleomycin.

The meta-analysis determined that chemical sclerosants are necessary for successful pleurodesis and supported the use of talc as the sclerosant of choice. Pleural effusions treated with talc had a relative risk of nonrecurrence of 1.34 compared with other agents based on 10 studies with 186 subjects.

Thoracoscopic pleurodesis was found to be more effective than tube thoracostomy with a relative risk of nonrecurrence of effusion at 1.68 based on five studies with a total of 145 participants.

Modified from Shaw P, Agarwal R: Pleurodesis for malignant pleural effusions, *Cochrane Database System Review* (1):CD002916, 2004.

***Procedural Considerations.*** The thoracostomy may not take place in an OR setting. The procedure is usually done with monitored anesthesia care and local anesthesia. A local anesthesia set, including syringes, needles, and an anesthetic agent of choice for local injection, will be needed. The minor instrument set is used, in addition to disposable chest catheters, water-seal drainage system, two aspirating needles, and culture tubes. The patient is placed in a lateral or sitting position. Despite the administration of local anesthetic, thoracostomy can be uncomfortable for the patient. The perioperative nurse should provide explanations and emotional support to the patient during the procedure.

### *Operative Procedure*

1. The correct depth of insertion is gauged; the catheter is marked. The operative site is anesthetized.
2. An aspirating needle attached to a syringe is introduced into the chest cavity to verify the presence of purulent drainage, air, or blood.
3. The skin is incised, and a clamp is introduced through the incision into the intercostal space and pleural cavity.
4. A catheter that fits the incision site without space around the circumference is inserted. The catheter is clamped to prevent egress of air as it is inserted into the cavity.
5. The incision site is sutured, and the catheter is secured.
6. The catheter is attached to water-seal drainage, and the tubing is secured. The clamp is removed, and a dressing is applied.

## Decompression for Thoracic Outlet Syndrome

Thoracic outlet syndrome is a compression of the subclavian vessels and brachial plexus at the superior aperture of the thorax (Figure 25-22). The first rib is the usual cause of the compression, because of either a congenital deformity or a traumatic injury that results in anatomic changes. Fibromuscular bands may also form between the cervical rib and other structures (i.e., scalenus tubercle) and cause compression. Symptoms depend on whether nerves, blood vessels, or both are compressed at the thoracic outlet. Decompression is accomplished through partial or entire removal of the rib using an open technique or video-assisted endoscopic techniques (Research Highlight).

***Procedural Considerations.*** Soft tissue and bone instrumentation is used. An ESU is required. The patient is positioned in a lateral decubitus position.

### *Operative Procedure (Open Technique)*

1. The skin and subcutaneous tissue are incised with the scalpel and electrodissection. Soft tissue dissection continues, to identify the neurovascular bundle.
2. The first rib is meticulously dissected subperiosteally using the periosteal elevator. The rib elevator, stripper, and rib raspatories may be required. Undue traction in the brachial plexus and damage to the subclavian artery or vein are avoided during the dissection.
3. A wedge is taken from the midportion, or the rib is removed in its entirety using rib shears.
4. A drain is placed, and the incision is closed. A dressing is applied.

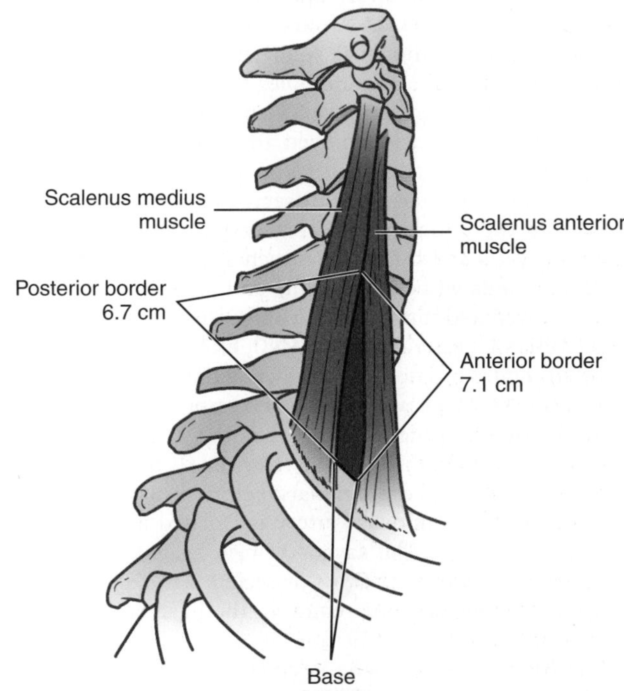


**FIGURE 25-22** The scalene (anterior) triangle showing its measurements and the narrow space through which the neurovascular bundle passes.

## Excision of Mediastinal Lesion

Excision of a mediastinal lesion involves removal of a lesion from the anterior, middle, and posterior sections. Identifying the compartment is important for planning a surgical approach to the resection, for optimal exposure and access. A mediastinoscopy should be performed to determine the diagnosis of an anterior mediastinal lesion. Indications for excision of a mediastinal lesion include miscellaneous cysts and tumors, thymoma, lymphoma, and neurogenic tumor.

***Procedural Considerations.*** The thoracic instrumentation is used. A procedure on the superior mediastinum might require use of thyroid instruments (see Chapter 16). The ESU and bone wax are needed. The patient is placed in a supine position for a median sternotomy incision (lateral position alternatively may be used).

## RESEARCH HIGHLIGHT

### Computer-Assisted Surgery for Thoracic Outlet Syndrome

One of the complications associated with open transaxillary first rib resection for thoracic outlet syndrome is temporary or permanent brachial plexus dysfunction. Video-assisted thoracoscopic surgery (VATS) has been an option for treating thoracic outlet syndrome since the 1990s and offers close range visual control over vital structures and requires less traction on the arm to enlarge the surgical field. An additional benefit of the VATS technique is the improved visualization of cervical bands. Cervical bands are classified according to clinical presentation and their anatomic insertion points.

The authors of this study sought to determine if using computer-assisted enhanced instrumentation would improve visualization over traditional VATS technique and therefore impact patient safety during transaxillary first rib resection. Over a 7-year period, 105 patients who had failed conservative treatment underwent surgery for thoracic outlet syndrome. The Aesop/Hermes voice-integrated instrumentation system was used for 89 endoscopic transaxillary first rib resections, and the da Vinci three-dimensional optical imaging surgical system was used for 42 procedures.

Analysis of the data demonstrated that 100% of the patients with a combination of neurogenic and arterial thoracic outlet syndrome requiring rib resection had cervical bands. Visualization and manipulation of the bands were enhanced in those patients who had their procedures with the da Vinci system. None of the patients in the study died or experienced any permanent neurovascular injury. The researchers acknowledge the learning curve associated with using the da Vinci technology currently evidenced by longer procedure times (i.e., mean surgical time for procedures with the Aesop/Hermes was less than 120 minutes whereas mean surgical time for the da Vinci technology was less than 180 minutes), but they note that the da Vinci system allowed better identification of cervical bands. Better identification of the cervical bands made more thorough excision and dissection possible, resulting in improved outcomes for the patients.

Modified from Martinez BD and others: Computer-assisted instrumentation during endoscopic transaxillary first rib resection for thoracic outlet syndrome: a safe alternate approach, *Vascular* 13(6):327-335, 2005.

*Operative Procedure (Thymectomy)*

1. The skin and subcutaneous tissue are incised with the scalpel and electrodissection.
2. The sternum is transected with a power saw or sternal knife. Bleeding is controlled at the bone edges with bone wax.
3. The thymus gland is dissected; vessels are clamped, ligated, and divided. The gland is removed.
4. The incision is closed. The sternum is reapproximated and closed with heavy wire (Figure 25-23). The skin is sutured closed. A dressing is applied.

## Lung Transplantation

Since the mid-1980s there has been growing experience with both single-lung transplantation (SLT) and double-lung transplantation (DLT). Since 1988 more than 13,000 lung transplants have been performed.[10] Indications for SLT include restrictive lung disease, emphysema, pulmonary hypertension, and other nonseptic end-stage pulmonary diseases. Bilateral lung transplantation is indicated for patients with cystic fibrosis or patients with a chronic infection in end-stage pulmonary failure. The procedure involves the allografting of one or both lungs from a cadaver or donor who has met clinical criteria for brain death. Developments in SLT include donor contribution from living relatives for patients who have chronic disease and a high risk for death while waiting on the donor transplantation list. Contraindications for a transplantation include multisystem disease other than the lung, history of carcinoma or sarcoma, current infection, significant renal or hepatic dysfunction, cigarette smoking within 3 or 4 months, drug or alcohol abuse, psychologic instability, or poor medication compliance. Although the surgical technique is increasingly successful, it is anticipated that future application of lung transplantation techniques may be limited by donor supply. As the field of lung transplantation continues to evolve, questions will need to be answered regarding quality of life after transplantation and whether the single or double procedure is ultimately best for patients with chronic obstructive lung disease and primary pulmonary hypertension. Issues include the shortage of suitable donors, improved methods for early detection of chronic rejection, and improved immunosuppressive agents and regimens.

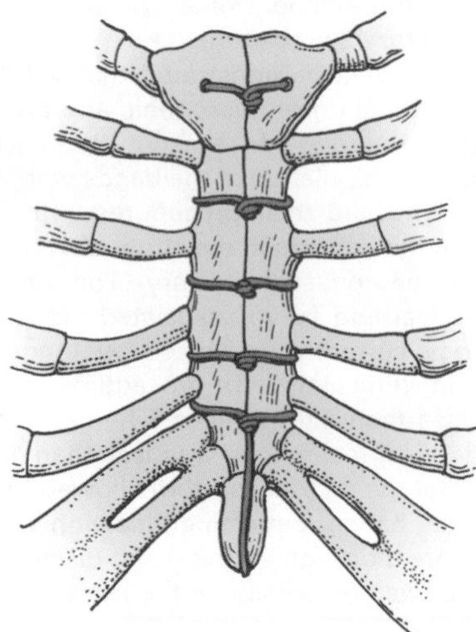

**FIGURE 25-23** Closure of median sternotomy with heavy-gauge wire.

***Procedural Considerations.*** Selection of the donor, recipients, lung preservation, and administration of anesthetic agents are considerations in this procedure. The nursing plan of care is modified considerably for each patient, since nursing personnel are caring for two patients with different needs. Recipient patients will have been started preoperatively on immunosuppressive therapy and infection prophylaxis. The patient's positioning will vary for the techniques being employed. The instrumentation is like that used for a thoracotomy. Cardiopulmonary bypass (CPB) may be required, as described in Chapter 27, along with the ESU, cold perfusion solution, and surgical stapling devices. The perioperative nurse will need to collaborate with the anesthesia provider, since continuous hemodynamic monitoring, oximetry, and ventricular function assessment by transesophageal echocardiography (TEE) are all performed intraoperatively.

*Operative Procedures (Single-Lung Transplantation)*

DONOR HARVESTING

1. The patient's skin is prepped from chin to knees and laterally to the midaxillary line. A median sternotomy incision or thoracotomy incision may be used.
2. The pleura is opened longitudinally posterior to the sternum, and the pericardium is divided back to the hilum on both sides. The inferior pulmonary ligament is taken down, pleural adhesions are incised, and the proximal pulmonary arteries are dissected at their origin.
3. After heparinization and hypotensive anesthesia, the superior vena cava is ligated and divided and heavy silk ties are placed around each vessel.
4. The aortic arch is dissected free, and the ligamentum arteriosum is divided. The anterior and inferior margins of the pulmonary artery are separated from the main artery and ascending aorta. Umbilical tapes are placed around the pulmonary artery and aorta. A purse-string suture is placed for infusion of the cardioplegia solution in the heart.
5. Once cardioplegia and pulmoplegia are accomplished, the heart is prepared for removal; veins and arteries are separated, and the heart is removed and placed in cold Collins solution.
6. The pulmonary arteries are dissected free from the mediastinum to the hilum anteriorly and then posteriorly to the anterior aorta and hilum. The trachea is dissected free. The lungs are inflated before stapling and dissection. The lungs are removed and immersed in cold Collins solution.

RECIPIENT PREPARATION AND TRANSPLANTATION

1. The patient is positioned laterally, and the skin is prepped for exposure of the chest and abdomen (nipple line to knees).
2. An incision is made for a thoracotomy. The procedure depends on which lung is to be removed. If the right lung is being removed, the pulmonary vein is isolated extrapericardially; the pulmonary artery is isolated as close to the lung as possible. The azygos vein is ligated and divided, and the pulmonary artery is dissected.
3. If the left lung is being removed, the ligamentum arteriosum is divided.
4. The lung to be removed is collapsed, and the proximal pulmonary artery is occluded. If instability occurs after occlusion, partial femoral arteriovenous bypass is initiated. If the patient remains stable, the pneumonectomy is performed.

5. Pulmonary veins are divided extrapericardially. The first branch of the pulmonary artery and descending branch are separated. One preserves the blood supply to the bronchus by not dissecting tissue around the bronchus.
6. The bronchus is divided, and the lung is removed. The pericardium is opened around the pulmonary veins to allow room for the atrial clamp.
7. Inferior and superior pulmonary veins are incised and joined.
8. Three anastomoses are completed for a single-lung transplant: bronchus to bronchus, pulmonary artery to pulmonary artery, and recipient pulmonary veins to donor atrial cuff. Techniques used to minimize bronchial anastomotic complications include shortening the donor bronchial stump, reinforcing the anastomosis with a vascularized tissue pedicle such as omentum or intercostal muscle pedicle flap, or using an intussuscepting bronchial anastomosis technique.
9. After anastomoses and restoration of circulation, the lung is fully inflated and observed.
10. After closure of the chest, the patient is examined with a bronchoscope to remove secretions and to ensure that the anastomosis is intact.

## REFERENCES


1. Barrera R and others: Smoking and timing of cessation: impact on pulmonary complications after thoracotomy, *Chest* 127(6):1873-1875, 2005.
2. Cerfolio RJ and others: The management of chest tubes in patients with pneumothorax and an air leak after pulmonary resection, *Chest* 128(2):816-820, 2005.
3. Coughlin AM, Parchinsky C: Go with the flow of chest tube therapy, *Nursing* 36(3):36-41, 2006.
4. Deslauriers J, Sirois C: Endoscopy: thoracoscopy for diagnosis and staging. In Pearson FG and others, editors: *Thoracic surgery,* ed 2, New York, 2002, Churchill-Livingstone.
5. Eisenach JH and others: Hyperhidrosis: evolving therapies for a well established phenomenon, *Mayo Clinic Proceedings* 80(5):657-666, 2005.
6. Ferguson JS, McLennan G: Virtual bronchoscopy, *Proceedings of the American Thoracic Society* 2:488-491, 2005.
7. Keller SM, Lin C: Surgical treatment of hyperhidrosis. In Selke FW and others, editors: *Sabiston & Spencer surgery of the chest,* ed 7, Philadelphia, 2005, Saunders.
8. Kolschmann S: Clinical efficacy and safety of thoracoscopic talc pleurodesis in malignant pleural effusions, *Chest* 128(3):1431-1435, 2005.
9. Lee RB: Benign pleural disease: empyema thoracis. In Selke FW and others, editors: *Sabiston & Spencer surgery of the chest,* ed 7, Philadelphia, 2005, Saunders.
10. Organ Procurement & Transplantation Network (OPTN): *Transplants by donor type 1988-2006.* Accessed April 8, 2006, on-line: www.optn.org/latestData/rptData.asp.
11. Rodrigue JR and others: Does lung transplantation improve health-related quality of life? The University of Florida experience, *Journal of Heart and Lung Transplantation* 24(6):755-763, 2005.
12. Scatarige JC, Fishman EK: Radiologic assessment of the chest. In Yang SC, Cameron DP, editors: *Current therapy in thoracic and cardiovascular surgery*, Philadelphia, 2004, Mosby.
13. Shander A, Rijhwani TS: Clinical outcomes in cardiac surgery: conventional surgery versus bloodless surgery, *Anesthesia Clinics of North America* 23(2):327-345, 2005.
14. Singhal S, Yang S: Lung volume reduction surgery—median sternotomy approach. In Yang SC, Cameron DP, editors: *Current therapy in thoracic and cardiovascular surgery*, Philadelphia, 2004, Mosby.
15. Takaoka ST, Weinacker AB: The value of preoperative pulmonary rehabilitation, *Thoracic Surgery Clinics* 15(2):203-211, 2005.

CHAPTER 26

# Vascular Surgery

PATRICIA WIECZOREK and KATHERINE STEGNER

Atherosclerosis continues to be one of the leading causes of death and disability in the Western world. It is estimated that peripheral atherosclerosis, including carotid, mesenteric, renal, and peripheral arterial disease (PAD) (also referred to as peripheral arterial occlusive disease [PAOD]), affects about 5% of Americans older than 60 years and up to 25% who are older than 75 years. This is particularly striking, given that by the year 2030 the percentage of the U.S. population older than 65 years will grow to 22%. Many of these people will require interventions for the syndromes of peripheral ischemia, aneurysm, and venous disease.

Interventional therapy for peripheral atherosclerosis has become common. Aortic operations are now routinely performed with less than 2% mortality. Carotid endarterectomy is also proven to be safe and effective, with a combined stroke-death rate of less than 2%. Peripheral angioplasty and bypass are initially technically successful in 98% of cases, but restenosis, graft failure, and progression of distal disease still lead to limb loss in approximately 30% of patients after 5 years. Thus emphasis has been placed on decreasing morbidity and hospital stay associated with revascularization. Minimally invasive methods and strategies, including endovascular aortic aneurysm repair,[23] carotid artery stenting (Research Highlight), stenting for lower-limb ischemia,[25] and percutaneous transluminal angioplasty, have been developed, and their application and popularity continue to increase. New technologies, such as miniature shavers for arterial plaque, are being developed.[22] Perioperative nurses must be prepared for the demands of patient care in vascular surgery. This chapter reviews surgical anatomy, perioperative nursing considerations, and surgical interventions for a variety of vascular procedures.

## Surgical Anatomy

Basic knowledge of anatomy is essential when caring for perioperative patients with a vascular disorder. Figure 26-1 depicts the principal arteries and veins of the body. Arteries and veins have three layers:

- Tunica intima (innermost layer)
- Tunica media (muscular middle layer)
- Tunica adventitia (fibrous outer layer)

Arteries differ from veins in function and slightly in structure (Figure 26-2). Structurally, arteries have a thicker muscle layer and more elastic fibers than veins. The properties of elasticity and distensibility enable the vessels to compensate for changes in blood pressure and volume. Because of the thicker muscle layer, severed arteries are capable of contracting and constricting enough to stop hemorrhage. In contrast, veins are more fragile than arteries, and whether its cause is traumatic or iatrogenic, venous bleeding may be difficult to control. Another difference is the presence of semilunar intimal folds, or valves, in veins that prevent backflow. Veins and arteries are nourished by a tiny network of vessels (the vasa vasorum), as well as from the intraluminal blood flow. Both are regulated by the autonomic nervous system, with veins having fewer nerve fibers than arteries have. The two systems are connected (except for the pulmonary artery and pulmonary venous system): major arteries carry oxygenated blood, they branch into smaller arteries and then arterioles, and then blood moves into capillaries to venules and to veins. The work of exchanging nutrients and metabolic waste is done at the capillary level.

Blood flow is a complex process that depends on many factors. Blood flows through arteries such that the blood in the center of the vessel moves faster than the blood at the periphery. Because the movement of the blood is in parallel lines, it is referred to as *laminar.* When flow is disrupted by an obstruction, stenosis, curve, or bifurcation the particle motion is referred to as *turbulent*. Turbulence may be evidenced by the presence of a bruit, detected by auscultation, or detected by a characteristic Doppler signal. Flow depends on blood viscosity, vessel wall resistance, and the peripheral resistance of the arterioles. There must be a difference in pressures, or a pressure gradient, to allow blood to flow. The gradient is provided by the contraction of the left ventricle. The negative pressure created by the relaxed right ventricle assists in venous return by creating a suctioning effect, and the skeletal and visceral muscles help propel venous return toward the heart.

## ARTERIAL DISEASE

### Aneurysmal Disease

The most common cause of an arterial aneurysm is atherosclerotic degeneration of the arterial wall.[1] The pathogenesis is a multifactorial process, involving atherosclerosis along with genetic predisposition, aging, inflammation, and localized activation of proteolytic enzymes.[1] A true aneurysm is a dilation of all layers of the artery wall. A dissecting aneurysm results from a tear in the artery wall, allowing blood to dissect between the layers of the vessel wall. A false aneurysm, or pseudoaneurysm, is not an aneurysm but a disruption through all the layers of a vessel wall with the escaping blood being contained by the perivascular tissues. False aneurysms may result from trauma, infection, or disruption of an arterial suture line after surgery. True aneurysms are most frequently found in the abdominal aorta but are also found in the thoracic aorta and iliac, femoral, and popliteal arteries. More men than women are affected, and aneurysmal disease tends to be a disease of

## RESEARCH HIGHLIGHT

### Does Carotid Artery Stenting Work in the Long Run: 5-Year Results in High-Volume Centers

This study was conducted on 2172 patients in four high-volume centers in Europe between February 1, 1993 and December 31, 2004. Both late-stroke rate and patency rates were analyzed as well as long-term restenosis and stroke-death rates. Of the 2172 patients in the study, 2165 (99.7%) underwent stent procedures that were technically successful. A Kaplan-Meier analysis of major stroke-death and of significant restenosis for the total population found stroke-death rates of 4.1% ($n$ = 1356), 10.1% ($n$ = 476), and 15.5% ($n$ = 138); and restenosis rates of 1% ($n$ = 1363), 2% ($n$ = 480) and 3.4% ($n$ = 139), after 1, 3, and 5 years, respectively. The authors concluded that carotid artery stenting is a valuable minimally invasive procedure. They recommended further studies that take into consideration preprocedural neurologic complications, risk factor distribution, procedural steps, and clinical outcomes.

Modified from Bosiers M: Does carotid artery stenting work in the long run: 5-year results in high-volume centers, *Journal of Cardiovascular Surgery* 46(3):241-247, 2005.

older persons. As early as 1977, a familial tendency was observed that subsequent research verified; as many as 18% of patients with abdominal aortic aneurysms have a first-degree relative with a similar diagnosis.

Abdominal aortic aneurysms (AAAs), which account for approximately 75% of all aneurysms, occur primarily between the renal arteries and the aortic bifurcation.[6] An aneurysm involves intimal damage of the aorta and weakening of the media[9] or elastic portion (collagen and elastin defects) of the arterial wall. Gradually the vessel wall in the damaged area expands and atheroma develops within the aneurysm sac (Figure 26-3). An AAA has minimal symptoms and is generally discovered on routine history and physical examination. Mortality is low with elective resection of the aneurysm. Dissection and rupture of the aneurysm (aortic dissection) dramatically increase operative mortality because of the abrupt and massive hemorrhagic shock that accompanies the rupture. Aortic dissection is believed to arise from a sudden tear in the aortic intima, opening the way for blood to enter the aortic wall.

## Acute Arterial Insufficiency

Arterial insufficiency may result from an acute occlusion, as in embolic disease, or the rupture of an unstable atherosclerotic plaque causing acute thrombosis of the vessel. Emboli usually arise from the heart from atrial fibrillation but may occasionally result from a myocardial infarction (MI), where a clot forms on the endocardium (the lining of the heart) in an area of muscle damage. Atherosclerotic plaque can also break loose from other areas and result in an acute arterial blockage. Patients with acute arterial occlusion usually present with the onset of the six Ps: sudden severe *p*ain, *p*ulselessness, *p*aresthesia, *p*aralysis, *p*allor, and *p*oikilothermia (coolness) of an extremity.[6] Heparin is the mainstay to prevent the enlargement of emboli while allowing time for collateral blood flow to develop. However, in the threatened limb there are basically two options: surgical removal of the clot (embolectomy) or chemical removal of the clot with the use of a thrombolytic drug. If the limb reaches the point where the muscle is rigid, the limb is not salvageable and amputation is a lifesaving procedure.

## Chronic Arterial Insufficiency

Chronic arterial insufficiency occurs because of the deposition of calcium and cholesterol within the wall of the artery. Arteriosclerosis is a natural part of the aging process whereby the walls of the arterial vasculature undergo changes such as increased thickness and hardening, reducing the elasticity of the arteries.[16] The decrease in elasticity should not be confused with atherosclerosis obliterans, which is a pathologic process that affects the intimal layer of the artery with the buildup of a fibrous plaque of lipids that can calcify and necrose. Atherosclerosis is the most common cause of PAOD, the probable mechanism being initial damage to the intima and subsequent activation and aggregation of the body's platelets. Inflammation follows, with the deposition of lipoproteins forming an atheroma. Calcification of this lesion leads to the development of an atherosclerotic plaque, resulting in inadequate muscle perfusion and ischemia.[17] The process is a gradual one, and a localized lesion usually indicates systemic disease. The body develops a network of collateral vessels as an adaptive mechanism to supply the tissues with oxygenated blood. Many theories have been postulated to explain the process of atherogenesis. The inflammatory process of intimal injury, as just described, seems to be the current and most widely accepted hypothesis. Box 26-1 presents risk factors for atherosclerosis. A large number of vascular surgical procedures revolve around the results of chronic arterial insufficiency.

## Arterial Insufficiency: Cerebrovascular Disease and Stroke

Cerebrovascular accident (CVA, or stroke) is a leading cause of death in the United States and most industrialized countries. In the United States, approximately 750,000 persons experience a stroke each year.[8] Cerebrovascular disease may manifest itself as a transient ischemic attack (TIA) or as a major or minor stroke. A TIA is an episode of neurologic dysfunction that resolves in 24 hours. It may be caused by atheromatous debris or a thromboembolism from a carotid artery or vertebral basilar system. Vascular lesions in the carotid artery occur primarily at the bifurcation of the common carotid artery into the internal and the external carotid arteries. The internal carotid artery supplies the brain with needed oxygenated blood. Obstruction in this arterial vessel leads to cerebrovascular insufficiency.

The right and the left carotid and vertebral arteries supply the brain (Figure 26-4). The first major branch of the internal carotid artery is the ophthalmic artery. Thromboembolic events that affect this artery may result in visual disturbances, ocular TIAs, or "amaurosis fugax" (complete or partial loss of vision). Patients will often describe amaurosis fugax as a curtain over a partial field of vision, usually the top. Clinical conditions that generally indicate the need for a carotid endarterectomy (CEA) are transient cerebral ischemia, asymptomatic severe stenosis, and stable strokes. Carotid disease may recur after a CEA. Redo surgery for restenosis poses the same complication risks as the original procedure (Research Highlight).

## Arterial Insufficiency: Peripheral Vascular Disease

The initial and most important symptom of vascular disease in the aortoiliac vessels and distal arteries is intermittent claudication. The term *claudication* is derived from the Latin word

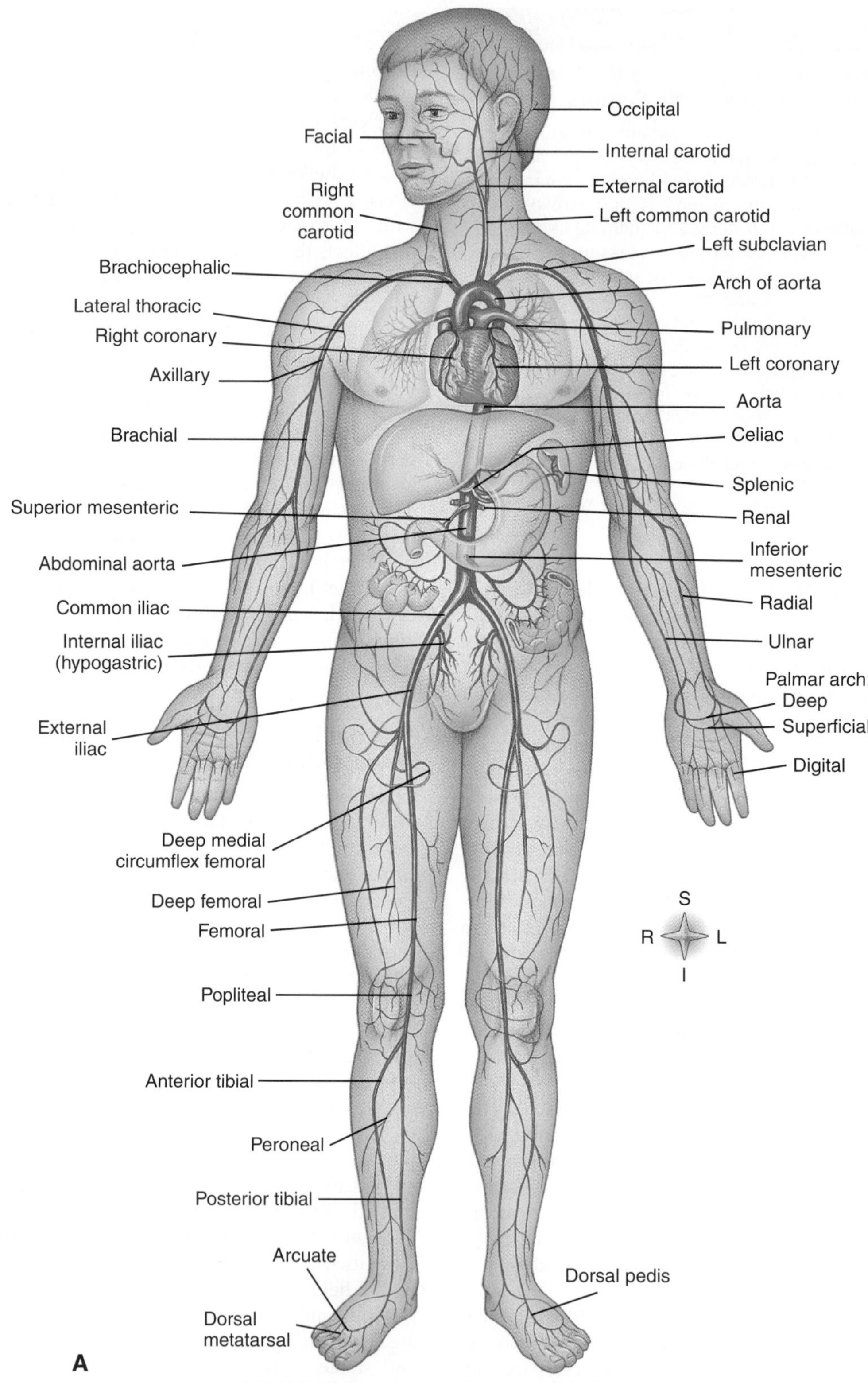
Occipital
Facial
Internal carotid
External carotid
Right common carotid
Left common carotid
Left subclavian
Brachiocephalic
Arch of aorta
Lateral thoracic
Pulmonary
Right coronary
Left coronary
Axillary
Aorta
Brachial
Celiac
Splenic
Superior mesenteric
Renal
Abdominal aorta
Inferior mesenteric
Common iliac
Radial
Internal iliac (hypogastric)
Ulnar
Palmar arch:
Deep
Superficial
External iliac
Digital
Deep medial circumflex femoral
Deep femoral
Femoral
S
R
L
I
Popliteal
Anterior tibial
Peroneal
Posterior tibial
Arcuate
Dorsal pedis
Dorsal metatarsal
A

FIGURE 26-1 **A,** Principal arteries of the body.

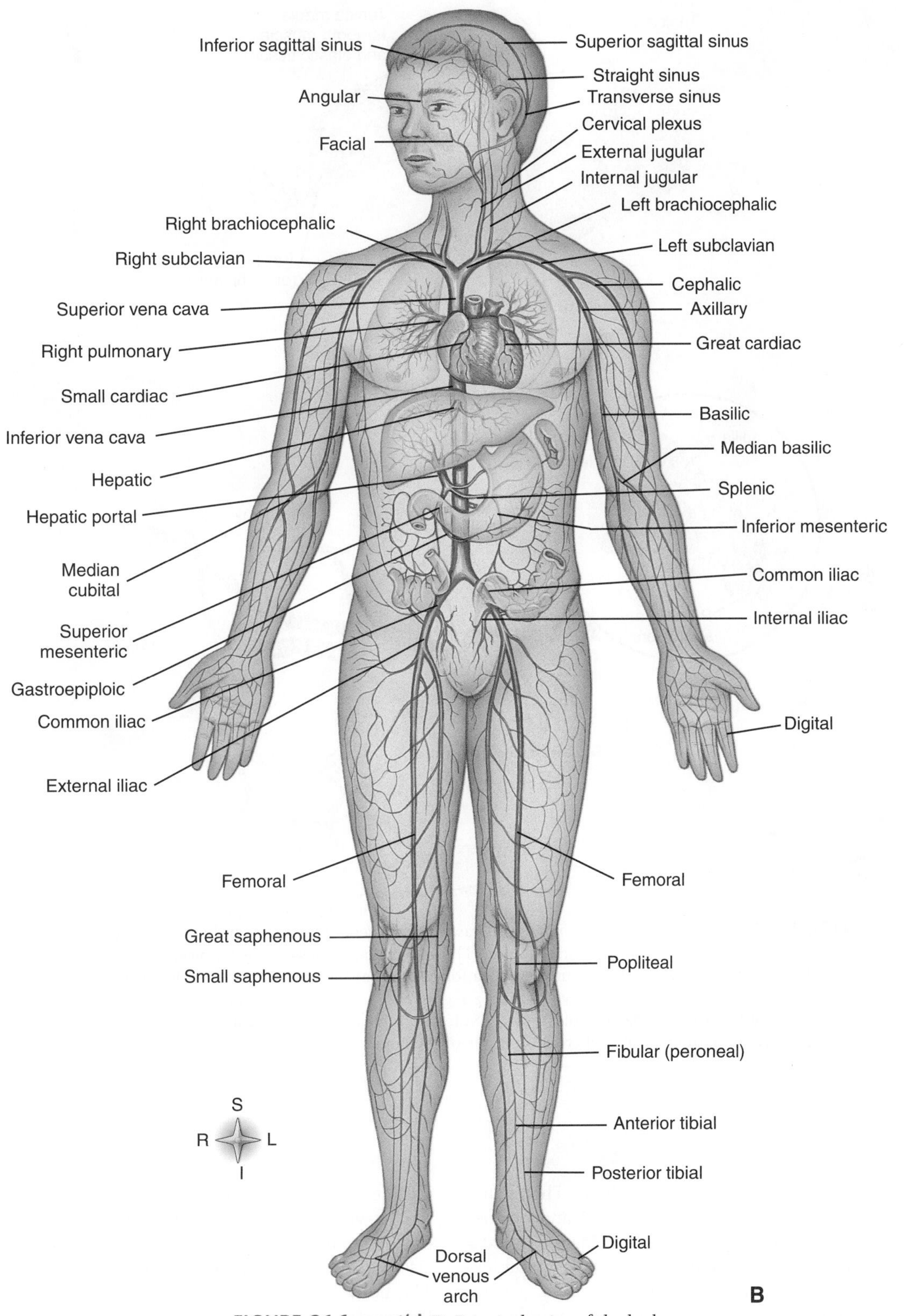


FIGURE 26-1, cont'd **B**, Principal veins of the body.

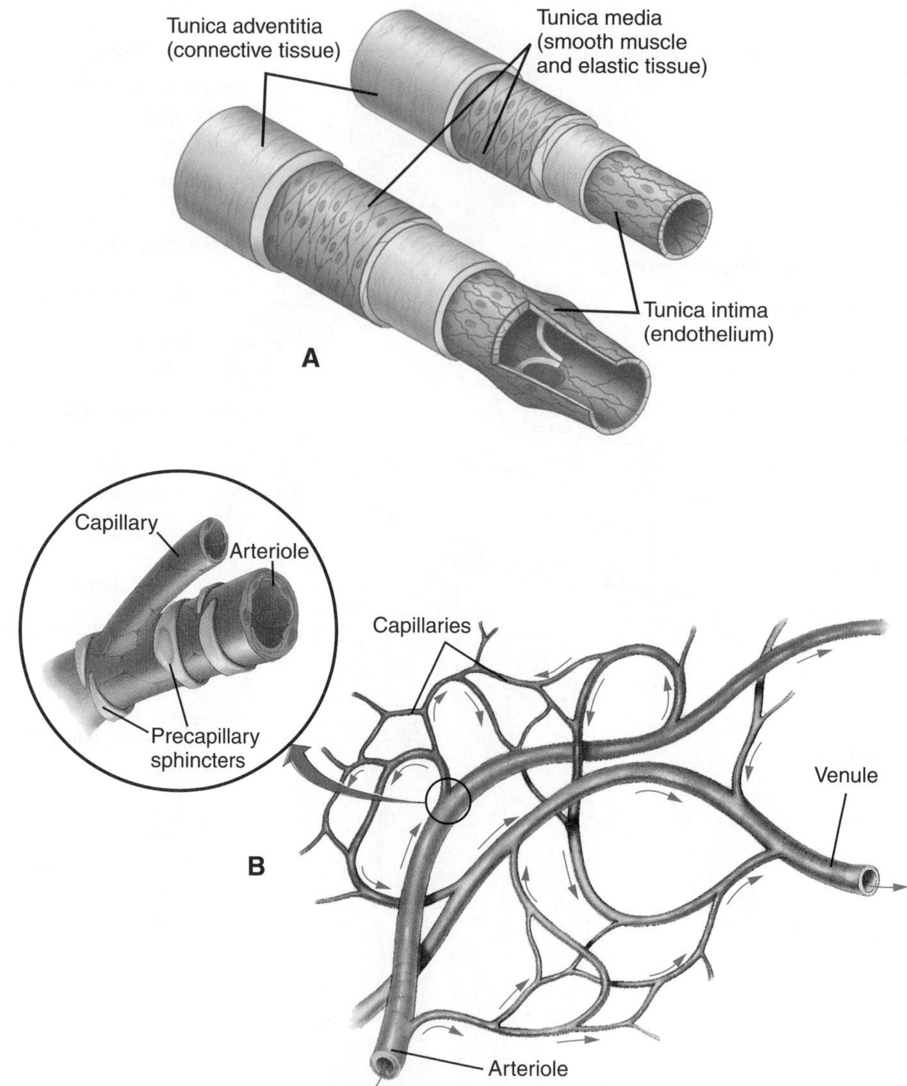


**FIGURE 26-2** **A,** Layers of artery and vein. Drawings of a sectioned artery and vein show the three layers of large vessel walls. **B,** Microcirculation. The smaller blood vessels—arterioles, capillaries, and venules—cannot be observed without magnification. Note that the control of blood flow through any particular region of a capillary network can be regulated by the relative contraction of precapillary sphincters in the walls of the arterioles *(inset)*. Note also that capillaries have a wall composed of only a single layer of flattened cells, whereas the walls of the larger vessels also have a smooth layer.

"claudicare," which means "to limp" (History box). This is the most common symptom of lower extremity PAD and occurs distal to the arterial obstruction on exercising. Many patients are asymptomatic and do not experience pain. When symptoms do appear it is typically located in the working muscle, occurs with the same amount of exercise each time, and is relieved with rest. This is referred to as functional ischemia; blood flow is adequate at rest but inadequate to sustain exercise. The increased muscle demand for oxygen with exercise cannot be met distal to the arterial obstruction. Anaerobic metabolism occurs, and muscle cramping develops. Surgery is not usually performed for claudication unless it is unusually disabling.

The second symptom, rest pain, which is located in the foot, develops as the vascular disease progresses. At this stage the ischemia is termed *critical*. Rest pain occurs without exercise and is a constant discomfort, often aggravated at night. The body is now unable to meet the oxygen needs of distal tissues even at rest. Rest pain may be somewhat relieved by analgesics or by lowering the legs off the bed. Gravity assists in increasing the tissue perfusion and oxygen supply to decrease the pain. Unless the vascular disease is corrected, nonhealing ulcers and gangrene can develop. Gangrene occurs when the arterial vessels are unable to meet the oxygen needs of distal tissues even at complete rest.

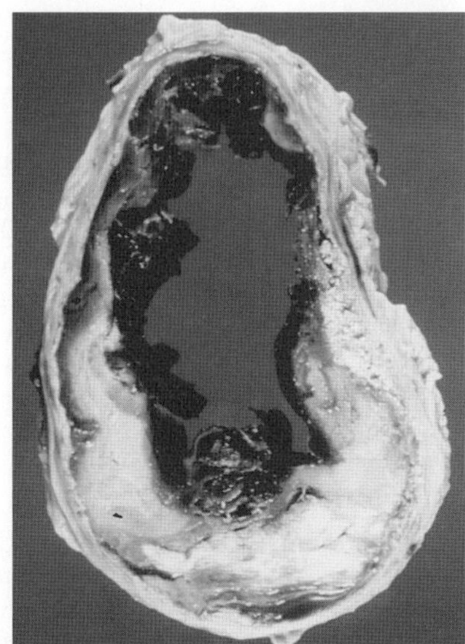

FIGURE 26-3 Cross section of an abdominal aortic aneurysm reveals dilated arterial wall with posterior atherosclerotic plaque and laminated mural thrombus.

BOX 26-1

### Risk Factors for Atherosclerosis

**FIRMLY ESTABLISHED FACTORS**
Hypercholesterolemia
Cigarette smoking
Hypertension
Diabetes mellitus

**RELATIVE FACTORS**
Advanced age
Male gender
Hypertriglyceridemia
Hyperhomocystinemia
Sedentary life-style
Family history

From Belkin M and others: Peripheral arterial occlusive disease. In Townsend CM and others: *Sabiston textbook of surgery*, ed 17, Philadelphia, 2004, Saunders.

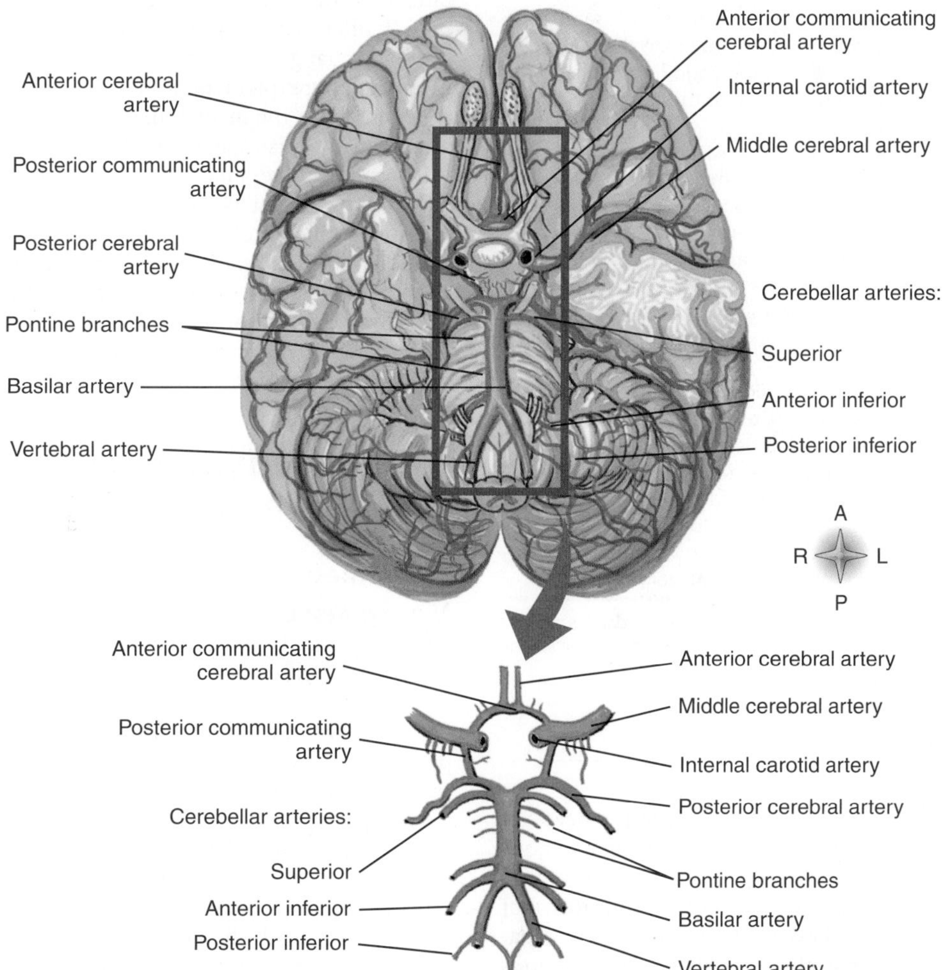


FIGURE 26-4 Arteries at the base of the brain. The arteries that compose the circle of Willis are the two anterior cerebral arteries joined to each other by the anterior communicating cerebral artery and to the posterior cerebral arteries by the posterior communicating arteries.

## RESEARCH HIGHLIGHT

### Carotid Redo Surgery: Both Safe and Durable

A retrospective cohort analysis of 1922 patients was undertaken by Harris and others to examine the outcomes and complications of surgery for recurrent carotid stenosis. The records identified 24 patients who underwent surgery for recurrent stenosis. The indications for redo surgery included severe or moderate symptomatic restenosis or severe asymptomatic restenosis. Within the 30-day perioperative period there were no deaths, strokes, or significant cardiac morbidity. The authors attributed the low surgical morbidity and mortality to selective reintervention for carotid restenosis. In conclusion, the study further supports documented evidence that surgery for carotid restenosis has similar results to surgery for initial carotid disease.

Modified from Harris R and others: Carotid redo surgery: both safe and durable, *Australian and New Zealand Journal of Surgery* 73(12):1000-1004, 2003.

## HISTORY

Operations on the vascular system have been performed since antiquity. In 1902, Osler described a theory of intermittent claudication. He noted that this phenomenon had been described by a French veterinarian in a horse. Later, the analogy was made between a male patient and a condition that corresponded to the intermittent claudication in the horse. The patient was unable to walk more than one quarter of a mile without experiencing cramps in the legs. After a period of rest, he would get better and be able to resume walking. This patient died, and on autopsy a ball was found encysted in the neighborhood of the iliac artery; a traumatic aneurysm was found as well that had obliterated the artery in its lower part. Osler went on to note that the circulation was carried by the collateral channels, which were ample to maintain nutrition while the patient was at rest and for a short period of exertion.

Since the early writings of Osler, significant advancements have occurred in vascular surgery. Contributing to this rapid forward march have been effective anticoagulants, availability of arterial allografts, expanded surgical techniques, improved suture materials, refined angiography, and the advent of noninvasive diagnostic methods. Current endovascular surgical devices continue to be modified, expanding the possibilities for their use and broadening the vascular surgery frontier.

Modified from Fye WB, editor: *William Osler's collected papers on the cardiovascular system*, Birmingham, Ala, 1985, The Classics of Cardiology Library.

## VENOUS DISEASE

### Acute Venous Insufficiency

Acute venous insufficiency is caused by a clot in the deep venous system, or deep venous thrombosis (DVT). Such venous insufficiency can be a diagnosis of DVT, phlebitis, thrombophlebitis, or phlebothrombosis, which merely indicates that there is a clot, usually in the lower extremity. Virchow, a pathologist, identified the three elements that trigger venous thrombosis. Referred to as Virchow's triad, these elements, or risk factors, are endothelial injury, venostasis, and hypercoagulability.[15] The cause of hypercoagulability is sometimes unknown but is seen in patients with tissue trauma (e.g., surgery, burns, or stroke), malignancy, sepsis, pregnancy or estrogen usage, and diabetes mellitus. The patient may be asymptomatic or present with limb swelling, pain, and a skin color change. The danger lies in the potential emboli migrating to the right ventricle and proceeding to the lungs. Pulmonary emboli (PEs) can be fatal. PE has been reported to be responsible for approximately 50,000 to 200,000 deaths and 300,000 hospitalizations per year. Approximately 95% of pulmonary emboli cases are caused by DVT. The majority of these originate in the lower extremities. The use of heparin and bed rest is the usual medical treatment. In cases that preclude the use of systemic heparin or in which heparin is ineffective, surgical insertion of a vena cava filter may be indicated.

### Chronic Venous Insufficiency

Patients with chronic venous insufficiency (CVI) have not been treated surgically as often as patients with arterial disease for several reasons. CVI is not life threatening or limb-threatening. Improved imaging techniques (e.g., duplex ultrasonography) allow better diagnoses of the precise problem. The treatment of the majority of venous disorders is nonsurgical and aimed at increasing venous return and decreasing edema. CVI, which presents with stasis ulcers from postphlebitic syndrome, usually occurs in one leg. The leg is usually very swollen with a cyclic edema, unlike lymphedema, which does not change visibly by morning from leg elevation. Stasis ulcers and hyperpigmentation usually are found in the "gaiter" area and above the medial malleolus on the leg. The condition is caused by incompetent perforator valves. The perforating veins connect the superficial and deep venous systems. The usual management is to apply 20 to 30 mm Hg of external pressure by means of special pressure stockings. Surgical interventions such as valvuloplasty (direct repair of the valve), valve transposition or transplantation (moving a valve from the arm to the leg), or perforator interruptions are occasionally performed but have had limited success. Patient selection is critical, and long-term results are mixed.

## *Perioperative Nursing Considerations*

### Assessment

***Nursing Responsibilities.*** A preoperative assessment is necessary for an adequate understanding of the patient's disease, the patient's response, and the proposed surgical procedure. Knowledge of vascular disease and its progression assists the perioperative nurse in performing a critical review of the comprehensive assessment and developing a plan of care for patients undergoing vascular surgical procedures.

The perioperative nurse should assess the patient, reviewing an already completed, current nursing assessment for the development and extent of vascular symptoms. Medical conditions, including cardiac, renal, and pulmonary disease, coagulation status, and allergies, must be assessed (Box 26-2) to ensure that the patient can tolerate a possible angiogram, since the contrast medium is toxic and increased fluid volumes are needed if angioscopy is planned. This is a shared responsibility of the nursing, surgical, and anesthesia team members. The patient's nutritional status, the patient's use of alcohol and to-

BOX 26-2

### Review of Patient's Medical Record

The perioperative nurse should review the patient's medical record, confirming or obtaining information for the following items:

- Correct and current medical record/chart
- Surgical consent
- History and physical examination
- Baseline vital signs (including height and weight)
- Mental status
- Medications
- Allergies or adverse reactions to drugs, topical agents, or other substances (e.g., latex)
- Skin tone and integrity
- Physical limitations
- Laboratory data (prescribed blood work, electrocardiogram [ECG] report, urinalysis, ultrasound or x-ray studies, other pertinent tests)
- Religious, cultural, ethnic preferences[14]
- Nursing plan of care or other notations from transferring nurse
- Presence or disposition of prosthetic devices (e.g., hearing aids, dentures, glasses)

bacco, and the existence of any skin lesions should also be noted. Preoperative location, grading, and marking of distal peripheral pulses assist the perioperative nurse with intraoperative and postoperative assessment of tissue perfusion.

The patient should be greeted by name and identified using two unique identifiers. When possible, the patient should confirm such identification. Identification must also be confirmed by the name band, medical record, surgical consent, operating room (OR) schedule, and marked surgical site. Safety is always the first priority. The surgical procedure must be confirmed and the patient's understanding of the procedure and associated risks assessed; inaccuracies or misconceptions must be clarified before proceeding with surgery. Written consent is designed to protect the patient by providing written clarification of the proposed procedure. The National Quality Forum (NQF) has identified Safe Practice 10 for informed consent, recommending that each patient (or legal surrogate) be asked to "teach back" what he or she has been told during the informed consent discussion.[26] Consents that are valid and obtained freely and from a competent person remain in effect for as long as the person still agrees to the surgery or procedure. This may vary by institutional modification.

It is important to assess comfort before continuing the interview and assessment. This reflects caring and will promote nurse-patient rapport and facilitate obtaining accurate and complete information. The acuity of the patient's condition will also affect the order of priority of the assessments and interactions. After reviewing the results of the patient's physical examination, the perioperative nurse should verify signs and symptoms of vascular disease that need to be considered during intraoperative care. Muscle and skin atrophy, the presence of tissue ulceration or necrosis, pain, neurovascular status, skin color and temperature, and other integumentary changes should be noted. Elderly, cachectic, and obese patients are at increased risk for pressure injuries.

The perioperative nurse should assess the patient's mental status and determine the level of understanding and emotional response to the surgery. Patients with vascular disorders usually have systemic disease, and the fear of a stroke (if the patient is having a CEA), amputation (if the patient has an ischemic limb), or other complications may be a realistic concern. A skin assessment should include notation of color, integrity, pain, and pulses. Any musculoskeletal problems that preclude patients moving themselves to the OR bed and any weaknesses that may have resulted from a stroke or that would modify the positioning for surgery should be noted. Correction of misunderstandings is possible only if the perioperative nurse identifies the patient's current level of knowledge. Identification of the patient's fears and concerns helps with planning supportive nursing interventions.

Vascular surgery can be lengthy. Attention to the maintenance of the patient's tissue and skin integrity as well as body temperature is important.[13] The patient's extremities should be assessed for color, temperature, and strength of pedal pulses before the surgical procedure so that baseline data will be available for comparison with perioperative assessment data. This assessment evaluates tissue perfusion distal to the arterial obstruction.

***Preoperative Tests.*** A variety of tests may be required to plan for surgical interventions. Segmental pressure measurements give partial anatomic information in that they assist in locating lesions. Hemodynamic tests provide information on the flow of blood, such as that to the brain or an extremity, and the effects on flow caused by a vascular lesion.

**ANGIOGRAPHY.** Invasive diagnostic tests may be performed preoperatively to identify the extent and location of the patient's peripheral vascular disease. The introduction of a contrast medium through a catheter into the arterial or venous system of the patient facilitates this visualization. Angiography also involves injecting a contrast medium into the patient's arterial system and taking serial radiographs of the movement of the dye through the arteries. Digital subtraction angiography (DSA) is one such technique that uses a computer along with contrast medium injection to make the image (Figure 26-5). Usually the left side of the film shows the bone for orientation, and the right side subtracts the density of the bone and soft tissue to allow a clearer view of the vessels. Arteriography provides information on arterial anatomy and the location of stenotic or occluded vessels and assists the surgeon in planning bypass procedures. A venogram (contrast venography) is performed to show venous abnormalities in extremities, the vena cava, and the hepatic and renal systems. Ascending venography can differentiate between acute and chronic thrombosis and can define anatomy. Descending venography assesses valve competence of lower extremities.

**DOPPLER SCANNING.** The Doppler effect, initially described by Christian Johann Doppler (1903-1953), is the change in the frequency of echo signals that occurs whenever there is a change in the distance between the sources of a sound and the receiving object. The probe, or transducer, is aimed toward the blood vessel at an angle of 45 to 60 degrees. This directs an ultrasound beam that is reflected back to the probe by moving red blood cells (RBCs). The velocity of the flow of cells is converted into an audible signal heard through a speaker. The signal is described as a swishing sound. The

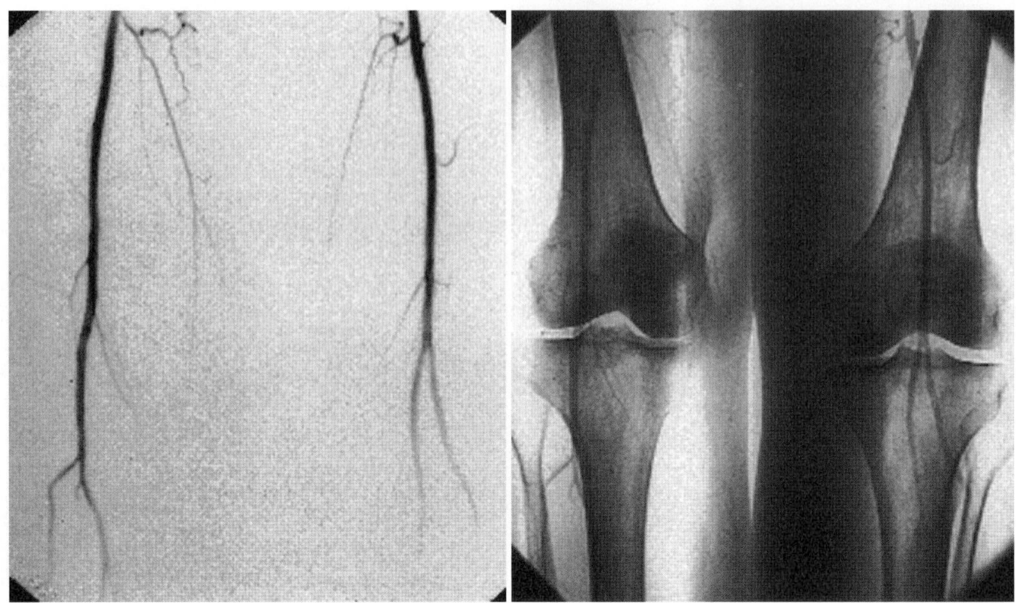

**FIGURE 26-5** Digital subtraction angiography.

sound is called a signal, not a pulse. The tip of the probe is made of an element called a ceramic piezoelectric crystal. This can send, receive, and convert signals when an electric current is applied. The element becomes thicker and thinner, thus resulting in a pressure wave converted to an audible signal. The simplest form is the continuous wave (CW) Doppler probe. It has two elements: one sends a high-frequency wave, and the other receives it. In a pulsed Doppler probe, the same element sends and receives signals. The pulsed Doppler probe has the advantage of being able to differentiate among vessels of different depths. A normal arterial Doppler signal is either biphasic or triphasic. The first sound corresponds to systolic flow and is forward-moving and of high velocity. The second sound is related to early diastole and has a lesser reversal of flow. The third is later diastole and is smaller, forward-flowing, and of a lower velocity. The pitch is described as rising quickly in systole and dropping quickly in early diastole. An abnormal signal, indicating stenosis or occlusion is heard as low-pitched and monophasic. These abnormal arterial signals may sound like venous signals.

The Doppler probe can provide information in three forms: the audible signal, a visible graph printout similar to an electrocardiogram (ECG) tracing, and a spectral analysis that appears on a screen and may be recorded on paper as well. The Doppler transducer is the most widely used instrument for vascular study. It has the advantages of being readily available, inexpensive, and easy to use. A small, portable battery unit is durable and can be transported and stored easily. When the probe is used on intact skin, a water-soluble gel is needed to conduct a signal. Probes can be used directly on a vessel intraoperatively. The probes are heat-sensitive and must either be sterilized according to manufacturer's instructions or inserted into a sterile sleeve or probe cover. If they are handled gently, the probes have a reasonable life span. Care must be taken to protect the sensitive tip from being dropped or crushed. The biggest drawback of the Doppler probe is a negative finding in the presence of a stenotic lesion pronounced enough to produce a flow disturbance that results in an altered signal.

A bruit is a sound disturbance that is sometimes described as a low-pitched, blowing sound. It can be heard through a stethoscope over an area of blood flow turbulence that occurs at points of vessel stenoses. Bruits do not provide information on the extent of a lesion—only that an abnormal flow may exist. They occur at points of significant stenosis and are not heard when severe flow restriction or total flow occlusion occurs. The Doppler probe is noninvasive and painless for patients. For a quick, inexpensive venous assessment with immediate results, the CW Doppler probe is a good screening tool.

**ULTRASONOGRAPHY.** Ultrasonography is done to obtain information about structures through the emission of high-frequency sound waves. These sound waves are reflected, or bounced back, to the probe or transducer that emits them and are electronically transformed into an image.

**B-Mode Ultrasonography.** B-mode is brightness modulation, a technique in ultrasound imaging that projects a two-dimensional image on an oscilloscope screen. The image appears as dots from the echoes of the signal. The strength of the echo is shown by the intensity and brightness of the dots on the screen.

**Duplex Ultrasonography.** A duplex ultrasound machine is a combination of the pulsed Doppler image and the so-called real-time B-mode image ultrasonogram. Real time simply refers to the image projecting current, undelayed information. B-mode image is best when the probe is perpendicular to the vessel, but the Doppler probe does not pick up signals at a perpendicular angle. Some manipulation of the probe angle is required to obtain the best results. Color duplex imaging converts the detected signals caused by blood flow into a color, depending on the direction of flow. Flow toward the probe may be displayed as red, away from the probe as blue, and turbulence as multiple colors. This imaging provides both hemodynamic and anatomic information. The technology is also used in transesophageal echocardiography (TEE) and is the diagnostic method of choice for venous insufficiency.

**PULSE VOLUME RECORDING (PVR), OR SEQUENTIAL VOLUME PLETHYSMOGRAPHY.** A plethysmograph measures and records the changes in the sizes and volumes in extremities by measuring the blood volumes at blood pressure cuffs placed at intervals along the extremity. The methods include electrical impedance, mercury in Silastic strain gauges, and air or fluid displacement. This test, which is used to determine the location of an arterial lesion and estimate the severity of the disease, requires careful limb positioning and a cooperative patient. A negative study is a good predictor of low risk for PE.

This test is inexpensive, has good predictive value, and is accurate in detecting thrombosis. It has the disadvantage of a high rate of false-positive results in the presence of old DVT, congestive heart failure (CHF), and external compression.

**MAGNETIC RESONANCE IMAGING.** Magnetic resonance imaging (MRI) measures the behavior of atoms in a strong magnetic field. This test provides detailed and three-dimensional images of anatomy for evaluation of carotid, aortic, and lower extremity disease. An MRI provides more detail than ultrasonography or computed tomography (CT) scan and avoids the complications of contrast medium injection and exposure to x-rays. MRI is contraindicated for patients with pacemakers or metal cerebral aneurysm clips, and vena cava filters may cause large image artifacts.

## Nursing Diagnosis

Nursing diagnoses related to the care of patients undergoing vascular surgery might include the following:

- Anxiety related to the surgical intervention and its outcomes
- Risk for Hypothermia related to surgical exposure and anesthesia[19]
- Risk for Deficient Fluid Volume related to loss of body fluids
- Risk for Impaired Skin Integrity and Ineffective Tissue Perfusion related to surgical positioning, presence of vascular disease, and vascular clamping

Based on the perioperative nurse's assessment, identification and prioritization of nursing diagnoses aid in the development of an individualized plan of care.

## Outcome Identification

Outcomes identified for the selected nursing diagnoses could be stated as follows:

- The patient will have all questions answered, will verbalize decreased anxiety and understanding of surgical procedure and perioperative routines, and will exhibit increased relaxation as shown by facial expression or other body language.
- The patient's body temperature will remain within normal limits as evidenced by postoperative temperature equivalent to preoperative level and absence of postoperative shivering.
- Fluid balance will be maintained as evidenced by postoperative pulses equivalent to preoperative level, hourly urine output of at least 30 ml, and good skin turgor.
- Skin integrity will be maintained. Skin temperature and color will be within normal limits. No skin injury lesions will be evident, and the electrosurgery unit (ESU) dispersive pad site will be intact.

## Planning

Before the patient is brought into the OR, the perioperative nurse should procure the necessary supplies and equipment for the intended surgical intervention. Because the need for an arteriogram or fluoroscopy for endovascular procedures is a possibility, the patient with a vascular disorder should be on an appropriate OR bed with x-ray capabilities. The perioperative nurse needs to coordinate the availability of x-ray department personnel. Appropriate contrast media, catheters, and impermeable sterile x-ray covers must be available. Radiation-protection devices, such as lead aprons and shields, should be used for the patient, when possible, and for surgical team members. A typical plan of care for a patient undergoing vascular surgery, using the suggested nursing diagnoses, is shown on p. 948.

Arterial procedures, especially those that involve the aorta, may place the patient at risk for significant blood loss. The perioperative nurse should confirm the availability of ordered blood-replacement products. The use of rapid infusion systems or blood salvage equipment should be determined and planned.

## Implementation

***Site Verification: "Time Out."*** Patient safety is of utmost importance. It is the entire surgical team's responsibility to verify that the correct patient is receiving the correct procedure on the correct site immediately before the start of any surgical procedure. The surgical site needs to be marked and visible after draping if laterality is involved. The "time out" is a requirement of the Joint Commission on Accreditation of Healthcare Organizations (JCAHO). During the time out, the patient's name, procedure, site verification, and laterality are reviewed. Other items that may be discussed include the consent, anesthesia plan/concerns, the patient's allergies, antibiotics ordered, the patient's position, required instruments and special equipment, availability of blood, and anticipated length of the procedure.[2] Such briefings improve team communication and intraoperative patient care.

***Intraoperative Monitoring.*** Intraoperative monitoring for patients with vascular disorders includes the use of the basic ECG, pulse oximeter, and blood pressure cuff. For patients undergoing saphenous vein stripping or amputation, these are usually adequate. For lengthy procedures, as in arterial bypass or reconstruction, an arterial line is usually placed percutaneously into the radial artery. This is kept open by a heparin drip line attached to a transducer, and a waveform monitor reads out the systolic and diastolic pressures. The monitor also calculates the mean arterial pressure (MAP), which aids in the evaluation of the perfusion of systemic and cardiac circulation. This arterial line also allows easy access for collecting specimens for arterial blood gas (ABG) analysis. The ECG and direct arterial lines are used for monitoring and assessment. Continuous assessment of the patient's arterial pressure is a critical part of the surgical procedure. Pulmonary capillary wedge pressure, as an index of left atrial pressure (LAP), may be monitored depending on the patient's physiologic status. A general anesthetic may be administered and the patient intubated; local or regional anesthesia may also be used, depending on the surgical intervention. Epidural catheters may be placed to provide intraoperative anesthesia that can be augmented to accommodate increased surgical time, as opposed to a spinal anesthetic, which provides a finite period of anesthesia. Epidural catheters may be left in place postoperatively for pain management as well. Since many patients undergoing vascular surgery have generalized atherosclerotic disease, the perioperative nurse should be constantly alert for cardiac dysrhythmias

## SAMPLE PLAN OF CARE

### NURSING DIAGNOSIS

**Anxiety** related to the surgical intervention and its outcomes

### OUTCOME

The patient will have all questions answered. The patient will verbalize decreased anxiety and understanding of surgical procedure and perioperative routines. The patient will exhibit increased relaxation as shown by facial expression or other body language.

### INTERVENTIONS

- Include the family, significant others, or both in explanations of perioperative routines.
- Allow time for patient's questions; provide explanations, or make appropriate referral.
- Observe verbal and nonverbal indications of anxiety; assist the patient with anxiety-reducing/coping techniques that have proven personally effective in the past, such as meditation, prayer,[4] rhythmic breathing, music, self-guided imagery, massage, and relaxation.[24]
- Encourage expression of concerns and fears; clarify any misperceptions, and reinforce information provided by other members of the health care team.
- Provide emotional support and comforting nursing measures (e.g., touch, a warm blanket).
- Demonstrate warmth, calmness, and acceptance of the patient's anxiety.
- Maintain a quiet environment; minimize distractions.[21]
- Document patient's reactions.

### NURSING DIAGNOSIS

**Risk for Hypothermia** related to surgical exposure and anesthesia

### OUTCOME

The patient's body temperature will remain within normal limits as evidenced by postoperative temperature equivalent to preoperative level and absence of postoperative shivering.

### INTERVENTIONS

- Limit the patient's physical exposure; expose only those body surfaces required for skin preparation.
- Cover the patient's head with a blanket or cap.
- Use warmed skin prep solutions (as applicable to agent being used).
- Use a warming device (e.g., a forced air–warming unit).
- Provide the anesthesia provider with a fluid warmer.
- Consult with the anesthesia provider regarding the patient's temperature.
- Use warm saline for irrigation.
- Provide warm blankets at the end of the surgical procedure.

### NURSING DIAGNOSIS

**Risk for Deficient Fluid Volume** related to loss of body fluids

### OUTCOME

Fluid balance will be maintained as evidenced by postoperative pulses equivalent to preoperative level, hourly urine output of at least 30 ml, and good skin turgor.

### INTERVENTIONS

- Determine the availability of replacement blood or blood products.
- Assist with the insertion of intravenous (IV) lines and fluid replacement therapy. Keep IV lines patent.
- Estimate blood loss on sponges and drapes; communicate to anesthesia provider and surgeon.
- Initiate autotransfusion or use of cell saver as required.
- Record the amount of irrigation used.
- Document the contents of the suction canisters.
- Monitor and document hourly urine output (as applicable); communicate results of measurements.
- Collaborate with the collection and interpretation of intraoperative blood analyses.

### NURSING DIAGNOSIS

**Risk for Impaired Skin Integrity and Ineffective Tissue Perfusion** related to surgical positioning, presence of vascular disease, and vascular clamping

### OUTCOME

Skin integrity will be maintained. Skin temperature and color will be within normal limits. No skin injury lesions will be evident, and the electrosurgery unit (ESU) dispersive pad site will be intact.

### INTERVENTIONS

- Assess and document the patient's preoperative skin condition and tissue perfusion.
- Position the patient on a pressure-reducing mattress on the operating room (OR) bed.
- Collaborate with anesthesia provider in modifications of surgical position required for access to airway and monitoring devices.
- Keep OR bed sheets dry and wrinkle-free.
- Pad all bony prominences.
- Maintain body alignment.
- Place restraining straps snugly but not tightly.
- Protect vulnerable neurovascular bundles from compression.
- Monitor and record tissue perfusion (color, temperature, pulses) as required.
- Elevate drapes off the patient's toes; use appropriate positioning accessories.
- Implement safety precautions for proper use of ESU.
- Reassess and document the patient's postoperative skin condition and tissue perfusion.

and blood pressure changes. Acid-base balance and pulmonary gas exchange are assessed from the ABG analysis.

A central venous pressure (CVP) catheter or pulmonary artery (PA) catheter may be inserted, usually by way of the right internal jugular vein. The CVP line allows assessment of blood volume and vascular tone. The PA catheter (e.g., Swan-Ganz) monitors cardiac output, fluid balance, and the cardiac response to drugs. PA catheters are commonly used for patients undergoing aortic surgery or for patients with cardiac disease.

TEE may be used to monitor the heart noninvasively during aortic surgery. The device looks similar to a bronchoscope and can be passed down the esophagus to provide an ultrasonic image. The cardiac structures, blood flow, wall motion, and great vessels can be observed. Use of TEE requires highly skilled personnel and may not be available in all surgical settings.

Electroencephalography (EEG) monitoring is used for patients undergoing a carotid endarterectomy and allows for immediate observation of the slowing of brain waves caused by cerebral ischemia or reduced perfusion. The surgeon may elect to place a temporary shunt in the artery if this occurs during clamping, potentially reducing the chances of perioperative stroke.

A urinary catheter should be inserted, especially if the proposed procedure involves the renal arteries or clamping of the aorta above the renal arteries; if considerable blood loss is anticipated; if the planned procedure time is lengthy; or whenever spinal or epidural anesthesia is used, because they delay the patient's ability to void voluntarily. Urinary catheterization facilitates accurate hourly measurements of urine during and after the surgical procedure and assists in the assessment of renal perfusion and fluid status.

***Positioning.*** Positioning of the patient undergoing vascular surgery is of particular importance because of restricted circulation distal to the area of arterial obstruction and a generalized state of poor circulation. Particular care must be exercised in positioning elderly patients (see Chapter 30). Awareness of joint range-of-motion limitations attributable to immobility or joint surgery is critical even for a procedure as routine as Foley catheter insertion. Again, preoperative assessment can prevent injury and decrease OR time. Whenever possible, the perioperative nurse should have the patient demonstrate the ability to assume the position for the proposed procedure while the patient is awake and able to provide feedback. A footboard may be applied to the OR bed to prevent the weight of drapes resting on the patient's lower extremities. A head support may be used to position the head. A roll may be placed between the scapulae. For surgical procedures involving a lower extremity, the patient's thigh may be externally rotated and abducted with the knee flexed. A small bolster may be used under the knee to support the patient's leg. Proper skeletal alignment during surgery prevents injury to the neuromuscular system. Attention to the skin overlying bony prominences, especially the heels, sacrum, and elbows, and the use of proper supports and pads prevent pressure and potential positioning injury to the patient.[18] If the procedure will be lengthy, a pressure-reducing mattress or pad can be placed on the OR bed to help prevent patient injury. For the same reasons, members of the surgical team should also be cognizant of heavy instruments and drapes resting on the patient's body and take measures to avoid pressure injuries. After the patient has been positioned, the ESU dispersive pad is then applied.

***Skin Preparation and Draping.*** Skin preparation for vascular surgery may be extensive. Hair should be removed preoperatively only if it interferes with the procedure; if hair removal is necessary, it should be done immediately before the surgical procedure using clippers, not a razor.[5] For abdominal aortic surgery, the patient's skin is prepped from the nipple line to the midthigh area. For peripheral vascular surgery on the lower extremities, the patient is prepped from the umbilicus to the feet. The patient's legs are prepped circumferentially. For carotid surgery, the patient is prepped from the ear and chin on the affected side to below the clavicle. It is important that alcohol-based prep solutions are dry before applying the surgical drapes and starting the surgical procedure.

Draping should permit the surgeon free access to involved areas. For example, abdominal surgery may also require exposure of the groin region for possible exploration of the femoral arteries. A femoral-popliteal bypass on one leg may require access to the other leg for harvesting of the saphenous vein. Impervious drapes should be used to prevent contamination of the surgical field from blood and irrigation fluids.

***Medications and Solutions.*** All medications and solutions on and off the sterile field must be labeled.[10] Heparin is the most common drug used in vascular surgery (Surgical Pharmacology). It may be given as an intravenous (IV) bolus by the anesthesia provider to provide systemic anticoagulation to the patient. When administered parenterally, it has a rapid onset of action and peaks in minutes. It has a 2- to 6-hour duration. Because it is metabolized in the liver and excreted by the kidneys, the effects of heparin may be prolonged in patients with liver and renal disease. The anticoagulant effects may be monitored by measurement of the activated partial thrombo-

## SURGICAL PHARMACOLOGY

### Heparin—A High-Alert Medication

Heparin sodium is an anticoagulant that interferes with blood coagulation by blocking conversion of prothrombin to thrombin and fibrinogen to fibrin. It has no effect on a blood clot that has already formed or on ischemic tissue injured as a result of inadequate blood supply caused by a clot.

It is considered a high-alert drug, so designated by the Joint Commission on Accreditation of Healthcare Organizations (JCAHO) and the Institute for Safe Medication Practices (ISMP) because, if administered incorrectly, it may cause life-threatening or permanent harm to the patient.

It is used for prophylaxis and/or treatment of vascular thromboembolic disorders, such as venous thrombosis and peripheral arterial embolism, and for prevention of thromboembolus during vascular surgical procedures. The number of units per milliliter varies in available dosage forms (supplied in vials). The most often used form is 5000 units/ml. One milligram of heparin is the equivalent of 100 units. Heparin may be administered by the anesthesia provider as an intravenous medication, administered by the surgeon as a full-strength injection during certain vascular procedures, or prepared as an irrigating solution by the scrub person. Standardized practices in the operating room (OR) should be used to reduce the risk of an adverse drug event from the administration of anticoagulants such as heparin.

*Sound-alike caution:* Hespan (institutions should identify and at a minimum annually review look-alike/sound-alike drugs to prevent errors involving the interchange of such drugs)

*Labeling requirements:* Any medication container, such as a syringe, medicine cup, or basin, containing heparin or a heparin solution must be labeled whether it is on or off the sterile field in perioperative or other procedural settings. Labels should be verified by two qualified individuals if the person preparing the medication is not the person administering it; this may be the case during relief of OR personnel.[10]

Modified from *Drug information handbook for perioperative nursing,* Hudson, Ohio, 2006, Lexi-Comp, Inc; Feix J: *Pharmacology handbook for the surgical technologist,* New York, 2005, Thomson Delmar Learning; Lilley LL and others: *Pharmacology and the nursing process,* ed 4, St Louis, 2005, Mosby.

plastin time (APTT) or partial thromboplastin time (PTT). Patients are given anticoagulants just before the placement of a vascular clamp to prevent a thromboembolic event. Systemic heparin may or may not need to be reversed at the end of the surgical procedure. Monitoring the activated clotting time (ACT) intraoperatively provides useful data for judging the need for reversal or additional heparin. Heparin can be reversed by protamine sulfate.

Since protamine sulfate is derived from fish sperm and testes, caution is advised when administering it to patients who are allergic to fish or who have received protamine-containing insulin. One milligram of protamine neutralizes 100 mg of heparin. The dose should be calculated to offset half of the last dose of heparin. Protamine must be given slowly, at a maximum of 50 mg in 10 minutes, or it may cause dyspnea, flushing, bradycardia, and severe hypotension. Another reason for monitoring heparin is that protamine, given in the absence of circulating heparin, acts as an anticoagulant and could delay hemostasis intraoperatively.

Heparinized saline solution is often used during vascular surgery for irrigation. It may be used to irrigate a blood vessel lumen during surgery, usually after the patient has been systemically heparinized. It is also commonly used to flush the lumen of tubes used to shunt blood. The probable mechanism is twofold—by creating a negative charge on the tubing wall and by interfering with platelet adherence. The strength of the heparin solution will vary according to the manufacturer's recommendations for certain implant devices or by the surgeon's preference. A reasonable range is 250 to 1000 units in 250 ml of normal saline.

Surgical preferences differ regarding solutions with which to distend, irrigate, or store vein grafts. Some surgeons prefer a cold solution to decrease the metabolic demands of the vessel, whereas others believe this may lead to spasm. Spasm may be of particular concern when working with the small vessels of the distal leg or foot. Papaverine HCl may be added to a heparinized saline solution for its direct antispasmodic effect on the smooth muscle of the vessel wall and for its vasodilating properties. A reasonable dose is 120 mg in 250 ml of saline. The pressure of a handheld syringe to distend vein grafts has been viewed as a potential cause of graft failure or graft stenosis because this causes endothelial damage. Papaverine HCl, as a smooth muscle relaxant, allows distention at a lower pressure and may decrease the risk of injury. Concentrations for infiltration range from 0.05 to 0.6 mg/ml, or 12.5 to 150 mg per 250 ml of solution.

Topical hemostatic agents may be needed. Absorbable hemostatics are effective by creating an environment that promotes the adhesion of platelets. For example, an absorbable gelatin sponge, such as Gelfoam, may be applied to a bleeding surface to provide a matrix into which clots form. It may be applied dry, moistened with saline, or soaked in a topical thrombin-saline solution. One hundred to two thousand NIH units of thrombin per 1 ml of saline or blood may be applied to control bleeding.

Infections of prosthetic vascular grafts are rare but are extremely serious. Infection may be life threatening for patients with aortic grafts or may be limb threatening in lower extremity procedures. Protecting the prosthetic graft from contact with the skin is essential to prevent bacterial contamination. Prophylactic IV antibiotics, using an appropriate antibiotic that provides coverage for any likely organisms to be encountered in the procedure, should be administered within 1 hour before the surgical incision.[7] In some institutions, medical staff–approved protocols are available for selection of the appropriate antibiotic.

***Vascular Prostheses.*** Vascular grafting materials and techniques are of major importance to the field of vascular surgery for bypass procedures and reconstruction. The understanding, study, and comparison of new prosthetic grafts; utilization and preparation of autogenous grafts; and knowledge of long-term patency rates are critical to improving patient outcomes. Grafts are made in various sizes and configurations; they may be conduits that are straight, tapered, or in the shape of a Y, called bifurcated; or they may be pieces of material cut for use as a patch. The arteriotomy of a CEA may be closed primarily or with a patch of either vein or synthetic fabric. In aortic surgery, a straight tube or a bifurcated synthetic graft is used. Dacron (polyester) grafts are the usual choice and have been used successfully for many years. Large vessels, such as the aorta, have high flow rates and thus have a low incidence of thrombus formation and excellent graft-patency rate. The search for the ideal vascular graft continues. Desired characteristics are that they are reasonably priced, readily available in a variety of sizes, suitable for use anywhere in the body, biocompatible and hypoallergenic, and able to survive repeated sterilizations. The surgeon's preference would also include ease of handling, that is, elastic, easy to sew, and nonfraying. An implanted graft should last a lifetime and permit blood passage without clotting or infection.

Prosthetic grafts are nonantigenic; tissue incorporates well, which helps prevent infection, and such grafts generally resist thrombosis. For years, knitted polyester grafts were preferred over woven polyester because they were easier to handle, although they had to be preclotted because of their high porosity. Woven grafts are somewhat stronger and bleed less through the fabric interstices but can be less flexible. Newer grafts have been developed to incorporate the best of both by using velour polyester. They are also being impregnated with albumin, collagen, or gelatin to provide ease in handling without the need to preclot. Preclotting is usually accomplished by submerging the graft into a basin containing a small quantity of the patient's own blood collected before systemic heparinization. This makes the graft impervious by allowing fibrin to fill in the fabric spaces.

The other popular prosthetic material is polytetrafluoroethylene (PTFE), which is available in straight, tapered, and bifurcated styles of varying lengths and may have external support rings to prevent compression. These grafts do not stretch, and needle-hole bleeding may be troublesome.

Human allografts were tried in the 1950s for aortic replacement but ultimately failed because of thrombosis, calcification, or aneurysm development. Human umbilical cord vein grafts and cryo-preserved saphenous vein grafts are commercially available for patients who have no veins available because of previous bypass procedures, saphenous vein stripping, or poor quality or size of available veins. Manufacturers' instructions must be followed to rid these grafts of preservative by being rinsed.

Volumes have been written on vascular grafts, and the reader should consider this chapter an introduction only. The American National Standards Institute (ANSI), the U.S. Food and Drug Administration (FDA), and the Association for the Advancement of Medical Instrumentation (AAMI) are a few of the organizations active in setting standards and regulating usage and development of grafts.

Autogenous vein grafting for infrainguinal bypass is considered the criterion standard. Undamaged endothelial cells inhibit the clotting mechanism by the natural release of fibrinolytic substances and plasminogen factors. Two methods of grafting veins have been extensively studied, and the results are not totally conclusive that one method is better than the other. These are the in situ graft and the reversed vein graft. The in situ method leaves the vein in its place, side branches are ligated to prevent arteriovenous fistulas, and the valves that would impede arterial flow are disrupted with instruments specifically designed to cut valves, called *valvulotomes* (Figure 26-6). Re-operation is more frequent with the in situ method because of missed valves and residual arteriovenous fistulas. Reversal of a vein graft is performed per the surgeon's preference or when it must be harvested from the contralateral limb. Vein grafts are used in below-knee (BK) bypass procedures. Above-knee (AK) bypasses may use PTFE or other synthetic grafts for vein sparing, or they may be used in high-risk patients who may not tolerate the longer vein harvesting or have a life expectancy of less than 3 years. *Atraumatic* clamps with rubber, plastic, or hydrostatic jaw clamps are used to protect vein grafts from injury. Distal bypasses, particularly those in persons with diabetes, are more successful today as a result of improved tissue handling. The pneumatic tourniquet as an alternative to clamping the vessels may also be considered by the surgeon.

***Sutures.*** Most vascular sutures are made of synthetic nonabsorbable materials, such as Dacron, polyester, PTFE, and polypropylene. Vascular sutures have swaged-on needles of various sizes and are available in sizes 0 to 10-0. The suture may be single-armed or double-armed (i.e., a needle on one or both ends). The size and curve of the needle depend on the vessel and its location. Teflon felt or leftover pieces of graft material (synthetic or vein) may be used as pledgets or buttresses under a suture. They are used when tissue is friable to keep the suture from tearing through or when an anastomosis leaks and needs a better seal. The pledget may be loaded onto the vascular suture or added by the surgeon to a suture already in use. The pledget remains on the suture line (Figure 26-7).

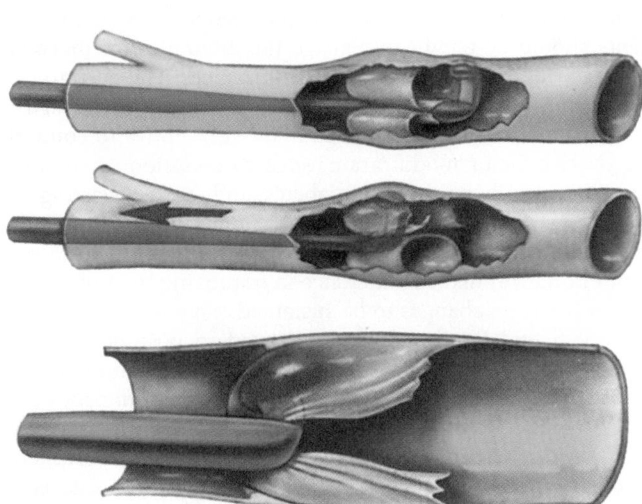

**FIGURE 26-6** Valve incision with valvulotome.

***Vascular Monitoring Equipment.*** Assessing blood flow through diseased vessels by palpation is often difficult. Physical assessment of the patient's hemodynamic status during surgery can be further complicated by spasm of the vessel walls, the cool environment of the OR, and alterations in blood pressure caused by hemorrhage. Therefore the surgeon often uses vascular monitoring equipment to evaluate tissue perfusion and flow. The Doppler device is critical when pulses cannot be palpated. With a coupling gel, the unsterile Doppler probe can be placed on the patient's skin distal to the surgical site. Some probes can be sterilized and used directly in the surgical wound to assess the flow in an arterial graft or determine whether the blood supply to the intestines or other structures is intact after aortic surgery. Besides providing an audible signal, the Doppler probe can provide a permanent record of the sound if a recorder is attached. The unit is inexpensive and easily transported. Perioperative nurses can similarly use the Doppler probe after minimal training.

An EEG accurately determines reduced cerebral perfusion during a CEA. This enables the surgeon to decide whether to use a temporary shunt in the carotid artery or if the patient can tolerate clamping. Sterile IV tubing connected to an arterial transducer can also be used to check pressure gradients intraoperatively. Stump pressure of unclamped carotid arteries before thromboendarterectomy can also determine the need for intraoperative shunting. Trained personnel are necessary to operate this equipment.

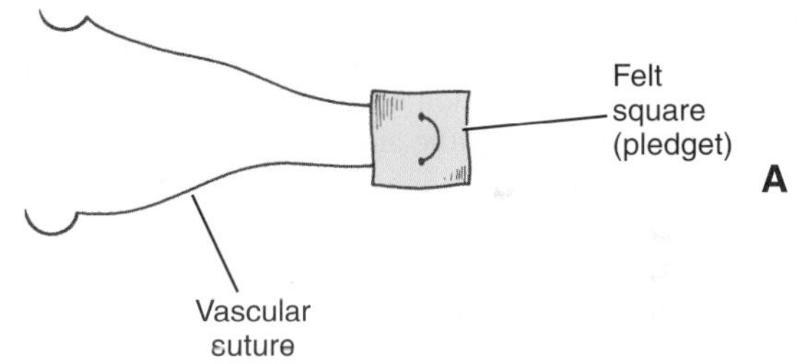



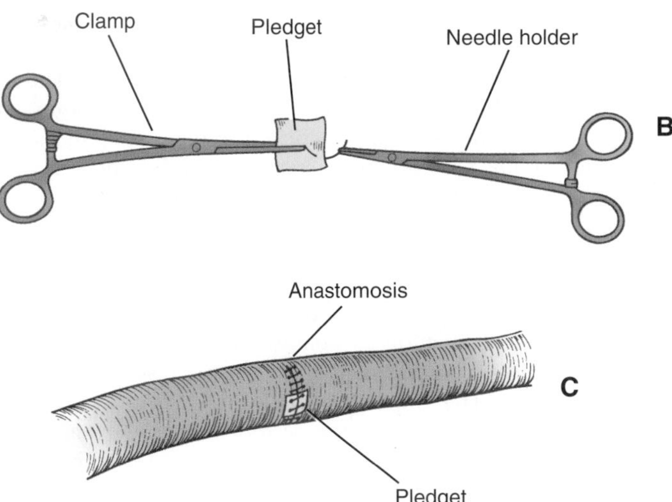



**FIGURE 26-7** Pledgeted suture. **A,** Double-armed vascular suture prepared with pledget. **B,** Technique for surgeon to add pledget to suture already in use. **C,** Appearance of suture line with pledget in place.

***Instrumentation.*** Most vascular procedures begin with a basic laparotomy set for scissors, clamps, and retractors and a vascular set. Items specific to each surgical procedure are then added. For abdominal surgery, a large self-retaining retractor (e.g., Omni-Tract, Thompson, Bookwalter) should be added. Additional individually wrapped, sterile aortic clamps, some long clamps (cystic duct and right angle), and long forceps for larger patients should be available in the OR. Smaller vascular clamps and vascular bulldog clamps should also be kept sterile in the operating room. For peripheral procedures, a variety of Weitlaner self-retaining retractors should be available. Carotid surgery requires carotid shunt clamps, shunts, microforceps, and dissectors for peeling plaque from the artery. One may use the saphenous vein as a graft conduit by removing and reversing it or by using it in situ. A variety of instruments are available for disrupting the valves to permit arterial flow in the in situ procedure. Amputations do not require vascular instrumentation. A minor basic set and appropriately sized bone instruments are needed.

***Documentation.*** During the implementation of perioperative nursing care, documentation of patient problems and nursing actions addressing these identified problems is important. Every patient is identified and assessed for allergies; the surgical procedure is verified; and any other interventions performed by the nurse for patient safety and mandated by institution policy are documented. A brief mental status assessment is especially important for vascular patients who are at risk for stroke. For a patient undergoing vascular surgery, documentation may include the preoperative and postoperative assessment of the integrity of the patient's skin, the presence or absence of peripheral pulses, the surgical position and positioning devices used, fluid intake and output, and the achievement of patient goals. During surgery, various local anesthetic drugs and irrigating solutions, such as thrombin, antibiotic, and heparin solutions, may be used. Each medication or solution container should be labeled with the medication name, strength, amount (if not apparent from the container), expiration date (if not used within 24 hours), and expiration time (if that occurs in less than 24 hours). Labels should be verified by two qualified individuals if the person preparing the medication is not the person administering it.[10] The circulating nurse maintains an accurate record of the solutions used and the amounts administered. The recording of ischemic times is captured when vascular clamps are applied and removed from arteries. The type, size, and serial and lot numbers of vascular implants should be documented according to institutional policy and procedure.

## Evaluation

Evaluation is an ongoing process during which the perioperative nurse determines the extent to which the patient goals are met. Patient evaluation is continuous as the perioperative nurse assesses, observes, and appraises the results of nursing interventions. The conclusion of the intraoperative phase is the transfer of the care of the peripheral vascular patient to colleagues in the postanesthesia care unit (PACU) or the intensive care unit (ICU). A nursing hand-off report should be given, which includes identification of the patient, the surgical procedure performed, any allergies or special needs, and the achievement of patient outcomes. If the patient is awake, introduce the patient to the PACU nurse.[20]

Some of the desired patient outcomes are achieved at the end of the intraoperative phase of surgical patient care. Others require ongoing evaluation during the postoperative phase. Because perioperative nursing practice is collaborative, the perioperative nurse develops a plan of care that extends from the admission to the surgical suite through safe recovery from surgery. Goals that can be measured are measured immediately on discharge from the OR; others require the collaboration of the PACU or unit nurse for final evaluation. The perioperative nurse thus develops and contributes to a comprehensive, holistic plan of patient care. Such planning and measurement of outcomes provide evidence of quality patient care and provide a mechanism of communication and continuity of care with other health care professionals.

Outcomes identified for the stated nursing diagnoses could be stated as follows:

- The patient verbalized an understanding of the surgical procedure and routines. All questions were answered to the patient's satisfaction. The patient appeared calmer as evidenced by facial expression and other body language.
- The patient's temperature remained within normal limits.
- The patient's fluid balance was maintained. Intake and output were documented.
- The patient's skin remained intact, with no lesions or reddened areas; skin color, temperature, and turgor were adequate.

## Patient and Family Education and Discharge Planning

All surgical patients need basic instruction on care of their wounds, identification of the signs and symptoms of infection, review of medications (Patient Safety), follow-up appointments, and a way to contact health care providers. Proper handwashing should be reviewed and emphasized to prevent wound infection. Patients who have undergone a lower-extremity arterial bypass are most interested in information that will assist them in recognizing, preventing, and managing complications. They need instruction on incisional care and bathing to optimize incisional healing. Many have had experience with slow healing of wounds because of their arterial disease. Pain, sleep disturbances, and fatigue have been identified as important areas for instruction. Patients are often capable of identifying their discharge learning needs in the preoperative period. Patients should be taught to manage the discomfort of incisions and leg swelling to prevent sleep disturbances. The need to balance activity and rest should be emphasized. Patients in the immediate postoperative period are often receptive to counseling on risk-factor modification, such as cessation of smoking and control of hypertension, diabetes, and stress. Assisting the patient in setting realistic goals without overwhelming demands is usually most productive. Patients must believe that their efforts will make a difference in improving their quality of life for life-style changes to be sustained.

Patient and family education related to postoperative activities and discharge planning for vascular procedures varies. Following an integrated care pathway improves efficiency and length of stay. Major vascular procedures, such as the resection of an AAA, have different educational concerns than peripheral vascular surgery. Patient and family education and discharge teaching for various procedures are presented in the Patient and Family Education box.

## PATIENT SAFETY

### Teaching the Patient Going Home on Anticoagulant Therapy

Anticoagulant therapy is prescribed to prevent the formation of blood clots. The time a patient remains on anticoagulant therapy depends on the underlying condition for which it is prescribed. It can be of short duration or lifelong. The patient and family or other caregiver should be provided with both verbal and written instructions. These should include the condition requiring anticoagulation therapy, reasons and benefits of therapy, name of the anticoagulant prescribed, dosage, time of administration and side effects, importance of follow-up monitoring, compliance issues, potential for any drug interactions, and safety precautions. After instructing the patient and family member or other caregiver, they should "teach back" information in their own words. In this way, the nurse can verify their understanding. Additional helpful information to provide includes the following:

- Use only an electric razor or hair removal cream; do not use a straight razor.
- Take precautions to avoid injury. For example, do not use tools such as saws or hammers, where an accident can occur. Avoid contact sports and other hazardous activities that can increase the risk of tissue injury.
- Report any signs and symptoms of bleeding, such as excessive bleeding from cuts; blood in urine, stool, or vomit; nosebleeds; bleeding from the gums; excessive menstrual bleeding; unusual bruising for unknown reasons; a change in mental status; dizziness; severe headache; or blurred vision.
- Take the prescribed dose of medication at the precise time it is prescribed to be taken.
- Do not stop taking the medication abruptly; the surgeon usually tapers this medication gradually.
- Carry or wear a Medic-Alert bracelet or tag, and carry information in your wallet naming the specific medication.
- Avoid eating foods high in vitamin K, such as tomatoes, dark leafy vegetables, bananas, and fish.
- In the event of a missed dose, do not make up for any missed dose or double up on doses. Call your physician if you are unsure about what to do in the event of a missed dose.

Modified from Blach DE, Ignatavicius DD: Interventions for clients with vascular problems. In Ignatavicius DD, Workman ML, editors: *Medical-surgical nursing: critical thinking for collaborative care*, St Louis, 2006, Saunders; Canobbio MM: *Mosby's handbook of patient teaching*, ed 3, St Louis, 2006, Mosby; Lilley LL and others: *Pharmacology and the nursing process*, ed 4, St Louis, 2005, Mosby.

## PATIENT AND FAMILY EDUCATION

**ABDOMINAL AORTIC ANEURYSM RESECTION**

Postoperative care procedures include the following:

- Intubation and ventilation continue for 12 hours (varies with setting and surgeon preference).
- Cardiac, respiratory, and renal function is monitored.
- Nothing-by-mouth (NPO) status and nasogastric tube are maintained until bowel signs and flatus return; diet is advanced as tolerated.
- Lower-extremity perfusion is assessed hourly.
- Pain is assessed, and pain relief is by means of epidural and/or patient-controlled analgesia (PCA); provide periods of rest.
- Patient is on bed rest but out of bed on postoperative day 1 and ambulating on postoperative day 2.

Discharge planning education includes the following:

- Reassure the patient that feelings of fatigue are normal and take weeks to resolve.
- Incision care: showering is permitted; use soap and water only, and pat dry. Protect incision from oils, lotions, and powder. If Steri-Strips are in place, showering is permitted. The strips will peel away in about 5 to 7 days.
- Activity is allowed with specific restrictions per surgeon:
  - Avoid lifting over 5 to 10 pounds for 6 weeks to allow abdominal healing.
  - Walk to increase strength and improve circulation; progress gradually.
  - Climb stairs and walk out-of-doors as desired.
  - Avoid sitting for more than 1 or 2 hours.
  - Avoid crossing legs.
  - Driving requires permission from surgeon, usually after first office visit and when patient is no longer taking pain medication.
- Smokers should be counseled about the profound effect of smoking on vascular disease and wound healing.
- Review all medications and any dietary recommendations.
- Antibiotics may be prescribed before any endoscopy procedures, surgery, or dental procedures.
- Instruct patient in foot care.
- Notify surgeon of the following: changes in wound (e.g., redness, swelling, increased tenderness, bleeding, drainage), fever, change in bowel habits.

**ENDOVASCULAR ABDOMINAL AORTIC ANEURYSM REPAIR**

Postoperative care procedures include the following:

- Transfer from operating room (OR) to postanesthesia care unit (PACU).
- Monitor cardiac, respiratory, and renal function.
- Peripheral pulse is checked every 15 minutes for 1 hour, every hour ×4, every 2 hours ×4, and then every 4 hours (in general).
- Checks are done for the presence of abdominal or back pain, sensation, and movement in lower extremities.
- Pain control is given as ordered (encourage patient to request pain medication).
- Within 2 hours, patient is transferred to a general unit.
- Patient advances from clear liquid to regular diet the first evening after surgery. Patient is NPO after midnight for ultrasound examination on day 2, with regular diet resumed after the examination.
- Patient ambulates gradually three times on day 1 (within 4 to 6 hours after surgery) and ambulates at will on day 2.
- Discharge to home is generally on day 2.

Discharge planning includes the following:

- Showers are okay but no soaking in tub.
- Sex is okay as comfortable, with no restrictions.
- Patient cannot drive until cleared by physician.
- No lifting more than 5 pounds is allowed for 6 weeks.
- It is okay to use soap and water on sterile wound closure tapes (Steri-Strips), which will gradually fall off.
- It is okay to take stairs.

*Continued*

PATIENT AND FAMILY EDUCATION—cont'd

**ARTERIAL RECONSTRUCTIVE PROCEDURES OF THE LOWER EXTREMITY**

Patient and family education and discharge planning include the following:

- Explain importance of control of diabetes and hypertension.
- Stress importance of smoking cessation.
- Teach signs and symptoms of graft failure; teach patient and family to assess pulses.
- Teach foot care and protection:
  - Inspect daily (use mirror-assistive methods, or have family member help).
  - Observe for cracks, ulcers, blisters, rashes, or discoloration.
  - Trim nails properly for prevention of ingrown toenails.
  - Shoes must fit properly (avoid walking barefoot).
  - Avoid tight socks or hose.
- Explain incisional care.
- Teach proper use and application of Ace wraps for leg swelling (normal after surgery).
- Discuss pain management, sleep disruption, fatigue.
- Driving with surgeon's approval is allowed after follow-up office visit (approximately 2 weeks postoperatively).
- No heavy lifting, vigorous exercise, or prolonged upright sitting is allowed; walking, stair climbing, and going out-of-doors are permissible as able.
- Gentle range-of-motion exercise of leg prevents flexion contractures.
- Showering is permitted.
- Diet: resume previous diet, review special diets with patient (e.g., diabetic, low salt, low fat); reinforce role of adequate nutrition in wound healing.
- Notify surgeon of the following: return of preoperative symptoms; wound changes (e.g., redness, swelling, drainage, pain); fever; change in color, temperature, sensation, or use of leg, foot, or toes.
- Antibiotics may be recommended before any dental or endoscopic procedures if a synthetic graft was implanted.

**CAROTID ENDARTERECTOMY**

- Teach patient about possibility of reperfusion headaches (patients may fear that they are having recurrent symptoms unless they know about this possibility).
- Explain that if there are no postoperative complications, discharge to home will occur within 24 to 48 hours after surgery.
- Explain that activity may return to normal as tolerated and driving may be resumed when neck discomfort no longer restricts range of motion and the surgeon has examined patient 2 weeks postoperatively.
- Explain that fatigue for 4 to 6 weeks after surgery is normal.
- Explain incision care: keep incision clean and dry, may shower with transparent dressing in place. Remove transparent dressing in 3 or 4 days. Wash incision with soap and water; pat gently to dry. Avoid the use of powder and lotion. Do not shave over incision until it is well healed.
- Explain that numbness around the incision and extending to the ear is normal, as well as mild swelling.
- Teach the patient about any cranial nerve deficits that he or she may experience as a result of manipulation of nerves during surgery. Assist the patient in understanding the difference between an intraoperative stroke and cranial nerve deficits; that is, nerve injury or trauma from surgical manipulation occurs on the same side as surgery except for eye symptoms. Use diagrams and pictures to review pertinent anatomy.
- Encourage relevant life-style changes as indicated, that is, low-cholesterol diet, review of diabetic diet, smoking cessation.
- Teach the patient and family to observe for and report any new symptoms, transient ischemic attacks (TIAs), mental-status changes, personality changes, or speech difficulties.
- If a synthetic patch is in place, explain that the patient will need antibiotics before dental procedures or scope procedures. Instruct the patient to notify dentists and other health care providers of this need.
- Explain that if a vein was used for a patch, occasional swelling in the leg may occur. If this occurs, elevate leg above the level of the heart. Swelling may take 4 to 6 weeks to completely resolve.

**VENA CAVA FILTER INSERTION (INFERIOR VENA CAVAL INTERRUPTION)**

Postoperative patient teaching for vena cava filter insertion includes the following:

- For a femoral vein insertion site, do not bend leg for about 8 hours.
- Avoid strenuous activity or lifting more than 5 pounds.
- Expect that bruising of the insertion site may occur because this is common in patients who are or have been receiving anticoagulant therapy.
- Inspect the incision site for bleeding; apply pressure using appropriate method if bleeding at insertion site occurs.
- Report signs of local infection or significant bleeding.
- Elevate affected leg and wear elastic stockings to relieve lower extremity swelling, which may be temporary side effect of the underlying deep venous thrombosis (DVT).
- Understand the purpose of and proper way to wear support stockings.
- Report sudden or severe leg swelling.
- Follow instructions for DVT prophylaxis.[12]

**VARICOSE VEIN SURGERY**

- Provide instruction on the proper way to wrap an Ace bandage, the timing of rest and leg elevation, and how to apply manual pressure if bleeding occurs.
- Walking is permitted, but sitting should be limited as should standing in one place. Legs should be elevated when sitting.

# *Surgical Interventions*

## ABDOMINAL AORTIC ANEURYSM RESECTION

Abdominal aortic aneurysmectomy is surgical obliteration of the aneurysm, which may or may not include the iliac arteries, with insertion of a synthetic prosthesis to reestablish functional continuity. The majority of AAAs begin below the renal arteries (infrarenal), and many extend to involve the bifurcation and common iliac arteries. Severe back pain, along with symptoms of hypotension, shock, and distal vascular insufficiency, usually indicates rupture and represents a true emergency condition. The prime surgical consideration when a rupture occurs is the control of hemorrhage by occlusion of the aorta proximal to the point of rupture. AAAs are usually asymptomatic and are found on routine physical examination. They occur more frequently in men than in women. Aneurysmal disease is caused by a disruption of the tunica media, which structurally weakens the aortic wall. Aneurysmal aortas are found to have a significantly decreased amount of collagen and elastin in the vessel wall. The risk of rupture is estimated at 1% to 2% per year for aneurysms less than 5 cm in diameter; 10% for 5- to 6-cm aneurysms; and 25% or higher for aneurysms larger than 6 cm.[1] Rupture carries less than a 50% mortality rate for patients in stable condition with a contained rupture. Risks from AAA surgery include massive hemorrhage and hypotension, injury to the ureters, renal failure, spinal cord ischemia, and death. Because peripheral vascular disease is a manifestation of a systemic disorder, it is not surprising that patients with aneurysms often have concomitant coronary artery disease. Patients are at risk of myocardial ischemia, myocardial infarction, hypotension, and hypertension. Myocardial infarction is the leading cause of death after AAA repair; therefore it is imperative that a patient with cardiac symptoms or ECG abnormalities have a thorough preoperative cardiac assessment.

The perioperative nurse must be alert to the fact that at the time the aortic clamp is released to permit distal flow, "declamping shock" or severe hypotension may occur. This may be attributable to inadequate volume replacement, the sudden reestablishment of flow to dilated distal vessels, or the release of acidic metabolites. Declamping shock and hemorrhage have been proposed as causes of renal failure from acute tubular necrosis.

### Procedural Considerations

The patient is placed in the supine position. General endotracheal anesthesia is used. A central venous catheter and arterial line are inserted as well as a Foley catheter. The skin is prepped for a midline abdominal incision, and draping is completed to permit access to the groin region for possible exploration of femoral arteries. The pedal pulses should be marked before the beginning of the procedure so that they may be located easily when the surgeon requests a check of the pulses. This assessment of pulses can be done manually or with a Doppler probe.

### Operative Procedure—Transperitoneal Approach

1. The abdomen is opened through a long midline incision (Figure 26-8, *A*) from the xiphoid process to the symphysis pubis. Hemostasis is achieved.
2. An abdominal self-retaining retractor is inserted into the wound. The small bowel, including the duodenum, is retracted to the right; it may be placed outside the abdomen and covered with moist laparotomy packs for better exposure.
3. The retroperitoneum overlying the aneurysm is incised and extended superiorly to expose the aneurysm and also inferiorly over the bifurcation and beyond the iliac arteries. Metzenbaum scissors, smooth forceps, and hemostats are used.
4. Careful blunt and sharp dissection is continued to expose the aorta above the aneurysm to permit placement of an aortic clamp. The renal artery and ureters are avoided. The iliac vessels and bifurcation are inspected for evidence of small aneurysms, thrombosis, and calcification.
5. The patient is given a dose of heparin intravenously, and an aortic clamp such as a DeBakey, Fogarty, or Satinsky is applied and closed. Distal runoff vessels are also clamped. Opening of the aneurysm is undertaken with a scalpel or electrosurgical blade and heavy scissors (Figure 26-8, *B*).
6. The aneurysm is completely opened, and all atheromatous and thrombotic material is removed. The aneurysm walls may be excised but usually are left in place for eventual coverage of the prosthesis. In either case, the posterior aspect of the aorta is left intact (Figure 26-8, *C*). Bleeding is controlled, especially from the lumbar vessels, which enter posteriorly, by oversewing their orifices with vascular suture.
7. A prosthetic graft of appropriate size is prepared for insertion. If the aneurysm does not involve the aortic bifurcation, a straight tubular graft is used; otherwise a bifurcated or Y-shaped graft is necessary. Preclotting of a knitted graft may be accomplished by immersing the graft into a small quantity of the patient's own blood before systemic heparinization or a manufactured graft impregnated with collagen, albumin, or gelatin may be used.
8. The aortic cuff is prepared for anastomosis by irrigating it with heparinized saline solution and by removing all fibrotic plaques. One or two vascular sutures (double-armed) are used to accomplish the anastomosis by a through-and-through continuous suture (Figure 26-8, *D*). Additional interrupted sutures may be needed if the anastomosis leaks on completion. A strip of Teflon felt may be used along the suture line for reinforcement.
9. The distal vessels are opened and inspected for backbleeding, and heparinized saline solution may be injected to prevent clotting.
10. Each limb of the graft is anastomosed to the iliac artery, using a smaller vascular suture and similar technique (Figure 26-8, *E*). After the first side of the anastomosis has been completed, blood is permitted to circulate and the remaining limb of the graft is clamped to prevent leaking during the last part of the anastomosis.
11. The aneurysm may be closed over the graft.
12. The peritoneum is closed to exclude contact of the intestine to the graft.
13. The abdominal wound is closed.

## ENDOVASCULAR ABDOMINAL AORTIC ANEURYSM REPAIR

Endovascular aneurysm repair (EVAR) differs from open surgical repair in that the prosthetic endograft or stent-graft is introduced into the aneurysm through a surgically exposed femoral artery and fixed in place to the nonaneurysmal infrarenal neck and iliac arteries with self-expanding or balloon-expandable stents rather than sutures (Figure 26-9). A major abdominal incision is thus avoided, and patient morbidity related to the procedure is much reduced. The benefits of this procedure are a hospital stay of 1 to 2 days, a rapid return to normal physical activity, and a reduction in the mortality and complication rates compared with those of the conventional surgical procedure. The procedure may also be applicable to high-risk patients.

A number of commercially manufactured stent-grafts have been developed since the first endovascular aneurysm repair was carried out in 1991, using a Dacron graft sutured onto balloon-expandable Palmaz stents. Early tubular grafts have

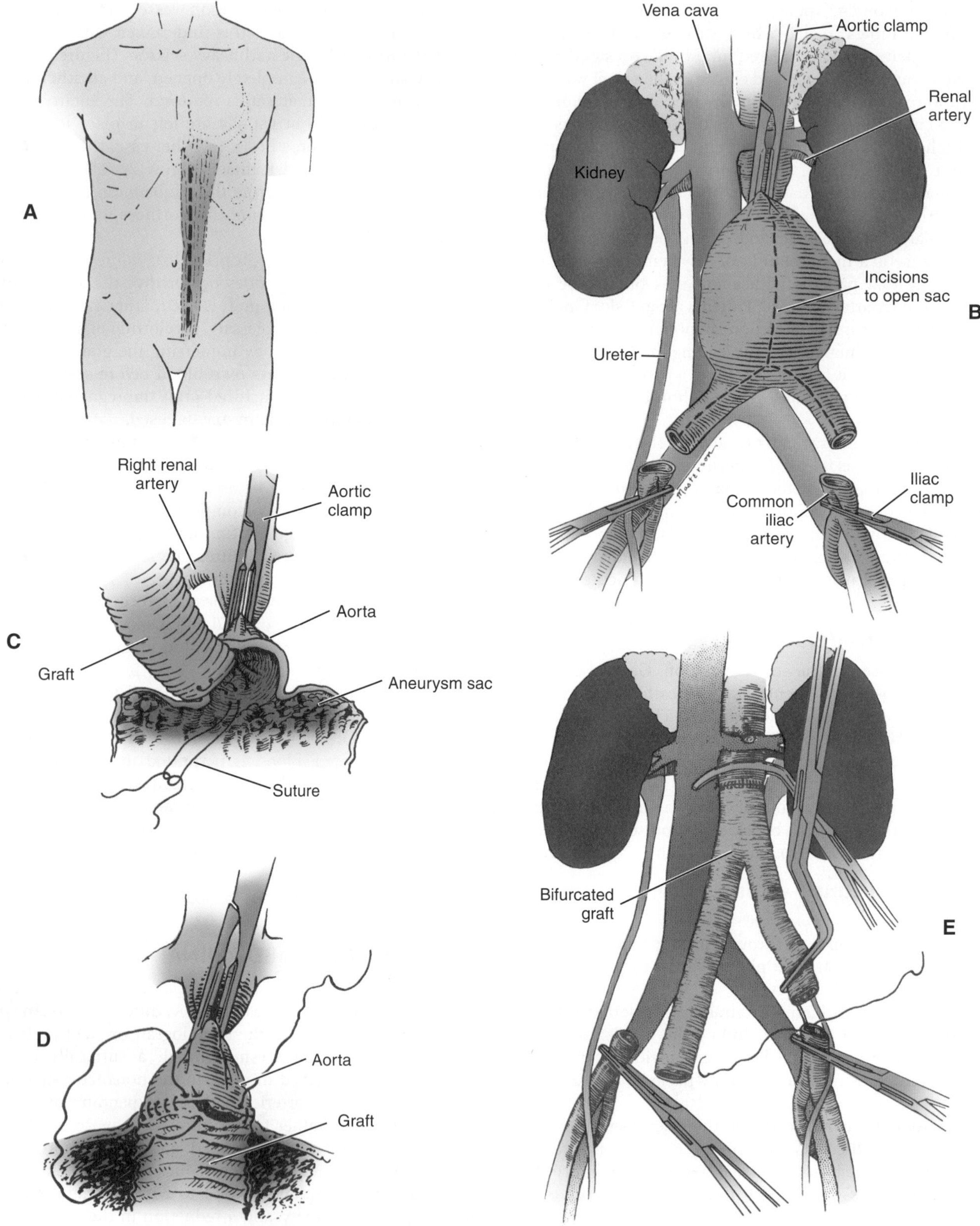


**FIGURE 26-8** Resection of abdominal aortic aneurysm. **A,** Midline abdominal incision. **B,** Aneurysm sac is opened. **C,** Prosthetic graft is sewn to back wall of aorta, creating a cuff. **D,** Completion of aortic graft anastomosis. **E,** Iliac artery anastomosis.

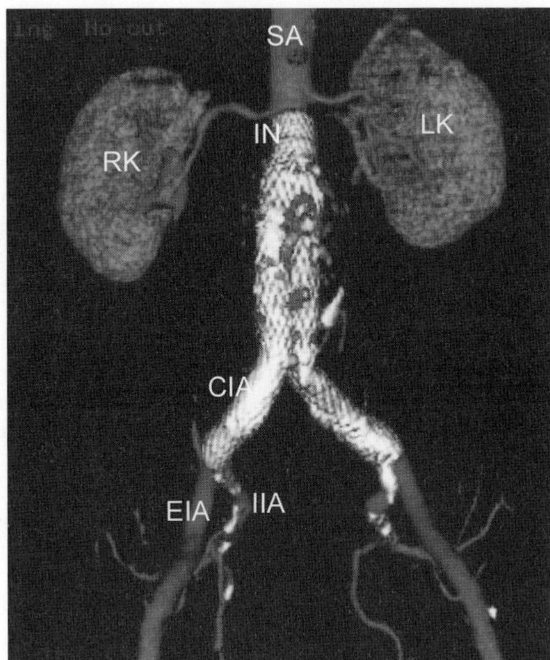


**FIGURE 26-9** Endovascular abdominal aortic aneurysm repair involves aneurysm exclusion with an endoluminal aortic stent-graft introduced remotely, usually through the femoral artery. An endovascular graft extends from the infrarenal aorta to both common iliac arteries, preserving the flow to the internal iliac arteries. *SA*, Suprarenal aorta; *IN*, infrarenal aortic neck; *CIA*, common iliac artery; *EIA*, external iliac artery; *IIA*, internal iliac artery; *RK*, right kidney; *LK*, left kidney.

largely been replaced by modular bifurcated grafts that have expanded the applicability of this therapy. Different graft configurations, depending on the anatomic problem, are available. For patients with an AAA that is limited to the aorta and in whom there is both a neck between the renal arteries and the aneurysm and a neck between the lower portion of the aneurysm and the iliac bifurcation, a graft of tubular configuration is available. For those patients in whom the abdominal aneurysm extends to the iliac bifurcation, a bifurcated or Y-shaped graft is available. For those patients who have both an AAA and an aneurysm of one or both iliac arteries, a tapered tube graft that excludes both the aortic aneurysm and one iliac aneurysm is usually selected. The technical details of endovascular repair vary with each specific device, but the general principles are similar. Candidates for this procedure include patients with a proximal infrarenal neck at least 1 to 2 cm in length and common iliac arteries for proximal and distal fixation of an endograft, without excessive tortuosity and with appropriate iliofemoral access. Long-term follow-up data are ongoing, and the procedure should be undertaken with the understanding that prolonged follow-up with periodic imaging will be required and that reintervention may become necessary. Nonetheless, the future of endoluminal grafting has the potential of significant rewards.

### Procedural Considerations

The patient is placed supine on a radiolucent OR bed with a special marker board. The board has remotely controlled radiopaque cursors that are used to fluoroscopically detect proximal and distal positions for graft deployment. An ample supply of lead gowns needs to be available. The patient may receive a general anesthetic or an epidural anesthetic. If an epidural anesthetic is used, mechanical ventilation is available in case conversion to the traditional surgical procedure is required. A central venous catheter and an arterial catheter are inserted for hemodynamic monitoring. A Foley catheter is inserted, and the patient's abdomen and groin areas are surgically prepped and draped to allow conversion to the traditional surgical technique if necessary.

### Operative Procedure

1. Both common femoral arteries are dissected through small cut downs.
2. After the administration of IV heparin, the right common femoral artery is clamped, an arteriotomy is performed, and an 8-Fr sheath is introduced into the right external iliac artery.
3. The left femoral artery is punctured, and a 12-Fr sheath is placed into the left external iliac artery. An angiocath is inserted, and an arteriogram is obtained to clearly mark the renal arteries and aortic bifurcation. The final length of the device to cover the aorta from the renal arteries to a suitable section of the common iliac arteries is chosen.
4. A snare is introduced into the aorta through the left femoral artery, and a pull wire is introduced into the aorta by way of the right femoral artery. The pull wire is snared above the aortic bifurcation and retracted into the left iliac artery. This step is done to help position the limbs of the graft into the iliac arteries.
5. The grafting device is then inserted into the right femoral artery, advanced into the proximal part of the aorta, and positioned above the aortic bifurcation. Fluoroscopy is used to determine proper position of the stent.
6. The device is exposed by retracting a covering jacket, and the graft limbs are positioned in the iliac arteries. The hooks of the graft become attached to the walls of the aorta and the iliac arteries as the attachment systems are deployed.
7. The balloon on the device is inflated to secure the proximal attachment system to the aorta and the contralateral and ipsilateral systems to the iliac arteries.
8. An arteriogram is obtained to confirm proper positioning and complete exclusion of the AAA. Ideally, the graft is positioned to occlude the inferior mesenteric artery to prevent persistent blood flow within the aneurysmal sac.
9. After all the sheaths are removed, the wounds are typically closed with subcuticular sutures.

## PERCUTANEOUS TRANSLUMINAL ANGIOPLASTY

During the 1990s, the indications for percutaneous transluminal angioplasty (PTA) became more liberal since the effectiveness of PTA of the iliac arteries was well documented. PTA is performed with local anesthesia with minimal sedation, as a day-surgery admission, with significantly less morbidity. Although initially performed only in the common iliac artery for stenosis, PTA is routinely used to treat short-segment occlusions as well as external iliac lesions. Iliac artery PTA may be particularly useful to help improve inflow before a more distal surgical reconstruction.

The use of iliac artery stents has also begun to play an increasing role in the management of patients with aortoiliac occlusive disease. Iliac artery stents are most useful after initial suboptimal results from PTA. Occasionally, however, they are used primarily in the treatment of complex lesions. Overall, reports from numerous series suggest that the results of percutaneous therapies for aortoiliac disease are more favorable for common (versus external) iliac lesions and less favorable for long occlusions as opposed to short stenoses. Stents appear to improve the results of isolated PTA in some situations, but these data are less clear. Five-year patency rates for common iliac PTA are typically in the range of 80% and are notably inferior (50% to 60%) for external iliac disease.

When PTA is not an option, a number of surgical alternatives are available. Depending on the condition of the patient and the patient's pathologic anatomy, the options include aortobifemoral bypass, aortoiliac thromboendarterectomy, axillofemoral bypass, iliofemoral bypass, and femorofemoral bypass.

## FEMORAL-POPLITEAL AND FEMORAL-TIBIAL BYPASS

Femoral-popliteal bypass is the restoration of blood flow to the leg with a graft bypassing the occluded section of the femoral artery. The bypass may be a saphenous vein or straight synthetic graft. The patency of an outflow artery must be demonstrated for a successful bypass procedure. If popliteal patency is doubtful, artery exploration is necessary as the first procedure. Involvement of the popliteal artery may necessitate the exposure and use of the tibial vessels for the lower anastomosis. If this occurs, the procedure could require the use of microvascular instruments and technique.

### Procedural Considerations

The patient is placed in a supine position. The hip is externally rotated and abducted with the knee flexed. Prepping and draping include the entire groin and leg. The instrument setup includes the basic minor and vascular sets, plus the following: Gelpi retractors, Garrett or Weitlaner retractors, a device to tunnel, and supplies and equipment for operative arteriograms.

### Operative Procedures

#### *Exploration of Common Femoral Artery*

1. A vertical incision, extending downward about 3 to 5 inches along the medial aspect of the thigh, is made over the femoral artery below the inguinal area, and a self-retaining retractor is inserted.
2. The common femoral artery is located, and the artery is dissected in both directions for complete exposure.
3. Moist umbilical tapes or vessel loops are passed around the common femoral, the superficial femoral, and the deep femoral arteries.

#### *Exploration of Above-Knee Popliteal Artery*

1. A vertical incision is made along the medial aspect of the lower area of the thigh. If the popliteal artery is diseased, an incision below the knee is necessary to expose the distal popliteal artery.
2. A Weitlaner retractor is used to retract the muscles and expose the artery.
3. The knee is flexed, the popliteal artery is dissected free, and a moist umbilical tape is passed around the popliteal artery. Arteriograms may be performed at this time if doubt exists about the patency of the popliteal artery or distal arterial tree.
4. The saphenous vein is exposed when the femoral and popliteal incisions the length of the thigh are joined or through multiple short incisions along the medial area of the thigh. If the vein is suitable, the necessary length is resected or prepared for in situ grafting. If a prosthesis is used, the length and size are determined and the graft may be preclotted as previously described.
5. The saphenous vein is prepared for use by carefully ligating side branches with fine silk. Finally, because of venous valves, the vein is reversed so that the end originally in the groin is anastomosed to the popliteal artery.
6. For a synthetic graft, the tunneling device is passed beneath the sartorius muscle from the popliteal fossa to the groin.
7. The graft is carefully pulled through the tunnel and positioned to prevent kinks or twists.
8. The patient is given IV heparin before applying a vascular clamp to the femoral artery. An incision is made into the femoral artery with a #11 knife blade and extended with a Potts angulated scissors.
9. The graft is anastomosed to the artery with fine vascular sutures.
10. The knee is flexed, and vascular clamps are placed on the popliteal artery at the site of the distal anastomosis.
11. An incision is made into the popliteal artery as explained for femoral arteriotomy.
12. The graft is sutured to the popliteal (or tibial) artery, and before completion the femoral occluding clamp is momentarily opened to eliminate air and debris.
13. All occluding clamps are removed, and the graft is assessed for anastomotic leaks.
14. The incision is closed as described previously.

## FEMORAL-POPLITEAL BYPASS IN SITU

In situ femoral-popliteal bypass is the restoration of blood flow to the leg, bypassing an occluded portion of the femoral artery with a patient's saphenous vein, which remains in place. The procedure includes incising the venous valves and interrupting the venous tributaries. The adequacy of the patient's saphenous vein may be validated before the surgical procedure by an ultrasound duplex scan. Varicose veins or a previous saphenous vein ligation and stripping are contraindications to the procedure. The advantages of a vein-bypass procedure include increased graft availability and improved patency. A disadvantage is the time-consuming aspect of this technique.

### Procedural Considerations

Valves can be incised with microvascular scissors, a Mills valvulotome, or a leather in situ valve cutter kit. An angioscope may be used to monitor the lysis of valve leaflets.

### Operative Procedure

1. The procedure is similar to that for a femoral-popliteal bypass. The groin incision is extended downward over the course of the saphenous vein. A skin bridge may be left between the groin and the popliteal incisions.

2. The saphenous vein is exposed and divided at its proximal and distal ends. Venous tributaries are occluded with vessel clips, such as hemoclips, or fine nonabsorbable sutures.
3. The valvulotome is passed from below to the top, usually through side branches. The valvulotome is used to incise the internal valve (see Figure 26-6). In angioscopically assisted bypass, valve lysis is done under direct vision.
4. The saphenous vein is distended with heparinized saline, papaverine, or heparinized blood to identify any valvular obstruction or open venous tributary. Another pass of the valve cutter alleviates the obstruction. Open branches of the saphenous vein can also be ligated with vessel clips or fine nonabsorbable sutures.
5. The incompetent saphenous vein is used to bypass the occluded segment of the femoral artery (see steps 8 through 14 of the femoral-popliteal bypass procedure described under "Exploration of Above-Knee Popliteal Artery").

## FEMOROFEMORAL BYPASS

Femorofemoral bypass is an extraanatomic (a route that is outside the normal path) bypass that is performed to restore blood flow to one leg when an inflow procedure is necessary but a major aortic procedure is not desired or surgical risks for the patient are high because of a complicated medical condition or technical problems with the procedure (Figure 26-10). Studies continue to examine the long-term patency rate and outcomes for this patient population (Research Highlight).

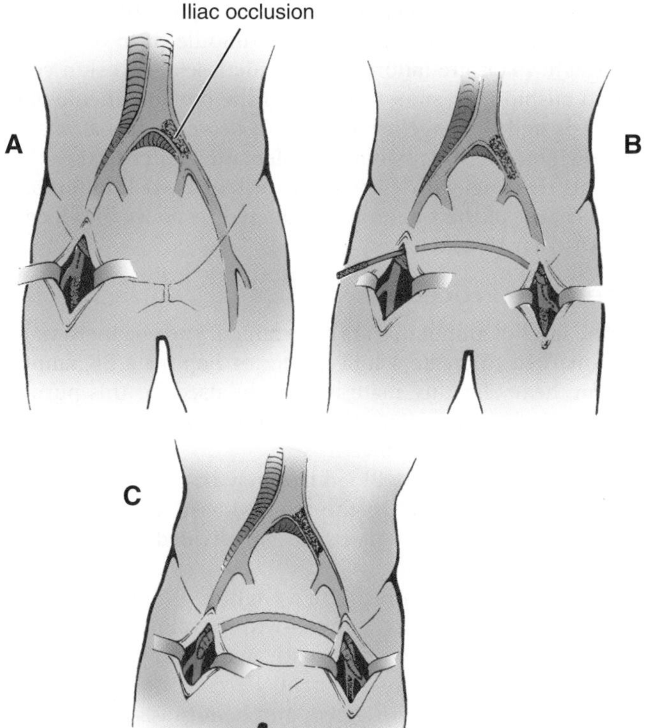


FIGURE 26-10 Femorofemoral bypass to restore blood flow to left leg. **A,** Left iliac artery occlusion and right femoral artery exposure. **B,** Exposure of the right and left femoral arteries: tunneling device creating a path for the graft in the subcutaneous tissue. **C,** Femorofemoral bypass graft in place.

Severe cardiac or pulmonary disease may prevent the patient from undergoing a more extensive procedure. Subcutaneous vascular grafting is an option in these conditions because the procedure bypasses normal vascular anatomy and can be done with local anesthesia with adjunct moderate sedation and analgesia. The patient must have one good iliac artery for inflow for a femorofemoral bypass to be considered. Another extraanatomic procedure that can be done in these instances is an axillofemoral bypass involving the subcutaneous placement of a prosthesis from the axillary artery to the femoral artery on the same side (Figure 26-11).

### Procedural Considerations

The patient is positioned on the OR bed in a supine position. For a femorofemoral bypass, a small pad is placed under each knee. The area prepped for surgery extends from the umbilicus to midthigh area. The genitalia are covered with a sterile towel.

## RESEARCH HIGHLIGHT

### Factors Influencing Long-Term Patency Rates in Femorofemoral Bypass Grafts

Crossover femorofemoral bypass graft (CFFBG) has been used in the past as a last resource for the treatment of critical limb ischemia. This retrospective study looked at a base of 228 patients. Of these patients, 154 patients presented a high surgical risk. The indication for operation was limb-threatening ischemia in 188 patients. All patients underwent CFFBG. The procedure was performed in 150 patients as the primary operation and in 78 patients after previous vascular graft failure or infection or both. Primary and secondary patency rates, as well as limb salvage and survival rates, were reviewed at 5 and 10 years. The researchers concluded that CFFBG allows early and long-term results similar to those obtained with reconstructions originating from the aorta when it is performed as a primary operation, when an adequate outflow is provided, and when externally supported prosthetic material is used.

Modified from Mingoli A and others: Femorofemoral bypass grafts: factors influencing long-term patency rate and outcome, *Surgery* 129(4):451-458, 2001.

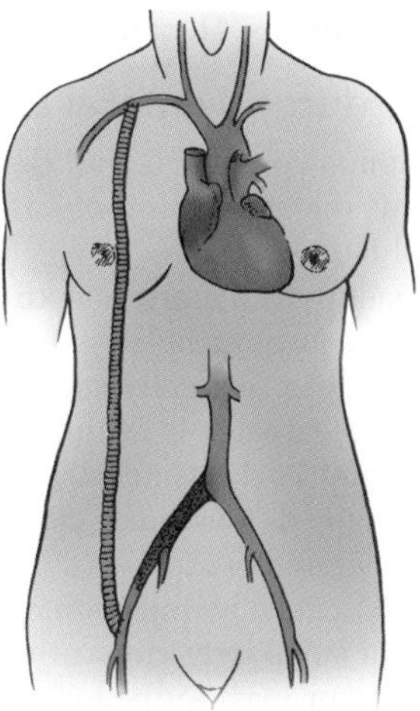

FIGURE 26-11 Axillofemoral bypass graft for right iliac artery occlusion.

### Operative Procedure

1. A longitudinal incision is made over each femoral artery from the inguinal ligament to just below the femoral bifurcation.
2. Each common femoral artery, superficial femoral artery, and deep femoral artery are dissected free, mobilized, and secured with umbilical tapes or vessel loops.
3. The graft tunnel between the two femoral arteries is created across the symphysis pubis in the subcutaneous tissue. This tunnel is created with digital dissection, scissors dissection, or the passage of a clamp or tunneling device across the preperitoneal space.
4. A Dacron or PTFE vascular graft is passed through the subcutaneous tunnel with care to prevent kinking of the graft.
5. The patient receives IV heparin, and vascular clamps are placed on the common femoral, superficial femoral, and deep femoral arteries. A longitudinal arteriotomy is made in the common femoral artery.
6. An end-to-side anastomosis using nonabsorbable vascular sutures is performed to join the graft with the common femoral artery. A similar anastomosis is done on the other side.
7. After the clamps are released and flow is restored, the patient's pulses are checked; the circulating nurse may be asked to assess the patient's feet for warmth and color.
8. The femoral incisions are closed.

## ARTERIAL EMBOLECTOMY

Arterial embolectomy entails an incision made in the affected artery to remove thromboembolic material and restore blood flow. Emboli may be clot particles, a foreign body, air, fat, or a tumor that circulates through the bloodstream and becomes lodged as the vessel decreases in size. More often the direct source is a cardiac mural thrombus, associated with cardiac or vascular disease. Pain or numbness distal to the obstruction is the initial symptom, accompanied by other signs of vascular occlusion, such as pallor and absence of pulses.

### Procedural Considerations

The patient is placed in the supine position, the skin area is prepped, and draping is completed to permit access to the affected area. The instrument setup includes the basic instrument and vascular sets, including Fogarty embolectomy catheters and irrigation catheters. Heparinized saline is required.

### Operative Procedure—Femoral Embolectomy

1. The initial incision is completed, and the artery is carefully exposed to permit the application of vascular clamps (Figure 26-12, *A* and *B*).
2. An incision is made into the artery with a #11 blade and a Potts scissors. A Fogarty catheter is carefully inserted beyond the point of clot proximally and distally. The balloon is inflated, and the catheter is withdrawn along with the detached clot (Figure 26-12, *C* and *D*).
3. As backflow is obtained, a vascular clamp is applied below the arteriotomy (Figure 26-12, *E*).
4. The artery may be flushed by injection of heparinized saline solution through a small irrigating catheter. Angioscopy or an arteriogram may or may not be requested at this time.
5. The arterial closure is completed with vascular sutures (Figure 26-12, *F*). The wound is closed, and dressings are applied.

## AMPUTATION

Amputations involving the lower extremity are performed to eliminate ischemic, gangrenous, necrotic, or infected tissue; relieve pain; and promote maximum independence. Amputations may be necessary because of trauma or malignancy or when the lower limb cannot be salvaged by arterial reconstruction. In the immediate postoperative period, patients may experience phantom limb pain, described as shooting, burning, throbbing, stabbing or squeezing. Phantom limb pain may recur, but less frequently, in the months following surgery.[11]

### Procedural Considerations

It is critical to verify the correct limb for this procedure. Because these are often performed with the patient under regional anesthesia, the perioperative nurse must be sure that the patient does not witness the wrapping or transport of the amputated limb. Toes or partial foot amputations may be done in certain instances, but often a below-knee (BK) or above-knee (AK) amputation is indicated. Syme's amputation, through the ankle, is seldom performed because of improved prosthetics and rehabilitation that favor midcalf amputation. The level is based on the patient's health, level of vascularity, and potential for healing and rehabilitation. Severe infection or toxemia may require amputation as a lifesaving procedure. Operative risks for amputation are higher than for reconstruction, possibly because of more extensive vascular disease. BK amputations are best done at the junction of the upper and middle thirds of the lower leg. This allows for an immediate postoperative prosthesis, aids in better healing, and may reduce phantom limb pain. AK amputations may be at the middle or lower third of the thigh. Flaps are tailored to provide fascial and skin coverage to cushion the smoothed end of the bone. Meticulous hemostasis and drainage are needed to decrease hematoma formation, since healing is both problematic and critical in these patients. Persons with diabetes are at highest risk for amputation because of their neuropathy, altered response to infection, and vascular insufficiency.

### Operative Procedure

1. The level of amputation is determined, and the incision line is marked to create a long posterior flap for a BK amputation; heavy ligature material may be used for this purpose. For an AK amputation, the anterior and posterior flaps are fairly equal (Figure 26-13).
2. The incision is made. Blood loss may be reduced by using a sterile tourniquet after the leg is raised to drain venous blood. Muscle and soft tissue are divided. Periosteum is raised with an elevator.
3. Bones are cut—the tibia with a Gigli or oscillating saw, and the fibula with a bone cutter—with beveling of their anterior aspect and smoothing with a rongeur and rasp. The specimen is handed off the field.
4. The stump is gently irrigated, and hemostasis is achieved.
5. A drain may be inserted.
6. Fascia is closed with interrupted sutures.
7. Skin is approximated and closed with interrupted suture or staples.
8. An immediate postoperative stump dressing may be applied to prevent flexion contracture.

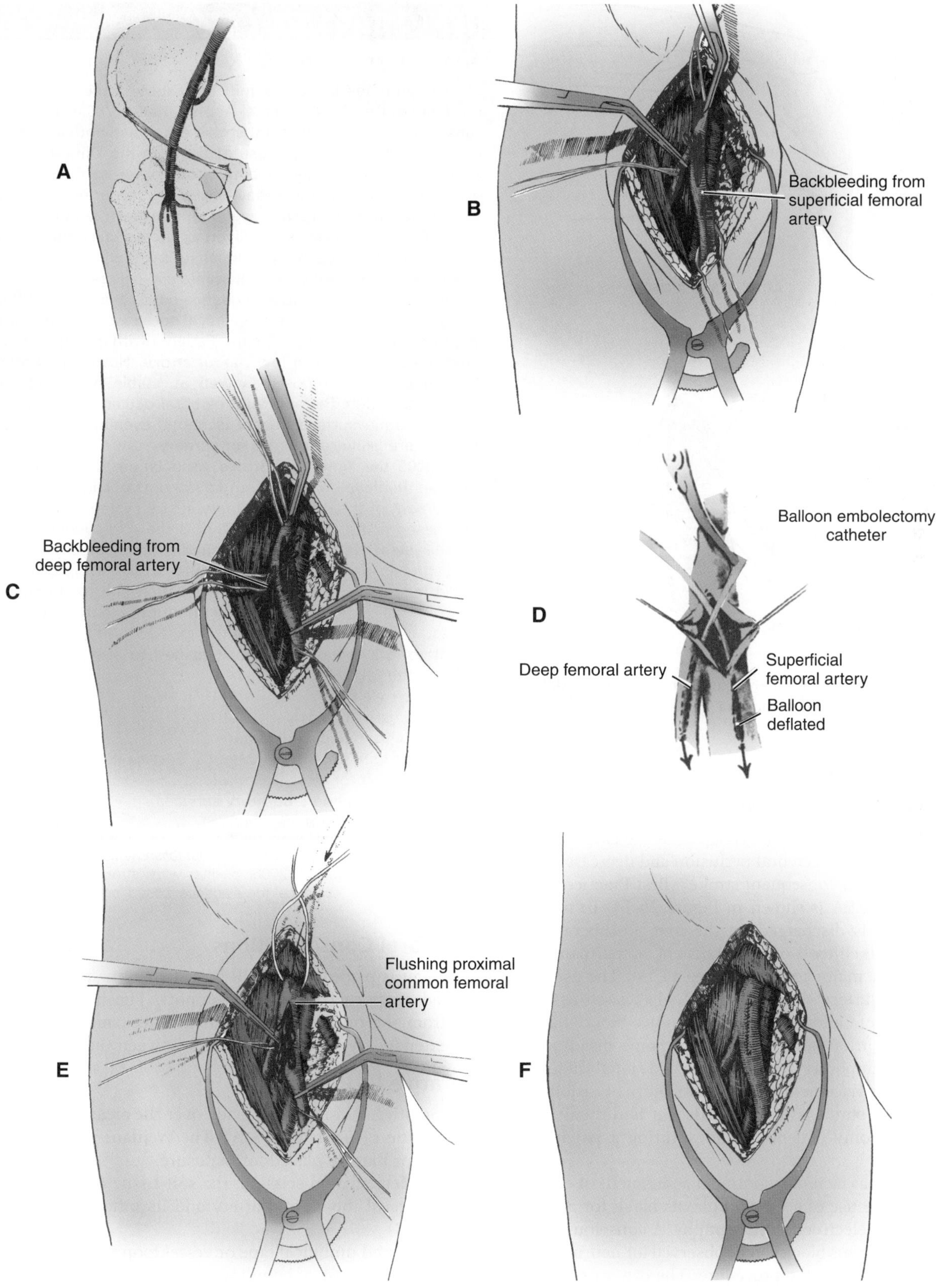


FIGURE 26-12 Femoral embolectomy. **A,** Femoral arteriotomy. **B,** Clamp on common femoral and deep femoral (profunda femoris) arteries. Backflow of blood from superficial femoral artery (SFA) is checked. **C,** Clamp on common femoral artery and SFA. Backflow of blood from deep femoral artery is checked. **D,** Balloon embolectomy catheters are passed into SFA and profunda. **E,** Proximal (common femoral) artery is unclamped and flushed. **F,** Arteriotomy is closed.

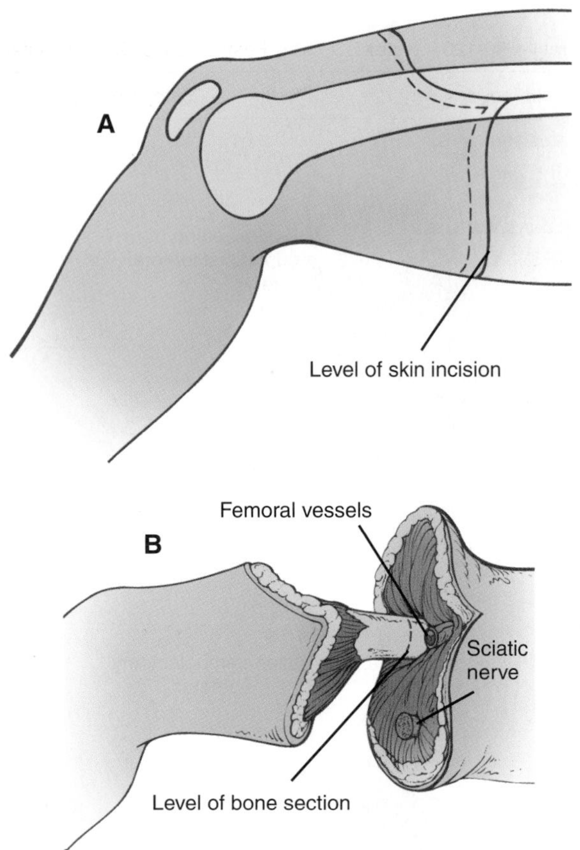


**FIGURE 26-13** Leg amputation, above knee, through the middle third of the thigh. **A,** Level of skin incision. **B,** Level of bone resection.

## BEST PRACTICE

### Acute Stroke Teams

Stroke continues to be a significant cause of morbidity and mortality in the United States. Approximately 700,000 Americans have a new or recurrent stroke each year, and stroke remains the third leading cause of death in the United States when considered independently from other cardiovascular diseases. Major advances have been made during the past several decades in stroke prevention, treatment, and rehabilitation. Despite successes in delivering effective new therapies, significant obstacles remain in ensuring that scientific advances are consistently translated into clinical practice. A best practice (often referred to as evidence-based practice [EBP]) is using "best evidence" to make clinical decisions and eliminate inappropriate or ineffective care. Patients with asymptomatic carotid stenosis have a low risk of stroke. However, carotid disease includes stenosis as well as stable and unstable plaque formation. Patients with cerebral ocular events, an irregular plaque surface, recent ischemic events, and carotid stenosis are likely candidates for surgery.

In 2005 the American Stroke Association formed a task force on the development of stroke systems of care. One critical element of the multidisciplinary stroke system is the hospital-based acute stroke team. This is the component of the stroke system that is prepared to handle the hyperacute phase of diagnosis and treatment of acute stroke events. Acute stroke teams facilitate the rapid evaluation and treatment of acute stroke patients that result in improved patient outcomes.

Part of the recommendations related to acute treatment includes the following:

- Acute stroke teams
- Written care protocols
- Continuing medical education
- Interface with Emergency Medical Service (EMS)
- A stroke unit for stroke admissions
- Neuroimaging and laboratory services
- Access to neurosurgical services

Modified from *Recommendations for the establishment of stroke systems of care.* Accessed April 27, 2006, on-line: www.stroke.ahajournals.org; Ross J: Finding the evidence for evidence based practice, *Breathline* 26(2):3, 2006.

## CAROTID ENDARTERECTOMY

CEA is the removal of an atheroma (plaque) at the carotid artery bifurcation to increase cerebral perfusion and decrease the risk of embolization and consequent stroke[3] (Best Practice). A clinical pathway for CEA is shown in Figure 26-14. In most settings, the patient is discharged on the first postoperative day. Lessening the likelihood of any transient or permanent neurologic deficit is a major concern during a CEA. The use of a temporary carotid artery shunt (Figure 26-15), such as an argyle or Javid shunt, allows for a continuous blood flow through the carotid artery and to the brain. Some disadvantages in using this temporary device are the additional dissection necessary for its placement and the possibility of dislodging debris when the shunt is inserted. Also, it is difficult to view the endarterectomy end point and suturing a patch is more difficult.

Two techniques that facilitate continual assessment of cerebral perfusion are the use of a cervical plexus block for anesthesia and the use of electroencephalography. A conscious patient with a cervical plexus block can be observed for neurologic deficits encountered during the procedure. The patient undergoing general anesthesia can be monitored with an EEG. If either method demonstrates reduced cerebral perfusion, the surgeon may decide to use a temporary carotid artery shunt. The shunting device should always be available and sterile at the beginning of the procedure.

### Procedural Considerations

The patient is placed on the OR bed in a supine position with the head supported on a head support. The head is turned away from the operative side, and the neck may be slightly hyperextended. A roll may be placed between the scapulae.

### Operative Procedure

1. A longitudinal incision is made over the area of the carotid bifurcation (Figure 26-16, *A*). The Weitlaner self-retaining retractor may be placed for exposure.
2. With Metzenbaum scissors, the soft tissue is dissected for exposure of the carotid artery and its bifurcation (Figure 26-16, *B*).
3. A moistened umbilical tape or vessel loop is passed around the vessel for ease of handling. Systemic heparin is given to the patient.
4. The external, common, and internal carotid arteries are clamped.
5. With a #11 scalpel blade, an arteriotomy is made over the stenotic area. The incision is lengthened with a Potts angu-

1. Focus of clinical path: Carotid endarterectomy
2. Timeline: Preoperative: 60-90 minutes | Intraoperative: 90-120 minutes | Postoperative: 60-90 minutes

| 3. Patient Care Problems | | Preoperative: | Intraoperative: | Postoperative: |
|---|---|---|---|---|
| A. Carotid stenosis<br>List existing neurodeficit ______<br>______<br>______<br><br>B. Risk for altered cerebral perfusion<br><br>C. Risk for fluid-volume excess<br><br>D. Risk for injury | 4.<br>INTERVENTIONS | • Identify patient<br>• Reinforce patient and family teaching<br>• Confirm operative site<br>• Secure results of diagnostic tests: arteriogram, laboratory studies, ECG<br>• Document baseline neuroassessment<br>• Assess skin integrity | • Use safety measures<br>• Safe transport/transfer<br>• Head/neck/arm positioning with appropriate aids<br>• Electrosurgical dispersive pad<br>• Containment of surgical prep solutions<br>• Assist anesthesia provider<br>— With induction<br>— With hemodynamic monitoring<br>• Prepare skin at surgical incision site<br>• Appropriate use of intraoperative medication/fluids/devices<br>— Heparin<br>— Surgicel<br>— Lidocaine<br>— IV fluids<br>— Shunts<br>• Create and maintain sterile field<br>• Perform counts<br>• Communicate with family | • VS q15min<br>• Neurocheck q30min<br>• Assess wound drainage q30min<br>• Observe for signs of tracheal edema q30min<br>• Assess skin integrity |

| 5. EXPECTED OUTCOMES | Immediate: | Discharge from PACU: |
|---|---|---|
| | • Free from physical, chemical, or electrical injury<br>• Normothermic<br>• Maintain preoperative level of neurofunction<br>• Free of hematoma at incision site | • Maintain VS within acceptable baseline limits<br>• Free of hematoma at incision site<br>• Freedom from or slight tracheal edema |

| 6. VARIANCES | For concurrent intervention: | For retrospective analysis: |
|---|---|---|
| | • Preoperative and postoperative neurofunction<br>• Impaired skin integrity<br>• Return to OR for hemostasis | • New postoperative onset of neurodeficit<br>• Impaired skin integrity<br>• Return to OR for hemostasis |

*ECG*, Electrocardiogram; *PACU*, postanesthesia care unit; *VS*, vital signs.

**FIGURE 26-14** Clinical pathway for carotid endarterectomy.

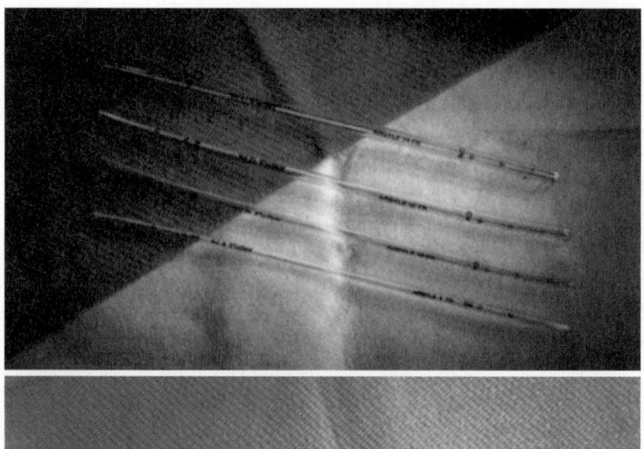

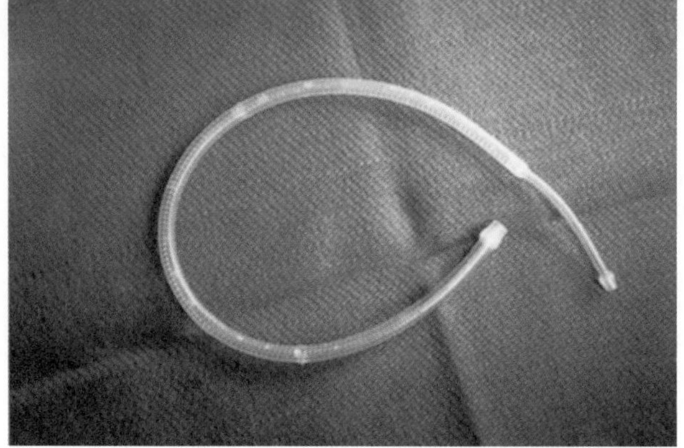

FIGURE 26-15 Example of temporary carotid artery shunts that are used to permit blood flow during carotid endarterectomy procedures.

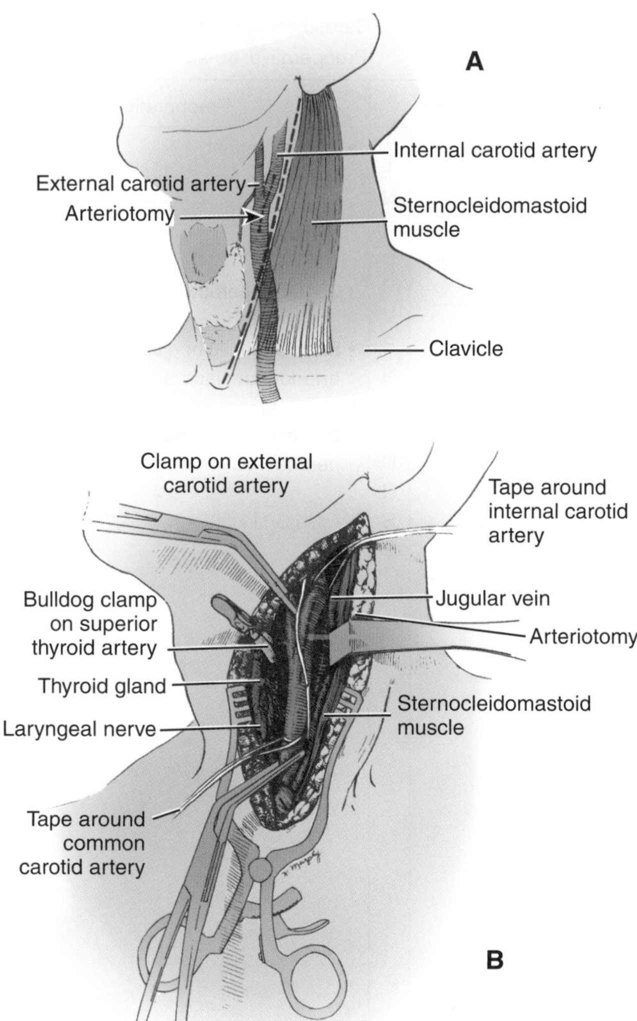


FIGURE 26-16 Left carotid endarterectomy. **A,** Incision and anatomy. **B,** Exposure of carotid bifurcation.

lated scissors to expose the full extent of the occluding plaque.

6. With a blunt dissector, the plaque or plaques are dissected free from the arterial wall. Heparin solution is used as an irrigant to clean the intima.
7. The arteriotomy is closed with fine vascular sutures. A synthetic (polyester or PTFE) or autogenous (vein) patch graft may be used to restore the arterial lumen if it is small (Figure 26-17). Before complete closure, blood flow is temporarily restored through the arteries to wash away any free plaques, air, or thrombi. For this to be done, the occluding clamps are opened and closed individually, with flushing of any debris away from the internal carotid artery. The closure of the arteriotomy is completed (Figure 26-18).
8. The occluding clamps are removed from the external and common carotid arteries; the internal carotid artery clamp is removed last. This sequence ensures that any minor debris missed will be flushed harmlessly into the external rather than the internal carotid artery.
9. Additional interrupted sutures may be needed to control leakage.
10. A drain is inserted by way of a separate stab incision.
11. The wound is closed, and dressings are applied.

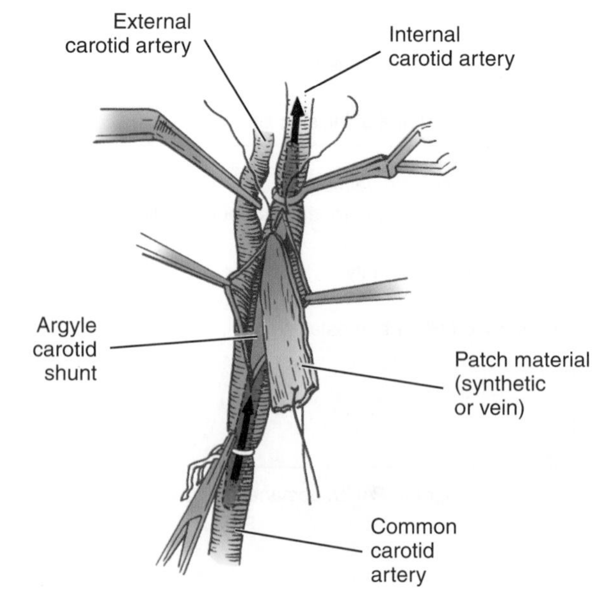


FIGURE 26-17 Left carotid endarterectomy illustrating initial placement and suturing of a patch (a shunt is in place).

## CAROTID ENDARTERECTOMY WITH SHUNT

### Operative Procedure

1-5. The first five steps as described for carotid endarterectomy are followed.

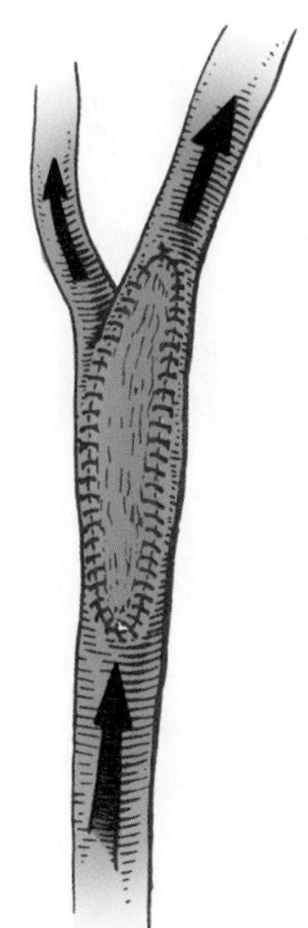

FIGURE 26-18 Left carotid endarterectomy (patch angioplasty) with patch sewn in place.

6. A piece of tubing (polyethylene or Silastic) with a suture tied around its center or a commercially prepared shunt device is inserted into the common carotid artery and the internal carotid artery to maintain cerebral blood flow and is held with vessel loops or shunt clamps (Figure 26-19).
7. The plaque is removed as described for carotid endarterectomy.
8. The arteriotomy is closed with or without a patch.
9. Before the arteriotomy closure is completed, the shunt clamp or vessel loop on the internal carotid artery is released and the shunt is removed. The external carotid occluding clamp is removed, followed by the common carotid artery clamp, and last, the internal carotid artery occluding clamp.
10. The wound is closed, and dressings are applied.

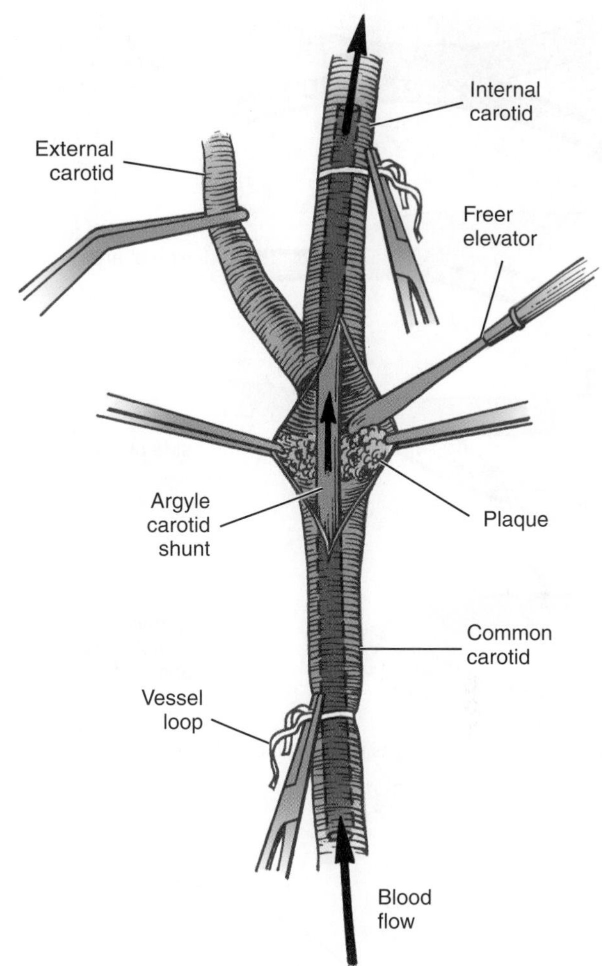


FIGURE 26-19 Left carotid endarterectomy. Argyle carotid shunt in place to allow blood flow to the brain. Stenotic plaque being removed with Freer elevator.

## ARTERIOVENOUS FISTULA

Arteriovenous fistulas—direct connections between an artery and a vein—are the standard means of vascular access for long-term renal dialysis. The dilated vein can then be used for direct cannulation with large-bore needles for hemodialysis. This method is preferable to an external shunt, which carries a high risk of thrombosis and infection. The best access is achieved using the patient's own vessels and creating a subcutaneous connection between the artery and vein, referred to as an arteriovenous shunt, or bridge fistula. Other choices include using a bovine carotid artery, human umbilical vein graft, or a synthetic vascular graft, usually PTFE. Four anastomoses that can be created between the artery and vein are side of artery to side of vein, end of artery to side of vein, end of vein to side of artery, and end of vein to end of artery (spatulated)[16] (Figure 26-20). The Brescia-Cimino fistula is a connection between the radial artery and cephalic vein at the wrist (Figure 26-21). A basic principle of creating a fistula is to start in the distal arm and move proximally with subsequent fistulas. These include ulnar artery to basilic vein and brachial artery to brachial or cephalic vein (Figure 26-22).

Arteriovenous shunts are indicated for long-term renal dialysis access. Patients with end-stage renal disease have their creatinine clearance levels observed. When the creatinine clearance falls to 10 ml/min, a Cimino fistula may be created in anticipation of the need for dialysis. A Cimino (or Brescia-Cimino) type of fistula has proved to have the longest patency and lowest infection rate. It is created to connect the patient's artery to a vein that will dilate and become thick-walled (its muscle layer hypertrophies). This occurs from the high rate of blood flow delivered by the connection to the artery. The arterialization, or maturation process, necessary to allow the fistula to withstand the repeated needle punctures of dialysis takes about 3 weeks.

Bridge fistulas do not need to mature and therefore are available for immediate dialysis use. For connections between an artery and a vein that are in proximity, a U-shaped graft is placed. Grafts that are far apart require a straight or slightly curved graft. Patency rates for bridge grafts using PTFE grafts

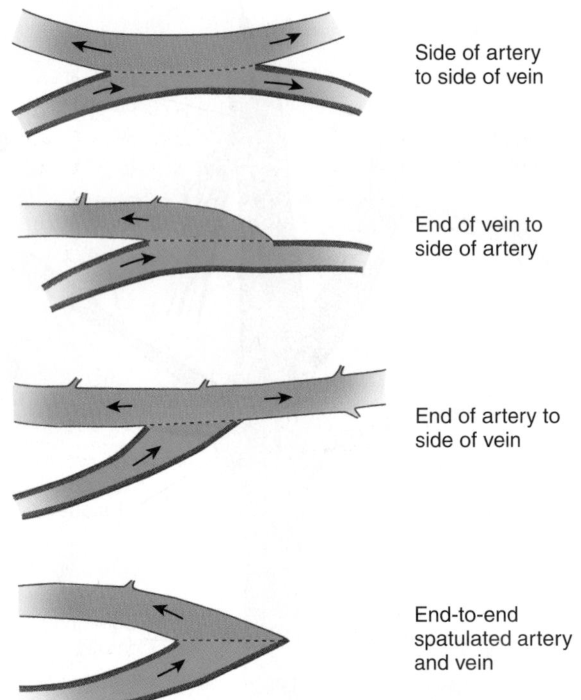


**FIGURE 26-20** Four types of anastomoses between radial artery and cephalic vein.

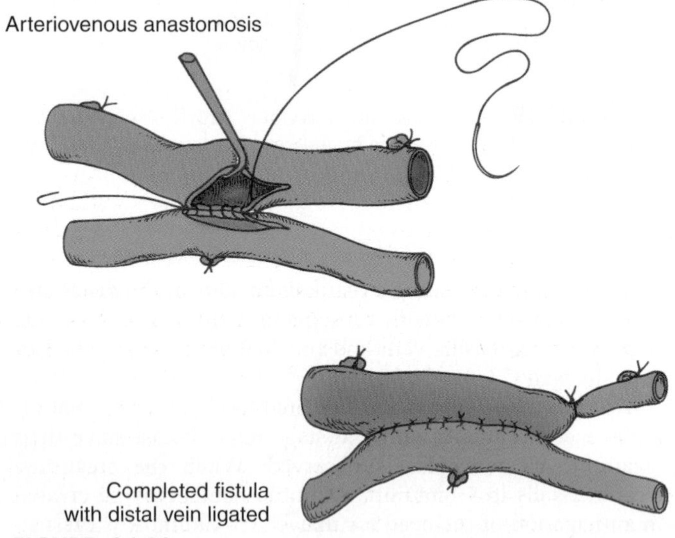


**FIGURE 26-21** Arteriovenous anastomosis. The artery is anastomosed to the vein.

are reported to be 70% to 80% at 1 year, which is comparable with the Cimino fistula in similar patients. Although saphenous vein, umbilical vein graft, and bovine carotid artery are used, the PTFE grafts work the best and are most commonly used for bridge fistulas. Some surgeons prefer to use a specially designed PTFE step-graft, or tapered graft. These have a short segment of 4 mm in diameter at one end and the majority of the graft with a 7-mm diameter. This graft may avoid an output or flow rate that is so high it causes cardiac overload. Primary

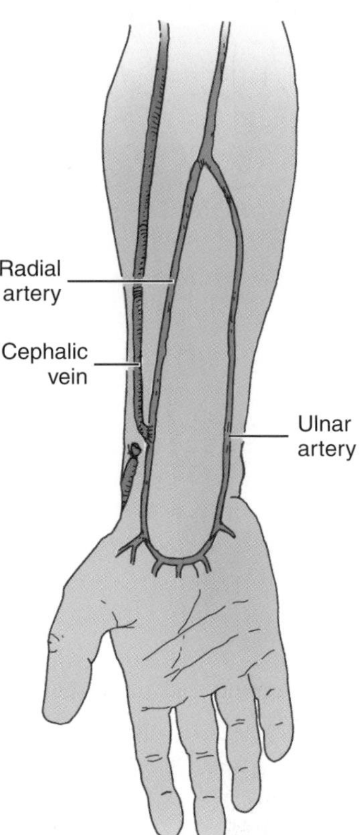


**FIGURE 26-22** End of the cephalic vein anastomosed to the side of the radial artery at a site superior to the usual location of the radiocephalic fistula. This technique can be useful if the distal radial artery is small or the cephalic vein at the wrist is thrombosed.

sites for bridge fistulas include the upper arm between the brachial artery and axillary vein and the forearm between the brachial artery and antecubital vein or brachial artery and basilic vein (Figure 26-23). The axillofemoral graft for dialysis is reserved for those patients who have exhausted other fistula sites. A regular-walled (versus a thin-walled) graft is placed from the axillary artery to the common femoral vein. PTFE grafts can be used immediately, but it may be better to wait 2 weeks for anastomotic healing to occur.

The side-to-side fistula was the original subcutaneous method introduced by Brescia in 1966. The side-to-side fistula is technically the easiest to perform and creates the highest flow rate. The arterial end-to-vein side fistula has a lower flow rate. The arterial side-to-vein end fistula is technically more difficult to create but has a lower incidence of venous hypertension. The end-to-end construction has the lowest rate of venous hypertension but also has the lowest flow rate. There is a trend toward performing fewer side-to-side fistulas and more artery side-to-vein end fistulas.

Since the patency of fistulas is limited, dialysis patients return for revision or embolectomy in attempts to salvage their function. Unfortunately, the success rate for salvage is low and access may be better managed by the creation of another site or a bridge fistula. Risk factors for complications include being female, African American, older than 65 years, and diabetic. Treatment for the most common complication, stenosis, is surgery. Stenosis usually results in thrombosis. Stenosis most

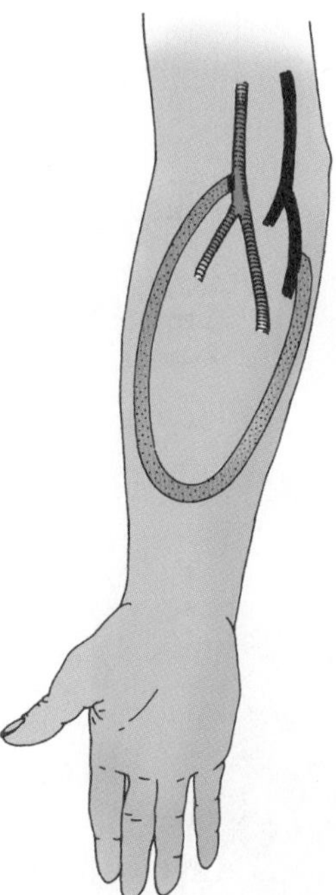

**FIGURE 26-23** An example of a loop fistula. A synthetic graft has been used to create a loop brachiocephalic fistula.

often involves the venous anastomosis, and a patch angioplasty is usually performed to revise a thrombosed fistula. Other complications include aneurysm and pseudoaneurysm formation, infection, steal syndrome, and high-output CHF.

## VENA CAVA FILTER INSERTION

Vena cava filter (VCF) insertion entails the partial occlusion of the inferior vena cava with an intravascular filter, such as a Greenfield filter, inserted under fluoroscopy with local anesthesia or moderate sedation and analgesia (monitored anesthesia care). VCFs are generally placed in the OR or angiography suite with fluoroscopic guidance. The Greenfield device offers the option of jugular or femoral vein insertion, and the correct kit must be selected. Box 26-3 gives indications for a caval filter. Several types of filters have been used during the past 20 years; Figure 26-24 gives examples. The Greenfield filter is the most successful and widely used device, and the mortality and morbidity have been extremely low. The device has progressed from an early design that required an incision and venotomy to the current percutaneous titanium vena cava filter. The filter maintains a patent vena cava but prevents PE by trapping the emboli at the apex of the device.

### Procedural Considerations

The patient is placed in the supine position on a radiopaque OR bed to permit fluoroscopic visualization at the level of the renal veins. This procedure may be performed in the OR, radiology suite, or ICU for critical patients. The head is turned to the left for jugular vein insertion, or the groin is exposed for femoral vein insertion. The right femoral vein is preferred over the left because the anatomy of the left vein often makes threading the filter more difficult. Local anesthetic, heparinized saline to flush device lumina, and contrast medium should be available. Because this is a percutaneous insertion, no instruments are needed.

**BOX 26-3**

**Indications for a Vena Cava Filter**

- Recurrent thromboembolism despite "adequate" anticoagulation
- Deep venous thrombosis in a patient with contraindications to anticoagulation
- Chronic pulmonary embolism and resultant pulmonary hypertension
- Complications of anticoagulation
- Propagating iliofemoral venous thrombus in anticoagulation

From Angle N, Freischlag JA: Venous disease. In Townsend CM and others: *Sabiston textbook of surgery*, ed 17, Philadelphia, 2004, Saunders.

### Operative Procedure

1. The right groin area is prepped and draped and infiltrated with local anesthetic.
2. An 18-gauge entry needle is used for right femoral venotomy.
3. The guidewire is inserted and advanced to a level above the renal veins under fluoroscopic guidance.
4. The sheath or dilator is inserted over the guidewire after all lumina have been flushed with heparin solution.
5. The sheath is removed, and the introducer catheter is inserted and advanced to the implantation site.
6. This catheter carries the preloaded, radiopaque carrier capsule. The sheath is retracted, the filter is discharged, and the sheath is removed.
7. Pressure is applied to the puncture site for approximately 5 minutes or until hemostasis is achieved.

## VARICOSE VEIN EXCISION AND STRIPPING

A series of cup-shaped valves maintain the venous blood flow in a direction toward the heart. Varicose veins are described as primary or secondary. Primary varicose veins are more prevalent and are not associated with a pathologic condition of the deeper venous system, that is, postthrombotic syndrome or a history of DVT. Secondary varicose veins are believed to be a result of insufficiency of the deep venous system. Disease may prevent the normal functioning of these valves, resulting in distention; as the vein wall weakens and dilates, venous pressure increases and the valves become incompetent. The veins gradually become dilated. Those in the lower extremities are most frequently affected, particularly the long saphenous vein. The incidence is estimated at 2% in Western populations, with women being affected 2.5 times as often as men are. Risk factors include female gender, increased age, pregnancy, geographic location, and race (more prevalent in Caucasians).

Dilation of the saphenous vein produces venous stasis, which may be followed by secondary complications, such as stasis ulcers. Venous obstruction causes an increase in venous pressure, which leads to an increase in capillary pressure. This causes fluid to leak from the capillaries and produce edema. The objective of surgical intervention is to remove the diseased

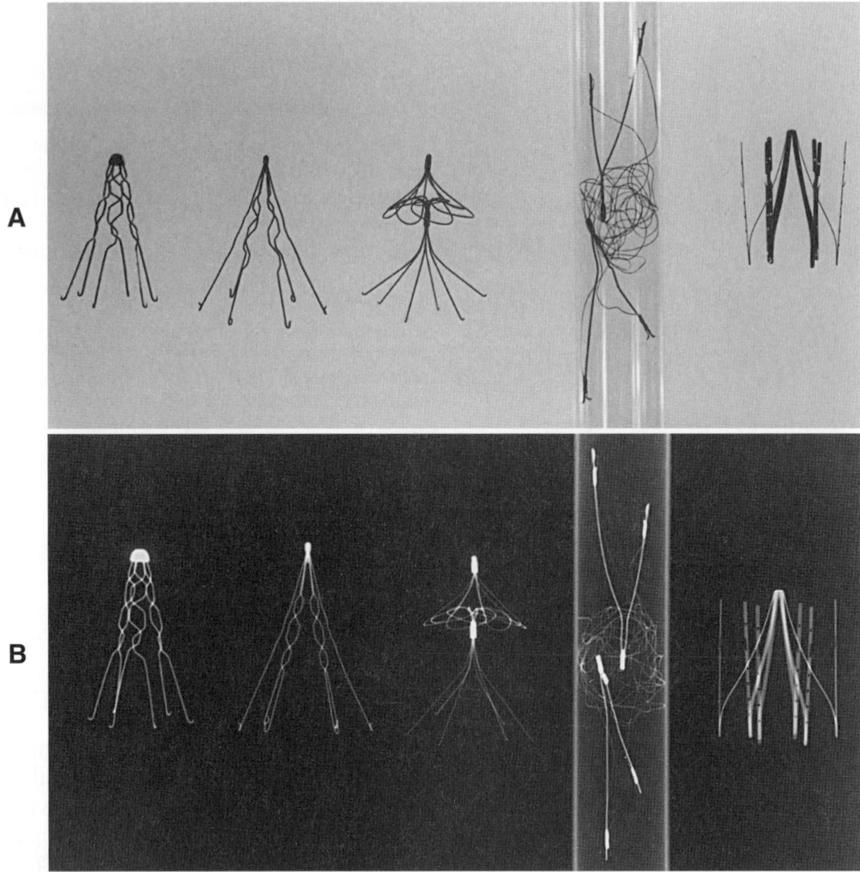


FIGURE 26-24 Vena cava filters. **A,** Actual filters. **B,** Radiographic images. *Left to right,* Kimray-Greenfield, titanium Greenfield, Simon nitinol, Gianturco bird's nest, and Vena Tech.

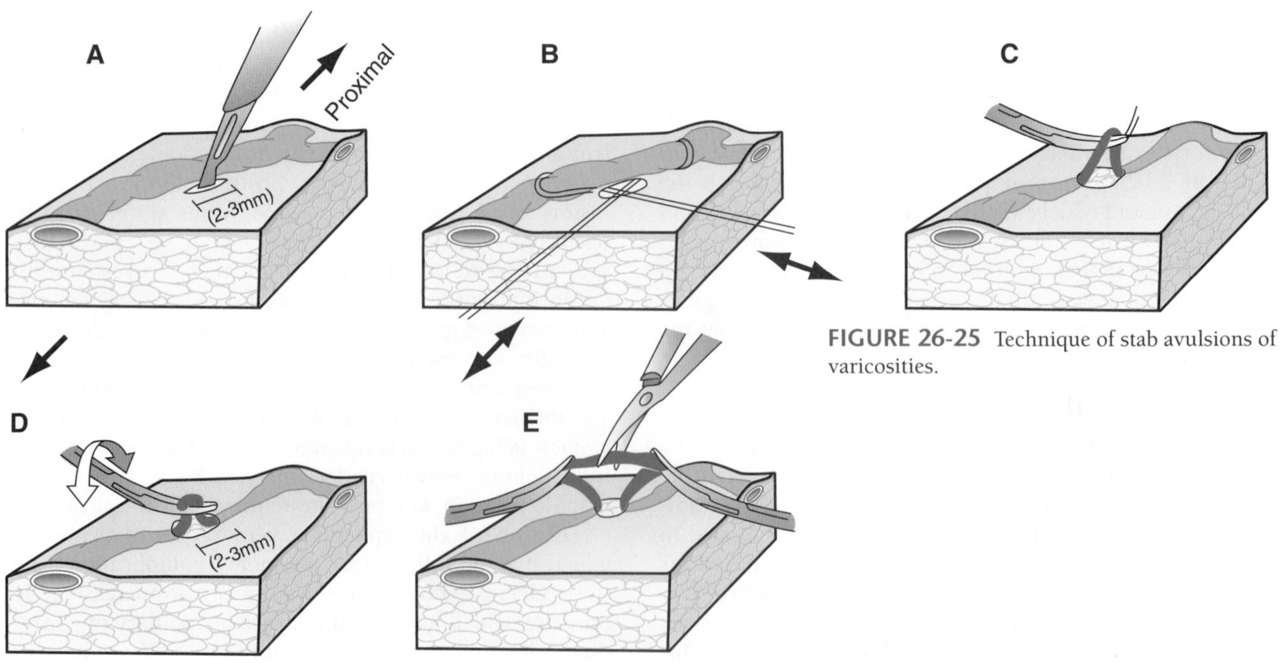


FIGURE 26-25 Technique of stab avulsions of varicosities.

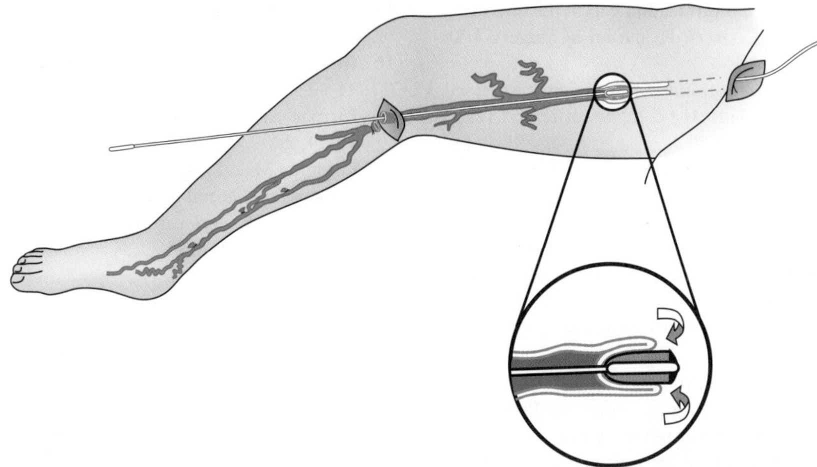

FIGURE 26-26 Inversion stripping of the saphenous vein for superficial venous reflux caused by an incompetent saphenofemoral junction.

veins, thus preventing ulceration, secondary edema, pain, and fatigue in the extremity.

## Procedural Considerations

Before sedation or entrance into the OR, the patient should stand and the varicose veins should be marked with an indelible marker. This ensures adequate visualization for complete removal of the varicosities, since the patient is often placed in the Trendelenburg position intraoperatively to decrease venous congestion, which could interfere with visualization of the varicosities. The patient is placed on the OR bed in a supine position with the legs slightly abducted. Ligation or stripping of the lesser saphenous veins and branches may require placing the patient in the prone position. In the stab avulsion technique, multiple small (2 to 3 mm) incisions are made over the identified varicosities, and the affected vein segments are removed (Figure 26-25). This is becoming the procedure of choice. Stripping indicates removal of a long segment of vein by means of a special device (Figure 26-26). Drapes are placed to enable flexing and lifting at the knee. Instruments include a basic minor instrument setup, plus the following: Weitlaner self-retaining retractors, #11 blades, skin hooks, mosquito hemostats, vein strippers with various tips available, and elastic bandages. Endovenous laser ablation (EVLA) is an innovative nonsurgical procedure for varicose veins and offers patients an alternative treatment to surgical vein stripping (Research Highlight).

## Operative Procedure

1. The incision is made in the upper area of the thigh, parallel to the crease in the groin. Bleeding vessels are clamped and ligated.
2. The saphenous vein is identified and isolated. Margins of the wound are separated with a Weitlaner self-retaining retractor.
3. The saphenous vein branches are doubly ligated with black silk ties, or they are transfixed, clamped, and divided. The proximal stump is dissected upward to the point at which it enters the femoral vein, where it is carefully ligated.
4. If the saphenous vein is to be excised, an incision is made at its distal portion at the ankle, and the vein is identified, ligated, and divided.
5. A vein stripper is inserted and advanced to the proximal end of the vein in the groin, where it is secured with a heavy suture, and the tip is attached.
6. As the stripper is pulled up the leg, external compression is applied.
7. Tributaries may be excised through numerous small incisions along the course of the vein.
8. The groin wound is closed in layers, and other small incisions are closed with skin sutures or staples. Dressings and circular compression bandages are applied.

## RESEARCH HIGHLIGHT

### Endovenous Laser Ablation for Varicose Veins

Endovenous laser ablation (EVLA) is an innovative nonsurgical procedure for varicose veins that offers an alternative treatment to the often painful surgical ligation (or stripping) of the veins, which is done with the patient under general anesthesia and often has a long recovery time. During EVLA a particular vein is sealed to prevent blood flow by delivering laser energy through a fiberoptic catheter. The catheter is inserted into the vein with ultrasound guidance. The entire procedure can be done in 1 hour as an ambulatory surgery procedure with the patient under local anesthesia. Having received U.S. Food and Drug Administration (FDA) approval in 2002, EVLA is seen as a more effective option than the surgical approach. Studies have noted a 96% success rate on more than 200 limbs using EVLA. Recurrence of preprocedure symptoms is less than 5% as opposed to 25% found with surgical ligation. Most candidates can undergo EVLA safely with the exception of pregnant women and those whose veins are too short or have sharp turns. These exceptions are more easily treated with traditional surgery.

Modified from Orenstein B: Replacing vein stripping, *Radiology Today* 6(12):22-27, 2005.

## REFERENCES

1. Arko FR, Zarins CK: Repair of infrarenal abdominal aortic aneurysms. In Souba WW and others: *ACS surgery principles & practice*, New York, 2006, WebMD.

2. Awad SS and others: Bridging the communication gap in the operating room with medical team training, *American Journal of Surgery* 190: 770-774, 2005.
3. Barclay L: *AAN updates guidelines on carotid endarterectomy.* Accessed October 4, 2005, on-line: www.medscape.com/viewarticle/513426_print.
4. Bensing K: Prayer and healing—part 1, *Advance for Nurses* 8(9):15, 2006.
5. Berry L, Schultz KJ: *Infection prevention for surgical site care.* Presentation at the AORN Congress, Washington, DC, March 19, 2006.
6. Blach DE, Ignatavicius DD: Interventions for clients with vascular problems. In Ignatavicius DD, Workman ML, editors: *Medical-surgical nursing—critical thinking for collaborative care,* St Louis, 2006, Saunders.
7. Bratzler DW and others: Antimicrobial prophylaxis for surgery: an advisory statement for the National Surgical Infection Prevention Project, *American Journal of Surgery* 189:395-404, 2005.
8. Choi JY and others: Using telemedicine to facilitate thrombolytic therapy for patients with acute stroke, *Joint Commission Journal on Quality and Patient Safety* 32(4):199-205, 2006.
9. Croft JA, Todd BA: Thoracoabdominal aneurysms, *Advance for Nurses* 7(20):16-17, 2005.
10. Crum BG: Revised National Patient Safety Goal on medication handling, *AORN Journal* 83(4):955-957, 2006.
11. D'Arcy Y: Managing phantom limb pain, *Nursing 2005* 35(11):17, 2005.
12. Decousis H: Eight year follow-up of patients with permanent vena cava filters in the prevention of pulmonary embolism, *Circulation* 12:416-422, 2005.
13. Farella C: While you were sleeping, *Nursing Spectrum—Perioperative Specialty Guide,* pp 24-26, 2006.
14. Galanti GA: Applying cultural competence to perianesthesia nursing, *Journal of PeriAnesthesia Nursing* 21(2):97-102, 2006.
15. Goldsmith C: Hidden danger—venous thromboembolism, *Nursing Spectrum* 14(11):17-19, 2005.
16. Gulczynski B: A question of homocysteine, *Advance for Nurses* 8(9): 41-42, 2006.
17. Kuznar KA: Peripheral arterial disease, *Advance for Nurses* 6(13): 19-24, 2004.
18. Lindgren M and others: Pressure ulcer risk factors in patients undergoing surgery, *Journal of Advanced Nursing* 50:605-612, 2005.
19. Mahoney CB: *Perioperative hypothermia—a clinical and financial risk.* Presentation at the AORN Congress, Washington, DC, March 19, 2006.
20. Mathias JM: Passing the baton for smooth handoffs, *OR Manager* 22(4):13, 2006.
21. Meola NM: Anesthesia awareness, *Advance for Nurses* 8(7):34, 45, 2006.
22. Neergaard L: *Tiny razor cleans out leg arteries.* Accessed November 1, 2005, on-line: news.yahoo.com/s/ap/20051031/ap_on_he_me/leg_arteries.
23. Pearce WH: The endovascular repair of abdominal aortic aneurysms, *What's New in ACS Surgery.* Accessed February 5, 2005, on-line: www.medscape.com.
24. Tracy S and others: Translating best practices in nondrug postoperative pain management, *Nursing Research* 55(2S):S57-S67, 2006.
25. Wolford JH, Davies MG: Endovascular procedures for lower-extremity disease, *What's New in ACS Surgery,* December 2005. Accessed December 9, 2005, on-line: www.facs.org.
26. Wu HW and others: *Improving patient safety through informed consent for patients with limited health literacy,* Washington, DC, 2005, National Quality Forum.

CHAPTER 27

# Cardiac Surgery

PATRICIA C. SEIFERT

Cardiac surgery has a history (History box) that reflects individual and collaborative innovation, risk-taking, and problem-solving abilities. The development of anastomotic techniques to join blood vessels, atraumatic vascular instruments, and myocardial protection strategies represents a few of the many advances that have led to remarkable achievements in the surgical repair of congenital and acquired cardiovascular diseases. From the repair of an atrial septal defect in a child to the implantation of a xenograft cardiac valve in an adult, cardiac surgeries continue to evolve, reflecting societal mandates for personal safety, enhanced functional outcomes, institutional efficiency, staff competence, and operational cost-effectiveness.[127]

These mandates can be seen in the rapid growth of endoscopic and video technology, minimally invasive techniques, the use of off-pump techniques, and molecular-level treatments for cardiovascular disease. This growing trend has not replaced the need for traditional techniques; rather, it has expanded the treatment options for coronary artery disease (CAD), valvular dysfunction, thoracic aneurysms, conduction disturbances, congenital abnormalities, and end-stage cardiac disease. Newer technologies employ laser, radiofrequency, and cryo energies; gene therapy is being used to induce cardiac neorevascularization at the cellular level; and heterograft replacement organs are becoming promising alternatives to allograft organs that are in scarce supply.[11,46,144]

## Surgical Anatomy

The heart (Figure 27-1) is a four-chamber muscular pump that propels blood into the systemic and pulmonary circulatory systems. It is enclosed in a pericardial sac within the mediastinum, which lies between the lungs, posterior to the sternum, and anterior to the vertebrae, esophagus, and descending portion of the aorta. The diaphragm is positioned below the heart (Figure 27-2). The cardiac wall is composed of three layers: the epicardium, the outer lining; the myocardium, or muscular layer, which is the important functional layer; and the endocardium, the inner lining (Figure 27-3). Two thirds of the heart is located to the left of the midline, and the remaining one third is to the right. Although functionally divided into right and left halves, the heart is rotated to the left, with the right side located anteriorly and the left side relatively posterior.

Each half of the heart contains an upper and a lower communicating chamber: the atrium and the ventricle. The right atrium receives desaturated blood from the inferior and superior venae cavae and from the coronary circulation by way of the coronary sinus. The left atrium receives oxygenated blood from the lungs by way of the pulmonary veins. From the atria, blood flows through the atrioventricular (AV) valves into the ventricles.

The left ventricle pumps blood into the major vessels of the *systemic circulatory system* by way of the aorta and its main branches to the head, upper extremities, abdominal organs, and lower extremities. The right and left internal (thoracic) mammary arteries, used as grafts during coronary bypass surgery, branch off the subclavian arteries and course behind and parallel to the edges of the sternum. The arteries of the circulatory system subdivide into arterioles and eventually into capillaries, where internal respiration and metabolic exchange occur. From the capillary beds, desaturated blood flows into the venules and veins and finally returns to the right atrium.

In the *pulmonary circulatory system,* blood is pumped from the right ventricle through the pulmonary valve into the main pulmonary artery. It divides into the right and left pulmonary arteries, which further subdivide into arterioles and the capillaries of the lungs. External respiration occurs in the capillary beds and the alveoli, where carbon dioxide is exchanged for oxygen. Freshly oxygenated blood from the lungs flows through the pulmonary veins into the left atrium.

The *coronary circulation* (Figure 27-4) supplies oxygen and nutrients to, and removes metabolic waste from, the myocardium; internal respiration occurs in the *myocytes.* The heart receives its blood supply from the left and right coronary arteries, which originate in the sinuses of Valsalva behind the cusps of the aortic valve in the ascending aorta. The left main coronary artery divides into the left anterior descending (LAD) coronary artery and the circumflex coronary artery; along with the right coronary artery (RCA), these arteries represent the three main vessels of the coronary arterial system. Depending on the severity of the lesion, atherosclerotic plaques within these arteries jeopardize myocardial blood flow and oxygenation, producing ischemic pain (in many cases). Given the progressive nature of CAD, irreversible damage (i.e., myocardial infarction) can result if untreated.

The main coronary arteries are situated in the epicardium, which facilitates their accessibility during coronary bypass procedures. From these arteries arise the septal perforators and other branches that penetrate the entire myocardium. The cardiac veins empty into the right atrium by way of the coronary sinus; the thebesian veins, prominent in the walls of the right atrium and the right ventricle, open directly into these chambers.

Nerve impulses to the heart travel from the medulla oblongata along the middle cervical nerve, which is composed of sympathetic fibers, and the vagus nerve, composed of parasympathetic fibers. The sympathetic nerves promote an increase in the force and rate of contraction, and the parasympathetic fibers control the heart rate. Running vertically along the

## HISTORY

### History of Cardiac Surgery

Although the notion of the heart as the seat of the soul is an ancient concept, cardiac surgery is one of the youngest clinical specialties, partly because of the religious restrictions and partly because of physiologic constraints. Rehn's suture repair of a right ventricular stab wound in 1896 opened the door to the specialty of cardiac surgery. The introduction of positive-pressure endotracheal anesthesia allowed surgeons to access the heart and enter the pleural cavities without causing the lungs to collapse; the introduction of electrical defibrillation and chemical arresting solutions made it possible to stop, and then restart, the heart with predictability. Diagnostic techniques to visualize the heart, record electrical activity, measure blood pressure and flow, and assess ventricular function expanded the opportunities to identify precisely the cardiac pathologic condition and to tailor the surgical intervention to the needs of the patient. The ability to isolate the heart and lungs from the circulation without producing irreversible cerebral anoxia was first demonstrated in 1953 when Gibbon repaired an atrial septal defect using extracorporeal circulation with a pump oxygenator that he and his wife had designed. Anastomotic techniques devised by Carrel in the early twentieth century made it possible for numerous advances, including DeBakey's and Cooley's innovations in the repair of aortic aneurysms in the 1950s, Favaloro's and others' direct myocardial revascularization with internal mammary artery and saphenous vein in the mid-1960s, and Barnard's and Shumway's cardiac transplantations in the late 1960s. The development of plastics, polyesters, and newer metal compounds fostered the creation of prosthetic implants for cardiac valve replacement, which was first performed in 1960 by Harkin and Starr, for the aortic and the mitral valves, respectively. Implantation of a long-term total artificial heart by DeVries in 1988 was possible in no small part because of developments in the chemical industry and laid the foundation for subsequent devices now widely employed to provide mechanical support to one or both failing ventricles. Perioperative nurses along with their surgeon colleagues contributed to these advances by actively participating in the design of equipment, supplies, and instruments (e.g., vascular clamps that would be both atraumatic and secure in clamping vascular structures). Nurses also made significant contributions by coordinating the complex operational and staffing requirements of a cardiac service, characteristic of the collaboration and team effort in delivering quality care to perioperative patients.

Data from Seifert PC: *Cardiac surgery,* St Louis, 1994, Mosby; Westaby S: *Landmarks in cardiac surgery,* Oxford, England, 1997, Isis Medical Media.

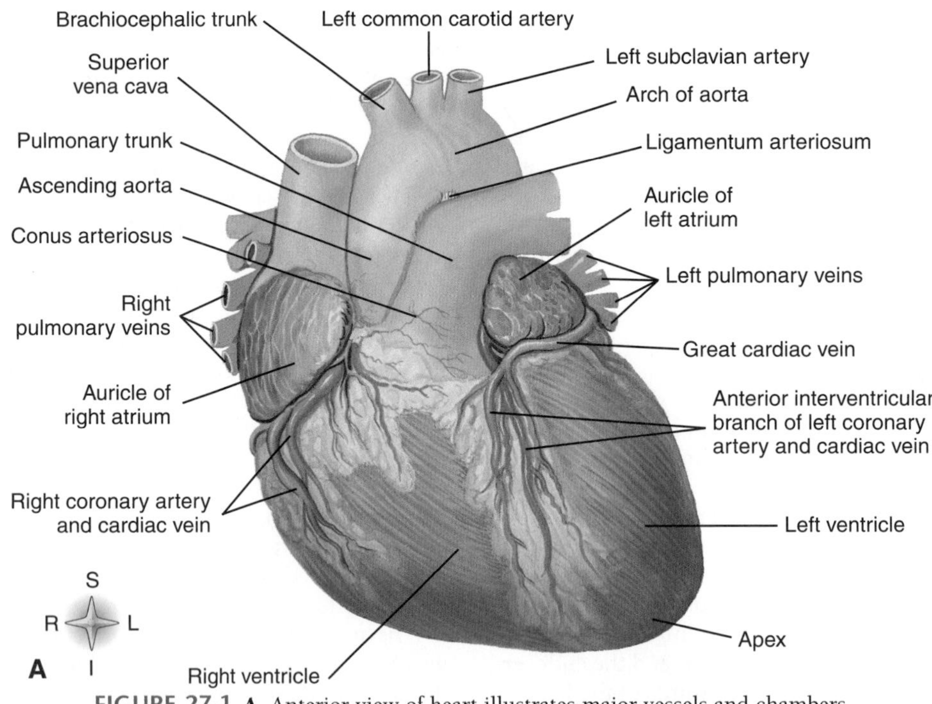


FIGURE 27-1 **A,** Anterior view of heart illustrates major vessels and chambers.

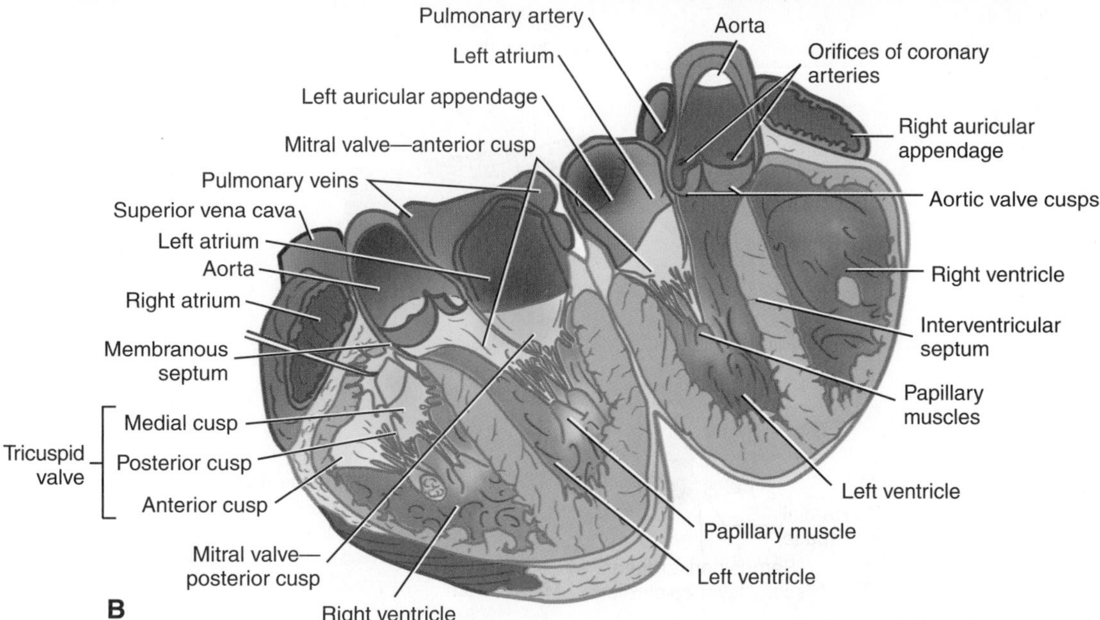


**FIGURE 27-1, cont'd** **B,** Drawing of a heart split perpendicular to the interventricular septum illustrates the anatomic relationships of the leaflets of the atrioventricular and aortic valves, and the receiving chambers (atria) and the pumping chambers (ventricles). Systemic venous blood returns to the heart by way of the inferior and superior venae cavae. It enters the right atrium, flows through the tricuspid valve into the right ventricle, and is ejected through the pulmonic valve (not shown) into the pulmonary circulation. The blood is oxygenated in the lungs and returns to the left atrium through the pulmonary veins. From the left atrium, it flows through the mitral valve into the left ventricle, where it is ejected through the aortic valve into the aorta and the systemic circulation.

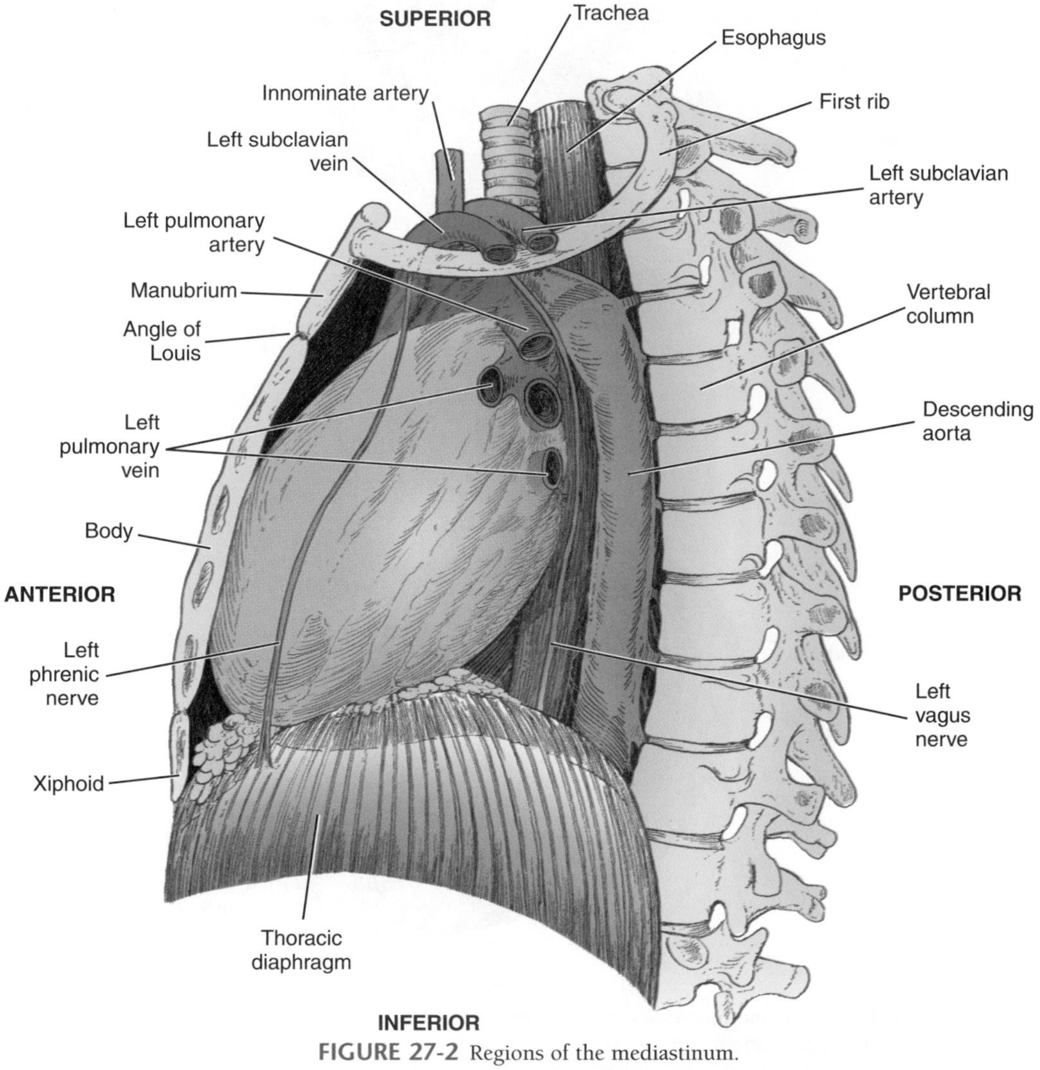

**FIGURE 27-2** Regions of the mediastinum.

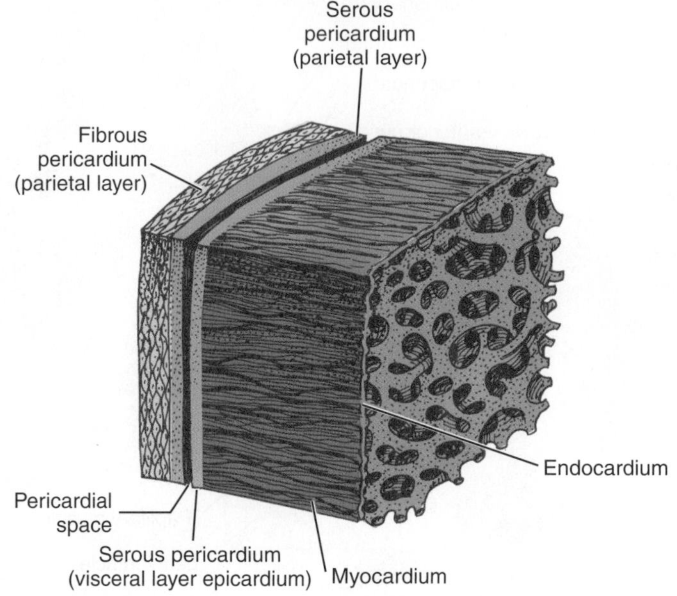


**FIGURE 27-3** Cross section of cardiac muscle showing its three layers (endocardium, myocardium, epicardium) and pericardium.

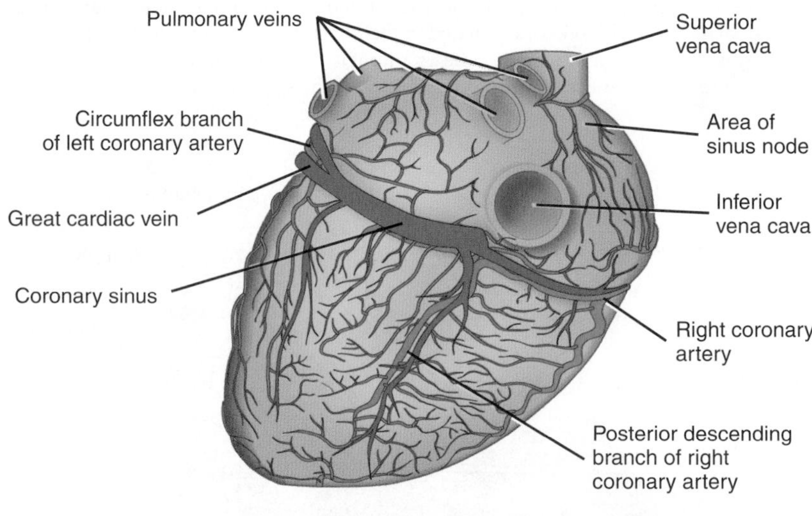


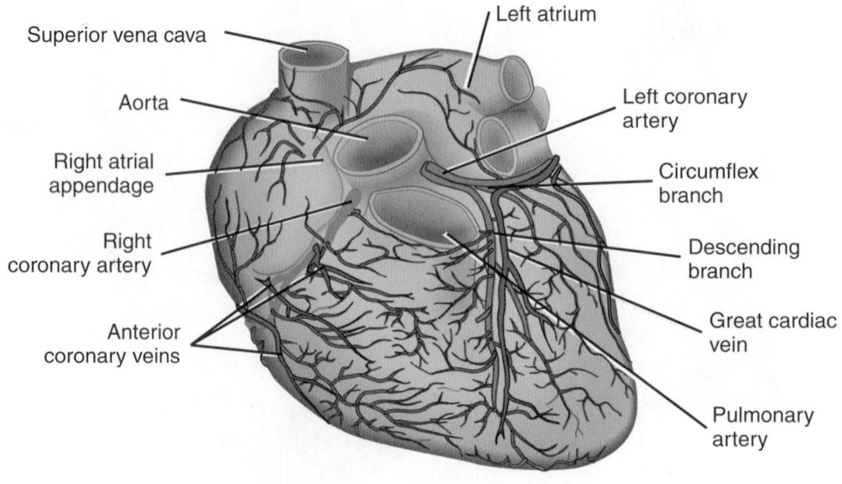


**FIGURE 27-4** Anterior and posterior surfaces of the heart, illustrating the location and distribution of the principal coronary arteries and veins.

right and left sides of the pericardium are major branches of the phrenic nerve, which innervate the diaphragm and stimulate it to contract. Identifying this nerve is important for protecting the diaphragm in procedures in which the lateral pericardium is incised or excised. Within the myocardium itself, certain areas of tissue are modified to form a *conduction system* (Figure 27-5). The process of excitation and contraction originates in the sinoatrial (SA) node, located in the area where the superior vena cava (SVC) meets the right atrium. The impulse spreads to the atria through the internodal pathways and travels to the AV junction (which contains the AV node) located medial to the entrance of the coronary sinus in the right atrium, close to the tricuspid valve. From the AV junction, the impulse spreads to the bundle of His, which extends down the right side of the interventricular septum. The bundle divides into the right and left bundle branches, which terminate in a network of fibers called the *Purkinje system*. The Purkinje fibers are spread throughout the inner surface of both ventricles and the papillary muscles, which when stimulated produce contraction of the heart muscle. The location of conduction tissue is clinically significant during surgical repair of atrial or ventricular septal defects.

During myocardial contraction and relaxation, the spiral fibers of the heart contract and relax (Figure 27-6, *A*). To prevent regurgitation of blood, the four cardiac valves (Figure 27-6, *B* and *C*, and Figure 27-7) open and close to maintain unidirectional blood flow. These AV valves are located between the atria and the ventricles. The right AV valve is called the *tricuspid valve* and contains three leaflets. The left AV valve, called the *mitral valve,* consists of two leaflets (see Figure 27-6). Each of these valves is a complex system consisting of a fibrous annulus surrounding the valve orifice, the valve cusps or leaflets, the chordae tendineae, and the papillary muscles, which anchor the valve to the inner ventricular wall (see Figure 27-1). When the ventricle contracts, these muscles and the chordae tendineae, connected to the valve leaflets, prevent the leaflets from everting into the atrium. All parts of the system must be functioning for the valve to work properly.

The semilunar valves are located at the outlets of the left and right ventricles. These valves are known as the *aortic* and *pulmonic* valves, respectively. They are less complex than the AV valves, and they open and close passively with the cyclic fluctuations in the blood pressure and volume that occur during systole and diastole.

Abnormalities such as stenosis, insufficiency, or a combination of both impair the mechanical function of the valves. Stenosed valves have leaflets that are fibrous and stiff, with uneven and adherent margins. Regurgitant, insufficient, or incompetent valves, such as those with leaflet degeneration or perforations, dilated annuli, or ruptured chordae tendineae, produce regurgitation of blood into the originating chamber. These conditions, or a combination of stenosis and insufficiency, strain the myocardium by increasing intracardiac pressure, volume, and workload. The sound of blood flowing through a narrowed or incompetent valve produces an abnormal sound called a *murmur*.

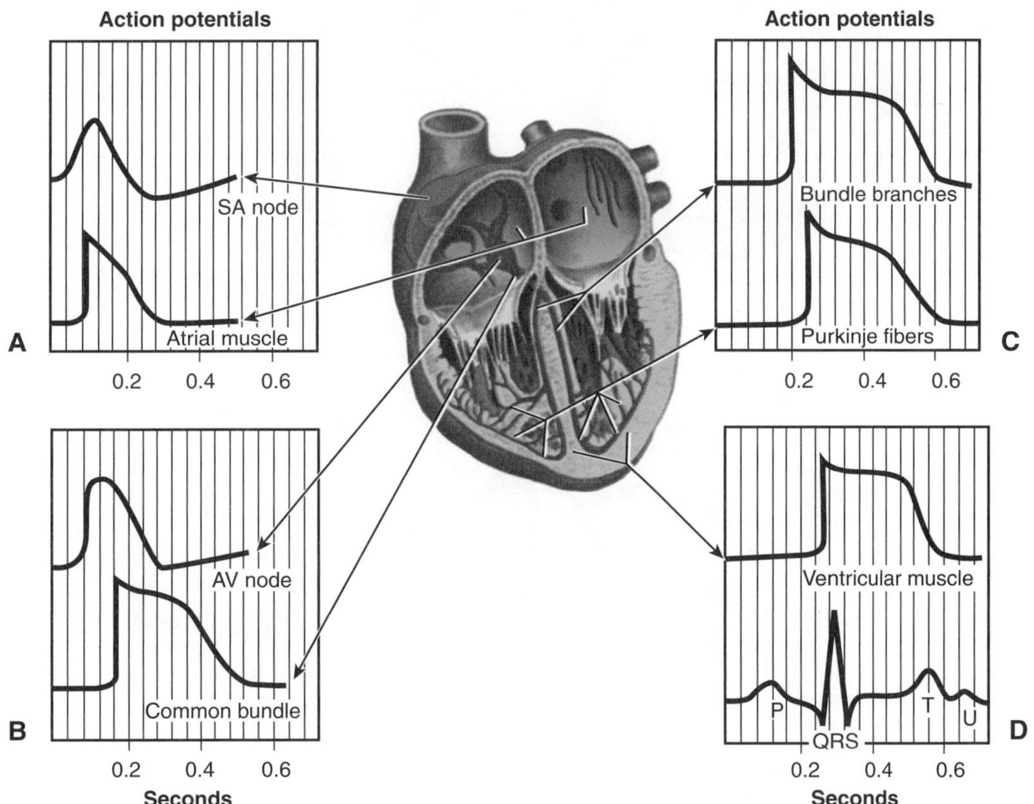


FIGURE 27-5 Heart with normal conduction pathways and transmembrane action potential of sinoatrial *(SA)* node, **A;** atrioventricular *(AV)* node (AV junction), **B;** bundle branches, **C;** and ventricular muscle, **D.**

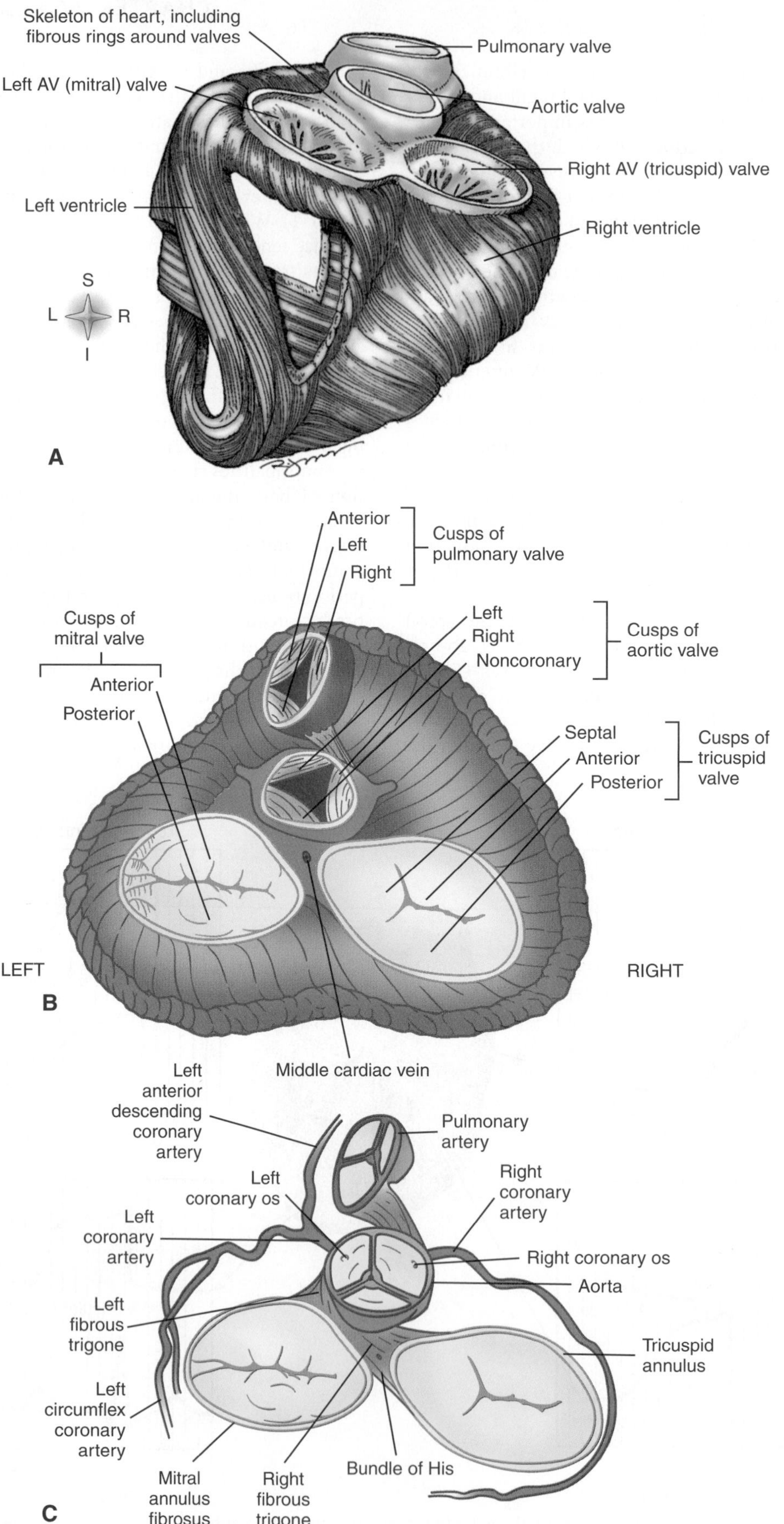


**FIGURE 27-6** **A,** Location of the heart valves in relation to the spiral fibers of the myocardium. *AV,* Atrioventricular. **B,** Superior view of cardiac valves: pulmonary *(top)*; aortic *(middle)*; mitral *(bottom left)*; and tricuspid *(bottom right)*. **C,** Superior view of valves in relation to coronary arteries and conduction tissue.

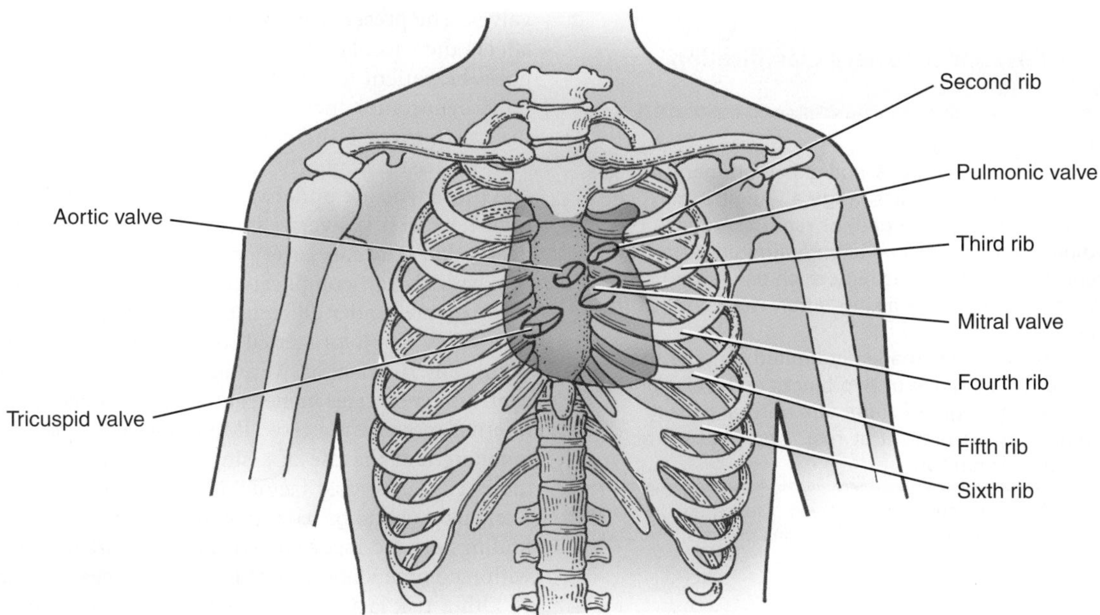


FIGURE 27-7 Anatomic position of cardiac valves. Note relationship of left ventricular apex to fourth and fifth ribs—a frequent site for minimally invasive incisions.

Any of the four valves may be congenitally deformed. Acquired valvular heart disease most commonly affects the mitral and aortic valves and is believed to be *exacerbated* by the increased stress associated with the higher pressures within the left chambers of the heart.

# *Perioperative Nursing Considerations*

Specialized nursing considerations that are indicated for thoracic surgery (see Chapter 25) also apply to cardiac surgical patients.

## Assessment

Because the severity of pathologic change varies among patients throughout the life span, knowledge of physical status, psychosocial concerns, and functional health patterns enables the perioperative nurse to plan and manage patient care. The perioperative nursing database should include the patient's biopsychosocial history, the physical examination, and results from laboratory and diagnostic imaging tests.

***History.*** The history includes information about the patient's health status as well as the response to the disease and the recommended intervention or interventions. Patients with cardiac disease may display symptoms including ischemic chest pain (angina pectoris), fatigue, dyspnea, and syncope. Depending on their severity, these symptoms affect the patient's functional status and ability to engage in activities of daily living; the New York Heart Association's Functional Classification System (Box 27-1) is often used to assess functional ability.[34] The Canadian Cardiovascular Society Classification System (Box 27-2) specifically grades the amount of activity producing angina pectoris.[18,23]

BOX 27-1

**New York Heart Association's Functional Classification System (NYHA Classes)**

| | |
|---|---|
| **Class I** | Patients with cardiac disease do not display symptoms of syncope, undue fatigue, dyspnea, or anginal pain with ordinary physical activity. |
| **Class II** | Patients with cardiac disease are comfortable at rest but display the above symptoms during ordinary physical activity. |
| **Class III** | Patients with cardiac disease, although comfortable at rest, are considerably limited functionally and display symptoms with less-than-ordinary exercise. |
| **Class IV** | Patients with cardiac disease are unable to engage in any physical activity without discomfort and may have symptoms of cardiac insufficiency even at rest. |

Modified from the New York Heart Association: *Diseases of the heart and blood vessels: nomenclature and criteria for diagnosis,* ed 6, Boston, 1964, Little, Brown.

Atypical ischemic chest pain is more likely in women than in men, and angina may be attributed to vasospastic angina, mitral valve prolapse, or psychologic factors. CAD is unusual in premenopausal women, but after cessation of menses the risk is similar to that of men.[136] Estrogen hormone replacement therapy is not recommended in postmenopausal women, according to the American Heart Association's "Guidelines for Cardiovascular Disease Prevention in Women."[98]

A cardiovascular disease risk factor profile (Box 27-3) is helpful in planning care for hospitalization and discharge by focusing on areas that might require further patient education. Mental stress has been increasingly implicated in the development of myocardial ischemia.[117] Recommended optimal cholesterol levels have been reduced to 100 mg/dl,[78] and obesity and the metabolic syndrome (central obesity, hypertension,

BOX 27-2

### Canadian Cardiovascular Society Classification System for Angina Pectoris

**Class 0** Patient has no angina.
**Class I** Walking, climbing stairs and other ordinary physical activity do not produce angina. Angina may occur with strenuous, prolonged, or rapid exertion.
**Class II** Ordinary activity may be slightly limited. Angina may occur with moderate activity, such as walking rapidly, walking uphill, or walking after meals or in cold weather.
**Class III** Ordinary activity is markedly limited. Angina may occur after walking one or two blocks on level ground or climbing one flight of stairs at a normal pace.
**Class IV** Angina may be present at rest. Any physical activity produces discomfort.

Modified from Zipes DP and others, editors: *Heart disease,* ed 7, Philadelphia, 2005, Saunders; Campeau L: Grading of angina pectoris, *Circulation* 54:522, 1975.

BOX 27-3

### Risk Factors for Coronary Artery Disease

**NONMODIFIABLE**
- Age
- Gender (postmenopausal women have risk similar to that of men)
- Heredity, genetic make-up, family history
- Race
- Menstrual status (estrogen levels may be modifiable; postmenopausal women have risk similar to that of men)

**MODIFIABLE**
- Elevated serum cholesterol and other lipids
- Hypertension
- Cigarette smoking
- Obesity, metabolic syndrome
- Diabetes mellitus
- Psychologic stress
- Personality type
- Physical inactivity

**ADDITIONAL CONTRIBUTING FACTORS**
- Elevated homocysteine levels (increase platelet aggregation)
- High C-reactive protein (CRP is a marker for inflammation associated with atherogenesis)

Modified from Zipes DP and others, editors: *Heart disease,* ed 7, Philadelphia, 2005, Saunders; Morton PG and others, editors: *Critical care nursing: a holistic approach,* ed 8, Philadelphia, 2005, Lippincott, Williams & Wilkins; Cushman M and others: C-reactive protein and the 10-year incidence of coronary heart disease in older men and women: the Cardiovascular Health Study, *Circulation* 112:25-31, 2005.

insulin resistance, and dyslipidemia) are increasingly scrutinized as risk factors for cardiovascular disease.[52]Additional contributing risk factors have been investigated: elevated homocysteine levels (which increase platelet aggregation),[59] and high C-reactive protein (CRP) levels (CRP is a marker for inflammation and is associated with increased risk for CAD).[35]

A history of rheumatic fever or frequent tonsillitis as a child is significant because the sequelae of rheumatic fever and streptococcal infections can lead to damage of the cardiac valves. The presence of diabetes is notable because this disease affects the vascular system and may retard healing and predispose the patient to infection. Hypertension and obesity (metabolic syndrome) increase the workload of the heart; obesity may also increase the risk for postoperative infection because adipose tissue is poorly vascularized. Patients who are obese and those who are underweight (compared with patients in the high-normal and overweight categories) have a higher risk of death after coronary artery bypass surgery.[66]

The risk for complications after cardiac surgery has also shown some gender differences.[43] Investigations of risk factors in men and women for sternal wound infection showed that three significant risk factors were identified and occurred at significantly different rates in men and women: smoking, use of a single internal mammary artery (IMA), and age more than 70 years. Smoking and the use of a single IMA for bypass grafting were more common risk factors in men compared with women; women tended to be older than men at the time of surgery. These findings can be incorporated into patient/family teaching plans with recommendations for life-style changes as indicated.[62]

Other risk factors associated with postoperative infection include previous cardiac surgery, duration of surgery and cardiopulmonary bypass (CPB), blood transfusion, postoperative blood loss, and length of preoperative hospitalization.[41] Female gender, obesity, and arterial occlusive disease of the legs are related to impaired wound healing at the saphenous venectomy site after coronary bypass surgery; bilateral IMA grafts, obesity, and postoperative inotropic support have also been implicated.[41,136] Of special concern is the epidemic growth of type 2 diabetes in particular and the role of hyperglycemia in general. Although type 2 diabetes was formerly considered an adult-onset disease, children are also vulnerable because of a greater incidence of increased body weight, sedentary life-style, and accelerated insulin resistance in this population.[118] Altered glucose metabolism (in the absence of diagnosed diabetes mellitus) has shown a significant correlation to atherosclerosis,[126] and control of hyperglycemia during coronary bypass surgery is an important strategy to reduce the risk of adverse clinical outcomes.[41,43,85] This information should become an integral component of patient assessment, especially in patients at risk.

In addition to risk factors and health status, the perioperative nurse reviews the patient's medication history with particular attention to vasoactive drugs and other medications that can affect the surgery. For example, patients taking aspirin and other antiplatelet drugs may require intraoperative replacement of platelets. Patients taking herbal medicines may be at risk for increased bleeding, hypoglycemia, or other complications, depending on the specific side effects of some herbal drugs (Surgical Pharmacology).

Patients' knowledge and understanding of cardiovascular disease and related risk factors and their effect on functional, physiologic, and psychologic status should also be part of the perioperative nursing assessment. The patient's personal strengths, external resources, and coping strategies should be determined. The perioperative nurse should note any cultural, ethnic, spiritual, or religious beliefs that are relevant to perioperative patient care.

***Physical Examination.*** The physical assessment provides the perioperative nurse with baseline data and information about potential problems that might require intervention. Table 27-1

## SURGICAL PHARMACOLOGY

### Perioperative Effects of Herbal Medicines

| Agent | Pharmacologic Action | Concerns and Considerations |
|---|---|---|
| Echinacea (purple coneflower root) | Activates cell-mediated immunity | Decreases effectiveness of immunosuppressants; should not be taken by organ transplant patients |
| Ephedra | Increases heart rate and blood pressure through sympathomimetic effects | Increases risk of stroke and myocardial ischemia; may cause intraoperative hemodynamic instability |
| Garlic | Inhibits platelet aggregation; increases fibrinolysis | Increases risk of bleeding, especially in combination with other platelet inhibitors |
| Gingko | Inhibits platelet activation | Increases risk of bleeding, especially in combination with other platelet inhibitors |
| Ginseng | Inhibits platelet activation; lowers blood glucose; has many diverse effects | Increases risk of bleeding; has potential to decrease anticoagulant effect of warfarin; may cause hypoglycemia |
| St. John's wort | Inhibits neurotransmitter reuptake | Induces enzymes that affect warfarin and many other drugs; may affect calcium channel blockers and decrease serum digoxin levels |

Modified from Ang-Lee MK and others: Herbal medicines and perioperative care, *JAMA: The Journal of the American Medical Association* 286(2):208, 2001; Liu EH and others: Use of alternative medicine by patients undergoing cardiac surgery, *Journal of Thoracic and Cardiovascular Surgery* 120:335, 2000; Brumley C: Herbs and the perioperative patient, *AORN Journal* 72(5):785, 2000; Association of periOperative Registered Nurses (AORN): *Safe medication administration tool kit,* Denver, 2005, AORN. Available at www.aorn.org.

**TABLE 27-1**

### Physiologic Features of the Very Young and the Very Old (Compared with Others)

| Very Young | Very Old |
|---|---|
| **CARDIOVASCULAR SYSTEM** | |
| **Myocardium** | |
| Less contractile tissue | Increased subendocardial fat |
| Less compliant | Increased heart weight |
| Cardiac output increased by faster heart rate | Reduced resting cardiac output |
| **Valves** | |
| Less tension created by papillary muscle | Fibrous thickening; calcification of leaflets and annulus |
| **Coronary Arteries** | |
| Rarely, anomalies of coronary arteries | Coronary arteriosclerosis, atherosclerosis; tortuous epicardial arteries |
| **CONDUCTION SYSTEM** | |
| Impulse conduction faster | Impulse conduction slower |
| **BLOOD VOLUME** | |
| Total circulating small amount; volume per kilogram of body weight relatively greater | Reduced plasma volume; reduced blood water content |
| **RESPIRATORY SYSTEM** | |
| Inadequate cough reflex | Decreased ability to eliminate secretions |
| Increased chest wall compliance; decreased pulmonary compliance | Increased chest wall rigidity; decreased lung compliance |
| Higher oxygen consumption | Reduced vital capacity, maximum ventilation volume |
| Short, narrow airway obstructed easily | |
| **RENAL SYSTEM** | |
| Glomeruli small and immature | Fewer functional glomeruli |
| Tubular concentration of fluids and electrolytes diminished | Reduced renal blood flow and glomerular filtration rate |
| Inability to excrete increased electrolytes and hydrogen ions (acids) | Impaired ability to excrete increased amount of water and electrolytes; reduced ability to secrete hydrogen ions |
| **OTHER** | |
| **Temperature Control** | |
| Immature regulating system: rapid heat loss | Decreased control |
| **Metabolic Rate** | |
| Higher | Lower |
| **Stress Response** | |
| Decreased phagocytic capability of leukocytes | Limited capability to retain homeostasis |
| Immature immunoglobulin synthesis | Decreased adrenal activity |
| **Physical Appearance** | |
| Good grooming suggests attentive care | Good grooming suggests positive mental status, ability to perform activities of daily living |

Modified from Association of PeriOperative Registered Nurses: *The geriatric patient. The neonate, infant, and toddler patients. The premature infant patient,* Denver, 1997, The Association; Betz CL, Sowden MN: *Mosby's pediatric nursing reference,* ed 4, St Louis, 2000, Mosby; Williams ME: Assessment of the geriatric patient: initial impressions, *Medscape (WebMD).* Released June 16, 2005, on-line: www.medscape.com/viewprogram/4179_pnt.

lists some normal, age-specific changes in the very young and the elderly populations that should be differentiated from pathologic conditions.[4-7,145] Chapter 29 describes pediatric cardiac surgery.

Before a review of systems is initiated, it is helpful to assess the patient's functional capacity. How are activities of daily living accomplished? What are the barriers that make independent living difficult? How are activities performed when there are disabilities? What support systems are available? These and other questions will alert the clinician to the need for referrals and other resources to help the patient achieve optimal outcomes.

The review of systems often starts with the skin. The appearance of the skin offers clues to cardiovascular status. Dryness, coolness, diaphoresis, paleness, edema, poor capillary refill, bruising, and petechiae can reflect impaired cardiovascular function. Visual problems and headaches may be related to inadequate cardiac output, atherosclerotic disease, peripheral vascular disease, aortic valve stenosis, or medications such as digitalis. The presence of chronic or local infection should be identified; if untreated, these may become potential sources of postoperative infection.

Nutritional status (including the metabolic syndrome) is assessed to determine increased risk for infection, skin breakdown, impaired wound healing, or other complications.

The patient's level of consciousness, memory, comprehension, and emotional status should be assessed. Confusion, restlessness, slurred speech, numbness, and paralysis can signal impaired perfusion. Their presence preoperatively should be noted by the perioperative nurse and communicated to the nurses receiving the patient postoperatively.

During respiratory assessment the perioperative nurse should note the use of accessory muscles or nostril flaring and should auscultate breath sounds. Adventitious sounds, such as crackles and wheezes, may point to pulmonary edema. Orthopnea, shortness of breath, or dyspnea may require elevation of the head of the stretcher and assistance during transfer onto the operating room (OR) bed. If the patient is receiving oxygen, the flow rate and method of administration should be observed. Alleviating pain is a prime consideration in the care of the cardiovascular patient because pain is a myocardial stressor. A patient with angina may come to the OR with nitroglycerin tablets or transdermal patches. Cold also increases the workload of the heart because the shivering that accompanies chilling elevates the metabolic rate; the patient should be kept warm.

Heart sounds, murmurs, and friction rubs provide clues to congenital, ischemic, or valvular heart disease or pericarditis. The patient may experience palpitations. Apical, radial, and femoral pulses also reflect cardiac function; their rate, rhythm, and quality should be determined. The presence of cyanosis or peripheral edema should be noted.

The blood pressure may be high, normal, or low. The hypertensive patient may have left ventricular hypertrophy, and the hypotensive patient may display changes in neurologic, gastrointestinal, and renal function. Blood pressures should be checked bilaterally. Unequal pressures in the arms may be a contraindication for the use of the IMA as a bypass graft on the side of the lower blood pressure, where perfusion may not be optimal. Radial and ulnar artery pulses should be checked bilaterally when the radial artery is to be used as a bypass graft. Patients with dissections or aneurysms may have unequal carotid, femoral, brachial, or radial artery blood pressures when the lesion occludes one or more of these vascular branches.

Because cardiac function affects all the body's organ systems, assessment of the patient should be comprehensive whenever possible. A thorough assessment also alerts the physician and perioperative nurse to the need for special diagnostic tests and laboratory procedures.

***Diagnostic Studies.*** Most patients referred for surgery have had clinical evaluations including both invasive and noninvasive studies (Box 27-4). After the history and physical assessment, a resting electrocardiogram (ECG) is ordered. An exercise ECG (stress test) is often performed because ST-segment changes indicating myocardial ischemia may be apparent only during or after exercise. In patients with intractable dysrhythmias, electrophysiology (EP) studies may be performed to locate the site of irritable atrial or ventricular foci that can be surgically ablated, excised, or controlled with pharmacologic therapy. EP studies are also performed to determine the need for internal defibrillators or antitachycardia devices. Bradycardia may be an indication for pacemaker insertion.

Chest radiography provides information about the size of the cardiac chambers, thoracic aorta, and pulmonary vasculature as well as the presence of calcium in valves, pericardium, coronary arteries, and aorta (Figure 27-8). Lateral chest radiographs of patients with prior sternal operations demonstrate the chest wires and extent of pericardial adhesions. Magnetic

**BOX 27-4**

**Diagnostic Tests Commonly Performed for Cardiovascular Disorders**

**NONINVASIVE***

- Resting ECG
- Exercise ECG (stress test)
- Chest radiography
- Echocardiogram
- Carotid Doppler echocardiogram
- Resting MUGA
- Exercise thallium
- Exercise MUGA
- CAT scan
- PET scan with stress
- CMRI, MRA

**INVASIVE**

- Aortography
- Arteriography
- Digital subtraction angiography
- Electrophysiology
- Cardiac catheterization
- Ventriculography
- Endomyocardial biopsy

Modified from Zipes DP and others, editors: *Heart disease,* ed 7, Philadelphia, 2005, Saunders.

*CAT,* Computerized axial tomography; *CMRI,* cardiovascular magnetic resonance imaging; *ECG,* electrocardiogram; *MRA,* magnetic resonance angiogram; *MUGA,* multiple uptake gated acquisition; *PET,* positron emission tomography.

*When dye is injected into the vascular system, the test is considered semiinvasive.

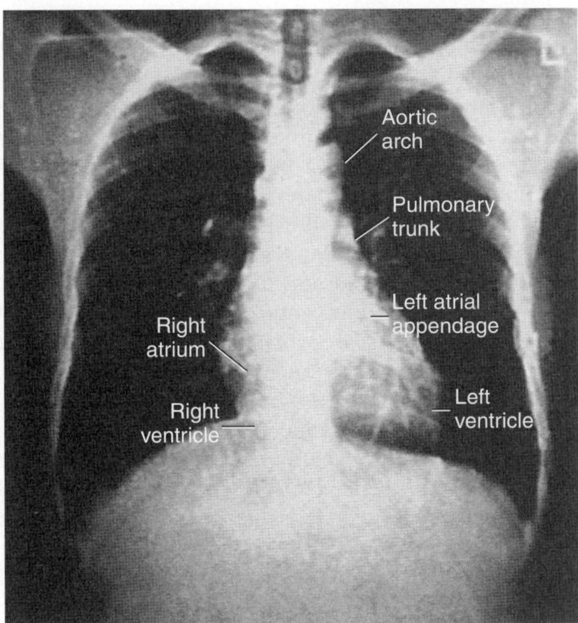


**FIGURE 27-8** Anteroposterior chest radiograph (normal).

resonance imaging (MRI) is used to assess myocardial viability[130]; MRI can also be employed to image vascular structures with MRI angiograms that provide great clarity (Figure 27-9, *A*). In patients with suspected aortic or other vascular abnormalities, a computerized tomography (CT) scan of the chest with intravenous injection of a contrast medium is used to create x-ray serial "slices" of the body area under study (Figure 27-9, *B*), and CT angiography is especially useful for imaging the aorta and great vessels. CT scans may be contraindicated in very unstable patients because the patient's position in the CT tubelike machine makes access to the patient difficult.[49,80] Less frequently performed is arteriography with radiographic contrast material (dye) to determine the size and location of the lesion and the site of the intimal tear in aortic dissections (Figure 27-10); digital subtraction angiography (DSA) provides clear images and requires less contrast material.

Echocardiography is a noninvasive test that evaluates both the structure and function of the heart by transmitting sound waves to the heart and measuring those sound waves reflected back to the transducer (Figure 27-11). They are processed by the transducer, which creates visual images of the structure's movements. This test is commonly used to assess ventricular and valvular function before, during, and after surgery and to determine the degree of valvular stenosis or regurgitation. It can also demonstrate a tumor, thrombus, or air in the ventricular or atrial cavities. Two-dimensional and color-flow Doppler techniques have greatly enhanced the functional assessment of valvular performance and carotid artery stenoses. Echocardiography is the gold standard for diagnosing mitral stenosis, and it is widely used to assess other valvular disorders and congenital heart disease.[12] Transesophageal echocardiography (TEE) is commonly used to evaluate the effectiveness of valve repairs and other surgical procedures.

Radionuclide imaging is employed to illustrate wall motion and blood flow through the heart and to quantify cardiac function. These noninvasive techniques are generally well tolerated by patients, especially when they may be too unstable to withstand a cardiac catheterization. These techniques may also be used as a complement to catheterization. Tests include the multiple uptake gated acquisition (MUGA) scan (also known

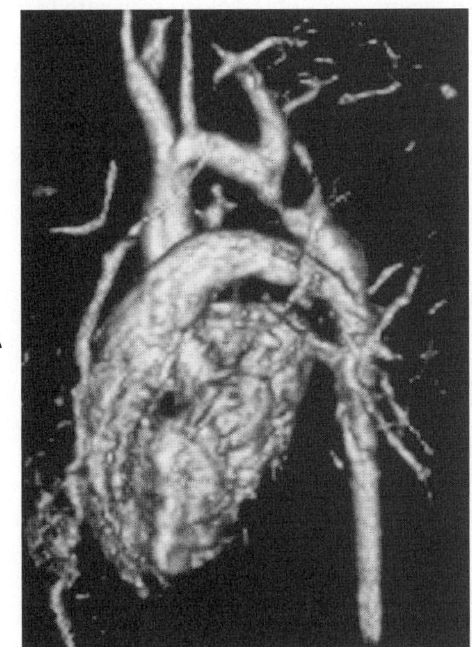


**FIGURE 27-9** **A,** Three-dimensional reconstruction of a contrast medium–enhanced magnetic resonance angiogram of the thoracic aorta, illustrating a severe coarctation (narrowing) of the aorta. **B,** High-resolution cross-sectional computed tomography (CT) scan of the heart illustrating calcification within the left anterior descending (LAD) coronary artery and left circumflex (LCX) coronary artery.

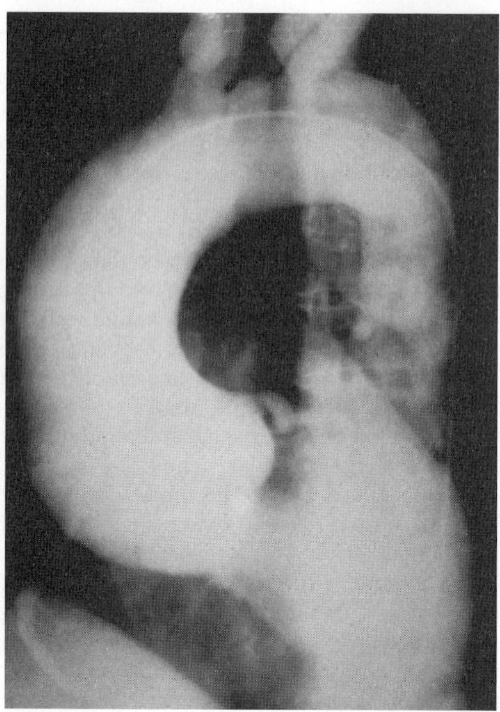

FIGURE 27-10 Aortogram of ascending aortic dissection, with aortic valve insufficiency. Note regurgitation of dye into left ventricle.

as *blood pool imaging*) and exercise thallium perfusion scintigraphy. In the MUGA, multiple images are viewed to evaluate regional and global wall motion of the heart and to determine the ejection fraction. Exercise thallium perfusion scintigraphy provides additional information about the function of the heart in patients with CAD by reflecting deficits in myocardial perfusion at rest and after exercise. The procedure is similar to a MUGA except that there is an exercise portion of the study. Patients unable to perform physical exercise may be stressed pharmacologically.[12]

Cardiac catheterization provides definitive information about the extent and location of ischemic heart disease and may be an adjunct to echocardiography for diagnosing valvular heart disease.[71] A radiopaque plastic catheter is inserted retrograde through the aortic valve into the left side of the heart by a percutaneous puncture or a cutdown to the vessels of the brachial artery (Sones technique) or the femoral artery (Judkins technique). The right side of the heart is approached percutaneously by the superior or inferior vena caval route. To perform coronary angiography that demonstrates coronary anatomy, a contrast medium is injected into the coronary ostia. Obstructions (Figure 27-12), flow, and distal perfusion can be assessed. Ventriculography illustrates contractile weaknesses of the ventricles as well as shunting and regurgitation of blood. These studies are used to assess the degree of myocardial dysfunction and to plan interventions such as coronary artery bypass grafting, valve repair or replacement, repair of congenital anomalies, and cardiac transplantation. The cardiologist can compute the orifice of a stenosed valve or determine the degree of regurgitation of an incompetent valve.

Ventricular, atrial, and pulmonary pressures are recorded, and cardiac output and ejection fraction are estimated (Box 27-5 and Table 27-2). Oxygen saturation of cardiac chambers and the ratio of pulmonary to systemic blood flow ($Q_p/Q_s$) are calculated for patients with shunts and congenital or acquired defects. Cinearteriograms record the movement of the heart, and cut films or digitized versions of the cines may be displayed during surgery.

The cardiac catheterization laboratory has also become the site for more aggressive percutaneous coronary interventional (PCI) therapies related to evolving and acute myocardial infarctions. Coronary thrombolysis with fibrinolytic drugs can dissolve fresh blood clots and reopen, or recanalize, the artery; antiplatelet agents such as aspirin, dipyridamole, and clopidogrel block platelet aggregation that can lead to restenosis.[73] Percutaneous transluminal coronary angioplasty (PTCA), with insertion of intracoronary stents, may be performed to dilate the artery. The introduction of drug-eluting, coated (with either sirolimus or paclitaxel) intraluminal coronary stents has significantly reduced the incidence of restenosis seen with bare metal stents.[99,108] Laser angioplasty and atherectomy to excise intraluminal plaque may also be employed. In many instances these interventions may obviate the need for surgical bypass grafting, although the progressive nature of CAD may eventually lead to patients requiring surgical revascularization. OR availability is recommended for unstable patients undergoing stent insertion and atherectomy. Not all institutions mandate a

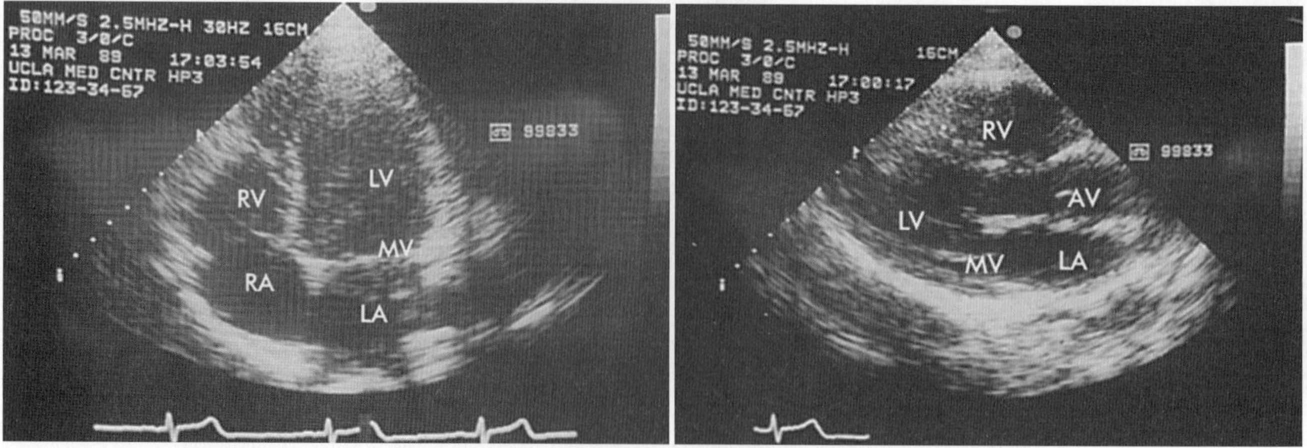


FIGURE 27-11 Two-dimensional echocardiography showing two views of the cardiac chambers. *LA*, Left atrium; *LV*, left ventricle; *MV*, mitral valve; *RA*, right atrium; *RV*, right ventricle.

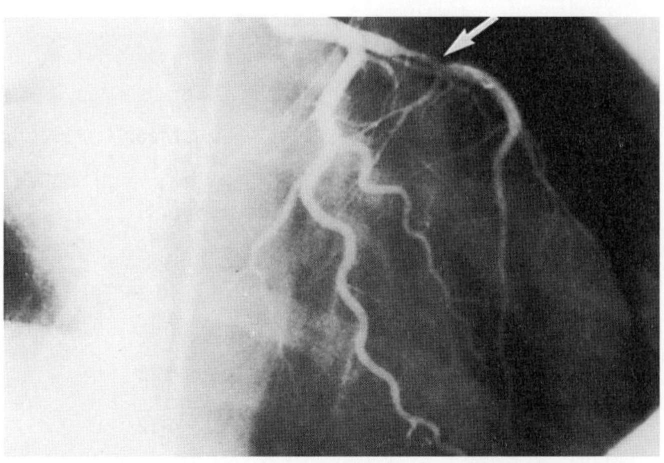

FIGURE 27-12 Right anterior oblique (RAO) view of left coronary artery injection demonstrating high-grade stenosis of the left anterior descending coronary artery *(arrow)* at the lead of the first septal perforator.

BOX 27-5

**Hemodynamic Concepts**

| | |
|---|---|
| **Cardiac Output** | The amount of blood (in liters) ejected by the left ventricle per minute; product of heart rate times the stroke volume. |
| **Cardiac Index** | The cardiac output corrected for differences in body size. |
| **Preload** | The volume and pressure of blood in the ventricle at the end of diastole. Central venous pressure (CVP) measures right-sided heart preload; pulmonary artery wedge pressure (PAWP) indirectly measures left-sided heart preload. |
| **Afterload** | The impedance, or resistance, the heart must overcome to pump blood into the systemic circulation; the left ventricular wall tension during systole; systemic vascular resistance. |
| **Contractility** | The inotropic state of the heart; the ability of the ventricle to pump. |
| **Ejection Fraction** | The percentage of end-diastolic volume ejected into the systemic circulation; indicator of ventricular function. |

TABLE 27-2

**Cardiac Catheterization Data**

| Hemodynamic Data | Normal Values | | |
|---|---|---|---|
| **FLOW** | | | |
| Cardiac output (CO) | 3.0-6.0 L/min | | |
| Cardiac index (CI) | 2.8-4.2 L/min/m$^2$ | | |
| Ejection fraction (EF) | 60%-70% | | |
| Left ventricular end-diastolic volume (LVEDV) | 90-180 ml | | |
| Stroke volume (SV) | 60-130 ml/beat | | |
| Stroke volume index (SVI) | 35-70 ml/beat/m$^2$ | | |
| | **Systolic** | **Diastolic** | **Mean** |
| **RESISTANCES** | | | |
| Systemic vascular resistance (SVR) | <20 Wood units | | |
| Total pulmonary resistance | <3.5 Wood units | | |
| Pulmonary vascular resistance (PVR) | <2.0 Wood units | | |
| **SHUNTS ($Q_p/Q_s$)** | | | |
| Pulmonary flow/systemic flow | | 1:1 | |
| **OXYGEN SATURATIONS** | | | |
| Venae cavae | | 70% | |
| Right atrium | | 70% | |
| Right ventricle | | 70% | |
| Pulmonary artery | | 70% | |
| Pulmonary veins | | 97% | |
| Left atrium | | 97% | |
| Left ventricle | | 97% | |
| Aorta | | 97% | |
| **VALVE ORIFICES (ADULT)** | | | |
| Aortic | 2-4 cm$^2$ | | |
| Mitral | 4-6 cm$^2$ | | |
| Tricuspid | 10 cm$^2$ | | |

Modified from Pagana KD, Pagana TJ: *Mosby's diagnostic and laboratory test reference,* ed 7, St Louis, 2005, Mosby; Kern MJ: *The cardiac catheterization handbook*, ed 4, Philadelphia, 2003, Mosby.

Continued

**TABLE 27-2**

## Cardiac Catheterization Data—cont'd

| Hemodynamic Data | Systolic | Diastolic | Mean |
|---|---|---|---|
| **PRESSURES (mm Hg)** | | | |
| Venae cavae | | | 0-5 |
| Right atrium (RA) | | | 2-6 |
| Right ventricle (RV) | 20-30 | 0-5 | |
| Pulmonary artery (PA) | 15-28 | 5-16 | 10-15 |
| Pulmonary artery wedge pressure (PAWP) | | | 4-12 |
| Left atrium (LA) | | | 4-12 |
| Left ventricle (LV) | 90-140 | 0-5 | |
| Left ventricular end-diastolic pressure (LVEDP) | | | 4-12 |
| Aorta | 120-140 | 60-80 | 70-90 |
| Brachial artery | 90-140 | 60-90 | |
| Femoral artery | 125 | 75 | |

| | Findings |
|---|---|
| **ANGIOGRAPHIC DATA** | |
| Coronary arteries | Anatomy/function of coronary vascular bed; distal coronary flow; arteriovenous (AV) fistula; atherosclerosis; anomalous origin of coronary arteries |
| Ventriculography | Anatomy/function of ventricles and associated structures; LV aneurysm; congenital abnormalities; valvular stenosis/regurgitation; shunts |
| Valvular angiography | Intact mitral/triscuspid complex; valvular incompetence/stenosis/regurgitation |
| Pulmonary angiography | Pulmonary embolism; congenital abnormalities |
| Aortography | Patency of aortic branches; normal mobility, competence, and anatomy of aortic valve; aneurysms: saccular, fusiform; origin of aortic dissection; shunts or anomalous connections; congenital defect or obstructions |

Modified from Pagana KD, Pagana TJ: *Mosby's diagnostic and laboratory test reference,* ed 7, St Louis, 2005, Mosby; Kern MJ: *The cardiac catheterization handbook,* ed 4, Philadelphia, 2003, Mosby.

cardiac OR standby policy,[131] but one study has demonstrated postprocedure mortality nearly twice as high as that in hospitals without onsite coronary bypass surgery.[143]

EP studies are performed to diagnose conduction disturbances and to provide therapeutic interventions, such as radiofrequency or cryologic ablation of accessory pathways seen in Wolff-Parkinson-White syndrome, or insertion of an internal cardioverter defibrillator for ventricular tachydysrhythmias.

***Laboratory Tests.*** Preoperative laboratory tests are used to assess physiologic function[105] (Table 27-3). Hematologic tests include a detailed coagulation profile to uncover hemorrhagic disorders. In patients who have been taking aspirin or dipyridamole, platelet activity is decreased; this alerts the perioperative nurse to anticipate prolonged bleeding necessitating infusion of this blood product. The patient's blood type is also determined, and the appropriate order is placed with the blood bank. Precautions are taken to test the blood for viral contamination and for cold antibodies that could produce agglutination of the patient's blood during surgery when the patient is cooled to hypothermic temperatures. Blood is brought to the OR suite before the start of surgery and stored in a monitored blood refrigerator. Although the use of bank blood products has been reduced with autotransfusion techniques, the occasional, emergent need for blood necessitates the immediate availability of bank blood packed red blood cells.

Liver and kidney function test results may be abnormal in patients with chronic heart failure, possibly because of congestion related to right heart failure in the former and reduced blood flow in the latter. Progressive improvement in hepatic and renal function is anticipated with successful operative intervention. The use of statins and other cholesterol-reducing drugs that can adversely impair hepatic function also alerts the nurse to check liver function laboratory results. Blood glucose levels are tested, monitored and controlled, especially in patients with impaired glucose metabolism and both type 1 and type 2 diabetes mellitus.

Additional perioperative laboratory examinations may include arterial blood gases and enzyme markers of myocardial damage (e.g., troponin I and troponin T; creatine kinase MB isoenzyme, known as *MB bands*), especially in the presence of persistent angina.[88] Pulmonary function tests are performed to determine baseline data and to plan postoperative care. Postoperative respiratory function may be impaired as a result of

**TABLE 27-3**
## Laboratory Data

| Test | Conventional Values |
|---|---|
| Arterial blood gases | |
| pH | 7.35-7.45 |
| $Po_2$ | 95-100 mm Hg |
| $Pco_2$ | 35-45 mm Hg |
| Blood chemistry | |
| Glucose (fasting) | 70-110 mg/dl |
| Protein (total) | 6.8-8.5 g/dl |
| Blood urea nitrogen (BUN) | 8.0-25 mg/dl |
| Uric acid | 3.0-7.0 mg/dl |
| Cardiac enzymes | |
| Creatine phosphokinase (total CPK) | Male: 55-170 units/L; female: 30-135 units/L |
| CPK-BB (isoenzyme, $CPK_1$) | 0% |
| CPK-MB (isoenzyme, $CPK_2$) | 0% |
| CPK-MM (isoenzyme, $CPK_3$) | 100% |
| Troponin T | $<$0.2 mcg/L |
| Troponin I | $<$0.03 mcg/L |
| Coagulation profile | |
| Platelet count | 150,000-400,000 /$mm^3$ |
| Prothrombin time (PT) | Depends on thromboplastin reagent used; typically 9.5-12.0 sec |
| Thrombin time | Depends on concentration of thrombin reagent used; typically 20-29 sec |
| Partial thromboplastin time (PTT) | Depends on phospholipid reagent used; typically 60-70 sec |
| Activated PTT (aPTT) | Depends on activator and phospholipid reagents used; typically 30-40 sec |
| Fibrinogen | 200-400 mg/dl |
| Fibrinogen split products | 10 mg/dl |
| Complete blood cell count | |
| Hemoglobin (Hgb) | |
| 1-3 days old | 14-24 g/dl |
| 2 mo old | 10-17 g/dl |
| 6-18 yr old | 10-15.5 g/dl |
| Adult | |
| Male | 14-18 g/dl |
| Female | 12-16 g/dl |
| Hematocrit (Hct) | |
| 2 days old | 44%-64% |
| 2 mo old | 35%-50% |
| Adult | |
| Male | 42%-52% |
| Female | 37%-47% |
| Red blood cells (RBCs) | |
| 1 wk old | 4.8-7.1 $\times$ $10^6/\mu l$ |
| 3-6 mo old | 3.5-5.5 $\times$ $10^6/\mu l$ |
| 2-6 yr old | 4.0-5.5 $\times$ $10^6/\mu l$ |
| Adult | |
| Male | 4.7-6.1 $\times$ $10^6/\mu l$ |
| Female | 4.2-5.4 $\times$ $10^6/\mu l$ |
| White blood cells (WBCs) | |
| 1 day old | 9000-30,000/$mm^3$ |
| 1 mo old | 6200-17,000/$mm^3$ |
| Adult | 5000-10,000/$mm^3$ |
| Creatinine (urine, 24-hr) | |
| Male | 107-139 ml/min |
| Female | 87-107 ml/min |
| Electrolytes | |
| Potassium ($K^+$) | 3.5-5.0 mEq/L |
| Sodium ($Na^+$) | 136-145 mEq/L |
| Chloride ($Cl^-$) | 98-106 mEq/L |
| Magnesium ($Mg^{++}$) | 1.3-2.1 mEq/L |
| Lipids | |
| Cholesterol | $<$100 mg/dl* |
| Triglycerides | 10-190 mg/dl |
| Phospholipids | 150-380 mg/dl |
| Free fatty acids | 9.0-15.0 mM/L |
| C-reactive protein | $<$1.0 mg/dl |
| Homocysteine | 4-14 $\mu$mol/L |
| Liver function | |
| Albumin (serum) | 3.5-5 g/dl |
| Alkaline phosphatase | 30-120 units/L |
| Globulin (serum) | 2.3-3.4 g/dl |
| Serum bilirubin (total) | 0.3-1.0 mg/dl |
| Pulmonary function | Normal values vary depending on the patient's age, gender, weight, and race. The following are generally calculated: Residual volume (RV) Tidal volume (TV) Expiratory reserve volume (ERV) Inspiratory reserve volume (IRV) Total lung capacity (TLC) Vital capacity (VC) |
| Urinalysis | |
| Color | Amber, yellow |
| Clarity | Clear |
| pH | 4.6-8 |
| Specific gravity (SG) | 1.005-1.030 |
| Protein | 0.0-8 mg/dl |
| Sugar, ketones, RBCs, WBCs, casts | Negative |

Modified from Pagana KD, Pagana TJ: *Mosby's diagnostic and laboratory test reference,* ed 7, St Louis, 2005, Mosby.
*Current recommendations are to target cholesterol levels below 100 mg/dl. See LaRosa JC and others: Intensive lipid lowering with atorvastatin in patients with stable coronary artery disease, *New England Journal of Medicine* 352:1425-1435, 2005.

the use of extracorporeal circulation and associated inflammatory response, and stasis of lung secretions that accompany prolonged surgery.

## Nursing Diagnosis

After a comprehensive review of individual patient data, the perioperative nurse identifies relevant nursing diagnoses, from which the perioperative plan for patient care is derived (see the Sample Plan of Care, pp. 986-987).

Nursing diagnoses related to the care of patients undergoing cardiac surgery might include the following[13,123]:

- Decreased Cardiac Output related to emotional (fear), sensory (pain), or physiologic (electrical, mechanical, or structural) factors
- Risk for Infection at the surgical site or sites related to surgical incision, catheters and intravascular lines, and altered cardiac function
- Risk for Perioperative Positioning Injury
- Deficient Knowledge related to the physiologic effects of the cardiac disorder, proposed surgical procedures, and immediate perioperative events
- Risk for Impaired Tissue Integrity (myocardial, peripheral, renal, and cerebral) related to surgery, hypothermia, CPB, or surgical particulate or air emboli

## Outcome Identification

Outcomes identified for the selected nursing diagnoses could be stated as follows:

- The patient's cardiac function will be consistent with or improved from baseline levels established preoperatively as evidenced by hemodynamic indicators (blood pressure, oxygenation, ECG) within expected range; warm, dry skin; and urine output more than 30 ml/hr.
- The patient will be free from signs and symptoms of infection as evidenced by absence of redness, edema, purulent incisional drainage, or untoward elevation of temperature postoperatively.
- The patient will be free from signs and symptoms of injury related to surgical position as evidenced by the absence of acquired neuromuscular impairment and tissue necrosis.
- The patient will demonstrate knowledge of the physiologic responses to the cardiac disorder (at his or her level of un-

## SAMPLE PLAN OF CARE

### NURSING DIAGNOSIS

**Decreased Cardiac Output** related to emotional (fear), sensory (pain), or physiologic (electrical, mechanical, or structural) factors

### OUTCOME

The patient's cardiovascular status is consistent with or improved from baseline levels established preoperatively as evidenced by hemodynamic indicators (blood pressure, oxygenation, electrocardiogram) within expected range; warm, dry skin; and urine output more than 30 ml/hr.

### INTERVENTIONS

- Identify baseline cardiac status.
- Use monitoring equipment to assess cardiac status.
- Identify and report the presence of implantable cardiac devices.
- Institute anxiety-reduction measures; address fear-producing concerns; clarify misconceptions, and answer questions.
- Measure pain level with pain scale; provide comfort measures and pharmacologic interventions as ordered; confirm and document degree of pain relief.
- Check clotting function, coagulation profile, and electrolyte values.
- Monitor blood pressures (arterial, central venous pressure [CVP], pulmonary artery wedge pressure [PAWP]) and electrocardiogram (ECG).
- Measure and report blood loss (e.g., suction, sponges).
- Maintain adequate supply and assist with administration of replacement blood or blood products.
- Follow institutional protocol for allergic blood reaction.
- Have topical hemostatic agents available.
- Have inotropic and antidysrhythmic medications available; assist with administration.
- Use autotransfusion system per protocol.
- Monitor, report, and record urine output and chest tube drainage; keep tubes and catheters patent.
- Have available defibrillator (with appropriate internal and external paddles and settings), fibrillator, external pacemaker, temporary epicardial pacemaker leads, and appropriate ECG cables for cardioversion and intraaortic balloon pump.
- Evaluate postoperative cardiac status.

### NURSING DIAGNOSIS

**Risk for Infection** at the surgical site or sites related to surgical incision, catheters, intravascular lines, and altered cardiac function

### OUTCOME

The patient is free from signs and symptoms of infection as evidenced by absence of redness, edema, purulent incisional drainage, or untoward elevation of temperature postoperatively.

### INTERVENTIONS

- Administer prescribed prophylactic treatments.
- Verify that prescribed preoperative prophylactic antibiotic has been administered within 1 hour of the surgical incision.
- Assess susceptibility for infection.
- Encourage/reinforce previous teaching regarding deep breathing and coughing exercises.
- Classify surgical wound.
- Implement aseptic technique.
- Initiate and maintain traffic control.
- Minimize length of invasive procedure by prioritizing, organizing, and planning care.
- Dress all invasive arterial and venous lines.
- Perform skin preparation.
- Use depilatories or electric clippers to remove hair at the surgical site; avoid razors if possible.
- Prepare anatomic area to knees (or lower if leg vein needed) with antimicrobial antiseptic agent.
- Monitor aseptic technique; correct breaks; accurately classify surgical wound on perioperative nursing record.

## SAMPLE PLAN OF CARE

**INTERVENTIONS—cont'd**

- Have available prescribed topical antibiotics.
- Manage culture specimen collection as indicated.
- Protect from cross-contamination.
- If the operating room (OR) bed is raised, lowered, or turned from side to side, take measures to maintain sterility of field.
- Confine and contain instruments used in groin or leg; change gown and gloves when moving from lower extremities to chest.
- Protect sterility of closed urinary drainage system.
- Maintain continuous surveillance.
- Provide/apply surgical dressings to wound and invasive device sites.
- Maintain sterility of instrument setup until patient discharged from the OR.
- Maintain documentation of all implants.
- During patient rewarming, avoid excessive heat loss: cover exposed areas, irrigate with warm solutions, increase room temperature.
- Monitor for signs and symptoms of infection.

**NURSING DIAGNOSIS**

**Risk for Perioperative Positioning Injury**

**OUTCOME**

The patient is free from signs and symptoms of injury related to positioning as evidenced by the absence of acquired neuromuscular impairment and pressure injury.

**INTERVENTIONS**

- Obtain and prepare appropriate positioning accessories; verify that these are clean and in working order.
- Identify physical alterations that require additional precautions for procedure-specific positioning.
- Verify presence of prosthetics or corrective devices.
- Position the patient by maintaining proper body alignment.
- Pad and protect vulnerable neurovascular bundles and dependent pressure areas.
- Prevent pooling of skin preparation agents at bed lines.
- Pad Thermia blanket.
- Keep all OR bed surfaces dry and wrinkle-free.
- Ensure patency and security of peripheral and central lines, catheters, and electrosurgical dispersive pad on positional changes.
- Have adequate personnel to assist with patient transfer to and from the OR bed and positional changes; lift (do not pull) patient during all positioning maneuvers.
- Safely secure patient to OR bed; ensure that safety straps are not too tightly placed yet maintain patient stability.
- Evaluate for signs and symptoms of injury as a result of positioning.

**NURSING DIAGNOSIS**

**Deficient Knowledge** related to the physiologic effects of the cardiac disorder, proposed surgical procedures, and immediate perioperative events

**OUTCOME**

The patient will demonstrate knowledge of the physiologic responses to the cardiac disorder (at his or her level of understanding), the proposed surgical treatment, and the immediate postoperative events as evidenced by verbalization of disease state, purpose of surgery, sequence of events, anticipated outcomes, and recovery process.

**INTERVENTIONS**

- Explain or describe the following events; solicit feedback from patient:
  - Purpose and expectations of surgery
  - Disease state producing need for surgery
  - Sequence of events during perioperative period
  - Recovery and rehabilitation process
  - Nothing-by-mouth (NPO) status
  - Administration and effects of preoperative medication
  - Transport to operating room
  - Holding area
  - Insertion of peripheral, arterial, and venous lines
  - OR environment (temperature, room furniture and equipment, sounds of monitors and other machines, staff functions, induction of anesthesia)
  - Skin preparation
  - Anticipated length of surgery
  - Minimally invasive versus standard cardiac procedures
  - Surgical intensive care unit and patient status (e.g., unable to talk while intubated and plans for alternative methods of communication)
- Assess knowledge regarding wound care and phases of wound healing.
- Provide information about wound care and anticipated phases of wound healing.
- Determine patient's desire for additional knowledge (respect denial).
- Answer questions; clarify misperceptions.
- Know where family or significant others will be waiting during surgery; provide communication per institutional protocol.
- Evaluate response to information about wound care and phases of wound healing.

**NURSING DIAGNOSIS**

**Risk for Impaired Tissue Integrity** (myocardial, peripheral, renal, and cerebral) related to surgery, hypothermia, cardiopulmonary bypass, and/or surgical particulate or air emboli.

**OUTCOME**

The patient's myocardial, peripheral, and cerebral tissue integrity will be adequate or improved as evidenced by absence of new electrocardiographic manifestations of infarction, the presence of palpable peripheral pulses, adequate urine output, and a clear or improving sensorium postoperatively.

**INTERVENTIONS**

- Identify baseline tissue perfusion.
- Assess factors related to risks for ineffective tissue perfusion.
- Place Thermia blanket on OR bed.
- Preoperatively, provide warm blankets as required.
- Expose only those body areas required for surgical intervention.
- Monitor patient's temperature (esophageal, pulmonary, rectal, bladder, or ventricular septal).
- Adjust room temperature as needed.
- Inspect cardiopulmonary bypass lines for patency and presence of particulate matter; alert surgeon as indicated.
- Use solutions of appropriate temperature when irrigating the heart (cold during hypothermia arrest; warm before and after arrest); warm throughout for "warm heart" surgery.
- Avoid large ice particles on heart.
- Evaluate postoperative tissue perfusion.
- Evaluate progress of wound healing as applicable.

derstanding), the proposed surgical treatment, and the immediate postoperative events as evidenced by verbalization of disease state, purpose of surgery, sequence of events, anticipated outcomes, and recovery process.
- The patient's myocardial, peripheral, renal, and cerebral tissue integrity will be adequate or improved as evidenced by absence of new electrocardiograph manifestations of infarction, the presence of palpable peripheral pulses, and a clear or improving sensorium postoperatively.

Additional nursing diagnoses, based on individual patient assessment, should have a corresponding outcome statement. The outcome should be measurable, with criteria by which to evaluate its achievement. For example, for the outcome "The patient's cardiac function will be consistent with or improved from baseline levels established preoperatively as evidenced by blood pressure within expected range; warm, dry skin; and urine output more than 30 to 50 ml per hour," the perioperative nurse might identify criteria such as vital signs and hemodynamic status consistent with or better than preoperative parameters; fluid and electrolyte balance consistent with preoperative levels; adequate urine output; normal temperature and pink mucosa; absence of rate, rhythm, or conduction defects; absence of iatrogenic injury to the heart; and normal clotting parameters. Each of these criteria becomes evidence that the outcome was achieved. When outcomes are evaluated, they should be documented in the perioperative record. Some outcomes will have been achieved at the conclusion of the surgical procedure; others require ongoing evaluation in the postoperative period to be adequately measured. The "Evaluation" section (see p. 1008) indicates the requirement for ongoing goal measurement by the use of "will" rather than stating the outcome as having been achieved.

The nursing interventions in the Sample Plan of Care incorporate data elements from the Association of periOperative Registered Nurses' (AORN's) Perioperative Nursing Data Set (PNDS).[13] The PNDS offers an exciting opportunity to demonstrate the nurse's ability to influence positive patient outcomes.

## Planning

Once the diagnoses and outcomes have been established, a plan of care (see the Sample Plan of Care) is devised that will enable the perioperative nurse to achieve the goals that have been set. Patient and family needs, elicited from interviews when possible, should be integrated into the planning. The perioperative nurse will need to identify criteria specific to the patient for each of the stated outcomes in the Sample Plan of Care.

## Implementation

Some considerations, in addition to those previously mentioned, can be useful in implementing the perioperative plan of care for patients undergoing cardiac surgery.

***Safety Considerations.*** The safety of the perioperative patient is a primary responsibility of the nurse. Equipment should be functioning properly and undergo routine testing by the biomedical engineering department. Supplies should be used according to manufacturers' instructions, and instruments should be regularly scrutinized to ensure that there are no burrs that could injure tissue, that the jaws of vascular and other clamps align properly, and that small items are accounted for at the end of surgery. Toxic material, such as the glutaraldehyde storage solution of bioprosthetic valves, should be thoroughly rinsed off before implantation. Monitoring the aseptic practices of team members as well as visitors is an important safety consideration.

Staff safety is also important. Protective personal equipment should be consistently and properly worn. Gloves should be used by personnel whenever coming into contact with blood or other body fluids. Electrical, chemical, and other potentially hazardous material within the OR can be minimized by reinforcing safe practices to minimize the risks of injury.

***Special Facilities.*** The OR must be large enough to accommodate bulky, highly specialized equipment while maintaining aseptic technique. Multiple electrical outlets, auxiliary lighting, and additional suction outlets should be available. Ceiling-mounted, mobile booms for housing electrosurgical units (ESUs), headlight sources, suction, medical gases, electrical outlets, and other items can reduce floor clutter and enhance the safety of the environment for patients and staff.[128]

***Instrumentation and Equipment.*** The basic setup described for thoracic procedures (see Chapter 25) is used, along with some specialized cardiovascular instruments and equipment.

Vascular clamps, which are designed to occlude blood flow partially or completely, must be maintained in good condition if they are to prevent fracture of the delicate tunica intima of the blood vessels and still retain their specific holding qualities. There are many variations in construction of vascular instruments. The jaws may consist of single or double rows of fine, sharp, or blunt teeth or special crosshatching or longitudinal serrations. The working angles of the clamps also vary. All clamps are designed to hold the vessels securely and without trauma (Figure 27-13).

Minimally invasive procedures require special instrumentation to access the heart by way of smaller incisions in the anterior and/or lateral aspects of the chest wall (Figure 27-14). Retractors, dissecting instruments, suturing devices, coronary artery stabilizers, and vascular clamps are available.

Sternal and rib retractors are available to meet specific needs. IMA retractors expose the retrosternal artery bed by elevating the sternal border (Figure 27-15). Some sternal retractors have attachments that provide improved exposure of

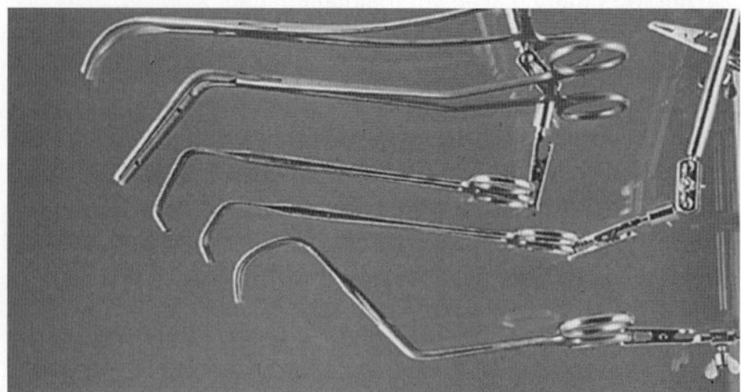

**FIGURE 27-13** Cardiovascular clamps *(top to bottom):* Semb suture passer, Fogarty cross-clamp (angled), Beck partial occlusion clamps (medium and small), Lambert-Kay partial occlusion clamp.

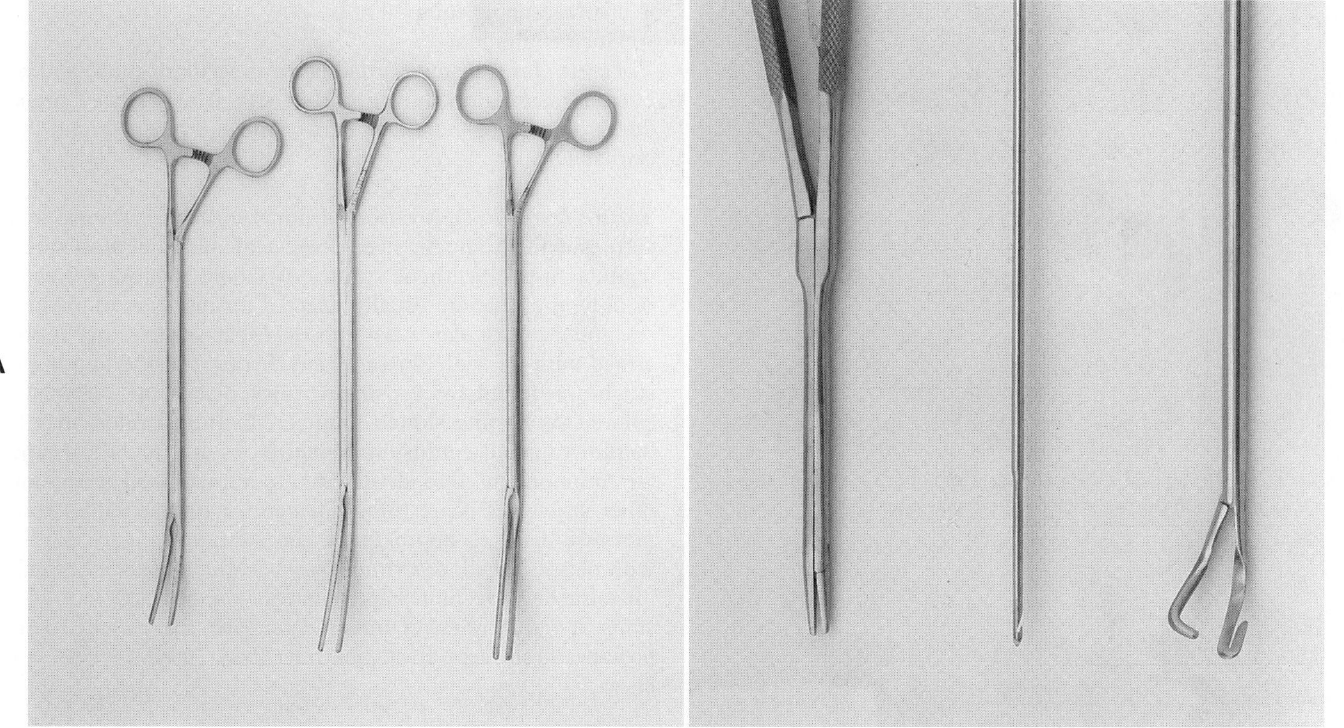


**FIGURE 27-14** **A,** Transthoracic DeBakey vascular clamps are designed to pass through the chest wall by way of smaller incisions for minimally invasive procedures. **B,** Close-up views of minimally invasive needle holder, trocar/suture puller, and knot slider.

the left atrium during mitral valve replacement (MVR) (Figure 27-16). Exposure of the left or right atrium or the aortic root may also be accomplished with handheld retractors. Special rib spreaders provide exposure for mini-thoracotomy procedures. Coronary artery stabilizer systems with left ventricular apical suction retractors (Figure 27-17) are widely employed for beating heart coronary bypass surgery.

Other equipment commonly used (or available) for cardiac surgery may include the following:

- Sternal saw and motor
- Irrigation fluid cooling/warming machine
- Autotransfusion/cell saver system
- Electrical fibrillator
- Direct current (DC) defibrillator with internal paddles (Figure 27-18) and adhesive external pads
- Thermia unit (mattress or forced air–warming)
- External and internal pulse pacemaker generator (single and dual chamber)
- Pump oxygenator/CPB machine
- Epicardial pacemaker leads (temporary and permanent)
- Fiberoptic headlight and light source
- Intraaortic balloon pump (IABP)
- Mechanical ventricular assist devices (VADs)
- Cryoablation energy sources (for atrial fibrillation [AF] surgery)
- Radiofrequency energy sources (for AF surgery)
- TEE probe and monitor
- Minimally invasive, video-assisted vein-harvesting system

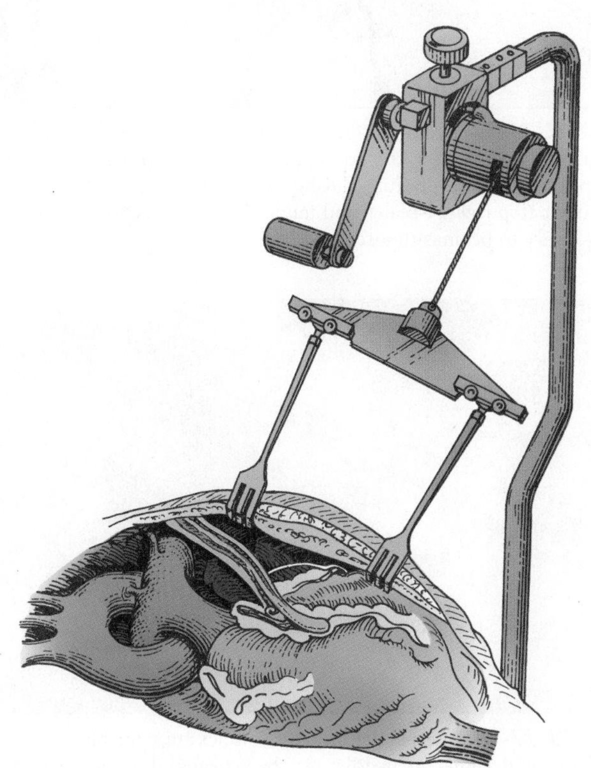

**FIGURE 27-15** Retractor used to elevate sternal border for exposure of the internal mammary artery.

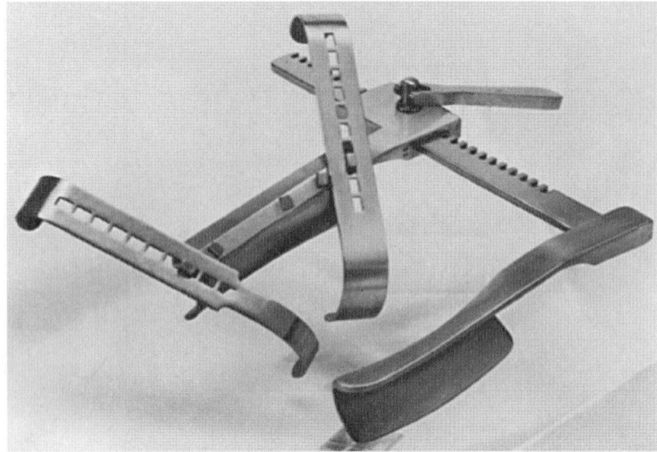

FIGURE 27-16 Sternal self-retaining retractor with attachments for left atrial retraction during mitral valve replacement.

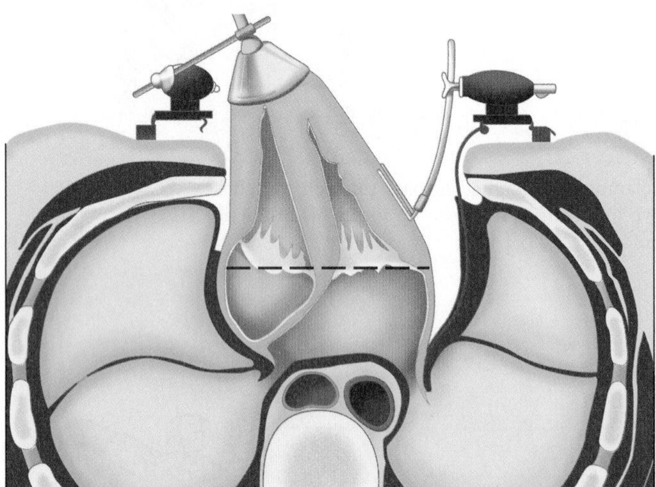

FIGURE 27-17 Cross-section of chest showing *(top left)* left ventricular apical suction cup to expose lateral and posterior coronary arteries for bypass grafting during off-pump surgery. The platform stabilizer *(top right)* isolates and immobilizes the section of the coronary artery to be anastomosed.

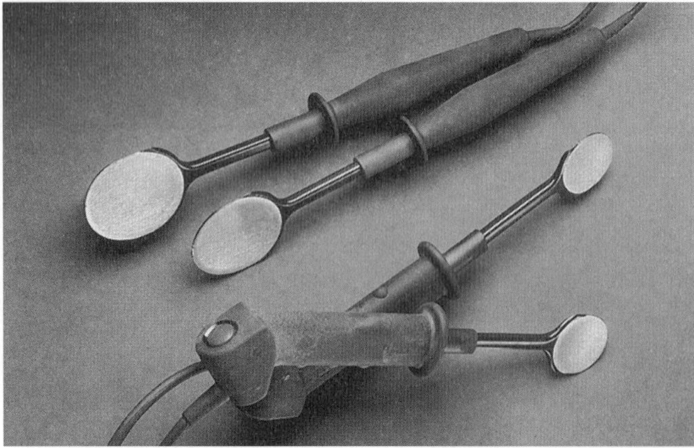

FIGURE 27-18 Internal defibrillator paddles are available in an array of sizes and designs: the paddles may be activated through the handles or by pressing the button on the defibrillator. Smaller internal paddles are used for infants and children.

- Thoracoscopic equipment
- Video equipment

Lasers (for transmyocardial laser revascularization) and robots (for retraction during port-access, video-assisted procedures) increasingly are also part of the equipment found in a cardiac OR.

***Suture Materials.*** A variety of nonabsorbable cardiovascular sutures with atraumatic needles are available from most suture manufacturers. Synthetic sutures of Teflon, Dacron, polyester, or polypropylene are usually selected for insertion of prostheses and for vascular anastomoses. Most sutures are double armed with a needle on each end. Because of the number of stitches required for prosthetic valve placement, alternately colored suture and slotted, numbered suture holders may be helpful to avoid confusion. Vessel loops and umbilical tapes are commonly used to identify and to retract blood vessels and other structures. Wire (monofilament or twisted cable) commonly is used to approximate the sternum (Figure 27-19), with plastic, metal, or nylon bands occasionally added to reinforce fragile bone. Skin staplers may be used to close skin incisions; a staple remover must accompany the patient to the postanesthesia area if staples have been used to close the chest.

***Supplies.*** The following supplies are generally used in most cardiac procedures. Depending on the surgeon's preference, other items may be added or substituted.

- Rubber shods
- Pill sponges (gauze dissectors)
- Various-sized Silastic or polyvinyl chloride tubing
- Tourniquet catheters

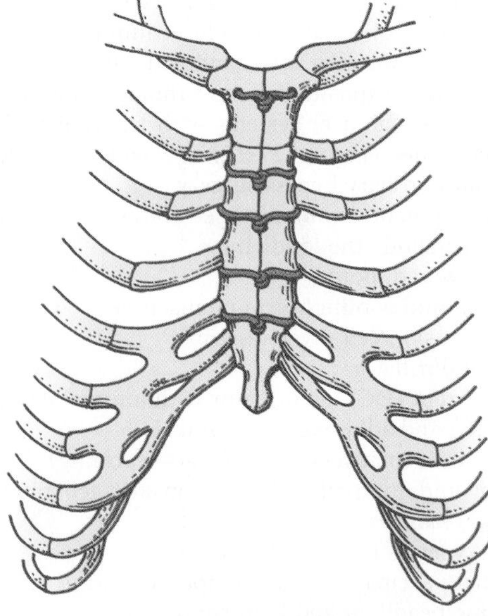

FIGURE 27-19 Technique for wire closure of the sternum. A variety of closing mechanisms have become available. These may consist of monofilament wire (shown), twisted wire cables, or in some instances, plates and screws. In selected patients in whom disruption may be anticipated, such as elderly, obese, or malnourished persons, two or more heavy bands of nylon may be passed around the sternum and secured by a twisted stainless steel wire in addition to the wire sutures. A figure-of-eight technique may also be employed.

- Disposable drapes
- Foot-control and hand-control ESU pencils, ultrasonic scalpel
- Adapters, connectors, stop cocks
- Extra syringes and needles for injections, infusions, and blood samples
- Marking pen to identify anastomotic sites and mark grafts
- Irrigation cannulas
- Disposable vascular (bulldog) clamps
- Coronary occluders and stabilizers
- Autotransfusion supplies
- Chest tubes, chest drainage system
- Topical hemostatic agents
- CPB and myocardial protection cannulas, tubing, connectors

***Prosthetic Material.*** In addition to these general supplies, special supplies are needed for repair or replacement of cardiovascular structures. Intracardiac patches, heart valves, and synthetic grafts should be handled with care to prevent damage or the introduction of foreign materials. Teflon, a fluorocarbon fiber, and Dacron, a polyester fiber, are available in a variety of meshes, fabrics, felts, tapes, and sutures and are also combined with other materials in prosthetic heart valves (Figure 27-20).

Teflon patches are made in a variety of forms for intracardiac and outflow tract use. Varying degrees of firmness, thickness, and porosity are available for specific uses. Low reactivity, strength retention, and tissue acceptance are important properties to be considered in the selection of such patches.

Dacron arterial grafts are commonly used in cardiac surgery, although reinforced expanded polytetrafluoroethylene (PTFE) grafts are also available. There are two types of Dacron grafts: knitted and woven. Woven prosthetic grafts are usually employed when the patient has been fully heparinized because the interstices of woven grafts are tighter than those in knitted grafts and bleeding is usually reduced. The advantages of knitted grafts are that they do not fray as readily as woven grafts when cut, they are easier to handle, and they reendothelialize more quickly than woven grafts do. Grafts are available in a variety of sizes and may be straight or bifurcated (Figure 27-21). Knitted and woven grafts impregnated with collagen to reduce interstitial bleeding are useful in the thoracic aorta and do not have to be preclotted, even when the patient is fully heparinized for cardiopulmonary bypass. Graft sizers are available for determining the correct size.

Endovascular, expandable stented tube grafts are available for both the abdominal aorta[111] and the thoracic aorta[63] (Figure 27-22). The endovascular graft is inserted percutaneously

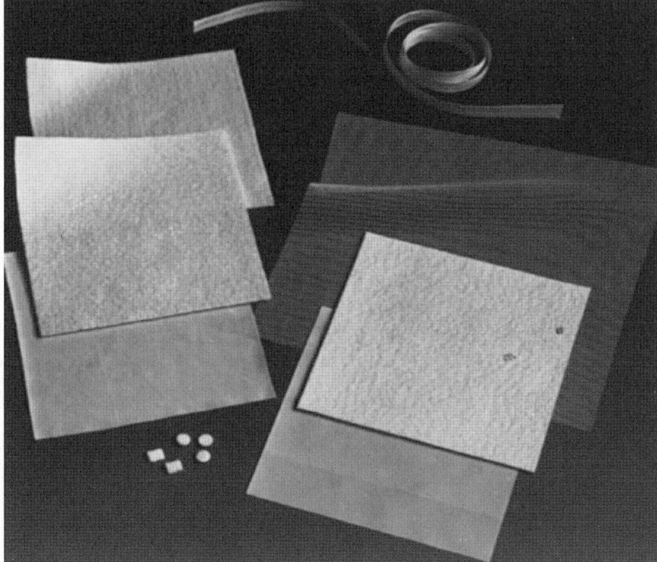

**FIGURE 27-20** Assorted prosthetic materials to repair intracardiac and extracardiac defects: tapes, Teflon and Dacron patches, and pledgets.

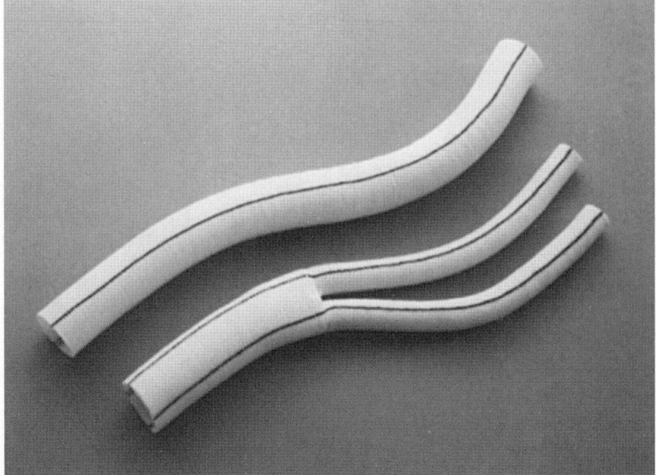

**FIGURE 27-21** Straight and bifurcated arterial tube grafts.

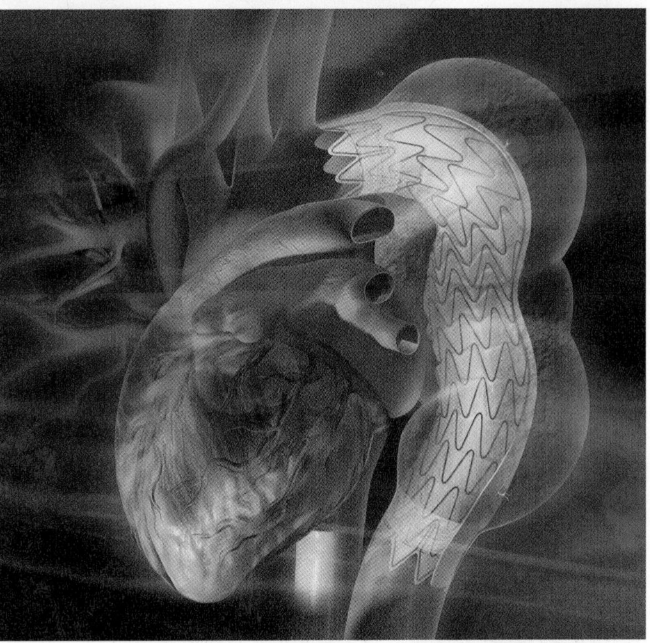

**FIGURE 27-22** Thoracic aortic endovascular stented prosthesis made from expanded polytetrafluoroethylene (PTFE). The compressed device is inserted percutaneously through the femoral artery by way of a delivery catheter and guided to the desired position in the thoracic aorta under fluoroscopy. When the correct position has been confirmed, the device expands automatically after it is deployed from the delivery catheter. The delivery catheter is then withdrawn, and hemostasis of the femoral incision site achieved.

into the femoral artery and advanced to the desired position in the abdominal or thoracic aorta where the prosthesis is opened and implanted.

***Valve Prostheses.*** Valve prostheses are selected according to their hemodynamics, thromboresistance, durability, ease of insertion, anatomic suitability, and patient acceptability. Cost, outcome, and value also have become important attributes.[28] Most mechanical prostheses employ a tilting disk or ball-and-cage design. Prosthetic valves allow complete closure with slight regurgitation to prevent stasis of blood (Figures 27-23 to 27-26). Biologic valves include porcine and bovine prostheses (Figures 27-27 to 27-29). Porcine valves consist of an aortic valve from a pig, which can be sutured to a Dacron-covered stent (see Figure 27-27, *A*), or the porcine aortic valve may be "stentless" (without a sewing ring) to enhance the hemodynamics, especially in patients with a small aortic root (i.e., orifice less than 21 mm) (see Figure 27-27, *B*). Bovine (calf) pericardial valves (see Figure 27-28) are created by cutting

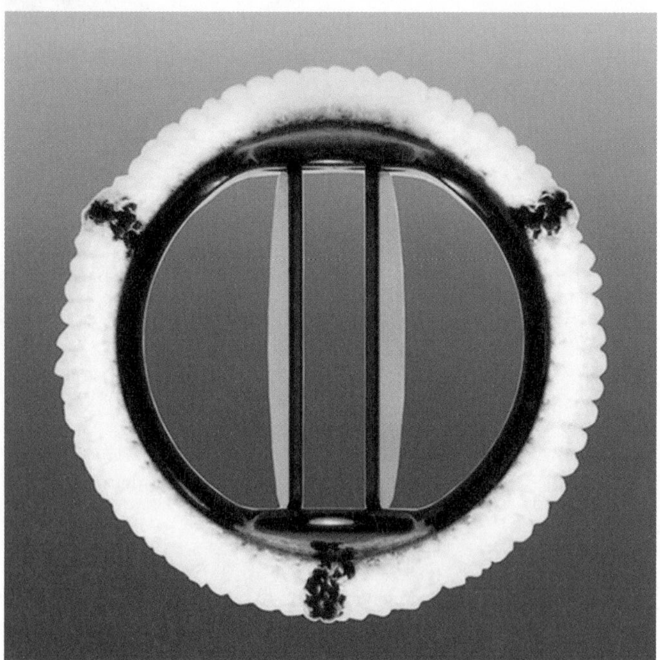

**FIGURE 27-23** St. Jude Medical bileaflet tilting disk valve prosthesis.

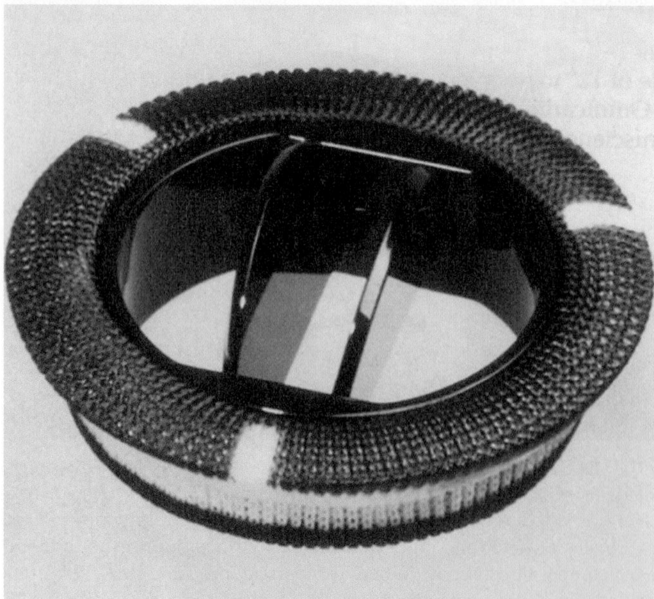

**FIGURE 27-24** Carbomedics supraannular aortic prosthesis designed for the small aortic root.

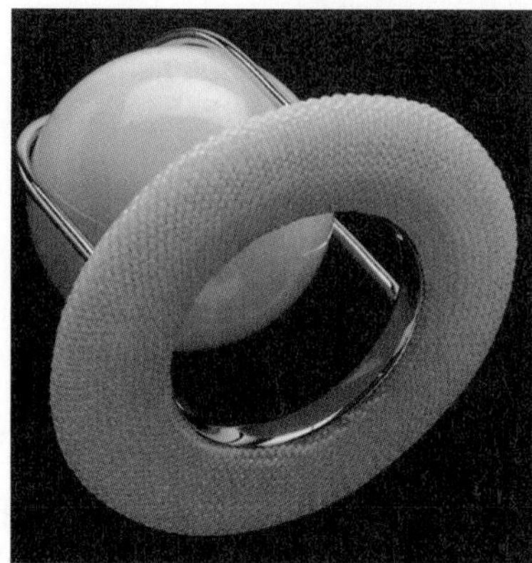

**FIGURE 27-25** Starr-Edwards ball and cage aortic valve prosthesis.

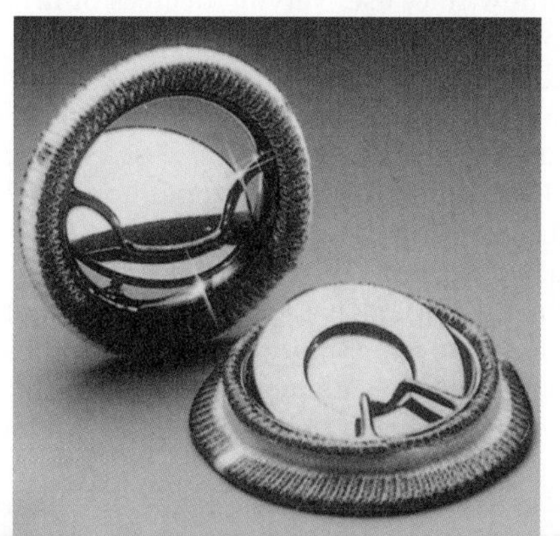

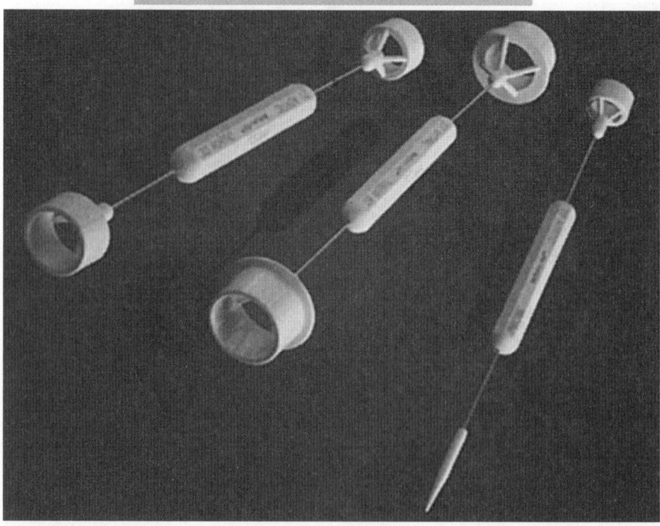

**FIGURE 27-26 A,** Medtronic-Hall tilting disk valve prosthesis. **B,** Double-ended sizing obturators for the Medtronic-Hall prosthesis *(left and center)* and probe *(right)* to test leaflet movement. All valve prostheses have sizing obturators specific to the prosthesis itself.

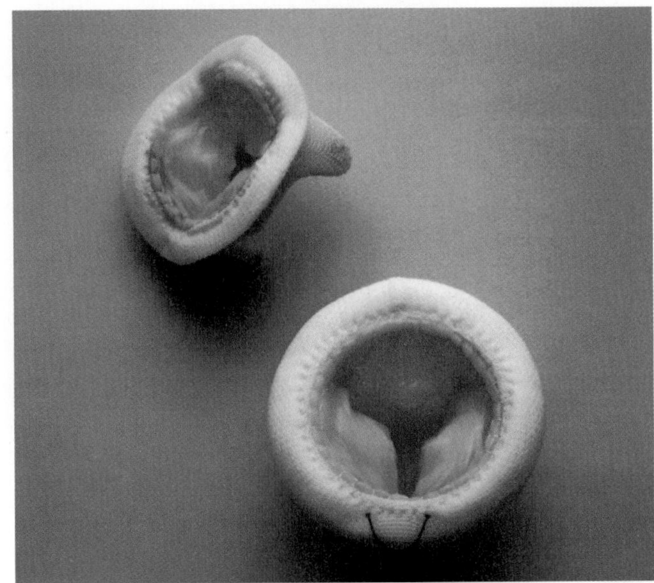



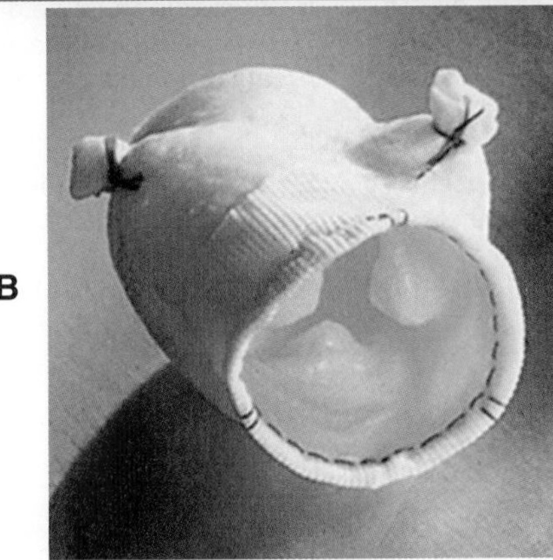



**FIGURE 27-27** **A,** Medtronic Mosaic porcine aortic *(top)* and mitral *(bottom)* bioprostheses. **B,** Stentless porcine aortic valve. The absence of a stent and sewing ring provides a greater orifice area through which blood can flow.

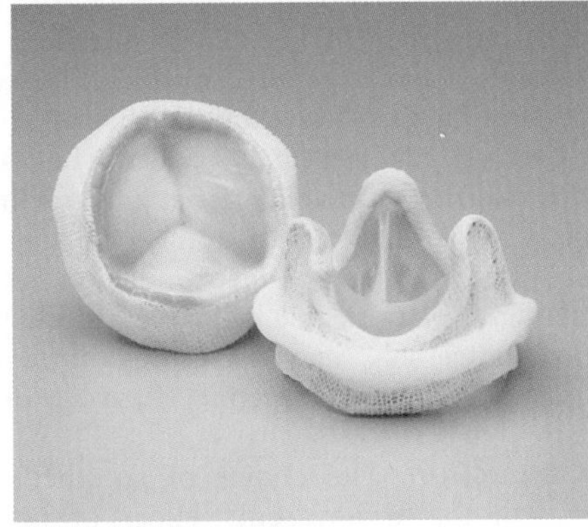

**FIGURE 27-28** Carpentier-Edwards bovine pericardial aortic bioprosthesis.

leaflet-shaped pieces from bovine pericardium and sewing them onto a stent. The advantage of these biologic valves is that long-term anticoagulants are not necessary in most patients. Obturators for sizing prosthetic valves as well as valve holders are specific to the prostheses (see Figures 27-26, *B,* and 27-29). Tables 27-4 and 27-5 compare mechanical and biologic prosthetic heart valves. Tissue-engineered heart valves may offer a future potential cure for valvular heart disease.[72]

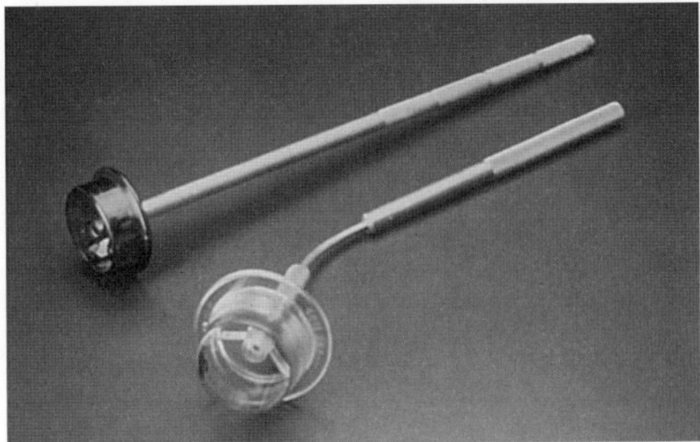

**FIGURE 27-29** Obturators for Carpentier-Edwards porcine bioprosthesis.

Aortic valve allografts (homografts) are also used with increasing frequency because of their advantages: little or no risk of thromboembolism, optimal hemodynamic function, no need for anticoagulation drugs, and no risk of sudden catastrophic failure. Moreover, they demonstrate a lower incidence of infective endocarditis than mechanical or biologic valves do and their long-term durability is comparable with that of bioprostheses. Allograft root replacement is also a valuable technique in the setting of prosthetic valve endocarditis.[74] The entire ascending aorta and valve (Figure 27-30) or the valve alone (Figure 27-31) may be inserted. Allografts are cyropreserved and must be thawed in saline according to the vendor's protocol before implantation.

Conduits consisting of mechanical or biologic aortic valves attached to a tube graft (Figure 27-32) are used in procedures such as repair of aortic dissections requiring replacement of the aortic valve and ascending aorta. If vein grafts must be inserted into the conduit or if a direct coronary ostial anastomosis is required, an eye cautery is used to make the opening into the graft and at the same time heat-seal the cut edges of the prosthesis. Conduits with *biologic* valves interposed between tube graft materials may be used when patients are at increased risk for bleeding complications from chronic anticoagulation. Allograft conduits may be used for these procedures as well.

In addition to the use of allografts to avoid the complications associated with prosthetic valve replacement, valve repair rather than replacement is preferred when possible, particularly with mitral and tricuspid valves. When repairing the native valve with an annuloplasty ring, obturators specific to various kinds of annuloplasty rings are used to size the annulus (Figure 27-33, *A* and *B*).

Safety considerations include storing prosthetic materials in a clean, protected environment and using them according to manufacturers' instructions. Before implantation, biologic valves must be rinsed in three saline baths to remove the glutaraldehyde storage solution. During insertion, they should be kept moist with saline. Mechanical valves should be protected from scratching and other injury.

**TABLE 27-4**

## Commonly Used Mechanical Valve Prostheses

| | Ball and Cage | Tilting Disk | |
|---|---|---|---|
| | **Starr-Edwards** | **Medtronic-Hall, Omniscience** | **St. Jude Medical, Carbomedics** |
| Model/description | 6120 Mitral<br>1260 Aortic | Spherical tilting disk | Bileaflet tilting disk |
| Advantages | Long-term durability<br>Good hemodynamics<br>Inaudible<br>Least risk of sudden thrombosis | Long-term durability<br>Good hemodynamics in all sizes<br>Low profile | Long-term durability<br>Good hemodynamics in all sizes<br>Low profile<br>Low TE rate for a mechanical valve |
| Disadvantages | Anticoagulation required<br>Higher incidence of TE than disk valves<br>Large profile<br>Suboptimal hemodynamics in small aortic sizes (less than 23 mm)<br>High profile not optimal in small LV or aortic root<br>Higher risk of TE in mitral position | Anticoagulation required<br>Potential for sudden thrombosis<br>Noisy<br>Higher risk of TE in mitral position<br>If Coumadin must be discontinued, there is increased risk of catastrophic thrombosis | Anticoagulation strongly recommended<br>Potential for sudden thrombosis<br>Some noise<br>Higher risk of TE in mitral position<br>If Coumadin must be discontinued, there is increased risk of catastrophic thrombosis |
| Special considerations | Sizers and handles specific to prosthesis; must be sterilized<br>Poppet of aortic valve removable to facilitate tying sutures; replaced before aorta closed; mitral poppet not removable<br>Aortic model has three struts; mitral has four | Sizers and handles specific to prosthesis; must be sterilized | Sizers and handles specific to prosthesis; must be sterilized<br>Frequently used in children needing prosthetic valve |
| Resterilization* | | | |

*TE,* Thromboembolism; *LV,* left ventricle.
*Follow manufacturer's instructions. All prostheses should be stored in a cool, dry, contamination-free area.

***Preinduction Care.*** The patient is brought to the OR suite, where a focused preoperative assessment is performed and the perioperative nurse reviews the chart for completion and documentation of informed consent, advance directives, laboratory results, diagnostic data, and other pertinent information. The nurse confirms the identity of the patient and the intended operation, including identification and confirmation of the site and side, as applicable. Verification of which leg (i.e., right or left) will be used for vein harvest in bypass patients may not be necessary if the choice of which leg to use depends on the operator's preference rather than a specific clinical indication. However, some institutions may require verification of bypass harvesting sites, and the nurse should follow institutional policy for guidance.

Preoperatively, cardiac surgical patients may exhibit more stress and anxiety than other types of patients. Perioperative nurses should anticipate and prepare for this reaction because anxiety increases myocardial oxygen consumption. Efforts to reduce the family's anxiety level are also important and result in less emotional stress being transmitted to the patient.

A peripheral arterial pressure line and venous infusion lines are inserted. A local anesthetic may be used at the insertion sites, and a sedative may be injected intravenously.

***Admission to the Operating Room.*** Depending on the amount of sedation received preoperatively, the patient may require assistance onto the OR bed. Warm blankets should be provided for comfort and to reduce shivering (Patient Safety). After application of the ECG leads and the pulse oximeter finger cot, the hands, elbows, and feet can be padded. The perioperative nurse confirms that the peripheral arterial pressure line is functioning properly and repositions the arm in collaboration with the anesthesia provider. Pulse oximetry function is confirmed. The nurse should be aware that skin pigment, especially in darker-skinned individuals, may overestimate arterial oxygen saturation measured by pulse oximetry[14] (Research Highlight).

***Anesthesia Induction.*** The choice of anesthetic agent or agents depends on the cardiovascular effects of the anesthetic (Table 27-6), the patient's hemodynamic status and general health, and the anticipated length of stay in the surgical intensive care unit (SICU). Newer, fast-acting anesthetic agents are used to "fast-track" patients postoperatively, whereby the patient is extubated in the OR, or very shortly after admission to the SICU, to speed the recuperation process.[2]

In addition to anesthetic medications, multiple other drugs are employed to vasodilate, constrict, enhance heart rate and

**TABLE 27-5**

## Commonly Used Biologic Valve Prostheses

| | Heterograft (Xenograft) | | |
|---|---|---|---|
| | **Carpentier-Edwards (CE) Medtronic Stentless Porcine Bioprostheses** | **Carpentier-Edwards Pericardial Valve Prosthesis** | **Allograft (Homograft)** |
| Model/ description | Porcine heterograft (from excised pig aortic valves)<br>CE: leaflets attached to sewing ring<br>Stentless (aortic): no sewing ring; includes porcine aortic root with coronary ostial branches | 2700 aortic bovine pericardium (cut and shaped into a trileaflet valve) | Aortic valve allograft (cadaver, organ donor, excised cardiomyopathic heart from transplant recipient; mitral valve allograft also available) |
| Advantages | Incidence of TE very low; anticoagulation rare after AVR<br>Stentless has excellent flow<br>No hemolysis<br>Good hemodynamics<br>Central flow<br>Gradual failure allows elective reoperation<br>Durability good after age 60 yr<br>Stentless graft has many advantages of allograft valves | Incidence of TE very low; anticoagulation rare after AVR<br>No hemolysis<br>Good hemodynamics in all sizes<br>Central flow<br>Gradual failure allows elective reoperation<br>Residual gradient minimal | Incidence of TE very low; anticoagulation rare; used for AVR and MVR<br>No hemolysis<br>Excellent hemodynamics, (especially with stentless technique)<br>Central flow<br>Gradual failure allows elective reoperation<br>No residual gradient |
| Disadvantages | Durability may be less than 15 yr<br>Stentless valve available only for AVR<br>Accelerated fibrocalcific degeneration in children, patients with hypertension, or patients on chronic renal dialysis<br>Suboptimal hemodynamics (except stentless model) and residual gradient in small sizes (less than 23 mm aorta or 29 mm mitral) may be contraindicated in small, hypertrophied LV | Durability not yet established<br>Available only for AVR<br>Accelerated calcification may be a problem in children, renal patients, or those with hypertension | Limited durability<br>Limited availability |
| Special considerations | Sizers and handles specific to prosthesis; must be sterilized before insertion; must be rinsed in saline to remove storage solution before insertion; frequent irrigation recommended to prevent drying<br>Diets low in calcium recommended for children, renal patients | Sizers and handles specific to prosthesis; must be sterilized before insertion; must be rinsed in saline to remove storage solution before insertion; frequent irrigation recommended to prevent drying<br>Diets low in calcium recommended for children, renal patients | No specific sizers; may use sizers for heterografts; cyropreserved allograft must be thawed per protocol; used for aortic or mitral valve replacement; stent can be attached if indicated for use in other positions |
| Resterilization | Not recommended | Not recommended | Not recommended |

Modified from Society of Thoracic Surgeons: *STS patient information.* Available at www.sts.org/doc/8786; Hammermeister K and others: Outcomes 15 years after valve replacement with a mechanical versus a bioprosthetic valve: final report of the Veterans Affairs randomized trial, *Journal of the American College of Cardiology* 36(4):1152-1158, 2000.
*TE,* Thromboembolism; *AVR,* aortic valve replacement; *MVR,* mitral valve replacement; *LV,* left ventricle.

contractility, anticoagulate, promote diuresis, and provide antibiotic prophylaxis (Table 27-7).

Because the period of induction is one of the most critical during the procedure, close monitoring of the patient is required, especially for patients with ventricular ischemia from congenital or acquired disease. Anesthetic management focuses on maintaining an adequate cardiac output by keeping myocardial oxygen demand low and the oxygen supply high.[2] (See Chapter 4 for additional considerations related to anesthesia care monitoring.)

***Monitoring.*** Extensive monitoring of hemodynamic and other variables is indicated during cardiac surgery (Surgical Pharmacology). After intubation (or before, depending on the anesthesia provider's preference), additional pressure lines may be inserted to measure central venous pressure (CVP) and pulmonary artery pressures (PAPs). Maximal sterile barriers should be used for insertion of central lines[60] (Best Practice). Peripheral and central arterial and venous pressures are usually monitored directly by means of a transducer and oscilloscope. Perioperative nurses may be required to collaborate in

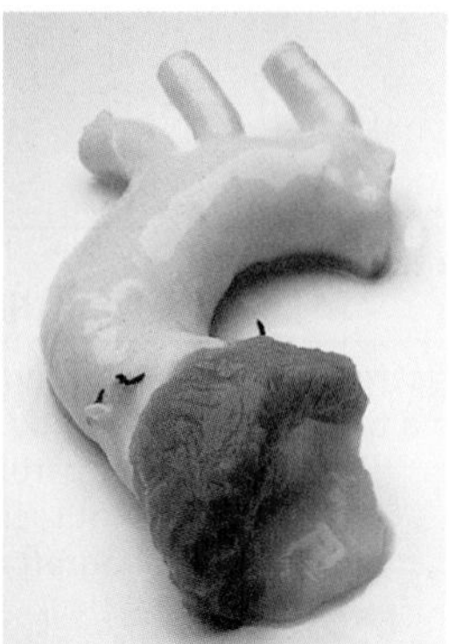

**FIGURE 27-30** Aortic allograft with aortic valve and arch vessels attached.

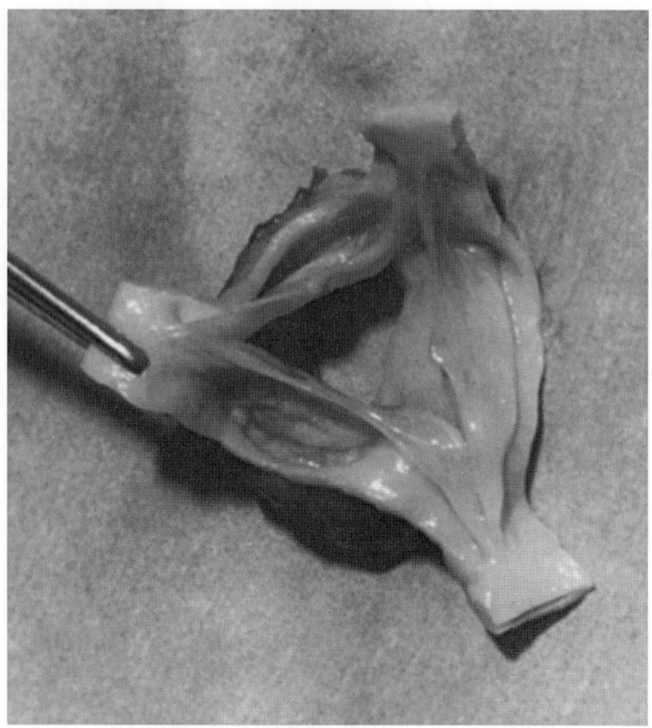

**FIGURE 27-31** Aortic valve allograft.

the preparation and placement of central lines; they should observe the ECG monitors for signs of ventricular irritability, such as ectopy or tachycardia, and be prepared to assist with defibrillation of the patient if necessary. If the patient cannot be resuscitated, the chest is opened rapidly and internal cardiac massage is performed to perfuse the circulatory system. An indwelling urinary catheter is inserted for monitoring renal function, especially during and after CPB. It may contain a thermistor temperature probe. Other temperature probes may be placed, usually in the esophagus, nasopharynx, or rectum. Temperatures can also be recorded from the pulmonary artery catheters and the arterial infusion line of the bypass circuit. Ventricular septal temperatures may be recorded while the patient's heart is arrested.

The skin is carefully inspected before ECG and ESU dispersive pads are placed. Bony prominences, such as the coccyx and the back of the head, are padded to prevent pressure necrosis resulting from hypoperfusion and hypothermia during bypass. Because elderly patients are especially vulnerable to skin breakdown, additional precautions to avoid pressure injuries are recommended.[4] Monitoring aseptic practice is an important infection control practice.

***Positioning.*** The supine position provides optimum exposure for the institution of CPB and the surgical repair of the heart and great vessels. In addition, there are less respiratory impairment and discomfort with this approach. When the su-

## PATIENT SAFETY

### Preventing Burns from Items Stored in Warming Cabinets

In cardiac surgery, as in other surgical specialties, attention is paid to keeping patients warm and avoiding inadvertent hypothermia. Warmth is associated with both patient comfort and preventing the physiologic consequences of even mild inadvertent hypothermia. For example, shivering increases the workload of the heart and this can have serious consequences in a patient with preexisting decreased cardiac reserve. Moreover, as early as 1997, a study by Sessler underscored the adverse outcomes of cardiac events, coagulopathy, surgical wound infections, and prolonged hospitalization associated with mild hypothermia. In a follow-up meta-analysis that examined the consequences of mild perioperative hypothermia, Mahoney noted adverse outcomes of patient discomfort, untoward cardiac events, adrenergic stimulation, impaired platelet function, altered drug metabolism, and impaired wound healing.

Because of these research findings, perioperative nurses direct many nursing care interventions toward actively keeping patients warm and maintaining normothermia. Most operating rooms (ORs) have warming cabinets for storing blankets and solutions. Solutions may include those used during surgery for irrigation, intravenous (IV) bags, or irrigation solution bags. Cotton blankets are frequently warmed and placed in layers on or under patients. To avoid burns from items stored in warming cabinets, the Emergency Care Research Institute (ECRI) recommends the following:

- Set the temperature of warming cabinets to 110°F (43°C), and ensure that the temperature setting cannot be changed. The engineering department should be consulted to ensure that warming cabinet temperature settings are accurately calibrated.
- Educate perioperative staff to the burn risk to unconscious patients. Items that do not feel overly hot to the perioperative nurse's hand can actually burn a patient who has received anesthesia, including regional anesthesia.
- Include responsibility for annual inspection of warming cabinets by the institution's engineering department.

Modified from ECRI hazard report: Limiting temperature settings on blanket and solution warming cabinets can prevent patient burns, *Health Devices* 34:168-171, 2005; Mahoney CB: Perioperative hypothermia: a clinical and financial risk. Presented at the 53rd annual AORN Congress, March 21, 2006, Washington, DC; Sessler DI: Current concepts: mild intraoperative hypothermia, *New England Journal of Medicine* 336:1730-1737, 1997.

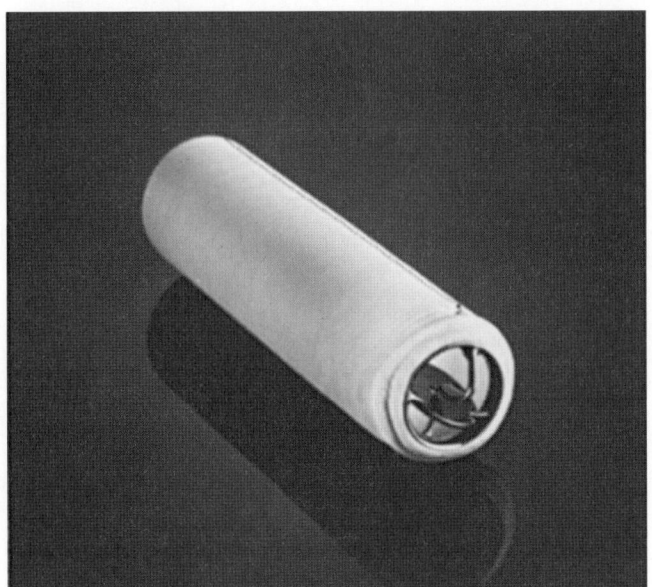

FIGURE 27-32 Valved conduit with Medtronic-Hall tilting disk valve prosthesis.

## RESEARCH HIGHLIGHT

### Skin Pigmentation and the Accuracy of Pulse Oximetry

Pulse oximetry is designed to compute accurately the arterial hemoglobin oxygen saturation independent of skin pigmentation. However, there have been cases of unacceptable errors in pulse oximetry at low saturation levels in pigmented subjects. The authors tested three types of pulse oximeters to determine whether errors at low arterial oxyhemoglobin saturation ($Sao_2$) correlate with skin color. Twenty-one healthy, nonsmoking subjects were studied; 11 subjects were very darkly pigmented individuals of African American descent, and 10 subjects were light-skinned individuals of northern European descent. Pulse oximeter probes were placed on the subjects' fingers; an indwelling 22-gauge radial artery line also was inserted to sample $Sao_2$. Study results showed that at all $Sao_2$ levels and with all three types of oximeters, $Spo_2$ (oxygen saturation measured by pulse oximetry) readings were approximately 1% higher in dark-skinned individuals than in light-skinned individuals ($P < 0.0001$). At lower oxyhemoglobin saturation levels (hypoxia), there were differences of up to 8% between light- and dark-skinned persons. The authors suggest that because most pulse oximeters have been designed and calibrated by manufacturers using light-skinned individuals at room air saturation levels, it has been assumed that skin pigment is unimportant. Accurate $Sao_2$ readings during surgery for acquired or congenital heart disease are necessary to anticipate, monitor, and treat hypoxic episodes. The authors recommend that there be a warning notice on devices to alert clinicians to the possibility of overestimation of arterial oxygen saturation in dark-skinned individuals, especially at low saturation levels.

Modified from Bickler PE and others: Effects of skin pigmentation on pulse oximeter accuracy at low saturation, *Anesthesiology* 102:715-719, 2005.

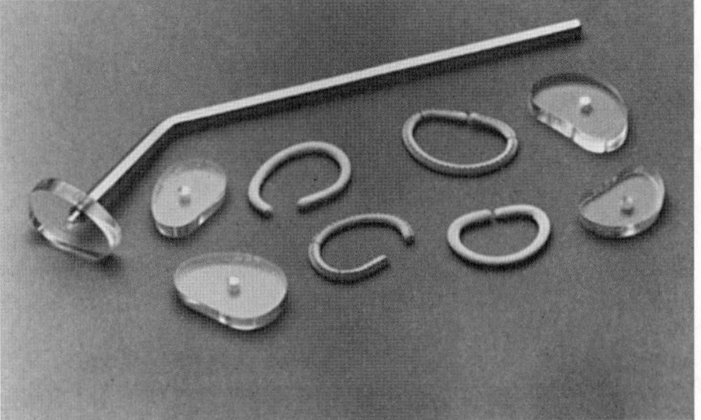

A

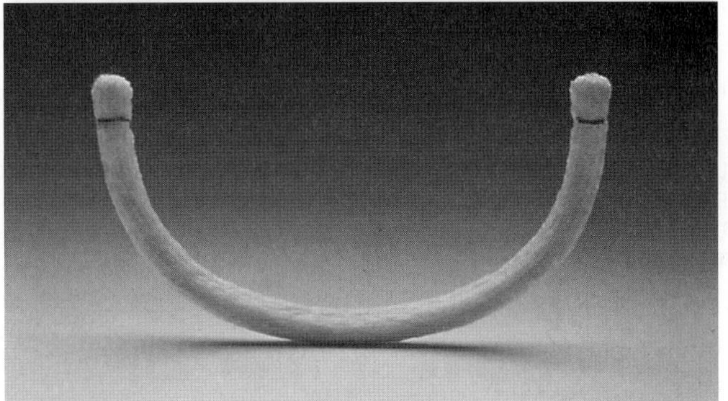

B

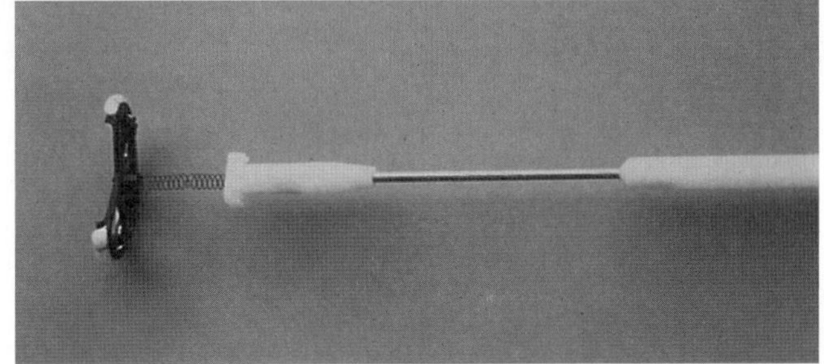

C

FIGURE 27-33 **A,** Carpentier-Edwards "classic" tricuspid and mitral annuloplasty rings, sizers, and sizer handle. The tricuspid rings are notched in the area corresponding to conduction tissue in the tricuspid annulus to avoid suture injury. **B,** Cosgrove annuloplasty ring. **C,** Ring attached to ring holder and handle.

pine position is used, the hands and arms are tucked along either side of the body. The legs may be slightly "frog-legged" to provide access to the femoral arteries for insertion of pressure lines and IABP lines or to excise the saphenous vein. Measures to avoid pressure injury (especially in the elderly, debilitated, or obese patient) include padding the coccyx and applying heel protectors. Measures to protect the occipital area from pressure ulcers include placing pillows under the head and repositioning the head during surgery. Significant factors associated with the development of pressure ulcers include diabetes mellitus; lower preoperative hemoglobin, hematocrit, and serum albumin levels; and the presence of intraaortic balloon pumps.[83]

A semilateral position may be employed for thoracoabdominal aneurysms in order to expose both the descending thoracic aorta and the abdominal aorta. A thoracotomy position is used for some minimally invasive procedures and surgery on the descending thoracic aorta. The presence of severe

**TABLE 27-6**

## Perioperative Patient Monitoring

| Monitoring Device | Location | Measures |
|---|---|---|
| Electrocardiogram (ECG) | Lateral, posterior electrode placement | Electrical activity of heart |
| Arterial line | Peripheral radial artery<br>Central femoral artery<br>Aorta (with needle attached to pressure tubing, or with sensor in bypass circuit) | Arterial blood pressure (direct) |
| Blood pressure (BP) cuff | Upper arm | Arterial BP (indirect) |
| Central venous pressure (CVP) | Right atrium (RA) | RA pressure (e.g., CVP) |
| Pulmonary artery (PA) catheter (Swan-Ganz) | RA (proximal port) | RA pressure (e.g., CVP) |
| | Right ventricle (RV) (midline port) | RV pressure |
| | Distal PA (distal port) | PA and pulmonary artery wedge pressure (PAWP)<br>Indirect measure of left atrial and left ventricular (LV) pressure<br>Cardiac output |
| Left atrial (LA) line | Left atrium | LA, LV pressure |
| Pulse oximeter | Finger, earlobe | Oxygen saturation of arterial hemoglobin |
| Urinary drainage catheter | Urinary bladder | Urine output, renal perfusion/function |
| Temperature probes | Esophagus<br>Urinary bladder<br>Rectum<br>Ventricular septum<br>Bypass circuit<br>Face/forehead (adhesive patch) | Temperature (core and peripheral) |
| Electroencephalogram (EEG) | Head | Electrical activity of brain; awareness |
| Transesophageal echocardiogram (TEE) | Esophagus | Cardiac function, presence of air |

**TABLE 27-7**

## Hemodynamic Effects of Anesthetic Drugs

| | Hemodynamic Effect | | | | | |
|---|---|---|---|---|---|---|
| **Drug** | **CI** | **BP** | **SVR** | **PLVED** | **HR** | **Contractility** |
| *d*-Tubocurarine | ↓ | ↓ | ↓ | ↓ | ↑ | ↔ |
| Diazepam | ↓ | ↓ | ↓ | ↓ | ↔ | ↔ |
| Dimethyl tubocurarine | ↑ | ↔↑ | ↔↓ | ↔↓ | ↑ | ↔ |
| Droperidol | ↔↑ | ↓ | ↓ | ↓ | ↑ | ↔ |
| Enflurane | ↓ | ↓ | ↓ | ↔↓ | ↔↓ | ↓ |
| Fentanyl | ↔ | ↓ | ↓ | ↔ | ↔ | ↔ |
| Halothane | ↓ | ↓ | ↔↓ | ↔↑ | ↔↑↓ | ↓ |
| Innovar | ↔↑ | ↓ | ↓ | ↓ | ↔ | ↔ |
| Isoflurane | ↔ | ↓ | ↓ | ↔ | ↑ | ↓ |
| Ketamine | ↑ | ↑ | ↑ | ↑ | ↑ | – |
| Methoxyflurane | ↓ | ↓ | ↓ | ↔ | ↔ | ↓ |
| Midazolam | ↔ | ↔ | ↔↓ | ↓ | ↑ | ↔↓ |
| Morphine | ↔↑ | ↔↓ | ↓ | ↔↑ | ↓ | ↔ |
| Nitrous oxide | ↓ | ↔↓ | ↔↑ | ↑ | ↔↓ | ↓ |
| Pancuronium | ↑ | ↑ | ↔ | ↓ | ↑ | ? |
| Succinylcholine | ↓ | ↔↓ | ↓ | ↓ | ↑↓ | ? |
| Thiopental | ↔↓ | ↔ | ↑ | ↔ | ↑ | ↓ |
| Vecuronium | ↔ | ↔ | ↔ | ↔ | ↔ | ↔ |

From Kouchoukos N and others: *Kirklin/Barratt-Boyes cardiac surgery,* ed 3, vol I, Philadelphia, 2003, Churchill Livingstone.
↓, decrease; ↑, increase; ↔, no change; ?, insufficient data; *BP,* blood pressure; *CI,* cardiac index; *HR,* heart rate; *PLVED,* left end-diastolic pressure; *SVR,* systemic vascular resistance.

## SURGICAL PHARMACOLOGY

### Medications Used in Adults During Cardiac Surgery

| Medication | Purpose/Description/Delivery |
|---|---|
| **ANALGESICS AND ANESTHETICS** | |
| Thiopental | Induction, ultra–short-acting barbiturate, intravenous bolus |
| Fentanyl (Sublimaze) | Synthetic narcotic, intravenous bolus and/or infusion |
| Sufentanil (Sufenta) | Synthetic narcotic, intravenous bolus and/or infusion |
| Alfentanil (Alfenta) | Synthetic narcotic, intravenous bolus and/or infusion |
| Morphine | Narcotic, intravenous bolus |
| Halothane (Fluothane) | Inhalation anesthetic, maintenance |
| Enflurane (Ethrane) | Inhalation anesthetic, maintenance |
| Isoflurane (Forane) | Inhalation anesthetic, maintenance |
| Methohexital (Brevital) | Three times more potent and faster clearance than thiopental |
| Remifentanil (Ultiva) | Synthetic narcotic, intravenous bolus and/or infusion |
| Propofol (Diprivan) | Intravenous anesthetic; bolus and/or infusion; very fast acting |
| Sevoflurane (Ultane) | Inhalation anesthetic, maintenance |
| Desflurane (Suprane) | Inhalation anesthetic, maintenance |
| **MUSCLE RELAXANTS** | |
| Vecuronium (Norcuron) | Intubation, maintenance of muscle relaxation |
| Pancuronium (Pavulon) | Maintenance of muscle relaxation |
| Pipecuronium | Maintenance of muscle relaxation; relatively free of circulatory effects |
| Rocuronium (Zemuron) | Fast-acting muscle relaxant; allows hemodynamic stability |
| **AMNESIACS** | |
| Midazolam (Versed) | Hypnotic; anxiety-reducing sedative |
| Scopolamine | Sedative; amnesic |
| Lorazepam (Ativan) | Hypnotic sedative; premedication |
| **CARDIOVASCULAR AGENTS** | |
| **Anticholinergics** | |
| Atropine | Decreases vagal tone; treats sinus bradycardia |
| Glycopyrrolate (Robinul) | Similar to atropine but has less incidence of dysrhythmias than atropine with slower onset |
| **Vasopressors** | |
| Norepinephrine (Levophed) | Increases force and velocity of contraction; increases systemic and pulmonary vascular resistance |
| Phenylephrine (Neo-Synephrine) | Arteriolar and venous vasoconstriction; increases blood pressure and systemic vascular resistance |
| **Vasodilators** | |
| Nitroglycerin (Tridil) | Dilates coronary arteries; reduces preload |
| Phentolamine (Regitine) | Decreases systemic and pulmonary resistance |
| Prostaglandin $E_1$ (Prostin VR) | Vascular smooth muscle dilator, potent pulmonary vascular dilator; used to maintain patency of ductus arteriosus in cyanotic neonates, patients with severe pulmonary hypertension |
| Nitroprusside (Nipride) | Arteriolar and venous vasodilation; reduces preload and afterload |
| **Inotropic Agents** | |
| Amrinone (Inocor) | Increases cardiac output, force and velocity of contraction |
| Calcium chloride | In iodized form, increases cardiac output, blood pressure (BP), and contractility |
| Dopamine (Intropin) | In low doses, increases renal and mesenteric perfusion; with moderate doses, increases heart rate, contractility, and cardiac output; in higher doses, increases systemic and pulmonary vascular resistance |
| Dobutamine (Dobutrex) | Increases contractility with less increase in heart rate than occurs with dopamine; has vasodilation effect on vascular bed |
| Ephedrine | Increases contractility, cardiac output, and BP |
| Epinephrine (Adrenalin) | Increases rate and strength of contraction, BP (effective bronchodilator) |
| Isoproterenol (Isuprel) | Increases heart rate, contractility, cardiac output; decreases systemic vascular resistance |
| Milrinone | Increases cardiac output, force and velocity of contraction |
| **Antidysrhythmics** | |
| Lidocaine (Xylocaine) | Acts on ventricles; decreases automaticity of ischemic ventricular tissue |
| Bretylium (Bretylol) | Prolongs duration of action potential and refractory period; useful for ventricular dysrhythmias refractory to therapy |

From Seifert PC: *Cardiac surgery,* St Louis, 2002, Mosby.

*Continued*

SURGICAL PHARMACOLOGY

**Medications Used in Adults During Cardiac Surgery—cont'd**

| Medication | Purpose/Description/Delivery |
|---|---|
| **Antidysrhythmics** | |
| Digoxin (Lanoxin) | Decreases ventricular rate in atrial fibrillation or flutter and other supraventricular dysrhythmias; avoid in patients with Wolff-Parkinson-White syndrome and other accessory atrioventricular pathways |
| Nifedipine (Procardia) | Calcium channel blocker; reduces coronary artery spasm; produces coronary vasodilation; extremely light sensitive; must be given orally or by way of nasal or oral mucosa; antihypertensive |
| Procainamide (Pronestyl) | Decreases automaticity and conduction in all cardiac tissue (normal and ischemic); stabilizes cellular membranes |
| Quinidine | Similar to procainamide; atrial and ventricular dysrhythmias |
| Verapamil (Calan, Isoptin) | Calcium channel blocker; used to treat atrial dysrhythmias; slows ventricular rate in atrial fibrillation or flutter; can be given intravenously |
| Adenosine | Supraventricular dysrhythmias |
| **DIURETICS** | |
| Furosemide (Lasix) | Decreases renal absorption of sodium and chloride; increases excretion of water and electrolytes, especially potassium, sodium, chloride, magnesium, and calcium |
| Mannitol | Osmotic diuretic; pulls free water out of organs (reducing cerebral edema); protects kidneys |
| **ANTICOAGULANTS/COAGULANTS** | |
| Heparin | Systemic anticoagulation during cardiopulmonary bypass (CPB); blocks activation of thrombin (and intrinsic clotting cascade) |
| Bivalirudin | Short-acting direct thrombin inhibitor |
| **ANTIBIOTICS** | |
| Cephalosporins (Mandol, Ancef, Keflex, Keflin, Cefadyl) | Broad-spectrum prophylaxis |
| Tobramycin (Nebcin) | Aerobic gram-negative and gram-positive bacteria |
| Vancomycin | Severe endocarditis |
| Bacitracin | Topical irrigation |
| **MISCELLANEOUS** | |
| Diazepam (Valium) | Sedative, induction of anesthesia |
| Nitric oxide (NO) | Vascular (especially pulmonary) relaxation; inhaled; reduces pulmonary hypertension |
| Lidocaine 1% (plain) | Local anesthesia |
| Papaverine | Reduces arterial spasm (e.g., mammary artery) |
| Potassium | Replaces electrolyte loss |
| Sodium bicarbonate | Corrects acidosis |
| Insulin (NPH, etc.) | Corrects hyperglycemia in diabetic patients |
| Topical hemostatic agents | Intraoperative control of bleeding |
| Desmopressin (DDAVP) | Pharmacologic hemostatic agent |

mediastinal adhesions may also necessitate this approach in some repeat valve operations. Thoracotomy positioning aids should be available to position arms and legs per the surgeon's protocol (see Chapter 5 for a discussion of positioning).

***Prepping and Draping.*** For procedures requiring excision of the saphenous vein, the prep extends from the jaw to the toes and includes the anterior (or lateral) area of the chest, abdomen, groin, and legs. The legs and feet are prepped circumferentially and the chest and abdomen from bedline to bedline.

In procedures not requiring saphenous vein excision, the prep extends to the knees to give the surgeon access to the femoral artery or saphenous vein in the thigh area. Femoral artery access may be required for arterial pressure monitoring or insertion of an intraaortic balloon. Saphenous vein exposure facilitates access if a bypass conduit is required. In the lateral position, the patient is prepped bedline to bedline anteriorly and posteriorly to the knees.

After the prep, the patient is draped so that the anterior areas of the chest, abdomen, and inguinal area are accessible. The perineum is covered, and a towel may be placed across the umbilicus to connect the side drapes. When the saphenous vein is to be excised, both legs remain exposed, with only the feet covered. When draping, the perioperative nurse should consider the placement of bypass lines so that they remain securely attached and do not become contaminated. A small drape or towel may be placed over the groin area when access to it is not immediately necessary. If the femoral artery needs to be accessed, the drape can be discarded.

## BEST PRACTICE

### Optimal Draping for Central Venous Catheters

Central venous catheters are associated with bacterial colonization of the catheter, local infection at the site of insertion, and bloodstream infection. The use of maximal barriers—although time-consuming, more expensive, and more cumbersome than other techniques employing minimal draping—may reduce the risk of infections. In addition, the researchers calculated the total direct medical costs and the incidence of catheter-related bloodstream infection, bacterial colonization of the catheter, and death. The use of maximal barriers resulted in lower costs ($369 versus $621 for minimal coverage), decreased bloodstream infections from 5.3% to 2.8%, decreased catheter colonization with local infection from 5.5% to 2.9%, and decreased death rates from 0.8% to 0.4%. The authors calculated that $68,000 would be saved with maximal barrier application for every 270 catheter placements, seven episodes of catheter-related infections would be avoided, and one death would be prevented. The results of this study support routine maximal draping for the insertion of central lines.

Modified from Hu KK and others: Use of maximal sterile barriers during central venous catheter insertion: clinical and economic outcomes, *Clinical Infectious Diseases* 39, November 15, 2004.

***Incisions.*** Either (1) standard median sternotomy or ministernotomy incisions or (2) full thoracotomy or mini-thoracotomy incisions may be used, depending on the surgeon's preference and type of procedure (Figure 27-34).

**MEDIAN STERNOTOMY.** The skin incision for full sternotomy extends from the sternal notch to the linea alba below the xiphoid process (Figure 27-35). For mini sternotomy, the sternum is partially divided starting from either the sternal notch or the xiphoid process (depending on the cardiac structures to be exposed). The sternum is divided with a saw, and a sternal retractor is inserted. If the IMA or the saphenous vein will be used, it is made available at this time. The pericardium is incised and retracted with sutures.

In repeat sternotomy, adhesions from a previous cardiac operation must be dissected. The sternum may be divided with an oscillating saw and the retrosternal tissue dissected free. Increased risk of fibrillation from manipulation of the heart and bleeding and laceration of the right ventricle should alert the perioperative nurse to the possibility of instituting femoral vein–femoral artery bypass (discussed later). In addition, disposable defibrillation patches are applied preoperatively to the left lateral chest and the right upper chest; these patches can be activated for defibrillation if the chest is not open. Sterile external paddles may also be available.

Anteroposterior and lateral chest radiographs are useful to determine the extent of retrosternal adhesions and to count the number of chest wires for removal. On occasion, a patient presents for repeat mitral valve surgery. If the initial operation was performed through a thoracotomy incision, sternal adhesions may be minimal or nonexistent and the special precautions associated with repeat sternotomy may not be necessary.

**MINI THORACOTOMY.** For minimally invasive cardiac procedures, a variety of smaller (up to approximately 4 to 8 cm) incisions and/or ports can be used. These include anterolateral chest incisions small enough for the insertion of specially designed instruments (see Figure 27-14), including video cameras and robotic arms. Minimally invasive cardiac procedures using smaller incisions may be performed under direct visualization or, increasingly, by means of video assistance.

**CARDIOPULMONARY BYPASS.** The temporary substitution of a pump oxygenator for the heart and lungs allows the surgeon to stop the heart to perform cardiac procedures under direct vision in a relatively dry, motionless field. It also allows the surgeon to manipulate the heart without the attendant risk of producing ventricular fibrillation and reduced cardiac output that jeopardize perfusion to the myocardial, peripheral, and cerebral tissues.

Under some circumstances, access to the anteroapical portion of the heart can be achieved without excess manipulation of the heart. Special retraction/stabilization devices (see Figure 27-17) allow the surgeon to create coronary artery bypass grafts (CABGs) to the anterolateral coronary arteries without the use of CPB and induced cardiac arrest. This forms the basis for minimally invasive procedures performed on a beating heart (discussed later).

In traditional CPB circuits, systemic venous return to the heart flows by gravity drainage through cannulas (Figure 27-36) placed in the superior and inferior venae cavae (Figure 27-37) or through a single two-stage cannula in the right atrium (Figure 27-38) into tubing connected to the bypass machine. Blood is oxygenated, filtered, warmed or cooled, and pumped back into the systemic circulation through a cannula placed in the ascending aorta or occasionally in the femoral artery (Figure 27-39). Because the CPB machine (Figure 27-40) oxygenates blood, the lungs do not need to function and can be deflated to provide better exposure of the mediastinal structures.

A percutaneous method of instituting femoral vein–femoral artery CPB can be used for minimally invasive (or conventional open) procedures (Figure 27-41) and in emergency situations where the environment is not conducive to traditional CPB methods (e.g., in the cardiac catheterization laboratory, the intensive care unit, and the emergency department). The system employs thin-walled, wire-reinforced catheters inserted into the femoral vein or artery or both. The resistance of the small-bore cannula used in the femoral vein can impede gravity drainage; to overcome this, a centrifugal pump may be used to actively siphon blood to the pump oxygenator. Other advances include the use of heparin-bonded bypass circuits and tubing; this reduces (but does not obviate altogether) the amount of heparin required to achieve systemic anticoagulation and can reduce bleeding and the associated need for blood products.

By diverting blood away from the heart, CPB also decompresses the ventricles, thereby reducing myocardial wall tension, which is a significant determinant of myocardial oxygen demand. This principle is evident when CPB or other means of ventricular support are employed to "rest" the heart. Further decompression is achieved by venting the left ventricle to remove air and accumulated thebesian and bronchial venous return as well as systemic return flowing around the venous cannulas (Figure 27-42). The venting catheter is inserted into the left ventricle by way of the right superior pulmonary vein or, less commonly, through the left ventricular apex. The venting line is connected to the suction lines of the bypass ma-

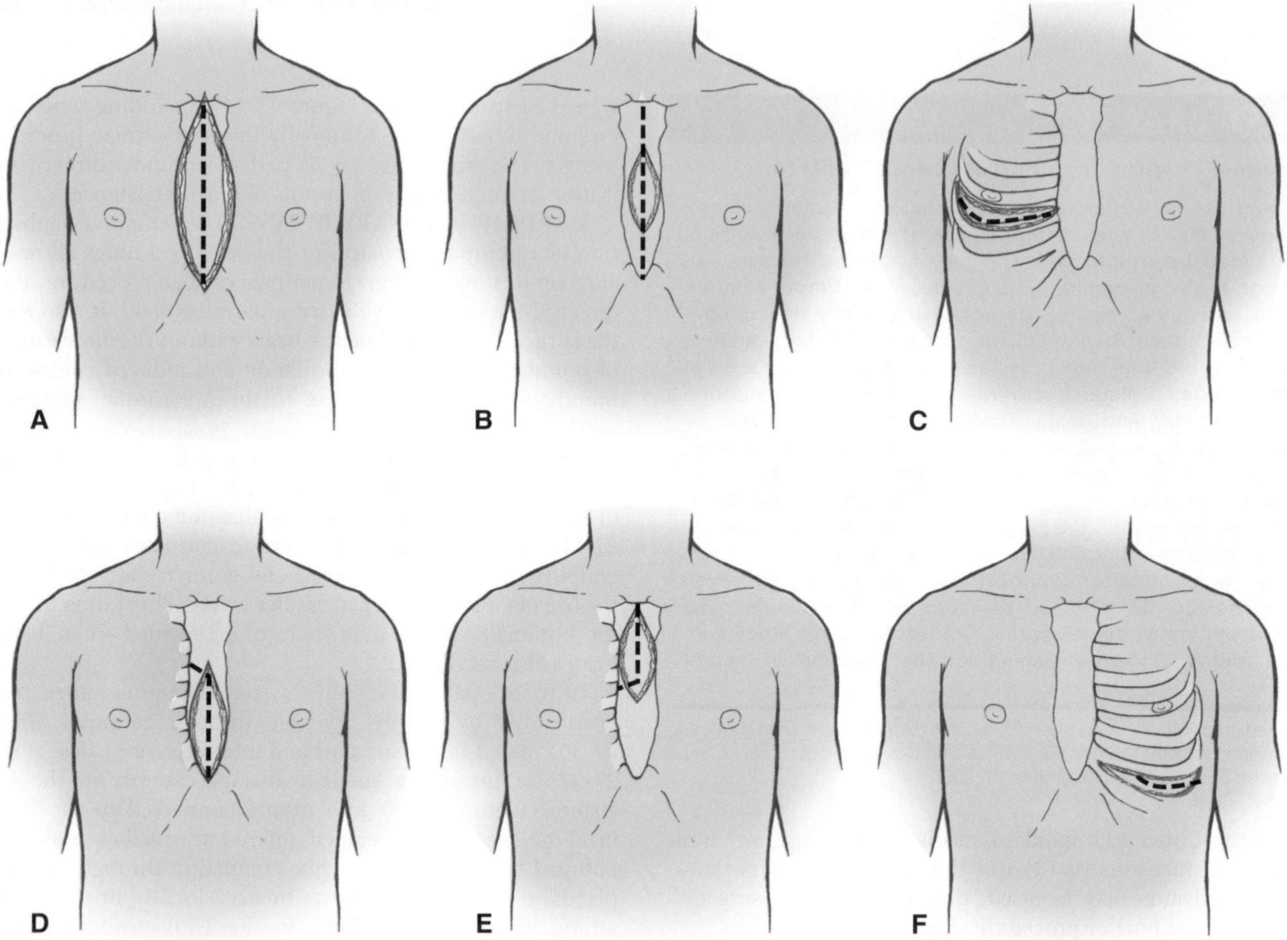

A B C

D E F

**FIGURE 27-34** Schematic representation of traditional incision and sternotomy, **A,** compared with a variety of less-invasive incisions (*dotted lines* represent chest wall incisions). Limited skin incision/full sternotomy, **B,** is gaining popularity because of improved cosmesis and reduced trauma from the limited chest wall retraction. The parasternal approach, **C,** is used less frequently because of the residual chest wall defect. Partial lower or upper sternotomy, **D** and **E,** have been used predominantly in valve procedures. Right anterior thoracotomy, **F,** is a useful approach, particularly in mitral valve reoperations.

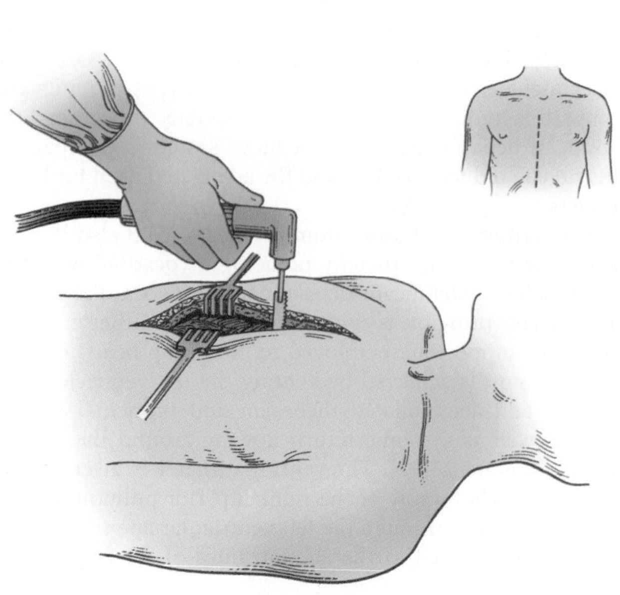

**FIGURE 27-35** Median sternotomy with sternal saw.

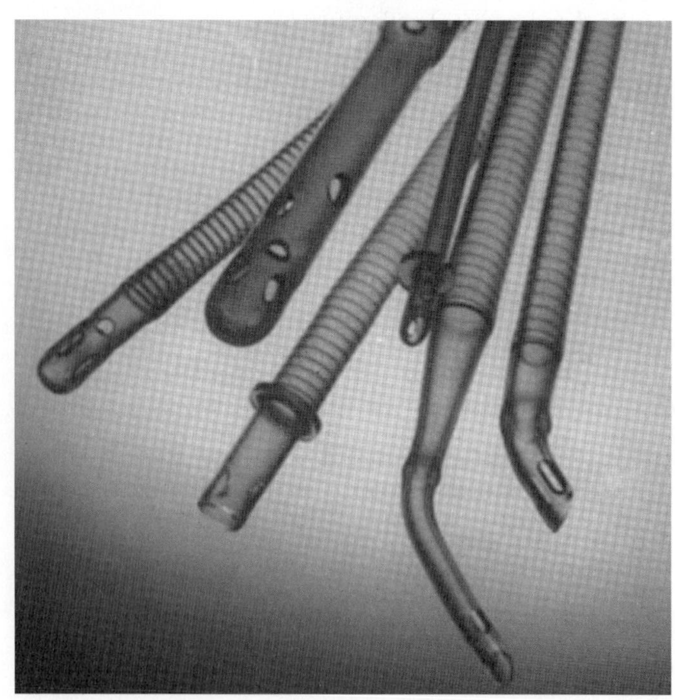

**FIGURE 27-36** Arterial and venous perfusion cannulas.

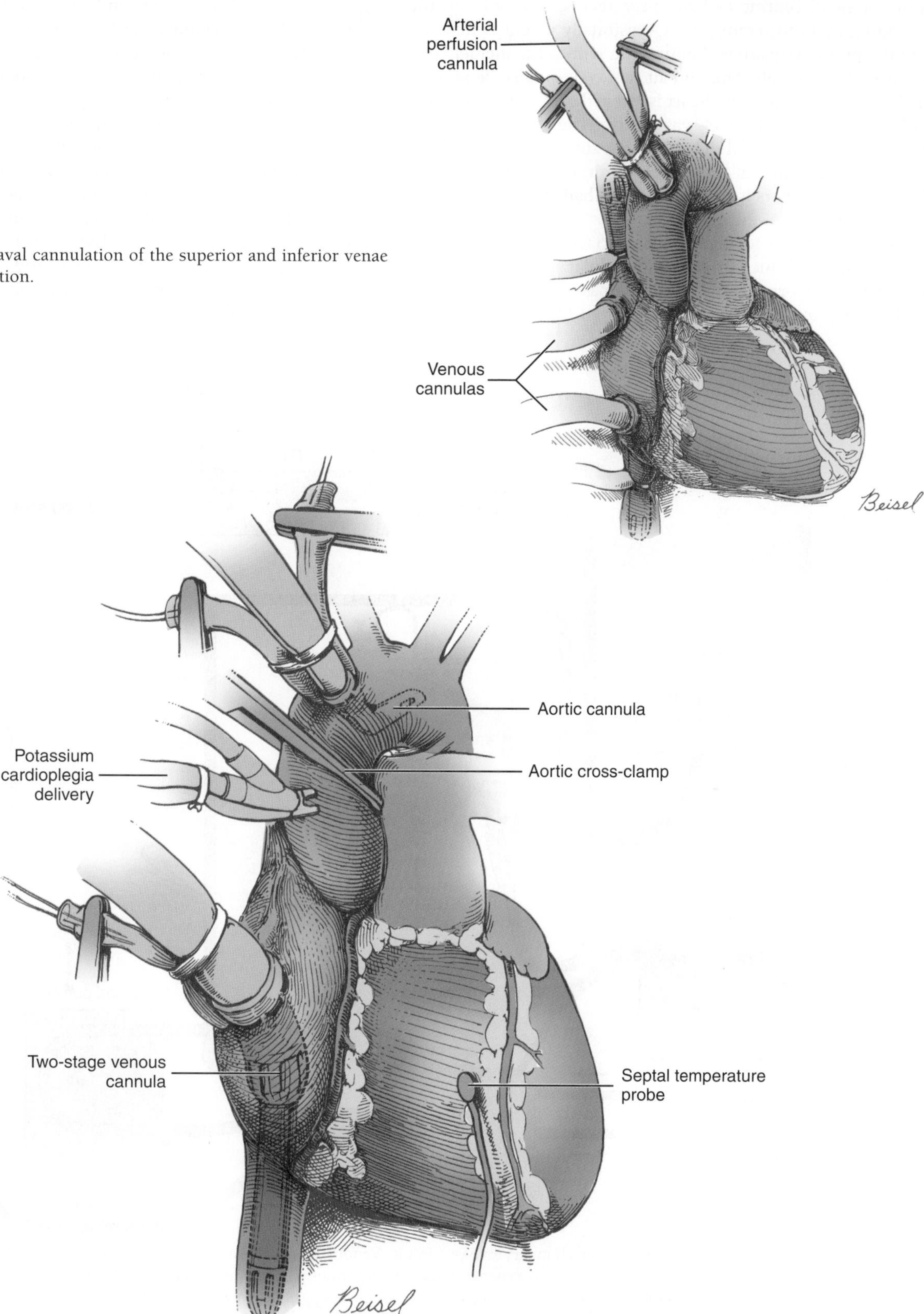


**FIGURE 27-37** Bicaval cannulation of the superior and inferior venae cavae; aortic cannulation.

**FIGURE 27-38** Diagram showing aortic and venous cannulas during aortic cross-clamping. Also shown is antegrade cardioplegic-solution delivery catheter in the aorta proximal to the cross-clamp and a temperature probe. The single (two-stage) venous cannula has openings in the distal end of the cannula to drain the inferior vena cava; the openings in the midportion (right atrial area) of the cannula drain the superior vena cava and the coronary sinus venous return.

chine. A small venting catheter may also be inserted into the ascending aorta to remove air. Occasionally a vent is inserted into the pulmonary artery. Venting can reduce the incidence of gaseous microemboli. Ambient air removal can also be accomplished in cases when the heart is opened (e.g., valve surgery) with the insertion of a $CO_2$ gas diffuser; the gas is insufflated into the pericardial well. The $CO_2$ gas dissolves in blood approximately 25 times faster than room air; $CO_2$ retained within the cardiac chambers is better tolerated than air and less harmful to tissue.[135]

Improved bypass technology has also reduced the incidence of bypass-related microemboli and cellular injury. Membrane oxygenators incorporated into the bypass circuit (see Figure 27-39) perform gas exchange (removing $CO_2$ and adding oxygen to the blood) more efficiently and less traumatically. Gases diffuse through a semipermeable membrane that separates the oxygenating gas and the venous blood. Although membrane oxygenators preserve platelet and red blood cell function better than the older "bubble" oxygenators, there does remain considerable morbidity associated with the use of CPB. Extracorporeal circulation causes fluid retention and intercompartmental fluid shifts, multiple organ dysfunction, showers of microemboli, inflammatory responses, and unique bleeding complications.[57] The mechanism of injury is believed to be related to the exposure of the blood to the abnormal surfaces of the bypass circuit, hypothermia, and altered blood flow. These can initiate a systemic inflammatory response (complement activation), which releases vasoactive substances.[42,44]

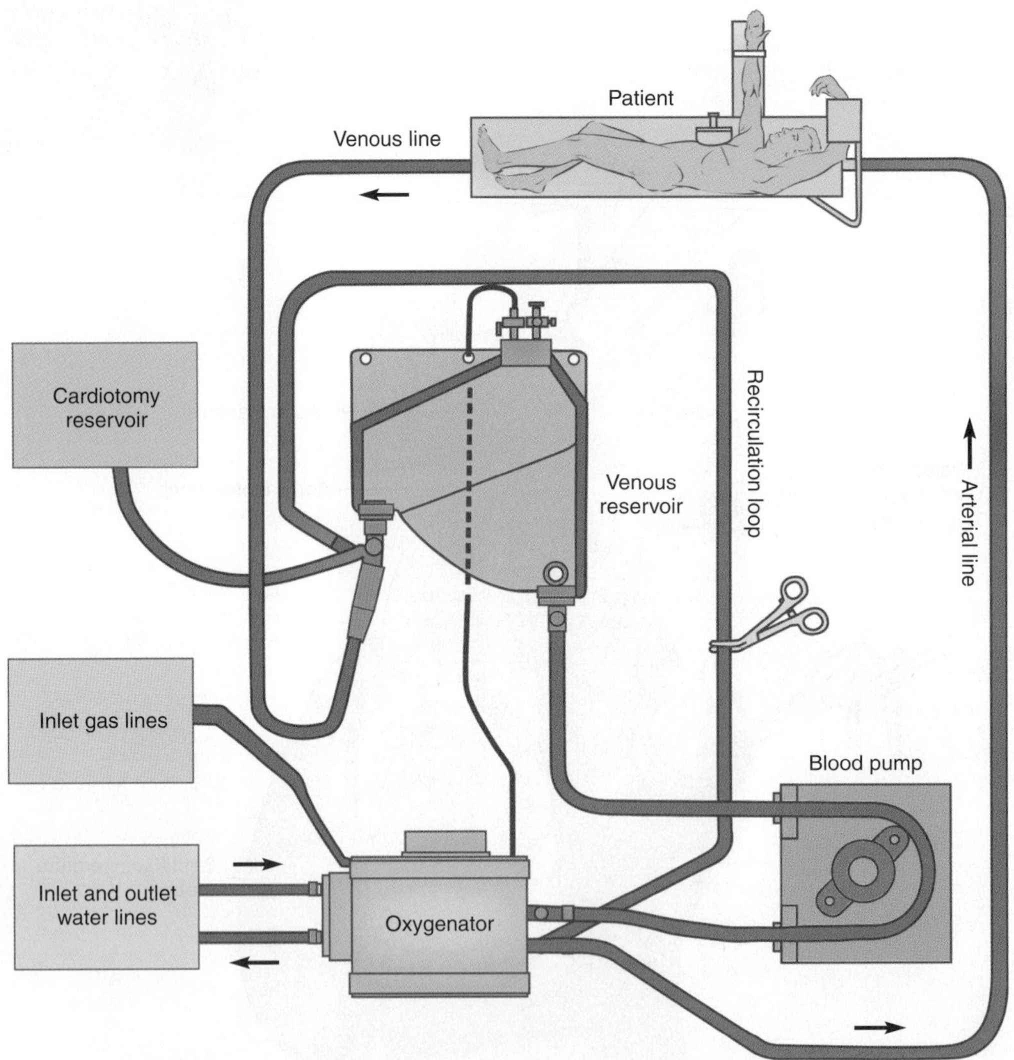


**FIGURE 27-39** Cardiopulmonary bypass circuit. Venous blood is drained by gravity from the right atrium or venae cavae into an oxygenator that incorporates a blood reservoir and a heat exchanger, which warms or cools the blood as needed. The ventilating gas flowing into the oxygenator removes carbon dioxide and adds oxygen to the blood. Saturated blood leaves the oxygenator and is pumped from the reservoir into the arterial system by the use of a roller pump. Filters and monitors are incorporated into the circuit. Additional roller pumps are used to suction shed blood from the pericardial well and the intracardiac chambers (cardiotomy suckers); the blood is returned to the cardiotomy reservoir. Another roller pump is used to vent air and blood through a right superior pulmonary venous catheter that is inserted into the left ventricle.

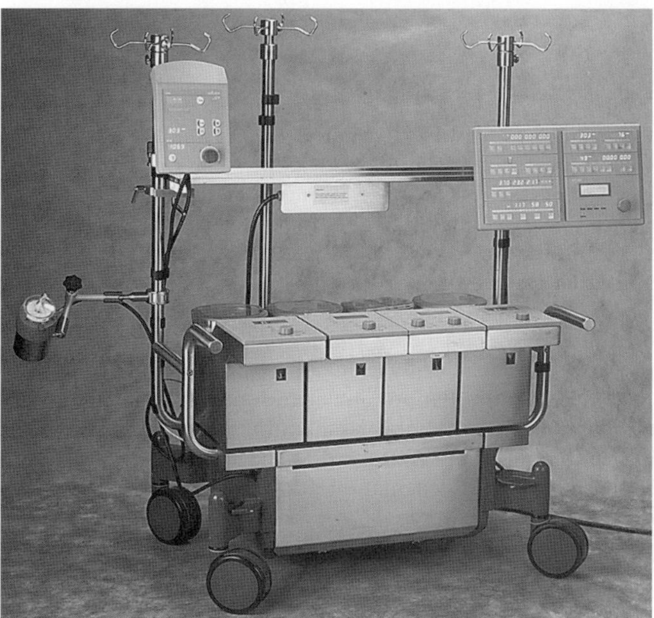

**FIGURE 27-40** Cardiopulmonary bypass pump. Modular system with integrated centrifugal pump driver.

Attempts to minimize the inflammatory reaction have focused on modifying the activation of platelets and blood factors that play a major role in initiating the response. To avoid the complications associated with CPB, clinicians have stimulated the development of "beating heart" ("off-pump") techniques for myocardial revascularization.

Two types of pumps are available: roller pumps and centrifugal pumps. Roller pumps have roller heads that propel blood forward by compressing blood-filled tubing against a smooth, metal housing. Centrifugal pumps use cones or blades that rotate at high speed to produce forward flow. All pumps produce some hemolysis from turbulence and shear forces, but careful calibration and minimal use of connectors can provide relatively atraumatic flow for short periods (e.g., less than 6 hours). Arterial blood flow on bypass is largely nonpulsatile, although some modifications to the pump can achieve a small degree of phasic (systolic/nonsystolic) flow; the arterial blood pressure is usually manifested by a mean arterial waveform on the oscilloscope during CPB.

Suction lines are ordinarily used during CPB to return shed blood to the venous reservoir and the oxygenator. These lines may combine conventional handheld suction tubes and ventricular decompression lines or sumps (see Figure 27-42). Before the initiation of CPB, the entire extracorporeal circuit must be primed and rendered free of air to prevent air emboli.

The priming solution is usually a combination of colloid and crystalloid fluids with a balanced electrolyte component. When the patient's blood volume mixes with the prime, there is some hemodilution and a subsequent reduction of the hematocrit (Hct). Advantages of hemodilution include reducing the number of homologous serum reactions and the incidence of hepatitis and human immunodeficiency virus (HIV) as well as providing better perfusion of the capillary beds because of reduced blood viscosity. Hct levels as low as 25% may be adequate during CPB, but once CPB is terminated, transfusion of red blood cells may be required to enhance the blood's oxygen-carrying capacity. In low-weight, low-hematocrit patients, hemodilution

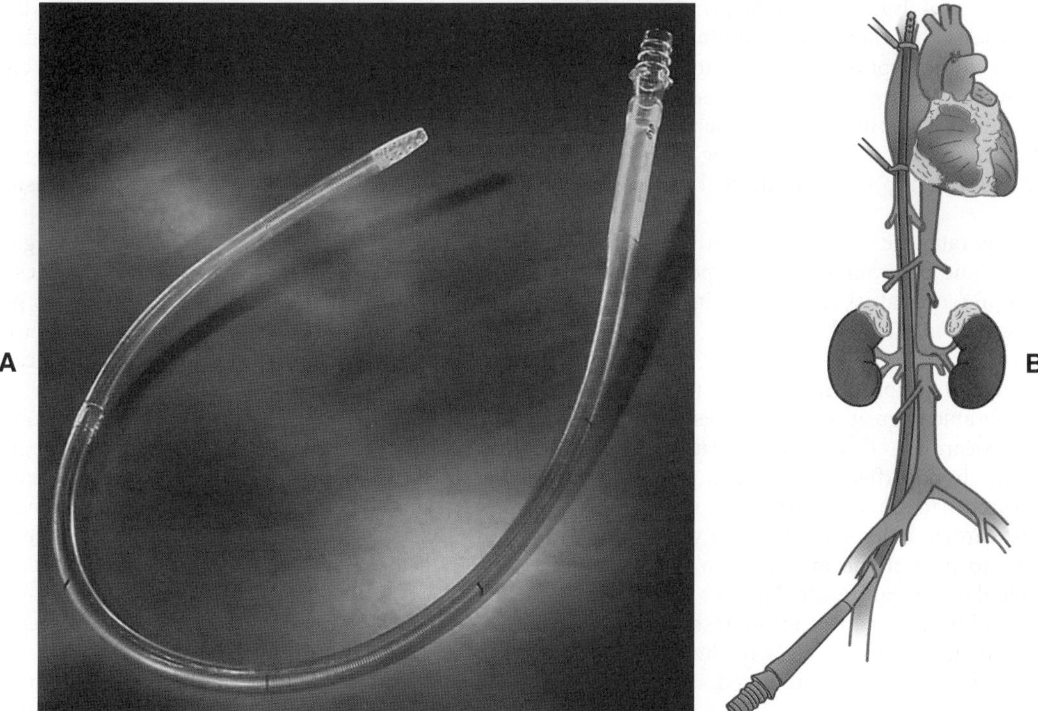


**FIGURE 27-41** **A,** Venous endovascular cannula. **B,** The catheter tip is inserted into the femoral vein and threaded to the right atrium; the distal tip is positioned in the superior vena cava (SVC) to drain the upper body.

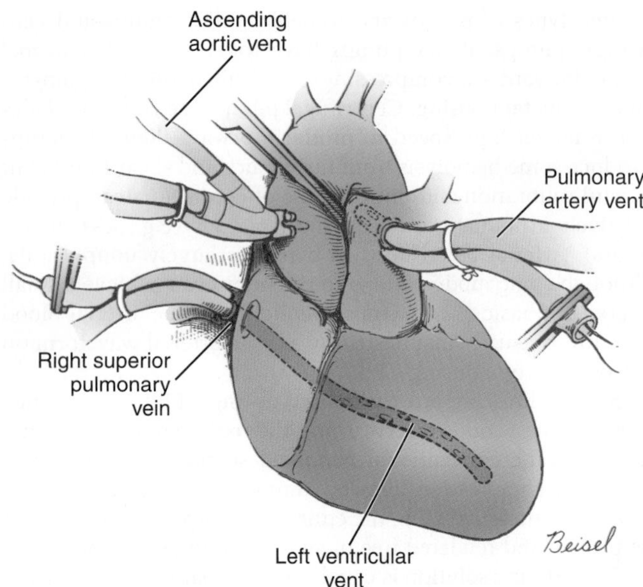


FIGURE 27-42 Types of venting catheters.

may not be tolerated. One method to decrease hemodilution is to employ the technique of *rapid-autologous-prime* (RAP). First, the perfusionist shortens the length of bypass tubing (thereby reducing the volume of prime solution). After the surgeon inserts the arterial cannula into the aorta and connects it to the arterial tubing leading to the bypass machine (but before initiation of bypass), the perfusionist allows a predetermined amount of the patient's arterial blood to drain from the line and fill part of the bypass circuit; the perfusionist then clamps the circuit. The clamps are removed at the initiation of bypass.[153]

The amount and kind of drugs used in the priming solution vary among institutions, but heparin is routinely added to block clot formation in the bypass circuit. Heparin-coated circuits are also available. Anticoagulation is routinely monitored during bypass, and more heparin is given as needed to maintain an activated clotting time (ACT) exceeding 600 seconds. Other ingredients are added to maintain normal pH and electrolyte status.

Arterial blood flow rates are estimated according to the patient's height, weight, and body surface area. Depending on the arterial and venous pressure values and the results of blood gas determinations, the flow is adjusted.

***Myocardial Protection.*** Improvement in the results of cardiac surgery is attributable in great part to progress made in the protection of the myocardium. Coronary circulatory interruptions, ischemia, and hypoperfusion accompanying induced cardiac arrest are often necessary to permit the surgeon sufficient time to repair cardiac lesions under direct vision. Unless measures are taken to protect the myocardium during these periods, irreversible damage can result. The two main protective strategies are cooling the heart (and the rest of the body) to reduce metabolic demand and rapidly arresting the heart so that myocardial energy resources are preserved.

**HYPOTHERMIA.** Hypothermia in cardiac surgery is the deliberate reduction of body temperature for therapeutic purposes. A moderate degree of hypothermia, to 28°C (82.4°F), permits reduction of oxygen consumption by 50%. At 20°C (68°F) there is a further reduction of about 25%. Systemic circulatory cooling is achieved with the heat exchanger of the heart-lung machine. When very cold temperatures (less than 20°C [68°F]) are desired for myocardial protection in prolonged, complex cases, additional surface cooling of the heart with topical application of cold saline/slush or continuous irrigation of the pericardial wall can be used. Large ice chips in pericardial irrigating fluids should be avoided to prevent injury to the phrenic nerve within the right and left lateral pericardia and other cardiac tissue.

Insulation pads placed behind the heart can reduce heat conduction from relatively warmer organs. Transmural cooling of the heart is achieved with cardioplegia (discussed later).

Ventricular fibrillation can occur during the cooling process although it is less likely at temperatures above 32°C (89.6°F). Other complications are related to the adverse effects that hypothermia has on coagulation and wound healing; this may delay hemostasis after heparin reversal and have an impact on recuperation.[42]

**CARDIOPLEGIC ARREST.** Rapidly arresting the heart during diastole is beneficial because an arrested heart uses less energy than a fibrillating or beating heart. Cardioplegia with hypothermia can reduce energy requirements even further.[75] Both "warm" and "cold" heart surgery proponents concur that infusing a warm initial bolus of cardioplegia acts as a form of active resuscitation in energy-depleted hearts. There is also concurrence that providing a warm terminal bolus of cardioplegia helps to avoid reperfusion injury (caused by oxygen-free radicals and lactic acid buildup) by providing oxygen and other nutrients to the heart.[20] The controversy lies in the use of normothermic cardioplegia during the period of arrest when the actual surgical repair or bypass construction occurs. Proponents of warm arrest techniques seek to avoid the complications associated with hypothermia; warm cardioplegia is delivered continuously while the surgical repair is performed. Opponents of continuous warm cardioplegia cite the technical difficulty associated with a constant flow of cardioplegia obscuring the surgical site. Some authors favor intermittent cold cardioplegia infusions because if cardioplegia infusions are even momentarily interrupted to enhance visualization, myocardial protection is jeopardized.[20,42]

**CARDIOPLEGIA DELIVERY.** Cardioplegic arrest is accomplished by infusing the coronary arteries with a 4°C to 10°C (39.2°F to 50°F) solution containing potassium (2 to 50 mEq/L) and buffering agents to counteract ischemic acidosis. Potassium acts by depolarizing the myocardial cell membrane and arresting the heart in diastole.

Delivery of the solution may be by the antegrade or the retrograde route (Figure 27-43). With antegrade delivery, a needle is inserted into the aortic root proximal to the aortic cross-clamp; the cardioplegic solution is infused under pressure that closes the aortic valve leaflets. The only remaining route for the solution is into the right and left coronary arteries and the coronary circulation (see Figure 27-38). If the aortic valve does not close properly, the cardioplegic solution will flow preferentially into the left ventricular chamber, causing distention; in these cases direct cannulation of the coronary ostia is performed. Direct infusion into vein grafts protects the myocardium distal to coronary lesions and enhances transmural cooling. Retrograde infusion is achieved with a catheter placed transatrially into the coronary sinus; the perfusate en-

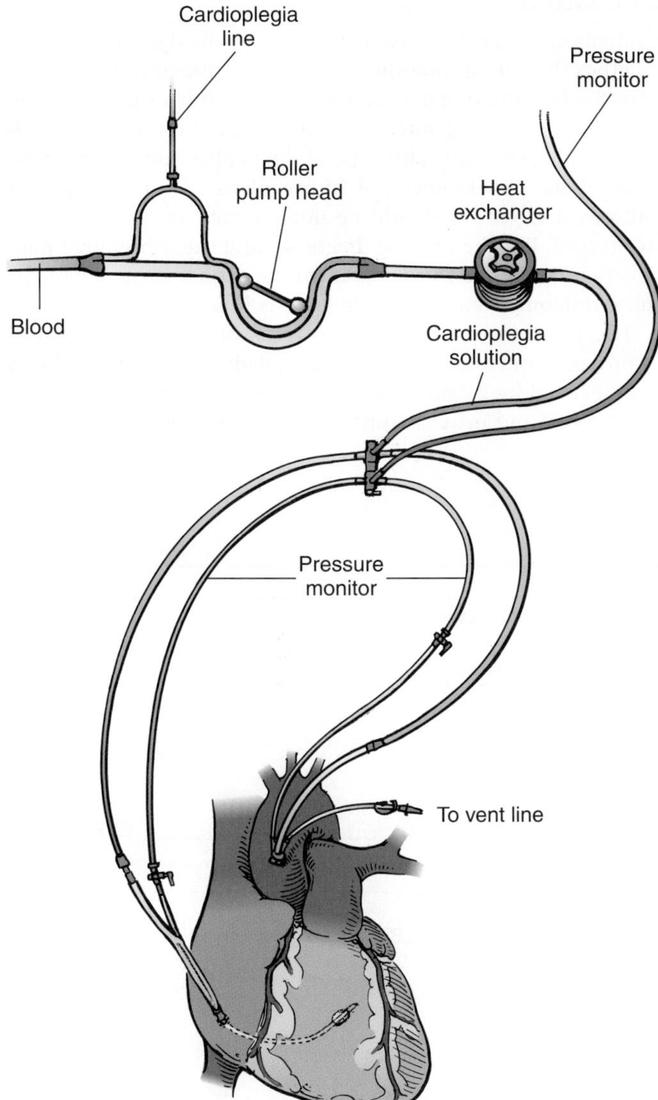


FIGURE 27-43 Antegrade-retrograde cardioplegia system. The antegrade cardioplegia catheter is inserted into the aorta proximally to the cross-clamp; the catheter is Y-ed into a vent line and into the retrograde cardioplegia catheter, which is inserted transatrially into the coronary sinus. The coronary sinus pressure is monitored; its pressure should remain under 50 mm Hg.

ters the coronary venous system and flows through the myocardial circulation, leaving through the coronary ostia. The retrograde route is especially useful in the presence of coronary artery obstructions and left ventricular hypertrophy.

When the heart is sufficiently arrested, the ECG reflects a straight line; when electrical activity is noted on the monitor (fine fibrillation), the cardioplegic solution is reinfused when continued cooling is desired (approximately every 15 to 20 minutes).

Minimally invasive techniques for myocardial protection have also been developed (described below). Percutaneously inserted catheters can infuse antegrade cardioplegic solution through a catheter threaded into the aortic root; retrograde cardioplegic solution is infused through a catheter inserted into the internal jugular vein and then passed into the SVC, the right atrium, and the coronary sinus.

**CIRCULATORY ARREST.** In some highly complex procedures, such as those involving the aortic arch, it may be impossible to place an occluding clamp across the aorta. In these cases, circulatory arrest may be used to maintain a dry operative site. Because all blood flow will be interrupted, additional protection is required to protect myocardial, cerebral, and other tissue from ischemia.

The patient is cooled with the heat exchanger to approximately 18°C (65°F), at which point the bypass pump is turned off. The incision is made, and the repair is performed. The small amount of collateral drainage entering the field can be removed with a suction catheter. When the repair is completed, air is removed and CPB is slowly reinstituted. Rewarming is performed at a rate of approximately 1°C every 3 minutes.[75]

**CEREBROPLEGIA.** Circulatory arrest poses additional risk to the brain. Cerebral protection, cerebroplegia, is provided by the infusion of oxygenated blood to the brain by means of antegrade perfusion. The aortic arch branches may be cannulated to perfuse the brain.[74]

***Termination of Cardiopulmonary Bypass.*** Near the end of the repair, the heart is allowed to rewarm while the perfusionist rewarms the patient systemically with the oxygenator's heat exchanger. Air is evacuated from the left ventricle and the proximal portion of the aorta. The cross-clamp is removed. The heart often converts spontaneously to sinus rhythm, but internal (or external) defibrillation may be necessary. Temporary epicardial pacing wires may be sutured to the right atrial appendage or the right ventricle; these are used postoperatively if the patient has transient bradycardia, supraventricular tachycardia, or other dysrhythmias. AF is a common postoperative complication that is associated with a greater risk of embolic events and increases the patient's length of stay.[41]

When the heart is contracting, the patient is gradually weaned from CPB. Ventilation of the lungs is restarted. Venous flow is gradually reduced by clamping the venous line or lines, and a commensurate reduction in arterial flow is made by the perfusionist. When heart action is sufficient and systemic and pulmonary blood pressures are stabilized, the bypass is terminated and the cannulas are removed.

Measures to actively promote body heat retention are implemented to enhance clotting mechanisms, immune function, and oxygenation. Maintenance of normothermia after the termination of CPB has also been recommended to reduce the risk of postoperative infection.[76,97]

***Closing.*** After hemostasis is achieved, catheters are inserted into the pericardium for mediastinal drainage of shed blood. If either or both pleura have been entered, chest tubes are inserted to drain shed blood entering from the pericardium and to create negative intrapleural pressure to facilitate lung expansion. The tubes are connected to straight or Y connectors to a water-seal drainage system or an autotransfusion drainage system.

Chest closure in median sternotomy is achieved with wire sutures (see Figure 27-19). The wire sutures are twisted, excess wire is cut, and the wire ends are buried into the sternal periosteum. Some surgeons use small metal crimpers to approximate and hold the wires (rather than twisting and burying the wire ends).

The linea alba is closed with suture. A layer of sutures is placed to approximate the fascia over the sternum; the subcutaneous tissue and skin are closed. If metal staples are used on the skin, a staple remover should accompany the patient to the recovery area. Thoracotomy incisions are closed in standard fashion.

Before transferring the patient, the perioperative nurse telephones a report to the recovery area, usually the cardiovascular SICU. Figure 27-44 lists information commonly supplied. The patient's special concerns and fears as well as significant physiologic alterations should be communicated.

Perioperative documentation follows the standard protocol and includes a description of the procedure performed and identification of medications and all implanted material (with lot and serial numbers). Hospital policy should be followed to ensure compliance with the Safe Medical Devices Act.

## Evaluation

Evaluation of perioperative care includes the determination of whether the patient met the outcomes identified in the plan of care. Such evaluation assists perioperative nurses to determine whether the nursing interventions designed for a specific patient were successful. This type of data collection becomes the basis of the development of future plans of care for similar patients. Evaluation should be documented in the perioperative record. For the nursing diagnoses and the subsequent plan of care presented in this chapter for the cardiac surgery patient, those outcome statements might be as follows[123]:

- The patient's cardiac function was consistent with or improved from baseline levels established preoperatively as evidenced by blood pressure within expected range; warm, dry skin; and urine output more than 30 ml/hr.

**Patient Transfer Report**

PROCEDURE (include source of autogenous grafts) on pump _____ off pump _____

Endoscopic vein harvest yes ___ no ___ N/A ___

**MONITORING DEVICES (LOCATION)**

CVP ________ Arterial Line ________ SWAN ________ Peripheral ________
LA ________ Other ________

**HEMODYNAMICS**

BP ____ PAP ____ PAD ____ PAWP ____ CO ____ CI ____ CVP ____ $Svo_2$ ____

**INTRAOPERATIVE OCCURRENCES**

BLOOD LOSS ________ URINE ________ DYSRHYTHMIAS ________ BYPASS
PROBLEMS ________ DEFIB X's ________ LO TEMP ________ HI TEMP ________
CROSS-CLAMP TIME ________ PUMP TIME ________

**BLOOD:** GIVEN ________ AVAILABLE ________ AUTOTRANSFUSION TOTALS: ________ ml ________ Units

**COMPONENTS:** FFP ________ PLATELETS ________ CRYO ________

ADDITIONAL ORDERED (TYPE) ________

**MEDICATIONS**

NEO ________ DOPAMINE ________ DOBUTAMINE ________ LIDOCAINE ________ NITRO ________
LEVOPHED ________ EPINEPHRINE ________ NITROPRUSSIDE ________ INOCOR ________
DDAVP ________ OTHER ________
TUBES/DRAINS: MEDIASTINAL ________ PLEURAL (Rt/Lt) ________

**EPICARDIAL LEADS:** ATRIAL ________ VENTRICULAR ________
PACING: YES/NO RATE ________

**LABS:**

K+ ________ Na+ ________ Glu ________ Hgb ________ Hct ________

**PATIENT CONCERNS** ________

**ADDITIONAL INFORMATION** ________
ICU BED # ________ ETA ________

REPORTED BY ________

To ________ TIME ________

*BP*, Blood pressure; *CI*, cardiac index; *CO*, cardiac output; *CRYO*, cryoprecipitate; *CVP*, central venous pressure; *DDAVP*, 1-deamino-8-*D*-arginine vasopressin (e.g., Desmopressin); *ETA*, estimated time of arrival; *FFP*, fresh frozen plasma; *Glu*, glucose; *Hct*, hematocrit; *Hgb*, hemoglobin; *K+*, potassium; *LA*, left atrial; *Na+*, sodium; *NEO*, Neo-Synephrine; *NITRO*, nitroglycerine; *PAD*, pulmonary artery diastolic pressure; *PAP*, pulmonary artery pressure; *PAWP*, pulmonary artery wedge pressure; $Svo_2$, percent saturation of mixed venous blood; *SWAN*, Swan-Ganz (pulmonary artery) catheter.

**FIGURE 27-44** Patient transfer report.

- The patient will be free from signs and symptoms of infection at the surgical site or sites as evidenced by absence of redness, edema, purulent incisional drainage, or untoward elevation of temperature postoperatively.
- The patient was free from signs and symptoms of injury related to surgical position as evidenced by the absence of acquired neuromuscular impairment and tissue necrosis.
- The patient demonstrated knowledge of the physiologic responses to the cardiac disorder (at his or her level of understanding), the proposed surgical treatment, and the immediate postoperative events as evidenced by verbalization of disease state, purpose of surgery, sequence of events, anticipated outcomes, and recovery process.
- The patient's myocardial, peripheral, and cerebral tissue integrity were adequate or improved as evidenced by absence of new electrocardiographic manifestations of infarction, the presence of palpable peripheral pulses, and a clear or improving sensorium postoperatively.

## Patient and Family Education and Discharge Planning

Many patients are admitted to the cardiac service on the day of surgery; teaching sessions can be scheduled before admission along with preoperative laboratory testing. Perioperative nurses should include details about the surgical procedure, sights and sounds that the patient may sense, and anesthesia care. With hospital length of stay shortened from 1 week or more to 4 or 5 days, patient education and preparation for home care maintenance have become even more critical for enhancing positive patient outcomes. The perioperative nurse acts to reinforce, review, clarify, and add to important information and instructions the patient and family or significant others need in planning for surgery, recovery, and discharge.[106] Although patients undergoing repeat operations have had experience with cardiac surgery, they still have significant learning needs because changes in surgical techniques and the introduction of newer devices alter the expectations of patients. Information about innovations such as endoscopic vein harvesting and off-pump coronary surgery should be provided (Table 27-8).

Additional resources (electronic, peer support) can supplement traditional education strategies.[8,102] An expanding array of Internet sites developed by professional organizations can be accessed for examples of patient information.[67,132] Electronic mail (e-mail) has also become more popular as a form of communication between patients and caregivers.[8,38]

In addition to specific information about the perioperative period, the cardiac patient's preoperative state of mind may be a significant factor. One study[54] showed that a negative (i.e., pessimistic) state of mind (compared with an optimistic state) may be predictive of an increased length of stay, stroke, and

**TABLE 27-8**

### Patient Teaching Considerations for Minimally Invasive Surgery (On/Off Pump)

| | Beating Heart/Off-Pump | Arrested Heart |
|---|---|---|
| Definition | CABG without CPB or induced cardiac arrest; HR and contractile force may be pharmacologically reduced; stabilizer used at anastomotic site; apical retractor used to expose lateral and posterior coronary arteries | CABG with CPB and endovascular technique for CPB and induced cardiac arrest |
| Indications | Multiple-vessel disease, angioplasty contraindicated, medical problems, poor anatomy, accessible target arteries, previous CABG with blocked grafts | Multiple-vessel disease, angioplasty contraindicated, need to stop the heart to enhance technical precision, accessible target arteries, mitral valve disease |
| Contraindications | Intramyocardial lesions, hemodynamic instability | Highly complex lesions, posterior targets |
| Incisions | Sternotomy or mini sternotomy (cephalad or caudad); 1-3 small right or left rib or submammary incisions | 1-4 small rib incisions, 1 or 2 groin incisions, 1 or 2 neck incisions |
| CPB | No, available on standby | Yes |
| Cardioplegia | No | Yes |
| Procedure time | 2 hr or more | 2 hr or more |
| Hospital LOS | 3-5 days (versus 4-6 for sternotomy) | 3-5 days (versus 4-6 for sternotomy) |
| Advantages | Avoids CPB, ischemic arrest, and hypothermia; may enable more complete revascularization with postoperative insertion of intracoronary stents into the posterolateral coronary arteries in the cardiac catheterization laboratory ("hybrid" procedure) | Allows repair of more complex lesions without the technical challenge of a moving heart; better able to produce more complete revascularization |
| Potential complications and disadvantages | Learning curve technically more challenging; may cause VF; may have to revert to standard sternotomy with CPB and induced arrest | Learning curve technically more challenging; may have to revert to standard sternotomy; potential for endovascular injury to cannulated blood vessels |
| Discharge planning | Anticipated faster recovery of 1-2 wk (versus 4-12 wk for sternotomy), earlier ambulation, need to identify reportable signs and symptoms (angina, difficulty breathing, infection) | Anticipated faster recovery of 1-2 wk (versus 4-12 wk for sternotomy), earlier ambulation, need to identify reportable signs and symptoms (angina, difficulty breathing, infection) |

Modified from Mack MJ and others: Improved outcomes in coronary artery bypass grafting with beating-heart techniques, *Journal of Thoracic and Cardiovascular Surgery* 124(3):598-607, 2002; Verma S and others: Off-pump coronary artery bypass surgery, *Circulation* 109:1206-1211, 2004.
*CABG*, Coronary artery bypass grafting; *CPB*, cardiopulmonary bypass; *HR*, heart rate; *LOS*, length of stay; *VF*, ventricular fibrillation.

prolonged ventilation time. Having the patient complete a preoperative mental health status questionnaire, or being aware of the results of a previously completed questionnaire, can provide insight into the patient's frame of mind and serve as an opportunity to alter pessimistic attitudes amenable to conversion to a more positive state of mind. Patient attitudes also may be affected by the anticipation of pain. Patients may be hesitant to complain of pain and to request pain medication; perioperative nurses can anticipate those fears and encourage patients to ask for pain medications.[51,116]

Specific information may be required. Patients undergoing prosthetic (i.e., mechanical) valve replacement can expect to require long-term anticoagulation. Important information includes drug dosage, reportable signs and symptoms of complications and side effects (e.g., bleeding, poor healing), and a follow-up protocol for monitoring bleeding times.

The patient's ability to cough and breathe deeply should be determined; the patient should be taught to use a cough pillow or splinting techniques. Required life-style changes should be reviewed and the patient's feelings about these modifications elicited. The perioperative nurse should verify that the patient knows reportable signs and symptoms associated with the specific procedure and understands prescribed medications, dosages and times, potential side effects, and signs and symptoms of complications. Any misconceptions should be clarified or referred to an appropriate source. The family or significant others' ability and willingness to assist the patient in home care maintenance should be queried; referrals to an agency for assistance at home may be required.

Quality of life is an important goal for patients. Although objective measures are often used by clinicians to determine the patient's level of satisfaction with the quality of care received, measuring the patient's quality of life experienced after surgery has been largely limited to evaluating angina relief and return to work. However, other important variables may reflect quality of life, and nurses can assist patients with recovery and recuperation by incorporating these variables into the discharge plan. Quality of life for family caregivers also needs to be considered because with shortened lengths of stay, patients increasingly depend on others to assist them in the recuperative process. Support for caregivers is an important adjunct in the patient's recovery. Nurses can help patients to set realistic postoperative goals and develop strategies for appropriate life-style changes. The nurse who knows that the subjective perceptions of patients can change over time can reassure patients that improvement in several aspects of life is a progressive process. Compared with objective measures, subjective perceptions of quality of life may be more precise in defining the experience of recovery from CABG.[110,122]

# *Surgical Interventions*

The following section describes operations for acquired forms of heart disease. Both traditional "open" procedures and minimally invasive techniques are described. Traditional procedures are performed through a median sternotomy incision using aortocaval CPB (see Figures 27-37 and 27-38) and antegrade-retrograde cardioplegia (see Figure 27-43) with routine chest drainage and closure. Minimally invasive procedures are described for CPB, saphenous vein harvesting, coronary artery bypass grafting, and MVR. These procedures may be performed through a median sternotomy or, less frequently, through an anterior left or right thoracotomy; some lesions may be approached through a cephalad or caudal mini sternotomy.

## EXTRACORPOREAL CIRCULATION PROCEDURES

### Operative Procedures

#### *Aortic-Caval Cannulation by Way of Sternotomy*

1. A longitudinal pericardial incision is made, and the pericardial edges are retracted by suture to the chest wall.
2. The aorta, if it is to be cannulated for arterial blood return to the patient, is partially dissected from the pulmonary artery.
3. Purse-string sutures are placed in the aorta (twice) and right atrium (or both venae cavae) for the eventual placement of the perfusion cannulas. Tourniquets are placed over the suture ends and held with a hemostat.
4. For ascending aortic cannulation, the aorta is incised inside the purse-string sutures with a knife (the surgeon places a finger over the aortotomy); the cannula is inserted, and the purse-string sutures are firmly secured with the tourniquet. It is important to have the distal end of the cannula clamped before it is inserted into the aorta to prevent backbleeding from the aorta. To prevent air emboli, the arterial connection is made under a saline drip or by having the perfusionist slowly pump priming solution out of the arterial line. Arterial cannulation is generally performed before the caval cannulation so that direct access for blood replacement is available if needed.
5. *Venous cannulation*
   a. Single, two-stage cannulation for venous return to the pump-oxygenator: An incision is made into the right atrial appendage and the two-stage cannula (see Figure 27-38) is inserted into the atrium. The distal end of the cannula is placed into the inferior vena cava (IVC). The purse-string suture is secured with a tourniquet, and the catheter is permitted to fill partially with blood before being connected to the venous line.
   b. Double cannulation: For double cannulation, a second incision is made into the atrial wall within the purse-string suture and the cannulas are placed in the inferior and superior venae cavae (see Figure 27-37). To force all venous return into the cannulas, umbilical tapes with tourniquets may be placed around each cava and then tightened. This forces systemic venous return to enter the cannulas, producing total CPB (see Figure 27-42).
6. In procedures where greater exposure of the right atrium is required (e.g., tricuspid valve surgery, closure of atrial septal defects in adults), a right-angle cannula may be inserted into the SVC (Figure 27-45).

#### *Femoral Vein–Femoral Artery Cannulation*

1. A vertical or oblique incision is made into the femoral triangle, and the femoral vein and artery are exposed. Umbilical compression tapes are passed around the vessels above and below the proposed venotomy and arteriotomy. Vascu-

lar clamps may be applied above and below the incision into each vessel.

2. A purse-string suture is placed in the femoral artery. A needle is inserted into the artery, followed by a guidewire. The needle is removed, and dilators are threaded over the guidewire to enlarge the artery. The dilators are removed, and the perfusion catheter (occluded distally with a tubing clamp) is inserted retrograde into the arteriotomy as the proximal clamp or tourniquet is released. The proximal tourniquet is tightened (Figure 27-46). The cannula is connected to the arterial line.
3. An incision is made into the femoral vein, and the venous catheter is inserted into the vein as the proximal clamp or tourniquet is released. After the cannula is in place, the proximal tourniquet is tightened to prevent bleeding from the venotomy. The cannula is occluded at the distal end with a tubing clamp to prevent bleeding from the cannula. The cannula is connected to the venous line, and the tubing clamp is removed.

**MINIMALLY INVASIVE CANNULATION.** Femoral cannulation techniques are employed. Femoral arterial cannulation is as just described. Venous drainage is achieved with an extended catheter inserted into the exposed femoral vein, and the distal tip is advanced to the SVC (see Figure 27-41). Side ports along the distal portion of the cannula allow drainage of blood from the SVC, the right atrium, and the IVC. Because of the higher resistance to drainage flow compared with right atrial cannulation, a centrifugal pump is used to augment venous drainage.

**PUMP-OXYGENATOR PREPARATION.** After the arterial and venous connections are completed and the lines secured, bypass is slowly begun and the desired flow rate is gradually achieved. Perfusion flow is adjusted as necessary during the operation.

### *Cardioplegic Delivery*

**ANTEGRADE CARDIOPLEGIA.** A purse-string suture and tourniquet are placed into the anterior ascending aorta proximal to the aortic cross-clamp, and a needle-tipped catheter is inserted. Both the catheter and the cardioplegic tubing are flushed to remove residual air. The catheter tubing is Y-ed into a vent line so that alternatively the needle can be used to infuse the cardioplegic solution into the aortic root or vent air and blood from the left ventricle. Individual lines incorporated into the antegrade infusion system can be used to selectively infuse the coronary bypass graft or grafts. Handheld cardioplegic cannulas may be used to infuse cardioplegic solution directly into the coronary ostia. Because of the risk of injuring ostial tissue with this technique, it is rarely used; retrograde delivery is the preferred alternative.

**RETROGRADE CARDIOPLEGIA.** A purse-string suture is placed into the lateral wall of the right atrium, and a tourniquet is applied to the suture. A stab wound is made into the atrium, and the retrograde catheter is inserted and palpated into the coronary sinus. Blood is aspirated from the catheter, and the catheter is connected to the flushed retrograde infusion line and to a pressure line. Infusion pressure should be less than 50 mm Hg.[20] Because a full right atrium facilitates insertion of the catheter, insertion is performed before the initiation of CPB when possible. If the patient is already on CPB, the surgeon can fill the atrium by clamping the venous drainage line momentarily, thereby diverting blood into the heart.

**MINIMALLY INVASIVE ENDOVASCULAR ANTEGRADE-RETROGRADE CARDIOPLEGIA.** A system of endovascular multilumen catheters designed to infuse solutions, vent air and blood, measure intravascular pressures, and occlude the aorta may be used (Figure 27-47). Fluoroscopy or TEE can be employed to confirm proper catheter placement.

The intravascular aortic catheter has three lumens. The first lumen has an inflatable balloon at the tip that, when inflated inside the vessel, occludes the aorta and serves as an internal "cross-clamp." The second lumen can be used either to infuse antegrade cardioplegic solution or to vent the ventricle. The third lumen is used to measure aortic root pressure. The catheter is introduced into the femoral artery and advanced into the ascending aorta. Either the femoral artery used for arterial inflow or the contralateral femoral artery is used.

A triple-lumen coronary sinus retrograde cardioplegic catheter is inserted percutaneously through the jugular vein into

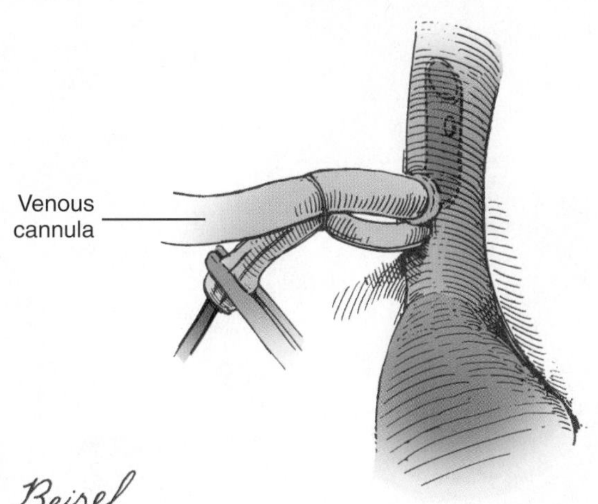


**FIGURE 27-45** Right-angle cannula in superior vena cava.

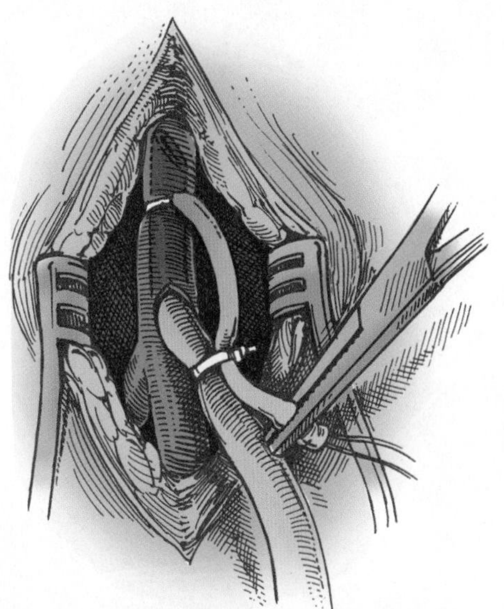

**FIGURE 27-46** Cannulation of femoral artery.

the SVC. The catheter is guided into the coronary sinus under fluoroscopy. One lumen allows manual catheter balloon inflation; another lumen is used to infuse retroplegic solution; and the third lumen measures coronary sinus pressure.

A third catheter is used as a venting-and-decompression device. It is inserted into the jugular vein (through a separate sheath from the retrograde catheter) and advanced into the main pulmonary artery.

These catheter systems allow surgeons to use minimally invasive techniques to treat lesions, such as mitral valve stenosis, that cannot be performed safely with a beating heart.

### *Termination of Cardiopulmonary Bypass*

1. After the intracardiac procedure has been completed, all air is evacuated from the left ventricle. A warm dose of cardioplegic solution may be given, after which the cross-clamp is removed.
2. Defibrillation is often spontaneous with removal of the aortic cross-clamp and the entry of warm blood into the coronary circulation. If not, internal defibrillation is necessary. Endovascular, minimally invasive procedures will require external defibrillation with sterile external paddles. Temporary epicardial pacing wires are attached to the atrium and to the ventricle.
3. Venous flow to the pump is reduced. Arterial flow is also reduced to equal the venous return. When heart action is sufficient and systemic arterial blood pressure is stabilized, venous return is further reduced and the patient is taken off bypass by clamping all lines and stopping the pump.
4. As the cannulation catheters are removed, the purse-string sutures are tightened and tied. Additional sutures may be required for hemostasis.
5. Chest tubes are inserted into the pericardium (and the pleural cavity if the pleura has been opened).
6. Protamine sulfate, a heparin antagonist, is administered.
7. The pericardium is usually left open so that accumulating drainage does not produce cardiac tamponade.

### *Closure of Femoral Incisions*

1. The femoral catheters are removed, and the arteriotomies are closed with nonabsorbable cardiovascular suture. Compression tapes and bulldog clamps, if used, are removed.
2. The incision is closed with absorbable sutures, and the skin is closed with interrupted or continuous sutures.
3. Dressings are applied to all incisions.

## PERICARDIECTOMY

Pericardiectomy is the partial excision of the adhered, thickened fibrotic pericardium to relieve constriction of compressed heart and large blood vessels. The adhered portions of the scarred, thickened pericardium restrict diastolic filling and myocardial contractility. As the pericardial space is obliterated and calcification of the pericardium occurs, the heart is further

A
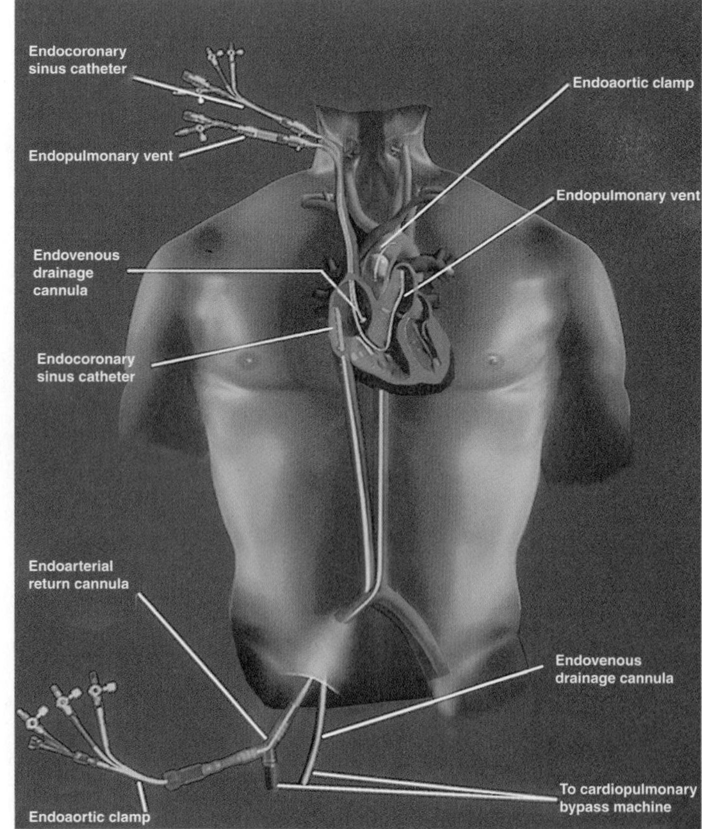


B
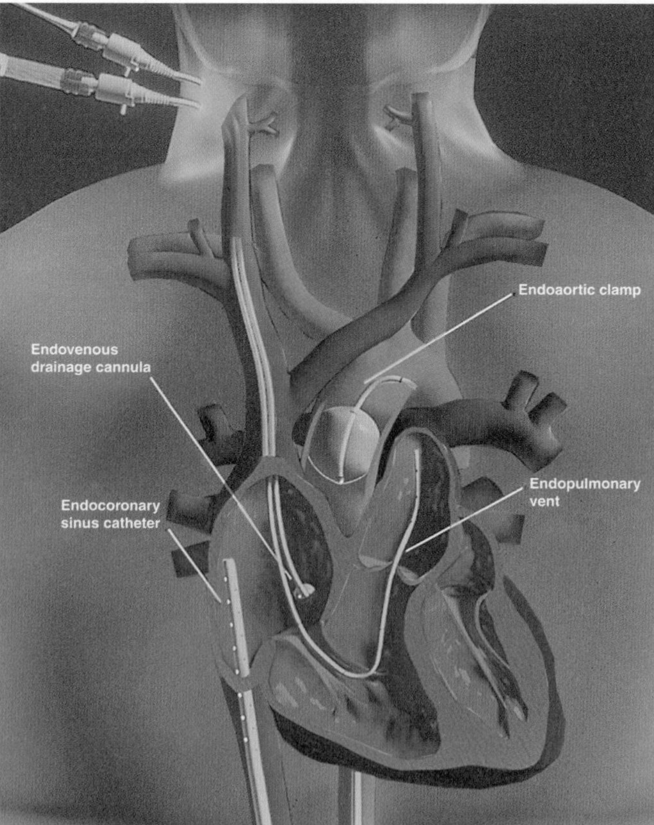


FIGURE 27-47 **A,** Endovascular cardiopulmonary bypass and myocardial protection system (see text). **B,** Intracardiac placement of catheters.

compressed. Ascites, elevated venous pressure, decreased arterial pressure, edema, and hepatic enlargement result. In most patients the etiology is unknown although there are documented cases caused by chronic pericarditis, which may be of tubercular, rheumatic, viral, or neoplastic origin.[74]

### Procedural Considerations

The use of CPB is rare, but it may be requested on a standby basis. The supplies and instruments for bypass should be available.

### Operative Procedure[142]

1. The lungs are hypoinflated to enhance exposure of the heart. The right and left phrenic nerves are identified and carefully protected. The pericardium is incised.
2. The outer, thickened pericardium is removed as indicated. Cartilage scissors may be required. The fibrous portions adhering to the atria and ventricles are carefully dissected with dry dissectors and scissors. Caution is exercised to prevent perforation of the atria and right ventricle; thus small islands of adherent pericardium may be retained.
3. Dissection is continued, and the large blood vessels are exposed and freed as indicated.
4. Drainage catheters are placed near the heart or through the pleural spaces, and connections to the water-seal drainage system are established.

## SURGERY FOR CORONARY ARTERY DISEASE

The growth of minimally invasive surgical techniques, increasingly accompanied by interventional cardiologic procedures, is most evident in the treatment of CAD. Revascularization of the ischemic myocardium can be achieved in new ways, thereby expanding treatment options for those patients in whom standard revascularization techniques are contraindicated. In addition to CABG, these techniques include transmyocardial laser revascularization[19] and percutaneous coronary interventions.[41] A variety of port-access, robotic, endoscopic, and video-assisted technology can be used with smaller thoracic[134] or sternal incisions or with median sternotomy (Table 27-9).[151] Another form of revascularization is left ventricular aneurysmectomy. Endoscopic saphenous vein[68,152] and radial artery[109] excision is performed with greater frequency.[3] Off-pump coronary artery bypass (OPCAB) is popular, and procedures employing CPB can be performed with minimally invasive systems. Table 27-10 lists revascularization procedures that can be performed in a variety of on- or off-pump techniques. Advantages of the minimally invasive techniques, with or without CPB, include more cosmetic incisions, less perioperative bleeding, fewer surgical wound infections, and earlier postoperative ambulation. Current disadvantages are that these procedures are more technically challenging, may prolong operative time, and may result in less complete revascularization.[129] Interestingly, in one randomized study, *patient-reported* outcomes after off-pump and on-pump procedures were similar for health status and overall quality of life.[90]

Distal and proximal anastomotic devices are being designed that have the potential to make it easier to perform bypass procedures in confined spaces on a beating heart. The design of these new vascular connectors employs a variety of grasping hooks that attach the vein to the aorta, magnets, U clips, and other coupling systems.[25]

Standard surgical treatment of CAD includes myocardial revascularization with CABG by use of the internal (thoracic) mammary artery (IMA), greater saphenous vein, radial artery, and other autogenous arterial and venous conduits. CABG often alleviates angina pectoris and can prolong life in certain subsets of patients, such as those with disease of the left main and left anterior descending coronary arteries.[21] The IMA demonstrates excellent long-term patency,[22,84] and this has promoted the use of arterial conduits such as the radial artery [124] the gastroepiploic artery,[138] and the inferior epigastric artery.[58] Table 27-11 compares different variables of arterial conduits, and the Research Highlight on p. 1015 reports 15-year patency rates for arterial conduits.[137] Saphenous vein remains an effective conduit when multiple grafts are needed. The increasing number of reoperations for CAD has also stimulated the use of alternative conduits (Box 27-6).

Dysrhythmias, and AF in particular, are common after CABG and can lead to hemodynamic compromise, systemic embolism, the need for extended anticoagulation (with its attendant risk of bleeding complications), cardiac pacing, patient discomfort and anxiety, and increased cost and length of stay. Preoperative or early postoperative administration of beta-blockers in appropriate patients may be given to reduce the incidence of postoperative AF; amiodarone may be used in patients who cannot receive beta-blockers.[37,41]

Increasing controversy over gender differences and their effect on outcomes after CABG has stimulated perioperative practice guidelines[43] for CABG in women (Best Practice). In particular, the guidelines focus on use of the IMA, glycemic control, avoidance of anemia and hypothyroid states, the questionable value of hormone replacement therapy, and off-pump CABG.

Other ischemia-related disorders that can require surgery include postinfarction ventricular septal defect (VSD), mitral regurgitation (MR), and certain ventricular (e.g., tachycardia) and supraventricular (e.g., AF) dysrhythmias.

### Coronary Artery Bypass Grafts with Arterial and Venous Conduits

***Operative Procedure.*** Coronary artery instruments are added to the basic setup for cardiac surgery.

1. A median sternotomy is performed as described.
2. Conduit preparation:
   a. *IMA.* The IMA is dissected free from its retrosternal bed (Figure 27-48). A special retractor, such as the one shown in Figure 27-15, can be used to expose the IMA until the necessary length is obtained. Occasionally, both right and left IMAs are used. Heparin is given before arterial grafts are clamped and cut to prevent intraluminal thrombosis.
   b. Endoscopic IMA dissection can be performed through thoracic ports (see Table 27-9) inserted into the left anterior thorax at the level of the fourth intercostal space. Ligation of arterial branches and venous tributaries is performed with hemostatic clips and electrocoagulation.
   c. *Radial artery.* A longitudinal incision is begun 3 cm distal to the elbow crease lateral to the biceps tendon and ends 1 cm before the wrist crease (Figure 27-49). The artery is exposed and mobilized with a vessel loop and harvested as a pedicle with adjacent veins and fatty tissue. The artery is ligated proximally and distally after systemic heparinization. Papaverine may be injected

**TABLE 27-9**

## Thoracic Incisions

| Incision | Position | Indications | Special Patient Needs |
|---|---|---|---|
| **Median sternotomy:** Incision along center of sternum | Supine | Most adult cardiac procedures except those on branch pulmonary arteries, distal transverse aortic arch, and descending thoracic aorta; OPCAB | Padding for hands, elbows, feet/heels, back of head, dependent bony prominences |
| **Mini sternotomy:** Partial upper or lower sternal incision starting either from sternal notch or xiphoid process and extending to midportion of sternum; lower-end sternal splitting (LESS) | Supine | MAS, or OPCAB procedures | Same as median sternotomy |
| **Parasternotomy:** Resection of right or left costal cartilages (from second to fifth cartilage, depending on surgical target) | Supine; small roll may be placed under affected side | Left: MAS CABG<br>Right: MAS CABG, valve procedures | Same as median sternotomy; risk of postoperative chest wall instability |
| **Anterolateral thoracotomy:** Curvilinear incision along subpectoral groove to axillary line | Supine with pad or pillow under operative site; arm supported in sling or overarm board; arm on unaffected side may be tucked along side | MAS, MIDCAB, trauma to anterior pericardium and left ventricle; repeat sternotomy | Padding for extremities; pillow or other device to elevate affected side; armboard or sling for arm on affected side |
| **Left anterior small thoracotomy (LAST); right anterior mini thoracotomy:** Curvilinear incision along subpectoral groove, right or left side | Supine with small roll under affected side<br>Right: MAS valve procedures or CABG | Left: MAS, MIDCAB | Same as anterolateral thoracotomy |
| **Lateral thoracotomy:** Curvilinear incision along costochondral junction anteriorly to posterior border of scapula | Placed on side with arms extended and axilla and head supported; knees and legs protected | Lung biopsies; first-rib resection; lobectomy | Armboard, overarm board, axillary roll, padding for extremities, pillow between legs; sandbags, straps, wide tape, or other devices to support torso |
| **Posterolateral thoracotomy:** Curvilinear incision from subpectoral crease below nipple, extended laterally and posteriorly along ribs almost to posterior midline below scapula (location of intercostal incision depends on surgical site); used less frequently with availability of VATS techniques | Lateral with arms extended and axilla and head supported; knees and legs protected | First-rib resection; lobectomy | Similar to needs for lateral thoracotomy |
| **Transsternal bilateral anterior thoracotomy ("clamshell"):** Submammary incision extending from one anterior axillary line to the other across sternum at fourth interspace | Supine | Bilateral lung transplant; emergency access to heart when sternal saw not available | Same as median sternotomy; requires transection of left and right IMA |
| **Subxiphoid incision:** Vertical midline incision from over xiphoid process to about 10 cm inferiorly (may divide lower portion of sternum to enhance exposure) | Supine | Pericardial drainage, pericardial biopsy, attachment of pacemaker electrodes, MAS | Same as median sternotomy |
| **Thoracoabdominal incision:** Low curvilinear incision on left side extended to anterior midline, continued vertically down abdomen | Anterior thoracotomy with chest at 45-degree angle to table; abdomen supine | Thoracoabdominal aneurysm | Same as anterolateral thoracotomy |

Data from Arom KV, Emery RW: Alternative incisions for cardiac surgery. In Yim APC and others: *Minimal access cardiothoracic surgery,* Philadelphia, 2000, Saunders; Arom KV, Emery RW: Ministernotomy for coronary artery bypass surgery. In Yim APC and others: *Minimal access cardiothoracic surgery,* Philadelphia, 2000, Saunders.

*CABG,* Coronary artery bypass graft; *IMA,* internal mammary artery; *MAS,* minimal access surgery; *MIDCAB,* minimal access direct coronary artery bypass; *OPCAB,* off-pump coronary artery bypass; *VATS,* video-assisted thoracoscopic surgery.

**TABLE 27-10**

## Types of Myocardial Revascularization

| Name | Description | Incision | Indication |
|---|---|---|---|
| MIDCAB | Minimally invasive direct coronary artery bypass (infrequent) | Left anterolateral thoracotomy | Single left anterior descending (LAD) and/or diagonal coronary artery anastomosis with left internal mammary artery (LIMA) |
| LATCAB | Lateral anterior thoracotomy coronary artery bypass | Anterolateral thoracotomy | Saphenous vein or radial artery from descending aorta to circumflex coronary artery system |
| OPCAB | Off-pump coronary artery bypass | Median sternotomy with full or limited skin incision | Multiple anastomoses |
| TECAB (also called ECABG) | Totally endoscopic coronary artery bypass; endoscopic coronary artery bypass graft (CABG) | Thoracic ports | Multiple anastomoses; on or off bypass |
| PACAB (also called port-access CAB) | Port-access coronary artery bypass | Thoracic ports | Multiple anastomoses; robot may or may not be used |
| Robotic CAB | Minimally invasive surgery (MIS) employing robotic assistance | Thoracic ports, small incisions | Multiple anastomoses |
| Robotic or nonrobotic LTMR | Laser transmyocardial revascularization | Thoracic ports, small incisions | Multiple anastomoses |
| Hybrid | Combined surgery and percutaneous coronary intervention (PCI) | Sternotomy (usually) | CABG: LAD and/or diagonal coronary artery; PCI: lateral and/or posterior coronary arteries |

Modified from Bridges CR and others: The Society of Thoracic Surgeons practice guideline series: transmyocardial laser revascularization, *Annals of Thoracic Surgery* 77:1494-1502, 2004; Mack MJ and others: Improved outcomes in coronary artery bypass grafting with beating-heart techniques, *Journal of Thoracic and Cardiovascular Surgery* 124(3):598-607, 2002; Verma S and others: Off-pump coronary artery bypass surgery, *Circulation* 109:1206-1211, 2004; Yuh DD and others: Totally endoscopic robot-assisted transmyocardial revascularization, *Journal of Thoracic and Cardiovascular Surgery* 130(1):120-124, 2005.

**TABLE 27-11**

## Comparison of Arterial Bypass Grafts

| Variable | ITA | GEA | IEA | Radial |
|---|---|---|---|---|
| Patency | Excellent | Good | Moderate | Good, short term |
| Versatility | Yes | No | Limited | Potentially yes |
| Complications | Fear of mediastinitis | Infrequent | Minor | Hand ischemia (rare) |
| Effect on survival and event-free survival | Excellent | Contributory with ITA | Unknown | Unknown |

From Loop FD: Coronary artery surgery, *Annals of Thoracic Surgery* 79:S2221-S2227, 2005.
*GEA,* Gastroepiploic artery; *IEA,* inferior epigastric artery; *ITA,* internal thoracic artery.

## RESEARCH HIGHLIGHT

### Patency of Arterial Coronary Bypass Grafts Over 15 Years

Given the excellent long-term patency of the left internal mammary artery (LIMA), there is an expectation that other arterial grafts—the right internal mammary artery (RIMA) and the radial artery (RA)—can provide similar patency rates that are superior to the saphenous vein. In this study, the consecutive postoperative angiograms of 2127 patients with arterial and venous coronary bypass grafts were reviewed. The postoperative angiograms were indicated for cardiac symptoms. The following patency rates were identified: LIMA, 96.4% (1296 of 1345); RIMA, 88.3% (534 of 605); RA (aortocoronary bypass), 89.3% (158 of 177). Patency of the LIMA to the left anterior descending (LAD) coronary artery was 97.1% (1131 of 1165); to the obtuse marginal (OM) branch of the circumflex coronary artery 91.7% (165 of 180, $P = 0.01$). Patency of the RIMA *pedicle* graft (i.e., remaining attached to the right subclavian artery) was 72.2% (275 of 381); the *free* RIMA (i.e., disconnected from the subclavian artery) had a patency of 91% (259 of 284, $P =$ not significant).

The researchers also observed that the degree of native coronary stenosis influenced patency rates: stenoses of greater than 60% were associated with higher patency rates. LIMA patency at 5 years was 98%, at 10 years 81%, and at 15 years 65%. RIMA patency was 96%, 81%, and 65% at 5 years, 10 years, and 15 years, respectively. RA patency was 96% at 1 year and 89% at 4 years. Of the 3714 vein grafts studied, 61% were open (2266 of 3714) overall. Vein graft patencies at 5 years, 10 years, and 15 years, respectively, were 95%, 71%, and 32%. The authors demonstrated in their study superior long-term patency of arterial grafts compared with vein grafts.

Modified from Tatoulis J and others: Patencies of 2,217 arterial to coronary conduits over 15 years, *Annals of Thoracic Surgery* 77:93-101, 2004.

BOX 27-6

### Alternative Conduits for Use as Coronary Bypass Grafts

- Splenic artery
- Lesser saphenous vein
- Cephalic vein
- Basilic vein
- Greater saphenous vein allografts (homografts)
- Synthetic grafts (e.g., Dacron, PTFE)

Modified from Buxton B and others: *Ischemic heart disease: surgical management*, London, 1999, Mosby.
*PTFE*, Polytetrafluoroethylene.

into the lumen to reduce spasm. The arm incision is closed over a small suction drain.[124]

d. *Gastroepiploic artery.* When an additional arterial conduit is needed, the gastroepiploic artery may be used, although the required entry into the peritoneum to dissect the artery increases the risk of postoperative complications (Figure 27-50).

e. *Saphenous vein.* The necessary length of saphenous vein is harvested from one or both legs either with video-assisted endoscopic techniques or (less commonly) by a traditional open incision (Figure 27-51). Tributaries on the leg side are ligated, cauterized, or clipped. After it is dissected free, the vein is removed and tributaries on the vein side are ligated. The distal end of the vein is identified to place the vein in a reversed position so that the semilunar valves do not interfere with the flow of blood. The vein is flushed with heparinized blood or saline and kept moist until needed.

3. With the endoscopic technique, saphenous vein harvesting is performed through one to three incisions over the vein at the knee and at the ankle and the groin if necessary. The vein is located under direct vision; the remaining length of vein is excised using a 5-mm angled endoscope and endoscopic scissors. An endoscopic clip applier or bipolar cautery can be used to seal tributaries on the leg side. To reduce postoperative tunnel dead space and minimize fluid accumulation, the leg is wrapped with a pressure bandage.
4. CPB with mild hypothermia is instituted. (If CABG is performed without CPB, the patient is not cooled.) CPB standby is usually available. Antegrade-retrograde cardioplegic solution is infused after the aorta is cross-clamped.
5. Coronary anastomoses using saphenous vein, free arterial grafts, and in situ arterial grafts (e.g., IMA and gastroepiploic artery) are performed.
   a. The affected coronary artery is identified, and a small incision is made into the artery. The graft conduit is beveled to approximate the incision (side-to-side jump grafts may be performed as well).
   b. The anastomoses are made with fine cardiovascular sutures (Figures 27-52). Before each anastomosis is completed, the distal coronary artery may be probed to ensure patency.
6. Steps 5.a and 5.b are repeated for each subsequent anastomosis.

## BEST PRACTICE

### Practice Guidelines for Females Undergoing Coronary Artery Bypass Surgery

In an effort to resolve the numerous inconsistencies surrounding the issue of gender-based differences between the outcomes of women and men undergoing coronary artery bypass grafts (CABG), the Society of Thoracic Surgeons (STS) Workforce on Evidence-Based Surgery reviewed published information on this subject. The following guidelines focus specifically on *perioperative* management and are based on the evidence available to the authors of the guidelines.

1. Use of the internal mammary artery (IMA)
   a. IMA underused in women
   b. Use of IMA associated with significant reduction in mortality (compared with CABG using venous conduits alone)
   c. At least one IMA used to bypass stenotic coronary artery
2. Management of hyperglycemia
   a. Diabetes more common in women than in men undergoing CABG
   b. Adverse effects of diabetes more pronounced in women
   c. Hyperglycemia produced incremental risk in CABG
   d. Maintain blood glucose levels at less than 150 mg/dl (range 100 to 150 mg/dl)
3. Intraoperative management of anemia
   a. Hematocrits below 22% associated with operative mortality
   b. Strategies to increase red blood cell concentration: hemoconcentration, ultrafiltration, minimizing pump prime volume, rapid autologous priming (see text)
   c. Maintain adequate hematocrit level at or greater than 22%
4. Use of off-pump CABG
   a. Improved outcomes after off-pump CAB versus on-pump CABG may be related to increased use of IMA with off-pump CAB
   b. No major differences in outcomes associated with *valve* surgery
   c. Absent of firm evidence that off-pump CAB is superior, the guidelines suggest that the indications for off-pump CAB are the same for women as for men
5. Optimization of thyroxine treatment for women with hypothyroidism
   a. Hypothyroidism associated with impaired contractility and increased risk of myocardial infarction
   b. Greater incidence of women with hypothyroidism (compared with men) undergoing CABG
   c. Maintain in a euthyroid state during surgery
6. Consideration of preoperative hormone replacement therapy (HRT)
   a. HRT not a significant predictor of mortality in multivariate analyses
   b. HRT associated with complications such as thromboembolism
   c. HRT not used for postmenopausal women undergoing CABG

Modified from Edwards FH and others: Gender-specific practice guidelines for coronary artery bypass surgery: perioperative management, *Annals of Thoracic Surgery* 79:2189-2194, 2005.

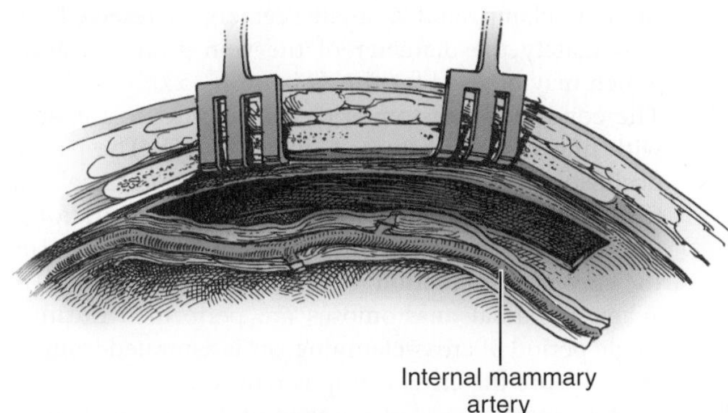


FIGURE 27-48 Dissection of internal mammary artery (IMA). Bleeding from side branches is controlled by vascular clips on the IMA side and electrocoagulation on the sternal side. Dilute solution of papaverine is sprayed onto or into lumen of IMA to dilate the artery and reduce muscular spasm. The IMA pedicle is placed in the pleural cavity until needed for anastomosis.

7. The distal anastomosis of the IMA to the coronary artery is done as described for the anastomosis of the saphenous vein graft to the coronary artery. No aortic (proximal) anastomosis is required because the IMA remains attached proximally to the subclavian artery. Because the IMA has demonstrated superior long-term patency—and the left anterior descending (LAD) coronary artery is a critical source of blood to the left ventricle—the IMA is commonly attached to the LAD.
8. Aortic anastomoses:
   a. Proximal aortic anastomoses are often all performed during a single aortic cross-clamping to avoid excessive manipulation of the aorta that could lead to intimal injury or dislodgment of atherosclerotic material. After the proximal anastomoses are completed, the aortic clamp is removed and the heart is defibrillated. Increasingly, the aorta is assessed with TEE before the anastomoses are performed to identify proximal anastomotic

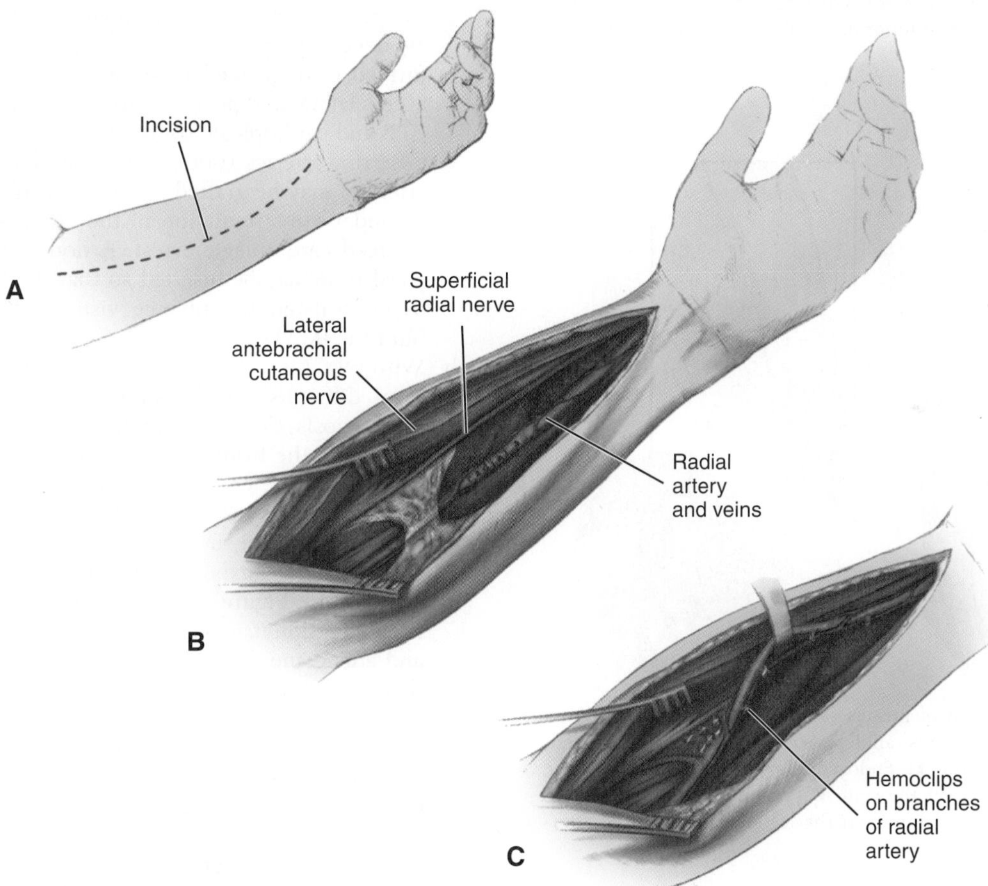


FIGURE 27-49 Dissection of radial artery. Before removal of the radial artery, Allen's test is performed to ensure that the ulnar artery will provide sufficient blood flow to the hand if the radial artery is excised: the radial and ulnar arteries are compressed to produce blanching of the hand. The ulnar artery is released while compression is maintained on the radial artery. The skin on the palm of the hand should immediately become red as blood flow is restored through the ulnar artery to the hand. **A,** Incision line. **B,** Deep forearm dissection exposes the radial artery and vein pedicle. **C,** Radial artery pedicle is mobilized, and the multiple side branches are clipped. The artery is removed and may be irrigated with a vasodilator. A continuous intravenous infusion of diltiazem helps to prevent vasoconstriction of the artery.

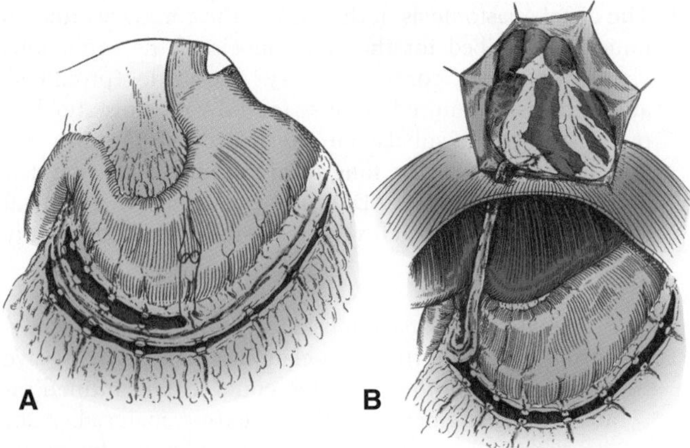


FIGURE 27-50 Right gastroepiploic artery mobilization. **A,** Branches to the stomach are divided with clamps and ties; omental branches may be divided with a staple gun. The gastroepiploic pedicle is isolated proximally to its origin from the gastroduodenal artery. **B,** The pedicle is brought up into the pericardium and anastomosed to the right coronary artery (shown here). The artery can also be grafted to the distal right and the left anterior descending coronary arteries.

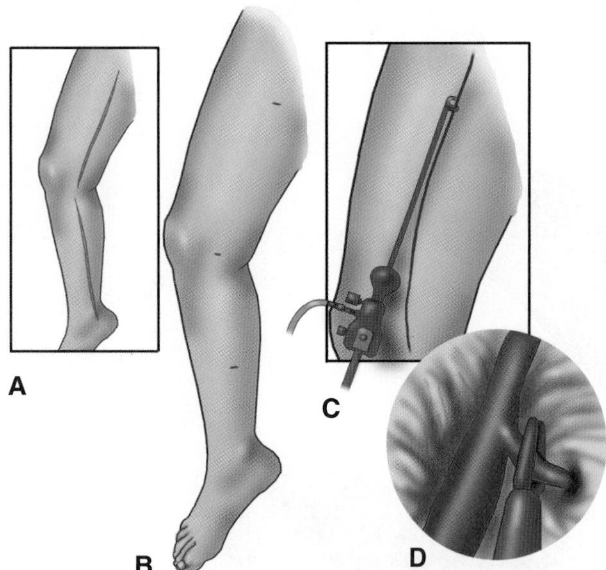


FIGURE 27-51 Excision of greater saphenous vein. **A**, Traditional open incision. **B**, Incision sites (ankle, knee, groin) for video-assisted, endoscopic vein harvesting. **C**, Endoscope inserted into medial knee incision and used to dissect the vein. **D**, Venous tributaries may be divided and cauterized or clipped on the leg side; silk ties are commonly used on the vein side.

sites that are relatively free of atherosclerotic plaque. This assessment is especially helpful during beating heart surgery (usually through a median sternotomy) that requires proximal aortic anastomoses (e.g., when a saphenous vein is used). After identification of a suitable site (i.e., relatively free of plaque), the proximal anastomoses may be performed with a partial-occlusion clamp. The aorta is partially occluded with an angled vascular clamp, and a small segment is resected, approximately the diameter of the vein graft. An aortic punch may be used for this (Figure 27-53).

b. The conduit is anastomosed, end to side, to the aorta with fine vascular sutures (Figure 27-54). The partial-occlusion clamp is removed, so that the proximal portion of the vein can fill with blood. Needle aspiration of the vein graft is performed to prevent air from entering the coronary circulation.
c. When proximal anastomoses are performed during a single period of cross-clamping, air is aspirated from the grafts before the cross-clamp is removed.

9. The aortic anastomoses of the vein grafts may be marked with clips or rings for future identification.
10. Cardiopulmonary bypass is discontinued, and the sternum is closed.
11. Minimally invasive procedures:
    a. Minimally Invasive Direct Coronary Artery Bypass (MIDCAB) may be performed, albeit less frequently, in patients with lesions easily accessible through an anterior thoracotomy (e.g., narrowings in the LAD and diagonal coronary arteries). Beating heart procedures performed through median sternotomy allow surgeons to access lateral and posterior arteries. When endovascular CPB and cardioplegic solution is used, more lateral and posterior arteries (obtuse marginal and right coronary arteries) may be grafted because ventricular fibrillation secondary to stimulation of the heart is obviated with induced cardioplegic arrest. A double-lumen endotracheal tube may be inserted so that the left lung can be hypoventilated to enhance visualization of the LAD (and the IMA).
    b. With OPCAB,[86,141,146] cardiac contraction poses a technical difficulty for the surgeon in creating a precise anastomosis. Coronary stabilizers are used to reduce the motion of the heart in the vicinity of the anastomosis (Figure 27-55). These attachments fit onto the retractor, thereby freeing the hands of the surgeon to sew. Left ventricular apical suction cups allow the apex to be retracted, thereby exposing lateral and posterior coronary arteries (see Figure 27-17). Pharmacologic cardiac motion reduction may be achieved with beta-blocker drugs and adenosine, but the newer stabilizers have reduced this need. Some surgeons may use bivalirudin (a short-acting direct thrombin inhibitor) in preference to heparin (and protamine) for anticoagulation because there is some evidence that graft flow is better with bivalirudin.[93] Bleeding from the arteriotomy (because of the continued beating of the heart) obscures the field; humidified $CO_2$ gas and elastic coronary artery tourniquets[104] may be used to control bleeding. Although a number of clinical trials have compared CABG with and without CPB, the superiority of one or the other has yet to be definitively established.[129]
    c. Port-access procedures (Figure 27-56) may be performed with a robot and the use of endovascular catheters (see Figure 27-47). Anastomoses are achieved with video-assisted thoracoscopic techniques. If better visualization is desired or required, the surgeon can convert to a median sternotomy.

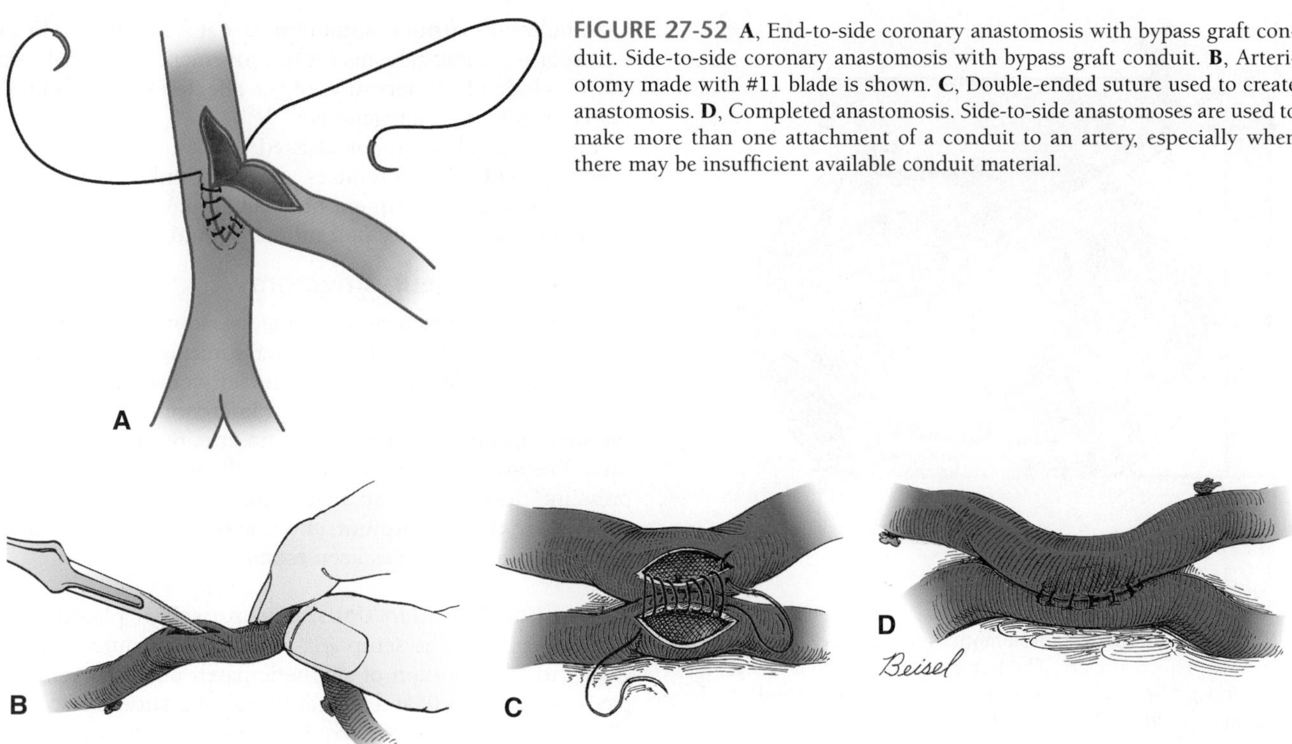


FIGURE 27-52 **A**, End-to-side coronary anastomosis with bypass graft conduit. Side-to-side coronary anastomosis with bypass graft conduit. **B**, Arteriotomy made with #11 blade is shown. **C**, Double-ended suture used to create anastomosis. **D**, Completed anastomosis. Side-to-side anastomoses are used to make more than one attachment of a conduit to an artery, especially when there may be insufficient available conduit material.

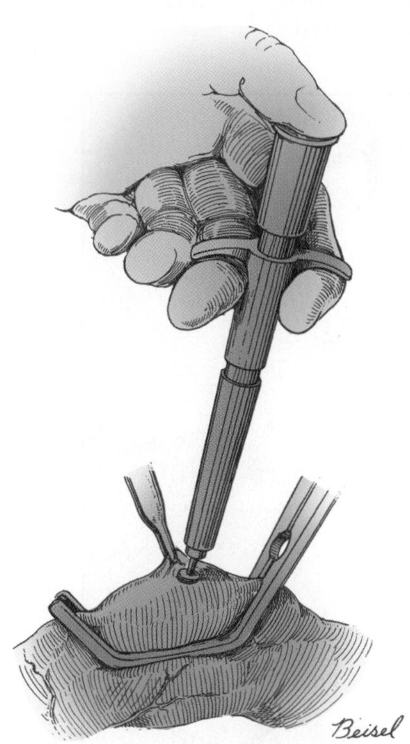


FIGURE 27-53 Proximal anastomosis of bypass graft. A partial occlusion clamp isolates the portion of the ascending aorta where the aortotomy is to be made with the punch.

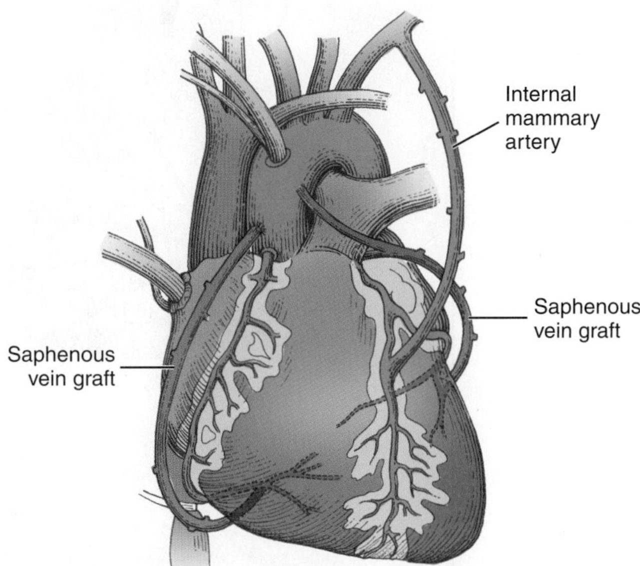


FIGURE 27-54 Coronary artery bypass grafts with reversed saphenous vein and the left internal mammary artery.

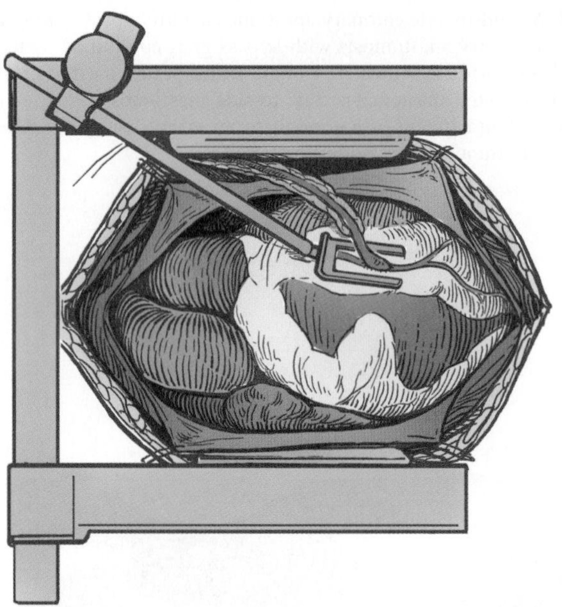

**FIGURE 27-55** Coronary anastomotic site stabilizer used during beating heart bypass surgery. The horseshoe-shaped foot has a non-smooth surface to provide an atraumatic grip on the epicardium, reduce the movement of the beating heart, and isolate the target coronary artery site for anastomosis.

## Laser Transmyocardial Revascularization

Patients with chronic, severe angina, who cannot be revascularized with either coronary bypass surgery or percutaneous catheter interventions (PCIs) may be appropriate candidates for laser transmyocardial revascularization (TMR). Channels are created in the left ventricular wall with laser energy (e.g., $CO_2$, holmium:yttrium-aluminum-garnet [Ho:YAG]). The current suggested mechanisms for improvement of anginal symptoms include (1) denervation of the affected myocardium and (2) laser-induced angiogenesis.[19,41]

Endoscopic, laser, robot-assisted TMR in the laboratory has been reported[151] and promises to further enhance the role of TMR as a surgical treatment or as an adjunct to percutaneous procedures. Laser safety precautions should be followed.

## Ventricular Aneurysmectomy

Ventricular aneurysmectomy is the excision of an aneurysmal portion of the left ventricle and reinforcement with synthetic patch material. An aneurysm of the left ventricle occasionally develops after a severe myocardial infarction in which part of the myocardium is replaced by thin scar tissue that can rupture. The scar may stretch as a result of the left ventricular pressure, thus forming an aneurysm. The aneurysm is usually adherent to the pericardium, and it may not be possible to dissect it free until CPB has been established.

***Procedural Considerations.*** The patient is placed in the supine position. The setup is as described for open-heart surgery, with the addition of synthetic patch material, Teflon felt pledgets, and 0, 3-0, and 4-0 cardiovascular sutures. Occasionally, Teflon felt strips are required to bolster the suture lines. Patch closure of the ventriculotomy (endoaneurysmorrhaphy) is performed more often than the traditional excision, plication, and oversewing of the ventricular tissue. Patch closure better preserves the geometry of the left ventricle.[74]

### *Operative Procedure*

1. A median sternotomy is performed, and CPB is begun as previously described.

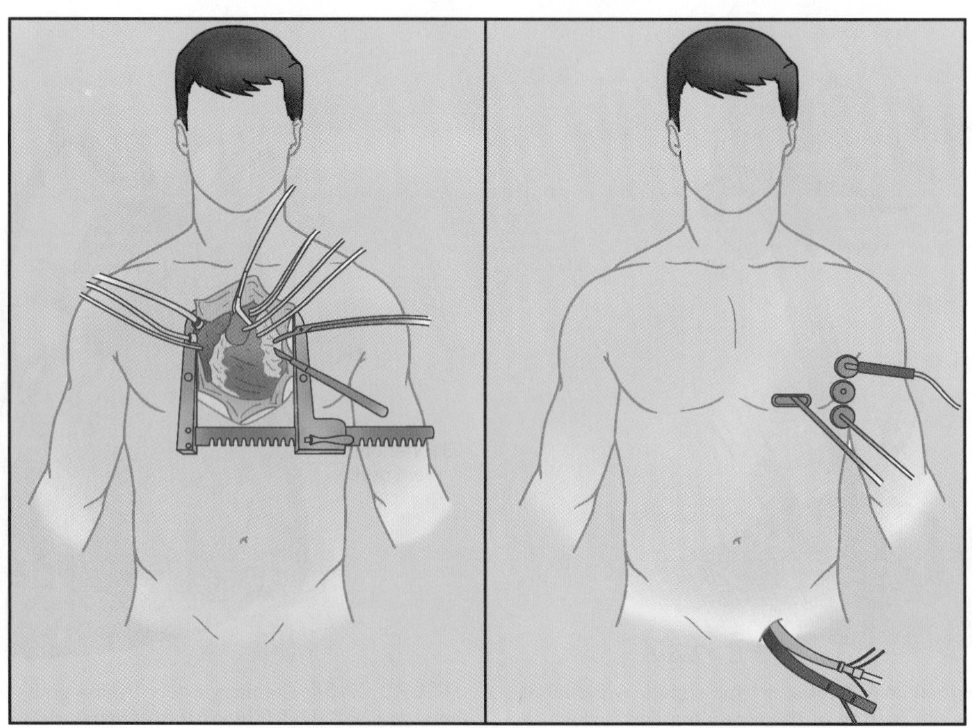

**FIGURE 27-56** Traditional sternotomy *(left)* compared with minimally invasive incisions *(right)* that provide access to the heart and to the femoral artery and vein.

2. The scar tissue of the ventricle is excised, and any clot is carefully removed (Figure 27-57, *A* and *B*).
3. A circular cuff of scar tissue is left, through which a purse-string suture with felt pledgets is placed through the rim of the scar (Figure 27-57, *C*).
4. A patch of woven Dacron is sewn to the rim with interrupted sutures (Figure 27-57, *D*). A second (internal) patch of pericardium may be placed for hemostasis.
5. The edge of the patch is reinforced with a running suture (Figure 27-57, *E*).
6. The left ventricle may be vented with a catheter inserted into the right superior pulmonary vein; after the ventricle is deaired, the catheter is removed and closure of the incision completed.

### Postinfarction Ventricular Septal Defect

Ventricular septal or free-wall rupture is a catastrophic complication of myocardial infarction, creating an acute left-to-right shunt and cardiac failure requiring early surgical repair. The defect is closed with a prosthetic patch and other materials commonly used for postinfarction ventricular aneurysm. Anterior VSDs are usually closed with felt strips and placating sutures.[15]

## SURGERY FOR CONGESTIVE HEART FAILURE

Other procedures, introduced by Batista[9] and modified by Dor,[40] were developed to remodel the left ventricle of patients with congestive heart failure (from CAD or other processes) by excising the dilated, hypokinetic portion of the ventricle and repairing it to produce a more efficient pumping chamber. These techniques of ventricular reconstruction are not widely performed, but they offer additional surgical options for patients with dilated cardiomyopathy.[94,150]

## SURGERY FOR THE MITRAL VALVE

Mitral *stenosis* (MS) is a narrowing of the valve orifice such that it causes impedance to forward blood flow. It is often caused by rheumatic fever. The normal opening in the valve is about 5 $cm^2$. As the disease progresses, the mitral valve becomes a narrow slit in a fibrotic plaque, severely limiting blood flow into the left ventricle. MS causes a rise in pressure and dilation of the left atrium. This pressure is transmitted throughout the pulmonary vascular bed, with subsequent pulmonary hypertension, right ventricular hypertrophy, and possibly tricuspid valve regurgitation.[17]

The major symptoms are dyspnea, fatigue, and orthopnea. Late findings are severe pulmonary congestion and right ventricular failure. A characteristic diastolic murmur is heard, and AF is not unusual. Thromboembolism may result from stasis of blood in the left atrial appendage. Later findings are severe pulmonary congestion and right ventricular failure.[74,82]

Mitral *regurgitation* (MR) occurs when the valve leaflets do not close properly or when the leaflets are perforated and blood escapes back into the left atrium during ventricular systole. Common causes of MR are myxomatous degeneration and secondary to aortic valve stenosis. In Western countries, other causes of MR are degenerative, ischemic, and dilated cardiomyopathy.[140] During ventricular diastole, the blood regurgitated into the left atrium augments blood volume entering the left ventricle. MR may accompany MS or be attributable to leaflet tears, annular dilation, or elongated or ruptured chordae. Ischemic heart disease may produce papillary muscle dysfunction, which prevents sufficient anchoring of the leaflets in the closed position. Symptoms are primarily dyspnea on exertion and easy fatigability.

The surgeon's selection of the procedure (repair or replacement) is determined by the stage of disease, presence or absence of calcification, history of thromboembolism and dysrhythmia, ability to tolerate long-term anticoagulation (required after insertion of a mechanical valve prosthesis), and any associated pathologic defects. Improvements in imaging capabilities with two-dimensional and three-dimensional echocardiography have enabled surgeons to diagnose more precisely and subsequently to identify the most appropriate reparative procedure.[148,149]

Reparative procedures that preserve the native valve are widely employed because the complications associated with prosthetic replacement and anticoagulation can be avoided. The technique selected must be tailored to the unique pathophysiologic findings; therefore the surgeon carefully evaluates the leaflets and related structures at the time of surgery before deciding on which procedure to perform. Because there is a possibility that the valve may have to be replaced, instruments (and prostheses) for replacement as well as repairs should be available. Also included are atrial handheld or self-retaining retractors, obturators for sizing prosthetic rings and valves, sizer or prosthesis handles, and special sutures if requested. Bicaval cannulation often is used to enhance exposure of the operative field and to decompress the heart (see Figure 27-37). TEE is used to establish a cardiac functional baseline and to confirm efficacy of the repair after the cross-clamp is removed and the heart resumes beating and again after bypass is discontinued. TEE is also used intraoperatively to assess left ventricular function and to detect the presence of air (seen as white specks) within the cardiac chambers.

### Mitral Valve Repairs

***Open Commissurotomy of the Mitral Valve for Mitral Stenosis.*** Open commissurotomy is the separation of fused, adherent leaflets of the mitral valve.

PROCEDURAL CONSIDERATIONS. The patient is placed in a supine position for a median sternotomy. The setup is as described for open-heart procedures, with mitral valve instruments.

OPERATIVE PROCEDURE

1. A median sternotomy is performed, and bicaval cannulation is performed for CPB.
2. The left atrium is incised, and the valve is inspected; in some cases, a transseptal approach (right atrium to left atrium) may be used.
3. Fused leaflets are separated with vascular forceps and scissors or a knife (Figure 27-58). A dilator may be used to enlarge the mitral valve orifice.
4. The valve is again inspected for any resultant insufficiency.
5. An annuloplasty ring may be inserted.
6. The left atrium is closed with a continuous cardiovascular suture.

***Mitral Annuloplasty for Mitral Regurgitation.*** Mitral annuloplasty is the reduction of a dilated annulus by inserting a prosthetic ring. Although it has been assumed that the poste-

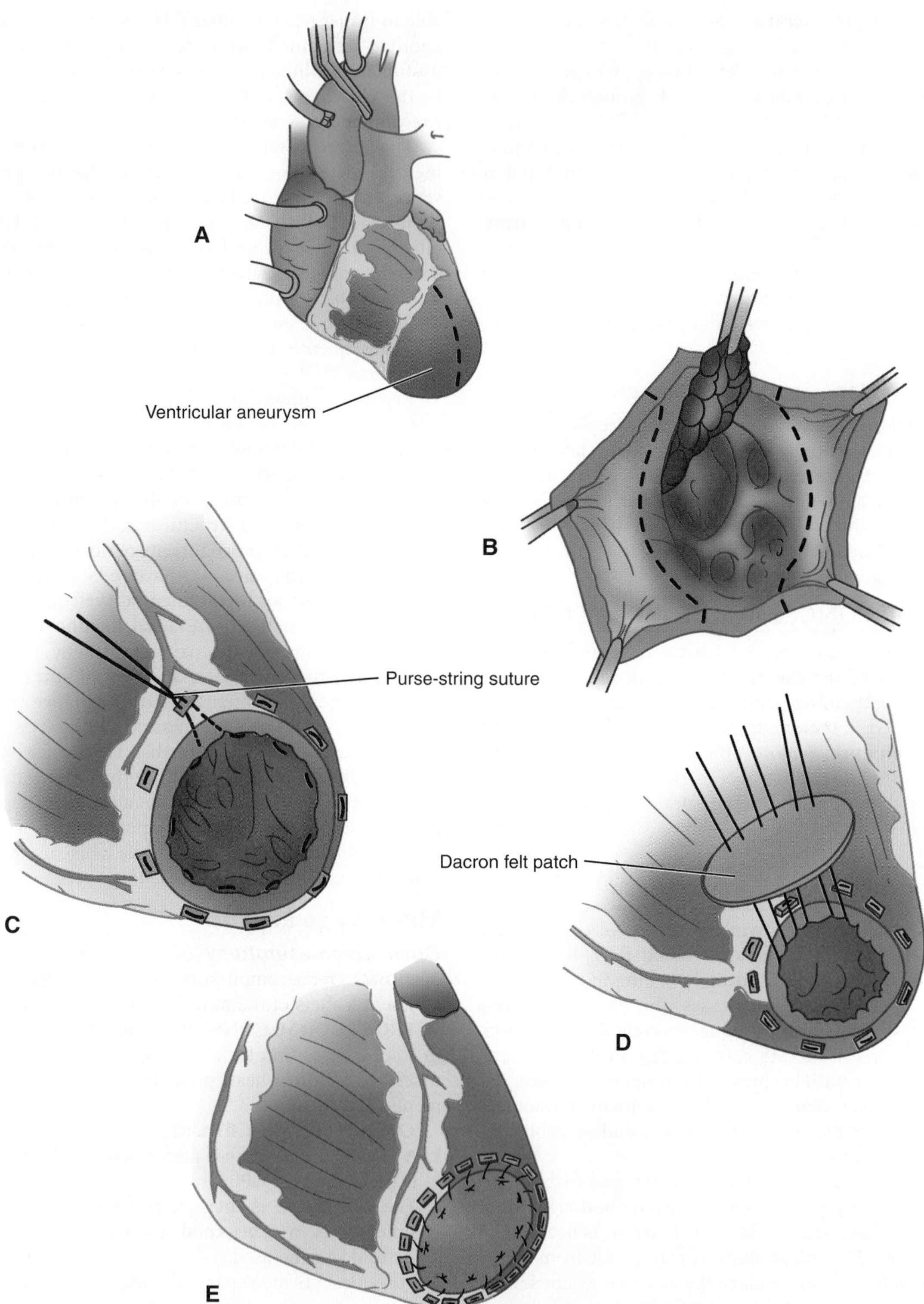


FIGURE 27-57 Repair of left ventricular aneurysm. **A**, Left ventricular apical aneurysm. **B**, Intracavitary clot is removed. **C**, Pledgeted sutures placed around the edge of the excised ventricular tissue. **D**, A patch is inserted. **E**, Completed repair.

rior leaflet only is subject to annular dilation, it has been demonstrated that the anterior portion can also be affected in certain groups.[50] The techniques (and associated prostheses) created by Carpentier[24] and others currently in wide use[149] undoubtedly will be expanded as more is learned about the dynamic nature of the mitral valve components in various disease states.

OPERATIVE PROCEDURE

1. The left atrium is incised, and sump suctions are inserted into the atrial cavity to remove blood.
2. The annulus, leaflets, chordae, and the rest of the mitral complex are inspected.
3. If generalized annular dilation is present, an annuloplasty ring is inserted; a C-shaped ring may be used for dilation affecting the posterior leaflet (see Figure 27-33). An obturator is used to determine the appropriate-size ring (Figure 27-59, *A*). Interrupted sutures are placed around the circumference of the annulus and then into the ring (Figure 27-59, *B*). When the stitches are tied, the excess annular tissue of the posterior leaflet is evenly drawn up against the prosthesis (Figure 27-59, *C*).

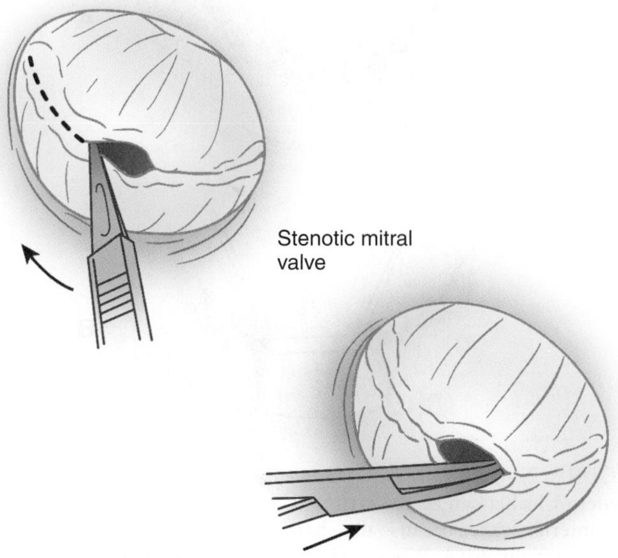


**FIGURE 27-58** Mitral commissurotomy (see text).

4. The valve is inspected for competency; a bulb syringe filled with saline may be used to distend the ventricle. The left atrium is closed.

### *Mitral Valvuloplasty Repairs for Mitral Regurgitation.*

Mitral valvuloplasty is the repair of the valve leaflets or related structures. Selection of the appropriate repair for perforated or redundant valve leaflets or for shortened or elongated chordae tendineae requires careful assessment and evaluation of the abnormalities present. Historically most mitral valve repairs have been performed on the posterior leaflet, but a number of anterior leaflet repairs have been developed (see steps 5 to 8 below).

OPERATIVE PROCEDURE

1. Perforated leaflets can be patched with pericardium.
2. Redundant, prolapsed *posterior* leaflet tissue can be resected (Figure 27-60). The cut edges of the posterior leaflet are sewn together, and the corresponding annular segment is plicated. An annuloplasty ring is inserted to reinforce the leaflet repair and reduce annular dilation.
3. Shortened, fused chordae tendineae can be lengthened and mobilized by their division into secondary chordae or by incising the tip of the papillary muscles.
4. Redundant tissue of elongated chordae may be implanted into the papillary muscle head or folded over itself and secured with a suture.
5. *Anterior* leaflet prolapse is a greater challenge and traditionally has been an indication for valve replacement. A small triangular resection of the anterior leaflet (reinforced with annuloplasty ring insertion) has been shown to be an alternative to valve replacement.[125]
6. Elongated or ruptured chordae may be replaced with polytetrafluoroethylene (PTFE) suture (Figure 27-61).
7. A chordal flip procedure (Figure 27-62) can be used to reestablish chordal attachment to the *anterior* leaflet. A section of the posterior leaflet with attached chordae is cut, swung over to the anterior leaflet, and sewn onto the anterior leaflet. The remaining posterior leaflet defect is closed with suture (no. 2 above).
8. The edge-to-edge technique introduced by Alfieri and colleagues[3] can be used to repair mitral valves with bileaflet prolapse (i.e., both the *anterior* and *posterior* leaflets are incompetent, producing severe MR). The free edges of the mitral leaflets are approximated, and a figure-of-eight suture is placed in the central portion of the apposed leaflets. This

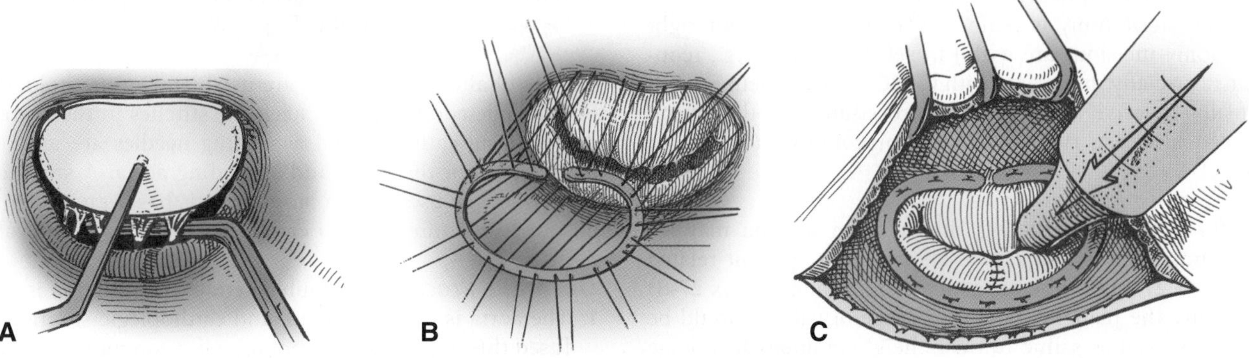


**FIGURE 27-59** Mitral valve annuloplasty (see text).

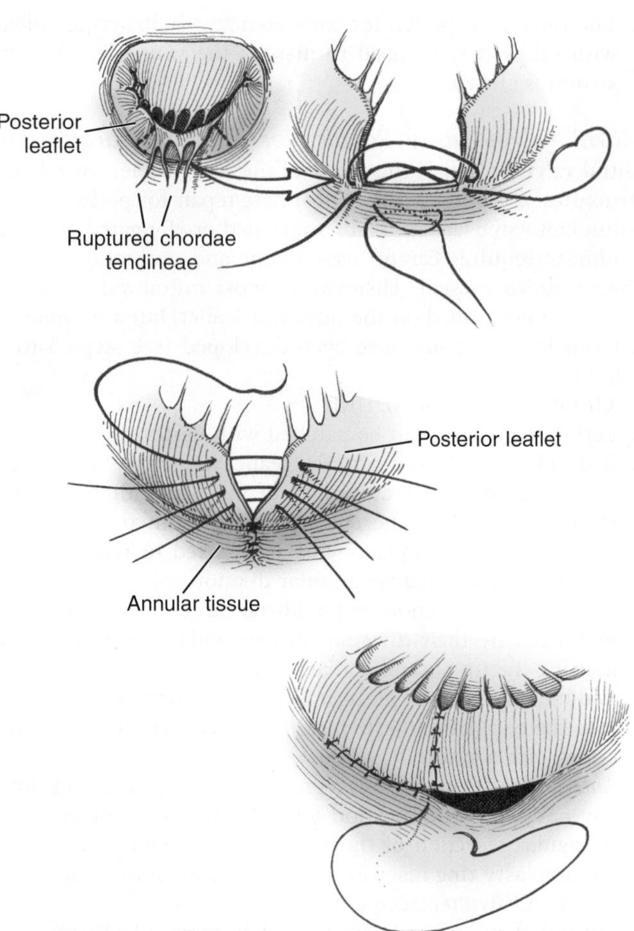


FIGURE 27-60 Quadrangular resection of nonsupported posterior leaflet tissue caused by ruptured chordae tendineae (see text). A similar technique can be used to resect *redundant* tissue causing mitral regurgitation.

creates a double orifice mitral valve that can eliminate MR and preserve the native valve.[89]

## Mitral Valve Replacement

Mitral valve replacement (MVR) is the excision of the mitral valve leaflets and replacement with a mechanical or biologic prosthesis. Generally, the mural (posterior) leaflet and associated chordae and papillary muscles are retained to maintain ventricular configuration, thereby enhancing postoperative ventricular function. If possible, the anterior leaflet is also retained if it is not too heavily calcified.

Median sternotomy is performed in most cases, but right thoracotomy incisions are useful in selected cases (e.g., reoperation, especially in patients with CABG IMA and vein grafts). Minimally invasive (and robotic) procedures on the mitral valve can also use right and left thoracotomy incisions or ports.

***Procedural Considerations.*** Although the surgeon may intend to implant a specific type of prosthesis, patient-related factors (Box 27-7) or prosthetic valve complications (Box 27-8) may modify the plan.[55] A complete range of valves should be available, as well as saline to rinse the glutaraldehyde storage solution from biologic prostheses if they are used. Pledgeted

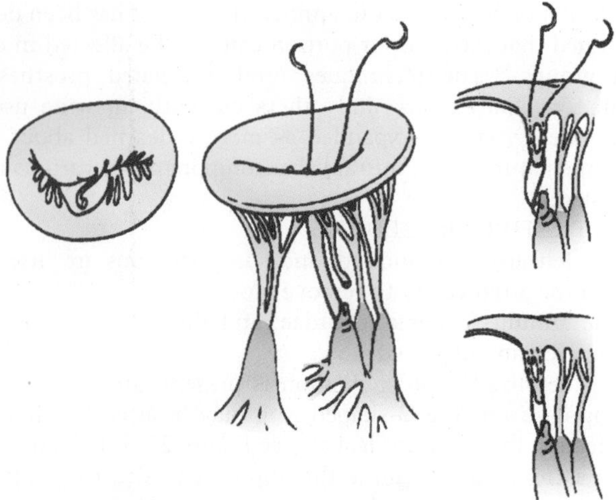

FIGURE 27-61 Chordal replacement with polytetrafluoroethylene (PTFE) (see text).

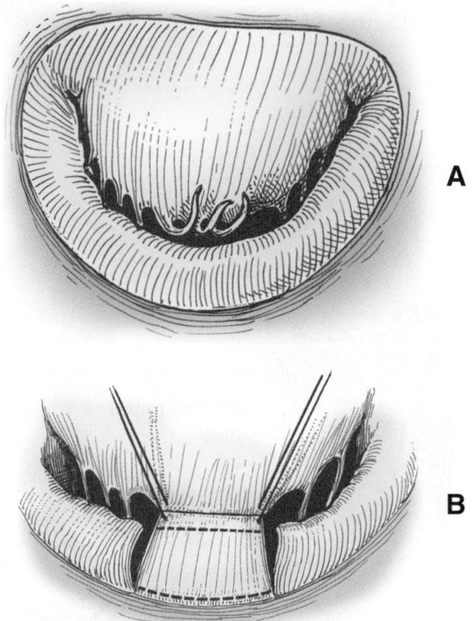


FIGURE 27-62 Chordal flip procedure. Although portions of the posterior leaflet can be resected with success, the same is not true of the anterior leaflet because the shape of the valve and the coaptation margin are altered. **A,** When there are ruptured chordae of the *anterior* leaflet of the mitral valve, the flip procedure can be used to reestablish chordal support for the anterior leaflet. **B,** A portion of normal posterior leaflet tissue with attached chordae is cut, swung over, and sewn onto the flail segment of the anterior leaflet. The posterior leaflet defect is repaired as illustrated in Figure 29-60.

sutures of alternating colors are used, and suture holders may be available additionally to keep the stitches in the correct order. Venting catheters and aspirating needles are used to remove air from the heart and ascending aorta. A small dental mirror may be used after a bioprosthesis has been implanted to ensure that sutures are not caught in the struts of the valve.

***Operative Procedure.*** Double venous cannulation is used.

1. The aorta is cross-clamped, and cardioplegic solution is infused through the aortic root or, more commonly, retrograde through the coronary sinus.

BOX 27-7

### Patient-Related Factors and Risks for Valve Surgery

- Age
- Gender
- Residence
- History of atrial fibrillation
- Endocarditis (preoperative)
- Connective tissue disorders (e.g., myxomatous changes)
- Congenital anomalies (e.g., bicuspid aortic valve)
- Enlarged left atrium
- Left atrial thrombus
- Left ventricular function (e.g., functional class, myocardial infarction, congestive heart failure)
- Syncope
- Anticoagulation compliance
- Preexisting medical problems (e.g., diabetes mellitus, hypertension, hepatic or renal disease)
- Valve lesion
- Previous cardiac surgery

Modified from Seifert PC: *Cardiac surgery*, St Louis, 2002, Mosby; Hammermeister K and others: Outcomes 15 years after valve replacement with a mechanical versus a bioprosthetic valve: final report of the Veterans Affairs randomized trial, *Journal of the American College of Cardiology* 36(4):1152-1158, 2000.

BOX 27-8

### Valve-Related Risks and Complications

- Thromboembolism
- Anticoagulation-related hemorrhage
- Prosthetic valve endocarditis
- Periprosthetic leak
- Prosthetic failure

Modified from Kincaid EH and others: Tissue engineered heart valves: a potential cure for valvular heart disease, *CTSNet.* Accessed January 14, 2005, on-line: www.ctsnet.org/sections/innovation/valvetechnology/articles/article-12.html; Seifert PC: *Cardiac surgery*, St Louis, 2002, Mosby; Hammermeister K and others: Outcomes 15 years after valve replacement with a mechanical versus a bioprosthetic valve: final report of the Veterans Affairs randomized trial, *Journal of the American College of Cardiology* 36(4):1152-1158, 2000.

2. The left atrium is incised along the interatrial groove to expose the mitral valve (Figure 27-63, *A*).
3. The valve is assessed, and the anterior leaflet is excised. The posterior leaflet is often retained to enhance the ventricular configuration and postoperative function. Occasionally the anterior leaflet is retained. Rongeurs may be used to debride heavy calcification; loose debris is removed. A margin of the valve annulus is retained to insert fixation sutures to the prosthesis (Figure 27-63, *B*).
4. A valve sizer is used to determine the correct size of the prosthesis, which is delivered to the field.
5. Nonabsorbable cardiovascular sutures (15 to 20 or more) are placed in the annulus of the valve and then placed into the sewing ring of the prosthesis.
6. The sutures are held taut (and moistened) as the prosthesis is guided into position and secured, and the sutures are tied and cut (Figure 27-63, *C*).
7. Continuous nonabsorbable sutures are used to partially close the atriotomy. The patient is placed in reverse Trendelenburg position, and the lungs are inflated to remove air from the pulmonary veins and atrium. Air is aspirated from the left ventricle through a hypodermic needle or vent catheter, and the atrial closure is completed.

Endoscopic, video-assisted, robotic mitral valve surgery has progressed from a technical curiosity to an acceptable (albeit with a significant learning curve) method of intracardiac, telemanipulated valve repair. Both mitral valve repair and replacement have been performed with these techniques (Figure 27-64), as well as procedures to correct other intracardiac structural lesions,[27,114,115] but robotic techniques currently are not widely employed.

## SURGERY FOR THE TRICUSPID VALVE

### Tricuspid Valve Annuloplasty

Tricuspid valve annuloplasty is the reduction of a dilated annulus with a suture technique[112] or a prosthetic ring. Tricuspid valve regurgitation may be caused by bacterial or viral endocarditis. It may be the functional result of mitral valve disease. After mitral valve correction, tricuspid valve function may return to normal. Preoperatively, if the tricuspid annular dilation is diagnosed to be severe, a repair similar to mitral annuloplasty may be performed. Caution is taken to avoid injury to the conduction tissue in the area of the AV node. A pulmonary artery catheter is usually not inserted preoperatively because it would interfere with the surgical field. A catheter may be inserted after the repair is completed.

Although tricuspid valve *replacement* is seldom performed, patients with tricuspid stenosis or regurgitation, or failed tricuspid annuloplasty may require insertion of a prosthetic biologic or mechanical valve.[26] There are no specific tricuspid prosthetic valves; rather, a mitral prosthesis would be implanted.

#### *Operative Procedure*

1. Double venous cannulas are inserted so that they do not cross one another in the right atrium, and occluding tapes are tightened around the cavae and cannulas to prevent venous return from entering the right atrium and obscuring the surgical site. A right-angled venous cannula may be placed into the superior vena cava to enhance exposure.
2. The right atrium is opened longitudinally to expose the tricuspid valve. Sump suctions are inserted to remove coronary sinus drainage.
3. In the DeVega technique[112] (Figure 27-65), a double-armed, felt-pledgeted suture is placed in the valve annulus, beginning at the anteroseptal commissure and continued around to the level of the coronary sinus orifice. The remaining arm of suture is similarly placed. The suture is tied over a pledget with sufficient tension to reduce the annular area to the size desired.
4. In the Carpentier[24] or Cosgrove[92] technique, a prosthetic ring is inserted in a manner similar to mitral valve annuloplasty (see Figure 27-59).
5. Saline may be injected into the ventricle to test the competence of the repair, and TEE is also employed.
6. The right atrium is closed with nonabsorbable suture.

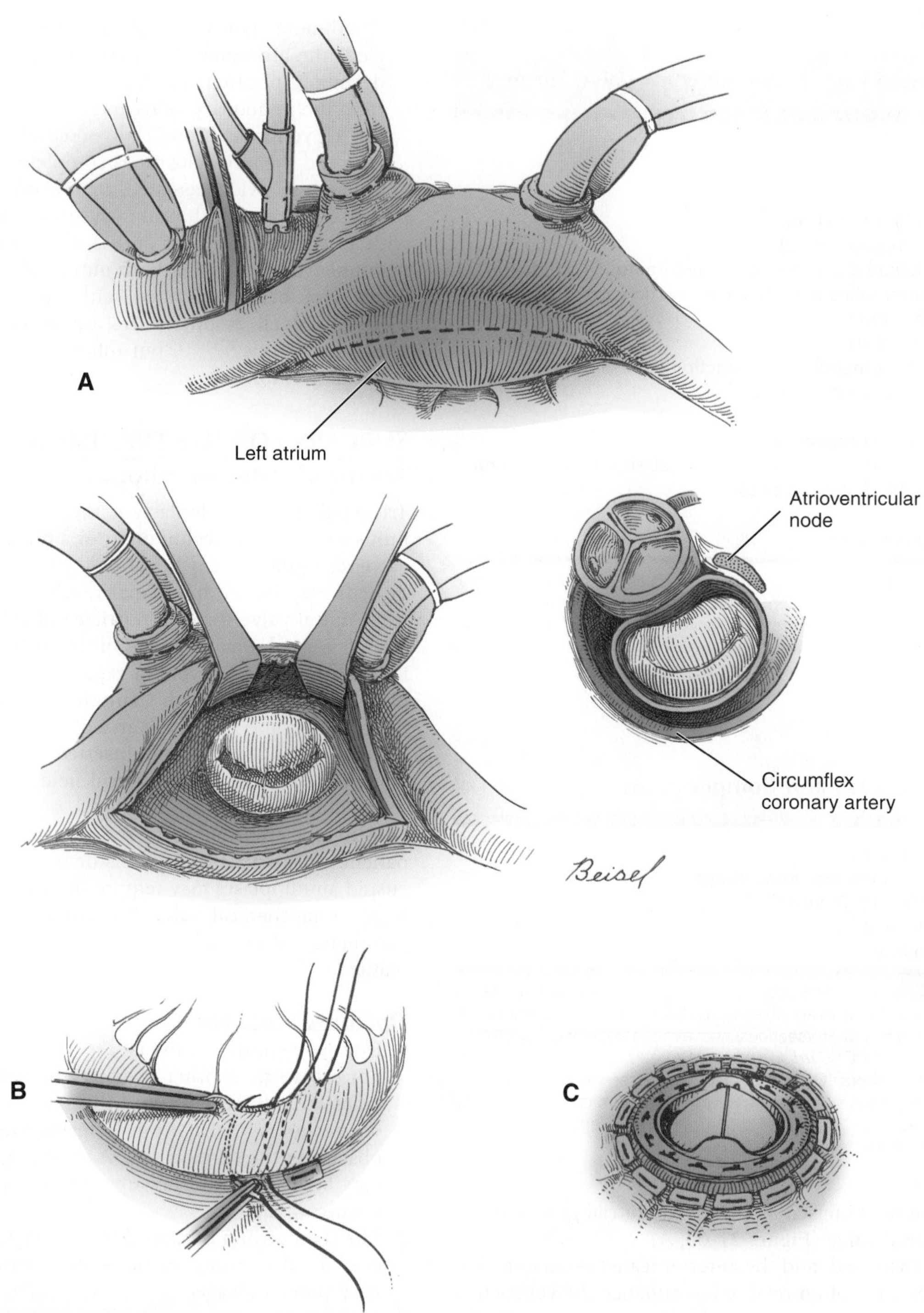


FIGURE 27-63 Mitral valve replacement. **A,** Line of incision and cannulation for bypass, anatomic relationship between mitral and aortic valves with location of conduction node, and exposure of valve. **B,** Placement of pledgeted double-armed sutures in native valve annulus. **C,** Completed valve replacement.

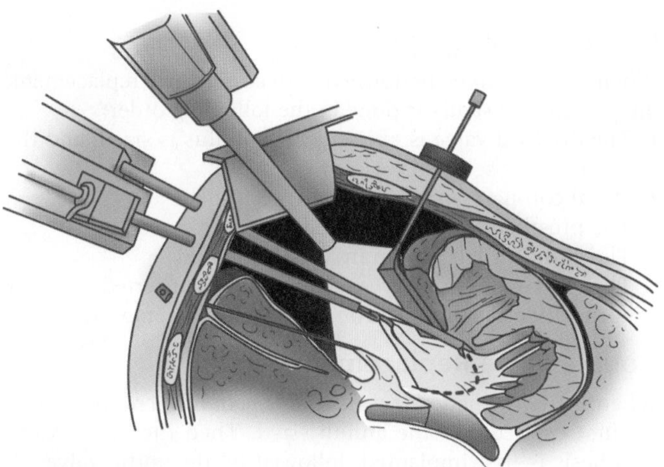

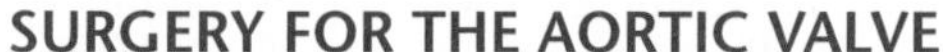

FIGURE 27-64 The 1-cm robotic instrument arms are placed through the chest wall. A transthoracic retractor arm elevates the interatrial septum toward the sternum. The three-dimensional camera is placed through a 4-cm incision, which also serves as a working port for the assistant.

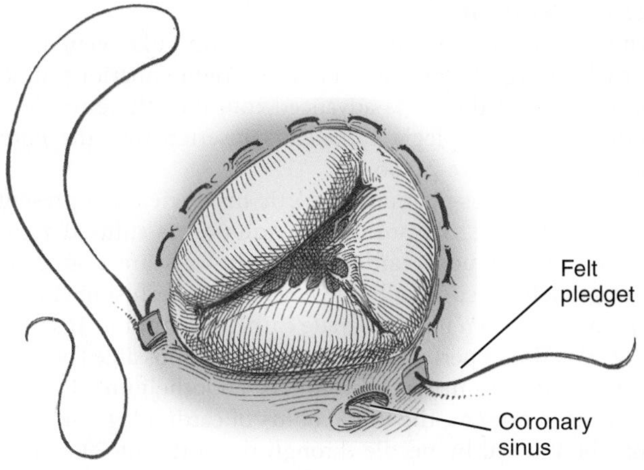


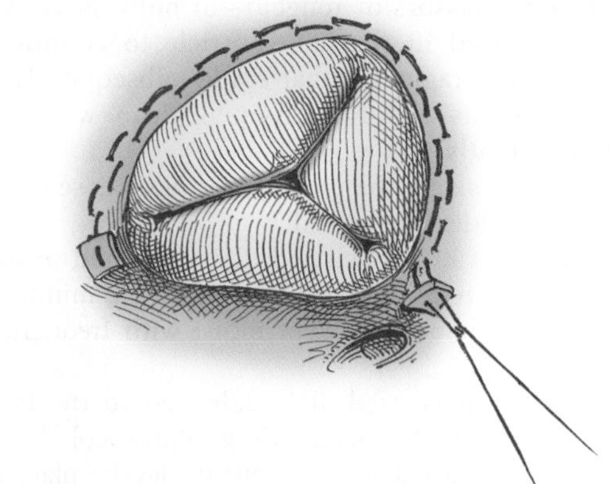

FIGURE 27-65 DeVega tricuspid valve suture annuloplasty.

## SURGERY FOR THE AORTIC VALVE

Aortic *stenosis* (AS) produces obstruction to left ventricular outflow. Whether caused by rheumatic fever, a congenital bicuspid valve, or calcification, the fused valve leaflets present an increasing resistance to left ventricular outflow, thus increasing the pressure inside the left ventricle. Recent histopathologic and clinical data suggest that calcified AS is not a "degenerative" passive process but, rather, an active,[47] possibly inflammatory[113] disease process.

To compensate for the increased pressure load, the ventricle hypertrophies so that it can generate sufficient pressure to eject blood through the narrowed opening. When disease is severe, large pressure gradients are often measured during cardiac catheterization, with differences in systolic pressures between the ventricle and the aorta reaching 50 mm Hg or more. In the early stages of the disease, a systolic ejection murmur may be heard, but patients are rarely symptomatic. Eventually, fatigue, exertional dyspnea, angina pectoris, syncope, and congestive heart failure may develop, presenting a grave prognosis. Sudden death may be the first sign of AS.[121]

Aortic *insufficiency (regurgitation)* is most often caused by rheumatic fever in developing countries and by congenital anomalies (commonly a bicuspid aortic valve) in developed countries.[45] Although *repair* of the aortic valve is challenging because of the precise closing mechanism of the valve leaflets, aortic valve reparative techniques have been employed successfully in selected patients.[96] Total valve excision and replacement with a prosthesis or an allograft are commonly performed.

The small aortic root (e.g., less than 21 mm) presents challenges to provide an adequate cardiac output. The choice and size of a prosthetic valve are based on achieving appropriate hemodynamic function in relation to body size. In patients with a small aortic annulus and large body mass (referred to as body/size mismatch), the surgeon selects a prosthesis that will provide optimum flow. The stentless aortic valve (see Figure 27-27, *B*) is frequently used because of the excellent hemodynamics. Patch enlargement of the small aortic root is another option,[142] and the patient's own pulmonary valve can be used as an autograft to replace the aortic valve; the pulmonary valve is then replaced with an allograft. Allografts may be used to replace the aortic valve as well.

### Aortic Valve Replacement

The aortic valve is excised and replaced with a mechanical or biologic prosthesis or an aortic valve allograft or autograft.

***Procedural Considerations.*** To the basic setup may be added the following:

- Aortic valve instruments
- Aortic valves, sizers, and holders
- Coronary sinus retrograde-infusion cannula and venting catheters
- Saline to rinse the glutaraldehyde storage solution from bioprostheses
- Saline bath to thaw frozen allografts

### Operative Procedure

1. After the institution of CPB, a left ventricular vent is inserted through a stab wound into the right superior pulmonary vein and the tip is advanced into the left ventricle. A retrograde cardioplegia catheter is inserted into the coronary sinus (Figure 27-66, *A*).
2. The aorta is cross-clamped. If aortic insufficiency is present, the initial bolus of cardioplegic solution is infused retrogradely; subsequent cardioplegic infusions are also given retrogradely. Occasionally, direct coronary perfusion (Figure 27-66, *B*) is given if a retrograde catheter cannot be inserted; however, direct perfusion is avoided when possible (because of the risk of injuring the coronary endothelium). If aortic stenosis is present, the initial bolus of cardioplegic solution may be infused by needle through the aorta into the aortic root. Once the heart is arrested, the aorta is opened.
3. The native valve is inspected. The valve is carefully excised to avoid injury to the annulus and underlying structures (Figure 27-66, *C*). Calcium is debrided from the annulus with scissors or rongeurs or both. Narrow packing may be used in the left ventricle to confine small, loose, calcified fragments that could subsequently embolize. Instruments should be wiped clean with a moist sponge frequently.
4. The annulus is sized, the proper prosthesis is selected, and a prosthesis holder is attached.
5. a. If a biologic valve is selected, it is delivered to the field and rinsed in three saline baths for at least 2 minutes each. Biologic valves should be kept moist with frequent saline rinsing.
   b. If an allograft is used, it is delivered to the field and thawed in saline baths according to protocol.[74]
   c. If a mechanical valve is chosen, it may be placed in an antibiotic solution until inserted (antibiotic solutions are not recommended for biologic valves).
6. a. The new valve is implanted (Figure 27-66, *D* and *E*) by use of a technique similar to that previously described for MVR.
   b. If the aortic annulus is too small to accept a prosthesis of adequate size, the annulus and proximal portion of the ascending aorta can be enlarged.[142] A patch of bovine pericardium or Dacron graft can be placed longitudinally in the proximal anterior ascending aorta where the aortic annulus has been incised (Figure 27-67, *A* and *B*). The valve prosthesis is sutured to the natural annulus and then to the patch (Figure 27-67, *C*). The patch is sutured to the remaining edges of the aortotomy (Figure 27-67, *D*).
7. The aorta is closed with nonabsorbable sutures, and the cross-clamp is removed.
8. The left side of the heart is deaired (by vent, by moving the OR bed side to side, or by other maneuvers chosen by the surgeon). The patient is placed in Trendelenburg position, and the lungs are inflated. The heart is not allowed to eject blood until the surgeon is satisfied that no air remains within the left ventricle. The heart is defibrillated if it does not resume beating spontaneously.
9. Rewarming of the heart continues, the venting catheter or catheters are removed, and the chest is closed in the routine manner.

### Combined Surgery

When CABG is to be performed with aortic valve replacement, the procedure usually is done in the following order:

1. The diseased valve is excised, the annulus is sized, and the prosthesis is selected.
2. Distal coronary anastomoses are performed.
3. The prosthetic valve is inserted.
4. The aorta (or left atrium in MVR) is closed.
5. The proximal coronary anastomoses are inserted into the aorta, after which the aortic cross-clamp is removed.

### Double Valve Replacement

When the *aortic and mitral valves are both replaced,* the valves are first excised and the annuli sized. Then the mitral valve prosthesis is first implanted, followed by the aortic valve. (If the aortic prosthesis were to be inserted first, the firm prosthetic aortic annular ring could make insertion of a mitral prosthesis difficult.) The aorta is closed, and after sufficient deairing of the left ventricle, the left atrium is closed.

## SURGERY FOR THE THORACIC AORTA

Thoracic aortic aneurysmectomy is excision of an aneurysmal portion of the ascending, arch, or descending thoracic aorta and replacement with a prosthetic graft, valve-graft conduit, or intraaortic prosthesis. Collagen-impregnated grafts have significantly reduced interstitial bleeding and obviated the need for preclotting techniques.

Aneurysms may be caused by atherosclerosis, trauma, infection, or cystic medial degeneration.[64] *Atherosclerosis* affects large and medium arteries with tunica intima deposits of plaques containing cholesterol, lipoid material, and lipophages. Atherosclerosis generally affects the smaller arteries rather than the aorta. *Arteriosclerosis* is a condition characterized by loss of elasticity and by thickening and hardening of the arteries. Both conditions may lead to aneurysm formation within an artery.

Aortic *dissection* is a unique entity and is related to degenerative changes in the tunica media layer of the artery. These changes predispose the artery to tearing of the tunica intima layer with subsequent dissection of the vessel wall by blood entering it through the tear.[103] As blood passes between the layers of the wall, it forms a false channel; as the channel extends and enlarges, the blood flow can be obstructed through the aorta and its branches, or the aorta can rupture causing severe hemorrhage (Figure 27-68, *A*).

Surgical intervention becomes necessary when presenting symptoms indicate a compromised circulation or danger of rupture; generally, medical management with hypotensive agents to reduce stress on the vessel is the preferred initial treatment until surgical repair can be performed.[64]

*Aneurysms* can be characterized morphologically as follows: (1) saccular—a sac type of formation with a narrowed neck projecting from the side of the artery and (2) fusiform—a spindle-shaped formation with complete circumferential involvement of the artery. Dissections can be characterized in at least two systems according to type, origin, and extent of the lesion (Table 27-12).

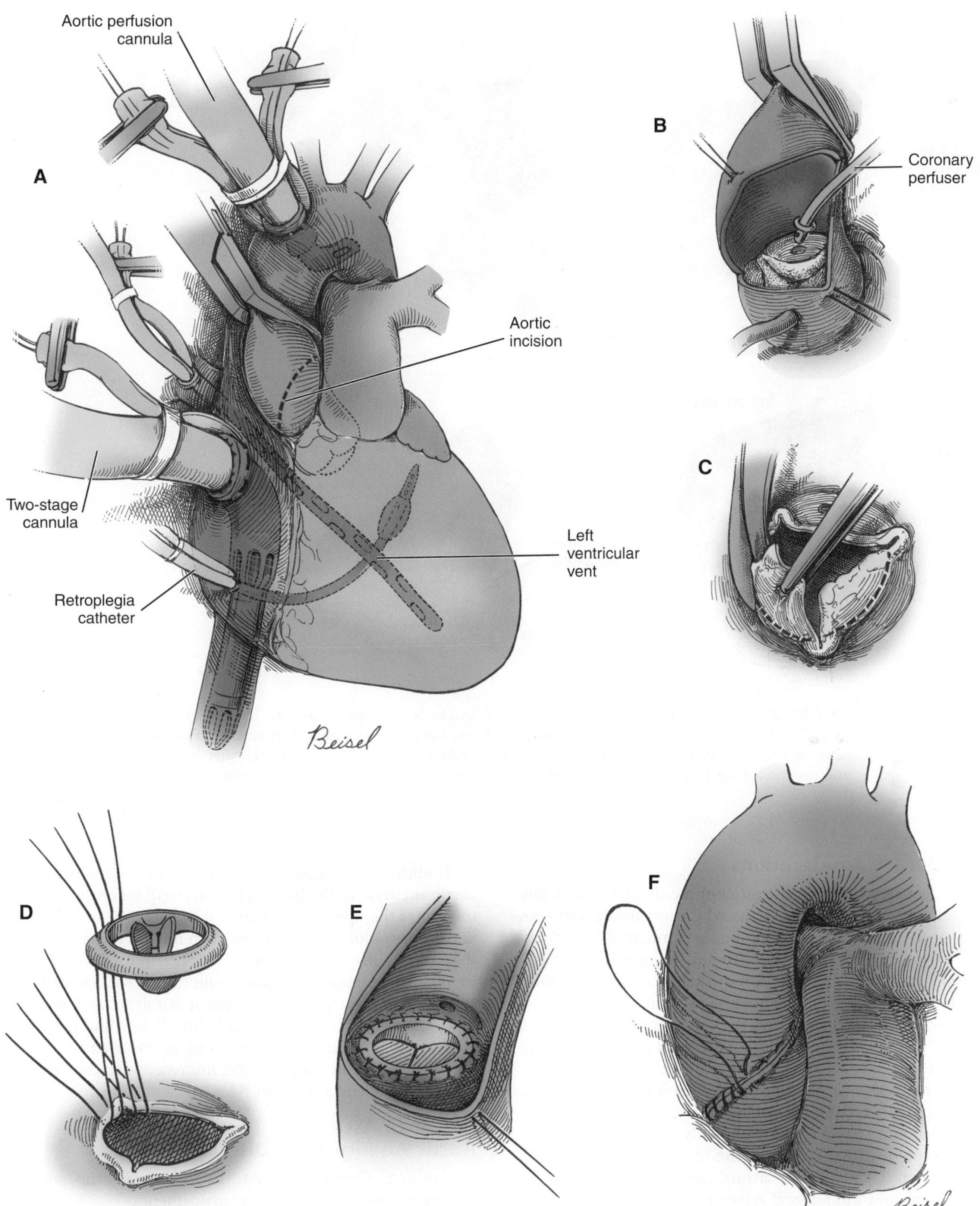


**FIGURE 27-66** **A,** Cannulation, retrograde cardioplegia, and vent sites for aortic valve procedures. Note incision line. **B,** If retrograde cardioplegia is not used, handheld coronary ostial catheters can deliver antegrade cardioplegic solution. **C,** Diseased valve is completely excised. **D,** Sutures are placed in the valve annulus and the prosthetic sewing ring. **E,** Stitches are tied and cut. **F,** Closure of the aortic suture line.

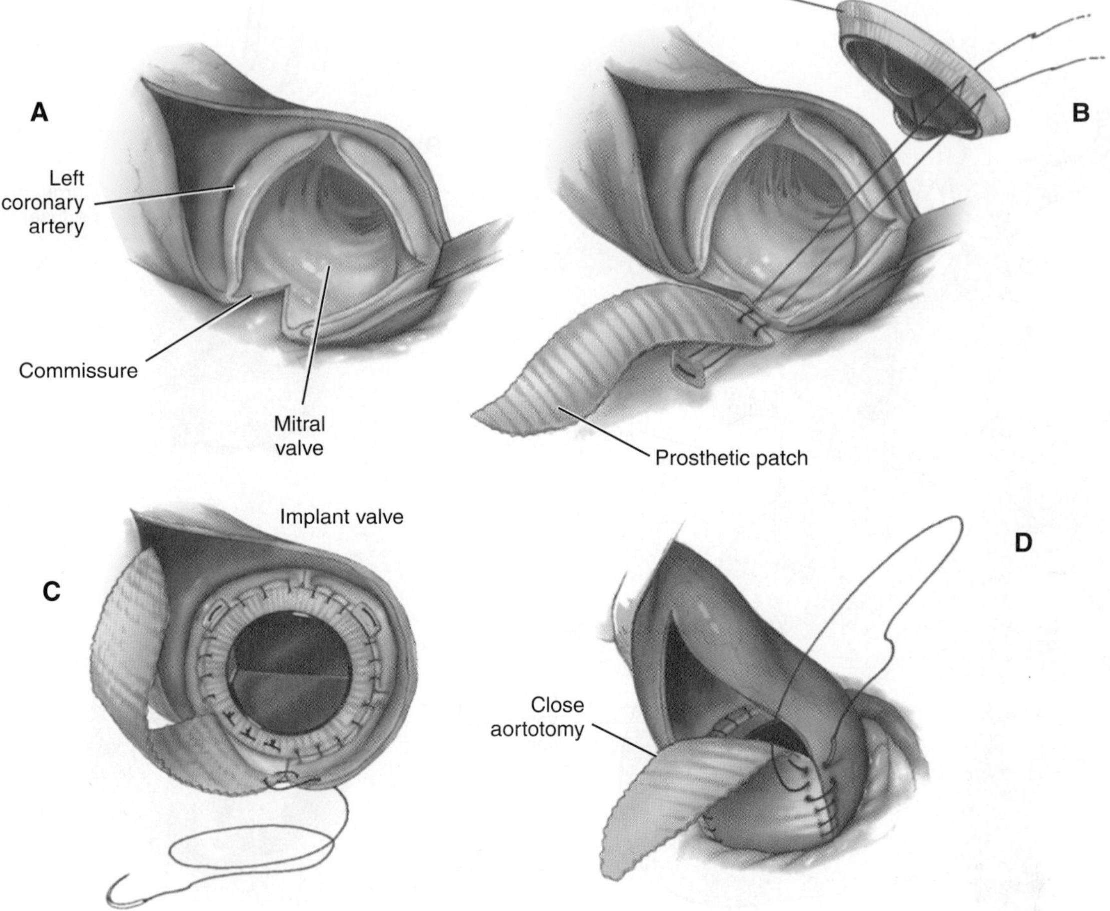


FIGURE 27-67 Technique for aortic enlargement (Nicks-Nuñez operation). **A,** The aortotomy is extended through the commissure separating the left and noncoronary cusps. **B,** A prosthetic patch is sewn into the cut portion of the aorta and into the prosthetic valve. **C,** The prosthetic valve is seated, and the stitches are tied and cut. **D,** The patch is incorporated into the aortotomy closure.

## Procedural Considerations

Several methods of surgical treatment are described in Crawford's classic study.[33] In situations where ascending aortic aneurysm or aortic dissection produces annular dilation with subsequent aortic valve insufficiency, a modified Bentall-DeBono procedure with a composite graft-valve conduit and reimplantation of the coronary ostia may be performed to replace the aortic valve and the aneurysmal aorta (Figure 27-69).[74] Retrograde cardioplegia is usually employed; if necessary, selective coronary infusion may be used. This procedure necessitates reimplanting the right and left coronary ostia into the prosthetic graft; in patients with CAD, vein grafts may be inserted and anastomosed proximally to the prosthesis.

The type of CPB depends on the location of the aneurysm or dissection. Generally, the atrium can be cannulated for venous return and the femoral artery is used for arterial inflow (because the weakened ascending aorta cannot be safely cannulated). Deep hypothermia with circulatory arrest and cerebroplegia may be needed to protect the heart and brain in particularly complex lesions of the aortic arch. In aneurysms involving the aortic arch, placement of a cross-clamp is difficult.

Traditionally, during the open repair of descending thoracic aortic aneurysms, the heart is not arrested; it continues beating to perfuse the upper body. Femoral bypass may be instituted to perfuse the kidneys and lower extremities; however, normothermia usually is maintained. Hypothermic CPB can be used to repair complex descending and thoracoabdominal aneurysms to provide protection against paralysis and renal, cardiac, and visceral organ system failure.[74] In some patients, an endovascular stented prosthesis can be inserted through the femoral artery and guided under fluoroscopy to the area of the descending aortic aneurysm.[39,87]

## Repair of Ascending Thoracic Aortic Aneurysm or Dissection

***Procedural Considerations.*** To the basic setup are added aneurysm instruments. Valve instruments, coronary instruments, and an array of tube grafts, valves, or valved conduits should be available. Bicaval cannulation for venous drainage is preferred, but if the cavae cannot be safely accessed, the femoral vein is used initially for venous drainage. Once the aneurysm is controlled, the femoral venous line can be Y-ed to a vena caval cannula.

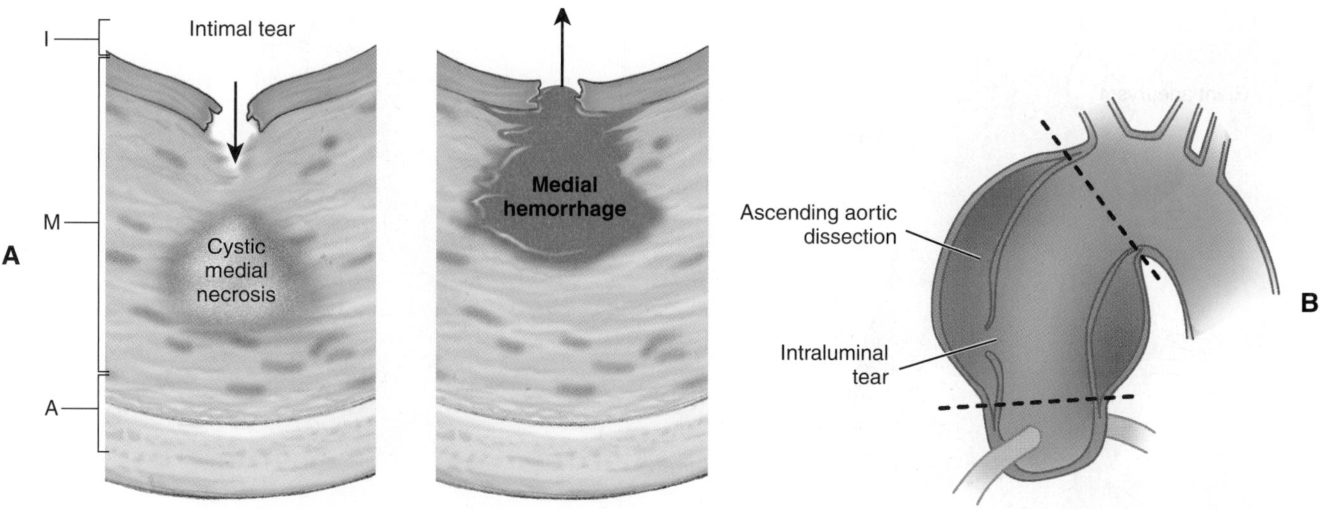


FIGURE 27-68 Aortic dissection. **A,** Proposed mechanism of the initiation of an aortic dissection (A= adventitia; M=media; I=intima). **B,** Intimal tear in the ascending aorta causing a dissection.

**TABLE 27-12**

**Commonly Used Classification Systems to Describe Aortic Dissection**

| Type | Site of Origin and Extent of Aortic Involvement |
|---|---|
| **DeBAKEY** | |
| Type I | Originates in the ascending aorta, propagates at least to the aortic arch and often beyond it distally |
| Type II | Originates in and is confined to the ascending aorta |
| Type III | Originates in the descending aorta and extends distally down the aorta or, rarely, retrograde into the aortic arch and ascending aorta |
| **STANFORD** | |
| Type A | All dissections involving the ascending aorta, regardless of the site of origin |
| Type B | All dissections not involving the ascending aorta |
| **DESCRIPTIVE** | |
| Proximal | Includes DeBakey types I and II or Stanford type A |
| Distal | Includes DeBakey type III or Stanford type B |

From Zipes DP and others: *Braunwald's heart disease*, ed 7, Philadelphia, 2005, Saunders.

### *Operative Procedure*

1. The patient is positioned for a median sternotomy.
2. Cannulation for CPB is performed.
3. The sternum is opened, and the aneurysm is inspected.
4. a. If the aortic annulus is not involved, the aneurysm is incised longitudinally and a woven graft is anastomosed proximally and distally to the healthy aorta (Figure 27-70). Felt strips incorporated into the anastomosis may be used to bolster friable tissue.

   b. If the aortic annulus is involved, the ascending aorta is incised to the annulus and the aneurysm may be excised. The leaflets are excised, and the annulus is measured. The proximal end of a valved conduit is inserted. An eye cautery is used to create openings in the graft at the location of the right and left coronary ostia, which are mobilized and anastomosed to the graft. (If the patient has concomitant CAD, saphenous vein grafts are inserted.) The distal end of the conduit is sutured to healthy aorta.
5. Bypass is discontinued, and all incisions are closed.

## Repair of Aortic Arch Aneurysm

***Procedural Considerations.*** Aneurysm instruments and woven grafts are available. If deep hypothermia is to be used, the patient's head may be covered with bags of ice at the beginning of the procedure. Precautionary measures (e.g., padding) to prevent frostbite are instituted. The location of the aneurysm will determine the positioning. Aneurysms of the proximal arch can be accessed through a median sternotomy; distal arch aneurysms may require a modified thoracotomy position to optimize exposure. Selective cerebral perfusion may be used during circulatory arrest to perfuse the brain; a piece of tubing is Y-ed off the arterial line and inserted into the cerebral vessel graft while the distal aortic anastomosis is performed.[133]

### *Operative Procedure*

1. Cannulation of the right atrium and femoral artery is performed.

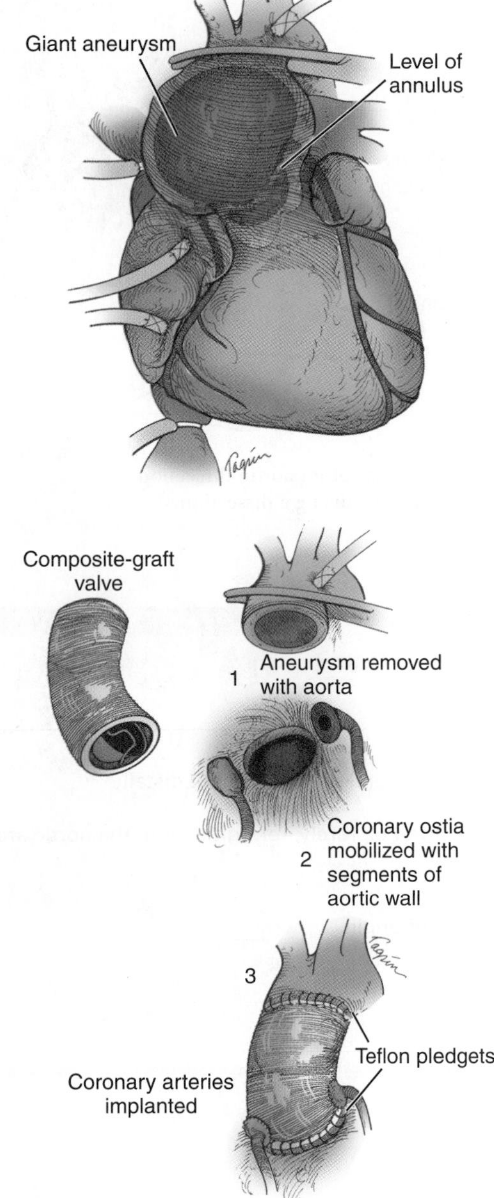


**FIGURE 27-69** Bentall-DeBono procedure (see text).

2. Once the patient is cooled to the desired temperature, the arch vessels are individually cross-clamped (Figure 27-71, *A* and *B*). (If circulatory arrest is indicated, cross-clamps are not used.) The aneurysm is incised, a tube graft is selected, and the anastomosis to the descending aorta is performed.
3. An opening is made into the side of the graft, and the graft is anastomosed to the common origin of the brachiocephalic, left carotid, and left subclavian vessels. The graft is cross-clamped proximally to the arch and deaired (Figure 27-71, *C*).
4. The proximal aorta is anastomosed to the graft while the patient is rewarming. The graft is deaired, and the patient is weaned from bypass (Figure 27-71, *D*).
5. All incisions are closed.

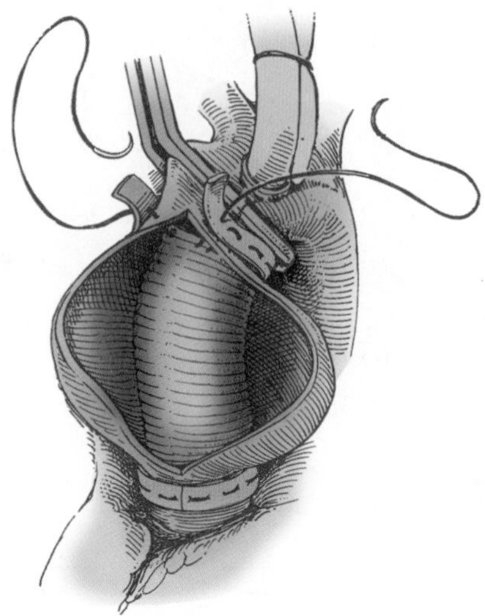

**FIGURE 27-70** Resection and graft repair of ascending aortic aneurysm.

## Repair of Descending Thoracic Aortic Aneurysm

***Procedural Considerations.*** Thoracotomy instruments and supplies are added to the basic setup; additional long aortic cross-clamps may be needed. Prosthetic grafts are available. The patient is positioned for a left posterolateral thoracotomy. Femoral vein–femoral artery bypass may be performed to perfuse the lower body. In this situation, the heart perfuses the upper body proximal to the aneurysm and normothermia is maintained. If an endovascular stent is used, additional supplies include guidewires, introducer sheath, dilators, pigtail catheters, and other related catheter delivery items.[39,87]

If hypothermic CBP with circulatory arrest is employed, instruments and supplies per the surgeon's request should be available. Protective covering for the patient's head, face, and extremities may be required to avoid frostbite.

### *Operative Procedure*

1. Cannulation for femoral vein–femoral artery bypass is performed.
2. A thoracotomy incision is made, the aneurysm is exposed, and the surrounding structures are inspected. (Occasionally the surgeon makes two thoracotomy incisions for better access to and control of the aorta.) Renal involvement is assessed; if indicated, measures to protect the kidneys are instituted (e.g., local cooling).
3. Normothermic femoral bypass is initiated.
4. The aneurysm is incised longitudinally, and the aorta is sized.
5. A woven graft (Figure 27-72) is inserted, and the aneurysmal remnants are wrapped around the graft.

## MECHANICAL AND BIOLOGIC CIRCULATORY ASSISTANCE

A small percentage of patients cannot be weaned from CPB after open-heart operations, even with the use of inotropic and vasodilator drugs. Other patients have end-stage cardiomyopathy. Various mechanical devices are available to support the circulation while the heart recovers or while the patient awaits

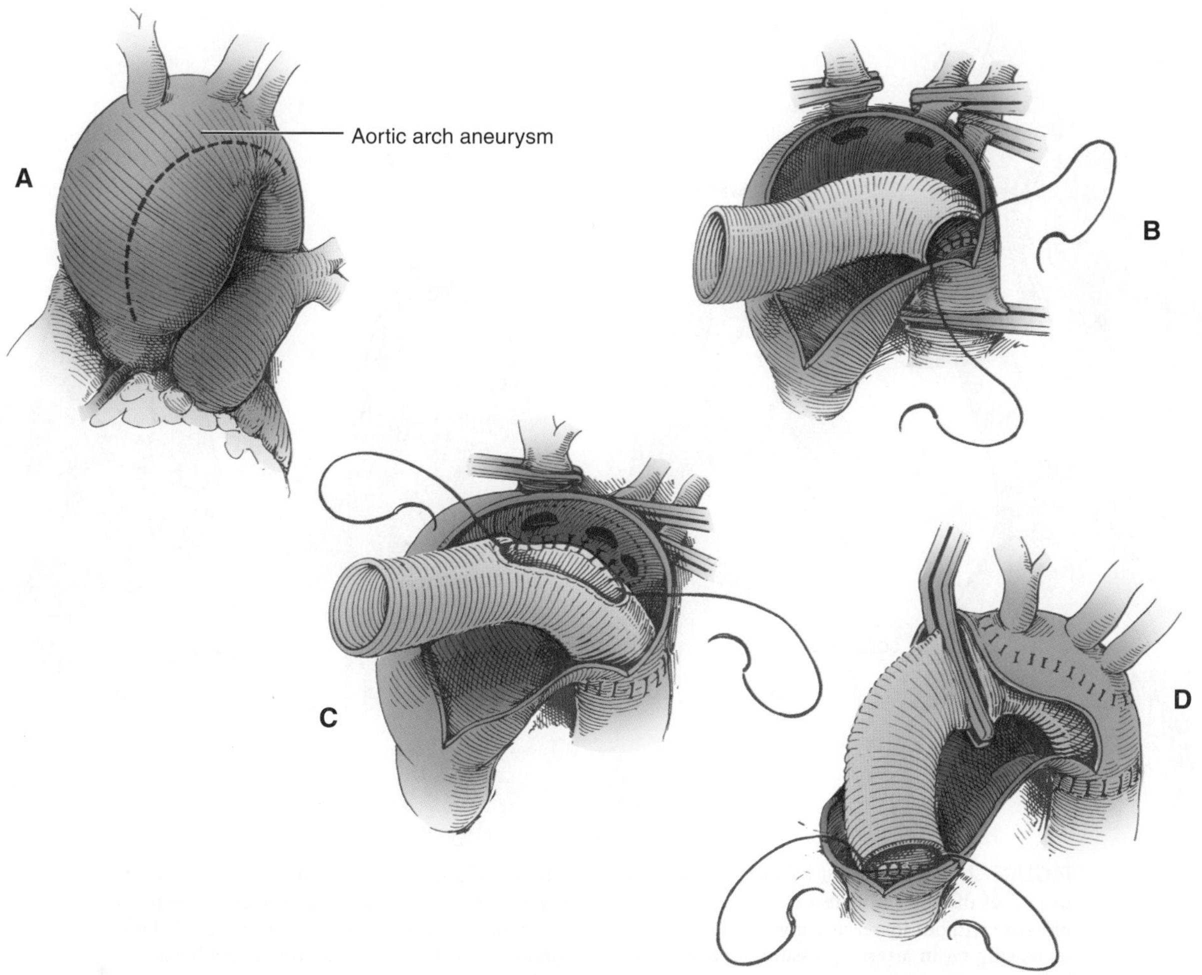

**FIGURE 27-71** Repair of aortic arch aneurysm. **A,** Incision. **B,** Distal anastomosis. **C,** Anastomosis of graft to common origin of arch vessels. **D,** Proximal anastomosis.

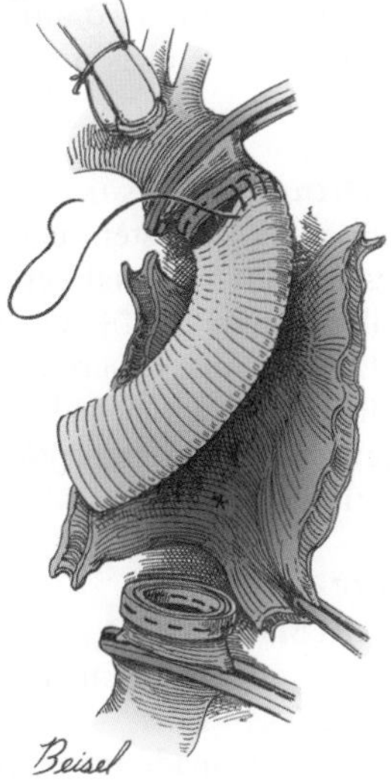


**FIGURE 27-72** Resection and graft replacement for descending thoracic aortic aneurysm.

cardiac transplantation.[48,101] Biologic assistance in the form of an autogenous muscle wrap is valuable in some patients who may not be candidates for transplantation.[74]

## Intraaortic Balloon Pump

The most widely used short-term device is the intraaortic balloon pump (IABP). The IABP (Figure 27-73) employs the principle of counterpulsation to increase coronary blood flow and decrease afterload (i.e., the resistance the ventricle must overcome to open the aortic valve).

### *Operative Procedure*

1. A flexible guidewire is passed through a percutaneous needle into the femoral artery. The needle is removed, and graduated dilators are inserted over the guidewire to dilate the overlying tissue and the artery wall.
2. The IABP catheter (with the furled balloon) is inserted into the artery and advanced to a position just distal to the left subclavian artery. The catheter can be marked at the proximal end with a silk tie to measure how far the catheter should be inserted.
3. The balloon is unfurled and activated.

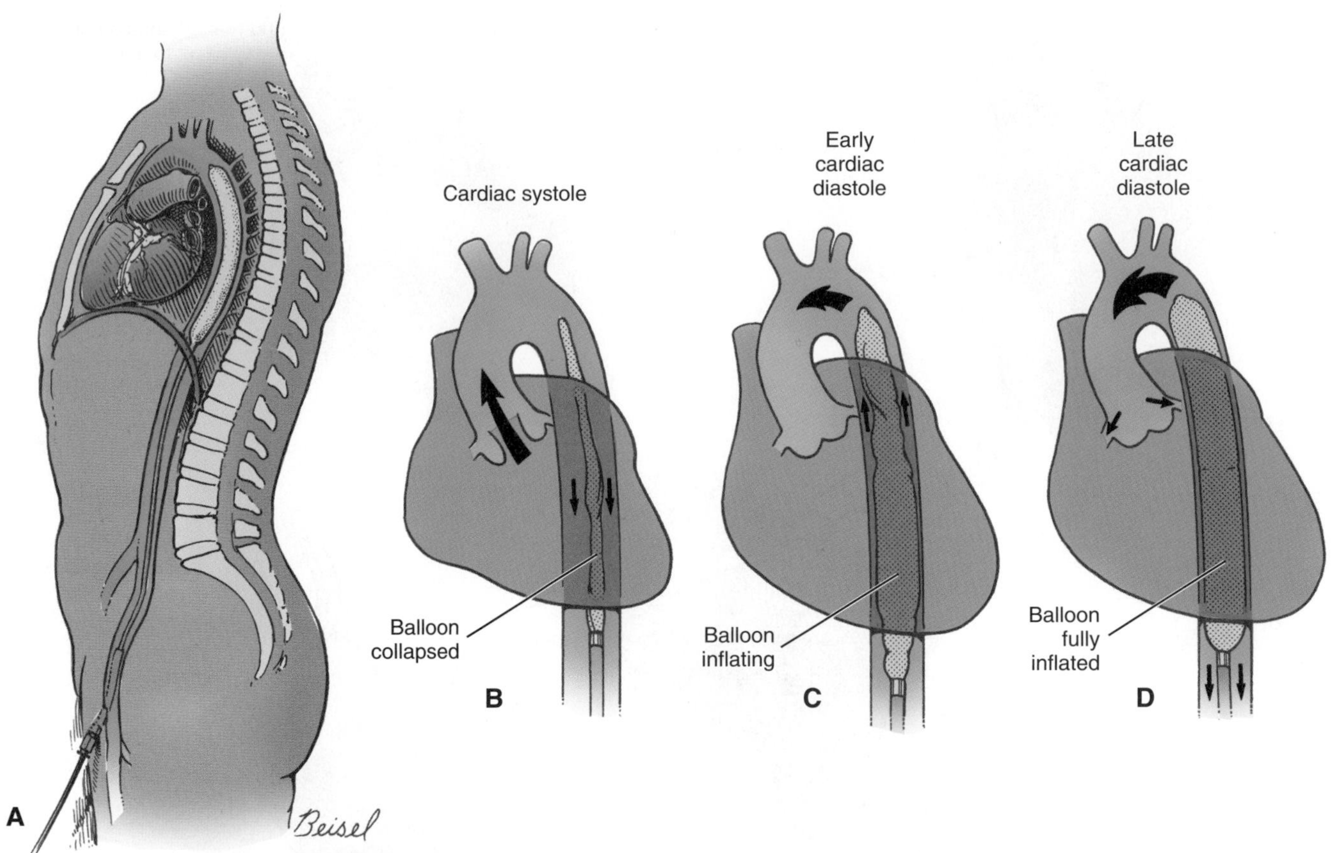


FIGURE 27-73 Phases of balloon pumping. **A,** Balloon inflation occurs from closure of aortic valve to end of diastole. Inflation causes retrograde flow of blood in aorta, increasing coronary perfusion pressure without increasing myocardial work or oxygen demand. Inflation also causes antegrade flow, increasing mean arterial pressure, renal flow, and cerebral flow. **B,** Balloon deflation occurs from just before opening of aortic valve to closure of aortic valve. Deflation encourages antegrade flow, decreasing afterload or resistance to left ventricular ejection. Deflation also decreases oxygen required by left ventricle, shortens systolic ejection, and increases stroke volume. **C** and **D,** When the balloon reinflates, the cycle is repeated.

## Ventricular Assist Device

Ventricular assist devices (VADs) are designed to augment cardiac output from the left (LVAD), right (RVAD), or both (biventricular—BiVAD) ventricles and to decrease the workload of the heart by diverting blood from the ventricle or ventricles to an artificial pump that maintains systemic perfusion. Patients with an LVAD can become better transplant candidates because the LVAD enhances anabolism, ambulation, and improved organ function. LVADs are employed as a bridge to cardiac transplantation by supporting the circulation while a suitable donor heart can be found. Based on the results of the Randomized Evaluation of Mechanical Assistance for the Treatment of Congestive Heart Failure (REMATCH) trial,[119,120] the use of the HeartMate (vented electric) LVAD (see below) was approved by the U.S. Food and Drug Administration in November 2002 for *destination therapy*/permanent replacement for the left ventricle.[107] Although complications (e.g., thromboembolism, infection) persist, they have been reduced.

An axial flow pump is a potentially valuable device that may be suitable for permanent use. The device is based on Archimedes' third-century screw pump that was used to raise well water for irrigation. The pump is inserted into the left ventricle to propel blood flow; the distal end is anastomosed to the descending aorta.[36]

***Procedural Considerations.*** If patients cannot be weaned from CPB with IAPB, an assist system may be indicated. Cardiac support devices include external centrifugal pumps and internal pneumatically (Figure 27-74) or electrically powered assist devices. The LVAD device described below is approved for support of the left ventricle when right ventricular function is normal.[107] Prosthetic valves are incorporated into the circuit to maintain unidirectional blood flow.

### *Operative Procedure*

THORATEC HEARTMATE LVAD

1. A median sternotomy incision is made and extended to the umbilicus (Figure 27-74, *A*).
2. A preperitoneal pouch is made for placement of the assist device.
3. CPB is established, and the aorta is cross-clamped. The atrial septum is inspected for defects, which if found are closed.

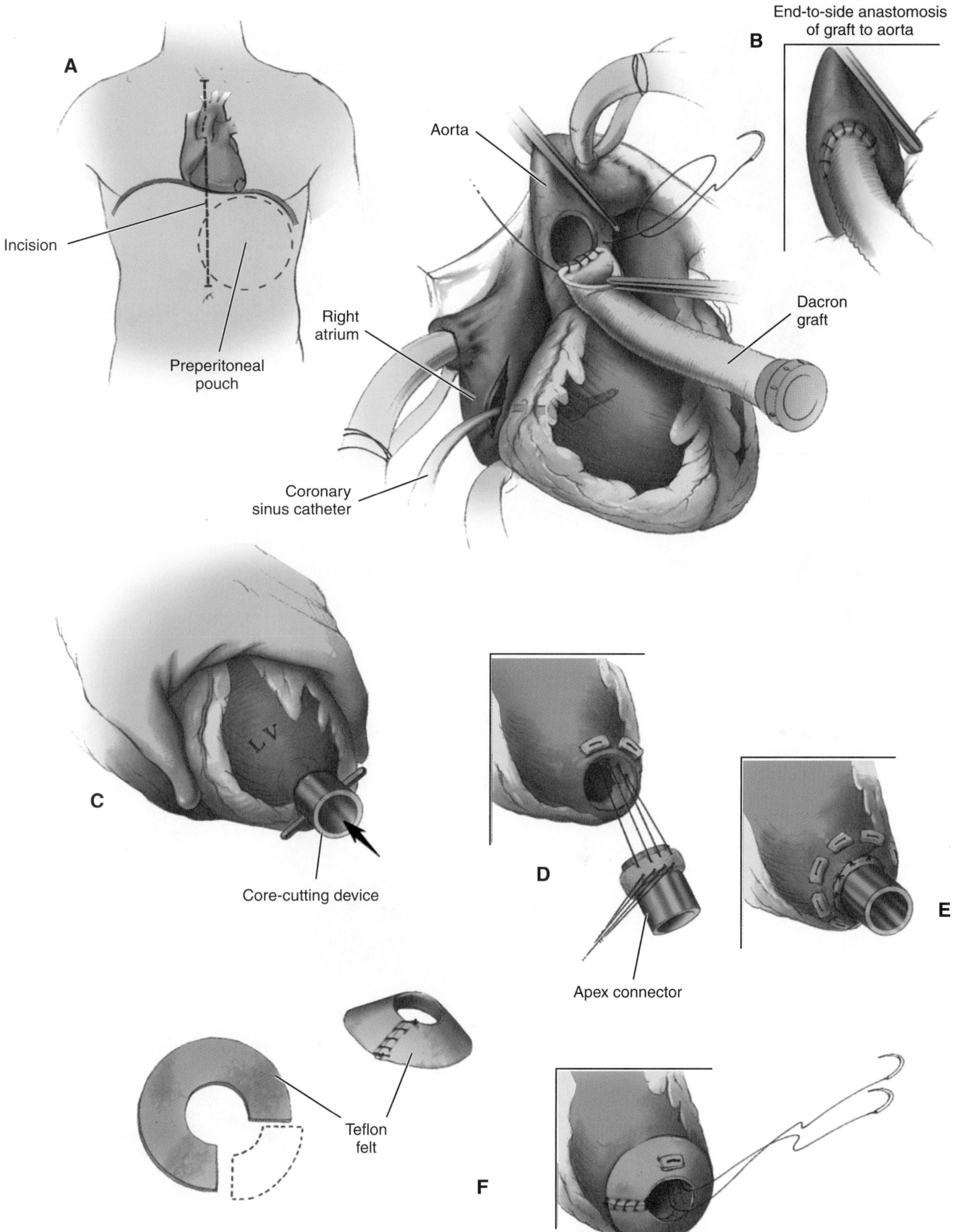


FIGURE 27-74 Left ventricular assist device (see text).

*Continued*

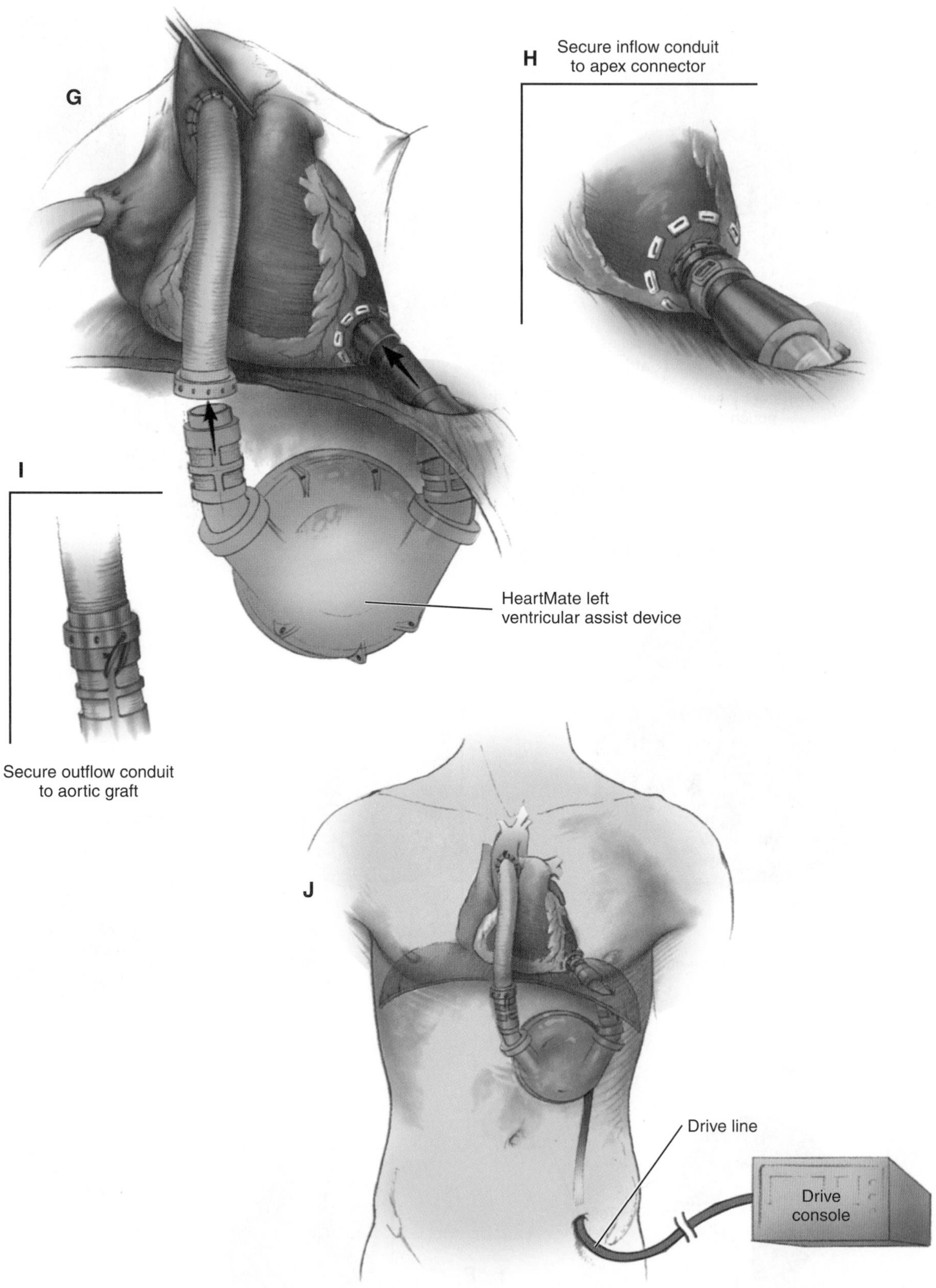


**FIGURE 27-74, cont'd** Left ventricular assist device (see text).

4. A Dacron graft is anastomosed to the aorta (Figure 27-74, *B*).
5. The left ventricular apex is mobilized, and an opening is created in the apex (Figure 27-74, *C*).
6. A connector is inserted into the apex, and the flange is sewn to the surrounding left ventricular myocardium with pledgeted sutures. The inflow conduit is attached to the apical connector (Figure 27-74, *D* to *G*).
7. An opening is made into the diaphragm near the location of the apical connector and inflow conduit. The conduit is passed through the diaphragm and attached to the assist device.
8. The aortic graft is attached to the outflow conduit, which is connected to the assist device (Figure 27-74, *H* and *I*).
9. The driveline is tunneled to the left lower quadrant, where it exits through the skin. The driveline can be connected to the drive console or to a battery pack. Blood flows from the left ventricular apex, to the device, and back into the body through the aortic conduit (Figure 27-74, *J*).
10. CPB is discontinued, and incisions are closed.

To remove the pump, the patient is returned to the OR, the sternotomy is reopened, and the cannulas are removed.

### Total Artificial Heart

The total artificial heart (TAH) continues to be refined and implanted in patients with end-stage biventricular failure. Complications associated with thromboembolism and infection have been reduced with technical and material refinements of VAD systems, but they remain. Long-term right or left VADs have been increasingly employed as a bridge to cardiac transplantation by supporting the circulation until a suitable donor heart can be found.[30,36]

### Biologic Ventricular Support

The use of latissimus dorsi muscle for cardiomyoplasty (Figure 27-75) is performed infrequently but may be used in patients considered unsuitable candidates for either heart transplantation or VAD support. The surgical procedure consists of using electrostimulated skeletal muscle to reinforce or partially replace the heart muscle.[74]

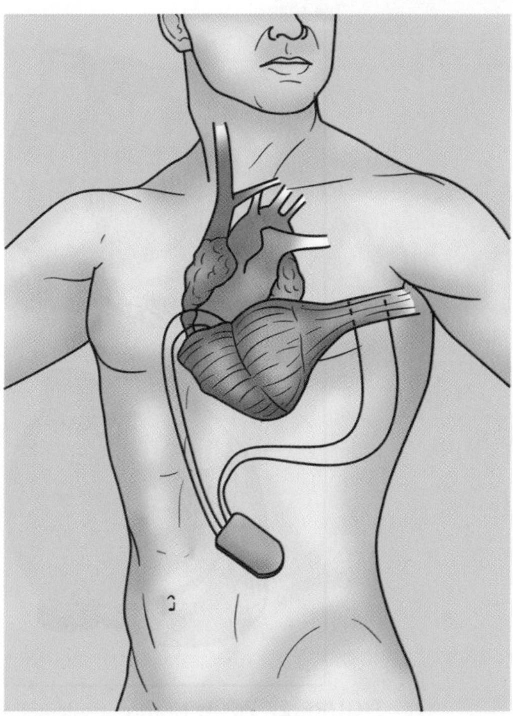

FIGURE 27-75 Cardiomyoplasty. The left latissimus dorsi muscle is dissected from the back and swung around to the heart, where it is sewn around the ventricle. This (skeletal) muscle is then transformed into a continuously beating muscle by a cardiomyostimulator that paces the muscle with increasing frequency, allowing the muscle to become fatigue-resistant. The muscle wrap squeezes the heart in synchronization with natural electrical impulses moving through the heart muscle.

## HEART AND HEART-LUNG TRANSPLANTATION

### Heart Transplantation (Figure 27-76)

Orthotopic transplantation (replacing one heart with another) is most commonly performed; less commonly, heterotopic (piggyback) and combined heart-lung procedures are performed. Important considerations continue to be recipient and donor selection, the immune response, and control of infection. Older recipients and donors (older than 60 years) have demonstrated acceptable morbidity and survival.[10,61]

Modification of the traditional transplantation technique (e.g., atrial-atrial anastomoses)[29] has reduced some of the dysrhythmias and valvular dysfunction associated with the traditional method of transplantation. End-to-end anastomoses between the donor and recipient SVC and the donor and recipient IVC are created, producing a more physiologic atrial contribution to ventricular filling and less distortion of the mitral and tricuspid annuli.[16] Tricuspid annuloplasty with the DeVega technique (see Figure 27-65) may be performed on the donor heart to minimize tricuspid insufficiency.[65] Revised pulmonary venous connections produce fewer dysrhythmias. These changes also lead to less AV valve regurgitation. Pulmonary artery and aortic anastomoses are performed in the traditional manner.[29]

***Procedural Considerations.*** Individual instrument setups are necessary for the donor and the recipient.

#### *Operative Procedures*

**DONOR HEART.** The donor heart is exposed through a median sternotomy. The aorta, pulmonary artery, and venae cavae are dissected. The venae cavae are occluded, the left atrium is opened to decompress the ventricle, and the heart is rapidly cooled and arrested.

The heart is excised by incision of the SVC and the IVC, the left atrium, the aorta, and the pulmonary artery. The donor heart is immediately placed into cold saline and transported to the site where it will be inserted into the recipient.[61]

**RECIPIENT HEART.** The recipient is placed on bypass with cannulation of the IVC and the SVC; caval tapes are placed around the cavae. The patient is cooled to approximately 32°C to 34°C (89.6°F to 93.2°F), and the caval tapes are tightened. The pulmonary trunk and aorta are dissected immediately above their respective semilunar valves; the left

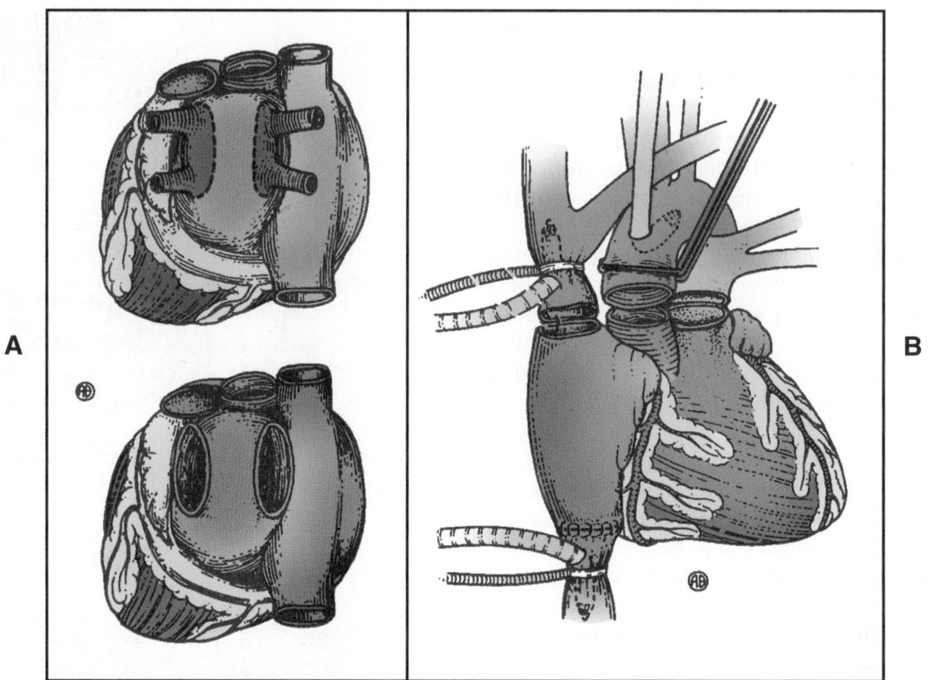


FIGURE 27-76 **A,** Heart transplantation with pulmonary venous anastomoses on right or left side, and caval anastomoses at the superior and inferior vena cavae. **B,** Aorta and pulmonary artery are joined last.

atrium is incised to leave intact portions of the left atrial wall and the atrial septum of the recipient; and the right atrium is incised, retaining the SVC and IVC for anastomosis to the donor heart. The recipient heart is then removed.

The donor heart is placed in the pericardial well. The pulmonary anastomoses are performed (see Figure 27-76, *A*). The SVC and IVC are anastomosed with running cardiovascular sutures (see Figure 27-76, *B*). The donor and recipient aortas and pulmonary arteries are similarly joined. Air is removed from the left side of the heart. Before the pulmonary artery is sutured, all caval and atrial suture lines are carefully inspected for significant bleeding areas, and the cross-clamp is removed. Figure 27-77 illustrates the traditional (but less frequently anastomosed) right atrial suture line; aortic and pulmonary anastomoses are similar to the technique just described.

Defibrillation of the ventricles is usually effected with a single DC shock. A needle vent in the ascending aorta allows residual air to escape. The patient is then gradually weaned from the bypass. Cannulas are removed from the venae cavae and the aorta. The incisions are closed as described previously.

## Heart-Lung Transplantation

Newer techniques for lung and heart-lung transplantation incorporate the bicaval anastomoses used for orthotopic heart transplantation and also employ a bibronchial anastomosis that reduces bleeding and enhances the integrity of the airway.[29] To maximize the allocation of scarce donor organs, transplantation procedures for the lungs may use a single lung or bilateral lungs; heart-lung transplantation is infrequent. Preservation of the *donor's* sinus node and the *recipient's* recurrent laryngeal, vagus, and phrenic nerves is an important surgical consideration.

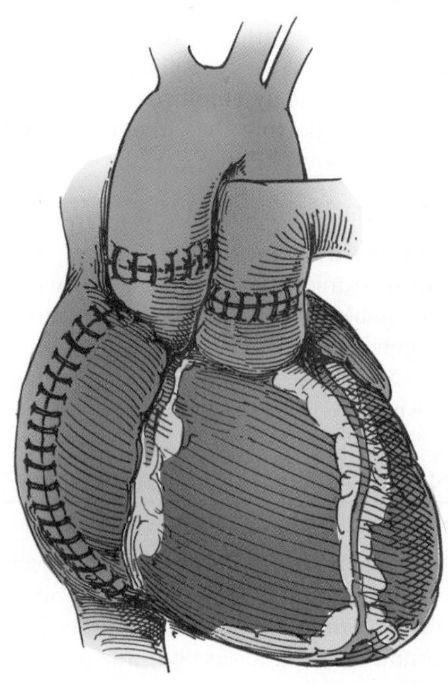

FIGURE 27-77 Traditional atrial anastomosis for heart transplantation.

***Operative Procedure.*** The recipient's diseased heart and lung or lungs are excised separately or en bloc, with care taken not to injure the major nerves listed previously. The recipient's right atrium, SVC, and IVC are saved to create bicaval attachments to the donor heart. The bronchi are transected. The donor heart and lungs are brought onto the field. The right lung is placed in the right pleural space, and the left lung is positioned in the left pleural space. The bronchial and the bicaval anastomoses are performed, and rewarming is begun. The aortic anastomosis is performed, the aorta is deaired, and the cross-clamp is removed.

## SURGERY FOR CONDUCTION DISTURBANCES

Disturbances of the conduction system affect the rate, rhythm, and effectiveness of the contracting heart. Surgical techniques have been developed to treat a variety of supraventricular dysrhythmias (e.g., atrial fibrillation [AF] and Wolff-Parkinson-White reentry tachycardia) and both ischemic and nonischemic ventricular tachydysrhythmias (e.g., ventricular tachycardia or fibrillation).[95] Preprocedural electrophysiologic mapping of the patient's conduction pathways identifies and locates aberrant pathways, tachydysrhythmias, the existence of additional pathways, as well as the effects of medications on a particular dysrhythmia. Indications for pacemaker implantation (including resynchronization therapy[79]) and antitachycardia-antifibrillation devices have been expanded.[81,100] Although many (but not all) pacemaker and internal cardioverter defibrillator (ICD) insertions are currently performed in the cardiac catheterization suite, newer procedures for AF are increasingly performed in the OR.

AF is receiving great attention because it is the most common cardiac dysrhythmia, affecting approximately 2.3 million adults in the United States, and accounts for 15% of all strokes.[32] Although *intermittent* AF commonly occurs after CABG, it is potentially preventable by treatment with beta-blockers, ACE inhibitors, and/or nonsteroidal antiinflammatory drugs.[90] If AF cannot be prevented, treatment includes restoration of sinus rhythm (when possible), control of the ventricular rate, and anticoagulants.[69,70,139,147]

Many new techniques to treat *continuous* AF are based on research demonstrating that the pulmonary veins are an important source of the ectopic beats that can initiate paroxysms of AF.[53] Surgical interventions for AF have expanded beyond Cox's original Maze procedures and been modified from the use of extensive atrial incisions that were sutured to create a maze through which electrical impulses were directed from the SA node to the AV node. The early research of Cox[31] demonstrated that electrical impulses are unable to cross incised and sutured tissue and consequently cannot regenerate the reentry circuits producing the dysrhythmia. Cox revised the cut-and-sew technique of the initial Maze procedures with a cryosurgical technique that ensures the creation of transmural lesions in the vicinity of the pulmonary veins and in other areas of the heart, generating impulses producing AF. This "mini-Maze" can be performed with sternotomy or through a minimally invasive thoracic route and requires placing fewer lesions in the left atrium and the right atrium.[32] Currently, the focus is on the selective ablation (with cryotherapy[1] or ultrasonic or radiofrequency energy sources) of tissues surrounding, for example, the pulmonary veins to reestablish normal conduction pathways.[32,91]

### Insertion of Permanent Pacemaker

A permanent pacemaker (pulse generator and electrodes) initiates atrial or ventricular contraction or both. Complete heart block and bradydysrhythmias (i.e., slow heart rates) are the most common indications for pacemaker implantation.[77] The development of multiprogrammable and physiologic pacemakers has made possible the treatment of many forms of dysrhythmias and neuroconductive disturbances as well as tachydysrhythmias. A temporary pacemaker may also be used for acute forms of heart block and dysrhythmias that occasionally occur during and after cardiac surgery.[56]

Dual-site pacing of both the right and the left ventricle is another treatment for patients with dilated cardiomyopathy and congestive heart failure.[79] *Cardiac resynchronization therapy* (CRT) employs leads placed on the right atrium and the right ventricle. Left ventricular pacing is achieved with an electrode introduced transvenously into the coronary sinus and extended into the great cardiac vein (or a tributary) to a position in the left side of the heart; this electrode functions as the second ventricular lead. The three electrodes are connected to the pacemaker generator (Figure 27-78). Resynchronization improves the mechanical pumping action between the right and left ventricles and optimizes AV synchrony; as a result, hemodynamic function is improved in heart failure patients.[79]

Two methods of placing electrodes for permanent cardiac pacing are the *transvenous* and the *epicardial* approach. The transvenous route is most commonly used because it does not require a major thoracotomy or a general anesthetic and is therefore safer for high-risk patients. Permanent epicardial electrodes may be placed during cardiac operations when the chest is opened and the heart is exposed; however, if a permanent pacemaker is required, it is likely to be inserted transvenously during the postoperative period (pacing is achieved with the temporary electrodes placed during surgery). A sub-

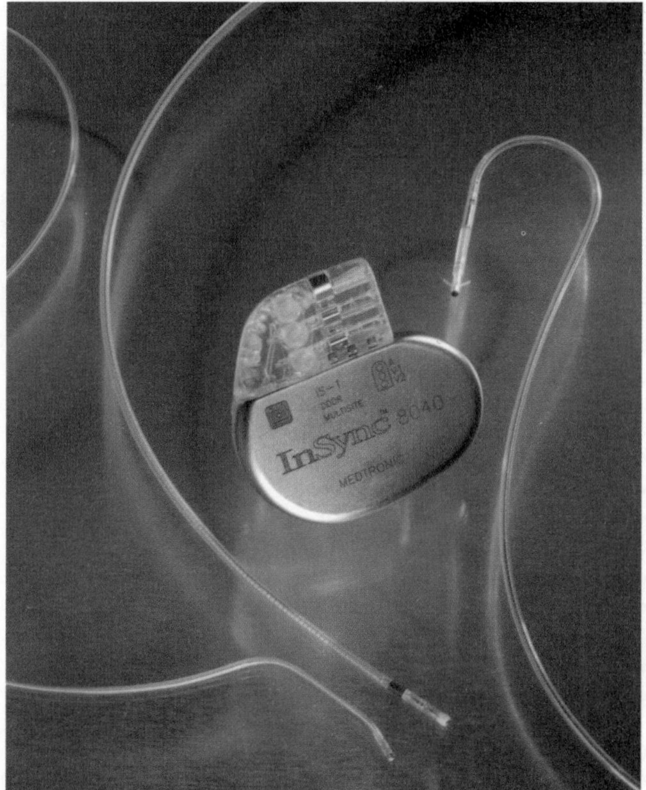


**FIGURE 27-78** Pacemaker and leads designed to resynchronize cardiac contraction. The three leads are implanted to carry impulses to the right atrium, the right ventricle, and the left ventricle (see text).

xiphoid approach may be used to place epicardial leads without having to open the sternum.[56]

Pulse generators are typically powered by lithium, which lasts 5 to 10 years. Life expectancy depends on the amount of power used and the frequency of demand. The generators are classified into three groups: fixed rate (or asynchronous), ventricular demand, and physiologic. The asynchronous was the first type implanted and fires at a fixed rate, independent of the electrical activity of the heart. A major disadvantage of this type of pacing is competition between the heart's intrinsic beat and the paced beat, possibly resulting in ventricular fibrillation if the paced beat occurs during the T-wave period of the ECG. Ventricular demand pacemakers were developed in response to this problem and fire at a fixed rate only if spontaneous ventricular activity fails. Adding a sensing mechanism to the existing stimulating mechanism makes this type of pacing possible. "Physiologic" pacemakers can stimulate both the atria and the ventricles, maintain AV synchrony, and enhance cardiac output by as much as 20%. Pacemakers are also capable of adjusting the rate of stimulation in response to increased metabolic activity (rate-responsive pacers).

The two types of electrodes are *myocardial (epicardial)*, which are attached to the heart muscle under direct vision; and *endocardial*, which are inserted transvenously. The stimulating and sensing electrodes are located at the tip of the lead, which attaches to the pulse generator.

Pacing systems are also available as *unipolar* or *bipolar*. A pacemaker with one stimulating electrode at the tip of the lead is unipolar. The electrical current flows between the electrode and the pulse generator. A bipolar pacemaker has two stimulating electrodes at the tip of the lead. Electrical current flows between the two electrodes.

## Insertion of Transvenous (Endocardial) Pacing Electrodes

***Procedural Considerations.*** The patient is placed in the supine position. Continuous ECG monitoring is essential. A defibrillator and emergency drugs should be available because lethal dysrhythmias can occur during catheter insertion. The patient should be made as comfortable as possible because this procedure can sometimes be lengthy and is frequently performed using local or local standby anesthesia (monitored anesthesia care).

Fluoroscopy is required; thus either a portable image intensifier is needed or the procedure is done in the special studies section of the radiology or cardiac catheterization department. A minor set of instruments is used, plus the following:

- Vascular dissecting instruments
- Tunneling instrument
- Sterile pacemaker and electrodes
- Introducer set
- External pacemaker (for testing) or a pacing system analyzer (PSA)
- Alligator test cables
- Screwdriver and other accessory items as needed

### *Operative Procedure (Figure 27-79)*

1. The skin and subcutaneous tissue are infiltrated with a local anesthetic, and the patient is placed in Trendelenburg position (to engorge the vein for easier access and to avoid air emboli).
2. A skin pocket is made close to the subclavian vein (Figure 27-79, *A*). The vessel may be encircled with a heavy suture.
3. A venotomy is performed with an introducer needle (Figure 27-79, *B*). A guidewire is threaded to the desired cardiac chamber, and the needle is removed. The pacing electrode is inserted through a peel-away dilator sheath, which is withdrawn after the lead insertion (Figure 27-79, *C*). The guidewire is withdrawn. A stylet is then inserted to help position the electrode.
4. The electrode is advanced under direct fluoroscopic vision into the right atrium, through the tricuspid valve, and into the right ventricle (Figure 27-79, *D*).
5. The surgeon attempts to entrap the tip of the electrode in the trabeculae carneae cordis of the right ventricular apex to stabilize it. Once the electrode is positioned and tested with alligator test cables and the pacing analyzer to confirm proper placement and function, the stylet is removed. If a dual-chamber pacemaker is inserted, the second lead is entrapped in the right atrial appendage (Figure 27-79, *D*).
6. The electrode or electrodes are brought down and attached to the pulse generator.
7. The pulse generator is placed into the pocket, and the incision may be irrigated with an antibiotic solution. If the pocket must be made farther away from the vein, a tunneling device may be used to thread the electrode to the pocket.
8. The incision is closed in layers with absorbable sutures.

## Insertion of Myocardial (Epicardial) Pacing Electrodes

A subxiphoid left anterior thoracotomy approach or sternotomy approach can be used; the setup is as described for placement of endocardial electrodes. The subxiphoid process and left upper quadrant area are infiltrated with the anesthetic agent. A small transverse incision is made below the xiphoid process and is carried down to the linea alba. A tunnel is created under the xiphoid process to the pericardium, which is incised to expose the heart. The pacing electrode, mounted on its carrier, is screwed into the ventricular myocardium, and the carrier is removed. The remainder of the procedure is as described for insertion of the endocardial electrode.

For the sternotomy approach, the mediastinum is opened for a concomitant cardiac procedure and an area of myocardium is chosen for placement of the pacing electrodes. The electrode tips are screwed into or are sutured to the myocardium and are attached by an appropriate cable to an external pulse generator or pacing analyzer for testing. The pocket and subcutaneous tunnel are created as described for insertion of the endocardial electrode.

## Insertion of Implantable Cardioverter Defibrillator

Surgery or pharmacologic intervention may not prevent malignant ventricular dysrhythmias (ventricular fibrillation and ventricular tachycardia) in persons who survive sudden cardiac death. The ICD is an electronic device designed to moni-

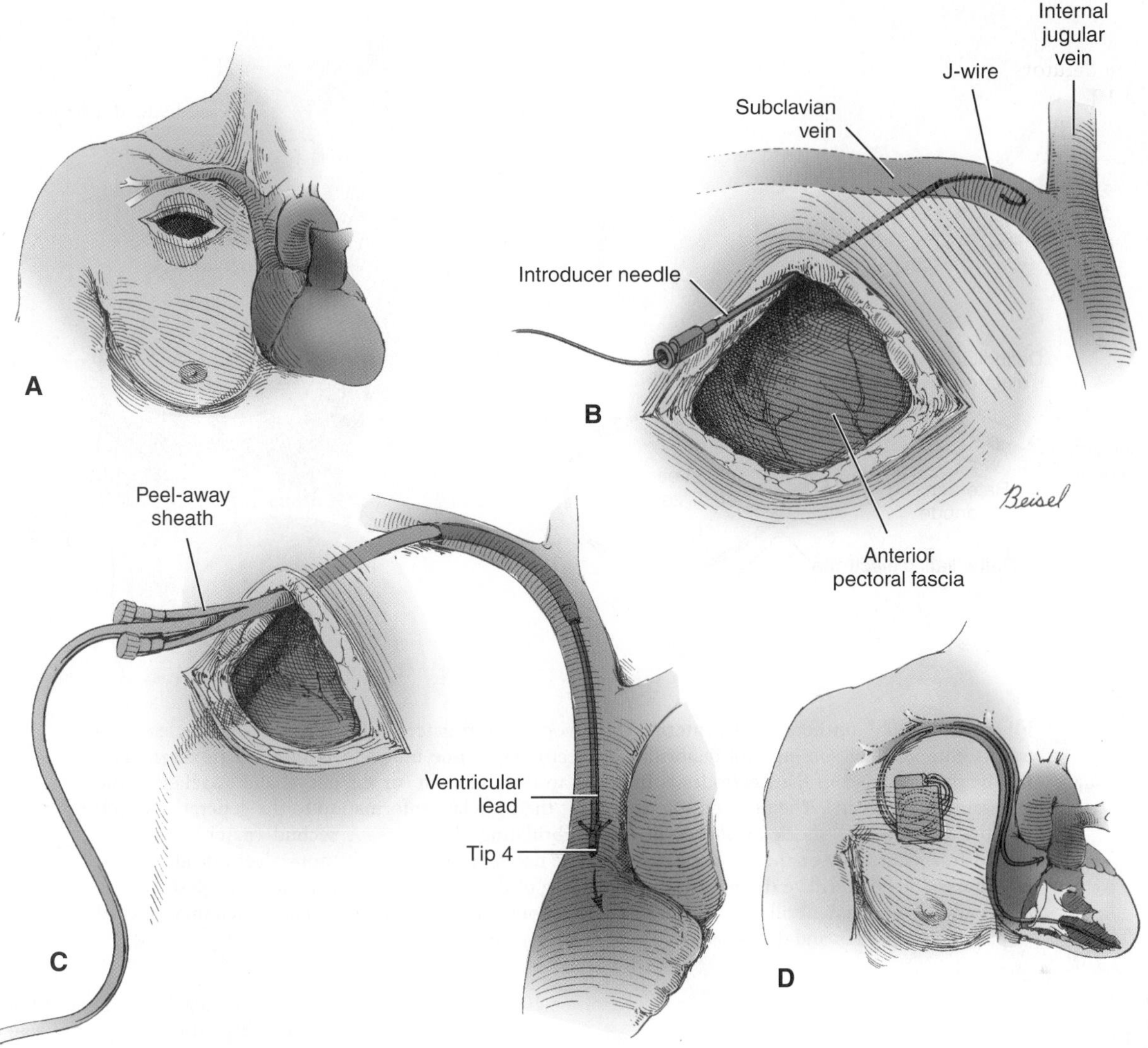


**FIGURE 27-79** Insertion of transvenous pacemaker (see text).

tor cardiac electrical activity and deliver prompt defibrillator shocks.[56] The ICD differs from a pacemaker in that the former senses ventricular tachycardia or fibrillation and the latter senses asystole. Current models are capable of tiered therapy, whereby increasingly stronger impulses are delivered depending on the underlying dysrhythmias; some devices can also be used to terminate AF. These devices are capable of pacing as well as defibrillating (pacing cardioverter defibrillators [PCDs]). The ICD device consists of a generator and sensing and defibrillator electrodes (Figure 27-80). Many ICD electrodes currently employed consist of transvenous electrodes inserted into the generator much like a transvenous pacemaker system. Myocardial or thoracic subcutaneous patches may be added if the transvenous catheters alone do not adequately defibrillate the heart. Patients with previously applied defibrillator patches may present for removal of a patch or patches; nurses should be prepared for emergency intervention if there is excessive bleeding or lethal dysrhythmia. EP studies are performed before and after insertion to diagnose the dysrhythmia and to evaluate device function, respectively.

The transvenous route with fluoroscopy is commonly employed, and insertion is similar to transvenous pacemaker insertion (Figure 27-80, *B*). The free ends of the lead system are tunneled to the generator, which is implanted in a subcutaneous pocket in the chest wall. The device is tested, and the incisions are closed.

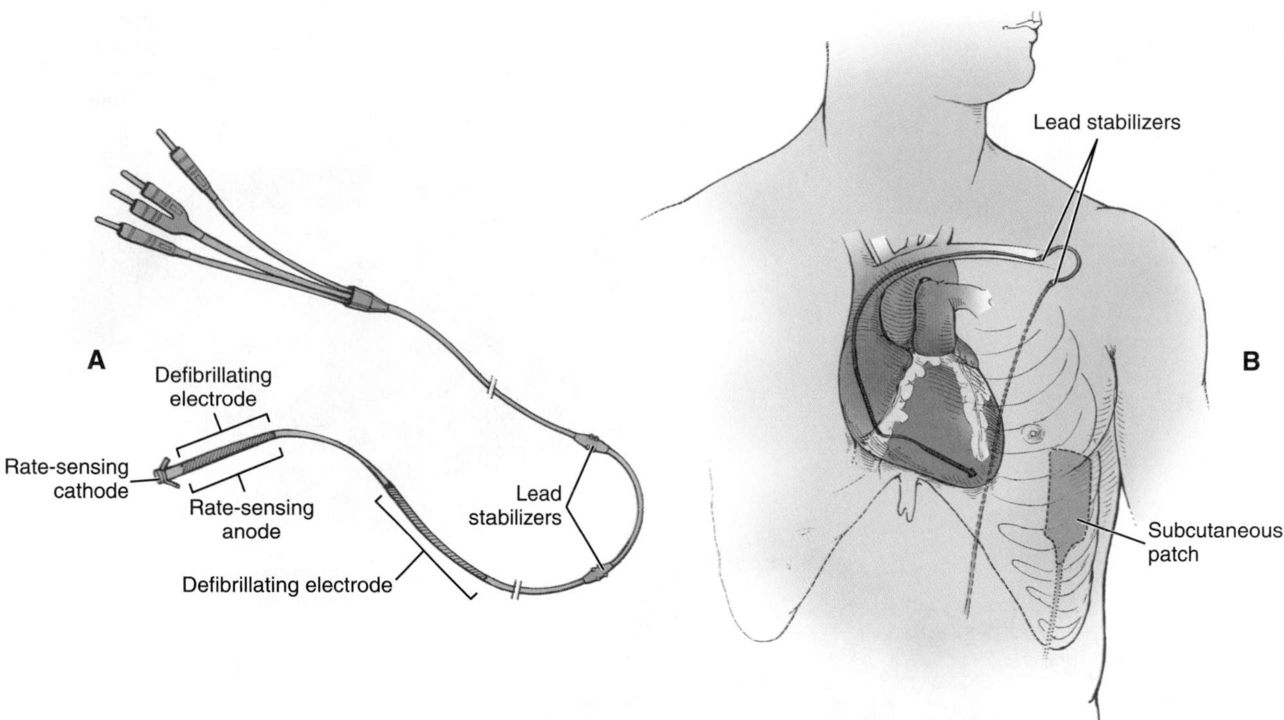


**FIGURE 27-80** Nonthoracotomy internal cardioverter defibrillator (ICD) insertion. **A,** The lead system is composed of sensing and defibrillating electrodes in one unit and is inserted transvenously. **B,** The proximal end of the electrodes is tunneled to the abdomen (or the chest) and attached to the generator (not shown). The rate-sensing cathode at the tip relays information to the generator, which initiates an electrical shock by means of the defibrillating electrodes. A second (patch) electrode, placed subcutaneously on the left chest wall, may be necessary if the transvenous electrode alone cannot successfully defibrillate the patient during testing of the unit. If the nonthoracotomy system does not result in suitable defibrillation thresholds, a left thoracotomy or subxiphoid approach may be used to place sensing leads and defibrillation patches directly on the heart.

## REFERENCES

1. Ad N: The cryosurgical MAZE procedure, *CTSNet*. Accessed March 18 2005, on-line: www.ctsnet.org.
2. Adams DH and others: Medical management of the patient undergoing cardiac surgery. In Zipes DP and others, editors: *Braunwald's heart disease*, ed 7, Philadelphia, 2005, Saunders.
3. Alfieri O and others: The double-orifice technique in mitral valve repair: a simple solution for complex problems, *Journal of Thoracic and Cardiovascular Surgery* 122(4):674-681, 2001.
4. Association of periOperative Registered Nurses: *The geriatric patient: AORN's age-specific competencies series,* Denver, 1997, The Association.
5. Association of periOperative Registered Nurses: *The neonate, infant, and toddler patient: AORN's age-specific competencies series,* Denver, 1997, The Association.
6. Association of periOperative Registered Nurses: *The premature infant patient: AORN's age-specific competencies series, Denver,* 1997, The Association.
7. Association of periOperative Registered Nurses: *The preschool, school-age, and adolescent patient: AORN's age-specific competencies series,* Denver, 1997, The Association.
8. Baker L and others: Use of the Internet and E-mail for health care information, *JAMA: The Journal of the American Medical Association* 289(18):2400-2406, 2003.
9. Batista RJV and others: Partial left ventriculotomy to improve left ventricular function in end-stage heart disease, *Journal of Cardiac Surgery* 11:96-97, 1996.
10. Baumgartner WA: Operative techniques used in heart transplantation. In Baumgartner WA and others, editors: *Heart and lung transplantation,* ed 2, Philadelphia, 2002, Saunders.
11. Baumgartner WA and others: Recommendations of the National Heart, Lung and Blood Institute Working Group on Future Direction in Cardiac Surgery, *Circulation* 111:3007-3013, 2005.
12. Beller GA: Relative merits of cardiac diagnostic techniques. In Zipes DP and others, editors: *Braunwald's heart disease*, ed 7, Philadelphia, 2005, Saunders.
13. Beyea SC: *Perioperative nursing data set: the perioperative nursing vocabulary*, ed 2, Denver, 2002, Association of periOperative Registered Nurses.
14. Bickler PE and others: Effects of skin pigmentation on pulse oximeter accuracy at low saturation, *Anesthesiology* 102:715-719, 2005.
15. Birnbaum Y and others: Ventricular septal rupture after acute myocardial infarction, *New England Journal of Medicine* 347(18):1426-1432, 2002.
16. Blanche C and others: Heart transplantation with bicaval and pulmonary venous anastomoses: a hemodynamic analysis of the first 117 patients, *Journal of Cardiovascular Surgery (Torino)* 38:561-566, 1997.
17. Bonow RO: Valvular heart disease. In Zipes DP and others, editors: *Braunwald's heart disease*, ed 7, Philadelphia, 2005, Saunders.
18. Braunwald E: The history. In Zipes DP and others, editors: *Braunwald's heart disease*, ed 7, Philadelphia, 2005, Saunders.
19. Bridges CR and others: The Society of Thoracic Surgeons Practice Guideline Series: transmyocardial laser revascularization, *Annals of Thoracic Surgery* 77:1494-1502, 2004.
20. Buckberg GD: Update on current techniques of myocardial protection, *Annals of Thoracic Surgery* 60:805-814, 1995.

21. CABRI Trial Participants: First-year results of CABRI (coronary angioplasty versus bypass revascularization investigation), *Lancet* 346: 1179-1184, 1985.
22. Cameron A and others: Coronary bypass surgery with internal-thoracic-artery grafts—effects on survival over a 15-year period, *New England Journal of Medicine* 334(4):216-219, 1996.
23. Campeau L: Grading of angina pectoris, *Circulation* 54:522, 1975.
24. Carpentier A: Cardiac valve surgery: the French correction, *Journal of Thoracic and Cardiovascular Surgery* 86:323, 1983.
25. Carrel TP and others: Clinical experience with devices for facilitated anastomoses in coronary artery bypass surgery, *Annals of Thoracic Surgery* 77:1110-1120, 2004.
26. Carrier M and others: Tricuspid valve replacement: an analysis of 25 years of experience at a single center, *Annals of Thoracic Surgery* 75: 47-50, 2003.
27. Chitwood WR: Current status of endoscopic and robotic mitral valve surgery, *Annals of Thoracic Surgery* 79:S2248-S2253, 2005.
28. Clarke DR: Presidential address: value, viability, and valves, *Journal of Thoracic and Cardiovascular Surgery* 124(1):1-6, 2002.
29. Cooper DKC: The surgical anatomy of experimental and clinical thoracic organ transplantation, *Texas Heart Institute Journal* 31(1):61-68, 2004.
30. Copeland JG and others: Cardiac replacement with a total artificial heart as a bridge to transplantation, *New England Journal of Medicine* 351:859-867, 2004.
31. Cox JL: New surgical and catheter-based modifications of the Maze procedure, *Seminars in Thoracic and Cardiovascular Surgery* 12(1): 68-73, 2000.
32. Cox JL: Surgical management of atrial fibrillation, *Medscape Cardiology* 9(1), 2005. Accessed April 29, 2006, on-line: www.medscape.com/viewarticle/503894.
33. Crawford ES: The diagnosis and management of aortic dissection, *JAMA: The Journal of the American Medical Association* 264(9):2537, 1990.
34. Criteria Committee of the New York Heart Association: *Nomenclature and criteria for diagnoses*, ed 9, Boston, 1994, Little Brown.
35. Cushman M and others: C-reactive protein and the 10-year incidence of coronary heart disease in older men and women: the Cardiovascular Health Study, *Circulation* 112:25-31, 2005.
36. DeBakey ME: Development of mechanical heart devices, *Annals of Thoracic Surgery* 79:S2228-S2231, 2005.
37. DeJong MJ, Morton PG: Predictors of atrial dysrhythmias for patients undergoing coronary artery bypass grafting, *American Journal of Critical Care* 9(6):388-396, 2000.
38. Delbanco T, Sands DZ: Electrons in flight—E-mail between doctors and patients, *New England Journal of Medicine* 350(17):1705-1707, 2004.
39. Demers P and others: Stent-graft repair of penetrating atherosclerotic ulcers in the descending thoracic aorta: mid-term results, *Annals of Thoracic Surgery* 77:81-86, 2004.
40. Dor V: Left ventricular aneurysms: the endoventricular circular patch plasty, *Seminars in Thoracic and Cardiovascular Surgery* 9:123-130, 1997.
41. Eagle KA and others: *American College of Cardiology/American Heart Association 2004 update for coronary artery bypass graft surgery,* 2004. Accessed April 29, 2006, on-line: www.acc.org/clinical/guidelines/cabg/index.pdf.
42. Edmunds LH: Cardiopulmonary bypass after 50 years, *New England Journal of Medicine* 351(16):1603-1606, 2004.
43. Edwards FH and others: Gender-specific practice guidelines for coronary artery bypass surgery: perioperative management, *Annals of Thoracic Surgery* 79:2189-2194, 2005.
44. Eikemo H and others: Markers for endothelial activation during open heart surgery, *Annals of Thoracic Surgery* 77:214-219, 2004.
45. Enriquez-Sarano M, Tajik AJ: Aortic regurgitation, *New England Journal of Medicine* 351:1539-1546, 2004.
46. Fazel S and others: Current status of cellular therapy for ischemic heart disease, *Annals of Thoracic Surgery* 79:S2238-S2247, 2005.
47. Freeman RV, Otto CM: Spectrum of calcific aortic valve disease: pathogenesis, disease progression, and treatment strategies, *Circulation* 111:3316-3326, 2005.
48. Gemmato CJ and others: Thirty-five years of mechanical circulatory support at the Texas Heart Institute, *Texas Heart Institute Journal* 32(2):168-177, 2005.
49. Goldin JG and others: Contemporary cardiac imaging, *Journal of Thoracic Imaging* 15(4):218-229, 2000.
50. Gorman GH and others: Annuloplasty ring selection for chronic ischemic mitral regurgitation: lessons from the ovine model, *Annals of Thoracic Surgery* 76:1556-1563, 2003.
51. Graling PR: Research review: coronary artery bypass patients' perceptions of acute postoperative pain, *AORN Journal* 66(2):337-338, 1997.
52. Gundy SM and others: Definition of metabolic syndrome: Report of the National Heart, Lung, and Blood Institute/American Heart Association Conference on Scientific Issues Related to Definition, *Circulation* 109:433-438, 2004.
53. Haissaguerre M and others: Spontaneous initiation of atrial fibrillation by ectopic beats originating in the pulmonary veins, *New England Journal of Medicine* 339(10):659-666, 1998.
54. Halpin LS, Barnett SD: Preoperative state of mind among patients undergoing CABG, *Journal of Nursing Care Quality* 20(1):73-80, 2005.
55. Hammermeister K and others: Outcomes 15 years after valve replacement with a mechanical versus a bioprosthetic valve: final report of the Veterans Affairs randomized trial, *Journal of the American College of Cardiology* 36(4):1152-1158, 2000.
56. Hayes DL, Zipes DL: Cardiac pacemakers and cardioverter-defibrillators. In Zipes DP and others, editors: *Braunwald's heart disease*, ed 7, Philadelphia, 2005, Saunders.
57. Henke K, Eigsti J: Bypass injury: implications of cardiopulmonary bypass, *Dimensions of Critical Care Nursing* 22(2):64-70, 2003.
58. Hlozek CC, Zacharias WM: The RN first assistant's role during inferior epigastric artery harvesting, *AORN Journal* 65(1):26-29, 1997.
59. The Homocysteine Studies Collaboration: Homocysteine and the risk of ischemic heart disease and stroke, *JAMA: The Journal of the American Medical Association* 288(16):2015-2022, 2002.
60. Hu KK and others: Use of maximal sterile barriers during central venous catheter insertion: clinical and economic outcomes, *Clinical Infectious Diseases* 39, November 15, 2004.
61. Hunt SA and others: Heart transplantation. In Zipes DP and others, editors: *Braunwald's heart disease*, ed 7, Philadelphia, 2005, Saunders.
62. Hussey LC and others: Risk factors for sternal wound infection in men versus women, *American Journal of Critical Care* 10(2):112-116, 2001.
63. Iannelli G and others: Thoracic aortic emergencies: impact of endovascular surgery, *Annals of Thoracic Surgery* 77:591-596, 2004.
64. Isselbacher EM: Diseases of the aorta. In Zipes DP and others, editors: *Braunwald's heart disease,* ed 7, Philadelphia, 2005, Saunders.
65. Jeevanandam V and others: A one-year comparison of prophylactic donor tricuspid annuloplasty in heart transplantation, *Annals of Thoracic Surgery* 78:759-766, 2004.
66. Jin R and others: Is obesity a risk factor for mortality in coronary artery bypass surgery, *Circulation* 111:3359-3365, 2005.
67. *JAMA: The Journal of the American Association: JAMA patient's page.* Available at www.jama.com.
68. Kappert U: Endoharvesting, *CTSNet.* Accessed January 16, 2005, on-line: www.ctsnet.org/sections/innovations/minimallyinvasive/articles/article-22.html.
69. Kellen JC: Implications for nursing care of patients with atrial fibrillation, *Journal of Cardiovascular Nursing* 19(2):128-137, 2004.
70. Kern LS: Postoperative atrial fibrillation: new directions in prevention and treatment, *Journal of Cardiovascular Nursing* 19(2):103-115, 2004.
71. Kern MJ: *The cardiac catheterization handbook*, ed 4, Philadelphia, 2003, Mosby.

72. Kincaid EH and others: Tissue engineered heart valves: a potential cure for valvular heart disease, *CTSNet*. Accessed January 14, 2005, on-line: www.ctsnet.org/sections/innovation/valvetechnology/articles/article-12.html.
73. Konkle BA, Schafer A: Hemostasis, thrombosis, fibrinolysis, and cardiovascular disease. In Zipes DP and others, editors: *Braunwald's heart disease*, ed 7, Philadelphia, 2005, Saunders.
74. Kouchoukos N and others: *Kirklin/Barratt-Boyes cardiac surgery*, ed 3, vol I, Philadelphia, 2003, Churchill Livingstone.
75. Kouchoukos NT and others: Safety and efficacy of hypothermic cardiopulmonary bypass and circulatory arrest for operations on the descending thoracic and thoracoabdominal aorta, *Annals of Thoracic Surgery* 72:699-708, 2001.
76. Kurz A and others: Perioperative normothermia to reduce the incidence of surgical wound infection and shorten hospitalization, *New England Journal of Medicine* 334:1209-1215, 1996.
77. Lamas GA and others: Evidence base for pacemaker mode selection: from physiology to randomized trials, *Circulation* 109:443-451, 2004.
78. LaRosa JC and others: Intensive lipid lowering with atorvastatin in patients with stable coronary artery disease, *New England Journal of Medicine* 352:1425-1435, 2005.
79. Leclercq C, Hare JM: Ventricular resynchronization: current state of the art, *Circulation* 109:296-299, 2004.
80. Lee TH, Boucher CA: Noninvasive tests in patients with stable coronary artery disease, *New England Journal of Medicine* 344(24):1840-1845, 2001.
81. Lee TH: Guidelines: cardiac pacemakers and cardioverter-defibrillators. In Zipes DP and others, editors: *Braunwald's heart disease*, ed 7, Philadelphia, 2005, Saunders.
82. Lee TH: Guidelines: management of valvular heart disease. In Zipes DP and others, editors: *Braunwald's heart disease*, ed 7, Philadelphia, 2005, Saunders.
83. Lewicki LJ and others: Patient risk factors for pressure ulcers during cardiac surgery, *AORN Journal* 65(5):933-942, 1997.
84. Loop FD and others: Influence of the internal-mammary-artery graft on 10-year survival and other cardiac events, *New England Journal of Medicine* 314:1, 1986.
85. Lorenz RA and others: Perioperative blood glucose control during adult coronary artery bypass surgery, *AORN Journal* 81(1):126-150, 2005.
86. Mack MJ: Coronary surgery: off pump and port access, *Surgical Clinics of North America* 80(5):1575-1591, 2000.
87. Makaroun MS and others: Endovascular treatment of thoracic aortic aneurysms: results of the phase II multicenter trial of the GORE TAG thoracic endoprosthesis, *Journal of Vascular Surgery* 41:1-9, 2005.
88. Malarkey LM, McMorrow ME: *Laboratory tests and diagnostic procedures*, ed 2, St Louis, 2000, Mosby.
89. Mascagni R and others: Edge-to-edge technique to treat post-mitral valve repair systolic anterior motion and left ventricular outflow tract obstruction, *Annals of Thoracic Surgery* 79:471-474, 2005.
90. Mathesin L and others: Patient-reported outcome after randomization to on-pump versus off-pump coronary artery surgery, *Annals of Thoracic Surgery* 79:1584-1589, 2005.
91. Mathew JP and others: A multicenter risk index for atrial fibrillation after cardiac surgery, *JAMA: The Journal of the American Medical Association* 291(14):1720-1729, 2004.
92. McCarthy JF, Cosgrove DM: Tricuspid valve repair with the Cosgrove-Edwards annuloplasty system, *Annals of Thoracic Surgery* 64:267-268, 1997.
93. Merry AF and others: Bivalirudin versus heparin and protamine in off-pump coronary artery bypass surgery, *Annals of Thoracic Surgery* 77:925-931, 2004.
94. Mickleborough LL and others: Left ventricular reconstruction: early and late results, *Journal of Thoracic and Cardiovascular Surgery* 128:27-37, 2004.
95. Miller JM, Zipes DP: Therapy for cardiac arrhythmias. In Zipes DP and others, editors: *Braunwald's heart disease*, ed 7, Philadelphia, 2005, Saunders.
96. Minakata K and others: Is repair of aortic valve regurgitation a safe alternative to valve replacement? *Journal of Thoracic and Cardiovascular Surgery* 127:645-653, 2004.
97. Mortensen N, Garrard CS: Colorectal surgery comes in from the cold, *New England Journal of Medicine* 334(19):1263-1264, 1996.
98. Mosca L and others: Evidence-based guidelines for cardiovascular disease prevention in women, *Circulation* 109:672-693, 2004.
99. Moses JW and others: Sirolimus-eluting stents versus standard stents in patients with stenosis in a native coronary artery, *New England Journal of Medicine* 349(14):1315-1323, 2003.
100. Moss AS and others: Prophylactic implantation of a defibrillator in patients with myocardial infarction and reduced ejection fraction, Multicenter Automatic Defibrillator Implantation Trial II (MADIT II) Investigators, *New England Journal of Medicine* 346:877-883, 2002.
101. Naka Y and others: Assisted circulation in the treatment of heart failure. In Zipes DP and others, editors: *Braunwald's heart disease*, ed 7, Philadelphia, 2005, Saunders.
102. Nguyen HQ and others: Supporting cardiac recovery through eHealth technology, *Journal of Cardiovascular Nursing* 19(3):200-208, 2004.
103. Nienaber CA, Eagle KA: Aortic dissection: new frontiers in diagnosis and management. 1. From etiology to diagnostic strategies, *Circulation* 108:628-235, 2003.
104. Okazaki Y and others: Coronary endothelial damage during off-pump CABG related to coronary clamping and gas insufflation, *European Journal of Cardiothoracic Surgery* 19:834-839, 2001.
105. Pagana KD, Pagana TJ: *Mosby's diagnostic and laboratory test reference*, ed 7, St Louis, 2005, Mosby.
106. Parent N, Fortin F: A randomized, controlled trial of vicarious experience through peer support for male first-time cardiac surgery patients: impact on anxiety, self-efficacy expectation, and self-reported activity, *Heart and Lung* 29(6):389-400, 2000.
107. Park SJ and others. Left ventricular assist devices as destination therapy: a new look at survival. *Journal of Thoracic and Cardiovascular Surgery* 129(1):9-17, 2005.
108. Park SJ and others: Paclitaxel-eluting stent for the prevention of coronary restenosis, *New England Journal of Medicine* 348(16):1537-1545, 2003.
109. Patel AM and others: Endoscopic radial artery harvesting is better than the open technique, *Annals of Thoracic Surgery* 78(1):149-153, 2004.
110. Perloff JK, Perloff M: Coronary artery bypass: a user's manual, *American Journal of Cardiology* 94:172-177, 2004.
111. Prinssen M and others: A randomized trial comparing conventional and endovascular repair of abdominal aortic aneurysms, *New England Journal of Medicine* 351(16):1607-1618, 2004.
112. Rabago G and others: The new DeVega technique in tricuspid annuloplasty, *Journal of Thoracic and Cardiovascular Surgery* 21:231, 1980.
113. Rahimtoola SH: The year in valvular heart disease, *Journal of the American College of Cardiology* 43(3):491-504, 2004.
114. Reade CC and others: Combining robotic mitral valve repair and microwave atrial fibrillation ablation: techniques and initial results, *Annals of Thoracic Surgery* 79:480-484, 2005.
115. Reichenspurner H and others: Video and robotic-assisted minimally invasive mitral valve surgery: a comparison of the port-access and transthoracic clamp techniques, *Annals of Thoracic Surgery* 79:485-491, 2005.
116. Reimer-Kent J: From theory to practice: preventing pain after cardiac surgery, *American Journal of Critical Care* 12(2):136-143, 2003.
117. Ridker PM, Libby P: Risk factors for atherosclerotic disease. In Zipes DP and others, editors: *Braunwald's heart disease*, ed 7, Philadelphia, 2005, Saunders.
118. Rizvi AA: Type 2 diabetes: epidemiological trends, evolving pathogenic concepts, and recent changes in therapeutic approach, *Southern Medical Journal* 97(11):1079-1087, 2004.
119. Rose E and others: Long-term mechanical left ventricular assistance for end-stage heart failure, *New England Journal of Medicine* 345:1435-1443, 2001.

120. Rose E and others: The REMATCH trial: rationale, design, and end points. Randomized evaluation of mechanical assistance for the treatment of congestive heart failure, *Annals of Thoracic Surgery* 67(3): 723-730, 1999.
121. Rosenhek E and others: Predictors of severe, asymptomatic aortic stenosis, *New England Journal of Medicine* 343(9):611-617, 2000.
122. Ross AC, Ostrow L: Subjectively perceived quality of life after coronary artery bypass surgery, *American Journal of Critical Care* 10(1): 11-16, 2001.
123. Rothrock JC, Seifert PC: Nursing diagnosis, outcomes, and plans for patient care. In Seifert PC: *Cardiac surgery: perioperative patient care,* St Louis, 2002, Mosby.
124. Sajja LR and others: Role of radial artery graft in coronary artery bypass grafting, *Annals of Thoracic Surgery* 79:2180-2188, 2005.
125. Sakamoto Y and others: Long-term assessment of mitral valve reconstruction with resection of the leaflets: triangular and quadrangular resection, *Annals of Thoracic Surgery* 79:475-479, 2005.
126. Sasso FC and others: Glucose metabolism and coronary heart disease in patients with normal glucose tolerance, *JAMA: The Journal of the American Medical Association* 291(15):1857-1863, 2004.
127. Seifert PC: *Cardiac surgery,* St Louis, 2002, Mosby.
128. Seifert PC, Hickman DS: Enhancing patient safety in a healing environment, *Topics in Advanced Practice eJournal* 5(1): 2005 (Medscape). Accessed April 29, 2006, on-line: www.medscape.com/viewarticle/499690.
129. Sellke FW and others: Comparing on-pump and off-pump coronary artery bypass grafting (American Heart Association Scientific Statement), *Circulation* 111:2858-2864, 2005.
130. Shan K and others: Role of cardiac magnetic resonance imaging in the assessment of myocardial viability, *Circulation* 109:1328-1334, 2004.
131. Shubrooks SJ and others: Urgent coronary bypass surgery for failed percutaneous coronary intervention in the stent era: is backup still necessary? *American Heart Journal* 142(1):109-196, 2001.
132. Society of Thoracic Surgeons: *STS patient information.* Accessed May 27, 2004, on-line: www.sts.org/doc/8747.
133. Strauch JT and others: Technical advances in total aortic arch replacement, *Annals of Thoracic Surgery* 77:581-590, 2004.
134. Subramanian VA and others: Robotic assisted multivessel minimally invasive direct coronary artery bypass with port-access stabilization and cardiac positioning: paving the way for outpatient coronary surgery? *Annals of Thoracic Surgery* 79:1590-1596, 2005.
135. Svenarud P and others: Effect of $CO_2$ insufflation on the number and behavior of air emboli in open-heart surgery, *Circulation* 109: 1127-1132, 2004.
136. Sweitzer NK, Douglas PS: Cardiovascular disease in women. In Zipes DP and others, editors: *Braunwald's heart disease*, ed 7, Philadelphia, 2005, Saunders.
137. Tatoulis J and others: Patencies of 2,217 arterial to coronary conduits over 15 years, *Annals of Thoracic Surgery* 77:93-101, 2004.
138. Tavilla G and others: Long-term follow-up of coronary artery bypass grafting in three-vessel disease using exclusively pedicled bilateral internal thoracic and right gastroepiploic arteries, *Annals of Thoracic Surgery* 77:794-799, 2004.
139. Van Gelder IC and others: Rate control versus electrical cardioversion for persistent atrial fibrillation study group—a comparison of rate control and rhythm control in patients with recurrent persistent atrial fibrillation, *New England Journal of Medicine* 347:1834-1840, 2002.
140. Vassiliades TA and others: The clinical development of percutaneous heart valve technology: a position statement of the Society of Thoracic Surgeons (STS), the American Association for Thoracic Surgery (AATS), and the Society for Cardiovascular Angiography and Interventions (SCAI), *Journal of Thoracic and Cardiovascular Surgery* 129(5):970-976, 2005.
141. Verma S and others: Off-pump coronary artery bypass surgery, *Circulation* 109:1206-1211, 2004.
142. Waldhausen JA and others: *Surgery of the chest,* ed 6, St Louis, 1996, Mosby.
143. Wennberg DE and others: Outcomes of percutaneous coronary interventions performed at centers without and with onsite coronary artery bypass graft surgery, *Journal of the American Medical Association* 292:1961-1968, 2004.
144. Westaby S: *Landmarks in cardiac surgery,* Oxford, England, 1997, Isis Medical Media.
145. Williams ME: Assessment of the geriatric patient: initial impressions, *Medscape (WebMD).* Accessed June 16, 2005, on-line: www.medscape.com/viewprogram/4179_pnt.
146. Woerth ST and others: A collaborative approach to minimally invasive direct coronary artery bypass, *AORN Journal* 66(6):994-1001, 1997.
147. Wyse DG and others (Atrial Fibrillation Follow-up Investigation of Rhythm Management [AFFIRM] Investigators): A comparison of rate control and rhythm control in patients with atrial fibrillation, *New England Journal of Medicine* 347:1825-1833, 2002.
148. Yacoub MH, Cohn LH: Novel approaches to cardiac valve repair: from structure to function. I, *Circulation* 109:942-950, 2004.
149. Yacoub MH, Cohn LH: Novel approaches to cardiac valve repair: from structure to function. II, *Circulation* 109:1064-1072, 2004.
150. Yamaguchi A and others: Left ventricular reconstruction benefits patients with dilated ischemic cardiomyopathy, *Annals of Thoracic Surgery* 79:456-461, 2005.
151. Yuh DD and others: Totally endoscopic robot-assisted transmyocardial revascularization, *Journal of Thoracic and Cardiovascular Surgery* 130(1):120-124, 2005.
152. Yun KL and others: Randomized trial of endoscopic versus open vein harvest for coronary artery bypass grafting: six-month patency rates, *Journal of Thoracic and Cardiovascular Surgery* 129(3):496-503, 2005.
153. Zelinka ES and others: Retrograde autologous prime with shortened bypass circuits decreases blood transfusion in high-risk coronary artery surgery patients, *Journal of the American Society of Extra-Corporeal Technology* 36:343-347, 2004.

CHAPTER 28

# Ambulatory Surgery

DONNA R. McEWEN

The concept of ambulatory surgery has revolutionized the delivery of surgical care, becoming a model for patient-centered perioperative care delivery models. Although phenomenal growth in ambulatory surgery has occurred since the early 1980s, writings from Egyptian scrolls have referred to the concept as early as 3000 BC. Ambulatory surgery is interwoven within medical and nursing history and is referred to in the Bible and in early Indian and Hindu literature. In the United States the initial concept of ambulatory surgery began in 1818 when Massachusetts General Hospital established the first outpatient department. It was not until the 1960s, however, that interest in ambulatory surgery became widespread (History box).

The first freestanding surgical center that was independently owned and operated was the Phoenix Surgicenter (in Phoenix, Arizona), founded by Drs. Wallace Reed and John Ford in 1970. Dr. Reed identified patient selection, types of procedures, anesthesia, careful surgery, well-defined discharge criteria, and appropriate patient follow-up examinations as key concepts in delivering safe care in ambulatory settings.[4] The Phoenix Surgicenter quickly became a prototype for other centers across the United States.

Since the advent of the Phoenix Surgicenter, market-driven forces have significantly influenced the resurgence of ambulatory surgery. Continued pressures to reform the health care system, at both federal and state levels, pressures of managed care, the increased presence of capitated payment systems, advances in technology, and public awareness and support of the concept have all been driving factors. In 1982 the federal government enacted the Tax Equity and Fiscal Responsibility Act (TEFRA), which included prospective payment for inpatient care with diagnosis-related groups (DRGs). As a result, Medicare reimbursement for outpatient procedures was higher than that for those performed on an inpatient basis. Third-party payers quickly followed suit, and financial incentives clearly favored surgical care delivery on an ambulatory basis.

Concurrently, an explosion of technology, such as minimally invasive techniques and new, shorter-acting anesthetic agents, contributed to the ability to meet criteria for ambulatory procedures. Public acceptance quickly followed as patients were drawn to the user-friendly environment created by successful ambulatory surgery centers. Highly effective marketing fostered public acceptance of the benefits of recuperation at home because the hospital had become the place for acutely ill patients. Many procedures that were once considered appropriate only for inpatient treatment are now being performed with great success as ambulatory surgery.

The shift to ambulatory surgery provided an opportunity for nurses to move their traditional practice skills to a new environment; the establishment of specialty centers (i.e., outpatient endoscopy, dermatology, oral/dental surgery) provided additional opportunities for perioperative nurses to grow and develop in new roles. In 1999 the Association of periOperative Registered Nurses (AORN) acknowledged the growth of ambulatory surgery as a significant facet of perioperative practice and published the first edition of *Ambulatory Surgery Principles and Practices.* Designed to supplement the *AORN Standards, Recommended Practices, and Guidelines,* the *Ambulatory Surgery Principles and Practices* recognizes the specialty of perioperative nursing practice in ambulatory surgery, outlining the significance and importance of a skilled perioperative nurse who is clinically and professionally competent to provide care to the ambulatory surgery patient in a short time frame. The care provided should be cost-effective, convenient, and efficient; should be consistent with established standards of perioperative nursing practice; and must include the patient and family or significant others throughout the surgical experience.[1]

## REGULATION AND ACCREDITATION

As the availability of ambulatory surgery has increased over the past 30 years, federal and state regulations have also increased, establishing guidelines for patient care, policies, safe practice, and physical plant standards. In the United States, a majority of individual states require ambulatory surgery centers (ASCs) to be licensed by the state. In addition to state licensure, 85% of all ASCs are Medicare-certified, and many centers go through additional voluntary accreditation.[3] Accreditation is an extra step many ASCs pursue to demonstrate their commitment to quality and excellence. The Joint Commission on Accreditation of Healthcare Organizations (JCAHO) provides guidelines and accreditation for ambulatory surgery, as does the American Association for Accreditation of Ambulatory Surgery Facilities (AAAASF) and the Accreditation Association for Ambulatory Health Care (AAAHC).

## FACILITIES

The success of ambulatory surgery has resulted in a proliferation of various models for ambulatory surgery. The business structure of an ASC is either not-for-profit or for-profit. Successful ambulatory surgery models include various types of facilities, such as hospital-based self-contained, hospital-integrated, freestanding, office-based, and recovery center. The Federated Association of Ambulatory Surgery (FASA) reports more than 8000 surgeries in approximately 4000 ASCs each year across the United States.[3] Regardless of the ownership or

## HISTORY

In the 1940s, ambulatory surgery was commonly performed in physicians' offices. The types of surgery performed in the ambulatory setting included lesion removal, abscess drainage, tonsillectomy, cystoscopy, anorectal procedures, podiatric procedures, injections for pain management, minor hernia repair, fracture reduction, and repair of lacerations. Advantages and disadvantages to ambulatory surgery cited in Ferguson's *Surgery of the Ambulatory Patient* were as follows:

> . . . the patient may continue his regular occupation with little or no disability. This combined with the fact that he may stay in his own home means a considerable saving of money and inconvenience. Also, the worry and dread of a hospital stay are avoided . . . . Surgery in the ambulatory patient is not always advisable even though possible. The patient should not be permitted to go home after an operation without a friend or relative to accompany him. Home care is sometimes required following operations. In the case of the patient who should be confined to his room for a day or two but who would have to go out for his meals, it is perhaps wiser to take advantage of the facilities of a hospital.

Within the arena of ambulatory surgery, the nurse worked very closely with the physician and often filled the role of preoperative nurse, circulating nurse, anesthesia provider, surgical assistant, and postanesthesia nurse. Before the patient arrived for surgery, the nurse ensured that the suite was clean by scrubbing the walls, floor, and all equipment. The nurse's duties included the preparation of instrumentation and needles. Instruments were first soaked in green soap and phenol, then rinsed in distilled water, followed by boiling for 30 minutes in a bleach solution and a rinse in ether. All needles were examined for burrs and sharpened by the nurse if necessary. If the surgeon's office had an electric dry-heat sterilizer, a limited number of instruments could be further sterilized after being prepared as described above. The sterilizers were typically small, having a length of only 16 to 18 inches, and had a 1-hour cycle. Preparation and sterilization of gauze bandages, muslin bandages, and flannel bandages in a variety of sizes were also the responsibility of the perioperative nurse. Dressings were cut and sewn to size by the nurse and sterilized in paper wrappings.

After preparing the room, instrumentation, and supplies, the perioperative nurse established the sterile field for the surgeon and prepared the patient. The patient removed only the amount or articles of clothing that were necessary to expose the surgical site. The nurse performed a shave prep on the site and positioned the patient on the operating room (OR) bed. If the procedure was to be performed with the patient under local anesthesia, the nurse supported the patient during the infiltration of the anesthetic agent and then assisted the surgeon during the procedure. If the procedure was to be performed with the patient under general anesthesia, often the nurse was responsible for the administration of ether by the drop method. Before beginning administration of the ether, the nurse and physician would ensure that everything was ready for the procedure and the surgeon would be poised over the site, scalpel ready for the moment the patient became unconscious. The nurse would either (1) have the patient count backwards from 100 and the surgeon would start the incision when the patient stopped counting or became confused or (2) instruct the patient to hold his or her arm in the air and when the patient's arm dropped, he or she was considered sufficiently anesthetized and the surgeon began. To assess the patient's respiratory status during the procedure, the nurse was instructed to tape a cotton ball to the patient's upper lip. The motion of the cotton over the nostril indicated respiratory changes. Additional ether was administered if the patient regained consciousness during the procedure. While administering ether and monitoring the patient, the nurse might also be required to assist the surgeon by holding retractors. After the procedure, the nurse was responsible for postoperative care of the patient. If the patient had local anesthetic, he or she might be discharged immediately to allow for arrival at home before the anesthesia wore off and postoperative pain ensued. Patients who were under general anesthesia were allowed to awaken and were administered morphine for pain control before discharge. The nurse and physician provided discharge instructions concerning postoperative bleeding, activity restrictions, and measures to take for emergencies. After the patient's discharge, the nurse cleaned the OR and reprocessed all items used.

The role of the perioperative nurse in ambulatory surgery has changed over the years, but the essence of patient advocacy has remained. Desirable qualities of the perioperative nurse of this era are described in Alexander's *Operating Room Technique* as follows:

> . . . physical strength and stamina are need to endure the strain and severity of this type of nursing . . . . the operating room nurse must be conscientious at all times. Her conscience should be of the type which will not allow her to take a chance at any time, even under the most pressing circumstances. Sincerity, tact, self control, the ability to think in a logical manner and to plan her work systematically are necessary qualifications . . . . above all, she should have a keen desire to be the best possible operating room nurse. Every nurse must be willing to practice and progress.

Modified from Alexander EL: *Operating room technique,* ed 2, St Louis, 1949, Mosby; Ferguson LK: *Surgery of the ambulatory patient,* Philadelphia, 1942, Lippincott.

physical location of the facility, several key issues must be considered to ensure success of the facility:

- Identification of a unique clinical niche based on an assessment of community need
- Active participation by a multidisciplinary surgical advisory committee with representation by all high-volume specialties targeted by the facility
- Effective, experienced manager with strong team-building skills
- Recruitment and retention of qualified, dedicated staff
- Participative governance structure allowing key-user input to decision making
- Sound financial management
- Efficient design
- Facility and equipment adequate to meet the demand, allowing for growth
- Design and decor that reflect a patient-oriented, user-friendly alternative to the traditional hospital environment

Patient condition and type of procedure assist the health care team (surgeon, anesthesia provider, perioperative staff) in determining the most appropriate facility. Questions often asked to determine appropriateness of patient selection and facility include the following:

- Is the facility equipped to deal with emergency situations related to the surgical procedure, patient's condition, and anticipated treatments?
- Can the procedure be performed without hospitalization?
- Is the risk to the patient minimal if the procedure is performed at the facility?
- Will extended recovery be necessary?
- Are quality standards adhered to at the facility?
- Does the patient need any special care (e.g., special equipment) that may not be available at the facility?
- Do the patient and family or significant others understand and accept the concept of ambulatory surgery?

The intent of ambulatory surgery is for safe, convenient, and cost-effective surgery to be provided at a facility and the patient to be discharged to a short-term recovery center or home. Patients are carefully screened to be healthy, with no unusual problems that cannot be managed in the facility, and the family or significant others need to be willing to monitor for signs and symptoms of complications, provide home treatments as necessary, and care for the patient once discharged.

## Hospital-Based Self-Contained Facility

The hospital-based facility is affiliated with the hospital but is a separate ambulatory surgery department with designated preoperative, intraoperative, and postoperative areas. The facility may be located within the hospital complex, adjacent to the hospital, or at a satellite location some distance from the hospital. In contrast to the hospital-integrated facility, the hospital-based self-contained facility has a dedicated staff, equipment, policies and procedures, and postanesthesia recovery care area for the ambulatory surgery patient. The facility is physically and organizationally separate from the hospital's main surgical suite and is exclusively for the ambulatory surgery patient population. Advantages of this type of facility include convenient scheduling, availability of hospital services, easy admission of the patient to the hospital if necessary, less likelihood of delay or cancellation as a result of scheduling complications, sharing of certain equipment and services with the main operating room (OR) suite, and use for more complicated procedures and higher-risk patients than at a freestanding or office-based facility.

## Hospital-Integrated Facility

The hospital-integrated facility uses the main OR suites for ambulatory as well as inpatient surgery. However, many hospitals have separate preoperative and postoperative areas that are designated specifically for ambulatory surgery patients. Ambulatory procedures may be either interspersed with inpatient procedures on any given day or done on a day or in an OR reserved solely for ambulatory patients. The admitting process for these patients may be handled by the hospital's admitting department or by the ambulatory unit itself. In this type of setting, family members of both inpatient and ambulatory surgery patients usually share a common waiting area. In addition to admitting ambulatory surgery patients, hospital-integrated facilities may handle the processing of day-of-surgery (DOS) patients or morning-admission patients, who are to be admitted to the hospital after surgery. Preoperative laboratory and diagnostic tests are usually done on an outpatient basis before the day of surgery, and these patients are admitted to the hospital after surgery.

The advantages of a hospital-integrated facility include shared personnel among the different areas, available equipment and supplies, rapid admission to the hospital if necessary, and sharing of cost related to capital budget. However, there is (1) less control of patient scheduling, (2) the potential for delays caused by scheduling ambulatory surgical patients after an inpatient procedure, and (3) the potential for the patient's procedure being canceled because of an inpatient surgical emergency.

## Freestanding Facility

A freestanding facility is usually independently owned and operated and may or may not be hospital-affiliated. These facilities are often operated on a for-profit basis and may be owned by entrepreneurs, physicians, and nurses. The types of ownership vary and generally include corporate, joint venture, or independent. A growing trend has been for health care corporation chains to own and operate such facilities. These facilities are conveniently located and attend to the desires and needs of the patient while providing safe, quality care that is cost-effective.

## Office-Based Facility

An office-based facility is much like a freestanding facility but is operated on a smaller scale, often using only one or two ORs. These facilities allow for ambulatory surgery to be provided safely and effectively in a surgeon's office. These for-profit facilities often have elaborate equipment, specially trained personnel, and an appropriate inventory of supplies and instrumentation. The concept of an office-based facility appeals to many physicians in terms of convenience of practice as well as for the financial opportunity such a structure presents. The physician owner is able to collect surgery fees as well as generate revenue from supply markup and facility fees. A mobile surgical services program can enhance office-based surgery by providing equipment, disposable supplies, staffing, and sterilization services to nontraditional surgical settings, such as offices. This allows the surgeon to provide services such as laser interventions to patients without the capital investment of equipment and the ongoing cost of specialized staff.

Advantages include more schedule flexibility for the surgeon and patient, cost-effectiveness of the procedure, and staff with clinical training and expertise specific to the procedures being performed. Limitations include strict patient selection criteria and the lack of nationwide regulations to assess and determine that standards of quality are being implemented. Approximately 50% of the 22 states have laws or regulations pertaining to office-based surgery. These regulations, which include administration, facility design, ancillary services, surgical care, and quality assurance, are intended to ensure and maintain superior quality of care for surgical patients undergoing procedures in office-based surgical facilities.[6]

## Recovery Center

The concept of a freestanding facility with an adjacent recovery center has become popular in many areas of the United States. The recovery center offers an alternative to the patient and family or significant others when skilled nursing care is desired but acute care is unnecessary. The center generally is equipped with private rooms designed with a decor similar to that of a hotel. A family member or significant other is allowed to stay with the patient if desired. The needs of the patient and visitors are catered to (e.g., meals, telephone, television, videos, vending machines). Such centers hold great appeal for patients desiring privacy and recovery in a nonmedical setting.

Hospital programs have also incorporated the concept of the recovery center into hospital-sponsored ambulatory surgery programs. The amenities are usually the same as those just mentioned, but the facility itself may be part of the hospital building. The patient is generally charged a reduced rate similar to a freestanding recovery center, but the appeal of the hospital program is the proximity to the hospital if these services are needed. Another advantage is that hospital-based recovery centers can be used for other procedural areas, such as cardiac catheterization and invasive radiology procedures, providing a more consistent patient volume. Consistent patient volume allows for cost-effective staffing and helps justify the overhead costs of the unit.

## PATIENT SELECTION

Criteria for appropriate patient selection are essential for safe ambulatory surgery. Because surgical intervention in an ambulatory facility does not decrease the risk for potential complications, each patient should be carefully evaluated. In the past, patients considered appropriate for ambulatory surgery were young and healthy, with no underlying illness. However, procedures performed today are more complex and the patients are older and have more coexisting health problems (Box 28-1).

Those responsible for determining appropriate patient selection include the surgeon, anesthesia provider, and perioperative nurse. The surgeon is responsible for assessing underlying problems that may lead to unexpected complications during the procedure. A patient with complex medical conditions unrelated to the procedure may be scheduled at a hospital-affiliated facility rather than a freestanding facility because of the potential for specific complications. Patients with complex medical conditions and underlying disease processes may be determined inappropriate for ambulatory surgery and scheduled in the main OR. Anesthesia providers are responsible for assessing any known or unknown problems related to the chosen anesthetic course. The perioperative nurse is responsible for assessing and evaluating the patient for factors that could lead to complications throughout the perioperative period.

A commonly used classification system is that of the American Society of Anesthesiologists (ASA) (see Chapter 4). The surgeon, anesthesia provider, or perioperative nurse assigns the patient an ASA physical-status classification. Patients classified as physical status 1 or 2 are perfect candidates for ambulatory surgery. These patients generally pose no great risk for procedures performed with general or local anesthesia or intravenous (IV) moderate sedation/analgesia. Patients classified as physical status 3 must be carefully evaluated and determined that no untoward event is likely to occur during the intraoperative and postoperative phases. Any concomitant disease must be well managed before the patient is acceptable for ambulatory surgery. Specific risk factors for ambulatory surgery include hypertension, heart disease or congestive heart failure, bronchopulmonary disease, diabetes, obesity, adrenocortical steroid therapy, alcohol or drug abuse, psychotropic drug therapy, psychiatric illness, and family or personal history of either malignant hyperthermia or pseudocholinesterase deficiency. The presence of one or more of these risk factors, or a classification of ASA 3, does not necessarily preclude a patient from ambulatory surgery; however, to minimize complications, these factors indicate that the patient must be carefully assessed preoperatively and home care must be planned.

## ANESTHESIA

Advances in anesthesia practice, which include the development and use of shorter-acting agents with fewer side effects, have made ambulatory surgery more feasible and helped foster its acceptance in both patients and caregivers. The anesthesia provider must understand the needs of the ambulatory patient population to facilitate anesthesia delivery that supports rapid recovery with adequate postoperative pain control (Research Highlight).

### Premedication

Preoperative medication may be prescribed to decrease the patient's anxiety and fear regarding the surgery, separation from family and significant others, pain, the unknown, diagnostic results, and perceived loss of control. Additional advantages include analgesia, amnesia effect (depending on drug and dosage), and a decreased incidence of postoperative nausea and vomiting (PONV). Before the administration of a premedication, the preoperative verification process should be complete and surgical site marking done. The patient should be offered the opportunity to void, since he or she will be limited to a bed, a stretcher, or a recliner after administration of the medication. Because the effects of premedication may generate a longer postoperative recovery period for the patient, use of premedication is often avoided. However, a patient experiencing anxiety and apprehension should never be denied premedication if necessary. Other preoperative medications may include antibiotics, anticholinergics, or oxytocin (Pitocin) for gynecologic procedures.

### General Anesthesia

General anesthesia renders patients unconscious, relaxed, and unable to perceive pain. For the ambulatory surgery patient receiving a general anesthetic agent, consideration of the anesthetic agent is based, in part, on readiness for timely discharge of the patient. The ideal anesthetic agent allows for quick induction, short duration of action, and few effects on the patient's vital signs (Surgical Pharmacology). Bispectral Index (BIS) monitoring may be used in the ambulatory setting. This offers the anesthesia care provider a method of assessing the depth of anesthesia, which allows for better control of emergence at the end of the procedure and the ability to titrate the anesthesia delivery to minimize the possibility of intraoperative awareness (IOA) (see Chapter 4). The BIS technology is based on electroencephalogram (EEG) monitoring and provides the anesthesia care provider a digital number that corresponds to brain activity (Table 28-1). The unit operates with

BOX 28-1

**Procedures Frequently Performed in Ambulatory Surgery**

**GENERAL SURGERY**
- Breast biopsy
- Hemorrhoidectomy
- Laparoscopic procedures
- Bariatric procedures
- Excisions of lesions
- Herniorrhaphy
- Vein stripping
- Mastectomy
- Temporal artery biopsy

**GYNECOLOGY**
- Tubal ligation
- Vaginal hysterectomy
- Dilation and curettage
- Laser conization
- Laser vaporization
- Hysteroscopy
- Laparoscopy
- Infertility procedures

**OPHTHALMOLOGY**
- Cataract extraction
- Keratotomy
- Photoreactive keratotomy, phototherapeutic keratectomy
- Muscle surgery (e.g., recession and resection)
- Vitrectomies
- Repair of entropion and ectropion
- Nasal lacrimal duct probe, irrigation, insertion of stents
- Yttrium-aluminum-garnet (YAG) laser treatment

**ORTHOPEDICS**
- Arthroscopy
- Anterior cruciate ligament repair
- Tendon release
- Removal of plates, screws
- Nerve repair
- Removal of ganglion cysts
- Hand surgery (e.g., carpal tunnel, open reduction with internal fixation [ORIF])
- Ulnar nerve transposition

**OTOLARYNGOLOGY**
- Tonsillectomy
- Adenoidectomy
- Nasal polypectomy
- Myringotomy
- Vocal cord biopsy
- Micro suspension laryngoscopy
- Laser surgery
- Otoplasty
- Sinus surgery
- Nasal fracture reduction
- Tympanomastoidectomy
- Excision submandibular masses
- Diagnostic bronchoscopy and laryngoscopy
- Phonosurgery

**PAIN MANAGEMENT**
- Trigger point injection
- Diskogram
- Placement of dorsal column stimulator
- Epidural steroid injection

**PLASTIC SURGERY**
- Rhinoplasty
- Skin graft
- Mammoplasty
- Liposuction
- Blepharoplasty
- Face-lift
- Mini abdominoplasty
- Endoscopic browlift
- Endoscopic transaxillary augmentation
- Laser skin resurfacing
- Excision of lesions, scar revisions

**UROLOGY**
- Cystoscopy
- Ureteroscopy
- Vasectomy
- Biopsy
- Circumcision
- Lithotripsy

**DENTAL SURGERY**
- Insertion of dental implants
- Extractions
- Children's dentistry/maintenance
- Temporomandibular joint (TMJ) procedures
- Gingival surgery

**CARDIOTHORACIC SURGERY**
- Arteriography
- Cardiac catheterization
- Endoscopic thoracic sympathectomy
- Bronchoscopy

**GASTROENTEROLOGY**
- Colonoscopy
- Esophagoscopy

an adhesive sensor that is applied to the patient's forehead and connected to the BIS monitor (Figure 28-1). BIS monitoring may be altered by factors that include cerebral ischemia from any cause, hypothermia (<35°C), and non-EEG electrical interference or artifact.[5]

## Regional Anesthesia

Regional anesthesia provides an additional option for the ambulatory surgical patient. Based on the procedure, patient history, or patient preference, regional anesthetics such as Bier blocks, sympathetic blocks (i.e., lumbar), peripheral nerve blocks (i.e., brachial plexus), and regional blocks (i.e. spinal, epidural) may be used. Regional anesthesia utilizes the agents used in local anesthesia and blocks the neural pathways impairing the communication between the central nervous system and the peripheral nervous system, resulting in loss of feeling to an entire region. Regional anesthesia is often supplemented with IV sedation to promote patient comfort and lessen anxiety. Nurses working in the ambulatory setting must be familiar with the variety of regional an-

## RESEARCH HIGHLIGHT

### Streamlining Efficiency in the Ambulatory Surgery Setting

Efficiency in the ambulatory surgery center (ASC) setting is paramount to successful completion of the surgical schedule. Improvements in anesthesia techniques have helped to foster this efficiency and facilitate timely emergence from anesthesia and earlier discharge. Use of the laryngeal mask airway (LMA) is a recognized means of simplifying airway management in the outpatient setting.

The purpose of this study was to show that efficiency of operating room (OR) times could be improved by using LMAs for airway management instead of endotracheal tubes (ETTs). Study candidates were aged 18 to 65 years with an American Society of Anesthesiologists (ASA) status of I, II, or III who were undergoing elective trauma-related orthopedic procedures expected to last less than 1 hour. A total of 72 patients were randomized into two groups; one group was managed by ETT, the other by LMA.

The researchers defined anesthesia induction as the time from the beginning of preoxygenation to the placement of the ETT or LMA. Emergence was defined as the time from the end of the procedure to extubation after the patient regained consciousness and was breathing spontaneously. Analysis of the data showed that anesthesia induction was 1.5 minutes shorter using the LMA than the ETT, but there was no difference in emergence times between the two devices.

Use of the LMA in the ASC is a safe and effective way to realize process efficiencies without compromising patient care.

Modified from Hartmann B and others: Laryngeal mask airway versus endotracheal tube for outpatient surgery: analysis of anesthesia controlled time, *Journal of Clinical Anesthesia* 16:195-1999, 2004.

**TABLE 28-1**

### The Bispectral (BIS) Index*

| Numeric Value of Bispectral Index | Clinical State of Patient |
|---|---|
| 85-100 | Awake, memory intact |
| 65-85 | Sedation |
| 45-65 | General anesthesia |
| 45 | Deep hypnosis |
| 35-40 | Near suppression |
| 0-35 | Increasing burst suppression |
| 0 | Cortical silence |

From Stanksi DR, Shafer SL: Measuring the depth of anesthesia. In Miller RD, editor: *Miller's anesthesia,* ed 6, Philadelphia, 2005, Churchill Livingstone.

*Maintaining the BIS index from 45-65 during general anesthesia appears to ensure unconsciousness with a hypnotic/opioid anesthetic technique while providing for rapid emergence.

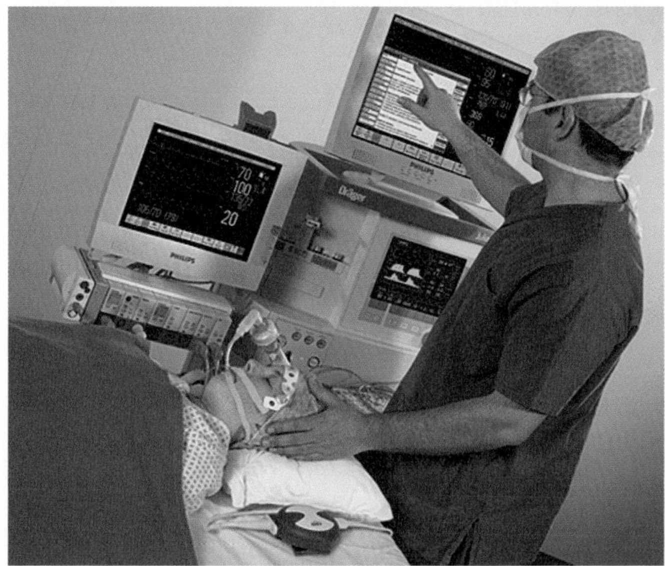

**FIGURE 28-1** Bispectral (BIS) sensors in place on patient's forehead. The electrical activity waveform will be tracked on the monitor by the anesthesiologist.

## SURGICAL PHARMACOLOGY

### Anesthetic Agents Commonly Used in the Ambulatory Surgery Setting

**INDUCTION AGENTS**

- Thiopental sodium
- Methohexital sodium
- Etomidate
- Ketamine
- Midazolam
- Propofol

**NEUROMUSCULAR BLOCKING AGENTS**

- Succinylcholine
- Mivacurium
- Atracurium
- Vecuronium
- Rocuronium
- Cisatracurium

**INHALATION AGENTS**

- Nitrous oxide
- Isoflurane
- Sevoflurane
- Desflurane

Guidelines established by the American Society of Anesthesiologists (ASA) for ambulatory anesthesia and surgery should be adhered to in all settings where general anesthetic agents are administered. Patients should have an appropriate preanesthesia evaluation and examination by an anesthesia provider; the provider must verify the information. An anesthesia plan should be developed by the anesthesia provider and discussed with (and accepted by) the patient.

Modified from *Guidelines for ambulatory anesthesia and surgery, American Society of Anesthesiologists (ASA),* last affirmed October 15, 2003. Accessed August 24, 2005, on-line: www.asahq.org.

esthetic techniques available to provide safe nursing care for these patients.

### Local Anesthesia

Local anesthesia is commonly used for the ambulatory surgery patient. Medication safety practices must be adhered to (see Chapter 2 for a full discussion of medication safety), such as the following:

- The circulating nurse and scrub person should visually and verbally review and confirm the medication ordered before transfer to the sterile field. Medication verification should include drug/solution/agent name, strength, dosage, and expiration date.
- All medications and containers with solutions (e.g., syringes, medicine cups, basins) both on and off the sterile field should be labeled, even if there is only one medication being used.
- Labeling should occur whenever any medication or solution is transferred from its original package to another container. Each medication should be labeled at the time it is delivered to the sterile field, *before* another product is prepared. Keep all original medication/solution containers in the room for reference until the procedure is concluded.
- Reverify all medications in use and their labels with relief staff (hand-off communication).

The surgeon administers the medication, and often the perioperative nurse is responsible for monitoring the patient throughout the procedure. Local anesthetics are classified as either amino esters or amino amides (Surgical Pharmacology). The surgeon chooses the local anesthetic based on its potency, desired duration of action, and surgery site. Local anesthetic agents are also available with epinephrine for vasoconstriction in the area injected, slowing the rate of absorption of the local anesthetic agent, prolonging its duration of action, and lowering the incidence of toxicity. The perioperative nurse checks the patient history for any allergies before dispensing the local anesthetic. Patients should be monitored (and monitoring results documented) for the presence of side effects such as central nervous system disturbances, cardiovascular problems, hypersensitivity to the medication, and toxic reaction resulting from high levels of the local anesthetic agent.

### Moderate Sedation/Analgesia

The perioperative nurse is responsible for monitoring and often administering medications to achieve IV moderate sedation/analgesia (Surgical Pharmacology). *Moderate sedation/analgesia* is defined as "a minimally depressed level of consciousness that allows a surgical patient to retain the ability to independently and continuously maintain a patent airway and respond appropriately to verbal commands and physical stimulation."[2] For optimal care of the patient receiving IV moderate sedation/analgesia, the perioperative nurse must be diligent in preoperative assessment and patient education, determining the patient's airway status and other conditions that may influence the administration of moderate sedation. Preoperative teaching should include explanations about what the patient will feel, hear, and see while sedated; the perioperative nurse should ensure that the patient understands that he or she will not be totally unconscious during the procedure and that the perioperative nurse will be closely monitoring him or her. Before the sedative is administered, the nurse may wish to establish gestures with the patient to allow for communication during the procedure, such as a hand squeeze or "thumb's up/thumb's down" to signal pain or discomfort. In addition, discharge instructions should be reinforced before the administration of sedation. The following parameters should be monitored and documented: respiratory rate, oxygen saturation, blood pressure, cardiac rate and rhythm, mental status, level of consciousness, pain, and skin condition. The perioperative nurse responsible for the management of the patient receiving IV moderate sedation/analgesia should provide uninterrupted monitoring. A second circulator should be assigned to assume the circulating responsibilities during the procedure so that the perioperative nurse administering moderate sedation/analgesia is not required to leave the patient or interrupt monitoring.

## APPEAL OF AMBULATORY SURGERY

With safety, efficiency, and cost-effectiveness well established, third-party payers not only support but also encourage (and in many procedures may require) the use of ambulatory surgery

### SURGICAL PHARMACOLOGY
#### Local Anesthetic Agents

**AMINO AMIDES***
- Bupivacaine
- Dibucaine
- Etidocaine
- Lidocaine
- Mepivacaine
- Prilocaine

**AMINO ESTERS†**
- Benzocaine
- Chloroprocaine
- Cocaine
- Procaine
- Proparacaine
- Propoxycaine
- Tetracaine

**MECHANISM OF ACTION**

Local anesthetics work by rendering a specific portion of the body insensitive to pain by interfering with nerve transmission. Nerve conduction is blocked in the area of application of the drug. Local anesthetics block both the generation and conduction of impulses through all nerve fibers (sensory, motor, and autonomic) by blocking movement of certain ions (sodium, calcium, and potassium). When the effects of the local anesthetic wear off, they do so in the following order: motor, sensory, and last autonomic activity.

Modified from Lilley LL and others: *Pharmacology and the nursing process,* ed 4, St Louis, 2005, Mosby.
*Metabolized in the liver by other enzymes to active and inactive metabolites.
†Metabolized by cholinesterase in the plasma and liver to para-aminobenzoic acid (PABA) compound, which is mainly responsible for allergic reactions.

## SURGICAL PHARMACOLOGY

### Conscious Sedation Drug Dosage Information

**The recommendations included here are generally acceptable guidelines and may require modification for individual patients at the discretion of the physician operator.** Dosages provided are generally acceptable but may need to be revised downward in a given patient to avoid serious cardiorespiratory depression or other undesired side effects. Further, many of these medications have synergistic respiratory depressant effects; when administered in combination, lower dosages may be required.

| Drug | Dose | Total | Onset | Duration | Nursing Consideration |
|---|---|---|---|---|---|
| | | | **Benzodiazepine Sedatives** | | |
| diazepam (Valium) | 2-10 mg into rapidly infusing IV line; may repeat @ 5 min intervals | 0.1 mg/kg to 0.2 mg/kg | 1 to 5 minutes | 15-60 minutes may be much increased in pts >60 y/o | Patient should remain supine until medication has worn off and risk of hypotension has passed. Hepatic and renal insufficiency increase duration of effect |
| midazolam (Versed) | <60 y/o 1.0 to 2.5 mg over 5 min (wait 2 min to evaluate) Titrate in small increments at 2 min intervals | Total maximum dose 2.5-5.0 mg | 1 to 5 minutes | 20 to 30 minutes | Too much or too little dose may cause cerebral hypoxia, agitation, combativeness. Hepatic insufficiency increases duration of effect; 30% dose reduction with concomitant use of opiate agonists or CNS depressants |
| | >60 y/o, debilitated, or chronically ill 0.5 mg (wait 3 min to evaluate) Titrate 0.5 mg increments at 2-3 min intervals | Total maximum dose 3.5 mg | | | 50% dose reduction with concomitant use of opiate agonists or CNS depressants |
| | | | **Opiate Agonists (Narcotics)** | | |
| morphine | 1-2 mg at 3-5 min intervals | up to 0.1 mg/kg– 0.15 mg/kg | 1 to 5 minutes | 3 to 5 hours | If respirations are 12/min or less, hold next dose. Hepatic or renal insufficiency increases duration of effect |
| fentanyl (Sublimaze) | Bolus of 1-2 mcg/kg then 1 mcg/kg hr | 1.5 mcg – 2.0 mcg/kg | 1 to 5 minutes | ½ to 1 hour | Hepatic insufficiency increases duration of effect |
| meperidine (Demerol) | 12.5 mg at 5-10 min intervals | up to 1 mg/kg | 1 to 5 minutes | 2 to 3 hours | Should not be used in patients with renal failure or pts on MAO inhibitors Caution with hepatic insufficiency |
| | | | **Opiate Antagonist (Patients who receive reversal agents should be observed closely for an additional 2 hours)** | | |
| naloxone (Narcan) | 0.4 mg to 2 mg IV prn at 2-3 min intervals until respiratory function is restored | | 1 to 2 minutes | 20-60 minutes | Narcotic effects may last longer than Versed. Must monitor at least 2 hours after Narcan |
| | | | **Benzodiazepine Antagonist** | | |
| flumazenil (Romazicon) | 0.2 mg over 15 sec into rapidly infusing IV line | Maximum dose 1 mg | 1-2 minutes | 60 minutes | Pts on chronic benzodiazepines or with acute head injury |

Modified from Hodgson BB, Kizior RJ: *Mosby's 2006 drug consult for nurses,* St Louis Mo, 2006, Elsevier Mosby.
*CNS,* Central nervous system; *IV,* intravenous; *MAO,* monoamine oxidase.

facilities by their subscribers. As an incentive for use, reimbursement has been higher for procedures performed at an ambulatory surgery facility.

Ambulatory surgery is appealing to the patient and family or significant others because there are fewer disruptions of normal daily activities, less separation, less time away from the workplace, and less worry about financial outlays because costly hospital stays are avoided. The use of an ASC may decrease the patient's risk for health care–associated (formerly known as *nosocomial*) infection because of the decreased exposure to critically ill patients. The ambulatory surgery patient and family or significant others are active participants in the patient's plan of care. Some ambulatory centers routinely schedule weekend surgery, further appealing to patients and their families or significant others who are unable to or desire not to interfere with their work schedules. Convenience and patient satisfaction are hallmarks of ambulatory surgery, making it a model for the health care industry's focus on customer-oriented service.

Ambulatory surgery offers many advantages for health care professionals. It is convenient for the surgeons and enables them to spend less time away from the office. It gives anesthesia providers an opportunity to enter into and specialize in a different arena in which anesthetic agents and techniques are continuously being improved to enhance rapid patient recovery and return to ambulation. Perioperative nurses have the opportunity to condense and refine nursing skills and to develop nursing practice models that focus on wellness, safety, comfort, patient education, and continuity of care. The emphasis on cross-training, productivity, versatility, and independence is appealing to the motivated perioperative nurse practicing in ambulatory surgery. The patient scheduled for ambulatory surgery is often awake and involved in nurse-patient interactions throughout the entire perioperative period. The opportunities for an expanded role are numerous for the nurse specializing in the care of the ambulatory surgery patient. Disadvantages for health care professionals may include less control over patient issues (e.g., lack of compliance with preoperative teaching/instruction, lack of transportation, failure to secure responsible adult supervision after discharge), exclusion of rural and uninsured patients (in some cases), and lack of resources that are associated with traditional hospital structures.

## NURSING CARE FOR THE AMBULATORY PATIENT

Perioperative nursing in the ambulatory surgery setting incorporates all elements of the AORN standards of perioperative nursing (Box 28-2) and safe patient care practices, including those established by JCAHO (Patient Safety). However, the paradigm from which the perioperative nurse manages care of the ambulatory patient is very different from that of the hospitalized patient. The ambulatory patient is essentially healthy, and the time spent in the ambulatory setting is relatively short, ranging from a few hours to 1 day (23-hour stay); therefore the plan of care for the ambulatory surgical patient must be organized and efficient. To achieve this, many health care facilities are incorporating concepts of case management into the planning and implementation of care for patients who are inpatient and ambulatory. Care delivered in ambulatory surgery lends itself well to the use of the principles of case management, which provides a framework for care that overlays traditional utilization review, resource management, care management, and outcomes management.

BOX 28-2

### AORN Standards of Perioperative Nursing

**STANDARDS OF PERIOPERATIVE CLINICAL PRACTICE**

- Assessment
- Nursing diagnosis
- Outcome identification
- Planning
- Implementation
- Evaluation

**STANDARDS OF PERIOPERATIVE PROFESSIONAL PERFORMANCE**

- Quality of practice
- Practice evaluation
- Education
- Collegiality
- Collaboration
- Ethics
- Evidence-based practice
- Resource utilization
- Leadership

Responsibility for most of the preoperative and postoperative care is assumed by the patient and family or significant others. Therefore their education and preparation are an integral part of ambulatory surgery. The education process is continuous; it begins preoperatively and continues even after the patient is discharged. This allows for both the patient and the caregiver to be prepared for discharge requirements and recovery at home. The ultimate goal of providing education to the patient and family or significant others is to ensure adequate preparation for meeting postoperative care needs and establishing plans for seeking additional assistance, if necessary.

### Preoperative Phase

The surgeon, anesthesia provider, perioperative nurse, and patient should jointly determine the appropriateness of surgical intervention at an ambulatory facility. The patient's or family's fears and concerns regarding ambulatory surgery should be discussed before the decision to perform the procedure; patients should not feel that they are receiving a lesser standard of care because the procedure is scheduled at an ambulatory surgery facility. Once the determination is made to have the procedure at the ambulatory surgery facility, the patient is contacted to ensure proper preoperative preparation.

The process and content of education of patients, families, or significant others may vary from facility to facility. Important characteristics of an ideal preoperative preparation program include an accessible physical setting, a standardized process, multidisciplinary involvement, and a program for patient education that enhances involvement in self-care. The following information is presented to the patient by the perioperative nurse, physician, or physician office staff; it is usually reinforced with printed teaching material:

- Time and nature of surgery
- Location, parking, and suggested time of arrival at the ambulatory surgery center

## PATIENT SAFETY

### National Patient Safety Goals for Ambulatory Surgery

The Joint Commission on Accreditation of Healthcare Organizations develops annual National Patient Safety Goals (NPSGs) designed to protect the health and well-being of the public and to foster quality care in all organizations. The NPSGs established for the ambulatory setting are similar to the goals for inpatient settings.

**2006 Ambulatory Care National Patient Safety Goals**

*Goal:* Improve the accuracy of patient identification.

- Use at lease two patient identifiers (neither to be the patient's room number) whenever administering medication or blood products; taking blood samples and other specimens for clinical testing; or providing any other treatments or procedures.

*Goal:* Improve the effectiveness of communication among caregivers.

- For verbal or telephone orders or for telephonic reporting of critical test results, verify the complete order or test result by having the person receiving the order or test result (receiver) "read back" the complete order or test result to the "sender."
- Standardize a list of abbreviations, acronyms, and symbols that are *not* to be used throughout the organization.
- Measure, assess, and, if appropriate, take action to improve the timeliness of reporting and the timeliness of receipt by the responsible licensed caregiver of critical test results and values.

*Goal:* Implement a standardized approach to "hand off" communications, including the opportunity to ask and respond to questions (see Chapter 2 for a Best Practice on Hand-off Communication).

*Goal:* Improve the safety of using medications.

- Standardize and limit the number of drug concentrations available in the organization.
- Identify and, at a minimum, annually review a list of look-alike/sound-alike drugs used in the organization, and take action to prevent errors involving the interchange of these drugs.
- Label all medications, medication containers (e.g., syringes, medicine cups, basins), or other solutions on and off the sterile field in perioperative and other procedure settings.

*Goal:* Reduce the risk of health care–associated infections.

- Comply with current Centers for Disease Control and Prevention (CDC) hand hygiene guidelines.
- Manage as sentinel events all identified cases of unanticipated death or major permanent loss of function associated with a health care–associated infection.

*Goal:* Accurately and completely reconcile medications across the continuum of care.

- Implement a process for obtaining and documenting a complete list of the patient's current medications on the patient's admission to the organization and with the involvement of the patient. This process includes a comparison of the medications the organization provides to those on the list.
- A complete list of the patient's medications is communicated to the next provider of service when a patient is referred or transferred to another setting, service, practitioner, or level of care within or outside the organization.

*Goal:* Reduce the risk of surgical fires.

- Educate staff, including operating licensed independent practitioners and anesthesia providers, on how to control heat sources and manage fuels, and establish guidelines to minimize oxygen concentration under drapes (see Chapter 2 for a discussion of fire prevention and safety).

Modified from JCAHO ambulatory care, 2006 ambulatory care national patient safety goals. Accessed August 24, 2005, on-line: www.jcaho.org/accredited+organizations/patient+safety/06_npsg/06_npsg_amb.

- Food and liquid restrictions
- Medication use before surgery (take essential medications as prescribed by surgeon with a sip of water)
- Suggested clothing for discharge
- Necessary items to bring (e.g., glasses, hearing aid)
- Instructions regarding valuables
- Identification of responsible adult escort for discharge
- Whom to call for any questions before the procedure
- Necessary insurance papers to bring
- Resources available in the home

To assist in data collection and plan individualized care, the patient is asked health-related questions pertaining to pertinent physical disabilities; existing health conditions; previous surgeries and anesthetics with associated responses; and vital information such as height, weight, allergies (e.g., foods, medications, latex), and current medications, including use of herbal remedies and dietary supplements (see Chapter 32). This preoperative assessment may be completed in various ways, including interviews conducted by telephone, in the preadmission clinic, at the time of admission to the facility, and through completion of written questionnaires. Many facilities have websites where patients can complete registration forms online and take a virtual tour of the surgery center. Some facilities offer preoperative tours for patients and may provide education through videotapes the patient takes home to review. When such preadmission information is obtained before the day of surgery, the admitting process is shortened. Regardless of how the data are collected, they should be documented on the record that will be used the day of surgery to prevent duplication of information. Accurate and thoughtful preoperative assessment and patient education can result in optimal patient care, comfort, and satisfaction and may reduce or eliminate procedural delays or cancellations.

After admission to the facility and correct identification of the patient, the patient and family or significant others should be given an orientation to the facility and be provided with an explanation of the expected sequence of events. The patient then changes into surgical attire (if appropriate), and provisions are made for the safekeeping of clothing and any valuables the patient may have brought. The following assessment parameters are then obtained and documented by the perioperative nurse:

- Observation and assessment of general physical and psychosocial behavior, sensory-perceptual alterations, emotional status, interaction with family, and compliance with preoperative instructions

- Baseline vital signs
- Preoperative verification process (required laboratory values, radiographs, history, physical examination, surgical and anesthesia consents, etc.) and surgical site marking
- Administration of preoperative medications as prescribed
- Assessment of anxiety and apprehension related to impending surgical procedure
- Assessment of patient knowledge regarding impending surgical procedure, recovery, and postoperative care
- Assessment of patient expectations regarding postoperative pain management
- Development of appropriate plan of care

An IV line or lock may be inserted as ordered. The family or significant others should be permitted to stay with the patient in the preoperative area, and provisions should be made for their comfort. These persons are an integral part of the patient's well-being and should be included as part of the patient's surgical experience. Colorful surroundings and the promotion of relaxation through means such as music, television, or videos should be provided.

The patient may walk to the surgical suite or be transported by wheelchair or stretcher. The mode of transportation depends on the patient's abilities, the effects of medications if administered, and the policies of the facility. The family or significant others are directed to the waiting area, informed of the approximate time for the procedure, and made comfortable with refreshments, reading material, music, or television.

## Intraoperative Phase

Intraoperative nursing care for the ambulatory surgery patient is consistent with the *AORN Standards, Recommended Practices, and Guidelines* for any patient undergoing an operative or other invasive procedure. Perioperative nursing care responsibilities include the following:

- Identify the patient, introduce self, review the chart, and complete the preoperative verification process and surgical site marking policy/checklist.
- Report to the physician any relative or absolute contraindications to intraoperative medications that may be used based on the patient's medication history or noted allergies.
- Safely transfer the patient to the OR bed.
- Properly position the patient, and maintain correct body alignment.
- Assist anesthesia personnel as appropriate.
- After positioning, prepping, and draping, conduct and document the "time out."
- Administer medications for IV moderate sedation/analgesia under the direction of a physician.
- Monitor the patient receiving IV moderate sedation/analgesia, and report any changes, such as restlessness, cyanosis, pallor, flushing, diaphoresis, nausea, low oxygen saturation, dysrhythmias, and allergic or toxic reaction.
- Monitor for safety precautions, aseptic technique, skin integrity, and fluid and electrolyte balance.
- Document patient care according to facility policy and procedure.

It is common practice in ambulatory surgery for the patient to receive IV moderate sedation/analgesia administered or monitored by the perioperative nurse. In addition to the preoperative assessment parameters previously described, the nurse responsible for managing the care of the patient receiving IV moderate sedation/analgesia during the intraoperative phase should conduct a thorough nursing assessment (Box 28-3). The goal of this assessment is to determine any contraindications to the administration of IV moderate sedation/analgesia medications and patient appropriateness for nurse management.

The AORN has developed recommended practices that specifically address monitoring parameters applicable to the ambulatory patient in the intraoperative phase. These include "Recommended Practices for Managing the Patient Receiving Moderate Sedation/Analgesia" and "Recommended Practices for Monitoring the Patient Receiving Local Anesthesia."[2] These recommended practices, intended for optimal patient care, along with the "Guidance Statements on Preoperative Care of the Patient in the Ambulatory Surgery Setting and Postoperative Care of the Patient in the Ambulatory Surgery Setting" should be utilized by the perioperative nurse.

Many institutions require specific credentialing for both nurses and physicians involved in the administration of moderate sedation/analgesia. Credentialing may include specific competency-based education. The perioperative nurse who monitors the patient during moderate sedation/analgesia should be able to demonstrate knowledge of anatomy, physiology, pharmacology of medications, cardiac dysrhythmia interpretation, complications related to the use of IV moderate sedation/analgesia, principles of oxygen delivery and transport, and respiratory physiology.[1] Policies and procedures should be developed and in place based on guidelines and recommendations set forth by external agencies, such as the state board of nursing and standards of national nursing associations.

The perioperative nurse monitoring the patient receiving moderate sedation/analgesia should "have no other responsibilities that would require the nurse to leave the patient unattended or compromise continuous patient monitoring during

**BOX 28-3**

### Nursing Assessment for the Patient Receiving Intravenous (IV) Moderate Sedation/Analgesia

The perioperative nurse's review of the patient should include the following:

- Relevant physical examination findings
- Current medications (including prescription, over-the-counter, illicit, and herbal supplements/remedies)
- Allergies and sensitivities to medications, latex, etc.
- Current medical problems, such as hypertension, diabetes, cardiopulmonary disease, liver disease, and renal disease
- Smoking history
- Alcohol intake history
- Recreational drug use
- Presenting medical problems
- Baseline vital signs
- Level of consciousness
- Emotional state
- Nothing-by-mouth (NPO) status
- Pain assessment scale
- Communication ability
- Perceptions of sedation/analgesia and the procedure itself.

Modified from Association of periOperative Registered Nurses: *AORN ambulatory surgery principles and practices*, ed 3, Denver, 2004, The Association.

the procedure."[1] The patient's vital signs are monitored by use of electrocardiogram (ECG), pulse oximetry, noninvasive blood pressure monitor, and general observation. The perioperative nurse must be familiar with the various types of monitoring equipment and have an understanding of ECG interpretation. Oxygen and suction lines should be readily available. A second perioperative nurse should be assigned to circulating responsibilities during the procedure.

## Postoperative Phase

After completion of the surgical procedure, the patient is transferred to the appropriate postanesthesia care unit (PACU). The perioperative nurse or anesthesia provider communicates a complete hand-off report on the status of the patient, procedure performed, medications administered, dressings, and allergies to the receiving nurse. Ambulatory surgery is followed by a rapid recovery period, which includes two distinct phases. The first phase is emergence from anesthesia. The second phase allows for readaptation to the environment, during which the patient is encouraged to sit up, stand, void, and ambulate. Although not always possible, many ambulatory surgery facilities have separate phase 1 and phase 2 recovery areas. The type of anesthetic administered determines the area to which the patient is transferred after surgery.

***Phase 1.*** Assessment during phase 1 should be determined and established as a policy and procedure. This ensures that nursing staff use a uniform method of assessing all patients in phase 1. The most common assessment parameters include respiration, circulation, level of consciousness, skin color, and level of voluntary activity. A variety of scoring systems that are simple to use allow for standardized reporting, such as the Aldrete score (see Chapter 9).

***Fast-Tracking.*** Some patients may be able to meet criteria for discharge from phase 1 (Box 28-4) while they are still in the OR and may be transferred directly to phase 2, bypassing phase 1 completely. This concept is known as *fast-tracking* and has been made possible through the advent of anesthetic, analgesic, and muscle relaxant agents that allow for quicker onset, easier titration, and more rapid metabolism and clearance, allowing patients early emergence from anesthesia. With fast-tracking, fewer patients arrive in the PACU deeply sedated and the time that they are at risk for airway obstruction or hemodynamic instability is lessened, reducing the need for one-on-one nursing care.[7] Patients meeting fast-track criteria may be discharged within 1 hour of their surgical procedure. There are many advantages and disadvantages to the fast-tracking concept for both the patient and the ASC (Box 28-5) and institutional policies with defined criteria must be developed to ensure quality outcomes (Best Practice).

***Phase 2.*** Patients who are fast-tracking or who have received only local anesthesia, moderate sedation/analgesia, or a regional anesthetic may be taken directly to the phase 2 recovery area. The patient is monitored for light-headedness, dizziness, bleeding at the surgical or drain sites, nausea, vomiting, significant changes from baseline vital signs, pain, and psychomotor and cognitive function. Methods that may be used to assess psychomotor and cognitive function include paper-and-pencil tests, single reaction time, coordination and attention tests, ability to walk in a straight line, Maddox wing test (measures imbalance of extraocular muscles), flicker fusion test, and psychomotor test. Postoperative nursing care and responsibilities applicable to both phase 1 and phase 2 include the following:

- Assess for inadequate respiration/ventilation related to anesthesia or airway obstruction.
- Monitor risk for deficient fluid volume related to anesthesia or hypovolemia.
- Monitor for injury related to emergence delirium.
- Monitor for pain (Research Highlight).
- Monitor for nausea and vomiting related to anesthesia or surgical procedure.

### BOX 28-4

#### Discharge Assessment—Phase 1

1. Airway patency, respiratory function, and oxygen saturation
2. Stability of vital signs
3. Hypothermia resolved
4. Level of consciousness and muscular strength
5. Adequate pain control
6. Mobility
7. Patency of tubes, catheters, drains, intravenous lines
8. Skin color and condition
9. Condition of dressing and surgical site
10. Intake and output
11. Comfort
12. Anxiety
13. Child-parent/significant others interactions
14. Numeric score, if used

From American Society of PeriAnesthesia Nurses, *2002 Standards of Perianesthesia Nursing Practice,* Cherry Hill, NJ: American Society of PeriAnesthesia Nurses, 2002.

### BOX 28-5

#### Advantages and Disadvantages of Fast-Tracking Outpatients Undergoing Elective Surgical Procedures

**ADVANTAGES**

- Cost savings
  - Postanesthesia care unit (PACU) phase 1 care is eliminated
  - Overall decreased length of stay
- Most patients feel better and want to be discharged earlier

**DISADVANTAGES**

- Focus is on short-term, nonacute care for the following purposes:
  - Discharge teaching
  - Reuniting patient with caregiver
- Therefore patients should not require the following:
  - Continuous monitoring
  - Aggressive pain or nausea management
- PACU phase 2 nurses may not have critical care skills needed to recognize and manage emergency situations

Modified from Redmond MC: Postanesthesia assessment phase II. In DeFazio-Quinn DM, Schick L, editors: *Perianesthesia nursing core curriculum,* Philadelphia, 2004, Saunders.

## BEST PRACTICE

### Criteria Used to Determine Fast-Track Eligibility After Ambulatory Anesthesia

Fast-tracking of patients directly from the OR to phase 2 of the recovery area can be safely accomplished provided the patient meets appropriate criteria. Determination of patient criteria should be collaboratively established by anesthesia providers and perianesthesia nurses. In this scoring system, the patient must have a score of 12 or higher, with no score less than 1 in the individual categories to be eligible for fast-tracking.

| Criteria | Score |
|---|---|
| **LEVEL OF CONSCIOUSNESS** | |
| Awake and oriented | 2 |
| Arousable with minimal stimulation | 1 |
| Responsive only to tactile stimulation | 0 |
| **PHYSICAL ACTIVITY** | |
| Able to move all extremities on command | 2 |
| Some weakness in movement of the extremities | 1 |
| Unable to voluntarily move the extremities | 0 |
| **HEMODYNAMIC STABILITY** | |
| Blood pressure <15% of the baseline mean arterial pressure (MAP) value | 2 |
| Blood pressure between 15% and 30% of the baseline MAP value | 1 |
| Blood pressure >30% below the baseline MAP value | 0 |
| **RESPIRATORY STABILITY** | |
| Able to breathe deeply | 2 |
| Tachypnea with good cough | 1 |
| Dyspneic with weak cough | 0 |
| **OXYGEN SATURATION STATUS** | |
| Maintains value >90% on room air | 2 |
| Requires supplemental oxygen (nasal prongs) | 1 |
| Saturation <90% with supplemental oxygen | 0 |
| **POSTOPERATIVE PAIN ASSESSMENT** | |
| None or mild discomfort | 2 |
| Moderate to severe pain controlled with intravenous (IV) analgesics | 1 |
| Persistent severe pain | 0 |
| **POSTOPERATIVE EMETIC SYMPTOMS** | |
| None, or mild nausea with no active vomiting | 2 |
| Transient vomiting or retching | 1 |
| Persistent moderate to severe nausea and vomiting | 0 |
| TOTAL SCORE | 14 |

Wherever fast-tracking of patients is practiced, there should be written guidelines addressing patient selection, preoperative patient education, selection and management of anesthetic agents, monitoring and reporting of patient outcomes, and discharge criteria.

Modified from AORN guidance statement: postoperative patient care in the ambulatory surgery setting. In Association of periOperative Registered Nurses: *AORN standards, recommended practices, and guidelines*, Denver, 2006, The Association; White PF, Freire AR: Ambulatory (outpatient) anesthesia. In Miller RD, editor: *Miller's anesthesia*, ed 6, Philadelphia, 2005, Churchill-Livingstone.

## RESEARCH HIGHLIGHT

### Postoperative Pain and Discharge from the Ambulatory Surgery Setting

Postoperative pain is one of the most frequently cited factors responsible for delayed discharge from ambulatory surgery units. This study sought to determine the severity of postoperative pain and analgesic use after six commonly performed outpatient procedures. Other goals of the survey were to analyze the role of pain and other side effects on return to activities of daily living and on patient satisfaction with the recovery process.

A total of 175 patients were enrolled in the study for a period of 6 months. Procedures included in the study were knee arthroscopy, inguinal hernia repair, pelvic laparoscopy, transvaginal uterine suspension, breast surgery, and plastic surgery. Baseline data were collected through assessment preoperatively and postoperatively before discharge. Follow-up assessment was conducted through phone calls to the patient's home. During the postdischarge period, the patients rated their pain on a 0 to 10 scale (0 = no pain, 10 = worse pain imaginable) for the first 24 and 48 hours after discharge from the center and also recorded the effect of pain on their sleep, number and type of pain medications used (and their estimated percent reduction in pain), and any side effects or symptoms attributable to the pain medications. Patients' postdischarge activity level was also assessed.

The results showed that 60% of patients reported pain of at least a moderate degree (>3/10) and that the pain interfered with sleep in 46% of patients surveyed. The researchers noted that nausea and vomiting and constipation reported as side effects from pain medication were also present in 45% to 46% of the patients. Activity level was reported at 33% of normal at 24 hours and 47% of normal at 48 hours. The reasons for activity limitation cited by patients were pain (54%), fatigue (17%), drowsiness (7%), and nausea (1%). Satisfaction decreased as pain and nausea increased.

This study, although relatively small in its sample size, provides baseline information that can be useful in designing pain protocols in the ambulatory surgery arena with a focus on prevention of pain and the side effects of analgesic use.

Modified from Pavlin DJ and others: A survey of pain and other symptoms that affect the recovery process after discharge from an ambulatory surgery unit, *Journal of Clinical Anesthesia* 16:200-205, 2004.

- Protect areas desensitized by the administration of a local anesthetic agent.
- Monitor for alteration in circulation related to surgical procedure, dressing, or cast.
- Encourage early ambulation and progressive fluid ingestion as appropriate.
- Document plan of care according to facility policy and procedure.
- Provide and review appropriate written discharge instructions.

The perioperative nurse documents the care given and progress of the patient throughout the postoperative phase (Figure 28-2). The patient and family or significant others review the discharge instructions with the perioperative nurse, receive clarification, and have the opportunity to ask questions. The patient is discharged when home readiness is determined.

Date: ____ / ____ / ____

Procedure suite: ❑ Cath Lab ❑ Radiology ❑ GI lab ❑ Derm

Other ____________________

Planned monitoring: ❑ EKG ❑ BP cuff ❑ Pulse oximeter

❑ Other ____________________

Procedure ____________________

Physician ____________________

RN performing conscious sedation ____________________

Other ____________________

**Time-Out**

Initiated by: __________ Initials of staff participating in "Time-Out" __________ Time: ______

❑ Identity of the patient

❑ Verification of procedure

❑ Verification of Site and Side .................. ❑ N/A

❑ Correct patient position...................... ❑ N/A

❑ Verification of implants or special equipment ..... ❑ N/A

❑ Radiological images ........................ ❑ N/A

❑ Patient Stable and appropriate for planned anesthetic

**Discrepancy noted, Surgeon notified** __________ date __________ time

Physician's final side/site directive with Physician's signature ____________________

**INTRAPROCEDURE**

| TIME | |
|---|---|
| MEDICATION | |
| | |
| | |
| | |
| | |
| | |
| IVF | |
| | |
| | |
| | |
| EBL/U.O. | |
| SEDATION | |
| PAIN | |
| $O_2$ Source | |
| $O_2$ SAT | |

**RECORD VITAL SIGNS OR ATTACH STRIP BELOW**

| | |
|---|---|
| V BP Λ | 180 |
| | 160 |
| | 140 |
| | 120 |
| • HR | 100 |
| | 80 |
| | 60 |
| • RR | 40 |
| | 20 |
| ECG Tracing | |

**NURSING PROCEDURE NOTES**

RN

FIGURE 28-2 Example of form for procedure and postprocedure recovery.

*Continued*

❑ Patient identified using two indicators ❑ N/A If no transfer of care

## POST PROCEDURE RECOVERY

| | | |
|---|---|---|
| V BP Λ | 180 | |
| | 160 | |
| | 140 | |
| | 120 | |
| ● HR | 100 | |
| | 80 | |
| | 60 | |
| ● RR | 40 | |
| | 20 | |
| ECG Tracing | | |
| $O_2$ SAT | | |
| PAIN | | |
| DRESSING | | |

## NURSING PROCEDURE NOTES

RN

| RECOVERY SCORE | TIME | | | PHASE 2 OUTPATIENT | TIME | | |
|---|---|---|---|---|---|---|---|
| ACTIVITY<br>Able to move 4 extremities voluntarily or on command 2<br>Able to move 2 extremities voluntarily or on command 1<br>Unable to move extremities voluntarily or on command 0 | | | | VITAL SIGNS<br>BP and pulse within 20% of preoperative baseline 2<br>BP and pulse 20%-40% of preoperative baseline 1<br>BP and pulse >40% of preoperative baseline 0 | | | |
| RESPIRATION<br>Able to breathe deeply and cough freel 2<br>Dyspnea, limited breathing or tachypnea 1<br>Apneic or on mechanical ventilator 0 | | | | ACTIVITY LEVEL<br>Steady gait, no dizziness, or meets preoperative level 2<br>Requires assistance 1<br>Unable to ambulate 0 | | | |
| CIRCULATION<br>BP plus or minus 20% of pre-anesthetic level 2<br>BP plus or minus 20% - 40% of pre-anesthetic level 1<br>BP plus or minus 40% of pre-anesthetic level 0 | | | | NAUSEA & VOMITING<br>Minimal to none 2<br>Moderate 1<br>Severe 0 | | | |
| CONSCIOUSNESS<br>Fully awake 2<br>Arousable on calling 1<br>Not responding 0 | | | | PAIN<br>Minimal to pain free 2<br>Moderate pain handled by oral medication 1<br>Severe pain requiring parenteral medication 0 | | | |
| $O_2$ SATURATION<br>Able to maintain $O_2$ saturation > 92% on room air 2<br>Needs $O_2$ inhalation to maintain $O_2$ saturation > 90% 1<br>$O_2$ saturation < 90% even with $O_2$ supplement 0 | | | | SURGICAL BLEEDING<br>Minimal to none 2<br>Moderate 1<br>Severe 0 | | | |
| TOTAL PAR / SCORE | | | | TOTAL PADS / SCORE | | | |
| SCORE = ≥ 8 RETURN TO INPATIENT UNIT. | | | | SCORE = 9 OR 10 DISCHARGE HOME. | | | |

**OUTPATIENT DISCHARGE CRITERIA**

- ❑ PADS score ≥ 9
- ❑ Able to void ❑ N/A
- ❑ Instructions reviewed
- ❑ Emergency contact given
- ❑ Patient demonstrates understanding
- ❑ Discharged with an adult escort
- ❑ Discharged Home

Time ______

- ❑ Transferred to unit report given

## NURSING DIAGNOSES AND PATIENT OUTCOMES

| OUTCOME CRITERIA MET | YES | NO | REASON |
|---|---|---|---|
| **1. Anxiety**<br>Outcome: The patient participates in decisions affecting his/her plan of care; the patient's right to privacy is maintained. | | | |
| **2. Alteration in Comfort: Pain**<br>Outcome: The patient demonstrates knowledge of pain management; the patient demonstrates and/or reports adequate pain control throughout the procedure. | | | |
| **3. Knowledge Deficit**<br>Outcome: The patient demonstrates knowledge of physiological and psychological responses to medications and procedure. | | | |
| **4. Potential for Injury**<br>Outcome: The patient is free from signs and symptoms of physical injury; The patient receives appropriately prescribed medications, safely administered by a qualified practitioner, during the procedure. | | | |
| **5. Ineffective Breathing Pattern**<br>Outcome: The patient's respiratory pattern is consistent with the baseline level established pre-procedure. | | | |

______________________ RN

FIGURE 28-2, cont'd

## Discharge

Each ambulatory surgery facility must have written guidelines that have been approved by the anesthesia and medical staff to outline criteria for patient discharge (see Figure 28-2). Regulatory agencies such as the JCAHO allow authorized personnel to discharge patients when the criteria are met. It is unlikely that a physician will be available to discharge every ambulatory surgery patient; therefore the registered nurse often has a greater responsibility in patient discharge in the ambulatory setting than in the inpatient arena. The nurse is the person most likely responsible for determining appropriateness of meeting the specified criteria and home readiness. The criteria may be predetermined as a set of standing discharge orders or written separately as an order by the surgeon. Criteria to determine home readiness are intended to meet the needs of the patient, nursing staff, and facility. The following is a list of common discharge criteria that may be applied to the ambulatory surgery patient:

- Order from the physician
- Stable vital signs
- No evidence of respiratory depression
- Oriented to person, place, and time
- Ability to void, as appropriate
- Ability to take fluids orally, as appropriate
- Ability to dress
- Ability to ambulate without assistance, as appropriate
- Minimal nausea, vomiting, and dizziness
- No excessive pain, as reported on a pain assessment scale
- No bleeding or excessive drainage
- Written discharge instructions that include possible complications, activity restrictions, diet, medications, wound care and hygiene, precautions, and plan for follow-up care
- Responsible adult escort

The ambulatory surgery patient should understand that recovery and convalescence are not complete on discharge. The patient is instructed not to plan to resume usual activities until at least 1 day after surgery and often longer. Discharge instructions related to possible complications, activity restrictions, diet, medications, pain management, wound care, and the plan for follow-up care are reviewed and reinforced with the patient and family or significant others. At the time of discharge, printed instruction forms, written in lay terms, are reviewed and signed and a copy is given to the patient, family member, or significant others. Any additional questions regarding postoperative care are answered. Instructions on how the patient or family should handle any questions, problems, or complications and information on what kind of problems and complications should be reported to the surgeon or back to the surgery center are provided.

Although it is anticipated that most patients will return home in the care of family or friends, some patients may not be able to be discharged to home without some additional form of assisted care. Options for care beyond the ambulatory surgery setting include admission to a 23-hour observation unit or short-stay unit; discharge to a recovery center, or release to home with home health care assistance. Many ambulatory surgery facilities contract with specific recovery centers or home care agencies to provide various types of assisted care. Possible indications for home health care follow-up referral after ambulatory surgery include a lack of support system, the need for complex postoperative care such as dressing change or IV medications, the need for assistance with activities of daily living, and pain management. Home health care personnel can assist in meeting the needs of the patient, thus avoiding a hospital stay.

On discharge from the facility, patients are often given a questionnaire to complete at their convenience. The questionnaire provides the facility feedback about its services, any postoperative complications the patient may experience, and any additional comments or suggestions from the patient. It is one way to measure the quality of services provided by the facility. In most ambulatory surgery programs, the perioperative nurse contacts the patient with a follow-up phone call 24 hours after surgery to evaluate recovery and general condition and to answer any questions regarding care (Box 28-6). The nurse should inform the patient and responsible adult that they will be contacted by a phone call for postoperative follow-up and should confirm the patient's telephone number and best time to call. The patient is advised to consult the surgeon for any complications related to the surgical procedure. In addition, the perioperative nurse may notify the surgeon regarding the complication. Postoperative calls are an important tool for the ambulatory facility to determine patient satisfaction and effectiveness of care (Research Highlight).

# CONTINUING EDUCATION AND PERFORMANCE MEASUREMENT

Continuing education and staff development for all staff members must be relevant, ongoing, and documented. Staff should annually attend educational programs on cardiopulmonary resuscitation (CPR), fire safety, emergency preparedness, and infection prevention and control practices (see Chapter 3). Other educational opportunities may include staff development programs related to technologic advances, new procedures, IV moderate sedation/analgesia, updated AORN standards and recommended practices, and performance measurement and improvement activities. Ongoing education

**BOX 28-6**

### Sample Questions for a Postoperative Phone Call

- Do you have any problems relating to your procedure?
- Is your pain controlled?
- What level of pain are you experiencing (scale of 0 to 10)?
- Have you taken any pain medications?
- Did you receive verbal and written instructions?
- Did you understand the instructions given?
- How did you find your stay on the unit?
- How could we improve the service we provide?
- Is there anything we could have done to make your stay better?

Allow questions to arise naturally during the conversation and respond accordingly.

Modified from Ontiveros JE, Schick L: Postprocedure follow up. In DeFazio-Quinn DM, Schick L, editors: *Perianesthesia nursing core curriculum*, Philadelphia, 2004, Saunders.

## RESEARCH HIGHLIGHT

### Patient Perceptions Following Day Surgery

This qualitative study used data collected from telephone interviews with 228 day surgery patients. Using a standard protocol that allowed the opportunity to answer questions and provide advice, the nurse researcher identified many misconceptions that patients held about their recovery process, pain management, and side effects from pain medications. Each patient was telephoned daily on the first 3 days after discharge.

During these phone calls, a number of findings related to discharge instructions were uncovered. All patients received written discharge instructions as well as verbal discharge instructions. Many patients did not recall verbal information they had been given at the time of discharge because they were too groggy or sleepy, had not been feeling well enough to be discharged, and therefore were not able to absorb the information provided. Even after the first phone call by the nurse researcher, patients did not remember those instructions on day 2 of the phone calls. By the third day, the patients anticipated the call and had questions to ask.

Several beliefs and misconceptions about pain and pain management were identified during the calls:

- Pain and activity: a number of patients thought they should experience some pain, were reluctant to take pain medication for fear they would "overdo it," and had numerous questions regarding appropriate activity level. For example, they were concerned that going up and down stairs might open their incision; if told not to lift, they needed more guidance about what kinds of lifting restrictions were to be enacted.
- Pain is to be endured: despite high levels of pain, some patients were reluctant to contact their surgeons. Others believed that taking a "lot of pain medication" should be avoided.
- Pain medication has side effects: many patients were very concerned about constipation (they had been told this might occur). Some maintained a light diet, such as "soup only," to avoid eating in bulk and then becoming constipated.
- Doing the right thing for themselves: Patients needed specific instructions on caring for themselves correctly. General instructions, such as "drink plenty of water" was imprecise. Specific advice was needed such as "Drink three glasses of water and/or fruit juice." Those who had undergone anal surgery had misconceptions about sitz baths, not understanding fully the role of the sitz bath in promoting healing and comfort.

The findings of this research emphasize the importance of providing specific, clear information to patients. In addition, questions developed over time in relationship to the surgery and pain. Thus information about contacting a physician or nurse with questions and concerns should be emphasized to patients and their families or significant others. Given the findings of attitudes toward pain, the researcher recommended that these attitudes be explored preoperatively as part of pain management education.

Modified from Dewar A and others: Telephone follow-up for day surgery patients—patient perceptions and nurse expectations, *Journal of PeriAnesthesia Nursing* 19(4):234-241, 2004.

should also be provided that addresses age-specific and cultural and ethnic aspects of the populations served. Observation and assessment skills are essential in ambulatory surgery nursing and should be updated periodically. Yearly assessment and verification of skills and competencies must be documented.

Performance measurement and improvement, along with continuing education, promote high-quality patient care. Standards used in quality-improvement activities include structure standards (management of the facility), process standards (what the nurse does for the patient), and outcome standards (what the patient can expect from the nursing care). The facility's performance measurement and improvement program must identify the scope of services provided and important aspects of care (Box 28-7). For effective monitoring and evaluation of care given, performance measurement and improvement activities must identify indicators that will be used to monitor the important aspects of care. Ongoing performance measurement and improvement activities are an important part of the care delivered in the ambulatory surgery setting and should look at the service aspect of the facility from the patient's perspective. Ambulatory surgery has led perioperative services in the delivery of efficient, cost-effective service. Patient satisfaction tools often lead to opportunities for operational improvement that promote efficiency and patient satisfaction.

The rapid shift to and acceptance of ambulatory surgery as an alternative to inpatient care has increased the pressure on ambulatory surgery facilities to demonstrate the best value to payers and patients alike. Outcomes measurement extends beyond traditional measures of quality of surgical programs such as patient satisfaction, morbidity and mortality, and infection rates to examination of quality and costs across the continuum of care for each patient.

## DOCUMENTATION

Medicolegal and risk management principles of documentation guide the manager and staff of an ambulatory surgery facility in the development and revision of existing patient records. Using the AORN recommended practices for documentation of perioperative nursing care as a guide, the following should be included in patient record forms:

- Face sheet (e.g., demographics)
- Consent for surgical procedure and anesthesia
- Advance directives
- History and physical examination reports
- Health history
- Applicable laboratory test results
- Preoperative and postoperative instruction sheets
- Preoperative nursing assessment sheet
- Preoperative verification process/checklist
- Physician order sheet
- Anesthesia record
- Local anesthesia and moderate sedation/analgesia records
- Intraoperative record
- Postoperative record
- Report of operation
- Pathology report, when applicable

It is important to streamline forms and documentation, allowing the attention of the team to be focused on the patient,

BOX 28-7

### Suggestions for Quality Measurement and Improvement: Ambulatory Surgery Patient Care

**Important Aspect of Care**: Preoperative assessment and patient education

*Indicators:*

- ◆ A preoperative nursing assessment is completed for each ambulatory surgical patient. The assessment includes the following:
  - Verification of the patient's identity using two identifiers
  - Review of the preadmission assessment/patient survey
  - Baseline physical assessment
  - Medication review
  - Notation of any allergies or sensitivities (medications, latex, etc.)
  - Nothing-by-mouth (NPO) status
  - Temperature assessment and management to prevent unplanned hypothermia
  - Confirmation of prescribed surgical preparation, such as preoperative shower, bowel prep, medications
  - Consents for surgery and anesthesia signed
  - Contact information for the patient's support person
- ◆ The learning needs of the patient, patient's family, and significant others are identified and recorded.
- ◆ Preoperative teaching and discharge planning/instructions are written and reviewed with the patient, family, significant others; demonstration of understanding is documented on the nursing plan of care.

**Important Aspect of Care**: Patient safety

*Indicator:*

- ◆ Patient is free from injury related to transfer/transport; perioperative positioning; extraneous objects; medication administration; hypothermia; fluid volume imbalance; and chemical, laser, radiation, and electrical hazards.

**Important Aspect of Care**: Discharge planning

*Indicators:*

- ◆ A physician is present until the patient has been assessed and determined to be medically ready for discharge after anesthesia has been administered.
- ◆ A responsible escort will accompany the patient when discharged and will be present before the start of surgery.
- ◆ Pain management and patient knowledge of pain and pain control are discussed.
- ◆ Appropriate referrals are made and communicated.
- ◆ There is written permission to leave postoperative follow-up telephone messages by voice mail or with a designated individual in accordance with Health Insurance Portability and Accountability Act of 1996 (HIPAA) privacy guidelines.

**Important Aspect of Care**: Skin integrity

*Indicators:*

- ◆ Skin is assessed preoperatively and postoperatively.
- ◆ Skin assessment is documented on nursing plan of care.

**Important Aspect of Care**: Management of physiologic functions for the patient receiving intravenous (IV) moderate sedation/analgesia

*Indicators:*

- ◆ Nasal cannula is in place for all patients.
- ◆ Vital signs are stable throughout the surgical procedure.
- ◆ Nausea and vomiting are evaluated.
- ◆ Level of consciousness and pulse oximetry readings are continually assessed.
- ◆ Management of pain is assessed and documented.

**Important Aspect of Care**: Patient satisfaction

*Indicators:*

- ◆ Patient surveys with comment cards are sent.
- ◆ All returned patient questionnaire complaints are recorded, and suggested improvements are noted.

**Important Aspect of Care**: Documentation

*Indicators:*

- ◆ A process is in place for procedure and surgical site verification, and the patient is involved in the process.
- ◆ The surgical site is marked by the person performing the procedure.
- ◆ The surgical team verifies the patient's identify, the intended procedure, and the correct surgical site and ensures that all equipment planned for use in the procedure is immediately available.
- ◆ A time out is conducted immediately before starting the procedure.
- ◆ Nursing record is completed according to established policy and procedures.
- ◆ Clinical records contain abbreviations and dose designations according to the standardized list approved by the facility.
- ◆ Patient response to IV moderate sedation/analgesia medications is documented.
- ◆ Consent form is correctly completed.
- ◆ Physician orders are documented and signed by the nurse.

Quality measurement and improvement activities should be delineated as part of a written program in the ambulatory surgery center. Goals and objectives should be identified and a process developed to identify problems and concerns that need to be addressed. The areas identified are then addressed through activities such as studies or benchmarking. Benchmarking is undertaken to compare key performance measures with other organizations or best practices.

Modified from AAAHC clarifies standards for 2005, *OR Manager* 21(4), 2005; AORN Guidance Statement: Preoperative care in the ambulatory surgery setting. In Association of periOperative Registered Nurses: *AORN standards, recommended practices, and guidelines*, Denver, 2006, The Association.

not on documentation. Many ambulatory surgery facilities have become leaders in the development and use of multidisciplinary records that prevent redundancy and duplication of information among caregivers. The same record often follows the patient through initial contact, preoperative preparation, intraoperative and postanesthesia care, and discharge planning. The shift away from paper records to computerized record keeping is an improvement that allows for easier access to patient data within the facility and also promotes streamlining of documentation. Storing the patient data in a computerized file accessible to all team members can eliminate duplicate charting and questioning.

All forms should be reviewed periodically and revised as needed. Interdisciplinary participation in review and revision will help ensure that the forms are easy to use and contain relevant information fields required by the staff.

## POLICIES AND PROCEDURES

The purpose of a policy and procedure manual is to provide a framework for daily operation of a facility. The manual should provide information that describes the expected course of action to be followed; as such, it becomes part of the institutional standard of care. A comprehensive policy and procedure manual is an effective tool for communication, education, and prevention of risks for injury if correctly followed. Policies and procedures for the ambulatory surgery facility may differ in form and content from institutional hospital regulations because of governing body, ownership, medical staff, accrediting and licensing bodies, and management.

## FUTURE TRENDS

Ambulatory surgery will continue to be a driving force in the growth of ambulatory care. As the health care system in the United States undergoes change, the ambulatory surgery arena will feel the effect. Key issues in health care reform include access to service, quality of care, and cost containment. Each affects ambulatory surgery facilities, and strategic plans to maintain continuity and success in the marketplace need to be developed with foci on consumer need, improving outcomes, and decreasing cost, without compromising safety or quality of care. With the continued expansion of technology, particularly in minimally invasive surgery, patients are provided with an alternative modality of treatment and surgery will continue to be performed outside the OR in areas such as the interventional radiology department, mobile surgery units, and physician offices. This will reshape the scope of ambulatory surgery services. Patient-centered care will remain an important component of patient satisfaction for the continued success of ambulatory surgery, as will the mandate to document outcomes of care from both a patient-satisfaction and cost perspective.

## SUMMARY

As ambulatory surgery continues to grow and flourish, perioperative nursing care is the most constant and pervasive part of the service. Care that was formerly spread over a period of several days is now completed in a few hours. Perioperative nurses practicing in ambulatory surgical care settings find themselves continuing to adapt to new technology, cross-training, working in an atmosphere of flexible professional roles and teamwork, and managing care across the surgical patient's continuum.

## REFERENCES


1. Association of periOperative Registered Nurses: *AORN ambulatory surgery principles and practices*, ed 3, Denver, 2004, The Association.
2. Association of periOperative Registered Nurses: *AORN standards, recommended practices, and guidelines*, Denver, 2006, The Association.
3. Federated Ambulatory Surgery Association, 2005. Accessed August 5, 2005, on-line: www.fasa.org.aschistory.html.
4. Odom-Forrester J: Evolution of perianesthesia care. In DeFazio DM, Schick L: *Perianestheisa nursing core curriculum*, St Louis, 2004, Saunders.
5. Stanksi DR, Shafer SL: Measuring the depth of anesthesia. In Miller RD: *Miller's anesthesia*, ed 6, Philadelphia, 2005, Churchill Livingstone.
6. Vila H and others: Comparative outcomes analysis of procedures performed in physician offices and ambulatory surgery centers, *Archives of Surgery* 138(9):991-995, 2003.
7. White PF, Freire AR: Ambulatory outpatient anesthesia. In Miller RD: *Miller's anesthesia*, ed 6, Philadelphia, 2005, Churchill Livingstone.

# CHAPTER 29

# Pediatric Surgery

JOANNE STOW

Pediatrics is a specialty focused on the health and well-being of neonates, infants, children, and adolescents. The pediatric patient's need for surgery is frequently because of congenital anomalies that threaten life or the child's ability to function. Trauma also impacts a child's health far more often than an adult's; injury is the number one cause of death in the pediatric population after the first year of life[21] and a common reason for surgical intervention. Pediatric surgery is an area of practice unto its own because the pediatric patient is so very different from an adult, and this field is even further subdivided into all the surgical specialties. It is important to recognize that the difference between pediatric care and adult care is not just a size issue; from birth onward, the body and organs exist in a continual state of development, and multiple physiologic changes occur with age. Major areas of distinction are the airway and pulmonary status, cardiovascular status, temperature regulation, metabolism, fluid management, and psychologic development. A thorough knowledge of these differences is integral to the provision of nursing care for the pediatric patient in the operating room (OR).

Advances in the surgical interventions for children have been phenomenal in the last 2 decades for many reasons. Improved diagnostic and interventional technology, the development of new anesthetics and pharmacologic agents for pain management, and the creation of even smaller and more delicate instrumentation have revolutionized perioperative care of the pediatric population. Numerous pediatric surgeries that were once performed as open cavity procedures are now being done endoscopically with minimally invasive techniques, resulting in shorter hospital stays and faster recovery times. Examples of procedures that are now being performed using these techniques include Nissen fundoplication, pectus excavatum repair, shoulder and ankle arthroscopies, and pyeloplasty. The expansion of high-risk pregnancy centers for mothers with problem pregnancies has resulted in earlier detection of malformations in fetuses, leading to the exciting frontier of fetal surgery. Improvements in the transport of critically ill children, neonatal and pediatric intensive care management, and the development of new surgical procedures are also saving more lives yet presenting medical professionals with a new and unique set of problems as complex, medically fragile children are now surviving into adulthood.

## PEDIATRIC SURGICAL ANATOMY

### Airway/Pulmonary Status

Respiratory mechanics alter dramatically from infancy to adulthood, resulting from increasing airway size, transformations in rigidity of airway and chest structures, and major neuromuscular changes. A proportionally large head, a short neck, and a large tongue in relation to jaw size create more of a challenge for airway management. The glottis is very anterior, moving from the level of the second cervical vertebrae to the level of the third to fourth vertebrae in the adult. The epiglottis is floppy and more curved, and the vocal cords are slanted anteriorly. The airway forms an inverse cone with the narrowest portion at the cricoid cartilage until 8 years of age; endotracheal tube size is therefore very important, since a tube that passes easily through the glottis may be too tight at the subglottic area, compromising the child's airway in the immediate postoperative period because of swelling. The infant is an obligate nasal breather, and the chest wall of an infant is very compliant, leading to increased work of breathing with any type of airway compromise. Infants also have type 2 respiratory muscle fibers until age 2 years, which fatigue more easily than type 1 muscle fibers. Premature infants are at risk for postanesthetic apnea until 60 weeks after conception age. There is a depression in the $CO_2$ response curve in infants; respiratory rate does not increase as readily in response to a rising $CO_2$ level as an adult, although all ages undergo a $CO_2$ response depression related to inhalational agents and narcotics. One of the most important considerations is that children have a much smaller pulmonary functional residual capacity; a child becomes hypoxic more quickly if the airway is lost. Alveolar maturation is not complete until 8 years of age. Smaller airways have higher resistance; airway resistance decreases approximately 15 times from infancy to adulthood, again with a major change occurring around 8 years of age. It is important to note that smaller airways can become compromised with even a minor amount of swelling. Be aware that loose teeth are common in children from ages 5 to 14 years; a dislodged tooth is a potential airway foreign-body risk.

### Cardiovascular Status

The most dramatic changes in the cardiovascular system occur at birth with the transition from fetal circulation. Even in full-term infants, persistent transitional circulation may occur. Heart rate is the predominant determinant of cardiac output in infants and children; bradycardia drastically decreases cardiac output and requires swift intervention. There is a decreased cardiac compliance because of a lower proportion of muscle to connective tissue until age 1 to 2 years, making infants preload insensitive. Young children are predisposed to parasympathetic hypertonia (increased vagal tone), which can be induced by painful stimuli such as laryngoscopy, intubation, eye surgery, or abdominal retraction. Attention to blood loss in young patients is very important because the patient's total blood volume is very small. Blood volume in neonates is 80 to 90 ml/kg;

at 1 to 6 years it is 70 to 75 ml/kg; and at age 6 years to adult it is 65 to 70 ml/kg. At birth, 70% to 90% of the hemoglobin is fetal hemoglobin with a high affinity for oxygen. It is normal for hemoglobin levels to fall at about 2 to 3 months of age (physiologic anemia) to a hematocrit of 29% and a hemoglobin of 10 mg/dl as the infant's body begins to produce its own blood cells. A cardiology evaluation is essential if a murmur is auscultated. A murmur can be from a patent foramen ovale, which normally closes at 3 to 12 months, a patent ductus arteriosus, which can be present for up to 2 months, a previously undetected cardiac anomaly, or an innocent flow murmur; the evaluation is critical because anesthetic agents cause vasodilation and are potentiators for cardiac dysrhythmias.

### Temperature Regulation

Infants and young children are most at risk of hypothermia because of their increased body surface area/weight ratio and thin fat layer. Cold stress leads to increased oxygen consumption, resulting in hypoxia, respiratory depression, acidosis, hypoglycemia, and pulmonary vasoconstriction. Hypothermia alters drug metabolism, prolongs the action of neuromuscular blockers, and delays emergence. The child's temperature must be monitored continuously throughout the intraoperative experience. An axillary temperature probe is acceptable for short procedures in healthy children; an esophageal or rectal temperature probe provides more accurate monitoring of the child's temperature for longer cases. Hyperthermia should also be avoided, leading to increased oxygen consumption and increased fluid losses.

Thermoregulatory interventions include altering the room temperature before the child enters the room, using a water-filled temperature-regulating blanket under the patient, or using a forced air–warming blanket over nonsurgical areas of the child. An overhead heater can be used during the anesthetic induction and patient preparation period immediately before prepping and draping. The anesthesia ventilation circuit can be heated and humidified. Warmed solutions should be provided at the sterile field for use instead of room temperature solutions for surgical procedures with large areas of exposure. Intravenous (IV) solutions can also be warmed before administration. It is vital to maintain normothermia in children.

### Metabolism

Infants have a higher basal metabolic rate than adults, and it is greatest at 18 months. Most importantly, children under age 2 years have immature liver function; pharmacologic response is altered, and there is slower hepatic clearance, decreased hepatic enzyme function, and decreased protein binding. Drug distribution is different in neonates and infants compared with older children and adults because of an increased percentage of total body weight and extracellular body fluid. Infants have an immature blood-brain barrier and decreased protein binding, which results in an increased sensitivity to sedatives, opioids, and hypnotics (Patient Safety).

### Fluid Management

Renal function at birth is immature, and the ability of the kidneys to concentrate urine is limited, so the infant is much more prone to dehydration. Complete maturation of renal function occurs at about 2 years. A child has a higher body water weight than an adult, a higher body surface area, and an increased metabolic rate, resulting in increased fluid requirements per kilogram of body weight. Despite these significant points, it is also important to remember that the body weight of the child, the length of time without fluids, and surgical losses are the primary factors in the calculations of the child's hydration needs.

## PSYCHOLOGIC DEVELOPMENT

A child's comprehension of and responses to the environment are based on his or her developmental age. A key factor is that a child's developmental age does not necessarily match the chronologic age. Nursing care should be tailored to the developmental age of the child to optimize the child's ability to understand what is going on, to minimize the child's and family's stress and anxiety, and to facilitate the development of a trusting and supportive medical relationship. The types of fears that a child has are also related to his or her level of psychologic development. Predictable stages mean predictable behaviors. The stages of growth have been described from a variety of different aspects; Dr. Jean Piaget described the stages by changes in cognition and the ability to think, and Dr. Erik Erikson based the stages on psychosocial and emotional needs. Their work provides an excellent guideline for assessing the pediatric patient's developmental level in order to use appropriate interventions (Table 29-1).

## *Perioperative Nursing Considerations*

### Assessment

The initial patient assessment provides information necessary to develop a plan of care specific to the needs of each particular pediatric patient related to age, developmental level, and diagnosis. The unique aspects of care of the pediatric surgical patient revolve around the fact that the child is constantly growing and changing. The perioperative nurse must have a good understanding of the normal physical and psychologic parameters for pediatric patients and be able to recognize deviations from these parameters. In addition, the perioperative nurse must be familiar with normal growth and development factors for each age-group. During any given day, the perioperative nurse may care for a variety of pediatric patients ranging from neonates through adolescents.

In some instances, children undergoing an ambulatory surgical procedure may visit the OR complex and ambulatory surgery area with their families 1 to 2 weeks before surgery, depending on the developmental level of the child and the availability of a preoperative pediatric education program. If the child has a complex medical history or an extensive surgical procedure is planned, the child and family members will meet with a member of the anesthesia team during this advance visit. A tour is provided by a child life specialist, along with pictures and age-appropriate explanations of what the child will see and experience. Visiting before the day of surgery can help decrease the anxiety related to the novelty of the experience.

Sometimes the child's history and physical, surgical consent, and any necessary tests or lab work are done in advance

## PATIENT SAFETY

### Safe Medication Administration in Pediatric Patients

Administering medications to children differs from medication administration for adults. Children metabolize medications at different rates and in some cases may require less or more medication than adults. Factors that influence metabolism of medication in children are often related to maturity and body composition. Premature and newborn infants have immature renal systems and liver enzyme systems. Lower plasma concentrations of protein influence drug binding. Children have less circulating volume than adults and are more vulnerable to dehydration, increasing the risk for overdosage.

The United States Pharmacopoeia (USP), a nongovernment organization that establishes quality standards for medications, identified improper dose (quantity), omission, and wrong time as the top three medication errors affecting pediatric patients. The responsibility for providing a timely and correct dose of medication to a child is a shared one between the physician who orders the medication and the nurse who administers it.

The perioperative nurse should carefully evaluate all pediatric dosages, and if the dose is out of range, or if there is any question about the validity of the dose, the nurse must consult with the physician who ordered the dose. Because many drugs are potentially hazardous or lethal, many institutions require certain critical medications to be double-checked by another individual before they are administered. Examples of these medications include digoxin, heparin, insulin, epinephrine, opioids, and sedatives.

Pediatric medication dosages are most accurately calculated using a formula that factors the child's age, weight, and body surface area (BSA). The BSA is determined by plotting the child's estimated weight and height on a nomogram, a device that uses graphic representation to predict an outcome. The BSA is then applied to a formula to arrive at the safest dose for the child.

A formula that uses BSA is:

$$\frac{\text{BSA of child}}{\text{BSA of adult}} \times \text{Adult dose} = \text{estimated child's dose}$$

In the perioperative setting many medications are given by the intravenous (IV) route. The nurse should consider the following factors when preparing and administering medications to infants and children by the IV route:

- Amount of medication to be administered
- Minimum dilution of the medication and if the child is fluid restricted
- Type of solution in which the medication should be diluted
- Length of time over which the medication can be safely administered
- Rate of infusion that the child and his or her vessels can safely tolerate
- IV tubing volume capacity
- Compatibility of all medications that the child is receiving intravenously and compatibility with the infusion fluids

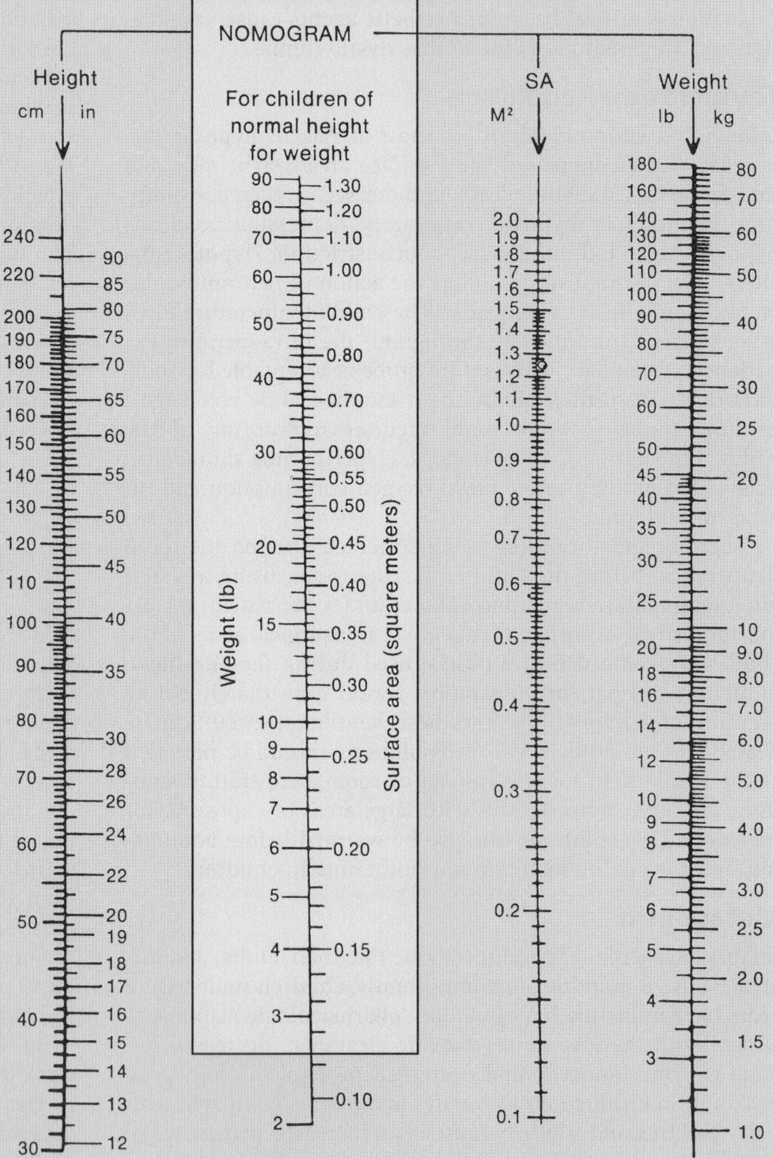


BSA is indicated where a straight line connecting the height and weight intersects the surface area (SA) or, if the patient is of normal proportion, from weight alone (tinted area).

Modified from Algren C, Arnow D: Pediatric variations of nursing interventions. In Hockenberry MJ and others, editors: *Wong's nursing care of infants and children,* ed 7, St Louis, 2003, Mosby; Pediatric medication safety position statement, *AORN Journal* 83(1):111-112, 2006.

**TABLE 29-1**

## Developmental Stages

| Approximate Ages | Piaget's Stage | Erikson's Stage | Developmentally Based Fears | Appropriate Nursing Interventions |
|---|---|---|---|---|
| Infancy–1 yr (Erikson)<br>Infancy–2 yr (Piaget) | Sensorimotor<br>Uses senses and motor skills to understand the world<br>Develops memory, begins to imitate others | Trust versus mistrust—develops belief that the world can be counted on to meet basic needs<br>Who to trust? Identifies strangers at 7-8 mo | Separation | Use soothing voice; sing, hold child, give child objects to hold to provide distractions. Meet child, family without touching child at first. Allow personal item into operating room (OR) for comfort/security. |
| Toddlerhood | Preoperational<br>Use of symbols, creative play (can pretend)<br>Is very egocentric | Autonomy versus shame, doubt<br>Develops free will; increasing control of their bodies<br>Feels regret, sorrow for inappropriate behavior | Separation<br>Forced dependence | Give only simple choices; involve child in actions when possible, use distractions, sing songs child may recognize. Allow personal item into OR for comfort/security. |
| Early childhood, preschool | Preoperational continues | Initiative versus guilt<br>Begins to explore, imagine<br>Feels remorse for actions<br>Thinking dominated by perceptions—distorted reasoning | Separation<br>Body mutilation | Magical thinkers—use stories during induction. Likes colorful Band-aids. Allow child to handle unfamiliar objects to decrease stress (i.e., mask, pulse oximeter probe). Allow personal item into OR for comfort/security. |
| Middle childhood, elementary school age (Erikson)<br>Ages 7-11 yr (Piaget) | Concrete operations<br>Uses symbols, logic, principles to solve problems<br>Classifies, sorts everything | Industry versus inferiority<br>Beginning to understand time and unseen body functions<br>Is cooperative, desires recognition for achievements | The unknown<br>Body mutilation<br>Inadequate performance | Provide simple information to decrease stress. Be honest at all times. Do not expect child to act like an adult yet. Allow personal item into OR for comfort/security. |
| Adolescence, puberty | Formal operations<br>Uses logical and abstract thinking<br>Understands hypothetical concepts | Identity versus role diffusion<br>Peer group has increased importance<br>Body image, clothing, activities help define identity | Altered body image<br>Death | Query patient about concerns; offer information to decrease fears. Provide as much privacy as possible if disrobing is necessary. Use mental imagery to decrease stress. Offer to hold hand to provide comfort; personal item still permitted. |

Modified from *Piaget's developmental theory.* Accessed April 28, 2006, on-line: www.psybox.com/web_dictionary/Developmentaltheory.htm; *Stages of social-emotional development in children.* Accessed April 28, 2006, on-line: www.childdevelopmentinfo.com/development/erickson.shtml.

in the surgeon's office setting, and the child and family have no introduction to the surgical experience until the day of surgery. Information related to the child's scheduled procedure is either sent home with the family from the surgeon's office or mailed to them the week before the surgery is scheduled. The facility where the surgery will be performed contacts the family on the day before the surgery to tell them when to bring the child in and to go over preoperative eating and drinking instructions. In these instances, the initial interview performed by the perioperative nurse in the day-surgery unit is especially crucial to provide a thorough, documented assessment of the child's growth (height and weight), current physical status (vital signs, heart and breath sounds, skin integrity), current medication history, allergies, nothing-by-mouth (NPO) status, recent illnesses, current medical concerns, and behavioral responses to the interview process. The day-surgery nurse confirms the intended surgical procedure with the child and family as it is written on the surgical consent and their understanding of the operation. This information is critical to the intraoperative nursing team's plan of care during the surgical procedure.

Children who are inpatients may be visited by a perioperative nurse in the hospital on the day before surgery. The patient's chart is reviewed, with particular attention given to the patient's age, developmental level, diagnosis, and intended surgical procedure. Current nursing diagnoses and ongoing plan of care are examined. A discussion with the primary nurse can facilitate data collection, assist in providing continuity of care, and provide the perioperative nurse with information regarding preoperative education done thus far. The perioperative nurse can meet the child and any family members present at the time of the visit. The interview can be used to gather information helpful to developing the intraoperative plan of care and decrease the anxiety related to the child's impending surgery by providing a familiar face on the day of the procedure. The focus of this visit is to discuss the perioperative process, not always to provide preoperative education regarding the surgery. In pediatric centers in the inpatient setting, preoperative education may be provided by the primary nurse, child life therapist, or clinical nurse specialist. During the preoperative visit the perioperative nurse can explain what the child will experience in the preoperative, intraoperative, and postoperative phases of care at a developmentally appropriate level. The perioperative nurse may briefly describe the roles of various staff members who will be a part of the team responsible for the child's care in the OR. Common concerns that families express are regarding the length of time that they are separated from their child and their child's pain management (Research Highlight). Explanations to children should be provided within a developmental framework, taking into account each one's cognitive and psychosocial abilities. Medical play items, audiovisual aids, puppets, and photographs are all helpful in the education process.

The circulating nurse who will be participating in the intraoperative care of the child will review the patient's information and meet with the patient and the family before the child is brought to the OR in the holding area. In addition to reviewing the documentation performed by the preoperative holding nurse, the circulating nurse validates the patient's identification using two patient identifiers and confirms that the surgeon has marked the child's surgical site per institutional protocol. If implants are to be used, availability must be confirmed before the patient's transport to the surgical suite. Frequently children will be given a premedication in the 20- to 45-minute period before their transportation to the OR. A premedication such as midazolam can greatly decrease a child's anxiety, minimizing the stress of separation for both child and family. The surgeon and anesthesia provider will each meet with the child and family, usually while the OR is being prepared for the patient. The circulating nurse will assess the child's psychologic state, review the intended surgical procedure with the child and family, and make sure that they have no additional questions or concerns. A final communication among the anesthesia provider, surgeon, and nursing staff for the room confirms the team's state of readiness for the delivery of care before the circulating nurse brings the child to the OR.

## RESEARCH HIGHLIGHT

### Improving Pain Management in Pediatric Patients

It is essential that pain be assessed and managed in all patients. In this study, researchers at Stanford University in California were interested in improving pain management interventions in pediatric patients undergoing liver transplantation, a very painful procedure. A program was developed consisting of pretransplant parental education, preoperative and postoperative behavioral consultation, postoperative physical and occupational therapy consultations, and implementation of a variety of nonpharmacologic pain management techniques.

The study compared the historical data of 13 children who underwent liver transplantation before the implementation of the program with 14 children who did participate in the pain management intervention program. Mean age at transplant was 53.8 months in the historical group and 63.6 months in the intervention group. There were no differences in intensive care unit (ICU) stay, total postoperative length of stay, total inpatient length of stay, time to extubation, or opioids used through postoperative day 6. The study did find differences between the two groups in pain scores and parental perception of pain. The intervention program group showed decreases in mean pain scores (2.12 compared with 2.82 in the historical group), decreases in parental pain perception scores (2.1 compared with 3.1 in the historical group), and an increase in pain assessments during a 12-hour shift (6.79 versus 3.43 in the historical group).

Modified from Sharek PJ and others: Improved pain management in pediatric postoperative liver transplant patients using parental education and non-pharmacologic interventions, *Pediatric Transplantation* 10(2):172-177, 2006.

***Informed Consent.*** Informed consent from the parent or legal guardian of the pediatric patient is required unless the patient is an emancipated minor. An emancipated minor is one who is legally under the age of majority but is recognized as having the legal capacity to consent. Minors may become emancipated by pregnancy, marriage, high school graduation, living independently, and military service. Collaboration from patients ages 7 years and older can involve the child or adolescent in the decision-making process and be a gesture of respect.[1] It is important for children to develop a trusting relationship with medical professionals and that these older children are in agreement (within their developmental capabilities) with their family's decision regarding surgery.

***Child Abuse and Neglect.*** Perioperative nurses are obligated to screen all pediatric patients for abuse or neglect. Child abuse and neglect are defined as "physical or mental injury, sexual abuse or exploitation, negligent treatment or maltreatment."[4] Child abuse is found in all segments of society, crossing cultural, ethnic, religious, socioeconomic, and professional groups. The perioperative nurse is in a unique situation to assess for the presence of abuse because the patient will be disrobed in the OR. Box 29-1 lists the clinical manifestations of child abuse. Every state has a child abuse law that spells out legal responsibility for reporting abuse and suspicion of abuse, and nurses are mandated reporters. Failure to report suspected child abuse could result in a fine or other punishment, according to individual statutes.[4]

## Nursing Diagnosis

Nursing diagnoses related to the care of pediatric patients undergoing surgery might include the following:

- Anxiety related to separation from family and friends
- Fear related to developmental level (fear of the unknown, fear of painful procedures and surgery)
- Risk for Infection related to surgical intervention and other invasive procedures
- Risk for Imbalanced Fluid Volume related to invasive surgery and accompanying blood loss
- Risk for Hypothermia related to loss of body surface heat to environment and immature temperature-control mechanism

## Outcome Identification

Perioperative nursing care is predicated on relevant nursing diagnoses and their corresponding desired outcome. Outcomes should be measurable with criteria by which to judge their attainment. Thus for the desired outcome "The patient will

BOX 29-1

**Clinical Manifestations of Child Abuse and Neglect**

**SKIN INJURIES**

Skin injuries are the most common and easily recognized signs of maltreatment of children. Human bite marks appear as an ovoid area with tooth imprints, suck marks, or tongue thrust marks. Multiple bruises in inaccessible places are indications that the child has been abused. Bruises in different stages of healing may indicate repeated trauma. Bruises that take the shape of a recognized object are generally not accidental.

**TRAUMATIC HAIR LOSS**

Traumatic hair loss occurs when the child's hair is pulled or used to drag or jerk the child. The result of the pulling on the scalp can cause the blood vessels under the skin to break. An accumulation of blood can help differentiate between abusive and nonabusive loss of hair.

**FALLS**

If a child is reported to have had a routine fall but has what appear to be severe injuries, the inconsistency of the history with the trauma sustained indicates suspected child abuse.

**EXTERNAL HEAD, FACIAL, AND ORAL INJURIES**

Cuts, bleeding, redness, or swelling of the external ear canal; facial fractures; tears or scarring of the lip; oral, perioral, and/or pharyngeal lesions; loosened, discolored, or fractured teeth; dental caries; tongue lacerations; unexplained erythema or petechiae of the palate; and bilateral black eyes without trauma to the nose may all indicate abuse.

**DELIBERATE OR UNEXPLAINED THERMAL INJURIES**

Immersion burns, with clear line of demarcation; multiple small circular burns, in varying stages of healing; iron burns (show iron pattern); diaper area burns; and rope burns suggest intentional harm.

**SHAKEN BABY SYNDROME**

A shaken baby may suffer only mild ocular or cerebral trauma. The infant may have a history of poor feeding, vomiting, lethargy, and/or irritability that occurs periodically for days or weeks before the initial health care consult. In 75% to 90% of the cases, unilateral or bilateral retinal hemorrhages are present but may be missed unless the child is examined by a pediatric ophthalmologist. Shaking produces an acceleration-deceleration (shearing) injury to the brain, causing stretching and breaking of blood vessels resulting in subdural hemorrhage. Subdural hemorrhage may be most prominent in the interhemispheric fissure. However, cerebral edema may be the only finding. Serious insult to the central nervous system may result, without evidence of external injury.

**UNEXPLAINED FRACTURES AND DISLOCATION**

Posterior rib fractures in different stages of healing, spiral fractures, or dislocation from twisting of an extremity may provide evidence of nonaccidental injury in children.

**SEXUAL ABUSE**

Abrasions or bruising of the inner thighs and genitalia; scars, tearing, or distortion of the labia/hymen; anal lacerations or dilation; lacerations or irritation of external genitalia; repeated urinary tract infections; sexually transmitted disease; nonspecific vaginitis; pregnancy in young adolescent; penile discharge; and sexual promiscuity may provide evidence of sexual abuse.

**NEGLECT**

The symptoms of neglect reflect a lack of both physical and medical care. Manifestations include failure to thrive without a medical explanation, multiple cat or dog bites and scratches, feces and dirt in the skinfolds, severe diaper rash with the presence of ammonia burns, feeding disorders, and developmental delays.

From Betz CL, Sowden LA: *Mosby's pediatric nursing reference,* ed 5, St Louis, 2004, Mosby.

demonstrate some ability to manage anxiety," measurable criteria (e.g., the child will have posture, facial expressions, gestures, and activity levels that reflect decreased anxiety and will demonstrate increased focus) might be identified.

Outcomes identified for the selected nursing diagnoses for the pediatric patient could be stated as follows:

- The child will demonstrate some ability to manage anxiety.
- The child will verbalize less fear.
- The child will remain free from signs and symptoms of surgical site and invasive procedure site infection.
- The child will be maintained in a state of fluid and electrolyte balance.
- The child will be maintained in a state of normothermia.

## Planning

Assessment data, combined with information about the planned surgical procedure, enable perioperative nurses to anticipate requirements for surgical positioning, instrumentation, equipment and supplies, medications, and activities necessary for the provision of safe, competent care for the pediatric patient. Knowledge of the child's developmental level allows the nurse to plan her or his approach and interactions with the child and family. The perioperative nurse identifies criteria appropriate to the child and surgical setting for each of the desired outcomes. A typical plan of care for the pediatric patient is shown on p. 1072.

## Implementation

Age-appropriate communication is important in implementing the pediatric nursing plan of care. Implementation begins during the perioperative nursing assessment and continues through discharge to the postanesthesia care unit (PACU) or other area. The presence of a parent during much of the preoperative period, including induction in the OR and in the PACU after emergence, can help decrease anxiety for both young children and their families.

Infants, reliant on family to meet their basic needs, are difficult to pacify when NPO for surgery. Provide rocking chairs, pacifiers, warm blankets, and simple distractions such as music or toys (Figure 29-1). Encourage the family to provide fluids for the infant right up to the deadline for NPO status. Unnecessary delays should be avoided at all costs. Parents may need reassurance and support during the period immediately before surgery.

The toddler or preschooler fears parental separation and abandonment. Toddlers fear, among other things, strangers,

## SAMPLE PLAN OF CARE

**NURSING DIAGNOSIS**

**Anxiety** related to separation from family and friends

**OUTCOME**

The child will demonstrate some ability to manage anxiety; a toy or other comfort/security object will remain with him or her, and he or she will cooperate with requests.

**INTERVENTIONS**

- Provide an atmosphere of warmth and acceptance for both child and family members.
- Maintain a calm and relaxed manner; try to smile at the child. Talking with the child, being calm, and smiling can provide comfort.
- Explain to the child when he or she will be reunited with parents.
- When speaking, try to get down to the child's eye level so he or she can see your face. Speak softly and slowly. Do not assume you were understood. Repetition may be necessary.
- Allow the child to keep familiar security objects (e.g., toy, blanket).
- Administer preoperative sedation as prescribed; note effects.
- Encourage parents to stay with the child as long as permitted and according to their wishes.
- Encourage parents to hold child until child falls asleep, if desired (may vary according to institution policy).
- Touch the child, and hold his or her hand.

**NURSING DIAGNOSIS**

**Fear** related to developmental level (fear of the unknown, fear of painful procedures and surgery)

**OUTCOME**

The child will verbalize less fear; he or she will respond in an age-appropriate manner to comfort measures and recognize that the perioperative nurse is there to help.

**INTERVENTIONS**

- Assess the child's growth and development, noting any variations from expected normal age-appropriate maturational levels.
- Provide preoperative education for the child and family, using audiovisual aids such as photographs, drawings, items for medical play, or a tour of the surgical suite.
- Provide explanations on the child's level and on the parent's level of understanding; use age-appropriate terminology that is familiar to the child, such as for body function.
- Place unfamiliar equipment out of the child's view to decrease fear.
- Encourage the child to handle items that may seem strange or threatening.
- Reassure the child that certain body parts can be removed without producing harm (e.g., blood, tonsils, appendix).
- Provide ongoing age-appropriate explanations for procedures/events during the perioperative period. Do not try to explain everything at once; explain procedure-by-procedure.
- Allow choices whenever possible, such as wearing pajamas or clothing to the operating room (OR).
- Respect need for modesty; expose only those body parts necessary.
- Provide diversional activities to decrease fear.
- Use pain assessment questions if the child is fearful of procedures (see Box 29-3).
- Do not lie to the child; be honest about the possibility of pain or discomfort.
- Reassure the child that you are there to help.

**NURSING DIAGNOSIS**

**Risk for Infection** related to surgical intervention and other invasive procedures

**OUTCOME**

The child will remain free from signs and symptoms of infection at the surgical site and invasive procedure sites; the surgical site will heal by first intention, and white blood cell count and differential will remain within normal limits.

**INTERVENTIONS**

- Administer antibiotic prophylaxis as prescribed.
- Follow Standard Precautions.
- Maintain aseptic technique, and monitor members of the surgical team for breaks in technique.
- Teach family members signs and symptoms of surgical site infection:
  - Redness
  - Swelling
  - Warmth
  - Tenderness
  - Pain
- Teach family members importance of and proper handwashing techniques.
- Apply dressing to surgical site before sterile drapes are removed to prevent contamination of incision.

**NURSING DIAGNOSIS**

**Risk for Imbalanced Fluid Volume** related to invasive surgery and accompanying blood loss

**OUTCOME**

The child will maintain fluid balance as evidenced by blood pressure within expected/acceptable range, palpable peripheral pulses, moist mucous membranes, and absence of peripheral edema.

**INTERVENTIONS**

- Maintain and protect patency of intravenous lines.
- Review laboratory analyses for results of total blood volume.
- Calculate estimated total blood volume using formula of 85 to 90 ml/kg of body weight if total blood volume has not been determined by laboratory tests.
- Provide gram scales for weighing sponges discarded from operative field; weigh sponges, and report estimated loss.
- Provide suction units with reservoirs that measure in 5-ml to 10-ml increments.
- Measure and record quantity of irrigating fluid used.
- Provide appropriate amounts of intravenous fluid replacement (e.g., 250-ml containers).
- Measure and record urinary output and output from other drainage tubes.
- Send laboratory specimens for analysis as indicated; review results indicating fluid status.

**NURSING DIAGNOSIS**

**Risk for Hypothermia** related to loss of body surface heat to environment and immature temperature-control mechanism

**OUTCOME**

The child will maintain normothermia as evidenced by body temperature within normal limits/expected range.

**INTERVENTIONS**

- Adjust room temperature approximately 1 hour before arrival of the child: 26°C to 27°C (78.8°F to 80.6°F) for infants and newborns; 23°C to 24°C (73.4°F to 75.2°F) for older children.
- Keep child covered as much as possible.
- Consider wrapping lower extremities in Webril or stockinette and encasing in plastic bag for newborns and infants.
- Provide radiant heat lamp for use during placement of monitoring lines, induction of anesthesia, positioning, skin prep, and draping.
- Warm blankets, skin prep solutions (according to manufacturer's instructions), and irrigation and other solutions to body temperature before use.
- Use warmers during administration of intravenous fluids and blood products; temperature settings should not exceed 38°C (100.4°F).
- Monitor body temperature by rectal, esophageal, tympanic membrane, or other automatic temperature-monitoring device.
- Document temperature at prescribed intervals; take appropriate action for temperature extremes.

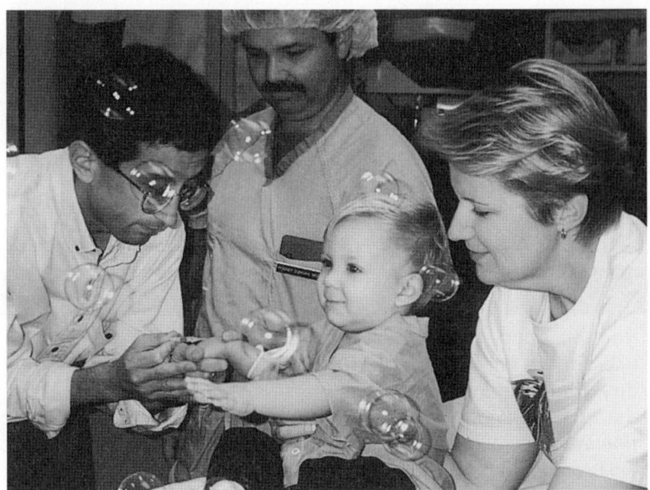

**FIGURE 29-1** The use of distraction technique during induction.

the dark, and machines. They attribute lifelike qualities to inanimate objects, believing that the objects, like them, have feelings. Thus a blood pressure cuff that squeezes the child's arm may be perceived to be doing so because it is angry with the toddler. Toddlers may also believe that their body is held together by their skin; anything that violates the skin integrity is feared. For this reason, bandages are very important. Toddlers and preschoolers interact with the environment using their senses. To integrate this into the patient's care, the perioperative nurse should give the toddler the opportunity to touch and play with objects that he or she will encounter. An example is to give the child a small anesthesia mask to put on his or her teddy bear. Sensory information should be provided in a soft, gentle voice: what things will look like and feel like and what the toddler will touch and hear. A security object is extremely comforting. The OR should be quiet; background noise should be controlled. Instruments that are frightening should be kept from view. The toddler should be brought into the room when everything is ready to allow quick induction of anesthesia.

The school-age child may still perceive hospitalization or surgery as a punishment but can evaluate painful intrusive actions in terms of logical function (e.g., getting an IV line hurts, but then I can get medicine in it to make me feel better). Feelings of inadequacy may be associated with something the child thinks he or she should be expected to do or know. Fear of body injury or mutilation, loss of control, and fear of the unknown characterize this developmental stage. These children benefit from simple, concrete explanations in familiar terms; a book or other teaching aid can be helpful. The concepts of time and unseen body functions can now be incorporated in the explanations. The child should be allowed to make choices when possible (e.g., letting the child decide which hand to place the IV line in or which flavor to add to the anesthetic mask).

Adolescents may fear altered body image, peer rejection, disability, and loss of control or status. The fear of death is more prevalent in this age-group than any other, and adolescents may find explanations of monitoring and safety measures reassuring. They need as much privacy as possible, and their attempts to be independent should be respected (e.g., walking into the OR instead of being wheeled in on a stretcher if the patient has not been sedated). The adolescent may not wish to show any fear; questions might not be asked while the parents are present. Information and explanations should be provided as reasonably and truthfully as possible. If appropriate, some choices should be allowed, such as wearing underwear to the OR. Patient care procedures that violate privacy, such as hair removal, skin preparation, or insertion of an indwelling urinary catheter, should be conducted after the patient is anesthetized.

Key points in providing perioperative care to pediatric patients include remaining alongside the child until the child is anesthetized, keeping the room quiet during induction, accepting a child's need to express fear and fearful behaviors (e.g., crying), and using simple words to explain care without double meanings (Table 29-2). Security objects should remain with the child until induction has been completed. A child's behavior during induction is likely to be the same during emergence; thus all attempts should be made to provide calm, reassuring care. Parents should be alerted to delays in the surgery schedule; in some instances, the child may be allowed to have fluids if the surgery is delayed by several hours.

Implementing the nursing plan of care includes continual reassessment of the patient's needs as well as the efficient execution of activities that facilitate the surgical intervention. Remaining with the child during induction, positioning, prepping the surgical site, creating and maintaining a sterile field, collecting, documenting and disposing of specimens, and administering medications, are all part of helping to provide a safe environment for the pediatric surgical patient. Making sure that the pediatric patient's family receives regular updates of the child's status is also a part of the perioperative nurse's responsibilities and will decrease their anxiety and help foster

**TABLE 29-2**

**Selecting Nonthreatening Words or Phrases**

| Word/Phrase to Avoid | Suggested Substitutions |
|---|---|
| Shot, bee sting, stick | Medicine under the skin |
| Organ | Special place in the body |
| Test | See how (specify body part) is working |
| Incision | Special opening |
| Edema | Puffiness |
| Stretcher, gurney | Rolling bed |
| Stool | Child's usual term |
| Dye | Special medicine |
| Pain | Hurt, discomfort, "owie," "boo-boo" |
| Deaden | Numb, make sleepy |
| Cut, fix | Make better |
| Take (as in "take your temperature, take your blood pressure") | See how warm you are; check your pressure; hug your arm |
| Put to sleep, anesthesia | Special sleep |
| Catheter | Tube |
| Monitor | TV screen |
| Electrodes | Stickers, ticklers |
| Specimen | Sample |

From Algren C, Arnow D: Pediatric variations of nursing interventions. In Hockenberry MJ and others, editors: *Wong's nursing care of infants and children*, ed 7, St Louis, 2003, Mosby.

a sense of trust in the health care professionals caring for their child.

***Instrumentation.*** The same types of instruments used in adult surgery are used in pediatric surgery. However, pediatric instruments are usually shorter, have more delicate or less pronounced curves, and are smaller. A complete range of instrument sizes is necessary to make the appropriate size available to each child, since pediatric patients can range in size from less than 1 kg to more than 100 kg. Fewer instruments are normally required because incisions in children are shorter and shallower than those in adults. Use of basic instrument sets, grouped according to types of surgery performed (e.g., minor, major), facilitates instrument counts. These sets are easily adapted to the patient's needs as well as the surgeon's needs and eliminate unnecessary instruments from the sterile field.

The following sets are examples of instrumentation used in pediatric surgery. The minor set is used for procedures such as inguinal hernia repair, head and neck procedures, and pyloromyotomy. The major set is used for major chest and abdominal cases, such as tracheoesophageal fistula (TEF) and diaphragmatic hernia repair, omphalocele repair, bowel resection, and pull-through for Hirschsprung's disease. Smaller and larger instruments should be in separate, additional sets to be dispensed to the surgical field as determined by the patient's size.

In addition to basic instruments, the minor pediatric instrument set should include curved Knapp iris scissors, both sharp and blunt; a Jacobsen curved clamp for delicate dissection; straight and curved Halstead mosquito clamps; sharp and blunt Senn retractors (two of each); 0.5-mm Castroviejo forceps; single-toothed Adson forceps; 6-inch fine DeBakey forceps; a small Weitlaner retractor; an Andrews-Pynchon 9½-inch suction; sizes 7 and 9 Fr Frazier suctions; a Castroviejo locking needle holder, and two Webster needle holders. The major pediatric instrument set should include the components of the minor set, slightly longer (7- to 8-inch) basic instruments (scissors, forceps, needle holders) and the following: curved Schnidt forceps; fine Kelly clamps; Gemini right-angled clamps; Army-Navy, small Deaver, and Richardson retractors (two of each size); Gerald forceps; Singley ring forceps; a set of malleable retractors; a grooved director; and a Poole suction.

***Sutures.*** A variety of sutures are used with the pediatric population because of the wide range of patient size; needles from size 0 to 7-0 are routinely stocked. Both absorbable and nonabsorbable sutures on cutting and tapered needles are employed. The most frequently used sizes are 3-0 to 5-0 with ½- and ⅜-circle needles. Staples, both pediatric and regular sizes, are oc-

## HISTORY

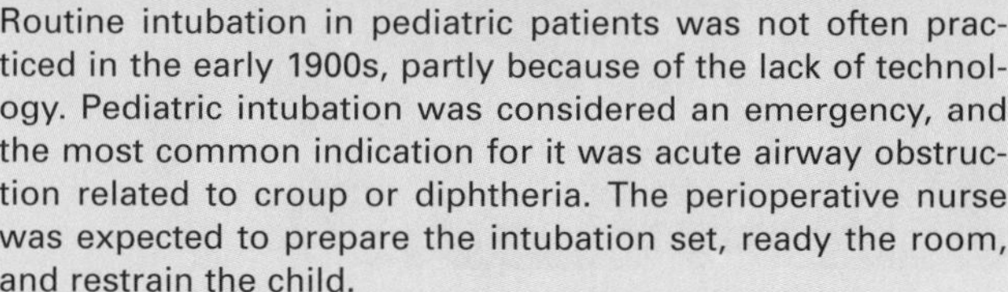

Routine intubation in pediatric patients was not often practiced in the early 1900s, partly because of the lack of technology. Pediatric intubation was considered an emergency, and the most common indication for it was acute airway obstruction related to croup or diphtheria. The perioperative nurse was expected to prepare the intubation set, ready the room, and restrain the child.

The intubation set consisted of a mouth gag, an introducer (known as the "intubator"), an "extubator" (used to remove the tube), and a graduated set of metal endotracheal tubes sized according to the age of the patient. Umbilical tape or heavy silk was threaded through the tube, and each tube was attached to an obturator.

The perioperative nurse was responsible for the position of the patient, and the success of the intubation depended largely on the nurse's ability to adequately restrain the child. The nurse placed a chair near a window to take advantage of natural light and arranged for a lamp to be used with the surgeon's head mirror. The nurse wrapped the child tightly in a sheet and sat in the chair with the child's feet held between her knees, the back of the child's head rested on her shoulder, and her arms encircled the child's torso. Another assistant held the child's head back and held the mouth gag in place. The tube was inserted, and the silk or umbilical tape was tied around the patient's ear or taped to the cheek.

The tube was left in place for 2 to 7 days, with the child often restrained to prevent self-extubation. The nurse assisted with removal of the tube and was then responsible for observing the patient afterward because edema and dyspnea were common after this procedure.

Modified from Allen GC, Stool SE: History of pediatric airway management, *Otolaryngologic Clinics of North America* 33(1):1-13, 2000; Harmer B: *Textbook of the principles and practice of nursing,* New York, 1925, Macmillan.

**TABLE 29-3**

**Recommended Sizes and Distance of Insertion Endotracheal Tubes and Laryngoscope Blades for Use in Pediatric Patients**

| Age | Internal Diameter of Endotracheal Tube (mm) | Recommended Size of Laryngoscope Straight Blade | Distance of Insertion (cm) |
|---|---|---|---|
| Premature (<1250 g) | 2.5 | 0 | 6-7 |
| Full term | 3.0 | 0-1 | 8-10 |
| 1 yr | 4.0 | 1 | 11 |
| 2 yr | 5.0 | 1-1.5 | 12 |
| 6 yr | 5.5 | 1.5-2 | 15 |
| 10 yr | 6.5 | 2-3 | 17 |
| 18 yr | 7-8 | 3 | 19 |

From Cote CJ: Pediatric anesthesia. In Miller RD: *Miller's anesthesia*, vol 2, ed 6, Philadelphia, 2005, Churchill Livingstone.

casionally used. Many skin incisions are closed with subcuticular techniques, over which adhesive strips or Dermabond (a type of skin adhesive) is then applied. The use of tape to apply dressings is done conservatively because of the delicate nature of children's skin; frequently either a small transparent or elastic net dressing is used to hold gauze dressings in place.

***Anesthetic Considerations.*** Anesthesia is approached differently in pediatric patients than it is in adults. The equipment and supplies are scaled down to match the size of the patient, and different anesthesia circuits and delivery systems may be used. The most common technique used in the pediatric population is a general inhalational anesthetic administered by facemask, laryngeal airway, or endotracheal tube. Selection of the endotracheal tube involves several considerations; the tube must be large enough to permit ventilation but small enough to minimize damage to the trachea while maintaining a seal to prevent aspiration (History box). Pressure from the cuff can cause tracheal damage.[7] Uncuffed endotracheal tubes are used in children up to 8 years of age. Table 29-3 provides a guide to choosing endotracheal tubes and laryngoscope blades for pediatric patients.

Microdrip IV tubing and burettes are commonly used to avoid the administration of excess fluids in pediatric patients under the age of 8 years, and only 500-ml bags of IV solution are used. The patient's IV line is usually started in the OR after induction with mask anesthesia, depending on the patient's diagnosis and medical history. Patients who require emergency surgery who have not been NPO; have increased intracranial pressure, an unusually difficult airway, or neuromuscular disease; or have been diagnosed with malignant hyperthermia require an IV placement before anesthetic induction. If the IV line is started before induction, measures should be taken to lessen the discomfort, such as an intradermal injection of 1% buffered lidocaine or saline at the site or the application of topical anesthetic creams (Best Practice). If possible, the surgical team should allow the child the option of sitting up or lying down during IV placement; hold the child's hand and tell him or her each step that will be done as the IV line is placed if developmentally appropriate.

Preoperative sedation is generally accomplished by the oral administration of midazolam. Midazolam is the most commonly used pediatric premedication used in the United States and can be given orally, nasally, rectally, intramuscularly, or intravenously.[7] Oral midazolam should be administered in a flavored base to mask the bitter taste. Relaxation is noted 15 to 45 minutes after administration; the child should be kept in a safe, observable environment after being medicated. Other agents used for premedication include fentanyl and, infrequently, ketamine.

Depending on institutional policy, a parent may be present during induction to comfort the child and decrease the child's anxiety. An explanation of what the OR will look like, who will be present in the room, how the child's anesthetic induction will be performed, and what the child will look like as the anesthesia takes effect should be provided to the parents. An additional staff person, such as a parent services provider or child life therapist, should be present to escort the parent to and from the OR so that the circulating nurse can focus on providing care for the patient once the child has been anesthetized.

## BEST PRACTICE

Eutectic mixture of local anesthetics (EMLA) cream is approved for children 37 weeks of gestational age and older. It may be used before procedures such as lumbar, venous, arterial, finger, heel, or earlobe punctures; implanted port access; peripherally inserted central catheter (PICC) line insertion; and intramuscular (IM) or subcutaneous (SC) injections. Best practice guidelines for the use of EMLA are listed as follows:

- Explain to the child that EMLA is like a "magic cream that takes hurt away." Tap or lightly scratch site of procedure to show child that "skin is now awake."
- Apply the "peel and stick" anesthetic disk or a thick layer (dollop) of EMLA cream over normal intact skin to anesthetize site (about one half of a 5-g tube; can use one third of tube if puncture site is localized and superficial, such as for intradermal injection or heel/finger puncture).
- For venous access, apply to two sites; place enough cream on antecubital fossa to cover medial and lateral veins. Do not rub the cream.
- If using the cream, place a transparent adhesive dressing, such as Tegaderm, over the EMLA. Make sure cream remains in a dollop or mound. A piece of plastic film, such as Saran Wrap, can be used with tape to seal the edges. Use only as much adhesive as needed to prevent leakage.
- To make the dressing less accessible to the child, cover it loosely with a self-adhering Ace-type bandage (e.g., Coban) or an intravenous (IV) protector. Label the dressing with "EMLA applied" and the date and time, to distinguish it from other types of dressings. Instruct older children not to disturb the dressing (covering the dressing with an opaque material may reduce the attraction and discourage "fingering"). Supervise younger or cognitively compromised children throughout the application time.
- Leave EMLA on the skin for at least 60 minutes for superficial puncture and 120 minutes for deep penetration (e.g., IM injection, biopsy). EMLA may be applied at home and may need to be kept on longer for children with dark or thicker skin. Anesthesia may last up to 4 hours after EMLA is removed.
- Remove disk or dressing before procedure, and wipe cream from skin. For transparent dressing, grasp opposite sides and, while holding dressing *parallel* to skin, pull sides away from each other to stretch and loosen. An adhesive remover may be used.
- Observe skin reaction (e.g., either blanched or reddened). If skin reaction is not obvious, EMLA may not have penetrated adequately. Test skin sensitivity, and reapply if needed.
- Repeat tapping or lightly scratch on skin to show child that "skin is asleep" and that it cannot feel a needle.
- After procedure, assess behavioral response. If child was upset, use a pain scale to distinguish between pain and fear.

| Age and Body Weight Requirements | Maximum Total Dose of EMLA | Maximum Application Area |
|---|---|---|
| 1-3 mo or < 5 kg | 1 g | 10 cm² (1.25 × 1.25 inches) |
| 4-12 mo and >5 kg | 2 g | 20 cm² (1.75 × 1.75 inches) |
| 1-6 yr and > 10 kg | 10 g | 100 cm² (4 × 4 inches) |
| 7-12 yr and > 20 kg | 20 g | 200 cm² (5.5 × 5.5 inches) |

Modified from Algren C: Family centered care of the child during illness and hospitalization. In Hockenberry MJ and others, editors: *Wong's nursing care of infants and children*, ed 7, St Louis, 2003, Mosby.

Distraction methods during the induction of anesthesia can help minimize a child's stress and anxiety. Singing softly, story telling, and, for the older child, providing a relaxing mental image are effective diversion techniques.

Malignant hyperthermia (MH), although very rare, may be more prevalent in the pediatric population as a result of the administration of inhalational anesthesia and succinylcholine (see Chapter 4). In addition, physiologic conditions present in some pediatric patients are associated with a higher risk of MH. These conditions are myotonia congenita, Duchenne's muscular dystrophy, Becker's muscular dystrophy, osteogenesis imperfecta, arthrogryposis, kyphoscoliosis, and King-Denborough syndrome.[12] Careful assessment of family history is essential to identify patients at risk for developing MH. The management of an MH crisis is described in Chapter 4.

***Pain Management.*** In the past, many common fallacies existed about pain in the pediatric population. Some of these mistruths were that infants do not feel pain; children have better pain tolerance than adults have; children cannot tell the health care provider where they hurt; children always tell the truth about pain; children become accustomed to pain or painful procedures; and narcotics are more dangerous for children than they are for adults. Research into this important area has revealed that infants do demonstrate behavioral and physiologic indicators of pain. Children have less pain tolerance than adults do; their pain tolerance increases as they mature. Children are able to indicate pain, and children as young as 3 years can use pain-rating scales. Often children may not admit to having pain; they may believe that others know how much they hurt, or they fear receiving an injection. Children may also feel that pain and suffering are punishment for some misdeed, or they may not know what the word *pain* means. Children do not become accustomed to pain or painful procedures. They actually may demonstrate increased behavioral signs of pain with repeated procedures. Many factors, such as development level, culture, coping ability, temperament, and activity levels, influence the behavioral manifestations of pain exhibited by the patient. Narcotics are no more dangerous for children than they are for adults and are not excluded as a treatment modality. The evaluation of a pediatric patient's level of pain is performed using a variety of assessment tools (pain scales) that are based on the age and developmental level of the child (Box 29-2). In infants and nonverbal children, evaluation is based on physiologic changes and observation of behaviors. Children with verbal skills are able to articulate pain. One assessment strategy to use with pediatric patients is the *QUESTT* method:

*Q*uestion the child.
*U*se pain-rating scales.
*E*valuate behavior and physiologic changes.
*S*ecure the parents' involvement.
*T*ake cause of pain into account.
*T*ake action, and evaluate results.

Questioning the child provides the most reliable indicator of pain. Children may not be familiar with the word *pain* and may be more comfortable with words like "ouch," "hurt," or "owie." It may also be helpful to ask the child to point to where it hurts. The FACES pain scale uses cartoon faces with a variety of expressions ranging from happy to crying. The child selects the face that best describes his or her pain (see Chapter 9). The Oucher scale has a numeric component and a component similar to the FACES scale but uses actual photographs of children. The adolescent pediatric pain tool (APPT) is a line drawing of a body; the child marks the drawing where he or she has pain.

Physiologic indicators of pain, such as increased blood pressure, respirations, and heart rate and restlessness, are the same for children as for adults but may not be of as much value except in neonates and nonverbal children. These indicators may also reflect anxiety or fear and should not be the sole indicator relied on to determine pain. Children may also tug or hold painful areas or show preference to a painful extremity.

BOX 29-2

### Developmental Characteristics of Children's Responses to Pain

**YOUNG INFANTS**

- Generalized body response of rigidity or thrashing, possibly with local reflex withdrawal of stimulated area
- Loud crying
- Facial expression of pain (brows lowered and drawn together, eyes tightly closed, mouth open and square shaped)
- Demonstrates no association between approaching stimulus and subsequent pain

**OLDER INFANTS**

- Localized body response with deliberate withdrawal of stimulated area
- Loud crying
- Facial expression of pain and/or anger (same facial characteristics as pain but eyes may be open)
- Physical resistance, especially pushing the stimulus away *after* it is applied

**YOUNG CHILDREN**

- Loud crying, screaming
- Verbal expressions of "Ow," "Ouch," or "It hurts"
- Thrashing of arms and legs
- Attempts to push stimulus away *before* it is applied
- Uncooperative; needs physical restraint
- Requests termination of procedure
- Clings to parent, nurse, or other significant person
- Requests emotional support, such as hugs or other forms of physical comfort
- May become restless and irritable with continuing pain
- All these behaviors may be seen in anticipation of actual painful procedure

**SCHOOL-AGE CHILDREN**

- May display all behaviors of young child, especially *during* painful procedure, but less in anticipatory period
- Stalling behavior, such as "Wait a minute" or "I'm not ready"
- Muscular rigidity, such as clenched fists, white knuckles, gritted teeth, contracted limbs, body stiffness, closed eyes, wrinkled forehead

**ADOLESCENTS**

- Less vocal protest
- Less motor activity
- More verbal expressions, such as "It hurts" or "You're hurting me"
- Increased muscle tension and body control

From Algren C: Family centered care of the child during illness and hospitalization. In Hockenberry MJ and others, editors: *Wong's nursing care of infants and children*, ed 7, St Louis, 2003, Mosby.

Parental involvement in pain management is important. Parents know their child's normal behavior and can give input into the behaviors being exhibited in the perioperative setting. Parents should be queried about the child's previous experiences with pain and be taught the nonverbal behaviors that may indicate pain.

Nurses should investigate all complaints of pain or discomfort and be sensitive to behavioral and nonverbal cues to determine treatment. Postoperative pain should be assessed after all surgical procedures, regardless of their nature (Box 29-3). It is also critical to assess and document the child's response to the interventions provided for relief of pain.

Effective pain management requires a willingness to use a variety of methods and modalities to achieve optimal results. Pharmacologic methods include the administration of analgesics, both narcotic and non-narcotic. Patient-controlled anesthesia (PCA) is an option for children. Children as young as 4 years have the cognitive and physical capabilities to successfully use this modality with appropriate instruction and support.[33] Nonpharmacologic methods include distraction, relaxation, guided imagery, behavioral contracting, and cutaneous stimulation. Nonpharmacologic methods should never be used as substitutes for appropriate medication administration but instead should be used to enhance the management of pain.

## Evaluation

The perioperative nurse evaluates care provided throughout the perioperative period. At the conclusion of the surgical intervention, the skin is inspected, especially at dependent pressure points and at the site of the electrosurgical dispersive pad. Inspection is carried out to detect any reddened, irritated areas or evidence of compression injury. If povidone-iodine (Betadine) was used for skin prep, the area needs to be checked for any signs of chemical irritation. The patient's temperature is reassessed. The cardiopulmonary status is closely monitored as the child emerges from anesthesia. The perioperative nurse should assist the anesthesia team during emergence, remaining at the patient's bedside. Warm blankets are provided; hydration status is evaluated as replacement fluids continue to be administered, and fluid output is noted. The child is transferred to and positioned on the stretcher, crib, neonatal intensive care unit (NICU) warmer or ICU bed; the airway and respiratory effort are reassessed before departing the OR. Tubes, IV lines, drains, and drainage devices must be carefully protected during the move from the operating table. Supplemental oxygen is always given during transport from the OR to PACU for pediatric patients.

The perioperative nurse provides a hand-off report to the PACU nurse, focusing on the condition of the child, the response to surgery and anesthesia, the presence of catheters and drains, the quality and amount of wound drainage, a description of the dressings applied, and any special needs. Part of this report should focus on the outcomes established in the perioperative plan of care. For the plan of care presented in this chapter, they might be as follows:

- The patient demonstrated decreased anxiety.
- The patient was protected from infection related to operative intervention; principles of asepsis and infection control were maintained.
- The patient remained free from injuries related to positioning for the surgery.
- The patient's temperature was maintained in the desired range during the perioperative period.

The perioperative nurse may receive further feedback on the child's progress after the child is discharged from the PACU; information may be relayed by the surgeon, unit nurse, or anesthesia team. This type of informal feedback helps the perioperative nurse collect additional data regarding effectiveness of the plan of care, providing information about the achievement of identified outcomes.

**BOX 29-3**

### Pain Assessment Questions

The following questions may be useful in pain assessment in the pediatric patient and will allow involvement of the parent or caregiver.

**QUESTIONS FOR THE CHILD**

- Tell me what pain is.
- Tell me about the hurt you have had before.
- Do you tell others when you hurt? If yes, who?
- What do you do for yourself when you are hurting?
- What do you want others to do for you when you hurt?
- What helps more to take your hurt away?
- Is there anything special that you want me to know about you when you hurt? (If yes, have child describe.)

**QUESTIONS FOR THE PARENT/CAREGIVER**

- What word or words does your child use in regard to pain?
- Describe the pain experiences your child has had before.
- Does your child tell you or others when he or she is hurting?
- How do you know when your child is in pain?
- How does your child usually react to pain?
- What do you do for your child when he or she is hurting?
- What does your child do for himself or herself when he or she is hurting?
- What works best to decrease or take away your child's pain?
- Is there anything special that you would like me to know about your child and pain? (If yes, describe.)

From Algren C: Family-centered care of the child during illness and hospitalization. In Hockenberry MJ and others, editors: *Wong's nursing care of infants and children,* ed 7, St Louis, 2003, Mosby.

## Patient and Family Education and Discharge Planning

Patient and family teaching varies significantly based on the type of surgery performed. Some hospitals provide special preoperative teaching and hospital tours for pediatric patients and their parents to help them prepare for the surgical experience. Sometimes information is discussed with the child and family at the time of the office visit, when the surgery is scheduled. For same-day procedures, the day-surgery nursing staff might teach postoperative care immediately before patient discharge. Basics of postoperative care are reviewed with the parents at this time. Parents should be advised to be alert for certain signs and symptoms during the postoperative recovery period that could indicate an infectious process, such as fever, pain, nausea, redness around the incisional area, drainage from the wound, or difficulty breathing. These signs and symptoms may develop days or even weeks after surgery. It is important that parents understand the necessity of not ignoring any of these signs and symptoms and of reporting them to the surgeon

PATIENT AND FAMILY EDUCATION

**Guidelines for Effective Teaching of Family Members**

- Establish rapport; reduce anxiety and fear.
- Assess what family members know and expect to learn, especially if they have concerns, and address their concerns before beginning teaching.
- Assess family's learning style; ask if the family prefers having everything explained in detail or knowing only the major facts.
- Direct teaching to family decision maker and/or primary caregiver.
- Use a variety of teaching materials (lecture, demonstration, video or slide presentation, written material).
- Speak family's language, avoid jargon, and clarify all terms.
- Be specific when giving information; divide information into small steps.
- Keep information short, simple, and concrete.
- Use "verbal" headings to organize information, such as, "There are two things you need to learn: how to give the medicine, and what side effects to look for. First, how to give . . . . Second, what side effects . . . ."
- Stress importance of instructions and expected benefits, and explain detrimental effects of inadequate treatment, but avoid fear tactics.
- Evaluate teaching by eliciting feedback to ensure that the family understands the information.
- Repeat information as needed.
- Reward family for learning through verbal praise.
- Use "teachable" moments—times when family is more apt to accept new information (e.g., when symptoms are present).
- Use "hands-on" demonstration and return demonstration to encourage mastery of skills and retention of information.

From Algren C: Family centered care of the child during illness and hospitalization. In Hockenberry MJ and others, editors: *Wong's nursing care of infants and children*, ed 7, St Louis, 2003, Mosby.

promptly so that an early diagnosis can be made and treatment prescribed. The Patient and Family Education box contains general guidelines for teaching family members. Although discharge information depends on the type of surgery performed, it typically includes recommendations about activity restrictions, return to school or day care, wound care, bathing or showering, diet, and follow-up appointments. The printed discharge instructions are reviewed with the parents, and their understanding is verified. This time should provide the family with an opportunity to ask questions or seek clarification of the instructions. Phone numbers for the surgeon and the main hospital are provided in case the family has concerns or questions during the child's recovery period at home. An appointment for the child's follow-up visit may be made before discharge, or the parents are instructed to call the physician's office to schedule an appointment.

# Surgical Interventions

As mentioned, children require surgery for congenital malformations, an acquired disease, or trauma. The field of pediatric surgery is further subdivided into all the specialties. Several surgical procedures that may be designated pediatric are presented in previous chapters of this text under particular specialty headings. The surgical interventions presented here represent procedures that are most commonly performed on children.

## VASCULAR ACCESS

Vascular access in pediatric patients may be established intraoperatively for short-term (weeks) or long-term (months, years) use. Examples of short-term use include peripherally inserted central venous catheters (PICC lines) for antibiotic therapy. Central venous lines or implanted ports are placed for long-term access to provide parenteral nutrition, chemotherapy, bone marrow transplantation, or multiple IV access lines for the critically ill patient. Common complications of vascular access include infection; thrombosis; catheter occlusion; extravasation/ migration; malposition/displacement; vascular stenosis; catheter fracture/embolization; surgical damage to nerves, lymphatics, vessels, or pleura; and poor cosmesis.[31]

### Central Venous Catheter Placement

The preferred site of placement is the external jugular vein. The internal jugular may be chosen if the external jugular has been used or is too small. From the cannulation site the catheter is tunneled under the skin about 5 to 10 cm. This is done to inhibit contamination of the bloodstream from frequent dressing changes. Subcutaneous ports are placed in a similar fashion. In cases where the internal or external vein sites are unavailable, the catheter may be placed into the external iliac vein by way of a cutdown in the greater saphenous vein. In these cases the catheter is tunneled out into the abdominal wall.

***Procedural Considerations.*** The manufacturer's instructions for handling and preparing the catheter must be followed. The catheter must not contact lint, glove powder, or other foreign matter. Before insertion, the catheter is flushed and filled with heparinized saline (concentration is determined by the size of the patient) to prevent air bubbles from entering the circulatory system and to eliminate blood clots in the catheter lumen. Fluoroscopy is used to confirm proper placement of the catheter; lead shielding must be provided for patient and staff, with appropriate signage on room doors. The use of a lead shield for the patient should be documented in the perioperative record.

The child is appropriately positioned as dictated by the site chosen for cannulation. The area is prepped and draped.

#### *Operative Procedure—External Jugular Vein Site*

1. A very small, transverse incision is made over the lower portion of the medial border of the sternocleidomastoid muscle.
2. The external jugular vein is exposed and prepared for cannulation.
3. Using a long, hollow needle with an obturator (a tendon passer or neuro tunneling device may be used on a larger

child), a subcutaneous tunnel is created, extending from the neck incision to the chest wall medial near the nipple.

4. The obturator is withdrawn, and the catheter is passed through the needle. The needle is removed, and the catheter then lies in the subcutaneous tunnel.
5. The external jugular vein is ligated distally and incised; the catheter is passed into the vein and advanced so that it lies at the point where the superior vena cava (SVC) enters the atrium.
6. The position of the catheter is then confirmed by radiography in the OR.
7. The catheter is secured at the exit site on the chest wall with nonabsorbable sutures, flushed with heparinized saline, and clamped.
8. Antimicrobial ointment is applied to the exit site, and an occlusive, transparent dressing is placed over this. The catheter is coiled under this dressing to avoid tension on the line and accidental displacement.

## MINIMALLY INVASIVE SURGERY

Improvements in instrumentation and the development of equipment in smaller sizes have made minimally invasive surgery a rapidly growing field in pediatric patients. Advantages of minimally invasive surgery include diminished postoperative pain, improved cosmetic results, decreased incidence of adhesion formation, and accelerated recovery periods and shorter hospital stays.

Laparoscopy is used to evaluate abdominal pain, malrotation, cancer, and for other diagnostic indications. Pyloromyotomy, splenectomy, gastric fundoplication, cholecystectomy, and nephrectomy are being performed laparoscopically in pediatric patients at present. Thoracoscopic approaches may be used for correction of pectus excavatum, lung biopsy, sympathectomy, and closure of a patent ductus arteriosus. Ventriculoscopy can be used to view the ventricles of the brain. The application of minimally invasive techniques for pediatric surgery is rapidly developing.

## BARIATRIC SURGERY

More than 15% of children and adolescents are obese, a prevalence that has more than tripled in the past 2 decades. Obesity in adolescents is defined as having a body mass index (BMI; kg/m$^2$) greater than the 95th percentile for age and weight. Overweight or "at risk" for overweight has been defined as a BMI greater than the 85th percentile for age and weight.[13] Risk factors that have been identified for pediatric obesity are low birth weight, bottle feeding, puberty, having a diabetic mother, and parental obesity.[13]

Bariatric surgery is gaining popularity as a treatment option for obesity in some adolescents (Research Highlight). The timing of the surgical procedure is critical. The patient must be physically mature. Skeletal maturation is generally complete by age 13 to 14 years in girls and age 15 to 16 years in boys. Bariatric surgery can be safely performed once the child has attained more than 95% of adult stature. Candidates undergo psychologic evaluation before surgery to ensure they are cognitively mature enough to participate in decision making and to comply with postoperative regimens. Box 29-4 details desirable attributes of the adolescent bariatric surgery candidate.

### RESEARCH HIGHLIGHT

#### Metabolic Changes After Gastric Bypass in Adolescents

Adolescents who are morbidly obese often suffer from issues such as hypercholesterolemia, diabetes mellitus, and hyperlipidemia in addition to their weight issues. Gastric bypass is an option to help some adolescents manage their weight and may also have an added benefit of improving preexisting metabolic abnormalities.

Researchers compared a group of nonsurgical patients with a group of adolescents undergoing Roux-en-Y gastric bypass to compare weight loss. The nonsurgical group had a 3% decrease in their body mass index (BMI) scores compared with the surgical group, who experienced a 37% decrease in BMI.

The surgical group demonstrated improvement in metabolic values, showing decreases in triglycerides (−65 mg/dl), total cholesterol (−28 mg/dl), and fasting blood glucose (−12 mg/dl). Researchers also evaluated complications. Sixty-one percent of the surgical patients had no complications, nine had minor complications, four had moderate complications, and two had severe complications resulting in one death. Based on the study results, the researchers concluded that bariatric surgery in adolescents allows patients to lose significant amounts of weight and improve their metabolic status with few complications.

Modified from Lawson ML and others: One-year outcomes of Roux-en-Y gastric bypass for morbidly obese adolescents: a multicenter study from the Pediatric Bariatric Study Group, *Journal of Pediatric Surgery* 41(1): 137-143, 2006.

### BOX 29-4

#### Characteristics of "Good" Adolescent Patients for Bariatric Surgery

- Patient is motivated and has good insight.
- Patient has realistic expectations.
- Family support and commitment are present.
- Family is compliant with health care commitments.
- Family and patient understand long-term life-style changes are needed.
- Patient and family agree to long-term follow-up.
- Decisional capacity is present.
- Well-documented and at least temporarily successful weight loss attempts have been made.
- No major psychiatric disorders that may complicate postoperative regimen adherence are present.
- No major conduct/behavioral problems are present.
- Patient has had no substance abuse in preceding years.
- Patient has no plans for pregnancy in upcoming 2 years.

From Inge TH and others: Bariatric surgical procedures in adolescence. In Ashcraft KW and others, editors: *Pediatric surgery*, ed 4, Philadelphia, 2005, Saunders.

### Procedural Considerations

The bariatric procedure most commonly performed in adolescents is the laparoscopic Roux-en-Y gastric bypass. The adjustable gastric band (i.e., lap band) has not been approved by the U.S. Food and Drug Administration for use in adolescents. The perioperative nurse must plan carefully for this surgical intervention with an emphasis on obtaining the appropriate-sized transport vehicle, monitoring devices (i.e., larger blood pressure cuff, possibly longer electrocardiogram [ECG] leads to accommodate placement on a larger patient), OR table rated for the patient's weight, and appropriate-length instruments in case conversion to an open procedure is necessary. Obesity places this patient group at risk for deep vein thrombosis (DVT); the nurse should ensure that elastic stockings and sequential compression devices are available.

### Operative Procedure

The operative procedure is described in Chapter 11.

## CORRECTION OF GASTROINTESTINAL DISORDERS

### Repair of Atresia of the Esophagus

Esophageal atresia is a congenital anomaly that may develop between the third and sixth weeks of fetal life. Several types are recognized, the most common being an upper segment of esophagus ending in a blind pouch and a lower segment of esophagus communicating by a fistula with the trachea (esophageal atresia with TEF). Ideally this defect is recognized in the first hours of life, but more often the diagnosis is made in the first 36 to 48 hours of life. Drooling, the need for frequent suctioning, and coughing or cyanosis during oral feeding are the most common presentations.[30] Prompt surgical intervention allows the child to breathe and eat without the danger of aspirating mucus, saliva, feedings, or stomach contents. Atresia of the esophagus is repaired through a right retropleural thoracotomy, with closure of the TEF and anastomosis of the segments of the esophagus.

***Procedural Considerations.*** A gastrostomy may be done first to decompress the air-distended stomach, thus facilitating chest movement and ventilation and preventing reflux of stomach contents into the trachea. The patient is then positioned for a right thoracotomy (sometimes rather posteriorly), prepped, and draped. The major instrument set is required with the appropriate size of chest tube and infant chest drainage system.

#### *Operative Procedure*

1. The chest is entered through the fourth intercostal space. Removal of the rib is not necessary (Figure 29-2, *A*).
2. The pleura is gently dissected off the chest wall (Figure 29-2, *B*).
3. As the dissection proceeds posteriorly, the azygos vein is encountered, which is reflected inferiorly after its highest intercostal branches are divided to expose the fistula beneath (Figure 29-2, *C*).
4. Tape or silk is passed under the fistula to apply traction gently (Figure 29-2, *D*). Dissection of the mediastinum begins with the TEF and distal end of the esophagus. The vagus nerve is an important landmark for the distal end of the esophagus.
5. The fistula is clamped and transected, leaving a thin cuff of esophageal tissue on the tracheal side to allow closure of the trachea without narrowing it and compromising the lumen of the airway (Figure 29-2, *E*).
6. To close the fistula, three or four interrupted atraumatic sutures of 5-0 nonabsorbable suture are used.

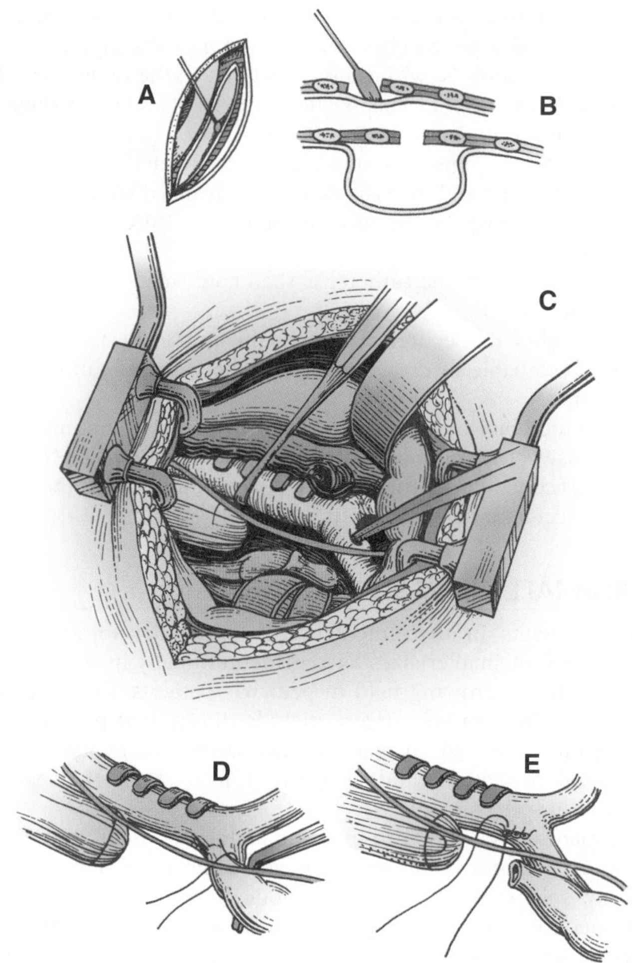


**FIGURE 29-2** Repair of atresia of the esophagus. **A,** Incision at fourth intercostal space. **B,** Dissection of pleura off chest wall. **C,** Identification and division of azygos vein to expose fistula beneath. **D,** Traction applied to fistula. **E,** Transection of fistula leaving 3-mm cuff on trachea.

7. The upper esophageal pouch is dissected; passage of a nasogastric tube by the anesthesia provider aids in its identification. The proximal pouch is identified and dissected as needed to allow it to reach the distal esophageal segment with minimal tension for anastomoses. At this point the surgeon decides whether to attempt primary anastomosis. If primary anastomosis is impossible, the distal esophagus is closed and tacked high on the prevertebral fascia. Infrequently the gap between the proximal and distal portions of esophagus is so long that esophageal replacement is required. In these cases the upper pouch is brought out to the neck in the form of a cervical esophagostomy.
8. Primary anastomosis is performed with 5-0 or 6-0 nonabsorbable suture, taking full-thickness bites along anterior and posterior borders (Figure 29-3). Some surgeons prefer the Haight, or two-layer, anastomosis (Figure 29-4). The inner layer is composed of the upper pouch mucosa sutured to the full thickness of the distal esophagus. The muscular sleeve of the upper esophagus is then pulled down over the inner anastomosis and sutured to the muscular layer of the inferior esophagus. The incision is irrigated with saline.

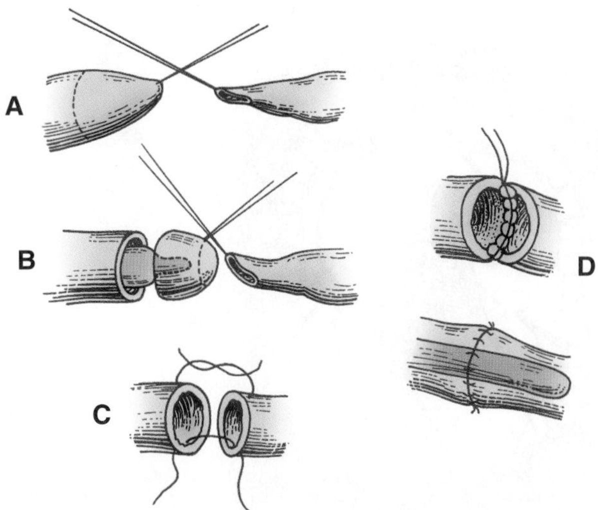


**FIGURE 29-3** Primary repair of atresia of the esophagus: single-layer repair. **A,** Traction applied to proximal and distal portions of esophagus. **B,** Blind proximal pouch transected. **C,** Full-thickness bites of anterior and posterior borders. **D,** Repair completed with Replogle tube in place to allow adequate lumen of esophagus.

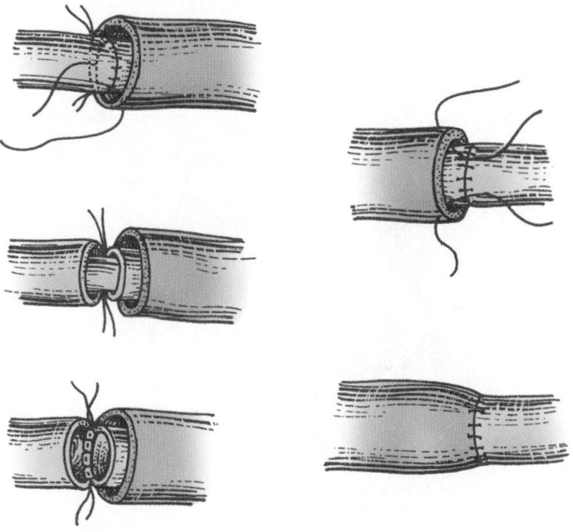

**FIGURE 29-4** Haight anastomosis. Mucosal layer of proximal pouch sutured to full thickness of distal esophagus. Muscular sleeve of upper pouch pulled down over inner anastomosis and sutured to muscle of distal esophagus.

9. Some surgeons place a 14-Fr or 16-Fr extrapleural chest tube near the anastomosis through a posterior stab wound. It is secured with sutures to prevent it from putting direct pressure on the anastomosis.
10. Muscle layers are closed with interrupted 5-0 or 6-0 nonabsorbable sutures or continuous 3-0 absorbable suture.
11. Skin is closed with a continuous 5-0 suture, and a collodion dressing or dressing of gauze and tape is applied.
12. The extrapleural chest tube is water-sealed after ensuring that the number of centimeters of water and the suction-control chamber are appropriate for the size of the infant. A chest x-ray examination is performed.

When the child reaches 1 year of age, esophageal replacement is attempted through colon interposition or construction of a reverse gastric tube (Figure 29-5).

## Repair of Congenital Diaphragmatic Hernia

A congenital diaphragmatic hernia is repaired by replacement of the displaced viscera into the abdominal cavity with surgical correction of the diaphragm defect (Figure 29-6). The conventional surgical repair is through the abdomen. The concurrence of intraabdominal abnormalities is somewhat high in infants with diaphragmatic hernia; therefore treatment is facilitated with an abdominal approach. It is technically easier to extract the viscera from below than to push them out of the thorax. The abnormal intrathoracic intrusion of the abdominal viscera usually causes severe compromise of intrathoracic pulmonary and vascular activities. Therefore urgent restoration of more normal intrathoracic and intraabdominal relationships is the rule in these newborns. The lung may be hypoplastic because of prolonged compression in utero by the displaced abdominal viscera. A residual intrapleural space usually remains for a few days after surgery.

***Procedural Considerations.*** A chest tube may be inserted and connected to water-seal drainage. Insertion of a gastrostomy tube minimizes postoperative distention and facilitates feeding. Direct suturing of the margins of the defect is usually possible. Insertion of prosthetic Silastic sheeting or Marlex mesh is occasionally required and should be available. The major instrument set is required. The infant is positioned supine.

### *Operative Procedure*

1. A contralateral chest tube may be placed in the anterior axillary line of the second intercostal space to prevent tension pneumothorax during surgery.
2. A subcostal incision going through all muscle layers is made on the side of the defect.
3. The abdominal viscera are withdrawn from the chest and held downward through the abdominal wound. Because abnormalities of abdominal viscera such as malrotation are associated with diaphragmatic hernia, the organs are carefully inspected at this time. If a malrotation is found, the surgeon may repair it if the clinical condition of the infant allows it.
4. The defect is then carefully inspected, including a search for a hernia sac, which is present in fewer than 5% of cases. If a sac is identified, it is excised. An ipsilateral chest tube is placed before the diaphragm is closed.
5. The posterior and anterior rims of the diaphragm are identified, and primary closure is performed with mattress sutures of 2-0 nonabsorbable material. If the rim of tissue is too small for mattress sutures, ample sutures of 2-0 or 3-0 nonabsorbable are used. Occasionally, reinforced Silastic sheeting or Marlex mesh may be needed if sufficient diaphragm is not available for primary closure.
6. Gastrostomy is then performed in most cases.
7. The abdominal wall is then closed. If the musculature cannot accommodate the abdominal viscera, it is left open and the skin is closed to leave a ventral hernia. In severe cases, the patient may be given extracorporeal membrane oxygenation (ECMO) for several days before repair of the defect. The infant is returned to the operating room within 7 days for repair of the ventral hernia.

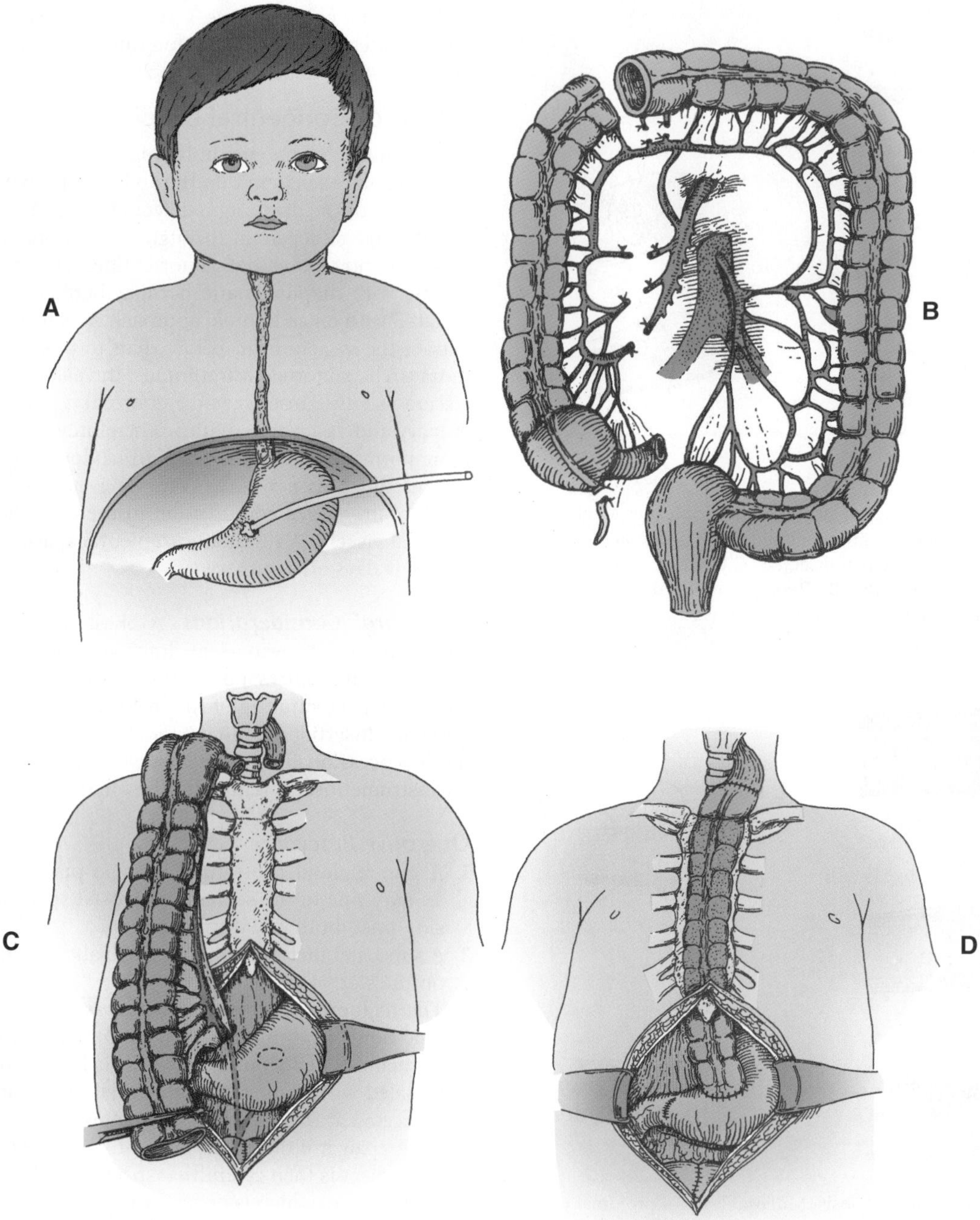

**FIGURE 29-5** Esophageal replacement. **A,** Gastrostomy. **B,** Isolation of right colon and ileum. **C,** Colon pedicle prepared for anastomosis. **D,** Anastomosis.

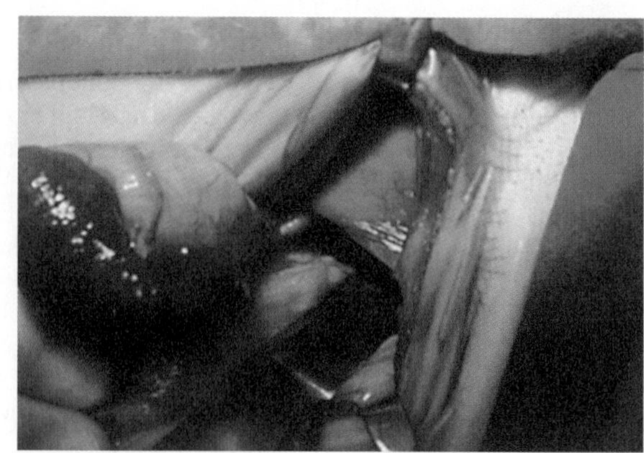

**FIGURE 29-6** Defect in the posterolateral aspect of the left diaphragm (diaphragmatic hernia).

## Nissen Fundoplication

Nissen fundoplication is the wrapping of the fundus of the stomach around the esophagus at the gastroesophageal (GE) junction. Nissen fundoplication is indicated for infants and children who experience severe GE reflux. The cause of GE reflux in these patients is believed to be an inadequate antireflux barrier. The antireflux barrier normally consists of a combination of anatomic and physiologic factors, including sufficient amount and strength of muscle fibers located in the lower esophageal sphincter, adequate length of the abdominal esophagus, and a high-pressure zone in the lower esophagus. An incompetent antireflux barrier can result in life-threatening complications, including obstructive apnea, aspiration pneumonia, esophagitis, and failure to thrive. The goal of the Nissen fundoplication is to create a competent antireflux barrier. The fundoplication may be performed laparoscopically or as an open procedure. A description of the open procedure follows.

***Procedural Considerations.*** The major instrument set is required. The patient is positioned supine. The surgeon passes the appropriate size of Maloney dilator into the esophagus to prevent the wrap from impinging on the lumen of the esophagus (Figure 29-7).

### *Operative Procedure*

1. A left subcostal incision is performed to allow exposure of the lower esophagus.
2. The esophagus is mobilized to create adequate intraabdominal length.
3. The stomach is mobilized to allow loose wrap of the fundus around the esophageal junction; it is used as the lower edge of the wrap.
4. Sutures of 3-0 or 4-0 nonabsorbable are placed through the seromuscular layers of both stomach and esophagus to fix the wrap.
5. Sutures are then placed to tack the fundus to the diaphragm (fundoplication); the posterior fundus is wrapped behind the esophagus and the anterior fundus in front. Two layers of sutures may be used. The first layer passes from the anterior fundus, through the right margin, to the posterior fundus. The second layer may be added between the anterior fundus and the posterior fundus for additional security.[5]
6. Some surgeons place clips at the level of the GE junction and the wrap to aid in follow-up radiographic studies. A gastrostomy is done in most cases. The incision is closed in layers, and a collodion dressing is applied.

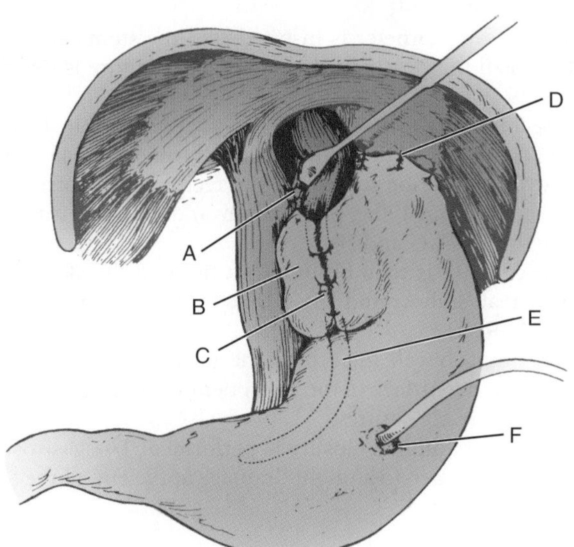


**FIGURE 29-7** Salient features of Nissen fundoplication in infants. *A*, Crural sutures to reduce hiatus. *B*, Generous loose, adequate tissue in wrap. *C*, Sutures placed through seromuscular depth of both gastric and esophageal walls. *D*, Sutures to fix fundus to diaphragm. *E*, Appropriate-sized mercury-filled dilator to ensure adequate lumen. *F*, Gastrostomy in all infants and whenever there is any question of gastric outlet problems.

## Fredet-Ramstedt Pyloromyotomy for Pyloric Stenosis

Pyloric stenosis is the most common cause of gastric outlet obstructions in children and is the most common condition requiring surgery in the newborn. Signs and symptoms of high gastrointestinal (GI) obstruction appear at 2 to 6 weeks of age. The first sign is projectile vomiting after feeds that is free of bile. The infant usually fails to gain weight adequately, and there may be a severe loss of body fluids and electrolyte imbalance, evidenced as hypochloremic, hypokalemic metabolic alkalosis. Once the diagnosis of hypertrophic pyloric stenosis is made, either through physical examination or imaging techniques, surgical intervention is planned. Electrolyte imbalances must be corrected before surgery. The Fredet-Ramstedt pyloromyotomy for pyloric stenosis involves the incision of the muscles of the pylorus to treat congenital hypertrophy of the pyloric sphincter that is obstructing the stomach. The open procedure is described below.

***Procedural Considerations.*** The stomach is emptied just before induction of anesthesia, and the nasogastric tube is removed to guard against reflux of gastric contents around the tube during induction. A minor instrument set and a pyloric spreader are used. The patient is prepped in the usual manner.

### *Operative Procedure*

1. The abdomen is opened through a right subcostal transverse skin incision. The rectus muscle is retracted or split longitudinally in the middle with spreading clamps, and the peritoneum is opened.
2. After the hypertrophied pylorus is delivered into the wound with a small vein retractor, the prepyloric area is grasped and rotated to expose the anterior superior border of the mass.
3. An incision is made in the serosa on the anterior wall of the pyloric mass from the duodenal junction proximally to a point proximal to the area of hypertrophied muscle (Figure 29-8, *A*). The circular muscle is spread with the pyloric spreader on the submucosal base, so that all muscle fibers are completely divided (Figure 29-8, *B*).
4. After completion of the separation, the pyloric end of the stomach is returned to the abdomen and the peritoneum and posterior rectus sheath are closed with a continuous 3-0 absorbable suture. The anterior rectus sheath is closed with a 4-0 absorbable suture.

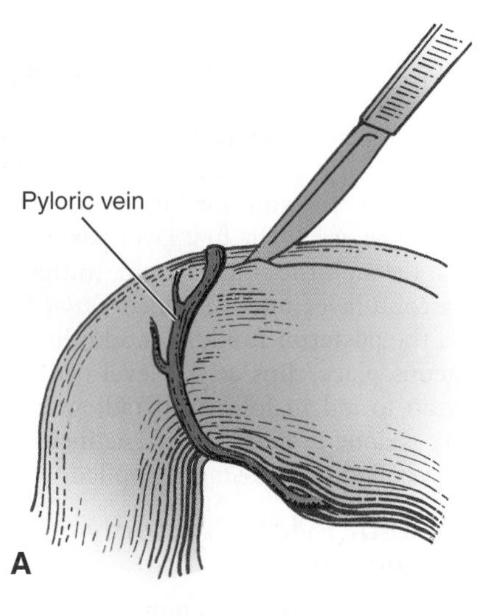


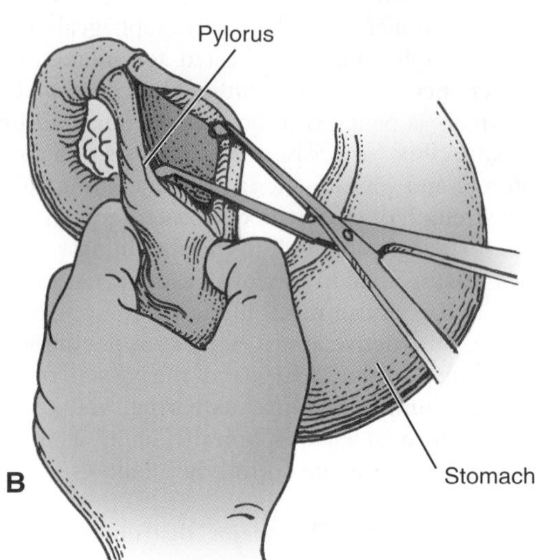


**FIGURE 29-8** Operative technique for pyloric stenosis.

5. The skin is closed with fine subcuticular sutures, and a dressing (adhesive strips or collodion) is applied.

## EMERGENCY GASTROINTESTINAL PROCEDURES

### Gastrostomy

Gastrostomy is establishment of a temporary or permanent channel from the gastric lumen to the skin to permit gastric emptying, liquid feeding, or retrograde dilation of an esophageal stricture. The procedure may be emergent in nature or performed with other surgical procedures to facilitate care of the infant or child after surgery. Placement of the gastrostomy tube may be through an abdominal incision (description follows) or percutaneously by means of an endoscope and local anesthesia. For children receiving long-term gastrostomy feedings, a skin-level device (e.g., button, Gastroport) may be inserted after the gastrostomy is well established. These devices, which protrude slightly from the abdomen, are more cosmetically acceptable and allow more mobility for the child. A gastrostomy tube can be placed in the OR as an open procedure, or it can be performed as a percutaneous procedure under fluoroscopy; both require the patient to receive a general anesthetic.

***Procedural Considerations.*** A minor instrument set is required, plus a gastrostomy feeding catheter (generally a 14 or 16 Fr for infants, or an 18, 20, or 22 Fr for older children) and a #11 knife blade on a knife handle. A variety of latex-free gastrostomy catheters are available. Routine prepping is done.

#### *Operative Procedure*

1. A short incision is made over the outer border of the left rectus muscle (Figure 29-9, *A*).
2. The subcutaneous tissues and rectus fascia are exposed with two small retractors (Figure 29-9, *B*).
3. The anterior rectus fascia is opened, and the rectus muscle is split for exposure of the posterior rectus sheath (Figure 29-9, *C*).
4. The peritoneum is opened for exposure of the liver edge and the greater curvature of the stomach (Figure 29-9, *D*).
5. The stomach is pulled out through the wound with Babcock forceps. A circular purse-string suture of 4-0 nonabsorbable suture is placed: in the center of this a very small incision is made with the #11 blade through the gastric wall (Figure 29-9, *E*).
6. The feeding catheter is inserted into the stomach through the small incision, and the purse-string suture is tied (Figure 29-9, *F*).
7. A second purse-string suture is placed outside the first one, and the same needle is then taken through the peritoneum and the posterior surface of the rectus fascia to place the stomach against the peritoneum and thus prevent leaks (Figure 29-9, *G* and *H*).
8. The catheter is then brought out through the skin by way of a small stab wound left, lateral to the skin incision (Figure 29-9, *A*).
9. The stomach wall adjacent to the gastrostomy site is tacked to the undersurface of the peritoneum with interrupted 4-0 nonabsorbable sutures.
10. Routine abdominal closure is performed. The gastrostomy tube is left open to straight drainage at the end of the surgical procedure.

### Omphalocele and Gastroschisis Repair

An omphalocele is the protrusion of abdominal viscera outside the abdomen through a defect in the umbilical ring into a sac of amniotic membrane and peritoneum at the base of the umbilical cord. There is no skin covering (Figure 29-10). Gastroschisis is the protrusion of the viscera through a defect in the

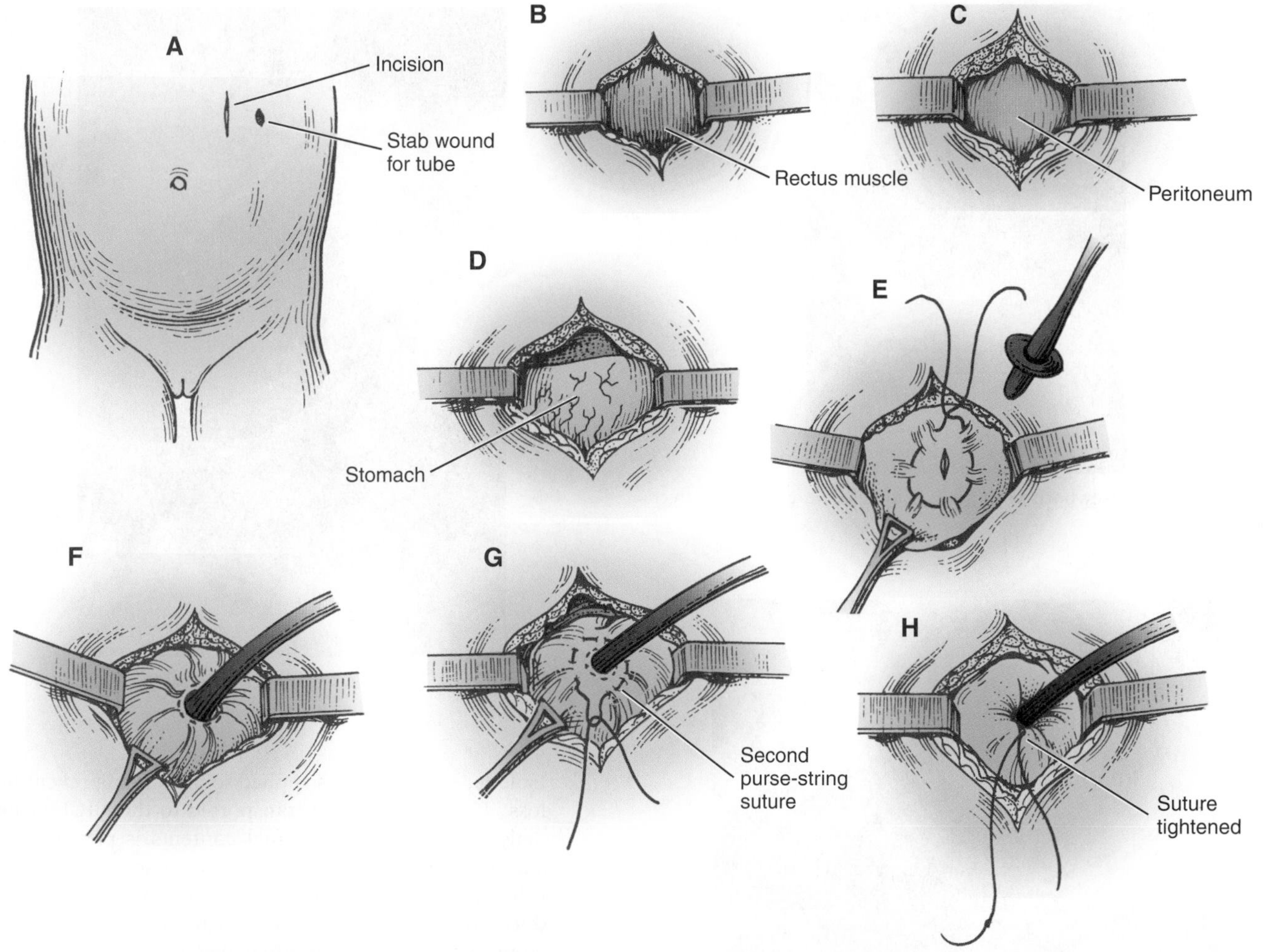


**FIGURE 29-9** Gastrostomy. **A,** Incision. **B,** Rectus muscle exposed. **C,** Posterior rectus sheath exposed. **D,** Peritoneum opened. **E,** Purse-string suture placed. **F,** Mushroom catheter inserted. **G,** Second purse-string suture placed. **H,** Suture tightened.

abdominal wall to the right of the umbilical cord. No amniotic membrane or peritoneum covers the defect.

Omphalocele occurs during the eleventh week of fetal life when the viscera fail to withdraw normally from the exocoelomic position to occupy the peritoneal cavity. The resulting abdominal wall defect can vary in size from 2 to 15 cm. The sac may contain only a few loops of bowel, to nearly all the intestines and the liver and spleen. Associated anomalies can include disorders of the cardiac, musculoskeletal, genitourinary, and nervous systems, along with malrotation and abnormal fixation of the bowel. Gastroschisis, on the other hand, is generally not associated with major congenital defects other than intestinal atresia[8] (Figure 29-11).

Because the infant is at risk for hypothermia, hypoglycemia, shock, sepsis, and vascular injury to the bowel, immediate management after birth is necessary.[15] Treatment consists of applying warm saline packs on the sac surface, inserting a nasogastric tube to prevent distention and aspiration, and beginning IV access with fluid resuscitation and antibiotic therapy. Surgical intervention is necessary to prevent rupture of the sac, infection, or both. If intrauterine rupture of the sac has occurred, the newborn is kept warm, the bowel is inspected for perforation and torsion, and moist, warm dressings are applied.

Omphaloceles and gastroschisis are repaired by placement of the viscera in the abdominal cavity, with reconstruction of the abdominal wall.

***Procedural Considerations.*** Particular attention to maintaining body temperature is essential because of the massive exposed surface area from which body heat can be lost. The use of nitrous oxide as an anesthetic agent is avoided during this procedure because it causes increased gas in the intestine, which in turn makes the reduction of abdominal contents into the peritoneal cavity very difficult. Repeated rectal irrigation with warm saline to evacuate meconium from the bowel may be carried out before the abdominal prep to aid in bowel decompression.

The major instrument set is required. The infant is positioned supine; and the abdomen, umbilical cord, and sac are gently prepped with a povidone-iodine solution.

### *Operative Procedure*

1. In the presence of small defects, primary closure is attempted. The skin edges are dissected free, and the sac is excised (if omphalocele). Abdominal contents are gently relocated into the peritoneal cavity. The abdominal cavity is closed in layers using 0, 2-0, and 3-0 nonabsorbable suture.

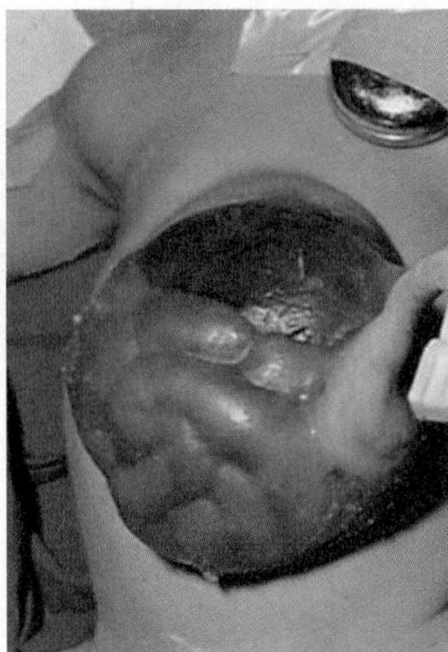

**FIGURE 29-10** Newborn with giant omphalocele containing liver and intestine.

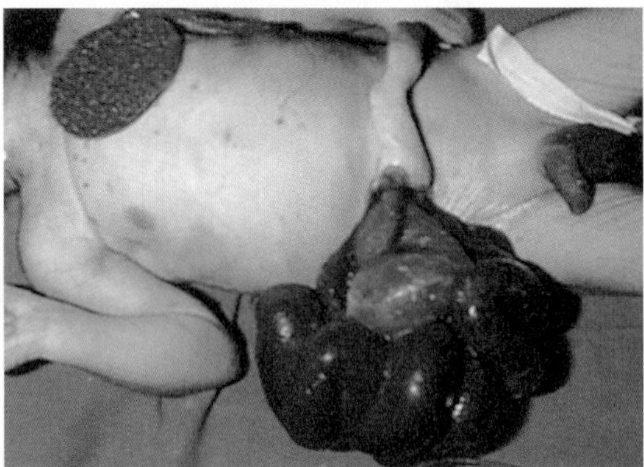

**FIGURE 29-11** Gastroschisis. A large amount of small intestine has eviscerated through a defect to the right of a normal-appearing umbilical cord. No sac is visible, and the intestine is thickened, edematous, and ischemic in areas.

2. In certain cases in which the defect is of medium to large size, a primary closure may not be accomplished. In these situations a staged procedure is done using prosthetic reduction. In the first stage the infant is brought to the OR and positioned and prepped as previously described, then:
   a. The sac is excised, and the umbilical vein and arteries are ligated.
   b. A gastrostomy may be performed at this time.
   c. A silo is then created with Silastic mesh. The mesh is secured through all layers of the edge of the defect using a continuous locking suture of 2-0 nonabsorbable. The open end of the silo is closed in the same manner; thus a cylinder of mesh is created extending upward from the abdomen (Figure 29-12).
   d. The open end of the cylinder is tied closed with umbilical tape or, alternatively, attached to a specifically designed roller clamp.
   e. The mesh silo suture line and edge of the defect are wrapped with Kling dipped in an iodophor solution to prevent infection. The infant is transferred to an open Isolette, and the silo is suspended from the top of the Isolette. Plastic wrap is applied to the silo to prevent heat loss. The infant is then transported to the NICU, where daily reduction of abdominal contents is performed by adding a lower tie of umbilical tape or adjustment of the roller clamp. The abdominal viscera are gradually reduced over several days, taking care to avoid respiratory compromise from abdominal distention. When reduction has successfully approached skin level, the infant is returned to the OR for the final stage of repair.
   f. The silo is removed, and the remaining abdominal contents are brought into the peritoneal cavity. The peritoneal fascia is closed with interrupted 2-0 or 3-0 nonabsorbable sutures. The skin is closed with interrupted 4-0 nonabsorbable suture. In an attempt to create the appearance of an umbilicus, a purse-string suture is used to close the inferior 2 cm of incision.

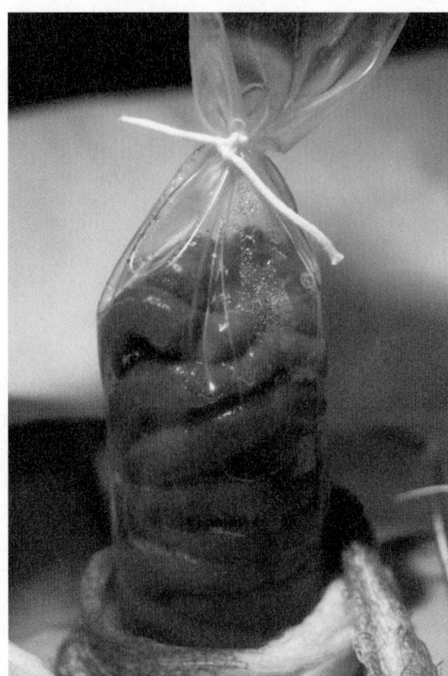

**FIGURE 29-12** Operative view of silo for the intestines.

3. Another technique for treating large omphaloceles is painting the sac and surrounding skin with silver sulfadiazine cream twice daily and applying external pressure with elastic bandages or abdominal binders. The sac membrane gradually contracts, and skin closes over the abdominal wall defect. Later surgery then repairs the abdominal musculature.

## REPAIR OF HERNIAS

### Umbilical Hernia Repair

Umbilical hernias are frequently seen in pediatric populations and are 10 times more common in African American children than in Caucasians.[11] These hernias are also common in premature infants and are corrected by repair of the defect where the intestine protrudes at the umbilicus. An umbilical hernia is always covered by skin. Small umbilical hernias may be left untreated. They usually close within a few months to 1 year. If surgical repair is required in a large fascial defect, it may be delayed until the child is at least 2 years of age; some surgeons delay repair until 4 years of age.

***Procedural Considerations.*** Surgical correction of umbilical hernia may be an ambulatory surgical procedure. General anesthesia is used. A minor instrument set is required. The child is prepped as discussed previously. Several variations in technique have been used; an infraumbilical approach is most common, and its description follows.

#### *Operative Procedure*

1. An incision is made below the umbilicus through the skin and subcutaneous tissue.
2. Flaps of skin and subcutaneous tissue are mobilized and held back with small retractors to expose the rectus fascia and hernial protrusion.
3. The hernia sac, which is between the rectus muscle sheaths in the midline, is completely freed from all surrounding structures.
4. The hernia sac may be invaginated, dissected free and ligated, or excised.
5. The peritoneum is closed with a continuous suture.
6. The two edges of the rectus fascia are brought together using interrupted 3-0 nonabsorbable sutures.
7. Subcuticular closure of the skin with a continuous fine absorbable suture is performed, and a pressure dressing is applied.

### Inguinal Hernia Repair

An inguinal hernia is a protrusion into the inguinal canal of a sac that contains the intestine. The testis develops high on the posterior wall of the abdomen. It gradually descends into the scrotum. Before the testis enters the inguinal canal, the processus vaginalis projects downward but retains a communication with the peritoneal cavity. The upper part of the processus does not; the remaining sac constitutes an indirect inguinal hernia. In a female child, a similar hernial sac is contiguous with the round ligament.

***Procedural Considerations.*** A minor instrument set is used, the child is positioned supine, and routine prepping is done.

#### *Operative Procedure*

1. An incision is made over the inguinal area in the direction of the skin crease.
2. The subcutaneous tissue is opened, and hemostats are placed on bleeding vessels, which are then ligated or electrocoagulated.
3. Right-angle retractors are placed inferiorly and medially.
4. The external ring is identified, and the external oblique fascia is cleaned and freed with small Metzenbaum scissors.
5. The external oblique fascia is opened with a #15 knife blade on a knife handle, and the upper flap is freed. The lower flap is freed to expose the inguinal ligament.
6. Cord structures are opened at the upper end of the cord. Two forceps are used to grasp tissues at the same level and to separate them.
7. The hernia sac is grasped with a hemostat, and structures of the cord are peeled downward and away from the sac with forceps until the sac is freed. Care is taken to protect the spermatic cord and major vessels as the sac is freed.
8. After the sac is opened, the surgeon's index finger is inserted and the sac is pulled upward. The upward traction is maintained with two or three hemostats.
9. The sac is ligated with 3-0 nonabsorbable suture, and excess sac is removed. Repair of the inguinal canal may be done with nonabsorbable sutures.
10. The subcutaneous tissue is closed with interrupted fine sutures; closure of the skin is with fine nonabsorbable subcuticular sutures. Collodion or adhesive strips are applied.

## REPAIR OF OBSTRUCTIVE DISORDERS

### Repair of Intestinal Obstruction

Repair of intestinal obstruction may include (1) correction of a volvulus, (2) division of a congenital band, (3) release of an internal hernia, (4) resection of bowel with an anastomosis, or (5) creation of an intestinal stoma.

Intestinal obstruction is the most common GI emergency requiring surgery in the newborn. Early recognition is essential to survival. Surgical intervention is usually within the first few hours after birth; delay may increase the risk of bowel necrosis. Intestinal obstruction can occur in the infant for a variety of reasons: atresia, stenosis, congenital aganglionosis (Hirschsprung's disease), meconium ileus, or malrotation. Lesions characterized by complete obliteration of the intestinal lumen are classified as *atresia.* Strictures characterized by a narrowing or partial obliteration of the lumen are classified as *stenosis.*

***Procedural Considerations.*** The major instrument set and pediatric bowel clamps are required. The infant is positioned supine, and routine prepping and draping of the abdomen are done.

#### *Operative Procedure*

1. An abdominal incision is made.
2. The intestines are explored to determine the location of the obstruction. The entire bowel must be examined to rule out multiple areas of involvement in infants with atresia or stenosis. If aganglionosis of the colon is suspected, sequential biopsy specimens are sent fresh immediately to pathology to determine the segment of large bowel to be resected.
3. Detorsion of bowel or resection is performed as indicated.

### Reduction of Intussusception

Intussusception is the telescopic invagination of a portion of intestine into an adjacent part, with mechanical and vascular impairment (Figure 29-13). It is relieved by reduction of invaginated bowel by the hydrostatic pressure of a barium enema or by laparotomy and manual manipulation. The highest incidence of intussusception occurs in infants between the ages of 5 and 9 months. More than half the cases occur within the first year of life, and only 10% to 25% of cases occur after the age of 2 years.[10] The most common site for intussusception is the ileocecal junction. Intussusception in most children is idiopathic; in others, causes may include Meckel's diverticulum, polyps, or hematoma of the bowel. Early diagnosis and reduction are essential to bowel viability.

***Procedural Considerations.*** The child is prepped for surgery as described previously. Reduction by barium enema is attempted only with the collaboration of the radiologist, sur-

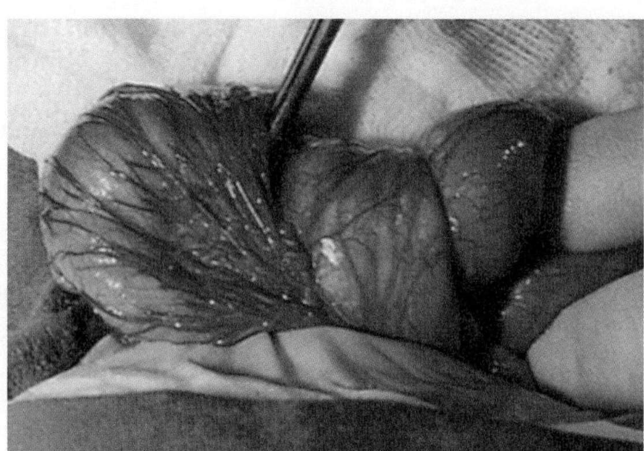

FIGURE 29-13 Operative view of intussusception.

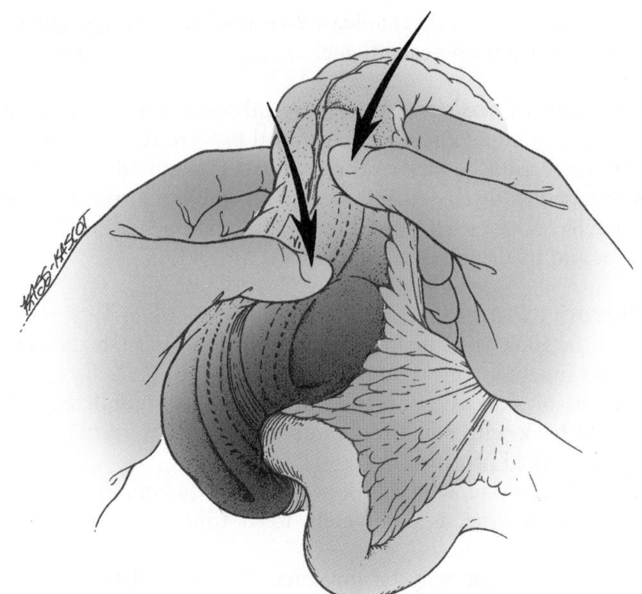

FIGURE 29-14 Manual reduction of intussusception.

geon, and pediatrician, with the OR team on standby. If reduction is unsuccessful, a laparotomy must be performed. The major instrument set is used with the addition of pediatric bowel clamps.

*Operative Procedure*

1. A right lower quadrant transverse or right paramedian incision is made, and the peritoneum is entered.
2. The cecum and ileum are identified; the intussusception is located and elevated with fingers.
3. If there is no evidence of bowel compromise, the bowel immediately distal to the intussusception is occluded with one hand and stripped proximally with the other in an attempt to achieve manual reduction (Figure 29-14). If the serosa splits during attempted reduction or if the mass cannot be reduced, bowel resection is done.
4. The abdomen is closed in layers, and the wound is dressed.

## Colostomy

Colostomy is the surgical construction of an artificial excretory opening from the colon. Most congenital anomalies that result in colonic obstruction require a temporary colostomy. These include imperforate anus and Hirschsprung's disease. Both conditions ultimately require further operative procedures, and proper construction of a colostomy is important. In Hirschsprung's disease the colostomy must be placed in a section of bowel containing ganglia.

*Procedural Considerations.* A major instrument set and pediatric intestinal clamps are used. The child is positioned supine and prepped as described previously.

*Operative Procedure*

1. A transverse incision usually is preferred, and the abdomen is entered in the right upper quadrant for a transverse colostomy or the left lower quadrant for a sigmoid colostomy.
2. The loop of colon is freed of peritoneal attachments until it can be brought easily through the abdominal wall without tension.
3. The edges of the mesentery are then sutured to the parietal peritoneum, and the serosa of the colonic loop is sutured with fine absorbable suture materials to the peritoneum and fascia as well as to the skin.
4. The colostomy may be sutured immediately. Some surgeons prefer to close the skin under a colostomy loop; others prefer to suture mucosa directly to skin edges. This decision may depend on the location of the colostomy. An important point is that each layer must be securely attached to the serosa of the colon to prevent evisceration and prolapse. The posterior wall of a loop colostomy may be divided by electrosurgery several days after surgery.

*Procedures Requiring Colostomy.* The following procedures require emergent colostomy at the time of presentation. Definitive repair of the anomaly usually occurs at about 1 year of age.

RESECTION AND PULL-THROUGH FOR HIRSCHSPRUNG'S DISEASE (RECONSTRUCTION). Hirschsprung's disease is characterized by the absence of ganglion cells in a distal portion of the bowel. The distal colon is more frequently involved, but the disease may encompass the entire colon, with a less favorable prognosis. The absence of ganglion cells results in a lack of peristalsis. The normal proximal colon becomes dilated with stool, since intestinal contents do not pass through the involved segment normally. The child presents with an abnormally distended abdomen. Barium enema reveals proximal distention of the colon and then a transition zone where the bowel appears funnel-shaped, followed by the distal aganglionic segment, which is narrowed. The child is taken to the OR for a leveling colostomy. Multiple frozen-section biopsy specimens from the muscularis of the proximal portion of the colon are taken to determine the presence of ganglion cells. The colostomy is performed at the most distal portion of the colon that contains ganglion cells. Some surgeons prefer a routine right transverse colostomy at this time and delay frozen-section biopsy specimens until the time of the definitive procedure. Resection and pull-through for Hirschsprung's disease, the definitive surgical procedure, consists of the removal of the aganglionic portion of the bowel and anastomosis of the normal colon to the anus. The child is returned to the OR for the definitive repair at 1 year of age if clinical and nutritional status permit.

Several surgical techniques have been devised. The procedure may be done laparoscopically or by an open approach. The Soave procedure of endorectal pull-through employs internal bypass of the involved segment. The internal sphincter muscle of the anus is kept intact for continence.

**Procedural Considerations.** The child is prepped and draped from the nipples down to and including the buttocks, genitalia, perineal area, and upper thighs to permit positioning for the perineal stage without redraping. (Before prepping, the rectum may be irrigated with warm saline solution.) An indwelling catheter is inserted to keep the bladder empty during the operation. The major instrument set, a minor instrument set, and pediatric intestinal clamps are needed.

**Operative Procedure**

1. A left paramedian incision that includes the sigmoid colonic stoma, if present, is made.
2. The stoma is freed from the abdominal wall, and the left portion of the colon is mobilized. (If there is no sigmoid colonic stoma, the extent of aganglionic intestine is established by biopsy and frozen section, and all involved colon is excised. If a stoma is present and the area has already been established as normal, the colon above it constitutes the proximal end of the resection.)
3. The mesocolon and the vessels of the intestine to be resected are divided close to the intestine, with care taken to preserve the blood supply to the rectum (Figure 29-15, *A*).
4. The mucosal tube is freed from the outer muscular layers by sharp dissection with Metzenbaum scissors and blunt dissection (Figure 29-15, *B*).
5. A muscular sleeve is transected, and traction sutures of 4-0 nonabsorbable are placed on the distal edge (Figure 29-15, *C*). The mucosa is stripped down to the anus. The depth of the dissection may be checked by inserting a finger into the anus (Figure 29-15, *D*).
6. When the mucosa is adequately freed, the perineal phase is started and the perineal instrument table is used.
7. The anus is dilated and retracted with Allis forceps. A circumferential incision is made, and the mucosal stripping is completed (Figure 29-15, *E*).
8. The proximal portion of the intestine is pulled through the rectal muscular sleeve and out the anus (Figure 29-15, *F*). If the portion of colon to be resected is large, it is excised

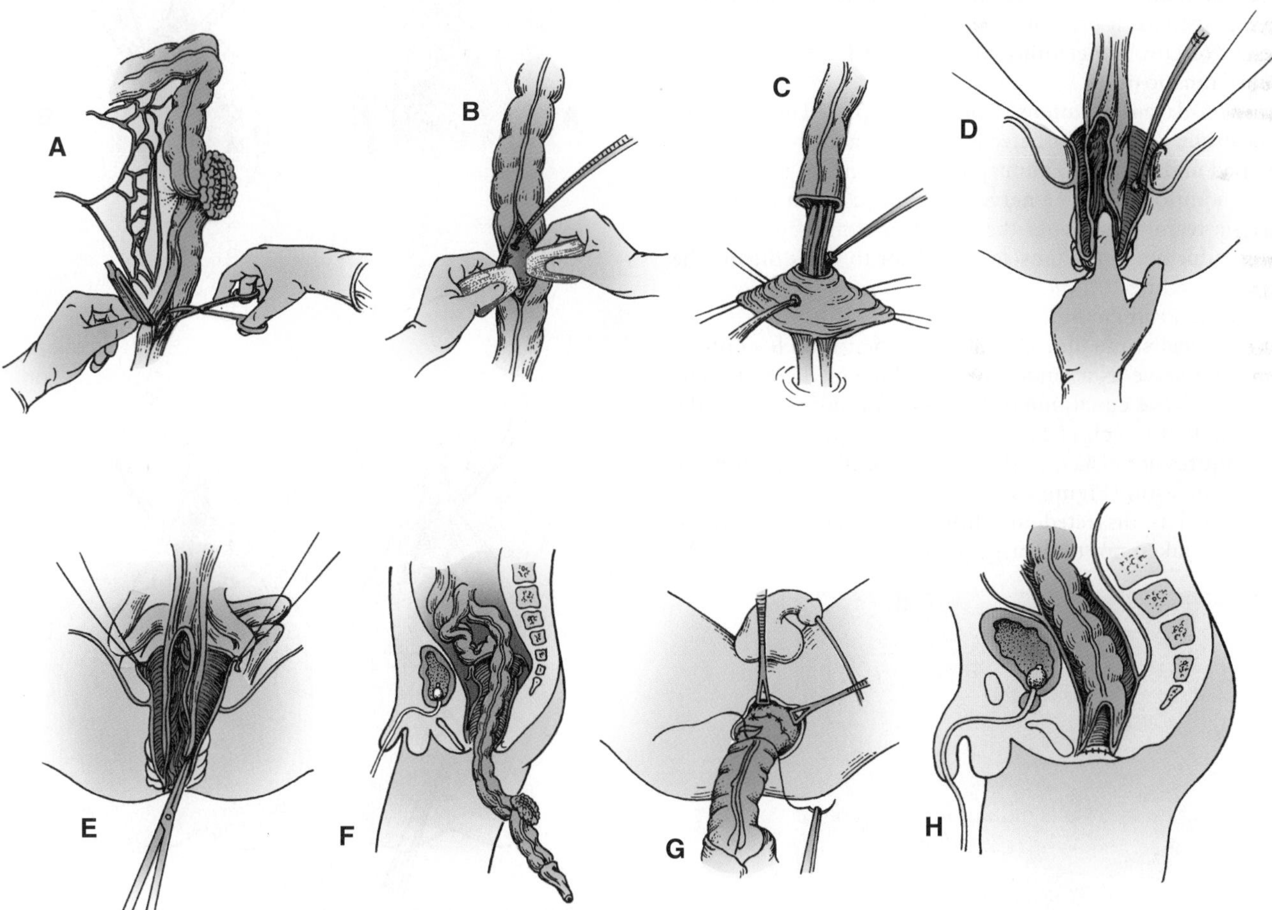


**FIGURE 29-15** Pull-through for Hirschsprung's disease. **A,** Dissection of mucosal tube begun through longitudinal incision. **B,** Gauze-tipped dissecting instrument used to dissect entire circumference of tube. **C,** Muscular sleeve transected. **D,** Depth of dissection determined by insertion of finger into anus. **E,** Circumferential incision made. **F,** Mucosal tube and proximal portion of colon and stoma pulled through rectal muscular cuff. **G,** Anastomosis performed among all layers of colon and anal mucosa. **H,** Anastomosis completed.

abdominally before the proximal portion of the intestine is pulled through the anus.

9. Absorbable sutures are used to secure the seromuscular layers of the intussuscepted colon to the rectal muscular cuff. The colon is divided into axial or longitudinal quadrants, and an anastomosis is performed with 3-0 absorbable sutures (Figure 29-15, *G*).
10. Gowns and gloves are changed, and abdominal instruments are used. The abdominal phase of the operation is completed by approximating the proximal edge of the muscular cuff to the seromuscular layer of the colon with 4-0 nonabsorbable sutures (Figure 29-15, *H*). The abdomen is closed in the routine manner, without the use of drains.

**REPAIR OF IMPERFORATE ANUS.** Congenital imperforate anus (Figure 29-16) presents in a variety of forms, classified as low, intermediate, and high lesions. Baby girls commonly have low lesions, and baby boys primarily exhibit high lesions. A covered anus and anovulvar fistula is an example of a low lesion. A high lesion consists of a blind rectal pouch, a "flat bottom," and a posterior urethral fistula or a fistula to the bladder. This type is the most prevalent and the most difficult to repair. An imperforate anus is repaired by establishing colorectoanal continuity through the external anal sphincter and closure of fistulas, if present.

**Repair of Low Imperforate Anus in a Girl: Anal Transposition**

*Procedural Considerations.* The infant is placed in the lithotomy position. A Foley catheter is inserted, and the perineum is prepped and draped. The major instrument set is required, with the addition of both a nerve and a muscle stimulator. The anesthesia team must avoid the use of neuromuscular blocking agents for the nerve/muscle stimulator to work during the surgical procedure.

*Operative Procedure*

1. An electrical stimulator is applied to elicit muscle contractions and serve as a guide to the midline of the anus. The goal is to leave equal innervated tissue on both sides of the anus, so that the child can be continent of stool.
2. Stay sutures are placed in the fistula, and it is excised using an oval incision (Figure 29-17, *A*).
3. The bowel is dissected free from surrounding structures, with care taken not to damage the vagina (Figure 29-17, *B*).
4. When the dissection is complete, a vertical midline incision is performed at the opening of the true anus and the fibers of the external sphincter are identified (Figure 29-17, *C*).
5. The mobilized rectum is pulled down through the subcutaneous tissue to its new location.
6. The end of the fistula is amputated. With interrupted sutures of 4-0 nonabsorbable, the external sphincter is sutured to the rectal serosa.
7. Using 4-0 absorbable suture, a new anus is constructed with interrupted sutures through all layers (Figure 29-17, *D*).
8. A drain may or may not be placed in the anterior incision before it is closed in layers with interrupted 4-0 absorbable sutures.
9. A Hegar dilator is used to calibrate the size of the new anus after closure.

**Repair of High Imperforate Anus: Posterior Sagittal Anorectoplasty.** When a high imperforate anal anomaly presents, surgical intervention is indicated within 24 to 48 hours of birth. A transverse or sigmoid colostomy is performed to

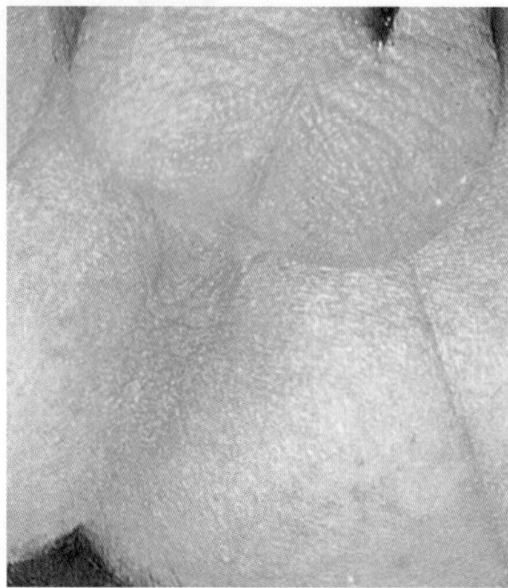

FIGURE 29-16 Imperforate anus.

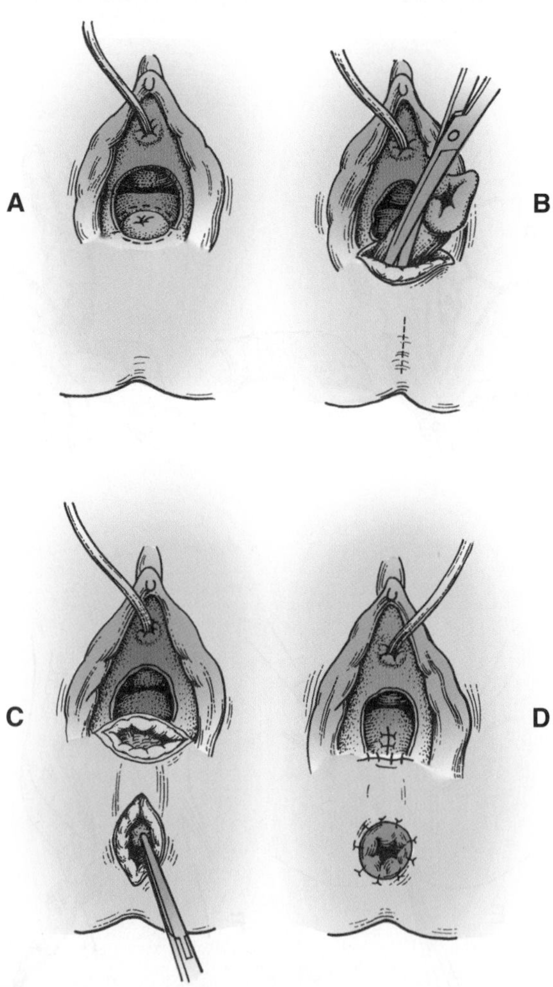


FIGURE 29-17 Anal transposition. **A,** Fistula excised by means of oval incision. **B,** Dissection of bowel from surrounding structures. **C,** Vertical midline incision at site of true anus; identification of external sphincter fibers; mobilized rectum pulled down through subcutaneous tissue to new location. **D,** External sphincter sutured to rectal mucosa; new anus constructed with interrupted sutures through all layers.

irrigate the hiatal lumen and to remove meconium plugs while allowing proximal colon function. After the colostomy, further diagnostic studies, such as cystogram and vaginograms, are done. The posterior sagittal anorectoplasty (PSARP) is the definitive surgical procedure and is performed when the condition and size of the child permit—usually around 1 year of age.

The PSARP is a highly technical procedure that uses electrostimulation throughout and may require position changes.

***Procedural Considerations.*** The child is placed in jackknife position with the hips flexed. Adequate padding must be placed under the hips to avoid compression injury to the femoral nerves. The major instrument set, nerve stimulator, and intestinal instruments are required.

*Operative Procedure (Figure 29-18)*

1. The electrostimulator is used to locate the true anus, and a midsagittal incision is made through the skin from the midsacrum to the anterior border of the anal site.
2. Dissection continues through subcutaneous tissue until the external sphincter muscle layers are identified.

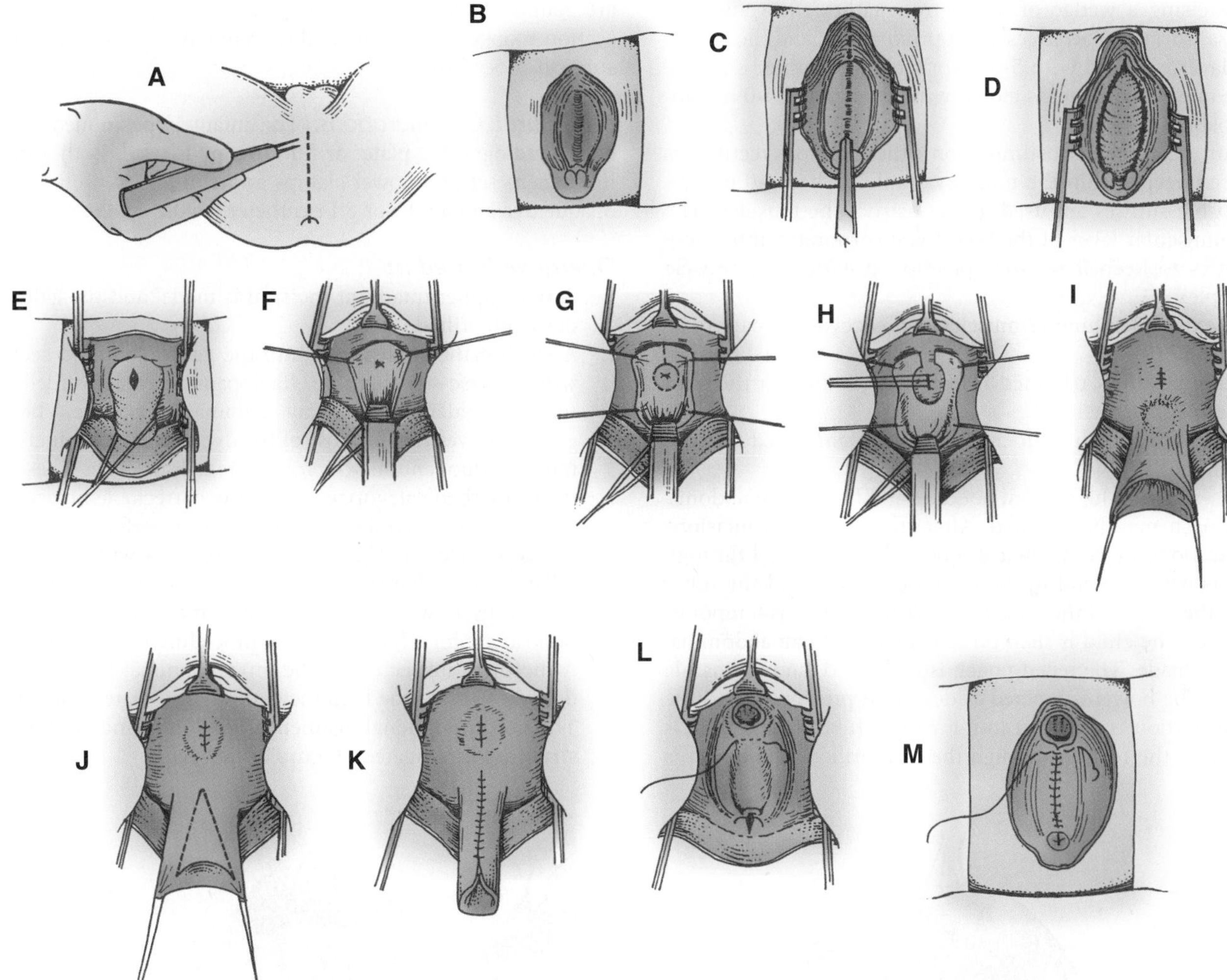


FIGURE 29-18 Posterior sagittal anorectoplasty. **A,** Line of incision and electrical stimulation to determine appropriate anal site. **B,** Midsagittal incision through coccyx and external sphincter fibers of anus, showing striated muscle complex deep to anal site; subcutaneous external sphincter extending about halfway to coccyx; superficial external sphincter inserting on coccyx; levator deeper in midline. **C,** Right-angled forceps beneath levator ani. **D,** All layers of striated muscle partially retracted laterally to expose visceral endopelvic fascia. **E,** Sagittal incision in terminal bowel after proximal dissection around rectum and placement of tape around rectum proximally. **F,** Retracted rectotomy showing fistula site. **G,** Semicircumferential incision through mucosa-submucosa for placement of first sutures to close fistula. **H,** Completed closure of fistula orifice. **I,** Stippled area where muscular bowel wall is left in place and clear area above where peritoneum may be encountered. **J,** Extent of anterior wedge resection for tapered repair of rectum *(dotted line)*. **K,** Approximation of tapered edges of rectum. **L,** First and deepest suture for approximation of levators to establish beginning of canal. **M,** After reapproximation of levator ani to coccyx, interrupted sutures are placed in edges of superficial external sphincter muscle.

3. With electrostimulation, these fibers are dissected midsagittally, exactly in the midline.
4. A midsagittal split of the coccyx is performed, and the striated muscle complex found beneath the coccyx is incised sagittally, along with the visceral endopelvic fascia. Electrostimulation is used to aid in identifying muscle complexes.
5. Next the rectal pouch and urethra are identified, and the bowel is incised vertically to expose the fistulae.
6. The fistula is closed in layers—first the mucosa with interrupted absorbable sutures and then the muscle layer with 5-0 nonabsorbable sutures.
7. The rectum is then mobilized and tapered to allow its placement within the muscle complexes. Tapering consists of excising a wedge of bowel from either the ventral or dorsal surface. The edges are approximated, and the mucosal layer is closed with 5-0 absorbable interrupted sutures. The muscularis layer is closed with interrupted 5-0 nonabsorbable sutures.
8. Again using electrostimulation, the tapered rectum is placed deep within the muscle complex. Then 5-0 nonabsorbable sutures are used to reconstruct the muscles. The seromuscular layer of the bowel is incorporated into these sutures to keep it securely positioned within the muscle complex.
9. The external sphincter muscles and coccyx are reapproximated.
10. Excess bowel is trimmed before it is secured to the skin edges of the anus.
11. Running absorbable subcuticular sutures are used to close the skin.

In cases of very high rectal pouches and fistulas, an abdominal approach may be required. After the midsagittal incisions and dissections are completed, a rubber drain is placed through the pelvis with one end in the peritoneal cavity and the other through the center of the anus to the skin, where it is temporarily sutured. The child is then turned supine, and an abdominal incision is made. The rectal pouch is mobilized, and the fistula is closed. The bowel is tapered as described previously, and the terminal portion is attached to the rubber tube, which then is used to pull the rectum through the anal orifice. The bowel is sutured to the muscle complex, and reapproximation of the coccyx and external sphincter muscle is done as described earlier.

## CORRECTION OF BILIARY ATRESIA

### Hepatic Portoenterostomy (Kasai Procedure)

Biliary atresia is a congenital defect that results from nonpatent extrahepatic bile ducts. Bile is unable to drain from the liver to the small intestine, leading to eventual cirrhosis and death. The Kasai procedure is the construction of a bile drainage system by use of an intestinal conduit. This procedure is indicated in patients with extrahepatic biliary atresia who are younger than 3 months. All atretic segments of the existing bile ducts are removed. An intraoperative cholangiogram and frozen-section biopsy of the hepatic duct remnant are included in the surgical procedure.

***Procedural Considerations.*** The infant is positioned supine over a radiographic plate, or fluoroscopy is used. Both a major instrument set and bowel clamps are required, as well as radiopaque dye and a 6 Fr or 8 Fr catheter for the cholangiography.

#### *Operative Procedure*

1. A right upper quadrant incision is made, and the gallbladder is identified.
2. A small catheter is placed into the gallbladder and secured with a purse-string suture. Radiopaque dye is instilled into the gallbladder, and an x-ray examination is done. The surgeon observes for free flow of the dye through the ducts and into the duodenum, which occasionally is seen. These patients are then categorized as having correctable biliary atresia. In such situations, a liver biopsy is performed and the incision is closed. The majority of patients with correctable biliary atresia demonstrate progressive improvement. More commonly, however, there is a very small amount of flow or none at all, for which the Kasai procedure is performed.
3. A thorough inspection of the intraabdominal organs is then done because of the high incidence of associated anomalies.
4. The hepatoduodenal ligament is explored, and all drainage structures are ligated (Figure 29-19, *A*).

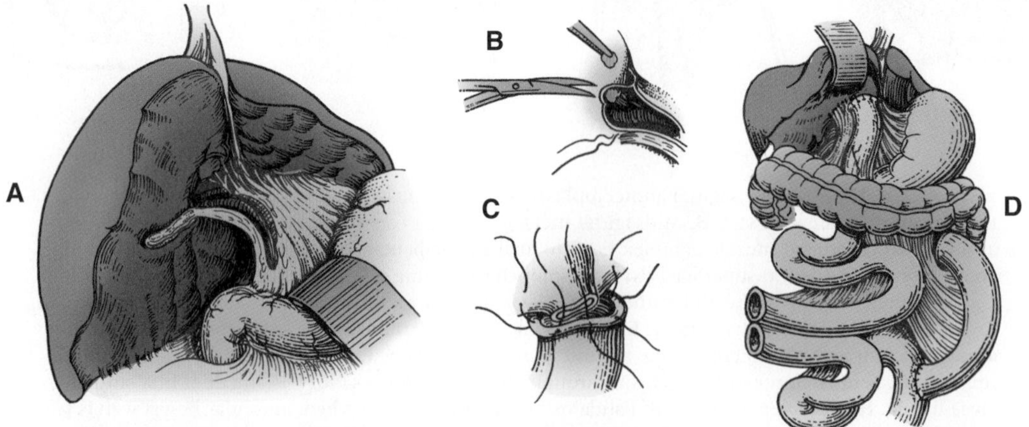


**FIGURE 29-19** Kasai procedure. **A,** Exploration of hepatoduodenal ligament and ligation of drainage structures. **B,** Transection of hepatic duct remnant using frozen-section biopsy specimens as a guide. **C,** Anastomosis of jejunal conduit at porta hepatis. **D,** Exteriorization of conduit using double-barreled Roux-en-Y approach.

5. The hepatic duct remnant is identified and traced to the liver hilum. The remnant is transected as high as possible using frozen-section biopsy specimens as a guide. Frozen-section biopsy specimens are also obtained at the porta hepatis to denote the presence of ductules. Precise identification of this location is essential (Figure 29-19, *B*).
6. The proximal portion of the jejunum is generally used as the intestinal conduit. A meticulous anastomosis is performed at the porta hepatis as previously identified, using a single running layer of absorbable sutures (Figure 29-19, *C*).
7. The conduit is exteriorized with a double-barreled Roux-en-Y approach (Figure 29-19, *D*).
8. A liver biopsy is then performed.
9. A drain is placed, and the incision is closed in layers.

The procedure just described is one approach of many. Others include exteriorization of the jejunal conduit as a cutaneous jejunostomy and use of double Roux-en-Y loops, avoiding any need for an enterostomy. If none of these procedures is successful, the child may be a candidate for liver transplantation.

## RESECTION OF TUMORS

Nearly two thirds of childhood cancers occur as solid tumor malignancies. As is always the case, the therapy administered depends on the type of tumor. Examination and judicious investigation of all unusual masses are imperative. Thorough diagnostic workup and prompt definitive treatment may result in cure, even if the tumor is malignant. Chemotherapy and radiation therapy are adjuncts to surgical excision of tumors.

### Wilms' Tumor

Wilms' tumor, also known as *nephroblastoma,* is the most common intraabdominal childhood tumor. It presents as a painless mass whose enlargement may laterally distend the abdomen (Figure 29-20). The child may be asymptomatic or may have weight loss, malaise, or abdominal pain. Nephroblastomas may cause obstruction of the vena cava, hepatic veins, or renal veins.

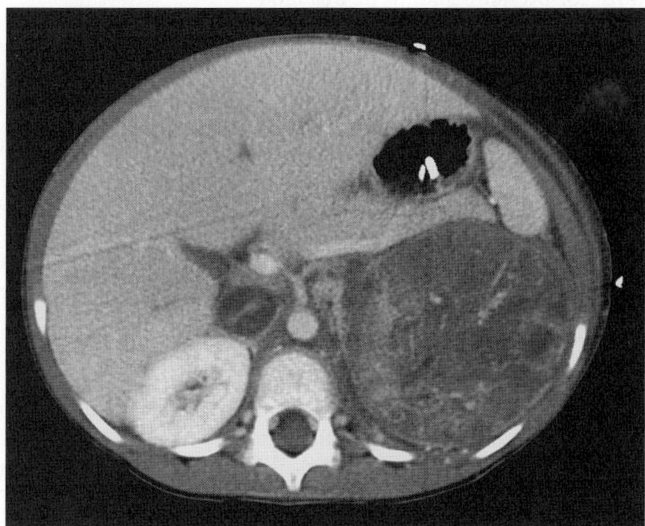

**FIGURE 29-20** Computerized tomographic scan showing left-sided Wilms' tumor with compression of the inferior vena cava.

***Procedural Considerations.*** The child is positioned supine with a roll under the affected side. Both chest and abdomen are prepped. Infrequently the tumor extends into the inferior vena cava as well as the atrium of the heart, and in such cases cardiopulmonary bypass (CPB) should be readily available. Lines are placed into the arms and neck to facilitate clamping of the inferior vena cava if needed. Separate sterile gloves and instruments should be available for inspection of the contralateral kidney. Careful attention should be given when handling tumor and lymph nodes to avoid tumor spillage.

***Operative Procedure.*** If the tumor is operable, the following aspects are important:

1. The transabdominal approach, which may be extended to a combined transabdominal-transthoracic approach, is used to inspect abdominal contents and clamp the vessels of the renal pedicle before tumor dissection.
2. All suspicious lymph nodes are removed, placed into separate containers, and labeled. If no suspicious nodes are present, biopsy specimens are obtained of those in adjacent areas.
3. The opposite kidney is explored before dissection of the tumor.
4. The extent of the tumor can be marked with hemostatic clips to facilitate radiation therapy.
5. The entire primary tumor is removed if doing so does not place the patient in jeopardy.
6. Any residual tumor is marked with clips.
7. Because of its proximity to the kidney, the adrenal gland is usually removed.
8. The abdominal cavity and viscera are thoroughly inspected for evidence of tumor extension or metastases. Extensive surgery may include partial colectomy or partial resection of the diaphragm.

### Neuroblastoma

Neuroblastoma is responsible for 7.4% of all childhood cancers and is the third most common childhood cancer after leukemias and brain and nervous system cancers.[2] It arises from neural crest tissue and can develop anywhere sympathetic nerve tissue is found; the most common sites are the retroperitoneum and adrenal medulla. The mass is usually firm, irregular, and nontender. It is a silent tumor in its early stages and metastasizes rapidly, often to the lymphatics, liver, skin, bone marrow, lung, brain, or orbits. Treatment includes an operation to ligate the tumor's blood supply and remove as much of the tumor as possible, as well as chemotherapy and radiation.

### Sacrococcygeal Teratoma

A sacrococcygeal teratoma is a tumor that originates early in embryonic cell division. The tumor is made up of cell types from more than one embryonic germ layer. Teratomas range from benign, well-differentiated cystic lesions to solid, malignant lesions. They are the most common tumor in newborns, occurring in 1:35,000 to 1:40,000 births.[16] The sacrococcygeal area is the most common extragonadal site of teratoma, usually presenting as a large protuberance rising from that site (Figure 29-21). It may be irregular or symmetric, may vary in size, and may be pedunculated.

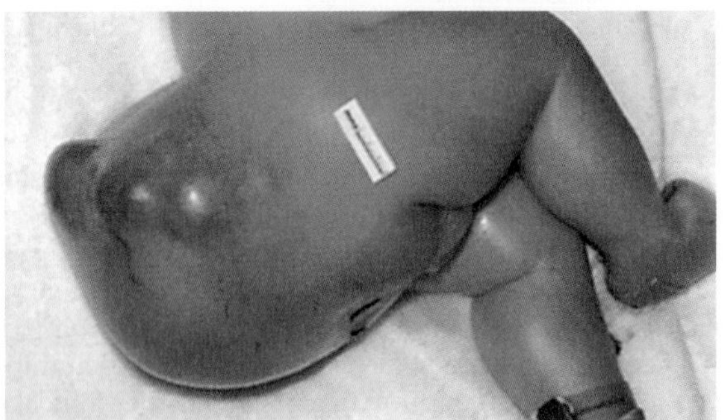

FIGURE 29-21 Infant with large sacrococcygeal teratoma.

A sacrococcygeal teratoma is usually resectable but may undergo malignant changes if not removed early in life. Tumors resected in the newborn period show microscopic evidence of malignant cells, but surgical cures have been achieved. Early surgical resection is important because these tumors are not sensitive to irradiation and are only temporarily responsive to chemotherapy.

The tumor is in the area of the sacrum and coccyx but may extend into the pelvis or abdomen. Resection is usually feasible by placing the patient in the jackknife position and excising the tumor mass and coccyx en bloc. In cases where the tumor extends high into the pelvis, an abdominal incision may also be required.

## GENITOURINARY SURGERY

### Pediatric Cystoscopy

Pediatric cystoscopy is endoscopic examination of the lower urinary tract of pediatric patients. The major difference between adult and pediatric cystoscopy is the size of the instruments used and consideration of the small, delicate orifices of the pediatric patient. Indications for pediatric cystoscopy include urinary tract infections, enuresis, urethral valves, vesicoureteral reflux, diverticula, bladder neck contractures, bladder tumors, and urinary tract obstructions. Pediatric cystoscopy may also be used in conjunction with Deflux injection for minimally invasive treatment of vesicoureteral reflux.

***Procedural Considerations.*** The cystoscopy setup will have the same type of components as those for the adult cystoscopy patient, except that the size of the cystourethroscope system will be specific to the pediatric patient's needs.

Each pediatric cystourethroscope is designed to fit specific component parts and is very delicate. Therefore the perioperative nurse must be familiar with the proper use of the system and handle the components carefully. The resectoscope loop is commonly used to resect urethral valves and occasionally bladder tumors. The cold knife may be used with the resectoscope to cut urethral strictures and occasionally to resect a urethral valve.

The most common anesthesia used for the pediatric patient is general anesthesia. After induction of anesthesia, the child is placed in a lithotomy or frog-leg position and prepped and draped according to established procedure.

***Operative Procedure*** The pediatric cystourethroscope is lubricated and inserted through the urethra into the bladder. The light cord and irrigation tubing are attached to the telescope and cystoscope, and the examination is performed. Most commonly the interior of the bladder is viewed on a video monitor by means of a camera attached to the cystoscope.

### Circumcision

Circumcision is the excision of the foreskin (prepuce) of the glans penis. Circumcision may be done for therapeutic reasons or for perceived prophylactic benefits; it may also be done for religious reasons, as is required in specific faiths. Provision should be made to observe the religious needs and preferences of the parents.

Therapeutic indications include correction of phimosis or paraphimosis or treatment of balanoposthitis. Phimosis is a condition in which the orifice of the prepuce is stenosed or too narrow to permit easy retraction behind the glans. Balanoposthitis is characterized by an inflamed glans and mucous membrane with purulent discharge and may require circumcision. Paraphimosis is a recurrent condition in which the prepuce cannot be reduced easily from a retracted position.

***Procedural Considerations.*** Newborns are generally positioned on a specially constructed board that facilitates restraint by immobilizing the limbs and exposing the genitalia. Although it was once thought that circumcision caused infants little pain, the neonatal foreskin contains mature nerve endings that allow for the transmission of pain. Measures to ameliorate the pain of the procedure include local dorsal penile nerve block, a ring block with buffered lidocaine and bupivacaine (Marcaine), or the topical application of eutectic mixture of local anesthesia (EMLA) cream. Older children require general anesthesia.

For infants, the setup includes fine plastic surgery instruments. A Gomco clamp of the appropriate size, a Plastibell, or the Hollister disposable circumcision device may be employed. The Hollister device includes sutures that are sealed in a sterile packet ready for use. The Plastibell technique uses a plastic ring and suture tied around the foreskin like a tourniquet. The excess tissue is trimmed, and in about 5 to 8 days the ring falls off. For older patients, the circumcision clamp is not needed, and only a plastic surgery instrument set is used. Petrolatum gauze for dressing should be available.

***Operative Procedure (Figure 29-22)***

1. If the prepuce is adherent, a probe or hemostat may be used to break up adhesions. The prepuce is clamped in the dorsal midline and incised toward the coronal mucosa margin, leaving about 5 cm of coronal mucosa intact. A similar procedure is performed ventrally. The two incisions are then joined circumferentially. Alternatively, a superficial circumferential incision is made in the skin with a scalpel at the level of the coronal sulcus and mucosa at the base of the glans. The redundant skin is undermined between the circumferential incisions and removed as a complete cuff.
2. Bleeding vessels are coagulated or clamped with mosquito hemostats and tied with fine absorbable ligatures. Before closure, the area may be cleansed with an appropriate antiseptic solution.
3. The raw edges of the skin incision are approximated to a coronal cuff of mucosal prepuce, generally with interrupted 4-0 or 5-0 absorbable sutures on fine plastic cutting

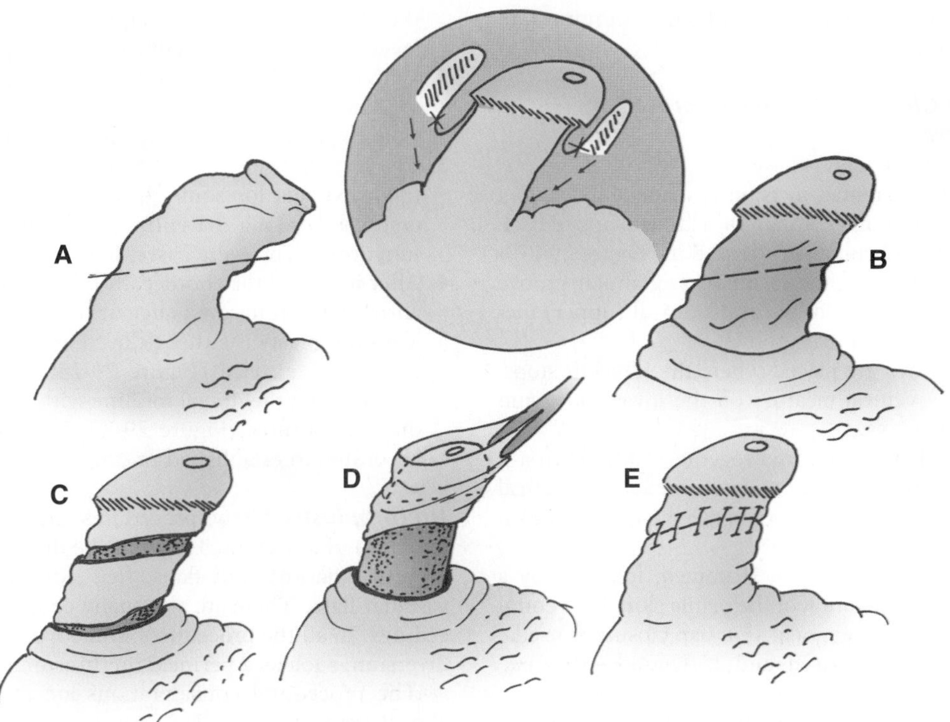


**FIGURE 29-22** Circumcision. **A,** Initial incision made in the shaft. **B,** Second incision made in subcoronal sulcus. **C,** Amount of tissue to be removed. **D,** Removal of tissue. **E,** Shaft skin sutured to subcoronal skin.

or GI needles. The wound is usually dressed with petrolatum gauze or an antibiotic ointment. A penile block with Marcaine is often done for immediate postoperative pain, thus providing a more comfortable emergence from anesthesia.

## Hypospadias Repair

Hypospadias is a developmental anomaly characterized by a urethral meatus that opens onto the ventral surface of the penis proximal to the end of the glans[20] (Figure 29-23). There are varying degrees of hypospadias. The meatus may be on the ventral surface of the glans, on the corona, anywhere along the shaft, in the scrotum, or even in the perineum. The more proximal the opening, the greater the degree of chordee (downward curvature of the penis). Chordee is caused by fibrous bands that extend from the hypospadiac urethral meatus to the tip of the glans and represent the abnormally developed urethra and its investing layer of Buck's fascia, dartos, and skin. In some cases of clinical curvature, however, these fibrous bands may not be present. Although these curvatures are still termed *chordee,* they are not true fibrous chordee.

The principal methods of hypospadias repair are meatoplasty and glanuloplasty, orthoplasty (release of chordee, thereby straightening the penis), urethroplasty (reconstruction of the urethra), skin cover, and scrotoplasty. These may be done in one- or two-stage repairs depending on the extent of the condition. Recently efforts have increased to relocate the meatus to the apex of the glans, especially in the more extensive one-stage repair.

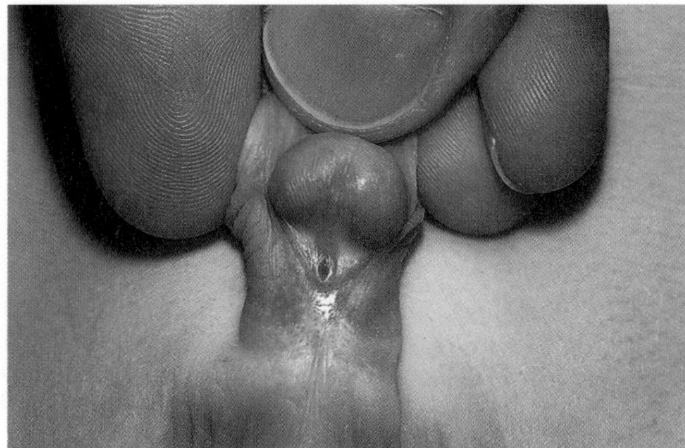

**FIGURE 29-23** Hypospadias.

One complication of hypospadias repair is urethral fistula formation, which can be repaired without much difficulty. Correction of strictures is more troublesome.

***Procedural Considerations.*** The patient (the majority are infants and young children) is placed in the supine position with legs apart. The urine may be diverted with a urethral catheter intraoperatively. The instrument setup varies according to the surgeon's preference. However, a minor set with fine plastic surgery instruments is generally required. Owens gauze, Elastomull, Coban, and Elastoplast, as well as adhesive tape, are generally required for the dressing, which is an important part of the hypospadias repair.

### *Meatoplasty and Glanuloplasty Incorporated (MAGPI) Procedure*

OPERATIVE PROCEDURE

1. A subcoronal circumferential incision is made about 8 mm proximal to the meatus and corona. The skin is stripped back from the phallus by subcutaneous dissection (Figure 29-24).
2. A bridge of tissue between the meatus and glanular groove is made, with a transverse closure of the dorsal (upper) meatal edge to the distal glanular groove.
3. Three traction sutures are placed where the foreskin stops, at the apex of the ventral meatus (on the lower side) and lateral areas of the glans.
4. The edges of the glans are sutured together ventrally in a V configuration, and the redundant edges are excised. Vertical mattress sutures are used to approximate the glans beneath the meatus.
5. If foreskin is excessive, it may be trimmed, followed by a sleeve style of reapproximation of the penile skin. If a ventral skin defect is present, a rotational skin flap closure is used.
6. An indwelling catheter is placed, and the wound is dressed.

***Orthoplasty.*** *Orthoplasty* is the proper designation for the plastic procedure performed to straighten the penis. *Chordee repair* is the more common term employed. In true fibrous chordee the penis is curved downward, with the meatus and glans in proximity to one another.

Artificial erection is achieved by injecting 0.9% preservative-free, injectable saline solution into the corpus cavernosum. Both corporal bodies fill, making it possible to determine the degree of curvature before and after the resection of the fibrous bands.

OPERATIVE PROCEDURE

1. An incision is made circumferentially around the corona and carried distally to the urethral meatus and well below the glans cap (Figure 29-25, *A*). Dissection continues to the level of the tunica albuginea of the corpora cavernosa.
2. With proximal dissection the adherent fibrous plaque is freed, working in a side-to-side fashion. The urethra is elevated from the corpora during this process (Figure 29-25, *B*).
3. The chordee generally surrounds the urethral meatus and often extends for some distance. It is important to free it completely along the entire penile shaft to the penoscrotal junction or, in severe cases, into the scrotum or perineum.
4. After release of the chordee, the glans penis is closed with 4-0 absorbable sutures in a circular manner (Figure 29-25, *C*).
5. If urethroplasty is either delayed or unnecessary, excess dorsal skin is excised (Figure 29-25, *D*) and the incision is closed along the dorsal midline with interrupted absorbable mattress sutures (Figure 29-25, *E*). The wound is dressed according to established protocol.

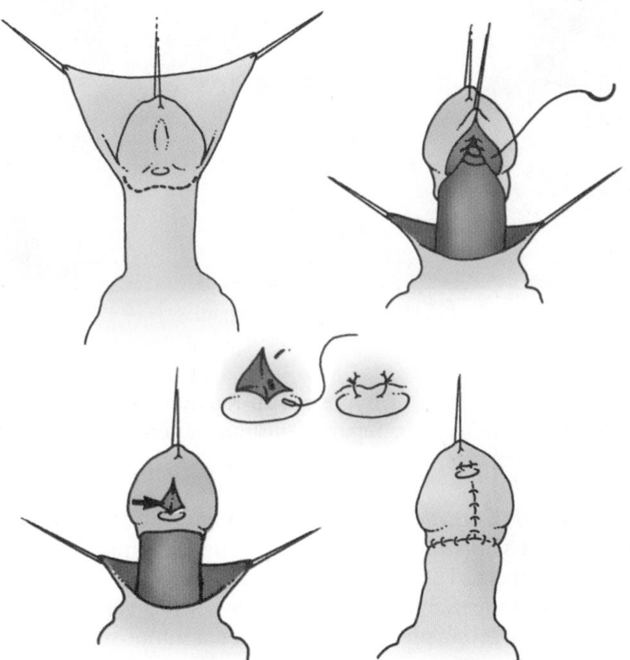

FIGURE 29-24 Meatal advancement and granuloplasty.

***Urethroplasty.*** Many procedures are described for reconstruction of a urethra. They may be divided into three general groups: adjacent skin flaps, free skin grafts, and mobilized vascular flaps. There are also many combinations of these procedures. In all the procedures, some type of temporary urinary diversion, such as a perineal urethrostomy, may be used.

The procedural considerations are the same as those for chordee repair.

ADJACENT SKIN FLAP. It is possible to tubularize skin adjacent to the meatus to create a neourethra in a one-stage repair. Transfer of dorsal skin to the ventrum will also provide graft material close to the meatus. However, this is generally done in two stages, and the vascularity of this thin rotational flap is less than optimum, with results that are prone to complication.

Operative Procedure

1. Traction sutures are placed in the tip of the penis and in the glans wings for stabilization and exposure.
2. The distance between the glans tip and the lower edge of the meatus is measured. An outline of the proposed incision is drawn on the penile shaft (Figure 29-26, *A*). In a one-stage approach the distal length must be increased to compensate for the added penile length after chordee release.
3. An incision is made around the outlined flap and carried proximally to a point on the shaft that corresponds to the distance required to reach the glans tip. A flap width of 14 to 16 mm is usually sufficient to ensure good circumference of the neourethra.
4. Once incised, the tube is rolled over an 8-Fr or 10-Fr catheter (Figure 29-26, *B*) with an inverted running stitch of 4-0 or 5-0 absorbable suture.
5. The glans penis is incised, and the glans wings are undermined and freed. The neourethra is carried to the distal portion of the glans and sutured in place (Figure 29-26, *C*).
6. The glans wings are sutured around the neourethra with absorbable interrupted mattress sutures. The redundant foreskin is split down the midline, and the flaps are brought around in a Z-plasty manner (Figure 29-26, *D*).
7. A dry, sterile, pressure dressing is applied. The patient can often be discharged on the same day, without the need for an indwelling catheter.

FREE SKIN GRAFT. Free skin grafts should be of full thickness. Because the free graft must be revascularized, it is important that it have a perfect skin cover of dorsal preputial

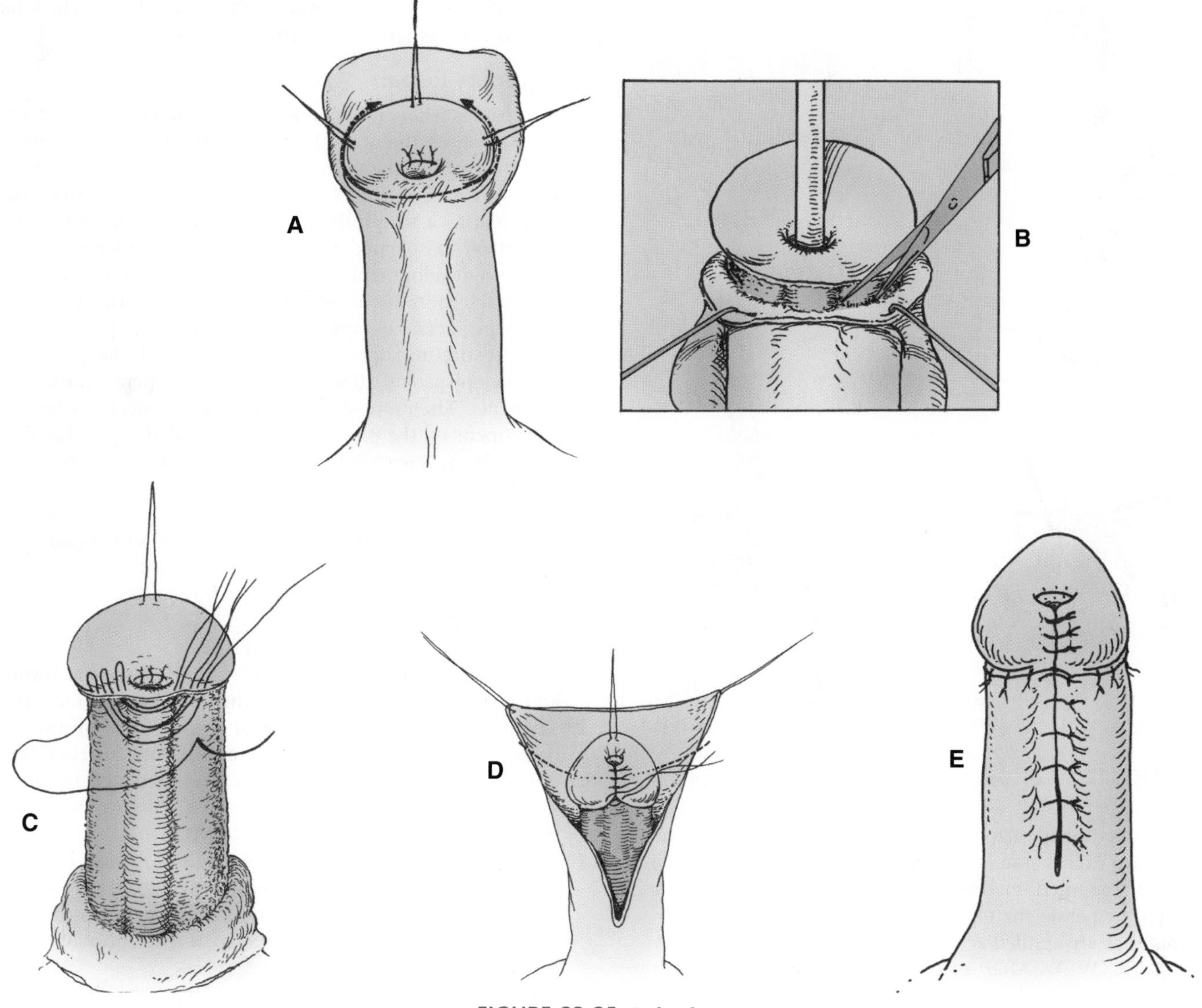


FIGURE 29-25 Orthoplasty.

penile skin that is well vascularized. This type of graft is generally used with a one-stage hypospadias repair.

**Operative Procedure**

1. A V-shaped incision is made on the glans, and the penile skin is mobilized after the chordee release (Figure 29-27, *A*).
2. Glans wings are developed in a triangular fashion, and ventral preputial skin is used for the full-thickness free graft (Figure 29-27, *B*).
3. The graft is formed into a neourethra over a stenting catheter (Figure 29-27, *C*).
4. The graft is anastomosed proximal to the urethra with the suture line of the graft next to the corpora. The middle glans dart is fixed to the corpora (Figure 29-27, *D*).
5. A meatoplasty with the dorsal glans dart is accomplished.
6. Fine absorbable interrupted sutures are placed around the meatus and glans and along the dorsal penile shaft (Figure 29-27, *E*).
7. The wound is dressed according to established protocol.

**MOBILIZED VASCULARIZED FLAPS.** Vascularized flaps of preputial penile skin may be mobilized to the ventrum by leaving them attached to the outer surface of the prepuce or as an island flap. One modification is the transverse preputial island-flap neourethra with glans-channel positioning for the meatus. Preputial skin seems to be preferred because of its rich, reliable blood supply.

**Operative Procedure**

1. The chordee is released (Figure 29-28, *A*).
2. Ventral preputial skin is dissected free and fanned out (Figure 29-28, *B*).
3. The rectangle of skin is rolled into the neourethra and measured (Figure 29-28, *C*).
4. The island flap is developed by dissection of the subcutaneous tissue from the dorsal penile skin (Figure 29-28, *D* and *E*).
5. A glans channel is created with fine scissors in a plane just above the corpora. The glans tissue is removed with the 14-Fr channel, and the island-flap urethra is spiraled to the ventrum (Figure 29-28, *F*).
6. The neourethra is anastomosed proximal to the urethra (Figure 29-28, *G*).
7. The neourethra is carried to the tip of the glans (Figure 29-28, *H*).

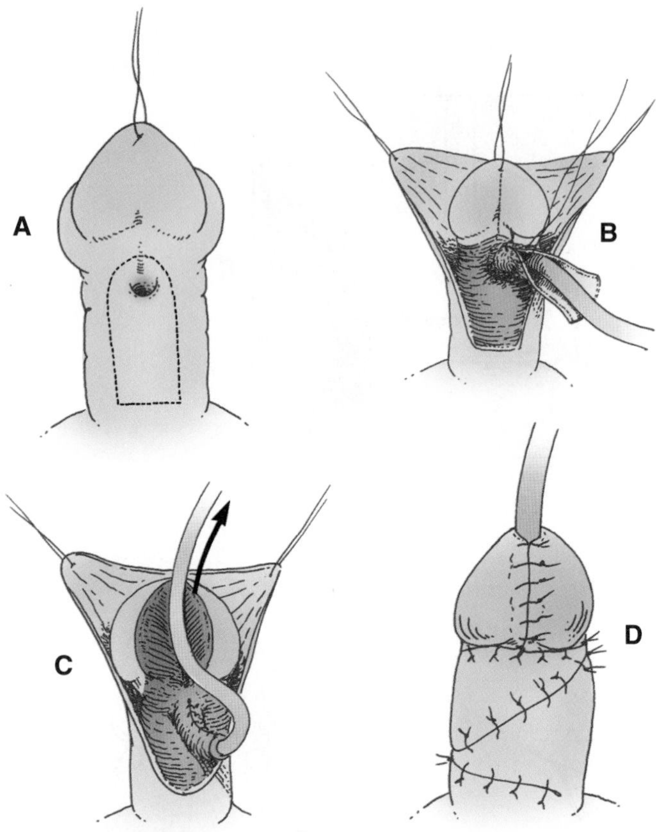


FIGURE 29-26 Urethroplasty with adjacent skin flap.

8. The dorsal penile flaps are transposed laterally to the midline, and excess skin is excised. Closure is with fine absorbable interrupted mattress sutures around the glans and down the penile shaft (Figure 29-28, *I*).
9. Dressings are applied according to established protocol.

SKIN COVER. After orthoplasty and urethroplasty, the penis must be resurfaced with skin. Abundant excess dorsal foreskin is usually adequate to achieve the desired results.

Operative Procedure

1. Preputial tissue is transposed through a small buttonhole opening in the midline (Figure 29-29, *A*).
2. The vasculature is spread laterally, and the glans penis is delivered through the hole (Figure 29-29, *B*).
3. The skin flap is then sutured with fine absorbable interrupted mattress sutures (Figure 29-29, *C*).

## Epispadias Repair

An epispadias is a congenital anomaly characterized by a urethral opening on the dorsum of the penis. The surgical procedures employed in the correction of epispadias depend on the extent of the deformity. In mild, incomplete defects the repair is the same as a simple hypospadias repair. Complete deformity is always associated with urinary incontinence because of little or no development of the bladder neck; thus the operation is much more involved. The least severe forms of the exstrophy-epispadias complex are (1) balanic epispadias, in which the urethra opens on the dorsum of the glans and (2) penile epispadias, in which the urethra opens on the shaft of the penis. The more severe variety, which occurs when the urethra opens on the proximal end of the shaft or in the penopubic position, is generally associated with severe dorsal chordee and urinary incontinence.

***Procedural Considerations.*** The setup for an epispadias repair is as described for hypospadias repair.

### *Operative Procedures*

FIRST-STAGE EPISPADIAS REPAIR

1. A vertical incision is made distal to the epispadial meatus and carried circumferentially to the dorsal coronal margin.
2. The foreshortened dorsal urethral strip is lifted off the corpora cavernosa, and the ventral prepuce (foreskin) is rotated dorsally to cover the dorsal skin defect created by penile straightening.

SECOND-STAGE EPISPADIAS REPAIR

1. A vertical suprapubic incision is made to expose the anterior bladder wall and widened vesical neck. A wedge section of the anterolateral prostatic urethra is removed on either side so that when it is reconstructed, a more normal-caliber prostatic urethra is formed.
2. The roof of the membranous urethra is removed.
3. The prostatic urethra is closed, including muscle that is sutured together in the midline, with absorbable sutures. The bladder is closed so that an indwelling suprapubic catheter is left. The abdomen is closed in layers.
4. The anterior urethra is closed after an appropriate size of octagonal strip of dorsal penile skin is outlined.

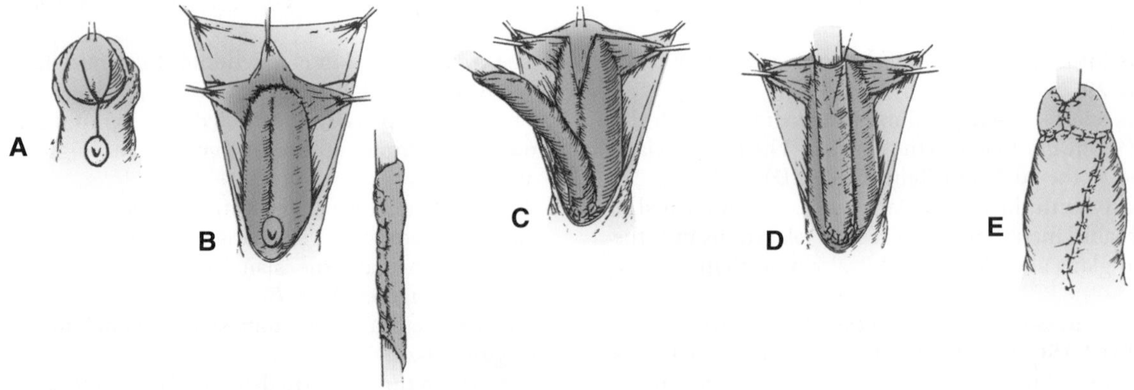


FIGURE 29-27 Urethroplasty with free graft.

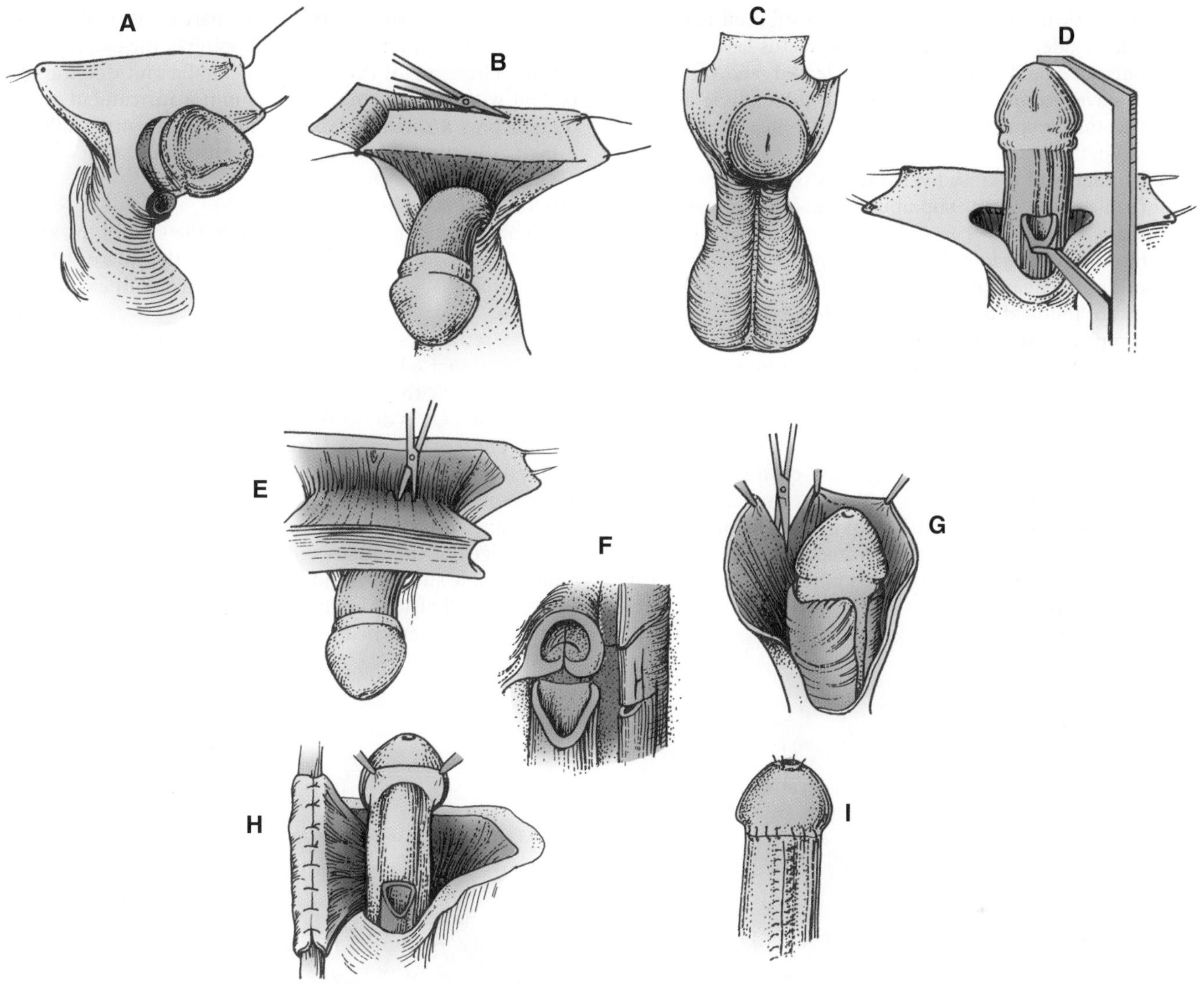

**FIGURE 29-28** Urethroplasty, island flap.

5. The remainder of the repair—the creation of the urethra and its coverage with lateral penile skin—is the reverse procedure of a second-stage hypospadias repair.

## Bladder Exstrophy Repair

Bladder exstrophy repair corrects a more severe form of epispadias, in which the anterior bladder wall as well as the roof of the urethra is absent. Bladder exstrophy is always accompanied by wide separation of the rectus muscles of the lower abdominal wall and by diastasis of the pubic bone with anterior displacement of the anus. Repair of bladder exstrophy requires an adequate size of bladder for ultimate continence to be achieved. It is preferable to perform this procedure in the neonatal period.

***Procedural Considerations.*** The infant is placed in a supine position, and the abdomen and thighs are prepped and draped. Instruments are as required for hypospadias repair.

### *Operative Procedure*

1. An incision is made around the exposed bladder medial to the paravesical neck mucosa. The incision is carried distally across the epispadial urethra distal to the verumontanum.

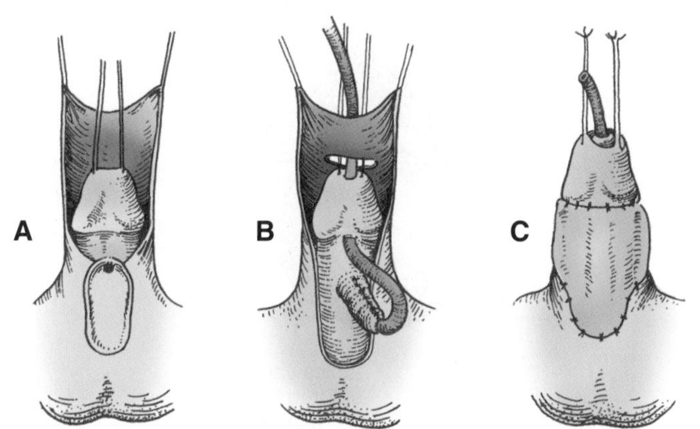


**FIGURE 29-29** Skin cover procedure.

The paravesical mucosa is preserved for urethral lengthening. The bladder is then freed from the rectus fascia and the peritoneum. The dorsal chordee is released, and the mobilized paravesical mucosa is apposed in the midline and sutured to the proximal end of the urethra just distal to the verumontanum.

2. The bladder wall is closed vertically in two layers with 3-0 absorbable sutures; a suprapubic tube is inserted for drainage.
3. The bladder neck is loosely reconstructed by approximating the interpubic ligament, which extends between the proximal end of the phallus and the pubic bone.
4. The symphysis pubis is approximated with a heavy nonabsorbable suture. During this step the assistant rotates the iliac bones anteriorly.

## Hydrocelectomy

A hydrocele is an abnormal accumulation of fluid within the scrotum. The fluid is contained within the tunica vaginalis. Excessive secretion or accumulation of hydrocele fluid may be the result of infection or trauma. A hydrocelectomy is the excision of the tunica vaginalis of the testis to remove the enlarged, fluid-filled sac. In older patients, the procedure is performed through a scrotal incision.

***Procedural Considerations.*** The patient is placed in the supine position. Preparation and draping of the patient include routine cleansing of the external genitalia and draping of the patient with a fenestrated sheet. A minor instrument set is required, plus a small drain, a 30-ml syringe with a 20-gauge, 2-inch aspirating needle, and a suspensory dressing.

### *Operative Procedure*

1. An anterolateral incision is made in the skin of the scrotum over the hydrocele mass by a scalpel with a #10 or #15 blade (Figure 29-30, *A*). Bleeding is controlled with electrocoagulation.
2. Small retractors may be placed, after which the fascial layers are incised to expose the tunica vaginalis (Figure 29-30, *B*). With fine scissors, forceps, and blunt dissection, the hydrocele is dissected free and delivered (Figure 29-30, *C*). The sac is opened, and the fluid contents are aspirated.
3. The sac is inverted so that it surrounds the testis, epididymis, and distal cord. Excess tunica vaginalis is excised, and the edges of the tunica are sutured with a continuous 4-0 absorbable suture behind the testicle (Figure 29-30, *D*). The testicle is "bottled" by the inverted tunica vaginalis, and this may then be returned to the sac.

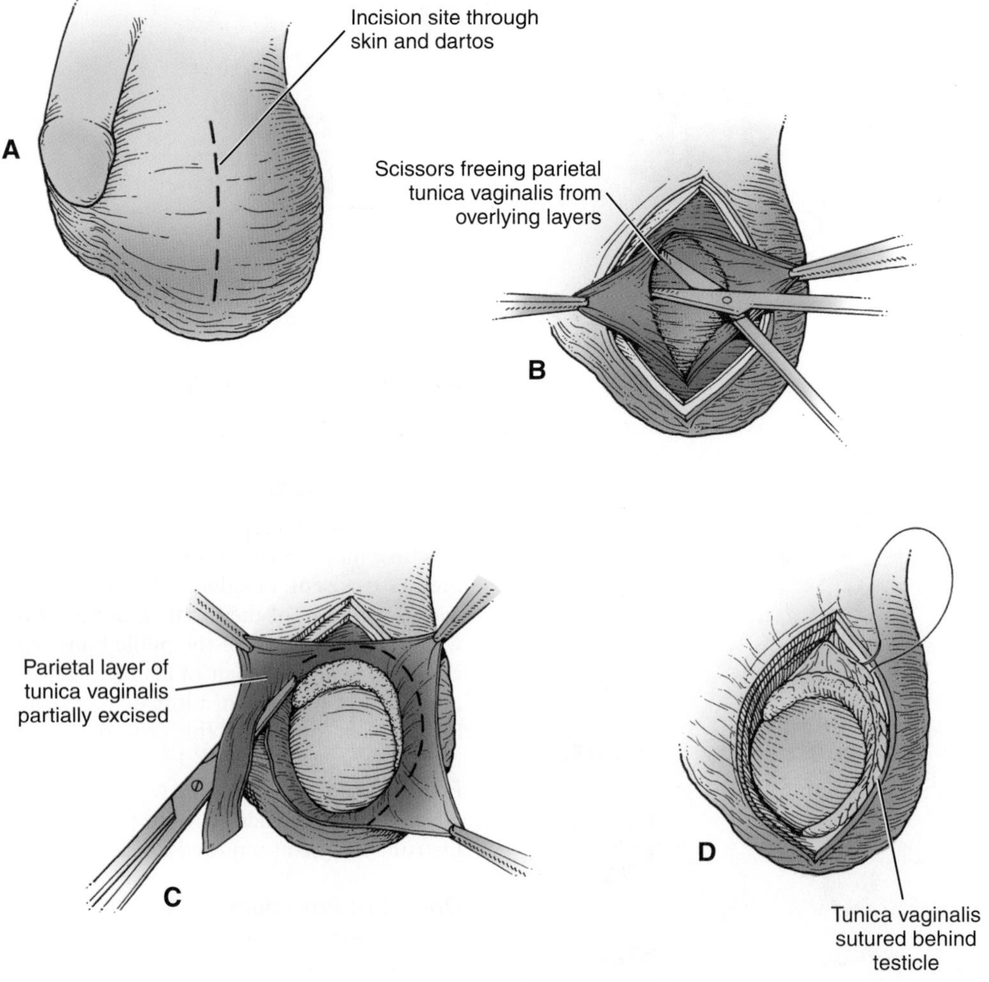


FIGURE 29-30 Hydrocelectomy.

4. A drain is placed within the scrotum and brought out through a stab wound in the most dependent portion of the scrotum. The scrotal incision is closed in layers with 3-0 and 4-0 absorbable sutures. A fluff compression dressing contained in a scrotal support (suspensory) helps reduce postoperative scrotal edema.

## Orchiopexy

An orchiopexy is the surgical placement and fixation of the testicle in a normal anatomic position in the scrotal sac. If the testis fails to descend into the scrotum during gestation, it is considered undescended. An undescended testis becomes arrested somewhere along its normal path of descent. If it is palpable in a position other than its normal path of descent, its position is considered to be ectopic.

A retractile testis has fully descended into the scrotum but retracts out of the scrotum as a result of contraction of the cremaster muscle. Gentle manipulation allows replacement of the testis in the most dependent portion of the scrotum. Retractile testes require no surgical or hormonal treatment.

All testes that are undescended after 1 year, including those that are unresponsive to hormone injections, require surgical placement in the scrotum for optimum maturation. Laparoscopic exploration may also be used to determine position, existence, or size of a "hidden" testis.

***Procedural Considerations.*** The setup is as described for hydrocelectomy. Prepping and draping include the lower abdomen, genitalia, and thighs. Because this operation is usually performed on children, a setup containing small, delicate instruments and sutures is required.

### *Operative Procedure*

1. An inguinal incision is generally employed for exploration of undescended testes (Figure 29-31, *A*). Most undescended testes are located in the superficial inguinal pouch or inguinal canal.
2. The external oblique aponeurosis is opened through the external inguinal ring to expose the inguinal canal; the gubernacular attachments of the undescended testis are dissected free as high as the internal inguinal ring or into the abdominal cavity (Figure 29-31, *B*).
3. All adhesions and the associated inguinal hernia sac are freed to lengthen the cord so that the testis is allowed to reach the scrotal cavity (Figure 29-31, *C*). The hernia sac is transected, twisted, and ligated with sutures.
4. To draw vessels into the inguinal canal, more proximal to the scrotum, the floor of the inguinal canal may have to be divided at the internal ring (Figure 29-31, *D*).
5. The lateral portion of the internal ring is closed to prevent herniation. A scrotal pocket is created, and the testis is anchored in a normal anatomic position within the scrotum with absorbable sutures (Figure 29-31, *E* to *K*).

NOTE: Orchiopexy may be accomplished by several surgical methods. The dependent portion of the undescended testis may be sutured to the base of the scrotum with absorbable or nonabsorbable sutures brought out through the scrotal wall and tied over a peanut dissector or pledget. The most popular method is to anchor the testis into a dissected subdartos pouch. In this procedure, a small midtransverse scrotal incision is made and the skin and dartos muscle are dissected to create a pouch. The testis is then brought through a small hole in the dartos into the subdartos pouch and anchored in position by the traction suture. The overlying skin of the subdartos pouch is closed with fine absorbable suture material. The inguinal incision is repaired in layers with 3-0 absorbable sutures. The skin is closed with a subcuticular suture, and Dermabond is used for dressing.

## Vesicoureteral Reflux

Vesicoureteral reflux (VUR) is defined as the retrograde flow of urine from the bladder to the ureter and even to the kidney pelvis. Children are usually initially diagnosed with the occurrence of a febrile urinary tract infection (UTI). The workup for reflux will include a renal bladder ultrasound with prevoid and postvoid views as well as a voiding cystourethrogram (VCUG). The VCUG is used to grade the reflux, with grade I being the least and grade V being the most extensive reflux. Children with VUR are given prophylactic antibiotics and checked yearly. Children with unresolved reflux or breakthrough infections will probably require repair of the reflux. Currently there are two types of repair. For lower-grade reflux the most common approach is the minimally invasive approach of cystoscopy with injection of Deflux at the ureteral orifice into the bladder wall (Research Highlight). If the reflux is more severe, the child may require reimplantation of the ureter into the bladder wall.

## RESEARCH HIGHLIGHT

### Treating Vesicoureteral Reflux

Vesicoureteral reflux (VUR) is a condition characterized by the retrograde flow of urine from the bladder into the ureters. The degree of reflux is rated on a grading scale of I to V. Grade I represents mild backflow up the ureter whereas grade V is severe backflow that causes dilation of the ureter and kidney. Low-grade VUR is treated conservatively with antibiotics and infection monitoring through urine cultures. Higher grades of the condition have traditionally required ureteral reimplantation for correction and management.

The use of dextranomer/hyaluronic acid co-polymer (Deflux) injection to the ureteral orifice offers a minimally invasive way to treat VUR. Researchers conducted a prospective study to determine the success factors influencing the effectiveness of using Deflux to treat VUR. The material is injected at the vesicoureteral junction in a "volcano" shape to provide a cushion that prevents the urine from returning to the ureter.

A total of 53 patients (50 females and 2 males; 80 ureters) were treated with a single injection of Deflux. The appearance (i.e., degree of mounding) of the injection was recorded. Researchers defined success as no reflux on postoperative voiding cystourethrography and were able to demonstrate success as 82% for grade I reflux, 84% for grade II, 78% for grade III, and 73% for grade IV. Their overall cure rate was 80% by ureter and 71% by patient.

In reviewing the data to determine success factors, they found a higher success rate (87%) in those injections with volcano-shaped mounds. Deflux offers a promising minimally invasive alternative to treat VUR.

Modified from Lavell MT and others: Subureteral injection of Deflux for correction of reflux: analysis of factors predicting success, *Urology* 65(3):564-567, 2005.

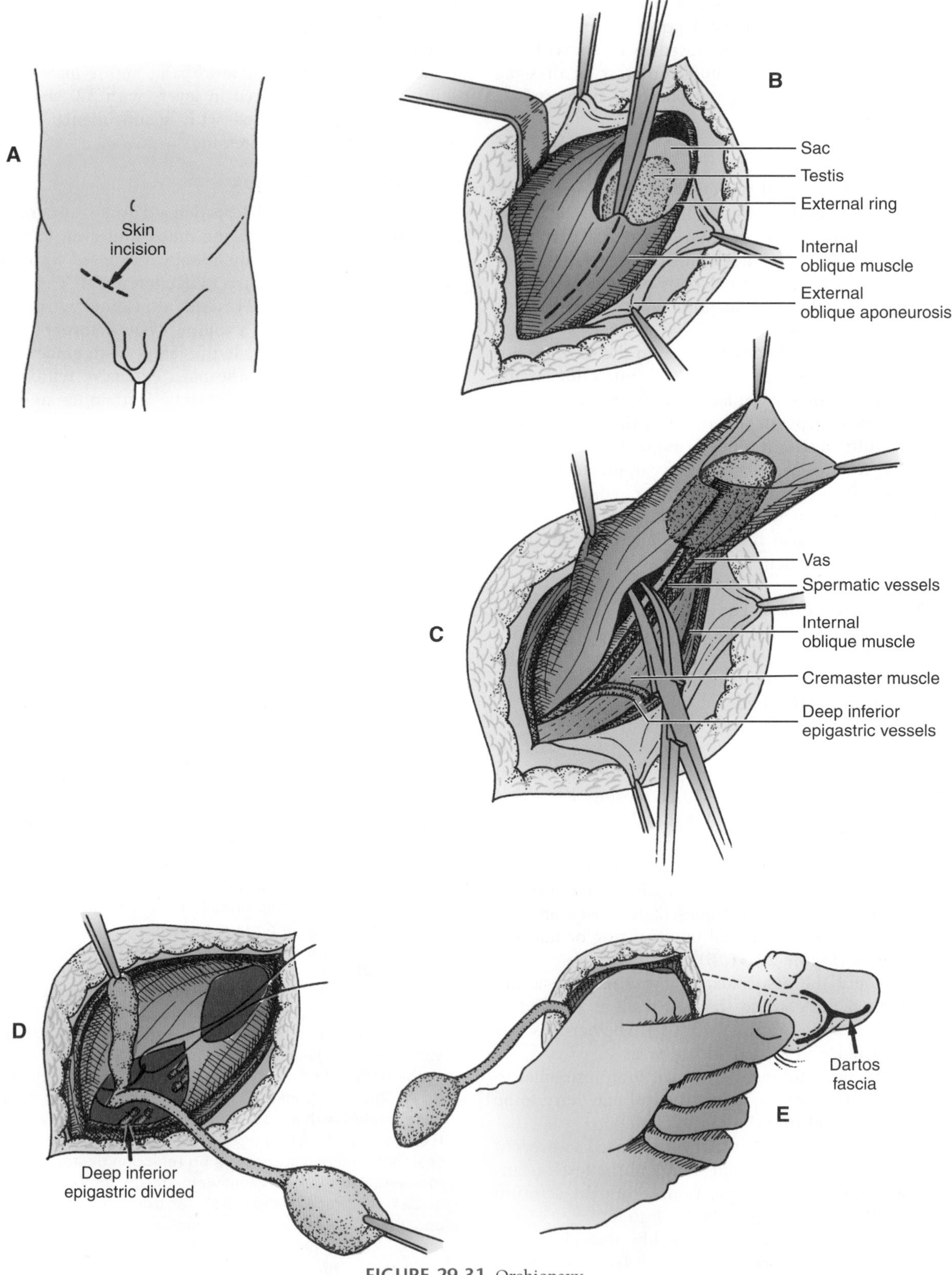


FIGURE 29-31 Orchiopexy.

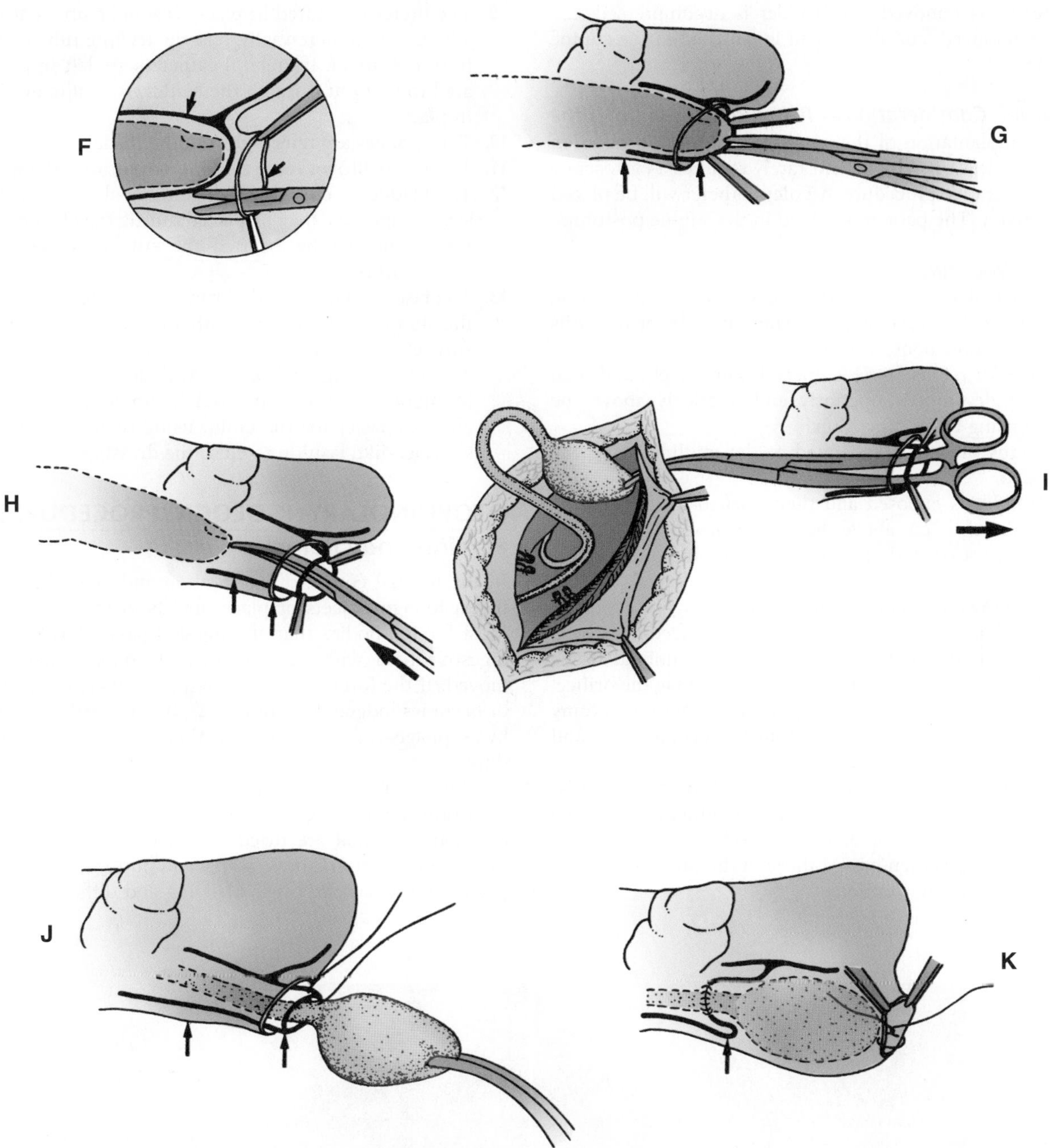


FIGURE 29-31, cont'd Orchiopexy.

***Procedural Considerations—Deflux.*** The setup for Deflux injection includes the same basic cystoscopy setup as described for cystoscopy including a 10-Fr offset cystoscope, light cord with a light source, cystoscopy fluid delivery tubing, Deflux needle, syringe of Deflux, and camera and monitor for the surgeon to view the procedure. The offset scope is the key to a good injection because the lens is offset at approximately a 45-degree angle and the port to insert the needle through the scope comes straight off the end of the scope. The patient is placed in dorsal lithotomy position for the procedure.

### *Operative Procedure*

1. The pediatric offset cystourethroscope is lubricated and inserted through the urethra into the bladder. The light cord, camera, and irrigation tubing are attached to the cystoscope, a urine specimen for culture is obtained, and then an examination is performed.
2. The bladder is partially filled, allowing good visualization of it.
3. The irrigation fluid is jetted into the ureteral orifice, opening it wide (hydrodistention), and then the needle is introduced under the mucosa of the midureteral tunnel at the 6-o'clock position. The needle tip is positioned just under the urothelium and is advanced 4 to 5 mm in the submucosal plane of the ureter. Deflux is then injected until a prominent bulge appears, and the orifice has assumed a volcano-like shape.
4. The needle is kept in position for 15 to 30 seconds after the injection to prevent extravasation of Deflux.

5. The needle is removed, the bladder is decompressed, the scope is removed, and the patient is returned to the supine position.

***Procedural Considerations—Reimplantation of the Ureter.*** Reimplantation of the ureter is indicated in children with high-grade VUR. The patient rarely requires a cystoscopy before the operative procedure. A Foley catheter will be placed intraoperatively. The patient is placed in the supine position.

*Operative Procedure*

1. A Pfannenstiel incision (a transverse skin incision along the pelvic skin crease, approximately two finger breadths above the pubic bone) is made.
2. The anterior rectus fascia is opened transversely, and then flaps are developed superiorly and inferiorly above the muscle using blunt dissection.
3. The rectus muscle is separated at the midline along the linea alba.
4. The bladder is exposed and then opened in the midline approximately 2 cm above the bladder neck. The bladder is decompressed and then packed with radio-detectable sponges.
5. A Denis-Brown retractor is placed, and the trigone exposed.
6. The ureter is identified, and a 6-Fr or 8-Fr feeding tube is placed; then the ureter is dissected with minimal tissue handling and an absorbable stitch is used to tag the orifice. The ureter is then further dissected sharply with tenotomy scissors, completely freeing it from the bladder wall and allowing it to move freely.
7. The original ureteral orifice is then used to begin the dissection for a tunnel leading to the new outlet between the bladder mucosa and the detrusor muscle.
8. The suture tag is then passed through the tunnel, bringing the ureter to its new outlet.
9. The ureter is sutured in place with interrupted absorbable stitches circumferentially, and the feeding tube is removed from the ureter. If ureteral catheters are left in place, they are brought out through the bladder and skin and sutured in place.
10. The sponges are removed from the bladder.
11. The Denis-Brown retractor is removed from the field.
12. The bladder is closed with a running absorbable suture (a suprapubic tube may be placed during the closure). A Penrose drain may be inserted and stitched in place with a nylon suture.
13. The fascia is closed with a running absorbable suture, and the skin is approximated with a running subcuticular closure. Dermabond is applied. If a drain is used, an absorbent wound dressing such as an ABD dressing is applied and Montgomery straps are used in order to make dressing changes easier for the child, using twill tape to string in shoelace-like fashion to close the dressing.

## OTORHINOLARYNGOLOGIC PROCEDURES

### Foreign Body Removal

In the normal course of exploration and play, children often ingest foreign objects or place objects in their noses or ears. Most foreign bodies that are ingested pass safely through the digestive tract without incident and do not need to be removed. If the foreign body is sharp, is caustic (i.e., batteries), or becomes lodged (Figure 29-32), it may need to be removed by esophagoscopy (see Chapter 21) or through an open procedure.

The external ear canal and nose are other areas of interest to curious children. Common objects placed in the nares and external ear canal are dried beans, buttons, plastic objects, metals, food, erasers, nuts, seeds, and button batteries.[17] Items placed in the ear can cause bleeding and difficulty with hear-

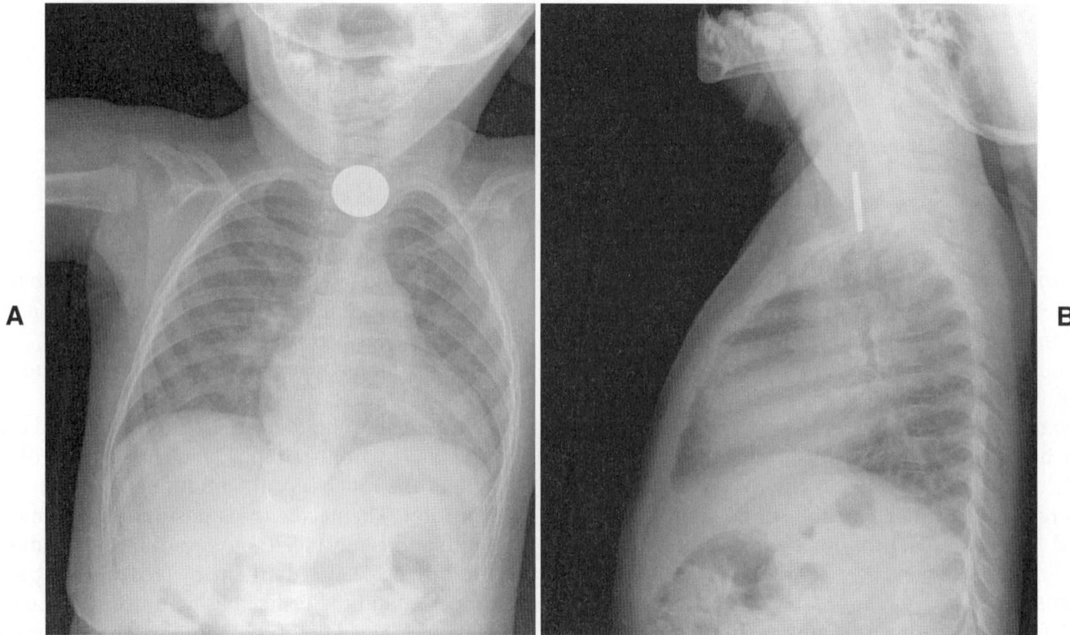


**FIGURE 29-32** **A,** Anteroposterior view of coin trapped in esophagus. **B,** Lateral view.

ing. A high index of suspicion should be raised in the child with unilateral rhinorrhea, nasal crusting, and air outflow obstruction because these symptoms are often caused by a nasal foreign body. Foreign bodies in the nose and ear may require removal in the OR setting with conscious sedation or general anesthesia.

The most significant risk of foreign-body ingestion is aspiration. Children are more prone to aspiration than adults because their laryngeal sphincters are immature, they do not have molars to chew all foods adequately, and they often run, shout, and play with objects in their mouths. The most commonly aspirated food products are candy/gum, peanuts and other nuts, seeds, popcorn, hot dogs, vegetable matter, meat matter, and fish bones. The most commonly aspirated nonfood items are coins, toy parts, crayons, pen tops, tacks, nails, needles, pins, beads, and screws.[17] Aspiration may produce a complete or partial airway obstruction (Figure 29-33). Foreign objects in the respiratory tree are removed by means of rigid or flexible bronchoscopy (see Chapter 25).

## Myringotomy with Ear Tube Placement

A myringotomy (incision of the tympanic membrane) with placement of a ventilation tube is performed as a short-term treatment for eustachian tube dysfunction resulting in otitis media (OM). This procedure is indicated when fluid has been present in the middle ear (serous OM) with conductive hearing loss for 8 to 12 weeks despite medical therapy, when the child has had numerous, frequent episodes of recurrent acute OM, or when significant tympanic membrane retraction is present with potential for fibrous adhesions or cholesteatoma formation.

OM is the second most common disease of childhood, after upper respiratory infection (URI); and OM is the most common cause for childhood visits to a physician's office. Annually, an estimated 16 million office visits are attributed to OM.[14] Risk factors for the development of OM include exposure to bacteria/viruses in a day care setting, exposure to passive (secondhand) cigarette smoke, bottle feeding (notably when the infant is fed lying down), and congenital abnormalities, such as cleft palate or Down syndrome. Although the majority of children with serous OM have spontaneous resolution, hearing loss caused by fluid in the middle ear can have a negative impact on a young child's speech development or on a school-age child's performance in class. Adults who may require this procedure can have it performed in an office setting; children require a general anesthetic to avoid moving while it is done. The procedure itself is very brief.

***Procedural Considerations.*** Myringotomy with tube placement is considered a clean procedure. The patient is usually not prepped or draped and receives a mask anesthetic only. The surgeon generally just wears gloves, depending on the policy related to Standard Precautions at the institution in which the procedure is performed. A microscope and suction are required.

The instrument setup includes the following: assorted sizes of aural speculums, wax curette, myringotomy knife, very delicate alligator forceps, Baron 5-Fr and 7-Fr suction tips, Rosen 18- to 22-gauge suction tips with suction tip adapter, and absorbent cotton. An alternate setup would be to use a disposable myringotomy set; several are available commercially. A very large number of ventilation tubes, made up of different materials and shapes (Figure 29-34), are available. The tubes are designed to remain in place for about 6 to 24 months and usually fall out on their own.

### *Operative Procedure*

1. An aural speculum is inserted into the ear canal, and the operating microscope is positioned. Excess cerumen is removed with a wax curette.
2. A small, radial incision is made in the anterior quadrant of the pars tensa with a myringotomy knife.
3. Fluid, if present, is suctioned from the middle ear space.
4. A tube is then inserted into the incision with an alligator forceps.

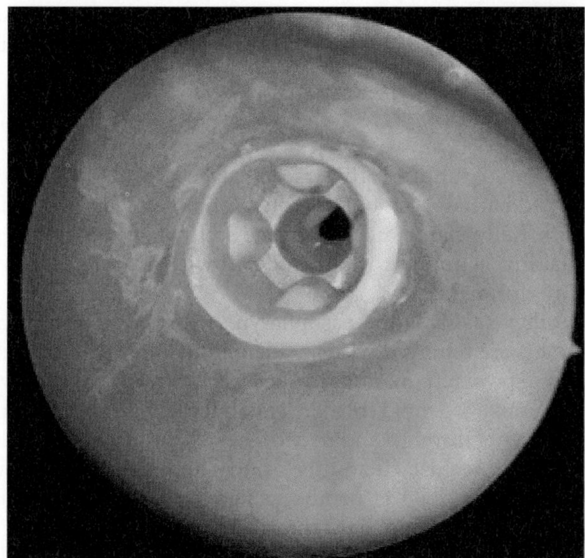

**FIGURE 29-33** Foreign body causing partial airway obstruction.

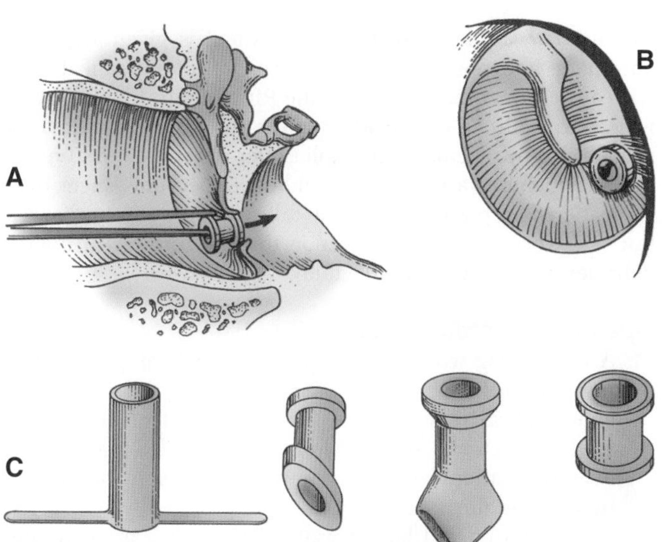


**FIGURE 29-34** **A,** Tube (placed on end of alligator forceps) being inserted into tympanic membrane. **B,** Tube in place. **C,** Several types of plastic tubes that may be inserted into tympanic membrane. Purpose of tubes is to aerate middle ear and reduce middle ear infections.

5. The lumen of the tube is gently suctioned with an 18- or 20-gauge suction tip.
6. Antibiotic drops may be instilled after the tube is positioned.

## Tonsillectomy and Adenoidectomy

Tonsillectomy and adenoidectomy are performed for two major reasons: either for multiple recurrent infections or for upper airway obstruction. Recurrent adenotonsillar infections may cause significant amounts of missed school and contribute to other medical problems, such as asthma, OM, and sinus disease. Upper airway obstruction caused by adenotonsillar hypertrophy can cause obstructive sleep apnea; children can have difficulties concentrating on schoolwork because of the chronic sleep disorder. A history and physical exam are usually sufficient to determine the need for surgery. Sometimes the surgical removal of just tonsils or adenoids needs to be done; the decision is based on the preoperative evaluation. A lateral neck film can indicate enlarged adenoids but is not helpful or necessary to evaluate the size of the tonsils. Occasionally a sleep study may be ordered to evaluate the degree of obstruction. The surgical procedure is particularly painful in the first 5 to 7 days of the postoperative period, because the eschar caused by the electrocoagulation of the surgical sites moves every time the patient swallows. The parents are instructed to keep a daily log of the child's drinking, eating, number of voids, and medication intake during the postoperative period until the child's activities return to normal, to help avoid dehydration and ensure adequate pain management. There is a small but significant risk (approximately 2% to 3%) of bleeding in the postoperative period that may necessitate emergent return to the OR for evaluation and additional electrocoagulation; families need to contact their surgeon immediately if there is any amount of bleeding, however small, in the recovery period.[9] Postoperative complications may include velopharyngeal insufficiency, nasopharyngeal stenosis, or pharyngeal stenosis.

***Procedural Considerations.*** The patient is given a general anesthetic and positioned supine. An oral endotracheal tube with a preformed bend, such as the Ring, Adair, Elwin (RAE), is used to facilitate visualization of the surgical field. The neck is extended by placing a small roll under the shoulders. Typical draping includes a head drape and an impervious sheet over the patient; no prep is used. The following description is of a hot (electrocoagulation) dissection tonsillectomy with microdebrider dissection adenoidectomy.

### *Operative Procedure (Figure 29-35)*

1. A mouth gag with an appropriately sized tongue blade is inserted in the mouth and opened, keeping the tongue and endotracheal tube midline. The distal end of the tongue blade retractor is stabilized on the edge of a Mayo stand over the patient's chest to prevent movement of the patient's head during surgery.
2. The posterior and lateral walls of the palate are carefully inspected and palpated to detect abnormally positioned vessels. The hard palate is palpated to detect the presence of a submucous cleft palate. A submucous cleft indicates the need to allow adenoid tissue to remain, to avoid the complication of velopharyngeal insufficiency.

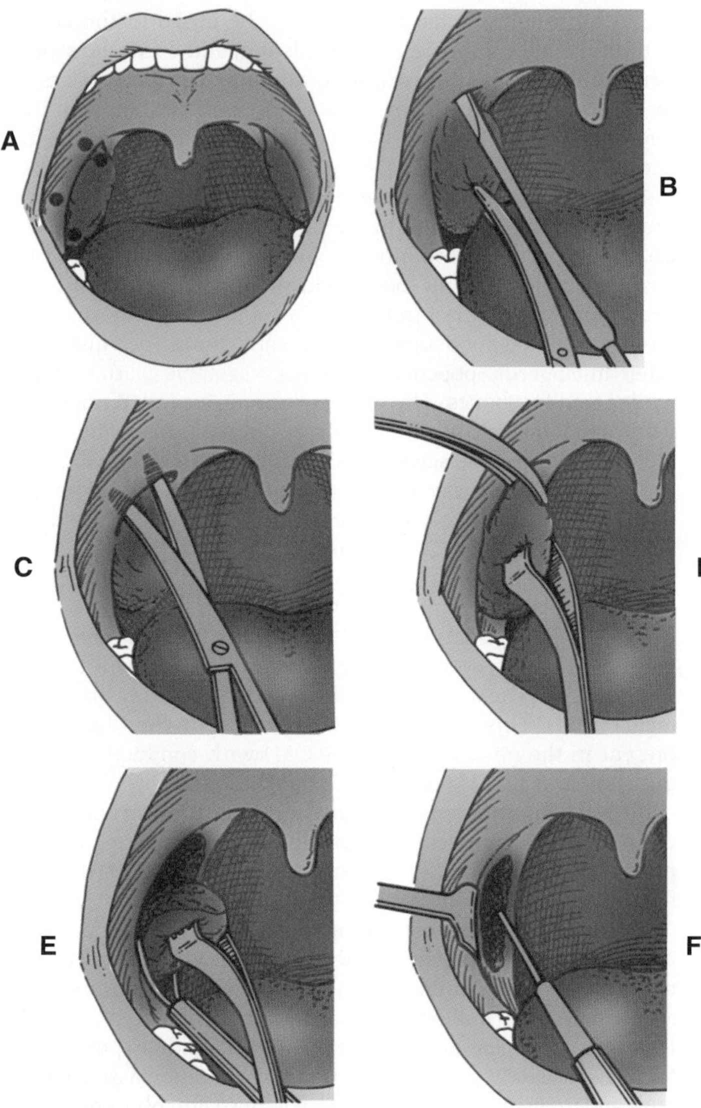


FIGURE 29-35 Surgical method of tonsillectomy. **A,** Local anesthesia infiltration points. **B,** Tonsil knife is used to make an incision at the tonsil anterior pillar superiorly. **C** and **D,** Scissors are used to dissect the superior pole of the tonsil. **E,** A snare is used to separate the tonsil from the lower pole. **F,** Hemostasis is achieved by electrocoagulation or tying of bleeding vessels.

3. 12-Fr red rubber catheters are placed through the nose, pulled partially out of the mouth, and then clamped snugly with Kelly clamps to retract the soft palate forward. A visual inspection of the adenoid bed with a laryngeal mirror is performed.
4. While visualizing the nasopharynx with the mirror, the adenoids are removed with an adenotome or curette or by using a powered microdebrider instrument with a curved, disposable adenoid blade. The microdebrider simultaneously cuts through and suctions away tissue. Care is taken to avoid the eustachian tube orifices and the torus tubarius.
5. The adenoid bed is firmly packed with moistened tonsil sponges. The sponges and the strings are thoroughly soaked in saline to avoid the risk of airway fire when electrosurgery is used in proximity to the sponges. The sponges

are left in place while the tonsils are removed. If the tonsils are so large as to impede visualization of the adenoids, then the tonsils must be removed first.

6. A tonsil suction is then inserted near the surgical field to remove the surgical plume (also referred to as "surgical smoke") from the electrosurgical active electrode and to help prevent pooling of oxygen in the pharynx from the endotracheal tube leak while the tonsils are removed.
7. The superior pole of the right tonsil is grasped with an Allis clamp, and the mucosal cuts on the anterior and posterior tonsillar pillars are outlined with electrosurgery using a guarded blade tip, preserving as much mucosa as possible.
8. Using careful dissection, the plane of the tonsillar capsule is located. The tonsil is removed by dissection with the electrosurgical unit as the tonsil is retracted medially with the Allis clamp. Larger vessels, when encountered, require additional cauterization.
9. The attachment of the inferior portion of the pharyngeal tonsil to the lingual tonsil is transected with the electrosurgical unit, and the tonsil is removed.
10. Residual bleeding vessels are coagulated with a suction/electrocoagulation device while the tonsil fossa is exposed using a Hurd dissector for retraction. The recessed superior pole of the tonsillar fossa is best visualized using a laryngeal mirror.
11. The procedure is repeated on the left side.
12. The sponges that were packed in the nasopharynx are then removed, and any remaining bleeding is stopped using the suction/electrocoagulation device with the mirror.
13. The mouth gag is released for a brief period, and then reopened to inspect the oral cavity and ensure that there is no further bleeding from vessels that might have been compressed by the mouth gag.
14. Oxymetazoline 0.05% in a nasal spray solution is sprayed in the nose and oropharynx at the end of the procedure to help decrease mucosal edema.
15. The mouth gag is closed and removed carefully to avoid accidental extubation of the patient as the tongue blade withdraws over the endotracheal tube.

### Excision of Branchial Cleft Cyst/Remnant/Sinus Tract

Congenital branchial cleft anomalies are remnants of the branchial arch apparatus that failed to disappear during early embryologic development. At approximately 5 weeks' gestation, the branchial arches are associated with an external cleft of ectodermal origin and an internal pouch of endodermal origin. Anomalies that remain from incomplete resolution can be in the form of a branchial cleft cyst, a sinus, or a fistula. The location of branchial cleft anomalies ranges from the preauricular area (type 1) to the lateral neck along the sternocleidomastoid muscle (types 2, 3, and 4). A cyst may not become apparent until later in childhood, typically during times of acute infection or possible abscess formation, and can occur anywhere along the course of a branchial sinus tract or fistulous tract. A sinus tract usually has an external opening to the neck, generally along the anterior border of the sternocleidomastoid muscle. A fistula has both an external opening and an internal opening; the internal opening is usually in the area of the pyriform sinus near the tonsil on that side. Excision of the branchial cleft anomaly is indicated if it is cystic in nature or if it has become infected. The infection must be treated before surgical excision; if an abscess is present an incision and drainage may be needed.

***Procedural Considerations.*** Imaging studies (computed tomography [CT], magnetic resonance imaging [MRI]) are helpful to determine the presence of an associated tract. The patient will be positioned supine with a roll under the shoulders to slightly extend the neck. A surgical drain, such as a rubber band, is frequently placed. Antibiotics are usually given intraoperatively before surgical incision. Description of a branchial cyst (type 2) excision follows.

#### *Operative Procedure*

1. A transverse skin crease overlying the lesion and 1.5 cm below the margin of the mandible is selected. The area of the incision is injected with 1% lidocaine with 1:100,000 epinephrine.
2. The area is prepped and draped in the usual fashion. The skin incision is made with a #15 blade through the skin and subcutaneous tissues.
3. The platysma muscle is divided with electrodissection.
4. The tissues overlying the cyst are gently dissected away with fine forceps and small scissors or a small gauze peanut.
5. The cyst is gently grasped with a Babcock clamp. Surrounding tissue is dissected free from the cyst using small scissors to spread between the cyst capsule and surrounding tissue and then to cut through fibrous attachments.
6. If a pedicle or fibrous tract is identified, it is followed as far cephalic as possible before it is clamped, cut, and tied with 3-0 absorbable suture.
7. A small rubber band drain is usually placed to prevent accumulation of fluid or blood in the dissected cavity. A safety pin or suture is attached to the distal end of the drain; the drain is removed within 24 hours.
8. The wound is closed in layers. The skin is closed with subcuticular sutures, and adhesive strips are applied to keep the wound edges approximated.

## NEUROSURGICAL PROCEDURES

Neuropathologic conditions requiring surgical intervention can be found in any age-group. The most common problems requiring neurosurgical procedures in infants and children include meningocele, myelomeningocele, encephalocele, craniosynostosis, hydrocephalus, brain tumors, and trauma. The surgical approach, instruments, and equipment required for brain tumors and trauma are relatively similar to those required for adults; consequently the majority of these procedures are as described in Chapter 23.

### Myelomeningocele/Meningocele

Myelomeningocele (Figure 29-36) is a form of spina bifida and is always associated with Chiari type II malformations. It occurs because of a congenital flaw in neural tube closure at approximately 8 to 12 days after conception. The failure of the neural tube to close correctly causes a defect in the posterior elements of the lumbar vertebrae, fascia, and dura, allowing the meninges, spinal cord, and nerve roots to protrude out in a sac or cyst through the skin. The exposed spinal cord is called the neural placode and is not properly developed; there

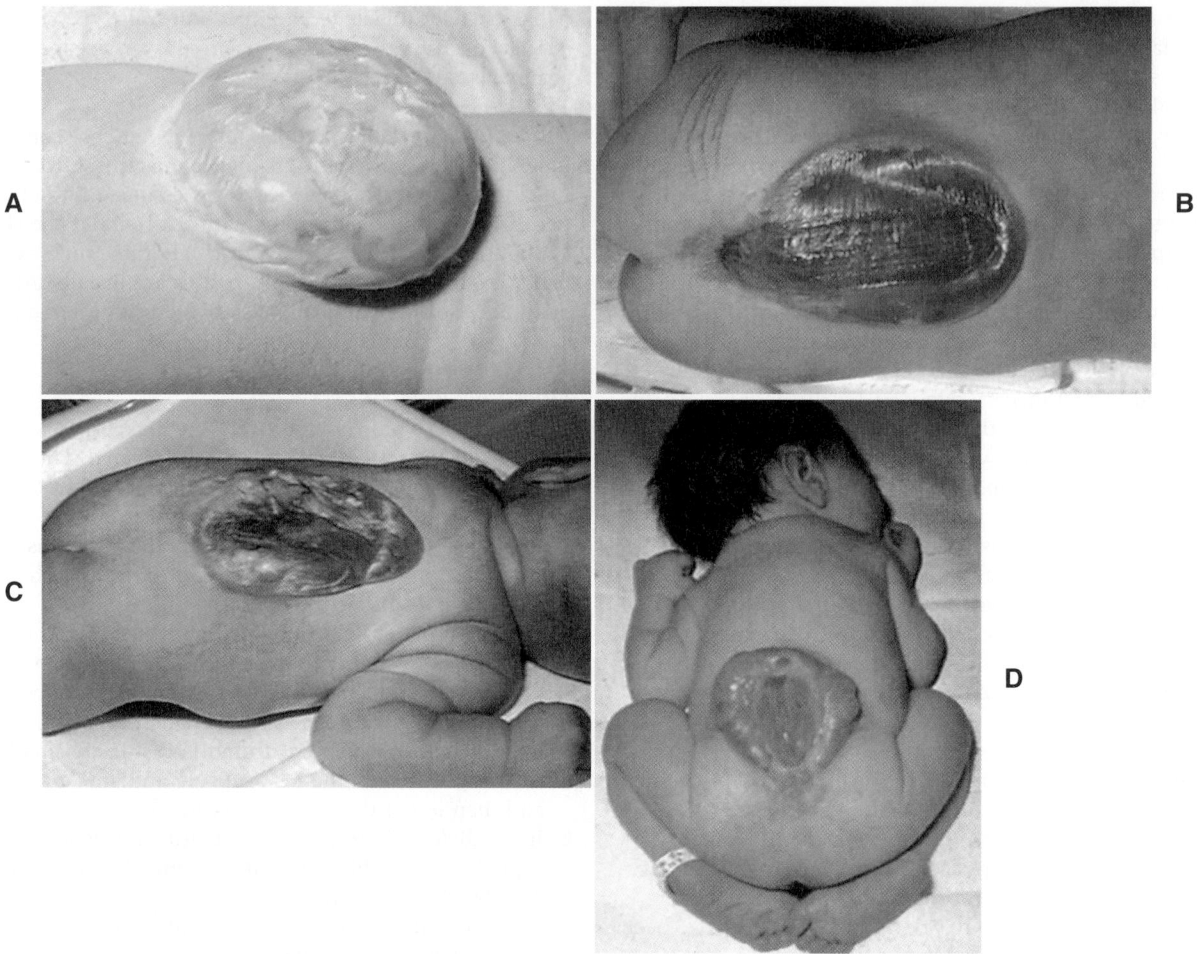


FIGURE 29-36 Examples of meningocele and myelomeningoceles. **A,** Meningocele. Lesion is covered by skin and meninges. **B,** Myelomeningocele. Neural component evident at central strip of lesion. **C,** Thoracolumbar myelomeningocele. **D,** Severe myelomeningocele. Neural tissue in center represents the open spinal canal.

is always some degree of paralysis and loss of sensation below the defect. The amount of disability depends on the vertebral level of the spina bifida and frequently includes loss of bladder and bowel function and hydrocephalus. Meningoceles are similar to myelomeningoceles but not as neurologically devastating: meninges and cerebrospinal fluid (CSF) protrude into the defect but not spinal cord.

***Procedural Considerations.*** Infants born with either of these defects need to be given broad-spectrum antibiotics immediately after birth and taken to the OR within 24 hours for closure of the defect. Nursing care includes keeping the area of the defect covered with sterile gauze kept moistened with normal saline solution; keeping the infant off the defect; and maintaining the infant's body temperature, a more difficult task because of the need to keep the exposed defect moist. A very high percentage of children with this defect develop an allergy to latex; surgical closure and all subsequent surgical procedures should be performed in a latex-free environment.

### *Operative Procedure*

1. An incision is made with a #15 blade in an elliptic fashion around the defect.
2. Metzenbaum scissors are used to remove the pearly epithelial tissue around the neural placode. Retention of the epithelial tissue can lead to formation of a postoperative epidermoid.
3. A blunt dissection is performed using Metzenbaum scissors, following the nerve tissue on the ventral side of the placode down to the spinal canal.
4. The dura is then separated from the fascia with the Metzenbaum scissors.
5. Using 4-0 braided nylon suture, the dura is closed over the neural placode.
6. A #11 blade and Metzenbaum scissors are used to free the fascia from the muscle layer.
7. Braided nylon suture is used to close the fascial layer over the dura.
8. The muscle layer is then closed, followed by skin closure.

## Craniectomy for Craniosynostosis

Craniosynostosis is the premature fusion of one or more cranial sutures. The condition can occur as part of a syndrome or as an isolated process. Craniosynostosis is characterized as "simple" when only one suture line is involved and "compound" when two or more suture lines are involved. The defect occurs in utero, and the exact etiology remains unknown. The purpose of the cranial sutures is to allow the calvaria to bend during the birth process and to allow the skull to expand to accommodate normal brain growth during infancy. The normal brain is finished growing by 2 years of age; at this time fusion of the cranial sutures normally begins. The fusion process is complete by 8 years of age.

Sagittal synostosis accounts for approximately 50% to 58% of all the synostoses and occurs more often in males than in females.[24] The sagittal suture runs in the midline of the skull, connecting the anterior fontanelle to the posterior fontanelle. Premature closure of this fontanelle produces an elongation of the skull in the anteroposterior plane. Surgical intervention involves a linear strip craniectomy to excise the sagittal suture line from the anterior fontanelle to the lambdoidal suture line. Surgery is generally performed on the infant between 6 weeks and 6 months of age, with the best cosmetic results coming from the earlier repair. A craniectomy for sagittal synostosis is described.

***Procedural Considerations.*** The infant will be positioned supine using a cerebellar headrest. Additional measures need to be taken to maintain the infant's normal body temperature; room temperature should be elevated, and forced air–warming blanket should be used. An overbed warmer should be used during the induction and IV placement.

### *Operative Procedure*

1. A sinusoidal incision is made midway between the anterior and posterior fontanelles from ear to ear, just posterior to the pinna.
2. The scalp is elevated off the skull anteriorly and posteriorly to expose the anterior fontanelle, posterior fontanelle, and asterion. Care is used to leave the pericranium attached to the skull to minimize bleeding.
3. A burr hole is made on each side of the sagittal suture on the lambdoidal suture.
4. A craniotome is used to cut anteriorly to the anterior fontanelle on each side of the sagittal suture. A Leksell or Lempert rongeur is used to cut across the sagittal suture and connect the burr holes.
5. A Cobb periosteal elevator is used to carefully dissect the sagittal suture off the underlying dura.
6. A burr hole is placed at the asterion on each side. The craniotome is used to make a curvilinear cut just posterior to the coronal suture.
7. The parietal bone is then "greensticked" (fractured but leaving the periosteum intact) laterally.
8. The skin is then closed with 3-0 and 4-0 absorbable sutures.

## Ventriculoatrial and Ventriculoperitoneal Shunts

Hydrocephalus may be a congenital or acquired condition in pediatric patients. It is characterized by excess production of CSF or is associated with a blockage in the ventricular drainage system. Congenital hydrocephalus is usually a result of a maldevelopment or an intrauterine infection. Acquired hydrocephalus can be caused by infection, neoplasm, or hemorrhage.[32] Early intervention is indicated in infants to prevent cranial distortion caused by the increasing size of the ventricles (Figure 29-37).

The two most widely used pediatric surgical procedures to divert excessive CSF from the ventricles to other body cavities from which it can be absorbed are ventriculoatrial (ventriculocardiac) (Figure 29-38) and ventriculoperitoneal shunts. See Chapter 23 for complete information related to these two procedures.

# ORTHOPEDIC PROCEDURES

## Developmental Hip Dysplasia

Until recently, dislocation of the hip seen in newborns was referred to as "congenital dislocation of the hip" (CDH). The term *developmental dysplasia of the hip (DDH)* has replaced the former

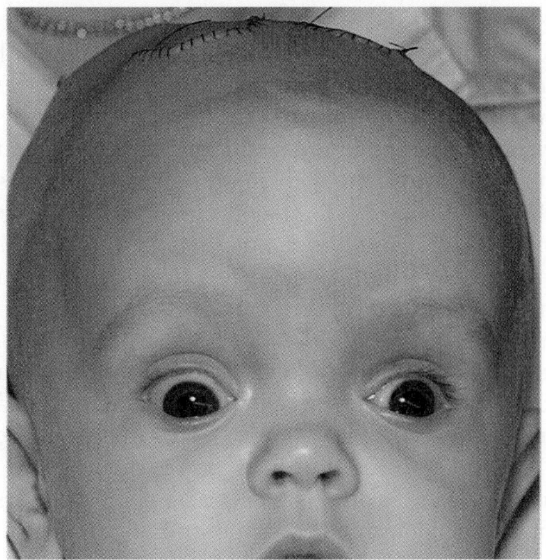

**FIGURE 29-37** Infant with hydrocephalus.

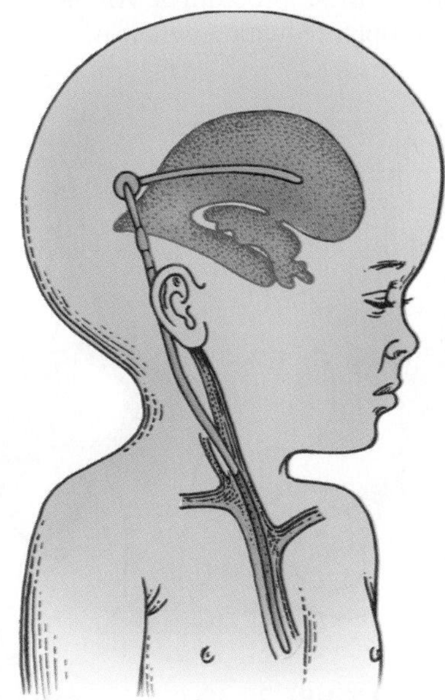

**FIGURE 29-38** Placement of ventriculoatrial shunt.

name to reflect the evolutionary nature of hip problems in the first few months of life. DDH is a progressive condition in which the hip structures fail to develop adequately. Because the pathologic process leading to hip dysplasia may not be present or identifiable at birth, periodic exams of every infant's hips are essential at each routine baby exam until the child is 1 year old. About 1% of infants have dislocated, dislocatable, or subluxatable hips. Eighty percent of DDH cases occur in females, and 60% of all cases involve only the left hip.[32] DDH encompasses the entire spectrum of abnormalities involving the growing hip, ranging from simple dysplasia to dysplasia with subluxation or dislocation of the hip joint. The goal of DDH management is to achieve and maintain a concentric reduction of the femoral head within the acetabulum, in order to provide the optimal environment for the normal development of both structures. When proper alignment is disrupted, soft tissue and bony changes cause contractures of the hip muscles, a shallow acetabulum, and possibly a deformed femoral head. Treatment of congenital dislocation of the hip varies depending on the age of the patient and the stability of the hip. A Pavlik harness is the most commonly used nonoperative device in infants. If the Pavlik harness fails, the infant is brought to the OR and anesthetized for a closed reduction of the hip (proper positioning of the femur head within the acetabulum) confirmed by intraoperative arthrogram and fluoroscopy, with application of a spica cast. Failure of closed reduction and immobilization necessitates an open reduction with an adductor tenotomy to allow adequate abduction to reduce the femoral head; after surgery children under 2 years are then placed in a postreduction spica cast. For children older than 3 years the surgeon may need to perform a shortening varus femoral osteotomy (derotational osteotomy) to facilitate reduction of the femoral head into the acetabulum. In addition, if the acetabulum coverage is inadequate, a pelvic realignment (pelvic osteotomy) procedure may be necessary. Many of the pediatric orthopedic plating systems offer congenital dysplastic hip implants, which can be used in the reconstruction.

***Procedural Considerations.*** The patient most often is in the lateral position for these procedures. An anterior incision is usually made for open reduction, whereas a lateral incision is made for the subtrochanteric femoral osteotomy. A soft tissue set and bone set (appropriate for age) are required as well as an oscillating saw, a wire driver, Steinmann pins, blade plate implants, and instrumentation.

### *Operative Procedures*

DDH OPEN REDUCTION (FIGURE 29-39)

1. The hip joint is opened, and the soft tissue in the acetabulum is excised.
2. The femoral head can then be reduced into the acetabulum and held by suturing of the capsule.

DEROTATIONAL OSTEOTOMY. A derotational osteotomy is performed when the head is improperly seated in the acetabulum.

1. The femur is placed in internal rotation and divided.
2. The distal fragment is rotated externally to place the knee and foot straight ahead.
3. If the patient is a young child, the osteotomy is frequently performed in the supracondylar region, and the patient is immobilized in a plaster spica cast.
4. For an older child, the osteotomy is frequently done in the subtrochanteric region and the osteotomized fragments are held with an osteotomy blade plate or an intermediate compression screw. Immobilization may not be necessary.

PELVIC OSTEOTOMY

1. A complete division of the wing of the ilium is made by an osteotomy from the sciatic notch to the anterior margin of the ilium, superior to the acetabulum.
2. The ilium is then wedged down to increase the depth of the acetabulum when the osteotomy site is opened and a bone graft is inserted.
3. Heavy suture is used to close the capsule, and a spica cast is applied for postoperative immobilization.

## PLASTIC AND RECONSTRUCTIVE SURGERY

### Cleft Lip Repair

The normal upper lip is composed of skin, underlying orbicularis oris muscle, and mucosa. Two skin ridges are situated near the midline of the central philtrum of the lip. The vermil-

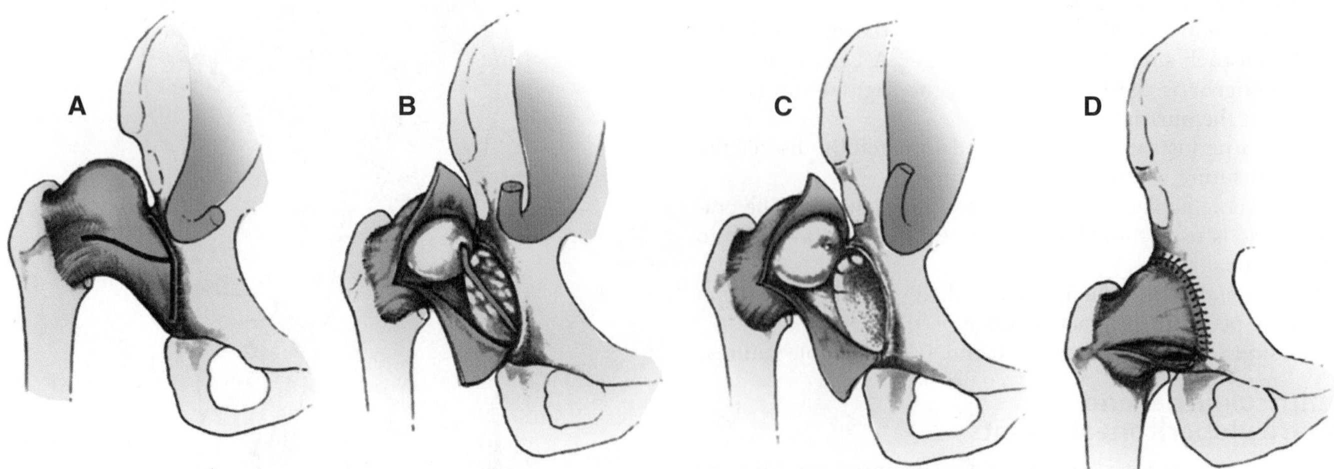


FIGURE 29-39 Repair of congenital hip disorder using open reduction. **A,** T-shaped incision of capsule. **B,** Capsulotomy of the hip and locating the true acetabulum. **C,** Removal of tissue from the depth of the acetabulum. **D,** Capsulorrhaphy.

ion (red portion of the lip) peaks at the philtral ridge on each side and gently curves downward as it reaches the midline to form the Cupid's bow. A deficiency in tissue (skin, muscle, and mucosa) along one or both sides of the upper lip or, rarely, in the midline results in a cleft at the site of this deficiency. The deficiency of tissue present with a cleft lip results in distortion of the Cupid's bow, absence of one or both philtral ridges, and distortion of the lower portion of the nose. Cleft lip is usually associated with a notch or cleft of the underlying alveolus and a cleft of the palate.

Cleft lip repair is most often performed when the infant is about 3 months of age. Timing of the repair follows the "rule of 10": the infant is 10 weeks of age, weighs 10 pounds, and has a hemoglobin of 10. Early surgical correction aids in feeding and infant-parent bonding. Lip repair is directed toward rearrangement of existing tissues to approximate the normal lip as closely as possible. Some considerations may also be given to correcting the nasal deformity at the time of the cleft lip repair.

***Procedural Considerations.*** A plastic surgery local instrument set is required, plus the following special instruments: Brown lip clamps; calipers; a Foment retractor; Beaver blades, #64 and #65; and a Logan bow. The OR bed is usually reversed to create more knee room if the surgeon performs surgery from a sitting position. The patient is placed in the supine position, with the head at the edge of the OR bed. The face is prepped, and the head drape is used. The surgeon may stand or sit at the patient's side or just above the patient's head during the operation.

***Operative Procedure.*** Many types of cleft lip repair are in common use, one of which is illustrated in Figure 29-40. The following steps are applicable to all lip repairs:

1. Normal landmarks are identified and marked or tattooed. Precise measurements, taken with calipers and a ruler, are made so that corresponding points can be marked along the cleft.
2. The lip may be infiltrated with epinephrine 1:200,000, or lip clamps may be used to aid hemostasis.
3. Incisions are made along the markings for the repair.
4. The abnormal musculature is dissected.
5. Additional dissection along the maxilla and nose may be performed.
6. Closure is done in three layers: muscle, skin, and mucosa. Adhesive strips may be used. A Logan bow is applied to the cheeks with tape strips, and elbow restraints are placed.

## Cleft Palate Repair

The palate is made up of the bony or hard palate anteriorly and the soft palate posteriorly. The alveolus borders the hard palate. A separation or cleft of the palate occurs in the midline and may involve only the soft palate or both hard and soft palates. The alveolus may be cleft on one or both sides.

The major function of the soft palate is to aid in the production of normal speech sounds. An intact hard palate is necessary to prevent escape of air through the nose during speech and to prevent the egress of liquid and food from the nose.

Cleft palate repair is usually performed when the child is 6 months of age and should be achieved before the beginning of speech. Variable factors, including the child's weight and the possibility of other disease processes, can affect the timing of the surgery. The various operations used to achieve surgical closure of the palate all employ tissue adjacent to the cleft (in the form of flaps), which is shifted centrally to close the defect.

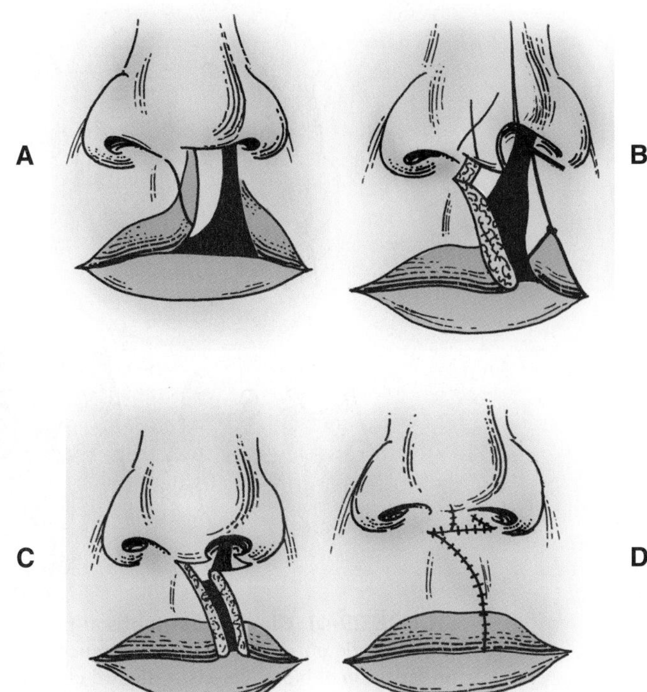


**FIGURE 29-40** Rotation-advancement method to correct complete unilateral cleft of lip. **A,** Rotation incision marked so that Cupid's bow–philtral dimple component will rotate down into normal position; flap advances into columella to form nostril sill. **B,** dimple component has dropped down, second flap has advanced into columella. **C,** Flap is being advanced into rotation gap, while skin-roll flap is interdigitated at mucocutaneous junction line. **D,** Scar is maneuvered into strategic position where it is hidden at nasal base and floor and philtrum column and interdigitated at mucocutaneous junction.

***Procedural Considerations.*** A basic plastic surgery instrument set is required, plus the following special instruments: Dingman mouth gag with assorted blades; Blair palate hook; palate knives; Blair palate elevators; and Fomon lower lateral scissors, short and long. The patient is placed in the supine position, with the head at the edge of the OR bed. The head drape is used. Many surgeons sit just above the patient's head and cradle the head on their lap (with the patient's neck hyperextended).

***Operative Procedure.*** One of the most frequently used cleft palate repairs is illustrated in Figure 29-41. The following steps are common to all palate repairs:

1. The Dingman mouth gag is inserted. Maintenance of the position of the endotracheal tube is crucial at this point. A throat pack may be inserted to absorb blood that may drain into the throat.
2. The outlines of the palatal flaps are marked.
3. The palate is injected with 1% lidocaine with epinephrine 1:100,000 for hemostasis.

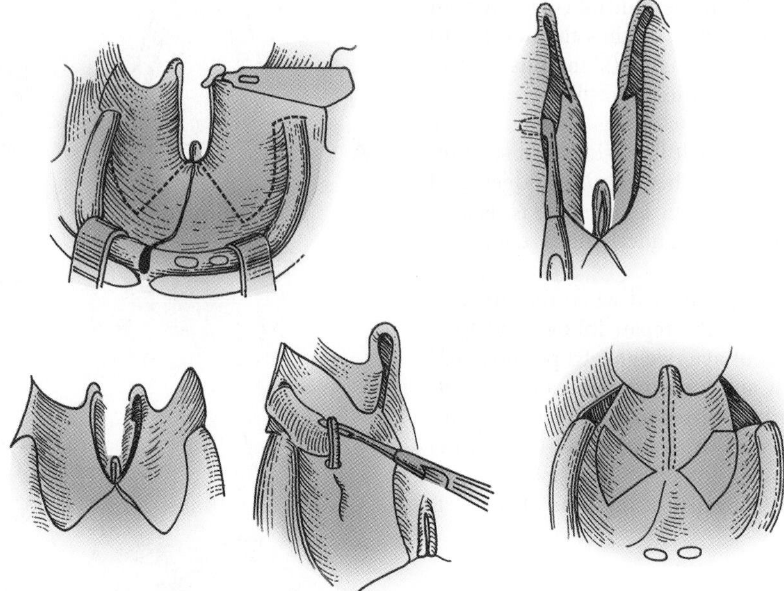

**FIGURE 29-41** Closure of cleft of soft palate by V-Y (Wardill-Kilner) palatoplasty. A V-shaped incision is made on oral side of palate; mucoperiosteal flaps are elevated on oral and nasal sides, with preservation of blood vessels; Y-shaped closure (in three layers) closes cleft and lengthens palate.

4. The flaps are incised and elevated.
5. Closure is in three layers: nasal mucosa, muscle, and palatal mucosa.
6. A large horizontal mattress traction suture is placed through the body of the tongue. If the patient experiences upper airway obstruction after extubation, traction is placed on this suture to pull the tongue forward, rather than insert an airway that might harm the palate repair. The throat pack is removed.

## Pharyngeal Flap

When abnormal speech (velopharyngeal insufficiency) results despite a cleft palate repair, a secondary surgical procedure may be necessary to improve speech. Primarily an excess of air escaping through the nose during speech characterizes typical "cleft palate speech." This hypernasality often results from insufficient bulk or movement of the muscles of the soft palate. To decrease or eliminate this problem, tissue from the pharynx, in the form of a pharyngeal flap, is added to the soft palate. This flap also reduces the size of the opening between the oropharynx and nasopharynx, thus decreasing or eliminating the nasal escape of air during speech.

A pharyngeal flap repair may be done at any age, but most are done before the patient is 14 years old. A pharyngeal flap also may be part of primary cleft palate repair.

***Procedural Considerations.*** Positioning, draping, and instruments are as described for cleft palate repair, with the addition of two 12-Fr red rubber catheters.

### *Operative Procedure*

1. The Dingman mouth gag is inserted. A throat pack may be inserted.
2. The palate and posterior wall of the pharynx are injected with 1% lidocaine with epinephrine 1:100,000 for hemostasis.
3. The palate is incised, and the pharyngeal flap is incised and elevated.
4. The pharyngeal wall donor site may be sutured or left open.
5. The pharyngeal flap is sutured to the palate, and the palate is closed.
6. A traction suture is placed through the body of the tongue. The throat pack is removed.

## Total Ear Reconstruction

An absent external ear presents the surgical team with the objective of developing or restoring a part of the appearance that will help with self-esteem and confidence in daily interactions as well as enhance hearing, since the external ear funnels sound waves from the environment into the inner ear. Emotional support is a key aspect of the plan of care for these patients.

The external ear comprises skin, subcutaneous tissue, and cartilage. The surgical procedure to create an external ear involves the retrieval of rib cartilage, carving the cartilage, placement of the newly fashioned ear on the side of the patient's head, and skin grafting and dressing of the operative sites, with continual assessment and reassessment of the preoperative sketches made of the patient's ear with relation to facial structure. This can be accomplished as a one-stage procedure or as a sequence of surgeries. For congenital defects, the ideal time for initiating the procedure is between 6 and 10 years of age. In the case of traumatic loss of the external ear (as from burns), the time is individually determined. The use of tissue expanders may be considered in some cases to stretch the skin surface required to cover the ear.

***Procedural Considerations.*** A basic plastic surgery instrument set is required, with the addition of rib graft instrumentation for autologous rib cartilage retrieval in total ear reconstruction. A Doppler probe with sterile conduction gel should be available for intraoperative use, and a small piece of unexposed x-ray film is used as a template. The patient is supine with the arms tucked securely at the sides. Appropriate padding and protection of vulnerable neurovascular bundles and pressure sites are critical. Use of a sequential compression device and a forced air–warming unit over the lower half of the patient's body should be considered because of the anticipated length of the procedure. A standard head drape and split drape (or U drape) for the patient's torso allow the team access to the auricular area and chest, respectively. Usually two instrument tables are used, with one designated for carving the rib cartilage. Because the procedure is lengthy (6 to 8 hours on average), rolling sitting stools should be provided for the team. Periodic progress of the procedure should be relayed to the patient's family members in the surgical waiting room.

### *Operative Procedure*

1. Preoperative sketches of the ear are done with the use of unexposed x-ray film. Symmetric and anatomic landmarks are vital considerations in the patterns developed for the reconstruction.
2. Assessment of the vascular integrity of the temporoparietal flap is done preoperatively with an unsterile Doppler pencil and conduction gel.
3. The donor skin graft site is identified and prepped with an antimicrobial scrub.
4. When the sketches are complete, the films are sterilized with care not to remove the markings made by the surgeon.
5. The operative site of the head and chest area are prepped and draped in the usual manner.
6. The temporoparietal fascia flap is lifted, and a sterile Doppler pencil and sterile conduction gel are used to assess the vascular integrity of the flap.
7. Infiltration of the operative sites with local anesthesia with epinephrine 1:200,000 can be used for hemostasis. Epinephrine in higher concentrations (e.g., 1:100,000) is not recommended for use in the area of the flap because of the possible obliteration of the vascular complexes present.
8. Costocartilage retrieval requires preoperative marking of the patient's chest wall (the area of the sixth, seventh, and eighth ribs). The chest wall is incised, and the rib cartilage segments are removed with care to preserve the perichondrium. This will encourage bone growth and help to prevent a chest wall defect. The assessment of intact pleura is critical before closure of the chest. Instillation of saline into the wound is done; if bubbles appear, the pleura is not intact; a chest tube is then inserted and attached to a chest drainage system. If the integrity of the pleura is in question, an intraoperative chest x-ray film may be taken to check for a pneumothorax. If the pleura is intact, closure of the wound is performed and the injection of 0.25% bupivacaine to the intercostal incision area is performed.
9. While one team closes the chest, another team begins the process of carving the rib cartilage for the ear reconstruction. The previously marked radiographs are crucial aids for the artistic abilities of the surgeon, providing a blueprint for the sculpting phase of the procedure. Surgical wire is used to connect the carved pieces of rib cartilage as it is shaped to resemble the external ear.
10. A skin graft is taken, and the donor site is covered with a dressing of choice.
11. Hemostasis is maintained with the use of electrocoagulation, topical thrombin, and infiltration of local anesthetic with epinephrine.
12. The flap covers the sculpted ear, and the skin graft is used to cover any exposed areas (this is a technique used especially with burn patients who have less available skin for coverage).
13. Drains are placed and attached to closed-wound suction, or gauze stents wrapped with nonadherent gauze are sutured in place behind the ear. Soft, bulky dressings are applied to the ear and secured with a head wrap of rolled gauze (e.g., Kerlix); standard dressings are applied to the chest wall.

## Otoplasty

A congenital deformity in which the ear protrudes abnormally from the side of the head is generally the result of an absent or insufficiently pronounced antihelical fold of the external ear. The various methods of otoplasty are an attempt at correction by creating an antihelical fold that positions the ear more normally (Figure 29-42). Protruding ears may be unilateral or bilateral. An otoplasty is generally performed for children who are uncomfortable or self-conscious about the deformity, usually in the elementary school–age years.

***Procedural Considerations.*** A plastic surgery instrument set is needed. The patient is placed supine on the OR bed, and a head drape is used, leaving both ears well exposed. The patient's head is turned with the affected ear up and with the lower ear well padded to avoid pressure injury.

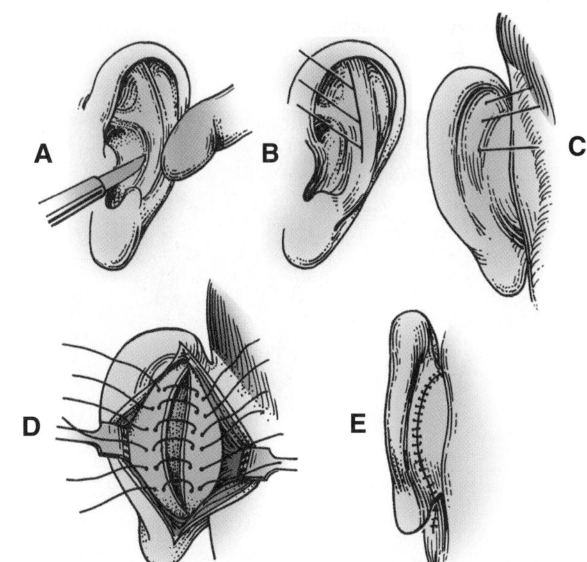


FIGURE 29-42 Otoplasty for correction of protruding ears. **A,** Antihelix defined by application of pressure to ear. **B,** Position of antihelical fold marked by the passage of straight needles through ear. **C,** Needle points visible along posterior surface of ear with ellipse of skin to be excised marked. **D,** Section of ear cartilage incised and scored or excised with sutures placed to hold cartilage back. **E,** Posterior ear incision sutured.

*Operative Procedure*

1. The antihelical fold is created when the external ear is bent backward. The position of the antihelical fold is marked by placing 25-gauge or straight needles through the ear from anterior to posterior, applying methylene blue to the tip of the needles, and withdrawing them to mark the cartilage within.
2. An ellipse of skin is excised from the posterior surface of the ear after it has been infiltrated with 1% lidocaine with epinephrine 1:100,000.
3. The ear cartilage is usually incised near the antihelical fold, and the anterior surface of the cartilage is scored to allow it to bend backward.
4. Sutures are usually placed to hold the cartilage in its new position.
5. The skin incision is closed.
6. A drain (TLS or butterfly cannula with red top tube) may be placed to aid in the skin's adherence to the cartilage framework beneath.
7. A nonadherent dressing, such as Xeroform or cotton coated with polysporin antibiotic ointment, is usually placed in front of and behind the ear, followed by fluffed gauze and a bulky dressing made of rolled gauze (e.g., Kerlix) to exert moderate compression on the ear.

## Repair of Syndactyly

*Syndactyly* refers to a congenital webbing of the digits of the hand or feet. It is occasionally seen in association with other abnormalities, such as extra fingers or toes (polydactyly), or with bony abnormalities. In syndactyly with normal digits, most commonly seen, a web of skin joins adjacent fingers (Figure 29-43) but each finger has its own tendons, vessels, nerves, and bony phalanges. Although the skin web may appear loose, a deficiency in skin is always present when surgical separation is performed. Plans for taking a skin graft (usually full thickness) should always be made. Surgical separation of syndactyly is performed at any time, usually after approximately 12 months of age.

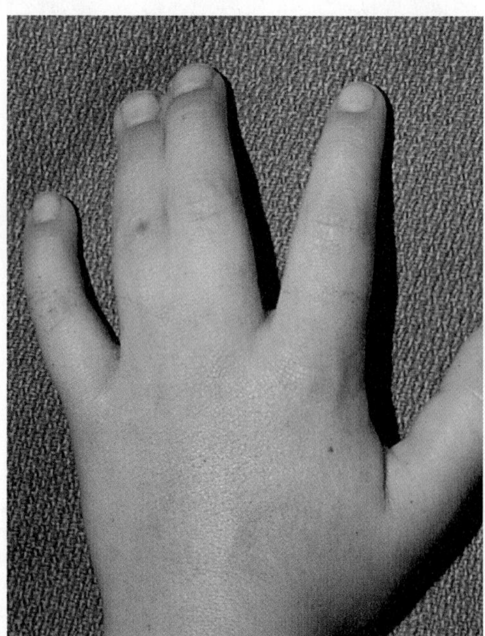

**FIGURE 29-43** Syndactyly involving third and fourth fingers.

Toe syndactyly is less often treated surgically than finger syndactyly because proper function of the foot does not require fine movements of individual toes. Although the setup and description that follow are for the repair of finger syndactyly, they can also be applied to the repair of toe syndactyly.

***Procedural Considerations.*** A plastic surgery local instrument set is required, plus a marking pen, unexposed x-ray film, a pediatric pneumatic tourniquet, and an Esmarch bandage. The patient is placed supine on the OR bed with the affected arm extended on a hand table. A hand drape is used, and the affected hand and wrist are prepped and draped as well as both inguinal areas (donor sites for full-thickness skin grafts). Some surgeons prefer to use the wrist or forearm as donor sites.

*Operative Procedure*

1. Skin incisions are marked, and the tourniquet is inflated.
2. The skin is incised, and small flaps at the sides of fingers and in the web are elevated.
3. After the flaps have been sutured into position, patterns of areas of absent skin on the sides of fingers are made and transferred to the skin-graft donor site.
4. The skin graft is taken; if a full-thickness skin graft is used, it must be defatted before the graft is sutured in place.
5. Skin grafts are sutured to fingers
6. Stent dressings are placed over the skin grafts. The entire hand is immobilized in a bulky dressing or in a long arm cast.

## Orbital-Craniofacial Surgery

Some congenital anomalies involve the orbital-craniofacial skeleton. These include hypertelorism, in which the distance between the orbits is increased as seen in Crouzon's disease and Apert's syndrome. Crouzon's disease (Figure 29-44) is characterized by premature closure of the cranial sutures, resulting in an abnormally shaped skull, exophthalmos and hypertelorism, parrot's beak nose, and maxillary hypoplasia. Apert's syndrome (Figure 29-45) includes the same craniofacial deformities as Crouzon's disease and also syndactyly or

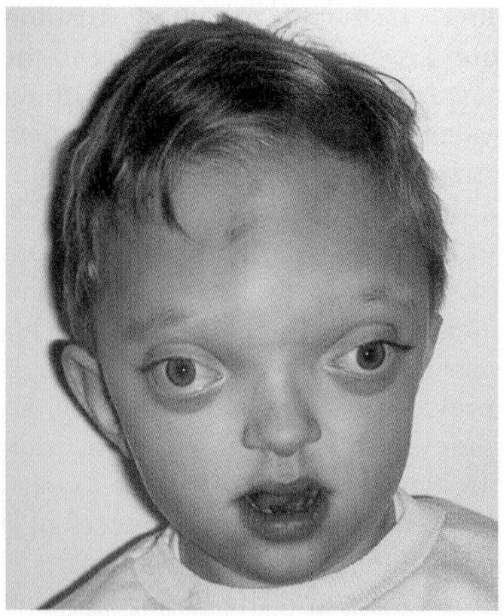

**FIGURE 29-44** Crouzon's disease.

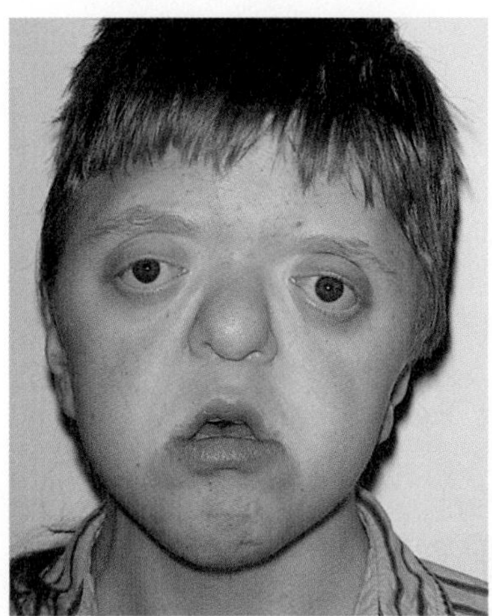

**FIGURE 29-45** Apert's syndrome.

other hand anomalies. Recent advances in plastic surgery make surgical correction of some of these deformities possible.

Binocular vision is normal in humans. It involves the coordinated use of both eyes to obtain a single mental impression of objects. Binocular vision is usually absent in craniofacial anomalies because of the increased distance between the orbits. The purposes of orbital-craniofacial surgery are to provide the patient with binocular vision by moving the orbits closer together and to provide the patient with a more acceptable appearance by moving the bones of the orbital-craniofacial skeleton into a more normal position. Correction of the deformity seen in Crouzon's disease and Apert's syndrome involves a surgically created Le Fort III maxillary fracture.

Although an extracranial approach may be used, an intracranial approach is used in most cases; therefore a neurosurgeon and a plastic surgeon perform these operations through a bifrontal (coronal) craniotomy. A tracheostomy may be done before the start of the procedure. Bone grafts from hips or ribs are necessary to augment areas of bone deficit, which result from movement of the craniofacial skeleton.

***Procedural Considerations.*** These operations are usually performed on children. They are very extensive procedures, often lasting 12 to 14 hours. Blood loss is considerable. Postoperative complications, such as cerebral edema or meningitis, can be formidable. The perioperative nurse must pay particular attention to the following important details: (1) insertion of a Foley catheter into the patient's bladder before the operation is started, (2) positioning of the patient on the OR bed so that all bony prominences are well padded, and (3) availability of accurate means for measuring blood loss. Use of a sequential compression device and forced air–warming units should also be anticipated.

A basic plastic surgery instrument set, craniectomy instruments and supplies (see Chapter 23), plastic hand instrumentation, and tracheostomy instruments and supplies are required. A high-speed drill, saws, and general orthopedic instrumentation are also needed. A separate setup is necessary for obtaining the bone graft.

The patient is positioned, prepped, and draped as described for bifrontal craniotomy (see Chapter 23). The entire face is left exposed, however, and may temporarily be covered with a plastic drape until the portion of the operation requiring access to the face is reached. The bone-graft donor site is also prepped and draped so that both iliac crests and the lower ribs are exposed.

### *Operative Procedure*

1. Tracheostomy, if required, is performed first, followed by application of arch bars (when indicated as in Crouzon's disease and Apert's syndrome).
2. The bifrontal craniotomy with craniectomy is performed.
3. Bilateral orbital osteotomies (Figure 29-46, *A*) into the anterior cranial fossa are performed. Bilateral conjunctival (lower eyelid) and labiogingival sulcus incisions (for Crouzon's disease and Apert's syndrome) are made for orbital and maxillary osteotomies.
4. The bones of the orbital-craniofacial region are now moved (Figure 29-46, *B*), based on measurement of the intercanthal distance (in hypertelorism) or occlusion of the teeth (in Crouzon's disease and Apert's syndrome).
5. Bone grafts may be taken from the calvaria, ribs, or hips to augment areas of bone deficit, which result from movement of the craniofacial skeleton.
6. Bone grafts are fixed in place with interosseous wires and by means of intermaxillary fixation applied to arch bars (for Crouzon's disease and Apert's syndrome) (Figure 29-46, *C*). Rigid plate-and-screw fixation is another option.
7. The craniotomy, conjunctival, intraoral, and bone-graft donor site incisions are closed and dressings applied.

## THORACIC PROCEDURES

### Correction of Pectus Excavatum

Pectus excavatum (funnel chest) is a visually obvious defect of the sternum, seen as a deep depression on the chest as a result of posterior displacement of the sternum (Figure 29-47). It is usually associated with kyphosis. The defect may be asymmetric, most often deeper on the right side, with sternal angulation. In a majority of cases, surgical treatment is cosmetic; impaired cardiorespiratory function is the underlying reason for surgical intervention in fewer cases. The procedure is most commonly performed in patients between 10 and 16 years of age, when children become embarrassed to undress in front of peers. Rigid fixation has become a choice for correction of the defect, wherein a metal retaining strut is added to gain chest wall stability and prevent recurrence. This strut must be removed 2 to 4 years later.[22] Other treatments may cosmetically correct the situation over the short term but usually result in progressive retraction of the sternum.

***Procedural Considerations.*** The thoracic instrument set is used, to which the following are added: Gigli saws and handles, osteotomes or chisels, bone hooks, bone-holding forceps, various periosteal elevators, and a fixation rod. The patient is positioned supine with a portion of the upper chest elevated on a soft roll or sheets. The surgical approach is by way of a median sternotomy or a bilateral inframammary incision.

### *Operative Procedure*

1. A vertical midline incision is made from the level of the manubrium to the point below the xiphisternum.
2. A pectoral muscle flap is raised, and origins of the pectoral muscles are detached from the sternum and costal carti-

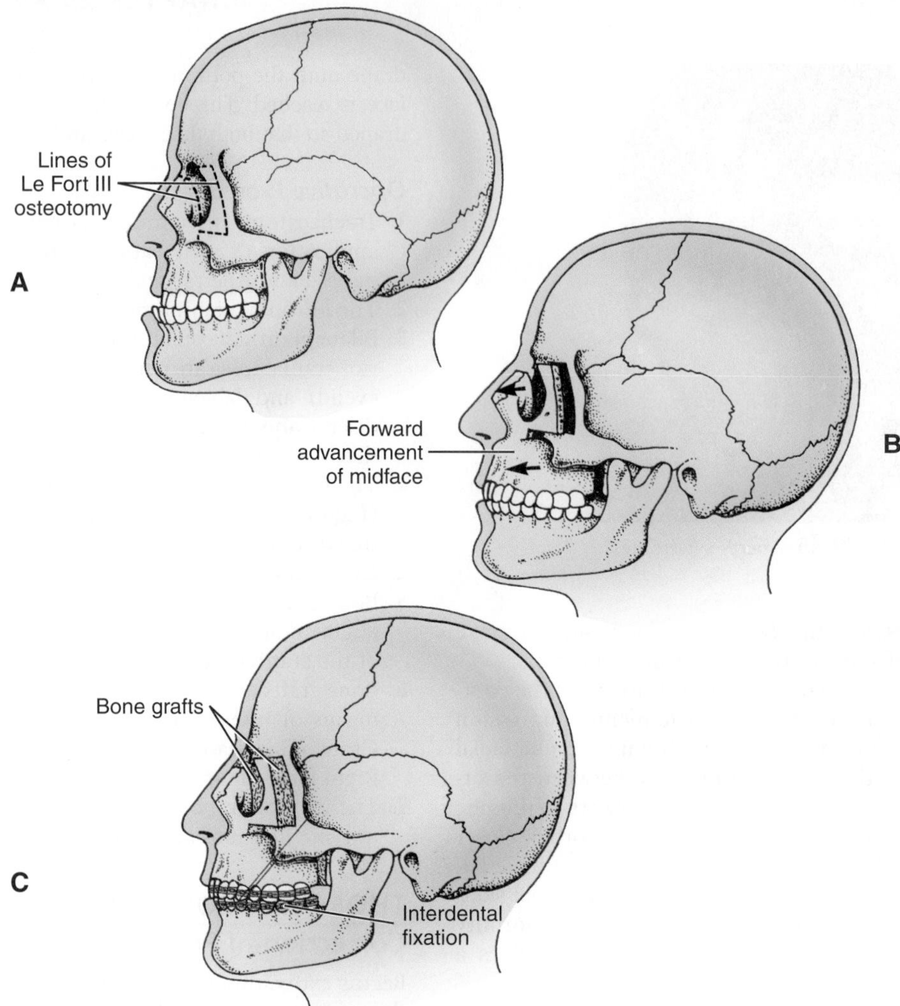


**FIGURE 29-46** Steps in surgical correction of Crouzon's disease deformities.

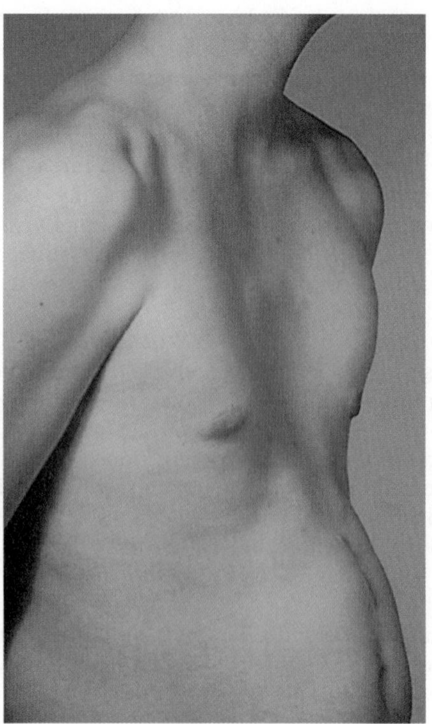

**FIGURE 29-47** Pectus excavatum.

lages. The origins of the rectus abdominis muscles are dissected off the lower end of the sternum and costal margins.

3. The deformed costal cartilages are removed completely, but the perichondrium is preserved.
4. The lower end of the sternum is elevated, and mediastinal structures and pleura are dissected free.
5. A transverse osteotomy is made through the anterior cortex of the sternum. The sternum is elevated, and the fixation rod is placed behind the sternum at the level of the anterior end of the fourth rib. Sutures are used to fixate the bar and adjacent rib.
6. A drain is passed into the anterior mediastinal space. The rectus muscles are sutured back to the perichondrium and to the lower end of the sternum.

## TRAUMA

Principles governing surgical care of trauma patients are discussed in Chapter 31. However, when caring for the pediatric trauma patient in surgery, the perioperative nurse must possess additional knowledge in order to develop a detailed plan of action that effectively drives the delivery of safe patient care. During all episodes of patient care, it is necessary for the perioperative nurse to communicate with members of the surgical and interdisciplinary team in a fashion that best supports positive patient outcomes. The urgency of injury will dictate the timeliness of surgical intervention. The perioperative nurse should be prepared to administer care to any type of injury in a safe and effective manner that is appropriate across all age levels.

Trauma is the leading cause of death in children from 1 to 14 years of age. Each year, another 100,000 children experience disability from trauma. Several factors, such as age, gender, behavior, and environment, influence the risk of traumatic injury. For instance, infants and toddlers are more prone to falls resulting in severe injury, which may be related to the pliable nature of the skeletal system. If broken bones are present, a severe force of injury must be assumed. Older children and adolescents are at higher risk for bicycle- and motor vehicle–related injuries. In this age-group, blunt injuries resulting from motor vehicle accidents or direct blows (as with contact sports or child abuse) along with falls are the most common mechanisms of injury.[6] Of note is the fact that approximately 35% of pediatric traumatic injuries occur in the home environment, stressing the importance of community awareness and education as it relates to trauma prevention.[21]

Throughout the pediatric population, neurologic injuries are the most common cause of traumatic death in children; their head is proportionately larger in relation to their body mass and especially vulnerable to injury. Table 29-4 gives a guideline for using the Glasgow Coma Scale for infants; children are scored using the same criteria as for adult trauma victims. Because children have a much smaller reserve than adults, once a decline in vital functions is noted, demise is rapid. Box 29-5 presents recommended resuscitation equipment for infants and children who are trauma victims. Information about commonly used medications in pediatric resuscitation is noted in the Surgical Pharmacology box.

IV access is often difficult in the pediatric patient, and an intraosseous line may be inserted by emergency rescue personnel before arrival at the hospital or in the emergency department (ED). These lines are inserted by use of an intraosseous needle or bone marrow aspirate needle and are placed slightly below the knee on the anterior aspect of the tibia at a 90-degree angle (Figure 29-48). Stabilization of the line may be difficult, but the line can remain for up to 24 hours and provides rapid access when other routes are too time-consuming or difficult to access.

Fluid resuscitation for children experiencing hemorrhage (Table 29-5) as well as types and dosages of medications are based on body weight, since weight provides a better mechanism of accuracy when calculating dosage. Because of the nature of the trauma, exact body weight may be unable to be

**TABLE 29-4**

### Glasgow Coma Scale

| Response | Adults and Children | Infants | Points |
|---|---|---|---|
| Eye opening | No response | No response | 1 |
| | To pain | To pain | 2 |
| | To voice | To voice | 3 |
| | Spontaneous | Spontaneous | 4 |
| Verbal | No response | No response | 1 |
| | Incomprehensible | Moans to pain | 2 |
| | Inappropriate words | Cries to pain | 3 |
| | Disoriented conversation | Irritable | 4 |
| | Oriented and appropriate | Coos, babbles | 5 |
| Motor | No response | No response | 1 |
| | Decerebrate posturing | Decerebrate posturing | 2 |
| | Decorticate posturing | Decorticate posturing | 3 |
| | Withdraws to pain | Withdraws to pain | 4 |
| | Localizes pain | Withdraws to touch | 5 |
| | Obeys commands | Normal spontaneous movement | 6 |
| **Total Score** | | | 3-15 |

From Rupp LA, Day MW: Children are different: pediatric differences and the impact on trauma. In Moloney-Harmon PA, Czerwinski SJ: *Nursing care of the pediatric trauma patient*, St Louis, 2003, Saunders.

BOX 29-5

### Recommended Resuscitative Equipment for Pediatric Patients

**AIRWAY MANAGEMENT**
- Clear oxygen masks (preterm, infant, child, and adult sizes)
- Nonrebreathing masks (infant, child, and adult sizes)
- Oral airways (sizes 00 to 5)
- Nasopharyngeal airways (12 Fr to 30 Fr)
- Bag/valve/mask resuscitator, self-inflating (450- and 1000-ml sizes)
- Nasal cannulas (infant, child, and adult sizes)
- Endotracheal tubes: uncuffed (sizes 2.5 to 8.5) and cuffed (sizes 5.5 to 9)
- Stylets (pediatric and adult)
- Laryngoscope handle (pediatric and adult)
- Laryngoscope blades, curved (sizes 2 and 3) and straight (sizes 0 to 3)
- Magill forceps (pediatric and adult)
- Nasogastric tubes (sizes 6 Fr to 14 Fr)
- Suction catheters, flexible (sizes 5 Fr to 16 Fr)
- Chest tubes (sizes 8 to 40 Fr)
- Tracheostomy tubes (sizes 00 to 6)

**MONITORING EQUIPMENT**
- Cardiac monitor with strip recorder
- Defibrillator with pediatric and adult paddles
- Pediatric and adult monitoring electrodes
- Pulse oximeter with varying sizes of sensors (newborn to adult)
- Blood pressure cuffs in varying sizes (newborn to adult)
- Doppler blood pressure device

**VASCULAR ACCESS**
- Butterfly needles (19- to 25-gauge)
- Catheter over needle devices (14- to 24-gauge)
- Infusion volume pumps and tubing
- Intraosseous needles (16- and 18-gauge)
- Fluid/blood warmers
- Umbilical vein catheters
- Pediatric vascular access kit

From Rupp LA, Day MW: Children are different: pediatric differences and the impact on trauma. In Moloney-Harmon PA, Czerwinski SJ: *Nursing care of the pediatric trauma patient*, St Louis, 2003, Saunders.

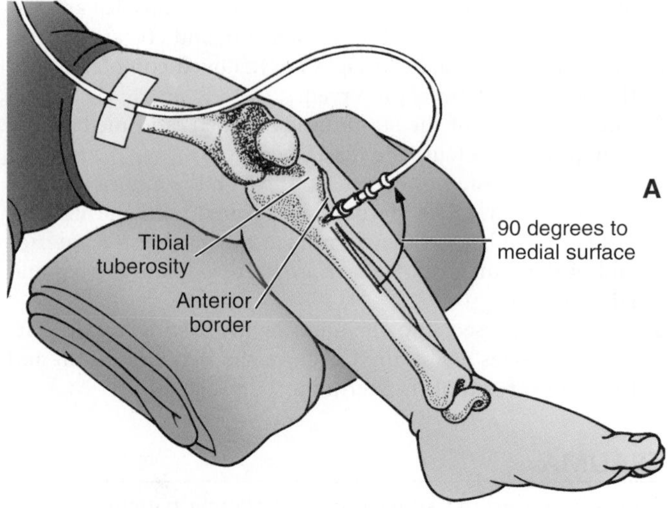


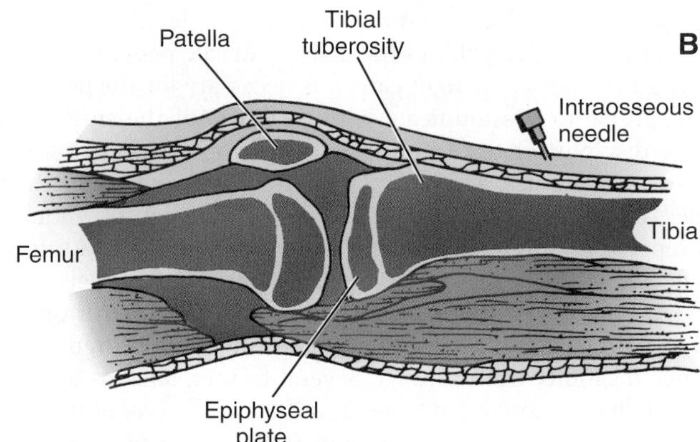


**FIGURE 29-48** **A,** Intraosseous infusion technique. **B,** Insertion.

obtained. In these instances, Broselow/Luten tapes, which are measuring tapes with spaces representing weight in kilograms instead of units of length, may be used to better estimate body weight.[29]

Body size of the patient determines the type of instrumentation required. Pediatric trauma instrument sets, including vascular clamps and retractors, and suture supplies should be available and organized in a fashion that promotes easy and timely access when urgent situations arise. Creative problem solving may be required of the perioperative nurse in adaptation of feeding tubes, drains, and other equipment.

Maintenance of body temperature is of utmost concern in the pediatric population, and undue skin exposure should be avoided. Fluids for irrigation and IV infusion may be warmed, depending on preferences of the surgeon and status of the child. Whenever possible, room temperature is elevated. Warming blankets and head coverings (stockinette) may be used to prevent heat loss; this is especially critical with children who have sustained burns.

The perioperative nurse should attempt to obtain a trauma history from ED personnel or the family if the patient comes directly to the OR. Initial vitals signs should be obtained and compared with those obtained during prehospital care or in the ED; Table 29-6 presents normal respiration and heart rate for infants and children. Box 29-6 gives a formula for blood pressure estimation. As the perioperative nurse obtains the initial assessment, it is important to use a developmental approach to pediatric trauma patients, who respond differently from adults (Box 29-7).Older infants (8 to 12 months of age) experience stranger anxiety; when their parents are not in sight, the perioperative nurse should use warm hands and a soothing voice and keep the room warm as comfort measures. Toddlers (1 to 3 years old) have fears of pain and separation from parents. Preschool children fear pain and disfigurement; the perioperative nurse should encourage expression of fears. School-age children (5 to 12 years old) also fear disfigurement, as well as loss of function and death. It is important to explain procedures, to stress the child's ability to master the situation with the nurse's help, and to project a positive demeanor. The adolescent fears loss of autonomy, loss of peer acceptance, and death. As much as possible, adolescents should be allowed choices and their autonomy respected. During traumatic events, it is also imperative to consider the well-being of patients, families, and caregivers. The perioperative nurse plays

## Medications Used in Pediatric Resuscitation

Perioperative nurses must always be prepared in the event of a cardiac event in the pediatric patient. The information contained in this section provides commonly used medications, their mode of action, and nursing implications for pediatric resuscitation.

| Drug | Dosage | Action | Nursing Implications |
|---|---|---|---|
| Epinephrine HCl | Intravenous/Intraosseous (IV/IO): 0.01 mg/kg (1:10,000)<br>Endotracheal (ET): 0.1 mg/kg (1:1000)<br>Repeat doses = 0.1 ml/kg (1:1000) | Adrenergic; acts on both alpha- and beta-receptor sites, especially heart and vascular and other smooth muscle | Most useful drug in cardiac arrest<br>Disappears rapidly from bloodstream after injection; instill 2-3 ml saline following ET administration<br>May produce renal vessel constriction and decreased urine output |
| Sodium bicarbonate | IV/IO: 1 mEq/kg<br>Newborn: 0.5 mEq/ml<br>2mg/kg | Alkalinizer, buffers pH | Infuse slowly and only when ventilation is adequate; flush with saline before and after administration<br>Do not mix with catecholamines or calcium<br>Incompatible with epinephrine |
| Atropine sulfate | 0.02 mg/kg dose<br>Minimum dose: 0.1 mg<br>Maximum single dose: infants and children, 0.5 mg; adolescents, 1.0 mg | Anticholinergic-parasympatholytic; increases cardiac output, heart rate by blocking vagal stimulation in heart | Used to treat bradycardia after ventilatory assessment; always provide adequate ventilation and monitor $O_2$ saturation<br>Produces pupil dilation, which constricts with light |
| Calcium chloride | 20 mg/kg IV<br>0.2 mg/kg/dose every 10 min | Electrolyte replacement; needed for maintenance of normal cardiac activity | Used only for hypocalcemia, calcium blocker overdose, hyperkalemia, or hypermagnesemia<br>Administer slowly, very sclerosing; administer in central vein<br>Incompatible with phosphate sodium |
| Lidocaine HCl | 1 mg/kg dose | Antidysrhythmic, inhibits nerve impulses from sensory nerves | Used for ventricular dysrhythmias only |
| Amiodarone | IV: 5 mg/kg over 30 min followed by continuous infusion starting at 5 mcg/kg/min; may increase to maximum 10 mcg/kg/min | Antidysrhythmic agent, inhibits adrenergic stimulation; prolongs action potential and refractory period in myocardial tissues; decreased atrioventricular (AV) conduction and sinus node function | Recommended as first choice for shock-refractory ventricular tachycardia<br>Contraindicated in severe sinus node dysfunction, marked sinus bradycardia, second- and third-degree AV block<br>Monitor for hypotension |
| Adenosine | 0.1-0.2 mg/kg<br>Maximum single dose: 12 mg<br>Follow with 2- to 3-ml normal saline flush | Antidysrhythmic, for supraventricular tachycardia (SVT)<br>Causes a temporary block through the AV node and interrupts reentry circuits | Administer rapid IV push, followed by saline flush<br>May cause transient bradycardia |
| Naloxone (Narcan) | 0.1 mg/kg/dose, may repeat every 2-3 min | Reverses respiratory arrest caused by excessive opiate administration | Evaluate level of pain after administration because analgesic effects of opioids are reversed with large dose of naloxone |
| Magnesium | 25-30 mg/kg<br>Maximum: 2 g | Inhibits calcium channels and causes smooth muscle relaxation | Given rapid IV infusion for suspected hypomagnesemia<br>Have calcium gluconate (IV) available as antidote |
| **IV INFUSIONS** | | | |
| Epinephrine HCl infusion | 0.1-1 mcg/kg/min | Adrenergic—see above | Titrate to desired hemodynamic effect |
| Dopamine HCl infusion | 2-20 mcg/kg/min | Agonist; acts on alpha receptors, causing vasoconstriction<br>Increases cardiac output | Titrate to desired hemodynamic effect |
| Dobutamine HCl infusion | 2.5-15 mcg/kg/min | Adrenergic direct-acting $beta_1$ agonist<br>Increases contractility and heart rate | Titrate to desired hemodynamic effect<br>Little vasoconstriction, even at high rates |
| Lidocaine HCl infusion | 20-50 mcg/kg/min | Antidysrhythmic<br>Increases electrical stimulation threshold of the heart | See above<br>Lower infusion dose used in shock<br>Used for ventricular tachycardia |

Modified from Winklestein ML: The child with disturbance of oxygen and carbon dioxide exchange. In Hockenberry MJ and others, editors: *Wong's nursing care of infants and children*, ed 7, St Louis, 2003, Mosby.

**TABLE 29-5**

## Classes of Hemorrhage for Children

| Class | Blood Loss | Signs | Treatment |
|---|---|---|---|
| I | 15% or less<br>40-kg child = 500 ml blood loss | Pulse: slight decrease<br>Blood pressure (BP): normal<br>Respiration: normal<br>Capillary refill: normal<br>Tilt test*: normal | Crystalloids |
| II | 20%-30%<br>40-kg child = 800 ml blood loss | Pulse: tachycardia >150<br>BP: decreased systolic; decreased pulse pressure<br>Respiration: tachypnea >35-40<br>Capillary refill: delayed<br>Tilt test*: positive<br>Urine output: normal (1 ml/kg/hr) | Crystalloids |
| III | 30%-35%<br>40-kg child = 1200 ml blood loss | BP: decreased<br>Narrow pulse pressure<br>Urine output: decreased | Crystalloids<br>Packed red cells |
| IV | 40%-50%<br>40-kg child = 1600 ml blood loss | Pulse: nonpalpable<br>BP: nonpalpable<br>No response to verbal or painful stimuli | Crystalloids<br>Packed red cells |

From Rupp LA, Day MW: Children are different: pediatric differences and the impact on trauma. In Moloney-Harmon PA, Czerwinski SJ: *Nursing care of the pediatric trauma patient*, St Louis, 2003, Saunders.

*A tilt test is done by sitting the child upright. The test is "normal" if the child can stay up for more than 90 sec and maintain blood pressure; it is "positive" if these criteria are not met.

**TABLE 29-6**

## Pediatric Vital Signs

| Age | Heart Rate (beats/min) | Respirations (breaths/min) | Systolic Blood Pressure (mm Hg) |
|---|---|---|---|
| Newborn | 100-160 | 30-60 | 50-70 |
| 1-6 wk | 100-160 | 30-60 | 70-95 |
| 6 mo | 90-120 | 25-40 | 80-100 |
| 1 yr | 90-120 | 20-30 | 80-100 |
| 3 yr | 80-120 | 20-30 | 80-110 |
| 6 yr | 70-110 | 18-25 | 80-110 |
| 10 yr | 60-90 | 15-20 | 90-120 |
| 14 yr | 60-90 | 15-20 | 90-130 |

From Rupp LA, Day MW: Children are different: pediatric differences and the impact on trauma. In Moloney-Harmon PA, Czerwinski SJ: *Nursing care of the pediatric trauma patient*, St Louis, 2003, Saunders.

an integral role in preparing those associated with the child for outcomes associated with trauma surgery and may help facilitate consults from the departments of child life, social work, and clergy.

Airway and breathing are part of the primary survey for pediatric trauma victims. Anatomic variations of the upper airway related to age must be considered. Airway patency must be assessed and secured. Initial assessment for all pediatric trauma patients may best be application of the head tilt chin-lift or jaw-thrust, depending on the age of the child and the nature of the injury. When integrity of the spinal cord is questionable, in-line cervical traction should be applied. Collars and stabilizing devices must remain in place until cervical fracture has been ruled out and the spine "cleared," or declared free of injury by a radiologist. Airway equipment sizes may be selected based on age as well as whether the child is breathing spontaneously and whether the child is unconscious. An assessment of relevant systems will be performed on stabilization of the pediatric airway, and surgery will progress as planned.

**BOX 29-6**

### Estimating Blood Pressure for the Pediatric Patient

Systolic BP (mm Hg) = (2 × Age in years) + 80
Diastolic BP (mm Hg) = ⅔ Systolic BP

**BOX 29-7**

### Specific Differences Between the Adult and Pediatric Trauma Patient

- Growth, development, and psychologic skills vary with age.
- Children have smaller airways with more soft tissue and a narrowing of the cricoid cartilage. The openings of the trachea and esophagus are closer together, which can make intubation more difficult.
- Children have faster respiratory rates and become hypoxic more quickly.
- The temperature control mechanism is immature in infants and small children.
- Children are easily dehydrated.
- Children have faster heart rates.
- Young children's extremities are likely to appear mottled. This may be a response to cold. Capillary refill may be a better indicator of circulatory status in the child.

## SURGERY FOR CONGENITAL HEART DISEASE

Congenital heart disease (CHD) occurs in approximately five to eight of 1000 live births. About two to three in 1000 infants will be symptomatic during their first year of life.[23] Structural abnormalities of the heart and great vessels result in an embryologic failure in septation, malalignment, failure to develop, and/or failure to progress.

The etiology of CHD varies, although certain factors are associated with increased incidence. For example, risk of CHD is increased secondary to environmental factors: rubella during the first 8 weeks of gestation may result in patent ductus arteriosus and pulmonary artery stenosis (along with other syndromes). Other risk factors include maternal chronic illnesses such as diabetes or poorly controlled phenylketonuria (PKU), alcohol consumption, and exposure to environmental toxins. Incidence of CHD is increased also in certain chromosomal defects; for example, atrial septal defects are seen in children with trisomy 21 (Down syndrome). In addition, an increased incidence is seen in small-for-gestational-age (SGA) babies and those where there is a positive family history, that is, those families with a sibling or parent having CHD.

Congenital cardiac abnormalities are classified as cyanotic or acyanotic as well as by their effect on pulmonary blood flow (Box 29-8). Of the acyanotic lesions, there are those that increase pulmonary blood flow, such as patent ductus arteriosus (PDA), atrial septal defect (ASD), ventricular septal defect (VSD), and atrioventricular canal defects (AVCs). With these, blood flows from the high-pressure left side of the heart to the low-pressure right side of the heart because of an abnormal connection either between the septum or in the great arteries. The resultant increase in pulmonary blood flow causes the right side of the heart and lungs to become overloaded. Congestive heart failure (CHF) may develop, pulmonary vascular resistance increases, the pulmonary vessel walls thicken, and if left untreated, the condition may become irreversible.

BOX 29-8

### Classification of Congenital Cardiac Defects

**ACYANOTIC WITH INCREASED PULMONARY BLOOD FLOW**
- Patent ductus arteriosus
- Atrial septal defect
- Ventricular septal defect
- Atrioventricular septal defect

**ACYANOTIC OBSTRUCTIVE LESIONS**
- Coarctation of the aorta
- Aortic stenosis
- Pulmonary stenosis

**CYANOTIC WITH DECREASED PULMONARY BLOOD FLOW**
- Tricuspid atresia
- Tetralogy of Fallot
- Pulmonary atresia with intact ventricular septum

**CYANOTIC WITH INCREASED PULMONARY BLOOD FLOW**
- Total anomalous pulmonary venous connection (return)
- Truncus arteriosus
- Hypoplastic left heart syndrome

**CYANOTIC WITH VARIABLE PULMONARY BLOOD FLOW**
- Transposition of the great arteries
- Double-outlet right ventricle
- Double-outlet left ventricle
- Single ventricle

Acyanotic obstructive lesions, such as aortic stenosis, pulmonary stenosis, or coarctation of the aorta, increase the workload of the chamber that pumps against the obstruction (increases afterload). Cardiomegaly and ventricular hypertrophy may be seen in response to the increased workload, and if the obstruction is severe, heart failure may ensue.

The presence of cyanosis implies that one of the following conditions is present: right-sided heart obstruction with blood traveling right to left without going to the lungs; the mixing of venous and arterial blood within the heart or great vessels; or the great vessels being in the wrong position. The degree of cyanosis depends on pulmonary blood flow and intracardiac mixing of blood through a shunt. This classification of lesions includes but is not limited to tetralogy of Fallot (TOF), pulmonary atresia with intact ventricular septum (PA/IVS), tricuspid atresia (TA), transposition of the great arteries (TGA), total anomalous pulmonary venous return (TAPVR), and hypoplastic left heart syndrome (HLHS). Treatment goals for these lesions include managing pulmonary blood flow and/or arterial oxygen saturation.

## Repair of Atrial Septal Defect

Congenital defects in the atrial septum occur in approximately 5% to 10% of CHD cases.[19] The classification within this group of defects is based on anatomic location and associated abnormalities (Figure 29-49). The ostium secundum defect is located in the superior and central portions of the septum. The ostium primum defect is in the lower portion of the atrial septum and is associated with other defects in the atrioventricular canal, usually with a cleft of the mitral valve or occasionally of the tricuspid valve. An accompanying VSD may also be present. The sinus venosus defect is located at the right atrium–superior vena cava junction and is associated with partial anomalous pulmonary venous return.

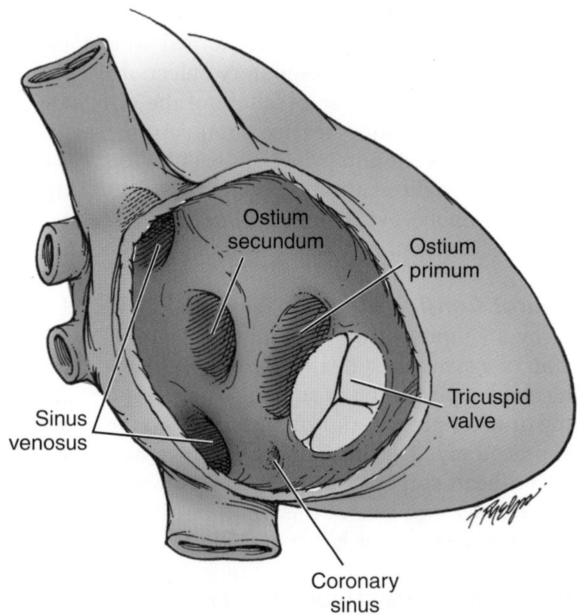


FIGURE 29-49 Various types of atrial septal defects (ASDs) viewed through the right atrium (ostium secundum, ostium primum, sinus venosus). An unroofed coronary sinus may also act as an ASD.

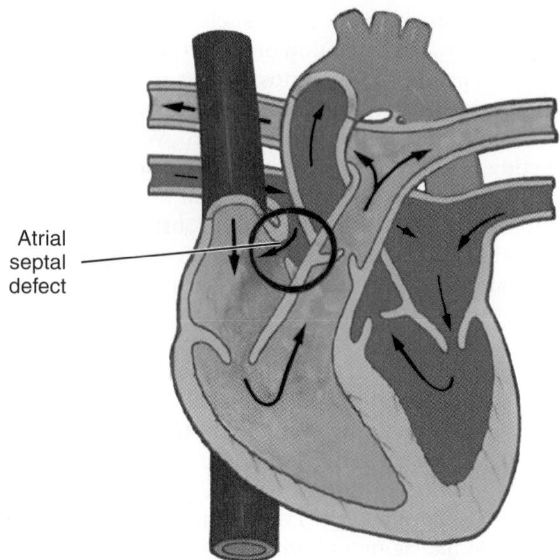


**FIGURE 29-50** Atrial septal defect.

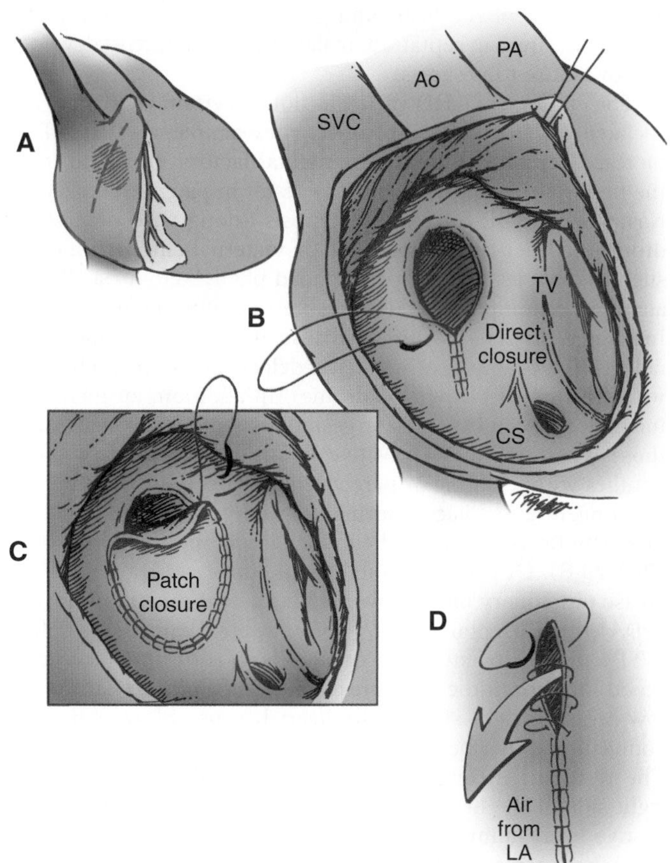


**FIGURE 29-51** Surgical procedure for atrial septal defect (ASD) closure. **A,** Incision through right atriotomy. Direct suture closure, **B,** and patch closure, **C,** of secundum ASD. **D,** Deairing of the left atrium. *Ao,* Aorta; *CS,* conduction system; *LA,* left atrium; *PA,* pulmonary artery; *SVC,* superior vena cava; *TV,* tricuspid valve.

An ASD results in a left-to-right atrial shunt whose direction and magnitude are determined by the size of the defect and relative resistance to flow into the ventricles and great vessels (Figure 29-50). ASDs are often tolerated well with no symptoms during childhood, especially if the defect is small. However, if the defect is large or of the ostium primum type, with a pronounced shunting of blood, the workload of the right side of the heart is increased. On assessment, there is a characteristic systolic pulmonary murmur at the second intercostal space at the left sternal border, and a fixed splitting of the second heart sound may also be heard. The right side of the heart and the pulmonary artery and its branches become enlarged. The vascularity of the lung field is increased, with resulting pulmonary hypertension and subsequent failure of the right side of the heart. At this point the shunt may reverse. The initial symptoms may include fatigue, retardation of normal weight gain, and increased susceptibility to respiratory infections. Later signs and symptoms include those of failure of the right side of the heart and cyanosis with a reverse shunt. Asymptomatic children whose ASD is left unrepaired until adulthood may develop right atrial and right ventricular hypertrophy, atrial dysrhythmias, CHF, embolic events, and pulmonary vascular disease. The defect is common in children with Down syndrome.

***Procedural Considerations.*** ASDs are closed, under direct vision, by a simple suture technique (primary closure) or by insertion of a synthetic prosthetic patch or pericardial patch.

The child is placed in the supine position for a median sternotomy or in a right anterior oblique position for an anterolateral thoracotomy. The instrument setup is as described for basic open-heart surgery (see Chapter 27), with consideration given to the age and size of the child, plus intracardiac patch material, 2 × 2 inches or larger.

### *Operative Procedure (Figure 29-51)*

1. A median sternotomy incision is performed, and CPB is instituted. (Infrequently, a right anterolateral incision is performed.) Many bypass strategies can be employed. With bicaval cannulation, the child remains on bypass during the repair and blood is directed away from the right atrium through cannulas in the superior and inferior venae cavae. Occasionally, in this method the cannulas may obstruct the view of the ASD. With single venous cannulation, a cannula is placed into the right atrium and the child remains on bypass during the repair. With this technique, the venous line is clamped immediately before the right atrium is incised and pump suctions are placed into the inferior and superior venae cavae during ASD closure. Deep hypothermic circulatory arrest is sometimes used in more complicated repairs, such as ostium primum ASD or sinus venosum defects associated with anomalous pulmonary venous return.
2. The right atrium is incised, and the pathologic defect is determined.
3. The defect is closed with a continuous suture, or a patch of pericardium or prosthetic material may be used. By filling the atrium with blood before the atriotomy is completely closed, the surgeon can express air from the atrium. For the ostium primum defect with a cleft mitral valve, repair of the cleft is accomplished by approximation, with use of interrupted (possibly pledgeted) sutures.

## Repair of Ventricular Septal Defect

One of the most common congenital cardiac anomalies, VSDs (Figure 29-52) occur in approximately two to six of every 1000 live births, with as many as 60% closing spontaneously.[3,23] Most VSDs are small with little physiologic importance. As with ASDs, the classification of VSDs depends on location and associated lesions (Figure 29-53). Perimembranous VSDs (also called *conoventricular, subaortic, infracristal,* or *membranous*) are most commonly found. These defects occur directly adjacent to the membranous septum and the fibrous trigone of the heart where the aortic, mitral, and tricuspid valves are in fibrous continuity. The tricuspid valve tissue sometimes forms an aneurysm of the membranous septum, which may be a mechanism of defect closure for this type of defect. The subpulmonary type of VSDs (also referred to as *supracristal, infundibular, intracristal, outlet, conoseptal,* or *conal*) are located above the crista supraventricularis within the outlet septum and border the semilunar valves. Muscular-type VSDs can be located anywhere in the muscular septum, including apical, anterior, or posterior, or the midseptum inlet and outlet. Malalignment-type VSDs are created by a malalignment between the infundibular septum and the trabecular muscular septum. Canal-type or inlet defects are located posteriorly within the area confined by the tricuspid valve septal leaflet papillary muscles. The defect borders the tricuspid valve annulus.

The hemodynamics depend on the size and location of the defect as well as the pulmonary vascular resistance (PVR) and systemic vascular resistance (SVR). Newborns are often asymptomatic until the PVR falls—then a left-to-right shunt occurs, and the corresponding murmur is auscultated. Small defects with moderate shunt and increased pulmonary blood flow but not increased pulmonary pressure may not produce any symptoms. A large VSD, however, may produce high pulmonary flow under high pressure and contribute to CHF. In this case the patient is at risk of developing pulmonary hypertension (Figure 29-54). Surgical closure of the defect should be performed to prevent increased pulmonary hypertension. If PVR further increases and rises above SVR, shunt reversal (Eisenmenger's syndrome, or shunting from right to left) and cyanosis may occur.

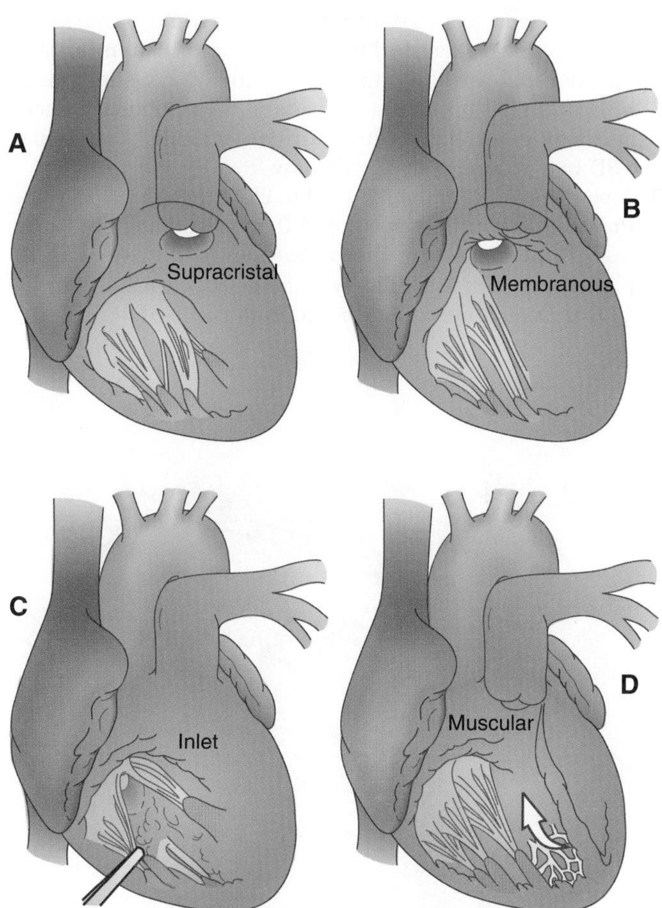


**FIGURE 29-53** Various types of ventricular septal defects viewed within the right ventricle. **A,** Infundibular (supracristal). **B,** Membranous. **C,** Inlet (AV canal). **D,** Muscular (trabecular).

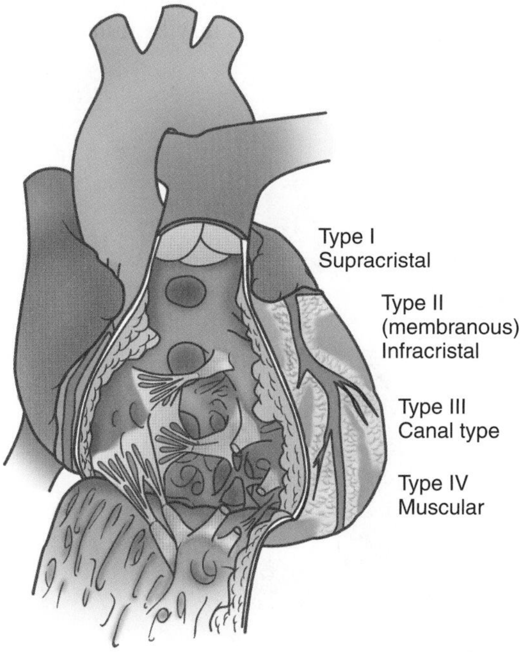

**FIGURE 29-52** Ventricular septal defects: anatomic classification.

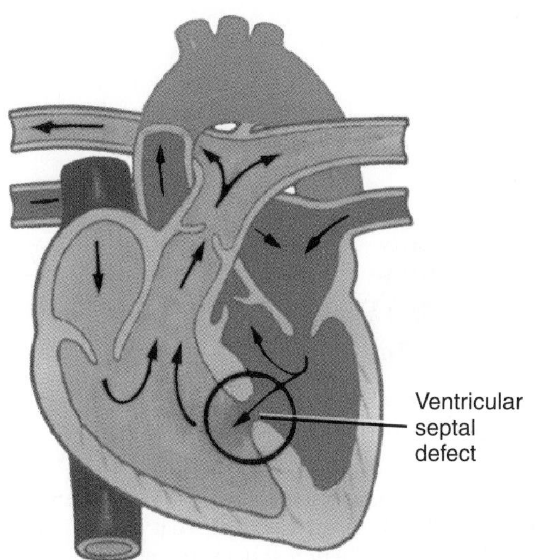


**FIGURE 29-54** Ventricular septal defect.

***Operative Procedure.*** Under direct vision, a congenital defect in the ventricular septum (Figure 29-55) is closed by a simple suture technique or, in most instances, by insertion of a synthetic prosthetic or pericardial patch.

1. A median sternotomy is performed, and CPB is instituted.
2. The location of the defect determines the location of the incision. For membranous and canal defects, an incision is usually made in the right atrium, the atrium is retracted, and the VSD is identified by use of a pump suction through the tricuspid valve into the right ventricle. For supracristal VSDs, an incision is usually made in the pulmonary artery and may be extended into the right ventricle. A muscular VSD may require a ventriculotomy.
3. A patch is most frequently used to close the defect. To place the patch, a continuous 6-0 or 5-0 nonabsorbable suture on a small needle or an interrupted suture with or without pledgets may be used. Rarely is the defect closed primarily.
4. CPB is discontinued, and the sternum is closed.

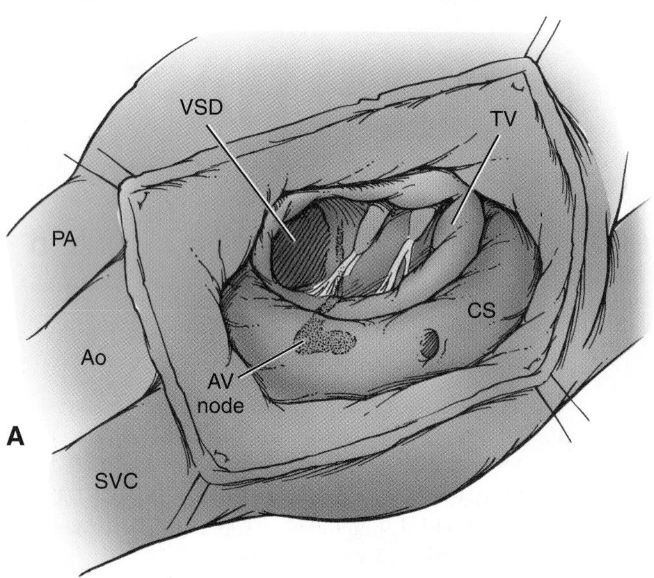


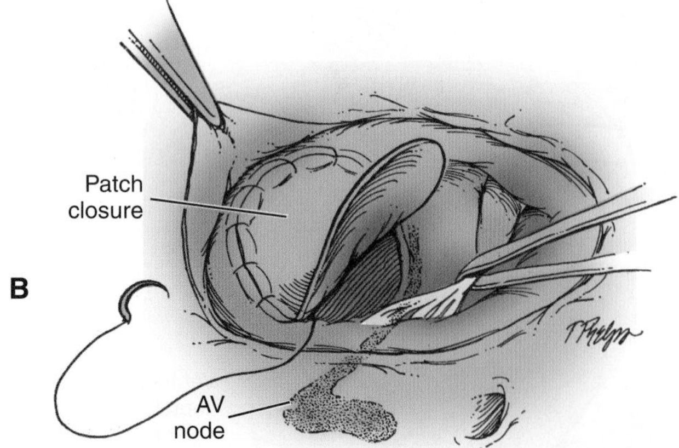


**FIGURE 29-55** Ventricular septal defect *(VSD)* closure through the tricuspid valve *(TV)*. **A,** Open site. **B,** Partial closure. *Ao,* Aorta; *AV,* atrioventricular; *CS,* conduction system; *PA,* pulmonary artery; *SVC,* superior vena cava.

## Repair of Common Atrioventricular Septal Defects

Atrioventricular (AV) septal defects (Figure 29-56) account for 4% to 5% of congenital cardiac malformations and represent 30% to 40% of cardiac defects seen in children with Down syndrome.[23] Also called *endocardial cushion defect,* the defect involves a single AV annulus that drains both atria (the common AV canal).

Partial AV canal defect (also called *incomplete* or *ostium primum defect*) is an interatrial communication associated with a cleft in the anterior leaflet of the left AV valve and usually some degree of left AV valve insufficiency. No interventricular communication exists, and two separate AV valves are present.

Transitional AV canal defects are those in which an ostium primum defect is present and the AV valves may be only partially separated into two valves. Dense attachments of the chordae to the crest of the muscular septum are such that the interventricular communication may be small or moderate, often with multiple individual communications.

Complete AV septal defects involve an ostium primum defect, a large interventricular communication, and a large common AV valve that straddles both ventricles.

The hemodynamics are determined by the differences between SVR and PVR as well as by the size of ASD and VSD. With a partial AV canal defect, signs of increased pulmonary flow under low pressure with a left-to-right shunt are seen—similar to those of a secundum ASD. In the complete form of AV canal, the pathophysiology resembles that of a VSD with an associated ASD, with left-to-right shunting at both atrial and ventricular levels leading to volume overload of the atria as well as the ventricles. With AV valve regurgitation, the ventricular volume overload worsens.

***Operative Procedure.*** The operative procedure depends on the type of common AV valve and the surgeon's preference.

1. A median sternotomy is performed, and CPB is instituted.
2. The right atrium is incised, and the cardiac anatomy is inspected. The AV valve leaflets may be tested at this time by

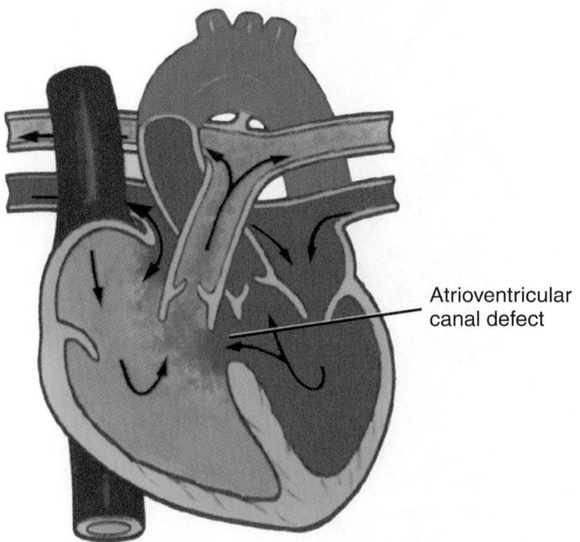


**FIGURE 29-56** Atrioventricular canal defect.

injection of cold saline into the ventricular chambers to float the AV leaflets into a closed position. Suture may be used to approximate the anterior and posterior bridging leaflets.

3. The superior and inferior bridging leaflets may be incised.
4. a. If a single-patch repair of a complete AV septal defect is used, a piece of synthetic patch material or the patient's own pericardium is cut to appropriate size and shape. Continuous or interrupted sutures are used to place the patch in the ventricular septum. The bridging AV valve tissues may be secured to the patch with interrupted pledgeted suture or running suture secured with a few interrupted pledgeted stitches. The right side of the AV valve may also be secured to the patch. The left AV valve is tested for competence by use of saline solution, and adjustments are made. The ASD is then closed by suturing the superior rim of the patch to the lower rim of the atrial septum.
   b. If a two-patch repair of the complete AV canal defect is used, the ventricular patch may be of synthetic material and the atrial patch may be of autologous pericardium. The synthetic material patch is often placed without division of the common AV valve leaflets. The leaflets are then attached to the crest of the synthetic patch, and the ASD is closed.
5. The atriotomy is closed using a running suture technique.

## Correction of Tetralogy of Fallot

TOF, described initially in the early nineteenth century, includes the association of four anatomic findings: VSD, subpulmonic stenosis, aortic override of the ventricular septum, and right ventricular hypertrophy (RVH) (Figure 29-57). Occurring in approximately 10% of congenital heart defects, TOF is actually the result of a single anatomic abnormality: anterior malalignment of the infundibular septum with the muscular septum.[8]

The preoperative hemodynamics or physiology depends mainly on the degree of pulmonary stenosis. In patients with minimal obstruction to pulmonary blood flow, the physiology is similar to that of a VSD with left-to-right shunting. These patients will have pulmonary overcirculation and symptoms of CHF. Occasionally labeled as "pink tets," these patients have little to no right-to-left shunting and do not exhibit cyanosis.

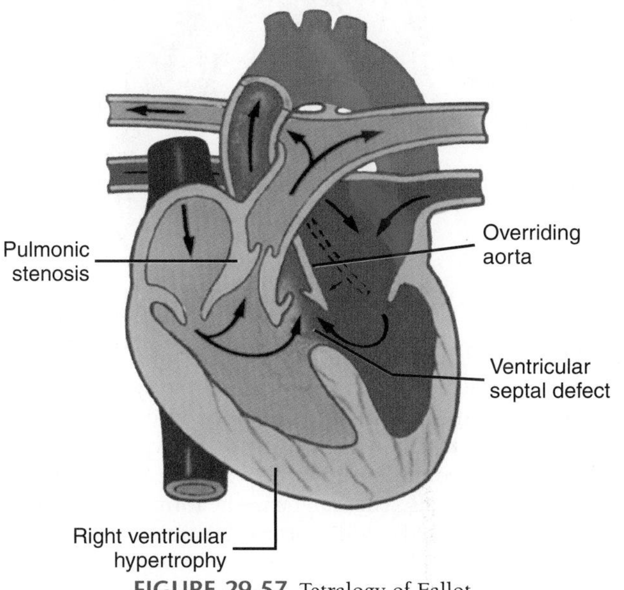

**FIGURE 29-57** Tetralogy of Fallot.

At the other end of the spectrum of this particular type of heart defect are children with severe pulmonary stenosis, who may have significant right-to-left shunting at the VSD level and exhibit hypoxemia with oxygen saturations in the 60% to 80% range. Cyanosis, as seen in the superficial vessels of the skin, is the result of shunting unoxygenated blood into the systemic circulation. Other clinical manifestations may include episodes of acute dyspnea with cyanosis, retarded growth, clubbing of extremities, reduced exercise tolerance, and increased incidence of "tet," or hypercyanotic spells. A systolic murmur and secondary polycythemia are usually present in the cyanotic child. Echocardiography is performed to confirm the diagnosis of TOF; occasionally a cardiac catheterization and angiography may be necessary in delineating other anatomic abnormalities, such as with the coronary arteries, before surgical repair.

The selection of a palliative or corrective procedure is based on the age and general condition of the child and the severity of the pulmonary stenosis. The treatment of choice is primary repair; contraindications for primary repair include anomalous origin of the anterior descending coronary artery and presence of pulmonary atresia. Complete or primary repair consists of closure of the VSD and repair of the pulmonic stenosis under direct vision.

***Procedural Considerations.*** The child is placed on the OR bed in a supine position. The setup is as described for open-heart surgery, with consideration given to the child's age and size. Additional items to be added to the basic open-heart setup include the following: intracardiac patch, 2 × 2 inch; outflow cardiac patch, 2 × 2 inch; and a felt or Gortex patch, 4 × 4 inch.

### *Operative Procedure*

1. A median sternotomy is performed, and CPB with hypothermia is instituted.
2. A vertical ventriculotomy over the infundibular area may be performed (Figure 29-58, *A*).
3. The VSD is identified. Closure requires an intracardiac patch in almost all instances. This can be of a synthetic material or a piece of pericardium.
4. Interrupted or continuous cardiovascular sutures are placed in the septum with caution because of the danger of suturing a branch of the neuroconductive system.
5. The hypertrophied infundibular muscle is excised, as completely as possible, from the right ventricular outflow tract. If the pulmonic valve is stenosed, the fused commissures are incised.
6. An estimate is made about whether the right ventricle can be closed primarily or if a patch is necessary. If the pulmonic stenosis cannot be relieved adequately by valvulotomy and infundibulectomy, an outflow patch of synthetic material or pulmonary homograft tissue may be needed to enlarge the outflow tract (Figure 29-58, *B*). If the pulmonary artery or valve annulus is quite small, it may be necessary to extend the patch across the valve ring to the proximal portion of the pulmonary artery (Figure 29-58, *C*).
7. CPB is discontinued, and the sternum is closed.

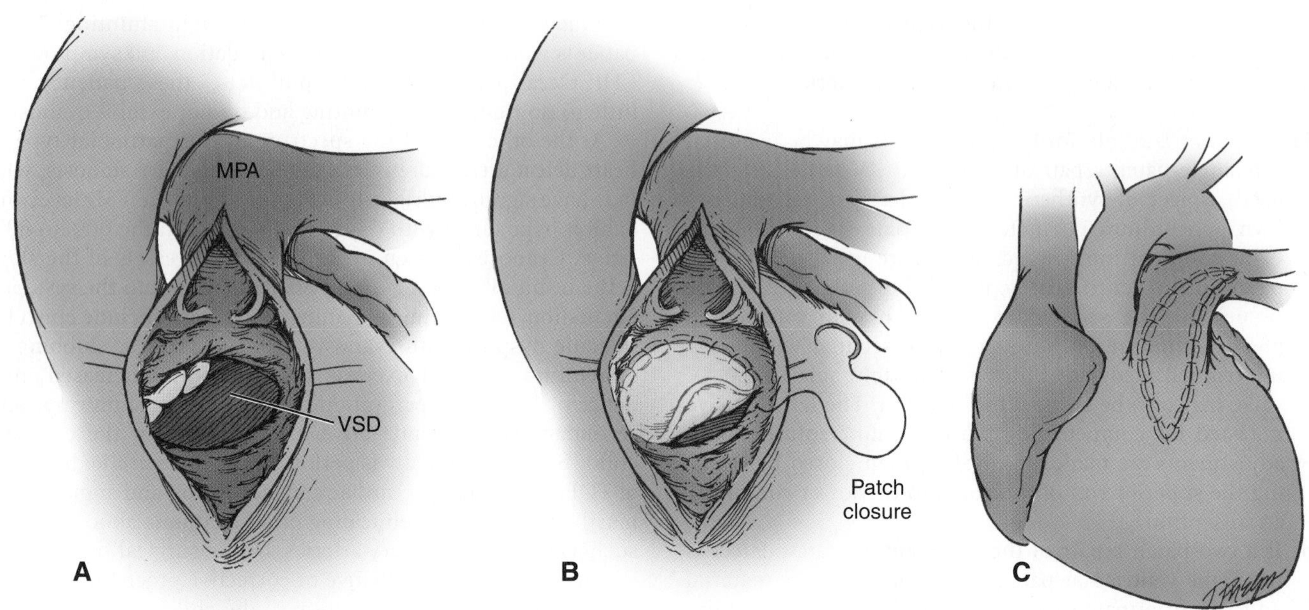


FIGURE 29-58 **A,** The most common ventricular incision used for repair of tetralogy of Fallot is vertical so that it can be extended as shown from the right ventricle across the pulmonary valve annulus and onto the main pulmonary artery *(MPA)*. It is possible to gain adequate exposure to the ventricular septal defect *(VSD)* by extending the incision a short distance beyond the infundibular septum. This "limited ventriculotomy" may help preserve late right ventricular function yet enable adequate enlargement of the hypoplastic area in the right ventricular outflow tract. **B,** The VSD is closed with a prosthetic patch. Right ventricular outflow obstruction is relieved when the outflow tract is enlarged with a patch as shown. **C,** In some cases it may be necessary to extend the incision onto the left pulmonary artery and to taper the patch at its most distal extent.

## Operation for Tricuspid Atresia

Occurring in approximately 1 per 10,000 live births, the failure of the tricuspid valve to develop results in an absence of communication between the right atrium and the right ventricle.[26] Blood flows from the superior and inferior venae cavae to the right atrium through a patent foramen ovale or ASD to the left atrium to the left ventricle to the aorta and body. Some of the left ventricular blood flows through a VSD to a small right ventricle and then to the lungs, as well as through a PDA when present (Figure 29-59). This disorder has hemodynamics similar to pulmonary atresia; there is no path for blood to enter the lungs. The infant displays cyanosis that worsens when the PDA closes, venous engorgement of the liver, periods of dyspnea, easy fatigability, growth retardation, and rapid progression of CHF.

Palliative operations (described later in this chapter) consist of the use of the Blalock-Hanlon procedure, which enlarges the ASD, or systemic-to-pulmonary artery shunts to relieve the cyanosis. A Fontan procedure, also described later, will then be performed after the newborn period.

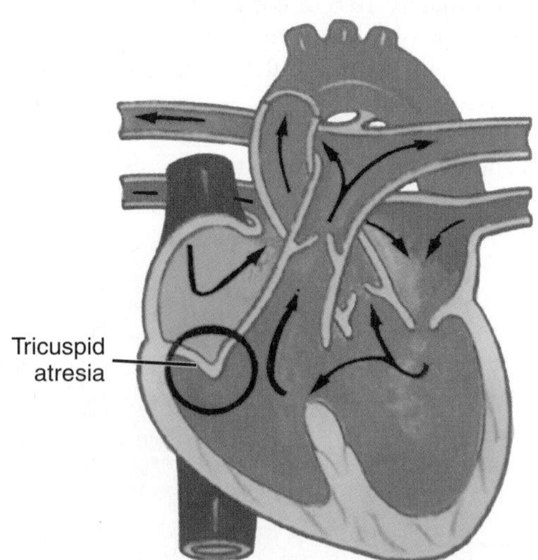


FIGURE 29-59 Tricuspid atresia.

## Operations for Transposition of the Great Arteries

TGA is a result of inappropriate separation and migration of the truncus arteriosus during cardiac development. The end result of this is the aorta arising from the anatomic right ventricle and the pulmonary artery arising from the anatomic left ventricle. Here the circulation is reversed (Figure 29-60); the blood from the right side of the heart goes to the body, and the blood from the left side of the heart goes to the lungs. In other words, desaturated blood is pumped into the systemic circulation, whereas saturated blood is pumped into the pulmonary circulation. For an infant with TGA to survive, there must be some mixing or communication between the two sides of the heart or major vessels. This can be in the form of a patent foramen ovale, PDA, ASD, VSD, or partial transposition of the pulmonary veins, all of which permit oxygenated blood to enter the systemic circulation.

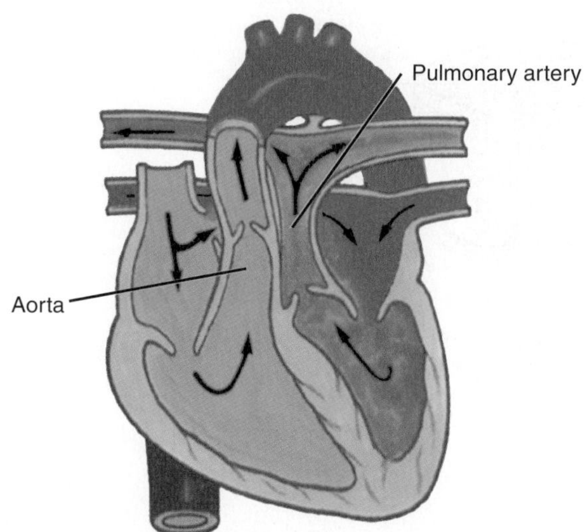


**FIGURE 29-60** Transposition of the great arteries.

The newborn with TGA is cyanotic at birth and becomes severely incapacitated with closure of the PDA; cardiomegaly is evident and progresses to CHF. Metabolic acidosis is also evident, and the mediastinum appears narrow on chest x-ray.

Corrective procedures include the arterial switch operation (ASO), the Senning atrial switch, the Mustard atrial switch, and the Rastelli procedure. The arterial switch procedure is the most common surgery performed for the TGA during the first week of life.

Palliative procedures that tend to improve intracardiac mixing, thereby increasing the oxygen content of the systemic blood, may be necessary if the surgeon chooses to do the Mustard or Senning procedure in the first few months of life. Palliative procedures include the Blalock-Hanlon procedure and the Rashkind atrial septostomy.

For each corrective procedure described, the child is placed on the OR bed in a supine position. The setup is as described for open-heart surgery, with consideration given to the age and size of the child.

***Arterial Switch Procedure.*** The surgeon performs anatomic repair of the transposition by switching the pulmonary artery to the right ventricle and the aorta to the left ventricle. The left ventricle must have developed sufficient contractile force to maintain systemic pressure once the procedure is completed. It occurs in patients with VSD and reversible hypertension or in patients in whom the procedure is performed during the newborn period while PVR is still high. In patients in whom the procedure is performed after the newborn period, pulmonary artery banding (described later) may first be performed to strengthen the left ventricle. Transfer of the coronary arteries must be accomplished without kinking, torsion, or tension.

*Operative Procedure (Figure 29-61)*

1. Median sternotomy is performed, and CPB is instituted.
2. The aorta is dissected away from the main and branch pulmonary arteries.
3. The coronary arteries are inspected, and the site for their transfer into the pulmonary artery is marked.
4. The aorta is cross-clamped and transected above the sinuses and aortic valve; the pulmonary artery is transected above the pulmonic valve.
5. The orifices of the coronary arteries with a rim of adjacent aortic wall are excised.
6. The corresponding sinuses of the pulmonary arteries are incised where previously marked. The cuff and coronary artery are then sutured into place. Care is taken not to kink the coronary arteries.
7. The distal aorta is brought behind the pulmonary artery (LeCompte maneuver). The distal aorta is anastomosed to the proximal pulmonary artery (neoaorta).
8. Pericardium or pulmonary homograft tissue is used to enlarge the aorta and patch the defects created by the excision of the coronary ostia.
9. The repair is completed by anastomosing the proximal pulmonary artery to the distal pulmonary artery.

***Senning and Mustard Procedures.*** The Senning and Mustard procedures are physiologic repairs (in contrast to an anatomic repair as seen with the arterial switch procedure) whereby the pulmonary and systemic venous return is rerouted through a baffle of Dacron or pericardium, causing each atrium to empty into the opposite ventricle. First successfully applied by Senning in 1959, the procedure was modified by Mustard in 1964. These procedures may be performed on children who are not candidates for the arterial switch procedure. Although the risk of mortality with either of these procedures is now low, long-term survival of patients with these repairs has been associated with late problems including systemic (right) ventricular dysfunction or failure, dysrhythmias, and obstruction of the superior vena cava by the baffle, causing superior vena cava syndrome.

SENNING OPERATIVE PROCEDURE (FIGURE 29-62)

1. A median sternotomy is performed, and CPB is instituted.
2. A right atrial incision is made longitudinally, extending to the insertion of the eustachian valve at the orifice of the inferior vena cava.
3. A lateral atrial septal flap is made and sutured above the left pulmonary veins.
4. The new systemic venous atrium is completed by suturing the edge of the original right atrial incision to the remnant of atrial septum between the mitral and tricuspid valves. This step creates a tube of right atrium containing the venae cavae at each end.
5. Pulmonary venous blood flows around this tube from an opening in front of the right pulmonary veins to the tricuspid valve.

MUSTARD OPERATIVE PROCEDURE. Under direct vision, the Mustard procedure allows excision of the remaining segments of the atrial septum; a pericardial or synthetic patch is sutured in place in the atrial cavities, creating a baffle so that the venous inflow is reversed. This permits the pulmonary venous return to be redirected into the right ventricle and the systemic venous return to be redirected into the left ventricle.

Previous creation of an ASD may serve as a first stage for this procedure. Pericardium or synthetic patch is used as a baffle.

1. A median sternotomy is performed.
2. A section of pericardium 2 × 3 inches is harvested.
3. CPB is instituted.

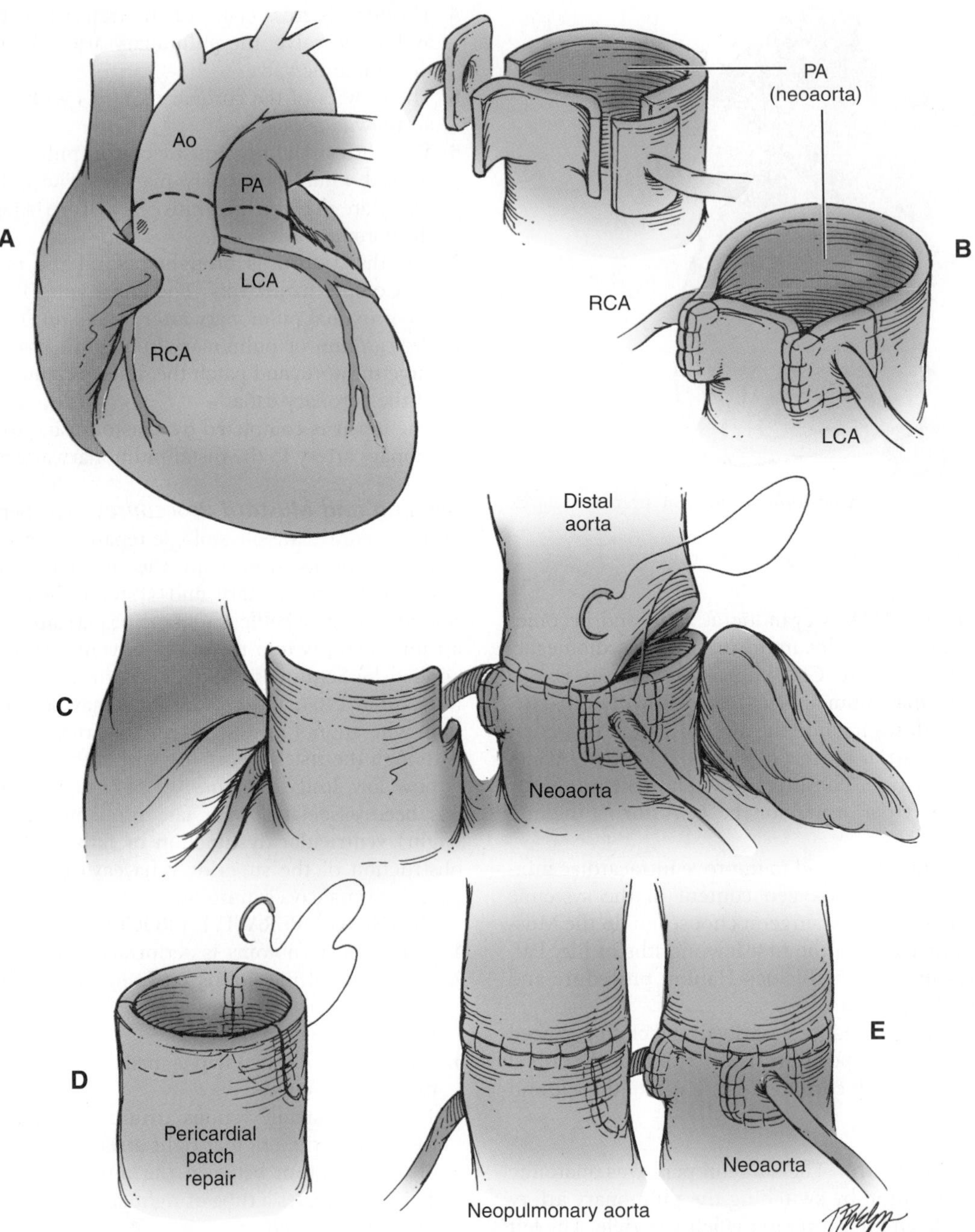


**FIGURE 29-61** Technique of the arterial switch operation. **A,** The great arteries are transected above the sinuses of Valsalva. **B,** The coronaries are excised from the aorta *(Ao)*, transposed posteriorly, and anastomosed to the pulmonary artery *(PA)* (neoaorta). **C,** The distal aorta is brought behind the pulmonary artery (LeCompte maneuver) and anastomosed to the neoaorta. **D,** Separate pericardial patches are sutured to fill in the defects in the aorta created by excision of the coronary arteries. **E,** Completed repair. *LCA,* Left coronary artery; *RCA,* right coronary artery.

4. A curved incision is made in the wall of the right atrium (Figure 29-63, *A*).
5. The entire atrial septum is excised. The orifice of the coronary sinus is enlarged (Figure 29-63, *B* and *C*).
6. Starting at the edge of the left pulmonary vein orifices, the surgeon sutures the baffle between the pulmonary veins and mitral valve, diverting the vena cava blood to the mitral valve and the pulmonary venous return to the tricuspid valve (Figure 29-63, *D*).
7. An additional section of pericardium or synthetic patch may be placed in the wall of the right atrium that enlarges the new left atrium.
8. CPB circulation is discontinued, and closures are completed.

**RASTELLI OPERATIVE PROCEDURE.** Initially described for correction of TGA with large VSD and significant left ventricular (pulmonary) outflow tract obstruction, the Rastelli procedure is an anatomic correction that has the advantage of

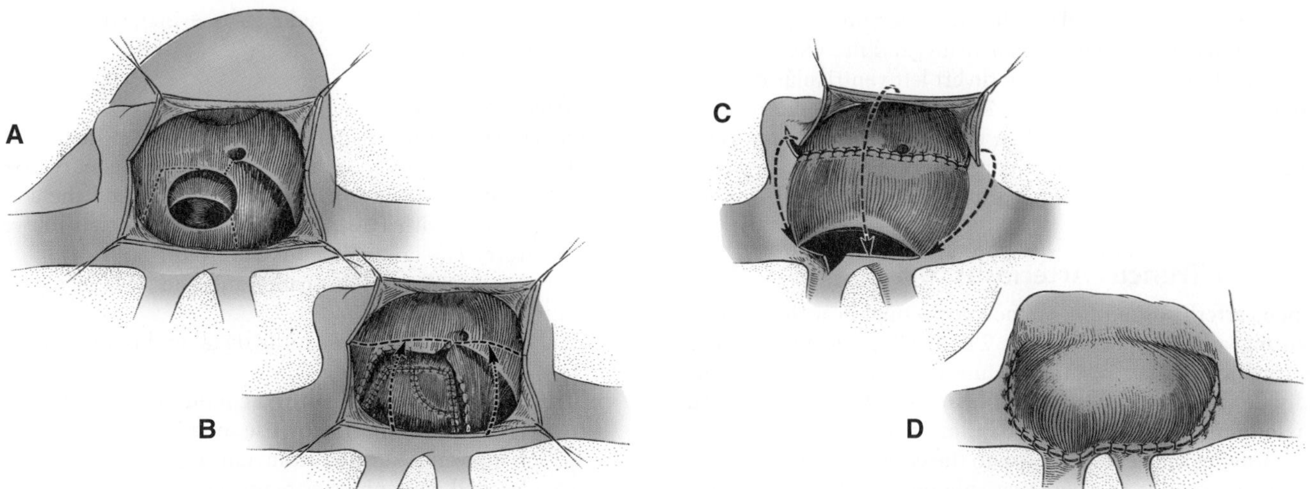


**FIGURE 29-62** The Senning procedure. **A,** The atrial septum is cut near the tricuspid valve, and the incision is extended down to the insertion of the eustachian valve at the orifice of the inferior vena cava. **B,** An atrial septal flap is developed and sutured to the anterior lip of the orifices of the left pulmonary veins, effectively separating the pulmonary and systemic venous channels. **C,** The posterior edge of the right atrial incision is sutured to the remnant of atrial septum, diverting the systemic venous channel to the mitral valve. **D,** The anterior edge of the right atrial incision (lengthened by short incisions at each corner) is sutured around the superior and inferior vena cava to the lateral edge of the left atrial incision, completing the pulmonary channel and diversion of pulmonary venous blood to the tricuspid valve area.

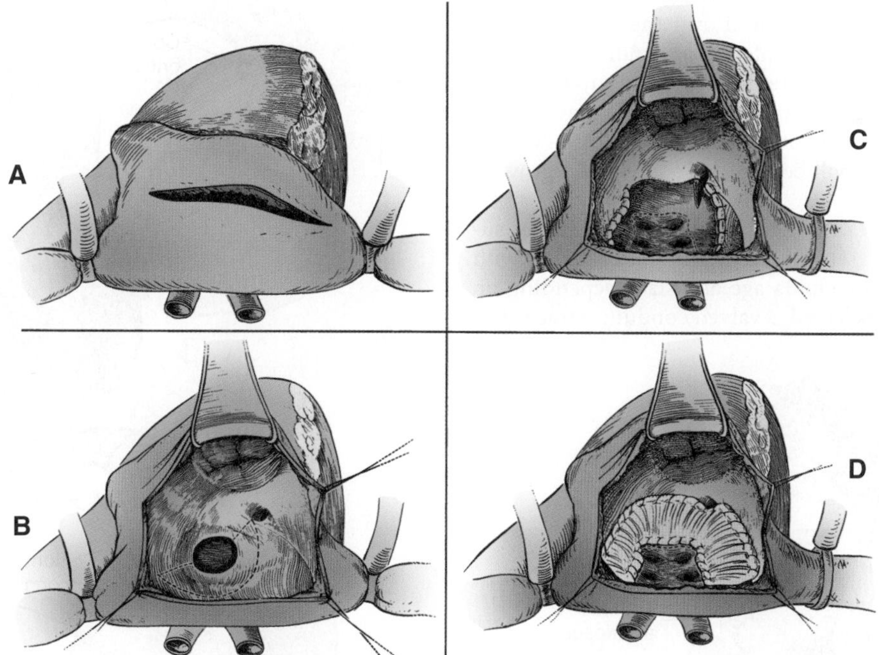


**FIGURE 29-63** The Mustard procedure. **A,** The right atrium is opened with a longitudinal incision well away from the sinoatrial node. **B,** The atrial septum is incised from the midpoint on the superior border of the atrial septal defect to the middle of the superior vena cava orifice. All the septum lateral to this incision is excised, with avoidance of the orifices of the right pulmonary veins. The ridge of septum medially is preserved. **C,** The coronary sinus is cut back into the left atrium, and all raw margins of atrial septum are oversewn. The dotted line indicates where the baffle will be sutured. **D,** Starting at the anterior lip of the left pulmonary vein orifices, the surgeon sutures the baffle in place, thus diverting the vena cava return to the mitral valve and the pulmonary venous return to the tricuspid valve.

converting the left ventricle to the systemic pumping chamber. A right ventriculotomy incision is made, and the VSD is closed with a patch in such a way as to divert left ventricular outflow through the VSD into the aorta. Either a valved conduit or an aortic valve homograft may then be used to connect the right ventricle and the main pulmonary artery. The Rastelli procedure is also sometimes modified for the correction of truncus arteriosus.

## Repair of Truncus Arteriosus

Truncus arteriosus, an uncommon congenital heart lesion representing approximately 1% to 2% of all congenital cardiac abnormalities, is the result of failure of the truncus arteriosus to divide into the aorta and pulmonary artery.[18] Characterized by retention of the embryologic bulbar trunk, the large single vessel leaving the heart gives rise to the coronary, systemic, and pulmonary arteries and contains only one valve. This vessel is situated just above the VSD and receives blood from both ventricles (Figure 29-64).

Although all infants with truncus arteriosus have a common outlet for right and left ventricular blood, the amount of blood flow to the lungs will vary and depends on the nature of the pulmonary arteries. Most infants with truncus arteriosus have well-developed branch pulmonary arteries and receive several times more blood flow in their pulmonary circulation than is normal. Because of this, infants who do not undergo repair show severe CHF with cyanosis and failure to thrive.

Correction is quite successful with a nonvalved conduit of polytetrafluoroethylene (PTFE). The left atrial appendage is opened and used as the floor of the conduit, with a patch of pulmonary homograft tissue as a roof over the conduit. With this technique, there is no circumferential conduit to replace and no further surgery is required as the child grows. Small (12-mm or 14-mm) extracardiac valved conduits may also be used to create a main pulmonary artery; in this instance, replacement of the conduit will be required as the child grows.

***Procedural Considerations.*** The child is placed in the supine position. The basic setup for a sternotomy is used, with consideration given to the child's age and size. Depending on the corrective approach selected, a valved conduit; intracardiac patch material, 2 × 2 inches; and a ½- × 4-inch strip of Teflon felt may be required.

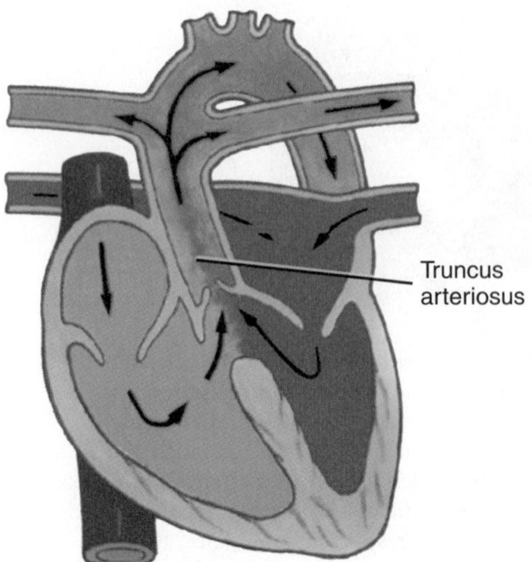


FIGURE 29-64 Truncus arteriosus.

### *Operative Procedure*

1. A median sternotomy is performed, and CPB is instituted.
2. A cross-clamp is placed on the aorta, the pulmonary artery is excised from the aorta (Figure 29-65, *A*), and the aortic defect is closed with a double layer of continuous cardiovascular suture. The cross-clamp is removed.
3. A right ventriculotomy is made, and the VSD is repaired (Figure 29-65, *B*).
4. a. If a valved conduit is used, the distal end is anastomosed to the pulmonary artery.
   b. The proximal end of the valved conduit is anastomosed to the right ventriculotomy by use of a Teflon felt buttress, which prevents sutures from cutting through the ventricular wall and enhances hemostasis (Figure 29-65, *C*).
5. CPB is discontinued, and chest closure is completed.

## Repair of Pulmonary Stenosis: Open Valvulotomy and Infundibular Resection

Pulmonary stenosis, accounting for approximately 8% to 12% of congenital heart defects, is the result of an obstructive lesion that interferes with blood flow from the right ventricle.[25] This

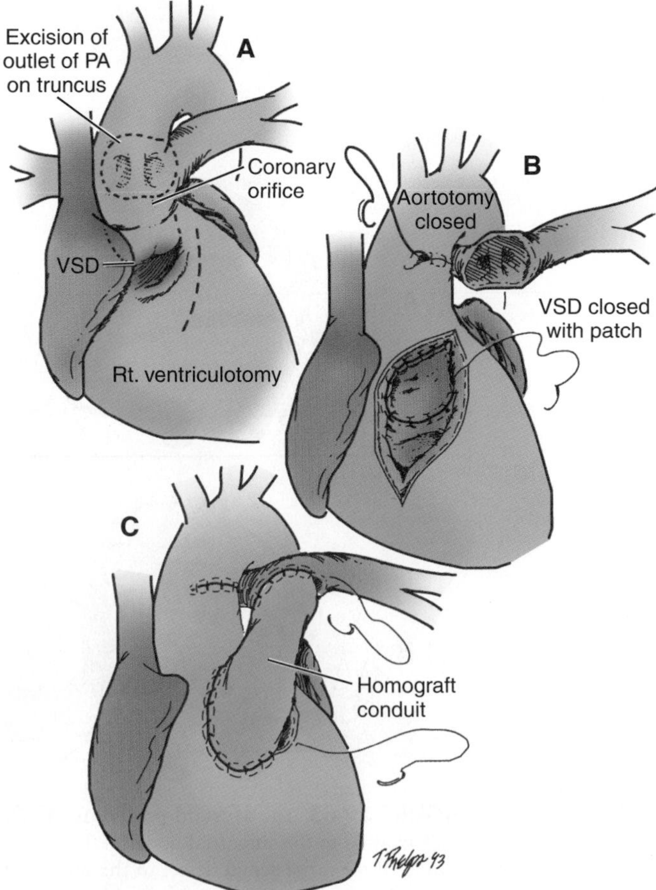


FIGURE 29-65 Complete surgical correction of truncus arteriosus. **A,** The pulmonary artery *(PA)* bifurcation is excised from the truncus. The ventricular septal defect *(VSD)* is exposed through a ventriculotomy. **B,** Aortotomy and VSD closed. **C,** A cryopreserved aortic homograft is anastomosed to the pulmonary artery and ventriculotomy.

lesion can occur at a number of different locations in the right ventricular outflow tract (RVOT), including valvular pulmonic stenosis, subvalvular pulmonic stenosis, and supravalvular pulmonic stenosis. The surgical repair depends on the degree and location of stenosis.

Open valvulotomy is the separation of the stenosed leaflets under direct vision; infundibular resection for pulmonary stenosis is excision of the hypertrophied infundibulum.

***Procedural Considerations.*** The child is placed in the supine position. The basic setup for a sternotomy is used, with consideration given to the child's age and size.

### *Operative Procedure*

1. A median sternotomy is performed, and CPB is instituted.
2. a. For open valvulotomy, the pulmonary artery is opened longitudinally and the stenotic valve is incised with a scalpel or scissors (Figure 29-66, *A*).
   b. For infundibular resection, the outflow tract of the right ventricle is opened, the resection is performed as described for TOF, and a patch of pericardium homograft tissue or synthetic patch material may be used to enlarge the pulmonary outflow tract (Figure 29-66, *B* and *C*).

***Other Procedures.*** Some surgeons use a valved conduit for the more severe forms of pulmonary stenosis and atresia. The Rastelli procedure (described previously) may be used to suture the conduit to the right ventricle and to the pulmonary artery, thus bypassing the atretic valve.

## Closure of Patent Ductus Arteriosus

PDA occurs because of persistence of the fetal ductus arteriosus, which connects the pulmonary artery to the aorta. The condition is common in premature infants. In fetal life, blood bypasses the lungs, traveling directly to the systemic circulation through the PDA. This vessel normally closes shortly after birth as a result of the onset of respiration causing an increase in $PaO_2$ and the release of circulating humoral substances. However, if this does not occur, the ductus arteriosus remains open (Figure 29-67), creating a shunt from the aorta through the ductus into the pulmonary circulation. This increases the work of the heart and causes subsequent enlargement and hypertrophy of the left atrium and ventricle. However, when persistent patency of the ductus is associated with other malformations such as TOF and extreme stenosis of the pulmonary orifice, it is a means of maintaining life. Surgery is not performed if the PDA is serving in a compensatory capacity.

Many children have few symptoms because of the small size of the shunt. A frequent clinical sign associated with this condition is a harsh, continuous murmur. Because the blood is oxygenated passing through the shunt, there is no cyanosis, clubbing, or reduction in peripheral arterial oxygen saturation. However, growth is retarded in children who have a large ductus. Other signs and symptoms may include dyspnea, frequent upper respiratory tract infections, palpitations, limited exercise tolerance, and cardiac failure.

***Procedural Considerations.*** Closure of the PDA is achieved by suture ligation or by division of the ductus. For newborn infants, the surgeon and anesthesia provider may elect to perform this procedure in the intensive care nursery bed because the operation is a short one. However, after the newborn period, the surgery is done in the OR. The child is placed in a right lateral position. The setup is as described, without items for CPB but with special patent ductus clamps. Generally a left posterolateral approach is used; in some cases, however, a left anterolateral approach is used.

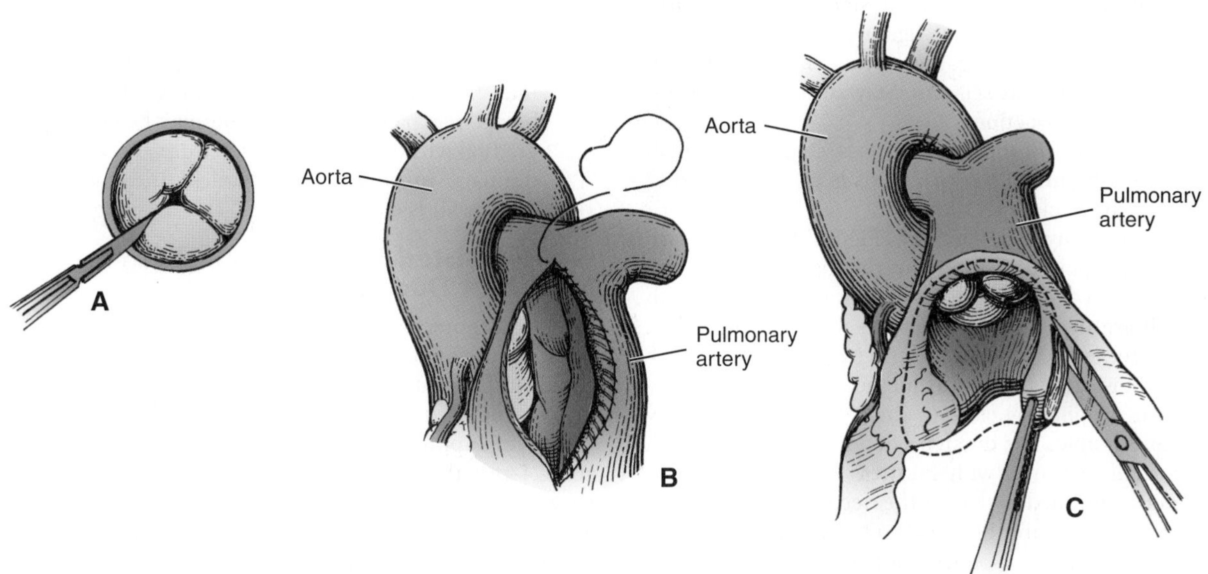


**FIGURE 29-66** **A,** Commissurotomy of stenotic valve. Knife is used, and care is taken to incise exactly on commissures. **B,** Diamond-shaped patch being used to enlarge pulmonary outflow tract and pulmonary valve annulus. If vertical pulmonary artery incision is made directly through anterior commissure of valve, three valve cusps remain intact and some valve competence is retained. **C,** Excision of obstructing infundibular tissue.

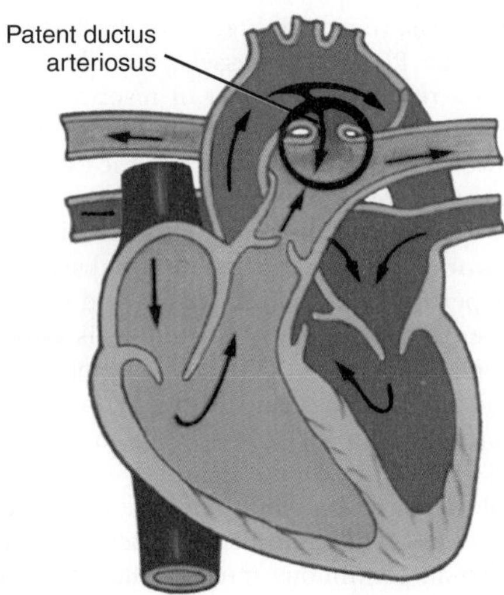


FIGURE 29-67 Patent ductus arteriosus.

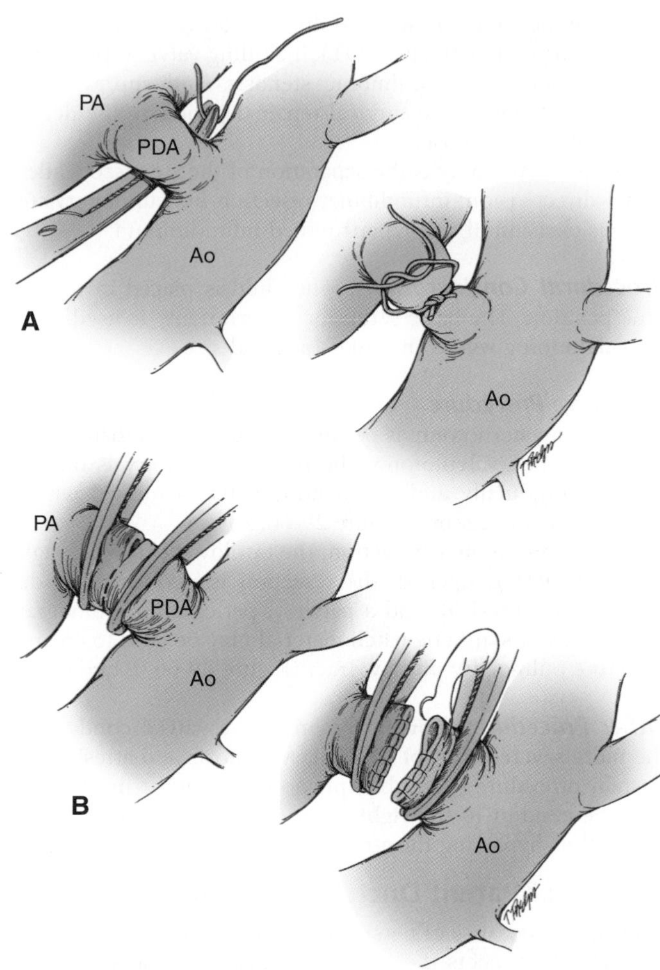


FIGURE 29-68 Surgical correction of patent ductus arteriosus (*PDA*). **A,** Ligation of ductus arteriosus. **B,** Division of ductus arteriosus. *Ao,* Aorta; *PA,* pulmonary artery.

### *Operative Procedure*

1. The incision is carried through the muscles over the fourth interspace. The chest wall is entered through the third or fourth intercostal space, with use of items as described for thoracotomy (see Chapter 25). The wound edges are protected and retracted with a Finochietto rib spreader.
2. The pleura is incised with Metzenbaum scissors, and the left lung is protected and retracted with a moist pack and a malleable retractor.
3. The mediastinal pleura is opened between the phrenic and vagus nerves over the region of the ductus. The pleura is retracted by insertion of stay sutures. The recurrent laryngeal nerve is identified and protected. The aortic arch and pulmonary artery are dissected with fine scissors and dry dissectors. Fine arterial branches are divided and ligated with curved Crile or mosquito hemostats and nonabsorbable ligatures and cardiac suture ligatures.
4. The parietal pleura overlying the ductus is dissected with fine vascular forceps and scissors. Stay sutures may be inserted to facilitate retraction.
5. The adventitial layer of the ductus is dissected free. A small portion of the obscure posterior ductus is carefully freed to admit a right-angle clamp.
6. a. For the suture-ligation method (Figure 29-68, *A*), two ligatures are placed around the ductus—one near the aorta and the other near the pulmonary artery side, both of which are tied in place. Between these two ligatures, two transfixion sutures may be inserted.
   b. For the division of the ductus method, the patent ductus clamps are applied as close to the aorta and pulmonary artery as possible. The ductus is divided halfway through and partially sutured with mattress cardiovascular sutures and continued back over the free edge with an over-and-over whip suture (Figure 29-68, *B*). After both openings are sutured, a sponge is held on the area for compression while the patent ductus clamps are removed.
   c. In premature infants, only a hemoclip may be applied to the ductus because of the friable nature of the ductal tissue. The mediastinal pleura is closed with interrupted sutures. The lung is reexpanded, and a chest catheter may be inserted to establish closed drainage. In newborns, reexpansion of the lung may be accomplished by gradual withdrawal of a catheter during closure; no chest drainage tube is required unless there is oozing. The chest wall is closed in layers, and dressings are applied.

## Video-Assisted Thoracoscopic Surgery for Patent Ductus Arteriosus

Although thoracoscopy was first described in 1910,[28] the application of video-assisted thoracoscopic surgery (VATS) to the pediatric population for cardiovascular repairs did not occur until recently. The procedure requires thoracoscopic equipment and supplies including 0-degree and 30-degree, 4.0-mm and 2.7-mm thoracoscopes, depending on the surgeon's preference and the patient's age and size. The endoscopic instruments, made smaller for the pediatric patient, include an electrocoagulation hook; Castroviejo type of scissors; graspers and right-angle clamps; fan lung retractors of varying sizes, either medium or medium-large; large endoscopic clip appliers; trocars with ports; and suction tip, preferably one that has a porthole to occlude when suction is required. Instrumentation for closure of PDA by thoracotomy is also set up in case the thoracoscopy fails or a complication arises and the chest needs to be opened emergently.

***Procedural Considerations.*** Before the procedure, the television cameras are set up on either side of the OR bed. The patient is placed in a right lateral position.

### *Operative Procedure*

1. Usually four small incisions are made along the line of the posterolateral thoracotomy incision and ports are introduced.
2. The thoracoscope is inserted. The first assistant holds the lung retractor while the second assistant holds the camera. Some institutions use a mechanical articulating arm.
3. A grasper is used to elevate the pleura overlying the aorta near the insertion of the PDA and pulmonary artery, and careful dissection is begun with electrocoagulation. Suction is required to keep the area of dissection clear to the surgeon's vision.
4. When the ductus has been clearly identified, a right-angle clamp may first be introduced and a tie applied to the duct. The clip applier is then inserted, and clips are applied.
5. Transesophageal or transthoracic echocardiography is usually performed by a cardiologist before closure of the porthole incisions to ensure closure of the ductus. Also, a chest tube will be inserted into the pleural space, the lungs are inflated, the chest tube is removed, or a chest tube may be left in place before porthole incision closures.

## Repair of Coarctation of the Aorta

Coarctation of the aorta (COA), responsible for approximately 5% to 10% of all congenital heart defects, is defined as a narrowing of the upper thoracic aorta caused by posterior infolding or indentation opposite ("juxtaductal") the region of the ductus arteriosus insertion.[27] The pathologic manifestations in this type of lesion vary. In the neonate, COA is a complex physiologic entity commonly associated with significant hypoplasia of the aortic arch and VSD, as well as other complex congenital heart diseases such as truncus arteriosus, double outlet right ventricle, and single ventricle. In older children, COA is usually an isolated lesion that may be associated with collateral formation. COA is also associated with Turner's syndrome. Depending on specific anatomy, COA (Figure 29-69) may be repaired by a number of different techniques: resection and end-to-end-anastomosis, subclavian flap angioplasty, patch aortoplasty, and bypass graft.

***Procedural Considerations.*** The child is placed in the right lateral position. Basic cardiac surgery instruments are required, plus Teflon or Dacron woven or knitted vascular prostheses in assorted sizes, to be used as necessary when primary anastomosis is not possible. Items for CPB are not needed.

### *Operative Procedure*

1. A left posterolateral incision is carried through the chest wall. Because collateral blood vessels are somewhat enlarged, bleeding may be profuse. Sponges may be weighed to determine accurate blood replacement, depending on the preference of the anesthesia provider. A Burford or Finochietto retractor is used.
2. The pleura is incised and the lung retracted. The mediastinal pleura is incised over the constricted portion of the aorta, and the edges are sutured to the chest wall.

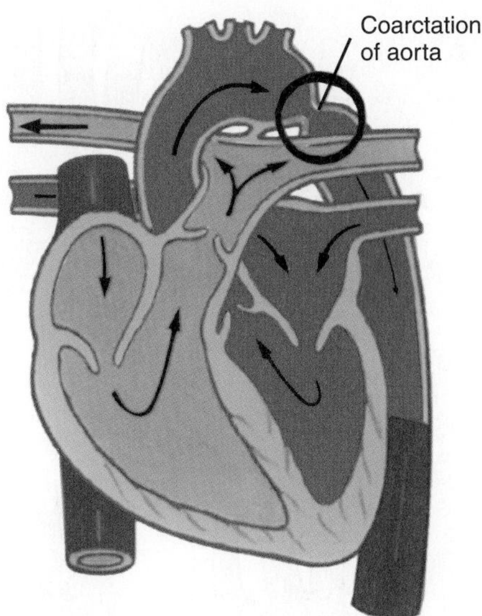


**FIGURE 29-69** Coarctation of aorta.

3. Careful dissection with fine vascular forceps and dry dissectors is continued to mobilize the aorta and the surrounding intercostal vessels. The laryngeal nerve is identified and protected. The ductus arteriosus is ligated and divided between ductus clamps.
4. a. For patch repair, the curved or angled vascular clamps are applied and a longitudinal aortotomy is performed with a #11 knife blade, Potts scissors, and vascular forceps.
   b. A piece of graft material is inserted, large enough to widen the aorta, by use of a continuous cardiovascular suture (Figure 29-70, *A*).
   c. The clamps are released slowly—the distal one first and then the proximal one. The blood pressure is noted at this time. Removal of clamps is not completed until the blood pressure is stabilized.
5. a. For resection, curved or angled vascular clamps are applied and the constricted segment is divided between them. A second set of clamps may be applied above and below, as a safety factor, in fashioning the cuffs for reapproximation.
   b. End-to-end anastomosis (Figure 29-70, *B*) is accomplished with a continuous, everting mattress technique for the posterior wall and interrupted, everting mattress sutures for the anterior row. If the stricture is long, a synthetic aortic prosthesis is used to bridge the defect (Figure 29-70, *C*)
   c. The clamps are removed, one at a time, as described in step 4c.
6. a. For subclavian flap repairs (Figure 29-70, *D*), the aorta above and below the patent ductus is dissected out, as is the subclavian artery. The subclavian artery is ligated at the origin of the vertebral artery, which is also ligated.
   b. The aorta is incised distally to the area of narrowing, through the coarctation to the subclavian artery.
   c. The aorta is opened, and the coarctation is excised.
   d. The tip of the subclavian flap is brought down into the aorta and sutured with absorbable or nonabsorbable ma-

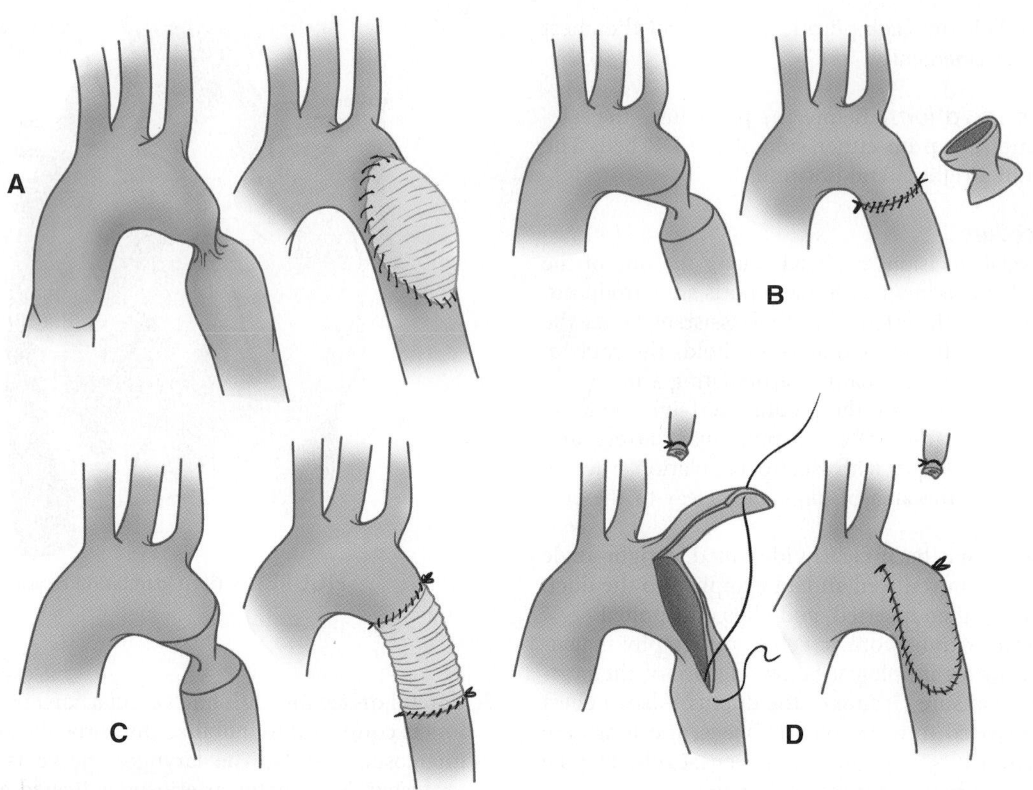


FIGURE 29-70 **A,** Prosthetic patch aortoplasty. **B,** Resection with primary end-to-end anastomosis. **C,** Prosthetic interposition graft. **D,** Subclavian flap aortoplasty.

terial. The parietal pleura is closed, with a small opening being left at the lower point; a chest tube is inserted; closed drainage is established; and the chest wall is closed in layers. A dressing is applied.

## Repair of Hypoplastic Left Heart Syndrome

Hypoplastic left-sided heart syndrome (HLHS) (Figure 29-71) is one of the most common forms of single ventricle. HLHS describes a range of congenital cardiac malformations that have in common underdevelopment of the left-sided heart structures, which include aortic valve atresia and stenosis with associated hypoplasia or absence of the left ventricle. The ascending aorta and arch are usually only a few millimeters in diameter and are functionally a branch of the ductus arteriosus–thoracic aorta continuum, with blood flowing retrograde through the aortic arch and into the small ascending aorta to the coronary arteries. Mitral valve atresia or stenosis also is present.

Survival in the newborn period depends on a PDA to maintain systemic circulation; therefore these infants are maintained on an infusion of prostaglandin $E_1$ ($PGE_1$) to maintain ductal patency before surgical intervention.

Newborns with HLHS typically present with cyanosis, respiratory distress, and variable degrees of circulatory collapse during the first few days of life. If left untreated, a majority of these neonates will die within the first month of life; without surgical intervention, HLHS is fatal.

It was not until the development of the Fontan procedure, a surgical correction for another form of single ventricle—tricuspid atresia—that long-term survival in patients with HLHS was considered possible. However, because of the neonate's high PVR, the Fontan procedure is not a surgical option in the newborn period. A palliative repair (stage I) was developed in the late 1970s by Norwood to prepare the heart for the Fontan procedure.

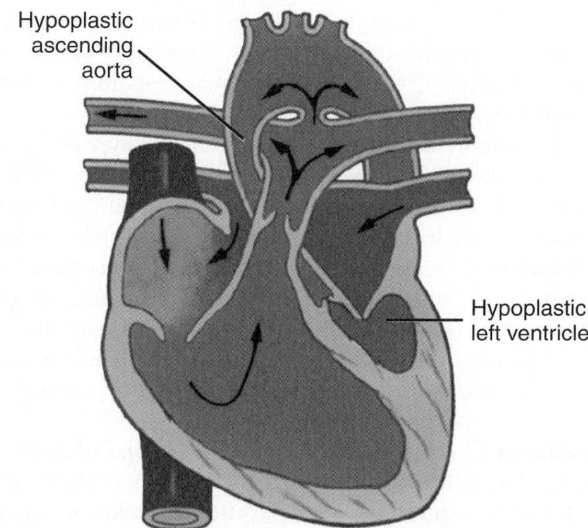


FIGURE 29-71 Hypoplastic left-sided heart syndrome.

Two surgical options for patients with HLHS exist: a series of reconstructive procedures or heart transplantation. The series of reconstructive procedures usually involves three stages. Stage I is performed during the newborn period. The goals of stage I are to (1) maintain systemic perfusion, (2) preserve the function of the only ventricle, and (3) allow normal maturation of the pulmonary ventricle. The first goal is met by creating an unobstructed communication between the right ventricle and the systemic circulation. This is accomplished by transecting the main pulmonary artery and creating a neoaorta from the main pulmonary artery, native aorta, and pulmonary homograft tissue. The other two goals are met by creating a right modified Blalock-Taussig (BT) shunt and a nonrestrictive interatrial communication. These measures allow for adequate pulmonary blood flow and for the PVR to decrease as the child grows while they limit the volume interposed on the single ventricle.

The modified Fontan procedure was initially performed on a child at approximately 18 months of age. However, since 1989 a staged approach to the Fontan procedure has been undertaken to minimize the effect of rapid changes in ventricular configuration and diastolic function that can be associated with a primary Fontan procedure and the postoperative complications associated with it. In the stage II procedure (hemi-Fontan or the bidirectional Glenn shunt), superior vena cava (SVC) blood flow is directed to the lungs and inferior vena cava (IVC) blood flow continues to flow to the right ventricle. The third and final stage, the modified Fontan procedure, separates the systemic and pulmonary circulations.

***Procedural Considerations.*** Additional items for the open-heart setup include the following:

- Stage I: PTFE tube graft, 3.5 or 4 mm, and pulmonary homograft tissue
- Stage II: oscillating saw and pulmonary homograft tissue
- Stage III: oscillating saw and PTFE tube graft, 10 mm; a higher-than-usual supply of blood should be available

### *Operative Procedures*

STAGE I (NORWOOD PROCEDURE) (FIGURE 29-72)

1. A median sternotomy is performed. The aortic cannula is placed into the main pulmonary artery rather than the diminutive aorta, and the venous cannula is placed into the right atrium. CPB is instituted, and the right and left pulmonary arteries are immediately occluded with tourniquets to force the blood through the ductus arteriosus to the systemic circulation.
2. When deep hypothermic circulatory arrest is about to be instituted, the innominate and left carotid arteries are occluded with tourniquets. The venous and aortic cannulas are removed.
3. The septum primum is excised through the venous cannulation site; occasionally a right atriotomy is necessary to facilitate the atrial septectomy.
4. The main pulmonary artery is transected immediately before the takeoff of the right and left pulmonary arteries.
5. The distal pulmonary artery is closed with a small patch of homograft tissue.
6. The ductus arteriosus is then exposed and closed using a 2-0 nonabsorbable tie. The tie is left long to better expose the thoracic aorta. The ductus is transected.
7. At the point where the ductus was attached to the aorta, the thoracic aorta is opened 1 to 2 cm, and the aortic arch and ascending aorta are opened to a point adjacent to the main pulmonary artery.
8. A gusset of homograft tissue is joined to the aorta starting at the thoracic end, and the pulmonary artery is incorporated at the proximal end of the ascending aorta. A continuous monofilament stitch is used. Occasionally interrupted sutures are used to attach the main pulmonary artery to the aorta.
9. To perform a right BT shunt, the innominate artery is cross-clamped and incised and a 3.5- or 4-mm PTFE tube graft is interposed.
10. CPB is instituted, and the pulmonary end of the shunt is performed by incising the pulmonary artery and interposing the distal end of the tube graft.
11. Immediately after the shunt is completed, the shunt is occluded with a bulldog clamp until termination of bypass.

STAGE II (HEMI-FONTAN PROCEDURE) (FIGURE 29-73)

1. Because these patients have had previous surgery, an oscillating saw is used for the median sternotomy.
2. The aorta, right atrium, and right BT shunt are exposed.
3. CPB is instituted, and the shunt is immediately occluded with a clip.
4. The branch pulmonary arteries are exposed.
5. Depending on the surgeon's preference, deep hypothermic circulatory arrest may be instituted.
6. An incision is made in the confluence of the pulmonary arteries, extending to the pericardial reflections.
7. An incision is made in the dome of the right atrium, extending to the SVC.
8. The pulmonary artery is then anastomosed to the SVC–right atrial junction.
9. The pulmonary arteries are augmented with a gusset of homograft tissue. In the hemi-Fontan procedure, part of the homograft tissue is incorporated intraatrially as a dam between the common atrium and the vena cava–pulmonary artery anastomosis. In the Glenn shunt, there is no intraatrial incorporation.
10. CPB is reinstituted until the patient is normothermic. CPB is then discontinued, and chest closure is completed.

STAGE III (MODIFIED FONTAN PROCEDURE) (FIGURE 29-74)

1. A median sternotomy is performed with an oscillating saw.
2. The aorta and right atrium are exposed.
3. CPB is instituted.
4. Deep hypothermic circulatory arrest may be used.
5. A lateral incision is made in the right atrium.
6. A 10-mm PTFE tube graft is cut in half lengthwise and is placed intraatrially by suturing the inferior end of the graft around the orifice of the IVC and up the right lateral free wall of the right atrium to the superior dome of the right atrium. This creates a tunnel in which the inferior blood flow is directed to the pulmonary arteries. The superior vena cava blood flow was directed to the pulmonary arteries during the stage II repair. (The surgeon may perform variations on this procedure, such as excluding a hepatic vein or doing a fenestrated Fontan by making a series of small openings in the PTFE tube graft or a single 4-mm opening with an aortic punch in the graft material.)
7. The atria are closed, and CPB is reinstituted until the patient is normothermic. CPB is then discontinued, and chest closure is completed.

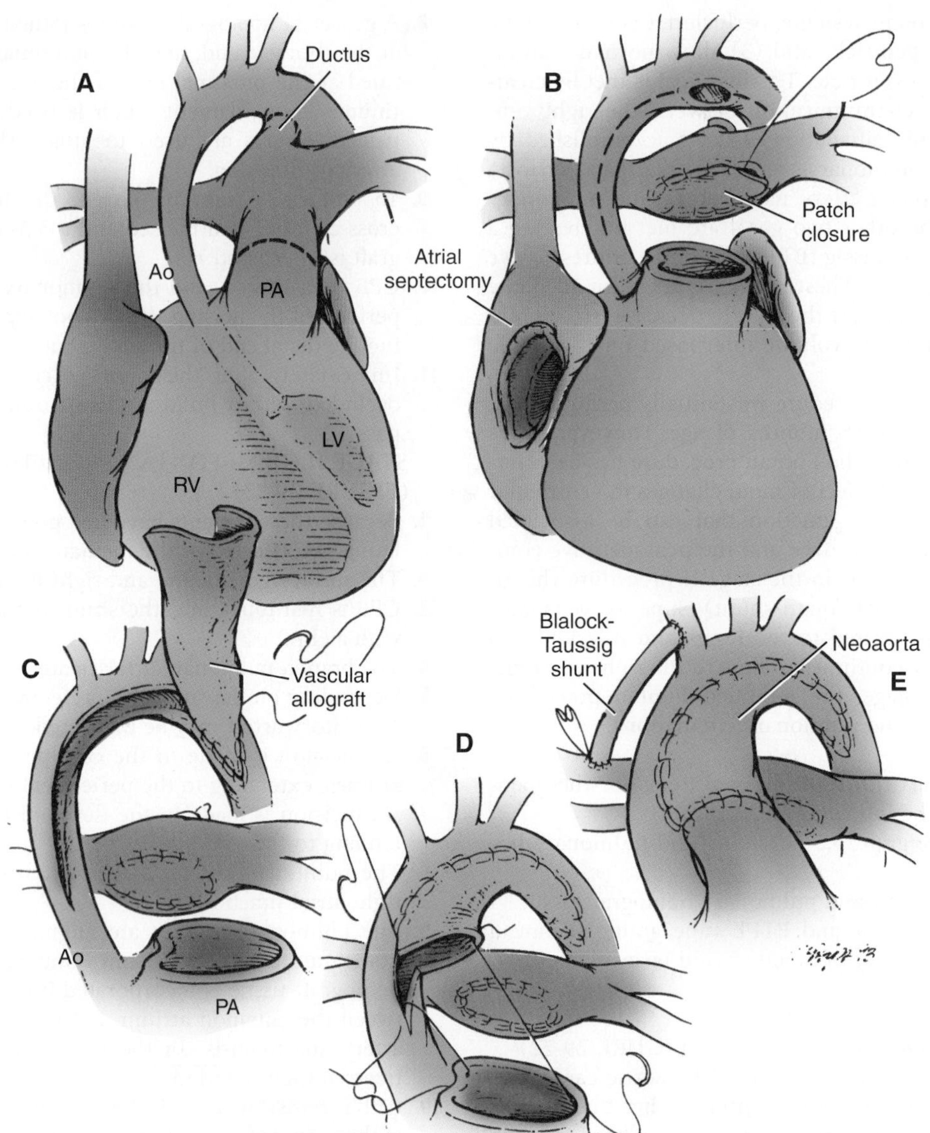


FIGURE 29-72 Stage I Norwood procedure. **A,** Transection points of the main pulmonary artery *(PA)* and ductus arteriosus. **B,** Atrial septectomy to avoid pulmonary venous hypertension. Patch closure of the distal main PA. Division and ligation of the ductus arteriosus. **C** and **D,** Construction of a "neoaorta" with use of the proximal main PA, diminutive ascending aorta, and vascular allograft. **E,** Pulmonary blood flow supplied by a right modified Blalock-Taussig shunt connecting the right subclavian artery to the right PA. *Ao,* Aorta; *LV,* left ventricle; *RV,* right ventricle.

## Repair of Severely Diseased Aortic Valves: Ross Procedure

There is an alternative to mechanical and allograft (homograft) replacement of aortic valves that cannot be repaired by valvuloplasty or annuloplasty (see Chapter 27). It involves using the patient's autologous pulmonary valve as a freestanding aortic root replacement and then replacing the patient's pulmonary outflow tract with pulmonary or aortic valve homograft tissue depending on size availability. Freestanding root replacement allows the valve to grow with the patient. The autograft operation provides a permanent aortic valve replacement for patients and avoids the threat of embolism and anticoagulant hemorrhage from mechanical valves.

***Procedural Considerations.*** Additional items for the open-heart setup include the following: pulmonary valve homograft tissue, Spencer plegia cannula, appropriate solution and basins to rinse homograft, and felt.

### *Operative Procedure*

1. A median sternotomy is performed with a sternal saw if the patient has had no previous surgery or with an oscillating saw if the patient has a former sternotomy incision.
2. The pericardium is opened, and the aorta, the coronary arteries, the pulmonary artery, and the superior and inferior venae cavae are exposed.
3. The aorta is cannulated close to the arch of the aorta. Superior and inferior venous cannulas are used.

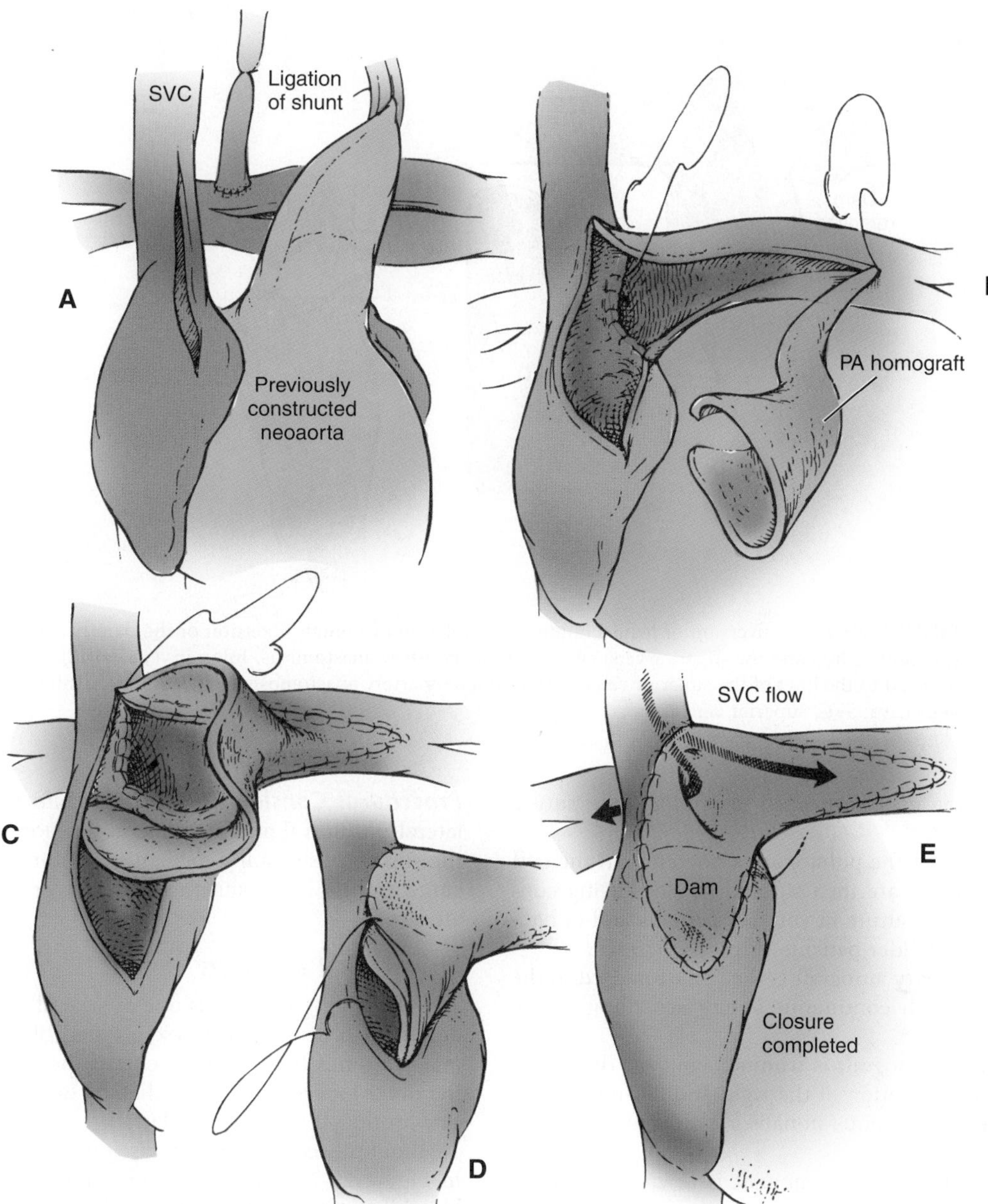


**FIGURE 29-73** Hemi-Fontan procedure in a patient with hypoplastic left-sided heart syndrome. **A** and **B**, Ligation of the systemic-to-pulmonary artery shunt and side-to-side anastomosis of the superior vena cava *(SVC)* to the confluence of the pulmonary artery *(PA)* with allograft augmentation. **C** to **E**, Placement of a dam to close the junction of the atrium with the SVC so that saturated pulmonary venous blood mixes in the common atrium with desaturated blood draining from the inferior vena cava. Pulmonary blood flow is supplied exclusively through the SVC.

4. Once on CPB, the patient is cooled to 28°C and the aorta is cross-clamped. Cardioplegia is given retrograde through the ascending aorta if the aortic valve is stenotic. If the aortic valve is regurgitant, the aorta is opened and the cardioplegia is administered directly into the coronary ostium.
5. The aorta is transected (Figure 29-75, *A*).
6. The pulmonary artery is transected (Figure 29-75, *B*).
7. The right ventricle is incised, and the pulmonary root is carefully dissected. Care is taken to avoid the first septal branch of the left anterior descending coronary artery (Figure 29-75, *C*).
8. The pulmonary artery allograft is placed in saline for use later in the repair.
9. Cardioplegia is administered intermittently before and during autograft implantation.
10. The orifice of the coronary arteries with a rim of adjacent coronary wall is excised.
11. The edges of the aortic commissures are exposed with 2-0 silk suture.
12. The aortic valve is excised.
13. The pulmonary autograft is trimmed and implanted in the aortic root position with absorbable suture being used in younger patients and nonabsorbable suture in older pa-

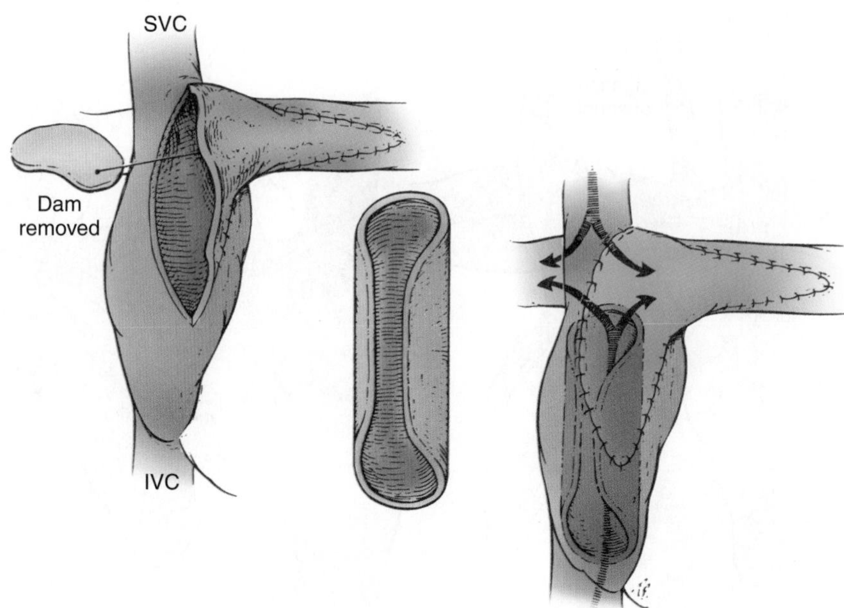


FIGURE 29-74 Conversion of hemi-Fontan to completion of Fontan. Excision of the dam between the right atrium and the superior vena cava–pulmonary artery anastomosis. Inferior vena cava flow is directed to the inlet of the superior vena cava–pulmonary artery anastomosis by a baffle. *IVC,* Inferior vena cava; *SVC,* superior vena cava.

tients. A felt ring may be needed to reinforce the suture (Figure 29-75, *D*).

14. Sinuses are made in the pulmonary autograft, and the cuff and coronary artery are then sutured in place using continuous absorbable suture in younger patients and nonabsorbable suture in older patients (Figure 29-75, *E*).
15. The distal pulmonary autograft is then anastomosed to the proximal aorta with continuous suture according to the patient's size and age.
16. The pulmonary homograft is trimmed, and the distal end is sewn to the bifurcation of the right and left pulmonary arteries with a continuous nonabsorbable suture (Figure 29-75, *F*).
17. The proximal end of the homograft is sewn to the right ventricle by means of a continuous nonabsorbable suture (Figure 29-75, *G*).
18. Suture lines are inspected. When the patient is fully rewarmed and hemodynamically stable, CPB is discontinued. Chest closure is completed after transesophageal echocardiographic confirmation of satisfactory results.

## Pulmonary Artery Banding

An infant with an enlarged heart in intractable failure and a large left-to-right shunt may be treated effectively by a palliative pulmonary artery banding operation. This procedure is designed to reduce the flow of blood through the pulmonary artery to approximately one half to one third of the existing rate. A tape is looped about the artery and secured in place by a simple suture technique. Pressures are measured by direct needle puncture before and after banding. A reduction of the distal pulmonary artery pressure by 50% to 70% is sought. Repair of the interventricular septal defect may be postponed until the child is clinically stable and can withstand an open-heart procedure.

***Procedural Considerations.*** The child is placed in the left lateral position if an anterolateral incision is to be used or in the supine position if a median sternotomy is to be used. The surgeon cuts Silastic sheeting or polyester tape to the appropriate size.

## Shunt for Palliation

The shunt for palliation is one of several palliative procedures designed to divert poorly oxygenated blood from one of the major arteries back through one of the pulmonary arteries to the lungs for reoxygenation, thereby increasing the total blood flow in the pulmonary circulation.

Shunt procedures that increase pulmonary flow are described in Figure 29-76, along with procedures to reduce pulmonary blood flow (pulmonary artery banding) and to increase intracardiac mixing of blood (Blalock-Hanlon ASD and Rashkind septostomy). The Blalock-Taussig (BT) procedure consists of making an end-to-side anastomosis between the proximal end of the subclavian and the side of the pulmonary artery. The procedure is performed on the side opposite the aortic arch. This shunt may be dismantled or ligated if a future operation for full correction is anticipated; however, the shunt has a tendency to decrease in size as the child grows. Currently the most commonly used form of shunt is a modification of the BT procedure in which a PTFE graft is used to connect pulmonary and systemic vasculature. It connects the subclavian artery to the ipsilateral pulmonary artery or the innominate artery to the right pulmonary artery. Occasionally, a central shunt is placed in which the PTFE graft connects the aorta and main pulmonary artery.

The Potts-Smith and Waterston procedures involve direct anastomosis of the aorta to the pulmonary arteries. These are rarely performed because of the potential for deformity of the pulmonary arteries, producing excessive pulmonary blood flow and CHF.

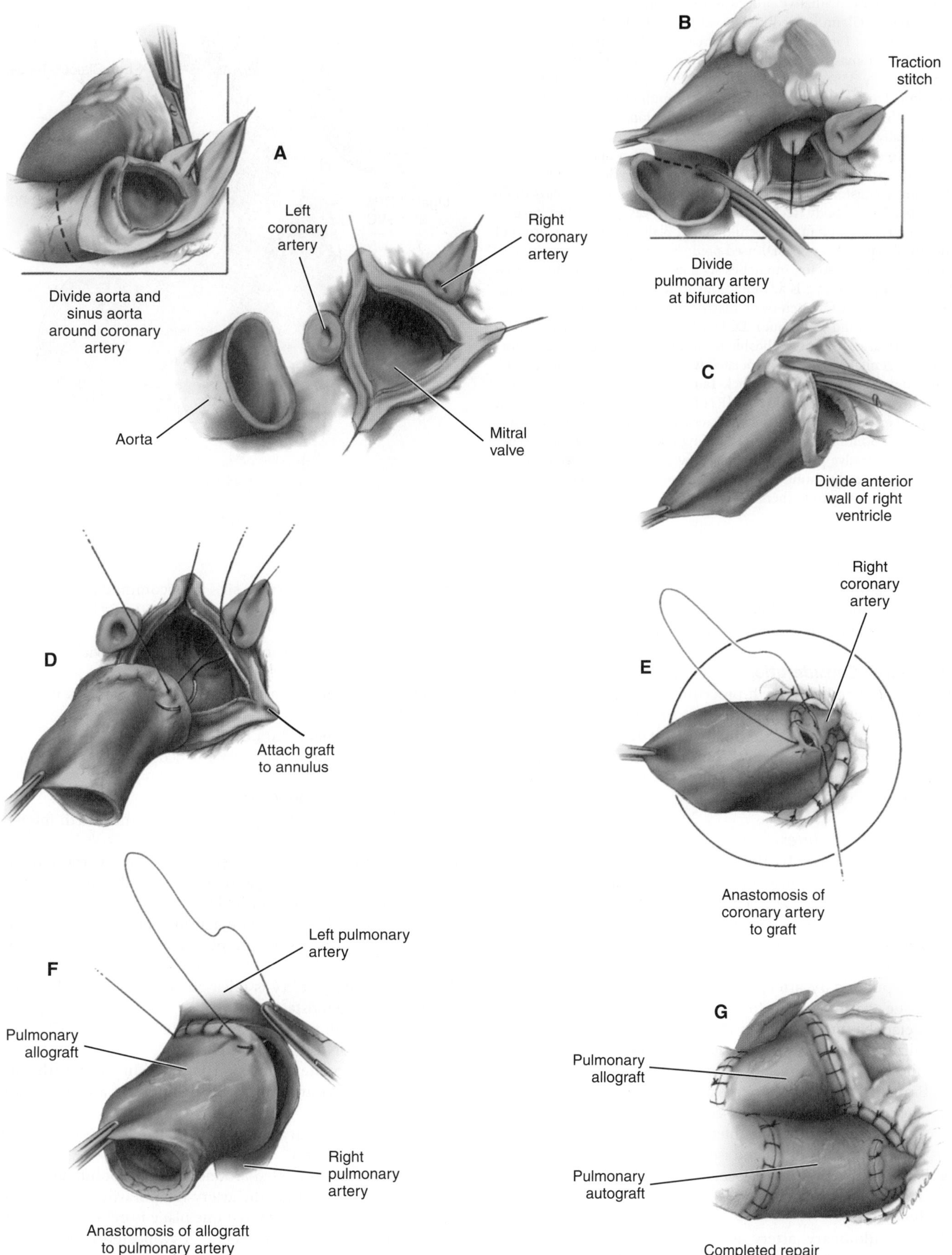
A
Divide aorta and
sinus aorta
around coronary
artery
Left
coronary
artery
Right
coronary
artery
Aorta
Mitral
valve
B
Traction
stitch
Divide
pulmonary artery
at bifurcation
C
Divide anterior
wall of right
ventricle
D
Attach graft
to annulus
E
Right
coronary
artery
Anastomosis of
coronary artery
to graft
F
Left pulmonary
artery
Pulmonary
allograft
Right
pulmonary
artery
Anastomosis of allograft
to pulmonary artery
G
Pulmonary
allograft
Pulmonary
autograft
Completed repair

**FIGURE 29-75** Ross procedure.

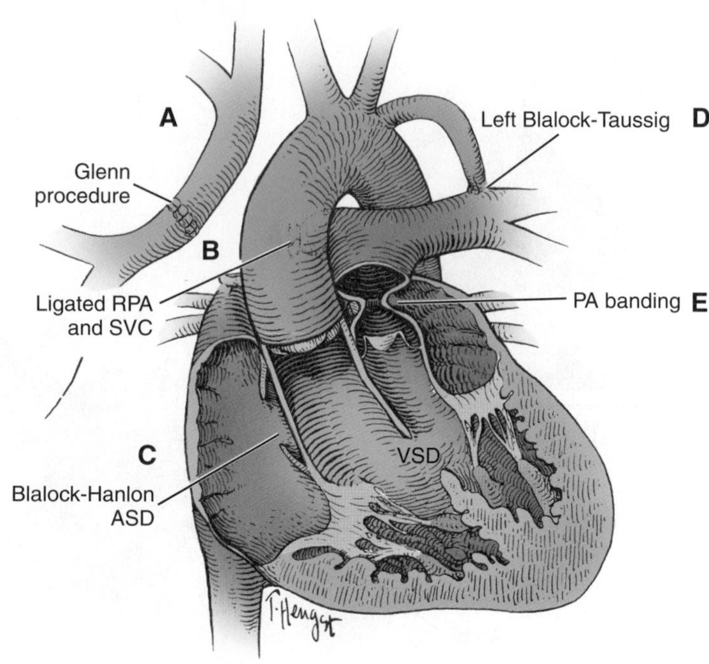


**FIGURE 29-76** Palliative procedures for congenital cardiac anomalies. **A** and **B,** Glenn procedure is used primarily for tricuspid atresia but is used also for transposition of great vessels. In **D,** superior vena cava *(SVC)* is anastomosed to right pulmonary artery *(RPA)* to direct approximately 35% of systemic venous return to right lung for oxygenation. This technique cannot be used if pulmonary vascular resistance is elevated, as often occurs in transposition. Glenn procedure, **E,** is usually performed by implantation of distal end of pulmonary artery into side of superior vena cava. Cava is then ligated at atriocaval junction. Ligation of azygos vein may enhance flow through cavopulmonary anastomosis but may also increase pressure in veins draining upper half of body. Techniques of delayed azygos ligation have been described in infants and children. **C,** Blalock-Hanlon creation of interatrial septal defect *(ASD)* used predominantly for transposition of great vessels but also for anomalies such as mitral or tricuspid atresia in which large opening is advantageous to reduce intraatrial pressure. Dilation of patent foramen ovale may be done with balloon-tipped catheter (Rashkind technique). **D,** Left Blalock-Taussig subclavian–to–pulmonary artery shunt applicable for tetralogy of Fallot and also for other congenital anomalies associated with insufficient pulmonary arterial flow. (Modification of Blalock-Taussig procedure consists of interposing polytetrafluoroethylene [PTFE] graft between the left subclavian artery and pulmonary artery, thereby preserving the subclavian artery.) **E,** Pulmonary artery *(PA)* banding used for anomalies associated with excessive pulmonary blood flow attributable to large intracardiac left-to-right shunt. These include ventricular septal defect, truncus arteriosus, and others.

The Glenn procedure consists of making an anastomosis of the SVC to the right pulmonary artery. This operation is employed frequently in the treatment of a single ventricle.

***Procedural Considerations.*** The child is placed in a position that is specific for each procedure (supine or right or left lateral position). Instruments are as previously described for open-heart surgery, plus the following, with appropriate sizes for infants and children: Potts-Smith aortic occlusion clamps, Johns Hopkins modified Potts clamps, Hendren ductus clamps, and Cooley anastomosis clamps.

### *Operative Procedures*

BLALOCK-TAUSSIG PROCEDURE

1. An anterolateral incision is made from the sternal margin to the midaxillary line. The chest cavity is opened, and the lung is retracted, as described previously.
2. The mediastinal pleura is incised and retracted with a stay suture.
3. The pulmonary artery is dissected from the surrounding tissue, with vascular forceps, dry dissector sponges, and Metzenbaum scissors. As the artery and branches are mobilized, heavy ligatures, moistened umbilical tapes, or fine silicone tubing is placed about them.
4. Branches of the vagus nerve are protected and retracted.
5. The subclavian artery is dissected completely from its origin to where it produces the internal mammary and costocervical branches. Its distal end is marked with a silk suture.
6. The subclavian artery is occluded with a vascular clamp, a ligature is placed at the distal segment, and the vessel is divided.
7. The pulmonary artery is occluded temporarily with a curved vascular clamp.
8. An incision of sufficient size to accommodate the subclavian artery is made with a scalpel with a #11 knife blade and Potts scissors.
9. An end-to-side anastomosis is completed with cardiovascular suture.
10. The clamps are released, and the suture line is inspected for hemostasis.
11. The mediastinal pleura is closed.
12. Closed-chest drainage is established, and the chest wound is closed.

POTTS-SMITH PROCEDURE

1. A left posterolateral incision is made in the fourth intercostal space.
2. The pulmonary artery is dissected from its surrounding tissue, and the descending aorta is mobilized. Occluding tapes and Blalock or Potts-Smith clamps are applied.
3. A longitudinal incision is made in each artery, and a side-to-side anastomosis is completed with cardiovascular sutures.
4. The pulmonary artery is released, and the suture line is inspected for hemostasis.
5. The aortic clamps are then removed.

WATERSTON PROCEDURE

1. A right anterolateral incision is made in the fourth interspace. The pericardium is opened, and the ascending aorta is exposed.
2. The right pulmonary artery is dissected as it passes beneath the ascending aorta.
3. A heavy suture is passed around the right pulmonary artery and is used to occlude the artery temporarily. A curved vascular clamp is placed so that one blade is behind the pulmonary artery and the other occludes a posterolateral portion of the ascending aorta.

4. On closure of the clamp, both the right pulmonary artery and a posterior portion of the ascending aorta are occluded.
5. Parallel incisions are made in the aorta and the right pulmonary artery.
6. An anastomosis is then made between the ascending aorta and the right pulmonary artery.

## Extracorporeal Membrane Oxygenation

Extracorporeal membrane oxygenation (ECMO) is a therapy used on pediatric patients who have reversible pulmonary or cardiac disease. Many patients are neonates with respiratory disease syndrome (RDS), persistent pulmonary hypertension (PPH), meconium aspiration (MA), or congenital diaphragmatic hernia (CDH) requiring adequate tissue oxygenation and waste removal from the body. In the cardiac patient, it may also be used as a bridge to heart or lung transplantation until donor organs are available. To perform ECMO, a facility must have an established ECMO service.

Most of the time children are placed on ECMO in the ICU. For venoarterial ECMO the surgical approach is usually through the right carotid artery and internal jugular vein. For the cardiac patient after surgical repair, cannulation of the carotid artery and jugular vein provides good venous drainage of the right atrium, and the incision site is remote from the sternotomy wound. However, the surgeon may choose to reopen the sternum on the postoperative patients and cannulate the aorta and right atrium. In the OR, for a patient who cannot be successfully weaned from bypass after surgery, the patient's bypass circuit may be switched to an ECMO circuit and the patient may be transferred on ECMO to the ICU.

***Procedural Considerations.*** An area by the patient's bedside should be provided for the ECMO pump, surgical table and instrumentation, electrosurgical unit (ESU), surgeon's headlight, and defibrillator with external and sterile internal paddles. A wall suction outlet should be available. Appropriate surgical attire should be provided for everyone involved with the procedure, and traffic should be limited.

### *Operative Procedures*

FOR NECK CANNULATION. A shoulder roll is placed under the patient, and the neck and chest to the nipple line are prepped and draped. The ears should also be exposed and prepped for use as reference points.

1. An incision is made in the neck, and the right common carotid artery and right internal jugular vein are exposed for venoarterial ECMO.
2. The surgeon may cannulate the vessels through a purse-string suture and then reconstruct these vessels at the time of decannulation.
3. After insertion of the arterial and venous cannulas, the clamped cannulas are connected to the ECMO circuit. All the air is eliminated (Figure 29-77).
4. The cannulas are secured to the skin. The neck incision is closed and dressed. The surgical instruments are kept sterile until proper positioning of the venous and arterial cannulas is confirmed by x-ray examination.

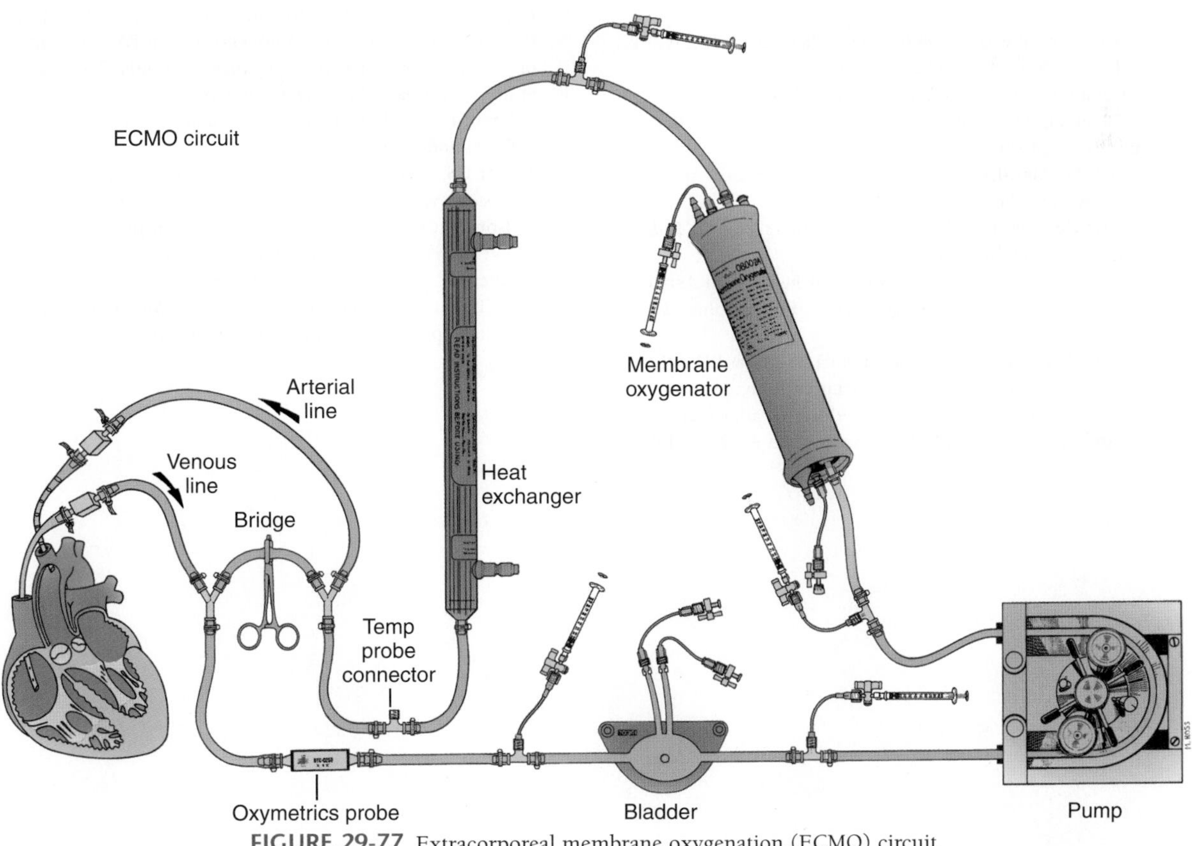


FIGURE 29-77 Extracorporeal membrane oxygenation (ECMO) circuit.

**FOR MEDIAN STERNOTOMY CANNULATION.** The patient is prepped from neck to umbilicus and draped.

1. The patient has usually had a prior sternotomy incision, and so the sternum is opened with wire cutters.
2. A chest retractor is inserted, and purse-string sutures for cannulation are placed in the aorta and right atrium.
3. The aorta and venous cannulas are inserted and clamped.
4. The clamped cannulas are connected to the ECMO circuit. All the air is eliminated.
5. The sternum is left open to prevent kinking of the cannulas and ECMO pump tubing. The wound is closed with a synthetic patch sutured to the skin. An antibiotic ointment may be applied and an "Open Chest" sign placed on top of the outer dressing to serve as a warning related to potential chest compressions.

## REFERENCES


1. Algren C, Arnow D: Pediatric variations of nursing interventions. In Hockenberry MJ and others, editors: *Wong's nursing care of infants and children*, ed 7, St Louis, 2003, Mosby.
2. American Cancer Society: *Cancer facts and figures 2005*, Atlanta, 2005, The Society.
3. Anbumani P and others: *Ventricular septal defect, general concepts*, November 25, 2004. Accessed April 25, 2006, on-line: www.emedicine.com/PED/topic2402.htm.
4. Betz CL, Sowden LA: *Mosby's pediatric nursing reference*, ed 5, St Louis, 2004, Mosby.
5. Boix-Ochoa J, Ashcraft KW: Gastroesophageal reflux. In Ashcraft KW and others, editors: *Pediatric surgery*, ed 4, Philadelphia, 2005, Saunders.
6. Cooper A: Early assessment and management of trauma. In Ashcraft KW and others, editors: *Pediatric surgery*, ed 4, Philadelphia, 2005, Saunders.
7. Cote CJ: Pediatric anesthesia. In Miller RD: *Miller's anesthesia*, vol 2, ed 6, Philadelphia, 2005, Churchill Livingstone.
8. Davis GT: Hemolytic disorders and congenital abnormalities. In Lowdermilk DL and others, editors: *Maternity and women's health care*, ed 8, St Louis, 2004, Mosby.
9. Drake A, Carr MM: *Tonsillectomy*, June 15, 2005. Accessed April 29, 2006, on-line: www.emedicine.com/ent/topic315.htm.
10. Fallat ME: Intussuception. In Ashcraft KW and others, editors: *Pediatric surgery*, ed 4, Philadelphia, 2005, Saunders.
11. Garcia VF: Umbilical and other abdominal wall hernias. In Ashcraft KW and others, editors: *Pediatric surgery*, ed 4, Philadelphia, 2005, Saunders.
12. Gronert GA and others: Malignant hyperthermia. In Miller RD: *Miller's anesthesia*, vol 2, ed 6, Philadelphia, 2005, Churchill Livingstone.
13. Inge TH and others: Bariatric surgical procedures in adolescence. In Ashcraft KW and others, editors: *Pediatric surgery*, ed 4, Philadelphia, 2005, Saunders.
14. Jones M: *Otitis media*, March 2, 2006. Accessed April 26, 2006, on-line: www.emedicine.com/ped/topic1689.htm.
15. Klein MD: Congenital abdominal wall defects. In Ashcraft KW and others, editors: *Pediatric surgery*, ed 4, Philadelphia, 2005, Saunders.
16. Laberge JM and others: Teratomas, dermoids and other soft tissue tumors. In Ashcraft KW and others, editors: *Pediatric surgery*, ed 4, Philadelphia, 2005, Saunders.
17. Lelli JL: Foreign bodies. In Ashcraft KW and others, editors: *Pediatric surgery*, ed 4, Philadelphia, 2005, Saunders.
18. McElhinney D: *Truncus arteriosus*, March 17, 2006. Accessed April 26, 2006, on-line: www.emedicine.com/PED/topic2316.htm.
19. Milliken JC: *Atrial septal defect*, November 21, 2004. Accessed April 25, 2006, on-line: www.emedicine.com/MED/topic3519.htm.
20. Murphy JP: Hypospadias. In Ashcraft KW and others, editors: *Pediatric surgery*, ed 4, Philadelphia, 2005, Saunders.
21. Nguyen TD: *Considerations in pediatric trauma*, October 2, 2003. Accessed April 25, 2006, on-line: www.emedicine.com/med/topic3223.htm.
22. Nuss D and others: Congenital chest wall deformities. In Ashcraft KW and others, editors: *Pediatric surgery*, ed 4, Philadelphia, 2005, Saunders.
23. O'Brien P, Baker AL: The child with cardiovascular dysfunction. In Hockenberry MJ and others, editors: *Wong's nursing care of infants and children*, ed 7, St Louis, 2003, Mosby.
24. Panchal J: *Craniosynostosis management*, July 23, 2004. Accessed April 30, 2006, on-line: www.emedicine.com/plastic/topic534.htm.
25. Pflieger K: *Pulmonary stenosis, valvular*, October 27, 2004. Accessed April 25, 2006, on-line: www.emedicine.com/PED/topic1953.htm.
26. Rao PS: *Tricuspid atresia*, March 6, 2006. Accessed April 25, 2006, on-line: www.emedicine.com/PED/topic2550.htm.
27. Reade C: *Coarctation of the aorta and interrupted aortic arch, surgical perspective*, January 4, 2006. Accessed April 24, 2006, on-line: www.emedicine.com/PED/topic2824.htm.
28. Rothenberg S: Thoracoscopy in children. In Ashcraft KW and others, editors: *Pediatric surgery*, ed 4, Philadelphia, 2005, Saunders.
29. Rupp LA, Day MW: Children are different: pediatric differences and the impact on trauma. In Moloney-Harmon PA, Czerwinski SJ: *Nursing care of the pediatric trauma patient*, St Louis, 2003, Saunders.
30. Spitz L: Esophageal atresia and tracheoesophageal malformations. In Ashcraft KW and others, editors: *Pediatric surgery*, ed 4, Philadelphia, 2005, Saunders.
31. Turner CS: Vascular access. In Ashcraft KW and others, editors: *Pediatric surgery*, ed 4, Philadelphia, 2005, Saunders.
32. Wilson D: Conditions caused by defects in physical development. In Hockenberry MJ and others, editors: *Wong's nursing care of infants and children*, ed 7, St Louis, 2003, Mosby.
33. Wu CL: Pain management. In Miller RD: *Miller's anesthesia*, vol 2, ed 6, Philadelphia, 2005, Churchill Livingstone.

CHAPTER 30

# Geriatric Surgery

SHEILA L. ALLEN

Aging is a process that can be described in chronologic, physiologic, and functional terms. Human aging from a physiologic perspective has changed little in the past 300 years. In general, we age neither faster nor slower than we did in Colonial America. Chronologic age, the number of years a person has lived, is an easily identifiable measurement. Average/median life span, or life expectancy, is the age at which 50% of a given population survives. Maximum life span potential (MLSP) is the age of the longest-lived member or members of the population or species. The average life span of humans has increased dramatically, yet our MLSP has not changed substantially. Although the number of people living beyond their 90s has increased more recently, the MLSP, estimated at 125 years for women and somewhat shorter for men, has not changed significantly in recorded history. Chronologic age or MLSP may not be the most meaningful measurement of age, however. Many people who have lived a long time remain physiologically and functionally young, whereas others are chronologically young but physiologically and functionally old.[17]

Many aspects of our society will be affected by the growth of the population that is 65 years old or older. Policymakers, families, businesses, and health care providers will be challenged to meet the needs of this growing age-group. With the aging of the baby boomers (born between 1943 and 1964), the gerontology boom will occur somewhere between 2010 and 2030, producing the most rapid increase in the older population. Nearly 36 million people age 65 years and older lived in the United States in 2003, accounting for more than 12% of the total population, and they can be divided into four subgroups (Box 30-1). The population considered oldest-old (age 85 years and older) increased from just more than 100,000 in 1900 to 4.2 million in 2000. In 2011, baby boomers will start turning 65 years old; and this segment of the population will increase at such a rate that the 2030 population is projected to be twice as large as it was in 2000. Numbers of the 65-year-old and older population will increase from 35 million to 71.5 million, representing nearly 20% of the total U.S. population.[6] The growth rate for this age-group is expected to slow after 2030 when the last of the boomers join the older population ranks. After 2030, the baby boomers will move into the oldest-old population (age 85 years and older), which will grow accordingly.[5] Figure 30-1 gives population data. The U.S. Census Bureau estimates that the population age 85 years and older could grow from 4.2 million in 2000 to nearly 21 million by 2050.[5] The proportion of the older population (age 65 years and older) varies by state. This proportion is partly affected by the state fertility and mortality levels and partly by the number of older and younger people who migrate to and from the state. In 2002, Florida had the highest proportion of people age 65 years and older: 17%. Pennsylvania and West Virginia also had high proportions: more than 15%. The proportion of the population age 65 years and older varies even more by county. In 2002, 35% of McIntosh County, North Dakota, was age 65 years and older, the highest proportion in the United States. In several Florida counties, the proportion was more than 30%. At the other end of the spectrum was Chattahoochee County, Georgia, with only 2% of its population age 65 years and older.[5]

As in most countries of the world, older women outnumber older men in the United States, and the proportion that is female increases with age. In 2003, women accounted for 58% of the older population and for 69% of the population age 85 years and older. The United States is fairly young by comparison with other countries, with just more than 12% of its population age 65 years and older. In most European countries, the older population made up more than 15% of the population, and it made up nearly 19% in both Italy and Japan in 2003.[5] Mirroring the total U.S. population, the elder population is more racially diverse than ever before. By 2050, programs and services for older people will require greater flexibility to meet the needs of a more diverse population. In 2003, non-Hispanic whites accounted for nearly 83% of the U.S. older population; African Americans, just over 8%; Asians, nearly 3%; and Hispanics (of any race), nearly 6%. Projections are that by 2050, the composition of the older population will change to 61% non-Hispanic white, 18% Hispanic, 12% African American, and 8% Asian. The older Hispanic population is projected to grow the fastest, from just over 2 million in 2003 to 15 million in 2050 and to be larger than the older African American population by 2028. In 2003, nearly 1 million older Asians lived in the United States; by 2050 this population is projected to be almost 7 million.[5] Figure 30-2 gives resident population by racial and ethnic composition.

Those older than 100 years are the fastest-growing age-group among the older-than-65-years U.S. population. The U.S. Census Bureau, generally conservative in its estimates of the aged population thus far, now estimates there will be more than 200,000 American centenarians in 2020 and 500,000 to 4 million by the year 2050. Translating these demographics into health care trends produces even more startling implications for perioperative patient care. As a result of the "graying" of America, health care will never be the same. Most older persons have at least one chronic condition, and many have multiple conditions. Chronic diseases that are rarely cured, such as heart disease, stroke, cancer, and diabetes, are among the most common and costly health conditions. These long-term health conditions negatively affect quality of life, contributing to declines in functioning and the inability to remain in

**BOX 30-1**

### Categorizing the Aging Population

65 to 74 years of age: the young old
75 to 84 years of age: the middle old
85 to 99 years of age: the old old
100 years of age or more: the elite old

From Ignatavicius DD: Health care of older adults. In Ignatavicius DD, Workman ML, editors: *Medical-surgical nursing: critical thinking for collaborative care,* ed 5, St Louis, 2006, Saunders.

the community. Although chronic conditions can be prevented or modified with behavioral interventions, five of the six leading causes of death among older Americans are chronic diseases.[5] Figure 30-3 gives the percentages of chronic diseases by gender. Between 1992 and 2001, the hospitalization rate in the older population increased from 306 hospital stays per 1000 Medicare enrollees to 365 per 1000; however, the average length of stay decreased from 8 days in 1992 to 6 days in 2001. The utilization rates for many services change based on changes in medical technology and physician practice patterns.[5] The dramatic growth in elderly surgical patients punctuates the necessity for perioperative nurses to recognize the special needs of these patients. Understanding how normal aging changes and chronic disease affect the successful outcome of any surgical procedure is critical and is therefore the emphasis of this chapter.

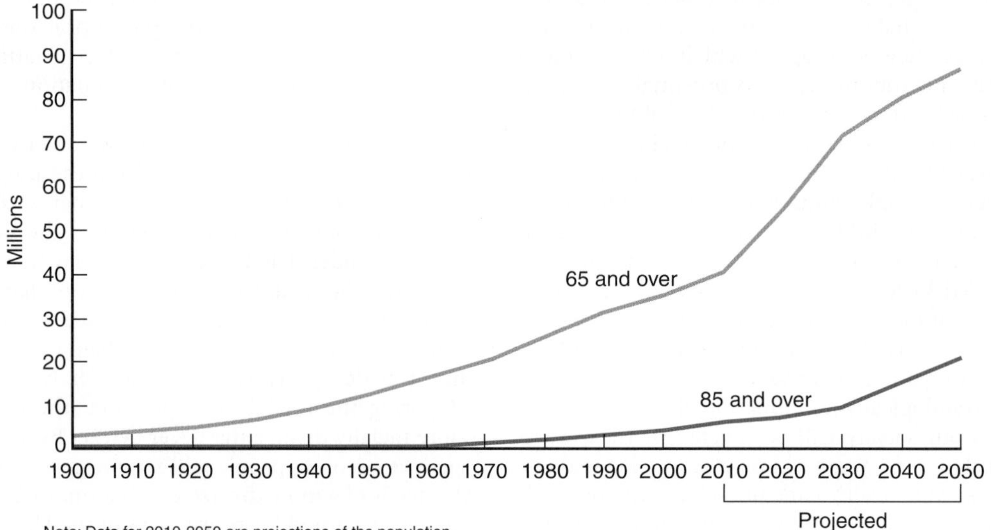


**FIGURE 30-1** Actual and projected population data for people age 65 years and older.

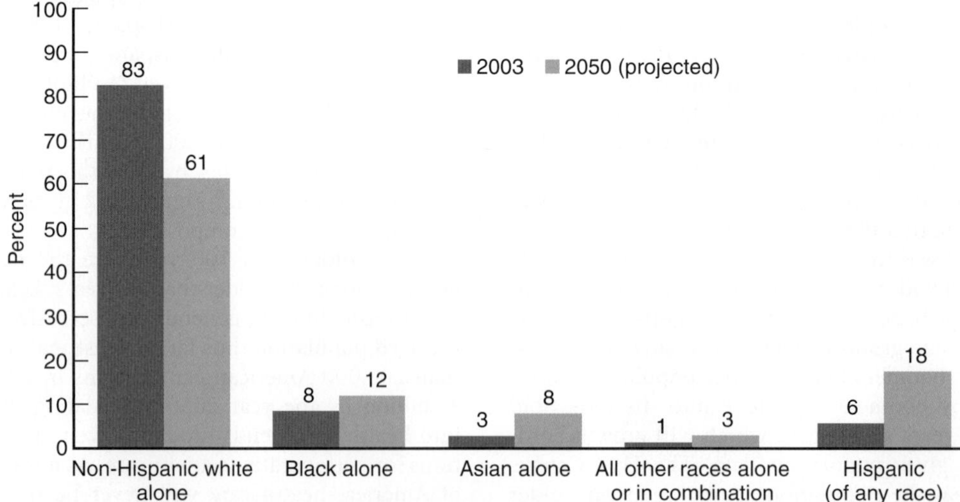


**FIGURE 30-2** Ethnic population data for people age 65 years and older.

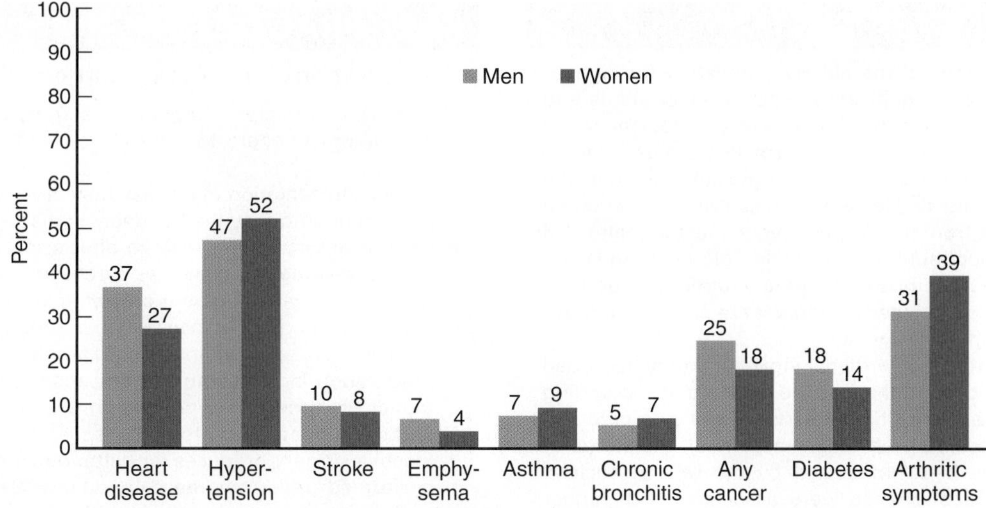


Note: Data are based on a 2-year average from 2001-2002. Data for arthritic symptoms are from 2000-2001.
Reference population: These data refer to the civilian noninstitutionalized population.

**FIGURE 30-3** Chronic disease by gender in people age 65 years and older.

# *Perioperative Nursing Considerations*

## Preliminary Evaluation

Before an elderly patient actually arrives in surgery, the physician considers many factors to determine whether the benefits outweigh potential risks. In the past, elders were not considered good candidates for surgery merely because of age (History box). Uncertainty about the value of surgery in elders and about the operative risks prevailed. Because surgical morbidity and mortality increase with age and complexity of disease conditions, a thorough understanding of the physiology of aging is necessary when considering surgery on older patients (Best Practice). Although improvements in technology, monitoring techniques, and anesthesia have made surgery safer for older patients, age remains a significant risk factor.

Occurrence of perioperative mortality in geriatric surgical patients is influenced by three factors—presence of coexisting disease, emergency surgery, and site of surgery[15]:

1. *Presence of coexisting disease as quantified by the American Society of Anesthesiologists (ASA) Physical Status Classification.* Patients with an ASA status of IV or V are consistently found to have greater mortality than those with a physical status of I or II.
2. *Emergency surgery.* Surgical risk in elders increases dramatically when the surgery is of an emergent nature.
3. *Site of surgery.* Major vascular, intrathoracic, and intraabdominal procedures are reported to have a higher surgical risk than other surgical procedures in elders.

Surgical decision making regarding elders can be a difficult task (Research Highlight). As the baby boomers become seniors, they will be very different from consumers of the past. They will tolerate less and expect more. They will expect to be partners in decision making regarding their care and will be more demanding in terms of quality and service.[16] A frequent mistake is to compare the risk in elderly patients with that of younger patients. Elderly patients have an increased tendency for slower metabolism, multiple chronic diseases, and a decreased reserve capacity of their organs to respond to stress.[11] What should be considered is the risk of not operating and the quality of life expected. Although the decision for surgery is within the purview of the physician, perioperative nurses should be aware of its implications. Surgical intervention and management should be tailored to the patient's symptoms, overall functional and health status, and the predicted advantage of palliative intervention. Important factors that need to be evaluated are (1) disease course versus life expectancy, (2) state of independence, (3) personal motivation, and (4) surgical risk versus nonoperative management:

*Disease course versus life expectancy:* Surgical intervention may not be appropriate if the prognosis of the disease is poor. However, if the patient has several years of life expectancy left and is likely to outlive the condition with minimal morbidity, surgical treatment may be the treatment of choice.

*State of independence:* The patient's right to self-determination and making health care decisions should always be considered. The need for independence is of utmost importance to elderly persons, and most of them are far more interested in maintaining health and independence than longevity. Complications of surgery are not well tolerated by elders and can quickly develop into life-threatening situations. If surgical intervention will further incapacitate an already debilitated person, alternative treatment should be considered. However, if surgery will help alleviate debilitating conditions and improve or maintain independence, it should be considered an appropriate modality of care.

*Personal motivation:* Evaluation of the elderly patient's level of motivation must be considered when surgery is planned. Many elderly patients are reluctant to undergo surgery. They are concerned that the surgery will not improve their quality of life and that it will make them depend more on others or destine them to a life in a care facility. In addition, they do not want to withstand the pain, discomfort, and rigors of surgery and the recuperative period necessary to treat a condition that really does not bother them very much or that they have "learned to live with." This lack of motivation will have a negative influence on the results of the surgery. Conversely, some elders expect and in some cases demand the best of care.

## HISTORY

Societal attitudes toward the elderly population throughout the world have had a significant impact on elder status and access to resources. Historically, respect and reverence for elders were not always the societal norm. In ancient times, the Romans had little respect for elders. Egyptians dreaded the thought of getting old, and leaders such as Aristotle prevented elderly individuals from having any involvement in matters of government. Throughout the Dark and Middle Ages, and even into the Industrial Age, those who were youthful and productive had higher status. Elderly people were seen as nonproductive and a drain on resources.

Cultures that had no written language highly regarded their elders and looked to them as the teachers of succeeding generations. The ancient Chinese saw old age as a great accomplishment, deserving of honor. In general, the status of older persons has been influenced by the rate of societal change; slow rates of change were associated with higher status for elders, whereas rapid change found elders "out of touch," only knowing how things were, not how they are. Today we are in the midst of a rapidly changing society. Unlike anything that has happened before, elders' influence and status are rising along with their numbers.

Nursing care of the elderly population has gone through similar changes. Caring for older persons was a very unpopular segment of nursing practice. Nurses who aspired to care for elders were regarded as being less capable. It was not until 1966 that the first Division of Geriatric Nursing was established in the American Nurses Association (ANA). Ten years later, in 1976, the Geriatric Division was changed to the Gerontological Nursing Division of ANA to more aptly reflect a broader scope of care. This change did much to focus nursing attention toward a more accurate view of the elderly population who were living life in all dimensions—not just as ill older adults.

In terms of surgical care of the aged, the definition of elderly has changed. The age that was considered too old for surgery has slowly moved up from 50 years old in the early half of the twentieth century, to the early twenty-first century, when elders well into their 80s, 90s, and even 100s are being successfully treated by surgical means. Perioperative nurses can expect to see the numbers of older and very old patients continue to rise in surgical settings. With the segmentation of age-specific competencies, perioperative nurses have more resources from which to base their care. Assisting the elders to achieve the maximum benefit from their surgery with more meaning and quality of life is an integral component of perioperative patient advocacy and patient safety.

They believe that the money they spend on taxes and health care entitles them to the very best that health care has to offer, regardless of its practicality. Nonetheless, patients who show a strong sense of determination in doing all that is necessary to get well and stay well are better candidates for surgery than those who believe illness is a prelude to death. Obviously, the outcome of surgery is enhanced if the patient is motivated to have a positive result.

*Surgical risk versus nonoperative management:* Deciding between the risks of nonoperative management and surgical intervention is particularly difficult for elderly patients. Surgical and anesthetic risks increase in proportion to the emergent nature of the patient's condition. When an acute emergency condition taxes an already overburdened physiologic state, survival is less likely. Patients may die even if the surgery was considered successful because of complications resulting from the complexity of the patient's co-morbid condition. Nonetheless, health care providers need to be sensitive to this possibility when communicating with family members. To increase the chances of survival from a surgical procedure, the elderly person must be in optimum condition and adequate preoperative assessment and preparation must precede an elective procedure.

## BEST PRACTICE

### Considerations for Geriatric Surgery

The following principles of geriatric surgery can be used as a guide for practitioners to improve care for elderly surgical patients:

- Clinical presentation of disease may differ from the general population and may lead to delay in diagnosis.
- Lack of organ system reserve affects the elder's ability to handle severe stress, such as extensive or emergency surgery, and may be apparent only after surgery.
- Perioperative risk increases when preoperative preparation is decreased or suboptimal. Examples of preoperative preparation include smoking cessation; perioperative antibiotics; treatment of hypertension, anemia, and bronchitis; and thromboembolic prophylaxis.
- Elective surgery produces far better outcomes than surgery performed under emergent conditions. Because of the elder's lack of reserve and the inability to do adequate preoperative preparation, the risk of emergency surgery is associated with at least a threefold increase in mortality and morbidity more than for planned or elective procedures.
- Meticulous attention to detail can help avoid minor complications that may escalate into major adverse events in elderly patients. Restoring and maintaining homeostasis, lowering the risk of septic complications, preventing anastomotic leaks, and hemodynamic monitoring greatly reduce the surgical risk.
- Physiologic age is a better indicator of risk in surgery on elderly people than is chronologic age. Most surgeons agree that age alone is not a contraindication to surgery. In fact, studies confirm that even the very old can have successful positive surgical outcomes when their physical health status is considered to be uncomplicated by chronic disease.

Modified from *American Society of Anesthesiologists syllabus on geriatric anesthesiology.* Accessed April 21, 2006, on-line: www.asahq.org/clinical/geriatrics/prean_eval.htm; Saufl NM: Preparing the older adult for surgery and anesthesia, *Journal of PeriAnesthesia Nursing* 19(6):372-378, 2004.

The following considerations should be included when deciding to proceed with surgery in elders[10]:

- Is there a clear indication for surgery, including a likelihood of disease progression?
- What practical limitations will be imposed on the patient with the progression of the disease?
- How much improvement can be expected after the surgical procedure?
- What is the expectation for quality of life with or without the surgery?
- How aware is the patient and his or her family about the problem and proposed solutions?
- What risks are there for negative outcomes related to the procedure and the presence of co-morbid conditions?
- Has an adequate preoperative assessment and preparation preceded an elective procedure?

## RESEARCH HIGHLIGHT

### Medical Decision Making in the Elderly

Age of patients alone is not a contraindication to most medical interventions. The increase in the elderly population has contributed to a sharp age-specific increase in health care costs. Vrakking and colleagues identified that by 2035 more than half of all health care costs will be incurred by people age 75 years and older.

This aspect of rising health care costs raises questions regarding justice and equity and must be considered with regard to policy and the role of age in medical decision making. Although some authors suggest that rationing should be employed, the aim of this study was to provide insights regarding medical decision making about life-prolonging interventions for different age-groups.

To provide these insights, researchers conducted a case-controlled study with face-to-face interviews using a structured questionnaire for nursing home physicians, cardiologists, and oncologists regarding clinical practices concerning elderly and nonelderly patients in potentially life-prolonging interventions. The selected cases were of seriously ill patients and interventions that are applied within a setting. All physicians were asked about nonelderly patients that did and did not receive the intervention, as well as elderly patients that did and did not receive the intervention.

The data were compared with elderly and nonelderly patient groups and were assessed using the Pearson chi-square test. The mean of the arguments from the data was calculated and compared using the likelihood ratio test. The results indicated no major differences in the determinants of decision making among nursing home, cardiology, and oncology patients. In patients with a relatively poor quality of life and those with no known preference for treatment, the chance of being treated was lower. In patients with similar patient characteristics, age was not the determinant of treatment, with one exception being that elderly patients were more likely to be treated against their will.

The authors identified the limitations of the study were that patients' perspectives were not included and that the results might not be applicable to other specialties. They did conclude that the increase in decision making will be influenced by patient characteristics that determine nontreatment for all age-groups and is more prevalent for the elderly population but is not based solely on age.

Modified from Vrakking AM and others: Medical decision-making for seriously ill non-elderly and elderly patients, *Health Policy* 75(1):40-48, 2005.

There are many important considerations related to the extent of surgical treatment. Therefore the decision for surgery relies heavily on the patient's physical status at the time of surgery and how extensively the disease has progressed. When treating patients who are nearing the end of life, attention should shift from solely maximizing survival to maximizing the quality of life and dignity while minimizing suffering. Early identification of problems with aggressive, preventive surgical treatment is considered more appropriate than waiting for problems to develop.

The preadmission visit may uncover possible elder abuse that could be one or a combination of the following:

- Physical (beating, sexual)
- Emotional (verbal threats, intimidation, humiliation)
- Neglect (withholding food or care)
- Material or financial

BOX 30-2

### Signs That May Indicate Elder Abuse

- The older person demonstrates *excessive* agreement or compliance with the caregiver.
- The older person shows signs of poor hygiene, such as body odor, uncleanness, or soiled clothing or underpants.
- The older person has malnutrition or dehydration.
- The older person has burns or pressure sores.
- The older person has bruises in various stages of healing that may indicate repeated injury.
- The older person lacks adequate clothing or footwear.
- The older person has had inadequate medical attention.
- The older person verbalizes lack of food, medication, or care.
- The older person verbalizes being left alone or isolated in some way.
- The older person verbalizes fear of the caregiver.
- The older person verbalizes his or her lack of control in personal activities or finances.

From Wold GH: *Basic geriatric nursing*, ed 3, St Louis, 2004, Mosby.

Perioperative nurses have a unique opportunity to assess and screen for the signs of emotional and physical abuse in elderly patients during their preoperative assessment and while assisting with surgical positioning. Box 30-2 lists signs that may indicate abuse. If such signs occur, the perioperative nurse should report the suspected abuse to the appropriate authority. Reporting laws and regulations vary by state and facility.

In elderly patients, the consent process may require additional time to ensure that the patient understands and adequately answers the questions posed. If the older adult patient is comatose, has some disease or level of brain injury that inhibits decision making, or is nondecisional, information must be relayed to the appropriate decision maker (designated family member or person with power of attorney for health care). In advocating for the older adult, the perioperative nurse should ensure any questions, concerns, or issues of the patient or the patient's decision maker are addressed before the surgery. The principles of bioethics are the underlying basis for the nurse's ethical actions. The six principles are as follows:

- Autonomy—respecting others and allowing individuals to make uncoerced, voluntary decisions
- Beneficence—acting in the best interests of the patient
- Fidelity—keeping promises by maintaining privacy and confidentiality of patient issues
- Justice—treating individuals according to what is owed to them or fair
- Nonmaleficence—directing health care providers to do no harm
- Veracity—telling the truth

Regardless of the age of the patient, the development of ethical competency is an important component of the practice of perioperative nursing.[12]

## Assessment

In elderly persons a preoperative medical assessment is conducted mainly to determine present physiologic functioning. An interdisciplinary approach is necessary to consider the complex health needs of the elderly patient in an effort to provide quality care. Application of these findings identifies operative risk, minimizes postoperative complications, and establishes the presence and status of any concomitant disease process that could negatively affect the outcome of the surgery. The preoperative nursing assessment is conducted to plan patient care throughout the perioperative period. In particular, assessment data are used to establish presurgical baseline data so that health status changes, primarily during the intraoperative and postoperative periods, are more readily recognized. Data collection includes the standard assessment information with considerations of coexisting conditions (Box 30-3).

Chronologic age as a valid predictor of a patient's response to surgery is not a reliable measurement. It gives little indication of the physiologic or biologic age and condition of a person. A 75-year-old person can be in better physical and mental condition for surgery than a 65-year-old person or even younger. Biologic age as a measurement criterion is much more reliable. Establishing biologic age, however, becomes the greatest challenge. Quality-of-life measurements that assess the abilities to perform activities of daily living (ADLs), including physiologic function and mobility, cognitive function, self-care, emotional status, sensory function, and pain, provide efficient parameters of assessment.[12]

Because of changes in biologic function of individuals over time, clinical pathways, rigid guidelines, algorithmic approaches, and other strategies of diagnostic investigation and resource allocation are likely to be less efficient for elders if based solely on age criteria. Health care providers, clinical investigators, and health policy makers must recognize that increasing variability becomes more important with chronologic age.[16] Chronic conditions may interfere with the elderly person's ability to distinguish between recent and long-standing ailments. Therefore the preoperative interview, especially in elderly persons, should be conducted in a quiet, relaxed environment with as few distractions as possible. The elderly person should be allowed to respond to each question independently without prompting from a spouse or other family members unless absolutely necessary (Figure 30-4). This helps to maintain the patient's dignity, independence, and control, which are extremely important to the older adult.

**BOX 30-3**

**Preanesthesia Evaluation Data**

Preanesthesia evaluation data include but are not limited to the following:

- Complete medical history with systems review and anesthetic history, including self or family difficulty with anesthesia
- Complete surgical history
- Proposed surgical procedure
- Allergies—drug, food, environmental, latex
- Routine medications—prescription, OTC (over the counter), herbal, diet, recreational
- Current physical information—height, weight, baseline vital signs
- Social history—cultural and religious beliefs, alcohol and tobacco use
- Mental status—emotional clues; learning barriers; sensory, sight, or speech impairments
- Prosthetics—dentures, glasses or contacts, hearing aids, assistive devices (walker, wheelchair), implanted devices, prosthetics, body piercings
- Socioeconomic issues—transportation, home support
- Advanced directives—living will, do-not-resuscitate (DNR) directive

Data from Saufl NM: Preparing the older adult for surgery and anesthesia, *Journal of PeriAnesthesia Nursing* 19(6):372-378, 2004; Asher ME: Surgical considerations in the elderly, *Journal of PeriAnesthesia Nursing* 19(6):406-414, 2004.

***Normal Age-Related Changes.*** Aging is a biologic process characterized by the inevitable, progressive, predictable evolution and maturation until death. Aging is not the accumulation of disease, although the two are related in subtle, complex ways. A fundamental principle is that biologic age and chronologic age are not the same. Different individuals age at different rates. Physical aging occurs in different organ systems at different rates, influenced by lifestyle choices and socioeconomic status.[16] In general, the aging process imposes a decline in organ functions, atypical responses to pain and temperature, alterations in pharmacokinetics (Surgical Pharmacology), and atypical signs and symptoms of disease, all of which may vary from one elderly person to the next. Having a clear understanding of normal age changes helps establish appropriate nursing diagnoses and develop a plan of care (Box 30-4). The following review of systems focuses on age-specific changes of particular importance to the perioperative plan of care.

PHYSIOLOGIC CHANGES

**Integumentary System.** The nails become thick and tough, and the circulation in the feet may decrease (Table 30-1). A nick or cut can lead to a serious infection. Color and texture of hair change, and the loss of pigmentation results in graying of hair. Decrease in oil content makes the hair dull and lifeless, and the amount of hair decreases. The skin loses elasticity and subcutaneous fat and becomes more prone to shear force and pressure injury. Because of the thinness of the skin and small-vessel fragility, bruising and hemorrhaging are quite common. Dry skin develops because of decreased oils and sweat glands. As a result, skin breakdown and pressure ulcers, as well as wound infections, develop more easily. The vascular system of the skin has nutritional and protective roles. It is necessary for body heat regulation, provides defenses against microbial and physical damage, provides nutrient supply to the avascular epidermis, and promotes wound healing. Having an intact vascular system to maintain these skin role character-

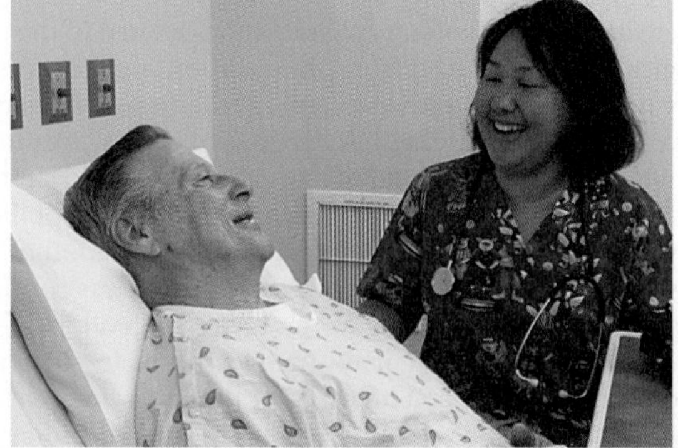

FIGURE 30-4 Allowing the elderly patient to respond to questions independently, without prompting from family members, helps to maintain a sense of dignity and control.

## SURGICAL PHARMACOLOGY
### Medication and the Elderly

Perioperative nurses caring for older adults must consider factors that affect the choice of medications and the effects of those medications on this population. Older adults may not tolerate the standard dosages used for younger adults and are at higher risk for side effects and toxicity. Dosages of drugs may initially be smaller than for the general adult population and then titrated based on the patient's response and therapeutic effect. Older adults have less reserve, and chronic disease may contribute to drug reactions. Physiologic changes may affect the absorption, distribution, metabolism, and excretion of medications. Older adults also have a higher incidence of nonprescription drug use (i.e., analgesics, antacids, laxatives, supplements, etc.). A thorough medication history is essential to provide safe care. The nurse should partner with the surgeon and anesthesia provider to ensure that drug therapy is individualized based on the patient's baseline condition, actual physiologic impairments, and severity of preexisting illness.

Common adverse drug reactions in older adults include the following:

- Edema
- Dizziness
- Nausea and vomiting
- Urinary retention
- Anorexia
- Diarrhea
- Dry mouth
- Constipation
- Fatigue
- Confusion
- Weakness

Age-related changes that may impact medication administration in the perioperative period are as follows:

**CHANGES IN ABSORPTION**
- Increased gastric pH
- Decreased gastric blood flow
- Decreased gastrointestinal motility

**CHANGES IN DRUG DISTRIBUTION**
- Decreased amounts of total body water
- Increased ratio of adipose tissue to lean body mass, causing storage of lipid-soluble drugs and decreased plasma drug levels
- Decreased albumin levels
- Decreased cardiac output

**CHANGES IN METABOLISM AND EXCRETION**
- Decreased liver size
- Decreased hepatic blood flow
- Decreased liver enzyme activity
- Decreased renal blood flow
- Reduced glomerular filtration rate, leading to slower excretion times for medications and allowing serum drug levels to rise

Modified from Hodgson BB, Kizior RJ: *Saunders nursing drug handbook 2006,* St Louis, 2006, Saunders; Ignatavicius DD: Health care of older adults. In Ignatavicius DD, Workman ML, editors: *Medical-surgical nursing: critical thinking for collaborative care,* ed 5, St Louis, 2006, Saunders.

istics is extremely important for a patient undergoing surgical intervention. However, papillary capillaries, responsible for epidermal nourishment and heat dissipation, degenerate with aging. What is left is only the horizontal arteriovenous plexus lying beneath the skin surface. This progressive impairment of vascular circulation and tissue nutrition and the loss of subcutaneous tissue predispose to a feeling of cold, especially in cool environments such as the operating room (OR). Therefore the ability to maintain thermoregulation is compromised in elders and must be controlled through external measures.

**Respiratory System.** Lungs lose elasticity, which contributes to a decrease in functional residual capacity, residual volume, and dead space. Lungs increase in size and are lighter in weight with aging. A rigid chest wall is the result of calcification of costal cartilages, osteoporosis, and dorsal kyphosis. Muscles responsible for inhalation and exhalation may be weakened, resulting in a diminished ability to increase and decrease the size of the thoracic cavity. All these changes contribute to a minimal tidal exchange, which makes the elderly patient more susceptible to pulmonary complications, such as adult respiratory distress syndrome (ARDS), pneumonia, and aspiration.[14] Lung changes are not usually obvious at rest. However, when the person becomes active, breathing may be more difficult. The ability to cough and clear the upper airway is lessened, and such reduction may increase the chance of respiratory infections and diseases. Some can be severe enough to threaten the elderly person's life.

**Cardiovascular System.** A decrease in coronary artery blood flow is more likely in elderly persons. Because of a shift in blood flow, there is a greater decrease in circulation to the kidneys and liver than to the brain and heart. Blood pressure rises as a result of increased arterial resistance. When the elderly person is at rest, the heart rate remains approximately the same as that of a younger person. However, the older heart requires a longer recovery time after each beat, which means that it reacts poorly to stress and anxiety-produced tachycardia. In general, the capacity of the cardiovascular system to tolerate and buffer insults is limited. Activity, exercise, excitement, and illness increase the body's need for oxygen and nutrients. The older heart may be unable to meet these needs. Arteries lose their elasticity and become narrow, causing a weakened heart to work harder. As a result, less blood flows through the arteries, causing poor circulation in many parts of the body. Elders have an increased risk for aortic arch disruption, myocardial contusion, and aneurysm development.[14]

**Digestive System.** The secretion of digestive glands decreases; mucus becomes thicker, causing dysphagia; and saliva becomes more alkaline. Loss of teeth or poorly fitted dentures make chewing difficult, resulting in digestion problems. Foods that are difficult to eat are avoided, and such avoidance can affect overall nutrition. Decrease in peristalsis and a reduction of gastric motility—the results of muscle tone loss—cause a delay in stomach emptying. Potential traumatic injuries to the bowel and mesenteric infarction are more likely to occur.[14] The absorption of drugs is affected because of a reduction of blood flow to abdominal viscera, a reduction of hydrochloric acid, and delayed gastric emptying. Decrease of total body water and plasma volume results in a smaller volume of distribution for

BOX 30-4

## Age-Related Physiologic Changes

**HEMATOPOIETIC AND LYMPHATIC SYSTEM**
- Increased plasma viscosity
- Decreased red blood cell production
- Increased immature T cells

**RESPIRATORY SYSTEM**
- Decreased tissue elasticity, resulting in pooling of secretions in lower lung bases
- Increased calcification of cartilage, leading to increased rigidity of the rib cage, decreased lung capacity, and reduced cough efficiency
- Less ciliary activity by bronchial lining
- Reduction in number of capillaries, resulting in decreased gas exchange and drying of mucous membranes

**CARDIOVASCULAR SYSTEM**
- Changes in cardiac muscle tone and blood vessel elasticity, leading to decreased tissue oxygenation and decreased venous return
- Dysrhythmias; rapid or slow heartbeat
- High blood pressure related to atherosclerosis
- Chest pain or shortness of breath on exertion
- Decreased cardiac output, causing decreased circulation to extremities

**DIGESTIVE SYSTEM**
- Dental issues (i.e., tooth loss, periodontal disease), leading to chewing issues
- Decreased saliva production
- Relaxation of esophageal muscle tone, increasing the incidence of esophageal reflux
- Decreased gastric secretions
- Bowel dysfunction from decreased peristalsis

**URINARY SYSTEM**
- Loss of nephron units
- Decline in renal tissue growth
- Reduced kidney size
- Reduced bladder capacity
- Increased prostate size in men
- Weakened bladder muscles with consequent postvoid residual

**MUSCULOSKELETAL SYSTEM**
- Progressive loss of muscle strength from decreased muscle mass
- Decreased fluid in intervertebral disks
- Postural changes, such as curvature of the spine from decreased bone calcium
- Joint and back pain/stiffness
- Bone breakdown overcomes bone building, with resultant osteoporosis
- Decreased tissue elasticity, resulting in decreased mobility and flexibility

**NERVOUS SYSTEM**
- Loss of neurons, leading to decreased reflexes
- Decreased reaction time from loss of nerve fibers
- Changes in sleep patterns; less rapid eye movement (REM) and deep sleep
- Decreased amounts of neuroreceptors resulting in decreased perception of stimuli

**SENSORY SYSTEM**
- Decreased tear production
- Increased lens discoloration, which decreases color perception
- Decreased muscle tone in eye, leading to decreased pupil diameter, decreased night vision, increased refractive errors, increased sensitivity to glare
- Loss of hair cells in inner ear, leading to balance problems
- Decreased joint mobility in bones of inner ear
- Decreased number of papillae on tongue

**ENDOCRINE SYSTEM**
- Decreased pituitary secretions (growth hormone), leading to decreases in muscle mass
- Reduction in the production of thyroid-stimulating hormone
- Decreased production of parathyroid hormone
- Increased incidence of diabetes mellitus

**REPRODUCTIVE SYSTEM**

**Female**
- Decreased estrogen levels
- Decreased tissue elasticity
- Increased vaginal alkalinity

**Male**
- Decreased testosterone levels
- Circulatory changes

Modified from Wold GH: *Basic geriatric nursing*, ed 3, St Louis, 2004, Mosby.

water-soluble drugs. A condition that increases the storage of lipophilic drugs, such as diazepam and lidocaine, occurs because the percentage of body fat increases and the lean body mass decreases. These factors are of particular importance for assessing the patient's response to preoperative, anesthetic, and postoperative medications.

**Urinary System.** Nephrons decrease in function with age, so by 75 years of age a person has probably lost one third to one half of original nephron function. Elasticity and tone are lost in the ureters, bladder, and urethra, which lead to incomplete emptying of the bladder. By age 50 years at least 50% of all men have some degree of benign prostatic hypertrophy (BPH) and the incidence increases with each decade of life.[4] Difficulty in voiding and retention are common with this condition. Total bladder capacity also declines, so elderly persons experience a more frequent and urgent need to urinate. Because blood flow to the kidneys is decreased, patients are at greater risk for fluid overload, fluid and electrolyte imbalance, and alterations in the elimination of medications. During the perioperative phase of the patient's hospital stay, the greatest number and variety of drugs are given; the cumulative effect increases the chances for adverse and consequential results.

**Musculoskeletal System.** Changes to the elderly person's skeleton, such as the loss of bone mass, contribute to skeletal instability and make fractures of the hip, rib, distal radius, and vertebrae very common. Curvature of the spine and arthritis of the joints are also common. Pain as a fifth vital sign is routinely evaluated for all patients. In elders, long-standing conditions

**TABLE 30-1**

## Age-Related Skin Changes

| Physiologic Change | Results |
|---|---|
| Decreased vascularity of dermis | Increased pallor in white skin |
| Decreased amount of melanin | Decreased hair color (graying) |
| Decreased sebaceous and sweat gland function | Increased dry skin; decreased sweating |
| Decreased subcutaneous fat | Increased wrinkling |
| Decreased thickness of epidermis | Increased susceptibility to trauma |
| Increased localized pigmentation | Increased incidence of brown spots (senile lentigo) |
| Increased capillary fragility | Increased purple patches (senile purpura) |
| Decreased density of hair growth | Decreased amount and thickness of hair on head and body |
| Decreased rate of nail growth | Increased brittleness of nails |
| Decreased peripheral circulation | Increased longitudinal ridges on nails, increased thickening and yellowing of nails |
| Increased androgen/estrogen ratio | Increased facial hair in women |

From Wold GH: *Basic geriatric nursing,* ed 3, St Louis, 2004, Mosby.

such as arthritis, neuralgia, and ischemic disorders produce chronic pain. Back pain is related to dehydration and decreased flexibility of the vertebral disks. These changes result in a gradual loss of height, loss of strength, and decreased mobility. Poor posture tends to be proportional to the degree of back pain experienced and may greatly compromise internal organ function. Joint range of motion is impaired to varying degrees and may affect surgical positioning.

**Nervous System.** Although not functionally significant, a steady loss of neurons begins at about 25 years of age. An inappropriate or slow response to stimuli is primarily a result of a decrease in some organ systems' ability to send reliable messages to the brain and spinal cord. Nerve cells are particularly sensitive to lack of oxygen. Because elderly persons may have, in varying degrees, cerebral arteriosclerosis and atherosclerosis, decreased blood flow and nervous system deficits, such as insomnia, irritability, visual motor deficits, and memory loss, may occur. These patients are more likely to experience subdural hematomas or closed head injuries from falls. Other neurologic changes significant to perioperative care include a loss of position sense in the toes, decreased tactile sense, and atypical response to pain. In addition, inadvertent hypothermia (temperature below 96.8°F [36°C]) is a common problem in elders (see Chapter 9 for a full discussion of preventing unplanned hypothermia in adult surgical patients). In the OR, maintaining balance between heat gain (metabolic production, muscular contraction, hot ambient temperature) and heat loss (radiation, convection, evaporation, ventilation, cold fluid infusion, blood loss, antithermoregulatory drugs, impaired heat production) can be difficult in older surgical patients.

**SENSORY CHANGES.** Sensory changes in vision, hearing, taste, smell, and touch may influence the patient's response to care. If preadmission communication is done, the perioperative nurse may ask about vision and hearing and remind patients to bring glasses and hearing aids to the facility with them.[1] Farsightedness, or presbyopia, in the aging person is a result of the lens becoming more rigid and less pliable with age. Consequently, visual acuity and accommodation are decreased. Color perception changes as a result of a yellowing of the lens, which makes distinguishing blue, green, and purple more difficult for the elderly person. Of particular importance in the OR is an awareness of the older person's difficulty in adapting to changes in light. Moving patients from a dimly lit holding area to the bright lights of the OR can cause momentary "blindness."

Presbycusis, or loss of hearing sensitivity, is irreversible, bilateral, and primarily sensorineural, although metabolic and mechanical causes are also possible. It is the most frequent cause of hearing loss in the geriatric patient. Hearing loss, which appears to be greater in men than in women, is mostly within the higher frequencies (above 1000 Hz). In addition, cerumen thickens and the eardrum becomes less pliable, and such changes also contribute to diminished hearing. Often geriatric patients are labeled "confused" or "senile" because they respond inappropriately to questions they did not hear or they describe what they see inaccurately because of poor vision.

Changes in taste and smell begin to occur at approximately 60 years of age and become more pronounced with advanced age. Older adults have two to three times more difficulty in detecting flavors than do young adults. Oral hygiene, dental disease and decreased salivary function may also alter tasting ability. There is a close association between the sense of smell and human behavior. Smell can affect emotions when a person recalls a particular odor. Other functions include protection of the individual by warning of danger in the air, such as smoke or gas fumes; assistance in digestion; and helping a person to remember or recollect. In elders, the sense of smell can be reduced, as well as the ability to identify odors.[17]

Changes in sensitivity to touch often accompany the aging process, but the degree of change varies among individuals. In some cases, losses can be related to neuropathy caused by disease, injury, or circulatory problems. Decreased sense of touch can affect the elderly person's ability to localize stimuli and can also reduce the speed of reaction to tactile stimulation. For example, an older person may have difficulty differentiating among coins, fastening buttons, or grasping small items.

**PSYCHOLOGIC CHANGES.** Physiologic and psychologic stress may result in an acute state of confusion or delirium in the geriatric patient that is analogous to convulsions as a stress reaction in the pediatric patient. In elders, mental change can be a warning of some underlying problem. Confusion or delirium should therefore not be dismissed as an expected behavior of the geriatric patient. The most important assessment factor is determining whether the confusion is chronic or acute. Chronic conditions, such as depression and Alzheimer's disease, can make communication with the patient difficult. Depending on the stage of disease, patients may or may not be able to understand explanations. Family members are the best resource to determine the patient's ability to comprehend and respond to questions and instructions. Behavioral changes, such as aggressiveness, agitation, and paranoia, are not uncommon. Soft restraints may be necessary during local procedures in the OR to ensure patient safety. Taking the time to talk slowly, being deliberate in movements, getting to know the patient, and developing a trusting relationship before surgery can help to lessen the patient's anxiety and control the combative outbursts that occur in some Alzheimer's patients.

Acute confused states or delirium in elders can be precipitated by a number of conditions and may be the sole manifestation of a life-threatening complication. Delirium in elders may be evidenced by alteration in their level of consciousness, inattention, disorganized thinking, or an acute onset of mental status change.

Some of the most common predisposing factors for confusion or delirium in hospitalized elders are increasing age, baseline brain damage, drug or alcohol addictions, fatigue, social and psychologic stressors, and sleep deprivation. Apparent confusion could be caused from drugs; infection (Research Highlight); withdrawal from alcohol; metabolic, cerebrovascular, or cardiac disorders; trauma; or cancer. Conditions such as fecal impaction, changes in routine, urinary bladder distention, dehydration, electrolyte imbalance, and stress can also affect cognition in elders.[11] Even the disruption of relocation into the hospital, which brings the patient into an unfamiliar environment, can cause acute confusion, particularly during the postoperative period. Validation of the patient's previous mental state with a relative or significant other can help to determine if the onset occurred since hospitalization.

## RESEARCH HIGHLIGHT

### Surgical Site Infections in the Geriatric Population

Surgical site infection (SSI) is a frustrating complication that can occur after any surgical procedure. When SSI occurs in the geriatric population, the outcome can be devastating. SSI caused by *Staphylococcus aureus* is associated with more than five times greater mortality, more than double the postoperative duration of hospitalization, and double the hospital charges of those rates for elderly operative patients without SSI.

Researchers sought to identify risk factors for SSI in older people by conducting a case-controlled retrospective study. They compared patients who developed SSI with a similar group who did not develop SSI. Patients were identified as having an SSI through microbiology reports, readmission after surgery, and clinical rounds. All SSIs were classified as deep or organ space, and superficial infections were excluded.

The mean age of the study groups was 73.9 years. The most common operative procedures were cardiothoracic (32%), orthopedic (18.3%), gastrointestinal (8%), and general (5%). The most common preoperative morbidities were obesity, diabetes mellitus, malignancy, and congestive heart failure. The most common baseline impairments in functional status were the inability to ambulate independently, the inability to bathe independently, and the inability to dress independently.

Analysis of the data identified the following risk factors for SSI in the elderly population: obesity, chronic obstructive pulmonary disease (COPD), and having a wound class score of 2 (contaminated or dirty). Researchers found that in 88% of the SSI cases, one or more SSI risk factors were present, and in 44% of the SSI cases, two or more risk factors were present.

The study recommends that measures such as optimizing medical regimens to reduce preoperative morbidity for identified factors should be undertaken.

Modified from Kaye KS and others: Risk factors for surgical site infections in older people, *Journal of the American Geriatric Society* 54(3):391-396, 2006.

***Routine Laboratory and Diagnostic Tests.*** The physiologic changes of aging do not significantly alter the diagnostic values of complete blood count (CBC), differential cell count, platelets, urinalysis, and blood chemistry results; therefore abnormalities should be evaluated. A slight increase may be noted in potassium levels, fasting blood glucose, postprandial blood glucose, oral glucose tolerance, total cholesterol, and thyroid-stimulating hormone. A decrease in vitamin $B_{12}$, folic acid, magnesium, creatinine clearance, and albumin may also be noted. The chest x-ray film may reveal increased anteroposterior diameter, osteopenia, and degenerative joint disease. The heart size should appear normal, even in elders. Cardiomegaly can contribute to postoperative complications and should be evaluated. The electrocardiogram (ECG) may show P-wave notching, ST-segment depression or left ventricular hypertrophy, and T-wave flattening or inversion that are associated with an increased risk of myocardial ischaemia.[8] An increase in bundle branch block, hemiblock, and first-degree block may also be noted, largely as a result of degenerative disease of the conduction system. Opinion about the number of preoperative laboratory tests to be ordered varies. Use of a focused history and physical examination yields important information regarding which preoperative tests are indicated. Preoperative testing should be based solely on the history, physical examination, and planned surgical procedure.

Because many elderly patients take several medications (also known as *polypharmacy*), assessing their drug history is important. Digoxin and nitroglycerin may be withheld during the perioperative period, whereas diuretics and antihypertensives may be taken as needed but not used routinely during the postoperative period. Any patient who had been receiving steroids within the previous 12 months should receive parenteral steroids starting the evening before surgery and continuing through the initial postoperative course.

Control of diabetes is often difficult during the perioperative period. For patients taking oral hypoglycemic agents, the medication is withheld and serum glucose and urinary glucose are closely monitored. Long-acting parenteral insulin is discontinued, and regular insulin is given during the preoperative period. Diabetic patients who are fasting the morning of surgery should take their insulin as directed by the anesthesia provider and have an intravenous (IV) line inserted for infusion of 5% dextrose and water on admission to the OR.

***Additional Assessment Data.*** Additional data regarding the patient can be gained from observation of appearance, behavior, dress, and language. For instance, does the patient's apparent age (how old the patient looks) match the chronologic age? Facial expressions and contradictory behaviors can help the nurse assess the patient's mental status. Perioperative nurses in the preoperative area can note the patient's clothing and dress for clues of signs of weight loss, stains on clothing, the presence of burns on clothing, or how the shoes are worn. The patient's use of language and communication skills should also be assessed when formulating a teaching plan.

Another very important but often overlooked area of assessment is dental/oral health evaluation. Disorders of the oral cavity, like any number of physiologic, psychologic, or social factors, can affect the nutritional condition of the patient. Many elderly persons simply do not care to eat because of ill-fitting dentures or poor oral health. In addition, the condition of the patient's temporomandibular joint and the presence of an oral disorder including loose teeth and dentures can make the difference between a smooth and safe anesthetic and a disastrous anesthetic outcome.

The risk for impaired nutritional intake is exacerbated by other factors, such as reduced salivary gland activity, receding gums, and thinner tooth enamel, with concomitant brittleness in the teeth. Esophageal mobility is reduced, and a more relaxed cardiac sphincter slows emptying in the esophagus. Moreover, weakened intestinal musculature and slower peristalsis in the lower gastrointestinal (GI) tract may lead to constipation. The confluence of these factors often results in poor nutrition. For the elderly surgical patient, this can have deleterious effects, especially for wound healing.

Life changes can also affect nutritional status. Of particular importance are the losses endured with aging, such as the loss of one's spouse, family, or friends through death or relocation; loss of a prior standard of living through retirement; and loss of physical or mental well-being. These changes can affect older persons to the point that they either cannot afford to buy nutritious foods or lose the ability or interest to prepare food. The ultimate effect, among other things, is a nutritionally debilitated patient. Any nutritional deficits should be corrected before surgery because the success of the operative procedure, the rate of wound healing, and the length of hospital stay are directly related to the nutritional state.

***Determination of Operative Risk.*** After assessment of the patient is completed, conditions that can add to the patient's operative risk may be identified (Box 30-5). Surgical procedures, including cardiac, abdominal, thoracic, and multiple operations performed on an emergency basis, significantly increase operative risk. Whenever possible, medical conditions are treated before surgery. Sometimes correction is not possible, and the risk of forestalling surgery outweighs any other medical problem. The determination of operative risk for the patient is generally based on the ASA physical status scale.[13] Although the anesthesia provider does the actual classification of the patient, familiarity with the parameters from which a decision is made is important:

- Class I: normal, healthy patient; no gross organic disease
- Class II: patient with mild to moderate systemic disease with functional impairment
- Class III: patient with severe systemic disease that limits activity but is not incapacitating
- Class IV: patient with incapacitating systemic disease that is a constant threat to life
- Class V: moribund patient not expected to survive 24 hours with or without the operation
- Class E: emergency procedure (applied to any classification above)

The most common surgical procedures in the elderly population that pose a greater risk of death are as follows:

- Acute intestinal vascular insufficiency
- Fracture of neck of femur
- Malignant neoplasm of colon
- Perforated diverticulum of colon
- Peripheral arterial occlusive disease
- Ruptured abdominal aortic or thoracic aneurysm[8]

Other factors that are considered in determining operative risk are the patient's cognitive and functional states. Surgeons and anesthesia providers can assess the patient's cognitive state through the use of tools such as the Folstein Mini Mental Status Evaluation (MMSE). The MMSE evaluates four areas: ori-

**BOX 30-5**

### Risk Factors for Surgery in Elders

**SURGICAL RISKS**
- Emergency surgery
- Site of surgery
- Vascular
- Aortic
- Intrathoracic
- Intraperitoneal
- Duration of procedure (more than 3.5 hours)

**ANESTHETIC RISKS**
- American Society of Anesthesiologists (ASA) classifications 3 to 5
- Age older than 75 years
- Preexisting medical disease (hypertension; diabetes mellitus; cardiac, renal, liver, or respiratory disease)

**DISEASE-RELATED RISKS**
- Cardiovascular
  - Angina
  - Previous myocardial infarction
  - Congestive heart failure
- Pulmonary
  - Bronchitis
  - Pneumonia
- Cigarette smoking
- Digestive
  - Poor nutritional status or malnutrition
  - Protein deficiency
  - Cirrhosis
  - Active peptic ulcer
- Endocrine
  - Adrenal insufficiency
  - Hypothyroidism

**COGNITIVE IMPAIRMENT**
- Dementia
- Acute confusional state (delirium)
- Alzheimer's disease

**OTHER FACTORS**
- Dehydration
- Anemia
- Recent stroke
- Malignancy
- Low albumin
- Impaired mobility
- Patient living in institutional care

Data from Barry PP and others: The elderly surgical patient. In Wilmore DW and others: *ACS surgery—principles and practice,* New York, 2002, WebMD Corp; Parker MJ and others: Surgery in elderly patients, *Current Orthopaedics* 18:333-344, 2004.

entation, registration, attention/calculation, and language. Points are assigned to each area; a perfect score is 30. A score below 24 indicates cognitive impairment, which may increase operative risk and increase the odds for postoperative complications. Functional status can be assessed through scoring the patient's ability to perform physical tasks. Each task is assigned a metabolic equivalent (MET). Tasks range from the ability to feed and dress oneself (1 MET) to the ability to participate in strenuous activity, such as football or skiing (10 METs). The inability to function above 4 METs is associated with increased perioperative cardiac events and long-term risk.[10]

## Nursing Diagnosis

In evaluating, synthesizing, and prioritizing the data collected during the preoperative assessment, the perioperative nurse can formulate nursing diagnoses that will form the basis of the plan of care.

Nursing diagnoses related to the care of geriatric surgical patients might include the following:

- Risk for Deficient Fluid Volume
- Ineffective Thermoregulation
- Risk for Impaired Skin Integrity
- Disturbed Sensory Perception (visual or auditory)
- Risk for Perioperative Positioning Injury
- Ineffective Therapeutic Regimen Management
- Risk for Infection

## Outcome Identification

Outcomes identified for the selected nursing diagnoses could be stated as follows:

- The patient will maintain age-appropriate fluid-volume levels intraoperatively and postoperatively.
- The patient will maintain normothermia ±1°F throughout the perioperative period.
- The patient's skin integrity will remain intact intraoperatively.
- The patient's perception and interpretation of environmental and sensory stimuli will be accurate throughout the perioperative period.
- The patient will be free from perioperative positioning injury.
- The patient receives appropriate medication or medications, safely administered during the perioperative period.
- The patient is free from signs and symptoms of infection.

## Planning

As a result of anatomic and physiologic effects of aging, geriatric patients have, in varying degrees, a general decline in organ function and an altered ability to recover from stressful events. In addition to normal age changes, many older adults experience one or more chronic conditions that influence the risk of surgery. Successful surgical outcomes in the geriatric patient depend on elective versus emergency surgical procedures, optimum physical condition of the patient, thorough preoperative assessment, close intraoperative and postoperative monitoring, and preventive measures to decrease the likelihood of complications. Collaboration with the entire surgical team can create an environment that is safe, efficient, and caring and provides for a positive patient outcome.

A typical plan of care for a geriatric surgical patient is shown on p. 1155-1156.

## Implementation

Perioperative geriatric patient care is very similar to the care provided to younger adults. However, modifications that involve consideration of age-specific differences between the two groups are made. The perioperative nurse who recognizes the special needs of the elderly patient during what may be the most critical period of hospitalization helps to enhance the course of surgical intervention and postoperative recovery (Patient Safety). All members of the surgical team must work together in all phases of the perioperative continuum to provide an environment that focuses on the needs of the patient.

***Preoperative Preparation.*** The preoperative period is an opportune time to evaluate the patient's psychosocial status and educational needs. As mentioned, the motivation of the patient can affect operative risk and successful surgical outcomes. Awareness of psychologic and emotional status is as important as awareness of physiologic status. Often the patient's concerns are focused on the spouse or other family members rather than on the impending surgery. An unexpected hospitalization can be very disruptive to an elderly patient who perhaps was the sole caretaker of an ill spouse, parent, or even a pet. In addition, the concern for quality of life and the fear of institutionalization after surgery can be extremely upsetting. This population has the highest morbidity and mortality rates in the adult population.[8] Using the assistance of the discharge planner or case manager to arrange for resources may help allay the patient's concerns.

Sensory deficits occurring either as a result of age-related changes or merely because eyeglasses and hearing aids are removed can make communication with geriatric patients more difficult. Unresponsive or uncooperative behavior may be inappropriately diagnosed as dementia, expected as part of aging, and ignored. As discussed, acute confusion or delirium in elders is the most important indicator of possible underlying conditions that could seriously and adversely affect surgical intervention and outcomes. Knowing whether the patient's cognitive impairment is recent or chronic will provide direction for planning postoperative care.

The perioperative nurse should take advantage of the time spent in the preadmission interview, presurgical care unit, preoperative holding, or the surgical corridor to introduce herself or himself and explain events to follow. Because a surgical mask is generally not required in these areas, this is the most opportune time for talking with the older adult. Once the patient is taken into the OR, a reassuring touch and remaining close to the patient, particularly during anesthesia induction, can help to decrease anxiety (Figure 30-5).

***Anesthesia Induction.*** Pertinent assessment data obtained by the perioperative nurse that may affect anesthesia are shared with anesthesia personnel. A medical history of asthma, previous patient or family anesthesia problems, abnormal laboratory data, and physical limitations affecting induction or airway management are important findings. The following anesthetic issues contribute to the morbidity and mortality of the older population:

- Active or unstable concurrent diseases
- Decreased mobility
- Intubation difficulties

## SAMPLE PLAN OF CARE

### NURSING DIAGNOSIS

**Risk for Deficient Fluid Volume** related to nothing-by-mouth (NPO) status and intraoperative blood and body fluid losses secondary to age-associated decrease in total body water and plasma volume

### OUTCOME

The patient will maintain age-appropriate fluid volume levels intraoperatively and postoperatively.

### INTERVENTIONS

- Review medical history for presence and number of chronic diseases.
- Review, document, and communicate significant abnormal laboratory findings.
- Monitor and record intraoperative intake and output.
- Monitor and calculate estimated blood loss on sponges and in suction canisters.
- Distinguish between blood and irrigation fluid amounts in suction canister or canisters.
- Ensure visibility of the urine drainage bag.
- Ensure availability of blood and fluid replacement products as needed.
- Monitor and report intake and output to anesthesia provider, surgeon, and postanesthesia care unit (PACU) nurse.

### NURSING DIAGNOSIS

**Ineffective Thermoregulation** related to poikilothermy secondary to age-associated physiologic decompensation

### OUTCOME

The patient will maintain normothermia (±1°F) throughout the perioperative period.

### INTERVENTIONS

- Identify risk factors for unplanned hypothermia.
- Use warm blankets during transport to the operating room (OR), and replenish as needed throughout the perioperative period (include the patient's feet within blanket covering).
- Adjust and maintain ambient room temperature at comfortable levels.
- Place warmed sheet on OR bed before patient transfer.
- Use active warming intraoperatively by applying forced air–warming system.
- Monitor patient's temperature.
- Provide additional head covering (cloth, plastic, or reflective) during surgical procedures.
- Minimize exposure of patient.
- Use warmed irrigation and preparation solutions (as recommended by manufacturer).
- Administer warmed blood and blood products and intravenous (IV) fluids at room temperature.
- Remove wet linens before transport to PACU.

### NURSING DIAGNOSIS

**Risk for Impaired Skin Integrity** related to preoperative and intraoperative procedures secondary to alterations in skin turgor, sensation, peripheral tissue perfusion, and skeletal prominence

### OUTCOME

The patient's skin integrity will remain intact intraoperatively.

### INTERVENTIONS

- Review risk factors for intraoperative pressure ulcer development.
- Assess potential pressure areas before anesthesia and positioning, noting bruises, sores, skin tears, rashes, lesions, and pressure ulcers.
- Avoid friction and shearing forces by using a four-person lift, a liftsheet, or lifting device when transferring patient to or from OR bed and turning patient into desired surgical position.
- Prevent wrinkling of linen under the patient or positioning devices.
- Place electrosurgical dispersive pad in the most appropriate area while avoiding bony prominences.
- Avoid pooling of solutions under the patient.
- Apply tape sparingly to prevent skin injury during removal. If tape must be used, consider paper tape or a nonadherent dressing on fragile skin. Gauze wrap, stockinette, or tape alternatives may also be considered.
- Position the patient.
- Evaluate for signs and symptoms of physical injury to skin and tissue.

### NURSING DIAGNOSIS

**Disturbed Sensory Perception** (visual or auditory) related to removal of eyeglasses or hearing aid in the OR secondary to age-associated changes in sensory organs

### OUTCOME

The patient's perception and interpretation of environmental and sensory stimuli will be accurate throughout the perioperative period.

### INTERVENTIONS

- If the patient uses an assistive device (e.g., hearing aid), leave in place as long as possible. Provide necessary information before removing assistive device.
- Remove OR mask to introduce self and explain procedures before surgery.
- Ask the patient to state his or her name, and continue to call the patient by stated name.
- Attract the patient's attention before speaking.
- Face the patient directly and on the same level (when possible) while speaking.
- Speak slowly and distinctly in a low-pitched, clear voice, frequently rephrasing and verifying communication.
- Control noise in the surgical setting.
- Use gestures to supplement words.
- Write instructions as needed to clarify information; use matte-finish paper.
- Allow ample time for patient to ask questions.
- Prepare patient for changes in light intensity, and allow time to adapt to lighting changes.
- Assist patient with transfers and mobility.
- Inform patient before positioning or procedures done before anesthesia.

### NURSING DIAGNOSIS

**Risk for Perioperative Positioning Injury** related to positioning procedures secondary to musculoskeletal changes and associated chronic pain

### OUTCOME

The patient will be free from perioperative positioning injury.

### INTERVENTIONS

- Assess pain and skeletal/range-of-motion limitations before anesthesia and positioning.

*Continued*

## SAMPLE PLAN OF CARE

**INTERVENTIONS—cont'd**

- Assess potential pressure areas before anesthesia and positioning.
- Place safety strap above the knees; prevent undue pressure on the popliteal space and heels.
- Provide adequate padding to protect potential pressure areas.
- Maintain body alignment within restrictions imposed by chronic pain and musculoskeletal age-related changes.
- Use gentleness during positioning and turning.
- Keep head and neck in a comfortable position that limits hyperextension.

**NURSING DIAGNOSIS**

**Ineffective Therapeutic Regimen Management**

**OUTCOME**

The patient receives appropriate medications, safely administered during the perioperative period.

**INTERVENTIONS**

- Administer prescribed antibiotic therapy and immunizing agents as ordered.
- Administer prescribed medications and solutions.
- Administer prescribed prophylactic treatments.
- Label all medications on the sterile field.
- Validate medication orders with perioperative team.

**NURSING DIAGNOSIS**

**Risk for Infection**

**OUTCOME**

The patient is free from signs and symptoms of infection.

**INTERVENTIONS**

- Implement aseptic technique.
- Monitor for signs and symptoms of infection.
- Initiate traffic control.
- Administer care to invasive device sites.
- Assess susceptibility for infection.
- Protect from cross-contamination.

## PATIENT SAFETY

### Prevention of Deep Vein Thrombosis in the Elderly

Providing safe care for older adults in the perioperative setting requires a thorough knowledge of the changes associated with aging and risk factors for surgical complications. One change associated with aging is the increased risk for the development of deep vein thrombosis (DVT). The chances for developing DVT increase with age and double each decade of life over the age of 40 years. For example, a person who is 80 years old is twice as likely to develop DVT as someone who is 70 years old and 16 times more likely as someone who is 40 years old.

DVT is triggered by the Virchow triad: venostasis, hypercoagulability, and vessel wall inflammation, which leads to intravascular coagulation and the formation of a structureless mass of red blood cells, fibrin, and other cellular components. Several risk factors may increase the likelihood of DVT in an older person and include the following:

- Immobility; physical limitations that influence ambulation and movement
- Congestive heart failure
- Hypertension
- Use of diuretics, which contribute to dehydration and hypercoagulability
- Obesity
- Smoking
- Varicose veins
- Atherosclerosis

Prevention of DVT in the older person begins in the preoperative phase of care. Whenever possible, the nurse should contact the patient well in advance of the planned procedure to begin education on DVT precautions. Before surgery, patients should avoid long airline travel or immobility. Walking and increasing the activity level before surgery can improve the patient's venous return as well as overall health state. Unless contraindicated by the patient's condition or physician's order, the nurse should advise patients to drink adequate fluids up until the time of their nothing-by-mouth (NPO) status to help maintain hydration. Whenever possible, the patient should be instructed on leg exercises (ankle rolls, leg lifts, etc.) to be performed before and after the surgery.

When the patient arrives in the preoperative area the nurse should consult with the surgeon to ensure that antiembolic stockings or sequential compression sleeves are ordered for the patient. Antiembolic stockings improve venous return by squeezing the valves of the vein closed, preventing pooling and stagnation of blood in the lower extremities. Sequential compression devices, which alternately inflate and deflate, serve to push the blood in the extremities back toward the heart. The nurse should demonstrate the leg exercises to be performed in the postoperative period and assess the patient's understanding and mastery through return demonstration and also discuss the benefits of early ambulation.

Before induction, the nurse ensures the patient's antiembolic stockings are placed correctly with no wrinkles or rolling that might impede venous return and verifies that the sequential compression device is functioning normally. If the patient's feet are accessible during long procedures, the nurse should perform periodic passive range-of-motion exercises to maximize venous blood return (if possible without compromising the sterile field).

The nurse encourages the patient to move his or her legs and perform the recommended exercises as soon as possible in the postanesthesia care unit (PACU). The PACU staff should reinforce the preoperative teaching about DVT prevention and ensure the patient's caregiver also understands the instructions.

Pharmaceutical prophylaxis for DVT may be a consideration in some patients. Medications used for DVT prophylaxis are described in Chapter 22.

Modified from Dunn D: Preventing perioperative complications in an older adult, *Nursing* 34(11):36-41, 2004; Koschel MJ: Pulmonary embolism, quick diagnosis can save a patient's life, *American Journal of Nursing* 104(6):46-50; 2004, *Understanding deep vein thrombosis.* Accessed April 22, 2006, on-line: www.clotcare.com/clotcare/dvt.aspx.

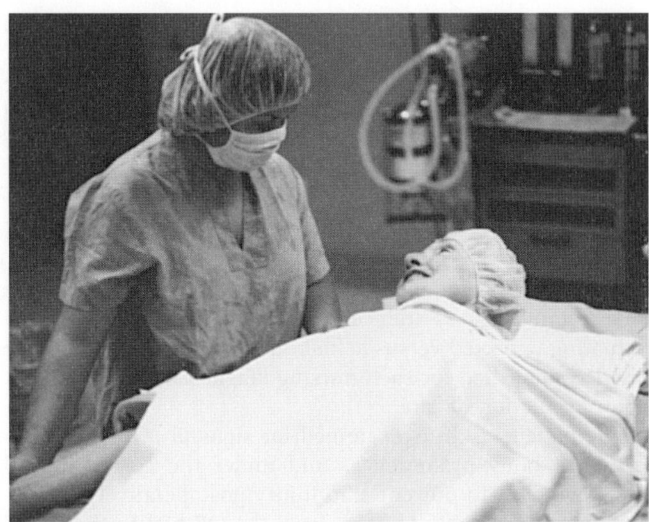

**FIGURE 30-5** Perioperative nurse's presence and reassuring touch help to allay the patient's anxiety before anesthesia induction.

- Gravity of the surgical procedure
- Myocardial depression from anesthetic agents
- Potentially altered respiratory and cardiac reserves

Elderly patients frequently have changes in airway anatomy that make appropriate ventilation difficult. Changes in facial contour from sunken cheeks or lack of dentition can result in an inadequately fitting anesthesia mask. Keeping dentures in place often offsets this problem; however, if intubation is planned, dentures are usually removed. The joints of the head and neck may exhibit limited range of motion, making intubation and airway management more difficult in elders. Identification of these potential problems before anesthesia administration facilitates a smooth induction period.

The choice of anesthesia in the elderly patient depends on physiologic status, length of the operative procedure, and preference of the anesthesia provider. IV sedation with local anesthesia may be selected for herniorrhaphy or other procedures that do not entail complicated manipulation of organs. Regional anesthesia (e.g., spinal, femoral, brachial, axillary, or peribulbar blocks) may be chosen over general anesthesia for specific surgical procedures (e.g., cataract extraction, transurethral resection of prostate [TURP]) because blood loss, deep vein thrombosis, and pulmonary embolism are less likely to occur.[13] Orthopedic surgical procedures, such as hip fractures or knee replacements, may be effective with the use of spinal anesthesia. Flexibility of the elderly patient or the presence of arthritic problems must be considered before attempting a spinal anesthetic. Geriatric patients undergoing vascular or abdominal surgical procedures may obtain positive results with epidural anesthesia postoperatively for the management of pain.[1]

Accurate predictions of how the elderly patient will respond to drugs or anesthesia are difficult to make because of a decrease in systems function. Older patients have both an altered pharmacodynamic (relation between plasma concentration and drug effect) and pharmacokinetic (distribution and elimination of drugs) response to drugs. These physiologic changes can affect medication administration because of a longer or shorter duration of action and less predictable effects. This is important in understanding the increased incidence of side effects. The increasing age of the patient decreases the dose requirement of anesthesia. This includes agents that induce anesthesia (e.g., thiopental sodium, etomidate, propofol) and narcotics. The induction dose of a barbiturate required for a 70-year-old patient will be less than that for patients 20 to 30 years old. Minimal blood levels of a drug may produce undesired side effects before therapeutic levels are reached. Likewise, reduced liver and kidney function, altered body composition, decreased albumin, and decreased cardiac output all modify the aged person's ability to eliminate drugs from the body. Age-related changes in homeostatic mechanisms affect the older adult's ability to deal with physiologic stresses of surgery, such as fluid depletion, volume overload, or hypoxemia. Mild hypothermia of only 1°C to 3°C below normal can increase postoperative myocardial ischemia and ventricular tachycardia. Incidence of hypothermia is greatest with combined epidural-general anesthesia.[13] The perioperative nurse should be prepared to respond quickly in assisting the anesthesia provider to stabilize the patient when adverse reactions occur.

***Positioning.*** Protection of skin integrity is of utmost importance. Loss of subcutaneous fat, poor skin turgor, and tissue fragility can worsen a postoperative skin problem. Elderly patients should be lifted into position, rather than slid or dragged, to prevent shearing injuries. Aging changes in the musculoskeletal system accentuate bony prominences and decrease the range of motion. These skeletal changes coupled with limitations imposed by chronic pain make positioning one of the most important considerations of care. The provision of appropriate positioning devices is pivotal to the protection from injury for this population of surgical patients.

Often, because of musculoskeletal deformity and chronic pain, elderly patients cannot fully extend the spine, neck, or upper and lower extremities. Using padding devices to compensate for these limitations not only makes the patient more comfortable during the procedure but also prevents residual pain or injury postoperatively (Figure 30-6). Depending on the

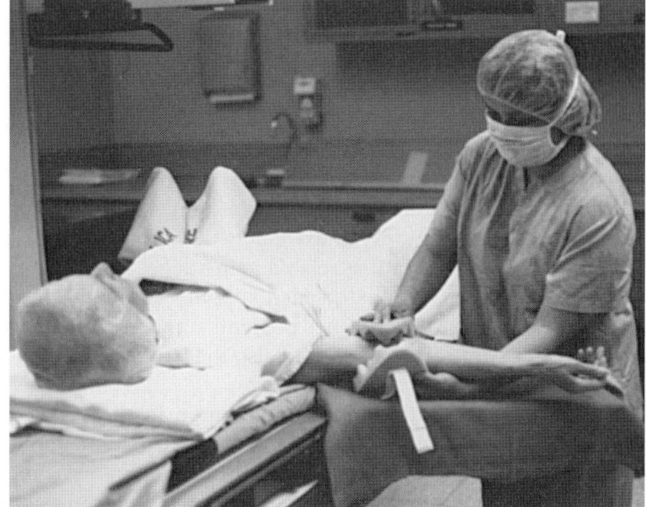

**FIGURE 30-6** Adequate padding aids patient comfort and prevents injury and residual postoperative pain.

situation, positioning the patient before anesthesia induction may be best so that the patient can direct positioning efforts in regard to comfort.

***Skin Preparation and Thermoregulation.*** Temperature fluctuations are common in elders as a result of impaired thermoregulation. Response to cold, including vasoconstriction and shivering, is diminished in elders, and the core temperature must be lower to trigger a response than that required in younger adults. Increasing the ambient OR temperature will help stabilize effects of heat loss. Devices such as warmed blankets or temperature-regulating blankets are highly recommended, particularly when a lengthy surgical procedure is expected. Special care should be taken by the perioperative nurse to prevent injury, such as burns, to the elderly patient with the use of such devices. Prepping solutions should be carefully chosen to prevent skin irritation and should be warmed (if recommended by the manufacturer) to help decrease hypothermic effects. Ensuring that the patient is not lying in a prep solution or on wet linens also helps to reduce skin injury and inadvertent lowering of body temperature.

When the body is exposed to cold temperatures, blood is shunted away from peripheral body parts to the head. Because the head lacks fat depots and vasoconstriction capabilities, heat loss from the head can be as much as 25% to 60% of total body heat loss. Elderly patients should therefore have some form of head covering to prevent additional effects of inadvertent hypothermia. The patient's feet should be kept warm with cotton socks or paper slippers and inspected frequently for signs of infection.

***Aseptic Techniques and Safety Measures.*** Age-related changes in the functioning of the immune system and some age-associated diseases have a detrimental effect on the aging body's ability to appropriately respond to infectious agents. Because of early discharge from acute-care facilities resulting in longer nursing home stays, it is reported that the risk of developing a nosocomial infection in a nursing home is comparable with the risk in an acute-care facility, with rates of 3% to 15%.[6] In the lungs, the diminished cough reflex and ciliary action weaken specialized defense mechanisms against foreign-body invasion. Pneumonia is the second most common nosocomial infection after urinary tract infections (UTIs).[6] Incomplete emptying of the bladder can cause UTI, which causes significant morbidity in older adults.

Immobility and drug therapy can alter flora in the intestines and make the body more vulnerable to infectious organisms. Infection and delayed healing of wounds are poorly tolerated and often fatal in the debilitated elderly patient, so strict adherence to aseptic technique is extremely important. Because length of surgical procedure is related to incidence of infection, the nurse should ensure that needed supplies and equipment are readily available. This practice prevents unnecessary delays and decreases surgical exposure and also the length of time the elderly patient is under anesthesia.

Fluctuations in fluid volume are common in the geriatric patient. Volume deficits occur as a natural course of aging, whereas volume excess can occur from intraoperative fluid replacement. Careful measurement of intake and output is essential. Collaboration among the surgical team members regarding blood loss during the procedure can enable caregivers to be alert to complications before they occur. The team should closely monitor discarded sponges, suction canister contents, and urinary drainage as part of the volume assessment. The nurse reports intraoperative fluid volumes, estimated blood loss, and other parameters to the postanesthesia care unit (PACU) staff to ensure continuity of care and provide a mechanism for continued assessment and evaluation.

## Evaluation

Before transporting the patient to the PACU, the perioperative nurse should assess the care provided intraoperatively by evaluating expected versus actual outcomes. Specific outcome criteria established for each nursing diagnosis provide the basis for evaluation of care.

The patient's skin is examined for signs of injury, particularly over bony prominences and under the electrosurgical dispersive pad. To prevent skin injury postoperatively the patient should be carefully lifted from the OR bed to the PACU transport vehicle. Pain is assessed and compared with preoperative levels. Evaluation of musculoskeletal pain will determine intraoperative positioning effectiveness. Postoperative pain levels are closely monitored and treated throughout the postoperative period. Anticipated frequency of dressing change, as in a draining wound, should govern the method used to secure the dressing. A minimal amount of tape should be used because its removal can cause additional skin trauma. Depending on the wound site and character, rolled gauze, stockinette, or similar bandaging over the primary dressing may be the best choice so that tape is not applied directly to the skin. Another alternative is Montgomery straps. For smaller wounds, the least possible amount of hypoallergenic tape should be used. Because infection is poorly tolerated, the choice of dressing should maximize wound protection while being the least irritating to the skin.

The nurse collaborates with the anesthesia provider to complete and record the patient's intake and output. Because of the consequences of postoperative dehydration or fluid volume overload in the elderly patient, fluids are increased or decreased accordingly. Blood loss is carefully evaluated, recorded, and reported. The wound is closely observed for bleeding before dressing application and postoperatively because the elderly person's ability to recover from hemorrhage and shock is extremely poor.

Evaluation of body temperature is particularly important in elders because postoperative hypothermia is quite common and can precipitate agitation and confusion or delirium. To prevent any adverse response, the patient should be covered with warmed blankets and a forced air–warming unit used throughout the recovery period.

Depending on the patient's level of consciousness, explanation should be given about the impending transfer to the PACU as a form of reality orientation. As appropriate, the patient should be introduced to the PACU nurse and told what to expect in the unit (Figure 30-7). Explanations should always precede any procedure. Often the elderly person is reluctant to cooperate simply because no one has taken the time to explain what is going to happen.

Because of the relatively fine line between stability and the development of postoperative complications, the elderly patient's response to surgery must be closely evaluated. Verbal communication between the perioperative and PACU nurses should include any pertinent preoperative and intraoperative information that could affect postoperative care outcomes. This information includes pain levels; physical and sensory limitations; intake and output; allergies; type and location of catheters, drains, packing, and implantable devices; anesthesia and medications received; and any unusual occurrences that could affect the patient's recovery (Figure 30-8). Perioperative nurses should be aware of the risk for the phenomenon known as postoperative delirium, a condition that can occur in elderly patients. Box 30-6 gives the most frequently identified preoperative risk factors for postoperative delirium.

Documentation of outcome evaluation can be phrased as follows:

- Skin integrity was maintained free from redness, bruises, and abrasions; patient reported no pain or impairment of the skin; and there were no apparent signs or symptoms of infection.
- Fluid balance was maintained; urinary output was within normal limits; the patient's forehead skin was checked and had good turgor; and vital signs were stable.
- Temperature was ±1°F of normal range; skin was warm to touch; and patient verbalized comfort.
- The patient accurately perceived and interpreted environmental stimuli, expressed and demonstrated understanding of procedures, and responded appropriately to auditory and verbal stimuli.
- Perioperative positioning injury was effectively prevented; and the patient had no complaints of increased pain and no compromise in musculoskeletal ability and range of motion from preoperative levels.
- Medications used during the intraoperative procedure caused no apparent adverse reaction.
- The type and extent of surgery may affect postoperative pain. Elderly persons may not complain of pain, but this does not indicate that pain does not exist. Those patients with cognitive impairment may experience pain but may be unable to verbalize it. Box 30-7 gives key elements of pain assessment and management in older adults.

Contemporary pain control delivery systems and techniques offer a variety of treatment routes and modalities. Various routes may be employed to deliver medication for pain control: oral, intramuscular, IV, regional (i.e., spinal or epidural), or patient-controlled analgesia (PCA). Cognitive modalities that may be employed are distraction, relaxation (i.e., biofeedback), or hypnosis. Physical modalities that may be used are cold, exercise, heat, immobilization/rest, massage, positioning, or transcutaneous electrical nerve stimulation (TENS).

Clinical management of pain should be multimodal and individualized for the patient, procedure, and circumstance. Evaluation of the balance between pain control and side effects

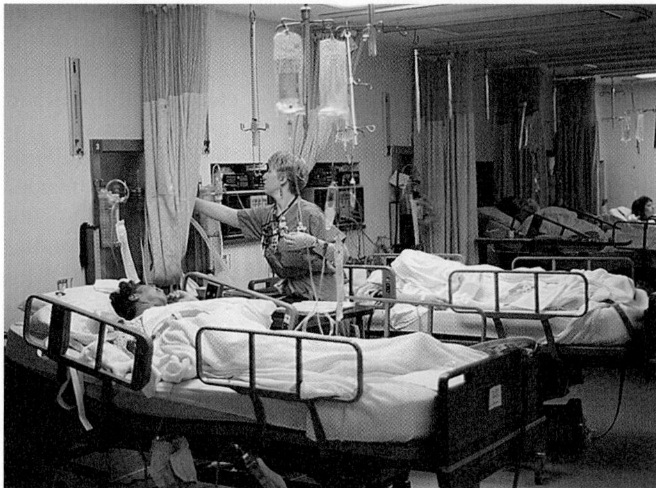

**FIGURE 30-7** Explanations of procedures and orientation to the environment are critical for the elderly patient in the busy postanesthesia care unit (PACU).

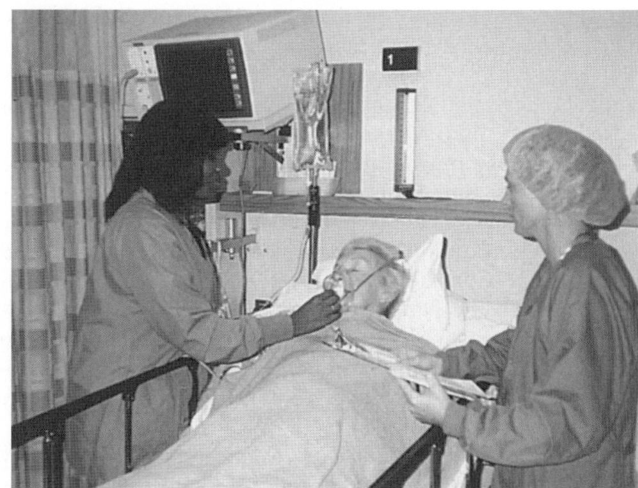

**FIGURE 30-8** Pertinent information that could affect postoperative care outcomes is communicated to the postanesthesia care unit (PACU) nurse.

**BOX 30-6**

### Preoperative Risk Factors for Postoperative Delirium in Elders

- Age 80 years or older
- Alcohol or sedative-hypnotic withdrawal
- Depression
- Drug interaction or polypharmacy; duration of anesthesia
- Endocrine and metabolic problems
- High stress or anxiety levels
- History of dementia-like symptoms
- Low mobility
- Presence of multiple diseases
- Sensory impairments
- Surgical procedures considered major in nature
- Dehydration
- Low serum albumin level
- Abnormal preoperative serum sodium, glucose, or potassium level
- American Society of Anesthesiologists (ASA) class III or IV
- Uncontrolled pain
- Urinary elimination problems

Modified from Saufl NM: Preparing the older adult for surgery and anesthesia, *Journal of PeriAnesthesia Nursing* 19(6):372-378, 2004; Sieber FE, Pauldine R: Anesthesia and the elderly. In Miller RD: *Miller's anesthesia,* vol 2, ed 6, Philadelphia, 2005, Churchill Livingstone.

BOX 30-7

**Pain and Older Adults**

**PREVALENCE OF PAIN**

Recognize that older adults are at great risk for undertreated pain.

**BELIEFS ABOUT PAIN**

In addition to receiving less analgesia, older adults tend to report pain less often than do younger adults. These findings may be related to beliefs and concerns about pain and the reporting of pain. Many older people hold the following beliefs and concerns about pain:

- Pain is something that must be lived with.
- Expressing pain is unacceptable or is a sign of weakness.
- Complaining of pain will result in being labeled as a "bad" patient.
- Nurses are too busy to listen to complaints of pain.
- Pain signifies a serious illness or impending death.

Nurses should be aware of the beliefs of older patients regarding pain management. Nurses and other caregivers often undermedicate these patients and are sometimes reluctant to administer the prescribed analgesics.

**ASSESSMENT**

- Ask about present pain only.
- Use a standard scale, such as the numeric faces or Iowa thermometer rating scale.
- Explain the scale each time it is used.
- Use verbal descriptions other than pain, such as "ache," "sore," and "hurt."
- Use visual representations of pain measures rather than mental images of pain rating scales, Be sure that the patient is wearing glasses and hearing aids if needed and available.
- Alter a written pain scale to include large lettering, adequate space between the lines, nonglossy paper, and color for increased visualization.
- Provide adequate lighting and privacy to avoid distracting background noise.

**CONSIDERATION FOR COGNITIVELY IMPAIRED PATIENTS**

- Assess for nonverbal indications of pain (facial expressions, grimacing, vocalizations, body movements, behavioral changes).
- Remember to "assume pain is present" in cognitively impaired patients in the perioperative setting.
- Consider an analgesic trial.

**MANAGEMENT OF PAIN**

- Beware of adverse effects of acetaminophen (hepatotoxicity and nephrotoxicity) and nonsteroidal antiinflammatory drugs (NSAIDs) (gastrointestinal [GI] bleeding and nephrotoxicity).
- Start low and go slow with opioid dosing.
- Avoid the use of meperidine, codeine, and propoxyphene.
- Use methadone and tramadol with caution.
- Older adults and those with renal disease should not take meperidine because of the prolonged half-life of its drug metabolite, normeperidine.
- Use nondrug pain relief measures.

Modified from McGuire L: Pain: the fifth vital sign. In Ignatavicius DD, Workman ML, editors: *Medical-surgical nursing: critical thinking for collaborative care,* ed 5, St Louis, 2006, Saunders.

should be documented, timely, routine, and specific. Patient and family education that begins in all phases of the care continuum decreases anxiety and improves patient outcomes and pain management.

## Patient and Family Education and Discharge Planning

Education should be conducted at a time when the patient is at rest rather than during preoperative or postoperative procedures. Too many stimuli from outside sources can interfere with the patient's ability to concentrate and motivation to learn. Physical comfort and privacy should be ensured. Education will be ineffective in the patient who is uncomfortable or in pain. Age-related changes can affect the elderly patient's ability to learn new material; therefore modification of traditional teaching approaches should be used to enhance effectiveness. Patient education should be individualized based on how the patient will best understand the information.

A comprehensive discharge plan should identify and address communication barriers, incorporate the patient's current mental and physical condition, address environmental issues that can be improved to support recovery, and diminish the social support challenges.[3] Sensory changes in vision and hearing, cognitive impairment, and literacy level can be communication barriers that interfere with the patient's ability to understand and retain information. Giving the patient postoperative instructions in written form helps with retention, and modifications using large, easy-to-read typeface on matte-finish paper of warm tones (yellow, tan) make them easier to read. It may be helpful to have a magnifying glass available and supplemental light on the object or surface involved in the teaching/learning activity. Family members or significant others who are present should be included in the educational session so that they can provide reinforcement at home.

The discharge plan should consider the patient's ability to perform ADLs, ambulate, and manage his or her preexisting medical condition after surgery. The older person's basic medical condition does not change because of surgery.[3] Content should focus only on relevant information about surgical procedures or postoperative recoveries; relating it to previous life experiences helps the patient grasp the concepts more readily. The nurse should provide the most important information first. If motor skills (i.e., crutch walking, dressing change) are involved, all steps should be taught one at a time and mastery should be demonstrated before moving to the next step. Increased time is often necessary when teaching motor skills.

Discharge planning begins during the preoperative assessment. Sufficient time is needed to make appropriate decisions about postdischarge care to prevent complications, reduce the risk of rehospitalization, and minimize stress to the patient and the caregivers. Consideration should be given to the environment to which the patient will go following the surgery. Although the plan should consider that older adults prefer to keep their autonomy, the postoperative care may require special facilities, such as a rehabilitation center or long-term care facility, at least for a time.

The type of surgery and expected postoperative recovery period determine the extent of resources and social systems needed, such as durable medical equipment, home health and homemaker services, extended care, social and community services, and physical rehabilitation. The success of postdischarge outcomes in elders is influenced by the patient's self-assessment of health as good or excellent, complexity of the patient's medical condition, history of being able to maintain responsibility for his or her own health, and family or social networks. Discharge needs of the patient should be evaluated as early as possible so that appropriate education, referrals, and home preparation can be completed before the patient leaves the hospital or ambulatory facility.

# *Surgical Interventions*

Surgical procedures that are common among the geriatric population are governed more by pathologic condition than by anatomy and are directly related to the common diseases affecting older adults. Healing is an important consideration in the decision to perform surgery on this population. The level of tissue oxygen is the main factor in determining wound healing and is influenced by factors such as cardiovascular status and anemia. Other factors are included in Box 30-8. In the text that follows, some surgical procedures that are commonly seen in elderly patients are briefly discussed. Reference is made to other sections of the text for a more in-depth description of the technical aspects of the procedures.

## COMMON SURGICAL PROCEDURES IN GERIATRIC PATIENTS

It is believed that the demographic structure of the population is a major influence on the numbers of surgical procedures performed on that population. In addition, a greater understanding and acceptance of the appropriateness of surgery in the older adult have affected the demand for and trending of surgical procedures in elders.

It is becoming common for patients well past 85 years of age to have surgery with relatively good outcomes. Decisions are no longer based solely on surgical risk but rather on optimal disease management and the preservation of quality of life. This shift in thinking has taken us beyond just getting the patient through the surgery and has produced a genuine concern about what the surgery will do for patients in the remaining years of life.

**BOX 30-8**

**Factors That Influence Wound Healing**

- Anemia
- Congestive heart failure
- Diabetes
- Hepatic failure
- Hypothyroidism
- Hypovolemia
- Malignancy
- Nutrition (protein, glucose, minerals, vitamins A and C)
- Peripheral vascular disease
- Renal failure
- Rheumatoid arthritis

Data from Parker MJ and others: Surgery in elderly patients, *Current Orthopaedics* 18:333-344, 2004.

### Thyroid Surgery

In the elderly population, thyroid gland dysfunction is common and associated with significant morbidity because the symptoms are often subtle, absent, or confused with co-existing diseases. Hypothyroidism occurs in 10% to 15% of patients older than 60 years and is more frequent in females than males.[9]

Typical symptoms of thyroid disorders may be absent or erroneously attributed to co-morbid conditions or normal aging. The polypharmacy used in the treatment of elderly patients can interfere with normal thyroid function. Drugs such as lithium or amiodarone may cause primary hyperthyroidism. For example, an elderly man taking medication for hypertension, congestive heart failure, and atrial fibrillation with complaints of fatigue, weakness, constipation, and weight gain may be considered to have these symptoms because of medication or medical conditions, whereas the symptoms could also be caused by hypothyroidism.

A rare complication of hypothyroidism, myxedema coma, affects patients older than 75 years. Confusion, disorientation, lethargy, thinning eyebrows and hair, hoarse voice, bradycardia, cardiomegaly, pericardial effusion, hypothermia, hyponatremia, and pseudomyotonic reflexes characterize this condition. The patient should receive support in the intensive care unit for ventilation and IV therapy with levothyroxine.

The great masquerader in the elderly population is hyperthyroidism and can easily be missed in patients older than 60 years. It can be severe and even life threatening. Elderly patients may not have a goiter, exophthalmos, or other ophthalmopathy. Hyperthyroidism may also cause osteoporosis. Almost any condition that can make a person ill can cause euthyroid sick syndrome; so elders are more susceptible because of their co-morbid conditions. Medication to suppress the gland, surgery to remove the hyperfunctioning tissue, and radioactive iodine (RAI) to destroy the gland are the three treatment options. Although surgery is a less attractive option, it must be employed when RAI is ineffective in the presence of a single nodule or multinodular toxic goiter or when the patient has dysphagia, tracheal compression, or suspected malignancy. Following surgery, the perioperative nurse must be aware of the possibility of a hyperthyroid storm that can be precipitated by the stress of the procedure, systemic infections, and anesthesia induction.

Until the treatment regimen is effective, patients require intensive care with close supervision.[9] (See Chapter 16 for an in-depth description of operations of the thyroid.)

### Abdominal Surgery

Accurate diagnosis of abdominal disease is important in elders to plan timely and appropriate surgical interventions. However, clinical signs of abdominal disease, such as tenderness, pain, muscle rigidity, and fever, are frequently less obvious in elderly patients. The common use of nonsteroidal antiinflammatory drugs (NSAIDs) may mask symptoms or even predispose elderly patients to acute abdominal disease.

The most common causes of acute abdominal complaints in older patients are biliary tract disease, intestinal obstruction,

GI hemorrhage, hernia, diverticulitis, and appendicitis. Thus common abdominal procedures in people older than 65 years include cholecystectomy, lysis of adhesions, appendectomy, and partial excision of the small bowel.[10]

Most often, surgery is performed for complications of calculus disease and less often for malignant obstruction of the bile ducts. The incidence of gallstones increases with age. Because laparotomy is a stressor in older ill patients, laparoscopic cholecystectomy is considered the preferred surgical approach in elderly patients with both symptomatic and asymptomatic gallstone disease. (See Chapter 12 for an in-depth description of operations of the biliary tract.)

The age-group older than 65 years has seen an increase of ulcer disease. Many believe that the higher incidence of *Helicobacter pylori* infection, prevalent use of NSAIDs, and prevalence of cigarette smoking in elders account for the age-related differences. Up to 80% of peptic ulcer–related deaths occur in patient older than 65 years.[10]

In selecting the procedure, the surgeon considers the patient's overall condition, history of chronic versus acute ulcer symptoms, and ulcer location. In poor-risk patients, suture plication with vagotomy and pyloroplasty can lessen the operative risk. Elderly patients tolerate a surgical procedure better than they tolerate prolonged or recurrent bleeding. (See Chapter 11 for an in-depth description of ulcer surgery.)

## Hernia

The estimated incidence of abdominal wall hernia in persons older than 65 years is 13 per 1000, with a fourfold to eightfold increase in the incidence in men. Fifty percent of all hernias are indirect inguinal, 20% are direct inguinal, 10% are ventral, 6% are femoral, 3% are umbilical, and 1% are esophageal hiatal.[10] The elective repair of inguinal and femoral hernias is strongly advised because of the risk of incarceration with subsequent emergency operation. Many hernia repairs in elderly patients are emergency procedures because of incarcerations and small bowel obstruction. When elective, the operation may be performed as an ambulatory procedure; IV sedation and local anesthesia provide a very satisfactory alternative to general or spinal anesthesia.

Laparoscopic techniques for hernia repair have gained popularity because of associated shorter hospital stay, minimal pain postoperatively, and early recovery. However, the necessity for general anesthesia makes this approach one that may not be advisable in elders. Decisions for local versus spinal or general anesthesia are made based on the patient's overall physiologic status and surgical risk.

In elderly men the coexistence of inguinal hernia and prostatism is fairly common. Depending on the size of the prostate, the hernia repair should be postponed until after the prostate surgery.

Not unusual in elders are large, neglected scrotal hernias. The repair of these hernias is not routine in that the abdominal wall defect may be so large that primary repair cannot take place without tension. Synthetic abdominal wall replacements are helpful in management of such large hernias. The repair of huge scrotal hernias can have a tremendous benefit on the personality of the geriatric patient, who is much relieved after removal of what can be considered an accessory appendage that is offensive, difficult to clean, and often an impedance to daily activities. (See Chapter 13 for an in-depth description of herniorrhaphy.)

## Genitourinary Surgery

The predominant reason for urologic surgery in elderly men is benign prostatic hypertrophy (BPH). BPH may be silent or have minimal symptoms in the presence of severe bladder decompensation. As part of history taking, it is important to determine if symptoms such as dysuria, strangury, and hematuria exist. Prostate surgery, especially transurethral prostatectomy (TURP), is relatively safe and generally well tolerated. The majority of BPH operations are performed to relieve symptoms, such as nocturia, slow stream, intermittency, and double voiding. TURP is indicated if the surgeon believes that total resection can be accomplished in 1 hour and that no bladder disease or impairment to urethral access is present.

A surgical alternative to TURP is transurethral incision of the prostate (TUIP). The resectoscope knife is used to make a full-thickness cut through the prostate from the bladder neck through the apex of the prostate with no tissue resection. The complications associated with TUIP are significantly fewer than those occurring after TURP, especially bleeding, retrograde ejaculation, and impotence. It is a more desirable alternative to TURP for patients with prostates weighing less than 30 g. Other alternatives are laser prostatectomy, transurethral vaporization of the prostate, microwave hyperthermia, and transurethral needle ablation. These techniques are gaining acceptance because they can be done as outpatient procedures using local anesthesia.[8] (See Chapter 15 for an in-depth description of prostate surgery.)

## Ophthalmic Surgery

Because of elders' long life span, undergoing eye surgery (most commonly for cataracts) is more likely than other surgical procedures. Most ophthalmic procedures are minimally invasive and have a high success rate. Because elderly patients may have concurrent systemic disease, even a low-stress procedure should not be treated lightly. Age-related changes, such as hearing loss and musculoskeletal disease, may pose a challenge during ophthalmic surgery where the patient must lie still for long periods and be able to follow verbal instructions. Patients with chronic lung disease lying in the supine position may experience coughing, which can increase intraocular pressure and jeopardize the outcome of the surgery.

Cataract surgery is among the most common ophthalmic surgical procedures performed in older adults. Some degree of cataract formation is expected in all people older than 70 years of age.[18] The majority of these procedures are performed in an ambulatory setting, with patients returning home the day of surgery. Cataracts are associated with factors including trauma, inflammation, genetic predisposition, metabolic disease, and cigarette smoking, but aging is by far the most common factor. Most eye surgery patients make the decision to have the procedure done after months of deliberation and slow, progressive loss of vision. The overall risk of death is low and does not change much whether local or general anesthetic is used. Intraocular lenses can be safely implanted in the majority of patients. Microsurgical wound closure ensures a secure incision that allows immediate ambulation. The surgical stress is considered so low and visual rehabilitation so rapid that severe visual impairment is considered a reasonable indication to perform surgery even if the elderly patient is debilitated. (See Chapter 18 for an in-depth description of cataract surgery.)

## Orthopedic Surgery

Osteoporosis is the most obvious skeletal change that occurs with advancing age. It leads to susceptibility to fracture, which doubles every 5 years after 50 years of age. An approximate loss of 25% to 40% of the mineral content of the bone must be present before detectable change is evident on x-ray films.[7] To some degree, osteoporosis is related to a lessening of physical activity, but other risk factors are female gender, Northern European ancestry, multiparity, lean body build, and excessive alcohol intake.[7] Osteoporosis is also related to decreased hormonal secretion; thus postmenopausal women are more prone to develop the condition and therefore more likely to sustain a hip fracture.

Age-related changes in bone increase the incidence of displaced femoral and intertrochanteric fractures of the upper femur. The incidence of hip fracture increases with advancing age, is more common in women, and is higher in institutionalized patients. Because the usual cause of death in patients with upper femur fracture is pulmonary embolus, surgery is designed to relieve the severe pain, allow movement in and out of bed, and return the patient to his or her former environment as quickly as possible with minimal debilitation. Between 25% and 50% of individuals who sustain hip fractures are more dependent after the fracture, with deterioration occurring more often in women over the age of 75 years, those with a poor clinical result, and those who were already dependent before the fracture.[15]

A displaced femoral neck fracture must be surgically repaired or healing will not occur. In elderly patients, 70 years and older, prosthetic replacement is usually done because it allows for early ambulation and will last throughout the remaining years of the patient's life. Intertrochanteric and subtrochanteric fractures are best treated with internal fixation. These methods also allow for early mobility.

Degenerative joint disease (osteoarthritis) and inflammatory polyarticular disease (rheumatoid arthritis) are the primary indications for total joint replacement in the hip and knee. In these patients, pain that disrupts normal daily activities and interrupts sleep is the major reason for surgery regardless of the patient's age. Octogenarians and nonagenarians achieve successful pain relief and report satisfaction after the procedure. Methylmethacrylate bone cement is often used in orthopedic procedures in spite of its cardiotoxic effect. Cardiac arrest from cement insertion is a risk that frail patients may be susceptible to. Supplemental inspired oxygen at the time of insertion, irrigation of the bone to remove excessive marrow elements, and insertion of the cement retrograde are methods to prevent the risk of adverse effects.[8] Usually knee replacement procedures are elective, and patients have better functional status and a higher bone mass than those with hip fracture. (See Chapter 22 for an in-depth description of hip and knee surgery.)

## Vascular and Cardiovascular Surgery

The most frequent vascular conditions treated surgically in the older population are abdominal aortic aneurysms, carotid artery disease, and peripheral vascular disease. In patients 65 years and older the mortality from elective aneurysm repair is less than 5% in spite of existing co-morbidities. Emergency repair for ruptured aneurysm carries an operative mortality of more than 50%.[10] Peripheral vascular surgery for limb salvage can be safely performed in patients older than 80 years of age and may be indicated for ischemic rest pain and nonhealing ulcers.

Cardiovascular disease is a significant cause of death in older patients. More than 55% of coronary artery bypass graft procedures are performed on patients older than 65 years of age. Several risk factors associated with increased mortality include emergency procedure, severe left ventricular dysfunction, mitral insufficiency requiring combined procedure, elevated preoperative creatinine level, chronic obstructive pulmonary disease (COPD), anemia, and prior vascular surgery. Factors associated with morbidity in the elderly population include obesity, diabetes mellitus, aortic stenosis, and cerebrovascular disease.[10]

(See Chapters 26 and 27 for a more in-depth description of vascular and cardiac surgery.)

# ADDITIONAL CONSIDERATIONS

Every surgical procedure carries with it a certain amount of risk no matter what the age of the patient. With increasing life expectancy, the number of surgical procedures on older adults will increase. Nonetheless, the physiologic deficits of aging increase surgical risk in the aged patient just as co-morbidity and emergent surgery do. Procedures that are performed in the thorax or the peritoneal cavity are considered high risk. Procedures of moderate risk include vascular and hip procedures, and low-risk procedures include prostatectomy and mastectomy. However, any procedure, even those considered low risk, can have poor outcomes, depending on the patient's overall condition. Caution is advised even with the ever-increasing numbers of minimally invasive surgeries (e.g., laparoscopy). It seems logical that elders would benefit from smaller incisions that produce less postoperative pain, atelectasis, and ileus. However, the extent of hemodynamic and pulmonary consequences of $CO_2$ pneumoperitoneum is still unclear. In patients with severe cardiac or pulmonary disease, recommendations include invasive monitoring to maintain adequate volume loading and alternate gas sources or gasless techniques.

When surgical intervention is being considered in elders, it is important to remember the following:

- Age alone should not be a barrier to surgery in elders.
- Elderly persons with conditions treatable by surgery have as much right to benefit from modern surgery, anesthesia, and medical and intensive care techniques as younger patients have.
- Medical and surgical techniques that can enhance the older person's life should be equally available to patients regardless of age.
- Elderly patients have special needs because of their atypical presentation of disease, multiple medical disorders or co-morbidity, impaired homeostasis, and altered drug response.
- Most elderly patients are mentally competent and should therefore always be involved in making decisions about their plan of care.

An ethical consideration with elderly surgical patients centers on the dilemma of do-not-resuscitate (DNR) orders. The organization's policy must give the patient a voice in the intraoperative area. Even though the patient may have made end-of-life decisions, the fact that the patient has signed the consent implies that he or she seeks to improve quality of life, which is incompatible with withholding cardiopulmonary resuscitation (CPR). It is difficult to differentiate between a cardiac arrest precipitated by the anesthesia and one that is spontaneous. The anesthetic agent itself promotes cardiovascular instability. Consideration should be given to the medical indications for the procedure with the goal of the treatment to alleviate pain and morbidity and provide for the patient's comfort. The guiding principle in the decision to maintain or suspend DNR orders should be respect for the patient's autonomy. Elderly patients have the right to participate in the process for making end-of-life decisions.

As more procedures are performed, there are ways to assist perioperative nurses to prepare for the care of the elderly population:

- Educate staff members by reviewing the special needs of this age-group.
- Develop a separate process for preoperative assessment, and use multiple screens for evaluation of older patients.
- Improve communication and collaboration among health care providers.

Understanding the age-specific needs of the older surgical patient will be critical to successful outcomes for these patients. The 2004 Institute of Medicine (IOM) report, *Keeping Patients Safe: Transforming the Work Environment of Nurses,* highlighted the critical connection between patient safety and the safe work environment. The report determined that a safe and supportive nurses' work environment reduces threats to patient safety in health care organizations. Numerous studies summarized in the report have linked inadequate staffing to negative clinical outcomes, such as cardiac arrests, death, increased length of stay, pneumonia, postoperative infections, and pressure ulcers. The recommendations from the report were knowledge based and centered on the four basic components of all organizations:

- Organizational management
- Workforce deployment practices
- Work design
- Organizational culture[2]

An organizational culture of safety must include a blame-free response to medical mistakes. Potential for errors must be recognized as opportunities to review process and policy to prevent future mistakes. Perioperative nurses have the responsibility to contribute to the creation of a culture of safety in the workplace to improve safety in the workplace for patients and nurses.

Future technical advances in surgery and anesthesia will continue to provide for beneficial surgery performed on older and older patients. The perioperative nurse who approaches the care of elders with this in mind not only will enhance the surgical outcome but also will significantly affect the patient's overall quality of life.

## REFERENCES


1. Asher M.:Surgical considerations in the elderly, *Journal of PeriAnesthesia Nursing* 19(6):406-414, 2004.
2. Beyea SC: A critical partnership—safety for nurses and patients, *AORN Journal* 79(6):1299-1302, 2004.
3. Burden N: Discharge planning for the elderly ambulatory surgical patient, *Journal of PeriAnesthesia Nursing* 19(6):401-405, 2004.
4. Ebersole P and others: *Toward healthy aging: human needs and nursing response*, ed 6, St Louis, 2004, Mosby.
5. Federal Interagency Forum on Aging-Related Statistics: *Older Americans 2004: key indicators of well-being. Federal Interagency Forum on Aging-Related Statistics,* Washington, DC, November 2004, U.S. Government Printing Office.
6. Goldrick BA: Infection in the older adult, *American Journal of Nursing* 105(6):31-34, 2005.
7. Murray CA: Interventions for clients with musculoskeletal problems. In Ignatavicius DD, Workman ML, editors: *Medical-surgical nursing: critical thinking for collaborative care,* ed 5, St Louis, 2006, Saunders.
8. Parker MJ and others: Surgery in elderly patients, *Current Orthopaedics* 18:333-344, 2004.
9. Rehman SU and others: Thyroid disorders in elderly patients, *Southern Medical Journal* 98(5):543-549, 2005.
10. Rosenthal R, Zenilman ME: Surgery in the elderly. In Townsend CM and others, editors: *Sabiston textbook of surgery*, ed 17, Philadelphia, 2004, Saunders.
11. Saufl NM: Preparing the older adult for surgery and anesthesia, *Journal of PeriAnesthesia Nursing* 19(6):372-378, 2004.
12. Schroeder K: Principles and applications. In Merriman JA and others, editors: *Ethics in perioperative practice*, Denver, 2004, AORN, Inc.
13. Sieber FE, Pauldine R: Anesthesia and the elderly. In Miller RD: *Miller's anesthesia*, vol 2, ed 6, Philadelphia, 2005, Churchill Livingstone.
14. Stevenson J: When the trauma patient is elderly, *Journal of PeriAnesthesia Nursing* 19(6):392-400, 2004.
15. Tobias JH, Sharif M: Bone and joint aging. In Tallis RC, Fillit HM, editors: *Brocklehurst's textbook of geriatric medicine and gerontology*, ed 6, Philadelphia, 2003, Churchill Livingstone.
16. Williams ME: *Physical diagnosis in elderly people.* Release date: March 23, 2005. Accessed April 21, 2006, on-line: www.medscape.com/viewprogram/3955_pnt.
17. Wold GH: *Basic geriatric nursing*, ed 3, St Louis, 2004, Mosby.
18. Workman ML: Assessment of the eye and vision. In Ignatavicius DD, Workman ML, editors: *Medical-surgical nursing: critical thinking for collaborative care*, ed 5, St Louis, 2006, Saunders.

CHAPTER 31

# Trauma Surgery

DIANE CATHERINE SAULLO

Trauma is ranked as one of the foremost public health issues in the United States today. Unintentional injury related to trauma is the fifth leading cause of death today.[15] Trauma is the leading nonobstetric cause of maternal mortality and accounts for at least 20% of maternal deaths each year.[4] Whether the injury is a result of a motor vehicle collision, violence, crime, or work-related injury, trauma occurs unplanned and without warning. The unpredictable nature of trauma poses a major challenge to the perioperative nurse and the patient care team.

The potential for injury has existed since the beginning of humanity. Most of the major advances in care of critically injured patients have been accomplished through experience in the military. Clearly, the shorter the response time is, the greater the survival rate for casualties. This was demonstrated by the success of the mobile army surgical hospitals (MASH) during the Korean conflict and again during the Vietnam conflict; MASH brought the necessary supplies, equipment, and personnel closer to the battlefields and, consequently, improved patient outcomes.

Eventually this concept was applied to the civilian population and is now commonly referred to as the "golden hour" of trauma care. More specifically, the golden hour refers to the time immediately after the injury when rapid and definitive interventions can be most effective in the reduction of morbidity and mortality. Traumatic deaths may occur in three phases, or time frames. The first occurs immediately after the injury. This accounts for about 50% of the deaths from trauma and is usually a result of lacerations to the heart or aorta or brainstem injury. These patients rarely survive to the hospital and die at the scene. The second phase occurs within the first 1 to 2 hours after the injury, representing about 30% of total fatalities. These patients have injuries to the spleen, liver, lung, or other organs that result in significant blood loss. This is the group in which definitive trauma care (i.e., appropriate and aggressive resuscitation with adequate volume replacement) may have the most significant effect (the golden hour). The third phase occurs days to weeks after the injury, often during the intensive care phase, and is usually caused by complications or a failure of multiple organ systems.

The war in Iraq (2003) has brought some changes in the way traumatic injuries are managed; the military has not set up convalescence centers as in Vietnam and Desert Storm. Rather, the doctrine of "essential care in theater" is followed. Physicians and nurses have been trained to provide immediate care, keeping in mind what will happen at the next level of care. Soldiers with upper body injuries are surviving because of body armor. However, there is not protection for upper extremities so there are many amputations being performed, including above-elbow and shoulder disarticulation. The new philosophy is to stress continuity of care with the goal of returning the soldier to the highest possible level of function. Physicians and nurses are using computer-assisted prostheses and different types of limbs that will become the standard of care.

Time is of the essence in providing definitive care to the critically injured person (History box). A significant number of deaths can be prevented if rapid transport is provided from the scene to a facility equipped to provide resuscitation and treatment in an efficient and timely manner. This concept is reflected in the national development of the Emergency Medical Services (EMS) system. Facilities and resources are allocated and coordinated to provide specific interventions for a group of patients. For example, facilities that meet certain criteria to accommodate the specialized needs of the critically injured patient are designated as *trauma centers*. Transfer and triage protocols are established that allow for a trauma patient to reach the appropriate facility with the least out-of-hospital time possible. This may be accomplished by a helicopter with a specially trained flight crew or by the use of ground transport with an advanced life support (ALS) ambulance team (Figure 31-1).

The American College of Surgeons (ACS) has published a position statement on criteria that defines the four specific levels of care that may be offered by designated trauma centers. A level I trauma center is committed to provision of qualified personnel and technologic equipment necessary for rapid diagnosis and treatment on a 24-hour basis. Level I trauma facilities are the receiving institution for severely injured patients in the region. In rural areas, transport time can be long in the absence of helicopter availability; therefore time is of the essence. A level II trauma center is able to treat seriously injured patients but lacks some of the specialized clinicians and resources required for the level I designation. Level II facilities may provide surgical intervention if resources match the patient's need or if the critical nature of the injury dictates immediate intervention before transfer to a major trauma facility.

A level III trauma center may be a community hospital in an area that does not have a level I or level II facility. The ACS recommends that in level II and III centers, an operating room (OR) team be readily available at all times. Depending on the population served and the volume of urgent cases, this requirement may be met with on-call staff. A level IV trauma center has the ability to provide advanced trauma life support before patient transfer. These facilities may be located in rural areas with limited access and may be a clinic or a hospital. Consequently, the designation of levels in the trauma system allows injured patients to be stabilized and transferred according to preestablished protocols that allow for the most efficient access to definitive care. Research has demonstrated that mortality

## HISTORY

In 1774, Dr. William Hawes and Dr. Thomas Cogan founded a group known as "The Institute for Affording Immediate Relief for Persons Apparently Dead from Drowning" in London. The group later became known as the Humane Society. Hawes and Cogan were interested in learning how to resuscitate drowning victims and positioned attendants at intervals along the banks of the river Thames and paid them two guineas to attempt resuscitation to anyone who had drowned (provided their attempts lasted longer than 2 hours!). Before this it was generally felt that the best thing you could do to drowned people was to pick their pockets.

At this time the function of the lungs was unknown. Oxygen had not yet been discovered, and Galen's idea that the function of the lungs was to cool the heart was widely accepted. The standard resuscitation regimen at the time was to dry and warm the body by applying friction to the skin and to administer tobacco smoke enemas.

There were recent clues as to the lung's function, however. William Harvey had described the circulation of the blood in 1628, and it had been noted that dark venous blood exposed to the air became bright red. In addition, there were reports of successful resuscitation of drowned people (and dogs) with bellows. Paracelsus (1493-1541), an alchemist and perhaps the greatest physician of his age, was said to have attempted the resuscitation of a corpse using bellows, a trick he perhaps picked up from Arabic medical writings. Andreas Vesalius (1514-1564), the father of modern anatomy, reported successfully using bellows to resuscitate asphyxiated dogs. By the 1740s, several cases of successful mouth-to-mouth resuscitation had been reported, the most famous of which was Tossach's 1744 report of the resuscitation of a clinically dead coal miner who had been suddenly overcome after descending into a burned-out mine.

Only 3 months after the society was founded, a member of the society was called to attend a 3-year-old child named Catherine Sophie Greenhill, who had fallen from an upper story window onto flagstones in nearby Pudding Lane and been pronounced dead. The society member, an apothecary (pharmacist) named Squires, was on the scene within 20 minutes, and history records that he proceeded to give the clinically dead child several shocks through the chest with a portable electrostatic generator. This treatment caused her to regain pulse and respiration, and she eventually (after a time in a coma) recovered fully.

Modified from *The first successful trauma resuscitation.* Accessed April 24, 2006, on-line: www.trauma.org/history/resuscitation.html.

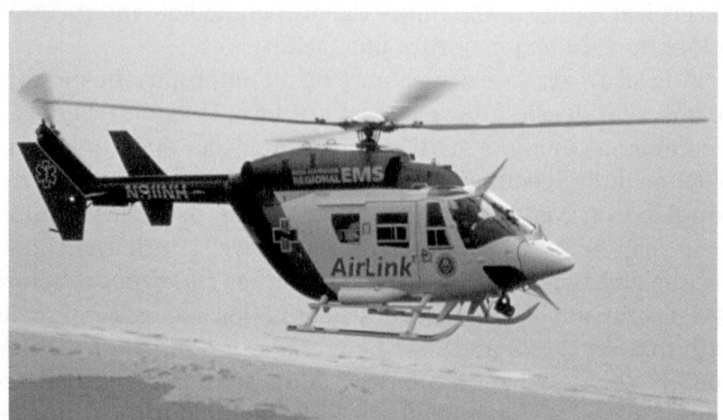


**FIGURE 31-1** New Hanover Health Network EMS Air Link. *EMS,* Emergency Medical Services, NC.

and length of stay are lower in high-volume trauma centers, which is an impetus for regionalizing trauma care and developing guidelines that recommend the number of trauma centers per unit population.[19]

Trauma patients require immediate access to the OR 24 hours per day, 365 days per year. A sudden influx of a large number of trauma patients to a trauma center may necessitate triage or classification of those less seriously injured as less urgent, allowing immediate access for the critically injured patients. The elective surgery schedule may need to be interrupted to expedite care for the trauma patient or patients. Scheduling policies and procedures are established collaboratively by the departments of surgery, trauma, anesthesia, and perioperative nursing services. Consequently, the perioperative nurse needs to be familiar with supplies and equipment located in the OR that are designated for trauma or in the ORs that are used most frequently for these patients.

# *Perioperative Nursing Considerations*

## Preliminary Evaluation: Mechanism of Injury

Because of the unpredictable timing of trauma, it is often the on-call perioperative nursing team who cares for injured patients requiring surgical intervention. In contrast to an elective surgical procedure, little information may be known about trauma patients and preparation time is often minutes at the most. A working knowledge of the mechanism of injury (MOI) is essential to assist the perioperative nurse in rapid patient assessment.

MOI, or kinematics, involves the action of forces on the human body and their effects. Knowing the forces applied provides valuable information in evaluation of the patient and injuries that may be present. On initial evaluation of the trauma patient at the scene of the injury, careful observations are made by the first responding EMS team. For example, the position of the victim in a car, whether the person was the driver or a passenger seated in the back seat or front seat, estimated velocity of the vehicle, location of impact, and use of a seat belt or air bag are all pieces of information used to determine the index of suspicion about the probable causes of injuries to the patient. After immediate threats to life are addressed, the MOI can provide valuable clues as to probable cause of injuries. This systematic approach can reduce morbidity and mortality (Table 31-1).

The MOI is a product of the type of injuring force and the resulting tissue response. The velocity of the collision, the shape of the object, and the tissue's flexibility influence the magnitude of the injury sustained. For example, long bone tissue has little or no flexibility. A strong collision involving a long bone most often results in a fracture of some type. In contrast, soft tissue injury from a colliding force may result in a contusion, since this tissue has greater flexibility.

Blunt trauma is injury resulting from a combination of forces, such as acceleration, deceleration, shearing, and compression, that does not result in a break of the skin. Morbidity and mortality may be greater than with penetrating trauma because identification of injuries is more difficult when injuries are less obvious. Causes of blunt trauma include motor

**TABLE 31-1**

## Biomechanics in Trauma

| | **Phases of Injury** |
|---|---|
| **Mechanisms of Injury** | **Examples** |
| Vehicle of transfer of energy from environment to human host | Falls<br>Motor vehicle crashes<br>Bullets<br>Stabbing instruments<br>Blasts/bombs |
| | **External Forces** |
| **DECELERATION FORCES**<br>Decrease in speed of a moving object or person | Victim strikes steering column<br>Victim impacts ground |
| **ACCELERATION FORCES**<br>Increase in speed of a moving object or person | Pedestrian thrown when struck by moving vehicle |
| **BLAST FORCES**<br>Heat, light, pressure<br>Low- and high-velocity missiles | Bomb explosion<br>Bullets<br>Stabbing instruments |
| | **Internal Forces** |
| Human body's response to kinetic energy load | Stress<br>Cells separate, stretch, compress, or shear<br>Strain<br>Tissue damage or deformation from stress |
| | **Types of Injuries** |
| Describing for clinical and diagnostic purpose | Blunt versus penetrating<br>Closed versus open<br>Primary versus secondary<br>Direct versus indirect |

From Emergency Nurses Association (ENA): *Trauma nursing core course,* ed 5, Des Plaines, Illinois, 2000, Emergency Nurses Association.

vehicle collisions (MVCs), contact sports, aggravated assault, and falls. Even low-energy trauma, such as that associated with low-level falls, can produce significant injuries.[6]

Acceleration and deceleration injuries occur most frequently in blunt trauma. A ruptured thoracic aorta is an example of an injury that occurs as a result of these types of forces. In an MVC the large vessels are stopped or decelerated rapidly, resulting in vessel damage caused by stretching that exceeds its elastic ability. This affects the aorta at the ligamentum arteriosum, the anatomic point where it is affixed tightly to the chest wall, just below the origin of the subclavian artery. This shearing below the attachment site causes a rupture as the aorta continues to move in a forward motion after the chest wall motion has stopped.

MVCs account for approximately 50% of blunt trauma. During an MVC, actually three collisions occur (Figure 31-2). The first collision is that of a car into another object. The second collision is the impact of the occupant's body on the vehicle's interior. The third collision occurs when an internal body structure hits a rigid bony surface. A coup-contrecoup injury of the brain, for example, is the result of an acceleration force to one area of the brain and a deceleration force to an opposite area. Front and side air bag deployment along with the use of seat belts can decrease the severity of traumatic injury (Best Practice). In addition, publicized information details many injuries in children related to the use of all-terrain vehicles (Research Highlight).

Falls also cause traumatic deaths in the United States. Injuries are most commonly associated with children experiencing falls more than twice their height. In adults, falls more than 10 to 15 feet are usually accompanied by significant injury. Deceleration forces in falls produce forces of stretching, shearing, and compression. Consequently, aortic injuries are also suspect in this group of patients. Skeletal injuries occur as well, because of the compressive forces present.

Penetrating trauma is a result of the passage of a foreign object through tissue. The degree or extent of tissue injury is a function of the energy that is dissipated to the tissue and the surrounding areas. The anatomic structures most often injured include the liver, intestines, and vascular system. Extent of the injury relates to the nature of the foreign object (e.g., bullet caliber, knife size), distance from the weapon, structures penetrated, and amount of energy dissipated to the structures.

The velocity of a bullet is responsible for the degree of injury or cavitation to the tissue. A low-velocity bullet is one that travels at a lower speed (1000 feet per second or less) and disrupts only the bullet tract and its immediate surrounding area. A high-velocity weapon, such as used by the military, fires

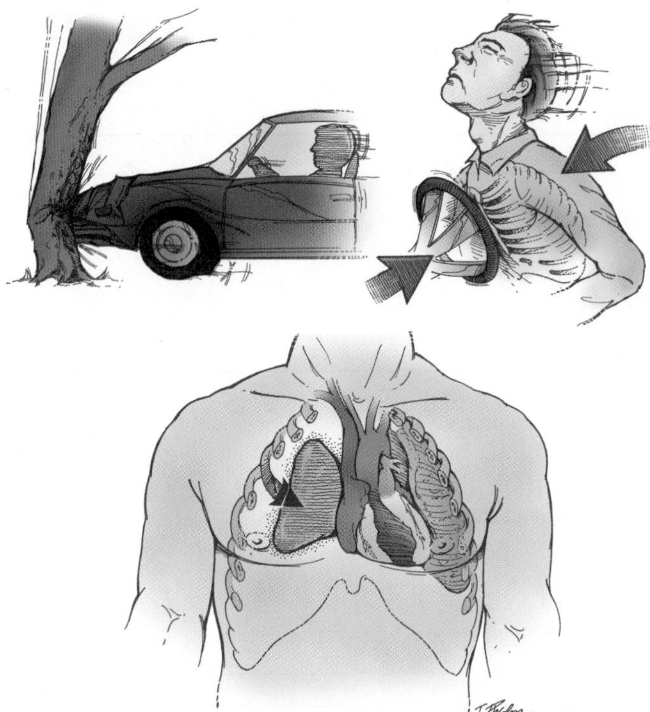

FIGURE 31-2 The three collisions of a head-on motor vehicle crash: the car hits an object; the occupant's body impacts on some surface within the motor vehicle; and the result is collision between internal tissues and the rigid body surface structures.

## BEST PRACTICE

### Safety Belt Enforcement

An estimated 3 million people are injured on U.S. roadways annually, resulting in more than 42,000 deaths. The use of safety belts has demonstrated significant reduction in morbidity and mortality following motor vehicle crashes, but in 2002, only 75% of occupants were using safety belts. It is estimated that increasing this to 90% compliance would prevent 5536 fatalities and 1,132,670 injuries and save almost $9 billion annually.

The American College of Surgeons has developed a position statement on the use of safety belts in which they support legislation standards for "primary" safety belt laws and their enforcement. The position statement makes the following points about safety belts and their use:

- They are the single most effective device for preventing serious injury and death.
- When used properly, they reduce the risk of injury/fatality by 45% to 50%.
- "Primary" laws allow a citation to be given if a driver or passenger is noted to be unbelted.
- "Secondary" laws require that a vehicle be stopped for another violation before a citation for being unbelted is given.

Therefore "The American College of Surgeons supports legislation enacting standards for 'primary' safety belt laws and their effective enforcement." Currently, all states but one have seat belt legislation, but the majority is "secondary" enforcement. All health care providers should support primary restraint legislation in their respective states.

Modified from American College of Surgeons: *Statement on safety belt laws and enforcement,* June 2003. Accessed April 24, 2006, on-line: www.facs.org/fellows_info/statements/st-43.html.

## RESEARCH HIGHLIGHT

### Dangers of All-Terrain Vehicles

Results of recently published studies show trends of injuries resulting from children's use of all-terrain vehicles (ATVs). The American Academy of Pediatrics issued a formal plea in November 2004 asking parents to prohibit children under the age of 16 years from riding the vehicles. The Consumer Product Safety Commission confirmed the injuries are a national trend and is considering the adoption of national rules similar to those of the American Academy of Pediatrics, which recommended that only people with a driver's license should operate the vehicles.

A research study in southeastern North Carolina looked at helmet use in ATV crash victims; there is no law in North Carolina requiring helmets. Head, face, and orthopedic injuries are the most common injuries requiring medical attention, with head injury being the primary cause of death in North Carolina and Pennsylvania riders under 16 years of age. The study looked at the rate of helmet use of victims admitted to New Hanover Regional Medical Center (NHRMC) and if outcomes of those wearing helmets were better than of those not wearing helmets. A retrospective review using the Trauma Registry looked at all crash victims admitted from 1994 to 2004. The results showed the following: most victims (77%) who were admitted were not wearing helmets; 100% of victims who died were not wearing helmets; 65% of victims sustained head or facial trauma, and, of those, 84% were not wearing a helmet. These results were congruent with national trends for trauma patients.

The results conclude that the study should be repeated at the state level; more outcome measures, such as the Injury Severity Score, should be included in the review; and the results should be shared with trauma leaders to elicit support for legislation requiring helmet use.

Modified from The American Trauma Society: Spivey, Christy, RN, BSN, CEN, EMT, SERAC Manager: *The effects of helmet use in all-terrain vehicle crash victims in southeastern North Carolina.* Poster session presented at Sigma Theta Tau International Annual Research Day, Wilmington, NC, April 2004.

a bullet traveling at a greater speed (3000 feet or more per second) and causes significantly more damage and tissue destruction, since the bullet tract involves more extensive surrounding tissue (Figure 31-3). The distance from the weapon also influences the degree of injury because the velocity is greatest when the bullet leaves the weapon and decreases as it travels. In addition, the type of bullet (e.g., shotgun shells with multiple pellets and hollow-point bullets, which mushroom on impact) influences the degree of injury. Commonly the entrance wound is smaller than the exit wound because of the dissipation of energy, but an exit wound may not always be present. If the bullet completely fragments or is lodged in an internal structure, there will not be an exit wound. Depending on the position of the bullet and any injury that could be caused by attempting to remove it, bullets are not always removed.

Stab and impalement wounds are considered to be low-velocity wounds. The associated injuries usually correspond to the path of the penetrating object. Factors such as the object's width and length assist in identification of the possible occurrence of injuries. A single injury site may penetrate several different organs or cavities. Penetrating injuries located at or be-

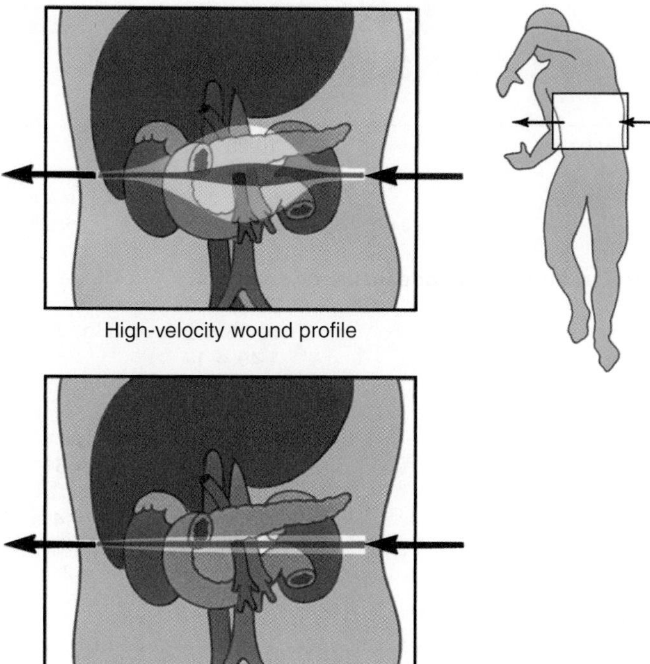


**FIGURE 31-3** Potential injury path of high- and low-velocity bullets.

low the nipple line may cause both chest and abdominal injuries. This is attributable to the diaphragmatic excursion that occurs with inspiration and expiration. Impaled objects should not be removed at the scene or in the emergency department (ED). The impaled object provides a tamponade effect to injured blood vessels and is removed only when the ability to control potential bleeding from those vessels is present. Wound debridement also may be necessary. These objects are removed in the OR where the needed supplies and instrumentation are.

Injuries that result from explosions are related to the effects of the blast. With the threat of domestic terrorism on the rise, the treatment of blast victims may become more frequent in trauma settings. Blast trauma inflicts injuries in a number of ways. Primary blast injury is the result of a direct pressure wave on the body. Secondary injury is associated with the impact of debris and fragments energized by the blast, which act like high-velocity missiles. Tertiary injuries result from the blast wind, since air is accelerated and may cause traumatic amputations or limb or skull fractures.[2] The type of injury sustained and its intensity are directly related to factors such as the size of the blast and the proximity of the victim or victims. Patients from a blast explosion may present with penetrating injury, contusions, lacerations, amputations, abrasions, avulsions, evisceration, and various degrees of burns.

Thermal and electrical tissue damage and inhalation injuries may occur from an explosion or as a sole mechanism of injury. These patients are usually resuscitated and require operative intervention for debridement on a nonemergent basis, unless the injury is limb- or life-threatening.

Injuries can be scored objectively according to their severity. This scoring system assists medical personnel in more effective triage and provides a universal method of communication among facilities, departments, and nursing personnel. The revised trauma score (RTS) incorporates physiologic criteria including head injury severity (Glasgow Coma Scale [GCS]). The GCS is used to evaluate head trauma, measuring the patient's best verbal, motor, and eye-opening capabilities.[9] The RTS may be calculated for both adult and pediatric patients (Tables 31-2 and 31-3).

## Assessment

The resuscitative process begins with arrival of emergency personnel on the scene and ends when the patient has been stabilized, received definitive care, and undergone a complete and thorough physical examination to determine all injuries sustained (Research Highlight). On arrival at the ED, the trauma team initiates a primary assessment. This is a logical, orderly process of patient assessment for potential life threats. These assessment activities are based on established protocols for advanced trauma life support (ATLS). The mnemonic "ABCDE," is used, representing assessment of the following:

- *A*irway (with cervical spine precautions)
- *B*reathing
- *C*irculation
- *D*isability (brief neurologic examination)
- *E*xposure (to reveal all life-threatening injuries) and *e*nvironmental control (thermoregulation)

Airway interventions may include manual maneuvers (chin-lift, jaw-thrust), insertion of oral or nasopharyngeal airways, or intubation. Emergent procedures, such as tracheotomy or needle cricothyrotomy, may also be used to obtain an airway. Pulse oximetry and capnography are also used. If cervical spine pre-

## RESEARCH HIGHLIGHT

### End Points of Resuscitation

Patients with severe trauma are at high risk for developing multiple organ dysfunction syndrome (MODS) or death. Treatment priorities must focus on resuscitation from shock, which leads to oxygen debt. Resuscitation is complete when oxygen debt is repaid and normal metabolism is restored. The standard markers of successful resuscitation include normal vital signs and urine output. However, up to 85% of patients still have evidence of inadequate tissue oxygenation after normalization of vital signs; this is described as compensated shock. An extensive literature search was done to look at other parameters that might be more predictive. Guidelines have been developed, based on this study, for end points of resuscitation. The recommendations are in part as follows:

- Level I: The initial base deficit, lactate level, or gastric pH can be used to stratify patients with regard to the need for ongoing fluid resuscitation. The ability of a patient to attain supranormal oxygen delivery parameters correlates with an improved chance for survival.
- Level II: The time to normalization of base deficit, lactate, and pH is predictive of survival. Persistently high base deficit or low pH may be an early indicator of complications.

The overall conclusion is that normalization of vital signs and urine output alone is not adequate to guarantee survival. More study of other end points, such as acid-base status, gastric tonometry, and measures of oxygen and carbon dioxide levels, need to be studied further.

Modified from Tisherman SA and others: *Clinical practice guideline: end-points of resuscitation*, 2003. Accessed April 24, 2006, on-line: Eastern Association for the Surgery of Trauma: www.east.org/tpg.html.

**TABLE 31-2**

## Revised Trauma Score

| Assessment | Method | Coding |
|---|---|---|
| Respiratory rate | Count respiratory rate in 15 sec and multiply by 4 | 10-29 = 4<br>>29 = 3<br>6-9 = 2<br>1-5 = 1<br>0 = 0 |
| Systolic blood pressure | Measure systolic cuff pressure in either arm by auscultation or palpation | >89 = 4<br>76-89 = 3<br>50-75 = 2<br>1-49 = 1<br>0 = 0 |
| Glasgow Coma Scale score<br>*Eye Opening*<br>Spontaneous = 4<br>To voice = 3<br>To pain = 2<br>None = 1 | <br>*Best Verbal Response*<br>Oriented = 5<br>Confused = 4<br>Inappropriate words = 3<br>Incomprehensible sounds = 2<br>None = 1<br><br>Convert Glasgow Coma Scale score as follows:<br>13-15 = 4<br>9-12 = 3<br>6-8 = 2<br>4-5 = 1<br><4 = 0 | <br>*Best Motor Response*<br>Obeys commands = 6<br>Localizes pain = 5<br>Withdraws to pain = 4<br>Flexion to pain = 3<br>Extension to pain = 2<br>None = 1 |

To obtain the trauma score, add the final scores for respiratory rate, systolic blood pressure, and converted Glasgow Coma Scale-score together.
Summary of Survival Probability in a Trauma Center

| **Trauma Score** | 12 | 11 | 10 | 9 | 8 | 7 | 6 | 5 | 4 | 3 | 2 | 1 | 0 |
|---|---|---|---|---|---|---|---|---|---|---|---|---|---|
| **Survival** | .995 | .969 | .879 | .766 | .667 | .636 | .630 | .455 | .333 | .333 | .286 | .259 | .037 |

From Galvin AA: Assessment of the trauma patient. In Newberry L, Criddle LM, editors: *Sheehy's manual of emergency care,* ed 6, St Louis, 2005, Mosby.

**TABLE 31-3**

## Pediatric Revised Trauma Score (RTS)

| Severity | +2 | +1 | −1 |
|---|---|---|---|
| Weight | >44 lb<br>(20 kg) | 22-44 lb<br>(10-20 kg) | <22 lb<br>(10 kg) |
| Airway | Normal | Oral or nasal airway | Invasive: intubation cricothyrotomy |
| Blood pressure | >90 mm Hg | 50-90 mm Hg | <50 mm Hg |
| Level of consciousness | Awake/alert | Obtunded: any loss of consciousness | Comatose |
| Open wound | None | Minor | Major or penetrating |
| Fracture | None | Single simple | Open or multiple |

From New Hanover Health Network, Trauma Services, Wilmington, NC.

cautions were not implemented before arrival at the hospital, they should be done before other procedures. A trauma team member can stabilize the head and neck, if necessary, until a cervical collar is placed. Once placed, the collar is not removed until a cervical radiograph clears the neck of injury.

During this time, the trauma surgeon or ED physician and trauma team identify and correct life threats that are present before progressing to the next part of the examination. A patient requiring immediate surgery is transported to the OR, undergoes surgical intervention, and then is transferred to the postanesthesia care unit (PACU) or intensive care unit (ICU), depending on his or her condition. On the other hand, a patient may have a penetrating wound with evisceration of abdominal contents. However, correcting the obvious defect, which is currently not life-threatening, is postponed until the trauma team is assured that the patient has a patent airway and an effective breathing pattern and that cervical spine precautions have been implemented. An evisceration needs to be corrected, but an inadequate airway is an immediate life threat and assumes priority.

If indicated by the injury, an arterial blood gas (ABG) measurement is also taken. This test provides an accurate assessment of the ventilatory status of the patient and also evaluates resuscitative airway and breathing interventions (Table 31-4) Metabolic acidosis or a large base deficit (pH < 7.35 or > 7.45), with all other causes ruled out, may indicate internal bleeding.

After completion of the primary assessment and correction of any immediate life threats (Surgical Pharmacology), the secondary assessment is completed. The purpose of the secondary assessment is to identify all injuries present. Sometimes the secondary assessment may be completed by the perioperative nurse, the PACU nurse, or the critical care nurse. This assessment is a more in-depth, head-to-toe evaluation of the patient. Inspection, palpation, percussion, and auscultation are used in the complete head-to-toe assessment to reveal any deformities, open injuries, tenderness, or swelling. The assessment begins at the head and face and then moves to the neck (including the spine), the chest, the abdomen, and the pelvis. The four extremities are next; distal pulses, motor function, and sensation are assessed. The final check is the back; the patient is carefully log-rolled to the side for a full visual and tactile assessment.

Vital signs, including a rectal or tympanic temperature, unless contraindicated, are obtained. Often during resuscitation a Foley catheter is inserted. The urinary meatus should be inspected for the presence of blood before insertion. If blood is noted, the surgeon should be notified and the catheter not inserted. The patient may have a ruptured bladder or a urethral injury, either of which is commonly associated with a fracture of the pelvis. The surgeon may wish to perform a retrograde urethrogram to examine the bladder and urethra for the presence of tears or disruption. After insertion, urine is obtained for a urinalysis and urine drug screen. The identification of specific drugs in the urine may assist in further diagnosis and treatment. The urine will also be tested to determine the presence of red blood cells (RBCs) (Box 31-1). Depending on the amount of hematuria present, a renal contusion or other renal injury may be present. In addition, a nasogastric tube may be inserted at this time.

A brief history is obtained from the family or significant others when possible. This history is referred to as the "AMPLE" history and may be obtained even after the patient is transferred to the OR by the ED personnel. The history includes the following:

- *A*llergies
- *M*edications
- *P*ast medical history
- *L*ast meal, *l*ast menstrual period (if appropriate)
- *E*vents or *e*nvironment leading to the accident or injury

If the history is obtained after the initiation of surgery, it is important to communicate it to the surgeon and the anesthesia team.

***Routine Laboratory Tests.*** Laboratory values aid in evaluating the trauma victim's status. Appropriate laboratory tests include a minimum of a complete blood count (CBC), hemoglobin and hematocrit (H&H), blood alcohol level (BAL), and a blood type and screen; other tests may be requested during evaluation. The results of the laboratory studies should be reviewed and communicated as appropriate (Box 31-2). An abnormal level of RBCs may signify dehydration, hypovolemia, or fluid overload (dilutional). An elevated white blood cell (WBC) count, indicating the presence of infection, may be related to inflammation, tissue necrosis, or immunocompromise. H&H values are also important to note. Caution is advised in evaluating an H&H drawn in the ED. The time delay between bleeding and a drop in H&H can be significant. It is only after hemodilution occurs (from shock compensation or crystalloid replacement) that hematocrit drops. Frequently, abnormal values in the patient with blunt trauma alert the team to the possibility of internal bleeding.

**TABLE 31-4**

## Laboratory Values: Arterial Blood Gases (ABGs)

| | | |
|---|---|---|
| **NORMAL VALUES** | | |
| $Pa_{O_2}$ | Amount of oxygen in arterial blood | 80-100 mm Hg |
| $Pa_{CO_2}$ | Pressure of carbon dioxide in arterial blood and a measurement of how well the lungs are getting rid of carbon dioxide ($CO_2$ is controlled by the lungs) | 34-45 mm Hg |
| pH | Acidity or alkalinity of arterial blood; a measurement of hydrogen-ion concentration | 7.35-7.45 |
| $HCO_3^-$ | Amount of bicarbonate in arterial blood; controlled by the kidneys | 21-28 mEq/L |
| $O_2$ saturation | Percentage of hemoglobin that is carrying oxygen | 95%-100% |
| **ABNORMAL VALUES** | | **POSSIBLE CAUSE** |
| $Pa_{O_2}$ | <50 mm Hg | Hypoxia |
| $Pa_{CO_2}$ | >45 mm Hg | Hypoventilation/$CO_2$ retention by lungs |
| pH | <7.35 | Acidosis |
| | >7.45 | Alkalosis |
| $HCO_3^-$ | <22 mEq/L | Renal excretion of too much bicarbonate |
| | >26 mEq/L | Renal retention of too much bicarbonate |

From Pagana KD, Pagana TJ: *Mosby's diagnostic and laboratory test references*, ed 7, St Louis, 2005, Mosby.

## SURGICAL PHARMACOLOGY

### Commonly Used Medications for Cardiac Arrest

Trauma patients may have undergone cardiac resuscitation in the field or in the emergency department before arriving in the operating room (OR). If the patient has been resuscitated, medications used as part of the advanced cardiac life support (ACLS) protocol may still be in use when the patient arrives. The perioperative nurse should have a working knowledge of the more commonly used ACLS medications to provide knowledgeable and safe care to the trauma patient.

| Medication | Usual Dosage | Nursing Implications | Rationale for Use |
|---|---|---|---|
| Epinephrine (Adrenalin) | 1-mg bolus followed by 20-ml saline flush q3-5min.<br>If this fails, consider 2- to 5-mg IV bolus q3-5min; 1-mg, 3-mg, and 5-mg IV boluses (3 min apart); or 0.1 mg/kg IV bolus q3-5min.<br>If necessary, give endotracheally with dose at least 2-2½ times the IV dose. | Monitor for return of rhythm and pulse when used for asystole or VF.<br>Assess for tachycardia, dysrhythmias, or hypertension.<br>Assess for the development of coarse VF when given during the VF. | Return of rhythm and pulse is the expected response.<br>Adverse reactions can occur with a dramatic response. This may improve the response to defibrillation. |
| Amiodarone hydrochloride (Cordarone) | 300-mg IV push for cardiac arrest in VF/pulseless VT.<br>150-mg IV push over 10 min (15 mg/min), followed by 360 mg IV over next 6 hr (1 mg/min), followed by 540 mg IV over next 18 hr (0.5 mg/min).<br>After first 24 hr, continue maintenance infusion of 720 mg/24 hr (0.5 mg/min). | Monitor for return of rhythm and pulse when used for recurrent, unstable VT or VF.<br>Use with extreme caution in patients receiving other antidysrhythmics.<br>Use caution in patients with pulmonary, hepatic, or thyroid disease.<br>Perform continuous cardiac monitoring while the patient is receiving the loading dose. | Return of rhythm and pulse is the expected response.<br>Amiodarone reduces the hepatic and renal clearance of certain antidysrhythmics, specifically procainamide, quinidine, and flecainide.<br>Amiodarone can cause fetal toxicity, especially in patients receiving more than 600 mg daily.<br>There is a slow onset of antidysrhythmic effect and a high risk of life-threatening dysrhythmias. |
| Dopamine hydrochloride (Intropin) | 2.5 mcg/kg/min IV infusion; titrate to desired clinical response.<br>1-2 mcg/kg/min for renal and mesenteric vasodilation.<br>2-10 mcg/kg/min for beta-adrenergic effects.<br>10-20 mcg/kg/min for alpha-adrenergic effects. | Assess patients for increased BP.<br>Monitor for tachycardia, dysrhythmias, or hypertension.<br>Monitor IV site for infiltration.<br>Assess for urine output <30 ml/hr, pallor, cyanosis, pain, or numbness in the extremities. | Increased BP is the expected response.<br>Adverse reactions may occur.<br>Extravasation of the drug can occur, causing necrosis.<br>Dosages >10 mcg/kg/min cause vasoconstriction of renal and peripheral vessels; dosages of 2-5 mcg/kg/min may improve urine output by causing renal vasodilation and improving renal blood flow. |
| Dobutamine hydrochloride (Dobutrex) | 2-20 mcg/kg/min IV infusion. | Assess for increased BP.<br>Assess for hypertension and dysrhythmias. | Increased BP is the expected response.<br>Adverse reactions may occur. |
| Norepinephrine (Levophed) | 0.5-1 mcg/min IV infusion; titrate to desired effect, up to 8-30 mcg/min. | Assess for increased BP.<br>Monitor for bradycardia.<br>Monitor for hypertension and dysrhythmias.<br>Administer drug through central IV line.<br>Assess for urine output <30 ml/hr, pallor, cyanosis, pain, or numbness in the extremities.<br>Assess for chest pain after resuscitation. | Increased BP is the expected response.<br>Reflex bradycardia may occur with a rise in BP.<br>Adverse reactions may occur with a dramatic response.<br>Extravasation can occur.<br>Norepinephrine is a powerful vasoconstrictor.<br>Norepinephrine increases myocardial oxygen demand. |
| Sodium bicarbonate | 1 mEq/kg IV bolus given after the first 10 min of cardiac arrest if necessary.<br>0.5 mEq/kg IV bolus q10min thereafter if necessary. | Assess arterial blood gas values for metabolic acidosis. | Administration without evidence of metabolic acidosis can result in metabolic alkalosis, which can hinder resuscitation efforts. |

Modified from Zickafoose PC: Interventions for clients with dysrhythmias. In Ignatavicius DD, Workman ML, editors: *Medical-surgical nursing: critical thinking for collaborative care*, ed 5, St Louis, 2006, Saunders.

*BP,* Blood pressure; *IV,* intravenous; *VF,* ventricular fibrillation; *VT,* ventricular tachycardia.

SURGICAL PHARMACOLOGY

## Commonly Used Medications for Cardiac Arrest—cont'd

| Medication | Usual Dosage | Nursing Implications | Rationale for Use |
|---|---|---|---|
| Isoproterenol (Isuprel) | 2-10 mcg/min IV infusion; titrate to desired clinical response. | Assess for increased heart rate.<br>Assess for tachycardia, hypotension, or hypertension.<br>Assess for chest pain after resuscitation.<br>Monitor for ventricular dysrhythmias. | Increased heart rate is the expected response.<br>Adverse reactions may occur with a dramatic response.<br>Isoproterenol increases myocardial oxygen demand.<br>Isoproterenol increases ventricular instability, especially in patients who are hypokalemic or who are receiving digitalis. |
| Calcium chloride ($CaCl_2$) | 2-4 mg/kg IV slowly; may repeat q10min if necessary. | Calcium chloride is indicated only for cardiac arrest associated with hyperkalemia, hypocalcemia, or calcium channel blocker toxicity. | Calcium chloride may cause cellular damage and cerebrovascular spasm. |
| Vasopressin | 40 units IV bolus, one time. | Monitor for return of rhythm and pulse when used for VF or pulseless VT. | Return of rhythm and pulse is the expected response. |

Modified from Zickafoose PC: Interventions for clients with dysrhythmias. In Ignatavicius DD, Workman ML, editors: *Medical-surgical nursing: critical thinking for collaborative care*, ed 5, St Louis, 2006, Saunders.

*BP*, Blood pressure; *IV*, intravenous; *VF*, ventricular fibrillation; *VT*, ventricular tachycardia.

BOX 31-1

## Laboratory Values: Urinalysis (UA)

A urinalysis is done to check for injury to the genitourinary system and for the presence of specific diseases.

### Normal Values

| | |
|---|---|
| **Color** | **amber yellow** |
| **Appearance** | **Clear** |
| **Specific gravity** | **1.005-1.030** |
| **pH** | **4.6-8.0** |
| **Protein** | **Negative** |
| **Glucose** | **Negative** |
| **Ketones** | **Negative** |
| **Microscopic findings** | |
| **• Red blood cells (RBCs)** | **0-2/high-power field (hpf)** |
| **• White blood cells (WBCs)** | **0-4/hpf** |
| **• Epithelial cells** | **Few** |
| **• Casts** | **0** |
| **• Crystals** | **0** |
| **• Bacteria** | **0** |
| **• Yeast** | **0** |

### Abnormal Values

| | | In Trauma, May Indicate |
|---|---|---|
| Color | Dark or red | Presence of blood |
| Appearance | Dark or red | Presence of blood |
| Specific gravity | >1.030 | Fluid volume deficit |
| pH | Alkaline: >8.0 | Alkalosis |
| | Acidic: <4.6 | Acidosis |
| Glucose | Present | Diabetes<br>Increased intracranial pressure |
| Protein | Present | Renal failure |
| Ketone | Present | Diabetes<br>Diarrhea and vomiting |
| Microscopic findings | | |
| • Red blood cells (RBCs) | >3/high-power field (hpf) | Kidney, ureteral, bladder trauma |
| • White blood cells (WBCs) | >4/hpf | Urinary tract infection |
| • Epithelial cells | ↑ | Renal tubular necrosis |
| • Casts | ↑ | Glomerular capsule trauma |
| • Bacteria | | Abnormalities not usually seen in early trauma |

Data from Pagana KD, Pagana TJ: *Mosby's diagnostic and laboratory test references,* ed 7, St Louis, 2005, Mosby.

BOX 31-2

## Laboratory Values: Blood and Serum Electrolytes

**RED BLOOD CELLS (RBCS, ERYTHROCYTES)**

RBC values vary, depending on age, gender, and geographic location (in relation to sea level) of the patient.

### Normal Values

| | |
|---|---|
| **CHILDREN** | |
| Newborn | 4.8-7.1 million/mcl |
| 2-8 wk | 4-6 million/mcl |
| 2-6 mo | 3.5-5.5 million/mcl |
| 6-12 mo | 3.5-5.2 million/mcl |
| 1-6 yr | 4-5.5 million/mcl |
| 6-18 yr | 4-5.5 million/mcl |
| **ADULTS/ELDERLY** | |
| Male | 4.7-6.1 million/mcl |
| Female | 4.2-5.4 million/mcl |
| Pregnant female | Decreased |

| Abnormal Values | Probable Cause |
|---|---|
| ↑ | Dehydration |
| ↓ | Hypovolemia |
| | Fluid overload (dilutional) |

**WHITE BLOOD CELLS (WBCS, LEUKOCYTES)**

A WBC count is obtained to identify the presence of an infection.

**Normal Value**

5000-10,000/μl (elevated in pregnancy)

| Abnormal Values | Probable Cause |
|---|---|
| >10,900/mcl | Infection/inflammation<br>Tissue necrosis<br>Immunocompromise |

**HEMATOCRIT (HCT)**

A hematocrit value is obtained to determine the percentage of RBCs in whole blood.

### Normal Values

| | |
|---|---|
| **CHILDREN** | |
| Newborn | 44%-64% |
| 2-8 wk | 39%-59% |
| 2-6 mo | 35%-50% |
| 6-12 mo | 29%-43% |
| 1-6 yr | 30%-40% |
| 6-18 yr | 3%-44% |
| **ADULT** | |
| Male | 42%-52% |
| Female | 37%-47% |
| Pregnant female | >33% |

**ABNORMAL VALUES IN TRAUMA**

| | |
|---|---|
| ↓ | Hemodilution<br>• From compensated hypovolemia<br>• From excessive volume replacement |
| ↑ | Hemoconcentration |

NOTE: When blood is lost acutely, the amount of hematocrit lost is in the same ratio as that of whole blood. Therefore the percentage of hematocrit in a whole blood sample would remain normal. It is only after hemodilution occurs (from shock compensation or crystalloid replacement) that hematocrit drops.

**HEMOGLOBIN (Hgb)**

A hemoglobin value is obtained to measure the amount of hemoglobin in whole blood. The amount of hemoglobin determines the oxygen-carrying capacity of blood.

### Normal Values

| | |
|---|---|
| **CHILDREN** | |
| Newborn | 14-24 g/dl |
| 0-2 wk | 12-20 g/dl |
| 2-6 mo | 10-17 g/dl |
| 1-6 yr | 9.5-14 g/dl |
| **ADULT** | |
| Male | 14-18 g/dl |
| Female | 12-16 g/dl |
| Pregnant female | >11 g/dl |
| Elderly | Values slightly decreased |

| Abnormal Value in Trauma | Possible Cause |
|---|---|
| ↓ | Hemorrhage |

NOTE: When whole blood is lost acutely, the amount of hemoglobin that is lost is proportionate. It is only after hemodilution occurs (as a result of shock compensation or crystalloid volume replacement) that hemoglobin drops.

**PLATELETS (THROMBOCYTES)**

A platelet count is obtained to test the amount of platelet function. Platelets play an essential role in coagulation. Particularly in vascular trauma, platelets are essential to hemostasis.

### Normal Values

| | |
|---|---|
| Newborn | 150,000-300,000/mcl |
| Infant | 200,000-475,000/mcl |
| Child | 150,000-400,000/mcl |
| Adult/elderly | 150,000-400,000/mcl |

| Abnormal Values | Probable Causes |
|---|---|
| ↑ | Splenectomy<br>Living at high altitude<br>Hemorrhage |
| ↓ | Disseminated intravascular coagulation |

**COAGULATION STUDIES: PROTHROMBIN TIME (PT, PRO TIME)**

A prothrombin time is evaluated in trauma patients to measure clotting time (caused by factors I [fibrinogen], II [prothrombin], V, VII, and X). This is important in determining the blood's ability to clot.

**NORMAL VALUE**

11.0-12.5 seconds

| Abnormal Value | Probable Cause |
|---|---|
| ↑ | Deficiency of factors I (fibrinogen), II (prothrombin), V, VII, and X; 2.5× normal values means that there is a bleeding tendency. |

NOTE: Clotting times may be prolonged in the presence of excessive alcohol ingestion or the use of anabolic steroids. Clotting times decrease with the use of antihistamines and diuretics.

BOX 31-2

## Laboratory Values: Blood and Serum Electrolytes

**COAGULATION STUDIES: ACTIVATED PARTIAL THROMBOPLASTIN TIME (APTT)**

An APTT is obtained to screen for problems with intrinsic clotting factors (except factors VII and XIII). It can be used also to monitor the effectiveness of anticoagulation with heparin. This laboratory test measures the amount of time it takes for fibrin to form a clot. In the trauma patient it is used to determine the patient's tendency to bleed.

**Normal value**
30-40 sec for the clot to form (after the clinical reagent is added)

| Abnormal Value | Probable Cause |
|---|---|
| >40 sec | Intrinsic factor deficiency |

NOTE: Be sure to fill the laboratory tube because the tube contains anticoagulant and the ratio of blood to anticoagulant may be altered if the tube is not filled, causing a false prolonged clotting time.

**SERUM ELECTROLYTES: SODIUM ($Na^+$)**

Sodium is one of the two major extracellular cations. It is the major cause of osmotic pressure in extracellular fluid. Sodium also plays a major part in both acid-base balance and neuromuscular function.

**Normal Value**
136-145 mEq/L

| Abnormal Values | Possible Causes |
|---|---|
| >145 mEq/L (hypernatremia) | ↓ Fluid intake/fluid loss<br>↑ Sodium intake |
| <136 mEq/L | ↓ Sodium intake<br>↑ Sodium loss |

**SERUM ELECTROLYTES: POTASSIUM ($K^+$)**

Because potassium is one of the two major cellular cations, it is essential for the maintenance of cellular osmosis. It plays a major role in the electrical conductivity of both cardiac and skeletal muscle. In addition, potassium plays a major role in both acid-base balance and kidney function.

**Normal Value**
3.5-5 mEq/L

| Abnormal Values | Possible Causes |
|---|---|
| >5 mEq/L (hyperkalemia) | Major burns<br>Renal failure<br>Major crush injuries |
| <3.5 mEq/L (hypokalemia) | Hypovolemia |

**SERUM ELECTROLYTES: CHLORIDES ($Cl^-$)**

Measurement of serum chlorides is important for the assessment of acid-base status. Chloride is a major extracellular anion that plays a role in the maintenance of oncotic pressure and thus blood volume and arterial pressure.

**Normal value**
98-106 mEq/L

| Abnormal Values | Possible Causes |
|---|---|
| >106 mEq/L (hyperchloremia) | Dehydration<br>Renal failure<br>Central nervous system (CNS) trauma with central neurogenic breathing |
| <98 mEq/L (hypochloremia) | Excess vomiting<br>Excess gastric suctioning |

BAL also assists the trauma team in their evaluation. If the level is significantly high, the physical examination and patient's response may be unreliable. In addition, the neurologic status of patients with high BALs is very difficult to assess. Abnormal clotting studies are of obvious significance in trauma patients. These results may be attributable to anticoagulant medication the patient is taking or the effects of profound hypothermia. Clotting times may also be prolonged in the presence of excessive alcohol ingestion or the use of anabolic steroids. Clotting times decrease with the use of antihistamines and diuretics.

A blood type and screen shorten the time for the blood bank to obtain a crossmatch if needed later. Most trauma centers have several units of type O–negative blood (universal donor) available in the event that a blood transfusion is required before a type and crossmatch (T&C) can be performed. Because of regional shortages of O-negative blood, O-positive blood can be used in male patients and adult female patients of non–childbearing age. Initially, trauma patients are fluid-resuscitated with warmed crystalloid solutions, such as lactated Ringer's solution or normal saline solution. If the patient's blood pressure responds, the diagnostic examination continues. However, if the hypotension returns, blood transfusions may be initiated and the patient may be transported immediately to the OR for exploratory surgery.

### *Diagnostic Procedures*

**RADIOLOGY.** Depending on the trauma center protocol, a blunt trauma radiographic series may be part of the resuscitative phase. This minimally includes a lateral view of the cervical spine and an anteroposterior (AP) view of the chest. In addition, lateral thoracic and lumbar spine films and an AP view of the pelvis are taken. Any area with deformity, swelling, or pain may also be examined by x-ray. Trauma patients are always treated as if they have a cervical spine injury until proved otherwise. When reviewing the cervical spine films for cervical spine injury clearance, the clinician should consider any existing factors that put the patient at high risk for spine injury. These include age over 65 years, a dangerous MOI, and paresthesias in the extremities. Patients with penetrating trauma injuries usually go straight to the OR for exploratory laparotomy.

If the resources are available, the trauma center protocol may also include a computerized axial tomography (CT) scan as a diagnostic or screening tool. Depending on the MOI, such as a fall, CT scans of the head and abdomen may be performed.

Because injuries in blunt trauma are very difficult to diagnose, the CT scan is frequently done before patient transfer to the OR. A high index of suspicion is maintained for other injuries until proved otherwise. Bowel injuries may be missed during initial scanning. A CT scan of the brain revealing an injury incompatible with life may alter the course of definitive treatment for a patient.

A CT-angiogram may be indicated in diagnosis of vascular injuries. If the patient is hemodynamically stable, this test is of great value in determining the extent of the injury. It is particularly beneficial in the diagnosis of a ruptured thoracic aorta, in which extravasation of the dye at the area of aortic fixation to the chest wall is noted. Other uses include evaluation of penetrating wounds, especially in the extremity. Vessel injury can be noted and the need for surgical intervention determined.

**OTHER DIAGNOSTIC TESTS.** Cardiac monitoring is another component of the initial phase of trauma care and is particularly important in blunt trauma. Early detection of ventricular dysrhythmias may indicate a myocardial contusion, or bruising of the heart. An electrocardiogram (ECG) is obtained when indicated by the mechanism of injury or the patient's symptoms. Undiagnosed heart disease, as evidenced by an abnormal ECG, is noteworthy in a patient requiring operative intervention.

The use of focused abdominal ultrasonography for trauma (FAST) has become a decision-making tool for aiding in triaging the trauma patient to appropriate care.[16] FAST allows for diagnosis of potentially life-threatening hemorrhage. It can determine need for further radiologic procedures or surgery if the presence of blood is in at least two of the four quadrants visualized. Its use began in Europe in the 1970s and in North America in the 1990s; data collected during that time supported its use as a definitive assessment tool. FAST is a rapid, bedside ultrasound examination performed to identify intraperitoneal hemorrhage or pericardial tamponade. FAST examines four areas for free fluid: the perihepatic and hepatorenal space, the perisplenic area, the pelvis, and the pericardium (Figure 31-4). FAST is an adjunct to the ATLS primary survey and is used after the "ABCDE" assessment is made. FAST is performed with a small portable ultrasound machine that should be immediately available to the trauma patient, thus allowing for prompt management of his or her injuries (Figure 31-5). One study looked at performance of abdominal ultraso-

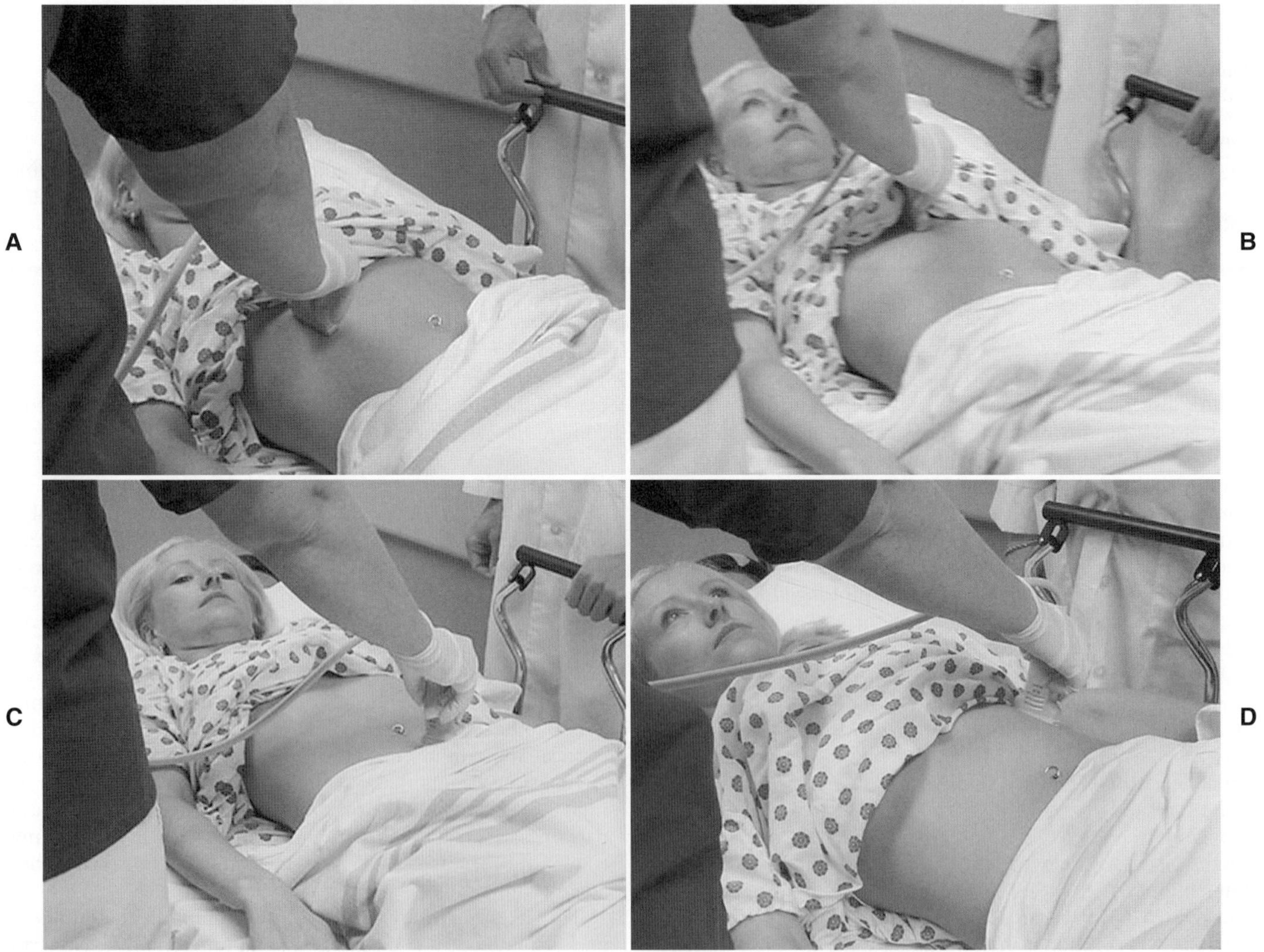


**FIGURE 31-4** Four areas examined by FAST. **A,** Perihepatic. **B,** Pericardium. **C,** Pelvis. **D,** Perisplenic. *FAST,* Focused abdominal sonography for trauma.

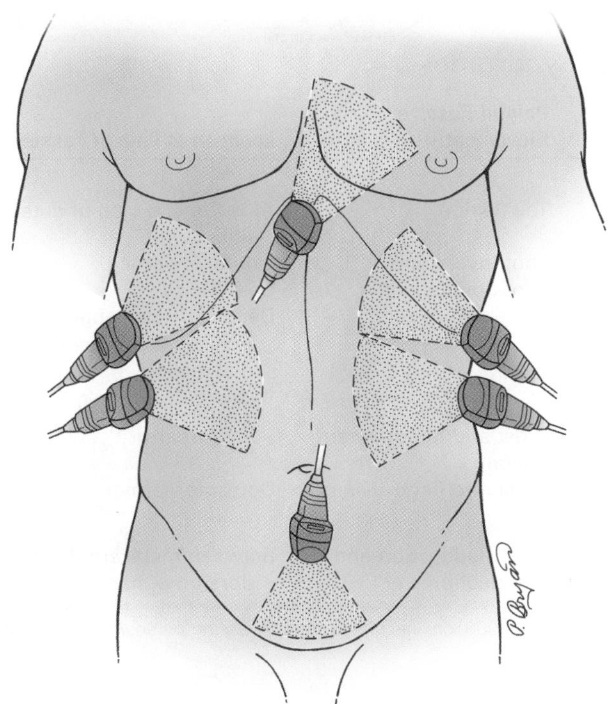

**FIGURE 31-5** FAST ultrasound examination performed to detect free intraperitoneal or pericardial fluid. *FAST,* Focused abdominal sonography for trauma.

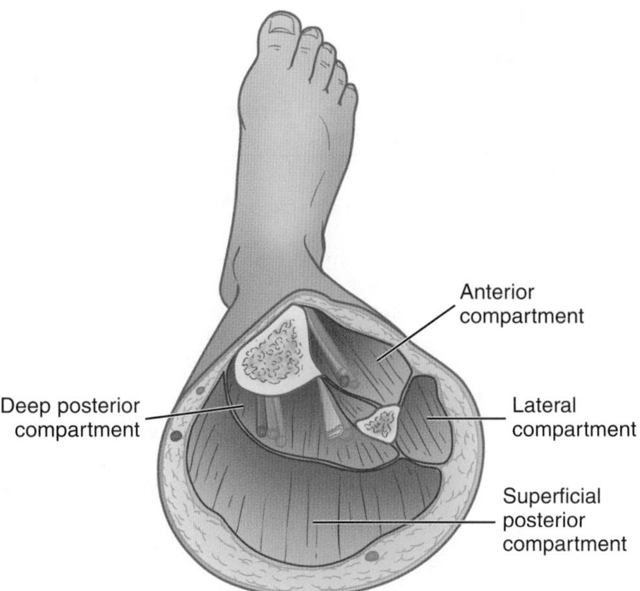


**FIGURE 31-6** Compartments of the lower leg.

nography in detecting hemoperitoneum in blunt trauma patients with hypotension.[11] Most patients with hemoperitoneum and intraabdominal injuries were identified. Patients with a negative ultrasound exam who remain hypotensive need further evaluation once stabilized.

Diagnostic peritoneal lavage (DPL) may be performed to determine the presence of abdominal injury. This tool is of particular benefit when evaluation of the abdomen is difficult, such as when the patient is intoxicated, unconscious, or hemodynamically unstable. DPL can be performed in the ED, OR, PACU, or ICU. Nonetheless, retroperitoneal blood may be missed with a DPL, whereas the FAST approach may be quicker and visualize more structures, even pericardium; it is also less expensive and noninvasive. Thus FAST may be used with patients who are unstable and need a quick approach without the risk of a false-positive tap.

Internal compartment pressures may be measured with an injury to the extremity as well as to the abdomen. Swelling of the muscles below the fascia covering may compromise circulation and result in the eventual loss of the extremity because of tissue necrosis. This is known as *compartment syndrome.* There are multiple compartments in the lower extremity that may be affected (Figure 31-6). Compartment pressures may be measured by the use of a manometer/stop cock/syringe or a commercial compartment pressure–measuring device. Normal compartmental pressures are less than 20 mm Hg. Pressures more than 30 mm Hg require a fasciotomy. Symptoms include severe pain, paresthesia, and a decrease in motor movement in the involved extremity, especially on passive movement (Table 31-5).

Massive intestinal edema may occur with trauma patients, causing compromise to internal organs and development of a different type of compartment syndrome. Abdominal compartment syndrome (ACS), also called abdominal hypertension, is characterized by increased intraabdominal pressure. High intraabdominal pressure increases systemic vascular resistance and impairs venous return. Common causes of ACS in trauma patients are ileus, bowel edema, bowel obstruction, postoperative hemorrhage, or as a result of abdominal distention secondary to resuscitation. Untreated ACS can progress to hypoxia, renal failure, fluid and electrolyte imbalance, and death. Management involves a decompressive laparotomy. After a decompression, the greatest nursing priority is wound management. The swelling may render the abdomen difficult or impossible to close. If the abdomen is closed, intraabdominal pressure may rise to a level greater than 25 cm of $H_2O$, at which point it may lead to significant organ dysfunction.[3] Intraabdominal pressure monitoring is accomplished with the use of a nasogastric tube in the stomach or a Foley catheter in the bladder. Simple water-column manometry is done at 2- to 4-hour intervals, although it is possible to connect a pressure transducer to a Foley catheter by way of the sampling port (Figure 31-7). By establishing a water column of urine in the Foley catheter with a clamp distal to the port, a pressure gradient is established. After zero-balancing the transducer, an 18-gauge needle is placed on the end of the pressure tubing and inserted into the sampling port. Using the pressure tubing and a 60-ml syringe, 50 to 60 ml of normal saline is then instilled into the Foley. On instillation of the saline, the waveform on the monitor is correlated to the existing bladder pressure. Normal intraabdominal pressure is zero or subatmospheric. A pressure of more than 25 cm of $H_2O$ is considered diagnostic of ACS.[3] After the pressure reading is obtained and recorded, the clamp is released from the distal port of the Foley catheter. Postoperatively, these patients are susceptible to fluid and heat loss. Continuous hemodynamic monitoring is essential in the critical care phase of treatment.

***Admission Assessment.*** The perioperative nurse may not obtain information concerning the trauma patient until the patient arrives in the OR for surgical intervention. If the pa-

TABLE 31-5

## Signs and Symptoms Associated with Compartmental Syndromes

| Compartment | Location of Sensory Changes | Movement Weakened | Painful Passive Movement | Location of Pain or Tenseness |
|---|---|---|---|---|
| **LOWER LEG** | | | | |
| Anterior | First web space | Toe extension | Toe flexion | Along lateral side of anterior tibia |
| Lateral | Dorsum (top) of foot | Foot eversion | Foot inversion | Lateral lower leg |
| Superficial posterior | None | Foot plantar flexion | Foot dorsiflexion | Calf |
| Deep posterior | Sole of foot | Toe flexion | Toe extension | Deep calf—palpable between Achilles tendon and medial malleoli |
| **FOREARM** | | | | |
| Volar | Volar (palmar) aspect of fingers | Wrist and finger flexion | Wrist and finger extension | Volar forearm |
| Dorsal | None | Wrist and finger extension | Wrist and finger flexion | Dorsal forearm |
| **HAND** | | | | |
| Intraosseous | None | Finger adduction and abduction | Finger adduction and abduction | Between metacarpals on dorsum of hand |

Modified from Matsen FA: *Compartmental syndromes,* February 10, 2005. Accessed April 24, 2006, on-line: www.orthop.washington.edu/faculty/matsen/compartmental.

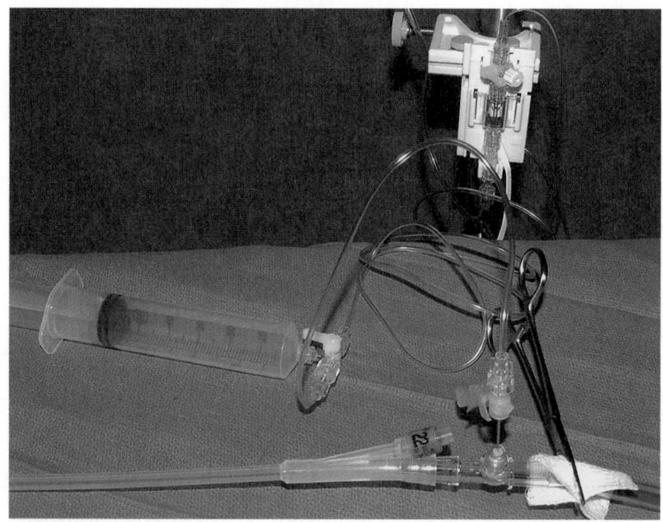

**FIGURE 31-7** Setup for measuring abdominal compartment syndrome using a two-way Foley catheter and a pressure monitoring system.

tient's condition permits, the perioperative nurse should obtain a brief, precise report from the ED nurse containing the following information: MOI, an AMPLE history (if available), condition on arrival (e.g., level of consciousness), availability of and prior administration of blood or blood products, spine clearance, injuries present, and any other pertinent information (e.g., family present, completion of secondary assessment). If the injury is life- or limb-threatening, implied surgical consent is assumed (i.e., if the patient were able, consent would be given).

Additional data are collected as the perioperative nurse accompanies the patient to the OR. The status of the airway, as well as breathing patterns and circulatory condition, can be observed. The ED record also provides information concerning amount and type of intravenous (IV) fluid received, vital signs, core temperature, and laboratory and other diagnostic examinations performed. A quick visual and physical survey of the patient when the perioperative nurse is preparing the patient for the procedure enables identification of other sites of injury that might require attention (Best Practice).

The patient's psychologic status can also be assessed. If the patient is awake, the perioperative nurse is challenged to allay fear and anxiety. The trauma patient has endured a very frightening experience and is in need of support. The perioperative nurse is often the best member of the surgical team to communicate with the patient and explain the interventions occurring before anesthesia induction. A touch or handhold is an important aspect of this communication process, demonstrating the nurse's caring behaviors and offering comfort.

## Nursing Diagnosis

Nursing diagnoses related to the care of trauma patients undergoing operative intervention might include the following:

- Anxiety and Fear (patient and family) related to unpredictable nature of condition
- Deficient Fluid Volume related to hemorrhage, fluid shifts, alteration in capillary permeability, alteration in vascular tone, or myocardial compromise
- Hypothermia related to rapid infusion of IV fluids, decreased tissue perfusion, and exposure
- Acute pain related to effects of trauma/injury agents, experience during invasive procedures or diagnostic tests
- Risk for Aspiration related to reduced level of consciousness secondary to injury or concomitant substance abuse; impaired cough and gag reflex; trauma to head, face, or neck; and secretions and debris in airway

## BEST PRACTICE

### Assessing Neurovascular Status in Patients with Musculoskeletal Trauma

Trauma patients frequently present to the operating room (OR) with fractures or other musculoskeletal injury. A thorough assessment of the patient's neurovascular status is imperative to establish a baseline for nursing and surgical interventions.

| Assessment Technique | Normal Findings |
|---|---|
| **SKIN COLOR** | |
| Inspect the skin distal to the injury. | There is no change in pigmentation compared with other parts of the body. |
| **SKIN TEMPERATURE** | |
| Palpate the area distal to the injury (the dorsum of the hands is the most sensitive to temperature). | The skin is warm. |
| **MOVEMENT** | |
| Ask the patient to move the affected area or the area distal to the injury (active motion). | The patient can move without discomfort. |
| Move the area distal to the injury (passive motion). | There is no difference in comfort compared with active movement. |
| **SENSATION** | |
| Ask the patient if numbness or tingling is present (paresthesia), | There is no numbness or tingling. |
| Palpate with a paper clip (especially in the web space between the first and second toes or the web space between the thumb and forefinger). | There is no difference in sensation in the affected and unaffected extremities. (Loss of sensation in these areas indicates perineal nerve or median nerve damage.) |
| **PULSES** | |
| Palpate the pulses distal to the injury. | Pulses are strong and easily palpated; no difference in the affected and unaffected extremities. |
| **CAPILLARY REFILL (LEAST RELIABLE)** | |
| Press the nail beds distal to the injury until blanching occurs (or the skin near the nail if nails are thick and brittle). | Blood return (return to usual color) is within 3 sec (5 sec for older people). |
| **PAIN** | |
| Ask the patient about the location, nature, and frequency of the pain. | Pain is usually localized and is often described as stabbing or throbbing. (Pain out of proportion to the injury and unrelieved by analgesics may indicate compartment syndrome.) |

From Evans MR: Interventions for clients with musculoskeletal trauma. In Ignatavicius DD, Workman ML, editors: *Medical-surgical nursing: critical thinking for collaborative care*, ed 5, St Louis, 2006, Saunders.

## Outcome Identification

Outcomes identified for the selected nursing diagnoses could be stated as follows:

- The patient and family will experience decreasing anxiety and fear, as evidenced by orientation to surroundings; ability to verbalize concerns and ask questions to health care team; decreased fear-related behaviors: crying, agitation; and use of effective coping skills.
- The patient will have an effective circulating volume as evidenced by strong, palpable peripheral pulses; skin normal color, warm, and dry; stable vital signs appropriate for age; maintenance of hematocrit of 30 ml/dl or hemoglobin of 12 to 14 g/dl or greater; and external hemorrhage controlled.
- The patient will maintain a normal core body temperature, as evidenced by a core temperature measurement of 36.6°C to 37.5°C (98°F to 99.5°F) and skin normal color, warm, and dry.
- The patient will experience relief of pain, as evidenced by diminishing or absent level of pain through patient's self-report, absence of physiologic indicators of pain: tachypnea, pallor, diaphoretic skin, increasing blood pressure, and ability to cooperate with care as appropriate.
- The patient will not experience aspiration, as evidenced by a patent airway; clear and equal bilateral breath sounds; regular rate, depth, and pattern of breathing; clear chest radiograph without evidence of infiltrates; and ability to handle secretions independently.

## Planning

Because of the unexpected nature of trauma, planning perioperative care is of the utmost importance. Equipment, instruments, and supplies that have a high probability of use must be immediately available. Autotransfusion or cell-saving devices should also be considered during patient care preparation, because blood salvage will be done if not contraindicated by the nature of the injury.

A typical plan of care for a trauma patient is shown on p. 1180.

## Implementation

***Multiple Operative Procedures.*** Depending on the severity of the injuries, the multiple trauma patient may require many surgical interventions. Some of these procedures may be performed simultaneously. This is determined through a collaborative effort among the trauma surgeon or surgeons, anesthesia provider, specialty surgeons, and perioperative nurse. If a patient has sustained severe head and abdominal trauma, a neurosurgeon will need to place an intracranial pressure (ICP) monitoring device. However, the abdominal exploration is also emergently indicated. Consequently, the severe condition of the patient may require performance of both of these procedures at the same time.

Multiple procedures, either simultaneously or in succession, require a great deal of preparation by the perioperative nurse and the trauma team. The order of procedures is determined by the presence or absence of life threats. The usual order of priority is chest, abdomen, head, and extremities. However, this priority is determined for each individual patient's situation and adjusted accordingly.

## SAMPLE PLAN OF CARE

### NURSING DIAGNOSIS

**Anxiety and Fear** (patient and family) related to unpredictable nature of condition

### OUTCOME

The patient and family will experience decreasing anxiety and fear, as evidenced by orientation to surroundings; ability to verbalize concerns and ask questions to health care team; decreased fear-related behaviors: crying, agitation; and use of effective coping skills.

### INTERVENTIONS

- Monitor the patient's level of anxiety by assessing the patient's state of alertness, ability to comprehend, and ability to comply with requests.
- Facilitate family's presence.
- Assist the family in identifying coping mechanisms; facilitate and support their use.
- Reassure patient and family during interactions by touch (when welcomed) and empathetic verbal and nonverbal communication.
- Explain perioperative environment to patient and what to expect to assist in reduction of anxiety.
- Discuss patient's postoperative appearance (i.e., drains, tubes, equipment) with the patient and family.

### NURSING DIAGNOSIS

**Deficient Fluid Volume** related to hemorrhage, fluid shifts, alteration in capillary permeability, alteration in vascular tone, or myocardial compromise

### OUTCOME

The patient will have an effective circulating volume as evidenced by strong, palpable peripheral pulses; skin normal color, warm, and dry; stable vital signs appropriate for age; maintenance of hematocrit of 30 ml/dl or hemoglobin of 12 to 14 g/dl or higher; and external hemorrhage controlled.

### INTERVENTIONS

- Control any uncontrolled bleeding by doing the following:
  - Applying direct pressure over bleeding site
  - Elevating extremity
  - Applying pressure over arterial pressure sites
- Ensure trauma profile laboratory work is complete.
- Verify that requested blood and blood replacement components are available in the operating room (OR).
- Prepare laboratory request slips as required; document time and type of analysis requested.
- Collaborate with anesthesia provider in monitoring cardiovascular changes suggestive of hypovolemia.
- Assist in accurate monitoring of intake and output during the surgical procedure.
- Administer blood and blood components as indicated.

### NURSING DIAGNOSIS

**Hypothermia** related to rapid infusion of intravenous (IV) fluids, decreased tissue perfusion, exposure

### OUTCOME

The patient will maintain a normal core body temperature, as evidenced by a core temperature measurement of 36°C to 37.5°C (96.8°F to 99.5°F) and skin normal color, warm, and dry.

### INTERVENTIONS

- Warm IV solutions and blood products using approved warming devices.
- Minimize body exposure during all phases of perioperative care.
- Use forced air–warming units and warm blankets to facilitate normothermia.
- Ensure irrigant solutions are warm.
- Monitor body temperature for signs of hypothermia, and report to anesthesia care provider.

### NURSING DIAGNOSIS

**Acute Pain** related to effects of trauma/injury agents, experience during invasive procedures or diagnostic tests

### OUTCOME

The patient will experience relief of pain, as evidenced by diminishing or absent level of pain through patient's self-report, absence of physiologic indicators of pain (tachypnea, pallor, diaphoretic skin, increasing blood pressure), and ability to cooperate with care as appropriate.

### INTERVENTIONS

- Collaborate with anesthesia provider and surgeon regarding pain management therapy to increase the patient's level of comfort if condition permits.
- Assess nonverbal cues regarding level of pain and discomfort.
- If the patient is unable to provide verbal or nonverbal cues, assume that pain is present or that procedures will cause pain.
- Use a visual or numeric pain scale to assess pain levels and change in comfort if patient is awake and able to respond.

### NURSING DIAGNOSIS

**Risk for Aspiration** related to reduced level of consciousness secondary to injury or concomitant substance abuse; impaired cough and gag reflex; trauma to head, face, or neck; and secretions and debris in airway

### OUTCOME

The patient will not experience aspiration, as evidenced by a patent airway; clear and equal bilateral breath sounds; regular rate, depth, and pattern of breathing; clear chest radiograph without evidence of infiltrates; and ability to handle secretions independently.

### INTERVENTIONS

- Ensure operation of suction apparatus preoperatively, and maintain one open suction line solely for the use of the anesthesia provider.
- Provide assistance with cricoid pressure under the direction of the anesthesia provider.
- Assist with placement of nasogastric or orogastric tube to evacuate stomach contents.

Performance of simultaneous procedures is preferable when physically possible. Anesthesia time is decreased for the critically ill patient, and definitive surgical interventions are accomplished more rapidly.

***Increased Risk for Infection.*** Many trauma patients have wounds that are contaminated with roadside debris, dirt, grass, or automobile parts. Others have a perforated full stomach, and food particles are released into the peritoneum, increasing the risk of peritonitis. Consequently, many patients are at high risk for infection. Sterile technique may be compromised secondary only to immediate life threat. Pouring an antimicrobial solution across the surgical site may be the only surgical skin prep undertaken when an immediate life threat exists. The use of antimicrobial prophylaxis shortly before skin incision has become the standard of care for surgical procedures. Perioperative nurses are in a position to ensure the timely administration of antibiotics (Research Highlight).

Wounds may be grossly decontaminated before the surgical skin prep. Sterile scrub brushes or a mechanical irrigation-under-pressure device may be used preoperatively and intraoperatively. Care must be exercised to remove as much contamination as possible, without creating further damage to the wound or body part. Perioperative personnel must wear personal protective equipment (PPE) during irrigation under pressure to prevent splashes and contamination from the lavage system.

Traffic in the OR should be limited to essential personnel. Increased traffic in the room increases chances for contamination in an already compromised patient, as well as potentially interferes with the delivery of expedient care.

***Procedure Preparation.*** Most level I trauma centers have a designated trauma operating room that contains all equipment and supplies potentially needed for trauma patients. Many hospitals maintain an emergency abdominal procedure set, craniotomy procedure set, and chest procedure set either within the OR's sterile supply area or immediately available in the central supply department. This streamlines preparation for the surgical procedure and allows for the possibility of rapid preparation in those instances where the patient bypasses the emergency room on arrival and is transported directly to the OR.

Once the perioperative nurse is notified of the surgical procedure, OR determination is made in consultation with the anesthesia staff and surgeon. Considerations include the following:

- Equipment required by the surgeon or surgeons to perform the surgical procedure
- Room availability
- Room size (to accommodate equipment, staff, and multiple procedures)
- Need for additional staff
- Capability for autotransfusion or cell-saver
- Availability of emergency procedure supplies (including power equipment)
- Selection of OR bed

Additional diagnostic procedures are often required during multiple trauma procedures. A fluoroscopic electric OR bed provides increased flexibility in patient management. The bed can be rotated on its base to facilitate two teams operating at once. The fluoroscopic capabilities allow for additional radiographs and arteriograms as needed. The bed should easily transform into different positions, such as lithotomy or lateral rotation. If a fluoroscopic bed is not available, arrangements must be made in advance to perform diagnostic radiologic procedures intraoperatively.

Before transfer of the patient to the OR bed, the perioperative nurse must ascertain if the spinal column has been cleared by the trauma surgeon or attending physician as free from injury. If the spine has not been cleared, the surgeon must be consulted before removal of the patient from the backboard. Safe transfer of the patient from the transport vehicle to the OR table can be accomplished using the log-rolling technique (Patient Safety).

Positioning of the patient is based on the surgical approach. Ascertaining the type and location of the wound (anterior or posterior) and type of operative procedure dictates the patient's position. For example, an aortic injury may be approached through a thoracotomy or a median sternotomy incision. The thoracotomy requires lateral positioning devices, and the sternotomy necessitates a supine position.

If several procedures are being performed, positioning may change intraoperatively. Changing the anesthetized patient's position is accomplished under the supervision of the anesthesia team. The patient is moved slowly, allowing for assessment of vital sign changes in response to the position movement. All precautions regarding positioning are reexecuted, with special attention given to the electrosurgical grounding pad. This pad may loosen during patient repositioning and require replacement to ensure adequate pad contact.

When the trauma patient is transferred to the OR, the extent of injury is not always known. The perioperative nurse should prep the patient from the suprasternal notch to the midthigh. This allows for rapid access to the chest to clamp the aorta should massive hemorrhage control be indicated; it also

## RESEARCH HIGHLIGHT

### Antimicrobial Prophylaxis

Evidence shows that antimicrobial prophylaxis is effective in reducing the risk of postoperative wound infections. Problems remain with the timing, selection, and duration of prophylaxis. This national study looked to determine the following: which patients received antimicrobial prophylaxis in a timely manner; which patients received antimicrobial prophylaxis based on published guidelines; and which patients had the prophylaxis discontinued after 24 hours. More than 34,999 patients having specified surgeries were reviewed. The findings showed that 55.7% of patients had timely administration and 92.6% of prophylaxis was based on published guidelines. Only 40.7% had the prophylaxis discontinued 24 hours after surgery. Postoperative infections were documented in 8.4% of the patients in the study group. These results suggest there is room for improvement in the timely administration and discontinuation of prophylaxis.

Modified from Bratzler DW and others: Use of antimicrobial prophylaxis for major surgery: baseline results from the National Surgical Infection Prevention Project, *Archives of Surgery* 140:174-182, 2005.

## PATIENT SAFETY

### Transferring and Intubating the Surgical Trauma Patient

Trauma patients may present to the operating room (OR) with actual or suspected cervical spine injuries. The perioperative nurse plays a key role in patient safety in these instances by assisting with transfer of the patient from the transport vehicle to the OR bed and by assisting with intubation.

The log-rolling technique is used to maintain cervical spine alignment. Even if the spine is cleared, initial radiographs are examined rapidly during initial evaluation and a very subtle injury to the vertebrae may be overlooked, so the use of the log-rolling technique during all patient transfers is advocated and should be documented as such.

The technique necessitates a minimum of four people—one positioned on each side and one each at the head and foot of the transfer cart. The person at the head of the patient is deemed in charge during transfer maneuvers. This person maintains manual in-line cervical spine immobilization at all times and counts aloud before the rolling and transfer of the patient. The nose of the patient is kept in line with the umbilicus and feet as the patient is rolled as one unit, avoiding any twisting of the spinal column.

Airway management of the spine-injured patient presents an additional challenge. The anesthesia provider will require assistance to secure the patient's airway because traditional direct laryngoscopy causes cervical motion, requiring adaptation of the usual techniques. Hyperextension of the neck is avoided, since an injury to the cervical spine is always presumed until proved otherwise in the trauma setting. At least three people are required for this type of intubation. The front of the cervical collar is removed while one person provides in-line cervical stabilization (not traction). This person must maintain stabilization until directed otherwise by the anesthesia provider. A second person holds cricoid pressure while the anesthesia provider ventilates, induces, and intubates the patient.

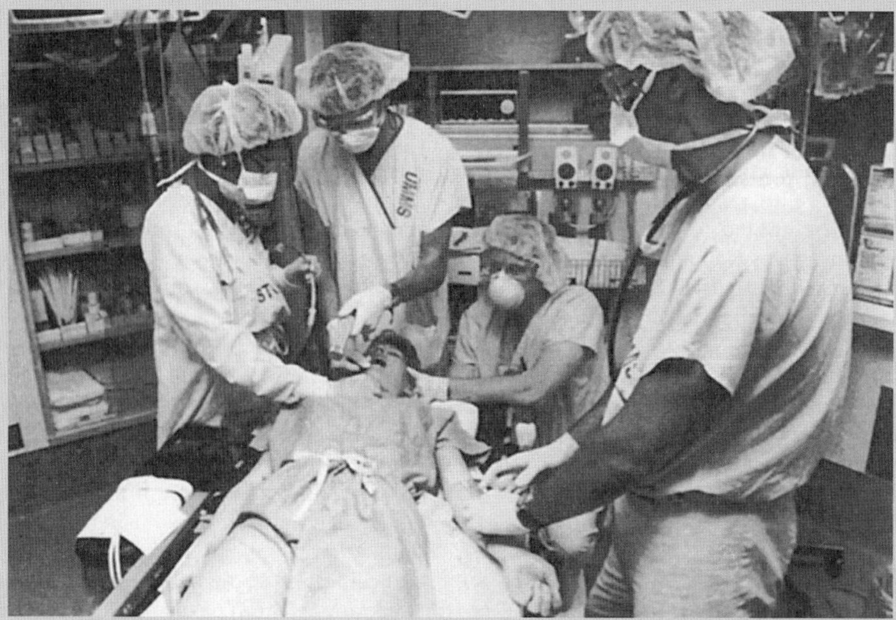

Technique of oral intubation performed by four-person team using laryngoscopy and manual, in-line axial traction in emergency trauma patient. Individual on left applies cricoid pressure (while also identifying landmarks for a cricothyroidotomy if it becomes necessary) and holds endotracheal tube ready. At center, intubator opens patient's mouth with right hand and holds laryngoscope with left hand. On right, assistant (ideally the neurosurgical consultant) uses both hands to stabilize head and neck. Note that anterior portion of cervical collar has been removed. Fourth person is responsible for administering intravenous induction agents.

From Dutton RP, McCunn M: Anesthesia for trauma. In Miller RD: *Miller's anesthesia,* ed 6, Philadelphia, 2005, Churchill Livingstone.

allows for exposure of the femoral arteries for potential cannulation and access to the thigh for harvesting a saphenous vein.

Established sponge, instrument, and sharp count policies should address surgical procedures of an emergent nature within the institution. Every attempt is made to verify appropriate numbers of counted items without compromising the timeliness of intervention in a life-threatening situation. If a preprocedural count is not performed, the perioperative nurse must document the occurrence and rationale used in accordance with established hospital policies and procedures. Some institutions require an x-ray examination postoperatively to examine the patient for the presence of a retained object. If counted sponges are intentionally left in the patient (e.g., in a damage control procedure at a level II, III, or IV center before transfer to a level I facility), the number and type of sponges left in the wound should be documented on the perioperative nursing record.[1] The operative dictation by the surgeon should also verify the presence of retained sponges, their type, and their number. This allows for accurate counts in subsequent procedures and prevents the potential for an inadvertent retained sponge.

In the presence of clotting difficulties or specific types of organ injuries with continuous oozing of blood, the surgeon may elect to pack the surgical site with laparotomy sponges and close the patient as a temporary measure. After a period of 24 to 48 hours, the patient returns to the OR for removal of the laparotomy sponges and primary closure if possible. In such instances the perioperative nurse must document and record accurately the number of sponges used for packing, as just noted. When the sponges are removed, the exact number is verified and the sponges are isolated and contained in accordance with established hospital policy and procedure.

***Autotransfusion.*** Considering the high blood loss associated with traumatic injuries, autotransfusion has become a vital asset in trauma care. Preoperative blood loss that is associated with an isolated hemothorax is collected in a designated chest-drainage device for reinfusion within 4 hours to avoid bacterial contamination. Intraoperative blood loss is collected, filtered, and reinfused to the patient. This provides immediate volume replacement, decreases the amount of bank blood used, and reduces the possibility of transfusion reactions or risk of transfusion with bloodborne pathogens.

The autotransfusion device, or cell-saver, requires specialized training for operation. Institutional policies vary regarding appropriate personnel designated for operation of the equipment. Capabilities for autotransfusion should be considered during procedure preparation, since additional qualified personnel may be required.

During cell-saver use the sterile scrub team member squeezes out additional blood and fluid from saturated sponges before discarding them from the surgical field. The cell-saver suction is used whenever possible to maximize the amount of blood salvaged. However, care must be taken to ensure that the blood collected in the cell-saver is free from contamination. For instance, if the abdomen is contaminated with free food particles or colonic perforation is present, the blood cannot be used. Similarly, once antibiotic irrigation is initiated, the cell-saver is not used.

***Evidence Preservation.*** If the injury to the patient is a result of a violent crime, attention must be given to preservation of evidence during the course of patient care. Physical evidence (bullets, bags of powder, weapons, pills, and other foreign objects), trace evidence (hair and fibers), biologic evidence (body fluids and blood), and clothing are considered types of evidence to be preserved. Specific procedures on handling of evidence may differ by institution and law enforcement agencies.

Clothing must be handled properly. When clothing is removed from the patient, it should be cut along the seams or around the bullet or stab wound holes. The shape of the hole may help identify the weapon used. Clothing is placed in paper bags, labeled appropriately, and given to law enforcement personnel. Plastic bags trap moisture and may facilitate growth of mold, which could destroy evidence. The transfer cart sheet should also be handled in a similar manner, since evidence may be present. Descriptions of wound appearances, body markings consistent with gang or cult activity, and statements from the patient must be accurately recorded.

The chain of custody for all evidence, including clothing, is followed. This process allows for identification of all people handling the evidence. Documentation must verify that the evidence has been in secure possession at all times. All evidence discovered must be recorded as to site of origin and when and to whom it was given. A system of documentation using receipts or a specific form should be established to ensure appropriate compliance.

Gunpowder residues, tissue, hair, or other valuable information may be present on the hands of a trauma patient. This evidence can be preserved by placing the patient's hands in a paper bag and securing it with tape. Washing the hands should be avoided. If the patient survives the injury, such avoidance may not be feasible.

Bullets and retained implements offer valuable evidence and may assist in identifying the assailant. The weapon firing the bullet and the bullet itself can be linked together by the specific grooves and markings placed on the bullet by the gun barrel when fired. Most bullets are composed of soft lead, and handling with metal instruments can interfere with the markings. Therefore using metal instruments to handle bullets should be avoided. Once a bullet is removed, it should be placed in dry, clean gauze in a plastic specimen container and passed off the sterile field to the circulator. The container is labeled appropriately. After the chain-of-custody procedures, the perioperative nurse should dispose of the bullet according to established institutional policies. Some of the newer exploding types of bullets can present a risk to perioperative team members during wound exploration. Care should be exercised to avoid sterile glove tears, since these types of bullets are extremely sharp.

***Deep Vein Thrombosis Prophylaxis.*** Because of the prolonged immobilization anticipated for the trauma patient, along with the frequency of orthopedic or lower extremity surgery performed on trauma patients, prevention of deep vein thrombosis (DVT) is an important concern.[18] Placement of sequential compression devices preoperatively is ideal. These pneumatic compression devices assist in decreasing the possibility of DVT, and their effect is optimized when applied before surgical intervention. Preoperative placement is subject to the physician's preference; clinical research regarding similar devices and demonstrated product effectiveness is ongoing. Subsequently, an inferior vena cava filter may be inserted in high-risk patients to prevent pulmonary embolus (PE). Risk factors for PE include prolonged immobility, multiple pelvic and lower extremity fractures, previous history of PE, or spinal cord injury with paralysis.

***Anesthesia Implications.*** Depending on institutional protocol, the anesthesia team may be directly involved in resuscitation of the trauma patient immediately after arrival at the ED. The anesthesia provider maintains the airway and intubates the patient if necessary. A critically injured patient may go directly to the OR, whereas some interventions may be performed in the ED of a trauma center. These interventions vary from insertion of an ICP monitor to an emergent exploratory thoracotomy.

However, if diagnostic evaluation can be accomplished without intubation and sedation, the patient may arrive in the OR awake. A trauma patient is assumed to have a full stomach. Thus these patients are at high risk for aspiration and resultant pneumonia. Under the direction of the anesthesia provider, cricoid pressure (Sellick maneuver) is provided by the perioperative nurse (Figure 31-8). This pressure is maintained over the cricoid area until the cuff on the endotracheal (ET) tube is inflated and tube placement verified by the anesthesia provider. This type of intubation is often referred to as a "crash induction."

In addition, the patient may require intubation for protection of the airway before radiologic examination of the cervical spine. If the cervical spine is not cleared or if the radiographic screening examination is not performed before intubation, ET intubation is done while cervical spine precautions (i.e., in-line intubation) are maintained (see Patient Safety). The trauma team may decide to use rapid-sequence intubation (RSI). RSI involves administration of 100% oxygen, analgesia, a neuromuscular relaxant, application of cricoid pressure, and insertion of a cuffed ET tube. Etomidate (Amidate) is the most commonly used induction agent.[13] It acts in about 1 minute and lasts about 5 minutes. It is often used in trauma patients because it does not cause an increase in ICP or worsening of hypotension. Succinylcholine (Anectine) is the most frequently used neuromuscular relaxant. The perioperative nurse can facilitate RSI by ensuring availability of all intubation and resuscitation equipment, assisting with monitoring devices, and confirming correct ET-tube placement.

In injuries of the face where midface fractures are present, nasal intubation and nasogastric tube placement are avoided. Tube placement in the brain through a fracture of the cribriform plate is a well-known complication. To avoid this, oral ET intubation is the technique of choice. Stomach decompression is achieved by placement of the gastric tube orally. An awake oral intubation is often necessary because anesthesia and muscle relaxants can result in the loss of any remaining airway in the presence of facial trauma.

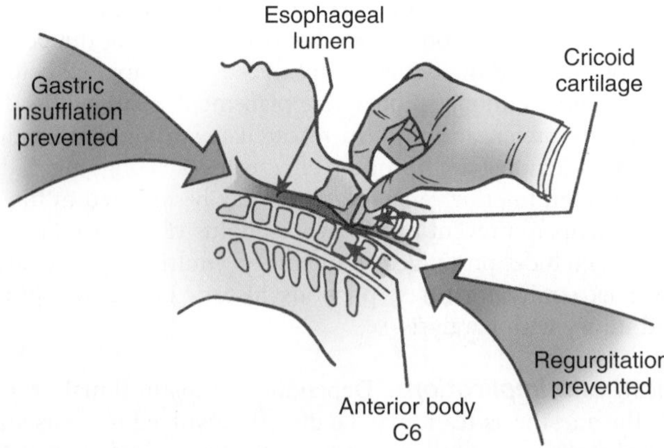


**FIGURE 31-8** Application of cricoid pressure. Thumb and forefinger are used to depress cricoid cartilage, causing it to impinge on lumen of esophagus and sealing it closed against anterior body of C6. As a result, gastric insufflation secondary to positive-pressure ventilation (bag-valve-mask apparatus) from above, as well as regurgitation of stomach contents from below, is largely prevented. *C6*, Sixth cervical vertebra.

Large-bore IV access used with rapid-infusion fluid warmers may be employed in the ED. These fluid warmers can deliver high volumes of crystalloid solution at body temperature (Figure 31-9). Use of the fluid warmer may continue during the intraoperative phase to facilitate volume replacement and help maintain normothermia. A number of factors may influence a trauma patient's response to fluid loss. These factors include age, severity of injury, type and location of injury, time lapse from injury to treatment, prehospital fluid therapy, prehospital use of a pneumatic antishock garment, and medications taken for chronic conditions. Fluid resuscitation should be initiated when early signs of blood loss are suspected. A classification system can be useful in determining the needs of the patient (Table 31-6).

***Pregnancy.*** The normal physiologic changes that occur during pregnancy increase the challenge of evaluation and treatment when these individuals are victims of trauma. It is most important to remember that two patients are being treated. The key to resuscitation of the fetus is to resuscitate the mother. One of the first physiologic changes to note is that the pregnant trauma patient has a much larger circulatory volume[4] (Table 31-7). The cardiac output may be increased by as much as 40%. Oxygen requirements are increased. Heart rate increases over the prepregnant state. The usual clinical indicators of hypovolemic shock are unreliable in the pregnant trauma patient (Table 31-8). It is imperative to assume that the pregnant trauma victim is in shock until proved otherwise. Early aggressive treatment is essential. The uterus is enlarged and no longer a pelvic organ, and it elevates the bladder out of the pelvis as well. Supine position for the pregnant patient can

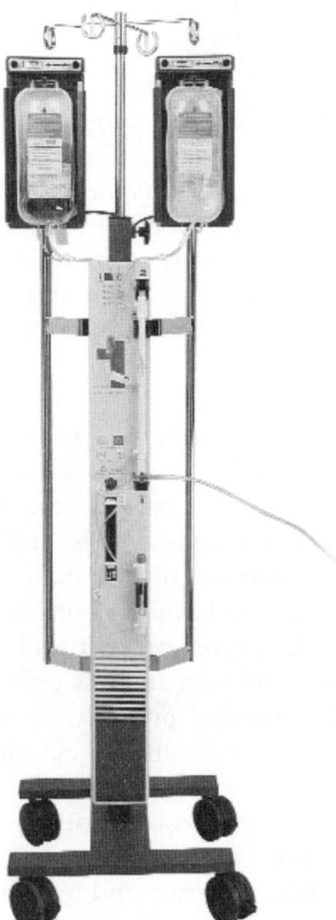

**FIGURE 31-9** Level I System 250 fluid warmer unit.

**TABLE 31-6**

## Estimated Fluid and Blood Losses Based on Patient's Initial Presentation*

| | Class I | Class II | Class III | Class IV |
|---|---|---|---|---|
| Blood loss (ml) | Up to 750 | 750-1500 | 1500-2000 | >2000 |
| Blood loss (% blood volume) | Up to 15% | 15%-30% | 30%-40% | >40% |
| Pulse rate (beats/min) | <100 | >100 | >120 | >140 |
| Blood pressure | Normal | Normal | Decreased | Decreased |
| Pulse pressure | Normal or increased | Decreased | Decreased | Decreased |
| Respiratory rate | 14-20 | 20-30 | 30-40 | >35 |
| Urine output (ml/hr) | >30 | 20-30 | 5-15 | Negligible |
| Central nervous system (CNS)/mental status | Slightly anxious | Mildly anxious | Anxious, confused | Confused, lethargic |
| Fluid replacement (3:1 rule) | Crystalloid | Crystalloid | Crystalloid and blood | Crystalloid and blood |

From American College of Surgeons: *ATLS program for doctors,* ed 7 Chicago, Illinois, 2004, American College of Surgeons.
*The guidelines are for a 70-kg man. They are based on the 3:1 rule. This rule derives from the empiric observation that most patients in hemorrhagic shock require as much as 300 ml of electrolyte solution for each 100 ml of blood loss. Applied blindly, these guidelines can result in excessive or inadequate fluid administration. For example, a patient with a crush injury to the extremity may have hypotension out of proportion to his or her blood loss and require fluids in excess of the 3:1 guidelines. In contrast, a patient whose ongoing blood loss is being replaced by blood transfusion requires less than 3:1. The use of bolus therapy with careful monitoring of the patient's response can moderate these extremes.

**TABLE 31-7**

## Maternal Adaptation During Pregnancy and Relation to Trauma

| System | Alteration | Clinical Responses |
|---|---|---|
| Respiratory | ↑Oxygen consumption<br>↑ Tidal volume<br>↓ Functional residual capacity<br>Chronic compensated alkalosis<br>↓$Paco_2$<br>↓Serum bicarbonate | ↑ Risk of acidosis<br>↑ Risk of respiratory mismanagement<br>↓ Blood-buffering capacity |
| Cardiovascular | ↑ Circulating volume, 1600 ml<br>↑ Cardiac output<br>↑ Heart rate<br>↓ Systemic vascular resistance (SVR)<br>↓Arterial blood pressure<br>Heart displaced upward to left | Can lose 1000 ml of blood<br>No signs of shock until blood loss >30% of total volume<br>↓ Placental perfusion in supine position<br>Point of maximal impulse, fourth intercostal space |
| Renal | ↑ Renal plasma flow<br>Dilation of ureters and urethra<br>Bladder displaced forward | ↑ Risk of stasis, infection<br>↑ Risk of bladder rupture |
| Gastrointestinal | ↓ Gastric motility<br>↑ Hydrochloric acid production<br>↓ Competency of gastroesophageal sphincter | ↑ Risk of aspiration<br>Passive regurgitation of stomach acids if head lower than stomach |
| Reproductive | ↑ Blood flow to organs<br>Uterine enlargement | Source of ↑ blood loss<br>Vena caval compression in supine position |
| Musculoskeletal | Displacement of abdominal viscera<br>Pelvic venous congestion<br>Cartilage softened | ↑ Risk of injury, altered rebound response; altered pain referral<br>↑ Risk of pelvic fracture<br>Center of gravity changed |
| Hematologic | Fetal head in pelvis<br>↑ Clotting factors<br>↓ Fibrinolytic activity | ↑ Risk of fetal injury<br>↑ Risk of thrombus formation |

From Dorman KF, Harvey MG: Obstetric critical care. In Lowdermilk DL, Perry SE, editors: *Maternity & women's health care,* ed 8, St Louis, 2004, Mosby.

result in a decrease in cardiac output as a result of compression of the inferior vena cava. If the patient is close to term, cardiac output can be reduced by as much as 30% as a result of compression on the inferior vena cava. Consequently, patients who are 20 weeks or more into their pregnancy should be placed in the left lateral decubitus position to avoid a hypotensive episode. If this is not possible, manual displacement of the uterus by lateral abdominal pressure should be attempted.

Ultrasound studies are conducted to determine viability of the fetus when possible. In the event of a ruptured uterus, a

**TABLE 31-8**

## Signs of Hypovolemic Shock in Pregnancy

| | Circulating Blood Volume Deficit | |
|---|---|---|
| | **Early (20%)** | **Late (25%)** |
| Pulse | <100 beats/min | >100 beats/min |
| Respiratory rate | 12-20/min | >20/min |
| Blood pressure | Normal | Hypotensive |
| Skin perfusion | Warm, dry skin | Cool, ashen skin |
| Capillary refill | <2 sec | >2 sec |
| Level of consciousness | Alert | Agitated, lethargic |
| Urine output | >30-50 ml/hr | <30-50 ml/hr |
| Fetal heart rate (normally 120-160 beats/min) | High, low, late decelerations | High, low, absent, late decelerations |

cesarean delivery and hysterectomy may be required if the fetus is viable. Neonatal resuscitation is of the utmost importance immediately on delivery of the fetus.

Fetuses of pregnant patients requiring surgery require fetal assessment intraoperatively. Any fetal movement should be noted. In addition, fetal monitoring is continuous. This includes fetal heart rate and uterine contractions. Fetal monitoring provides information on the condition of the fetus and response to uterine contractions if present. Fetal heart rate can usually be obtained after 10 weeks of gestation. Abnormalities in fetal heart rate can be an early sign of maternal compromise because the pregnant uterus is viewed as a nonessential peripheral organ in states of hypovolemic shock. Personnel qualified in the interpretation of fetal heart rate patterns must be present. This expertise may be provided by the obstetric nursing staff.

Perimortem (postmortem) cesarean delivery may be performed in the event of the sudden death of the mother and presence of a viable fetus.

***Pediatric Trauma Patients.*** Special considerations related to the care of infants and children who have sustained a trauma are described in Chapter 29.

***Elderly Trauma Patients.*** As the number of adults older than 65 years continues to grow, so does the number of elderly patients requiring surgical intervention related to trauma. The physiologic effects of aging, combined with the preinjury health status of many elderly patients, significantly affect their ability to respond to initial treatment for traumatic injuries and subsequent surgical intervention. Consequently, the mortality rate for elderly trauma patients is significantly higher than that in younger patients with the same level of injury. Preexisting medical conditions, decreased physiologic reserves, and the physical and psychologic stress experienced during surgical interventions place elderly trauma victims at increased risk for perioperative complications.[14] (See Chapter 30 for the physiologic and psychologic changes that occur in elderly patients.)

***Invasive Emergency Department Interventions.*** If a patient has had very recent loss of vital signs, either en route to the hospital or on arrival at the ED, the trauma surgeon may elect to perform an emergency thoracotomy in the ED. A left-sided approach is usually performed because this allows rapid access to the heart for external cardiac massage and exposure of the great vessels for clamping in the event of severe blood loss. The incision can be extended to the right side by cutting across the sternum. This procedure can be used to gain control in hemorrhage of the great vessels, to access the heart, or in a grave situation, as a final effort to save a life (Figure 31-10). The procedure is used more often in penetrating injuries where a laceration to a ventricle or other potentially treatable, life-threatening injury may be present.

Because of the perioperative nurse's knowledge of surgical instrumentation and procedures, his or her assistance in this procedure in the ED is often required. Rapid access to the heart and great vessels is the goal. The patient is then transported to the OR for additional interventions once hemorrhage is controlled.

In a similar fashion, an exploratory laparotomy can be initiated in the ED to control abdominal hemorrhage, especially when a splenic rupture is suspected and the patient is severely compromised.

If all other techniques of airway access are unsuccessful, a cricothyrotomy is performed. A vertical incision is made through the skin, and the cricothyroid membrane is incised. An ET or tracheostomy tube can be inserted through the membrane to create an airway. In the event a tube is not immediately available, a large-bore needle can be inserted into the membrane and the catheter left in place. This provides a temporary airway access measure but is inadequate to effectively ventilate the patient without a jet oscillating ventilator.

***Successive Surgical Interventions.*** Often the multiple trauma patient requires a multitude of surgical procedures—either specialty-related or as a stepwise progression in the primary treatment of the initial injury. Acalculous cholecystitis is often a secondary complication of the trauma patient's postoperative course that requires cholecystectomy. Secondary wound closures, debridements, and fixation of initially undiscovered fractures make up the majority of follow-up procedures. Ini-

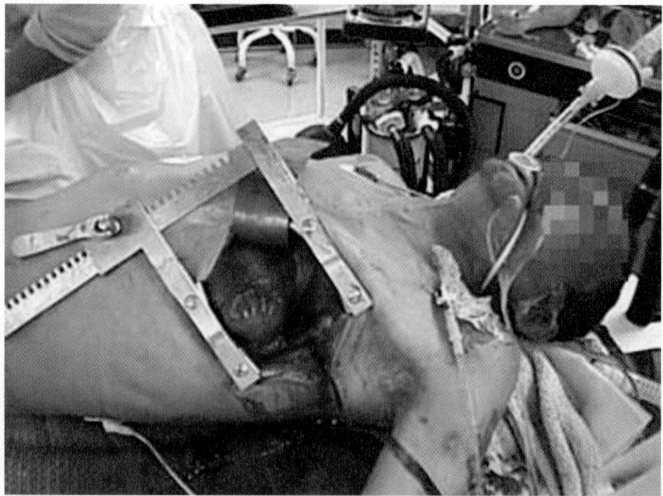

**FIGURE 31-10** Emergency exploratory thoracotomy performed in the emergency department.

tially the trauma patient is critically ill and requires intensive care facilities. When surgery is scheduled, the perioperative nurse may need additional assistance in transport of the patient as transport monitoring of the ECG, arterial line, and blood pressure monitoring is performed. Oxygen and mechanical ventilation with an Ambu bag are necessary for the intubated patient.

## Evaluation

The evaluation of the patient should reflect the effectiveness of the interventions. Did the patient remain free from untoward complications? Was there progress toward the expected outcomes as described in the perioperative plan of care? The following are examples of evaluation statements in relation to the Sample Plan of Care:

- The patient demonstrated a decreased level of anxiety; he or she verbalized less apprehension, maintained eye contact, and was able to comply with requests even though anxiety persisted.
- The patient remained hemodynamically stable; fluid resuscitation was undertaken, blood pressure and pulse were adequate considering the patient's status, and the H&H were within acceptable ranges.
- The patient achieved and maintained normothermia in the OR.
- The patient reported reasonable relief from pain during preparatory maneuvers in the OR.
- The airway was maintained, and induction of anesthesia proceeded without complication.

On completion of the procedure or procedures, the perioperative nurse is afforded an opportunity to further assess the trauma patient as well as evaluate the plan of care implemented. If the patient sustained numerous injuries and remains critically injured, the PACU may be bypassed and the patient may be transferred directly to the ICU. The perioperative nurse should accompany the patient, along with the anesthesia team, to the ICU. Once the anesthesia report is given, the perioperative nurse can provide a wealth of information to the critical care nurse. At this point, family members may have been contacted or are present, allowing more specific medical history information to be obtained. However, the mechanism of injury and events surrounding the trauma are still significant. A high index of suspicion remains during postoperative care of the patient sustaining multiple injuries. Attention can be diverted from a less significant injury in the presence of a highly visible or obvious trauma. Once the obvious trauma undergoes intervention, pain or discomfort from other injuries becomes more apparent. In the care of a patient with neurologic deficit, physical assessment and continued evaluation are essential because patient self-report is nonexistent.

Status of progress in the secondary assessment should also be reported. Any additional laboratory work or interventions that have yet to be completed should be discussed. It is imperative in a thorough examination to view the back of the patient in an effort to locate all injuries.

Additional diagnostic procedures may be required after completion of the surgical procedure if the patient's condition is stable. The perioperative nurse may be requested to accompany the patient to the diagnostic department with the anesthesia team. In addition, respiratory care personnel may assist in patient transport and maintenance of the airway.

## Critical Incident–Stress Debriefing

Unfortunately, some accidental injuries result in death. This can be particularly difficult for the perioperative team, since most surgical interventions are of a curative or restorative nature. In many emergency medical systems, a critical incident–stress debriefing team exists. It is composed of mental health professionals and specially trained volunteers who are also professionals and peers in the health care field. Police officers, firefighters, paramedics, ED nurses, and ICU nurses can also be on the team. In the event of a particularly tragic death of a patient, the team can be contacted, and a meeting with that patient's care providers is arranged. The benefit of this team is enhanced when intervention is timely for the care providers. Opportunity for them to discuss their feelings and emotions is provided and encouraged as each provider discusses feelings related to personal participation in the care of the patient. Critical incident–stress debriefing teams enhance coping mechanisms and can provide a healthy professional growth from what may otherwise be felt to be a tragedy.[7]

## Patient and Family Education and Discharge Planning

Traumatic injury to a family member or significant other occurs without warning. Patients may be traveling or visiting out of town or state at the time of injury. Families or friends involved in a motor vehicle collision may be triaged to several different facilities based on severity of injury or age. A family member or significant other may not be contacted until several hours or even days after the injury. Sometimes the patient's identity is either unknown or must be kept confidential to prevent further harm. Both the patient and family member are truly victims of traumatic injury. Consequently, patients and family members are in a time of crisis.

Some families may handle the crisis with ease, whereas others become dysfunctional. Coping strategies may be inappropriate at times as the patient and family attempt to reestablish patterns of function. A family system already taxed before the event may be overwhelmed with the additional stress of a sudden traumatic event. On the other hand, family members may wish to be present during resuscitation efforts. Family presence requires a facilitator to explain to the family procedures to be performed, sights, sounds, and smells. Rules are often established about time restrictions and family behavior to protect the patient, staff, and family members themselves. In instances of disruptive behavior or overwhelming grief, family members may be escorted out. These rules and restrictions must be explained to the family in advance.[8]

The perioperative nurse must be prepared for a variety of responses, both from the patient and the family or significant others. Interaction with the patient before surgical intervention may be impossible because of the severity of the injury, prior intubation, or hemodynamic instability. The perioperative nurse will need to offer brief, simple instructions and explanations if the patient is awake enough. These may include the following:

- Background noise as caregivers prepare for emergent intervention
- Perception of cold within the OR room
- Placement of safety and restraining straps, armboards, warming devices, pneumatic compression stockings, and so on
- Invasive interventions, such as additional IV access or arterial line monitoring

A reassuring touch or holding the patient's hand may be the only communication possible. Touch, placement of warm blankets, a gentle squeeze of the hand, and softly spoken words of reassurance are important comfort measures.

In accordance with hospital policies and procedures, the perioperative nurse may call the surgical waiting room with periodic updates on the patient's condition. The information shared is subject to the trauma surgeon's discretion and is usually concise in nature, such as, "at this time the extent of injury is unknown; his/her condition is critical." When implemented, these contacts with family members are appreciated because frequently they were unable to see or speak with the patient before the operation.

Many facilities have a chaplain or social worker available to assist family members during this time of crisis. These caregivers assist in the initial family contact and provide immediate support. The chaplain may act as the facilitator for family presence.

All injuries and possible subsequent complications may not be known at the time of operative intervention. The multiply injured patient frequently requires rehabilitation or an extended stay in a skilled nursing facility before discharge to home. Continued therapy, such as neuropsychology (for cognitive impairment) or occupational and physical therapy, may be on an outpatient basis. Consequently, information regarding recovery and rehabilitation is limited on admission to the hospital. Many facilities have access to or provide support groups for patients and families related to the type of injury and its subsequent lifelong effects.

# Surgical Interventions

## DAMAGE CONTROL SURGERY

The central tenet of damage control surgery is that patients die from a triad of coagulopathy, hypothermia, and metabolic acidosis. Once this metabolic failure has become established, it is extremely difficult to control hemorrhage and correct the trauma triad. The principles of the first damage control procedure are control of hemorrhage, prevention of contamination, and protection from further injury. Once this has been achieved, the definitive surgical procedure can be carried out as necessary—often referred to as the "staged procedure." Damage control surgery is the most technically demanding and challenging surgery a trauma surgeon can perform.[3]

Damage control surgery is somewhat unique to the field of trauma surgery. The principles of damage control were originally slow to be accepted by surgeons around the world, because they contradict most standard surgical teaching practices—that the best operation for a patient is one definitive procedure. However, it is now well recognized that multiple trauma patients are more likely to die from their intraoperative metabolic failure than from a failure to complete a specific operative repair. Patients with major exsanguinating injuries will not survive complex procedures, such as formal hepatic resection or pancreaticoduodenectomy.

## INJURIES OF THE HEAD AND SPINAL COLUMN

Trauma to the head is responsible for one half of all trauma deaths. Brain injury occurs either as a direct result of the trauma to the tissue or as a complication. Often, forces of energy from the impact are tolerated by the rigid skull, but the soft tissue of the brain is traumatized. This results in formation of subdural (Figure 31-11), epidural, or intracerebral hematomas. In addition, cerebral swelling can result in herniation of the brain despite treatment (Figure 31-12).

A baseline neurologic examination is extremely important. The pupils are examined, and the presence or absence of posturing is noted. The Glasgow Coma Scale (Table 31-9) provides a universally accepted mechanism to assess the baseline data for the trauma team. However, in the presence of alcohol or drug intoxication or chemical paralysis, the scale cannot be used. For patients with a score of 8 or less, intubation with controlled ventilation is the immediate treatment of choice. In the highly combative patient, intubation may also be performed to allow adequate assessment of the extent of injury.

Previously, hyperventilation was routinely used in initial management of patients with neurologic deterioration to decrease ICPs. No studies have shown improved outcome for these patients, and other methods of assessment have shown that this can cause significant constriction of cerebral vessels and may reduce cerebral blood flow to an ischemic level. One study has shown long-term improvement when hyperventilation was not used. Occasionally, hyperventilation may be necessary with persistently high ICP unresponsive to other treatment modalities.

An osmotic diuretic, such as mannitol, can be used in the treatment of ICP. Osmotic effects take place in 15 to 30 minutes[10] and set up an osmotic gradient to draw out water from neurons. Osmotic diuretics such as mannitol have shown benefits in lowering ICP without reducing cerebral blood flow. They are given by bolus administration to create an acute re-

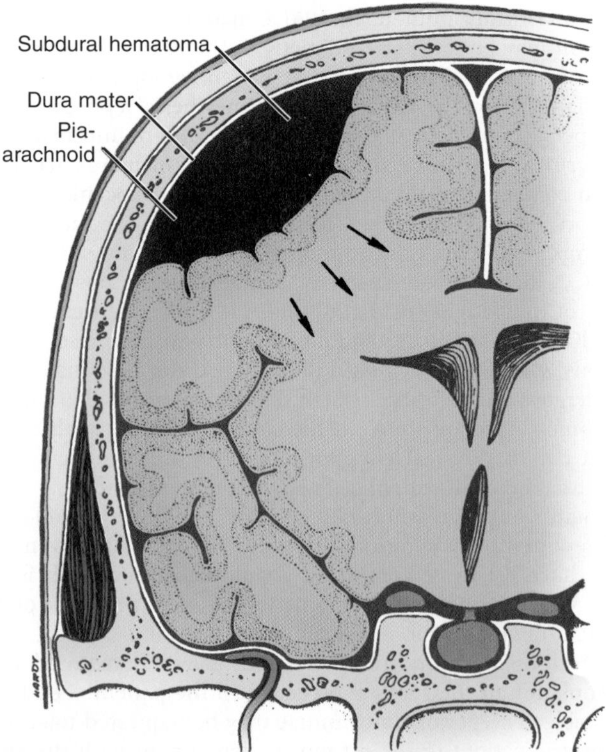


FIGURE 31-11 Subdural hematoma causing increased intracranial pressure with shifting of tissue.

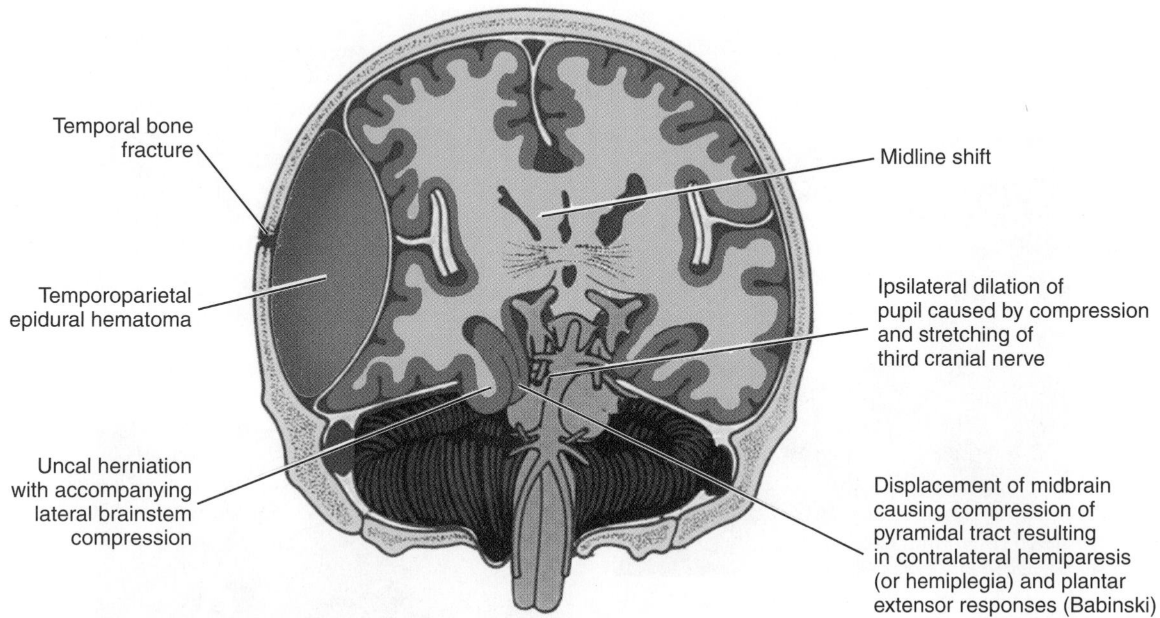


**FIGURE 31-12** Cross section showing herniation of lower portion of temporal lobe (uncus) through tentorium caused by temporoparietal epidural hematoma. Herniation may occur also in cerebellum. Note mass effect and midline shift.

**TABLE 31-9**

## Glasgow Coma Scale

| | Points |
|---|---|
| **EYE OPENING** | |
| Spontaneous | 4 |
| To speech | 3 |
| To pain | 2 |
| None | 1 |
| **VERBAL COMMUNICATION** | |
| Oriented | 5 |
| Confused conversation | 4 |
| Inappropriate words | 3 |
| Incomprehensible sounds | 2 |
| None | 1 |
| **MOTOR RESPONSE** | |
| Obeys commands | 6 |
| Localizes to pain | 5 |
| Withdraws to pain | 4 |
| Abnormal flexion | 3 |
| Abnormal extension | 2 |
| None | 1 |

From Hausman KA: Assessment of the nervous system. In Ignatavicius DD, Workman ML, editors: *Medical-surgical nursing: critical thinking for collaborative care,* ed 5, St Louis, 2006, Saunders.

duction phase in ICP. These agents are excreted in the urine and cause a rise in serum urine and osmolality. Patients with serum osmolalities higher than 320 mOsm/kg[3] are at risk of acute tubular necrosis. Hypovolemia should be avoided with the infusion of isotonic fluids as necessary. Because such agents act quickly, fluid intake and output and the potential for fluid and electrolyte imbalances mandate close hemodynamic monitoring. Elevation of the head of the bed at 30 degrees and keeping the head midline (to promote venous drainage) can also be beneficial.

Skull fractures usually do not require operative intervention when there is no displacement and the fracture is linear. Depressed fractures or the presence of bone in the brain frequently requires elevation and debridement (Figure 31-13). Hematoma evacuation is based on the location of the hematoma, size, and number present. Before a craniotomy or burr hole is performed, the CT scan, the neurologic status of the patient, morbidity or mortality associated with the procedure, other injuries present, and any underlying medical problems, if known, are evaluated. An ICP monitor may be placed in the patient who is at risk for increased ICP. Chapter 23 discusses neurosurgical procedures.

The patient with a cervical spine injury at or near C3 to C5 is at great risk for respiratory difficulties because this is the area of diaphragmatic innervation. There is also the possibility of swelling above the area of injury, and the perioperative nurse should be alert for the potential of respiratory distress even if not initially present. A 24- to 48-hour dose of methylprednisolone (Solu-Medrol), calculated by body weight, is considered to decrease initial cord swelling.

The standard indicators of possible cord injury are absence of rectal tone and bradycardia in the presence of hypotension. The body's normal response is to increase heart rate in the presence of decreased blood flow or hypotension. These responses are not present in injury of the spinal cord, and vagal control results in bradycardia.

Injuries involving the spinal cord can range from complete transection, without hope of recovery, to a contusion of the cord. Fractures or dislocation of the vertebra can result in the protrusion of small pieces into the spinal canal. This is known as a *burst fracture.* Several vertebrae may be fractured or have fractured components. Generally, in compression fractures, if the loss of vertebral height is more than 20%, surgical treatment may be indicated. Spinal bracing can be considered an

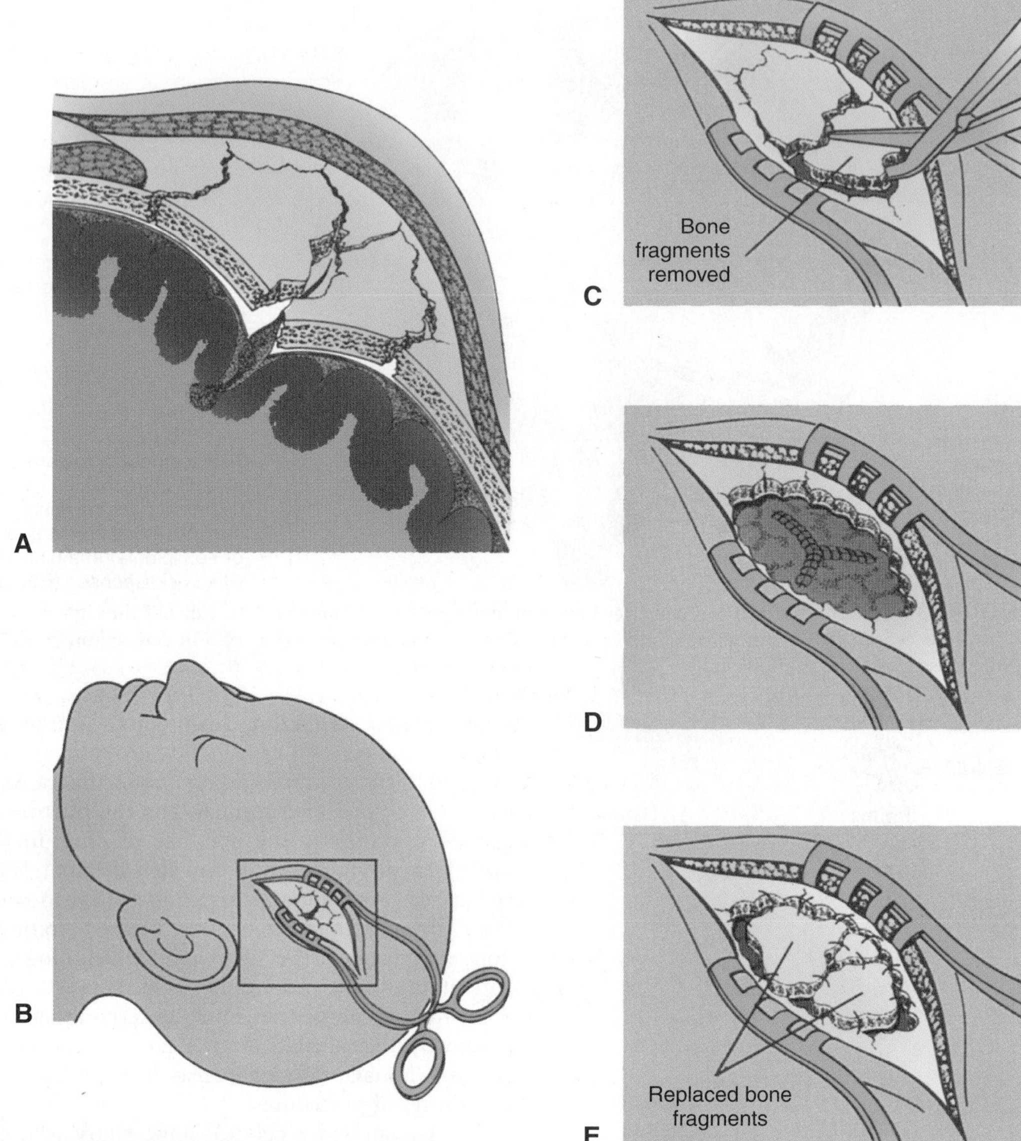


**FIGURE 31-13** Treatment of compound depressed fracture of skull. **A,** Depressed skull fracture and scalp injury. **B,** Incision to expose fracture and remove the portion of the scalp that is devitalized. **C,** Removal of impacted bone by burr hole to locate and identify normal dura, followed by resection of bone fragments. **D,** Watertight closure of dura after brain debridement. **E,** Replacement and fixation of bone fragments.

option if the compression is less than 20% and no neurologic signs or symptoms are present. Cerebral arteriography may be used to screen patients with cervical vertebral fractures for blunt vertebral artery injuries (BVIs). Patients who sustain blunt trauma with unilateral headache or posterior neck pain, particularly if it is sharp, sudden, and severe, should be screened for BVIs and treated with anticoagulant therapy if not contraindicated.[12]

Treatment of spinal column fractures can involve surgery. Stabilization of the fracture may be necessary, depending on the severity of the injury. For cervical spine fractures, traction may be used initially to reduce the fracture, followed by surgical intervention as soon as the patient's condition permits. Internal fixation devices are discussed in Chapter 22.

## INJURIES OF THE FACE

Motor vehicle crashes account for about 60% of maxillofacial injuries. Mandibular fractures alone are highly associated with assault as the MOI. In the patient who presents with facial injury, the airway must be secured. This requires ensuring patency and removing any items that pose the threat of aspiration. If a midface fracture is present, nasogastric tube placement and nasotracheal intubation are avoided. A tracheostomy may need to be performed before initiation of the operative procedure. Control of scalp or facial hemorrhage can be achieved through a pressure dressing until surgical intervention is possible, since exsanguination can occur. Treatment of the fracture may be delayed until the immediate life threats have been successfully managed. Goals of operative intervention are to reduce and immobilize the fracture, prevent infection, and restore facial cosmesis and function.

Facial fractures can be categorized into Le Fort I, II, or III (Figure 31-14). A Le Fort I fracture is the most common maxillary fracture. It involves a horizontal interruption of the anterior and lateral wall of the maxillary sinus. Le Fort II is a pyramidal fracture along the maxilla and lacrimal bones and through the infraorbital rim. Le Fort III is otherwise known as *craniofacial disjunction.* The midface is completely disengaged from the cranial base, resulting from a fracture across the frontomaxillary sutures. Specific information regarding these injuries is in Chapter 24.

## INJURIES OF THE EYE

Injuries to the eye can result from blunt or penetrating types of trauma. Penetrating objects in the globe are stabilized and not removed until the patient is in the OR. These injuries threaten loss of vision because of the injury itself, inflammation, or infection. Blunt injury to the eye can result in hematomas and accompanying fractures. A blowout fracture is the result of a blunt force to the eye that pushes soft tissue through the thin bony orbital floor. The patient has recession of the eye into the orbit and loses the ability to gaze upward. Surgical repair is often indicated. Chapter 18 discusses ophthalmic procedures.

## INJURIES OF THE NECK

Injury to the neck and soft tissue structures is most commonly a result of penetrating trauma. The neck can be divided into three zones with respect to injury and consequence. Zone I is the base of the neck below the clavicles. Anatomic structures located in this region are the great vessels and aortic arch, innominate veins, trachea, esophagus, and lungs. Zone II is the area in the middle of the neck between the clavicles and the mandible. Structures located in this area include the carotid artery, internal jugular vein, trachea, and esophagus. Zone III is located between the angle of the mandible and the base of the skull. The primary target of evaluation in these injuries is vascular structures.

Zone II injuries may necessitate an otorhinolaryngology specialist. Penetrating injuries to the larynx and trachea can be primarily repaired. Blunt force to the larynx can result in a fracture and impose immediate airway obstruction. These patients require immediate tracheotomy followed by repair of the fracture when it is unstable or displaced. Chapter 21 gives specific information concerning otorhinolaryngologic procedures.

## INJURIES OF THE CHEST AND HEART

Trauma to the chest area is the primary cause of death in approximately 25% of trauma victims. Blunt trauma is most often associated with high-speed motor vehicle crashes. Penetrating trauma may be associated with an increase in violent crime. Penetrating injuries at or immediately below the nipple line or level of the scapular tips are evaluated for both chest and abdominal involvement. Diaphragmatic injury is also a possibility.

Deceleration injury, such as that from a fall or striking the steering wheel in a motor vehicle crash, may cause contusions of the chest wall, rib or sternal fractures, cardiac or pulmonary contusions, or rupture of the aorta and other major vessels. Rib fractures are also associated with a hemothorax or pneumothorax (Figure 31-15). A flail-chest segment may result when two or more adjacent ribs are broken in two or more places (Figure 31-16). This results in a paradoxic chest wall movement as a result of loss of bony support. The segment of chest wall will move in the opposite direction. If there are respiratory distress and diminished breath sounds, a chest tube is indicated immediately; an autotransfusion chest-drainage device is also considered. Chest tube output must be closely monitored intraoperatively because accumulation of 1000 to 1500 ml of

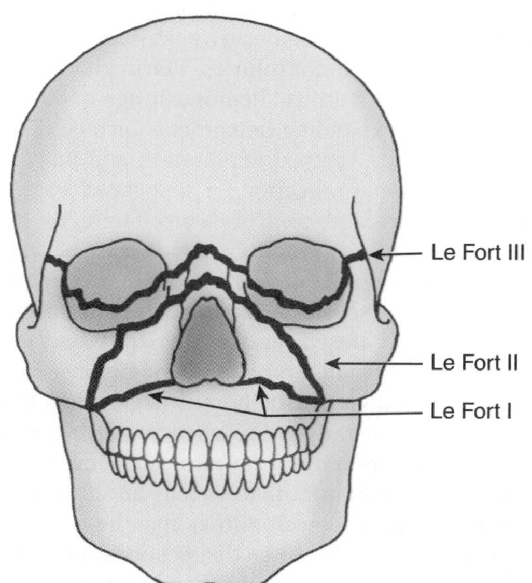


**FIGURE 31-14** Le Fort classification of maxillary fractures.

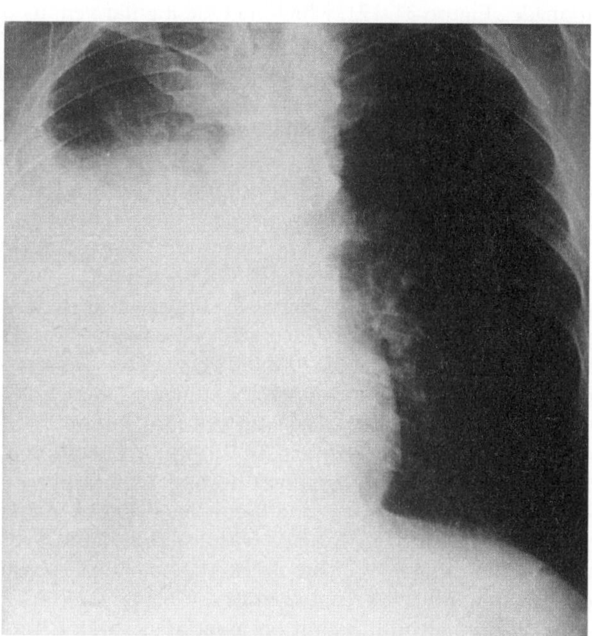

**FIGURE 31-15** Right hemithorax on chest x-ray.

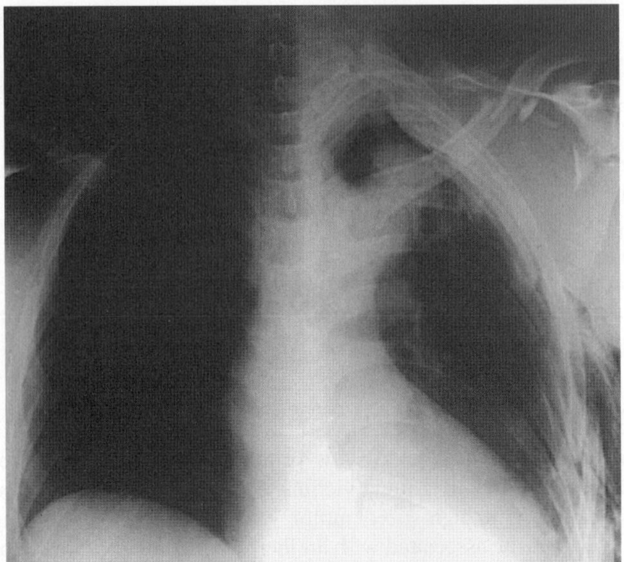

**FIGURE 31-16** Flail chest.

blood is an indication for chest exploration. Penetrating wounds, either as a result of gunshot or stab injuries, may cause hemothorax and pneumothorax as well. Lacerations or perforation of the lung, heart, great vessels, trachea, esophagus, and bronchus is possible.

Myocardial contusion usually involves the right ventricle and can be evidenced by dysrhythmias on patient arrival or shortly thereafter. The patient is monitored on a telemetry unit, and surgical intervention is not required. Rupture of a heart valve can occur, depending on which part of the cardiac cycle the heart is in at the time of contusion. If valve rupture has occurred, surgical repair is necessary. Heart sounds should be evaluated during the secondary assessment to document the presence or absence of murmurs. Heart valve rupture can occur as a late complication of myocardial contusion. Pericardiocentesis is performed for signs and symptoms of pericardial tamponade (Figure 31-17), which include jugular venous distention, muffled heart sounds, and a narrowing pulse pressure. Patients may present to the OR for a pericardial window either emergently or during the recovery phase.

An emergency thoracotomy may be indicated in the patient with penetrating trauma to the chest in full arrest or pulseless electrical activity on ECG. If a laceration to the heart is suspected and the patient is rapidly deteriorating, a thoracotomy may be performed in the ED. The laceration may be primarily repaired and the patient taken to the OR for irrigation, wound debridement, and closure. Otherwise, surgical intervention is begun in the OR. Wounds located across the mediastinum accompanied by hemodynamic instability, massive penetrating lung injuries, and disruption of the trachea, bronchus, or esophagus also require surgical intervention. Rupture of the thoracic aorta is another injury requiring an operation and includes the use of extracorporeal bypass. This injury is an obvious life threat but may be difficult to diagnose. An arch aortogram is indicated in patients with trauma that may have caused such an injury. Rupture of the thoracic arch is associated with first rib or sternal fractures. Chapters 25 and 27 provide additional information on associated surgical procedures in thoracic and cardiac surgery.

## INJURIES OF THE ABDOMEN

The spleen is the most common organ injured in blunt trauma, and the liver, because of its large size, is the most common organ injured in penetrating trauma. Historically, initial efforts were aimed at performing splenectomy with splenic injury. However, because of the role of the spleen in the body's defense against infection, every effort is made to control hemorrhage in the spleen and avoid its removal. Treatment is determined by the condition of the spleen and of the patient. Injury to the spleen occurs with deceleration injuries resulting in fracture of the organ because of its multiple fixation points. Splenic injury may be associated with fractures of the left tenth through twelfth ribs. The patient may exhibit left shoulder pain (Kehr's sign), upper left quadrant tenderness, abdominal wall muscle rigidity, spasm or involuntary guarding, and/or signs and symptoms of hemorrhage and hypovolemic shock. Splenic injuries range from laceration of the capsule (Figure 31-18) to ruptured subcapsular hematomas or parenchymal laceration (Table 31-10). The most serious injury is a severely fractured spleen or vascular tear, producing massive blood loss, and splenic ischemia. Rupture of the spleen can be immediate or delayed. Splenic lacerations may be treated nonoperatively by close monitoring and bed rest or operatively for those lacerations of a more severe nature. A midline incision is used, which allows for exposure of all abdominal contents. Topical hemostatic agents are also used with success, as well as suturing and the argon laser in some instances. A laceration involving the splenic hilum or complete shattering of the organ usually results in splenectomy.

The severity of hepatic injury ranges from controlled hematoma to severe vascular injury of the hepatic veins or hepatic avulsion (Table 31-11). Because liver tissue is so friable and has an extensive blood supply as well as blood storage capacity, hepatic injuries often result in profuse hemorrhage and require surgical control of bleeding. The patient usually exhibits upper quadrant pain, abdominal wall muscle rigidity, involuntary guarding, rebound tenderness, hypoactive or absent bowel sounds, and signs of hemorrhage or hypovolemic shock. Nonoperative treatment is indicated in minor capsular and subcapsular injuries. This can be accomplished with bed rest and close monitoring. Topical hemostatic agents and suturing are used in management of minor injuries. Fibrin glue is also used in some institutions as a topical hemostatic agent. More severe injuries with active expanding hematomas or lobe disruption (Figure 31-19) require surgical exploration and may necessitate hepatic resection or ligation of associated vasculature. With massive hemorrhage, control of bleeding is the primary concern. Packing with laparotomy sponges may be indicated, along with manual compression of the organ if intraoperative hypotension becomes severe. A pressure dressing may be applied and the wound closed temporarily until associated coagulopathies, hypothermia, and hemodynamic instability can be corrected. The patient is usually returned to the OR within 24 to 72 hours postoperatively or when his or her condition permits for further exploration and removal of the sponges.

Injuries to the gastrointestinal system are also associated with abdominal trauma. Bowel injuries may be missed on abdominal CT scan during the initial diagnostic period. The small bowel is frequently injured because deceleration may lead to shearing, which causes avulsion or tearing. The most com-

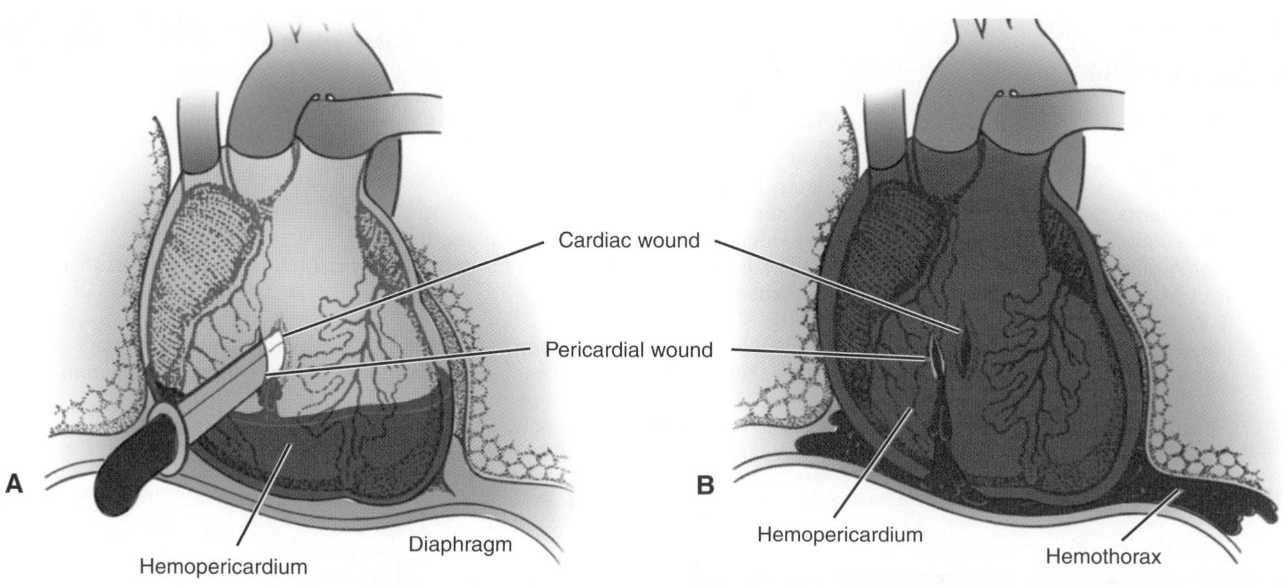


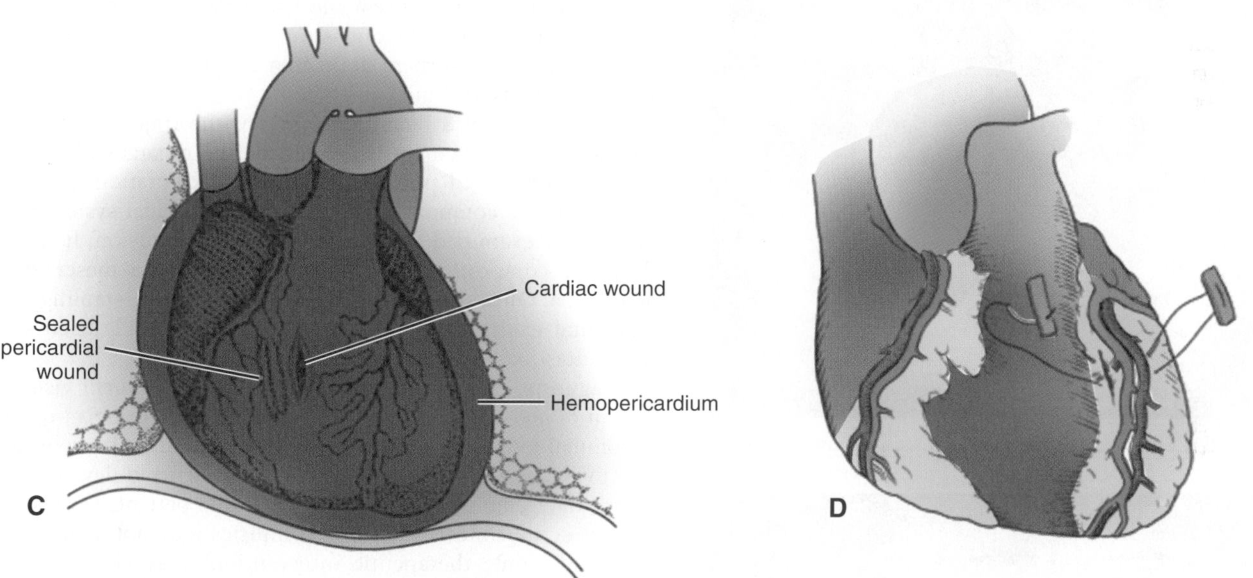


**FIGURE 31-17** **A,** Cardiac injury with pericardial disruption. **B,** Bleeding from heart through pericardial tear into pleural space. **C,** Self-sealing of pericardial wound resulting in pericardial tamponade. **D,** Sutured cardiac wound.

**TABLE 31-10**

## Splenic Injury Scale

| Grade | Type of Injury | Description of Injury |
|---|---|---|
| I | Hematoma | Subcapsular: <10% of surface area |
| | Laceration | Capsular tear: <1 cm parenchymal depth |
| II | Hematoma | Subcapsular: 10%-50% of surface area; intraparenchymal: <5 cm in diameter |
| | Laceration | Capsular tear 1-3 cm; parenchymal depth that does not involve a trabecular vessel |
| III | Hematoma | Subcapsular: >50% of surface area or expanding; ruptured subcapsular or parenchymal hematoma; intraparenchymal hematoma >5 cm or expanding |
| | Laceration | >3 cm parenchymal depth or involving parenchymal vessels |
| IV | Laceration | Laceration involving segmental or hilar vessels producing major devascularization (>25% of spleen) |
| V | Laceration | Completely shattered spleen |
| | Vascular | Hilar vascular injury that devascularizes spleen |

From Hoyt DB and others: Management of acute trauma. In Townsend CM and others, editors: *Sabiston textbook of surgery*, ed 17, Philadelphia, 2004, Saunders.

**TABLE 31-11**

## Liver Injury Scale

| Grade | Type of Injury | Description of Injury |
|---|---|---|
| I | Hematoma | Subcapsular: <10% of surface area |
| | Laceration | Capsular tear: <1 cm parenchymal depth |
| II | Hematoma | Subcapsular: 10%-50% of surface area; intraparenchymal: <10 cm in diameter |
| | Laceration | Capsular tear; 1 to 3 cm parenchymal depth; <10 cm in length |
| III | Hematoma | Subcapsular: >50% surface area of ruptured subcapsular or parenchymal hematoma; intraparenchymal hematoma: >10 cm or expanding |
| | Laceration | >3 cm parenchymal depth |
| IV | Laceration | Parenchymal disruption involving 25%-75% of hepatic lobe or 1-3 of the 8 Couinaud segments |
| V | Laceration | Parenchymal disruption involving >75% of hepatic lobe or >3 of the 8 Couinaud segments within a single lobe |
| | Vascular | Juxtahepatic venous injuries (i.e., retrohepatic vena cava/central major hepatic veins) |
| VI | Vascular | Hepatic avulsion |

From Hoyt DB and others: Management of acute trauma. In Townsend CM and others, editors: *Sabiston textbook of surgery*, ed 17, Philadelphia, 2004, Saunders.

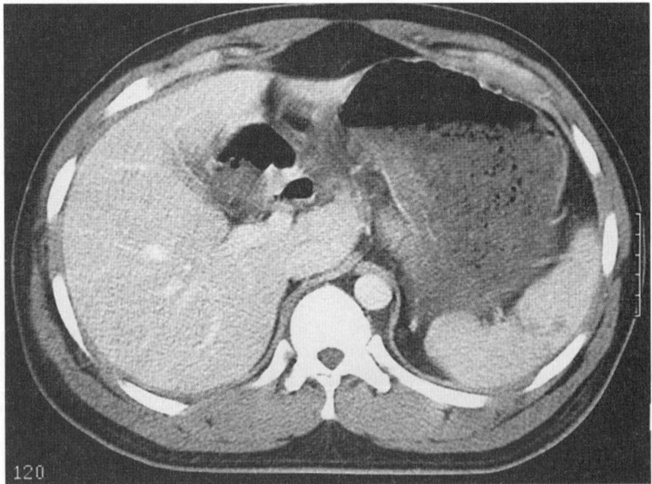


**FIGURE 31-18** Computed tomography (CT) scan showing splenic laceration.

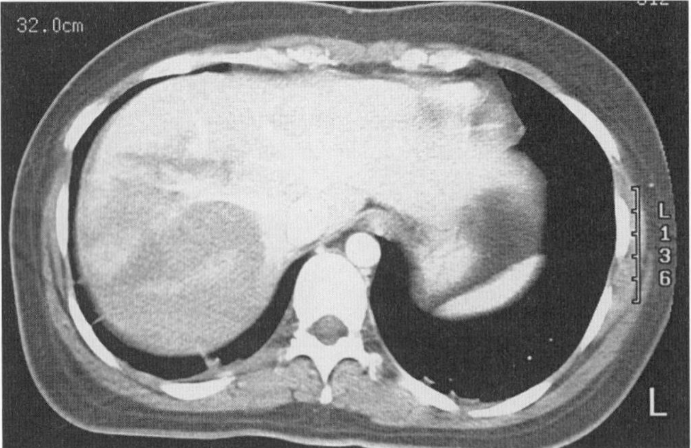


**FIGURE 31-19** Grade IV liver laceration.

monly affected areas of the small bowel are areas relatively fixed or looped. Any perforation of the gastrointestinal tract carries with it a chance for peritonitis and sepsis or compartment syndrome from increased pressure. Crystalloid resuscitation and capillary leakage contribute to tissue swelling. The resulting abdominal edema creates a pressurized compartment that must be explored to render relief to the compromised organs.

If the abdomen is difficult to close, alternative wound closure techniques may be used to prevent the occurrence of ACS. One such method is to use a silo-bag closure, in which heavy plastic is trimmed to fit and sutured to skin edges (Figure 31-20). A sterile absorbent drape may also be placed inside the abdomen to absorb fluid.

In the event of a penetrating injury, the trajectory of the missile or the implement is examined, and organs within the area are considered potentially injured. Exploration is indicated, and the components of the gastrointestinal system are thoroughly examined for any perforations, contusion, hemorrhage, or compromise of vasculature, such as a mesenteric hematoma. Once the injury is identified, suturing, stapling, or segmental excision may be indicated. Chapter 11 discusses gastrointestinal surgery.

Diagnostic laparoscopy is frequently used for direct visualization of abdominal organs to decrease the need for an open abdominal exploration. This procedure allows the surgeon to effectively evaluate the presence of any injury and develop an appropriate plan of treatment in the stable patient. However, there is some concern that bowel injuries may not always be identified. Some therapeutic interventions may also be performed through the laparoscope so that the more invasive open approach is avoided. Increased intraabdominal pressure required in laparoscopic insufflation may create an adverse ventilatory effect. In the presence of abdominal vein injury with low pressures, $CO_2$ could leak into the vasculature and result in $CO_2$ emboli to the heart or lungs. Tension pneumothorax may be created in patients with a diaphragmatic injury. Consequently, indications for these procedures in the trauma setting continue to be evaluated.

## INJURIES OF THE GENITOURINARY SYSTEM

Laceration of the kidney is closely associated with fracture of the ribs and transverse vertebral processes. Because the kidney is retroperitoneal, the presence of bleeding may not be observed on diagnostic peritoneal lavage. Renal contusions often produce hematuria. Gross clots may also be seen in more serious injury, but it should be noted that hematuria is not present in a complete avulsion injury. Management of renal contusions can be nonoperative with monitoring of hematuria. Lacera-

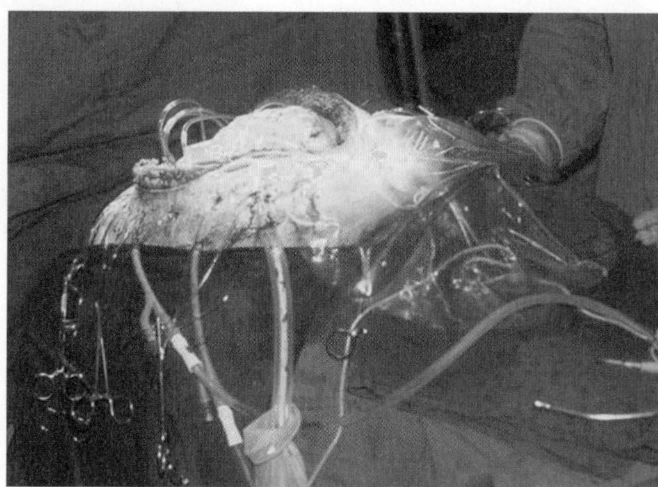

**FIGURE 31-20** Alternative technique using plastic for temporary closure of the abdomen.

tions involving the collecting system, severe crush injuries, or pedicle injuries necessitate surgical intervention (Figure 31-21). Nephrectomy may be indicated with severe injury of the pedicle or massive hemorrhage.

Rupture of the bladder and urethral injury are most often associated with pelvic fractures. Both blunt trauma and penetrating trauma are causative factors. The type of bladder injury is a direct result of the amount of urine present in the bladder at the time of injury. Blunt forces applied to a full bladder result in an intraperitoneal rupture. This type of rupture is closely associated with alcohol consumption because of alcohol's diuretic effect. Pelvic fracture is associated with an extraperitoneal bladder rupture. Most often these patients present with gross hematuria. A small extraperitoneal rupture may be managed by urinary catheter drainage. A large extraperitoneal rupture and intraperitoneal rupture require surgical intervention. A suprapubic cystostomy tube may be placed, and the bladder is repaired. Pelvic fracture reduction and fixation are also performed.

Urethral injuries require exploration and primary repair. These types of injuries are more common in the male because the male urethra is longer and less protected than the female urethra (Figure 31-22). A fall or straddle type of injury is usually responsible. This injury is detected by the presence of blood at the urinary meatus. In these instances an indwelling urethral catheter should not be inserted. Blood at the urinary meatus may indicate a tear in the anterior urethra. A retrograde urethrogram may be performed to evaluate for extravasation of urine and potential injury. Suspicion of a pelvic fracture raises the index of suspicion of a concomitant urethral injury. Chapter 15 provides additional information on urologic procedures.

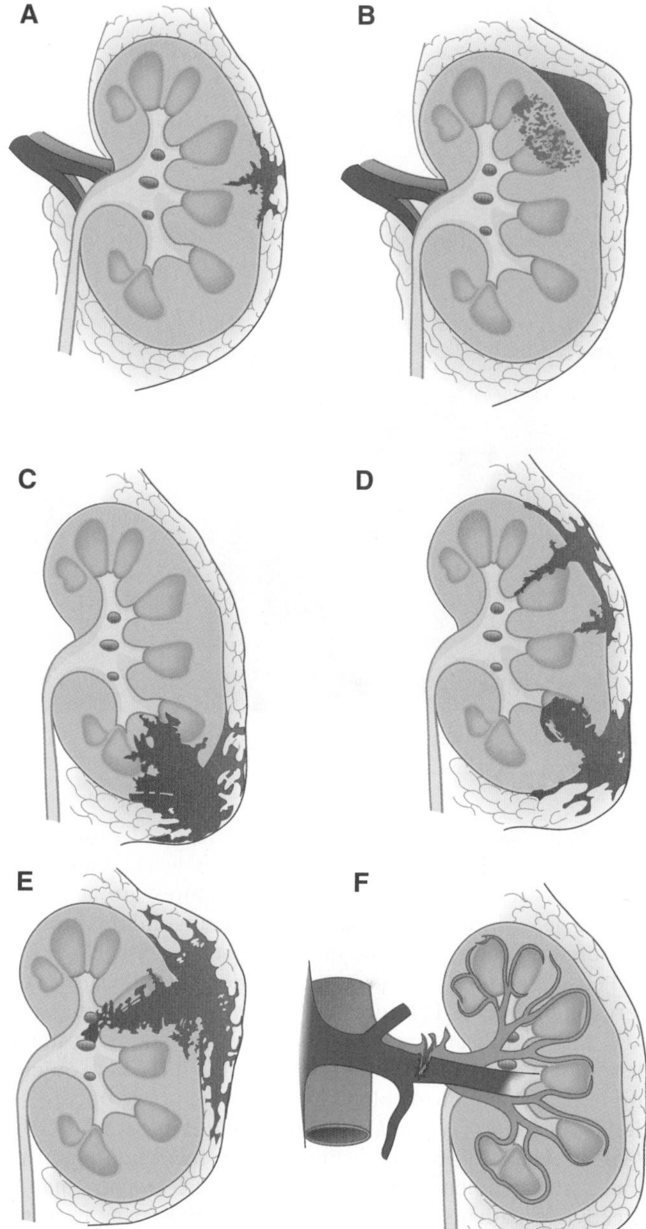


**FIGURE 31-21** Renal injuries. **A,** Small renal laceration with contained subcapsular hematoma. **B,** Minor subcapsular and parenchymal hematoma. **C,** Parenchymal laceration extending through the renal cortex without involvement of the collecting system. **D,** Multiple parenchymal lacerations; the inferior one extends through the cortex and collecting system. **E,** Parenchymal laceration extending through the cortex, medulla, and collecting system with subcapsular hematoma and extravasation of urine. **F,** Injury to the renal vessels at the hilum with extravasation of urine.

## SKELETAL INJURIES

Trauma to the skeletal system usually results in contusion or fracture. After stabilization of the patient, radiographs are taken of any body part that is distorted, edematous, painful, or highly suspicious for fracture or dislocation. Treatment of fractures is aimed at restoring function with a minimum of complications. Immobilization of fractures can be accomplished by casting, bracing, splinting, and application of traction or hardware fixation. Femur fractures in particular can be associated with a high risk of hemorrhage and require traction before surgical repair. Closed and open reductions, application of internal and external fixators, and some types of traction may be performed in the OR. The perioperative nurse involved in care of the trauma patient must have a working knowledge of the

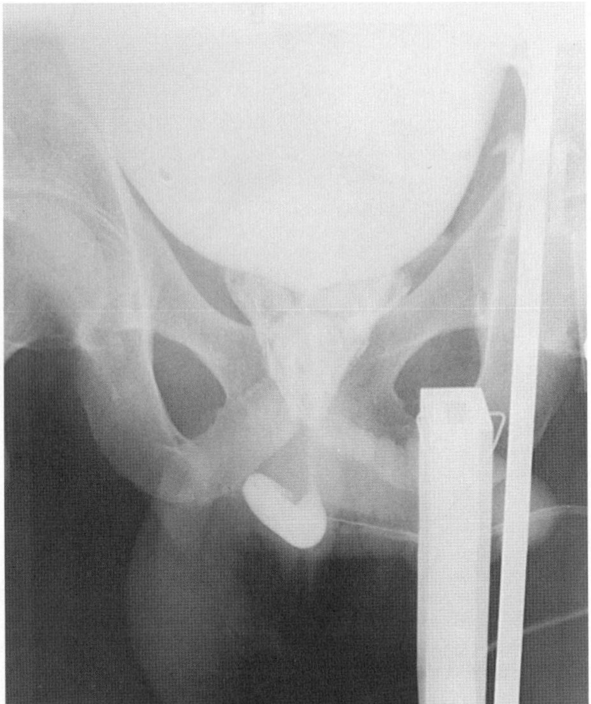

**FIGURE 31-22** Complete urethral injury as demonstrated on urethrogram.

orthopedic specialty. Fractures must be repaired in a timely manner to avoid untoward complications; however, immediate life threats are corrected first. Open fractures are at an increased risk of infection. Chapter 22 contains information on the surgical procedures used in fracture management.

Pelvic fractures may pose an additional challenge to the perioperative team. Fractures within the pelvic ring are associated with significant internal blood loss and shock. Systemic peripheral vascular resistance is increased. A method to quickly minimize or tamponade blood loss in severe pelvic fractures is the application of a pneumatic antishock garment (PASG) or PASG trousers to provide stabilization of the fracture and reduce associated hemorrhage. The use of PASG trousers may be effective in patients who are 20 to 40 minutes away from the hospital and have unstable pelvic fractures and decompensated shock.[17] If a pneumatic garment is applied, the patient may be transported to the OR with the trousers still inflated. The perioperative nurse must be familiar with deflation procedures. The attending anesthesia provider directs deflation in collaboration with the surgeon. Blood pressure and other vital signs are closely monitored. The abdominal compartment is deflated first. Deflation continues slowly while IV fluids are infused to maintain blood pressure. A 5–mm Hg drop in blood pressure requires fluid resuscitation of approximately 200 ml before deflation of the next compartment. If the patient remains stable, each leg compartment is deflated slowly, one at a time.

Some trauma centers apply external fixator devices in the ED during initial resuscitation. A pelvic C-clamp may also be used in initial management. A more recent development is the pelvic corset device, which consists of a power unit/pulley system that affixes to a support binder made of radiolucent material.[5] This allows evaluation of the patient by means of radiography, ultrasound, CT scan, and peritoneal lavage; when evaluation is completed, definitive open reduction and internal fixation can be performed. Severe hemorrhage associated with the fracture may be controlled by arterial embolization performed in the radiology department if surgical intervention for fracture fixation must be delayed.

Soft tissue injuries of an extremity are subject to compartment syndrome. This is a result of swelling of the soft tissues and muscles encased in the fascia. With a significant amount of swelling, pain is increased and the surrounding circulation may be compromised. The patient may experience a decrease in motor and sensory function. This injury must be treated surgically by a fasciotomy. Incising the fascia allows space for tissue swelling. Several days later, the patient returns to the OR for closure, which may require skin grafting for complete coverage.

## HYPOTHERMIA

The trauma patient may experience prolonged environmental exposure and be subject to a decrease in core temperature. Immersion victims or patients whose accident occurred several hours before discovery may be hypothermic despite the ambient temperature. The perioperative nurse needs to be aware of several effects on the body when hypothermia is present. For purposes of definition, generalized hypothermia is considered to be present when the core temperature is below 36°C (96.8°F). (See Chapter 9 for discussion of a clinical guideline to prevent inadvertent hypothermia in adult surgical patients.) Trauma patients are subject to prolonged bleeding and clotting times. Coagulopathies of this sort become clinically significant in a multiple trauma patient undergoing surgical intervention. Viscosity of the blood is also increased. Thrombocytopenia has been noted. Many facilities use a thermistor Foley catheter to monitor core temperature.

Hypothermia can be classified into three types. *Mild hypothermia* is a core temperature between 32°C and 36°C (89.6° F and 96.8° F). These patients may appear gray and are cool to the touch. Some alterations in level of consciousness can be present. If the patient's clothing is wet, it should be removed and the patient covered with warm blankets. Treatment is aimed at passive rewarming of the patient by means of warm ambient room temperature, warm fluids, and infrared radiant energy lights. *Moderate hypothermia* is characterized as core temperatures between 30°C and 32°C (86°F and 89.6°F). Warmed fluids are given by IV line and also by gastric or peritoneal lavage. In addition, a warming blanket, such as a forced air–warming device, may be used. Immersion in a Hubbard tank filled with warm water has also been successful. An irritable myocardium may cause dysrhythmias to be present. Shivering may or may not be present. If the patient is intubated, warmed, humidified gases can be administered. *Severe hypothermia* is diagnosed in the patient with a temperature below 30°C (86°F). The heart rate and the respiratory rate are greatly decreased. This patient is comatose, often appears deceased, and requires active rewarming processes. It is advisable to warm the core first to avoid complications associated with rewarming. This can best be accomplished by core heating using cardiopulmonary bypass (CPB), which directly warms internal vital organs, including the heart. The patient should be handled gently during transfers to avoid further tissue injury and stimulation of an irritable myocardium.

It should be noted that severe cases of hypothermia mimic death, and no patient can be pronounced dead until he or she is rewarmed and pronounced dead. Resuscitation measures are ceased if the patient is rewarmed to at least 35°C (95°F) and cardiac functions remain nonexistent.

## THERMAL INJURIES

Heat and cold exposure injuries require prompt initial management in the ED setting. Some institutions transfer pediatric burn patients and severely burned adult patients to a burn center for treatment once the patients' conditions are stabilized. In addition to treatment of the site of injury to decrease further tissue damage, fluid management is of the utmost importance in these patients. After hemodynamic stabilization of the patient, burn and frostbite wounds usually require a series of procedures. These patients may have multiple surgical debridement procedures before skin grafting and cosmetic interventions. Restoration of function is important. Circumferential burns may restrict the neurovascular structures during eschar formation. Chest burns with eschar may restrict movement of the chest wall and ventilatory function. An escharotomy (incision of the eschar) may be performed to alleviate the constriction. If necessary, this procedure may be performed at the bedside and the perioperative team may be asked to assist.

## ORGAN AND TISSUE PROCUREMENT

As previously noted, trauma affects primarily young people. In the event that resuscitation efforts or surgical interventions are not successful, the patient may be declared dead. Depending on the cause of death and preexisting medical conditions, the patient may be an organ-donor candidate. Both federal and state laws mandate that local organ-procurement facilities are notified of potential donors and that families are informed that organ-donation exists as an option. Organ-donation agencies can be contacted early and will assist in assessing the potential donor, as well as providing a protocol for donor management once the patient is declared dead. Definition of brain death is not uniform throughout the United States. The perioperative nurse should be familiar with the state's definition of brain death and the institution's criteria for the declaration. Once a patient is declared dead and becomes a potential organ donor, the patient's family does not incur any financial costs acquired from that point. The patient is not disfigured in any way that will interfere with bereavement rituals.

A transplantation coordinator assists in managing the organ-donor patient in the ICU setting until the procurement teams arrive. The perioperative nurse must prepare for the organ-procurement procedure. The harvesting of organs and tissue may take several hours and additional members of the perioperative team. Different organ-procurement agencies will provide a surgical team, but additional scrub and circulating personnel are needed. The transplantation coordinators actively seek tissue and organ recipients during the harvest procedure. Most organ-transplantation agencies contact the institution and provide follow-up information regarding the ultimate success of the transplantation procedures and information about the recipients.

The heart is removed first, followed by the lungs, pancreas, liver, and kidneys. Tissue dissection is performed in such a manner as to allow for optimal organ transplantation. Sterile technique remains important. In addition, traffic control is of concern during these procedures. Traffic should be limited to essential personnel. Bone, skin, and corneas can also be removed. Some procurement agencies remove bone and corneas in the morgue rather than in the OR.

## SUMMARY

Nowhere is the team concept more important than in the provision of definitive care to the multiple trauma patient. The perioperative nurse is a vital member of the trauma team. Through the application of principles of trauma care as outlined in this chapter, perioperative nurses can significantly contribute to positive outcomes for trauma patients.

## REFERENCES


1. Association of periOperative Registered Nurses: *AORN standards, recommended practices, and guidelines*, Denver, 2006, The Association.
2. Born CT: Blast trauma: the fourth weapon of mass destruction, *Scandinavian Journal of Surgery* 94(4):279-285, 2005.
3. Dayton MT: Surgical complications. In Townsend CM and others, editors: *Sabiston textbook of surgery*, ed 17, Philadelphia, 2004, Saunders.
4. Dorman KF, Harvey MG: Obstetric critical care. In Lowdermilk DL, Perry SE, editors: *Maternity & women's health care*, ed 8, St Louis, 2004, Mosby.
5. Frakes MA, Evans T: Major pelvic fractures, *Critical Care Nurse* 24(2):18-30, 2004.
6. Galvin AA: Assessment of the trauma patient. In Newberry L, Criddle LM, editors: *Sheehy's manual of emergency care*, ed 6, St Louis, 2005, Mosby.
7. Gray MJ, Litz BT: Behavioral interventions for recent trauma: empirically informed practice guidelines, *Behavior Modification* 29(1):189-215, 2005.
8. Halm MA: Family presence during resuscitation: a critical review of the literature, *American Journal of Critical Care* 14(6):494-511, 2005.
9. Hausman KA: Assessment of the nervous system. In Ignatavicius DD, Workman ML, editors: *Medical-surgical nursing: critical thinking for collaborative care,* ed 5, St Louis, 2006, Saunders.
10. Hodgson BB, Kizior RJ: *Mosby's 2006 drug consult for nurses*, St Louis, 2006, Mosby.
11. Holmes JF and others: Performance of abdominal ultrasonography in blunt trauma patients with out-of-hospital or emergency department hypotension, *Journal of the American College of Emergency Medicine* 43(3):354-361, 2004.
12. Inamasu J, Guiot BH: Vertebral artery injury after blunt cervical trauma: an update, *Surgical Neurology* 65(3):238-245, 2006.
13. Jagim M: Airway management: rapid-sequence intubation in trauma patients, *American Journal of Nursing* 103(10):32-35, 2003.
14. Kuhne CA and others: Mortality in severely injured elderly patients—when does age become a risk factor? *World Journal of Surgery* 29(11):1476-1482, 2005.
15. *National vital statistics report,* March 17, 2005. Accessed April 23, 2006, on-line: www.cdc.gov/nchs/data/nvsr/nvsr53/nvsr53_17.pdf.
16. Rose JS: Ultrasound in abdominal trauma, *Emergency Medicine Clinics of North America* 22(3):581-589, 2004.
17. Salomone JP and others: Opinions of trauma practitioners regarding prehospital interventions for critically injured patients, *Journal of Trauma* 58(3):509-515, 2005.
18. Schuerer DJ and others: Evaluation of the applicability, efficacy, and safety of a thromboembolic event prophylaxis guideline designed for quality improvement of the traumatically injured patient, *Journal of Trauma* 58(4):731-739, 2005.
19. Utter GH and others: Inclusive trauma systems: do they improve triage or outcomes of the severely injured? *Journal of Trauma* 60(3):529-535, 2006.

CHAPTER 32

# Integrated Health Practices: Complementary and Alternative Therapies

SUSAN M. CRAIG AND WENDELYN A. VALENTINE

## HISTORY AND BACKGROUND

Any accurate presentation of the history of medicine in the United States needs to include influences from the botanic traditions of Easterners, Europeans, and Native Americans. Our current medical system, called *biomedicine,* began to dominate sometime in the mid-1800s with the discovery that microorganisms were responsible for disease and pathologic damage and that antitoxins and vaccines could improve the body's ability to fend off the effects of pathogens. Armed with this knowledge, scientists and clinicians began to refine surgical procedures and defeat previously serious and fatal infections.

As biomedicine dominated the health care system, it became the mainstream or "conventional" approach, establishing the standards for diagnosis and treatment of illness. By the 1990s, however, consumer faith and trust in this conventional system began to falter and many Americans sought complementary or alternative treatments for their health care. Complementary and alternative medicine (CAM) grew to constitute a significant percentage of American health care dollars and visits. This growth was accompanied by a plethora of media information about the many alternatives to the mainstream, traditional Western biomedical approach to medicine.

Myths and misconceptions initially prevented the investigation and development of promising therapies outside the biomedical regimen. In response to growing consumer pressure, anecdotal evidence, and a small body of published scientific results, the U.S. Congress established the Office of Alternative Medicine (OAM) within the office of the Director, National Institutes of Health (NIH) in 1992. This office was given responsibility for (1) facilitating fair, scientific evaluation of alternative therapies that showed promise in health promotion and (2) reducing barriers to the acceptance and utilization of those alternative therapies that showed promise.[13]

In 1998 the OAM became the National Center for Complementary and Alternative Medicine (NCCAM). This expansion into a center allowed more substantial funding for and initiation of research projects, providing more sound information about CAM therapies and systems. The annual budget for NCCAM has grown significantly, as has the sophistication of research design of studies being funded by the center. Nonetheless, much CAM therapy and intervention stem from a philosophy of wholeness, with intent to treat the entire person (body-mind-spirit) (Best Practice). This is in contrast to the current "gold standard" of randomized, control-led clinical trials, which may not be the best, or indeed appropriate, way to measure the effectiveness of many CAM therapies.

Hence a debate between conventional scientists and physicians and the proponents of CAM exists concerning the appropriate forms of research to determine efficacy and safety of these therapies. A reason for this disparity stems from divergent theoretic models. The *comprehensive approach* takes into account multidimensional factors that may not easily or appropriately be studied independently. The comprehensive approach is more congruent with the philosophic underpinnings of most CAM. The *biomedical approach,* on the other hand, is concerned with a disease orientation, suggesting that a specific agent or variable is responsible for a specific disorder or illness. The major components of this approach are hypothesis, linear reasoning with logic, and causation.[19]

In 2003 the Integrated Health Practices Special Assembly (IHP-SA) was created. A dedicated group of perioperative nurses met for several years at Association of periOperative Registered Nurses (AORN) congresses to discuss how they integrated CAM and preventive health into their practices. The title of the IHP-SA evolved as clearer description and an affirmation for a desired reality (Box 32-1). In the future, perioperative nurses may expect newer research methodologies that will permit the full integration of complementary therapies into current conventional perioperative patient care (Box 32-2).

The NCCAM has categorized the many CAM modalities into five major domains: alternative medical systems, mind-body interventions, biologically based therapies, manipulative and body-based methods, and energy therapies. Numerous treatments and systems are within each category. The remainder of this chapter discusses the major domains and some examples within each.

BEST PRACTICE

### Evaluating Complementary and Alternative Medicine Therapies

In a recent survey of 31,000 Americans, the Centers for Disease Control and Prevention (CDC) estimated that 36% use some form of complementary and alternative medicine (CAM). In discussing the use of CAM with perioperative patients, nurses have a unique opportunity to advise patients on best practices to adopt when considering the use of CAM therapies. Talking points to use when counseling patients about choosing CAM therapies are listed below.

- Take charge of your health by being an informed consumer. Investigate the therapy to see what studies have been done on its safety and effectiveness.
- The Internet is a good source to find information about CAM. In evaluating information on the Internet you should always ask:
  - Who runs the website? Is it a government, university, or reputable medical or health-related association? Is it sponsored by a manufacturer of products, drugs, and so on? It should be easy to clearly identify the sponsor.
  - What is the purpose of the site? Is it to educate the public or sell a product? The purpose should be clearly stated.
  - What is the basis of the information? Is it based on scientific evidence with clear references?
  - How current is the information? Is it reviewed and updated frequently?
- If you do not have access to the Internet, contact the NCCAM Clearinghouse at 1-888-644-6226 for assistance.
- Visit your local library or medical library to search for scientific information about CAM.
- Discuss the CAM with your health care provider before making any decision about care. Ask questions about any possible interactions with medications you currently take or therapy you are undergoing. If your physician cannot answer your questions, he or she may be able to refer you to someone who can.
- Before taking herbal supplements:
  - Talk to your physician before starting to take herbal supplements.
  - Talk to a licensed pharmacist if you have questions about the supplement, and discuss any potential reactions with any prescription or nonprescription medication (over the counter [OTC]) you currently take.
  - Read labels carefully. Buy only supplements that are approved by the American Botanicals Council's Commission E.
  - Buy products from a reputable herbal company. Be cautious about products for sale through magazines, TV, radio, or the Internet.

Modified from *Are you considering using complementary and alternative medicine (CAM)?* Accessed April 30, 2006, on-line: nccam.nih.gov/health/decisions/index.htm#; Herbal supplements, *Nursing* 34(12):52, 2004; More Americans than ever use CAM, says CDC, *Nursing* 34(9):73, 2004.

BOX 32-1

### Symbolism Behind the Integrated Health Practices (IHP) Logo*

The IHP logo was designed by Norrie MacIlraith, RN, MS, CNS.

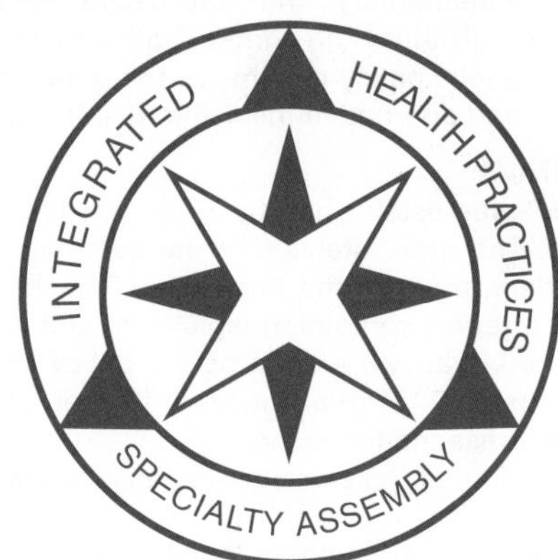


1. Outer circle represents life continuity.
2. Inner circle represents the binding of the health care continuum.
3. The dark triangle represents the individual's mind, body, and spirit. It touches both circles because of direct interaction.
4. The darker star represents traditional medical practices.
5. The gold star represents all the integrated practice applications.
6. Both stars are superimposed on one another to indicate the meshing of philosophies.
7. Lettering identifies the Integrated Health Practices Specialty Assembly within the outer circle binding all processes.

*Color for the logo lapel pin is dark blue and gold.

## MAJOR CATEGORIES OF COMPLEMENTARY AND ALTERNATIVE MEDICINE

### Alternative Medical Systems

An estimated 10% to 30% of human health care is delivered by practitioners such as surgeons and nurses who have been trained in the mainstream, traditional Western biomedical model. The remaining 70% to 90% involves care given in a health care system that is based on an alternative tradition—self-care based in folk practice or many practices that range somewhere between. Many of these therapies are culturally, ethnically, spiritually, or religiously derived (Figure 32-1). Among the diverse values, beliefs, and practices found in the many cultural groups in the United States are those relating to health, illness, professional health care, and folk health care (Box 32-3). They include well-known and respected Asian systems of medicine. Many Asian medicine techniques or systems are widely known here in the United States. The most well-known and popular of these include herbal medicines, massage, energy therapy, acupressure, acupuncture, and qigong. This alternative medicine system has a wide range of applications from health promotion to the treatment of illness. A significant aspect of Asian medicine is an emphasis on diagnosing and treating disturbances of *qi* (pronounced "chee"), or vital energy, and restoring its proper balance.[11]

Ayurveda is a traditional system from India that strives to restore the innate harmony of the individual while placing equal emphasis on body, mind, and spirit. Native American, Middle Eastern, Tibetan, Central and South American, and African cultures have developed other traditional medical systems.[2] Other examples of complete alternative medicine systems are naturopathic and homeopathic medicine systems. Homeopathic medicine is based on the principle that

BOX 32-2

## Ten Guiding Principles for Legislative and Administrative Recommendations

Following are 10 guiding principles from the White House Commission on Complementary and Alternative Medicine Policy (WHCCAMP) for legislative and administrative recommendations that will ensure public policy maximizes the potential benefits of complementary and alternative medicine (CAM) to all citizens.

**EXECUTIVE SUMMARY**

The WHCCAMP was established by Executive Order No. 13147 in March 2000. The order states that the commission is to provide the President, through the Secretary of Health and Human Services, with a report containing legislative and administrative recommendations that will ensure public policy maximizes the potential benefits of CAM to all citizens. The report of the commission is to address the following:

- The coordination of research to increase knowledge about CAM products
- The education and training of health care practitioners in CAM
- The provision of reliable and useful information about CAM practices and products to health care professionals
- Guidance regarding appropriate access to and delivery of CAM

The commission's 20 presidentially appointed members represented an array of health care interests, professional backgrounds, and knowledge. Health care expertise was provided by both conventional and CAM practitioners.

Based on its mission and responsibilities, the commission endorsed the following 10 guiding principles to shape the process of making recommendations and to focus the recommendations themselves:

1. *A wholeness orientation in health care delivery.* Health involves all aspects of life—mind, body, spirit, and environment—and high-quality health care must support care of the whole person.
2. *Evidence of safety and efficacy.* The commission is committed to promoting the use of science and appropriate scientific methods to help identify safe and effective CAM services and products and to generate evidence that will protect and promote the public health.
3. *The healing capacity of the person.* People have a remarkable capacity for recovery and self-healing, and a major focus of health care is to support and promote this capacity.
4. *Respect for individuality.* Each person is unique and has the right to health care that is appropriately responsive to him or her, respecting preferences and preserving dignity.
5. *The right to choose treatment.* Each person has the right to choose freely among safe and effective care or approaches, as well as among qualified practitioners who are accountable for their claims and actions and responsive to the person's needs.
6. *An emphasis on health promotion and self-care.* Good health care emphasizes self-care and early intervention for maintaining and promoting health.
7. *Partnerships as essential to integrated health care.* Good health care requires teamwork among patients, health care practitioners (conventional and CAM), and researchers committed to creating optimal healing environments and to respecting the diversity of all health care traditions.
8. *Education as a fundamental health care service.* Education about prevention, healthy life-styles, and the power of self-healing should be made an integral part of the curricula of all health care professionals and should be made available to the public of all ages.
9. *Dissemination of comprehensive and timely information.* The quality of health care can be enhanced by promoting efforts that thoroughly and thoughtfully examine the evidence on which CAM systems, practices, and products are based and make this evidence widely, rapidly, and easily available.
10. *Integral public involvement.* The input of informed consumers and other members of the public must be incorporated in setting priorities for health care and health care research and in reaching policy decisions, including those related to CAM, within the public and private sectors.

CAM is a heterogeneous group of medical, health care, and healing systems other than those intrinsic to mainstream health care in the United States. Although "complementary and alternative medicine" is the term used in this report, the commission recognizes that the term does not fully capture all the diversity with which these systems, practices, and products are being used by consumers, CAM practitioners, and mainstream health care institutions.

From the *White House Commission on Complementary and Alternative Medicine Policy,* 2002. Accessed April 28, 2006, on-line: www.whccamp.hhs.gov/es.html.

"like cures like," (i.e., a substance that, in large doses, produces the symptoms of a disease will, in a very diluted dose, cure it). Small doses of plant extracts and minerals specially prepared are given to stimulate the body's defense mechanisms and encourage healing processes. A careful evaluation of symptoms enables the practitioner to determine a patient's specific sensitivity and to select the appropriate remedy.

Naturopathic medicine emphasizes health restoration as well as disease treatment based on the belief that disease is a manifestation of alterations in the body's natural healing processes. Naturopathic physicians use multiple modalities, including clinical nutrition and diet; acupuncture; herbal medicine; homeopathy; spinal and soft tissue manipulation; physical therapies involving ultrasound, light, and electric currents; therapeutic counseling; and pharmacology.[17]

## Mind-Body Interventions

A growing scientific movement has explored the mind's ability to affect the body. The clinical application of this relationship is categorized as *mind-body medicine.* Some mind-body interventions, formerly categorized as CAM therapies, have been assimilated into conventional mainstream medicine. Cognitive-behavioral approaches have a well-documented theoretic basis with supporting scientific evidence and are examples of mind-body medicine. Other mind-body interventions still considered CAM include meditation, some applications of hypnosis, music, dance, art therapy, prayer, and mental healing.[10]

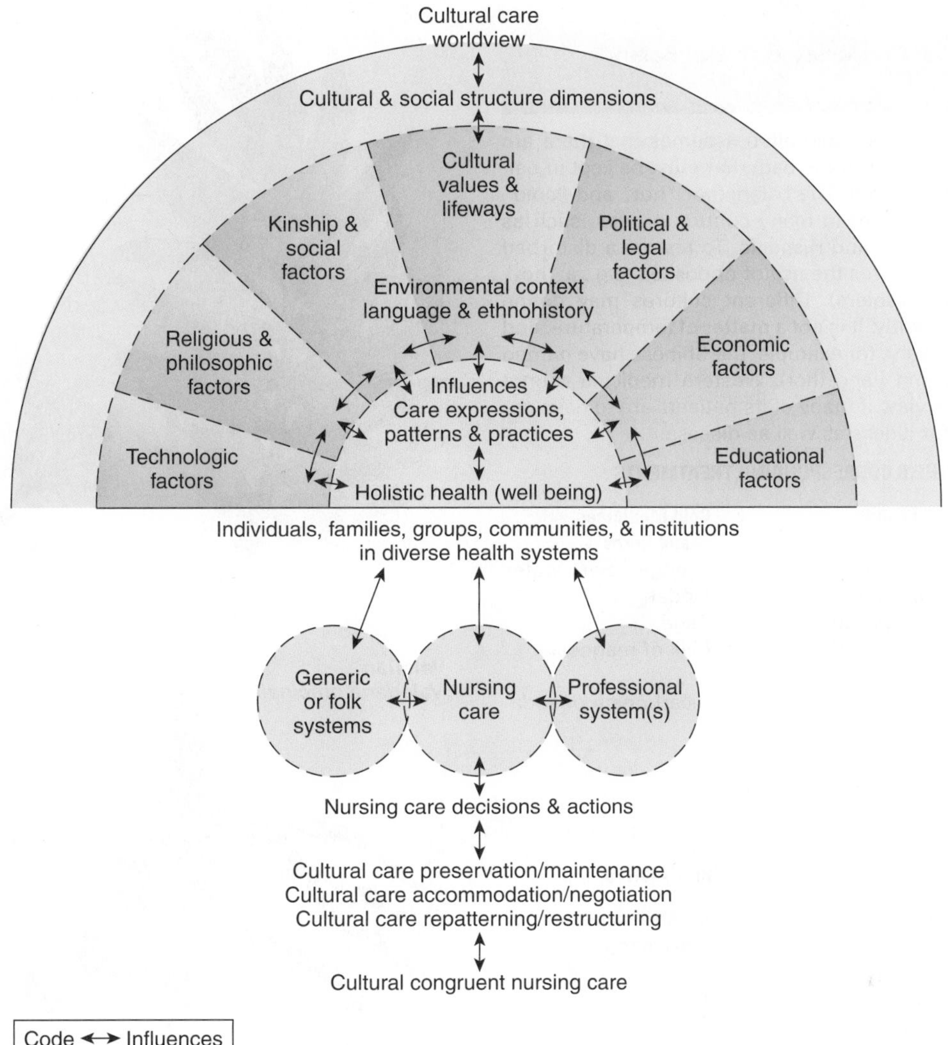


**FIGURE 32-1** The Leininger Sunrise Model. From a holistic, worldview stance, the Sunrise Model serves as a map depicting the cultural, social, and environmental dimensions affecting individuals, families, communities, and institutions.

## Biologically Based Therapies

The CAM category of biologically based therapies includes biologically based and natural-based practices, products, and interventions, some of which overlap with mainstream medicine's use of dietary supplements. Herbal, orthomolecular, individual biologic therapies and special dietary treatments are encompassed in biologically based therapies.

Herbs are plants or parts of plants that contain and produce chemical substances that act on the body (Figure 32-2). Some diet therapies are believed to promote health and prevent and/or control health. Proponents of diet therapies include Drs. Atkins, Pritikin, and Weil. Orthomolecular therapies use differing concentrations of chemicals such as magnesium, melatonin, and megadoses of vitamins aimed at treating disease. Many biologic therapies are available that are not currently accepted by mainstream medicine, such as the use of cartilage products from cattle, sheep, or sharks for treatment of cancer and arthritis or the use of bee pollen to treat autoimmune and inflammatory diseases.[10]

## Manipulative and Body-Based Methods

Methods that are based on the movement or manipulation of the body include chiropractic, osteopathy, and massage. Touch and manipulations with the hands have been used in healing and medical practice since the beginning of the history of medicine. At one time, the physician's hands were considered the most important diagnostic and therapeutic tool. This remains true today, despite sophisticated diagnostic equipment and modalities (Box 32-4). Manual healing methods are based on the principle that dysfunction of a part of the body often affects secondarily the function of other discrete, possibly indirectly connected body parts. Theories have developed for correction of these secondary dysfunctions by realigning body parts or manipulating soft tissues. Chiropractic science is concerned primarily with the relationship between structure (spine primarily) and function (nervous system primarily) of the human body to preserve and restore health. Osteopathic medicine incorporates an extensive body of work that supports the use of osteopathic techniques for both musculoskeletal and nonmus-

BOX 32-3

### Cultural Characteristics Related to the Balance of "Hot" and "Cold"

A naturalistic or holistic approach often assumes that there are external factors (some good, some bad) that must be kept in balance if we are to remain well. The balance of "hot" and "cold" is a part of the belief system in many cultural groups, such as the Arab, Chinese, Filipino, and Hispanic. To restore a disturbed balance (i.e., to treat) requires the use of opposites (e.g., a "hot" remedy for a "cold" problem). Different cultures may define "hot" and "cold" differently. It is not a matter of temperature, and the words used might vary; for example, the Chinese have named the forces yin (cold) and yang (hot). Western medicine cannot ignore the naturalistic view if many of its patients are to have appropriate treatment for illness as well as disease.

**HOT CONDITIONS AND THEIR CORRESPONDING TREATMENTS**

| Hot Conditions | Cold Foods | Cold Medicines and Herbs |
|---|---|---|
| Fever | Fresh vegetables | Orange flower water |
| Infection | Tropical fruits | Linden |
| Diarrhea | Dairy products | Sage |
| Kidney problem | Meats such as goat, fish, chicken | Milk of magnesia |
| Rash | Honey | Bicarbonate of soda |
| Skin ailment | Cod | |
| Sore throat | Raisins | |
| Liver problem | Bottle milk | |
| Ulcer | Barley water | |
| Constipation | | |

**COLD CONDITIONS AND THEIR CORRESPONDING TREATMENTS**

| Cold Conditions | Hot Foods | Hot Medicines and Herbs |
|---|---|---|
| Cancer | Chocolate | Penicillin |
| Pneumonia | Cheese | Tobacco |
| Malaria | Temperate-zone fruits | Ginger root |
| Joint pain | Eggs | Garlic |
| Menstrual period | Peas | Cinnamon |
| Teething | Onions | Anise |
| Earache | Aromatic beverages | Vitamins |
| Rheumatism | Hard liquor | Iron preparations |
| Tuberculosis | Oils | Cod liver oil |
| Cold | Meats such as beef, water fowl, mutton | Castor oil |
| Headache | Goat's milk | Aspirin |
| Paralysis | Cereal grains | |
| Stomach cramps | Chili peppers | |

From Seidel HM and others: *Mosby's guide to physical examination*, ed 5, St Louis, 2003, Mosby.

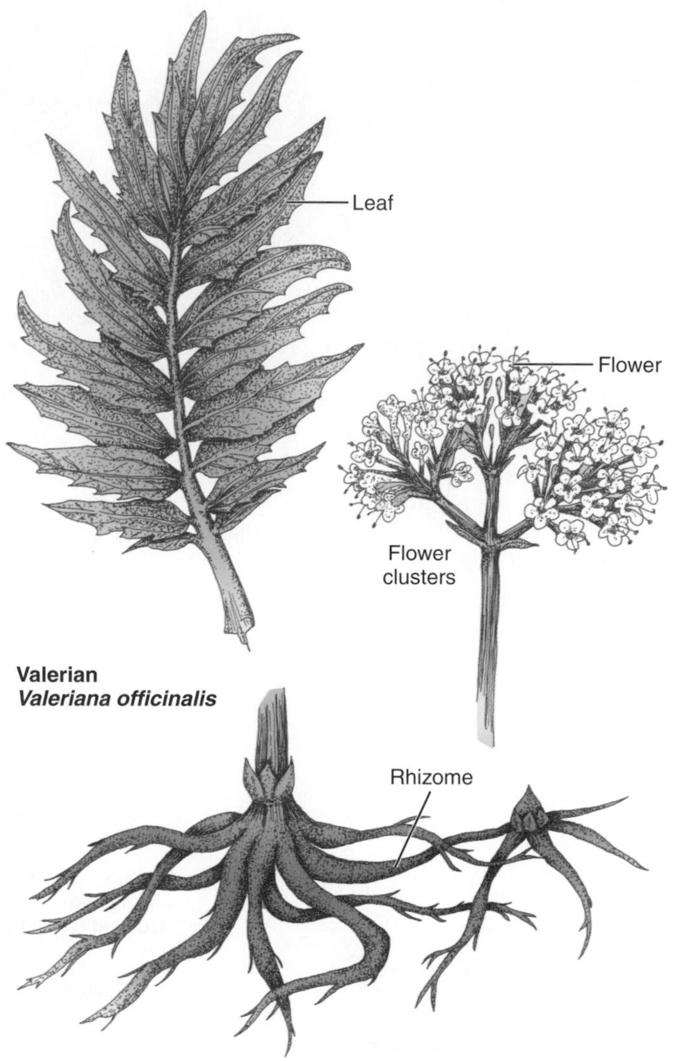


FIGURE 32-2 Valerian is a perennial plant cultivated throughout the world. Its reported uses include treatment of nervous disorders such as anxiety, restlessness, and insomnia. The plant rhizomes and roots are used to produce valerian in the forms of capsules, crude tea, extracts, and tinctures and in combination with products containing other herbs.

culoskeletal problems. Massage therapy is one of the oldest methods known in the practice of health care. Many different massage techniques are aimed at helping the body heal itself through the use of manipulation of the soft body tissues.

## Energy Therapies

Energy therapies have been categorized into two groups: biofield therapies (those that focus on fields believed to originate within the body) and electromagnetic fields (those that originate from other sources). The existence of energy fields that originate within and around the body has not yet been proven experimentally. However, many studies have examined the experience of recipient or healer and the outcomes of this type of energy therapy. Examples of therapies with a biofield basis include acupuncture, Reiki, qigong, therapeutic touch (TT) (described on p. 1205), and healing touch. Therapies that involve electromagnetic fields use unconventional pulsed fields, magnetic fields, alternating current fields, or direct current fields. These therapies have been clinically applied with patients who have arthritis, cancer, and pain.[10]

# COMPLEMENTARY AND ALTERNATIVE MEDICINE USE AND SURGERY

## Energy Therapies

Patients have choices in how to manage their health care. However, surgery is the most invasive of all options (History box). As health care consumers become more knowledgeable about their health they may seek out complementary modalities to augment traditional Western medical therapies (Patient Safety).

BOX 32-4

### The Use of Palpation in Physical Examination

Palpation involves the use of your hands and fingers to gather information through the sense of touch. Certain parts of your hands and fingers are better than others are for specific types of palpation. The palmar surface of the fingers and finger pads is more sensitive than the fingertips and is used whenever discriminatory touch is needed for determining position, texture, size, consistency, masses, fluid, and crepitus. The ulnar surface of the hand and fingers is the most sensitive area for distinguishing vibration. The dorsal surface of the hands is best for estimating temperature; of course, this estimate provides only a crude measure and is best used to detect temperature differences in comparing parts of the body.

Touch is in many ways therapeutic, and palpation is the actuality of the "laying on of hands." It is the moment at which we begin our physical invasion of the patient's body. Our much-repeated advice that your approach be gentle and your hands be warm is not only practical but symbolic of your respect for the patient and for the privilege the patient gives you.

From Seidel HM and others: *Mosby's guide to physical examination,* ed 5, St Louis, 2003, Mosby.

## HISTORY

Nursing has long been known as both an art and a science. The medical condition of a patient has consequently been just as important as the "rest" of the patient as nurses seek to tend to emotional needs and individual patient concerns. In this excerpt from a 1918 textbook, the following recommendations are provided for preparing the surgical patient:

> The general preparation of the patient begins from the time that the surgical condition is recognized. Patients should be treated in such a manner as to maintain, and indeed increase, their confidence in a successful solution of their trouble. Anything tending toward discouragement should be obviated. As a rule, the nearer the individual's normal manner of living is imitated, the more satisfactory the result. If the patient is not ill enough to be confined to bed it is well for him to walk about, read, go to the toilet, take his own bath, and at the time set for the operation walk to the operating room. By so doing not only is the patient's mind kept active but especially in hospital work a not inconsiderable amount of nurse's time saved. Nervous patients should be insured a good rest the night prior to the operation by the administration of a sedative, preferably a combination of the bromids. Any concomitant disease should receive appropriate treatment.

From Fowler RS: *The operating room and the patient—a manual of pre- and post-operative treatment,* Philadelphia, 1918, Saunders.

## PATIENT SAFETY

### Supporting CAM in the Perioperative Setting

Awareness of the various forms of complementary and alternative medicine (CAM) that might be used by perioperative patients is vital to provide safe care. The roles of advocate and educator become very important in integrating therapies.

As advocates using the holistic approach, perioperative nurses play an important role in supporting the patient who desires to use CAM in the perioperative setting. It is important to balance the use of conventional and nonconventional interventions in respecting the patient's wishes and providing safe care. Reasonable accommodations, planned with safety in mind, can be made in many instances to allow the patient to supplement traditional medical approaches. The nurse should determine if there is any potential for the CAM to interfere with any other planned treatment modality when planning accommodations. Examples of such accommodation might be providing massage without using an oil that could compromise the surgical skin prep or ensuring that any CAM practitioners or healers who wish to treat the patient in the perioperative setting do so under the institution's policies and procedures. The nurse should document any use of CAM in the perioperative nursing record along with the patient's response.

In the educator role, the nurse may be able to partner with patients to empower them to research the safety and efficacy of the techniques they are using. The preoperative assessment offers a prime opportunity for the nurse to identify possible safety risks for the perioperative patient. Whenever possible the preoperative assessment should be conducted a few days before the planned surgical procedure to allow ample time to gather data and begin patient teaching in a controlled, unhurried setting. The nurse can use this time to educate patients about the impact of CAM therapies in the perioperative period and beyond. For example, patients who take certain herbal supplements are at increased risk for perioperative coagulopathy and other anesthesia-related adverse events (see Table 32-6). By obtaining information in advance on the patient's use of these medications, the nurse can impact safe care by advising the patient to consult with the surgeon and modify the treatment regimen to avoid anesthetic complications.

The preoperative assessment also allows a forum to educate patients about the need to obtain reliable information about CAM. In discussing the patient's use of CAM, the nurse should remind him or her that results should be supported by clinical trials and that information on the Internet may be commercial in nature rather than scientific. Patients who use CAM should also be encouraged to notify their physician if any side effects occur.

Modified from Dossey BM, Guzzetta CE: Holistic nursing practice. In Dossey BM and others: *Holistic nursing, a handbook for practice,* ed 4, Boston, 2005, Jones & Bartlett; Fetrow CW, Avila JR: *Professional's handbook of complementary and alternative medicines,* ed 3, Philadelphia, 2004, Lippincott, Williams & Wilkins; Herring M: Guidelines for advising patients about CAM. In Herring MA, Roberts MM: *Complementary and alternative medicine, fast facts for medical practice,* Williston, VT, 2002, Blackwell Scientific.

To use the term *alternative* is actually misleading. Many progressive medical facilities embrace a holistic patient focus, exploring and integrating nontraditional healing modalities to support an individualized surgical experience. Biofield therapeutics are nonpharmacologic anxiolytics for surgical patients that may be integrated with an allopathic treatment plan (Research Highlight).

## RESEARCH HIGHLIGHT

### Electroacupuncture for Postoperative Nausea and Vomiting

Postoperative nausea and vomiting (PONV) can present a challenging situation for the patient and the health care practitioner and has the potential to negatively impact the patient's outcome. Many techniques to prevent PONV involve pharmaceutical intervention, such as the administration of ondansetron and dopamine antagonists. Although generally effective, the use of these pharmaceuticals to prevent PONV may be associated with unpleasant side effects.

Researchers at Duke University sought to determine the usefulness of electroacupuncture, a complementary and alternative medicine (CAM) that uses electrostimulation applied to acupuncture points to treat PONV. They conducted a study with 77 patients who were undergoing major breast surgery. The patients were randomized into three groups. One group received electroacupuncture delivered through the application of a small electrical pulse through the skin by means of an electrode at P6, a point proximal to the wrist; the second group received ondansetron, 4 mg intravenously, and the third group received a placebo in the form of a sham control (placement of the electrodes without stimulation). The electroacupuncture technique for the first group was begun before induction of anesthesia and continued for 30 to 60 minutes to the end of surgery. The ondansetron group received the medication at the point of induction.

Outcomes evaluated were the number of PONV episodes, the patient's subjective rating of PONV on a 0 to 10 point scale, use of rescue antiemetics, and patient satisfaction at 24-hour follow-up. Subjective rating of PONV was assessed at 0, 30, 60, 90, and 120 minutes; rescue antiemetics were given at the patient's request, when the subjective score was 5 or more for 15 minutes or longer, or when the patient had two or more emetic episodes in 15 minutes.

Seventy-seven percent of the electroacupuncture group had no PONV compared with 64% in the ondansetron group and 42% in the placebo group. The electroacupuncture group needed fewer antiemetics (19%) than the ondansetron (28%) and placebo (54%) groups. Patient satisfaction was highest in the electroacupuncture group. A secondary outcome of the study was the reduction of postoperative pain. The electroacupuncture group had less pain compared with the ondansetron and placebo groups.

Electroacupuncture was more effective in relieving the patient's nausea than it was in relieving vomiting, but it was a very well-received CAM. The authors of the study note that the technique is very convenient to use in the busy perioperative setting and offers a viable alternative to traditional pharmaceutical treatment of PONV.

Modified from Gan TJ and others: A randomized controlled comparison of electro-acupoint stimulation or ondansetron versus placebo for the prevention of postoperative nausea and vomiting, *Anesthesia and Analgesia* 99(4):1070-1075, 2004.

Many ancient cultures refer to a human biofield (Table 32-1) or "life force." Sometimes referred to as "energy work," biofield therapeutics are a range of interventions sharing common threads. First is the existence of a "universal force" or "healing energy" arising from God (as the person understands this being), the cosmos, the earth, or another supernatural source. Second, the human biofield, as part of the "universal field," is dynamic, open, complex, and pandimensional. Human biofields are constantly changing, interacting with each other, the environment, and the universal force field. Third, the ability to use one's biofield for healing is considered to be universal, although few people are aware of it without specific training. Last, practitioners intend to positively affect the patient's biofield, either by direct contact or by using the hands in proximity, akin to the ancient practice of "laying on of hands"[8] (Table 32-2).

***Therapeutic Touch.*** TT is the contemporary interpretation of several ancient healing modalities. Dolores Krieger and Dora Kunz developed TT in the early 1970s. The practice, like others that form part of the body of CAM, consists of learned skills for the conscious manipulation of human energies (Table 32-3). In practice it is not necessary for the practitioner (healer) to actually touch the recipient (healee), because the energy field can be "felt" several inches away from the physical body. TT describes a process of healing with clear definitions of the required skills and knowledge for successful practice. Explanations of the assumptions, the concepts, and the background of the practice follow.

ASSUMPTIONS[8]

- *A human being is an open energy system.* This assumption implies that the transfer of energy is natural and continuous. When a healer transfers energy to a healee using TT, it is without effort and guided by conscious, mindful action. The healer adds intentionality within a compassionate context.
- *A human being is bilaterally anatomically symmetric.* Symmetry is apparent in several anatomic systems, most clearly

**TABLE 32-1**

**Biofield Terms and Source Culture**

| Term | Source Culture |
|---|---|
| Ankh | Ancient Egyptian |
| Bioenergy | American, European |
| Ki | Japanese |
| Life force | General use |
| Oki, Orenda, Ton, Wakan | American Indian: Huron, Iroquois, Dakota, Lakota |
| Pneuma | Ancient Greek |
| Prana | Sanskrit, Ancient Hindu Indian |
| Qi | Chinese |
| Subtle energy | American, European |
| Sila | Inuit |
| Tane | Hawaiian |

Modified from *Alternative medicine: expanding medical horizons—a report to the National Institute of Health on Alternative Medical Systems and Practices in the United States.* From the Workshop on Alternative Medicine held in Chantilly, Va, on September 14-16, 1992 (p. 134); Cassidy CM: Social and cultural factors. In Micozzi MS: *Fundamentals of complementary and integrative medicine,* ed 3, St Louis, 2006, Saunders.

TABLE 32-2

## Comparisons of Selected Biofield Therapies

| Therapy | Practice Initiated | Developers | Hand Placement | Theoretic Basis and Intent |
|---|---|---|---|---|
| Healing Science Hands of Light | 1978 | Barbara Brennan | Both on and near the body | Human body as "open" system, incorporates *chakras* (energy wheels) and psychic layers to treat the whole person and specific disorders. |
| Healing Touch | 1981 | American Holistic Nurses Association | Both on and off the body | Uses elements of Healing Science and Therapeutic Touch in conjunction with crystal and dowsing to treat the whole person and specific disorders. |
| Huna | Traditional | Hawaiian | Both on and near the body | Involves *mana* (universal force) and *aka* (universal substance) to heal body and mind. |
| Qigong | Traditional | Chinese | At meridian points or a short distance from the body | Qi follows meridians and body patterns to heal biologic disorders. |
| Reiki | Traditional<br>1800s<br>1936 | Buddhist<br>Japan—Hawayo Takata<br>United States—Mikao Usui | A few standardized hand placements on the physical body | Spiritual energy from the universe is channeled by "masters" to heal the spiritual body, which in turn heals the physical body. |
| Shen | 1977 | Richard Pavek | Sequence of paired-hand placements, according to flux patterns | Biofield conforms to natural laws of physics; practitioner uses conventional medical and psychotherapy questioning to discover and resolve primarily emotional disorders and somatopsychic dysfunctions. |
| Therapeutic Touch | 1972 | Dolores Krieger and Dora Kunz | Primarily off the body 2-4 inches | Aligning Kunz's Human Energy Field Model with Martha Rogers' Science of Unitary Human Beings, the centered practitioner assesses, directs, and modulates biofield energy to achieve relaxation response for healing of the whole person. |

Modified from *Alternative medicine: expanding medical horizons—a report to the National Institute of Health on Alternative Medical Systems and Practices in the United States.* From the Workshop on Alternative Medicine held in Chantilly, Va, on September 14-16, 1992 (pp. 137-138).

seen in the skeleton. This symmetry is the rational basis for the inference that there is also a pattern in the underlying human energy field. This provides the background for the TT practitioner's assessment of the healee's energy state.

- *Illness is an imbalance in an individual's energy field.* With TT, the healer manipulates the energy field by directing or modulating using the sense of touch much like the other four major senses of the body. All these senses are able to act from a distance without direct connection. The human energy field extends a few inches away from the body surface, and the practitioner senses fine energetic cues such as changes in pattern.
- *Humans have natural abilities to transform and transcend their conditions of living.* These functions are, in a sense, prerequisites for healing to occur.

CONCEPTS AND CONSTRUCTS[8]

- *Laying on of hands.* This is a healing practice found in multiple ancient cultures as well as contemporary religious groups.
- *Vital energy fields.* All persons share in a unity with nature and all living things, which includes universal energies. Most Eastern and ancient cultures have words and concepts for this phenomenon; the Western culture does not. This concept was derived from Chinese, Indian, and Native American cultures and other ancient religions; it supports or demonstrates some of the theories of quantum physics and nurse theorist Martha Rogers, but it is not derived from these sources.
- *Energy transfer.* This is described as a method by which one individual can transfer or send energy to another.
- *Energy congestion.* When energy is not flowing from head to toe but seems to be localized, or *stuck* at a certain level of the body, it is considered congested. Although energy flow is not only head to toe, this is considered the major flow pattern.
- *Energy imbalance.* When the energy field does not appear to be symmetric, there seems to be some disturbance or difference in the field on one side and not another.
- *Inner healer.* With TT, persons in the role of healer have to be more than masters of techniques—they must become masters of themselves. This concept, like the laying on of hands, was derived from multiple sources including cultural and religious and the martial arts, as well as personal observation and experience.
- *Intentionality.* This concept addresses the focused and inner intent to help another achieve the maximum level of whole-

**TABLE 32-3**

## Complementary and Alternative Medical Practices

| Alternative Practice | Uses | Education | Technique(s) | Background |
|---|---|---|---|---|
| Therapeutic Touch | Stress relief<br>Pain relief<br>Promotion of wellness | Level I: 12-hr seminar<br>Level II: 1 yr of practice and seminar<br>Level III: 1 yr of mentoring<br>Level IV: 5 yr of practice twice weekly, two advanced workshops, and 1 yr of teaching with a mentor | Contact, or "laying on of hands"<br>Noncontact, or working in the subtle energy field surrounding the body (aura) | Developed by Dolores Krieger, PhD, RN<br>Beginning in early 1970s<br>Official organization: Nurse Healers—Professional Associates International |
| Healing Touch | Stress relief<br>Pain relief<br>Promotion of wellness | Level I: 15-hr seminar<br>Level II: two 15-hr seminars<br>Level III: two 3-hr sections with 100 client sessions and a case study<br>Level IV: instructor training | Therapeutic Touch, penduluming, hand scanning, magnetic unruffling, chakra connection, headache technique, ultrasound laser, chakra spread, and Scudder technique | Techniques gathered by Janet Mentgen, RN, BSN<br>Offered since 1989; American Holistic Nursing Association (AHNA) certification since 1993<br>Sponsored by Healing Touch International |
| Reiki | Promotion of mental, physical, emotional, and spiritual well-being | Level I: 2-day seminar<br>Level II: 6- to 12-mo experience and 1-day seminar<br>Level III: 2-yr experience, mentorship, 2- to 3-day seminar, each level student receives an attunement | Laying on of hands<br>Reiki Circle<br>Distance Healing | Taught master to student from Master Mikao Usiu in mid-nineteenth century Japan to present day<br>Based on healing modalities found in ancient Tibetan Sanskrit |
| Reflexology | Promotion of balance and wellness through nerve stimulation | Multiple courses available with ability to attain certification<br>Videotapes also available | Application of pressure to sites on the foot, hands, ears, and so on that correspond with organs and nerves to cause a reflex arc of stimulation to the area in need | Ancient method of treatment for ailments dating back to Egyptians and beyond |

From Scales B: CAMPing in the PACU: using complementary and alternative medical practice in the PACU, *Journal of PeriAnesthesia Nursing* 16(5):325-334, 2001.

ness or well-being that he or she is capable and desirous of attaining.

- *Centered consciousness.* This concept describes the act of self-searching—a going within to explore the deeper levels of oneself. Centered consciousness is a concept derived from ancient cultures and religions.

**BACKGROUND.** The Upanishads in the Vedas, the oldest literature of the East Indian people, describe chakras (Table 32-4). Although the most detailed descriptions are in the Upanishads, the attributes are found in the teachings of other cultures as widely geographic as the Sufis of the Middle East to the Native Americans, particularly from the North American Southwest (Figure 32-3)

• • •

TT practice lends itself well to the fast-paced surgical environment. The skills learned through study of TT provide a nurse healer with the ability to center quickly and use intention to calm themselves and those around them in stressful situations.

Research design, methods, techniques, and sample sizes are considerations for future studies into how biofield therapeutics may benefit surgical patients. Replicating past studies, as well as new research based on physiologic data and quantitative studies, is necessary. It has become evident that the concepts involved in energy therapies need consistent definitions. If the concepts do not have agreed-on definitions, they cannot be quantified or measured in meaningful ways. However, interest is high and research continues in an effort to better understand a phenomenon that seems to provide meaningful relief to the patient as well as to often-stressed nurse (or other health care) colleagues.

## Perioperative Medical Hypnotherapy

Use of medical hypnotherapy in hospitals and clinics for perioperative care is becoming more common. Patients are seeking an active role in their treatment and are better informed regarding surgical options. Participating in perioperative medical hypnotherapy allows patients to take shared responsibility for their healing process, giving them a measure of control, because all hypnosis is self-hypnosis. Meaningful and active participation empowers a patient to enter into anesthesia and surgery with confidence.

Surgery is a life-changing event, and each perioperative medical hypnotherapy patient is unique. The initial assessment serves to determine goals and explore questions relative

**TABLE 32-4**

**Chakra Chart**

| Chakra | Color | Frequency | Location | Section Control | Characteristics | As a Tool |
|---|---|---|---|---|---|---|
| Root | Red | 500 Hz | Base of spine Perineum | Spine, feet, legs, kidneys, stress response | Governs will to survive, will to live, survival | Used to ground, to stay present in the here and now, to strengthen, to fortify, to purge by fire |
| Sacral | Orange | 600 Hz | Lower abdomen below umbilicus | Reproductive system, intestines | Controls desire, emotions, will to feel | Regulation of menstruation, reproduction, gastrointestinal (GI) system, kidneys, bladder |
| Solar plexus | Yellow | 400 Hz | Midabdomen, above umbilicus | Liver, pancreas, stomach, gallbladder | Seat of ego, the self, ability to think, willpower, controls laughter and anger | Eases digestion, calms emotion, correction of an action, access knowledge, self-empowerment |
| Heart | Pink, green | 300 Hz | Midthorax | Heart, blood, circulatory system, hands, arms, vagus nerve, thymus | Center for physical love and unconditional love, balance | Opening to love, harmony, contentment, circulatory and lymph and breast cleansing; to resolve conflicts to enhance harmony, empathy, compassion, healing |
| Thyroid | Blue | 200 Hz for muscle; 700 Hz for other | Base of throat | Lymphatic system, vocals, respiratory system, ears, thyroid | Communication, stroke prevention, cleansing of lymphatics, aids circulation | Will to express, communication, grieving, higher emotions, cooling and soothing for inflammation, reduce worry, tranquility, state of grace, self-reflection |
| Third eye or brow | Purple | 800 Hz | Space above and between eyes | Pituitary gland, low brain, eyes | Growth, regulation of body functions, eyes | Relaxation, ability to "see" things (i.e., intuition), wisdom to stimulate endorphins for pain control |
| Crown | Pale violet, cream, white | 1000 Hz | Caput | Pineal gland, upper brain | Brain development | Thought processing, clarity, connection to cosmic consciousness; to balance left and right hemispheres place hands on sides of head |

From Scales B: CAMPing in the PACU: using complementary and alternative medical practice in the PACU, *Journal of PeriAnesthesia Nursing* 16(5):325-334, 2001.

to emotional as well as physical concerns. The hypnotherapist, working within the patient's belief system, helps acknowledge areas of the patient's concern as a multidisciplinary partnership of healing is forged in a patient-centered manner.

As the hypnotherapist guides the patient into relaxation and induces hypnosis, they journey into the body, together addressing predetermined issues. Fear of the unknown, preprocedure anxiety, changes in body image, anticipated pain or nausea, loss of organs, and transplantation of new ones are some examples.[10]

Hypnosis compassionately allows a patient to explore emotions without judgment or expectation of those feelings. The practice of emotional awareness, of being present with feelings, and of holding those feelings sacred can bring a sense of peace and healing insights during a time of profound stress, such as that experienced by many surgical patients. Predetermined suggestions or affirmations may increase confidence in the health care team, increase compliance with the treatment plan, decrease blood loss, maintain intraoperative homeostasis, reduce need for sedation or pain medication, decrease postoperative nausea or vomiting, and increase patient satisfaction.[20]

Postoperative hypnotherapy sessions reinforce continued participation of patients in their healing process. This may take the form of establishing metabolic gauges in the "control room" or a symbolic shield of protection, holding or sending color, light, or a certain feeling of safety to a specific part of the body. It may be expressing gratitude to and confidence in the medical and nursing community. Follow-up sessions allow both patient and hypnotherapist to evaluate attainment of preoperative goals, consider postoperative outcomes, and explore issues relevant to the ongoing healing process.

## Guided Imagery

Another therapy closely related to hypnosis is guided imagery (Research Highlight). Imagery, or thinking in pictures, is the natural language of the unconscious mind and is used by the autonomic nervous system as a primary mode of communication. The autonomic nervous system controls unconscious body functions such as heart rate, immune function, digestion, blood flow, smooth muscle tension, and pain perception (Figure 32-4). Guided imagery for surgical patients may be in the form of pre-scripted tapes that lead the patient through relax-

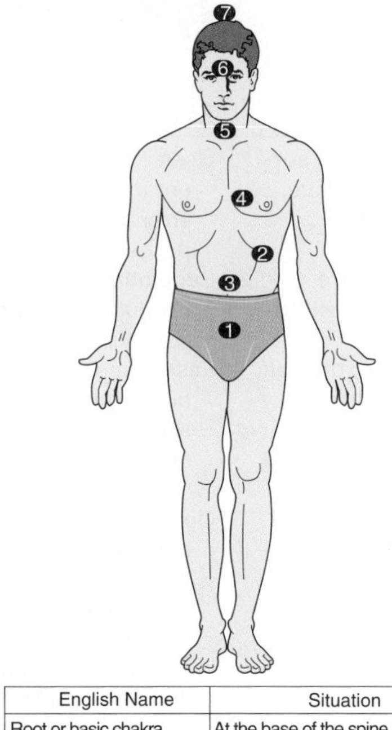

| | English Name | Situation |
|---|---|---|
| 1 | Root or basic chakra | At the base of the spine |
| 2 | Spleen or splenic chakra | Over the spleen |
| 3 | Navel or umbilical chakra | At the navel, over the solar plexus |
| 4 | Heart or cardiac chakra | Over the heart |
| 5 | Throat or laryngeal chakra | At the front of the throat |
| 6 | Brow or frontal chakra | In the space between the eyebrows |
| 7 | Crown or coronal chakra | On the top of the head |

**FIGURE 32-3** Chakras.

ation exercises and provide healing suggestions. In other instances, the perioperative nurse may assist the patient with guided imagery through the use of a calming, monotone voice; a smooth speaking delivery; and the use of relaxing images, such as a place in nature. The perioperative nurse coaches the patient to see, feel, smell, sense, and hear the imagined scene. Benefits of guided imagery with surgery patients may include the following[9,16]:

- Decreased anxiety
- Decreased pain perception
- Faster recovery
- Increased sense of control

## Aromatherapy in Perioperative Services

The use of complementary and holistic therapies in health care facilities is going through a renaissance. Long before Western medicine, aromatherapy and herbs were part of physicians' practice and prescriptive use. Florence Nightingale recognized the need to create a "healing environment." Some progressive health care facilities across the United States subscribe to a holistic, patient-focused model known as the *Planetree model.* The name of this model is taken from the tree under which Hippocrates taught his medical students that patients should be the focus of care and that the environment was an important factor in healing.

This model, instituted in 1985 under the guidance of Angelica Thieriot, embodies the commitment of Hippocrates. It was created as a philosophy of caring that personalizes, humanizes, and demystifies the health care experience for patients and their families. All participants, both caregivers and patients, seek to optimize health care outcomes by integrating complementary medical therapies, such as clinical aromatherapy and therapeutic massage, with conventional medical therapies.[18] Potential uses for perioperative services include reducing anxiety for patients and their families in the waiting area and ameliorating nausea and vomiting during the immediate postoperative phase.

Clinical aromatherapy is gaining acceptance with consent and participation of patients. It is practiced by certified clinical aromatherapy practitioners (CCAPs), knowledgeable about the specific properties of essential oils and how they interact with patients and the therapeutic environment. CCAPs use clinical-grade essential oils in a controlled way for specific, measurable outcomes. These may affect the patient on a psychologic, physiologic, or cellular level. The choice of essential oil is based on the chemistry of that essential oil and its proven effects (Table 32-5).

As pharmacology combines medications to potentiate effect, aromatherapy may act synergistically with traditional treatment; or it may be offered in concert with other complementary modalities to relieve discomfort, thereby reducing dosages of analgesics or sedatives.[6]

## RESEARCH HIGHLIGHT

### Guided Imagery and Pain Descriptors

Imagery has been used in the healing arts since treatments for disease have been recorded. Interest in the use of guided imagery for chronic pain has increased as the limits of traditional medicine have been recognized. Because pharmacologic and invasive procedures do not alleviate all pain, the efficacy of guided imagery with persons experiencing chronic pain is worthy of scientific inquiry. Although research findings indicate that guided imagery is effective in reducing the intensity of pain, there has been no attempt to systematically describe how the overall experience, especially the meaning it holds for the person, changes with its use.

The purpose of this study was to determine how verbal descriptions of pain changed with the use of a guided imagery technique. A mixed method, concurrent nested design, was used. Participants were randomized to either the treatment group, which used guided imagery, or the control group (no guided imagery). Verbal descriptions of pain were obtained before the study started and at intervals over a consecutive 4-day period. A total of 210 pain descriptions were obtained across the five time points. Data were analyzed using content analysis. Six categories emerged from the data: pain is never-ending, pain is relative, pain is explainable, pain is torment, pain is restrictive, and pain is changeable. The meaning of pain as never-ending was a prominent theme for participants before randomization to treatment and control groups. It remained a strong theme for participants in the control group throughout the 4-day study period; however, pain as never-ending did not resurface for participants in the treatment group. For participants in the treatment group, pain became changeable.

An appreciation of how pain language changes with the use of guided imagery can help perioperative nurses understand how the meaning of pain is altered by interventions such as guided imagery. This study provides a foundation for initiating guided imagery techniques for patients with chronic pain as part of a holistic approach to pain management.

Modified from Lewandowski W and others: Changes in the meaning of pain with the use of guided imagery, *Pain Management Nursing* 6(2):58-67, 2005.

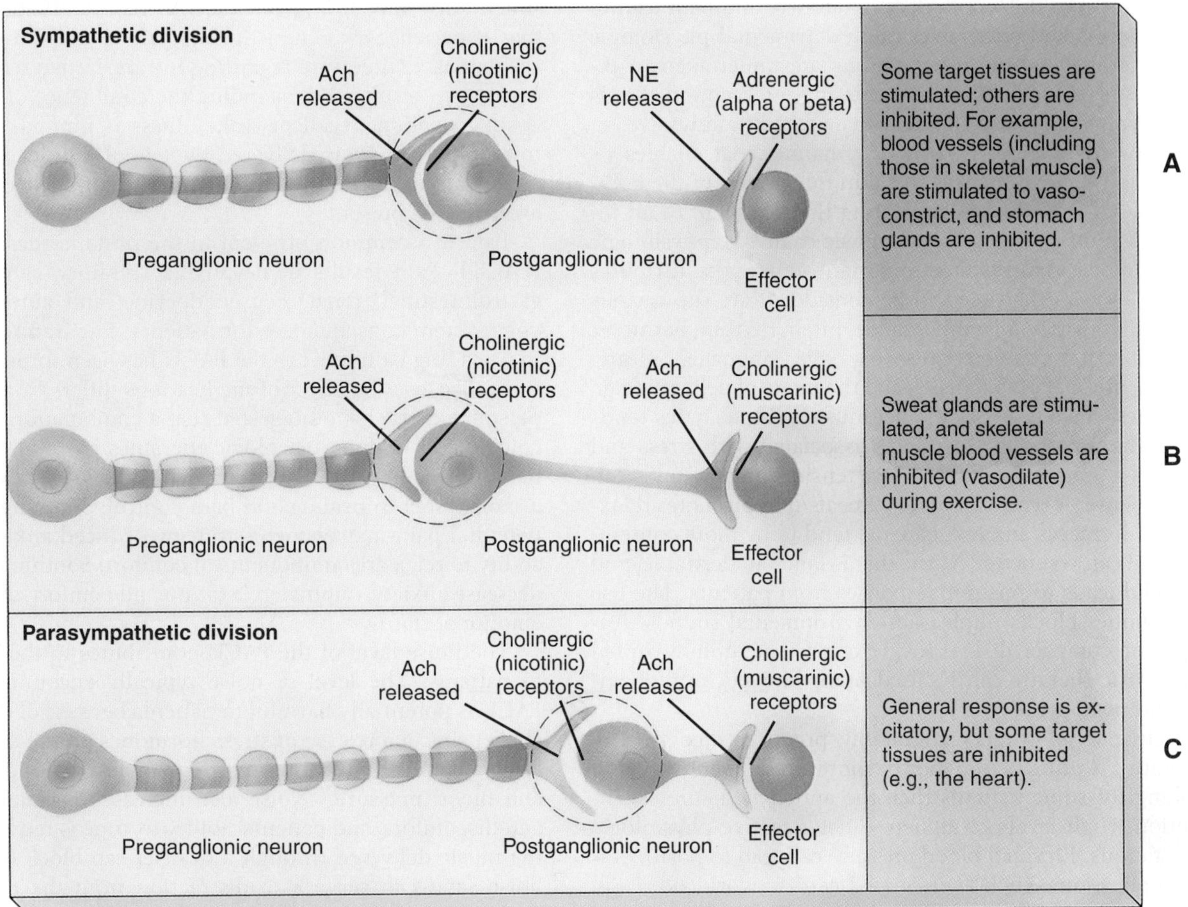


**FIGURE 32-4** Locations of neurotransmitters and receptors in the autonomic nervous system. In all pathways, preganglionic fibers are cholinergic, secreting acetylcholine *(Ach)*, which stimulates nicotinic receptors in the postganglionic neuron. Most sympathetic fibers are adrenergic, **A,** secreting norepinephrine *(NE)*, thus stimulating alpha- or beta-adrenergic receptors. A few sympathetic postganglionic fibers are cholinergic, stimulating muscarinic receptors in effector cells, **B.** All parasympathetic postganglionic fibers are cholinergic, **C,** stimulating muscarinic receptors in effector cells.

The nursing process of aromatherapy begins with obtaining consent for use of aromatics and collecting pertinent information. Assessment of the patient, the physical environment, and the team of caregivers defines the Healing Environment. Along with review of the medical and nursing histories, allergies, vital signs, and laboratory values, subjective data are relevant, such as how to offer treatment. The plan of therapy may include direct inhalation (on a cotton ball or through a diffuser), compresses, topical application, or with massage. As with all nursing interventions, postprocedure follow-up with the patient is imperative to assess efficacy of this intervention.

Further, well-designed research is required to provide data substantiating the value of clinical aromatherapy as another component of holistic perioperative nursing practice.

## Music and Surgery

Music is recognized as a way to decrease anxiety and discomfort. The therapeutic and healing properties of music have been recognized throughout history. Over time, studies have validated the positive psychologic and physiologic effects of music. Music has been shown to increase metabolism; increase or decrease muscular energy, breathing, blood volume, pulse rate, and blood pressure; and lower sensory stimuli thresholds. Music can touch patients deeply and thus transform their anxiety and discomfort into relaxation and healing.

Anxiety and pain are common perioperative nursing diagnoses identified in the sample plans of care in Unit II ("Surgical

**TABLE 32-5**

**Essential Oils and Their Properties**

| Property | Essential Oils |
|---|---|
| Antiemetic | Chamomile, lavender, lemon, peppermint |
| Antiseptic | Bergamot, clove, eucalyptus, lavender, juniper, thyme, tea tree |
| Anxiolytic | Benzoin, bergamot, chamomile, jasmine, lavender, neroli, rose, sandalwood, verbena, ylang-ylang |
| Pain relieving | Birch, blue chamomile, black pepper, clove, ginger |
| Sedating | Bergamot, chamomile, jasmine, lavender, neroli, rose, ylang-ylang |
| Stimulating | Basil, black pepper, eucalyptus, peppermint, rosemary |

Interventions") in this book. Because anxiety and pain lead to increased stress and stress may cause detrimental physiologic reactions, many nursing interventions are undertaken to reduce patients' anxiety. Music is a nursing intervention that is easy to administer, relatively inexpensive, and noninvasive.

Music is therapeutic if used in a manner that enables its elements and their influences to aid in integration of the body, mind, and spirit of the patient during the treatment of an illness or disability. When selecting music to invoke physiologic and psychologic changes, it is important to note the attributes of music. Factors that need to be considered are the various elements of music (e.g., tempo, mode, pitch, rhythm, harmony, melody); listener characteristics (e.g., age, language, culture, education, musical preferences); and the mode of delivery (e.g., headphones, speakers). Slow, quiet music without lyrics tends to lower the physiologic responses associated with stress and anxiety. Fast tempos tend to increase tension. Slow tempos can cause suspense. A tempo of 60 to 72 beats/min promotes relaxation and decreases anxiety; patients tend to be more contemplative and can rest better. Music that is familiar, desirable, and meaningful leads to positive responses from patients. The use of headphones blocks unpleasant environmental sounds. Audiotapes or compact disks provide consistent, uninterrupted music. Music therapy can be used preoperatively, intraoperatively, and postoperatively.

Anticipation of surgery commonly produces anxiety. The preoperative waiting period may be more stressful and anxiety-provoking for some patients than the anticipated surgical intervention. High levels of anxiety cause negative physiologic manifestations. Elevated blood pressure can lead to postoperative complications, such as increased cardiac workload. High levels of depression, fear, and anger are psychologic postoperative complications that may be related to preoperative anxiety. Using music during the preoperative phase can decrease anxiety. Emotions are altered, apprehension and tension are reduced, and sympathetic stimulation and adrenocortical activation are more controlled. Therefore changes in vital signs, such as elevated blood pressure and increased heart rate, are minimal. Studies have verified that patients listening to music had a significant decrease in anxiety when compared with patients in a control group who did not listen to music.[3]

Patients undergoing surgery under local or regional anesthesia have an acute awareness of the environment of the operating room (OR). The OR may appear threatening, with unfamiliar machines, equipment, noises, and smells. Physical positioning and exposure of body parts intensify anxiety. Unfamiliar sounds, bright lights, and technical language add to the stressors of the surgical experience. During surgery, music serves as a distractor, as well as reduces anxiety. The music not only blocks the various sounds in the room but also provides an escape through imaginative thought. Daydreaming, imagery, escape, and fantasizing are common to listeners. This creates a release of tension and is a way of focusing attention away from threats. Intraoperative music may decrease the patient's anxiety and consequently minimize the need for patient-controlled conscious sedation and analgesia. Music can have a positive effect during general anesthesia when delivered through headphones. Researchers support the idea that musical vibrations have an effect on the subconscious mind. The subject of patient awareness during anesthesia and surgery continues to receive much attention (see Chapter 7). Auditory functioning may be largely intact. As many as 1% of all patients may experience awareness during general anesthesia. Much of the extensive literature regarding intraoperative recall is anecdotal. As a result, understanding the confluence of factors relevant to patient recall or wakefulness is limited. The use of intraoperative music delivered by way of a headset can minimize fear and facilitate a more pleasant experience if recall or awareness is present.

Pain is a common problem in the postanesthesia care unit (PACU). Pain results in negative respiratory, cardiovascular, gastrointestinal, renal, neuroendocrine, and autonomic nervous system consequences for patients. The traditional means to providing pain relief in the PACU has been through medications. Because the effect of medications differs from person to person, experts have suggested that a combination of pharmacologic and nonpharmacologic therapies has a greater potential for providing optimal pain relief.[14] Music has a long history as an adjunct to healing and pain control. Soothing music is a potential pain-management strategy. Reduced anxiety and the ability to relax are components of comfort. Soothing music can decrease anxiety, improve relaxation and comfort, and improve emotional status.

The noise level of the PACU contributes to the discomfort of patients. The level of noise typically encountered in the PACU is potentially harmful to patients because of the undesirable effects of a release of stress hormones on the cardiovascular system, including increased vasoconstriction, heart rate, and blood pressure.[7] Noise also increases psychologic stress and discomfort, and patients' ability to cope is reduced. Soothing music delivered through a headset can block out external noises and can serve as a distraction from the noise of the PACU.

When using music as a nursing intervention to promote physiologic and psychologic well-being, it is important to prepare the patient and the environment. Inform the patient of the purpose of the music experience. Interview the patient about musical preferences, and document this in the medical record. A library of different types of music selections should be available. When compiling these collections, it is important that attention is given to the tempo, rhythm, melody, and harmony of the music (as noted earlier). In addition to implementing the music intervention, nurses must monitor patients' responses to ensure that intended outcomes are achieved, making adjustments as necessary.

## Psychoneuroimmunology

A great deal of change has transpired in health care as sophisticated techniques have been developed to define intricate biologic systems and underlying connections among these systems. Psychoneuroimmunology theory and research have insights for all complementary and alternative therapies.[12]

Psychoneuroimmunology seeks to analyze the relationship between the brain and immune function. Thus perioperative nursing interventions that seek to reduce stress influences have the potential to improve immune system function.

Early animal conditioning studies show links on a molecular level (immune regulators: neurotransmitters and hormones) that act to stimulate nerves or trigger physiologic changes. Further, the perception of stress is known to lead to a reduced ability to fight infection. Because measurement of immune function is a complicated process, much remains to be learned about the precise mechanism of how psychosocial or emotional factors affect susceptibility to disease.

## Herbs and Surgery

The use of herbal and botanic products is common today. Studies suggest that one third or more of patients having surgery are taking herbal supplements.[1] However, many patients do not communicate this information to their conventional medical physicians or nurse caregivers, because they are unsure of the reaction of conventional caregivers to their use of alternative substances.

Botanicals are marketed as food supplements in the United States. Manufacturers are not allowed to make claims about health benefits for these products because they are not FDA-approved. Since 1994, when the Dietary Supplement Health and Education Act (DSHEA) was passed, the definition of dietary supplements was broadened. A product that contains a vitamin, mineral, herb, amino acid, or other botanic or dietary substance used to supplement the diet is considered a dietary supplement; this includes concentrates, metabolites, constituents, extracts, and combinations of listed ingredients. These supplements are no longer subject to premarket safety evaluations by the FDA. Once a supplement is marketed, under the DSHEA, the FDA can restrict its use only if it can be shown that the product is unsafe.[4] There are no regulations establishing criteria for purity, manufacturing procedures, or identification of ingredients for these supplements. Therefore the potential exists for high variability in the potency of different batches of the same botanic product. In addition, impurities and unknown substances may also be present in these products. Because herbal products are so readily available and have such widespread media attention, many people think that they can safely self-medicate. Another mistaken assumption is that dietary supplements are safer than prescribed or over-the-counter drugs (see Patient Safety).[4]

Botanicals may initiate a pharmacologic response within the body (Table 32-6). Because this is the reason they are taken by many people, these products should be considered "drugs" from a medical or nursing perspective.[4] Many herbal products have actions that could be dangerous during surgery. Some herbal supplements may accentuate the toxicity of anesthetics or interfere with drug metabolism or clearance (Surgical Pharmacology).

***Coagulation Interactions.*** Anesthesia providers are concerned about the potential increased risk of instability intraoperatively resulting from inhibition of coagulation with the use of ginger, ginseng, feverfew, ginkgo, and garlic.[1] One difficulty

**TABLE 32-6**

### Potential Herb-Pharmaceutical Interactions

| Herb | Pharmaceutical | Unfavorable Herbal Interaction |
|---|---|---|
| Garlic, feverfew, ginger | Warfarin | May *increase* anticoagulant effect |
| *Astragalus* and licorice | Corticosteroids, cyclosporine | Immunosuppressive effects may be inhibited |
| Echinacea | Corticosteroids | Immunosuppressive effects may be inhibited |
| | Anabolic steroids, methotrexate, or other hepatotoxic drugs | Hepatotoxicity |
| Hawthorne | Digoxin | May potentiate effect |
| Siberian ginseng | Warfarin | May *inhibit* anticoagulation |
| | Digoxin | May interfere with assays |
| All ginsengs, yohimbe | Monoamine oxidase inhibitors (MAOIs) Phenelzine and others | May cause headaches, tremors, and insomnia |
| Licorice | MAOIs Phenelzine and others | May act as inhibitors and potentiate effects |
| | Digoxin | May cause hypokalemia |
| Chromium | Hypoglycemics | May decrease insulin requirements and potentiate effects |
| Chamomile, feverfew, and St. John's wort | Iron | May inhibit iron absorption |
| Borage, evening primrose oil | Phenobarbital Phenytoin | May lower seizure thresholds |
| Ephedra (banned by U.S. Food and Drug Administration [FDA]) | Cardiac glucosides or halothane | Cardiac dysrhythmias |
| | MAOIs, guanethidine | Enhanced sympathomimetic effects |
| | Oxytocin | Hypertension, potentiates contractile effects |
| Gingko | Aspirin (ASA), nonsteroidal antiinflammatory drugs (NSAIDs), warfarin, or heparin | Increased bleeding risk |
| Valerian | Sedative/hypnotic or anesthetic agents | Potentiated or prolonged effects |
| St. John's wort | Cyclosporine | Posttransplant complications |
| | MAOIs, steroids, warfarin, sympathomimetics, antidepressants | Alters drug metabolism for unpredictable results |
| Goldenseal | Oxytocin | Potentiates contractile effect |

Modified from Flanagan K: Preoperative assessment: safety considerations for patients taking herbal products, *Journal of PeriAnesthesia Nursing* 18(1):19-26, 2001; Norred CL: Herbs and anesthesia, *Alternative Therapies in Women's Health* 3(4):26-30, 2001; Skidmore-Roth L: *Mosby's handbook of herbs & natural supplements,* ed 3, St Louis, 2006, Mosby; Mills S, Bone, K: *The essential guide to herbal safety,* Philadelphia, 2005, Churchill Livingstone.

## SURGICAL PHARMACOLOGY

### Herbs: Effects and Precautions/Recommendations

The use of herbal supplements has become increasingly popular as people become more educated consumers and take a more active interest in their health. Because herbal supplements and other nutriceuticals are available without prescription, patients may not reveal their use of these therapies unless specifically questioned. The perioperative nurse must always consider the possibility that the patient is taking supplements and assess for their use. As with other medications the patient may be taking, the nurse is responsible to know the potential for interaction with medications used in the perioperative period. The information that follows offers a source for broadening the perioperative nurse's knowledge of commonly used herbal supplements.

| Herb (Scientific Name) and Other Names | Uses and Desired Effects | Potential Side Effects | Precautions and Recommendations |
|---|---|---|---|
| Garlic<br>*(Allium sativum)*<br>Clove garlic<br>Ajo<br>Poor man's penicillin | Antioxidant; antibiotic; lowers low-density lipids (LDLs) to prevent atherosclerosis; has antihypertensive, antiplatelet, and antithrombolytic properties | May prolong bleeding or clotting time, potentiate effects of antihypertensive or anticoagulant drugs | Large doses (>5 cloves) may cause gastrointestinal (GI) upset, garlic breath/flatus.<br>Discontinue use at least 7 days preoperatively. |
| Ginkgo<br>*(Ginkgo biloba)*<br>Duck foot<br>Kew tree<br>Maidenhair tree<br>Silver apricot<br>Fossil tree | Antioxidant; anticlotting; enhances blood flow (especially to the brain); reduces cellular lesions, retinal edema; treats symptoms of peripheral vascular disease and dementia; inhibits platelet-activating factors; used to enhance brain function and memory; treats headaches, depression, vertigo, and tinnitus | Headache, GI upset, palpitations, dizziness, or skin reactions | Increased bleeding risk by inhibiting platelet activity, lowering fibrinogen levels, and decreasing plasma viscosity. May potentiate anticoagulant therapy.<br>Discontinue use at least 36 hr preoperatively. |
| Ginseng<br>American ginseng<br>*(Panax quinquefolius)*<br>Chinese ginseng or Korean ginseng<br>*(Panax ginseng)*<br>Siberian ginseng<br>*(Eleutherococcus ginseng)* | Antioxidant; enhances memory and immune function; increases stamina; decreases fatigue; reduces stress response; lowers blood glucose; inhibits clotting | Usually mild and dose-related: nervousness, dizziness, mastalgia<br>"Ginseng abuse syndrome" (>15 g/day) = insomnia, hypotonia, and edema<br>Siberian ginseng may falsely elevate digoxin levels; potentiate monoamine oxidase inhibitors (MAOIs) | Contraindicated for patients with hypoglycemia, hypertension, and cardiac disorders.<br>Avoid with other stimulants; may lead to tachycardia or hypertension.<br>May decrease effectiveness of warfarin (decreased international normalized ratio [INR]).<br>May cause postmenopausal bleeding.<br>Discontinue use at least 7 days preoperatively. |
| Ephedra<br>*(Ephedra sinica)*<br>Ma huang<br>Mexican or Mormon tea<br>Dessert tea<br>Natural ecstasy<br>Natural fen-phen<br>Ephedrine<br>Chinese joint fir | Stimulant; bacteriostatic; antitussive; decongestant; bronchodilator; used for weight loss | Hypertension (HTN), tachycardia, dysrhythmias, cardiac arrest, myocardial infarct, nausea, vomiting, decreased GI motility, mydriasis, diuresis, anxiety, constipation, dizziness, headache, insomnia, psychosis, urine retention, seizure, stroke, uterine contractions | Do not use with cardiac glycosides, guanethidine, MAOI medications.<br>Do not use for patients with anxiety, HTN, glaucoma, enlarged prostate, or heart disease.<br>Discontinue use at least 24 hr preoperatively.<br>Limit use to 7 days. |
| Echinacea<br>*(Echinacea purpurea, E. pallida, E. angustifolia)*<br>Purple coneflower | Antiinfective; antiinflammatory; enhances immune function; may prevent or minimize symptoms and duration of common cold, upper respiratory infection (URI); enhances wound- and burn-healing process | May activate T-cells<br>Cross-allergic reaction<br>Immune suppression if taken long term | Discontinue as far in advance as possible. Should not be used by patients with autoimmune diseases.<br>Should not be used by patients with allergy to sunflower.<br>Avoid use for transplant patients or those with liver dysfunction. |

Modified from Flanagan K: Preoperative assessment: safety considerations for patients taking herbal products, *Journal of PeriAnesthesia Nursing* 18(1):19-26, 2001; Norred CL: Herbs and anesthesia, *Alternative Therapies in Women's Health* 3(4):26-30, 2001; Skidmore-Roth L: *Mosby's handbook of herbs & natural supplements,* ed 3, St Louis, 2006, Mosby; Mills S, Bone K: *The essential guide to herbal safety*, Philadelphia, 2005, Churchill Livingstone.

## SURGICAL PHARMACOLOGY

### Herbs: Effects and Precautions/Recommendations—cont'd

| Herb (Scientific Name) and Other Names | Uses and Desired Effects | Potential Side Effects | Precautions and Recommendations |
|---|---|---|---|
| St. John's wort (*Hypericum perforatum*) Amber touch-and-heal Goatweed Klamath weed | Anxiolytic; antidepressant (mild to moderate symptoms), may take 4-6 wk for effect; relieves dyspepsia and insomnia; mechanism: inhibits uptake of neurotransmitters | Photosensitization, skin irritation, restlessness, fatigue May prolong effects of anesthesia and potentiate meperidine or other narcotics Possible peripheral neuropathy, serotonergic crisis | May alter metabolism of other drugs: cyclosporine, warfarin, steroids, protease inhibitors. Do not combine with ephedra. Discontinue use at least 5 days preoperatively. |
| Cayenne (*Capsicum annuum*) Hot chili pepper Paprika | External use: muscle spasm or soreness Internal use: GI disorders | External: skin irritation, especially if used longer than 2 days Internal: lower GI discomfort, overdose may cause hypothermia | Avoid use preoperatively. |
| Feverfew (*Tanacetum parthenium*) Featherfew Midsummer daisy | Antipyretic; relieves arthritis, fever, headache, and migraine pain; increases fluidity of respiratory mucus; promotes menses and uterine contractions | Oral lesions, GI tract irritation Rebound headache with sudden cessation Hypersensitive reaction in those allergic to ragweed, asters, chrysanthemums, or daisies May increase clotting time | Increased bleeding risk. Avoid use preoperatively. |
| Goldenseal (*Hydrastis canadensis*) Orange or yellow root Ground raspberry Tumeric root Eye root | Antibacterial, antiinflammatory properties; diuretic (no sodium excreted); laxative; improves immune function; aids digestion; regulates menses | Hypotension, nausea, vomiting, abdominal cramping May exacerbate edema or hypertension May potentiate effects of insulin | May cause electrolyte imbalance, seizures, respiratory paralysis. Avoid use preoperatively. |
| Valerian (*Valerian officinalis*) All heal Setwell Vandal root | Mild anxiolytic, muscle relaxant, hypnotic, and sedative; may ease symptoms of benzodiazepine withdrawal | Headache, excitability, nausea, visual disturbance Potentiates sedative/hypnotics Long-term use may increase anesthesia tolerance Sudden cessation may cause withdrawal symptoms | Potential prolonged anesthesia recovery time. Treat withdrawal symptoms with benzodiazepines. If possible, taper dose over 1-2 wk preoperatively. If not, continue use until surgery. |
| Ginger (*Zingiber officinale*) African ginger Black ginger | Prevents nausea caused by motion sickness, pregnancy, chemotherapy, and anesthesia; antispasmodic | Heartburn Inhibition of platelet aggregation | Increased bleeding risk. Avoid use preoperatively. |
| Kava Kava (*Piper methysticum*) Awa, kawa Intoxicating pepper Tonga | Anxiolytic; mild sedative; muscle relaxant; sleep aid | Adverse effect on motor reflexes and judgment | Potentiates sedative/hypnotics. Discontinue use at least 24 hr preoperatively. |
| Licorice (*Glycyrrhiza glabra*) Sweet root | Antipyretic; antiviral; demulcent; expectorant; beneficial for chronic fatigue, allergies, asthma, bronchitis, depression, emphysema, herpes, and hypoglycemia; treats gastritis and gastric and duodenal ulcers | May cause headache, muscle flaccidity, lethargy, edema, HTN, hypokalemia, or other electrolyte imbalance and electrocardiogram (ECG) changes (prolonged QT interval) Pseudoprimary aldosteronism a possible complication | Contraindicated for chronic liver conditions, renal insufficiency, hypertonia, or existing hypokalemia. Avoid use for more than 7 consecutive days. |
| Saw palmetto (*Serenoa repens*) Sabal cabbage palm | Relieves benign prostatic hypertrophy; has antiandrogenic and antiexudative properties | Headache, increased appetite | Additive effects with other hormone therapies. |
| Dong quai (*Angelica polymorpha*) | Relieves menstrual disorders; increases effects of ovarian and testicular hormones | Dizziness, headache, nausea, miscarriage, dermatitis, GI upset, photosensitivity | Avoid use in pregnancy. |

*Continued*

SURGICAL PHARMACOLOGY

**Herbs: Effects and Precautions/Recommendations—cont'd**

| Herb (Scientific Name) and Other Names | Uses and Desired Effects | Potential Side Effects | Precautions and Recommendations |
|---|---|---|---|
| Huang qi *(Astragalus membranaceous)* | Antibacterial; increases production of white blood cells (WBCs); immunostimulant; cardiotonic; energy tonic (strengthens *wei qi*); regulates water metabolism | Inhibits platelet aggregation, and fibrinolysis | Increased bleeding risk. |
| Black cohosh *(Cimicifuga racemosa)* Rattle root Squaw root | Antihypertensive; lowers cholesterol; reduces mucus production; induces labor to aid in childbirth; relieves menopausal symptoms (hot flashes) | May lead to premature labor if used in pregnancy | Avoid use in pregnancy. |
| Senna *(Cassia senna)* | Stimulating laxative | Abdominal cramping, affects absorption in the GI system | Potential electrolyte imbalance. |
| Vitamin E (*d*-alpha-tocopherol) | Antioxidant used for cardiovascular disease | Reduced platelet adhesion and aggregation | Increased bleeding risk. |
| Yohimbe *(Pausinystalia yohimbe)* | Increases blood flow (particularly to genitalia) and libido | Anxiety, hallucinations, HTN, elevated heart rate, headache, dizziness, flushing | Avoid use by patients with psychologic or renal disorders. |
| Hawthorn *(Crataegus oxyacantha)* May bush May blossom Whitethorn | Antihypertensive; dilates coronary blood vessels; improves cardiovascular function (inotropic and beta-blocking effect); lowers cholesterol | Nausea, fatigue, sweating, headache, hypotension, mild central nervous system (CNS) depression | Use caution with cardiac glycosides, CNS depressants, antihypertensives, and nitrates. |

Modified from Flanagan K: Preoperative assessment: safety considerations for patients taking herbal products, *Journal of PeriAnesthesia Nursing* 18(1):19-26, 2001; Norred CL: Herbs and anesthesia, *Alternative Therapies in Women's Health* 3(4):26-30, 2001; Skidmore-Roth L: *Mosby's handbook of herbs & natural supplements*, ed 3, St Louis, 2006, Mosby; Mills S, Bone K: *The essential guide to herbal safety*, Philadelphia, 2005, Churchill Livingstone.

with analyzing case reports is the lack of laboratory analysis of the purported botanicals. In some reported cases in which prolonged or excessive bleeding occurred, the patient had been taking multiple herb supplements and drugs. Many plants contain anticoagulant components, including ginger, ginseng, feverfew, and others; however, it is unknown if the danger posed is clinically significant.

***Sedative Interactions.*** Some botanicals have significant sedative actions. Anesthesia providers are concerned about the potential for valerian and St. John's wort to prolong or potentiate the sedative effect of anesthetic agents. Valerian has been associated with central nervous system (CNS) depression and muscle relaxant effects in animals; large doses of valerian may contribute to delirium and high-output cardiac failure on emergence from general anesthesia. Although St. John's wort has been found to inhibit the binding of naloxone, to date no cases have been reported of excessive sedation when combined with narcotics. In addition, there is concern about the monoamine oxidase inhibitor (MAOI) activity of St. John's wort, although no cases of MAOI effects in humans have been reported.[15]

***Cardiovascular Interactions.*** Hypertension and cardiac dysrhythmias are potential adverse events that may result from the sympathetic stimulation that occurs during intubation and surgery. Ephedra has been associated with cardiovascular effects, including hypertension, palpitations, tachycardia, stroke, and seizures.[15] The long-term use of licorice may cause hypertension, dysrhythmias, or hypokalemia, which can potentiate muscle relaxants and cause adverse cardiovascular effects.[15]

Because the use of botanic supplements may increase the risk of adverse herb-drug interactions, patients should be counseled to discontinue herbs preoperatively (Box 32-5). The American Society of Anesthesiologists (ASA) recommends that patients stop taking any herbal supplement at least 2 weeks preoperatively.[1] Most patients, however, do not see an anesthesia provider until the day of surgery or a few days before surgery; so the implementation of this recommendation is challenging. Clinical research is insufficient to quantify the actual dangers of these herbal supplements. However, because individuals vary in their absorption, distribution, and clearance of the drugs administered during anesthesia, adding unknown chemicals into an already complex and fast-acting mix of drugs is likely an unnecessary risk.[15]

## Integrative Health Therapies in Cardiothoracic Surgery

At the Columbia University Medical Center, a program explores CAM safety, efficacy, and appropriateness for treatment of cardiothoracic surgery patients. Their philosophy states that cardiothoracic patients should experience "complementary healing approaches that are equally ambitious, novel, and promising as any new technology that is offered." The following therapies are recommended for cardiothoracic patients based on clinical observations and research[5]:

BOX 32-5

**Surgical Patient Assessment and Education on the Use of Dietary Supplements and Herbal Remedies**

**PREOPERATIVE**

- Identify all dietary supplements and herbal remedies the patient regularly takes. Patients are sometimes fearful of disclosing this information to physicians but may be more willing to divulge it to a nurse.
- Indicate the agent's brand name and description of the contents, using proper botanic names for herbs rather than common names. For example, there are many different kinds of ginseng. Ask the patient or family member to bring the package or container, and transcribe the details from the label.
- Note the dosage, in terms of amount, frequency, and history of usage. Also note the form of the remedy. For example, 300 mg of dried St. John's wort herb is very different from 300 mg of standardized extract of St. John's wort (the former has no verified constituent levels; the latter is prepared as a standardized extract).
- Check the list of supplements against a list of potentially serious interacting agents. The two primary areas of preoperative concern are interactions affecting blood coagulation and other hematologic parameters and interactions with anesthetics that may affect sensitivity to sedation or recovery times.
    - Examples of herbs that may affect coagulation include garlic, ginkgo, ginger, and cayenne. Herbs that may affect the central nervous system (CNS) include valerian, kava kava, and St. John's wort.
- If you discover a potential interaction, notify the anesthesia provider and surgeon. They will assess whether the scheduled procedure should be postponed while the supplement is withdrawn from use. This may involve additional laboratory tests.

**POSTOPERATIVE**

- Postoperatively, natural remedies may have positive effects.
- Preoperative consumption of capsules containing 1 g of dried ginger root can reduce nausea and vomiting during recovery. Ginger also has anticoagulant effects, but a single preoperative dose is unlikely to alter coagulation.
- Several folk and natural remedies are considered to speed the healing process, reduce bruising and soreness, and minimize scar formation. These include topical *Calendula* (marigold) or homeopathic *Arnica* or *Staphisagria* (some agents, such as herbal *Arnica,* are not suitable for internal use in high doses).
- Postoperative patients discharged with pain medication prescriptions should be advised about possible additive interactions with natural agents acting on the central nervous system (CNS) that may be consumed to enhance sleep, reduce anxiety, or help pain relief, such as valerian, hops (*Humulus*), or passion flower *(Passiflora).*

Modified from Stargrove MB: *Are herbs safe before surgery?* Accessed April 28, 2006, on-line: www.healthwwweb.com/overview/surg.html.

- Yoga
- Walking
- Guided imagery
- Stress-management techniques
- Relaxing body-work modalities, such as massage, reflexology, and acupressure/shiatsu
- Dietary modifications and micronutrient supplementation
- Aromatherapy
- Energy work
- Other noninvasive therapies for which patients may express interest

## INTEGRATIVE HEALTH THERAPIES AND PERIOPERATIVE NURSING

A variety of factors influence the perioperative patient's experience. Well-informed health care consumers increasingly choose a blend of traditional and nontraditional healing modalities with sensitivity to cultural, spiritual, and health education needs. Public involvement and legislative policy decisions are just beginning to equalize emphasis between the traditional biomedical model of care and a holistic comprehensive focus. Integrating health and wholeness incorporates elements of self-responsibility for wellness and self-awareness to inner changes on the part of the patient.

A collaborative partnership of professionals involved in an individual's care optimizes resources that promote comprehensive, effective, less-invasive/nonpharmacologic adjuncts to allopathic medical treatment. Perioperative nurses using available resources on interactions among prescriptions, dietary supplements, and herbals ensure preoperative medication safety. Seeking out and participating in appropriate research methodologies are essential for grounding the diverse components of our practice in evidence-based knowledge.

Integrative health therapies have a place in each perioperative nurse's practice. Nursing history demonstrates a philosophic attitude of altruism and compassion, founded in creating an environment of healing. Awareness of how vital self-care practices are to sustaining a caregiver role may ultimately benefit our practice. Self-care learning and experiences may come full circle by enhancing the caregiver's therapeutic use of self through presence, compassion, and holistic assessment skills.

## REFERENCES


1. American Society of Anesthesiologists: *What you should know about your patients' use of herbal medicines,* 2003. Accessed April 28, 2006, on-line: www.asahq.org/patientEducation.htm.
2. Bodeker GC: Global dimensions. In Micozzi MS: *Fundamentals of complementary and integrative medicine*, ed 3, St Louis, 2006, Saunders.
3. Cooke M and others: The effect of music on preoperative anxiety in day surgery, *Journal of Advanced Nursing* 52(1):47-55, 2005.
4. Flanagan K: Preoperative assessment: safety considerations for patients taking herbal products, *Journal of PeriAnesthesia Nursing* 18(1):19-26, 2001.
5. Frishman WH and others: *Complementary and integrative therapies for cardiovascular disease*, St Louis, 2005, Mosby.
6. Gedney JJ and others: Sensory and affective pain discrimination after inhalation of essential oils, *Psychosomatic Medicine* 66(4):599-606, 2004.
7. Ikonomidou E and others: Effect of music on vital signs and postoperative pain, *AORN Journal* 80(2):269-277, 2004.
8. Keegan L, Shames KH: Touch: connecting with the healing power. In Dossey BM and others: *Holistic nursing, a handbook for practice,* ed 4, Boston, 2005, Jones & Bartlett.
9. Lindquist R, Synder M: Introduction to complementary and alternative therapies in nursing. In Ignatavicius DD, Workman ML, editors: *Medical-surgical nursing: critical thinking for collaborative care*, ed 5, St Louis, 2006, Saunders.

10. McCann JA: *Nurse's handbook of alternative and complimentary therapies*, ed 2, Philadelphia, 2003, Lippincott, Williams & Wilkins.
11. Micozzi MS: Translation from conventional medicine. In Micozzi MS: *Fundamentals of complementary and integrative medicine*, ed 3, St Louis, 2006, Saunders.
12. Micozzi MS, Amri H: Neurohumoral physiology and psychoneuroimmunology. In Micozzi MS: *Fundamentals of complementary and integrative medicine*, ed 3, St Louis, 2006, Saunders.
13. National Center for Complementary and Alternative Medicine: *Important events in NCCAM history.* Accessed April 28, 2006, on-line: www.nih.gov/about/almanac/organization/NCCAM.htm.
14. Nilsson U and others: Analgesia following music and therapeutic suggestions in the PACU in ambulatory surgery; a randomized controlled trial, *Acta Anaesthesiologica Scandinavia* 47(3):278-283, 2003.
15. Norred CL: Herbs and anesthesia, *Alternative Therapies in Women's Health* 3(4):26-30, 2001.
16. Pellino TA and others: Use of nonpharmacologic interventions for pain and anxiety after total hip and total knee arthroplasty, *Orthopedic Nursing* 24(3):182-190, 2005.
17. Pizzorno JE, Snider P: Naturopathic medicine. In Micozzi MS: *Fundamentals of complementary and integrative medicine*, ed 3, St Louis, 2006, Saunders.
18. Planetree: *Planetree components.* Accessed April 28, 2006, on-line: www.planetree.org/about/components.htm.
19. Spencer JW, Jacobs JJ: *Complementary and alternative medicine: an evidence-based approach*, ed 2, St Louis, 2003, Mosby.
20. Valente SM: Hypnosis for pain management, *Journal of Psychosocial Nursing and Mental Health Services* 44(2):22-30, 2006.

APPENDIX

# Illustration Credits

## CHAPTER 1

**1-1**, Courtesy University of Pennsylvania School of Medicine, Philadelphia; **1-3**, **1-6**, Reprinted with permission from AORN: *Perioperative nursing data set,* ed 2. Copyright 2002 © AORN, Inc, 2170 S Parker Rd, Suite 300, Denver, Colo 80231; **1-4**, From Wojner AW: *Outcomes management: applications to clinical practice*, St Louis, 2001, Mosby; **1-5**, From Haynes RB and others: Clinical expertise in the era of evidence-based medicine and patient choice, *ACP Journal Club* 136:A11-A14, 2002.

## CHAPTER 2

**2-1**, **2-2**, **2-3**, **2-4**, **2-6**, Courtesy Christiana Care Health Services, Newark, Del; **2-5**, From Beare PG, Myers JL: *Principles and practices of adult health nursing*, ed 3, St Louis, 1998, Mosby.

## CHAPTER 3

**3-1**, Courtesy Charleston Area Medical Center, Charleston, West Virginia; **3-2**, From Wong D: *Whaley & Wong's nursing care of infants and children*, ed 5, St Louis, 1995, Mosby; **3-3**, **3-6**, Courtesy STERIS Corp, Mentor, Ohio.

## CHAPTER 4

**4-4**, Redrawn from Whitten C: *Anyone can intubate*, ed 4, San Diego, 1997, K-W Publications.

## CHAPTER 5

**5-1**, **5-7**, **5-8**, Courtesy Kendall-LTP; **5-10**, Courtesy Skytron, Grand Rapids, Mich; **5-18**, **5-19**, Courtesy Allen Medical Systems, Acton, Mass.

## CHAPTER 6

**6-2**, **6-5**, **6-6**, **6-7**, **6-9**, **6-10**, From Davis & Geck: *Surgical atlas and suture guide*, ed 2, Wayne, NJ, 1992, American Cyanamid Co; **6-3**, Courtesy 3M, St Paul, Minn; **6-4**, From Atkinson LJ, Fortunato NM: *Berry & Kohn's operating room technique*, ed 8, St Louis, 1996, Mosby; **6-14**, **6-21**, From Phillips N: *Berry & Kohn's operating room technique*, ed 10, St Louis, 2004, Mosby; **6-15**, Courtesy Miltex Instrument Co; **6-16**, **6-17**, **6-19**, **6-20**, Courtesy Codman & Shurtleff, Inc, Randolph, Mass.

## CHAPTER 7

**7-2**, **7-5**, **7-6**, **7-9**, **7-10**, **7-13**, **7-17**, **7-20**, **7-38**, **7-39**, **7-47**, **7-48**, **7-59**, **7-60**, **7-76**, **7-77**, From Ball KA: *Endoscopic surgery*, St Louis, 1997, Mosby; **7-3**, **7-44**, **7-45**, **7-50**, **7-51**, Courtesy Gyrus-ACMI, Southborough, Mass; **7-4**, Courtesy HGM Medical Laser Systems, Santa Clara, California; **7-7**, **7-36**, **7-40**, **7-43**, Courtesy Olympus Surgical America, Orangeburg, NY; **7-8**, Courtesy Endoscopy Support Services, Inc, Brewster, New York; **7-11**, **7-12**, **7-15**, From Brooks-Tighe SM: *Instrumentation for the operating room*, ed 6, St Louis, 2003, Mosby; **7-14**, **7-18**, **7-19**, **7-21**, **7-24**, **7-27**, Copyright © 2005 United States Surgical, a division of Tyco Healthcare Group LP. All rights reserved. Reprinted with the permission of United States Surgical, a division of Tyco Healthcare Group LP; **7-22**, **7-23**, Courtesy Ethicon Endo-Surgery, Cincinnati; **7-29**, Courtesy STERIS Corp, Mentor, Ohio; **7-67**, Courtesy Megadyne, Draper, Utah; **7-68**, **7-69**, **7-70**, Copyright © 2005 Valleylab, a division of Tyco Healthcare Group LP. All rights reserved. Reprinted with the permission of Valleylab, a division of Tyco Healthcare Group LP; **7-72**, **7-73**, Courtesy Encision, Boulder, Colo.

## CHAPTER 8

**8-1**, **8-3**, From Bryant RA: *Acute and chronic wounds*, ed 2, St Louis, 2000, Mosby; **8-2**, **8-4**, From Ignatavicius DD, Workman ML: *Medical-surgical nursing: critical thinking for collaborative care*, ed 5, St Louis, 2006, Mosby; **8-5**, Courtesy KCI, San Antonio; **8-7**, Courtesy CR Bard, Inc, Murray Hill, NJ.

## CHAPTER 9

**9-1**, **9-2**, From Litwack K: *Post anesthesia care nursing*, ed 2, St Louis, 1995, Mosby; **9-3**, Courtesy Forrest General Hospital, Hattiesburg, Miss; **9-4**, **9-5**, From Phipps WJ and others: *Medical-surgical nursing: concepts and clinical practice*, ed 5, St Louis, 1995, Mosby; **9-6**, Copyright © 2005 Arizant Healthcare; **9-7**, From Acute Pain Management Guideline Panel: *Acute pain management in adults: operative procedures: quick reference guide for clinicians, AHCPR pub no. 92-0019,* Rockville, Md, 1992, Agency for Health Care Policy and Research; **9-8**, ***A-C***, From Acute Pain Management Guideline Panel: *Acute pain management in adults: operative procedures: quick reference guide for clinicians. AHCPR pub no. 92-0019,* Rockville, Md, 1992, Agency for Health Care Policy and Research; ***D***, From Wong DL: *Whaley & Wong's nursing care of infants and children,* ed 5, St Louis, 1995, Mosby; **9-9**, Data from McCaffery M, Pasero C: The Agency for Health Care Policy and Research and the American Pain Society. Chris Pasero, MS, RN, Pain Management Educator and Consultant, reviewed and advised the development of this algorithm; **9-10**, From Long BC and others: *Medical-surgical nursing: a nursing process approach*, ed 3, St Louis, 1993, Mosby.

## CHAPTER 10

**10-1**, From McHatton M: A theory for timely teaching, *American Journal of Nursing* 85:799, 1985; **10-3**, **10-4**, From Lorig K: *Patient education: practical approach*, ed 2, Thousand Oaks, Calif, 1992, Sage Publications.

## CHAPTER 11

**11-4**, **11-5**, **11-16**, **11-17**, **11-18**, **11-21**, **11-22**, **11-29**, From Thompson JC: *Atlas of surgery of the stomach, duodenum, and small bowel*, St Louis, 1992, Mosby; **11-7**, **11-15**, **11-30**, **11-31**, **11-32**, **11-33**, **11-34**, **11-35**, **11-36**, **11-37**, From Bauer JJ: *Colorectal surgery illustrated,* St Louis, 1993, Mosby; **11-10**, From Thibodeau GA: *Anthony's textbook of anatomy and physiology,* St Louis, 1990, Mosby; **11-23**, Courtesy of Inamed Health, Inc, Santa Barbara, Calif. In Townsend CM and others: *Sabiston textbook of surgery: the biological basis of modern surgical practice*, ed 17, Philadelphia, 2004, Saunders; **11-24**, **11-25**, **11-26**, From Townsend CM and others: *Sabiston textbook of surgery: the biological basis of modern surgical practice*, ed 17, Philadelphia, 2004, Saunders; **11-27**, **11-28**, From Marceau P and others: Malabsorptive obesity surgery, *Surgical Clinics of North America* 81:1113-1127, 2001. In Townsend CM and others: *Sabiston textbook of surgery: the biological basis of modern surgical practice*, ed 17, Philadelphia, 2004, Saunders.

## CHAPTER 12

**12-6**, From Townsend CM and others: *Sabiston textbook of surgery*, ed 16, Philadelphia, 2001, Saunders; **12-7**, From Daly JM, Cady B: *Atlas of surgical oncology*, St Louis, 1993, Mosby; **12-19**, **12-20**, From Cerilli GJ: *Organ transplantation and replacement*, Philadelphia, 1998, Lippincott; **12-21**, **12-22**, **12-23**, Copyright © 1990 Lahey Clinic, Burlington, Mass; **12-24**, From Anscher NL and others. In Simmons RL and others, editors: *Manual of vascular access, organ donation, and transplantation*, New York, 1984, Springer-Verlag.

## CHAPTER 13

**13-1**, From Ignatavicius DD, Workman ML: *Medical-surgical nursing: critical thinking for collaborative care*, ed 5, St Louis, 2006, Mosby; **13-2**, From Harkreader H, Hogan M: *Fundamentals of nursing*, ed 2, St Louis, 2004, Mosby; **13-12**, From Zollinger RM, Zollinger RM, Jr: *Atlas of surgical op-*

*erations*, ed 7, New York, 1993, McGraw-Hill; **13-14**, From Schumpelick V: *Atlas of hernia surgery*, Toronto, 1990, BC Decker; **13-16**, From Liechty RD, Soper RT: *Synopsis of surgery*, St Louis, 1985, Mosby.

## CHAPTER 14

**14-1, 14-27, 14-28**, From Lowdermilk DL and others: *Maternity and women's health care*, ed 6, St Louis, 1997, Mosby; **14-2, 14-8**, From Lowdermilk DL: *Maternity and women's health care*, ed 8, St Louis, 2004, Mosby; **14-7, 14-9, 14-10, 14-24, 14-32, 14-40, 14-43**, From Hacker NF, Moore JG, Gambone JC: *Essentials of obstetrics and gynecology*, ed 4, Philadelphia, 2004, Saunders; **14-11, 14-42**, From Townsend CM and others: *Sabiston textbook of surgery: the biological basis of modern surgical practice*, ed 17, Philadelphia, 2004, Saunders; **14-12, 14-37**, From Ignatavicius DD, Workman ML: *Medical-surgical nursing: critical thinking for collaborative care*, ed 5, St Louis, 2006, Mosby; **14-13, *B*, 14-14, *B*, 14-15**, From Seidel HM and others: *Mosby's guide to physical examination*, ed 5, St Louis, 1999, Mosby; **14-16**, Redrawn from Symmonds RE: Relaxation of pelvic supports. In Benson RC, editor: *Current obstetric and gynecologic diagnosis and treatment*, ed 5, Los Altos, Calif, 1984, Lange Medical Publications; **14-17, 14-18**, From Herbst AL and others: *Comprehensive gynecology*, ed 2, St Louis, 1992, Mosby; **14-23, 14-26, 14-36, 14-44**, From Ball TL: *Gynecologic surgery and urology*, ed 2, St Louis, 1963, Mosby; **14-29**, From Emond RT: *Colour atlas of infectious diseases*, ed 3, St Louis, 1995, Mosby; **14-30, *A***, From Brooks-Tighe SM: *Instrumentation for the operating room*, ed 6, St Louis, 1999, Mosby; ***B***, From Baggish MS and others: *Diagnostic and operative hysteroscopy: a text and atlas*, ed 2, St Louis, 1999, Mosby; **14-33, 14-34, 14-35**, From Edwards SK and others: Surgery in the pregnant patient, *Current Problems in Surgery* 38(4):213-292, 2001; **14-38, 14-45, 14-46, 14-47**, From Nichols DH: *Gynecologic and obstetric surgery*, St Louis, 1993, Mosby; **14-48, 14-49, 14-50**, Courtesy Conceptus Inc, San Carlos, Calif; **14-53**, From Ashcraft KW, Holcomb GW, Murphy JP: *Pediatric surgery*, ed 4, Philadelphia, 2005, Saunders. **14-54**, From Cortes RA, Farmer DL: Recent advances in fetal surgery, *Seminars in Perinatology* 28(3), 2004; **14-55**, From Adzick NS and others: Successful fetal surgery for spina bifida, *The Lancet* 352(9141):1675-1676, 1998; **14-56, 14-57**, Courtesy Marjorie Pyle, RNC, Lifecircle, Costa Mesa, Calif. In Lowdermilk DL: *Maternity and women's health care*, ed 8, St Louis, 2004, Mosby.

## CHAPTER 15

**15-1, 15-6, 15-7**, Modified from Seidel HM and others: *Mosby's guide to physical examination*, ed 5, St Louis, 1995, Mosby; **15-3, 15-9, 15-15, 15-25, 15-30, 15-32, 15-40, 15-49, 15-50, 15-51, 15-52, 15-65, 15-79**, From Nagle GM: *Genitourinary surgery*, St Louis, 1997, Mosby; **15-4**, From Schumpelick V: *Atlas of hernia surgery*, Toronto, 1990, BC Decker; **15-10, 15-12**, Courtesy Jeffrey Rosenblum, MD; **15-13**, Courtesy CR Bard, Urological Division, Covington, Ga. In Nagle GM: *Genitourinary surgery*, St Louis, 1997, Mosby; **15-14, 15-17, 15-31, 15-61**, From Williamson MR, Smith AY: *Fundamentals of uroradiology*, Philadelphia, 2000, Saunders; **15-16, 15-33, 15-56, 15-57**, Courtesy Gyrus-ACMI, Southborough, Mass; **15-18**, Courtesy Circon Corp, Santa Barbara, Calif. In Nagle GM: *Genitourinary surgery*, St Louis, 1997, Mosby; **15-20, 15-21, *B*, 15-77**, From Brooks-Tighe SM: *Instrumentation for the operating room*, St Louis, 1994, Mosby; **15-24, 15-27, 15-28, 15-71, *A***, Courtesy American Medical Systems, Minnetonka, Minn; **15-26, 15-42, 15-43, 15-44, 15-53, 15-54, 15-69, 15-70, 15-71, *B*, 15-78, 15-80**, From Droller MJ: *Surgical management of urologic disease*, St Louis, 1992, Mosby; **15-37, 15-38**, Courtesy Ethicon, Inc, Somerville, NJ; **15-41, 15-47**, Courtesy Omni-Tract Surgical, St Paul, Minn; **15-56, 15-57, 15-58**, Reprinted with the permission of Medtronic, Inc © 2005; **15-60**, Courtesy Circon Corp, Santa Barbara, Calif; **15-62, 15-64**, From Raz S: *Atlas of transvaginal surgery*, ed 2, Philadelphia, 2002, Saunders; **15-63**, Courtesy Bard Urological, Covington, Ga; **15-72, 15-73, 15-75**, From Gillenwater JY and others: *Adult and pediatric urology*, ed 3, vol 2, St Louis, 1996, Mosby; **15-74**, From Gray M: *Genitourinary disorders*, St Louis, 1992, Mosby; **15-76**, Copyright © Karl Storz Endoscopy America, Inc.

## CHAPTER 16

**16-2, 16-7**, From Healy J, Hodge J: *Surgical anatomy*, ed 2, Philadelphia, 1990, BC Decker; **16-6**, From Kukora JS and others: Thyroid nodule. In Cameron JL, editor: *Current surgical therapy*, ed 7, St Louis, 2001, Mosby; **16-8**, Photograph courtesy Josie Reyes.

## CHAPTER 17

**17-1, 17-2, 17-3**, From Isaacs JH: *Textbook of breast disease*, St Louis, 1992, Mosby; **17-4, 17-8**, From Townsend CM: *Sabiston textbook of surgery*, ed 16, Philadelphia, 2001, Saunders; **17-5**, Copyright 1997 United States Surgical Corp. All rights reserved. Reprinted with the permission of United States Surgical Corporation. Trademark of United States Surgical Corp; **17-6**, Image redrawn courtesy of Ethicon Endo-Surgery, Inc; **17-7, 17-9, 17-10**, From Ignatavicius DD, Workman ML: *Medical-surgical nursing: critical thinking for collaborative care*, ed 5, St Louis, 2006, Mosby.

## CHAPTER 18

**18-1, 18-3**, From Thompson JM and others: *Mosby's clinical nursing*, ed 4, St Louis, 1997, Mosby; **18-2**, From Seidel HM and others: *Mosby's guide to physical examination*, ed 6, St Louis, 2006, Mosby; **18-4**, From Phipps WJ and others: *Medical-surgical nursing: concepts and clinical practice*, ed 5, St Louis, 1995, Mosby; **18-7, 18-45, 18-46**, From Federman JL and others: *Retina and vitreous*, London, 1994, Mosby; **18-10**, Modified from Thibodeau GA: *Anthony's textbook of anatomy and physiology*, ed 13, St Louis, 1990, Mosby; **18-12**, From Elkin MK and others: *Nursing interventions and clinical skills*, ed 3, St Louis, 2004, Mosby; **18-17**, Courtesy Carl Zeiss; **18-18, 18-21, 18-39**, From Ignatavicius DD, Workman ML: *Medical-surgical nursing: critical thinking for collaborative care*, ed 5, St Louis, 2006, Mosby; **18-20, 18-22, 18-23, 18-24**, From Tenzel RR: *Textbook of ophthalmology*, vol 4. *Orbit and oculoplastics*, London, 1993, Gower; **18-25**, From Swartz MH: *Textbook of physical diagnosis*, ed 5, Philadelphia, 2006, Saunders; **18-27**, Courtesy Kolberg Ocular Prosthetics, Escondido, Calif; **18-32**, From Wilson TS: LASIK surgery, *AORN Journal* 71(5):977-978, 2000; **18-33, 18-34, 18-35, 18-36, 18-37**, From Lindquist TD, Lindstrom RL: *Ophthalmic surgery: looseleaf and update service*, St Louis, 1990, Mosby; **18-40**, From Glaser BM, Michels RG: *Retina*, vol 4. *Surgical retina*, St Louis, 1994, Mosby.

## CHAPTER 19

**19-1, 19-2, 19-4**, From Ignatavicius DD, Workman ML: *Medical-surgical nursing: critical thinking for collaborative care*, ed 5, St Louis, 2006, Mosby; **19-3, 19-13, 19-17**, From DeWeese DD and others: *Otolaryngology: head and neck surgery*, ed 7, St Louis, 1988, Mosby; **19-5**, From Seidel HM and others: *Mosby's guide to physical examination*, ed 5, St Louis, 1999, Mosby; **19-6, 19-9, 19-11, 19-12**, Courtesy Medtronic Xomed; **19-7, 19-8**, Courtesy Carl Zeiss; **19-10**, From Brooks-Tighe SM: *Instrumentation for the operating room*, ed 6, St Louis, 2003, Mosby; **19-14**, From Saunders WH and others: *Nursing care in eye, ear, nose, and throat disorders*, ed 4, St Louis, 1979, Mosby; **19-18, 19-19**, Courtesy Cochlear, Ltd; **19-20, 19-21, 19-22, 19-23**, Courtesy Entific Medical Systems; **19-24, 19-25**, Courtesy Symphonix.

## CHAPTER 20

**20-2**, From Saunders WH and others: *Nursing care in eye, ear, nose, and throat disorders*, ed 4, St Louis, 1979, Mosby; **20-5, 20-11**, From DeWeese DD, Saunders WH: *Textbook of otolaryngology*, ed 6, St Louis, 1982, Mosby; **20-6, 20-8**, From Schuller DE, Schleuning AJ: *Otolaryngology: head and neck surgery*, ed 8, St Louis, 1994, Mosby; **20-7**, From Cummings CW and others: *Otolaryngology: head and neck surgery*, ed 3, St Louis, 1993, Mosby; **20-9**, From Thawley SE, Garrett H: Endoscopic sinus surgery; an outpatient procedure that minimizes tissue removal, *AORN Journal* 47:902, 1988. Copyright © AORN, Inc, Denver, Colo.

## CHAPTER 21

**21-1, 21-2, 21-3**, From Marino LB: *Cancer nursing*, St Louis, 1981, Mosby; **21-4, 21-5, 21-6, 21-7, 21-16, 21-17, 21-21, 21-22**, From Cummings CW and others: *Otolaryngology: head and neck surgery*, ed 3, St Louis, 1993, Mosby; **21-8**, From Lewis SM and others: *Medical-surgical nursing: assessment and management of clinical problems*, ed 6, St Louis, 2004, Mosby; **21-9**, From Luckmann J: *Medical-surgical nursing*, ed 3, Philadelphia, 1987, Saunders; **21-10, 21-12**, From Ignatavicius DD, Workman ML:

*Medical-surgical nursing: critical thinking for collaborative care*, ed 5, St Louis, 2006, Mosby; **21-11, 21-18,** From Shah JP, Patel SG: *Head and neck surgery and oncology,* ed 3, London, 2003, Mosby Ltd; **21-19,** From DeWeese DD: Saunders WH, *Textbook of otolaryngology,* ed 6, St Louis, 1982, Mosby.

## CHAPTER 22

**22-1, 22-2, 22-4, 22-5, 22-6, 22-8, 22-9,** From Thibodeau GA, Patton KT: *Anatomy and physiology*, ed 5, St Louis, 2003, Mosby; **22-3,** Redrawn from Lewis RC: *Primary care orthopedics*, New York, 1988, Churchill Livingstone; **22-7,** *A*, **22-12, 22-100,** From Thibodeau GA, Patton KT: *Anatomy and physiology*, ed 3, St Louis, 1996, Mosby; **22-11, 22-19, 22-44, 22-77, 22-81,** Courtesy Zimmer, Inc, Warsaw, Ind; **22-13,** Courtesy Franciscan Hospital, Mount Airy Campus, Cincinnati, Ohio; **22-14,** Courtesy Tenet Medical, Dallas; **22-15,** Courtesy Innomed, Savannah, Ga; **22-16, 22-66,** Courtesy Acufex Microsurgical, Inc, Mansfield, Mass; **22-17,** Courtesy OSI, Union City, Calif; **22-18, 22-28, 22-31, 22-40, 22-42, 22-51, 22-62, 22-83, 22-85,** From Gregory B: *Orthopaedic surgery*, St Louis, 1994, Mosby; **22-20, 22-55,** Courtesy Zimmer Traction Handbook, 1989, Zimmer, Inc., Warsaw, Ind; **22-22,** From Mourad LA: *Orthopedic disorders*, St Louis, 1991, Mosby; **22-24,** From Ignatavicius DD, Workman ML: *Medical-surgical nursing: critical thinking for collaborative care*, ed 5, St Louis, 2006, Mosby; **22-25, 22-87, 22-88, 22-89, 22-90, 22-93,** Courtesy ConMed Linvatec, Utica, NY; **22-26,** From Phipps WJ and others: *Medical-surgical nursing*, ed 5, St Louis, 1995, Mosby; **22-27,** Courtesy EBI, Parsippany, NJ; **22-29, 22-53, 22-54,** From Gustilo RB and others: *Fractures and dislocations,* vol 2, St Louis, 1993, Mosby; **22-30, 22-67,** Courtesy Synthes, West Chester, Penn; **22-32,** Courtesy Synthes U.S.A., Paoli, Penn; **22-33,** Courtesy Prototech AS, Bergen, Norway; **22-35,** Courtesy LTI Medica and the UpJohn Co. Illustration by Beverly Kessler, 1982, Learning Technology, Inc; **22-36, 22-46, 22-47, 22-49,** From Crenshaw AH: *Campbell's operative orthopaedics,* ed 8, St Louis, 1992, Mosby; **22-37,** Courtesy Biomet, Inc, Warsaw, Ind; **22-39,** Redrawn from Rockwood CA and others: *Fractures in adults,* ed 2, Philadelphia, 1984, Lippincott; **22-41,** Courtesy of The Anspach Effort, Palm Beach Gardens, Fla; **22-43,** Redrawn from Neer CS: *Journal of Bone and Joint Surgery* 52-A:1007, 1970; **22-48,** From Knight RA: *AAOS Instructional Course Lecture* 14:123, 1957; **22-50, 22-69,** From Muller ME and others: *Manual of internal fixation: techniques recommended by AO-ASIF group*, ed 3, Berlin, 1990, Springer-Verlag; **22-52,** Redrawn from Sprague HH, Howard FM: *Contemporary Orthopedics* 16:18, 1988; **22-56,** Courtesy OsteoMed, Addison, Tex; **22-57, 22-68,** From Canale ST: *Campbell's operative orthopaedics*, ed 9, St Louis, 1998, Mosby; **22-58,** Courtesy Exactech, Inc, Gainesville, Fla; **22-59,** From Gustilo RB: *The fracture classification manual,* St Louis, 1991, Mosby; **22-60,** Redrawn from Muller ME and others: *The comprehensive classification of fractures of long bones,* Berlin, 1990, Springer-Verlag; **22-61,** Redrawn from Schatzker J and others: *Clinical Orthopedics* 138:94, 1979; **22-63,** From DePuy ACE Medical Co, El Segundo, Calif; **22-64, 22-72, 22-73, 22-78,** Courtesy Stryker, Kalamazoo, Mich; **22-65,** Redrawn from Cox JS: *American Journal of Sports Medicine* 4:72, 1976; **22-70,** From Richards V: *Surgery for general practice*, St Louis, 1956, Mosby; **22-74, 22-76, 22-82,** Courtesy Howmedica, Inc, Rutherford, NJ; **22-79,** Redrawn from Gristina AG, Webb LX: *Proximal humeral and monospherical glenoid replacement: surgical technique*, Rutherford, NJ, 1983, Howmedica, Inc; **22-80,** Courtesy Smith & Nephew, Memphis; **22-84,** Courtesy College of Southern Idaho, Twin Falls; **22-84,** From Brooks-Tighe SM: *Instrumentation for the operating room*, ed 6, St Louis, 2003, Mosby; **22-94,** Courtesy Johnson & Johnson; **22-98,** Courtesy Smith & Nephew Dyonics, Andover, Mass; **22-99,** Courtesy NuVasive, Inc, San Diego; **22-101,** From Bradford DS and others: *Moe's textbook of scoliosis and other spinal deformities*, ed 2, Philadelphia, 1987, Saunders; **22-102,** Courtesy Medtronic Sofamor Danek, Memphis; **22-103, 22-104, 22-105, 22-106,** Reprinted with permission from Synthes Spine LP.

## CHAPTER 23

**23-1,** From Thibodeau GA, Patton KT: *Structure and function of the human body*, ed 12, St Louis, 2004, Mosby; **23-2, 23-3, 23-4, 23-6,** From Thibodeau GA, Patton KT: *Anatomy and physiology*, ed 3, St Louis, 1996, Mosby; **23-5,** Photograph by Sarah-Jane Smith. Artwork modified from Lumley JSP: *Surface anatomy,* ed 3, Edinburgh, 2002, Churchill Livingstone. In Standring S: *Gray's anatomy,* ed 39, Edinburgh, 2005, Churchill Livingstone; **23-7, 23-9, 23-10, 23-12, 23-29,** From Conway-Rutkowski BL: *Carini and Owens' neurological and neurosurgical nursing*, ed 8, St Louis, 1982, Mosby; **23-8, 23-15, 23-16, 23-22,** From Anthony CP, Thibodeau GA: *Textbook of anatomy and physiology,* ed 11, St Louis, 1983, Mosby; **23-11,** Photograph by Kevin Fitzpatrick on behalf of GKT School of Medicine, London. In Standring S: *Gray's anatomy,* ed 39, Edinburgh, 2005, Churchill Livingstone; **23-13,** Modified from Thibodeau GA, Patton KT: *Anatomy and physiology*, ed 5, St Louis, 2003, Mosby. In McCance KL, Huether SE: *Pathophysiology: the biologic basis for disease in adults and children,* ed 5, St Louis, 2006, Mosby; **23-14,** From Nolte J: *The human brain: an introduction to its fundamental anatomy*, ed 2, St Louis, 1988, Mosby; **23-17, 23-18, 23-19, 23-20, 23-31, 23-32, 23-47, 23-48, 23-49, 23-50, 23-54,** From Rengachary SS, Wilkins RH: *Principles of neurosurgery*, London, 1994, Wolfe/Mosby Europe Ltd; **23-21,** From Thibodeau GA, Patton KT: *Anatomy and physiology*, ed 5, St Louis, 2003, Mosby; **23-23,** From Standring S: *Gray's anatomy*, ed 39, Edinburgh, 2005, Churchill Livingstone; **23-24, 23-25,** From Mettler FA: *Neuroanatomy*, ed 2, St Louis, 1948, Mosby; **23-27,** Modified from Thibodeau GA, Patton KT: *Structure and function of the human body*, ed 12, St Louis, 2004, Mosby. In McCance KL, Huether SE: *Pathophysiology: the biologic basis for disease in adults and children*, ed 5, St Louis, 2006, Mosby; **23-33,** Provided by Shaun Gallagher, GKT School of Medicine, London; photograph by Sarah-Jane Smith. In Standring S: *Gray's anatomy*, ed 39, Edinburgh, 2005, Churchill Livingstone; **23-34, 23-46, 23-52, 23-57,** From Rengachary SS, Ellenbogen RG: *Principles of neurosurgery,* ed 2, Edinburgh, 2005, Mosby Ltd; **23-35,** Courtesy Dr Justin Lee, Chelsea and Westminster Hospital, London. In Standring S: *Gray's anatomy*, ed 39, Edinburgh, 2005, Churchill Livingstone; **23-36,** Courtesy Integra LifeSciences Corp, Plainsboro, NJ; **23-38,** Courtesy Cordis Corp, Miami; **23-40,** Courtesy Zimmer-Reed, Midlothian, Va; **23-41,** Courtesy Midas Rex Corp, Fort Worth, Tex; **23-43, 23-44, 23-45,** Courtesy Codman, a Johnson & Johnson Co, Raynham, Mass; **23-51,** *A*, Courtesy Codman & Shurtleff, Inc, Randolph, Mass Courtesy Omi Surgical Products, a division of Ohio Medical Instrument Company, Cincinnati; *B*, Courtesy Holco Instrument Corp, New York; **23-53,** From Sachs E: *Diagnosis and treatment of brain tumors and the care of the neurosurgical patient*, ed 2, St Louis, 1949, Mosby; **23-55, 23-56,** From Carini E, Owens G: *Neurological and neurosurgical nursing*, ed 6, St Louis, 1974, Mosby.

## CHAPTER 24

**24-1,** From Townsend CM and others, editors: *Sabiston textbook of surgery*, ed 16, Philadelphia, 2001, Saunders; **24-2, 24-5, 24-15, 24-21, 24-22, 24-28, 24-37, 24-38,** From Fortunato N, McCullough SM: *Plastic and reconstructive surgery*, St Louis, 1998, Mosby; **24-4, 24-13,** From Ignatavicius DD, Workman ML: *Medical-surgical nursing: critical thinking for collaborative care*, ed 5, St Louis, 2006, Mosby; **24-7,** Courtesy Carl Zeiss, Oberkochen, Germany; **24-8,** Courtesy Burton Medical, Chatsworth, Calif; **24-9, 24-10,** From Swartz MH: *Textbook of physical diagnosis: history and examination*, ed 5, Philadelphia, 2006, Saunders; **24-11,** From Habif TP: *Clinical dermatology*, ed 4, St Louis, 2004, Mosby; **24-12, 24-14,** From Thibodeau GA, Patton KT: *The human body in health and disease*, ed 2, St Louis, 1997, Mosby; **24-19,** Courtesy Inamed Aesthetics, Santa Barbara, Calif; **24-23,** From McCarthy J, editor: *Plastic surgery*, Philadelphia, 1990, Saunders. In Semer NB: *Practical plastic surgery for nonsurgeons*, Philadelphia, 2000, Hanley & Belfus; **24-25,** From Weinzweig N, Weinzweig J: *The mutilated hand*, St Louis, 2005, Mosby; **24-26,** From Neff JA, Kidd PM: *Trauma nursing: the art and science*, St Louis, 1993, Mosby; **24-27,** From Fonseca RJ and others: *Oral and maxillofacial trauma*, ed 3, Philadelphia, 2005, Saunders; **24-29, 24-30,** From Wang T: *The facelift: an issue of facial plastic surgery clinics*, Philadelphia, 2005, Saunders; **24-35, 24-39,** From Wilkinson TS: *Atlas of liposuction*, Philadelphia, 2005, Saunders.

## CHAPTER 25

**25-4, 25-6,** From Schottelius BA, Schottelius DD: *Textbook of physiology,* ed 18, St Louis, 1978, Mosby; **25-5,** From Townsend CM and others: *Sabiston textbook of surgery*, ed 16, Philadelphia, 2001, Saunders; **25-8,** From Johnson J, Kirby CK: *Surgery of the chest*, ed 4, Chicago, 1970, Year Book;

**25-9**, *A*, From Thompson JM and others: *Mosby's clinical nursing*, ed 4, St Louis, 1993, Mosby; *B*, Courtesy Teleflex Medical, Research Triangle Park, NC; **25-11**, From Damjanov I, Linder J, editors: *Anderson's pathology*, ed 10, St Louis, 1996, Mosby; **25-12**, From McCance KL, Huether SE: *Pathophysiology—the biologic basis for disease in adults and children*, ed 5, St Louis, 2006, Mosby; **25-18**, Modified from Des Jardins T, Burton GG: *Clinical manifestations and assessment of respiratory disease*, ed 3, St Louis, 1995, Mosby. In McCance KL, Huether SE: *Pathophysiology— the biologic basis for disease in adults and children*, ed 5, St Louis, 2006, Mosby; **25-21**, From Sellke F and others: *Sabiston & Spencer surgery of the chest*, ed 7, Philadelphia, 2005, Saunders.

## CHAPTER 26

**26-1**, **26-2**, **26-4**, From Thibodeau GA, Patton KT: *Anatomy and physiology*, ed 5, St Louis, 2003, Mosby; **26-3**, **26-9**, **26-25**, **26-26**, From Townsend CM and others: *Sabiston textbook of surgery*, ed 17, Philadelphia, 2004, Saunders; **26-5**, From Dettenmeier PA: *Radiographic assessment for nurses*, St Louis, 1995, Mosby; **26-10**, From Haimovici H: *Vascular surgery: principles and technique*, Norwalk, Conn, 1984, Appleton-Century-Crofts; **26-12**, From Hershey FB, Calman CH: *Atlas of vascular surgery*, ed 3, St Louis, 1973, Mosby; **26-13**, From MacVittie BA: *Vascular surgery*, St Louis, 1998, Mosby; **26-14**, Reprinted with permission, *AORN standards, recommended practices, and guidelines 2002*, pp. 110-111. © AORN, Inc, 2170 S Parker Rd, Suite 300, Denver, Colo, 80231; **26-15**, From MacVittie BA: *Vascular surgery*, St Louis, 1998, Mosby; **26-16**, From Hershey FB, Calman CH: *Atlas of vascular surgery*, ed 3, St Louis, 1973, Mosby; **26-18**, Reprinted with permission from *AORN clinical path template*, 1997, pp. 14-17. Copyright AORN, Inc, Denver, Colo; **26-20**, **26-22**, **26-23**, From Wilson SE: *Vascular access: principles and practice*, ed 3, St Louis, 1996, Mosby; **26-21**, From Calne R, Pollard SG: *Operative surgery*, London, 1992, Gower; **26-24**, From Ballinger PW: *Merrill's atlas of radiographic positions and radiologic procedures*, ed 8, vol 2, St Louis, 1995, Mosby.

## CHAPTER 27

**27-1**, *A*, **27-6**, *A*, From Thibodeau GA, Patton KT: *Anatomy and physiology*, ed 5, St Louis, 2003, Mosby; **27-2**, **27-6**, *B*, *C*, From Seifert PC: *Cardiac surgery*, St Louis, 1994, Mosby. Drawings by Peter Stone; **27-4**, From Berne RM, Levy MN: *Cardiovascular physiology*, ed 8, St Louis, 2001, Mosby; **27-5**, From Thompson JM and others: *Mosby's clinical nursing*, ed 4, St Louis, 1997, Mosby; **27-8**, **27-11**, From Canobbio M: *Cardiovascular disorders*, St Louis, 1990, Mosby; **27-9**, *A*, **27-34**, **27-54**, From Braunwald E and others, editors: *Heart disease*, ed 6, Philadelphia, 2001, Saunders; **27-9**, *B*, **27-33**, *B*, *C*, **27-41**, *A*, From Seifert PC: *Cardiac surgery*, St Louis, 1994, Mosby; **27-10**, Courtesy Edward A Lefrak, MD, Annandale, Va; **27-12**, From Kinney M, Packa D: *Andreoli's comprehensive cardiac care*, ed 7, St Louis, 1995, Mosby; **27-13**, From Brooks-Tighe SM: *Instrumentation for the operating room*, ed 4, St Louis, 1994, Mosby; **27-14**, Courtesy Scanlan International, St Paul; **27-15**, Courtesy Rultract, Inc, Cleveland; **27-16**, Courtesy Pilling Co, Fort Washington, Penn; **27-17**, **27-51**, **27-68**, From Zipes DP and others: *Braunwald's heart disease: a textbook of cardiovascular medicine*, ed 7, Philadelphia, 2005, Saunders; **27-18**, Courtesy Hewlett-Packard Co, Medical Products Group, Andover, Mass; **27-19**, **27-35**, **27-37**, **27-38**, **27-42**, **27-44**, **27-45**, **27-47**, **27-48**, **27-50**, **27-52**, *A*, **27-57**, **27-58**, **27-59**, **27-61**, **27-62**, **27-63**, **27-65**, **27-67**, **27-69**, **27-70**, **27-71**, **27-72**, **27-76**, **27-77**, **27-79**, From Waldhausen JA and others: *Surgery of the chest*, ed 6, St Louis, 1996, Mosby; **27-20**, **27-21**, Courtesy Meadox Medicals, a division of Boston Scientific Co; **27-22**, Courtesy WL Gore & Associates, Inc, Flagstaff, Ariz; **27-23**, Courtesy of St Jude Medical, Inc, St Paul; **27-24**, Courtesy Sulzer Carbomedics, Inc, Austin, Tex; **27-25**, **27-28**, **27-29**, **27-33**, Courtesy Baxter Healthcare Corp, Edwards CVS division, Santa Ana, Calif; **27-26**, **27-27**, **27-32**, **27-46**, **27-74**, **27-78**, Copyright Medtronic, Inc, Minneapolis; **27-30**, **27-31**, Courtesy CryoLife, Inc, Marietta, Ga; **27-36**, Courtesy Bard Cardiopulmonary GTC, Haverhill, Mass; **27-39**, From Buxton B and others: *Ischemic heart disease surgical management*, London, 1999, Mosby. **27-40**, Courtesy Stockert Instrumente, Gmbh, Munich; Courtesy of US distributor: COBE CV, division of Sorin Biomedica, Arvada, Colo; **27-49**, From Lytle BW and others: Coronary artery bypass grafting with the right gastroepiploic artery, *Journal of Thoracic and Cardiovascular Surgery* 976:826, 1989; **27-52**, *B-D*, From Fuller JK: *Surgical technology: principles and practice*, ed 4, St Louis, 2005, Saunders; **27-55**, Courtesy Heartport, Inc, Redwood City, Calif; **27-60**, Reprinted from the *Journal of Thoracic and Cardiovascular Surgery*, Vol 115, David TE and others: Long-term results of mitral valve repair for myxomatous disease with and without chordal replacement with expanded polytetrafluoroethylene sutures, 1279-1286, 1998, with permission from the American Association for Thoracic Surgery. **27-66**, **27-73**, From Doty DB: *Cardiac surgery: operative technique*, St Louis, 1997, Mosby.

## CHAPTER 28

**28-1**, Courtesy Philips Medical Systems, Bothell, Wash; **28-2**, From Odom-Forren J, Watson DS: *Practical guide to moderate sedation/analgesia*, ed 2, St Louis, 2005, Mosby.

## CHAPTER 29

**29-1**, From Kirby RR and others: *Clinical anesthesia practice*, ed 2, Philadelphia, 2002, Saunders; **29-2**, **29-3**, **29-4**, **29-17**, **29-19**, From Coran AG and others: *Surgery of the neonate*, Boston, 1978, Little, Brown; **29-5**, **29-14**, **29-20**, **29-22**, **29-24**, **29-31**, **29-32**, **29-77**, From Ashcraft KW and others: *Pediatric surgery*, ed 3, Philadelphia, 2002, Saunders; **29-6**, **29-10**, **29-11**, **29-13**, **29-21**, **29-36**, From Spitz L and others: *A colour atlas of paediatric surgical diagnosis*, London, 1990, Mosby Ltd; **29-7**, From Randolph JG: *Annals of Surgery* 198:579, 1985; **29-8**, From Benson CD: *Infants' hypertrophic pyloric stenosis*. In Mustard WT and others: *Pediatric surgery*, ed 2, Chicago, 1969, Year Book; **29-9**, Modified from Gross RE: *An atlas of children's surgery*, Philadelphia, 1970, Saunders; **29-12**, Courtesy Dr David Clark, NeoPIX, Albany, NY; **29-15**, Modified from Boley SJ: An endorectal pull-through operation with primary anastomosis for Hirschsprung's disease, *Surgery, Gynecology and Obstetrics* 127(2):253, 1986; **29-16**, From Chessell G and others: *Diagnostic picture tests in clinical medicine*, vol 2, St Louis, 1984, Mosby; **29-18**, From DeVries PA: Posterior sagittal anorectoplasty. In Holmann von Kap S, editor: *Anorektale Fehlbildungen*, Stuttgart, 1984, Gustav Fischer-Verlag; **29-23**, Courtesy H Gil Rushton, MD, Children's National Medical Center, Washington, DC. In Hockenberry MJ and others: *Wong's nursing care of infants and children*, ed 7, St Louis, 2003, Mosby; **29-25**, **29-26**, **29-30**, Modified from Droller MJ: *Surgical management of urologic disease*, St Louis, 1992, Mosby; **29-27**, From Devine CJ, Jr: Chordee and hypospadias. In Glenn JF, Boyce WH, editors: *Urologic surgery*, ed 3, Philadelphia, 1983, Lippincott; **29-33**, From Fuhrman BP, Zimmerman J: *Pediatric critical care*, ed 3, Philadelphia, 2006, Mosby; **29-34**, From Saunders WH and others: *Nursing care in eye, ear, nose and throat disorders*, ed 4, St Louis, 1979, Mosby; **29-35**, From Luckmann J, Sorenson KC: *Medical-surgical nursing*, ed 3, Philadelphia, 1987, Saunders; **29-37**, Courtesy Albert Biglan, MD, Children's Hospital of Pittsburgh. In Zitelli BJ, Davis HW: *Atlas of pediatric physical diagnosis*, ed 4, St Louis, 2002, Mosby; **29-38**, From Neurosurgery wound closure, Ethicon, Inc; **29-43**, **29-44**, **29-45**, From Zitelli BJ, Davis HW: *Atlas of pediatric physical diagnosis*, ed 4, St Louis, 2002, Mosby; **29-46**, Courtesy Emory University School of Medicine, Atlanta; **29-47**, From Swartz MH: *Textbook of physical diagnosis: history and examination*, ed 5, Philadelphia, 2006, Saunders; **29-48**, *A*, Redrawn from Chameides L: *Pediatric advanced life support*, Dallas, 1988, American Heart Association; **29-48**, *B*, From Barkin RM, Rosen P: *Emergency pediatrics: a guide to ambulatory care*, ed 3, St Louis, 1990, Mosby; **29-49**, **29-51**, **29-55**, **29-58**, **29-61**, **29-65**, **29-68**, **29-72**, **29-73**, **29-74**, From Nichols DG and others: *Critical heart disease in infants and children*, St Louis, 1994, Mosby; **29-50**, **29-54**, **29-56**, **29-57**, **29-59**, **29-60**, **29-64**, **29-67**, **29-69**, **29-71**, From Wong DL: *Whaley & Wong's nursing care of infants and children*, ed 5, St Louis, 1995, Mosby; **29-52**, **29-76**, From Cooley DA, Norman JC: *Techniques in cardiac surgery*, Houston, 1975, Texas Medical Press; **29-53**, From Lappe DG and others: *Critical heart disease in infants and children*, St Louis, 1995, Mosby; **29-62**, **29-63**, **29-70**, From Mavroudis C, Backer CL: *Pediatric cardiac surgery*, ed 2, St Louis, 1994, Mosby; **29-66**, From Effler DB: *Blades' surgical disease of the chest*, ed 4, St Louis, 1978, Mosby; **29-75**, From Doty DB: *Cardiac surgery operative technique*, St Louis, 1997, Mosby.

## CHAPTER 30

**30-1**, **30-2**, **30-3**, From Federal Interagency Forum on Aging-Related Statistics: *Charts from older Americans 2004: key indicators of well-being*; **30-4**, From Lewis SM and others: *Medical-surgical nursing: assessment and management of clinical problems*, ed 6, St Louis, 2004, Mosby; **30-7**, From Potter PA, Perry AG: *Fundamentals of nursing*, ed 6, St Louis, 2005, Mosby.

## CHAPTER 31

**31-1**, Courtesy New Regional Medical Center, Hanover, Md; **31-2**, From McQuillan KA and others: *Trauma nursing*, ed 3, St Louis, 2002, Saunders; **31-3**, **31-14**, **31-17**, From Neff JA, Kidd PS: *Trauma nursing: the art and science*, St Louis, 1993, Mosby; **31-5**, From Trunkey DD, Lewis FR: *Current therapy of trauma*, ed 4, St Louis, 1999, Mosby; **31-8**, From Grande CM: *Textbook of trauma anesthesia and critical care*, St Louis, 1993, Mosby; **31-10**, From Brohi K: www.trauma.org, June 2001, www.trauma.org/thoracic/EDToperative.html; **31-11**, From Cosgriff H, Jr, Anderson DL: *The practice of emergency care*, ed 2, Philadelphia, Lippincott; **31-12**, Redrawn from Kintzel KC: *Advanced concepts in clinical nursing*, ed 2, Philadelphia, 1997, Lippincott; **31-13**, Redrawn from Becker DP and others: Diagnosis and treatment of head injury. In Youman JR, editor: *Neurological surgery*, ed 3, Philadelphia, 1990, Saunders; **31-15**, **31-16**, **31-18**, **31-19**, **31-22**, From Townsend CM and others: *Sabiston textbook of surgery*, ed 17, Philadelphia, 2004, Saunders; **31-20**, Courtesy Haim Paran, MD; **31-21**, From Peterson NE: Genitourinary trauma. In Feliciano DV and others, editors: *Trauma*, ed 3, Norwalk, Conn, 1996, Appleton & Lange, p. 667, with permission of the McGraw-Hill Cos.

## CHAPTER 32

**32-1**, From Rothrock JC: *Perioperative care planning*, St Louis, 1996, Mosby; **32-2**, From Skidmore-Roth L: *Mosby's handbook of herbs and natural supplements*, ed 3, St Louis, 2006, Mosby; **32-3**, From Jonas WB: *Mosby's dictionary of complementary and alternative medicine*, St Louis, 2005, Mosby; **32-4**, From McCance KL, Huether SE: *Pathophysiology—the biologic basis for disease in adults and children*, ed 5, St Louis, 2006, Mosby.

# Index



Page numbers followed by f indicate figures; t, tables; b, boxes.

## D

# Special Features

## BEST PRACTICE



## HISTORY



## SAMPLE PLAN OF CARE



*Continued*

# Special Features—cont'd

## PATIENT AND FAMILY EDUCATION



## SURGICAL PHARMACOLOGY



## PATIENT SAFETY